D0161862

Maxcy-Rosenau-Last

Public Health & Preventive Medicine

13th Edition

Maxcy-Rosenau-Last

Public Health & Preventive Medicine

Editors

John M. Last, MD, DPH
Professor
Department of Epidemiology and Community Medicine
University of Ottawa
Ottawa, Ontario, Canada

Robert B. Wallace, MD, MSc
Professor of Preventive and Internal Medicine
Head, Department of Preventive Medicine and Environmental Health
University of Iowa College of Medicine
Iowa City, Iowa

Associate Editors

Elizabeth Barrett-Connor, MD
Professor and Chairman
Division of Epidemiology
Department of Community and Family Medicine
University of California, San Diego
La Jolla, California

Jonathan E. Fielding, MD, MPH
Professor of Public Health and Pediatrics
Schools of Public Health and Medicine
University of California, Los Angeles
Los Angeles, California

Arthur L. Frank, MD, PhD
Professor and Chairman
Department of Preventive Medicine and Environmental Health
University of Kentucky College of Medicine
Lexington, Kentucky

F. Douglas Scutchfield, MD
Professor and Director
Graduate School of Public Health
College of Health and Human Services
San Diego State University
San Diego, California

Carl W. Tyler, Jr., MD
Assistant Director for Academic Programs
Public Health Practice Program Office
Centers for Disease Control
Atlanta, Georgia

Richard P. Wenzel, MD, MSc
Professor
Departments of Medicine and Preventive Medicine and Environmental Health
University of Iowa College of Medicine
Iowa City, Iowa

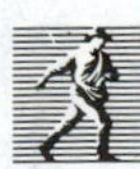

APPLETON & LANGE
Norwalk, Connecticut/San Mateo, California

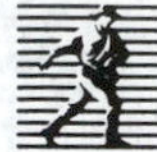

92 93 94 95 96 / 10 9 8 7 6 5 4 3 2 1

Prentice Hall International (UK) Limited, *London*
Prentice Hall of Australia Pty. Limited, *Sydney*
Prentice Hall Canada, Inc., *Toronto*
Prentice Hall Hispanoamericana, S.A., *Mexico*
Prentice Hall of India Private Limited, *New Delhi*
Prentice Hall of Japan, Inc., *Tokyo*
Simon & Schuster Asia Pte. Ltd., *Singapore*
Editora Prentice Hall do Brasil Ltda., *Rio de Janeiro*
Prentice Hall, *Englewood Cliffs, New Jersey*

Library of Congress Cataloging-in-Publication Data

Maxcy-Rosenau-Last public health and preventive medicine. — 13th ed.
/ editors, John M. Last, Robert B. Wallace : associate editors,
Elizabeth Barrett-Connor . . . [et al.]
p. cm.
Rev. ed. of: Maxcy-Rosenau public health and preventive medicine.
12th ed. / editor, John M. Last. c1986.
Includes bibliographical references and index.
ISBN 0-8385-6188-8
1. Public health. 2. Medicine, Preventive. I. Last, John M., 1926– . II. Wallace, Robert B., 1942– . III. Public health and preventive medicine. IV. Maxcy-Rosenau public health and preventive medicine.
[DNLM: 1. Preventive medicine. 2. Public Health. WA 100 M4635]
RA425.M382 1992
614.4'4—dc20
DNLM/DLC
for Library of Congress 91-18031

ISBN 0-8385-6188-8

Acquisition Editor: R. Craig Percy
Production Service: CRACOM Corporation
Designer: S. M. Byrum

PRINTED IN THE UNITED STATES OF AMERICA

The editors wish to make the following dedications:

John M. Last: To Wendy
Robert B. Wallace: To Maureen
Elizabeth Barrett-Connor: To her family
Jonathan E. Fielding: To Karin
Arthur L. Frank: To Joanne
F. Douglas Scutchfield: To Phyllis and Alex
Carl W. Tyler, Jr: To Elma
Richard P. Wenzel: To JoGail

In addition, this book is dedicated to all others who sustained and inspired the contributors

Preparation of this edition was sponsored by the Association of Teachers of Preventive Medicine. An advisory board approved by the Association of Teachers of Preventive Medicine included the following:

[†]*Deceased*

CONTRIBUTORS

Richard D. Andersen, MD
Consultant, Infectious Diseases
Children's Hospital of St. Paul
St. Paul, Minnesota

Thomas J. Armstrong, PhD, MPH
Professor
Division of Occupational Health
Department of Environmental and Industrial Health
The University of Michigan
Ann Arbor, Michigan

Mary Jane Ashley, MD, DPH, MSc
Professor
Division of Community Health
Faculty of Medicine
Department of Preventive Medicine and Biostatistics
University of Toronto
Toronto, Ontario, Canada

Robert Austrian, MD, DSc [Hon]
Professor Emeritus and Chairman
Department of Research Medicine
University of Pennsylvania School of Medicine
Attending Physician
Division of Infectious Disease
Department of Medicine
Hospital of the University of Pennsylvania
Philadelphia, Pennsylvania

Patricia A. Baird, MD, CM
Professor
Department of Medical Genetics
University of British Columbia
Vancouver, British Columbia, Canada

James F. Bale, Jr., MD
Professor
Division of Pediatric Neurology
Department of Pediatrics and Neurology
University of Iowa College of Medicine
Iowa City, Iowa

William H. Barker, MD
Associate Professor
Department of Community and Preventive Medicine
University of Rochester
Rochester, New York

Harold M. Barnhart, PhD
Associate Professor
Department of Food Science and Technology
University of Georgia
Athens, Georgia

Elizabeth Barrett-Connor, MD
Professor and Chairman
Division of Epidemiology
Department of Community and Family Medicine
University of California, San Diego
La Jolla, California

J. George Bekesi, MD, PhD
Professor of Neoplastic Diseases
Cancer Center
Mount Sinai School of Medicine
New York, New York

A. E. Benjamin, PhD
Associate Professor-in-Residence
Department of Social and Behavioral Sciences
Institute for Health and Aging
School of Nursing
University of California, San Francisco
San Francisco, California

Stephan A. Billstein, MD, MPH
Director, Medical Marketing
Roche Laboratories
Nutley, New Jersey

Eula Bingham, PhD
Professor
Department of Environmental Health
University of Cincinnati School of Medicine
Cincinnati, Ohio

Robert E. Black, MD, MPH
Professor and Chairman
Department of International Health
Johns Hopkins University School of Hygiene and Public Health
Baltimore, Maryland

Henry Blackburn, MD, MS
Mayo Professor of Public Health
Division of Epidemiology
School of Public Health
University of Minnesota
Minneapolis, Minnesota

Paul A. Blake, MD, MPH
Chief, Enteric Diseases Branch
Division of Bacterial and Mycotic Diseases
Center for Infectious Diseases
Centers for Disease Control
Atlanta, Georgia

Robert F. Breiman, MD
Chief, Epidemiology Section, Respiratory Diseases Branch
Division of Bacterial and Mycotic Diseases
Center for Infectious Diseases
Centers for Disease Control
Atlanta, Georgia

Joel G. Breman, MD, DTPH
Deputy Chief, Malaria Branch
Division of Parasitic Diseases
Centers for Disease Control
Atlanta, Georgia

Edward W. Brink, MD, DTPH
Epidemiologist
Division of Immunization
Center for Preventive Services
Centers for Disease Control
Atlanta, Georgia

Evelyn J. Bromet, PhD
Professor of Psychiatry
Department of Psychiatry and Behavioral Science
State University of New York at Stony Brook
Health Sciences Center
Stony Brook, New York

Claire V. Broome, MD
Chief, Department of Meningitis and Special Pathogens Branch
Centers for Disease Control
Atlanta, Georgia

Alfred A. Buck, MD, DrPH
Tropical Disease Advisor
Office of Health, Science and Technology
Agency for International Development
Washington, D.C.

Joanna Burger, PhD, MSc
Professor of Biology
Director, Graduate Program of Ecology
Division of Biology/Ecology
Rutgers University
New Brunswick, New Jersey

Department of Biological Sciences
Environmental and Occupational Health Sciences Institute
Piscataway, New Jersey

Ann W. Burgess, RN, DNSc
van Ameringen Professor of Psychiatric Mental Health Nursing
University of Pennsylvania
Philadelphia, Pennsylvania

C. M. G. Buttery, MD, MPH
Commissioner
Virginia Department of Health
Richmond, Virginia

Adjunct Professor of Community Medicine
Department of Family Medicine
Eastern Virginia Medical School
Norfolk, Virginia

Department of Preventive Medicine
Medical College of Virginia
Richmond, Virginia

Department of Preventive Medicine and Biometrics
Edward F. Hébert School of Medicine
Uniformed Services University of the Health Sciences
Bethesda, Maryland

Willard Cates, Jr., MD, MPH
Director, Division of Training
Epidemiology Program Office
Centers for Disease Control

Adjunct Professor
Division of Epidemiology and Biostatistics
Emory University School of Medicine
Atlanta, Georgia

Stephen L. Cochi, MD
Chief, Infant Immunization Section
Division of Immunization
Centers for Disease Control
Atlanta, Georgia

Judith M. Conn, MS, MBA
Statistician
Division of Injury Control
Center for Environmental Health and Injury Control
Centers for Disease Control
Atlanta, Georgia

Denny G. Constantine, DVM, MPH
Public Health Veterinarian
Infectious Disease Branch
California Department of Health Services
Berkeley, California

David B. Coultas, MD
Associate Professor of Medicine
Pulmonary Division
Department of Internal Medicine
University of New Mexico School of Medicine
Albuquerque, New Mexico

Linda D. Cowan, PhD
Associate Professor
Department of Biostatistics and Epidemiology
College of Public Health
University of Oklahoma
Oklahoma City, Oklahoma

Robert B. Craven, MD
Chief, Epidemiology Section
Division of Vector-borne Infectious Diseases
Centers for Disease Control
Fort Collins, Colorado

Alan W. Cross, MD
Associate Professor
Departments of Social Medicine and Pediatrics
University of North Carolina at Chapel Hill School of Medicine
Chapel Hill, North Carolina

Mark R. Cullen, MD
Associate Professor of Medicine and Epidemiology
Director, Yale Occupational/Environmental Medicine Program
Department of Internal Medicine
Yale University School of Medicine
New Haven, Connecticut

James W. Curran, MD, MPH
Director, Division of HIV/AIDS
Center for Infectious Diseases
Centers for Disease Control
Atlanta, Georgia

Roy L. DeHart, MD, MPH
Professor and Director
Division of Occupational and Environmental Medicine
Department of Family Medicine
University of Oklahoma College of Medicine
Oklahoma City, Oklahoma

Bradley N. Doebbeling, MD, MS
Assistant Professor
Division of General Medicine, Clinical Epidemiology and Health Services Research
Department of Internal Medicine
University of Iowa College of Medicine
Iowa City, Iowa

Janice S. Dorman, PhD
Assistant Professor of Epidemiology
Graduate School of Public Health
University of Pittsburgh
Pittsburgh, Pennsylvania

D. Peter Drotman, MD, MPH
Assistant to the Director
Division of HIV/AIDS
Center for Infectious Diseases
Centers for Disease Control

Clinical Assistant Professor
Department of Community Health
Emory University School of Medicine
Atlanta, Georgia

Vladimir Dvorak, MD, PhD
Assistant Professor
Department of Preventive Medicine and Environmental Health
University of Kentucky College of Medicine
Lexington, Kentucky

L. K. Eveland, PhD
Professor and Chairman
Department of Microbiology
California State University, Long Beach
Long Beach, California

George D. Everett, MD
Director, Internal Medicine Residency Program
Orlando Regional Medical Center
Orlando, Florida

Laura J. Fehrs, MD
Medical Epidemiologist
Division of Immunization
Centers for Disease Control
Atlanta, Georgia

Nancy Fiedler, PhD
Assistant Professor
Division of Occupational Medicine
Department of Environmental and Community Medicine
University of Medicine and Dentistry of New Jersey
Robert Wood Johnson Medical School
Piscataway, New Jersey

Jonathan E. Fielding, MD, MPH
Professor of Public Health and Pediatrics
Schools of Public Health and Medicine
University of California, Los Angeles
Los Angeles, California

David Finkelhor, PhD
Family Violence Research Program
Department of Sociology
University of New Hampshire
Durham, New Hampshire

Alf Fischbein, MD
Visiting Professor
The Institute for Occupational Health
Sackler Faculty of Medicine
Tel Aviv University
Tel Aviv, Israel

Stacey C. FitzSimmons, PhD
Associate Scientific Director, Cystic Fibrosis Foundation
Medical Affairs Department
Cystic Fibrosis Foundation
Bethesda, Maryland

Anne H. Flitcraft, MD
University of Connecticut Health Center
Farmington, Connecticut

Co-Director, Domestic Violence Training Project
New Haven, Connecticut

William H. Foege, MD, MPH
Executive Director
The Carter Center of Emory University
Atlanta, Georgia

Arthur L. Frank, MD, PhD
Professor and Chairman
Department of Preventive Medicine and Environmental Health
University of Kentucky College of Medicine
Lexington, Kentucky

Joseph F. Frank, PhD
Professor
Department of Food Science and Technology
University of Georgia
Athens, Georgia

Susan Frankel, PhD
Family Research Laboratory
University of New Hampshire
Durham, New Hampshire

David W. Fraser, MD
President
Swarthmore College
Swarthmore, Pennsylvania

Adjunct Professor
Department of Medicine
University of Pennsylvania
Philadelphia, Pennsylvania

Cedric F. Garland, DrPH
Associate Professor
Department of Community and Family Medicine
Director, Cancer Center Epidemiology Program
School of Medicine
University of California, San Diego
La Jolla, California

Frank C. Garland, PhD
Head, Epidemiology Department
Naval Health Research Center
San Diego, California

Assistant Adjunct Professor
Department of Community and Family Medicine
School of Medicine
University of California, San Diego
La Jolla, California

H. Jack Geiger, MD, MSciHyg
Arthur C. Logan Professor of Community Medicine
Department of Community Health and Social Medicine
City University of New York Medical School
New York, New York

Michael Gochfeld, MD, PhD
Director, Division of Occupational Health
Department of Environmental and Community Medicine and Environmental and Occupational Health Sciences Institute
University of Medicine and Dentistry of New Jersey
Robert Wood Johnson Medical School
Piscataway, New Jersey

Leon Gordis, MD, DPH
Professor and Chairman
Department of Epidemiology
Johns Hopkins University School of Hygiene and Public Health
Baltimore, Maryland

Edward D. Gorham, MPH
Epidemiologist, Epidemiology Department
Naval Health Research Center
San Diego, California

Staff Research Associate
Department of Community and Family Medicine
School of Medicine
University of California, San Diego
La Jolla, California

Philippe Grandjean, MD, PhD
Professor of Environmental Medicine
Institute of Community Health
Odense University
Odense, Denmark

Lawrence W. Green, DrPH
Professor and Director
Institute of Health Promotion Research
Faculty of Graduate Studies
University of British Columbia
Vancouver, British Columbia, Canada

Patricia M. Griffin, MD
Assistant Chief, Epidemiology Section, Enteric Diseases Branch
Division of Bacterial and Mycotic Diseases
Center for Infectious Diseases
Centers for Disease Control
Atlanta, Georgia

Carol R. Hartman, RN, DNSc
Professor of Psychiatric Mental Health Nursing
Boston College School of Nursing
Chestnut Hill, Massachusetts

D. Gray Heppner, MD
Fellow in Infectious Diseases and Geographic Medicine
Department of Internal Medicine
University of Maryland
Baltimore, Maryland

Joan M. Herold, PhD
Assistant Professor
Department of Behavioral Science and Health Education and International Health
Emory University School of Public Health
Atlanta, Georgia

Alan R. Hinman, MD, MPH
Director
Center for Prevention Services
Centers for Disease Control

Adjunct Professor
Emory University School of Public Health
Atlanta, Georgia

Marc C. Hochberg, MD, MPH
Associate Professor of Medicine
Joint Appointment in Epidemiology
Department of Medicine, School of Medicine
Department of Epidemiology, School of Hygiene and Public Health
Johns Hopkins Medical Institutions
Baltimore, Maryland

King K. Holmes, MD, PhD
Director, Center for AIDS and STD
Professor of Medicine
Adjunct Professor of Microbiology and Epidemiology
University of Washington
Seattle, Washington

Cyrus C. Hopkins, MD
Physician and Hospital Epidemiologist
Infection Control Unit
Massachusetts General Hospital

Associate Professor
Department of Medicine
Harvard Medical School
Boston, Massachusetts

Sanford W. Horstman, MS, PhD
Associate Professor
Department of Preventive Medicine and Environmental Health
University of Kentucky College of Medicine
Lexington, Kentucky

Wendy E. Hoy, MB, BS, BScMed
Center for Health and Population Research
Lovelace Medical Foundation
Albuquerque, New Mexico

S. Y. Li Hsü, PhD
Professor Emeritus
Department of Preventive Medicine and Environmental Health
University of Iowa College of Medicine
Iowa City, Iowa

James Huff, PhD
Associate Director for Risk Evaluation
Division of Biometry and Risk Assessment
National Institute of Environmental Health Sciences
National Institutes of Health
United States Public Health Service
Research Triangle Park, North Carolina

Yoshinori Itokawa, MD
Department of Hygiene
School of Medicine
Kyoto University
Kyoto, Japan

Karl M. Johnson, MD
Professor of Epidemiology
School of Hygiene and Public Health
Johns Hopkins University
Baltimore, Maryland

Arnold F. Kaufmann, DVM, MS
Chief, Mycotic Diseases Branch
Division of Bacterial and Mycotic Diseases
Center for Infectious Diseases
Centers for Disease Control
Atlanta, Georgia

Jennifer L. Kelsey, PhD
Professor
Department of Health, Research and Policy
Stanford University
Stanford, California

W. Monroe Keyserling, BIE, MSE, MS, PhD
Associate Professor
College of Engineering
Department of Industrial and Operations Engineering
The University of Michigan
Ann Arbor, Michigan

M. Marlyne Kilbey, PhD
Professor and Chairperson
Department of Psychology
Wayne State University School of Medicine
Detroit, Michigan

Edwin M. Kilbourne, MD
Assistant Director for Science
Epidemiology Program Office
Centers for Disease Control
Atlanta, Georgia

Kaye H. Kilburn, MD
Ralph Edgington Professor of Medicine
Environmental Sciences Laboratory
Department of Internal Medicine
University of Southern California School of Medicine
Los Angeles, California

Dean G. Kilpatrick, PhD
Crime Victims Center
Medical University of South Carolina
Charleston, South Carolina

Jeffrey P. Koplan, MD, MPH
Director, Center for Chronic Disease Prevention and Health Promotion
Centers for Disease Control
Atlanta, Georgia

Jess F. Kraus, PhD
Professor
Department of Epidemiology
School of Public Health
University of California, Los Angeles
Los Angeles, California

Darwin R. Labarthe, MD, PhD
James W. Rockwell Professor of Public Health
School of Public Health
University of Texas Health Science Center at Houston
Houston, Texas

Philip J. Landrigan, MD, MSc
Professor and Chairman
Department of Community Medicine
Director, Division of Environmental and Occupational Medicine
Professor
Department of Pediatrics
Mount Sinai School of Medicine
New York, New York

Ronald E. LaPorte, PhD
Associate Professor of Epidemiology
Graduate School of Public Health
University of Pittsburgh
Pittsburgh, Pennsylvania

John M. Last, MD, DPH
Professor
Department of Epidemiology and Community Medicine
University of Ottawa
Ottawa, Ontario, Canada

Jennifer Leaning, MD, MScHyg
Instructor in Medicine
Harvard Medical School
Boston, Massachusetts

Director of Medical Program Evaluation
Chief of Emergency Services
Harvard Community Health Plan

Attending Physician
Emergency Service
Brigham and Women's Hospital
Brookline, Massachusetts

Philip R. Lee, MD
Professor of Social Medicine
Director, Institute for Health Policy Studies
School of Medicine
University of California, San Francisco
San Francisco, California

Llewellyn J. Legters, MD, MPH
Professor and Chairman
Department of Preventive Medicine and Biometrics
Edward F. Hébert School of Medicine
Uniformed Services University of the Health Sciences
Bethesda, Maryland

William C. Levine, MD, MSc
Enteric Diseases Branch
Division of Bacterial and Mycotic Diseases
Center for Infectious Diseases
Centers for Disease Control
Atlanta, Georgia

Alan Leviton, MD, SM
Associate Professor
Department of Neurology
Harvard Medical School
Boston, Massachusetts

Ruth Lilis, MD
Professor
Division of Environmental and Occupational Medicine
Department of Community Medicine
Mount Sinai School of Medicine
New York, New York

Craig H. Llewellyn, MD, MS, MPH
Professor and Chair
Department of Military and Emergency Medicine
Professor, Department of Preventive Medicine and Biometrics
Edward F. Hébert School of Medicine
Uniformed Services University of the Health Sciences
Bethesda, Maryland

William W. Lockwood, MD
Associate
Division of General Medicine, Clinical Epidemiology and Health Services Research
Department of Internal Medicine
University of Iowa College of Medicine
Iowa City, Iowa

Russell Luepker, MD
Professor of Epidemiology and Medicine
Head, Division of Epidemiology
School of Public Health
University of Minnesota
Minneapolis, Minnesota

Harold S. Margolis, MD
Chief, Hepatitis Branch
Division of Viral and Rickettsial Diseases
Centers for Disease Control
Atlanta, Georgia

Lauri E. Markowitz, MD
Medical Epidemiologist
Division of Immunization
Center for Prevention Services
Centers for Disease Control
Atlanta, Georgia

James A. Merchant, MD, DrPH
Professor of Preventive and Internal Medicine
Department of Preventive Medicine and Environmental Health
Director, Institute of Agricultural Medicine and Occupational Health
University of Iowa College of Medicine
Iowa City, Iowa

James A. Mercy, PhD
Chief, Epidemiology Branch
Division of Injury Control
Center for Environmental Health and Injury Control
Centers for Disease Control
Atlanta, Georgia

Aage R. Møller, PhD, DMedSci
Professor of Neurological Surgery
Department of Neurological Surgery
University of Pittsburgh School of Medicine
Pittsburgh, Pennsylvania

Thomas P. Monath, MD
Chief, Virology Division
Department of the Army
United States Army Medical Research Institute of Infectious Diseases
Fort Detrick
Fredrick, Maryland

Arnold S. Monto, MD
Professor of Epidemiology
Department of Epidemiology and International Health
The University of Michigan
Ann Arbor, Michigan

Marion Moses, MD
Assistant Clinical Professor
Department of Family and Community Medicine
School of Medicine
University of California, San Francisco
San Francisco, California

Karin B. Nelson, MD
Medical Officer
Neuroepidemiology Branch
National Institute of Neurological Disorders and Stroke
Bethesda, Maryland

Marion Nestle, MD, MPH
Professor and Chair
Department of Nutrition, Food and Hotel Management
New York University
New York, New York

Eli H. Newberger, MD
Director, Family Development Study
Children's Hospital

Assistant Professor
Department of Pediatrics
Harvard Medical School
Boston, Massachusetts

Patrick W. O'Carroll, MD, MPH
Chief, Intentional Injuries Section
Division of Injury Control
Center for Environmental Health and Injury Control
Centers for Disease Control
Atlanta, Georgia

Daniel A. Okun, MS, ScD
Kenan Professor of Environmental Engineering, Emeritus
Department of Environmental Sciences and Engineering
School of Public Health
University of North Carolina at Chapel Hill
Chapel Hill, North Carolina

Erol Onel, BA
Albert Einstein College of Medicine
Bronx, New York

Trevor J. Orchard, MD
Associate Professor of Epidemiology
Graduate School of Public Health
University of Pittsburgh
Pittsburgh, Pennsylvania

Diana L. Ordin, MD, MPH
Adjunct Assistant Professor
Department of Epidemiology and Biostatistics
Case Western Reserve University

Consultant, Occupational/Environmental Medicine
St. Vincent Charity Hospital and Health Center
Cleveland, Ohio

Walter A. Orenstein, MD
Director, Division of Immunization
Center for Prevention Services
Centers for Disease Control
Atlanta, Georgia

Michael T. Osterholm, PhD, MPH
State Epidemiologist and Chief, Acute Disease Epidemiology Section
Minnesota Department of Health
Minneapolis, Minnesota

David K. Parkinson, MD
Professor of Preventive Medicine
Department of Preventive Medicine
State University of New York at Stony Brook
Health Science Center
Stony Brook, New York

Peter A. Patriarca, MD
Chief, Epidemiologic Research Section
Division of Immunization
Centers for Disease Control
Atlanta, Georgia

Herbert B. Peterson, MD
Chief, Women's Health and Fertility Branch
Division of Reproductive Health
Center for Chronic Disease Prevention and Health Promotion
Centers for Disease Control
Atlanta, Georgia

Michael A. Pfaller, MD
Professor and Vice Chair
Division of Clinical Pathology
Department of Pathology
Oregon Health Sciences University School of Medicine
Portland, Oregon

Karl Pillemer, PhD
Family Research Laboratory
University of New Hampshire
Durham, New Hampshire

Jack D. Poland, MD, MPH
Research Associate
Department of Environmental Health
Colorado State University
Fort Collins, Colorado

Susan H. Pollack, MD
Instructor
Department of Community Medicine
Division of Environmental and Occupational Medicine
Instructor
Department of Pediatrics
Mount Sinai School of Medicine
New York, New York

Stephen R. Preblud, MD[†]
Medical Epidemiologist
Division of Immunization
Centers for Disease Control
Atlanta, Georgia

David P. Rall, MD, PhD
Director, Retired
National Institute of Environmental Health Sciences
Research Triangle Park, North Carolina

James G. Rankin, MB
Professor
Faculty of Medicine
Departments of Preventive Medicine and Biostatistics and Medicine
University of Toronto

Head of Medicine
Division of Clinical Research and Treatment Institute
Addiction Research Foundation of Ontario
Toronto, Ontario, Canada

Robert L. Rausch, DVM, PhD
Division of Animal Medicine
Health Sciences Center
University of Washington School of Medicine
Seattle, Washington

Jonathan I. Ravdin, MD
Department of Medicine
Case Western Reserve University

Veterans Administration Medical Center
Cleveland, Ohio

[†]Deceased

Arthur L. Reingold, MD
Professor of Epidemiology
Department of Biomedical and Environmental Health Sciences
School of Public Health
University of California, Berkeley
Berkeley, California

Leon S. Robertson, PhD
Lecturer
Department of Epidemiology and Public Health
Yale University
New Haven, Connecticut

Mark L. Rosenberg, MD, MPP
Director, Division of Injury Control
Center for Environmental Health and Injury Control
Centers for Disease Control
Atlanta, Georgia

R. Gary Rozier, DDS
Associate Professor
Department of Health Policy and Administration
School of Public Health
University of North Carolina at Chapel Hill
Chapel Hill, North Carolina

Harriet L. Rubenstein, JD, MPH
Assistant Professor
Division of Occupational and Environmental Health
Department of Community and Preventive Medicine
Medical College of Pennsylvania
Philadelphia, Pennsylvania

Thomas G. Rundall, PhD
Professor
Department of Social and Administrative Health Sciences
School of Public Health
University of California, Berkeley
Berkeley, California

Jonathan M. Samet, MD
Professor of Medicine
Pulmonary and Critical Care Division
Department of Medicine
University of New Mexico School of Medicine
Albuquerque, New Mexico

Julius Schachter, PhD
Professor of Epidemiology
Chlamydia Laboratory
Department of Laboratory Medicine
University of California, San Francisco

Director, World Health Organization Collaborating Center for Reference and Research on *Chlamydia*
San Francisco, California

C. Roberts Schuster, PhD
Director, National Institute on Drug Abuse
Alcohol, Drug Abuse, and Mental Health Administration
United States Public Health Service
Department of Health and Human Services
Rockville, Maryland

Charles R. Scriver, MDCM
Professor of Biology/Human Genetics/Pediatrics
Department of Biology/Human Genetics/Pediatrics
McGill University
Montreal, Quebec, Canada

F. Douglas Scutchfield, MD
Professor and Director
Graduate School of Public Health
College of Health and Human Services
San Diego State University
San Diego, California

Victor W. Sidel, MD
Distinguished University Professor of Social Medicine
Department of Epidemiology and Social Medicine
Montefiore Medical Center/Albert Einstein College of Medicine
Bronx, New York

George A. Silver, MD
Professor Emeritus
Institute for Social and Policy Studies
Yale University
New Haven, Connecticut

Louis Slesin, PhD
Editor and Publisher
Microwave News and *VDT News*
New York, New York

Alfred Sommer, MD, MHSc
Dean
Johns Hopkins School of Hygiene and Public Health
Baltimore, Maryland

Evan Stark, PhD, MSW
Graduate Department of Public Administration
Rutgers University
Newark, New Jersey

Co-Director, Domestic Violence Training Project
New Haven, Connecticut

Paul A. Stehr-Green, DrPH, MPH
Medical Epidemiologist
New Zealand Communicable Disease Centre
Porirua, New Zealand

Zena A. Stein, MA, MB, BCh
Associate Dean of Research
Professor of Public Health (Epidemiology)
G. H. Sergievsky Center
Columbia University

Co-Director, HIV Center for Clinical and Behavioral Studies
New York State Psychiatric Institute
New York, New York

Richard W. Steketee, MD, MPH
Chief, Malaria Epidemiology and Control Activity
Malaria Branch
Division of Parasitic Disease
Center for Infectious Diseases
Centers for Disease Control
Atlanta, Georgia

Mervyn W. Susser, MD
G. H. Sergievsky Professor of Epidemiology and Director
G. H. Sergievsky Center
Columbia University
New York, New York

Roland W. Sutter, MD, MPH
Medical Epidemiologist
Infant Immunization Section
Division of Immunization
Centers for Disease Control
Atlanta, Georgia

S. Leonard Syme, PhD
Professor of Epidemiology
School of Public Health
University of California, Berkeley
Berkeley, California

Hiroshi Takatsuki, PhD
Environmental Conservation Center
Kyoto University
Kyoto, Japan

Masaru Tanaka, PhD
Chief
Solid Waste Management Office
Department of Sanitary Engineering
The Institute of Public Health
Tokyo, Japan

Robert V. Tauxe, MD, MPH
Chief, Epidemiology Section, Enteric Diseases Branch
Division of Bacterial and Mycotic Diseases
Center for Infectious Diseases
Centers for Disease Control
Atlanta, Georgia

David B. Thomas, MD, DrPH
Professor
Department of Epidemiology
School of Public Health and Community Medicine
University of Washington

Program Head
Program in Epidemiology
Division of Public Health Sciences
Fred Hutchinson Cancer Research Center
Seattle, Washington

Dennis D. Tolsma, MPH
Assistant Director for Public Health Practice
Centers for Disease Control
Atlanta, Georgia

Theodore F. Tsai, MD, MPH
Assistant Director for Medical Sciences
Division of Vector-borne Infectious Diseases
Centers for Disease Control
Fort Collins, Colorado

Peter Tsang, MD, PhD
Assistant Professor of Neoplastic Diseases
Cancer Center
Mount Sinai School of Medicine
New York, New York

Carl W. Tyler, Jr., MD
Assistant Director for Academic Programs
Public Health Practice Program Office
Centers for Disease Control
Atlanta, Georgia

Robert B. Wallace, MD, MSc
Professor of Preventive and Internal Medicine
Head, Department of Preventive Medicine and Environmental Health
University of Iowa College of Medicine
Iowa City, Iowa

Steven G. F. Wassilak, MD
Medical Epidemiologist, Epidemiologic Research Section
Division of Immunization
Centers for Disease Control
Atlanta, Georgia

Jonathan B. Weisbuch, MD, MPH
Medical Director
Medical Administration, Department of Health Services
Los Angeles County
Los Angeles, California

Jay D. Wenger, MD
Medical Epidemiologist, Meningitis and Special Pathogens Branch
Centers for Disease Control
Atlanta, Georgia

Richard P. Wenzel, MD, MSc
Professor
Departments of Medicine and Preventive Medicine and Environmental Health
University of Iowa College of Medicine
Iowa City, Iowa

S. Benson Werner, MD, MPH
Chief, Central Infectious Disease Unit
Infectious Disease Branch
Preventive Medical Services Division
California Department of Health Services

Lecturer
University of California School of Public Health
Berkeley, California

Stephen J. Williams, ScD
Professor and Head
Division of Health Services Administration
Graduate School of Public Health
San Diego State University
San Diego, California

Mary E. Wilson, MD
Assistant Professor
Department of Internal Medicine
University of Iowa College of Medicine
Iowa City, Iowa

Robert G. Yaeger, PhD
Professor, Retired
School of Public Health and Tropical Medicine and the Department of Medicine
Tulane University
New Orleans, Louisiana

CONTENTS

PREFACE

With the appearance of this edition, we are about to enter the ninth decade of this book's existence. Readers will be applying its lessons in the 21st century. The changes in substance and style since the first edition of 1913 are impressive: new vistas of public health and preventive medicine then undreamed of have come into prominence, and instead of a single author assisted in a couple of places by a friendly colleague, we have a volume to which 165 experts have contributed. Yet the essential knowledge about public health and preventive medicine can still be encompassed within a single volume—and we are pleased to observe that this volume is not as large as were the 11th and 12th editions. Though communicable diseases continue to occupy a large proportion of the total number of pages, environmental and behavioral factors that can influence health each have an increased share.

Several new chapters reflect the changing emphasis and new priorities of public health. Human immunodeficiency virus infection was considered in the 12th edition, but much new information is contained in the corresponding chapter in this edition. The appearance of chapters on the global environment and on prison health services and the reappearance of a chapter on military medicine are recognition that these issues have increased in importance and relevance to public health practice since the mid-1980s. In addition to this new material, every chapter in the book has been rewritten, many of them entirely rewritten, some by authors who appear for the first time in this edition. Although contributors come predominantly from North America, they all are aware of the fact that we live in one world, so that, with the exception of a few details about health care organization and administration, the substance of public health theory and practice contained in this book is universal in its application.

John M. Last
Ottawa

Robert B. Wallace
Iowa City

ACKNOWLEDGMENTS

Members of the Editorial Board gave generously of time and expertise to the editors and to many contributors. Individual authors and editors acknowledge in addition much help they have received. The following list is arranged in alphabetical order and does not specify who helped with what, but each of the people named here will know. If names are inadvertently omitted, we apologize in advance, because there have been so many helpers that keeping track of them is probably beyond the competence even of well-organized record-keepers, which we are not.

Martha Dehaven Carmel
Terry K. Gray
Paul Hasselback
Isra Levy
Ian MacDowell
Mark MacLean
Brent Moloughney
Stan Music
Charles Mustard
Rebecca Payne
Delite Sharp

Craig Percy of Appleton & Lange, and Mary Espenschied of CRACOM Corporation, have been unfailing in support and good advice.

HISTORICAL NOTE

Milton J. Rosenau was a Harvard man, as was his principal collaborator, George C. Whipple. His successor, Kenneth Maxcy, moved to Johns Hopkins. When Maxcy was in turn succeeded as editor by Philip E. Sartwell and the size of the team began to grow, the center of gravity of "Maxcy-Rosenau" was decisively located in Baltimore: 20 of the 39 contributors to the 10th edition were Johns Hopkins staff (D. A. Henderson was temporarily with the World Health Organization in Geneva), and all but two or three contributors were associated with schools of public health. In 1976, the Publisher invited the Association of Teachers of Preventive Medicine to assume responsibility for the 11th and subsequent editions. After a search, John M. Last, Professor of Epidemiology and Community Medicine at the University of Ottawa, was selected as editor. From the 11th edition onward, the character of the book has changed: the team has grown in size and its composition has become more diverse, though it is still predominantly American. A smaller proportion of contributors come from schools of public health and more from medical schools and health departments, and there is strong representation from the Centers for Disease Control. Believing there is strength in diversity, the editors and Editorial Board look forward to continuation of this trend onward into future editions of this book.

PUBLISHER'S NOTE

John M. Last has guided the course of this book through three editions. Each has involved extensive revisions that have focused and fine-tuned this leading textbook on the topic, the standard work in the field. John Last has brought to his editorship the characteristics he brings to everything in his professional life: his immense scope of knowledge, his insight and wisdom, his sense of humor, and his tact. In recognition of his outstanding contributions, the Publisher is proud to announce that this text will henceforth be known eponymously as *Maxcy–Rosenau–Last Public Health and Preventive Medicine.*

Maxcy-Rosenau-Last

Public Health & Preventive Medicine

SECTION ONE

Public Health Methods

Edited by John M. Last and Carl W. Tyler, Jr.

1

Scope and Methods of Prevention

John M. Last

As we approach the twenty-first century, the challenges facing public health services remain as daunting as at any time in the past. For a brief period around the middle of the twentieth century, humanity seemed set on a course toward steadily improving health, and as we entered the final quarter, the optimistic World Health Organization (WHO) slogan, Health for All by the Year 2000, seemed an attainable goal, at least to some quite realistic health planners at the national and international level. It still could be if we define targets and priorities for health care in all nations and focus our energies on achieving them. But in addition to many long-standing unresolved public health problems, we face new and challenging difficulties. The epidemic of HIV infection has the highest profile, but other public health problems are no less troublesome. Unprecedented environmental damage endangers all of us and the other living creatures with which we share our planet. We have not found a way to deal effectively with many behavioral aberrations that threaten to impair good health. Even the provision of health care carries risks, as well as ever-rising costs for diminishing returns.

SUCCESSES AND FAILURES OF PUBLIC HEALTH

Public health has had many encouraging successes, dating back to about 100 years ago when the sanitary revolution and improved standards of personal hygiene began to reduce the toll of diarrheal diseases in the industrial nations. About the same time, improved living conditions, including better housing and enhanced nutritional status, better education, especially of the mothers of the generation being born, and indeed of each subsequent generation, began to produce sustained improvements in infant mortality rates. Immunizing agents, some of which were developed in the early twentieth century, others more recently, led to better control of communicable diseases. The most spectacular victory over a deadly contagious disease, aided by epidemiological insights, surely has been the eradication of smallpox.[1] But many other communicable diseases, notably tuberculosis, diphtheria, measles, scarlet fever, whooping cough, typhoid, pneumococcal pneumonia, meningococcal meningitis, and poliomyelitis, have been almost or entirely controlled, at least in the affluent industrial nations, by a combination of vaccines and antibiotics. In the 1980s and 1990s the WHO Expanded Programme on Immunization is striving to repeat this achievement in the developing nations, with varying degrees of success.

But there are some failures. The common cold is undefeated, and so to a large extent is influenza. Sexually transmitted diseases are rampant; AIDS is mainly a sexually transmitted disease of course. Among the communicable diseases of the tropics, we are not much nearer controlling malaria than we were half a century ago; both parasites and vectors are often resistant to the agents we deploy against them. Schistosomiasis too continues to challenge us.

There are other failures. Many Western industrialized nations appear to be experiencing a rising prevalence of what Durkheim called anomie, a form of social disorganization that is especially prevalent among young people. Families are unstable; young people are restless and rootless, easily addicted to tobacco and, worse, to illicit drugs, and prone to violent behavior within their own families and among their peers. In the United States, teenage pregnancy is epidemic among unmarried, poorly educated girls; this problem has been much better controlled in many other nations where sex education is more vigorously conducted in schools and contraceptives are easily available.[2]

Among middle-aged and older people we are perhaps beginning to make progress toward control of ischemic heart disease and, in men anyway, lung cancer. But ways to prevent most other cancers continue to elude us. Chronic obstructive lung disease remains a common end result of addiction to tobacco smoking. We have failed to find the causes of or means to prevent most serious mental disorders and uncommon but devastating neurological conditions such as multiple sclerosis, amyotrophic lateral sclerosis, and muscular dystrophy. Premature death and permanent disability in traffic crashes seem likely to afflict us as long as there is abundant cheap gasoline and we remain addicted to the automobile as a means of personal transport. Many of our industrial areas are so heavily polluted with toxic wastes that it is surprising to find any form of life surviving in them.

Above all, the human population continues to increase exponentially. The population doubled from 2.5 billion to 5 billion in less than 40 years from 1950 to 1989; if the trend continues without change, it will double again to 10 billion before 2030. Cities in many parts of the world and especially in the developing nations are increasingly unworkable. There is nowhere to put the waste, and human and other services are stretched beyond the limit. The misery and absence of health care and social support for many millions in periurban slums in developing nations are a harbinger of what might soon be in store for millions more in overcrowded cities in the industrially developed, affluent nations. All these people consume energy and generate waste products, including the gaseous products of combusted fossil fuels, and thus contribute to the greenhouse effect, which may raise the temperature of the biosphere enough in the next 100 years to change our environment beyond recall. The highest priority is the need to achieve sustainable development,[3] in contrast to our present mindless looting of nonrenewable resources, which will leave our descendants a bitter legacy. Sustainable development requires among other things that we limit families everywhere to replacement level. Almost nothing is being done in most nations to promote effective family planning programs, and there is widespread ideological, political, and religious resistance to contraception, aggravated in many developing countries by female illiteracy and restrictions on the rights of women.

FAILURES OF SUCCESS[4]

Sometimes our apparent success in dealing with intractable problems has brought failure in its train. The revolution in care of mental disorders is an example: psychoactive drugs and physical methods of treating the mentally ill encouraged psychiatrists to minimize custodial care, but the result has been the pathetic spectacle of hundreds of thousands of homeless mentally ill people across the United States and other nations with similar policies. Other failures of success include the tragic consequences of resuscitating extremely low birthweight infants, who remain alive but severely mentally retarded, blind, palsied, and a burden to their families, to health services, and to themselves if they are sentient. At the upper end of the age scale, our success in treating previously lethal respiratory infections and other conditions of advanced middle and early old age has led to a rise in the number of the very old (85 years and over), most of whom require institutional care, often at considerable expense and often with no close kin who care for or about them.

PUBLIC HEALTH METHODS

We can promote, preserve, and restore health by any of several methods or by combinations of them.

Safe Environment. Environmental threats to health were described by Hippocrates in *Airs, Waters, Places;* the threats are physical, biological, and social. In the past the greatest dangers came from pathogenic organisms; many of the worst of these have been controlled by sanitary engineering, improved housing, and so forth. We face new physical hazards, for instance, exposure to dangerously increased levels of ultraviolet irradiation if the stratospheric ozone layer becomes more attenuated. We do not fully comprehend the health-endangering factors in our social environment. How is health affected by crowding, by the sensory bombardment we receive from television? Intuitively we may consider these influences to be harmful, but evidence is elusive.

Enhanced Immunity. Development of methods to immunize persons and populations against infectious disease began with Jenner's discovery of vaccination 200 years ago. This has been the greatest single triumph of the science of preventive medicine. The priorities now are for vaccines against the family of malaria parasites and for a vaccine to prevent the transmission of AIDS.

Behaving Sensibly. The diseases of life-style, that is, diseases attributable to the ways we behave, include ischemic heart disease, tobacco-induced cancers, and traffic-related injury—the three leading causes of premature death in industrial nations. The behaviors that public health workers seek to change in the people to control these conditions are all pleasurable or profitable or both, and our efforts are therefore often resented and resisted. Public health has not yet found a satisfactory way to deal with this dilemma.

Maintaining Good Nutrition. Throughout history, and for much of the world's population today, food shortages have been the rule, rather than the exception; nutritional deficiency diseases have been pervasive. Nutritional deficit reduces resistance to infection, and infection raises the metabolic demand for nutriment, so a vicious circle exists. In the affluent industrial nations the opposite problem—overnutrition—contributes to the risk of ischemic heart disease, diabetes, probably certain cancers, and, of course, obesity. Members of religious sects that adhere to vegetarian diets consistently have lower death rates from these conditions than do persons belonging to other faiths who live in the same environment but who are not vegetarians.

Having Well-born Children. As birth rates fall, it becomes increasingly important to ensure that the babies who are born are the best possible. Good prenatal care, including attention to maternal health, contributes to this. Avoiding exposure of the developing fetus to toxic substances such as tobacco, alcohol, and drugs, especially illicit addictive drugs, is very important. Genetic screening and counseling seem likely to become increasingly important in the future. Genetic engineering offers hope of controlling lethal genetic defects such as cystic fibrosis and Huntington's disease.

Providing Health Care Prudently. The medical profession has a depressing history of uncritical enthusiasm for fads and fashions. We tend to be more cautious now than formerly but still employ surgical procedures of dubious efficacy, such as tonsillectomy. It seems difficult also to find a good reason why cesarean delivery is the mode for up to a third of all the babies born in places where facilities for the procedure are abundant and why perinatal mortality rates are no better in such places than in others of similar economic and medical development where cesarean delivery is less often done. In public health practice we need to be rigorous in critically appraising the efficacy and adverse effects of mass medication such as vaccines and fluoridation of municipal water supplies. In this respect, public health practice has lagged behind clinical practice, where critical appraisal is increasingly often applied to guide decisions about appropriate application of health care technology.

Primary, Secondary, and Tertiary Prevention

We customarily distinguish several levels of prevention. The aim of primary prevention is to preserve health by removing the precipitating causes and determinants of departures from good health. To put it in epidemiological terms, the aim of primary prevention is to reduce the incidence of disease and injury. This can be done by eliminating causative agents such as the smallpox virus, by pasteurizing raw milk to kill the pathogenic organisms found in it; by rendering people and populations immune by artificially immunizing them; by safeguarding workers against exposure to toxic substances and hazardous processes in the workplace; and by using seat belts in automobiles and all sorts of industrial safety equipment.

The aim of secondary prevention is to detect and correct departures from good health as early as possible; in other words, to reduce the prevalence of disease and disability. We can often accomplish this with screening procedures that detect disease before it is manifested by symptoms or signs. Examples include tests to detect congenitally dislocated hips and metabolic or endocrine aberrations such as phenylketonuria and hypothyroidism at birth and cervical cytology to detect preinvasive cancer of the cervix. Screening needs to be combined with counseling about reduction of risks to health if it is to be fully efficacious. The U.S. Preventive Services Task Force has rigorously examined the current state of knowledge and technology for dealing with a wide range of conditions that lend themselves to secondary prevention.[5] Table 1–1 is an example of tables that set out the successful strategies and tactics and summarize the measures of proven efficacy.

TABLE 1–1. GUIDE TO CLINICAL PREVENTIVE SERVICES[a]

Birth to 18 Months (Schedule: 2, 4, 6, 15, 18 Months[b])

Screening	***Parent Counseling***	***Immunizations and Chemoprophylaxis***	***Leading Causes of Death***	***First Week***	***Remain Alert For***
Height and weight Hemoglobin and hematocrit[c] *High-Risk Groups* Hearing[d] (HR1) Erythrocyte protoporphyrin (HR2)	▪ **Diet** Breastfeeding Nutrient intake, especially iron-rich foods ▪ **Injury Prevention** Child safety seats Smoke detector Hot water heater temperature Stairway gates, window guards, pool fence Storage of drugs and toxic chemicals Syrup of ipecac, poison control telephone number ▪ **Dental Health** Baby bottle tooth decay ▪ **Other Primary Preventive Measures** Effects of passive smoking	Diphtheria-tetanus-pertussis (DTP) vaccine[e] Oral poliovirus vaccine (OPV)[f] Measles-mumps-rubella (MMR) vaccine[g] Haemophilus influenzae type b (Hib) conjugate vaccine[h] *High-Risk Groups* Fluoride supplements (HR3)	Conditions originating in perinatal period Congenital anomalies Heart disease Injuries (nonmotor vehicle) Pneumonia/influenza	Ophthalmic antibiotics[i] Hemoglobin electrophoresis (HR4[i]) T4/TSH[i] Phenylalanine[i] Hearing (HR1)	Ocular misalignment Tooth decay Signs of child abuse or neglect

▪ **HIGH-RISK CATEGORIES**

HR1: Infants with a family history of childhood hearing impairment or a personal history of congenital perinatal infection with herpes, syphilis, rubella, cytomegalovirus, or toxoplasmosis; malformations involving the head or neck (e.g., dysmorphic and syndromal abnormalities, cleft palate, abnormal pinna); birthweight below 1500 g; bacterial meningitis; hyperbilirubinemia requiring exchange transfusion; or severe perinatal asphyxia (Apgar scores of 0–3, absence of spontaneous respirations for 10 minutes, or hypotonia at 2 hours of age).

HR2: Infants who live in or frequently visit housing built before 1950 that is dilapidated or undergoing renovation; who come in contact with other children with known lead toxicity; who live near lead processing plants or whose parents or household members work in a lead-related occupation; or who live near busy highways or hazardous waste sites.

HR3: Infants living in areas with inadequate water fluoridation (less than 0.7 parts per million).

HR4: Newborns of Caribbean, Latin American, Asian, Mediterranean, or African descent.

Footnotes on page 9.

(continued)

TABLE 1-1. GUIDE TO CLINICAL PREVENTIVE SERVICES[a] (Continued)

Ages 40–64 (Schedule: Every 1–3 Years[k])				
Screening	***Counseling***	***Immunizations***	***Leading Causes of Death***	***Remain Alert For***
▪ **History** Dietary intake Physical activity Tobacco/alcohol/drug use Sexual practices ▪ **Physical Exam** Height and weight Blood pressure Clinical breast exam[l] *High-Risk Groups* Complete skin exam [HR1] Complete oral cavity exam [HR2] Palpation for thyroid nodules [HR3] Auscultation for carotid bruits [HR4] ▪ **Laboratory/ Diagnostic Procedures** Nonfasting total blood cholesterol Papanicolaou smear[m] Mammogram[n] *High-Risk Groups* Fasting plasma glucose [HR5] VDRL [HR6] Urinalysis for bacteriuria [HR7] Chlamydial testing [HR8] Gonorrhea culture [HR9] Counseling and testing for HIV [HR10] Tuberculin skin test (PPD) [HR11] Hearing [HR12] Electrocardiogram [HR13] Fecal occult blood/sigmoidoscopy [HR14] Fecal occult blood/colonoscopy [HR15] Bone mineral content [HR16]	▪ **Diet and Exercise** Fat (especially saturated fat), cholesterol, complex carbohydrates, fiber, sodium, calcium[o] Caloric balance Selection of exercise program ▪ **Substance Use** Tobacco cessation Alcohol and other drugs: Limiting alcohol consumption Driving/other dangerous activities while under the influence Treatment for abuse *High-Risk Groups* Sharing/using unsterilized needles and syringes [HR19] ▪ **Sexual Practices** Sexually transmitted diseases: partner selection, condoms, anal intercourse Unintended pregnancy and contraceptive options ▪ **Injury Prevention** Safety belts Safety helmets Smoke detector Smoking near bedding or upholstery *High-Risk Groups* Back-conditioning exercises [HR20] Prevention of childhood injuries [HR21] Falls in the elderly [HR22] ▪ **Dental Health** Regular tooth brushing, flossing, and dental visits ▪ **Other Primary Preventive Measures** *High-Risk Groups* Skin protection from ultraviolet light [HR23] Discussion of aspirin therapy [HR24] Discussion of estrogen replacement therapy [HR25]	Tetanus-diphtheria (Td) booster[p] *High-Risk Groups* Hepatitis B vaccine [HR26] Pneumococcal influenza vaccine [HR27] Influenza vaccine [HR28][q]	Heart disease Lung cancer Cerebrovascular disease Breast cancer Colorectal cancer Obstructive lung disease	Depressive symptoms Suicide risk factors [HR17] Abnormal bereavement Signs of physical abuse or neglect Malignant skin lesions Peripheral arterial disease [HR18] Tooth decay, gingivitis, loose teeth

Footnotes on page 9.

TABLE 1-1. GUIDE TO CLINICAL PREVENTIVE SERVICES[a] (Continued)

▪ **HIGH-RISK CATEGORIES**

HR1: Persons with a family or personal history of skin cancer, increased occupational or recreational exposure to sunlight, or clinical evidence of precursor lesions (e.g., dysplastic nevi, certain congenital nevi).

HR2: Persons with exposure to tobacco or excessive amounts of alcohol, or those with suspicious symptoms or lesions detected through self-examination.

HR3: Persons with a history of upper-body irradiation.

HR4: Persons with risk factors for cerebrovascular or cardiovascular disease (e.g., hypertension, smoking, coronary artery disease [CAD], atrial fibrillation, diabetes) or those with neurologic symptoms (e.g., transient ischemic attacks) or a history of cerebrovascular disease.

HR5: The markedly obese, persons with a family history of diabetes, or women with a history of gestational diabetes.

HR6: Prostitutes, persons who engage in sex with multiple partners in areas in which syphilis is prevalent, or contacts of persons with active syphilis.

HR7: Persons with diabetes.

HR8: Persons who attend clinics for sexually transmitted diseases, attend other high-risk health care facilities (e.g., adolescent and family planning clinics), or have other risk factors for chlamydial infection (e.g., multiple sexual partners or a sexual partner with multiple sexual contacts).

HR9: Prostitutes, persons with multiple sexual partners or a sexual partner with multiple contacts, sexual contacts of persons with culture-proven gonorrhea, or persons with a history of repeated episodes of gonorrhea.

HR10: Persons seeking treatment for sexually transmitted diseases; homosexual and bisexual men; past or present intravenous (IV) drug users; persons with a history of prostitution or multiple sexual partners; women whose past or present sexual partners were HIV-infected, bisexual, or IV drug users; persons with long-term residence or birth in an area with high prevalence of HIV infection; or persons with a history of transfusion between 1978 and 1985.

HR11: Household members of persons with tuberculosis or others at risk for close contact with the disease (e.g., staff of tuberculosis clinics, shelters for the homeless, nursing homes, substance abuse treatment facilities, dialysis units, correctional institutions); recent immigrants or refugees from countries in which tuberculosis is common (e.g., Asia, Africa, Central and South America, Pacific Islands); migrant workers; residents of nursing homes, correctional institutions, or homeless shelters; or persons with certain underlying medical disorders (e.g., HIV infection).

HR12: Persons exposed regularly to excessive noise.

HR13: Men with two or more cardiac risk factors (high blood cholesterol, hypertension, cigarette smoking, diabetes mellitus, family history of CAD); men who would endanger public safety were they to experience sudden cardiac events (e.g., commercial airline pilots); or sedentary or high-risk males planning to begin a vigorous exercise program.

HR14: Persons aged 50 and older who have first-degree relatives with colorectal cancer; a personal history of endometrial, ovarian, or breast cancer; or a previous diagnosis of inflammatory bowel disease, adenomatous polyps, or colorectal cancer.

HR15: Persons with a family history of familial polyposis coli or cancer family syndrome.

HR16: Perimenopausal women at increased risk for osteoporosis (e.g., Caucasian race, bilateral oophorectomy before menopause, slender build) and for whom estrogen replacement therapy would otherwise not be recommended.

HR17: Recent divorce, separation, unemployment, depression, alcohol or other drug abuse, serious medical illnesses, living alone, or recent bereavement.

HR18: Persons over 50, smokers, or persons with diabetes mellitus.

HR19: Intravenous drug users.

HR20: Persons at increased risk for low back injury because of past history, body configuration, or type of activities.

HR21: Persons with children in the home or automobile.

HR22: Persons with older adults in the home.

HR23: Persons with increased exposure to sunlight.

HR24: Men who have risk factors for myocardial infarction (e.g., high blood cholesterol, smoking, diabetes mellitus, family history of early-onset CAD) and who lack a history of gastrointestinal or other bleeding problems, and other risk factors for bleeding or cerebral hemorrhage.

HR25: Perimenopausal women at increased risk for osteoporosis (e.g., Caucasian, low bone mineral content, bilateral oophorectomy before menopause or early menopause, slender build) and who are without known contraindications (e.g., history of undiagnosed vaginal bleeding, active liver disease, thromboembolic disorders, hormone-dependent cancer).

HR26: Homosexually active men, intravenous drug users, recipients of some blood products, or persons in health-related jobs with frequent exposure to blood or blood products.

HR27: Persons with medical conditions that increase the risk of pneumococcal infection (e.g., chronic cardiac or pulmonary disease, sickle cell disease, nephrotic syndrome, Hodgkin's disease, asplenia, diabetes mellitus, alcoholism, cirrhosis, multiple myeloma, renal disease, or conditions associated with immunosuppression).

HR28: Residents of chronic care facilities and persons suffering from chronic cardiopulmonary disorders, metabolic diseases (including diabetes mellitus), hemoglobinopathies, immunosuppression, or renal dysfunction.

(continued)

TABLE 1–1. GUIDE TO CLINICAL PREVENTIVE SERVICES[a] (Continued)

Ages 65 and Over (Schedule: Every Year[k])

Screening	*Counseling*	*Immunizations*	*Leading Causes of Death*	*Remain Alert For*
▪ **History** Prior symptoms of transient ischemic attack Dietary intake Physical activity Tobacco/alcohol/drug use Functional status at home ▪ **Physical Exam** Height and weight Blood pressure Visual acuity Hearing and hearing aids Clinical breast exam[r] *High-Risk Groups* Auscultation for carotid bruits (HR1) Complete skin exam (HR2) Complete oral cavity exam (HR3) Palpation for thyroid nodules (HR4) ▪ **Laboratory/ Diagnostic Procedures** Nonfasting total blood cholesterol Dipstick urinalysis Mammogram[s] Thyroid function tests[t] *High-Risk Groups* Fasting plasma glucose (HR5) Tuberculin skin test (PPD) (HR6) Electrocardiogram (HR7) Papanicolaou smear[u] (HR8) Fecal occult blood/Sigmoidoscopy (HR9) Fecal occult blood/Colonoscopy (HR10)	▪ **Diet and Exercise** Fat (especially saturated fat), cholesterol, complex carbohydrates, fiber, sodium, calcium[t] Caloric balance Selection of exercise program ▪ **Substance Use** Tobacco cessation Alcohol and other drugs: Limiting alcohol consumption Driving/other dangerous activities while under the influence Treatment for abuse ▪ **Injury Prevention** Prevention of falls Safety belts Smoke detector Smoking near bedding or upholstery Hot water heater temperature Safety helmets *High-Risk Groups* Prevention of childhood injuries (HR12) ▪ **Dental Health** Regular dental visits, tooth brushing, flossing ▪ **Other Primary Preventive Measures** Glaucoma testing by eye specialist *High-Risk Groups* Discussion of estrogen replacement therapy (HR13) Discussion of aspirin therapy (HR14) Skin protection from ultraviolet light (HR15)	Tetanus-diphtheria (Td) booster[v] Influenza vaccine[w] Pneumococcal vaccine *High-Risk Groups* Hepatitis B vaccine (HR16)	Heart disease Cerebrovascular disease Obstructive lung disease Pneumonia/influenza Lung cancer Colorectal cancer	Depressive symptoms Suicide risk factors (HR11) Abnormal bereavement Changes in cognitive function Medications that increase risk of falls Signs of physical abuse or neglect Malignant skin lesions Peripheral arterial disease Tooth decay, gingivitis, loose teeth

Footnotes on page 9.

TABLE 1-1. GUIDE TO CLINICAL PREVENTIVE SERVICES[a] (Continued)

▪ **HIGH-RISK CATEGORIES**

HR1: Persons with risk factors for cerebrovascular or cardiovascular disease (e.g., hypertension, smoking, CAD, atrial fibrillation, diabetes) or those with neurologic symptoms (e.g., transient ischemic attacks) or a history of cerebrovascular disease.

HR2: Persons with a family or personal history of skin cancer, or clinical evidence of precursor lesions (e.g., dysplastic nevi, certain congenital nevi), or those with increased occupational exposure to sunlight.

HR3: Persons with exposure to tobacco or excessive amounts of alcohol, or those with suspicious symptoms or lesions detected through self-examination.

HR4: Persons with a history of upper-body irradiation.

HR5: The markedly obese, persons with a family history of diabetes, or women with a history of gestational diabetes.

HR6: Household members of persons with tuberculosis or others at risk for close contact with the disease (e.g., staff of tuberculosis clinics, shelters for the homeless, nursing homes, substance abuse treatment facilities, dialysis units, correctional institutions); recent immigrants or refugees from countries in which tuberculosis is common (e.g., Asia, Africa, Central and South America, Pacific Islands); migrant workers, residents of nursing homes, correctional institutions, or homeless shelters; or persons with certain underlying medical disorders (e.g., HIV infection).

HR7: Men with two or more cardiac risk factors (high blood cholesterol, hypertension, cigarette smoking, diabetes mellitus, family history of CAD); men who would endanger public safety were they to experience sudden cardiac events (e.g., commercial airline pilots); or sedentary or high-risk males planning to begin a vigorous exercise program.

HR8: Women who have not had previous documented screening in which smears have been consistently negative.

HR9: Persons who have first-degree relatives with colorectal cancer; a personal history of endometrial, ovarian, or breast cancer; or a previous diagnosis of inflammatory bowel disease, adenomatous polyps, or colorectal cancer.

HR10: Persons with a family history of familial polyposis coli or cancer family syndrome.

HR11: Recent divorce, separation, unemployment, depression, alcohol or other drug abuse, serious medical illnesses, living alone, or recent bereavement.

HR12: Persons with children in the home or automobile.

HR13: Women at increased risk for osteoporosis (e.g., Caucasian, low bone mineral content, bilateral oopherectomy before menopause or early menopause, slender build) and who are without known contraindications (e.g., history of undiagnosed vaginal bleeding, active liver disease, thromboembolic disorders, hormone dependent cancer).

HR14: Men who have risk factors for myocardial infarction (e.g., high blood cholesterol, smoking, diabetes mellitus, family history of early-onset CAD) and who lack a history of gastrointestinal or other bleeding problems, or other risk factors for bleeding or cerebral hemorrhage.

HR15: Persons with increased exposure to light.

HR16: Homosexually active men, intravenous drug users, recipients of some blood products, or persons in healh-related jobs with frequent exposure to blood products.

[a] This list of preventive services is not exhaustive. It reflects only those topics reviewed by the U.S. Preventive Services Task Force. Clinicians may wish to add other preventive services after considering the patient's medical history and other individual circumstances.

[b] Five visits are required for immunizations. Because of lack of data and differing patient risk profiles, the scheduling of additional visits and the frequency of the individual preventive services listed in this table are left to clinical discretion, except as indicated in other footnotes.

[c] Once during infancy; [d] at age 18-month visit, if not tested earlier; [e] at ages 2, 4, 6, and 15 months; [f] at ages 2, 4, and 15 months; [g] at age 15 months; [h] at age 18 months; [i] at birth; [j] days 3 to 6 preferred for testing.

[k] The recommended schedule applies only to the periodic visit itself. The frequency of the individual preventive services listed in this table is left to clinical discretion, except as indicated in other footnotes.

[l] Annually for women; [m] every 1 to 3 years for women; [n] every 1 to 2 years for women beginning at age 50; [o] for women; [p] every 10 years; [q] annually.

[r] Annually for women until age 75, unless pathology detected; [s] every 1 to 2 years for women until age 75, unless pathology detected; [t] for women; [u] every 1 to 3 years; [v] every 10 years; [w] annually.

From U.S. Preventive Services Task Force: Guide to Clinical Preventive Services. Baltimore: Williams & Wilkins, 1989.

Health Promotion

A conference sponsored by WHO in Ottawa, Canada, in 1986 produced a Charter on Health Promotion[6] that called for a new approach to building healthy public policy. Health promotion is defined as the process of enabling people to increase control over and improve their health. An individual or a group must be able to identify and to realize aspirations, to satisfy needs, and to change or cope with the environment. Health is a resource for everyday life, a positive concept emphasizing social and personal resources as well as physical capabilities.

Prerequisites for health are peace, shelter, education, food, income, a stable ecosystem, sustainable resources, social justice, and equity. Improvement of health requires a secure foundation in these basic prerequisites.

The Ottawa charter calls for building healthy public policy, creating supportive environments, strengthening community action, developing personal skills, and reorienting health services.

The Scientific Basis of Public Health

Public health specialists use the natural, biological, and behavioral sciences; dependence upon particular fields of science varies from one specialty to another. All have in common dependence upon epidemiology as the principal basic science of public health. The uses and methods of epidemiology are described and discussed in Chapter 2. Epidemiology provides most of the facts that are the basis for decisions about health policies. We must be aware of the limitations imposed upon the validity of decisions by imperfect knowledge and by misinterpretation of the evidence—a common problem, especially when competing interests lead to different degrees of emphasis on particular items of evidence. The conclusions that shape health policy can vary, depending on whether the health worker making the interpretation is employed by a university department, by government, a labor union, a public interest lobby group, an industrial corporation, or a private consultant firm that accepts contracts from the highest bidder. Problems of uncertainty and conflict of interest are considered in the final chapter of this book.

The Politics of Public Health

Steps necessary to protect and improve the public health may not be universally welcomed. Sometimes they are vigorously opposed by powerful lobby groups, such as the tobacco industry and the National Rifle Association. The meat and dairy industries have opposed the suggestion that their products are implicated as risk factors in ischemic heart disease. Sometimes the campaigns mounted against public health measures are based on emotion more than reason, as was the case with the antivaccinationists of the nineteenth century and the antifluoridationists in the second half of the twentieth century. In the latter instance the catch phrase "Keep the water pure" is a difficult aspiration for ill-informed voters to resist.

It is essential for public health workers who are in the public eye, especially for prominent officials such as medical officers or commissioners of health, to be politically astute. Even junior public health workers can be thrust into situations where their ability to marshall the facts and debate the issues will be severely tested. An important role for national organizations such as the American Public Health Association is advocacy of health-protecting action in contentious situations such as disposal of hazardous waste or the control of indoor air pollution due to tobacco smoke. The opposition to actions sought by public health workers at the local level is often powerful and well organized. It is wise to call on experienced advocates if situations of this sort arise.

At every level from local to national and international, public health professionals always need to marshall their arguments carefully, to be thoroughly in command of the necessary facts, and to use communication skills effectively to ensure that the political decision-makers are apprised of the priorities that will ensure the enhancement of health for which public health services exist. The remaining chapters in this book contain the necessary facts and often the arguments that can be used to help achieve leadership and to implement effective public health policies.

REFERENCES

1. Fenner F, Henderson DA, Arita I, Jezek Z, Ladnyi ID: Smallpox and its eradication. Geneva: World Health Organization, 1988
2. Jones EF, Forrest JD, Goldman N, Henshaw S, Lincoln R, Rosoff JI, Westoff CF, Wulf D: Teenage Pregnancy in Industrialized Countries. New Haven: Yale University Press, 1986
3. World Commission on Environment and Development: Our Common Future (the Brundtland Report). Oxford and New York: Oxford University Press, 1987
4. Gruenberg EM: The failures of success. Milbank Mem Fund Q 55:3, 1977
5. U.S. Preventive Services Task Force: Guide to Clinical Preventive Services: An Assessment of the Effectiveness of 169 Interventions. Baltimore: Williams & Wilkins, 1989
6. Ottawa Charter for Health Promotion: Can J Public Health 77:425–430, 1986

2
Epidemiology

Carl W. Tyler, Jr.
John M. Last

We can study health and disease by observing their effects on individuals, by laboratory investigation of experimental animals, and by measuring the distribution of health problems in the population. The third method is epidemiology—the basic science and most fundamental practice of public health and preventive medicine.

The word *epidemiology* derives from *epidemic,* which literally translated from the Greek means "upon the people." The word reminds us that the first concern of the epidemiologist was to investigate, control, and prevent epidemics. This chapter is about epidemiology. It deals with the sources and characteristics of information used to assess the health of populations, how this information can be analyzed, and ways in which epidemiology may be useful in controlling and preventing health problems.

HISTORY

Like much of Western medicine, epidemiology has roots in the Bible and in the writings of Hippocrates. The *Aphorisms* of Hippocrates (fourth to fifth century BC) contain many generalizations that can have been based only on prolonged and careful observation of large numbers of cases. The introductory paragraph of *Airs, Waters, Places* offers timeless advice on good environmental epidemiology:

> Whoever would study medicine aright must learn of the following subjects. First he must consider the effect of each of the seasons of the year and the differences between them. Secondly he must study the warm and the cold winds, both those which are common to every country and those peculiar to a particular locality. Lastly, the effect of water on the health must not be forgotten. . . . When, therefore, a physician comes to a district previously unknown to him, he should consider both its situation and its aspect to the winds. . . . Similarly, the nature of the water supply must be considered. . . . Then think of the soil, whether it be bare and waterless or thickly covered with vegetation and well-watered; whether in a hollow and stifling, or exposed and cold. Lastly consider the life of the inhabitants themselves; are they heavy drinkers and eaters and consequently unable to stand fatigue or, being fond of work and exercise, eat wisely but drink sparely?[1]

Physicians in ancient times were much concerned with epidemics, although often they could do little more than observe the victims and record mortality. Their limited knowledge rarely permitted effective intervention. Until the Renaissance the approach of physicians was essentially nonnumerical: generalizations were based on impressions rather than on real numbers. John Graunt is often regarded as the founder of vital statistics, because he was the first to describe the use of numerical methods, in *Natural and Political Observations on the Bills of Mortality* (1662).

The control of communicable diseases was the first application of epidemiology to public health and was carried out through quarantine and isolation, even though ideas about disease transmission and microbiology as well as epidemiology were rudimentary. In the eighteenth century, Johann Peter Frank, a physician who became "director-general of public health" (in modern terminology) to the Hapsburg Empire, produced a massive work, *System einer vollständigen medicinischen Polizey* (1779), in which he systematized and codified many rules for personal and communal behavior that contributed to health.

Careful clinical observation, precise counts of well-defined cases, and demonstration of relationships between cases and the characteristics of the populations in which they occur all combine in the method on which epidemiology depends. This method was first developed in the nineteenth century. Modern epidemiologists hold John Snow[2] in high esteem because he painstakingly collected the facts about sources of drinking water and related these to mortality rates from cholera in London, thus demonstrating the mode of transmission about 30 years before Koch isolated and identified the cholera *Vibrio*. Snow's great contemporary, William Farr,[3] defined and clarified many basic concepts of vital statistics and epidemiology: the scope of epidemiology, the concept of person-years, the relationship between mortality rate and probability of dying, standardized mortality ratios, dose-response relationships, herd immunity, the relationship between incidence and prevalence, and the concepts of retrospective and prospective study. He also developed the first effective classification of disease, the direct ancestor of the nosology that we still use today. *Vital Statistics* (1885), an edited volume of excerpts from Farr's annual reports to the registrar-general, is perhaps the best textbook of epidemiology ever written, graced by beautiful writing and well-chosen tables to illustrate the text.

Methods of epidemiological investigation have evolved since the mid-nineteenth century. The case-control study reentered medicine from the social sciences in the third decade of the twentieth century. The cohort study came into use after World War II as a means of identifying risks associated with heart disease, lung cancer, and other emerging public health problems. Epidemiological "experiments" as now conducted in randomized trials are essentially a modern innovation. Statistical methods and the electronic computer add greatly to the power of epidemiological analysis. Present indications suggest expanding potential and an exciting future for epidemiology. There is an increasingly broad interface between clinical medicine and epidemiology. Case-control studies are adding rapidly to our understanding of cause-effect relationships in many chronic and disabling disorders. Epidemiological methods are also increasingly used to evaluate health services.

DEFINITION

Science. Epidemiology was originally defined as the scientific study of epidemics. More recently, however, the definition has been broadened to recognize the application of epidemiology to the control and prevention of health problems. A recent definition, agreed upon by an international panel, is the following:

> Epidemiology is the study of the distribution and determinants of health-related states and events in specified populations and the application of this study to the control of health problems.[4]

Some terms in this definition require discussion. *Distribution* is considered in relation to time, place, and person, that is, the relationship between the disease or health problem and the population in which this exists. The relevant population characteristics include location, age, sex, and race distribution; occupational and other social characteristics; living places; susceptibility; and exposure to specific agents. In addition, the distribution of the exposure under study to this population over time is concerned with trends, cyclic or secular patterns, clusters, and intervals between exposure to inciting factors and the onset of disease.

Determinants include both causes and factors that influence the risk of disease. Diseases are said to have a single necessary cause, for example, the agent of disease such as the tubercle bacillus, the lead in lead-based paint to which children with lead poisoning are exposed, or the radiation from an atomic bomb to which persons with leukemia might have been exposed. In addition, there are usually many other determinants. These fall into two broad groups: (1) host factors, which determine the susceptibility of the individual, and (2) environmental factors, which determine the host's exposure to the specific agent. Host factors include age, sex, race, genetic or constitutional makeup, physiologic state, nutritional condition, and previous immunologic experience. Environmental factors include all conditions of living—family size and composition, crowding, hygienic conditions, occupation, geographic, climatic, and seasonal circumstances, and those qualities of individuals or populations (such as use of tobacco, alcohol, and automobiles) that are identified by the term *life-style.* Past as well as present environment—including the period of intrauterine life—may influence exposure and susceptibility to disease.

Practice. The practice of a science can best be defined in terms of the tasks a scientist performs. As Langmuir[5] put it, "the basic operation of the epidemiologist is to count cases and measure the population in which they arise" so that rates can be calculated and the occurrence of a health problem compared in different groups of people. Developing this fundamental idea in more detail, the practice of epidemiology is the scientific process by which health problems are detected, investigated, analyzed, and applied to the control and prevention of these problems. This practice requires that health problems be the subject of public health surveillance, epidemiological investigation, and analysis. The findings of this analysis are linked to health policy and programs intended to control and prevent recurrence of the problem. Evaluation of these control and prevention measures is also the responsibility of the practicing epidemiologist, as is the clear and persuasive communication of the scientific findings to policy makers, program personnel, and the public.

USES OF EPIDEMIOLOGY

The most important use of epidemiology is to improve our understanding of health and disease—a goal shared by all the disciplines and branches of the biomedical sciences. Morris[6] defined seven uses of epidemiology: historical study, community diagnosis, working of health services, individual chances, completing the clinical picture, identification of syndromes, and the search for causes (Table 2-1). Each deserves brief comment.

Historical Study. Is community health improving? We can decide only by comparing experience (rates) over time; this is one essential routine activity in all health services. Sometimes unexpected trends appear when the data are closely examined, for example, the unexpected occurrence of rare opportunistic infections in Los Angeles, New York, and Miami that marked the beginning of the AIDS epidemic.

Community Diagnosis. What are the health problems? This question can be answered in many ways. For example, what proportion of school children have become regular cigarette smokers by various stages of their progress through school? What proportion of people always or never use seat belts when driving or when passengers in cars? Answers to such questions have prognostic as well as diagnostic value; it is possible to predict the impact of future health problems on the basis of known effects of many risk factors.

Working of Health Services. Are all needed services available, accessible, and used appropriately? Are children receiving necessary immunizations? Are pregnant women beginning to receive prenatal care before the end of the first trimester of pregnancy? Are known contacts of persons with sexually transmitted diseases followed up and treated? Information on these and many other questions is often gathered routinely or by special survey. Health service administrators should not think always of

TABLE 2-1. USES OF EPIDEMIOLOGY

- Historical study: Is community health getting better or worse?
- Community diagnosis: What actual and potential health problems are there?
- Working of health services
  - Efficacy
  - Effectiveness
  - Efficiency
- Individual risks and chances
  - Actuarial risks
  - Health hazard appraisal
- Completing the clinical picture: Different presentations of a disease
- Identification of syndromes: "Lumping and splitting"
- Search for causes: Case control and cohort studies
- Evaluation of presenting symptoms and signs
- Clinical decision analysis

these simple routine questions but should be alert to less obvious potential gaps in coverage. For example, the census will disclose the numbers of elderly persons who live alone. Are all or only a small portion of such persons known to the public health nurses and others who provide home services and care?

Individual Chances. What is the risk that you will die before your next birthday? Actuaries who risk-rate persons seeking life insurance have calculated answers based on probabilities derived from past experience. This has become a prominent activity of epidemiologists who work on risk assessment and has led to many new insights, for example, about occupational and environmental risks, the hazards associated with immunizations.[7]

Completing the Clinical Picture. One of Morris's original illustrations of this use for epidemiology was the demonstration that myocardial infarction does, indeed, occur commonly among women as well as among men, but at older ages, and appears more often as a "ruptured ventricle"—which, of course, causes sudden death. The technique of "completing the clinical picture" has been used in many other ways, for example, to construct a model[8] of what might occur in the average general practice population in the course of a year—what is known to and seen by the physician, and what else is there but unidentified, undiagnosed—whether overt disease or precursor states that, if detected early, could be corrected before they cause irreversible harm (i.e., the submerged part of the iceberg of disease).

Identification of Syndromes. Epidemiologists have been called "lumpers and splitters" because our investigations sometimes make it possible to group together several differing manifestations of a condition or to separate seemingly identical diseases into more than one category. The latter is more common than the former; examples include the differentiation of hepatitis A from hepatitis B and the distinction between several varieties of childhood leukemia. Examples of "lumping" include the identification of many manifestations of tuberculosis that were once known each by a different name, for example, phthisis, consumption, pleurisy, and the efforts now in progress to identify addiction to tobacco as the underlying cause of several outcomes, notably respiratory cancers, chronic obstructive pulmonary disease, and at least a proportion of cases of coronary heart disease. All of these could be called results of "tobaccoism."

The Search for Causes. The search for causes is the most obvious use for epidemiology. Most hypothesis-testing studies (discussed later) have the primary aim of identifying causal factors or at least risk factors for disease. Examples of many such studies are mentioned throughout this book.

Other Uses. Clinical epidemiologists have defined other uses of epidemiology outside the scope of Morris's original seven. One important use of epidemiology is the evaluation of presenting symptoms and signs of disease, which can be done by analyzing the data in hospital charts and relating presenting symptoms and complaints to final diagnoses. This makes it possible to produce algorithms showing the probability that a particular cluster of presenting symptoms and signs is due to any of several possible underlying disease processes. A related use is clinical decision analysis,[9] a technique whereby rigorous quantitative methods and logic are applied to arrive at decisions about the best method of managing patients with particular diseases or, more commonly nowadays with aging populations and multiple pathologic conditions, constellations of diseases. This procedure involves the use of "decision trees"—algorithms in which probabilities of outcomes for each alternative choice are predicted on the basis of past experience. Some of this fits more or less into the category of "individual chances," but for the most part it is a sufficiently specialized use of epidemiology and clinical logic to merit a name of its own.

THE EPIDEMIOLOGICAL METHOD

Epidemiology applies all available pertinent methods and tools to ascertain the distribution and determinants of health-related states and events in a population and to synthesize the derived information to acquire understanding of health problems and disease processes for the purpose of controlling and preventing them. Clinical, laboratory, and field observations are all used. Ultimately, it is the reasoning of the epidemiologist that ties these facts together.

Epidemiological reasoning is based on a group of fundamental and straightforward actions. First, the epidemiologist defines the events or clinical cases to be studied, using careful, specific, and objective observations. Next, these events or cases must be counted and oriented to time, place, and person. After this orientation, the epidemiologist determines the population at risk and calculates rates using methods little more complicated than long division, that is, putting the events or cases in the numerator according to their relevant characteristics and using a denominator of (the portion of) the population at risk characterized in a manner similar to that of the numerator. These rates are then compared with the rates of occurrence in other population groups. Finally, using this information, the epidemiologist draws inferences about the events that define the health problem, the agent or agents that cause it, the host and environmental factors that influence the risk of its occurrence, and the means by which it is transmitted. Using this information and collaborating with other health professionals, the epidemiologist proposes control measures and then continues the observations required to assess the proposed control program.

In identifying a health problem or case, many kinds of clinical examination may be employed. The patient's history may reveal information about exposure to risk, incubation period, susceptibility, occupation, residence, course of disease, or other factors. Physical examination can classify individuals not only as to whether they have the condition under study but also as to type, stage, and duration of disease. Laboratory tests are valuable for a similar purpose. In addition, they are essential in revealing clinically unapparent cases, and they often shed light on the pathogenesis of the condition. Field observations are the sine qua non of the epidemiological method.

As an example of the fruitfulness of interlocking clinical, laboratory, and field studies, let us consider viral hepatitis. Epidemic jaundice was mentioned by Hippocrates and has occurred in wars from ancient times to the present. When needle biopsy was developed in the 1940s, the acute disease was found to be accompanied by generalized parenchymal inflammation of the liver. Hepatitis A ("infectious hepatitis") was soon distinguished through epidemiological study from hepatitis B ("syringe jaundice"). Both were shown to be due to filterable agents, presumably viruses, but hepatitis A had the epidemiological features of fecal-oral transmission, while hepatitis B was clearly blood borne and transmitted by inadequately sterilized hypodermic needles or other medical equipment; there was no cross-immunity. Krugman's studies with volunteers showed further differences: hepatitis A had a shorter incubation period, was more contagious, and had a briefer period of abnormal serum transaminase activity than hepatitis B.[10] Later epidemiological studies revealed the pattern of sexual transmission of hepatitis B among male homosexuals. In 1965 Blumberg and colleagues[11] found Australia antigen in the serum of patients who had had multiple transfusions, and in 1967 this was unequivocally associated with hepatitis B. Blumberg subsequently received the Nobel Prize for his work. In 1970, Dane and coworkers[12] identified and described the virus, and in 1971 Almeida and colleagues[13] found that the surface particles, HBsAg, represented Australia antigen. HBsAg was soon found to be of great value in screening carriers for hepatitis B and also in developing a vaccine. Vaccines developed independently in the late 1970s in France and in the United States have been rigorously tested in laboratory and field trials and are of proven efficacy and safety in preventing hepatitis B in susceptible individuals, such as patients and staff members in renal dialysis units, infants born to mothers carrying hepatitis B, and male homosexuals. The virus of hepatitis A was identified in 1973 and successfully grown in tissue culture in 1979; this led to preparation of hepatitis A viral antigen, paving the way for serological tests for hepatitis A antibody. This antibody was found in some 70% of adult urban Americans, indicating a high prevalence of subclinical cases. Vaccine preparation is made possible by these advances; as hygiene and sanitation improve, infants and children are spared, and more serious cases occur among adults in contrast to the previous pattern of subclinical and mild cases among children. Vaccination against the disease is therefore more desirable than ever.

Finally, the epidemiological features of hepatitis B among homosexual men have provided a useful model to follow in the investigation of acquired immunodeficiency syndrome (AIDS). Both conditions have the same pattern of distribution in this subset of the population. Case-control studies have shown that many of the persons who contract AIDS, like those who have hepatitis B, are male homosexuals who engage in anal intercourse and have numerous partners.[14]

The tools employed in this illustration of the epidemiological method are clinical, immunological, microbiological, pathological, demographic, sociological, and statistical. None could be considered uniquely epidemiological; it is their employment in particular ways with particular objectives that constitutes the epidemiological method.

In epidemiology, unlike clinical medicine, the concern is not with individual cases but with all the cases in a defined population. Furthermore, the entire range of manifestations of the condition must be considered in relation to the population from which the cases arise.

THE EPIDEMIOLOGICAL SEQUENCE

There is an orderly sequence in epidemiology: (1) Observation, (2) counting cases or events, (3) relating cases or events to the population at risk, (4) making comparisons, (5) developing the hypothesis, (6) testing the hypothesis, (7) making scientific inferences, (8) conducting experimental studies, and (9) intervention and evaluation. This sequence describes the actions we take whenever a "new" condition occurs. The stages in this sequence can be illustrated by several examples. One of these is the relationship between cigarette smoking and lung cancer:

1. **Observation:** Scientific observations on smoking and cancer appeared in the *Journal of the American Medical Association*[15] in 1920 and in the *New England Journal of Medicine*[16] in 1928. In the following decade, *Science*[17] documented that smokers had a shorter life expectancy than nonsmokers.
2. **Counting cases or events:** Vital statistics trends showed an increase in deaths caused by lung cancer in the United States beginning in the 1930s.
3. **Relating cases or events to the population at risk:** Even though population growth increased in the United States, increasing death rates attributable to lung cancer were reported in national vital statistics and remarked on in annual reports of health departments and offices of vital statistics in other countries where smoking was an established life-style characteristic.
4. **Making comparisons:** Studies of British physicians reported by Doll and Hill,[18] and of contacts of American Cancer Society volunteers reported by Hammond and Horn[19] in the 1950s provided definitive comparisons between groups of smokers and nonsmokers, demonstrating an association between smoking and lung cancer. (These studies led to the establishment of contemporary criteria for epidemiological associations[20] in addition to identifying an important threat to the health of the public.)
5. **Developing the hypothesis:** Since cigarette smoke contains more than 2000 chemical components, some of which are carcinogenic in animals,[21] only a small logical step was required to develop the hypothesis that smoking might cause lung cancer.
6. **Testing the hypothesis:** The hypothesis that smoking caused lung cancer lent itself to testing by means of a case-control study. Although a small case-control study was actually done in Germany in 1938-1939, the report was overlooked in the turmoil of World War II. Epidemiological studies designed to test the hypothesis were conducted in postwar Britain by Doll and Hill[18] and in the United States by Hammond and Horn.[19] Both showed consistent relationships between the present occurrence of lung cancer and a past history of cigarette smoking, with a dose-response relationship. Subsequent case-control studies produced similar results. These studies were soon followed by cohort studies. Studies of both kinds have confirmed the association and demonstrated other adverse effects.[22]
7. **Making scientific inferences:** Clinical observations, national trends in mortality from several countries associated with the increased prevalence of cigarette smoking, epidemiological comparisons made in large groups representing different segments of national populations in more than one country, and the biological effects of tobacco smoke all led to the inference that smoking caused or at least increased the risk of dying from this disease.
8. **Conducting experimental studies:** Laboratory animal studies with beagles have shown that exposure to tobacco smoke produces the precancerous lesions that are followed by squamous cell carcinoma in both animals and humans.
9. **Intervention and evaluation:** Action by public health and voluntary health agencies has been followed by a reduction in cigarette smoking rates with a subsequent decline in mortality rates from smoking-related causes in the United States and other countries. An important step in this process was the Surgeon General's annual *Report on Smoking and Health,* which began in 1964 and commemorated its twenty-fifth issue in 1989.[22]

THE FOUNDATIONS OF EPIDEMIOLOGICAL PRACTICE

Putting the epidemiological method into practice requires the epidemiologist to be skilled and experienced in a unique set of tasks.

Surveillance. Surveillance as an element of epidemiological practice is "the ongoing systematic collection, analysis, and interpretation of health data essential to the planning, implementation, and evaluation of public health practice, closely integrated with the timely dissemination of these data to those who need to know. The final link in the surveillance chain is the application of these data to prevention and control." This definition is part of the plan for the national coordination of disease surveillance of the Centers for Disease Control (CDC)[23] and is based in part on that proposed by Langmuir[24] in 1963.

The surveillance of public health problems is the first important task for the practicing epidemiologist, because it is the means of detecting problems on an ongoing basis. Public health surveillance makes use of established data-collection procedures and existing data sets, uses a minimum of data items, and is intended to detect changes in the occurrence of health events in a timely manner, so that problems can be found, confirmed quickly, investigated, analyzed and brought under control without delay. Surveillance focuses on descriptive information, the analysis of time trends, the estimation of rates, and the feedback of analysis to the health personnel of the community from which the data originated, as well as to other health-policy makers who need this information.

Investigation. Epidemiological investigations may be triggered by public health surveillance information or by any of a number of other initiating factors, including news articles, telephone calls, other health departments, or colleagues in epidemiology who share similar responsibilities.

The investigation of an epidemiological problem, whether it is an epidemic of acute infection or a long-term condition such as cancer, begins with careful observation and a detailed description. The basic steps of an epidemiological investigation have been worked out in detail and are discussed below.

Analysis. The analysis of epidemiological data proceeds through a series of orderly steps beginning with a careful, detailed description of cases or events. The description should include direct observations of persons influenced by the health event, the environment in which they live and work, the risk factors relevant to the event, and information about the agents that might have caused the health problem. The observations need to be quantified. The analysis progresses to comparison groups. The epidemiologist then compares rates of occurrence among groups by specific characteristics of the groups (e.g., looking for a dose-response relationship) and may ultimately reach the point of complex and sophisticated quantitative analysis.

Evaluation. Evaluation addresses problems that are well defined, such as the effectiveness of a drug or vaccine. It involves the assessment of problem-solving action. For this reason, the first essential step is a detailed description of the problem to be solved and of the action intended to resolve it. Evaluation not only includes assessment of the effectiveness of specific agents, but it can also be applied in many other situations (e.g., contraceptive effectiveness, smallpox eradication, effectiveness of screening for cervical cancer).

Other Essential Tasks. Communication, management, consultation, and human relations tasks are essential but not unique to the practice of epidemiology.

Communication. Communicating epidemiological information clearly and persuasively is essential to effective practice. Just as a clinician must persuade a patient to take pills or to undergo surgery, an epidemiologist must persuade professional colleagues, public officials, and the public that epidemiological findings warrant action to control and prevent a health problem.

Management. Because they rarely work alone, epidemiologists also need to develop management skills. Even in the investigation of a small outbreak, the assistance of a public health nurse may be essential. Subsequent analytic work often requires collaboration with statistical personnel, computer staff, or secretarial professionals. In these circumstances, basic concepts of management are needed to do the work of epidemiology, beginning with planning and including organizing, team building, directing, and management evaluation.

Consultation. Consultations with colleagues in epidemiology, other fields of public health, clinical medicine, or public groups is part of the professional practice. Consultation requires a special kind of communication skill; it is difficult to offer scientifically sound advice in a persuasive yet dispassionate manner, especially when past experience indicates that the advice may not be followed. Nonetheless, that is what is required of a consultant. An epidemiologist who excludes this role from professional practice diminishes the satisfaction gained from epidemiology. Not only will the excitement of exchanging ideas be diminished but so will the availability of others whose consultation might be valuable.

Presentation Skills. The ability to present epidemiological findings to professional and public groups is as much a part of epidemiology as doing a case count or computing a relative risk. This skill differs from that of consultation because a presentation is most often a single event in which epidemiological information is discussed and often presented orally and visually to a large group. Consultation, on the other hand, is a process that requires information gathering, often involves interviewing, and may conclude with a presentation. Distinguishing between these two is important because it emphasizes skill in presentation. Without this skill, important epidemiological work may have little health or scientific impact.

Human Relations. Human relations cannot be ignored in any profession. Skills in human relations are best learned by practice and observation. The classroom may not be the best place to learn these skills, but it is often an important place to start by listening to the person giving instruction and by also practicing and observing the interactions of those in the classroom.

Relationship to Other Public Health Professions. The unique discipline of epidemiology interacts with a host of other professions.

Statistics. Statistics is the discipline most closely allied with epidemiology. Epidemiologists need to know enough statistics to calculate rates and to determine how likely it is that differences in comparison groups could be due to chance. Statisticians support epidemiological studies in many ways, for example, by helping determine sample size, choosing samples, ensuring data quality, selecting the correct approach to complex analysis, and interpreting findings.

Laboratory Science. Laboratory science is often the key to correctly identifying a disease agent and an environmental exposure. Laboratory determinations help characterize host susceptibility and assess carrier and preclinical disease states. Perhaps most important, the laboratory provides the greatest predictive capability possible in arriving at a case definition.

Health Policy. Epidemiologists optimize their contribution to public health when the problems they address influence health policy. Policy decisions often seem remote from the practice of epidemiology because epidemiologists may equate policy with politics. However, the fact is that epidemiologists influence policy to some degree almost every time they issue a report.

Health Service and Program Management. Epidemiology often provides the information that sets the standards of care in health service programs. Epidemiological evaluation of effectiveness may determine the product used in nationwide programs and the schedule for administering preventive agents, such as vaccines, or conducting screening examinations, such as cervical cytology.

SURVEILLANCE

Definition

Because it often marks the beginning of the epidemiologic sequence, the definition of surveillance, as put forth by CDC and the Council of State and Territorial Epidemiologists (CSTE) in the United States, warrants reinforcement: "Surveillance is the ongoing systematic collection, analysis, and interpretation of health data essential to the planning, implementation, and evaluation of public health practice, closely integrated with the timely dissemination of these data to those who need to know. The final link in the surveillance chain is the application of these data to prevention and control."[23] This link leads to the formation of a cycle. This cycle brings together the evaluation of prevention and control and the detection of subsequent epidemics through the continued collection, analysis, and interpretation of data into a system of public health surveillance.

While the concept of surveillance in epidemiology goes back centuries—at least to Graunt and Farr—the practice of surveillance has continued to evolve. Its most important modern milestone was the clear and precise definition given to this practice by Langmuir[24] in 1963. He stated that surveillance was "the continued watchfulness over the distribution and trends of incidence through the systematic collection, consolidation, and evaluation of morbidity and mortality reports and other relevant data" and the reporting of this information to all of those who needed to know, implicitly including health officials, clinical physicians, and the public.

Surveillance is not the same as epidemiological research. The definition used by CDC and CSTE explicitly points out the need for timeliness and for dissemination; at the same time, it clearly links surveillance to public health action. While surveillance may identify problems in need of research, it is better described as a problem-finding process with an immediate relationship to public health action.

Surveillance systems also differ from health-information systems. Health information systems include the registration of births and deaths, the routine abstraction of hospital records, and general health surveys. Most often these systems differ from surveillance systems in that health information systems may not be ongoing, they may not be integrated with timely dissemination, or they may not be specifically applied to prevention and control efforts. Nonetheless, data from health-information systems can be important components of the practice of surveillance, depending on how the information is used. For example, birth weight as recorded on a birth certificate is an important element in the case definition in a surveillance system for the birth of premature, high-risk infants.

Purpose

In the practice of epidemiology and public health, surveillance has the following specific purposes: (1) to describe trends and the natural history of a health condition, (2) to detect epidemics, (3) to provide details about patterns of disease occurrence, (4) to monitor change in disease agents through laboratory testing, (5) to plan and set priorities for health programs, (6) to evaluate control and prevention measures, (7) to detect changes in health practices, (8) to evaluate hypotheses about disease occurrence, and (9) to detect rare but significant cases of diseases, such as botulism.

To assure that a surveillance system fulfills its purpose, the problem surveillance is intended to address needs to be clearly defined. Objectives for the system need to be established in terms of the case (or event) definition and the timeliness and completeness with which it is reported. Because of its role in initiating public health action, and to make the difference between surveillance and epidemiological research more distinct, Thacker and Berkelman[25] propose that this practice be referred to as "public health surveillance" rather than epidemiological surveillance.

The Surveillance Cycle

Public health surveillance embodies a systematic cycle of public health actions. The cycle includes (1) collection of pertinent data in a regular, frequent, and timely manner, (2) its orderly consolidation, evaluation, and descriptive interpretation, and (3) prompt dissemination of the findings (Table 2–2). Dissemination must focus on the distribution of information to those who provided the data so that they can confirm or correct them and to those who are in a position to take action on the data. The cycle is ongoing. The data may be updated and corrected, because new data may lead to a response by the public health system. Under rare circumstances, surveillance may be terminated, as was done when smallpox was eradicated, because the public health problem under surveillance is resolved.

The surveillance cycle is applicable to a wide range of public health problems, depending on the purpose and objective of the system. Initially, surveillance focused on the detection of epidemics and the characterization of seasonal fluctuations in infections. At present, the surveillance cycle is also used for injury control, a select group of cancers, certain cardiovascular diseases, and high-risk and unintended pregnancies, to cite a few illustrations.

Characteristics of a Surveillance System

An effective system of public health surveillance has seven essential attributes:

1. Simplicity
2. Sensitivity
3. Flexibility
4. Acceptability
5. Timeliness
6. Representativeness
7. High predictive value positive

Simplicity is essential if the quality of the data is to be maintained and the data are to be consolidated, interpreted, and dis-

TABLE 2–2. THE SURVEILLANCE CYCLE

- **Collection of Data**
  - Pertinent
  - Regular
  - Frequent
  - Timely
- **Consolidation and Interpretation**
  - Orderly
  - Descriptive
  - Evaluative
  - Timely
- **Dissemination**
  - Prompt
  - All who need to know
    - Data providers
    - Action takers
- **Action to Control and Prevent**

seminated promptly. *Acceptability* is essential because most public health surveillance systems rely on the cooperation of individuals and organizations to provide data. *Sensitivity* is important because public health surveillance is used as a screening test for health problems in a population. Just as screening tests must be highly sensitive if they are to detect abnormalities, a public health surveillance system must be highly sensitive if it is to detect and characterize epidemics, new disease trends, and changing patterns in health. A surveillance system must also have a *high predictive value positive,* that is, those persons reported to have the condition under surveillance must have a very high probability of actually having that condition. A system with a low predictive value positive wastes valuable public resources by collecting inadequate data and by requiring unproductive effort on incorrectly identified epidemics or other health problems. *Timeliness* is an important characteristic of a surveillance system for two reasons. First, reports based on information obtained must be disseminated with a very short lag time if the response is to occur soon enough to minimize additional morbidity or mortality. Second, information must be collected and processed on a regular basis because data that are edited, revised promptly, and put to use are more likely to be of consistent quality. *Flexibility* is important because such systems are often called on to accommodate to new health problems, as they were when penicillinase-producing *Neisseria gonorrhoeae* infections were first detected and when the first clusters of AIDS cases were found. Finally, surveillance systems need to be *representative;* that is, the data collected by the system must correctly portray the occurrence of a health event over time and characterize its geographic distribution and its distribution in the population.[26]

Data Sources

Vital Statistics. Information about births and deaths (i.e., vital events) has been collected, classified, and published at least since the middle of the seventeenth century in several European countries. At present the *International Classification of Diseases*[27] provides the standard nomenclature by which causes of death, disease, and injury are categorized.

Mortality. Death is, for the epidemiologist, the most definitive measure of ill health. A death certificate is a public document of legal, medical, and health importance. It provides information about time, date, and place of death; place of residence; sex, race, birth date, birthplace; marital status and usual occupation; as well as cause of death for each individual. Moreover, a unique number identifies individual certificates in many countries. It is the basic document for determining the number of deaths, calculating death rates, and estimating the probability of mortality and life expectancy by each of the variables included on the death certificate.

In developed countries the occurrence of mortality in a population is almost completely reported, but specific items on the death certificate may not be accurate. Sex and age are recorded with close to 100% accuracy, but race, marital status, and occupation are not. The greatest problems arise in certifying the cause of death. While in most cases in which persons die of an injury or of cancer the cause of death is correctly certified, that may not be true of persons who die of other causes. Cause-of-death certification may change according to current medical interests, perceptions, and philosophies. Moreover, autopsy information may not be received before the death certificate is completed and therefore may not be included on the certificate. The result is that secular and international comparisons are difficult to carry out and some conditions may be difficult to study unless the cause of death is confirmed by (1) interviewing individuals who knew the decedent, (2) reviewing medical records, or (3) verifying death-certificate information through comparison with autopsy reports.

Fertility. Information from birth certificates is increasingly important as epidemiologists place more emphasis on reproductive health problems. These documents characterize births by sex of infant, place of residence, place of occurrence, birth date, birth weight, length of gestation, and other characteristics of both parents. Birth data are essential for estimating pregnancy rates and perinatal, neonatal, and infant mortality. They are also often the most appropriate denominator in estimating the occurrence of events, such as rates of birth defects.

Birth registration is more complete than death registration, but some items are not as well reported as others. Those items that deserve special care from an epidemiological standpoint include race, ethnicity, marital status, and length of gestation.

Vital Record Linkage. Vital record linkage provides a broad base of information important to the practice of public health. By linking birth and infant or maternal death certificates, for example, it is possible to describe trends in more detail over a longer period and a broader geographic area than would otherwise be possible.

Until recently, the utility of separate sets of health statistics was limited by an inability to relate members of populations included in one set (e.g., hospital discharge statistics) to members of the same population who may appear in mortality statistics also. Thus it has often been impossible to obtain complete survival statistics for a large series of patients who were treated and discharged alive from a hospital but who have later been lost to follow-up and have subsequently died. At a seemingly simpler level, it has usually not been possible to relate information contained in a series of birth certificates to information on the death certificates of some of the same infants, even when death occurs on the same day, let alone when it occurs many months later. What has been needed is a method of assembling the information contained in several different sets of medical charts or other records, such as employment history, augmenting this with vital records—birth and death certificates—and a procedure to ensure that the same person is counted only once. The term *record linkage* is used to describe this method and procedure. Acheson[28] quotes Dunn as the source for the original definition:

> Each person in the world creates a book of life. This book starts with birth and ends with death. Its pages are made up of the records of the principal events in life. Record linkage is the name given to the process of assembling the pages of this book into a volume.

Dunn's definition does not include the additional step of summarizing the experience of many such books in the form of statistical tables; if this is done, the result is among the most powerful tools available for epidemiological studies. The prerequisites are a procedure for uniquely identifying individuals, even if they change their names, a method of abstracting and storing relevant information about them from health and vital records, and a technique for error-free matching of bits of information obtained from different sites and settings over prolonged periods. The final step is output of statistical tables. Record linkage systems with these qualities have been operational for some years in the Oxford region of England, in Scotland, in Sweden, and in Canada.

In Canada, the national mortality data base is the central element in many successful record linkage studies. Details of all deaths in Canada since 1950—personal identifying information and cause of death—have been coded and stored in computers. All the death certificates have been preserved on microfiche.

Canada has made effective use of record linkage, in part by using simple, standard, readily available documents for the origin of the data. If all items of information are available from two sources (e.g., a past medical record or employment history and a death certificate), the two can be matched precisely, with an extremely high probability that they relate to the same person.

Similar procedures to set up a national mortality data base began in the United States in 1979. The resulting system, the National Death Index (NDI), uses magnetic tapes of death records sent to the National Center for Health Statistics (NCHS) by the individual states. These tapes contain standard identifying information, comprising the decedent's first and last names and middle initials, father's last name (especially for females), Social Security number, birth date, sex, state of birth and of residence, marital status, race, and age at death. Names can be matched with other records to be linked with NDI records, either by exact spelling or Soundex Code, a system based on phonetic spelling that has been found efficacious in other record linkage systems. A match is possible with any of the following criteria:

1. Social Security number and first name match on both records.
2. Social Security number and last name match on both records.
3. Social Security number and father's last name match on both records.
4. If the subject is female, Social Security number matches and the last name on the user request record matches the father's last name on the NDI record.
5. Month and year of birth and first and last name match on both records.
6. Month and year of birth and first name and father's last name match on both records.
7. If the subject is female, month and year of birth and first name match and the last name on the user record matches the father's last name on the NDI record.

Technically, a record linkage system makes it possible to relate significant health events that are remote from one another in time and place. For example, a patient who received a particular antibiotic drug may be treated elsewhere some time later for a blood dyscrasia, or a temporary worker in the nuclear energy industry may die of cancer many years and several occupations later. As an isolated sequence, this would have no significance; however, if appropriate analytical techniques are applied to large data files in a comprehensive linked record system and many such sequences are identified, it becomes possible to demonstrate a significant association between an event and its underlying cause. As medical care has become more complex, we have become aware that it may have occasional untoward consequences. The chances of identifying potentially or actually hazardous diagnostic and therapeutic procedures are enhanced if surveillance is maintained by means of an information system with linked records. More fundamental epidemiological studies aimed at elucidating environmental and occupational associations and underlying causes of such conditions as cancer are also possible. An important advantage of epidemiological studies that make use of record linkage is the very large number of observations available.

Record linkage studies have successfully identified a number of previously unknown or doubtful occupational cancers[29] and can assess other occupational risks (e.g., exposure to formaldehyde).[30] They have made it possible to calculate the risks associated with exposure to ionizing radiation, both in medical and in occupational settings.[31,32] This epidemiological method is a form of historical cohort study (see below). The investigation usually begins by using the personal identifiers to identify accurately and precisely those members of the population who have been exposed to the risk being examined. Past medical records or records from employment are used for this purpose. The computerized mortality data base is searched to find the causes of death of these individuals, whose cause-specific death rates can then be calculated. The microfiche death certificates are used to verify the identity of the individuals in the study. This and certain other aspects of the method require access to personal information that is normally strictly confidential; this access is limited to staff members of the national agency, Statistics Canada, who have signed an oath to preserve the confidentiality of the documents.

Other Certified Events. Marriage and divorce are legally certifiable events which are often relevant to health. They describe changing characteristics of human populations and human relationships.

Health Reports. Estimates of morbidity, particularly those for infectious disease reporting, are based on a national system of notifiable diseases that has been operating in the United States since at least 1920. Reports from physicians sent to CDC through health departments make up most of the entries in this data base, but information provided by hospitals and laboratories is also important. This approach to surveillance has proved effective at national, regional, and local levels in characterizing seasonal trends, demonstrating temporal relationships to explain trends, finding small numbers of urgently important cases (such as botulism or meningitis), and detecting epidemics even though notification of this kind is incomplete. Thacker and Berkelman[25] cite a series of national surveillance systems that include some of those mentioned above, as well as others that are based on information from medical examiners, emergency rooms, and public clinics.

Hospital Records. Well over 130 years have passed since Florence Nightingale effectively used hospital statistics to point out the serious problems faced by patients in hospitals.[33] Subsequently, hospital records have proved essential to the acquisition of clinical data, demographic information, sociological data, information about the quality of medical care, economic data, and administrative information such as site of care and type of service. Few data sources offer such a rich spectrum of information.

Nonetheless, hospital records are associated with unique problems. Items of key importance to studies of past events may not have been collected consistently or at the same level of detail for each subject. Moreover, some recorded information may not be legible. Of greatest seriousness, however, is the fact that in some institutions it may not be possible to retrieve the entire record for a given person.

Summary information about hospital discharges can be analyzed from survey data. The National Hospital Discharge Survey (NHDS) has been published for every year since 1965.[34] Nongovernmental organizations, such as the Commission on Professional and Hospital Activity (CPHA), which is responsible for the Professional Activity Study (PAS),[35] and McAuto, a hospital discharge abstract system operated by the McDonnell-Douglas Corporation, are also useful sources of data on hospital discharges. These systems have their own special set of problems, particularly with regard to their representation of a definable population. The NHDS is based on a stratified probability sample of hospital discharges; since not all strata are represented in the same way, interpretation of NHDS reports requires a detailed understanding of the sampling procedures. Other hospital discharge abstraction systems exist, including ones for Medicare and a number of states. Since they represent different geographic areas and have been gathered by different data-collection procedures, their approaches to gathering information need to be clearly understood before they can be correctly interpreted.

Registries. There are two kinds of registry: (1) population-based and (2) disease-case registries. Population-based registries provide the data most useful for epidemiological purposes. This kind of registry has information about all cases of a specific disease in a geographically defined area that relates to a specific population. Data of this kind can be used to calculate rates of occurrence, and they are also useful for estimating survival rates and rates of disease progression and of mortality from a specific cause. The Surveillance, Epidemiology, and End Results (SEER) centers supported by the National Cancer Institute illustrate this kind of population-based registry for cancer.

Disease-case registries are most often kept at a hospital or treatment facility. They provide detailed documentation of diseases that are treated in that facility. For two reasons, however, they usually are not population based. First, rarely does a single facility ascertain all of the cases that occur in a specific area; second, a population residing in the catchment area for a health care facility is even more rarely counted or characterized in detail.

Health Surveys. Health surveys provide extremely valuable information. NCHS has conducted nationwide household interview surveys since 1957. These interviews are taken from a probability sample of the civilian population of the United States who are not residing in institutions. They are carried out annually and gather a core of information on disability, the characteristics of health problems, and the kinds of care the respondent has undergone. In addition, detailed questions are added to each survey to explore health problems related to a specific system of the body, a group of diseases, or personal health practices in greater depth.[36]

In 1959, NCHS augmented its household interview surveys by conducting a series of health-examination surveys. These surveys involved physical and biological measurements, such as height, weight, blood pressure, visual acuity, hemoglobin determinations, and more detailed laboratory tests; a valuable follow-up element has recently been added. In 1970, a nutrition-examination survey was included in the NCHS battery of periodic sample surveys.[37] Additional information about these surveys is given in the chapter on Public Health and Population.

The need for information about risk factors related to chronic diseases led CDC to initiate the Behavioral Risk Factor Surveillance System (BRFSS).[38] This system uses telephone interviews on chronic disease risk factors, such as obesity, treatment for blood pressure, alcohol use, and exercise. The monthly collection of information about these risk factors permits both CDC and state health departments to characterize the occurrence of long-term trends, seasonal variations, and population distribution of chronic disease risk factors, giving health professionals and the public current information about them.

The National Survey of Family Growth (NSFG) conducted by NCHS assesses the use of family-planning services, contraceptive practice, and surgical sterilization.[39] It also gathers information about the determinants of family size and composition. Information from this survey has proved useful in epidemiological studies of human reproduction and the safety of widely used methods of fertility control.

Data Collection

Public health surveillance relies on three approaches to data collection. The first is used in urgent situations, such as active and ongoing epidemics. Under these circumstances, health agencies initiate surveillance by contacting those data sources most likely to have current information, for example, clinicians who see sick children or public health nurses who make home visits. Referred to by some as "active" surveillance, this approach ensures that reporting will be timely and characterized by simplicity, acceptability, and sensitivity. This approach has the possibility of sacrificing representativeness by weighting responses toward a preselected group of reporting sources. It may also limit the predictive value if those who report the occurrence of illness need to identify cases before a diagnostic work-up is complete, thereby leading to the reporting of cases that do not fulfill the definition.

A second approach—disease or event reporting by individual health care practitioners—is most frequently used by the national notifiable-disease surveillance system. Referred to by some as "passive" surveillance, this approach is simple, acceptable, and flexible. It is rarely as sensitive as health agency–based surveillance, and it may not be timely or representative. Nonetheless, its value in describing seasonal and long-range trends and promoting the detection of epidemics has withstood the test of time for public health professionals.

Finally, the sentinel approach has its roots in the surveillance of occupational health problems and is now being applied more widely. The use of canaries to detect lethal levels of odorless gases, such as carbon monoxide, in mines may have been the earliest form of sentinel surveillance. Concern about epidemic infections has led to the use of sentinel animal flocks to detect arthropod-borne viruses that cause encephalitis and herald the occurrence of epidemics of this infection in humans. Rutstein and his colleagues have proposed that this concept be extended to a broader range of occupational health problems[40] and to the health care system more generally.[41]

Computers permit surveillance information to be transmitted widely, in great detail, and in a timely manner. Notifiable-disease reporting relied for decades on information about the aggregate numbers of cases of infectious diseases being reported on postcards mailed each week from health departments. Computers now permit cases to be characterized individually and yet confidentially. Telecommunication ensures that the information is available in a timely manner. Computer networks have the potential of making this information available to a wide range of skilled epidemiological analysts and of eliciting a timely public health response. CDC has developed a software package called EPI INFO[42] (which assists in the collection, recording, and transmission of surveillance information) and a network, the National Electronic Surveillance System (NETSS) (which now reaches every state and a number of major local health departments in the United States).[43]

Data Quality

The quality of health data becomes an increasingly important issue as information becomes more important to the detection of epidemics and other public health problems, the development of health policy, the assurance of effective and accessible preventive services, and the evaluation of public health programs. Just as epidemiologists are concerned about the quality of information they receive from others, they also want to know that the data they collect themselves are of good quality. Four dimensions of data quality are of key importance.

First, data input must be of high quality. This can be brought about by careful questionnaire design, training of interviewers, the use of technology such as CATI (computer-assisted telephone interviewing), and meticulous data verification. To illustrate some of the basic procedure, epidemiologists should know that in a one-dimensional check of data input, all variables should be within an appropriate range. A surveillance system concerned with childhood lead poisoning, for example, ought not to include a 50-year-old person. A two-dimensional check of input would ensure that pairs of variables were reasonable, so that, for example, a surveillance system concerned with the nutritional status of pregnant women ought not to report a 17-year-old woman with 10 children. Moreover, data should be logically consistent so that a child with measles reported to have a date of onset in the year *1988* ought not to have a reported birth date of *1998*.

Second, the management of data records is essential to ensure data quality. Records must be uniquely identified and carefully tracked so that they can be retrieved and verified. The status of record completion must be documented, particularly in household and telephone interview surveys. Confidentiality is a point of tension in records management. Striking the balance between ensuring the privacy of an individual and permitting a public agency to meet an urgent public need, such as controlling the transmission of AIDS, will always be difficult. Many conflicts may be resolved by using identification numbers instead of names. In some instances, however, events are rare enough that individuals might be identified simply by the disease they have and their demographic characteristics, such as age, sex, and county of residence, especially if the county is not a populous one.

Third, data output must be of excellent quality. One-dimensional, two-dimensional, and logic checks are as important in handling data output as they are in checking data input. Computer programs that produce the output should create totals for columns and rows that are added up for each table rather than being brought forward from an earlier computation. Procedures for handling incomplete data should be subjected to critical examination so that they are relevant to the way the output will be interpreted and used. In short, epidemiologists need to examine every piece of relevant data and to ask, ''Will this make sense to the people who need to know this information?''

Finally, data archives must be of good quality. Keeping an archive of public health information requires that an epidemiologist not only file the final output so that it can be retrieved but also retain enough of the intermediate computations so that questions raised by other researchers, the media, or the public can be answered quickly, intelligently, and responsibly. In keeping an archive of epidemiological data, three questions must be addressed: First, how will the issues of public accountability and individual confidentiality be addressed? Second, if an important question is asked, can the answer be retrieved in 3 seconds? . . . an hour? . . . 2 days? . . . not at all? Finally, since data collected by health agencies are in the public domain, what measures are appropriate for a public agency to take to preserve individual confidentiality and to make data accessible to others, such as researchers, journalists, and individual citizens?

Data Reporting

The reporting of public health surveillance data should consider four approaches.

The first is tabular. A typical issue of the *Morbidity and Mortality Weekly Report* (*MMWR*)[44] illustrates this point. The *MMWR* reports case counts of the diseases that are nationally notifiable. Each week aggregated case reports are entered into tables for each state and a few additional major reporting areas, such as the District of Columbia.

Second, graphs of surveillance data permit a visual display. A histogram that shows the distribution of cases of a given disease in a specific area over a stated period is often referred to as an ''epidemic curve'' (Fig. 2–1). Line graphs that display cases over time help characterize temporal relationships in disease occurrence. (Fig. 2–2 shows surveillance data for malaria in the United States.) More recently, graphs that contrast current with historical data to signal the occurrence of unexpected changes in disease trends have been introduced (Fig. 2–3).

Third, maps often provide an effective presentation of the geographic distribution of a disease (Fig. 2–4). Spot maps illustrate the distribution of individual cases or small groups of cases. Shading differentiates the relative intensity with which a disease or other public health problem occurs over a wide area. Sequences of maps illustrate changing disease distributions over time. Three-dimensional maps may also demonstrate differing intensities of health problems over an area. Computer mapping with data that give the distribution of cases by county of occurrence and residence helps determine whether epidemics are being transmitted across jurisdictional boundaries.

Finally, the mathematical analysis of surveillance data may help detect important changes in the trends of health events. Use of a moving average in analyzing national trends in fertility is a regular part of the *Monthly Vital Statistics Report*[45] published by NCHS. Epidemics may be detected when time-series analysis is used. Presentation of trends in influenza mortality in graphs that use either periodic regression analysis or the autoregressive, integrated-moving-average approach is yet another way of identifying epidemics of this disease.[46] Excess mortality among the aged during periods of unusual heat waves has been detected with these methods.[47]

Dissemination

The findings from public health surveillance must be disseminated to two groups immediately: (1) those who are the source of the data so that the information can be verified and their interest maintained and (2) those responsible for taking actions on the

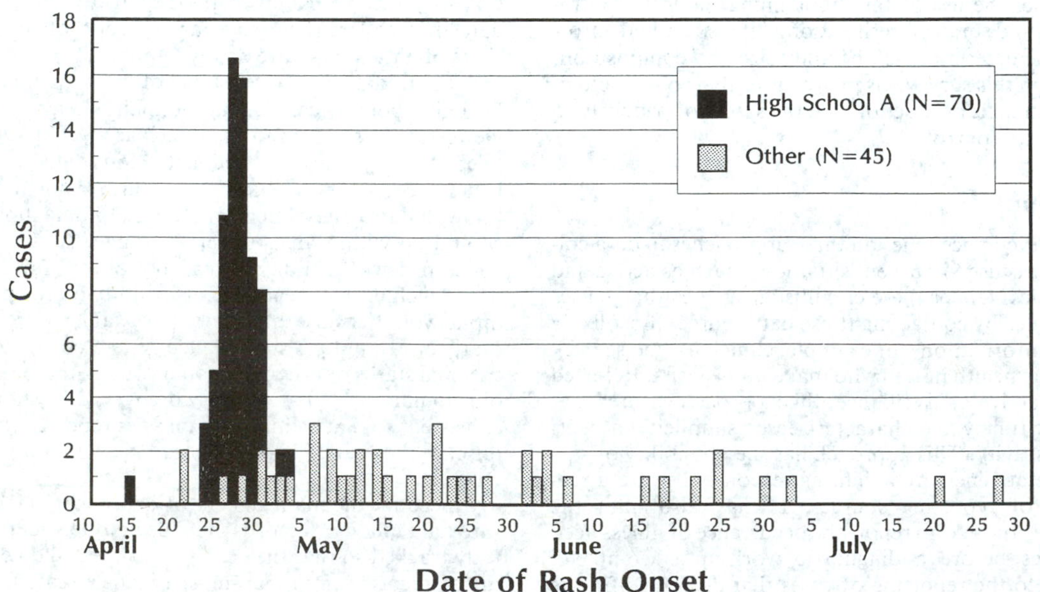

Figure 2–1. Reported measles cases by date of rash onset, Elgin, Illinois, April 15 to July 28, 1985.

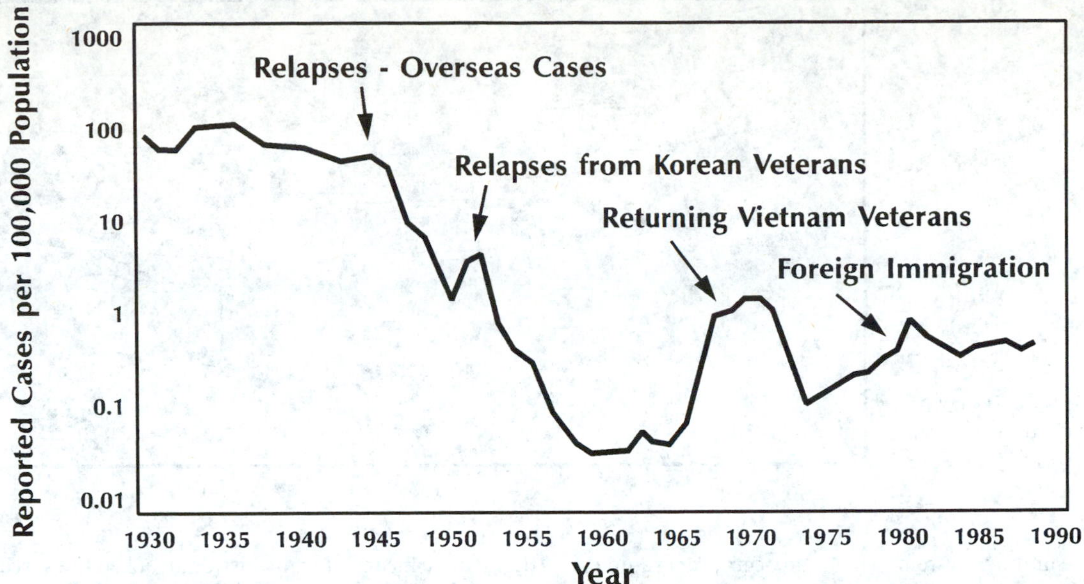

Figure 2-2. Malaria, by year, United States, 1930–1988.

findings. When surveillance detects urgent public health problems, an immediate response is required. For years, CDC has sent data on notifiable-disease surveillance and on epidemic field investigations to state and local health officials before the information is published in *MMWR*.[44]

CDC's surveillance information is now disseminated in *MMWR,* in an additional series of special *MMWR* reports, in an annual summary of notifiable diseases,[48] and in numerous other professional publications. Surveillance data are also used to characterize historical trends and project those trends into the future. Many other nations have surveillance and reporting systems similar to those of the CDC. WHO maintains worldwide a similar reporting system, *WHO Weekly Epidemiological Record,* augmented by quarterly, annual, and occasional special reports.

A Case Study of Surveillance: The AIDS Epidemic

In mid-1981, an epidemiologist at the Los Angeles County Health Department realized that the five reports he had received of a rare kind of pneumonia caused by a microorganism named *Pneumocystis carinii* might be indicative of an epidemic. The disease reports had come from three different hospitals and had involved men 29 to 36 years of age. Typically this kind of pneumonia occurs among people who have

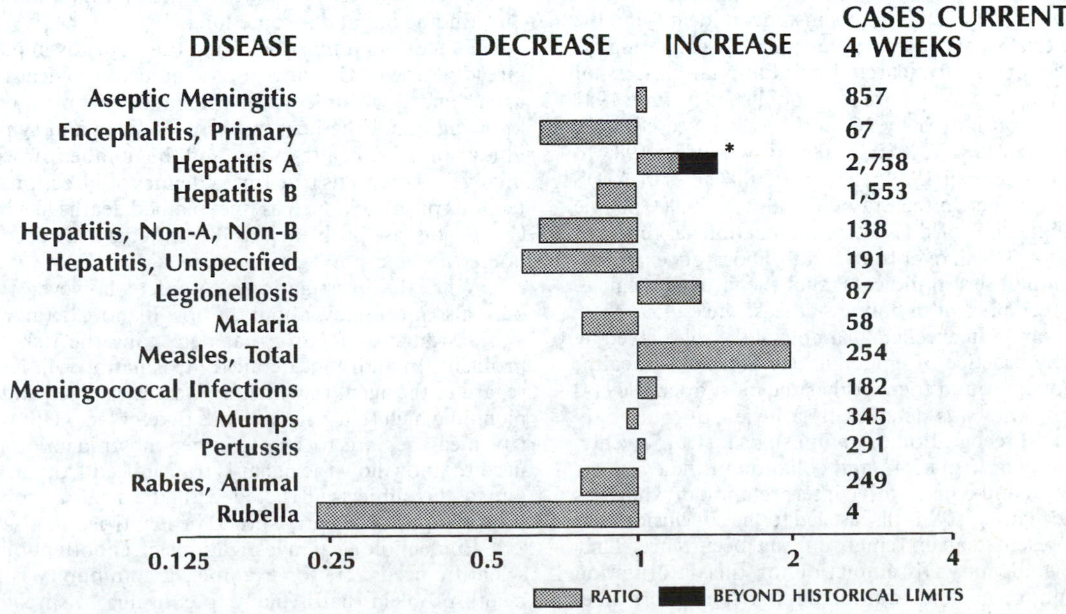

Figure 2-3. Notifiable-disease reports; comparison of 4-week totals, ending 11/25/89, with historical data, United States.

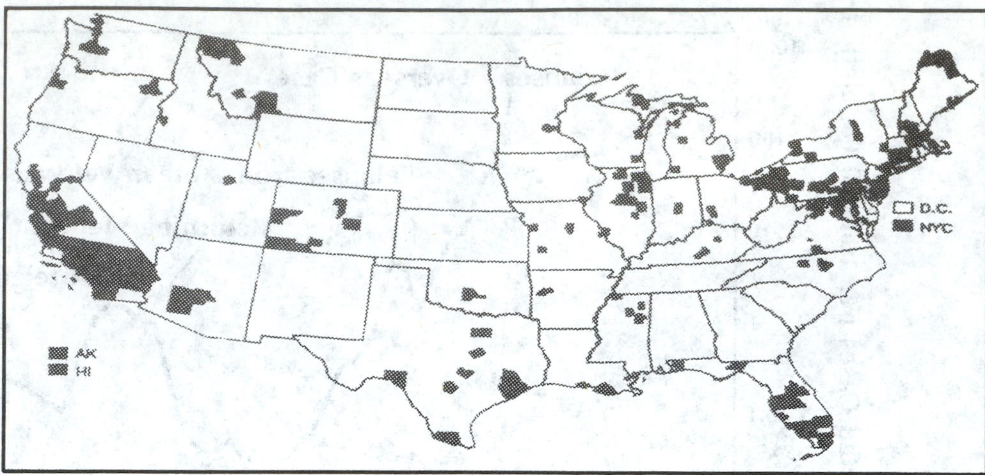

Figure 2-4. Measles [Rubeola], counties reporting cases, United States, 1988.

depression of the immune system, which can occur, for example, when patients receive cancer chemotherapy. At one hospital, a large university medical center, the clinician caring for these patients had already recognized this unusual occurrence.[49]

A month later, a report from another part of the United States documented the occurrence of this same kind of pneumonia. In addition, some patients in this group had other unusual infections and a rare form of cancer, Kaposi's sarcoma. This group of 26 individuals ranged in age from 26 to 51 years. Twenty of them lived in New York City, six in California; eight had died within 24 months after diagnosis of Kaposi's sarcoma; all were homosexual men.[50] Within the next year, 355 additional cases were reported to CDC. Five states—California, Florida, New Jersey, New York, and Texas—accounted for 86% of the reported cases.

This was the beginning of the AIDS epidemic.

A cluster of cases of an unusual infection affecting previously well individuals was picked up by an astute clinician and an observant epidemiologist who knew that even five cases of this kind represented an unusual occurrence, perhaps even an epidemic. Confirming each case; providing a clear, brief (no more than seven lines of text in the original report) description to a central reporting source (CDC, in this instance); identifying the common characteristics of the individuals; and disseminating the report stimulated others to search for additional clusters of cases. The original group of five reports published in June 1981 and augmented a month later by 26 more cases increased more than 10-fold by June 1982 to 355 cases and by August 1983 to 1972 cases. As of December 1989, almost 120,000 cases of AIDS had been reported in the United States and almost 70,000 people had died of AIDS. The World Health Organization has reported the occurrence of AIDS all over the world. Laboratory examination of frozen human serum indicates that the virus that causes this disease has been present in humans at least since 1959.

The AIDS story is an excellent example of the role played by surveillance in the practice of epidemiology and public health. What is now known around the world as the most dramatic epidemic of modern times was detected by a review of routine reports of disease and recognition of an unusual cluster of events. The consolidation, confirmation, and collation of these reports followed by careful and conservative interpretation of what was known about the history of this disease led to the conclusion that these reports represented an extremely unusual occurrence. They represented an epidemic. Dissemination of this information throughout the nation elicited additional reports in a short time. Ultimately, this one cluster of five cases triggered intense surveillance, which resulted in identifying the extent of the epidemic, defined the means of transmission, tracked the spread of disease across the nation, showed which groups in our country carried the greatest burden of this feared disease, provided the basis for distributing public funds, and permitted the course of the epidemic and its associated demand for health care to be forecast.[51]

INVESTIGATION

An investigation is "an examination for the purpose of finding out about something," according to a current dictionary. It differs from a surveillance, which is a continuing and reiterative activity. An investigation is an action of limited duration, out of the ordinary, and carried out because one assumes that a problem already exists. Moreover, an investigation may use information from an established data-collection system, but an investigation goes farther and gathers new information. Analysis, on the other hand, involves the study of a problem by breaking it down into its constituent parts. In carrying out an investigation, therefore, an epidemiologist must have some idea as to what analysis will ultimately be necessary, but the investigation itself focuses on "finding out about something."

Exactly what must be found out depends in part on what is already known. Considering the epidemiological triad of host, agent, and environment, the epidemiologist most often starts by knowing about the host in terms of signs and symptoms of an illness, or other health event, and the number of people who are involved. This holds true for epidemics of infection, acute noninfectious problems (such as unexplained deaths in a hospital), and chronic disease problems, as illustrated by the occurrence of endometrial cancer and estrogen use.

When the investigation is complete, however, the epidemiologist also must know about the host in more detail with regard to a wide range of factors that determine the risk of the health problem. In addition, detailed information will be needed with regard to the agent to which the host is exposed and the environment in which that exposure has taken place. Ultimately, if control measures are to be effective, the epidemiologist will also need to know how the agent is transmitted from its point of origin to the subjects afflicted with the health problem, and, if possible, portal of entry should be identified.

Epidemiological investigations meet both public service and scientific needs. If, for example, a community is faced with a health problem that is likely to continue to spread and the approach to control is uncertain, then the epidemiologist has an important role to play. Epidemics of viral infections that affect presumably immunized young people—as has been the case with measles epidemics on college campuses—illustrate this problem. Moreover, public concern may also require the epidemiologist to provide assurance that no epidemic exists and that none is threatening. Exposure to medical waste on beaches, for example, creates genuine fear that AIDS might be transmitted this way, even though there is no epidemiological evidence that this occurs.

Scientific need is a second important reason for an epidemiologist to do a detailed field investigation. This kind of investigation has led to the discovery of Lyme disease and Legionnaire's disease. Field investigation also led to the discovery that vinyl chloride was causally associated with angiosarcoma of the liver and oral contraceptive use with hepatocellular adenoma.

Preparing for an Investigation

After determining the need for an epidemiological field investigation, preparation has three general elements: (1) notifying essential people and organizations, (2) identifying materials needed for the investigation, and (3) planning travel. While the notification process will have begun before the epidemiologist departs for the field, consideration must be given to documentation of the date and place of investigation as well as its purpose with supervisory personnel, health officials in the area where the investigation is to occur, and other officials whose jurisdiction may include that area. Failure to notify these individuals can bring the investigation to a halt, limit access to people who have essential information, or lead to a withdrawal of support personnel needed to complete the investigation.

Before the epidemiologist goes to the field, materials must be assembled to assist with the investigation. Depending on the nature of the problem, the epidemiologist may want reprints of scientific articles, copies of sample questionnaires, paper for line lists or the coding of data, a hand-held calculator, a portable computer, a camera, the materials with which to collect laboratory specimens, and pocket references on disease agents.

Basic Steps of an Investigation

Ten steps are essential considerations in every epidemiological investigation. While the sequence of these tasks may differ, it is this list to which practicing epidemiologists return more than any other (Table 2-3). From the beginning, however, the public health practitioner must not lose sight of the ultimate purpose of an epidemiological investigation, which is to control and prevent a health problem for the people in the community.

1. Ensure the existence of an epidemic: The first important decision to be made is that an epidemic does exist. This decision is often based on a preliminary count of people with similar symptoms. Laboratory confirmation may be absent. It may even be inappropriate because of the urgent need to begin an investigation.

2. Confirm the diagnosis: The epidemiologist needs to know the diagnosis of the health problem being addressed. The number of cases is sometimes too great to permit a history and physical examination of every person. Nonetheless, information about the signs and symptoms must be obtained early in the investigation and as soon after the event as possible; it must be verified in a few key individuals. The collection of laboratory specimens must then follow as soon as possible.

On the basis of this preliminary information, the epidemiologist must formulate a case definition of the health problem. Symptoms must be explicitly defined. Physical signs must be described in detail. Measurements of levels of severity of the health problem or disease must be determined. It may not be possible to confirm every reported case, and laboratory specimens may be obtained in only 15% to 20% of the cases. In some large epidemics (e.g., milk contamination with *Salmonella* in Illinois in 1985, which involved more than 200,000 people) a sample of cases yielded information about the agent, the host, the method of transmission, the portal of entry, and the environment of the disease more quickly than an exhaustive ascertainment of every ill individual could have.[52]

The absence of a satisfactory case definition is frequently the Achilles heel of field investigations. Each case report is much like a problem-oriented medical record. It contains subjective and objective criteria. Symptoms (e.g., a complaint of diarrhea) may be the one complaint common to all those who are ill, but such a complaint may be made by others who are not part of the epidemic. Objective criteria, such as a stool culture with growth of an organism such as *Salmonella typhimurium,* ensure that each of those presumed to be part of the epidemic actually has the health problem that is being investigated.

Objective information (e.g., laboratory data), has high priority at the beginning of every investigation. Specimens may have to be collected, and provision may be needed for preservation and transportation to a distant laboratory. Samples for chemical analysis may also be needed. In other situations, photographs may help describe the surroundings as they were at the beginning of the investigation. The epidemiologist may need the advice of a microbiologist, a toxicologist, a pathologist, or even a skilled photographer at this point.

Case finding may begin with a single report or with a small cluster of cases. The epidemiologist must begin the investigation by casting a wide net that will bring in all of the cases and identify all of those in the population who are at risk. The preliminary case definition must, therefore, be a sensitive one that will exclude as few of the true cases as possible. Once the total number of cases has been estimated, the problem may be so large that the epidemiologist must determine whether to study all of them or a sample. If only a sample is selected, then those cases that are the most severe are the ones of greatest value in determining the agent, the characteristics of the host, the environment, and the means of transmission. Outlying observations require special attention at this point because their relationship to the epidemic may be the key to understanding the mode of spread or other key factors.

3. Estimate the number of cases: Given a workable definition, the epidemiologist must count the cases, collect data about them, and determine the features they have in common. The demographic characteristics of each individual; the characteristics of the illness from beginning to the present; the places where the ill people live, work, and have traveled to; and the possible exposures that might lead to health impairment all must be documented. Among the questions the epidemiologist may want to answer are the following: What signs and symptoms are the most important? Are any of them pathognomonic? What laboratory test is most likely to confirm the diagnosis, and what specimens

TABLE 2-3. STEPS IN AN EPIDEMIOLOGICAL INVESTIGATION

1.	Ensure the existence of an epidemic
2.	Confirm the diagnosis
3.	Estimate the number of cases
4.	Orient the data in terms of time, place, and person
5.	Determine who is at risk of having the health problem
6.	Develop an explanatory hypothesis
7.	Compare the hypothesis with the established facts
8.	Plan a more systematic study
9.	Prepare a written report
10.	Propose measures for control and prevention

will the laboratory need? Can both the exposure to the presumed source and the severity of the illness be characterized at different levels? What must be done to identify the people with these problems, should long-term follow-up be necessary? Are there any inapparent or subclinical cases? What role do they play in determining the future size of this epidemic or the susceptibility of the people in this community?

4. Orient the data in terms of time, place, and person: Data on each case must include the date of onset of the illness; the place where the person lives or became ill; and the characteristics of each person, including age, sex, and occupation. A histogram, often referred to as "the epidemic curve," is a clear, simple way to show the relationship between the occurrence of cases and their time of onset. (See Fig. 2–1.)[53] The spatial relationships of cases is often shown best on a spot map, based on case counts and, depending on the stage of analysis, population-based rates for each area. Maps, for instance, help show that the cases occurred close to a body of water, a sewage-treatment plant, or its outflow. Characterizing individuals by personal traits such as age, sex, and other relevant attributes permits the epidemiologist to estimate rates of occurrence and compare them to other appropriate community groups.

5. Determine who is at risk of having the health problem: The epidemiologist calculates rates at which a health problem or a disease occurs, using the population at risk as the denominator, while those individuals with the problem form the numerator. If the original reports of an illness come from a state surveillance system, then the first estimations of rates may be based on a state's population. If the epidemic is eventually shown to occur only in school-age children from a particular school, the population at risk may prove to be only the children who attend that school. Those groups of people who are not ill must be characterized by the same attributes as those who are ill (i.e., age, sex, grade in school, or classroom). In some instances, immunized children or those who have already had the illness might be excluded so that the population at risk was made up only of those susceptible to the disease.

6. Develop an explanatory hypothesis: Comparing the frequency of occurrence of the health problem among those who are at greatest risk with that of other groups in the population at risk and with comparison groups outside the population helps the epidemiologist develop hypotheses that may explain the cause of a health problem and how it is transmitted.

7. Compare the hypothesis with the established facts: The hypothesis that explains the epidemic must be consistent with all the facts the epidemiologist knows. If it is not, then it must be reexamined. It should do more than just strengthen speculation explaining the cases at the peak of the epidemic. The epidemiologist may need to repeat the interviews with case subjects, reassess medical records, gather additional laboratory specimens, and repeat calculations.

8. Plan a more systematic study: When the initial field investigations and preliminary calculations are complete, the investigator may need to conduct one or more systematic studies using either case-control or cohort methods, which are discussed in more detail later. The data for such studies may be in hand, but more often additional information is needed. It may be collected either by interviewing subjects in more detail or by surveying the population at risk. In some instances, a serological survey, extensive sampling of the environment for chemical or biological agents, or perhaps even more extensive photographing or videotaping of a work process will be required. In the event of a food-borne infection, a detailed food history may be necessary. If a water-borne infection is suspected, a history of the number of glasses of water drunk by each person will permit the epidemiologist to estimate a dose-response relationship. An occupational illness might be determined by a specific machine that each worker used and the number of hours that each one used it.

9. Prepare a written report: Preparation of a written document is an essential step in any epidemiological investigation. It need not be a publishable paper, but it should be regarded as a benchmark in the conduct of an investigation, just as a hospital discharge summary is for patient care, or a thesis is for the academic advancement of a scholar. It is an essential public health document because it may be the basis for action by health officials, or it may be a record of performance for the epidemiologist working at a place far from a customary work site. For the public, it may provide information for those concerned about the epidemic, its spread, and the likelihood that other persons will be involved. A report may have scientific epidemiological importance in documenting the discovery of a new agent, a new route of transmission, or a new and imaginative approach to epidemiological investigation. Moreover, many investigative reports are useful in teaching.

10. Propose measures for control and prevention: The ultimate purpose of an epidemiological investigation is to control a health problem in a community. The epidemiologist is part of the team that develops the approach to control and prevention.

The establishment of a surveillance system for the population at risk is an important element in assuring the effectiveness of the control program. Although epidemiological evaluation is dealt with in detail later, it must be recognized as one element of an epidemiologist's responsibility in fulfilling a public need and carrying out a scientific study.

Designing an Investigation

Descriptive Studies. Epidemiological investigations often begin with case reports, evolve to become a series of cases, and then go on to include ecological studies, cross-sectional studies, or surveys. Working with information from case reports or a series of cases is often the first step in a field or community investigation. For an epidemiologist concerned with the clinical details of an illness, as well as the causal agent, the environmental and other risk factors, added information will be needed. Demographic, social, and other behavioral characteristics, as well as possible exposures to biological, physical, or chemical agents are also essential.

At a more complex level of study design, ecological studies compare the frequency of events in different groups. Because they compare groups rather than individuals, caution is required in drawing conclusions and identifying associations. The hazard in interpreting studies of this kind is "the ecological fallacy."[54] It is a bias or error in inference that occurs when an association observed between variables on an aggregate level is assumed to exist at an individual level. For example, a person's risk of heart attack is not related to the fact that he drinks "hard" or "soft" water, although there are several studies linking quality of drinking water and mortality from heart disease. This correlation is not a causal association because the criteria for such an association (discussed later) are not fulfilled. On the other hand, ecological studies generate or support new hypotheses, are usually quick, easy to do, and use existing data.

Cross-sectional studies simultaneously evaluate exposure and outcome in a population. Although this approach is often useful at the time of an epidemic investigation to determine the extent of the epidemic in a population and to assess the susceptibility of those in the population at risk, it is not an appropriate way to study rare events, events of short duration, or events related to rare exposures. Moreover, cross-sectional studies are not appropriate for assessing the temporal relationship between exposure and a health event or outcome.

Analytical Studies. Analytical studies may be observational or experimental. In an observational study, the epidemiologist observes and assigns subjects to case and comparison groups after an event has occurred. The investigation of an epidemic (such as infections following childbirth) or a study based on clinical observation (e.g., the occurrence of angiosarcoma of the liver in persons who work with vinyl chloride) is typically observational. In these instances, the epidemiological study had to be confined to observations about events that had already taken place, use data that had already been collected, and assign people to groups based on the presence of disease or exposure that had already occurred.

In an experimental study, subjects may be observed under predetermined conditions, using carefully designed approaches to data and specimen collection, the observations to be made can be stated and categorized before the study begins, and the individuals being observed may be allocated to different groups on a probabilistic basis.

This section addresses the design of epidemiological studies, only mentioning analytic approaches. The following section deals with analytical issues in more detail and gives examples of ways in which they might be handled.

Observational studies can be categorized as case-control or cohort studies. In a case-control study, the risk of exposure to a presumed cause by those with a health problem (the case group) is compared with the risk of exposure of those who do not have that problem (the control group). The frequency with which the exposure occurs is compared in the two groups, and the strength of association is measured in terms of a relative risk. The likelihood that such a risk could occur because of chance is evaluated by using statistical confidence intervals.

Case-control studies begin with a case group of individuals who have the health problem under investigation. The outcomes typically studied with this design are those that are rare or have a long latent or incubation period, such as cancer. Conditions for which there are detailed records, such as hospital records, pathology reports and specimens, and laboratory documentation (e.g., electrocardiograms, x-rays, or other imaging techniques), are well suited to this design. For health problems that are rare or that develop over long periods, the case-control design yields findings in a short time and with a minimum resource requirement. In addition, the case-control design permits comparisons to be made with appropriate subjects, even when the entire population at risk cannot be precisely determined. The Cancer and Steroid Hormone Study, which investigated the association between cancer in some key sites of the female reproductive system, illustrates the use of the case-control study design in dealing with an important worldwide public health problem.[55]

Cohort studies begin with a case group made up of individuals exposed to the hypothesized cause of a health problem. The comparison group is one that is not so exposed but has similar demographic, behavioral, and biological characteristics. The groups are compared and characterized according to the rates at which the health problem occurs in each group. The strength of association is measured by means of relative rates; its occurrence due to chance is evaluated statistically by using confidence intervals.

Cohort studies may look back in time by reviewing recorded events, or they may require that subjects be observed in the future. Those done by reconstructing records of exposure and health outcome are called *retrospective cohort studies* because they look back over time. Studies of acute disease outbreaks caused by exposure to infectious agents often use this design. Those that follow similar groups with different exposures into the future are referred to as *prospective cohort studies.* The study of American veterans of the Vietnam War who were exposed to Agent Orange is an example of a retrospective cohort study,[56] while many of the reports on cardiovascular disease in Framingham, Massachusetts,[57] illustrate prospective cohort studies. The most difficult problems posed for epidemiologists wishing to do cohort studies is, if retrospective, finding records that are comparable for both the exposed and the unexposed subjects and, if prospective, finding the resources and motivating the staff conducting the study to carry out the careful observations that must be made over a long period, often many years or even decades.

A comparison of these two study design approaches is shown in Table 2-4. Case-control studies are especially advantageous when the epidemiologist is studying a rare condition (one that occurs no more often than once in every 100 people in the population under study, although this design approach is also useful in studying more frequently occurring conditions, (e.g., up to 20% in the population at risk). Case-control studies evaluate an association between disease and exposure relatively quickly, require limited resources, and deal with health problems that have a long latency or incubation period. Of the advantages for cohort studies, on the other hand, the most important are that this approach provides an opportunity to describe the natural history of a health problem, directly estimate the rate at which the health problem is occurring, and communicate the findings to people who are not epidemiologists.[58]

The findings of any study, regardless of approach to design, can be distorted if bias occurs. Bias is the "deviation of results, or inferences from the truth, or processes leading to such deviation."[4] The most generic categories of this kind of deviation are selection bias and information bias. Selection bias occurs when comparison groups differ from each other in some systematic way that influences the outcome or exposure being investigated. This form of bias is a more frequent problem in case-control studies, but it can occur in both approaches to study design. As an illustration, any study of oral contraceptive safety in which case subjects were exposed to pills manufactured in the 1960s (which contained large amounts of steroid hormones to protect against unintended pregnancy) were compared with control subjects using current brands of low-dose contraceptive pills would be biased toward finding an association of inappropriately large magnitude. The bias would be introduced by the way in which subjects were selected for the two study groups.

The role of information bias is important when exposure or health outcome is measured systematically in different ways for subjects in the case and control groups. This can be related to the inability to collect comparable information, to systematically

TABLE 2-4. STRENGTHS AND WEAKNESSES OF CASE CONTROL AND COHORT STUDIES

Case Control Studies	Cohort Studies
▪ Advantages	
Excellent way to study rare diseases and diseases with long latency	Provides complete data on cases, stages
Relatively quick	Allows study of more than one effect of exposure
Relatively inexpensive	Can calculate and compare rates in exposed and unexposed
Requires relatively few study subjects	Choice of factors available for study
Can often use existing records	Quality control of data
Can study many possible causes of a disease	
▪ Disadvantages	
Relies on recall or existing records about past exposures	Need to study large numbers
Difficult or impossible to validate data	May take many years
Control of extraneous factors incomplete	Circumstances may change during study
Difficult to select suitable comparison group	Expensive
Cannot calculate rates	Control of extraneous factors may be incomplete
Cannot study mechanism of disease	Rarely possible to study mechanism of disease

different approaches to observing the two groups, or to differences in the quality of information that is collected. A comparison of surgical complications in two groups, one of which underwent the study procedure in a hospital with hourly observation for 3 days while the other had the operation performed in an ambulatory facility with observation only during the first 4 hours after surgery, illustrates one way in which information bias can occur. In this instance the bias favors the detection of more postoperative complications in the hospitalized subjects than in the others.

Gathering Information. Data gathering is an essential part of "finding out about something." Investigations most often involve interviewing people and reviewing records. Any time an interview is required, a friendly, persuasive introduction should precede questioning. Training of interviewers, therefore, should include practicing both the introduction and the questions.

The form in which information is gathered may differ from one investigation to another. In straightforward field investigations of disease outbreaks, or even in surveys that deal with clearly defined problems (e.g., childhood immunizations), a line listing of responses may suffice. (This approach is illustrated in Table 2–5.) In more complex investigations a detailed interview form, sometimes using visual memory aids (e.g., pictures of medication packaging by brands), will be more suitable.

Identifying the respondent and recording information that can be used for follow-up or for record retrieval are among the first items to be gathered. If follow-up or verification of information is needed, then information about family, friends, and neighbors may also be important.

Responses to questions, both for interview and for record abstraction, should be simple and in a form that is easy to code. Data collection about items should not be grouped into intervals but gathered in terms of individual years. Age, for example, is best collected by individual years (ideally, date of birth should be collected to prevent the bias people have for digits ending in 5 or 0 or an even number), and grouping is done at the time of tabulation and analysis. Open-ended questions must be avoided as far as possible because of the difficulties in tabulating and analyzing the resulting information.

Pretesting of the data-gathering form or interview is essential. Simulation of an interview with a respondent or abstracting of a chart that represents a typical case should be followed by simulation of some of the unlikely circumstances. Training the individuals who will fill out the form is also essential and might include scenarios used in pretesting.

Case finding (i.e., searching for and gathering information from subjects for the case and comparison groups) is essential to an investigation. Initially, a study should include a wide range of those at risk of the health problem, because it is generally easier to be sure that the entire population at risk is being considered at the beginning of the investigation than it is to make a second trip to the community.

If members of the comparison group are matched to specific individuals in the case group by, for example, age, sex, or place of residence, then the forms for both case and comparison individuals must be identified in such a way that they can be linked at the time of analysis. Choosing comparison groups is not easy, and the epidemiologist must think carefully before selecting the easiest way. For example, if the case subjects are all hospitalized, the question of using control subjects from the hospital or from the neighborhoods where the case subjects normally lived must be examined carefully.

TABLE 2–5. ILLUSTRATIVE PARTIAL LINE LISTING OF MEASLES EPIDEMIC IN A HIGH SCHOOL

ID No.	Grade	Sex	Date of First Rash	Fever?	Cough?
SA04	09	M	April 24	Yes	Yes
DA10	12	F	April 22	Yes	Yes
B020	09	F	April 25	Yes	Yes
DB06	09	M	April 27	Yes	Yes
SB04	10	F	April 22	Yes	Yes

Illustrative Investigative Study: Unexplained Deaths in Hospital[59]

Case Data. Four infants on a pediatric cardiology ward in a 700-bed university affiliated hospital died unexpectedly. They were found to have unusually high tissue levels of digoxin, a medication used to treat heart failure. This drug had never been prescribed for one of these infants. High tissue levels of digoxin were subsequently found in several additional infants. Hospital authorities sought consultation with several epidemiologists, as well as specialists from other fields.

Descriptive Epidemiology

Time. The epidemiological investigators determined that for a 5-year period before the epidemic there were 49 deaths on the cardiology ward, and the death rate had been 11.0/10,000 patient days. For the 9 months defined as the epidemic period, however, 34 such deaths had occurred with a resulting rate of 43.1/10,000 patient days, giving a relative risk of death equal to 3.9 (the 95% confidence intervals ranged from 2.6 to 5.9).

Place. Three months before the epidemic period, the cardiology service had been moved from a single ward to two adjacent wards. Twenty-six of the deaths occurred on one of the new wards (74.5/10,000 patient days) whereas only eight (18.2/10,000 patient days) occurred on the other, giving a relative rate of 4.1, with a 95% confidence interval ranging from 2.0 to 8.5.

Person. Most (92%) of those who died were children less than 1 year of age. Moreover, a large proportion had begun to deteriorate clinically during the midnight to 6 AM period, which was unusual when compared to deaths that occurred during other months. An expert clinical cardiology consultant judged that the timing of a significant number of deaths among 1-year-olds cared for on this ward was unexpected and inconsistent with their clinical conditions during the epidemic period as compared to the nonepidemic period. In addition, there was a particularly strong association of clinical digoxin intoxication with death during the epidemic period. Because these infants were cared for by teams of physicians and nurses, identifying a specific individual who might be associated with the unexpected deaths during the epidemic period was extremely difficult.

Systematic Study. Nonetheless, by imaginative use of duty rosters and call schedules, as well as hospital records, the epidemiologists excluded an association between physicians and deaths and then computed relative risks for each member of the nursing team. One nurse in particular was associated with a high relative risk of death, even though another nurse had been the subject of criminal charges.

When this investigation began, the epidemiologists knew of the epidemic, and the cases had clinical diagnoses that were confirmed by laboratory findings. The investigators were able to define the epidemic period, calculate mortality rates, and identify the specific hospital ward and age group of patients in which the epidemic had occurred. In this instance, determining the population at risk (patients in the pediatric cardiology wards in a large university-affiliated hospital) was easy, and so was hypothesizing the cause since criminal charges had already been made. Nonetheless, it was essential for the epidemiologists to avoid preconceptions about digoxin intoxication and to consider all possible causes for an increase in death rates. Comparing this hypothesis with the facts required creativity, good judgment, and courage because the epidemiological and legal evidence led to different conclusions. (The epidemiologists on the team were questioned by more than 15 attorneys, who represented a diverse group of clients, including the nurses, physicians, parents, and police.) The ingenious use of carefully documented data sources (duty rosters and call schedules) and the assessment of cardiology ward deaths with relative risks derived from incidence density ratios showed skill and judgment of a very high level. The epidemiologists were in a particularly difficult situation because they knew that their findings would be part of legal proceedings.[60] Careful observation and meticulous data collection made an important contribution to this investigation.

Using Judgment

The judgment of experienced epidemiologists regarding investigations rests on a series of questions. The first is "When do you do a field investigation?" Public need and scientific importance are the most frequent determinants of this answer. If the community is faced with a health problem that is difficult to control and whose cause is not known or a problem that has created public alarm, the community may have an urgent need that can be satisfied only by doing an epidemiological investigation. Scientific importance, while rarely isolated from public need, is more often determined by the nature of the problem, as was the case in Legionnaire's disease,[61] the initial studies of penicillinase-producing *Neisseria gonnorrhoeae* infection,[62] or the more recent epidemic of Brazilian purpuric fever caused by a form of *Haemophilus aegyptius* with a new plasmid type.[63] In each of these instances, the etiological agent required that an epidemiological investigation be done in the field with intensive and highly technical laboratory support.

Once in the field, when does an epidemiologist ask for help? Since epidemic investigations are rarely carried out by a single health professional, key questions must be asked before the field work begins. Among the foremost are the following: Will there be enough people available to ensure a successful investigation? Will these people have the necessary skills? What kind of technical support in terms of data collection and analysis, specimen gathering, computer science, and laboratory science will be required? Since the answers to these questions will change as the investigation evolves, the epidemiologist must re-ask each of them repeatedly.

How detailed should an investigation be? This question is best answered by considering the reasons for undertaking the investigation. If public need is the principal determinant, once this has been met, in terms of recommending control measures and addressing information needs, the epidemiologist must assess the overall scientific importance of the investigation and its value in the context of changing health policy for a larger population group. At this point, the advice of a more experienced epidemiologist or a colleague with specialized experience may be of help.

Before leaving the site of a field investigation, the epidemiologist should have affirmative answers to the following questions:

1. Is it possible to do a quantitative analysis of the data?
2. Is the analysis sufficient to permit the epidemiologist to make preliminary recommendations about control measures to the local officials?
3. Is it possible to give local officials a report that would permit them to initiate control measures and provide a credible explanation of the occurrence of the health problem to the public?
4. Will the person responsible for supervising the investigation from its institutional base find the report of the investigation acceptable?

If these questions cannot be answered satisfactorily, the investigation may have to be continued. Epidemiologists who do field investigations always should be prepared to *go back for the facts,* but it is preferable to get all of the facts in the first place.

Clearly communicating the investigative findings is essential, particularly when the epidemiologist feels that the field work has been completed. Who needs to know these findings? As a rule, those who reported the first cases in the epidemic are the first who must be informed, as are those who permitted, enabled, or facilitated the fieldwork. If the official and professional personnel responsible for control of the health problem are not part of these groups, then they, too, must be informed of the findings and of the rationale that is the scientific basis for control and prevention. Finally, the public and the media must be informed. Since the action to be taken in a community is the responsibility of public officials in that community, it is those officials rather than the investigating epidemiologist who should discuss the problem, the investigative findings, and the approach to control and prevention with the community and the media.

ANALYSIS

Epidemiological analysis is the identification, separation, and study of the component parts of a health problem for the purpose of describing the health problem, the population in which it occurred, and the factors that explain its occurrence. Analysis requires that each component be correctly identified and separated into its parts and that the relationship of the parts be determined. Analysis is built on a foundation of careful investigation, but it goes beyond investigation in that analysis focuses on comparisons and relationships while investigation emphasizes careful observation. In some cases, analysis identifies the need to return to vital statistics, another source of existing health information, or further field investigation. The process of analysis can be applied to descriptive studies, case-control studies, and cohort studies.

The process of analysis must be orderly. It interacts with the investigation of an epidemiological problem; the issues that will be met during the analytical process must be anticipated during the design of an epidemiological study.

Analysis proceeds from the simple to the complex. Starting with careful description by counting cases, analysis proceeds to percentage distributions, risk and rate estimation, and comparison, and then to more sophisticated, quantitative techniques.

Description

Detailed description is the foundation of epidemiology. Characterizing the persons who are the case subjects in an epidemic or who have health problems is important because these cases are essential in calculating rates and risks needed to solve an epidemiological problem. A line listing (Table 2–5) is one approach that shows relevant characteristics of the cases and helps determine how the population at risk should be characterized.[53] A graphic description of the cases, using an "epidemic curve" (see Fig. 2–1) for health problems with a short latent period and time trends for health problems with a longer latent period, will strengthen the description.

The population at risk provides the denominator for calculation of rates. It must be categorized by the same characteristics (e.g., grade in school, sex), with the same time interval of risk, as the cases in the numerator of the rate estimates. The first estimate of the rate is, therefore, usually made by putting the number of cases or events that occurred in a given period and in a given population within a geographic area in the numerator. The population at risk for the same period and area is the denominator.

The population at risk must be determined as precisely as possible. In an epidemic reported from a large area, the initial estimate of the population at risk is likely to include many people who are not really at risk of the reported condition (e.g., *all* students of high school age rather than only those attending the school in which the epidemic occurred). Subsequent study of the case characteristics may identify the communities in which many of those who are ill reside. Further inquiry may show that only the ones who attend a particular school or work in a single factory are really at risk. This same general idea applies to a wide variety of conditions other than infectious diseases. If, for example, a form of cancer is found only in workers using a particular chemical (e.g., vinyl chloride) or menopausal women, then only people who work with that chemical or women of menopausal age should be included as part of the epidemiological problem.

Selection of a comparison group, usually part of the study design and investigative process, warrants review during analysis. An initial study that covered an entire community may not be sufficiently sensitive, or even appropriate, if those with the health problem under analysis prove to reside in a specific area of the community (e.g., downwind or downstream from an industrial effluent) or can be shown to have eaten at specific restaurants that have been found to serve contaminated food. Under such circumstances, it may be necessary to restrict the analysis only to those at risk, even though it may seem like effort has been wasted or statistical power might be lost.

Two measures often used to describe the frequency of occurrence are *cumulative incidence* and *incidence density*. Cumulative incidence, often called the attack rate in an epidemic, is the proportion of a population initially free of a health problem who then develop the health problem. When applied to an epidemic, the cumulative incidence refers to the average population at risk and to the time during which the epidemic occurred. Cumulative incidence is a measure of the probability, or risk, of developing a particular condition during a specified period for the individuals in the population.

An explosive epidemic of 70 cases of measles illustrates how cumulative incidence is measured, as well as how a graph of the "epidemic curve" (see Fig. 2-1) can be used. In this outbreak the person with the index case had onset of rash on April 15. Investigation in the school where the epidemic occurred showed that there were 70 students who met the case definition (i.e., rash, fever, and at least one other symptom) in a school with an enrollment of 1873 students, of whom 43 students in a special program were not at risk. For this epidemic the cumulative incidence was 3.8% [70/1830 × 100 = 3.8%].[53]

A particular type of incidence density, the case-fatality rate, can be estimated, with the deaths as the numerator and the total number of cases as the denominator, once the number of cases or events of a particular problem are known and those who died of it have been identified. For example, during the years 1970 to 1986, an estimated 790,500 ectopic pregnancies occurred in women who live in the United States; 752 of them died. The case-fatality rate for ectopic pregnancy during this period can be calculated, therefore, as 9.5/10,000 ectopic pregnancies.[64]

Incidence density, on the other hand, is a measure of the rate at which a particular health problem develops in those in a population who were initially free of that problem per unit of *population and time,* most often expressed as person-years. Incidence density is often calculated for annual periods using standard health information, such as vital statistics or notifiable-disease data for the numerator and midyear population for the denominator. Alternatively, incidence density may be estimated in a cohort study from enrollment in the study to a predetermined point in time, such as the onset of the health problem, the end of a study, death from some cause not related to the study, or loss to follow-up.

In dealing with the unexplained deaths in the neonatal intensive care unit cited earlier,[59] incidence density (i.e., deaths per 10,000 patient-days) was used because those at risk of death were newborn infants (defined as infants 28 days old or younger) whose duration of exposure to risk varied. (Some were born recently; others were discharged after varying lengths of stay in the unit, and still others died.) On the other hand, cumulative incidence was the appropriate measure in the measles outbreak in a school since the same group of students was at risk each day during a relatively brief epidemic period.

The unexplained neonatal deaths, moreover, were spread out over a 9-month period. In that period of 9 months, or 274 days, an average of 28.8 newborn infants were in the unit each day, and 34 infants died. The incidence density was, therefore, [34/(274 days × 28.8 patients)] ×10,000 = 43.1/10,000 patient-days.

The epidemiologists compared the rate of death during the epidemic period with the comparable rate during the preceding 5 years and 6 months. They found that the epidemic period rate (or, more precisely, the incidence density ratio) was 3.9 times greater, a figure significantly beyond the limits of chance.

Comparison. Calculation and comparison of rates is the key to determining the strength of association between risk factor and the health problem. (It is important to realize that case counts, not rates, describe the magnitude of a problem. Rates describe the frequency with which events occur.) Rates for different groups may be compared to help identify the group in which a health problem is most intense. Age- and sex-specific rates, for example, can be compared to characterize the population groups at greatest risk of having the disease or health problem.

Quantitative comparisons of rates and risks can be made by means of the 2 × 2 table (Table 2–6). Summarizing epidemiological data by distributing it into the four cells of such a table according to the relevant exposure and the health problem or disease enables the epidemiologist to assess the occurrence of disease in relation to exposure, using a number of measures.

Arranging data in a 2 × 2 table as shown in Table 2–7 permits the information to be used for the analysis of a cohort study, yielding the information needed to calculate cumulative incidence. These are then used to compare the risk that a person will experience the health problem under investigation, depending on that person's exposure to the presumed risk factor. The ratio of these rates in the exposed and unexposed populations can be compared as a ratio, referred to as the relative risk. When

TABLE 2–6. FEATURES OF THE 2 × 2 TABLE

		Health Event or Disease		
		Present	***Absent***	***Total***
Exposure	***Present***	a	b	a+b
	Absent	c	d	c+d
	Total	a+c	b+d	a+b+c+d

a = Those with both disease and exposure
b = Those exposed who have no disease
c = Those diseased but not exposed
d = Those neither diseased nor exposed

a+c = All those with disease
a+b = All those with exposure
b+d = All those free of disease
c+d = All those without exposure
A+b+c+d = All those at risk

TABLE 2–7. FEATURES OF A COHORT STUDY IN A 2 × 2 TABLE USING DATA FROM A MEASLES EPIDEMIC IN A SCHOOL

		Disease (Measles)		
		Present	*Absent*	*Total*
Exposure	*Present (10th grade)*	21 [a]	453 [b]	474 [a + b]
	Absent (not 10th grade)	49 [c]	1,307 [d]	1,356 [c + d]

- **Cumulative Incidence in the Exposed Group**

$$\frac{a}{a+b} = \frac{21}{21+453} = 0.044 \text{ or } 4.4\%$$

- **Cumulative Incidence in the Unexposed Group**

$$\frac{c}{c+d} = \frac{49}{49+1{,}307} = 0.036 \text{ or } 3.6\%$$

$$\textbf{Relative Risk} = \frac{a/[a+b]}{c/[c+d]} = \frac{21/474}{42/1{,}356} = \frac{0.044}{0.036} = 1.2$$

*95% confidence interval is between 0.7 and 2.0 = 0.4.

the relative risk is equal to 1.0, indicating identical risks in the exposed and unexposed groups, there is no evidence of an association between health problem and exposure. However, if the relative risk is greater than 1.0, the epidemiologist has evidence that there may be an association between exposure and event. If, on the other hand, the ratio is significantly less than 1.0, the exposure presumably protects against the occurrence of the health problem.

In the measles epidemic in a school, the index case was a student in the tenth grade, as were 474 other students, 21 of whom were ill.[53] Therefore the cumulative incidence for measles in the grade with the index case is 21/474, or 4.4%. It is reasonable to hypothesize that students in this class might have greater risk of measles than those in the other classes. This latter group includes 49 students with measles and 1356 in the three other classes. The cumulative incidence in the other classes is 49/1356, or 3.6%. The ratio of the cumulative incidence for these two groups of students is 1.2 (4.4/3.6 = 1.2), a figure that could have occurred because of chance alone, since the confidence interval (0.7, 2.0) includes 1.0. (See Chance discussion below.) Being a classmate of the person who is the index case is, therefore, not a risk factor.

In case-control studies, the frequency of exposure to a risk factor in a group with the health problem under investigation is compared to the frequency of the same exposure in a group that does not have that problem. The *odds ratio* can then be computed (Table 2–8, panel A). Confidence limits are interpreted for odds ratios as they were for relative rates; those greater than 1.0 with confidence limits that do not include 1.0 indicate that an association is likely, while those significantly less than 1.0 indicate a protective effect.

The use of this measure to demonstrate both a causal and a protective effect is illustrated by studies of oral contraceptive (OC) use and tumors in women. A study of OC use in women with benign tumors of the liver (hepatocellular adenomas) by Rooks and her colleagues[65] shows a causal association. (This work will be discussed in more detail later.) Of the 79 women with this rare tumor, 72 had used OCs at some time in their lives. In a group of 220 control subjects (i.e., comparable women without the tumor), however, 99 had used OCs at some time (Table

TABLE 2–8. FEATURES OF CASE CONTROL STUDIES IN A 2 × 2 TABLE

- **A. Causal, or Positive, Association**

		Disease (Liver Tumor)	
		Present	*Absent*
Exposure (Oral Contraception)	*Present*	72 [a]	99 [b]
	Absent	7 [c]	121 [d]

$$\text{Odds ratio} = \frac{a/c}{b/d} = \frac{ad}{bc} = \frac{(72)(121)}{(99)(7)} = 12.6^{a}$$

- **B. Protective, or Negative, Association**

		Disease (Ovarian Cancer)	
		Present	*Absent*
Exposure (Oral Contraception)	*Present*	197 [a]	2,335 [b]
	Absent	242 [c]	1,532 [d]

$$\text{Odds ratio} = \frac{(197)(1{,}532)}{(2{,}335)(242)} = 0.5^{b}$$

[a]95% confidence interval is between 5.5 and 28.6; $P < 0.0001$.
[b]95% confidence interval is between 0.4 and 0.7; $P < 0.0001$.

2–8, panel A). The odds ratio is 12.6; it is significantly greater than 1.0 and has confidence limits that do not include 1.0.

A study of OC use as related to ovarian cancer uses the same measure to demonstrate a protective effect.[66] There were 242 women with ovarian cancer who had not used OCs for even as long as 3 months, whereas 197 of those with this cancer had used OCs; of the control subjects, 1532 had never used OCs and 2335 had used them. Table 2–8, panel B, shows that the odds ratio is 0.5, a figure significantly lower than 1.0, thereby indicating a protective effect by OCs against ovarian cancer.

Comparisons can also be used to estimate the potential impact of a health problem. The *risk difference,* also referred to as excess risk, can be used as a measure of impact as well as of association. The risk difference is the risk for the exposed group minus the risk for the unexposed group. The use of this measure is illustrated in its application to the lung cancer and smoking data of Doll and Hill[18] (Table 2–9). These data show that three

TABLE 2–9. MEASURES OF ASSOCIATION AND IMPACT: AN ILLUSTRATION BASED ON SMOKING AND LUNG CANCER

Cigarettes Smoked Daily	Lung Cancer Cases	Person-Years of Risk	Incidence Density (per 100,000 person-years)
None	3	42,800	7
1–14	22	38,600	57
15–24	54	38,900	139
25+	57	25,100	227
All smokers	133	102,600	130
Total	136	145,400	94

persons had lung cancer during a total of 42,800 person-years of observation of people who did not smoke cigarettes. The lung cancer rate for these subjects is 7/100,000 person-years. Among individuals who smoked cigarettes, 133 had lung cancer in 102,600 person-years, an incidence density of 130/100,000 person years. Since the risk difference is the risk for the exposed (smokers) minus the risk for those not exposed, the risk difference for smoking and lung cancer in this study is 130–7, or 123/100,000 person-years.

Other measures of potential impact include the attributable risk percent, the population attributable risk, and the population attributable risk percent. The *attributable risk percent* is a measure of the percentage of all deaths that can be attributed to the exposure being studied. This measure is also referred to as the etiological fraction. With use of the data on lung cancer and smoking of Doll and Hill,[18] the attributable risk is divided by the risk for those who smoke (then multiplied by 100) to calculate this measure. The attributable risk percent of smoking for death caused by lung cancer, therefore, is (123/130) × 100, or 95%. The data from this study are interpreted to mean that 95% of all deaths due to lung cancer among smokers can be attributed to cigarette smoking.

The *population attributable risk* is a measure of the excess disease rate in the total population. It can be estimated by subtracting the incidence density in the population not exposed to a causal risk factor from the incidence density for the total population. If, for example, the risk of death from lung cancer as a result of smoking is 54/100,000, as is stated in a recent estimate for the United States,[67] and the risk of death from lung cancer is 7/100,000, as Doll and Hill reported, the population attributable risk of death from lung cancer caused by smoking is 54–7, or 47/100,000.

The *population attributable risk percent* is the proportion of the rate of a disease that exists in a community, or population, because of a specific exposure. In the case of lung cancer deaths and smoking in the United States, for example, the population attributable risk is estimated to be 47 and the rate of death caused by lung cancer is 54/100,000; the population attributable risk percent is, therefore, 87% since (47/54) × 100 = 87. This percent differs from attributable risk percent because it considers the characteristics of exposure (i.e., smoking) for the entire population rather than those of a special group of individuals who are the subjects of a study.

These measures, their formulas, and examples are discussed in more detail in textbooks on epidemiology.[4,58,75,81]

Epidemiological analyses can measure the strength of the association between exposures and outcomes. These associations are characterized as direct and causal if they are positive or direct and protective if they are negative. Associations which appear direct but result from the interaction of another variable are indirect; they can result from confounding. Associations may also be artifactual. Distinguishing different forms of association requires knowledge of bias, confounding, effect modification, and chance, as well as the other criteria for judging epidemiological associations.

Bias. Bias, defined as "deviation of results or inferences from the truth, or processes leading to such deviation,"[4] may create either indirect or artifactual associations. It may also exaggerate or obscure associations. While some authorities identify many forms of bias,[67] often it can be classified as selection bias or information bias.

Selection Bias. Selection bias is error due to systematic differences between subjects selected for study and those who are excluded. Refusal to participate in a study or to respond to a questionnaire may introduce selection bias if those who refuse or are not able to respond differ in certain ways from those who participate. Selection of case and comparison subjects from hospitalized groups may also introduce bias if, for example, the hospitalized patients used as control subjects do not represent the same population from which those with the problem being studied have come. Comparison of subjects who have died with living subjects may introduce bias. Selection bias includes, and is sometimes used synonymously with, ascertainment bias, detection bias, sampling bias, or design bias.

Information Bias. Information bias is error that is due to systematic differences in the way data have been gathered from controls and cases. If, for example, one set of questions is used to evaluate the exposure or the health condition affecting the comparison subjects and another set is used for the case subjects, there may be information about the two groups that is systematically different, thereby leading to a distorted inference. If, in a clinical study, one group is observed more frequently than another, the probability of making a diagnosis will be greater for the group that is observed more frequently. This kind of bias could occur in a study evaluating the effectiveness and safety of two approaches to patient care, one conducted on subjects seen in an ambulatory clinic and the other conducted on subjects who required hospitalization. Information bias may include or be referred to as observer, interviewer, measurement, recall, or reporting bias. These terms are defined more precisely and discussed in detail in other writings.[4,68]

Confounding. Comparisons may differ from the truth and, therefore, may be biased when the association between exposure and the health problem varies because a third factor confounds or distorts the association. A confounding factor may distort the effect of the risk factor under study when the factor is associated with the outcome that is being studied and is unequally distributed among the exposed and unexposed groups being compared. Age can be a confounding variable when the age distribution of two populations differs. Age adjustment, or stratification, is used to examine the confounding effect of age differences. There are many other commonly encountered confounding variables. For example, in studies of the effects of occupational exposure on respiratory disease, smoking often must be evaluated as a confounding variable.

Confounding can be illustrated with the use of mortality data from two counties in Florida. The data are shown in Table 2–10 (see total population comparison). The cumulative incidence of mortality is greater in Pinellas County than in Dade County by 70%, as indicated by the relative risk of 1.7. When the relative risk is adjusted for age, however, it approximates 1.0 (the Mantel-Haenszel summary relative risk ratio is 0.95), a better representation of the risk of mortality at each age since these two areas have substantially different age structures.

Stratification of data helps evaluate the effect of a third factor on an epidemiological association. In using stratification to assess the effects of confounding, the epidemiologist constructs two or more 2 × 2 tables. Each table includes subjects and controls who are comparable in terms of the confounding factor. The other 2 × 2 tables include subjects who have all been exposed to the confounding factor and who may have varying levels of exposure to it. Stratification thereby controls the effects of confounding. Using the Florida example and developing separate 2 × 2 tables shows how stratification adjusts for confounding (see Table 2–10, Comparison by Age Groups). While comparing two strata does not adjust for confounding as fully as the summary approach involving 10 strata mentioned above, even this simple modification to the use of a single, unstratified measure illustrates the importance of this approach.

Effect Modification. Effect modification is a change in the measure of association between a risk factor and the epidemiological outcome under study by a third variable. The third variable is an effect modifier. An effect modifier provides added information about an association by helping to describe an association in more detail.

TABLE 2-10. EVALUATING COMPARISONS BIASED BY CONFOUNDING: AN ILLUSTRATION USING MORTALITY DATA FROM FLORIDA

A. Overall Comparison with Confounding Population

	Dead	*Alive*	*Total*
Pinellas County	5,726	368,939	374,665
Dade County	8,332	926,725	935,047

Mortality Rate*

Pinellas County	15.3
Dade County	8.9

Relative Rate = 15.3/8.9 = 1.7

B. Stratified Comparison Adjusted for Confounding

Age Range: birth to 54 years

	Dead	*Alive*	*Total*
Pinellas County	737	228,461	229,198
Dade County	2,463	745,572	748,035

Mortality Rate*

Pinellas County	3.2
Dade County	3.3

Relative Rate = 3.2/3.3 = 1.0

Age Range: 55 years and older

	Dead	*Alive*	*Total*
Pinellas County	4,989	140,158	145,147
Dade County	5,898	182,087	187,985

Mortality Rate*

Pinellas County	34.4
Dade County	31.2

Relative Rate = 34.4/31.2 = 1.1

*Deaths per 1,000 population.

Effect modification can be illustrated by the association between intentional injury and the sex of the children and adolescents in a study from Massachusetts.[69] For the entire population, defined as all individuals younger than 20 years of age in a specified geographic area, the incidence density for intentional injury is half as great for girls as for boys (Table 2-11). Nonetheless, age modifies this main effect (Table 2-11). For children younger than 5 years, girls have an incidence density 60% greater than that for boys. In the age interval from 5 to 9 years the rate for girls becomes just one third that for boys. The overall association, or main effect (i.e., intentional injury associated with male sex), therefore, is not uniform for all age intervals in this study. The effect is modified by age.

Both effect modification and confounding are concerned with the way in which a third variable influences an epidemiological association; nonetheless, these two concepts are different. Effect modification gives the epidemiologist more information about the association and the group in which it is found; confounding distorts the association. Effect modification is inherent in the nature of the association. Confounding is not; a confounding factor is not a consequence of exposure to the risk factor and can occur even in the absence of the risk. A confounding

TABLE 2-11. EVALUATING COMPARISONS WITH EFFECT MODIFICATION: AN ILLUSTRATION USING INTENTIONAL INJURIES AMONG CHILDREN AND ADOLESCENTS IN MASSACHUSETTS

Effects	Male	Female	Relative Risk
By Incidence Density*			
All Ages	97.9	53.6	0.5
By Age (y)			
0–4	10.6	17.0	1.6
5–9	21.8	7.4	0.3
10–14	59.7	40.5	0.7
15–19	259.8	131.0	0.5

*Intentional injuries per 10,000 person-years.

factor exerts its influence by being unevenly distributed between the study groups. It is possible, therefore, for a variable to be an effect modifier, a confounding factor, both, or neither. Moreover, a single variable may both modify and confound the same main effect in a single study.

Stratifying an epidemiological analysis by an effect modifier adds knowledge about the association because it describes the effects of such a factor. Stratification also adjusts for, or neutralizes, the effects of a confounding factor.

Many analyses require the epidemiologist to stratify for a number of effect modifiers or confounding factors. Analytical complexities of this kind require the use of multivariate analysis. This analytic approach permits the epidemiologist to adjust simultaneously for a number of potential confounding variables. These analytic approaches are dealt with in detail in specialized textbooks.[58,75,81]

Chance. Chance can play two roles in epidemiology. It may account for an apparent association and make it appear real when it is not. (This is referred to as a type I, or alpha, error.) Alternatively, chance may lead to an association being overlooked, or missed, when it truly exists. (This is called a type II, or beta, error.) Statistical significance testing of epidemiological data helps evaluate the role of chance by permitting an epidemiologist to determine the probability that an association actually exists. Assessing the statistical power of a study evaluates the probability that an association would be detected if it were present.

In epidemiology, as in other sciences, we must often decide whether a difference between observations is statistically significant. Two questions arise: What is meant by "statistically significant?" How can we test for statistical significance? A complete answer to these questions demands a thorough understanding of statistics, which can be acquired in courses and textbooks on the subject. The following discussion assumes familiarity with the terms and concepts of elementary statistics.

When data have a normal or Gaussian distribution, 5% of the observations lie more than two standard deviations from the mean or central value. This fact leads to the arbitrary decision that the 5% level is a suitable point to set for observed differences to be described as statistically significant. In the conventional notation, the probability of an observation falling in this range is less than 5%, or $P < 0.05$. This level of statistical significance is suitable for many purposes in epidemiology, but sometimes we are justified in insisting on higher levels, for example, a difference that could occur by chance less often than once in 100 times (i.e., $P < 0.01$) or less often than once in 1000 times (i.e., $P < 0.001$). When we set a 5% level (i.e., $P < 0.05$), one observed difference in 20 tests can be expected to be "statistically significant" just by chance when many comparisons are being made in sets of data (e.g., in multivariate analysis, when on the average 1 in 20 of the correlations will be "statistically significant" because of chance alone).

TABLE 2-12. CASE CONTROL STUDY OF LUNG CANCER AND PAST HISTORY OF SMOKING

History of Smoking	Cases of Lung Cancer	Controls
Yes	647	622
No	2	27
Total	649	649

Significance Tests. The most widely used tests of statistical significance in epidemiology are the chi-squared and the *t* test, the correlation coefficient, and the analysis of variance. A detailed description of ways to perform these tests and their underlying mathematical theory can be found in the reference books listed at the end of this chapter; here is a brief and necessarily oversimplified account of the circumstances under which each should be used.

The chi-squared test is used to determine whether two or more series of proportions or frequencies are significantly different from one another, or whether a single series of proportions differs from a theoretically expected distribution. There are a number of variations on the chi-squared test (e.g., the Mantel-Haenszel test, widely used in epidemiology to test for statistically significant differences in 2 × 2 tables when confounding variables are present).

The *t* test is used when we want to compare the means of two or more populations or groups of data in which the standard deviation is not known, which is often the case when one is dealing with small numbers. The *t* test is based on the assumption that the data are normally distributed; in many biomedical data sets, the distribution is skewed rather than normal, but if the skewing is not extreme, the assumption of normal distribution is considered approximately valid.

The correlation coefficient is used to detect a trend in the relationship of two variables (e.g., heights and weights of a sample of schoolchildren, national per capita consumption of dietary fats, and mortality rates from coronary heart disease or cancer of the large bowel). These relationships are often represented visually as scatter diagrams that reveal how two variables are related but do not fully describe the nature of the statistical relationship, which is provided by calculation of the correlation coefficient.

If we know the means of two or more distributions, we can use analysis of variance to compare these and detect statistical differences or similarities. When we use analysis of variance, we could search for close similarity or parallelism of trends. In interpreting the results of these tests, it must be remembered that observed parallelism of trends does not necessarily imply a causal relationship. For example, the death rate from coronary heart disease in the United States rose in the period from the 1940s to the mid-1960s at about the same rate as the number of licensed automobiles per 1000 population, but this does not mean, of course, that automobile use causes coronary heart disease. There are many such "nonsense correlations." Common sense as well as logic must be brought to bear in interpreting data and the statistical significance tests that are applied to the data.

Confidence Intervals. A confidence interval is defined as the range of possible values for the attribute that is being measured or assessed, constructed so that this range has a specified probability, usually greater than 95%, of including the true value. While the results of hypothesis-testing studies have conventionally been evaluated in terms of significance tests used expressed in a single value, this assumes that the populations in the study groups are truly representative of the universe and that the data have a normal or other known distribution. Often neither assumption is true. Several authorities have argued cogently that scientific papers must show the confidence intervals rather than, or in addition to, the *P* values derived from statistical significance testing.

Reporting single values of this kind focuses undue attention on statistical, rather than clinical or epidemiological, significance. For instance, in an early case-control study of cigarette smoking and occurrence of lung cancer, Doll and Hill[18] observed the distribution of cigarette smoking in the cases and controls cited in Table 2-12 (male patients only). The probability that this distribution would occur by chance, according to Fisher's exact test, was 0.00000064. However, this test which gives a single point of statistical significance, provides less information than the confidence intervals because this interval measure gives information about sample size that a point value cannot. According to the odds ratio method of estimation, the relative risk of lung cancer among smokers, compared to nonsmokers, is 14 (i.e., smokers had about 14 times higher risk of lung cancer than nonsmokers). This figure is consistent with the relative risks derived from distributions observed in later, more carefully conducted case-control studies (and also with the risks calculated from cohort studies). Confidence intervals are related to sample size, as Table 2-13 clearly shows. Methods of calculating confidence intervals vary according to the nature and quality of the data and represent a branch of applied biostatistics beyond the scope of this book. Details are given in some of the references cited at the end of this chapter.

Statistical Power. If a real difference exists between case and control groups, there is a chance that this difference may not be detected on statistical analysis, thereby leading to a type II, or beta, error. Statistical power states the probability that this chance occurrence will be avoided and is expressed as (1-beta), the complement of the type II, or beta, error. Its computation is relevant only when the confidence interval of the measure of association does not include the value 1.0. Conventional practice is to design studies with a sample size that will give a type II, or beta, error no greater than 0.10 and a type I, or alpha, error no greater than 0.05, given the hypothesized risk for the exposed group.

TABLE 2-13. INFANT MORTALITY RATE: SAMPLE SIZE AND CONFIDENCE INTERVAL

Sample Size: Number of Persons	Number of Births Observed	Number of Infant Deaths Observed	95% Confidence Interval for the Infant Mortality Rate
1,000	40	4	4-196
5,000	200	20	58-142
10,000	400	40	70-130
50,000	2,000	200	87-113
100,000	4,000	400	91-109
250,000	10,000	1,000	94-106
500,000	20,000	2,000	96-104

Adapted from Development of Indicators for Monitoring Progress Towards Health for All by the Year 2000. Geneva: WHO, 1981.

Interpretation

Although we have focused on the measurement of association, the identification of bias, and the role of chance up to this point, interpretation of epidemiological data requires that causal associations between exposure and outcome be correctly identified by using specific objective criteria. The initial criteria used to distinguish causal associations from indirect and artifactual ones were applied to epidemic infections by Henle and Koch and can be stated as follows[70]:

1. The causative agent must be recovered from all individuals with the disease.
2. The agent must be recovered from those with the disease and grown in pure culture.
3. The organism grown in pure culture must replicate the disease when introduced into susceptible animals.

Such rigorous criteria ensure that studies which adhere to them are likely to correctly identify causal associations. Nonetheless, they are restrictive, and, had they been adhered to inflexibly, some important epidemiological associations would not have been found. The association between smoking and lung cancer is one.

Criteria more suited to contemporary health problems were first proposed in the mid-1960s. The Advisory Committee on Smoking and Health convened by the Surgeon General of the U.S. Public Health Service[71] and Sir Austin Bradford Hill[20] in his first presidential address to the Section of Occupational Medicine of the Royal Society of Medicine in England both proposed criteria that can be summarized as follows:

1. **Chronological relationship:** Exposure to the causative factor must occur before the onset of the disease.
2. **Strength of association:** If all those with a health problem have been exposed to the agent believed to be associated with this problem and only a few in the comparison group have been so exposed, the association is a strong one. In quantitative terms, the larger the relative risk, the more likely the association is causal.
3. **Intensity or duration of exposure:** If those with the most intense, or longest, exposure to the agent have the greatest frequency or severity of illness while those with less exposure are not as ill, then it is more likely that the association is causal. This is also referred to as a biological gradient, or a dose-response relationship.
4. **Specificity of association:** If an agent, or risk factor, can be isolated from others and shown to produce changes in the frequency of occurrence or severity of the disease, the likelihood of a causal association is increased.
5. **Consistency of findings:** An association is consistent if it is confirmed by different investigators, in different populations, or using different methods of study.
6. **Coherent and plausible findings:** This criterion is met when a plausible relationship between the biological and behavioral factors related to the association support a causal hypothesis. Evidence from experimental animals, analogous effects created by analogous agents, and information from other experimental systems and forms of observation are among the kinds of evidence to be considered.

Interpretation of epidemiological data, therefore, requires two major steps: First, each criterion for a causal association must be carefully evaluated. The second step is an equally careful assessment of the association to identify bias and evaluate the role of chance. Undue emphasis may be given to the role of chance. As a result, Hill[20] said of tests of statistical significance, "Such tests can, and should, remind us of the effects that the play of chance can create, and they will instruct us in the likely magnitude of those effects. Beyond that they contribute nothing to the 'proof' of our hypothesis."

Illustrative Epidemiological Study

Less than a decade after oral contraceptives were approved for use in the United States, a report was published about seven women who developed a benign but extremely rare tumor of the liver while using oral contraception. On the basis of this report, Rooks and her colleagues[65] hypothesized an association between oral contraceptive use and the occurrence of this tumor, hepatocellular adenoma. A review of the literature in 1944 reported only 67 histologically confirmed cases as of that date. However, records at the Armed Forces Institute of Pathology (AFIP) documented 105 such tumors in females in the 20 years after 1957. No similar increase was found for males.

Collaborating with the AFIP, Rooks and her coworkers identified 79 women for whom histological confirmation of this tumor was on file. Each subject was matched with three women of similar age who lived in the same neighborhood. They were all interviewed about exposures that might influence their risk of liver disease, including liver tumors, and about their obstetric history and contraceptive use. The interview provided a detailed description of both case and control women.

The analysis of this case-control study showed a very strong association between the exposure (oral contraceptive use) and the health problem (hepatocellular adenoma). An overall odds ratio derived from the analysis of a 2 × 2 table was 12.6 (see Table 2–8, panel A). Separation of the exposure to oral contraceptive use (measured by months of use) into five levels showed that the odds ratio increased as months of oral contraceptive use increased. The odds ratio estimation done while the matching of cases with their controls was retained showed an even greater relative risk, so that when oral contraceptive use was 7 years or longer, the relative risk estimate changed from 50 for the unmatched analysis to more than 500 for the matched analysis (see Table 2–14).

This study meets each of the criteria for a causal association between oral contraceptive use and the occurrence of hepatocellular adenoma in women. The interviews ensured that oral contraceptive use started before any signs or symptoms of liver disease appeared. The strength of association documented by the odds ratio was so great that statistical testing was hardly necessary. Separation of oral contraceptive use into five different levels by duration of use showed that as the degree of exposure increased so did the risk of disease (i.e., there was a strong dose-response relationship). Interview information permitted Rooks and her colleagues to identify oral contraception as the specific agent, rather than some other agent used during the same time. Further analysis showed that low-potency oral contraceptive hormones were associated with a lower risk of disease, while high-potency preparations had a higher relative risk, thereby

TABLE 2–14. ODDS RATIOS BY DURATION OF ORAL CONTRACEPTIVE USE ASSOCIATED WITH BENIGN LIVER TUMORS

Duration of Use (mo)	Cases	Controls	Odds Ratios	
			Unmatched	Matched
0–12	7	121	[referrent]	[referrent]
13–36	11	49	4	9
37–60	20	23	15	116
61–84	21	20	16	129
≥85	20	7	49	503
Total	79	220		

supporting the specificity of the association. This association was consistent with the original case series and with other scientific reports. Moreover, it was coherent and plausible because animal studies also showed that hormones of the kind used in oral contraceptives led to an increased frequency of liver tumors in rats. In addition, two women in the series studied by Rooks and her associates, as well as nine others reported elsewhere, experienced regression of their tumors when the use of oral contraceptives was stopped.

Further analysis of potentially confounding variables did not influence risk estimates, and all of these estimates were unlikely to have occurred from chance alone. Moreover, bias was not a likely explanation for these findings because of the use of neighborhood controls, uniform interviewing methods, and a special recall aid (i.e., pictures of oral contraceptive packages). The evidence to support this association between oral contraceptive use and the occurrence of hepatocellular adenoma in women is, therefore, causal and not likely to be due to chance or bias.

Using Judgment in Analysis

The following points are important when judgment is applied to epidemiological analysis:

1. Start with data of good quality and know the strength and weakness of the data set in detail.
2. Make careful description of the epidemiological problem the first step.
3. Determine the population at risk as precisely as possible.
4. Selection of the comparison, or control, group is one of the most difficult judgments to make. As a rule, try to choose for comparison subjects who are as similar to the case group as possible.
5. Taking the time to reduce the data analysis to a 2 × 2 table whenever possible will clarify both the decisions that the analyst must make and the communication of the findings.
6. The strongest case for an epidemiological association is one that meets all of the causal criteria (listed earlier).
7. Carefully determine the role that bias, including confounding, may have played in distorting an association.
8. In assessing an association, do not rely on tests of statistical significance alone. Remember the words of Hill, who stated: "There are innumerable situations in which they [tests of statistical significance] are totally unnecessary—because the difference is grotesquely obvious, because it is negligible, or because, whether it be formally significant or not, it is too small to be of any practical importance."

EVALUATION

For an epidemiologist, evaluation is the scientific process of determining the effectiveness and safety of a given measure intended to control or prevent a health problem. Evaluation can involve a clinical trial that tests effectiveness of a drug, vaccine, or medical device and determines the occurrence of adverse side effects. Evaluation can be used to assess intervention programs in communities, as was done with water fluoridation and its effect on the prevention of dental caries. Evaluation may also assess the effectiveness of measures to control an epidemic.

Those who work in evaluation differentiate the terms *effectiveness, efficacy,* and *efficiency*. *Effectiveness* is defined as "the extent to which a specific intervention, procedure, regimen, or service, when deployed in the field, does what it is intended to do for a defined population."[4] *Efficacy* is "the extent to which a specific intervention, procedure, regimen, or service produces a beneficial result under ideal conditions."[4] Under the best of circumstances, efficacy is determined by a carefully controlled trial. *Efficiency* is defined as "the effects or end-results achieved in relation to the effort expended in terms of money, resources, and time."[4] Efficiency assumes that therapeutic or preventive agents and intervention procedures are effective and safe. Stated in another way, efficiency is "a measure of the economy (or cost in resources) with which a procedure of known efficacy and effectiveness is carried out."[4]

Characteristics of Epidemiological Evaluation. The epidemiological evaluation of a health problem has special characteristics. First, the health problem is usually well defined; this means that the epidemiologist does not need to be deeply concerned with such questions as "is there an epidemic?" as is the case with investigation of an outbreak. Second, because the problem definition is clearer, epidemiological evaluation customarily has specific, explicit, and quantifiable objectives. Third, a case definition for the health problem has often been formulated in detail before the epidemiologist begins fieldwork. Finally, careful planning of an evaluation study is often essential, so that a complex set of study design issues can be carefully addressed.

Epidemiologists are called on to evaluate a wide range of issues. Investigating an epidemic of measles may require an evaluation of vaccine effectiveness when one is considering hypotheses about the cause of disease occurrence. An unusual group of abnormal cytology reports may suggest either a cluster of cancer cases or a problem with screening procedures. The epidemiologist may also be called on to evaluate therapeutic and preventive measures in carefully designed clinical trials. Such measures may include an assessment of the effectiveness of a surgical procedure such as contraceptive sterilization,[72] a formal field trial of vaccine effectiveness,[73] as was done with polio vaccine, or a study of low-dose acetyl salicylate and its effects on the occurrence of myocardial infarction.[74] Epidemiologists may also conduct program evaluations to assess organized efforts intended to improve the health of entire communities, regardless of the specific method of intervention used. Such worthwhile efforts have been made in controlling epidemics of infection and in programs to prevent unplanned pregnancy. In addition, carefully organized community trials have been used to evaluate the prevention of cardiovascular disease, nutritional deficiencies, and dental health problems.

The need for carefully designed clinical and community trials to evaluate prevention programs and agents has led some writers to characterize this as "experimental epidemiology."[75] The scientific desirability of carrying out a randomized, blinded, controlled clinical trial of a therapeutic or preventive intervention is undeniable. Nonetheless, epidemiologists may need to evaluate health problems because a presumably effective form of intervention did not lead to adequate prevention or treatment of a health problem in a community.

Meta-analysis. Meta-analysis is the systematic process of combining results from different research studies with the use of statistical methods to obtain a numerical estimate of an overall effect. Its primary aim is to enhance the statistical power of research findings when numbers in the available studies are too small. It is intended to be more objective and quantitative than a narrative review. In public health and clinical medicine, meta-analysis is often applied by pooling results of small randomized controlled trials when no single such trial has large enough numbers to demonstrate statistical significance.

The steps in carrying out a meta-analysis begin with an explicit and detailed definition of the problem for which research studies are to be reviewed. The full sequence of steps (Table 2-15) was reviewed recently by Thacker.[76] Although *meta-analy-*

TABLE 2-15. STEPS IN META-ANALYSIS

1. Define the problem
2. Establish the criteria for including individual studies in the meta-analysis
3. Locate the individual research studies
4. Classify and code each study by characteristics relevant to the meta-analysis
5. Aggregate the results of the individual studies
6. Relate the aggregated results to the characteristics of the meta-analysis
7. Report the results of the meta-analysis

sis is a term that originated in the field of educational psychology, it has been widely used in behavioral and policy science and is the topic of several books. Applications of this approach have made important contributions to the use of ultrasound[77] and of fetal monitoring[78] in obstetrics, the use of β-blockers in cardiology,[79] and in defining the role of adjuvant therapy for women with breast cancer.[80]

Although meta-analysis is an important new tool for the epidemiologist, it has some pitfalls. The problems with bias take on new dimensions. One, referred to as publication bias, results from the tendency of authors and editors to put into print studies that have positive findings in preference to those that demonstrate no association between factors being studied. Moreover, authors tend to select or emphasize studies that confirm their own viewpoint by applying the criteria for inclusion in a meta-analysis that vary from one study to another, thereby supporting their own beliefs.

It is essential, therefore, to ensure the meticulous use of the methods and procedures of each meta-analysis, as it is the individual studies that are the subject of a meta-analysis. If there are uncertainties about comparability of individual studies because the results of one study differ greatly from the findings of others or the methods and procedures cannot be easily understood, the original investigators may be of help in providing more details about research procedures or access to unpublished data. Nonetheless, it may be better to include studies of uncertain methods in a different category, or stratum, of studies than to group their findings with those for which the methods have been published in detail.

The process of aggregating, or pooling, follows the classification of all the individual studies eligible for inclusion in the meta-analysis. Pooled data are then analyzed by application of appropriate statistical methods to evaluate the association under investigation. As with any epidemiological analysis, it is as important to search for bias and assess the role of chance as it is to evaluate the strength of the association.

Design Issues. Two issues in the design of epidemiological evaluation that warrant explicit mention are restriction and randomization. Restriction minimizes potential confounding by limiting the study to a group with characteristics for which a confounding variable is either absent or can be clearly identified and measured. In an evaluation of the effectiveness of a vaccine, for example, those included in the evaluation might be restricted by age. The youngest age at which a child would be included would be that at which children first became eligible for vaccination. The older age limit would be that at which natural immunity is so prevalent that the role of vaccine-induced immunity is negligible. Restriction of this kind minimizes confounding by natural immunity. Similarly, a study of the association between the use of hormones and a tumor, such as that of oral contraception and a liver tumor cited earlier, might restrict admission by age, depending on how the hormone was used.

Randomization is the assignment of people who are eligible for the research trial into study and control groups so as to ensure that each has a known (usually equal) chance of allocation to any group. Randomization minimizes both selection bias and confounding and ensures the comparability of the groups being studied. Randomization is a powerful strategy. Its use controls selection bias, but it does not replace the need for blinding of observers or the use of a placebo control group as a means of minimizing observer bias.

Analytical Approaches. Measuring the preventive effect of an agent or program can be done by computing the prevented fraction in the exposed group. Comparison of the cumulative incidence, or attack rate, of the condition to be prevented in the group that received the preventive procedure with that for the group that did not permits the relative risk to be computed. Setting the cumulative incidence in the comparison group equal to 1.0 and subtracting from it the relative risk of occurrence in the population receiving the intervention procedure gives the prevented fraction in the exposed group as the difference. This approach assumes that the frequency at which the condition occurs in the group with no intervention is the true one. Presumably, the lower frequency of occurrence (i.e., < 1.0) reflects the effects of the intervention. A more detailed discussion of this topic is given by Miettinen[81] and by Orenstein and his colleagues,[82] who address the measurement of preventive effect specifically as it applies to vaccine efficacy.

The use of modified approaches to the life table is often important for epidemiological evaluation. Studies of contraceptive use and effectiveness that focus on the intrauterine device illustrate this method, as discussed above. This analytical approach permits estimates to be made of effectiveness and also of specific reasons for discontinuing the use of a device. In addition, the use of ordinal months permits study subjects to be admitted on different dates and to be excluded when lost to follow-up.

Program/Community Evaluation. Evaluation of program or community intervention differs from clinical trials in important ways. Community interventions address an intervention approach introduced into a population group, whereas a clinical trial involves the treatment of individuals—usually a group of carefully selected subjects. The evaluation of the influence of water fluoridation on the occurrence of dental caries compared the communities of Newburgh (the trial community) and Kingston (the comparison community) in New York State, so that the public health policy for fluoridation of water to improve dental health had a solid epidemiological basis.[83]

Illustrative Case. Epidemiological evaluation is called for almost any time a new approach to prevention is to have widespread use. The introduction of new plastics and the global concern about uncontrolled fertility led to new developments in intrauterine contraception. While this approach to fertility control was not new, it had never been evaluated for either effectiveness or safety. Under the direction of Christopher Teitze, a network of researchers from around the world began a trial of intrauterine contraceptive devices (IUDs) to assess their effectiveness and side effects and to find out whether they could be used safely and effectively. A report on nine such devices describes their work.[84] The trial was restricted to women of childbearing age who stated they were sexually active. Each woman was characterized by age, parity, outcome of last pregnancy, date IUD use began, and clinical center attended. Effectiveness was measured in terms of pregnancies that occurred while an IUD was in place. Side effects were categorized as expulsions, removals, and pregnancies. The removals were further classified as being done because of bleeding, pain, other medical indications, planning pregnancy, or other personal choice. The dates on which expulsions and removals occurred and on which pregnancies were diagnosed were recorded. The use of life table techniques permitted the investigators to report the average duration of IUD use and the reason for discontinuation of use. Discontinuation of use is analogous to death; discontinuation for a particular reason is analogous to death from a particular cause, such as heart disease. This is referred to as a multiple-decrement life table. After 2 years of use the researchers had accumulated data on a total of more than 380,000 woman-months of IUD use, ranging from 7000 to 136,000 woman-months for each device (Table 2–16). Their results showed that pregnancy rates ranged from 2.2 to 16.1/100 woman-months of use, depending on the device. Expulsion rates had a range of 1.8 to 33.4, while removal rates fell between 11.9 and 20.5. Overall continuation rates did not differ significantly among the devices, and one (the size D loop) was judged to offer the best overall combination of pregnancy prevention and lack of serious side effects. More recent trials compared this IUD and a copper-carrying device, applying a similar but more refined life table method.

The international evaluation of IUDs makes important points about study design and shows how life table analysis can be used imaginatively. Using an approach referred to as restriction, these investigators confined their study participants to sexually active women of reproductive age, thus reducing distortion, which would result if women not yet able to become pregnant or postmenopausal women were included. Life table analysis, particularly the use of ordinal months of study participation, and the careful categorization of events enabled the researchers to use as much of their data as possible and to interpret them precisely and quantitatively. In subsequent reports these workers were able to calculate standard errors for the life table rates.

Using Judgment

Ethics and Doubt. Ethics and scientific doubt are the base from which epidemiological judgment on evaluation must begin. The most fundamental decision is determination of the need for an epidemiological evaluation of the kind done for IUD effectiveness, water fluoridation, or poliovirus vaccine use. Nonetheless, the entire body of scientific knowledge must be given careful consideration (thus the need for meta-analysis) if this judgment is to be acceptable to scientists and to the public. This contrast is highlighted by the fact that, while these studies were instrumental in setting public health policy for contraception, the control of dental caries, and the control of poliomyelitis, no similar trial of the effectiveness and safety of smallpox vaccine was ever carried out; yet smallpox remains the only disease eradicated by an organized public health program.[85]

Establishment of rules for stopping evaluation studies before their scheduled completion also poses ethical problems. If the intervention being evaluated is so effective that the outcome of the trial is obvious before its scheduled completion, what must be done? On the other hand, if there are unexpected problems concerning the safety of the intervention, such as rare, extremely grave side effects, how will the decision be made about continuing the trial? More particularly, what should be done if the adverse effects are only mild ones, or if they are extremely rare but unexpectedly serious? The role of a scientifically competent, publicly acceptable advisory group becomes very important under circumstances of this kind. (See Chapter 75 for further discussion.)

Selection of the Study Population. The selection of subjects for study is critical to both clinical and community trials. The following three factors are among the most important selection criteria: First, the experimental subjects must be sufficiently representative of the larger population that changes in policy as a result of the findings will be scientifically acceptable and credible to the public. Second, the number of subjects estimated to be eligible for and likely to consent to the study must be sufficient that interpretable results can be obtained. Third, the health problem under investigation must occur frequently enough in the groups being studied that the results will be statistically significant.

Ascertainment of Outcome. The outcome of concern in an epidemiological evaluation must meet clear and explicit criteria. Moreover, it must be as free of observer bias as possible. Mortal-

TABLE 2-16. NET CUMULATIVE RATES OF EVENTS AND CLOSURES PER 100 CASES, BY TYPE OF TERMINATION: ALL DEVICES BY TYPE AND SIZE, TWO YEARS OF USE

	Loops				Spirals		Bows		
Type of Termination	**A**	**B**	**C**	**D**	**Small**	**Large**	**Small**	**Large**	**Steel Ring**
Events:									
Pregnancies	9.3	4.8	4.0	4.1	4.5	2.2	16.1	7.1	9.0
Expulsions									
First	22.9	17.7	15.1	11.0	33.4	23.5	4.7	1.8	18.1
Later	4.9	4.4	5.7	4.2	10.0	7.1	1.3	1.1	4.5
Removals									
Bleeding and/or pain	13.0	16.8	15.1	16.5	13.2	20.5	16.5	15.7	11.9
Other medical	6.7	6.3	4.7	5.7	5.5	11.4	4.1	5.6	3.2
Planning pregnancy	4.0	2.2	3.3	2.8	3.4	3.0	4.4	2.6	4.3
Other personal	6.6	2.9	2.4	3.8	12.1	5.8	7.0	3.0	3.3
Closures:									
Pregnancies	8.0	4.6	3.7	3.5	3.2	1.7	13.7	6.0	8.2
Expulsions									
First	6.9	4.7	4.1	3.4	9.7	7.6	1.0	0.7	5.3
Later	2.5	2.1	2.1	2.2	3.5	2.1	0.3	0.4	2.2
Removals									
Bleeding and/or pain	8.6	15.3	13.6	14.6	8.8	13.8	9.5	13.3	10.1
Other medical	3.1	4.8	3.6	4.1	3.9	6.3	3.2	4.6	2.9
Planning pregnancy	2.3	2.2	3.0	2.2	1.8	2.6	4.1	2.2	3.4
Other personal	5.1	2.7	2.3	3.4	10.0	4.7	6.2	2.6	3.2
Total Closures	36.5	36.4	32.4	33.4	40.9	38.8	38.0	29.8	35.3
Active at End of 2nd Year	63.5	63.6	67.6	66.6	59.1	61.2	62.0	70.2	64.7
Woman-months of Use	13,428	8,045	43,474	109,946	5,883	28,890	18,987	40,411	25,163

ity is, therefore, a more desirable end point for study than morbidity. The availability of the National Death Index in the United States now permits researchers to identify consistently and completely all persons who die from a specified cause. Morbidity is not similarly indexed, for example, because subjects may be lost to follow-up. Moreover, morbidity may recur so that duplication of data entries and analytic problems become more complex.

APPLYING EPIDEMIOLOGY TO PUBLIC HEALTH

Epidemiology, as the scientific basis for the practice of public health, has important applications to the resolution of high-priority contemporary health problems. This closing section highlights three illustrative case studies on this topic.

Epidemic Control. Epidemiology and the control of epidemics remain relevant to contemporary public health practice. While the AIDS pandemic is well recognized, many other epidemics still occur; several thousand epidemics occur in the United States each year.

A 1986 mumps epidemic that afflicted 840 persons in one metropolitan area almost 20 years after mumps vaccine had been licensed illustrates the importance of applying epidemiology to the understanding of disease outbreaks. In this incident, epidemiologists showed that 332 students from a single public high school contracted mumps and that a pep rally held early in the school year may have contributed to widespread transmission. The infection also involved an additional 126 students in middle schools and 28 elementary school students in feeder schools to that high school. Fifty-five high school students made visits to hospital emergency rooms, and six were hospitalized with complications of mumps, including orchitis, meningitis, and pancreatitis. The administration of vaccine through a high school-based immunization clinic may have helped bring the epidemic under control.[86]

Program Operations. Preventive health service programs that affect the health of large population groups and geographic areas are also influenced by the work of epidemiologists. The package inserts for oral contraceptive pills have information for women in their reproductive years that is taken directly from the findings of epidemiological studies. Safeguards against the risks of environmental and occupational exposures, such as those of radon, asbestos, vinyl chloride, and tobacco smoke, are based on epidemiological research. Immunization policy also rests on the scientific work of epidemiologists.

The events that followed the mumps epidemic discussed earlier illustrate how epidemiology may influence the direction of public health programs. Analysis of surveillance data for the entire state in which the 1986 epidemic occurred showed that mumps outbreaks had spread across the state and that most cases affected persons 10 to 19 years of age, rather than persons 5 to 9 years of age as had occurred before 1986. Detailed studies showed that the mumps problem was related not to vaccine failure but to the failure to vaccinate. Moreover, nationwide data indicated that mumps epidemics were confined to states, like this one, that did not have laws requiring proof of immunity for school attendance.

In 1987 the total number of mumps cases in the state declined, but epidemics still occurred in specific areas. In one county more than 10% of the 15- to 19-year-olds contracted mumps, a rate almost 100 times greater than that for all state residents in that age range. Shortly thereafter, the public media reported more information about the problem and commented editorially on the disease burden carried by people dependent on public immunization programs.[87]

Public officials responded effectively, using extraordinary means to add $300,000 to the state immunization program's funds. No unexpected recurrences of this disease have been reported. The effort that began as an investigation of a single epidemic at a high school culminated in a statewide change in an important preventive health service program, thereby solving a problem that kept children from school and parents from work and that caused serious but preventable complications of a virus infection.

Policy Development. Epidemiology is essential to the development of scientifically responsible public health policy. Within the past two decades the countries of North America have analyzed the health problems faced by their citizens and have proposed important new approaches to policy development, focusing on nationwide health objectives.[88,89] If these objectives are to be met, professionals throughout the many disciplines involved in public health and preventive medicine will play essential parts. The role of epidemiology and its practicing professionals is not always clearly recognized, however. Nonetheless, epidemiologists will be involved in carrying out every essential task of the profession. Surveillance will be required to provide a baseline description of the epidemiology of each health problem and the ways in which it changes and evolves. Investigations will be carried out in communities as unexpected clustering occurs of uncontrolled infections, emerging new infections, automotive and other vehicular injuries, suicides, homicides, workplace fatalities, disabling exposures to chemical and physical agents, and persisting problems of neoplasia and cardiac and other vascular diseases. Analysis will uncover previously unknown risk factors and ineffective prevention measures. Evaluation will lead to the development of new community preventive services and improved clinical treatment. Effective communication will be increasingly important to epidemiology as complicated scientific studies influence the behavior of individuals and the laws and regulations that govern communities.

What evidence is there that epidemiology can have this kind of impact on the health of a population? The eradication of smallpox is one such bit of evidence. The role of epidemiology in this worldwide effort is now well documented. The development of the Planned Approach to Community Health (the PATCH process) has already begun to show how communities can use public health surveillance to define the baseline of the health problems they face.[90] The provision of epidemiological assistance by local, state, and national public health agencies illustrates the ways in which investigations influence public health. The elegant analyses of complicated health risks, such as the relationship between ovarian cancer and oral contraceptive use,[66] are likely to have a favorable impact on important groups of people. The epidemiological evaluation of personal health practices (e.g., administration of low-dose acetyl salicylate as it relates to myocardial infarction),[74] will determine their effects on lengthening life expectancy. How the sum of all these actions will influence the health and quality of life of current and future populations will be determined by the policies, programs, and practices through which they act. Epidemiology plays an important part in developing the scientific base for this kind of societal change. It seems fitting that epidemiologists play a leading role in ensuring that the outcome of these changes is a desired one.

REFERENCES

1. Lloyd GER (ed): Hippocratic Writings, Harmondsworth, England: Penguin, 1978
2. Snow J: On the Mode of Transmission of Cholera, 2 edt. London: Churchill, 1855 (reprinted New York: Commonwealth Fund, 1936)
3. Farr W: Vital Statistics. In Humphreys NA (ed): London, The Sanitary Institute, 1885 (reprinted New York: New York Academy of Medicine, 1975)

4. Last JM (ed): A Dictionary of Epidemiology. New York: Oxford, 1983
5. Langmuir AD: The territory of epidemiology: pentimento. J Infect Dis 155:3, 1987
6. Morris JN: Uses of Epidemiology, 3 edt. Edinburgh, London: Churchill-Livingstone, 1975
7. Task Force on Health Risk Assessment: Determining Risks to Health: Federal Policy and Practice. Dover, Mass: Auburn, 1986
8. Last JM: The iceberg: completing the clinical picture in general practice. Lancet 2:28–31, 1963
9. Feinstein AR: Clinical Epidemiology: The Architecture of Clinical Research. Philadelphia: Saunders, 1985
10. Krugman S, Giles JP, Hammon J: Infectious hepatitis: evidence for two distinctive clinical and immunological types of infection. JAMA 200:365–373, 1967
11. Blumberg BS, et al: A serum antigen (Australia antigen) in Down's syndrome, leukemia and hepatitis. Ann Intern Med 66:924–931, 1967
12. Dane DS, Cameron CH, Briggs M: Virus-like particles in serum of patients with Australia-antigen-associated hepatitis. Lancet 1:695–698, 1970
13. Almeida JD, Rubenstein D, Stott EJ: New antigen-antibody system in Australia-antigen-positive hepatitis. Lancet 2:1225–1226, 1971
14. Jaffe HW, et al: National case-control study of Kaposi's sarcoma and Pneumocystis carinii pneumonia in homosexual men. Part I. Epidemiologic results. Ann Intern Med 99:145–151, 1983
15. Broders AC: Squamous-cell epithelioma of the lip: a study of five hundred and thirty-seven cases. JAMA 74:10, 1920
16. Lombard HL, Doering CR: Cancer studies in Massachusetts. 2. Habits, characteristics and environment of individuals with and without cancer. N Engl J Med 198:10, 1928
17. Pearl R: Tobacco smoking and longevity. Science 87:2253, 1938
18. Doll R, Hill AB: The mortality of doctors in relation to their smoking habits: a preliminary report. Br Med J 1:1451–1455, 1954
19. Hammond EC, Horn D: Smoking and death rates: report on forty-four months of follow-up of 187,783 men. II. Death rates by cause. JAMA 166:1159–1172; 1294–1308, 1958
20. Hill AB: The environment and disease: association or causation? Proc R Soc Med 58:295–300, 1965
21. U.S. Department of Health, Education, and Welfare: Smoking and health: a Report of the Surgeon General. Washington, D.C.: U.S. Department of Health, Education, and Welfare, Public Health Service. U.S. Government Printing Office, 1979
22. U.S. Department of Health and Human Services: Reducing the Health Consequences of Smoking: 25 Years of Progress: a Report of the Surgeon General. DHHS Publication No. (CDC) 89–8411, 1989
23. Centers for Disease Control: Comprehensive Plan for Epidemiologic Surveillance. Atlanta: Centers for Disease Control, 1986
24. Langmuir AD: The surveillance of communicable diseases of national importance. N Engl J Med 268: 182–192, 1963
25. Thacker SB, Berkelman RL: Public health surveillance in the United States. Epidemiol Rev 10, 1988
26. Centers for Disease Control: Guidelines for evaluating surveillance systems. MMWR 37 (Suppl S-5), 1988
27. World Health Organization: International Classification of Disease, 9th Rev (ICD-9), Geneva, 1975
28. Acheson ED: Medical Record Linkage. London: Oxford, 1967
29. Smith ME, Newcombe HB: Use of the Canadian mortality data base for epidemiological follow-up. Can J Public Health 73:39–46, 1982
30. Acheson ED, et al: Formaldehyde in the British chemical industry. Lancet 1:611–616, 1984
31. Epidemiology of radiogenic breast cancer. In Boice JD, Fraumeni JF (eds): Radiation Carcinogenesis: Epidemiology and Biological Significance. New York: Raven, 1984, pp 119–130
32. Hewitt D: Radiogenic Lung Cancer in Ontario Uranium Miners, 1955–74. In Ham Jr (Commissioner): Report of the Royal Commission on the Health and Safety of Workers in Mines. Toronto: Ministry of the Attorney-General of Ontario, 1976
33. Nightingale F: Notes on Hospitals. London: JW Parker, 1859
34. NCHS Vital and Health Statistics, Series 1, 13. Washington, DC: US Department of HEW (published annually)
35. Length of Stay in PAS Hospitals. Ann Arbor, Michigan: Commission on Professional and Hospital Activities (published annually)
36. NCHS Vital and Health Statistics, Series 1, 10. Washington, DC: US Department of HEW (published annually)
37. NCHS Vital and Health Statistics, Series 1, 11. Washington, DC: US Department of HEW, 1971
38. Centers for Disease Control: Behavioral risk factor surveillance, 1981–1983. MMWR CDC Surveillance Summaries 33:1SS, 1984
39. NCHS Vital and Health Statistics. Series 1, 23. Washington, DC: US Department of HEW (published annually)
40. Rutstein DD, et al: Sentinal health events (occupational): a basis for physicians' recognition. Am J Public Health 75:11, 1985
41. Rutstein DD, et al: Measuring the quality of medical care (second revision of tables, May 1980): A clinical method. N Engl J Med 294:582–588, 1976
42. Dean AD, Dean JA, Burton AH, Dicker RC: Epi Info, version 5: a word processing, database, and statistics program for epidemiology on microcomputers. Atlanta: Centers for Disease Control, 1990
43. Graitcer PL, Burton AH: The epidemiologic surveillance project: a computer-based system for disease surveillance. Am J Prev Med 3:123–127, 1987
44. Centers for Disease Control: Cigarette advertising—United States, 1988. MMWR 39:16, 1990
45. NCHS Monthly Vital Statistics Report 39:2, 1990
46. Choi K, Thacker SB: An evaluation of influenza mortality surveillance, 1961–1979. Am J Epidemiol 113:3, 1980
47. Jones TS, et al: Morbidity and mortality associated with the July 1980 heat wave in St Louis and Kansas City, Mo. JAMA 247:24, 1982
48. Centers for Disease Control: Summary of notifiable diseases, United States. MMWR 36:2–3, 1987
49. Centers for Disease Control: Pneumocystis pneumonia-Los Angeles. MMWR 30:250–252, 1981
50. Centers for Disease Control: Kaposi's sarcoma and Pneumocystis pneumonia among homosexual men—New York City and California. MMWR 30:305–308, 1981
51. Buehler JW, et al: Reporting of AIDS: tracking HIV morbidity and mortality. JAMA 262:20, 1989
52. Ryan CA, et al: Massive outbreak of antimicrobial-resistant salmonellosis traced to pasteurized milk. JAMA 258:22, 1987
53. Chen RT, et al: An explosive point-source measles outbreak in a highly vaccinated population, modes of transmission and risk factors for disease. Am J Epidemiol 129:1, 1989
54. Morgenstern H: Uses of ecologic analysis in epidemiologic research. Am J Public Health 72:12, 1982
55. Wingo PA, et al: The evaluation of the data collection process for a multicenter, population-based, case-control design. Am J Epidemiol 128:1, 1987
56. Centers for Disease Control: Serum 2,3.7,8-tetrachlorodibenzo-p-dioxin levels in US army Vietnam-era veterans. JAMA 260:9, 1988
57. Kannel WB, Wolf PA, Garrison RJ, eds. The Framingham Study: an epidemiologic investigation of cardiovascular disease. Section 35. Washington, DC: National Technical Information Service, 1988. (DHHS publication No. (NIH) 88–2969.)
58. Schlesselman JJ: Case Control Studies. New York: Oxford University Press, 1982
59. Buehler JW, et al: Unexplained deaths in a children's hospital; an epidemiologic assessment. N Engl J Med 313:4, 1985
60. Grange SGM: Report of the Royal Commission of Inquiry into Certain Deaths at the Hospital for Sick Children and Related Matters. Ontario: Ontario Ministry of the Attorney General, Canada, 1984
61. Fraser DW, McDade JE: Legionellosis. Sci Am 241:4, 1979
62. Centers for Disease Control: Penicillinase-producing *Neisseria gonorrhoeae*—United States, worldwide. MMWR 28:8, 1979
63. Fleming DW, Berkley SF, Harrison LH, the Brazilian Purpuric Fever Group: Epidemic purpura fulminans associated with anteced-

ent purulent conjunctivitis and *Haemophilus aegyptius* bacteremia in Brazilian purpuric fever. Lancet 2:757–763, Oct. 3, 1987

64. Centers for Disease Control. CDC Surveillance Summaries. MMWR 38 (No. SS-2), 1989
65. Rooks JB, et al: Epidemiology of hepatocellular adenoma: the role of oral contraceptive use. JAMA 242:7, 1979
66. Lee NC, et al: The reduction in risk of ovarian cancer associated with oral-contraceptive use. N Engl J Med 316:11, 1987
67. NCHS Monthly Vital Statistics Report 39:2, 1990
68. Sackett DL: Bias in analytic research. J Chron Dis 32:51–63, 1979
69. Guyer B, et al: Intentional injuries among children and adolescents in Massachusetts. N Engl J Med 321:23, 1989
70. Koch R: Über bacteriologische Forschung, Verh Ten Internat Med Cong Berlin 1:35, 1891
71. US Department of Health, Education, and Welfare: Smoking and Health: A Report of the Surgeon General. Washington, DC: US Government Printing Office, 1964
72. Peterson HB, Grubb GS, DeStefano F: Complications of tubal sterilization. In Siegler AM (ed): The Fallopian Tube: Basic Studies and Clinical Contributions. Cincinnati: Futura Publications, 1986, pp 329–346
73. Francis T, et al: Evaluation of the 1954 Field Trial of Poliomyelitis Vaccine. Ann Arbor: University of Michigan Press, 1957
74. Steering Committee of the Physicians' Health Study Research Group: Final report of the aspirin component of the ongoing physicians' health study. N Engl J Med 321:129, 1989
75. Lilienfeld AM, Lilienfeld DE: Foundations of Epidemiology, 2 edt. New York: Oxford, 1980
76. Thacker SB: Meta-analysis: a quantitative approach to research integration. JAMA 259:11, 1988
77. Thacker SB: Quality of controlled clinical trials: the case of imaging ultrasound in obstetrics: a review. Br J Obstet Gynaecol 92:437–444, 1985
78. Thacker SB: The efficacy of intrapartum electronic fetal monitoring. Am J Obstet Gynecol 156:1, 1987
79. Blackburn BA, Smith H, Chalmers TC: The inadequate evidence for short hospital stay after hernia for varicose vein stripping surgery. Mt Sinai J Med 49:383–390, 1982
80. Himel HN, et al: Adjuvant chemotherapy for breast cancer: a pooled estimate based on published randomized control trials. JAMA 256:1148–1159, 1986
81. Miettinen OS: Theoretical Epidemiology: Principles of Occurrence Research in Medicine. New York: John Wiley & Sons, 1985
82. Orenstein WA, Berner RH, Hinman AR: Assessing vaccine efficacy in the field; further observations. Epidemiol Rev 10:212–241, 1988
83. Dunning JM: Principles of Dental Public Health. Chap 16. Cambridge, Mass: Harvard University Press, 1986
84. Tietze C, Lewit S: Evaluation of intrauterine devices: ninth progress report of the cooperative statistical program. Stud Fam Plann 55:1–40, 1970
85. Fenner F, et al: Smallpox and Its Eradication. Geneva: World Health Organization, 1988
86. Wharton M, et al: A large outbreak of mumps in the postvaccine era. J Infect Dis 158:6, 1988
87. Milner L: Prevention's the cure officials should seek. Sunday Tennessean, Jan. 17, 1988
88. Lalonde M: A New Perspective on the Health of Canadians: a Working Document. Ottawa: Government of Canada, 1974
89. Department of Health and Human Services, Public Health Service: The 1990 Health Objectives for the Nation: A Midcourse Review, 1990
90. Fuchs JA: Planning for community health promotion: a rural example. Health Values 12:6, 1988

GENERAL REFERENCES

Biostatistics

Colton T: Statistics in Medicine. Boston: Little, Brown, 1974

Fleiss JL: Statistical Methods for Rates and Proportions, 2 edt. New York: John Wiley & Sons, 1981

Kahn HA, Sempos, CT: Statistical Methods in Epidemiology. New York: Oxford University Press, 1989

Epidemiology

Hennekens CH, Buring JE, Mayrent SL (eds): Epidemiology in Medicine. Boston: Little, Brown, 1987

Kelsey JL, Thompson WD, Evans AS: Methods in Observational Epidemiology. New York: Oxford University Press, 1986

Kleinbaum DG, Kupper LL, Morgenstern H: Epidemiology—Principles and Quantitative Methods. Belmont, Calif: Lifetime Learning Publications, 1982

Kramer MS: Clinical Epidemiology and Biostatistics: A Primer for Clinical Investigators and Decision-Makers. New York: Springer-Verlag, 1988

Lilienfeld AM, Lilienfeld DE: Foundations of Epidemiology. New York: Oxford, 1980

Miettinen OS: Theoretical Epidemiology: Principles of Occurrence Research in Medicine. New York: John Wiley & Sons, 1985

Morris JN: Uses of Epidemiology, 3 edt. London: Churchill-Livingstone, 1975

Schlesselman JJ: Case-Control Studies—Design, Conduct, Analysis. New York: Oxford, 1982

Susser MW: Causal Thinking in the Health Sciences. New York: Oxford, 1973

Historical Background

Farr W: Vital Statistics: A memorial volume of selections from the reports and writings of William Farr, with an introduction by Mervyn Susser and Abraham Adelstein. Metuchen, New Jersey: Scarecrow Press, 1975 (published under auspices of New York Academy of Medicine)

Frost WH: Collected Papers, Maxcy KF (ed). New York: The Commonwealth Fund, 1941

Greenwood M: Medical Statistics From Graunt to Farr. Cambridge, England: Cambridge University Press, 1935

Panum PL: Observations Made During the Epidemic of Measles on the Faroe Islands in the Year 1846. Hatcher AS (translator). New York: American Public Health Association, 1940

Snow J: The Mode of Communication of Cholera (1855) (reprinted New York: The Commonwealth Fund, 1936)

Terris M: Goldberger on Pellagra. Baton Rouge: Louisiana State University Press, 1964

3

Public Health and Population

Carl W. Tyler, Jr.
Joan M. Herold

Public health focuses on health issues in populations. Carrying out the mission of public health and achieving its goals therefore depend on the factors that change the size and characteristics of the population whose health is at stake.

The relationship between health and the dynamics of population change guides the need for changes in public health practice. Changes in health influence vital events (births and deaths) that lead to population change. These events, accompanied by a third demographic force, migration (the movement of people from place to place), lead to new health issues and problems.

Four such issues illustrate the relationship between public health and population:

1. *Teenage pregnancy.* Teenage pregnancy is a serious public health issue because it creates preventable health problems for both infant and mother, is often unintended, and may interfere with education, personal development, and socioeconomic advancement for the young mother and father. In addition, teenage pregnancies have an important demographic impact on future generations.
2. *Aging.* As the death rate declines in most parts of the world, life expectancy increases, and therefore so do the number and ages of older people. Moreover, when low or declining fertility accompanies the decline in mortality, the proportion of older persons and the median age of the population also increase. The result for public health is a drastic change in the spectrum of health problems and health care needs.
3. *Urbanization.* In 1950 less than 30% of the world's population lived in cities. By the year 2000, more than 40% will be found in urban areas.[1] Urbanization creates health problems related to the need for housing and sanitation, improved food supply, better urban transportation, and the redistribution of preventive and other health services.
4. *Refugees and Other Migrants.* An estimated 15 million refugees are dispersed throughout the world.[2] Refugees and other migrants may bring with them serious public health problems such as severe malnutrition and infections, and their settlements may have high levels of violence.

This chapter should enable a public health practitioner to achieve the following:

1. Identify useful sources of information about population and vital statistics
2. Calculate basic measures of population change
3. Identify determinants of population change
4. Understand four contemporary critical issues related to population change.

POPULATION DATA AND MEASUREMENTS

Data Sources

Population data are essential for defining and measuring public health problems and the groups of people associated with them. Nonetheless, public health practitioners often find that although the need for information of this kind is great, their lack of familiarity with data sources prevents them from calculating the measurements required to evaluate public health problems. Census, survey, and vital registration statistics are the most fundamental sources of population data.

Census. A census is an enumeration of a population that has the following essential characteristics:

- Each individual is enumerated separately.
- The characteristics of each individual are recorded separately.
- Those enumerated reside in a precisely defined area.
- Enumeration takes place within a defined and reasonably brief period and in reference to a well-defined time period.
- Enumeration is repeated at regular intervals.[3]

In the United States the census enumerates people first by mail and later by personal interviews of those not responding to mail inquiry. It covers the nation and its territories, and makes data public for areas as small as groups of city blocks. (There are certain limits on the information provided in these tabulations because of the need to protect the privacy of individuals.) By law the census is conducted every 10 years. Because of its importance to political representation, as specified in the Constitution, and because of public concern about use of data by governing bodies, the census in the United States has been a source of controversy. Nonetheless, its importance to the health of the public is undiminished.

Population-based Surveys. A survey differs from a census in that it is not an enumeration of individuals and it need not include all members of the population. Nonetheless, most surveys characterize individuals separately rather than in groups, and the sample represents a precisely defined group of people from a specific area. The distinction between a census and a survey is not always clearly defined. In some instances a sample of those persons included in an enumeration are asked more questions than the total population, and the sample is still considered part of the census. In other cases, data from a national census may be used to establish the sampling frame at a later time for surveys of health status, fertility, the use of health services, or some other issue of importance to the population, such as employment or education.

Current Population Surveys. A series of national population-based surveys, called the Current Population Survey, is conducted each month in the United States. Although this series focuses more on economic than on other issues, its information describes important characteristics of the national population, such as family composition (including births and ages of children), mobility, school enrollment, marital status, living arrangements, work experience, and multiple job holdings.

Health Surveys. In the United States the National Health Care Survey is conducted by the National Center for Health Statistics (NCHS) of the Centers for Disease Control. This survey has five components, including health care providers (see the National Master Facility Inventory), hospital and surgical care (see the National Hospital Discharge Survey [NHDS]), ambulatory care (see the National Ambulatory Medical Care Survey), and long-term care (see the National Nursing Home Survey), and will provide data based on patient follow-up. In addition, NCHS provides data to health officials, their agencies, researchers, and the public through a series of population-based surveys. These include the National Health Interview Survey (NHIS, reported annually and based on surveys that began in 1957), the National Medical Care Utilization and Expenditure Survey (NCUES, first conducted in 1980 and 1981), the National Health and Nutrition Examination Survey (NHANES, a series of five surveys, the first of which was conducted in 1960–1962), and the Hispanic Health and Nutrition Examination Survey (HHANES, conducted in 1984). Each of these surveys measures a different aspect of health in the population of the nation by interview responses (NHIS), physical measurements, laboratory testing, and interviews (NHANES), and hospitalization and its accompanying diagnoses and surgical procedures (NHDS). Plans have been formulated for surveys of follow-up and long-term care on a sample of individual consenting respondents to these surveys. In addition, the National Survey of Family Growth (NSFG) gathers information on family formation, some of the determinants of infant health, and health practices of women between and during pregnancies. Other surveys, such as the National Maternal and Infant Health Survey, based on samples from the national vital registration system assess fetal, neonatal, and infant health.[4]

Other Surveys. Internationally, the World Fertility Survey and the Demographic and Health Surveys have collected data from many (mostly developing) countries around the world. They focus on interview responses from women in their childbearing years and are based on population samples of several thousand women in each country. Data collection is confined to a few months. For example, a recent survey report for Ghana characterized vital rates, population growth, life expectancy, economic and social status, childbearing desires and accomplishments, and contraceptive use.[5]

Vital Data (Birth, Death, Marriage, and Divorce). The registration of vital events, specifically births and deaths, provides important data for defining public health problems at almost every level of society, including cities, counties, states, nations, and the world. In the United States, vital registries are maintained at the national level by NCHS, at the state level by state health departments and centers for health statistics, and for some metropolitan areas by the health departments for the immediate jurisdiction, for example, New York City. The registration of other events of health and social importance, specifically, marriage and divorce, also is done at the national, state, and local levels.

Other Sources. Migration is an important determinant of population size and distribution. Census information is often available to study internal migration and evaluate its effects. Assessing international migration is, however, more complex. In the United States, annual reports from the Immigration and Naturalization Service provide the official information. For a wider range of countries, special studies by the United Nations and certain issues of the *Demographic Yearbook* give useful data. Unfortunately, the rules for movement across geographic boundaries, especially international borders, make the collection of reliable data much more difficult than that done by census, survey, or vital registration.

Some areas of the world, such as northern and eastern Europe, maintain national population registries based on unique individual identification numbers assigned to each person at birth. This type of registry offers opportunities to study problems that require knowledge of the demographic, social, and economic events experienced by individuals over their lifetime.

Demographic Measures

The relation between health problems and the populations in which they occur needs to be measured if the problems are to be controlled and prevented.

Rates. A rate is a quotient in which time is an essential element and a distinct relationship exists between the numerator and denominator.

Crude Rates. A crude rate is one in which all of the events that occurred in a given time and population comprise the numerator and in which the population of the specific area at the midpoint of that time period comprises the denominator. By convention, it also contains a constant multiplier of 1000. A death rate, for example, might have a numerator of 75 people who died during a given year and a denominator of the midyear population, 10,000, of the community in which they lived; therefore the death rate for the community in that year would be 7.5/1000 population. This rate is the crude death rate (CDR). If the same community had 150 births during the same year, the crude birth rate (CBR) would be 15.0/1000. The crude rate of natural increase (CRNI) is equal to the CBR minus the CDR; in this illustration the CRNI would be 7.5/1000 or 0.75%.

Standardized Rates. Comparing rates among different populations is often difficult if the demographic characteristics are not known in detail. Following the trend in mortality for the United States over several decades beginning in 1940 illustrates this point (Fig. 3–1). The CDR was nearly 10.8/1000 population at the beginning of that period and decreased to 8.78 by 1980. This comparison, however, masks the real decline in mortality over the 40-year period because the U.S. population had an older age composition in 1980 and therefore had more people exposed to the high mortality rates of older ages than it had in 1940.

By using a population with the same age composition as that in 1940 as the standard of comparison, the age standardized

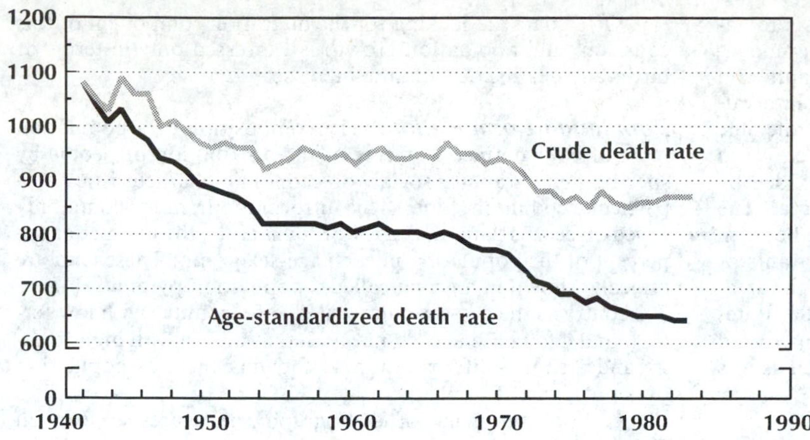

Figure 3-1. Crude and age-standardized death rates, United States, 1940–1987. Rates are for the total population. They have been calculated as deaths per 100,000 population and are standardized on the United States population of 1940. Vertical axis: Rate per 100,000.

death rate for the United States in 1980 is computed to be 5.85. The comparison using the standardized death rate more accurately reflects the mortality decline in the United States that has occurred in all age groups since 1940 than the CDR does because of the change in age composition, that is, the higher proportion of older people in the population in the more recent years. Standardization is dealt with in more detail in other studies.[6]

Period and Cohort Rates. A period rate is one in which the events of concern occur in the population being observed during a specified time interval. The CDR for the United States in the year 1987 of 5.36/1000 population is an example of a period rate. Most often the period for demographic rates is 1 year. Figure 3-1 shows the trend of mortality in the United States since 1940 using period rates.

A cohort is a group of people who experience a major event in the same short, clearly defined period, usually a year. The most common demographic cohorts are birth and marriage cohorts. Cohort rates are concerned with events that occur (subsequent to the defining event) to a cohort of people over subsequent periods. Population studies often are based on birth cohorts, as was done in the cohort analysis of fertility reported by the National Center for Health Statistics.[7] The analysis of fertility by marriage cohorts helps us to understand changes in fertility or family structure. Epidemiologists use cohort analysis to study groups according to their exposure to a specific agent hypothesized to cause, or prevent, a health problem. If the problem is related to occupational exposure, the cohort may be analyzed by date of employment. Frost's study[8] of mortality caused by tuberculosis is a classic public health report using cohort analysis.

Fertility. The CBR, which uses all births as the numerator and the total population (regardless of gender or age) as the denominator, is the most fundamental fertility measure. The general fertility rate (GFR) also uses all births as the numerator, but is based on a denominator comprising all women of childbearing age, most often defined as women 15 to 44 years of age, although 49 years is used as the older age limit in other circumstances. The age-specific fertility rate (ASFR) is calculated using births to women in a specific age interval (usually 5 years but sometimes single years of age) as the numerator and women in the same age interval as the denominator. Each of these measures is a period rate and customarily is multiplied by a constant of 1000.

The total fertility rate (TFR) is the sum of all of the age-specific fertility rates by single years of age. This measure characterizes a synthetic cohort of women of reproductive age. By using data for a short period, usually 1 year, it addresses the question, "If the women in this population continued to have children at the rate they did this year, how many would they have, on average, when they finished bearing their children?" If the sum of age-specific fertility rates totaled 3000 live births per 1000 women in a given year, each woman would average three children if these rates continued unchanged for the remainder of her reproductive years. (The total fertility rate may be expressed per 1000 women or per woman.) The true cohort rate for fertility is referred to as the completed fertility rate and customarily is based on surveys, rather than vital data.

Mortality. The CDR, which uses all deaths as the numerator and the total midyear population as the denominator, is the most fundamental mortality measure. The age-specific death rate (ASDR) is calculated using deaths that occur among those in a specific age interval as the numerator and the population in the same age interval as the denominator. Each of these measures is a period rate and customarily is multiplied by a constant (1000 or 100,000). Rates for specific causes of death add an important dimension to mortality analysis. Most often the cause of death is based on vital registration and the International Classification of Diseases (ICD) coding system; deaths classified by cause are the numerator, while the population, or an appropriate segment, is the denominator. The rate usually is multiplied by a constant of 100,000.

Some special measures that are not true rates deserve mention. Among them are the infant mortality rate (IMR) and maternal mortality rate (MMR). The IMR is the number of children who die before their first birthday in a year divided by the number of live births in that year. The MMR indicates the risk of death from causes associated with childbirth. Deaths during pregnancy, labor and delivery, or postpartum in a year make up the numerator, and live births in the same year are the denominator. Their measurement has been defined succinctly elsewhere.[9]

A life table is based on ASDRs that are converted to probabilities of death for each age interval. Life table data describe the mortality or survival of a person or a group over a lifetime. Life table analysis addresses the question, "What would be the mortality experience and life expectancy of a group of people who had these probabilities of death at each age for the rest of their lives?" Using ASDRs for a specific period (usually 1 year) permits a current, or period, life table to be calculated for a synthetic cohort. Using ASDRs over the lifetime of a group born in the same year or interval (often 5 years) permits a real (rather than synthetic) cohort life table to be constructed. Cohort life tables more often are referred to as generation, or longitudinal, life tables.

Migration. The measurement of migration is conceptually similar to that for fertility and mortality. Defining terms requires that a distinction be made between internal migration (movement by in-migrants and out-migrants across borders that are within a nation's bounds) and international migration (movement across international boundaries by immigrants and emigrants). The crude in-migration rate is the number of in-migrants or immigrants who enter a specified geographic area during a stated time interval, divided by the population of the area at the midpoint of the time interval. Similarly, the crude out-migration rate is the measure in which the number of out-migrants or emigrants is divided by population of the area at the midpoint of the time interval. The crude net migration rate is one in which the difference between the number of in-migrants or immigrants and out-migrants or emigrants is the numerator divided by the population of the area. All these rates are multiplied by a constant, usually 1000. Rates specific for age, gender, and national origin may be constructed using appropriate migrant and population groups much as was described for measures of fertility and mortality.

Population Growth. Population growth is a function of births, deaths, and migration. Growth measured by births and deaths alone is referred to as natural increase; it is measured by the CRNI, such that

$$CRNI = CBR - CDR$$

When growth also includes changes resulting from migration, the relation between these events and population growth is expressed in terms of the following equation, which often is referred to as the demographic equation. It states that the difference in population from time 1 to time 2 is equal to the births in the time interval, minus the deaths in the interval, plus in-migration in the interval, minus out-migration in the interval.

$$P_2 - P_1 = B - D + IM - OM$$

Often data are lacking for the migration component of this equation, and population growth is expressed only in terms of births and deaths, i.e., natural increase.

Population Composition. The composition of a population most often is defined in terms of the distribution of people by specific demographic, social, or economic characteristics at a particular point in time. This information, most commonly based on census data, may show, for example, the number or the percent of the population in each age-sex group. These data are typically shown in a graph called a population pyramid. Figure 3-2 contrasts the age-sex composition of a country with low fertility and a long life expectancy with that of one with high fertility and a shorter life expectancy, showing them as population pyramids.

A brief summary of demographic measures appears in Table 3-1.

FERTILITY

Fertility is important to public health, population change, and the quality of human life. Its role in determining the size, composition, and growth of populations and in the health of women and the offspring of families is a powerful factor governing the course of public health practice.

Fertility, in its most specific sense, refers to the actual birth of living offspring. (The capacity to bear children is termed fecundity and the probability of conceiving in a given month is

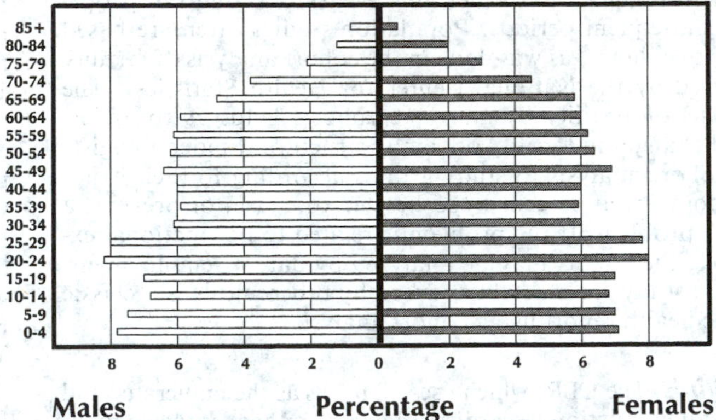

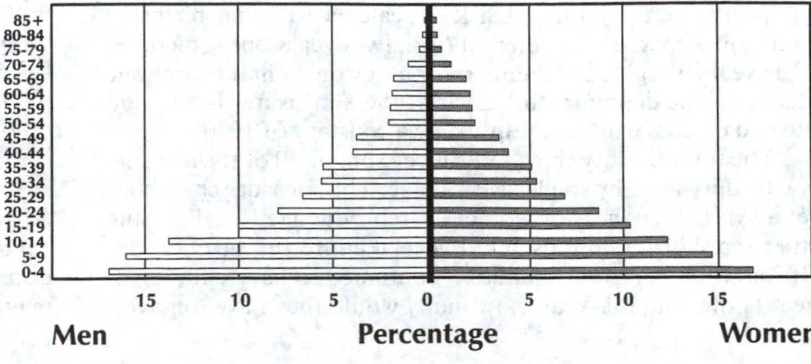

Figure 3-2. Percentage distribution of populations of Sweden [*upper panel*] and Mexico [*lower panel*] by age and sex in 1970. Vertical axis: Age.

TABLE 3-1. BASIC FERTILITY AND MORTALITY MEASURES

Measurement	Numerator	Denominator	Constant[a]
CBR	All births	Total population	1,000
GFR	All births	Women aged 15–44	1,000
ASFR	Births in age group	Women in age group	1,000
CDR	All deaths	Total population	1,000
ASDR	Deaths in age group	Population in age group	1,000
IMR	Infant deaths in year	All births in same year	1,000
MMR	Maternal deaths in year	All births in same year	10,000 *or* 100,000

KEY: *CBR*, Crude birth rate; *GFR*, general fertility rate; *ASFR*, age-specific fertility rate; *CDR*, crude death rate; *ASDR*, age-specific death rate; *IMR*, infant mortality rate; *MMR*, maternal mortality rate.

[a]The constants shown in this column are those used most often. Others may be used in special demographic or public health reports.

called fecundability.) Natality often is used synonymously for fertility. Natural fertility describes the level of fertility found in populations in which neither contraception (temporary or permanent) nor induced abortion is used.

The factors that determine fertility in a population may be readily identified as biological and behavioral. These determinants can be aggregated into a structure that permits a quantitative appraisal of the factors influencing fertility change in a population.

Biological Determinants

Menarche and Menopause. Menarche, the beginning of menstruation, defines the youngest end of the age limit within which women begin to ovulate and are able to conceive; in the twentieth century as compared to the nineteenth, it is occurring earlier in life in developed countries. Menopause, the cessation of menstruation, signals the end of the reproductive years; the age at menopause has increased slightly in recent decades in developed countries. Since fertility usually is controlled in societies that have experienced the widened span of reproductive years created by changes in the ages at menarche and menopause, these changes are not of primary importance in determining contemporary fertility.

Ovulation. In demographic terms, ovulation influences fertility most by influencing waiting time until conception or ovulatory interval. This interval is greatest at the extremes of the reproductive years, either when regular ovulation is not established or when it is waning. Although this aspect of ovulation is not a consequential determinant of current fertility levels, the delay in ovulation after childbirth is. The length of postpartum anovulation may vary from 1 1/2 months to as long as 2 years, depending on the frequency and duration of lactation.[10]

Age Within Reproductive Span. Once intercourse is an established practice, natural fertility declines with age. This has been shown for several societies that have differing fertility levels. Figure 3-3 (*left panel*) illustrates this by showing marital fertility rates by age for two societies with high fertility (Hutterites and Nepal), one with low fertility (United States), and a standard model population (Coale and Trussel); in each instance fertility declines steadily, although the shape of the curves may differ. Figure 3-3 (*right panel*) shows the same data; in this graph the fertility level for women 20 to 24 years of age is set at an index of 100 for four different populations.[11]

Spontaneous Intrauterine Mortality. The influence on fertility of spontaneous abortions, or miscarriages, and stillbirths is difficult to assess because of the problems in ascertaining these events in a representative population. Current evidence indicates that the risk of spontaneous pregnancy loss is greatest early in pregnancy and declines steadily throughout. It is probably greatest among women in their later childbearing years. Since the evidence suggests little variation in this biological factor among communities, it is not likely to be an important determinant of differing levels of fertility.

Involuntary Infertility. Involuntary infertility, also referred to as sterility or infecundity, is measured, in demographic terms, as the incapacity of a woman to bear a living child during the span of reproductive years. (Although involuntary infertility in males is a serious health concern, it has not been shown to have influenced fertility in a population.) Involuntary infertility in

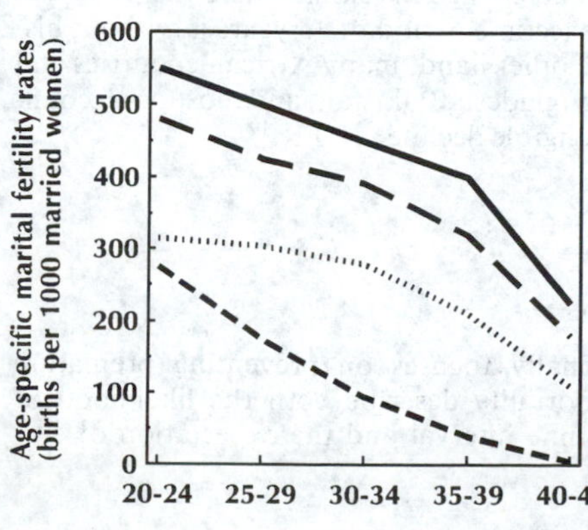

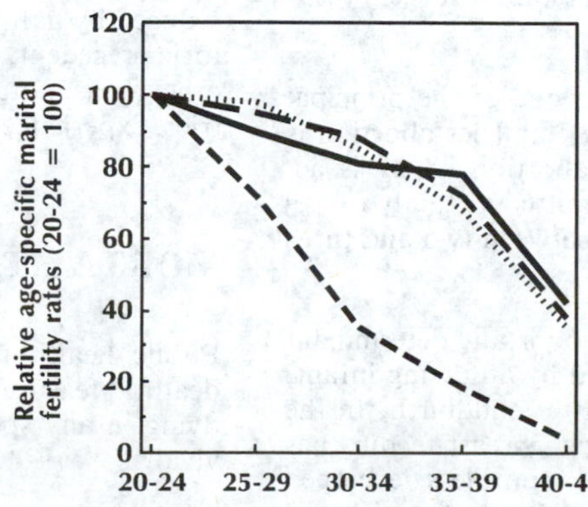

Hutterites (1921-1930)
Coale-Trussel standard schedule
Nepal 1975
U.S. 1967

Figure 3-3. Absolute and relative age-specific marital fertility rates of selected populations. Horizontal axis [both panels]: Age. [From Bongaarts J, Potter RG: Fertility, Biology, and Behavior: An Analysis of the Proximate Determinants. New York: Academic Press, 1983.]

women may result from anatomical abnormalities of the reproductive tract, malfunction of ovulation so that conception does not occur, recurrent intrauterine loss of pregnancy, or specific diseases that are associated with infertility, such as gonorrhea and genital tuberculosis.[12] The first three categories are presumed to occur to a similar extent in all populations although the evidence for this is not entirely satisfactory. The last group is presumed to account for the occurrence of a high proportion of childlessness among groups in Africa where fertility is otherwise quite high.[13]

Behavioral Determinants[11,14]

Marriage or Sexual Union. Age at first marriage or consensual union is a principal determinant of the number of children a woman will bear. It marks the beginning of socially approved exposure to the probability of conception. The association between increase in the age at marriage and concurrent decline in fertility has been shown in several societies.

Frequency of Intercourse. Frequency of sexual intercourse is related directly to the capacity to bear children, assuming that the menstrual cycle is ovulatory and insemination occurs in midcycle. Studies of the frequency of intercourse (short of abstinence) and probability of ovulation in a specific cycle are insufficient to suggest that these factors account for differences in fertility levels from one population to another.

Abstinence, whether voluntary or involuntary, is an important determinant of fertility. In some cultures abstinence is required during lactation. In other situations it is related to religious beliefs and the role an individual or group plays within a religion. In economic circumstances that require couples to separate because of employment, abstinence may result from a work situation.

Contraception. Use of contraceptives is one of the principal determinants of fertility. The prevalence of contraceptive use varies widely among nations, ranging from approximately 10% to more than 75%. Modern contraception is highly effective and safe. The variation in patterns of use by method among different countries is substantial. China, for example, is reported to have a high incidence of intrauterine device use, whereas oral contraceptives are widely used in the United States, and condoms play a particularly important role in Japan.[15]

Voluntary Sterilization. Voluntary surgical sterilization is an important determinant of fertility because it limits the span of years during which reproduction is possible. This approach to fertility regulation is highly effective and safe. Although some studies treat this method of fertility control as if it were a method of contraception, the fact that this method requires surgery justifies its placement in a separate category.

Induced Abortion. Induced abortion is one of the principal determinants of human fertility. In some countries abortion is prohibited legally, and the practice of abortion rarely is acknowledged.[16] Elsewhere abortion is permitted virtually on request, and women may have on average between two and three during their reproductive years.[17]

Breast-Feeding. Breast-feeding is an important determinant of fertility. Lactation, which is stimulated by a nursing infant, influences the duration of anovulation after childbirth. In the United States and other developed countries, breast-feeding has little influence on the level of fertility, but in some less developed areas in which infants are breast fed frequently, on demand, and have almost no other source of nutrition, no other form of fertility control is used, yet fertility levels are nearly the same as those in developed countries.

The determinants of fertility[11] are shown in Table 3–2.

TABLE 3–2. DETERMINANTS OF FERTILITY

▪ BIOLOGICAL
Menarche
Menopause
Ovulation
Age within reproductive span
Intrauterine mortality
Postpartum anovulation
Involuntary infertility
▪ BEHAVIORAL
Frequency of intercourse
Age at marriage or first union
Contraception
Voluntary sterilization
Induced abortion
Breast-feeding

Status and Trends

United States. A review of official birth statistics for the twentieth century shows that after reaching a peak number of births early in the 1960s of more than 4.25 million, the United States experienced a decline to less than 3.25 million in the early 1970s and was at 3.8 million in 1987. The CBR was more than 30.0 early in this century but had a peak of 25.0 in 1955, the high point since 1950. The low point (14.6) for the century was in 1975; the CBR was 15.7 in 1987.[18]

Estimates of the total fertility rate (TFR) indicate that this measure of fertility declined throughout the history of the United States until the period between 1947 and 1961, referred to as the "Baby Boom." Official vital statistics show that the TFR increased from 2.3 in 1940 to 3.7 in 1960, remained more than 3.0 until 1965, then declined to below 2.0 in 1973. Demographers estimate that current fertility is such that each woman is unlikely to replace herself with a daughter. If these fertility levels continue and are accompanied by current trends in migration, continued growth of the national population would be determined more by migration than by natural increase.

International. Fertility around the world has undergone striking changes in the last several decades. Because the TFR is standardized for age and the age structure of individual countries differs substantially, the most informative comparisons use the TFR. In the 30 years from 1950 to 1980 the estimated TFR for the world decreased from 4.99 to 3.54, a decline of 29%. Individual regions showed decrements that ranged from 59% for east Asia to 2% (Africa). The change in China where the TFR was reduced by half in a peacetime period of 15 years is without historic precedent. On the other hand, many African countries and other areas, notably Bangladesh, Pakistan, and most Arab countries, experienced a negligible decline in TFR.[19]

MORTALITY

Public health traditionally focuses on preventing premature death. Measures of mortality describe both the likelihood of dying in any specific time interval and the expectation of survival.

Determinants

The factors that determine differences and changes in the levels of mortality among populations are biological or behavioral.

Age. Age is a principal determinant of mortality. Starting at a high level in infancy, mortality declines precipitously in childhood, remains at a low level through adolescence and early adulthood, and then increases inexorably in adulthood and older ages. This pattern holds true for both males and females in both developed and developing countries and is illustrated by data from the United States in Figure 3-4.

Sex. Throughout life, and perhaps even from conception, males have a higher risk of mortality than females. Figure 3-4 also illustrates this point. For this reason published life tables separate computations for each sex.[20] Exceptions exist under special circumstances, for example, in societies that may value the survival of male offspring over females and situations of low levels of economic development where childbearing increases the risk of mortality for women of reproductive age. Specific causes of death, as illustrated by breast cancer, also may carry greater risk for women than men. When all causes of death are considered together, the risk of mortality is less, the likelihood of survival is greater, and life expectancy is longer for females than for males.

Race/Ethnicity. Differences in racial and ethnic characteristics within a population often are associated with differences in mortality. These differences are recognized in population data from major regions of the world, including Asia, Africa, and North America, and in large part are considered to be the result of social and economic differences among racial or ethnic groups in a population. In the United States, differences in the mortality for blacks and whites are sufficiently important that official life tables are published for all causes of death by race, as well as by sex, and official public health policy focuses on approaches to resolve these differences.

Region/Area. Mortality may differ by geographic region both within and across national boundaries. This can be most readily recognized by reviewing United Nations publications, especially the *Demographic Yearbook*. Model life tables constructed to estimate mortality in areas where population data are incomplete reflect this fact by having four sets of models based on regional differences in the risk of death.[21] In North America data published by region, province, or state show differences in key parameters of mortality such as life expectancy.[18] The reasons for these differences presumably are related to social, economic, and health service factors.

Cause of Death. Although the specific cause of death is important to each individual and often to a specific public health program, population changes are determined by the spectrum of disease causes prevalent in a community and whether the means are available to control such causes. Diarrheal diseases, for example, are an important cause of mortality in developing countries, while cardiovascular disease deaths are more prevalent in modernized nations. See discussion of the epidemiological transition below.

Social and Economic Conditions. Economic development, measured by per capita national income and other indicators of economic advancement, is related to the increase in life expectancy in most parts of the world; moreover, this one factor accounts for between 10% and 25% of the improvement in life expectancy, depending on the region and time period over which the change occurs.[22] The mortality decline of the nineteenth century is ascribed to improvements in living standard and diet, sanitation, and improved working conditions.[23]

Public Health. Public health measures have played a leading role in reducing mortality through preventing the transmission of infection. Even before the discovery of specific microorganisms, epidemiologists identified the ways in which diseases, such as childbed fever and cholera, were transmitted and promoted measures for prevention. Vaccination has led to the worldwide eradication of smallpox[24] and brought about a substantial decline in measles in the United States.[25] Studies of tobacco use and its attendant health problems have led to a reduction in cigarette smoking.[26] Screening for cervical cancer has in all likelihood led to a decline in mortality caused by this condition.[27] More recent improvements in mortality, the likely result of collective individual modifications in lifestyle, such as dietary improvements and exercise, have been aided by public health promotion efforts.

Medicine and Technology. Medical and technological discoveries are important determinants of mortality, although their contribution is reflected in changes during the twentieth century rather than in earlier times. The discovery of insecticides and antibiotics, the introduction of anesthesia, the control of hospital-acquired infection, and the organization of health services are all presumed to have made important contributions to improving mortality.

Status and Trends

United States. Life expectancy at birth has increased substantially over the past century: from 47 to 75 years. Although life expectancy has reached a historic high point (78.9 years) for white females, this measure for black males crested in 1984 at 65.6 years; provisional data show a life expectancy of 65.1 for black males in 1988. In the past two decades the CDR has declined steadily and the age-standardized death rate has decreased

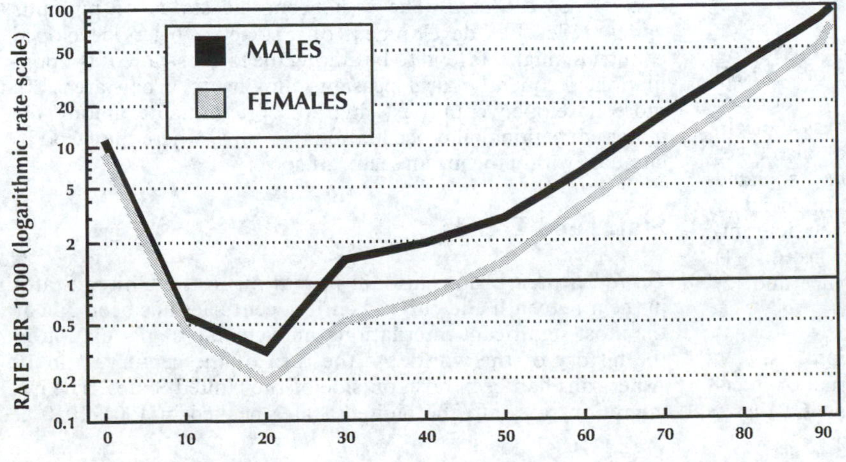

Figure 3-4. Death rates from all causes for females and males, United States, 1976. Rates are deaths per 1000 population, by age at death, and shown on a logarithmic scale. Horizontal axis: Age.

even more. For the most recent year available (1987), the death rate by sex-race group is lowest for black females and highest for black males. The age-standardized rate, however, is lowest for white females, next lowest for black females, and highest for black males. The ranking of death rates by cause during the mid-1980s consistently shows diseases of the heart to be the leading, albeit a declining, cause of death. It is followed by malignant neoplasms (all organ systems taken together), cerebrovascular diseases, accidents and adverse effects, and pneumonia and influenza. In the national population overall, death resulting from human immunodeficiency virus infection is the only cause ranked in the top 20 that has advanced its rank (from 19 in 1985 to 15 in 1987). Homicide is the most important cause that differs for a specific group compared to national rankings; homicide is the fifth leading cause of death for black males and ranks twelfth for the nation.[18]

International. Mortality for the world generally is declining. In recent years Japan has become the country with the highest life expectancy at birth for males, reaching 73.8 years in 1981 and 75.5 by 1986, among 40 nations for which current information is available. (For these same years, male life expectancy in Canada was 71.9 and 73.1 years and in the United States was 70.4 and 71.3 years.) For females, four countries reported life expectancy at birth that reached or exceeded 80 years in 1986 (Japan, 81.6; Switzerland, 80.6; Sweden, 80.2; and France, 80.0). Several other nations were very near that level (Canada had a life expectancy for females of 79.9 years).[18] In contrast, mortality in developing countries is at much higher levels. Some of the highest mortality rates are found in Africa. For example, life expectancy for both sexes combined in the late 1980s is 41 years in Ethiopia and Sierra Leone, 43 years in The Gambia, 45 years in Somalia, and 48 years in Nigeria.[28]

MIGRATION

Migration is an important component of population change but often is neglected in calculations of population growth because of the difficulty in measuring and collecting accurate migration information. Migration may be defined as movement of people involving a change of residence between two clearly defined geographic units.[29] The definition of residence and the choice of geographic units vary, depending on the particular use of the migration data.

The study of migration is divided into two subdisciplines: internal migration and international migration. Internal migration refers to changes of residence within national borders; the movers are called in-migrants and out-migrants. International migration refers to residence changes across national boundaries, with movers termed immigrants and emigrants.

Determinants

Lee's "push-pull theory"[30] explains that migration comes about as the result of individuals responding to negative or "push" factors at place of origin and positive or "pull" factors at place of destination. In addition to the positives and negatives at origin and destination, the decision of the potential migrant also takes into account "intervening obstacles," that is, factors associated with the migration process itself, such as distance, financial or psychic costs of the move, or immigration laws. The determinants of migration therefore can be divided into two groups: (1) characteristics associated with the places of residence and (2) characteristics of the migrants themselves.

Characteristics of Places of Origin or Destination

Economic Conditions. Most migration, whether internal or international, occurs in response to economic conditions. Of these, *employment* is the foremost factor. In a less developed setting, peasants leave the farm for the city because of poor income, loss of work, or soil depletion. In developed countries, professional workers make interurban moves seeking better jobs. *Education* also is considered an economic factor in that it represents an investment in human capital that will bring later reward in the marketplace. In both less and more developed societies, adolescents and young adults migrate for access to educational institutions.

Family and Kinship. Family and kinship factors are important determinants in less developed countries but also can be found in developed settings. In many parts of the world, people migrate on entering marriage and also to follow kin who had migrated at an earlier time.

Retirement. Retirement has both an economic and social nature in that it pushes people away from places where their work has ceased and can pull them toward destinations where other family members live. Substantial retirement migration can be observed in both developing and developed nations.

Political Events. The political determinants of migration act primarily as push factors, driving people away from their places of origin because of political, religious, or other persecution. Politically determined migration is found mostly in international movements.

Environment. In addition to the economic effects of environment on employment conditions, the natural and man-made environments also play an important role as they affect the psychological or physical well-being of people. Migration as a response to purely environmental factors is found primarily in developed societies, where people can afford to make "consumption-oriented" moves.[31]

Characteristics of Migrants

Age. Age is the single characteristic found to have the same association with migration universally. Throughout the world, peak migration rates are found between the ages of 15 and 29 years. In less developed countries, the age of men and women at migration clusters around 15 to 24; in more developed countries, the peak age is found between 20 and 29.

Marital Status. In many societies migration is associated with the event of marriage; this is not consistent across cultures. In certain traditional settings, migration may be necessary when marriage occurs between persons from different towns or villages. In more modern cultures, marriage may precipitate a migration to obtain improved employment or living conditions. In much of the world, however, migration is more frequent among unmarried persons who find it easier to move without the encumbrance of a family.

Socioeconomic Status. The socioeconomic status of migrants varies by level of development of a society. In less developed countries, migrants tend to be among the lower strata of the population, frequently rural peasants moving to urban areas. In more developed countries, migrants predominate among the upper educational and occupational groups, where they tend to circulate within the urban sector of society.

Status and Trends

United States. International migration to the United States in the nineteenth and early twentieth centuries has been one of the most significant international movements of population in the history of the world. At the turn of the century, 1 in 10 Americans had been born outside of the United States. The immigration rate into the United States peaked in 1901–1910 at

10.4/1000 population, when 92% of the immigrants were from Europe. As a result of restrictive immigration laws, migration into the United States later declined. Today the legal immigration rate is 2.5/1000, with 85% arriving from Asian and Latin American countries. In addition, demographic estimates of illegal migration suggest that we receive 100,000 to 300,000 "permanent" illegal immigrants annually.[32]

International. In addition to the movement to the United States, in the nineteenth and twentieth centuries European migration to South America and Australia in the nineteenth and twentieth centuries also was significant. Other, more recent, major international migrations include the movement of populations between India and Pakistan after the partitioning of the Indian subcontinent, the movement of Chinese into Hong Kong, the migration of Jews and Palestinians into and out of Israel, Southeast Asian refugee movements, and both political and environmental refugees in Africa.[33]

Internal migration is probably of greatest impact in less developed countries, where the pace of movement into urban areas often is too rapid for the urban infrastructure to absorb the new residents. In developed countries, internal migration is not viewed as a problem because it tends to be more balanced across many urban areas and involves movement of people who have the resources for successful adaptation to the new place of residence.

DETERMINANTS OF POPULATION GROWTH

The determinants of demographic change for the world's population, that is, fertility and mortality, have been the subject of theoretical concepts at least since Malthus published his first essay, *On The Principle of Population as It Affects the Future Improvement of Society,* in 1798.[34] Subsequently, careful examination of population data has led to the formulation of other concepts of population change.

Theory of Demographic Transition. The original theory of the demographic transition describes the historical experience of population growth of Western countries that accompanied economic development.[35] The transition can be divided into three stages. During the first stage, birth and death rates both are high but at similar levels so that population growth is minimal. This stage is referred to as the stage of high growth potential because if mortality were to decline without a concurrent decline in fertility, the size of the population would increase rapidly. The second stage is called the transition stage because it describes the transition from high to low birth and death rates that result from economic development. It is characterized by an initial decline in mortality while fertility remains high, followed by a decline in fertility until both fertility and mortality meet at low levels. During the first part of this stage the high growth potential is realized, while at the latter part of this stage growth has tapered off. The third and final (theoretical) stage is called incipient decline and describes both birth and death rates at low and relatively stable levels, with fertility at times falling below death rates and thus at times producing a decline in population.

Although the classic theory of the demographic transition provides a perspective for interpreting the historical change in Western populations, it does not describe or explain patterns of population change in non-Western societies nor those in developing countries.[36,37] Over the years, the theory has been examined and reexamined in light of new data and knowledge of variation in cultural conditions.[38,39] Today, reformulated versions of the theory, which depend more on social structural explanations for changes in birth and death rates, are being considered. The basic relationship between mortality decline, fertility decline, and population growth, however, is still used as a framework for comparing population trends.

Epidemiological Transition. In 1971 the theory of epidemiological transition was proposed, which built on the demographic transition theory. Accepting the assumption that mortality is a fundamental factor in population change, this theory identified three stages through which the causes of mortality evolved: the first was a period of widespread epidemics and famine; the second was a stage of receding epidemics associated with increasing population growth; and the third was a stage of degenerative diseases and those related to individual life-style. In terms of fertility, this concept identified a classic or Western model in which change is related to social factors, an accelerated model in which change is related to medical factors (including antibiotics, steroid contraceptive pills, and induced abortion), and a delayed model in which mortality is influenced by the medical factors of the accelerated model but in which fertility decline is delayed.[23]

This theory is susceptible to some of the same criticisms as the demographic transition theory because both have difficulty adapting to less developed countries and both ignore migration. Moreover, the epidemiologic transition model has not been subjected to the detailed scholarly review given the theory of demographic transition. The concept of epidemiologic transition, however, is an important idea that builds appropriately on the theory of demographic transition.

Relative Role of Determinants in United States. If demographic trends were evaluated for the United States to assess its status in terms of demographic and epidemiological transitions, it would be in the latest stage of each model. The population of the United States, estimated to be 243.4 million in 1987, grew by nearly 17 million people since the 1980 census. Natural increase accounts for most (74%) of this change and the remaining portion is due to migration. Mortality is caused in greatest part by chronic, degenerative diseases (diseases of the heart, cerebrovascular diseases, and malignant neoplasms). Fertility is maintained at a low level for more than a decade, and in 1987 the TFR was 1.8.[18]

Relative Role of Determinants Internationally. Examining demographic trends for the world in terms of demographic and epidemiological transitions is not as easy. Population growth is persistent: the planet's population reached 2.5 billion in 1950, and 5 billion in 1989. The rate of increase reached a peak of 2.04% between 1965 and 1970 and has declined since. The downturn has not been sufficiently great to be associated with a decrease in the absolute number of people being added to the world's population. Indeed, the downturn does not reflect a universal decline in growth rates. Most of the decline is a result of low growth and even negative growth in developed countries that have passed through the demographic transition and have been in the final stage for several decades. Applying the demographic transition model to less developed countries would place most of them in the middle stage, in which death rates are declining and birth rates are declining less rapidly or not declining at all. Thus the world growth rate in 1989 of 1.8% reflects a growth rate of 0.5% for developed countries and 2.1% for less developed countries. (The growth rate for less developed countries excluding China was estimated at 2.4% in 1989.[28])

A decline in global mortality is taking place. Between 1950–1955 and 1980–1985 the estimated life expectancy at birth increased worldwide more than 13 years, reaching 59.5 years of age. Less developed countries increased by 16.2 years, while more developed countries increased 7.3 years to a total of 73.1 years of life expected at birth.[19] Given the success in eradicating smallpox and reducing the burden of other infections such as malaria, polio, and measles, the transition from death chiefly caused by acute infectious diseases to death more often caused by chronic diseases and injuries should continue.

CONSEQUENCES OF POPULATION GROWTH

Projecting Change. Projecting population growth in terms of size and composition is an important starting point in trying to determine the consequences of population change. Using age- and sex-specific probabilities of death, age-specific fertility probabilities and the sex ratio at birth, and reported or assumed migration rates permits demographers to project, but not to forecast, population into the future. The distinction between projecting and forecasting is important because a projection uses an explicit set of assumptions, and is intended to be an illustrative calculation based on these assumptions. A forecast, on the other hand, includes an element of subjective judgment to set the levels of mortality, fertility, and migration for specific times in the future. Projections usually are based on a single set of mortality probabilities. Fertility, on the other hand, because it varies over shorter intervals, often is projected using three or four different sets of assumed probabilities, thereby generating different projections. Migration is based on current data and estimates; projections assume numbers of migrants will remain stable unless specific changes in policy or other determinants of population mobility are known.

Projections based on the assumptions judged by the U.S. Bureau of the Census to be most likely to hold true in the near future indicate that by the year 2000 the population of the United States will be 267.7 million people, which will increase to 282.1 million by 2010. Although the largest proportion of the population will live in the South, the most rapid increase is projected for the West (13.7%). Growth in the Northeast (2.4%) and Midwest (−0.3%) is calculated to be negligible. Most of the increase is expected to be the result of natural increase (72%) rather than net migration (28%). The median age is projected to increase from 33.0 years in 1990 to 36.5 in 2000, and 39.0 by 2010; the median age in the Northeast is anticipated to exceed 40 years by 2010 for the first time in any major region of the United States.[40]

Population Growth and Economic Change. The role of population growth in relation to economic change is a central global concern, especially of bodies such as the World Bank and the United Nations Fund for Population Activities (UNFPA). The work of Coale and Hoover[41] in 1958 was instrumental in pointing out that "A reduction in fertility would make the process of modernization more rapid and more certain. It would accelerate the growth in income, provide more rapidly the possibility of productive employment, . . . make the attainment of universal education easier—and . . . [provide] women of low-income countries some relief from constant pregnancy, parturition, and infant care." Pursuing a course of lower fertility would, according to these scholars, create this advantageous effect by reducing the number of dependent children, that is, those aged 15 years and younger, with only minor effects on the size of the labor force or its increase until 30 years later.

Reviewing this work 30 years later, Coale[42] emphasized, as he had stated in his earlier writings, that no relationship existed between the rate of growth of the total population and an increase in the rate of per capita income, but current data did show that annual per capita income increased as TFR decreased in developing countries. In addition, he pointed to a positive relationship between the rate of growth in per capita income and increase in life expectancy at birth. Moreover, productive employment is a more realistic prospect in those countries that immediately initiate measures to reduce high rates of fertility. The importance of these observations has not been lost on most world leaders.

Population, Environment, Resources, and Food. Around the beginning of the nineteenth century Malthus recorded his views on population growth and its consequences, specifically inadequate food supplies. In more recent years others have emphasized and extended these observations, linking environmental degradation to uncontrolled population growth. Among the important contributions to this debate was the publication of *The Limits to Growth* in 1972.[43] Supported by an informal group of international professionals who called themselves The Club of Rome, a research team at the Massachusetts Institute of Technology investigated the state of the world in terms of population growth, agricultural productivity, environmental pollution, industrial output, and nonrenewable resources. After determining the status of each and the trends of change from 1900 to 1970, they projected the effects of these trends into the future and reached the following conclusions: (1) If these trends persist unchanged, the limits to growth on the earth would be reached within the next 100 years; (2) the trends could all be altered so that economic and ecological stability might be reached and sustained; and (3) the sooner governments and citizens around the world undertake the measures to alter current trends in all five of these areas of social and ecological concern, the greater would be the chances of attaining global equilibrium. A flurry of criticism followed the publication of *The Limits to Growth.* Nonetheless, it heightened the intensity of debate over global issues important to the present and future of human well-being, and many of the issues, including continued population growth, remain important today.

Concern about the environment and its importance to humanity has rekindled awareness of population growth.[1] Ehrlich and colleagues[44] have reemphasized the gravity of environmental degradation as a consequence of population growth. Specifically, they draw attention to the human impact on land use, desertification, deforestation of moist tropical areas, and "anthropogenic climate change." In the United States, citizen groups concerned about these issues, such as the National Audubon Society, have also become more active.[45,46] (See Chapter 39.)

PUBLIC HEALTH ISSUES

Teenage Fertility. Teenage pregnancies are a profound population issue because children born to young women may lead to unanticipated momentum in population growth by increasing total family size over a lifetime and by shortening the time between generations of future children. Moreover, they are a serious public health problem because teenage pregnancies may be at high risk of preventable infant mortality and pregnancies in very young women of reproductive age often are not intended. (See Chapter 68.)

Demographic Trends and Effects. What are the current trends in fertility for teenaged women? In the United States the number of births to women 15 through 19 years of age increased nearly 8% from an estimated 361,000 in 1973 to 389,000 in 1982, while the total number of births to all women in the childbearing age group declined nearly 20%. Moreover, this estimate does not include the legal abortions (232,000 in 1973 and 418,000 in 1982) that women in this age group underwent, or the births and abortions to those younger than age 15, which accounted for more than 24,000 pregnancies in 1973 and in 1982.[47]

Birth rates for teenaged women in the United States have not declined substantially since 1982. Compared with other nations for which data on teenage pregnancy are available, the U.S. rate (95 pregnancies per 1000 women aged 15 to 19) is among the highest. The pregnancy rate for Canada (46/1000) is less than half that for the United States, and the Netherlands has a teenage pregnancy rate of 15/1000, the lowest reported.[15]

These patterns have important demographic implications. Age at first sexual union is a principal determinant of lifetime fertility and family size. Women who begin having children at an early age therefore are likely to have larger families, births at shorter intervals, and contribute proportionately more to increasing growth of a community or population than women who begin having children at later ages. In terms of long-term demographic change, couples who have offspring while the mother is still in her teens have a short generation. The result is that the female children of these couples are at risk of childbearing in a shorter span of years than are the female children of mothers who defer childbearing until their twenties or thirties.

Health Effects. Although the children of teenaged mothers are at higher risk of death than children of women in their twenties, the risk to the health of pregnant women under age 20 is more difficult to assess because first births and births to women in social minorities are thought to carry a higher risk of mortality. The most recent analysis of maternal mortality by age of mother for the United States did not show any appreciable differences in age-specific mortality ratios.[48] The reasons for the greater risk among minorities are not entirely clear, but they may be related to marital disruption, access to care, compliance with care standards, or the unintendedness of pregnancies of women in their teen years.

Urbanization. The movement of people to cities (urbanization) is one of the dominant characteristics of population change of the twentieth century. At the beginning of the century, fewer than one of every seven persons in the world lived in a city; as we near the year 2000, more than 40% of the world's population is found in urban areas.[1]

The growth of cities is determined by three factors: (1) migration, (2) natural increase, that is, the number of births in excess of the number of deaths, and (3) the reclassification of areas from rural to urban as they rapidly become more populous. Urban growth at the global level has been 2.5% annually in recent years or about 50% greater than that of the total population. Urbanization is most profound in developing countries where the annual urban growth rate is 4.4%. As a result, São Paulo, Brazil, is projected to have 25.8 million residents and Mexico City 31.0 million by the year 2000.[49]

The health problems of city life are not caused directly by urban living as much as they are by the extent to which the infrastructure of society is overwhelmed by the size of the population. Rapid urban growth resulting primarily from rural-to-urban migration creates health problems related to the need for housing and sanitation, improved food supply, transportation within the city, and the distribution of preventive and curative health services. In many developing countries the vast numbers of people leaving rural areas for urban places reside in the unsanitary conditions of shantytowns or squatter settlements on the fringe of the capital cities, where public health problems are exacerbated.

Refugees and Other Migrants. An estimated 15 million refugees are dispersed throughout the world.[2] An additional 50 million people have been displaced by natural disasters such as drought or by war or civil unrest. While most are in Africa and have come from other countries on that continent, refugees can be found in almost every nation. Although many such people leave their homelands for political reasons, others do so for reasons that have led Brown to identify them as "ecological refugees."[33] He cites food shortages and sharp increases in food prices (generally or for specific staples) as events that trigger ecological refugee movements. In other situations migrants move to find better employment opportunities and an improved quality of life. Even in areas where people from other nations are welcome or when migration takes place within a single country, the difficulties of geographic displacement may be augmented by occupational displacement, environmental change, social disruption, and economic hardship.

Refugee movements may bring with them serious public health problems such as severe malnutrition as in the Horn of Africa. In other instances refugees and other migrants may carry infections to areas in which such diseases are under control or where they have not previously existed, thereby necessitating new or intensified public health screening efforts followed by treatment or other control measures.

Health problems also are encountered by migrants as a consequence of their move to a new environment. Psychological stress and physical deprivation associated with living in an unfamiliar environment, such as a refugee camp or squatter settlement, can bring about high levels of violence, including suicide, homicide, and other behavioral disturbances. Language and other cultural differences between refugees or migrants and the inhabitants of their place of destination produce serious barriers to health care information and services at the new location.

Aging. As the death rate declines in most parts of the world, life expectancy increases, and the number and ages of older people increase. This change is more characteristic in developed countries where life expectancy often exceeds 70 years. A shift in the age of a population has important implications for the health problems a society must face and the health services that must be provided.

The United States illustrates how aging has become an important issue and how it is developing momentum for the future. From 1950 to 1980, while the world population growth created alarm as it increased at the rate of approximately 2% each year, portending a doubling of the global population every 30 years, the number of people aged 65 and older increased 2.3% annually; the number of those aged 85 years and older increased at a rate of 4.2% yearly. The result is that the number of people in this country aged 65 and older increased to 29 million by 1987 (compared with 3 million in 1900), and those 85 and older numbered 3 million (in 1900 only 122,000 Americans were in this age group). The combined demographic dynamics of an increase in life expectancy and a decline in fertility has profoundly changed the proportion of the U.S. population who are age 65 and older. Recent estimates indicate that people who are 65 years and older comprised 12% of the national population in 1987; in 1900 they were 4% of the nation's people. Current projections show this trend will persist into the next century. Between 1990 and 2010 the number of people 65 and older is likely to increase by at least 7 million, while those between 25 and 44 years of age could decrease by 9 million. By 2030 there are likely to be 59.2 million Americans aged 65 and older; 6.3 million of them will be 85 years and older.[50]

The spectrum of health problems facing the public with an aging population will change profoundly. Heart disease, cancer, and cerebrovascular disease, which already account for nearly two thirds of the deaths in the United States, will be more prevalent. The need to prevent disability and injury in the aging, intensified needs for long-term care, and other special health services have reached a new level of importance that will persist well into the next century. A 1984 survey of people in the United States who were between 55 and 74 years of age showed that more than half (54%) had difficulty walking a quarter of a mile; more than three fifths of them had difficulty lifting 25 pounds (62%) or stooping, kneeling, or crouching (65%). Moreover, health reasons were given for retirement from the work force by one of every six respondents, and the role of health became increasingly important as the age of the respondents increased. Health measures, public policy on retirement, and the desire of the older members of the population to continue working will be important determinants of the quality of living in the future.[51]

REFERENCES

1. World Commission on Environment and Development: Our Common Future. Oxford: Oxford University Press, 1987
2. World Health Organization, Division of Epidemiological Surveillance: Global estimates for health situation assessment and projections, 1990. Geneva: WHO/HST/90.2 Official Publication, 1990
3. United Nations: Principles and recommendations for the 1970 population censuses. Statistical Papers, Series M, No. 44, 1967, pp 3–4
4. Kovar MG: Data systems of the National Center for Health Statistics. Hyattsville, Md.: NCHS Vital and Health Statistics, Series 1, No. 23, March 1989; DHHS Publication No. (PHS) 89-1325, 1989
5. Brown GF, Bongaarts J, Churchill EP, et al (eds): Ghana 1988: Results from the demographic and health survey. Studies in family planning. New York: Population Council 21:236–240, 1990
6. Palmore JA, Gardner RW. Measuring Mortality, Fertility, and Natural Increase: A Self-teaching Guide to Elementary Measures. Honolulu: East-West Center, 1983
7. Heuser RL: Fertility tables for birth cohorts by color: United States, 1917–73. Rockville, Md.: National Center for Health Statistics, DHEW Publication No. (HRA) 76-1152, 1976
8. Frost WH. The age selection of mortality from tuberculosis in successive decades. Am J Hyg 30:90–96, 1939
9. Peavy JV, Dyal WW, Eddins DL: Descriptive statistics rates, ratios, proportions and indices. Atlanta: DHHS, Centers for Disease Control, 1989
10. Leridon H: Human Fertility: The basic Components. Chicago: University of Chicago Press, 1977
11. Bongaarts J, Potter RG: Natural fertility and its proximate determinants. In Fertility, Biology, and Behavior: An Analysis of the Proximate Determinants. New York: Academic Press, 1983
12. Mishell DR. Infertility. In Droegemueller W, Herbst AL, Mishell DR, Stenchever MA (eds): Comprehensive Gynecology. St. Louis: C. V. Mosby, 1987
13. Brass W: The demography of French-speaking territories covered by special sample inquiries: Upper Volta, Dahomey, Guinea, North Cameroon, and other areas. In Brass W, Coale AJ, Demeny P, et al (eds): The Demography of Tropical Africa. Princeton, N.J.: Princeton University Press, 1968, pp 342–449
14. Davis K, Blake J: Social structure and fertility: An analytic framework. Econ Dev Cult Change 4:211–235, 1956
15. Hatcher RA, Kowal D, Guest F, et al: Contraceptive Technology, international edt. Atlanta: Printed Matter, 1989
16. Jacobson JL: The global politics of abortion. Worldwatch Paper 97. Washington, D.C.: Worldwatch Institute, 1990
17. Tietze C: Induced abortion: A world review 1981. In A Population Council Fact Book. New York: Population Council, 1986
18. Health United States 1989 and prevention profile. Washington, D.C.: National Center for Health Statistics, DHHS Publication No. (PHS) 90-1232, 1990
19. Demeny P: The world demographic situation. In Menken J, (ed): World Population and U.S. Policy—The Choices Ahead. New York: W.W. Norton, 1986, pp 27-66
20. Lancaster HO: Expectations of Life: A Study in the Demography, Statistics, and History of World Mortality. New York: Springer-Verlag, 1990
21. Coale AJ, Demeny P, Vaughan B: Regional Model Life Tables and Stable Populations, 2 edt. New York: Academic Press, 1983
22. Preston SH: Mortality Patterns in National Populations. New York: Academic Press, 1976
23. Omran AR: Epidemiologic transition in the United States—the health factor in population change. Washington, D.C.: Population Reference Bureau. Population Bulletin 32(2), 1980
24. Fenner F, et al: Smallpox and Its Eradication. Geneva: World Health Organization, 1988
25. Centers for Disease Control: Summary of notifiable diseases, United States, 1988. MMWR 37(54), 1988
26. U.S. Department of Health and Human Services: Reducing the health consequences of smoking: 25 years of progress. A report of the Surgeon General. Washington, D.C.: Public Health Service, DHHS Publication No. (CDC) 89-8411, 1989
27. Worth AJ: The Walton report and its subsequent impact on cervical cancer screening programs in Canada. Obstet Gynecol 63:135–139, 1984
28. Population Reference Bureau: 1990 World population data sheet, April 1990
29. Shryock HS, Siegel JS, et al: The methods and materials of demography. Washington, D.C.: U.S. Bureau of the Census, 1971
30. Lee ES: A theory of migration. Demography 3:47–57, 1966
31. Kuznets SS: Introduction. In Eldridge HT, Thomas DS (eds): Demographic Analyses and Interrelations. Vol. 3: Population Redistribution and Economic Growth, United States, 1870–1950. Philadelphia: American Philosophical Society, 1964
32. Bouvier LF, Gardner RW: Immigration to the U.S.: The unfinished story. Washington, D.C.: Population Reference Bureau. Population Bulletin 41(4), Nov 1986
33. Jacobson JL: Abandoning homelands. In Brown LR, et al (eds): State of the World, 1989. New York: W.W. Norton, 1989
34. Malthus TR: On population. Himmelfarb G, ed. New York: Random House, 1960
35. Notestein FW: Population—the long view. In Schultz TW (ed): Food for the World. Chicago: University of Chicago Press, 1945
36. Hauser PM, Duncan OD: Demography as a body of knowledge. In Hauser PM, Duncan OD (eds): The Study of Population: An inventory and an Appraisal. Chicago: University of Chicago Press, 1959
37. Notestein FW, Kirk D, Segal S: The problem of population control. In Hauser PM (ed): The Population Dilemma. Englewood Cliffs, N.J.: Prentice-Hall, 1963
38. Coale A: The demographic transition. In Proceedings of the International Population Conference, vol. 1. Liege, Belgium: International Union for the Scientific Study of Population, 1973
39. Caldwell J: Toward a restatement of demographic transition theory. Popul Dev Rev 2(3–4):321–366, 1976
40. Wetrogan SI: Projections of the population of states, by age, sex, and race: 1988 to 2010. Washington, D.C.: U.S. Bureau of the Census, Current Population Reports, Series P-25, No. 1017, 1988
41. Coale AJ, Hoover E: Population Growth and Economic Development in Low-Income Countries. Princeton, N.J.: Princeton University Press, 1958
42. Coale AJ: Population trends and economic development. In Menken J (ed): World Population and U.S. Policy—The Choices Ahead. New York: W.W. Norton, 1986, pp 96–104
43. Meadows DH, Meadows DL, Randers J, Behrens WW: The Limits to Growth. New York: Potomac Associates, 1972
44. Ehrlich PR, et al: Global change and carrying capacity: Implications for life on earth. In DeFries RS, Malone TF (eds): Global Change and Our Common Future. Washington, D.C.: National Academy Press, 1989
45. Baldi PA, Spivey-Weber F, Snyder K, et al: A message to Congress on sustainable developments in United States foreign assistance. Washington, D.C.: National Audubon Society, 1989
46. Maize KP: Blueprint for the environment: Advice to the President-elect from America's environmental community. Washington, D.C.: Blueprint for the Environment, 1988
47. Henshaw SK, Kenney AM, Somberg D, Van Vort J. Teenage Pregnancy in the United States: The Scope of the Problem and State Responses. New York: Alan Guttmacher Institute, 1989
48. Centers for Disease Control: Maternal mortality surveillance, United States, 1980–1985. MMWR 37:19–29, 1988
49. World Bank Development Report, 1984: New York: Oxford University Press, 1984

50. Spencer G: Projections of the population of the United States, by age, sex, and race: 1988 to 2080. Washington, D.C.: U.S. Bureau of the Census. Current Population Reports, Series P-25, No. 1018, U.S. Government Printing Office, 1989
51. Kovar MG, LaCroix AZ: Aging in the eighties, ability to perform work-related activities. Data from the Supplement on Aging to the National Health interview survey, United States, 1984. Advance Data from Vital and Health Statistics, No. 136. Hyattsville, Md.: Public Health Service, DHHS Publication No. (PHS) 87-1250, 1987

SECTION TWO

Communicable Diseases

Edited by Richard P. Wenzel

4

Control of Communicable Diseases

Overview

Richard P. Wenzel

The most important function of public health in its broadest sense is to seek an optimal harmony between groups of people in society and their environment. This goal can be approached in three ways: (1) by methods to improve host resistance of populations to environmental hazards, (2) by effective plans to improve the safety of the environment, and (3) by improving health care systems designed to increase the likelihood, efficiency, and effectiveness of the first two goals. With respect to infectious diseases there are special elements within each of the three categories (Table 4-1). One might then view communicable diseases as an imbalance in the relationship of people and their environment which favors microbial dominance in populations.

It is often argued that improved host resistance is the purview of clinical medicine and that both environmental safety and public health systems are public health efforts. However, improved resistance in populations cannot be divorced from necessary educational and effective health delivery systems. For that reason it may be considered an essential component of public health. In this schema of public health, the infectious agent is considered not as a separate focus but as one important component of the environment. This organization is designed to integrate the schema with a concept of health, and of public health in particular. The implication is that the organism is a necessary but not sufficient cause of ill health; it is only one of many risk factors. Moreover, humans constantly encounter myriads of potential microbial pathogens, and removing all such organisms is untenable. It seems more fruitful to develop effective barriers between humans and problematic environmental microbes or at the very least to create pathways for peaceful coexistence. In addition, to many authors it has seemed that public health has focused excessively on environmental controls and too little on the health care system. Yet all of these categories are interrelated; a change in any aspect of the three areas perturbs the entire system and has a direct effect on public health.

With respect to improved host resistance, McKeown[1] has argued that improved nutrition, personal hygiene, and public sanitation have more to do with the control of infectious diseases than vaccines and health care. There is no question, however, that vaccines and new antibiotics have greatly reduced morbidity and mortality from infectious diseases.[2] Furthermore, with respect to smallpox, the vaccine—in concert with a public health system for identifying and isolating cases and contacts—was essential for its eradication.[3]

Recently it has been proposed that exercise may improve both mental and physical health[4,5] and that there may be important interactions between psychological factors and immunity.[6] Lastly, with the explosion of activities in the field of molecular biology[6] and the prospect of cloning the human genome,[7] it is not farfetched to think that within a decade, genetic alteration of cells will enable us to enhance host resistance to adverse environmental challenges.[8]

The environment has long been a primary focus of public health, with efforts to improve the cleanliness of food and water, upgrade public sanitation, and clean the air of toxic pollutants. Efforts to remove infectious agents by reducing animal reservoirs and vectors or efforts to reduce their numbers have been another focus for public health in general and in veterinary medicine in particular. Recently many have postulated that adequate personal space is important for prevention of many urban problems. It has long been recognized that control of streptococcal infections in the military could be minimized by increasing space between the bunks of recruits and that crowding is a major risk factor.[9] In addition, since large droplets are known to be important for many viral respiratory agents,[10] it is generally accepted that spatial considerations are important for the prevention and control of communicable diseases.

A third method for public health control of infectious diseases involves the systems approach or management aspects. The social, economic, legal, and administrative forces important for health must operate in the interest of the public. Progress toward such goals must begin with access not only to health care but also to preventive health services and to health education. To do that, resources must be made available and important public health problems given sufficient priority—usually a political process—to demand necessary resources. Proper management at federal, state, and local levels needs to be operative for efficiency, effectiveness, and cost-effective delivery of care and education. Moreover, surveillance needs to be developed and maintained to detect new problems, new epidemics, and the efficacy of control measures.[11]

MAJOR PROBLEMS

There is always risk in attempting to prioritize the most important infectious agents, and readers may construct a different list from that of the author (Table 4-2). Nevertheless, the agents listed are important and serve as a focus for discussion of public health issues. An example of how one might apply the proposed

TABLE 4–1. METHODS TO IMPROVE PUBLIC HEALTH CONTROL OF COMMUNICABLE DISEASES

- **Improved Resistance to Environmental Hazards**

Hygiene
Nutrition
Immunity
Antibiotics
Psychological factors
Exercise
Genetic alteration

- **Improved Environmental Safety**

Sanitation
Air
Water
Food
Infectious agents
Vectors
Animal reservoirs

- **Public Health Systems**

Access
Efficiency
Resources
Priorities
Containment
Contact tracing for prophylaxis and therapy
Education
Social forces
Laws
Measurement of problems and of the efficiency and effectiveness of control

schema to a communicable disease is discussed below with the example of acquired immunodeficiency syndrome (AIDS).

There is no question that AIDS—caused by the human immunodeficiency viruses 1 and 2 (HIV-1 and HIV-2)—is the principal viral problem today. It is a global epidemic that affects the young in our society. Therapy is in its infancy, there is no cure in sight, and it involves the strongest of human emotions. Few drugs are available to assist in its control, and only one is known to prolong life[12]; the efficacy of educational programs has not been proven, and many problems have been related to health care delivery. With respect to improving host resistance, prophylactic aerosolized pentamidine has been shown to reduce the incidence of *Pneumocystis* infections, but no effective drugs directly affecting the immune system are available. Most patients attempt to maintain a high level of nutrition and personal hygiene, and some engage in exercise, support groups, and reading, which appear to provide a positive psychological outlook.

With respect to improved environmental safety, the office of the surgeon general of the United States has recommended barrier protection, that is, safer sexual practices and the Centers for Disease Control has recommended universal precautions for health care workers to minimize transmission in hospitals and clinics.[13] Since patients with HIV infection are at high risk for infections of all kinds, especially intracellular parasites, obviously it is prudent for them to avoid environments with high risk (e.g., exposure to tuberculosis, *Legionella,* or obviously infected people and animals). Nevertheless, specific guidelines are not yet available.

From a public health systems point of view, a great deal of discussion has occurred regarding access to medical care for AIDS victims and efficient testing of new drugs, and there has been unprecedented political pressure by homosexual activists for continued priority and use of national resources to prevent and control this infection. Similar pressures have been applied to create equitable and compassionate laws to protect the interests of high-risk groups and infected patients. One can apply the proposed paradigm to HIV infection (Table 4–1) and understand not only the illness but also the disease in populations as a function of the three components of public health control.

Other illnesses needing special attention in the 1990s (Table 4–2) are discussed elsewhere in this text. One could easily expand the list and include other classes of agents such as fungi (which include *Pneumocystis*). Little work has been done internationally on the rickettsial infections despite continuing problems with several species, and much remains to be learned about Q fever, the newly recognized problem with *Ehrlichia* species,[14] and the pathogenesis of the so-called spongioform encephalopathies.[15] Within each infectious disease class one might easily include other agents that have recently caused public health problems.

TABLE 4–2. CHIEF INFECTIOUS DISEASES IN THE 1990s

Infectious Disease Class	Major Problem	Other Major Problems
Virus	AIDS	Measles Hepatitis
Bacterium	Staphylococci	Streptococci Nosocomial infections Pathogens
Spirochete	Lyme disease	Syphilis
Parasite	Malaria	Onchocerciasis *Leishmania*

A NEW ROLE FOR PUBLIC HEALTH

With the spiraling costs of medical care and the corresponding interest in cost containment and accountability,[16] it is reasonable to avoid duplications. We need a closer link of clinical and public health disciplines and activities. In medical schools it is propitious for these disciplines to develop curricula and research projects collaboratively.

In the health service arena, closer ties between clinicians and public health officials will be efficient and effective for the good of the population. A special role for public health officials could be to "translate" important epidemiological data for clinicians giving primary care. This could be particularly important and useful in enhancing prevention. Examples of useful data would be the risk ratios for becoming an alcohol abuser for persons with and without a family history of abuse; cigarette smoking for the smoker, those nearby, and the unborn fetus; and for fatal vs nonfatal injury in persons driving with and without a seat belt. In the field of communicable diseases it is useful to know the risk of AIDS in those practicing intravenous drug abuse or unprotected sexual activities, the relative risk of Lyme disease in those using effective insect repellants vs those not using such agents, and the relative risk of hepatitis B in health care workers who have received the vaccine and those who have not. An epidemiological approach to community-wide education about local health risks, perhaps with a well-designed periodical, would further link the clinician and public health official. The Centers for Disease Control (CDC) has done this successfully with the *Morbidity and Mortality Weekly Report*. A community-wide modification for consumption by local practitioners would be helpful. Such networking is feasible and desirable.

Networking with schools, businesses, health clubs, and senior citizen groups might increase compliance with behavior designed to enhance resistance to environmental hazards. Fundamentals of general and dental hygiene, nutrition, exercise, and stress control would be essential components. It would be reasonable to reinforce such basic principles as maintaining immunizations and proper use of antibiotics. In summary, we need a proactive and integrative role in education, one that involves networking with clinicians and the public directly.

Improving environmental safety has been the focus and strength of public health. Essentially, the goal has been to reduce the microbial hazards to humans. For the most part this is carried out by systematic measurement or a series of inspections of the environment. Good general sanitation and safe air, water, and food are hallmarks of public health. Environmental activist groups have heightened interest in environmental safety. This is an opportune time to build a coalition between informed public health officials and interested and energetic activists genuinely concerned with improving the environment.

From an infectious diseases point of view, an important goal would be to reduce the degree of exposure while preserving the vitality of the ecosystem. The government of Brazil was reported to have instituted a $200 million program to control malaria in the Amazon region by spraying DDT in thousands of rain forest huts. As McCoy and Thompson[17] pointed out, however, the chemical has been banned in over 40 countries because of its lethal effect on birds and fish. Moreover, in India, although it had a remarkable short-term effect initially (75 million annual cases of malaria reduced in the 1950s to 50,000), the number of cases rose to 6.5 million by 1976, the result of resistance in mosquito vectors. Moreover, bottled milk sampled in India in April 1990 had 10 times the permissible limit of DDT. DDT is fat soluble and has been carried in food chains to countries all over the world.[17] The lesson we have learned from the Russian nuclear accident at Chernobyl, the AIDS epidemic, and the DDT experience is that radiation, viruses, and pollutants respect no national borders.

The response to such lessons needs to be an enhanced commitment by individuals, communities, and nations to solve the problems of others and to view the world as a global village. Limiting the survival of important infection agents, their animal reservoirs, or hosts requires careful examination of the implications of such approaches in collaboration with veterinarians, entomologists, and toxicologists.

PUBLIC HEALTH SYSTEMS

Of the 10 proposed public health systems important for control of communicable disease (Table 4–1), containment, contact tracing for prophylaxis and therapy, education, and measurement (surveillance) have been the mainstay of public health. Public health should become more involved with the rest as well.

The CDC has taken the lead by suggesting an epidemiological approach to priorities, listing adjusted mortality rates for various conditions and years of productive life lost (YPLL) for leading causes of death.[18,19] Ideally there would also be separate measures of morbidity and economic burdens so that in a country with limited resources, leaders of the public health system could make more informed decisions and have the general community "buy into" their decisions.

It would seem prudent and desirable to have public health become more visible in terms of medical care access and efficiency of care. Great optimism can be appreciated, however, by the effort of the CDC to show the real risk of AIDS and the low (but not zero) probability of incurring an infection while taking care of an AIDS patient. Surely this contributes to the access of AIDS victims to the health care system.

With respect to efficiency of care, it has primarily been a function of the individual physician and more recently of hospitals interested in cost containment. Such activities are often subsumed under the umbrella term "quality assurance."[20,21] Accrediting agencies in the United States such as the Joint Commission for Accreditation of Healthcare Organizations (JCAHO) also are interested in the efficiency of health care services. It is not unreasonable to expect that public health officials working with hospital epidemiologists would lend their expertise to this aspect of quality care of populations.

The legal process is paying attention to epidemiological data. Public health workers may need to "translate" public health findings that may have an impact on the legal system in a beneficial way for the population. Finally, social forces are often more effective than education alone in beneficially modifying health-related behavior. The facts on the hazards of smoking have been available for decades, but only in the last 10 years have substantial numbers of the population in the United States avoided smoking. It has become socially unacceptable in many situations to smoke; applause is often heard when the pilot of a commercial airline announces a smoke-free flight. In addition, lucrative business enterprises have made healthy behavior and exercise fashionable. These social forces need to be exploited and tested for use in control of infectious diseases. Patients in hospitals could be advised to request that all their health care providers wash their hands before touching them. This would reduce nosocomial infection rates, especially those due to staphylococci. It is not far-fetched to imagine safer sex as a result of social pressure to ask a partner to use barrier protection. Similar social pressures are operating when both passengers and drivers use a seat belt or when friends drive an intoxicated friend home after a party. Such social forces are powerful.

A corollary would be a suggestion for marketing good public health. An effective marketing campaign was carried out by former surgeon general of the United States C. Everett Koop. He was perceived as caring, knowledgable, and honest. An expanded approach to increasing the acceptance of vaccines, avoiding unsafe travel, and avoiding unsafe sex could be promoted just as consumer products are promoted—by use of effective peer groups and role models. This is a testable hypothesis for the 1990s.

In summary, a unified approach to public health is suggested involving clinicians, public health officials, and interested members and groups in the community. Networking, clarity in the presentation of epidemiologically important data, and a sense of the global community at risk with its environment are important. A sensitivity for the side effects of public health measures is essential and the use of effective education, social forces, and marketing practices may be the new tools of public health.

Travelers' Health

Elizabeth Barrett-Connor

Travel or residence in developing countries carries a risk of diverse infections, some of which are rarely or never encountered in more socioeconomically advanced countries.[1] Many of these infections are preventable through immunization, chemoprophylaxis, or other measures. Physicians who advise travelers should help them tread the line between caution and neurosis. The advice given and the emphasis with which it is presented should be weighed according to the personality and itinerary of the traveler.

IMMUNIZATIONS

Immunization for travelers can be divided into the required and the recommended. Although an immunization required by international health regulations may be essential to enter or leave a country, immunizations in the second group often are more important for the traveler's health.[2]

Required Immunizations. An annually updated list of required immunizations by country is provided by the World Health Organization.[3] Until recently immunization could be legally required against three diseases: smallpox, cholera, and yellow fever. Countries requiring immunization against any of these diseases could refuse the right of entry to travelers who did not have either a valid immunization recorded on the International Certificate of Vaccination or (in some cases) a written statement by a physician indicating why immunization was not given.

Smallpox has been eradicated officially (the last reported endemic case was in October 1977). No country now requires smallpox vaccination for entry.

Cholera is widespread around the world, but infection in travelers is rare. The available killed cholera vaccine is not particularly effective, protecting perhaps half of recipients for 3 to 6 months. In 1973 the twenty-sixth World Health Assembly recommended that vaccination against cholera should no longer be required as a condition of admittance to any country, and in 1988 the World Health Organization dropped this requirement. Some countries still require proof of cholera vaccination for travelers entering or leaving an area with cholera. If cholera vaccine is given, one injection of either 1.0 ml subcutaneously or 0.2 ml intradermally will meet international requirements. The latter causes fewer reactions. After a 6-day waiting period, a cholera vaccination certificate is valid for 6 months. Cholera immunization is not recommended or required for infants less than 6 months of age.

Yellow fever, limited to tropical Africa and Central and South America, can be prevented by a single subcutaneous injection of 0.5 ml of live attenuated 17-D virus vaccine. To ensure that effective vaccine is given, it must be stored at less than 5° C and used within 1 hour of reconstitution. A certificate of yellow fever vaccination is valid for 10 years after a 10-day waiting period although protection probably lasts for life. The vaccine is not recommended for infants less than 9 months of age. Like all other live virus vaccines, it should be avoided during pregnancy and is contraindicated in immunocompromised patients. Because the vaccine is grown in chick embryo, it should not be given to persons clearly hypersensitive to eggs. A letter from the physician stating that the immunization is contraindicated may permit travel if the patient cannot be immunized safely.

Recommended Immunizations. Accidents are the second most common cause of death in international travelers and nonfatal trauma is presumably even more common. Tetanus immunization must be kept up to date; it is protective for at least 10 years. In the absence of a wound, boosters are necessary only every 10 years; more frequent boosters increase the probability of vaccine reactions. Tetanus immunization should be given in combination with diphtheria vaccine, either tetanus and diphtheria (dT) for adults or diphtheria-pertussis-tetanus (DPT) vaccine for children less than 6 years of age, because diphtheria is endemic in many countries.

Poliomyelitis remains endemic in many parts of the world. All travelers to warm climates should be immunized adequately. The person who has had a complete immunization series (three or four doses of either live oral or killed parenteral poliomyelitis vaccine at appropriate intervals) should have a booster dose if the last immunization was given 10 or more years previously. Oral poliomyelitis vaccine recipients have a small (1 in 11 million doses) risk of vaccine-virus paralysis. Therefore adults with no or an uncertain history of poliomyelitis immunization should receive parenteral vaccine, as should immunocompromised patients and their families. Three doses of an enhanced potency inactivated polio vaccine, which has replaced the conventional Salk vaccine, are said to provide protection similar to three doses of trivalent oral polio vaccine. When time does not permit three doses, two should be given.

In recent years at least a quarter of measles cases in the United States were imported or epidemiologically associated; half were in returning residents and the other half in foreign visitors. Measles vaccine therefore is recommended for persons traveling abroad. Children may be immunized as early as 6 months of age with monovalent measles vaccine.[4] If so immunized, they should receive measles-mumps-rubella vaccine at 15 months and again when they reach school age. In adults no immunity from natural infection is likely in those born after 1956, nor is acquired immunity common in those vaccinated before 1980 or those who received live vaccine before 15 months of age. Such persons also should be immunized. Pregnant women and immunocompromized patients should not be given the measles vaccine.

Typhoid fever is endemic in many parts of the world; imported cases represent over half of those diagnosed in the United States. Current strains of *Salmonella typhi* often are resistant to antimicrobials. Immunization against typhoid therefore is appropriate for persons traveling to countries where sanitation is poor. The heat-phenol-inactivated vaccine contains killed whole typhoid bacilli. A new oral typhoid vaccine made from attenuated *S. typhi* Ty 21a bacteria probably is equally effective and may cause fewer side effects. The first dose of parenteral vaccine should be followed by a second dose 4 weeks later; this is followed by a single booster if 3 or more years have elapsed since immunization. One oral vaccine capsule is given on 3 alternate days as a primary series of three capsules and also requires a booster after 3 years. Oral typhoid vaccine should not be given concurrently with the antimalarials chloroquine or mefloquine.

Meningococcal meningitis poses a sporadic or epidemic risk—most notably to trekkers in Nepal and travelers to Saudi Arabia, the New Dehli region of India, and sub-Saharan Africa and Brazil. A single dose of quadrivalent vaccine (serogroups A, C, Y, and W-135) appears to be protective for about 3 years in adults and older children. Meningococcal vaccine is not effective in children less than 2 to 3 years of age.

Preexposure rabies vaccine is appropriate for adults and

children planning extended stays in much of the developing world and for persons who work with animals. The human diploid-cell culture vaccine, a killed vaccine that is more immunogenic and less reactogenic than earlier rabies vaccines, is given on days 1, 7, and 28. A series of three doses almost always yields a satisfactory antibody titer of $\geq 1{:}16$, and routine measurement of antibody titers is no longer recommended after the third dose of vaccine. Travelers should be advised that preexposure vaccination eliminates the need for rabies immune globulin after rabies exposure but does not eliminate the need for additional postexposure rabies vaccine.

Immunization against plague is recommended rarely except for travelers to rural Southeast Asia whose occupation or plans may lead them to direct exposure to wild animals. Three injections of the formaldehyde-inactivated vaccine are given at 4-week intervals, with booster doses every 6 to 12 months. Plague vaccine should not be given to infants less than 12 months of age.

Japanese encephalitis virus is transmitted in summer and fall in many parts of rural Asia. Travelers to high risk areas should consider obtaining the killed virus vaccine, currently available in Japan, Hong Kong, Korea, and Sri Lanka. The primary series is two or three injections and takes at least 1 week.

Typhus is seen rarely in travelers, and routine immunization is not recommended. Typhus vaccine is not available in the United States.

Tuberculosis is common in developing countries, and persons who will live and work there are at an increased risk of exposure. The efficacy of bacille Calmette-Guérin (BCG), a live vaccine derived from a strain of *Mycobacterium bovis,* is still debated in the United States. In most other countries it is recommended for persons with a negative tuberculin skin test who are planning an extended stay in a developing country. Side effects, ranging from draining abscesses at the site of immunization (common) to disseminated infection (rare), must be weighed against the risk of exposure to active tuberculosis for the traveler—a risk that varies directly with the intimacy and duration of contact with the indigenous population.

In sub-Saharan Africa, Southeast Asia, China, Korea, Indochina, the South Pacific Islands, Haiti, and the Dominican Republic 5% to 20% of the population are hepatitis B virus (HBV) carriers. Effective (but expensive) vaccines are available against hepatitis B. Vaccination is not recommended routinely except for travelers who will have an extended stay (6 months or longer) in a high-risk area and be in intimate contact with the local population. The full vaccine series of three doses takes 6 months; some protection probably is afforded by fewer doses if time constraints require.

There is an increased risk of hepatitis A in travelers to Africa, Asia, and Central and South America. The risk increases with the duration of stay. Passive immunization using immune globulin is recommended for most travelers who will spend more than 3 to 4 weeks in a developing country or any amount of time in the Middle East. The recommended dose for preexposure prophylaxis, 0.05 ml/kg (3 to 5 ml for adults), must be repeated every 4 to 6 months. For a trip of less than 6 weeks, 2 ml constitutes an adequate adult dose.

Many travelers come to the physician only a short time before the anticipated date of departure. When necessary, all active immunizations can be given concurrently. Febrile reactions are probably no more common with concurrent immunizations, but often it is difficult to determine which vaccine was responsible. If vaccines are administered concurrently, they should be given at different sites, using separate syringes. Ideally, immune globulins should not be given until at least 2 weeks, preferably 4 weeks, after the last active immunization because passively acquired antibody theoretically could interfere with response to immunization. Both required and optional immunizations should be recorded in the International Certificate of Vaccination booklet and carried with the passport.

CHEMOPROPHYLAXIS

Malaria is the most important disease for which chemoprophylaxis should be recommended.[5] Although many travelers come to physicians for immunizations, relatively few actively request antimalarials. When physicians obtain the itinerary on which to base immunization recommendations, they have obtained the information essential to ascertain malaria risk. Current information on malaria transmission by country is provided by the World Health Organization and by the Centers for Disease Control in the United States. In recent years nearly half of all reported malaria infections in U.S. travelers were caused by *Plasmodium falciparum,* a potentially fatal infection.

Chloroquine is still recommended for travelers to most parts of Asia, Africa, and Central and South America despite the widespread (and rapid) emergence of chloroquine-resistant falciparum malaria. In addition to being the best drug for chloroquine-sensitive malaria, it may reduce the severity of illness due to resistant strains.[6] Chloroquine should be begun before departure to ascertain intolerance and taken after a meal to reduce gastrointestinal side effects. It is taken weekly throughout the entire period of exposure and for 6 weeks thereafter. There are no contraindications to chloroquine prophylaxis, which can be given safely to children and pregnant women. The difference between a prophylactic dose and a potentially fatal toxic dose is, however, relatively small, and there is no antidote. Therefore chloroquine tablets and the pediatric elixir (often chocolate-flavored) should be kept in closed, child-proof containers.

Travelers to rural Southeast Asia and to expanding parts of South America and Africa are at high risk of chloroquine-resistant falciparum malaria. Resistance has been found (in some places) to nearly all available regimens. All drugs also carry some risk of serious or fatal reactions, including pyrimethamine and sulfadoxine in fixed combination (Fansidar), amodiaquine, pyrimethamine, dapsone, mefloquine, and doxycycline. Concerns about toxicity have led to recommendations for a "curative dose" when malaria is first suspected instead of prophylaxis. In this regimen the traveler takes chloroquine as above and carries a therapeutic dose of the best other antimalarial for the location, to be taken presumptively if immediate medical care is not available. For example, Fansidar has been associated with Stevens-Johnson syndrome, agranulocytosis, and death in a few persons without previously known sulfa allergy. Mefloquine has been associated with serious and sometimes irreversible neurotoxicity. In areas of heavy transmission, however, many experts still recommend prophylactic antimalarials rather than presumptive antimalarials when the risk of drug toxicity is less than the risk of malaria. Known or suspected falciparum malaria, whether or not on prophylaxis, is a medical emergency.

Chemoprophylaxis against trypanosomiasis is not recommended for the usual safari visitor who is most likely to be exposed in East Africa and South Africa to Rhodesian trypanosomiasis. It is sometimes recommended for workers living in endemic areas in rural West or Central Africa, where they may be exposed to Gambian trypanosomiasis. A single intramuscular injection of 250 mg of pentamidine provides protection for about 6 months. Pentamidine may not be available in parts of Africa where it is needed and travelers should be so advised.

Most travelers to areas endemic for filariasis will not have sufficient exposure to acquire disease. For some persons planning an extended stay, however, prophylactic diethylcarbamazine may be recommended.

There are no suitable drugs presently available for the chemoprophylaxis of other parasitic diseases, including amebiasis and schistosomiasis.

TRAVELERS' DIARRHEA

The most common infection acquired by travelers is a self-limited diarrhea, usually caused by enterotoxigenic *Escherichia coli.*[7] Several prophylactic agents, including a nonabsorbable sulfonamide, neomycin, doxycycline, and bismuth subsalicylate (Pepto-Bismol), have been shown in double-blind, placebo-controlled trials to reduce the frequency and severity of traveler's diarrhea. Prophylactic antimicrobials generally are not recommended for two reasons: resistance to antimicrobial agents is widespread, and their use carries a risk of untoward drug reaction or superinfection with more pathogenic microorganisms. Pepto-Bismol prophylaxis can be initiated at departure for a short trip or begun as early as possible in the course of illness for a longer trip. Tablets, which are easier to carry, are nearly as effective as the liquid. Some travelers prefer self-treatment to prophylaxis; early treatment does reduce the severity and duration of illness.[8]

Health Maintenance. The background, itinerary, and life-style of the traveler determine the risk of illness during travel abroad. Long-term visitors are at highest risk because their activities usually are more adventuresome and because their longer stay increases opportunities for exposure.

Precautions are not always practical for travelers who go by overland routes, when it is not possible to choose food, drink, or sleeping facilities. Some travelers, such as missionaries, deliberately may choose to adopt the native life-style when it is impossible to practice most of the advocated protective measures. Similarly, immigrants who return to visit their countries of origin may not insist on different food, drink, or sleeping facilities in order not to seem culturally alienated from their relatives. They may not realize that their acquired immunity to most bacteria and parasites has waned.

Water and Food Precautions. Although careful attention to what is ingested may not prevent traveler's diarrhea, such precautions theoretically reduce the risk of more serious fecal-oral infections such as salmonellosis, amebiasis, and hepatitis. Outside of North America, the United Kingdom, and northwestern Europe, the local water supply should be considered suspect. Travelers should avoid tap water and ice; boiled water is safer than water treated with iodine or chlorine. Raw fruits and vegetables should be avoided unless they can be peeled at the table. Ingestion of raw mollusks carries a risk of cholera, hepatitis, and other enteric infections.

Exposure to Vectors. The risk of insect-borne diseases can be reduced by the proper use of mosquito netting and insect repellants and by remaining inside screened dwellings from dusk to dawn. Travelers to areas endemic for schistosomiasis should be warned that freshwater bathing is dangerous.

Sexually Transmitted Disease. Travelers who are sexually active in any country increase their risk of acquiring one or more sexually transmitted diseases. The risk is increased by exposure to multiple or professional partners. Safe sexual behavior, including the use of condoms throughout intimacy, is particularly important in the era of AIDS.

Illness After Return. Physicians may forget to ask, "Where have you been?" of travelers who become ill after their return. Travelers should be warned before departure that if they become ill after return, they must take the initiative to inform their physician about their travel history, regardless of how carefully they have followed recommended precautions.

REFERENCES

Overview

1. McKeown T: The Role of Medicine: Dream, Mirage, or Nemesis? Oxford: Basil Blackwell, 1979
2. Plotkin SA, Mortimer EA Jr (eds): Vaccines. Philadelphia: W.B. Saunders, 1988
3. Henderson DA: Smallpox and vaccinia. In Plotkin SA, Mortimer EA Jr (eds): Vaccines. Philadelphia: W.B. Saunders, 1988
4. Farmer ME, Locke BZ, Moscicki EK, et al: Physical activity and depressive symptoms: The NHANES I Epidemiologic follow-up study. Am J Epidemiol 128:1340–1351, 1988
5. Paffenburger RS Jr, Wing AL, Hyde RT: Physical activity as an index of heart attack risk in college alumni. Am J Epidemiol 108:161–175, 1978
6. Locke S. Mind and Immunity. New York: Praeger: Institute for the Advancement of Health, 1985
7. Watson JD: The human genome project: Past, present and future. Science 248:44–48, 1990
8. Culliton BJ: Gene therapy proposed [note in Research News]. Science 247:1181, 1990
9. Quinn RW: Streptococcal infections. In Evans AS, Feldman HA (eds): Bacterial Infections of Humans Epidemiology and Control. New York: Plenum Medical Book Co., 1982, pp 538–539
10. Knight V: Airborne transmission and pulmonary deposition of respiratory viruses. In Viral and Mycoplasma Infections of the Respiratory Tract. Philadelphia: Lea & Febiger, 1973, pp 1–9
11. Thacker SB, Choi K, Brachman PS: The surveillance of infectious diseases. JAMA 249:1181–1185, 1983
12. Fischl MA, Richman DD, Grieco MH, et al: The efficacy of azidothymidine (AZT) in the treatment of patients with AIDS and AIDS-related complex. N Engl J Med 317:185–202, 1987
13. Centers for Disease Control: Update: Universal precautions for prevention of transmission of human immunodeficiency virus, hepatitis B virus, and other bloodborne pathogens in health-care settings. MMWR 37(24):377–387, 1988
14. Saah AJ. *Ehrlichia* species (human ehrlichiosis). In Mandel GL, Douglas RG, Bennett JE (eds): Principles and Practice of Infectious Diseases, 3 edt. New York: Churchill-Livingstone, 1989, pp 1482–1483
15. Prion disease—spongioform encephalopathies unveiled [Editorial]. Lancet 336:21–22, 1990
16. Relman AS: Assessment and accountability: The third revolution in medical care. N Engl J Med 319:1220–1222, 1988
17. McCoy TM: Brazil enlists DDT against malaria outbreak. World Watch 3:9–10, 1990
18. Centers for Disease Control: Mortality trends—United States, 1986–1988. MMWR 38:117–118, 1989
19. Centers for Disease Control: Premature mortality in the United States. MMWR 35(25), 1986
20. Wenzel RP, Carlson BB: Hospital epidemiology: Beyond infection control and toward quality assurance. Clin Microbiol Newsletter 10:60–62, 1988
21. Wenzel RP: Quality assessment: An emerging component of hospital epidemiology. Diagn Microbiol Infect Dis 13:197–204, 1990

Travelers' Health

1. Jong EC: Infectious diseases: The changing scene. V. Travel-related infections: Prevention and treatment. Hosp Pract 24(11):145–172, 1989
2. Hill DR, Pearson RD: Health advice for international travel. Ann Intern Med 108:839–852, 1988

3. World Health Organization: Vaccination Certificate Requirements and Health Advice for International Travel. Geneva: WHO (revised annually)
4. Preblud SR, Tsai TF, Brink EW, Nahlen BL, Parsonnet J: International travel and the child younger than two years. I. Recommendations for immunization. Pediatr Infect Dis J 8:416–425, 1989
5. Keystone JS: Advantages and disadvantages of antimalarials for chemoprophylaxis. In Steffen R, Lobel HO, Haworth J, Bradley DJ (eds): Travel Medicine. Proceedings of the first conference on international travel medicine, Zürich, April 1988. Berlin: Springer-Verlag, 1989, pp 102–112
6. Lobel HO, Campbell CC, Roberts JM: Fatal malaria in U.S. civilians. Lancet 1:873, 1985
7. DuPont HL, Ericsson CD: Travelers' diarrhea—its prevention and treatment. In Steffen R, Lobel HO, Haworth J, Bradley DJ (eds): Travel Medicine. Proceedings of the first conference on international travel medicine, Zürich, April 1988. Berlin: Springer-Verlag, 1989, pp 291–295
8. Ericsson CD, DuPont HL, Mathewson JJ, et al: Treatment of traveler's diarrhea with sulfamethoxazole and trimethoprim and loperamide. JAMA 263:257–261, 1990

5

Diseases Controlled Primarily by Vaccination

Measles

Walter A. Orenstein
Lauri E. Markowitz
Alan R. Hinman

Measles has been recognized as a distinct clinical disease for more than 10 centuries and in the developing world is associated with high mortality rates in early childhood. The epidemiology of measles is markedly affected by population size, density, movement, and social behavior. In the absence of vaccination, the disease infects essentially everyone at some time during life except in isolated populations. Beginning in 1963 the availability and increasing use of live attenuated measles vaccines have made prevention possible. Countries in the Americas and Europe have undertaken the elimination of measles.[1,2]

Measles is one of the most contagious of infectious diseases. Mathematical models suggest that in a totally susceptible population the average case of measles may result in transmission of measles to 12 to 18 persons.[3] Thus it is estimated that the immunity level needed to interrupt transmission is on the order of 94% or higher. However, although high levels of immunity substantially reduce the likelihood that susceptible persons within a population will be exposed to disease, measles transmission can occur in unusual circumstances,[4,5] and there is no level of immunity short of 100% that will absolutely guarantee absence of transmission.

Clinical Characteristics. Following an incubation period averaging 10 to 12 days (range 8 to 16 days) the patient typically has fever and malaise, followed shortly thereafter by cough, coryza, and conjunctivitis.[6] An exanthem, characterized by small bluish white spots on a red background (Koplik's spots), may be seen on the buccal mucosa within the 2 days before and after the onset of rash. The characteristic maculopapular rash of measles usually appears an average of 14 days after infection begins and typically 2 to 4 days after the onset of the prodromal symptoms. The exanthem classically starts on the face and hairline and then spreads to the trunk and extremities. The patient's temperature usually peaks 1 to 3 days following the onset of rash. The rash, areas of which fade in order of appearance, typically lasts 5 to 7 days, and the illness is entirely gone by 10 to 14 days after the onset of symptoms. Clinically apparent primary infections are the rule.

The patient is infectious during the prodromal period and for the first few days of rash. The infectious period is usually considered to stretch from 4 days before to 4 days after the onset of rash. Measles is usually transmitted in large respiratory droplets, requiring close contact between patients and susceptible persons. However, measles virus can survive for at least 2 hours in fine droplets, and airborne spread has been documented.[7,8] Neither a long-term infectious carrier state nor an animal reservoir are known.

Complications. The risk of complications and death is highest in young children and adults. The most common complications of measles are otitis media and pneumonia, which occur in 5% to 9% and in 1% to 6% of cases, respectively. Pneumonia, the most common cause of death, may be caused by the measles virus itself or by secondary bacterial infection.[9] These complications frequently require specific antibiotic therapy. Secondary viral infections may play a prominent role in measles pneumonia-related deaths in the developing world.[10] Severe diarrhea and malnutrition may result from measles infection, particularly in the developing world.[11] A substantial proportion of patients in less developed countries who survive during the first month after measles succumb during the ensuing year.[12]

Measles encephalitis, which occurs typically 4 to 7 days after the onset of rash (range generally 1 to 15 days), is reported approximately once in every 1000 cases of measles.[13] Approximately 15% of patients with measles encephalitis die, and another 25% to 35% have permanent neurologic residua. Less common complications include bronchiolitis, sinusitis, mastoiditis, myocarditis, keratoconjunctivitis, mesenteric adenitis, hepatitis, and thrombocytopenic purpura. In the United States, the reported death-case ratio has been 1 or 2 deaths per 1000 cases. In contrast, the death-case ratio in the developing world, particularly where malnutrition and crowding are common, frequently ranges from 5% to 10% or higher.[14]

Atypical measles syndrome, characterized by high fever, pneumonia, pleural effusions, edema of the hands and feet, hepatic abnormalities, and an unusual rash, is a rare manifestation of measles infection sometimes seen in persons who received killed measles vaccine in the past and who were subsequently exposed to measles virus. An estimated 600,000 to 900,000 persons received the killed vaccine between 1963 and 1967, when it was available in the United States.

Measles infection during pregnancy is associated with spontaneous abortion and with delivery of low birth weight infants.[15] Although there have been rare reports of congenital malformations associated with measles infection during the first trimester, there is no good evidence for the existence of a congenital measles syndrome.

In addition to the acute complications noted above, approximately once in every 100,000 cases, measles virus can cause a rare degenerative disorder of the central nervous system known as subacute sclerosing panencephalitis (SSPE).[16] This illness begins insidiously an average of 7 years following the initial infection and is characterized by progressively severe personality changes, myoclonic seizures, motor impairment, coma, and death over the course of several months to years. There is no convincing evidence of a causal association between measles and multiple sclerosis.

Etiological Agent, Immunology, and Diagnosis. Measles is caused by a single-stranded RNA virus of the paramyxovirus group. It is very sensitive to acid conditions, drying, and light but can survive well in aerosolized droplets. Three glycoproteins appear to play critical roles in the pathogenesis.[17] The hemagglutinin, which projects from the virion, attaches to cell surfaces. The F protein allows cell-to-cell spread. Finally, the M protein, associated with the inner surface of the viral envelope, appears important for successful generation of intact viral particles. Abnormalities in the synthesis of M proteins have been postulated to play an important role in the pathogenesis of SSPE.

Measles virus infection induces the production of a variety of antibodies. The most frequently used assays for measles antibodies include neutralization (Nt), hemagglutination inhibition (HI), complement fixation (CF), enzyme immunoassay (EIA), and immunofluorescence (IF). Antibodies detected by Nt and HI tend to appear with rash onset and peak 2 to 4 weeks later.[18] In the absence of reexposure with subclinical reinfection and titer boosts, HI antibodies, measured by standard assays (screening dilution 1:8 to 1:10) persist in approximately 85% of patients for at least 16 years.[19] Persons who lose detectable antibody by standard tests usually have antibody measurable by more sensitive tests such as plaque-reduction neutralization. IgM antibodies are usually detectable shortly after rash onset in primary infections and peak 7 to 11 days later; IgM falls to nondetectable levels approximately 1 month after appearance of the rash. Immunity following measles disease appears to be lifelong.

Although the virus can be cultured from respiratory secretions, tears, or urine, the clinical diagnosis is more easily confirmed by documenting a significant rise in antibody titer. Alternatively, the presence of IgM antibodies in a single specimen is evidence of primary measles infection.

Occurrence

Prevaccine Period. Before the introduction and widespread use of measles vaccine, measles infection was essentially universal in the United States. Approximately 95% of persons living in urban areas were infected by age 15 years.[1] The disease typically appeared in cycles with major peaks every 2 to 3 years. A marked seasonal pattern was apparent with peaks during the late spring months. The highest recorded age-specific incidence rates were in children 5 to 9 years old. In the decade from 1950 to 1959, an annual average of more than 500,000 cases was reported. The true number of infections was estimated to be nearly 10 times as high. During the same period, nearly 500 measles deaths were recorded each year.

Postvaccine Period. The licensure and widespread use of live-virus vaccine, beginning in 1963, have brought about both a dramatic reduction in the reported occurrence of measles and a substantial alteration in its epidemiological characteristics. By 1968 the reported level dropped by 95%, reaching a low of 22,000 cases (Fig. 5-1). Between 1968 and 1978 the reported occurrence varied from a low of 22,000 cases to a high of 75,000 cases. In 1978 an effort began to eliminate indigenous measles in the United States. In 1983 measles reached a record low with only 1497 cases reported, a reduction of greater than 99% from the years preceding vaccine licensure. However, since that time measles incidence has increased, averaging 3700 cases annually from 1984 through 1988. In 1989 a provisional total of more than 14,000 cases were reported, the highest number since 1978. Despite the recurrence of measles in 1989, the current morbidity rate is still a fraction of the reported morbidity rate in the prevaccine era. Current morbidity rates have three major patterns: preschool, school, and college.[20] The preschool pattern consists of high proportions of cases in unvaccinated preschoolers (primarily in the inner cities), many of whom are younger than 15 months—the routine age for measles vaccination. In the school-age pattern, the majority of patients generally have histories of appropriate vaccination. In the larger outbreaks among school-age children, up to 90% of patients have histories of vaccination on or after the first birthday. Most of these vaccine failures are thought to result from an initial seroconversion failure (primary vaccine failure), although in some cases, seroconversion may have occurred but immunity was lost later (secondary vaccine failure).

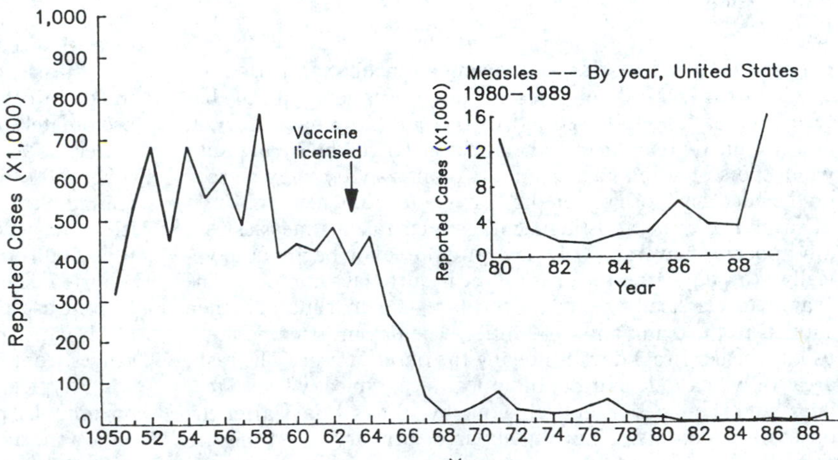

Figure 5-1. Reported measles cases, United States, 1950–1989 [1989 provisional data].

The remaining major problem is measles in college students. Although immunization records are often lacking in these populations, the vaccination status of most of the infected college students is likely to be similar to that of infected school-age children.

Immunization

Passive Immunity. Passive immunity against measles disease can be induced by the administration of commercially prepared immune globulin (IG) (formerly called immune serum globulin [ISG]), which typically has a high measles antibody titer. Administration of 0.25 ml of IG (maximum dose 15 ml) per kilogram can modify or prevent the development of measles in the exposed person.[21] The IG preparation is most effective if administered within 6 days of exposure, preferably as soon after the exposure as possible. IG is particularly indicated for susceptible household contacts, especially those who are less than 1 year of age and those who are immunocompromised. Persons in the latter groups are at greatest risk of complications from measles.

Almost all infants acquire passive immunity against measles from the transfer of maternal antibodies across the placenta. Such infants are usually immune to measles for at least the first 6 months of life. Immunity gradually wanes thereafter, and by 15 months essentially 100% of infants are susceptible.

"Modified" measles is a mild form of illness occasionally seen in persons with passively acquired antibody. The incubation period may be prolonged up to 20 days. Immunity after modified measles is believed to be permanent.

Active Immunity. In 1963, two types of measles vaccine were licensed in the United States. One was a vaccine prepared from live-attenuated virus grown in chick embryo tissue culture (Edmonston B strain). Because there was a high rate of reactions to this vaccine, including fever, rash, and catarrhal symptoms, the concomitant administration of IG was recommended.[21]

A second vaccine used the same virus, but the virus had been inactivated (killed) by formaldehyde. Immunity to the killed measles virus (KMV), or to KMV vaccine followed by live measles vaccine within 3 months, was short lived and induced hypersensitivity to measles virus in some persons, resulting in the atypical measles syndrome (see above).

Beginning in 1965, vaccines prepared from further-attenuated strains of measles virus and not requiring the concomitant administration of IG became available and quickly became the most common vaccines in use in the United States (Schwarz strain licensed in 1965 and Moraten strain licensed in 1968). From 1963 through 1988, more than 170 million doses of live measles vaccines have been distributed in the United States.

The proportion of vaccine recipients who developed antibodies to measles virus is inversely related to the age at administration up to 15 months of age, presumably because of the persistence of passively acquired maternal antibodies in the infant and young child.[22] The recommended age for measles vaccination was changed as disease control improved and as information accumulated showing increasing efficacy with increasing age. When measles vaccine was first licensed, it was recommended for infants as young as 9 months of age because complication rates were highest in younger infants and because passively acquired antibody could not be detected by the techniques available at the time. In 1965 the Immunization Practices Advisory Committee (ACIP) recommended administration beginning at 12 months of age.

In 1976 the ACIP changed the age for routine administration of vaccine to 15 months after serologic and clinical vaccine efficacy determinations indicated that the risk of vaccine failure in persons vaccinated at 12 months of age was higher than in persons vaccinated at 15 months of age. Administration of further-attenuated live measles vaccine to children at 15 months of age or older can be expected to produce measurable circulating antibodies in 95% or more of recipients.[19] The vast majority of persons with seroconversion have long-term, probably lifelong, immunity, although waning immunity may occur in a small percentage.[23]

Measles vaccine is indicated for all persons without contraindications who are at least 12 months of age, who were born after 1956, and who lack documented proof of the receipt of live measles vaccine on or after the first birthday, proof of physician-diagnosed measles, or laboratory evidence of immunity.[21] Whenever such proof is lacking, persons should be vaccinated. Vaccination causes no harm if the person is already immune to measles. The preferred age for administration of measles vaccine in most areas of the United States is 15 months.

In 1989, to prevent measles transmission among vaccine failures, both the Committee on Infectious Diseases of the American Academy of Pediatrics (AAP) and the ACIP recommended a change from a one-dose schedule to a routine two-dose schedule for measles vaccination. The two-dose schedule will generally be implemented in one age group at a time, although some localities may elect to revaccinate multiple age groups to achieve more rapidly the goal of vaccinating all the school children with two doses. The first dose should generally be administered at 15 months of age except as noted above. The ACIP recommends that the second dose be given at school entry (4 to 6 years of age), whereas the AAP recommends that the second dose be given at entry to middle school or junior high school (12 to 14 years of age). Both the ACIP and the AAP recommend that both doses of the two-dose schedule be measles-mumps-rubella (MMR) vaccine. The ACIP recommendation is based on feasibility of implementation. Children already receive a dose of diphtheria and tetanus toxoids and pertussis (DTP) vaccine and oral polio vaccine (OPV) at school entry, so additional visits are unnecessary. In addition, school systems already have extensive tracking systems at this grade level to ensure that children are vaccinated. The major disadvantage of the ACIP approach is the time interval required for impact. Most outbreaks in vaccinated persons occur in persons 12 to 18 years of age. Thus substantial impact would not be seen for 7 to 13 years. Vaccination at entry to middle school or junior high school may have a more rapid impact but may be more difficult to implement, particularly in the public sector.

Both the AAP and the ACIP give some flexibility to localities, however, to choose ages for the second dose. Both groups recommend that college entrants have two doses or other evidence of measles immunity (i.e., documented prior physician-diagnosed measles or laboratory evidence of immunity). In addition, in controlling school-based outbreaks, both groups recommend that school-age persons and school staff at risk be revaccinated if they have not previously received two doses of live vaccine on or after the first birthday or do not have other evidence of measles immunity.

A substantial proportion of remaining measles morbidity occurs in young preschool children, particularly those residing in inner city areas. Many of the cases occur in children younger than 15 months of age. In areas at high risk of preschool measles, both the ACIP and the AAP recommend that the first dose of vaccine be given routinely at 12 months of age instead of 15 months. During measles outbreaks, vaccine can be given even as young as 6 months of age with subsequent revaccination.

Fever $\geq 103°$ F ($\geq 39.4°$ C) and fleeting rash are reported in 5% to 15% of recipients of measles vaccine.[21] Encephalitis has been reported after the use of measles vaccine. Comparing the number of cases reported to have occurred within the 30 days after immunization to the number of doses distributed in the United States yields an estimate of approximately one case of encephalitis per million doses of vaccine distributed.[16] This rate is similar to that of reported encephalitis of unknown cause seen in a comparable period in the general population in the same age group. SSPE has been reported in recipients of measles vaccine, but the incidence rate is approximately 5% of that following natural illness. Case-control and cohort analyses have not suggested any relationship between measles vaccine and SSPE.[16]

Measles vaccine should not be given to persons with anaphylactic hypersensitivity to eggs (hives, swelling of the mouth and throat, difficulty breathing, hypotension, or shock). Protocols have been developed for vaccinating such egg-allergic children.[24] Children with allergies to eggs who are not anaphylactic may be vaccinated without problems. Persons with a history of anaphylactic hypersensitivity to neomycin should not be vaccinated. On theoretical grounds, vaccine should not be administered to a woman known to be pregnant. Measles vaccine is contraindicated in persons with immunodeficiency or immunosuppression. However, since measles disease may be severe or fatal in such persons, it should be administered to persons with asymptomatic human immunodeficiency virus (HIV) infection and considered for those with symptomatic infection (acquired immunodeficiency syndrome [AIDS] or AIDS-related complex [ARC]).

Vaccination of persons who received IG, whole blood, or other antibody-containing blood products should be postponed for 3 months to avoid potential interference with seroconversion. Vaccination should be postponed in persons with severe febrile illnesses. Persons with mild illnesses such as upper respiratory tract infections may be vaccinated.

Measles Elimination in the United States. In 1978 the goal to eliminate indigenous measles from the United States was established. The elimination strategy had three components: (1) achieving and maintaining high immunization levels, (2) strong surveillance, and (3) aggressive outbreak control. The most important component was high immunization levels. The enactment and enforcement of comprehensive school immunization laws covering all students, from kindergarten through high school, have been instrumental in achieving high levels. States with strict enforcement policies had significantly lower incidence rates than states without those policies.[25] Careful surveillance included establishing active surveillance systems in which persons likely to see students with measles were queried periodically. A national case definition was instituted. A probable case of measles was defined as an illness with (1) fever (≥101° F [≥38.3° C], if measured), (2) generalized rash of ≥3 days' duration, and (3) either cough, coryza, or conjunctivitis. A confirmed case was one that met the definition given above and that was epidemiologically linked to another case or to any case with laboratory confirmation. Aggressive outbreak control consisted of defining zones of risk for transmission, establishing a target population, and vaccinating that population. In school-based outbreaks, exclusion of students lacking proof of immunity played a key role in terminating transmission.[16] Despite the major success in measles control, indigenous measles still occurs in the United States.

Measles elimination has proved to be more difficult than initially anticipated. However, elimination remains the goal, and new strategies recommended by the ACIP and the AAP should eventually lead to elimination. Full implementation of the two-dose schedule should prevent measles in school- and college-age populations. Modification of school laws and prematriculation immunization requirements for college students will need to be vigorously pursued if the two-dose schedule is to be successfully implemented. However, elimination will not be accomplished unless means are found to deliver a first dose of vaccine at the recommended age to all children. Immunization levels for measles at 2 years of age, particularly those in inner city populations, have been found to be as low as 49% in some inner city populations.[20]

Worldwide Control and Elimination. Measles poses a substantial health problem in both the developing and the developed world. Factors predisposing infected persons to complications and death are young age, crowding, malnutrition, and coincident respiratory or gastrointestinal illness. Before immunization, almost 2.5 million children died from measles or measles-related complications annually.[26] In the developed world, measles vaccine is usually recommended during the second year of life, typically at 12, 15, or 18 months of age, depending on the country. In contrast, in the developing world, measles vaccine is generally administered in a single dose at 9 months of age. This younger age was chosen for two reasons. First, measles attack and complication rates are often high during the first year of life in the developing world. Waiting until the second year would result in substantial morbidity and mortality rates. Second, seroconversion rates after measles vaccination at 9 months of age are higher in developing countries than in developed countries.

In developing countries it is particularly important to vaccinate sick children. Often, they are at greatest risk of measles complications, and nosocomial spread of disease is common.

A major problem with measles in the developing world is its occurrence in infancy, when standard Schwarz and Moraten vaccines are not maximally effective because of interference by maternal antibody. Recent data show that the Edmonston-Zagreb (EZ) strain of measles vaccine, a strain attenuated in human diploid cells, may be as effective at 6 months of age as the Schwarz vaccine at 9 months of age.[27] In the future, there will likely be increasing use of the EZ vaccine, particularly in high-risk areas of the developing world, at 6 months of age and perhaps at younger ages.

In the developed world, measles control is dependent on motivation of national health care providers. In the developing world, limited financial resources and managerial skills are problems.

European health authorities have set the year 2000 as a goal for measles elimination in Europe. The English-speaking Caribbean countries have set a goal of elimination by 1995. In addition to the United States, substantial success in measles control has been achieved in such countries as Czechoslovakia, Cuba, Canada, Finland, Sweden, Germany, and Costa Rica.

Mumps

Paul A. Stehr-Green
Stephen L. Cochi

Hippocrates described mumps (epidemic parotitis) as a distinct clinical entity in the fifth century BC. Knowledge of the clinical illness has improved over the past two centuries with the awareness that orchitis and meningoencephalitis are relatively common complications. Isolation of the virus and development of a safe, effective vaccine have led to a dramatic decline in mumps-associated morbidity and mortality rates in the United States. When given in combination with measles and rubella vaccines, mumps vaccine reduces the costs associated with mumps by more than 86%.[1]

Etiological Agent, Immunology, and Diagnosis. Mumps is caused by an RNA virus of the myxovirus group. Man is the only known reservoir. Transmission occurs after direct contact with, or droplet spread from, an infected person. The incubation period ranges from 14 to 21 days, with an average of 18 days. Virus may be excreted from 7 days before to 9 days after clinical onset of disease. Infections (up to one third of which are subclinical) induce apparently long-lasting immunity; reports of second attacks have lacked epidemiological, virological, or serological, confirmation.

Diagnosis is usually made on clinical grounds. Assay for neutralization antibody is both sensitive and specific but is time-consuming and not readily available. Similarly, radial hemolysis and enzyme-linked immunoassay (EIA) tests provide accurate results but are not widely available. For both screening and diagnosis of acute infection, the complement fixation (CF) antibody test may be nonspecific (cross-reaction with parainfluenza) and the hemagglutination inhibition (HI) antibody test has been shown to be insensitive. The mumps skin test has also been shown to be an unreliable diagnostic or screening tool. For epidemiological purposes, the use of serologic tests with established reliability (neutralization, enzyme immunoassay, and radial hemolysis antibody tests) is recommended. Recently, experimental techniques have become available to distinguish vaccine from wild mumps viruses.[2]

Clinical Characteristics. Mumps is a generalized viral infection. The most common clinical manifestations are mild to moderate fever and painful unilateral or bilateral parotid gland swelling[3]; however, other viruses (such as parainfluenza and coxsackie virus) and bacteria may also cause parotitis. Prodromal symptoms—including anorexia, headache, vomiting, and myalgia lasting for 12 to 48 hours—are present in some cases. Inflammation of other salivary glands may occur alone or in combination with the parotitis. The usual uncomplicated illness resolves completely in approximately 10 days.

Complications. Among the reported mumps-associated complications, strong epidemiological and laboratory evidence for an association with meningoencephalitis, deafness, and orchitis has been reported.[4] Meningeal signs appear in up to 15% of cases. Reported rates of mumps encephalitis range as high as 5 cases per 1000 reported mumps cases, and adults are at higher risk than children. Permanent sequelae are rare, but the reported encephalitis death-case ratio has averaged 1.4%. Although the overall mortality rate is low, death caused by mumps infection is much more likely to occur in adults; about half of mumps-associated deaths have been in persons ≥ 20 years of age.[4] Sensorineural deafness is one of the most serious of the rare complications involving the central nervous system (CNS). It occurs with an estimated frequency of 0.5 to 5.0 per 100,000 reported mumps cases. Orchitis (usually unilateral) has been reported as a complication in 20% to 30% of clinical mumps cases in postpubertal males.[3] Some testicular atrophy occurs in about 35% of cases of mumps orchitis, but sterility rarely occurs. Symptomatic involvement of other organs has been observed less frequently. There are limited experimental, clinical, and epidemiological data suggesting that mumps infection may rarely result in permanent pancreatic damage from direct viral invasion. Further research is indicated to determine whether mumps infection contributes to the pathogenesis of diabetes mellitus. Mumps infection during the first trimester of pregnancy may increase the rate of spontaneous abortion (reported to be as high as 27%).[5] There is no evidence that mumps during pregnancy causes congenital malformations, although mumps virus has been shown to cross the placenta and infect the fetus.

Occurrence. There appear to be no geographical differences in the clinical presentation or epidemiology of mumps infection, nor has a clear-cut epidemic cycle been observed for mumps. Cases follow a seasonal pattern, with the peak occurrences in winter and spring. After the introduction of the live mumps virus vaccine in 1967 and recommendation of its routine use in 1977, there was a steady decrease in the incidence rate of reported mumps cases in the United States (Fig. 5–2). In 1985 a record low of 2982 cases was reported, representing a 98% decline from the 185,691 cases reported in 1967. However, the recent epidemiology of mumps has been characterized by a change in the age distribution of reported cases. Between 1985 and 1987 the annual reported incidence rate rose almost fivefold. In 1988 a total of 4866 cases was reported, representing a 62% decrease compared with the 12,848 cases reported in 1987.[6]

As in the prevaccine era, the majority of reported mumps cases still occur in school-aged children (5 to 14 years of age); at least 85% to 90% of persons in the United States are thought to acquire mumps antibody by 15 years of age. However, for the first time since mumps became a reportable disease, the reported peak incidence rate shifted, in 1986, 1987, and 1988, from 5- to 9-year-old children to 10- to 14-year-old children. The increased occurrence of mumps in susceptible adolescents and young adults has been demonstrated in several recent outbreaks in high schools, on college campuses,[7,8] and in occupational settings.[9] Both the shift in risk to older persons and the relative resurgence of reported mumps activity noted in recent years are attributable primarily to the relatively underimmunized cohort of children born between 1967 and 1977.[10] Although primary vaccine failure undoubtedly has played some role, there is no evidence of waning immunity in persons vaccinated previously, estimates of mumps vaccine effectiveness from outbreak investigations having ranged from 75% to 91%.[10]

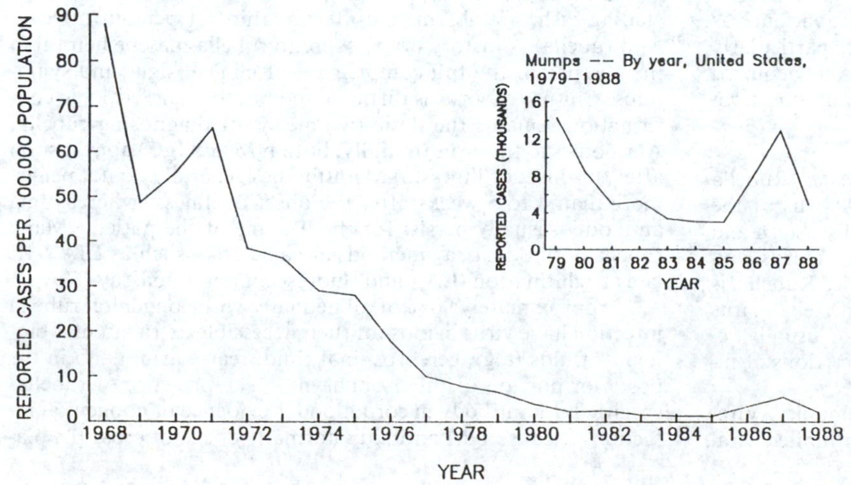

Figure 5–2. Number of cases of mumps, by year, in the United States, 1968–1988.

Lower incidence rates have been demonstrated in states with laws requiring mumps immunization for school attendance. In 1987 the lowest incidence rates (1.1 cases per 100,000 population) were reported from the District of Columbia and from the 14 states with comprehensive laws requiring proof of immunity to mumps for school attendance from kindergarten through grade 12, and the highest rates (11.5 cases per 100,000 population) were in the 14 states that had no requirements for mumps vaccination.[6]

Strategy for Prevention. There is no worldwide agreement regarding the necessity of preventing mumps infection. The principal strategy to remove the burden of mumps illness employed in the United States is through achieving and maintaining high immunization levels. Programs aimed at vaccinating children with mumps as well as measles and rubella vaccines (preferably as combined MMR vaccine) should be established. In the United States, mumps vaccine as part of MMR vaccine has been demonstrated to be highly cost-effective.[11]

A killed virus vaccine was developed in 1948 but did not provide lasting protection. In 1967 the Jeryl Lynn strain of live attenuated vaccine was licensed.[12] It induced seroconversion in more than 95% of recipients in clinical trials and was found to be noncommunicable and safe. Minimal side effects were reported during large-scale field trials. Epidemiological studies have generally shown vaccine effectiveness in excess of 85%.[13,14] Vaccine-induced immunity is expected to be lifelong.[15,16]

In the United States, mumps vaccine is recommended to be given to all susceptible persons born after 1956 at any age after 12 months, unless vaccination is contraindicated.[15] When given with measles vaccine, it should be given generally at 15 months of age. Persons should be considered susceptible to mumps unless they have documentation of (1) physician-diagnosed mumps, (2) adequate immunization with live mumps virus vaccine on or after their first birthday, or (3) laboratory evidence of immunity. Persons who are unsure of their mumps disease history and mumps vaccination history should be vaccinated; there is no evidence that persons who have previously either received mumps vaccine or had mumps are at any increased risk of local or systemic reactions from live mumps vaccine. Serological and skin tests for immunity may be misleading, unreliable, or simply unavailable and should not be routinely performed before immunization.[17]

There is no evidence that vaccination with mumps vaccine given after exposure provides protection in persons already infected, nor is there any contraindication to the vaccine's use.[8] The vaccine has not been observed to increase the severity of disease, and if the exposure did not result in infection, it should induce protection against subsequent infection. IG given after exposure to mumps will not reliably prevent infection or viremia and is not recommended. Mumps IG is not available or licensed for use in the United States.

Contraindications to vaccination include pregnancy, recent administration of IG, altered immunity, severe febrile illnesses, and anaphylactic allergy to eggs or to neomycin. Egg allergy is not an absolute contraindication to vaccination; such persons can be vaccinated with caution if published protocols are followed.[18,19]

Further decline in mumps incidence can be achieved by maintaining high immunization levels, primarily in infants and young children. However, a greater emphasis on vaccinating susceptible adolescents and young adults and more aggressive outbreak control measures have been recommended in light of the recent relative resurgence of mumps in the United States.[17] It is of special interest that transmission has been documented in health care settings, indicating the need to incorporate routine mumps vaccination programs for health care personnel into similar programs to prevent measles and rubella transmission.[20]

Rubella

Paul A. Stehr-Green
Stephen L. Cochi

In 1941 an epidemic of congenital cataracts in Australia was observed in the wake of a large outbreak of rubella. A usually mild and self-limited illness assumed new importance because of its ability to induce congenital defects in infants of women who acquire rubella during pregnancy. Subsequent success in developing and making available an effective vaccine to prevent rubella has been a major public health achievement. Because vaccine has not been administered to all susceptible persons, particularly women of childbearing age, a low level of postnatally acquired and congenital rubella infection, with its full array of long-term sequelae, persists in the United States.

Etiological Agent, Immunology, and Diagnosis. Rubella (German or 3-day measles) is caused by an RNA virus of the togavirus group. Other agents in this group include eastern and western equine encephalomyelitis viruses, yellow fever virus, and dengue viruses. Man is the only known reservoir. Rubella is highly communicable but less so than measles or varicella. Virus is transmitted by the respiratory route, and infection usually occurs as a result of contact with nasopharyngeal secretions of infected persons by droplet spread.

Primary rubella infection induces lifelong immunity. Viremia and infection of nasopharyngeal tissues with limited viral shedding has been rarely detected after reinfection with rubella virus in persons with either natural or vaccine-induced immunity. However, there is no demonstrable risk of communicability, and such reinfection in a pregnant woman apparently poses minimal, if any, risk to the unborn fetus.[1]

Clinical diagnosis is often unreliable because symptoms, including rash, are absent in up to one third of persons infected with rubella. A history of exposure to rubella may be helpful in the absence of the full complement of clinical signs and symptoms. Culture of virus is difficult and unreliable. Serologic confirmation remains the definitive means of diagnosing rubella. Antibodies to the virus (initially, both IgM and IgG) appear soon after the onset of illness. IgM antibodies generally do not persist more than 4 to 5 weeks after the onset of illness, whereas IgG antibodies usually persist for the lifetime of the patient. Many rubella antibody assay methods are available, such as EIA, HI, latex agglutination (LA), and fluorescent immunoassay (FIA).

Approximately 90% of all neonates with congenital rubella infection have virus in most of their accessible extravascular biological fluids (e.g., cerebrospinal fluid, tears, urine) and in the posterior portion of the oropharynx.[2] The presence of rubella-specific IgM antibody in cord blood is evidence of congenital infection, because IgM antibody normally does not cross the placenta. The presence and persistence of rubella-specific IgG at higher-than-expected levels post partum (the half-life of maternal antibodies is 1 month) are also suggestive of intrauterine infection.

Clinical Characteristics

Postnatal Infection. Rubella is an acute, mild disease in children and young adults. The first symptoms occur after an incubation period ranging from 14 to 21 days. Communicability begins about 7 days before onset of rash and persists at least 4 days after rash onset. The cardinal manifestations of the disease are a nonspecific maculopapular rash lasting 3 days or less (hence the term "3-day measles"), although rubella may occur without a rash, and generalized lymphadenopathy, particularly of the postauricular, suboccipital, and posterior cervical lymph nodes. The rash, which is often the first sign of illness, appears first on the face and then spreads downward rapidly to the neck, arms, trunk, and extremities; pruritus is not unusual. In adolescents or adults, the rash may be preceded by a 1- to 5-day prodrome of low-grade fever, headache, malaise, anorexia, mild conjunctivitis, coryza, sore throat, and lymphadenopathy. The manifestations rapidly subside after the first day of the rash. Exanthems comparable to that observed with rubella infection have been described in infections with echovirus and coxsackievirus, fifth disease, other enteroviral infections, and mild measles; these infections, however, are not commonly associated with postauricular or suboccipital adenopathy.

Prenatal Infection. The major disease burden of rubella virus is congenital infection. Primary rubella infection during pregnancy, whether clinical or subclinical, carries a significant risk of fetal infection. Congenital rubella is often associated with a disseminated and chronic infection that may persist throughout fetal life and for many months after birth. Spontaneous abortion, stillbirth, or congenital rubella syndrome (CRS) can result from chronic infection and inhibition of cell multiplication in the developing fetus. Delayed and deranged organogenesis and hypoplastic organ development lead to the characteristic structural defects; Table 5-1 lists manifestations associated with congenital rubella infection. Transplacental infection is not always reflected by immediately apparent disease; as many as 50% to 70% of infants with congenital rubella infection may appear normal at birth. Deafness is the most common later-onset manifestation. Other, relatively less frequent effects, including delayed developmental milestones to learning, and speech, behavioral, and psychiatric disorders, have been described.[3] Endocrinopathies such as thyroiditis with hypothyroidism or hyperthyroidism, diabetes mellitus, and Addison's disease have also been occasionally reported to be late sequelae.

Congenital infection is not inevitable, however, and the fetal response to infection is not uniform; the gestational age of the conceptus at the time of primary maternal infection is the principal factor influencing the outcome of pregnancy. The risk of CRS as a consequence of maternal infection in the first trimester may be as high as 70%,[4] but the risk decreases sharply after the eighth week and is absent after the twentieth week of gestation.

TABLE 5-1. MANIFESTATIONS OF CONGENITAL RUBELLA INFECTION

- Spontaneous abortions
- Stillbirths
- Bone lesions
- Cardiac defects
  - Patent ductus arteriosus
  - Pulmonary stenosis and coarctation
  - Myocardial necrosis
- CNS defects
  - Encephalitis
  - Mental retardation
  - Microcephaly
  - Progressive panencephalitis
  - Psychomotor retardation
  - Spastic quadriparesis
- Deafness
- Endocrinopathies
  - Adrenal disorders
  - Diabetes mellitus
  - Precocious puberty
  - Growth retardation
  - Growth hormone deficiency
- Eye defects
  - Cataracts
  - Glaucoma
  - Microphthalmos
  - Retinopathy
- Genitourinary defects
- Hematologic disorders
  - Anemia
  - Thrombocytopenia
  - Immunodeficiencies
- Hepatitis
- Interstitial pneumonitis
- Psychiatric disorders

Complications. Although rubella is a mild disease in children, it may be more significant with complications in adults.[5] Arthralgia and arthritis may occur in adults, particularly women, at a reported rate as high as 70%. Joint involvement usually occurs after the rash fades and typically lasts 5 to 10 days, although it occasionally may persist to chronic arthritis. Rare complications include optic neuritis, thrombocytopenic purpura, and myocarditis. Postinfectious encephalitis of short duration may occur 1 to 6 days after the appearance of rash; its incidence rate is estimated at 1 in 5000 to 16,000 cases.

Occurrence. In temperate climates, rubella is endemic year-round, with a regular seasonal peak during springtime. In tropical areas, rubella is widespread. Before the advent of rubella vaccination, major epidemics of rubella tended to occur at 6- to 9-year intervals. The last major epidemic of rubella in the United States occurred in 1964 and 1965 (Fig. 5-3), and resulted in an estimated 31,000 cases of rubella and congenital rubella infection in an estimated 12,500,000 pregnancies; of these cases, 11,000 resulted in fetal death or therapeutic abortion and 20,000 infants were born with CRS. However, the incidence of rubella has declined by >99% since 1969, the year that rubella vaccine was licensed. Long-term trends of rubella incidence indicate that rates have declined by ≥95% for all age groups, with the greatest decreases occurring among persons <20 years of age. In 1988 a total of only 225 cases of rubella were reported.[6] As of September 1989, only three cases of CRS in children born in 1988 were reported, although the actual number of CRS cases may be as much as tenfold higher.[7] Despite the marked drop in incidence, it is estimated that up to 15% of adolescents and young adults remain susceptible.[8-10] Transmission of rubella has continued to occur in the postpubertal population, with more than half of all cases occurring among persons ≥20 years of age in recent years.[6]

Strategy for Prevention. Since licensure of live attenuated rubella virus vaccines in 1969, efforts to control rubella in the United States have been directed primarily at preschool and ele-

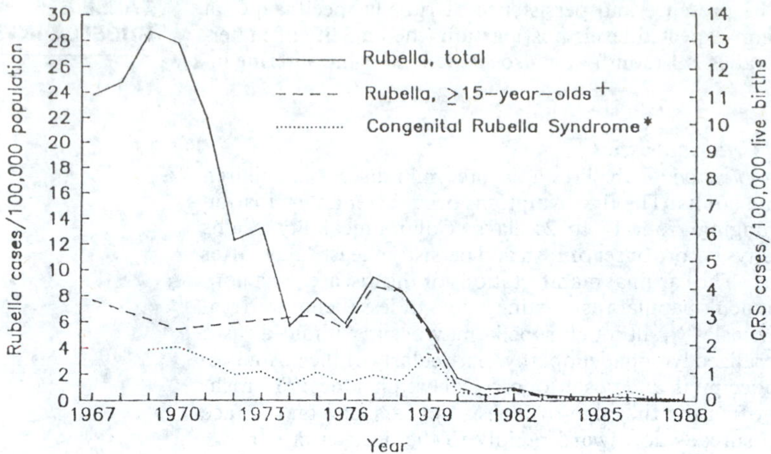

+Includes proration of patients ≥15 years old for whom age was unreported. Average annual U.S. estimate based on data from Illinois, Massachusetts, and New York City for the 3-year periods 1966–1968, 1969–1971, and 1972–1974.
* Confirmed and compatible cases, by year of birth. Provisional data due to delayed diagnosis and reporting.

Figure 5-3. Incidence rates of reported rubella and congenital rubella syndrome [*CRS*] cases, United States, 1967–1988.

mentary schoolchildren of both sexes. It was reasoned that, in addition to protection of children, circulation of the virus would be greatly reduced or interrupted, and susceptible pregnant women would be protected indirectly by virtually eliminating the risk of exposure. As noted above, although this strategy has substantially reduced the incidence of rubella and congenital rubella infection in the United States, elimination has not been attained and serological surveys of postpubertal populations have shown rates of rubella susceptibility only slightly lower than in prevaccine years. An alternative approach to the universal immunization of children to prevent congenital rubella infection that has been implemented elsewhere (e.g., in the United Kingdom*) prescribes immunization of only girls at approximately 11 to 14 years of age, accompanied by vaccination of all susceptible adult women of childbearing age. It was anticipated that this approach would not reduce the total number of cases of rubella but would have a direct protective effect as these girls enter their childbearing years. Indeed, there was little change in the reported occurrence of rubella and CRS in the United Kingdom through the mid-1980s, and major epidemics occurred in 1978, 1979, 1982, and 1983; however, serological evidence indicates that the proportion of young adult women who are susceptible has declined in recent years. Any approach to the control of rubella and the elimination of CRS requires special attention to currently susceptible women of childbearing age.

In 1969, three rubella vaccines were licensed for use in the United States: the HPV-77 strain, prepared in duck embryo cell culture; the HPV-77, prepared in dog kidney cell culture; and the Cendehill strain, prepared in rabbit kidney cell culture. In 1979 the RA 27/3 strain, which is prepared in human diploid cells, was introduced and has since been the only rubella vaccine that is distributed for use in the United States. In ≥95% of vaccinees, all these vaccines induce antibodies that have been shown to persist for >16 years,[12] indicating that immunity is durable and probably lifelong. Most of those persons who lack detectable antibody by standard tests have been shown to have antibody by more sensitive tests and have almost always shown laboratory evidence of secondary infection without detectable viremia when exposed to either natural disease or revaccination.

In the United States, rubella vaccine is recommended for all susceptible persons at any age after 12 months, unless vaccination is contraindicated.[13] Rubella vaccination is most cost-effective when offered as MMR vaccine. When given with measles vaccine, it should routinely be given at 15 months of age. Persons should be considered susceptible to rubella unless they have documentation of (1) adequate immunization with rubella virus vaccine on or after their first birthday or (2) laboratory evidence of immunity. Persons who are unsure of their rubella disease or vaccination history or both should be vaccinated.

Rubella vaccine given after exposure may not provide protection, but there is no contraindication to its use. The vaccine has not been observed to increase the severity of disease, and if the exposure did not result in infection, it should induce protection against subsequent infection. Immune globulin (IG) given after exposure to rubella will not reliably prevent infection or viremia but may only modify or suppress symptoms. Infants with congenital rubella have been born to women given IG shortly after exposure. The routine use of IG for postexposure prophylaxis of rubella in early pregnancy is not recommended unless abortion would not be considered under any circumstances.

Children sometimes have vaccine side effects, such as low-grade fever, rash, and lymphadenopathy. As many as 40% of vaccinees in large-scale field trials had joint pain, usually of the small peripheral joints, but frank arthritis has generally been reported in fewer than 2% of subjects. As with natural disease, vaccine-associated arthralgia and transient arthritis occur more frequently and tend to be more severe in women than in men or children. As many as 3% of susceptible children have been reported to have arthralgia, and arthritis has been reported only rarely in these vaccinees; in contrast, 10% to 15% of susceptible female vaccinees have been reported to have arthritis-like symptoms. With both natural and vaccine-associated disease, these symptoms usually have not caused disruption of activities and most often have not persisted. However, "wild" rubella infection in adults is associated with a higher incidence, greater severity, and more prolonged duration of joint manifestations than are seen after rubella immunization.[13] Transient peripheral neuritic complaints, such as paresthesias and pain in the arms and

**Beginning in October 1988 the United Kingdom instituted a policy of vaccinating all children with MMR vaccine at 1 to 2 years of age, in addition to vaccinating all girls with single-antigen rubella vaccine at 10 to 14 years of age.[11] This change in strategy was intended to circumvent several of the problems inherent in the original strategy—namely, the need for mass serological screening of postpubertal females, the risk of multiple exposures of pregnant women to rubella, and the continued high rate of therapeutic abortions as a result of exposure.*

legs, have also very rarely occurred. Reactions such as these usually occur only in susceptible vaccinees; persons who are already immune to rubella, either because of rubella vaccine or natural disease, are not at increased risk of local or systemic reactions as a result of receiving live rubella vaccine.

Because of the theoretical risk to the fetus after exposure to attentuated rubella vaccine virus, 1221 women who inadvertently received rubella vaccine within 3 months before or 3 months after their presumed date of conception were examined between 1971 and 1988.[14] All 290 infants born to 538 women vaccinated during pregnancy with either Cendehill or HPV-77 rubella vaccine through April 1979 were free of defects compatible with CRS, although eight infants had serological evidence of intrauterine infection. Through Dec. 31, 1988, the vaccination of 683 women with the RA 27/3 rubella vaccine within 3 months of conception was also reported. Among the 272 women who were known to be susceptible at the time of vaccination, outcomes of pregnancy are known for 254 (93%); 83% delivered living infants, all 212 of whom were free of defects associated with CRS. Rubella-specific IgM was detected in three infants, but all three were normal on physical examination. These data are consistent with results reported from other countries in that they show no evidence that rubella vaccine can cause defects associated with CRS.

Nonetheless, although no CRS-like defects have been noted, rubella vaccine should not be given to women known to be pregnant. In view of the importance of protecting women of childbearing age, however, reasonable practices in a rubella immunization program should include (1) asking women if they are pregnant, (2) excluding from the program those who say they are, and (3) explaining the theoretical risks to the others before vaccinating.[13,14] The vaccine should also not be given to those with immunodeficiency diseases or compromised immune systems as a result of disease or treatment because of the theoretical possibility that replication of the vaccine virus can be potentiated. Other contraindications to vaccination are recent administration of IG, and severe febrile illness.

Indigenous rubella and CRS can be eliminated from the United States. Much of the success in rubella control in the United States can be attributed to comprehensive school immunization laws; all 50 states have enacted laws requiring rubella vaccination at school entry, and in 41 states and the District of Columbia the students at all grade levels are included. The major problem remaining is to reduce the persisting susceptibility levels in postpubertal females. Vaccination of women not known to be pregnant and without a history of vaccination is justifiable without serological testing, particularly when the costs of testing are high and follow-up of identified susceptible women for vaccination is not ensured. Programs to identify and vaccinate high-risk groups might include premarital screening and vaccination of susceptible women, prenatal screening followed by postpartum vaccination of susceptible women, establishment of requirements for proof of rubella immunity for college entry, and routine vaccination of all hospital employees, volunteers, trainees, and physicians, both male and female.

Rubella remains uncontrolled in much of the developed as well as the developing world. As described earlier, two basic strategies exist for the prevention of congenital rubella infection: (1) vaccination of only girls at about the time of puberty to provide individual protection during their childbearing years and (2) vaccination of all children of both sexes at an early age to interrupt transmission as well as to provide protection during girls' subsequent childbearing period. Combinations of these strategies have been undertaken in some countries, with vaccination of all children at age 1 year, combined with vaccination of adolescent girls to reduce rubella transmission and to provide future protection of those about to enter the childbearing period. Other countries have combined vaccination of children of both sexes at age 1 year and at ages 6 to 12 years to shorten the period necessary to achieve a fully immunized childhood population and to interrupt transmission. If rubella is added to a country's childhood immunization schedule, it is most cost-effective when offered as combined MMR vaccine.

Pertussis

Stephen L. Cochi
Steven G. F. Wassilak
Alan R. Hinman

Pertussis is a highly communicable, vaccine-preventable disease that lasts for many weeks and is typically manifested in children with paroxysmal spasms of severe coughing, whooping, and vomiting. It is caused by infection with *Bordetella pertussis,* a bacillus first isolated in 1906 by Bordet and Gengou. Because other etiological agents may also cause the symptom complex suggestive of pertussis and because clinical pertussis is frequently not confirmed by laboratory means, the constellation of symptoms is often referred to as the "whooping cough syndrome." Whooping cough also may be caused infrequently by *Bordetella parapertussis* and by the animal pathogen *Bordetella bronchiseptica.* Evidence that adenoviruses can cause the syndrome has been disputed.

Clinical Characteristics. The main clinical feature of classic pertussis is spasmodic, paroxysmal coughing (i.e., the sudden onset of repeated violent coughs without intervening respirations). The onset of illness is insidious. During the first 1 or 2 weeks of illness, coryza is accompanied by shallow, irritating, nonproductive coughing, which gradually changes into deep spasms of paroxysmal coughing. The child generally remains well and free from cough between paroxysms. As the coughing attacks become more severe, they are commonly followed by inspiratory whooping or vomiting. After a week or so of paroxysmal coughing, the disease peaks in severity and begins to subside, although convalescence is protracted. Leukocytosis and lymphocytosis are generally present during the early paroxysmal stage of the disease.

Adults, partially immunized persons, and infants younger than 6 months of age do not commonly have the repeated typical paroxysms, but a clinical diagnosis may be suggested by a history of a severe or persistent cough before or after exposure to a known case. Asymptomatic infection can be demonstrated in a small minority of household contacts of a patient, but whether long-term carriage occurs is not known.

Complications. The major complications, including hypoxia, pneumonia, malnutrition, seizures, and encephalopathy, are most common in younger patients. The following rates of complications were estimated from a large population-based study in the United Kingdom.[1] Fifteen percent of children younger than 5 years of age with pertussis are hospitalized (60% of those younger than 6 months). Pneumonia (primary or secondary) complicates the course of at least 2% of patients; seizures, possibly caused by hypoxia or toxin-mediated events or both, occur in 0.4%. Encephalopathy occurs in 2 to 6 per 10,000 patients. Patients who die of encephalopathy generally had evidence of hypoxic damage or hemorrhage without inflammation. Death occurs in 0.17% of patients (0.7% of patients younger than 1 year of age). In the developing world, it is estimated that 1.5% of patients die.

Long-term complications include residual neurological deficits and, both in the preantibiotic era and currently in the developing world, substantial permanent lung damage.

Bacteriology and Pathogenesis. *B. pertussis* is a small, fastidious, gram-negative coccobacillus. Isolation requires a complex medium that contains blood or charcoal or both, on which it appears as a small, pearly colony.

The presence of agglutinogens permits serotyping of *B. pertussis* strains. The possible role of agglutinogens as virulence factors and in the acquisition of immunity against pertussis is controversial. Pili possessing the agglutinogens are apparently responsible for the specific attachment of *B. pertussis* organisms to the site of infection.

Pathologically, pertussis is a superficial respiratory infection, primarily of the subglottic respiratory tract. Systemic invasion does not occur. Pathological specimens from patients demonstrate focal bronchial epithelial necrosis and inflammation. Pertussis appears to be a toxin-mediated disease resulting from local infection.[2] The products or antigens of *B. pertussis* that may be responsible for the local or systemic pathophysiological events, or both, include endotoxin, tracheal cytotoxin, extracytoplasmic adenylate cyclase, filamentous hemagglutinin (FHA), and pertussis toxin (PT), an inhibitor of cellular adenylate cyclase regulation that has many physiological effects and that is also known as lymphocytosis-promoting factor (LPF), islet cell-activating factor, or histamine-sensitizing factor. PT is considered responsible for the lymphocytosis and hypoglycemia that may be seen in whooping cough. PT and adenylate cyclase are considered important mediators of altered immunological and phagocytic function. FHA is derived from the pili (fimbriae) of the organism and may mediate its attachment to respiratory epithelial cells.

Diagnosis. Laboratory confirmation of the clinical diagnosis can be difficult. Culture specimens are best obtained by passing a fine wire tipped with Dacron or calcium alginate through the patient's nose to the posterior portion of the nasopharynx. Swabs are streaked on Bordet-Gengou, Regan-Lowe, or other appropriate agar medium. A selective antimicrobial agent, such as cephalexin, greatly enhances recognition of pertussis colonies by suppressing the overgrowth of normal flora. The plates must be incubated for at least 3 to 5 days.

Recovery of *B. pertussis* from patients is affected by prior vaccination or antimicrobial therapy and by the stage of illness. If nasopharyngeal specimens are collected from children during the early stages of the disease and cultured on proper media, an experienced laboratory technician can isolate *B. pertussis* from up to 80% of patients with clinical disease who have had no prior vaccination or antimicrobial therapy. The frequency of positive cultures diminishes rapidly beginning with the third week after onset of paroxysmal cough.

During acute infection, increases in antibody titer of agglutinins (antibodies to the specific surface agglutinogens of *B. pertussis*) or of class-specific antibodies (as measured by EIA) to several cellular components, including PT and FHA, can be useful in diagnosis. However, the first of paired serum specimens must be collected soon after cough onset for these tests to be of value.[3]

Diagnosis can also be made by direct fluorescence antibody (DFA) staining of mucous smears from nasopharyngeal swabbings. Specific adsorbed antisera, the inclusion of positive and negative controls, and experienced personnel are needed to maximize the reliability of this method. Rates of false-positivity and false-negativity can be high.

Immunity. The mechanism of immunity in pertussis is not well understood. After natural infection, a rise in serum antibody levels in most patients can be observed by agglutination testing or EIA measurement of class-specific antibodies to PT or FHA. The timing of the appearance of humoral antibody and local IgA corresponds roughly to the disappearance of culturable organisms from the nasopharynx. Immunity against clinical whooping cough induced by natural infection is believed to be long lasting. Neonates are apparently generally susceptible to pertussis, suggesting short-term or no protection from immunoglobulins that cross the placenta.

The components of *B. pertussis* that induce protective antibody in humans have not been precisely identified. The protective effect of whole-cell pertussis vaccine in humans, as measured by its effect on the secondary attack rate in household contacts, correlates well with its potency in protecting mice against intracerebral challenge with the organism. In the mouse potency test, mice are inoculated intraperitoneally with dilutions of the vaccine being tested or with the U.S. standard pertussis vaccine. Fourteen days later the mice are challenged intracerebrally with live pertussis bacteria and then observed for 14 days. Protection is determined by comparing the survival rates in recipients of the test vaccine and of the standard vaccine.

Persons with titers of circulating agglutinins of 1:320 or higher are usually protected against pertussis; however, persons with lower or nondetectable titers may also be protected.[3] Current speculation regarding immunity is that protective antibody may either prevent attachment of *B. pertussis* to ciliated epithelial cells by combining with surface components, such as FHA, or neutralize circulating PT or other toxin(s) produced by virulent organisms.[2]

Transmission. Pertussis is spread from person to person by respiratory droplets and is among the most contagious of diseases. The secondary attack rate in unimmunized susceptible household contacts averages 90%.

The incubation period is usually 7 to 10 days (range 4 to 21 days). The period of communicability probably begins approximately 1 week after effective exposure. A child is considered most infectious during the early stages of the disease. By 3 weeks after onset of paroxysmal coughing, culture positivity rapidly declines.

Occurrence. Pertussis occurs worldwide. The Expanded Programme on Immunization of the World Health Organization (WHO) estimates a global total of 60 million cases of pertussis per year, with approximately 700,000 deaths. In countries without an immunization program, WHO estimates that 80% of surviving newborn infants acquire pertussis in the first 5 years of life. In a longitudinal study in Machakos, Kenya, an annual incidence rate of 13 per 1000 total population was observed; the case-fatality rate was 1.2% (3.2% among infants).

Pertussis is widely underrecognized and underreported in the United States. During the period from 1986 through 1988, on the average, 3500 cases were reported annually in the United States. Approximately two thirds were confirmed by laboratory testing, by either culture or DFA. Among laboratory-confirmed cases, 40% were confirmed by culture and the remaining 60% by DFA alone. Of patients whose ages were known, 42% were less than 1 year of age and 25% were 1 to 4 years of age. There is no striking geographical or seasonal distribution in U.S. cases. Twenty-six deaths from pertussis were recorded from 1986 through 1988 in the United States. The case-fatality ratio was 0.3% overall; for infants younger than 6 months of age, the ratio was 0.5%.

The reported incidence of pertussis in the United States has decreased >99% since 1940 (Fig. 5-4), in large part because of the use of whole-cell pertussis vaccines. However, morbidity and mortality rates for pertussis had begun falling, although at a slower rate, before the introduction of pertussis vaccine, indicating that other factors may affect the occurrence of *B. pertussis* in the community.

With the introduction and widespread use of vaccine, the age-specific incidence and clinical manifestations of reported pertussis have changed; the incidence of the disease is now highest in infants too young to receive adequate immunization (i.e., at least three doses) (Fig. 5-5). In addition, recent outbreaks have highlighted the important role that older children and adults (in whom pertussis often is unrecognized) play in transmitting the agent. Several outbreaks have been centered in hospitals, indicating that young professional staff, even though immunized in childhood, can act either as the source or as the recipients of nosocomial pertussis.

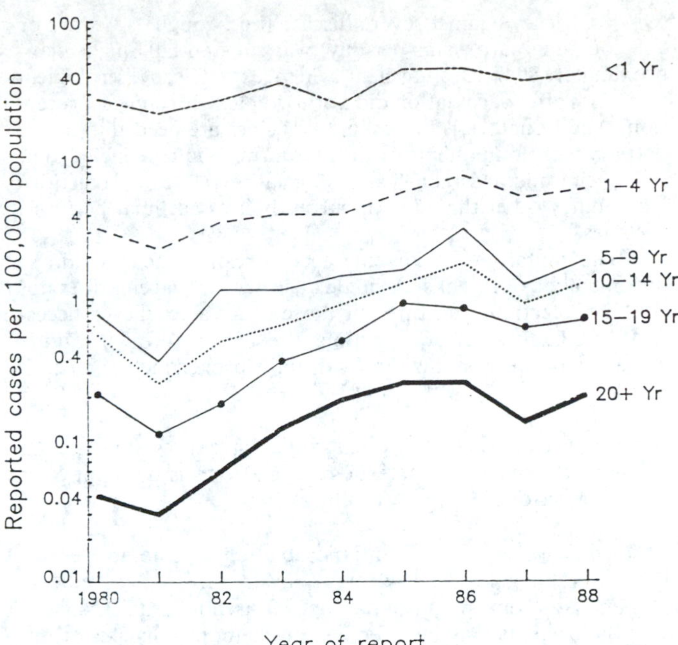

Figure 5-5. Incidence of reported cases of pertussis (MMWR data) by age group in the United States, 1980–1988.

Strategy for Prevention and Control

Active Immunization. Active immunization is the only method of proven value in the prevention of pertussis. Since the mechanisms of disease and immunity are unclear, current vaccines continue to consist of formaldehyde-treated or heat-treated whole cell preparations. Aluminum salt adsorbents have been used to decrease side effects of vaccine preparations, generally without affecting immunogenicity. Although immunogenicity of the vaccine in young infants is not as good as in older children, it is recommended that immunization begin at 6 to 8 weeks of age because the disease is most often life-threatening in young infants. Pertussis vaccine is generally available and is given in combination with diphtheria and tetanus toxoids (DTP vaccine). Three doses are given 4 to 8 weeks apart, and a reinforcing dose is given approximately 9 to 12 months later. A booster is recommended at 4 to 6 years of age.[4] The efficacy of immunization in preventing disease in household contacts of a patient with pertussis is good initially (70% to 90%) but apparently begins to wane in several years. One study showed efficacy to be 79% in the first 3 years, 53% after 4 to 7 years, 35% after 8 to 11 years, and essentially nil 12 years after immunization.[5] When pertussis does occur in immunized persons, it tends to be milder than in the unimmunized.[1]

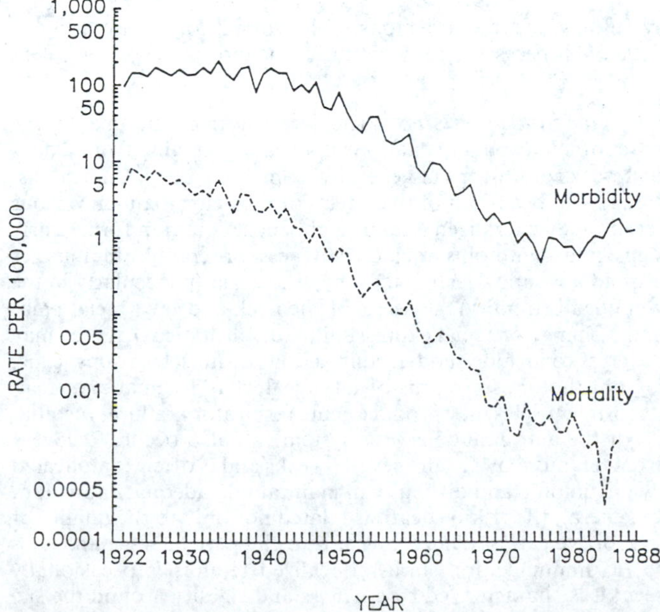

Figure 5-4. Morbidity and mortality rates for pertussis cases in the United States, 1922–1988. Mortality data are not available for 1987 and 1988.

Fever (temperature ≥38° C [≥100° F]) or local reactions (pain and swelling) occur in approximately half of vaccinees after pertussis or DTP immunization. Seizures or a peculiar shocklike reaction characterized by pallor, unresponsiveness, and spontaneous recovery ("hypotonic-hyporesponsive episodes") have followed the administration of pertussis vaccine; in a recent large cohort study the rate of either seizures or the shocklike state was 1 in 1750 injections each.[6] Other studies have not found as high a rate of seizures. Unusually high-pitched, persistent screaming has been reported in 0.1% of vaccinees. Permanent brain damage has rarely been reported after pertussis immunization; from a case-control study in the United Kingdom, that occurrence has been estimated at 1 in 330,000 injections.[7] However, several methodological questions have raised doubts about the accuracy of this estimate, or even whether any measurable risk exists.

When the mechanisms of pathophysiology and immunity are better understood, a highly purified-component, acellular vaccine may be feasible. In the interim, several products high in FHA, moderately high in PT, and low in endotoxin, and some containing measurable quantities of immunogenic outer membrane protein, have been used in Japan. These products are effective and have been associated with fewer common adverse reactions than whole cell vaccines.[8] However, these vaccines have not been used routinely in children younger than 2 years of age.

Two Japanese acellular pertussis vaccines (one with PT and FHA and the other with PT only) have been evaluated in infants in a placebo-controlled, randomized clinical trial in Sweden.[9] The results indicated clinical efficacy of two doses of each vaccine, but the level of protection was less than anticipated (54% to

69%). Efficacy against severe disease (i.e., cough >30 days or >8 coughing paroxysms per day) was substantially higher, approximately 80%. Despite clear evidence of efficacy, serological responses after vaccination did not correlate with clinical protection. Additional trials of acellular vaccines are needed to better define which components of the organism should be included in the vaccine and to establish a serological correlate of protection. No country other than Japan currently uses acellular pertussis vaccines.

The limitations of current vaccines restrict their usefulness in controlling outbreaks. A single dose of DTP vaccine does not confer protection, and three or more doses are believed necessary to reliably confer protection. Prevention through routine age-appropriate immunization is the only proven method of control.

Passive Immunization. Controlled studies have shown that human pertussis IG given for postexposure prophylaxis does not alter the incidence or the severity of illness.

Chemoprophylaxis. Several antimicrobial agents, notably erythromycin (50 mg/kg per day for 14 days), consistently eradicate *B. pertussis* from the nasopharynx. Household studies suggest that these agents may be effective for chemoprophylaxis of unimmunized persons exposed to pertussis; however, no prospective studies have confirmed this observation. Similarly, it has been suggested that these agents may be of some benefit when given in the earliest, catarrhal phase of the illness; they have no clear beneficial effect when given after the onset of paroxysmal coughing. The major role of antimicrobial agents is to decrease communicability and therefore shorten the period of isolation. In general, children may be permitted to return to school during the fourth week after the onset of paroxysmal coughing. Children treated with effective antimicrobial agents probably become noninfectious within 5 days.

Risks and Benefits of Pertussis Vaccine. In the United States, as in some other industrialized nations, the lay and scientific media have recently paid increased attention to pertussis vaccine risks. In the United Kingdom, media portrayals of children in whom neurological impairments occurred after they received pertussis vaccine led to a substantial decline in public acceptance of the vaccine. This decline was followed by two large pertussis epidemics before vaccine coverage again increased to levels that prevented additional such epidemics. In Japan, when all pertussis vaccine was rapidly removed from use as a precautionary measure after deaths associated temporally with vaccine administration, a similar experience occurred. These experiences have helped prevent exaggerated negative public responses in the United States. However, as the number and cost of claims against U.S. manufacturers have increased, the cost of available vaccine has increased greatly and the number of manufacturers has declined. It is hoped that a recently enacted vaccine injury compensation program may stabilize prices and supply.

Benefit-cost analyses of pertussis vaccine have repeatedly demonstrated the advantages of continuing pertussis vaccination.[10] The quest for safer and yet equally effective vaccines continues.

Tetanus

Steven G. F. Wassilak
Edward W. Brink

Although tetanus is not a communicable disease, its prevention has high public health priority throughout the world because the disease has a high case-fatality ratio and because, with the wide availability of an effective and safe toxoid, it is almost completely preventable. Tetanus is now an uncommon disease in developed countries but is still common in developing countries, particularly among neonates.[1]

Etiological Agent, Pathogenesis, and Diagnosis. *Clostridium tetani,* the etiological agent, was identified by Kitasato in 1889. It is an anaerobic, gram-positive rod that exists in both vegetative and sporulated forms. The spores are highly resistant to heat and chemical agents but can be destroyed by sterilization procedures.

Tetanus spores can survive for years if not exposed to deleterious influences. As a result, spores are ubiquitous in nature and are found in soil, dust, animal feces, and, less commonly, human feces, and on human skin. Germination and multiplication of tetanus bacilli are favored by the presence of necrotic tissue and the lack of oxygen at the site of inoculation.

The *C. tetani* bacillus produces an exotoxin, tetanospasmin, a potent selective neurotoxin responsible for clinical tetanus. Tetanospasmin travels along motor nerves generally after being disseminated through the bloodstream. It fixes to gangliosides in skeletal muscle, the spinal cord, the brain, and the autonomic nervous system. Tetanus infection may not confer immunity.

The diagnosis of tetanus depends on clinical signs and symptoms. Neither a demonstrable wound nor the isolation of *C. tetani* is necessary for a definitive diagnosis.

Clinical Characteristics. The interval from trauma to the onset of clinical manifestations is variable, ranging from 2 days to 3 weeks or longer but generally from 6 to 8 days. Clinical disease is wholly a result of the effects of the neurotoxin on various receptors. Generalized tetanus is the most common form. Early signs and symptoms include stiffness or cramps in muscles around a wound, deep tendon hyperreflexia (particularly in the wounded extremity), stiffness of the neck and jaw, facial pain, and a change of facial expression (risus sardonicus). These may progress to include sudden contractions of muscle groups, causing opisthotonos. Spasms of laryngeal, diaphragmatic, and intercostal muscles may produce acute respiratory failure. Instability of the autonomic nervous system can also occur. Recovery from tetanus may require several weeks and is often complicated by pneumonia and difficulty in maintaining adequate nutrition. In general, the risk of death is related not only to the quality of supportive care provided but also to the patient's age and, less so, to immunization status. Localized tetanus is occasionally seen; it is characterized by stiffness and rigidity around the site of injury and usually resolves without sequelae.

Neonatal tetanus occurs after contamination of the umbilical stump at or following delivery, usually in the circumstance of an unattended delivery or of one attended by an untrained midwife. In some areas of the world, the cord is cut with an unclean object or the umbilical stump is traditionally covered with contaminated materials.

Occurrence. Tetanus can occur as a complication of puncture wounds, compound fractures, abrasions, burns, injections, surgery, animal bites, gastrointestinal infections, abortions, childbirths, and infections of the umbilical stump. Puncture and deep wounds are more hazardous than superficial abrasions. Abscesses and chronic skin ulceration may permit infection and lead to tetanus. Illicit injectable drug use carries a risk of this disease. Tetanus has occurred not uncommonly after innocent-appearing wounds and in instances where no wound could be recalled.

The incidence rate of tetanus in the United States declined substantially from 1947 through the early 1970s.[2] Since then, there has been a more gradual decline in the annual incidence rates. A total of 101 cases were reported in 1987 and 1988; 92% of cases occurred in persons 20 years of age or older and 67% in persons 50 years of age or older. In recent years the incidence rates of tetanus in blacks and other minority groups were twice the rate in whites. Both age and ethnic differences tend to reflect the disparities in the immunization status of these groups. A recent limited serosurvey in the United States indicated that as many as two thirds of persons 60 years of age or older lacked protective levels of circulating antitoxin against tetanus.[3] The case-fatality ratio has declined in the last decade but remains 20% to 30% in reported cases, with a poorer prognosis for tetanus in elderly patients and in neonates.

In many developing countries, mortality rates for tetanus neonatorum have been estimated at 10 to 30 or higher per 1000 live births. Worldwide neonatal tetanus currently accounts for approximately 800,000 deaths annually and represents 90% of the total deaths from tetanus in developing countries.[1]

Prevention. Preexposure active immunization with tetanus toxoid offers the best and most efficient method of preventing tetanus. Tetanus toxoid is one of the most effective of the immunobiologic agents and has been used on an increasing scale since the mid-1930s. The results of active immunization of U.S. Army personnel during World War II showed the value of the toxoid. Only 12 cases occurred among 2.73 million wounded or injured personnel (0.44/100,000) compared with 70 cases among 0.52 million wounded or injured during World War I (13.4/100,000).[4]

Both aluminum phosphate adsorbed (4 to 10 Lf) and fluid single-antigen tetanus toxoid (4 to 5 Lf) preparations are available. Tetanus toxoid is available alone or combined with 10 to 15 Lf of diphtheria toxoid and pertussis vaccine, adsorbed, as DTP, combined with 10 to 15 Lf of diphtheria toxoid, adsorbed, as DT, for use in children less than 7 years of age, and combined with less than 2 Lf of diphtheria toxoid, adsorbed, as Td, for use in older persons. The adsorbed toxoid preparations are currently recommended for primary immunization and booster doses.[5] In general, tetanus toxoid should be given as DTP, DT, or Td to provide concurrent protection against diphtheria with or without protection against pertussis. Because of the declining risk of serious cases of pertussis and the increasing frequency and severity of reactions to diphtheria toxoid with increasing age, neither DTP nor DT is routinely recommended for persons 7 years of age or older.

Although two doses of single-antigen, adsorbed tetanus toxoid provide temporary protection, a third dose should be given at least 6 to 12 months later to complete the primary series. When given as DT or Td, a primary series should consist of three doses, and when it is combined with both diphtheria toxoid and pertussis vaccine as DTP vaccine, a primary series should ideally consist of four doses of DTP vaccine. The interval between the first and second doses of DT or Td and between the first, second, and third doses of DTP should be 4 to 8 weeks. The last dose of the primary series should be given approximately 1 year later.

Available evidence indicates that a complete primary series with a tetanus toxoid–containing preparation provides long-lasting protective levels of circulating antitoxin—10 years or more—in most recipients. Rarely has a case of tetanus been reported in a person with a documented primary series of toxoid injections. Consequently, after complete primary tetanus immunization, booster doses of tetanus toxoid need be given only once every 10 years.[6]

Although immediate hypersensitivity to tetanus toxoid does occur infrequently, a history of such a reaction should be confirmed by skin testing with appropriately diluted toxoid before a decision is made to discontinue further tetanus toxoid immunization.[7] Major local reactions have been reported, particularly in adults who have received doses more frequently than is generally recommended.[8]

The management of wounds includes evaluation of the wound, adequate wound cleaning and débridement, and evaluation of immunization status.[5,9] A careful attempt should be made to determine how many doses of toxoid a person has received previously.

The major obstacle to appropriate active and passive prophylaxis in wound management is the difficulty of obtaining an accurate immunization history. A record of immunizations carried by each person would obviate this problem. Patients with unknown or uncertain previous immunization histories should be considered to have received no previous tetanus toxoid. Patients who have not completed a primary series require tetanus toxoid at the time of wound cleaning and débridement and may require passive immunization, preferably with human tetanus immune globulin (TIG) (Table 5-2).

If the patient has completed a primary series or received a booster dose within the preceding 10 years, and if the wound is judged to be clean and minor, no further toxoid is necessary. A small proportion of vaccinees do not maintain a protective level of antitoxin for 10 years. If a patient sustains a wound that is judged to be other than clean and minor, and if the tetanus toxoid primary series was completed or a booster dose received more than 5 years before, a booster dose is required. Persons with a clean, minor wound and less than three known previous doses of toxoid need only a dose of toxoid at the time of initial treatment. For patients with wounds with an increased risk of tetanus and less than three known previous doses of toxoid, appropriate passive immunization is indicated at the time of wound treatment in addition to a dose of toxoid. Subsequently, all inad-

TABLE 5-2. SUMMARY GUIDE TO TETANUS PROPHYLAXIS IN ROUTINE WOUND MANAGEMENT

History of Absorbed Tetanus Toxoid Doses	Clean, Minor Wounds		All Other Wounds[a]	
	Td[b]	TIG	Td[b]	TIG
Unknown or less than 3	Yes	No	Yes	Yes
3 or more[c]	No[d]	No	No[e]	No

[a] Such as, but not limited to, wounds contaminated with dirt, feces, soil, saliva; puncture wounds; avulsions; and wounds resulting from missiles, crushing, burns, and frostbite.

[b] For children less than 7 years old, DTP (DT, if pertussis vaccine is contraindicated) is preferred to tetanus toxoid alone. For persons 7 years of age and older, Td is preferred to tetanus toxoid alone.

[c] If only three doses of fluid toxoid have been received, a fourth dose of toxoid, preferably an absorbed toxoid, should be given.

[d] Yes, if more than 10 years since last dose.

[e] Yes, if more than 5 years since last dose.

From MMWR 34:405–414, 419–426, 1985.

equately immunized patients should receive complete primary immunization.

When passive protection is indicated, 250 to 500 units of TIG given intramuscularly and concurrently with toxoid is an appropriate regimen for protection against tetanus.[10] Tetanus toxoid and TIG should be given at separate sites. Protection from TIG can be expected to last about 3 weeks. The use of equine antitoxin has serious disadvantages compared with the use of TIG, including short-lived protection, serum sickness, and occasionally anaphylaxis.

The treatment of tetanus includes TIG in dosages of 3000 to 6000 units intramuscularly to neutralize circulating tetanus toxin, antibiotics, and débridement to help eliminate the organism and thereby prevent further toxin production. In addition, intensive primary medical and supportive care is critical.

Neonatal Tetanus Prevention. Neonatal tetanus is currently unusual in the United States because the vast majority of deliveries are appropriately attended and because routine immunization in childhood for several decades has resulted in a high percentage of immunized women of childbearing age.[11] Active immunization of unimmunized pregnant women with two doses of appropriately timed toxoid prevents tetanus neonatorum. In the developing world an effective strategy of preventing tetanus neonatorum includes increasing the proportion of attended births and providing two or more doses of tetanus toxoid to women of childbearing age, pregnant or not. Additional doses can be given with each pregnancy. Five adult doses are likely to provide lifelong protection against neonatal tetanus.[12]

Summary. All persons should receive active primary tetanus immunization, preferably combined with diphtheria toxoid (and, if appropriate for age, pertussis vaccine), and booster doses once every 10 years. Health care providers should use every encounter a person has with a health service to evaluate immunization status and administer needed immunizations.

Diphtheria

Edward W. Brink
Steven G. F. Wassilak

Bretonneau first defined diphtheria as a distinct clinical entity in 1826. Even with the availability of an effective and safe toxoid, diphtheria continues as an important cause of morbidity and death in developing countries, particularly among children, and as a cause of occasional small outbreaks in developed countries.

Etiological Agent, Pathogenesis, and Diagnosis. The causative organism of diphtheria is *Corynebacterium diphtheriae,* a gram-positive, nonmotile bacillus and obligate parasite of man that was first described as the etiologic agent by Loeffler in 1884. The organism is killed if held at 60° C for 20 minutes but survives freezing and desiccation for months when enclosed in proteinaceous materials.

C. diphtheriae causes disease by first establishing a superficial infection. Necrotic debris, exudate, and bacteria coalesce to form the membrane. The toxin acts by inhibiting protein synthesis; this facilitates local cell destruction and invasion and causes the systemic manifestations of infection.[1] With further multiplication of the bacteria, the membrane extends and the absorption of toxin into the bloodstream increases. Only circulating, unbound toxin can be neutralized by diphtheria antitoxin. Lysogeny of diphtheria strains with the coryneform bacteriophage carrying the toxin structural gene confers the ability to produce toxin. Strains that are not in a lysogenic state (i.e., nontoxigenic) are generally less virulent. Lysogenic conversion of nontoxigenic strains to toxigenic probably can occur within a colonized person.[2]

Diphtheria transmission is generally by droplet spread from either active cases or carriers. Untreated, a patient generally remains infectious for 2 weeks or less. Chronic carriage may occur rarely and even after antimicrobial therapy. Transmission from cutaneous cases can be a result of environmental contamination or of skin contact.

The characteristic features of a fully developed diphtheritic membrane suggest the possibility of the disease in most instances. Specific diagnosis depends on the recovery of the organism. Methylene blue or other stains may not be reliable because of inexperienced personnel or the presence of nonpathogenic corynebacteria in the normal flora. If the patient has not been receiving antibiotics, the bacillus can be recovered by culture on a tellurite-containing medium, Loeffler's medium, or a blood agar plate. For transport, Loeffler's medium can be used, but if a long delay is anticipated, swabs should be transported in silica gel. Toxigenicity of the diphtheria organism may be determined by in vivo and in vitro tests of isolates.

Clinical Characteristics. The incubation period of diphtheria is 1 to 7 days. Both respiratory tract and cutaneous infections occur. In uncomplicated disease, mild local symptoms occur and systemic symptoms such as fever and tachycardia are usually mild. In more severe forms of the disease, respiratory obstruction or toxin-induced complications or both occur.

Respiratory tract forms of diphtheria consist of pharyngotonsillar, laryngotracheal, nasal, and combinations thereof. Patients with pharyngotonsillar diphtheria usually have a sore throat, difficulty in swallowing, and low-grade fever at presentation. Examination of the throat may show only mild erythema, localized exudate, or a membrane. The membrane may be localized to a patch of the posterior pharynx or tonsil, may cover the entire tonsil, or, less frequently, may spread to cover the soft and hard palates and the posterior portion of the pharynx. In the early stage a membrane may be whitish and may wipe off easily. The membrane may extend and become thick, blue-white to gray-black, and adherent. Attempts to remove the membrane result in bleeding. A minimal area of mucosal erythema surrounds the membrane. Patients with severe disease may have marked edema of the submandibular areas and the anterior portion of the neck, along with lymphadenopathy, giving a characteristic "bullnecked" appearance. Pseudomembranes may occur in infectious mononucleosis and other viral pharyngitides, as well as in streptococcal or monilial pharyngitis.

Laryngotracheal diphtheria most often is preceded by pharyngotonsillar disease, usually is associated with hoarseness and a croupy cough at presentation, and, if the infection extends into the bronchial tree, is the most severe form of disease. Initially it may be clinically indistinguishable from viral croup or epiglottitis. Nasal diphtheria, the mildest form of respiratory diphtheria, usually is localized to the septum or turbinates of one side of the nose. Occasionally a membrane may extend into the pharynx.

Nonrespiratory mucosal surfaces (i.e., the conjunctivae and genitals) may also be sites of infection.

Cutaneous diphtheria is common in tropical areas. It often appears as a secondary infection of a previous skin abrasion or infection. The presenting lesion, often an ulcer, may be surrounded by erythema and covered with a membrane. Patients are generally seen because of the chronicity of the skin lesion.

Complications. Antimicrobial therapy has significantly reduced the incidence of secondary bacterial complications. Heart and nervous system complications caused by the toxin are the most common and serious. Both toxigenic and nontoxigenic diphtheria strains can cause airway obstruction by extension or sudden displacement of the membrane into the larynx and the bronchial tree.

In cutaneous disease, infections with nontoxigenic strains are more common than with toxigenic strains. In all forms of the disease, toxigenic strains produce more severe local symptoms and can produce myocarditis and neuritis. In severe cases the toxin may cause interstitial nephritis with proteinuria or thrombocytopenia. Primary endotoxic manifestations of shock with disseminated intravascular coagulation rarely can occur.

Although the likelihood of toxin-induced myocarditis or neuritis is probably related directly to the extent of the local infection and therefore to the amount of toxin absorbed, either complication can occur after an otherwise clinically mild infection. Myocarditis may begin in the first through the sixth week of clinical illness. As many as one fourth of the patients may have electrocardiographic changes; a smaller proportion have clinically evident cardiac impairment with decreased heart sounds to overt congestive heart failure. Recovery may be complete, or, less frequently, persistent cardiac disturbances may result.

Cranial or peripheral neuritis, primarily involving motor loss, can develop 1 to 8 weeks or longer after onset of disease. Loss of visual accommodation, diplopia, nasal-sounding voice, and difficulty in swallowing are the most frequent manifestations of cranial nerve involvement. Complete recovery of neurologic impairment is the rule.

Mechanical airway obstruction and toxigenic myocarditis are the major causes of death.

Occurrence. The occurrence of diphtheria in the United States has fallen dramatically from 147,000 cases in 1920 to an annual average of three reported cases of respiratory diphtheria from 1980 through 1988. Twenty-one of the twenty-six cases reported in the United States during 1980 through 1988 affected persons 20 years of age or older. Limited serosurveys in the 1970s and 1980s in the United States indicated that 40% or more of adults lacked protective circulating antibody levels against diphtheria, and that the percentage lacking protection increased with increasing age.[3]

Although data from developing countries on the occurrence of diphtheria are incomplete, low immunization coverage, unfavorable socioeconomic conditions, and occasional reported outbreaks suggest that diphtheria remains an important, preventable disease in much of the world. Many persons show evidence of immunity in spite of having had neither overt disease nor toxoid immunization; their immunity was probably acquired as a result of mild or inapparent infection. As a result of frequent cutaneous infections, many children in tropical areas develop diphtheria antitoxin titers at a very early age; thus such persons are protected and epidemic potential is minimized.[4] With improvements in immunization coverage of children, the occurrence of the disease in children can be expected to decline.

Prevention and Control. In 1923, Ramon showed that formalin-treated toxin (now called toxoid) is effective in producing active immunity. With the development of a safer and more potent alum-precipitated toxoid in 1931, a sound basis for mass immunization campaigns was established.[4] By the early 1940s, diphtheria toxoid had achieved wide use in the United States.

Active Immunization. The rationale for active immunization is to induce and maintain adequate levels of circulating antitoxin that will neutralize exotoxin and minimize the extent of local invasion of the organism, thus preventing life-threatening systemic complications. Diphtheria toxoid, when given as a three-dose series, significantly reduces both the risk of diphtheria and the severity of clinical illness. Although the toxoid does not prevent or eliminate carriage of the organism in the pharynx or on the skin, its widespread use appears to have decreased diphtheria transmission in the United States. Diphtheria toxoid is available in combination with tetanus toxoid or pertussis vaccine or both as DTP, DT, or Td to provide concurrent protection against tetanus or pertussis or both. For children less than 7 years of age, DTP is recommended.[5] When contraindications to the use of pertussis vaccine exist, DT should be used. Both DTP and DT are prepared to contain 10 to 15 Lf of diphtheria toxoid per 0.5 ml dose. Three doses of DTP or DT are recommended at 4- to 8-week intervals beginning, when possible, at 2 months of age. A fourth dose is recommended approximately 12 months after the third dose. Because with increasing age the frequency and severity of local reactions increase, Td, which contains less than 2 Lf of diphtheria toxoid per dose, is the recommended agent for immunizing persons 7 years of age or older against diphtheria. For such persons a primary series consists of three doses, the first two given at an interval of 4 to 8 weeks and the third 6 to 12 months later. Protection after a primary series lasts for at least 10 years.[6] Booster doses are recommended at 10-year intervals. There is no need to restart a primary series regardless of the time elapsed between doses.

Treatment. Treatment of cases of respiratory tract diphtheria requires the use of diphtheria antitoxin (produced in horses) to neutralize circulating toxin. Antibiotic treatment with penicillin or erythromycin rapidly eliminates the organism and terminates toxin production. In addition, antibiotic treatment stops transmission to others. Treatment of clinically suspected noncutaneous diphtheria should begin promptly and without awaiting bacteriologic confirmation. Before administration of the antitoxin, the patient should be tested for sensitivity to horse serum and desensitized if necessary. Antitoxin dosage and route depend on the severity of disease, the interval between the onset of signs and symptoms and administration, and the recommendations of the manufacturer. Antitoxin doses range between 20,000 and 120,000 units. Serum sickness develops in approximately 5% of antitoxin recipients. It is important to point out that patients should also receive toxoid and, if unimmunized or inadequately immunized, should complete a primary series.

Management of Contacts of Patients With Suspected Disease. All household and other close contacts of patients with noncutaneous diphtheria should receive a dose of a diphtheria toxoid–containing preparation appropriate for their age unless they have received a booster dose or completed a primary series within the preceding 5 years. After bacteriologic culture, previously unimmunized or inadequately immunized symptom-free close contacts should receive prompt chemoprophylaxis with either intramuscularly administered benzathine penicillin (600,000 units for persons less than 6 years old and 1.2 million units for those 6 years old and older) or a 7- to 10-day oral course of erythromycin (30 to 50 mg/kg not to exceed 2 g/d). Primary immunization should be completed in persons who have received less than the recommended number of doses. Identified untreated carriers of toxigenic strains should receive antibiotics as described above. Bacteriologic cultures before and after receipt of antibiotics may aid in management of close contacts and carriers. Patients in whom antibiotic treatment with penicillin or erythromycin has failed should receive an additional 7- to 10-day oral course of erythromycin.

Conclusion. Even without evidence of substantial toxigenic *C. diphtheriae* circulation in the United States currently, high levels of immunization need to be maintained in all age groups of the general population because (1) toxoid confers individual protection against complicated disease; (2) asymptomatic carriage of the organism occurs; (3) lysogenic changes of nontoxigenic strains to toxigenic can occur in vivo, and (4) introduction by international travelers will continue. To accomplish the goal of high immunization levels, health care providers must consider every professional encounter with a patient as an opportunity to review and update the patient's immunization status.

Poliomyelitis

Peter A. Patriarca
Roland W. Sutter

Poliomyelitis, or infantile paralysis, is an acute infection caused by three serotypes of poliovirus that can range in severity from inapparent illness to flaccid paralysis or death. Although there is considerable evidence that poliomyelitis has afflicted mankind for thousands of years, the disease was not recognized as a distinct clinical entity until the late 1700s. Epidemic paralytic poliomyelitis became a notable public health problem in the United States and Western Europe in the late nineteenth and early twentieth centuries, with tens of thousands of cases reported annually.

Etiology. In 1908, Landsteiner and Popper experimentally induced paralytic disease in monkeys by intraperitoneal inoculation of spinal cord material from a patient with fatal poliomyelitis. It soon was shown in other experiments that the infectious agent was present in the nasopharyngeal secretions and stools of patients with symptomatic disease and of their symptom-free contacts.

In 1931, Burnet and Macnamara established that more than one virus strain can cause poliomyelitis. These closely related but antigenically distinct viruses were eventually designated as poliovirus types 1, 2, and 3 and are classified as picornaviruses belonging to the enterovirus group.[1] A major laboratory breakthrough occurred in 1949, when Enders, Weller, and Robbins successfully propagated polioviruses in tissue culture, paving the way for efficient growth of virus for ultimate production of vaccines.[2]

Pathogenesis. After introduction into the mouth, polioviruses replicate initially in the oropharyngeal mucosa and in Peyer's patches in the ileum after attachment to specific poliovirus receptors.[3] The virus then enters the bloodstream and disseminates to the central nervous system (CNS), where it preferentially attacks the motor neurons of the spinal cord and occasionally the brain stem. Infection of these cells results in death of the lower motor neurons and flaccid paralysis of the muscles they innervate. Death is usually a result of bulbar involvement with respiratory paralysis.

Infections with only limited involvement of the CNS may not produce the characteristic flaccid paralysis of poliomyelitis. Rather, they may cause illness with fever and evidence of meningeal irritation—stiff neck and back and elevated protein and leukocyte levels in the spinal fluid—followed by complete recovery. This syndrome is clinically identical to aseptic meningitis caused by other viral agents such as mumps virus, echoviruses, and coxsackieviruses. Most patients have no infection of the CNS and are symptom-free or have mild illness consisting of any combination of fever, malaise, headache with nausea, vomiting, constipation, diarrhea, and sore throat. The ratio of asymptomatic to symptomatic infection in most studies has varied from 100:1 to 1000:1.

Several factors appear to provoke or increase the likelihood of paralysis. These include the age of the patient at the time of infection, stress, pregnancy, tonsillectomy, adenoidectomy, exercise during the acute stages of infection, and injections.[4] Poliovirus type 1 is most commonly associated with paralytic illness, followed in order by types 3 and 2.

Epidemiology. After the development and widespread use of effective poliovirus vaccines in the United States and other industrialized countries, paralytic poliomyelitis has largely been eliminated as a public health concern.[5] The same success has yet to be achieved in much of the developing world, however, where an estimated 250,000 cases continue to occur each year.[6] Most of these cases are reported from tropical and subtropical regions, where crowding, poor sanitation, inadequate hygiene, and other factors are believed to facilitate transmission of wild polioviruses and other enteric pathogens.

Humans are the only known reservoir of poliovirus infection and harbor the agent in pharyngeal secretions and feces. The incubation period is most commonly 7 to 24 days, with a range of 3 to 36 days. Patients can be infectious for up to several weeks before symptoms develop; virus is subsequently excreted in pharyngeal secretions for a few days and in the stool for several weeks. Transmission occurs primarily via the oral-fecal route, particularly in settings where sanitation and personal hygiene are poor. In developing countries, poliomyelitis primarily afflicts infants less than 2 years of age, with boys being affected more often than girls.

During the past several years, considerable information has been obtained on the epidemiologic features of poliovirus transmission by using molecular techniques.[7] In contrast to influenza viruses, which tend to spread globally on an annual basis, most polioviruses appear to circulate within relatively small geographic areas, with only occasional instances of spread to adjacent countries. Furthermore, the advent of techniques combining polymerase chain reaction (PCR) and DNA probe technology will allow for enhanced detection of wild virus in sewage, water, and other environmental samples as an additional means of surveillance at the national, regional, and global levels.

Prevention and Control

Vaccine Development and Use. After Enders' successful propagation of poliovirus in human tissue culture, Salk used this method to prepare an inactivated poliovirus vaccine (IPV), which, after major field trials in 1954, was shown to be highly effective in preventing paralytic disease. Sabin and others soon developed live, attenuated strains of the three poliovirus types, which were ultimately incorporated into an orally administered, trivalent vaccine (OPV). Because of the ease of administration of OPV and improved effectiveness in preventing gut infection with wild polioviruses, Sabin's vaccine largely supplanted IPV for use in the United States beginning in the early 1960s.

The apparent elimination of indigenous spread of wild-poliovirus infections in the United States during the past decade can be attributed to the high degree of effectiveness of widespread immunization with poliovirus vaccines. After licensure of IPV in 1955, more than 450 million doses were administered to children and adults during the next 5 years. During this period the incidence of poliomyelitis declined precipitously from 18 cases per 100,000 total population to less than 2 cases per 100,000. After licensure of OPV in 1961, the incidence declined further to less than 1 case per 10 million population by 1970, with no known cases of indigenously acquired wild-virus infection after 1979.[8] Similar success has been achieved in other industrialized nations, as well as in a number of developing countries that have achieved high levels of coverage with three or more doses of OPV.[6]

Although both IPV and OPV are effective in preventing poliomyelitis, OPV continues to be the vaccine of choice for primary immunization of children in the United States.[9] Primary immunization with trivalent OPV consists of three doses at approximately 2, 4, and 15 to 18 months of age. A new, more potent inactivated vaccine was licensed for use in the United States in 1988 and is recommended primarily for persons with congenital or acquired immunodeficiency disorders.[10] A primary series of the new IPV also consists of three doses, which are usually administered on the same schedule as the OPV schedule. A supplementary dose of either vaccine should be given at school entry. The need for routine administration of additional doses of OPV or IPV has not been established, but immunity after a complete series of OPV is believed to be lifelong. However, one dose of either vaccine should be given to previously immunized adults who may be at increased risk of exposure to wild viruses.[10]

Regional and Global Eradication Initiatives. The apparent elimination of wild-poliovirus infection in the United States and other industrialized countries, coupled with the continued progress of the Expanded Programme on Immunization (EPI) toward achieving the goal of universal vaccination services for all children by 1990 (see Chapter 70), has engendered considerable interest in both regional and global elimination of poliomyelitis.[5] A formal initiative began in the western hemisphere in 1985 under the auspices of the Pan American Health Organization, which called for regional elimination in the Americas by the end of 1990. In view of substantial progress towards this goal—with only 279 (1.9%) of some 14,700 geopolitical units in the region having confirmed cases in 1988[11]—the forty-first World Health Assembly (1988) called for global eradication of poliomyelitis by the year 2000.[12] It is hoped that this goal can be achieved with a combination of strategies, including the achievement and maintenance of high immunization levels; the development of a standardized surveillance system to detect polio cases in a timely manner; assurances of vaccine quality control and the availability of adequate laboratory services to all countries; adequate training and supervision of in-country personnel; social mobilization; provision of rehabilitation services for affected patients; and additional research and development to maximize the effectiveness of polio vaccination, particularly in tropical and subtropical regions.[6]

Vaccine-associated Poliomyelitis. In spite of the apparent elimination of naturally occurring poliovirus infection in the United States and other industrialized nations, an epidemiologically distinct but rare clinical occurrence of vaccine-associated poliomyelitis has been observed since the introduction of OPV. Although the absolute numbers of vaccine-recipient or contact-associated cases have remained small—no more than 14 per year, with an average of approximately eight per year since 1980—such cases now account for the vast majority of all reported cases of poliomyelitis in the United States.[8] Although the exact risk of contracting vaccine-associated poliomyelitis is not known, it has been estimated that one case of vaccine-associated disease occurs for every 2.6 million doses of OPV distributed.[13] However, the relative frequency of paralysis associated with the first dose in the OPV series appears to be higher (1 case per 520,000 doses) than for subsequent doses (1 case per 12.3 million doses distributed). The type 3 vaccine strain causes paralysis most frequently, followed by type 2 and, more rarely, type 1.

The emergence of OPV-associated disease as the major form of paralytic poliomyelitis in the United States has generated considerable debate about current polio vaccination recommendations. Whether elimination of naturally occurring disease could be maintained with increased or exclusive use of the new, more potent IPV remains controversial, although such an approach would presumably reduce or even eliminate OPV-associated disease. A special Institute of Medicine panel convened by the U.S. Public Health Service in 1987 recommended that no change in vaccination policy be made at the present time.[14] However, in the hope of minimizing the number of cases of OPV-associated paralysis, the panel also recommended that a sequential schedule using both OPV and IPV be considered in the future when a combined preparation of DTP vaccine and IPV becomes available.

Influenza

William W. Lockwood

Influenza is an acute respiratory illness caused by influenza virus A, B, or C. Although frequently a mild or asymptomatic disease, influenza can be severe and even fatal. Influenza A or B usually occurs in epidemic outbreaks every winter. Worldwide outbreaks, which occur less frequently, are termed pandemics. Type C influenza is uncommon and has not been associated with epidemics. Unlike other classic viral diseases—smallpox, plague, yellow fever, and typhus—which have been eradicated or greatly controlled, influenza remains uncontrolled. Vaccination can decrease the attack rate and severity of disease, but because the virus regularly alters its two major surface proteins, elimination of the disease through vaccination directed at these antigens is at present unachievable.

History. Recurrent epidemics of influenza occur on an average of once every 1 to 3 years and can be traced back hundreds of years. As early as the fourteenth century, widespread outbreaks of rapidly spreading febrile respiratory diseases with high morbidity but a low case-fatality ratio were probably outbreaks of influenza. The term "influenza" resulted from an epidemic in 1357, which Buonissequi referred to as the "grande influenza."[1] The Italian word for "influence" was used as a collective term for various causes of widespread epidemics. Among them, cold weather, "influenza di freddo," was regarded for many years as a causal factor. Although conjecture on origin was lively when influenza was prevalent, interest waned between the major epidemics.

The pandemic of 1918–1919 demonstrated the potential devastation caused by influenza. Worldwide, an estimated 500 million persons were infected and 20 million persons died. In the era of AIDS, it is easily forgotten that influenza caused the most deadly epidemic of disease in recorded history. Although this pandemic is the foremost example, many other epidemics show the severe consequences of influenza on public health and economics.

The rapidity of the spread of influenza was probably best documented in the epidemic of 1957. A distinctive strain of influenza A was recovered in Hong Kong and Singapore in early April. The virus spread rapidly through the South Pacific, Southeast Asia, and the Middle East by June, and into Europe and North America by midsummer. By the end of 1957 the "Asian" strain of the virus had spread worldwide. In the United States, primary and secondary waves of cases resulted in nearly 70,000 deaths.

In contrast to earlier epidemics, the epidemic of the "Russian" strain of influenza A in 1977–1978 was remarkable in that the illness was largely confined to persons born after about 1955. Most adults in 1977 appeared to have possessed immunity as a result of infection with similar strains that had been present beginning in the late 1940s. Even so, major outbreaks occurred in children and young adults in the rest of the world during the next few months, and the rate of spread was parallel to that of earlier pandemic viruses.

The first influenza virus isolated was a type A virus from ferrets in 1933 by Smith et al.[2] Influenza B was first isolated in 1939 by Francis[3] and influenza C in 1950 by Taylor.[4]

Public health control measures such as widespread use of inactivated vaccines began in the 1950s. Since then, vaccines have been directed at selected segments of the population. Chemotherapy and prophylaxis with amantadine began in the United States in 1966.

Clinical Characteristics. Influenza usually occurs as an abrupt respiratory illness with fever, chills, fatigue, headache, myalgias, and nonproductive cough. Fever appears early (within 12 to 24 hours) and may reach 40° C (104° F). Early laboratory studies reveal a normal leukocyte count with a relative lymphopenia. The chest x-ray film usually shows only enlarged hilar shadows. Commonly, symptoms including fever last 3 days, after which convalescence begins. Recovery is usually rapid, although cough sometimes lasts for weeks.

Complications. Complications of influenza, although relatively uncommon, are usually pulmonary in nature. Either primary influenza virus pneumonia or a complicating bacterial pneumonia can occur, both of which can be severe, with an associated high mortality rate. Complicating bacterial pneumonias are reported in less than 1% of all patients with influenza and are most common in persons older than 60 years of age. Pneumococci, *Staphylococcus aureus,* and *Haemophilus influenza* are the most common causes of complicating bacterial pneumonias.

Nonpulmonary complications are less common. Cardiac complications, including pericarditis and myocarditis, although unusual, occur primarily in patients with pneumonia. Neurological syndromes such as encephalitis, transverse myelitis, and Guillain-Barré syndrome have followed influenza, but no definitive causal relationship has been proved. Children will occasionally acquire myositis after influenza. Reye's syndrome has been associated with influenza B more commonly than with influenza A.[5]

The effects of influenza infection on the fetus are controversial. Information regarding congenital defects and spontaneous abortion suggests that the fetus may be at increased risk, but the exact risk is unknown. The case-fatality ratio during pregnancy has been reported to be greater than that of the general population.

In the United States each year an excess 10,000 to 20,000 deaths are attributed to influenza, primarily in elderly persons. Deaths caused by pneumonia and influenza average about 5% to 6% of the total U.S. deaths and peak in the winter.[6] When deaths from pneumonia and influenza exceed the threshold for epidemics, influenza is almost always the cause (Fig. 5–6).

Etiology. Influenza virus is a medium-sized virus (80 to 120 nm) and is a member of the family Orthomyxoviridae. Usually spherical, the virus consists of single-stranded ribonucleic acid (RNA) enclosed in a helical protein shell, or capsid (9 to 10 nm in diameter), and covered by a lipid envelope.[7] Influenza viruses can be divided into three distinct types, A, B, and C, on the basis of their ribonucleoprotein (RNP), or soluble protein. Influenza A viruses have been isolated from humans, horses, swine, and avian species. Types B and C are almost exclusively recovered from humans, although type C influenza reportedly has now been isolated in pigs in China. Influenza C virus, which almost always causes a common cold–like illness, differs biochemically from types A and B and may eventually be assigned to another genus.

Projecting from the surface of the envelope are two distinct polypeptide "spikes," 8 to 14 nm long, both of which are highly antigenic. The more common of the spikes, the hemagglutinin (H), is the attachment site of the virus to human cells before phagocytosis and can cause agglutination of erythrocytes (hemagglutination). The second species, the neuraminidase (N), is about one fourth as frequent as the hemagglutinin and is an enzyme that splits neuraminic acid from mucoproteins. Neuraminidase is involved in releasing newly formed viruses from the host cell surface. Whether it provides other functions for the virus is less clear. Hemagglutinin can be subdivided into 12 or 13 distinct subtypes, and neuraminidase into nine.[8] Subtypes are numbered sequentially H1 through H13 and N1 through N9, respectively.

The nomenclature system for influenza virus in general use is from the World Health Organization (WHO) and consists of a strain designation followed by a description of the hemagglutinin and neuraminidase antigens. The strain designation for types A, B, and C includes, in order, the virus type, geographical origin, laboratory reference number, and year of occurrence. For example, the first type B strain isolated in Oregon in 1965 would be designated B/Oregon/1/1965. In influenza A viruses, a parenthesized description of the H and N antigens follows the strain designation: A/Mississippi/1/85 (H3N2). The WHO system is periodically revised as necessary to accommodate new information.[8]

Strains in any particular H or N subtype are interrelated, but relationships may differ widely, depending on the interval between isolation. For example, the H3N2 viruses isolated in 1968 and those isolated in 1983 can be readily distinguished in serological comparisons of their H or N antigens, although both cross-react with H3N2 strains isolated during the intervening years.

The influenza virus has the ability to change its surface antigens by either antigenic "drift" or "shift." Minor changes in either the H or N antigen is called antigenic drift.[9] In influenza A this occurs frequently and is responsible for the nearly annual epidemics. Although antigenic drift occurs in type B influenza, it is less common than in influenza type A. Major changes in the H or N antigen of type A strains is termed antigenic shift. Antigenic shifts are associated with influenza pandemics such as the pandemic that occurred in 1957, when type A "Asian" (H2N2) replaced type A (H1N1) influenza. Antigenic shift of the hemag-

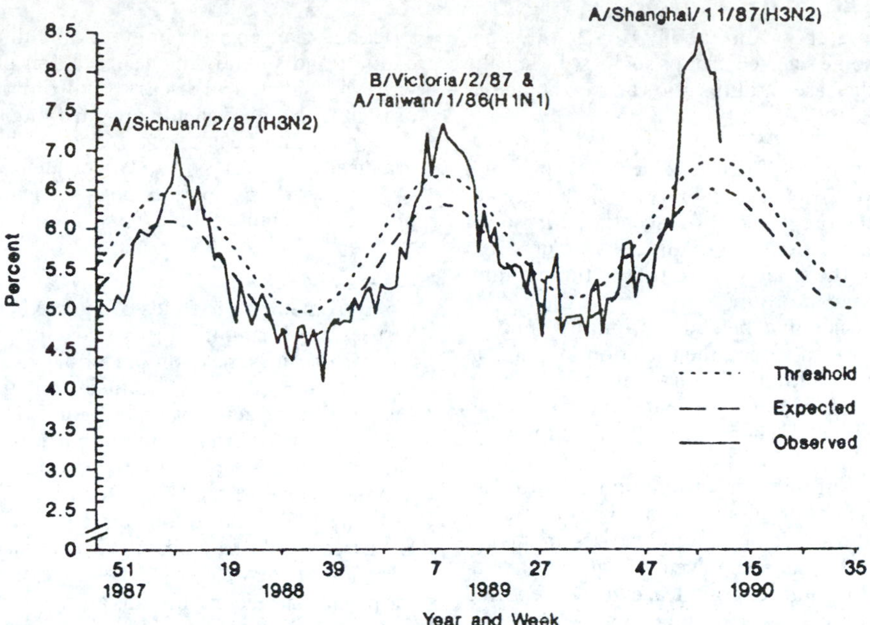

Figure 5-6. Pneumonia and influenza deaths as a percentage of total deaths in the United States, from October 1988 to March 3, 1990. Data were reported to the Centers for Disease Control from 121 U.S. cities. Pneumonia and influenza deaths include all deaths for which pneumonia is listed on the death certificate as a primary or underlying cause or for which influenza is listed on the death certificate. The predominant strains are shown above the peak mortality rate for each season. The epidemic guideline (threshold) for each season is 1.645 standard deviations above the expected baseline, estimated by using a periodic regression model applied to observed percentages since 1983. This baseline was estimated by using a robust regression procedure.

glutinin has occurred several times in the last century, but a shift of the neuraminidase has occurred only once—in 1957.

After the emergence of a new H or N subtype, antigenic drift occurs infrequently. New variants appear more and more frequently until the next major change or antigenic shift occurs. Antigenic drift is therefore thought to result from selection of preexisting mutants because of pressure from increasing immunity in the population to previous strains. When there is sufficient immunity in the population as a result of minor viral changes (antigenic drift) to allow the virus to escape the immunity, then major antigenic changes (antigenic shift) occur with a resultant pandemic. The most popular explanation of antigenic shift is a genetic recombination of human and animal strains.[10]

It has been thought by some that newer strains "replace" older strains in a continual, linear fashion. For example, H1N1 strains were commonly isolated until 1957, when H2N2 strains appeared. The H2N2 strains were the predominant strains isolated until they were replaced in 1968 by H3N2 strains. Recently, however, several strains have coexisted at the same time and mixed infections have occurred but are not common.

The virus is thought by others to "recycle" its surface antigen by having a previously predominant strain that has disappeared return as the common isolate.[11] There is no evidence that recycling is predictable.

Influenza Virus Surveillance. Because of frequent changes in the surface antigens of the influenza virus and the resultant epidemics, the WHO established in 1947 an international network to collect and disseminate laboratory and epidemiological data. The laboratory surveillance effort is aimed primarily at (1) monitoring influenza infection in humans and animals, (2) characterizing antigenic changes in prevalent viruses to trace their evolution, and (3) detecting antigenic changes that may signal an updated formulation of influenza vaccines.

Virus can be isolated from throat swabs, nasal swabs and washes, and sputum. Cultures can be grown in primary monkey kidney cell culture and in certain continuous cell lines.[12] Successful virus recovery is dependent on early collection of specimens (up to 72 hours from the onset of illness), proper transport to the laboratory, and proper culture techniques. The isolation can be confirmed with hemadsorption inhibition, hemagglutination inhibition, or serum neutralization. Direct or indirect fluorescent antibody staining of nasal mucosal cells aspirated from patients have also been used for rapid diagnosis. Serological tests are available and consist of type-specific complement fixation, tests using ribonucleoprotein antigen, and strain-specific hemagglutination inhibition tests employing selected viral antigens. Positive test results require a fourfold rise between paired acute and convalescent serum drawn 2 to 3 weeks apart. Since such tests require a delay in processing, serologic findings are not helpful in making an early diagnosis. Thus a diagnosis of influenza is usually a clinical diagnosis based on history, physical examination, season, and known presence of influenza in the community.

Epidemiology

General Characteristics. Influenza occurs worldwide. In the tropics, influenza occurs year-round in an endemic pattern, but epidemics can also occur (in any season). In temperate climates, cases usually occur in an epidemic pattern in winter and early spring. Physical conditions such as ambient temperature, low humidity, relative intactness of mucous membranes, and closeness of personal contact are believed to contribute to the seasonality of cases of influenza. Pandemics can occur at any time and follow a major antigenic shift.

Influenza A epidemics are more common than influenza B epidemics. The reason is the slower rate of antigenic variation of type B strains. The virus is transmitted by respiratory secretions via an airborne route. The incubation period is short, only 1 to 3 days. Viral shedding usually begins 1 to 2 days before symptoms begin and generally lasts about 1 week, most predominantly during the acute illness, when fever is present.

Although frequently a mild disease, influenza can cause

death. It has a low case-fatality ratio, about 1 or 2 deaths per 2000 cases; however, in some selected groups such as chronically ill and elderly persons, the case-fatality ratio can be as much as 30%.

Epidemic-Pandemic Potentiality. Influenza occurs in epidemics and pandemics because of the high mutability of the surface antigens of the virus and the prevalence of susceptible persons in the population. Thus the infectiousness of any new variant strain depends on the novelty of the strain with respect to the immunologic experience of the exposed groups.

Influenza infects susceptible persons, primarily children and young adults, who in turn spread the infection to adults in their homes and in the community.[13] Transmission between adults occurs but is less important than that from younger to older persons, except, perhaps, when distinctly new strains appear.

The first evidence of influenza in a community is often an explosive outbreak in a school or nursing home. The outbreak is often found to have been preceded by sporadic cases or clusters of cases either overlooked or unrecognized. Frequently a dramatic increase in the number and geographical extent of reported outbreaks and visits to physicians or hospital emergency clinics for medical care confirms the spread of the disease. In circumscribed geographical areas, epidemics reach peak levels within 2 to 3 weeks and resolve for the next month.

Attack rates show that 10% to 25% of the population in a community encounter the influenza virus during mild to moderately brisk epidemics in the United States. Some population subgroups have markedly differing experiences, however, because of enhanced susceptibility or increased chances of exposure. For example, while 40% to 60% or more of children who ride crowded school buses may be having cases of influenza, suburban adults without children can appear to be completely uninvolved in the same outbreak.

The "influenza season" usually lasts about 3 to 4 months during winter and early spring. Occasionally the season is prolonged or shortened depending on the causative viruses or cocirculation of both A and B strains.

Social Impact. There are few data on the average cost of a case of influenza. Estimates of total U.S. expenditures on influenza are in the range of 1 to 3 billion dollars per year.[14] Industrial absenteeism usually increases by less than 1% to 2% during the average epidemic, but at times it can be extremely disruptive. Of special concern are cases of influenza in nursing homes, where attack rates up to 80% and case-fatality rates of 30% have been reported.

Immunity. Antibodies to surface antigens of the influenza viruses are important in preventing infection.[15] Most patients convalescing from influenza develop specific antibodies in 2 to 4 weeks. Whereas adults have a high degree of resistance to reinfection with the same virus strain or its subsequent variants for many years, children can be reinfected frequently. Immunity to influenza is a complex function of antibody, host resistance, and changes in the biological and antigenic characteristics of prevalent viruses.

Antibody against the hemagglutinin is the primary mechanism for virus neutralization, and its relative abundance provides the best index of protection. Nonetheless, antibody against neuraminidase also plays a role in ameliorating disease and decreasing virus transmission. The roles of secretory antibody in local immunity and of cytotoxic T cells in cell-mediated immunity are not yet fully understood.

Control. Traditional efforts to control epidemics on a global or community scale, such as quarantine, isolation, or travel restrictions, are generally impractical and not worthwhile because of the rapid spread, short incubation period, and shedding of virus with subclinical disease. Environmental approaches such as ultraviolet irradiation and air-purifying or sterilizing techniques have either not been tested or are too inefficient to be put into practical use. Efforts to control influenza have been successful in two areas, (1) vaccination and (2) chemotherapy or chemoprophylaxis with amantadine.

Influenza Vaccines. Commercially available vaccines are prepared from allantoic fluids of infected embryonated hens' eggs. Viruses are formalin inactivated and purified by a variety of means. Vaccines may contain whole virions, "split" virus products, or purified surface antigens created by disrupting the viruses with detergents or lipid solvents. Live attenuated vaccines are in use in several countries but remain experimental in the United States. Vaccines work by inducing production of serum antibodies against the H and N antigens.

The WHO makes recommendations yearly to the Centers for Disease Control and the vaccine manufacturers on the formulation of the vaccine.[16] Their efforts are made to ensure that the proposed vaccine contains antigens similar to those of strains already in circulation. Thus the formulations are necessarily changed frequently. Such data as recent and expected strains in the community, antigenicity of strains, and in vitro strain similarities are used to determine which strains of viruses to include in the vaccine. Recently, antigenically similar strains with good growth characteristics have been substituted for strains with poor growth to ensure adequate production of strains for manufacture of the vaccine.[17] The most common recent vaccines are trivalent and have contained two A strain viruses and one B strain virus.

Vaccination is protective against both disease and death. Elderly residents of nursing homes are protected from disease by about 30%, and all other groups are protected by about 70%.[18] Vaccination of high-risk groups reduces mortality rates by 60% to 87%.

The side effects of inactivated vaccines are usually minor and can be local or systemic. They are most frequent in persons younger than age 20 years and in those given whole virus vaccines. During general use of a "swine" influenza virus vaccine in 1976 in the United States, the Guillain-Barré syndrome (GBS) was reported to affect one in 120,000 vaccinees. Recomputation of attributable risk data suggests that there was, in fact, a lesser degree of association (4.0 to 5.9 cases per million vaccinees).[19] An increased incidence of GBS has not been observed with influenza vaccines administered after 1976.

Antiviral Drugs. Amantadine hydrochloride is licensed in the United States for treatment or prophylaxis of influenza A.[20] Its analogue, rimantadine hydrochloride, is in use in other countries. Neither has been shown to be effective against influenza B. These drugs are most effective when given before exposure and reduce both the frequency of infection (attack rate) and the severity of illness. When the drugs are used prophylactically, from 70% to 90% of cases can be prevented. When they are used therapeutically, symptoms such as fever have been reduced by about 50% if administration is within 48 hours of the onset of symptoms. Amantadine is reported to have a higher frequency of neurological side effects than rimantadine and should be used cautiously in elderly patients and in persons with renal failure. Studies continue to accumulate showing the efficacy of amantadine in specialized situations, including protection of high-risk patients in acute care hospitals and long-term care facilities.[21]

Public Health Implications. Not only can epidemic influenza cause significant increases in morbidity and mortality rates, but the social and economic consequences are sometimes devastating. Nationwide epidemics have affected millions of persons, with frequently greater than 10,000 excess deaths. Such epidemics could cost billions of dollars. How our knowledge of the epidemiology, virology, and use of vaccines can best be applied to national policy development, when knowledge of the mutability of influenza viruses remains largely descriptive and our skill in forecasting epidemics is limited, continues to be problematic.

The difficulties of epidemiological forecasts and the complexities of developing a national influenza-prevention strategy were demonstrated in 1976 when a focal outbreak of "swine" influenza A occurred in a New Jersey military camp. Since this strain resembled the one thought to have caused the great epidemic of 1918 and 1919, scientists promptly agreed on the need for a national vaccination program using a swine influenza–specific vaccine. Congress voted funds for vaccine production and program development and eventually insured manufacturers against vaccine-associated risks so that the program could be implemented. The vaccination program for swine influenza begun in December 1976 was a major undertaking distributing 85.4 million doses of vaccine. In that program, 37.7% and 32.1% of elderly and young high-risk patients, respectively, were vaccinated.

Although expected to become epidemic, the swine influenza outbreak did not reach epidemic proportions. Furthermore, the vaccination program had to be abandoned after 3 months when there appeared to be an excess number of Guillain-Barré syndrome cases after vaccination. The remarkable achievement of implementing a coordinated national influenza vaccination program (conducted at the state and local health department level) was overshadowed by challenges to the soundness of scientific judgment and public health policy in responding to the prospects of epidemic influenza.

Despite an effective, safe, and reasonably inexpensive vaccine, except for the swine influenza vaccine, fewer than 25% of persons for whom the vaccine was recommended received the vaccine yearly from 1968 to 1985.[22] Studies have generally suggested three ways to improve immunization compliance: (1) educational programs of the general public and health care providers, (2) administrative direction, such as highly visible immunization programs or mandated vaccination for some clinics and hospitals, and (3) financial incentives or disincentives for health care providers by institutions and reimbursement providers.

Current Recommendations. The Immunization Practices Advisory Committee of the Centers for Disease Control makes recommendations for the use of influenza vaccine in the United States.[23] Generally, the goals are to reduce influenza-associated mortality rates. Traditionally this program has been accomplished by recommending that the vaccine be given annually to persons at greatest risk of death: persons of all ages with chronic cardiovascular, bronchopulmonary, renal, or metabolic diseases; residents of nursing homes; persons older than 65 years of age; immunosuppressed persons, including those with HIV infection; and persons who are receiving long-term aspirin therapy and are therefore at risk of Reye's syndrome. In 1984 the recommendations were expanded to include the immunization of persons capable of transmitting influenza to those high-risk patients: all health care workers of acute and long-term care facilities, members of high-risk patients' households and providers of home care to high-risk persons.

Influenza immunization practices differ in different countries. In the United States, inactivated vaccines are generally recommended only for those at greatest risk of severe and fatal consequences of disease; in Japan, inactivated vaccines are widely used for schoolchildren in an attempt to reduce transmission of the virus.

Currently it is thought that immunizing the entire U.S. population is neither feasible nor desirable for technical and logistical reasons and because of costs. Despite evidence showing the vaccines' efficacy in reducing morbidity and mortality rates in certain populations, such data do not support their use in the general population.

Thus the major elements of current influenza prevention and control policy for the civilian population of the United States remain (1) recognition of the seriousness of epidemic influenza and the need to plan how best to use community and personal health resources; (2) annual immunization of high-risk groups and of persons capable of transmitting influenza to high-risk groups with the best available vaccine; and (3) monitoring of influenza cases and influenza vaccine efficacy as a basis for immunization program evaluation, research, and future planning.

Haemophilus influenzae Infections

Jay D. Wenger
David W. Fraser
Claire V. Broome

Haemophilus influenzae was advanced by Pfeiffer in 1892 as the etiologic agent of influenza because of its recovery from the respiratory tract of many persons with that disease. Although later shown not to cause influenza, it has been identified as a major cause of invasive bacterial disease in children, and of significant morbidity in adults with chronic respiratory disease. It is the most common cause of bacterial meningitis in the United States.

Bacteriology. *H. influenzae* usually appears as a small pleomorphic gram-negative coccobacillus on Gram-stained clinical specimens. However, it can be difficult to stain and may occasionally appear as gram-positive diplococci in the spinal fluid.

H. influenzae strains may be either encapsulated or nonencapsulated. Among the encapsulated strains there are six distinct capsular types, designated a, b, c, d, e, and f. Most invasive *H. influenzae* disease is due to encapsulated strains, with type b organisms predominating.

Until recently, *H. influenzae* consistently demonstrated in vitro susceptibility to ampicillin and chloramphenicol. Since plasmid-mediated ampicillin resistance associated with β-lactamase activity was first reported in 1974, resistance among *H. influenzae* organisms has become widespread. In 1986, 33% of *H. influenzae* type b strains were resistant to ampicillin.[1] Resistance to chloramphenicol is much rarer but has been observed in type b and nonencapsulated strains.

Clinical Characteristics and Pathophysiology. Meningitis is the most common life-threatening illness caused by *H. influenzae* and is caused almost exclusively by encapsulated type b strains. Bacteremia has been documented in about 70% of meningitis cases but probably occurs in all as a necessary step as the bacteria pass from the nasopharynx to seed the meninges.[2] The case-fatality rate averages 3% to 6%; 20% to 30% of survivors may have significant residual neurological deficits, including blindness, severe retardation, hydrocephalus, seizures, or hearing loss.

Acute epiglottitis—with cellulitis and edema of the epiglottis, aryepiglottic folds, and surrounding soft tissue—is most commonly caused by *H. influenzae* type b. Because of respiratory obstruction, it can be rapidly fatal.

H. influenzae pneumonia caused by type b strains affects children more commonly than adults and is often accompanied by bacteremia and less often by empyema or pericarditis. Nontypeable *H. influenzae* is a common cause of pneumonia or exacerbations of chronic bronchitis in adults with chronic lung disease; bacteremia is uncommon in such cases.

H. influenzae, together with the pneumococcus, is one of the two most common causes of acute otitis media and is therefore a major cause of deafness in the world. Ninety-five percent of *H. influenzae* strains causing otitis media are nonencapsulated. *H. influenzae* may cause facial or orbital cellulitis, septic arthritis, or bacteremia without a detectable focus.

Diagnosis of *Haemophilus* infection is by culture of the organism from normally sterile body fluids or by demonstration of capsular antigens in those fluids by counterimmunoelectrophoresis, latex particle agglutination, or staphylococcal coagglutination. Nasopharyngeal cultures are of limited assistance in making a specific diagnosis because this organism can frequently be found in the absence of disease.

Initial therapy for life-threatening *H. influenzae* infections may include both ampicillin and chloramphenicol or a third-generation cephalosporin; antibiotic therapy can be simplified when it is shown that the infecting strain does not produce β-lactamase. Otitis media is best treated with ampicillin unless it is refractory; trimethoprim-sulfamethoxazole is a useful alternative.

Immunity. In 1933 Fothergill and Wright described an inverse relationship between serum bactericidal activity against *H. influenzae* type b and the incidence of *H. influenzae* meningitis at various ages. A nadir in bactericidal activity from age 3 months to 2 years roughly corresponded to the age of peak incidence of *H. influenzae* meningitis. The prevalence of antibody to polyribosylribitol phosphate (PRP), the type b capsular material, roughly parallels that of bactericidal activity. Experimental studies have shown that anti-PRP antibodies may be protective against *H. influenzae* type b infection in animal models and in humans.

Several stimuli have been identified that lead to serum antibodies directed against *H. influenzae* type b. Systemic disease or nasopharyngeal colonization of children older than 1 year is typically associated with an antibody response. Of great interest is the observation that infants with *H. influenzae* meningitis may not develop specific antibodies during convalescence,[3] apparently because of immunologic immaturity. Parenterally administered PRP will induce serum antibodies to PRP in children older than 2 years of age or in adults.

The role of serum antibody is uncertain in protection against diseases usually caused by nonencapsulated *H. influenzae,* such as otitis media or pneumonia, or against epiglottitis, which occurs typically at an age when most patients have antibodies to PRP.

Transmission. *H. influenzae* is carried primarily in the nasopharynx. The prevalence of *H. influenzae* in healthy children less than 6 years of age averages 12% and that of type b about 1%. Type b carriage is most common in the third and fourth years of life. During episodes of respiratory illness in individual children, the prevalence of *H. influenzae* carriage may increase threefold and that of type b, sixfold.[4]

Little is known about the dynamics of the spread of *H. influenzae* from one person to another, although it probably occurs via contact with respiratory secretions or respiratory droplets. Culture surveys of family or day care center contacts of children with *H. influenzae* type b disease have generally shown high rates of carriage of the organism. Whether the index case is usually the cause or the victim of active transmission has not been defined.

Occurrence. *H. influenzae* causes disease most commonly in young children. Ninety-five percent of *H. influenzae* meningitis cases occur in children less than 5 years of age. That age group has an average incidence of 40 per 100,000 per year. The peak incidence (150/100,000 per year) is in children 6 to 7 months old.[1] Epiglottitis is distinctive among illnesses caused by encapsulated strains in that most cases occur in children 2 to 5 years of age. Pneumonia caused by nonencapsulated strains is probably most common in older adults. The incidence of *H. influenzae* meningitis is three times as high for black as for white persons. The incidence for Alaskan natives is 10 times the national average. Recent studies suggest that some of this increased risk may be due to risk factors such as socioeconomic status or day care attendance, rather than genetic predisposition.[5] The incidence of *H. influenzae* infection is lowest in the summer, with peak incidence from October to December and a second peak in March and April.[6]

Children with disorders of immunoglobulin synthesis are at increased risk of *H. influenzae* disease, as apparently are those with sickle-cell disease. Chronic lung disease has been mentioned as predisposing patients to pneumonia caused by nonencapsulated strains.

Epidemics of *H. influenzae* disease have not been observed, although clusters of cases are seen in households, day care centers, and facilities for the care of chronically ill children. The risk of systemic *H. influenzae* disease in household contacts during the month after the onset of *H. influenzae* meningitis in an index case has been estimated as 0.3% overall, and 2% in contacts younger than 4 years of age. Other studies have suggested that the risk of disease in day care classroom contacts younger than 2 years of age may be as high as 1%.[7]

Prevention. Initial efforts to develop a vaccine for prevention of *H. influenzae* disease focused on evaluation of a purified PRP antigen. A randomized, double-blind field trial conducted in Finland showed 90% efficacy in children vaccinated older than 24 months of age, and no efficacy in children younger than 18 months of age, apparently because of marked age-dependent variation in immunogenicity of PRP.[8] After this vaccine was licensed for use in the United States in children 18 to 24 months of age and older, a series of postmarketing studies showed vaccine efficacy in this age group ranging from 52% to 80%, with four of five such studies demonstrating efficacy between 42% and 80%.[9]

In the meantime, efforts proceeded to develop vaccines that would be more immunogenic, especially in the younger children. A number of promising candidate vaccines were prepared by covalently binding PRP with a protein carrier. Initial immunogenicity results with several of these "conjugate vaccines" showed marked increases in anti-PRP antibody in children immunized at 18 months of age and older,[10] and on the basis of immunogenicity data three conjugate vaccines have been licensed for use in this age group in the United States. In addition, enhanced immunogenicity in younger children has been demonstrated. A second field trial in Finland showed greater than 90% efficacy of a conjugate vaccine in children immunized between 2 and 6 months of age, although a randomized trial in Alaska of a similar vaccine demonstrated much lower efficacy. Additional field trials of conjugate vaccines in 2- to 6-month-old infants will be completed in the United States in 1991. If efficacy is demonstrated, subsequent licensure of these vaccines for use in infants at 2 months of age should drastically reduce the incidence of *H. influenzae* type b disease in the United States.

Although secondary cases represent only 1% to 3% of *H. influenzae* disease, the elevated rate in contacts indicates the need for effective prophylaxis. A national collaborative study has examined whether chemoprophylaxis for contacts of patients with *H. influenzae* disease might prevent secondary cases in households and day care centers. A randomized, controlled trial showed a significant effect of rifampin in preventing disease.[11] Among day care contacts alone, the study suggested that prophylaxis provided protection, but with the limited size of the study the trend was not statistically significant. Later studies evaluating risk of secondary *H. influenzae* disease in day care centers also showed a significant protective effect of rifampin prophylaxis.[7] Therefore chemoprophylaxis with rifampin at a dosage of 20 mg/kg (maximum dosage 600 mg/d) once daily for 4 days has been recommended for household contacts of *H. influenzae* disease when a child less than 4 years of age is a member of the household. Because a significant risk of secondary disease exists in day care contacts who are less than 2 years of age, prophylaxis for day care classmates and teachers is recommended if children less than 2 years of age are present in the classroom.[12]

Pneumococcal Infections

Robert Austrian

The pneumococcus (*Streptococcus pneumoniae*) is a component of the normal bacterial flora of the human nasopharynx and commonly enjoys a commensal relationship with its host. Injury to any region of the respiratory epithelium may disturb the relationship between host and parasite and be followed by clinical illness. The pneumococcus is the commonest cause of community-acquired bacterial pneumonia[1,2] and otitis media[3] and a major cause of bacterial meningitis.

The organism is a nonmotile, facultatively anaerobic, gram-positive, encapsulated coccus growing in pairs and short chains. The capsule of a given strain is composed of high-molecular-weight polysaccharide, of which more than 80 varieties are now recognized and which gives a strain its type specificity. Although nontoxic, the capsular polysaccharide plays an essential role in the virulence of pneumococci by inhibiting phagocytosis of the organism by polymorphonuclear leukocytes in the absence of type-specific anticapsular antibody. When the latter is present, the efficiency of phagocytosis is increased markedly. The pathogenicity of the soma of the pneumococcal cell can be demonstrated in the agranulocytic animal in which usually avirulent noncapsulated pneumococci can produce progressive and fatal disease.[4] Although several toxic products of the pneumococcus have been identified, including pneumolysin, neuraminidase, and components of the cell wall, the precise mechanisms whereby pneumococci injure the hosts they infect remain obscure.

In evaluating studies of the various associations of pneumococci with humans, it is important to recognize the methods employed in the collection of data. In the first half-century after the discovery of pneumococci, the number of capsular types identified and reagents for their recognition were limited. Between 1930 and 1945, when the most prevalent types had been identified and sera were used for treatment of infections caused by them, very sensitive methods were employed for isolating and typing pneumococci; epidemiologic data from this period are likely to have a high level of validity.[5] With the advent of chemotherapeutic and antibiotic therapy, treatment before material has been obtained for bacteriologic study and the abandonment of sensitive laboratory techniques have resulted in data that may reflect minimal rather than true findings relating to pneumococcal infection. In an assessment of such data, it is critically important to know the methods used in each study scrutinized.

Pneumococcal Colonization and the Carrier State. Colonization of the human nasopharynx with pneumococci may occur on the day of birth, the type acquired usually being that carried by the mother.[6] Adherence of pneumococci to respiratory epithelial cells is mediated by a bacterial adhesin, thought to be protein in nature, that attaches to a specific glycoprotein receptor of the epithelial cell.[7] In the first years of life, rates of pneumococcal carriage are high, and children observed for several years, with specimens cultured repeatedly, have been found to be colonized sequentially with as many as 12 distinct serotypes.[8] Carefully executed studies have shown approximately half of all children to carry two pneumococcal types simultaneously, and simultaneous carriage of as many as four serotypes has been demonstrated.[9] Rates of pneumococcal carriage tend to decline with age.

Carriage of a single pneumococcal serotype may extend over periods exceeding a year, both in children and in adults; carriage of a single serotype for a period exceeding 3 years has been demonstrated in adults.[10] Few data are available concerning the acquisition of new types by adults with the passage of time, but limited findings suggest the number to be one or two per year.[11]

Colonization with a given pneumococcal type may be followed by the development of homotypic anticapsular antibody in the absence of overt signs of clinical illness.[12] The presence of circulating anticapsular antibody will not eliminate an established carrier state, but it will reduce by approximately half the likelihood of being colonized with the homotypic strain.[13]

The ability of antimicrobial drugs to eliminate the pneumococcal carrier state seems limited. Neither penicillin, sulfonamides, nor a variety of other antimicrobial agents have been successful in ridding the nasopharynx of pneumococci from all carriers.[14]

Ecology of Pneumococcal Types. The wide geographical distribution of pneumococci was presaged by the two initial isolates of the organism in 1880, one in North America[15] and the other in Europe.[16] Data on its recovery from persons living on all five continents were reviewed by Heffron in his monograph published in 1939[17]; in the ensuing half century, isolates of the organism have been identified in a number of additional regions, suggesting its presence in any area inhabited by humans.

The distributions of pneumococcal types causing infection

differ between children and adults, in different geographic areas, and with the passage of time. At the present time, 85 pneumococcal capsular types have been identified. All are not equally invasive. Approximately half the invasive infections are caused by six types, an additional one fourth by six different types, and an additional one eighth by six other types. Although the rank order of frequency of these invasive types may change with time[18] and may vary somewhat from one place to another, studies of isolates from blood, cerebrospinal fluid, and the middle ear have shown considerable overall stability among the 12 capsular types accounting for the preponderance of such infections.[19]

The distribution of pneumococcal types that cause the majority of infections in infancy and early childhood is more limited than in adults. Pneumococcal types 6A, 6B, 14, 19F, 19A, and 23F cause approximately 50% to 60% of such illnesses in this age group. Noteworthy is the observation that immunologic responsiveness to the capsular antigens of these types is among the last to develop with maturation.[20]

Among adults in the United States, types 3, 4, 6B, 9V, 14, and 23F have been the most frequent causes of bacteremic infections in the past 5 years, accounting for 53% of such illnesses. This distribution of types represents a significant change from 25 years ago, when types or groups 1, 3, 4, 7, 8, and 12 predominated. In 1989, infections with pneumococcus type 1 were the cause of a significantly smaller proportion of pneumococcal infections in North America than elsewhere, and those caused by capsular types 2 and 5 were virtually unknown in this area. In contrast, infections with these latter serotypes are still common in South America, Africa, and Asia.

Epidemiologic data suggest that genetic constitution may influence susceptibility to infection with certain pneumococcal types. Infections with capsular types 45 and 46 have been frequent among black gold miners in South Africa since these capsular types were first identified, whereas they have been isolated only rarely from white persons in the same region. These same types have been recognized also in some Melanesian populations.

Pneumococcal Resistance to Antimicrobial Drugs. Although the first drug-resistant bacterium recovered from a human was a pneumococcus isolated from a patient being treated with Optochin in 1916,[21] the observation was made so long in advance of the introduction of safe and effective antibacterial agents as to have been largely forgotten when the latter became available two decades later. Pneumococci resistant to sulfonamide drugs were recognized within a few years of the advent of sulfapyridine, but clinical isolates of this organism that were resistant to antibiotics did not prove to be an early cause for concern.

It is of interest that pneumococci manifesting decreased susceptibility to penicillin G, the antimicrobial agent of choice for treating pneumococcal infection caused by sensitive strains, were isolated both in vitro and in vivo as early as 1943.[22] Noteworthy also is the fact that if such phenomena can be demonstrated experimentally, it can be predicted that bacterial variants resistant to the drug in question will emerge eventually in therapeutic settings. One reason for the slow development of pneumococcal resistance to antibiotics of the β-lactam class may be the fact that such resistance results from the cumulative effect of multiple mutations affecting the penicillin-binding proteins of the organism.[23]

Since the late 1970s, pneumococci resistant to one or all of the following antimicrobial agents have been described: penicillin, tetracyclines, chloramphenicol, macrolides, aminoglycosides, and trimethoprim-sulfamethoxazole. Isolated initially in South Africa, these multiple drug-resistant pneumococcal strains have been identified in a number of additional geographical areas.[24] Monitoring of pneumococcal isolates both in South Africa[25] and in Spain[26] has shown a significant and steady increase in isolates with resistance to penicillin, and such strains have been recovered in most parts of the world. Manifestation of drug resistance is independent of capsular type. Such resistance, however, tends to be found most commonly in the pneumococcal types that most frequently infect children and to be manifested specifically to the drugs most widely administered to the population at risk.[27]

To date, no pneumococcal strain manifesting resistance to vancomycin has been described, and it remains the agent of choice for the initial treatment of pneumococcal infection in areas where strains resistant to other antimicrobial drugs have been identified. An alternative method of dealing with the problem of drug resistance is prophylactic vaccination with polyvalent pneumococcal vaccine.

Pneumococcal Infection. Infections with the pneumococcus arise when the normal commensal relationship with the organism's host is disturbed, most commonly by injury to the epithelial lining of the respiratory tract. Such injury may be physical or chemical but is thought to result in most instances from viral infection. Studies in experimental animals have shown both the normal lung[28] and the normal middle ear[29] to be resistant to pneumococcal infection, but both areas are vulnerable to bacterial multiplication when viral injury has antedated exposure to the bacterium. Three clinical syndromes result from disturbance of the usual host-parasite relationship: pneumococcal otitis media (and, less commonly, paranasal sinusitis), pneumococcal pneumonia, and pneumococcal bacteremia unassociated with evidence of primary pneumococcal infection.

The pneumococcus remains the commonest cause of community-acquired bacterial pneumonia.[1,2] The clinical features of the disease are described in detail by Heffron.[17] The precise incidence of pneumococcal pneumonia is unknown because of the difficulty in establishing the exact cause of bacterial pneumonia in the absence of bacteremia.[30] On the basis of available evidence, the incidence of putative pneumococcal pneumonia in developed countries is estimated to be between 1 and 5/1000 persons per year. Retrospective study of pneumococcal bacteremia in the United States has yielded rates of approximately 10/100,000 persons per year,[31] but passive prospective surveillance suggests a minimum rate of 25 to 30/100,000 persons per year.[30] In Alaska a bacteremia rate of 105/100,000 persons per year in persons of all ages in the native population has been reported.[32] Rates of pneumococcal bacteremia in infancy and in persons older than 60 years of age exceed those in older children and younger adults.[33] Case-fatality rates of bacteremic pneumococcal pneumonia remain significant even with optimal therapy, being in the vicinity of 17% for bacteremic pneumococcal pneumonia treated with penicillin in the absence of extrapulmonary foci of infection.[34] When metastatic foci of infection are present, case-fatality rates may exceed 40%.

The pneumococcus is the commonest cause of otitis media, a disorder that afflicts three fourths of American children at least once in their first 6 years of life. Although now rarely followed by serious or lethal sequelae, pneumococcal otitis media is the cause of considerable morbidity and expenditure for medical services. Recurring attacks caused by a succession of pneumococcal types are not infrequent.[3]

Like *Neisseria meningitidis* and *Haemophilus influenzae* type b, the pneumococcus appears capable of invading the epithelium of the nasopharynx and spreading to the regional lymph nodes, where, if unchecked, it finds its way to the systemic circulation, giving rise to bacteremia. Pneumococcal bacteremia in the absence of an identifiable focus of infection is now a well-recognized syndrome in infants and, more recently, has been identified in adults.[35]

Pneumococcal meningitis, a sequela of bacteremia or an extension of infection from the paranasal sinuses or mastoid to the cranial cavity, has an incidence of approximately 1.6/100,000 persons per year[36] and remains one of the three commonest forms of bacterial meningitis. The case-fatality rate is high, exceeding 40% in persons more than 40 years of age.

Treatment of Pneumococcal Infections. Penicillin G (benzyl penicillin) remains the drug of choice for the treatment of infections caused by pneumococci sensitive to it and occurring in patients lacking hypersensitivity to this antibiotic. Most pneumococcal strains are sensitive to other drugs of the β-lactam class and to macrolides, tetracyclines, chloramphenicol, and trimethoprim-sulfamethoxazole. Because pneumococcal mutants resistant to most or all of these agents have been identified, it is desirable to determine the level of sensitivity of the causal organism to the drug to be employed for therapy. In areas where multiply resistant strains have been identified, therapy with vancomycin should be initiated and continued until the foregoing information is available. Limited data suggest that ceftriaxone may be used successfully to treat pneumococcal meningitis caused by strains manifesting increased resistance to penicillin G.[37]

Immunoprophylaxis of Pneumococcal Infections. The continuing morbidity resulting from pneumococcal infections in all societies and the significant case-fatality rates unamenable to further reduction by antimicrobial drugs make prevention of such illnesses highly desirable.[38] In addition, the slow but steady increase in the number of pneumococcal strains resistant to therapeutic agents poses an additional impediment to treatment.[25,26] These circumstances provide the basis for immunoprophylactic measures to prevent pneumococcal infections.

Mammalian responses to polysaccharide antigens are complex. In the mouse, initial response to an injected, purified bacterial capsular polysaccharide is manifested by the formation of antibodies of the IgM class (which persist for a limited time) and is unaccompanied by evidence of immunologic memory. If, however, the same polysaccharide chemically conjugated to a protein is injected, antibodies of both the IgM and IgG classes are formed, and antibodies of both classes are "boosted" if the polysaccharide antigen is reinjected either in purified form or conjugated chemically to protein.[39]

In analogous fashion, the human infant, immunologically immature at birth, responds only transiently to purified polysaccharide antigens with antibodies of the IgM class. In addition, responsiveness to all such antigens is not present in the first year of life and may be delayed for several years. By contrast, as has been shown with the capsular polysaccharide of *Haemophilus influenzae* type b chemically linked to diphtheria toxoid, infants respond to this antigen at the age of 3 to 6 months with the formation of antibodies of both the IgM and IgG classes and manifest a "booster" response, or immunologic "memory," when reexposed to the same capsular polysaccharide in either purified or complexed form.[40] Experimental studies in animals with pneumococcal capsular polysaccharides complexed to similar proteins have shown analogous results, and conjugates of the pneumococcal capsular polysaccharides of the several types responsible for the preponderance of infections in early childhood are being developed.[41]

Probably because of exposure to the commoner pneumococcal types during childhood, adults respond to many purified pneumococcal polysaccharide antigens with the formation of antibodies of the IgM and IgG classes. Studies in children have shown that type-specific antibodies may be stimulated by colonization with the homologous organism in the absence of overt illness.[12] These circumstances and the fact that 80% to 90% of invasive pneumococcal infections are caused by 23 of the 85 known capsular types have led to the introduction of a 23-valent vaccine containing 25 μg each of the pneumococcal capsular polysaccharides of types 1, 2, 3, 4, 5, 6B, 7F, 8, 9N, 9V, 10A, 11A, 12F, 14, 15B, 17F, 18F, 19F, 19A, 20, 22F, 23F, and 33F. In an assessment of the efficiency of a vaccine of this complexity, it is of critical importance to recognize that the vaccine is designed to prevent 23 immunologically distinct infections and that its aggregate efficacy can never equal that of a monovalent vaccine.

Several methods have been used to assess the aggregate efficacy of polyvalent pneumococcal vaccines, including randomized, double-blind, controlled trials,[42] quasi-cohort studies,[43] and case-control studies.[44,45] Trials of all three designs have found the aggregate efficacy of polyvalent pneumococcal vaccines to be between 60% and 80%. This finding is compatible with observations of 90% efficacy of monovalent capsular polysaccharide vaccines in adults[46] and of exposure during a 2-year period to four pneumococcal types represented in the vaccine (i.e., 0.9^4, or 64%). Pneumococcal vaccine is accompanied rarely by untoward reactions, and no permanent injuries or deaths have resulted from its administration. Limited studies in older children and in adults of all ages so far have shown no age-related differences in the vaccine's aggregate efficacy, and limited data have not revealed a decline in protection by the vaccine in the 6 years following immunization.[45] Currently there is no recommendation to revaccinate.

Recommendations for the administration of pneumococcal vaccine have been promulgated by the Immunization Practices Advisory Committee of the Centers for Disease Control[47] and by the American College of Physicians in its *Guide for Adult Immunization.*[48] The vaccine should be administered to all persons 65 years of age and older and to those over 10 to 15 years of age with any of a variety of chronic systemic illnesses associated with increased risk of a fatal outcome from bacteremic pneumococcal infection. Although the vaccine may be given to immunocompromised persons who are at increased risk of pneumococcal infection, it must be administered with the foreknowledge that its efficacy will be limited in those whose antibody responses are impaired. All persons with anatomical or functional asplenia, including recipients of 14 valent pneumococcal vaccine, should be given the 23 valent pneumococcal vaccine because of their high risk of death if infected with any pneumococcal type.

Chickenpox

Laura J. Fehrs
Stephen R. Preblud

Public Health Significance. In the nontropical countries, chickenpox (varicella) is a ubiquitous disease of childhood. More than 90% of adults have immunity to varicella. However, although chickenpox is generally regarded as a mild childhood illness with few complications,[1] it may have more serious consequences for newborn infants, immunocompromised children, and all adults.[1,2] Complications of varicella such as pneumonia and encephalitis can occur even among normal children. Complications among normal children comprise more than 80% of all complications of the disease.[3] Substantial burdens of school absenteeism, costs of parental leave, and medical costs are associated with childhood chickenpox. A live attenuated varicella vaccine is likely to be licensed soon in the United States for use in healthy children and adolescents. Medical and home care costs associated with varicella in normal children could be reduced by 66% with a strategy of routine vaccination of children.[3] Routine use of varicella vaccine in childhood may affect the epidemiology of chickenpox in the United States. Depending on vaccine coverage levels and duration of immunity, the incidence of varicella should decrease, but infection may shift into older age groups, with a resultant increased risk of complications.

Etiological Agent, Immunology, and Diagnosis. Chickenpox is caused by the varicella-zoster (VZ) virus, a DNA-virus of the herpesvirus group. Infection usually produces a typical clinical illness; inapparent primary infection is estimated to occur in no more than 5% of susceptible children.[23] Immunity after inapparent infection is believed to be as permanent and protective as the immunity after overt infection. Although subclinical reinfections are common, second clinical infections rarely occur.[24,25]

The most accurate and sensitive antibody tests currently available for immunity screening are the fluorescent antibody to membrane antigen (FAMA) test, immune adherence hemagglutination (IAHA) test, and enzyme immunoassay (EIA). Commercially available tests include EIA and complement fixation (CF) test, the latter being relatively insensitive, although generally specific. In normal persons the presence of antibody detectable by one of these assays can be considered as evidence of past infection with VZ virus and hence evidence of immunity. The specificity of these assays may, however, be diminished in immunocompromised persons. Clinical varicella has developed in persons with a carefully obtained history of no previous illness but with detectable antibodies presumed to be a result of transfusion in the preceding months.[26] Therefore the results of laboratory tests in the immunocompromised should be interpreted cautiously.[27]

Clinical Characteristics. The incubation period of chickenpox ranges from 10 to 21 days (average of 14 to 15 days) and may be prolonged in patients passively immunized against VZ virus.[4]

The exanthem, which initially is pruritic and may require symptomatic treatment, may be preceded for 1 to 2 days by low-grade fever and malaise. The prodrome in children is usually very mild or absent, with the eruption being the first indication of illness; adults are more likely to suffer prodromal symptoms. The rash quickly evolves from macules to papules to clear, fluid-filled vesicles approximately 2 to 4 mm in diameter. The vesicles are initially surrounded by an erythematous base, which fades during the process of crusting. Unruptured vesicles sequentially become purulent and dry and crust over. Drying starts at the center of the lesion, giving it an umbilicated appearance. The crust, which is not infectious, may remain intact from 1 to 3 weeks. Early in the illness all stages of the rash can coexist. The rash is most concentrated on the central portions of the body, predominantly the face and trunk. Lesions are not confined to the skin and can develop on any mucosal surface. They can also develop on the cornea[5] and tympanic membranes.

Fever (approximately 38° to 39° C [100° to 102° F]) is present during the peak of rash evolution and disappears by the time all the vesicles have either dried or crusted over.

Complications. Most children have a relatively benign course, but approximately 5% may suffer from some complication, most commonly secondary bacterial infection of the cutaneous lesions.[1] Bacteremia with infection of other sites may occur. A higher rate of complications occurs in adults. Systemic involvement is more prominent, with primary varicella pneumonia a frequent, life-threatening complication. It has been estimated that 16% to 33% of adults with chickenpox have clinical or radiologic evidence of pneumonitis.

Some, but not all, studies have indicated that pregnant women may have a higher risk of complications than do nonpregnant adults of childbearing age. Because available studies included small numbers of subjects, there is a need for population-based estimates of complications of varicella in pregnancy.[6]

Neurological Complications. Varicella-associated encephalitis is a postinfectious condition similar to that seen after measles. The actual frequency of this complication is unknown, but estimated rates based on reported data are 1 to 4 per 10,000 reported chickenpox cases.[1,7] There is a slight predominance among males. Adults more than 20 years of age are 6 to 12 times more likely to have encephalitis after varicella than are children less than 14 years of age.[8] Symptoms generally begin 2 to 14 days after the appearance of the rash. Cerebellar involvement occurs in approximately 35% of encephalitis cases and is usually associated with a relatively mild course, with complete recovery. Corticocerebral involvement carries a higher rate of neurologic sequelae (up to 15%) and death (5% to 25%). Encephalitis accounts for 90% of all CNS involvement; transverse myelitis, peripheral neuritis, and optic neuritis have also been reported.

Chickenpox was also circumstantially implicated as a cause of 20% to 30% of all cases of Reye's syndrome reported annually in the 1970s.[1] More recently, there has been a dramatic decrease in the incidence of Reye's syndrome, presumably because of decreased use of aspirin in children.[9] At the same time, the proportion of cases that are associated with VZ virus infection has decreased to 5%.[3,9]

Deaths. Between 1980 and 1987, approximately 40 to 90 chickenpox-associated deaths were reported annually. In adults the course of varicella infection is usually more severe than it is in normal children.[1,8] The estimated death-to-case ratio in normal adults aged 25 to 55 years without cancer or other underlying cause of immune system dysfunction is approximately 11 per 100,000 varicella cases. This rate is approximately 20 times that estimated for normal children—0.6 per 100,000 varicella cases.[10] Septic complications, pneumonia, and encephalitis are the usual causes of death in children,[1] whereas pneumonia is most often the cause in adults.[2] Case-fatality rates of 7% to 14% have been reported for immunocompromised children, but the case-fatality rate may be decreasing with the use of antiviral agents to treat chickenpox in this group.[11]

Immunocompromised Patients. In immunocompromised patients, such as children with acute lymphocytic leukemia, all expressions of the infection may be markedly enhanced.[12] In approximately one third of these patients the rash covers the entire body and involves multiple organ systems, often becoming fulminant and hemorrhagic. Death occurs in more than 5% of such cases, usually within a few days.

Serious complications, disseminated disease, and chronic skin infections have been reported in persons with HIV infection who then acquired primary varicella or herpes zoster (shingles, see below).[13] In one series of children with perinatally acquired HIV infection and subsequent primary varicella, seven had evidence of visceral dissemination, including pneumonia (seven children) and hepatitis (three children), and one died.[14] From June 1983 to March 1985, a period during which the Centers for Disease Control AIDS report form collected information on herpes zoster, 5% of reported AIDS patients were reported to have this condition.[15] Acyclovir has been used to treat primary varicella and shingles in persons with HIV disease. Acyclovir-resistant varicella infections have been reported in this group and may become an increasing problem with the use of prolonged acyclovir therapy for patients with chronic or recurrent herpes zoster infections.[16]

Neonatal Varicella. Neonatal varicella is associated with visceral involvement and a high case-fatality rate. As many as 30% of infected infants whose mothers had a chickenpox rash within 5 days before delivery may die of the disease.[17] The risk of serious illness is highest when maternal onset of varicella is from 5 days before delivery to 2 days afterward. Disease earlier in pregnancy is associated with the passage of protective maternal antibody to the fetus; disease onset more than 2 days after birth does not result in intrauterine infection. Infants who are infected postnatally are not at increased risk for complications.[18]

Congenital Varicella Syndrome. Maternal infection within the first 16 weeks of gestation can lead to congenital varicella syndrome, a recognized constellation of congenital defects including hypoplasia of an extremity, cicatricial skin scarring, localized muscular atrophy, encephalitis, cortical atrophy, ocular abnormalities, mental retardation, and low birth weight.[19] This syndrome has been estimated to occur in about 2% of first-trimester infections.[20]

Shingles. Herpes zoster, or shingles, is a painful rash that occurs when VZ virus is reactivated after having been latent in nervous system ganglia for many years after primary VZ virus infection.[21] Under certain environmental conditions (e.g., stress, trauma, sunlight) and host conditions (e.g., advancing age, malignancy, immunosuppression), the virus may become reactivated and produce herpes zoster. Because this reactivation can occur in the presence of circulating antibodies against the VZ virus, cellular immunity probably plays an important role in this process. The annual incidence of herpes zoster has been estimated at 131 per 100,000 persons, with the highest rates reported for older adults (more than 400 per 100,000 for persons more than age 75 years).[22] For children younger than age 20 years, the annual incidence has been estimated to be 42 per 100,000 and the incidence among those with prior clinical varicella has been estimated to be 68 per 100,000.[7] Herpes zoster usually is limited to a painful, vesicular, pustular eruption localized in the distribution of one or more sensory nerve roots and lasting 2 to 3 weeks. Immunocompromised patients, including persons with HIV disease, can have chronic herpes zoster or disseminated zoster illness with visceral or neurologic involvement. Antiviral drugs can be used when acute, serious complications of herpes zoster occur.[11]

Epidemiology. Chickenpox is endemic in the United States and has a striking seasonal distribution.[1] Low levels are recorded in summer and fall with a peak in the winter and spring. Although the total number of U.S. cases reported annually to the Centers for Disease Control has varied only slightly between 150,000 and 225,000, local areas may experience more variation. Nationally reported cases represent only an estimated 4% to 6% of the actual number of cases that occur. If it is assumed that virtually all persons are infected by the time they reach adulthood, the equivalent of a birth cohort (approximately 3.6 million) of persons is infected annually.

At least 80% of all reported cases of varicella occur in children less than 10 years of age.[1,23] The highest reported attack rate is in 5- to 9-year-old children.[7] By adulthood, 90% to 95% of the U.S. population has antibodies to chickenpox.[21] There are no known race or sex differences in either susceptibility to or expression of the disease.[23]

The epidemiology of varicella in tropical regions is poorly understood, but varicella infection appears to be more common among adults living in the tropics than in those living in temperate areas,[28] suggesting that there is decreased transmission in younger age groups. The reasons for this difference in the age-specific epidemiology of varicella, including the possible roles of population size, population density, crowding, and higher ambient temperatures in the tropics, are not clear.

Varicella is highly contagious, with secondary attack rates among susceptible household contacts approaching 90%.[29] The virus can readily be cultured from vesicular fluid; it is infrequently isolated from respiratory secretions. The virus is transmitted primarily by direct contact with an infected person. Airborne transmission can also occur. Indirect exposure may occur through contact with articles freshly soiled by discharges from an infected person. The path of entry of virus into the susceptible host is assumed to be the upper respiratory tract.[30]

The period of communicability extends from 1 to 2 days before to 5 to 6 days after the onset of the varicella rash. Patients with altered immunity may have a prolonged period of infectivity because new lesions may develop for an extended period. The virus cannot be cultured from the lesions once they have crusted over.

Control and Prevention. In normal populations the only means currently available for control of varicella lies in isolation of infected patients and separation of high-risk persons from those clinically ill or susceptible and recently exposed.

The current approaches for susceptible high-risk patients who are exposed to persons with varicella or zoster are early prophylaxis with VZ immune globulin (VZIG) and prompt treatment with antiviral drugs once illness is recognized. Seropositive persons are, in general, not at risk for primary chickenpox infection, except in the case of the immunocompromised patient or the newborn infant whose mother develops rash between 5 days before and 2 days after delivery. Antibody in the absence of a history of previous infection should not be considered indicative of immunity in immunocompromised patients (see above). A carefully obtained history of previous clinically apparent chickenpox may be regarded as reliable, and patients may be considered to be immune and at minimal risk for clinical reinfection.

Patients at higher risk for serious illness with varicella should receive passive immunization shortly after an exposure to chickenpox or zoster.[24,26,27] Persons at higher risk for serious illness who should be considered include immunocompromised patients, the newborn infant whose mother develops rash between 5 days before and 2 days after delivery, premature infants, and, possibly, pregnant women. VZIG should be administered as soon as possible—no later than 96 hours—after exposure. In most cases the patient will be susceptible to future infection once antibody levels have declined. VZIG is a licensed product and is available through the Red Cross.[27]

VZIG has been shown also to reduce the risk of complications from neonatal varicella. The newborn infant whose mother develops varicella rash between 5 days before and 2 days after delivery should be given VZIG.[27] VZIG can also be considered for the pregnant woman because she may be at higher risk for complications while pregnant. VZIG should not be administered to prevent fetal infection, because there is no evidence that it is effective for this use.[27]

Acyclovir and adenine arabinoside (Ara-A) are used for treatment of chickenpox in the immunocompromised host and serious disease in other patients, including newborn infants.[11] Interferon and other experimental antiviral compounds are currently being evaluated.[24,31]

A live attenuated vaccine developed and extensively tested in Japan has been field tested in the United States and Europe in both normal and immunocompromised children and adults.[32–35] It is currently licensed in Japan and some European countries for use in immunocompromised children and may be licensed soon in the United States for routine use in normal children and adolescents. The vaccine is safe and effective in normal children and adolescents. Studies of normal children show seroconversion rates of 94% or greater after a single dose of vaccine, and vaccine efficacy has been reported to be 100% 1 year after vaccination[36] and slightly lower (95%) in the second year (personal communication, Merck Sharp & Dohme Research Laboratories, Rahway, N.J.). When varicella occurs in vaccinees, the illness is milder; rash lesions are usually fewer and often maculopapular rather than vesicular. Herpes zoster may follow vaccination of children, but the reported incidence is lower for vaccine recipients than for control subjects with natural disease.[37-39]

Seroconversion rates are lower after vaccination of immunocompromised children—88% after one dose of vaccine but 98% after two doses.[40] Seroconversion rates are also lower for normal adults—82% after one dose and 94% after two doses.[41] Two or more doses of vaccine may be necessary to provide adequate protection in these populations. The efficacy of two doses of vaccine is 80% or greater for immunocompromised persons[42] and only 50% or greater for normal adults.[41] Vaccine-related rashes are more common after vaccination of immunocompromised persons than of normal persons. However, adverse events after vaccination are usually mild, even in immunocompromised persons. Transmission of vaccine virus resulting in secondary rash illnesses among household contacts has been documented, but only from immunocompromised persons with rash. Tertiary transmission has also been reported.[43]

Selective administration of VZIG and antiviral agents is available for the prevention of serious disease in high-risk persons. A safe and effective live attenuated vaccine should be available soon in the United States for routine use in children. Recent interest has focused on the sizable health impact of childhood varicella in developed countries.[1,3] The impact of varicella on developing countries has not yet been examined. Once varicella vaccine is licensed, the availability of resources for local vaccine programs, the benefits of immunity to varicella, and the potential impact of vaccination on the epidemiology of varicella will need to be considered in recommendations for the use of the vaccine.

REFERENCES

Measles

1. Hinman AR, Brandling-Bennett AD, Nieburg PI: The opportunity and obligation to eliminate measles from the United States. JAMA 242:1157–1162, 1979
2. Centers for Disease Control: The feasibility of measles elimination in Europe. MMWR 32:523–524, 530, 1983
3. Anderson RM, May RM: Directly transmitted infectious diseases: Control by vaccination. Science 215:1053–60, 1982
4. Gustafson TL, Lievens AW, Brunell PA, et al: Measles outbreak in a fully immunized secondary school population. N Engl J Med 316:771–4, 1987
5. Chen RT, Goldbaum GM, Wassilak SG, et al: An explosive point-source measles outbreak in a highly vaccinated population: Modes of transmission and risk factors for disease. Am J Epidemiol 129:173–82, 1989
6. Robbins FC: Measles: Clinical features. Am J Dis Child 101:266–72, 1962
7. DeJong JG, Winkler KC: Survival of measles virus in air. Nature 201:1054–5, 1964
8. Bloch AB, Orenstein WA, Ewing WM, et al: Measles outbreak in a pediatric practice: Airborne transmission in an office setting. Pediatrics 75:676–83, 1985
9. Barkin RM: Measles mortality: Analysis of the primary cause of death. Am J Dis Child 129:307–9, 1975
10. Kaschula ROC, Druker J, Kipps A: Late morphologic consequences of measles: A lethal and debilitating lung disease among the poor. Rev Infect Dis 5:395–404, 1983
11. Morley D: Severe measles: Some unanswered questions. Rev Infect Dis 5:460–2, 1983
12. Hull HF, William PJ, Oldfield F: Measles mortality and vaccine efficacy in rural West Africa. Lancet 1:972–5, 1983
13. Bloch AB, Orenstein WA, Wassilak SG, et al: Epidemiology of measles and its complications. In Gruenberg E, Lewis C, Goldston SE, (eds.): Vaccinating Against Brain Syndromes: The Campaign Against Measles and Rubella. New York: Oxford University Press, 1986, pp 5–20
14. Aaby P: Malnutrition and overcrowding/intensive exposure in severe measles infection: Review of community studies. Rev Infect Dis 10:478–91, 1988
15. Amler RW: Measles in pregnancy. In Amstey MS (ed): Virus Infection in Pregnancy. Orlando, Fla.: Grune & Stratton, 1984, pp 159–68
16. Measles surveillance report. No. 11, 1977–1981. Atlanta: Centers for Disease Control, Sept. 1982
17. Choppin PW, Richardson CD, Merz DC, et al: The functions and inhibition of the membrane glycoproteins of paramyxoviruses and myxoviruses and the role of the measles virus M protein in subacute sclerosing panencephalitis. J Infect Dis 143:352–63, 1981
18. Centers for Disease Control: Serologic diagnosis of measles. MMWR 31:396, 401–2, 1982
19. Krugman S: Further attenuated measles vaccine: Characteristics and use. Rev Infect Dis 5:477–81, 1983
20. Markowitz LE, Preblud SR, Orenstein WA, Rovira EZ, Adams NC, Hawkins CE, Hinman AR: Patterns of transmission in measles outbreaks in the United States. N Engl J Med 320:75–81, 1989
21. Centers for Disease Control: Measles prevention: Recommendations of the Immunization Practices Advisory Committee (ACIP). MMWR 38(No. S-9)1–18, 1989
22. Orenstein WA, Markowitz LE, Preblud SR, Hinman AR, Tomasi A, Bart KJ: Appropriate age for measles vaccination in the United States. Dev Biol Stand 65:13–23, 1986
23. Markowitz LE, Preblud SR, Fine PE, et al: Duration of live measles vaccine-induced immunity. Pediatr Infect Dis J 9:101–10, 1990
24. Herman JJ, Radin R, Schneiderman R: Allergic reactions to measles (rubeola) vaccine in patients hypersensitive to egg protein. J Pediatr 102:196–9, 1983
25. Robbins KB, Brandling-Bennett AD, Hinman AR: Low measles incidence: Association with enforcement of school immunization laws. Am J Public Health 71:270–4, 1981
26. Henderson RH, Keja J, Hayden G, et al: Immunizing the children of the world: Progress and prospects. Bull World Health Organ 66:535–43, 1988
27. Markowitz LE, Sepulveda J, Diaz-Ortega JL, et al: Immunization of six-month-old infants with different doses of Edmonston-Zagreb and Schwarz measles vaccines. N Engl J Med 322:580–7, 1990

Mumps

1. Koplan JP, Preblud SR: A benefit-cost analysis of mumps vaccine. Am J Dis Child 136:362–4, 1982
2. Forsey T, Mawn JA, Yates PJ, Bentley ML, Minor PD: Differentiation of vaccine and wild mumps viruses using the polymerase chain reaction and dideoxynucleotide sequencing. J Gen Virol 71:987–90, 1990
3. Philip RN, Reinhard KR, Lackman DB: Observations on the mumps epidemic in a "virgin" population. Am J Hyg 69:91–111, 1959
4. Mumps surveillance, January 1977–December 1982. Atlanta: Centers for Disease Control, Sept. 1984
5. Siegel M, Fuerst HT, Peress NS: Comparative fetal mortality in maternal virus diseases: A prospective study on rubella, measles, mumps, chickenpox, and hepatitis. N Engl J Med 274:768–71, 1966
6. Centers for Disease Control: Mumps in the United States—1985-1988. MMWR 38:101–5, 1989
7. Sosin DM, Cochi SL, Gunn RA, Jennings CE, Preblud SR: The changing epidemiology of mumps and its impact on university campuses. Pediatrics 84:779–84, 1989
8. Wharton M, Cochi SL, Hutcheson RH, Bistowish JM, Schaffner

WA: A large outbreak of mumps in the post-vaccine era. J Infect Dis 158:1253–60, 1988
9. Kaplan KM, Marder DC, Cochi SL, Preblud SR: Mumps in the workplace. JAMA 260:1434–8, 1988
10. Cochi SL, Preblud SR, Orenstein WA: Perspectives on the relative resurgence of mumps in the United States. Am J Dis Child 142:499–507, 1988
11. White CC, Koplan JP, Orenstein WA: Benefits, risks, and costs of immunization for measles, mumps, and rubella. Am J Public Health 75:739–44, 1985
12. Hilleman MR, Buynak EB, Weibel RE, Stokes J Jr: Live, attenuated mumps-virus vaccine. N Engl J Med 278:227–32, 1968
13. Chaiken BP, Williams NM, Preblud SR, Parkin W, Altman R: The effect of a school entry law on mumps activity in a school district. JAMA 257:2455–8, 1987
14. Kim-Farley R, Bart S, Stetler H, et al: Clinical mumps vaccine efficacy. Am J Epidemiol 121:593–7, 1985
15. Weibel RE, Buynak EB, McLean AA, Hilleman MR: Follow-up surveillance of antibody in human subjects following live attenuated measles, mumps, and rubella virus vaccines. Proc Soc Exp Biol Med 162:328–32, 1979
16. Weibel RE, Buynak EB, McLean AA, Roehm RR, Hilleman MR: Persistence of antibody in human subjects for 7 to 10 years following administration of combined live attenuated measles, mumps, and rubella virus vaccines. Proc Soc Exp Biol Med 165:260–3, 1980
17. Immunization Practices Advisory Committee. Mumps vaccine. MMWR 38:388–92, 397–400, 1989
18. Herman JJ, Radin R, Schneiderman R. Allergic reactions to measles (rubeola) vaccine in patients hypersensitive to egg protein. J Pediatr 102:196–9, 1983
19. Greenberg MA, Birx DL. Safe administration of measles-mumps-rubella vaccine in egg-allergic children. J Pediatr 113:504–6, 1988
20. Wharton M, Cochi SL, Hutcheson RH, Schaffner W: Mumps transmission in hospitals. Arch Intern Med 150:47–9, 1990

Rubella

1. Balfour HH Jr, Groth KE, Edelman CK, et al: Rubella viremia and antibody responses after rubella vaccination and reimmunization. Lancet 1:1078–80, 1981
2. Preblud SR, Serdula MK, Frank JA Jr, et al: Rubella vaccination in the United States: A ten-year review. Epidemiol Rev 2:171–94, 1980
3. Ziring PR: Congenital rubella: The teenage years. Pediatr Ann 6:762–70, 1977
4. Miller E, Cradock-Watson JE, Pollock TM: Consequences of confirmed maternal rubella at successive stages of pregnancy. Lancet 2:781–4, 1982
5. Preblud SR, Alford CA: Rubella. In Remington JS, Klein JO (eds): Infectious diseases of the fetus and newborn infant, 3 edt. Philadelphia: WB Saunders Co., 1991.
6. Centers for Disease Control: Rubella and congenital rubella—United States, 1985–1988. MMWR 38:173–8, 1989
7. Cochi SL, Edmonds LE, Dyer K, et al: Congenital rubella syndrome in the United States, 1970–1985: On the verge of elimination. Am J Epidemiol 129:349–61, 1989
8. Crowder M, Higgins HL, Frost JJ: Rubella susceptibility in young women of rural East Texas: 1980 and 1985. Texas Med 83:43–7, 1987
9. Witte JT, Karchmer AW, Caes G, et al: Epidemiology of rubella. Am J Dis Child 118:107–11, 1969
10. Bart KJ, Orenstein WA, Preblud SR, Hinman AR: Universal immunization to interrupt rubella. Rev Infect Dis 7(suppl 1): S177–84, 1985
11. Miller C: Introduction of measles/mumps/rubella vaccine. Health Visit 61:116–7, 1988
12. Chu SY, Bernier RH, Stewart JA, et al: Rubella antibody persistence after immunization: Sixteen-year follow-up in the Hawaiian Islands. JAMA 259:3133–6, 1988
13. Centers for Disease Control: Rubella prevention: Recommendation of the Immunization Practices Advisory Committee. ACIP MMWR 39(No.RR-15), 1990
14. Centers for Disease Control: Rubella vaccination during pregnancy—United States, 1971–1988. MMWR 38:289–93, 1989

Pertussis

1. Miller CL, Fletcher WB: Severity of notified whooping cough. Br Med J 1:117–9, 1976
2. Pittman M: Pertussis toxin: The cause of the harmful effects and prolonged immunity of whooping cough—a hypothesis. Rev Infect Dis 1:401–12, 1979
3. Onorato IM, Wassilak SGF: Laboratory diagnosis of pertussis: The state of the art. Pediatr Infect Dis J 6:145–51, 1987
4. Immunization Practices Advisory Committee: Diphtheria, tetanus and pertussis: Guidelines for vaccine prophylaxis and other preventive measures. MMWR 34:405–14, 419–26, 1985
5. Lambert HJ: Epidemiology of a small pertussis outbreak in Kent County, Michigan. Public Health Rep 80:365–9, 1965
6. Cody DL, Baraff LJ, Cherry JD, et al: Nature and rates of adverse reactions associated with DPT and DT immunizations in infants and children. Pediatrics 68:650–60, 1981
7. Miller D, Wadsworth J, Diamond J, Ross E: Pertussis vaccine and whooping cough as risk factors in acute neurological illness and death in young children. Dev Biol Standard 61:389–94, 1985
8. Noble GR, Bernier RH, Esber EC, et al: Acellular and whole-cell pertussis vaccines in Japan: Report of a visit by U.S. scientists. JAMA 257:1351–6, 1987
9. Ad Hoc Group for the Study of Pertussis Vaccines: Placebo-controlled trial of two acellular pertussis vaccines in Sweden: Protective efficacy and adverse events. Lancet 1:955–60, 1988
10. Hinman AR, Koplan JP: Pertussis and pertussis vaccine: Reanalysis of benefits, risks, and costs. JAMA 251:3109–13, 1984

Tetanus

1. Galazka A, Gasse F, Henderson RH: Neonatal tetanus in the world and the global Expanded Programme on Immunization. In Nistico G, Bizzini B, Bytchenko R, Triau R (eds): Eighth International Conference on Tetanus, Leningrad, USSR, 25–28 Aug. 1987. Rome: Pythagora Press, 1989
2. Centers for Disease Control: Morbidity Mortality Summary of Notifiable Diseases United States. 36(54):41, 1987–1988
3. Crossley K, Irvine P, Warren JB, Lee BK, Mead K: Tetanus and diphtheria immunity in urban Minnesota adults. JAMA 242:2298–300, 1979
4. Long AP, Sartwell PE: Tetanus in the U.S. Army in World War II. Bull US Army Med Dept 7:371–85, 1947
5. U.S. Public Health Service Advisory Committee on Immunization Practices: Diphtheria, tetanus, and pertussis: Guidelines for vaccine prophylaxis and other preventive measures. MMWR 34:405–14, 419–26, 1985
6. Peebles TC, Levine L, Eldred MC, Edsall G: Tetanus toxoid emergency boosters: A reappraisal. N Engl J Med 280:575–81, 1969
7. Jacobs RL, Lowe RS, Lanier BQ: Adverse reactions to tetanus toxoid. JAMA 247:40–2, 1982
8. Edsall G, Elliot MW, Peebles TC, Levine L, Eldred MC: Excessive use of tetanus toxoid boosters. JAMA 202:111–3, 1967
9. Brand DA, Acampora D, Gottlieb LD, Glancy KE, Frazier WH: Adequacy of antitetanus prophylaxis in six hospital emergency rooms. N Engl J Med 309:636–40, 1983
10. McComb JA: The prophylactic dose of homologous tetanus antitoxin. N Engl J Med 270:175–8, 1964
11. Hinman AR, Foster SO, Wassilak SGF: Neonatal tetanus: Potential for elimination in the USA and the world. Pediatr Infect Dis J 6:813–6, 1987
12. Expanded Programme on Immunization: Issues in Neonatal Tetanus Control. EPI/GAG/87/WP. 11. Geneva: World Health Organization, 1987

General References

Alfrey DD, Rauscher LA: Tetanus: A review. Crit Care Med 7:176–81, 1979

Bleck TP: Pharmacology of tetanus. Clin Neuropharmacol 9:103–20, 1986

Nistico G, Bizzini B, Bytchenko R, Triau R (eds): Eighth International Conference on Tetanus, Leningrad, USSR, 25–28 Aug. 1987. Rome: Pythagora Press, 1989

Nistico G, Mastroeni P, Pitzurra M (eds): Seventh International Conference on Tetanus, Copanello, Italy, 10–15 Sept. 1984. Rome: Gangemi Publishing Co., 1985

Diphtheria

1. Uchida T: Diphtheria toxin. Pharmacol Ther 19:107–22, 1983
2. Pappenheimer AM Jr, Murphy JR: Studies on the molecular epidemiology of diphtheria. Lancet 2:923–6, 1983
3. Crossley K, Irvine P, Warren JB, Lee BK: Tetanus and diphtheria in urban Minnesota adults. JAMA 240:1198–200, 1978
4. Griffith AH: The role of immunization in the control of diphtheria. Dev Biol Stand 43:3–13, 1979
5. U.S. Public Health Service Advisory Committee on Immunization Practices: Diphtheria, tetanus, and pertussis: Guidelines for vaccine prophylaxis and other preventive measures. MMWR 34:405–14, 419–26, 1984
6. Scheibel I, Bentzon MW, Christensen PE, Biering A: Duration of immunity to diphtheria and tetanus after active immunization. Acta Pathol Microbiol Scand 67:380–92, 1966

General References

Dobie RA, Tobey DN: Clinical features of diphtheria in the respiratory tract. JAMA 242:2197–201, 1979

Hodes HL: Diphtheria. Pediatr Clin North 26:445–59, 1979

McCloskey RV, Eller JJ, Green M, et al: The 1970 epidemic of diphtheria in San Antonio. Ann Intern Med 75:495–503, 1971

Naiditch MJ, Bower AG: Diphtheria: A study of 1,433 cases observed during a 10-year period at Los Angeles County Hospital. Am J Med 17:229–45, 1945

Poliomyelitis

1. Evans AS (ed): Viral Infections of Humans: Epidemiology and Control. New York: Plenum, 1982
2. Enders JF, Weller TH, Robbins FC: Cultivation of the Lancing strains of poliomyelitis virus in cultures of various human embryonic tissue. Science 109:85–7, 1949
3. Mendelsohn CL, Wimmer E, Racaniello VR: Cellular receptor for poliovirus: Molecular cloning, nucleotide sequence, and expression of a new member of the immunoglobulin superfamily. Cell 56:855–65, 1989
4. Cherry JD: Enteroviruses: Polioviruses (poliomyelitis), coxsackieviruses, echoviruses, and enteroviruses. In Feigin RD, Cherry JD (eds): Textbook of Pediatric Infectious Diseases, 2 edt. Philadelphia: WB Saunders, 1987, pp 1764–5
5. Hinman AR, Foege WH, deQuadros CA, Patriarca PA, Orenstein WA, Brink EW: The case for global eradication of poliomyelitis. Bull World Health Organ 65:835–40, 1987
6. Expanded Programme on Immunization. Poliomyelitis in 1986, 1987, and 1988. Weekly Epidemiol Rec 64:273–9, 1989
7. Rico-Hesse R, Pallansch MA, Nottay BK, Kew OM: Geographic distribution of wild poliovirus type 1 genotypes. Virology 160:311–22, 1987
8. Sutter RW, Brink EW, Cochi SL, et al: A new epidemiologic and laboratory classification system for paralytic poliomyelitis cases. Am J Public Health 79:495–8, 1989
9. Advisory Committee on Immunization Practices: Poliomyelitis prevention. MMWR 31:22–6, 1982
10. Advisory Committee on Immunization Practices: Poliomyelitis prevention: Enhanced-potency inactivated poliomyelitis vaccine: Supplementary statement. MMWR 36:795–8, 1987
11. Centers for Disease Control: Progress toward eradicating poliomyelitis from the Americas. MMWR 38:532–5, 1989
12. World Health Organization: Global eradication of poliomyelitis by the year 2000. Weekly Epidemiol Rec 63:161–2, 1988
13. Nkowane BM, Wassilak SGF, Orenstein WA, et al: Vaccine-associated paralytic poliomyelitis: United States, 1973 through 1984. JAMA 257:1335–40, 1987
14. Institute of Medicine: An evaluation of poliomyelitis vaccine policy options. Washington, D.C.: National Academy of Sciences, 1988 (publication No. IOM 88-04)

Influenza

1. Skinner HA: The Origin of Medical Terms. Baltimore: Williams & Wilkins, 1949, pp 191–2
2. Smith W, Andrews CH, Laidlaw PP: A virus obtained from influenza patients. Lancet 2:66, 1933
3. Francis T Jr: A new type of virus from epidemic influenza. Science 92:405, 1940
4. Taylor RM: A further note on 1233 ("influenza C") virus. Arch Gesamte Virusforsch 4:485, 1951
5. Varma RR, Riedel DR, Komorouski RA, et al: Reye's syndrome in non-pediatric age groups. JAMA 242:1373, 1979
6. Centers for Disease Control: Influenza—United States, 1989-90. MMWR 39(10):157–9, 1990
7. Kilbourne ED: The influenza viruses and influenza: An introduction. In Kilbourne ED (ed): The Influenza Viruses and Influenza. New York: Academic Press, 1975, pp 1–14
8. World Health Organization: A revision of the system of nomenclature for influenza viruses: A WHO memorandum. Bull World Health Organ 1980;58:585–91
9. Webster RG, Laver WG: Antigenic variation of influenza viruses. In Kilbourne ED (ed): Influenza Viruses and Influenza. New York: Academic Press, 1975, pp 269–314
10. Webster RG, Hinshaw VS, Naeve CW, Bean WJ: Pandemics and animal influenza viruses: In Stuart-Harris CH, Potter CW (eds): The Molecular Virology and Epidemiology of Influenza. New York: Academic Press, 1984, pp 17–38
11. Masurel N, Marine WM: Recycling of Asian and Hong Kong influenza A virus hemagglutinin in man. Am J Epidemiol 97:44–9, 1973
12. Kendal A, Harmon MW: Orthomyxoviridae: The influenza viruses. In Lennette EH, Halonen P, Murphy FA (eds): Laboratory Diagnosis of Infectious Diseases (Principles and Practices), Vol. II. New York: Springer-Verlag, 1988, pp 602–25
13. Glezen WP, Six HR, Perotta DM, Decker M, Joseph W: Epidemics and their causative viruses: Community experience. In Stuart-Harris CH, Potter CW (eds): The Molecular Virology and Epidemiology of Influenza. New York: Academic Press, 1984, pp 17–38
14. Schoenbaum SC: Economic impact of influenza: The individual's perspective. Am J Med 82(s6A):26–30, 1987
15. Askoras BA, McMichael AJ, Webster RG: The immune response to influenza viruses and the problem of protection against infection. In Beare AS (ed): Basic and Applied Influenza Research. Boca Raton, Fl.: CRC Press, 1982, pp 157–88
16. Centers for Disease Control: Recommendations of the Immunization Practices Advisory Committee (ACIP): Prevention and control of influenza. I. Vaccines. MMWR 38(17):297–311, 1989
17. Centers for Disease Control: Update: Influenza activity—worldwide and recommendations for influenza vaccine composition for the 1990–1991 influenza season. MMWR 39(17):293–6, 1990
18. Ruben FL: Prevention and control of influenza: Role of vaccine. Am J Med 82:31–4, 1987
19. Langmuir AD, Bregman DJ, Kurland LT, Nathanson N, Victor M: An epidemiologic and clinical evaluation of Guillain-Barré syndrome reported in association with the administration of swine influenza vaccines. Am J Epidemiol 119:841–79, 1984
20. Douglas RG: Antiviral drugs. Med Clin North Am 67:1163–9, 1983

21. Couch RB, Kasel JA, Glezen WP: Influenza: Its control in persons and populations. J Infect Dis 153:431–40, 1986
22. Fedson DS: Influenza prevention and control: Past practices and future prospects. Am J Med 82(s6A):42–7, 1987
23. Centers for Disease Control: Prevention and control of influenza: Recommendations of the Immunization Practices Advisory Committee. Ann Intern Med 107:521–5, 1987

Haemophilus influenzae Infections

1. Wenger JD, Hightower AW, Facklam RR, Gaventa S, Broome CV, and the Bacterial Meningitis Study Group: Bacterial meningitis in the U.S., 1986: Report of a multistate surveillance project. J Infect Dis (in press)
2. Moxon ER, Glode MP, Sutton A, Robbins JB: The infant rat as a model of bacterial meningitis. J Infect Dis 136(suppl);5186–90, 1977
3. Nordon CS, Melish M, Overall JC Jr, Baum J: Immunologic responses to *Haemophilus influenzae* meningitis. J Pediatr 80:209–14, 1972
4. Sell SHW, Turner DJ, Federspiel CF: Natural infections with *Hemophilus influenzae* in children. I. Types identified. In Sell SHW, Karzon DT (eds): *Hemophilus influenzae.* Nashville, Tenn.: Vanderbilt University Press, 1973, pp 3–12
5. Cochi SL, Fleming DW, Hightower AW, et al: Primary invasive *Haemophilus influenzae* type b disease: A population-based assessment of risk factors. J Pediatr 108:887–96, 1986
6. Schlech WF III, Ward JI, Band JD, et al: Bacterial meningitis in the United States, 1978–1981: The National Bacterial Meningitis Surveillance Study. JAMA 253:1749–54, 1985
7. Broome CV, Mortimer EA, Katz SL, Fleming DW, Hightower AW: Use of chemoprophylaxis to prevent the spread of *Hemophilus influenzae* b in day-care facilities. N Engl J Med 316:1226–8, 1987
8. Peltola H, Kayhty H, Virtanen M, Makela PH: Prevention of *Haemophilus influenzae* bacteremia infections with the capsular polysaccharide vaccine. N Engl J Med 310:1561–6, 1984
9. Ward JI, Broome CV, Harrison LH, Shinefeld H, Black S: *Haemophilus influenzae* type b vaccines: Lessons for the future. Pediatrics 81:886–92, 1988
10. Wenger JD, Ward JI, Broome CV: Prevention of *Haemophilus influenzae* type b disease: Vaccines and passive prophylaxis. In Remington JS, Swartz MN (eds): Curr Clin Top Infect Dis 10:306–339, 1989
11. Band JD, Fraser DW, Ajello G: Prevention of *Hemophilus influenzae* type b disease. JAMA 251:2381–6, 1984
12. Immunization Practices Advisory Committee: Update: Prevention of *Haemophilus influenzae* type b disease. MMWR 35:170, 1986

Pneumococcal Infections

1. Research Committee of the British Thoracic Society: Community-acquired pneumonia in adults in British hospitals in 1982–1983: A survey of aetiology, mortality, prognostic factors and outcome. Q J Med 62:195, 1987
2. Macfarlane J: Community-acquired pneumonia. Br J Dis Chest 81:116, 1987
3. Austrian R, Howie VM, Ploussard JH: The bacteriology of pneumococcal otitis media. Johns Hopkins Med J 141:104, 1977
4. Rich AR, McKee CM: The pathogenieity of avirulent pneumococci for animals deprived of leukocytes. Bull Johns Hopkins Hosp 64:434, 1939
5. Hodges RG, MacLeod CM, Bernhard WG: Epidemic pneumococcal pneumonia. III. Carrier studies. Am J Hyg 44:207, 1946
6. Gundel M, Schwarz FKT: Studien über die Bakterienflora der obern Atmungswege Neugeborener (im Vergleich mit der Mundhöhlenflora der Mutter und des Pflegepersonals) unter besonderer Berucksichtigung ihrer Bedeutung für das Pneumonie- problem. Z Hyg Infectionskir 113:411, 1932
7. Andersson B, Dahmen J, Frejd T, et al: Identification of an active disaccharide unit of a glycoconjugate receptor for pneumococci attaching to human epithelial cells. J Exp Med 158:559, 1983
8. Loda FA, Collier AM, Glezen WP, et al: Occurrence of *Diplococcus pneumoniae* in the upper respiratory tract of children. J Pediatr 87:1087, 1975
9. Gundel M, Okura G: Untersuchungen über das gleichzeitige Vorkommen mehrer Pneumokokkentypen bei Gesunden und ihre Bedeutung fur die Epidemiologie. Z Hyg Infektionskr 114:678, 1933
10. Webster LT, Hughes TP: The epidemiology of pneumococcus infection: The incidence and spread of pneumococci in the nasal passages and throats of healthy persons. J Exp Med 53:535, 1931
11. Bliss EA, McClaskey WD, Long PH: A study of pneumococcus carriers. J Immunol 27:95, 1934
12. Gwaltney JM, Sande MA, Austrian R, et al: Spread of *Streptococcus pneumoniae* in families. II. Relation of transfer of *S. pneumoniae* to incidence of colds and serum antibody. J Infect Dis 132:62, 1975
13. MacLeod CM, Hodges RG, Heidelberger M, et al: Prevention of pneumococcal pneumonia by immunization with specific capsular polysaccharides. J Exp Med 82:445, 1945
14. Koornhof HJ, Jacobs MR, Ward JL, et al: Therapy and control of antibiotic-resistant pneumococcal disease. In Schlessinger D (ed): Microbiology—1979. Washington, D.C.: American Society for Microbiology, 1979
15. Sternberg GM: A fatal form of septicaemia in the rabbit produced by subcutaneous injection of human saliva: An experimental research. Natl Bd of Health Bull 2:781, 1881
16. Pasteur L: Note sur la maladie nouvelle provoquée par la salive d'un enfant mort de la rage. Bull Acad Natl Med (Paris) 10:94, 1881
17. Heffron R: Pneumonia, With Special Reference to *Pneumococcus* Lobar Pneumonia. New York: Commonwealth Fund, 1939. Reprinted: Cambridge, Mass.: Harvard University Press, 1979
18. Finland M, Barnes MW: Changes in the occurrence of capsular serotypes of *Streptococcus pneumoniae* at Boston City Hospital during selected years between 1935 and 1974. J Clin Microbiol 5:154, 1977
19. Austrian R: Some observations on the pneumococcus and on the current status of pneumococcal disease and its prevention. Rev Infect Dis 3(suppl):S1, 1981
20. Paton JC, Toogood IR, Cockington RA, et al: Antibody response to pneumococcal vaccine in children aged 5 to 15 years. Am J Dis Child 140:135, 1986
21. Moore HF, Chesney AM: A study of ethylhydrocuprein (Optochin) in the treatment of acute lobar pneumonia. Arch Intern Med 19:611, 1917
22. Schmidt LH, Sesler CL: Development of resistance to penicillin by pneumococci. Proc Soc Exp Biol Med 52:353, 1943
23. Jabes D, Nachman S, Tomasz A: Penicillin-binding protein families: Evidence for the clonal nature of penicillin resistance in clinical isolates of pneumococci. J Infect Dis 159:16, 1989
24. Applebaum PC: World-wide development of antibiotic resistance in pneumococci. Eur J Clin Microbiol 6:367, 1987
25. Klugman KP, Koornhof HJ: Drug resistance patterns and serogroups or serotypes of pneumococcal isolates from cerebrospinal fluid or blood, 1979–1986. J Infect Dis 158:956, 1988
26. Casal J, Fenoll A, Vicioso MD, et al: Increase in resistance to penicillin in pneumococci in Spain. Lancet 1:735, 1989
27. Klugman KP, Koornhof HJ, Kuhnle V: Clinical and nasopharyngeal isolates of unusual multiply resistant pneumococci. Am J Dis Child 140:1186, 1986
28. Harford CG, Hara M: Pulmonary edema in influenza pneumonia of the mouse and the relation of fluid in the lung to the inception of pneumococcal pneumonia. J Exp Med 91:245, 1950
29. Giebink GS: The pathogenesis of pneumococcal otitis media in chinchillas and the efficacy of vaccination in prophylaxis. Rev Infect Dis 3:342, 1981
30. Austrian R: Pneumococcal pneumonia: Diagnostic, epidemiologic, therapeutic and prophylactic considerations. Chest 90:738, 1986
31. Broome CV, Facklam RR, Allen JR, et al: Epidemiology of pneu-

mococcal serotypes in the United States, 1978–1979. J Infect Dis 141:119, 1980

32. Davidson M, Schraer CD, Parkinson AJ, et al: Invasive pneumococcal disease in an Alaska native population. JAMA 261:715, 1989
33. Filice GA, Darby CP, Fraser DW: Pneumococcal bacteremia in Charleston County, South Carolina. Am J Epidemial 112:828, 1980
34. Austrian R, Gold J: Pneumococcal bacteremia with especial reference to bacteremic pneumococcal pneumonia. Ann Intern Med 60:759, 1964
35. Austrian R: Untreated pneumococcal bacteraemia of cryptic origin in the human adult with spontaneous recovery. S Afr Med J 70(suppl):46, 1986
36. Fraser DW, Geil CC, Feldman RA: Bacterial meningitis in Bernalillo County, New Mexico: A comparison with three other American populations. Am J Epidemiol 100:29, 1974
37. Viladrich PF, Gudiol F, Linares J, et al: Characteristics and antibiotic therapy of adult meningitis due to penicillin-resistant pneumococci. Am J Med 84:839, 1988
38. Hook EW III, Horton CA, Shaberg DR: Failure of intensive care unit support to influence mortality from pneumococcal bacteremia. JAMA 249:1055, 1983
39. Beuvery EC, van Rossum F, Nagel J: Comparison of induction of immunoglobulin M and G antibodies in mice with purified pneumococcal type 3 and meningococcal group C polysaccharides and their protein conjugates. Infect Immun 37:15, 1982
40. Anderson P, Pichichero ME, Insel RE: Immunization of 2-month-old infants with protein-coupled oligosaccharides derived from the capsule of *Haemophilus influenzae* type b. J Pediatr 107:346, 1985
41. Schneerson R, Robbins JB, Parke JC Jr, et al: Quantitative and qualitative analysis of serum antibodies elicited in adults by *Haemophilus influenzae* type b and pneumococcus type 6A capsular polysaccharide–tetanus toxoid conjugates. Infect Immun 52:519, 1986
42. Austrian R, Douglas RM, Schiffman G, et al: Prevention of pneumococcal pneumonia by vaccination. Trans Assoc Am Physicians 89:184, 1976
43. Broome CV, Facklam RR, Fraser DW: Pneumococcal disease after pneumococcal vaccination. N Engl J Med 303:549, 1980
44. Shapiro ED, Clemens JD: A controlled evaluation of the protective efficacy of pneumococcal vaccine for patients at high risk of serious pneumococcal infections. Ann Intern Med 101:325, 1984
45. Bolan G, Broome CV, Facklam RR, et al: Pneumococcal vaccine efficacy in selected populations in the United States. Ann Intern Med 104:1, 1986
46. Artenstein MS, Gold R, Zimmerly JG, et al: Prevention of meningococcal disease by group C polysaccharide vaccine. N Engl J Med 282:417, 1970
47. Immunization Practices Advisory Committee: Pneumococcal polysaccharide vaccine. MMWR 38:64, 1989
48. Committee on Immunization: Guide for Adult Immunization. Philadelphia: American College of Physicians, 1985, pp 66–9

Chickenpox

1. Preblud SR, Orenstein WA, Bart KJ: Varicella: Clinical manifestations, epidemiology, and health impact. Pediatr Infect Dis 3:505–9, 1984
2. Oxman MN, Richman DD, Spector SA: Management at delivery of mother and infant when herpes simplex, varicella-zoster, hepatitis, or tuberculoses have occurred in pregnancy. In Remington JS, Swartz MN (eds): Curr Clin Top Infect Dis 4:224–80, 1983
3. Preblud SR: Varicella: Complications and costs. Pediatrics 78:S728–35, 1986
4. Gershon AA, Steinberg S, Brunell PA: Zoster immune globulin: A further assessment. N Engl J Med 290:243–5, 1974
5. Jordan DR, Noel L-P, Clarke WN: Ocular involvement in varicella. Clin Pediatr 23:434–6, 1984
6. Stagno S, Whitley RJ: Herpesvirus infections of pregnancy. II. Herpes simplex virus and varicella-zoster virus infections. N Engl J Med 313:1327–30, 1985
7. Guess HA, Broughton DD, Melton LJ, et al: Population-based studies of varicella complications. Pediatrics 78:S723–7, 1986
8. Preblud SR: Age-specific risks of varicella complications. Pediatrics 68:14–7, 1981
9. Centers for Disease Control: Reye Syndrome Surveillance—United States, 1986. MMWR 36:689–91, 1987
10. Fehrs LJ: Update on varicella vaccine. Proceedings of the 24th Immunization Conference (in press).
11. Strauss SE, Ostrove JM, Inchauspe G, et al: Varicella-zoster virus infections: Biology, natural history, treatment, and prevention. Ann Intern Med 108:221–37, 1988
12. Feldman S, Hughes WT, Daniel CB: Varicella in children with cancer: Seventy-seven cases. Pediatrics 56:388–97, 1975
13. Cohen PR, Grossman ME: Clinical features of human immunodeficiency virus–associated disseminated herpes zoster virus infection: A review of the literature. Clin Dermatol 14:273–6, 1989
14. Jura E, Chadwick EG, Josephs SH, et al: Varicella-zoster virus infections in children infected with human immunodeficiency virus. Pediatr Infect Dis J 8:586–90, 1989
15. Selik RM, Starcher ET, Curran JW: Opportunistic diseases reported in AIDS patients: Frequencies, associations, and trends. AIDS Res Ther 1:175–82, 1987
16. Jacobson MA, Berger TG, Fikrig S, et al: Acyclovir-resistant varicella zoster virus infection after chronic oral acyclovir therapy in patients with the acquired immunodeficiency syndrome (AIDS). Ann Intern Med 112:187–91, 1990
17. Meyers JD: Congenital varicella in term infants: Risk reconsidered. J Infect Dis 129:215–7, 1975
18. Preblud SR, Bregman DJ, Vernon LL: Deaths from varicella in infants. Pediatr Infect Dis 4:503–7, 1985
19. Brunell PA: Fetal and neonatal varicella zoster infections. Semin Perinatol 7:47–56, 1983
20. Preblud SR, Cochi SL, Orenstein WA: Letter to the Editor. N Engl J Med 315:1415–8, 1986
21. Weller TH: Varicella and herpes zoster: Changing concepts of the natural history, control, and importance of a not-to-benign virus. N Engl J Med 309:1362–8, 1434–40, 1983
22. Ragozzino MW, Melton LJ, Kurland LT, Chu CP, Perry HO: Population-based study of herpes zoster and its sequelae. Medicine 61:310–6, 1982
23. Gordon JE: Chickenpox: An epidemiologic review. Am J Med Sci 224:362–89, 1962
24. Gershon AA: Immunoprophylaxis of varicella-zoster infections. Am J Med 76:672–7, 1984
25. Gershon A, Steinberg SP, Gelb L: Clinical reinfection with varicella-zoster virus. J Infect Dis 149:137–42, 1984
26. Zaia JA, Levin MJ, Preblud SR, et al: Evaluation of varicella-zoster immune globulin: Protection of immunosuppressed children after household exposure to varicella. J Infect Dis 147:737–43, 1983
27. Immunization Practices Advisory Committee: Varicella-zoster immune globulin for the prevention of chickenpox. MMWR 33:84–90, 95–100, 1984
28. Venkitaraman AR, Seigneurin J-M, Baccard M, et al: Measurement of antibodies to varicella-zoster virus in a tropical population by enzyme-linked immunosorbent assay. J Clin Microbiol 20:582–3, 1984
29. Ross AH: Modification of chickenpox in family contacts by administration of gamma globulin. N Engl J Med 267:369–76, 1962
30. Brunell PA: Interview with Philip A. Brunell: Contagion and varicella-zoster virus. Pediatr Infect Dis 1:304–7, 1982
31. Preblud SR, Arbeter AM, Proctor EA, Starr SE, Plotkin SA: Susceptibility of vaccine strains of varicella-zoster virus to antiviral compounds. Antimicrob Agents Chemother 25:417–21, 1984
32. Takahashi M: Clinical overview of varicella vaccine: Development and early studies. Pediatrics 78:S736–41, 1986
33. Arbeter AM, Starr SE, Plotkin SA: Varicella vaccine studies: Healthy children and adults. Pediatrics 78:S748–55, 1986

34. Gershon AA, Steinberg SP, Gelb L, et al: Live attenuated varicella vaccine use in immunocompromised children and adults. Pediatrics 78:S757–62, 1986
35. Gershon AA, Steinberg SP, NIAID Varicella Vaccine Collaborative Study Group: Live attenuated varicella vaccine: Protection in healthy adults compared with leukemic children. J Infect Dis 161:661–6, 1990
36. Weibel RE, Neff BJ, Kuter BJ, et al: Live attenuated varicella virus vaccine: Efficacy trial in healthy children. N Engl J Med 310:1409–15, 1984
37. Plotkin SA, Starr SE, Connor K, et al: Zoster in normal children after varicella vaccine. J Infect Dis 159:1000, 1989
38. Lawrence R, Gershon AA, Holzman R, et al: The risk of zoster after varicella vaccination in children with leukemia. N Engl J Med 318:543–8, 1988
39. Hammerschlag MR, Gershon AA, Steinberg SP, et al: Herpes zoster in an adult recipient of live attenuated varicella vaccine. J Infect Dis 160:535–7, 1989
40. Gershon AA, Steinberg SP, Varicella Vaccine Collaborative Study Group: Persistence of immunity to varicella in children with leukemia immunized with live attenuated varicella vaccine. N Engl J Med 320:892–7, 1989
41. Gershon AA, Steinberg SP, LaRussa P, et al: Immunization of healthy adults with live attenuated varicella vaccine. J Infect Dis 158:132–7, 1988
42. Gershon AA, Steinberg SP, Gelb L, et al: Live attenuated varicella vaccine: Efficacy for children with leukemia in remission. JAMA 252:355–62, 1984
43. Tsolia M, Gershon AA, Steinberg SP, et al: Live attenuated varicella vaccine: Evidence that the virus is attenuated and the importance of skin lesions in transmission of varicella-zoster virus. J Pediatr 116:184–9, 1990

6

Sexually Transmitted Diseases

Willard Cates, Jr.
King K. Holmes

Few areas of public health have been more dynamic in recent years than the field of sexually transmitted diseases (STDs). During the past decade, this discipline has evolved from one emphasizing the traditional venereal diseases of gonorrhea and syphilis, to one concerned with the bacterial and viral syndromes associated with *Chlamydia trachomatis,* herpes simplex virus (HSV), and human papillomavirus (HPV), and to one dominated by the fatal systemic infection caused by human immunodeficiency virus (HIV).[1] Over 20 organisms (Table 6–1) and countless syndromes (Table 6–2) are now recognized as being sexually transmitted. All these STDs are historically, biologically, behaviorally, economically, and programmatically interrelated.[2]

HISTORY OF STDS AND PUBLIC HEALTH

Social Attitudes. Throughout history, STDs have caused society to wrestle with its moral feelings about this public health problem. In recent years, the human tragedies suffered by persons with STDs have led to more effective social and political responses designed to interrupt transmission and reduce complications rather than to stigmatize those with disease.

Before 1900, physicians were known to withhold treatment for STDs, fatalistically regarding infection as evidence of (and even punishment for) "promiscuous" behavior.[3] Before World War I, the increasing professionalization of medicine coincided with the rise of venereology as an established specialty. Syphilis became the disease on which the skills of twentieth-century physicians were judged. Knowledge in this field rapidly progressed from acceptance of the germ theory to fascination with serological tests and use of toxic cures. The foundations were laid for a medical, rather than a moralistic, approach to STD control.

In the New Deal era, Surgeon General Thomas Parran seized an opportunity to dramatize the plight of those with STDs. With penicillin available and the higher national imperative of winning a war, the image of STD shed a portion of its stigmatic cloak during the 1940s. The diagnosis and treatment of sexually transmitted infections could be performed on an outpatient basis, thus allowing a more positive attitude toward finding and treating both patients and partners alike.

Finally, during the most recent decades, the changing social role of women and minorities and the greater acceptance of homosexuality have been accompanied by a slow shift in the nation's attitude toward human sexuality. The population at risk of STDs has increased, creating a growing constituency that demands personal and public health solutions. Feminists, realizing that women and children bear the brunt of the sexually related complications, have become increasingly active in politics. Homosexual organizations, spurred by the availability of a hepatitis B virus (HBV) vaccine and the tragedy of HIV and acquired immunodeficiency syndrome (AIDS), lobbied for a greater share of political resources for their health concerns. Finally, those interested in minority health are increasingly acknowledging STDs and HIV as priorities for their constituencies. Thus, society has apparently become more concerned about STD as the scope of the problem has increased and public health interventions have become more available.

Control Programs. U.S. current public health approaches to STDs and HIV greatly resemble those used for syphilis in the preantibiotic era. National programs to control STD were established during the early days of World War I.[3] For the next half century, the focus was almost exclusively on controlling syphilis and its complications. Diagnosis was complex, and treatments were dangerous, which stimulated the continued development of the specialty of venereology. Federal grants to support venereal disease control initiatives were begun in 1939. Rapid-treatment centers for syphilis and gonorrhea were established during World War II.

After World War II, the widespread availability of penicillin led to a dismantling of the rapid-treatment centers and a decline of the clinical specialty of venereology. However, particularly during the 1960s, federal assistance continued to support sex partner tracing, serological testing for syphilis, and health education. The STD "epidemiologist" emerged as a central figure in syphilis control efforts, focusing on locating and treating individuals exposed to syphilis.

By the late 1960s, officials became concerned with the rapidly escalating number of gonorrhea cases. The gonorrhea epidemic, together with the development of selective culture media for isolating the gonococcus, stimulated the implementation of a national gonorrhea control strategy. Beginning in 1968, pilot projects had been initiated to evaluate casefinding of infected women both by using culture diagnosis and by identifying sex partners of infected men. During the 1970s, gonorrhea control gradually received a larger portion of the STD federal dollar, at the expense of syphilis control. By 1980, expenditures for gonor-

TABLE 6–1. TWENTY-FOUR SEXUALLY TRANSMITTED PATHOGENS AND THE DISEASES THEY CAUSE

Agent	Associated Disease or Syndrome
▪ BACTERIA	
Neisseria gonorrhoeae	Urethritis, epididymitis, proctitis, cervicitis, endometritis, salpingitis, perihepatitis, bartholinitis, pharyngitis, conjunctivitis, prepubertal vaginitis, ?prostatitis, accessory gland infection, disseminated gonococcal infection (DGI), chorioamnionitis, premature rupture of membranes, premature delivery, amniotic infection syndrome
Chlamydia trachomatis	All of above except DGI, plus otitis media, rhinitis, and pneumonia in infants and Reiter's syndrome
Mycoplasma hominis	Postpartum fever, ?salpingitis
Ureaplasma urealyticum	Nongonococcal urethritis, ?chorioamnionitis, ?premature delivery
Treponema pallidum	Syphilis
Gardnerella vaginalis	Bacterial ("nonspecific") vaginosis (in conjunction with *Mycoplasma hominis* and vaginal anaerobes, such as *Mobiluncus* spp)
Haemophilus ducreyi	Chancroid
Calymmatobacterium granulomatis	Donovanosis (granuloma inguinale)
Shigella spp	Shigellosis in homosexual men
Campylobacter spp	Enteritis, proctocolitis
Group B streptococcus	Neonatal sepsis, neonatal meningitis
▪ VIRUSES	
Human immunodeficiency virus, types 1 and 2	AIDS
Herpes simplex virus	Initial and recurrent genital herpes, aseptic meningitis, neonatal herpes
Human papilloma virus (57 separate types described as of early 1990)	Condyloma acuminata, laryngeal papilloma, cervical intraepithelial neoplasia and carcinoma, vaginal carcinoma, anal carcinoma, vulvar carcinoma, penile carcinoma
Hepatitis B virus	Acute hepatitis B, chronic active hepatitis, persistent (unresolved) hepatitis, polyarteritis nodosa, chronic membranous glomerulonephritis, ?mixed cryoglobulinemia, ?polymyalgia rheumatica, hepatocellular carcinoma
Hepatitis A virus	Acute hepatitis A
Cytomegalovirus	Heterophil-negative infectious mononucleosis; congenital CMV infection with gross birth defects and infant mortality, cognitive impairment (e.g., mental retardation, sensorineural deafness); protean manifestations in the immunosuppressed host
Molluscum contagiosum virus	Genital molluscum contagiosum
Human T-lymphotrophic retrovirus, type I	Human T cell leukemia or lymphoma
▪ PROTOZOA	
Trichomonas vaginalis	Trichomonal vaginitis
Entamoeba histolytica	Amebiasis in homosexual men
Giardia lamblia	Giardiasis in homosexual men
▪ FUNGI	
Candida albicans	Vulvovaginitis, balanitis
▪ ECTOPARASITES	
Phthirus pubis	Public lice infestation
Sarcoptes scabiei	Scabies

rhea control accounted for almost three quarters of federal STD grant dollars.

Simultaneously, the growing variety and recognition of other syndromes causing patients to seek STD care produced a need for major improvements in clinical skills, clinic services, and physical facilities. This upgrading was necessary both to encourage infected individuals to obtain treatment and to provide additional capability to diagnose the broad array of STDs. Once again, technological change required hard choices. In the 1980s, increased availability of laboratory diagnostic testing for chlamydial infection created opportunities for chlamydia control, requiring further tradeoffs among resources primarily directed to gonorrhea and syphilis control. By the late 1980s, the need to provide testing and counseling for HIV infection has placed additional demands on STD personnel and facilities and has contributed to a delay in implementing chlamydia control programs.

KEY FACTORS AFFECTING STDS

Populations at Risk. During the past 3 decades, various sociosexual changes in the United States dramatically influenced those at highest risk for STD[4]: (1) the baby boomers' passed through the most active and highest-risk sexual years; (2) continuing high birth rates changed the composition of teenagers and young adults toward greater proportions of those with the highest rates of STD, low-income minority heterosexuals; (3) national and international migration patterns and economic shifts led to an increasing concentration of low-income minority groups in the inner cities; (4) the percentage of sexually experienced young persons increased during the 1970s and 1980s; and (5) sexual behaviors of specific high-risk STD populations—primarily homosexual men and those using illicit drugs—have varied. These behavioral changes have measurably decreased STD

TABLE 6-2. SELECTED SYNDROMES AND COMPLICATIONS WITH ASSOCIATED SEXUALLY TRANSMITTED AGENTS[a]

Syndrome	Associated Sexually Transmitted Agent
▪ MEN	
AIDS	Human immunodeficiency virus, types 1 and 2
Urethritis	*Neisseria gonorrhoeae, Chlamydia trachomatis,* herpes simplex virus, *Ureaplasma urealyticum*
Epididymitis	*C. trachomatis, N. gonorrhoeae*
Intestinal infections	
Proctitis	*N. gonorrhoeae,* herpes simplex virus, *C. trachomatis*
Proctocolitis or enterocolitis	*Campylobacter* spp, *Shigella* spp, *Entamoeba histolytica*
Enteritis	*Giardia lamblia*
Hepatitis	Hepatitis A and B viruses, cytomegalovirus, *Treponema pallidum*
▪ WOMEN	
AIDS	Human immunodeficiency virus, types 1 and 2
Lower genitourinary tract infection	
Vulvitis	*Candida albicans,* herpes simplex virus
Vaginitis	*Trichomonas vaginalis, C. albicans*
Vaginosis	*Gardnerella vaginalis, Mobiluncus* spp, other anaerobes, *Mycoplasma hominis*
Cervicitis	*N. gonorrhoeae, C. trachomatis,* herpes simplex virus
Urethritis	*N. gonorrhoeae, C. trachomatis,* herpes simplex virus
Pelvic inflammatory disease	*N. gonorrhoeae, C. trachomatis, M. hominis,* anaerobes, Group B streptococcus
Infertility	
Postsalpingitis, postobstetrical, postabortion	*N. gonorrhoeae, C. trachomatis, ?M. hominis*
Pregnancy morbidity	Several STDs have been implicated in one or more of these conditions
Chorioamnionitis, amniotic fluid infection, prematurity, premature rupture of membranes, preterm delivery, postpartum endometritis, ectopic pregnancy	
▪ MEN AND WOMEN	
Neoplasia	
Cervical, vulvar, vaginal, anal, and penile intraepithelial neoplasia, carcinoma	Human papilloma virus
Hepatocellular carcinoma	Hepatitis B virus
Kaposi's sarcoma, non-Hodgkin's lymphoma	Human immunodeficiency virus, types 1 and 2
Genital ulceration	Herpes simplex virus, *T. pallidum, Haemophilus ducreyi, Calymmatobacterium granulomatis, C. trachomatis* (LGV strains)
Acute arthritis with urogenital or intestinal infection	*N. gonorrhoeae, C. trachomatis, Shigella* spp., *Campylobacter* spp.
Genital warts	Human papilloma virus
Molluscum contagiosum	Molluscum contagiosum virus
Ectoparasite infestations	*Sarcoptes scabiei, Phthirus pubis*
Heterophil-negative mononucleosis	Cytomegalovirus, Epstein-Barr virus (some evidence for sexual transmission)
▪ NEONATES AND INFANTS	
TORCHES syndrome[b]	Cytomegalovirus, herpes simplex virus, *T. pallidum*
Conjunctivitis	*C. trachomatis, N. gonorrhoeae*
Pneumonia	*C. trachomatis, ?U. urealyticum*
Otitis media	*C. trachomatis*
Sepsis, meningitis	Group B streptococcus
Cognitive impairment, deafness	Cytomegalovirus, herpes simplex virus, *T. pallidum*

[a] For each of the above syndromes, some cases cannot yet be ascribed to any cause and must currently be considered idiopathic.
[b] TORCHES is an acronym for toxoplasmosis, rubella, cytomegalovirus, herpes, and syphilis. The syndrome consists of various combinations of encephalitis, hepatitis, dermatitis, and disseminated intravascular coagulation (DIC).

rates among white homosexual males, but little impact has been observed in teenagers and low-income, minority, heterosexual populations.[4]

In addition, the role of the so-called STD core group in sustaining high levels of these infections in their communities is better understood. Mathematical models have demonstrated that sustained endemicity of various STDs can be maintained by a relatively small subgroup of the population's engaging in high-risk sexual practices with a large number of partners. This concept has been supported by considerable empirical evidence showing the entrenchment of particular gonococcal strains in demographically and behaviorally identifiable subgroups within cities such as Rochester, N.Y., Miami, Fla., Colorado Springs, Seattle, and Baltimore. Similar patterns for syphilis have been demonstrated in New York State. Recent investigations have highlighted the role of illicit drugs—especially the exchange of sex for crack cocaine—as a factor both enlarging the core population and facilitating risky sexual behaviors.

Governmental Responsibilities for STD Control and HIV Prevention. National, regional, and local tiers of government have different responsibilities for STD control and HIV prevention. At the federal level, in the United States, the Centers for Disease Control (CDC) coordinates STD (including HIV) control strategies, provides surveillance for STD/HIV/AIDS, and undertakes epidemiological and laboratory research. The National Institutes of Health (NIH) supports both basic science and applied clinical investigations.

State and local health departments are responsible for controlling many communicable diseases, including STD. States (and the largest metropolitan areas) receive federal project grants (numbering 63 in 1990) from CDC for STD control activities, including disease reporting, health promotion, training, and program evaluation. They also receive support through federal cooperative agreements for HIV surveillance and prevention. Local health departments are charged with providing direct clinical services, including diagnosis, treatment, patient counseling, and sex partner notification activities.[5]

These different responsibilities require federal, state, and local health officials to cooperate closely to ensure an integrated STD/HIV prevention program. Crucial factors include (1) identifying local priorities based on well-defined epidemiological indicators and (2) applying the prevention and control strategies most likely to halt disease. Emphasis has been placed on evaluating standard STD interventions because of rapid expansion of STD control efforts in many directions. Moreover, each of the three governmental tiers has increasingly had to create a matrix of activities both within and outside the traditional health sphere to gain further leverage on preventing STD/HIV. For example, STD control programs require close integration with programs for family planning, maternal and child health, and adolescent health; school health and education programs have required collaboration with education officials, substance abuse programs with law endorsement officials, and so on.

Resources for STD Control and HIV Prevention. National budgets allocated to preventing STDs other than HIV have not kept pace with the worsening problem in most countries. For example, in the United States, after adjusting for effects of inflation, the peak year for funding STD control programs was 1947. In that year, over $130 million (in 1990 dollars) were focused on the control of a single STD, syphilis. By 1973, even with the boost of a national gonorrhea control program, *total* federal grant resources for these two diseases was $64 million. By 1990, this aggregate amount had risen slightly to $68 million, although it was spread across the full spectrum of STDs described earlier.[5]

Resources for HIV prevention have grown rapidly throughout the world, especially after the HIV antibody test was developed. Before 1985, the U.S. government had invested less than $50 million in AIDS research and prevention. However, since mid-1985, federal spending for HIV/AIDS prevention and research has risen every year, up to $1400 million in 1990; approximately 30% of this is allocated for HIV surveillance and prevention activities coordinated by CDC. State and local health departments are also increasing their resources for HIV prevention; in 1989, an estimated $249 million was available from state and local legislatures for a variety of programs, including surveillance, prevention, research, and patient care.[6]

STD Clinical Preventive Services. The phrase usually goes "an ounce of prevention is worth a pound of cure"—for a 1:16 ratio. However, in the STD arena, cure is part of prevention. Proper treatment of persons infected with curable STD serves several preventive functions. First, reservoirs for sexual transmission are eliminated; this represents primary prevention. Second, the more severe complications are prevented; this represents secondary prevention. Third, patients can be counseled to reduce high-risk sexual behavior and to refer sex partners for treatment (primary and secondary prevention). Fourth, treatment of curable STD (e.g., syphilis and chancroid) may reduce concurrent transmission of certain incurable STD, such as HIV infection.

For these reasons, STD prevention strategies employ approaches—such as diagnosis and treatment—that have typically been considered in the realm of the clinician rather than the public health practitioner. Simplified diagnosis of persons with symptoms ensures rapid treatment; Gram's stain for gonorrhea is an example. Single-dose therapy reduces problems with compliance; penicillin for gonorrhea and metronidazole for *Trichomonas* spp infection are examples. Attractive clinical settings allow those with stigmatizing conditions to obtain dignified health care. Thus, curative and preventive medicine are complementary in STD control.

To assist clinicians in deciding which STD services might be most useful for their patients, the U.S. Preventive Services Task Force[7,8] has provided recommendations for preventing STDs (Table 6-3). Screening cultures and serological tests are primarily recommended only for those patients practicing high-risk behaviors. Prophylactic treatment for the partner(s) of a known infected person has a strong scientific basis for efficacy and should be integral to clinical practice. Although the evidence supporting other STD interventions is less conclusive, those providing clinical preventive services should be aware of the role of such strategies as STD reporting, partner notification, and patient education.

Public Interest in STDs. Because the public's perception of the STD problem influences both policymakers and program planners, the public has a strong impact on the resources available for STD control. However, the public's interest in STD has varied. The press has ignored (or denied) the importance of these infections in some years and then has overreacted in others. For example, the news media first focused on the problem of genital herpes in 1982, nearly 10 years after the initial rise in number of cases. A media lag of about one year occurred with AIDS. Over the past several years, STDs, especially AIDS, made frequent headlines, although some have perceived a recent waning of media attention.

Different interest groups also affect public policy. One private voluntary organization, the American Social Health Association, has a mission to increase attention toward preventing STD. Other public health organizations are now recognizing the necessity of controlling STD at both the national level and in their own communities. Recent networking among private health-interest organizations, AIDS-service groups and other community-based organizations serving minorities, and federal, state, and local government will help ensure more efficient use of this increasing public interest in STD.

BACTERIAL INFECTIONS

Syphilis

Syphilis remains an important sexually transmitted disease because of (1) its public health heritage, (2) its effect on perinatal morbidity and mortality, (3) its association with HIV transmission, (4) its escalating rate among inner-city minority heterosexuals, and (5) its preventability. After penicillin was introduced in the late 1940s, the number of U.S. cases of primary and secondary syphilis declined by 99%.[9] However, in recent years, infectious syphilis trends have followed specific patterns (Fig. 6-1). In white males, the number of reported cases has been affected by homosexual behavior: steadily increasing during the 1970s but decreasing in the 1980s; presumably, this decline reflects behavior changes to reduce the risk of transmitting HIV, which in turn affects the incidence of other STDs.[4]

During the second half of the 1980s, infectious syphilis increased dramatically, to its highest level in 40 years.[10] This increase has largely occurred in low-income, minority, heterosexual populations (see Fig. 6-1). An important contributor to this

TABLE 6–3. RECOMMENDATIONS FOR PREVENTION OF SEXUALLY TRANSMITTED DISEASES

Disease	Intervention	Grade of Evidence[a]	Recommendations[b]
General recommendations	Epidemiological treatment	I	A
	Contact tracing	II-2	B
	Disease reporting	III	B
	Barrier methods	II-3	B
	Patient education	III	C
Gonorrhea			
Gonococcal ophthalmia neonatorum	Erythromycin	I	A
	Ophthalmic ointment		
	Postpartum		
	Culture of pregnant women	III	C
Gonorrhea	Culture of high-risk group members	II-1	A
Syphilis			
Syphilis	Epidemiological treatment of sexual contacts of established infection	I	A
	VDRL testing of high-risk group members	III	B
Congenital syphilis	VDRL testing of pregnant women	II-3	Risk group B No risk group C
HIV infection	HIV antibody testing	III	Risk group B No risk group C Pregnant women B
	Use of heat-treated blood products	II	A
	Blood and needle precautions for persons exposed to infected secretions	II	A
Hepatitis A	Immune serum globulin	I	A
Genital warts	Physical examination of risk group members	III	C
Neonatal herpes	Caesarean section in women with active genital herpes during labor	III	B
Chlamydia trachomatis			
Ophthalmia neonatorum	Erythromycin eye ointment	I	A
Neonatal chlamydial infection	Culture screening of pregnant women	III	Risk group B

[a]Effectiveness of interventions:
I: Evidence obtained from at least one properly randomized controlled trial.
II-1: Evidence obtained from well-designed controlled trials without randomization.
II-2: Evidence obtained from well-designed cohort or case-control analytic studies, preferably from more than one center or research group.
II-3: Evidence obtained from multiple time series studies with or without the intervention. Dramatic results in uncontrolled experiments could also be regarded as this type of evidence.
III: Opinions of respected authorities, based on clinical experience, descriptive studies, or reports of expert committees.
[b]Classification of recommendations:
A: There is good evidence to support the recommendation that the condition be specifically considered in a periodic health examination.
B: There is fair evidence to support the recommendation that the condition be specifically considered in a periodic health examination.
C: There is poor evidence regarding the inclusion of the condition in a periodic health examination, but recommendations may be made on other grounds.
Data from CDC[7] and Hymes et al.[8]

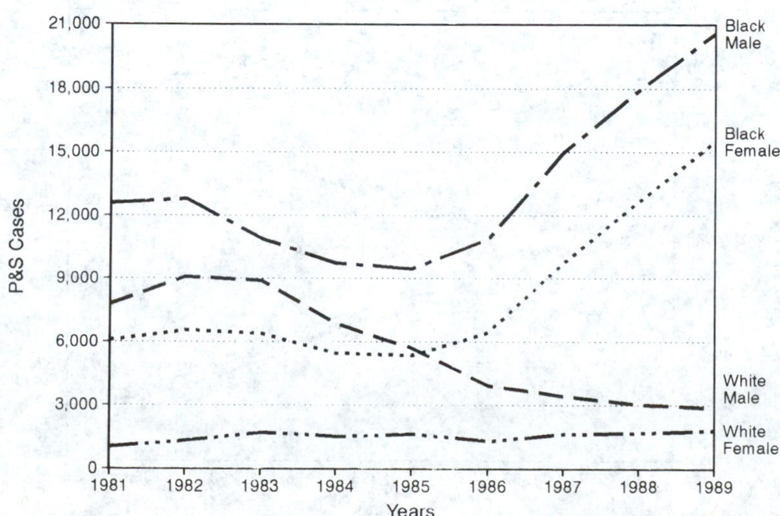

Figure 6–1. Primary and secondary syphilis by gender and race in the United States, 1981 to 1989.

rise has been the exchange of sexual services for drugs, especially crack cocaine.[11] The increasing syphilis rate in this traditional STD "core" population has important implications: (1) rises in heterosexual adult syphilis predict similar trends in congenital syphilis (CS), (2) community health education messages—generated by concerns about HIV—to reduce risky sexual behavior have not yet permeated minority heterosexual populations, and (3) because of the association of genital ulcers with HIV transmission,[12] control of syphilis could reduce HIV spread in this population.

Trends in CS reflect both recent heterosexual syphilis rates and also varying definitions of the condition. Although the incidence of CS declined steadily in the 1950s and 1960s, substantial increases have been reported in recent years.[13] Part of the rise observed since 1984 may be attributed to changing surveillance definitions, particularly for stillbirths.[13] In addition, increased vertical transmission may also be related to underutilization and inadequacy of prenatal care.[14] With escalating rates of female syphilis occurring in many areas of the United States, early prenatal care must be provided to the high-risk populations, with serological testing in both the first and third trimester encouraged.[15]

Gonorrhea

Recent gonorrhea trends reveal two major themes: (1) a sustained decrease in cases caused by penicillin-sensitive organisms and (2) the continued increase in the number and variety of antibiotic-resistant strains.[16] From 1975 to 1988, reported gonorrhea in the United States declined 30%, with nearly all the decrease occurring since 1981 (Fig. 6–2). In 1989, no further decline occurred. As with the decreasing rate of syphilis cases, white males accounted for most of the gonorrhea decrease, apparently a result of safer sexual practices.[4] Gonorrhea also decreased in white females. Unfortunately, black populations did not share in the decline of gonorrhea during the 1980s.

However, part of the decrease in gonorrhea may be an artifact of evolving tradeoffs in U.S. gonorrhea control strategy. First, in the interests of cost effectiveness, public health policy has focused gonorrhea screening on the populations that have yielded the highest percentage of positive cultures. This focusing of effort has decreased the overall number of asymptomatic persons tested and thus reduced the total number of infected persons identified. Second, as a cost-saving measure, a number of public STD clinics have either shut down satellite facilities or shortened the hours of their central clinics. Finally, because the amount of clinical care required for a typical STD patient in 1990 is greater than it was a decade earlier (e.g., HIV counseling, pelvic examinations, therapy for genital warts), fewer symptomatic persons can be evaluated in the same interval of time. As a result, fewer persons with gonorrhea are being diagnosed, further contributing to an artifactual decline.

In the face of the generally declining rates, whether real or artifactual, gonorrhea trends in teenagers and racial minorities are disturbing.[17] Adolescents have not shared in the decade-long gonorrhea decrease. Gonorrhea rates for black teenagers actually increased between 1981 and 1989. The disturbing disease rates among the teenage population may mean that gonorrhea control programs are not reaching this key risk group. Equally worrisome, reports of drug-associated gonorrhea transmission into young, inner-city, minority populations may possibly be the harbinger of future national gonorrhea increases, akin to trends in syphilis.[18]

Gonococcal antibiotic resistance further clouds the gonorrhea scene. The discovery of beta-lactamase-producing *Neisseria gonorrhoeae* (penicillinase-producing *N. gonorrhoeae* [PPNG]) in 1976 marked the beginning of an accelerated trend toward greater antibiotic resistance.[19] Since the emergence of PPNG, clinically significant resistance has been described for the three most widely used classes of drugs—the penicillins, tetracyclines, and aminoglycosides (spectinomycin). Furthermore, the variety of mechanisms involved is cause for increasing concern. Since 1980, and especially in the last 4 years, the incidence of PPNG has increased dramatically.[20] In 1989, PPNG strains accounted for almost 7% of national gonococcal morbidity. This led to current recommendations to change from penicillin to a third-generation cephalosporin as the drug of choice for treating patients with gonorrhea in most areas.[21]

Plasmid-mediated resistance to tetracycline has become common in gonococci in many U.S. cities, as has lower-level chromosomally mediated resistance to the penicillins and tetracycline. Surveillance of chromosomally mediated resistance is severely hampered by the lack of a simple, standardized, inexpensive, and sensitive screening test that can be performed outside of reference laboratories.[22]

Chlamydia

Genital infections caused by *C. trachomatis* are the most common bacterial sexually transmitted syndromes in the United States today.[23] Nongonococcal urethritis (NGU) rates in men serve as a surrogate measure for *C. trachomatis* infection rates.

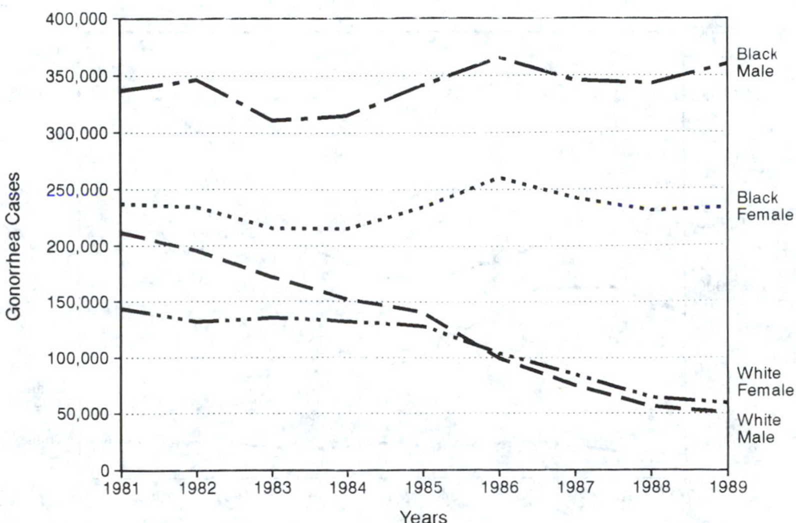

Figure 6–2. Gonorrhea by gender and race in the United States, 1981 to 1989.

In 1972, NGU surpassed gonorrhea as a diagnosis for patient visits to private physicians' offices; the gap has widened in recent years, with NGU now being twice as common as gonococcal urethritis (Fig. 6–3). This pattern of increasing NGU (contrasted with the decreasing gonococcal urethritis) is consistent with trends in other developed countries.

Besides its role in male infections, *C. trachomatis* also plays an important role in causing mucopurulent cervicitis—the female equivalent of NGU.[24] This condition predisposes either to acute pelvic inflammatory disease (PID) in nonpregnant women or to perinatal infection of infants and puerperal infections in pregnant women. Those at highest risk are unwed teenagers living in urban areas, precisely the group at highest risk both for other STDs and for adverse pregnancy outcomes.

In 1986, using gonorrhea as an index, chlamydia was estimated to cause over 4 million infections in the United States.[25] An estimated 2.6 million infections occurred in women, 1.8 million in men, and one quarter million in infants. The ratio of *C. trachomatis* to *N. gonorrhoeae* infection was influenced by at least five variables besides gender and age: race, pregnancy status, choice of contraception, the presence or absence of symptoms, and sexual preference. Considerably higher ratios of chlamydia to gonorrhea were found among whites, pregnant women, oral contraceptive users, and asymptomatic individuals; lower ratios were found among homosexual men.

Efforts to control chlamydia have been hampered by the *relative* difficulties, compared with gonorrhea, of diagnosis.[26] National chlamydia control guidelines were developed by the CDC in 1985.[27] To make maximum use of limited STD funds, recommendations for chlamydia control were primarily based on treating syndromes rather than specific infections. The effectiveness of this strategy remains uncertain. However, in areas that can provide such usual STD strategies as diagnosis, screening, and partner notification services for chlamydia, apparent declines in sexually transmitted chlamydial infections have occurred.[28]

PERSISTENT VIRAL INFECTIONS

Human Immunodeficiency Virus

The epidemiology of HIV—and its fatal sequela AIDS—is well known. In fact, even before the virus was discovered, epidemiological analysis of persons with AIDS allowed development of landmark AIDS prevention guidelines in March 1983 that remain relevant today. Risky behaviors had been identified, a virus was felt to be the causative agent, routes of transmission were understood, and the "core" population of asymptomatic infected persons capable of transmitting the agent was assumed.

In 1989, the number of reported AIDS cases broke the 100,000 barrier.[29] Based on a variety of studies and mathematical models, an estimated 1 million persons appear to be already infected with HIV,[30] with an estimated annual incidence of 80,000 infections. Various risk markers predict higher levels of HIV seropositivity. Because the virus initially became widely transmitted within the homosexual community, the male-female ratio among populations routinely screened in the United States ranges from 3 to 10:1. In addition, minorities have higher HIV antibody rates than do whites, a discrepancy that further increases when men who acquired HIV by having sex with other men are excluded.[30] Finally, geography also strongly influences HIV seropositivity levels. Persons on the Atlantic Coast, South Florida, Puerto Rico, and San Francisco have higher rates.

Although these markers are useful for directing public health resources, they do not identify which individual persons are infected. Thus, clinicians must evaluate specific risk behaviors for HIV and other sexually transmitted infections as a routine part of the medical history. A recent survey[31] of physicians revealed: (1) about one tenth routinely (though briefly) took sexual and drug histories from their patients, (2) more than half did so when the clinical diagnosis suggested these behaviors might be important, (3) most tended to underestimate the proportion of their patients who might be at higher risk of infection, and (4) over 80% felt their colleagues were unprepared to deal with HIV-infected patients. (See also pp 115–121.)

Genital Herpes

Genital herpes, although now less publicized than AIDS, still accounts for sizable morbidity. It is the main cause of genital ulcers in the United States, probably accounting for at least 10 times as many cases as syphilis. The total number of physician-patient consultations for genital herpes increased 15-fold between 1966 and 1989, from 30,000 to almost 450,000 (Fig. 6–4). First office visits—a more likely indicator of first genital infections—also increased eightfold over this same period, from 18,000 in 1966 to 176,000 in 1989. Adults aged 20 to 29 continued to account for most consultations; women visited physicians' offices more frequently than men for genital herpes.

The most recent finding on the epidemiology of genital herpes is that symptomatic infections are merely a tip of the iceberg.[32] Only one fourth of those with antibodies to HSV type 2 (HSV-2) give histories compatible with genital herpes infection.

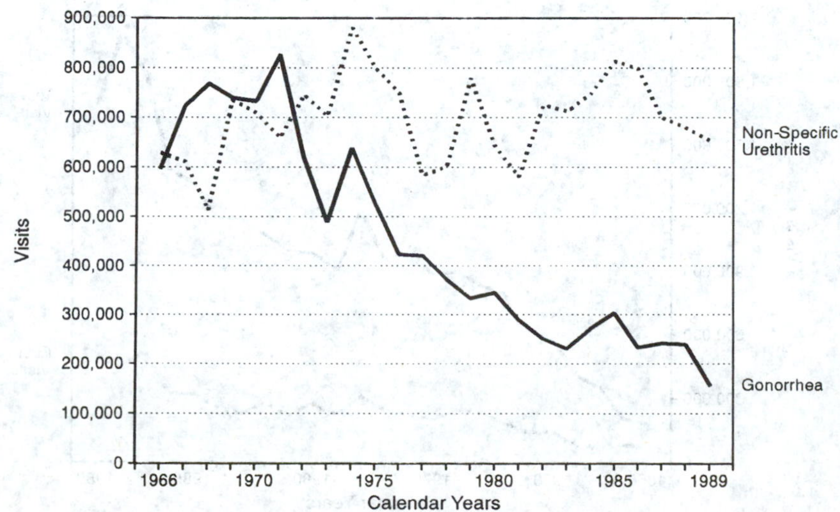

Figure 6–3. Nonspecific urethritis and gonorrhea for males. Number of visits to private physicians' offices in the United States, 1966 to 1989.

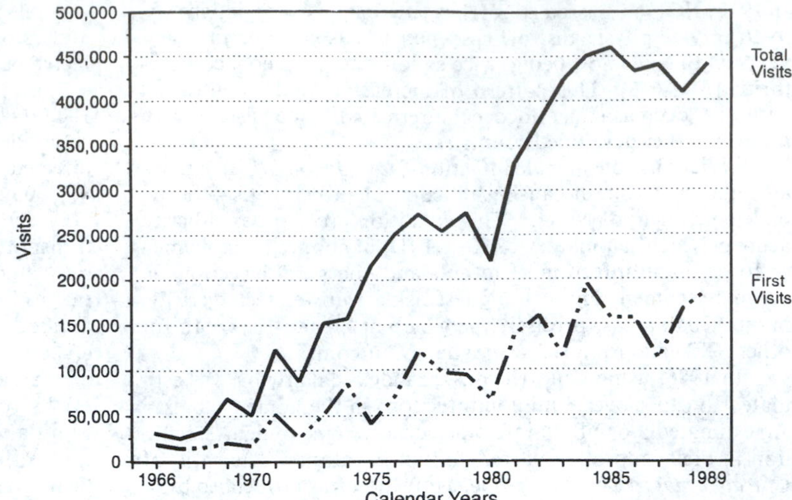

Figure 6–4. Genital HSV infections. Number of visits to private physicians' offices in the United States, 1966 to 1989.

Based on data from a national sample in 1978, over 30 million Americans are probably infected with HSV-2 today. Blacks are more likely to have HSV-2 antibodies than whites, and HSV-2 antibody prevalence was higher in women than in men.

Asymptomatic individuals are primarily responsible for sexual transmission of HSV.[33] Three fourths of those who had been the sources of infection for patients with documented primary HSV-2 infections gave no histories of genital lesions at the time of contact. Although all source contacts had HSV antibodies indicating prior infection, only one third had ever noticed any symptoms compatible with genital herpes.

Infection with HSV-2, as with syphilis, has been linked to higher risks of HIV infection among homosexual men.[34,35] Presumably this is due to either genital or anorectal herpetic lesions (both recognized and unrecognized), which act as the portal of entry (or egress) for HIV.

A serious consequence of genital herpes is neonatal herpes. Although the United States has no national surveillance on which to calculate incidence, in several regions the incidence of neonatal herpes reported between 1966 and 1988 rose more than fourfold.[36] This increase is undoubtedly mostly attributable to the epidemic increase in genital herpes noted above. To what extent these reports also reflect an improved ability to diagnose the disease is uncertain.

Genital Human Papillomavirus (HPV) Infections

The frequency of consultations for symptomatic genital warts is nearly threefold higher than that for genital herpes,[37] and the key consequence associated with this infection, cervical neoplasia, is more severe. In the United States, the number of physician-patient consultations for genital warts increased over ninefold between 1966 and 1989, from 179,000 to 1,700,000 (Fig. 6–5). First visits also increased nearly ninefold over the same period from 54,000 in 1966 to 480,000 in 1989. Persons from 20 to 24 years of age had more frequent consultations for genital warts than did patients in other age groups; visits for women outnumbered those for men.

Even more than for genital herpes, genital warts represent only the symptomatic tip of the iceberg of HPV infections. As physician awareness and availability of diagnostic methods increase, subclinical papillomavirus infections of the male and female genital tract are becoming commonly recognized.[37] At present, serological tests are still under development, and the virus cannot be grown in cell culture. Subclinical infection may be suspected on the basis of koilocytes on a cytological smear, by certain morphological features on colposcopy, by immunochemical strains for HPV antigen, or by detection of HPV nucleic acid sequences. A commercial kit is now available for detection of

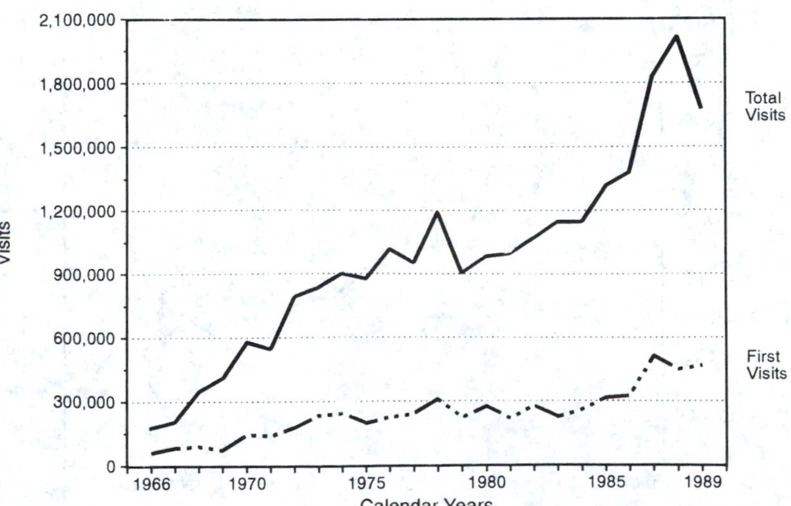

Figure 6–5. Genital warts. Number of visits to private physicians' offices in the United States, 1966 to 1989.

HPV sequences using radioactive RNA probes; the polymerase chain reaction (PCR) technique is being widely used for detection of HPV DNA in research. From 1983 to 1988, evidence of cervical HPV lesions was found in 1% to 3% of all Papanicolaou smears in U.S. Planned Parenthood clinics, especially in women under 20 years of age.[38] However, HPV DNA is now being detected by PCR in the cervixes of a much higher percentage of sexually active women, many of whom have had normal cervical cytological smears.

By 1990, 57 types of HPV had been described, each type differing on DNA homology by more than 50% determined by hybridization. Over 10 HPV types are associated with genital infection, of which types 16 and 18 are most closely associated with cervical cancer. Even these so-called high-risk types seem to be highly prevalent. For example, HPV type 16 has been detected by polymerase chain reaction (PCR) in cervical specimens from more than 10% of college students and over 20% of STD clinic patients in Seattle.

The prevalence of HPV infection in men has been less well studied, but subclinical penile infection is thought to be common. Subclinical penile HPV infection has been detected by non-PCR DNA hybridization methods in nearly 10% of young healthy men. Based on extrapolations from a variety of selected studies to the population aged 15 to 49 years, an estimated 12.2 million HPV infections were prevalent in the United States in 1987,[37] of which only one tenth were symptomatic. More recent studies using the PCR method suggest that the level of prevalent subclinical cases is substantially greater.

Hepatitis B Virus (HBV) Infections

Nationwide, the incidence of hepatitis B has increased steadily over the last decade despite both effective blood screening programs and the availability of a vaccine. New infections have risen from about 200,000 in 1978 to 300,000 in 1989.[39] Approximately half of those infected suffer symptomatic acute hepatitis. However, the more serious concerns involve the effects of chronic HBV infection. Between 6% and 10% of those infected with HBV become chronic carriers. Chronic active hepatitis develops in more than 25% of carriers, and studies in Taiwan of persons infected at birth have shown a high risk of progression to cirrhosis and hepatocellular carcinoma.[40] The natural history of HBV infection acquired sexually by adults has not yet been well studied.

Most HBV infections in the United States with known routes of transmission result from sexual exposure. Unfortunately, U.S. vaccination programs have focused only on three risk groups—health care workers who are exposed to blood, staff and residents of institutions for the developmentally disabled, and staff and patients in hemodialysis units.[39] These groups, however, account for fewer than 10% of acute HBV cases and have played a small role as further transmitters of infection. The populations that account for most HBV cases[41]—intravenous (IV) drug users, persons acquiring the disease through heterosexual exposure, and homosexual men—are not being reached effectively by current HBV vaccine programs. These groups have also been responsible for spreading the most HBV infection. Therefore, vaccination of seronegative members of these risk groups would be the most efficient method of interrupting transmission.

The behavior changes of homosexual men to reduce their risk of HIV have already led to striking decreases in the number of HBV cases (along with the other STDs) among this group. However, the number of cases of HBV caused by heterosexual exposure has increased over the past several years, not surprisingly, primarily among inner-city minority heterosexuals.[41] Of similar concern is the large rise in the proportion of HBV patients with a history of IV drug use.[42] Because of the implications of HBV for chronic hepatitis, cirrhosis, and hepatocellular carcinoma, the recent trends of sexual transmission carry long-term risks to STD core populations. Public health authorities in many countries now urge higher-priority use of HBV vaccine to interrupt sexual transmission of HBV.

SYNDROMES CAUSED BY STDS

Pelvic Inflammatory Disease

Pelvic inflammatory disease (PID) is one of the most severe complications of lower genital tract infections in women and one with the greatest public health consequences. Trends in PID are more difficult to interpret, however, than trends in gonorrhea in women. Results of two national data bases generated from physician office visits have demonstrated a consistent falloff from the peak number of PID cases in the mid-1970s. The decline was greater in black and oriental women than in white women. However, the rate of PID visits has been quite stable through the 1980s.

Rates for patients hospitalized for PID have followed a different course. Overall, rates increased slightly during the 1970s, with nearly all the increase occurring in young white women. However, in the 1980s, rates fell in all age and racial categories. This is consistent with trends in hospitalization for all causes during the same interval. A unifying hypothesis for these trends is that the changing spectrum of sexually transmitted organisms (i.e., a decline in the incidence of gonorrhea relative to the incidence of chlamydial infection) has led to a greater proportion of subclinical PID. Although chlamydial PID is less clinically severe, it smolders to produce subsequent tubal damage and reproductive sequelae.

The cumulative impact of PID affects a substantial portion of the female population. In 1988, one in seven American women of reproductive age reported having had PID. The syndrome was reported twice as frequently among blacks as among whites; one in four black women and one in eight white women reported having received treatment for PID. As expected, the condition increased with age up to 35 and then plateaued.

Infertility

Involuntarily infertility, as well as requests for infertility services, also increased during the 1970s but stabilized thereafter. By 1988 an estimated 2 million American families wished to have more children but were unable to conceive. Over 900,000 visits to physicians' offices in 1988 were for infertility counseling and treatment.

The exact proportion of those infertile couples whose status is secondary to the consequences of STD is unknown; estimates have ranged from 15% to 30%, depending on the populations involved and the types of infertility attributed to STD. Extrapolating from the number of PID cases, and assuming a 15% risk of infertility due to tubal occlusion after PID, between 100,000 and 150,000 women would be rendered involuntarily infertile each year because of pelvic infection after STD. This estimate does not include causes of infertility that might also be related to STD (e.g., cervical factor infertility, chronic endometritis, epididymal occlusion).

Reproductive Outcomes

Prenatal STDs also produce adverse effects on both pregnancy outcome and maternal-infant health. The obstetrical consequences of syphilis are well known. Nearly 40% of pregnant women with recently acquired but untreated syphilis suffer a spontaneous abortion, a stillbirth, or a perinatal death. About half the infants who survive will be infected with *Treponema pal-*

lidum and develop congenital syphilis. Gonococcal infection during pregnancy has been associated with an increased risk of chorioamnionitis, premature rupture of membranes, and prematurity in several retrospective studies. In Nairobi, Kenya, gonorrhea at delivery was associated with a threefold increased risk of low-birthweight, premature infants.

The effects of other bacterial STDs on pregnancy outcome are not yet certain. *C. trachomatis,* bacterial vaginosis, *Ureaplasma urealyticum,* and group B streptococcus each have been associated with abnormal outcomes, including chorioamnionitis, premature rupture of membranes, preterm delivery, and low birth weight. However, studies in different populations have shown differing results, and the reasons for the differences are not yet well understood.

Finally, genital HSV and systemic HIV infection influence both pregnancy management and outcome. The risk of neonatal herpes is greatest when the mother experiences an initial attack of genital herpes at delivery. In women with visible ulcers during labor, cesarean deliveries have been recommended to reduce the risk of neonatal herpes. Although a large proportion of neonatal herpes cases occur without any history of maternal genital lesions, screening before delivery for maternal genital HSV shedding is not a cost-effective way to prevent neonatal herpes. Moreover, cesarean delivery solely to prevent neonatal herpes is not indicated for asymptomatic women who simply have a history of genital herpes. Primary HSV infection during pregnancy has also been associated with spontaneous abortion. Recent studies suggest an association between maternal HIV infection and increased risk of preterm delivery and low birth weight.

Ectopic Pregnancy

Ectopic pregnancy has increased dramatically during the last 15 years. Since 1965, the number of ectopic pregnancies has quadrupled in the United States, reaching almost 90,000 cases in 1987. Although some of this alarming rise may be attributable to improved detection of subclinical ectopic pregnancies, the increased incidence of PID with the resultant tubal scarring has contributed to the incidence of ectopic implantation. Women with a history of PID are over eight times more likely to suffer ectopic pregnancy than those without such a history. If one assumes that 15% of U.S. women of childbearing age have experienced PID, then more than 50% of ectopic pregnancies can be attributed to it.

STD-related Neoplasia

At least five squamous cell neoplasias—carcinomas involving the cervix, vagina, vulva, anus, and penis—have been strongly associated with HPV infection, particularly with HPV types 16 and 18. Squamous cell carcinoma of the cervix has also been strongly correlated with both the number of sexual partners and (in some but not all studies) with smoking and HSV-2 infection. Squamous cell carcinoma of the anus is greatly increased among homosexual men. Hepatocellular carcinoma is usually caused by HBV, another sexually transmitted virus. Finally, the tumors associated with AIDS, namely, Kaposi's sarcoma and non-Hodgkins lymphomas, are in some way related to the profound immunosuppression caused by HIV and may themselves have a viral etiology.

PREVENTION AND CONTROL STRATEGIES FOR STDS

The recent trends in STDs have stimulated new directions in prevention and control programs. Previously successful approaches to controlling syphilis and gonorrhea have relied on diagnosis, therapy, and partner notification.[43] In the future, more emphasis will be needed on primary prevention of STDs through behavioral messages and vaccine development.

Many simultaneous activities are necessary to reduce STD. In the current approach to STD prevention, an understanding of two fundamental concepts is helpful: (1) the dynamics of STD spread and (2) the growing importance of STD core groups.

First, the forces responsible for sustaining transmission of any sexually transmitted infection can be represented in a simple equation, $R_0 = \beta \times C \times D$.[44] R_0 represents the reproductive rate of an infection, that is, the number of new infections produced by an infected individual. β is the average probability that an infected individual will infect a susceptible partner given exposure. C is the average number of new partners acquired by an infected individual per unit of time. D is the average duration of infectiousness of the specific infection. Public health interventions to prevent STD are targeted at reducing the magnitude of β, C, or D by (1) reducing the probability of infecting a susceptible partner, (2) limiting the number of partners who have sex with infected persons, and (3) reducing the duration of infectiousness.

The probability of infecting a susceptible partner can be reduced by promoting condom use and safe sex practices (e.g., masturbation is the most safe and receptive anal intercourse is the least safe with respect to acquiring HIV or HBV). The efficiency of transmitting HIV may also be reduced by controlling STDs that have been implicated as risk factors for transmitting or acquiring HIV. Promoting circumcision might reduce the acquisition of chancroid in countries where chancroid is now endemic. Prophylactic antibiotics can protect susceptible partners, and vaccination can lower the susceptibility of the available partner pool.

The average number of new partners acquired by an infected individual can be lowered if everyone in the population chooses to have fewer sexual partners. Alternatively, reducing sexual contact among persons who engage in high-risk behaviors would more specifically target this behavioral approach. In the case of chronic, incurable, viral STDs, identifying those who are infected and encouraging them to have fewer partners and to employ measures to reduce STD transmission, are essential.

The duration of infectiousness, for the patient with a curable STD, can be reduced by early diagnosis and curative treatment. This in turn can be improved by screening for asymptomatic infections, by improving recognition of STD symptoms, by motivating early health care seeking, by increasing access to good health care, and by notifying and treating sex partners.

Second, the role of "core groups" (involving "high-frequency transmitters") in sustaining the spread of STD within a community is again becoming recognized for its importance. In terms of the above equation, such individuals may be more effective transmitters of HIV because they have concurrent problems of other STDs, may have larger numbers of sex partners, and may have longer duration of infection (because of poor health care). Clearly, preventing a case of STD in a high-frequency transmitter will have a much greater impact on reducing subsequent transmission of STD than preventing a case in an individual who is not a high-frequency transmitter. Thus, public health interventions should include efforts to identify and reach members of STD core groups.

Public health interventions should be designed and delivered differently, according to target groups. Health promotion and behavioral intervention messages can move from generalities to greater specificity as one approaches the target groups at highest risk.

We will group the available strategies for STD prevention into eight somewhat overlapping categories: organization of STD control, health promotion, clinical skills, STD detection, STD treatment, patient counseling, partner notification, and use of vaccines.

Organization, Implementation, and Evaluation of an STD Control Program. Wherever STD control programs are part of the health care bureaucracy, overall program organization and levels of specific functional responsibilities must be clearly defined. A model program would include a program manager, one or more special STD centers, and a health care infrastructure to provide STD program interventions (Table 6-4). The program manager is responsible for setting quantifiable objectives for the program, developing an overall strategy for STD control, and helping evaluate the program at regular intervals. This involves setting both process indicators (e.g., are services being provided at the level indicated?) and outcome indicators (e.g., is the incidence of STD falling?).

Health Promotion. Health promotion, an integral part of STD intervention activities, is based on three principles: advocacy, enabling, and mediating. Broadly defined, health promotion encompasses five strategic areas: promoting healthy public policy, promoting a supportive environment, strengthening community action, promoting healthy personal behavior and skills (by providing information, education, and counseling), and orienting health services toward meeting all the patient's health needs, including health education. Health promotion thus is not limited to health education directed to society as a whole or to groups, but certainly includes individual health education, person-to-person counseling, and partner notification. Counseling and partner notification are nonetheless considered separately below to highlight the importance of each strategy in STD control.

TABLE 6-4. ORGANIZATION AND LEVEL OF FUNCTIONAL RESPONSIBILITIES OF AN STD CONTROL PROGRAM

- **SINGLE ADMINISTRATIVE DIRECTOR FOR STD/HIV**
- **STD/HIV Program Management and Planning**

Set quantifiable objectives and plan for STD/HIV program (e.g., 3–5 years)
Coordinate planning with managers of related programs
Develop STD program guidelines for:
Health promotion/behavioral intervention
Laboratory services
Patient management
Counseling, testing, partner notification
STD surveillance
Surveillance of risk behaviors
Evaluation, replanning of STD program, including all components of the program (e.g., health services)
Coordinate community involvement, coordinate training program
Resource development and financial management, public relations

- **Model STD/HIV Centers**

Implementation and feedback reporting to management
Health promotion
Clinical services (diagnosis and treatment), consultations
Laboratory services
Training (clinicians, technicians, counselors, managers)
Surveillance
Operational research
  Monitor treatment outcome
  Monitor antimicrobial resistance
  Evaluate new diagnostic tests
  Evaluate new treatments
  Evaluate health promotion

- **Other STD/HIV Services**

STD Clinics
  Health promotion
  STD diagnosis and treatment
  Counseling and partner notification
  Contraceptive counseling and services
  Laboratory services
  STD reporting for surveillance
Family planning clinics
Maternal and child health clinics
Hospital clinics
Primary health care providers
Laboratories
Pharmacies

Specific community health education efforts usually encourage primary prevention (preventing acquisition of an STD) in persons at risk. Traditionally, judgmental messages have not been an effective method of changing behavior.[3] In fact, stigmatizing infected individuals by widespread social disapproval may hinder STD control through delaying care or increasing denial of high-risk behaviors. Given today's concerns about AIDS, public health officials are continually trying to balance their messages between creating excessive fear or excessive reassurance. Fear can provide necessary stimulation for preventive actions, but it can also lead to less rational responses that undermine constructive programs.[45]

Health education interventions that promote early health care seeking, avoidance of sex after onset of STD symptoms, treatment compliance, and partner notification can result in both primary prevention (prevention of further transmission) and secondary prevention (prevention of complications). Recent experience with videotapes to promote such actions as follow-up cultures, treatment compliance, and condom use have been encouraging.[46] Current emphasis on providing HIV counseling and testing for persons with other STDs will also reinforce appropriate preventive behaviors.

School education strategies to increase students' knowledge of the full spectrum of STDs (including HIV) have recently been encouraged by the World Health Organization (WHO). Unfortunately, this nation's past heritage of teaching about "VD" in high schools has generally consisted of didactic biomedical lectures concentrating only on syphilis and gonorrhea. As a result, in 1987, tenth graders' knowledge of ways to prevent common STDs was inadequate.[47] To correct this situation, prototype AIDS and STD curriculum materials for both teachers and students in grades 6 through 12 have been widely circulated. These curricula use a self-instructional format and emphasize behavioral skill building.[48] It is to be hoped that they will facilitate systematic STD and AIDS education in courses dealing with family life, quality of life, sex education, and health education throughout the country and will upgrade students' knowledge about preventive behaviors.

Hotlines for both STD and AIDS provide general information and specific answers to questions of callers nationwide. These hotlines are funded by the CDC and operated by the American Social Health Association. In 1989, almost 80,000 calls were answered on the STD hotline, and over 1 million were answered on the AIDS hotline.[5] A large proportion of callers are referred to confidential medical services in either the public or private sector. Many local hotlines for AIDS and STD are also operated throughout the United States, and AIDS hotlines are being used in other countries.

In the future, public health personnel must make better use of the mass media for health promotion and prevention of STDs, including HIV infection. Awareness of herpes and AIDS is widespread largely because of the attention given these conditions by the media. Teenagers are a special audience for the broadcast media; they spend an average of 23 hours a week listening to radio or watching television.[49] Public service announcements are increasingly being aired to encourage condom use in high-risk settings and to publicize hotline numbers for further questions.

STD Clinical Services. U.S. medical schools have been slow to respond to the increasing magnitude of the STD problem. In 1980, fewer than one in six American medical schools had a specific STD clinic available for STD training.[50] A survey conducted in 1985 showed some improvement, but still only one in five medical schools provided even half its students with STD clinical training. Paradoxically, this occurred just when American physicians need STD training the most; the majority enter specialties requiring knowledge of STD diagnosis and treatment. In 1989, nearly two thirds of first-year residents chose internal medicine, pediatrics, obstetrics and gynecology, family practice, emergency medicine, and dermatology. Without training in STD problems, the medical community cannot be effectively mobilized to support control programs.

Recent STD training initiatives have taken three approaches. First, to respond to immediate needs, clinical practice guidelines were developed by CDC to assist STD services in improving patient management.[51] For STD clinicians, national STD treatment recommendations are regularly reviewed to reflect changing diagnostic capabilities, antibiotic susceptibilities, and pharmaceutical innovations.[21] In addition, a variety of useful clinical publications are aimed at primary care physicians to allow a syndromic approach to STD patient management.[52]

Second, federally funded regional STD prevention and training centers integrate a university medical school with a model public STD clinic to provide training for mid-career clinicians as well as for medical, nursing, and paramedical students. In 1990, specific courses were included to address clinical management of the HIV-infected patient. By 1989, 11 such multidisciplinary centers were in operation; over 14,000 students have been trained in these facilities since 1979.[5]

Third, clinical and research training support has been provided directly by CDC, NIH, and the American Social Health Association to medical schools to train a cadre of medically qualified clinicians and researchers who have a career commitment to the STD discipline. Faculty role models and challenging clinical clerkships are the most important influences on students' choice of their specialty.[53] Once interested in STD, these individuals are able to establish their own STD academic programs, thus multiplying the effect of the training efforts. However, despite these efforts, as of 1989, STD research or STD clinical training centers existed in fewer than 10% of American medical schools.

Physicians interested in STD must complement their traditional diagnostic and therapeutic skills with training in social and behavioral sciences and epidemiology. Most clinicians are incapable of taking an adequate sexual history; inquiring about the intimate details of their patient's sexual practices and partners does not come naturally. These skills must be taught. Clinicians could include a brief sexual history while patients are being asked about such behaviors as smoking, alcohol and other drugs, exercise, sleep patterns, and so on. Further, eliciting a history of STD is important as an index of sexual risk-taking behavior. Regarding psychosocial training, the increasing emphasis on behavioral factors in STD control is part of the general growing awareness in medicine of the importance of behavior in both producing and preventing disease and in promoting health.[54] The role of life style in STD is obvious; the transition from curable bacterial STD to incurable viral STD makes it particularly important that physicians shift their emphasis toward educating individuals to adopt a healthy sexual life style.

STD Detection. Early detection of infection is crucial to STD intervention strategies. Early detection affects primary prevention (by decreasing the duration of infectiousness) and secondary prevention (by leading to treatment before complications). Casefinding methods include presumptive clinical diagnosis based on symptoms and signs, confirmatory laboratory testing in patients with suggestive symptoms or signs, targeted laboratory diagnostic testing in individuals at high risk, broader screening without regard to likelihood of STD (e.g., premarital testing, testing of blood donors), and locating sex partners of persons with STD.

Whether for making specific diagnoses in those with symptoms or for screening persons without symptoms, tests for STD ideally should be inexpensive, rapid, simple, and accurate. Current U.S. methods for diagnosing the common STDs incorporate these principles (Table 6–5). However, in many developing countries, constraints on expense, rapidity, and simplicity are so great that few of these tests can be used, except in specialized central laboratories. For example, if cultures are not available to detect gonorrhea in women, the control of gonorrhea becomes problematic. In developed countries, constraints on expense have delayed introduction of some diagnostic tests—for example, *C. trachomatis*—even in settings where such tests are considered cost-effective.

The usual parameters for assessing diagnostic techniques—sensitivity, specificity, and predictive value—have certain unique implications for STD control. STD treatment is generally shorter and safer than therapy for many chronic conditions. Moreover, as discussed earlier, curing STD in one individual frequently prevents infection in others. Consequently, achieving high sensitivity by reducing false-negative results becomes a priority. Achieving high specificity by reducing false-positive results is less important from the public health perspective when treatment is safe, simple, and inexpensive. However, when false-positive tests trigger partner notification, additional expenses must be considered. Furthermore, from the individual's perspective, the human and emotional costs of erroneously stigmatizing someone as having an STD means specificity is also crucial.

Deficiencies in sensitivity causes particular problems in populations with a high prevalence of a disease with serious morbidity. For example, a new test for gonorrhea with a sensitivity of 80% in women would fail to identify 20% of infected women. If the prevalence of gonorrhea in women at an STD clinic is 30%, then six women out of 100 tested would not be identified and would be at risk for developing salpingitis and further spreading the infection.

Deficiencies in specificity can also cause difficulties, especially in low-prevalence populations. For example, a new test for *N. gonorrhoeae* with a specificity of 90% and sensitivity of 100%, when used in a low-prevalence population (1%), would produce almost 10 times as many false-positive tests as true-positive tests. Referring and evaluating 11 individuals and their sex partners to identify one infected person and that person's exposed partner(s) would tax clinical personnel and cause unnecessary anxiety. In public health terms, testing 20,000,000 women using the new test would increase the follow-up burden from approximately 200,000 with culture diagnoses to 2,200,000 individuals from the new test. Such an increase could overwhelm clinical resources.

Even with highly specific tests (specificity ≥99%), screening for STD of very low prevalence (<0.1%) creates many false-positive results. Thus, tests such as the fluorescent treponemal antibody absorption (FTA-ABS) or *Treponema pallidum* hemagglutination assay (TPHA) test for syphilis, although highly specific and having high positive predictive value in patients with positive reagin tests for syphilis, are not recommended for screening the general population for syphilis. In the United States, the prevalence of syphilis has become so low in many areas that the cost effectiveness of serological screening and casefinding with the less expensive and less specific reagin tests (e.g., in premarital examinations, blood banking services, and new admissions to hospitals) is being debated. Because yield and cost considerations are particularly important to screening activities, selection of the target population directly influences these factors. For example, in the United States during the 1970s, the cost per gonorrhea case detected varied from a low of $25 in metropolitan STD clinics to a high of $350 in low-prevalence areas.

To make most effective use of resources, targeted casefinding and screening have been recommended in (1) high-prevalence groups such as prostitutes, homosexual men, and illicit drug users, (2) facilities (e.g., jails, emergency rooms) where high levels of STD might be expected, and (3) pregnant women, because

TABLE 6–5. CURRENT METHODS FOR DIAGNOSING COMMON SEXUALLY TRANSMITTED DISEASES

Presumptive Diagnosis	Definitive Diagnosis
▪ **Neisseria gonorrhoeae**	
Microscopic identification of typical gram-negative intracellular diplococci on smear of urethral exudate (men) or endocervical material (women) *or* Growth on selective medium demonstrating typical colonial morphology, positive oxidase reaction, and typical gram-stain morphology.	Growth on selective medium demonstrating typical colonial morphology, positive oxidase reaction, and typical gram-stain morphology; confirmed by sugar utilization, coagglutination, or antigonococcal fluorescent antibody (FA) testing. A definitive diagnosis is required if specimen is (1) extragenital, (2) from a child, or (3) medicolegally significant.
▪ **Chlamydia trachomatis**	
Mucopurulent cervicitis The presence of yellow mucopurulent endocervical exudate or the finding of this exudate on a white cotton-tipped swab of endocervical secretions. In women without visible mucopus, the presence of >10 polymorphonuclear leukocytes per $\times 1000$ field on a gram-stained specimen of endocervical mucus (without contamination by vaginal cells) also allows a presumptive diagnosis.	Definitive diagnosis is made by growth on cycloheximide-treated McCoy cells. Fluorescent monoclonal antibody stains or enzyme immunoassay (EIA) tests are also widely available. If confirmatory tests are not available, empirical therapy can be given on clinical grounds.
Nongonococcal urethritis (NGU) Symptomatic men are presumed to have NGU when their gonorrhea tests are negative and they have either white blood cells on Gram's stain of urethral discharge or sexual exposure to an agent known to cause NGU. Asymptomatic men with negative gonorrhea tests are also presumed to have NGU if they have >4 polymorphonuclear leukocytes per $\times 1000$ field on an intraurethral smear.	Same as above.
▪ **Treponema pallidum**	
Primary: Patients have typical lesion(s) and a newly positive serological test for syphilis (STS), or their present STS titer is at least fourfold greater than the last, or there has been syphilis exposure within 90 days of lesion onset. *Secondary:* Patients have the typical clincial presentation and a strongly reactive STS. *Latent:* Patients have serological evidence of untreated syphilis without clinical signs.	Primary and secondary syphilis are definitively diagnosed by demonstrating *T. pallidum* with darkfield microscopy or FA techniques in material from a chancre, regional lymph node, or other lesion. A definitive diagnosis of latent syphilis cannot be made under usual circumstances.
▪ **Herpes Simplex Virus**	
When typical genital lesions are present or a pattern of recurrence has developed, herpes infection is likely. A presumptive diagnosis is further supported by direct identification of multinucleated giant cells with intranuclear inclusions in a clinical specimen prepared by Papanicolaou or other histochemical stain, by typical HSV morphology by electron microscopy, or by detection of HSV antigens by monoclonal or polyclonal antibody detection systems.	An HSV virus tissue culture demonstrates the characteristic cytopathogenic effect (CPE) following inoculation of a specimen from the cervix, the urethra, or the base of a genital lesion. The isolates can be identified as type 1 or type 2 by FA, neutralization, or other serological techniques.
▪ **Human papillomavirus**	
A diagnosis may be made on the basis of the typical clinical presentation. Colposcopy may also aid in the diagnosis of certain cervical lesions. Exclude the possibility of condylomata lata by obtaining a darkfield or serological test for syphilis.	A biopsy, although usually unnecessary, is required to make a definitive diagnosis. Very atypical lesions, where neoplasia is a consideration, should be biopsied before initiating therapy. A Pap smear of cervical lesions shows typical cytological changes.
▪ **Human Immunodeficiency Virus**	
A presumptive diagnosis of HIV infection usually is based on clinical evidence.	A diagnosis of asymptomatic HIV infection usually is made on the basis of a repeatedly reactive EIA (enzyme immunoassay) test followed by a reactive supplemental test (e.g., Western blot or immunofluorescent assay or IFA). Polymerase chain reaction (PCR) is a gene amplification technique that has been used as a research tool to detect infection before detectable levels of antibody are found by EIA or Western blot techniques. Although isolation of the virus from body fluids is the most highly specific means to make a definitive diagnosis of HIV infection, such testing is not widely available.

STD could harm the fetus. In the United States, testing prostitutes for syphilis, chancroid, and PPNG has proved particularly useful for stemming specific outbreaks in Los Angeles and New York City. Recent experience using mobile vans to provide STD screening to those visiting crack houses in Philadelphia has also been encouraging.

STD Treatment. Treatment based on presumptive diagnosis should be inexpensive, simple, safe, and effective. Early and adequate treatment of patients and their sexual partners is an effective means of preventing the community spread of STD. National treatment recommendations are an essential part of the STD control strategy in any country.[21] Initially, in the United States these recommendations covered syphilis and gonorrhea but were expanded in the 1980s to include 18 other sexually transmitted organisms and syndromes. Current regimens for treating common STDs have been derived from clinical consensus among a group of experts (Table 6-6).

Selective prophylactic (preventive or "epidemiological") treatment also has a major role in STD control strategies.[55] In certain clinical instances, as with many other infectious diseases, it is preferable to offer treatment on the basis of presumptive diagnosis or exposure, before the specific diagnosis is confirmed. In addition, based on epidemiological indications, antibiotics can be administered to high-risk individuals when infection is considered likely, in the interest of public health gains. This approach interrupts the chain of transmission and prevents complications that might occur between the time of testing and treatment, ensures treatment for infected individuals with false-negative laboratory tests, and guarantees treatment for those who might not return when notified of positive tests.

Most recently, this approach of selective preventive treatment has helped to limit outbreaks of syphilis, PPNG, and chancroid in metropolitan areas. In addition, within certain closed communities with a high prevalence of infection, selective mass penicillin treatment has been useful. The same philosophy underlies the recommendation for giving tetracycline concurrently with penicillin to patients with confirmed gonococcal infection, since a relatively high proportion are likely to be harboring coexistent *C. trachomatis*.[56]

Counseling of Patients. Because of HIV and other incurable viral STDs, individual counseling (e.g., educating) of patients to facilitate changes in their behavior has taken on a new importance. Patients who are seen in any clinical setting with an STD are by definition a high-risk group; because of their own or their partner's behavior, they are most in need of counseling. The behaviors sought include (1) responding to suspected disease by promptly seeking appropriate medical evaluation, (2) taking oral medication as directed, (3) returning for follow-up tests when applicable, (4) promoting concern for sex partners and ensuring examination and treatment of partners when indicated, (5) avoiding future sexual exposure while infectious, and (6) preventing exposure by using condoms in high-risk settings.

Risk-reduction counseling to prevent acquisition or transmission of STD is increasingly becoming ingrained as a standard part of STD clinical care, whether provided in public STD clinics, other public health facilities, or private physician offices. In those areas of the world and population groups where health care is provided by nurses, pharmacists, and traditional practitioners (e.g., traditional birth attendants, who attend the majority of deliveries in rural areas in developing countries), these individuals should be trained to provide such counseling. The emergence of persistent viral infections has lessened the role of curative treatment and simultaneously raised the need for risk reduction counseling (primary prevention). The concept of "safer sex" has captured worldwide attention because of HIV infection.

Risk-reduction counseling is much more than emphasizing condom use. Patients must understand the importance of knowing the risk behaviors of their partners if they are to avoid high-risk partners. They need to know which sexual practices reduce the potential risk of infection and which practices carry highest risk. They should be introduced to the social skills essential to negotiating safer behaviors with their partners.[57] This is especially important for those known to be carriers of HIV, HBV, and genital HSV-2 infection. Counselors must maintain nonjudgmental attitudes in discussing potential life style changes.

TABLE 6-6. CURRENT REGIMENS FOR TREATING COMMON SEXUALLY TRANSMITTED DISEASES

Recommended Treatment
▪ **Neisseria gonorrhoeae**
Ceftriaxone, 250 mg IM once, *plus* doxycycline, 100 mg orally 2 times a day for 7 days.
▪ **Chlamydia trachomatis**
Doxycycline, 100 mg orally 2 times a day for 7 days, *or* tetracycline, 500 mg orally 4 times a day for 7 days.
▪ **Treponema pallidum**
Primary, secondary, or early syphilis of less than 1 year's duration: Benzathine penicillin G, 2.4 million units IM. Syphilis of indeterminate length or of more than 1 year's duration: Benzathine penicillin G, 7.2 million units total, administered as 2.4 million units IM given 1 week apart for 3 consecutive weeks. Neurosyphilis (inpatient therapy recommended; see STD Treatment Guidelines for outpatient regimen[21]): Aqueous crystalline penicillin G, 12–24 million units total, administered as 2–4 million units q4h IV, for 10–14 days.
▪ **Herpes Simplex Virus**
No known cure. Systemic acyclovir treatment may reduce symptoms and signs of herpes episodes and may accelerate healing but does not eradicate the infection or effect subsequent recurrence.
First Clinical Episode of Genital Herpes
Acyclovir, 200 mg orally 5 times daily for 7 to 10 days or until clinical resolution occurs.
Recurrent Episodes
Acyclovir, 200 mg orally 5 times daily for 5 days initiated within 2 days of onset, *or* acyclovir, 800 mg orally 2 times a day for 5 days.
Suppression of Recurrent Genital Herpes Infection
Continuous treatment reduces the frequency of active disease by at least 75% among patients with frequent (at least 6/y) recurrences. Dosage must be individualized for each patient. Acyclovir, 200 mg orally 2 to 5 times daily, *or* acyclovir, 400 mg orally 2 times daily.
▪ **Human Papillomavirus**
Cryotherapy with liquid nitrogen (or cryoprobe for external genital/perianal warts).
Alternative Treatments for External Genital/Perianal/Vaginal Warts
Podophyllin, 10%–25% in compound tincture of benzoin; trichloroacetic acid, 80%–90%. NOTE: For women with cervical warts, dysplasia must be excluded before treatment is begun. Management should therefore be carried out in consultation with an expert.
▪ **Human Immunodeficiency Virus**
For persons with HIV infection, zidovudine (ZDV, formerly called AZT) has been shown to be effective in preventing the clinical conditions associated with AIDs; in persons with AIDS, it has been shown to prolong life. Aerosolized pentamidine has been shown to be effective in preventing *Pneumocystis carinii* pneumonia. Both these drugs have serious side effects and require careful monitoring by knowledgable clinicians. For persons in whom AIDS has been diagnosed, standard therapy consists of treating opportunistic diseases aggressively as they occur. See N Engl J Med 323:1009–10014, 1990. (See also p 119.)

Unrealistic recommendations will either be ignored or will only lead to short-term changes. Patients must find the counseling messages comprehensible, acceptable, and attainable.

Counseling has additional meaning in HIV testing programs. Persons wishing an HIV antibody test should understand the meaning and implications of test results and be prepared to accept the test results.[58] Posttest counseling should be delivered by well-trained professionals, one-on-one, face-to-face, not by letter or telephone. Information imparted should build altruistic motivations in seropositive persons and self-protective motivations in seronegative persons. Moreover, HIV-infected individuals should be offered or referred for appropriate medical and psychosocial follow up.[59]

Partner Notification. Traditionally, STD control programs in the developed countries have emphasized active intervention by health providers to interview the patient, to identify the sex partners, and to ensure that these individuals are evaluated and treated. The privacy of original patients and partners is rigorously protected. During the 1970s in the United States, in large part due to the expanded spectrum of infections, a process of active notification was modified in many settings to encourage the patient to assume responsibility for locating and referring his or her sexual partners.[60]

This patient referral method actively involves the patient in the disease control effort, is relatively inexpensive, is acceptable to many patients, and reserves scarce staff time for targeted provider referral. Potential shortcomings of patient referral methods, however, include limited effectiveness with noncompliant patients and difficulty in evaluating its outcomes.

Active provider referral (i.e., contact tracing by the public health staff) is more labor-intensive, time-consuming, and expensive; therefore, active provider referral frequently concentrates on high-yield cases or on high-risk "core" environments.[61] Despite the initial costs, provider referral can also be economical because of its greater yield of infected persons and because these persons tend to be high-frequency transmitters of STD.[62] Special situations where this strategy has been useful include (1) partners of persons infected with HIV who might not otherwise realize they have been exposed to infection,[63] (2) introduction of a serious disease (e.g., syphilis or PPNG infection) into a community previously unaffected, (3) men and women with repeated STD infections, (4) female partners of men with infectious syphilis, and (5) STD infections in children.

Clinicians providing clinical preventive services may find it especially difficult to notify the sexual partner(s) of their longstanding patients, not only because such issues as infidelity, homosexuality, and child abuse generate anxiety, but also because the clinician may not have the skills or time to provide needed marital counseling. To avoid addressing this situation, more than half of primary care clinicians said they would lie to a spouse about the implications of a sexually transmitted infection if requested to do so by their infected patient.[64] Clearly more training in this delicate area is necessary to provide private clinicians with skills and incentive for partner notification.

Vaccines. HBV vaccine has been available for several years but has not yet been efficiently deployed to prevent sexual transmission of HBV. Since sexual transmission has been implicated as the principal route of transmission of HBV in the developed countries, vaccination strategies for preventing sexual transmission are probably overdue. Increasingly, health officials in industrialized countries are turning to development of such strategies.

STDS IN DEVELOPING COUNTRIES

Magnitude of the Problem. Although population-based information on STDs is generally lacking, sexually transmitted infections appear to be common problems in nearly all developing countries. Health care visits for lower genital tract complaints are extremely numerous, adding more stress to developing nations' already overburdened health care services. As in the United States, HIV commands center stage as the "international STD." Gonorrhea, syphilis, and chancroid are of next greatest concern.

The prevalence of gonococcal infections in non-STD clinic populations has been as high as 20% in the general population and as high as 50% among female prostitutes. In a Nairobi community hospital, 3% to 5% of all newborns developed gonococcal conjunctivitis, a potentially blinding infection. Gonorrhea incidence estimates have ranged from as high as 3% to 10% per year in selected population groups in Asia, Africa, and Latin America.

Chancroid and syphilis are also endemic. In many of the developing countries of Asia, Africa, and the Americas, chancroid may be as frequent as gonococcal infection. The prevalence of reactive serological tests for syphilis among antenatal clinic attendees has been as high as 15% in some countries of Africa and the Western Pacific. Because of this extremely high prevalence of untreated early syphilis among pregnant women in some urban centers in developing countries, the risk of stillbirth or perinatal death due to syphilis is also elevated. In two countries, Ethiopia and Zambia, studies have shown that at least 1% of all pregnancies are lost as a result of maternal syphilis, and about one third of all stillbirths are attributable to syphilis.

A growing awareness exists of the importance of chlamydial infections in causing infertility and infant morbidity. In addition, some countries are concerned about the potentially oncogenic viruses, such as HBV and HPV, in causing high rates of hepatocellular carcinoma and genital cancers, respectively.

Antimicrobial Resistance. To an even greater extent than in the United States, increasing resistance to antimicrobial agents has become a worldwide problem for many infectious agents, including the organisms causing STD. The dose of penicillin required to cure gonococcal infection has increased more than 100-fold since this agent was first introduced to treat patients with gonorrhea. PPNG isolates constitute over 10% of gonococcal infections in nearly all Southeast Asian and African country settings where this problem has been explored. PPNG has accounted for up to two thirds of all gonococci isolated in some regions of Africa and Asia during the 1980s. On these continents the prevalence of chromosomally mediated gonococcal resistance to penicillins, tetracyclines, and other antimicrobial agents also was high, making the problem of gonorrhea therapy even more difficult. Similar drug-resistance problems have been identified for chancroid infections in Africa, Asia, and Latin America.

As a result of rising antimicrobial resistance, penicillins have been replaced by alternative therapies for gonorrhea in many settings. Unfortunately most of these other antimicrobial agents (e.g., spectinomycin, newer cephalosporins) are either prohibitively expensive or not available in developing countries. This is especially true at the primary health care level. The majority of women seen for symptoms of gonorrhea or chlamydial infection in Africa probably do not receive effective treatment for either of these infections. Even if such economic and administrative barriers could be overcome with altered national or international pharmaceutical policies, practical issues of how to distribute the new drugs and how to ensure that practitioners use them effectively are substantial.

Demographic Pressures. During the next 2 decades, certain demographic and behavioral factors will further influence STD in developing countries. The number of young people—the group at highest risk for STD—and their proportion in the population will increase because of the existing high fertility levels. Moreover, continued decreases in infant and childhood mortality from successful immunization and diarrhea control programs will reinforce this trend. Population shifts from rural to urban areas, where STD rates are higher, are proceeding rapidly in most of the developing world. The growing use of contraceptives may further alter patterns of sexual behavior, particularly among women. In addition, increasing educational opportunities for women in some developing countries may delay marriage, also increasing STD risks.

Worldwide communication and transportation patterns affect STD. The rapid social transition in less developed countries has produced corresponding changes in values between generations. Diffusion of cultural values from developed countries to less developed countries introduces new social concepts. Migration, particularly temporary labor migration, expanded mass communications, and educational exchanges are substantial and further broaden the generation gap, since youth are more receptive to riskier sexual values.

STD Control in Developing Countries. Because of the relationship between ulcerative STD and transmission of HIV, increased attention is being given to establishing effective STD control programs in developing countries. Thus, the time is ripe for creative strategies. The goals of developing world STD control should be oriented toward (1) eliminating the principal reservoirs of bacterial STD infection, so costly to the countries themselves and so important to the spread of HIV and (2) decreasing maternal and perinatal infection to create an atmosphere where fecundability and life expectancy are sufficiently great that voluntary birth control will be acceptable.

Not all the STD control strategies currently used in the developed countries are appropriate for the developing world. Resources and facilities do not allow the type of intensive efforts through categorical STD programs that can be applied in developed countries. Simplified STD services must be provided at the primary health care level and other sources of health care (e.g., family planning clinics, pharmacies) to ensure effective management of the greatest number of cases. Such management limits further disease transmission and reduces STD complications. These providers can also perform important preventive services by encouraging treatment of steady sex partners and informing communities about the health effects of, and ways to avoid, STDs, including HIV infection.

The highest priority for preventing the serious consequences of STDs in developing countries should be given to the least expensive and most effective programs. Thus, health care planners concerned with maternal and child health in developing countries should provide effective ocular prophylaxis against gonorrhea in all neonates and serological testing for syphilis in all pregnant women.

Even where more complex laboratory tests, such as cultures for *N. gonorrhoeae* or *C. trachomatis,* are not widely accessible, their use on a limited scale can clarify disease epidemiology and improve approaches to patient care. Definition of the usual etiology of common genital syndromes allows the development of simple management algorithms suitable for settings where diagnostic tests are not available. If coexisting gonococcal and chlamydial infection are common, dual treatment for these conditions can be employed even before testing for gonorrhea and chlamydial infection becomes widespread. Similarly, dual therapy for syphilis and chancroid can be provided for patients with genital ulcers in areas where both diseases are common. Thus, improved appreciation of the epidemiology of STDs leads to more effective application of existing technologies.

A number of new antimicrobial agents have broadened the options for treatment of resistant gonococcal and chancroid infections. For example, safe, effective, and affordable alternatives to the penicillins for treatment of gonorrhea are being used in Africa and Asia. HBV vaccines are effective and safe and are increasingly available in the developing world economies. Although no other STD vaccines have proved effective, extensive work characterizing the immunogens of other STD agents is ongoing.

Finally, STD control activities provide an opportunity for enhancing other high-priority health programs. For example, HIV-prevention strategies are partly based on controlling other STDs. In addition, family planning clinics that provide optimal diagnosis and treatment for gonorrhea and chlamydia will prevent infertility. Conversely, interaction with the young adult population that has STD can be used to promote acceptance of immunization and diarrhea treatment programs for children and contraceptive programs for young adults.

FUTURE DIRECTIONS

First, reducing the transmission of HIV and controlling its progression to AIDS will become even more integral to public health and preventive medicine. Activities will evolve from emphasis on public and professional education to actual disease intervention through person-to-person HIV counseling and testing and confidential partner notification. Physician skills will increasingly involve supportive counseling to help persons with potentially lethal infections maintain safer sexual behaviors.

Second, clinicians will increasingly provide STD services to the high-risk populations, in facilities other than STD clinics, for example, drug treatment centers and adolescent health, maternal and child health, and family planning clinics. Diagnosis and treatment of STD in these settings will be funded by public and private resources and will be justified as part of essential medical services provided to these population groups.

Third, clinicians and patients alike will increasingly learn about the medical problems of STDs, the need for compliance with therapeutic recommendations, and the responsibility toward sexual partners of infected patients. The ability to take and provide an accurate sexual history will become part of routine medical examinations. Postgraduate education programs will increasingly involve developing skills in patient counseling.

Fourth, the private medical sphere will increasingly underwrite the costs and delivery of modern diagnostic and therapeutic methods for STDs in private patients. Care of patients with STDs will be paid for by private insurance and understood by patients and providers alike to be cost-effective. As emphasized earlier, with STD, curative medicine equals preventive medicine.

CONCLUSION

In the United States today, over 12 million new cases of STD occur in the young adult population each year. Globally, the number probably exceeds 250 million per year. Up to 40 million persons in the United States are currently infected with at least one organism. Conservative estimates of the total cost of STD to the United States exceed $3 billion annually, with the cost of gonorrhea alone exceeding $1.1 billion. Internationally, the costs are exponentially higher. Moreover, the magnitude of the STD problem appears to be expanding. There is an urgent need for both the public and private medical sectors to recognize the implications of the STD problems confronting us in the 1990s. The United States' 1990 STD objectives have been achieved with only one bacterial agent—gonorrhea. The others are nowhere in sight. The growing complexity and incidence of viral STDs requires all those providing clinical care to employ the most current diagnostic and treatment methods. The entrenchment of STD in inner-city "core" populations, already succumbing to urban decay and illicit drugs, makes patient recruitment a herculean task. Without the professional community's support and simultaneous involvement of the public and private health care sectors, the incidence of STD will continue to increase. The opportunity for promoting health, preventing human suffering, and reducing societal costs is great.

Epidemiology and Prevention of Acquired Immunodeficiency Syndrome

D. Peter Drotman
James W. Curran

AIDS is arguably the chief public health issue of the late twentieth century. AIDS not only is a leading cause of morbidity and mortality throughout the world but also involves topics that capture the public's attention and imagination such as sex, drugs, premature death, and intimate personal relationships. AIDS also has prompted changes in public health departments, private practices, and research, and it may ultimately affect the financing of medical care in the United States. A textbook chapter cannot adequately address all these biomedical, social, economic, and other AIDS issues, especially since they change so rapidly in response to new data, research, and public attitudes. Therefore, knowing sources of current information is important.

HIV infection and AIDS are among the most heavily researched topics of our time with hundreds of scientific reports being published monthly in biomedical and other professional or academic journals, including several devoted entirely to AIDS. Recommendations for prevention, treatment, counseling, testing, infection control, laboratory safety, clinical monitoring, and other topics are published frequently by WHO, the U.S. Public Health Service, and professional medical, dental, nursing, public health, and hospital associations all over the world. Several large textbooks on AIDS have been published, but these often become outdated rapidly. Computer-based information retrieval systems devoted to AIDS and HIV citations have proliferated and are readily available to users with appropriate hardware and minimal skills.

Many factors explain why AIDS became a worldwide epidemic during the 1980s. A former surgeon general of the U.S. Public Health Service, C. Everett Koop, MD, deserves considerable credit for promoting understanding of both the disease and persons afflicted with HIV infection and AIDS. By preparing his 1986 Surgeon General's Report on AIDS to be readable by the lay public and then distributing it widely, Dr. Koop promulgated sound scientific public health policies in the face of severe criticism. He received support from and in turn supported public health scientists. Although many AIDS controversies persist, many have been overcome. Dealing with new ones, including assigning proper public health priority to HIV infection control efforts, will be an issue for public health practitioners the world over in the 1990s. AIDS and HIV infection are irrevocably on the public health agenda. AIDS is prominently listed by the Preventive Services Task Force as part of comprehensive preventive health care[1] (Table 6–7), and is the only single disease chapter in the U.S. Public Health Service's Year 2000 Objectives for the Nation[2] (Table 6–8).

Although sporadic AIDS cases have been diagnosed by

TABLE 6-7. CLINICAL INTERVENTIONS FOR HIV RECOMMENDED BY THE U.S. PREVENTIVE SERVICES TASK FORCE

Counseling and testing for HIV should be offered to:

- Persons seeking treatment for sexually transmitted diseases
- Homosexual and bisexual men
- Past or present IV drug users
- Persons with a history of prostitution or multiple sexual partners
- Women whose past or present sexual partners were HIV-infected, bisexual, or IV drug users
- Persons with long-term residence or birth in an area with high prevalence of HIV infection
- Persons with a history of transfusion between 1978 and 1985
- Women in the above categories who are contemplating pregnancy.
- Pregnant women in these categories, as soon as the woman is known to be pregnant [If the initial test is negative, repeat testing may be indicated near delivery.]

Testing should not be performed in the absence of informed consent and pretest counseling, which should include the purpose of the test, the meaning of reactive and nonreactive results, measures to protect confidentiality, and the need to notify persons at risk.

A positive test requires at least two reactive enzyme-linked immunosorbent assay tests and a follow-up Western blot test. Clinicians should have these tests performed only at qualified laboratories that perform frequent test runs, use appropriate controls, and receive regular external proficiency testing.

Persons found to be seropositive should receive information regarding the meaning of the results, the distinctions between casual nonsexual contact and proven modes of HIV transmission, measures to reduce risk to themselves and others, symptoms requiring medical attention, and the availability of medical treatments [including experimental therapies] and community resources to provide psychological counseling, support groups, and other forms of assistance. Seropositive persons also should be evaluated for other infectious diseases, particularly tuberculosis. Arrangements for follow-up medical care are especially important for IV drug abusers, who may require assistance in achieving entrance to a drug-treatment program.

All seropositive individuals should be informed of the need to notify sexual partners, persons with whom IV drug needles have been shared, and others at risk of exposure. If it cannot be ensured that partners will be properly notified, physicians or health department personnel should use confidential procedures to alert these individuals.

All seropositive cases should be reported confidentially or anonymously to public health officials.

Persons with nonreactive test results should be informed that the risk of acquiring subsequent HIV infection can be prevented by maintaining monogamous sexual relationships with uninfected partners. Other measures to reduce the risk of infection, such as avoiding anal intercourse, using condoms, and not using unsterilized needles and syringes, should be specifically mentioned. The frequency of repeat testing of seronegative individuals is a matter of clinical discretion; persons with recent [less than 3 months] high-risk exposure are in greatest need of repeat testing to rule out false-negative results from low antibody titers.

Adapted from the Public Health Service.[2]

TABLE 6-8. NATIONAL HEALTH PROMOTION AND DISEASE PREVENTION OBJECTIVES FOR THE YEAR 2000 FOR SPECIAL POPULATION TARGETS

▪ HEALTH STATUS OBJECTIVES

1. Confine annual incidence of diagnosed AIDS cases to no more than 98,000 cases. [Baseline: An estimated 44,000 to 50,000 diagnosed cases in 1989.]

Diagnosed AIDS Cases	1989 Baseline	2000 Target
Homosexual and bisexual men	26,000–28,000	48,000
Blacks	14,000–15,000	37,000
Hispanics	7,000–8,000	18,000

NOTE: Targets for this objective are equal to upper bound estimates of the incidence of diagnosed AIDS cases projected for 1993.

2. Confine the prevalence of HIV infection to no more than 800/100,000. [Baseline: An estimated 400/100,000 in 1989.]

Estimated Prevalance of HIV Infection (per 100,000)	1989 Baseline[a]	2000 Target
Homosexual men	2,000–42,000[b]	20,000
Intravenous drug abusers	30,000–40,000[c]	40,000
Women giving birth to live-born infants	150	100

▪ RISK REDUCTION OBJECTIVES

3. Reduce the proportion of adolescents who have engaged in sexual intercourse to no more than 15% by age 15 and no more than 40% by age 17. [Baseline: 27% of girls and 33% of boys by age 15 and 50% of girls and 66% of boys by age 17 were reported in 1988.] Baseline data sources: National Survey of Family Growth; National Survey of Adolescent Males.

4. Increase to at least 50% the proportion of sexually active, unmarried people who used a condom at last sexual intercourse. [Baseline: 19% of sexually active, unmarried women aged 15 through 44 reported that their partners used a condom at last sexual intercourse in 1988.]

Use of Condoms	1988 Baseline[d]	2000 Target
Sexually active young women (by their partners) aged 15–19	26%	60%
Sexually active young men aged 15–19	57%	75%
IV drug abusers	—	60%

Baseline data sources: National Survey of Family Growth; National Survey of Adolescent Males.

NOTE: Strategies to achieve this objective must be undertaken sensitively to avoid indirectly encouraging or condoning sexual activity among teens who are not yet sexually active.

5. Increase to at least 50% the estimated proportion of all IV drug abusers who are in drug abuse treatment programs. [Baseline: An estimated 11% of opiate abusers were in treatment in 1989.] Baseline data source: National Institute on Drug Abuse.

6. Increase to at least 50% the estimated proportion of IV drug abusers not in treatment who use only uncontaminated drug paraphernalia ("works"). [Baseline: 25% to 35% of opiate abusers in 1989.] Baseline data source: National Institute on Drug Abuse.

7. Reduce the risk of transfusion-transmitted HIV infection to no more than 1/250,000 units of blood and blood components. [Baseline: 1/40,000 to 150,000 units in 1989.]

▪ SERVICE AND PROTECTION OBJECTIVES

8. Increase to at least 80% the proportion of HIV-infected people who have been tested for HIV infection. [Baseline: An estimated 15% of approximately 1 million HIV-infected people had been tested at publicly funded clinics in 1989.] Baseline data source: Center for Prevention Services.

9. Increase to at least 75% the proportion of primary care and mental health care providers who provide age-appropriate counseling on the prevention of HIV and other STDs. [Baseline: 10% of physicians reported that they regularly assessed the sexual behaviors of their patients in 1987.]

HIV Counseling by	1987 Baseline	2000 Target
Primary care and mental health care providers who practice in areas of high AIDS and STD incidence	—	90%

NOTE: Primary care providers include physicians, nurses, nurse practitioners, and physician assistants. Areas of high AIDS and STD incidence are cities and states with incidence rates of AIDS cases, HIV seroprevalence, gonorrhea, or syphilis that are at least 25% above the national average.

10. Increase to at least 95% the proportion of schools that have age-appropriate HIV education curricula for students in grades 4 through 12, preferably as part of quality school health education. [Baseline: 66% of school districts required HIV education, and 5% of school districts required HIV education in each year for grades 7 through 12 in 1989. Data source: General Accounting Office.]

NOTE: Strategies to achieve this objective must be undertaken sensitively to avoid indirectly encouraging or condoning sexual activity among teens who are not yet sexually active.

11. Provide HIV education for students and staff in at least 90% of colleges and universities. [Baseline data available in 1995.]

12. Increase to at least 90% the proportion of cities with populations over 100,000 that have outreach programs to contact drug abusers (particularly IV drug abusers) to deliver HIV risk reduction messages. [Baseline data available in 1995.]

NOTE: HIV risk reduction messages include messages about reducing or eliminating drug use, entering drug treatment, disinfection of injection equipment if still injecting drugs, and safer sex practices.

13. Increase to at least 50% the proportion of family planning clinics, maternal and child health clinics, STD clinics, tuberculosis clinics, drug treatment centers, and primary care clinics that screen, diagnose, treat, counsel, and provide (or refer for) partner notification services for HIV infection and bacterial STDs (gonorrhea, syphilis, and *Chlamydia*). [Baseline: 40% of family planning clinics for bacterial STDs in 1989. Data source: State Family Planning Directors.]

14. Extend to all facilities where workers are at risk for occupational transmission of HIV regulations to protect workers from exposure to blood-borne infections, including HIV infection. [Baseline data to be available in 1992.]

NOTE: The Occupational Safety and Health Administration (OSHA) is expected to issue regulations requiring worker protection from exposure to blood-borne infections, including HIV, during 1990. Implementation of the OSHA regulations would satisfy this objective.

[a] Data source: Centers for Infectious Diseases, Centers for Disease Control (CDC).
[b] Per 100,000 homosexual men aged 15 through 24 based on men tested in selected STD clinics in unlinked surveys; most studies find HIV prevalence of between 2,000 and 21,000/100,000.
[c] Per 100,000 IV drug abusers aged 15 to 24 in the New York City vicinity; in areas other than major metropolitan centers, infection rates in people entering selected drug treatment programs tested in unlinked surveys are often under 500/100,000.
[d] Data source: Center for Biologic Evaluation and Research, Food and Drug Administration.

using preserved autopsy specimens from as early as 1959 and 1968,[3,4] AIDS was first recognized as a distinct clinical syndrome in 1981. Initially, five cases of *Pneumocystis carinii* pneumonia among homosexual men were diagnosed and reported by clinical investigators in June 1981.[5,6] Shortly after, cases of Kaposi's sarcoma, a neoplasm that previously had been reported in the United States only rarely, were reported in young homosexual men.[7,8] Support for the recognition of AIDS as a new syndrome could be found in the increased demand for pentamidine isethionate, a then unlicensed antiparasitic drug used for the treatment of *P. carinii* pneumonia and a few other indications. This drug was only available in the United States through the CDC. Reviews of requests for pentamidine from 1976 to 1980 revealed only one request for the drug to treat an adult without an underlying immune disorder,[9] and by 1985, most requests were for treatment of *P. carinii* pneumonia associated with AIDS.

Investigations into the increase of opportunistic diseases, which were occurring in previously healthy young adult males, led to the "discovery" of AIDS in 1981. By 1985, a basic understanding of the etiology, immunopathogenesis, and epidemiology of HIV infection and AIDS had been developed[10] as the result of immense research efforts directed to this syndrome.

Case Definition. Since its recognition in 1981, cases of AIDS reported in the United States to the CDC have increased steadily (Fig. 6-6), a trend that has been projected to continue into the 1990s.[11] The epidemic curve includes only patients whose illnesses meet the criteria of the CDC case definition used for surveillance[12] and is adjusted for delays in case reporting. The case definition was originally designed to be highly specific, as is frequently the situation with new and serious epidemics, but it has become more sensitive to serious morbidity and mortality caused by HIV infection. Thus, more leading manifestations of HIV infection have been incorporated into the CDC case definition. The primary AIDS indicator diseases are listed in Table 6-9.[13] Since AIDS cases are often reported after the first diagnosis of an opportunistic disease, the frequency percentages are biased toward diseases that occur early in the course of AIDS; later diagnoses tend not to be reported. *P. carinii* pneumonia is the most frequent opportunistic disease reported. AIDS cases are only the tip of an iceberg representing the full clinical spectrum of infection with HIV. This spectrum includes asymptomatic HIV infection, mild illness with such nonspecific symptoms as fever, fatigue, loss of appetite and weight, diarrhea, and lymphadenopathy; other conditions not always associated with AIDS, such as idiopathic thrombocytopenic purpura and, perhaps, malignant neoplasms such as anal and cervical carcinomas; and probably other manifestations.

The surveillance definition has proved very useful in assisting public health officials in carrying out their responsibilities. The consistent use of a specific case definition resulted in accurate trend monitoring. AIDS has always represented the most severe end of a very wide disease or clinical spectrum, but the restrictive (highly specific) case definition caused some underestimation of the magnitude of this problem. To address this issue the CDC has revised the case definition to reflect more accurately the range of severe morbidity due to HIV infection and to maintain consistency with contemporary diagnostic practice. Changes have increased both the sensitivity of the case definition by including such conditions as HIV encephalopathy and wasting syndrome and its specificity by encouraging use of laboratory tests for HIV infection.

Etiological Agent and Modes of Transmission. By discerning that the main modes of transmission of the causative agent of AIDS are sexual contact, sharing contaminated needles, and receipt of blood or certain blood products, epidemiologists provided direction for laboratory investigators seeking the etiology of the disease. In 1983 and 1984, researchers at the Institut Pasteur (Paris) and the National Cancer Institute isolated HIV, a retrovirus, and demonstrated it to be the cause of AIDS.[14-18] In 1985, a genetic variant of the AIDS virus was isolated and has been named HIV-2.[19-20] Serological tests to detect antibody to HIV were rapidly developed.

HIV preferentially infects T-lymphocytes because a glycoprotein (gp) of the viral envelope (termed gp120 because of its molecular weight of about 120 kilodaltons) strongly binds to the CD-4 molecule, a marker found on the surface of the T-helper lymphocytes and a few other cell types. HIV eventually destroys the host cells. This destruction results in the characteristic decrease in T-helper and total lymphocyte counts, inversion of the normal helper-to-suppressor cell ratio, anergy to skin tests with recall antigens, and the cellular immunodeficiency that characterize AIDS.[21]

Natural History of HIV Infection. As with other viral infections, potential outcomes occupy a wide clinical spectrum, ranging from "CDC case definition" AIDS to asymptomatic HIV carriers. Classification systems have been proposed to assist in clinical management, prognosis, and epidemiological study of the natural history of HIV infection.[22-24] Because clinical decisions regarding use of antiviral drugs and chemoprophylaxis for opportunistic infections correlate best with declining absolute T-helper lymphocyte counts, clinically useful systems are heavily dependent on laboratory results such as measures of immune status and viral replication. These classification systems are often impractical for use in surveillance or HIV reporting, especially in

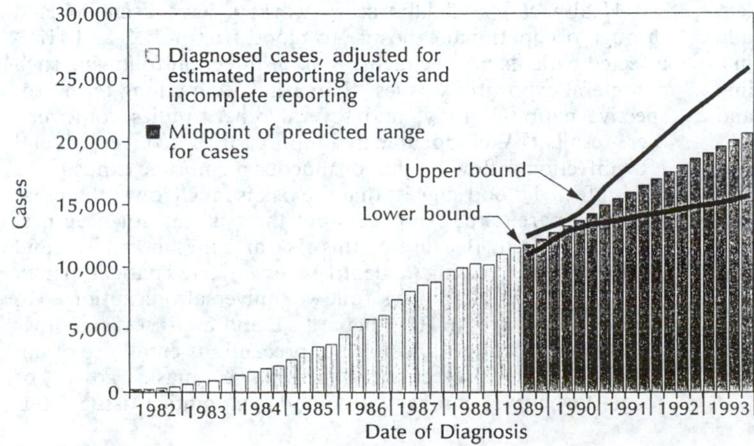

Figure 6-6. Reported and predicted AIDS cases in the United States. Predictions were made using back-calculation and extrapolation from recent trends, based on cases diagnosed through June 1989 and reported through September 1989. *[From Karon JM, Green T: AIDS case projections for the United States. 6th International Conference on AIDS: Final program and abstracts. Abstract F.C.213, 2:127, 1990]*

TABLE 6-9. PERCENTAGES[a] OF AIDS CASES REPORTED WITH VARIOUS AIDS-INDICATIVE DISEASES AMONG CASES DIAGNOSED SINCE THE 1987 REVISION OF THE CASE DEFINITION AND REPORTED THROUGH 1988 IN THE UNITED STATES AND U.S. TERRITORIES.

AIDS-indicative Disease	Percentage (N = 28,920)	AIDS-indicative Disease	Percentage (N = 28,920)
Bacterial infections, multiple or recurrent, serious pyogenic (counted in children only)	0.3	Lymphoma, Burkitt's or equivalent (other than in brain)	0.7
Candidiasis of bronchi, trachea, or lungs	3.0	Lymphoma, immunoblastic or equivalent (other than brain)	1.7
Candidiasis of esophagus		*Mycobacterium avium* complex or *M. kansasii* disease, disseminated or extrapulmonary	
Definitive diagnosis	6.7	Definitive diagnosis	2.5
Presumptive diagnosis	5.2	Presumptive diagnosis	0.2
Coccidioidomycosis, disseminated or extrapulmonary	0.2	*Mycobacterium tuberculosis,* extrapulmonary disease	
Cryptococcosis, extrapulmonary	5.7	Definitive diagnosis	1.6
Cryptosporidiosis, causing chronic diarrhea	1.6	Presumptive diagnosis	0.3
Cytomegalovirus disease other than retinitis	3.0	Mycobacterial disease caused by other or unidentified species, disseminated or extrapulmonary	
Cytomegalovirus retinitis (presumptive or definitive)	1.4	Definitive diagnosis	0.9
HIV encephalopathy (dementia)	5.8	Presumptive diagnosis	0.3
Herpes simplex, causing esophagitis, pneumonitis, or chronic mucocutaneous ulcers	3.2	*Pneumocystis carinii* pneumonia	
Histoplasmosis, disseminated or extrapulmonary	0.9	Definitive diagnosis	45.1
Isosporiasis, causing chronic diarrhea	0.2	Presumptive diagnosis	11.5
Kaposi's sarcoma		Progressive multifocal leukoencephalopathy	0.6
Definitive diagnosis	8.2	*Salmonella* septicemia, recurrent (counted separately in adults only)	0.5
Presumptive diagnosis	1.6	Toxoplasmosis of brain	
Lymphoid interstitial pneumonia (in children only)		Definitive diagnosis	1.2
Definitive diagnosis	0.1	Presumptive diagnosis	2.5
Presumptive diagnosis	0.1	HIV wasting syndrome	14.6
Lymphoma, primary in brain	0.4		

[a]The sum of percentages exceeds 100%, because some cases had more than one disease reported.

From Selik RM, Buehler JW, Karon JM, Chamberland ME, Berkelman RB: Impact of the 1987 revision of the case definition of acquired immune deficiency syndrome in the United States. AIDS 3:73–82, 1990.

patients who are poor or live in rural or underdeveloped nations or who otherwise lack access to health care or laboratory services.

It is unknown how many HIV-infected individuals will develop AIDS. Observations by early 1990 suggest that at least 50% of seropositive homosexual men develop AIDS within 10 years of follow-up study and that a similar fraction of HIV-infected transfusion recipients will develop AIDS within 7 years.[25] Because early treatment of HIV-infected persons seems to prevent the onset of AIDS-related opportunistic infections, the prognosis will be subject to variation as treatments improve and become more widely available and applied. The duration of infection is presumed to be indefinite in all infections since few if any persons have had a well-documented loss of HIV infection. Other similar lentivirus infections in animals, such as feline leukemia virus or simian immunodeficiency viruses, are typically lifelong. The virus titer and potential infectiousness of HIV in a given individual may vary according to many factors, including the infected person's clinical status, T-lymphocyte count, and possibly the strain of the infecting virus.

Factors that may contribute to variations in development of clinically severe manifestations of HIV infection include repeated viral exposures, basic health and nutritional status of the host, route of exposure to the virus, and exposure to possible environmental or infectious cofactors (which may help to explain, for instance, why Kaposi's sarcoma is far more common among homosexual male AIDS patients than other AIDS patients[26,27]).

Modes of Transmission and Distribution of Infection. HIV has been recovered from peripheral blood, semen, vaginal secretions, and numerous other fluids and anatomical sites.[28–30] It is transmitted sexually or through injection or transfusion of blood or its components or clotting-factor concentrates. Epidemiological observations and controlled studies have confirmed these routes of transmission in homosexual and bisexual men,[31] heterosexual men and women,[32,33] and IV drug users.[34] The previously documented risks to persons with hemophilia[35–37] and transfusion recipients[38] have been remarkably well controlled by education of donors and testing of all donations of blood and plasma for HIV antibody.[39] In addition, AIDS has been recognized in infants as a result of transmission of HIV from infected mothers before, at, or shortly after birth.[40–42] Estimates of the rate of transmission of HIV infection to such infants are 20% to 40%.[43]

Health care and laboratory workers have been infected through occupational exposure to blood from AIDS and HIV-infected patients or specimens. Risk of infection following such parenteral exposures was less than 1 in 250 in a long-term prospective national study, and several other studies confirmed these results.[44] Well-documented reports of seroconversion and HIV infection following skin or mucous membrane exposure to HIV-infected blood suggest that the risk is much lower than that following parenteral exposures, but the risk has not been precisely quantified. Because of this risk and the uncertainty and ineffectiveness of trying to identify every infected patient, health care workers should always follow "universal precautions" to minimize exposures to HIV, hepatitis B and C viruses, and other blood-borne pathogens. Universal precautions entail use of appropriate barrier protection (such as gloves, masks, gowns, or goggles) whenever contact with blood or nonintact tissue seems probable.[45] The possibility of transmission of HIV from infected dentists or surgeons to their patients has prompted further revisions in guidelines for infection control during invasive procedures.[46,47] Reviews of recommended precautions and guidelines proposed for hospital settings are available from the National Institute for Occupational Safety and Health of the CDC or the Occupational Safety and Health Administration of the U.S. Department of Labor, which has proposed regulating health care workplaces with regard to HIV and other blood-borne pathogens.

Studies with HIV antibody tests have elucidated the national epidemiology of HIV infection and have provided information on the future of AIDS. A series of retrospective seroprevalence surveys using frozen serum samples from a high-risk cohort of homosexual men in San Francisco documented a rapid increase in seroprevalence rates from 0.3% in 1978 to 28% in 1981 before plateauing at about 50% by 1983.[48] In New York City, 57% of IV drug users had antibody detected.[49] Of 860 hemophilia A patients tested in California, 62% were infected with HIV.[50] These high seropositivity rates show that infection with HIV is quite common among persons who have been in high-risk groups for many years and that there is a substantial and increasing risk to those exposed through heterosexual contact[51] but a decreasing risk to those receiving transfusions.[40] Seroprevalence rates in childbearing women ranged from 0.02% in New Mexico to 1.4% in New York City in blind surveys.[49]

There has been no epidemiological evidence to suggest that HIV is spread by air, water, food, or casual contact. If such modes of transmission did exist, cases would appear in the "other or no-identified-risk" category in Table 6–10. Only a small fraction of the reported cases, however, do not fall readily into a characteristic patient group. This fraction includes patients from whom information was not available because of severe illness, rapid death, or refusal to cooperate and patients for whom further investigation is incomplete.[52] Extensive follow-up of household contacts of both adults and children with AIDS has failed to demonstrate any evidence of HIV transmission via shared living space, kitchens, or bathrooms or through casual contact.[53]

Although the number of patients has increased markedly and steadily since the first cases were reported in 1981, the epidemiological pattern has evolved somewhat gradually. While it is reasonable to expect some shifts in risk categories to be identified on the basis of past epidemiological patterns, expectations of explosive new epidemic patterns, as would occur with airborne transmission of HIV, are not warranted. Data from sentinel hospitals that anonymously tested all non-AIDS-related admissions for antibody to HIV showed infection rates ranging from 0.1% to 7.8% with the highest rates clustered in northeastern U.S. cities, in blacks and Hispanics, in men, and in young adults, reflecting the patterns of AIDS.[54] In AIDS, as in other public health arenas, judicious application of scarce resources must be based on sound epidemiological data.

International Patterns. The geographic origin of HIV is not documented, but sub-Saharan Africa seems to fit most observations.[55] By 1990, AIDS cases had been reported from all 44 countries in sub-Saharan Africa.[56] It also has not been established when AIDS first occurred in Africa, but from the limited data available, it has been hypothesized that HIV may have evolved no more recently than the 1940s.[57] Large numbers of AIDS cases and HIV infections are now being diagnosed in many countries the world over. Studies are in progress to delineate the epidemiology of HIV infection in Africa, Latin America, and Asia, where the male-to-female ratio of patients is about equal, in contrast to the male preponderance seen in more industrialized countries. Homosexual transmission and IV drug abuse do not appear to be significant factors for the spread of AIDS in Africa, where heterosexual transmission is likely to account for the vast majority of HIV infections. An epidemic in intravenous drug users and prostitutes in Southeast Asia and India has allowed HIV to gain a foothold on that populous part of the world.

As of mid-1990, about 300,000 cases of AIDS had been reported to WHO from more than 150 countries. The clinical and epidemiological patterns of western European cases are similar to those seen in the United States, except for the relatively large number of cases occurring among persons originating from central Africa and the lower proportion of cases among IV drug users and persons born in Haiti. With the opening of eastern Europe, HIV is being noted as a public health problem there, especially in health settings where transfusions are not screened and injection equipment is reused and in places where sexual contact with infected travelers is more frequent. Most notable was the major epidemic of HIV and AIDS among children in Romania reported in 1989. Over 1000 children and infants apparently acquired HIV while living in overcrowded orphanages and other health facilities, probably largely through receipt of unscreened blood transfusions and reuse of injection equipment.

Therapy. Prospects for effective treatment for patients with AIDS or symptomatic or asymptomatic HIV infection are steadily increasing. Although the immunodeficiency that underlies AIDS has been resistant to treatment, several agents are able to inhibit viral replication in infected persons and stimulate lymphocyte function in laboratory systems. Zidovudine (formerly known as azidothymidine, or AZT) was licensed in the United States and other countries in 1987. Although it has become a mainstay of antiviral therapy, it is not curative and has serious toxic effects, such as severe anemia. Clinical trials are continuing, and progress in therapy may be expected once carefully organized trials are completed using different dosage schedules and various combinations of therapeutic agents (such as other nucleotide analogues and interferons or other immune modulators) in different stages of illness and in patients with asymptomatic viral infection.

Monitoring asymptomatic HIV-infected patients with serial T-helper lymphocyte counts and other clinical and laboratory markers is the standard of care in developed nations. Use of prophylactic AZT and antibiotics (trimethoprim-sulfamethoxazole orally or monthly inhalation treatments with aerosolized pentamidine) to prevent *P. carinii* pneumonia is well recognized.[58] Progress in prophylaxis of other opportunistic infections can be expected. As more HIV-infected persons perceive the specific medical benefits of early HIV diagnosis, the medical care system may be faced with the care of the hundreds of thousands of asymptomatically infected persons in the United States alone. This has become a serious issue for health care services and economic resources in many cities where HIV and AIDS are highly prevalent.

Until more effective antiviral therapy becomes available, the main goal of existing therapies will be to treat the manifestations of AIDS. Trimethoprim-sulfamethoxazole is the drug of choice for *P. carinii* pneumonia, the most common and among the more severe manifestations of AIDS; pentamidine isethionate is the second choice (the drugs are equally efficacious, but not equally toxic).[59] Other agents are becoming available. Kaposi's sarcoma might be treated in some stages with interferon, chemotherapy, or radiation. Several manifestations such as cytomegalovirus (CMV) retinitis and cryptococcosis have been partially controlled by newer agents (ganciclovir and fluconazole, respectively), while others such as *Cryptosporidium* enteritis have been resistant to virtually all treatments. Many patients with severe HIV infection need to take some of these expensive and often toxic medicines for prolonged periods, even indefinitely.

The case-fatality ratio is extremely high for cases meeting the CDC surveillance definition, reaching about 85% 3 years

TABLE 6–10. AIDS CASES BY AGE GROUP, EXPOSURE CATEGORY, AND SEX, REPORTED JULY 1988 THROUGH JUNE 1989, JULY 1989 THROUGH JUNE 1990; AND CUMULATIVE TOTALS, BY AGE GROUP AND EXPOSURE CATEGORY, THROUGH JUNE 1990, UNITED STATES

	Males		Females		Totals		
	July 1988–June 1989	July 1989–June 1990	July 1988–June 1989	July 1989–June 1990	July 1988–June 1989	July 1989–June 1990	Cumulative total[a]
	No. (%)	No. (%)	No. (%)	No. (%)	No. (%)	No. (%)	No. (%)
▪ **ADULT/ADOLESCENT EXPOSURE CATEGORY**							
Male homosexual/bisexual contact	18,927 (64)	22,103 (63)	—	—	18,927 (58)	22,103 (56)	82,304 (60)
Intravenous (IV) drug use (female and heterosexual male)	6,003 (20)	7,116 (20)	1,793 (52)	2,111 (49)	7,796 (24)	9,227 (23)	29,487 (21)
Male homosexual/bisexual contact and IV drug use	2,121 (7)	2,271 (6)	—	—	2,121 (6)	2,271 (6)	9,370 (7)
Hemophilia/coagulation disorder	310 (1)	287 (1)	7 (0)	8 (0)	317 (1)	295 (1)	1,234 (1)
Heterosexual contact:	677 (2)	921 (3)	1,119 (32)	1,417 (33)	1,796 (5)	2,338 (6)	6,952 (5)
Sex with IV drug user	*335*	*410*	*723*	*895*	*1,058*	*1,305*	*3,627*
Sex with bisexual male	—	—	*86*	*115*	*86*	*115*	*415*
Sex with person with hemophilia	*2*	*2*	*10*	*26*	*12*	*28*	*66*
Born in Pattern-II[b] country	*232*	*313*	*126*	*138*	*358*	*451*	*1,861*
Sex with person born in Pattern-II country	*12*	*17*	*9*	*20*	*21*	*37*	*101*
Sex with transfusion recipient with HIV infection	*10*	*15*	*23*	*28*	*33*	*43*	*109*
Sex with HIV-infected person, risk not specified	*86*	*164*	*142*	*195*	*228*	*359*	*773*
Receipt of blood transfusion, blood components, or tissue[c]	461 (2)	494 (1)	335 (10)	340 (8)	796 (2)	834 (2)	3,273 (2)
Other/undetermined[d]	947 (3)	1,834 (5)	192 (6)	407 (10)	1,139 (3)	2,241 (6)	4,765 (3)
Adult/adolescent subtotal	29,446 (100)	35,026 (100)	3,446 (100)	4,283 (100)	32,892 (100)	39,309 (100)	137,385 (100)
▪ **PEDIATRIC (<13 YEARS OLD) EXPOSURE CATEGORY**							
Hemophilia/coagulation disorder	33 (10)	26 (7)	1 (0)	—	34 (5)	26 (4)	119 (5)
Mother with/at risk for HIV infection:	262 (77)	294 (82)	256 (92)	307 (90)	518 (84)	601 (86)	1,966 (83)
IV drug use	*137*	*139*	*114*	*138*	*251*	*277*	*991*
Sex with IV drug user	*52*	*75*	*56*	*70*	*108*	*145*	*415*
Sex with bisexual male	*5*	*6*	*4*	*9*	*9*	*15*	*46*
Sex with person with hemophilia	—	—	*1*	*1*	*1*	*1*	*8*
Born in Pattern-II country	*28*	*24*	*26*	*22*	*54*	*46*	*197*
Sex with person born in Pattern-II country	*1*	*2*	*2*	*2*	*3*	*4*	*10*
Sex with transfusion recipient with HIV infection	*3*	—	*4*	*2*	*7*	*2*	*10*
Sex with HIV-infected person, risk not specified	*11*	*13*	*13*	*18*	*24*	*31*	*83*
Receipt of blood transfusion, blood components, or tissue	*3*	*6*	*9*	*4*	*12*	*10*	*40*
Has HIV infection, risk not specified	*22*	*29*	*27*	*41*	*49*	*70*	*166*
Receipt of blood transfusion, blood components, or tissue	38 (11)	23 (6)	16 (6)	15 (4)	54 (9)	38 (5)	233 (10)
Undetermined	8 (2)	14 (4)	6 (2)	18 (5)	14 (2)	32 (5)	62 (3)
Pediatric subtotal	341 (100)	357 (100)	279 (100)	340 (100)	620 (100)	697 (100)	2,380 (100)
Total	**29,787**	**35,383**	**3,725**	**4,623**	**33,512**	**40,006**	**139,765**

[a] Includes three patients known to be infected with HIV-2.

[b] Pattern II countries defined by WHO include several Caribbean and sub-Saharan African nations where heterosexual HIV transmission predominates.

[c] Includes 12 transfusion recipients who received blood screened for HIV antibody, and 1 tissue recipient.

[d] "Other" refers to three health care workers who seroconverted to HIV and developed AIDS after occupational exposure to HIV-infected blood. "Undetermined" refers to patients whose mode of exposure to HIV is unknown. This includes patients under investigation; patients who died, were lost to follow-up study, or refused interview; and patients whose mode of exposure to HIV remains undetermined after investigation.

From Centers for Disease Control: HIV/AIDS Surveillance Report, July 1990:8.

after AIDS diagnosis; the 5-year rate is well over 95%. Although this interval is likely to lengthen as more and better treatments are developed, the severe clinical course of AIDS, the uncertain efficacy of treatment, and the toxicity of available treatments serve to stress the importance of prevention.

Problems and Prospects for Control and Prevention. Future prospects for the prevention of HIV infection and AIDS are not completely predictable. Since infection with the AIDS virus is persistent and the period of communicability is long, the prevalence of infected individuals probably will continue to increase. AIDS likely will become the leading cause of severe morbidity and mortality in many high-risk populations.[60] It is the only disease that is rapidly increasing as a cause of "years of potential life lost" (YPLL)[61]—increasing from eleventh to sixth place during the 1980s and projected to equal cancer for third place in the 1990s.

The search for HIV vaccines and for specific therapies will be very high priorities during the next few years. Although recent advances in molecular virology and antiviral agents provide some reason for optimism, there is no guarantee that either of these technologies will be available to improve infection control substantially. The prevention focus remains on health promotion and education efforts aimed at all segments of the population but specifically targeted toward infected individuals and those at increased risk. Evidence that many homosexual men changed their sexual practices in the early 1980s to avoid infection with HIV is indicated by a decline in the incidence of STDs with short incubation periods, such as syphilis and rectal or pharyngeal gonorrhea.[62] This behavior change may in part be responsible for the change in the shape of the AIDS epidemic curve in 1987 to a less steep slope.[11]

Serological tests to screen donated blood and to aid in the diagnosis of patients were licensed for use in the United States in March 1985. Sensitive and specific antibody tests are now standardized and part of clinical prevention-oriented practices and public health services throughout the United States.[63] Additional tests, perhaps including tests for viral antigens or nucleic acid sequences,[64] may become available and allow for earlier diagnosis of asymptomatic HIV infection in adults and children and improved counseling and prevention programs.

The development and availability of serological tests for antibody to HIV promised further protection for the blood supply. The development of earlier medical interventions, such as AZT and *P. carinii* pneumonia prophylaxis, rendered many concerns about counseling and testing individuals secondary to preserving the health and lives of infected persons. Nonetheless, many concerns about HIV testing deserve to be addressed by public health practitioners and include the following: What may be the ramifications to populations screened for HIV? Will seropositive individuals be unjustly excluded from employment or housing? How well can confidentiality of test results be assured? What are the benefits vs costs of requiring reporting of serological test results by name to health departments? These and other equally difficult issues must be resolved while the nation continues to address HIV infection and AIDS as current public health problems.

AIDS differs from other public health problems in at least one other respect—the degree of public concern it has generated over a prolonged period. On the positive side, this has resulted in support for productive research, public information programs, and school health education. Some concern, however, has been misplaced, resulting in fear, panic, prejudice, and discrimination. Public health personnel have expended considerable effort to sidetrack nonuseful approaches and allay inappropriate concerns. Housing, employment status, and other community participation have all been scrutinized for HIV-infected persons and persons with AIDS. Increased testing for HIV antibodies probably will raise these issues anew, especially in communities with few reported AIDS cases.

Many groups have been formed to educate homosexual men and others about these issues, what the risks truly are, and how to avoid infection with the virus. On first consideration, the recommendations for preventing HIV infection are deceptively easy: avoid sex with others known or thought to be infected, stop using IV drugs or avoid sharing drug administration equipment, and eliminate infectious blood from use in transfusions or biopharmaceutical manufacturing processes. Sexual behavior is extraordinarily difficult to change, however, and changing sexual practices or giving up drugs are often beyond an individual's control without strong social support systems. Not surprisingly, the greatest progress has occurred in influencing sexual activity among homosexual men in cities where AIDS has the highest reported incidence, such as New York and San Francisco, where a leveling off of new AIDS cases among homosexual men has occurred.[65] Independent community-based organizations, often working with official health agencies but with a greater degree of freedom and perhaps more credibility in some of the communities they serve, have taught "safer sex practices" to homosexual men that supplement, in easy to understand language, those recommended by the U.S. Public Health Service. The premise of the guidelines promulgated by community organizations is that sexual expression and pleasure are attainable without engaging in activities likely to transmit HIV and other pathogens. Current and proposed health promotion approaches must be assessed and their ability to prevent HIV infection evaluated. Innovative approaches to IV drug users show some progress.[66] The innovations include use of nontraditional outreach workers (such as former drug users), reducing or eliminating charges for services, and repeated counseling and follow-up contacts. The hope, of course, is to provide a solid basis on which to make further recommendations and to pattern prevention activities.

In the years since its discovery, AIDS has generated extraordinary interest and sustained publicity, often characterized by fear and hysteria. There are many reasons for this reaction, including the public's fear and prejudice toward the groups comprising nearly all of the first AIDS patients and the misperceptions that AIDS was uniformly fatal and highly contagious. Fear also resulted from the belief that little was known about the disease, although AIDS was characterized clinically, epidemiologically, immunologically, etiologically, and serologically within 3 years of its discovery. School health education guidelines have been promulgated.[67] Their application holds the best hope for the future of AIDS prevention. Future progress in treatment and prevention can be anticipated. Now and in the future, public health officials at all levels will continue to be called on for leadership and direction in attempts to control HIV infection and AIDS. There remains much for all of us to do.[68]

REFERENCES

Sexually Transmitted Diseases

1. Holmes KK, Mardh P-A, Sparling PF, et al (eds): Sexually Transmitted Diseases, 2 edt. New York: McGraw-Hill, 1990
2. Cates W Jr: The "other STD"—do they really matter? JAMA 259:3606–3608, 1988
3. Brandt AM: No Magic Bullet: A Social History of Venereal Disease in the United States since 1880. New York: Oxford University Press, 1985
4. Turner CF, Miller HG, Moses LE (eds): AIDS: Sexual Behavior and Intravenous Drug Use. Washington, DC: National Academy Press, 1989, pp 73–185
5. Centers for Disease Control: Division of Sexually Transmitted Diseases, annual report, 1989. Atlanta: CDC, January 1990
6. Rowe MJ, Ryan CC: A National Survey of State-Only Spending for

AIDS Program. Washington, DC: Intergovernmental Health Policy Project, George Washington University, 1989

7. Horsburgh CR Jr, Douglas JM, LaForce FM: Preventive strategies in sexually transmitted diseases for the primary care physician. JAMA 258:814–821, 1987
8. Berg AO: The primary care physician and sexually transmitted disease control. In Holmes KK, et al (eds): Sexually Transmitted Diseases, 2 edt. New York: McGraw-Hill, 1990, pp 1095–1098
9. Fichtner RR, Aral SO, Blount JH, et al: Syphilis in the United States, 1967–1979. Sex Transm Dis 10:77–80, 1983
10. Centers for Disease Control: Syphilis and congenital syphilis—United States, 1985–1988. MMWR 37:486–489, 1988
11. Rolfs RT, Cates W Jr: The perpetual lessons of syphilis. Arch Dermatol 125:107–109, 1989
12. Pepin J, Plummer FA, Brunham RC, et al: The interaction of HIV infection and other sexually transmitted diseases: An opportunity for intervention. AIDS 3:3–9, 1989
13. Zenker PN, Berman SM: Congenital syphilis: Reporting and reality. Am J Public Health 80:271–272, 1990
14. Mascola L, Pelosi R, Blount JH, et al: Congenital syphilis. Why is it still occurring? JAMA 252:1719–1722, 1984
15. Centers for Disease Control: Policy guidelines for the prevention and control of congenital syphilis. MMWR 37(S-1):1–13, 1988
16. Barnes RC, Holmes KK: Epidemiology of gonorrhea—current perspectives. Epidemiol Rev 6:1–30, 1984
17. Rice RJ, Aral SO, Blount JH, Zaidi AA: Gonorrhea in the United States, 1975–1984: Is the giant only sleeping? Sex Transm Dis 14:83–87, 1987
18. Handsfield HH, Rice RJ, Roberts MC, Holmes KK: Localized outbreak of penicillinase-producing *Neisseria gonorrhoeae:* A community. JAMA 261:2357–2361, 1989
19. Jaffe HW, Biddle JW, Johnson SR, et al: Infections due to penicillinase-producing *N. gonorrhoeae* in the U.S., 1976–1980. J Infect Dis 144:191–196, 1981
20. Whittington WL, Knapp JS: Trends in resistance of *Neisseria gonorrhoeae* to antimicrobial agents in the United States. Sex Transm Dis 15:202–210, 1988
21. Centers for Disease Control: 1989 Sexually Transmitted Diseases Treatment Guidelines. MMWR 38(S-5):1–43, 1989
22. Centers for Disease Control: Sentinel surveillance system for antimicrobial resistance in clinical isolates of *Neisseria gonorrhoeae.* MMWR 36:585–592, 1987
23. Thompson SE, Washington AE: Epidemiology of sexually transmitted *Chlamydia trachomatis* infections. Epidemiol Rev 5:96–123, 1983
24. Brunham RC, Paavonen J, Stevens CE, et al: Mucopurulent cervicitis—the ignored counterpart in women of urethritis in men. N Engl J Med 311:1–6, 1984
25. Washington AE, Johnson RE, Sanders LL, et al: Incidence of *Chlamydia trachomatis* infections in the United States: Using reported *Neisseria gonorrhoeae* as a surrogate. In Oriel D, Ridgway G, Schachter J, et al (eds): Chlamydial Infections. Cambridge: Cambridge University Press, 1986, p 487
26. Schachter J: Why we need a program for the control of *Chlamydia trachomatis.* N Engl J Med 320:802–803, 1989
27. Centers for Disease Control: *Chlamydia trachomatis* Infections: Policy Guidelines for Prevention and Control. Atlanta: CDC, 1985
28. Handsfield HH: Control of sexually transmitted chlamydial infections. JAMA 257:2073–2074, 1987
29. Centers for Disease Control: Update: Acquired immunodeficiency syndrome—United States, 1981–1988. MMWR 38:229–236, 1989
30. Centers for Disease Control: AIDS and human immunodeficiency infection in the United States: 1988 update. MMWR 38(S-4):1–14, 1989
31. Lewis C, Freeman H: The sexual history taking and counseling practices of primary care physicians. West J Med 147:165–167, 1987
32. Johnson RE, Nahmias AJ, Magder LS, Lee FK, Brooks CA, Snowden CB: Distribution of genital herpes (HSV-2) in the United States: A seroepidemiological national survey using a new type-specific antibody assay. N Engl J Med 321:7–12, 1989
33. Mertz GJ, Coombs RW, Ashley R, et al: Transmission of genital herpes in couples with one symptomatic and one asymptomatic partner: A prospective study. J Infect Dis 157:1169–1175, 1988
34. Holmberg SD, Stewart JA, Gerber AR, et al: Prior herpes simplex virus type 2 infection as a risk factor for HIV infection. JAMA 259:1048–1050, 1988
35. Stamm WE, Handsfield HH, Rompalo AM, Ashley RL, Roberts PL, Corey L: The association between genital ulcer disease and acquisition of HIV infection in homosexual men. JAMA 260:1429–1433, 1988
36. Sullivan-Bolyai J, Hull HF, Wilson C, et al: Neonatal herpes simplex virus infection in King County, Washington. JAMA 250:3059–3062, 1983
37. Koutsky LA, Galloway DA, Holmes KK: Epidemiology of genital human papillomavirus infection. Epidemiol Rev 10:122–163, 1988
38. Stone KM: Epidemiologic aspects of genital HPV infection. Clin Obstet Gynecol 32:112–116, 1989
39. Centers for Disease Control: Protection against viral hepatitis. MMWR 39(RR-2):1–2, 1990
40. Beasley RP: Hepatitis B virus as the etiologic agent in hepatocellular carcinoma: Epidemiologic considerations. Hepatology 2:21S–26S, 1982
41. Alter MJ, Hadler SC, Margolis HS, et al: The changing epidemiology of hepatitis B in the United States. JAMA 263:1218–1222, 1990
42. Lettau LA, McCarthy JG, Smith MH, et al: Outbreak of severe hepatitis due to delta and hepatitis B viruses in parenteral drug abusers and their contacts. N Engl J Med 317:1256–1262, 1987
43. World Health Organization: WHO Expert Committee on Venereal Diseases and Treponematoses: Sixth Report. Geneva, Switzerland, World Health Organization, 1986
44. May R, Anderson R: Transmission dynamics of HIV infection. Nature 326:137–142, 1987
45. Allard R: Beliefs about AIDS as determinants of preventive practices and of support for coercive measures. Am J Public Health 79:448–452, 1989
46. Solomon MZ, DeJong W: Preventing AIDS and other STDs through condom promotion: A patient education intervention. Am J Public Health 79:453–458, 1989
47. Centers for Disease Control: Results from the national adolescent student health survey. MMWR 38:147–150, 1989
48. Yarber WL: AIDS: What young adults should know. Reston, Virginia: American Alliance for Health Physical Education, Recreation and Dance, 1987
49. Brown JD, Childers KW, Waszak CS: Television and adolescent sexuality. J Adolesc Health Care 11:62–70, 1990
50. Stamm WE, Kaetz S, Holmes KK: Clinical training in venereology in the United States and Canada. JAMA 248:2020–2025, 1982
51. Centers for Disease Control: Quality Assurance Guidelines for STD Clinics—1986. Atlanta: CDC, 1986
52. Stamm WE, Kaetz SM, Beirne MB, Ashman JA: The practitioner's handbook for the management of STDs. Seattle: University of Washington, 1988
53. Babbott D, Baldwin DC Jr, Killian CD, Weaver SO: Trends in evolution of specialty choice: Comparison of US medical school graduates in 1983 and 1987. JAMA 261:2367–2373, 1989
54. Johns MB, Hovell MF, Ganiats T, et al: Primary care and health promotion: Model for preventive medicine. Am J Prev Med 3:346–357, 1987
55. Hart G: Epidemiologic treatment for syphilis and gonorrhea. Sex Transm Dis 7:149–160, 1980
56. Stamm WE, Guinan ME, Johnson C, et al: Effect of treatment regimens for *Neisseria gonorrhoeae* on simultaneous infection with *Chlamydia trachomatis.* N Engl J Med 310:545–551, 1984
57. Becker MH, Joseph JG: AIDS and behavioral change to reduce risk: A review. Am J Public Health 78:394–410, 1988
58. Centers for Disease Control: Public Health Service guidelines for counseling and antibody testing to prevent HIV infection and AIDS. MMWR 36:509–515, 1987
59. Francis DP, Anderson RE, Gorman ME, Fenstersheib M, Padian

NS, Kizer KW, Conant MA: Targeting AIDS prevention and treatment toward HIV-1-infected persons. JAMA 262:2572–2576, 1989

60. Potterat JJ, Rothenberg RB: The casefinding effectiveness of a self-referral system for gonorrhea: A preliminary report. Am J Public Health 67:174–179, 1977
61. Association of State and Territorial Health Officials: Guide to public health practice: HIV partner notification strategies. Washington, DC: Public Health Foundation, 1988, pp 1–15
62. Katz BP, Danos CS, Quinn TS, Caine V, Jones RB: Efficiency and cost-effectiveness of field follow up for patients with *Chlamydia trachomatis* infection in a sexually transmitted diseases clinic. Sex Transm Dis 15:11–16, 1988
63. Toomey KE, Cates W Jr: Partner notification for the prevention of HIV infection. AIDS 3(suppl 1):S57–S62, 1989
64. Novack DH, Detering BJ, Arnold R, Forrow L, Ladinsky M, Pezzullo JC: Physicians' attitudes toward using deception to resolve difficult ethical problems. JAMA 261:2980–2985, 1989

Epidemiology and Prevention of Acquired Immunodeficiency Syndrome

1. Public Health Service: Guide to Clinical Preventive Services: Report of the U.S. Preventive Services Task Force. Washington, DC: Public Health Service, 1989, pp 93–98
2. Public Health Service: Healthy People 2000: National Health Promotion and Disease Prevention Objectives. Washington, DC: Public Health Service, 1990, pp 476–491
3. Corbitt G, Bailey AS, Williams G: HIV infection in Manchester, 1959. Lancet 336:51, 1990
4. Garry RF, Witte MH, Gottlieb AA, et al: Documentation of an AIDS virus infection in the United States in 1968. JAMA 260:2085–2087, 1988
5. Centers for Disease Control: *Pneumocystis* pneumonia—Los Angeles. MMWR 30:250–252, 1981
6. Gottlieb MS, Schroff R, Schanker HM, et al: *Pneumocystis carinii* pneumonia and healthy homosexual men. N Engl J Med 305:1425–1431, 1981
7. Centers for Disease Control: Kaposi's sarcoma and *Pneumocystis* pneumonia among homosexual men—New York City and California. MMWR 30:305–308, 1981
8. Hymes K, Cheung T, Greene JB, et al: Kaposi's sarcoma in homosexual men. Lancet 2:598–600, 1981
9. CDC Task Force on Kaposi's Sarcoma and Opportunistic Infections: Epidemiologic aspects of the current outbreak of Kaposi's sarcoma and opportunistic infections. N Engl J Med 306:248–252, 1982
10. Scientific American: The Science of AIDS. New York: W. H. Freeman, 1989
11. Centers for Disease Control: Estimates of HIV prevalence and projected AIDS cases: Summary of a workshop, October 31–November 1, 1989. MMWR 39:110–112, 1990
12. Centers for Disease Control: Revision of the CDC surveillance case definition for acquired immunodeficiency syndrome. MMWR 36:1–155, 1987
13. Selik RM, Buehler JW, Karon JM, Chamberland ME, Berkelman RL: Impact of the 1987 revision of the case definition of acquired immunodeficiency syndrome in the United States. J AIDS 3:73–82, 1990
14. Barre-Sinoussi F, Chermann JC, Rey F, et al: Isolation of a T-lymphotropic retrovirus from a patient at risk for acquired immunodeficiency syndrome (AIDS). Science 220:868–871, 1983
15. Popovic M, Sarngadharan MG, Read E, et al: Detection, isolation, and continuous production of cytopathic retroviruses (HTLV-III) from patients with AIDS and pre-AIDS. Science 224:497–500, 1984
16. Gallo RC, Salahuddin SZ, Popovic M, et al: Frequent detection and isolation of cytopathic retroviruses (HTLV-III) from patients with AIDS and at risk for AIDS. Science 224:500–503, 1984
17. Schupbach J, Popovic M, Gilden RW, et al: Serological analysis of a subgroup of human T-lymphotropic retroviruses (HTLV-III) associated with AIDS. Science 224:503–505, 1984
18. Sarngadharan MG, Popovic M, Bruch L, et al: Antibodies reactive with human T-lymphotropic retroviruses (HTLV-III) in the serum of patients with AIDS. Science 224:506–508, 1984
19. Barin F, M'Boup S, Denis F, et al: Serological evidence for virus related to simian T-lymphotropic retrovirus III in residents of West Africa. Lancet 2:1387–1389, 1985
20. Clavel F, Guetard D, Brun-Vezinet F, et al: Isolation of a new human retrovirus from West African patients with AIDS. Science 233:343–346, 1986
21. Fauci AS: The human immunodeficiency virus: Infectivity and mechanisms of pathogenesis. Science 239:617–622, 1988
22. Centers for Disease Control: Classification system for human T-lymphotropic virus type III/lymphadenopathy associated virus infections. MMWR 35:334–339, 1986
23. Redfield RR, Wright DC, Tramont EC: The Walter Reed staging classification for HTLV-III/LAV infection. N Engl J Med 314:131–132, 1986
24. World Health Organization: Acquired Immunodeficiency Syndrome (AIDS): Interim proposal for a WHO staging system for HIV infection and disease. Weekly Epidemiol Rec 65:221–224, 1990
25. Ward JW, Bush TJ, Perkins HA, et al: The natural history of transfusion-associated infection with human immunodeficiency virus: Factors influencing the rate of progression to disease. N Engl J Med 321:947–952, 1989
26. Haverkos HW, Pinsky PF, Drotman P, Bregman DJ: Disease manifestation among homosexual men with acquired immunodeficiency syndrome: A possible role of nitrites in Kaposi's sarcoma. Sex Transm Dis 12:203–208, 1985
27. Beral V, Peterman TA, Berkelman RL, Jaffe HW: Kaposi's sarcoma among persons with AIDS: A sexually transmitted infection? Lancet 335:123–128, 1990
28. Ho DD, Schooley RT, Rota TR, et al: HTLV-III in the semen and blood of a healthy homosexual man. Science 226:451–453, 1984
29. Bernard DZJ, Leibowitch J, Safai B, et al: HTLV-III in cells cultured from semen of two patients with AIDS. Science 226:449–451, 1984
30. Hollander H: Transmission of HIV in body fluids. In Cohen PT, Sande MA, Volberding PA (eds): The AIDS Knowledge Base: A Textbook on HIV Disease from the University of California, San Francisco, and the San Francisco General Hospital. Waltham, Mass: The Medical Publishing Group, 1990, pp 1.2.1:1–3
31. Auerbach DM, Darrow WW, Jaffe HW, et al: Cluster of cases of acquired immunodeficiency syndrome: Patients linked by sexual contact. Am J Med 76:487–492, 1984
32. Peterman TA, Stoneburner RL, Allen JR, et al: Risk of human immunodeficiency virus transmission from heterosexual adults with transfusion-associated infections. JAMA 259:55–58, 1988
33. Redfield RR, Markham PD, Salahuddin SZ, et al: Frequent transmission of HTLV-III among spouses of patients with AIDS-related complex and AIDS. JAMA 253:1571–1573, 1985
34. Guinan ME, Thomas PA, Pinsky PF, et al: Heterosexual and homosexual cases of acquired immunodeficiency syndrome: A comparison of surveillance, interview, and laboratory data. Ann Intern Med 100:213–218, 1984
35. Centers for Disease Control: *Pneumocystis carinii* pneumonia among persons with hemophilia A. MMWR 31:365–367, 1982
36. Stehr-Green JK, Holman RC, Jason JM, Evatt BL: Hemophilia-associated AIDS in the United States, 1981 to September 1987. Am J Public Health 78:439–442, 1988
37. Goedert JJ, Kessler CM, Aledort LM, et al: A prospective study of human immunodeficiency virus type 1 infection and the development of AIDS in subjects with hemophilia. N Engl J Med 321:1141–1148, 1989
38. Curran JW, Lawrence DL, Jaffe HW, et al: Acquired immunodeficiency syndrome (AIDS) associated with transfusions. N Engl J Med 310:69–75, 1984
39. Ward JW, Holmberg SD, Allen JR: Transmission of human immunodeficiency virus (HIV) by blood transfusions screened as negative for HIV antibody. N Engl J Med 318:473–477, 1989

40. Centers for Disease Control: Unexplained immunodeficiency and opportunistic infections in infants—New York, New Jersey, and California. MMWR 31:665–667, 1982
41. The European Collaborative Study: Mother-to-child transmission of HIV infection. Lancet 2:1039–1043, 1988
42. Rogers MF, Ou C-Y, Rayfield M, et al: Use of the polymerase chain reaction for early detection of the proviral sequences of human immunodeficiency virus in infants born to seropositive mothers. N Engl J Med 320:1649–1654, 1989
43. Oxtoby MJ: Perinatally acquired HIV infection. In Pizzo PA, Wilfert CM (eds): Pediatric AIDS: The Challenge of HIV Infection in Infants, Children and Adolescents. Baltimore: Williams & Wilkins, in press
44. Marcus R, CDC Cooperative Needlestick Study Group: Surveillance of health-care workers exposed to blood from patients infected with the human immunodeficiency virus. N Engl J Med 319:1118–1123, 1988
45. Centers for Disease Control: Update: Universal precautions for prevention of transmission of human immunodeficiency virus, hepatitis B virus, and other bloodborne pathogens in health-care settings. MMWR 37:377–388, 1988
46. Centers for Disease Control: Possible transmission of human immunodeficiency virus to a patient during an invasive dental procedure. MMWR 39:489–493, 1990
47. Rhame FS: The HIV-infected surgeon. JAMA 264:507–508, 1990
48. Hessol NA, Lifson AR, O'Malley PM, Doll LS, Jaffe HW, Rutherford GW: Prevalence, incidence, and progression of human immunodeficiency virus infection in homosexual and bisexual men in hepatitis B vaccine trials, 1978–88. Am J Epidemiol 130:1167–1175, 1989
49. Centers for Disease Control: AIDS and human immunodeficiency virus infection in the United States: 1988 update. MMWR 38 (S4):1–38, 1989
50. Holman RC, Gomperts ED, Jason JM, Abildgaard CF, Zelasky MT, Evatt BL: Age and human immunodeficiency virus infection in persons with hemophilia in California. Am J Public Health 80:967–969, 1990
51. Holmes KK, Karon JM, Kreiss K: The increasing frequency of heterosexually acquired AIDS in the United States, 1983–88. Am J Public Health 80:858–863, 1990
52. Castro KG, Lifson AR, White CR, et al: Investigations of AIDS patients with no previously identified risk factors. JAMA 259:1338–1342, 1988
53. Friedland G, Kahl P, Saltzman B, et al: Additional evidence for lack of transmission of HIV infection by close interpersonal (casual) contact. AIDS 4:639–644, 1990
54. St. Louis ME, Rauch KJ, Petersen LR, et al: Seroprevalence of human immunodeficiency virus infection at sentinel hospitals in the United States. N Engl J Med 323:213–218, 1990
55. Osmond D: AIDS in Africa. In Cohen PT, Sande MA, Volberding PA (eds): The AIDS Knowledge Base: A Textbook on HIV Disease from the University of California, San Francisco, and the San Francisco General Hospital. Waltham, Mass: The Medical Publishing Group, 1990, pp 1.1.4:1–10
56. World Health Organization: Acquired immunodeficiency syndrome (AIDS)—data as of 31 July 1990. Weekly Epidemiol Rec 65:240–241, 1990
57. Smith TF, Srinivasan A, Schochetman G, Marcus M, Myers G: The phylogenetic history of immunodeficiency viruses. Nature 333:573–575, 1988
58. Centers for Disease Control: Guidelines for prophylaxis against *Pneumocystis carinii* pneumonia for persons infected with human immunodeficiency virus. MMWR 38(S-5):1–9, 1989
59. Leoung GS, Hopewell PC: *Pneumocystis carinii* pneumonia: Therapy and prophylaxis. In Cohen PT, Sande MA, Volberding PA (eds): The AIDS Knowledge Base: A Textbook on HIV Disease from the University of California, San Francisco, and the San Francisco General Hospital. Waltham, Mass: The Medical Publishing Group, 1990, pp 6.5.4–1–15
60. Chu SY, Buehler JW, Berkelman RL: Impact of the human immunodeficiency virus epidemic on mortality in women of reproductive age, United States. JAMA 264:225–229, 1990
61. Centers for Disease Control: Years of potential life lost before ages 65 and 85—United States, 1987 and 1988. MMWR 39:20–22, 1990
62. Centers for Disease Control: Declining rates of rectal and pharyngeal gonorrhea among males—New York City. MMWR 33:295–297, 1984
63. Centers for Disease Control: Interpretation and use of the Western blot assay for serodiagnosis of human immunodeficiency virus type 1 infections. MMWR 38(S7):1–7, 1989
64. Ou C-Y, Kwok S, Mitchell SW, et al: DNA amplification for direct detection of HIV-1 in DNA of peripheral blood mononuclear cells. Science 239:295–297, 1988
65. Centers for Disease Control: Update: Acquired Immunodeficiency syndrome—United States, 1989. MMWR 39(5):81–86, 1990
66. Centers for Disease Control: Update: Reducing HIV transmission in intravenous-drug users not in drug treatment—United States. MMWR 39:529, 535–538, 1990
67. Centers for Disease Control: Guidelines for effective school health education to prevent the spread of AIDS. MMWR 37(S-2):1–14, 1988
68. Valdiserri RO: Preventing AIDS: The Design of Effective Programs. New Brunswick, N.J.: Rutgers University Press, 1989

7

Diseases Spread by Close Personal Contact

Acute Respiratory Infections

Arnold S. Monto

Acute respiratory diseases are the most common illnesses suffered by humans. The Health Interview Survey has estimated that more than 122 million respiratory episodes that involve restricted activity or medical consultation occur annually in the United States. The pathogens involved are multiple, and reinfection with the same agent is common. In this chapter, only the situation in developed countries and the principal pathogens involved there are discussed. Infection with influenza virus is discussed on pages 81 to 85. Agents reviewed in detail are parainfluenzaviruses, respiratory syncytial (RS) virus, the rhinoviruses, coronaviruses, adenoviruses, *Mycoplasma pneumoniae,* and *Chlamydia pneumoniae.* Additional agents, such as *Coxiella burnetti,* the cause of Q fever, and a number of other viruses, such as coxsackie and echoviruses, are less frequent or limited causes of acute illness. These pathogens and other agents, such as the measles virus, which produce respiratory manifestations as one component of a more generalized disease, are considered elsewhere.

Although there are certain well-defined clinical syndromes associated with specific agents, such as croup or bronchiolitis, it is not possible on the basis of clinical characteristics of most illnesses to classify them etiologically in the absence of laboratory tests. An illustration of the situation is seen in Figure 7–1. In each portion of Figure 7–1 is shown the frequency with which ill individuals, infected with a particular agent, exhibit a specific respiratory symptom or restriction of daily activity. The agents are those most frequently encountered in a normal population. No clearly distinguishing characteristics are present. In spite of the overlap, however, certain differences are apparent. With the exception of coryza, symptoms are less abundant with the rhinoviruses. RS virus and parainfluenza-associated illnesses are similar in characteristics, although cough is more common with the parainfluenzaviruses, and activity restriction is more common with RS virus. Hemolytic streptococcal illness is included for completeness, and as expected, sore throat is its most prominent symptom. Influenza produces the most severe illnesses, with a greater frequency of symptoms and activity restriction for type A than for type B.

Because of the inability to determine etiology on clinical grounds, it is usual for illnesses to be enumerated simply as common or undifferentiated respiratory disease. The distribution of these illnesses has been defined in a number of different populations, and determinants of their frequency have been identified. Illness rates are highest in youngest children and decrease with increasing age, except in the third decade of life when young adults are exposed to infection by their own young children. The actual number of illnesses reported per year has varied not only with age but also with the population studied and the methods used to ascertain their occurrence. In the Cleveland family study,[1] which was carried out in a group of upper middle class households, infants had more than four such annual episodes. In the Tecumseh study,[2] in which a larger number of households of all social groups were followed, this figure was 6.1. In young adults age 20 to 24 years, it was 2.8. The difference is related not only to social group, since better educated people are known to perceive more illness as occurring than less well educated individuals, but also to the method of ascertainment. In Cleveland, illness was recorded by medical personnel who actually visited the household, but in Tecumseh, frequency and characteristics of acute episodes were determined by a weekly telephone call.

Illness frequency is affected by sex as well as by age and social group: adult women experience more illness than men. This observation has been confirmed by laboratory investigations documenting that infections are more common in women. The greater exposure of women to small children may be responsible for this. Although there has been disagreement about the small sex difference in frequency of illness and infection in older children, there is agreement that in young children, especially under age 3 years, boys are affected more often and more severely.

Familial factors also influence the frequency of respiratory illnesses. Schoolchildren, including preschoolchildren, most often introduce infection into the family, fathers least often. The position of children in the family also determines their frequency of infection. Youngest children suffer more frequent illness earlier in life than their siblings did, mainly because of exposure to and introduction of infection by their older siblings.

The discussion of the principal agents involved focuses on their microbiology, the pathogenesis and spectrum of diseases they cause, the potential severity and frequency of these diseases, and the possibility of prevention and control. The order selected for consideration is not based simply on the relative importance of an agent but rather on a combination of factors, including potential severity and prospects for prevention.

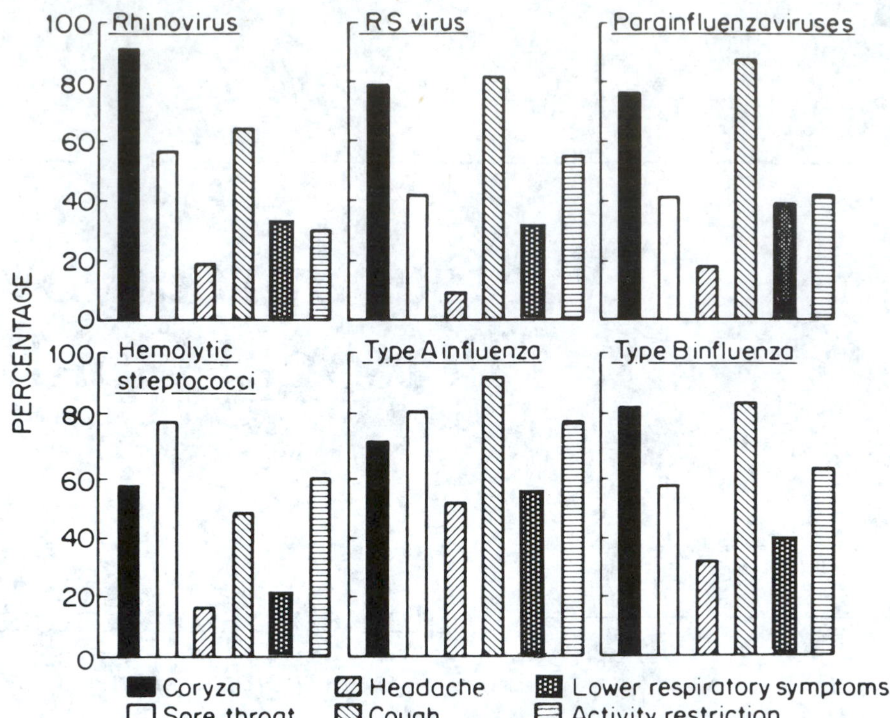

Figure 7-1. Characteristics of illnesses associated with isolation of viruses and hemolytic streptococci; percentage of those infected experiencing five symptoms and activity restriction.

RESPIRATORY SYNCYTIAL VIRUS

Characteristics, Pathogenesis, and Distribution. This virus was isolated originally from chimpanzees and was termed the "chimpanzee coryza agent." When it was associated with disease in humans, it was renamed respiratory syncytial (RS) virus on the basis of the appearance of its cytopathic effect in cell culture. It is a medium-sized (120 to 200 nm), lipid-containing pleomorphic RNA virus and has been classified as a member of the pneumovirus group. The virion possesses spikelike projections, which in similar viruses would be associated with a hemagglutinin. However, RS virus never has been found to hemagglutinate, and identification of the virus and antibody against it must rely on different methods, such as complement fixation, neutralization, and enzyme linked immunosorbent assay (ELISA). The virus can be identified directly by the last technique and by fluorescent antibody methods. Minor antigenic variation among RS viral isolates has been recognized for many years.[3] Monoclonal antibody has permitted separation into two subgroups, generally termed A and B. The significance of these subgroups in terms of cross-protection is unclear.[4]

RS virus is considered the most important agent of respiratory infection among infants and young children because of its capacity to cause life-threatening bronchiolitis and pneumonia. In a number of large cities in different parts of the world, it is possible to determine when RS viral transmission is occurring simply by observing the sharp increase in pediatric admissions for lower respiratory disease.[5] A number of theories have been offered to explain the pathogenesis of the disease. Since all except young children have been infected many times in life by RS virus, mothers always pass RS antibodies transplacentally to their children. RS-associated bronchiolitis and pneumonia are more severe when they occur in the first 6 months of life, when infants usually still have detectable circulating IgG antibodies against RS. Thus, it was postulated that these antibodies, through antigen-antibody complex formation, are involved, at least in part, in the pathogenesis of the disease. The theory was difficult to prove epidemiologically, and it has now largely been discounted, since maternally derived antibody actually appears to be protective when present at sufficient titer.[6,7]

Certain facts about RS illnesses are well documented. The virus is transmitted mainly during the winter and spring, and the duration of this transmission period is longer in large cities than in small communities.[8] Major outbreaks occur in the winter of alternate years. Then, in the next year, a smaller outbreak takes place in the spring.[3,5] Although a small proportion of young children when initially infected become ill enough to be hospitalized or seek medical attention, by age 4 or 5 years, all have antibodies against RS virus, indicating that infection with the agent has occurred. Severe manifestations of the initial infection are more common among residents of densely populated urban areas, probably as a result of crowding and greater likelihood of infection early in life.[9] Severe illnesses are more common in small boys than in girls. Protection is relative, and reinfection with the virus throughout life is common, occurring at least every 5 years in childhood and less frequently thereafter. When reinfection occurs in partially immune adults or older children, it may result in asymptomatic infection that can be detected only serologically or mild illness that does not resemble the severe disease in infants. However, it is these individuals who frequently are responsible for transmitting severe infection to young children in a family group or introducing infection in newborn nurseries.

Prevention and Control. RS virus was given high priority for attempts at prevention by immunization after recognition of its association with severe lower respiratory illness in infants. It was decided first to use a formalinized concentrated cell culture preparation because of the known protective value of inactivated influenza vaccine. Not only did this vaccine not prevent infection when infants and children subsequently were naturally exposed to wild virus, but the disease they experienced was more severe than otherwise would have been expected.[10] The vaccine had stimulated production of high levels of circulating IgG antibodies. A number of theories have been developed to explain this phenomenon, including an antibody response not balanced between the F and G glycoprotein antigens of the virus.

As a result of this experience, efforts at development turned toward a live attenuated vaccine, usually for intranasal inoculation. A live vaccine would be more similar to natural infection, without the danger of inducing a paradoxical antibody response. The intent would be to modify, not necessarily to prevent, the first infection in life so that it would resemble in severity that seen on reinfection. More recently, recombinant technology has been employed to produce preparations containing F and G glycoproteins, those antigens thought to be associated with protection. Work has proceeded with caution, based in part on past adverse experience with inactivated vaccines. Another problem with any kind of vaccine is that the target age group, young infants, may have difficulty in mounting a good antibody response. In view of the importance of RS virus in potentially lethal disease of infants, further evaluation of candidate vaccines is of great importance.

Antiviral therapy is an accepted approach for treatment of at least a portion of hospitalized patients. It has been found that ribavirin will modify the severity of RS viral disease when administered by aerosol. The effect has been most marked in children with preexisting illnesses or disabilities.[11]

PARAINFLUENZAVIRUSES

Characteristics and Pathogenesis. These viruses are members of the paramyxovirus group. The virions contain RNA, and essential lipids are relatively large and pleomorphic, with spike-like projections. Each spike incorporates both the hemagglutinin and neuraminidase enzyme of the virus. There are four different types of parainfluenzaviruses. Their presence in cell culture usually is detected through the hemadsorption technique, the result of viral budding from the cell surface. Type 1 and type 3 viruses originally were detected by hemadsorption, the latter originally called HA (hemadsorption agent) 1 and the former HA 2.[12] Type 2 parainfluenzavirus was first detected by virtue of its cytopathic effect, and it previously was called the croup-associated, or CA, virus. Type 4 viruses were described somewhat later and have been divided into two subtypes, type 4A, originally called M25, and type 4B, originally called 19503. Although it is relatively easy to separate isolates of the parainfluenzaviruses into types, it is difficult to determine serologically the specific virus involved in an illness, other than very early in life during primary infection.

As with RS virus, initial infections with parainfluenzavirus are more likely to produce severe disease than are subsequent reinfections in later years. However, in these initial infections, the different parainfluenzavirus types produce quite distinct syndromes. Both types 1 and 2 are responsible for a large proportion of croup (laryngotracheobronchitis) in the first years of life, type 1 more frequently than type 2. In contrast, type 3 is more likely to produce bronchiolitis and pneumonia in infants.[13] Type 4 viruses normally do not produce severe disease at all and have been associated mainly with mild upper respiratory infection. The pathogenesis of the severe infections with types 1 and 2 and that with type 3 appear to differ. As with RS virus, bronchiolitis seen with type 3 parainfluenzavirus occurs in the first 6 months of life. In contrast, initial infection with types 1 and 2 usually is delayed until at least past the first 4 months of life.

Occurrence of Infection. The seasonality of the different parainfluenzavirus types is not uniform. Type 3 virus is transmitted year around, usually with a late autumn and sometimes a spring peak. Type 2 is transmitted for a limited period in the late autumn into the winter. Parainfluenza type 1 participates with type 3 in the autumn peak of infection. However, two patterns of occurrence of this virus have been observed. In the early 1960s, parainfluenza 1 virus was isolated year around, resembling parainfluenza type 3. In the late 1960s into the 1970s, type 1 virus began to exhibit a different prevalence and, like type 2, was isolated only during a period each year. In fact, for a period, type 1 virus was being seen every other year, and in the alternate years, type 2 virus was being transmitted. It is not clear why the change in viral prevalence occurred, but it has been repeated in recent years.[9,14]

Reinfection of older children and adults with the parainfluenzaviruses is at least as common as with RS virus. When infections were evaluated serologically, it was found that each year 28.6% of individuals were reinfected with one or more of the parainfluenzaviruses. This rate varied from 42.9% in children 5 to 9 years of age to 16.1% in adults. A most important feature of these reinfections is that they serve as a means to introduce the infection into a family group, so that mild or asymptomatic infection in an adult may have as its consequence severe croup or pneumonia in an infant.[14]

Prevention and Control. Vaccines for parainfluenza types 1,2, and 3 are currently under development. Type 4 has not been included because it is involved only with mild sporadic disease. As with RS virus, the aim of vaccine prophylaxis would be to make an initial infection in an infant or small child more like a reinfection. Thus, the intent is not to prevent the infection but rather to modify it. Inactivated vaccines, similar to those produced against influenza, were studied initially. They induced high levels of antibody but neither protected against infection nor made the subsequent disease more severe.[10] There appears to be an essential difference between parainfluenza types 1 and 2 and parainfluenza type 3 in time of occurrence. With the former agents, initial infection is not frequent until after the first 4 to 6 months of life. This observation means that immunization against types 1 and 2 can be delayed, but immunization for type 3, like that for RS, would have to be given to an infant shortly after birth. A variety of methods, including live attenuated and recombinant antigens, are being explored without any major success as yet. The development of immunoprophylaxis is encouraged by evidence that vaccine against the bovine parainfluenza virus, related to type 3 virus, is associated with protection in calves.

RHINOVIRUSES

The Agent and Its Pathogenesis. Although similar to the previously described agents in possessing RNA, the rhinoviruses are different in being small, capsomeric viruses without essential lipid. They are members, along with the enteroviruses, of the picornavirus family. The rhinovirus genus is made up of a very large number of serotypes. The total number of types is unknown but is in excess of 110. However, an isolate can be identified as a rhinovirus by its growth characteristics in cell culture and its acid and ether lability without the necessity of actually typing it. This is of some importance, since sera to most types are not readily available. There is some evidence of cross-reactions among certain types,[15] but protection appears mainly to be type specific, and, thus, sequential infection with different rhinoviruses occurs throughout life. As with most respiratory viruses, antibody is only partially protective against reinfection. The higher the titer of antibody, the greater the likelihood of protection.[16]

Rhinoviruses are the principal etiological agent of common colds in all age groups. There is no evidence that disease caused by initial infection in small children is more severe than that observed later in life. Minor alterations in lung function values can be seen in healthy individuals, but only in persons with altered host defenses, such as those with chronic bronchitis or asthma, is rhinoviral infection associated with symptomatic disease of the lower respiratory tract.[17] The major site of viral replication appears to be in the nasal mucosa, where extrusion of ciliated epithelial cells is observed. The resulting symptoms of sneezing and nasal obstruction are well-known characteristics of the common cold. Secretory IgA antibody, if present in sufficient titer in nasal secretion, protects against infection. In the absence of antibody, a very small dose of infectious virus, about the lowest amount that can be detected by the most sensitive cell culture system, is sufficient to initiate infection. When infection does occur, it is accompanied by disease in approximately 70% of cases.

Distribution of Infection. Rhinoviruses are the most commonly involved viruses in respiratory infections. This relationship holds not only in adults, where other agents such as the parainfluenzaviruses are not frequently isolated, but also in young children, who actually have the highest rhinoviral isolation rates. For this reason, many of the observations made on total respiratory illnesses not of specified etiology apply directly to the rhinoviruses. Infection rates are highest in the younger age groups and fall with increasing age. School and home are important sites for transmission of rhinoviral infection. Rhinoviruses can be isolated year round but peak in frequency in the autumn. After the opening of school, there is typically a sharp increase in respiratory illness in general, which is accompanied by a parallel increase in rhinoviral isolations. This increase is not restricted to one type of rhinovirus, but instead up to 20 different types can be recovered during this period.[18] Transmission in the school clearly is responsible for the mixing of the different types and their subsequent introduction into the home, where secondary cases then occur. Secondary cases are more frequent in more crowded surroundings, and mothers experience more infections than fathers, presumably because of closer contact with their infected children. The mechanisms that have been suggested for rhinoviral transmission are large droplet and indirect contact via autoinoculation. The relative importance of these two mechanisms has been a matter of debate.[19]

The existence of multiple serotypes is a major problem both in describing the epidemiology of the rhinoviruses and in developing strategies for control. Sera must be prepared for each type in order to identify and track occurrence of a strain. Thus, only a limited number of investigations have been carried out on the relative importance of each type. It appears that some may cause more infections than others. There also have been suggestions that new rhinoviral types may be evolving or that old strains never before identified are recycling, but new evidence suggests that this may not be the case.[20]

Protection and Control. An important portion of common colds is rhinoviral in origin, and it is useful to consider prevention of rhinoviral infection as prevention of the common cold. The technology is available for production of vaccines against a single rhinoviral type, and such a vaccine would be protective. However, the multiplicity of different rhinoviral types makes the feasibility of immunoprophylaxis questionable. Certain rhinoviruses are encountered more commonly than others, and there may be more sharing of antigens than previously realized. Both of these factors might make the development of vaccines more attractive.

Rhinoviruses are sensitive to interferon, and it has been shown experimentally that intranasal interferon at relatively low doses can prevent rhinoviral infection. However, this approach has been limited by the occurrence of side effects. Chemoprophylaxis of rhinoviral infections also has been studied, and, although there have been some encouraging results with certain compounds, large-scale trials have not yet demonstrated efficacy and safety. The attractiveness of chemoprophylaxis is that a suitable compound ideally would be effective against many or all rhinoviral types.

Vitamin C has been used for common cold prophylaxis, and, as noted above, most common colds are rhinoviral in origin. The data from controlled trials to date have not been conclusive, especially in those involving viral isolation.[21] There remains the possibility of environmental control. When schoolchildren have a cold, it is common sense to keep them at home, but whether doing so limits the transmission to other children is debatable. It is also common sense for adults to absent themselves from work when they have a cold. Again, the value of thus limiting contact in controlling the spread of infection is uncertain.

CORONAVIRUSES

The Virus and Occurrence of Disease. The coronaviruses are another group of RNA-containing agents heavily involved in the etiology of respiratory infections. The name of the group was adopted to describe the typical fringelike projection seen on electron microscopy. This appearance clearly distinguishes them from the paramyxoviruses with which they were initially confused because both are approximately of the same size and possess essential lipid. Coronaviruses infect a number of domestic animals, and the entire group originally was designated the infectious bronchitis-like viruses, named after the prototype coronavirus of chicken.

The greatest problem with the human viruses is that, aside from one strain, 229E, they cannot be isolated in cell culture. One additional strain, OC43, although originally isolated in organ culture, has been adapted to growth in a number of cell systems.[22,23] The majority of the human strains can be isolated and propagated in human embryonic tracheal organ culture, with subsequent visualization of the virus on electron microscopy. This fact has hampered the determination of the number of types of coronaviruses, their behavior, and relative importance in human infections. Much of the work on epidemiology of the agents has been carried out by serological studies using 229E and OC43 as antigens. Molecular studies of the viruses themselves generally have used the animal agents.

The animal coronaviruses are similar to the human strains from a virological standpoint and cause a variety of disease syndromes, including hepatitis, gastroenteritis, and encephalitis. In contrast, the human agents have as yet not been associated convincingly with any illnesses except those involving the respiratory tract. The disease is generally similar to that produced by the rhinoviruses, with more profuse nasal discharge and somewhat less frequent sore throat. The mean duration of coronaviral colds is shorter, 6 1/2 days, than that seen with rhinoviruses, 9 1/2 days. There is no clear evidence that coronaviruses are involved in lower respiratory tract infection in infants and young children. There have been reports of identification of the virus in association with a few instances of lower respiratory diseases in both hospitalized children and military recruits, but these associations should be viewed as tentative. Infection is associated with production of clinical disease in approximately 50% of cases.

All information on the behavior of coronaviruses in human populations is based on serological studies using two strains, OC43 and 229E. Occurrence of infection by age is similar to that seen with the other respiratory agents, with the highest rates of infection in children, decreasing in frequency with increasing age. Reinfection in the face of preexisting antibody has been demonstrated. In contrast to the rhinoviruses, a single coronavirus type is capable of producing outbreaks of infection in a community over a limited period of time, which suggests that coronaviruses may be transmitted by the small droplet or airborne route. The principal season of such transmission is late winter and early spring, at the time when rhinoviral isolation rates decrease but respiratory illnesses in general still are occurring at relatively high frequency. A particular coronaviral type exhibits a cyclical pattern of occurrence. The 229E virus reappears every 2 to 3 years, but with OC43, although cycling does occur, its periodicity is difficult to define. This problem is related to the existence of other, as yet not properly studied, coronaviruses that are serologically related to OC43. Such viruses have been identified in investigations using organ culture.[24] The cycling phenomenon and the involvement of coronaviruses in outbreaks have led to the conclusion that, as compared to the rhinoviruses, there are a relatively limited number of coronaviral serotypes.

Prevention and Control. It is premature to think in terms of prevention or control of coronaviral infections. The initial need is not control but rather the development of techniques for isolation and cultivation of the coronaviruses so that more can be determined on the epidemiological behavior. Data now suggest that ELISA techniques might be used for recognition of these noncultivable viruses.[25] Until this is accomplished, it is impossible to plan for vaccine or chemoprophylaxis. From animal data, it appears that vaccine can be protective.

ADENOVIRUSES

Characteristics and Resultant Diseases. Unlike all previously described viruses, the adenoviruses contain DNA, which is double stranded. The size of the virion is 60 to 90 nm, and it is capsomeric in structure. Adenoviruses are much more stable to acid pH and adverse environmental conditions, a fact that has important implications for transmission patterns. They can be isolated easily in a number of cell systems, and infection can be identified serologically using a common antigen that all share. The adenoviruses are divided into more than 40 types, which can be grouped together by virtue of the species of red cells that they hemagglutinate and nucleic acid homology. Adenoviruses of different types behave epidemiologically in very different fashions, so that such identification is of great importance, especially when outbreaks are being investigated. Certain adenoviral types cause enteric, not respiratory, disease and are described below.

The clinical types of respiratory illness produced by adenoviruses are summarized in Table 7–1. Several of the lower numbered types produce common respiratory disease in family settings. It has been estimated that about 5% of all respiratory disease occurring under age 5 can be attributed to adenoviruses. No clear syndromes, such as croup or bronchiolitis, are associated in this situation with adenoviruses, but a portion of these infections do involve the lower respiratory tract, with infrequent production of pneumonia.[26] All adenoviruses can infect the intestinal as well as the respiratory tract and may be shed in the stool for prolonged periods. Fecal-oral transmission often is of considerable importance in acquisition of infection by young children. Secondary spread in this situation can take longer than would be expected if only respiratory transmission were involved.[27] Few infections can be documented during the first 6 months of life, indicating that passively acquired maternal antibody exerts a protective effect. Initial infection is acquired during the first years of life, especially in crowded situations and in East Asia, and is associated half of the time with symptomatic disease.

TABLE 7–1. CHARACTERISTICS OF ADENOVIRUS-ASSOCIATED DISEASE

Disease	Principal Types Involved	Characteristics
Common respiratory disease	1, 2, 5, 3, 6	Endemic infections of childhood
Acute respiratory disease	4, 7, 21, 14, 3	Febrile disease of military recruits
Epidemic keratoconjunctivitis	8	"Shipyard eye," iatrogenic spread
Pharyngoconjunctival fever	3, 7	Epidemic spread; may involve water
Pneumonia	7, 12	Unusual

Acute respiratory disease (ARD) is an entity confined to military recruits in many nations of the world. In North American forces, it has been an important cause of morbidity, second only to influenza. Clinical characteristics include fever, sore throat, cough, headache, and chest pain. Pulmonary infiltrates in chest x-ray have been found in approximately 10% of those with typical illness. Deaths from the syndrome have been rare, but they do occur.[28] Transmission is by the respiratory route. Of great concern to the military is the high attack rate over a short period of time and the incapacity that results.

Epidemic keratoconjunctivitis (EKC) was described during World War II in Hawaii and on both coasts of the U.S. mainland.[29] Outbreaks have since been observed in families, especially in East Asia and in crowded settings. In the United States, iatrogenic spread also has occurred, usually involving improperly sterilized tonometers in ophthalmologists' offices. This suggests that direct inoculation of the agent into the eye is the important route of transmission. Typically, clinical keratitis is produced, and the conjunctivitis may be follicular.

The clinical features of pharyngoconjunctival fever are incorporated into the name of the syndrome. It was initially described in 1955 in association with adenovirus type 3.[30] It may occur in sporadic or in epidemic form in children and their families. However, it is most dramatically associated with common source outbreaks involving swimming pools and small lakes. Children directly exposed to the water usually exhibit the most severe disease. Secondary spread to contacts does occur, generally resulting in milder illness. The fact that common source outbreaks are possible with the adenoviruses is a good indication of their relative stability.

Prevention and Control. Unlike the previously described viruses, there is clear evidence that vaccines can protect against adenoviral infection. However vaccine development and use have been limited to situations in which the illness produced is viewed as being of particular importance. Military recruits are an identifiable population at high risk of ARD, a disease of high morbidity. Thus, it was decided early to be worthy of prevention. Initial inactivated vaccines against types 4 and 7 were used extensively and were protective. However, for reasons not related to efficacy, their use was discontinued, and ARD returned to recruit camps. Subsequently, live preparations of types 4 and 7 have been administered orally in enteric-coated capsules. The route of inoculation is possible in view of the ability of adenovirus to multiply in the intestinal tract.[31] This unusual approach has again been successful in prevention of ARD.

A number of candidate vaccines have been developed against the adenoviral types involved in common respiratory disease of children, but there is some question as to the need for these preparations because of the low frequency of illness of significant severity. Prevention of EKC in opthalmologists' offices can be accomplished easily by proper sterilization of equipment. Pharyngoconjunctival fever can be prevented by proper chlorination of pools and monitoring of other places used for swimming. Bacteriological testing can be used as an indirect indication of the safety of water.

MYCOPLASMA PNEUMONIAE

This agent and *Chlamydia pneumoniae,* although not viruses, are included in a discussion of acute respiratory disease because both can produce an undifferentiated upper respiratory tract illness and lower respiratory illness previously called "viral pneumonia." As a mycoplasma, *M. pneumoniae* can be grown in artificial media, but for efficient isolation, there are rather rigid cultural requirements. In addition, *M. pneumoniae* is susceptible to a number of antibiotics that sometimes are incorporated into media used for collecting specimens for viral isolation. Needless to say, these must be omitted.[32]

Mycoplasma pneumoniae is the agent principally responsible for primary atypical pneumonia (PAP). The responsible pathogen formerly was called Eaton agent and was thought to be a virus.[33] The clinical description of the pneumonic disease has remained unchanged. Typically, there is abrupt onset and a protracted course. Symptoms of fever, cough, headache, chills, and malaise may be present for 5 days before x-ray evidence of pneumonitis develops. The nonspecific cold agglutinin test, when positive in a person with pneumonic disease, correlates well with laboratory confirmation of true *M. pneumoniae* infection. However, in only half of cases of PAP documented to be of mycoplasmal etiology is the cold agglutinin test positive. As the laboratory tests for identification of the agent became available, it was quickly realized that, as with other respiratory pathogens, there was a wide spectrum of clinical manifestations associated with *M. pneumoniae* infection. This varies from asymptomatic infection through a common coldlike syndrome to lower respiratory illness. Reinfection with the agent also was identified, and the question of the role of antibody in the pathogenesis of the condition was investigated.

The distinct patterns of behavior of *M. pneumoniae* can be identified, that observed in families and the community and that seen in the military and in closed populations. Infections move slowly through families because, unlike the situation with most other respiratory pathogens, the incubation period of *M. pneumoniae* infection is relatively long, from 14 to 21 days. By seroepidemiology, the age groups most frequently involved are children and adolescents, indicating again the importance of school-age children in introducing infections to the family. Most of the infections seen in the family are mild, but it has been estimated that pneumonitis of some degree occurs in approximately 10% of infections. *M. pneumoniae* does not exhibit any clear seasonality, but there is, at least in certain geographic areas of the United States, cyclical waxing and waning of prevalence. In the eastern and central portions of the country, periods of near absence of the agent have been observed, but in the Seattle area, such a pattern has not been seen.[34]

In the military, *M. pneumoniae* has been involved in periodic outbreaks of illness with a relatively high attack rate. Such outbreaks were carefully documented at Camp Lejeune, North Carolina, in the 1960s. Often, they occurred at the same time as outbreaks of ARD caused by adenoviruses, and it was difficult to differentiate between them clinically. Outbreaks have been documented in other military situations and in civilian institutions.[35] The hypothesis has been advanced that crowding is responsible for the different frequency of transmission from that seen in families.

Prevention and Control. An inactivated vaccine was developed against *M. pneumoniae* primarily for use in the military, where the agent may be a serious problem. It was shown to protect, but the protective efficacy was approximately 50%, which limited its practical usefulness.[36] Because of the nature of disease in the civilian population, no serious efforts at prevention have been attempted. As a bacterium, *M. pneumoniae* is susceptible to certain broad-spectrum antibiotics. The principal drugs in use, erythromycin and tetracycline, are quite effective in speeding recovery from this usually protracted illness. Once the drug is stopped, however, it is common for the agent to return and persist in the now asymptomatic individual. Thus, drug therapy has only limited usefulness in control of further transmission.[37]

CHLAMYDIA PNEUMONIAE

Chlamydia pneumoniae strain TWAR can now be considered an important cause of infections similar in general characteristics to those produced by *Mycoplasma pneumoniae.* The species designation is new, and the strain designation comes from the combined laboratory identification numbers of two original isolates, one of which was recovered in Taiwan in 1965.[38] The exact nature of the organism and its relation to disease remained in question for so long because of the problem of cross-reaction with other chlamydia, resolved only with the availability of monoclonal antibodies. It can be grown in cell culture. The most satisfactory line has been found to be HL cells, by chance also used to identify RS virus. The organisms are identified by the fluorescent antibody technique. Most epidemiological studies have relied on serological tests, and for this purpose, the microimmunofluorescent method is most sensitive and specific. This technique allows recognition of two kinds of antibody response, one associated with primary infection and the second with reinfection.

Knowledge of the behavior of *C. pneumoniae* strain TWAR in populations is not complete because of its relatively recent characterization. It clearly is an important cause of pneumonia, accounting for 6% to 10% of those hospitalized with the diagnosis. The characteristics of these illnesses do not allow recognition of the etiological agent on clinical grounds, since so much overlap in symptoms exists. There are insufficient data to determine the organism's importance in milder illness in the community, although it appears to be involved in producing bronchitis and pharyngitis. Asymptomatic or nonpneumonic infection must be common, since by age 20, half of the population can be shown to have acquired antibodies.[39]

The transmission is clearly person to person, not involving birds (as with *Chlamydia psittaci,* a much less common cause of pneumonia) or other animal reservoirs. No seasonality has been demonstrated, but there may be cycling over a period of years. Outbreaks among military recruits have been documented in Finland, lasting over periods of months.[40]

Prevention and Control. No vaccines are available for this agent, nor are any likely to be developed in the near future. Work on prevention of diseases caused by other chlamydia, however, ultimately may have implications for *C. pneumoniae.* No controlled trials of treatment have been carried out, but as with other chlamydial infections, antibiotics are useful in therapy. Tetracycline and erythromycin are the drugs of choice, and therapy must be at high dosage and maintained for up to 2 weeks.

Viral Hepatitis

Harold S. Margolis

The existence of hepatitis as an infectious entity has been recognized for many centuries, and two major forms were characterized by their means of transmission. Infectious hepatitis produced large epidemics in various settings, was transmitted by the fecal-oral route and by person to person contact, and probably represented both hepatitis A and enterically transmitted non-A, non-B hepatitis (hepatitis E). The inoculation or injection of materials produced from human lymph or serum produced outbreaks of hepatitis due to bloodborne transmission and probably included both hepatitis B and parenterally transmitted non-A, non-B hepatitis.

Human volunteer studies conducted in the mid-1940s and early 1950s firmly established the viral etiology of hepatitis, the routes of transmission of the two major types, and the specificity of the immunity induced by each infection. Studies conducted by Krugman and colleagues[1] showed that short incubation period hepatitis (31 to 38 days) could be transmitted either orally or parenterally using a serum pool (MS-1) collected before the onset of illness. A second serum pool (MS-2) obtained from the same child following a second episode of hepatitis was shown to transmit disease parenterally only after a longer incubation period (41 to 83 days). Subsequently, MS-1 hepatitis was shown to be caused by hepatitis A virus (HAV) and MS-2 hepatitis by hepatitis B virus (HBV).

In 1965, studies of isoantibodies by Blumberg and associates led to the discovery of Australia antigen, which was shown to be the surface antigen of HBV.[2] Characterization of HBV led rapidly to the development of diagnostic tests, the routine screening of blood for hepatitis B surface antigen (HBsAg) and the virtual elimination of this form of posttransfusion hepatitis, and the development of hepatitis B vaccines. In 1973, HAV was identified in the stools of volunteers inoculated with MS-1 and in the stools of patients involved in a foodborne outbreak of hepatitis.[3,4] This led to the development of serological tests that differentiated acute HAV infection from past infection, propagation of HAV in cell culture, and the development of prototype vaccines.

In 1977, Rizzetto and colleagues described second episodes of hepatitis in patients chronically infected with HBV and a new antigen detectable in patients with chronic HBV liver disease.[5] Studies showed that this form of hepatitis (hepatitis delta) could be transmitted only in the presence of HBV infection and that the hepatitis delta virus (HDV) was defective and required HBsAg to produce infection.[6]

The availability of sensitive and specific tests for both HAV and HBV infection and the occurrence of posttransfusion hepatitis in spite of routine testing for HBsAg led to the identification of another bloodborne type of hepatitis termed non-A, non-B (NANB) hepatitis.[7] Subsequent studies showed that parenterally transmitted NANB (PT-NANB) hepatitis also occurred outside the transfusion setting.[8] Molecular cloning techniques were required to identify hepatitis C virus (HCV), which appears to be the major cause of PT-NANB hepatitis.[9] The ability to make the serological diagnosis of acute HAV infection also led to identification of a form of NANB hepatitis that produced large epidemics and was transmitted by the fecal-oral route.[10] This was termed enterically transmitted NANB (ET-NANB) hepatitis, and the causative virus was identified in the stools of patients but was not characterized further until it was cloned and sequenced.[11]

Each of the major agents of viral hepatitis belongs to a different viral class. Their only common characteristic is that they are hepatotropic. The enterically transmitted agents (HAV and HEV) produce acute, self-limited infections, and the bloodborne agents (HBV, HDV, and HCV) have the ability to produce persistent infections and chronic liver disease.

HEPATITIS A

Etiological Agent. HAV is a small (27 nm), nonenveloped, single-stranded, positive sense RNA virus whose genomic organization and replication scheme are similar to poliovirus and other members of the family Picornaviridae. HAV is more heat stable than other picornaviruses, retains its infectivity in feces for at least 2 weeks, is resistant to pH 3, and remains viable for many years at −20° C. It is completely inactivated by formalin or heating at 100° C for 5 minutes but is somewhat more resistant to inactivation by hypochlorite than are enteroviruses and is only partially inactivated at 60° C for 1 hour.[11]

There is a single serotype, but significant genomic heterogeneity exists in the region coding for the viral capsid, and this has been used to define strains that are geographically distinct.[12] Besides humans, the host range of HAV includes several species of nonhuman primates (marmosets and chimpanzees), as shown by experimental infections, and several genetically distinct strains of HAV have been identified in both old and new world monkeys.[13] It is not known whether the viruses isolated from monkeys can infect humans, but it is doubtful that such reservoirs are of importance in human infections.

Primary cell culture of HAV has been difficult because of the very long adaptation period (27 to 33 days) and lack of a cytopathic effect. HAV has now been adapted to growth in a number of cell lines, and rapidly replicating strains have been used for development of both attenuated and inactivated vaccines.[14]

Clinical Illness, Pathogenesis, and Immune Response. The manifestations of HAV infection include age-dependent expression of clinical illness, low rates of fulminant disease, and absence of chronic disease. Children under age 6 generally have mild, nonspecific symptoms that include nausea and vomiting, malaise, diarrhea, fever, and dark urine. Jaundice is uncommon in this age group, being present in less than 5% of children under age 3 and in 10% of those age 4 to 6 years.[15] Among adolescents and adults infected with HAV, most develop the classic symptoms of malaise, nausea and vomiting, and loss of appetite, and 50% to 90% have dark urine or jaundice or both.

Clinical symptoms due to hepatitis A are indistinguishable from those due to other types of viral hepatitis and should not be used to establish an etiological diagnosis. Fulminant hepatitis is infrequent, and the risk of this outcome among clinical cases is between 0.1% and 0.5%.[16] The highest case fatality ratio is in persons over age 40 years (1.3% to 2.2%) and often is associated with other forms of chronic liver disease. There is no evidence that HAV causes either chronic disease or persistent infection, although about 15% to 20% of infected persons may have a relapse of illness.[17]

The pathogenetic events that occur during the course of infection have been determined through studies in nonhuman primates and from naturally acquired infection in humans. The incubation period for HAV infection has ranged from 14 to 45 days, with a median of 28 days.[11] Virus is found in liver cells before appearing in feces and persists in the liver throughout the period of liver enzyme elevations. HAV is excreted in the feces and is present in high quantity from 1 to 2 weeks before the onset of clinical illness. It begins to decrease at the time symptoms appear and, in most persons (66%), is not detectable by the first week after the onset of clinical illness. However, children may excrete virus for longer periods than adults.[18] Viremia occurs late in the incubation period and during early clinical illness.[1] Available data suggest that the pathogenesis of liver injury is immune mediated rather than due to direct cytotoxicity and that it probably involves cell-mediated immune responses. A specific IgM immune response to HAV develops before the onset of clinical illness, and neutralizing IgG antibodies usually are detectable at or before the onset of illness. The specific antibody response is accompanied by a nonspecific rise in serum IgM.

Diagnosis. Acute HAV infection can be diagnosed by detecting IgM anti-HAV using commercially available solid-phase immunoassays. This antibody response usually is detectable 1 week before the onset of symptoms and remains detectable for 3 to 6 months after infection. Previous HAV infection can be detected by the presence of IgG anti-HAV, which probably persists for life. HAV can be detected in feces by a number of methods, including immune electron microscopy, solid-phase enzyme immunoassay, and nucleic acid hybridization, but these methods are not used routinely.

Epidemiology. Hepatitis A is an important cause of illness throughout the world. The endemicity of infection is directly related to hygienic standards and inversely related to socioeconomic conditions. In the majority of developing countries, including most of Africa, South and Central America, and Asia, almost all adults and older children have been infected with HAV, usually by age 10 years.[19] In more advanced developing countries, such as Greece, Taiwan, and parts of China, improved sanitation has reduced the endemic rate of infection significantly. In these countries, a significant decrease in the prevalence of HAV infection has occurred among children, and the greatest increase in infection is among young adults. However, the potential for outbreaks remains as long as HAV is present in food sources or in the environment. The effect of these shifts in HAV infection patterns was observed recently in Shanghai, China, where 300,000 young adults became ill with hepatitis A due to the consumption of contaminated shellfish that were not cooked adequately.[20]

In Europe and the United States, the prevalence of infection in adults varies from 30% to 70% but is less than 10% in young children. In the United States, low socioeconomic status has been associated with higher prevalence of infection, and certain populations, such as American Natives, Alaskan Natives, and Hispanics, have been shown to have high rates of infection.[21] A significant increase in the incidence of hepatitis A has occurred in the United States since 1986, and an epidemic cycle similar to those previously observed may be developing (Fig. 7-2). Over the last 3 decades, the predominant age groups have changed from 5 to 14 years in the 1961 epidemic to 15 to 24 years in the 1971 epidemic to 20 to 29 years recently. Currently, about 60% of cases occur in young adults age 15 to 39 years, and 25% occur in children under age 15 years.[16] Within the national pattern, community-wide outbreaks affecting primarily lower socioeconomic classes remain common and occur in 5- to 10-year cycles.[22]

The most important factors for acquiring hepatitis A in the United States include contact with a recognized case (30% of cases), enrollment or contact with children in day care centers (12% of cases), drug abuse (12%), and travel to developing countries (5%). Fewer than 10% of cases are associated with food or waterborne outbreaks, and in about 50% of cases, a source cannot be identified. Susceptible household contacts have about a 10% risk of acquiring disease from a family member with acute illness. Hepatitis A outbreaks in centers enrolling children in diapers involve transmission not only among young children but also to adult contacts, who make up 70% to 80% of recognized cases. Contact with children less than 5 years of age has emerged as a risk factor in recent community-wide outbreaks of hepatitis A, suggesting that these patients may have acquired their infections from asymptomatically infected young children.

Common source outbreaks due to contaminated water, shellfish, and food continue to play a role in disease transmission. Implicated foods usually are eaten raw and have been handled extensively or have been handled after being cooked. These include salads, sandwiches, and glazed or iced pastries. Shellfish-associated outbreaks usually are associated with eating raw or partially cooked clams, mussels, or oysters harvested from sewage-contaminated water. Fruits or vegetables that are normally eaten raw and that have been contaminated during picking or packing have accounted for some outbreaks.[23,24]

Hepatitis A represents a rare cause of posttransfusion hepatitis, although a number of outbreaks have been recognized in recent years. Infection in the transfused patient usually is not recognized, and transmission to hospital staff, and rarely to other patients and their contacts, has involved up to 50 clinical cases. The largest outbreaks have occurred in neonatal intensive care units, with silent transmission among the infants but high attack rates among hospital staff and patients.[25]

Control and Prevention. Since transmission of HAV is associated primarily with close personal contact and fecal contami-

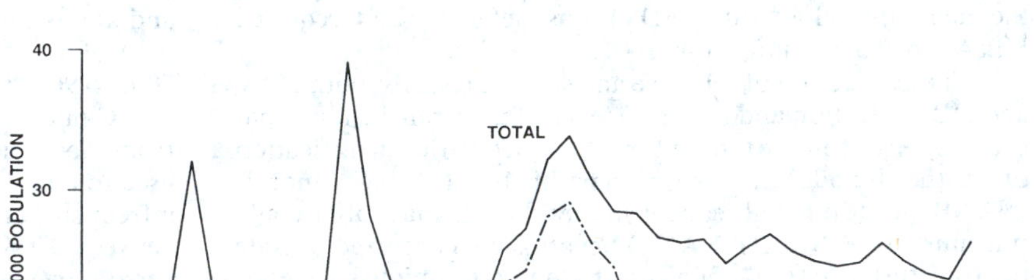

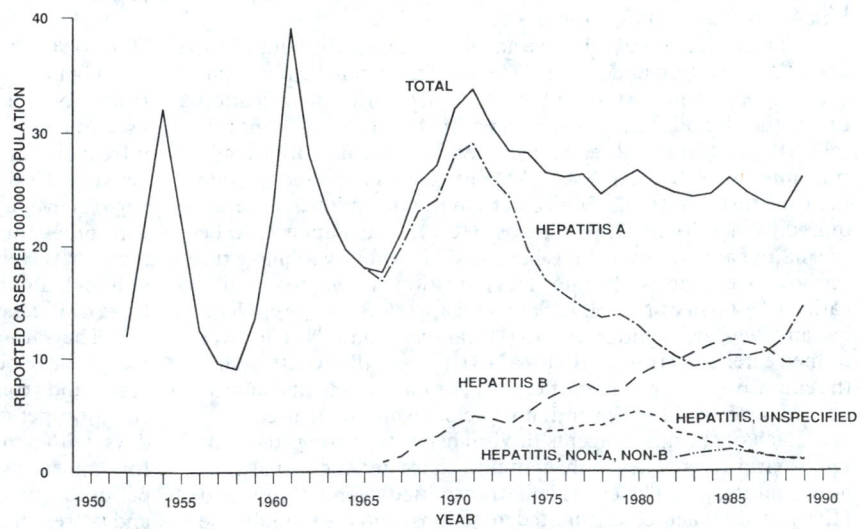

Figure 7-2. Incidence of viral hepatitis in the United States, 1952–1989.

nation of food or water, improved personal hygiene and environmental sanitation have been the basis for control. Improved sanitation in developed countries is presumed to have caused the decrease in disease frequency. However, these improvements in less developed countries would be expected to shift infection to older age groups and result in increases in clinical disease rates, since the clinical syndrome is not specific in infants and young children.

Numerous studies have confirmed that human immunoglobulin that contains detectable anti-HAV (IG, also immune serum globulin, ISG) is 75% to 85% effective in preventing symptomatic hepatitis A infection if given before exposure or within 2 weeks after exposure to HAV.[26] The nature of protection is not fully documented but probably involves prevention of infection if given before exposure and modification of symptoms when given after exposure. IG currently is recommended for postexposure prophylaxis for household and sexual contacts of acute cases, for children and staff exposed in day care settings, and for institutions for the mentally disabled. Preexposure prophylaxis is recommended for persons traveling to endemic areas.[26]

Hepatitis A vaccines that could provide long-term protection are under evaluation. Inactivated vaccines obtained from cell culture-propagated virus have been developed and have been shown to be immunogenic in marmosets and chimpanzees and to protect against challenge with wild-type virus. Immunogenicity trials have shown rapid induction of anti-HAV activity after two doses of vaccine.[14] Clinical trials to evaluate the protective efficacy of these vaccines are now underway.

Candidate live attenuated HAV vaccines have been developed through serial passage of HAV in cell culture and have been shown not to produce disease in marmosets and chimpanzees.[14] Several such strains have been tested in humans and have induced antibody to HAV. Further evaluation will determine whether a vaccine to induce long-term protection against hepatitis A will become available. Use of hepatitis A vaccines might be targeted initially at high-risk groups, including children in day care centers, residents of institutions for the mentally retarded, overseas travelers to developing areas, homosexual men, and other groups, such as military populations and food handlers. General vaccination in childhood might be considered if an inexpensive vaccine offering long-term protection is developed.

HEPATITIS B

Etiological Agent. Hepatitis B virus is a member of the family Hepadnaviridae, which includes viruses infecting woodchucks, ducks, ground squirrels, and herons. The genome consists of a small circular DNA that is partly single stranded and has a viral coded DNA polymerase and a replication mechanism that is retroviral in nature.[27] The primary site of replication is the liver, and all cause persistent infection, have a potential for integration into host cells, and are oncogenic. The hepatitis B surface antigen (HBsAg), which is the coat of HBV, exists both associated with the complete virion and independently and circulates as 22 nm spheres and tubules. HBV has been shown to retain infectivity for at least 1 month when stored at either room temperature or frozen. Infectivity is destroyed at 90° C after 1 hour.[28]

The only natural host for HBV appears to be humans. Propagation of HBV in cell culture generally has been unsuccessful, although HBV is easily purified from infected hosts and has been characterized extensively. A number of antigen and antibody systems have been characterized and have been used to identify various stages of infection (Table 7–2). HBsAg is the most useful marker of viral presence, and subtypes of HBsAg have been used in epidemiological studies to show patterns of disease transmission.[29]

TABLE 7–2. HEPATITIS B VIRUS TERMINOLOGY

HBV	Hepatitis B virus: a 42-nm double-shelled virus, originally known as the Dane particle
HBsAg	Hepatitis B surface antigen: the hepatitis B antigen found on the surface of the virus and on the accompanying unattached spherical (22 nm) and tubular particles
HBcAg	Hepatitis B core antigen: the hepatitis B antigen found within the core of the virus
HBeAg	The e antigen that is closely associated with hepatitis B infection
anti-HBs	Antibody to hepatitis B surface antigen
anti-HBc	Antibody to hepatitis B core antigen
anti-HBe	Antibody to the e antigen

Clinical Illness, Pathogenesis, and Immune Response. HBV infection can be asymptomatic, cause clinically evident hepatitis, result in fulminant hepatitis and death, or become persistent. Acute hepatitis B cannot be differentiated from other viral causes of hepatitis on the basis of signs or symptoms, and the diagnosis can only be made by serological testing. The clinical onset of hepatitis B usually is insidious, with malaise, weakness, and anorexia being the most common findings. Myalgia and arthralgia without other clinical signs have been described in 10% to 30% of patients, and in one third of these patients, an urticarial or maculopapular rash appears with joint symptoms. Jaundice develops in 20% to 30% of infected individuals and may persist for several weeks. Liver enzyme elevations usually occur before the onset of jaundice.

HBsAg becomes detectable 1 to 2 months before the onset of clinical symptoms and is soon followed by the appearance of both IgM anti-HBc and anti-HBc. In those infections that resolve, HBsAg will disappear, and anti-HBs then becomes detectable. During late convalescence, a window phase may occur during which neither HBsAg or anti-HBs is detectable, but IgM anti-HBc will remain positive. HBeAg is present during acute infection and disappears as the infection resolves. In persons who completely resolve their HBV infection, anti-HBs and anti-HBc persist as evidence of the previous infection. Among individuals in whom HBV infection persists, both HBsAg and anti-HBc remain detectable indefinitely. HBeAg initially will be detectable in all individuals, but each year, approximately 10% of chronic carriers will lose HBeAg.[30] In a small number of individuals (2% to 3%), HBsAg and anti-HBs may cocirculate. A modest proportion of chronic HBV carriers (1% to 2% per year) may naturally lose HBsAg and resolve infection.

HBV must gain access to the circulation by direct inoculation, breaks in the skin, or passage through mucous membranes. Primary replication occurs in hepatocytes, and although HBsAg has been detected in other tissues, there is little evidence to suggest replication. The number of cells affected during the acute phase of infection is variable, and during persistent infection, the number of affected cells can vary from 1% to 100%.

Hepatocellular injury during HBV infection appears to be immune mediated, and clinical studies have suggested a role for cytotoxic T cells. Extrahepatic manifestations of infection (arthritis, urticaria) are immune mediated and are attributable to immune complex formation. Vasculitis and glomerulonephritis also have been associated with chronic HBV infection. The mechanisms associated with the establishment of viral persistence in HBV infection are not known. However, this phenomenon is strongly age related. Infants infected with HBV at birth have a 90% chance of becoming chronic carriers. This decreases to approximately 30% at age 5 years and 6% to 10% in older children and adults. Persistent infection usually results in chronic active hepatitis and cirrhosis. The mechanisms that initiate these inflammatory sequelae are not known. However, HBeAg, HBV-DNA, and HBcAg are present more often in individuals with chronic active hepatitis and chronic persistent hepatitis than in asymptomatic chronic carriers. Thus, it appears that active replication of the virus and its circulation initiate the ongoing chronic inflammatory response. The association of primary hepatocellular carcinoma (PHC) with chronic HBV infection is well established in both demographic and prospective studies.[31] HBV-DNA has been found in tissue of tumor cells, although not all PHC patients have active HBV infection. The frequent association of PHC in woodchucks and Pekin ducks chronically infected with their species-specific hepadnavirus has provided additional evidence that these hepadnaviruses may be etiological factors in tumor formation.

Diagnosis. Currently, solid-phase radioimmunoassay and enzyme immunoassay are the most widely used methods to detect HBsAg. A serum sample positive for HBsAg indicates the presence of HBV infection, but it does not fully determine the stage of the disease. An individual is classified as a chronic carrier of HBV if HBsAg remains positive for longer than 6 months. Although all HBsAg-positive persons should be considered potentially infectious, the relative degree of infectivity can be assessed by the presence of HBeAg or HBV-DNA. Anti-HBs testing is used to determine the immune status of an individual to determine appropriate prophylactic therapy following HBV exposure or in follow-up after hepatitis B vaccination. Specific antibodies to hepatitis B core antigen (anti-HBc) develop during acute infection, persist in persons after infection, and are present in all individuals with chronic HBV infection. IgM anti-HBc can be used in the differential diagnosis of acute versus chronic hepatitis B, as well as for diagnosing acute NANB hepatitis in those individuals with chronic HBV infection. IgM anti-HBc becomes detectable almost coincident with the appearance of HBsAg during acute HBV infection and persists for 2 to 6 months. It is present also during that period of resolving clinical illness, the window phase. In a small proportion of cases of chronic HBV infection, IgM anti-HBc remains elevated but at relatively low titers. Most of the commercially available diagnostic tests are configured in such a way as to minimize the likelihood of a positive result in this situation.[32]

Epidemiology. The endemicity of HBV infection throughout the world varies greatly[33] (Fig. 7-3). Endemicity is considered high in those areas of the world where the prevalence of HBsAg is ≥8% and where 70% to 90% of the population have serological evidence of previous infection. In these areas, perinatal and early childhood HBV infection account for the high rates of chronic infection and the high rates of PHC found in these countries. In most developed parts of the world, the prevalence of HBV infection is low, with HBsAg chronic carrier rates of less than 1% (Fig. 7-3). In these areas, most infections occur among adults, and populations at high risk of infection usually can be identified. These include homosexual men, intravenous drug abusers, persons with multiple heterosexual partners, heterosexual contacts of cases or carriers, health care workers, residents of institutions for the developmentally disabled, and chronically transfused patients. Within these areas of low endemicity, however, the prevalence of infection can vary widely. For example, within North America, Eskimo populations have been shown to have high rates of infection (Fig. 7-3), and first generation immigrant populations continue to transmit HBV infection at high rates.[34] In areas with intermediate endemicity of infection, transmission in infancy, childhood, and adulthood maintains the high rates of infection.

The principal modes of HBV transmission are shown in Table 7-3. Direct transmission via blood products has been essentially eliminated through the use of donor screening except in areas where this is not done routinely. In developed countries, transmission with inadequately sterilized medical instruments

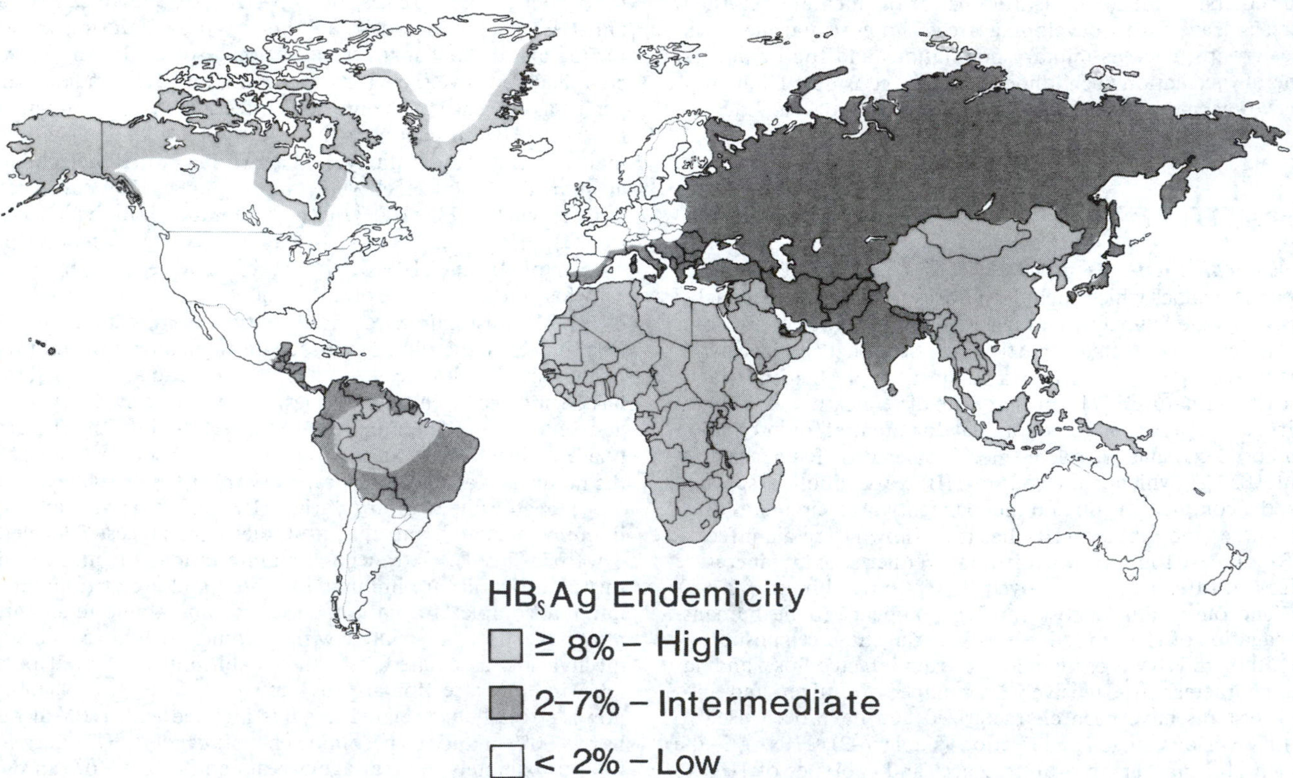

Figure 7-3. Worldwide pattern of incidence of chronic hepatitis B infection. *[Adapted from Maynard et al.[33]]*

TABLE 7-3. PRINCIPAL MODES OF HEPATITIS B VIRUS TRANSMISSION

Direct percutaneous inoculation by needle contaminated with serum or plasma, or transfusion of infective blood or blood products
Nonneedle percutaneous transfer of infective serum or plasma
Introduction of infective serum or plasma onto mucosal surfaces
Introduction of infective secretions other than serum or plasma onto mucosal surfaces
Indirect transfer of infective serum or plasma via vectors or inanimate environmental surfaces

has not been a significant mode of transmission, although occasional outbreaks have occurred through the contamination of multidose vials or from the improper use of multiple-use devices. Transmission from contaminated needles remains a problem in developing countries because of the lack of disposable supplies or the lack of means of sterilization. Sharing of needles among intravenous drug abusers accounts for a large proportion of cases in the United States.

One of the most effective routes of transmission is from infected mothers to newborns at the time of birth.[35] In utero infection is rarely observed, and the presumed mechanism of perinatal transmission is mucous membrane penetration by HBV at the time of delivery. HBV in semen and vaginal secretions provides a mechanism for transmission through both heterosexual and homosexual activity. Person to person spread can occur in settings involving interpersonal contact over a long period of time, such as from mother to infant, between siblings, and between adults. The precise mechanisms of transmission are unknown, but it is presumed that transmission occurs when secretions, such as blood or possible saliva, contaminate a nonintact skin barrier or repeatedly contact mucous membranes. HBsAg contamination of surfaces has been demonstrated in homes of HBV chronic carriers.[36]

Epidemics of hepatitis B are unusual and usually signal transmission through direct parenteral exposure. Outbreaks have been reported among intravenous drug abusers, and more recently these have been associated with high mortality rates due to coinfection with hepatitis delta virus.[37] Outbreaks of nosocomial hepatitis B continue to occur and usually represent lapses in well-defined infection control techniques. Transmission of disease from chronically infected health care workers to their patients during the course of invasive procedures also has occurred. The risk factors associated with these infections have been the blind palpation of suture needles and not using gloves for dental or other procedures.[38]

Sexual transmission is the source of the majority of HBV infections in U.S. communities and includes homosexual activity (9% to 12%) and heterosexual activity with multiple partners (20% to 25%). Cases among intravenous drug abusers (25% to 30%) and persons with multiple heterosexual partners have increased significantly since 1985, when the proportion of cases due to homosexual activity dropped because of changes in sexual practices secondary to AIDS.[39] The proportion of cases among health care workers (2%) also has declined because of the use of hepatitis B vaccine. However, approximately 33% of cases have no known source for their infection.[39]

Control and Prevention. The control and prevention of hepatitis B now are feasible with the widespread availability of hepatitis B vaccine. The finding that inactivated HBsAg could serve as an immunogen and that anti-HBs was protective against infection led to the development of plasma-derived hepatitis B vaccines.[40] All have been shown to be safe and highly immunogenic and to have high protective efficacy following preexposure immunization of children and various groups of adults.[41,42] Recently, recombinant DNA technology has been used to produce a new generation of hepatitis B vaccines with immunogenicity and efficacy comparable to that of the plasma-derived vaccines.

Strategies for the use of hepatitis B vaccine have been based on the endemicity of infection within a given country or region.[33] In areas of high endemicity of HBV infection, prevention of both perinatal and early childhood transmission is required to reduce the high rates of chronic infection. This can be accomplished by giving the first dose of vaccine at birth and integrating the remaining doses into the routine childhood immunization schedule. A number of studies have shown that hepatitis B vaccine given in this manner will effectively prevent perinatal HBV infection and the subsequent chronic carrier state.[43,44] The feasibility of these approaches has been shown in Taiwan, Indonesia, China, and a number of other countries.

In areas of low endemicity, such as the United States, the strategy has been to prevent infant and early childhood infections as well as infections among individuals belonging to high-risk groups.[26] Providing postexposure prophylaxis to infants born to HBsAg-positive mothers requires identification of these women during pregnancy. Selective screening of pregnant women whose ethnic background and behavioral or sexual history placed them at risk of having acquired HBV infection has been shown to have poor sensitivity. Universal screening of pregnant women has been shown to be cost-beneficial, and HBsAg screening during an early prenatal visit currently is recommended.[26] Inoculation of infants born to HBsAg-positive mothers with hepatitis B immune globulin (HBIG) and hepatitis B vaccine soon after birth is 90% to 95% effective in preventing infection and in preventing the HBV chronic carrier state.[45,46] To prevent childhood infection in other well-defined populations, such as Alaskan natives, Pacific Islanders, and first generation immigrant populations from areas of high endemicity of HBV infection, universal hepatitis B vaccination as part of the routine childhood immunization schedule has been recommended.[26]

Selective immunization of groups at high risk of infection has been recommended to prevent adult infection. However, the rate of vaccine use has been low and has not appreciably affected the rate of hepatitis B. The feasibility of this approach, therefore, has been called into question.[39] Hepatitis B vaccination of children as a part of their routine childhood immunization schedule has been suggested as the most effective approach to eliminate the transmission of hepatitis B among adults. The long-term duration of vaccine-induced protection from chronic infection makes this strategy feasible, and it currently is being evaluated.[47]

Follow-up studies of adults and children receiving hepatitis B vaccine have shown that 16% to 60% have lost antibody after 5 to 7 years. However, protection from chronic HBV infection persists among those who have lost antibody. Some individuals became infected, as demonstrated by seroconversion to anti-HBc or by increases in titer in anti-HBs. However, these infections were considered benign, since there was no evidence of hepatitis or of antigenemia.[48] Antibody persistence in children appears even better, and vaccine efficacy similar to that in adults has been found.[49]

The secondary prevention of PHC among chronic HBV carriers has been accomplished in limited studies by screening for elevated levels of alpha-fetoprotein and resection of small tumors.[50] Recent clinical trials have shown that interferon-alfa therapy following induction with steroids will induce HBsAg in selected populations of chronic HBV carriers.[51]

DELTA HEPATITIS

Etiological Agent. The hepatitis delta virus (HDV) is a 35 to 38 nm enveloped particle containing a small, circular, single-stranded RNA of 500,000 daltons, the delta antigen, and an outer coat of HBsAg.[52] The virus appears most closely related to the satellite viruses of plants, or viroids, and requires HBsAg as a surface protein in order to replicate.[53]

Clinical Illness, Pathogenesis, and Immune Response. HDV infection can occur either as a coinfection with HBV or as a superinfection of an HBV carrier. Coinfection follows exposure to an inoculum containing both HDV and HBV and has an incubation period similar to that of HBV infection. A biphasic illness, which is not common in other types of hepatitis, is observed in 15% to 20% of patients. HDV replication is limited by resolution of the HBV infection. Chronic HDV infection only occurs when the patient progresses to the HBV carrier state. HDV superinfection follows exposure of an HBV carrier to an HDV inoculum and may appear within 2 to 6 weeks.[6] Acute HDV infection may partially suppress HBV replication and occasionally terminate the HBV carrier state. However, in the majority of cases, persistent HBV infection allows HDV infection to persist indefinitely.[54]

The spectrum of clinical disease in acute HDV infection, whether coinfection or superinfection, varies from no illness to acute hepatitis, including fulminant hepatitis. HDV augments the severity of both acute and chronic HBV infection. Most HDV infections of either type cause an episode of acute hepatitis with jaundice, in contrast to about 30% of HBV infections. The risk of fulminant disease may reach 10% for clinical HDV-HBV coinfections and 20% in HDV superinfections.[37] HDV infection has been found in 30% to 50% of fulminant cases of HBsAg-positive fulminant hepatitis.[55]

During coinfection, serological markers of acute HBV infection are accompanied by the presence of delta antigen and antibodies to HDV (total or IgM anti-HDV). Delta antigen is usually present during early acute illness, whereas IgM antibodies appear within days to weeks after onset.[56] The antibody response is not strong, and accurate diagnosis is best accomplished during acute illness or early convalescence. In acute superinfection, serological markers of chronic HBV infection are present, and delta antigen may be present early in the illness. Both IgM and IgG specific antibodies appear rapidly. In cases of fulminant hepatitis, HDV markers in serum may be negative in spite of demonstrable delta antigen in the liver.[37] In chronic HDV hepatitis, HBsAg is present along with IgM anti-HDV in the serum and delta antigen in the liver.

Chronic HDV infection can be asymptomatic or manifest as chronic active hepatitis and progress rapidly to cirrhosis and death due to liver failure.[57] HDV superinfection markedly increases the risk of chronic liver disease, and it is estimated that 50% to 90% of these patients develop chronic hepatitis. There is no evidence that HDV infection is associated with a higher risk of primary hepatocellular carcinoma (PHC).

Diagnosis. Both IgG and IgM antibodies to HDV develop during the course of HDV infection, and serological tests to detect these antibodies are available commercially. Tests for HDV antigen in serum specimens also are available, have modest sensitivity because they require treatment with detergent to disrupt the viral particles, and are positive only during the acute phase of infection. Immunoperoxidase and immunofluorescence assays for HDV antigen in liver are more sensitive and can be used in cases of chronic HDV hepatitis. Hybridization assays for HDV-RNA in serum have proven more sensitive in detecting HDV than assays for HDV antigen and appear useful in determining infectivity of people with chronic HDV infection.

The diagnosis of acute coinfection is made by demonstrating serological markers of acute HBV infection (IgM anti-HBc and HBsAg), accompanied by either HDV antigen in serum or total or IgM anti-HDV or both. Acute HDV superinfection is diagnosed by demonstrating either HDV antigen or total or IgM anti-HDV or both in a person with acute hepatitis and evidence of chronic HBV infection (HBsAg positive, IgM anti-HBc negative). In cases of fulminant hepatitis, HDV markers in serum may be negative in spite of demonstrable delta antigen in the liver.

Patients with chronic HDV hepatitis have serological evidence of chronic HBV infection (HBsAg positive and IgM anti-HBc negative) and antibodies to HDV. Often, IgM anti-HDV is positive, and HDV antigen can be found in the liver.

Epidemiology. HDV is found in highest concentration in the blood of persons with acute or chronic infection. HDV is presumed to be present in serum-derived fluids, such as wound exudates. Its presence in other body fluids has not been studied. Transmission of HDV, like HBV, occurs by percutaneous exposure to blood, either directly or indirectly, and by sexual contact. Perinatal transmission from mother to infant can occur but is of minimal importance in this disease. Casual contact does not result in viral transmission, but HBsAg-positive household contacts of HBV-HDV carriers are at significant risk of infection over long periods of time.

The age-specific frequency of delta infection depends on the predominant age of HBV infection in the region, and the transmission patterns and epidemiology of HDV closely parallel those of hepatitis B, with several notable departures. In low HBV endemicity areas, such as the United States and Western Europe, the prevalence of HDV infection is low (0 to 5%) in HBV carriers but reaches 10% to 25% in persons with HBV-associated chronic hepatitis. Certain risk groups, such as drug abusers and hemophiliacs, have a uniformly high risk (30% to 50%) of infection. However, the prevalence of infection is much lower in other HBV risk groups, such as homosexual men (5%), persons with multiple heterosexual partners, and household contacts of HBV carriers.[58] This suggests that HDV is transmitted less efficiently by sexual contact than by blood exposure. In the United States, HDV infection is found in about 5% of cases of acute hepatitis B and in up to 25% of cases of fulminant hepatitis.[58]

Delta prevalence tends to be higher, reaching 15% in HBV carriers and 30% to 50% in persons with hepatitis B-associated chronic liver disease in moderate and high endemicity areas, such as southern Italy, parts of Eastern Europe, the Middle East, Africa, and some Pacific Islands groups. The highest levels (20% in HBV carriers and up to 90% in chronic hepatitis B cases) have been found in parts of the Amazon Basin, parts of Africa, and Romania. HDV has been identified as the cause of fulminant hepatitis in northern Colombia since the 1930s and is the cause of Labrea hepatitis, which is found in the Amazon Basin.[59] Curiously, HDV prevalence is uniformly low in East and Southeast Asia despite high HBV endemicity throughout this region.[60]

Outbreaks of HDV infection have been recognized among drug abusers and in certain high HBV endemicity populations. Outbreaks among drug abusers usually involve coinfection of HBV and HDV, may cause high mortality due to fulminant hepatitis, and result in secondary transmission to sexual contacts.[37] Outbreaks of superinfection in HBV carriers have been recognized in populations in Brazil, Venezuela, Colombia, and the Central African Republic.[61] These outbreaks characteristically affect children and young adults and cause high acute mortality and chronic morbidity. Transmission occurs primarily via open skin wounds and sexual contact. The risk is highest for those HBV carriers who live with an index case, accounting for the familial clustering of cases of fulminant hepatitis observed in these regions.[61]

Control and Prevention. Control and prevention of HDV infection are dependent on the control of HBV infection. General measures, which include sterilization of needles and instruments that penetrate the skin in a medical care setting and screening of blood for HBsAg, are effective in preventing both HBV and HDV infection. However, the risk for recipients of pooled plasma products (e.g., hemophiliacs) remains high. Hepatitis B vaccine will prevent HBV-HDV coinfection, and vaccination of persons at risk of HBV infection is the best protective measure against HDV coinfection. No specific treatment or prevention can be offered for HBV carriers at risk of HDV superinfection. Counseling to avoid exposure to contaminated needles, occupational exposure, or sexual exposure to HBV-HDV carriers should be undertaken.

PARENTERALLY TRANSMITTED NON-A, NON-B HEPATITIS

Etiological Agent. The term non-A, non-B hepatitis has been applied to those cases of acute hepatitis for which other specific viral etiologies (hepatitis A and B, Epstein-Barr virus, cytomegalovirus) and a variety of other infectious and noninfectious agents that can cause liver inflammation have been reliably excluded. Parenterally transmitted non-A, non-B (PT-NANB) hepatitis has been recognized after blood transfusion or other direct blood exposure but also occurs outside the transfusion setting. Until very recently, no agent had been identified that could be associated with this form of viral hepatitis. Recently, cDNA was cloned and sequenced from the plasma of a chimpanzee experimentally infected with plasma products that produced PT-NANB hepatitis in human recipients,[6] and this same genome has been sequenced from a patient with PT-NANB hepatitis acquired following transfusion. This virus, designated hepatitis C virus (HCV), has not been visualized, but its genome is known to consist of single-stranded, positive sense RNA approximately 10,000 base pairs in size. Its genomic organization has characteristics of both flaviviruses and pestiviruses, but its coded antigens have not been characterized. Previous experiments demonstrated that this agent contained lipid and was 50 to 80 nm in size. Infectivity can be eliminated by treatment with formalin (1:1000) or heating at 100° C for 60 minutes or at 60° C for 10 hours.

It now appears that the majority of PT-NANB hepatitis is due to HCV infection, although it has been shown in chimpanzee infectivity studies that there may be another agent that produces a clinical picture indistinguishable from HCV infection.[62]

Clinical Illness, Pathogenesis, and Immune Response. The spectrum of illness due to PT-NANB ranges from asymptomatic infection to acute fulminant hepatitis. Among adults who acquired PT-NANB hepatitis from transfusion, 14% to 33% of those with elevated liver enzymes developed clinical hepatitis with jaundice. The fatality rate among reported clinical cases of PT-NANB hepatitis in the United States has been approximately 2.0%. In Western Europe and the United States, 27% to 44% of cases of fulminant hepatitis are due to NANB hepatitis.

Prospective studies of patients with acute PT-NANB hepatitis have shown that at least 50% continue to have elevated liver enzymes irrespective of the source of their infection.[63] The majority of patients who progress to chronic liver disease have evidence of HCV infection, and the histological spectrum of disease ranges from chronic persistent hepatitis to cirrhosis. In Japan, a high prevalence of antibody to HCV has been found among patients with PHC who are not HBsAg positive.

The full picture of the immune response to HCV infection is not known at this time. The antibody test currently available is derived from an antigen expressed using recombinant DNA technology. This antigen (C-100) comes from that part of the genome coding for nonstructural viral proteins.[64] Antigens representing the nucleocapsid portion of the virus currently are being evaluated, and the antibody response to this part of the virus may be quite different from that to the nonstructural proteins. Among patients with acute PT-NANB hepatitis, approximately 50% are anti-HCV positive at the onset of clinical illness, but 6 months after the onset of illness, antibody has been detected in 70% to 90%.[64] Following acute infection, anti-HCV appears to persist in patients with chronic hepatitis, as well as in patients with no evidence of chronic liver disease. However, there have been some reports of patients not having detectable antibody following the resolution of their acute hepatitis. Within 1 week of transfusion, HCV can be detected in the serum of patients who subsequently had acute hepatitis and became anti-HCV positive.[65]

Diagnosis. Since it is not known whether all PT-NANB hepatitis is due to HCV infection, the diagnosis of acute NANB hepatitis must first be established in persons with signs and symptoms consistent with acute hepatitis by ruling out acute HAV and HBV infection. Currently, only immunoassays for antibodies to part of the nonstructural region of HCV (anti-HCV) are available, as well as supplemental tests used to confirm anti-HCV positive results. The supplemental tests represent antigens from the same region of the virus that are used in a different assay format (Western blot or competitive inhibition assay) to improve the specificity of the test. The presence of anti-HCV during the acute phase of the illness most likely represents acute infection. However, since there is not a specific test for acute HCV infection (e.g., IgM anti-HCV), the presence of antibody could represent a preexisting infection. Patients with acute PT-NANB hepatitis who are anti-HCV negative at the onset of illness should be tested 6 months later, and if they are anti-HCV positive, the diagnosis of acute HCV infection can be made.

Among persons with chronic liver disease, the diagnosis of chronic HCV infection is strongly suggested if they are anti-HCV positive. The long-term prognostic meaning of a positive test for anti-HCV in a person with no evidence of chronic liver disease is not known at this time. It is not known what proportion of these persons are chronically infected or whether they are at risk for development of chronic liver disease. Tests for HCV antigen are not available, but identification of HCV-RNA using techniques to amplify low levels of virus-specific nucleic acid (polymerase chain reaction) have demonstrated HCV in serum.[65]

Epidemiology. Most of the descriptive epidemiology of PT-NANB is limited to serological studies of the etiology of acute hepatitis, outbreaks of NANB hepatitis, prospective studies among persons exposed to blood products, and prospective natural history studies of persons with acute PT-NANB hepatitis. The serum specimens from many of these studies are being tested for anti-HCV and are beginning to provide a better picture of the epidemiology and natural history of PT-NANB hepatitis and HCV infection. It is apparent that PT-NANB hepatitis and hepatitis C are diseases of worldwide distribution and an important cause of acute and chronic hepatitis among adults. A study with complete serological testing of all cases of acute hepatitis in four U.S. counties has shown that PT-NANB hepatitis accounts for 15% to 40% of acute viral hepatitis and appears to be the most poorly reported type of viral hepatitis[66] (Fig. 7-4). Risk factors associated with PT-NANB hepatitis include antecedent blood transfusion (5% to 17% of cases), parenteral drug abuse (21% to 42%), occupational exposure (2%), multiple heterosexual partners (3% to 9%), and hemodialysis (less than 1%). No identifiable source of infection can be found in 40% to 50% of cases (Fig. 7-4).

The risk of PT-NANB hepatitis and hepatitis C is well documented in persons exposed to blood or blood products through transfusion. Prospective studies in the 1970s showed that 5% to 12% of persons receiving blood screened for HBsAg developed acute hepatitis, and 25% to 50% of these became jaundiced. The risk was lower among recipients of volunteer rather than commercial blood. Recently, testing of blood donors for alanine aminotransferase (ALT) levels and anti-HBc was instituted after

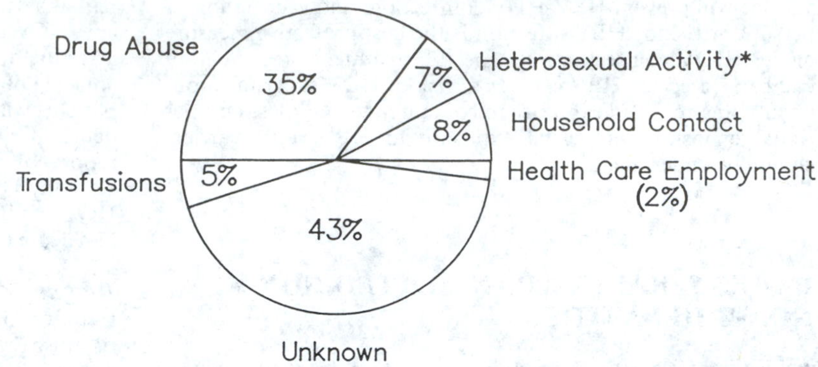

Figure 7-4. Reported sources of infection among patients with non-A, non-B hepatitis in the United States. *[Adapted from Alter et al.[66]]*

it was shown that these surrogate markers potentially could lower the risk of PT-NANB hepatitis by about 50%.[67] In a limited examination of patients with transfusion-associated NANB hepatitis, 79% were found to seroconvert to anti-HCV when followed prospectively.[68] Preparations of pooled clotting factors pose a markedly higher risk for infection except for those treated by wet heat pasteurization.

Outbreaks of PT-NANB have been documented among hemodialysis patients and, occasionally, staff and among groups of patients having common exposure to blood components. Secondary transmission to household contacts (attack rate 2%) has occurred in some of these outbreaks but is usually limited.

The most significant mechanism for transmission of HCV is via blood. No other body fluids have been studied for possible infectivity or presence of virus. Risk of PT-NANB hepatitis and HCV infection from occupational exposure to blood appears to occur but probably at a lower rate than in HBV infection. Transmission via blood contamination of the environment has been demonstrated in outbreaks among nontransfused hemodialysis patients. The extent to which HCV infection is transmitted from anti-HCV-positive mothers to their infants during the perinatal period is not clear. The only definite infections appear to occur in infants born to human immunodeficiency virus (HIV)-positive mothers.

HCV infection and PT-NANB hepatitis appear to be sexually transmitted but not as efficiently as HBV. A low rate of secondary transmission to household contacts of cases of PT-NANB hepatitis has been recognized, but transmission has not been widely recognized among sexual contacts of cases. NANB hepatitis was documented to occur among active homosexual men at a rate of 2.9% per year compared to hepatitis A (5.2%) and B (25%) in these same men. Heterosexual exposures have consistently accounted for approximately 10% of reported cases of PT-NANB hepatitis, and a recent study found that patients with NANB hepatitis were more likely than controls to have had multiple sexual partners during the appropriate risk period.[69] The prevalence of anti-HCV among persons with multiple heterosexual partners (5% to 16%) is greater than that among blood donors or persons without multiple partners (0.5% to 3%). Surprisingly, the prevalence of anti-HCV among homosexual men (8% to 15%) has been lower than rates of HBV infection, suggesting that sexual transmission of HCV is not efficient.[70]

Studies in chimpanzees and humans have shown frequent progression of HCV infection to chronicity. Studies of HCV-infected chimpanzees, of patients with acute posttransfusion NANB hepatitis subsequently shown to be due to HCV, and of patients with acute, nontransfusion-acquired PT-NANB hepatitis due to HCV have shown that 30% to 70% will develop persistent liver enzyme abnormalities and histological evidence of chronic liver disease.

Several lines of epidemiological and laboratory evidence suggest that at least two different agents cause PT-NANB hepatitis. Multiple attacks of non-A, non-B have been reported among patients with multiple transfusions and among parenteral drug abusers. Cross-challenge experiments in chimpanzees have suggested that two different agents, with different physical-chemical characteristics are responsible for infection.[62] Although not all patients with PT-NANB hepatitis are anti-HCV positive after appropriate follow-up, this may be due to the poor sensitivity of the assay. Resolution of the question of the number of agents responsible for PT-NANB hepatitis must await further studies.

Control and Prevention. Elimination of paid blood donors was shown to decrease the risk of posttransfusion NANB hepatitis. Further reduction of this disease will be achieved with screening of donors for anti-HCV and the use of elevated ALT and anti-HBc as surrogate markers of other forms of NANB infection.[67] However, transfusion-transmitted infection accounts for only a small proportion of the annual disease burden. General measures used to prevent transmission of other bloodborne pathogens in hospital settings are important in preventing NANB hepatitis and HCV transmission. The prevention of infection among intravenous drug abusers is more problematic. Prevention of infection among persons with multiple heterosexual partners should be achieved with the use of condoms, similar to HIV and HBV prevention. A recent study has suggested that interferon may ameliorate the course of chronic NANB hepatitis.[71] Whether it also alters infectivity is not known.

HEPATITIS E

Etiological Agent. The development of specific serological tests for acute HAV infection resulted in the retrospective examination of serum samples obtained from large outbreaks of hepatitis that resembled hepatitis A. The tests indicated that the vast majority of the cases were not attributable to HAV infection.[72] This new form of non-A, non-B hepatitis with a fecal-oral mode of transmission was initially called epidemic NANB hepatitis and then enterically transmitted non-A, non-B hepatitis. Laboratory investigations demonstrated viruslike particles having a diameter of 27 to 32 nm in the feces of patients. These viruslike particles have been demonstrated consistently by immune electron microscopy to aggregate with serum obtained from persons in the late acute and early convalescent phase of ET-NANB hepatitis.[73] Reproducible animal models of disease have been established in nonhuman primates. Studies have demonstrated the immunological relatedness of both virus and antibody from geographically unrelated outbreaks and suggest that the virus may have only a single dominant serotype. Recently, cDNA was cloned from virus isolated from cynomolgus macaques experimentally infected with ET-NANB hepatitis, and the genome of hepatitis E virus (HEV) has been partially characterized.[10]

Clinical Illness, Pathogenesis, and Immune Response. The incubation period is longer than for hepatitis A, with a range of 22 to 60 days and a mode of 40 days. A prodromal phase lasting 1 to 10 days has been described, followed by nausea (46% to 84%), dark urine (92% to 100%), abdominal pain (41% to 87%), vomiting (50%), pruritis (13% to 55%), joint pain (28% to 81%), rash (3%), and diarrhea (3%). Fever and hepatomegaly have been present in over 50% of patients.[74] Clinical and biochemical presentations cannot differentiate cases of hepatitis A and hepatitis E. A human volunteer study showed that transmission of the ET-NANB agent can occur via the enteral route. In the nonhuman primate model and the human volunteer study, the relationship of viral excretion in feces to liver enzyme elevations was similar to that observed in hepatitis A, with the peak of viral excretion occurring before the onset of biochemical evidence of hepatitis.[75] Histopathological examination of liver biopsies from nonfulminant cases has demonstrated a cholestatic form of viral hepatitis with glandlike transformation and preserved lobular structure. Liver cell necrosis has varied from single cell degeneration to more severe forms with bridging necrosis.[76]

A high case fatality rate among pregnant women has been a consistent feature of ET-NANB hepatitis and has ranged from 17% to 33%.[77] High rates of perinatal death have been associated with fulminant disease among pregnant women. However, termination of pregnancy does not appear to improve their clinical status. Follow-up studies of persons with ET-NANB hepatitis indicate that chronic liver disease is not a consequence of this infection.

Diagnosis. The key to diagnosis of hepatitis E is an increased awareness that the disease may exist in a particular region. Currently, no diagnostic reagents are available commercially. Exclusion of acute hepatitis A and hepatitis B must include demonstration of the absence of IgM anti-HAV and IgM anti-HBc. Patients in countries where hepatitis E has not been identified should raise the possibility of imported cases, and a complete travel history should be obtained to determine if the individual had been in an area of known endemicity for the disease.

Visualization of virus in the feces of infected persons by immune electron microscopy can be done in some research centers. An immunofluorescent blocking assay for anti-HEV recently has been reported but requires substrate obtained from nonhuman primates infected with HEV.[73] It would be expected that solid-phase immunoassays would be developed following the cloning of HEV.

Epidemiology. Identification of numerous outbreaks of ET-NANB hepatitis and identification of sporadic cases in many parts of the world have been the result of more widespread use of IgM anti-HAV testing for hepatitis A. Several epidemiological features of ET-NANB are quite distinct from those of hepatitis A, namely, a high attack rate among adults and an unusually high case fatality rate among pregnant women.[77] The mean age for infection has been 29 years, and the highest age-specific prevalence of infection has been between 20 and 30 years of age.[74,77] In both epidemic and nonepidemic situations, symptomatic cases are seen among children and usually contribute 5% to 10% of the total clinical cases observed.[74]

Hepatitis E is clearly transmitted by the fecal-oral route. The endemicity among groups at risk for infection, however, is not well defined because of the lack of serological markers. Epidemics have occurred in areas where drinking water has been contaminated with feces, usually during periods of extensive rain. Sporadic cases of ET-NANB hepatitis probably occur within all the countries where epidemics have been reported, but the extent to which sporadic disease occurs is not known. Several characteristics of this disease distinguish it from hepatitis A but cannot be fully explained until further diagnostic capabilities are available. These include the observation that the majority of cases occur among young adults, an unexpected finding in areas where enteric diseases are highly endemic. This observation suggests either age-specific differences in the clinical response to infection or that this is a relatively new virus. Another unusual characteristic is the high case fatality rate among pregnant women with hepatitis E.

Epidemics of hepatitis E have been reported from central Soviet Asia, India, Pakistan, Burma, Nepal, Somalia, Sudan, Algeria, and Mexico.[73] More recently, epidemics have been reported from Northwest China, Bangladesh, Borneo, the Ivory Coast, Indonesia, and Ethiopia. To date, outbreaks have not been recognized in the United States, Canada, Northern Europe, or Australia, although there are confirmed reports of sporadic cases in Mediterranean countries. With widespread air travel throughout the world, imported cases have now been recognized in the United States.[76]

Dramatic epidemics have been produced by this agent, including one in New Delhi, India, in 1955–1956 with an estimated 29,000 icteric cases, in other parts of India, in Burma, and in Nepal with 5 to 10,000 cases. Smaller epidemics and outbreaks also have been reported from many parts of the world. The settings of these epidemics have included large urban areas, rural villages, small towns, and refugee camps. In all instances, there has been inadequate disposal of feces and contamination of water supplies with fecal material, often by heavy seasonal rains. High rates of disease often have persisted through two rainy seasons, followed by an end to the epidemic. Clinical attack rates have been 0.7% to 10%, and secondary attack rates in households have ranged from 0.7% to 2.2%. Cases have occurred among health care workers caring for patients during epidemic periods.

Control and Prevention. The most important means of preventing hepatitis E is protection of water systems from contamination with fecal material. Epidemiological evidence suggests that boiling water will interrupt disease transmission. Data concerning chlorination of water are not available, although this strategy also should be used to interrupt disease transmission in epidemic situations. Since pregnant women are particularly vulnerable to fulminant hepatitis from ET-NANB, they should be advised of these sanitary requirements, and travelers to epidemic areas should be particularly cautious with regard to these recommendations.

The prophylactic effect of immunoglobulins has not been ascertained, and it is not known what the protective immunological parameters are for preventing hepatitis E.

Aseptic Meningitis and Enteroviral Infections

Cyrus C. Hopkins

ASEPTIC MENINGITIS

"Aseptic meningitis" is a nonspecific clinical term that describes an acute febrile lymphocytic meningitis with negative bacterial cultures. Most strictly defined cases are caused by viral agents, especially the enteroviruses, but a wide variety of illnesses can cause the same syndrome. On the other hand, enteroviral infections produce a variety of clinical illnesses not involving the meninges or central nervous system.

Aseptic meningitis in its strictest form is definable as an acute febrile illness, with meningeal signs, in which an examination of the spinal fluid shows lymphocytic pleocytosis and in which bacterial cultures, appropriately obtained, are negative. The differential diagnosis, however, can be significantly affected by minor differences in interpretation of each of these variables. For example, some chronic conditions of the central nervous system, such as fungal or mycobacterial infection, brain abscess or tumor, can produce a long chronic illness with subtle symptoms that are not recognized initially. The history obtained may then feature only the aspects of recent deterioration, making the illness appear to be acute. In more acute disease, a variety of nonviral infections, especially Lyme disease, syphilis, and leptospirosis, can have a similar presentation. Other nonenteroviral viral infections can cause aseptic meningitis, especially other encephalitides (e.g., herpes simplex), lymphocytic choriomeningitis, mumps, and mononucleosis. An important confusion is often raised by partially treated bacterial meningitis, since the characteristic acute polymorphonuclear response can be blunted by preceding antibiotics. On the other hand, viral infections early in their course can cause a polymorphonuclear pleocytosis in the cerebrospinal fluid (CSF), mimicking, in some respects, bacterial infection. The interpretation of CSF glucose concentrations sometimes may help resolve these two conditions.

Diagnosis of this clinical picture can be made with increasing security only with an accurate history of the temporal course of disease, of prior treatment and contacts, the passage of time, and a response demonstrating a self-limited disease. The selection and use of additional studies, especially serological tests, will vary with the specific clinical and epidemiological setting. Fortunately, the nonviral diagnoses still represent infrequent occurrences and are epidemiologically insignificant.[1]

ENTEROVIRUSES

Aseptic meningitis as strictly defined will have an etiological agent identified only infrequently. Most is due to enteroviral infection, and the majority of the remainder are presumed to have a similar etiology. On the other hand, aseptic meningitis is only one of many common presentations of enteroviral infections.[2] Among the most common clinical conditions are several well-defined febrile illnesses: lymphonodular pharyngitis, pharyngitis with a shallow vesicular exanthem on the anterior tonsillar pillars (herpangina), or pharyngitis with both an enanthem and a macular to papulovesicular rash on the distal extremities (hand-foot-and-mouth disease). Syndromes with prominent pleuritic chest pain can occur (epidemic pleuritis, pleurodynia). Pericarditis or myocarditis often can occur with coxsackie B infections. Since the enteroviruses colonize and proliferate within the intestinal tract, they often may be grown from patients with gastroenteritis of other cause; only a few strains cause gastroenteritis. Many diseases of the central nervous system have been associated with enteroviral infections, among which aseptic meningitis is by far the most common. Encephalitis is very infrequent with these agents. Poliovirus, discussed elsewhere, is associated with aseptic meningitis or, characteristically, with paralytic disease. Specific strains have been associated with some cases of epidemic conjunctivitis (coxsackie 24 and enterovirus 70), with the hemolytic-uremic syndrome (several strains, especially coxsackie B), and perhaps with diabetes, at least in persons of specific HLA type.[3] A wide variety of other clinical manifestations have been observed, although less frequently, in acute enteroviral infection.

The enteroviruses are a diverse group of dozens of strains of small RNA viruses, which were originally classified by their differential behavior in laboratory animals into echoviruses or coxsackie viruses (separable into types A and B). They are, as a rule, remarkably stable to many chemical and lipid solutions, especially to acid, and can be relatively protected from destruction by heat in some chemical environments. These features permit passage through gastric acid and contribute to a potential mode of spread involving either the fecal-oral route or an environmental common source. Generally, close person to person contact is required, which occurs via respiratory droplets during acute illness or, for longer periods, by fecal-oral spread, depending in part on the strain and the site of infection.[4]

Infection may appear after an incubation period of only 2 to 5 days, although acute illness occurs only in about half of all infected persons. The inapparent/apparent infection ratio may vary from 2:1 to as high as 20:1 (as in poliovirus). Viral excretion begins with the onset of illness and appears acutely in pharyngeal secretions, but it can continue in the feces for weeks. In temperate regions, transmission and disease are more common in the summer and early fall. Summer epidemics, sometimes very prominent, often involve only a few strains each summer. Although the clinical manifestations of a specific strain may be quite diverse, the epidemic appearance of a single clinical syndrome, especially aseptic meningitis, is common. In tropical areas, transmission occurs year round, and more people become infected at a younger age, often in infancy. Except for the neonate, infection at an early age results in an even higher prevalence of inapparent infection.

Nearly all enteroviral infections are short, self-limited illnesses, with fever and acute symptoms of only a few days, although persistent or recurrent infections, especially of the nervous system, can occur in immunocompromised patients.[5] Secondary complications are infrequent, although some stigmata, especially myocarditis, can result in permanent damage.

Infection with a single strain leads to both systemic and mucosal immunity, probably for life. Any heterologous protection is very weak. Accordingly, vaccination could be provided for single strains. The only enteroviruses that are of sufficient significance to warrant such attention are the three poliovirus strains.

There is no specific treatment.

Prevention of transmission can be accomplished by elimination of close personal contact with infected persons, but since so many infected persons are asymptomatic, this is virtually impossible. Mass immunization with either oral (live, attenuated) or parenteral (inactivated) poliovaccine has been successful in eliminating poliovirus as an epidemic disease in western developed countries (see Chapter 5) but is not used for the prevention of other enteroviral infection.

Epstein-Barr Virus and Infectious Mononucleosis

Cyrus C. Hopkins

The Epstein-Barr virus (EBV) is a member of the herpesvirus family. It commonly occurs in this country as infectious mononucleosis but has a strong epidemiological association with certain tumors, especially nasopharyngeal carcinoma and Burkitt's lymphoma, in Africa.

Like other members of the herpesvirus group, the virus is a DNA virus and has the ability to persist in living cells for long periods of time both in vitro and in vivo. In vitro, it is capable of transforming lymphocytes, allowing them to persist immortalized in tissue culture. Unlike some other members of the herpesvirus group, recurrent clinical infections with this agent do not occur in spite of evidence that the virus can persist in human cells. After convalescence from acute illness, however, the genome often can be identified within cells, particularly in association with later malignancies.[1]

Pathogenesis. Infection is primarily a disease of humans, and its significant epidemiology is confined to human transmission, although the cells of some animals have viral receptors. Outside of cells, the virus is labile and does not survive well in the environment. In humans, the virus is capable of infecting nasopharyngeal and oropharyngeal epithelial cells and lymphocytes, primarily B lymphocytes. Infection begins with attachment to specific receptors in the nasopharyngeal epithelium, and infection of nasal and oropharyngeal cells is subsequently maintained. B lymphocytes subsequently acquire the virus, and at least some lymphocyte lines maintain viral infection for long periods of time. During illness, a complex immunological reaction occurs in the normal host, involving both cellular and humoral immunity. Activated B cells produce antibody, and T cell immunity also is enhanced. This complex phenomenon controls infection in the normal host, but in the immunocompromised host, prolonged viral excretion and progressive infection can occur, sometimes with a progressive lymphoproliferative disease.

The immune response includes a sequential appearance of cellular reactions and antibodies of various types. The initial clinical diagnosis often is suggested by characteristic atypical lymphocytes, which do not represent the infected cell lines but are a mixture of reactive and noninfected T and B cells. The heterophil antibody generally is used to make the specific diagnosis. These heterogeneous antibodies agglutinate sheep red blood cells and are differentially absorbed by beef RBCs but not by guinea pig kidney. Specific viral antibodies appear in a characteristic sequence. Early in infection, with or without symptoms, antibody to viral capsid and envelope appear. Accordingly, early IgM antiviral capsid antibody (VCA) can permit the diagnosis of acute infection. Similar IgG antibody persists for life. On the other hand, nuclear antibody (EBNA) and soluble complement-fixing antibody (anti-S) appear later in the course of illness, often after 3 to 4 weeks, persist for life, and occasionally can be helpful in establishing a later diagnosis.[2]

Epidemiology. Serological surveys have demonstrated that the virus is ubiquitous and in all human populations studied. The age of acquisition of infection and, accordingly, the patterns of clinical disease vary in different populations. In tropical regions and under lower socioeconomic conditions, infection tends to be acquired earlier in childhood and is more often asymptomatic. In temperate and developed industrialized countries, up to half the infections are not acquired until adolescence or young adulthood. When disease is acquired later, it is more likely to produce clinical disease. By adulthood, 90% to 95% of all populations have serological evidence of prior infection.

Spread of infection is primarily by direct contact with infected oropharyngeal secretions. Virus appears in the throat during infection and persists for up to 18 months thereafter. Infection is often asymptomatic. Accordingly, viral excretion can be found in 10% to 20% of healthy young adults, even without a history of antecedent illness. Contact with infected patients must be close or sustained to cause infection. College roommates of clinically ill students do not become more readily infected than does the general population. Infection in college or military settings can occur at up to 12% per year. The reservoir is most likely the asymptomatic healthy adult.[3]

Clinical Course. After acquisition of the virus, there is a 30 to 50 day incubation period, during which viral replication in epithelial cells and lymphocytes occurs, with dissemination and the progressive immunological response. The clinical spectrum of disease is highly variable. In most persons, the infection is inapparent, particularly in very young children, who often lack heterophil antibody as well. The ratio of inapparent to clinically evident infection decreases with age. By college age, nearly half may be symptomatic.

The symptoms are those of a febrile illness, usually with a prominent sore throat. Malaise, fatigue, and myalgias are prominent but nonspecific. On examination, virtually all patients show a prominent lymphadenopathy. Splenomegaly is found in about half the cases, mildly abnormal liver function tests are frequent, and hepatomegaly is found less often, though frank hepatitis can occur. Laboratory studies include a significant increase in lymphocytes (generally >50% to establish the diagnosis) with atypical lymphocytes (usually requiring >10% to be diagnostic).

The serological finding of the heterophil antibody generally is used to make the diagnosis, either by formal testing (including a diagnostic pattern of differential absorption) or, with a high degree of specificity, by commercially prepared kits or cards. Specific EBV antibodies are less readily available and rarely are necessary to make the diagnosis acutely. They can be helpful in those cases (perhaps 10% of adults and up to 50% of children) that lack the heterophil antibody.

Complications are infrequent but can be serious and include an autoimmune hemolytic anemia, usually in the presence of an IgM cold agglutinin. Thrombocytopenia can occur but is usually mild. Splenic rupture can occur, especially in the second or third week. A wide variety of neurological manifestations can occur, ranging from encephalitis through myelitis, aseptic meningitis, and peripheral neuropathy. Serious sequelae and death are very uncommon in the immunocompetent host. Most infections resolve within 2 to 3 weeks, although some patients have a period of persistent fatigue and weakness that may persist for months (postviral asthenia). In spite of this, there are no convincing data that EBV is related to the chronic fatigue syndrome.

In addition to these patterns of acute disease, EBV has been found in association with various neoplasias. In some immunocompromised patients, whether natural, as in the X-linked lymphoproliferative syndrome, or induced, as in AIDS or transplant recipients, primary infection may progress to produce a progressive lymphoproliferative syndrome.[4] In a quite different setting, EBV is strongly associated with two tumors, Burkitt's lymphoma in tropical Africa and nasopharyngeal carcinoma. Tissues of both tumors can contain the EBV genome, and VCA titers in serum are increased significantly. Neither tumor may be exclusively caused by EBV. Burkitt's lymphoma in this country seems to lack this association, and a selective epidemiological distribution of nasopharyngeal carcinoma in certain ethnic groups in the tropics suggests that although EBV is involved, some other risk factor or causative factor must also be required to initiate malignant transformation.

The differential diagnosis of clinical mononucleosis generally is quite clear, when atypical lymphocytes and the heterophil antibody are both present. The lack of either one changes the differential diagnosis. Infectious mononucleosis can occur without the heterophil antibody in 10% of EBV-infected persons (more so in young children), but the nearly identical pattern, including atypical lymphocytosis, is equally likely to be caused by cytomegalovirus (CMV). Similar patterns of illness can occur with other viruses (especially hepatitis), though with far fewer atypical lymphocytes, and these patients will always lack the true heterophil reaction.

Treatment. There is no specific treatment currently available. Corticosteroids are used only for amelioration of some of the most severe complications, especially upper airway obstruction from lymphoproliferation in Waldeyer's ring, for hemolytic anemia, or for severe thrombocytopenia.

Prevention. There is no vaccine or preventive form of therapy. Most transmission occurs as the result of close contact with oropharyngeal secretions, but since the largest reservoir is in asymptomatic patients, only complete avoidance of such contact can be expected to decrease or delay the risk of acquisition of the virus. This cannot be expected to be applied as an effective public health measure.

Herpes Simplex Virus

Richard D. Andersen

Herpes simplex virus (HSV) causes a variety of infections in humans worldwide. Most individuals will become infected with HSV at some point in life, a fact that is critical in planning preventive strategies. The agent is ubiquitous, and HSV acquisition usually results in asymptomatic infection, followed by a latent state. By far the most common manifestation is the common cold sore or fever blister. The spectrum of disease with HSV extends from this relatively minor problem to more serious and life-threatening disease in special circumstances.[1,2]

HSV occurs as two relatively distinct biological types, type 1 and type 2. Whereas the genetic homology and antigenic similarity of the two types are considerable, the prevalence and anatomical affinities differ. Most oral HSV infections are caused by type 1, and most genital infections are caused by type 2.

Epidemiology. HSV infection is ubiquitous, but because most infections are asymptomatic, tracking human to human spread is difficult, and the source of virus is often obscure. Serological evidence suggests a cumulative rate of HSV-1 infection of 60% to 80% of humans worldwide and of 10% to 20% for HSV-2 infection in adults. Sexual behavior greatly affects the likelihood of HSV-2 seropositivity,[3] evidenced by exceedingly low seroprevalence in nuns and very high seroprevalence in prostitutes. Up to 1% of pregnant women may be colonized with HSV in the cervix and at time of delivery. The relative infrequency of neonatal HSV disease (perhaps 1 case per 3000 to 5000 live births) suggests that well below 5% of natally exposed neonates experience clinical illness.

Transmission of the virus depends on direct contact with HSV-infected lesions or with secretions containing the virus. Nosocomial newborn to newborn transmission has been suspected, presumably via adult contacts.[4] Nosocomial acquisition of HSV from hospital personnel is a concern, particularly from those with oral HSV lesions.[5]

The sporadic character of primary gingivostomatitis and herpes encephalitis implies that host factors are more important than epidemiological issues with most HSV-1 infections. Although child to child HSV-1 transmission undoubtedly occurs frequently, especially in the preschool years, outbreaks per se are not usual.

In selected circumstances, such as a young child with genital lesions or in nosocomial clustering, the epidemiological questions are more critical. Although both types 1 and 2 can cause genital lesions, viral typing may be of value in weighing the probability of child abuse. With nosocomial clustering of HSV infection, restriction endonuclease mapping may be used to prove whether viral isolates are identical.

Pathogenesis. Primary HSV infection acquired orally usually is asymptomatic, and the virus takes up residence in neural ganglia. If disease results from this encounter, it may be as a primary gingivostomatitis, with intraoral ulceration and perioral vesiculation. Systemic symptoms, such as fever, may arise as viremia occurs, and lymphadenopathy reflects regional extension of virus.

Similarly, genital HSV infection may be asymptomatic, evidenced by the common isolation of HSV from the uterine cervix in asymptomatic females. When primary genital HSV infection is symptomatic, inguinal adenopathy and fever again reflect regional and distant viral spread. Females appear more prone to clinically significant primary genital HSV disease.

Rarely, HSV extends to the central nervous system in the form of HSV encephalitis.[6] The focality and temporal lobe affinity suggest direct extension of virus along neural tracts. Necrosis of brain tissue occurs as cell to cell viral spread ensues, resulting in high morbidity or mortality, even with antiviral therapy. HSV may infect the fetus and neonate in several ways.[7] Most perinatal HSV infection apparently takes place around the time of birth, following (primary) maternal viremia or infection of the neonate by direct contact with cervical or vaginal HSV. Viremic spread may yield multisystem neonatal disease in deep viscera, especially liver, lung, and brain, often sparing the skin. In other newborns, viral progression is limited to the skin, eyes, mucous membranes, or the central nervous system only. In the last circumstance, brain disease is more diffuse, and virus is more likely to be present in cerebrospinal fluid than it is in older children and adults. Occasionally, in utero transmission of HSV occurs, usually resulting in neurocutaneous localization in the fetus.

Clinical Manifestations. Primary encounters with HSV, if symptomatic, are more likely to yield fever, malaise, and constitutional symptoms than are reactivations. Primary gingivostomatitis may produce intraoral ulceration, perioral vesiculation, anorexia, fever, and regional lymphadenopathy. Young children with this manifestation often are sufficiently dehydrated or anorexic to warrant hospitalization. Untreated, such individuals may remain symptomatic for 10 days or more.

Genital HSV often begins with fever, malaise, and painful vesiculation of genital lesions, with subsequent regional adenopathy. Ulcerations may occur in the mucous membranes of the female genitalia. Primary genital HSV tends to be more severe in the female and also may be accompanied by dysuria or even anuria. Patients with primary genital HSV may remain symptomatic for more than a week untreated.

Reactivations of oral and genital HSV are generally less severe than primary disease. The common cold sore or fever blister, also known as herpes labialis, usually occurs without fever after a prodrome of tingling and localized pain, followed by a small vesicular focus at the lip margin. Genital reactivations evolve in a similar fashion, with one or more vesicular skin lesions or ulcerative mucous membrane lesions.

In patients with burns or eczematoid skin disease, the onset of painful vesiculation in areas of abnormal skin should prompt consideration of HSV. The underlying skin condition and lack of dermatomal distribution help differentiate HSV infection from herpes zoster. In the severely compromised host, widely disseminated HSV disease may resemble varicella and often is accompanied by fever and malaise. The presence of organomegaly in such instances suggests ominous visceral dissemination.

Herpes encephalitis generally begins with fever and headache and may proceed over days or hours to include seizures, lethargy, disorientation, or coma. Focality of clinical symptoms or signs and the absence of seasonal meningoencephalitis warrant an increased suspicion of herpes encephalitis. Early diagnosis and treatment are especially critical with this clinical entity.

Similarly, neonatal HSV infection necessitates prompt diagnosis and therapy. Fever in the first several weeks of life may be a more consistent occurrence in neonatal HSV or enteroviral infection than in the more common generalized bacterial infections of newborns. Patients with superficial disease (skin, eyes, mucous membranes) usually are diagnosed early due to the characteristic vesicular lesions in any site, but particularly at loci of minor trauma, such as scalp monitor sites, forceps abrasions, and so on. Natally acquired disease may occur at any time in the first several weeks of life, but those with rapid visceral dissemination tend to occur in the first week of life, often without cutaneous lesions and generally with fever and obtundation. Both this group and those with localized central nervous system disease—which occurs later in the first month of life—pose more difficult diagnostic issues.

Diagnosis. Diagnosis of HSV infections usually is based on visual inspection of skin lesions. In some clinical situations, especially where antiviral therapy is contemplated, precise virological diagnosis is desirable. HSV is readily grown in tissue culture, reliably producing cytopathic effects within a few days in a wide variety of mammalian cell lines. HSV survives transport to viral culture facilities better than do other more labile viral pathogens.

Rapid presumptive diagnosis is possible with the Tzanck preparation, wherein characteristic multinuclear giant cells are observed in skin or other tissue on slides stained with the Wright or Giemsa stain. Varicella or zoster may produce identical histological changes, however, which limits the diagnostic value of the Tzanck preparation. In the past decade, virus-specific and type-specific monoclonal antibodies with fluorescent labels have allowed more precise distinction of HSV from varicella-zoster virus and of type 1 from type 2 lesions.

In patients with herpes encephalitis, definitive diagnosis has been possible only by obtaining tissue from brain biopsy for cytological analysis and culture. Studies of HSV antigen detection or HSV antibody analysis in cerebrospinal fluid have not resulted in well-standardized, widely available rapid diagnostic reagents. The use of computed axial tomography (CT) and magnetic resonance imaging (MRI) may be of great value in defining the likelihood of HSV encephalitis, as is electroencephalography (EEG). The increasing frequency of empiric antiviral therapy without biopsy reflects a reasonable concern over the morbidity of biopsy. It also reflects the presumption of safety of acyclovir in treatment. Nevertheless, in patients with compromised immunity and in those with atypical presentation, biopsy remains as an important tool.

Treatment. Serious or life-threatening infections with HSV usually are treated with intravenous acyclovir, a nucleoside analog requiring thymidine kinase specified by herpes viruses. Acyclovir is widely distributed in the body, including the cerebrospinal fluid, and is effective in the treatment of HSV encephalitis and HSV disease with involvement of other deep viscera.

Management of neonatal HSV disease also includes intravenous antiviral therapy. A recent comparative trial between the older agent, vidarabine, and acyclovir failed to demonstrate the superiority of acyclovir that has been seen in virtually all other HSV disease. Most investigators believe that this reflects the inadequacy of the previously recommended dose (30 mg/kg/d) of acyclovir and suggest consideration of a higher dosage in newborns.

Oral acyclovir has some role in prophylaxis of HSV infections in the compromised host, for example, following bone marrow transplantation.[8] Oral acyclovir also may have a role in the treatment of primary gingivostomatitis or recurrent oral lesions, as well as in management of genital HSV. Some investigators have cautioned against extensive or prolonged use of oral acyclovir for minor disease, noting the emergence of HSV acyclovir resistance in several patients.

Topical therapy with one of several antiviral ophthalmic preparations is appropriate with HSV keratoconjunctivitis. In other HSV infections, topical antiviral therapy has limited value, with some reduction of viral shedding in recurrent skin lesions but minimal clinical benefit.

Prevention and Control. HSV-1 ultimately infects most of the human race, and its relative benignancy and its latency argue against infection control measures. There is little rationale for attempting to control HSV transmission in the general population. However, some efforts are appropriate to minimize nosocomial HSV transmission and genital HSV transmission in the general population, taking into account the special vulnerability of the newborn and of certain immunocompromised patients.

Prevention of genital HSV transmission in the general population requires responsible sexual behavior. The asymptomatic character of many female genital HSV infections makes less effective any precautions taken only when overt lesions are present. Further, condoms are probably less effective in preventing HSV (and syphilis) transmission than they are in preventing gonorrhea and HIV transmission, where semen is the principal source of transmission.

In the perinatal situation, the presence of overt maternal genital herpetic lesions is considered an indication for cesarean section to prevent natal acquisition. Prolonged rupture of membranes or primary maternal viremia may reduce the benefit of this procedure. Furthermore, most neonatal HSV arises following asymptomatic, unsuspected maternal colonization. No rapid, reliable, inexpensive, universal screening for HSV appears practical as yet, in part because of intermittent maternal excretion. Moreover, recent studies have shown that serial antenatal maternal cervical cultures are a poor predictor of HSV presence in the birth canal at the time of delivery.[9] Until cost-effective, reliable screening procedures are practical, meaningful preventive measures in the perinatal setting are unlikely to emerge. Fortunately, the vast majority of HSV-exposed neonates do not experience clinical infection.

Prevention of nosocomial transmission depends on recognizing the role of direct contact and the awareness that both patients and health care personnel with active HSV lesions pose a potential threat to newborns, to burn patients, and to the severely compromised host. Patients with herpetic disease should be isolated appropriately, with an emphasis on the use of gloves and gowns. Hospital personnel with oral herpes and, to a lesser degree, with genital herpes, should be aware of the mode of transmission and should be diverted temporarily from care of high-risk patients until their lesions subside, usually no more than a few days. Finally, HSV may be present in asymptomatic patients or personnel, a fact that underscores the ever-present need for frequent handwashing in hospitals.

Cytomegalovirus Infections

James F. Bale, Jr.

Human cytomegalovirus (HCMV), first isolated in the early 1950s, can produce severe, life-threatening disease when the virus infects the developing fetus or patients with immunocompromising conditions, such as the acquired immunodeficiency syndrome (AIDS).[1-4] Studies worldwide indicate that 0.5% to 3.0% of infants excrete HCMV in their urine at birth, and most adults over the age of 40 years possess antibody to HCMV, evidence of prior infection.[2] Fortunately, few infected persons experience serious complications of HCMV infection.

Approximately 10% of congenitally infected infants have symptomatic infections characterized by petechial rash, jaundice, hepatosplenomegaly, microcephaly, chorioretinitis, thrombocytopenia, or anemia. Infants who survive such infections frequently have neurological sequelae consisting of vision loss, sensorineural hearing loss, seizures, or developmental and intellectual retardation.[5] Asymptomatically infected newborns are at risk for hearing loss but not for other neurological complications.

Acquired HCMV infection occasionally produces a heterophil-negative infectious mononucleosis syndrome that mimics disease due to the Epstein-Barr virus.[6] Patients have low grade fever, malaise, lymphadenopathy, pharyngitis, hepatitis, or occasionally pneumonitis. Although the course of HCMV-induced mononucleosis can be protracted, lasting several weeks, nearly all patients recover without sequelae.

By contrast, HCMV can be a particularly virulent pathogen in immunocompromised hosts, causing fatal pneumonitis, severe gastroenteritis, encephalitis, and necrotizing retinitis.[2,3] Conditions associated with an increased risk for such complications include congenital immunodeficiency syndromes (involving cell-mediated immunity), immunosuppression for organ or bone marrow transplantation, chemotherapy for malignancy or connective tissue disorders, and AIDS.[3] In patients with AIDS, HCMV is the most frequently recognized secondary infectious complication, affecting 40% or more of such individuals.

Direct contact with an HCMV-excreting individual serves as the natural mode of transmission. In infected persons, HCMV can be detected in urine, saliva, circulating leukocytes, tears, breast milk, semen, or cervical secretions. During childhood, ingestion of HCMV-infected breast milk or contact with the urine or saliva of infected playmates accounts for most infections. After puberty, sexual contact (heterosexual or homosexual) with HCMV-infected persons contributes substantially to transmission. Infected persons excrete HCMV in urine for extended periods, typically 4 or more years after congenital infection[7] or as long as 1 year after acquired infection.[8] Prolonged excretion, particularly by young children, contributes substantially to spread of HCMV.

HCMV can be acquired also via transfusion of blood products or transplantation of tissues or organs from seropositive donors. The risk of infection after blood transfusion, greatest when patients receive blood from multiple donors, ranges from 0.14% to 2.7% per unit transfused.[2] Several studies performed during the late 1970s and early 1980s clearly indicate that kidney or bone marrow transplants from seropositive donors can also transmit HCMV to seronegative recipients.[9,10] Such infections usually result from transmission of latent HCMV contained within certain leukocyte subpopulations or, possibly, tissue macrophages.

Culturing the urine remains the most widely used and specific means to detect HCMV infection.[3] Serological studies, employing any of several methods, have important adjunctive roles. Seroconversion or detection of HCMV-specific IgM in the absence of HCMV-specific IgG supports recent primary infection, whereas detection of fourfold or greater rises in HCMV-specific IgG levels suggests reactivation or, possibly, reinfection. Molecular techniques can be used to identify HCMV nucleic acids in tissues or body fluids and to determine genetic similarities between HCMV isolates.

Prevention and Therapy. At present, congenital or acquired HCMV infections cannot be prevented by vaccination. Several live virus vaccines, prepared from attenuated laboratory strains of HCMV (Towne or AD169), have been studied during the past two decades.[2,4] These candidate vaccines induce cellular and humoral immune responses against both wild and laboratory HCMV strains but have not prevented infection in such patients as renal transplant recipients. Some studies, however, suggest that vaccination reduces the severity of disease induced by HCMV.[11] Other strategies, such as the use of subunit vaccines, require further investigation.

Several critical factors that contribute to natural HCMV transmission, such as the minimum infectious dose or the exact nature of the contact necessary to transmit the virus, have not been determined with certainty. Thus, measures that uniformly interrupt natural routes of HCMV transmission have not been established. When compared with other viral pathogens, HCMV is not highly contagious. Because infection usually results from direct contact with fresh, HCMV-infected secretions, attention to hygienic principles, such as good handwashing and the adoption of universal precautions in hospital environments, probably diminishes the risk of transmission to exposed individuals. Similarly, condoms may diminish the potential risk of sexual transmission of HCMV.

Fomites presumably contribute to HCMV transmission in day care or nursery environments,[12] and the potential for transmission can be reduced by prompt disposal of soiled diapers and disinfection of environmental surfaces. In child care environments, mouthing toys can be disinfected by immersion in a bleach and water solution, prepared fresh daily by adding 1/4 cup household bleach to 1 gallon of water. Items that cannot be immersed or washed with disinfectant solutions should be thoroughly air-dried, a practice that usually renders HCMV noninfectious.

In seronegative patients who are at high risk for severe HCMV disease (e.g., marrow or organ transplant recipients), certain strategies may reduce the risk of primary HCMV infection. The most effective is to avoid transfusion of blood products or transplantation of tissues from HCMV-seropositive donors.[13] The same approach can prevent transmission of HCMV to small (< 1500 g) premature infants or infants undergoing large volume exchange transfusions.[14] When seronegative blood is unavailable, leukocyte depletion of seropositive red cell units may reduce the risk of HCMV infection.[15] However, further studies are necessary to confirm the efficacy of the latter approach.

When blood products or tissues (such as matched organs or marrow) from HCMV-seropositive donors cannot be avoided or when patients are seropositive before transplantation and at risk for HCMV reactivation, therapeutic strategies that may potentially prevent infection or reduce the severity of disease include passive immunotherapy or prophylaxis with antiviral drugs. These strategies remain experimental and must be tailored to the underlying clinical disorder and the associated risk for HCMV disease. We caution that infectious disease experts should be consulted to obtain updated information about HCMV prophylaxis or treatment in immunocompromised patients.

The role for cytomegalovirus immune globulin in preventing or treating HCMV infections has not been characterized fully. Studies in marrow or renal transplant recipients, however, suggest that although immune globulin therapy may not prevent infection, such therapy can modify or prevent certain HCMV-related complications, such as pneumonitis.[16] Various regimens of immune globulin have been used, but common to all is an attempt to provide passive protection during the high-risk period for HCMV infection, typically the first 3 to 4 months after transplantation. Immune globulin therapy usually has been initiated before marrow transplantation or within 72 hours of renal transplantation and has been continued at weekly or monthly intervals for up to 120 days. Thus far, the side effects of immune globulin therapy have been minor, consisting of headache, fever, nausea and vomiting, or flushing.

Of the various prophylactic antiviral drugs investigated to date, only acyclovir, a 2′-deoxyguanosine analogue, has been moderately effective in preventing HCMV infections in patients undergoing marrow or renal transplantation. In a study of HCMV-seropositive marrow recipients, acyclovir given intravenously at 500 mg/m^2 q8h. for 5 days before and continued for up to 30 days after transplantation reduced the incidence and severity of HCMV disease.[17] Similarly, acyclovir diminished the risk for HCMV disease in a controlled study of renal transplant recipients.[18] In this study, the drug was given orally at daily doses ranging from 800 to 3200 mg beginning 6 hours before and continuing for 30 days after transplantation. In contrast to the potential prophylactic benefits of acyclovir, the drug has been ineffective when used to treat established HCMV infections.

Although several different antiviral agents, including cytarabine, vidarabine, ribavirin, and the interferons, possess anti-HCMV activity in vitro, none has clinical utility for symptomatic HCMV infections. Recent trials suggest that two other agents, ganciclovir (9-[1,3-dihydroxy-2-propoxy)methyl]guanine; DHPG) and foscarnet (trisodium phosphonoformate), can be used to treat HCMV pneumonitis, retinitis, gastroenteritis, or CNS infections.[19-21] Despite encouraging results with these agents, successful therapy of HCMV infections in immunocompromised hosts remains a major clinical challenge.

Ganciclovir, a 2′-deoxyguanosine analogue that inhibits HCMV DNA synthesis, has been used at doses of 2.5 mg/kg t.i.d. or 5.0 mg/kg b.i.d. given intravenously over 1 hour for 10 to 14 days.[19,20] Patients with AIDS and serious HCMV disease, such as retinitis, must be maintained subsequently on ganciclovir, 25 to 35 mg/kg/wk, indefinitely to prevent relapses.[3] Potential adverse effects of ganciclovir therapy include bone marrow suppression (neutropenia, thrombocytopenia; present in 20% to 40% of patients), rash, nausea and vomiting, and central nervous system complications (seizures, altered mental status).[20] Among more than 200 immunocompromised patients reported by the Syntex Collaborative Ganciclovir Treatment Study Group, nearly 80% improved or stabilized during ganciclovir therapy for HCMV-induced retinitis, gastroenteritis, or pneumonitis.[19]

Foscarnet interferes with HCMV replication by binding with the viral DNA polymerase and possesses anti-HCMV activity in vitro and in vivo.[19] HCMV-infected marrow or renal transplant recipients, treated with foscarnet in doses ranging from 20 to 200 mg/kg/d intravenously for 1 to 4 or more weeks, frequently have shown favorable clinical responses, as measured by resolution of fever, clearance of HCMV from blood or urine, and improved survival.[20,21] Potential toxic effects consist of altered serum calcium levels, decreased renal function, elevations of hepatic enzymes, hallucinations, and tremor.[20]

Marrow transplant recipients with HCMV pneumonitis have not responded favorably to single-drug or combination therapy with the available antiviral agents.[22] Such therapeutic failures led to a novel strategy—using antiviral agents in concert with immunoglobulin. Recent studies suggest that combined therapy with ganciclovir and intravenous immunoglobulin (IVIG) enhances survival in marrow transplant patients with HCMV pneumonitis.[22-24] The regimens reported to date vary but typically consist of an induction phase (ganciclovir 7.5 to 10 mg/kg/d for 10 to 21 days and IVIG 400 to 500 mg/kg q.o.d. for up to 21 days) and a maintenance phase (ganciclovir 5 mg/kg/d for approximately 30 days and IVIG 100 to 500 mg/kg given 1 to 5 times per week).[22] Combined antiviral drug and IVIG therapy appears highly promising and requires further controlled clinical trials.

Acute Gastrointestinal Infections

Arnold S. Monto

Enteric illnesses are second only to respiratory illnesses in causing acute disease in the U.S. population. Based on the Household Interview Survey, it has been estimated that 21 million episodes involving restricted activity or medical attention occur annually. Enteric disease is of even greater consequence in the developing countries. There, in an interplay with malnutrition and acute respiratory infection, it is responsible for a major portion of infant mortality. Until the last decade, there were few studies of frequency and patterns of occurrence in developed country populations of the common enteric illnesses, self-limited diseases with symptoms of vomiting, diarrhea, and abdominal pain, alone or in combination. This reflects the lack of knowledge of the principal etiological agents involved. Now, an increasing number of viral and bacterial pathogens have been identified as etiological agents, and greater attention is being paid to the problem.

As with respiratory disease, enteric illnesses are most common in young children, and incidence falls with increasing age. The actual annual number of episodes experienced has varied from study to study, depending on population evaluated and methods used to ascertain occurrence. In the Cleveland Family Study, it was found that children under the age of 10 years experienced approximately two episodes a year, whereas young adults had somewhat more than one such acute attack each year. School attendance was associated with an increase in illness frequency, as was increasing family size.[1] In the Tecumseh Study, with different methods of ascertaining occurrence of illness and a broader population group, illness frequency again varied with age. Mean annual incidence was 1.9 in the under 5 year olds, 1.2 in the 5- to 19-year age group, and 1.0 in adults.[2] The episodes occurred mainly in the colder months of the year, with 28.3% occurring in autumn, 36.7% in winter, 18.3% in spring, and 16.7% in summer.

In Tecumseh, as in Cleveland, a problem in interpretation arose from the overlap of respiratory and gastrointestinal symptoms in the same illness. Approximately 25% of people with gastrointestinal illness observed during 6 years of study in Tecumseh also had respiratory symptoms, with the highest overlap in children under 5 years of age. In the Cleveland Study, the combined respiratory-gastrointestinal syndrome made up 20% of all cases of gastrointestinal illness, and the frequency of association of the two types of symptoms in the same illness was much higher than would be expected by chance alone. Thus, it appears that certain specific agents may be responsible for this combined illness.

Studies of the common enteric illnesses have determined if specific agents can be associated with particular syndromes or certain seasons of the year. It is now known that at least three groups of viruses, the rotaviruses, the Norwalk-like agents, and certain adenoviruses, are significantly involved in such illnesses. The adenoviruses are discussed elsewhere as etiological agents of respiratory disease. The ones involved in gastrointestinal disease were identified by electron microscopy more often from hospitalized children with enteric illness than from controls. These viruses could not be grown in standard cell culture.[3] Other studies confirmed the etiological role of these agents, which have been identified also in a number of outbreaks, especially among infants. These particular adenoviruses belong to a limited number of serotypes, share nucleic acid characteristics in common (subgroup F), and have been grown in a special cell culture, 293.[4]

Other viruses, including astroviruses, caliciviruses, reoviruses, and coronaviruses, have been reported in some enteric illnesses and outbreaks. In most cases, they have been identified by electron microscopy from cases of illness. It is not yet clear if any or all of them are truly etiologically associated with disease, since the necessary controlled or experimental investigations have yet to be performed. However, association with disease has been most convincingly demonstrated with the astroviruses and caliciviruses. Certain bacteria, other than the salmonella and shigella, are known to be involved in enteric illnesses. These are toxigenic, invasive, and enteropathogenic strains of *Escherichia coli*. They are described on page 178.

ROTAVIRUSES

The rotaviruses are double-stranded RNA-containing viruses belonging to the family Reoviridae. The name "rotavirus" was suggested for the group on the basis of the wheel-like appearance of complete virions on electron microscopy. They can be distinguished on the basis of morphology and other characteristics from true reoviruses and orbiviruses and have been variously termed in earlier descriptions human reovirus-like agents and duoviruses. The rotaviruses cause diarrhea in humans and in several species of domestic animals.[5,6] The animal agents can be grown readily in a number of generally available cell systems. However, this is not true of the human rotaviruses, which cannot be grown in cell culture except under special circumstances, such as pretreatment of specimens with trypsin. Other methods must, therefore, be employed in most laboratories to detect the human agents. Initially, all studies used electron microscopy to identify the virus. It is now known that this was possible because it is so abundant in stool, with a titer of 10^8 or 10^9 particles per gram. A number of alternate techniques have been developed for detection of virus. The enzyme-linked immunosorbent assay (ELISA) has the greatest use, since it is sensitive and can be done without special equipment.[7] It is also useful, with modification, for detection of antibody.

Much of the information on the pathogenesis of the disease comes from work with animal agents.[8] Microscopically, the sides and tips of the villi are most affected, especially in the lower part of the small intestine. In severe cases, there is almost complete destruction of the villi. Damage to the brush-bordered epithelium produces a local decrease in disaccharidases, which results in accumulation of lactose and other disaccharides in the bowel. Fluids accumulate in the lumen osmotically, resulting in diarrhea and a degree of malabsorption. Immunity to rotaviruses is acquired at an early age and is transmitted transplacentally. Infants in newborn nurseries are infected frequently but usually do not experience disease, even if not breast fed, which suggests that circulating IgG antibody may protect.[9]

The rotavirus genome contains 11 segments. The genes coding for the various antigens of biological importance have been identified, and the complex antigenic structure of the virus has been clarified. This structure is of importance in view of work in vaccine development. There is a group antigen, as well as subgroup and serotype antigens. Most rotaviruses of humans are in group A. Nongroup A viruses have been isolated in China from outbreaks of unusual characteristics.[10]

Distribution of Disease. Aside from the outbreaks described above, rotavirus diarrhea is mainly a disease of infants and small children. Characteristically, the children ill enough to be hospitalized are febrile, and half have vomiting in addition to diarrhea. Dehydration is a typical feature of these illnesses. The incidence of diarrheal disease associated with rotaviruses resulting in a visit to a physician can be estimated to be 15/100 children under the age of 1 year.[11] It is also known that in developed countries close to 50% of children age 1 to 3 years, hospitalized for severe diarrhea, are infected with rotaviruses.[12] A similar frequency of rotaviruses in severe dehydrating diarrhea has been found in several developing countries. Since the total incidence of such illnesses is higher there than in developed countries and the events are associated with mortality and malnutrition, it is apparent that rotaviruses are of critical importance in the Third World.[13]

In the temperate zone, rotaviruses exhibit a distinct seasonal pattern, with infections most common in the colder months of the year. During peak months, more than 75% of children hospitalized with diarrhea are infected with the agent.[14] Studies in families have not been carried out extensively, but it is already clear that transmission does occur, with reinfection of older children and adults.[15]

Prevention and Control. Rotaviruses are stable agents, relatively resistant to adverse environmental conditions. They are not inactivated by lipid solvents, are acid stable, and can remain on surfaces and in water for prolonged periods. Since fecal-oral transmission is the likely method of acquisition, interruption of this mechanism by appropriate interventions is a possible means of prophylaxis, recognizing the possible persistence of the agent. Since rotaviruses possess a segmented genome, it should be possible through reassortment recombination to create an attenuated variant for vaccine purposes. Vaccines prepared by this method and those using viruses of animal origin are currently under study. These studies, although generally encouraging, occasionally have produced conflicting results, in part reflecting prior antibody status of diverse populations and differing antigenic makeup of the preparation. Such a vaccine could be especially useful in the developing countries where, interacting with malnutrition, the virus is responsible for considerable childhood mortality.

Norwalk-like Agents

Characteristics, Pathogenesis, and Distribution. This distinct group of agents is responsible for outbreaks of enteric disease with diarrhea, vomiting, and systemic symptoms. Disease has occurred among residents of institutions and individuals of all ages living in families. The etiological agents have never been grown in cell culture but have been visualized on electron microscopy. On the basis of appearance and size, they have been termed the 27 nm, parovirus-like, or Norwalk agent, the latter referring to an outbreak from which the most thoroughly studied strain was isolated.[16] The viruses are acid and ether stable and relatively resistant to heat.[17] Thus, it is not surprising that they have been involved in waterborne outbreaks.

There are a number of different serotypes of the agent, some of which are quite distinct antigenically from the others.[18] No animal strains with shared antigens have been identified. These facts have presented great difficulties in the study of the behavior of the agents in population groups. In addition, the virus is present in relatively small quantities in the stool. Thus, it may not be visualized easily without the use of immune serum for clumping of the virus (immune electron microscopy).[19] It also means that stool is not as rich a source of virus that can then be used as a reagent in seroepidemiology.

In spite of the problems posed by these observations, valuable information has been gathered on the Norwalk-like agents. Antibody is not acquired very early in life, as is the situation with the rotaviruses. Its later acquisition indicates that widespread exposure to these viruses is somewhat delayed. In keeping with this finding, when adults are challenged experimentally, disease often results. Typically, illness consists of combinations of diarrhea, vomiting, low-grade fever, abdominal cramps, and malaise. Upper gastrointestinal symptoms usually predominate, and the illness has a relatively short duration. Microscopically, in the proximal intestine, there is mucosal inflammation, villous shortening, crypt hypertrophy, and absorptive cell abnormalities.[20] When a group of volunteers was challenged with this virus, half experienced self-limited illness with characteristic vomiting or diarrhea or both after an incubation period of approximately 1 to 2 days. On rechallenge of the same volunteers 2 or more years later, the same individuals who had initially experienced illness again were sick. On further rechallenge 4 to 8 weeks thereafter, most of those who previously had developed illness were protected.[21] Thus, immunity to the Norwalk-like agents is complicated, and there may be specific receptors involved that could well be genetically determined.

Prevention and Control. Work with these viruses has been hampered by technical difficulties, and any conclusions on control must be regarded as tentative. The principles of environmental control discussed for the rotaviruses probably apply to the Norwalk-like agents. These viruses do affect adults and are stable, and they have occurred in familial and institutional-propagated outbreaks. They also have been associated with waterborne outbreaks in which large numbers of cases have occurred. In the former situation, prevention of the opportunity for fecal-oral transmission will be useful. In the latter, proper handling of sources of water has been associated with cessation of outbreaks. Coliform counts can be useful as an indication of the effectiveness of treatment of the water. Until more is known of the precise nature of the virus and until it can be cultivated in some way, vaccine development will be impossible.

Trachoma and Inclusion Conjunctivitis

Julius Schachter

Trachoma, a chronic inflammation of the mucous membranes lining the eyelid and eyeball, is the leading cause of preventable blindness in the world. Inclusion conjunctivitis is an acute infection of newborns and sexually active adults that usually heals spontaneously without sequelae even if not treated. Trachoma and inclusion conjunctivitis may, in fact, be two forms of eye diseases caused by the same organism or may be different aspects of the same clinical spectrum. These two diseases, however, have different epidemiological patterns and present very real differences in terms of relevance to public health and control measures.

Etiology. The etiological agents of trachoma and inclusion conjunctivitis, formerly referred to as the "TRIC" agents and originally believed to be viruses, now are classified as chlamydiae. Some human chlamydial diseases, such as trachoma, have been known since antiquity, but the recognized clinical spectrum still is expanding. The current human diseases attributed to chlamydiae are summarized in Table 7–4.

Trachoma and inclusion conjunctivitis are caused by *Chlamydia trachomatis.* This species also includes the causative agent of lymphogranuloma venereum (LGV). These organisms are obligatory intracellular bacteria that are placed in an order (Chlamydiales) separated from other microorganisms because of a unique developmental cycle. The other organisms in the same genus are *Chlamydia psittaci,* the causative agent of psittacosis and a variety of mammalian and avian infections, and *Chlamydia pneumoniae,* a human respiratory pathogen.

Chlamydia trachomatis may be separated into 15 related serotypes. Three (designated L1, L2, and L3) comprise the LGV strains, which may be differentiated from the others by biological properties. Trachoma in the endemic and blinding form has been associated with types A, Ba, B, and C, whereas types D, E, F, G, H, I, J, and K have been associated with inclusion conjunctivitis and genital tract disease. It is not known whether these differentiations represent sampling limitations or geographical distribution or reflect biological properties of the organism. The trachoma-associated serotypes are rarely, and in some cases have never been, recovered from genital tract infections. The genital strains have been associated with eye disease (inclusion conjunctivitis) and, in some instances, with a disease clinically indistinguishable from trachoma.

Extraocular infections with trachoma organisms do occur, and many children in endemic trachoma areas have infections of the upper pulmonary or gastrointestinal tracts. Relevance of this observation to pathogenesis of trachoma or to *C. trachomatis*-

TABLE 7-4. HUMAN DISEASES CAUSED BY *CHLAMYDIA*

Species	Serotype[a]	Disease
Chlamydia psittaci	Many unidentified serotypes	Psittacosis
Chlamydia trachomatis	L1, L2, L3	Lymphogranuloma venereum
	A, B, Ba, C	Hyperendemic blinding trachoma
	D, E, F, G, H, I, J, K	Inclusion conjunctivitis (adult and newborn), otitis, nongonococcal urethritis, cervicitis, salpingitis, proctitis, epididymitis, and pneumonia of newborns
Chlamydia pneumoniae	One	Pneumonia, other respiratory disease

[a]Predominant but not exclusive association of serotype with disease.

induced extraocular disease is not clear. Persistence of extraocular infection may well have implications for the efficacy of topical chemotherapy.

TRACHOMA

Distribution and Public Health Significance. Trachoma is usually more severe in poorer populations. With increased economic development, it becomes milder and may disappear in time. Blinding trachoma is a major public health problem in developing countries in North Africa, sub-Saharan Africa, the Middle East, and the drier regions of the Indian subcontinent and Southeast Asia. Small areas with blinding trachoma are recognized in Australia, the Pacific Islands, and Latin America.

Trachoma was once a major problem in the United States. The last pockets of blinding trachoma were found on the American Indian reservations. Control programs and improved environmental conditions have reduced the consequences, but mild trachoma can still persist. Active trachoma cases may be imported from endemic areas, and although they should be treated, they are not a major public health problem because hygienic conditions in the United States are not conducive to spread.

Clinical Description. In areas where blinding trachoma is endemic, the onset of the disease is usually in young children. Trachoma is a chronic follicular conjunctivitis with varying degrees of papillary hypertrophy and inflammatory infiltration of the conjunctiva and corneal pannus. Bacterial superinfection contributes significantly to the pathogenesis of the disease. As trachoma progresses, scarring of the conjunctiva may develop, with progression from fine linear scars to broader confluent scars. As a result of scarring, the major potentially blinding sequelae slowly develop. These lesions, called trichiasis and entropion (distortion of the lids in the inward direction so that the eyelashes abrade the cornea), cause the corneal damage that ultimately results in visual loss. The end result of blindness usually develops many years after active inflammatory disease has waned. Active disease peaks in the early childhood years, whereas the blinding lesions resulting from contraction of scars and tear deficiencies may occur 25 or more years later.

Classification. Trachoma cases usually are classified in stages according to the McCallan classification, which scores conjunctival findings of follicles and scars. This classification has not been useful in evaluating the impact of trachoma on a community, since it does not identify the potentially disabling lesions. A modification that classifies intensity of active inflammatory diseases and potentially disabling, irreversible lesions recently has come into use.

Transmission. Trachoma usually is transmitted from child to child and occurs in families. Concomitant bacterial infections increase the severity of the disease and the quantity of ocular discharges. These discharges are spread by contact and also by moisture-seeking flies, which act as mechanical vectors of chlamydiae in traveling from eye to eye.

Treatment and Control. Trachoma responds more to improved hygiene, sanitary conditions, and economic development than to specific measures. In hyperendemic areas, virtually all children are infected in the first months of life, and active disease progresses for several years. It is almost impossible to institute mass systemic treatment with any antichlamydial drug under such conditions. Thus, the thrust of trachoma control has been not to eradicate the disease but to prevent blinding complications. Periodic intermittent topical treatment with tetracyclines has been recommended by the World Health Organization (WHO) as the method of choice. This probably works in reducing the load of *Chlamydia* as well as minimizing the secondary bacterial infections, thus decreasing the severity of the disease and minimizing the development of blinding sequelae.

INCLUSION CONJUNCTIVITIS

Distribution and Public Health Significance. Inclusion conjunctivitis occurs in two distinct age groups and generally is considered to be a sporadic disease occurring in industrialized societies. The disease, which is not considered a cause of blindness, affects neonates and sexually active adults. The incidence of inclusion conjunctivitis is a reflection of the larger genital tract reservoir of the agent. Incidence of the adult form is not known, but it is considered one of the most common forms of follicular conjunctivitis. Cohort studies indicate that 30% to 50% of infants exposed to the organism during the birth process will develop chlamydial conjunctivitis. Prevalence rates in maternal cervix cover a wide range, with rates from 2% to 30% being reported.

Clinical Description. The adult form (AIC) is an acute follicular conjunctivitis that is usually self-limited. Keratitis is common, and occasionally the disease is chronic. In infants, inclusion conjunctivitis of the newborn (ICN) is usually a mucopurulent conjunctivitis that occurs 1 to 2 weeks after birth. The disease generally is considered to be self-limiting, although conjunctival scarring may develop, and chronic forms, with visual debility resulting later in life, have been identified.

Transmission. AIC results from inoculation of the conjunctiva with infective genital tract discharges. Before the introduction of chlorination this was one of the forms of swimming pool conjunctivitis. ICN results from infection of the neonate during passage through an infected birth canal. The chlamydiae are spread through the population by sexual activity. Genital tract infections are very common, eye disease is relatively uncommon, and eye to eye transmission is rare.

Treatment and Control. Inclusion conjunctivitis in the infant is not prevented by Credé prophylaxis (silver nitrate drops), used for the prevention of gonococcal ophthalmia neonatorum.

Inclusion conjunctivitis in adults always calls for systemic treatment because the individuals almost always have genital tract infection. Three-week courses with tetracycline, erythromycin, or sulfonamides at full doses are recommended. Neonatal inclusion conjunctivitis may be treated topically, although high failure rates are observed. It is not known whether this failure is due to inadequate administration of the drug or reflects inadequate treatment. With the recent recognition that *C. trachomatis* is a cause of pneumonia in infants, it seems prudent to recommend systemic treatment with erythromycin (50 mg/kg in divided doses given four times daily for 2 weeks).

Chlamydial Pneumonia

Julius Schachter

Chlamydia trachomatis is a common sexually transmitted pathogen. It is the major identifiable cause of nongonococcal urethritis in men and is commonly found in the cervices of sexually active women. The infant born through an infected birth canal is at risk of acquiring the infection. A neonatal conjunctivitis (inclusion conjunctivitis of the newborn) has been recognized since early in this century. Only since 1975 has it been known that the same agent is capable of producing systemic disease in such exposed infants.

A characteristic pneumonia syndrome in infants has been shown to be caused by these organisms. The disease is characterized by a chronic afebrile course, a staccato cough (without the inspiratory whoop of pertussis) and tachypnea, marked elevation of immunoglobulins, and a relative eosinophilia. Chlamydial pneumonia is found often in infants infected with other potential pulmonary tract pathogens.

History or presence of inclusion conjunctivitis of the newborn (ICN) is common. Minor upper respiratory signs often precede the development of pneumonia. Some of the children have otitis. These infants do not appear to be severely ill, although x-rays may show the appearance of extensive interstitial pneumonia. Biopsies have demonstrated both interstitial pneumonitis and a rather severe necrotizing bronchiolitis. The disease usually develops in the second month of life, although incubation periods ranging from 3 weeks to 4 months have been observed. In the absence of treatment, the course tends to be prolonged, but ultimately the infants recover. Systemic treatment with sulfonamides or erythromycin does not provide dramatic response but does result in more rapid recovery. Most infected infants have decreased respiratory function and many become asthmatic.

This disease appears to be relatively common. Preliminary surveys indicate it may represent 30% to 50% of of pneumonias seen in infants less than 6 months of age.

Approximately 10% to 20% of the exposed infants do develop pneumonia. In settings where there is a high maternal carrier rate for *C. trachomatis,* it seems reasonable to screen for these infections and to treat the pregnant woman to prevent transmission to the newborn.

Streptococcal Disease

Leon Gordis

Streptococcal infections are among the most frequent bacterial infections in human populations. Their importance lies in both the immediate morbidity associated with these infections and in the nonsuppurative sequelae they produce—acute rheumatic fever and glomerulonephritis. A basic understanding of the biology of the streptococcus is essential for understanding the epidemiology of these infections and of their nonsuppurative sequelae and for developing a rational program of treatment and prevention.

Streptococci are classified as hemolytic or nonhemolytic. When grown on blood agar plates, beta-hemolytic strains are surrounded by a clear zone of hemolysis, whereas alpha-hemolytic strains are surrounded by green zones of hemolysis. The beta-hemolytic strains can be subdivided into groups designated A, B, C, and so on on the basis of serologically specific carbohydrates in their cell wall. Over 90% of human streptococcal infections are caused by group A strains. Current evidence indicates that rheumatic fever can follow only group A streptococcal infections.

As seen in Figure 7–5,[1] the cell wall of the streptococcus is a three-layered structure: the outer layer contains the protein antigens, the middle layer the group-specific carbohydrates, and the inner layer the peptidoglycan (mucopeptide). The cell wall encloses a central core of cytoplasm surrounded by a distinct cytoplasmic membrane.

The protein layer of the cell wall contains M, T, and R proteins. The M protein is most important for several reasons. It is antigenic and immunologically distinct and stimulates production of type-specific antibodies in the infected person. The M protein appears to be localized in hairlike fimbriae that may facilitate the adherence of the streptococcus to epithelial linings. On the basis of their M proteins, the group A strains can be subdivided into serological types, and these types are designated types 1, 2, 3, and so on. Well over 60 types have now been identified. The antibodies produced in response to the M antigen of each type are type-specific bactericidal antibodies that confer long-lasting immunity, possibly for life, to the particular serological type causing the infection. Since the antibodies are type-

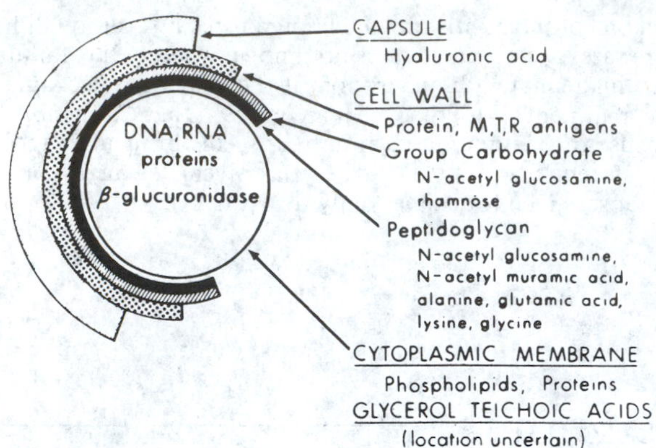

Figure 7-5. Schematic representation of cellular components of beta-hemolytic streptococci. [*From Krause.*[1]]

specific, they do not protect against infection with other types. Consequently, successive streptococcal infections in the same person are usually caused by different serological types, although under certain circumstances, there may be cross-protection. Formation of these antibodies may be suppressed by treatment with antibiotics, in which case reinfection by the same serotype is possible.[2]

The group A streptococci secrete a number of important extracellular products, including streptolysin O, streptolysin S, erythrogenic toxin, NADase, several DNAases, hyaluronidase, streptokinase, and proteinase. Several of these are antigenic and can, therefore, be used in antibody tests for streptococcal infections. For example, streptolysin O is the basis for the anti-streptolysin O (ASO) test, which is the best standardized antibody test for streptococcal infections thus far available. The anti-DNAse B test is another useful serological test for detecting streptococcal infections. Erythrogenic toxin is the cause of the rash of scarlet fever and stimulates a specific antitoxin. There is no evidence to suggest that any of the specific extracellular products produced by the streptococcus is the etiological factor in rheumatic fever.

The human oropharynx appears to be the main natural reservoir for hemolytic streptococci. Streptococci have also been transmitted from nasal, anal, and vaginal streptococcal carriers. The incubation period is approximately 24 to 48 hours. After infection, antibodies to the antigenic extracellular products of the streptococcus develop relatively rapidly and reach a maximum level at about 3 to 4 weeks, following which they gradually decline. The type-specific antibodies to M proteins take longer to rise and persist for protracted periods of time.

In many of the early reports of streptococcal transmission through food outbreaks, milk and milk products were responsible. Foods contaminated during preparation, such as egg salad, also have been implicated. Droplet transmission does not appear to play a major role in person to person transmission. Infection is caused primarily by intimate or direct contact.

STREPTOCOCCAL PHARYNGITIS

Streptococcal pharyngitis has been called "an occupational disease of schoolchildren." In addition, as the number of day care centers has increased in recent years, the group A streptococcus has been shown to be an important pathogen in this setting as well.[3]

The sudden onset of fever, pain, swelling, or beefy redness of the pharynx, with exudate and tender cervical nodes, represent a characteristic syndrome of the streptococcal sore throat. A scarlatinal rash is diagnostic when it occurs, but it is much less frequent today than it was in the past. The classic findings of streptococcal disease are more likely to be present during epidemics, and the diagnosis of streptococcal pharyngitis during endemic periods is extremely difficult on a clinical basis. The diagnosis is even more difficult when tonsils are absent and when the patient is seen only once during the course of the illness. Several studies have shown that physicians can correctly diagnose streptococcal infections clinically in 55% to 75% of cases.

A major problem is in distinguishing mild streptococcal illnesses from viral infections of the upper respiratory tract. Conjunctivitis, coryza, hoarseness, and tracheitis are more likely to be caused by viral infections. Pharyngeal redness alone is not enough to distinguish a streptococcal infection. Even an exudate may not be a sufficiently reliable sign, since exudative pharyngitis also has been described in adenoviral and coxsackie viral infections. Appropriate laboratory tests must, therefore, be carried out for diagnosing streptococcal infections.

Throat cultures are an important technique for diagnosing streptococcal infection. Although such cultures are often available in public health laboratories, they can be readily done also in the physician's office using inexpensive prepared media and a low cost incubator. Sheep blood agar is superior for recognizing beta-hemolytic streptococci and is available in disposable plastic plates from many commercial laboratories. The technique for streaking a blood agar plate in order to identify streptococci has been well described by Wannamaker.[4] When necessary, swabs well moistened with pharyngeal secretions may be kept for several hours at room temperature before inoculation. The plates can be read after overnight incubation at 37° C. Beta-hemolytic streptococci hemolyze the blood cells in the medium completely and are, therefore, completely surrounded by a clear halo in contrast to the greenish area visible around alpha-streptococci.

Grouping is generally not necessary, since most streptococcal infections are caused by group A organisms, but when grouping is indicated, several approaches are possible. Antisera are available commercially for grouping streptococci by the Lancefield precipitin method. Fluorescent antibody techniques also are available. A simple practical method for identifying group A streptococcal strains was developed by Maxted in 1953.[5] He showed that a 0.02 unit bacitracin disk applied to a culture of streptococci growing on blood agar will inhibit group A but not nongroup A strains. The fluorescent antibody technique and the bacitracin disk method are 90% accurate when compared with the Lancefield method.

Physicians should be encouraged to take and read their own throat cultures. Not only is this approach economical, but a number of studies have shown that physicians can read such cultures with considerable accuracy after minimal training. This approach also eliminates the delay inherent in sending cultures to a laboratory and waiting for the report. When this is not feasible, however, state and other laboratories should be used appropriately.

In recent years, with the decline in the nonsuppurative sequelae of group A streptococcal infections, the value of throat cultures has been called into question. However, a negative throat culture has a high negative predictive value and thus can contribute to avoiding needless use of antibiotic treatment in children with acute pharyngitis.[6] Furthermore, in view of the reported outbreaks of rheumatic fever in several U.S. cities in recent years, as well as the high risk in many developing countries, throat cultures remain important for the prompt diagnosis of streptococcal infection and the prevention of rheumatic fever.

In addition to attempting to isolate streptococci from throat cultures of individuals suspected of having had streptococcal infections, it is possible to obtain serological confirmation of streptococcal infections even when the organism can no longer be isolated from the throat or the skin. The most frequently employed antibody test is the ASO test, which has been well standardized. The antigen, streptolysin O, is readily available commercially, and the procedure can be performed by most laboratories with reliable results. The highest dilution of the patient's serum that inhibits lysis of red blood cells by 1 unit of streptolysin O is the end point. The ASO titer is expressed in units as the reciprocal of the end point dilution. The series of dilutions most commonly used results in the following progression of titers: 12, 50, 100, 125, 166, 250, 333, 500, 625, 833, 1250, and 2500.

The ASO titer increases from infancy, and highest levels are found in school-age children. Titers as high as 250 units are common in well children ages 6 to 14 years in the north temperate part of the United States. In this age group, a single titer of 333 units is considered borderline, and a titer of 500 units is considered indicative of a recent streptococcal infection. A single low or borderline titer does not exclude a streptococcal infection. Regardless of the initial level, a rise or fall in titer of two or more increments (tube dilutions) in serial specimens is considered significant. It is best to perform the test on serial specimens simultaneously. In cases where the ASO is negative, additional antistreptococcal antibody determinations may be useful. These include the anti-DNAse B and the antihyaluronidase tests. Recent years have seen the marketing of rapid antigen tests for group A streptococci. In general, these tests have high specificities, but their sensitivities have not been as good, particularly when the amount of streptococcal antigen present is small.[7] Technology in this area is progressing rapidly, so that these tests may be of considerable value in the diagnosis and prevention of streptococcal infections and their sequelae.

STREPTOCOCCAL PYODERMA

Although pharyngitis is one of the most common manifestations of streptococcal infection, streptococcal pyoderma and, specifically, impetigo skin infections have been shown to precede the development of glomerulonephritis. Impetigo is primarily a disease of the summer, a time when respiratory infections are infrequent. It often will follow some type of skin trauma. Streptococci can be transferred to the skin from the respiratory tract but rarely in the reverse direction. Different serological types can coexist in the skin lesions and in the throat. Streptococcal infections of the skin differ in a number of ways from streptococcal pharyngitis, as shown in Table 7-5.

Since it appears that treatment of pyoderma, even when effective, may not prevent subsequent glomerulonephritis, attempts have been made at prophylaxis of skin infections. However, such attempts have produced only temporary control of streptococcal infections at best, so that mass prophylaxis does not appear feasible.

SCARLET FEVER

Scarlet fever results from infection with strains of beta-hemolytic streptococci that produce erythrogenic toxin. The illness occurs primarily in children between the ages of 2 and 8 years. It is most frequent during the winter and spring months. The clinical findings generally include those symptoms seen in streptococcal sore throat plus a classic skin rash. The rash usually is erythematous and punctate and blanches on pressure. The rash is often most visible on the neck, chest, and skin folds and does not involve the face. Desquamation of the skin, particularly the tips of the fingers and the toes, is characteristic during convalescence. In the United States, the incidence of scarlet fever seems to have declined in recent years, and in particular the severity of the disease has decreased. As with other forms of streptococcal infection, nonsuppurative sequelae may follow this condition.

STREPTOCOCCAL TOXIC SHOCK-LIKE SYNDROME

In recent decades, streptococci generally have not caused very serious infections in developed countries, but in the late 1980s, severe streptococcal infections producing a toxic shock-like syndrome were reported. For example, Cone and associates[8] reported two patients with such a syndrome in California, and Stevens and colleagues[9] reported 20 cases of streptococcal infection in the Rocky Mountain region that were characterized by considerable tissue destruction and systemic disease, including renal impairment and a respiratory distress syndrome with a high case fatality rate. The disease seems to be linked to a streptococcal pyrogenic exotoxin and has again focused attention on the extracellular toxic products of the streptococcus that for many years attracted relatively little interest. The appearance of this condition over a relatively short period of time suggests that there has been an increase in the virulence of the streptococcal strains prevalent in many communities.

TREATMENT

The principal aim of treating streptococcal infections is to eliminate the organism from the nasopharynx. Clinical recovery alone is not sufficient and may occur even when the organism persists in the nasopharynx. The basic principles of antistreptococcal therapy are (1) selecting an appropriate antimicrobial agent, (2) administering it in sufficient dosage, and (3) maintaining therapeutic blood levels for 10 days. Penicillin is the drug of choice, and erythromycin is a satisfactory substitute when penicillin sensitivity precludes its use. Although sulfonamides have been shown to be effective in preventing streptococcal infection, they are not effective in treating streptococcal infection and should not be used for this purpose.

The most effective treatment procedure is a single intramuscular injection of benzathine penicillin, 600,000 to 900,000 units in children and 1.2 million units in adolescents and adults.[10] Such treatment will eliminate the streptococci in 95% of patients. Since benzathine penicillin may cause painful local reactions, it is useful to combine it with procaine penicillin. When this is done, it is essential that the total dose the patient receives contain the full recommended amount of benzathine penicillin G.

Oral penicillin, 200,000 to 250,000 units four times daily, also may be used, or twice-daily doses of 400,000 units for a full 10 days. Although the oral preparations of different penicillins appear to be equally effective when given in proper dosages, it is generally recommended that oral penicillin G be taken only under fasting conditions.

When patients are allergic to penicillin, erythromycin in a dose of 125 to 250 mg four times daily for 10 days is effective. Tetracyclines should probably be avoided because of reports of increasing numbers of tetracycline-resistant strains of group A streptococci.

Although oral medication has a number of advantages—it can be stopped if the culture is negative or if there is an allergic reaction, it is less likely to produce an allergy, and it is preferred by many patients over an injection—it has a major disadvantage, and that is the potential problem of patient noncompliance. A number of studies have shown that many children prescribed 10 days of penicillin failed to complete the course of therapy.[11] It is, therefore, essential that each patient and family be individually assessed regarding the likelihood that the patient will comply for a full 10 days. If the patient seems unlikely to comply, the intramuscular route should probably be selected.

Streptococcal Carriers. In certain patients, streptococci may persist in the nasopharynx for a long period after an untreated

TABLE 7-5. GENERAL FEATURES OF STREPTOCOCCAL INFECTIONS AT DIFFERENT SITES

Feature	Streptococcal Pharyngitis and Tonsillitis	Streptococcal Impetigo and Pyoderma
▪ Clinical		
Erythema	Usually present and generalized	Often minimal and localized to immediate area around lesion
Vesicular stage	Absent	Type of early lesion but transient
Pustular stage	Patchy exudate—sometimes confluent	Usually discrete; flora often mixed
Crusted stage	Absent	Frequent and characteristic
Local pain	Common—may be intense	Usually absent
Systemic reaction	Fever, headache, and malaise occur commonly	Unusual
Regional adenitis	Common	Less common, but adenopathy frequently seen
Course	Typically acute, except in infants	Often chronic
▪ Laboratory		
Leukocytosis	Usually present	Often absent
Bacteriological species	Group A streptococci usually predominate	Often also contain large numbers of staphylococci
Serological types of group A streptococci	Many different types	Few types predominate
Antistreptolysin O response	Common	Uncommon
▪ Epidemiology		
Seasonal occurrence	Winter and spring	Late summer and early fall
Common source epidemics	May occur	Not described
Geographical distribution	More common in temperate or cold climates	Common in hot or tropical climates
Age	Young school-age children	Children of preschool age
Sex	Equal	Equal
Transmission	Direct spread from human reservoirs, particularly nasal carriers	Unknown; insects may be mechanical vectors
Carrier state	Common in pharynx of many populations	Unusual in skin, except in certain situations
Preceding trauma	Not present	May predispose to natural or experimental infection
▪ Complications		
Acute nephritis	Occurs; preventability unknown	Occurs; preventability unknown
Acute rheumatic fever	Occurs; preventable	Does not occur
▪ Treatment		
Local	Not important	Removal of crusts and scrubbing with hexachlorophene soap
Systemic	Single injection of intramuscular benzathine penicillin or oral penicillin for 10 days	May not be necessary; extensive lesions may require intramuscular benzathine penicillin.

Adapted from Wannamaker LW: N Engl J Med 282:23–31, 78–85, 1970.

infection and occasionally even after several courses of antibiotics. Such carriers are usually only lightly colonized and not dangerous to others and also are unlikely to develop complications themselves. Such carriers, however, have posed therapeutic dilemmas in view of the failure of different antibiotic regimens to eradicate the organism. Because of the generally declining risk of nonsuppurative sequelae of streptococcal infections in developed countries, it would appear wise not to pursue the treatment of streptococcal carriers vigorously unless they are members of a family with a prior history of rheumatic fever.

Treatment of Family Contacts. A number of studies have shown that there is a relatively high rate of spread of streptococci when there is an active infection in a household. Although some physicians prescribe prophylactic doses of penicillin for several days for children and adults who have been in contact with the infected individual, some of these family contacts often already have positive cultures at the time the diagnosis is made in the index case. Consequently, prophylactic doses of penicillin in such individuals would be potentially dangerous, since they might suppress an overt infection but not eradicate the organism.[12] Although it might be desirable ideally to culture all members of the family, this often is not possible, particularly when patients lack a continuous relationship with a physician. A study showing that the risk of secondary cases was greater in low-income families with many children suggests that antibiotic therapy should be considered for asymptomatic siblings in such families.[13]

MASS CULTURING OF SCHOOLCHILDREN

A number of projects have been undertaken in different cities in the United States to culture the throats of schoolchildren, identify infected individuals, and exclude them from school until a negative culture is obtained.[14] Although there is some appeal to the idea of identifying such children in school populations and thereby preventing transmission to other children in order to prevent rheumatic fever and nephritis as well as the morbidity associated with streptococcal infections themselves, there does not appear to be sufficient justification for community-wide programs for culturing schoolchildren in most areas of the United States today. A case might be made, however, for conducting culturing programs on a limited basis in certain high-risk populations, such as inner-city schools, if they are shown to have had high streptococcal infection rates during the preceding years. In any such program, it is essential that the culturing go hand in hand with the provision of follow-up services and that an ongoing evaluation of the effectiveness of such a program be an integral component.

INFECTIONS WITH NONGROUP A ORGANISMS

Although the group A streptococci are by far the most important from the standpoint of human infections, particularly the subsequent development of rheumatic fever and nephritis, in recent years infections with streptococci of other serological groups have gained increasing prominence. Group B streptococci have been recognized to be important human pathogens.[15] Group B infections in early infancy are particularly serious. Neonatal meningitis as a result of group B infection is a major concern. Neonatal sepsis is another complication of group B infection. Aggressive antibiotic treatment is essential, and intravenous gamma globulin may be a useful adjunct.

Infection in early infancy seems to be associated with maternal colonization, prematurity, low birthweight, and prolonged rupture of the membranes. In one study, 19% of nonpregnant women were found to be vaginal carriers of group B organisms, and the carrier rate in pregnancy in another study was 28%. Group B streptococci have been isolated also from the throat, perianal skin, and urethra of the mothers. There is evidence that neonatal group B infections can be prevented in infants receiving an intramuscular injection of 50,000 units of aqueous penicillin immediately upon delivery.[16] Although it is potentially possible to develop a polyvalent vaccine, this does not appear to be a practical solution in the immediate future.

Group C streptococci also have been found to colonize newborns and to produce neonatal meningitis. Glomerulonephritis has been reported following group C streptococcal infection.

RHEUMATIC FEVER

A major sequel of group A streptococcal infections is rheumatic fever. In the past, the attack rate of rheumatic fever following streptococcal infections was about 3% in military populations and 0.3% in populations of schoolchildren. In the United States today, the attack rate may be much lower, but valid data are not available.

The diagnosis of rheumatic fever is made using the modified Jones criteria (Table 7-6). It is important to emphasize that the diagnosis is suspect in the absence of evidence of a preceding streptococcal infection. Most cases of rheumatic fever in the United States today are manifested by arthritis. Since carditis is the only manifestation that can lead to permanent sequelae, interest in prevention of rheumatic fever largely focuses on this manifestation. The arthritis seen in rheumatic fever invariably clears without any permanent damage. The carditis, on the other hand, may often lead to the development of rheumatic heart disease, particularly of the mitral valve.

There is no satisfactory animal model for rheumatic fever, and usually the streptococcus can no longer be isolated from the patient by the time acute rheumatic fever develops, since there is a latent period of several weeks between the streptococcal infection and the development of rheumatic fever. The evidence linking the streptococcus to rheumatic fever is of three general types. First, epidemiological data suggest that outbreaks of streptococcal infection often are followed by outbreaks of rheumatic fever.[17] Second, if the sera of children with acute rheumatic fever are examined for at least three streptococcal antibodies, evidence of a recent streptococcal infection can be obtained in 95%. Third, chemotherapeutic agents that prevent beta-hemolytic streptococcal infections have been observed also to reduce the attack rate of acute rheumatic fever.

TABLE 7-6. JONES CRITERIA (REVISED) FOR GUIDANCE IN THE DIAGNOSIS OF RHEUMATIC FEVER

Major Manifestations	Minor Manifestations
Carditis	▪ **Clinical**
Polyarthritis	Fever
Chorea	Arthralgia
Erythema marginatum	Previous rheumatic fever or rheumatic heart disease
Subcutaneous nodules	
	▪ **Laboratory**
	Acute phase reaction
	Erythrocyte sedimentation rate, C-reactive protein, leukocytosis
	Prolonged PR interval
	Plus

Supporting evidence of preceding streptococcal infection (increased ASO or other streptococcal antibodies; positive throat culture for group A streptococcus; recent scarlet fever).

The presence of two major criteria, or of one major and two minor criteria, indicates a high probability of the presence of rheumatic fever. Evidence of a preceding streptococcal infection greatly strengthens the possibility of acute rheumatic fever. Its absence should make the diagnosis doubtful except in Sydenham's chorea or long-standing carditis.

The epidemiology of rheumatic fever results from an interaction of the agent, the group A streptococcus, a susceptible host, and the environment. Available data suggest that the environment operates primarily by facilitating transmission of the streptococcus from one person to another primarily through crowding.[18] No genetic characteristics have been found consistently in children who develop rheumatic fever. A familial pattern is observed in rheumatic fever, but in contrast to glomerulonephritis, multiple cases in the same family are rarely seen simultaneously. Both the familial pattern and the high rates seen in childhood could be due either to increased exposure to streptococcal infections or to an increased susceptibility to their rheumatogenic potential once they have occurred.

It is difficult to obtain reliable data regarding temporal changes that have taken place in the incidence of rheumatic fever. In developed countries, morbidity rates are far more important than mortality rates as indices of rheumatic fever. Because of a variety of problems, including incomplete ascertainment of cases, inclusion of diseases other than rheumatic fever, and the highly selected populations that often are studied, valid incidence rates are difficult to generate. However, a study of rheumatic fever in Nashville, Tenn., from 1963 to 1965, using intensive case finding yielded an estimated incidence of 12.6 per 100,000 population of all ages. Rates among blacks were almost twice as high as rates among whites.[19] A study in Baltimore from 1960 to 1964 yielded annual attack rates of 13.3 per 100,000 for initial attacks, 2.3 for recurrences, and 15.6 for all attacks for the age group 5 through 19.[20] Rheumatic fever rates were two and one half times as high in blacks as in whites and appeared highest in low-income areas. These observations appeared to be due primarily to increased crowding in these groups.

Despite all the methodological difficulties, it seems quite clear that both the incidence and the severity of rheumatic fever have significantly declined in the United States. A comparison of data from the National Health Survey from 1935–1936 and the data from Baltimore in 1960–1964 shows a decline in the incidence of both first and recurrent attacks of rheumatic fever, with the greatest drop being seen in recurrent attacks. This may be attributable to a change in the disease itself over time, or more likely to the effectiveness of secondary prevention programs.

Studies of the changing incidence rates of rheumatic fever in Baltimore from 1960–1964 to 1968–1970, showed a dramatic decline in incidence in black children in Baltimore, but during this time the rates in white children remained relatively unchanged. Analysis of these comparative data indicated that the declining incidence in Baltimore resulted entirely from a reduction in preventable cases that were preceded by clinically overt pharyngitis. The findings suggested that comprehensive care programs were the critical factor in reducing the incidence of rheumatic fever in the inner city during this period.[21] From 1968–1970 to 1977–1981, incidence rates in Baltimore declined dramatically in both blacks and whites to a rate of only 0.5 per 100,000 in both races[22] (Figs. 7-6 and 7-7). These findings appear comparable to the experience in most areas of the United States.

The clinical spectrum of the disease also has changed, so that chorea, for example, is a highly unusual clinical finding today. In addition, the disease appears to be generally milder in the United States. Studies of the prevalence of rheumatic heart disease in schoolchildren have shown significant declines over time. Whereas prevalence rates varied from 4.3 to 5.0 per 1000 in New York, Boston, and Philadelphia in the 1920s and 1930s, later studies in Chicago, Michigan City, and Los Angeles reported prevalence rates of 0.7 and 0.5 per 1000.

In the mid-1980s, however, rheumatic fever outbreaks unexpectedly were reported from communities in many parts of the United States, including Utah, Ohio, and Pennsylvania, and from several military installations.[23] The Centers for Disease Control reported a doubling of incidence rates in 6 of 24 states with passive surveillance for rheumatic fever. The epidemiological characteristics of these new outbreaks are of particular interest, since the disease was found to occur not in impoverished urban minority populations as in the past but rather in white, middle class children, many from suburban areas. Although the explanation for these outbreaks is not completely clear, a mucoid type 18 streptococcus has been implicated. In any case, the most reasonable explanation is that the observed outbreaks are the result of some biological change in the organism that led to the emergence of rheumatogenic strains of streptococci in these populations. It is not clear at this time whether these outbreaks

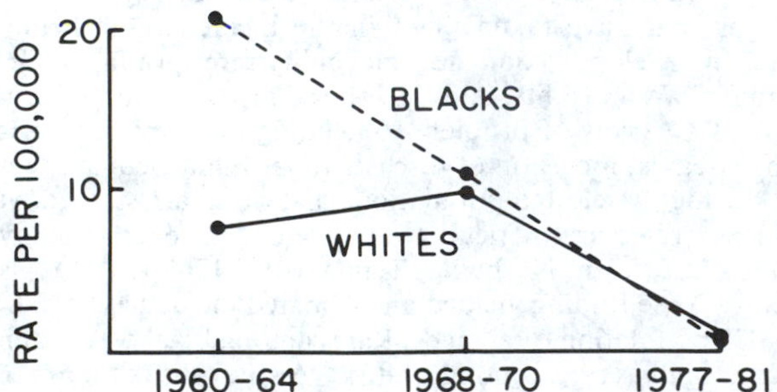

Figure 7-6. Average annual incidence of first attacks of rheumatic fever for ages 5 to 19, by race, in Baltimore from 1960 to 1981.

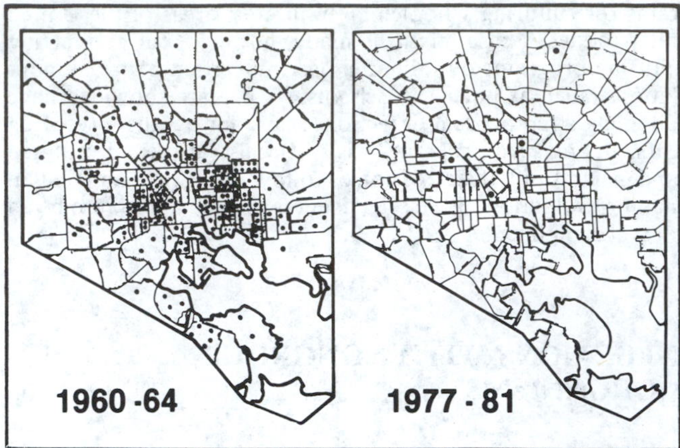

Figure 7-7. Spot maps showing distributions of residence of hospitalized cases of rheumatic fever in Baltimore in 1960 to 1964 and 1977 to 1981.

portend a general resurgence of rheumatic fever in the United States or whether these outbreaks are only relatively isolated phenomena in the face of a continuing general decline in rheumatic fever incidence.

Mortality rates from rheumatic fever have also declined. Although mortality rates from rheumatic heart disease have not shown as sharp a drop, any decline in these rates resulting from improved treatment of streptococcal infections would be expected to follow the decline in rheumatic fever death rates by several decades, since in the past, most mortality from acute rheumatic fever has occurred in childhood and that from rheumatic heart disease in adult life. Thus, if the members of a given birth cohort benefit from antistreptococcal treatment, reduction of mortality from rheumatic fever would occur when they are children and from rheumatic heart disease when they reach adult life.

Rheumatic fever is a worldwide disease, which, although more prevalent in temperate climates, is also found in tropical areas. Thus, countries with warm climates, such as Egypt and India, have relatively high incidence rates of rheumatic fever, and this fact may well reflect inadequate living conditions of much of the population in developing countries.

The incidence of rheumatic fever is highest in children. There is a seasonal pattern to rheumatic fever occurrence. The peak in the eastern United States is in March and April, and on the west coast of the United States, the peak appears to be in January and February. The seasonal pattern appears to parallel the seasonal pattern of streptococcal pharyngitis and differs from that of poststreptococcal glomerulonephritis (Fig. 7-8).

A latent period occurs between the acute pharyngitis and the clinical appearance of acute rheumatic fever or glomerulonephritis. The latent period for nephritis is shorter than that for rheumatic fever, and although the difference in length of latent period probably is related to the pathogenetic mechanisms involved, the nature of such mechanisms is not yet understood (Fig. 7-9). It is important to emphasize, however, that while streptococcal infections are contagious, there is no communicability of rheumatic fever or nephritis.

Rheumatic Fever Recurrences

One of the most striking characteristics of rheumatic fever is its tendency to recur. Before the introduction of preventive measures, 60% to 75% of patients with an initial attack of rheumatic fever had one or more recurrences. In recent years, the recurrence rate appears to have dropped significantly. Virtually every

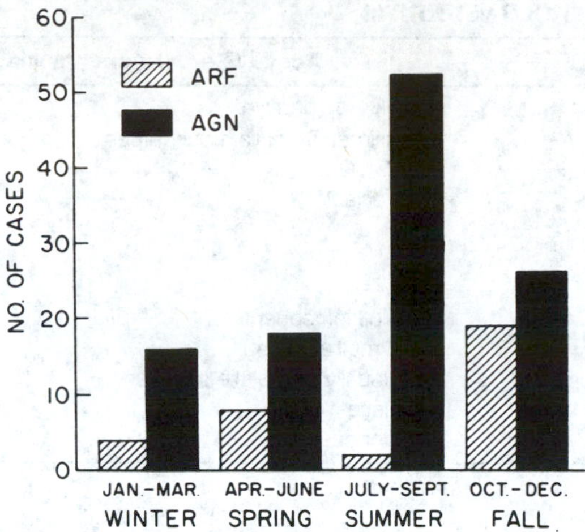

Figure 7-8. Seasonal distribution of acute rheumatic fever [ARF] and acute glomerulonephritis [AGN] admission at the City of Memphis Hospital from September 1965 to August 1968. [*From Bisno AL, et al: N Engl J Med 283:561-565, 1970.*]

recurrence of rheumatic fever appears to be associated with a preceding streptococcal infection. The risk of a recurrence after streptococcal infection appears related to the magnitude of the immune response. Recurrences are more common when the initial attack occurs early in life, when this attack includes carditis, and when the interval since the last attack is short. Recurrences are more frequent in childhood than in adult life, and the risk of recurrences rises in proportion to the number of previous recurrences and the severity of heart disease.

Because of the concern over recurrent attacks of rheumatic fever and particularly because of the likelihood of a recurrence aggravating the cardiac damage from preceding attacks, continuous antistreptococcal prophylaxis is essential. This can be accomplished by using oral penicillin, the recommended prophylactic dose being 200,000 units (125 mg) twice daily. If oral penicillin G is used, it should be given before meals. Sulfadiazine may be used in doses of 0.5 g daily for patients weighing 27 kg (60 lb) or less and 1.0 g daily for patients weighing over 27 kg. An alternate route is to use a single monthly intramuscular injection of 1.2 million units of benzathine penicillin G. Hypersensitivity reactions to benzathine penicillin G occur at a rate of less than 1% in adults and even lower in children.

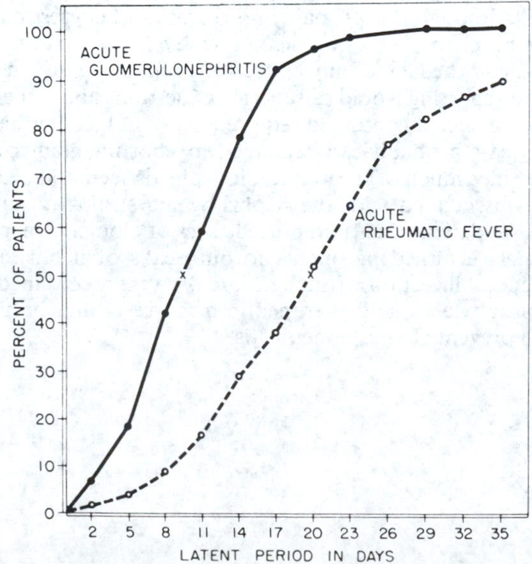

Figure 7-9. Latent period between onset of acute pharyngitis and clinical appearance of acute glomerulonephritis and acute rheumatic fever.

All children and adolescents who have had a documented attack of rheumatic fever or chorea or who have rheumatic heart disease should be started on prophylactic treatment as soon as the diagnosis is made. Most investigators believe that every rheumatic individual should be started on prophylaxis whether or not carditis is demonstrated. The American Heart Association has suggested that the safest general procedure is to continue prophylaxis indefinitely, particularly if rheumatic heart disease is present. At a very minimum, prophylaxis should be maintained for 5 years after the most recent attack, and individuals with a high risk of exposure to streptococcal infection, such as young men in military service, mothers of young children, school teachers, physicians, nurses, and allied medical personnel, should be protected. In addition, individuals with high recurrence rates of streptococcal infection, including those with rheumatic heart disease, those with a recent previous attack of rheumatic fever, or those with multiple attacks, also should receive prophylaxis. Low socioeconomic groups are at high risk, and special efforts should, therefore, be made to ensure that regular prophylaxis is maintained in all these groups.

Adolescents are particularly likely to be delinquent in their prophylaxis, so that careful follow-up of compliance is essential in this age group, and intramuscular prophylaxis should be strongly considered. The reader should consult the excellent statements issued by the American Heart Association regarding prevention of rheumatic fever, a method for culturing beta-hemolytic streptococci from the throat, and the Jones criteria (revised) for guidance in the diagnosis of rheumatic fever.

Historically, registries of patients who have had rheumatic fever or currently have rheumatic heart disease and require continuous antistreptococcal prophylaxis were established in many communities in the United States. The main purpose of such registries was to facilitate follow-up of rheumatic fever patients so that regular prophylaxis could be maintained. All too often, however, registries remained lists of names without any follow-up program. Reporting was often inadequate, and invalid cases were often reported. Thus, overascertainment and underascertainment of cases occurred simultaneously. These problems, together with the marked decline in the incidence of rheumatic fever and in the prevalence of rheumatic heart disease in the United States, have led to the discontinuation of many community registries, although the concept of registries may still be of value in developing countries where rheumatic fever remains a major problem.

ACUTE GLOMERULONEPHRITIS

Acute glomerulonephritis may follow a group A beta-hemolytic streptococcal infection but may also be associated with bacterial endocarditis, pneumococcal lobar pneumonia, staphylococcal infections, viral infections, systemic diseases, and drug exposures. The poststreptococcal form of the disease follows the infection after a latent period that is shorter than that of rheumatic fever (Fig. 7-9). Nephritis is characterized by hematuria, proteinuria, and red blood cell casts. Edema and hypertension are frequent. Acute heart failure, hypertensive encephalopathy, and convulsions may occur. The disease is of sudden onset, and serological evidence of a recent streptococcal infection can generally be obtained. Although the ASO response is generally weak, responses to DNAse B often can be demonstrated.

Although the data are equivocal, available evidence sug-

TABLE 7-7. DIFFERENCES BETWEEN RHEUMATIC FEVER AND GLOMERULONEPHRITIS

	Rheumatic Fever	Acute Glomerulonephritis
Infection site	Pharynx	Skin or pharynx
Serological types of streptococcus	Any of over 60	Primarily certain serotypes
Usual latent period	2–3 wk	7–10 d
Attack rate	Fairly constant	Variable
Immune response		
ASO	+	±
Anti-DNAse B	+	+
Age <3 y	Rare	Not infrequent
Familial attacks	Staggered	Simultaneous
Prognosis	May leave residual cardiac damage	Usually complete recovery
Recurrent attacks	May be frequent	Rare
Antistreptococcal prophylaxis	Mandatory	Unnecessary

gests that the vast majority of patients with acute glomerulonephritis recover completely without residual renal disease, provided there was no underlying renal disease to begin with. The prognosis may be worse in adults who contract nephritis than in children.

In contrast to rheumatic fever, acute poststreptococcal glomerulonephritis is seen in epidemic form. Large epidemics have been seen in hot areas, such as Israel, Trinidad, and the southern United States, generally following skin infections rather than pharyngitis or tonsilitis. Heat, humidity, arthropod bites, and crowded living conditions are all important risk factors. Streptococcal pyoderma is often seen in low-income families with many children. There appears to be a male preponderance over age 6, and this may be a result of increased trauma to the skin.

In many areas today, most cases of poststreptococcal glomerulonephritis occur after skin infections rather than throat infections. This accounts for the observation that the anti-DNAse B response is present whereas the ASO response is weak. Nephritis follows infections with specific serological types of streptococci. It is seen after respiratory infections with types 1, 4, 12, 49, and possibly other types. Skin infections with types 2, 49, 52, 55, 57, 59, 60, and 61 are also followed by nephritis. Since there are specific nephritogenic strains, epidemics of nephritis associated with outbreaks of streptococcal infections due to specific strains are observed.

It has been shown that prophylaxis of streptococcal infections can prevent acute glomerulonephritis. When military recruits were routinely administered 1.2 million units of benzathine penicillin upon arrival at a naval base, nephritis was virtually eliminated. However, there is insufficient evidence to suggest that prompt treatment of streptococcal infections will also prevent nephritis. Further studies are needed to document such a possible effect.

Persons who have had glomerulonephritis do not require continuous antistreptococcal prophylaxis because nephritis is caused by relatively few serological types. Patients who have been infected by another nephritogenic strain and have developed type-specific immunity are unlikely to be infected by another nephritogenic strain to which they are susceptible and, therefore, are at low risk of developing a second attack of glomerulonephritis. This is in contrast to the situation in rheumatic fever, where there is no clear-cut evidence to indicate that only a few types of streptococci are rheumatogenic. Consequently, any serological type of streptococcus may cause rheumatic fever, and a patient who has had an acute attack of rheumatic fever may be at high risk for a recurrent attack on infection with another strain of streptococcus of any type. Some of the major contrasts between rheumatic fever and glomerulonephritis are seen in Table 7-7.

DISEASE REPORTING

For many years, there has been a policy of requiring reporting of streptococcal infections and of rheumatic fever in many communities in the United States. With the decline in rheumatic fever incidence and that of other serious complications of streptococcal infections, there generally has been a relaxation of reporting policy. It would be difficult to justify routine reporting of streptococcal infections and rheumatic fever today in the United States. In a recent 5-year period in Baltimore, for example, only five new hospitalized cases of rheumatic fever could be documented. Although this probably represents an underestimate of the true number of cases of rheumatic fever, the small number reported and the lack of any concerted program of action in response to reporting would raise serious questions about the justification for such a continued requirement. On the other hand, a stronger case probably can be made for reporting glomerulonephritis. Since much of the glomerulonephritis seen in the United States is associated with the nephritogenic strains of streptococci, a sudden increase in reported cases of glomerulonephritis could alert health departments to outbreaks of nephritogenic streptococcal infection. If such outbreaks were ascertained, vigorous prophylactic and therapeutic measures could be undertaken to prevent glomerulonephritis.

Meningococcal Meningitis

David W. Fraser
Claire V. Broome
Jay D. Wenger

Vieusseaux described the clinical characteristics of epidemic cerebrospinal meningitis as it occurred in Geneva, Switzerland, in 1805. In 1887, Weichselbaum demonstrated that *Neisseria meningitidis*—the meningococcus—was the cause of this disease. The high mortality and epidemic potential of meningococcal disease has led to intensive study of control methods in the last 70 years.

Bacteriology. *Neisseria meningitidis* is a nonmotile, nonspore-forming gram-negative coccus. The organisms usually are arrayed in pairs that are flattened along the axis joining them. Isolation of meningococci from the nasopharynx in Mueller-Hinton agar is facilitated by addition of vancomycin, colistin, and nystatin, to which they are resistant. Addition of blood or other detoxicants to agar also facilitates growth, as does incubation in 5% to 10% CO_2. All *Neisseria* species are oxidase positive. The meningococcus can be differentiated from other *Neisseria* by its fermentation of glucose and maltose but not of sucrose or lactose, by its lack of pigmentation, and by its failure to grow at room temperature.

Strains of *N. meningitidis* can be divided on the basis of specific capsular polysaccharides into several serogroups, including A, B, C, D, X, Y, Z, Z′, W-135, and 29E. Serogrouping of strains is accomplished easily by agglutination with specific antisera. Other strains lack capsular polysaccharide and cannot be serogrouped. The vast majority of cases of invasive meningococcal disease are caused by groupable strains, with group A, B, C, or W-135 predominating in most populations. Other typing schemes have been proposed. Protein antigens in the outer cell-envelope membrane can be used to define 12 serotypes, one of which (serotype 2) is associated with more than half of all cases of serogroup B disease and has been postulated as a virulence factor.[1] Development of isoenzyme typing methods has allowed estimates of genetic relatedness between strains of meningococci. Recent studies using these methods suggest that certain clonal groups of meningococci may be responsible for waves of epidemic disease.[2]

The sensitivity of meningococci to sulfonamides has shown important shifts over time. When first introduced, these agents were remarkably effective in the treatment of meningococcal disease and eradication of nasopharyngeal carriage. Resistance was not a problem until 1963, when widespread sulfonamide resistance developed in meningococcal strains in U.S. military recruits. By 1968, the majority of cases in the U.S. civilian population were caused by strains resistant to sulfadiazine 10 μg/ml, and resistance was widespread throughout the world. The proportion of resistant strains has decreased since that time. In 1980, only 12% of U.S. strains tested were resistant.[3] Although penicillin resistance has been reported, it is extremely rare and apparently is mediated by a beta-lactamase.

Clinical Characteristics. The most common infection caused by *N. meningitidis* is of the oropharynx or nasopharynx and is primarily asymptomatic. Specific immunity may be induced, but carriage is not eradicated by the serological response.

In an occasional person, meningococci penetrate respiratory epithelium and cause bacteremia. Clinical manifestations then vary according to the intensity of bacteremia, the organs seeded from the blood, and perhaps the strain involved. Overwhelming septicemia can cause death within 2 to 8 hours of the first symptoms and can be associated with vasculitis, irregular petechial, purpuric, or maculopapular skin eruption, cutaneous infarction, and bilateral adrenal hemorrhage (Waterhouse-Friderichsen syndrome).

Although arthritis, pericarditis, and pneumonia occur, meningitis is the most common systemic manifestation of meningococcal disease. The incubation period is often difficult to assess but apparently ranges from 2 to 10 days. Symptoms of meningitis include sudden onset of malaise, followed rapidly by fever, headache, nausea, vomiting, and stiff neck.

The diagnosis of acute fulminant meningococcemia often can be made clinically, although bloodstream infection with other bacteria or rickettsiae can be close mimics. Specific diagnosis can be made by recovery of meningococci from blood, spinal fluid, or other normally sterile sites or by demonstration of capsular polysaccharide in those sites by counterimmunoelectrophoresis or latex particle agglutination. A presumptive diagnosis may be made by demonstration of gram-negative diplococci in gram-stained smears of blood buffy coat or normally sterile body fluids. However, these observations do not exclude the role of *Neisseria gonorrhoeae* or other organisms of similar appearance.

Penicillin is the drug of choice for meningococcal disease except for persons who are allergic to it. Up to 20 million units per day (300,000 U/kg/d for children) may be given intravenously in divided doses. Several third-generation-cephalosporin antibiotics appear effective. Chloramphenicol is a satisfactory alternative in patients allergic to penicillin. Sulfonamides are very effective against susceptible strains but are rarely used now in the United States for treatment because of resistance and the availability of alternative agents.

Carriers. Pharyngeal carriage of meningococci is common. The proportion of carriers may vary from 5% to 80% depending on the population, season, age, and living conditions.[4] Carriage tends to be greatest in the winter and spring and under crowded conditions, such as among military recruits.

In many populations, carriage of nongroupable strains is more common than that of groupable strains. Carriage tends to persist for a long time. In one study, the average was 10 months. The carriage rate in a population is of little value in predicting whether an outbreak will occur, probably because of the great variation in virulence of strains, susceptibility of the population, and the difficulty in assessing incidence of infection from a prevalence measurement, such as the carriage rate.

Immunity. Immunity to the meningococcus is mediated primarily by bactericidal antibodies directed against capsular or noncapsular antigens. Goldschneider and colleagues showed that bactericidal antibody probably resulted most commonly from asymptomatic meningococcal infection in the nasopharynx.[5] The presence of serum bactericidal antibodies is common in neonates, reflecting transplacental transfer of maternal antibodies, and decreases rapidly in the first 3 months of life, increasing again toward the end of the first year. The prevalence of bactericidal antibodies thus mirrors the incidence of meningococcal disease, which peaks at 6 to 7 months of age in endemic periods. Following asymptomatic infection or disease, antibodies commonly develop to capsular polysaccharide—although less strikingly to group B than to other serogroup antigens—and to protein serotype antigens. The presence of complement is necessary for the full protection of bactericidal antibody.

A number of bacteria share antigens with various strains of meningococci and may be important inducers of protective antibody. Serogroup A meningococcal polysaccharide cross-reacts with certain strains of *Bacillus pumilis* and enterococcus, group B polysaccharide with *Escherichia coli* K1, and group C polysaccharide with other *E. coli* strains. Meningococci can cleave secretory IgA, but whether this function assists pathogenesis is unknown.

Transmission. Meningococci are found only in humans. They are spread from the nasopharynx of one person to that of another, probably by respiratory droplets, although airborne spread may play a role under certain conditions.[6] Transmission is most intense in closed, crowded conditions—in the home, barracks, or jail. In sub-Saharan Africa, where seasonal epidemics are typical, disease occurs primarily in the dry season and decreases abruptly with the first rains. However, transmission of carriage occurs during both the dry and rainy seasons. A study of a Nigerian village has shown high rates of seroconversion to serogroup A during an epidemic period, even among people without clinical disease.[7]

Studies of meningococcal carriage in case contacts have shown that persons who sleep overnight in the house of a person with meningococcal disease are more likely to be colonized than those who visit only during the day or are neighbors.[8] Roommates are no more likely than other family contacts to carry the organism. Typically, the meningococcus is introduced into the household by an adult and spreads first to older children and then to infants.[9] Hospital contacts are colonized infrequently.

Occurrence. Meningococcal disease occurs endemically at a rate of 1 to 3 cases per 100,000 population per year, with a peak in late winter and early spring. Serogroups B and C have been responsible for most endemic disease, although variations in the proportion of disease due to each serogroup are observed. The peak incidence is at 6 to 7 months of age. Group B is relatively more common in cases in young infants. Race and economic level do not appear to be major risk factors for endemic disease. The risk of meningococcal disease is increased 1000-fold among household contacts of a person with meningococcal disease. In endemic periods, 0.4% of such contacts, if not given chemoprophylaxis, develop meningococcal disease in the month after the index case.[10] Day care center contacts also are at increased risk for at least a month.[11]

Most large epidemics of meningococcal disease are caused by serogroup A, although epidemics of group B or C have been observed in recent years. Epidemics may be community-wide or confined to only parts of the population. In the latter situation, crowded or impoverished groups seem particularly susceptible, for example, military recruits, prisoners, and skid row residents. Until 1945, meningococcal epidemics occurred about every 10 years in the United States. For unknown reasons, no major epidemic has occurred in the United States since 1945. Periodic epidemics continue to occur in sub-Saharan Africa, where incidence rates may increase to more than 700 cases per 100,000 population per year. Although introduction of new strains, concurrent viral infections, socioeconomic status, and other factors may be important in epidemic disease, additional study is needed to define the relative importance of these factors.[12]

Prevention. The use of mass prophylaxis with sulfadiazine was shown to be more than 95% effective in preventing cases of meningococcal disease in troops during an outbreak.[13] The dosage used was 1 g twice a day for 2 days. Mass sulfadiazine prophylaxis has been used once in a civilian population to control a group B meningococcal disease outbreak.[14] With the emergence of sulfonamide-resistant strains in the early 1960s, a search was made for alternative chemoprophylactic agents. Rifampin and minocycline enter nasopharyngeal secretions in high concentrations and are effective in eradicating meningococcal carriage. Because use of minocycline has been associated with vestibular reactions, rifampin has been recommended for chemoprophylaxis of household and nursery school contacts of cases of meningococcal disease not known to be caused by sulfonamide-sensitive strains. In addition, persons with very intimate contact with respiratory secretions of cases—such as giving mouth-to-mouth resuscitation—should receive prophylaxis. The dosage of rifampin is 600 mg b.i.d. for 2 days for adults, 10 mg/kg b.i.d. for 2 days for children over 1 month of age, and 5 mg/kg b.i.d. for 2 days for neonates.[15] A single intramuscular dose of ceftriaxone (250 mg for adults and 125 mg for children) has been shown to be significantly more effective in clearing meningococcal carriage than rifampin and may be useful as an alternative agent for chemoprophylaxis.[16] Observational studies suggest that chemoprophylaxis of household contacts is effective.[10] Respiratory isolation of patients with meningococcal disease is widely practiced but is of unproven value, and secondary cases in hospital contacts are rare.

Serogroup C vaccine was first tested in military recruits, for whom it was 90% effective in preventing disease.[17] A subsequent study in Brazil has shown it to be effective in children as young as 2 years of age. Serogroup A vaccine was first shown to be effective in Egyptian schoolchildren.[18] In widespread immunization of the Brazilian population to control an outbreak, it appeared to be effective in children as young as 1 year of age. A trial of group A meningococcal vaccine in children 3 months to 5 years of age in Finland also showed efficacy, but the numbers of cases observed were too few to permit a judgment as to whether the vaccine was effective for children less than 1 year of age to whom a booster had been given to improve immunogenicity.[19] A subsequent study in Burkina Faso demonstrated substantial protective efficacy for as long as 3 years after a single dose of group A meningococcal vaccine given to persons older than 4 years. However, protective efficacy declined rapidly in children vaccinated at less than 4 years of age. Efficacy in this group was estimated to be 8% 3 years after vaccination.[20]

In the United States, a licensed vaccine for groups A, C, Y, and W-135 is available. Use is recommended for control of localized outbreaks known to be due to serogroups included in the vaccine. Group A vaccine has been used for control of epidemic meningococcal meningitis in sub-Saharan Africa. Vaccine also has been used with some success in protecting household contacts of group A meningococcal cases in the 5 weeks after onset of the index case.[21] Since immunogenicity of group A and C vaccines in very young children is poor and, in children less than 4, of short duration, several investigators have attempted to enhance immunogenicity by developing covalent protein-polysaccharide conjugates. Although these vaccines appear promising, efficacy has not been demonstrated in humans. Vaccine for group B meningococcus has not been available because of the poor immunogenicity of the polysaccharide antigen. A number of strategies similar to those being used for groups A and C conjugates, as well as the use of outer membrane proteins, are being investigated to develop an effective group B vaccine.

Tuberculosis

D. Gray Heppner

Tuberculosis, the "white plague," remains a scourge of mankind.[1] Worldwide it is a leading cause of death and disability, with an estimated 10 million new cases each year.[2] In the United States the incidence, which had been decreasing since the beginning of the twentieth century, began to level off in 1984. If the previous 3-year rate of decline had continued, the Centers for Disease Control estimates that 14,768 fewer cases would have occurred between 1985 and 1988 (Fig. 7-10).[3] There were 22,436 new cases of tuberculosis reported in the United States in 1988. Recognition of this disturbing trend led the Department of Health and Human Services to establish the Advisory Committee for the Elimination of Tuberculosis (ACET) in 1987. The ACET has published a plan for the elimination of tuberculosis in the United States.[4]

History. Tuberculosis is an ancient disease, as evidenced by the skeletal remains of neolithic, pre-Columbian and Old Kingdom Egyptian persons. This disease referred to as "a consumption" in early Hindu writings, and as "phthisis" by the Greeks, is characterized by hemoptysis, cough, wasting, and chronic fever. Not until the rise of cities, with the attendant crowded conditions conducive to the transmission of tuberculosis, did this disease exact its greatest toll.[5] By about 1650, tuberculosis is thought to have caused 20% of all deaths in England and Wales,[1] leading John Bunyan to write "The Captain of all these men of death that came against him to take him away, was the Consumption." A modern understanding of the disease was ushered in by the discoveries of Laennec, Villemin, and Koch. Laennec in 1826 correlated the presence of the characteristic lesion of tuberculosis, the tubercle, with the disease but failed to recognize the infectious nature of tuberculosis.[6] Villemin established the infectiousness of tuberculosis by transmitting infection with lung tissue and fluids of humans to rabbits and guinea pigs.[7] Koch, in one of the seminal discoveries of science, first demonstrated the tubercle bacillus as the causative agent of tuberculosis and in so doing fulfilled his now famous postulates for the proof of pathogenicity.[8] Later, A. Conan Doyle and subsequently Von Pirquet proposed that tuberculin, a culture filtrate of *Mycobacterium tuberculosis,* might be used as a diagnostic indicator of the presence of infection.[9] Calmette and Guérin, working at the Pasteur Institute, attenuated *Mycobacterium bovis* between 1908 and 1922 to make the first live vaccine against tuberculosis, known as bacille Calmette-Guérin (BCG).

Although the incidence of tuberculosis declined during the last 2 centuries, the disease continued to exact a heavy toll. Therapy consisted of iatrogenic collapse of the lungs, fresh air, and exercise, modalities popularized by the sanatorium movement.[10] However, the advent of specific chemotherapy (streptomycin in 1944, isoniazid in 1952) obviated both sanatoria and the long-term quarantine of patients. Moreover, the emergence of antituberculous chemotherapy provided an impetus to renewed efforts at case finding. As a result, the incidence of tuberculosis fell dramatically in the United States until 1985. Recently, a number of factors have led to an increased incidence in this country. These factors include decreased case finding, immigration of persons from areas with a high prevalence of infection, and increasing numbers of persons who are unusually susceptible to disease, particularly those with human immunodeficiency virus (HIV) infection.

Microbiology. The causative agents of human tuberculosis are *M. tuberculosis* and *M. bovis.* Of the numerous species of *Mycobacterium,* only these two are designated tubercle bacilli. The other *Mycobacterium* of major public health importance is *Mycobacterium leprae,* the etiological agent of leprosy. The rest of the mycobacteria are referred to as nontuberculous or atypical mycobacteria.

Tubercle bacilli are nonsporebearing, acid-fast, rod-shaped microorganisms with generation times on the order of 18 to 24 hours. They are distinguished from each other and from other mycobacteria on the basis of biochemical tests and growth in artificial media.[11] *M. tuberculosis* accumulates niacin and reduces nitrate, whereas *M. bovis* does neither. Disease due to *M. bovis* is rare, and the term "tubercle bacillus" generally refers to *M. tuberculosis.* Humans are the only reservoir of *M. tuberculosis,* although domestic animals may become infected.

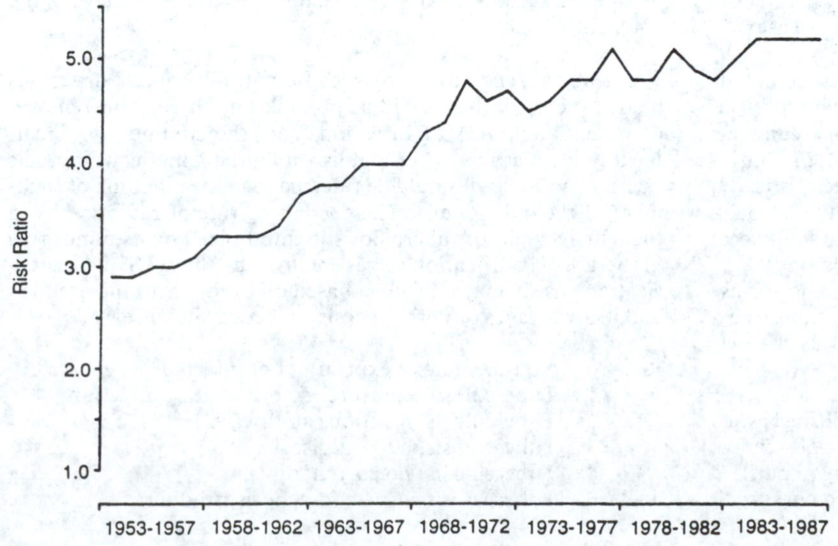

Figure 7-10. Ratio of tuberculosis risk among other-than-whites to whites from 1953 to 1987.

Many other mycobacteria of lesser pathogenicity have been isolated from humans. These nontuberculous mycobacteria have been classified into four groups by Runyon on the basis of pigment production, growth rates, and virulence in animals. Nontuberculous isolates may cause serious disease in the immunocompromised host, particularly persons with concomitant HIV infection. Pending definitive identification, they may be confused clinically with *M. tuberculosis* in these patients.[12]

Tubercle bacilli are destroyed by exposure to direct sunlight, ultraviolet light, heat, and such disinfectants as phenol or tricresol. They are more resistant to chemical agents, such as acid and alkalis, and to antibacterial agents, such as penicillin, than are most pathogenic microorganisms. Tubercle bacilli may remain viable for years in dried sputum, but for the most part, only airborne bacilli are infectious.

Pathogenesis. Persons with active pulmonary tuberculosis constitute the major reservoir of infection. The predominant mode of infection is by the inhalation of airborne tubercle bacilli, contained within droplet nuclei, which may be produced by talking, coughing, sneezing, or even singing.[13,14] Transmission by transfusion or by direct inoculation is rare and not of epidemiological significance. Inspired droplet nuclei that avoid the mucociliary blanket deliver bacilli to the terminal airspaces, where they multiply both within and outside of macrophages. Initial spread causes a local pneumonitis and involvement of the regional lymphatics. Pending the development of hypersensitivity (tuberculin reactivity), a silent lymphohematogenous dissemination occurs with unimpeded growth, which later may give rise to pulmonary and extrapulmonary foci of disease. The infection may progress to active clinical pulmonary tuberculosis or may become latent for many years. Host factors favoring progression to active disease include immunosuppression, extremes of age, poor nutritional status, other infection, underlying pulmonary disease (e.g., silicosis), diabetes mellitus, and pregnancy. In most cases, the acute infection is self-limited, and the tubercle bacilli lie dormant, contained by the host's immune defenses. Factors favoring breakdown of dormant foci of infection (reactivation) are similar to those that favor initial disease progression. Subsequent infection may become manifest in numerous sites, including the lung, the skeleton, the brain, and the meninges.

In understanding the pathogenesis of this disease, it is critical to appreciate the distinction between asymptomatic infection with *M. tuberculosis,* on the one hand, and the progression of such infection to disease, that is, tuberculosis, on the other.

Mycobacterium bovis infection in humans is acquired by ingesting unpasteurized milk from infected cows. It generally occurs as a systemic illness rather than as a pulmonary disease.

Incubation Period and Symptoms. The primary tuberculous infection most often is asymptomatic. The time from establishment of infection to the development of a positive tuberculin test is between 2 and 8 weeks. Pulmonary tuberculosis often is insidious in onset and variable in progression. Characteristically, there is low-grade fever, night sweats, fatigue, weight loss, cough productive of small amounts of nonpurulent sputum, and occasional slight hemoptysis. Except with advanced pulmonary disease, physical examination findings are minimal and not of use in diagnosis or management. The protean manifestations of extrapulmonary tuberculosis are beyond the scope of this chapter, and the reader is referred to an excellent review.[5]

Diagnosis. The diagnosis of tuberculosis is established when tubercle bacilli are demonstrated in sputum or other body fluids. Intracutaneous tuberculin testing for hypersensitivity to purified protein derivative (PPD) of the tubercle bacillus and chest radiography are important adjuncts to diagnosis.

Sputum Examination. At least three adequate sputum samples for culture should be examined before making a preliminary judgment as to the presence or absence of pulmonary tuberculosis. An optimal specimen is collected in early morning, before eating, and is stained by the Ziehl-Neelsen or Kinyoun method. Fluorescent techniques, using auramine-rhodamine or phenolic auramine staining, offer increased sensitivity and speed but require a fluorescence microscope and are less specific. Sputum may be induced by inhalation of nebulized saline if none is produced spontaneously. Sputum smears are not as sensitive as sputum cultures for detecting tubercle bacilli but may provide a rapid working diagnosis. A pitfall in the diagnosis of TB is the false positive smear caused by the presence of nonpathogenic acid-fast bacilli. Positive cultures may be obtained as soon as 3 weeks, but almost always by 6 weeks.

PPD. The PPD skin test, the intracutaneous inoculation of antigen from the tubercle bacillus, is an indicator of lymphocyte sensitivity to mycobacteria, and its clinical importance is due to the fact that a positive test generally indicates infection with *M. tuberculosis.* Induration of greater than 10 mm at the test site at 48 hours is considered presumptive evidence of prior infection by the tubercle bacillus. False positive skin tests may occur as a result of past, often occult, infection by atypical mycobacteria or previous vaccination with BCG. Persons with infections caused by atypical mycobacteria usually tend to have quantitatively less induration compared with those infected with *M. tuberculosis,* but there is overlap between the two populations with regard to extent of induration. Such background reactivity is endemic in some parts of the United States, particularly the southeast, and should be kept in mind when borderline skin test results are interpreted.

Immunocompromised persons, especially those with HIV infection, who harbor tubercle bacilli may exhibit less or no induration.

A *booster effect* may be seen on repeat skin testing and is the term used to describe recall of reactivity to tuberculin by the second dose. Such test results are true positives. In elderly patients, some authorities recommend that initial PPD testing be repeated at a 1-week interval and that the second result be used to classify the patient. Subsequent surveillance or diagnostic skin testing is then accomplished by a single test on a yearly or as needed basis.

Radiology. The lungs are the initial site of infection, and thus the chest radiograph may be quite helpful in determining active or latent infection. The value of the chest radiograph in asymptomatic tuberculin responders is disputed,[15] but radiology has been used with success in mass screening programs in developing countries.

Treatment. The advent of specific antituberculous drugs has made the cure of the individual possible and thereby the removal of potential sources of infection from the community. Treatment guidelines have been published by the American Thoracic Society (ATS), and should be referred to in the planning of treatment of the individual.[16] The decreasing role of radiography in the management of tuberculosis is emphasized by its minor role in the 1981 classification of tuberculosis by the ATS. The classification has six major groups, based on exposure to tuberculosis and its two stages of pathogenesis, infection and disease.[17]

- **0** No tuberculosis exposure, not infected
- **1** Tuberculosis exposure, no evidence of infection
- **2** Tuberculosis infection, no disease
- **3** Tuberculosis, current disease
- **4** Tuberculosis, no current disease
- **5** Tuberculosis suspect (diagnosis pending)

Inpatient vs Outpatient. Most persons with tuberculosis can be treated outside the hospital. The two exceptions to this rule are (1) the brief quarantine necessary during initiation of therapy, pending sterilization of the sputum, and (2) the enforced hospitalization for treatment necessitated by patient noncompliance with prescribed therapy.

Duration of Therapy. Combination chemotherapy for as little as 6 months has proven efficacious in uncomplicated cases caused by sensitive strains. Extensive pulmonary or extrapulmonary disease or infection with drug-resistant strains may require treatment for a year or more. Pregnancy, breast-feeding, and extremes of age are not contraindications to the treatment of tuberculosis.

Compliance. Most treatment failures are due to noncompliance with therapy rather than to resistant organisms. Chemotherapy may be administered biweekly in an observed setting on an outpatient basis without apparent loss of therapeutic efficacy.

Drugs. To be effective, chemotherapy must include at least two drugs to which the strain is susceptible. A combination of three or four drugs is used initially in those with a heavy infectious burden. Current first-line drugs against the tubercle bacillus are isoniazid (INH), rifampin, pyrazinamide, streptomycin, and ethambutol. However, ethambutol is not bactericidal. The treatment supervisor should be aware of the side effects of the antituberculous drugs and, at a minimum, clinically assess the patient on a monthly basis. Isoniazid is the cornerstone of therapy for sensitive strains. The major side effect is hepatitis, which is more common in older persons and in those who abuse alcohol. Peripheral neuropathy may occur and can be prevented by the coadministration of pyridoxine. Ethambutol, which may cause optic neuritis, should not be administered to children, since accurate ophthalmological assessment is not feasible.

Infectiousness of Sputum. The treatment time required to render the sputum noninfectious is not exactly known, but a classic study by Riley suggests that 2 weeks is adequate.[18] It should be remembered that tubercle bacilli may persist in the sputum for weeks during successful therapy, and their persistence may not necessarily indicate infectivity or treatment failure.

Relapse. Relapse is uncommon after an adequate course of antimicrobial therapy. Posttreatment follow-up is reserved for special cases, such as those in which there is a slow response to treatment, extensive clinical disease, or suspected poor compliance with medications.

INH Prophylaxis. Individuals with latent tuberculous infection are at risk for developing active disease. Large-scale, randomized, prospective trials have established the efficacy of monotherapy with INH in decreasing the risk of their developing active disease.[19,20] The risk of active disease is greatest in the first year after development of tuberculin hypersensitivity as manifested by a positive PPD. Despite the benefits of INH, the risk of drug toxicity limits its use prophylactically in those persons at high risk; such as recent PPD converters, persons with HIV infection, and persons receiving immunosuppression. Persons from areas where *M. tuberculosis* is drug resistant may not benefit from INH prophylaxis.

Epidemiology. The two most important factors in determining the spread of tuberculosis are airborne transmission, favored by crowded living conditions, and host susceptibility. Droplet nuclei are the major vehicle for the spread of tuberculosis infection. Droplet nuclei are produced by breathing, sneezing, or coughing. Theoretically, a single tubercle bacillus, once having gained access to the terminal airspaces, could establish infection. However, since not all inspired bacilli reach the terminal airspaces, the likelihood of infection is related to the intensity of exposure, which is proportional to the airborne concentration of droplet nuclei and the duration of exposure.

Certain conditions, including bronchogenic carcinoma, silicosis, and corticosteroid use, heighten individual susceptibility to developing active disease. The higher incidence seen in blacks, native Americans, and Hispanics vs whites is due to socioeconomic class and attendant crowded living conditions rather than to innate racial differences in susceptibility to disease.[21]

The importance of infectious droplet nuclei in the airborne spread of tuberculosis was proved by Wells and colleagues, who infected rabbits by exposing them to aerosols of tubercle bacilli in suspension.[13] Riley and others demonstrated the relevance of this animal model to the spread of tuberculosis between humans in a series of experiments at the Baltimore Veterans Hospital.[18] Air from a tuberculosis ward was circulated to one of two test groups of guinea pigs. The system was designed so that only buoyant particles suspended in air would reach the test animals. The air to the control group was exposed continuously to ultraviolet light; the air to the test group was not. Over the course of 2 years, tuberculosis developed only in the 135 guinea pigs exposed to untreated air. There were no cases of tuberculosis in the control group. The rate of infection was about three guinea pigs per month. Riley and coworkers thus demonstrated the presence and significance of infectious droplet nuclei in the air of buildings containing humans with tuberculosis.

Tuberculosis in Correctional Institutions. Recent studies have demonstrated consistently a higher incidence of TB in prisons than in the general population. In a 1988 CDC survey of 15,379 TB cases from 29 states, the incidence of TB among inmates was 30.94 cases per 100,000, and the relative risk of TB in prisoners compared with that of the general population was 3.9.[22] The reason is twofold: prisoners often are from populations at high risk for TB, and subsequent transmission of TB within the prison occurs more readily because of overcrowding. As Stead has pointed out, the failure to identify and treat infected inmates before their release from correctional facilities constitutes a risk to the community and increases the cumulative lifetime risk of the individual developing active TB.[23]

Nosocomial Transmission of Tuberculosis. The major reservoir of the spread of TB within hospitals is the undiagnosed case.[24,25] This problem often is due to the failure of the physician to consider it in the differential diagnosis as well as to unusual presentations in the elderly or chronically ill.

The risk of nosocomial spread may be limited by frequent room air changes with exhaust to the outside, ultraviolet sterilization of air, and limiting procedures that might produce infectious droplet nuclei, such as suctioning. Persons in contact with the patient, as well as the patient, should wear masks. Autopsy rooms pose a special hazard to medical personnel, and even more stringent precautions are warranted.

HIV and Tuberculosis. HIV infection is a significant, independent risk factor for the development of TB. The exact contribution of HIV-related TB morbidity to the total U.S. morbidity is unknown, but comparison of HIV and TB patient registries shows significant overlap. The immunosuppression of HIV infection leads to the reactivation of latent TB, and such doubly infected patients often present with TB before or at the time of their AIDS defining illness. Clinician recognition of TB cases in HIV-infected patients is impeded by the unusual and often extrapulmonary manifestations of disease. Conversely, the new diagnosis of active TB should prompt consideration of coinfection with HIV, particularly in persons belonging to groups at risk for HIV infection.[26] Case finding in HIV-infected persons is more difficult than in normal hosts because of a diminished reactivity to PPD. Tuberculin testing is especially important at places that treat those who might be infected with HIV, particularly substance abuse treatment centers, sexually transmitted disease clinics, and HIV counseling and testing sites. CDC guidelines suggest that tuberculin reactions greater than 5 mm of induration should be considered indicative of TB infection in an HIV-infected person. INH prophylaxis for the development of TB should be given to any untreated previous or current PPD reactor with HIV infection for 12 months or more. Public health concerns and optimal care of the individual have prompted the CDC to suggest that the recovery of any acid-fast bacilli from the respiratory tract of an HIV or potentially HIV-infected individual be treated with INH, rifampin, and pyrazinamide pending definitive identification of the organism as a tubercle bacillus or atypical mycobacterium.[27,28]

Intravenous Drug Abuse and Tuberculosis. The incidence of TB infection among intravenous drug users is higher than in the general population. Tuberculosis infection is more likely to progress to active disease in the drug users who are HIV infected.[29] Case finding and treatment in this high-risk group are important goals of the ACET.

Tuberculosis and the Elderly. Demographic shifts in the U.S. population are reflected in an increasing number of institutionalized elderly. Tuberculous disease in this group most often represents reactivation, although new TB infection does occur.[30] The benefit of prophylaxis with isoniazid must be weighed against the age-related risk of hepatitis and other side effects. For these reasons, Stead and associates have concluded that isoniazid should be administered only to documented recent converters.[31]

Tuberculosis and the Homeless. Incidences of latent TB of 18% to 51% and active disease of 1.6% to 6.8% have been found among indigents in shelters. Although the surveys cited may not be indicative of all homeless persons, they do illustrate the need for active screening measures and follow-up among this underserved group.[32]

Bovine Tuberculosis. As a result of pasteurization of milk supplies in the United States and the removal of infected cows under a nationwide program of tuberculin testing, bovine TB is no longer a public health menace in the United States.

Tuberculosis Public Health Measures. The need for more vigorous public health measures is underscored by the CDC's estimate that only 1% of the 10 million TB-infected people in the United States were identified and treated in 1988.[3] Reactivation in this reservoir of latently infected persons is thought to account for more than 90% of the current active cases. The 1987 ACET plan is designed to serve as a blueprint for the TB elimination effort in the United States.[4] Its goal is the reduction of TB incidence to less than one case per million population by the year 2010. It is predicated on a three-step plan of action. The first step is the more effective use of existing prevention and control technologies, with special attention to high-risk groups. Step two calls for the development of new technologies for diagnosis, treatment, and prevention. Step three involves prompt transfer of new technologies into clinical and public health practice.

Elimination of tuberculosis must begin with the identification and screening of groups at high risk for infection and disease. In 1991, the groups at highest risk include persons with HIV infection, the homeless, immigrants and refugees from countries with a high incidence of TB, intravenous drug abusers, prison inmates, residents of nursing homes, close contacts of persons with known or suspected disease, and members of lower socioeconomic groups, particularly blacks, Hispanics, and Native Americans. Once those at high risk are identified, appropriate decisions regarding prophylaxis and treatment need to be made. The plan advocates the use of short-course regimens and, to ensure compliance, supervised therapy. Health care providers would be responsible not only for therapy and follow-up of their individual cases but also for the education, screening, and treatment of their case contacts.

New technology priorities include the development of a more effective TB vaccine, alternative means of preventing disease in infected individuals, and more accurate tests for identifying persons harboring live tubercle bacilli.

Integral to the implementation of this plan is the establishment of a nationwide public education effort by medical, nursing, and public health schools, professional societies, voluntary agencies, and minority advocacy groups to educate health care providers and members of high-risk groups.

The current vaccine against TB, BCG vaccine, is an attenuated strain of *M. bovis.* Its major role has been in preventing severe tuberculous disease in children residing in endemic areas. Once inoculated, persons often remain reactive to PPD. There is a practical consideration against administering this live attenuated vaccine to people in areas of the world where there is a significant incidence of HIV infection, since there are isolated reports of subsequent disseminated BCG infection. There has been no documented harm, however, from administering this vaccine to persons previously infected by the tubercle bacillus.[33,34]

Leprosy

Bradley N. Doebbeling

Leprosy (Hansen's disease) is a chronic mycobacterial infection affecting millions of people worldwide, primarily in the rural tropics and subtropics. Significant physical disability occurs in up to one third of untreated cases. The diagnosis also carries a profoundly negative social stigma in many societies. In the United States the prevalence of reported cases steadily increased in the early 1980s among recent immigrants from endemic areas.[1]

Since the advent of effective chemotherapy in 1941, new cases of leprosy, when diagnosed early and treated adequately, should no longer pose a significant public health problem. The potential for crippling and disfigurement remains, however, because of incomplete physician knowledge or experience or patients' failure to seek early medical care. In this age of rapid international travel, every health worker should be alert for leprosy and familiar with the appropriate preventive measures for cases and contacts.

Etiological Agent. Leprosy is caused by *Mycobacterium leprae,* a bacillus first described in 1873 by Hansen in Norway. This gram-positive, minimally curved bacillus is acid-alcohol-fast by the Ziehl-Neelsen stain and is more easily decolorized by acids than is *Mycobacterium tuberculosis,* which it resembles morphologically. It can be grown in the footpads of certain mice, in thymectomized congenitally athymic nude mice and rats, and in the nine-banded armadillo. *M. leprae* has not yet been cultivated in vitro.

Clinical Description. Clinically, the disease is characterized by (1) lesions of the skin (infiltration, macules, papules, nodules) with decreased sensation to light touch and (2) involvement and often palpable enlargement of peripheral nerves, causing anesthesia, muscle weakness, and paralysis, followed by trophic changes in skin, muscle, and bone. Two distinct major clinical types occur, tuberculoid and lepromatous, with a clinical spectrum of overlap between the two types.[3,4]

Lepromatous leprosy (LL) is characterized by diffuse skin lesions (which may ulcerate and mimic other diseases), thickened facial skin and ear lobes, nasal congestion, epistaxis, brawny edema of the extremities, and occasionally, erythema nodosum. Iritis and keratitis are common, sometimes leading to blindness. LL tends to progress if inadequately treated, since there is a defect in cell-mediated immunity.

Tuberculoid leprosy (TL) usually displays localized, discretely demarcated anesthetic skin lesions (erythematous plaques), often with relatively early peripheral neuropathy (typically involving the ulnar nerve at the elbow, the peroneal nerve at the upper end of the fibula, or the greater auricular nerve in the neck). Tuberculoid skin lesions often heal spontaneously in 1 to 3 years, but permanent nerve damage is common. Residual paralysis and anesthesia leading to trophic ulcers and other complications may result from either form of leprosy if treatment is not started early and continued for an appropriate period.

Leprosy displaying characteristics intermediate between these two extremes are described as borderline (BB), often further subdivided into borderline tuberculoid (BT) or borderline lepromatous (BL).[4]

Clinical spectrum: LL→BL→BB→BT→ TT

An indeterminate form represents the earliest manifestations and often occurs as a skin macule in a young child, frequently is missed by clinicians, and usually is self-limited.

Diagnosis. In endemic areas, primary health personnel can be taught to identify leprosy suspects accurately and make the presumptive diagnosis by physical examination and a slit-skin smear. Leprosy is almost certain if two of the following three criteria are present: (1) a skin lesion (any kind) anesthetic to light touch, (2) the presence of acid-fast bacilli in an incised smear or biopsy of such a lesion, and (3) a palpable enlarged superficial nerve. A skin biopsy or slit-skin smear interpreted by a pathologist or dermatologist familiar with leprosy usually confirms the diagnosis.[5,6] Biopsies of lepromatous or borderline lepromatous skin lesions contain large numbers of *M. leprae* (multibacillary), whereas biopsies of most tuberculoid or borderline tuberculoid cases contain small numbers (paucibacillary).

The lepromin, or Mitsuda, test is an intradermal skin test of cellular immunity, useful for classification and to determine prognosis. Heat-treated, emulsified material derived from bacilli-rich leprosy tissue is used as an antigen.[6] A delayed hypersensitivity reaction characterized by a nodule appearing at the injection site, reaching a maximum diameter 3 to 4 weeks after injection, is found in many unexposed or bacille Calmette-Guérin (BCG)-immunized individuals. The lepromin test is positive in approximately one half of paucibacillary cases. A negative lepromin test in clinically confirmed leprosy is evidence of a specific cellular immune defect and indicative of multibacillary leprosy. A negative lepromin test in a person exposed to lepromatous leprosy is associated with an increased risk of multibacillary disease. However, the positive and negative predictive values of the test for the development of leprosy are low.[7]

An enzyme-linked immunosorbent assay (ELISA)-detectable rise in a nonprotective serum antibody against a *M. leprae*-specific cell wall surface component (phenolic glycolipid I) occurs in many patients after infection.[7,9] This antibody often is detectable transiently in early paucibacillary disease and at a higher and more persistent titer in multibacillary disease. The ELISA is limited by cross-reactivity with other mycobacterial organisms (low specificity), depending on the technique used and gives negative results in up to 80% of paucibacillary disease (low sensitivity).[7-9] Monoclonal antibodies may be useful in early diagnosis.[7]

Distribution. Leprosy has existed in eastern Mediterranean and Asian populations since ancient times. During the Middle Ages, leprosy became widespread in Europe. It declined in most of Europe after the sixteenth century but peaked in Norway during the nineteenth century, followed by a rapid decline for unknown reasons. The disease is now endemic primarily only in tropical Africa, southeast Asia, India, certain Pacific islands, and parts of Latin America. There were 12 million cases estimated worldwide in 1985,[9] mostly in developing countries, with only a fraction under adequate therapy.

Leprosy apparently was introduced to the Americas through African and European immigration. Leprosy was reported in French Polynesia as the eighteenth century ended. Ethnic links among these islands, Easter Island, and Hawaii probably helped spread the disease.[10] North American endemic foci are now limited to Louisiana, Texas, California, and Hawaii.[1] New cases in North America now occur primarily among immigrants, with secondary cases extremely rare.[1] Approximately one half of imported cases in the United States come from Southeast Asia, and one-fourth come from Mexico.

Since leprosy usually becomes evident before marriage, those cultures with a strong historical religious or social stigma against leprosy (Europe and east Asia) may have managed to prevent, through early ostracism, the reproductive activities of a large proportion of severe (LL) cases. Transmission was largely intrafamilial, since close extrafamilial contact was strongly discouraged. Children in infected families who were able to reproduce presumably were those with sufficient cellular immune competence to avoid the development of leprosy, at least in its severe, recognizable forms. Thus, leprosy-resistant populations may have been selected over many generations. The disease is currently a problem in only two largely tropical populations: (1) those who historically have not practiced rigid social rejection and (2) those introduced to leprosy for the first time only in recent generations, during the era of European colonialism, slavery, and contract labor. The disease also persists among impoverished populations, perhaps reflecting a lowering of resistance because of malnutrition.

Long-term surveillance in China, India, Japan, Nigeria, Venezuela, Norway, and the United States has demonstrated a gradual decline in the incidence of indigenous leprosy.[11] Secular trends of increasing age at onset, increasing male excess, and an increasing proportion of multibacillary disease have been cited as evidence of rapid decline in a disease, such as leprosy, with a long and variable incubation period.[11]

Transmission. Infection apparently is transmitted from person to person by close contact, most likely through nasal secretions that often have high bacillary loads. Cohort studies among poor, overcrowded children and spouses of leprosy patients in endemic areas have suggested that untreated multibacillary leprosy is the major source of human transmission. Household contacts of untreated multibacillary cases have a relative risk of leprosy 3 to 6 times that of the general population.[12] Incidence rates are highest in children, peaking at 5 to 9 years of age.[12] Contacts of untreated, paucibacillary cases have a lower relative risk, approximately two to four times the local population.[12] Recent data from a case-control study suggest that intrahousehold leprosy contact increases the risk of developing leprosy 2.5 times that of age- and sex-matched controls.[13] Corresponding rates are much lower among similarly exposed people in developed countries.

Untreated lepromatous women rarely transmit the infection to unborn infants, although infants exposed after birth to an untreated lepromatous parent have a 10% to 40% risk of infection, peaking 6 to 9 years after their first exposure.[12]

Observations that 50% to 70% of sporadic cases occur in the absence of known contact with human leprosy suggest that nonhuman environmental sources may also be important.[2] Several series have recently noted an association between armadillo exposure or handling and development of leprosy. Other environmental sources including soil, water, vegetation, and arthropods (flies, mosquitoes) have been studied.[2] The epidemiological importance of these sources for leprosy in humans remains to be demonstrated.

Natural History. At any time, close contact with an untreated or inadequately treated person may lead to transmission. The risk of infection is predominantly influenced by environmental conditions such as (1) the prevalence of untreated cases in that environment, (2) crowding within households, and (3) social rules governing close contact. Once a person has been exposed, the risk of developing actual disease is dependent on that person's resistance. Most exposed persons (90% to 95%) have a subclinical infection and remain healthy. Factors that may enhance the development of disease include the following:

1. *General factors:* Childhood exposure, malnutrition, physiological stress (e.g., clinical flares during pregnancy are not unusual), and possibly the route of entry or size of the infective "dose"
2. *Genetic factors:* Impaired immune response of the infected person, nonimmunologically induced susceptibility

Adequate treatment renders cases rapidly noninfective but may not halt the signs and symptoms of disease promptly because of tissue reaction to dead or dying bacilli.

Treatment and Rehabilitation. The treatment of leprosy is problematic for a number of reasons.[3] Only a limited number of drugs are available, including diaminodiphenylsulfone (dapsone or DDS), clofazamine (Lamprene), rifampin, ethionamide, and prothionamide. Testing of antimicrobial agents against *M. leprae* is difficult because of the necessity to test the agent in living mice over an 8-month period. Frequently, compliance with oral therapy is poor because of the long treatment duration and minimal symptoms of active infection reinforcing compliance. Furthermore, resistance to DDS is increasing because of its extensive use as monotherapy. Finally, recent reports of rifampin resistance underscore the importance of multidrug regimens for all leprosy patients.[3]

The World Health Organization (WHO) began recommending multidrug therapy for all forms of leprosy in 1982 to shorten treatment duration and minimize the emergence of resistance.[14] Therapy should be continued for a minimum of 2 years, ideally until all skin biopsies and smears are negative for acid-fast bacilli.[3] Consulting an experienced clinician may be useful before therapy is begun, since experiments with new drugs and drug combinations are underway. New cases should be reported to public health officials. Over the next decade, development and testing of alternative drugs for the treatment and chemoprophylaxis of leprosy will be critical for its control.[15]

Prevention has always been an important issue in the management of leprosy. The best measure, obviously, is to prevent the case from occurring (primary prevention). Alternatively, an environment may be created in which cases are reported early and the diagnosis is not missed or delayed. If leprosy is diagnosed early and treated at home, there is an improvement in patients' attitudes and more effective medical care and use of resources.[16] Typically, patients suffer neither unemployment nor the social stigma associated with segregation, long institutionalization, or disfigurement. Most properly handled cases do not develop permanent nerve damage or trophic changes. Tuberculoid cases with early and severe nerve involvement, however, may develop some permanent muscular paralysis or anesthesia. In such cases, physical therapy, patient education, and occasionally muscle transplantation are beneficial. The National Hansen's Disease Center at Carville, La., maintains a special unit for restorative surgery, and consultation or treatment may be obtained there.

Control. Control measures encompass three general approaches:

1. Active case finding for early diagnosis and treatment of multibacillary cases to render them noninfective as quickly as possible and effective treatment protocols to keep them noninfectious
2. Preventive treatment during the incubation period of those at high risk (children with known exposure to untreated multibacillary cases or those with high or rising titers of humoral antibody)
3. Immunization of potentially exposed people with an effective vaccine (not yet available)

Active case finding and prompt, adequate ambulatory therapy complement all preventive programs. In no other way can we control source cases and obtain the necessary public cooperation. The traditional approach first used in medieval Europe was to segregate leprosy patients into leprosaria or leprosy villages. Although this approach may have had some unexpectedly favorable long-term genetic selection, it is socially and medically unnecessary today.[16] Segregation may cause delay or postponement of treatment, increasing the likelihood of irreversible nerve damage and providing greater opportunity for transmission of leprosy to close contacts. It also, of course, delays prophylaxis for those exposed. A policy of "chemical isolation" through prompt and adequate treatment of the ambulatory patient avoids these delays.

Prophylaxis with DDS protects children under the age of 16 years who have close household contact with patients likely to shed large numbers of organisms, that is, those with lepromatous or borderline lepromatous leprosy.[17] Prophylaxis is not recommended for adults with household exposure because clinical infection is unlikely. Household contacts should be examined closely for evidence of leprosy, and any suggestive skin lesions should be biopsied. Individuals exposed to patients with tuberculoid or borderline tuberculoid leprosy should be evaluated annually but do not require chemical prophylaxis.[3]

A new leprosy case apparently quickly loses the ability to transmit the disease to others once therapy is started. This conclusion is based on loss of normal appearance microscopically, loss of the ability of the organism from biopsy specimens to multiply in the mouse footpad, and human evidence of reduced transmission following initiation of treatment.

BCG immunization to protect against leprosy has been studied in three large randomized controlled trials with varying results.[18] One, in Uganda, where most of the cases are tuberculoid, showed a reduced incidence in the BCG group to approximately one fifth the rate in the control group.[19] A study in New Guinea, in a tribe without tuberculosis (which confounds such studies), demonstrated an incidence rate of leprosy approximately one half that in the control group.[20] BCG was most effective in BT leprosy and in children under 15 years of age, although the protection did not appear until after several years of observation in most subgroups. A much larger study in Burma with a relatively high proportion of lepromatous leprosy and considerable tuberculosis showed only a slight advantage to the BCG group (20% reduction) and only among the very young.[21] It appears from these data that BCG may protect those who are relatively immunocompetent and either have not yet been infected or who are early in their incubation period when they receive it.

Trials of a vaccine combining heat-killed whole *M. leprae* (armadillo-derived) and live BCG are now underway in Venezuela and Malawi.[18] The Malawi trial is also evaluating repeated BCG dosing.[22] Additionally, a clinical trial is underway in India to evaluate leprosy prophylaxis with killed atypical mycobacterial vaccines.[18] However, firm conclusions regarding the vaccines' effectiveness and safety will require many years of follow-up.

Conclusion. Long-term secular trends suggest that leprosy had been decreasing gradually in many countries, such as Norway, even before treatment became available. Early diagnosis and effective treatment eventually may eradicate the disease in areas where it persists. Drug resistance is an increasing problem, and new antimycobacterial drugs are needed to improve the efficiency of treatment and prophylaxis. Worldwide control of leprosy requires patient, conscientious, persistent work on many fronts but appears to be an achievable goal.

REFERENCES

Acute Respiratory Infections

1. Dingle JH, Badger GF, Jordan WS Jr: Illness in the home: A study of 25,000 illnesses in a group of Cleveland Families. Cleveland: The Press of Western Reserve University, 1964
2. Monto AS, Ullman BM: The Tecumseh study. Acute respiratory illness in an American community. JAMA 227:164–169, 1974
3. Monto AS, Bryan ER, Rhodes LM: The Tecumseh study of respiratory illness. VII. Further observations on the occurrence of respiratory syncytial virus and *Mycoplasma pneumoniae* infections. Am J Epidemiol 100:458, 1975
4. Mufson MA, Belshe RB, Orvell C, Norrby E: Respiratory syncytial virus epidemics: Variable dominance of subgroups A and B strains among children, 1981–1986. J Infect Dis 157:143–148, 1988
5. Mufson MA, Levine HD, Wasil RE, et al: Epidemiology of respiratory syncytial virus infection among infants and children in Chicago. Am J Epidemiol 98:88, 1973
6. Glezen WP, Paredes A, Allison JE, et al: Risk of respiratory syncytial virus infection for infants from low-income families in relationship to age, sex, ethnic group, and maternal antibody level. J Pediatr 98:708, 1981
7. Chanock RM, Kapikian AZ, Mills J, et al: Influence of immunological factors in respiratory syncytial virus disease. Arch Environ Health 21:347, 1970
8. Kim HW, Arrobio JO, Brandt CD, et al: Epidemiology of respiratory syncytial virus infection in Washington, D.C. I. Importance of the virus in different respiratory tract disease syndromes and temporal distribution of infection. Am J Epidemiol 98:216, 1973
9. Glezen WP, Denny FW: Epidemiology of acute lower respiratory disease in children. N Engl J Med 288:498, 1973
10. Chin J, Magoffin RL, Shearer LA, et al: Field evaluation of a respiratory syncytial virus vaccine and a trivalent parainfluenza virus vaccine in a pediatric population. Am J Epidemiol 89:449, 1969
11. Hall CB, McBride JT, Walsh EE, et al: Aerosolized ribavirin treatment of infants with respiratory syncytial viral infection. A randomized double-blind study. N Engl J Med 308:1443, 1983
12. Chanock RM, Parrott RH, Cook K, et al: Newly recognized myxoviruses from children with respiratory disease. N Engl J Med 258:207, 1958
13. Chanock RM, Parrott RH, Johnson KM, et al: Myxoviruses: Parainfluenza. Am Rev Respir Dis 88:152, 1963
14. Monto AS: The Tecumseh study of respiratory illness. V. Patterns of infection with the parainfluenza viruses. Am J Epidemiol 97:338, 1973
15. Cooney MK, Kenny GE, Tam R, Fox JP: Cross relationships among 37 rhinoviruses demonstrated by virus neutralization with potent monotypic rabbit antisera. Infect Immun 7:335, 1973
16. Hendley JO, Edmondson WP Jr, Gwaltney JM Jr: Relationship between naturally acquired immunity and infectivity of two rhinoviruses in volunteers. J Infect Dis 125:243, 1972
17. Minor TE, Dick EC, De Meo AN, et al: Viruses as precipitants of asthmatic attacks in children. JAMA 227:292, 1974
18. Monto AS, Cavallaro JJ: The Tecumseh study of respiratory illness. IV. Prevalence of rhinovirus serotypes, 1966–1969. Am J Epidemiol 96:352, 1972
19. Hendley JO, Wenzel RP, Gwaltney JM Jr: Transmission of rhinovirus colds by self-inoculation. N Engl J Med 288:1361, 1973
20. Monto AS, Bryan ER, Ohmit S: Rhinovirus infections in Tecumseh, Michigan: Frequency of illness and number of serotypes. J Infect Dis 156:43–49, 1987
21. Coulehan JL, Eberhard S, Kapner L, et al: Vitamin C and acute illness in Navajo schoolchildren. N Engl J Med 295:973, 1976
22. Hamre D, Beem M: Virologic studies of acute respiratory disease in young adults. V. Coronavirus 229E infections during six years of surveillance. Am J Epidemiol 96:94, 1972
23. McIntosh K, Becker WB, Chanock RM: Growth in suckling-mouse brain of "IBV-like" viruses from patients with upper respiratory tract disease. Proc Natl Acad Sci USA 58:2268, 1967
24. Monto AS, Lim SK: The Tecumseh study of respiratory illness. VI. Frequency of and relationship between outbreaks of coronavirus infection. J Infect Dis 129:271, 1974
25. McNaughton MR: Occurrence and frequency of coronavirus infections in humans as determined by enzyme-linked immunosorbent assay. Infect Immun 38:419, 1982
26. Benyesh-Melnick M, Rosenberg HS: The isolation of adenovirus type 7 from a fatal case of pneumonia and disseminated disease. J Pediatr 64:83, 1964
27. Fox JP, Brandt CD, Wassermann FE, et al: The virus watch program: A continuing surveillance of viral infections in metropolitan New York families. VI. Observations of adenovirus infections: Virus excretion patterns, antibody response, efficacy of surveillance, patterns of infection, and relation to illness. Am J Epidemiol 89:25, 1969
28. Dudding BA, Wagner SC, Zeller JA, et al: Fatal pneumonia associated with adenovirus type 7 in military trainees. N Engl J Med 286:1289, 1972
29. Jawetz E: The story of shipyard eye. Br Med J 1:873, 1959
30. Bell JA, Rowe WP, Engler JI, et al: Pharyngoconjunctival fever: Epidemiological studies of a recently recognized disease entity. JAMA 175:1083, 1955
31. Top FH Jr, Grossman RA, Bartelloni PJ, et al: Immunization with live types 7 and 4 adenovirus vaccines. I. Safety, infectivity, and potency of adenovirus type 7 vaccines in humans. J Infect Dis 124:148, 1971
32. Slotkin RI, Clyde WA Jr, Denny FW: The effect of antibiotics on *Mycoplasma pneumoniae* in vitro and in vivo. Am J Epidemiol 86:225, 1967
33. Eaton MD, Meiklejohn G, Van Herick W: Studies on etiology of primary atypical pneumonia. I. Filterable agent transmissible to cotton rats, hamsters and chick embryos. J Exp Med 79:649, 1944
34. Foy HM, Kenny GE, McMahan R, et al: *Mycoplasma pneumoniae* pneumonia in an urban area. Five years of surveillance. JAMA 214:1666, 1970
35. Sawyer R, Sommerville RG: An outbreak of *Mycoplasma pneumoniae* infection in a nuclear submarine. JAMA 195:958, 1966
36. Wenzel RP, Craven RB, Davies JA, et al: Field trial of an inactivated *Mycoplasma pneumoniae* vaccine. I. Vaccine efficacy. J Infect Dis 134:571, 1976
37. Smith CB, Friedewald WT, Chanock RM: Shedding of *Mycoplasma pneumoniae* after tetracycline and erythromycin therapy. N Engl J Med 276:1172, 1967

38. Grayston JT, Kuo CC, Campbell LA, Wang SP: *Chlamydia pneumoniae* sp. nov. for *Chlamydia* sp. strain TWAR. Int J Syst Bacteriol 39:88–90, 1989
39. Grayston JT, Campbell LA, Kuo C-C, et al: A new respiratory tract pathogen: *Chlamydia pneumoniae* strain TWAR. J Infect Dis 161:618, 1990
40. Kleemola M, Saikku P, Visakorpi R, et al: Epidemics of pneumonia caused by TWAR, a new *Chlamydia* organism, in military trainees in Finland. J Infect Dis 157:230–236, 1988

Viral Hepatitis

1. Krugman S, Giles JP, Hammond J: Infectious hepatitis: Evidence for two distinctive clinical, epidemiological, and immunological types of infection. JAMA 200:95–103, 1967
2. Blumberg BS, Alter HJ, Visnich S: A "new" antigen in leukemia sera. JAMA 191:541–546, 1965
3. Feinstone SM, Kapikian AZ, Purcell RH: Hepatitis A: Detection by immune electron microscopy of a virus-like antigen associated with acute illness. Science 182:1026–1028, 1973
4. Gravelle CR, Hornbeck CL, Maynard JE, et al: Hepatitis A: Report of a common source outbreak with recovery of a possible etiologic agent. II. Laboratory studies. J Infect Dis 131:167, 1975
5. Rizzetto M, Canese MG, Arico S, et al: Immunofluorescence detection of a new antigen-antibody system (delta/anti-delta) associated to the hepatitis B virus in the liver and in the serum of HBsAg carriers. Gut 18:997–1003, 1977
6. Rizzetto M, Canese MG, Gerin JL, et al: Transmission of the hepatitis B virus associated delta antigen to chimpanzees. J Infect Dis 141:590–601, 1980
7. Purcell RH, Walsh JH, Holland PV, et al: Seroepidemiologic studies of transfusion-associated hepatitis. J Infect Dis 123:406, 1971
8. Alter MJ, Gerety RJ, Smallwood LA, et al: Sporadic non-A, non-B hepatitis: Frequency and epidemiology in an urban United States population. J Infect Dis 145:886–893, 1982
9. Choo Q-L, Kuo G, Weiner AJ, et al: Isolation of a cDNA clone derived from a blood-borne non-A, non-B viral hepatitis genome. Science 244:359–362, 1989
10. Reyes GR, Purdy MA, Kim JP, et al: Isolation of a cDNA from the virus responsible for enterically transmitted non-A, non-B hepatitis. Science 247:1335–1339, 1990
11. Lemon SM: Type A viral hepatitis: New developments in an old disease. N Engl J Med 313:1059–1067, 1985
12. Jansen RW, Siegl G, Lemon SA: Molecular epidemiology of human hepatitis A virus defined by an antigen-capture polymerase chain reaction method. Proc Natl Acad Sci USA 87:2867–2871, 1990
13. Brown EA, Jansen RW, Lemon SA: Characterization of a simian hepatitis A virus (HAV); antigenic and genetic comparison with human HAV. J Virol 63:4932–4937, 1989
14. Purcell RH: Approaches to immunization against hepatitis A virus. In Hollinger BF, Lemon SA, Margolis HS (eds): Viral Hepatitis and Liver Disease. Baltimore: Williams & Wilkins, 1991
15. Hadler SC, McFarland L: Hepatitis in day care centers. Epidemiology and prevention. Rev Infect Dis 8:548–557, 1985
16. Centers for Disease Control: Hepatitis Surveillance Report No. 52. Atlanta: CDC, 1989
17. Sjogren MH, Tanno H, Fay O, et al: Hepatitis A virus in stool during clinical relapse. Ann Intern Med 106:221–226, 1987
18. Tassopoulos NC, Papavangelou GJ, Ticehurst JR, Purcell RH: Fecal excretion of Greek strains of hepatitis A virus in patients with hepatitis A and in experimentally infected chimpanzees. J Infect Dis 154:231–237, 1986
19. Hadler SC: Global impact of hepatitis A virus infection: Changing patterns. In Hollinger BF, Lemon SA, Margolis HS (eds): Viral Hepatitis and Liver Disease. Baltimore: Williams & Wilkins, 1991
20. Xu ZY, Fu T-Y, Margolis HS, et al: The impact and control of viral hepatitis in China. In Hollinger BF, Lemon SA, Margolis HS (eds): Viral Hepatitis and Liver Disease. Baltimore: Williams & Wilkins, 1991
21. Shapiro CN, Shaw FE, Mandel EJ, Hadler SC: Epidemiology of hepatitis A in the United States. In Hollinger BF, Lemon SA, Margolis HS (eds): Viral Hepatitis and Liver Disease. Baltimore: Williams & Wilkins, 1991
22. Shaw FE, Sudman JH, Williams SM, et al: A community-wide outbreak of hepatitis A in Ohio. Am J Epidemiol 123:1057–1065, 1986
23. Rosenblum LS, Mirkin IR, Allen DT, et al: A multifocal outbreak of hepatitis A traced to commercially distributed lettuce. Am J Public Health 80:1075–1079, 1990
24. Reid TMS, Robinson HG: Frozen raspberries and hepatitis A. Epidemiol Inf 98:109–112, 1987
25. Noble RC, Kane MA, Reeves SA, Roeckel I: Posttransfusion hepatitis A in a neonatal intensive care unit. JAMA 252:2711–2715, 1984
26. Centers for Disease Control: Protection against viral hepatitis: Recommendations of the Immunization Practices Advisory Committee (ACIP). MMWR 39:5–22, 1990
27. Tiollais P, Charnay P, Vyas GN: Biology of hepatitis B virus. Science 213:406–411, 1981
28. Kobayashi H, Tsuzuri M, Koshimizi K, et al: Susceptibility of hepatitis B virus to disinfectants or heat. J Clin Microbiol 20:214–216, 1984
29. Courouce AM, Holland PV, Muller JY, Soulier JP: HBs antigen subtypes. Proceedings of the International Workshop of HBs Antigen Subtypes. Bibl Haematologica 42:1–158, 1976
30. Alward WLM, McMahon BJ, Hall DB, et al: The long-term serological course of asymptomatic hepatitis B virus carriers and the development of primary hepatocellular carcinoma. J Infect Dis 151:604–609, 1985
31. Beasley RP: Hepatitis B virus. The major etiology of hepatocellular carcinoma. Cancer 61:1942–1956, 1988
32. Chau KH, Hargie MP, Decker RH, et al: Serodiagnosis of recent hepatitis B infection by IgM class anti-HBc. Hepatology 3:142–149, 1983
33. Maynard JE, Kane MA, Hadler SC: Global control of hepatitis B through vaccination: Role of hepatitis B vaccine in the Expanded Programme on Immunization. Rev Infect Dis 11(suppl 3):s574–578, 1989
34. Franks AL, Berg CJ, Kane MA, et al: Hepatitis B infection among children born in the United States to southeast Asian refugees. N Engl J Med 321:1301–1305, 1989
35. Beasley RP, Hwang LY, Lee GCY, et al: Prevention of perinatally transmitted hepatitis B virus infections with hepatitis B immune globulin and hepatitis B vaccine. Lancet 2:1099–1102, 1983
36. Petersen NJ, Barrett DH, Bond WW, et al: Hepatitis B surface antigen in saliva, impetiginous lesions, and the environment in two remote Alaska villages. Appl Environ Microbiol 32:572–574, 1976
37. Lettau L, McCarthy JG, Smith MH, et al: An outbreak of severe hepatitis due to delta and hepatitis B viruses in parenteral drug abusers and their contacts. N Engl J Med 317:1256–1261, 1987
38. Lettau L, Smith JD, Williams D, et al: Transmission of hepatitis B with resultant restriction of surgical practice. JAMA 255:934–937, 1986
39. Alter MJ, Hadler SC, Margolis HS, et al: The changing epidemiology of hepatitis B in the United States. Need for alternative vaccination strategies. JAMA 263:1218–1222, 1990
40. Purcell RH, Gerin JL: Hepatitis B subunit vaccine: A preliminary report of safety and efficacy tests in chimpanzees. Am J Med Sci 270:395–399, 1975
41. Francis DP, Hadler SC, Thompson SE, et al: Prevention of hepatitis B with vaccine. Report from the Centers for Disease Control multicenter efficacy trial among homosexual men. Ann Intern Med 97:362–366, 1982
42. Yvonne B, Coursaget P, Petat E, et al: Immunogenic effect of hepatitis B vaccine in children. J Med Virol 14:137–139, 1984
43. Xu ZY, Liu CB, Francis DP, et al: Prevention of perinatal acquisition of hepatitis B virus carriage using vaccine: Preliminary report of a randomized, double-blind placebo-controlled and comparative trial. Pediatrics 76:713–718, 1985
44. Poovorawan Y, Sanpavat S, Pongpuniert W, et al: Protective effi-

cacy of a recombinant DNA hepatitis B vaccine in neonates of HBe antigen-positive mother. JAMA 261:3278–3281, 1989
45. Stevens CE, Toy PT, Tong MJ, et al: Perinatal hepatitis B virus transmission in the United States. Prevention by passive-active immunization. JAMA 253:1740–1745, 1985
46. Stevens CE, Taylor PE, Tong MJ, et al: Yeast-recombinant hepatitis B vaccine. Efficacy with hepatitis B immune globulin in prevention of perinatal hepatitis B virus transmission. JAMA 257:2612–2616, 1987
47. Margolis HS, Alter MJ, Krugman S: Strategies for controlling hepatitis B in the United States. In Hollinger BF, Lemon SA, Margolis HS (eds): Viral Hepatitis and Liver Disease. Baltimore: Williams & Wilkins, 1991
48. Hadler SC, Francis DP, Maynard JE, et al: Long-term immunogenicity and efficacy of hepatitis B vaccine in homosexual men. N Engl J Med 215:209–214, 1986
49. Wainwright RB, McMahon BJ, Bulkow LR, et al: Duration of immunogenicity and efficacy of hepatitis B vaccine in a Yupik Eskimo population. JAMA 261:2362–2366, 1989
50. Heyward WL, Lanier AP, McMahon BJ, et al: Early detection of primary hepatocellular carcinoma. JAMA 254:3052–3054, 1985
51. Perrillo RP, Schiff ER, Davis GL, et al: A randomized, controlled trial of interferon alfa-2b alone and after prednisone withdrawal for the treatment of chronic hepatitis B. N Engl J Med 323:295–301, 1990
52. Bonino F, Hoyer BH, Shih JW-K, et al: Delta hepatitis agent: Structural and antigenic properties of the delta associated particle. Infect Immun 43:1000–1005, 1984
53. Wang K-S: Structure, sequence and expression of the hepatitis delta virus genome. Nature 323:508–513, 1986
54. Smedile A, Dentico P, Zanetti A, et al: Infection with the HBV-associated delta agent in HBsAg carriers. Gastroenterology 81:992–997, 1981
55. Smedile A, Farci P, Verme G, et al: Influence of delta infection on the severity of hepatitis B. Lancet 2:9–15, 1982
56. Caredda F, Antinori S, Re T, et al: Course and prognosis of acute HDV infection. Prog Clin Biol Res 234:267–276, 1986
57. Rizzetto M, Verme G, Recchia S, et al: Chronic hepatitis in carriers of hepatitis B surface antigen with intrahepatic expression of the delta antigen. An active and progressive disease unresponsive to immunosuppressive treatment. Ann Intern Med 98:437–441, 1981
58. Maynard JE, Hadler SC, Fields HA: Delta hepatitis in the Americas: An overview. Prog Clin Biol Res 234:493–505, 1986
59. Buitrago B, Popper H, Hadler SC, et al: Specific histologic features of Santa Marta hepatitis: A severe form of hepatitis delta virus infection in northern Colombia. Hepatology 6:1285–1291, 1986
60. Ponzetto A, Forzani B, Parravicini PP, et al: Epidemiology of delta virus infection. Eur J Epidemiol 1:257–263, 1986
61. Hadler SC, De Monson M, Ponzetto A, et al: Delta virus infection and severe hepatitis. An epidemic in the Yucpa Indians of Venezuela. Ann Intern Med 100:339–344, 1984
62. Bradley DW, Krawczynski K, Ebert JW, et al: Parenterally transmitted non-A, non-B hepatitis: Virus-specific antibody response patterns in hepatitis C virus infected chimpanzees. Gastroenterology 99:1054–1060, 1990
63. Alter HJ, Hoofnagle JH: Non-A, non-B: Observations on the first decade. In Vyas GN, Dienstag JL, Hoofnagle JH (eds): Viral Hepatitis and Liver Disease. Orlando, FL: Grune & Stratton, 1984, pp 345–354
64. Kuo G, Choo QL, Alter HJ, et al: An assay for circulating antibodies to a major etiologic virus of human non-A, non-B hepatitis. Science 244:362–364, 1989
65. Cristiano K, Baker B, DiBisceglie A, Feinstone S: Detection of hepatitis C viral RNA by the polymerase chain reaction. In Hollinger BF, Lemon SA, Margolis HS (eds): Viral Hepatitis and Liver Disease. Baltimore: Williams & Wilkins, 1991
66. Alter MJ, Hadler SC, Judson FN, et al: Risk factors for acute non-A, non-B hepatitis in the United States and association with hepatitis C virus infection. JAMA 264(17):2231–2235, 1990
67. Stevens CE, Aach RD, Hollinger BF, et al: Hepatitis B virus antibody in blood donors and the occurrence of non-A, non-B hepatitis in transfusion recipients: An analysis of the Transfusion Transmitted Virus Study. Ann Intern Med 101:733–738, 1984
68. Alter HJ, Purcell RH, Shih JW, et al: Detection of antibody to hepatitis C virus in prospectively followed transfusion recipients with acute and chronic non-A, non-B hepatitis. N Engl J Med 321:1494–1500, 1989
69. Alter MJ, Coleman PJ, Alexander WJ, et al: Importance of heterosexual activity in the transmission of hepatitis B and non-A, non-B hepatitis. JAMA 262:1201–1205, 1989
70. Alter MJ: Epidemiology of community acquired hepatitis C. In Hollinger BF, Lemon SA, Margolis HS (eds): Viral Hepatitis and Liver Disease. Baltimore: Williams & Wilkins, 1991
71. Hoofnagle JH, Mullen KD, Jones B, et al: Treatment of chronic non-A, non-B hepatitis with recombinant human alpha interferon: A preliminary report. N Engl J Med 315:1575–1578, 1986
72. Wong DC, Purcell RH, Sreenivasan MA, et al: Epidemic and endemic hepatitis in India: Evidence for a non-A, non-B hepatitis virus aetiology. Lancet 2:876–878, 1980
73. Bradley DW: Enterically transmitted non-A, non-B hepatitis. Br Med Bull 46:442–461, 1990
74. Velazquez O, Stetler HC, Avila C, et al: Epidemic transmission of enterically transmitted non-A, non-B hepatitis in Mexico, 1986–1987. JAMA 263:3281–3285, 1990
75. Balayan MS, Andjparidze AG, Savinskaya SS, et al: Evidence for a virus in non-A, non-B hepatitis transmitted via the fecal-oral route. Intervirology 20:23–31, 1983
76. DeCock KM, Bradley DW, Sandford NL, et al: Epidemic non-A, non-B hepatitis in patients from Pakistan. Ann Intern Med 106:227–230, 1987
77. Kane MA, Bradley DW, Schrestha SM, et al: Epidemic non-A, non-B hepatitis in Nepal. Recovery of a possible etiologic agent and transmission studies in marmosets. JAMA 252:3140–3145, 1984

Aseptic Meningitis and Enteroviral Infections

1. Meyer HM, Johnson RT, Crawford IP: Central nervous syndromes of "viral" etiology: A study of 713 cases. Am J Med 29:334–347, 1960
2. Modlin JF: Coxsackieviruses, echoviruses, and newer enteroviruses. In Mandell GL, Douglas RG Jr, Bennett JE (eds): Principles and Practice of Infectious Diseases, 3 edt. New York: Churchill Livingston, 1990, pp. 1367–1383
3. Barrett-Connor E: Is insulin-dependent diabetes mellitus caused by coxsackie virus B infection? A review of the epidemiologic evidence. Rev Infect Dis 7:207–215, 1985
4. Melnick JL: Enteroviruses: Polio viruses, coxsackieviruses, echoviruses, and newer enteroviruses. In Fields BN (ed): Virology, 2 edt. New York: Raven Press, 1990, pp. 549–605
5. Wilfert CM, Buckley RH, Mohanakumar T: Persistent and fatal central-nervous-system echovirus infections in patients with agammaglobulinemia. N Engl J Med 296:1485–1489, 1977

Epstein-Barr Virus and Infectious Mononucleosis

1. Miller G: Epstein-Barr virus. In Fields BN (ed): Virology, 2 edt. New York: Raven Press, 1990, pp. 1921–1958
2. Chin TD: Diagnosis of infectious mononucleosis. South Med J 69:654–658, 1976
3. Schooley RT, Dolin R: Epstein-Barr virus (infectious mononucleosis). In Mandell GL, Douglas RG Jr, Bennett JE (eds): Principles and Practice of Infectious Diseases, 3 edt. New York: Churchill Livingston, 1990, pp. 1172–1185
4. Purtilo DT, Bhawan J, Hutt LM, et al: Epstein-Barr virus infections in the X-linked recessive lymphoproliferative syndrome. Lancet 1:798–801, 1978

Herpes Simplex Virus

1. Corey L, Spear PG: Infections with herpes simplex viruses. Parts 1 and 2. N Engl J Med 314:686–691, 749–757, 1986
2. Nahmias AJ, Roizman B: Infection with herpes simplex viruses 1 and 2. N Engl J Med 289:667–674, 719–725, 781–789, 1973
3. Corey L, Adams HG, Brown ZA, Holmes KK: Genital herpes simplex virus infections: Clinical manifestations, course and complications. Ann Intern Med 98:958–972, 1983
4. Francis DP, Hermann KL, MacMahon JR, et al: Nosocomial and maternally acquired herpesvirus hominis infections. Am J Dis Child 129:889, 1975
5. Linnemann CC Jr, Buchmann TG, Light IJ, et al: Transmission of herpes simplex type 1 in a newborn nursery: Identification of viral isolates by DNA "fingerprinting." Lancet 1:964, 1978
6. Whitley RJ, Soong SJ, Linneman C Jr, et al: Herpes encephalitis: Clinical assessment. JAMA 247:317–320, 1982
7. Whitley RJ, Nahmias AJ, Visintine AM, et al: The natural history of herpes simplex virus infection of mother and new born. Pediatrics 66:489, 1980
8. Saral R, Burns WH, Laskin OL, et al: Acyclovir prophylaxis of herpes-simplex-virus infections: A randomized, double-blind, controlled trial in bone-marrow-transplant recipients. N Engl J Med 305:63–67, 1981
9. Arvin AM, Hensleigh PA, Prober CG, et al: Failure of antepartum maternal cultures to predict the infant's risk of exposure to herpes simplex virus at delivery. N Engl J Med 315:796–800, 1986

Cytomegalovirus Infections

1. Weller TH: The cytomegaloviruses: Ubiquitous agents with protean clinical manifestations. N Engl J Med 285:203–214, 267–274, 1971
2. Ho M: Cytomegalovirus: Biology and Infection. New York and London: Plenum, 1982
3. Drew WL: Cytomegalovirus infection in patients with AIDS. J Infect Dis 158:449–456, 1988
4. Alford CA, Britt WJ: Cytomegalovirus. In Fields BN, Knipe DM, et al (eds): Virology, 2 edt. New York: Raven Press, 1990
5. Bale JF Jr, Jordan MC: Cytomegalovirus infections. In Vinken PJ, Bruyn GW, Klawans HL (eds): Handbook of Clinical Neurology. Amsterdam: Elsevier, 1989
6. Jordan MC, Rousseau WE, Stewart JA, et al: Spontaneous cytomegalovirus mononucleosis: Clinical and laboratory observations in nine cases. Ann Intern Med 79:153–160, 1973
7. Pass RF, Stagno S, Britt WJ, et al: Specific cell-mediated immunity and the natural history of congenital infection with cytomegalovirus. J Infect Dis 148:953–961, 1983
8. Murph JR, Bale JF Jr: The natural history of acquired cytomegalovirus infection among children in group day care. Am J Dis Child 142:843–846, 1988
9. Fiala M, Payne JE, Berne TV, et al: Epidemiology of cytomegalovirus after transplantation and immunosuppression. J Infect Dis 132:421–433, 1975
10. Zaia JA: The biology of human cytomegalovirus infection after bone marrow transplantation. Int J Cell Clon 4:135–154, 1986
11. Plotkin SA, Friedman HM, Fleisher GR, et al: Towne-vaccine-induced prevention of cytomegalovirus disease after renal transplants. Lancet 1:528–530, 1984
12. Hutto C, Little EA, Ricks R, et al: Isolation of cytomegalovirus from toys and hands in a day care center. J Infect Dis 154:527–530, 1986
13. Meyers JD: Prevention and treatment of cytomegalovirus infection after marrow transplantation. Bone Marrow Trans 3:95–104, 1988
14. Yeager AS, Grumet FC, Hafleigl EB, et al: Prevention of transfusion-acquired cytomegalovirus infections in newborn infants. J Pediatr 98:281–287, 1981
15. Tegtmeier GE: Transfusion-transmitted cytomegalovirus infections: Significance and control. Vox Sang 51(suppl 1):22–30, 1986
16. Snydman DR, Werner BG, Heinze-Lacey B, et al: Use of cytomegalovirus immune globulin to prevent cytomegalovirus disease in renal-transplant recipients. N Engl J Med 317:1049–1054, 1987
17. Meyers JD, Reed EC, Shepp DH, et al: Acyclovir for prevention of cytomegalovirus infection and disease after allogeneic marrow transplantation. N Engl J Med 318:70–75, 1988
18. Balfour HH Jr, Chace BA, Stapleton JT, et al: A randomized, placebo-controlled trial of oral acyclovir for the prevention of cytomegalovirus disease in recipients of renal allografts. N Engl J Med 320:1381–1387, 1989
19. Buhles WC, Mastre BJ, Tinker AJ, et al: Ganciclovir treatment of life- or sight-threatening cytomegalovirus infection: Experience in 314 immunocompromised patients. Rev Infect Dis 10 (suppl 3):S495–S506, 1988
20. Verheyden JPH: Evolution of therapy for cytomegalovirus infection. Rev Infect Dis 10(suppl 3):S477–489, 1988
21. Klintmalm G, Lonnqvist B, Oberg B, et al: Intravenous foscarnet for the treatment of severe cytomegalovirus infection in allograft recipients. Scand J Infect Dis 17:157–163, 1986
22. Emanuel D: Treatment of cytomegalovirus disease. Semin Hematol 27:22–27, 1990
23. Emanuel D, Cunningham I, Jules-Elysee K, et al: Cytomegalovirus pneumonia after bone marrow transplantation successfully treated with the combination of ganciclovir and high-dose intravenous immune globulin. Ann Intern Med 109:777–782, 1988
24. Reed EC, Bowden RA, Dandliker PS, et al: Treatment of cytomegalovirus pneumonia with ganciclovir and intravenous cytomegalovirus immunoglobulin in patients with bone marrow transplants. Ann Intern Med 109:783–788, 1988

Acute Gastrointestinal Infections

1. Dingle JH, Badger GF, Jordan WS Jr: Illness in the Home: A study of 25,000 Illnesses in a Group of Cleveland Families. Cleveland: The Press of Western Reserve University, 1964
2. Monto AS, Bryan ER, Rhodes LM: The Tecumseh study of respiratory illness. VII. Further observations on the occurrence of respiratory syncytial virus and *Mycoplasma pneumonaie* infections. Am J Epidemiol 100:458, 1975
3. Brandt CK, Hyun WK, Rodriguez WJ, et al: Pediatric viral gastroenteritis during eight years of study. J Clin Microbiol 18:71, 1983
4. Takiff HE, Straus SE, Garon CF: Propagation and in vitro studies of previously noncultivable enteral adenoviruses in 293 cells. Lancet 2:832, 1981
5. Bishop RF, Davidson GP, Holmes IH, Ruck BJ: Virus particles in epithelial cells of duodenal mucosa from children with acute non-bacterial gastroenteritis. Lancet 2:1281, 1973
6. Flewett TH, Woode GN: The rotaviruses: Brief review. Arch Virol 57:1, 1978
7. Yolken RH, Kim HW, Clem T, et al: Enzyme-linked immunosorbent assay (ELISA) for detection of human reovirus-like agent of infantile gastroenteritis. Lancet 1:263, 1977
8. Hall GH, Gridger JC, Chandler RL, Woode GN: Gnotobiotic piglets experimentally inoculated with neonatal calf diarrhea reovirus-like agent (rotavirus). Vet Pathol 13:197, 1976
9. Murphy AM, Albrey MB, Crewe EB: Rotavirus infections of neonates. Lancet 2:1149, 1977
10. Wang S, Cai R, Chen J, et al: Etiologic studies of the 1983 and 1984 outbreaks of epidemic diarrhea in Guangxi. Intervirology 24:140, 1985
11. Koopman JS, Turkish VJ, Monto AS, et al: Patterns and etiology of diarrhea in three clinical settings. Am J Epidemiol 119:114, 1984
12. Birch CJ, Lewis FA, Kennett ML, et al: A study of the prevalence of rotavirus infection in children with gastroenteritis admitted to an infectious diseases hospital. J Med Virol 1:69, 1977
13. Paniker CKJ, Mathew S, Dharmarajan R, et al: Epidemic gastroenteritis in children associated with rotavirus infection. Indian J Med Res 66:525, 1977
14. Kapikian AZ, Kim HW, Wyatt RG, et al: Human reovirus-like agent as the major pathogen associated with "winter" gastroenteritis in

hospitalized infants and young children. N Engl J Med 294:965, 1976

15. Monto AS, Koopman JS, Longini IM, Isaacson RE: The Tecumseh study. XII. Enteric agents in the community. J Infect Dis 148:284, 1983
16. Thornhill TS, Kalica AR, Wyatt RG, et al: Pattern of shedding of the Norwalk particle in stools during experimentally induced gastroenteritis in volunteers as determined by immune electron microscopy. J Infect Dis 132:28, 1975
17. Dolin R, Blacklow NR, DuPont H, et al: Biological properties of Norwalk agent of acute infectious nonbacterial gastroenteritis. Proc Soc Exp Biol Med 140:578, 1972
18. Wyatt RG, Dolin R, Blacklow NR, et al: Comparison of three agents of acute infectious non-bacterial gastroenteritis by cross-challenge in volunteers. J Infect Dis 129:709, 1974
19. Thornhill TS, Wyatt RG, Kalica AR, et al: Detection by immune electron microscopy of 26- to 27-nm viruslike particles associated with two family outbreaks of gastroenteritis. J Infect Dis 135:20, 1977
20. Schreiber DS, Blacklow NR, Trier JS: The mucosal lesion of the proximal small intestine in acute infectious nonbacterial gastroenteritis. N Engl J Med 288:1318, 1973
21. Parrino TA, Schreiber KDS, Trier JS, et al: Clinical immunity in acute gastroenteritis caused by Norwalk agent. N Engl J Med 297:86, 1977

Trachoma and Inclusion Conjunctivitis

General References

Dawson CR, Jones BR, Darougar S: Blinding and non-blinding trachoma: Assessment of intensity of upper tarsal inflammatory disease and disabling lesions. Bull WHO 52:279–282, 1975

Jones BR: The prevention of blindness from trachoma. Trans Ophthalmol Soc UK. 95:16–33, 1975

Schachter J: Chlamydial infections. N Engl J Med 298:428–435, 490–495, 540–549, 1978

Schachter J, Dawson CR: Human Chlamydial Infections. Littleton, MA: Publishing Sciences Group, 1978

Chlamydial Pneumonia

General References

Schachter J, Lum L, Gooding CA, Ostler B: Pneumonitis following inclusion blennorrhea. J Pediatr 87:779–780, 1975

Beem MO, Saxon EM: Respiratory-tract colonization and a distinctive pneumonia syndrome in infants infected with *Chlamydia trachomatis*. N Engl J Med 296:306–310, 1977

Harrison HR, English G, Lee K, Alexander R: *Chlamydia trachomatis* infant pneumonitis (comparison with matched controls and other infant pneumonitis). N Engl J Med 298(13):702–708, 1978

Schachter J: Chlamydial infections. N Engl J Med 298:428–435, 490–495, 540–549, 1978

Streptococcal Disease

1. Krause RM: Symposium on relationship of structure of microorganisms to their immunologic properties. IV. Antigenic and biochemical composition of hemolytic streptococcal cell wall. Bacteriol Rev 27:369, 1963
2. Benenson AB (ed): Control of Communicable Diseases in Man. An Official Report of the American Public Health Association, 14 edt. Washington, DC: American Public Health Association, 1985, p 370
3. Smith TD, Wilkinson V, Kaplan EL: Group A *Streptococcus*-associated upper respiratory tract infections in a day-care center. Pediatrics 83:380–384, 1989
4. Wannamaker LW: A Method for Culturing Beta-Hemolytic Streptococci from the Throat. New York: American Heart Association, 1965
5. Maxted WR: The use of bacitracin for identifying group A hemolytic streptococci. J Clin Pathol 6:224, 1953
6. Bisno AL: Where has all the rheumatic fever gone? Clin Pediatr 22:804–806, 1963
7. Kaplan EL: The rapid identification of group A beta-hemolytic streptococci in the upper respiratory tract—Current status. Pediatr Clin North Am 35:535–542, 1988
8. Cone LA, Woodard DR, Schlievert PM, Tomory GS: Clinical and bacteriologic observations of a toxic shock-like syndrome due to *Streptococcus pyogenes*. N Engl J Med 317:146–149, 1987
9. Stevens DL, Tanner MH, Winship J, et al: Severe group A streptococcal infections associated with a toxic shock-like syndrome and scarlet fever A. Infectious Disease Service, Veterans Administration Medical Center, Boise, Idaho. N Engl J Med 321:1–7, 1989
10. Taranta A, Markowitz M: Rheumatic Fever, 2 edt. Boston: Kluwer Academic Publishers, 1989, p 87
11. Charney E, Bynum R, Eldredge D, et al: How well do patients take oral penicillin? A collaborative study in private practice. Pediatrics 40:188, 1967
12. Markowitz M, Gordis L: Rheumatic Fever, 2 edt. Philadelphia: Saunders, 1972, p 222
13. Rosenstein BJ, Markowitz M: Unpublished observations cited by Gordis L and Markowitz M: Environmental determinants in rheumatic fever prevention. In Wannamaker LW, Masters JM (eds): Streptococci and Streptococcal Diseases: Recognition, Understanding, and Management. New York: Academic, 1972
14. Jackson H: Streptococcal control in grade schools. Am J Dis Child 130:273–279, 1976
15. Wilkinson HW: Group B streptococcal infection in humans. Annu Rev Microbiol 32:41–57, 1978
16. Baker CJ: Group B streptococcal infection in neonates: Is prevention possible? South Med J 69:1527, 1976
17. Paul JR: Epidemiology of Rheumatic Fever. New York: American Heart Association, 1957
18. Gordis L, Lilienfeld A, Rodriguez R: Studies in the epidemiology and preventability of rheumatic fever. II. Socioeconomic factors in the incidence of acute attack. J Chronic Dis 21:655, 1969
19. Quinn RW, Downey FM, Federspiel CF: The incidence of rheumatic fever in metropolitan Nashville, 1963–65. Public Health Rep 82:673, 1967
20. Gordis L, Lilienfeld A, Rodriguez R: Studies in the epidemiology and preventability of rheumatic fever. I. Demographic factors and the incidence of acute attacks. J Chronic Dis 2:645, 1969
21. Gordis L: Effectiveness of comprehensive-care programs in preventing fever. N Engl J Med 289:331–335, 1973
22. Gordis L: The virtual disappearance of rheumatic fever in the United States: Lessons in the rise and fall of disease. T. Duckett Jones Memorial Lecture. Circulation 72:1155–1162, 1985
23. Bisno AL: The resurgence of rheumatic fever in the United States. Annu Rev Med 41:319–329, 1990

Meningococcal Meningitis

1. Frasch CE: Role of protein subtype antigens in protection against disease due to *Neisseria meningitidis*. J Infect Dis 136:584–590, 1977
2. Olyhoek T, Crowe BA, Achtman M: Clonal population structure of *Neisseria meningitidis* serogroup A isolated from epidemics and pandemics between 1915 and 1983. Rev Infect Dis 9:665–692, 1987
3. Band JD, Chamberland ME, Platt T, et al: Trends in meningococcal disease in the United States. J Infect Dis 148:754–758, 1983
4. Broome CV: The carrier state: *Neisseria meningitidis*. J Antimicrob Chemother 18(suppl A):25–34, 1986
5. Goldschneider I, Gotschlich EC, Artenstein MS: Human immunity to the meningococcus. I. The role of humoral antibodies. J Exp Med 129:1307–1326, 1969
6. Ghipponi P, Darrigol J, Skalova R, Cvjetanovic B: Study of bacterial air pollution in an arid region of Africa affected by cerebrospinal meningitis. Bull WHO 45:95–101, 1971
7. Blakebrough IS, Greenwood BM, Whittle HC, et al: The epidemiol-

ogy of infections due to *Neisseria meningitidis* and *Neisseria lactamica* in a Northern Nigerian community. J Infect Dis 146:626-637, 1982

8. Munford RS, Taunay ADE, Morais JS, et al: Spread of meningococcal infection within households. Lancet 1:1275-1278, 1974
9. Greenfield S, Sheehe PR, Feldman HA: Meningococcal carriage in a population of "normal" families. J Infect Dis 123:67-73, 1971
10. Meningococcal Surveillance Group: Analysis of endemic meningococcal disease by serogroup and evaluation of chemoprophylaxis. J Infect Dis 134:201-204, 1976
11. Favorova LA, Sokova IN, Chernyshova TF, et al: Results of controlled epidemiological trial on the use of placental gamma globulin in foci of meningococcal infection. Zh Mikrobiol Epidemiol Immunobiol 6:15-18, 1975
12. Schwartz B, Moore PS, Broome CV: Global epidemiology of meningococcal disease. Clin Microbiol Rev 2:S118-S124, 1989
13. Kuhns DM, Nelson CT, Feldman HA, Kuhn LR: The prophylactic value of sulfadiazine in the control of meningococcic meningitis. JAMA 123:335-339, 1943
14. Jacobson JA, Chester TJ, Fraser DW: An epidemic of disease due to serogroup B *Neisseria meningitidis* in Alabama: Report of an investigation and community-wide prophylaxis with a sulfonamide. J Infect Dis 136:104-107, 1977
15. Immunization Practices Advisory Committee: Meningococcal vaccines. MMWR 34:255-259, 1985
16. Schwartz B, Al-Tobaiqi A, Al-Ruwais A, et al: Comparative efficacy of ceftriaxone and frifampicin in eradicating pharyngeal carriage of group A *Neisseria meningitidis*. Lancet 1:1239-1242, 1988
17. Artenstein MS, Gold R, Zimmerly JG, et al: Prevention of meningococcal disease by group C polysaccharide vaccine. N Engl J Med 282:417-420, 1970
18. Wahdan MH, Rizk R, El-Akkad AM, et al: A controlled field trial of a serogroup A meningococcal polysaccharide vaccine. Bull WHO 48:667-673, 1973
19. Peltola H, Makela PH, Kahty H, et al: Clinical efficacy of meningococcus group A capsular polysaccharide vaccine in children 3 months to 5 years of age. N Engl J Med 297:686-691, 1977
20. Reingold AL, Broome CV, Hightower AW, et al: Age-specific differences in duration of clinical protection after vaccination with meningococcal polysaccharide A vaccine. Lancet 2:114-118, 1985
21. Greenwood BM, Hassan-King M, Whittle HC: Prevention of secondary cases of meningococcal disease in household contacts by vaccination. Br Med J 1:1317-1319, 1978

Tuberculosis

1. Dubos R, Dubos J: The White Plague: Tuberculosis, Man and Society. Boston: Little, Brown, 1952
2. Gracey DR: Tuberculosis in the world today. Mayo Clin Proc 63:1251, 1988
3. Rieder HL, Cauthen GM, Kelly GD, et al: Tuberculosis in the United States. JAMA 262:385, 1989
4. Centers for Disease Control: A strategic plan for the elimination of tuberculosis in the United States. MMWR 38(suppl S-3):1-25, 1989
5. Des Prez RM, Heim CR: Mycobacterium tuberculosis. In Mandell GL, Douglas RG, Bennett JE (eds): Principles and Practice of Infectious Diseases, 3 edt. New York: Churchill Livingstone, 1989, pp 1877-1906
6. Laennec RTH: Traite de L'Auscultation Mediate et des Maladies des Poumons et du Coeur, 2 edt. Paris: JS Chaude, 1826
7. Villemin JA: Cause et nature de la tuberculose. Bull Acad Med Paris 31:211, 1865
8. Koch R: Die etiologie der tuberkulose. Berlin Klin Wochenschr 17:1189, 1882
9. Von Pirquet C: Der diagnostischen wert der kutanen tuberculin reaktion bei der tuberculosis des kindersalters auf grund von 100 sektionen. Wien Klin Wochenschr 20, 1907
10. Caldwell M: The Last Crusade: The War on Consumption 1862-1954. New York: Atheneum, 1988
11. Wayne LG, Kubica GP: Genus *Mycobacterium*. In Sneath PHA (ed): Bergey's Manual of Systematic Bacteriology, Vol 2. Baltimore: Williams & Wilkins, 1986, pp 1436-1457
12. Modilevsky T, Sattler FR, Barnes PF: Mycobacterial disease in patients with immunodeficiency virus infection. Arch Intern Med 149:2201-2205, 1989
13. Wells WF, Ratcliffe HL, Crumb C: On the mechanics of droplet nuclei infection. II. Quantitative experimental air-borne tuberculosis in rabbits. Am J Hyg 47:11-28, 1948
14. Riley RL: Disease transmission and contagion control. Am Rev Respir Dis 125:16-19, 1982
15. Gottridge J, et al: The nonutility of chest roentgenographic examination in asymptomatic patients with positive tuberculin test result. Arch Intern Med 149:1660, 1989
16. American Thoracic Society and Centers for Disease Control: Treatment of tuberculosis and tuberculous infection in adults and children. Am Rev Respir Dis 134:355-366, 1986
17. American Thoracic Society: Diagnostic standards and classification of tuberculosis and other mycobacterial diseases. Am Rev Respir Dis 123:343, 1981
18. Riley RL, et al: Infectiousness of air from a tuberculosis ward: Ultraviolet irradiation of infected air: Comparative infectiousness of different patients. Am Rev Respir Dis 85:511, 1962
19. Ferebee SH: Controlled chemoprophylaxis trials in tuberculosis. A general review. Tuberc Med Thorac 76:78-106, 1970
20. Snider DE, Caras GJ, Koplan JP: Preventive therapy with isoniazid: Cost-effectiveness of different durations of therapy. JAMA 255:1579, 1986
21. Hinman AR, Judd JM, Kolnick JT, Daitch PB: Changing risks in TB. Am J Epidemiol 103:487-497, 1976
22. Snider DE, Hutton MD: Tuberculosis in correctional institutions. JAMA 261:436-437, 1989
23. Stead WW: Undetected tuberculosis in prison (source of infection for community at large). JAMA 240:2544-2547, 1978
24. Counsell SR, Tan JS, Dittus RS: Unsuspected pulmonary tuberculosis in a teaching hospital. Arch Intern Med 149:1274, 1989
25. Kantor HS, Poblete R, Pusateri SL: Nosocomial transmission of tuberculosis from unsuspected disease. Am J Med 84:833, 1988
26. Rieder HL, et al: Tuberculosis and acquired immunodeficiency syndrome—Florida. Arch Intern Med 149:1268, 1989
27. Centers for Disease Control: Screening for tuberculosis and tuberculous infection in high-risk populations and the use of preventive therapy for tuberculous infection in the United States. MMWR 39:No. RR-8, 1989
28. Centers for Disease Control: AIDS and human immunodeficiency virus infection in the United States: 1988 update. MMWR 38:No. S-4, 1989
29. Selwyn PD, Hartel D, Lewis VA, et al: A prospective study of the risk of tuberculosis among intravenous drug abusers with human immunodeficiency virus infection. N Engl J Med 320:545-550, 1989
30. Stead WW, Lofgren JP, Warren E, et al: Tuberculosis as an epidemic and nosocomial infection among the elderly in nursing homes. N Engl J Med 312:1483-1487, 1985
31. Stead WW, To T, Harrison RW: Benefit risk considerations in preventive treatment of tuberculosis in elderly persons. Ann Intern Med 107:843-845, 1987
32. Schieffelbein CW, Snider DE: Tuberculosis control among homeless populations. Arch Intern Med 148:1843, 1988
33. Use of BCG vaccines in the control of tuberculosis: A joint statement by the ACIP and the advisory ACIP Committee for elimination of tuberculosis. JAMA 260:2983, 1988
34. Boudes P, Sobel A, Deforges L, Leblic E: Disseminated *Mycobacterium bovis* infection from BCG vaccination and HIV infection. JAMA 262:2386, 1989

Leprosy

1. Neill MA, Hightower AW, Broome CV: Leprosy in the United States, 1971-1981. J Infect Dis 152:1064-1069, 1985

2. Blake LA, West BC, Lary CH, Todd JR IV: Environmental nonhuman sources of leprosy. Rev Infect Dis 9:562–577, 1987
3. Bullock WE: *Mycobacterium leprae* (leprosy). In Mandell GL, Douglas RG Jr, Bennett JE (eds): Principles and Practice of Infectious Diseases, 3 edt. New York: Churchill Livingstone, 1990, pp 1906–1914
4. Ridley DS: Review of the five-group system for the classification of leprosy according to immunity. Int J Lepr 40:102, 1972
5. Sehgal VN, Joginder MBBS: Slit-skin smear in leprosy. Int J Dermatol 29(1):9–16, 1990
6. Nakamura K: Leprosy. In Balows A, Hausler WJ Jr, Lennette EH (eds): Laboratory Diagnosis of Infectious Diseases: Principles and Practices, 1 edt. New York: Springer-Verlag, 1988, pp 333–343
7. Fine PE: Immunological tools in leprosy control. Int J Lepr Other Mycobact Dis 57(3):671–686, 1989
8. Desforges S, Bobin P, Brethes B, et al: Specific anti-*M. leprae* PGL-I antibodies and Mitsuda reaction in the management of household contacts in New Caledonia. Int J Lepr Other Mycobact Dis 57(4):794–800, 1989
9. Nordeen SK: Current global strategy for leprosy control. In Proceedings of the First International Leprosy Symposium in China. Beijing, PRC: The China Leprosy Association, 1985, pp 18–23
10. Vigneron E: The epidemiological transition in an overseas territory: Disease mapping in French Polynesia. Soc Sci Med 29(8):913–922, 1989
11. Irgens LM, Skjaerven R: Secular trends in age at onset, sex ratio, and type index in leprosy observed during declining incidence rates. Am J Epidemiol 122:695–705, 1985
12. Sundar RPS, Jesudasan K, Mani K, Christian M: Impact of MDT on incidence rates of leprosy among household contacts. Part 1. Baseline data. Int J Lepr Other Mycobact Dis 57(3):647–651, 1989
13. George K, John KR, Muliyil JP, Joseph A: The role of intrahousehold contact in the transmission of leprosy. Lepr Rev 61(1):60–63, 1990
14. WHO Study Group: Chemotherapy of leprosy for control programmes. WHO Tech Rep Ser 625:7, 1982
15. Baker RJ: The need for new drugs in the treatment and control of leprosy. Int J Lepr Other Mycobact Dis 58(1):78–97, 1990
16. Loretti A: Leprosy control: The rationale of integration. Lepr Rev 60(4):306–316, 1989
17. Filice GA, Fraser DW: Management of household contacts of leprosy patients. Ann Intern Med 88:538, 1978
18. Fine PEM, Rodrigues LC: Modern vaccines: Mycobacterial diseases. Lancet 335(1):1016–1020, 1990
19. Stanley SJ, Howland C, Stone MM, Sutherland I: BCG vaccination of children against leprosy in Uganda: Final results. J Hyg (Camb) 87:233–248, 1981
20. Bagshawe A, Scott GC, Russell DA, et al: BCG vaccination in leprosy: Final results of the trial in Karimui, Papua New Guinea, 1963–1979. Bull WHO 67:389–399, 1989
21. Lwin K, Sundaresan T, Gyi MM, et al: BCG vaccination of children against leprosy: Fourteen-year findings of the trial in Burma. Bull WHO 63:1069–1078, 1985
22. Fine PEM: Background, design and prospects of the Karonga prevention trial, a leprosy vaccine trial in northern Malawi. Trans R Soc Trop Med Hyg 82:810–817, 1988

8

Diseases Spread by Food and Water

Typhoid Fever

William C. Levine
Paul A. Blake

Typhoid fever is an acute bacterial disease caused by *Salmonella typhi*. Although it was initially confused with typhus, the disease was clinically and pathologically differentiated from typhus, and control of typhoid fever was first attempted with a killed-cell vaccine in the late nineteenth century. Although the other *Salmonella* species with which it is grouped bacteriologically have many natural animal hosts, *S. typhi* is a natural pathogen only of humans.

Bacteriology. *S. typhi,* like other *Salmonella* species, is a gram-negative, flagellated, non-lactose-fermenting bacillus and is identified by its biochemical properties and its somatic (O) and flagellar (H) antigens. Most freshly isolated strains have a capsular (Vi) antigen. In the Kauffman-White schema, *S. typhi* is a member of *Salmonella* group D, characterized by O antigens 1, 9, and 12. *S. typhi* is readily killed by pasteurization. The organism survives well in water and sewage. Phage typing is a useful epidemiological tool.[1] Organisms resistant to antibiotics, including chloramphenicol, have been reported. Organisms with multiple resistance now occur, and determining antimicrobial resistance patterns may be useful in epidemiological studies.[2]

The organism is present in the blood most commonly in the first week of fever, but in a high percentage of cases it is also present in the second and third weeks of illness. During clinical relapse the organism can be isolated from the blood almost as regularly as during the acute phase of the disease, although usually for a shorter time. Fecal cultures are positive in approximately half of the cases during the first week of fever and are more frequently positive in the second and third weeks of untreated disease. Bacteria may be passed in the urine, especially during the first weeks of illness. Infection of the gallbladder is common; organisms are also likely to be present in duodenal aspirates.[3] Bone marrow cultures are more likely to yield *S. typhi* than are cultures of other sites and may be especially useful when the patient has undergone antimicrobial therapy.[4]

Clinical Characteristics. The onset of typhoid fever is normally insidious and is characterized by fever, malaise, chills, headache, and generalized aches in the muscles and joints.[5] The spleen is usually enlarged, leukopenia is generally present, and small, discrete, rose-colored spots caused by bacterial emboli in the skin capillaries may appear on the trunk early in the illness. Diarrhea is uncommon, and vomiting, which may occur toward the end of the first week, is not usually severe. Abdominal distention and tenderness are common. Many patients cough for the first few days of illness, and some complain of sore throat or joint pain. Although typhoid fever is typically a septicemic, febrile illness, the presenting symptoms vary widely. After the first weeks, untreated persons may be confused and delirious even when the fever is not high. In children the disease is often atypical and occurs as a short febrile illness rather than a long septicemic one. Respiratory symptoms are often present.[6]

In studies of volunteers, incubation periods have been as short as 3 days and as long as 56 days after oral challenge.[7] In the majority of cases the incubation period ranges from 7 to 21 days, with an average of 14 days. The infective dose and the incubation period are inversely related. Immunity follows clinical illness, but reinfection and illness can occur with a large (10^9 organisms) oral challenge. Antibody titers are not correlated with resistance to reinfection or occurrence of relapse.

Treatment. Antimicrobial therapy terminates the clinical illness; significant clinical symptoms subside within 48 hours and fever recedes within 5 days. Chloramphenicol is the drug of choice for treatment of the acute illness in the absence of antimicrobial resistance.[8] Trimethoprim-sulfamethoxazole, ampicillin, and amoxicillin are effective alternatives. Newer agents, the third-generation cephalosporins and quinolones, may also be effective and are useful for treating infection with resistant strains, but few clinical trials have compared their efficacy with that of chloramphenicol.[9,10] Without antimicrobial therapy the illness may continue for 3 to 4 weeks. Relapses, characterized by a somewhat less severe but otherwise typical illness, occur in 10% to 20% of patients with typhoid fever, usually after an afebrile period of 1 to 2 weeks. The frequency of relapse does not appear to have been changed dramatically by antimicrobial therapy.[11]

Intestinal hemorrhage, perforation, and the other complications of typhoid fever are less likely if effective antimicrobial therapy is begun early. Occasionally, late sequelae such as periosteal abscess of the tibia or ribs occur. The case-fatality rate for treated patients is often less than 5% but depends on the patient's condition when treatment begins.

Serological Diagnosis. During the course of typhoid fever, serological responses occur to cell wall (O), flagellar (H), and capsular (Vi) antigens. The Widal test, which measures responses to

H and O antigens, can suggest the diagnosis, but the results must be interpreted with care. High-titer, single serum specimens from adults in areas of endemic disease have little diagnostic value. Even when paired sera are used, the results must be interpreted in light of the patient's history of typhoid immunization and previous illness, the stage of the illness when the first serum specimen was obtained, the use of early antimicrobial therapy, and the reagents used. Agglutinins usually appear in the blood by the end of the first week of illness.[12]

Carriers. Following treated or untreated infection, carriage of *S. typhi* in the stool often persists for 1 to 2 months, but cultures are negative for nearly all patients by 3 months. The likelihood of a chronic carrier state, that is, excretion of the organism for more than 1 year, is related to age at onset of disease and sex. In both men and women with onset under 20 years of age, chronic enteric carriage is infrequent (0.3%), whereas in women with onset over 40 years of age, chronic enteric carriage is common (13.3%).[13] Antimicrobial treatment of typhoid fever may not significantly decrease the occurrence of chronic fecal carriage.[10] Urinary excretion is common in the first months after illness, but chronic urinary carriage is usually associated with preexisting pathological changes in the kidneys or bladder, as occur in patients with schistosomiasis and in the elderly.[14] Elimination of a chronic carrier state requires prolonged use of ampicillin or other antimicrobial agents in high doses. Results of recent trials with orally administered quinolones have been more promising, with cure rates of approximately 80% at 1 year of follow-up.[10] In patients with chronic gallbladder or urinary tract disease, antimicrobial agents alone may be ineffective, and surgery may be necessary.

Antibody to the Vi antigen is often present in serum samples from persons who are chronic carriers and can be used as a screening test for identification of chronic carriers during investigation of sporadic cases and outbreaks and in certain high-risk groups.[15–18]

Transmission. Since *S. typhi* has no animal reservoirs, isolated cases and outbreaks must originate from a human carrier. Most typhoid outbreaks are traced to ingestion of food or water contaminated with human waste. Studies of common-source outbreaks have rarely revealed secondary spread in families, a finding compatible with Hornick and coworkers' observation[7] that the usual infective dose for humans is large (10^6 to 10^9 bacilli).

Of 1013 cases of typhoid fever reported in the United States from 1975 to 1984 in persons with no history of foreign travel,[19] 28% were related to outbreaks. The source of exposure was unknown in most cases, but 21% were associated with newly discovered typhoid carriers, 9% with previously identified carriers, and 3% with exposures to laboratories.

Health departments have developed routine methods of monitoring known chronic typhoid carriers. These persons are asked to supply periodic stool specimens for culture, are instructed concerning personal hygiene, and are prohibited from preparing food for anyone except members of their families.

Occurrence. Typhoid fever has worldwide distribution but varies widely in incidence, seasonality, and vehicles of infection. The steady decrease in incidence of the disease in western Europe and the United States in the first half of the twentieth century was associated with the development of protected water supplies, pasteurization of milk, and improved sewage systems. As with many infectious diseases, the best epidemiological data about typhoid fever come from studies of outbreaks, whereas endemic disease has been studied less. In the United States fewer than 500 clinical cases are reported each year, and approximately 62% of these are associated with foreign travel,[20] although large outbreaks still occur.[20] For cases acquired in the United States, the incidence is equal for both sexes and the median age is 20 years. In the early 1970s, resistance of *S. typhi* to chloramphenicol appeared in the United States among travelers returning from Mexico, where there was a prolonged epidemic of chloramphenicol-resistant *S. typhi.*[2] Outbreaks of chloramphenicol-resistant *S. typhi* in Vietnam, Peru, and India have also been reported.[21–23]

Prevention. Although vaccines against typhoid fever have been available for more than 80 years, the first controlled field trials were carried out by the World Health Organization in 1954 to 1967. In these trials the heat- and phenol-inactivated vaccine provided 51% to 67% efficacy, and the acetone-inactivated vaccine 56% to 88% efficacy.[24] Studies in volunteers from areas where typhoid fever is rare have shown that vaccine-induced immunity is protective (65% to 70% effective) against low to moderate infecting doses (10^5 organisms) but, like natural immunity, it provides no protection against very large (10^9 organisms) challenge doses.[7]

Because of the unpleasant side effects of the killed-cell vaccines, which include fever, headache, myalgia, malaise, localized pain, and swelling, other vaccines have been developed. A mutant *S. typhi* strain, Ty2la, which lacks the enzyme UDP-galactose-4-epimerase, has been an effective and safe oral immunizing agent in adult volunteers in the United States and in field trials in Egypt and Chile.[25] The liquid formulation used in Egypt, although cumbersome, was highly effective (96% efficacy). In the trials in Chile, three doses of an enteric-coated capsule given within 1 week had an efficacy of 69% for at least 4 years, with additional protection conferred by a fourth dose. Serum levels of IgG antibodies to *S. typhi* O antigen correlated well with vaccine efficacy. This vaccine has recently been approved for use in the United States. Further studies in Chile and Indonesia will directly compare the efficacy of a liquid formulation with that of enteric-coated capsules. Another vaccine, a parenteral polysaccharide formula based on purified Vi antigen, is being field tested in Nepal and South Africa. This vaccine appears safe, and after 17 to 21 months its efficacy is 64% to 72%.

Immunization has been advised for persons going to or residing in areas where typhoid incidence is high and when circumstances make exposure difficult to avoid. It is sometimes advised for household contacts of a carrier. No evidence indicates that immunization is necessary or effective after earthquakes, floods, and other disasters.

Although effective vaccines with minimal side effects are expected to become more widely available and may assist in controlling typhoid fever in areas of endemic disease, avoidance of exposure to the organism remains the primary means of prevention. As the level of community and personal hygiene rises, the incidence of typhoid fever in susceptible areas will undoubtedly decrease.

Shigellosis

Patricia M. Griffin
Paul A. Blake

In past decades, epidemics of dysentery caused by shigellae have been problems of the military, displaced persons, and, occasionally, crowded urban and rural poor populations. The term "bacillary dysentery," used to describe a diarrheal illness with fever, abdominal pain, and blood and pus (leukocytes) in the stool, is often used as a synonym for diarrhea caused by *Shigella*. Although shigellae do not usually cause epidemic diarrhea in the United States, they commonly cause endemic diarrhea.

Bacteriology. At the end of the nineteenth century, bacillary dysentery was clearly distinguished from dysentery caused by amebae. At that time the bacillary illness was found to be caused by a fairly homogeneous group of aerobic, nonmotile, non-lactose-fermenting, gram-negative bacilli, divided serologically and biochemically into four species, which are both named and given an alphabetical serologic designation. *S. dysenteriae* (group A) has 13 serotypes; type 1 (the Shiga bacillus) remains a cause of epidemic severe dysentery. *S. flexneri* (group B) has six serotypes, some of which are subdivided. *S. boydii* (group C) is divided into 18 serotypes. *S. sonnei* (group D) has only one serotype. Determinations of serotypes, antibiotic resistance profiles, phage types, plasmid profiles, and colicin types have been useful in epidemiological studies.

Many *Shigella* organisms are present in the intestinal mucus or feces early in the illness. When feces are alkaline, the bacilli may survive for days, whereas in acidic stools they remain viable for only a few hours. Therefore, if direct inoculation of culture media is not possible, placing fecal material or rectal swabs in Cary-Blair transport media is suggested. Isolation of *Shigella* from the blood is rare.

Antimicrobial-resistant organisms have been reported frequently in recent years. Resistance to sulfonamides was reported first, followed by tetracycline, and then ampicillin. Resistance of *Shigella* to trimethoprim-sulfamethoxazole has been reported worldwide,[1] and nalidixic acid resistance has also occurred. Multiple drug resistance is common.

Clinical Characteristics. Shigellosis often begins with fever, abdominal pain, and watery diarrhea without blood. At this stage the diarrhea is difficult to distinguish from that caused by other agents. With invasion of the colonic mucosa, stools often become bloody, mucoid, and of low volume. The usual incubation period is about 48 hours but ranges from less than 12 hours to 6 days. The clinical illness associated with *S. dysenteriae* type 1 (Shiga bacillus) is often severe. In the major outbreak in Central America in the late 1960s, case-fatality ratios were 8% to 15% in untreated persons.[2] The death rate was highest in children up to 4 years of age.

Extraintestinal infections are rare, but the disease has some important noninfectious extraintestinal manifestations. Convulsions may occur in children, but the mechanism has not been established.[3] Reiter's syndrome is a late complication of *S. flexneri* infection, especially in HLA-B27-positive persons. Hemolytic-uremic syndrome can occur after *S. dysenteriae* infection.[4]

Asymptomatic infections occur, but an asymptomatic excreter is less likely than a clinically ill person to transmit infection.[5] Prolonged carriage is uncommon in healthy people, but carriage for more than 1 year has been reported.[6] With repeated infections by the same serotype, clinical illness becomes milder or absent. In volunteers prior infection has resulted in reduced proliferation of virulent organisms, apparently because of local gut immunity.

Treatment and Diagnosis. Treatment with ampicillin, trimethoprim-sulfamethoxazole, tetracycline, and quinolone agents reduces the duration of symptoms and the excretion of shigellae.[7,8] *Shigella* organisms, however, are often resistant to the commonly used antimicrobial agents. In a community with endemic disease, monitoring the local antimicrobial resistance patterns can help in selecting an effective drug with which to begin therapy. Since the illness is often mild and self-limited, in areas with endemic shigellosis a policy of reserving antimicrobial treatment for very ill and high-risk persons may delay the emergence of resistant strains. Without a positive culture, diagnosis is often difficult, although the presence of large numbers of polymorphonuclear leukocytes and blood in the stool suggests bacillary dysentery.

Transmission. The primary reservoir for *Shigella* organisms is humans, although shigellae occasionally infect other primates. A small number (10 to 200 organisms) is sufficient to cause infection. As a result, person-to-person spread is easy and more common than transmission by food and water. The incidence of *S. flexneri* infections has increased among homosexual men, in whom the organisms may spread by direct oral-anal contact. Outbreaks are infrequently caused by contaminated food or water. The most common vehicle in foodborne *Shigella* outbreaks in the United States is salad, in which contamination is attributed to poor hygiene practices of the food handler.[9] Drinking or swimming in contaminated water has also led to outbreaks.

Occurrence. *Shigella* infections are most common in preschool children but may occur at any age. In the United States the highest attack rates are in children 1 to 4 years of age, with the peak rate in 2-year-olds. The isolation rates by sex are approximately equal, except for a female predominance in the age groups 10 to 29 and 60 to 79 years.[10] The seasonality of infections varies from country to country. In the United States, *S. sonnei* infections are common in the late summer. The serotype pattern of *Shigella* isolates changes as a region develops, with *S. dysenteriae* being replaced by *S. flexneri* and in turn by *S. sonnei.*[10] In the past 10 years in the United States, *S. sonnei* has been isolated more than twice as frequently as *S. flexneri*. Isolation of *S. dysenteriae* and *S. boydii* is infrequent in the United States, whereas these species are common in developing countries. Epidemics of multiply resistant *S. dysenteriae* type 1 infections still occur in developing areas.[11] Such infections in U.S. residents are often traced to travel to these areas.[12]

Groups with an increased risk of shigellosis include children in day care centers,[13] American Indians,[1] travelers, homosexual men, persons in custodial institutions where personal hygiene is difficult to maintain,[14] and those in homes with inadequate water for handwashing. Secondary attack rates are high in homes of preschool children with clinical shigellosis.

Prevention and Control. Outbreaks of shigellosis are difficult to control.[13,15] Efforts have included isolation of patients, handwashing, improved sanitation, antimicrobial treatment of ill persons and occasionally those with asymptomatic infection, and, rarely, prophylactic treatment of all members of a household or closed institution. Often these measures are only minimally successful. Attempts to control outbreaks with antimicrobial agents may be compromised by the development of antimicrobial-resistant strains. Efforts have been directed to the development of *Shigella* vaccines,[16] but an effective commercially available vaccine is still years in the future.

Shigella infections are least common in communities and institutions where water is easily available and used frequently for handwashing and where an adequate system exists for disposal of human wastes. Handwashing is an effective control measure even in areas with poor sanitation.[17] Protected food supplies and adequate refrigeration are important in reducing the possibility of common-source infection.

Cholera

Robert E. Black

Cholera, an acute infection of the small intestine by *Vibrio cholerae,* is manifest as watery diarrhea. It has been known and feared for centuries because of its propensity to occur in epidemics resulting in high mortality and social disruption.

History. Cholera has probably afflicted humankind since prehistoric times but was not clearly distinguished from other diarrheal illness in ancient medical writings. As a result, the ancestral home of the cholera vibrio is unclear, although Portuguese explorers' descriptions of diarrhea epidemics in India from the late fifteenth century suggest that the Bengal region of India and Bangladesh has been a continuous endemic region for cholera.[1]

The worldwide spread of cholera began in 1817, and by 1823 the first pandemic of cholera had spread from the Ganges River delta to much of Asia and Africa. During the nineteenth century, cholera repeatedly spread along routes of trade and travel from India to Europe, Africa, and North America. Five periods of pandemic spread occurred before 1900: from 1817 to 1823; 1826 to 1837; 1846 to 1862; 1864 to 1875; and 1887 to 1896. In each country involved, thousands were affected, with case-fatality rates often approaching 50%. The fear of this disease can be appreciated from a description written in 1831. Its victims

> were in a manner stricken down at once, and exhibited more the appearances of a corpse than a living being; with the eyes sunk in the sockets, the skin dark as if from nitrate of silver, the toes and fingers shrivelled, and the tendons standing out like rigid cords along the limbs; while the very breath was cold, and the pulse scarcely to be felt.[2]

The sixth pandemic (1902 to 1923) also involved severe epidemics, especially in Asia, but outbreaks in Africa and Europe were more limited than in previous pandemics and the Western Hemisphere was not involved. The sixth pandemic and presumably the previous pandemics were due to the classic biotype of *V. cholerae.* Classic cholera has recently reappeared in a major epidemic in Bangladesh.[3]

The seventh pandemic, which continued through the 1980s, is generally considered to have started in 1961. The causative agent of this pandemic was first isolated in 1905 by Gotschlick from pilgrims returning from Mecca at the El Tor quarantine camp in Egypt. Although this organism was initially considered nonpathogenic, outbreaks of severe disease between 1937 and 1958 confirmed its ability to cause epidemic disease.[4] An outbreak caused by *V. cholerae* biotype El Tor in Sulawesi in 1961 was the beginning of the seventh pandemic. From there it quickly spread to Java, Sarawak, Borneo, the Philippines, and most of Southeast Asia. Between 1963 and 1969 this organism continued its spread across the Asian mainland. In India and later in Bangladesh the El Tor biotype eventually replaced classic *V. cholerae.* In 1970 the pandemic continued its westward progression and involved the Middle East, the Soviet Union, and large areas of Africa. Since 1970 serious outbreaks have occurred in Spain, Portugal, and Italy.

North America had no indigenous cases of cholera from 1911 until a single case was detected in Texas in 1973. In August 1978 a case in Louisiana led to an investigation that ultimately detected infection in 11 persons.[5] In this outbreak *V. cholerae* El Tor serotype Inaba was recovered from sewage and canal water and from crabs, which were implicated as the vehicle of infection. In 1981 cholera was found in two residents of the Gulf Coast of Texas and another 17 persons on an oil rig in the gulf near Texas. Other than in the United States, no recent cases of cholera were recognized in any country of North, Central, or South America until 1983 when a U.S. tourist apparently became infected with *V. cholerae* while visiting the Caribbean coast of Mexico and developed cholera after returning home.

Agent and Pathogenesis. In 1883 Koch first isolated *V. cholerae* from the stools of patients with cholera. It is a small, curved, motile aerobic gram-negative organism best identified by inoculating stool into taurocholate-tellurite-gelatin (TTG) agar or thiosulfate–citrate–bile salts–sucrose (TCBS) agar. *V. cholerae* colonies are relatively small on TTG agar after 24 hours and are translucent with a dark center and a cloudy zone surrounding the colonies. On TCBS agar *V. cholerae* are easily recognized as large yellow colonies on a blue-green medium. The species is identified on the basis of cultural and biochemical tests; the O group determination requires agglutination with type-specific antisera.[6]

Cholera vibrios, which have been associated with pandemic disease, are assigned to O group 1. They are further separated into three serotypes—Ogawa, Inaba, and Hikojima—based on three somatic, or O, antigens. Closely related vibrios that do not agglutinate in cholera antiserum are assigned to other O groups. They may be isolated from persons with sporadic and even epidemic diarrhea but have not occurred in pandemics as has *V. cholerae* O group 1. *V. cholerae* is differentiated from classic *V. cholerae* by its ability to agglutinate chick cells and by its resistance to phage IV and to polymyxin.[7]

The organism produces a protein enterotoxin that increases the activity of adenylate cyclase in the intestinal mucosa, resulting in increased levels of cyclic 3′:5′ adenosine monophosphate (cAMP). This in turn leads to inhibition of sodium chloride absorption by villus cells and secretion of chloride and bicarbonate by secretory cells in the crypts of Lieberkühn. The bacteria do not invade or structurally damage the intestinal mucosa.

Clinical Characteristics. The clinical spectrum of cholera is broad, ranging from inapparent infection to cholera gravis, which may be fatal in a few hours. The incubation period of 24 to 48 hours is followed by an abrupt onset of watery, generally painless, diarrhea. Vomiting often follows the diarrhea in the early stages of illness.

In severe cases the loss of diarrheal stool can be extreme. The appearance of the stool as a nonoffensive, sometimes fishy-smelling, clear fluid with flakes of mucus has resulted in the descriptive term "rice water stool."

The symptoms and signs of cholera are entirely due to the loss of large volumes of isotonic fluid and resultant depletion of intravascular and extracellular fluid, metabolic acidosis, and hypokalemia. In addition to the diarrhea and vomiting, symptoms include lightheadedness, anxiety, thirst, and muscle cramps. Signs include cyanosis, tachycardia, hypotension, tachypnea, and loss of skin turgor. In those who survive, the disease subsides spontaneously in 2 to 7 days. Excretion of the organism may continue for days and occasionally weeks after recovery from the illness; a chronic gallbladder carrier state is rare. Both the duration of diarrhea and the persistence of the organism can be greatly reduced by tetracycline therapy.[8] However, the emergence of *V. cholerae* strains resistant to multiple antibiotics, including tetracycline, in East Africa and Bangladesh complicates antimicrobial therapy.

The severity of illness caused by classic cholera and *V. cholerae* El Tor differs greatly. In classic cholera about 60% of infections are inapparent but 20% of infected persons have severe cholera requiring hospitalization. In El Tor cholera 80% of infections are inapparent and less than 3% are severe. This milder disease has important public health implications because, for each severe case, many more undetected infections are present in the community.

Therapy has improved dramatically during the last 20 years, so that with prompt treatment few persons die of cholera, regardless of severity. Therapy is based simply on the prompt and complete replacement of water and electrolytes.[9] This can be done intravenously or more simply by the oral route in those not vomiting.[10] Intravenous therapy is necessary for patients in shock and for those with an exceptionally high rate of stool output. In these settings, the rapid administration of a large volume of fluid may be lifesaving. Since glucose-facilitated sodium absorption is not disturbed in cholera, all but the most severe disease can be treated with oral administration of glucose (or even sucrose) electrolyte solution. The oral solution currently recommended by WHO contains (in milliequivalents or millimoles per liter) sodium 90, potassium 20, chloride 80, citrate 30, glucose 111. This oral form of therapy has great importance because in many areas where cholera occurs a sufficient supply of intravenous fluid is too expensive or too difficult to obtain. The ingredients for oral rehydration can be readily packaged, transported, and reconstituted on site. In the absence of any immediately available method of prevention in many areas of the world that are infected with cholera, this simplified treatment is critically important.

Susceptibility and Immunity. Lower socioeconomic groups have a higher incidence of cholera for a variety of reasons: (1) occupational exposures (e.g., boatmen in several areas have a high incidence of cholera, probably because they often drink raw river water); (2) unsanitary conditions in low-income housing areas, primarily reflected in inadequate sewage disposal and contaminated water sources; and (3) high population density in low-income areas, increasing the risk of introduction of *V. cholerae* and possibly enhancing transmission of the organism after it has been introduced. Malnutrition among low-income people may aggravate the risk of infection. Although some studies suggest that poor nutrition increases duration of diarrhea from *V. cholerae*, there is no convincing evidence of an increased incidence of disease.[11]

Many studies have demonstrated an increased rate of infection among the household contacts of persons with cholera.[12] Although the techniques varied in sensitivity, these studies reveal that 6% to 27% of family contacts are also infected with *V. cholerae* within 10 to 14 days after the person whose disease was initially recognized. The onset of disease at almost the same time in the initial patient and household contacts suggests that the family contacts have "coprimary" cases; that is, they are infected from the same common source rather than by "secondary" infection from the first patient.

Studies in India, Italy, Israel, and Bangladesh, as well as volunteer challenge studies, have shown that diminished gastric acid increases risk of infection and of more severe illness.[13] The protection afforded by gastric acid is probably due to the sensitivity of *V. cholerae* to the low pH. In addition, for unknown reasons, severe disease is more common in persons with blood group O.

The relationship between age and cholera has been extensively studied. In newly infected areas, cholera characteristically affects more adults than children. The earliest cases often occur in men, who may have more frequent exposure because of their greater mobility. In endemic areas such as Bangladesh, cholera has a higher attack rate in children than in adults, with a peak incidence in the 2- to 9-year-old group.[14] Breast-feeding provides some protection from illness in younger children.[15]

One possible explanation for the difference in age distribution of cholera between newly infected and endemic areas is acquired immunity. Studies in Bangladesh demonstrated that, with increasing age and a fall in cholera incidence, the serum vibriocidal titer rises. Serum vibriocidal antibody is thought to reflect the immune state but does not itself provide protection. Animal experiments and volunteer challenge studies suggest that immunity to *V. cholerae* is long lasting and is mediated by the local intestinal immune system.[16] The way in which these defenses operate is not yet clearly understood, but intensive work is being aimed at exploiting these mechanisms for the development of a more protective cholera vaccine.

Breast-feeding protects infants against cholera in areas of both endemic and epidemic disease. Breast-feeding, especially exclusively, reduces exposure to *V. cholerae* in food or water. In addition, IgA antibodies in breast milk protect children from diarrhea, although not from infection.

Seasonality. Cholera occurs in a seasonal pattern; however, the season differs among countries and even among regions of the same country. Moreover, the season may change with time in the same area. Thus the waning of an epidemic may be a natural occurrence and not the result of control measures.

Pattern of Spread. The spread of cholera during the seventh pandemic has been facilitated by modern transportation. Now, as observed in 1931, "It travels as man travels, stops where he stops, and proceeds again at the time, and in the direction, in which he resumes his journey."

Humans are the usual reservoir of *V. cholerae*. These organisms reach the environment through the stool of infected persons, but *V. cholerae* poorly tolerates exposures such as drying and sunlight. On moist, fecally contaminated clothing *V. cholerae* El Tor survives 1 to 3 days, but on dry surfaces it dies quickly; thus fomites are not a dangerous vehicle of cholera. Cholera vibrios may remain viable for up to 7 days on the surface of fruits, vegetables, and meat under favorable conditions, and up to 3 weeks in nonacidic fish and shellfish.[1]

In water the survival time is enhanced by a temperature of 18° to 23° C (60° to 70° F), pH between 6 and 9, and sodium chloride content 1% to 4%. Many other factors, such as the presence of nutritives and the deposition of a large number of organisms, may favor survival. In contrast, competitive organisms, sunlight, chemicals such as chlorine and iodine, and rapidly flowing water shorten survival. *V. cholerae* El Tor probably cannot survive for more than 4 weeks in water and usually survives for less than 1 week. The cases of cholera in the Gulf Coast area of Texas and Louisiana since 1973, however, may have been due to a strain of *V. cholerae* that has persisted as a free-living organism in the estuarial environment.[17] In this area and possibly others, it appears that the organism has a free-living cycle with a natural reservoir in the environment.

Since the investigations of John Snow (see Chapter 2) and the waterborne epidemic in Hamburg in 1892, water has been considered an important vehicle in transportation.[2] Water is probably the primary vehicle of infection in endemic areas such as Bangladesh.[18] Even in this setting, however, the exposures are varied and complex. Epidemiological studies in rural Bangladesh have failed to demonstrate lower cholera infection rates in persons taking drinking water from bacteriologically safe tube wells than in persons drinking contaminated surface water. This unexpected finding has led to the speculation, supported by several studies, that the protection afforded by drinking better quality water may be overwhelmed by frequent exposure to polluted surface water through bathing, food preparation, and utensil washing.[19] Avoidance of tube well water by children, who have a high incidence of cholera, may also contribute to the apparent lack of protection noted in these areas when such safe drinking water was provided.

In endemic areas, outbreaks can sometimes be related to a common food source. In addition, contaminated foods have been the source of explosive outbreaks in newly infected areas. During the seventh pandemic, careful epidemiological investigation of outbreaks has frequently led to the identification of a responsible food item. These have included raw vegetables in Israel (1970), mussels in Italy (1973), salted fish in Guam (1974), raw cockles and commercially bottled water in Portugal (1974), raw shellfish in the Gilbert Islands (1977), and inadequately steamed crabs in Louisiana (1978).[5] The commonly implicated foods, such as shellfish, either come from polluted water or are "freshened" with contaminated water before being sold. In arid, inland areas of Africa that should be hostile to marine vibrios, the organism seems to survive under environmental conditions. Person-to-person transmission can occur under special circumstances. For example, transmission during burial ceremonies has been reported, particularly in Africa. In these settings transmission may be from person to person or via food or drinks served at the time of the burial. Hospitals are another setting in which person-to-person spread has been reported. Although flies may transport a small number of vibrios from excreta to food, the lack of multiplication of vibrios in such contaminated food makes it unlikely that flies play an important role in transmission. Fomites probably play only a limited role in transmission, although fecally contaminated bedlinen or clothing may pose a risk if measures to avoid further contaminating the environment are not taken during laundering.

Prevention. The provision of safe water and adequate disposal of excreta would reduce the high rate of cholera and other diarrheal diseases in many developing countries. Certainly in an epidemic, steps should be taken to ensure uncontaminated or treated water and proper disposal of excreta.

Surveillance, including systematic identification, investigation, and reporting of cases, is a vital aspect of any cholera control program. Appropriate use of laboratory diagnostic facilities facilitates identification of cases. A rectal swab or stool sample should be obtained from persons with suspected cholera to confirm the presence of *V. cholerae.* Communities threatened by cholera can easily institute bacteriologic surveillance for the introduction of *V. cholerae* by culturing feces from the community sewage system. Complete reporting of cases and suspected cases to appropriate public health authorities is important. Repressive control measures such as quarantine should be avoided, since they serve little purpose and may inhibit reporting of cases. Epidemiologic investigation of cases and analysis of information are critical for the formulation of specific control measures.

Surveillance also suggests where to establish treatment facilities in an affected area. With proper warning and preparation, supplies can be ordered and staff trained or shifted to the area. This must remain the first priority of a control effort because adequate treatment can prevent deaths from cholera.

Antibiotic prophylaxis of household contacts of persons with cholera decreases the risk of transmission.[20] However, such an approach has little application for the community at large, where individual risk of infection is much lower, is harder to define, and is spread over a longer period. Treating hundreds of persons would be necessary to prevent a single case.

Mass immunization with parenteral cholera vaccine, although frequently done, offers little in a cholera control program. The current vaccine does not prevent transmission of the organism, and the 50% to 60% protection, lasting for less than 5 months, that is conferred is not enough to justify the cost and difficulty of its delivery. Thus an immunization program may create a false sense of security among both recipients and health administrators and should not supplant more effective control measures. WHO no longer recommends cholera vaccine as a requirement for travel from country to country in any part of the world, but some countries continue to require evidence of immunization. New killed or live *V. cholerae* vaccines may offer greater efficacy and duration of protection.[21]

Escherichia coli Diarrhea

Robert E. Black

Escherichia coli is a gram-negative bacillus that can be found in the normal intestinal flora of humans and animals but can also be an important cause of enteric illness.[1] *E. coli* can be typed biochemically and serologically. The serotypes are described by letter and number on the basis of three antigenic groups, O, K, and H (e.g., *E. coli* O111, K58, and H12).

E. coli organisms are important causes of diarrhea in residents and visitors of developing countries, but *E. coli* diarrhea is relatively uncommon in the United States and northern Europe. Disease with which *E. coli* has been associated has a variety of pathogenic mechanisms, including the ability of the bacteria to produce toxins (enterotoxigenic), penetrate the gut (enteroinvasive), or adhere to the membrane of the enterocyte, resulting in destruction to the microvilli (enteroadherent). Some *E. coli* strains appear to cause diarrhea by as yet unknown mechanisms.

Enteropathogenic **Escherichia coli.** Nursery epidemics of watery diarrhea associated with *E. coli* were first reported in the 1940s. The *E. coli* identified in these outbreaks commonly belonged to specific serotypes that subsequently became known as "enteropathogenic serotypes."[2] Nursery epidemics associated with enteropathogenic serotypes have decreased in the United States in recent years but continue to be reported in other countries, such as the United Kingdom.

Enteropathogenic serotypes of *E. coli* rarely produce the enterotoxins associated with enterotoxigenic *E. coli*. The ability of some enteropathogenic *E. coli*, isolated during an outbreak, to cause diarrhea when given to volunteers suggested that other mechanisms of action may exist. In fact, with the recent discovery that many of the *E. coli* belonging to the so-called enteropathogenic serotypes adhere in a seemingly pathognomonic way to the intestinal epithelium (see the discussion of enteroadherent *E. coli*), this category of pathogenic *E. coli* based on serotype will probably disappear from use.

***Enterotoxigenic* Escherichia coli.** In the late 1960s it was first recognized that some *E. coli* strains produced enterotoxins that caused diarrhea in many animals and in humans. Research in the following decade led to the recognition that these organisms are a major cause of diarrhea in developing countries. The illness caused by enterotoxigenic *E. coli* ranges from mild diarrhea to a dehydrating, cholera-like illness but is usually characterized by watery, nonbloody diarrhea lasting from 1 to 3 days and little or no dehydration. Replacement of water and electrolytes by either the oral or the parenteral route is the only treatment usually required.

Enterotoxigenic *E. coli* organisms are now known to produce two plasmic-mediated enterotoxins: one heat labile and the other heat stable. The heat-labile toxin is structurally similar to cholera toxin and causes loss of fluid and electrolytes in the intestine as a result of adenylate cyclase stimulation.[3] The heat-stable toxin acts in a similar way through stimulation of adenylate cyclase. The relative frequency with which *E. coli* produces the heat-labile toxin, the heat-stable toxin, or both varies in different regions of the world. Analysis of *E. coli* from various areas suggests that strains producing both toxins are largely restricted to a small number of serotypes that are different from the so-called enteropathogenic serotypes.[2] The ability to produce only heat-stable toxin or only heat-labile toxin seems to occur in a broader range of serotypes. Colonizing factors, also plasmid mediated, are probably essential for the *E. coli* to establish itself in the small intestine.

Enterotoxigenic *E. coli* has been shown to cause diarrhea worldwide but seems to be more common in developing countries. Since few community-based studies have been performed, the epidemiology of this illness is only partially understood. In Bangladesh the incidence of diarrhea associated with enterotoxigenic *E. coli* was highest during the first 2 years of life, when one to two episodes per year per child were noted.[4] Although *E. coli* diarrhea also occurs in adults, partial immunity does appear to develop after childhood and the incidence declines after the first 5 years of life.

Transmission of enterotoxigenic *E. coli* is thought to be primarily in water and food. Water was the vehicle for an outbreak in a national park in the United States.[5] Foodborne outbreaks have also been reported in a hospital nursery and on a cruise ship, and enterotoxigenic organisms have been isolated from foods in Bangladesh and the United States. Rarely, person-to-person transmission occurs, particularly in hospital nurseries.

Because of the association of contaminated water and food with occurrence of this disease, avoidance of fecally contaminated water and attention to hygienic food-handling help prevent illness. More specific prevention measures, including immunization, may be possible after further epidemiological and laboratory studies.

Travelers' Diarrhea. Travelers' diarrhea, or "turista," commonly affects travelers within 1 to 2 weeks after they arrive in a foreign country, particularly a developing country. The illness usually consists of watery diarrhea with abdominal cramps; vomiting and high fever are unusual. The diarrhea lasts from 1 to 8 days and is self-limited in most cases.

Diarrhea in travelers may be caused by a variety of bacteria (such as shigellae, salmonellae, and vibrios), viruses (such as calicivirus and rotavirus), and parasites (such as *Giardia lamblia* and *Entamoeba histolytica*). Enterotoxigenic *E. coli* strains appear to cause most cases, however.[6] Travelers apparently acquire the *E. coli* from fecally contaminated water or food, such as salads containing raw vegetables.

Travelers should be advised to avoid water and ice of dubious safety, uncooked foods, and partially cooked shellfish and meats. Perishable or cooked foods that have been left at room temperature should also be avoided. Raw fruits the traveler peels are generally safe, but raw, leafy vegetables (if consumed at all) should be disinfected in chlorine solution. Drinking water may be purified by boiling or by adding 2 to 4 drops of 5% chlorine bleach or 5 to 10 drops of 2% tincture of iodine per quart of water 30 minutes before drinking. Carbonated drinks may be considered safe, but noncarbonated drinks should be avoided.

Daily prophylaxis with doxycycline or trimethoprim-sulfamethoxazole prevents most travelers' diarrhea, primarily by preventing infection with enterotoxigenic *E. coli*.[7] Norfloxacin is also effective in preventing travelers' diarrhea. The antibiotics, however, may have side effects and may promote the emergence of bacteria with multiple drug resistance.

Iodochlorhydroxyquin (Entero-Vioform) should not be used in therapy for diarrhea; it is of dubious value and is dangerous (associated with subacute myelooptic neuropathy). Limited studies have shown little or no value in using most antidiarrheal agents, such as kaolin-pectin or diphenoxylate-atropine, to treat diarrheal illness. Preparations containing bismuth subsalicylate (e.g., Pepto-Bismol), however, may reduce gastrointestinal fluid loss. Furthermore, several studies with trimethoprim-sulfamethoxazole or other drugs indicate that antibiotic treatment of diarrhea caused by enterotoxigenic *E. coli* decreases the duration of illness and reduces the total volume of diarrheal fluid lost.[8] Although replacement of stool fluid and electrolyte losses during enterotoxigenic *E. coli* diarrhea is usually sufficient, as in cholera,[8] antibiotic therapy may be indicated for persons with particularly severe diarrhea or those with cardiac, renal, or other diseases, in whom management of fluid and electrolyte imbalance is difficult. Some other types of diarrhea occurring in travelers, such as shigellosis, giardiasis, and amebiasis, may require more specific antimicrobial treatment.

***Enteroinvasive* Escherichia coli.** In 1971 an outbreak of disease caused by enteroinvasive *E. coli* involved almost 400 persons in the United States. This outbreak was caused by imported French cheese contaminated with *E. coli* O124:B17.[9] These *E. coli* organisms cause a dysenteric diarrheal illness with tenesmus, fever, abdominal cramps, and sometimes bloody stools. The *E. coli* strains associated with this illness produce keratoconjunctivitis in guinea pigs, which serves as a marker for the capability of these organisms to invade the intestinal mucosa.

The global importance of enteroinvasive *E. coli* organisms as a cause of disease is unknown, but they have not been common in several studies in the United States, Bangladesh, and other areas of the world. Because of limited knowledge about the transmission of these organisms, specific preventive measures are unknown.

***Enterohemorrhagic* Escherichia coli.** In 1982 two outbreaks of illness characterized by severe abdominal cramps, grossly bloody diarrhea, and little or no fever occurred.[10] The outbreaks were due to *E. coli* of a rare serotype (O157:H7), which was acquired from inadequately cooked, contaminated ground beef eaten at a fast food restaurant. The *E. coli* strains were not invasive or toxigenic by standard tests; they did appear, however, to produce a cytotoxin that may be identical to Shiga toxin and may play a role in the pathogenesis of the bloody diarrhea. Since these outbreaks sporadic cases of hemorrhagic colitis associated with O157:H7 *E. coli* have been reported in many areas of the world.

***Enteroadherent* Escherichia coli.** Largely because of a search for pathogenic mechanisms of the so-called enteropathogenic *E. coli,* several new categories of *E. coli* pathogens have recently been formed.[11] Some enteropathogenic *E. coli* strains cause characteristic histopathological changes in the intestine involving close adherence to the enterocyte membrane with cupping of the membrane around the bacterium and destruction of the microvilli.[12] Furthermore, most of the enteropathogenic *E. coli* adhere to Hep-2 tissue culture cells with either a localized or a diffuse pattern. After the adherence property was shown to be plasmid mediated, DNA probes were developed as diagnostic tests for research purposes. Enteroadherent *E. coli* organisms manifesting both the localized and diffuse forms of adherence to Hep-2 cells have been shown to be prevalent and to be associated with diarrhea in limited studies in developing countries. Illness caused by these organisms is characterized by fever, malaise, vomiting, and diarrhea, with fecal mucus but not gross blood. The enteroadherent forms of *E. coli* may be more associated than most other enteropathogens with persistent diarrhea lasting beyond 14 days. Since these organisms largely constitute what heretofore have been called enteropathogenic *E. coli,* the epidemiology and control measures known for the latter organisms should pertain.

With the use of the Hep-2 tissue culture assay to identify types of *E. coli,* a third pattern of adherence, different from the localized and diffuse patterns, has been identified.[13] In this pattern the *E. coli* organisms autoagglutinate and have a "stacked-brick" appearance on the microscope slide. This type of *E. coli* was initially called enteroadherent-aggregative, which has been simplified to enteroaggregative. One strain was shown to cause diarrhea in North American adult volunteers, but the pathogenesis of the illness is unknown. Although these organisms have been associated with persistent diarrhea in India, their global importance is not clear.

Yersiniosis

Robert E. Black

Yersinia enterocolitica and *Y. pseudotuberculosis* became widely recognized as human pathogens only in the 1960s. Subsequently these organisms have been implicated in a wide variety of clinical syndromes.

Clinical Characteristics. Illnesses associated with *Yersinia* infection include mesenteric adenitis, terminal ileitis, diarrhea, nonsuppurative arthritis, erythema nodosum, septicemia, and hepatic or splenic abscesses.[1,2] The type of illness varies with age and the presence of underlying disease. The most common syndrome, an acute abdominal illness simulating appendicitis, has been reported in older children in many areas of the world.[1–5] In these cases the appendix is usually normal; but mesenteric adenopathy and inflammation of the terminal portion of the ileum are characteristically present. Diarrhea, as the predominant manifestation of yersiniosis, has been reported primarily in young children in northern Europe but is uncommon in the United States. Arthritis and erythema nodosum, most common in adults, are sequelae of infection reported in Scandinavia and occasionally other countries. Systemic infections, such as septicemia, occur predominantly in persons who are compromised by debilitating disease. Complications of disseminated infections include suppurative hepatic, renal, and splenic lesions, osteomyelitis, wound infections, and meningitis.

Bacteriology. *Y. enterocolitica* and *Y. pseudotuberculosis* are difficult to isolate from stool with routine laboratory procedures. Holding specimens at 4° C (39° F) for several weeks increases the possibility of isolation because *Yersinia,* unlike many other bacteria, grows at this temperature. Cold enrichment may not be necessary to isolate the organism from the stool during acute illness caused by most serotypes of *Y. enterocolitica* but can increase the yield of cultures from asymptomatic persons or convalescent patients and furthermore may be helpful in recognizing some serotypes that cause acute illness. Biotyping and serotyping can further identify these bacteria and are particularly useful in the investigation of an epidemic to document the same *Yersinia* type in ill persons and in the suspected vehicle. Of the serotypes of *Y. enterocolitica,* types O:3, O:5, 27, O:8, O:9, and O:13 are the most frequently associated with human disease in Europe, and type O:8 is the most common in North America.[2–4] Although the pathogenesis of *Yersinia* infections is not well understood, some strains isolated from humans are invasive and some strains produce a heat-stable enterotoxin.

Epidemiology and Prevention. *Yersinia* is frequently isolated from wild and domestic animals, including pigs, dogs, cats, and hares.[6] *Yersinia* is thought to be primarily a zoonotic pathogen with humans as accidental hosts. Several small, family outbreaks of *Y. enterocolitica* infection in the United States have apparently resulted from contact with infected dogs.[3] In many countries swine are a major reservoir for the organisms and human disease has been associated with contact with swine or infected meat. The importance of wild animals as reservoirs or in transmission of disease to humans is unknown.

Transmission of *Yersinia* in food has been suggested because the organisms have been isolated from a variety of foods, including raw beef, poultry, fish, mussels, oysters, milk, and ice cream.[7] Transmission in contaminated milk was documented in the largest outbreak of *Y. enterocolitica* disease in the United States[4] and in several subsequent outbreaks.

Y. enterocolitica has been found in drinking water (usually nonchlorinated well water) in the United States, Canada, and Norway; however, most isolates from water have not been associated with human illness. Waterborne transmission has been hypothesized but, apart from a single case in New York State, is poorly documented. Human-to-human transmission has been implicated in a hospital outbreak of *Y. enterocolitica* infection. Since a large oral inoculum has been needed to cause illness in studies of volunteers, the opportunities for direct fecal-oral spread may be limited.

The demonstration that *Y. enterocolitica* can result in foodborne outbreaks and that foods are sometimes contaminated with *Yersinia* suggests that attention to hygienic food-handling practices may be an important preventive measure, especially with foods of animal origin. Similarly, avoidance of contact with excreta from domestic pets or other animals that potentially harbor the organisms should reduce direct fecal-oral transmission. Although the role of water in human infection is unknown, *Y. enterocolitica* is sensitive to chlorination, which presumably would eliminate the risk of infection from drinking water.

Legionellosis

Robert F. Breiman
David W. Fraser

Legionellosis occurs most often as either of two clinically and epidemiologically divergent syndromes: Legionnaires' disease, a serious, potentially fatal disease that often includes pneumonia, and Pontiac fever, a self-limited, influenza-like disease without pneumonia.[1] Legionellosis was first recognized during an epidemic of pneumonia that largely affected persons attending an American Legion convention in Pennsylvania in 1976.[2] Five months after the outbreak McDade identified the etiologic agent, *Legionella pneumophila,* a bacterium that had not been recognized as a cause of human disease.[3] Testing of stored specimens associated with earlier investigations demonstrated that sporadic cases and epidemics of pneumonia occurring as early as 1947 were due to species in the genus *Legionella.* Since the initial description of legionellosis, considerable knowledge has been gained about the causal bacteria and the epidemiology, treatment, and prevention of the disease.

Bacteriology. Since the recognition of the first species of *Legionella* in 1977, 30 species and 48 serogroups have been identified from clinical and environmental specimens. Members of the genus have common characteristics, including failure to grow on blood agar and a nutritional requirement for L-cysteine. *L. pneumophila* accounts for more than 75% of cases of documented legionellosis. Although 15 serogroups of *L. pneumophila* have been described, serogroup 1 causes the greatest number of clinical infections, followed by serogroups 4 and 6. Other legionellae associated most frequently with clinical infections include *L. micdadei, L. dumoffi, L. bozemanii, L. feelei,* and *L. longbeachae.*

Legionella species are widely distributed in water, both in natural sites such as lakes and ponds and in constructed sources such as cooling towers and plumbing systems.[4] The bacteria do not survive desiccation and have never been isolated from dry soil.

Legionella grows slowly on agar media supplemented with ferric salts and L-cysteine but not at all on most other bacteriologic media. Buffered charcoal yeast extract agar supports growth particularly well. The ideal temperature range for growth of *Legionella* is 25° to 42° C. *L. pneumophila* is a facultative intracellular bacterium because it multiplies avidly inside various human cells, including monocytes and alveolar macrophages,[5,6] as well as within ciliated protozoa and amebae, and it does not multiply if supporting cells are removed from tissue culture medium.[7] Amebae, also ubiquitous in water supplies, appear to support *Legionella* multiplication in aquatic environments where the bacteria's strict nutritional requirements cannot otherwise be met.

Molecular epidemiologic tests, including monoclonal antibody subtyping, restriction endonuclease analysis, isoenzyme analysis, and ribosomal DNA hybridization to *E. coli* RNA (ribotyping), can be helpful in outbreak investigations by demonstrating whether isolates from patients are similar to isolates from suspected sources of transmission.[8]

Clinical Characteristics. Legionnaires' disease begins with headache, myalgia, and fever. The disease progresses relatively rapidly with chills (often rigors), cough, and pleuritic chest pain, which may be accompanied by diarrhea or obtundation. The physical examination typically shows few abnormalities except pulmonary rales and sometimes confusion. The white blood cell count is mildly elevated with a preponderance of early forms. Proteinuria and microscopic hematuria are common. Chest roentgenograms taken early in the course of the disease show patchy infiltrates that may progress to nodular consolidation and, in severe cases, coalescence. Pleural effusions are common but small; fluid usually has a high protein concentration. Lung abscess is a rare occurrence. Renal failure with or without antecedent shock occurs occasionally; temporary dialysis has been necessary for about 3% of patients.

Since the clinical presentation of *Legionella* pneumonia is not distinct from infections caused by a number of other pathogens, the diagnosis is based on laboratory evidence of infection. This includes (1) recovery of *Legionella* spp. from lung tissue or respiratory secretions, or use of a direct fluorescent antibody (DFA) test to demonstrate reacting bacteria, or (2) a fourfold rise in paired acute- and convalescent-phase serum antibody reciprocal titer to ≥128 by use of an indirect immunofluorescent IgG antibody (IFA) assay. Detection of *L. pneumophila* serogroup 1 antigens in urine by means of a radioimmunoassay can be helpful for early diagnosis and treatment, but conventional diagnostic tests should be used for confirmation. Although culture is the "gold standard" and appears to be 100% specific, sensitivity depends greatly on the quality, handling, and processing of the specimen. The DFA test generally is not sensitive (25%) but is highly specific (99.9%) when experienced personnel use standardized reagents.[9] For infection caused by *L. pneumophila* serogroup 1, the sensitivity of the IFA assay is 75% and the specificity is 99% if *L. pneumophila* serogroup 1 is the only antigen used but is lower (96%) if additional antigens are used.[9] Although the urinary antigen radioimmunoassay appears highly specific (99.6%) for *L. pneumophila* serogroup 1 infections,[9] its sensitivity has not been established. The usefulness of a DNA probe to detect *Legionella* in respiratory secretions has not been fully evaluated. The sensitivity and specificity of diagnostic tests for legionellae other than *L. pneumophila* serogroup 1 are not well defined.

Erythromycin with or without rifampin is generally effective therapy. Quinolone agents, including ciprofloxacin, also appear effective, but they have been evaluated in only a small number of patients with Legionnaires' disease.[10]

Death from progressive pneumonia or shock occurs in 10% to 15% of patients. Extreme fatigue and chronic respiratory symptoms may persist for several months after recovery from acute infection. Repeat episodes of legionellosis rarely occur; exposure to *L. pneumophila* has been shown to provide protective immunity against a subsequent lethal dose of the bacteria in an animal model.[11]

Pontiac fever is a self-limited illness in which fever, headache, and myalgia are prominent symptoms; pleuritis has been observed, but not pneumonia.[1] Illness generally resolves within 5 days without antibiotic therapy.

Legionella infections that do not fit the clinical syndromes of Legionnaires' disease or Pontiac fever have also been reported and include peritonitis, endocarditis, and wound infections.

Transmission. Legionellosis is transmitted to persons who inhale *Legionella* organisms in droplet nuclei or droplets of water from aerosol-producing devices. Cooling towers and evaporative condensers, heat-rejection devices that produce sizable volumes of aerosol, have been sources of several outbreaks.[12,13] Ducts and vents of air-conditioning systems can be conduits for passage of aerosol containing *Legionella* organisms from nearby contaminated cooling towers. Although most studies have indicated that aerosol from contaminated cooling towers can transmit disease within a limited range (< 200 m), data from one investigation of a community-wide outbreak suggested that the range may be several miles.[14] Air-conditioning systems based on direct exchange of heat from refrigerant to air, without use of water evaporation (such as window and most other home air-conditioning units), are not intrinsically capable of transmitting disease.

Use of showers that produce droplets of respirable size containing *L. pneumophila* serogroup 1 was epidemiologically linked to Legionnaires' disease in one outbreak[15] and has probably played a role in others.[16,17] An ultrasonic humidifier, contaminated with *L. pneumophila* serogroup 1 and used as a misting machine for produce in a grocery store, was implicated in a large community-wide outbreak.[18] The role of home humidifiers in sporadic cases of Legionnaires' disease is unknown. Respiratory therapy equipment containing contaminated tap water[19] and whirlpool spas have been shown to transmit disease.[20,21] A large outbreak of Pontiac fever at an automobile engine assembly plant resulted from aerosolization of an industrial grinding fluid containing *L. feelei*.[22] The infectious dose for *L. pneumophila* is unknown, but data from an outbreak investigation suggest that disease can be transmitted to susceptible persons exposed to 1 colony-forming unit of bacteria per 50 L of air.[13]

No evidence has shown person-to-person transmission or persistent colonization of humans with the bacteria. Although early epidemiologic studies suggested an association between Legionnaires' disease and exposure to construction sites, transmission has not been demonstrated to occur via inhalation of dust. Links between disease and ingestion of contaminated water or aspiration of upper respiratory secretions or gastric contents have been hypothesized but not established. In rare instances legionellosis results from direct inoculation with *Legionella* via hemodialysis or contaminated surgical wound dressings.

Occurrence. From 600 to 1000 cases of Legionnaires' disease are reported annually in the United States. However, the actual incidence is probably much higher because the disease is often undetected. Although incidence rates are unknown, Legionnaires' disease has been found worldwide in areas where diagnostic tests are available. *Legionella* spp. are the etiologic agents in 1% to 15% of community-acquired pneumonias in adults.[23-26]

Legionnaires' disease occurs predominantly in middle-aged and elderly adults, cigarette smokers, and persons who have underlying medical conditions, including chronic renal failure, organ transplantation, use of immunosuppressive agents (e.g., corticosteroids), malignancy, chronic pulmonary disease, diabetes mellitus, and alcohol addiction. The incubation period is generally 2 to 10 days. In outbreaks of disease the attack rate is often 1% to 5%, reflecting the importance of host susceptibility to developing disease. In contrast, Pontiac fever often occurs in young, healthy people, has a brief (12 to 48 hours) incubation period, and has a very high (up to 100%) attack rate. The basis for the divergence of the two syndromes is not established; however, one possibility is that Pontiac fever represents a toxic or inflammatory response to nonviable *Legionella* antigens or other antigens (e.g., amebae) that may be inhaled along with *Legionella*. This theory is based on the observation that Pontiac fever does not progress to systemic *Legionella* infection but consistently has a self-limited course.

Legionnaires' disease occurs in both epidemic and sporadic form. Some epidemics have been brief and explosive, whereas others have smoldered for several years. Explosive outbreaks occur most commonly in summer months and are often associated with point sources, such as cooling towers or evaporative condensers. Prolonged outbreaks have often been documented in institutional settings, such as hospitals and hotels, and have frequently been attributed to contaminated potable water. The source of infection for sporadic cases is generally unknown. Pontiac fever is recognized only in epidemic form; sporadically occurring disease would probably be misclassified as the viral syndrome.

Prevention and Control. An intensive epidemiologic investigation is frequently necessary to identify the source of a legionellosis outbreak. Since the bacteria are often found in aquatic environments, identification of *Legionella* spp. in the water in an aerosol-producing device does not implicate that device as the source of disease. Interviews of patients can help generate hypotheses about possible exposure risks, and case-control or cross-sectional studies are necessary to evaluate the hypotheses. Comparing isolates from patients and from aerosol-producing devices by molecular epidemiologic techniques, including monoclonal antibody subtyping, and restriction endonuclease and isoenzyme analyses, can confirm epidemiologic findings.[8] Particle-sizing microbial air samplers can help to demonstrate that a device suspected of transmitting *Legionella* is capable of generating an aerosol containing viable bacteria within droplets of respirable size (1 to 5 μm in diameter).[13,15]

Once a source of bacteria-laden aerosol is identified, intervention by decontamination procedures depends on the type of source and the institution in which it is located. For a potable water source (e.g., tap water, showers, or hot water heaters), flushing the entire system with superheated (>60° C) or hyperchlorinated water (> 10 mg free residual chlorine per liter) may reduce the concentration of *Legionella* spp. to undetectable levels.[27,28] In addition, contaminated water heaters require drainage and mechanical cleaning, particularly if they contain sediment. These procedures must be followed by a regular maintenance program to decrease the likelihood that *Legionella* will recolonize the system. Possible strategies include continuous infusion of chlorine (generally 1 to 2 mg free residual chlorine per liter), maintenance temperatures >50° C, or intermittent superheating or hyperchlorination. Drawbacks to these approaches include expensive damage to plumbing fixtures as a result of persistent exposure to chlorine[29] and the risk of scalding, particularly among elderly persons and young children.

Cooling towers and evaporative condensers that are sources of legionellosis should be drained, mechanically cleaned with a dispersant (such as automatic dishwasher detergent), and hyperchlorinated.[30] Maintenance strategies include regular cleaning and infusion of chlorine or other biocides that inhibit *Legionella* growth.

Monitoring the source of *Legionella* for the presence of the bacteria and surveillance for new cases of legionellosis are necessary for 6 to 12 months to evaluate the effectiveness of the intervention and make changes in the maintenance strategy.

The value of routine bacterial monitoring and maintenance of natural and constructed aquatic environments in preventing epidemics of legionellosis has not been shown, in part because legionellae are so widespread and frequently do not cause disease.[4] The bacteria have been found in water of aerosol-producing devices without being associated with known cases of disease, even in hospital settings where susceptible persons are potentially exposed.[31] Use of biocides, in conjunction with periodic drainage and cleaning, recommended for efficient operation of cooling towers and evaporative condensers, may prevent proliferation of legionellae to high concentrations in those devices. Some institutions maintain hot water temperatures at >50° C. Ultraviolet light and ozone in potable water systems are promising approaches that require further study to evaluate effectiveness. Humidifiers should be drained and cleaned regularly, although their role in sporadic and epidemic Legionnaires' disease is not fully defined.[17] Several studies have demonstrated that tap water should not be used in the operation, rinsing, or cleaning of respiratory care equipment.[19,32]

Better understanding of the relationship between *Legionella* and amebae may lead to exciting new approaches in prevention and control. Sampling water from aerosol-producing devices for the presence of both *L. pneumophila* and certain species of amebae may detect sites likely to support *Legionella* multiplication to high concentrations. Based on available information, intervention should focus on eliminating both amebae and *Legionella* from the outbreak source and on altering environmental factors that promote their interaction.

Vaccination of susceptible persons represents an entirely different approach for prevention of Legionnaires' disease. Two vaccine preparations provide protective immunity in animals but have not yet been tested in humans.[33,34]

Amebiasis and Amebic Meningoencephalitis

Jonathan I. Ravdin

AMEBIASIS

Amebiasis refers to human infection by the enteric protozoan *Entamoeba histolytica. E. histolytica* infects 10% of the earth's population, with the percentage higher in poor developing areas, and is estimated to be the third leading parasitic cause of death worldwide.[1] Infection with *E. histolytica* readily follows ingestion of the cyst form; however, only a small minority of those infected manifest the symptoms of invasive amebiasis, colitis, and liver abscess. Recognition of amebic infection requires knowledge of the epidemiology of the parasite, the varied clinical presentations, and the available diagnostic methods. Therapy for amebiasis requires use of multiple antiparasitic drugs that act against amebae in the bowel lumen or invading host tissues. Prevention of amebic infection depends on adequate sanitation with availability of safe water supplies and avoidance of direct fecal-oral contamination among family members or sexual partners.

Life Cycle and Epidemiology. Infection is contracted by ingestion of the cyst form, which by virtue of its chitinous cell wall resists desiccation in the environment and destruction by stomach acid. Cysts contain one to four nuclei; excystation occurs in the small bowel, and the trophozoite form proceeds downstream to colonize the colon. Encystment of trophozoites followed by fecal excretion of cysts completes the life cycle; trophozoites rapidly disintegrate in the environment and if immediately ingested would most likely be killed by the acid pH of the stomach.

Risk factors for acquisition of *E. histolytica* infection and increased susceptibility to aggressive invasive amebiasis are summarized in Table 8-1. Infection is most prevalent in developing areas of the world such as Mexico, Africa, India, and South America. In developed countries amebic infection and disease are concentrated in high-risk groups, such as those with prior exposure to an endemic environment or more likely to have direct fecal-oral contamination because of unhygienic living conditions or sexual practices. Although *E. histolytica* is one of the treatable causes of diarrhea in patients with the acquired immunodeficiency syndrome (AIDS),[2] aggressive fulminant amebiasis has not been reported in this group, despite their profound defects in host immunity. Severe invasive amebiasis with increased mortality has been reported in the very young, during pregnancy, in association with corticosteroid administration, and in malnourished individuals. A careful epidemiological history is essential for recognition of amebic disease.

Pathogenesis and Host Immune Response. The low frequency of invasive clinical disease complicating widespread *E. histolytica* infection appears to be due to the existence of distinct pathogenic and nonpathogenic strains and a complex interplay between parasite and host factors that regulate expression of invasive pathogenic activities. Isoenzyme analysis of *E. histolytica* isolates has been used to demonstrate electrophoretic patterns uniquely associated with invasive amebiasis or asymptomatic noninvasive infection.[3] Asymptomatic intestinal infection with pathogenic-type *E. histolytica* does occur and is distinguished from nonpathogenic infection by the presence of serum antiamebic antibodies during pathogenic infection. However, in vitro shifting of isoenzyme pattern from nonpathogenic to pathogenic has been demonstrated, which raises doubts about the stability of *E. histolytica* virulence properties.

Pathogenesis of invasive amebiasis requires adherence of amebae to the colonic mucus blanket, disruption of the colonic epithelial barrier, parasite attachment to and lysis of host epithelial and acute inflammatory cells, and resistance of trophozoites to host humoral and cell-mediated immune defense mechanisms present in tissues.[4] Amebic adherence to colonic mucins is mediated by a surface lectin inhibitable by galactose or *N*-acetyl-D-galactosamine (Gal/GalNAc); binding of this Gal/GalNAc-inhibitable adherence lectin to cell surface carbohydrates is required for *E. histolytica* cytolytic activity. Amebic proteinases can degrade epithelial basement membranes and cell-anchoring proteins, disrupting epithelial cell layers. Amebae lyse responding host neutrophils, resulting in release of neutrophil nonoxidant constituents that are toxic to host tissues. *E. histolytica* cytolytic activity is apparently regulated by a parasitic protein kinase C enzyme, involves amebic phospholipase A enzyme and acid pH vesicles, and results from an irreversible toxic increase in target cell free intracellular calcium ion concentration, possibly mediated by an amebic pore-forming protein.[5] Invasive *E. histolytica* trophozoites are resistant to the lytic effects of complement,

TABLE 8-1. EPIDEMIOLOGIC RISK FACTORS THAT APPARENTLY PREDISPOSE TO *ENTAMOEBA HISTOLYTICA* INFECTION AND INCREASED SEVERITY OF DISEASE

▪ INCREASED PREVALENCE

Lower socioeconomic status in endemic area, including crowding and lack of indoor plumbing
Immigrants from endemic area
Institutionalized population, especially mentally retarded
Communal living
Promiscuous homosexual men

▪ INCREASED SEVERITY

Children, especially neonates
Pregnancy and postpartum states
Corticosteroid use
Malignancy
Malnutrition

Reproduced with permission from Ravdin JI [ed]: Amebiasis: Human Infection by Entamoeba histolytica. New York: Churchill Livingstone, 1988, p. 496.

despite their activation of both alternative and classic pathways. In a nonimmune host, *E. histolytica* trophozoites are capable of killing host lymphocytes and macrophages.

In humans, asymptomatic nonpathogenic *E. histolytica* infection usually ends within 8 to 12 months; whether this results from a specific host immune response or is associated with even brief immunity to subsequent intestinal infection is unknown. In contrast, cure of invasive amebiasis in humans or experimental animals is followed by resistance to a recurrence of invasive amebic disease. This is apparently due to development of an amebicidal cell-mediated immune response, although antibodies that block the amebic adherence lectin are also present in the serum of immune individuals.[5] Immunization of experimental animals with total amebic protein or purified Gal/GalNAc-inhibitable adherence lectin provides effective immunity against liver abscess through amebicidal cell-mediated mechanisms.

Clinical Characteristics. The clinical syndromes associated with *E. histolytica* infection are listed in Table 8–2. As discussed, 90% to 99% of individuals infected with *E. histolytica* are asymptomatic and without evidence of ill health related to the parasite. Many infected persons have nonspecific gastrointestinal symptoms, such as abdominal pain, bloating, or watery diarrhea, but are without evidence of invasive disease. Although the reason for their complaints may not be clear or detectable, their amebic infection should be eradicated. Amebic dysentery has a subacute onset over days to weeks and is manifest as abdominal pain and bloody diarrhea; only a minority of patients are febrile.[6] Stool almost always contains occult blood; despite the inflammatory nature of the lesion, fecal leukocytes may not be present because the trophozoites can lyse neutrophils. The differential diagnosis includes invasive bacterial causes of colitis such as *Campylobacter, Shigella,* and *Salmonella* infection or toxin-mediated *Clostridium difficile* colitis.

Amebic colitis may be fulminant, especially in the high-risk groups summarized in Table 8–1, with high fever, peritonitis, and colonic perforation resulting in a high mortality. Conversion of amebic dysentery to toxic megacolon is clearly associated with corticosteroid administration, often resulting from the misdiagnosis of amebic colitis as idiopathic inflammatory bowel disease. A chronic nondysenteric syndrome is characterized by intermittent bouts of inflammatory diarrhea over a period of years.

TABLE 8–2. CLINICAL SYNDROMES ASSOCIATED WITH *ENTAMOEBA HISTOLYTICA* INFECTION

- **INTESTINAL DISEASE**
  - Asymptomatic infection
  - Symptomatic noninvasive infection
  - Acute rectocolitis (dysentery)
  - Fulminant colitis with perforation
  - Toxic megacolon
  - Chronic nondysenteric colitis
  - Ameboma
  - Perianal ulceration
- **EXTRAINTESTINAL DISEASE**
  - Liver abscess
  - Liver abscess complicated by:
    - peritonitis
    - empyema
    - pericarditis
  - Lung abscess
  - Brain abscess
  - Genitourinary disease

Reproduced with permission from Mandell GL, Douglas RG Jr, Bennett JE (eds): Principles and Practices of Infectious Diseases, 3 edt. New York: Churchill Livingstone, 1989.

These patients have invasive amebic colitis that can be diagnosed by biopsy and the presence of serum antiamebic antibodies, yet their disease is frequently mistaken for idiopathic ulcerative colitis.[7] Ameboma is a chronic segmental lesion, usually in the cecum or ascending colon, that is characterized by abdominal pain and mass and is often confused with colonic carcinoma. Perianal ulcerative amebic lesions may develop in patients with skin maceration caused by diarrhea; squamous epithelium is usually resistant to amebic invasion.

Extraintestinal disease is overwhelmingly due to liver abscess and its spread to contiguous body spaces. Common symptoms of amebic liver abscess are acute right upper quadrant pain and fever, necessitating differentiation from biliary tract disease. Alternatively, liver abscess may become manifest over a period of weeks with pain and weight loss but without fever, a presentation more suggestive of abdominal malignancy.[8] Knowledge of epidemiological risk factors and early use of hepatic imaging are essential for diagnosis. Occasionally an amebic liver abscess, especially an abscess of the left lobe, which may be less symptomatic, ruptures into the peritoneum. The liver abscess can also penetrate through the diaphragm into the pleural space, resulting in an empyema. Extension of a left lobe abscess into the pericardium is a rare but often fatal complication that usually occurs because the clinical presentation is fulminant and confusing. Lung and brain abscesses are rare examples of hematogenous dissemination; amebiasis of the penis and of the uterine cervix has been reported.

Diagnosis. Diagnosis of intestinal amebiasis usually rests on microscopic findings of *E. histolytica* in the stool. The occurrence of invasive colitis is indicated by the finding of trophozoites (often containing ingested erythrocytes) in stool, a positive serological test for antiamebic antibodies, and the presence of ulcerative mucosal lesions observed by lower gastrointestinal endoscopy.[9] For reliable exclusion of amebic disease from the diagnosis, at least three separate stool samples should be examined using permanently stained slides; alternatively, total colonoscopy with biopsy is highly sensitive and definitive. At minimum, serological tests for *E. histolytica* should be performed before a diagnosis of idiopathic inflammatory bowel disease leads to use of corticosteroids. Gastrointestinal barium roentgenograms are useless and make parasitological examinations of the stool unreliable for weeks.

Patients with a clinical syndrome and epidemiological risk factors consistent with amebic liver abscess should immediately undergo ultrasonography to look for a nonhomogeneous defect in the liver or evidence of biliary tract disease.[10] Ultrasonography is highly sensitive, nontoxic, and relatively inexpensive; computed tomography (CT) and magnetic resonance imaging are not more specific and are only slightly more sensitive.[11] Amebic liver abscess is usually difficult to distinguish from bacterial liver abscess or hepatoma by imaging. Amebic liver abscess may occur at any age in persons who do not have the risk factors commonly associated with pyogenic abscess or hepatoma; however, if amebic serological testing is unavailable, ultrasonography or CT-guided fine-needle aspiration can be helpful. Gram's stain and culture for bacteria establish the diagnosis; in amebic abscesses a yellow proteinase debris without white blood cells is found. Trophozoites are not usually seen in the abscess aspirate, since they commonly reside in tissue only at the lesion's periphery. Virtually all persons with amebic liver abscess develop serum antiamebic antibodies but often not until the seventh day of symptoms.[8] Thus an initial negative serological test for *E. histolytica* can be misleading early in the course of the abscess. *E. histolytica* trophozoites or cysts can be found in the stool of only a small number of patients with amebic liver abscess.

Treatment. Therapy for *E. histolytica* infection is complicated by the necessity for different agents to treat intraluminal and tissue infestation. Tables 8–3 and 8–4 summarize the drugs in use, their respective sites of activity, and recommendations for drug dosage and duration of therapy. In a nonendemic area, most experts would treat asymptomatic cyst passers, especially given the difficulty differentiating pathogenic from nonpathogenic isolates. I recommend that in a highly endemic area, asymptomatic infection be treated only if serum antiamebic antibodies are present. Diloxanide furoate is highly efficacious and relatively nontoxic; unfortunately, in the United States this drug is available only from the Centers for Disease Control Drug Service in Atlanta.[12] Paromomycin is a nonabsorbable aminoglycoside that is efficacious and often better tolerated than the combination of tetracycline and diiodohydroxyquin.[13]

The nitroimidazoles are the drugs of choice for treatment of invasive amebiasis; metronidazole is the only one available in the United States. In the regimens outlined in Table 8–4, metronidazole is highly effective in treating amebic colitis or liver abscess; however, treatment with an intraluminal agent should follow to ensure that intestinal infection is eradicated. Use of metronidazole may be limited by side effects such as nausea and vomiting and by concerns regarding carcinogenesis and teratogenesis. Long-term clinical follow-up has not indicated a carcinogenic effect of metronidazole, but if possible the drug should be avoided during pregnancy. The emetines are second-line agents rarely used in the United States. Adding these cardiotoxic agents to metronidazole has not been found to enhance clinical outcome. Patients with amebic liver abscess respond to metronidazole with gradual defervescence and decreased symptoms over a 3- to 5-day period. Progression of symptoms during therapy or failure of metronidazole treatment is an indication for drainage of the liver abscess by needle aspiration and continued treatment with metronidazole.[14] Open surgical drainage or addition of emetine therapy may be considered. Some authorities routinely add chloroquine to metronidazole in treatment of liver abscess, but I know of no studies that support this practice.

Prevention. Prevention of *E. histolytica* infection rests on availability of safe water supplies, adequate disposal of fecal material, and avoidance of practices that promote direct fecal-oral contamination. Boiling of water is the only certain means of killing *E. histolytica* cysts; use of halide tablets is generally inadequate. No vaccine or reasonable form of chemoprophylaxis is available; however, recent research on pathogenesis and host immunity has suggested that numerous amebic proteins are viable candidates for vaccine development.

TABLE 8–3. ANTIMICROBIAL AGENTS FOR USE IN TREATING AMEBIASIS

- **Luminal Agents**
  Diloxanide furoate
  Paromomycin
  Diiodohydroxyquin
- **Tissue Agents**
  Bowel wall only
    Tetracycline
    Erythromycin
  Liver only: chloroquine
- **Agents Active in All Tissues**
  Metronidazole
  Tinidazole
  Emetine hydrochloride
  2-Dehydroemetine

Reproduced with permission from Mandell GL, Douglas RG Jr, Bennett JE (eds): Principles and Practices of Infectious Diseases, 3 edt. New York: Churchill Livingstone, 1989.

TABLE 8–4. THERAPEUTIC REGIMENS FOR TREATMENT OF AMEBIASIS*

- **CYST PASSERS**

Diloxanide furoate 500 mg tid × 10 d
Paromomycin 30 mg/kg/d in 3 divided doses × 5–10 d
Tetracycline 250 mg qid × 10 d then diiodohydroxyquin 650 mg tid × 20 d
Metronidazole 750 mg tid × 10 d

- **INVASIVE RECTOCOLITIS**

Metronidazole 750 mg tid × 5–10 d
  or 2.4 g qd × 2–3 d
  or 50 mg/kg × 1 dose
  plus diloxanide furoate or paromomycin
Tetracycline 250 mg qid × 15 d plus chloroquine (base) 600 mg, 300 mg, then 150 mg tid × 14 d
Dehydroemetine 1–1.5 mg/kg/d × 5 d plus diloxanide furoate or paromomycin

- **LIVER ABSCESS**

Metronidazole 750 mg tid × 5–10 d or 2.4 mg qd × 1–2 d plus diloxanide furoate or paromomycin
Dehydroemetine 1–1.5 mg/kg/d × 5 d plus diloxanide furoate or paromomycin
Chloroquine (base) 600 mg qd × 2 d, 300 mg base qd × 2–3 w (can be added to other regimens)

*All dosages are for oral administration except that of dehydroemetine, which is given intramuscularly; metronidazole can be given intravenously.

Reproduced with permission from Mandell GL, Douglas RG Jr, Bennett JE (eds): Principles and Practices of Infectious Diseases, 3 edt. New York: Churchill Livingstone, 1989.

AMEBIC MENINGOENCEPHALITIS

Amebic meningoencephalitis is a rare clinical syndrome caused by acquisition of free-living amebae from the environment. *Naegleria fowleri* causes a primary amebic meningoencephalitis (PAM) in otherwise healthy individuals; infection with *Acanthamoeba* spp. is manifest as a subacute granulomatous amebic encephalitis (GAE) in patients already having serious underlying diseases. The diagnostician must be familiar with the epidemiology and clinical manifestations of amebic meningoencephalitis to avoid overlooking this infection in the differential diagnosis of patients at risk, despite the low frequency of occurrence. Diagnosis ultimately rests on finding the amebae in cerebrospinal fluid or brain tissue. Unfortunately, treatment is usually ineffective for either syndrome if it is diagnosed, or the diagnosis is not made until postmortem examination.

Life Cycle and Epidemiology. *N. fowleri* can exist in a trophozoite or a flagellate form; cell division is restricted to trophozoites. The organism grows best at higher temperatures (46° C) and is acquired from fresh water.[15] Encystment does occur and allows prolonged survival of the parasite at low temperatures. PAM is a rare disease despite the frequent occurrence of warm fresh water exposure during swimming, diving, or boating. The disease occurs in all areas of the world, especially in tropical regions.

Acanthamoebae exist in only the trophozoite and cyst forms, grow best at normal ambient temperatures (25° to 35° C), and may be transmitted by an airborne or a droplet route.[16] As with *Naegleria,* despite broad exposure to the *Acanthamoeba* species, *A. culbertsoni, A. polyphaga,* and *A. rhysodes,* GAE is found mainly in individuals with serious underlying conditions such as diabetes mellitus, AIDS, or recent organ transplantation.

Pathogenesis and Host Immune Response. *N. fowleri* apparently enters the central nervous system by penetrating the nasal mucosa and cribriform plate. Trophozoites can be found in nerves and perivascular spaces.[16] Amebic cell lytic activity has been demonstrated in vitro. Invasion of gray matter results in purulent meningitis. Trophozoites are susceptible to complement-mediated lysis, which is potentiated by agglutinating antibody to *N. fowleri.* Humoral and cell-mediated mechanisms limit the occurrence of PAM despite the ubiquitous exposure to this parasite.

In GAE granulomatous lesions can occur throughout the central nervous system, suggesting a hematogenous route of dissemination. Further evidence for this route of spread is the frequent occurrence of skin lesions before spread to the nervous system and other organ systems. *Acanthamoeba* can be differentiated from *Naegleria* by the presence of cysts in tissue. The opportunistic nature of *Acanthamoeba* infection suggests that cell-mediated mechanisms are important in resistance to disease; however, GAE in immunologically competent hosts has been reported.

Clinical Characteristics. PAM is often first manifest as alterations in taste or smell, followed by abrupt onset of headache, fever, and meningismus.[15,16] A fulminant illness ensues with depressed mental status and focal neurologic signs ending in death within 1 week. Other than the olfactory involvement in PAM, the disease is difficult to distinguish from community-acquired bacterial meningitis.

GAE is a subacute disease that becomes manifest over a period of weeks with focal neurologic signs, mental status changes, seizures, headache, and fever.[17] The occurrence of nodular or ulcerative skin lesions containing *Acanthamoeba* can be helpful in establishing the diagnosis. Most patients do not have meningismus, and the disease must be differentiated from brain abscess or other opportunistic infection such as toxoplasmosis.

Diagnosis. PAM is characterized by a neutrophilic cerebrospinal fluid (CSF) pleocytosis; elevated protein levels in the CSF and hypoglycorrhachia are not uncommon. A Gram stain of CSF negative for bacteria and an India ink test negative for cryptococcal disease in a young healthy person should suggest the need to examine the CSF for motile *N. fowleri* trophozoites, which are 10 to 30 μm in diameter. In contrast, in GAE, amebae are not found in the CSF, and brain biopsy is necessary for diagnosis. CT scans of the brain reveal nonspecific findings in PAM but may show focal lucencies in GAE.[18] In GAE the CSF undergoes nonspecific changes such as lymphocytic pleocytosis and alterations in protein and glucose levels. A biopsy specimen should be obtained from any suspect skin lesion and examined for *Acanthamoeba.*

Treatment. No effective treatment for amebic meningoencephalitis has been established. The two known survivors of PAM were treated with systemic and intrathecal amphotericin B.[17] One patient also received systemic rifampin, sulfisoxazole, and miconazole by the intravenous and intrathecal routes. Successful therapy for GAE also is undetermined; *Acanthamoeba* is generally susceptible in vitro to ketoconazole, miconazole, 5-flucytosine, and pentamidine, although isolates vary substantially.[19] If GAE is diagnosed, in vitro susceptibility should be studied, and therapy with the above agents and amphotericin B considered.

Prevention. PAM and GAE are such rare infections that in general preventive measures are unnecessary. A small risk of PAM may be associated with repeated episodes of having water forced into the nose under pressure, as in diving or waterskiing in warm freshwater lakes. However, the level of risk is impossible to define. Opportunistic infections other than GAE are more common and of paramount importance in immunocompromised individuals.

Giardiasis

Mary E. Wilson

Giardia lamblia is a flagellated protozoan that causes subacute or chronic diarrheal disease in humans. Giardiasis occurs worldwide, particularly where people do not adhere strictly to hygienic standards. In the United States giardiasis has been documented as a cause of waterborne outbreaks, epidemics in day care centers, and sporadic disease of overseas travelers, family members, and campers or hikers who ingest untreated surface water. The disease can be associated with acute or chronic malabsorption and has caused failure to thrive in children.

Life Cycle and Epidemiology. The life cycle of *G. lamblia* includes two stages: the cyst and the trophozoite. Giardiasis is acquired by ingestion of the dormant cyst from contaminated environmental sources. The parasite excysts while passing through the acidic stomach environment, and out of each cyst emerge two trophozoites that colonize the proximal portion of the small intestine. As the parasite passes through to the proximal colon it once again encysts and undergoes one cell division before it is passed in the stool. Trophozoites are fragile motile forms with four pairs of flagella, a ventral surface disc involved in attachment to intestinal mucosa, central axonemes, and two nuclei, which give the parasite a facelike appearance. Cysts are oval and thin walled with four nuclei. During severe bouts of diarrhea both stages of the parasite can be seen in fresh stool specimens because of rapid transit of bowel contents. Usually, however, only cysts are detected in stool samples. Furthermore, because cysts are excreted intermittently, the presence of the organism is frequently difficult to document by stool examination. Such diagnosis may require a small bowel aspirate and biopsy, or examination of small intestinal contents by a string test (Enterotest).[1] Noninvasive diagnostic techniques such as enzyme-linked immunosorbent assay (ELISA) of the stool and counterimmunoelectrophoresis are being investigated.

Several aspects of the parasite's life cycle are important determinants in the epidemiology of the disease. First, giardial cysts are immediately infectious for humans when passed in the stool, allowing person-to-person transmission of infection in settings of frequent interpersonal contact. This accounts for epidemic outbreaks in day care centers and institutions and for transfer of infection between family members. Second, *Giardia* cysts can survive for long periods in the environment, up to 16 days at 8° C, so that waterborne spread of infection is possible. Third, most infected patients are asymptomatic carriers, providing a large reservoir of infection in some populations. In combination these factors produce efficient fecal-oral spread of the organism, particularly where hygienic practices are poor.

Pathogenesis and Clinical Characteristics. The spectrum of giardial infection includes asymptomatic cyst passage; subacute, noninflammatory, usually self-limited diarrhea; and a chronic diarrheal syndrome with malabsorption and weight loss. The incubation period is 1 to 2 weeks, after which typical symptoms of abdominal bloating, flatulence, eructation, crampy abdominal pain, malaise, and greasy foul-smelling diarrhea may develop. Tenesmus, vomiting, and fever are less common, and leukocytes are generally absent from the stool. The symptoms are often present for a prolonged period, averaging 17 days in one study, and approximately half of patients have a significant weight loss. Laboratory examinations may reveal increased fecal fat content, as well as impaired absorption of D-xylose, lactose, and vitamin B_{12}. Protein-losing enteropathy and vitamin A deficiency have also been documented.[2]

Histological studies often show flattening of intestinal villi and varying degrees of cellular infiltration. According to one study these changes relate to symptoms and are reversible with eradication of the organism. Assays of brush border disaccharidases show deficient levels in patients with giardiasis, leading to theories that enzymatic deficiencies, abnormal lipolysis, and other factors may contribute to the pathogenesis of disease.[2] Partial immunity to reinfection with *G. lamblia* probably occurs, and secretory IgA may be an important determinant of the local immune response. In this vein African children who are breast fed have an apparent lower susceptibility to giardiasis than those who are not, presumably because of secretory IgA in their mothers' breast milk.[3] A systemic IgG antibody response to giardiasis occurs, but this is not reliable as a diagnostic tool and probably is most useful in epidemiological surveys. Finally, the importance of humoral immunity in giardiasis is apparent because of an increased susceptibility of hypogammaglobulinemic patients to giardial infection.[1]

Epidemiology. Transmission of giardiasis occurs by the fecal-oral route, either through direct contact with an infected individual or by ingestion of contaminated water or (less often) food. Giardial infection is more common in young children, probably because of their poorer hygienic practices. Prevalence rates for the organism vary widely depending on location. In the United States 3.9% of stool specimens submitted for examination have contained the organism, and prevalence among 1- to 3-year-olds in Washington State was 7.1%. Children in Queensland, Australia, were found to harbor the organism in 5.7% and 2.1% of random stool samples from households serviced by septic tanks or city sewage lines, respectively.[4] A study of 1000 adults in South Australia undergoing upper endoscopy for abdominal pain revealed *G. lamblia* trophozoites in 2.1%.[5] The annual incidence of symptomatic disease has been 9.8, 11.6, and 45.7 per 100,000 population in Minnesota, Colorado, and Vermont, respectively.[6] Prevalence rates were higher in developing countries, estimated at 19.4% in Zimbabwe and 42% in rural Egypt.[7] Surveillance of travelers to the Soviet Union revealed that 22.8% of 1419 tourists were ill with giardiasis and that infection was strongly associated with consumption of tap water in Leningrad.[8]

Cases of giardiasis can be divided into those occurring sporadically in high-risk individuals and those associated with outbreaks. The former group includes travelers to countries where the organism is endemic and hikers or campers who ingest untreated surface water in areas where the streams and lakes are contaminated, such as Minnesota or Colorado. Up to 20% of homosexual men harbored the organism in surveys of stool examinations, presumably because of habits that facilitate fecal-oral transmission. The presence of the organism in this population, however, does not correlate well with symptomatic disease. In addition, children who attend day-care centers frequently pass giardial cysts, and rates of giardiasis among household contacts of infected children range from 12% to 27%.

Several large outbreaks of giardiasis have resulted from contamination of municipal water supplies with human waste. One such outbreak, affecting 11.3% of 1094 skiers, occurred in an Aspen ski resort during the 1965–1966 season when well water was contaminated with leaking sewage.[9] A large outbreak in Rome, N.Y., affected 10.6% of the population (5300 persons). This outbreak was possibly due to contamination of the water supply with human waste from settlements in the watershed area. Investigators discovered a giardial cyst in a water sediment sample from a city water inlet.[10] In addition, in several waterborne outbreaks human waste was not thought to be the source of contamination. Notably, a Camas, Wash., outbreak was traced to the city water supply, and cysts were found in three beavers in the watershed area for the water system, implying that they might constitute a reservoir for the parasite.[11] During another outbreak, in Pittsfield, Mass., *Giardia* cysts were found in one of three city reservoirs and again the surrounding area contained *Giardia*-positive animals that may have been the source.[12] Although chlorine may be sufficient to kill *Giardia* cysts in the laboratory, other factors such as temperature, pH, and contact time with chlorine may result in less than optimal killing of cysts in water treatment systems that use chlorination alone. Thus, of 21,990 cases of waterborne giardiasis caused by contaminated surface water sources in the United States between 1965 and 1984, 10.1% were due to cross-contamination of water supplies with sewage lines and 54.6% of cases (56% of outbreaks) were due to water sources treated with chlorination alone. In contrast, only 33.8% of cases (21% of outbreaks) were associated with water supplies that had also undergone filtration. Thus systems that include a filtration step as well as chlorination seem to be more effective in eliminating the organism.[9]

Outbreaks in day-care centers have affected between 17% and 47% of the children attending. In general, ambulatory diapered children harbor the organism most frequently.[13] Several recurrent outbreaks have been documented, sometimes despite extensive efforts to improve personal and environmental hygiene among children and staff.[14] Other situations that have facilitated outbreaks of giardiasis include a contaminated cistern providing water to several families and a swimming pool contaminated by feces of a mentally retarded child. Finally, several foodborne outbreaks have been documented, usually traced to a dish consumed by the majority of affected individuals. These usually have occurred when food was mixed by the bare hands of an individual carrying *G. lamblia* cysts.[15]

Humans are the main reservoir of *G. lamblia;* thus giardiasis is a cosmopolitan disease. As mentioned above, however, several wild animals also harbor the organism and may constitute a reservoir for human outbreaks. These include most notably beavers, but *G. lamblia* cysts have also been found in muskrats, cows, goats, and sheep. Whether all of these strains are pathogenic for humans is unclear.

Control of giardiasis includes identification and treatment of colonized or infected individuals and screening of their household members for cyst passage. Treatment of water supplies by both chlorination and filtration is most effective for clearing the organism. In addition, water supplies should be routinely screened for coliform bacteria and turbidity to monitor for contamination with sewage or other sources. Although treatment of asymptomatic cyst passers is recommended in developed countries to decrease *G. lamblia* transmission, this is probably impractical in developing countries where giardiasis is endemic, because the incidence of reinfection from environmental sources after treatment is high.

REFERENCES

Typhoid

1. Nicolle P: The geographical distribution of *Salmonella typhi* and *Salmonella paratyphi* A and B phage types during the period 1 January 1966 to 31 December 1969. J Hyg (Camb) 71:59–84, 1973
2. Baine WB, Farmer JJ III, Gangarosa EJ, Hermann GT, Thornsberry

C, Rice PA: Typhoid fever in the United States associated with the 1972–1973 epidemic in Mexico. J Infect Dis 135:649–653, 1977
3. Wilson GS, Miles AA, Parker MT: Topley and Wilson's Principles of Bacteriology, Virology and Immunity. 7 edt. Baltimore: Williams & Wilkins, 1984
4. Gilman RH, Terminel M, Levine MM, Hernandez-Mendoza P, Hornick RB: Relative efficacy of blood, urine, rectal swab, bone-marrow, and rose-spot cultures for recovery of *Salmonella typhi* in typhoid fever. Lancet 1:1211–1213, 1975
5. Huckstep RL: Typhoid fever and other *Salmonella* infections. London: E & S Livingstone, Ltd, 1962
6. Ferreccio C, Levine MM, Manterola A, Rodriguez G, Rivara I, Prenzel I, Black RE, Mancuso T, Bulas D: Benign bacteremia caused by *Salmonella typhi* and *paratyphi* in children younger than 2 years. J Pediatr 104:899–901, 1984
7. Hornick RB, Greisman SE, Woodward TE, DuPont HL, Dawkins AT, Snyder MJ: Typhoid fever: Pathogenesis and immunologic control. N Engl J Med 283:686–691, 739–746, 1970
8. Snyder MJ, Perroni J, Gonzalez O, Woodward WE, Palomino C, Gonzalez C, Music SI, DuPont HL, Hornick RB, Woodward TE: Comparative efficacy of chloramphenicol, ampicillin, and co-trimoxazole in the treatment of typhoid fever. Lancet 2:1155–1157, 1976
9. Islam A, Butler T, Nath SK, Alam NH, Stoeckel K, Houser HB, Smith AL: Randomized treatment of patients with typhoid fever by using ceftriaxone or chloramphenicol. J Infect Dis 158:742–747, 1988
10. Rodriguez-Noriega E, Andrade-Villanueva J, Amaya-Tapia G: Quinolones in the treatment of *Salmonella* carriers. Rev Infect Dis 11(suppl 5):S1179–S1187, 1989
11. Christie AB: Infectious diseases: Epidemiology and clinical practice. 4 edt. New York: Churchill Livingstone, 1987
12. Levine MM, Grados O, Gilman RH, Woodward WE, Solis-Plaza R, Waldman W: Diagnostic value of the Widal test in areas endemic for typhoid fever. Am J Trop Med Hyg 27:795–800, 1978
13. Ames WR, Robbins M: Age and sex as factors in the development of the typhoid carrier state, and a method for estimating carrier prevalence. Am J Public Health 33:221–230, 1943
14. Bassily S, Farid Z, Lehman JS, Kent DC, Sanborn WR, Hathout SD: Treatment of chronic urinary *Salmonella* carriers. Trans R Soc Trop Med Hyg 64:723–729, 1970
15. Nolan CM, White PC Jr, Feeley JC, Brown SL, Hambie EA, Wong KH: Vi serology in the detection of typhoid carriers. Lancet 1:583–585, 1981
16. Engleberg NC, Barrett TJ, Fisher H, Porter B, Hurtado E, Hughes JM: Identification of a carrier by using Vi enzyme-linked immunosorbent assay serology in an outbreak of typhoid fever on an Indian reservation. J Clin Microbiol 18:1320–1322, 1983
17. Lanata CF, Ristori C, Jimenez L, et al: Vi serology in detection of chronic *Salmonella typhi* carriers in an endemic area. Lancet 2:441–443, 1983
18. Lin F-Y C, Becke JM, Groves C, Lim BP, Israel E, Becker EF, Helfrich RM, Swetter DS, Cramton T, Robbins JB: Restaurant-associated outbreak of typhoid fever in Maryland: Identification of carrier facilitated by measurement of serum Vi antibodies. J Clin Microbiol 26:1194–1197, 1988
19. Ryan CA, Hargrett-Bean NT, Blake PA: *Salmonella typhi* infections in the United States, 1975–1984: Increasing role of foreign travel. Rev Infect Dis 11:1–8, 1989
20. Taylor JP, Shandera WX, Betz TG, Schraitle K, Chaffee L, Lopez L, Henley R, Rothe CN, Bell RF, Blake PA: Typhoid fever in San Antonio, Texas: An outbreak traced to a continuing source. J Infect Dis 149:553–557, 1984
21. Brown JD, Mo DH, Rhoades ER: Chloramphenicol-resistant *Salmonella typhi* in Saigon. JAMA 253:162–166, 1975
22. Goldstein FW, Chumpitaz JC, Guevara JM, Papadopoulou B, Acar JF, Vieu JF: Plasmid-mediated resistance to multiple antibiotics in *Salmonella typhi*. J Infect Dis 153:261–266, 1986
23. Anand AC, Kataria VK, Singh W, Chatterjee SK: Epidemic multiresistant enteric fever in eastern India [letter]. Lancet 1990; 335:352.
24. Levine MM, Taylor DN, Ferreccio C: Typhoid vaccines come of age. 8:374–381, 1989
25. Levine MM, Ferreccio C, Black RE, Tacket CO, Germanier R, Chilean Typhoid Committee: Progress in vaccines against typhoid fever. Rev Infect Dis 11(suppl 3):S552–S567, 1989

Shigellosis

1. Griffin PM, Tauxe RV, Redd SC, Puhr ND, Hargrett-Bean N, Blake PA: Emergence of highly trimethoprim-sulfamethoxazole-resistant *Shigella* in a Native American population: An epidemiologic study. Am J Epidemiol 129:1042–1051, 1989
2. Mendizabal-Morris CA, Mata LJ, Gangarosa EJ, Guzman G: Epidemic Shiga-bacillus dysentery in Central America: Derivation of the epidemic and its progression in Guatemala, 1968–1969. Am J Trop Med Hyg 20:927–933, 1971
3. Barrett-Connor E, Connor JD: Extraintestinal manifestations of shigellosis. Am J Gastroenterol 53:234–245, 1970
4. Butler T, Islam MR, Azad MAK, Jones PK: Risk factors for development of hemolytic uremic syndrome during shigellosis. J Pediatr 110:894–897, 1987
5. Ross AI: The role of the symptomless excreter in the spread of Sonne dysentery. Month Bull Min Health 16:174–179, 1957
6. Levine MM, DuPont HL, Khodabandelou M, Hornick RB: Long-term *Shigella* carrier state. N Engl J Med 288:1169–1171, 1973
7. Nelson JD, Kusmiesz H, Shelton S: Oral or intravenous trimethoprim-sulfamethoxazole therapy for shigellosis. Rev Infect Dis 4:546–550, 1982
8. Gotuzzo E, Oberhelman RA, Maguina C, et al: Comparison of single-dose treatment with norfloxacin and standard 5-day treatment with trimethoprim-sulfamethoxazole for acute shigellosis in adults. Antimicrob Agents Chemother 33:1101–1104, 1989
9. Black RE, Craun GF, Blake PA: Epidemiology of common-source outbreaks of shigellosis in the United States, 1961–1975. Am J Epidemiol 108:47–52, 1978
10. Blaser MJ, Pollard RA, Feldman RA: *Shigella* infections in the United States, 1974–1980. J Infect Dis 147:771–775, 1983
11. Ebright JR, Moore EC, Sanborn WR, Schaberg D, Kyle J, Ishida K: Epidemic Shiga bacillus dysentery in Central Africa. Am J Trop Med Hyg 33:1192–1197, 1984
12. Parsonnet J, Greene KD, Gerber AR, Tauxe RV, Aguilar OJV, Blake PA: *Shigella dysenteriae* type 1 infections in US travelers to Mexico, 1988. Lancet 2:543–545, 1989
13. Tauxe RV, Johnson KE, Boase JC, Helgerson SD, Blake PA: Control of day care shigellosis: A trial of convalescent day care in isolation. Am J Public Health 76:627–630, 1986
14. DuPont HL, Gangarosa EJ, Reller LB, et al: Shigellosis in custodial institutions. Am J Epidemiol 92:172–179, 1970
15. Centers for Disease Control: Multistate outbreak of *Shigella sonneii* gastroenteritis—United States. MMWR 36:440–449, 1987
16. Formal SB, Hale TL, Kapfer C: *Shigella* vaccines. Rev Infect Dis 11:S547–S551, 1989
17. Khan MU: Interruption of shigellosis by hand washing. Trans R Soc Trop Med Hyg 76:164–168, 1982

Cholera

1. Pollitzer R: Cholera Monograph No. 43. Geneva: World Health Organization, 1959
2. Schoenberg BS, Mann RJ, Kurland LT: Snow on the water of London. Mayo Clin Proc 49:680–684, 1974
3. Samadi AR, Huq MI, Shahid N, et al: Classical *Vibrio cholerae* biotype displaces El Tor in Bangladesh. Lancet 1:805–807, 1983
4. Barua D, Burrows W (eds): Cholera. Philadelphia: Saunders, 1974
5. Blake PA, Allegra DT, Snyder JD, et al: Cholera—a possible endemic focus in the United States. N Engl J Med 302:305–309, 1980
6. Wachsmuth IK, Morris GK, Feeley JC: *Vibrio*. In Lennette EH,

Balows A, Hausler WJ, Truant JP (eds): Manual of Clinical Microbiology, 3 edt. Washington, DC: American Society for Microbiology, 1980. Chapter 18

7. Bart IJ, Huq Z, Khan M, Mosley WH: Seroepidemiologic studies during a simultaneous epidemic of infection with El Tor Ogawa and classical Inaba *Vibrio cholerae.* J Infect Dis 121:S17–S24, 1970
8. Greenough WB, Gordon RS, Rosenberg IS, et al: Tetracycline in the treatment of cholera. Lancet 1:355–357, 1964
9. Black RE: The prophylaxis and therapy of secretory diarrhea. Med Clin North Am 66:611–621, 1982
10. Nalin DR, Cash RA, Islam R, et al: Oral maintenance therapy for cholera in adults. Lancet 2:370–375, 1968
11. Palmer DL, Koster FT, Alam AKMJ, Islam MR: Nutritional status: A determinant of severity of diarrhea in patients with cholera. J Infect Dis 134:8–14, 1976
12. Oseasohn R, Ahmed S, Islan MA, Rahman ASMM: Clinical and bacteriologic findings among families of cholera patients. Lancet 1:340–341, 1966
13. Nalin DR, Levine RJ, Levine MM, et al: Cholera, nonvibrio cholera, and stomach acid. Lancet 2:856–859, 1978
14. Merson MH, Black RE, Kahn M, Huq I: Epidemiology of Cholera and Enterotoxigenic *Escherichia coli* Diarrhoea: Cholera and Related Diarrheas, 43rd Nobel Symposium, Stockholm, 1978. Basel: Karger, 1980, pp 34–45
15. Glass RI, Srennerholm A-M, Stoll BJ, et al: Protection against cholera in breast-fed children by antibodies in breast milk. N Engl J Med 308:1389–1392, 1983
16. Levine MM, Black RE, Clements ML, et al: Duration of infection-derived immunity to cholera. J Infect Dis 143:818–820, 1981
17. Kaper JB, Bradford HB, Roberts NC, Falkow S: Molecular epidemiology of *Vibrio cholerae* in the US Gulf Coast. J Clin Microbiol 16:129, 1982
18. Spira WM, Khan MU, Saeed A, Sattar MA: Microbiological surveillance of intra-neighbourhood El Tor transmission in rural Bangladesh. Bull WHO 58:731–740, 1980
19. Hughes JM, Boyce JM, Levine RJ, et al: Epidemiology of El Tor cholera in rural Bangladesh: Importance of surface water in transmission. Bull WHO 60:395–404, 1982
20. MacCormack WM, Chowdhury AM, Jahangir N, et al: Tetracycline prophylaxis of families of cholera patients. Bull WHO 38:787–792, 1968
21. Clemens JD, Sack DA, Harris JR, et al: Field trial of oral cholera vaccines in Bangladesh: Results from three-year follow-up. Lancet 1:270–273, 1990

Escherichia coli Diarrhea

1. Gorbach SL: Intestinal microflora. Gastroenterology 60:1110–1129, 1971
2. Robins-Browne RM: Traditional enteropathogenic *Escherichia coli* of infantile diarrhea. Rev Infect Dis 9:28–53, 1987
3. Richards KL, Douglas SD: Pathophysiological effects of *Vibrio cholerae* and enterotoxigenic *Escherichia coli* and their exotoxins in eucaryotic cells. Microbiol Rev 42:592–613, 1978
4. Black RE, Brown KH, Becker S, et al: Longitudinal studies of infectious diseases and physical growth of children in rural Bangladesh. II. Incidence of diarrhea and association with known pathogens. Am J Epidemiol 115:315–324, 1982
5. Rosenberg ML, Kaplan JP, Wachsmuth IK, et al: Epidemic diarrhea at Crater Lake from enterotoxigenic *E. coli:* A large waterborne outbreak. Ann Intern Med 86:714–718, 1977
6. Merson MH, Morris GK, Sack DA, et al: Traveler's diarrhea in Mexico: A prospective study of physicians and family members attending a congress. N Engl J Med 294:1299–1305, 1976
7. Sack DA, Kaminsky DC, Sack RB, et al: Prophylactic doxycycline for travelers' diarrhea: Results of a prospective double-blind study of Peace Corps volunteers in Kenya. N Engl J Med 298:758–763, 1978
8. Black RE: The prophylaxis and therapy of secretory diarrhea. Med Clin North Am 66:611–621, 1982
9. Marier R, Wells JG, Swanson RC, et al: An outbreak of enteropathogenic *Escherichia coli:* Foodborne disease traced to imported French cheese. Lancet 2:1376–1378, 1973
10. Riley LW, Remis RS, Helgerson SD, et al: Hemorrhagic colitis associated with a rare *Escherichia coli* serotype. N Engl J Med 308:681–685, 1983
11. Levine MK: *Escherichia coli* that cause diarrhea: Enterotoxigenic, enteropathogenic, enteroinvasive, enterohemorrhagic, and enteroadherent. J Infect Dis 155:377–388, 1987
12. Ulshen MH, Rollo JL: Pathogenesis of *Escherichia coli* gastroenteritis in man—another mechanism. N Engl J Med 302:99–101, 1980
13. Vial PA, Robins-Browne R, Lior H, et al: Characterization of enteroadherent-aggregative *Escherichia coli,* a putative agent of diarrheal disease. J Infect Dis 158:70–79, 1988

Yersiniosis

1. Nilehn B: Studies on *Yersinia enterocolitica* with special reference to bacterial diagnosis and occurrence in human acute enteric disease. Acta Pathol Microbiol Scand [Suppl] 206:1–48, 1969
2. Black RE, Slome S: *Yersinia enterocolitica.* Infect Dis Clin North Am 2:625–641, 1988
3. Gutman LT, Ottesen EA, Quan TJ, et al: An inter-familial outbreak of *Yersinia enterocolitica* enteritis. N Engl J Med 288:1372–1377, 1973
4. Black RE, Jackson RJ, Tsai T, et al: Epidemic *Yersinia enterocolitica* infection due to contaminated chocolate milk. N Engl J Med 298:76–79, 1978
5. Saari TN, Triplett DA: *Yersinia pseudotuberculosis* mesenteric adenitis. J Pediatr 85:656–659, 1974
6. Hubbert WT: Yersiniosis in mammals and birds in the United States. Am J Trop Med Hyg 21:458–463, 1972
7. Morris GK, Feeley JC: *Yersinia enterocolitica:* A review of its role in food hygiene. Bull WHO 54:79–85, 1976

Legionellosis

1. Glick TH, Gregg MB, Berman B, et al: Pontiac fever—epidemic of unknown etiology in a health department: Clinical and epidemiologic findings. Am J Epidemiol 107:149–160, 1978
2. Fraser DW, Tsai TF, Orenstein W, et al: Legionnaires' disease: Description of an epidemic of pneumonia, N Engl J Med 297:1189–1197, 1977
3. McDade JE, Shepard CC, Fraser DW, et al: Legionnaires' disease: Isolation of a bacterium and demonstration of its role in other respiratory disease. N Engl J Med 297:1197–1203, 1977
4. Redd SC, Cohen ML: *Legionella* in water: What should be done? JAMA, 257:1221–1222, 1987
5. Horwitz MA, Silverstein SC: Legionnaires' disease bacterium (*Legionella pneumophila*) multiplies intracellularly in human monocytes. J Clin Invest 66:441–450, 1980
6. Nash TW, Libby DM, Horwitz MA: Interaction between the Legionnaires' disease bacterium (*Legionella pneumophila*) and human alveolar macrophages. J Clin Invest 74:771–782, 1984
7. Fields BS, Sanden GN, Barbaree JM, et al: Intracellular multiplication of *Legionella pneumophila* in amoebae isolated from hospital hot water tanks. Curr Microbiol 18:131–137, 1989
8. Edelstein PH, Nakahama C, Tobin JO, et al: Paleoepidemiologic investigation of Legionnaires' disease at Wadsworth Veterans Administration hospital by using three typing methods for comparison of legionellae from clinical and environmental sources. J Clin Microbiol 23:1121–1126, 1986
9. Edelstein PH: Laboratory diagnosis of infections caused by legionellae. Eur J Clin Microbiol 6:4–10, 1987
10. Unertl KE, Lenhart FP, Forst H, et al: Ciprofloxacin in the treatment of legionellosis in critically ill patients including those cases unresponsive to erythromycin. Am J Med 87:128S–131S, 1989
11. Breiman RF, Horwitz MA: Guinea pigs sublethally infected with aerosolized *Legionella pneumophila* develop humoral and cell-medi-

ated immune responses and are protected against lethal aerosol challenge. J Exp Med 164:799–811, 1987

12. Dondero TJ, Rentdorff RC, Mallison GF, et al: An outbreak of Legionnaires' disease associated with a contaminated air-conditioning cooling tower. N Engl J Med 302:365–370, 1980
13. Breiman RF, Cozen W, Fields BS, et al: Role of air-sampling in an investigation of an outbreak of Legionnaires' disease associated with exposure to aerosols from an evaporative condenser. J Infect Dis 161:1257–1261, 1990
14. Addiss DG, Davis JP, LaVentura M, et al: Community-acquired Legionnaires' disease associated with a cooling tower: Evidence for longer-distance transport of *Legionella pneumophila.* Am J Epidemiol 130:557–568, 1989
15. Breiman RF, Fields BS, Sanden G, Volmer L, Meier A, Spika J: An outbreak of Legionnaires' disease associated with shower use: Possible role of amoebae. JAMA 263:2924–2926, 1990
16. Hanrahan JP, Morse DL, Scharf VB, et al: A community hospital outbreak of legionellosis; transmission by potable hot water. Am J Epidemiol 1987; 125:639–649, 1987
17. Tobin JO, Dunnill MS, French M, et al: Legionnaires' disease in a transplant unit: Isolation of the causative agent from shower baths. Lancet 2:118–121, 1980
18. Centers for Disease Control: Legionnaires' disease outbreak associated with a grocery store mist machine—Louisiana, 1989. MMWR 39:108–110, 1990
19. Arnow PM, Chou T, Weil D, Shapiro EN, Kretzschmar C: Nosocomial Legionnaires' disease caused by aerosolized tap water from respiratory devices. J Infect Dis 146:460–467, 1982
20. Vogt RL, Hudson PJ, Orciari L, Heun EM, Woods TC: Legionnaires' disease and a whirlpool spa [letter]. Ann Intern Med 107:596, 1987
21. Goldberg DJ, Collier PW, Fallon RJ, et al: Lochgoilhead fever: Outbreak of nonpneumonic legionellosis due to *Legionella micdadei.* Lancet pp 316–318, 1989
22. Herwaldt LA, Gorman GW, McGrath T, et al: A new *Legionella* species, *Legionella feelei* species nova, causes Pontiac fever in an automobile plant. Ann Intern Med 100:333–338, 1984
23. Foy HM, Hayes PS, Cooney MK, Broome CV, Allan I, Tobe R: Legionnaires' disease in a prepaid medical-care group in Seattle 1963–75. Lancet pp 776–770, 1979
24. Renner ED, Helms CM, Hierholzer WJ, et al: Legionnaires' disease in pneumonia patients in Iowa. Ann Intern Med 90:603–606, 1979
25. MacFarlane JT, Ward MJ, Finch RG, Macrae AD: Hospital study of adult community acquired pneumonia. Lancet 1:767–770, 1982
26. Schurmann D, Ruf B, Fehrenbach FJ, Jautzke G, Pohle HD: Fatal Legionnaires' pneumonia: Frequency of legionellosis in autopsied patients with pneumonia from 1969–1985. J Pathol 155:35–39, 1988
27. Sanden GN, Fields BS, Barbaree JM, Feeley JC: Viability of *Legionella pneumophila* in chlorine-free water at elevated temperatures. Curr Microbiol 18:61–65, 1989
28. Bartlett CLR, Macrae AD, Macfarlane JT: Surveillance, control, and prevention. In *Legionella* Infections. London: Edward Arnold, 1986, pp. 134–138
29. Helms CM, Massanari RM, Wenzel RP, et al: Legionnaires' disease associated with a hospital water system: A five-year progress report on continuous hyperchlorination. JAMA 259:2423–2427, 1988
30. Control of *Legionella* in cooling towers—summary guidelines. Madison: Wisconsin Department of Health and Human Services, 1987
31. Vickers RM, Yu VL, Hanna SS, et al: Determinants of *Legionella pneumophila* contamination of water distribution systems: 15 hospital prospective study. Infect Control 8:357–363, 1987
32. Mastro TD, Fields BS, Breiman RF, Sharp TW, Campbell J, Spika JS: Nosocomial legionellosis associated with nebulized medication use. In Program of the 29th Interscience Conference on Antimicrobial Agents and Chemotherapy, Houston, September 1989
33. Blander SJ, Horwitz MA: Vaccination with the major secretory protein of *Legionella pneumophila* induces cell-mediated and protective immunity in a guinea pig model of Legionnaires' disease. J Exp Med 169:691–705, 1989
34. Blander SJ, Breiman RF, Horwitz MA: A live avirulent mutant *Legionella pneumophila* vaccine induces protective immunity against lethal aerosol challenge. J Clin Invest 83:810–815, 1989

Amebiasis and Amebic Meningoencephalitis

1. Walsh JA: Prevalence of *Entamoeba histolytica* infections. In Ravdin JI (ed): Amebiasis: Human Infection by *Entamoeba histolytica.* New York: Churchill Livingstone, 1988, pp 93–105
2. Smith PD, Lane HC, Gill VJ, et al: Intestinal infections in patients with the acquired immunodeficiency syndrome (AIDS): Etiology and response to therapy. Ann Intern Med 108:328–333, 1988
3. Sargeaunt PG: The reliability of *Entamoeba histolytica* zymodemes in clinical diagnosis. Parisitol Today 3:40–43, 1987
4. Ravdin JI: *Entamoeba histolytica,* from Adherence to Enteropathy. Infectious Diseases Society of America plenary presentation. J Infect Dis 159:420–429, 1989
5. Ravdin JI: *Entamoeba histolytica:* Pathogenic mechanisms, human immune response, and vaccine development. Clin Res 38:215–225, 1990
6. Adams EB, MacLeod IN: Invasive amebiasis. I. Amebic dysentery and its complications. Medicine (Baltimore) 56:315–323, 1977
7. Schleupner CJ, Barritt AS III: Differentiation and occurrence of amebiasis in inflammatory bowel disease. In Ravdin JI (ed): Amebiasis: Human Infection by *Entamoeba histolytica.* New York: Churchill Livingstone, 1988, pp 582–593
8. Katzenstein D, Rickerson V, Braude A: New concepts of amebic liver abscess derived from hepatic imaging, serodiagnosis, and hepatic enzymes in 67 consecutive cases in San Diego. Medicine (Baltimore) 61:237–246, 1982
9. Ravdin JI: Intestinal disease caused by *Entamoeba histolytica.* In Ravdin JI (ed): Amebiasis: Human Infection by *Entamoeba histolytica.* New York: Churchill Livingstone, 1988, pp 495–509
10. Reed SL, Braude AI: Extraintestinal disease: Clinical syndromes, diagnostic profile, and therapy. In Ravdin JI (ed). Amebiasis: Human Infection by *Entamoeba histolytica.* New York: Churchill Livingstone, 1988, pp 511–532
11. Ralls PW, Henley DS, Colletti PM, et al: Amebic liver abscess: MR imaging. Radiology 165:801–804, 1987
12. Drugs for parasitic infections. Med Lett 30:15–24, 1988
13. Sullam PM, Slutkin G, Gottlieb AB, et al: Paromomycin therapy of endemic amebiasis in homosexual men. Sex Transm Dis 13:151–155, 1986
14. Thompson JE Jr, Forlenza S, Verma R: Amebic liver abscess: A therapeutic approach. Rev Infect Dis 7:171–179, 1985
15. Sotelo-Avila C: *Naegleria* and *Acanthamoeba:* Free-living amebas pathogenic for man. Perspect Pediatr Pathol 10:51–85, 1987
16. Martinez AJ: Free-Living Amebas: Natural History, Prevention, Diagnosis, Pathology and Treatment of Disease. Boca Raton, Florida: CRC Press, 1985
17. Petri WA, Ravdin JI: Free living amebas. In Mandell GL, Douglas RG, and Bennett JE (eds): Principles and Practices of Infectious Disease, 3 edt. New York: Churchill Livingstone, 1989, pp 2049–2055
18. Wiley CA, Safrin RE, Davis CE, et al: *Acanthamoeba* meningoencephalitis in a patient with AIDS. J Infect Dis 155:130–133, 1987
19. Duma RJ, Finley R: In vitro susceptibility of pathogenic *Naegleria* and *Acanthamoeba* species to a variety of therapeutic agents. Antimicrob Agents Chemother 10:370–376, 1976

Giardiasis

1. Smith PD: Pathophysiology and immunology of giardiasis. Annu Rev Med 36:295–307, 1985
2. Hartong WA, Gourley WK, Arvanitakis C: Giardiasis: Clinical spectrum and functional-structural abnormalities of the small intestinal mucosa. Gastroenterology 77:61–69, 1979

3. Gendrel D, Lenoble DR, Kombila M, Gendrel C, Baziomo JM: Giardiasis and breast-feeding in urban Africa. Pediatr Infect Dis J 8:58–59, 1989
4. Boreham PFL, Dondey J, Walker R: Giardiasis among children in the city of Logan, South East Queensland. Aust Pediatr J 17:209–212, 1981
5. Kerlin P, Ratnaike RN, Butler R, Gehling N, Grant AK: Prevalence of giardiasis: A study at upper-gastrointestinal endoscopy. Dig Dis 23:940–942, 1978
6. Birkhead G, Vogt RL: Epidemiologic surveillance for endemic *Giardia lamblia* infection in Vermont. Am J Epidemiol 129:762–768, 1989
7. Sullivan PS, DuPont HL, Arafat RR, Thornton SA, Selwyn BJ, El-Alamy MA, Zaki AM: Illness and reservoirs associated with *Giardia lamblia* in Egypt: The case against treatment in developing world environments of high endemicity. Am J Epidemiol 127:1272–1281, 1988
8. Brodsky RE, Spencer AC, Schultz MG: Giardiasis in American travelers to the Soviet Union. J Infect Dis 130:319–323, 1974
9. Fishel S, Webster J, Jackson P, Faratian B: Waterborne giardiasis in the United States 1965–84. Lancet 2:513–514, 1986
10. Shaw PK, Brodsky RE, Lyman DD, Wood BT, Hibler CP, Healy GR, MacLeod KIE, Stahl W, Schultz MG: A community-wide outbreak of giardiasis with evidence of transmission by a municipal water supply. Ann Intern Med 87:426–432, 1977
11. Dykes AC, Juranek DD, Lorenz RA, Sinclair S, Jakubowski W, Davies R: Municipal waterborne giardiasis: An epidemiologic investigation. Ann Intern Med 92:165–170, 1980
12. Kent GP, Greenspan JR, Herndon JL, Mofenson LM, Harris JS, Eng TR, Waskin HA: Epidemic giardiasis caused by a contaminated public water supply. Am J Publ Health 78:139–143, 1988
13. Pickering LK, Woodward WE: Diarrhea in day care centers. Pediatr Infect Dis 1:47–52, 1982
14. Steketee RW, Reid S, Cheng T, Stoebig JS, Harrington RG, Davis JP: Recurrent outbreaks of giardiasis in a child day care center, Wisconsin. Am J Publ Health 79:485–490, 1989
15. Common-source outbreak of giardiasis—New Mexico. MMWR 38:405–407, 1989

9

Food Poisoning

S. Benson Werner

Although the expression "food poisoning" is generally applied to any disease caused by food, a more appropriate rubric is "foodborne disease." This designation includes not only true "poisonings," such as from the metabolic products (toxins) produced by certain microorganisms while they multiply in food (e.g., *Staphylococcus aureus*), but also foodborne "infections" such as salmonellosis. While foodborne diseases are a worldwide problem, this chapter is restricted to the perspective of the situation in the United States and other developed countries.

The potential for large-scale foodborne outbreaks has never been greater. A major reason is our increasing reliance on massive, centralized food production and processing, combined with extensive distribution. Any contamination in that chain could result in the exposure of thousands, whereas contamination of foods processed in the home, where foods were primarily processed a generation ago, exposed relatively few individuals. The technological advances in industry that freed homemakers from food production and processing have not always been coupled with advances that assured food safety.

CLASSIFICATION OF FOODBORNE DISEASES

The extensive variety of foodborne diseases can be classified into several major categories based on the type of agent that causes illness. These are outlined below:

1. *Infection, bacterial:* Salmonellosis is an example. As with other infections, and in contrast to poisons, fever is common.
2. *Poisons, bacterial:* Staphylococcal or botulinal toxin poisoning. As with other poisons, these produce no fever.
3. *Infection, viral:* Hepatitis A is an example. Because of its long incubation period of approximately 30 days, identification of the responsible food vehicle can pose a problem.
4. *Infection, parasitic:* Trichinosis, taeniasis, and anisakiasis.
5. *Poisons, chemical:* Salts and oxides of such chemicals as arsenic, antimony, copper, and lead. Symptoms generally begin just minutes after ingestion.
6. *Poisons, plant and fungal origin:* Mushroom poisoning, ergot alkaloids, hemlock poisoning, jimsonweed.
7. *Poisons, animal (including marine) origin:* Ciguatera (ichthyosarcotoxism), scombroid, and paralytic shellfish poisoning.
8. *Radionuclides:* Strontium-90 from nuclear weapon testing.

Bryan's monograph[1] reviews the many etiological agents, their nature, sources, and important reservoirs, epidemiology, foods frequently involved, specimens to study, and control measures.

SURVEILLANCE AND INVESTIGATION OF FOODBORNE DISEASES

The surveillance of foodborne diseases has traditionally aimed at disease control through (1) identification and removal of contaminated products from the commercial market, (2) identification and correction of improper food handling practices both in commercial establishments and in the home, and (3) the identification and treatment of cases and carriers of foodborne disease. Surveillance also contributes to knowledge of disease causation and new etiologic agents and their food vehicles.

In the data published by the Centers for Disease Control (CDC) summarizing foodborne diseases in the United States in recent years, about 500 outbreaks have been reported annually. In only about 40% of these was a cause identified; it was bacterial in about 75% of the cases, chemical in 20%, parasitic in 3%, and viral in 2%. Most cases of bacterial origin involve *Salmonella, Staphylococcus,* and *Clostridium perfringens*. Accordingly, an appreciation of the different clinical features and incubation periods of these three diseases (Table 9–1) is important in the investigation of foodborne outbreaks. If a judgment as to probable cause can be made early in an epidemic investigation, then one can better decide on the most appropriate specimens to select for study, whether studies should be performed aerobically or anaerobically, and how far back in time to inquire about food exposures.

Procedures for the investigation of foodborne disease outbreaks are detailed in a monograph published by the International Association of Milk, Food, and Environmental Sanitarians, Inc.[2] Some general points merit emphasis. Interviews with food handlers, cases, and controls should be conducted as soon as possible: memories fade, people scatter, and the suspect foods

TABLE 9-1. DISTINCTIVE FEATURES OF THREE COMMON CAUSES OF FOODBORNE ILLNESS[a]

Entity	Incubation Period (h)	Fever	Vomiting	Diarrhea
Staphylococcal poisoning	3	–	+	±
Clostridium perfringens poisoning	12	–	–	+
Salmonella infection	24	+	±	+

[a]Applicable as a group phenomenon; no great reliance as to probable etiology should be placed on a single case of illness.

NOTE: These features offer practical guidelines for provisional identification of the etiology in foodborne disease outbreaks; they help to decide the most appropriate specimens for study and how far back to inquire about food exposure. Laboratory confirmation is necessary for definitive diagnosis.

may be discarded and unavailable for study or, worse, consumed by others. The investigator should appreciate the urgent necessity to collect the facts and materials that may not be practical or sometimes even possible to obtain at a later time.

In a relatively small outbreak an effort should be made to question all who were exposed, whether ill or not, for symptoms and food consumption history. To identify the responsible food(s), a method analogous to a cohort study design is commonly used. Rates of illness in those who ate specific food items (the "attribute" or "characteristic") are calculated and compared with the rates of illness in those who did not eat those items (Table 9–2). The implicated foods generally have the highest attack rates. More important, however, is that when rates for eaters and noneaters are compared, the implicated foods show the greatest differences in attack rates. The difference is called the "attributable risk," or the rate of disease that can be attributed to the food under consideration. In Table 9–2, barbecued chicken appears to be implicated (see last column), while those eating fried chicken might appear to have been spared from illness (probably by choosing that item instead of barbecued chicken). The necessity of interviewing well people in order to incriminate a particular food is illustrated by the item root beer, which might have been suspected as the cause of the outbreak. More ill people had root beer than any other item; in fact, all ill people had drunk some. However, it is evident that root beer was also consumed by nearly all those who remained well. The reason it was so popular is that it was the only drink available.

One might think that the association of illness with a particular implicated food should be "perfect" (i.e., all those who ate it must have become sick, and all those who got sick must have eaten it), but there are several reasons why this is rarely so:

1. The implicated food may not be contaminated throughout.
2. Host susceptibility varies.
3. Dosage (the quantity consumed) varies.
4. Food histories may contain reporting errors through faulty recall, uncertainty, or lying; there may also be errors in recording.
5. Those who report illness but no exposure to the incriminated food may have coincidental, unrelated illness or secondary infection when the outbreak is due to infection (e.g., *Salmonella*); alternatively, illness may be due to trace contamination of other foods or utensils by the implicated food.

If an outbreak is large and it is not possible to interview all participants, a random sample should be selected and questioned for symptoms and food exposure history. The data can be arranged in prospective fashion, as in Table 9–2, and similarly analyzed.

On the other hand, outbreaks can also be studied in a case-control fashion, and in fact there may be no alternative to case-control studies when the overall attack rate is low and the exposed population large, as exemplified by the occurrence of 13 cases of trichinosis aboard a luxury liner carrying 1300 passengers and crew.[3] In such situations the frequencies with which specific food items were selected by patients are compared with the frequencies in controls; that is, the so-called "food preference" rates are compared. Food preference rates can also be effectively used when recall for specific food items is compromised, as can occur in patients ill with diseases that have especially long incubation periods, such as hepatitis A.[4]

The remainder of the chapter describes the most frequently encountered foodborne diseases and comments briefly on newly identified ones.

STAPHYLOCOCCAL FOOD POISONING

History. The work of Dack et al,[5] in 1930 established staphylococci as a cause of food poisoning. They isolated *Staphylococcus aureus* in pure culture from a cake implicated in an outbreak; when cell-free filtrates prepared from broth cultures of the isolate were fed to volunteers, symptoms like those in the outbreak resulted. Five enterotoxins have been identified, and a sixth may

TABLE 9-2. DIFFERENCES IN FOOD-SPECIFIC ATTACK RATES IN AN OUTBREAK OF FOODBORNE ILLNESS

	Persons Who Ate Specified Food				Persons Who Did Not Eat Specified Food				Difference in Attack Rates
	Ill	*Well*	*Total*	*Attack Rate (%)*	*Ill*	*Well*	*Total*	*Attack Rate (%)*	
Shrimp salad	8	4	12	67	15	21	36	42	+25
Olives	19	13	32	59	5	13	18	28	+31
Fried chicken	10	33	43	23	4	2	6	67	−44
Barbecued chicken	17	1	18	94	3	27	30	10	+84
Baked beans	12	13	25	48	12	10	22	55	− 7
Potato salad	17	20	37	46	8	6	14	57	−11
Macaroni salad	9	15	24	38	15	10	25	60	−22
Root beer	23	23	46	50	0	2	2	0	+50
Bread	8	9	17	47	18	13	31	58	−11
Neapolitan cream pie	1	2	3	33	21	21	42	50	−17

exist. These toxins easily resist boiling for 30 minutes or more. It is the heat-stable, preformed toxin, not *S. aureus* organisms per se, that causes staphylococcal food poisoning. The target organ is the gut.

Symptoms. Symptoms usually appear 2 to 4 hours after ingestion; the range is 1 to 6 hours. Onset is generally abrupt and may be violent. Salivation, nausea, vomiting, abdominal cramps, prostration, diarrhea (diarrhea less often than vomiting), and occasionally hypertension occur. There is generally no fever or chills, but patients may experience a subjective feeling of fever from the flushing and perspiration that accompany vomiting, and a subsequent chilly sensation as perspiration evaporates. Acute gastrointestinal symptoms commonly last several hours but generally less than a day; weakness may persist for another 1 or 2 days. Death in otherwise healthy individuals is rare. The intensity of symptoms has prompted surgical exploration (for suspected appendicitis) in sporadic, severe cases.

Diagnosis. Staphylococcal food poisoning is generally suspected when a number of people develop acute, predominantly upper gastrointestinal tract symptoms a few hours after eating some food item in common. Isolation of coagulase-producing staphylococci from epidemiologically implicated food, vomitus, or stool specimens confirms the diagnosis. Rarely, coagulase-negative *S. aureus* has been implicated. The implicated food generally contains at least 10^6 *S. aureus* organisms per gram to produce sufficient enterotoxin to cause human disease. A small amount of *S. aureus* in food is not unusual, and so it is incumbent on the investigator to refrigerate food specimens promptly until testing can be done, so that any *S. aureus* present will not multiply to levels that did not exist when the food was obtained. On the other hand, if staphylococci are not recovered from the epidemiologically implicated food, the food may have been heated by someone apprised of an imminent visit by local public health authorities and aware that heating can destroy bacteria. In this case a Gram stain may be useful in demonstrating sheets of gram-positive cocci, and an assay is available at special laboratories (such as the Food and Drug Administration's [FDA]) to identify the presence of heat-resistant enterotoxin. Isolates of *S. aureus* from patients and from foods can be compared to those recovered from food handlers, either by antibiogram typing or by phage typing, to complete the epidemiological connection.

Sources of Contamination. Staphylococci are widely distributed in nature, and humans are a natural reservoir. *S. aureus* can colonize normal, healthy skin as well as the normal oronasopharynx, but the organism can be especially abundant in purulent discharges of an infected finger, hangnail, cut, burn, eye, or chronic infections of the nasal sinuses. Individuals with acne, boils, carbuncles, and common colds may be heavy shedders as well. Cows with infected udders also pose a health hazard if their milk is not promptly refrigerated. Foods implicated in staphylococcal food poisoning generally require much handling and are characteristically rich in protein (e.g., custards and cream fillings, sliced and chopped meats). Occasionally, surprising foods are implicated such as the extensive, widespread 1989 outbreak due to canned mushrooms imported from the People's Republic of China.[6]

Prevention. The three principal requirements for the production of sufficient enterotoxin to cause disease are: (1) the food must be contaminated with enterotoxin-producing staphylococci; (2) the food must be a good growth medium, and (3) the food must be held at an improper temperature (such as ambient room) for several hours. Prevention depends on eliminating sources of contamination and practicing safe food handling: workers with purulent discharges, common colds, etc., should be excluded from food preparation. The actual food handling time should be reduced to an absolute minimum. Foods should be at room temperature no longer than necessary and then should be kept hot (≥140° F, 60° C) or cold (≤40° F, 4° C) and covered to exclude dust.

SALMONELLA INFECTION

The epidemiology of salmonellosis is discussed in Chapter 12; this discussion will focus on aspects of salmonellae as a cause of foodborne disease. Salmonellae are among the most prevalent of zoonotic infectious agents. Raw meat and raw meat products frequently harbor salmonellae (poultry more commonly than pork; pork more commonly than beef). Foodborne *Salmonella* infection, however, can be prevented by adequate heating to destroy these pathogens and avoidance of cross-contamination after heating. Occasionally, infected food handlers are implicated in outbreaks as sources of contamination, but more often they represent additional cases, having eaten the same foods as their customers. Any "responsibility," however, lies in their not having eradicated (through proper heating etc.) the salmonellae introduced into their establishments in the raw meat and meat products that were implicated.

While low-level contamination of foods with *S. aureus* is unavoidable and, in itself, poses no threat, there can be no tolerance of any level of *Salmonella* contamination in foods ready for serving.

The infective dose for *Salmonella* infection is most commonly given as 10^5 organisms but can be as high as 10^9 or 10^{10}, depending on the serotype and the host. However, past volunteer studies to determine the infectious dose were limited by several factors: they were often done on healthy young males with laboratory strains that could have lost their virulence; they failed to assess minimal infective doses; and they used few volunteers at the lower dose levels. Much lower infective doses, of $\leq 10^3$ total organisms ingested, have been estimated from observations in the "more natural" setting of recent foodborne outbreaks. Specifically, 60 to 2300 organisms per 100 g of food were estimated in raw hamburger that caused *S. newport* infection,[7] less than 100 organisms per 100 g of chocolate candy that caused *S. eastbourne* infection,[8] and less than 1 organism per 100 g of cheddar cheese that caused *S. heidelberg* infection.[9] A comprehensive review of the infective dose of *Salmonella* in both volunteers and outbreak settings has been published.[10]

It is recognized that gastric acid protects against ingested enteric pathogens such as salmonellae. This can explain why infants (and the aged) can be infected by relatively low doses: they may normally lack stomach acid. The reason why the foods listed above may have caused disease in presumably healthy, young adults despite low-level *Salmonella* contamination, probably relates to their high fat content, which protects the salmonellae from gastric acid and allows salmonellae to reach the less hostile, alkaline duodenum. Milk has a high fat content and, if contaminated, poses an additional risk. Since it is fluid, it quickly passes into the duodenum (unless consumed with solid food) and escapes acid contact. The large Riverside, California, waterborne outbreak of 1965[11] was due to low-level contamination (MPN of 17 salmonellae per liter) of water, which, as a fluid, could similarly reach the duodenum after short gastric contact time.

CLOSTRIDIUM PERFRINGENS FOOD POISONING

History. While it was suggested earlier in this century that *C. perfringens* (*C. welchii*) caused foodborne disease, it was not until the classic paper by Hobbs et al. in 1953[12] that *C. per-*

fringens received attention. Since then it has become recognized as one of the most frequent causes of foodborne disease in developed countries.

The organism is a common, anaerobic, spore-forming rod that exists widely in nature and can frequently be recovered from raw meats and meat products. Five toxicological types (A to E) are recognized; types A and C cause human gastroenteritis. Type A also causes gas gangrene, and type C, necrotic enteritis ("pigbel"). Of the several toxins and enzymes produced by *C. perfringens* type A, the important one appears to be alpha toxin, which includes the enzyme lecithinase. This acts on the substrate lecithin in food to liberate phosphorylcholine, which was suspected for a time of being the true cause of *C. perfringens* food poisoning. Animals given only phosphorylcholine developed diarrhea; however, similar studies in human volunteers were negative. In 1977, several outbreaks[13] were attributed to lecithinase-negative *C. perfringens.* Accordingly, the exact pathophysiology of *C. perfringens* poisoning remains to be elucidated. *C. perfringens* produces both heat-resistant spores and heat-sensitive spores; the latter predominate in nature, but it is the heat-resistant strains that are most often associated with outbreaks of foodborne poisonings.

Typical Setting of* C. perfringens *Poisoning. With rare exceptions the implicated food is a meat dish prepared in bulk for a large group, for example, a banquet or institutional population, in such a way that anaerobic and thermal conditions exist to permit germination of spores that survive initial cooking. These spores are heat shocked (activated) to germinate as soon as the cooling mass reaches a suitable temperature. Young vegetative cells continue to multiply, depending on temperature, storage time, and the nature of the food (liquid masses of meat can provide especially good anaerobic conditions). With generation times as short as 9 minutes under optimal conditions, a critical dose of disease-producing *C. perfringens* (several million organisms or a concentration of organisms $\geq 10^5$/g of food) can readily result. If the mass is too large to cool quickly during subsequent refrigeration, multiplication can continue in the refrigerator and can also resume on subsequent rewarming if not carried out at temperatures inhibitory to growth ($\geq$ 140° F, 60° C). In summary, the cooking of meats and poultry in huge quantities, prolonged storage at room temperature, slow cooling, and insufficient reheating are typical features in *C. perfringens* outbreaks.

The Disease. After an incubation period of approximately 12 hours (range: 6 to 24), abdominal cramps and diarrhea develop. Occasionally, nausea is reported, but vomiting and fever are typically absent. The disease is so mild that medical consultation is rarely sought; for most the illness lasts only a day or less. In elderly debilitated patients, however, the disease can be severe, and deaths have been reported.

Diagnosis. As in any foodborne outbreak, laboratory study of the epidemiologically implicated food is most important; for *C. perfringens,* the organism concentration criterion is $\geq 10^5$/g. A direct smear of the implicated food typically shows square-ended, gram-positive bacilli almost exclusively. Stool cultures also should be obtained from cases and controls for anaerobic study. Although healthy adults may harbor *C. perfringens* in their intestinal tracts, many different serotypes are represented and the concentration of *C. perfringens* is much less than in those who are ill. *C. perfringens* enterotoxin can also be detected in the feces of patients but not in the feces of controls. Environmental cultures from the kitchen and fecal cultures from food handlers may also be obtained but are not encouraged. Since *C. perfringens* is so commonly found in raw meat and poultry, the human carrier or unsanitized kitchen equipment and working surfaces represent relatively unimportant sources of contamination.

Prevention. Outbreaks of *C. perfringens* foodborne disease would not occur if cooked foods were eaten after initial cooking, while still hot. If it is absolutely necessary to prepare large amounts of food several hours or days before its intended use, the cooked food should not be held at room temperature to cool. It should be chilled rapidly to a temperature of 40° F (4° C), preferably in a walk-in refrigerator with forced air circulation. To speed the cooling process, the meat, gravy, or stew, for example, should be placed in a freezer compartment or divided into shallow containers to induce more rapid heat transfer in the refrigerator. The meat may be served cold, but if it is to be served hot, it should be rewarmed to 165° F (74° C) as quickly as possible. Cold meat slices may be covered with boiling-hot gravy immediately before serving, but the habit of pouring warm gravy on sliced meat and putting both in a warming oven with temperature below 140° F (60° C) is to be condemned. The expression "Keep hot foods hot and cold foods cold" is worth emphasizing for *C. perfringens,* as well as for other organisms responsible for foodborne diseases.

BOTULISM

History. Botulism was first recognized as a disease entity early in the nineteenth century and was named for sausage (from the Latin *botulus*), which was often implicated in the earliest outbreaks. Since then a host of other improperly preserved foods (fish, vegetables, fruit) have caused disease, but the name has been retained. Van Ermengem first identified the causative organism in 1895. Its neurotoxins (simple proteins) are among the most deadly of all known poisons.

Three forms of botulism are now recognized according to the site of toxin production by *Clostridium botulinum* (although a fourth category, "undetermined," exists for those cases not easily categorized):

1. Classic foodborne botulism, the form with which most health workers are familiar, results from the ingestion of preformed botulinal toxin in improperly preserved food. Interest in foodborne botulism far exceeds its importance as a cause of extensive illness (less than 2000 cases reported in the United States since 1900 and only about 10 cases per year in recent decades), yet foodborne botulism continues to pose an ever-present threat of widespread, often fatal disease.
2. Wound botulism results from local tissue infection and in situ toxin production of *C. botulinum.* This form of botulism is rarely documented; only 50 to 60 cases have been reported worldwide.
3. Infant botulism results from colonization of the gut lumen by *C. botulinum* with subsequent in vivo production of toxin. This third form of botulism was first recognized in 1976, and by 1990 approximately 900 cases had been identified worldwide. Some "undetermined" cases of botulism in adults have been considered adult forms of infant botulism, occurring particularly in those who have had altered intestinal anatomy and physiology.[14–16]

Clostridium botulinum is a gram-positive, strictly anaerobic, spore-forming bacillus whose natural habitat is the soil. Seven toxigenic types (A to G) have been identified, but in humans the disease is almost always caused by A, B, or E toxins and rarely by F or G. These toxins prevent the release of acetylcholine at cholinergic synapses and therefore interrupt transmission of nerve impulses. The effect is most noted at myoneural junctions because of resultant flaccid paralysis. The spores of *C. botulinum* are ubiquitous, and except for those infants who develop the third type of botulism for reasons still unknown, the spores are not otherwise dangerous when ingested. Indeed, since spores are so widely distributed in soil and dust, they could be ingested every time fresh produce is eaten. Toxin is elaborated, however, when spores that survive improper food preservation germinate in anaerobic conditions. Botulinal toxin, once formed, is readily destroyed by boiling, but most botulinum spores are not promptly destroyed by boiling; they require temperatures of 240° F (116° C) for destruction.

The Disease. In classic foodborne botulism, signs and symptoms of intoxication appear 6 hours to 8 days (most typically 12 to 48 hours) after ingestion of contaminated food. Those with the shortest interval to onset (< 24 hours) generally are most severely affected. The initial symptoms are frequently ptosis, blurred or double vision, and dry, sore throat. Progressive descending paralysis, usually but not always symmetrical, may then develop. After impairment of cranial nerve function (which causes diplopia and poor accommodation, dysphagia, dysphonia, and inability of neck muscles to support the head), paralysis of the respiratory muscles and of the extremities may ensue. Conspicuously absent are objective sensory abnormalities, altered mental status, and fever. Gastrointestinal symptoms are frequently but not necessarily present and may precede or accompany neurological symptoms; constipation is common after paralysis develops. The case fatality ratio for classic foodborne botulism was formerly about 60%, but in recent years it has been less than 30%. Respiratory paralysis is generally the immediate cause of death. If vital functions can be maintained, full neurological recovery can be expected, although convalescence may be slow and weakness may last for months.

The clinical picture in *wound* botulism is like that in foodborne botulism, but there is more likely to be fever (secondary to wound infection) and less likely to be early gastrointestinal complaints. With some exceptions, cases to date have primarily involved wounds of an extremity, and the median interval between injury and symptoms of botulism has been 6 days. An increasing proportion of recent cases has been reported in drug abusers, with sinusitis or rhinitis infection occurring in cocaine "sniffers" and skin abscesses in skin "poppers" and intravenous drug users (*Archives,* California Department of Health Services).

In the typical case of *infant* botulism requiring hospitalization, the child is 3 months old, and the first symptom is usually constipation, followed by lethargy, poor sucking and swallowing, and then generalized weakness and hypotonia. The infant appears "floppy." In less than 3% of infant botulism cases requiring hospitalization in the United States has the child died; however, it has been shown that some cases of sudden infant death syndrome (SIDS) can be attributed to infant botulism.[17]

Foods Involved. Most cases of classic botulism are caused by preserved foods that received some preliminary heat treatment such as canning or smoking. More recently, however, major restaurant-associated outbreaks have involved foods that were not preserved in the usual sense, for example, previously baked potatoes used for potato salad, chopped garlic in oil, and sauteed fresh onions. Inadequately rewarmed foods have also been implicated, such as commercial pot pies and home-prepared meat loaf that were kept in gas ovens, with only the pilot light on, for many hours after initial cooking. Despite the publicity given to commercial foods, about 90% of all outbreaks in recent years have been due to improper home canning rather than commercial canning. Home canning at temperatures insufficient to destroy spores is the usual problem. For vegetables a pressure cooker that can reach temperatures of 240° F (116° C) is necessary. Resistance of spores to heat sterilization is reduced at a low pH, and this is why highly acid fruits are rarely implicated in outbreaks and why acidification of home-canned vegetables (with vinegar or lemon juice) is recommended before pressure cooking as an extra measure of protection.

In the United States, most botulinal poisonings are due to home-canned vegetables or fruits, rarely meats; but in Europe, most cases are due to sausages, smoked or preserved meats, and fish. Foods spoiled by some types of *C. botulinum* are frequently foul smelling and vile tasting, especially when proteolytic strains of the organism are involved. Jar lids or can tops may be swollen from gas produced by *C. botulinum,* but this is not invariably the case.

For those infants who develop botulism, it is likely that there are multiple sources of gastrointestinal colonization since botulinal spores are ubiquitous in the environment. To date, toxin has not been found in any food fed to infants with botulism. *C. botulinum* spores, however, have been found in up to 10% of honey samples surveyed and in honey that had been fed to patients.

Distribution. Spores of *C. botulinum* exist in soil throughout the world, and botulism occurs worldwide. In nations where home canning is discouraged (e.g., England) or where fresh fruits and vegetables are available year round and there is little home canning (as in tropical Third World countries), botulism outbreaks are rare. Additionally, some cases may go undiagnosed in some developed and in most developing countries because laboratory tests to diagnose the disease are not generally available.

In the United States, more than 50% of outbreaks have been reported from five western states. California alone has reported 33% of the national total. There is a distinct geographical distribution of botulinal toxin types: type A outbreaks predominate west of the Mississippi River, type B occurs primarily in eastern states, and type E is reported primarily from Alaska and the Great Lakes area. This correlates with the types of spores found in these respective regions. Most outbreaks in Europe are due to type B, and in Japan most are due to type E.

Wound botulism has been reported primarily from the United States but undoubtedly occurs worldwide. The diagnosis should be considered when characteristic features of botulism develop in a person (often a youth) with a wound, particularly of an extremity (not necessarily suppurative), where food cannot be incriminated.

Infant botulism, as of January 1990, has been recognized on all inhabited continents except Africa. More than 850 laboratory-confirmed cases have been identified in the United States, where it was first recognized. As medical awareness of this disease entity increases throughout the world, the incidence and importance of infant botulism worldwide will probably exceed that of classic foodborne botulism, as it has in the United States.

Diagnosis. Botulism is confirmed by demonstrating that the patient's serum or stool contains a heat-labile substance toxic for mice that is specifically neutralized by botulinal antitoxin. Parallel studies should be performed on leftover, suspect food or, if none is available, on food from the same lot or batch. Stool cultures for *C. botulinum* should also be obtained. Despite the routine ingestion of *C. botulinum* spores on fresh fruits and vegetables, neither *C. botulinum* nor its toxins are normally found in feces. For this reason the presence of *C. botulinum* toxin or organisms in the stools of patients with suspected foodborne botulism can be considered diagnostic. In wound botulism an effort should be made to culture *C. botulinum* from the wound as well as to test the serum for toxin.

Electromyography is a useful diagnostic tool. In botulism the muscle action potential is diminished after a single nerve stimulus, but repetitive supramaximal stimulation at rates of 20 to 50 per second can result in facilitation (augmentation) of the action potential. This may not be present early, however, and it is not pathognomonic. In infant botulism a characteristic electromyographic pattern termed "brief, small, abundant, motor unit action potentials" (BSAPs) can be observed and has been seen to persist for as long as clinical evidence of blocked neuromuscular transmission is present.[18]

Treatment. Most important in all forms of botulism is high-quality supportive care with immediate access to an intensive care unit, so that respiratory failure—the usual cause of death—can be anticipated and promptly treated. Polyvalent antitoxins of equine origin are available that neutralize circulating toxin but not the toxin already fixed to nerve tissue. If treatment is clinically indicated, antitoxin should be administered without delay and without waiting for results of mouse neutralization tests (which are usually not available for at least 24 hours). The role of antitoxin in infant botulism, however, is not clear: circulating toxin has been demonstrated only rarely, and virtually all hospitalized patients have recovered completely without antitoxin treatment. A study to evaluate the efficacy of botulism immune globulin (of human origin) in infants is underway in California. Antibiotics have not been of value in either classic or infant botulism. Antibiotics certainly have not prevented continued excretion of *C. botulinum* toxin and organisms. In classic botulism the gastrointestinal tract should be emptied of still unabsorbed toxin by emesis or gastric lavage (if foods were eaten recently) and by cathartics and high enema (if ileus is absent). In those who are suspected of having ingested contaminated food but are not symptomatic, evacuation of gastrointestinal contents as described is also indicated. In wound botulism, thorough debridement, wound irrigation, and antibiotic therapy are indicated along with administration of antitoxin. Trivalent botulinal antitoxin is available around-the-clock from the Centers for Disease Control, Atlanta, Georgia: (404)639-3753 daytime and (404)639-2888 nights and holidays.

Prevention. For foods canned at home, attention must be given to the necessary time, pressure, and temperature to ensure destruction of *C. botulinum* spores. Vegetables should generally be acidified before they are pressure cooked and should be reboiled for at least 3 minutes, with stirring, before serving. Although the toxin is readily destroyed by boiling, foods with off-odors should not be consumed or "taste tested," and cans or bottles with bulging lids, whether home canned or commercial, should not be opened. Classic foodborne botulism is a public health emergency; local public health authorities should be notified immediately of any presumed case so that efforts can be initiated to confirm the diagnosis, locate other cases and impending cases, determine the food source, and confiscate all existing food containers. Notification of even suspected cases is a legal requirement in most states. Until the epidemiology of infant botulism is better delineated, no recommendations can be given except that honey should not be fed to infants, especially since this is not an essential food.

MISCELLANEOUS

Other important foodborne diseases as well as those recently identified deserve comment. *Vibrio parahaemolyticus* is one of the leading causes of foodborne disease in Japan, but it was not identified in the United States until 1969. Most outbreaks have been traced to crustaceans taken from warm coastal marine waters that were either inadequately cooked or subsequently recontaminated by raw shellfish or surfaces and implements that had contact with raw fish or shellfish. The incubation period is about 12 hours; onset is generally acute; and symptoms resemble those of salmonellosis. Recovery is usually complete in 2 to 5 days. Special media (thiosulfate citrate bile salts agar—TCBS) should be used in tests when this disease is suspected. Other *Vibrio* species (which contaminate 5% to 10% of shellfish in the U.S. market) cause disease too. The most virulent is *V. vulnificus,* which is fatal in more than 50% of those who develop bacteremia. At greatest risk of serious *V. vulnificus* infection are those with liver disease (such as from alcoholism), reduced stomach acid (naturally occurring or therapeutically induced), acquired immunodeficiency syndrome (AIDS), and other conditions with compromised immunity. These individuals, especially, should avoid eating raw or undercooked shellfish.

Scombroid fish poisoning results from the ingestion of spoiled fish, primarily of the suborder *Scombroidei* (e.g., tuna, mackerel). Inadequate or delayed refrigeration at sea of fish taken from temperate and tropical waters results in overgrowth of bacteria (*Proteus morganii,* among others) that normally comprise the microflora of fish. These bacteria metabolize histidine and degrade the protein of fish flesh to produce scombrotoxin, which consists of histamine and other amines. Since orally administered histamine has no effect in humans, it may be co-contaminants like cadaverine, putrescine, and other products of fish decomposition that enhance the toxic action of histamine by inhibiting histaminases in the human intestine.[19] (Similarly, drugs such as isoniazid, which inhibit histamine-detoxifying enzymes, have evoked reactions to low levels of histamine normally found in such foods as cheese.) Scombroid fish poisoning is sometimes misdiagnosed as "fish allergy." Symptoms develop about 30 minutes after eating and include a peppery sensation of the tongue, rash, flushing (sometimes urticaria), pruritus, headaches, dizziness, periorbital edema, thirst, nausea, vomiting, diarrhea, and abdominal cramps. Some of these symptoms resemble histamine reaction and appear to respond to antihistamine therapy. Laboratory studies of implicated fish frequently show "honey-combing" (a sign of decomposition), bad odor, and histamine levels ≥ 50 mg/100 g. Scombrotoxin is heat stable and can withstand the temperatures used in canning; commercially canned fish has been implicated in several international outbreaks.

Ciguatera poisoning can be caused by more than 400 species of fish that are primarily bottom-dwelling shore fish caught near reefs between 35° N and 35° S latitude. In the United States, 90% of outbreaks are reported from Hawaii and Florida and are due mostly to grouper, red snapper, and barracuda. Ciguatoxin is actually produced by certain dinoflagellates attached to algae on coral reefs. Small fish feed on the algae and are, in turn, eaten by larger bottom-dwelling shore fish and so on up the food chain. The larger fish are more toxic than smaller ones; organs such as liver, intestines, and gonads are the most toxic parts. The median latency period is 5 hours, and the median duration of symptoms is 8 days. Besides gastrointestinal symptoms of abdominal cramps, nausea, vomiting, and diarrhea, there may be numbness and paresthesia of lips and tongue, paresthesias of the extremities, metallic taste, arthralgia, myalgia, blurred vision, temporary blindness, and paradoxical temperature sensation. In those with life-threatening disease there may be hypotension, bradycardia, cranial nerve palsies, and respiratory paralysis. Therapy is primarily supportive, although intravenous mannitol has been reported to produce dramatic improvement.[20] Tocainide, an orally effective lidocaine analogue, has also been reported of value (presumably by blocking the toxic effect of ciguatoxin).[21] Prevention is difficult; ciguatoxic fish do not appear or taste spoiled, and ordinary cooking does not destroy the heat-stable toxin. Unusually large reef fish should be avoided, especially their liver and roe.

Paralytic shellfish poisoning is caused by the ingestion of filter-feeding bivalve mollusks (e.g., mussels and clams) that had previously ingested (without adverse effect) toxic dinoflagellates of *Gonyaulax* sp. and concentrated the neurotoxin saxitoxin in their tissues. Symptoms in humans usually begin about 30 minutes after eating with paresthesias of the mouth, lips, face, and fingertips; then, in more severe cases, dysphagia, dysphonia, ataxia, weakness, paralysis, and occasionally respiratory arrest occur. Treatment is supportive and should include efforts to remove unabsorbed toxin from the gut. Fortunately, even in severe cases, symptoms disappear completely in 1 to 2 days. A standardized mouse bioassay is used for demonstrating and quantifying toxin in shellfish. Toxic dinoflagellates bloom in waters above 30° N and below 30° S latitude and sometimes impart a reddish color to the water—the so-called red tide.

Bacillus cereus poisoning has been recognized for decades in Europe, but the first fully documented episode in the United States occurred in 1969. At least two clinical syndromes exist. The first is like staphylococcal food poisoning in that it has a median latency period of only 2 hours and produces primarily upper gastrointestinal symptoms. The vehicle for this form has most commonly been fried rice served in Chinese restaurants, where the rice had previously been steamed or boiled and then left unrefrigerated for hours or days before it was mixed with egg or pork and quickly stir-fried before serving. The second syndrome resembles *C. perfringens* poisoning in that it has a median latency period of 10 hours and produces primarily lower gastrointestinal symptoms. A variety of foods has been implicated in this type of illness. In both syndromes, disease is generally mild and lasts only a few hours. Diagnosis can be confirmed by the isolation of $\geq 10^5$ *B. cereus* organisms per gram of food from epidemiologically implicated food and also by fecal culture. The prevalence of *B. cereus* in controls will be much less than in cases. The organism produces at least two enterotoxins—one is heat stable and causes vomiting, and the other is heat labile and causes diarrhea. *B. cereus* is widely distributed in soil and in raw, dried, and processed foods. In one survey, 52% of 1500 food ingredients were positive for *B. cereus*.[22] Foods with low colony counts (e.g., $\leq 10^3$/g) probably pose no problem if they are handled properly and refrigerated promptly after cooking.

Listeria monocytogenes is commonly found in the environment and in food, the primary mode of transmission to humans. Studies in the United States and Europe have shown it to be present in 15% to 20% of ground beef, in 15% to 80% of poultry, and in a small percentage of ready-to-eat processed foods including such dairy products as soft cheeses and ice cream. Moreover, unlike other foodborne pathogens, this organism continues to grow at refrigerated temperatures (4° C, 39° F), and so the degree of contamination increases with storage. The infectious dose is unknown, but it is presumably less for immunosuppressed persons, pregnant women, and the elderly. Although most cases are sporadic (1 to 10 per million people per year), common-source outbreaks have occurred and have implicated several commercial foods: cole slaw, pasteurized milk, and soft cheeses. Case-control studies have implicated uncooked hot dogs and undercooked chicken. A World Health Organization (WHO) informal working group on foodborne listeriosis concluded in 1988 that total elimination of *Listeria* from all food is impractical, if not impossible, but that control procedures should be carried out at all stages of the food chain. It indicated that pasteurization of milk "reduces the number of *Listeria monocytogenes* in raw milk to levels that do not pose an appreciable risk to human health" and that the contamination of cheeses from pasteurized milk commonly reflects contamination during manufacturing and handling. The group recommended withdrawal of foods from market in two situations: (1) when the contents of sealed packages are contaminated despite treatment to eliminate *Listeria* and (2) when foods have been implicated in human cases of listeriosis.

Escherichia coli can be grouped into four categories by differences in virulence properties, epidemiology, and clinical syndromes. These are enteropathogenic *E. coli* (EPEC), enteroinvasive *E. coli* (EIEC), enterotoxigenic *E. coli* (ETEC), and enterohemorrhagic *E. coli* (EHEC). The latter is most commonly represented by *E. coli* 0157:H7. Symptomatic and asymptomatic human carriers are believed to be a principal reservoir and source of EPEC, EIEC, and ETEC strains involved in human illness, whereas the primary reservoir for *E. coli* 0157:H7 appears to be dairy cattle. Ground beef (hamburger) and, less commonly, rare roast beef and raw cow's milk have been implicated in most outbreaks due to *E. coli* 0157:H7. Secondary person-to-person transmission also occurs. In limited population-based studies done to date the incidence of *E. coli* 0157:H7 disease (which commonly presents as afebrile bloody diarrhea) slightly exceeds that of shigellosis. Occasionally, infection with *E. coli* 0157:H7 is followed by hemolytic uremic syndrome. Studies of retail meat and poultry in the United States and Canada have revealed *E. coli* 0157:H7 in 4% to 30% of ground beef and in about 2% of pork, poultry, and lamb samples. Accordingly, concern about *E. coli* 0157:H7 disease should provide one additional reason to avoid consumption of raw milk and raw or partially cooked meats and poultry.

Yersinia enterocolitica infection has been recognized for years in other areas of the world, especially Scandinavia and Japan. While outbreaks have suggested the possibility of foodborne transmission, specific food items have not been incriminated until recently. These include not only unprocessed "natural" products such as tofu,[23] raw milk,[24] and raw pork[25] but also pasteurized milk[26] and pasteurized products probably contaminated by the addition of ingredients after pasteurization (chocolate milk).[27] Generally, *Y. enterocolitica* is destroyed by standard pasteurization[28,29]; but if it is present in great numbers, some *Yersinia* may survive pasteurization and multiply during refrigeration.[24,28,30] In one large multistate outbreak due to pasteurized milk, symptoms in children included abdominal pain (suggestive of acute appendicitis which prompted appendectomies), fever, and diarrhea; many adults, however, presented with pharyngitis and had throat cultures positive for *Y. enterocolitica*.[31] Since this pathogen grows best at 75° to 77° F (24° to 25° C), it may be missed when stools, foods, and pharyngeal swabs are cultured at the usual 99° F (37° C).

Campylobacter jejuni, formerly known to veterinarians as *Vibrio fetus,* has become recognized as an important cause of enteritis in humans.[32,33] In developed countries it has been isolated from the stools of 3% to 14% of patients evaluated for diarrhea, but it is rarely isolated from healthy individuals.[33] Transmission occurs through contaminated food and water, as well as from person to person. The apparent incubation period is 2 to 10 days. The organism has been found in pets, domestic livestock, and fowl (live and dressed). Investigations in the United States have implicated raw milk, raw clams, raw hamburger, raw and undercooked chicken, untreated water, and even municipal water supplies.[33] The epidemiology of this pathogen is similar to that of *Salmonella* (with chicken also a common vehicle), and where reporting is compulsory, the incidence of *C. jejuni* infection rivals and sometimes surpasses that of salmonellosis.[34] Selective media, vacuum jar, and an incubator set at 109° F (43° C) have made this zoonotic infection an important addition to the growing list of enteric pathogens.

Mushroom poisoning can be produced by 50 species among the 2000 that are known. Even trained mycologists confuse toxic varieties with edible ones because of the extensive variations and intergradations between species; contrary to popular belief, there are no simple field tests to aid in differentiation. Mushroom poisons are conveniently divided into two categories based on their latency period: the delayed onset group and the rapid onset group. The most deadly types tend to have delayed onsets of at least 6 hours. These include *Amanita phalloides, Amanita verna,* and certain *Galerina* species, which cause 90% of all deaths from mushrooms and produce heat-stable cyclic polypeptides toxic to kidneys and liver. Typically a biphasic illness is seen. There may be sudden onset of severe nausea, vomiting, bloody diarrhea, abdominal pain, and cardiovascular collapse 6 to 20 hours after ingestion. After a short phase of improvement, painful, tender hepatomegaly with jaundice and oliguria may develop. Confusion, coma, and convulsions are common. Death ensues in 30% to 50% of cases. There is no specific antidote for *Amanita* intoxication; treatment is mostly supportive but should include purgation and high enemas to remove unabsorbed toxin. Experimental or invasive treatment including hemodialysis or hemoperfusion, repeated doses of activated charcoal given orally, cytochrome C, penicillin, corticosteroids, or thioctic acid (which is available from the FDA) have not been subjected to controlled studies to confirm effectiveness.[35] An algorithm for treating mushroom poisoning has been proposed.[36]

The rapid onset group (2 hours or less) includes mushrooms that contain hallucinogens that produce psychotropic, LSD-like effects that begin minutes after eating as well as mushrooms with muscarinic effects of salivation, perspiration, lacrimation, increased bronchial secretions, abdominal pain, miosis, nausea, vomiting, diarrhea, and bradycardia beginning about 1 hour after ingestion. Atropine is a specific antidote for this intoxication. Other mushroom poisons primarily cause gastric irritation, produce disulfiram-like effects, or produce states resembling alcoholic intoxication.

Chemical food poisoning may result from eating foods that have been contaminated accidentally or deliberately with toxic chemicals. The contaminant may be inorganic or organic, naturally occurring or human made. The soluble salts or oxides of such heavy metals as antimony, cadmium, copper, tin, and zinc can cause abrupt and severe gastrointestinal symptoms, typically in a setting where foods or beverages of high acid content have reacted chemically with the metal containers in which they were prepared or stored. The latency period is characteristically short (about 15 minutes). The explosive vomiting that occurs generally eliminates enough of the chemical from the gastrointestinal tract so that systemic toxicity is rarely a problem. Treatment is symptomatic and supportive; antiemetics should be avoided to prevent gastrointestinal retention of toxic ions and potential systemic absorption. A greater threat to life is posed by foods poisoned with *insecticides* and *rodenticides*. These chemicals are all too often kept in kitchens where they are mistaken for flour, salt, sugar, baking powder, and other food ingredients. Such chemicals include arsenic, barium carbonate, sodium fluoride, and silver polishes containing cyanide and mercury. Preventive measures are obvious; such chemicals should be labeled poisonous and kept out of food handling areas and away from children.

Contamination with heavy metal salts occurs occasionally in commercial food items with catastrophic consequences. In 1955 more than 12,000 Japanese children were poisoned by arsenic-tainted Morinaga dry milk, and more than 130 died. A study of survivors 15 years later showed them to be shorter and to have lower IQs, more central nervous system disorders (epilepsy, brain damage, reduced hearing), and other mental and physical defects than control subjects had. Another catastrophic incident due to a commercial product occurred in Morocco in 1960 when 10,000 people became ill (6000 suffered paralysis of the legs) after they had consumed cooking oil adulterated with turbo-jet lubricating oil containing 3% triorthocresyl phosphate.

Chinese Restaurant Syndrome sometimes follows ingestion by those susceptible to monosodium glutamate (MSG), a flavor enhancer especially popular in Chinese restaurants. Illness typically begins 20 to 30 minutes after exposure and can include a flushed or burning sensation of the neck and face, perspiration, a heavy feeling in the precordial area, palpitations, headache, and lacrimation. Since absorption of MSG is rapid when the stomach is empty, the first course of a meal—typically soup—is a common vehicle. Susceptible individuals, who can be sensitive to just 2 g of MSG, should avoid eating foods containing MSG, especially on an empty stomach.

In 1981 an epidemic of a new illness tentatively designated "toxic oil syndrome" (TOS) occurred in Spain and resulted in 20,000 cases and 300 deaths. It was traced to the ingestion of unlabeled, illegally marketed rapeseed oil that had been denatured with aniline and further treated to remove the aniline before it was fraudulently sold to the public as pure olive oil. As yet unidentified toxic agents were probably produced during the illegal refining process, but the resulting disease, which affected multiple organ systems in progression, suggested either a continued body burden of toxin(s) or, more probably, the triggering of a chronic autoimmune process. Unique was the common progression of disease through an initial phase of febrile pneumonia-like symptoms sometimes with rash, followed late in the first month by gastrointestinal problems and striking eosinophilia, and about 100 days after onset in severely affected cases by profound neuromuscular manifestations (myalgia, atrophy of major muscle groups, and contractures). The suggestion that an immunological mechanism is at least partially responsible for the syndrome is based on the fact that scleroderma-like skin thickening, Raynaud's phenomenon, sicca syndrome, dysphagia, and pulmonary hypertension have been common in those who progressed to neuromuscular disease. In addition, histopathological changes of vasculitis were seen, and high antinuclear antibody titers were prevalent, as were high levels of IgE.[37,38] In late 1989 a new disease, tentatively designated *eosinophilia myalgia syndrome* (EMS), was identified. It shares many clinical features of the intermediate and chronic phases of TOS. In EMS a striking association has been found with oral preparations of L-tryptophan-containing products, but like toxic oil syndrome, the apparent contaminant in processing that causes this disease has not yet been identified (as of early 1991).[39]

The hazard of *methylmercury poisoning* was dramatized in Japan. Those who consumed fish taken from Minamata Bay, which had received direct factory discharges of methylmercury, subsequently developed Minamata disease, which was frequently fatal. Methylmercury poisoning may take weeks, months, and possibly even years before symptoms are manifest, and unlike poisoning from inorganic mercury, it primarily affects the central nervous system, especially the cerebellum and cerebrum, where damage is usually irreversible. Symptoms can include paresthesia, ataxia, emotional lability, blindness, deafness, and in those most severely affected, stupor, coma, and death. It is not generally appreciated that discharges of even relatively inoffensive metallic mercury can be converted via biological methylation to methylmercury by bottom-dwelling bacteria. These bacteria are then consumed by plankton, which are consumed by small fish, and these by larger fish, and so on up the food chain until humans fall victim. Human exposure can sometimes be more direct. Alkyl mercury compounds have been used for years as a fungicidal seed dressing. Although such seeds are meant for planting purposes only, they have occasionally been consumed by people who were unaware of the danger or were driven by starvation. In 1971, 80,000 tons of methylmercury-treated wheat and barley were imported by Iraq for planting. Some of the grain was used, however, in the preparation of homemade bread and resulted in 6000 hospital admissions and 400 deaths. Similar outbreaks were reported from Pakistan and Guatemala.

Foodborne viral infections are uncommonly reported. Poliomyelitis appears to have been the first human viral disease for which a food vehicle was reported (in 1914, in association with raw milk), but there have been none since 1949.[40] Though hepatitis A is an uncommon cause of foodborne disease, a 1988 outbreak associated with cockles from the Shanghai area of China that affected nearly 300,000 gives hepatitis A the distinction of causing the "largest" foodborne outbreak recorded.[41] Other foodborne illnesses of proven viral etiology include tickborne encephalitis virus, ECHO 4, and, most importantly of late, Norwalk agent and small round viruses resembling Norwalk agent.[40] The Norwalk group probably caused many past outbreaks previously designated as "gastroenteritis of undetermined etiology" or "acute infectious nonbacterial gastroenteritis (AING)" but was not identified until modern diagnostic methods, particularly immune electron microscopy, became available. The incubation period for Norwalk agent disease is 24 to 48 hours; onset is abrupt; symptoms can include nausea, vomiting, abdominal cramps, diarrhea, headache, and sometimes low grade fever; the duration is generally 1 to 2 days. The secondary attack rate among contacts of cases is notably higher than in other foodborne infections. While viruses belonging to about seven groups (rotaviruses, parvoviruses, adenoviruses, caliciviruses, enteroviruses, astroviruses, and coronaviruses) can cause human gastroenteritis, are shed in stools, and have the potential to contaminate food, only the Norwalk group has been repeatedly identified in common-source outbreaks of gastroenteritis.[40]

The two basic mechanisms for the contamination of food by viruses that infect the intestinal tract are (1) "indirect" contamination by growing of filter-feeding shellfish in fecally contaminated waters or by irrigation of produce by polluted water and (2) "direct" contamination of food, primarily by feces, by a food handler with poor personal hygiene. Once contamination has occurred, the question is whether the virus will retain infectivity. Unlike bacterial pathogens, no virus can replicate outside living cells.

REFERENCES

1. Bryan FL: Diseases Transmitted by Foods (a classification and summary), 2 edt. Atlanta: HHS Pub. No. (CDC)83-8237. USPHS, Centers for Disease Control, 1982
2. Committee on Communicable Diseases Affecting Man, Food Subcommittee: Procedures to Investigate Foodborne Illness, 4 edt. Ames, Iowa: International Association of Milk, Food, and Environmental Sanitarians, Inc., 1987
3. Singal M, Schantz PM, Werner SB: Trichinosis acquired at sea. Am J Trop Med Hyg 25:675–681, 1976
4. Joseph PR, Millar JD, Henderson DA: An outbreak of hepatitis traced to food contamination. N Engl J Med 273:188–194, 1965
5. Dack GM, Cary WE, Woolpert O, Wiggers HJ: An outbreak of food poisoning proved to be due to a yellow hemolytic staphylococcus. J Prevent Med 4:167–175, 1930
6. Centers for Disease Control: Multiple outbreaks of staphylococcal food poisoning caused by canned mushrooms. MMWR 38:417–418, 1989
7. Fontaine RE, Arnon S, Martin WT, et al: Raw hamburger: An interstate common source of human salmonellosis. Am J Epidemiol 107:36–45, 1978
8. D'Aoust JY, Aris BJ, Thisdele P, et al: *Salmonella eastbourne* outbreak associated with chocolate. J Inst Can Sci Technol Aliment 8:181–184, 1975
9. Fontaine RE, Cohen ML, Martin WT, Vernon TM: Epidemic salmonellosis from cheddar cheese: Surveillance and prevention. Am J Epidemiol 111:247–253, 1980
10. Blaser MJ, Newman LS: A review of salmonellosis: I. Infective dose. Rev Inf Dis 4:1096–1106, Nov-Dec 1982
11. Collaborative Report: A waterborne epidemic of salmonellosis in Riverside, California, 1965—epidemiologic aspects. Am J Epidemiol 93:33–48, 1971
12. Hobbs BC, Smith ME, Oakley CL, et al: *Clostridium welchii* food poisoning. J Hyg 51:75–101, 1953
13. Pinegar JA, Stringer MF: Outbreaks of food poisoning attributed to lecithinase-negative *Clostridium welchii.* J Clin Pathol 30:491–492, 1977
14. Bartlett JC: Infant botulism in adults. N Engl J Med 315:254–255, 1986
15. Chia JK, Clark JB, Ryan C, Pollack M: Botulism in an adult associated with food-borne intestinal infection with *Clostridium botulinum.* N Engl J Med 315:239–241, 1986
16. McCroskey LM, Hatheway CL: Laboratory findings in four cases of adult botulism suggest colonization of the intestinal tract. J Clin Microbiol 26:1052–1054, 1988
17. Arnon SS, Midura TF, Damus K, et al: Intestinal infection and toxin production by *Clostridium botulinum* as one cause of sudden infant death syndrome. Lancet 1:1273–1276, 1978
18. Arnon SS, Midura TF, Clay SA, et al: Infant botulism—epidemiological, clinical, and laboratory aspects. JAMA 237:1946–1951, 1977
19. Taylor SL: Histamine food poisoning: Toxicology and clinical aspects. CRC Crit Rev Toxicol 17:91–128, 1986
20. Palafox NA, Jain LG, Pinano AZ, Gulick TM, Williams RK, Schatz IJ: Successful treatment of ciguatera poisoning with intravenous mannitol. JAMA 259:2740–2742, 1988
21. Lange WR, Kreider SD, Hattwick M, Hobbs J: Potential benefit of tocainide in the treatment of ciguatera: Report of three cases. Am J Med 84:1087–1088, 1988
22. Nygren B: Phospholipase C-producing bacteria and food poisoning. Acta Pathol Microbiol Scand 160(suppl):1–89, 1962
23. Tacket CO, Ballard J, Harris H: An outbreak of *Yersinia enterocolitica* infections caused by contaminated tofu (soybean curd). Am J Epidemiol 121:705–711, 1985
24. Schiemann DA, Toma S: Isolation of *Yersinia enterocolitica* from raw milk. Appl Environ Microbiol 35:54–58, 1978
25. Tauxe RV, Vandepitte J, Wauters G, et al: *Yersinia enterocolitica* infections and pork: The missing link. Lancet 1:1129–1132, 1987
26. Tacket CO, Narain JP, Sattin R, et al: A multistate outbreak of infections caused by *Yersinia enterocolitica* transmitted by pasteurized milk. JAMA 251:483–486, 1984
27. Black RE, Jackson RJ, Tsai T, et al: Epidemic *Yersinia enterocolitica* infection due to contaminated chocolate milk. N Engl J Med 298:76–79, 1978
28. Francis DW, Spaulding PL, Lovett J: Enterotoxin production and thermal resistance of *Yersinia enterocolitica* in milk. Appl Environ Microbiol 40:174–176, 1980
29. Lovett J, Bradshaw JG, Peeler JT: Thermal inactivation of *Yersinia enterocolitica* in milk. Appl Environ Microbiol 44:517–519, 1982
30. Hughes D: Isolation of *Yersinia enterocolitica* from milk and a dairy farm in Australia. J Appl Bacteriol 46:125–130, 1979
31. Tacket CO, Davis BR, Carter GP, et al: *Yersinia enterocolitica* pharyngitis. Ann Intern Med 99:40–42, 1983
32. Skirrow MB: *Campylobacter* enteritis: A "new" disease. Br Med J 2:9–11, 1977
33. Blaser MJ, Reller LB: *Campylobacter* enteritis. N Engl J Med 305:1444–1452, 1981
34. Finch MJ, Riley LW: *Campylobacter* infections in the United States. Arch Intern Med 144:1610–1612, 1984
35. Olson KR, Pond SM, Seward J, et al: *Amanita phalloides*-type mushroom poisoning. West J Med 137:282–289, 1982
36. Hanrahan JP, Gordon MA: Mushroom poisoning-case reports and a review of therapy. JAMA 251:1057–1061, 1984
37. Kilbourne EM, Rigau-Perez JG, Heath CW Jr, et al: Clinical epidemiology of toxic-oil syndrome—manifestations of a new illness. N Engl J Med 309:1408–1414, 1983
38. Toxic Epidemic Study Group: Toxic epidemic syndrome, Spain, 1981. Lancet 2:697–702, 1982
39. Kilbourne EM, Swygert LA, Philen RM, et al: Editorial. Interim guidance in the eosinophilia-myalgia syndrome. Ann Intern Med 112:85–86, 1990
40. Cliver DO: Manual of food virology. Geneva: WHO, 1983
41. WHO: Weekly Epidemiologic Record, No. 38:290–291, Sept 22, 1989

10

Control of Infections in Institutions

Nosocomial Infections

Bradley N. Doebbeling

Nosocomial, or hospital-acquired, infections occur at a rate of 5 to 10 per hundred admissions in U.S. hospitals.[1] While precise national mortality data are unavailable, an estimated 30,000 patients die each year as a direct result of nosocomial bloodstream infection.[2] Furthermore, many nosocomial infections are associated with an extended length of stay, substantial morbidity, and prolonged therapy.[2–4] Because of these factors, it has been estimated that nosocomial infections have a direct cost of $5 billion to $10 billion annually in this country.[5]

In the era of prospective reimbursement based on the patients' diagnosis (diagnosis related groups, or DRGs), hospitals typically receive no additional reimbursement to care for patients with nosocomial infections.[5] Data from the Study on the Efficacy of Nosocomial Infection Control (SENIC) suggest that up to one third of nosocomial infections could have been prevented in the mid-1970s if an effective infection control program were in place.[1] Thus there are strong financial incentives and benefits for hospitals to implement and maintain an efficacious infection control program.[5] Although little data exist on the frequency of nosocomial infection in developing countries, rates may be as high as 65% on certain services, with nosocomial diarrhea particularly prevalent.[6] In Third-World countries with limited economic resources the importance of preventing nosocomial infections is even more evident.

DESCRIPTIVE EPIDEMIOLOGY

An individual's risk of nosocomial infection is determined by three major factors: the host, agent, and environment. First, intrinsic host susceptibility to infection is clearly important and is influenced by characteristics such as age, nutritional status, and severity of underlying disease. Second, a variety of organisms are especially important nosocomial pathogens by virtue of intrinsic virulence. Finally, the hospital environment contains a variety of risks. Diagnostic procedures and medical or surgical therapy may breach the normal host defenses and predispose to infections. Potent immunosuppressives, chemotherapy, and antibiotics may affect the host's normal colonizing flora, cause skin and mucosal membrane breakdown, and impair the function of the immune system. Exposure to infected or colonized patients, asymptomatic health care workers, and various medical devices may transmit infecting microorganisms as well.

Currently, little can be done to decrease individual patient's intrinsic susceptibility to infection. Prospective hospital surveillance may identify clusters of a particular type of infection or specific infectious agent at an early stage. Importantly, investigation of the reservoirs of organisms and modes of transmission may allow effective intervention to be planned and implemented. Appropriate use of diagnostic procedures, invasive devices, and medical therapy may also decrease the likelihood of nosocomial infection. Likewise, the hospital environment may be modified to prevent nosocomial infections. Proper use of isolation materials, strategies to increase handwashing, and other approaches to prevent transmission may be particularly beneficial.

Infection rates differ considerably among hospitals. Referral hospitals generally have higher rates than community hospitals have, a difference primarily attributed to the more complex patient mix and more aggressive modes of therapy used at referral centers.[1,7] Infection rates also differ among hospitals of the same type, however; these differences are influenced by the effectiveness of the hospital infection control program.[1] Within an institution, rates also vary by the service caring for patients.[7]

Infection Categories

Virtually any infection that occurs in the community may be acquired within the hospital. Certain infections, however, are particularly common because of the unique susceptibility and exposure of the hospitalized patient (Fig. 10–1).[8]

Urinary Tract Infections. Urinary tract infections (UTIs) are the most common infections acquired in the hospital, responsible for 35% of nosocomial infections.[8] Most (70% to 80%) nosocomial UTIs are related either to the use of urinary catheters or urinary tract manipulation. The typical UTI prolongs hospital stay by an average of 1.2 days.[9] Risk factors for bacteriuria include duration of catheterization, microbial colonization of the drainage bag, diabetes mellitus, no antibiotic use, female gender, abnormal serum creatinine, errors in catheter care, failure to use a urinemeter, and indications other than drainage during surgery or measurement of output.[10] The daily incidence of bacteriuria in the presence of a short-term (< 30 day) catheter ranges from 3% to 10%.[11,12] More than 70% of catheter-associated bacteriuria cases appear to be due to movement of bacteria up the urethra on the external catheter surface.[12] The major complications of short-term catheterization are symptomatic UTI and bacteremia. Although only 3% to 5% of nosocomial UTIs develop secondary bacteremia overall, up to 16% of patients with UTIs

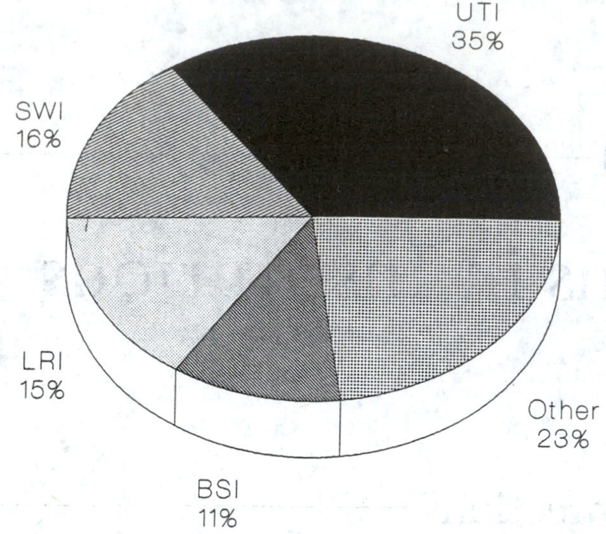

Figure 10-1. Frequency distribution of nosocomial infections at each of the major sites, 1986-1990. *UTI* = urinary tract infection, *LRI* = lower respiratory tract infection, *SWI* = surgical wound infection, *BSI* = bloodstream infection. *(From Gaynes R: National Nosocomial Infections Surveillance System, CDC, November 1, 1990.)*

due to *Serratia marcescens* become bacteremic.[13] UTI is the single most important source of nosocomial bacteremia.[11]

Prevention of UTI has been proposed and studied in a variety of ways. Prevention of catheterization, if possible, is simple and extremely effective. Alternative approaches to catheterization have included intermittent catheterization, external collection devices (condom catheters), suprapubic catheterization, and urinary diversions. Each approach has its relative merits and disadvantages.[14] If a urinary catheter must be used, most authorities would recommend minimizing the duration of catheterization and maintaining the closed drainage system as important preventive measures. The single measure likely to prevent cross transmission of urinary pathogens is good handwashing after caring for each patient.

Surgical Wound Infections. Surgical wound infections (SWIs) are now the second most common hospital-acquired infections, accounting for 16% of nosocomial infections.[8] Infection rates vary with the level of contamination of the operative site, although ideally rates should be compared for specific operative procedures. Operative wounds have traditionally been classified as clean, clean-contaminated, and contaminated based upon the degree of bacterial contamination expected during a particular procedure. In the era of routine preoperative antibiotics, infection rates have ranged from 0.8 to 1.3 and 10.2 per hundred, respectively, for each of the classes of procedures above in one large series.[15] SWIs contribute substantially to patient morbidity, prolonged hospital stay, and increased direct costs.[16] Although a variety of sources of microbial contamination of the surgical wound have occasionally been implicated, important sources include direct inoculation from the patient's residual flora, contaminated host tissues, and surgical team members' hands at the time of surgery; postoperative drains or catheters; and airborne contamination at the time of surgery.

A variety of host factors have been shown to predispose to surgical wound infection: age, obesity, current infection at another site, and prolonged preoperative hospitalization. Effective preoperative measures in preventing wound infection include not shaving the operative site with a razor, disinfection of the skin at the incision site, and preoperative antibiotics when indicated.[17] Perioperative antibiotics started immediately before surgery and continued for up to 48 hours are effective in clean-contaminated and contaminated surgery.[17] Perioperative antibiotics may also be beneficial in certain clean procedures when the occurrence of a postoperative wound infection would be potentially catastrophic, for example, implantation of prosthetic devices and open-heart surgery, or when it is consistently shown to be beneficial in prospective trials.[18] Important intraoperative measures include good surgical technique, minimizing the duration of surgery, and possibly, the appropriate use of surgical drains.[17] Aseptic technique in changing dressings on a postoperative wound left open also seems important. Feedback of surgeon-specific infection rates for clean procedures to each member of the surgical staff has been shown to reduce the rates of SWI, presumably through more meticulous attention to surgical technique.[19]

Lower Respiratory Tract Infections. As a group, lower respiratory tract infections (LRTIs) are responsible for approximately 15% of nosocomial infections.[8] The incidence of nosocomial LRTI is estimated to be approximately 6 per 1000 discharges in acute care hospitals.[7] Nosocomial LRTIs are associated with a case fatality rate of 30%,[20] ranging from 20% to 50% in some series. A matched cohort study of nosocomial pneumonia recently demonstrated that the pneumonia itself accounts for one third of the crude mortality observed and is associated with an excess length of stay of 1 week.[20] Stepwise logistic regression demonstrated that age, time from admission to pneumonia, prior use of mechanical ventilation, and neoplastic disease were significant risk factors for mortality. Similarly, prior mechanical ventilation, posttracheotomy status, nasogastric intubation, immunosuppression or leukopenia, and prior bacteremia were significantly associated with prolonged hospital stay.[20]

Endotracheal intubation has consistently been shown to predispose to nosocomial pneumonia.[21] Both tracheostomy and endotracheal intubation bypass the normal upper respiratory tract defense mechanisms, lead to drying of the lower respiratory mucosa, and provide a direct portal for the introduction of exogenous microorganisms. Ventilator and other respiratory equipment may also transmit infection. Contaminated aerosols from fluid nebulizers, as well as inadequately cleaned equipment, have been shown to cause nosocomial LRTIs.[22] The condensate in disposable ventilator tubing may also become contaminated with bacteria and predispose to LRTI. Routine changing of ventilator tubing every 48 hours rather than every 24 hours may actually decrease the risk of pneumonia.[23]

Prevention of nosocomial LRTI has been approached in several different ways. General hygienic measures encouraging handwashing, the use of barrier isolation materials when appropriate, and routine decontamination of respiratory equipment have been widely used. The normal gastric acidity is an important natural barrier that kills bacteria that otherwise would colonize the upper gastrointestinal tract. Maintenance of the stomach's acidity through avoidance of histamine type 2 blockers and antacids in intubated patients may also be protective.[24] Compliance with glove and gown isolation precautions was recently shown to decrease the nosocomial spread of respiratory syncytial virus.[25] Topical broad-spectrum antibiotics or "selective decontamination" of the gastrointestinal tract has been used in several European centers and occasionally in the United States in an attempt to prevent nosocomial pneumonia. Although nosocomial pneumonia rates were decreased in several series,[26,27] concern about the emergence of resistant bacteria has limited the approach in this country. Additionally, larger controlled studies of prophylactic antibiotics are needed. Immune system modulation is the final area of potential intervention. The single immunologic measure likely to decrease nosocomial respiratory infections is annual influenza immunization of hospital staff members. The immunocompromised host is at risk for a broad range of respiratory infections; preventive measures in this population have been recently reviewed.[28]

Bloodstream Infections. The next most frequent hospital-acquired infections are bloodstream infections (BSIs), which are responsible for 11% of nosocomial infections.[8] Rates of nosocomial bacteremia have ranged from 1.5 to 4 per 1000 admissions in most series, although higher rates have occasionally been reported.[2] At least 120,000 episodes of nosocomial bacteremia occur annually in this country.[29] A primary bacteremia is defined as the isolation of a bacterial bloodstream pathogen in the absence of an infection at another site. Secondary bacteremia occurs when bacteria are isolated from the blood during an infection at another site with the same organism, that is, a UTI, SWI, or LRTI. Independent predictors of true bacteremia from a prospective cohort of hospitalized patients include temperature of 38.3° C or higher, presence of a rapidly or ultimately fatal disease, shaking chills, intravenous drug abuse, acute abdominal examination, and major comorbidity.[30] The mortality rate for nosocomial bacteremia is higher than for community-acquired bacteremia and increases with the isolation of more than one organism (polymicrobial) in some series. A controlled study of nosocomial BSI demonstrated that independent predictors of death (excluding parameters of septic shock) included increased age, severity of underlying disease, and infection with either *Pseudomonas aeruginosa* or *Candida* spp.[31] The attributable mortality (the crude mortality in carefully matched controls subtracted from that of infected individuals) for nosocomial BSI has ranged from 21% to 31% in several studies.[2]

The chief sources of primary bacteremia or fungemia include IV catheters, intrinsic IV fluid contamination, and multidose parenteral (IV) medication vials. A number of outbreaks of pseudobacteremia have been reported, related either to contamination of the blood culture medium or skin at the bedside or to contamination at different points in the microbiology laboratory. Vascular catheter-related infection appears to be the most important source of BSI and may be due to contaminated antiseptics used to disinfect the skin, contamination from the hands of health care workers, autoinfection following hematogenous seeding, or most importantly to external colonization of the catheter. Risk factors for peripheral catheter infection include duration longer than 72 hours, cutdown placement (rather than percutaneous), lower extremity site, emergent placement, and poor handwashing.[32]

Effective preventive measures have not been well studied. Minimizing the duration of intravascular catheterization appears to be important. The catheter should be routinely changed to a new site every 72 hours if possible. Although somewhat controversial, vascular catheters should not be routinely changed over a wire, particularly if there is any concern about infection.[32] Careful handwashing prior to catheter placement or manipulation, minimizing entry into the system, and careful observation for the development of any signs or symptoms of infection should be performed.[32]

Major Pathogens

The spectrum of microbial organisms causing nosocomial infections continues to evolve. Gram-positive organisms now represent the top three nosocomial bloodstream pathogens: the coagulase-negative staphylococci, *Staphylococcus aureus,* and the enterococci together now account for approximately one half of nosocomial BSIs.[33] A variety of gram-negative bacteria remain important causes of nosocomial BSI, UTI, LRTI and SWI. Other bacteria have been recognized as important causes of nosocomial infection as our ability to isolate organisms improves, particularly *Legionella pneumophila,* the agent of Legionnaire's disease, which causes sporadic and occasionally epidemic LRTIs in certain hospitals.[34]

The fungi have emerged as major nosocomial pathogens, primarily as a result of increasing host susceptibility and therapeutic practices in recent years. Chemotherapy and immunosuppression predispose to a variety of microorganisms. Additionally, widespread antibiotic use appears to reduce the host's indigenous flora and predispose to colonization and infection. The *Candida* species as a group have shown the most rapid growth and are now the fourth most common cause of bloodstream infection.[33] The *Candida* species are responsible for over 10% of nosocomial BSIs and have an attributable mortality of 38%.[35]

The changing bacterial and fungal spectrum in hospitals presumably reflects increased antibiotic use, particularly of the newer broad-spectrum antimicrobial agents (Fig. 10–2). Additionally the development of antibiotic resistance by certain bacteria, increased use of invasive devices, and profound immunosuppressive agents used may also affect the secular trends of microorganisms in hospitals.

Certain viruses, particularly cytomegalovirus, varicella-zoster virus, and herpes simplex viruses are common causes of infection in immunocompromised hosts. The hepatitis viruses, particularly A and B, may be transmitted in the hospital between patients and occasionally to health care workers. Preventive measures, including the use of hepatitis B vaccine, have been recently reviewed.[36]

The acquired immunodeficiency syndrome (AIDS) virus is increasingly prevalent among hospitalized patients, and occasional transmission has occurred.[36] The routine use of universal precautions has been recommended to attempt to decrease the likelihood of exposure to potentially infectious blood and body fluids.[37] Measures designed to decrease the likelihood of exposure from contaminated sharp objects should be equally important in prevention of transmission.[38]

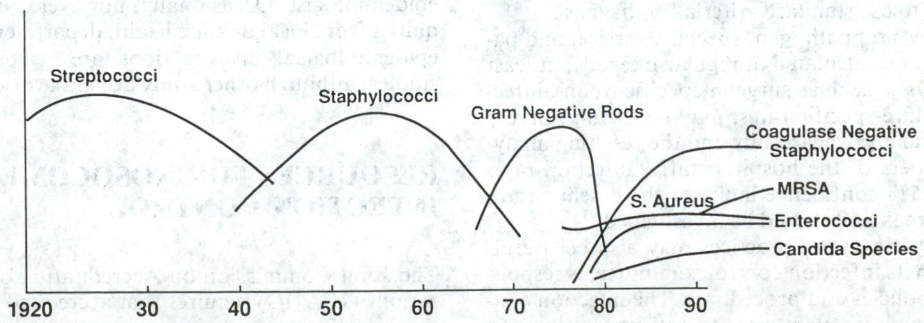

Figure 10–2. A schematic representation of the relationship between time and usage of antibiotics and the emergence of "new" pathogens responsible for most nosocomial infections. MRSA = methicillin-resistant *S. aureus.* *[From Wenzel RP: Epidemiology of hospital-acquired infection. In Manual of Clinical Microbiology, 5 edt. Washington, D.C.: American Society for Microbiology, 1991.]*

PREVENTION AND CONTROL PROGRAMS

During the late 1960s the need for a more vigorous approach to the prevention and control of nosocomial infections became apparent. A model infection control program,[39] widely publicized by the Centers for Disease Control (CDC), American Hospital Association, and Joint Commission on the Accreditation of Healthcare Organizations was adopted in principle by many U.S. hospitals by the mid-1970s.[40] The CDC conducted the SENIC in the late 1970s to evaluate the effectiveness of hospital infection control programs.[1] The SENIC project evaluated a random sample of 338 hospitals, stratified by size, medical school affiliation, and type of infection control program, assessing the effect of infection control programs on rates of UTI, LRTI, SWI, and BSI in adult patients.

The study demonstrated that hospitals with active surveillance and control programs had significantly fewer infections than did hospitals without such programs. The SENIC study also found that four elements were associated with effective programs: (1) an active infection surveillance system with reporting of results to staff members, (2) presence of vigorous control measures designed to eliminate recognized hazards, (3) at least one full-time infection control practitioner for every 250 beds, and (4) a physician on the staff knowledgable about nosocomial infections who took an active part in the infection control program.[1]

Components of Effective Programs

Surveillance. An infection control program may include surveillance of patient infections, patient-care practices, and microbial contamination of the environment. Evaluation of patient disease is the most important activity because the incidence of nosocomial infection is the ultimate measure of program effectiveness.

Surveillance of patient illness should be conducted prospectively, before patients are discharged. Typical surveillance is conducted by an infection control practitioner who actively seeks nosocomial infections by making regular, frequent visits to patient-care areas. The practitioner may review patient-care plans, microbiology laboratory results, medical charts, radiographic reports, and lists of patients receiving antibiotics or on isolation precautions.[41] Once an infection is identified, the practitioner uses standard criteria to determine whether it is nosocomial.[42] Other techniques such as questionnaires or serosurveys may be useful in the evaluation of specific problems or clusters of cases. Retrospective case-finding is difficult to perform effectively and does not provide current information upon which to base decisions about intervention. Although some hospitals require that nosocomial infections be listed as discharge diagnoses, surveillance based upon these diagnoses is ineffective because of underreporting and failure to use standard criteria for diagnosis.

Infection rates by site, pathogen, specialty service, and patient-care area should be calculated at regular intervals, at least monthly. Other analyses, such as surgeon-specific wound infection rates and procedure-specific rates, may be useful. Surveillance data should be analyzed carefully and the resulting analyses reported to members of the hospital staff.[1] Infection rates that lie beyond the 95% confidence limits of the baseline rates may identify an outbreak and should be investigated.[43]

Surveillance of patient-care practices may also be useful. The hospital, through its infection control committee, is responsible for developing policies and procedures. The infection control practitioner, through frequent visits to patient-care areas to review patient-care practices, can do much to assure their implementation.

Microbiological surveillance of the inanimate hospital environment may also be elected. Except for monitoring the effectiveness of sterilization and disinfection procedures, or investigation of a specific problem, routine microbiological surveillance of the environment adds little to the infection control program and is not recommended.

Control Measures. Most preventable nosocomial infections are related to specific patient-care practices. A substantial proportion of urinary tract, respiratory, and bloodstream infections are related to instrumentation, and guidelines are available to minimize their risks.[14,32,37] In addition, the hospital should develop and implement policies for isolation of patients with potentially communicable diseases,[44] use of antimicrobial agents, and control of the hospital environment.[45]

Infection Control Practitioner. Hospitals have traditionally employed infection control practitioners to provide day-to-day coordination of surveillance and control programs. Practitioners have occasionally been laboratory technicians, nonphysician epidemiologists, or sanitarians, although over 90% of U.S. hospitals have employed nurses to function as infection control practitioners.[1] Their duties have included collection and analysis of surveillance data, assisting in the development of infection control policies and procedures, and providing education and consultation to other hospital personnel.

The SENIC project demonstrated that the presence of at least one full-time infection control nurse (ICN) for every 250 hospital beds significantly improved the effectiveness of infection control programs.[1] The effectiveness of these programs decreased as the ratio of beds-to-ICNs increased, suggesting that a single ICN is not sufficient in large hospitals.

Hospital Epidemiologist. A physician who takes responsibility for the infection control program also appears to be integral to the program's success.[1] This physician usually serves as the hospital epidemiologist, although nonphysician epidemiologists have occasionally filled this role. The physician supervises the infection control nurses and practitioners, provides liaison with other members of the medical staff, and provides advice about surveillance methods, analysis of surveillance data, methods of conducting epidemiologic studies, and development of control measures. The physician plays a critical role in advising the hospital's medical staff and administration about the clinical implications of patient-care practices, infection problems, and prevention and control measures.

Investigation of Problems. Even in hospitals with exemplary infection control programs, epidemic and endemic infections continue to occur. The infection control committee is responsible for assuring that problems are investigated effectively. Usually these investigations are conducted by the hospital's infection control team, the infection control practitioner(s), and hospital epidemiologist. Occasionally, however, outside assistance is required from local or state health departments or the CDC. Most epidemiological investigations are retrospective case-control studies, although other study designs are occasionally needed.

RESOURCES FOR NOSOCOMIAL INFECTION CONTROL

The Joint Commission on Accreditation of Healthcare Organizations (JCAHO) requires that accredited hospitals have an active infection control program, an infection control committee, as well as specific written infection control policies and procedures for each of the hospital's departments.[46] The JCAHO also requires written definitions of nosocomial infections, a system for reporting of infections, laboratory support for infection control, an active employee health program, and review of antibiotic use.[46] The American Hospital Association's (AHA) Committee on Infections within Hospitals has published guidelines for establishing infection control programs.[47] The Association of Practitioners in Infection Control and the Society for Hospital Epidemiology in America (the professional organizations for persons working in infection control) have developed training courses in infection control. Additionally, a number of state health departments, universities, and the CDC also provide training courses and advice or assistance in conducting epidemiological investigations. Several major textbooks[48–50] and the proceedings of two recent international symposia on infection control are available as important resources.[51–52]

Infectious Diseases and Child Day Care

Michael T. Osterholm

The first known facility for the care of children outside of their home in the United States was opened in Boston in 1828. Since that time the number and type of facilities providing child day care have reflected both the economic conditions of the time, which require both parents to work, and the increase in the proportion of single-parent families. By 1986 it was estimated that more than 5.3 million children were in out-of-home, nonrelative child day care.[1] This included 2.1 million children that attended approximately 63,000 licensed child-care centers. An additional 500,000 children received care in 105,000 regulated day-care homes. Since the total regulated child-care slots available in centers and homes is only about 2.6 million, some 2.7 million additional children were likely attending unregulated family day-care homes.

As recently as 1984, mothers who had delivered a child in the past year comprised over 50% of the female work force, and 75% of preschool children had full-time working mothers.[2] With the clustering of infants and preschool-age children (most of whom are susceptible to virtually all infectious disease agents) into child-care facilities that often lack adequate toilet and washing facilities and that are staffed by individuals with little or no training in infection control, outbreaks of common respiratory and enteric diseases are to be expected. Although placing children in out-of-home care should not pose health or safety risks to the child, the family, or the community, patterns of childhood disease in the past decade indicate that child care has had a significant influence on the incidence of certain diseases.

Most epidemiological studies of infectious disease in child day care have been conducted in the United States. Limited information for studies carried out in the Scandinavian countries is also available. In the Peoples Republic of China, child-care facilities, which often involve boarding care of children starting from about 2 years of age, reported severe outbreaks of adenovirus pneumonia. This epidemic disease problem previously had been observed only in military recruits. However, scant information is available on child day care throughout the world, making it difficult to evaluate infectious disease problems in such a setting on a worldwide basis.

Much progress has been made in the recognition of the out-of-home child care setting and the potential for increased occurrence of infectious diseases and unintentional injuries. As a result of this concern, in 1987 the American Academy of Pediatrics and the American Public Health Association initiated a nationwide project, The Development of National Health and Safety Standards for Out-of-Home Child Care Programs.[2] This project, funded by the Bureau of Maternal and Child Health and Resources Development of the Department of Health and Human Services, resulted in the writing of standards for health, safety, nutrition, and sanitation in out-of-home child care. The standards, finalized in late 1990, address the needs of infants, toddlers, preschoolers, and school-age children through 12 years of age in child-care centers, family child-care homes, and group child-care homes. Although the standards are not regulations, they delineate professional criteria between minimum requirements and the ideal. Specifically, recommendations regarding infectious disease control have been promulgated by the Infectious Disease Technical Panel of the National Child Care Standards Project. This panel is composed of individuals with expertise in pediatric infectious disease, public health, state licensing, medical and legal aspects of child care, and child-care service.

In addition to the report of the Infectious Disease Technical Panel, two other comprehensive reviews of the status of infectious diseases in child day care have been published in recent years. The first, published in 1986, represents the proceedings of the first symposium related to infectious diseases in child day care held in Minnesota in 1984.[3] The second, published in 1990 in *Seminars in Pediatric Infectious Diseases,* was devoted to providing a comprehensive and current review of this issue by a group of national experts.[4]

This review describes the pathogens most frequently associated with infections in child day-care settings in the United States and the patterns of these infections. It discusses current aspects of control and prevention of these infectious diseases and the controversies related to infectious diseases in child day care and outlines aspects of this problem that warrant further attention.

AGENTS AND PATTERNS OF OCCURRENCE

Nearly all infectious agents associated with common illnesses in young children have been observed in children in day-care settings. Agents listed in Table 10–1 represent common causes of infectious disease, although a variety of other agents have also been reported in day-care settings.

Most early studies of infectious diseases in child day care focused on the role of specific pathogens or investigated recognized outbreaks. Only recently have investigators recognized the need for prevalence and longitudinal studies to define the occurrence of certain infections in day care. More importantly, few studies have concurrently compared the risk of infections among cohorts of children attending day care with those not attending day care. Thus, for most diseases it remains unclear as to the relative risk of acquiring a specific infectious agent in day-care programs compared to the risk in other care settings.

Four patterns of infectious disease occurrence among children in day-care facilities are characterized (Table 10–2) in the following discussions.

Haemophilus influenzae, Type B

Few infectious disease issues related to the child-day-care environment are more complex and controversial than natural history in management of invasive bacterial diseases. The occur-

TABLE 10-1. CAUSES OF INFECTION IN CHILDREN IN DAY CARE

Organ System of Condition	Common Agents
Respiratory tract[5,6]	Viruses: Respiratory syncytial virus, parainfluenza virus, adenovirus, rhinovirus, enterovirus, influenza viruses. Bacteria: Group A *Streptococcus, Mycoplasma pneumoniae.*
Gastrointestinal tract and liver[7-10]	Viruses: Rotavirus, caliciviruses, Norwalk and Norwalk-like viruses, hepatitis A virus, hepatitis B virus. Bacteria: *Shigella, Salmonella, Campylobacter, Escherichia coli* 0157:H7, *E. coli* 0114:HM, *E. coli* 0111:K58, *Clostridium difficile.* Parasites: *Giardia lamblia, Cryptosporidium.*
Invasive bacterial disease[11]	*Haemophilus influenzae,* type B, *Neisseria meningitidis, Streptococcus pneumoniae*
Skin	*Streptococcus pyogenes, Staphylococcus aureus,* scabies [*Sarcoptes scabiei* var *hominis*], lice [*Pediculus humanus* var *corporis* and *capitis*]
Multiple organ systems[12-14]	Cytomegalovirus, varicella zoster

rence of *Haemophilus influenzae* type B disease in children attending day care is of great public health interest because of its seriousness and incidence. One area of confusion regarding the epidemiology of *H. influenzae* type B infection is estimating the risk of primary disease in the day-care environment.[11] The question of whether children who attend day care are at an increased risk of primary *H. influenzae* type B disease compared with children who do not attend day care is of considerable importance because of the potential for public health intervention. In contrast, other recognized primary disease risk factors for *H. influenzae* type B disease that are host related and include age, gender, race, and the presence of other selected underlying health conditions cannot be affected at this time by public health intervention other than vaccination.

To date, seven studies have addressed the issue of risk of primary disease and day-care attendance.[11] Six of these studies employed case-control methodology to assess independent day-care-associated risk factors. In the seventh study the incidence of *H. influenzae* type B among children attending licensed day-care facilities was compared with the incidence among children who reportedly did not attend day care. All the studies were conducted between 1981 and 1989; six of the studies were conducted in the United States and one in Finland. Six of these studies employed a similar definition of child day-care attendance; it was defined as any regular (more than 4 hours per week) supervised care of at least two unrelated children. No definition of day-care attendance was provided for the remaining study.

TABLE 10-2. PATTERNS OF OCCURRENCE OF DISEASES IN CHILD DAY CARE

Patterns of Occurrence	Examples
Manifestations of infection primarily in children attending day-care facilities	*Haemophilus influenzae,* type B disease
Infection affects children, day-care staff, and close family members	Shigellosis, giardiasis
Infection is inapparent in children attending day-care facilities, but is likely to be apparent in the adult contacts	Hepatitis A virus
Infection is inapparent or mild in children attending day-care facilities and in adult contacts, but may have serious consequences for the fetus of a pregnant contact	Cytomegalovirus

From Goodman RA, Osterholm MT, Granoff DM, Pickering LK: Infectious diseases in child day care. Pediatrics 74:134, 1984.

In general, the studies found a significantly increased risk of *H. influenzae* type B disease among children attending day care independent of other possible risk factors. However, there was a significant variation in the presence and magnitude of the increased risk by age of the child, type of day-care facility attended, and geographic location of the study.

It is reasonable to believe that day-care attendees might be at increased risk for primary *H. influenzae* disease. Day-care attendance may increase the likelihood of exposure to individuals who may be asymptomatic pharyngeal carriers of *H. influenzae* type B. In addition, factors such as crowding previously have been demonstrated to play a role in the increased risk in the family setting, and they are likely to play a role in the day-care environment. It has been suggested that the development of invasive *H. influenzae* type B disease may be facilitated by concomitant infection with other microorganisms such as cytomegalovirus; these infections may impair immune responses and possibly increase the susceptibility to *H. influenzae* type B disease. Further studies of *H. influenzae* type B primary disease in child day care should take into consideration these hypotheses.

Few topics in the area of infectious diseases in child day care remain more controversial than the risk of subsequent or secondary *H. influenzae* type B infection and the appropriate contact management follow-up. Since 1984 the results of five investigations defining the risk of subsequent disease among day-care attendees exposed to an attendee with *H. influenzae* type B infection have been reported.[11] The incidence of subsequent *H. influenzae* type B disease among contacts who were not treated with chemoprophylaxis within 60 days of a primary case varied significantly by age and study. A 2-year, population-based prospective follow-up with children in day care exposed to a primary case of *H. influenzae* type B disease was conducted in Minnesota. During the study, 1086 children 47 months of age or younger who did not receive rifampin chemoprophylaxis were observed for 60 days after exposure to 1 of 185 primary cases of *H. influenzae* type B disease. None of the 370 day-care contacts from 0 to 23 months of age or 716 contacts from 24 to 47 months of age subsequently developed disease. In contrast, in a multicenter study conducted by the CDC, children 0 to 47 months of age who were contacts of 1 of 129 children with primary *H. influenzae* type B disease who attended day care in King County, Washington, and in the states of Oklahoma and Georgia were surveyed. Contacts did not receive rifampin prophylaxis. Of classroom contacts who were 23 months of age or younger, 10 of 632 (1.6%) subsequently developed disease compared with 0 of 738 contacts who were 24 to 47 months of age. None of the 10 children who subsequently developed disease took rifampin compared with 232 (of 598) contacts aged 0 to 23 months who were given rifampin and who did not subsequently develop disease ($P < 0.1$). Because there was a strong correlation between rifampin administration to an individual and rifampin compliance in a classroom, it could not be determined which of these factors was more closely linked with disease prevention.

The risk of subsequent disease for the remaining three studies fell between those demonstrated in Minnesota and the CDC multicenter study. Attempts to reconcile the difference in findings of these five studies has been unsuccessful. Although subsequent *H. influenzae* disease accounts for less than 1% of all invasive *H. influenzae* type B disease, a single case in the day-care setting raises both important logistic and resource issues related to appropriate follow-up and the need for chemoprophylaxis.

Diarrheal Disease

Studies of diarrheal disease in the child-care setting conducted in the early 1980s described outbreaks of diarrhea involving many children within the same child-care setting.[6-9] Recent advances in laboratory methods and the identification of additional enteropathogens have made it possible to greatly expand our knowledge of these diseases in this setting during the past 5 years. In addition, recognition of the transmission of enteropathogens from children to their adult contacts is becoming more widespread.

Numerous enteropathogens have been shown to cause acute infectious gastrointestinal illness among children in the day care setting (Table 10–1). Transmission of these agents was facilitated by close person-to-person contact among children and by environmental contamination associated with young children who are not yet toilet trained. Infections caused by *Shigella, Escherichia coli* 0157:H7, *Giardia lamblia,* and rotavirus are more common than other enteropathogens because of the low inoculum necessary to produce disease. Diarrheal illness associated with day care may affect both infants and children in the facility, their immediate family contacts, and adult personnel. Contamination of hands, communal toys, and other classroom objects may be important in transmission of enteropathogens and outbreaks of diarrhea in day-care facilities. Additionally, day-care personnel may transmit enteric pathogens through diapering and meal preparation. Although mortality associated with diarrheal illness in the United States is generally low, acute infectious diarrhea is a major cause of hospitalization in young children and results in a substantial economic burden for parents and day-care providers. Recently several outbreaks have been associated with enteropathogenic or enterohemorrhagic *E. coli* that resulted in significant morbidity and mortality in the day-care setting. Future outbreaks with these organisms may need to be approached with more stringent infection control practices than previously proposed for dealing with enteropathogens in the day-care environment.

Hepatitis A Virus

Hepatitis A is typically a mild illness in infants and young children but can cause substantial morbidity in adults. Transmission for hepatitis A among asymptomatic children in day care may result in subsequent spread of infection to and occurrence of symptomatic disease in older family members, day-care personnel, and other adults in the community.[10] A major mode of hepatitis A virus transmission is fecal-oral, with infection spread most commonly by person-to-person transmission, often between household and sexual contacts. Fomites may play a role in infection transmission; hepatitis A virus is environmentally stable and can survive on environmental surfaces for at least 1 month. (See also p 131.)

National hepatitis surveillance data for 1983 through 1987 show that between 12.9% and 14.8% of persons with hepatitis A reported to the CDC were either children or employees in a day-care facility or were in contact with a child or employee in a day-care facility. Studies of large series of outbreaks in Phoenix and New Orleans have provided important descriptive information as well as data to support control strategy. The size and characteristics of reported outbreaks vary, but they share several features. First, outbreaks may follow one of two patterns. Some outbreaks were explosive with infection spreading rapidly and often unrecognized among day-care children. Within several weeks many cases occur among adult contacts of those children. Other outbreaks may be prolonged with cases occurring intermittently among children and contacts over several months. Second, infection among children attending child-day-care facilities is usually mild or nonspecific or asymptomatic, and outbreaks usually are recognized when adult contacts of children become ill.

Finally, perhaps the most important factor associated with the transmission of hepatitis A virus in child-day-care facilities is the presence of diaper-wearing children, particularly toddlers.

Cytomegalovirus Infection

Cytomegalovirus (CMV), the leading cause of congenital viral infection, occurs commonly among children in day care.[13,14] CMV is found in body secretions, including urine, saliva, feces, blood and blood products, semen, and cervical secretions. Most CMV infections are mild or asymptomatic. Numerous studies have shown that the incidence of CMV infection is highest among infants and young children, especially those in group day-care settings. Recent studies, based in day-care centers, show that young children shed the virus chronically after acquiring CMV and often transmit the virus to other children with whom they have daily close contact. Of even greater medical importance, evidence indicates that young, CMV-excreting children are an important source of virus for women in daily close contact with them.[14] This type of transmission of virus in day-care facilities is of significance because it can potentially increase the exposure of pregnant women (mothers or day-care workers) and thus increase the incidence of fetal infections. Two studies have reported annual seroconversion rates for CMV of 11% and 20% from cohorts of seronegative day-care workers, whereas the expected incidence of infection from a study of large numbers of pregnant women or hospital workers would be approximately 2% per year. Women of childbearing age need to be informed that CMV is a prevalent infection of all children, but especially those in group day care. The prevention of CMV infection from infants and young children in any home or day-care setting is best accomplished by observing good personal hygiene in handling saliva and urine of children whether or not they are known to be shedding CMV.

APPROACHES TO PREVENTION

Both primary measures that prevent infections from occurring and secondary measures that minimize spread of infection or reduce the clinical severity of a disease can be adapted to the day-care setting. Examples of primary measures include the use of vaccines and immune globulin preparations for susceptible persons who previously have not been exposed, routine handwashing, and environmental decontamination. Immunization against measles and other vaccine-preventable diseases is an established method of primary prevention. Vaccines under development against hepatitis A virus, rotavirus, and other pathogens also offer the prospect of primary prevention. Evidence suggests that handwashing programs in child-day-care facilities reduce the occurrence of diarrheal diseases.[16]

Secondary prevention is best illustrated by the use of antibiotics to treat infections that are established or the use of chemoprophylaxis or immune globulin preparations among exposed contacts.

CONTROVERSIES

Controversies regarding infectious diseases in child-day-care programs include regulatory and socioeconomic concerns as well as biomedical issues. Regulatory mechanisms that enable the detection, management, and prevention of infectious diseases in day-care settings vary considerably by locality and by their intent and scope. It is intended that the development of the national standards for infection control in out-of-home child care will greatly improve the uniform application of state and local regulations.

Resistance to regulations may arise from conflicts inherent between socioeconomic concerns and the effects of regulations. For example, a working parent may have little alternative to taking a child who is ill to a day-care facility; at the same time, that facility may benefit economically by providing day care for that child even though the child may have an acute illness. The issue of providing sick-child day care and the implementation of exclusion policies deserve special attention since it is inevitable that children experience illnesses caused by infectious agents, regardless of whether they attend day care. Available information on the provision of day care for a sick child, the economic costs and benefits of providing such care, and the risk to healthy children in the same facility of developing illness is limited.[17]

FUTURE DIRECTIONS

As child-day-care utilization continues to increase, physicians, other health-care providers, preventive medicine specialists, public health authorities, day-care providers, regulators, and parents will need to become more familiar with infectious disease problems that occur in day-care settings. Effective control and prevention of these infections require prompt reporting of disease by health-care providers and day-care management and rapid response by physicians and public health authorities. In addition, day-care and health-care providers and day-care regulators should increase efforts to characterize the epidemiological features of infectious diseases in day-care facilities and to develop more effective strategies of control and prevention in this setting.

The following efforts might be considered for future development:

1. Improvement of the denominator data base for children attending day-care centers and home day care and for those not in day-care programs; such data are fundamental to the conduct of reliable epidemiological studies.
2. Development of more complete prevalence and incidence data for different infectious diseases in children attending day-care programs.
3. Education for day-care providers in the principles of disease transmission and in methods of infectious disease prevention in the day-care setting.
4. Promulgation of uniform local and state regulations as well as guidelines for management of day-care contacts exposed to different infectious diseases (such regulations should be based on the National Health and Safety Standards for Out-of-Home Care Programs).
5. Development of surveillance systems that enable the evaluation of the effectiveness of educational and training programs in decreasing the risk of disease.
6. Development of safe and effective immunizing agents to prevent common causes of infectious diseases in children attending day-care facilities.

Many state and local health departments have recognized the need to address these issues and have taken initiatives directed at baseline data collection and disease surveillance, special epidemiological studies, intervention trials, protocols for disease management, and training programs. As the use of child day care continues to increase, however, preventive medicine specialists and other health-care professionals will face an even greater responsibility to define the impact of infectious diseases on this setting and to develop the best methods for their prevention.

REFERENCES

Nosocomial Infections

1. Haley RW, Culver DH, White JW, et al: The efficacy of infection surveillance and control programs in preventing nosocomial infections in US hospitals. Am J Epidemiol 121:182–205, 1985
2. Wenzel RP: The mortality of hospital-acquired bloodstream infections: Need for a new vital statistic? Internat J Epidemiol 17:225–227, 1988
3. Donowitz LG, Wenzel RP: Endometritis following cesarean section: A controlled study of the increased duration of hospital stay and direct costs of hospitalization. Am J Obstet Gynecol 137:467–469, 1980
4. Townsend TR, Wenzel RP: Nosocomial bloodstream infections in a newborn intensive care unit: A case-control matched study of morbidity, mortality, and risk. Am J Epidemiol 114:73–80, 1981
5. Wenzel RP: Nosocomial infections, Diagnosis-Related Groups, and Survey on the Efficacy of Nosocomial Infection Control: Economic implications for hospitals under the prospective payment system. Am J Med 78(suppl 6B):3–7, 1985
6. Ponce de Leon S: Nosocomial infection control in Latin America: We have to start now. Infect Control 5:511–512, 1984
7. Centers for Disease Control: National Nosocomial Infections Study Report. Annual Summary. MMWR 35:17s–29s, 1986
8. Gaynes R: Personal communication. National Nosocomial Infections Surveillance System, November 1, 1990
9. Dixon RE: Effect of infections on hospital care. Ann Intern Med 89(2):749–753, 1978
10. Platt R, Polk BF, Murdock B, et al: Risk factors for nosocomial urinary tract infection. Am J Epidemiol 124:977–985, 1986
11. Garibaldi RA, Mooney BR, Epstein BJ, et al: An evaluation of daily bacteriologic monitoring to identify preventable episodes of catheter-associated urinary tract infection. Infect Control 3:466–470, 1982
12. Garibaldi RA, Burke JP, Dickman ML, Smith CB: Factors predisposing to bacteriuria during indwelling urethral catheterization. N Engl J Med 291:215–219, 1974
13. Krieger JN, Kaiser DL, Wenzel RP: Urinary tract etiology of bloodstream infections in hospitalized patients. J Infect Dis 148:57–62, 1983
14. Warren JW: Nosocomial urinary tract infections. In Mandell GL, Douglas RG Jr, Bennett JE (eds): Principles and Practice of Infectious Diseases, 3 edt. New York: Churchill Livingstone, 1990, pp 2205–2215
15. Olson M, O'Connor M, Schwartz ML: Surgical wound infections: A five-year prospective study of 20,193 wounds at the Minneapolis VA Medical Center. Ann Surg 199:253–259, 1984
16. Green JW, Wenzel RP: Postoperative wound infection: A controlled study of the increased duration of hospital stay and direct cost of hospitalization. Ann Surg 185:264–268, 1977
17. Mayhall CG: Surgical infections including burns. In Wenzel RP (ed): Prevention and Control of Nosocomial Infections. Baltimore: Williams and Wilkins, 1987, pp 344–384
18. Platt R, Zaleznik DF, Hopkins CC, et al: Perioperative antibiotic prophylaxis for herniorrhaphy and breast surgery. N Engl J Med 322:153–160, 1990
19. Cruse PJE, Foord R: A five-year prospective study of 23,649 surgical wounds. Arch Surg 107:206–210, 1973
20. Leu HS, Kaiser DL, Mori M, Woolson RF, Wenzel RP: Hospital-acquired pneumonia: Attributable mortality and morbidity. Am J Epidemiol 129:1258–1267, 1989

21. Cross AS, Roup B: Role of respiratory assistance devices in endemic nosocomial pneumonia. Am J Med 70:681–685, 1981
22. Pierce AK, Sanford JP, Thomas GP, et al: Long-term evaluation of decontamination of inhalation-therapy equipment and the occurrence of necrotizing pneumonia. N Engl J Med 282:528–531, 1970
23. Craven DE, Kunches LM, Kilinsky V, et al: Risk factors for pneumonia and fatality in patients receiving continuous mechanical ventilation. Am Rev Respir Dis 133:792–796, 1986
24. Driks MR, Craven DE, Celli BR, et al: Nosocomial pneumonia in intubated patients given sucralfate as compared with antacids or histamine type 2 blockers. N Engl J Med 317:1376–1382, 1987
25. Leclair JM, Freeman J, Sullivan BF, et al: Prevention of nosocomial respiratory syncytial virus infections through compliance with glove and gown isolation precautions. N Engl J Med 317:329–333, 1987
26. Unertl K, Ruckdeschel G, Selbmann HK, et al: Prevention of colonization and respiratory infections in long-term ventilated patients by local antimicrobial prophylaxis. Intensive Care Med 13:106–113, 1987
27. Ledingham IM, Alcock SR, Eastaway AT, McDonald JC, McKay IC, Ramsay G: Triple regimen of selective decontamination of the digestive tract, systemic cefotaxime, and microbial surveillance for prevention of acquired infection in intensive care. Lancet 1:785–790, 1988
28. Doebbeling BN, Wenzel RP: Prevention of respiratory disease in immunosuppressed patients. In Shelhamer J, Pizzo PA, Parillo JE, Masur H (eds): Respiratory Disease in the Immunosuppressed Host. Philadelphia: J.B. Lippincott 1990
29. Haley RW, Culver DH, White JW, et al: The nationwide nosocomial infection rate: A new need for vital statistics. Am J Epidemiol 121:159–167, 1985
30. Bates DW, Cook F, Goldman L, Lee TH: Predicting bacteremia in hospitalized patients: A prospectively validated model. Ann Intern Med 113:495–500, 1990
31. Miller PJ, Wenzel RP: Etiologic organisms as independent predictors of death and morbidity associated with bloodstream infection. J Infect Dis 156:471–477, 1987
32. Henderson DK: Bacteremia due to percutaneous intravascular devices. In Mandell GL, Douglas RG Jr, Bennett JE (eds): Principles and Practice of Infectious Diseases, 3 edt. New York: Churchill Livingstone, 1990, pp 2189–2199
33. Horan T, Culver D, Jarvis W, et al: Pathogens causing nosocomial infections. Preliminary data from the National Nosocomial Infections Surveillance System. Antimicrobic Newsletter 5:65–68, 1988
34. Doebbeling BN, Wenzel RP: The epidemiology of *Legionella pneumophila* infections. Semin Respir Infect 2:206–221, 1987
35. Wey SB, Mori M, Pfaller MA, Woolson RF, Wenzel RP: Hospital-acquired candidemia: The attributable mortality and excess length of stay. Arch Intern Med 148:2642–2645, 1988
36. Doebbeling BN, Wenzel RP: Nosocomial viral hepatitis. In Mandell GL, Douglas RG Jr, Bennett JE (eds): Principles and Practice of Infectious Diseases, 3 edt. New York: Churchill Livingstone, 1990, pp 2215–2221
37. Mullan RJ, Baker EL, Bell DM, et al: Guidelines for prevention of transmission of the human immunodeficiency virus and hepatitis B virus to health-care and public-safety workers. MMWR 38(S-6):1–37, 1989
38. Doebbeling BN, Wenzel RP: The direct costs of universal precautions in a teaching hospital. JAMA 264:2083–2087, 1990
39. Stamm WE: Elements of an active, effective infection control program. Hospitals 50:60–66, 1976
40. Haley RW, Shachtman RH: The emergence of infection surveillance and control programs in US hospitals: An assessment, 1976. Am J Epidemiol 111:574–591, 1980
41. Wenzel RP, Osterman CA, Hunting KJ, Gwaltney JM Jr: Hospital-acquired infections: I. Surveillance in a university hospital. Am J Epidemiol 103:251–260, 1976
42. Garner JS, Jarvis WR, Emori TG, Horan TC, Hughes JM: CDC definitions for nosocomial infections, 1988. Am J Infect Control 16:128–140, 1988
43. Wenzel RP: Epidemics-identification and management. In RP Wenzel (ed): Prevention and Control of Nosocomial Infections. Baltimore: Williams and Wilkins, 1987, pp 94–108
44. Streed SA, Wenzel RP: Isolation. In Mandell GL, Douglas RG Jr, Bennett JE (eds): Principles and Practice of Infectious Diseases, 3 edt. New York: Churchill Livingstone, 1990, pp 2180–2182
45. Martin MA, Wenzel RP: Sterilization, disinfection, and disposal of infectious waste. In Mandell GL, Douglas RG Jr, Bennett JE (eds): Pr inciples and Practice of Infectious Diseases, 3 edt. New York: Churchill Livingstone, 1990, pp 2182–2189
46. Wenzel RP: Organization for infection control. In Mandell GL, Douglas RG Jr, Bennett JE (eds): Principles and Practice of Infectious Diseases, 3 edt. New York: Churchill Livingstone, 1990, pp 2176–2180
47. Committee on Infections within Hospitals, American Hospital Association: Infection Control in the Hospital, 4 edt. Chicago: The Association, 1979
48. Wenzel RP: Handbook of Hospital Acquired Infections. Boca Raton, Fla: CRC Press, 1981
49. Bennett JV, Brachman PS: Hospital Infections, 2 edt. Boston: Little, Brown, 1986
50. Wenzel RP (ed): Prevention and Control of Nosocomial Infections. Baltimore: Williams and Wilkins, 1987
51. Proceedings of the Second International Hospital Infection Society Conference: London, England. J Hosp Infect (suppl). In press, 1991
52. Abstracts of the third International Conference on Nosocomial Infections: Atlanta, GA: Am J Med (suppl). In press, 1991

Infectious Diseases and Child Day Care

1. Aronson SS: Political and social aspects of child care. Sem Pediatric Infect Dis 1:195–203, 1990
2. Giebink GS: National standards for infection control in out-of-home child care. Sem Pediatric Infect Dis 1:184–194, 1990
3. Osterholm MT, Klein JO, Aronson SS, Pickering LK (eds): Infectious Diseases in Child Day Care: Management and Prevention. Chicago: University of Chicago Press, 1986
4. Pickering LK (ed): Infections in day care centers. Semin Pediatric Infect Dis 1:181–292, 1990
5. Denny IW, Collier AM, Henderson FW: Acute Respiratory Infections in Day Care. In Osterholm MT, Klein JO, Aronson SS, Pickering LK (eds): Infectious Diseases in Child Day Care: Management and Prevention. Chicago: University of Chicago Press, pp 15–20, 1986
6. Frenck RW, Glezen WP: Respiratory tract infections in children in day care. Sem Pediatric Infect Dis 1:234–244, 1990
7. Pickering LK, Bartlett AV, Woodward WE: Acute infectious diarrhea among children in day care: Epidemiology and control. In Osterholm MT, Klein JO, Aronson SS, Pickering LK (eds): Infectious Diseases in Child Day Care: Management and Prevention. Chicago: University of Chicago Press, pp 27–35, 1986
8. Pickering LK: Bacterial and parasitic enteropathogens in day care. Sem Pediatric Infect Dis 1:263–269, 1990
9. O'Ryan M, Matson DO: Viral gastroenteritis pathogens in the day care center setting. Sem Pediatric Infect Dis 1:252–262, 1990
10. Shapiro CN, Hadler SC: Significance of hepatitis in children in day care. Sem Pediatric Infect Dis 1:270–279, 1990
11. Osterholm MT: Invasive bacterial disease and child day care. Sem Pediatric Infect Dis 1:222–233, 1990
12. Brunell PA, Taylor-Wiedeman J, Lievens AW: Varicella in day care centers. In Osterholm MT, Klein JO, Aronson SS, Pickering LK (eds): Infectious Diseases in Child Day Care: Management and Prevention. Chicago: University of Chicago Press, pp 77–78, 1986
13. Pass RF: Day care centers and transmission of cytomegalovirus: New insight into an old problem. Sem Pediatric Infect Dis 1:245–251, 1990

14. Pass RF, Hutto C, Lyon D, Cloud G: Increased rate of cytomegalovirus infection among day care center workers. Pediatr Infect Dis J 9:465–470, 1990
15. Goodman RA, Osterholm MT, Granoff DM, Pickering LK: Infectious diseases in child day care. Pediatrics 74:134–139, 1984
16. Black RE, Dykes AC, Anderson KE, et al: Handwashing to prevent diarrhea in day-care centers. Am J Epidemiol 113:445–451, 1981
17. MacDonald KL, White KA, Heiser J, Gabriel L, Osterholm MT: Evaluation of a sick child day care program: Lack of detected increased risk of subsequent infections. Pediatr Infect Dis J 9:15–20, 1990

11

Diseases Transmitted Primarily by Arthropod Vectors

Viral Infections

Thomas P. Monath
Karl M. Johnson

The term *arbovirus* (a contraction of *arthropodborne virus*) refers to a group of taxonomically diverse animal viruses that are unified by an epidemiological concept, that of transmission between vertebrate host organisms by the agency of blood-feeding (hematophagous) arthropod vectors, such as mosquitoes, ticks, sandflies, and midges. True arboviruses have the capacity to multiply in arthropod tissues, including the salivary glands; this provides a mechanism for transmission of the virus to susceptible hosts by bite and distinguishes *biological* and *mechanical* transmission, in which virus is simply transported between hosts by insects with externally contaminated mouth parts. A significant delay is required between ingestion of an infectious blood meal and sufficient viral replication in salivary tissues of the vector for transmission to occur; this interval is referred to as the *extrinsic incubation period.* Arboviruses are distinguished from viruses of insects and many viruses of plants, which also replicate in and are transmitted by arthropods, in their capacity to infect vertebrate animal hosts. After infection, vertebrate host species, which are essential to maintenance of the arboviral transmission cycle, circulate virus in their blood at levels (titers) sufficiently high to infect arthropod vectors. The arboviral transmission cycle is determined by important quantitative variables, which include (1) the susceptibility of individual vector species or populations to infection and (2) the susceptibility of individual vertebrate species to mount an infection-effective viremia. Variables that affect the extent to which arboviruses are amplified in vector-host cycles in natural communities will be discussed further below.

Certain vertebrates respond to infection without developing overt signs of illness. If such *inapparent infections* are accompanied by an effective viremia in a high proportion of infected individuals, the species is well suited as an epidemiologically important host in the transmission cycle. In general, the primary hosts for arboviruses have silent infections, representing an evolved and balanced host-parasite relationship. This is not invariably the case, since for some infections (e.g., yellow fever and dengue in humans, Venezuelan equine encephalitis in equines) the primary viremic hosts are also clinically involved. Since arthropod vectors rarely confine their blood feeding to single vertebrate species, hosts other than those involved in transmission occasionally become exposed to arboviruses. In this instance, infection may be abortive, resulting in no illness or viremia but often leaving a detectable record in the form of serum antibodies. On the other hand, infection may produce clinically apparent disease, such as encephalitis or febrile illness. Because of the individual variability within host species, severe or medically recognizable disease generally occurs in only a small fraction of the total number infected. The ratio of clinically inapparent or mild to apparent or severe infections is a distinctive and measurable quality of a given arboviral infection and often may be dependent on age.

The disease patterns produced by arboviruses are fairly simple and provide a basis for a classification that is most useful to the epidemiologist. Arboviruses produce infections in clinically susceptible hosts that are characterized predominantly or in their classic form by:

1. *Acute central nervous system disease* (aseptic meningitis, encephalitis, encephalomyelitis)
2. *Undifferentiated febrile illness* with or without rash
3. *Hemorrhagic fever* (febrile systemic illness with hemorrhagic manifestations, cardiovascular instability, and varying degrees of hepatic and renal insufficiency)

Specific infections manifested by these syndromes may be transmitted by mosquitoes, ticks, or other arthropod vectors. In addition to arthropodborne infections, certain other viral infections will be included in this chapter. These are non-arthropodborne (often rodent-associated) zoonotic diseases, most of which produce the hemorrhagic fever syndrome.

ETIOLOGICAL AGENTS

At present 520 viruses are registered in the *International Catalogue of Arboviruses.*[1] Of these, only approximately 100 viruses are known to produce disease in humans and only about 25 are known or suspected to cause illness in domestic livestock. Those viruses that are of true medical importance, because the disease produced is either unusually severe or of high incidence, are much fewer in number. It is on these epidemiologically important diseases that we shall focus in this section; the reader is referred to more exhaustive reviews[2,3] for information about the full spectrum of arboviral infections.

The arboviruses and hemorrhagic fever viruses are divided into families on the basis of morphological and physicochemical properties. Within each family further groupings are made on the basis of shared serological and, in some instances, morphological characteristics. Some ungrouped viruses and serologically related groups of viruses remain taxonomically unclassified. Most medically important viruses are included in seven families of RNA viruses; the *Togaviridae, Flaviviridae, Bunyaviridae, Reoviridae, Arenaviridae, Filoviridae,* and *Rhabdoviridae* (Table 11-1). The virological properties that distinguish these families are reviewed elsewhere.[4-7] Within the *Togaviridae* the genus alphavirus contains agents among which are the important mosquitoborne encephalitis viruses that cause eastern, western, and Venezuelan equine encephalitides. The *Flaviviridae* comprise registered virus infections, including mosquitoborne encephalitides (e.g., St. Louis encephalitis and Japanese encephalitis), undifferentiated febrile illnesses (e.g., dengue), and hemorrhagic fevers (e.g., yellow fever), as well as tickborne diseases characterized by these syndromes. Each of the other major families of arboviruses is similarly represented by medically important viruses within the classification by disease category and arthropod vector (Table 11-1).

EPIDEMIOLOGICAL PATTERNS

Arboviral epidemiological patterns may be simple as exemplified by dengue and urban yellow fever, which are transmitted in a human–*Aedes aegypti*–human cycle (Fig. 11-1), or more complex, with enzootic cycles involving one or more vector species and wild animal hosts (Fig. 11-2). Many epidemiological, ecological, and biological factors play a role in determining the distribution and incidence of infections.

Geographical Distribution. The distribution of an arbovirus is determined by the presence of competent arthropod vectors, susceptible vertebrate hosts, efficient means of virus survival through periods (winter or dry season) adverse to continued transmission, and other more poorly understood factors. Barriers to spread of a virus may be geophysical (e.g., a water mass or a mountain range) or biological. A possible example of the latter is the absence of yellow fever in Asia despite presence of established vector species (*A. aegypti*), susceptible hosts, and ample opportunities for introduction; possible explanations include cross-protection of the human population by immunity to heterologous flaviviruses, such as dengue, or relative susceptibility of Asian *A. aegypti* to yellow fever viral infection. The distribution of a virus may also be much wider than that of the associated disease. For example, St. Louis encephalitis (SLE) virus is distributed throughout the western hemisphere but causes epidemics only in North America. In this and other examples, one or more explanations may apply: among them (1) the vector(s) in the silent, enzootic part of the virus's distribution may be only weakly attracted to clinically apparent hosts (humans); (2) the virus may circulate only in remote, inaccessible areas rarely visited by humans or under minimal medical surveillance; (3) viral strains in the epidemiologically silent area have reduced virulence for humans. In general, viruses that have birds as hosts are more evenly distributed than agents with such hosts as small terrestrial mammals that are restricted in their movements and migrations.

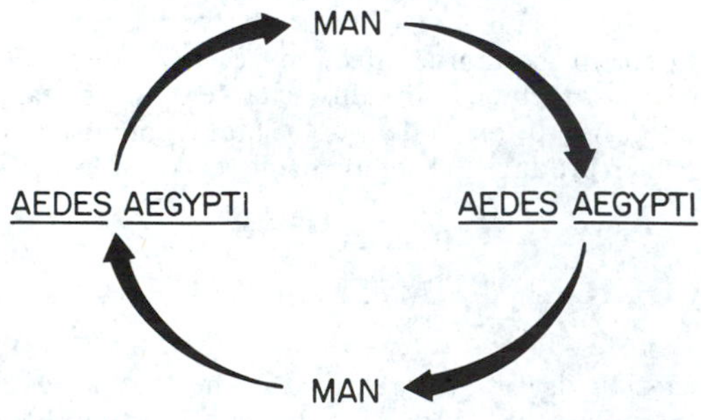

Figure 11-1. Schematic transmission cycle of urban yellow fever and dengue. Man serves as source of virus for *Aedes aegypti* mosquito vectors.

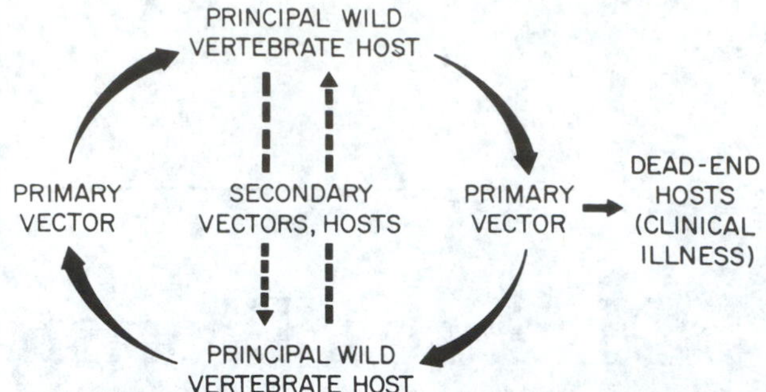

Figure 11-2. Schematic transmission cycle of arboviruses with complex natural histories involving wild vertebrate hosts (birds, rodents, etc.) and hematophagous arthropod vectors. Enzootic transmission occurs during the spring and summer in the silent cycle and may spill over tangentially to (dead-end) hosts (such as man or horses), which are clinically susceptible but do not serve as a source of infection for vectors.

Seasonal Distribution and Chronology of Epidemics. In the temperate zone, viral transmission is limited to seasons of the year, principally late spring through early fall, when arthropod vectors are active. This period of activity often corresponds to the breeding period and peak population density of immunologically susceptible wild vertebrate hosts, thereby assuring amplification of virus in the natural cycle. In tropical regions, dry seasons with low vector density correspond to wintertime periods in the temperate zone: the transmission cycle is retarded or interrupted, risk of infection of clinically apparent hosts is reduced, and virus survival is challenged. The known and speculative mechanisms for viral recrudescence after adverse seasonal periods are discussed briefly later.

The seasonal distributions of individual arboviral diseases vary. For example, in the western United States, western equine encephalitis (WEE) and SLE viruses share the same mosquito vector (*Culex tarsalis*) and the same wild bird hosts; however, human and equine WEE infections occur in early summer, whereas human SLE cases occur in late summer and fall. The greater temperature dependence of SLE virus for replication and the longer extrinsic incubation period in the vector, plus the lower, briefer, and relatively delayed viremia in avian hosts retard amplification of the virus. In addition, exposure of *C. tarsalis* larvae to high temperatures appears to reduce their ability to transmit WEE but not SLE virus.

In general, since arboviruses with complex transmission cycles (Fig. 11-2) must amplify by progressive and cumulative infection of wild vertebrates and vectors before the virus can spill over to humans or domestic livestock, the appearance of an outbreak reflects intense viral transmission weeks or more earlier. This forms the basis for surveillance of viral activity in the natural cycle.

Viruses transmitted by arthropods often cause sharply defined outbreaks with a rapid accumulation of cases, a relatively sharp peak, and a rapid decline as conditions unfavorable to vector breeding, host seeking, or survival develop or as susceptible hosts are depleted.

VECTORS AND VERTEBRATE HOSTS: VARIABLES AFFECTING VIRAL TRANSMISSION

The principal vectors and hosts for medically important arboviruses and the reservoir hosts of rodentborne zoonoses are listed in Table 11–1. General concepts regarding their biology and interactions will be presented here, and special references will be given in the sections on individual diseases. Mosquitoes require aquatic habitats for oviposition and larval development; the exact requirements vary from species to species and include such diverse conditions as tree holes, man-made receptacles, or floodwaters. In general, mosquitoes adapted to breeding in habitats created or modified by humans reach high densities in close association with humans, and viruses transmitted by them are responsible for the major epidemic diseases. Examples include (1) SLE virus transmitted in the eastern United States by *Culex pipiens,* a species that breeds in polluted wastewater in urban-suburban environments, and in the West by *C. tarsalis,* a species adapted to richly irrigated croplands and pasturelands, and (2) dengue and urban yellow fever viruses transmitted by *A. aegypti,* a peridomestic breeder in water-storage pots, discarded automobile tires, and other man-made containers. In contrast, viruses such as La Crosse encephalitis virus, carried by vector species with natural, sylvan breeding sites, cause endemic infections and sporadic disease more often than well-defined outbreaks.

Most mosquitoborne arboviruses are transmitted by one primary vector species or, at most, one primary and several secondary species. This phenomenon probably reflects constraints of evolved and specialized relationships between virus, vector, and reservoir host. However, there are a few examples of viruses that are transmitted by a wide array of taxonomically and ecologically different vectors. These viruses, such as those that cause Venezuelan equine encephalitis and Rift Valley fever, have the common feature of producing exceedingly high viremias in vertebrate hosts, surpassing the threshold for infection of many and diverse arthropod species.

Ticks have terrestrial immature stages that, like the adult, feed on blood; in some species, such as *Dermacentor andersoni,* the vector of Colorado tick fever, the larval, nymphal, and adult stages seek different hosts, adding complexity to the transmission cycle. In general, because of lower vector densities, specialized or focal ecological requirements, and other factors, tickborne infections are more often endemic than epidemic; certain infections, notably Kyasanur Forest disease and tickborne encephalitis, nevertheless, reach high incidence in regions conducive to intense viral transmission.

Some tickborne infections may be amplified by a curious phenomenon that bypasses the need for virus replication in the vertebrate host. Attached, infected ticks may transfer virus (e.g., certain tickborne orthomyxoviruses and nairoviruses) directly to cofeeding uninfected ticks via the host's bloodstream without the need for viral replication in vertebrate host tissues.

Several factors related specifically to the vector determine the rate of viral transmission and the risk of epidemics. One of these, *vector abundance,* is also an important variable, in turn dependent on favorable climatic and environmental conditions for breeding and survival. In the western United States, for example, Reeves[8] has shown that human and equine cases of WEE appear only when the density of *C. tarsalis* vectors reaches ten adult females per light trap night. Yet extremely high vector densities may actually inhibit viral transmission, since host avoidance behavior is increased or host-selection patterns are altered. *Longevity* of the vector is also a critical factor, since even a brief prolongation may increase the proportion of the vector population capable of transmitting virus and able to take a second blood meal. The *host preference* of vector species is also epidemiologically important; vectors that are strongly attracted to virus reservoir hosts but are also highly anthropophilic are ideal vectors. Host preference may change during the viral transmission season. The vectors of WEE and SLE viruses shift from predominant avian feeding in early summer to mammals (including humans) in late summer, a situation that is obviously ideally suited to amplification and spillover to humans.

Wild birds are important vertebrate hosts in transmission cycles of most of the mosquitoborne encephalitides and several mosquitoborne undifferentiated febrile diseases; some ground-dwelling kinds may also play a role in tickborne infections. Birds are abundant, often present in large numbers in close association with humans and livestock. Moreover, because they readily move and migrate, they may transport, disseminate, and reintroduce viruses over considerable distances. Nestling birds, present in large numbers during spring and summer, are relatively defenseless against mosquito bites and often support higher viremic infections than adults; they are considered important hosts for some viruses. In general, birds develop viremia within 18 to 48 hours after being bitten by an infected arthropod; viremia lasts 2 to 5 days and is followed by the appearance of specific antibodies. Antibodies to certain viruses (e.g., SLE) are passed transovarially to hatchlings but wane rapidly. Most avian species show no outward signs of infection. However, in the case of eastern equine encephalitis in exotic penned birds (chukar partridges, pheasants), severe outbreaks sustained by direct bird-to-bird viral transmission through pecking may provide an indication of viral activity in advance of human or equine cases. Clinical disease caused by the eastern equine encephalitis virus in the whooping crane (an endangered species) has caused concern.

Rodents are the principal hosts for (1) a number of viruses transmitted by ticks, including tickborne encephalitis, Colorado tick fever, Powassan, Crimean-Congo hemorrhagic fever, and Kyasanur Forest disease viruses; (2) viruses that cause some important mosquitoborne infections such as La Crosse encephalitis; and (3) viruses responsible for certain zoonotic hemorrhagic fevers. General characteristics of rodent hosts that affect viral transmission rarely include high reproductive capacity and population turnover, limited movements and dispersal, and, often, specific requirements for habitat. These factors favor restricted or focal viral transmission, which, however, can be quite intense. In general, rodents are hosts for the larval and nymphal stages of tick vectors, whereas the adult forms generally feed on large animals, including humans.

Domestic animals are effective viremic hosts for a limited number of arboviruses. Those viruses of epidemiological importance (and their amplifying hosts) include those that cause Venezuelan equine encephalomyelitis (Equidae), Rift Valley fever (sheep, cattle), and Japanese encephalitis (swine). In each case the hosts show signs of illness in addition to serving as sources of infection for arthropod vectors that may transmit the virus to humans. Since viral amplification in livestock necessarily precedes spillover to humans, occurrence of an epizootic often provides warning of an impending epidemic. Unlike agents with rodent or avian hosts that have high reproductive potential, epizootics caused by these viruses often deplete the population of immunologically susceptible large animal hosts; several more years may be required to attain susceptible host population densities allowing a high rate of viral transmission.

TABLE 11–1. SELECTED ARBOVIRAL AND ZOONOTIC INFECTIONS OF EPIDEMIOLOGICAL IMPORTANCE

Predominant Syndrome	Transmission	Etiology: Virus	Etiology: Family (Genus)	Pattern or Frequency of Recognized Human Disease	Associated Animal Disease	Known Geographical Distribution of Virus
Central nervous system infection	Mosquitoborne	Eastern equine encephalitis	*Togaviridae* (alphavirus)	Endemic-epidemic	Equids, penned exotic birds	U.S.A., Canada, Caribbean, South America
		Western equine encephalitis	*Togaviridae* (alphavirus)	Endemic-epidemic	Equids	U.S.A., Canada, Mexico, Guyana, Argentina, Brazil, Uruguay
		St. Louis encephalitis	*Flaviviridae* (flavivirus)	Endemic-epidemic	—	U.S.A., Canada, Mexico, Caribbean, Guatemala, South America
		Japanese encephalitis	*Flaviviridae* (flavivirus)	Endemic-epidemic	Swine, equids	East and Southeast Asia (see text)
		Murray Valley encephalitis	*Flaviviridae* (flavivirus)	Endemic-epidemic	—	Australia
		Rocio encephalitis	*Flaviviridae* (flavivirus)	Epidemic	—	Brazil
		California serogroup viruses (e.g., La Crosse and Jamestown Canyon)	*Bunyaviridae* (bunyavirus)	Endemic	—	U.S.A., Canada
	Tickborne	Tickborne encephalitis	*Flaviviridae* (flavivirus)	Endemic	—	Eastern Europe, Soviet Union, Scandinavia
		Powassan	*Flaviviridae* (flavivirus)	Rare, sporadic	—	U.S.A., Canada, Soviet Union
		Louping ill	*Flaviviridae* (flavivirus)	Rare, sporadic	Sheep	British Isles
	Rodentborne	Lymphocytic choriomeningitis	*Arenaviridae*	Endemic-epidemic	—	Worldwide (see text)
Undifferentiated febrile illness (with or without rash)	Mosquitoborne	Barmah forest	*Togaviridae* (alphavirus)	Endemic	—	Australia
		Bwamba	*Bunyaviridae* (bunyavirus)	Endemic-epidemic	—	West, East Africa
		Carapuru, Marituba, Oriboca, and five other related viruses	*Bunyaviridae* (group C bunyavirus)	Rare, sporadic	—	Central and South America
		Chikungunya	*Togaviridae* (alphavirus)	Endemic-epidemic	—	Sub-Saharan Africa, Asia
		Dengue	*Flaviviridae* (flavivirus)	Endemic-epidemic	—	Worldwide (see text)
		Guama, Catu	*Bunyaviridae* (Guama group bunyavirus)	Rare, sporadic	—	South America
		Mayaro	*Togaviridae* (alphavirus)	Endemic-epidemic	—	South America
		O'nyong-nyong	*Togaviridae* (alphavirus)	Epidemic	—	Sub-Saharan Africa
		Orungo	*Reoviridae* (orbivirus)	Endemic-?epidemic	—	West, East Africa
		Rift Valley fever	*Bunyaviridae* (phlebovirus)	Epidemic	Sheep, cattle	South Africa, East Africa, Nigeria, Mauritania, Madagascar, Egypt
		Ross River	*Togaviridae* (alphavirus)	Endemic-epidemic	—	Australia, Oceania

TABLE 11–1. SELECTED ARBOVIRAL AND ZOONOTIC INFECTIONS OF EPIDEMIOLOGICAL IMPORTANCE (Continued)

Predominant Syndrome	Transmission	Etiology: Virus	Etiology: Family (Genus)	Pattern or Frequency of Recognized Human Disease	Associated Animal Disease	Known Geographical Distribution of Virus
		Semliki forest	*Togaviridae* (alphavirus)	Epidemic	Equid	Sub-Saharan Africa
		Sindbis	*Togaviridae* (alphavirus)	Endemic-epidemic	—	Africa, Asia, Europe
		Spondweni	*Flaviviridae* (flavivirus)	Rare, sporadic		Africa
		Tataguine	*Bunyaviridae*	Endemic	—	West Africa
		Usutu	*Flaviviridae* (flavivirus)	Rare, sporadic	—	Africa
		Venezuelan equine encephalitis	*Togaviridae* (alphavirus)	Endemic-epidemic	Equids	Venezuela, Colombia, Ecuador, Trinidad, Peru, Central America, Mexico, U.S.A.
		Wesselsbron	*Flaviviridae* (flavivirus)	Rare, sporadic	Sheep	South and West Africa, Asia
		West Nile	*Flaviviridae* (flavivirus)	Endemic-epidemic	Equids (rare)	Africa, Asia, Europe
		Zika	*Flaviviridae* (flavivirus)	Rare, sporadic	—	Africa, Asia
	Culicoidesborne	Oropouche	*Bunyaviridae* (bunyavirus)	Endemic-epidemic	—	Brazil, Panama, Guianas, Trinidad
	Phlebotomine-borne	Phlebotomus fever, Sicilian and Naples	*Bunyaviridae* (phlebovirus)	Endemic-epidemic	—	Mediterranean, Syria, Iran, Pakistan, India, Afghanistan, Sudan, Soviet Union
		Toscana	*Bunyaviridae* (phlebovirus)	Endemic-epidemic	—	Italy
		Alenquer	*Bunyaviridae* (phlebovirus)	Endemic-epidemic	—	Brazil
		Punta Toro, Chagres, Candiru	*Bunyaviridae* (phlebovirus)	Endemic-epidemic	—	Central America
	Tickborne	Colorado tick fever	*Reoviridae* (orbivirus)	Endemic	—	U.S.A.
	Vector unknown	Vesicular stomatitis	*Rhabdoviridae* (vesiculovirus)	Rare, sporadic	—	North Central and South America
Hemorrhagic fever (HF)	Mosquitoborne	Yellow fever	*Flaviviridae* (flavivirus)	Endemic-epidemic	Certain monkey species	Tropical America, Africa
		Dengue HF	*Flaviviridae* (flavivirus)	Endemic-epidemic	—	Southeast Asia, Caribbean
	Tickborne	Kyasanur Forest disease	*Flaviviridae* (flavivirus)	Endemic-epidemic	Monkeys	India
		Omsk HF	*Flaviviridae* (flavivirus)	Endemic-epidemic	—	Soviet Union
		Crimean HF-Congo	*Bunyaviridae* (nairovirus)	Endemic-epidemic	—	Soviet Union, Pakistan, East and West Africa, Iraq, Saudi Arabia, Dubai
	Rodentborne	Junin (Argentine HF)	*Arenaviridae*	Endemic-epidemic	—	Argentina
		Machupo (Bolivian HF)	*Arenaviridae*	Endemic-epidemic	—	Bolivia
		Lassa fever	*Arenaviridae*	Endemic-epidemic	—	West Africa
		Hantaan, Seoul, and Puumula (hemorrhagic fever with renal syndrome)	*Bunyaviridae* (hantavirus)	Endemic-epidemic	—	Far eastern Soviet Union, Korea, Japan, eastern Europe, Scandinavia
	Mode of natural transmission unknown	Marburg, Ebola	*Filoviridae* (filovirus)	Epidemic	—	Sub-Saharan Africa, Asia

Overwintering is an important concept in the epidemiology of vectorborne diseases, since the annual recrudescence of viral activity after periods (winter, dry season) adverse to continual transmission depends on a mechanism for local survival of virus or its reintroduction from outside the endemic area. To some extent, the risk of a summertime epidemic may be determined by the relative success of virus survival in the local winter reservoir. Since overwinter survival may, in turn, depend on the level of viral activity during the preceding summer and fall, arboviral outbreaks sometimes occur for 2 or more successive years.

For a comprehensive review of the many possible explanations of overwintering, see Reeves.[9] Briefly, the mechanisms for survival of virus may be summarized as follows:

1. *Survival in primary arthropod vector through adverse period (e.g., by hibernating).* This mechanism has been well documented for a nonpathogenic alphavirus (Fort Morgan virus), transmitted and maintained by avian bedbugs,[10] and Colorado tick fever and tickborne encephalitis viruses, which persist in hibernating nymphal and adult ticks. In the case of viruses transmitted by mosquitoes of the genus *Culex* (which hibernate in the adult stage), the situation is much less clear, despite reports of midwinter isolations of SLE virus from hibernating *C. pipiens* and of WEE virus from *C. tarsalis.* In general, female mosquitoes that have taken a blood meal (required for acquisition of the infection) appear to be physiologically poorly prepared for hibernation and rarely survive the winter. Other observations[11] suggest that this may not always be the case.
2. *Survival in persistently infected vertebrate reservoirs.* Chronic arboviral infections, sometimes spanning periods of hibernation, have been experimentally demonstrated in a variety of vertebrates, including bats (SLE and Japanese encephalitis virus) and small mammals (tickborne encephalitis and Tahyna virus, a member of the California encephalitis group). Long-term virus persistence and congenital infections have been demonstrated in laboratory models (mice, monkeys) of several flaviviruses. In general, evidence that chronically infected, intermittently viremic animals maintain arbovirus *in nature* is lacking. A possible exception requiring confirmation may be blue tongue, an important pathogen of sheep and cattle, in which congenitally acquired, immunotolerant latent infection may occur. In this instance, viremic relapses may be stimulated nonspecifically by bites of uninfected *Culicoides* gnats. Persistent viral carriage assures that maintenance of some zoonotic infections of rodents in nature. LCM virus in *Mus musculus,* machupo virus in *Calomys callosus,* Lassa fever virus in *Mastomys natalensis,* and several hantaviruses in their rodent hosts are principal examples; moreover, chronic shedding of large amounts of virus in the urine by specific rodents harboring these and related agents is the most important element in transmission of disease to humans (see the following).
3. *Inherited infection in the arthropod vector.* Transovarial infection, first demonstrated for a human pathogen and a dipteran insect vector in the case of vesicular stomatitis virus, has been shown to account for local survival of California encephalitis group viruses in their *Aedes* mosquito vectors. The vector-host relationships of these viruses explain the evolution of this mechanism. The vertebrate hosts for these viruses are small forest rodents unsuited for dispersal or reintroduction of virus from afar, and the vector *Aedes* overwinters only in the egg stage. Transovarial transmission is biologically efficient: a high proportion (70% to 90%) of progeny from infected female *Aedes* mosquito acquire the virus, and as many as 1% of mosquitoes reared from overwintering ova collected in nature have been found infected.[12] Evidence has now been obtained to show that a number of flaviviruses, notably those that cause St. Louis encephalitis (SLE), Japanese encephalitis (JE), dengue, and yellow fever, may also be vertically transmitted by *Aedes* spp. Unlike the California encephalitis group of bunyaviruses, rates of inherited infection are often lower (1:100 or less). Obviously, high rates of summertime amplification are required for the virus to successfully survive the winter as a low-incidence infection of mosquito ova. Certain tickborne infections (e.g., tickborne encephalitis and Crimean-Congo hemorrhagic fever) are also transovarially transmitted in their tick vectors.
4. *Reintroduction of virus by migratory vertebrates.* Transport of viruses over long distances by migratory birds has occasionally been documented, but it is generally not considered to be an important mechanism for the annual recrudescence of viral activity.

SURVEILLANCE AND DIAGNOSIS OF VECTORBORNE VIRAL DISEASES

Recognition of disease in the community and definition of the incidence, geographical extent, and chronology are essential if control measures are to be applied and their effectiveness assessed. In the case of dengue fever, surveillance of human cases is the only applicable method, but viral infections involving wild vertebrate hosts lend themselves to other approaches. A classic example is jungle yellow fever, which may be monitored in neotropical forests by observing wild monkey populations or sentinel monkeys for deaths or antibody conversions. Similarly, epizootics of encephalitis in equids or epornitics in penned exotic birds may provide warning of human outbreaks of certain equine encephalitides.

Viruses with clinically silent enzootic transmission cycles, such as the SLE virus, require sophisticated studies to determine the level of viral activity in nature. Serologic surveillance of wild bird populations, periodic antibody tests on individually marked, sentinel chickens, determination of vector population density and age structure, and viral assays of vector mosquitoes have all been used to detect viral activity. Experience over the years has allowed quantitative estimates of the risk of an impending human outbreak. For example, cases of human western equine encephalitis in California appear only when adult female *C. tarsalis* mosquitoes are present at densities reflected by 10 captures per light trap night and when minimum infection rates in *C. tarsalis* exceed 3/1000. SLE outbreaks in the eastern United States seem to occur only when the prevalence of antibodies in wild bird populations exceeds about 3%.[13]

Surveillance of human or equine cases or of wild hosts and vectors requires the availability of a competent virus laboratory. In the case of human surveillance, the need for laboratory diagnosis is underscored by the nonspecific nature of the clinical illness caused by most arboviruses. Dengue fever may be confused with influenza or rubella; yellow fever with hepatitis, malaria, leptospirosis, or the other viral hemorrhagic fevers; and acute arboviral infections of the central nervous system with those caused by enteroviruses or childhood infections.

Diagnosis of arboviral infection (in humans or lower vertebrates) is achieved either directly by viral isolation or antigen detection or indirectly by demonstration of specific serum antibodies. Certain viruses, such as dengue, yellow fever, West Nile, group C bunyaviruses, Rift Valley fever, Lassa, Marburg, Ebola, Crimean-Congo hemorrhagic fever, Argentine hemorrhagic fever, and VEE viruses, may be isolated from serum during the first few days of illness; certain other viruses are not readily recovered, probably because viremia is of low magnitude and occurs only during the incubation period. Similarly, in many of the encephalitides, infectious virus is no longer present in detectable form in brain tissue at autopsy. Viral isolation techniques vary from laboratory to laboratory. Intracerebral inoculation of infant mice has long been a standard method, but cell cultures have come into increased use. Certain viruses are quite difficult to isolate (because of insensitivity of the usual assay systems), notably dengue virus, the phlebotomus fever viruses, and O'nyong-Nyong virus. The advantage of inoculation of live mosquitoes or mosquito cell cultures for isolation of dengue virus from human serum has been recognized.[14] The presence of virus in the assay systems mentioned is detected by the appearance of illness (mice), cytopathic effect or plaques (cell cultures), or specific immunofluorescence (cell cultures or mosquitoes). Viral isolates are further identified and characterized by physicochemical and serologic techniques. Use of specific monoclonal antibody reagents has facilitated this task. Advances in antigen detection in serum by enzyme-linked immunosorbent assay (ELISA) have allowed rapid diagnosis of yellow fever, dengue, Crimean-Congo hemorrhagic fever, Ebola, and other virus infections without the need for viral isolation. Recent development of the polymerase chain reaction (PCR) for detecting viral genome in clinical samples provides extremely sensitive and specific diagnostic approaches; application has been reported for detection of dengue, Ebola, and Dugbe viruses (a nairovirus).

Serological diagnosis is achieved by use of one or more tests, including hemagglutination inhibition (HI), complement fixation (CF), neutralization (N), fluorescent antibody (FAT), ELISA, or radioimmunoassay (RIA). The bases for these techniques and their relative sensitivity and specificity are reviewed elsewhere.[15] Generally accepted criteria for the serological diagnosis of a case are as follows:

- *Confirmed case.* A fourfold or greater rise or fall in antibody titer in appropriately timed paired sera or demonstration of virus-specific IgM antibodies in a single serum.
- *Presumptive cases.* (1) High antibody titers in a single convalescent serum, (2) stable high serum titers in paired sera obtained during convalescence, or (3) a case that is fatal 5 days or more after onset, with presence of detectable antibody in serum and postmortem findings consistent with the presumed infection.
- *Inconclusive case.* Antibody present but at titers that do not satisfy above criteria.
- *Negative case.* No antibodies, or stable minimally detectable titers in appropriately timed paired sera.

PREVENTION AND CONTROL

Effective vaccines have been produced for a number of arbovirus infections, including yellow fever, tickborne encephalitis, Japanese encephalitis, Rift Valley fever, Crimean-Congo hemorrhagic fever, Hantaan, dengue, VEE, and western and eastern equine encephalitis, but only one (yellow fever) is licensed for human use in the United States. Immunization of equids with VEE, WEE, and EEE vaccines is widely practiced. Both live attenuated and inactivated VEE vaccines are available, and their use is especially relevant, since nonimmune equids are the principal source of VEE virus for arthropod vectors in epizootics or epidemics. Tickborne encephalitis, Japanese encephalitis, and yellow fever vaccines have been responsible for reduced morbidity in regions where these vaccines have been effectively employed. Since all arboviruses and hemorrhagic fever viruses have transmission cycles involving wild animals, vaccination of clinical hosts must be continued indefinitely. Immunization of wildlife may, however, be a practical approach in the future.

Prophylaxis of disease in persons accidentally exposed in the laboratory to the viruses included in this section represents a minor, if important, public health problem. Transfusion of plasma or globulin containing specific neutralizing antibodies may successfully abort infection in such cases, especially if given early (within 24 hours) after exposure. Immune globulin is also used for postexposure (tick bite) prophylaxis of tickborne encephalitis and for treatment of Crimean-Congo hemorrhagic fever.

Prevention of epidemics may be achieved by reduction of arthropod vector populations. In the case of mosquitoborne infections, this is most efficiently done by reducing the sources of vector breeding and by killing the larvae. In the event of an impending outbreak (viral activity at a high level detected in nature) or an established outbreak, measures must be taken to eliminate the adult female mosquitoes themselves, since source reduction and killing of larvae will not rapidly reduce the infected, transmitting segment of the vector population. The use of insecticide space sprays, applied by ground or aerial equipment by the ultralow-volume (ULV) technique, may be effective. It is essential that the effectiveness of such vector control efforts be monitored. Factors to be measured include (1) susceptibility of the target vector population to the insecticide used; (2) reduction in target vector populations; and (3) effects on the viral transmission cycle (vector infection rates, sentinel flock seroconversions, incidence of human disease, etc.).

VIRUSES CAUSING ACUTE CENTRAL NERVOUS SYSTEM INFECTIONS

Mosquitoborne Viral Infections

The Equine Encephalitides. Viruses causing outbreaks of encephalitis in equids and humans are most important in the Western Hemisphere.

Eastern equine encephalitis (EEE) occurs east of the Mississippi River, in the Caribbean, and throughout much of South America. Epizootics or epidemics have been reported from Massachusetts (1938, 1956, 1973, 1983), Louisiana (1947), Maryland (1968), New Jersey (1959), Michigan (1982), Georgia (1982), Gulf and Atlantic states (1989), the Dominican Republic (1949, 1978), Jamaica (1962), Panama (1969), Venezuela (1977), and Argentina (1981). Epornitics in penned exotic birds are a feature of the disease in the United States. Outbreaks in the United States occur in the late summer and early fall. Sporadic equine and human EEE cases occur annually in enzootic areas of the eastern United States (Fig. 11-3). A total of 194 human cases

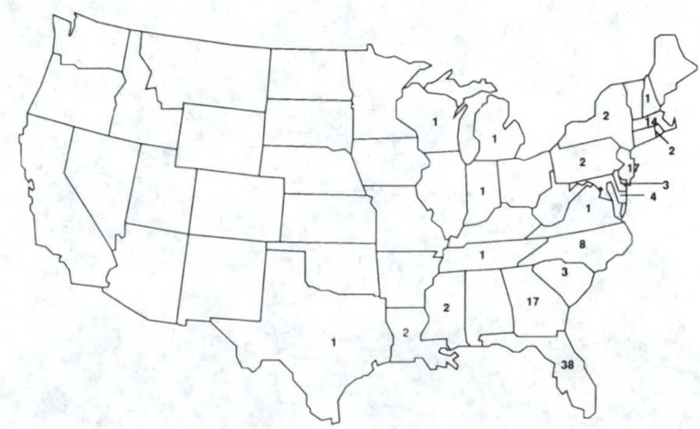

Figure 11-3. Human cases of eastern equine encephalitis, United States, 1964–1989.

have been reported between 1955 and 1989, with fewer than 10 cases in most years (Table 11-2). The clinical disease is severe, with case-fatality rates in humans approaching 50%. Young children and elderly persons are primarily affected. The inapparent/apparent infection ratio in these age groups is estimated at 1:10 and 1:20, respectively, but is about 1:50 in young adults. Illness is characterized by fever, signs of severe neurological dysfunction, high cell counts in cerebrospinal fluid with early granulocytic predominance, and a high incidence of residual neurological damage. In the United States the virus is sustained in freshwater swamps in a cycle involving wild birds and *Culiseta melanura* mosquito vectors. This species only rarely bites horses and humans, and the epidemic vectors vary from place to place; *Aedes sollicitans* and *Coquillettidia perturbans* have been implicated in the spread of EEE virus to clinical hosts. Horses apparently contribute to the cycle only rarely as viremic hosts, although this point deserves further study.

The epidemiology in tropical areas is less well known; *Cx. taeniopus* and wild birds constitute the enzootic cycle in Trinidad, Brazil, and Panama. Two serotypes of the virus are distinguishable, designated North American and South American subtypes. The North American subtype, present in the United States, is also responsible for outbreaks in the Greater Antilles. It is unknown whether this virus is enzootic in these islands or is periodically introduced by southward-migrating birds. A rough coincidence has been noted between outbreaks in the Caribbean and in the Atlantic seaboard states. The overwintering mechanism of EEE virus in the United States is unknown; midwinter isolations of the virus have been made from *Culiseta melanura* larvae and small rodents, but the significance of these observations is disputed. Surveillance techniques applied to detect early EEE viral activity include the use of sentinel fowl, virologic testing of mosquitoes, and indices of vector populations. In coastal New Jersey, the vector potential of *Aedes sollicitans* is routinely measured by the number of parous mosquitoes landing on human bait in 1 minute.

In pheasants and other penned birds and in equids the disease is controlled with the use of a formalin-inactivated vaccine, usually in the form of a bivalent (EEE/WEE) or trivalent (EEE/WEE/VEE) vaccine. Vector control affords the only available means of controlling established epidemics.

Western equine encephalitis (WEE) virus is distributed throughout western North America (Fig. 11-4), and the virus has been isolated in Brazil, Argentina, and Guyana. Outbreaks have occurred in the western United States, Canada, Uruguay, and Argentina. Large epizootics/epidemics occurred in the United States in 1941, with more than 3000 human cases in the north central region and neighboring Canadian provinces, and in 1952 in the Central Valley of California (375 cases). Between 1955 and 1983, 1031 human cases were officially reported to the Centers

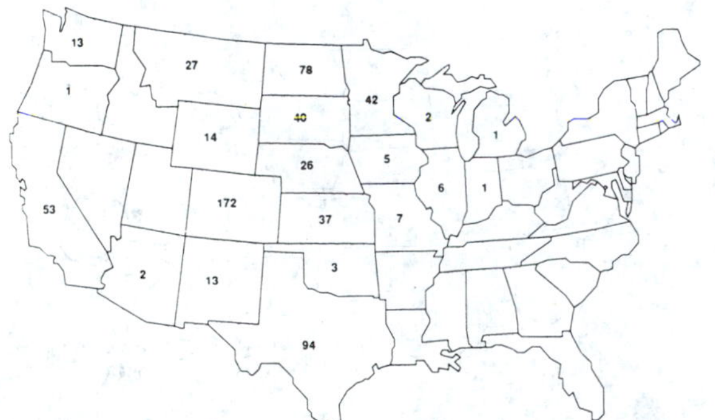

Figure 11-4. Distribution of human cases of western equine encephalitis in the United States, 1964–1989.

TABLE 11-2. ARBOVIRAL CENTRAL NERVOUS SYSTEM INFECTIONS IN THE UNITED STATES, 1955–1989

	SLE	WEE	EEE	CE	VEE	POW	Total
1955	107	37	15				159
1956	563	47	15				625
1957	147	35	5				187
1958	94	141	2				237
1959	118	14	36				168
1960	21	21	3				45
1961	42	27	1				70
1962	253	17	0				270
1963	19	56	0	1			76
1964	470	64	5	42			581
1965	58	172	8	59			297
1966	323	47	4	64			438
1967	11	18	1	53			83
1968	35	17	12	66	1		131
1969	16	21	3	67	1		108
1970	15	4	2	89		1	111
1971	57	11	4	58	19		150
1972	13	8	0	46	2		72
1973	5	4	7	75			91
1974	74	2	4	30		1	111
1975	1815	133	3	160		3	2114
1976	379	1	0	47			427
1977	132	41	1	65		1	240
1978	26	3	5	109		1	144
1979	32	3	3	139			177
1980	125	0	8	49			182
1981	15	19	0	91			125
1982	34	9	12	130			185
1983	20	7	14	64			105
1984	33	2	5	89			129
1985	21	1	0	68			90
1986	43	7	1	64			115
1987	17	41	3	87			148
1988	4	1	3	41			49
1989	34	0	9	65			108
Total	5171	1031	194	1918	23	7	8348

SLE = St. Louis encephalitis; WEE = western equine encephalitis; EEE = eastern equine encephalitis; CE = California (La Cross) encephalitis; VEE = Venezuelan equine encephalitis; POW = Powassan encephalitis

for Disease Control in Fort Collins, Colorado (Table 11-1). During this interval, small outbreaks, involving 25 to 68 human cases, occurred in Kansas, Utah, and California (in 1958), western Texas (1963–1964), Colorado (1965 and 1987), and the Red River basin of Minnesota and North Dakota (1975). On a statewide basis, the attack rates in these outbreaks were in the range of 4 to 6 per 100,000 population; however, rates in severely affected counties (such as Kern County, California, in 1952 or Hale County, Texas, in 1963–1964) have been higher, 50 to 125 per 100,000. The disease occurs in midsummer, and the appearance of equine outbreaks often precedes the occurrence of human cases by several weeks. Human factors, including the practice of watching television indoors and the use of screens and air conditioners, have been partly responsible for a declining incidence of infection in the United States.

The virus causes clinical encephalitis in equids and in humans; it is an especially severe infection in infants, producing neurological sequelae. The case-fatality rate approximates 3%. Infection most often is abortive or mild and undifferentiated; the ratio of inapparent infection to overt central nervous system infection is approximately 50:1 in children under the age of 5 years and more than 1000:1 in adults. Surveys in endemic areas have demonstrated an antibody prevalence of about 5% in young children, rising to 20% in adults.

In the western United States, the virus circulates between wild birds (especially house finches and house sparrows) and *C. tarsalis* mosquitoes. Since the primary enzootic vector also bites horses and humans, it is responsible for disease transmission. *C. tarsalis* may feed exclusively on birds in the spring and then shift to mammalian hosts in midsummer, coinciding with the appearance of equine and human infections. Horses and humans do not have viremias sufficient to infect mosquito vectors. *C. tarsalis* breeds predominantly in irrigated pastureland, and the incidence of human infections is correlated with rural residence and agricultural pursuits. Flooding of riverine basins, heavy snow melt, and riverflows yield high vector populations and may accelerate rates of viral transmission. The WEE viral transmission cycle is shared with that of SLE virus in the western United States; mixed WEE-SLE outbreaks have occurred, although in general one of the two viruses predominates in a given year. In the eastern United States, a virus (highlands J) closely related to WEE virus is enzootically maintained in freshwater swamps in a cycle identical to that of EEE. Only rare equine and human cases have been reported, and the viral strains in this region may have reduced virulence characteristics.

Various means of surveillance of WEE viral activity have been applied. As previously noted, measurements of adult female *C. tarsalis* populations provide an index of risk, but more direct information on rates of viral transmission may be obtained by use of sentinel fowl or determination of viremia rates in wild nestling house sparrows. The latter indices appear to correlate well with risk of human disease[16] and appear to have predictive value.

Mosquito control provides the only available means of reducing human infections. Survey data on mosquito-breeding sites are used to direct efforts in source-reduction campaigns and the use of biological and chemical agents to eliminate larvae. Aerial ULV applications of chemical adulticides may be used to control outbreaks. An effective formalinized vaccine is licensed for equine use.

Venezuelan equine encephalitis (VEE) occurs in the form of focal or extensive epizootics and epidemics in northern South America, from Venezuela south to Peru. In 1969 the disease appeared on the Pacific coast of Guatemala, whence it spread southward to Costa Rica in 1970 and northward through Mexico, reaching Texas in 1971. The equine morbidity associated with VEE outbreaks has been high. For example, the 1967 epizootic in Colombia is estimated to have killed more than 100,000 horses and burros, that in 1969 in Ecuador approximately 30,000, and that in Central American and Mexico between 1969 and 1971 more than 20,000. A total of 1426 horses died in Texas in 1971. The disease in humans is usually mild and grippelike, characterized by sudden onset, fever, chills, headache, myalgia, and gastrointestinal disturbances; pharyngitis is a feature of the infection in about 25% of the cases. The illness lasts 4 to 6 days, but a small proportion of cases have a biphasic illness pattern, with return of signs and symptoms several days to a week after initial onset. Overt signs of encephalitis occur in only about 4% of the cases; the incidence of encephalitis is highest in children under 15 years of age. The overall case-fatality rate is under 1%, but it is higher (15%) among cases with encephalitis. Subclinical infections are rare. More than 20,000 human cases have been associated with individual major equine epizootics in South America. The disease appears during the rainy season; equine outbreaks precede epidemics by several weeks or longer.

The epidemiology of VEE is complicated by the existence of multiple antigenic subtypes and variants, only two of which (designated IAB and IC) have been associated with epizootics.[17] Other, enzootic subtypes are widespread in tropical regions of the hemisphere (including Florida), where they produce a high prevalence of infection but only sporadic disease. The epizootic subtypes (IAB, IC) differ not only in their virulence but also in their vector-host relationships. Equidae are the principal viremic hosts in the cycle, and transmission is effected by a wide variety of mosquito vectors, including species of the genera *Aedes, Psorophora,* and *Mansonia.*[18] In contrast the enzootic subtypes are transmitted in a silent cycle involving primarily small rodents and *Culex (Melanoconion)* mosquitoes. Several enzootic subtypes (ID, IE, IF, II, III) cause sporadic disease in humans but not in Equidae.

In tropical America, outbreaks occurred at intervals of approximately 10 years, generally in dry tropical forests and coastal plains. The periodicity of outbreaks was in part due to the high infection rates and consequent exhaustion of immunologically susceptible equines. The maintenance cycle of VEE virus during interepizootic periods is unknown. No VEE epizootics have been recorded since 1973. Disappearance of the disease may be linked to the discontinued manufacture and use of formalinized vaccines prepared from epizootic (IAB) virus, which often contained residual infectivity.

Surveillance techniques are rudimentary in much of tropical America, and specific laboratory diagnosis of equine and human central nervous system infections is rarely achieved. Potentially useful techniques for surveillance of the infection include use of sentinel equines or sentinel laboratory rodents, such as hamsters or guinea pigs.

Prevention of epizootics and epidemics may be achieved by use of VEE vaccine in Equidae. Both an effective, live, and attenuated vaccine (TC-83) and killed vaccines prepared from TC-83 are available. Development of immunity is rapid following use of the live vaccine, and it therefore has a role in limiting the spread of an ongoing epizootic. Aerial ULV applications of organophosphate insecticide have been used in several outbreaks.

St. Louis Encephalitis. St. Louis encephalitis (SLE) is the most important epidemic arboviral disease in the United States, and it is widely distributed (Fig. 11-5).[19] In certain epidemic years the incidence of SLE exceeds that of all other viral encephalitides of known etiology combined (Table 11-2). Between 1955 and 1989, 5171 cases of SLE were reported to the Centers for Disease Control, representing 62% of the total cases of arboviral encephalitis in the United States. The virus also is widespread in tropical America, but only rare, sporadic clinical infections are recognized.

Two epidemiological patterns of SLE are evident in the United States. In the West, SLE is an endemic infection, generally of low incidence; small epidemics of fewer than 100 cases occur periodically, usually associated with outbreaks of WEE.

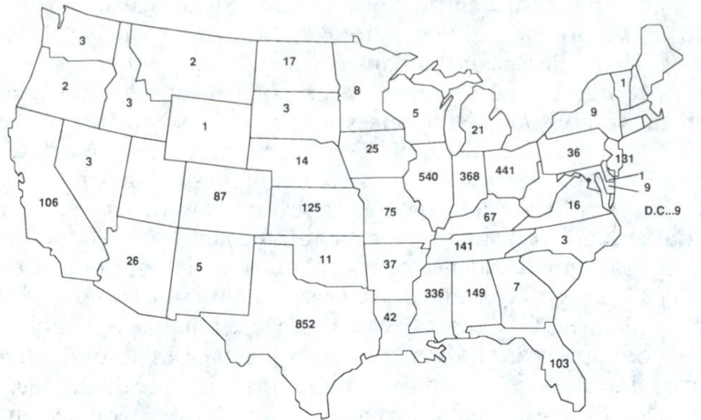

Figure 11-5. Distribution of human cases of St. Louis encephalitis in the United States, 1964–1989.

In 1989 the largest outbreak in California in 30 years struck the Central Valley. Morbidity is generally higher in rural or suburban populations living in irrigated farmland districts than in urban populations. Most cases occur in children because older age groups have acquired high levels of immunity. The disease appears to be less severe than in the eastern United States; the case-fatality rate in persons over 60 years of age is about 9%, compared to 20% in age-matched patients in the East, suggesting a difference between geographic virus strains in human virulence. The virus circulates in a bird-*C. tarsalis*-bird cycle. Human infections occur in late summer. *C. tarsalis* (and possibly *C. pipiens*) are responsible for virus transmission to humans. Horses develop antibodies but not overt signs of illness.

In the eastern United States, the disease occurs in epidemic form at approximately 10- to 20-year intervals. Outbreaks have varied in size from a few clustered cases to more than 2000 cases in a multifocal pattern throughout the Ohio-Mississippi basin and eastern Texas. Attack rates in individual outbreaks have been as high as 800/100,000. The economic cost of these epidemics has been high; the 1966 Dallas, Texas, outbreak was estimated to have resulted in direct costs (resulting from hospital charges, investigation, and vector control) and indirect costs (loss of work output) of $10 million (1990 dollars). The disease strikes urban-suburban areas and affects primarily older persons. Antibody surveys conducted after outbreaks have shown that this age distribution is due to an increased susceptibility of the elderly to overt encephalitis, rather than to an increased rate of exposure to the virus. The inapparent-apparent infection rate is approximately 800:1 in children under 10 years, 400:1 in young adults, and 80:1 in persons over 60 years. In some large urban outbreaks attack rates have been highest in predominantly black, low socioeconomic areas of the city. This and other epidemiological features of the disease are based on the virus-vector relationships. SLE in the eastern United States (except Florida) is transmitted by the household mosquito *C. pipiens,* which breeds in polluted wastewater. High vector populations are associated with poor sanitary conditions and weather patterns (low rainfall, high temperatures) that favor pooling and stagnation of water. Wild birds, especially species abundant in the urban-suburban environment (house sparrows, pigeons, blue jays, robins) constitute the principal reservoirs. In Florida the tropical mosquito *Culex nigripalpus* is the vector.

Although many epidemics have been limited to a single year, reappearance of outbreaks in successive years has been a feature of SLE in some localities. Although the overwintering mechanism of the virus has not been elucidated, it is likely that these successive occurrences may be due to "priming" dependent on a high rate of local maintenance of SLE virus during the intervening winter season. SLE virus may be carried through the winter by infected hibernating adult *C. pipiens.*[11] Vertical transmission of virus from infected female *Culex* mosquitoes to their progeny promotes this phenomenon, since mosquitoes may not feed on blood before hibernation.

The interval between the date of onset of the first human case and the recognition of an epidemic has been between 2 and 8 weeks. Much attention has been paid in recent years to development of systems for early detection of SLE viral activity in nature. Monitoring antibody prevalence in juvenile wild birds and serologic conversion rates in sentinel fowl have provided reasonably accurate predictions.[13]

No vaccine is available for human use. The principles of prevention and control by reduction of vector populations have been discussed above. Reduction of *C. pipiens* breeding is extremely difficult, and the growth of cities with attendant problems of man-made mosquito breeding sites has increased the potential for outbreaks of this disease in the United States.

California Encephalitis. A group of 11 antigenically distinct but related viruses constitutes the California virus group, of which three (La Crosse, Jamestown Canyon, and California encephalitis viruses) are established human pathogens in the United States. A subtype of La Crosse virus designated snowshoe hare virus is also associated with human disease in North America. La Crosse virus is responsible for nearly all recognized infections. It is an important cause of endemic disease of children under the age of 15 years in the north central states, primarily Ohio, Minnesota, Wisconsin, eastern Iowa, Illinois, and upstate New York. The disease is also reported from the southern and southeastern states and California (Fig. 11-6). From 50 to 75 cases are reported to the Centers for Disease Control in years of average viral activity, and they occur in July, August, and early September. A total of 1918 cases have been reported between 1963 and 1989 (Table 11-2). The pattern is one of scattered clinical infections; viral activity tends to be quite focal, associated with residence in small valleys with deciduous hardwood forests. The true clinical disease spectrum is poorly understood, but mild, undifferentiated febrile illness, perhaps with respiratory symptoms, occurs in addition to full-blown encephalitis. Encephalitis may be clinically severe during the acute phase, but full recovery is the rule, and the occurrence of neuropsychiatric sequelae has not been well established, although seizure disorders seem linked to the disease. The case-fatality rate is less than 1%. La Crosse virus has been isolated from brain tissue in two fatal cases.

Antibody surveys have shown increasing rates of immunity with age, from 5% in children under 5 years to more than 30% in adults over 40 years of age. Serosurveys are complicated by the presence of other California-group viruses in La Crosse endemic areas, which cause cross-reacting antibody responses. La Crosse

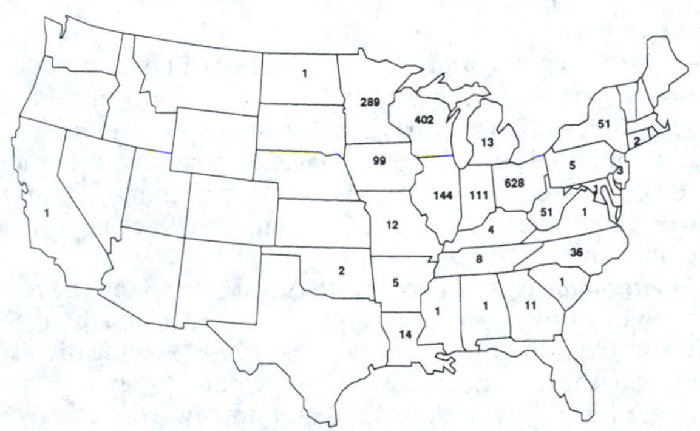

Figure 11-6. Distribution of California encephalitis in the United States, 1964–1989. Most cases are caused by the La Crosse serotype, but others also contribute to human morbidity.

virus is transmitted by woodland *Aedes* mosquitoes, primarily *A. triseriatus* and *A. canadensis.* The vectors breed in tree holes and artificial containers (e.g., tires) and transmit the virus to small rodents, such as chipmunks and tree squirrels. La Crosse virus is transovarially transmitted in *A. triseriatus,* and the virus can apparently survive in an area for up to 4 years without amplification by horizontal spread in vertebrate hosts.[12] The phenomenon of vertical transmission through many generations of the mosquito vector assures its survival and undoubtedly contributes to the focality of the human disease.

Surveillance has consisted mainly of human case finding, but detection of the virus with the use of sentinel rabbits is feasible. Control measures are not well established. Elimination of tree holes (by filling with cement) and other sites of vector mosquito breeding (artificial containers) may be locally effective. Because of the sporadic pattern of cases and the vertical transmission of the virus, spraying to reduce adult vector populations would be expected to have limited and transient usefulness.

The Jamestown Canyon serotype has been mainly associated with disease (febrile illness, aseptic meningitis, encephalitis) in adults in the north central United States and Ontario.

California-group viruses have a wide distribution. Snowshoe hare virus has been implicated in human disease in China, and Tahyna virus with febrile and neurological syndromes in Europe and the Soviet Union.

Japanese Encephalitis. Japanese encephalitis (JE) virus, a close relative of SLE virus, causes endemic/epidemic disease in parts of Asia, including Japan, Korea, Taiwan, Okinawa, Guam, China, and Vietnam, the Philippines, Malaysia, Thailand, and eastern India. Morbidity in some outbreaks has been high, with thousands of cases; case-fatality rates of 50% or more have been reported but reflect poor recognition of nonfatal cases. Children and older persons are at higher risk of clinical infection than young adults; in endemic areas, however, where immunity prevalence increases with age, the disease occurs primarily in preschool children. Since 1960 the disease has declined as a problem in Japan (as a result of immunization and changing agricultural practices that have limited vector breeding), but elsewhere (China, northern Thailand, and India) recurrent outbreaks account for more than 50,000 cases annually. In tropical parts of Asia (e.g., southern Thailand, Indonesia), human infections are prevalent, but only sporadic disease occurs. RNA sequence data indicate that these tropical strains differ genetically, and it is likely that their human virulence may be less than epidemic virus strains.

JE is generally a more severe disease than SLE. Neurological sequelae have been noted in as many as 75% of survivors and are more severe in affected children under 10 years of age; sequelae include motor disturbances, parkinsonism, and psychiatric abnormalities.

The disease has a summer-fall distribution in temperate areas, but in tropical areas no clear seasonal pattern is evident. The principal epidemic vector differs by geographical region, but overall *Culex tritaeniorhyncus,* a rice paddy breeder, is the most important. This species principally bites large animals but also feeds on birds. Other *Culex* species implicated include *C. pseudovishnui* (in India), *C. gelidus* (Malaysia, Thailand), *C. annulus* (Guam, Taiwan), and *C. fuscocephalus* (Taiwan, Thailand). The virus has also been isolated from certain *Aedes* species, which may play a role in enzootic viral transmission and overwintering. Wild birds, especially black-crowned night herons, are effective viremic hosts in the cycle, may be important in dispersal of the virus, and probably represent its original vertebrate reservoir. With the expansion of human populations in Asia and the increased popularity of the pig as a source of food, swine have become the principal vertebrate hosts for JE virus. Pigs are abundant (especially in rural areas), circulate the virus at high titers in their blood, and have a high population turnover as a result of slaughtering. Intrauterine infection of pigs with JE virus, however, causes abortion and stillbirth; consequently, pig breeding is timed to avoid infection. This imposed schedule assures that young pigs will have lost maternal antibodies by the time of peak viral transmission and also limits the usefulness of immunization of sows. Horses are susceptible to overt encephalitic infection but do not contribute to circulation of the virus.

The mechanism of overwinter survival of JE virus in temperate zones is not known; recent experimental observations suggest that the virus may be transmitted transovarially by certain *Aedes* mosquitoes.

A formalin-killed mouse brain vaccine has been widely used to immunize children in Japan.[20] The vaccine is available in the United States but is not yet licensed, and it is administered to travelers who give voluntary informed consent. Both live, attenuated and inactivated cell culture vaccines are produced and widely used in China. Larviciding, residual insecticide house spraying, and ULV aerial application of adulticides have been suggested for the prevention and control of JE.

Rocio Encephalitis. In 1975 Rocio encephalitis emerged as a new arboviral disease of humans. A series of severe outbreaks occurred in the coastal zone of São Paulo State, restricted to a 1000 km^2 area south of Santos. In 1975 and 1976 approximately 1000 cases occurred in several discrete outbreaks, with attack rates of up to 3.8%.[21] The highest incidence was in young men engaged in rural agricultural work. The clinical illness resembled that of JE. The case-fatality rate was 4%, and sequelae were noted in 20% of survivors. Rocio virus, isolated in fatal human cases and in a wild bird, was shown to be a new flavivirus serologically related to SLE and JE viruses. Cross-reactivity among flaviviral antigens in tests for antibody complicates serologic diagnosis, since human infections with other viruses (SLE and Ilheus) related to Rocio virus are prevalent in Brazil. Since the distribution of the virus may not be limited to southern Brazil, the diagnosis of Rocio viral infection should be considered in all cases of central nervous system infection from tropical America. The transmission cycle is known, but birds are believed to be the principal hosts and *Aedes scapularis* mosquitoes the vector.

No vaccine is available. Since the virus-vector relationships are not understood, specific preventive and control measures cannot be formulated accurately, but emergency spraying to reduce mosquito populations would seem warranted in the event of future epidemics.

Tickborne Viral Infections

Tickborne encephalitis (TBE), also known as Russian spring-summer encephalitis, central European encephalitis, and diphasic meningoencephalitis, is an important endemoepidemic disease in eastern Europe and the Soviet Union; imported infections have been rarely documented in the United States. Between 500 and 1000 cases are reported annually in Europe, with peak incidence during June and July. Infection is acquired both by tick bite and by ingestion of unpasteurized milk from infected goats or sheep.

The ecology and clinical features of the disease in Europe and the far eastern Soviet Union differ. In Europe the typical case has a biphasic course with an early, viremic influenza-like stage, followed in 7 to 8 days by the appearance of signs of meningoencephalitis. The central nervous system disease is generally mild, but occasional severe motor dysfunction and permanent disability are described. The case-fatality rate is 0 to 2%. In the far eastern form, severe encephalomyelitis and residual damage are much more frequent and the case-fatality rate is high (20% to 30%).

Ixodes ricinus in Europe and *I. persulcatus* in the far eastern Soviet Union are the principal vectors. Small mammals, especially rodents and insectivores, and larval and nymphal ticks constitute the basic viral transmission cycle. As infected ticks molt, the virus is passed transstadially (to the next stage). Large animal species (goats, sheep, cattle, deer) are susceptible to infection, may shed virus in their milk, develop antibodies, and serve as important sources of food and means of dispersal of ticks, but they are not effective viremic hosts. Humans are infected accidentally when exposed to nymphal or adult ticks, generally during recreational or vocational pursuits in wooded areas or field margins supporting the elements of the natural transmission cycle or during clearing and settlement of uninhabited natural foci. Human infections acquired from milk account for 8% to 25% of cases.

The virus overwinters in hibernating ticks and possibly also in hibernating insectivores and rodents with prolonged viremias. Tickborne encephalitis is also passed transovarially in the ixodid tick vectors, a phenomenon that assures its survival and replenishes the small mammal–immature tick cycle. Surveillance is primarily directed at mapping foci of TBE viral activity in a given area and determining the extent of contact of tourists and agricultural workers with such foci.

Prevention is aimed at public health measures to reduce human contact with ticks, pasteurization of milk, reduction of natural habitats for viral transmission, selective use of insecticides, and immunization. An effective killed vaccine is produced commercially in Austria and a licensed vaccine is available in the Soviet Union. Mass immunization of the Austrian population has significantly reduced the incidence of TBE. Passive immunization with globulin from vaccines is used for post–tick bite prophylaxis.

Powassan encephalitis is a rare flaviviral infection of humans in the northeastern United States and adjacent regions of Canada. Recognized cases have occurred in children and adults, with a case-fatality rate of approximately 50%. Antibody prevalences in residents of the affected area are less than 1%, indicating that human exposure to the cycle is a rare event. The transmission cycle involves ixodid ticks and small mammals (squirrels, woodchucks).

VIRUSES CAUSING UNDIFFERENTIATED FEBRILE ILLNESS

Mosquitoborne Infections

Dengue fever (breakbone fever) outbreaks have occurred on every continent between 30° and 40° north and south of the equator, coinciding with the range of the principal vector mosquito, *A. aegypti.* The disease was a major affliction of troops in the Pacific theater of World War II. In the last two decades pandemics involving millions of cases have occurred in the Caribbean, eastern Africa, southeast Asia, and the Pacific Islands. Dengue is not a single virus but, rather, consists of four distinct serotypes (dengue type 1, type 2, etc.) within the flavivirus genus of the *Flaviviridae.* Infection with one serotype confers long-lasting specific immunity but only incomplete and short-lived cross-protection to infection with heterologous serotypes. Consequently, recurrent outbreaks may occur in a geographical region on introduction of a new serotype.

Classic dengue fever is an acute, self-limited disease characterized by abrupt onset, a biphasic febrile course, anorexia, weakness, prostration, arthralgia, rash, leukopenia, lymphadenopathy, and, in a small proportion of cases, minor hemorrhagic manifestations (petechiae, epistaxis). A prolonged convalescence with asthenia and depression is not uncommon. No fatalities have been recorded. This syndrome is in marked contrast to that of dengue hemorrhagic fever, described in the following section.

The public health significance of dengue fever may be appreciated by a brief review of events in the Americas since 1977. Before this time, outbreaks of dengue types 2 and 3 infection had occurred repeatedly in Caribbean islands and major epidemics of type 2 infection had swept the Atlantic coast of Colombia. In March 1977 a dengue type 1 outbreak occurred in Jamaica, the agent possibly being introduced from western Africa or southeast Asia. This virus was spread to other islands by infected humans, reaching Barbados and Trinidad by late 1977 and coastal Central America by 1978. In the fall of 1980 it arrived in the continental United States at Brownsville, Texas, but failed to cause a major epidemic there or to spread to neighboring cities.[22] A rather similar geographical movement of dengue type 4 virus, which had never been isolated in the region, subsequently occurred. Millions of cases were reported, and attack rates of 500 to 5000 per 100,000 population were registered. The costs were very high in terms of investigative and vector-control efforts and losses of work and tourist revenues. In Cuba in 1981, dengue hemorrhagic fever occurred in epidemic form for the first time in the Americas, with 116,143 hospitalized cases and 158 deaths. The epidemic followed the introduction of dengue 2 virus 4 years after a major outbreak of dengue 1; the severe form of the disease occurred in persons sustaining sequential infections (see Dengue Hemorrhagic Fever below). Between 1982 and 1985, 25,000 to 68,000 cases of dengue fever were reported in the Americas annually. In 1986 the city of Rio de Janeiro and other areas of coastal Brazil were struck by epidemic dengue 1, with at least 300,000 cases (and perhaps as many as 1 million). Over the next several years, large outbreaks of dengue appeared in Paraguay, Bolivia, Ecuador, and Peru, signaling the recrudescence of *A. aegypti*–borne disease in areas of the Americas from which the vector had long been eradicated. At present three serotypes of dengue (types 1, 2, and 4) are circulating in the Americas, raising the specter of further outbreaks of dengue hemorrhagic fever (DHF). Indeed, Venezuela experienced an epidemic of DHF in 1989, with 3108 cases of severe disease and 73 deaths; once again the offending serotype was dengue 2.

The virus is transmitted from person to person, principally by *A. aegypti* mosquitoes. Infected humans circulate the virus in their blood for several days. *A. aegypti* is a daytime-biting, peridomestic mosquito, which breeds in any container holding fresh water. It is also the urban vector of yellow fever virus, and occurrence of dengue outbreaks in the Caribbean and northern South America is prima facie evidence of the receptivity of these areas to introduction and spread of yellow fever from the jungle cycle.

Prevention depends on avoiding mosquito bite (use of screening, repellents, protective clothing) and reduction of *A. aegypti* by elimination of breeding sites and use of larvicides. Eradication of *A. aegypti* has been a goal of member states of the Pan American Health Organization since 1947 and was successful in a few areas, notably Brazil, Argentina, Chile, Paraguay, Uruguay, Peru, and Ecuador. By the 1980s, however, nearly all countries that had succeeded in eradication had become reinfested, with resulting introduction and spread of dengue. Areas of the southern United States have high *A. aegypti* populations, but, despite importation of dengue patients from the Caribbean, only limited secondary transmission has occurred. Prophylaxis by immunization is feasible, and experimental live attenuated vaccines are under study. Epidemic measures are based on use of space insecticides applied by the ULV technique.

Chikungunya virus (an alphavirus) is a generally benign disease that clinically resembles classic dengue fever. The Swahili name means "that which bends up," referring to the severe arthralgia that accompanies the illness. Deaths and hemorrhagic phenomena are extremely rare and poorly documented features of the disease. The virus is endemic in sub-Saharan Africa and the Asian tropics. Major outbreaks have occurred in Africa and Asia, with high attack rates. The infection is now hyperendemic in areas of Africa and Asia infested with *A. aegypti,* the principal viral vector to humans. An enzootic, sylvan transmission cycle in Africa, however, involves subhuman primates and forest mosquitoes, including *Aedes furcifer,* and is analogous to that of jungle yellow fever.

Various experimental chikungunya viral vaccines have been investigated, but none are commercially available. Control measures applicable to the epidemic disease are similar to those described for dengue.

Tickborne Infections

Colorado tick fever (CTF) occurs in mountainous areas of the United States within the distributional range of the vector, *Dermacentor andersoni* (Colorado, Wyoming, Idaho, Montana, Utah, and parts of South Dakota, New Mexico, California, Oregon, Washington, Alberta, and British Columbia). Several hundred human cases are recorded annually, but the actual incidence of the disease is probably tenfold higher. Infections are acquired during recreational and occupational pursuits that bring humans into contact with infected ticks; campers, foresters, telephone line workers, and the like are thus affected. Infections occur from early spring to October, but the highest incidence is in May and June, representing the seasonal peak of adult tick vector feeding activity. In focal areas of high viral activity, such as some campsites within the Rocky Mountain Park (Colorado), as many as 20% of adult tick vectors are found to be infected; the risk of acquiring the disease is approximately one case per 400 camper days.

The clinical illness is characterized by an incubation period of 3 to 6 days, abrupt onset of biphasic febrile course, chills, weakness, prostration, headache, myalgia, photophobia, gastrointestinal complaints, leukopenia, and thrombocytopenia. Rash is uncommon (5% to 10% of cases) but may lead to confusion with Rocky Mountain spotted fever. Meningoencephalitis, pericarditis, orchitis, and pleuritis are rare manifestations. Hemorrhagic phenomena have been described in the two reported fatal cases, both involving children.

The virus is amplified in a cycle involving immature *D. andersoni* ticks and small rodents, especially ground squirrels and chipmunks. These species develop prolonged viremias. The virus survives the winter in infected hibernating nymphal and adult ticks, which reinitiate the cycle in the spring. Adult ticks feed on large mammals, including humans, but humans are dead-end hosts and do not serve as a source of tick infection. Infected persons have prolonged viremias, however, and antibodies appear quite late. Consequently, the possibility of transfusion-induced CTF is recognized.

Viruses Transmitted by Phlebotomine Flies

Phlebotomus (sandfly) fever is caused by at least six serologically distinct viruses (designated Sicilian and Naples phlebotomous fever, Alenguer, Candiru, Chagres, Punta Toro, and Toscana viruses) which belong to a group of 38 related viruses comprising the genus phlebovirus, family *Bunyaviridae* (Table 11-1). Naples and Sicilian viruses cause disease in the Mediterranean region, the Middle East, Iran, India, Pakistan, southern Soviet Union, and the Sudan. Immunity rates are generally high, and infection is usually acquired early in life, when disease is mild or escapes notice. Explosive outbreaks with high attack rates have nonetheless occurred, involving as many as 1 million persons. The epidemic disease has occurred with wartime disturbances, displacement of populations, and movements of nonimmune armies. The clinical infection is characterized by a denguelike syndrome but without rash. Toscana virus has been associated with febrile disease and aseptic meningitis in Italy.

Phlebotomus papatasii is the vector. This terrestrial breeding species is mainly nocturnal, is found in close association with humans, and has a very limited flight range. The phlebotomus fever viruses are transmitted transovarially by the vector, and this apparently represents their main means of survival, since adult sandflies do not overwinter. Humans probably contribute little to the transmission cycle (because of low and brief viremias); no other vertebrate reservoir has been unequivocally demonstrated, although serologic evidence suggests that certain rodents (gerbils) may be involved.

Several phleboviruses in tropical America (Alenguer, Candiru, Chagres, Punta Toro viruses) cause sporadic undifferentiated febrile illness in humans but are of no public health consequence. Control is by reduction of vector populations through use of insecticides.

Culicoidesborne Infections

Oropouche fever (febre du Mojui), caused by a bunyavirus of the Simbu group, is responsible for at least 15 major epidemics in cities and towns of the Amazon region of Brazil. As many as 102,000 persons were infected in individual outbreaks, at rates as high as 30%. The disease is self-limited, characterized by sudden onset, high fever, severe headache, myalgia, gastrointestinal symptoms, leukopenia, and prostration, sometimes requiring hospitalization. Aseptic meningitis is not uncommon. The virus has been isolated from *Culicoides paraensis* gnats (suspected to be the epidemic vector) and from mosquitoes. Experimental studies show conclusively that *C. paraensis* is a biologically competent vector of Oropouche virus.[23] Wild birds or monkeys may play a role in the forest transmission cycle. Although the ecological relationships are not completely understood, reduction of *C. paraensis* populations appears to be a justifiable approach in future outbreaks.

VIRUSES CAUSING HEMORRHAGIC FEVER

Mosquitoborne Infections

Dengue Viruses. In addition to the classic syndrome of breakbone fever, all four dengue virus serotypes are capable of producing a more severe, sometimes fatal syndrome variously called dengue hemorrhagic fever or dengue shock syndrome. Although there is historical evidence that this disease occurred during major dengue outbreaks in Greece and Australia more than 70 years ago, it has been recognized since 1948 only in certain areas of Southeast Asia, some islands of the western Pacific Ocean, and in parts of the Americas (Cuba and Venezuela), a geographical distribution far smaller than that of dengue virus infection.

A fundamental problem is clinical definition of dengue hemorrhagic fever (DHF). Persons with dengue virus infections who have a positive tourniquet test reaction have been included in this taxon by many authors. Many patients with otherwise self-limited illnesses may have scattered petechiae in the skin, and these phenomena are frequently recorded during dengue outbreaks in parts of the world where the more serious form of the disease is rare or absent. The fully developed clinical picture consists typically of the abrupt onset, after a 2- to 7-day incubation period, of fever and myalgia, significant thrombocytopenia, hepatomegaly, and various bleeding manifestations, including hemorrhagic petechiae, epistaxis, and gastrointestinal bleeding. There is loss of intravascular protein with attendant hemoconcentration, metabolic acidosis, and in 10% to 40% of cases there is both objective and clinical evidence of shock. The mortality rate during the shock crisis ranges from 1% to 20%, depending on the vigor and efficacy of supportive therapy.

The basic virus cycle, the seasonal pattern of occurrence, and the arthropod vectors of DHF do not differ from those of classic dengue infection; hemorrhagic fever is seen either in annual rainy season outbreaks in large metropolitan areas in Southeast Asia where all dengue serotypes are endemic or during epidemics on islands where a given serotype is introduced after a variable period of absence.

Extensive work on this problem has been done in Bangkok, Thailand, where the vector is *A. aegypti.* There the majority of hemorrhagic fever patients are children under 10 years of age. Annual hospitalization rates on an age-specific basis may reach 5 to 8 per 1000, or about one case per 60 to 100 serologically estimated dengue virus infections in this age group.[24] Females are affected more often than males, 1.2:1 to 1.4:1, despite the fact that dengue virus infection rates in this population do not differ by sex. There are no differences in attack rates between the major ethnic groups: Thai and Chinese.

Hemorrhagic fever occurred significantly more often in children with immunological evidence of secondary dengue virus infection than in those who had a "primary" response. From this observation it has been postulated that DHF is an immunopathological process selectively occurring among persons experiencing a second dengue infection in a rather short interval.[25]

Recent work appears to both strengthen and modify this hypothesis. In vitro and in vivo experimental studies demonstrated that dengue virus replication in mononuclear phagocytic cells, the apparent primary target cells for infection, was enhanced in the presence of small amounts of heterologous dengue antibody.[26] Such antibodies have been found in cord blood of infants born in virus-endemic areas of Southeast Asia. In addition, the first recorded epidemic of DHF in the Americas occurred in Cuba in 1981. This outbreak was caused by dengue 2 virus just 4 years after a major epidemic of type 1 infection that was the first dengue experience on that island in more than 30 years. In contrast, it has also been shown that primary dengue infection can cause DHF[27]; however, the risk of DHF following primary infection is 0.25% compared with 3.1% after secondary infection. Complex variables, including virus stain differences and host genetic factors, remain to be elucidated before a clear understanding of the relative risk factors influencing DHF emerges. In Cuba the risk of contracting DHF was greater in whites than in blacks, despite similar rates of secondary infection with dengue 2 virus. Methods for surveillance and control of DHF are the same as those described earlier for classic dengue fever.

Yellow Fever. Yellow fever is the prototypical viral hemorrhagic fever. It now occurs only in tropical and subtropical regions of Africa and the Americas, but historically it was an important passenger during the burgeoning European colonial period of the eighteenth and nineteenth centuries, causing urban epidemics in major seaport cities of the United States, the United Kingdom, and Europe. Indeed, the roots of our current system of quarantine, infection disease control, and a now defunct chain of national marine hospitals can be traced to attempts to understand and control yellow fever in the past century. Yellow fever is caused by a flavivirus closely related to the dengue virus and several other arthropod-transmitted agents of the flavivirus genus. A single infection confers lifelong immunity; thus the modern pattern of disease occurrence consists of recurrent outbreaks with intervals of several years in areas where an extrahuman virus cycle is maintained.

Clinical response to infection with yellow fever virus ranges from mild, undifferentiated fever to severe illness in which hemorrhagic, hepatic, and renal manifestations predominate.[28] In patients who survive or do not manifest an early fulminating hemorrhagic syndrome, jaundice typically develops after 4 to 6 days of illness, when viremia wanes and humoral antibodies appear. Renal tubular necrosis may occur during the second week of illness and, before the advent of peritoneal or hemodialysis, it accounted for nearly one third of fatalities. Notwithstanding these various clinical forms of disease, it is the clustering of jaundice cases with fatality rates of 10% to 50% that usually brings yellow fever outbreaks to public health attention, a feature of fundamental value in differential diagnosis between this disease and most other viral hemorrhagic fevers.

Attack rates during urban epidemics of yellow fever in the eighteenth and nineteenth centuries were often staggering, ranging to 20 cases per 100 persons, with up to a 5% mortality rate. In the past 30 years one of the largest epidemics on record was in southwestern Ethiopia, where an estimated 100,000 cases occurred in a population of 2 million, with 30,000 deaths. More recently, an epidemic in Gambia caused 2.5 severe illnesses per 100 inhabitants of nine villages with a case-fatality rate of 19%.[29] Serological studies carried out before an emergency immunization campaign revealed that about 12 persons had been infected for each severe clinical case; this ratio was 8:1 where yellow fever infection was the first apparent exposure to a flavivirus but 45:1 where the infection was secondary to a previous experience with a yellow fever–related virus. Between 1986 and 1988, Nigeria sustained a series of sylvatic and urban outbreaks, with several thousand officially notified cases and a case-fatality rate exceeding 50%.

Humans of all ages and both sexes are equally susceptible to yellow fever virus infection. Although frequently suggested, there is no scientific evidence that blacks are more resistant clinically to this virus than members of other races.

Observed patterns of human yellow fever are based on enzootic cycles of virus maintenance; despite decades of investigation, several major ecological mysteries persist. Classic urban yellow fever is transmitted in a human-mosquito cycle by the Stegomyia mosquito *A. aegypti.* African in origin, this species has been disseminated throughout the tropics and subtropics of the entire world. Yet yellow fever has never occurred in India or in the densely populated countries of southeast Asia. Control of this mosquito and of urban yellow fever during the 1920s in the Americas led to the recognition of a forest cycle causing "jungle" yellow fever. Each year 50 to 300 cases are reported from the countries comprising the Amazon, Orinoco, and Magdalena River systems of South America, and the virus makes additional periodic incursions into Panama and the island of Trinidad. Mosquito vectors are arboreal, diurnally active species of the genera *Haemagogus* and *Sabethes,* which oviposit in tree holes. Monkeys are the only proven nonhuman vertebrate hosts in this cycle, and certain species incur high mortality, which is frequently an early signal of human outbreaks. Although attack rates in humans are usually low, disease is concentrated in adult males involved in road building, lumbering, or agriculture where destruction of forest is in progress. The virus appears to wander about the vast tropical rain forest, returning to cause human disease at intervals of 5 to 10 years.

Yellow fever ecology in Africa is more complex. Monkeys and arboreal *Aedes* species, such as *A. africanus,* appear to maintain enzootic cycles with only scattered cases of human disease in the rain forests of central and eastern Africa. Larger outbreaks in rural and semiurban settings take place in the savannah and savannah-transition belts around the forests with extensions into western Africa. Here human-mosquito cycles are important and vectors include *A. luteocephalus, A. simpsoni,* and *A. furcifer,* which breed in tree holes. Recent experimental documentation of transovarial mosquito transmission of virus indicates that many questions concerning yellow fever ecology require reexamination. African monkeys are generally not susceptible to fatal yellow fever virus infection and thus do not provide an early signal of human outbreaks.

There is no specific treatment for human yellow fever, but prevention and control of epidemics can be achieved by use of one of the most successful live attenuated vaccines known to science. The 17D vaccine is highly immunogenic and has a very low incidence of clinical reaction. Rates for serious side effects are so low as not to have been accurately calculated. The vaccine confers long-lasting (perhaps lifetime) immunity, although international requirements for persons traveling to endemic or epidemic areas call for reimmunization every 10 years. No untoward effects on the human fetus have been reported, but in the absence of definitive data prudence requires due exercise of judgment regarding degree of potential exposure before immunization of pregnant women.

Adjuncts to mass vaccine programs during urban epidemics of yellow fever include destruction of *A. aegypti* breeding sites (sanitary engineering and cleanup efforts) and the use of insecticides to reduce both adult and larval mosquito populations. These measures are futile where virus transmission is of the "jungle" type.

Rift Valley Fever. Until 1977, outbreaks of Rift Valley fever (RVF) were limited to small numbers of cases observed in eastern and southern Africa in association with major epizootics among large wild and domestic animals. In that year, however, portions of the lower Nile River delta in Egypt were struck by an explosive epidemic-enzootic in which an estimated 200,000 cases with at least 598 deaths were recorded.[30]

RVF virus is a member of the phlebovirus genus, family *Bunyaviridae.* Clinical illness in humans as observed in eastern and southern Africa is usually an undifferentiated acute febrile illness marked by high but brief fever and no sequelae. Serious complications of clinical ocular serous retinopathy with central scotomata are seen in about 1% of cases, and in another 1% fulminant acute, usually nonicteric, hepatitis and hemorrhage with death develop. Nothing resembling the Egyptian epidemic had ever occurred before, however. In this outbreak patients with seemingly typical self-limited illnesses suddenly had hemorrhagic manifestations (gastrointestinal and other mucous membrane bleeding and skin petechiae) and died within 1 to 3 days. Infection-morbidity rates were not accurately determined, but it is estimated that up to 20% of persons of all ages and both sexes were infected in the Ismailia district.

Although the ecology of RVF virus in Africa is still not clear, there is evidence suggesting that biological transmission of the agent may be principally attributed to mosquitoes of the genus *Aedes*. In eastern and southern Africa, the association of RVF maintenance cycles with specific breeding habitats of *A. mcintoshi* (shallow depressions called "dambos") has been elucidated in Kenya.[31] During periods of high rainfall, flooding of dambos results in an abundance of *Aedes* and recrudescence of virus in transovarially infected mosquitoes. The latter initiate infection in domestic livestock, with secondary cycles of virus transmission being effected by *Anopheles, Culex,* and *Erethmapodites* vectors. Mechanical transmission by biting arthropods seems likely in addition because of the very high viremia levels (10^6 to 10^9 infectious units) reached in many domestic animals, and direct transmission to humans handling infected large animals or their carcasses is a recurrent phenomenon. Both contact with infectious blood and infectious aerosols are suspected as mechanisms.

The vectors involved in the Egyptian epidemic-epizootic, which affected a previously "virginal" human population and probably virginal animal herds, have not been conclusively elucidated; the principal candidate is the mosquito *Culex pipiens quinquefasciatus* which was present in large numbers in houses and environs during the months of October and November, when most cases occurred. After a pause during the winter months, renewed virus transmission to domestic animals and humans was documented during the spring and summer of both 1978 and 1979, but subsequently the virus has disappeared by virtue of the absence of critical elements for virus maintenance described above.

Retrospective evidence now suggests that the virus may have reached Egypt from the Sudan, where animal epizootics were documented during the 5-year period before 1977. Recent outbreaks involving animals and humans have been reported in Mauritania (1987) and Madagascar (1990). National and international concern over this emergent disease is not limited to public health workers. RVF virus causes a serious pantropic infection in domestic animals with significant mortality and high rates of abortion. Since it occurs naturally only in Africa, other nations are vitally interested in preventing its introduction into their animal industries. Thus work with this virus in the United States and many other countries is either totally proscribed or limited to facilities with a maximum containment configuration.

To date there is no treatment for the human disease, although the antiviral drug ribavirin, as well as interferon and interferon inducer, shows promise in preclinical studies. Inactivated vaccines provide immunity for 2 years after two or three doses and have been used to immunize livestock. Such products, however, are of little use should an outbreak occur in a previously uninfected country. The dynamics of virus transmission revealed in Egypt are so strikingly similar to those of VEE virus in the Americas that a live vaccine for animals that will confer rapid protection and curtail arthropod virus transmission is urgently needed. A live vaccine developed in South Africa has been associated with abortion in sheep. More recently, a live vaccine (MP-12) developed in the United States appears safe and highly effective but requires field testing. Such a vaccine, together with emergency mosquito-control measures, forms a rational armamentarium against a major tragedy, which could strike inside or away from Africa. Killed vaccines for human use have been used to protect laboratory workers and military populations.

Tickborne Infections

Kyasanur Forest Disease. Kyasanur forest disease (KFD) was first recognized in 1957 in a forest area of the state of Mysore in southwestern India. Attention of health authorities was drawn to a dramatic epizootic among monkeys in this forest, and it was feared that yellow fever had at last arrived in India. The causative agent was, indeed, shown to be a flavivirus, but it proved to be immunologically related to tickborne flaviviruses causing encephalitis and Omsk hemorrhagic fever in the Soviet Union.

The incubation period of human disease is 5 to 8 days. Clinical forms characterized by gastrointestinal hemorrhage, mild encephalitis, or both are commonly observed. Case-fatality rates vary between 3% and 10%, and the apparent-inapparent infection rate has been estimated at about 1:1. Within the slowly expanding endemic region in the state of Karnataka, the disease occurs in a strongly focal pattern, and the number of cases recorded annually ranges from 50 to more than 1000. Attack rates in given villages may reach 5/100 in a given year, but it is clear that variables related to the natural virus cycle, rather than immunity in human populations, are responsible for the large swings in disease occurrence.

KFD is strongly seasonal, most cases being recorded during the intermonsoon drier spring months from February through June. Adults are attacked more commonly than children, males slightly more often than females. This pattern reflects the seasonal activity of both the forest-dwelling tick vectors and humans. Larval and nymphal stages of *Haemaphysalis spinigera* and *H. turturis* are most active at this time, and people enter the forest to gather wood and wild plants for food during this annual pause in their agricultural year. Domestic livestock serve as an important source of blood for adult *Haemaphysalis* ticks but do not take part in the virus transmission cycle.

Human infection is most commonly acquired after the bite of tick nymphs. Although there is no evidence of transovarial tick transmission of KFD virus, the agent has been recovered frequently from forest monkeys, rodents, and squirrels. Birds are infected by KFD virus, although there is no conclusive proof that they serve as a source of tick infection. Thus the mechanism of overwintering for this virus has not been elucidated.

Hospital-based surveillance of acute febrile disease with hemorrhagic or neurological manifestations is maintained in the endemic area. Diagnoses are made principally by serologic procedures. An inactivated vaccine was tested in the affected region about 20 years ago. Although the vaccine was not highly immunogenic, a trial in villagers in the state of Karnataka showed efficacy. Research on improved vaccine is required.

Omsk Hemorrhagic Fever. Omsk hemorrhagic fever (OHF) is restricted to the mixed forest-steppe region of western Siberia. First recognized during World War II, clinical cases reported per year ranged from the teens to a few hundred during the next 2 decades but have apparently decreased dramatically in recent years, with only sporadic cases in muskrat trappers and their families. OHF is caused by a virus closely related to that of Russian spring-summer encephalitis, and the geographical areas of occurrence of these agents overlap, rendering many epidemiological aspects of OHF rather imprecise in the absence of a laboratory method for clear differentiation of these infections.

The disease resembles KFD. The incubation period of OHF in humans ranges from 3 to 7 days. Fever is typically present in two distinct waves. During the first interval of 5 to 12 days there are signs of bronchopneumonia and hemorrhagic manifestations, while mild neurological signs appear during the second febrile period of 2 to 7 days. Case-fatality rates are less than 5%. No data are available regarding human attack rates or inapparent/apparent infection ratios. Transmission of infection to humans occurs either by tick bite, the principal vector being the adult form of *Dermacentor pictus,* or by direct contact with infected muskrats, *Ondatra,* introduced into this region from Canada about 1929 to generate a fur industry. A variety of small mammals and tick species of the genus *Ixodes* have been incriminated by Soviet workers to explain the evidently complex natural virus cycle.[32]

Although there is no doubt that muskrats experience serious disease with high viremia when infected by OHF virus, it is not clear how they acquire the infection. Experimental studies show that this mammal is readily infected orally and that the OHF virus is naturally present in water frequented by muskrats and other rodents.[33] Persons trapping and skinning these animals formerly accounted for many cases during the winter and early spring months, and the possibility of aerosol transmission exists, since several laboratory infections have been recorded from such exposure. Muskrat populations have declined dramatically for unknown reasons in recent years, so that today the few cases reported occur mainly in May, June, and August, are all secondary to tick bite, and affect principally young women who work on farms.

Cross-protection against OHF may be afforded by tickborne encephalitis vaccines. However, given the low incidence of infection, vaccination is not a practical measure except for laboratory workers and, perhaps, muskrat hunters.

Crimean-Congo Hemorrhagic Fever (CCHF). Although compatible clinical accounts of Crimean-Congo hemorrhagic fever (CCHF) in central Asia date to the thirteenth century, epidemics occurring during World War II in the Crimea provided the first modern recognition and the name for this clinically serious syndrome. The causative agent of the disease was finally isolated in newborn mice in 1968. It was found to be a member of the large *Bunyaviridae* family, genus nairovirus, and, surprisingly, was antigenically indistinguishable from a virus of African origin, Congo virus, originally discovered in 1956.[34] This virus was subsequently proved to be responsible for previously independent nosologic hemorrhagic entities termed Bulgarian and central Asia hemorrhagic fever and has been designated as Crimean-Congo hemorrhagic fever (CCHF) virus.

The clinical disease caused by CCHF outside Africa is one of the most virulent viral hemorrhagic fevers. The incubation period is brief (2 to 9 days), and the onset of fever and nonspecific symptoms is sudden. Hemorrhagic manifestations, often with severe blood loss, appear after 3 to 7 days of illness. There are various mild neurological manifestations as well, and surviving patients occasionally suffer peripheral neuritis, emotional disturbances, or both for months or even years. The disease is acquired by exposure to infected ticks or by close contact with persons who have the disease. Case-fatality rates average 13% to 25% for tick-transmitted disease, but nearly 40% for contact infection, which is frequently nosocomial where strict isolation of patients and use of protective clothing are not practiced. Attack rates in certain areas of the Soviet Union have reached 14/1000 in "epidemic" years. The infection morbidity ratio in the Astrakhan and Rostov regions has been estimated at about 6:1.[35]

Depending on the geographical area, a large variety of tick species has been incompletely incriminated in the natural cycle and transmission to humans of CCHF virus. In Bulgaria and the valleys of the lower Don and Volga rivers of the Soviet Union, *Hyalomma marginatum,* a two-host species, is the principal vector. Immature stages parasitize hares, small rodents, and ground-feeding birds, while adults favor large domestic animals, such as cattle and sheep, and also attack humans. Persons engaged in pastoral and agricultural activities are most often attacked, and most cases occur during April to July, the period of peak activity of the adult ticks. Outbreaks of disease in central Asia are less strongly seasonal but tend to occur most often during summer months and are thought to be transmitted by ticks of the genera *Hyalomma, Rhipicephalus,* and *Boophilus,* which have life cycles ranging from single to as many as three hosts, most of which are large domestic animals. This epidemiological pattern extends from Dubai, Iraq, and Iran as far east as Pakistan.

To date approximately 70 human cases have been recognized in Africa, including temperate South Africa and tropical areas of eastern, western, and central Africa. The virus has been recovered on numerous occasions from ticks, cattle, and hedgehogs in these areas. The case-fatality rate (30% in South America) is similar to that in eastern Europe and the Soviet Union, and there is no evidence of a difference in virulence between virus strains.

The dynamics of virus maintenance in nature are not clear. CCHF in the Soviet Union has decreased significantly since 1970, but the biological correlates of this phenomenon were not elucidated. There is good evidence that CCHF virus is maintained serially in *H. marginatum* ticks by overwintering in infected nymphs and by both transtadial and transovarial passage.[36] Hares experience viremia and can, therefore, infect larval and nymphal ticks, but birds apparently serve only as hosts for tick reproduction. Viral biology in ticks and vertebrate hosts in Asia and Africa is even less well known.

Soviet workers state that virus-specific passive antibodies are of value in therapy of CCHF if given during the initial 3 days of illness. An immune globulin formulation for intravenous administration is used in Bulgaria, with good results reported. A formalinized mouse brain vaccine has been produced and tested in more than 150,000 persons in Bulgaria, but no definitive conclusions as to efficacy have been reported. Prevention of disease is stressed in the Soviet Union through use of personal measures, such as special clothing, tick repellants, and the systematic dipping of livestock to control adult stages of tick vectors. Whether these measures or natural forces are responsible for the observed decline in disease in the Volga and Don River basins during this decade is not known.

The lack of an animal model of CCHF disease is an obstacle to development of a vaccine and an antiviral drug. Ribavirin may be an effective therapeutic agent. In uncontrolled trials in South Africa, early initiation of intravenous therapy is said to be lifesaving. Given orally, the drug may also be useful for postexposure prophylaxis of case contacts. Future work on this disease is dependent on construction of more maximum containment laboratories since CCHF virus is a class IV pathogen, and it is well to remember that CCHF is the hemorrhagic fever most likely to be confused with a noninfectious cause of acute gastrointestinal hemorrhage, with potentially devastating consequences to patient and medical staff alike.

DISEASES ACQUIRED FROM RODENTS OR FROM UNIDENTIFIED SOURCES

Undifferentiated and Central Nervous System Infection

Lymphocytic Choriomeningitis. Human illness due to infection with lymphocytic choriomeningitis (LCM) virus has occurred in sporadic small outbreaks only in Europe, Asia, and the Americas, despite the fact that the reservoir-vector of this infection is the peridomestic wild mouse *Mus musculus,* which is found on all continents of the earth. The peculiar biology of the rodent-virus relationship, together with the initially unrecognized infection of animals other than *Mus* housed in medical research facilities, is responsible for the epidemiological patterns of human infection described here. The virus is the historical prototype of the *Arenavirus* family, and some of the LCM relatives produce acute hemorrhagic fever as described subsequently.

Human disease due to LCM is almost never fatal or hemorrhagic. Clinical syndromes range from an acute undifferentiated febrile illness to forms characterized by aseptic meningitis and mild encephalitis, the neurological symptoms and signs usually appearing during a second febrile period that begins 1 to 5 days after termination of an initial febrile episode of 3 to 7 days' duration. The virus is maintained in nature by chronic infection in feral *Mus* mice which arises from both horizontal and vertical contact among individuals of this species. Mice infected in utero or from maternal milk excrete significant quantities of virus in the urine for weeks, months, or throughout their entire lives. Transmission to humans occurs on exposure to infectious rodent urine, most commonly in the form of aerosols associated with the moving of hay or other detritus accumulated near mouse nests. An alternate host of significance in recent years in both Europe and the United States is the Syrian hamster. Outbreaks have occurred among personnel in medical research institutions where hamsters were housed, as well as among persons keeping hamsters as pets. These animals are also chronically infected with continuous viruria.

Because of this very specific transmission pattern, attack rates in human populations are almost impossible to determine. Infection is probably more common than is realized, since specific viral techniques are needed to make the diagnosis. Over 30 years ago about 10% of aseptic meningitis and encephalitis cases studied in one U.S. center over a period of several years were caused by LCM virus.[37] The accumulated literature suggests that adults are infected more often than children and that most *Mus*-related infections occur in fall and winter. Between 1965 and 1975, hamster-related outbreaks totaling 7, 48, and 181 proven cases occurred in New York, California, and 10 other states.[38]

There is no specific treatment and no vaccine is available for LCM infection. Good standards of environmental sanitation and testing of hamster colonies for endemic LCM virus infection represent available methods for avoiding human contact with this agent.

Hemorrhagic Fevers

Arenaviridae

Argentine and Bolivian Hemorrhagic Fevers. The clinically similar syndromes of Argentine and Bolivian hemorrhagic fevers were recognized during the decade between 1953 and 1963 and are restricted in occurrence to the countries for which they are named. They are caused by antigenically related but immunologically distinct arenaviruses called Junin and Machupo, respectively. Argentine hemorrhagic fever (AHF) is an endoepidemic disease found on the rich agricultural pampas of Buenos Aires, Córdoba, and Santa Fe provinces. From about 50 to more than 2000 cases occur per year during the autumn months of February through July, and the great majority of victims are men. Case-fatality rates are 5% to 15%. Bolivian hemorrhagic fever (BHF) is limited to the sparsely populated subtropical savannah of Beni province. Cases occur in adults and children, and there is no sex difference; the mortality rate is about 20%. Peak incidence of the disease usually occurs during the late rainy season and early dry season months of February to July. About 2000 cases were recorded during the years 1960 to 1964, but only sporadic small outbreaks have been observed since that time. Attack rates of both diseases may be high in circumscribed, small communities; they reached 20/100 per year in San Joaquin, Bolivia, and 10/100 in 1953 at O'Higgins, Argentina.

Inapparent infections rarely occur in either AHF or BHF. Clinical disease may be mild (resembling flu), or it may progress to a hemorrhagic form with acute shock and paradoxical hemoconcentration or a neurological form marked by intention tremors, other signs of cerebellar and brain stem dysfunction, and generalized convulsions. Viremia is sporadic or of low titer in these diseases, and nosocomial infection, although reported, is unusual.

Chronic viremic and viruric infection of rodents has been shown to be the principal means of virus maintenance and, by strong inference, of transmission to humans. The main host of AHF is the wild mouse *Calomys musculinus.* Similar in size to *Mus musculus,* this indigenous rodent invades crops during the fall from permanent harborage along roadsides and railways. Population densities are highest in fields of maize. Migratory workers harvesting maize by hand were the principal victims during the 1950s and early 1960s. The number of cases has not diminished, despite recent mechanization of maize harvesting in the region. Combine and truck operators now have attack rates estimated as 20 to 50 times those of the earlier migrant laborers. Aerosols as well as blood and fluids from mice crushed in the combines are now thought to be primary sources of infection.

BHF ecology is different from that of AHF in several ways. The reservoir host is *Calomys callosus,* a larger rodent that is naturally found at the edge of riverine forest-savannah formations. When humans cut the forest to plant gardens, *C. callosus* invades these plots and the houses of humans as well. Thus, disease transmission by the continual excretion of virus in the urine of this species occurs in and near homes, resulting in disease among all members of the population.

Argentine workers have proved in a double-blind clinical trial that human plasma containing Junin virus antibodies reduces mortality from 15% to 1% if given during the first 8 days of illness.[39] This mode of therapy should work equally well for BHF. Outbreaks of BHF have been controlled and prevented by vigorous rodent-control programs in affected towns and ranches. Machupo virus–infected *Calomys* mice have chronic splenomegaly, and this marker has been absent for some time. For example, no BHF has been documented in San Joaquin since 1965, despite the fact that a few infected splenomegalic mice have been captured on several occasions. Rodent control does not appear feasible in the vast cultivars of Argentina, and work on Junin virus vaccine is being actively pursued.

A live, attenuated Junin vaccine developed in the United States is in phase III clinical trials in Argentina. The vaccine cross-protects against BHF in monkey models.

Lassa Fever. First recognized during 1969 in Nigeria, Lassa fever has focused worldwide attention on problems related to the management and control of class IV pathogens. This was a result of several west African nosocomial outbreaks in rural hospitals in Nigeria, Liberia, and Sierra Leone, where direct secondary transmission with high mortality occurred. Moreover, at least 20 persons known to be suffering from this disease have flown on commercial aircraft to large urban centers in Europe, North

America, Israel, and Japan. Imported cases have occurred in the United States and Great Britain.

The disease appears to be restricted to western Africa, occurring principally in savannah landscapes or tropical forest areas severely modified by human agricultural activity. In its severe form, Lassa fever is a protean febrile disease that attacks many vital organs, including the heart, lungs, liver, pancreas, and kidneys. Onset is nonspecific; the clinical triad of pharyngitis, retrosternal pain, and proteinuria appear useful diagnostically. Jaundice is unusual, but pulmonary and peritoneal effusions are commonly observed. A fulminating episode with shock occurs in only about 20% of hospitalized cases. Virus is present in blood and abnormal effusions for many days and has been recovered from throat washings and urine. The agent also attacks the human fetus, and abortion with increased mortality is a common feature of infection among pregnant women.

Prospective laboratory-based studies of Lassa fever in eastern Sierra Leone have demonstrated that transmission is endemic, with peak activity in the dry season months of January through May. The disease is of major public health importance, accounting for more than one third of all deaths on medical wards of hospitals in the endemic region.[40] Attack rates range up to 5/1000 per year. The case-fatality rate is 16% in hospitalized cases. Epidemiological investigations conducted in villages, however, show that up to one half of the population has been infected with the virus, and annual infection rates as high as 12% have been documented, giving an infection/case ratio of about 16:1. Persons of all ages and both sexes are infected and suffer severe clinical illness; why only certain persons become very sick is not known.

Lassa virus, most closely related immunologically to LCM virus among the *Arenaviridae,* is maintained and transmitted naturally by the rodent *Mastomys natalensis.*[41] This large mouse, which resembles a juvenile *Rattus rattus* in appearance, is widely distributed over much of Africa south of the Sahara. In western Africa it is chronically infected and sheds virus in the urine for many weeks. Recent work has shown there are at least two distinct genetic species of *Mastomys,* one having 32 chromosomes, which is found principally in and close to houses in wet forested areas, and another with 38 chromosomes, which predominates in the savannah bushland. Lassa virus infection occurs in both rodents, but the ecological adaptation of the 32-chromosome *Mastomys* results in greater transmission of Lassa virus to man in areas with wet climates. Whether and how much person-to-person transmission occurs in villages has not been determined, but it is noteworthy that little or no nosocomial spread has taken place in two hospitals where nearly 400 patients were treated in a 2-year period.

Surveillance for Lassa fever presents a difficult challenge. Geographical surveys in western Africa have disclosed significant foci of infection in areas where the disease has never been clinically detected. Because the clinical spectrum observed in laboratory-documented infection is so wide, it is now clear that only the most severe cases could be clinically suspected, and probably then only if a cluster of such cases occurred with transmission to the hospital staff. Thus specific diagnosis is essential and best made by measurement of immunofluorescent or enzyme-immunosorbent virus-specific IgM antibodies, which appear in nearly all patients within 7 to 10 days after the onset of symptoms. It has been found that mortality in Lassa fever is directly related to virus concentration in blood. The potential hazards associated with such laboratory work and the paucity of virological laboratories in western Africa have limited the application of this technology.

The occurrence of imported cases in the United States and other countries emphasizes the need to include Lassa fever in the differential diagnosis of severe febrile illness. Containment of the patient, with the use of standard barrier nursing techniques and effective decontamination procedures is essential. Treatment of patients consists of intravenous administration of ribavirin, which has proved effective in trials in Africa. Fever surveillance, but not quarantine, for 3 weeks is indicated for all persons who have been in face-to-face contact with Lassa fever patients before their effective isolation. Persons at highest risk (e.g., those with direct blood contact) may be given oral ribavirin prophylactically.

Control of Lassa fever represents a major biological challenge. Development of a vaccine is in an early stage. Rodent-control trials in villages where 32-chromosome *Mastomys* mice predominate have reduced virus transmission to humans, but it seems unlikely that this approach can be systematically applied throughout the immense endemic area of west Africa.

African Hemorrhagic Fever: Marburg and Ebola Disease. Among the most severe and mysterious viral pathogens to emerge in this century, Marburg and Ebola viruses have burst on an unprepared world only since 1967. Knowledge of these agents is largely restricted to a few distinct human outbreaks: Marburg, Germany, and Belgrade, Yugoslavia (1967), Zimbabwe, and South Africa (1975), Nairobi, Kenya (1980), and the Mt. Elyon area of Kenya (1987) for Marburg virus; northern Zaire and southwestern Sudan (1976 and 1979) for Ebola virus.

The viruses are morphologically similar but immunologically distinct. They are long pleomorphic rods reminiscent of but distinguishable from rhabdoviruses, such as rabies virus, and now placed in a new family, the *Filoviridae.* Clinical disease seen during each of the outbreaks involving 3 to 400 persons was very severe and was similar in all instances. The incubation period averaged 1 week, and fatal infections were uniformly marked by the advent of a hemorrhagic diathesis after 4 to 7 days of generalized symptoms. Disseminated intravascular coagulation was documented in most such cases where it was sought. A maculopapular rash, necrotizing nonicteric hepatitis, and chemical pancreatitis are common findings. Case-fatality rates range from 25% to 88%, and person-to-person transmission, largely nosocomial, occurred in each epidemic. Serologic studies in Zaire suggest that the mild illness or inapparent infection rate for Ebola virus was about 5:1 when the population for the entire region centered on Yandongi was considered, but about 1:1 when only villages in which there were acute clinical cases were considered. Clinical attack rates during this outbreak of more than 300 cases ranged from 2/1000 in young children to 7 to 12/1000 adults.

The ecology of both Marburg and Ebola viruses is unknown. The singular German-Yugoslavian outbreak occurred among workers in laboratories in which kidney cells from *Cercopithecus* monkeys were processed for use in the preparation of poliovirus vaccine, and secondary cases resulted among medical staff and family members. Subsequent work, however, failed to disclose any evidence of natural infection in this or other monkey species in the region of Uganda, where the infected animals had been captured. The source of infection in the index case during the small outbreak in southern Africa could not be established. Likewise, the precise origin of the Sudan and Zaire epidemics of 1976, which occurred nearly concurrently, was not elucidated. Secondary direct transmission in both of these epidemics, however, was a significant feature and may have accounted for all or nearly all of the cases. Contaminated needles and syringes were very important means of infection in Zaire, and close, continued contact with patients was responsible for many infections in both countries.[42] Overall secondary attack rates ranged between 3% and 14%, and the institution of simple isolation together with the use of protective clothing was sufficient to terminate virus transmission. Although the blood of patients contains large amounts of virus, there is little to suggest that infectious aerosols played a major role in these dramatic epidemics. Had this been the case, the worst modern human pandemic imaginable would surely have occurred.

Prospective and retrospective work in Zaire since 1976 has disclosed that Ebola virus is endemic and presumably enzootic in the rain forest of the Zaire (Congo) River basin.[43] Sporadic cases occurring in 1972 and 1977 were documented, the former leading to a secondary case in a physician who suffered a laceration while performing an autopsy. Efforts are in progress to search for vertebrate reservoirs of infection in this region where serosurveys disclose that 1% to 10% of persons have antibodies to the agent.

In 1989–1990, Ebola virus was responsible for several epizootics of fatal hemorrhagic fever in captive macaques imported from the Philippines into the United States.[44] At least four human infections occurred among monkey handlers, but there was no overt disease; this suggests that the responsible virus strains differ biologically from those in Africa. The epizootics resulted in several new restrictions on importation and quarantine of monkeys for research. Studies showed that Ebola-like viruses have a wider geographic distribution than previously recognized and appear to be strongly associated with nonhuman primates.

No vaccines or antiviral drugs are yet available for prevention or treatment.

Hemorrhagic Fever with Renal Syndrome (HFRS). Synonyms for HFRS are Korean hemorrhagic fever, epidemic hemorrhagic fever, hemorrhagic fever, hemorrhagic nephrosonephritis, and nephropathia epidemica. HFRS occurs across a wide belt of northern Eurasia from Japan and Korea to northern Scandinavia, including portions of China, the Soviet Union, Yugoslavia, Czechoslovakia, Bulgaria, Hungary, Finland, Norway, and Sweden. After more than 40 years of effort, the causative agent of this syndrome was finally isolated during 1976 and 1977 in Korea.[45] The virus, named Hantaan, is a member of the *Bunyaviridae* and represents the prototype of a probably new genus.[46] Several other viruses, related by immunofluorescence but distinct by neutralization, have been described.

HFRS appears to have a rather long incubation period of up to 4 weeks, and the severe clinical form of illness, seen mostly in Asia east of the Ural Mountains, comprises three distinct phases: toxic-hemorrhagic, uremic with renal shutdown, and diuretic with major abnormalities in fluid and electrolyte balance. Milder forms are seen in Europe, but some degree of renal impairment is a unique feature of this hemorrhagic syndrome. Attack rates are frequently difficult to calculate. More than 2000 cases occurred among United Nations and Korean soldiers during the Korean War, but the denominator of persons exposed was not accurately measured. During a notable epidemic at Ufa in the Soviet Union in the 1960s, about 1000 cases occurred in a population of 400,000, or 2.5 cases per 1000 population. Inapparent infection rates remain to be determined. Case-fatality rates vary from 1% to 10% in Asia to less than 1% in Europe. Nosocomial infections have not been documented.

Adults are everywhere attacked clinically more often than children. Most cases occur during the northern spring and again in the fall. There is strong temporal association between illness and recent contact with field or forest; thus farmers, construction crews, hikers, campers, and soldiers are the predominant victims. Investigation of many focal disease outbreaks repeatedly pointed toward contact with rodents or their excreta as probable sources of infection, and many authors suggested that ectoparasites of wild rodents, particularly mites, were important as vectors for transmission of the agent to humans. Thus it was not surprising that the initial recovery of the causative agent of HFRS was made from tissues of the healthy wild-caught field mouse *Apodemus agrarius* in Korea. This was accomplished with the use of indirect immunofluorescence employing convalescent human serum to detect antigen in frozen sections of rodent lung, liver, and kidney.

Intensive work in an endemic region of Korea has revealed that only *A. agrarius* seems to be infected, that infection is at least semichronic, and that annual population peaks of this species precisely precede the observed spring-fall peaks in human disease. The role ectoparasites may play in the cycle is under study. The agent causing the milder clinical syndrome in Scandinavia was recently recovered from the vole, *Clethrionomys glariolus* and named Puumala virus. Another virus (Seoul virus) distinguishable from Hantaan has been obtained from both wild and laboratory rats in several countries, and acute disease in laboratory workers and urban residents has been documented.[47] Recent evidence suggests that Seoul virus may be responsible for chronic renal disease and hypertension in a small proportion of the inner city populations of Baltimore (and possibly other rat-infested urban areas).

Surveillance of this syndrome has classically consisted of a clinical search for patients with compatible illness during the spring and fall in areas of known endemic activity. Now that specific immunological methods are available, it is certain that surveillance and the elucidation of many fundamental epidemiological parameters will rapidly improve.

Control of HFRS is in its infancy. Reduction of certain rodent populations during years of high reproduction may prove to be of value, and the protection from rodent contamination of foodstuffs to be consumed without cooking is a reasonable recommendation. Formalinized rat and mouse brain vaccines have been produced in both North Korea and South Korea; the former has undergone large-scale field trials and is said to be effective. Efforts to develop molecularly based vaccines are under way in the United States, China, and the Soviet Union.

A placebo-controlled trial of intravenous ribavirin conducted in 1986–87 in China showed that initiation of treatment early in the course of the disease reduced mortality and the incidence of renal failure, hemorrhage, and hypertension.

Rickettsial Infections

Bradley N. Doebbeling

There are at least 11 major rickettsial diseases of man, which are caused by six antigenically related groups of organisms (Table 11-3). Most of the rickettsioses are characterized by the syndrome of severe headache, fever, myalgias, and rash of a specific pattern. There is no rash with Q fever. The epidemiological and public health aspects of rickettsial diseases are emphasized in this account. More comprehensive reviews of the historical, clinical, microbiological, and diagnostic aspects of the rickettsial infections are available elsewhere.[1–6]

The Rickettsiaceae that are pathogenic for humans are classified in four genera: *Rickettsia* (including the typhus, scrub typhus, and spotted fever groups), *Rochalimaea, Coxiella,* and *Ehrlichia.* The latter organisms have only recently been shown to be important causes of human disease. Numerous other rickettsiae occur as parasites of vertebrates and arthropods. Although a few of these may be of minor importance as human pathogens, they are not considered here.

Considerable progress has been made in the past decade in

TABLE 11-3. RICKETTSIAL DISEASES OF MAN

Disease	Etiological Agent	Geographical Distribution	Vector(s)	Natural Hosts
▪ TYPHUS GROUP				
Epidemic typhus	*Rickettsia prowazekii*	Africa, Central and South America, Asia, potentially worldwide	Human body louse (*Pediculus humanus corporis*)	Man; flying squirrel; others(?)
Brill-Zinsser disease	*Rickettsia prowazekii*	Worldwide	None	Man (recurrent attacks)
Murine typhus	*Rickettsia typhi* (formerly *L. mooseri*)	Temperate zones, worldwide	Oriental rat flea (*Xenopsylla cheopis*); others(?)	Rats (*Rattus rattus, Rattus norvegicus*) cats, opossums; other peridomestic mammals(?)
▪ SCRUB TYPHUS GROUP				
Scrub typhus	*Rickettsia tsutsugamushi*	Asia, Australia, Pacific Islands	Larval trombiculid mites (*Leptotrombidium* species)	Small wild rodents; birds
▪ SPOTTED FEVER GROUP				
Rocky Mountain spotted fever (and related spotted fevers)	*Rickettsia rickettsii*	Western hemisphere	Numerous tick species (*Dermacentor, Amblyomma, Rhipicephalus, Haemaphysalis*)	Numerous small mammals (rodents, rabbits, hares and dogs)
Mediterranean spotted fever	*Rickettsia conorii*	Mediterranean region, Black Sea region, Middle East, Africa, India	Numerous tick species (*Rhipicephalus, Hyalomma, Amblyomma, Dermacentor*[?], *Ixodes*[?])	Small mammals (rodents, dogs); birds(?)
North Asian tick typhus	*Rickettsia sibirica*	Siberia, central Asia, China, Mongolia, Pakistan (?)eastern Europe	Various tick species (*Dermacentor, Haemaphysalis, Rhipicephalus*)	Small mammals (rodents); domestic animals(?)
Queensland tick typhus	*Rickettsia australis*	Australia	Ticks (*Ixodes holocyclus, Ixodes tasmani*)	Small marsupials, rodents
Rickettsialpox	*Rickettsia akari*	North America, Soviet Union, Korea, South Africa	Gamasid mite (*Liponyssoides* [= *Allodermanyssus*] *sanguineus*)	House mouse (*Mus musculus*), other rodents(?)
▪ MISCELLANEOUS				
Ehrlichiosis	*Ehrlichia canis*	U.S.A., unknown	*Rhipicephalus sanguineus*(?)	Canids
Sennetsu fever	*Ehrlichia sennetsu*	Japan	Unknown	Humans(?)
Q fever	*Coxiella burnetii*	Worldwide	Inhalation, ingestion(?), numerous ixodid and argasid tick species	Cattle, sheep, goats, other domestic animals; numerous wild mammals; birds(?)
Trench fever	*Rochalimaea quintana*	Potentially worldwide	Human body louse (*Pediculus humanus corporis*)	Man

clarifying the taxonomy, biochemistry, genetics, and morphology of the Rickettsiaceae. The rickettsiae are obligate intracellular parasites that can propagate only in living cells. They are small coccoid to rod-shaped bacteria, usually 0.3 to 0.5 μm in diameter and up to 2.0 μm in length. The Rickettsiae have typical bacterial cell walls and cytoplasmic membranes, contain both DNA and RNA, and divide by binary fission. They may be cultured and isolated in several laboratory animal species, arthropod vectors, embryonated eggs, and some cell cultures; however, this is a time-consuming, expensive, and occasionally dangerous process.

Serology is the mainstay of laboratory diagnosis, although diagnostic titers are not achieved until the second week of illness or later. Indirect fluorescent antibody (IFA) tests are the most widely accepted serological diagnostic techniques; they are now available for all the human rickettsioses except trench fever.[1] The complement-fixation (CF) test using acute- and convalescent-phase sera and the nonspecific Weil-Felix (WF) reaction for agglutinating antibodies against certain *Proteus* strains are still widely used, although both tests lack sensitivity.[1] A fourfold rise in titer by any technique other than the WF reaction is considered diagnostic. Direct immunofluorescence, if available, may demonstrate *R. rickettsii* in the skin lesions of Rocky Mountain spotted fever or *R. conorii* in the lesions of Mediterranean spotted fever. For most rickettsial infections, however, therapy must be initiated on the basis of clinical presentation and epidemiological setting.

The natural life cycles of rickettsiae involve arthropod vectors (lice, fleas, mites, or ticks) and various vertebrate hosts. In ticks and mites, transovarial transmission of the agent to the offspring frequently occurs. The vector transmits the rickettsiae to animals or man by fecal contamination of the bite wound, scratches or other skin breaks; occasionally direct bite inoculation or inhalation of aerosols may occur. Man is an incidental host and not important in the life cycle of the rickettsial organism, with the exception of louseborne typhus. In the latter disease, man is the major reservoir.

Rickettsial infections cause a generalized capillary and small vessel vasculitis, with consequent damage in the host's skin, brain, lungs, kidneys, and heart. Chronic infection or late relapse (especially in epidemic typhus and trench fever) and long-term persistence of rickettsiae in lymph nodes or other tissues is common. Antibiotic treatment with tetracyclines or chloramphenicol is usually effective if started early. Most available drugs inhibit the organisms rather than kill them; general supportive measures and the host's immune response are also important factors in recovery. Prevention and control of rickettsial diseases depend on avoidance of vector-infested sites, vector and vertebrate host control by habitat modification or use of appropriate pesticides, and specific immunization.

TYPHUS GROUP

Epidemic Typhus. *Rickettsia prowazekii* has been responsible for millions of cases of epidemic or louseborne typhus (typhus exanthematicus, classic typhus fever) and uncounted deaths throughout history. This disease has disappeared from much of the world except remote areas of Africa, Asia, Central, and South America. It may, however, recur under conditions of famine, war, or other disasters.

Gerhard defined the disease clinically in 1836, and Brill described a milder (recrudescent) form unassociated with body lice in 1910. After an incubation period of 1 to 2 weeks, there is an abrupt onset of fever, chills, malaise, muscle ache, and severe headache. Approximately 5 days later a faint pink macular rash usually develops over the upper trunk. The rash may become darker, maculopapular, and confluent, covering the entire body but usually sparing the face, palms, and soles, or it may gradually fade away. High fever becomes constant early, typically lasting up to 2 weeks, terminating by lysis. Changes in mental status occur frequently, occasionally with delirium or coma. Mortality ranges from 5% to 40% if the disease is untreated, increasing with age. Tetracycline or chloramphenicol is usually curative if given early. Recovery is complete, with immunity to reinfection. Epidemic typhus may recur decades later, however, as Brill-Zinsser (BZ) disease, which is usually milder with little or no rash.

Man is the host and long-term reservoir. The body louse, *Pediculus humanus corporis,* is infected by a blood meal from a rickettsemic patient. *R. prowazekii* replicates in the louse's intestinal tract and then is excreted in its feces within 1 week. After a blood meal, the louse defecates, contaminating the broken skin of the host. Other potential mechanisms of infection include either mucosal contact or inhalation of dried louse feces. The louse dies of its rickettsial infection within a few weeks. *R. prowazekii,* however, may remain viable for months to years in the dried state. Lice can be infected by feeding on persons with BZ disease as well as those with acute typhus, thus ensuring the perpetuation of *R. prowazekii.* Head lice, crab lice, and some fleas may be experimentally infected, although their role as natural vectors is uncertain. Transmission between humans usually requires close personal contact or exposure to contaminated clothing or bedding. Rickettsia are not present in human secretions, so there is no direct person-to-person spread.

Extrahuman reservoirs have been suspected in ticks and certain animal species; yet most of the evidence is tenuous. The southern flying squirrel, *Glaucomys volans,* found in the eastern United States has recently been implicated as an animal reservoir for *R. prowazekii.* Human infections have been linked to the flying squirrel, although the mode of transmission has yet to be demonstrated.[4] This flying squirrel–associated typhus agent appears to have a lower virulence than the louseborne variant. While human body lice may be experimentally infected with *R. prowazekii* from flying squirrels, the general scarcity of body lice in the United States may explain the lack of outbreaks in this country.[1]

Certain social factors that predispose to epidemic typhus, including overcrowding, poverty, and infrequent bathing or changing of clothes, are especially common during cold weather or periods of war. Most cases occur in the winter or spring. Epidemic typhus nearly disappeared from Europe, Asia, and areas in Africa, where it was once common, coincident with improved sanitation, delousing measures, antibiotics, and better medical care after World War II. Under international sanitary regulations, louseborne typhus ceased to be a quarantinable disease in 1971, although the World Health Organization (WHO) continues to monitor the disease because of its epidemic potential. Endemic foci still produce thousands of cases annually in highland areas of central Africa (particularly Rwanda, Burundi, and Ethiopia) and southern Africa, the Himalayas and Asian highlands, eastern Europe, Mexico, and Central and South America. Case reporting is incomplete because of inadequate surveillance and often undocumented by specific laboratory tests, particularly in the areas of highest endemicity. The presence of the vector, as determined by social, cultural, and climatic conditions affects the geographic distribution of cases. No epidemics have occurred in the United States since 1893, and the last recorded small outbreak occurred in 1921. Brill-Zinsser disease is reported sporadically from many countries, particularly in southeastern Europe.

Prevention of epidemic typhus is accomplished primarily by application of residual insecticide powder to the individual, the clothing, and the bedding on which the eggs are laid and lice reside. Several applications may be required periodically, since the eggs are resistant to most insecticides and continue to hatch. A pediculicide, such as DDT or lindane, that is effective on the local body louse population should be used. Alternatively, malathion or carbaryl may be effective in resistant settings. Washing clothes in hot water kills lice and eggs. Head lice and pubic lice should also be eradicated with effective chemical agents. Similar treatment of family or other close contacts is advisable. Once deloused, the patient need not be quarantined, but others who have been exposed should remain under surveillance for the disease for 2 weeks. In epidemics, treatment of the entire community is often the most practical and effective approach.

As a secondary measure, immunization of all susceptible persons during an outbreak may also be useful. A formaldehyde-inactivated vaccine prepared from infected chicken eggs is commercially available. The vaccine is administered in two subcutaneous injections 4 or more weeks apart, with yearly boosters thereafter for persons at continued high risk. Although not completely protective, the vaccine reduces the severity and mortality of epidemic typhus. Persons working in areas endemic for the disease, as well as laboratory personnel working with *R. prowazekii,* should receive the vaccine.

Murine Typhus. In 1926 Maxcy differentiated murine or endemic typhus (fleaborne typhus, shop typhus, urban typhus) from epidemic typhus in the eastern United States on clinical and epidemiological grounds. The rodent reservoir and flea vector of the agent, *Rickettsia typhi* (formerly *R. mooseri*), were demonstrated in the early 1930s.

Murine typhus is usually milder than epidemic typhus, with an incubation period of 1 to 2 weeks. Fever lasts 1 to 2 weeks, often accompanied by persistent headache, myalgia, nausea and vomiting, abdominal pains, conjunctivitis, splenomegaly, and pneumonitis; delirium, stupor, or coma occurs rarely. On the fourth day a macular rash usually appears (in 70% of the cases) on the chest and abdomen, becoming maculopapular and persisting 4 to 8 days without significant limb involvement. Permanent sequelae are rare, and no BZ-like phenomenon has been observed. Death is uncommon (<2% of cases) and a single attack usually confers reliable immunity.

Murine typhus occurs in temperate zones throughout the world, principally in Malaysia, southeast Asia, Africa, Central America, and the Mediterranean region. In the United States, it is most prevalent in the southeastern and Gulf states. During the 15-year period prior to 1946 approximately 42,000 cases occurred. Subsequently, a sharp decrease occurred; this was attributed primarily to improved rat control. Fewer than 80 cases are now recorded annually in the United States, although the disease is probably greatly underreported. Murine typhus occurs primarily in urban areas and certain rural settings infested by wild rats (e.g., grain-storage facilities). A seasonal incidence peak occurs in late summer and fall, although the disease may peak in early summer along the Gulf coast. Cases tend to be sporadic or to occur in clusters or small outbreaks related to common exposure to a rat-flea focus. The infection is relatively frequent in southern Texas, particularly among older adults and Hispanics.[7] There is no documented person-to-person spread.

The main life cycle involves a reservoir of rats (*Rattus rattus* and *Rattus norvegicus*) and other rodents and the vector *Xenopsylla cheopis* (tropical rat flea). The rat flea is infected by the blood of a rickettsemic host, remains infected for life, and readily infects other rats and man. *R. typhi* infects the intestinal tract of the flea, and transovarial transmission may occur. Flea feces or crushed fleas apparently contaminate skin breaks or the mucous membranes; direct flea bites or inhalation of aerosols may also cause infection. The human flea, *Pulex irritans*, and the human body louse may play a role in transmission. Numerous wild vertebrates (mice, voles, squirrels, rabbits, skunks, opossums) are natural hosts and may bring infected fleas into close proximity. Dog and cat fleas have been suspected as occasional vectors for man.

Prevention requires ongoing control of the natural host and vector: rodent-control measures and use of organophosphorous or carbamate insecticides. Local public health authorities should be consulted for advice on approved residual-action insecticides to apply to rat habitats. Flea control should be achieved initially, followed by rat poisoning and trapping, rodent-proofing of buildings, and elimination of rodent shelter and food attractants. Failure to control the flea population initially may lead to human outbreaks as the infected fleas move from dying rats to man. There is no specific vaccine. Epidemic typhus vaccine does not protect against murine typhus; nevertheless, there may be some reciprocal cross-protection following a natural attack of each disease.

Scrub Typhus. Although scrub typhus (tsutsugamushi disease, miteborne typhus, Japanese river fever, tropical typhus, rural typhus) was first described by Li Shi-Zhen in sixteenth-century China, definitive studies were first reported by Japanese workers in the late nineteenth century. The ancient name for scrub typhus in China was *sha shi du*, meaning chigger fever.[8] The disease is known in Japan as tsutsugamushi disease, which, roughly translated, means "noxious mite."[9] Fletcher first differentiated between murine typhus and scrub typhus in 1926. A rickettsial agent (*Rickettsia orientalis*) was described in 1930, and the current name (*R. tsutsugamushi*) was assigned in 1931. There is marked antigenic and pathogenic diversity of the agent, with three major and multiple minor serotypes recognized.

The clinical spectrum of scrub typhus is broad, with most infections of mild to moderate severity. Significant morbidity occurs regularly, however, and mortality rates may range from 0 to 30% if the disease is untreated. The first sign of disease after an incubation period of 6 to 21 days is a vesicular lesion at the site of mite attachment, which later becomes an eschar or ulcer, with tender lymphadenopathy common. Although an eschar develops in 85% to 90% of patients,[9] in its absence the disease may be misdiagnosed as fever of unknown origin.[10] Fever lasts up to 2 weeks, accompanied by headache, myalgia, and occasionally conjunctivitis or cough. In one third of the patients a central macular rash may appear on the trunk and in the axillary folds around the fifth day, spreading to involve the proximal arms and legs. The rash usually becomes maculopapular, lasting only a few days. Myocarditis, pneumonitis, cardiac failure, disseminated intravascular coagulation, and cerebritis may occur.

Infection with one strain does not assure immunity against subsequent infection by others. Nevertheless, repeat attacks may be milder or atypical. No person-to-person transmission has been documented. Tetracyclines and chloramphenicol are relatively effective, but relapses are common, often requiring another course of treatment. Doxycycline appears to be particularly reliable, and relapses are rare following its use.[8]

R. tsutsugamushi strains are widespread throughout much of the Far East and the western Pacific, including Malaysia, India, Pakistan, Indonesia, southern China, eastern Soviet Union, Korea, Japan, the Philippines and the South Pacific islands, and northern Australia. It remains a leading cause of illness in indigenous populations throughout endemic areas. World War II brought the disease to the attention of the Western world; 18,000 cases occurred in U.S. troops, with up to a 35% mortality rate. Similarly, scrub typhus was a frequent source of illness in U.S. troops during the Vietnam conflict. Scrub typhus is seen in North America primarily among returning travelers. A well-defined seasonal occurrence that peaks during the hot, wet months occurs in many areas, although the disease may peak in the winter or occur year-round in other regions. Seasonal incidence varies by region but is related to the presence of the larval mite. The incidence of scrub typhus in Japan has markedly increased since 1975, predominantly during the winter.[9]

The basic life cycle is complex and only partly understood. Larval mites ("chiggers") of the Family Trombiculidae, subgenus *Leptotrombidium*, are the vectors and reservoirs. Although approximately 150 species have been described, only a few are known to be important human pathogens (e.g., *L. deliensis, L. akamushi, L. fletcheri, L. arenicola, L. scutellaris, L. pallida,* and *L. pavlovskyi*). The larval mite feeds just once on the lymph and tissue juice of a mammalian host and transmits the agent by fecal contamination. Other life stages of the mite are free living only; transovarial or vertical transmission occurs regularly, with nearly all offspring affected.[9] The natural reservoir includes many species of wild rats, monkeys, tree shrews, and birds, although natural infection occurs in multiple animal species.[9]

The ecological niches of *R. tsutsugamushi* are highly variable, being especially common in wet tropical and subtropical areas, including equatorial rain forests, along riverbanks and seashores, and occasionally in semideserts, Himalayan alpine meadows, and areas with harsh, cold winters.[8] The agent may persist or amplify in hyperendemic foci of vector mites as small as a few square feet.[9] The limited mobility of unfed larvae, the clustering of broods of larvae within a localized area, and the clustering of hundreds of larvae at a few sites on an individual animal, where they may be brushed off at one time, favor the focal distribution of larvae on the ground.[9] Endemic foci usually occur where secondary or transitional vegetation (e.g., abandoned farmland or man-made forest clearings) has created a habitat attractive to the natural hosts of the vector mites. The chiggers or mites are not host-specific and will attack any animal, including man, that invades their limited territory.

Focal areas known to be endemic should be avoided. Alternatively, vertebrate hosts and protective vegetation can be eliminated and the area can be treated with chlorinated hydrocarbons (e.g., lindane, dieldrin, or chlordane). Personal prophylaxis with protective clothing, treatment of clothing with insecticides such as benzyl benzoate, and application of mite repellants (diethyltoluamide) to the skin is useful. Prophylactic antibiotic use for heavily exposed persons has been studied but requires further evaluation. There is no commercial vaccine.

SPOTTED FEVER GROUP

Rocky Mountain Spotted Fever. Rocky Mountain spotted fever (RMSF) and related spotted fevers of the western hemisphere are the best-known and most severe of the tickborne typhus diseases. Although various names are used (São Paulo typhus, fiebre manchada), there is basically a single clinical entity and a single agent, *R. rickettsii.* Closely related species and diseases occur in Europe, Africa, and Asia (see below). RMSF has been recognized as a distinct entity in the United States since the late 1800s; various workers, most notably Ricketts in Montana (1906), defined the disease and described the natural cycle of the agent.

Illness usually begins abruptly 2 to 12 days after tick exposure. A high, persistent fever of 2 to 3 weeks' duration, severe headache, and myalgias are characteristic, while nausea, vomiting, abdominal pain, and conjunctivitis occur frequently. The maculopapular rash, present in about 90% of the cases, usually does not appear until the fourth day or later. The rash begins on the ankles or wrists (50%) or on the palms and soles (25%) and spreads rapidly to the rest of the body; it becomes petechial and often is accompanied by edema and cyanosis. Headache is typically severe; meningismus or focal neurologic deficits may result, occasionally with permanent neurological sequelae. Necrosis of the skin lesions or gangrene of extremities may occur. Thrombocytopenia, anemia, coagulopathy, renal failure, pulmonary edema, and involvement of all organ systems may be seen. The overall fatality rate is about 20% untreated, higher in the very young, in adults over 30, in males, and in persons who are inadequately treated. Treatment should be initiated promptly on the basis of epidemiological setting and clinical suspicion. Direct immunofluorescence of skin lesions, if available, may provide immediate confirmation; however, most laboratory diagnoses are made retrospectively by means of serological studies. Supportive care is important in the management of the complications of RMSF. The disease is not contagious except by direct inoculation of contaminated blood.

The incidence of RMSF in the United States increased unexpectedly over the past 2 decades. Cases have been reported from across the country, with the highest prevalence in the south Atlantic states. Cases also occur in western Canada, from British Columbia to Saskatchewan. Variants of *R. rickettsii* produce a very similar disease in Mexico and Central and South America, but less is known of their natural life cycles. The incidence of RMSF peaks during late spring and summer, although the disease continues to occur in temperate climates through the winter. Disease is most common among people exposed occupationally or recreationally to tick-infested areas. However, RMSF has been demonstrated in areas as unlikely as a public park in New York City.[10]

The vectors and major hosts of *R. rickettsii* include various ixodid ticks, particularly the dog tick, *Dermacentor variabilis* in the East, and the wood tick, *Dermacentor andersoni* in the West. *Amblyoma cajennense* and *Rhipicephalus sanguineus* have been implicated in Central and South America. Various other species may help maintain the wildlife chains of infection. Ticks transmit the agent among vertebrate hosts (ground squirrels, chipmunks, mice, rabbits, etc.) by blood feeding, with the hosts apparently remaining unharmed. Dogs are also infected, sometimes developing clinical disease, and can readily transport ticks to within close proximity to man.[11] The tick gut and tissues become heavily infected with rickettsiae, which are maintained through transstadial (larva, nymph, adult) and transovarial transmission through repeated generations. During attachment and blood feeding, the tick fecally contaminates the skin with rickettsial organisms, which then enter abraded or possibly even normal skin. The tick bite or even contact with crushed ticks may be hazardous since the salivary glands, tissues, and coxal fluid may contain organisms.

A commercial RMSF vaccine previously available in the United States is no longer produced. Experimental cell culture vaccines are under study but require further evaluation.

Other Spotted Fever Rickettsioses. The etiological agents and clinical manifestations of spotted fevers in the eastern hemisphere are sufficiently different to separate them from RMSF of the western hemisphere. Mediterranean spotted fever or tick typhus (boutonneuse fever, Kenya tick typhus, South African tick typhus, Indian tick typhus, Marseilles fever), caused by *Rickettsia conorii,* occurs in the Mediterranean countries of Europe (Italy, France), Asia, and Africa, the Middle East, Pakistan, India, and central and southern Africa. Tick typhus is the most ubiquitous of the spotted fever group of diseases and the most commonly seen rickettsial disease among travelers returning to North America.[12] The disease is transmitted by tick bite. Important vectors include numerous tick species of the genera *Rhipicephalus, Dermacentor, Amblyomma, Haemaphysalis,* and *Ixodes.* Many small rodents and other mammals, including urban and rural rats and mice, are natural hosts. In the Mediterranean countries, where the disease has seen a recent resurgence, the common dog tick, *Rhipicephalus sanguineus,* is particularly important.[13,14] Returning travelers usually give a history of exposure to a dog in an endemic area or of a tick bite in areas of high grass or bush.[12]

A mild to moderately severe illness, with high fever lasting a few days to 2 weeks, is typical. The name *boutonneuse fever* is derived from the buttonlike maculopapular rash, which is similar in timing and distribution to RMSF. The rash appears on about the third day and is usually generalized. Three fourths of patients develop a characteristic eschar ("tache noir") at the site of tick attachment.[14] Abrupt onset of headache, arthralgia, and myalgia is common. The rash persists 6 to 7 days and is unassociated with the progressive, hemorrhagic tendency of RMSF. Antibiotic therapy shortens the course of the illness, although the disease is usually self-limited.

North Asian tick typhus (Siberian tick typhus, North Asian tickborne rickettsiosis) is clinically similar to boutonneuse fever but is caused by a separate species, *Rickettsia sibirica.* It occurs in Siberia, other parts of Asiatic Soviet Union, Mongolia, China, Central Asia, Pakistan, and parts of eastern Europe. The vectors include ticks of the genera *Dermacentor, Haemaphysalis,* and *Rhipicephalus;* reservoirs include various rodents, other wild mammals, and possibly domestic animals. Other rickettsioses of the spotted fever group have recently been described in both China[8] and Japan.[15]

North Queensland tick typhus is clinically similar, although the etiological agent is *Rickettsia australis,* which has been recognized only in eastern Australia. The natural life cycle involves *Ixodes holocyclus* and *I. tasmani* ticks and various small marsupials and rodents.

Avoidance of tick-infested areas is the only reliable method for prevention of the tickborne rickettsioses. Obviously, eradication of the vectors, the natural hosts, or the rickettsiae from their well-established niches in nature is not feasible. Protective clothing, tick repellents on skin or clothing, regular searching of the body for ticks and removal of them with tweezers, and chemically impregnated collars or shampoos for domestic pets are often useful.

Rickettsialpox. Rickettsialpox (vesicular rickettsiosis) was first recognized as a distinct clinical entity in tenement dwellers in New York City. *Rickettsia akari,* the causative agent, is closely related to other members of the spotted fever group.

The disease is relatively mild. Early in the incubation period of 7 to 21 days, a firm, red 1 to 3 cm papular lesion with surrounding erythema develops at the site of mite attachment, accompanied by regional lymphadenopathy. The papule ulcerates centrally, forming an eschar and a permanent scar. Systemic symptoms, including fever, chills, sweats, headache, myalgias, and occasionally photophobia, last approximately 1 week. A generalized maculopapular rash develops within a few days of the onset of symptoms on the face, trunk, and extremities. The rash becomes vesicular, eventually forming black crusts that heal without scarring. Recovery is complete, and death is rare.

Cases were subsequently also detected in Boston, West Hartford, Philadelphia, Cleveland, Pittsburgh, and Utah, with an annual incidence of nearly 200 cases. Recently only a few cases have been confirmed in the United States; the disease may be misdiagnosed as chickenpox or other rash diseases, or it may have actually decreased in frequency. Rickettsialpox has also been recognized in the Soviet Union, in Korea, and in South Africa.

The vector in the United States is the mouse mite, *Allodermanyssus sanguineus,* a small colorless parasite of the house mouse, *Mus musculus.* The life cycle is not completely understood: all stages of the mite except the larvae ingest blood through a painless bite. Transstadial and transovarial transmission occur. As with scrub typhus, rickettsial-laden feces of the mite are the source of infection. A recent outbreak confirms the importance of control of the mouse and mite populations.[16] Disinfestation with residual insecticides and rodent-control measures may limit or temporarily eliminate the vector and the reservoir.

TRENCH FEVER

Epidemics of trench fever (Wolhynian fever, five-day fever, quintana fever) during World Wars I and II in troops living under crowded, unhygienic conditions brought this disease to prominence. Subsequently it has nearly disappeared, although it has been reported in Mexico. The etiological agent is *Rochalimaea* (formerly *Rickettsia*) *quintana,* which is genetically related to the typhus-group agents. *R. quintana* is an unusual species with the ability to grow on blood agar at 37° C (98° F) under 5% carbon dioxide. In addition, it can be isolated from feeding lice on the patient (xenodiagnosis).

The incubation period ranges from 9 to 17 days. Trench fever is self-limited, but patients may be severely ill for 6 to 8 weeks. Headache, malaise, myalgias, and single or multiple episodes of fever occur, and splenomegaly is common. A transient, macular rash may develop on the trunk and recur. Trench fever has a striking tendency to relapse, similar to Brill-Zinsser disease, and recurrences 20 to 30 years after primary infection have been documented. Rickettsemia may persist for many months, even when the patient is entirely free of symptoms.

The natural cycle had been thought to involve only man and the human body louse, *Pediculus humanus corporis.* However, an agent (*Rochalimaea vinsonii*), which is similar or identical to *R. quintana* from a vole in Canada, suggests the possibility of a wildlife cycle. Lice remain infectious for life and appear unharmed by infection. Infected louse feces contaminate breaks in the skin, transmitting infection to man. Transovarial transmission of *R. quintana* does not occur. Preventive measures include improvement in hygiene and living conditions and delousing if cases occur, as described for epidemic typhus.

Q FEVER (QUERY FEVER)

In the 1930s, Derrick studied cases of "abattoir fever" in Brisbane, Australia, describing the agent, *Rickettsia burnetii,* now renamed *Coxiella burnetii.* In 1935, an agent isolated from *Dermacentor andersoni* ticks in Montana was found to be identical. *C. burnetii* is a pleomorphic organism that differs from the *Rickettsia* species in its ability to grow in host cell cytoplasmic vacuoles rather than in the cytoplasm or nucleus. The organism is also smaller than the *Rickettsia* species, is usually gram-negative, but may appear gram-positive or acid-fast. The unusual resistance of *C. burnetii* to ultraviolet light, drying, heat, and chemical agents and its ability to persist in the environment may be due to its endospore-like differentiation.

Many infections are asymptomatic or mild, self-limited, febrile illnesses. After an incubation period of 2 to 4 weeks, Q fever often manifests as fever, malaise, myalgias, headache, weakness, anorexia, and weight loss, lasting a few days to several weeks or longer. Q fever is a systemic, generalized disease, frequently accompanied by pneumonitis. Convalescence is slow, although mortality is rare. In patients with protracted illness, such complications as hepatitis, endocarditis, osteomyelitis, hemorrhage, thromboses, and rarely encephalitis or aseptic meningitis, may occur. Tetracyclines and chloramphenicol are useful but are less efficacious than in the other rickettsioses. Relapses may occur, requiring repeated treatment. The organism may remain latent in tissues for years, and treatment of chronic disease is difficult. Person-to-person transmission is rare.

The diagnosis is confirmed serologically. A fourfold rise in convalescent titers or a single IFA titer of 256 or greater is usually considered diagnostic. The organism can be isolated from blood, sputum, urine, or spinal fluid, but this is rarely practical.

Q fever is essentially worldwide in distribution, with the apparent exceptions of Iceland and Scandinavia. *C. burnetii* is the most frequent and important cause of rickettsiosis in many areas, although it is uncommon in the United States. Q fever caused major epidemics during World War II ("Balkan grippe") in southern and eastern Europe. Sporadic or focal outbreaks occur wherever contact with domestic animals (predominantly cattle, sheep, and goats) occurs, particularly on farms, dairies, and abattoirs.

Many animals and various birds are natural hosts for the agent. Ticks develop a generalized, massive infection and appear to be important vectors. More than 40 species of naturally infected ixodid and argasis ticks are known, particularly of the genera *Amblyomma, Dermacentor, Haemaphysalis,* and *Ixodes.* Domestic animals, including cattle, sheep, and goats, are the main source of human illness. The agent persists in the environment for months or years, particularly in wool, hides, feces, dried placental detritus, dried tick feces, and soil. Inhalation is the usual route of infection for man. Airborne transmission over long distances or from animal products transported from endemic sites may account for epidemiologically puzzling cases. Raw milk from infected cattle and goats contains *C. burnetii* and may transmit infection; however its role in causation of disease is less clear. Sheep used in medical research facilities have caused outbreaks, and special control measures have been advised.[17]

Control of the natural life cycles of *C. burnetii* in ticks and wild animals is clearly impossible. However, the main sources of human infection can be partially controlled by aerosol reduction, location of dairy and other livestock operations away from population centers, and disinfection and appropriate disposal of infected animal tissues. Regular spraying of cattle, sheep, and goats with persistent insecticides for control of ectoparasites may be beneficial. Milk pasteurization should eliminate that mode of transmission. Experimental vaccines for domestic animals and occupationally exposed workers are currently being evaluated.

EHRLICHIOSIS

The only member of the genus *Ehrlichia* previously known to cause disease in man was *E. sennetsu,* which caused a mononucleosis-like syndrome called Sennetsu fever, described in 1954. *Ehrlichia canis* was eventually shown to cause a puzzling syndrome of tropical canine pancytopenia in military working dogs in Vietnam, which was often fatal.[18] Other species of *Ehrlichia,* particularly *E. risticii* (potomac horse fever), *E. equi* (equine ehrlichiosis), and *E. phagocytophilia* (tickborne fever) have been shown to be animal pathogens. In 1986 an acute febrile syndrome similar to RMSF was first recognized in man.[18] The Ehrlichiae differ from the *Rickettsia* species because they replicate within the host cell phagosome and are tropic for white blood cells.

The clinical course of human ehrlichiosis usually begins with tick attachment, followed by a mean incubation period of 9 days. Acute onset of fever, malaise, myalgia, fatigue, and headache develops, occasionally with vomiting, cough, or dyspnea. Encephalopathy, coagulopathy, and azotemia occur in severe cases. The clinical presentation is remarkably similar to that of RMSF; however, a macular (nonpetechial) rash is present in less than one half of the patients and leukopenia is common.[18-20] Diagnosis is based on clinical and epidemiological risk factors. IFA serologic study is usually confirmatory.

Human ehrlichiosis has been recognized primarily in the south central and southeastern United States, although it has occurred sporadically in the West. The disease is apparently tickborne with a peak incidence in May through July.[19,20] Most patients (80%) are male and are exposed occupationally or recreationally to ticks. In a prospective study in Georgia, 11% of hospitalized patients with fevers unexplained after the first day had serological findings diagnostic for *E. canis.*[21] The natural reservoirs of *E. canis* include dogs, foxes, coyotes, and jackals. Canine ehrlichiosis is transmitted by *Rhipicephalus sanguineus* ticks from infected to uninfected dogs. The importance of this vector for human disease remains to be demonstrated.

Preventive measures have yet to be defined. It would seem appropriate to recommend the same measures mentioned earlier to avoid exposure to ticks, as well as prompt removal of ticks when found.

Plague

Robert B. Craven
Jack D. Poland

Human plague, historically known as "the plague" or "the Black Death," continues to produce panic and irrational responses, even though this infection is readily responsive to antibiotic therapy. Although concurrent mortality in rats was noted during plague epidemics of earlier centuries, the ecological and epidemiological significance was not appreciated until late in the nineteenth century. An appropriate public health response to human plague involves clinical, epidemiological and environmental factors.

History. Four plague pandemics have been recognized since the sixth century A.D. An estimated one fourth of the European population perished in the fourteenth century, and in England approximately half the total population died (2 million persons). The origins of public health quarantine measures date from these plague epidemics.

Although it remained endemic in some of the world, plague then disappeared from Europe. The modern pandemic era began in 1894 in China. Spread from there was probably by steamships capable of transporting infected rats between ports on different continents. Millions died in India, and most countries of the world were affected.

During the modern pandemic, plague did not persist in some areas more than a few years (gulf and eastern coastal areas of North America) or a few decades (Hawaii and the Philippine Islands). Whether it will also die out in other areas remains to be seen. Introduction of plague into North America may have been by commercial shipping or by vertebrate hosts crossing the Bering strait.

Plague in Nature. The causative organism of plague, *Yersinia pestis,* is maintained in a natural reservoir of infected small rodents and their fleas. Naturally occurring plague is either enzootic or epizootic. Enzootic plague maintains the organism in relatively resistant rodent populations. Partly because of the virtual absence of overt disease, plague in reservoir hosts is not readily noticed. Their low mortality also produces low human risk, since vector fleas tend to remain on their preferred hosts.

Epizootic plague results when the organism is introduced into more susceptible rodent populations. In epizootic hosts with high mortality (e.g., prairie dogs and rock squirrels), infected fleas leave their dead hosts to seek other hosts, and interspecies spread, including to humans, is then possible. The high mortality of epizootic plague is more likely to be noticed, especially among diurnal rodents.[1]

The Plague Organism. *Y. pestis* is a bipolar staining, gram-negative, nonsporulating, nonmotile coccobacillus. It grows slowly in most nutrient bacteriological media at the optimum temperature of 28° C (82° F). On agar plates incubated at 37° C (98.6° F), colonies are barely discernible at 24 hours and are small (1 to 3 mm in diameter) at 48 hours. Stained smears of *Y. pestis* grown in a liquid medium may reveal pleomorphic cells occurring singly, in pairs, or in chains. Since several other gram-negative rods may appear to be bipolar, identification of *Y. pestis* by staining characteristics alone is unreliable. A positive fluorescent antibody (FA) test for fraction I antigen provides a presumptive identification, but FA does rarely produce falsely positive results. When corroborated by other results, lysis by a specific bacteriophage provides definitive identification of *Y. pestis.*[2]

Arthropod Vectors. Fleas are the only arthropod hosts known to transmit *Y. pestis* in nature. The vector efficiency of fleas varies by species, environmental effects such as temperature, flea population density, and flea-host biological interaction. Although fleas vary in their propensity to bite humans, any flea can be a potential vector. When a susceptible flea feeds on a bacteremic host, multiplication of *Y. pestis* in the flea's foregut and stomach blocks the proventriculus so that subsequent feedings do not pass into the stomach. Subsequent feeding attempts by the blocked flea result in regurgitation of *Y. pestis* organisms into the bite wound, producing the host infection. The vector efficiency of the oriental rat flea (*Xenopsylla cheopis*) is markedly affected by ambient temperature. When the mean daily temperature reaches or exceeds 28° C, enzymatic lysis of the flea's enteric blockage renders the flea noninfective.[3,4]

Vertebrate Hosts. Rodents serve as the primary hosts for both enzootic (maintenance) and epizootic plague and also as the primary source of human exposure. Other naturally involved mammals, such as rabbits, hares, carnivores, and humans, are incidental hosts, but occasionally they may serve as a direct (not vector-mediated) source of infection to other animals or humans.[3]

Epidemic plague is historically associated with domestic rats and their fleas and still constitutes the most serious hazard to humans. Epizootic plague among wild rodents may produce sporadic human infections, but an epizootic plague among commensal rats often produces multiple human cases because of their close association with humans and the propensity of the oriental rat flea to bite humans.

In most areas of the world, enzootic hosts for plague have not been defined. Epizootic plague among ground squirrels (*Spermophilus beecheyi,* the California ground squirrel, and *S. variegatus,* the rock squirrel) and their fleas has been implicated as a frequent source of fleaborne plague to humans in North America. Even when other rodents or domestic pets, such as cats or dogs, are implicated as the source of infected fleas affecting humans, the ultimate source of the fleas often has been the California ground squirrel or the rock squirrel. Wild carnivores or predatory birds may transport infected rodents or fleas to susceptible rodent populations, and wild rodent fleas may be transported to humans by dogs, cats, or other vertebrates and possibly by brush or nest material from the burrow system of an infected rodent.

Lagomorphs (rabbits and hares) may be infected by extension from adjacent wild rodent plague. Humans have been infected when dissecting infected mammals, including lagomorphs, rodents, and carnivores, with the organism apparently gaining entry through breaks in the skin.[5] Most carnivores, although readily infected by ingestion of infected prey, rarely develop a bacteremia and seldom, if ever, serve as a source of *Y. pestis* to their fleas. Experimental infection of felines and epidemiological evidence of plague mortality in cats[6,7] indicate that these carnivores are more susceptible to illness with *Y. pestis* infection than are other carnivores studied.[3]

Since 1977, diseased cats have been recognized as significant sources of infection to humans; three cats with plague pneumonia transmitted the infection to humans, resulting in two cases of primary pneumonic plague (one death) and one case of pharyngeal plague.[3,6,7]

Current World Distribution. Plague persists as a public health problem in many areas of the world because of continued human contact with potentially infected domestic and wild rodents. Wild rodent plague exists in the western third of the United States. Human plague in the United States is sporadic, with only single cases or small common-source clusters in an area, usually following exposure to fleas of wild rodents. In 1989, four human cases were reported. During the 1980s the greatest numbers of cases were reported in 1983 (40) and 1984 (31), most from New Mexico and Arizona. In the United States virtually all diagnosed cases of human plague are reported, in contrast to most other areas of the world, where reported cases reflect only a small percentage of actual occurrence.

In 1988, 1364 cases of human plague with 134 deaths were reported to the World Health Organization from nine countries. In South America, wild rodent plague foci exist in northeastern Brazil and the Andean regions, producing sporadic human cases and outbreaks. In 1988, 52 human cases were reported from four American countries: Bolivia, Brazil, Peru, and the United States of America. Wild rodent plague is also present in north central, eastern, and southern Africa. In 1988, 1100 cases were reported from three African countries: Madagascar, Tanzania, and Zaire. In the Near East, rodent plague persists in Iranian Kurdistan and along the frontier between Yemen and Saudi Arabia. Plague foci are also present in central and southeast Asia and Indonesia. In 1988, 202 human cases were reported from two Asian countries: Vietnam and China.

Urban plague, associated with domestic rodents, essentially has been controlled in most parts of the world, although human cases likely associated with domestic rodents have been reported recently from several countries in Africa. Plague continues to be endemic in Burma and in South Vietnam, where thousands of human cases of bubonic plague, both urban and rural, and scattered outbreaks of pneumonic plague were reported between 1962 and 1985. Recognition of plague in areas of the world where it has not been previously recognized is to be expected when long-standing, relatively stable ecological features are disrupted by major industrial and agricultural developments. For example, intensive irrigation projects of deserts for agricultural purposes, particularly for grain production, may produce burgeoning rodent populations close to human activity or residences. In such settings, epizootic plague and exposure of humans may result from the opportunistic amplification of existing known or even unrecognized enzootic plague, or expansion from adjacent enzootic-epizootic plague foci, or by transport of plague-infected rodents or fleas. Public health authorities should be alert to the possibility that human plague cases may arise in what may appear to be new foci in countries making such major ecological changes.

Surveillance. According to international sanitary regulations, known plague activity in animals or humans must be reported to the WHO with an evaluation of its potential for international spread via shipping, air transport, or by humans. Consequently in the United States, reporting of suspect human plague cases to local, state, and federal authorities (Centers for Disease Control, Fort Collins, Colorado) is mandatory.

Surveillance for plague activity and investigation of human and animal plague should be carried out in areas where plague has occurred in recent decades. Direct surveillance is accomplished by bacteriological testing of rodents found dead from natural causes (not poisoned, shot, or road killed). Indirect evidence of plague activity may be obtained by testing wild carnivore sera for antibody to *Y. pestis.* When evidence of plague activity in a broad area is found, further studies may include field observations to detect rodent mortality and selective collection and testing of rodents and fleas for evidence of plague infection. The collected data should then be evaluated to determine the relative risk to humans and whether control measures are needed.

HUMAN PLAGUE

The classic form of *Y. pestis* infection in humans is bubonic plague. Other clinical forms (e.g., septicemic, pneumonic, meningeal) usually occur as complications of bubonic plague. Rarely, local ulceration, similar to lesions seen with tularemia (eschar), occurs at the site of entry of *Y. pestis* organisms. In addition to flea bites, entry sites can include mucous membranes of the eye and oropharynx as well as broken skin. Within 2 to 7 days after exposure, onset of illness is heralded by fever, chills, pain in the area of the lymph nodes, and eventually lymph node enlargement (the bubo). In untreated, progressive disease, plague septicemia develops.

Septicemia in the absence of lymph node involvement is referred to as *primary septicemic plague.* Plague septicemia, if untreated, generally causes septic shock and rapid death; in patients who do not quickly succumb, metastatic involvement of other organ systems may lead to such complications as pneumonia, meningitis, multiple lymphadenopathy, endophthalmitis, arthritis, or other focal abscesses. Clinical problems are compounded in primary septicemic plague because absence of a classic bubo reduces the likelihood that plague would be suspected, and resistance factors that would be stimulated by reactive lymph nodes are circumvented.

Plague pneumonia resulting from hematogenous spread from bubonic or septicemic plague is referred to as *secondary plague pneumonia.* In contrast, *primary pneumonic plague* results from inhalation of fine droplets of *Y. pestis* organisms, usually originating from a mammal (primarily humans) with plague pneumonia. *Y. pestis* does not survive well saprophytically, and fomite or true airborne transmission has not been recognized. Instead, respiratory infection is transmitted to close contacts (within 2 m) by their inhaling fine droplets ejected by a pneumonic plague victim during forceful coughing.

Before antibiotic therapy was available, approximately 5% of cases during outbreaks developed plague pneumonia. In the United States a few instances of limited respiratory infection spread to contacts were reported, and two major outbreaks of pneumonic plague were reported in the first 2 decades of this century: in 1919 and 1924. From 1925 to 1974, 4 of 91 plague patients developed secondary pneumonia, with no spread to contacts. In the years from 1975 through 1989, 33 of 247 patients (13%) developed secondary pneumonia, and four patients had primary pneumonic plague acquired primarily from domestic pets[3,6-9] (Fig. 11-7). Over 2000 known or possible contacts of these patients with respiratory involvement were given chemoprophylaxis; no secondary spread was recognized. The reason for the increase of secondary plague pneumonia in the United States is unknown. Two possible factors are (1) a basic change in *Y. pestis* and (2) initial therapy with inappropriate antibiotics (e.g., ampicillin), which may have some effect on the plague organism but are not curative. If the recent trend of increased secondary plague pneumonia continues, the unfortunate circumstance of secondary spread to medical personnel or household contacts may occur before the index case is identified.

Pharyngeal or tonsillar plague has been associated with oral contamination from either infected exudates of patients or aerosolized particles from pneumonic patients or animals.[6,9,10]

Diagnosis and Therapy. A careful epidemiological history is essential to consider plague in the differential diagnosis. When plague is suspected, it is imperative to obtain appropriate diagnostic specimens promptly and, if the clinical and epidemiological evidence is sufficiently strong, to initiate specific therapy without awaiting laboratory confirmation. Bubonic plague is best diagnosed by culture of material aspirated from a fluctuant bubo; if aspiration is "dry," sterile saline should be injected into the node, and then the node should be aspirated again. Multiple blood cultures and, if indicated, throat and sputum cultures should also be obtained. Materials for culture should be taken before specific antibiotics are given. Paired sera obtained 3 weeks apart should be tested for antibody to *Y. pestis.* Smears of bubo aspirates, exudates, and suspect growth in bacteriological media should be stained by a polychromatic stain, such as Wayson's or Giemsa, to demonstrate the characteristic bipolarity of *Y. pestis.* Thick smears or primary material from bubo aspirates should be forwarded to a reference laboratory for examination by the fluorescent antibody technique for presumptive evidence of *Y. pestis.* Suspect cultures should also be forwarded for confirmatory identification.

The most effective antibiotic against *Y. pestis* is streptomycin. Other effective drugs include tetracycline, gentamicin, kanamycin, chloramphenicol, and certain sulfonamides (e.g., sulfadiazine). The penicillins are not effective against *Y. pestis,* although these drugs frequently show in vitro activity and some synthetic penicillins have some, although inadequate, in vivo activity. Since streptomycin is bacteriolytic, it must be given in adequate but not excessive doses to avoid massive release of plague endotoxin. Chloramphenicol, a highly effective drug for *Y. pestis,* is the agent of choice for plague meningitis or endophthalmitis because of its greater permeability into those organs.

Hospital Procedures and Care of Contacts. Because secondary pulmonary infection may develop, all patients with suspected bubonic plague should be placed in respiratory isolation for at least 48 hours of specific antibiotic therapy. Additional isolation time is not necessary unless the patient has pulmonary involvement or drainage from open lesions. Personnel caring for pneumonic plague cases must observe strict respiratory isolation techniques, including the use of eye protection. All patients should have an initial chest x-ray regardless of whether they have respiratory symptoms.

Community associates of bubonic plague patients should be kept under surveillance because of the possibility of other zootic exposures to the same source as the index case; prophylaxis is *not* indicated as a routine practice. All persons who had close contact with pneumonic plague patients before they were isolated should be given chemoprophylaxis for 6 days. It should consist of 30 mg/kg/d of tetracycline in four doses. These persons should also be kept under close observation, including temperature measurement at least twice daily. Should fever develop, the person should be immediately hospitalized in isolation for evaluation, and streptomycin therapy should be given if indicated. Sputum

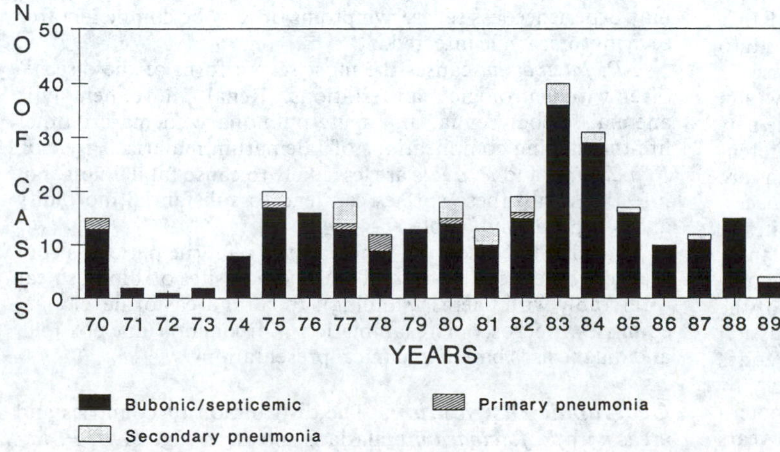

Figure 11-7. Reported human plague cases by year, 1970–1989. *[From Plague Section, Bacterial Zoonoses Branch, DVBID, CID, CDC, USPHS.]*

and throat cultures and paired sera should be obtained from these suspect contact cases in an effort to document whether *Y. pestis* infection occurred.

Prevention and Control. Immunization with either killed or live vaccines has met with apparent success in certain circumstances,[11] but when feasible, rodent control and avoidance of flea bites are much more effective public health measures. Plague vaccine should be used for persons working regularly with the agent in laboratories or in situations (e.g., war conditions, field exercises, and Peace Corps service) where the risk of infection may be high and environmental control measures cannot be constantly applied.[12]

Methods of preventing human infection vary considerably, depending on the social and ecological features of the plague problem.[13-15] In general, prevention of human disease revolves sequentially around (1) public health education, (2) vector control, and (3) rodent host management. During an epizootic plague, rodent host reduction should never precede vector control, although they may be done concurrently. Vectors may be controlled by selective target-oriented application of insecticides approved for flea control. Rodent control requires elimination of both food and harborage, since pesticidal control alone will produce an ecological void, which will promptly be reinvaded, often by young, susceptible rodent hosts.

Although plague is still not entirely preventable in humans, sanitary practices and appropriate antibiotic therapy have made feasible a rational approach to epidemic and epizootic plague incidents and to individual human infections.

Malaria

Joel G. Breman
Richard W. Steketee

Malaria remains one of the most prevalent and serious diseases in the world, with endemic transmission occurring in 102 countries that together contain more than one half of the world's population.[1,2] The major malarious areas are in sub-Saharan Africa, Central and South America, Hispaniola (the Dominican Republic and Haiti), the Middle East, the Indian subcontinent, other Asian countries, and Oceania. All developed countries are at risk because of importations from immigrants, refugees, and travelers to malaria-endemic countries. The World Health Organization (WHO) estimates that more than 270 million people are infected with malaria parasites at any one time and that more than 100 million episodes of clinical malaria occur yearly. More than 80% of these people live in Africa, where more than 1 million children die yearly from the direct and indirect effects of malaria infection.

Agent and Life Cycle. Human malaria is caused by any of four species of the genus *Plasmodium* (*P. falciparum, P. vivax, P. malariae,* and *P. ovale*). The infected female *Anopheles* mosquito inoculates malaria sporozoites into a human while feeding, and within 30 minutes these enter hepatocytes, initiating the exoerythrocytic stage of development. Primary tissue schizogony of parasites takes 7 to 15 days in the liver. The schizont then ruptures, and the resulting circulating merozoites enter red blood cells (RBCs). The erythrocytic schizogonic cycle leads to maturation of blood stage parasites, with ring stage parasites in RBCs becoming schizonts, which rupture and release merozoites into the bloodstream. These merozoites invade RBCs, and the erythrocytic cycle is continued. The parasite development cycle within RBCs takes 48 to 72 hours, depending on the species of the parasite. Most blood stage parasites are asexual, but some differentiate into male and female gametocytes. These sexual forms are ingested by another feeding mosquito and develop into, successively, gametes, zygotes, ookinetes, oocysts, and sporozoites in the gut of the mosquito before migrating to the salivary glands. Development of the parasite within the female mosquito (sporogonic cycle) takes 8 to 25 days, depending on the species of the parasite and on environmental temperature. The transmission cycle is continued when the female mosquito injects sporozoites into another human while taking a blood meal (Fig. 11–8).

P. vivax and *P. ovale* are relapsing species, with the potential to initiate renewed cycles of RBC infection months or years after the initial sporozoite inoculation. Some dormant forms (hypnozoites) of these parasites reside in the liver and can develop into liver schizonts. When the schizonts rupture, merozoites enter RBCs, initiating the erythrocytic cycle once again. When these continuing infections manifest themselves parasitologically or clinically, they are called relapses. *P. falciparum* and *P. malariae* do not relapse.

Strains of *P. falciparum* may be "cleared" by antimalarial drugs and then reappear after an interval during which they persist in RBCs but are subpatent (not detected by standard microscopic techniques); the reappearance is termed a recrudescence and may be asymptomatic or manifest itself as clinical illness. *P. malariae* may recrudesce after many years of asymptomatic parasitemia.

Clinical Features and Diagnosis. The diagnosis of malaria must be considered in all febrile patients who have traveled to or lived in malaria-endemic areas or who have received blood transfusions or blood products from persons who have been in such areas.[3,4] The classic malaria illness occurs in a person with no prior exposure to the parasite; the patient experiences fever, chills, sweats, and nonspecific symptoms and signs, such as headache, back pain, muscle pain, and malaise. Infants may be only lethargic, irritable, and anorectic. Persons who have had frequent exposure to the parasite develop partial immunity and may experience less severe symptoms or may be completely free of symptoms while infected.

P. falciparum causes the most severe form of the disease, often with neurologic manifestations.[5] Renal failure, hemolytic anemia, hypoglycemia, and acute pulmonary edema are other life-threatening complications of falciparum malaria. *P. vivax, P. malariae,* and *P. ovale* are less likely to cause fatal illness, but infections with these species can lead to substantial morbidity and complications (Table 11–4).

Ideally, the diagnosis of malaria in a febrile patient is confirmed by the identification of malaria parasites on blood smear (preferably with Giemsa staining). In rural areas of developing countries, microscopic examination is frequently not possible, and diagnosis is based on clinical presentation.

Geographic Distribution. The distribution of countries and areas with *P. falciparum* malaria is shown in Fig. 11–9. *P. fal-*

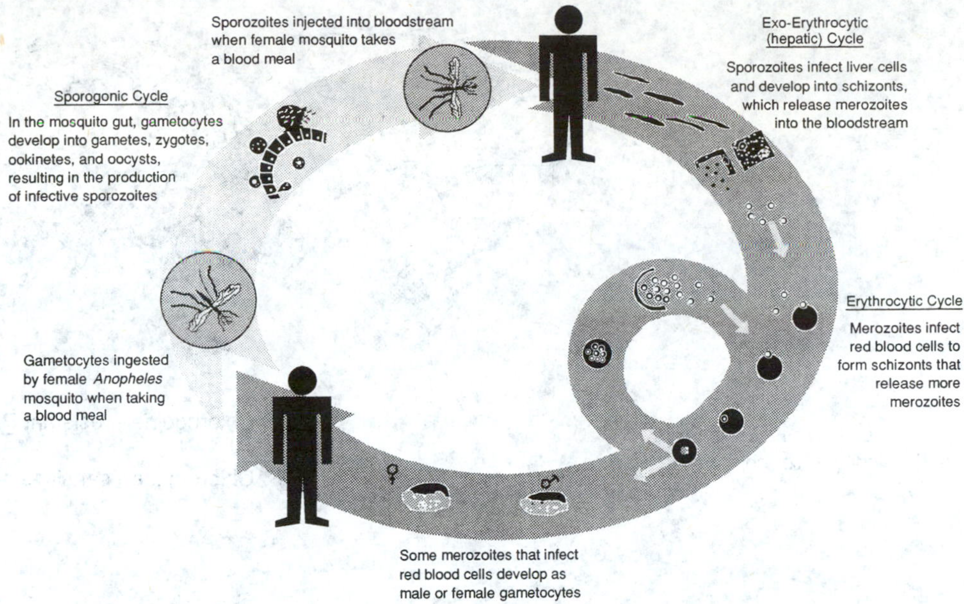

Figure 11-8. The malaria transmission cycle.

ciparum is found only in tropical or subtropical regions because the development of the parasite in the mosquito is reduced greatly when the temperature is below 20° C; *P. falciparum* thus predominates in sub-Saharan Africa. *P. vivax* is prevalent throughout all malarious areas except sub-Saharan Africa. *P. ovale* is found chiefly in tropical areas of western Africa and is transmitted occasionally in areas in the western Pacific and southeast Asia. *P. malariae* has a wide global distribution but occurs in localized "patches" in many areas; it is prevalent in areas of western and eastern Africa, Guyana, and parts of India.[3,6]

Although many countries are not entirely malarious, WHO estimates that about 2.1 billion persons, more than 40% of the world's population, live in malarious areas. In certain areas of Africa, virtually 100% of the population may acquire a malaria infection each year.[7] In the 1980s, between 7 and 15 million malaria cases were recorded yearly at WHO, with tropical Africa recording about 50% of the reported cases (Fig. 11-10).

In addition to the estimated 80% of all malaria episodes that occur in Africa, four fifths of the remaining 20% of cases are concentrated in nine countries (India, Brazil, Afghanistan, Sri Lanka, China, Thailand, Papua New Guinea, Mexico, and the Philippines) (WHO, unpublished data, 1990). Of these, the first four countries reported 63% of all cases in 1987. Localization of malaria within countries has been done, but it may reflect variability in reporting. In India, only 6 of 31 states and union territories reported two thirds of all cases. Likewise, more than 80% of the cases reported in Brazil in 1987 occurred in 3 of 12 states.

Table 11-5 indicates the number of cases of malaria reported by each administrative region of WHO.[1,2] These data underestimate true incidence because of incomplete recording, particularly in Africa. Recent increases in the incidence of malaria have been recorded in the Amazon basin of South America, Madagascar, several countries in continental Africa (Malawi, Rwanda, Togo, Zaire), and parts of Asia and the western Pacific. With increasing air travel and immigration throughout the

TABLE 11-4. CHARACTERISTICS OF THE HUMAN MALARIAS

	P. falciparum	*P. vivax*	*P. ovale*	*P. malariae*
Exoerythrocytic cycle (days)	6–7	6–8	9	14–16
Prepatent period (days)	9–10	11–13	10–14	15–16
Incubation period, days (mean)	9–14 (12)	12–17 (15) to 6–12 m	16–18 (17) or longer	18–40 (28) or longer
Periodicity, asexual cycle (days)	2	2	2	3
Primary attack[a]				
Severity	+ + +	+ to + + +	+	+
Duration (hours)	16–36 or longer	8–12	8–12	8–10
Duration of untreated infection (years)	1–2	1½–5	1½–5	3–50
Relapse	No	Yes	Yes	No
Complications[a]				
Central nervous system	+ + +	+	+	+
Anemia	+ + +	+ +	+	+
Renal insufficiency	+ +	+	+	+ + Nephrotic syndrome
Effects on pregnancy	+ + +	+	?	?
Hypoglycemia	+ + +	?	?	?

[a]Influenced by immunity: + infrequent, + + common, + + + frequent; documentation of complications for species other than *P. falciparum* are limited.
Modified from Bruce-Chwatt.[3]

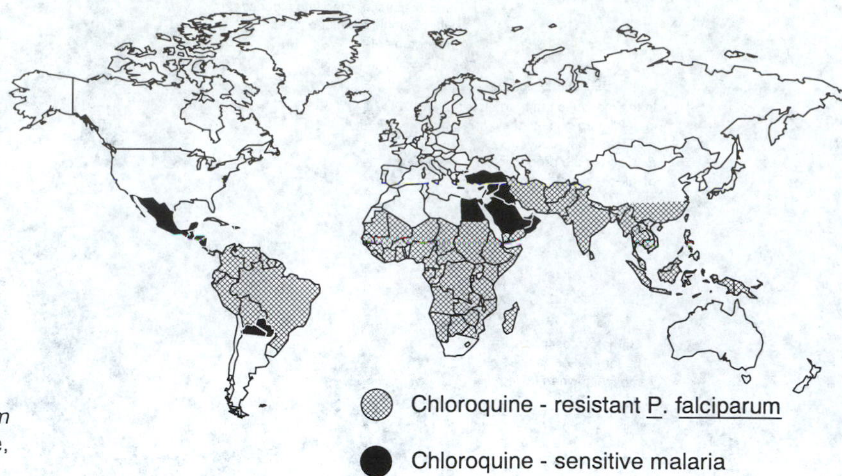

Figure 11-9. Malarious areas with *Plasmodium falciparum* resistant and sensitive to chloroquine, 1990. *[From CDC, 1990.]*

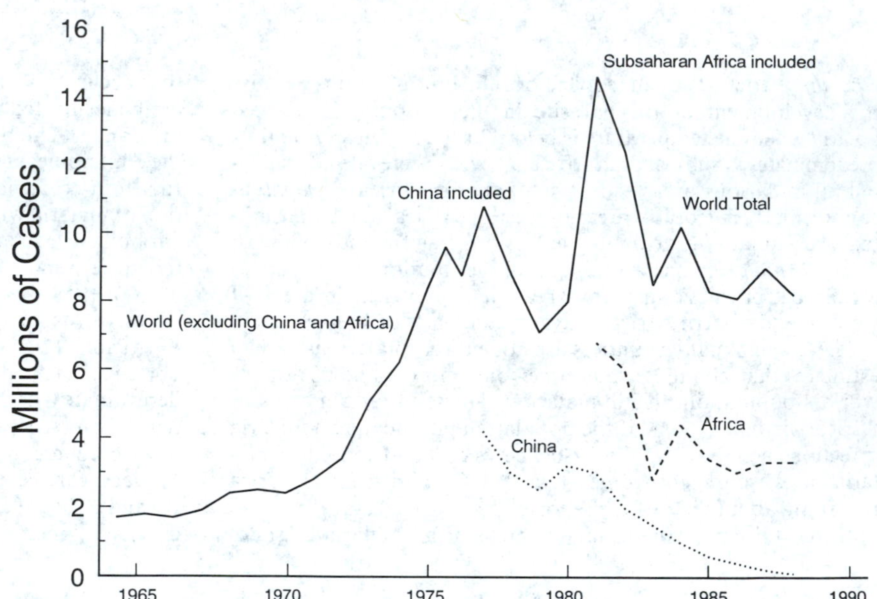

Figure 11-10. Malaria reported to the World Health Organization, 1965–1988. *[From WHO, 1987, 1990.]*

TABLE 11-5. NUMBER OF MALARIA CASES REPORTED (IN THOUSANDS), BY WHO REGION, 1981–1988[a]

WHO Region	1981	1982	1983	1984	1985	1986	1987	1988
Africa[b]	6,754	6,042	2,726	4,420	3,373	3,046	3,309	3,385
Americas	638	718	831	931	911	951	1,109	1,110
Southeast Asia	3,566	2,964	2,731	3,004	2,521	2,689	2,823	2,645
Europe	60	66	71	60	32	45	27	8
Eastern Mediterranean	207	308	305	335	391	610	564	602
Western Pacific	3,464	2,487	1,839	1,839	1,066	758	758	704
Total	14,689	12,585	8,503	10,111	8,294	8,127	8,500	8,344

[a]The information provided does not always cover the total population at risk.[1,2]
[b]Mainly clinically diagnosed cases; incomplete figures.

world, many developed countries have had regular importations of malaria[8]; some of these have threatened to reestablish transmission in malaria-free areas.[9]

Africa. Special studies in some areas of Africa indicate that at least six febrile episodes are experienced annually by children under 5 years.[10] Because almost 25% of the sub-Saharan African population (500 million) is under 5 years of age, well over 750 million episodes of fever occur in African children, about one half of which are due to malaria.[11] It is estimated that about 1% of all malaria episodes are severe, requiring hospitalization, and that 15% to 20% of hospitalized pediatric malaria patients will die. Thus 563,000 to 750,000 deaths of African children each year are due to acute malaria.

In Africa 10% to 35% of newborn infants have low birth weight (<2500 g), and this condition is more common in first-born infants. Placental malaria infection is associated with an increased risk of low birth weight and, in some areas of Africa, up to two thirds of the placentas of primigravida women are malarious.[12] While not the only factor affecting birth weight, malaria is one of the few preventable infectious causes of low birth weight. Of the approximately 20 million pregnancies yearly, at least 2 to 7 million infants will have low birth weight, and it is estimated that 233,000 to 817,000 of them will die before the age of 1 year. When low birth weight and anemia (which can be due to the acute or chronic effects of malaria) are considered, along with malaria-related deaths in older children, there are probably at least 1 million malaria-related deaths of African children each year, or 2700 deaths daily.

Central and South Americas. Malaria in the Americas seems to have stabilized during the 1980s. There have been steadily increasing trends in Brazil, Mexico, Ecuador, and Peru.[1,2] Of the 911,000 cases of malaria reported from Central and South America in 1985, 45% were registered in Brazil (where about one half of the cases are due to *P. falciparum*), 13% in Mexico, and 17% in four countries of Central America (El Salvador, Guatemala, Honduras, and Nicaragua). The epidemic situation in northwest Brazil is related to a large influx of nonimmune workers from other areas of the country who have been attracted by economic opportunities.

Asia and Western Pacific. In Asia, India and China recorded the highest number of cases in 1985, with 1,855,840 and 563,400 cases, respectively.[1,2] In China, the incidence of malaria is decreasing (Fig. 11-10). Excluding Africa, the highest incidence of malaria in the world in 1985 was reported from the Solomon Islands (151 cases per 1000 population) and Vanuatu (177 cases per 1000 population). In these countries in the western Pacific, *P. falciparum* is responsible for more than 50% of recorded cases, whereas in China and the Indian subcontinent *P. vivax* predominates.

Malaria in the United States. In the United States, transmission of malaria was interrupted in the mid-1950s. Numbers of cases have increased at specific times, such as when military personnel returned from Korea and Vietnam and when immigration accelerated in the late 1970s (Fig. 11-11).

Since World War II, there have been 16 episodes of introduced malaria (transmission from imported cases), all due to *P. vivax.* The most recent outbreaks occurred in southern California in 1986, 1988, and 1989, with malaria affecting 59 migrant workers and five residents in those episodes.[13] Other sources of malaria are also important in the United States. Congenital malaria (31 cases), transfusion-associated malaria (28 cases), laboratory-acquired malaria (1 case), and transplant-associated malaria (1 case) were reported to the Centers for Disease Control (CDC) from 1980 through 1989.

In 1989, 1102 malaria cases and two deaths in the United States were reported to CDC. Approximately one half of the cases were in U.S. citizens who were permanent residents, and the remainder were in foreign citizens.[14] In U.S. citizens, approximately 65% of imported malaria was acquired in Africa, 15% in Asia, and 5% each in Mexico, other Central American countries combined, and Oceania; 5% of cases were acquired elsewhere.

Transmission. Malarious areas have been classified in two ways, with some overlap between them: (1) qualitatively by stability of malaria transmission and (2) quantitatively by the degree of endemicity.

Stability of Malaria. In stable malaria there is high and continual transmission without major changes over several years, although there may be seasonal variations. In unstable malaria the amount of transmission varies from year to year. The concept of the stability of malaria transmission was first proposed by MacDonald[15] and rests on the efficiency of the local anophelines as malaria vectors and on environmental characteristics that are conducive to anopheline reproduction and longevity. A highly efficient vector is one that is highly susceptible to the full development of the malaria parasite, prefers to feed on humans, rests and bites in human dwellings, and lives for a relatively long time. The optimal conditions for establishing stable transmission include a geographic setting with warm temperatures, high humidity, and frequent rains to create abundant breeding sites in collections of standing water. Environments or vector characteristics and habits that vary from this ideal will decrease the stability of transmission. An efficient vector is the African *Anopheles gambiae* complex, which breeds in any fresh water collection exposed to sunlight, is highly susceptible to the *P. falciparum* par-

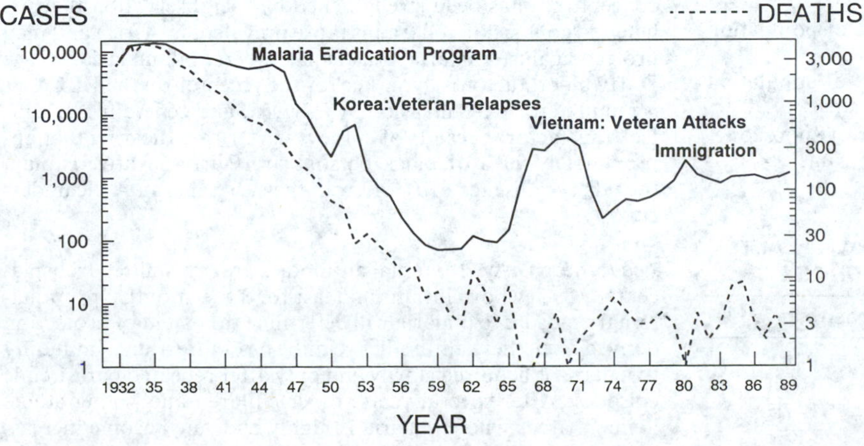

Figure 11-11. Reported cases and deaths from malaria in the United States, 1932–1989.

TABLE 11-6. DISTRIBUTION AND SUSCEPTIBILITY OF THE MAJOR VECTORS OF HUMAN MALARIA—*ANOPHELES*

Species	Distribution	Susceptibility to Malaria	Host Preference	Typical Breeding Sites
A. albimanus	Western hemisphere from southeast Texas, Mexico, Central America, to Ecuador, Venezuela, and Carribean	Low	Animal	Wide range from temporary collections of water to ponds, streams, and lakes
A. culicifacies	Indian subcontinent	Low	Animal	Sunlit collections of fresh water, including rice fields
A. darlingi	South America east of the Andes	Moderate	Human	Clear, fresh, partially shaded lagoons or marshes
A. dirus	Southeast Asian forests	High	Human	Shaded water collections
A. gambiae, A. funestus	Tropical Africa	High	Human	Fresh water collections exposed to sunlight
A. maculatus	Foothills of southeast Asian countries and Indian subcontinent	Moderate	Human	Sunlit hilly streams
A. minimus	Southeast Asian hills	Moderate	Human	Margins of slow-moving sunlit streams
A. stephensi	Urban areas of Indian subcontinent	Moderate	Human	Shaded wells, cisterns, cans, roof gutters

asite, bites humans primarily, and tends to rest indoors. In contrast, the Central American and Haitian vector *Anopheles albimanus* tends to feed on cattle and has low relative susceptibility to *Plasmodium;* this species is a less efficient transmitter of malaria. An overview of the ecology of the major vectors of malaria is shown in Table 11-6.

Endemicity. Epidemic malaria describes intense and rapid spread of infection in the human population in an area where little or no malaria is usually transmitted. With the uncommon occurrence of heavy rainfall, followed by an abundant increase of *Anopheles* vectors, high levels of transmission may occur in a nonimmune population. Endemic malaria refers to continual natural transmission at varying levels of intensity. In the classification of endemicity developed by WHO in 1950, the rate of spleen enlargement detected by palpation and the rate of parasitemia in children 2 through 9 years of age were used as the major measurements (Table 11-7). These indices were used extensively during malaria-eradication activities. Spleen palpation, an indirect measure of malaria prevalence, has decreased as emphasis has switched to control. The different levels of endemicity (Table 11-7) are often cited, sometimes in a less rigorous way without actual surveys for spleen rates, to describe approximate levels of malaria importance in a given area or country.

Indices. Other important quantitative indices to describe the potential for malaria transmission and endemicity have been used to monitor control efforts.[3,6] These indices are usually determined by special field surveys and include:

- Incidence rate: Number of cases per unit of population per unit of time
- Prevalence rate: Number of cases per unit of population at a point in time
- Entomological inoculation rate: Number of sporozoite-positive mosquito bites per person per time unit

TABLE 11-7. LEVELS OF ENDEMICITY BY SPLEEN AND PARASITE RATES IN CHILDREN 2-9 YEARS OF AGE

Endemicity	Spleen Rate (%)	Parasite rate (%)
Hypoendemic	0–10	≤10
Mesoendemic	11–50	11–50
Hyperendemic	>50 (>25 in adults)	51–75
Holoendemic	>75 (low in adults)	>75

- Vectorial capacity of a mosquito population: The expected number of inoculations of humans originating from one infective case in 1 day
- Basic reproduction rate of the malaria parasite: The potential number of secondary cases originating from one case throughout its duration

The most frequently used descriptive measure of the level of endemicity has been the prevalence of malaria parasites in a population as determined by blood smear examination; this information is reported most usefully by age group, species of parasite, and season and in relation to the timing of malaria-control interventions.

Host Factors Affecting Distribution. Within areas of endemic malaria, the distribution of infection and clinical illness is determined mainly by transmission forces as reflected by the entomological inoculation rate, the genetic susceptibility of the humans at risk, and the level of innate and acquired immunity in the population.

Genetic Susceptibility. Humans are susceptible to the four species of malaria, with exceptions due to specific genetic characteristics.[6] Sickle cell trait, hereditary ovalocytosis, and other inherited traits that alter RBC structure or function confer a degree of protection from parasite invasion or growth; persons with β-thalassemia, hemoglobin E, fetal hemoglobin, and glucose-6-phosphate dehydrogenase deficiency may have some degree of protection from *Plasmodium* infections. The protection of populations by their genetic makeup is ''balanced polymorphism,'' a concept that has been strengthened by the observation that the heterozygous sickle cell trait is more prevalent in Africa and may protect against malaria, particularly cerebral malaria.[16] The Duffy blood factor is a marker for the receptor on the RBC that is required for RBC invasion by *P. vivax,* and generally Africans lack this factor[17]; results of surveys in Africa indicating that approximately 90% of black persons are Duffy-negative explain the relative absence of *P. vivax* in the sub-Saharan African desert.

Acquired Immunity. Maternal antibodies are transmitted transplacentally to newborn infants and last for 3 to 9 months; prior maternal exposure to malaria will determine the extent of protection derived from these antibodies. Unlike most infections, immunity to malaria is acquired slowly and only after repeated parasitemic episodes. After several years, older children and young adults living in areas where malaria is highly endemic become increasingly resistant to clinical illness, despite frequent malaria infections. In contrast, residents of areas with low levels of malaria transmission and infrequent infections may never develop adequate levels of acquired immunity. Hence, in areas of stable transmission and high malaria endemicity, the high-risk groups are young children, especially between 6 and 23 months of age, and pregnant women, particularly primigravidas. The increased susceptibility of these two groups is due to absent or incomplete immunity in children and, probably altered immunity in pregnancy. However, all segments of the population are at risk of illness in malarious areas with unstable transmission.

While parasitological indices indicate the current prevalence of malaria, serological testing reflects past exposure to infection. Serological surveys to measure malaria-specific antibodies use the indirect fluorescent antibody test (IFA) or the enzyme-linked immunosorbent assay test (ELISA). Except where measures to interrupt transmission are operative, serological study is not often useful for direct comparisons of endemicity between populations or within populations over time; this applies especially to areas with stable transmission, where all segments of the population may maintain high levels of antibody because of frequent reinfection.

Impact

Case Definition. Malaria surveillance has been incomplete in many areas because standard precise definitions for diagnosis and reporting have not been developed. *Plasmodium* infection is defined as the presence of the parasite in the peripheral blood of an individual. Febrile illness in association with *Plasmodium* parasitemia is considered malaria illness when no other cause for the fever can be identified. Because excluding other potential causes of fever may be difficult in many settings, particularly in the developing world, the case definition of malaria illness can lack both sensitivity and specificity.

Effect on Groups at Risk. The impact of malaria infection in a population has three different manifestations: (1) the acute febrile illness, which may lead to severe disease and risk of death; (2) the chronic persistent "asymptomatic" malaria, which may lead to anemia or contribute to chronic undernutrition; and (3) perinatal malaria infection leading to maternal death, abortion, or stillbirth in women with little or no immunity, or low birth weight in babies born to women with higher levels of immunity (Fig. 11-12).

The acute illness leading to severe and complicated malaria takes its toll primarily in the most susceptible segments of the population, including children in malaria-endemic areas, all persons in areas with epidemic potential, and nonimmune travelers. At any point in time in areas where malaria is highly endemic, some children will have asymptomatic parasitemia, others will have mild illness associated with their parasite infection, and a few will have severe disease. Work is currently under way to determine which factors place children at risk of the severe, life-threatening form of the disease and what interventions can limit this risk.

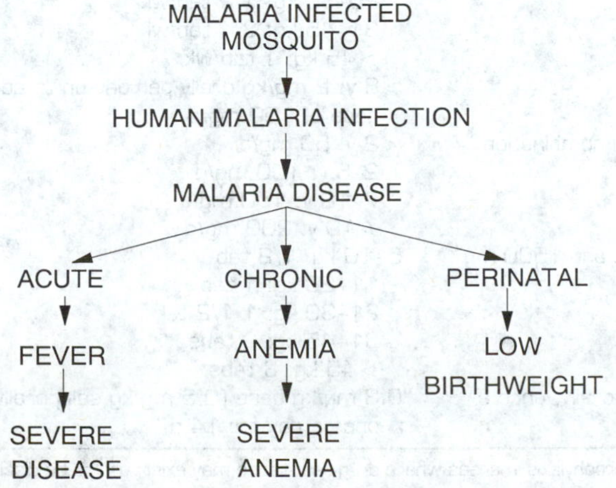

Figure 11-12. Scheme of malaria impact on populations.

Chronic malaria manifests itself most commonly as recurrent infection leading to anemia. In community studies in Africa, 25% to 60% of children under the age of 5 years are anemic, and parasitemic children are more likely to be anemic than children without malaria parasitemia.[11] Severe anemia (hemoglobin <5g/dl) is associated with an in-hospital mortality rate of 5% to 10%. Thus anemia in young children in malaria-endemic areas is often linked to malaria parasitemia, and severe anemia may be associated with a high rate of childhood death.

Perinatal malaria, although frequently more silent in its manifestations, may play an equally important role in causing disease and death. Malaria infection during pregnancy in areas of low endemicity leads to maternal illness, abortions, and stillbirths. In areas of high endemicity, malaria infection in pregnancy leads to low birth weight and its consequent risk of neonatal and early infant mortality. Compared with rates for infants with normal birth weights (≥ 2500 g), neonatal mortality rates for infants with birth weights of 2000 to 2499 g and of less than 2000 g are 3.5 and 22 times higher, respectively. In addition, anemia in pregnant women is frequently associated with malaria and with low-weight newborn infants. Thus malaria infection in pregnancy can contribute either to fetal loss or to an increased risk of neonatal or early infant mortality.

Economic Impact. The economic toll from malaria is measured mainly by the effects of mortality, morbidity, and disability on reduced productivity.[18,19] It is estimated that hospitalization for an acute malaria attack in the United States may cost $10,000. In the developing world, where malaria is often the leading cause of outpatient visits and inpatient admissions, the malaria-related treatment costs to families and countries are considerable. Seven days of work are commonly lost to disability for each bout of nonfatal malaria, so that tens of millions of days are lost to productivity each year because of acute attacks of the disease. Benefits from educational programs can be compromised severely by malaria, particularly in areas where young schoolchildren are affected by frequent febrile attacks; when an epidemic of malaria occurs, all segments of the population are affected.

Control

Historical Perspective. After the discovery of the effectiveness of DDT (dichloro-diphenyl-trichloroethane) against insects in the first half of the century, a malaria-eradication program relying mainly on vector control began in the mid-1950s under the aegis of the WHO. Despite excellent progress in many countries, including elimination of endemic transmission in several nations located in temperate areas, eradication worldwide was not achieved because of several factors. Anopheline resistance to insecticides, parasite resistance to antimalarial drugs, and inadequate health infrastructure, resources, and commitment proved formidable obstacles to malaria-eradication efforts. In western Africa, spraying of households with residual pesticides was accompanied by a decrease in the entomologic inoculation rates, but this decrease was not sufficient to bring about a proportionate decrease in malaria incidence in that environment that could lead to eradication.[7] However, it has been demonstrated that mortality could be reduced substantially in an eastern African community participating in a pilot project that also relied on spraying of residual pesticides on the walls of houses.[20]

The above factors, coupled with the integration of all health programs into the general health services—the primary health care movement—were the basis for the termination of the global malaria-eradication program at the end of the 1960s. While eradication has not been achieved, several areas of the world, mainly in the temperate areas of southern Eu-

TABLE 11-8. COMPONENTS OF COMPREHENSIVE MALARIA CONTROL[a]

Type of Control	Effect
▪ Antiplasmodial Measures[a]	
Treatment of acute cases	Elimination of malaria parasites and prevention of transmission
Prophylaxis and suppression of infection	
Radical treatment of relapses	
Vaccination (projected)	
▪ Individual Protection[b]	
Mosquito repellents	Reduction of human-mosquito contact
Bed nets and curtains (impregnated with pesticide)	
House screening	
House location	
Antimosquito sprays, fumigants	
▪ Vector Control[b]	
Environmental modification and manipulation	Reduction of vector breeding habitats
Chemical and biological larvicides	
Insecticide spraying of open spaces	Reduction of vector density
Residual insecticide spraying	Reduction of longevity of vector population

[a]Factors reducing the parasite reservoir.
[b]Factors reducing the vectorial capacity.
Modified from Bruce-Chwatt.[3]

rope and the Americas, eliminated malaria; approximately 1.5 billion people live in malaria-free areas that were malarious in the mid-1950s.

Principles of Malaria Control. The objective of control is to decrease morbidity and mortality—and ultimately infection and transmission—by effective intervention at the key areas of the parasite-vector-human cycle. Table 11-8 indicates that the control of malaria disease is achieved by measures directed toward acute illness (mild to severe), chronic infection, and the effects of disease on the mother, fetus, and newborn. The control of malaria transmission is achieved mainly through prevention of mosquito-human contact (termed "personal protection") or through reduction of the number of mosquito vectors, either by altering breeding sites through environmental modification or by killing adult or preadult stages of the mosquito. A key element to the control of malaria in every country is the proper use of surveillance to describe the epidemiological conditions where control actions are initiated to determine the needed resources for control operations.

Disease Control and Drug Use. The designation of priority groups for targeted control efforts is based on low altered levels of immunity and other host and environmental factors that render individuals susceptible to the severe consequences of malaria; priority groups include young children, pregnant women, migrants, and travelers to malarious areas from areas with minimal or no malaria transmission. The control measures may include primary prevention (preventing human-vector contact by barrier methods or repellents) or secondary prevention using chemoprophylaxis (in pregnant women, migrants, and travelers) and prompt chemotherapy of acute illness in children and all other groups.

Antimalarial drugs have specific characteristics in terms of parasite stage-specific efficacy, rapidity and duration of action, parasite resistance, adverse effects, and cost. Frequent or long-term drug use by the resident partially immune population exposes large populations of parasites to low levels of drug for prolonged periods and may foster development of resistance to those drugs. Consequently, the ideal cost-effective treatment of residents of malarious areas is a full therapeutic dose to provide the highest likelihood of elimination of the parasite from the individual. The use of prophylaxis should be limited to target groups, such as pregnant women. Table 11-9 indicates the drugs that can be used for chemoprophylaxis of malaria.[21]

Malaria provides an excellent example of premunition, a condition in which the infecting organism is present along with

TABLE 11-9. DRUGS FOR PROPHYLAXIS OF MALARIA

Drug	Adult Dose	Pediatric Dose
Chloroquine phosphate (Aralen)[a]	300 mg base (500 mg salt) orally, once a week	5 mg/kg base (8.3 mg/kg salt) orally once a week, up to maximum adult dose of 300 mg base
Hydroxychloroquine sulfate (Plaquenil)[a]	310 mg base (400 mg salt) orally, once a week	5 mg/kg base (6.5 mg/kg salt) orally, once a week, up to maximum adult dose
Mefloquine (Lariam)	228 mg base (250 mg salt) orally, once a week	15–19 kg:1/4 tab/wk 20–30 kg: 1/2 tab/wk 31–45 kg: 3/4 tab/wk >45 kg: 1 tab/wk
Doxycycline	100 mg orally, once a day	>8 y: 2 mg/kg orally per day up to adult dose of 100 mg/d
Proguanil[a]	200 mg orally, once a day in combination with weekly chloroquine	<2 y: 50 mg/d 2–6 y: 100 mg/d 7–10 y: 150 mg/d >10 y: 200 mg/d
Pyrimethamine-sulfadoxine (Fansidar)	3 tab (75 mg pyrimethamine and 1500 mg sulfadoxine), orally as a single dose	5–10 kg: 1/2 tab 11–20 kg: 1 tab 21–30 kg: 1 1/2 tab 31–45 kg: 2 tabs >45 kg: 3 tabs
Primaquine[b]	15 mg base (26.3 mg salt) orally, once a day for 14 days	0.3 mg/kg base (0.5 mg/kg salt) orally once a day for 14 d

[a]It is advised that Fansidar be carried as treatment dose by travelers using antimalarial prophylaxis in areas where drug resistance may exist; use to be discussed with a physician.
[b]Begin after departure from endemic area.

partial immunity. While this condition may have substantial benefit for populations living in malaria-endemic areas,[22] the host response, even in partially immune persons, is not always capable of limiting the infection and preventing the parasite proliferation that leads to clinical illness.

Treatment of acute malaria and its complications (Table 11–10) should be based on an accurate diagnosis, clinical status of the patient, an awareness of the pathophysiological mechanisms that can lead to severe illness, knowledge of the patterns of resistance of local parasites, and available drugs and supportive measures.[3,5,23] The objectives of therapy are the rapid reduction or elimination of parasitemia and the prevention of severe complications. Drugs that are effective against the asexual parasite within RBCs include the 4-aminoquinolines (i.e., chloroquine and amodiaquine), the combination of pyrimethamine and sulfonamides or sulfones (i.e., pyrimethamine-sulfadoxine, pyrimethamine-dapsone), the cinchona alkaloids (i.e., quinine and quinidine), and the tetracyclines. Newer and promising antimalarial compounds under continuing assessment include mefloquine, halofantrine, and the class of artemisinin compounds.[24]

TABLE 11–10. DRUGS FOR TREATMENT OF SEVERE *P. FALCIPARUM* MALARIA

Chloroquine-sensitive	Chloroquine-resistant or Sensitivity Unknown[a,b]
1. Chloroquine: base 10 mg/kg in isotonic fluid by constant rate intravenous infusion over 8 h, followed by 15 mg/kg over 24 h	1. Quinine: dihydrochloride salt 7 mg/kg [loading dose] IV by infusion pump over 30 min, followed immediately by 10 mg/kg diluted in 10 ml/kg isotonic fluid by intravenous infusion over 4 h, repeated q8h [maintenance dose] until patient can swallow; then quinine tablets salt 10 mg/kg q8h, to complete 7 d of treatment
Or	Or
2. Chloroquine: base 5 mg/kg in isotonic fluid by constant rate IV infusion over 6 h to a total dose of base 25 mg/kg over 30 h	2. Quinine: salt 20 mg/kg [loading dose] by infusion over 4 h; then 10 mg/kg over 4 h, q8h until patient can swallow; then quinine tablets [as in 1] to complete 7 d of treatment
Or	Or
3. Quinine [see right-hand column]	3. Quinidine: gluconate base 10 mg/kg [loading dose] by infusion over 1–2 h, followed by 0.02 mg/kg/min by infusion pump for 72 h or until patient can swallow; then quinine tablets [as in 1] to complete 7 d of treatment
	Or
	4. Quinidine: gluconate base 15 mg/kg [loading dose] by IV infusion over 4 h; then 7.5 mg/kg over 4 h, q8h until patient can swallow; then quinine tablets [as in 1] to complete 7 d of treatment

[a] In areas of significant drug resistance [Thailand], 250 mg tetracycline 250 mg four times a day for 7 days should be added, except for children under 8 years of age and pregnant women. Patients receiving more than 48 hours of parenteral therapy should receive a one-third reduction in the maintenance dosage of quinine or quinidine [i.e., 5 to 7 mg/kg q8h].
[b] Loading dose not used if patient received quinine, quinidine, or mefloquine in preceding 12 to 24 hours.
From WHO, 1990.[5]

Objectives of management of the acutely ill patient with malaria include rapid elimination of parasitemia with specific therapy and attention to complicating conditions that can lead to severe illness and death. Renal failure, pulmonary edema, hypoglycemia, disseminated intravascular coagulation, hyperpyrexia, and unrousable coma are conditions that require special attention. Table 11–11 indicates the scheme used in the United States for treating patients actively ill with malaria. Recent studies have shown that quinidine is as effective as quinine for the treatment of acute severe malaria.[5,25] The use of exchange transfusions for patients with cerebral malaria and hyperparasitemia (>10% of RBCs infected) has been supported recently.

If *P. vivax* or *P. ovale* malaria is diagnosed, an 8-aminoquinoline compound is given to the patient, after the initial treatment is completed, to eliminate relapses. In countries outside the United States, variations of these treatment regimens are based on available and affordable drugs and available methods of drug delivery.

Parasite Resistance to Drugs. Parasite resistance to antimalarial drugs was first recognized in South America in 1961 with chloroquine-resistant *P. falciparum* (CRPF). Subsequently, CRPF was recognized in southeast Asia (1962) and in Africa (1978).[26] *P. falciparum* has also become resistant to other 4-aminoquinolines, to pyrimethamine and other antifolate compounds, and to sulfonamide-antifolate combinations. In Africa, chloroquine resistance has spread from the initial focus in Kenya and Tanzania in 1978 across central, southern, and now western Africa to include virtually all areas where *P. falciparum* is transmitted. Except for some malarious countries in the Middle East, north Africa, and Central America, Haiti, and the Dominican Republic, CRPF has been identified in all other malarious nations (Fig. 11–9). Resistance to pyrimethamine-sulfadoxine is widespread in Thailand and Brazil, and a few instances of such resistance have been reported from Africa. Reports of decreased sensitivity of *P. falciparum* to quinine and mefloquine from some areas of Thailand indicate that no drug offers complete protection. A recent report has indicated that strains of *P. vivax* resistant to chloroquine may be emerging in the western Pacific (Papua New Guinea).[27]

Sensitivity of *P. falciparum* to antimalarial drugs is measured by standard in vivo and in vitro testing methods.[24] The in vivo scheme assesses the parasitological and clinical response to treatment; there are three levels of resistance (I = low, II = moderate, III = high) based on the parasitological response (Fig. 11–13). The in vitro assay determines the level of drug that impedes parasite maturation. In vitro testing is useful for comparing the sensitivity of isolates from different areas to several drugs at once. Many developing countries are relying on in vivo methods to assess their antimalarial treatment strategies because objectives of their control programs are to decrease severe illness and mortality, and laboratory support for in vitro testing is limited.[28] Hence, in vitro assays are not critical, but serve as a complement to the in vivo assessments for program planning and development.

The mechanisms by which antimalarial drug resistance develops and spreads are not fully understood, although parasite mutation and exposure to suboptimal levels of drug are important factors in selecting for resistant parasites. Parasites resistant to chloroquine may not be exposed to lethal amounts of this drug because the membrane of the host RBC and the parasite membrane become impermeable to the drug; this is due to the abnormally high pH of the metabolic products of the parasite.[24] Resistant parasite mutants may survive by using alternative metabolic pathways to those blocked by the particular drug, and continual

TABLE 11-11. DRUGS FOR THE TREATMENT OF UNCOMPLICATED MALARIA INFECTIONS

Chemical Setting	Drug(s) of Choice[a]	Dosage [b]
Uncomplicated attacks of malaria **Except** *P. falciparum* acquired in areas of chloroquine resistance	Chloroquine phosphate (Aralen)	10 mg/kg base (up to maximum of 600 mg base), then 5 mg/kg base (maximum of 300 mg base for follow-up doses) 6 h later, then 5 mg/kg base per day for 2 d
Uncomplicated attacks of *P. falciparum* acquired in areas of chloroquine resistance	Quinine sulfate	25 mg/kg/d in 3 divided doses for 3 d (maximum of 650 mg/dose)
	plus pyrimethamine/sulfadoxine (Fansidar)[c]	2–11 mo: 1/4 tab 1–3 y: 1/2 tab 4–8 y: 1 tab 9–14 y: 2 tab >14 y: 3 tab Above as a single dose
	or Quinine sulfate plus tetracycline[d]	Same as above 5 mg/kg qid for 7 d (maximum of 250 mg per dose)
After treatment of acute attack of *P. vivax* or *P. ovale* to prevent further relapses ("radical cure")	Primaquine phosphate[e]	0.3 mg/kg/d base for 14 d (maximum dose: 15 mg/d base)

[a]Consult experts, including the Malaria Branch of the Centers for Disease Control, Atlanta, GA 30333 (404-488-4046; nights and weekends 404-639-2888) for information regarding alternative regimens. Note that quinidine may be substituted for quinine according to dosages given in Table 11–10.

[b]Dosages are oral unless otherwise stated.

[c]Fansidar should not be given to persons with known allergy to sulfonamides or pyrimethamine.

[d]For the treatment of malaria, the U.S. Food and Drug Administration considers tetracycline an investigational drug. Tetracycline has been shown to be effective in the treatment of *P. falciparum* strains resistant to Fansidar and acquired in southeast Asia. Physicians must weigh the benefit of tetracycline therapy against the possibility of known adverse effects in children under 8 years of age.

[e]As primaquine may cause severe hemolysis in persons with a G6PD deficiency, patients should be tested for this trait before the drug is given. Congenital malaria and transfusion malaria do not require treatment with primaquine.

drug pressure promotes the selection of these mutants. Although anopheline vectors can then transmit the resistant parasites, the observation that spread has occurred from country to contiguous country indicates that human travel contributes to the dispersion of drug-resistant parasites. Introduction of resistant mutant *P. falciparum,* use of suboptimal drug dosages, and placement of persons with drug-resistant parasites are the major factors responsible for the appearance, selection, intensification, and spread of parasites with reduced susceptibility to drugs.

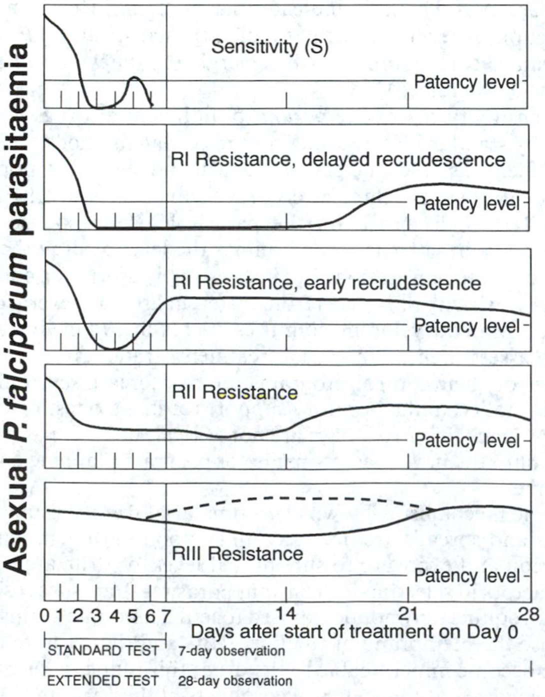

Figure 11-13. *Plasmodium falciparum* response to treatment. (*From Bruce-Chwatt, 1986.*[24])

Protection of Travelers. Nonimmune travelers to malarious areas can reduce vector-human contact by using insect repellents, bed nets, and protective clothing. Travelers should also use chemoprophylaxis with a safe and effective antimalarial drug. In only a few areas of the world is chloroquine still effective as a prophylaxis against *P. falciparum* (Fig. 11-9). Mefloquine chemoprophylaxis is advised by the CDC to protect travelers to areas where *P. falciparum* is resistant to chloroquine. Drug use in short-term travelers has little epidemiologic effect on parasite sensitivity to drugs in the area. Because the malaria situation and corresponding recommendations for prevention can change periodically, travelers are advised to contact their physicians before going to malarious areas. Updated information for United States travelers is available in the guidelines "Prevention of Malaria in Travelers" which is published annually as a supplement to the *Morbidity and Mortality Weekly Report (MMWR)* and can be requested from the Malaria Branch, Centers for Disease Control, Atlanta, GA 30333.[21] The CDC also maintains an updated 24-hour malaria hot line that can be accessed by Touch-Tone telephone (404-332-4555).

Persons with no previous exposure or immunity are highly susceptible to severe illness and death, especially with *P. falciparum;* therefore, when treating patients with fever, health workers need to include malaria in the differential diagnosis and take a comprehensive travel history. Laboratory diagnosis with Giemsa-stained thick and thin blood smears is necessary.

Vector Control

Personal Protection. The use of protective clothing, insect repellents, and bed nets, particularly during the mosquito biting hours, can be extremely effective in preventing malaria infection.

Similarly, the use of insecticide-impregnated bed nets and curtains has been shown to be highly effective in reducing transmission.[29]

Insecticides [Larviciding, Adulticiding]. Programs focused on decreasing transmission emphasize decreasing mosquito larvae by covering breeding areas with insecticidal agents and indoor house spraying with a residual insecticide to eliminate safe resting sites on house walls for the indoors mosquito that bites and rests.[30,31]

Environmental Source Reduction. The elimination of anopheline mosquito breeding sites by drainage of standing water is an important control measure that is cost-effective in the urban setting and can be used on a smaller scale in rural communities, depending on the mosquito species and the distribution of breeding sites in the environment.

Biological Control. Biological control measures, such as the introduction of larvivorous fish into collections of water or the use of microbiological toxins (*Bacillus thuringiensis,* serotype H-14), have potential for mosquito control.[32] In addition, the introduction of mosquitoes refractory to parasite multiplication or of sterile male mosquitoes into the population could lead to lower breeding efficiency. While such biological control measures are attractive and are being studied, they have not yet been shown to be effective or ready for widespread use in the community setting.

Research and Control. The chief areas of research in malaria that can have the greatest impact on control strategies are (1) understanding host-parasite-vector interactions, including the immunological response to the parasite in both the human and vector hosts; (2) developing new or improved technologies for control; (3) improving delivery of current or new technologies; (4) monitoring changes in the epidemiological patterns and the disease impact; and (5) assessing interrelationships with other childhood and adult diseases.

More information is needed on the mechanisms by which malaria parasites cause disease and by which humans and vectors respond to infection. Recent work has been directed at the pathophysiology of cerebral malaria, with emphasis on the molecular basis of cytoadherence of malaria parasites within postcapillary venules.[33] The immunological mechanisms required for cellular and antibody responses and for protection against malaria are not completely understood; only when these mechanisms are more fully understood will it be possible to develop a suitable vaccine.[34]

The major recent developments in control technology have involved antimalarial drugs. The process of developing new drugs is long and time-intensive. At the Walter Reed Army Institute of Medical Research, more than 250,000 compounds were screened for antimalarial activity during the three decades following World War II. One product from this program is mefloquine, a quinoline-methanol compound that resembles quinine structurally and has excellent blood schizonticidal activity against *P. falciparum* strains resistant to chloroquine and pyrimethamine-sulfadoxine. This drug has recently been licensed for use in the United States and is now recommended as chemoprophylaxis for U.S. travelers to areas with parasite resistance to other drugs.[21] Other recently tested drugs with promise include halofantrine and a variety of artemisinin compounds (e.g., Quing hao tsu, derived from the plant *Artemesia annua*), while still other drugs are in the development phase[24] awaiting more complete data on their pharmacokinetics, efficacy, side effects, and formulations.

The use of pesticide-impregnated mosquito nets and curtains to protect communities in malarious areas has been studied recently in Asia and Africa.[29,35] Initial results indicate that the entomologic effect of these interventions is excellent, but their parasitological, clinical, and epidemiological impact remains to be clarified. Assessment of the feasibility and cost-effectiveness of personal protection measures and integration of malaria-control activities into other disease control programs are major challenges in health services delivery research.

Although no vaccine is available, much progress has been made in the development of malaria vaccine over the past 2 decades; antigen production has been aided by developments that allow for the identification and synthesis of protein sequences from various stages of the parasite. Great attention was given initially to the sporozoite antigens.[36] Following the successful in vitro cultivation of *P. falciparum* in the mid-1970s,[37] large amounts of blood stage antigens have been produced for characterization and study. More recently, asexual blood stage vaccine development research has accelerated. It is likely that an effective vaccine will include sporozoite and asexual blood stage components to prevent acute illness. Antigamete vaccines may be included to help block the emergence of immunological variants and possibly help to interrupt transmission. Research on combining antigens against *P. falciparum* and *P. vivax* (and possibly other species) will be needed for areas where these parasites coexist.

Research continues to be needed to understand further the population at risk for acute malaria and to develop appropriate control measures, particularly for young children. Because the case fatality rates for cerebral malaria continue to be in excess of 20%, methods for prevention of this syndrome need urgent attention; such work will need to include the evaluation of control measures at the community level.

Further work is required to understand better the role of malaria chemoprophylaxis in preventing low birth weight. While chemoprophylaxis for pregnant women exposed to malaria has been advised, parasite resistance to drugs (especially to chloroquine), the potential side effects of antimalarial drugs, and the difficulty in assuring compliance among pregnant women have prompted the reevaluation of this strategy. Research in areas with chloroquine-resistant parasites has been aimed at assessing drugs other than chloroquine for chemoprophylaxis for pregnant women. Studies are required to determine the pathological and immunological processes that affect the mother, the placenta, and the fetus.[38] Investigations are also necessary to evaluate the relative contribution of malaria to low birth weight in settings with multiple causes of low birth weight, such as malnutrition, other infectious diseases, and anemia.[39]

Research is needed to evaluate the role of repeated or chronic malaria infections that may become accentuated if antimalarial drugs that do not clear parasitemia are used. Studies of the effects of various drug treatment strategies on anemia and of the effects of transfusions given for malaria-induced anemia are needed.[40] The transmission of HIV infection in malarious areas has been associated with blood transfusions to treat anemia caused by malaria.[41] HIV-infected patients do not appear to be predisposed to severe episodes of malaria[42]; however, evaluation of control measures to prevent malaria-associated anemia may be important in the control of HIV transmission.[41]

While routine surveillance is used to monitor health indicators at some health units, special studies are needed often to describe more precisely the medical and economic actions required in communities to sustain control successfully. Other research priorities include studies to define the contribution of malaria to the overall disease burden in the developing countries and to characterize the interrelationships between malaria, low birth weight, anemia, HIV infection, acute respiratory illness, and other conditions.

Once new and improved drugs, vector-control approaches, and immunological interventions are available, the major challenges will be to ensure that these products and services are being used by target populations. Effective delivery of services to communities and health units requires well-designed training and health education programs, integration of malaria interventions into other health activities by employment of sound management principles, and well-designed operations research to measure the effect of the interventions.

Conclusion. While malaria infection and disease have been eradicated or controlled in many parts of the world, the situation in Africa and the increase in cases in many areas of South America and Asia merit intensified efforts. To strengthen malaria control, a more comprehensive understanding of the biology and epidemiology of malaria will be required, as will increased efforts to use available technologies more effectively and to develop new ones.

REFERENCES

Viral Infections

1. Karabatsos N (ed): International Catalogue of Arboviruses, Including Certain Other Viruses of Vertebrates, 3 edt. San Antonio: American Society of Tropical Medicine and Hygiene, 1985
2. Monath TB (ed): The Arboviruses: Ecology and Epidemiology, Vol. I-V, Boca Raton: CRC Press, 1988
3. Fields RN, Knipe DM (eds): Virology, 2 edt, Vols I-II. New York: Raven, 1990
4. Elliott RM: Molecular biology of the Bunyaviridae. J Gen Virol 1990;71:501-522
5. Strauss JH, Strauss EG (eds): The Togaviridae and Flaviviridae. New York: Plenum, 1986
6. Bishop DHL: The Bunyaviridae. In Fraenkel-Comrat H, Wagner RR (eds): Comparative Virology, Vol 14. New York: Plenum, 1986
7. Bishop DHL. The Rhabdoviruses. West Palm Beach, Fla: CRC Press, 1979
8. Reeves WC. Factors that influence the probability of epidemics of western equine, St. Louis, and California encephalitis in California. Calif Vector Views 14:13-18, 1967
9. Reeves WC. Overwintering of arboviruses. Prog Med Virol 17:193-220, 1974
10. Hayes RO, Francy DB, Lazuick JS, Smith GS, Gibbs EPJ: Role of the cliff swallow bug (*Oeciacus vicarius*) in the natural cycle of a western equine encephalitis-related arborvirus. J Med Entomol 14:257-262, 1977
11. Bailey CL, Eldridge BF, Hayes DE, et al: Isolation of St. Louis encephalitis virus from overwintering *Culex pipiens* mosquitoes. Science 199:1346-1349, 1978
12. Miller BR, DeFoliart FR, Yuill TM: Vertical transmission of La-Crosse virus (California encephalitis group): transovarial and filial infection rates in *Aedes triseriatus* (Diptera: *Culicidae*). J Med Entomol 14:437-440, 1977
13. Bowen GS, Francy DB: Surveillance. In Monath TP (ed): St. Louis Encephalitis. Washington, DC: American Public Health Association, 1979
14. Rosen L, Gubler D: The use of mosquitoes to detect and propagate dengue viruses. Am J Trop Med 23:1153-1160, 1974
15. Calisher CH, Monath TP. Alphaviruses and flaviviruses. In Lennette E, Halonen PE, Murphy FA (eds): The Laboratory Diagnosis of Infectious Diseases: Principles and Practices. New York: Springer Verlag, 1989
16. Holden P, Hayes RO, Mitchell CJ, et al: House sparrows, *Passer domesticus* (L.), as hosts of arbovirus in Hale County, Texas. I. Field studies, 1965-1969. Am J Trop Med Hyg 22:244-253, 1971
17. Young NA, Johnson KM: Antigenic variants of Venezuelan equine encephalitis virus: their geographic distribution and epidemiologic significance. Am J Epidemiol 89:286-307, 1969
18. Sudia WD, Newhouse VF: Venezuelan equine encephalitis in North America: a summary of virus-vector-host relationships. Am J Epidemiol 101:1-13, 1975
19. Monath TP, Tsai TF: St. Louis encephalitis: lessons from the last decade. Am J Trop Med Hyg 37:40S-59S, 1987
20. Hammon WMcD, Kitaoka M, Downs WG (eds): Immunization for Japanese Encephalitis. Baltimore: Williams & Wilkins Co, 1971
21. Lopes OS, Sachetta L de A, Coimbra TLM, Pinto GH, Glasser CM: Emergence of a new arbovirus disease in Brazil. II. Epidemiologic studies on 1975 epidemic. Am J Epidemiol 108:394-401, 1978
22. Hafkin B, Kaplan JE, Reed C, et al: Reintroduction of dengue fever into the continental United States. I. Dengue surveillance in Texas, 1980. Am J Trop Med Hyg 31:1222-1228, 1982
23. Pinheiro FP, Travassos da Rosa AP, Gomes ML, LeDuc JW, Hoch AL: Transmission of Oropouche virus from man to hamster by the midge *Culicoides paraensis*. Science 215:1251-1253, 1982
24. Halstead SB, Scanlon JE, Umpaivit P, Udomsakdi S: Dengue and Chikungunya virus infection in man in Thailand, 1962-1964. IV. Epidemiological studies in the Bangkok metropolitan area. Am J Trop Med Hyg 18:997-1021, 1969
25. Halstead SB: Observations related to pathogenesis of dengue hemorrhagic fever: hypotheses and discussion. Yale J Biol Med 42:350-362, 1970
26. Halstead SB: The pathogenesis of dengue: molecular epidemiology in infectious disease. Am J Epidemiol 114:632-648, 1981
27. Barnes WJS, Rosen L: Fatal hemorrhagic disease and shock associated with primary dengue infection on a Pacific island. Am J Trop Med Hyg 23:495-506, 1974
28. Monath TP: Yellow fever—a medically neglected disease. Rev Infect Dis 9:165-176, 1987
29. Monath TP, Craven RB, Adjukiewicz A, et al: Yellow fever in the Gambia, 1978-1979: epidemiologic aspects with observations on the occurrence of Orungo virus infections. Am J Trop Med Hyg 29:912-928, 1980
30. Meegan JM: The Rift Valley fever epizootic in Egypt 1977-1978. I. Description of the epizootic and virological studies. Trans R Soc Trop Med Hyg 73:618-623, 1979
31. Linthicum KJ, Davies FB, Kairo A: Rift Valley fever virus (Bunyaviridae, Phlebovirus): isolations from Diptera collected during an interepizootic period. J Hyg (Cambr) 95:197-209, 1985
32. Casals J, Henderson BE, Hoogstraal A, Johnson KM, Shelokov A. A review of Soviet viral hemorrhagic fevers. J Infect Dis 122:437-453, 1970
33. Kharitonova NN, Leonov YuA: Infection of small mammals with Omsk hemorrhagic fever (OHF) virus by alimentary route. Simposium Itogi 6 Virus Ekoh Svyazan, 114-117, 1971 (English translation NAMRU 3-T676)
34. Casals J: Antigenic similarity between the virus causing Crimean hemorrhagic fever and Congo virus. Proc Soc Exp Biol Med 131:233-236, 1969
35. Goldfarb LG, Chumakov MP, Myskin AA, Kondratenko VF, Resnikova OYu: An epidemiological model of Crimean hemorrhagic fever. Am J Trop Med Hyg 29:260-264, 1980
36. Kondratenko VF: Importance of ixodid ticks in transmission and preservation of Crimean hemorrhagic fever agent in infection foci. Parazitologiia. 10:297-302, 1976 (English translation NAMRU3-T1116)
37. Meyer HM Jr, Johnson RT, Crawford IP, Dascomb HE, Rogers NG: Central nervous syndromes of "viral" etiology: a study of 713 cases. Am J Med 29:334-341, 1960
38. Gregg MB: Recent outbreaks of lymphocytic choriomeningitis in the United States of America. Bull World Health Organ 52:549-554, 1975
39. Maiztegui JI, Fernandez NJ, Damilano AJ. Efficacy of immune plasma in treatment of Argentine hemorrhagic fever and association between treatment and a late neurological syndrome. Lancet 2:1216-1217, 1979
40. McCormick JB, Webb PA, Krebs JW, et al: A prospective study of the epidemiology and ecology of Lassa fever. J Infect Dis 155:445-455, 1987
41. Keenlyside RA, McCormick JB, Webb PA, et al: Case-control study of *Mastomys natalensis* and humans in Lassa virus-infected households in Sierra Leone. Am J Trop Med Hyg 32:829-837, 1983
42. Anonymous: Ebola haemorrhagic fever in Zaire, 1976: report of an international commission. Bull World Health Organ 56:271-293, 1978

43. Heymann DL, Weisfeld JS, Webb PA, Cairns J, Berquist H. Ebola hemorrhagic fever: Tandala, Zaire, 1977–1978. J Infect Dis 142(3): 372–376, 1980
44. Jahrling PB, Geisbert TW, Dalgard DW, Johnson ED, Ksiazek TG, Hall WG, Peters CJ. Preliminary report: isolation of Ebola virus from monkeys imported to USA. Lancet 335:502–505, 1990
45. Lee HW, Lee PW, Johnson KM: Isolation of the etiologic agent of Korean hemorrhagic fever. J Infect Dis 137:298–308, 1978
46. Schmaljohn CS, Dalrymple JM: Analysis of Hantaan virus RNA: evidence for a new genus of Bunyaviridae. Virology 131:482–491, 1983
47. Desmyter J, LeDuc JW, Johnson KM, et al: Laboratory rat associated outbreak of hemorrhagic fever with renal syndrome due to Hantaan-like virus in Belgium. Lancet 2:1445–1448, 1983

General References

Blascovic D (ed): Studies on tick-borne encephalitis. Bull World Health Organ 36(suppl 1):5–94, 1967

Calisher CH, Thompson WH (eds): California Serogroup Viruses. Progress in Clinical and Biological Research, Vol 123. New York: Alan R. Liss, 1983

Hoogstraal H. The epidemiology of tick-borne Crimean-Congo hemorrhagic fever in Asia, Europe, and Africa. J Med Entomol 15:307–417, 1979

International symposium on arenaviral infections of public health importance. Bull World Health Organ 52:307–417, 1975

Lehmann-Grube F. Lymphocytic Choriomeningitis Virus. Virology Monograph No. 10. New York: Springer-Verlag, 1971

McKee KT, Jr, LeDuc JW, Peters CJ: Hantaviruses. In Belshe R (ed): Human Virology, 2 edt. Littleton, Mass: PSB Publishing Co, 1990

Monath TP (ed): St. Louis Encephalitis. Washington, DC: American Public Health Association, 1979

Monath TP (ed): The Arboviruses: Ecology and Epidemiology. Vols. I-V. Boca Raton: CRC, 1988

Peters CJ: Arenaviruses. In Belshe R (ed): Human Virology, 2 edt, Littleton, Mass: PSB Publishing Co, 1990

Reeves WC, Hammon WMcD: Epidemiology of the Arthropod-Borne Viral Encephalitides in Kern County, California, 1943–1952. Berkeley: University of California Press, 1962 (University of California Publication in Public Health, Vol. 4)

Schlesinger RW: Dengue Viruses. Virology Monographs, Vol 16. New York: Springer-Verlag, 1977

Strode GK (ed): Yellow Fever. New York: McGraw-Hill Book Co, 1951 1951

Theiler M, Downs WG: The Arthropod-Brone Viruses of Vertebrates. New Haven: Yale University Press, 1973

Venezuelan Encephalitis: Proceedings of the Workshop-Symposium on Venezuelan Encephalitis Virus. Washington, D.C., Sept 14–17, 1971. Washington, D.C.: Pan American Health Organization Scientific Publication 243, 1972

Rickettsial Infections

1. McDade JE, Fishbein DB. Rickettsiaceae: The Rickettsiae. In Balows A, Hausler WJ Jr, Lennette EH (eds): The Laboratory Diagnosis of Infectious Diseases: Principles and Practice, Vol. 2. New York: Springer-Verlag, 1988, pp 864–890
2. Krieg NR (ed): Bergey's Manual of Systematic Bacteriology. Vol. 1. Baltimore: Williams & Wilkins Co, 1984, pp 687–704
3. Raoult D, Walker DH: *Rickettsia rickettsii* and Other Spotted Fever Group Rickettsiae (Rocky Mountain Spotted Fever and Other Spotted Fevers). In Mandell GL, Douglas RG Jr, Bennett JE (eds): Principles and Practice of Infectious Diseases, 3 edt. New York: Churchill Livingstone, 1989, pp 1465–1471
4. Saah AJ: *Rickettsia prowazekii* (Epidemic or Louse-borne Typhus). In Mandell GL, Douglas RG Jr, Bennett JE (eds): Principles and Practice of Infectious Diseases, 3 edt. New York: Churchill Livingstone 1989, pp 1476–1478
5. Saah AJ: *Rickettsia tsutsugamushi* (Scrub Typhus). In Mandell GL, Douglas RG Jr, Bennett JE (eds): Principles and Practice of Infectious Diseases, 3 edt. New York: Churchill Livingstone, 1989, pp 1480–1482
6. Marrie TJ: *Coxiella burnetii* (Q Fever). In Mandell GL, Douglas RG Jr, Bennett JE (eds): Principles and Practice of Infectious Diseases, 3 edt. New York: Churchill Livingstone, 1989, pp 1472–1476
7. Taylor JP, Betz TG, Rawlings JA: Epidemiology of murine typhus in Texas, 1980 through 1984. JAMA 255:2173–2176, 1986
8. Ming-yuan F, Walker DH, Shu-rong Y, Qing-huai L. Epidemiology and ecology of rickettsial diseases in the People's Republic of China. Rev Infect Dis 9:823–840, 1987
9. Rapmund G: Rickettsial diseases of the Far East: new perspectives. J Infect Dis 149:330–338, 1984
10. Salgo MP, Telzak EE, Currie B, et al: A focus of Rocky Mountain spotted fever within New York City. N Engl J Med 318:1345–1348, 1988
11. Gordon JC, Gordon SW, Peterson E, Philip RN: Rocky Mountain spotted fever in dogs associated with human patients in Ohio. J Infect Dis 148:1123, 1983
12. McDonald JC, MacLean JD, McDade JE: Imported rickettsial disease: clinical and epidemiologic features. Am J Med 85:799–805, 1988
13. Mansueto S, Tringali G, Walker DH: Widespread simultaneous increase in the incidence of spotted fever group rickettsiosis. J Infect Dis 154:538–540, 1986
14. Font-Creus B, Bella-Cueto F, Espejo-Arenas E, et al: Mediterranean spotted fever: a cooperative study of 227 cases. Rev Infect Dis 7:635–642, 1985
15. Uchida T, Tashiro F, Funato T, et al: Isolation of a spotted fever group rickettsia from a patient with febrile exanthematous illness in Shikoku, Japan. Microbiol Immunol 30:1323–1326, 1986
16. Brettman LR, Lewin S, Holzman RS, et al: Rickettsialpox: report of an outbreak and a contemporary review. Medicine 60:363–372, 1981
17. Bernard KW, Parham GL, Winkler WG, Helmick CG: Q fever control measures: recommendations for facilities using sheep. Infect Control 3:461–465, 1982
18. Maeda K, Markowitz N, Hawley RC, Ristic M, Cox D, McDade JE. Human infection with *Ehrlichia canis,* a leukocytic Rickettsia. N Engl J Med 316:853–856, 1987
19. McDade JE: Ehrlichiosis—a disease of animals and humans. J Infect Dis 161:609–617, 1990
20. Rohrbach BW, Harkess JR, Ewing SA, Kudlac J, McKee GL, Istre GR. Epidemiologic and clinical characteristics of persons with serologic evidence of *E. canis* infection. Am J Public Health 80:442–445, 1990
21. Fishbein DB, Kemp A, Dawson JE, Greene NR, Redus MA, Fields DH: Human ehrlichiosis: prospective active surveillance in febrile hospitalized patients. J Infect Dis 160:803–809, 1989

Plague

1. Barnes AM: Surveillance and control of bubonic plague in the United States. Symp Zool Soc Lond 50:237–270, 1982
2. Quan TJ: Plague. In Wentworth BB (ed): Diagnostic Procedures for Bacterial Infections, 7 edt. Washington, D.C.: American Public Health Association, 1987, pp 445–453
3. Poland JD, Barnes AM: Plague. In Steele J (ed): Handbook of Zoonoses. Boca Raton: CRC Press, 1979, pp 515–559
4. Cavanaugh DC: The specific effect of temperature upon the transmission of the plague bacillus by the oriental rat flea (*Xenopsylla cheopis*). Am J Trop Med Hyg 20:264, 1971
5. Von Reyn CF, Barnes AM, Weber NS, Hodgrin UG: Bubonic plague from exposure to a rabbit: a documented case and a review of rabbit-associated plague cases in the United States. Am J Epidemiol 104:81, 1976
6. Kaufman AF, Mann JM, Gardiner TM, et al: Public health implications of plague in domestic cats. J Am Vet Med Assoc 179:875–878, 1981
7. Eidson M, Tierney LA, Rollag AJ, et al: Feline plague in New Mex-

ico: risk factors and transmission to humans. Am J Public Health 78:1333–1335, 1988

8. Barnes AM, Poland JD: Plague in the United States, MMWR 32(5):1955–1958, 1982
9. Quan TJ, Poland JD, Barnes AM: Winter plague. MMWR 33:145–148, 1984
10. Marshall JD, Quy DV, Gibson FL: Asymptomatic pharyngeal plague infection in Vietnam. Am J Trop Med Hyg 16:175, 1967
11. Cavanaugh DC, Elisberg BL, Llewellyn CH, et al: Plague immunization. V. Indirect evidence of the efficacy of plague vaccine USP. J Infect Dis 129:537–540, 1974
12. Recommendations of the Public Health Service Advisory Committee on Immunization Practices: plague vaccine. MMWR 31:301–304, 1982
13. Barnes AM: Surveillance and control of bubonic plague in the United States. Symp Zool Soc Lond 50:237–270, 1982
14. World Health Organization: Plague surveillance and control. WHO Chron 34:139–143, 1980
15. Beard ML, Montman CE, Maupin GE, et al: Field trials of the rodenticide cholecalciferol against *Spermophilus variegatus* (rock squirrel), a source of human plague in the southwestern United States. J Environ Health 51(2):69–75 (revised version), 1988

Malaria

1. World Health Organization: Weekly epidemiologic record. 65: No. 25, 189–190; No. 26, 200–202, 1990
2. World Health Organization. World Malaria Situation 1985. World Health Stat Q 40:142–170, 1987
3. Bruce-Chwatt LJ: Essential Malariology, 2 edt. New York: John Wiley & Sons, Inc., 1985
4. Bruce-Chwatt LJ: Transfusion malaria. Bull World Health Organ 50:337–346, 1974
5. World Health Organization: Severe and complicated malaria, 2 edt. Trans R Soc Trop Med Hyg 84 (suppl 2):1–65, 1990
6. Molineaux L: The epidemiology of human malaria as an explanation of its distribution, including some implications for its control. In Wernsdorfer WH, McGregor IA (eds): Malaria, Principles and Practice of Malariology. Vol 2. London: Churchill Livingstone, 1988, pp. 913–998
7. Molineaux L, Gramiccia G: The Garki Project, Research on the epidemiology and control of malaria in the Sudan Savannah of West Africa. Geneva, Switzerland: World Health Organization, 1980
8. Bruce-Chwatt LJ: Imported malaria: an uninvited guest. Br Med Bull 38:179–186, 1982
9. Maldonado YA, Nahlen BL, Roberto RR, Ginsberg M, Orellana E, Misrahi M, McBarron K, Lobel HO, Cambell CC: Transmission of *Plasmodium vivax* malaria in San Diego County, California, 1986. Am J Trop Med Hyg 42:3–9, 1990
10. Dabis F, Breman JG, Roisin A, Haba F: Monitoring selective components of primary health care: methodology and community assessment of vaccination, diarrhoea, and malaria practices in Conakry, Guinea. Bull World Health Organ 67:675–684, 1989
11. Greenwood BW, Bradley AK, Greenwood AM, Byass P, Jammeh K, Marsh K, Tulloch S, Oldfield FSJ, Hayes R: Mortality and morbidity from malaria among children in a rural area of the Gambia, West Africa. Trans Soc Trop Med Hyg 81:478–486, 1987
12. McGregor IA, Wilson ME, Billewicz WZ: Malaria infection of the placenta in Gambia, West Africa: its incidence and relationship to stillbirth, birthweight, and placental weight. Trans R Soc Trop Med Hyg 77:232–244, 1983
13. Centers for Disease Control: Transmission of *Plasmodium vivax* malaria, San Diego County, California, 1988 and 1989. MMWR 39:91–94, 1990
14. Centers for Disease Control: Malaria Surveillance, Annual Summary 1988. Atlanta, Ga: US Department of Health and Human Services, 1990
15. MacDonald G: Dynamics of Tropical Disease. In Bruce-Chwatt LJ, Glanville LJ (eds): London: Oxford University Press, 1973
16. Allison AC: Protection afforded by sickle cell trait against subtertian malarial infection. Br Med J 1:290–294, 1954
17. Miller LH, Mason SJ, Clyde DF, McGinniss MH: The resistance factor to *Plasmodium vivax* in blacks: the Duffy blood group genotype, Fy-Fy. N Engl J Med 295:302–304, 1976
18. Barlow R, Grobar RW: Costs and Benefits of Controlling Parasitic Diseases. Washington, D.C.: The World Bank, PHN Technical Note 85-17, 1986
19. Conly GN: The Impact of Malaria on Economic Development: A Case Sudy. Washington, D.C.: Pan American Health Organization, Scientific Publication No. 297, 1975
20. Payne D, Grab B, Fontaine RE, Hempel JHG: Impact of control measures on malaria transmission and general mortality. Bull World Health Organ 54:369–377, 1976
21. Centers for Disease Control: Recommendations for the prevention of malaria among travelers. MMWR 39/No. RR-3:1–10, 1990
22. Greenwood BM: Asymptomatic malaria infections—do they matter? Parasitol Today 3:206–213, 1987
23. Aikawa M, Iseki M, Barnwell JW, Taylor D, Oo MM, Howard RJ: The pathology of human cerebral malaria. Am J Trop Med Hyg 43 (suppl): 30–37, 1990
24. Bruce-Chwatt LJ: Chemotherapy of Malaria; WHO Monograph Series No. 27, Rev 2 edt. Geneva, Switzerland: World Health Organization, 1986
25. Miller KD, Greenberg AE, Campbell CC: Treatment of malaria in the United States with a continuous infusion of quinidine gluconate and exchange transfusion. N Engl J Med 321:65–70, 1989
26. Bjorkman A, Phillips-Howard PA: The epidemiology of drug-resistant malaria. Trans R Soc Trop Med Hyg 84:177–180, 1990
27. Rieckmann KH, Davis DR, Hutton DC: *Plasmodium vivax* resistant to chloroquine? Lancet 2:1183–1184, 1989
28. Breman JG, Campbell CC: Combating severe malaria in African children. Bull World Health Organ 66:611–620, 1988
29. Rozendaal JA: Impregnated mosquito nets and curtains for self-protection and vector control. Trop Dis Bull 86(No. 7): R1-R41, 1989
30. Gratz NG, Pal R: Malaria vector control: larviciding. In Wernsdorfer WH, McGregor IA (eds): Malaria, Principles and Practice of Malariology. Vol. 2. London: Churchill Livingstone, 1988, pp 1213–1226
31. Pant CP: Malaria vector control: Imagociding. In Wernsdorfer WH, McGregor IA (eds): Malaria, Principles and Practice of Malariology. Vol. 2. London: Churchill Livingstone, 1988, pp 1173–1212
32. Rishikesh N, Dubitski AM, Moreau CM: Malaria vector control: biological control. In Wernsdorfer WH, McGregor IA (eds): Malaria, Principles and Practice of Malariology. Vol. 2. London: Churchill Livingstone, 1988, pp 1227–1249
33. Howard RJ, Handunneti SM, Hasler T, Gilladoga A, de Aguiar JC, Paslooske BL, Morehead K, Albrecht RR, van Schravondijk MR. Surface molecules on *Plasmodium falciparum*-infected erythrocytes involved in adherence. Am J Trop Med Hyg 43(suppl):15–29, 1990
34. Miller LH, Howard RJ, Carter R, et al: Research toward malaria vaccines. Science 234:1349–1356, 1986
35. Snow RW, Lindsay SW, Hayes RJ, Greenwood BM: Permethrin-treated bed nets (mosquito nets) prevent malaria in Gambian children. Trans R Soc Trop Med Hyg 82:838–842, 1988
36. Clyde DF, Most H, McCarthy V, et al: Immunization of man against sporozoite-induced falciparum malaria. Am J Med Sci 266:166–177, 1973
37. Trager W, Jensen JB: Human malaria parasites in continuous culture. Science 193:673–675, 1976
38. Steketee RW: Recent findings in perinatal malaria. Int J Pediatr 10:418–433, 1989
39. Kramer M: Determinants of low birth weight: methodological assessment and meta-analysis. Bull World Health Organ 65:663–737, 1987

40. Schmutzhard E, Rainer J, Rwechungura RI: Treatment of severe malarial anemia in East Africa's underfives—an unsolvable problem since the advent of AIDS. Trans R Soc Trop Med Hygiene 82:220, 1988
41. Greenberg AE, Nguyen-Dinh P, Mann JM, Kabote N, Colebunders RL, Francis H, Quinn TC, Baudoux P, Lyamba B, Davachi F, Roberts JM, Kabeya M, Curran JW, Campbell CC: The association between malaria, blood transfusions, and HIV seropositivity in a pediatric population in Kinshasa, Zaire. JAMA 259:545–549, 1988
42. Nguyen-Dinh P, Greenberg AE, Mann JM, et al: Absence of association between *Plasmodium falciparum* malaria and human immunodeficiency virus infection in children in Kinshasa, Zaire. Bull World Health Organ 65:607–613, 1987

12

Diseases Transmitted Primarily from Animals to Humans (Zoonoses)

Rabies

Denny G. Constantine

Rabies, an acute viral infection of the central nervous system, is known to have occurred in animals and humans since ancient times. The major reservoir of rabies is wildlife, but in much of the world it is a public health hazard because of its endemicity in dogs. Humans are only incidental hosts. The etiological agent is a bullet-shaped virus that belongs to the Rhabdoviridae, a family that includes over 100 viruses of vertebrates, invertebrates, and plants. Rabies has a worldwide distribution and exists enzootically on every continent except Australia. Many islands or peninsular countries, such as Hawaii, New Zealand, and Cyprus, have never experienced rabies, or they have eliminated the infection and remain free of it through the application of rigid control and quarantine measures, as in Japan, Norway, Sweden, the United Kingdom, and Iceland.

Occurrence. The incidence of human rabies in the countries of western Europe, Canada, and the United States has been reduced to about one or two cases per year but is much higher in other parts of the world. Each year, about 50,000 persons and millions of animals are said to die of rabies worldwide, and some 3.7 million people take rabies prophylaxis.[1] The diagnosis and reporting of human and animal rabies in developing countries of Asia, Africa, and South America is grossly deficient, and information on the incidence of the disease in these areas is not reliable. Other diseases may cause greater mortality or morbidity, but the impact of rabies remains very significant in most parts of the world, causing great discomfort, sometimes serious side effects, and incalculable anxiety in the individuals and families concerned. The number of persons treated for potential rabies exposure each year in the United States is probably much higher than the 20,000 persons estimated because this estimation is based on a study of treatment in 21 states, where strict consultation likely reduced the numbers of persons treated to one fifth or less compared to the numbers treated in other states.[2]

Epidemiological Patterns and Distribution. Rabies in nature exists in two epidemiological forms: (1) the urban type in dogs and (2) wildlife rabies, principally in wild Canidae (jackals, wolves, coyotes, foxes), Viverridae (mongoose, civet cat, meerkat), Mustelidae (weasel, polecat, skunk), and Chiroptera (bats). Urban (canine) rabies is the more noticeable epidemiological pattern in most parts of the world and usually constitutes the main source of human infections. The true character or extent of the wildlife reservoir in many countries remains unexamined, however.

Fox rabies is a serious problem in North America and has resulted in widespread and current epizootics in Europe since at least 1803. In Africa and Asia, the jackal is a prominent source of virus for other species, and in western Asia, the wolf has long been known as a dangerous source of the virus. The mongoose is an important transmitter of rabies in certain Caribbean islands, India, and South Africa. In Central and South America, the vampire bat is a principal vector of rabies for both humans and domesticated animals and is estimated to cause losses in cattle exceeding $40 million annually. In Canada, where canine rabies was the primary problem from 1920 to 1950, a shift to wildlife rabies, primarily in skunks and foxes, was reported following widespread disease in foxes in Arctic areas.

In the United States, there is a complex epidemiological pattern of disease, with widespread terrestrial animal rabies (skunk, fox, raccoon) overlaid by the disease in insectivorous bats. A shift in the distribution of rabies cases, by species, has been reported in the United States during the last 50 years (Table 12–1), but the early lack of surveillance in certain animals, such as bats, may have distorted this recorded pattern. In recent years, skunk rabies has comprised over half of all wildlife rabies reports. There has been a marked increase in raccoon rabies cases in the eastern portion of the United States since 1982. The decrease in dog and cat cases is a true diminution of the disease in these species and is related to widespread canine immunization and the application of rabies control measures. Cat cases are generally sporadic and peripheral to cycles in dogs and wild carnivores. Although the actual number of reports of rabies-positive bats has increased markedly since the disease was first described in this species in 1953, the proportion of those found to have the disease in comparison to the total number of submitted specimens apparently has not changed. Thus, no real increase in bat disease has occurred. On rare occasions, a rodent has been found infected with rabies virus, but no rodent species has been implicated as a source of the virus for other mammals.

Associated with the decrease of rabies seen in the dog and cat are a marked decrease of the disease in humans and a shift in

TABLE 12-1. REPORTED RABIES CASES IN THE UNITED STATES (1938–1987)

Year	Dogs	Cats	Farm Animals	Foxes	Skunks	Bats	Raccoons	Other Animals	Humans	Total
1938	8,452	207	662	—	—	—	—	44	47	—
1946	8,384	455	1,055	—	—	—	—	956	33	10,883
1954	4,083	462	1,032	1,028	547	4	—	118	8	7,282
1962	565	232	614	594	1,449	157	62	52	2	3,727
1970	185	135	399	771	1,235	296	181	71	3[a]	3,276
1978	119	96	254	148	1,657	567	404	49	4	3,298
1987	170	166	223	119	2,033	629	1,311	77	1	4,729

[a]One patient recovered.

the species responsible for causing human disease. Since 1974, all but 1 of the 7 cases of human rabies in the continental United States that could be attributed directly to dogs occurred in persons who were exposed elsewhere. During this period, only 2 cases were associated with cats. The human cases not associated with a dog or cat were attributed to bats (2), laboratory exposure (1), infective corneal transplant (1), and unknown sources (11). Animal rabies in the United States and its territories in 1987 was widespread except in Hawaii, Guam, and the Virgin Islands. The relative importance of different animal species (i.e., fox, skunk, raccoon, and bat) varies according to area, but since 1976, close to 90% of all reported animal rabies in the United States has been in wildlife species.[3]

Transmission. Virus may be present in saliva 7 days before the onset of symptoms in dogs and for longer intervals in wildlife. Skunks may secrete virus 8 days and bats 12 days before the development of symptoms. The bite route is the main rabies transmission mechanism among animals and from animals to humans, but in recent years, nonbite routes have been documented. Respiratory transmission of rabies virus was implicated in the deaths of two men who had been working in a bat cave that contained millions of bats.[4] Two laboratory workers contracted rabies, apparently as a consequence of accidentally inhaling aerosolized virus during experimental procedures. Both oral and respiratory transmission routes have been demonstrated experimentally in animals. Whether such nonbite routes play an important role in maintaining the virus in nature is speculative.[5]

The Disease in Animals

Rabies has a prolonged and highly variable incubation period and is remarkable in the variety of symptoms it may evoke in any species of animal. A dog bitten by a rabid animal may develop rabies within 9 days, or it may show no symptoms for 8 1/2 months or longer. The incubation period usually ranges from 20 to 60 days.

The dog manifests symptoms in either or both of two forms: (1) furious rabies and (2) dumb or paralytic rabies. The form the disease assumes may depend on the dose of the virus, the strain of virus, the resistance of the animal, and the sequence of nerve cells involved as the virus invades the brain and central nervous system. Furious rabies is frequent and more likely to lead to infection of other animals or humans. During the early stages, the dog may appear more affectionate than usual but is easily irritated and, if picked up, may bite. It exhibits restlessness and a tendency to snap at anything that comes its way.

In dumb rabies, the animal is not observed to be irritable and usually hides and becomes somnolent. Paralysis of the jaw is followed rapidly by general paralysis, and death occurs 1 to 3 days after onset. Dogs with this form present much less hazard, but exposure may result from attempting to look in the animal's throat or to administer medication.

Rabid cats may hide and may viciously attack anyone who comes near. The cat's voice becomes hoarse and is soon lost as paralysis sets in. Prostration and death follow in a few days. Most other animals show similar syndromes, with the furious and aggressive behavior slowly giving way to gradually developing uncoordination and paralysis.

The disease in bats, including vampire bats, is nearly always paralytic. In the United States, colonial bats, such as the free-tailed bat, show the paralytic form, whereas some noncolonial bat species rarely show furious signs before becoming paralytic. Most human bites are due to the handling of sick or paralyzed bats.

The signs of rabies may resemble those of other infectious diseases or toxic syndromes that affect the central nervous system, and clinical diagnosis is uncertain. Laboratory tests must be performed to be certain of the diagnosis. There is increasing evidence that rabies in animals may not necessarily have a fatal outcome. Live skunks, foxes, and raccoons have been found with serological evidence of past infection, and clinical rabies has been described in the vampire bat, followed by recovery.[5] Serological studies in the gregarious free-tailed bats have shown that 15% to 80% have evidence of serum antibody. Abortive clinical rabies has been demonstrated in laboratory animals and has been followed by recovery.[6]

The Disease in Humans

The virus, after inoculation into a wound, travels along the nerves from the peripheral site of inoculation to the central nervous system. The incubation period in humans is highly variable and is determined in part by the location of the bite and the distance the virus must travel to the brain. The incubation period usually is rather short after facial bites and longer after bites on the extremities. The typical incubation period is about 6 weeks, but extremes of 10 days to 15 months have been recorded. In animals and presumably in humans, the incubation period also is influenced by the viral dose and the type of tissue exposed.[7]

The disease in humans usually runs its course within 1 week. The term "hydrophobia" derives from the fact that swallowing is difficult and produces painful contraction of the muscles of deglutition, leading to a reflex contraction at the sight of liquids and an aversion to them. There are alternate periods of excitability (sometimes reaching the point of mania) and quiet. Paralytic manifestations usually are late and may not appear. Prolonged survival of up to 133 days has been reported after the use of intensive respiratory care to prevent hypoxia.[8] Three cases are on record of recovery from probable clinical rabies after the use of such therapy, but in only one has recovery been complete.

Diagnosis. The diagnosis of rabies is based on the consideration of as many factors as are available, including the history of exposure, clinical symptoms, and course. If a seemingly healthy dog or cat has bitten someone, it should be held under veterinary supervision for at least 10 days unless clinical symptoms of rabies develop, at which time it may be killed and its brain examined. Ordinarily, symptomatic rabid dogs or cats succumb within 7 days. However, wild rabid animals may live for 18 days or longer after the appearance of disease signs, so those that have bitten humans should be destroyed immediately and tested as quickly as possible.

There should be no delay in submitting the head for diagnosis. Following decapitation, the head should be placed in a watertight container, which in turn is immersed in ice in a larger watertight container for shipping. Alternatively, the brain may be removed with aseptic precautions and either quick-frozen in dry ice or preserved in 50% glycerol saline. The laboratory diagnosis of rabies may consist of one or more of several types of examinations.

The fluorescent rabies antibody (FRA) test is the test of choice in the United States and many other countries. The test is highly specific and requires only a few hours to perform. It is based on identification of rabies antigen in a slide of brain or salivary gland tissue by direct staining so as to visualize the antigen-antibody reaction. The FRA test on a corneal smear taken from a living patient is sometimes positive and thus may be useful to confirm a diagnosis of rabies. The demonstration of Negri bodies in brain neurons is a method decreasingly used throughout the world because the inclusions are not always present or may be atypical or confused with other inclusions.

The mouse inoculation test can take 7 to 14 days or more before results are apparent. The virus can be identified by a positive FRA test or a positive serum virus neutralization test. In comparative trials, the mouse inoculation test and the FRA test proved equally sensitive as diagnostic procedures. Antibody level in blood serum can be determined by serum virus neutralization tests performed either by a mouse inoculation technique or the rapid fluorescent focus inhibition test (RFFIT), which can measure antibody levels in 24 hours. Because it can be done quickly, the latter is the test of choice for antibody, but its performance requires a well-equipped laboratory and well-trained technicians. A greater than fourfold rise in titer in the serum neutralization (RFFIT), complement-fixation (CF), or indirect FRA tests in patients who have not received rabies vaccine is considered diagnostic of rabies.

Rabies viral strains have been considered similar antigenically, only minor differences being demonstrable. Recently, certain rabies-related viruses, discovered in African shrews and bats and in European bats, have been observed to produce rabieslike diseases in humans, dogs, and cats. These viruses may be mistaken for rabies or missed altogether in FRA tests. Rabies vaccines and globulins provide little, if any, protection, and no specific biologicals are available for immunization against these rabieslike viruses.[9]

Postexposure Treatment. Prompt and adequate treatment of all skin wounds possibly contaminated with rabies virus is of paramount importance. Local treatment of animal bites and scratches should include thorough cleansing with a 20% soap solution or a detergent and flushing of the wound. Although cauterization with nitric acid in puncture wounds has its advocates, there is no available evidence that this procedure is more effective than soap solutions. The wound should not be sutured immediately if this can be avoided. Use of antibiotics and tetanus prophylaxis may be indicated.

Prophylactic Immunization. Pasteur developed a method of postexposure rabies prophylaxis using desiccated nerve tissue in 1883. Agents, such as phenol (the basis of Semple vaccine), formalin, and ultraviolet light, have been reported to inactivate the virus in brain or spinal cord tissue while allowing it to retain its antigenicity.

Allergic reactions may occur after administration of vaccine made from such nerve tissue. Much more serious are the occasional neurological complications—encephalitis, peripheral neuritis, and various paralytic phenomena—that have been attributed to sensitization to brain tissue. These occur more often in persons who previously have received rabies vaccine. The frequency of paralysis during and after administration of a course of Semple vaccine containing nervous tissue has varied considerably in different countries. Some estimates of incidence have ranged between 1:600 and 1:6000 individuals immunized. The Semple vaccine, despite these reactions, continues in wide use in many countries. A suckling mouse brain vaccine is used widely in South America. In the United States, a duck embryo vaccine (DEV) was in routine use from 1957 until about 1980–1981. This vaccine was used in a manner similar to the Semple vaccine (14–21 doses at daily intervals).

A human diploid cell vaccine (HDCV), which first became available in the late 1970s, represents a major advance in the prevention of human rabies. Antibody response is more rapid, and titers are approximately 10 times higher than with DEV. Conversion rates also are higher, and the vaccine is well tolerated. Initially, only minimal reactions were noted, with virtually no reports of anaphylactic, neuroparalytic, or systemic reactions. Since 1984, however, with the steady increase of persons who began to receive booster doses of this inactivated vaccine, a systemic allergic reaction (mainly type III immune complex) has been reported in 5% to 10% of recipients.[10] Although sometimes intense, all reactions have had a favorable outcome. Most occurred after a preexposure booster dose of vaccine was given. Only a few of these reported reactions were severe enough to require hospitalization, but the full implications of these reactions for the future receipt of HDCV for these persons are not clear.

The WHO postexposure prophylaxis regimen with this vaccine consists of a total of six 1-ml doses of vaccine given intramuscularly in the deltoid region on days 0, 3, 7, 14, 28, and 90. Studies in the United States by the Centers for Disease Control have indicated that a five-dose regimen achieves adequate antibody response and has provided protection against rabies in over 500 persons bitten by proven rabid animals. The recommended postexposure prophylaxis regimen in the United States is five doses on days 0, 3, 7, 14, and 28.[11]

Use of Rabies Immune Globulin or Antirabies Serum. Rabies immune globulin (RIG) of human origin or antirabies serum (ARS) of equine origin should be given to all persons bitten by animals in whom rabies cannot be excluded and for nonbite exposures to animals suspected or proved to be rabid. The only exceptions to this recommendation are those persons who have received preexposure rabies immunization. RIG or ARS should be given as soon as possible after exposure and should be used regardless of the interval between exposure and the onset of treatment. If RIG or ARS was not given when rabies vaccine was started, however, these globulins can be given up to the eighth day after the first vaccine dose was given. RIG is the product of choice in the United States, where ARS is to be used only if RIG is not available. For either product, up to half the dose may be given intramuscularly and the rest thoroughly infiltrated around the wound. The first dose of vaccine should be given at the same time at a separate site.

General Guide to Postexposure Treatment. The U.S. Public Health Service's Advisory Committee on Immunization Practices has published a guide[11] for specific postexposure treatment (Table 12–2). These recommendations are subject to modification depending on the circumstances of the bite, species of animal involved, type of exposure, and prevalence of rabies in the biting species. Knowledge of the last condition requires adequate surveillance.

TABLE 12-2. POSTEXPOSURE RABIES PROPHYLAXIS GUIDE

Animal Species	Condition of Animal at Time of Attack	Treatment of Exposed Person[a]
Domestic dog and cat	Healthy and available for 10 days of observation	All bites and wounds should immediately be cleaned thoroughly with soap and water None, unless animal develops rabies[b]
	Rabid or suspected rabid	RIG[c] and HDCV
	Unknown (escaped)	Consultation with public health officials. If treatment is indicated, give RIG[c] and HDCV
Wild: skunk, bat, fox, coyote, raccoon, bobcat, and other carnivores	Regard as rabid unless proven negative by laboratory test[d]	RIG[c] and HDCV
Other: livestock, rodents, and lagomorphs, such as rabbits and hares	Consider individually. Local and state public health officials should be consulted about questions that arise about the need for rabies prophylaxis. Bites of squirrels, hamsters, guinea pigs, gerbils, chipmunks, rats, mice and other rodents, or rabbits and hares almost never call for antirabies prophylaxis.	

Note: The recommendations in this table are only a guide. They should be applied in conjunction with knowledge of the animal species involved, circumstances of the bite or other exposure, immunization status of the animal, and presence of rabies in the region. Local or state public health officials should be consulted if questions arise about the need for rabies prophylaxis.

[a]If antirabies treatment is indicated, both RIG and HDCV should be given as soon as possible, regardless of the interval from exposure. Local reactions to vaccines are common and do not contraindicate continuing treatment. Discontinue vaccine if fluorescent antibody tests of animals are negative.

[b]Begin treatment with RIG and HDCV at first sign of rabies in biting dog or cat during the usual holding period of 10 days. The symptomatic animal should be killed immediately and tested.

[c]If RIG is not available, use antirabies serum (ARS) of equine origin. Do not use more than the recommended dosage.

[d]The animal should be killed and tested as soon as possible. Holding for observation is not recommended.

From U.S. Public Health Service's Advisory Committee on Immunization Practices, 1984.[11]

Preexposure Immunization. For persons with special risks of exposure to rabies, such as veterinarians, laboratory staff working with rabies virus, dog handlers, field naturalists, or those living or working in parts of the world where rabies is a constant threat, it is desirable to provide active immunization in advance of possible exposure. For this purpose, three doses of HDCV are recommended on days 0, 7, and 21 or 28. Because the antibody response following the recommended preexposure regimen with HDCV has been so satisfactory, routine postimmunization serological study is not generally recommended. It needs to be pointed out that preexposure immunization does not eliminate the need for postexposure prophylaxis after an exposure. It only reduces the postexposure regimen. Booster doses of vaccine or periodic (generally about every 2 years) antibody testing should be scheduled for those who remain at continued risk of exposure to rabies.

Because HDCV is a very expensive vaccine, the intradermal route of administration using 0.1 ml per dose has been explored for preexposure immunization. Results generally have been good, but the mean antibody response is somewhat lower and may be of shorter duration than with the 1.0-ml dose given intramuscularly. Poor antibody titers resulted when the technique was used on subjects during antimalarial chemoprophylaxis with chloroquine.[12]

Animal Vaccines. Vaccines for dogs and cats contain either inactivated virus or modified live virus. Some of these vaccines must be administered annually, whereas the other vaccines, which produce an immunity lasting at least 3 years, are generally vaccines of choice.

A compendium for animal rabies vaccines and recommendations for immunization procedures has been developed and is available through the National Association of State Public Health Veterinarians. This compendium reviews all the licensed animal rabies vaccines and provides information on dosage, species, age at immunization, and reimmunization schedules. For many species, specific contraindications concerning particular vaccines exist, so caution should be used in selecting vaccines for animal use. Although uncommon, certain live virus rabies vaccines have been known to cause rabies in some species, especially wildlife species.

Control. It has been demonstrated in many parts of the world that rabies can be controlled, even eradicated, in limited geographical areas by quarantine measures applied to the dog population, provided wild animals are not involved in the propagation of the disease. Where rabies has become established in wildlife, control depends basically on measures that are directly or indirectly effective in reducing stray dogs to below the critical number required to maintain continuous propagation of the virus by serial biting. By the enforcement of ordinances designed to accomplish this reduction, rabies frequently has been temporarily eliminated from urban and suburban communities in the United States.

The prophylactic immunization of dogs is one of the most important methods for rabies control. Where the disease is enzootic in wildlife, routine immunization of both dogs and cats should be practiced. Although it is effective where it is used, such immunization does not reach stray dogs or feral cats, however. Therefore, it is essential to maintain other measures of dog control, designed to "prevent any dog from biting another for a period of the longest latency of the disease."[7] Licensure of dogs and collection of all stray, ownerless, or unwanted dogs should be carried out routinely. Where there is any threat of canine rabies, all dogs in urban areas should be restrained on a leash or kept on the owner's premises. Restraint of cats is indicated as well. Cats bring home the majority of bats that bite or are handled by people. Animal bites should be reported to an official agency, and if rabies is present in a community, any dog or cat biting a person must be confined and observed for signs of rabies. Biting wildlife should be killed and tested without delay.

A permanent solution to the enzootic rabies problem in humans and animals would require the control and eventual elimination of the disease in wildlife. Rabies control in wildlife is exceedingly difficult or impossible, however, depending on the host species. The current and only available method for carnivores is population reduction. This is highly controversial, meeting great resistance from ecologists and conservationists.

Except for vampires, bats should not be killed or molested, since this will likely increase exposures as people and animals handle the fallen animals. Housebat colonies do not experience rabies outbreaks. Only a fraction of 1% are infected, and the infected bat does not bite unless handled. Unwanted colonies should be excluded from buildings by sealing them out after summer, when young bats can fly. Massive reduction of carnivores (skunks, foxes, coyotes, bobcats) in North America and vampire bats in Latin America has effectively reduced the immediate threat to the local animal or human population. The programs are expensive, however, and unless they are intensively carried out to the extent of at least 80% reduction of the target species over a wide area, the effects are short-lived.

For maximum effectiveness, reduction programs should be undertaken only by professional predator-control specialists. The choice of techniques depends on local conditions and may include poisoning or gassing or the more expensive methods of trapping and shooting. In areas where human or domestic animal populations are heavily concentrated, poisoning must be used with great care. Other methods under study include interrupting the reproductive cycles of wild carnivores and the immunization of wildlife populations. The former has been unsuccessful to date, and the latter is undeveloped or controversial. Compared to the cost of trapping and killing predators, immunizing the trapped animals with an inactivated vaccine and releasing them would be more productive in rabies control. The procedure requires a yet undevised trap, however, that will capture the more wary carnivores without injury. Immunization of foxes (but not other species) by feeding them baits that contain large doses of live attenuated rabies vaccine virus has been used in Europe as one method of rabies control where foxes constitute the predominant wildlife species. Native rodents and some nontarget carnivores, however, can develop the infection after consuming these vaccine strains, and they can spread at least one of the strains among themselves. A cat was similarly infected during a field trial. Recombinant oral vaccines show promise of effectiveness in skunks and raccoons, but safety testing is indicated.

Until these problems can be resolved, the control of wildlife rabies will continue to be an immense problem and challenge in most areas, and the occasional human case of rabies from this vast reservoir also will continue to occur.

Psittacosis

Julius Schachter

Psittacosis is a zoonosis first described approximately 100 years ago. The causative agent is an obligatory intracellular bacterium, *Chlamydia psittaci.* Virtually all avian species may be naturally infected with *C. psittaci.* When these agents infect humans or psittacine species, the resulting diseases are called psittacosis. Similar infections in other birds are called ornithosis. In infected birds, the infection is mainly in the gastrointestinal tract, with a secondary respiratory involvement. The agent is shed in feces or respiratory secretions and usually is transmitted to humans in an aerosolized form.

Clinical Description. Human psittacosis usually is described as a severe febrile pneumonitis. It is commonly associated with severe headache, and there often is a pulse rate much lower than would be predicted in patients with high fever. The x-rays show extensive pneumonic involvement even in the absence of severe respiratory symptoms. Although a cough is common, it is dry, hacking, and nonproductive. In addition to the respiratory syndrome, a form of psittacosis without marked respiratory involvement is recognized, in which patients are febrile and appear toxic, often having a severe headache. Hepatosplenomegaly may occur in either form of the disease. Complications, such as hepatitis, myocarditis, endocarditis, and meningitis, are known. Milder flu-like disease and asymptomatic infections also occur.

Human psittacosis may be diagnosed by demonstrating rising titers of complement-fixing or fluorescent antibodies to chlamydial antigens in paired acute convalescent sera. Isolation of chlamydiae is feasible, but it is best left to specialized laboratories because of the danger of laboratory infection. Chlamydial infection in birds may be demonstrated by finding characteristic intracytoplasmic inclusions in smears from involved organs.

Public Health Significance. Human psittacosis is relatively uncommon. In recent years, less than 100 cases have been reported in the United States. Because correct diagnosis requires a high index of suspicion by the physician and specialized laboratory tests, it is likely that the true incidence is considerably higher.

Psittacosis is a common occupational hazard to workers in the pet bird industry and in turkey-processing plants. The major threat for mass outbreaks is an industrial one. Sporadic cases commonly are associated with ownership of pet birds. Often, smuggled birds are implicated. Psittacosis occurs worldwide, but reliable data on distribution are not available.

Control and Treatment. As a public health measure, all imported psittacine species are required to undergo a quarantine period, during which they receive a chemoprophylactic regimen of chlortetracycline in their feed for 30 days. Since the efficacy of this program is not monitored, it has been found that infected birds often escape adequate treatment and are released into commerce. Specific methods of treating birds according to the feeding habits of different species have been developed and have been shown to be efficacious both in artificially infected birds and in treatment centers where adequate intake of the chlortetracycline has been documented.

Mass treatment of infected turkey flocks by incorporation of tetracyclines in their feed has been shown to suppress the infection.

For treatment of human psittacosis, tetracycline is considered the drug of choice, and the recommended regimen is 250 mg four times daily for 21 days. Short-term treatment is not indicated and may result in relapse. Response to treatment often is not dramatic, and there may be a prolonged convalescent period. The infection does not confer immunity.

Tularemia

Arnold F. Kaufmann
Jay D. Wenger

Tularemia derives its name from Tulare County, California, where McCoy and Chapin, in 1911 and 1912, discovered that *Francisella tularensis* was the cause of a plaguelike illness in California ground squirrels. In 1914, Wherry and Lamb reported the first documented instance of human infection with *F. tularensis.* Their patient had acquired tularemia from contact with a rabbit. In 1919, *F. tularensis* was isolated from patients in Utah suffering from deerfly fever, a condition described 9 years earlier by Pearse but for which an etiology had not been determined. Several years later, ticks also were implicated in the transmission of *F. tularensis* to humans. Since these early discoveries, many animal species, water, and other inanimate objects contaminated with *F. tularensis* have been reported to be of importance in the epidemiology of tularemia.[1]

The Agent. *Francisella tularensis* is a small pleomorphic, gram-negative, nonsporeforming bacillus. The organism may demonstrate bipolar staining with Giemsa stain but can be identified more readily in tissues by fluorescent antibody techniques.

For isolation and cultivation, *F. tularensis* requires a higher concentration of cysteine than is present in most media used in hospital laboratories. Glucose-cysteine blood agar is the medium of choice for isolating *F. tularensis* from clinical specimens. Inoculation of mice or guinea pigs is used to isolate the organism from environmental and contaminated specimens.

The disease is diagnosed in most patients by serological tests rather than by culture. By the third week of illness, agglutinating antibody is detectable with the standard tube agglutination test.[1]

Francisella tularensis can be subdivided into two types, A and B. Type A strains ferment glycerol and are highly virulent for laboratory rabbits; type B strains have the opposite characteristics. Type A strains are associated with the tick–rabbit cycle of infection found in North America. Type B strains are associated with rodent and waterborne infections throughout most of the northern hemisphere. Human illness generally is more severe with type A strain infections.[2]

The Disease. A variety of clinical syndromes has been associated with *F. tularensis* infection. Differentiation of these syndromes is important because they may provide clues to the source of infection.

Ulceroglandular tularemia comprises about 70% to 80% of reported cases. After an incubation period of 3 to 4 days (range 1–10 days), the illness begins with sudden onset of fever, chills, sweating, myalgia, and headache. Either concurrent with or shortly after clinical onset, a papule develops at the skin site through which infection occurred. The papule progresses through a pustular stage to formation of a small skin ulcer. As the ulcer forms, the regional lymph nodes become swollen, inflamed, and painful. The skin lesion is not present in all patients. In uncomplicated illness, symptoms resolve in 2 weeks to several months in untreated patients. Therapy results in prompt clinical improvement and shortens the duration of illness.

In typhoidal tularemia, skin lesions and localized lymphadenitis are not apparent. The illness is nonspecific, with fever, chills, profuse sweating, and headache being predominant symptoms. The diagnosis of typhoidal tularemia often is delayed because of its nonspecific features.

Tularemic pneumonia may be either primary due to inhalation of *F. tularensis* or secondary to one of the other clinical forms. The pneumonia often is associated with pleuritic chest pain, reflecting the frequent occurrence of inflammatory pleural involvement.[3]

The treatment of choice for tularemia is streptomycin or gentamicin. Tetracycline and chloramphenicol are used as alternatives but are associated with a higher relapse rate. In the United States, untreated ulceroglandular tularemia has a case fatality rate of 5% to 6%, whereas typhoidal and pulmonary tularemia cases result in a mortality rate of 40% to 60%. Mortality rates are lower in other countries where infections are caused by type B strains of *F. tularensis.* Appropriate therapy markedly reduces the case fatality rate.

Tularemia in animals is a nonspecific febrile illness. At necropsy, small white-to-yellow necrotic foci are found in the liver, spleen, and lymph nodes. The disease is associated with high mortality in rodents, rabbits, grouse, pheasants, and sheep.

Mode of Transmission. *Francisella tularensis* is a highly infectious organism. As few as 10 organisms inoculated under the skin or inhaled will produce human disease. For persons ingesting contaminated food or water, however, the infectious dose is much higher, being in the range of 100 million organisms.

Arthropod vectors are the single most important factor in the epidemiology of tularemia. Hard-bodied ticks and deerflies are of particular importance in the United States. In other countries, mosquitoes and biting horseflies also may play a role.

Some infected tick species pass the infection transovarially to succeeding generations, thus serving as both reservoir and vector. Ticks most commonly associated with human cases in the United States are the western or Rocky Mountain wood tick (*Dermacentor andersoni*), the American dog tick (*Dermacentor variabilis*),[4] and the lone star tick (*Ambylomma americanum*). Biting flies, such as the deerfly, mechanically transport the infection on their mouth parts after feeding on an infected host. Human tularemia associated with fly bites occurs only in the presence of a wild animal epizootic in the area. Arthropod bites usually result in ulceroglandular disease, although typhoidal tularemia cases also may result.

Although the rabbit tick (*Haemaphysalis leporispalustris*) does not directly transmit tularemia to humans, it is extremely important as a reservoir and vector of tularemia in rabbits. Rabbit lice and fleas, as well as biting flies, also transmit tularemia among rabbits.

Contact exposure to infectious animal tissue, crushed ticks, and contaminated water and mud is another important mode of transmission.[5] Although infections occur more readily through the broken skin, the tularemia bacillus can invade through apparently unbroken skin. Rubbing or spraying of infectious material in the eyes will result in oculoglandular tularemia. The rabbit, particularly the cottontail (*Sylvilagus*), is directly or indirectly related to more human cases in the United States than any other species. Human infections, however, have followed contact with sheep, pheasants, muskrats, and numerous other animal species. On rare occasions, infections following a cat bite have been reported.

Airborne transmission is particularly important in the laboratory, where reports of accidental human tularemia infections are common.[6] In Sweden and Russia, extensive pulmonary tularemia outbreaks have followed processing of agricultural products, such as sugar beets. Smaller outbreaks and isolated cases have been associated with infectious aerosols inadvertently generated during the handling of dead animals, the shearing of sheep, and road grading.[7]

Water and mud of streams and wells may become contaminated by animals dying of tularemia. Outbreaks of human disease have followed ingestion and contact exposure to contaminated water. Animals drinking the water also may be infected.

Occurrence. Beginning in 1927, when tularemia became a notifiable disease in the United States, the annual number of cases steadily increased from 219 to a peak of 2291 in 1939. The number of reported cases subsequently has declined, with less than 300 cases being reported annually in the past decade. The greatest number of cases generally occur in Arkansas, Missouri, Oklahoma, Tennessee, and Texas. Another area of high incidence incorporates Utah, Wyoming, and southeastern Montana.

A similar pattern of rising and falling incidence has been noted elsewhere, most notably in Russia. Human tularemia reached its peak incidence in Russia during World War II, when large waterborne epidemics occurred.

The seasonal distribution of onset is bimodal, with winter and summer peaks. The winter peak primarily represents cases associated with animal tissue contact, and the summer peaks represent insect vectorborne disease. In recent years, a greater proportion of the cases has been reported in the summer months.

Tularemia is primarily a disease of adult males. This skewed age-sex distribution probably reflects differences in occupational and leisure activities. As might be expected, tularemia is a disease of rural rather than urban residents.

Certain occupations traditionally have been associated with high risk of infection. These include laboratory workers, trappers, hunters, farmers, sheep shearers, and meat market employees who handle wild rabbits.

Prevention and Control. Prevention of tularemia is based primarily on minimizing exposure to infected animals and insect vectors. Any contact with sick or dead wild animals should be avoided. Trappers and hunters should wear rubber gloves while dressing wild rabbits and rodents and avoid rubbing any blood or tissues on their face. Meat from any game animal should be cooked thoroughly before being eaten.

In tick-infested areas, frequent self-examination for and removal of ticks is an important protective measure. Removal of tick harborage, such as vegetation along sidewalks, may be of benefit. Limited insecticide applications along commonly used walkways also has been used when infestations are severe. The wearing of slacks with the cuffs tucked into socks will provide some protection in brush and wooded areas.

Public health agencies should maintain surveillance of tularemia to identify any unusual occurrence of cases. Case investigation may identify possible sources of common source outbreaks, which are amenable to control. News releases at appropriate seasons can be used to inform the public how to prevent tularemia and other vectorborne diseases.

An experimental live tularemia vaccine is available on a limited basis and is recommended primarily for laboratory workers.[8] The vaccine provides protection against systemic infection but not against ulceroglandular disease. A similar degree of immunity is provided by natural infection. In high-risk exposures, chemoprophylaxis with tetracycline has been documented to be effective in preventing disease.

Anthrax

Arnold F. Kaufmann
Jay D. Wenger

Anthrax has been recognized as an infectious disease of humans and animals for many centuries. Perhaps the first recorded anthrax epizootic was the Fifth Plague described in the Book of Exodus. Anthrax apparently was a common disease of both humans and animals in Rome during the last five centuries BC. In his description of an animal outbreak, Virgil observed that eating meat or wearing clothes made from wool or hides of infected animals resulted in human anthrax. Unfortunately, Virgil's admonition that the contagion be controlled by burial of carcasses was not widely practiced.

In nineteenth century Europe, anthrax occurred in panzootic proportions. The magnitude of the losses of livestock to anthrax created widespread apprehension that agriculture was doomed in Europe. In France, 20% to 30% of the sheep and cattle died of anthrax each year. The need to control the disease stimulated the work of Davaine, Koch, and Pasteur. As a result, anthrax became the first disease conclusively proved to be caused by a microorganism as well as the first bacterial disease for which an effective vaccine was developed.

The Agent. *Bacillus anthracis,* the etiological agent of anthrax, is a large, gram-positive, nonmotile, sporeforming bacterial rod. The bacillus grows well on a variety of bacterial culture media. On blood agar plates, the bacillus forms large, nonhemolytic, ground glass-appearing colonies. The tenacious character of these colonies can be demonstrated by drawing an inoculation needle through them.

Virulence factors of *B. anthracis* include capsule production and two toxins (edema factor and lethal factor).[1] The toxins are of the AB type and share a common binding moiety (protective antigen). The genes coding for the production of the toxins and capsule are found on separate plasmids. DNA probes for detection of the plasmids can be used for rapid, specific identification of the bacillus.

Diagnosis of anthrax may be made by culture of clinical or autopsy specimens or by serological evaluation using a western blot technique for detection of antibody to the toxins. Fluorescent antibody examination of tissues may also be useful.

Human Anthrax. Human anthrax has three major clinical forms, cutaneous, inhalation, and gastrointestinal,[2] which directly reflect the route of infection. Any of these forms may lead to complications, such as septicemia and meningitis.

Cutaneous anthrax is associated with a characteristic skin lesion developing 2 to 7 days (range 1–12 days) after infection. The lesion develops at the site where the anthrax bacillus is introduced beneath the skin, for example, by rubbing or through a cut. Most cutaneous anthrax lesions occur on exposed areas of the body. The lesion usually is first noted as a papule resembling a pimple or insect bite. Blistering or vesiculation of the papule occurs within 3 days, and the vesicle ruptures shortly after its formation, revealing an underlying ulcer. A scab or eschar then develops over the surface of the ulcer. The lesion usually is surrounded by edematous swelling out of proportion to the magnitude of the central lesion. Although death occurs in 5% to 20% of untreated patients, treatment with penicillin or other appropriate antibiotics virtually eliminates fatalities.

Inhalation anthrax usually occurs only in persons exposed to certain industries, such as goat hair processing.[3] This form of the disease results from inhaling aerosols of anthrax spores generated during the manufacturing process. After an incubation period of 1 to 5 days, the initial illness is characterized by low-grade fever, malaise, fatigue, myalgia, nonproductive cough, and, occasionally, a sensation of precordial oppression. After 2 to 4 days, the second stage of acute toxicity begins with sudden onset of dyspnea, cyanosis, and profuse sweating. On x-ray, widening of the mediastinum due to swollen lymph nodes and surrounding edema often is apparent. Even with therapy, death usually ensues within 24 hours.

Gastrointestinal anthrax develops 2 to 5 days after meat from infected animals is eaten. The clinical course is variable. Many patients have fever and cervical and submental swelling, apparently due to profound cervical lymphadenopathy or subcutaneous edema. Other patients have a gradual onset of nausea, vomiting, anorexia, and fever. This mild prodromal illness is followed by abdominal pain, intensification of vomiting with the vomitus changing to red or black, rising temperature, and diarrhea that may be blood-tinged. In less severe cases, only mild diarrhea and abdominal pain may be noted. The entire clinical course lasts 1 to 5 days, and mortality ranges from 25% to 75%.

Animal Anthrax. Anthrax has been described as an experimental or naturally occurring disease in numerous animal species,[4] but primarily in mammals. Birds are more resistant, with some exceptions, such as the duck and ostrich. Anthrax in animals resembles the gastrointestinal form of the disease in humans. The inhalation and cutaneous forms of human anthrax do not occur naturally in animals.

In domestic livestock, the incubation period is typically 3 to 7 days but may range from 1 to 14 days or more. The clinical course ranges from acute to chronic. Sudden death in animals that appeared normal a few hours earlier is common.

In cattle, sheep, and goats, the acute illness is characterized by abrupt onset of fever, variably followed by anorexia, ruminal stasis, signs of abdominal pain, hematuria, and blood-tinged diarrhea. Pregnant animals may abort, and milk production in lactating animals often abruptly decreases, with the milk being abnormal or blood-tinged. Subcutaneous edematous swellings may occur, particularly on the ventral side of the neck. Death usually occurs 1 to 3 days after onset. Occasionally, animals survive infection without treatment, but this is uncommon. Chronic infection, characterized by localized edematous subcutaneous swelling, rarely occurs in cattle. In swine, the disease is similar to that in ruminants, except that both acute and chronic infections more commonly localize in the tonsils and cervical lymph nodes.

Mode of Transmission. The natural reservoir of *B. anthracis* is soil.[5] The organism is a part of the normal flora of numerous soil types having a pH higher than 6. Although naturally contaminated soil is the usual reservoir of infection, animal anthrax outbreaks have been traced to a variety of sources, such as animal-origin feed and fertilizer, river water contaminated by wastes from animal-product processing, and even crops raised on contaminated soil. Anthrax is not communicable directly between animals, although infection can be acquired by scavengers feeding on carcasses.

Animal anthrax tends to be restricted to certain regions, such as the lower Mississippi River Valley in the United States. Outbreaks, however, can occur virtually anywhere. Anthrax occurs irregularly. In some areas, anthrax occurs annually, whereas, in other regions, intervals of many years between outbreaks are typical.[6]

Outbreaks in grazing animals occur primarily when the minimum daily temperature is above 16° C (61° F), but documented cases have occurred even in midwinter in cold climates. Epizootics tend to occur after periods of marked climatic or ecological change, such as heavy rainfall, flooding, or drought.

Human anthrax is secondary to the disease in animals. Infection may occur through direct contact with animal tissues at necropsy or during attempts to salvage parts of the carcass. Less obvious risk occurs when hides, hair, and wool are removed from the carcass and sold for processing, a practice that has made anthrax an occupational disease in the tanning, gelatin, and animal hair and wool-processing industries. Occasional human cases have resulted from contaminated animal-origin products sold at the retail level, such as shaving brushes, yarn, and goatskin-topped drums.

Occurrence. Except in underdeveloped areas, human anthrax is an uncommon to rare disease. Fewer than 10 cases have occurred in the United States during the past decade. In some countries, such as Haiti, however, several hundred cases still occur each year. In Zimbabwe, an epidemic of almost 10,000 human cases occurred in the period 1978 to 1980 when political instability disrupted animal anthrax control activities.

Cases associated with industrial processing of animal products may occur at any season. Agriculture-related cases, however, occur in a seasonal pattern parallel to that of animal anthrax in the area.

Animal anthrax has a worldwide distribution. In the United States, multiple small outbreaks occur each year, but epizootics are uncommon.

Prevention and Control. Prevention of human anthrax associated with agriculture is dependent on control of animal anthrax. Annual immunization of livestock in areas of endemic anthrax is recommended. The animal anthrax vaccine that is used almost universally is a live spore suspension of the avirulent Sterne strain.[7] Livestock should be vaccinated 2 to 4 weeks before the season when outbreaks may be expected.

Reporting of animal anthrax outbreaks to agriculture and public health officials should be mandatory. Affected premises or areas should be quarantined to prevent infected animals from being marketed, and all susceptible livestock on affected and surrounding premises should be immunized. Investigation for sources of infection other than contaminated pastures should be initiated and, if found, eliminated. Carcasses of animals that die of anthrax should be either buried deeply or burned completely. Bedding and other contaminated material also should be burned or buried.

Dairy herds in an outbreak area should be placed under surveillance if the herd has not been immunized previously.[8] The rectal temperature of each animal should be determined just before milking; a febrile animal should be isolated immediately and its milk discarded. All afebrile animals should be vaccinated when surveillance is initiated. The surveillance period can be terminated 10 days after immunization.

A human anthrax vaccine is available in the United States for protection of persons with ongoing risk of infection.[9] The vaccine is recommended for employees of high-risk industries, such as those processing imported animal hides, hair, and wool, as well as for laboratory personnel working with *B. anthracis* cultures.

Disinfection of materials and surfaces contaminated with *B. anthracis* is complicated by the resistance of the spore. A variety of procedures, however, are effective. These include dry heat, steam under pressure, formaldehyde soaking or vapor exposure, ethylene oxide gas exposure, hypochlorite solution soaking, and gamma-irradiation. Regardless of the procedure used, the effectiveness of the disinfection should be verified by appropriate cultures and quality control procedures.

Brucellosis

Arnold F. Kaufmann
Jay D. Wenger

Brucellosis was first recognized as a vague febrile illness occurring in Mediterranean countries. Mediterranean fever, as it was then known, was a major cause of illness in the British soldiers garrisoned on Malta. In 1887, the cause of the illness was first reported to be *Brucella melitensis* by Sir David Bruce, a British army surgeon. Nearly 20 years elapsed before the role of the goat and its milk in the epidemiology of brucellosis was uncovered by Sir Themistokles Zammit, a Maltese physician.

Brucella abortus and *Brucella suis* were first isolated from cattle and swine, respectively. In contrast to *B. melitensis,* the ability of *B. abortus* and *B. suis* to cause human disease was seriously questioned until the mid-1920s. Alice Evans, a U.S. Public Health Service bacteriologist, deserves much of the credit for gaining acceptance of this fact by the medical community. Miss Evans contracted brucellosis in the course of her pioneering work and suffered relapsing illness for over 20 years, once being hospitalized for 14 months.

The Agent. *Brucella* organisms are small, nonmotile, gram-negative bacilli. The various *Brucella* species are slow-growing, fastidious organisms that vary in their nutrient requirements.[1]

All *Brucella* species and biotypes appear to be partially host-adapted. The species having known human health significance and their usual reservoir hosts are *B. abortus* (cattle), *Brucella canis* (dogs), *B. melitensis* (goats and sheep), and *B. suis* (swine).

Definitive diagnosis of brucellosis can be made only by culture, and blood cultures are most useful. Cultures of bone marrow or other infected tissues may be valuable, especially for patients with chronic disease.

A variety of serological tests for brucellosis are available.[1,2] The standard tube agglutination test, which uses a *B. abortus* antigen, is used most commonly in the United States and can detect infections due to *B. abortus, B. melitensis,* and *B. suis.* Detection of *B. canis* antibody requires use of a *B. canis* antigen. Enzyme-linked immunosorbent assay (ELISA) tests for *Brucella* antibody are now available and appear to be more useful than the tube agglutination test.

The Disease. Human illnesses caused by the various *Brucella* species tend to be quite similar, although *B. melitensis* and certain *B. suis* biotypes tend to produce more severe disease. The incubation period is usually from 5 to 21 days but may be as long as several months. The onset of illness often is insidious but may be abrupt.

Brucellosis is most consistently characterized by fever (constant or intermittent), chills, sweats, malaise, weakness, headache, muscle aches, loss of appetite, and loss of weight.[3,4] Pregnant women may abort spontaneously. Less common findings include aching joints, pneumonia, meningitis, epistaxis, and enlarged lymph nodes, spleen, and liver.

The course of illness is variable, ranging from a few days to years in duration. Untreated, the illness often lasts months. Even with treatment, a patient often is ill for a month or more. Relapsing illness is common. Five percent of the patients receiving appropriate therapy have one or more relapses within 3 years of initial onset, and the relapse rate is higher in the absence of appropriate therapy. Death due to brucellosis is rare but is more common with *B. melitensis* infections.

Chronic brucellosis is rare in appropriately treated patients. Chronic manifestations include spondylitis, osteomyelitis, and granulomas in a variety of sites, such as the liver, spleen, kidney, heart, and abdominal aorta. Prolonged mental depression is an infrequent sequel of brucellosis.

The drugs of choice for treating brucellosis are tetracycline and streptomycin. In many countries, a combination of doxycycline and rifampin has been adopted as the standard therapy. Therapy should be continued for at least 3 weeks to minimize rates of relapse.

The disease in animals causes infertility and abortion.[4] When brucellosis is first introduced into a group, an abortion epizootic often ensues. Endemic disease is less dramatic, since abortion occurs primarily in animals undergoing their first pregnancy. The birth of weak offspring, retained placentas, and diminished milk production also may occur. In males, chronic inflammation of the testicle and epididymis may result in infertility. Infection of the bones and joints may occur and may result in chronic lameness and, occasionally, posterior paralysis.

Mode of Transmission. In the animal reservoir hosts, brucellosis is transmitted by several mechanisms. Venereal transmission can occur as the result of infected semen. This is thought to be of minor importance except with artificial insemination, when it could be significant. The most important mechanism of transmission is the shedding of *Brucella* organisms in the uterine discharges after abortion or, on occasion, normal parturition in infected animals. Other animals in the herd become infected by ingesting *Brucella* organisms from the contaminated environment or directly from the infected animal's genitals. Fetal membranes and aborted fetuses may serve as sources of infection. *Brucella* organisms are capable of surviving for months in moist environments and manure.

Brucella organisms also may be shed in milk. This shedding may occur for several months, in multiple successive lactation periods, in otherwise apparently healthy dairy cows. The period of shedding is shorter for goats but still lasts for weeks and may recur in the next lactation period.

Human infections result primarily from exposure to *Brucella* organisms by one of three routes—ingestion, direct contact, and inhalation.[5] *Brucella* species also vary in their virulence for humans. For example, *B. melitensis* can produce disease with fewer organisms than *B. abortus* when ingested in dairy products.

Worldwide, ingestion of unpasteurized dairy products is the primary source of human brucellosis. Cheese made from raw goat's milk is particularly hazardous.

Contact with infectious materials, such as uterine discharges or blood, is an important source of infection for livestock raisers, veterinarians, and abattoir workers. The intact skin is an effective barrier against invasion by *Brucella* organisms under experimental conditions. The persons at primary risk of contracting infection, however, frequently have skin abrasions and cuts as a result of their occupation. *Brucella* organisms can readily invade the body through the conjunctiva if infectious material is rubbed or sprayed into the eyes.

Infection via inhalation also occurs under certain circumstances. This route of infection is only slightly less effective than parenteral challenge for inducing brucellosis in laboratory animals. Occupational groups at risk of infection via inhalation include laboratory and abattoir workers.

Reports of person to person transmission of brucellosis are rare. Transmission via whole blood transfusions has been reported but is very rare.

Occurrence. Brucellosis occurs worldwide. The reporting of cases is far from complete. Nonetheless, more than 20,000 cases are reported each year. Brucellosis is considered an important public health problem in Western and Central Asia, the Mediterranean region of Europe and Africa, and a number of countries in Central and South America.

In the United States, the reported incidence of brucellosis rose rapidly from slightly more than 100 cases in 1927 to a peak of 6321 cases in 1947. The virtually universal requirement for dairy product pasteurization and efforts to eradicate the disease from livestock have resulted subsequently in a progressive reduction in incidence. Less than 100 cases are now reported annually.

The relative importance of the various reservoir hosts and their associated *Brucella* species differs from region to region. *Brucella melitensis* infections associated with ingestion of unpasteurized goat cheese and milk remain a serious public health problem in most hyperendemic countries. *Brucella suis* biotype 4 infections are associated predominantly with ingestion of raw bone marrow and other tissues from caribou in Arctic regions.

In the United States, *B. abortus* infections associated with consumption of raw dairy products or contact with infected cattle constituted the majority of cases until the late 1950s. Brucellosis subsequently has been primarily an occupational disease of abattoir workers, livestock producers, veterinarians, and laboratory workers. The primary source of infection has changed to swine, and *B. suis* is now the predominant infecting species.[6] Cases associated with ingestion of unpasteurized dairy products continue to be reported, but these are now mostly *B. melitensis* infections associated with eating dairy products while traveling in Mediterranean countries and Mexico.

Brucellosis occurs throughout the year. Seasonal variations in incidence do occur, but the reasons for seasonality are not always clear. In regions where *B. melitensis* infections predominate, peak season incidence tends to coincide with the months when goats give birth. Cases in the United States tend to occur more frequently in April, May, and June and least frequently in November and December.

In the United States, brucellosis usually is a disease of adult males, reflecting their occupational exposure. Adult male predominance, although less marked, also tends to occur in other countries, reflecting increased risk due to occupational exposure of livestock raisers.

First reported as a cause of reproductive disease in dogs, *B. canis* now is known to cause human disease. Infections caused by this organism are widespread in the dog and, possibly, the cat populations of many countries. In contrast, only a small number of human infections have been reported. Less than 40 human infections have been reported in the United States through 1989.

Prevention and Control. The ideal method of preventing brucellosis is to eradicate the disease from domestic livestock. Bovine brucellosis reportedly has been eradicated from the British Channel Islands, Norway, Sweden, Finland, Denmark, Czechoslovakia, the Netherlands, Belize, and the Isle of Man. Other countries, including the United States and England, have made substantial progress toward eradication of bovine brucellosis, but the disease persists in swine and other domestic species.

Eradication programs are cost-beneficial to a country's economy in the long run because of increased livestock productivity. The short-term capital expenditure and disruption of agricultural routines, however, have dampened enthusiasm for undertaking eradication programs. When eradication is not feasible, control and reduction of incidence in livestock can be achieved with immunization.

A safe, effective vaccine is not available for use in humans. Persons who have fully recovered from an initial infection are resistant to reinfection. The protection afforded by a prior infection appears to be in the range of 90%.[7]

Pasteurization of milk and dairy products is an effective control procedure. Pasteurization will simultaneously control other milkborne diseases, such as salmonellosis and tuberculosis.

For persons with occupational exposure, some steps can be taken to reduce risk of infection and ameliorate the impact of the disease. An educational program should inform these persons about the disease, its symptoms, how it is acquired, and the need for early diagnosis and treatment. The use of appropriate protective equipment should be encouraged. For example, shoulder-length rubber gloves should be worn during obstetrical procedures on livestock.

Brucellosis should be considered routinely in the differential diagnosis of febrile illnesses in persons having occupational exposure to the disease. All such persons with fever of unknown origin lasting more than 3 days should be evaluated appropriately to avoid undue delay in diagnosis. Brucellosis patients for whom therapy is initiated within 30 days of onset have, as a group, a shorter course of illness and fewer complications.

Leptospirosis

Arnold F. Kaufmann
Jay D. Wenger

Leptospirosis was first recognized in 1883 as an occupational disease of sewer workers, an association still true.[1] Soon thereafter, the disease was reported in widely separated geographical areas. Whether leptospirosis was a variant of viral hepatitis or a truly distinctive disease soon became a controversial topic. The issue was resolved when the infecting leptospires were isolated in Japan about 1914 and shortly thereafter in Germany.

The initial confusion as to whether leptospirosis and viral hepatitis were distinct diseases was later repeated with yellow fever. The isolation of leptospires from jaundiced patients in yellow fever endemic areas led to this controversy, which continued until the viral etiology of yellow fever was established in 1928.

The Agent. The genus *Leptospira* comprises pathogenic and saprophytic strains. Although now subdivided into at least 12 species on the basis of DNA relatedness,[2] the older taxonomic system based on the serological relatedness of strains continues to be used. More than 250 pathogenic serovars are recognized currently. A leptospiral serogroup is a collective term for antigenically related serovars, but members of a serogroup may belong to multiple species as defined by DNA relatedness.

The parasitic leptospires are fastidious, slow-growing spirochetes.[3] They are small, thin, threadlike organisms tightly coiled about their long axis. Actively motile, leptospires rotate on their long axis, often with a whiplike motion.

Most leptospiral serovars have their primary reservoir in wild mammals, although some appear to be adapted to certain domestic and peridomestic animals. For example, *canicola* is associated with dogs, *pomona* with cattle and swine, and both *ballum* and *icterohaemorrhagiae* with rats and mice.

Leptospirosis is definitively diagnosed by culture of the organism from clinical or autopsy specimens using a semisolid medium. Culture of leptospires from environmental specimens, such as water, is best done by inoculation of laboratory animals.

In practice, serological tests, such as the microscopic agglutination procedure, are used more frequently than cultures for diagnostic purposes.[4] Direct microscopic examination of patient specimens with darkfield and fluorescent-antibody techniques also is used but is considered unreliable.

The Disease. Leptospirosis was described originally as a severe disease characterized by fever, jaundice, hemorrhage, and liver and renal failure. Subsequently, leptospirosis was recognized to occur much more frequently in a variety of often mild clinical forms. The protean manifestations of leptospirosis frequently result in its being misdiagnosed. Some common symptoms of the disease include influenza-like illness, fever of unknown origin, generalized enlargement of lymphoid glands resembling infectious mononucleosis, a macular to maculopapular rash, particularly with a pretibial distribution, abdominal pain, and aseptic meningitis and encephalitis.[5]

To some extent, specific clinical syndromes more commonly occur after infection with certain leptospiral serovars. The severe icteric form is associated with *icterohaemorrhagiae* infections, a prominence of gastrointestinal complaints with *grippotyphosa* infections, and aseptic meningitis with *pomona* and *canicola* infections. These associations are generalizations at best, and any leptospiral serovar can cause the various signs and symptoms associated with leptospirosis.

The incubation period is 4 to 19 days, usually 10 days. The illness often is biphasic, with an initial febrile (septicemic) stage lasting 3 to 7 days followed by a second (immune) stage lasting from 0 to 30 days or more.[6] Disease referable to specific organs, such as the kidneys, liver, eye, and meninges, becomes apparent in the immune stage. Mortality generally is low but is higher for older persons and those with jaundice.

Animal leptospirosis, as in the human disease, is often subclinical. Leptospirosis in dogs is characterized by febrile jaundice with liver and renal failure or by renal infection alone. In cattle and sheep, hemolytic anemia, hemoglobinuria, abortion, atypical mastitis, and production of thick, yellow, blood-tinged milk are common manifestations. Leptospirosis in swine is a nonspecific illness, with abortions late in pregnancy being the most important single sign.

Leptospiruria, the shedding of leptospires in urine, is a common and epidemiologically important aspect of the disease. Leptospiruria frequently continues for months after initial infection, particularly in animals. Leptospiruria is more transient in humans and seldom lasts more than 60 days.

Mode of Transmission. Human leptospirosis is contracted almost exclusively from direct or indirect exposure to urine of leptospiruric animals. Direct exposure appears to be a mode of transmission for pet owners and certain occupational groups, such as farm workers and veterinarians. Indirect exposure through vehicles, such as contaminated water and soil, is more common, however. Humans are a dead-end host for practical purposes, and person to person transmission is rare.

Leptospires can gain entry into the body through breaks in the skin as well as via mucous membranes. Most common source outbreaks in the United States have been associated with swimming in contaminated water. Persons in occupations that involve exposure to water and mud, such as sewer workers and rice field workers, have a high risk for leptospiral infections. Partial or total immersion in water or mud seems to play a role in facilitating infection.

Milkers are another high-risk group. In herring-bone milking parlors, persons milking cows frequently are spattered in the face with urine, with resultant infection via the conjunctiva.

Infections following animal bites are reported occasionally. Most of these cases involve rodent bites. Infection following consumption of contaminated food and water has been reported, and because leptospires cannot survive in the acid gastric environment, the route of infection in these cases presumably is the mucous membranes of the mouth and esophagus.

Occurrence. Leptospirosis occurs worldwide. Although it is considered more common in tropical countries, the majority of cases are reported from countries with temperate climates. The geographical distribution of reported cases reflects the availability of diagnostic facilities and the interests of individual investigators.

Of the 1500 to 2000 cases reported annually worldwide, about 100 are from the United States. In contrast to many infectious diseases, leptospirosis has been reported with increasing frequency over the past five decades in the United States. Sixteen cases were reported in the period 1925–1934, 230 in 1935–1944, 267 in 1945–1954, 705 in 1955–1964, 791 in 1965–1974, and more than 800 in 1975–1984.

The incidence of leptospirosis varies by season, with most cases occurring in the late summer and early fall. In the United States, more than 50% of cases occur in the months July through October.

In most countries, leptospirosis is predominantly a disease of adult males, reflecting the importance of occupational exposure. In the United States, a trend toward more cases in females and at younger ages has developed. This reflects changing social roles and the increasing importance of exposure during leisure activities. Almost one half of the cases in the period 1978–1987 were associated with recreational exposures.

A shift has occurred in the predominant infecting serogroup in the United States. Before 1948, only infections by *icterohaemorrhagiae* (90%) and *canicola* (10%) were recognized. In the period 1949–1961, infections by members of the *pomona, grippotyphosa, autumnalis, hebdomadis, bataviae, ballum,* and *pyrogenes* serogroups were recognized, and less than 40% of the cases were ascribed to *icterohaemorrhagiae* infections. In the period 1978–1987, infections by members of all the foregoing serogroups plus *tarassovi, javanica, cynopteri, andamana, australis,* and *shermani* were detected, and only 32% of the cases were ascribed to *icterohaemorrhagiae* infections.

Prevention and Control. All leptospirosis cases should be investigated to detect potential common source outbreaks and implement appropriate control measures to prevent occurrence of further cases. Control, unfortunately, is not a simple matter.

Human leptospirosis vaccines have been used in countries other than the United States for selected high-risk populations, such as rice field workers in Italy. These vaccines are serovar specific.

A recent field study demonstrated that 200 mg of doxycycline administered once weekly was effective in the prevention of leptospirosis. Chemoprophylaxis is recommended when the exposure period is short term and the expected attack rate is greater than 1%.

Animal vaccines are available that protect against illness but not against infection and leptospiruria. Human infections have been acquired from asymptomatic dogs that were immunized but nonetheless shed leptospires in their urine.

Treatment with antibiotics, such as streptomycin and tetracycline, has been recommended as a method of eliminating renal shedding in swine, cattle, and dogs. The effectiveness of this approach is equivocal. In cattle, concurrent administration of streptomycin and vaccine has been recommended to control acute outbreaks.

Use of protective equipment is of value in certain circumstances. The wearing of rubber boots is recommended for sewer workers and agricultural workers who frequently wade in rodent urine-contaminated water. Environmental hygiene measures, such as rodent control and work surface decontamination, also may be of benefit. Swimming should not be permitted in streams where risk of infection is high.

Salmonellosis

Robert V. Tauxe
Paul A. Blake

The *Salmonella* genus of bacteria was identified in 1885 by Salmon and Smith. There are now over 2000 specific antigenic types of *Salmonella,* and new ones are still being identified. Salmonellosis is a convenient etiological term to describe a variety of conditions that affect humans and many animal species. The clinical results of *Salmonella* infection in humans range from symptomless carriage to septicemia, with infection often the result of ingestion of contaminated foods. In contrast to *Salmonella typhi,* infection and illness with the nontyphoid *Salmonella* are increasing in areas with adequate sanitation and are now an important cause of morbidity and expense in many developed and developing countries (Fig. 12–1).

Characteristics of the Bacteria. Bacteria of the genus *Salmonella* are gram-negative bacilli that have many cultural properties and antigens in common with other members of the family Enterobacteriaceae. Individual serotypes are characterized by their somatic (O) and flagellar (H) antigens. Salmonellae are grouped and subgrouped (A, B, C_1, C_2, C_3, D, E_1, E_2, E_3, E_4, and so on) by O antigens. Within each group, individual serotypes are distinguished by their H antigens. Although over 2000 serotypes are known, 10 serotypes accounted for about 70% of the total human isolates in the United States in 1986[1] (Table 12–3).

Temperatures used in routine pasteurization of milk destroy salmonellae. Salmonellae within meat or other products, however, may survive if cooking temperatures and time of cooking are adequate only to cook the surface of the food. Refrigeration does not destroy *Salmonella,* and growth has been recorded at 10° C (50° F). Once in the environment, salmonellae survive for long periods in water and soil and on or within foods. Phage typing of many individual serotypes is possible and has been used in epidemiological studies, most often with *Salmonella typhimurium.*[2] Analysis of the plasmid profiles of *Salmonella* isolates in investigations of salmonellosis has contributed greatly to the understanding of the epidemiology of these organisms.[2,3] Use of antimicrobials in animal feeds has led to antimicrobial-resistant salmonellae, often with transferable drug-resistant plasmids, and antimicrobial-resistant salmonellae from animal sources have been shown to have caused outbreaks in humans.[4] Transfer of the antimicrobial resistance from *Salmonella* to other bacteria has been documented.[5] Strains that are particularly invasive and multiply-resistant have appeared in the nosocomial setting in developing countries.[6,7]

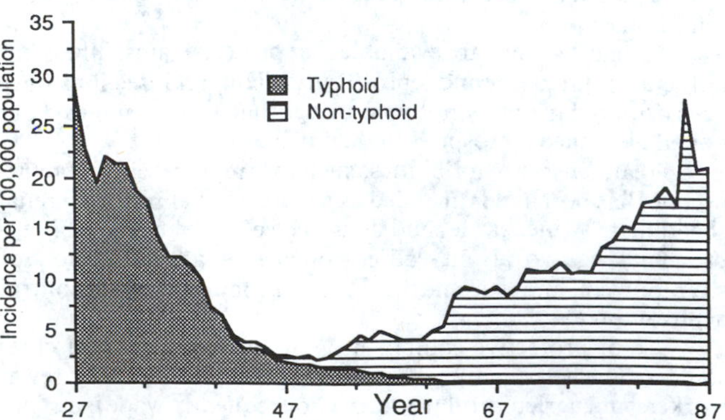

Figure 12–1. Reported combined incidence of typhoid fever and nontyphoid salmonellosis in the United States from 1927 to 1987.

Clinical Characteristics. The most frequent symptoms of salmonellosis—diarrhea, abdominal cramps, pain, fever, headache, nausea, and vomiting—do not easily distinguish salmonellosis from many other causes of gastroenteritis. The illness results from bacterial invasion, predominantly of the ileum, which explains the frequent occurrence of fever and generalized symptoms. In addition to gastroenteritis, *Salmonella* infections occasionally may result in a septicemic illness resembling typhoid and described as enteric fever. Persons with human immunodeficiency virus (HIV) infections are particularly prone to develop severe bloodstream infections, which may recur after apparently adequate therapy. Occasionally, localization of the *Salmonella* may lead to an abscess, meningitis, osteomyelitis, and other inflammatory conditions. Many infections are not associated with clinical illness. Following gastrointestinal infection, the median duration of enteric carriage is approximately 5 weeks.[8] Children, especially infants, have longer periods of carriage than other age groups. Antimicrobial treatment of the acute gastrointestinal illness is ineffective and may prolong the duration of enteric carriage.[9] Antimicrobials are indicated in the treatment of systemic illness, however. Case fatality rates usually are low, but infants, the aged, and the immunosuppressed often become seriously ill.

The incubation period is most often between 6 and 48 hours, although long incubation periods (over 10 days) have been documented.

Diagnosis. The laboratory diagnosis is made by culture of feces on one of the standard selective media, followed by determination of biochemical reactions and by specific agglutination with polyvalent and monovalent typing sera by the simplified method described by Edwards and Ewing. Instead of using fecal specimens as a source, rectal swab cultures facilitate diagnosis in survey work. In the septicemic, typhoidal, and other extraintestinal forms, the organism may be recovered from the blood or from a site of focal infection. Although serological responses may occur to the O and H antigens of the infecting *Salmonella,* they are not useful routinely in diagnosis.

Transmission. Infections in humans often are related directly or indirectly to infection in animals. Before its distribution was banned in 1975, the small pet turtle was the single most commonly identified source of salmonellosis in the United States.[10] Infections in animals may be initiated or perpetuated when animal feed or feed supplements are contaminated with salmonellae. Infections in animals, often restricted to the intestinal tract, occasionally also involve systemic lymph nodes, which can lead to human infection if meat is cooked only superficially. Infections may be amplified when herds are stressed during moving or holding before slaughter and, subsequently, within the slaughterhouses themselves.[11] Salmonellae infect cattle, pigs, fowl, and other vertebrates and enter the human food chain on raw meat brought into the kitchen. Cross-contamination by uncooked food or inadequate cooking of food may then lead to human infection. Salmonellae often are found in unpasteurized milk.[12] Although vegetables have been shown to be contaminated, they are rarely incriminated as the source of infection in human outbreaks. Salmonellae frequently are found on the external surfaces of freshly laid eggs, and contamination of bulk eggs is frequent, whether spray dried, liquid, or frozen. Pasteurization of bulk egg products has effectively controlled this contamination. In the 1980s, a large number of outbreaks caused by the serotype

TABLE 12-3. THE 10 MOST FREQUENTLY REPORTED *SALMONELLA* SEROTYPES FROM HUMAN AND NONHUMAN SOURCES IN 1987

Human 1987			Nonhuman 1987		
Serotype	**Number**	**%**	**Serotype**	**Number**	**%**
typhimurium[a]	10,462	23.5	*typhimurium*[a]	1,246	13.5
enteritidis	6,950	15.6	*heidelberg*	1,124	12.2
heidelberg	5,714	12.8	*choleraesuis*[b]	667	7.2
newport	2,858	6.4	*reading*	438	4.8
hadar	2,170	4.9	*hadar*	352	3.8
infantis	1,136	2.5	*senftenberg*	331	3.6
agona	1,080	2.4	*newport*	302	3.3
montevideo	1,037	2.3	*montevideo*	301	3.3
thompson	635	1.4	*enteritidis*	270	2.9
braenderup	548	1.2	*anatum*	266	2.9
Subtotal	32,590	73.1	Subtotal	5,297	57.5
Total	44,609		Total	9,208	

[a]*typhimurium* includes var. *copenhagen*.
[b]*choleraesuis* includes var. *kunzendorf*.

Salmonella enteritidis were traced to grade A shell eggs, which can be contaminated internally before the shell forms as a result of ovarian infection in the hen.[13]

The oral dose of *Salmonella* necessary to initiate a human infection has often been low ($<10^3$) in outbreaks, in which only a small proportion of exposed persons may be infected.[14] Volunteer studies, however, have suggested that a large dose ($<10^6$ or more organisms) generally is necessary to initiate infection in a high proportion of the recipients. This may explain the low frequency with which secondary illness occurs within households in which a primary case is identified. The virulence of the organisms, the nature of the vehicle, and host factors, such as reduced gastric acidity in infants and the elderly and underlying disease, may increase the risk of infection, even with a low infecting dose. Use of antibiotics for other reasons shortly before or during exposure increases the susceptibility of the host to infection with resistant strains by reducing competitive flora and lowering the infectious dose.[4]

A mean of 60 foodborne outbreaks of salmonellosis was reported to CDC each year during the period 1978–1987, 37% occurring in restaurants or cafeterias. Poultry, meat, eggs, and dairy products are the most commonly reported food vehicles. These outbreaks typically result from mishandling foods of animal origin. Inadequate cooking, cross-contamination, and prolonged holding at inappropriate temperatures are the usual contributing foodhandling errors. Although foodhandlers often are found to be infected in the course of investigation, this is generally because they ate the contaminated foods. They are more likely to be victims than sources of the contamination.[15]

Nosocomial Salmonellosis. Outbreaks of salmonellosis in hospitals and nursing homes are associated with especially high mortality.[16] Such outbreaks appear to have become less common in recent years and, when they occur, are often the result of foodborne transmission. Good routine infection control and handwashing procedures can reduce transmission from caregivers to patients, and thus make person to person transmission less likely. Because of the extreme susceptibility of newborns, intensive care patients, and those with immunosuppressive conditions, special precautions are warranted to prevent transmission to these patients (Fig. 12-2).

Salmonellae can spread among patients in a ward, either by person to person contact or occasionally by fomites. Fomites have included dust, delivery room resuscitators, bedside tables and cribs, thermometers, waterbaths, suction tubing, and endoscopes. The common vehicles identified in institutional outbreaks are most often foods but occasionally have included medicinal and pharmaceutical products of animal origin, such as carmine dye, pancreatin, pepsin, bile salts, gelatin, vitamins, extracts of various tissues, and transfused platelets. Outbreaks in nurseries often are preceded by an episode of diarrhea in the mother of the index case infant.[17]

Occurrence. Approximately 45,000 *Salmonella* isolations are reported annually in the United States.[1] The highest reported infection rates occur in children 2 to 4 months of age.[1] Approximations of the number of cases actually occurring in the United States, extrapolated from data developed during studies of outbreaks, suggest that there are 30 to 100 persons clinically ill for every *Salmonella* isolate reported. Thus, it is probable that 1 to 4 million cases of salmonellosis actually occur annually in the United States.

Regular seasonal changes in the incidence of salmonellosis

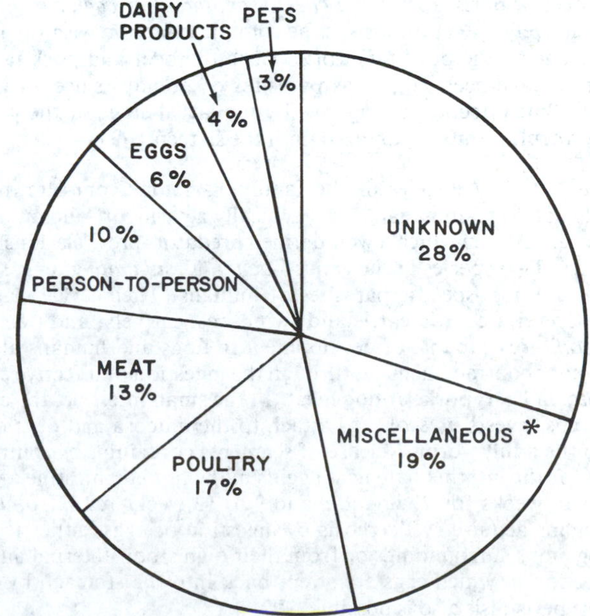

Figure 12-2. Mode of transmission in 500 human salmonellosis outbreaks in 1966 to 1975.

generally have been observed in all countries studied, but the pattern varies with the serotype, vehicle, mode of spread, and local circumstances.[18] The reasons for seasonality are poorly understood but include more transmission among food animals, heavier contamination at slaughter plants, and greater opportunity for rapid bacterial growth should refrigeration be inadequate in the warmer months. The age-specific incidence varies considerably by serotype, probably because different serotypes contaminate different food vehicles.[18] The annual frequency of individual serotypes is not stable, since single serotypes can rapidly gain importance after introduction into the food chain. *Salmonella agona* emerged as a dominant serotype worldwide after it was introduced into poultry feed on contaminated fishmeal in the early 1970s.[19] *S. enteritidis* currently is increasing rapidly on four continents as a result of widespread infection of poultry flocks.[20]

Some salmonella serotypes are highly host specific (*Salmonella dublin* in cattle, *Salmonella cholerae-suis* in pigs, *Salmonella pullorum* in poultry, and *S. typhi* in humans), whereas others have very broad host ranges. Some salmonellae are restricted to certain geographical areas, whereas others are cosmopolitan. Some serotypes are frequent in a particular region or state in the United States (*S. enteritidis* in the northeast, *Salmonella javiana* in the southeast, *Salmonella weltevreden* in Hawaii).

Prevention. Since the majority of human infections occur directly or indirectly through food, control measures are most effective when applied somewhere along the food chain or in the controlling of the entry of *Salmonella* into the kitchen.

Salmonellae are frequent contaminants of animal feeds, and efforts have been made to control *Salmonella* before they infect food animals. The high cost of such efforts has limited their use in the past except in a few Scandinavian countries, but the steady increase in salmonellosis in many countries has led to increased interest in these methods and to a reevaluation of this position.[17] Prohibiting the sale of *Salmonella*-contaminated pet turtles in the United States led to reduction in disease associated with this vehicle.[10] However, beyond the pasteurization of milk and the regulation of precooked beef, the control of *Salmonella* contamination in foods has not yet been generally effective in the United States. Attempts to reduce the frequency of antimicrobial-resistant *Salmonella* have been initiated in many countries in Europe by restricting the use of antimicrobials in animal feed.

Inspecting foodservice areas to ensure that foodhandling procedures are well understood, refrigeration is adequate, storage facilities are appropriate, and handwashing is frequent is a critical part of preventing salmonellosis outbreaks. Control of *Salmonella* in foodhandlers is difficult to effect because excretion of *Salmonella* may be prolonged, and no treatment regimen has been shown to reduce carriage. Although many health departments recommend special preventive measures, control of salmonellosis by procedures directed at foodhandlers is probably most effectively addressed by educating them in good personal hygiene and proper foodhandling practices. In infected persons working in hospitals, restriction of their contact with patients is prudent, although transmission from hospital personnel to patients is rarely documented. Patients excreting *Salmonella* should be managed with routine enteric precautions.

It is unlikely that the incidence of salmonellosis in humans can be reduced significantly with the control measures currently available. Irradiation of foods of animal origin has been suggested by the World Health Organization as a future general control measure.[21]

Taeniasis and Cysticercosis

Robert L. Rausch

Taeniasis refers to an intestinal infection with the adult stage of the beef or pork tapeworm (*Taenia saginata* and *Taenia solium,* respectively). Cysticercosis is the somatic infection with the larval stage of the pork tapeworm. Both the beef and pork tapeworms have been known as parasites of humans since ancient times, but infection of humans by the larval stage of the pork tapeworm was not recognized until the sixteenth century.

Life Cycle. Cestodes of the family Taeniidae complete their cycle in two mammalian hosts, typically a carnivore and an herbivore, between which a well-defined predator–prey relationship exists.[1] Two species in the genus *Taenia, T. saginata* and *T. solium,* are host-specific parasites of humans. Their larval stages (cysticerci) occur in cattle and swine, respectively, and that of *T. solium* is capable of development in dogs and humans also. Humans contract taeniasis through the ingestion of infective cysticerci in beef, pork, or dog meat. In the small intestine, the cysticercus invests its scolex to attach to the mucosa and develops into the adult worm. Release of segments containing eggs infective for the intermediate host begins in the human intestine after 8 to 10 weeks for *T. saginata* and 9 to 13 weeks for *T. solium.* Humans acquire cysticercosis by ingestion of eggs, either from exogenous surroundings or from their own stool. Internal autoinfection in which eggs are swept back into the stomach by reverse peristalsis also is possible.

Distribution. According to recent estimates, about 45 million people worldwide are infected by *T. saginata* and about 3.5 million by *T. solium.* The former occurs widely in Europe, where its prevalence is increasing. *Taenia saginata* is common in some regions of the USSR, in Southeast Asia, and in some South American countries. Highest rates have been reported in Africa among nomadic herders and their cattle. *Taenia saginata* is uncommon in North America north of Mexico, but its prevalence seems to have increased locally in the southwestern United States. In that region, workers harboring the adult worms or sewage used in irrigation appear to be sources of infection for cattle.[2] The distribution and prevalence of this cestode have been reviewed in detail by Pawlowski and Schultz.[3] *Taenia solium* is a rare cestode in most of the developed countries, but it is relatively common in some regions of Africa, southern Asia, Mexico, and Central and South America.

Clinical Picture. The presence of these cestodes in the human intestine often is undetected, but disorders manifested by diarrhea, flatulence, and vague abdominal pain are sometimes attributed to taeniasis.

The larval *T. solium* is the usual cause of cysticercosis in humans. This cestode is unique in the family Taeniidae in that both stages of its cycle are capable of development in a single mammalian host. Larvae in skeletal muscle usually are asymptomatic unless present in large numbers. Severe functional disturbances may result when cysticerci localize in tissues of the central nervous system. Clinical manifestations, however, usually are delayed until severe tissue responses are evoked by the degeneration of dead larvae.

Diagnosis. The diagnosis of taeniasis is made usually on the basis of the characteristic eggs found by fecal examination. The eggs of *T. solium* and *T. saginata* are indistinguishable, but they can be differentiated by examination of the gravid proglottis. The number of main uterine branches of *T. saginata* is 15 to 20 and that of *T. solium* is 7 to 13.

Diagnosis of cysticercosis involving the central nervous system is often difficult. This condition should be considered in the differential diagnosis of epilepsy, basilar meningitis, obstructive hydrocephalus, and other disorders in patients with a history of residence or travel in regions where *T. solium* is endemic. Radiological diagnosis may be possible after the death and calcification of the larvae. Imaging techniques, such as computed tomography scan and nuclear magnetic resonance, are the main diagnostic tools in neurocysticercosis.[4–7] Cysticerci localized in subcutaneous tissues or skin, where they form palpable nodules, are identified readily after biopsy. Immunodiagnostic tests for cysticercosis are available. Both antibody and antigen have been detected in serum or cerebrospinal fluid by ELISA or a combination of other immunochemical techniques based on ELISA.[8–10] Highly purified specific antigens are required for reliable results. The new enzyme-linked immunoelectrotransfer blot method (EITB), using lentil-lectin affinity-purified glycoprotein antigens for immunodiagnosing human cysticercosis, has been reported to be 98% sensitive, 100% specific, highly reproducible, and simple to perform.[11]

Treatment. In the treatment of taeniasis, good results have been obtained with niclosamide and dichlorophen, both of which cause some disintegration of the strobilae. Praziquantel (Bayer AG, Leverkusen) is 100% effective against *T. saginata* and other cestodes when administered as a single dose of 10 mg/kg. Transient side effects occur in only a small proportion of patients and are considered of negligible importance.

Treatment of neurological cysticercosis has been limited mainly to use of anticonvulsive drugs to control epileptiform attacks. Disorders attributable to interference with the flow of cerebrospinal fluid by racemose cysticerci sometimes can be alleviated surgically. Recently, praziquantel has been found to be effective in the treatment of neurocysticercosis.[4,12] Preliminary results indicate that flubendazole also may have therapeutic value.[13]

Prevention and Control. Requisite conditions for the infection of humans by *T. saginata* and *T. solium* are poor sanitation and consumption of beef and pork insufficiently cooked to kill the cysticerci. The best preventive measures include strict attention to personal hygiene, environmental sanitation, and protection of cattle and hogs from contact with human excretions. Individual infection is prevented by thorough cooking of beef and pork at 55° C or freezing at −17° C for 5 days. In endemic regions, educational programs are needed to alert the public to the risks of eating inadequately cooked beef and pork. In the United States, federal meat inspection includes direct examination for the presence of cysticerci (i.e., looking for "measly" meat).

Trichinosis

Robert L. Rausch

Trichinosis, or trichinelliasis, is caused by the larval stage of nematodes of the genus *Trichinella,* of which until recently a single species, *Trichinella spiralis,* was known. At least seven gene pools—*T. spiralis, Trichinella nativa, Trichinella nelsoni, Trichinella pseudospiralis, Trichinella 3, Trichinella 5,* and *Trichinella 6*—have now been identified. They are distinguished, now, by genetic, immunological, and ecological differences.[1] Of these nematodes, however, *T. spiralis* is the most important medically.

Life Cycle. All stages of the cycle of *Trichinella* species occur in individual mammalian hosts. When skeletal muscle containing the infective larvae is ingested by another mammal, the larvae are released by the action of gastric fluids and pass into the small intestine. There, the nematodes molt four times before becoming sexually mature. After copulation, the females begin to expel larvae about 6 or 7 days after exposure. This process continues for the life of the female, about 5 weeks. Most of the first-stage larvae penetrate to the submucosa and are carried to various organs, including the myocardium, brain, lungs, retina, lymph nodes, pancreas, and cerebrospinal fluid. Finally, they relocate inside the skeletal muscle, where they gradually encyst and develop into the infective stage about 30 days after penetration of muscle fibers. Infectivity can be retained for many years, depending on the species of mammalian host. The larvae appear to be nonpathogenic for the natural hosts (excluding humans) unless very large numbers are involved.

Epidemiology. Trichinosis is a cosmopolitan disease that occurs commonly in Europe and the United States. More than 100 different animals can be infected with trichinella. There are two transmission patterns. Salvatic trichinosis is a disease cycling among wild carnivores, and urban trichinosis cycles among humans, rats, and pigs. The most important source of infection by *T. spiralis* for humans is the flesh of swine. Pigs and rats become infected by feeding on infected pork waste in garbage. Dead or dying infected rats are eaten by pigs, rats, and other animals, serving as an important source of infection.[2,3] In recent years, bear, horse, and walrus, rather than swine, have been found to be responsible for small outbreaks in certain endemic areas.[4–6]

The prevalence of trichinosis in humans and in swine has diminished steadily during the last 30 years in the United States, where fatal cases are now rare. The number of cases reported to the Centers for Disease Control declined markedly from an average of 400, with 10 to 15 deaths, reported each year in the late 1940s to 57 per year, with 3 deaths, in the 5 years 1982–1986. This decline can be attributed to improvement in the quality of commercially produced pork and to national and state efforts toward prevention of trichinosis.[7] A comparable decline has occurred in most countries. The incidence of the infection in Northern Italy decreased from 32% in 1980 to 4% in 1988. Most human infections there are caused by wild bear or by imported horse meat. The urban cycle has disappeared in many European countries, such as Italy, Switzerland, France, and Austria, where wild animals, especially bear and fox, are the only source of infection. In Yugoslavia, however, there are still many human cases caused by both domestic and sylvatic cycles.[4] In the USSR, the study of trichinosis in the Ternopol Province (Ukraine) in 1954–1979 showed that there were 39 cases of trichinosis in humans, with 4 deaths. There have been no cases reported since 1980 in either humans or domestic pigs. Trichinosis invasion of wild, domestic, and synanthropic mammals also has decreased.[8]

In the Arctic, *T. nativa* is a common parasite of terrestrial carnivores and, less frequently, of marine mammals (Pinnipedia).[9] One characteristic of this form is its ability to retain infectivity after long exposure to freezing temperatures. The flesh of bear has been a common source of infection for humans. Outbreaks usually have been confined to indigenous populations. Small-scale epidemics sometimes occur because of the traditional sharing of large marine mammals. In 1975, 29 persons at Barrow, Alaska, became ill after consumption of meat from an infected walrus.[5]

Clinical Picture. The clinical course of trichinosis in humans is variable, depending on numbers of larvae ingested and other factors. Light infections often are asymptomatic, or the symptoms and signs are nonspecific. With more severe infections, three clinical stages may be discerned. The intestinal phase, with onset 2 to 7 days after exposure, is characterized by malaise, vomiting, diarrhea and other intestinal disorders, and abdominal pain. The second phase, overlapping the first, begins with migration of the larvae and usually is more constant in its manifestations, which typically include facial edema, myalgia, weakness, fever, and eosinophilia. In severe infections, other organs may be involved, resulting in neurological disorders, myocarditis, nephritis, and pneumonia.

Death may occur from the fourth to the sixth week. The phase of convalescence usually begins from the third to the fourth week, with subsidence of fever and muscular symptoms and diminution of edema and toxic or allergic manifestations. Convalescence may be slow, and muscular dysfunction, weakness, fatigue, and other disorders may persist for several months. The prognosis usually is good in cases involving light infections.

Diagnosis. Mild infections often escape detection, particularly when they are sporadic. Clinical findings during the intestinal phase are nonspecific. During invasion of the musculature, edema of the eyelids and face, eosinophilia, and myalgia are characteristic. A positive diagnosis can be made by finding larvae in biopsied muscle. When antibodies appear 2 to 4 weeks after exposure, various immunodiagnostic tests can be used, such as enzyme-linked immunosorbent assay (ELISA), bentonite flocculation test (BFI), counter electrophoresis (CEP), and indirect latex agglutination test (LAT). The ELISA appears to have high specificity and sensitivity. Diagnosis usually is based on the combination of epidemiological information, clinical findings, biopsy, and results of immunodiagnostic tests.

Treatment. There is no established specific treatment for trichinosis. Amelioration of clinical signs and prevention of severe complications may be obtained through the use of corticosteroids. Thiabendazole may be beneficial, but its effects have not been fully evaluated. This drug produces rapid symptomatic improvement but may cause side effects, such as nausea, vomiting, and dermatitis.[10] Mebendazole has been shown to have a lethal effect on both the invasive and encapsulated phases of *Trichinella* in mice and rats[11] and was reported to be effective for human treatment in an outbreak of trichinosis in eastern Siberia.[12]

Prevention and Control. Infection by *Trichinella* species can be prevented by thorough cooking of meat of swine and carnivorous animals or by freezing below $-20°$ C for 3 days or $-15°$ C for 3 weeks. Conditions defined for the treatment of pork, however, are inadequate to kill the larvae of the more cold-resistant *T. nativa* in carcasses of Arctic mammals. Bear or raccoon meat must be cooked before consumption to destroy the larvae. Microwave cooking of pork, especially roasting, should be avoided until specifications for time and temperature for disinfecting the larvae are established. Prohibitions against feeding of raw garbage have contributed significantly to the decreasing prevalence of *T. spiralis* in swine in North America. Trichinoscopy has been an effective means for detecting infected swine in European countries and in some republics of the Soviet Union. In Germany, federal law requires inspection of carcasses of wild boar or of any carnivorous mammals intended for human consumption. Transmission of the disease from domestic swine to sylvatic hosts has been recognized, and any control or eradication efforts must take into account the potential for reinfection of hogs from wild animals.

Paragonimiasis

Alfred A. Buck

Paragonimiasis (lung fluke disease, endemic hemoptysis, pulmonary distomiasis) is caused by various species of the trematode *Paragonimus.* Humans and a great variety of crab-eating and crayfish-eating mammals are definitive hosts and act as reservoirs. Until about 1950, human paragonimiasis was thought to be endemic only in the Far East and in Southeast Asia. Since then, there has been clear evidence of its endemicity in other parts of the world, notably West and Central Africa and New Guinea.

Life Cycle. All species of *Paragonimus* that infect humans have similar life cycles, which require two intermediate hosts, a snail and a freshwater crab or crayfish. There are now at least eight different species of lung fluke diseases in humans, of which *Paragonimus westermani* is the most widespread in the endemic areas of the Orient.

Infection with the human lung fluke is acquired by ingestion of raw or partially cooked freshwater crabs and crayfish that contain the encysted stages of the parasite, the metacercariae. After ingestion of the viable cysts by the definitive host, excystation occurs in the duodenum. The young worm migrates through the peritoneal cavity, penetrates the diaphragm, enters the lung, and finally settles down near a bronchiole. The large number of eggs and the metabolites produced by the fluke cause injury to the surrounding lung tissue and walls of the bronchioli. The circuitous migration from the intestinal tract to the lungs provides abundant opportunity for the worms to become sidetracked or to wander into organs and tissues far removed from the typical intrapulmonary residence of the adult worm.

Eggs are excreted either by expectoration or, if swallowed, with the stools. When they reach fresh and clear water, they embryonate and usually hatch within 16 to 20 days. The free-swimming larva, or miracidium, then must enter a suitable snail host of several species of *Semisulcospira, Tarebia, Thiara,* and *Assimenia,* where development to the cercarial stage takes place in approximately 3 months of maturation. The cercariae emerge from the snail and penetrate into the second intermediate host, one of various species of freshwater crabs or crayfish of the genera *Potamon, Eriocheir, Sesarma,* or *Astacus.* In the flesh of these crustaceans, they encyst and form metacercariae.

In addition to humans, the other mammalian hosts that serve as reservoirs for human paragonimiasis are cats, dogs, pigs, tigers, leopards, wolves, wildcats, opossums, mongoose, and bandicoots.

Geographic Distribution. Areas of relatively high endemicity of paragonimiasis usually are confined to foci near streams, especially mountain streams, and rivers, where the intermediate hosts are abundant. Endemic areas with a high prevalence of lung fluke disease are in the Far East in Korea, Taiwan, China, and Japan; in Southeast Asia in the Philippines, Indonesia, Thailand, Vietnam, Laos, India, and New Guinea; in Africa in Cameroon, Congo, Chad, Gabon, Guinea, Liberia, Zaire, Nigeria, Senegal, and Gambia; and in South America in Peru, Ecuador, Venezuela, and Colombia. Sporadic cases are reported from Bokina Faso, Ivory Coast, and Solomon Islands.

Clinical Illness. The clinical picture of paragonimiasis depends on the organs involved and on the extent to which the tissue is parasitized. Paragonimiasis occurs primarily as a chronic lung disease characterized by chronic cough and hemoptysis. Its onset usually is insidious. Later, chest pain, dyspnea, and constitutional symptoms may be present. Pleurisy with effusion, empyema, and pleural adhesions are common complications. Extrapulmonary paragonimiasis occurs more often than is usually thought. Most important are cerebral lesions. Other sites include the liver, mesenteric lymph nodes, genitourinary system, the eye, and the subcutaneous tissue.

Diagnosis and Screening. Recognition is the first step toward prevention. A specific diagnosis can be made readily by the recovery of *Paragonimus* eggs from patients having the typical rusty, blood-tinged sputum. Nevertheless, a correct diagnosis of pulmonary paragonimiasis is often missed, owing to the similarity of the symptoms to those of pulmonary tuberculosis and an inability to find the eggs in the sputum. In extrapulmonary paragonimiasis, surgical means may be the only way to recover the eggs from the tissue lesions. Sputum examination for the presence of acid-fast bacilli by appropriate staining methods can deform and even destroy *Paragonimus* eggs beyond recognition. Therefore, unstained sputum specimens should be examined wherever paragonimiasis is suspected. Recovery of eggs can be improved by including a routine stool examination. *Paragonimus* eggs are large (18–120 by 40–60 μm) and yellow-brown with a thick shell with a visible operculum.

Chest x-rays may be helpful in making a tentative diagnosis. The use of intradermal and serological tests with purified antigens of *P. westermani* can be regarded as a valuable aid both for the differential diagnosis against tuberculosis and for epidemiological surveys. A highly purified antigen has been produced that does not cross-react with other parasites commonly found in areas where paragonimiasis exists.[1]

Community Patterns of Infection. In endemic areas, the prevalence of the disease and the infection continues to rise with age up to about 40 years, when the prevalence levels off. In some areas, as in Korea, there is a significant sex difference, with male preponderance. This is related to the habit of eating raw, marinated, or pickled crabs and crayfish while consuming alcoholic beverages in public bars. The common practice of pickling crabs in wine, vinegar, or brine does not always kill the infective metacercariae of the parasite. By contrast, in some African foci, women are more frequently affected than men because the eating of raw crayfish and crabs is thought to enhance fertility.

In time of famine, the incidence of paragonimiasis often rises significantly because many new infections occur in persons who eat raw freshwater crabs and crayfish when other food is unavailable.

Small, single-source epidemics of paragonimiasis have occurred after the consumption of crab and crayfish meat heavily infected with the metacercariae of *P. westermani.*

The reported frequency of cerebral paragonimiasis appears to be much higher in the Far East than in any of the other endemic foci.

Control and Prevention. There are three effective new drugs for treatment of paragonimiasis. They are praziquantel [2-cyclohexyl carbonyl 1,2,3,6,7,116-hexahydropyrazino (2,1-a) isoquinolin-4-a], bithionol (2, 2′thiobis[4, 6,-dichloro phenol]), and menichlopholan (niclofan) (2,2′-dihydroxy-3,3′-dinitro-5, 5-dichlordiphenyl).[2] Praziquantel is the drug of choice, with close to 95% cure rates when given orally in three doses of 25 mg/kg over 3 days. Bithionol proved effective in about 80% of cases when given in a single dose of 2 mg/kg body weight.

Temporary control of snails by molluscicides as well as destruction of crabs is feasible but requires careful consideration of the effects of the chemicals on local nontarget fauna. Significant results of controlling paragonimiasis by sanitary disposal of sputum and feces can be expected only if the maintenance of the life cycle of *Paragonimus* does not depend on other mammalian reservoir hosts. Education of people in endemic areas concerning the life cycle of the parasite is one of the most important methods for preventing paragonimiasis. The present method of preparing uncooked crabs and crayfish by keeping them in brine for several days is not sufficient to kill the infective metacercariae, especially when the time of aging in these salt solutions is short. Cooking the crabs and crayfish is a safe way to prevent infection. It requires continued and intensive efforts to convince the people that a change in their food habits is the best safeguard against new infections with the lung fluke.

In Korea, mass treatment of paragonimiasis using a single dose of menichlopholan has been effective, with few side effects.[2]

The fertility of the adult trematodes may be as long as 20 years or more, during which eggs may be discharged by the human host. Even after destruction of the mollusks and crustaceans involved in the life cycle of the lung fluke, therefore, transmission may begin again as soon as the intermediary hosts repopulate the rivers and streams in the area.

Clonorchiasis

Alfred A. Buck

Clonorchis sinesis, a trematode of the family Ophisthorchiidae, is responsible for the production of chronic disease of the liver and bile ducts. Human infections are common and widely distributed in countries of the Far East and Southeast Asia. They present serious public health problems in certain localized areas of Japan, Korea, and China. With the increased travel and migration of Asians to other parts of the world, imported cases of clonorchiasis are being found with increasing frequency in many nonendemic areas.

Life Cycle. The parasite, *C. sinensis,* requires two intermediate hosts and a definitive host for the completion of its life cycle. In addition to humans, dogs, cats, and other fish-eating mammals serve as reservoir hosts. When the eggs of *C. sinensis* are passed with the stools, they are fully embryonated. They do not hatch spontaneously when they reach fresh water. The miracidium is set free only after the eggs are ingested by an operculate snail, the first intermediate host. Appropriate species of these snails are among those of *Parafossarulus, Bulinus, Semisulcospira, Alcocinma,* and *Thiara.* In these intermediate hosts, further development from the stage of miracidium to cercariae takes place. The cercariae emerge into water, and on contact with a suitable freshwater fish of the minnow and carp family (Cyprinidae), they penetrate the skin of the fish, discard their tails, and encyst in the flesh as metacercariae. When infected raw freshwater fish containing the encysted stages of *C. sinensis* are eaten, the young worms are set free in the duodenum of the final host, and the larvae enter the bile ducts within a few hours after being ingested. In about 3 weeks, the flukes reach maturity and begin to shed eggs into the bile ducts. The complete life cycle, from person to person, requires at least 3 months.

Geographic Distribution. The geographic distribution of endemic clonorchiasis is determined by two factors: (1) the presence of suitable intermediate hosts and (2) the preference of the people in these areas to eat raw fish. Human infections are common in Korea, China, parts of Japan and Taiwan, the Red River Valley in Indochina, and among refugees from Vietnam and Cambodia. Clonorchiasis infection in humans is long-lived (up to 25 years) and has been found in Asians in all parts of the world. Nevertheless, no new endemic foci are known to have been introduced by such migrants into their new environment.

Clinical Illness. The flukes cause injury to the bile ducts and produce chronic cholangitis characterized by marked hyperplasia of the cylindrical epithelium, frequently associated with numerous mitoses. Eventually, the nonspecific changes due to chronic inflammation and subsequent reinfections lead to a progressive fibrous thickening of the walls, causing partial or complete obstruction of terminal bile ducts, pressure necrosis of the surrounding parenchyma, and in severe cases, biliary cirrhosis. Development of cholangitic cirrhosis is enhanced by intermittent, acute episodes of complicating bacterial cholangitis, which also produces abscesses that lead to chronic cholecystitis. A causal relationship between chronic clonorchiasis and biliary tract carcinoma (cholangiocarcinoma) has been established.[1,2]

The signs and symptoms of clonorchiasis are neither characteristic nor pathognomonic. Mild infections and the earlier phases of the disease may pass unnoticed. Complaints and symptoms during later stages are common to so many diseases of the liver and the bile ducts of various etiologies that they provide poor clues to establishing a firm clinical diagnosis of clonorchiasis.

Diagnosis. Diagnosis is based on recovery of the typical eggs from stool specimens. There is a new quick Kato technique for field examinations. Sometimes, eggs may be found only in the bile or duodenal contents after intubation. The eggs of *C. sinensis* are among the smallest produced by trematodes that are pathogenic for humans and measure only 27 by 16 μm. They are yellow-brown and have a characteristic operculum fitting into the rim of the shell like a lid on a sugar bowl and a small knoblike protuberance located at the opposite pole.

Intradermal and complement-fixation tests with purified antigens prepared from *C. sinensis* are helpful in establishing the diagnosis. Among the modern immunodiagnostic tests, an enzyme-linked immunosorbent assay (ELISA) gives highly predictive results. The test combines a high degree of sensitivity with specificity and is a good tool in epidemiological investigations.

Community Patterns of Infection and Disease. In hyperendemic areas, there is a rapid increase in the prevalence of infection from the age of 1 to about 20 years. Thereafter, the rate of increase becomes much smaller, until at about 40 years, a plateau is reached. In rural areas of the Republic of Korea, along the Naktong River, it is not unusual to find as many as 80% of the villagers infected with *C. sinensis.* Although raw fish is eaten by both sexes, males are more often infected. This sex difference probably is related to local customs of serving raw fish with alcoholic beverages at the many social gatherings, which are the exclusive privilege of the males.

Community studies in rural areas of China, Korea, and Indochina may yield age-specific prevalence rates of close to 100%. The disease has a pronounced focal distribution, depending on the availability and the habit of eating uncooked fish containing the metacercariae of the fluke.

The full public health importance of chronic clonorchiasis in relation to the prevalence and intensity of infection, the frequency of reinfections, and the risks of developing chronic disability or even cancer of the bile ducts has not yet been determined. Answers to these questions can be obtained only from prospective epidemiological studies of residents in endemic and nonendemic areas.

Treatment and Control. Praziquantel [2-cyclohexyl carbonyl1-1,2,3,6,7,116-hexahydropyrazino(2,1-a) isoquinolin-4-a] and hexachloroparaxylene are the most effective drugs for the treatment of human chlonorchiasis. The recommended doses are 25 mg/kg body weight of praziquantel twice daily given either on a single day or spread over 2 days. Cure rates as high as 90% have been reported in mass treatment campaigns. The recommended safe dose for hexachloroparaxylene for mass treatment of clonorchiasis is 60 to 70 mg/kg for 5 consecutive days.[3]

Thoroughly cooking all fish in endemic areas safeguards the population against infection without the need to remove an important, and often the only available, source of animal protein from the diet. In areas where night soil is used as a fertilizer in fish ponds, treatment of the feces with a 0.7% solution of ammonium sulfate kills the miracidia in the eggs and prevents infection of the snail host. Because shipments of dried or pickled fish may be sources of infection in nonendemic areas and lead to small epidemics, the control of imported fish and fish products from endemic areas is recommended.

Related Liver Flukes. Besides *C. sinensis,* two other members of the family Opisthorchiidae are of public health importance in some parts of the world: *Opistorchis viverrini* and *Opisthorchis felineus.* The life cycles of these two flukes are similar to that described for *C. sinensis,* and the liver is the principal site of the mature worms in their final host. In Thailand, *O. viverrini* has significant influence in the development of several cholestatic diseases, such as hilar intrahepatic cholangiocarcinoma, biliary calculi, opisthorchiatic intrahepatic cysts, and aggregated dead opisthorchiatic worms blocking the biliary system.

The quick modified Kato technique for stool examination and an ELISA with purified antigens of *O. viverrini* are new diagnostic tools for epidemiological studies. Praziquantel is highly effective against *O. viverrini.* There are numerous reservoir hosts in endemic areas, the most important of which are cats, dogs, and civets. Human infections with *O. viverrini* are common in Thailand, and endemic foci of *O. felineus* infection are found in eastern Europe, Asiatic USSR, and Indochina. Hexachloroparaxylene also is effective against *O. viverrini.*[3]

Fascioliasis hepatica

Alfred A. Buck

Liver fluke disease (liver rot) caused by *Fasciola hepatica* is a cosmopolitan and enzootic parasite of sheep, cattle, goats, and hogs. Human fascioliasis is not infrequent in sheep-raising and cattle-raising areas, where the infection is caused by consumption of raw watercress to which the infective cysts of the fluke, the metacercariae, are attached. In addition to the many reports in the medical literature of sporadic cases, there have been small epidemics of fascioliasis. A major outbreak of liver fascioliasis occurred in Britain in 1968.[1]

Life Cycle. The relatively large, operculated eggs of *F. hepatica* are excreted in the feces of infected mammals, especially sheep and cattle. When they reach fresh water, they mature within 9 to 15 days. Within 24 hours, the larva, or miracidia, must find snails of the genus *Lymnaea,* especially *Lymnaea truncatula,* and other species of the family Lymnaeidae. Within the snail host, the miracidia multiplies and develops into many mature cercariae, which, after leaving the snail, encyst on water vegetation. A moist environment is favorable for their survival, and even short periods of drying can kill the metacercariae. Ingestion of viable cysts attached to grass and water plants, predominantly free watercress (*Nasturtium officinale*), leads to infection. Humans are accidental hosts. The young fluke migrates through the peritoneal cavity, entering the liver from its surface. It reaches the bile ducts after about 6 to 8 weeks and begins to produce eggs approximately 3 months after the infective cysts were ingested.

Pathology and Symptoms. During the period of invasion the fluke can cause traumatic damage and toxic necrosis along its pathway through the liver. This may be accompanied by fever and eosinophilia. After reaching the bile ducts, *F. hepatica* causes chronic inflammation leading to symptoms similar to those described earlier for clonorchiasis. In addition, fascioliasis hepatica can cause constitutional and systemic symptoms, including fever, malaise, anemia, and urticaria. There may be night sweats, weight loss, and pain under the right costal margin. Occasionally, severe and persistent coughing may occur. From time to time, the fluke is recovered from atypical locations such as the lungs, brain, and subcutaneous tissues.

Diagnosis. The diagnosis is based on the recovery of the typical eggs in stool specimens. Their similarity to those of *Fasciolopsis buski,* the giant intestinal fluke, can cause difficulties in differential diagnosis. Duodenal intubation and recovery of eggs of *Fasciola hepatica* from bile can help to establish a firm diagnosis. False fascioliasis occurs in individuals who, following the ingestion of livers of sheep, goats, and cattle infected with the trematode, excrete eggs of the fluke in their stools. Serological tests, such as ELISA and skin tests with purified antigens from *F. hepatica,* are helpful diagnostic tools. There is eosinophilia and increased erythrocyte sedimentation rate. Even after an outbreak there can be difficulties in reaching a firm diagnosis. In the early stages of an epidemic, many other conditions may be considered in the differential diagnosis, such as diaphragmatic pleurisy, cholecystitis, ambebiasis, and peptic ulcer. The mimicry of fascioliasis ranging from symptom-free cases to severe illness is remarkable.

Community Patterns of Infection. Most infections result from the ingestion of the encysted metacercariae attached to watercress. Because humans are only occasional hosts of this infection, most cases are sporadic. However, epidemics of human fascioliasis have been reported from many countries in the world where the dietary habits of the population favor consumption of raw watercress. The infections occur equally frequently in males and females and involve persons of all ages. Although consumption of watercress as salad greens is the most common means of acquiring the infection, occasionally apples and pears dropped from the trees into ponds and pools and subsequently contaminated with metacercariae can serve as vehicles of infection.

Treatment. Drug treatment of fascioliasis is unsatisfactory. Patients involved in recent outbreaks were treated with intramuscular emetine hydrochloride and chloroquine.[1] Although praziquantel is still in the stage of clinical trials, promising results of its use in treating this liver fluke disease have been reported by Rim.[2]

Prevention and Control. Even where eggs of *Fasciola* are found, one has to make sure that these are not spurious infections of eggs in transit following the ingestion of infected liver of cattle or sheep.

At the present time, radical and fundamental control of fascioliasis, including natural infections in herbivorous animals, is not possible. Field trials in sheep and cows with oxyclozanide show this compound to be highly effective against *F. hepatica* in animals.[3] Prevention of human disease can be achieved by omitting watercress and other freshwater plants from the diet, particularly in areas where sheep and cattle are raised and where liver fluke infection is known to occur.

OTHER LIVER FLUKES

Human infection with *Fasciolopsis buski* is widely distributed in the Orient, especially in China. In addition to humans, pigs and dogs are definitive hosts of the adult flukes. The life cycle of *Fasciolopsis* is similar to that of *Fasciola hepatica.* Raw water chestnuts infected with the metacercariae are the source of infection. The symptoms may be quite severe. Diarrhea usually alternates with constipation; vomiting and anorexia are frequent in massive infections; generalized toxic and allergic symptoms may appear, often in the form of edema, particularly of the face, abdominal wall, and legs. Ascites may be present in heavy infections. There is pronounced eosinophilia and leukopenia. Drying of the aquatic plants that harbor the infective stages of the parasite, or dipping them into boiling water for a few seconds if eaten fresh, is sufficient to kill the metacercariae.

Diphyllobothriasis

Robert L. Rausch

Among members of the cestode genus *Diphyllobothrium,* the two species, *Diphyllobothrium latum* and *Diphyllobothrium dendriticum,* occur most commonly in humans.

Life Cycle. The life cycle of these cestodes requires three hosts for completion, but additional paratenic hosts may be involved. After hatching of the egg in water, the motile embryo (coracidium) is ingested by a minute crustacean, in which the first-stage larva (procercoid) develops. When the procercoid is ingested by the second intermediate host, a fish, further development leads to the plerocercoid, infective for the final host. The site of localization of the plerocercoid in the second intermediate host differs with species of *Diphyllobothrium* and, to some extent, species of fish.

After the final host ingests the plerocercoid, the adult worm develops comparatively rapidly. Depending on species, the adult worm ranges from less than 1 m long to 12 m or more. The largest have thousands of segments, each of which produces large numbers of eggs. Eggs may be present in great numbers in the feces of the final host, but detached segments are not often observed. Host specificity is little developed in these cestodes.

Epidemiology. *D. latum* occurs in most parts of the world but is most prevalent in subarctic and temperate regions of the northern hemisphere, including Scandinavia, Northern Italy, Switzerland, Hungary, parts of Germany, Finland, North America, and the western Soviet Union. It is found also in the Middle East, Chile, Argentina, Peru, and Japan. In North America, several foci have been known, particularly western Alaska, the lake regions of northern Minnesota, southeastern Manitoba, and the Lake Nippigon district of Ontario, but some of these areas may no longer be endemic.[1,2] Pleroceroids are found commonly in a variety of fresh water fish, such as pike, salmon, trout, sugar, ruff, and whitefish. Up to 70% of walleye pike found in some small lakes in the northern United States and Canada are infected. Although a number of fish-eating mammals—dogs, bear, cats, martins—may act as reservoir hosts, humans are the primary definitive host and are mainly responsible for establishing and maintaining endemicity in human populations through contamination of water with feces.

Clinical Picture. In a high proportion of human cases, infections are asymptomatic and remain undetected. Conditions, such as weakness, diarrhea, and abdominal discomfort, frequently are attributed to these cestodes. In a small proportion of persons infected by *D. latum* (1%–2%), depletion of vitamin B_{12} produces a macrocytic anemia resembling pernicious anemia. The cestode apparently interferes with absorption of vitamin B_{12} by the host and at the same time takes up a large quantity of the vitamin. Factors contributing to development of the deficiency include inadequate supply of vitamin B_{12} in the diet, deficiency of intrinsic factor attributable to endogenous or exogenous damage to the gastric mucosa, location of the cestodes proximally in the small intestine or the presence of a large mass of worm tissue, and an increased requirement for the vitamin.[3] Other species of *Diphyllobothrium* are not known to be associated with macrocytic anemia.

Diagnosis. Diagnosis of infection by *D. latum* and other diphyllobothriid cestodes usually depends on finding the eggs in the feces of the host. Clinically, vitamin B_{12} deficiency caused by *D. latum* is diagnosed from the combination of macrocytic anemia with leukopenia, thrombocytopenia, and increased hemolysis, signs of neurological disorders, and reduced serum levels of vitamin B_{12}.

Treatment. Of the various anthelmintics used to expel diphyllobothriid cestodes from the human host, niclosamide and desaspidin have been used most in endemic regions. In a clinical test in Finland, 33 patients were treated successfully with a single oral dose of 25 mg/kg of praziquantel.[4] After expulsion of the cestodes by anthelmintic treatment, therapeutic use of vitamin B_{12} may be indicated.

Prevention and Control. The infection of humans by *Diphyllobothrium* species depends on the consumption of fish containing plerocercoids. Thorough cooking or freezing at −18° C for 24 to 48 hours will make fish safe for consumption. Drying or brine curing also will render the plerocercoid in fish noninfective. Fish from endemic areas should be frozen for at least 24 hours before being shipped. Dumping of human excreta into local ponds and streams should be prohibited. Proper treatment of sewage can have a major impact on preventing infection. Programs conducted in various countries have been reviewed by von Bonsdorff.[3] It is not practicable to attempt control of *D. dendriticum* and other species for which fish-eating birds and mammals also serve as final host.

Larva Migrans

Robert L. Rausch

Various disorders are produced in humans by the incidental invasion by larval stages of nematodes that occur naturally in carnivorous or fish-eating mammals. In an unfavorable parasite-host relationship, the nematodes may migrate extensively in the human body, sometimes causing severe lesions, but they rarely complete development to sexual maturity. The resulting disorders are designated cutaneous larva migrans (creeping eruption), visceral larva migrans, and herring worm disease, depending on the species of nematodes involved.

CUTANEOUS LARVA MIGRANS

Cutaneous larva migrans, or creeping eruption, is caused by larvae of hookworms, including *Ancylostoma braziliense* and *Ancylostoma caninum,* and of *Strongyloides stercoralis.* The eggs of the hookworms are expelled in the feces of dogs, after which hatching occurs, and the larvae develop to the infective third stage after about 1 week. On contact with soil on which the larvae are present, the skin is penetrated and the larvae migrate about, usually at the upper level of the dermis. The larvae evoke an inflammatory response, accompanied by severe pruritus. Diagnosis is based on the presence of the typical cutaneous lesions. The filiform larvae of *S. stercoralis* penetrate the skin and enter the corium. Erythema with pruritus develops within 24 hours. A more severe, allergic response occurs in persons sensitized by previous infections. Recovery is spontaneous after death of the larvae. Mild cases of cutaneous larva migrans can be treated by spraying the affected area with ethyl chloride. Thiabendazole usually is used for treatment of more severe cases. It has been reported recently, however, that albendazole is the drug of choice, with high efficacy and few side effects.[1]

ANISAKIASIS

Herring worm disease, or anisakiasis, is caused by larvae of *Anisakis simplex, Terranova* spp, or related nematodes of the family Anisakidae, the adults of which occur naturally in marine mammals. First recognized in Holland, herring worm disease is especially prevalent in Japan and may be expected to occur wherever marine fish are eaten raw or otherwise prepared without cooking. Such nematodes have been obtained from Alaskan Eskimos, either expelled spontaneously or after anthelmintic treatment. The cycles of these nematodes involve two intermediate hosts, of which the second is a fish. When the infected fish are ingested by humans, the nematodes penetrate the wall of the stomach or intestine, causing formation of severe eosinophilic granulomata. Gastric anisakiasis usually produces upper abdominal pain. Involvement of the intestine produces acute abdominal pain, often accompanied by nausea and vomiting. Intestinal infections may take a more chronic course, with recurrent diarrhea and lower abdominal pain. Radiological findings in such cases often are indicative of stenosis. Herring worm disease rarely is correctly diagnosed clinically, but surgical treatment usually is undertaken for suspected gastric carcinoma or ulcer, appendicitis, intussusception, and other disorders. Segmental resections frequently are required for the treatment of intestinal lesions. The diagnosis of herring worm disease usually is made microscopically after surgery.

VISCERAL LARVAL MIGRANS

Visceral larva migrans is caused most frequently by the larvae of *Toxocara canis,* a ubiquitous parasite of dogs in temperate and warm climates, or of the closely related *Toxocara cati.* At high latitudes, *Toxascaris leonina* is the indigenous ascarid in canine animals. This nematode does not produce significant lesions in humans. *Toxocara canis* has been widely introduced into northern regions by the importation of infected dogs from the south. When the infective eggs of *T. canis* are ingested by a dog, the larvae hatch and penetrate the intestinal wall, after which they are carried via the liver to the lungs. In dogs less than 3 months old, the larvae emigrate from the lungs via the trachea and make their way down the esophagus via the stomach to the small intestine, where they become sexually mature.

Visceral larva migrans occurs most commonly in children less than 5 years old. When eggs containing infective (second-stage) larvae are ingested, the larvae are released in the small intestine, after which they migrate extensively. The majority localize in the liver, but other organs, including tissues of the central nervous system and eyes, may be invaded. The larvae evoke an inflammatory response, usually leading to the formation of eosinophilic granulomata. According to Beaver, the clinical manifestations of visceral larva migrans depend on numbers of larvae ingested, site of localization, duration of infection, and other factors that are not understood.[2] With hepatic or pulmonary involvement, clinical findings may include hepatomegaly, bronchitis, bronchopneumonia, febrile episodes, transient gastrointestinal disorders, and various other conditions. Ocular involvement is a frequent and serious manifestation of infection, resulting in such conditions as retinal granulomata, retinal detachment, optic neuritis, and diffuse endophthalmitis. Invasion of the central nervous tissues may cause muscular weakness, sensory abnormalities, convulsions, and coma.

Clinical and laboratory findings are important in the diagnosis of all forms of visceral larva migrans caused by the larval *T. canis.* A history of geophagia or pica or of association with dogs may be helpful in conjunction with clinical findings. A comparison of immunodiagnostic tests by Glickman and associates showed that indirect hemagglutination, bentonite flocculation, double diffusion in agar, and enzyme-linked immunoabsorbent assay (ELISA) were highly specific, but the ELISA was the most sensitive and was considered to be the test of choice for diagnosis of visceral larva migrans caused by the larval *T. canis.*[3]

There is no specific treatment for visceral larva migrans, but corticosteroids may be beneficial in cases of severe disease. The efficacy of thiabendazole has not been established, although its use has been recommended.

Under the most favorable conditions, ingestion by children of eggs containing the infective larvae of *T. canis* can be prevented by high sanitary standards and appropriate management of dogs. Small children should not be permitted contact with potentially infected dogs, nor should they be allowed access to areas contaminated by canine feces. A program of anthelmintic treatment of dogs under veterinary supervision would be effective in keeping the animals essentially free of infection, but often it is not a realistic possibility.

Hydatid Disease

Robert L. Rausch

Hydatid disease (sensu lato) is the infection of humans by the larval stages of taeniid cestodes of the genus *Echinococcus.* Four species of *Echinococcus* are recognized, of which three cause distinctive forms of disease: *Echinococcus granulosus* (cystic hydatid disease), *Echinococcus multilocularis* (alveolar hydatid disease), and *Echinococcus vogeli* (polycystic hydatid disease). As a cause of morbidity in humans, *Echinococcus* species rank high among the helminths.

Life Cycle. The life cycles of *Echinococcus* species involve carnivores as final host and ungulates or rodents as intermediate host. In their adult stage, these cestodes are small, ranging from about 2 to 12 mm in length, with three to six segments. They typically localize in the lower duodenum and jejunum of the final host. Embryophores containing infective embryos are expelled in large numbers in the feces of the final carnivorous host. After ingestion by the intermediate host, the embryo is released into the small intestine and soon enters the portal circulation. The site of localization and development of the embryo to the larval or hydatid stage differs with species of *Echinococcus* and may be influenced as well by species of the intermediate host. Humans are an incidental intermediate host, since further development of these cestodes depends on ingestion of their larvae (hydatids) by a carnivore.

Distribution and Transmission Patterns. Cystic hydatid disease is caused by the larval stage of *E. granulosus,* of which two biologically distinct forms are recognized. The northern form is indigenous to the Holarctic zones of tundra and boreal forest. It is propagated via a sylvatic cycle, which involves the wolf and deer (mainly reindeer and moose) as final and intermediate hosts, respectively. In some regions of North America where the wolf has been wiped out, the cycle is completed in coyotes and deer. Attempts to infect domestic ungulates with cestodes of this form have been unsuccessful. Wild ungulates are an important source of infection for dogs when viscera of animals killed by hunters are fed directly or are discarded in accessible places. This has been an important pattern of transmission to dogs in northern North America, where subsistence hunting is widely practiced. Nonindigenous populations may be at risk in rural areas, as in southcentral Alaska.

The European form of *E. granulosus* has a nearly cosmopolitan distribution other than in arctic and subarctic regions and is propagated via a pastoral cycle, which involves almost exclusively synanthropic animals (dogs and domestic ungulates). This cestode is prevalent in some regions of Eurasia, in several South American countries, and in Africa. The European form of *E. granulosus* is endemic in apparently disjunct regions of the western United States. Populations at risk include Basque-Americans in California, Mormons in central Utah, and Navajo and Zuni Indians in New Mexico.[1] Humans become infected through association with dogs that have been fed viscera from slaughtered animals or have had access to carcasses or discarded offal of domestic ungulates in which the larvae are present.

Alveolar hydatid disease is caused by *E. multilocularis,* which has an extensive geographical range in the northern hemisphere. The natural cycle involves foxes and small rodents as final and intermediate hosts, respectively. This cestode appears to have a continuous distribution in the zone of tundra, from the White Sea in the west to Hudson Bay in the east. Alveolar hydatid disease is most prevalent in indigenous populations in the arctic and subarctic, with the highest known rates reported in northeastern Siberia. A disjunct endemic region exists in central Europe, where the larval stage was first identified in the human liver in 1854. *Echinococcus multilocularis* occurs widely at low latitudes in the Soviet Union, and the reports of alveolar hydatid disease in India[2] and China[3] suggest that its occurrence in Eurasia is more extensive than has been realized. This cestode has become established in Japan (Hokkaido) and in central North America. Since its recognition in North Dakota in 1964, the cestode has been recorded in nine of the surrounding states and in the three adjacent provinces of Canada. The first autochthonous case of alveolar hydatid disease in the United States outside Alaska was diagnosed in Minnesota in 1977.[4]

The infection of humans by the larval *E. multilocularis* is usually the result of association with dogs and perhaps cats that have eaten infected rodents. Villages within the zone of tundra may constitute hyperendemic foci because of the interaction between dogs and wild rodents that live as commensals in and around dwellings. In central Europe, rodents inhabiting cultivated fields and gardens become infected by ingesting embryophores expelled by foxes and, in turn, may be a source of infection for dogs and cats. In rural regions of central North America, the cycle involves foxes and rodents of the genera *Peromyscus* and *Microtus.* Keeping uncontrolled dogs and cats in these regions may be hazardous.

Polycystic hydatid disease, caused by *E. vogeli,* has been reported infrequently from Central and South America. The natural hosts of this cestode are the bush dog, *Speothos venaticus,* and the paca, *Cuniculus paca.* The larval stage occurs occasionally in rodents of other species. Little is known of the epidemiology of polycystic hydatid disease. The natural final host of *E. vogeli,* the bush dog, is a wary and rarely seen animal that could hardly be a source of infection for humans. The intermediate host, the paca, is widely hunted for food in northern South America. In eastern Colombia, local hunters routinely feed the viscera of pacas to their dogs.[5] Many of the animals are unrestrained and have free access to the doorless dwellings typical of this region.

Clinical Picture

Cystic Hydatid Disease. In humans, uncomplicated cysts of *E. granulosus* are slowly enlarging masses comparable to benign neoplasms. The larval stages of the two biological forms exhibit well-defined differences in the human host. That of the northern form occurs almost exclusively in the lungs and liver, with a ratio of frequency in the two organs of about 6:4. In the lungs, cysts of this form are relatively small, with an average diameter of about 40 mm. Spontaneous rupture of pulmonary cysts, with evacuation of larval membranes and fluid, occurs rather frequently. Secondary spread after spontaneous rupture or rupture at surgery is unknown, nor have anaphylaxis or other serious complications been observed. The disease in humans is benign and usually asymptomatic and has a low mortality. The larval stage of the European form is more pathogenic, and up to about 90% of cases are symptomatic. The localization of cysts is different, with a ratio in lungs and liver of about 3:5.5. Cysts in the lungs are larger. In about 15% of cases, the cysts occur in organs other than the lungs and liver. In addition to the severe effects produced by larvae in such loci as the cranium, orbit, or myocardium, conditions such as anaphylaxis, secondary spread following rupture, pathological fracture of bones, infected cysts with empyema, formation of hepatopulmonary fistulae, and other complications are frequent. The characteristics of the larval stages of the two forms of *E. granulosus* have been compared in detail by Wilson and associates.[6]

Alveolar Hydatid Disease. The embryo of *E. multilocularis* seems to localize invariably in the liver of the intermediate host, including humans.

Development of the larval *E. multilocularis* is inhibited in humans, so that it persists indefinitely in the proliferative phase. As a result, the hepatic parenchyma is gradually invaded and replaced by fibrous tissue in which great numbers of vesicles, many microscopic in size, are embedded. Proliferation continues peripherally, with the result that an entire hepatic lobe may be replaced over a period of years. As the lesion enlarges, it usually undergoes degenerative changes that lead to central necrosis, often with liquefaction, and abscesses having a volume of several liters may be produced. Uneven calcification of necrotic tissues is typical in lesions of long standing. Hepatomegaly is characteristic and may be extreme. The disease takes a chronic course, with deterioration of health often occurring around middle age. Patients eventually succumb to hepatic failure, invasion of contiguous structures, or, less frequently, metastases to the brain. However, instances of spontaneous death of the cyst during its early stage of development have been reported in people with asymptomatic infection.[7]

Polycystic Hydatid Disease. In human cases, hepatomegaly or tumorlike masses in the liver have been typical findings. Proliferation of vesicles may lead to destruction of much of the liver, and involvement of adjacent structures by extension does not appear to be unusual. The prognosis in polycystic hydatid disease is poor. The known cases have been described by D'Alessandro and associates.[5]

Diagnosis. X-ray examination is effective in detecting hydatid cysts, caused by the northern form of *E. granulosis,* especially for revealing calcified cysts. Various ultrasound procedures may locate noncalcified hepatic cysts. Serological tests usually are nondiagnostic, since sera from patients infected by this form are rarely reactive. For diagnosis of infections by the European form, various immunodiagnostic tests have been employed. In the United States, the indirect hemagglutination test (IHA) is routinely combined with more specific tests, such as bentonite flocculation (BF), latex agglutination (LA), or gel diffusion. Among various serological tests, enzyme-linked immunoassay (ELISA) has been reported to be the most sensitive, based on the results of examination of blood samples with screening tests—IHA, LA, and ELISA—and confirmatory tests—complement fixation (CF), countercurrent electrophoresis (CCEP), and immunoelectrophoresis (IEOP)—from 443 suspected cases of hydatid disease.[8] The specificity of ELISA has been found to be 100% and sensitivity 85%.[9] It may reach 91% if the new isolated antigen with an apparent molecular weight of 8 kDA is used.[10] For purposes of surveys, the Casoni intradermal test usually is employed in conjunction with serological tests, such as the IHA and BF. A high rate of nonspecific reactions prevents use of the intradermal test alone.

Diagnosis of alveolar hydatid disease may be difficult, particularly in regions where its possible occurrence is not known to clinicians and pathologists, as in central North America. The combination of hepatomegaly, typical diffuse calcification as seen in x-rays, and a high serological titer is characteristic of advanced disease. Sonography has a very high accuracy in detecting the type, size, number, and location of hepatic hydatid cysts. It also indicates whether they are alive or dead. The presence of hydatid cysts in the rest of the peritoneal cavity and their complications also can be detected.[11] ELISA usually gives reliable results. Exploratory laparotomy with biopsy may be necessary to confirm the diagnosis and to determine the feasibility of surgical intervention. Microscopic diagnosis may be difficult, since the readily identifiable protoscolices rarely are produced in larvae developing in humans. Staining of sections by the PAS method permits recognition of the larval membranes. Inoculation of susceptible rodents with larval membranes from humans provides a further means of identification. The diagnostic features of polycystic hydatid disease have not been defined, and none of the confirmed cases has been diagnosed correctly clinically. Limited information suggests that immunodiagnostic tests may be useful.

Treatment. A policy of conservative management has been adopted generally in the treatment of infections by the northern form of *E. granulosus,* and surgical intervention is considered only in cases of uncertain diagnosis (i.e., possible neoplasms) or in rare cases of symptomatic disease. Surgical intervention is routine in the treatment of cystic hydatid disease caused by the European form of *E. granulosus.* Total excision of cysts often is possible, but other approaches may be required because of the wide range in sites of localization and the frequency of complications. In the surgical treatment of hepatic infections, postoperative mortality ranges from about 7% to 12%. Success in the treatment of cystic hydatid disease with albendazole or mebendazole has been reported by many investigators, although the degrees of success vary.[12-16] Since there are different strains in several species of *Echinococcus,* notably *E. granulosus,* the chemotherapeutic regimen effective against one strain may not be effective against others. In one study of over 500 cases (with 269 hepatic, 86 pulmonary, 50 peritoneal, and 5 cysts at other sites) treated with an average of 2.5 cycles of 800 mg albendazole daily for 28 days, with 14-day intervals, 28% was regarded as cured, 51% as improved, 18.1% as unchanged, and 2.4% as worse.[13] The results indicate that this compound can be effective in the treatment of cystic hydatid disease. Ultrasonography and changes in IgE levels provide the means for evaluating results of chemotherapy.[12] A new therapeutic approach for the treatment of hepatic hydatid cysts by aspiration and injection of sterile 95% ethanol, under sonographic guidance, has been reported most recently to be very successful. Five patients were treated without any complications or relapses during a follow-up period ranging from 10 to 26 months.[17]

Until recently, surgery has offered the only possibility for treatment of alveolar hydatid disease. The usual procedure has involved removal of the lesion with part or all of the affected hepatic lobe. Cases of advanced disease and those involving multiple lesions often are inoperable. With or without surgery, alveolar hydatid disease has a very high mortality rate. With metastases to the brain, death occurs within a few months after onset of neurological disorders. The efficacy of mebendazole or albendazole in the treatment of inoperable or repeatedly recurrent cases of hydatid disease and for prophylaxis before surgery has been well recognized. Destruction of the cysts and improvement, or at least stabilization, of the disease have been reported frequently. In a clinical trial involving long-term treatment of four patients with inoperable disease, 40 mg mebendazole/kg/d was administered orally. Progressively enlarging thoracic metastases in two patients regressed, and all four exhibited symptomatic improvement.[18] In the WHO-coordinated studies of chemotherapeutic effect with 54 cases of *E. multilocularis* echinococcosis, it has been confirmed that mebendazole therapy may arrest development of the lesions. In another study of the effect of albendazole in the treatment of 35 cases of *E. multilocularis* infection, 2 cases were cured, 4 were improved, 24 were stabilized, and 4 worsened. Praziquantel may be found to have application in the treatment of alveolar hydatid disease. Experience in the treatment of polycystic hydatid disease is limited. Surgery has been employed, but cases of advanced disease usually seem to be inoperable.

Prevention and Control. Infection of humans by larval cestodes of the genus *Echinococcus* is contingent on ingestion of embryophores distributed in the feces of dogs and perhaps other carnivores that harbor the adult worms. Control of hydatid disease in humans depends on means to prevent or to eliminate infection of dogs. These objectives, so simple in concept, generally have been unattainable and will probably remain so in many regions because of human attitudes and other factors that defy change.

Little effort has been made to control the northern form of *E. granulosus,* in part because of the benign nature of the infection and perhaps also because the disease affects mainly scattered indigenous peoples. The significant decrease in incidence observed in recent years in Alaskan Eskimos and Indians has been attributable mainly to replacement of dogs by mechanized vehicles for winter travel. Some advantage, however, is being lost with the growing tendency of these people to adopt the European practice of keeping dogs as pets.

Few countries have shown significant accomplishment in attempts to control the European strain of *E. granulosus* in synanthropic animals. In most regions where hydatid disease is a serious medical and economic problem, the combination of uncontrolled slaughter, indiscriminate disposal of carcasses and offal, and an abundance of free-ranging dogs provides near-optimal conditions for the completion of the life cycle of this cestode. Large-scale programs of control have had noteworthy success only in Iceland, New Zealand, Australia, and Cyprus, which have in common the features of insularity, literate populations, satisfactory economies, and effective political organizations. In these countries, the programs have been based on public education combined with strict regulations directed particularly toward control of dogs. Cyprus accomplished nearly complete control of *E. granulosus* during the period between 1971 and 1975 through elimination of excess dogs, destruction of all dogs found to be infected, and regulation of slaughter.[19] With the development of praziquantel, the effective use of an anthelmintic in conjunction with other measures for the control of hydatid disease has become possible for the first time. Tests have shown that a single oral dose at the rate of 5 mg/kg removes all adult worms of *E. granulosus* and *E. multilocularis* from dogs.[20] The mass treatment of dogs and strict control of slaughter would be effective under some conditions but of little value where early reinfection is probable.

Control of *E. multilocularis* presents a difficult problem of potentially increasing importance. Measures for control of the cestode have involved anthelmintic treatment of dogs and destruction of stray animals. In Alaska, the general reduction of numbers of dogs probably has had some effect on the prevalence of *E. multilocularis*. The implications of the spread of *E. multilocularis* in central North America are not now predictable. Since the control of this cestode in its natural hosts does not appear to be possible, preventive measures must be directed toward domestic carnivores. Keeping of dogs and cats as pets in the endemic areas would be best avoided. Regular anthelmintic treatment of such animals might be practicable under some conditions.

Other Cestodes and Intestinal Trematodes

Robert L. Rausch

CESTODES

Hymenolepis nana is a common parasite of humans, estimated to infect about 44 million people worldwide. It differs from almost all other tapeworms in being able to complete its entire life cycle in a single host. *Hymenolepis nana* is a small, filamentous tapeworm ranging up to about 100 mm in length. When ingested by humans or rodents, eggs disseminated in the feces of the final host hatch in the small intestine. The released embryos penetrate into the villi, where development to the infective larval stage (cysticercoid) takes place within a few days. The cysticercoids then reenter the lumen and attach to the mucosa of the ileum, where the worms develop. Eggs appear in the feces about 30 days after exposure. The cycle may involve an intermediate host if eggs are ingested by grain beetles or larvae of fleas. The embryo penetrates to the hemocoelom of the insect, where the cysticercoid develops. Infection of the final host follows ingestion of insects containing cysticercoids.

Children are infected more commonly by *H. nana* than are adults. The cestodes have little apparent effect when present in small numbers, but infections involving hundreds to thousands of tapeworms are typically symptomatic. Symptoms in patients infected by *H. nana* are reported to include restlessness, diarrhea, abdominal pain, irritability, and anal and nasal pruritus. Eosinophilia exceeded 5% in a third of the patients. More severe disorders commonly attributed to infection by *H. nana* include enteritis, epileptiform convulsions, laryngeal spasm, and strabismus.

Infection by *H. nana* is diagnosed by finding the eggs in the feces. Niclosamide has been used most frequently to expel this cestode, but satisfactory results are obtained only with repeated treatment. Recent trials indicate that a single oral dose of 15 to 25 mg/kg of praziquantel is highly efficacious against *H. nana*. Preliminary results indicate that a single dose of 50 mg/kg of nitazoxanide also is effective.[1]

Hymenolepis nana is a common parasite of humans in warmer regions, wherever poor sanitation, inadequate storage of grain, and an abundance of rats and mice provide the requisite conditions for completion of its life cycle. It would appear that eggs disseminated on grain products and other foods by murine rodents provide the most important source of infection for humans. The ingestion of small grain beetles, such as *Tribolium*, could result in massive infections. Implementation of large-scale measures to control *H. nana* does not now seem practicable in most regions where this cestode is a prevalent parasite of humans.

Cestodes that occasionally or rarely infect humans include *Hymenolepis diminuta, Dipylidium caninum,* and species of such diverse genera as *Bertiella, Raillietina, Inermicapsifer,* and *Mesocestoides*. Infections are usually asymptomatic, and diagnosis depends on identification of the characteristic eggs or gravid segments in the feces. Treatment is as for other cestodes.

INTESTINAL TREMATODES

The most important trematodes that occur in the human intestine are *Fasciolopsis buski, Heterophyes heterophyes, Metagonimus yokogawai, Gastrodiscoides hominis,* and *Echinostoma* species. The eggs of these trematodes are expelled in the feces of the final host, after which the motile miracidium hatches in water. After penetration of the tissues of a snail by the miracidium, a complex process of asexual reproduction leads to the development of cercariae. The cercariae escape from the snail and encyst in a second intermediate host or on vegetation, where the infective metacercariae develop. Use of human excreta to fertilize aquatic vegetation or discharge of sewage into water ensures completion of the cycles of these trematodes.

Fasciolopsis buski is a parasite of humans and pigs in southeast Asia, including Japan and the Philippine Islands. Its occurrence in humans is restricted by the distribution of certain aquatic plants, particularly water caltrop, *Trapa* species, on which the metacercariae encyst. The cultivation of such plants usually involves fertilization with feces of humans or pigs. Humans usually become infected by ingesting metacercarial cysts attached to the seedpods of water caltrop, which are peeled with the aid of the teeth, or to the bulbs or roots of other edible plants. The ingested metacercariae excyst in the intestine and attach to the mucosa of the duodenum and jejunum, where they attain full development in about 3 months. The trematodes may cause ulceration and an inflammatory response at the site of attachment and may produce diarrhea and abdominal pain. When large numbers are present, absorption of metabolic products may cause severe toxic or allergic reactions, manifested by facial or generalized edema, ascites, and other disorders. Diagnosis usually is based on clinical findings and identification of the eggs in the feces. The prognosis is good in light infections, which often are asymptomatic, or when early diagnosis is made. Massive infections may be fatal. The trematodes can be expelled by treatment with hexylresorcinol or with tetrachlorethylene followed by a saline purge.[2]

Heterophyes heterophyes is a very small trematode that may occur in large numbers in the intestine of humans and other fish-eating mammals in southern Asia, Egypt, Turkey, and perhaps in southern Europe. The metacercariae encyst beneath the scales or in the superficial musculature of fishes of various species. Following ingestion by the final host, the metacercariae excyst and attach to the intestinal mucosa, where they attain full development in about a week. Light infections are typically asymptomatic, but large numbers of trematodes may cause mucous diarrhea and abdominal discomfort. The trematodes sometimes penetrate the intestinal wall to the extent that eggs find their way into the systemic circulation. Such eggs may localize in tissues, such as the myocardium or brain, where they seem to act as minute emboli. They evoke little inflammatory response, but focal fibrosis may be observed. Diagnosis of heterophyiasis is best made after treatment, since the eggs in the feces of the host closely resemble those of other trematodes. The trematodes are expelled by treatment with hexylresorcinol, tetrachlorethylene, or biphenium hydroxynaphthoate.

Metagonimus yokogawai is another small trematode that occurs in humans as well as in other fish-eating mammals and certain birds in southern Asia and in the Balkan region. The metacercariae localize in the gills, in the musculature, and on the scales of fishes that serve as second intermediate host. In humans, this trematode typically localizes in the jejunum, where its effects are similar to those of *H. heterophyes*. Diagnosis is best made after treatment, for which praziquantel or tetrachlorethylene is suitable.

Gastrodiscoides hominis is a relatively large, thick-bodied trematode that inhabits the caecum and ascending colon of humans. It also occurs in pigs. The cercaria is believed to encyst on vegetation, but the cycle has not been fully elucidated. The trematodes attach firmly by drawing a small mass of mucosa into the ventral sucker, around which a superficial, craterlike lesion is formed. Infections are usually asymptomatic, but large numbers of trematodes may cause a mucoid diarrhea. Diagnosis is made from eggs expelled in the feces. Tetrachlorethylene is recommended for treatment.

Trematodes of the genus *Echinostoma,* including *Echinostoma ilocanum, Echinostoma malayanum,* and others, occur in the small intestine of humans in southern Asia and less commonly in other regions, such as southern Europe and the Soviet Union. Infections are acquired through consumption of mollusk containing the metacercariae. Large numbers of trematodes may cause diarrhea and abdominal pain, but most infections are asymptomatic. Diagnosis depends on identification of eggs in the feces. Treatment is usually with tetrachlorethylene or praziquantel.

Trematodes of several other species occur occasionally or rarely in the human intestine. Most have been recorded from populations among which traditional dietary habits favor exposure to infection by trematodes that occur typically in other animals. Most are of minor medical importance.

Toxoplasmosis

Robert G. Yaeger

The etiological agent of toxoplasmosis is *Toxoplasma gondii,* one of the most common protozoan parasites of humans. Although the organism was described and named early in this century, human infection was not recognized until 3 decades later. Before 1969, numerous surveys demonstrated that this parasite was found worldwide and in a wide range of warm-blooded hosts. Furthermore, it was shown that infection in humans was highly prevalent in many areas. Yet it was not until the late 1960s that the taxonomic position and the life cycle of *T. gondii* were elucidated.[1]

Life Cycle and Modes of Transmission. The three forms of the parasite—the tachyzoite, the bradyzoite, and the sporozoite—are similar in appearance, being crescent shaped and 4 to 8 μm long. The tachyzoites (Fig. 12-3) are the rapidly proliferating intracellular forms seen in many tissues and organs during the acute phase of infection. Bradyzoites occur in cysts (Fig. 12-4) and are formed primarily in brain, eye, heart muscle, and skeletal muscle. Bradyzoites multiply slowly and persist in tissues for many years, possibly for the life of the host. The sporozoite occurs in the mature oocyst (Fig. 12-5). It is the stage resulting from the sexual reproduction phase, which takes place in the small intestine of cats. Tachyzoites and bradyzoites occur in all hosts susceptible to this infection, but oocysts occur only in felines, where they develop during the sexual phase of the enteroepithelial cycle.

Cats can acquire infection by ingesting tachyzoites or bradyzoites in fresh tissue or sporulated oocysts. Kittens are more susceptible than older cats. The prepatent period of infection, that is, the time between ingestion of infective stages and the passage of oocysts in the feces, may be as short as 1 to 5 days when bradyzoites are ingested, 9 to 11 days if tachyzoites are ingested, and up to 3 weeks or longer if mature oocysts are eaten. Cats that have recovered from toxoplasmosis may become reinfected if exposed, but their immunity may arrest the infection before oocyst formation.

Hosts other than cats usually become infected in the same manner—by ingestion of infective stages. However, there is no enteroepithelial cycle leading to the production of oocysts in

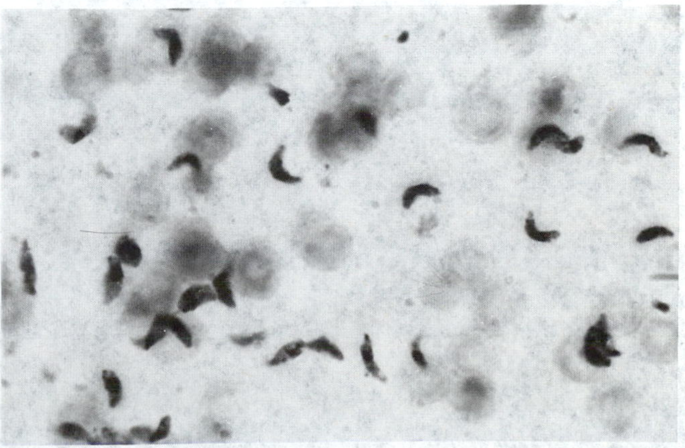

Figure 12-3. Tachyzoites of *Toxoplasma gondii* in smear of mouse peritoneal fluid. Giemsa stain. (×1200.)

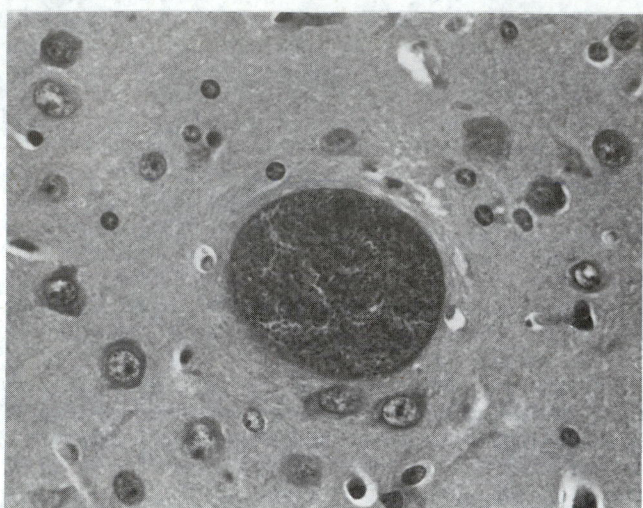

Figure 12-4. Section of mouse brain showing a cyst of *Toxoplasma gondii* containing hundreds of bradyzoites. H & E stain. (×480.)

nonfelines. After initial infection of the intestinal wall, the parasites spread to extraintestinal sites, where intracellular multiplication of tachyzoites takes place. Rupture of infected cells releases tachyzoites, which infect nearby cells or are carried to other sites by body fluids to repeat the cycle. Hosts whose immune system has not been compromised usually survive the acute phase, with or without specific therapy, whereupon tachyzoites disappear and bradyzoite-containing cysts form in the tissues, mainly the brain and muscle. This chronic or latent infection may persist for the life of the host.

Although ingestion of infective material is the principal mode of transmission for toxoplasmosis in humans, others are known. In fact, transplacental transmission was the first to be recognized and may have serious consequences. Parasitemia occurs primarily during the acute stage of toxoplasmosis, and although transmission via blood transfusion can be considered possible, the risk from normal donors apparently is slight.[1] Acquisition of *T. gondii* infection from donor organs has been reported in transplant recipients and probably resulted from persistence of cysts in tissues.[2]

Clinical Characteristics. Postnatally acquired toxoplasmosis usually is asymptomatic or has such mild transient manifestations as to go unrecognized. This is substantiated by the high prevalence of seropositive individuals with no history of a diagnosed infection with this parasite. The most common feature in the immunocompetent host is local or generalized lymphadenopathy, which must be differentiated from lymphomas and Hodgkin's disease.[3] Tender cervical nodes often are accompanied by fever, sore throat, myalgia, a maculopapular rash sparing the palms and soles, abdominal pain from enlarged retroperitoneal nodes, hepatosplenomegaly, and atypical lymphocytosis suggestive of infectious mononucleosis. With rare exceptions and without drug therapy, symptoms resolve over a period of several weeks, although lymphadenopathy may persist for many months. Studies in laboratory animals have demonstrated the persistence of cysts in brain and skeletal muscle for long periods after the initial mild acute stage, but data on the proportion of recovered human cases with persistent cysts are not available. In a few instances there have been severe complications, including pneumonitis, myocarditis, pericarditis, hepatitis, polymyositis, encephalitis, meningoencephalitis, and ocular complications. The immunocompetency of the patient was not reported in many of these cases. It has been estimated that only 10% to 20% of immunocompetent individuals are symptomatic during mild acute infections. In adults, chorioretinitis may be the only manifestation of toxoplasmosis, and most of these infections are believed to have been congenitally acquired. The lesions, which may be unilateral or bilateral, occur as inactive scars or as recurrent active infection consisting of an active lesion without a scar or old scars with active satellite lesions.

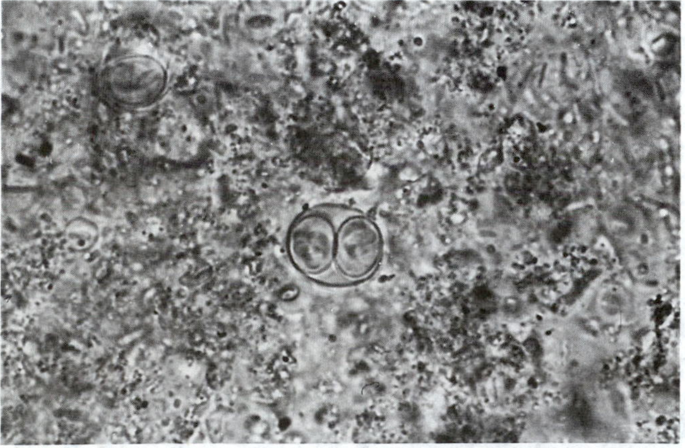

Figure 12-5. Sporulated oocyst of *Toxoplasma gondii* containing two sporocysts, each with four sporozoites. (×1200.)

Congenital toxoplasmosis occurs when a woman acquires her initial infection during pregnancy. Although the disease usually is mild in the woman, the lesions show a wide degree of severity in the conceptus, depending on the gestational age at which transplacental transmission occurs. Results can be (1) a spontaneous abortion of a severely damaged fetus, (2) a fully developed stillborn infant with evidence of severe infection, (3) a live infant with classic signs, such as hydrocephalus or microcephalus, cerebral calcifications, and chorioretinitis, or (4) an apparently normal infant in whom chorioretinitis or other symptoms of central nervous system involvement develop later.[4] Evidence suggests that if a woman becomes infected a few weeks before conception, it is unlikely that a live, infected infant will be born. Since physical examinations and antibody titers of infants born to women who acquired toxoplasmosis during pregnancy may be inconclusive, these infants should be observed over a period of up to 10 years for evidence of the disease, such as chorioretinitis, cerebral calcifications, or a rise in antibody titer. If necessary, prompt therapy should be given to prevent more serious injury to the brain and retina.

The persistence of *T. gondii* in the tissues of individuals who have recovered from a primary infection, together with the high percentage of such individuals in most populations, has become another problem associated with AIDS patients. The low levels of resistance in these individuals may result in a recrudescence, and the infection reverts from latent or chronic to the acute stage. It has been estimated that toxoplasmic encephalitis will develop in at least 30% of AIDS patients who are seropositive for the parasite.[5] Furthermore, individuals who acquire HIV infection and who have not been infected previously with *Toxoplasma* are more likely to develop a severe primary infection with this parasite. In addition to ocular toxoplasmosis from newly acquired infection, dissemination from nonocular sites of infection may occur.[6] Toxoplasmic encephalitis is a life-threatening complication, which has been seen more frequently in AIDS patients in recent years.[5] In some instances the CNS symptoms occurred before a diagnosis of HIV infection was made. The prognosis is poor if the patient is in a coma when first seen.

Epidemiology. Most *Toxoplasma* infections are acquired by the ingestion of infective stages; that is, tissue forms in raw or undercooked meat and oocysts passed into the environment by cats from 4 to 15 days after infection. Cats usually bury their feces, thus protecting the oocysts, which measure 10 by 13 μm and may remain viable for at least a year. An area where cats abound may be contaminated continually with infective oocysts as generations of cats inhabit an area. Although cats can become reinfected, evidence suggests that in subsequent infections oocysts are not passed or only a few are passed if a previous infection resulted in oocyst production. Thus older cats that were infected previously have some degree of immunity. Parasitemia is transient during acute toxoplasmosis. Hence, infection via transfusion of whole blood or cells is of lesser significance. Patients who receive organ transplants may acquire *T. gondii* infection from the donor organ, but it is more likely that recrudescence will occur from a latent infection as a result of immunosuppressive therapy.[7]

Surveys have shown that up to 95% of various populations have been infected with *Toxoplasma* based on serological tests. Such studies have shown that the percentage of seropositive individuals increases with age, indicating continued exposure throughout life. The presence of cats has also been associated with a higher percentage of seropositive individuals. Prevalence of infection is highest in hot, humid climates and lowest in dry or cold climates as well as at high altitudes. A 10-year study in Panama showed that antibody prevalence rose from 25% at 5 years of age to 50% at 10 years and increased gradually, reaching 90% by 60 years of age.[8] In a collaborative project involving 12 university medical centers located throughout the United States an analysis of antibody titers to *Toxoplasma* for 22,845 pregnant women was conducted in relation to clinical and laboratory findings in the mothers and children through 7 years of age.[9] Based on more than 900 observations considered for each mother and child, the major findings were in children and included a predicted doubling in frequency of deafness and a predicted 60% increase in microcephaly among children born to women with antibody to *Toxoplasma*. A 30% increase in low IQ (<70) was associated with a high antibody titer (256 to 512) in the mothers.

Toxoplasma is one of the most common protozoan parasites of humans. Survival as a species is assured because (1) it does not usually kill its host; (2) it infects a wide range of hosts; (3) it can remain in its host for many years so that predators can acquire infection; (4) its natural hosts, various members of the cat family, produce large numbers of oocysts, which remain infective in the environment for long periods; and (5) it can be transmitted transplacentally (Fig. 12-6).

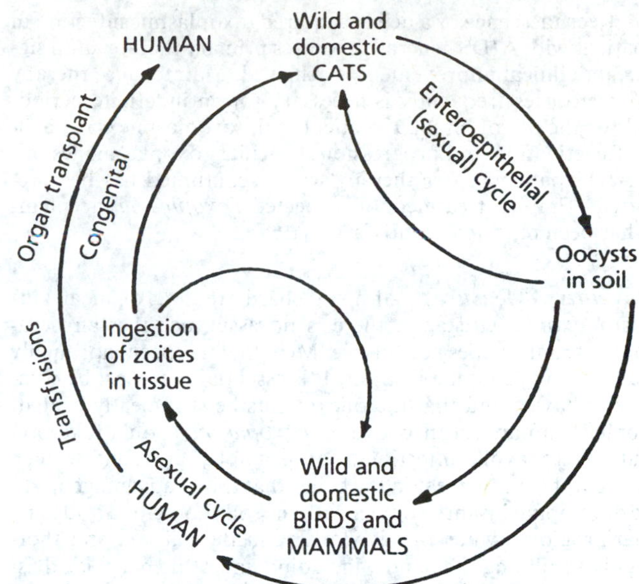

Figure 12-6. Transmission of *Toxoplasma* in nature involves two main cycles: [1] from cats to intermediate hosts and back to cats and to humans through fecal contamination of the environment with oocysts that are generated during the enteroepithelial cycle in the cat, mature in the outside environment, and are taken up in contaminated foods or water, and [2] from intermediate hosts to cats and to intermediate hosts [and humans] when zoites [tachyzoites and bradyzoites, generally the latter] that are generated in extraintestinal tissues by asexual reproduction [endodyogeny] are ingested. Except for congenital transmission, blood or cell transfusion, or organ transplant, the place of humans in either of these two cycles is that of a dead-end intermediate host. Predation and cannibalism among intermediate hosts, though not essential to enzooticity, are factors of great significance.

Diagnosis. A diagnosis can be made by demonstrating the characteristic crescent-shaped zoites in material from the patient. Bone marrow, biopsies of tissue such as lymph node or brain, placenta, cerebrospinal fluid, and other materials have been used. The various preparations such as tissue sections and smears or smears of CSF sediments can be stained with Giemsa or other suitable stain. Material can be inoculated into cell cultures or weanling mice in an effort to isolate the parasite. In most instances serological tests are employed because of the difficulty of locating a laboratory equipped to isolate the organism and the time that may be required to accomplish the task. The dye test (DT), conventional indirect fluorescent antibody test (IFAT), and direct agglutination test (DAT) detect IgG antibody. Titers rise sooner and reach higher levels (>1000). Usually, peak titers are reached within 3 months, begin to fall within a year, and reach a stable, low level in 2 or 3 years. Occasionally a patient will maintain a high titer (>1000) for a number of years.

In all suspected cases of acute toxoplasmosis a test for IgM *Toxoplasma* antibody should be performed.[10] If the test is positive, if it is confirmed by a test for IgG *Toxoplasma* antibody, and if the clinical course is compatible with toxoplasmosis, further tests probably are unnecessary. The indirect fluorescent antibody test for IgM (IgM-IFAT) can give false positive and false negative results. Purification of the IgM fraction before testing gives more reliable results but makes the test less practical. The double sandwich IgM enzyme-linked immunosorbent assay (DS-IgM-ELISA) has been recommended for acquired and congenital toxoplasmosis. A modification of the test, claimed to be more sensitive and specific than the immunofluorescence assay, requires only 2 hours to complete.[11] False negative results are obtained when rheumatoid factor or antinuclear antibody is present. If the serological test results are equivocal, the test should be repeated after 2 weeks or more. A serial two-tube or greater rise in titer with any serological test establishes the diagnosis of acute infection. In some instances it may be advisable to submit a serum sample to a second testing facility.

Treatment. Most immunologically competent individuals recover from the acute phase of toxoplasmosis without chemotherapy. A combination of pyrimethamine with either sulfadiazine or trisulfapyrimidines has been shown to be effective in most cases, although it may not eliminate the parasite completely. Specific inhibition of the parasite's folate-metabolizing enzymes is the mode of action of this combination. Frequent complete and differential blood counts are required to check for bone marrow toxicity. Folinic acid (not folic acid), given in dosages of 5 to 15 mg/d or higher if necessary, has been recommended.[5] If the patient has an adverse reaction to the pyrimethamine-sulfonamide combination, most often it is to the sulfonamide component, and the use of pyrimethamine plus clindamycin has been shown to be efficacious.[12] Spiramycin has been used to prevent in utero transmission of *Toxoplasma*.[4]

Recrudescence or a newly acquired toxoplasmic infection in a patient with AIDS generally requires primary therapy until significant clinical improvement is achieved. Maintenance therapy at lower doses frequently is necessary for an indefinite period, and for the life of an AIDS patient with toxoplasmic encephalitis. Reactivation and progression of ocular toxoplasmic lesions in AIDS patients after therapy was discontinued has been reported.[6] Empiric treatment of suspected *Toxoplasma* encephalitis has been reported as satisfactory.[12]

Preventive Measures. Although hard freezing of meat kills most *Toxoplasma* stages, there is no assurance that an occasional organism does not survive. Meat that has been thoroughly heated during cooking is safest. It is essential that meat be completely thawed and that the thicker cuts be sufficiently heated. Women who are seronegative to *Toxoplasma* should take precautions to avoid infection. For example, pregnant women should not eat raw meat in the belief that this is advantageous to the developing infant. Contact with the soil should be avoided by wearing gloves when one is working in the garden, and thoroughly scrubbing the hands, including under the nails, is advisable. Cats do not recognize property lines, and a neighbor's cats may use the yard of another, especially if the soil is well cultivated for flowers or vegetables. Children's sandboxes should be covered when not in use. If a cat, especially a kitten, shows signs of an enteric illness, it should be checked by a veterinarian. Ideally, cat box litter should be bagged daily for disposal. Only cooked meat, dried food, or canned food should be fed to cats. Stray cats should be controlled, and if possible, house cats should be prevented from hunting rodents and birds. Although much research is underway to find a vaccine to protect against *Toxoplasma* infection, a reliable vaccine for cats is not yet commercially available.[13] The problem of transmission through blood transfusion or organ transplant is of concern because the recipient may be immunocompromised, and vigilance is essential.

REFERENCES

Rabies

1. Kuwert E, Merieux C, Koprowski H, Bogel K (eds): Rabies in the Tropics. Berlin: Springer-Verlag, 1985
2. Helmick GG: The epidemiology of human rabies postexposure prophylaxis, 1980–1981. JAMA 250:1990–1996, 1983
3. Centers for Disease Control: Rabies Surveillance, United States, 1987. In CDC Surveillance Summaries, September 1988. MMWR 37(No. SS-4), 1988
4. Constantine DG: Rabies Transmission by Air in Bat Caves. Public Health Service Publication No. 1617. Washington, DC: U.S. Government Printing Office, 1967
5. Baer GM (ed): The Natural History of Rabies, Vol. II. New York: Academic Press, 1975
6. Bell JF: Abortive rabies infection. J Infect Dis 114:249–257, 1964
7. Johnson HN: Rabies. In Horsfall FL, Tamm L (eds): Viral and Rickettsial Infections of Man. Philadelphia: Lippincott, 1965
8. Emmons RW, Leonard LL, De Gennaro F Jr, et al: A case of human rabies with prolonged survival. Intervirology 1:60–72, 1973
9. WHO Expert Committee on Rabies: Seventh Report. WHO Tech Rep Ser 709, 1984
10. Dreesen DW, Bernard KW, Parker RA, et al: Immune-complex-like disease in 23 persons following a booster dose of rabies human diploid cell vaccine. Vaccine 4:45–49, 1986
11. Recommendation of the Immunization Practices Advisory Committee (ACIP): Rabies prevention. MMWR 33:393–402, 407–408, 1984
12. Pappaioanou M, Fishbein DB, Dreesen DW, et al: Antibody response to preexposure human diploid-cell rabies vaccine given concurrently with chloroquine. N Engl J Med 314:280–284, 1986

Psittacosis

General References

Meyer KF: Ornithosis. In Biester HE, Schwarte LH (eds): Diseases of Poultry, 5 edt. Ames, Iowa: Iowa State University Press, 1965, pp 675–770

Page LA: Chlamydiosis (ornithosis). In Hofstad MS (ed): Diseases of Poultry, 6 edt. Ames, Iowa: Iowa State University Press, 1972, pp 414–447

Schachter J, Dawson CR: Human Chlamydial Infections. Littleton, Mass.: Publishing Sciences Group, 1978

Schachter J, Sugg N, Sung M: Psittacosis: The reservoir persists. J Infect Dis 137:44–49, 1978

Tularemia

1. Jellison WL: Tularemia in North America. Missoula: University of Montana, 1974
2. Rausmeir JC, Ewing CL: The agglutination reaction in tularemia. J Infect Dis 69:193–205, 1941
3. Miller RP, Bates JH: Pleuropulmonary tularemia: A review of 29 patients. Am Rev Respir Dis 99:31–41, 1969
4. Saliba GS, Harmston FC, Diamond BE, et al: An outbreak of human tularemia associated with the American dog tick, *Dermacentor variabilis*. Am J Trop Med Hyg 15:531–538, 1966
5. Young LS, Bicknell DS, Archer BG, et al: Tularemia epidemic: Vermont, 1968: Forty-seven cases linked to contact with muskrats. N Engl J Med 280:1253–1260, 1969
6. Overholt EL, Tigertt WD, Kadull PJ, et al: An analysis of forty-two cases of laboratory-acquired tularemia. Am J Med 30:785–806, 1961
7. Halsted CC, Kulasinghe HP: Tularemia pneumonia in urban children. Pediatrics 61:660–662, 1978
8. Burke DS: Immunization against tularemia: Analysis of the effectiveness of live *Francisella tularensis* vaccine in prevention of laboratory acquired tularemia. J Infect Dis 135:55–60, 1977

Anthrax

1. Turnbull PCB (ed): Proceedings of the International Workshop on Anthrax. Salisbury Med J 68:1–105, 1990
2. Dutz W, Kohout E: Anthrax. Pathol Ann 6:209–248, 1971
3. LaForce FM: Woolsorters' disease in England. Bull NY Acad Med 54:956–963, 1978
4. Lincoln RE, Walker JS, Klein F, Haines BW: Anthrax. Adv Vet Sci 9:327–368, 1964
5. Van Ness GL: Ecology of anthrax. Science 172:1303–1307, 1964
6. Fox MD, Kaufmann AF, Zendell SA, et al: Anthrax in Louisiana, 1971: Epizootiologic study. J Am Vet Med Assoc 163:446–451, 1973
7. Kaufmann AF, Fox MD, Kolb RC: Anthrax in Louisiana, 1971: An evaluation of the Sterne strain anthrax vaccine. J Am Vet Med Assoc 163:442–445, 1973
8. Tanner WB, Potter ME, Teclaw RF, et al: Public health aspects of anthrax vaccination of dairy cattle. J Am Vet Med Assoc 173:1465–1466, 1978
9. Brachman PS, Gold H, Plotkin SA, et al: Field evaluation of a human anthrax vaccine. Am J Public Health 52:632–645, 1962

Brucellosis

1. Alton GG, Jones MJ, Pietz DE: Laboratory Techniques in Brucellosis. Geneva: World Health Organization, 1975
2. Araj GF, Kaufmann AF: Determination by enzyme-linked immunosorbent assay of immunoglobulin G (IgG), IgM, and IgA to *Brucella melitensis* major outer membrane proteins and whole-cell heat-killed antigens in sera of patients with brucellosis. J Clin Microbiol 27:1909–1912, 1989
3. Young EJ, Corbel MJ: Brucellosis: Clinical and Laboratory Aspects. Boca Raton, Fla.: CRC Press, 1989

4. Spink WW: The Nature of Brucellosis. Minneapolis: University of Minnesota Press, 1956
5. Kaufmann AF, Fox MD, Boyce JM, et al: Airborne spread of brucellosis. Ann NY Acad Sci 353:105–114, 1980
6. Fox MD, Kaufmann AF: Brucellosis in the United States, 1965–1974. J Infect Dis 136:312–316, 1977
7. Buchanan TM, Hendricks SL, Patton CM, Feldman RA: Brucellosis in the United States, 1960–1972. An abattoir-associated disease. III. Epidemiology and evidence for acquired immunity. Medicine (Balt) 53:427–439, 1974

Leptospirosis

1. Alston JM, Broom JC: Leptospirosis in Man and Animals. Edinburgh and London: Livingstone, 1958
2. Yasuda PH, Steigerwalt AG, Sulzer KR, et al: Deoxyribonucleic acid relatedness between serogroups and serovars in the family Leptospiraceae with proposals for seven new Leptospira species. Int J Syst Bacteriol 37:407–415, 1987
3. Turner LH: Leptospirosis III. Maintenance, isolation and demonstration of leptospires. Trans R Soc Trop Med Hyg 62:623–646, 1970
4. Turner LH: Leptospirosis II. Serology. Trans R Soc Trop Med Hyg 62:880–899, 1968
5. Feigin RD, Anderson DC: Human leptospirosis. Crit Rev Clin Lab Sci 5:413–467, 1975
6. Turner LH: Leptospirosis I. Trans R Soc Trop Med Hyg 61:842–855, 1967

Salmonellosis

1. Hargrett-Bean N, Pavia AT, Tauxe RV: *Salmonella* isolates from humans in the United States, 1984–1986. In CDC Surveillance Summaries, June 1988. MMWR 37(No. SS-2):SS25–SS31, 1988
2. Holmberg SD, Wachsmuth IK, Hickman-Brenner FW, Cohen ML: Comparison of plasmid profile analysis, phage typing, and antimicrobial susceptibility testing in characterizing *Salmonella typhimurium* isolates from outbreaks. J Clin Microbiol 19:100–104, 1984
3. Riley LW, DeFerdinando GT Jr, DeMelfi TM, Cohen ML: Evaluation of isolated cases of salmonellosis by plasmid profile analysis: Introduction and transmission of a bacterial clone by precooked roast beef. J Infect Dis 148:12–17, 1983
4. Cohen ML, Tauxe RV: Drug-resistant *Salmonella* in the United States: An epidemiologic perspective. Science 234:964–969, 1986
5. Tauxe RV, Holmberg SD, Cohen ML: The epidemiology of gene transfer in the environment. In Levy SB, Miller RV (eds): Gene Transfer in the Environment. New York: McGraw-Hill, 1989, pp 377–403
6. Riley LW, Ceballos BSO, Trabulsi LR, et al: The significance of hospitals as reservoirs for endemic multi-resistant *Salmonella typhimurium* causing infection in urban Brazilian children. J Infect Dis 150:236–241, 1984
7. LePage P, Bogaerts J, Nsengumuremyi F, et al: Metastatic focal infections due to multi-resistant *Salmonella typhimurium* in children: A 34-month experience in Rwanda. Eur J Epidemiol 2:99–103, 1986
8. Buchwald DS, Blaser MJ: A review of human salmonellosis: II. Duration of excretion following infection with nontyphi *Salmonella*. Rev Infect Dis 6:345–356, 1984
9. Aserkoff B, Bennett JV: Effect of antibiotic therapy in acute salmonellosis on the fecal excretion of salmonellae. N Engl J Med 281:636–640, 1969
10. Cohen ML, Potter M, Pollard R, Feldman RA: Turtle-associated salmonellosis in the United States: Effect of public health action, 1970 to 1976. JAMA 243:1247–1249, 1980
11. Schwabe CW. Veterinary Medicine and Human Health, 3 edt. Baltimore: William & Wilkins, 1984
12. Marth EH: Salmonellae and salmonellosis associated with milk and milk products: A review. J Dairy Sci 52:283–312, 1969
13. St. Louis ME, Morse DL, Potter ME, et al: The emergence of grade A eggs as a major source of *Salmonella enteritidis* infections: New implications for the control of salmonellosis. JAMA 259:2103–2107, 1988
14. Blaser MJ, Newman LS: A review of human salmonellosis: I. Infective dose. Rev Infect Dis 128:1096–1106, 1982
15. Cruickshank JG, Humphrey TJ: The carrier foodhandler and non-typhoid salmonellosis. Epidemiol Infect 98:223–230, 1987
16. Baine WB, Gangaros EJ, Bennett JV, Barker WH: Institutional salmonellosis. J Infect Dis 128:357–360, 1973
17. Weikel CS, Guerrant RL: Nosocomial salmonellosis [editorial]. Infect Control 6:218–220, 1985
18. Martin SM, Hargrett-Bean N, Tauxe RV: An Atlas of *Salmonella* in the United States: Serotype-specific surveillance 1968–1986. Atlanta: Centers for Disease Control, 1989. Stock No. PB89-213441-AS, National Technical Information Service, Springfield, VA 22161
19. Clark GM, Kaufmann AF, Gangaros EJ: Epidemiology of an international outbreak of *Salmonella agona*. Lancet 2:490–493, 1973
20. Rodrigue DC, Tauxe RV, Blake PA, Rowe B: International increase in *Salmonella enteritidis:* A new pandemic? Epidemiol Infect 105(1):21–27, 1990
21. World Health Organization: Wholesomeness of irradiated foods. Technical Report Series 659, Geneva, 1981

Taeniasis and Cysticercosis

1. Rausch RL: On the ecology and distribution of *Echinococcus* spp (Cestoda: Taeniidae), and characteristics of their development in the intermediate host. Ann Parasit 42:19–63, 1967
2. Slonka GF, Matulich W, Morphet E, et al: An outbreak of bovine cysticerocosis in California. Am J Trop Med Hyg 27:101–105, 1978
3. Pawlowski Z, Schultz MG: Taeniasis and cysticercosis (*Taenia saginata*). Adv Parasitol 10:269–343, 1972
4. Earnest MP, Reller LB, Filley CM, et al: Neurocysticercosis in the United States: 35 cases and a review. Rev Infect Dis 9:961–979, 1987
5. Rodriguez-Carbajal J, Boleaga-Duran B, Dorfsman J: The role of computed tomography (CT) in the diagnosis of neurocysticercosis. Childs Nerv Syst 3(4):199–202, 1987
6. Pau A, Turtas S, Brambilla M, et al: Computed tomography and magnetic resonance imaging of cerebral cysticercosis. Surg Neurol 27:548–552, 1987
7. Lotz J, Hewlett R, Albeit B, et al: Neurocysticercosis: Correlative pathomorphology and MR imaging. Neuroradiology 30:35–41, 1988
8. Plancarte A, Espinoza B, Flisser A: Immunodiagnosis of human neurocysticercosis by enzyme-linked immunosorbent assey. Childs Nerv Syst 3(4):203–205, 1987
9. Nunez R, Munoz A, Nunez C, Gomez B: A micro ELISA for the diagnosis of cerebral cisticercosis. J Immunoassay 10(2–3):169–176, 1989
10. Estrada JJ, Estrada JA, Kuhn RE: Identification of *Taenia solium* antigens from patients with neurocysticercosis. Am J Trop Med Hyg 41(1):50–55, 1989
11. Tsang VC, Brand JA, Boyer AE: An enzyme-linked immuno-electrotransfer blot assay and glycoprotein antigens. J Infect Dis 159(1):50–59, 1989
12. Botero D, Castaño S: Treatment of cysticercosis with praziquantel in Colombia. Am J Trop Med Hyg 31:811–821, 1982
13. Téllez-Girón E, Ramos MC, Dufour L, et al: Treatment of neurocysticercosis with flubendazole. Am J Trop Med Hyg 33:627–631, 1984

Trichinosis

1. Pozio E: Present knowledge of the taxonomy, distribution and biology of genera of *Trichinella* (*Nematoda, Trichinelledase*). Ann 1st Super Sanita 25:615–623, 1989
2. Schad GA, Duffy CH, Leiby DA, et al: *Trichinella spiralis* in an agricultural ecosystem: Transmission under natural and experimentally modified on-farm conditions. J Parasitol 73:95–102, 1987
3. Murrell KD, Stringfellow F, Dame JB, et al: *Trinchinella spiralis*

spiralis from domestic swine to wildlife. J Parasitol 73:103–109, 1987

4. De Carneri I, Di Matteo L: Epidemiology of trichinellosis in Italy and in neighboring countries. Ann 1st Super Sanita 25:625–633, 1989
5. Margolis HS, Middaugh JP, Burgess RD: Arctic trichinosis: Two Alaskan outbreaks from walrus meat. J Infect Dis 139:102–103, 1979
6. Ferraccioli GF, Mercadanti M, Salaffi F, et al: Clinico-biological aspects of myositis due to *Trichinella* T3 with special regard to a rheumatologic study. Ann 1st Super Sanita 25:641–647, 1989
7. Bailey TM, Schantz PM: Trends in the incidence and transmission patterns of trichinosis in humans in the United States: Comparisons of the periods 1975–1981 and 1982–1986. Rev Infect Dis 12:5–11, 1990
8. Kulikova NA, Ialuga EP: Trichinelliasis in Western Podolial. Med Parasitol 6:51–54, 1989
9. Rausch FL: Trichinosis in the Arctic. In Gould SE (ed): Trichinosis in Man and Animals. Springfield, Ill.: Charles C Thomas, 1970, pp 348–373
10. Hawking F: Chemotherapy of tissue nematodes. In Hawking F (ed): Chemotherapy of Helminthiasis. New York: Pergamon, 1973, pp 437–500
11. McCracken RO, Taylor DD: Mebendazole therapy of parenteral trichinellosis. Science 207:1220–1222, 1980
12. Morenels TM, Bronshiteen AN, Tikhonova EV: Treatment with vermosl of trichinellosis. Science 50:43–48, 1981

Paragonimiasis

1. Paragonimiasis. In Parasitic Zoonoses. WHO Tech Rep Series, 1979, p 637
2. Chemotherapy of paragonimiasis: Clonorchiasis and liver flukes. Arzeimittelforschung Symposium Proceedings Trematode Infections and Chemotherapy of Southeast and East Asia. 34:1115–1242, 1984

Clonorchiasis

1. Chou ST, Chan CW: Mucin-producing cholangiocarcinoma: An autopsy study in Hong Kong. Pathology 8:321–328, 1976
2. Purtilo DT: Clonorchiasis and hepatic neoplasms. Trop Geogr Med 28:21–27, 1976
3. Loscher T, et al: Praziquantel in clonorchiasis and opisthorchiasis. Tropenmed Parasitol 32:234–236, 1981

Fascioliasis Hepatica

1. Hardman EW, Jones RL, Davis AH: Fascioliasis—A large outbreak. Br Med J 3:502–505, 1970
2. Rim HJ: Praziquantel in the treatment of *Fascioliasis hepatica* infections. Proc Int Congr Parasitol Warsaw, Poland, 1978
3. Lammler G: Chemotherapy of trematode infections. Adv Chemother 3:200–207, 1968

Diphyllobothriasis

1. Rausch RL, Scott EM, Rausch VR: Helminths in Eskimos in western Alaska, with particular reference to Diphyllobothrium infection and anaemia. Trans R Soc Trop Med Hyg. 61:351–357, 1967
2. Peters L, Davis D, Robertson J: Is *Diphyllobothrium latum* currently present in northern Michigan? J Parasitol 64:947–949, 1978
3. von Bonsdorff B: Diphyllobothriasis in Man. New York: Academic Press, 1977
4. Apajalahti J: Tratamiento de infecciones por *Diphyllobothrium latum* can una dosis oral uńica de praziquantel. Bol Chil Parasitol 32:43, 1977

Larva Migrans

1. Jones SK, Reynolds NJ, Oliwiecki S, Harman RR: Oral albendazole for the treatment of cutaneous larva migrans. Br J Dermatol 122:99–101, 1990
2. Beaver PC: The nature of visceral larva migrans. J Parasitol 55:3–12, 1969
3. Glickman L, Schantz P, Dombroske R, Cypess R: Evaluation of serodiagnostic tests for visceral larva migrans. Am J Trop Med Hyg 27:492–498, 1978

Hydatid Disease

1. Pappaioanou M, Schwabe CW, Sard DM: An evolving pattern of human hydatid disease transmission in the United States. Am J Trop Med Hyg 26:732–742, 1977
2. Aikat BK, Bhusnurmath SR, Cadersa M, et al: *Echinococcus multilocularis* infection in India: First case report proved at autopsy. Trans R Soc Trop Med Hyg 72:619–621, 1978
3. Jiang C: Liver alveolar echinococcosis in the Northwest. Report of 15 patients and a collective analysis of 90 cases. Chin Med J 94:771–778, 1981
4. Gamble WB, Segal M, Schantz PM, Rausch RL: Alveolar hydatid disease in Minnesota: First human case acquired in the contiguous United States. JAMA 241:904–907, 1979
5. D'Alessandro A, Rausch RL, Cuello C, Aristizabal N: First observation of *Echinococcus vogeli* in man, with a review of human cases of polycystic hydatid disease in Colombia and neighboring countries. Am J Trop Med Hyg 28:303–317, 1979
6. Wilson JF, Diddams AC, Rausch RL: Cystic hydatid disease in Alaska. A review of 101 autochthonous cases of *Echinococcus granulosus* infection. Am Rev Respir Dis 98:1–15, 1968
7. Rausch RL, Wilson JF, Schantz, PM, et al: Spontaneous death of *Echinococcus multilocularis:* Cases diagnosed serologically (by EM_2 ELISA) and clinical significance. Am J Trop Med Hyg 36:576–585, 1987
8. Moir IL, Ho-Yen DO: The use of serology in patients with suspected hydatid disease. Scott Med J 34:466–468, 1989
9. Njerug FM, Okelo GB, Gathuma JM: Usefulness of indirect haemagglutination (IHA) and enzyme-linked immunosorbent assay (ELISA) in the diagnosis of human hydatidosis. East Afr Med J 66:310–314, 1989
10. Maddison SE, Slemenda SB, Schantz PM, et al: A specific diagnostic entigen of *Echinococcus granulosus* with an apparent molecular weight of 8 kDA. Am J Trop Med Hyg 40:337–383, 1989
11. Jain AK, Gupta NC, Gupta PD, Saha MM: Sonographic appearance of hepatic hydatid disease. Australas Radiol 33:373–375, 1989
12. Bekhi A, Schaaps JP, Capron M, et al: Treatment of hepatic hydatid disease with mebendazole: Preliminary results in four cases. Br Med J 2:1047–1051, 1977
13. Horton RJ: Chemotherapy of *Echinococcus* infection in man with albendazole. Trans R Soc Trop Med Hyg 83:97–102, 1989
14. Guleria R, Dhaliwal RS, Malik SK: Pulmonary hydatid disease presenting as non-resolving bilateral consolidations. Indian J Chest Dis Allied Sci 31:129–131, 1989
15. Cossetto D, Gruenewald S, Antico V, Little JM: Albendazole treatment of recurrent hydatid disease: Serial evaluation with ultrasound. Aust NZ J Surg 59:933–936, 1989
16. Davis A, Pawlowski ZS, Dixon H: Multicentre Clinical Trials of Benzimidazole Carbamates in Human Echinococcosis. Geneva, Switzerland: World Health Organization, 64:383–388, 1986
17. Filice C, Pirola F, Brunetti E, et al: A new therapeutic approach for hydatid liver cysts. Aspiration and alcohol injection under sonographic guidance. Gastroenterology 98(5 Pt 1):1366–1368, 1990
18. Wilson JF, Davidson M, Rausch RL: A clinical trial of mebendazole in the treatment of alveolar hydatid disease. Am Rev Respir Dis 118:747–757, 1978
19. Polydorou K: The anti-*Echinococcus* campaign in Cyprus. Trop Anim Health Prod 9:141–146, 1977

20. Thakur AS, Prezioso U, Marchevsky N: Efficacy of droncit against *Echinococcus granulosus* infection in dogs. Am J Vet Res 39:859–860, 1978

Other Cestodes and Intestinal Trematodes

1. Rossignol JF, Maisonneuve H: Nitazoxanide in the treatment of *Taenia saginata* and *Hymenolepis nana* infections. Am J Trop Med Hyg 33:511–512, 1984
2. Cavier R, Erhardt A: The Chemotherapy of Trematodes Other than schitosomes. In Hawking F (ed): Chemotherapy of Helminthiasis. New York: Pergamon, 1973, pp 1–28

Toxoplasmosis

1. Frenkel JK: Toxoplasmosis. Parasite life cycle, pathology, and immunology. In Hammond DM, Long PL (eds): The Coccidia. Baltimore: University Park Press, 1973, pp 343–410
2. Wreghitt TG, Hakim M, Gray JJ, et al: Toxoplasmosis in heart and lung transplant recipients. J Clin Pathol 42:194–199, 1989
3. McCabe RE, Brooks RG, Dorfman RF, Remington JS: Clinical spectrum in 107 cases of toxoplasmic lymphadenopathy. Rev Infect Dis 9:754–774, 1987
4. Desmonts G, Couvreur J: Congenital toxoplasmosis. A prospective study of 378 pregnancies. N Engl J Med 290:1110–1116, 1974
5. Dannemann BR, Remington JS: Toxoplasmic encephalitis in AIDS. Hosp Pract 139–154, March 15, 1989
6. Holland GN, Engstrom RE, Glasgow BJ, et al: Ocular toxoplasmosis in patients with the acquired immunodeficiency syndrome. Am J Ophthalmol 106:653–667, 1988
7. Luft BJ, Naot Y, Araujo FG, et al: Primary and reactivated *Toxoplasma* infection in patients with cardiac transplants. Clinical spectrum and problems in diagnosis in a defined population. Ann Intern Med 99:27–31, 1983
8. Sousa OE, Saenz RE, Frenkel JK: Toxoplasmosis in Panama: A 10-year study. Am J Trop Med Hyg 38:315–322, 1988
9. Sever JL, Ellenberg JH, Ley AC, et al: Toxoplasmosis: Maternal and pediatric findings in 23,000 pregnancies. Pediatrics 82:181–192, 1988
10. Brooks RG, McCabe RE, Remington JS: Role of serology in the diagnosis of toxoplasmic lymphadenopathy. Rev Infect Dis 9:775–782, 1987
11. Tomasi JP, Schlit AF, Stadtsbaeder S: Rapid double-sandwich enzyme-linked immunosorbent assay for detection of human immunoglobulin M anti-*Toxoplasma gondii* antibodies. J Clin Microbiol 24:849–850, 1986
12. Cohn JA, McMeeking A, Cohen W, et al: Evaluation of the policy of empiric treatment of suspected *Toxoplasma* encephalitis in patients with the acquired immunodeficiency syndrome. Am J Med 86:521–527, 1989
13. Hermentin K, Aspock H: Efforts towards a vaccine against *Toxoplasma gondii:* A review. Zentralbl Bakteriol Mikrobiol Hyg [A] 269:423–436, 1988

13

Opportunistic Fungal Infections

Michael A. Pfaller

Fungal infections, or mycoses, may be broken into two broad categories: (1) endemic and (2) chiefly opportunistic. The endemic mycoses are those in which susceptibility to the infection is acquired by living in a geographic area constituting the natural habitat of the particular fungus. The most commonly encountered endemic mycoses in North America are due to *Histoplasma capsulatum, Coccidioides immitis, Blastomyces dermatitidis,* and *Sporothrix schenkii.* Infection due to these agents is usually acquired by inhalation of conidia from an environmental source. Although infections with these fungal pathogens are clearly important, a more pressing problem now is that of the opportunistic mycoses, which carry a particularly high mortality and appear to be increasing significantly.

The opportunistic mycoses occur primarily in immunocompromised patients, particularly those with malignancies and acquired immune deficiency syndrome (AIDS), and after major surgery, severe burn injury, and bone marrow and solid organ transplantation. Contributing factors include exposure to broad spectrum antibacterial agents, adrenal corticosteroids, cytotoxic chemotherapy, and prolonged use of indwelling catheters. The most important agents of the opportunistic mycoses are *Candida* spp., *Cryptococcus neoformans, Aspergillus* spp., and the *Zygomycetes.*

The prevention, diagnosis, and therapy of opportunistic mycoses remain extremely difficult. Increased recognition of the importance of these infections has spurred efforts to develop new diagnostic and therapeutic approaches as well as to expand our knowledge of the epidemiology and pathogenesis of the mycoses.

CANDIDIASIS

Clinical and Epidemiological Features. *Candida* species are commonly found as part of the endogenous microbial flora of the oropharynx, gastrointestinal tract, and vagina of a variable proportion of normal persons. Although *C. albicans* remains the most common cause of local and disseminated infection, there has been an increase in infections caused by *C. tropicalis, C. parapsilosis, C. krusei,* and *C. lusitaniae.*[1-3]

The clinical manifestations of candidiasis include local mucocutaneous infection and hematogenously disseminated candidiasis.[1-4] Local mucocutaneous candidiasis is most commonly caused by *C. albicans* and may involve the oropharynx (thrush) and the entire gastrointestinal tract, including esophagus, stomach, and large and small bowel. Genitourinary tract involvement includes cystitis and vulvovaginal candidiasis. Superficial infections of the skin are less common but may involve the axillae, groins, inframammary folds, perianal region, and other warm moist areas, particularly following antimicrobial therapy. Although vulvovaginitis commonly occurs in otherwise normal, healthy women, mucocutaneous candidiasis most commonly occurs in immunocompromised patients: neonates, the elderly, patients with AIDS, and patients hospitalized with various malignancies and following organ transplantation and major surgery. Prolonged exposure to multiple broad spectrum antibiotics may promote mucosal overgrowth of *Candida* spp., and thus predispose these patients to superficial candidiasis.[2,4]

Chronic mucocutaneous candidiasis is a rare syndrome associated with defects in T cell mediated immunity. These patients have persistent superficial *Candida* infection of skin, scalp, nails, and mucous membranes.[2] Disease onset may begin at any age, be associated with various endocrinopathies (diabetes mellitus, hypoparathyroidism, hypothyroidism, or hypoadrenalism), and the clinical manifestations may be limited or quite extensive.

Hematogenously disseminated candidiasis is a serious infection of hospitalized and immunocompromised patients which appears to be increasing markedly over the past 10 to 15 years.[1-5] Candidemia and disseminated candidiasis occur most commonly in hospitalized patients with neutropenia, malignancies, and severe burn injuries, and following major surgical procedures.[1-4] Disseminated candidiasis is also a frequent, serious problem in infants hospitalized in neonatal intensive care units. Hematogenously disseminated candidiasis is generally thought to originate from an endogenous, usually gastrointestinal, source and is most commonly caused by *C. albicans* followed by *C. tropicalis, C. parapsilosis,* and *C. krusei.* Infection of peripheral and central venous catheters may result from endogenous or exogenous contamination of the catheter surface. The infected catheter may serve as a nidus for subsequent hematogenous dissemination. The clinical manifestations of hematogenously disseminated candidiasis are nonspecific, and infection may present with candidemia or focal involvement of specific "target organs" such as skin, liver, lung, bone, eye, or central nervous system.

Crude mortality rates reported for patients with candidemia

and disseminated candidiasis have been as high as 90%; however, because these infections occur in patients with serious underlying disease, the actual contribution of the infection to the death of the patients has been difficult to estimate. One study has estimated the mortality directly attributable to nosocomial candidemia to be approximately 38%.[6] This estimate of attributable mortality is comparable to data reported for primary aerobic gram-negative bacteremia and considerably higher than the 13.6% reported for nosocomial bloodstream infections due to another opportunistic pathogen, *Staphylococcus epidermidis.*

The identification of risk factors for disseminated candidiasis has been difficult because of the complex nature of the patients at risk for these infections. Significant independent risk factors for disseminated candidiasis identified by multivariate analysis include prior colonization by *Candida* spp., central catheterization (including Hickman catheters), neutropenia, hemodialysis, and chemotherapy for hematological malignancies.[7,8] These factors may be important in the development of serious candidal infection independent of the underlying disease state or other confounding factors and should serve as the focus for future studies concerning methods of prevention, diagnosis, and therapy.

Microbiology. *Candida* organisms are small (4 to 6 μm), oval, thin-walled cells that reproduce by budding and may also form pseudohyphae and hyphae (*C. albicans* only) in tissue. Although over 80 species of *Candida* have been identified, only a few have been isolated from humans, including *C. albicans, C. tropicalis, C. parapsilosis, C. krusei, C. guilliermondii, C. pseudotropicalis,* and *C. lusitaniae. Candida* species grow well on most laboratory media and appear as white, creamy colonies and may be smooth, wrinkled, or fuzzy in appearance. Blastospores (yeasts), hyphae, or pseudohyphae may be seen directly in gram-stained (gram-positive) or potassium hydroxide (KOH)–treated preparations of clinical material. Special stains, such as the Gomori methenamine silver stain, may be used to visualize the organisms in tissue sections. Identification of *Candida* isolates to species level is accomplished by employing a series of biochemical and physiological tests. A number of prepackaged identification kits are commercially available and allow species identification within 48 to 72 hours. The germ tube test is a simple and rapid means of presumptively identifying isolates of *C. albicans.* This test takes advantage of the fact that most *C. albicans,* but not other species of *Candida,* will form germ tubes (hyphal evaginations) within 2 hours in the presence of serum.

Diagnosis. One of the major problems in the prevention and therapy of candidiasis in hospitalized patients is the difficulty in diagnosing infection vs colonization in these frequently complex patients.[1–4] The clinical signs and symptoms associated with both local and disseminated candidiasis are nonspecific and generally not helpful in distinguishing bacterial from candidal infection. The most common clinical presentation of superficial candidiasis is that of white or gray pseudomembranous plaques overlying the mucosal surface. Removal of the plaques reveals a red, painful base with ulcerations and necrosis. Oropharyngeal and esophageal involvement may be quite painful with considerable dysphagia and pain on swallowing. Vaginal and cutaneous involvement may be both painful and pruritic. Two major clues to diagnosis of hematogenously disseminated candidiasis are the presence of endophthalmitis and macronodular skin lesions. *Candida* endophthalmitis is marked by single or multiple raised, white, fluffy chorioretinal lesions, with or without an overlying vitreous haze. The lesions are usually in the macular area and are easily detected by ophthalmoscopic examination. Unfortunately they are rarely observed in neutropenic patients. In addition to endophthalmitis and macronodular skin lesions, several additional clinical presentations of disseminated candidiasis have been described in recent years including suppurative thrombophlebitis, hepatitis, purpura fulminans and bullous dermatitis, epiglottitis, and osteomyelitis.[1–4]

The laboratory diagnosis of candidiasis has been limited because available methods are insensitive and nonspecific. Superficial infection may be diagnosed by direct microscopic examination of 10% KOH-treated or gram-stained material obtained from infected lesions. The most reliable means of documenting disseminated candidiasis is by histopathological demonstration of tissue invasion on biopsy or recovery of *Candida* spp. from normally sterile body fluids such as pleural fluid, peritoneal fluid, or cerebrospinal fluid. Isolation of *Candida* spp. from urine or sputum may be helpful but frequently only represents colonization or contamination of the specimen. Isolation of *Candida* spp. from blood is also helpful; however, fungemia may occasionally be transient and is not indicative of widespread dissemination, particularly when associated with a removable intravascular focus such as an infected catheter. Conventional broth blood cultures are positive for *Candida* spp. in less than 50% of patients with documented disseminated candidiasis and frequently are positive only immediately preceding or after death. Therefore they are rarely helpful in making diagnostic and therapeutic decisions. The usefulness of blood cultures in diagnosing disseminated candidiasis is significantly improved when biphasic media or lysis-centrifugation (Isolator, DuPont) methods are employed to optimize the detection of candidemia.[9] Serological methods have also been disappointing.[10] Measurement of antibody titers has been unsuccessful in delineating colonization and local infection from disseminated candidiasis. Likewise detection of circulating fungal antigens, with few exceptions, has not been successful in providing an accurate, early diagnosis of disseminated infection.

Therapy. Deeply invasive infection such as severe esophagitis and disseminated candidiasis requires systemic therapy with amphotericin B. Prompt removal of potentially contaminated devices such as intravenous catheters is important. The addition of 5-fluorocytosine may provide synergistic candidacidal activity; however, improved clinical efficacy has not been proven in properly designed clinical trials. Although newer antifungal compounds, including a wide array of azole antifungal agents, have been developed, their usefulness in treatment of disseminated candidiasis remains to be established. Amphotericin B remains the drug of choice. Topical antifungal agents such as nystatin, clotrimazole, or miconazole may be useful in the treatment of superficial mucocutaneous infections. Occasionally oral therapy with ketoconazole may be indicated, such as in patients with chronic mucocutaneous candidiasis. Attempts at prophylaxis with oral or systemic administration of antifungal agents have met with limited success in preventing invasive disease despite a reduction in the extent of local colonization.

CRYPTOCOCCOSIS

Clinical and Epidemiological Features. Cryptococcosis is a mycosis caused by the encapsulated yeast *Cryptococcus neoformans,* which may present as a localized acute or chronic pulmonary infection or, more importantly, with hematogenous dissemination and meningitis. Although the incidence and prevalence of cryptococcosis is unknown, the disease occurs worldwide.[1–3] Pulmonary infection is most common; however, symptoms may be mild and self-limited and thus less likely to be reported than cryptococcal meningitis. There are four capsular serotypes of *C. neoformans* (A–D), with serotype A being responsible for most disease worldwide.[3] Serotype D is common only in Europe, whereas serotypes B and C are found predominantly in the tropics and subtropics including a focus in southern California.

C. neoformans serotypes A and D are commonly recovered in large numbers from environmental sources contaminated with the droppings of pigeons and other birds. Serotypes B and C are rarely recovered from the environment, suggesting a unique, and as yet unknown, environmental niche. Despite the strong association of *C. neoformans* with pigeon droppings, most patients infected with *C. neoformans* do not give a history of contact with pigeons or other birds. Thus, infection most likely results from inhalation of aerosolized organisms. Infection due to direct implantation has been reported but is extremely rare.

Cryptococcosis, particularly meningitis, commonly occurs in patients with underlying immunodeficiency; however, both local and disseminated infections are observed in patients with no known immunological defect. Immunosuppressed patients at particular risk for cryptococcal infection include those with lymphoreticular malignancies or sarcoid, and those receiving corticosteroid therapy, organ transplants, or immunosuppressive therapy. The most common immunological defect in patients with cryptococcal infection is a defect in cell-mediated immunity. The importance of cell-mediated immunity as a host defense mechanism is underscored by the fact that cryptococcosis is the fourth most common infection complicating AIDS.[4,5] It is estimated that 7% to 10% of patients with AIDS are infected with *C. neoformans.* Because of persistent immunological defect in patients with AIDS, cryptococcal infection is extremely difficult to manage and generally requires life-long suppressive therapy.

Primary cryptococcal disease is generally considered to occur in the lungs. The presentation of pulmonary cryptococcal infection is variable, ranging from asymptomatic airway colonization without parenchymal invasion to an acute pneumonic process with lobar infiltrates, cough, and fever. Chronic pulmonary infection may occur with progressive involvement over several years. Although only about 10% of all patients with pulmonary cryptococcosis have evidence of immunological deficiency, this group of patients is at high risk for dissemination and development of cryptococcal meningitis.

Central nervous system lesions are the most common and important clinical manifestation of extrapulmonary cryptococcosis. It is estimated that approximately 300 cases of cryptococcal meningitis occur in the United States each year; however, this number is likely to increase dramatically with the increasing number of immunocompromised patients and the emergence of *C. neoformans* as a major pathogen complicating AIDS.[1,2,4,5] Central nervous system infection may present as either a focal or diffuse process, and chronic meningitis with disease presenting over weeks to months has been observed. Although meningitis is the most common manifestation of systemic cryptococcosis, disseminated infection may present with cryptococcemia and involvement of skin and mucous membranes, bone, liver, lung, kidneys, prostate, adrenals, spleen, lymph nodes, or testes with or without clinically apparent central nervous system involvement.

Microbiology. *C. neoformans* is a ubiquitous, encapsulated soil yeast that reproduces asexually by budding. The perfect or sexual stage of *C. neoformans* can be produced by mating the fungus *in vitro;* however, the role of this stage in infectivity and pathogenesis is unknown. The yeast cell may vary from 4 to 20 μm in diameter and is surrounded by a polysaccharide capsule ranging from 1 to 30 μm. The narrow-based buds are usually single. The capsule may be visualized indirectly by the India ink or nigrosin technique and more specifically in clinical material with mucicarmine, which stains capsular mucopolysaccharide. In tissue, cryptococci stain poorly with hematoxylin-eosin but well with methenamine silver and periodic acid–Schiff.

C. neoformans grows well on most bacterial and fungal media used in the routine clinical microbiology laboratory. A rapid presumptive identification of an encapsulated yeast as *C. neoformans* may be accomplished by demonstration of urease and phenoloxidase enzyme activity.[1,6] *C. neoformans* is strongly urease positive and possesses a membrane-bound phenoloxidase enzyme that converts phenolic compounds to melanin. Phenoloxidase activity is readily demonstrated on media such as bird-seed agar or caffeic acid agar, which contains 3,4 dihydroxycinnamic acid. Oxidation of the *O*-diphenol in the medium produces dark colonies suggestive of *C. neoformans.* Confirmatory identification is accomplished by employing standard biochemical and physiological tests.

Diagnosis. The clinical presentation of pulmonary cryptococcosis may mimic a number of acute and chronic infectious processes as well as malignancies. Signs and symptoms include fever, malaise, pleuritic pain, cough, scanty sputum, and hemoptysis. Chest roentgenograms may reveal lobar infiltrates, single or multiple nodules, or tumor-like masses. Sputum cultures are positive in only 20% of cases, and the diagnosis is frequently made at thoracotomy for suspected malignancy. Patients with pulmonary cryptococcosis should be thoroughly evaluated for systemic infection, with cultures of blood, urine, and cerebrospinal fluid (CSF).

Central nervous system cryptococcosis may present as either meningitis (most common), encephalitis, or a more focal process suggestive of malignancy. Signs and symptoms in patients without AIDS include fever, headache, mental status changes, ocular symptoms, meningismus, nausea, vomiting, cranial nerve palsies, and seizures. Aside from fever and headache these signs and symptoms may be significantly less common in patients with AIDS. The chest roentgenogram may or may not be abnormal in patients with central nervous system or systemic cryptococcosis. Extraneural dissemination may present as cryptococcemia or focal involvement of one of several target organs.

The laboratory diagnosis of cryptococcosis requires the isolation of cryptococci from normally sterile body fluids, histopathology showing encapsulated organisms, or detection of cryptococcal antigen in serum or CSF. A rapid diagnosis of extraneural infection may be facilitated by biopsy and staining with methenamine silver and mucicarmine. Examination of the CSF in patients with meningitis usually suggests a chronic lymphocytic meningitis with a low-grade ($<500/mm^3$) lymphocytic pleocytosis, elevated protein, and low glucose. Microscopic examination of CSF mixed with India ink or nigrosin may reveal encapsulated organisms in approximately 50% of cases. Cultures of CSF and other clinical material are usually positive. Occasionally repeated lumbar punctures, cisternal taps, or sampling of large volumes (up to 10 ml) of CSF may be necessary to establish the diagnosis. In patients with AIDS, cryptococci are present in large numbers, but the CSF shows fewer abnormalities.

Detection of cryptococcal antigen in serum and CSF is extremely valuable in the diagnosis of cryptococcal infection. Antigen titers are particularly high in patients with AIDS. Several latex agglutination assays are commercially available and are rapid, sensitive, and specific.[7] Antigen is detected in the serum in approximately 50% and in CSF in greater than 90% of patients with cryptococcal meningitis. High titers of cryptococcal antigen in CSF or serum are associated with a poor prognosis. False-positive results are rare but may be due to rheumatoid factor or, more recently, cross-reactivity in patients infected with *Trichosporon beigelii.*[8]

Therapy. Pulmonary cryptococcosis may not require therapy as long as the process appears to be resolving and the patient is intact immunologically. Long-term follow-up is necessary in patients whose infection is diagnosed at thoracotomy because there is a 3% to 10% risk of meningitis for up to 3 years after surgery. Patients with progressive pulmonary infection, particularly those who are immunocompromised, and all patients with extrapulmonary infection require systemic antifungal therapy. At present such therapy consists of intravenous amphotericin B. The efficacy of ketoconazole or other azoles in the treatment of pulmonary cryptococcosis remains to be documented in appropriate clinical trials.

Cryptococcal meningitis and extrapulmonary cryptococcosis always require systemic antifungal therapy. Cryptococcal meningitis is almost universally fatal without therapy, but approximately 80% to 90% of patients (non-AIDS) can be cured with current therapeutic regimens. Current therapeutic recommendations are restricted to amphotericin B alone or in combination with 5-fluorocytosine.[1,2,9] The combination of amphotericin B and 5-fluorocytosine provides synergistic fungicidal activity and is favored by many clinicians; however, the added toxicity of 5-fluorocytosine (bone marrow suppression, gastrointestinal, and liver toxicity) may limit its application, particularly in AIDS patients.

Treatment of cryptococcal meningitis in patients with AIDS has been difficult. Initial response to both combination and single-drug therapy has been poor, and relapses are common.[4,5] In general, patients with AIDS cannot be cured of their cryptococcal infection and require chronic maintenance therapy with either weekly amphotericin B or one of the newer triazoles such as itraconozole or fluconazole.

ASPERGILLOSIS

Clinical and Epidemiological Features. The term *aspergillosis* refers to any one of a number of disease states caused by members of the genus *Aspergillus*. *Aspergillus* species are ubiquitous fungi that may be isolated from a variety of environmental sources including insulation and fireproofing materials, soil, grain, leaves, grass, and air.[1] The aerosolized conidia are present in large numbers and are constantly being inhaled. Although several hundred species of *Aspergillus* have been described, relatively few are known to cause disease in humans. *Aspergillus fumigatus* remains the most common cause of aspergillosis, followed by *A. flavus, A. terreus, A. niger, A. glaucus,* and *A. nidulans.*[1-3]

Aspergillus infections occur worldwide and appear to be increasing in prevalence, particularly among patients with chronic pulmonary disease and among the immunocompromised population.[2,3] Recent data from the M.D. Anderson Cancer Center documented a 23% increase in *Aspergillus* spp. as a cause of systemic fungal infection, rising from 12% of all systemic fungal infections in the 1966–1970 period to 35% in 1981–1985.[2] *Aspergillus* spp. are particularly important causes of nosocomial infections in patients who are immunocompromised secondary to burn injury, malignancy, leukemia, and bone marrow and other organ transplantation. Several major outbreaks of invasive nosocomial aspergillosis have been described in association with exposure to *Aspergillus* conidia aerosolized by hospital construction, contaminated air-handling systems, and insulation or fireproofing materials within walls or ceilings of hospital bed units.[4-6] The crude mortality associated with these infections is high, approximately 90% in most series.[2]

The clinical manifestations of aspergillosis include pulmonary colonization with bronchitis and aspergilloma formation, allergic syndromes such as allergic bronchopulmonary aspergillosis (ABPA), and invasive aspergillosis.[1-3] Intoxication or neoplasm secondary to ingestion of aflatoxin or other toxins produced by *Aspergillus* spp. contaminating grain and other foods is also a serious problem worldwide.

Pulmonary colonization by *Aspergillus* spp. may involve the bronchial mucosa or may become localized in a preexisting cavity, resulting in the formation of an aspergilloma. Superficial colonization of the tracheobronchial mucosa produces little inflammation and is not associated with tissue invasion. The expectoration of bronchial casts containing mucus and hyphal elements may be observed. Patients in whom mucosal colonization is observed are those with preexisting pulmonary disease including cystic fibrosis, chronic obstructive pulmonary disease, and chronic asthma requiring administration of corticosteroids.

Aspergillomas are masses of mycelia and amorphous debris localized in preexisting pulmonary cavities, usually in the upper lobes. The cavities usually are lined with modified bronchial epithelium and have been formed secondary to other disease processes such as tuberculosis, infarcts, or neoplasms. There is little surrounding inflammation, and invasion of the pulmonary parenchyma by *Aspergillus* spp. is rare. Aspergillomas may be clinically silent; however, hemoptysis secondary to ulceration of the epithelial lining of the cavity is observed in 50% to 80% of cases.[2] The lesions may be stable, grow, or shrink with the surrounding cavity. Spontaneous lysis occurs in approximately 10% of cases within 3 years.[7]

The allergic manifestations of aspergillosis are the result of tissue hypersensitivity to conidia or other antigens of *Aspergillus* spp., (almost always *A. fumigatus*).[3] The clinical picture may vary from mild asthma to fibrosis and bronchiectasis secondary to allergic bronchopulmonary aspergillosis. Exposure to aerosolized *Aspergillus* conidia may produce bronchospasm in individuals with atopic asthma. Repeated and heavy inhalation of *Aspergillus* conidia and other antigens may result in extrinsic allergic alveolitis in nonatopic patients. Prolonged exposure may lead to micronodular changes and fibrosis. Allergic bronchopulmonary aspergillosis (ABPA) is the result of type I (IgE-mediated), type III (immune complex-mediated), and possibly type IV (cell-mediated) hypersensitivity reactions to *Aspergillus* antigens. This condition occurs in up to 20% of individuals with asthma and is associated with colonization of the bronchial mucosa by *Aspergillus* spp. These patients experience recurrent bouts of severe asthma, wheezing, fever, weight loss, chest pain, and cough productive of blood-tinged sputum. Eventually the disease becomes chronic, with the development of fibrosis, bronchiectasis, and mucous plugging with subsequent atelectasis or cavitation. This condition may be associated with nasal polyps and chronic sinusitis.

Invasive aspergillosis occurs most commonly in patients who are severely immunocompromised secondary to hematological and lymphoreticular malignancies. Major risk factors include neutropenia, broad spectrum antibacterial therapy, and administration of corticosteroids.[1-4] Patients undergoing bone marrow transplantation are at particularly high risk. Although invasive aspergillosis may be acquired either in the community or in the hospital, most cases are nosocomial in origin. The disease process is most commonly localized to the lungs, followed by the paranasal tissues. The infectious process is typified by mucosal ulceration and direct extension of hyphae into surrounding tissues. Vascular invasion results in thrombosis, embolization, and infarction. Hematogenous dissemination occurs in 35% to 40% of cases of invasive pulmonary aspergillosis and may involve brain, liver, kidneys, gastrointestinal tract, thyroid, heart, skin, and other sites.[1,8] Extension of paranasal infection into the orbit and brain may mimic rhinocerebral zygomycosis. Although the pulmonary process may occasionally be inapparent, it most commonly presents as a necrotizing, patchy bronchopneumonia with or without hemorrhagic infarction. In all infected foci the infection is characterized by vascular invasion, tissue infarction, and necrosis. Massive hemoptysis, gastrointestinal bleeding, and cerebral infarcts and abscesses may occur.

Chronic necrotizing aspergillosis, a more indolent pulmonary infectious process, occurs predominantly in middle-aged patients with mildly compromised host defenses or preexisting pulmonary lung damage.[9] The locally invasive infection is slowly progressive and results in cavitation and aspergilloma formation. The infectious process is usually confined to the upper lobes but occasionally may involve an entire lung.

Microbiology. *Aspergillus* species are molds that reproduce by means of spores or conidia. The conidia germinate to form hyphae, which are the forms most commonly found in infected tissue. *Aspergillus* species grow well on most media and are identified to species level based on the microscopic identification of specific morphologic features. Over 600 different species of *Aspergillus* have been described; however, most clinical infections are due to *A. fumigatus* and *A. flavus.*[1] *Aspergillus niger* is the most common cause of otomycosis. At present there are no commercially available kits to aid in the identification of *Aspergillus* spp. In tissue, *Aspergillus* hyphae stain well with Gomori methenamine silver stain and are uniform, 2 to 7 μm in diameter, septate, and dichotomously branched with angles of approximately 45 degrees. These features are not diagnostic and are shared by several other opportunistic fungal pathogens.

Diagnosis. The clinical signs and symptoms of pulmonary aspergillosis are nonspecific and range from mild asthma to severe hemoptysis, acute bronchopneumonia, and pulmonary infarct. Extrapulmonary involvement may present as cellulitis, hemorrhage, or infarction depending on the specific site of infection. Chest radiographs may be useful in the diagnosis of aspergilloma with the appearance of a freely movable intracavitary mass surrounded by a crescent of air (Monod's sign). The radiographic appearance of allergic bronchopulmonary aspergillosis varies with the stage and chronicity of the disease but may appear as bronchiectasis with bronchial thickening or dilation, consolidation, and atelectasis. The most common radiographic picture of invasive pulmonary aspergillosis is that of a patchy density or well-defined nodule, which may be single or multifocal with progression to diffuse consolidation or cavitation.[10]

The laboratory diagnosis of aspergillosis is generally unsatisfactory. Definitive diagnosis of invasive aspergillosis usually requires biopsy of the involved tissue. Unfortunately the severe underlying diseases and associated bleeding diatheses commonly seen in these patients often preclude such an invasive approach. Sputum cultures are nondiagnostic and may be positive in patients with simple colonization and negative in patients with invasive disease.[1,2,8] The usefulness of surveillance cultures in high-risk patients remains to be confirmed.[11] Blood, urine, and CSF cultures are rarely positive in patients with invasive disease. Detection of *Aspergillus* antigen in blood, urine, and lung washings is a promising noninvasive means of diagnosing invasive aspergillosis but is restricted to the research laboratory at present.[12] Skin tests and demonstration of serum precipitins have been useful in diagnosing ABPA; however, they are of no use in diagnosing invasive infection. Additional laboratory features of ABPA include elevated serum IgE and peripheral blood eosinophilia.

Therapy. Treatment of aspergillosis is difficult and is probably not indicated for aspergilloma unless life-threatening hemoptysis occurs, in which case segmental resection or lobectomy is indicated. Systemic antifungal therapy has been of no value. Likewise, neither systemic nor aerosolized antifungal therapy has been effective in treatment of the allergic syndromes such as ABPA. Corticosteroids are considered the treatment of choice.

Given the high mortality associated with invasive aspergillosis, an aggressive approach to diagnosis and treatment is required. In addition, return of bone marrow function or reversal of neutropenia is essential for survival. Amphotericin B is the only antifungal agent with established activity in this infection. Concomitant reduction or elimination of immunosuppressive therapy may also be necessary. The efficacy of granulocyte transfusions, 5-fluorocytosine, or rifampin in combination with amphotericin B is unproven. Azole antifungal agents such as miconazole or ketoconazole have no role in the treatment of invasive aspergillosis.

Prophylaxis of invasive aspergillosis is most important in immunocompromised patients. Laminar airflow facilities provide the only means of preventing this infectious complication. Prophylactic antifungal drugs lack proven efficacy. Intranasal instillation of amphotericin B has been used with promising results; however, more studies will be necessary.

ZYGOMYCOSIS

Clinical and Epidemiological Features. Zygomycosis is a general term that includes infections caused by fungi in the order Mucorales and order Entomophthorales (class Zygomycetes). The Zygomycetes are ubiquitous worldwide in soil and decaying vegetation. Zygomycosis is not communicable and is acquired by inhalation, ingestion, or contamination of wounds with conidia from the environment. Although *Rhizopus arrhizus* is the most common agent of human zygomycosis, additional species of *Rhizopus, Mucor, Absidia, Mortierella, Cunninghamella* and *Saksenaea* have been causing infection with increasing frequency.[1-3]

Clinically zygomycosis is a fulminant infectious process that produces rhinocerebral disease in patients with diabetic ketoacidosis; rhinocerebral, pulmonary, or disseminated disease in immunocompromised patients; local or disseminated disease in patients with burns or open wounds; and gastrointestinal disease in patients with malnutrition or preexisting gastrointestinal disorders. In each case the progression of disease may be rapid, with invasion and destruction of key anatomic structures in a matter of days. This is particularly true with rhinocerebral infection, where death may occur within 3 to 10 days in untreated patients.[3-5] Although classically the major risk factor for zygomycosis is diabetic acidosis, it is now clear that neutropenia, hematological malignancy, and cytotoxic or immunosuppressive therapy place patients at risk for these infections.[1-5]

The hallmark of zygomycosis is vascular invasion with thrombosis, hemorrhage, infarction, and tissue necrosis.[6] The disease usually extends locally across tissue planes; however, hematogenous dissemination may also occur. Mortality is directly related to rapidity of diagnosis (extent of disease), aggressiveness of therapy, and underlying disease state. Estimates of crude mortality in patients with rhinocerebral zygomycosis are 40% in patients with diabetes and 80% in patients with other underlying diseases (malignancy, organ transplantation, neutropenia). The prognosis is poor in cases of pulmonary zygomycosis: only about 15 patients have been reported to have survived the infectious process.[3,5,7]

Focal outbreaks of zygomycosis have been related to the use of certain adhesive bandages or tape on open wounds. The resulting cutaneous infections were due to *Rhizopus* species, which were also isolated from the bandage material.[8]

Microbiology. The agents of zygomycosis are molds that reproduce by means of spores or conidia. All of the Zygomycetes appear identical in tissue and are seen microscopically following staining with hematoxylin-eosin or Gomori methenamine silver as broad (6 to 50 μm), irregular, branching, usually aseptate hyphae. Definitive identification requires isolation on agar medium and subsequent microscopic examination. Following primary isolation the Zygomycetes grow well on most media; however, primary isolation from clinical material is frequently difficult. Isolates are identified to genus and species level based on the microscopic identification of specific morphological features.

Diagnosis. The clinical signs and symptoms of zygomycosis are dependent on the site of infection. Rhinocerebral disease may present with nasal stuffiness, blood-tinged nasal discharge, facial swelling, and facial or orbital pain. Major diagnostic clues are the presence of a black eschar on the nasal or palatine mucosa and drainage of "black pus" from the eye.[1-3,5] Radiographic examination of the sinuses may reveal clouding, thickening of the mucous membranes, and bony destruction. Progression of the disease is manifested by orbital cellulitis, proptosis, and cranial nerve defects. Cerebral infarction caused by vascular compromise is common. Examination of the CSF may reveal an elevated protein, normal glucose, and a modest pleocytosis. Culture and microscopic examination of CSF is uniformly negative. Pulmonary zygomycosis may resemble invasive pulmonary aspergillosis presenting as an acute bronchopneumonia or pulmonary infarction. Radiographic findings are nonspecific and include a patchy, nonhomogeneous infiltrate progressing to consolidation and cavitation.[9] Life-threatening hemoptysis may occur. Gastrointestinal infection may present with abdominal pain, diarrhea, and bleeding. Vascular invasion results in infarction and perforation of the bowel with subsequent hemorrhage and peritonitis. Cutaneous infection may present as chronic ulceration, papules, or black, necrotic areas of infarction.

The fulminant and life-threatening nature of these infections precludes the use of culture in the diagnosis of zygomycosis.[1,5] Cultures are positive in only 20% of cases and are rarely positive antemortem. Serological tests are not reliable, and microscopic examination of sputum or wound drainage rarely is positive for fungal elements. The key to diagnosis is the demonstration of the characteristic hyphae in tissue obtained on biopsy.[5] A negative histopathological examination does not rule out infection, and additional material should be obtained if clinically indicated.

Therapy. Successful therapy of zygomycosis requires early diagnosis, systemic antifungal therapy with amphotericin B, aggressive surgical debridement of the involved area, and control of the underlying disorder. Local instillation of amphotericin B into infected paranasal sinuses may be useful. There is no proven role for additional antifungal agents such as 5-fluorocytosine or the azoles.

Prevention of zygomycosis involves control of underlying disease and conservative use of immunosuppressive agents. As seen with invasive aspergillosis, the use of laminar airflow facilities may be necessary to protect severely immunocompromised patients from infections with the Zygomycetes.

REFERENCES

Candidiasis

1. Bodey GP, Fainstein V (eds): Candidiasis. New York: Raven, 1985
2. Odds FC (ed): Candida and Candidosis. 2nd edt. London: Baillière Tindall, 1988
3. Meunier F: Candidiasis. Eur J Clin Microbiol Infect Dis 8:438, 1989
4. Crislip MA, Edwards JE: Candidiasis. Infect Dis Clin N Am 3:103, 1989
5. Horan T, Culver D, Jarvis W, Emori G, Banerjee S, Martone W, Thornsberry C: Pathogens causing nosocomial infections: Preliminary data from the National Nosocomial Infections Surveillance System. Antimicrob Newsletter 5:65, 1988
6. Wey SB, Mori M, Pfaller MA, Woolson RF, Wenzel RP: Hospital-acquired candidemia: The attributable mortality and excess length of stay. Arch Intern Med 148:2642, 1988
7. Wey SB, Mori M, Pfaller MA, Woolson RF, Wenzel RP: Risk factors for hospital-acquired candidemia: A matched case-control study. Arch Intern Med 148:2642–2647, 1988
8. Pfaller MA: Opportunistic fungal infections – the increasing importance of *Candida* species. Infect Cont Hosp Epidemiol 10:270, 1989
9. Bille J, Edson R, Roberts G: Clinical evaluation of the lysis centrifugation blood culture system for the detection of fungemia and comparison with a conventional biphasic broth blood culture system. J Clin Microbiol 19:126, 1984
10. DeRepentigny L: Serological techniques for diagnosis of fungal infections. Eur J Clin Microbiol Infect Dis 8:362, 1989

Cryptococcosis

1. Perfect JR: Cryptococcosis. Infect Dis Clin N Am 3:77, 1989
2. Patterson TF, Andriole VT: Current concepts in cryptococcosis. Eur J Clin Microbiol Infect Dis 8:457, 1989
3. Bennett JE, Kwon-Chung KJ, Howard DH: Epidemiological differences among serotypes of *Cryptococcus neoformans*. Am J Epidemiol 105:582, 1977
4. Kovacs JA, Kovacs AA, Wright WC, Gill VJ, Tuazon CV, Gelmann EP, Lane HC, Longfield R, Parrillo JE, Bennett JE, Magur H, Polis M: Cryptococcosis in the acquired immunodeficiency syndrome. Ann Intern Med 103:533, 1985
5. Zuger A, Louie E, Holzman RS, Simberkoff MS, Rahal JJ: Cryptococcal disease in patients with the acquired immunodeficiency syndrome. Ann Intern Med 104:234, 1986
6. Zimmer BL, Roberts GD: Rapid, selective urease test for presumptive identification of *Cryptococcus neoformans*. J Clin Microbiol 10:380, 1979
7. Wu TC, Koo SY: Comparison of three commercial latex kits for detection of cryptococcal antigen. J Clin Microbiol 18:1127, 1983
8. McManus EJ, Jones MJ: Detection of a *Trichosporon beigelii* antigen cross-reactive with *Cryptococcus neoformans* capsular polysaccharide in serum from a patient with disseminated *Trichosporon* infection. J Clin Microbiol 21:681, 1985
9. Bennett JE, Dismukes WE, Duma RJ, Medoff G, Sande MA, Gallis H, Leonard J, Fields BT, Bradshaw M, Haywood H, McGee ZA, Cate TR, Cobbs CG, Warner JF, Alling DW: A comparison of amphotericin B alone and combined with flucytosine in the treatment of cryptococcal meningitis. N Engl J Med 301:126, 1979

Aspergillosis

1. Rinaldi MG: Invasive aspergillosis. Rev Infect Dis 5:1061, 1983
2. Bodey GP, Vartivarian S: Aspergillosis. Eur J Clin Microbiol Infect Dis 8:413, 1989
3. Levitz SM: Aspergillosis. Infect Dis Clin N Am 3:1, 1989
4. Perraud M, Piens MA, Nicoloyannis N, Girard P, Sepetjan M, Garin JP: Invasive nosocomial pulmonary aspergillosis: risk factors and hospital building works. Epidemiol Infect 99:407, 1987
5. Sherertz RJ, Belani A, Kramer BS, Elfenbein GJ, Weiner RS, Sullivan ML, Thomas RG, Samas GP: Impact of air filtration on nosocomial aspergillosis infections. Am J Med 83:709, 1987
6. Rotstein C, Camminges KM, Tidings J, Killion K, Powell E, Gustafson TL, Higby D: An outbreak of invasive aspergillosis among allogeneic bone marrow transplants: a case–control study. Infect Cont 6:347, 1985
7. Fahen PJ, Utell MJ, Hyde RW: Spontaneous lysis of mycetomas after acute cavitating lung disease. Am Rev Resp Dis 123:336, 1981
8. Pennington JE: *Aspergillus* pneumonia in hematologic malignancy: improvements in diagnosis and therapy. Arch Intern Med 137:769, 1977
9. Binder RE, Faling LJ, Pugatch RD, Mahasaen C, Snider GL: Chronic necrotizing pulmonary aspergillosis: a discrete clinical entity. Medicine 61:109, 1982
10. Libshitz HI, Pagoni J: Aspergillosis and mucormycosis: two types of opportunistic fungal pneumonia. Radiology 140:303, 1981
11. Aisner J, Murillo J, Schimpff SC, Steere AC: Invasive aspergillosis in acute leukemia: correlation with nose cultures and antibiotic use. Ann Intern Med 90:4, 1979
12. DeRepentigny L: Serological techniques for diagnosis of fungal infections. Eur J Clin Microbiol Infect Dis 8:362, 1989

Zygomycosis

1. Rinaldi MG: Zygomycosis. Infect Dis Clin N Am 3:19, 1989
2. Lehrer RI, Howard DH, Sypherd PS: Mucormycosis (UCLA Conference). Ann Intern Med 93:93, 1980

3. Mayer RD, Armstrong D: Mucormycosis-changing status. CRC Crit Rev Clin Lab Sci 4;412, 1973
4. Berger CS, Disque FC, Tapazion RG: Rhinocerebral zygomycosis. Diagnosis and treatment. Oral Surg 40:27, 1975
5. Parfrey NA: Improved diagnosis and prognosis of mucormycosis. A clinicopathologic study of 33 cases. Medicine 65:113, 1986
6. Chandler FW, Kaplan W, Ajello L: Atlas and Text of the Histopathology of Mycotic Diseases. Chicago: Year Book, 1980, pp 122–127, 294–301
7. Medoff G, Kobayashi GS: Pulmonary mucormycosis. N Engl J Med 286:86, 1972
8. Mead JH, Lupton GP, Dillavou CL, Odom RB: Cutaneous *Rhizopus* infection: Occurrence as a postoperative complication associated with an elasticized adhesive dressing. J Am Med Assoc 242:272, 1979
9. Bartum RJ Jr, Watnick M, Herman PG: Roentgenographic findings in pulmonary mucormycosis. Am J Roentgenol Radium Ther Nucl Med 117:810, 1973

14

Other Communicable Diseases

Lyme Disease

Theodore F. Tsai

Lyme disease (Lyme borreliosis) is a tickborne bacterial infection caused by the spirochete *Borrelia burgdorferi.*[1,2] An epidemiological investigation of arthritis cases of unknown cause clustered in Lyme, Connecticut, led Steere to suspect a tickborne disease. Clinical features of the illness, usually heralded by a distinctive rash, erythema chronicum migrans (ECM), suggested a relationship to the tickborne eruption known in Europe since early in the century. Laboratory investigations eventually isolated the etiological agent from *Ixodes dammini* ticks, proving the deer tick as the principal vector in the northeastern United States. Lyme disease is a newly recognized but not a new infection in the United States. Genomic sequences of *B. burgdorferi* have been identified by polymerase chain reaction in museum specimens of *I. dammini* collected from Long Island, New York, in the 1940s.

Lyme disease can manifest a broad range of clinical symptoms with acute, subacute, or chronic features. Early localized infection is characterized by an acute or subacute febrile grippe with ECM. Early disseminated infection is manifested by multiple skin lesions, polyarthralgias and polyarthritis, inflammation of the myocardium and cardiac conduction system, or aseptic meningitis and cranial or peripheral polyneuritis. Other organ systems may be involved as well. The infection may become chronic, often with a relapsing and remitting course, leading to erosive arthritis, central and peripheral nervous system symptoms, and acrodermatitis chronica atrophicans (ACA), a destructive dermatological condition. Manifestations of Lyme disease in Europe and the United States qualitatively are similar; however, the frequency of arthritis and ACA are relatively lower in the respective continents. Horses, dogs, cats, and certain wild animals may develop symptomatic infections as well.

The laboratory diagnosis of Lyme disease relies principally upon immunofluorescent and enzyme-linked immunosorbent assay (ELISA) serological tests. *B. burgdorferi* is not readily recovered from blood, cerebrospinal fluid, and skin biopsies. The detection of spirochetes in silver stained tissue specimens requires considerable experience and interpretation, and the sensitivity and specificity of antigen capture ELISA to detect *B. burgdorferi* antigen in urine is unproven. Polymerase chain reaction is a promising approach to direct identification of the spirochete in clinical samples and ticks, but further clinical evaluations are needed.

The sensitivity, specificity, and reproducibility of serological assays for Lyme disease remain in doubt. Several studies indicate the need to standardize reagents and procedures. Improvements will accompany the development of antigens more specific than the whole cell sonicate in common use. Although immunoblotting has been reported to be more sensitive or specific than other serological assays, standardization of antigens and criteria for interpreting Western blots also are needed. Until these issues are resolved, the diagnosis of Lyme disease will rely heavily on clinical and epidemiological criteria, and seroepidemiological studies should be interpreted cautiously.

Treatment with tetracycline, doxycycline, or amoxicillin in early stages of the illness usually prevents progression to chronic symptoms. Parenteral penicillin, ceftriaxone, cefuroxime, chloramphenicol, or doxycycline have been used to treat disseminated and chronic infections.

Lyme disease is recognized throughout Europe, parts of the Soviet Union and China, and in the United States and Canada. Isolates of *Borrelia* closely related to *B. burgdorferi* have been identified in Egypt, and clinical cases of Lyme disease have been reported from Australia. Serological cross reactions with other spirochetes, especially *Borrelia* associated with relapsing fever and certain commensal treponemes, limit the interpretation of seroepidemiological studies.

The epidemiology of Lyme disease reflects the regional ecology of tick vectors in their respective enzootic cycles. The principal tick vectors are members of the *Ixodes ricinus* complex, hard ticks that require relatively moist habitats. On the Eurasian continent, *I. ricinus* and *I. persulcatus,* respectively, are the chief vectors in Europe and Asia. In the United States, *I. dammini* is the principal vector in the Northeast and the Upper Midwest, and *I. pacificus* occupies this role in the Far West (Fig. 14–1). *I. scapularis,* which is not clearly differentiable as a species from *I. dammini,* is the principal vector in the Southeast. Isolated Lyme disease cases have been attributed to infection with *I. angustus. I. dentatus* contributes to enzootic maintenance of the spirochete in nature and probably plays no role in transmission to humans. *Amblyomma americanum* ticks and other blood sucking insects probably occupy minor roles as vectors of Lyme disease.

Lyme disease is now the leading vectorborne disease in the United States (Fig. 14–2). Nationally, reported cases have risen from approximately 500 in 1983 to 7500 cases in 1989. However, the national distribution is far from uniform, with endemic counties located principally in the Northeast, Upper Midwest, and the Pacific Coast (Fig. 14–1). In 1987 to 1988, over 95% of the nation's cases were reported from just nine states (Table

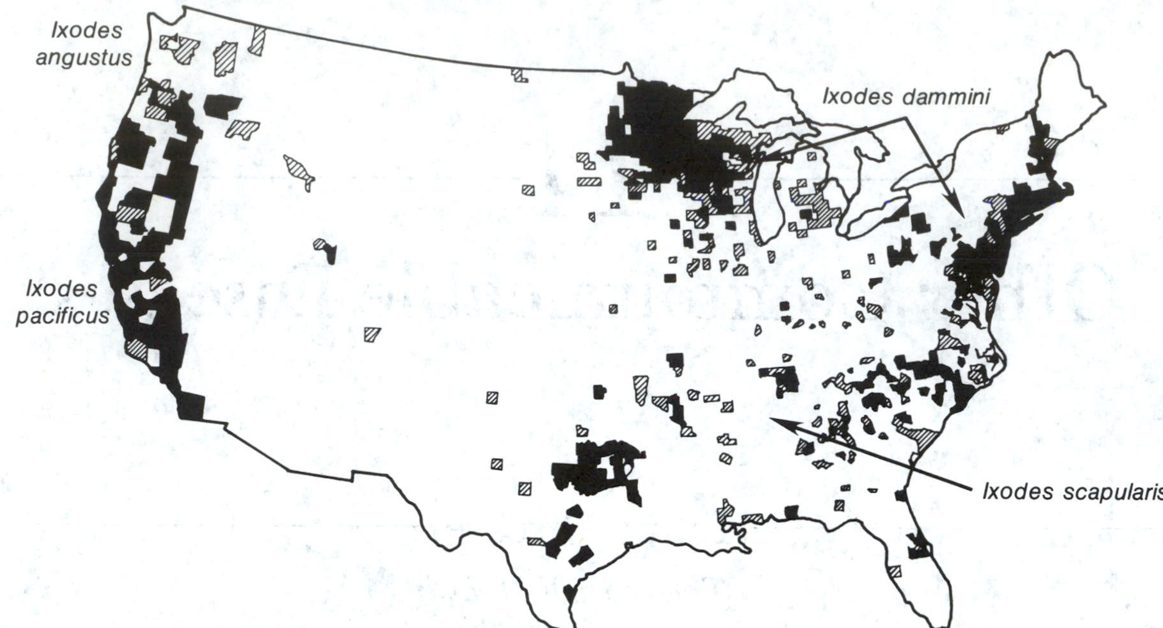

Figure 14-1. County distribution of Lyme disease cases, 1983-1988. The geographic distribution of the principal tick vectors of Lyme disease corresponds roughly to the county distribution of cases.

14-1), and in 1988, New York alone reported 54% of the nation's cases; two suburban New York city counties, Westchester and Suffolk, accounted for 45% of the nation's cases. The public health importance of Lyme disease varies by region. Compared with Rocky Mountain spotted fever, the next most prevalent tickborne infection in the United States, Lyme disease occupies a secondary position in the Southeast and Southwest; in the Plains and Mountain states, Lyme disease remains a rare and possibly misdiagnosed infection (Fig. 14-3).

In the Northeast and Upper Midwest, *B. burgdorferi* is transmitted in *I. dammini* ticks transtadially but not transovarially. Larval ticks emerge in early summer and feed upon small rodents, especially *Peromyscus leucopus,* the white footed mouse, from which they may become infected. The infected larvae overwinter and emerge as infected nymphs from April to July. The nymphs feed on mice, providing the infected reservoir for the next generation of larvae that emerge later in the summer. Nymphs also are the principal vectors transmitting infections to humans. After feeding, the nymphs overwinter and emerge as adults, which feed in the fall principally on deer and large mammals in preparation for egg laying. Adult females also may feed on and transmit infections to humans.

The epidemiological characteristics of cases reflect the circumstances of exposure to infected vectors. The seasonal distribution of cases peaks in May and June, during the period when *I. dammini* nymphs are questing. In the Far West the onset month of cases lacks this distinct peak, reflecting the broader period during which *I. pacificus* ticks are active. The age distribution of cases in the East is bimodal, with the highest risk in children under 15 years and in adults from 35 to 55 years. The sex distribution of cases differs regionally; in the Upper Midwest a slightly higher proportion of cases occurs in males, perhaps reflecting greater outdoor exposure as a risk factor. Certain occupational groups, such as forestry workers, appear to be at high risk in Europe and in China. In the United States the role of outdoor occupation as a risk factor has varied in different regions.

In the northeastern United States, Lyme disease probably is transmitted in a peridomestic setting. Trends toward preserving

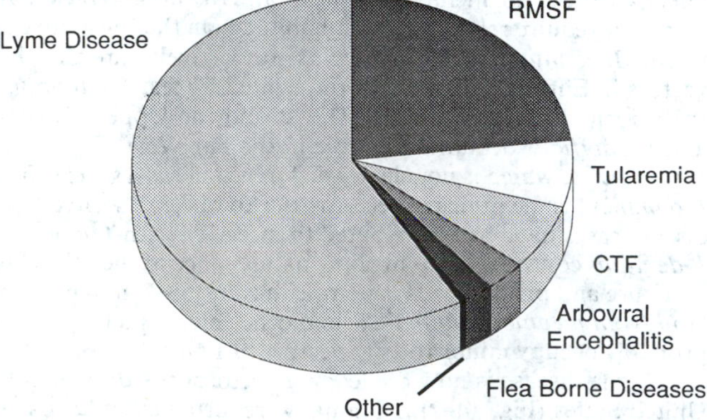

Figure 14-2. Cases of vectorborne infections reported to the CDC, United States, 1983-1988, by etiology. Tickborne diseases now constitute more than 95% of all reported vectorborne infections, and Lyme disease cases account for nearly 60% of the total. RMSF, Rocky Mountain spotted fever; CTF, Colorado tick fever.

TABLE 14-1. STATE REPORTS OF LYME DISEASE IN LEADING 9 STATES 1987-1988

	1987	1988	Total	Average Annual Incidence/100,000
New York	877	2553	3430	9.86
New Jersey	257	550	807	4.93
Wisconsin	358	246	604	6.28
Connecticut	215	362	577	8.98
Pennsylvania	65	306	371	1.55
Rhode Island	74	121	195	9.89
California	182	—*	182	0.66
Massachusetts	95	80	175	1.49
Minnesota	94	67	161	1.90
Subtotal	2217	4285	6502	
National Total	2367	4483	6850	1.42

*unavailable

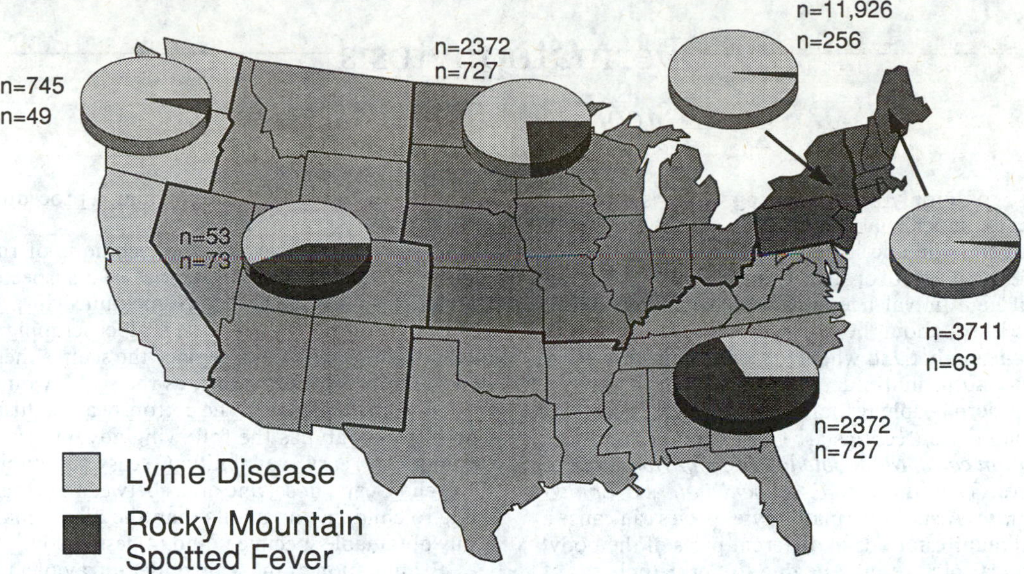

Figure 14–3. Regional incidence of Rocky Mountain spotted fever (RMSF) and Lyme disease, United States 1983–1989. Lyme disease is clearly the most important vectorborne disease in the Northeast, but in the Southeast, RMSF predominates, and even in the Midwest and Mountain states, RMSF remains an important public health concern.

the natural environment and the reversion of agricultural lands to fields and forest have led to unprecedented numbers of white tailed deer, which increasingly are observed in residential locations. In areas where houses are surrounded by dense vegetation or forest, providing suitable habitat for white tailed deer, mice, and vector ticks, all the elements of the transmission cycle are present.

Tickborne diseases are "diseases of place," and people must travel to these often sylvatic locations to encounter ticks and acquire the infections they transmit. Usually these encounters are sporadic, during occupational or avocational activities. In these circumstances, personal protection is the logical approach to prevention. Appropriate dress, the use of repellents, and frequent inspections to remove ticks are practical approaches for a limited period of time (Table 14–2).

In the Northeast the peridomestic environment is the "place" where Lyme disease is transmitted. In these circumstances the possibility of daily and perennial exposure limits the feasibility of personal protective measures. Modifying landscaping to create inhospitable habitats for ticks (e.g., minimizing shaded, heavily vegetated areas) is one approach to prevention.[3] Area application of acaricides such as Dursban to lawns and surrounding areas may be effective if applications are timed with the emergence of nymphs. Evaluations of the effectiveness of Damminix in reducing abundance of *I. dammini* have been inconsistent. A long-term solution to controlling Lyme disease in the peridomestic setting probably will require an integrated approach combining management of vertebrate hosts, ticks, and their environment. A canine vaccine is under evaluation, but for the moment the possibility of a human vaccine is remote.

The use of prophylactic antibiotics after a documented tick bite is controversial. The only controlled study, which was limited by a small sample size, found that side effects of antibiotic prophylaxis in the treated group occurred with the same frequency as Lyme disease in the untreated group. The infection rate in local tick populations, if known, is essential information to guide the decision to use prophylactic antibodies. Infection rates may approach 40% in many areas of the northeast, but infection rates vary widely even in restricted locations.

TABLE 14–2. PERSONAL PROTECTION TO REDUCE THE RISK OF ACQUIRING LYME DISEASE

- Avoid tick-infested areas.
- Open, sunlit, and sparsely vegetated locations are less likely to be infested.
- Wear long pants and overlap socks with pant cuffs.
- Avoid open-toed shoes and sandals.
- Wear light-colored clothing to facilitate identification of attached ticks.
- Inspect clothing and skin frequently (at least daily) to remove attached ticks. Nymphal *I. dammini* are no bigger than a poppy seed and may be difficult to detect.[a]
- Wash clothing and inspect hiking and other equipment after returning from tick-infested areas.
- Use deet-containing repellents on exposed skin; avoid excessive use, and in small children do not use on the hands and face.[b]
- Treat clothing, shoes, and equipment with permethrin (0.5%), an acaricide and repellent.[c]

[a]In animal experiments, deer ticks attached for less than 48 hours were unlikely to transmit infection.
[b]Percutaneous exposure and ingestion of deet have been associated with seizures and other neurological side effects in rare cases.
[c]Permethrin spray (Permanone) is approved for use only in certain states. Check with state environmental agencies.

Dermatophytosis

Stephen A. Billstein

Dermatophytosis, commonly known as ringworm, is a general term used to describe superficial mycotic infections of the dead, cornified layers of the skin and its appendages (hair and nails). These infections are not severe ordinarily and rarely become systemic. Because of high prevalence, however, they are of public health significance throughout the world, especially in areas with a warm, moist environment and where personal hygiene is poor.

Three genera and a multitude of species of fungi, known collectively as the dermatophytes, are the etiological agents of ringworm. Most human infections are caused by the following species: *Microsporum canis, M. audouinii, Trichophyton rubrum, T. mentagrophytes, T. tonsurans, T. schoenleinii,* and *Epidermophyton floccosum.* A single dermatophyte species can cause a variety of clinical manifestations in different parts of the body, and the same clinical picture may be due to dermatophytes of different species and different genera.

Clinical Presentation and Pathogenesis. Clinically, ringworm is classified according to the body area involved. The Latin word *tinea,* meaning gnawing worm, is used with the designated site of infection to describe ringworm of the scalp (tinea capitis), body (tinea corporis), feet (tinea pedis), and so on. It has been postulated that some ringworm strains are more virulent than others. These may occur naturally or may develop selectively whenever better nutrition is afforded by opportunity for invasion deep into the skin or hair follicles. Dermatophytes seek the areas of newly forming keratin deep in the skin or hair follicles for maximum development.

Infection with dermatophytes most often appears on the skin as red, scaly patches. These patches become progressively larger if untreated; the border extends while the center area clears, and this process gives rise to a ringlike, wormy-appearing lesion. Although the fungi invade only the dead, keratinized layers of the skin, hair, and nails, the resulting signs and symptoms—which may include erythema, scaling, and vesiculation—are more than would be expected from such a superficial infection. Much of the disease is a result of the host's reaction to the fungus.

Tinea capitis (ringworm of the scalp) is seen in elementary school epidemics. The usual clinical presentation is hair loss, erythema, and scaling. Pruritus is rare.

Tinea corporis (ringworm of the body) presents with erythematous, scaling, round patches on any part of the body. These annular lesions have a central scaly area and an advancing active periphery, which is usually studded with crusting vesicles and pustules. Most lesions are relatively asymptomatic, although some of them cause itching.

Tinea pedis (athlete's foot) most often presents as scaling or cracking between the toes and vesicular lesions on the soles of the feet. The dorsal areas of the feet are rarely involved at the onset. Poor hygiene, hyperhidrosis, inadequate drying of the feet, and immunoincompetence are factors that contribute to disease. Once infection has been acquired, it may remain throughout life and exhibit periods of exacerbation and remission.

Diagnosis. The existence of these fungal infections is often suspected by the morphology of the individual lesions and their anatomical distribution. A presumptive diagnosis can be made by treating scrapings from skin lesions with a 10% potassium hydroxide solution and examining this preparation under a microscope for the presence of arthrospores or for segmented, branched filaments. Confirmation of the diagnosis is made by culture on Sabouraud's agar medium, a procedure requiring 1 to 4 weeks.

It has been shown that the technique of rubbing a sterile, moist cotton swab over the surface of a suspected ringworm lesion and then onto the culture medium will produce a similar positive yield of cultures as the scalpel scraping technique. This method will probably not replace the scalpel method for potassium hydroxide examinations, as the scales would have to be removed from the fibers of the cotton swab, a difficult procedure. The cotton swab has the following advantages over the scalpel technique: (1) easy availability; (2) easy adaptability to lesions of the eyelids, ears, nose, and areas between the toes; (3) less frightening to children and adults than the blade, making for a more easily obtainable specimen; and (4) less costly.[1]

Examination of the scalp under ultraviolet light (Wood's filter) for yellow-green fluorescence is helpful in diagnosing tinea capitis caused by *M. canis* or *M. audouinii.* Ringworm of the scalp caused by *Trichophyton* species will not show fluorescence.

Tinea pedis, tinea corporis, and tinea unguium are common in patients with human immunodeficiency virus (HIV) disease. Despite being immunocompromised, an inflammatory response to the fungus is often quite pronounced. Therefore, in patients who present with marked inflammatory lesions, which are diagnosed dermatophyte infections, it is prudent to evaluate for an underlying disease such as acquired immunodeficiency syndrome (AIDS), or diabetes mellitus.

Source of Infection. The source of human infections can be infected persons (anthropophilic fungi), infected animals (zoophilic fungi), or soil (geophilic fungi). It is speculated that the dermatophytes arose from two or three related genera among the ascomycetes, which grew as saprophytes in the soil. The initial saprophytic species probably used shed hair and dander as preferential nutritional substrates. From these, other species evolved, which acquired progressively greater pathogenicity and dependence on the living skin of animal hosts until, as in the case of *M. audouinii* and *T. tonsurans,* a high degree of host specificity and an apparently intimate biochemical relationship developed between the parasite and the host.

A multiplicity of sources of dermatophyte infections exists. Fomites such as combs, towels, blankets, and barber shears can disseminate the fungus from the primary source to contacts. Tinea capitis, when caused by *M. canis* or *M. audouinii,* usually has as its source a human or an animal host, especially a dog or kitten. The source of tinea corporis due to *M. canis* is frequently a dog or kitten, but this fungus can also be spread from human to human. In addition, various *Trichophyton* species can cause tinea corporis, and these may be animal or human in origin. Tinea pedis is most often caused by *T. rubrum* or *T. mentagrophytes* in the United States; the source of these fungi can be anthropophilic or geophilic.

Epidemiology. The geographic distribution and the prevalence of dermatophytes are influenced by climate, social and antisocial activities, cultural habits, migrations, and developments in therapy[2–5] and thus are constantly changing. The endemic or most prevalent species of dermatophyte can differ strikingly from one locality to another. Some species are widely distributed, and others have a limited geographic range.

The incidence and distribution of dermatophyte infections by area, season, age, sex, and race have not been well delineated because extensive epidemiological surveys of these infections have not been carried out. Dermatophytoses are not reportable diseases, and most of the available data have been obtained from patients who seek medical care. From these data it has been estimated for developed countries that 5% of patients with dermatological conditions have ringworm, and more than 90% of the male population have had at least a transient ringworm infection by age 40.

Reported epidemics of tinea capitis or corporis occur in school children predominantly. The causative dermatophyte in these outbreaks has most often been *M. canis* or *M. audouinii.* The military is another population group in which ringworm epidemics have been prominent. Soldiers especially are prone to acquisition of these infections in hot, humid climates when hygiene is poor and clothing is inappropriate to climactic conditions.[6] Outbreaks in the military are most often caused by *T. mentagrophytes* or *T. rubrum.*

Prevention and Control. Public health departments usually are not involved in the routine control of dermatophytosis but are frequently called upon when an outbreak is suspected. It is difficult to define an outbreak precisely, however, because the baseline or endemic level of these infections varies greatly by area and population involved.

Outbreaks of tinea pedis (athlete's foot) are rarely related to a common source. Usually, a noticeable increase in cases results from poor hygiene, coupled with hot, humid climatic conditions. Outbreaks most often occur among persons who participate in vigorous sports and among military personnel who have been on training exercises or in combat conditions where personal hygiene and climate control are poor. Efforts to control tinea pedis are primarily directed toward education of the affected population about the need to maintain strict personal hygiene. Careful drying of the toes after bathing and an application of dusting powder containing an effective fungicide will prevent most infections.

In contrast to the treatment of athlete's foot, treatment of tinea capitis or tinea corporis by topical medications is usually ineffective. Topical application medications often misses incubating lesions, which are not easily visible yet are still contagious. Therefore, griseofulvin is the treatment of choice for these infections together with a topical agent.[7] Griseofulvin given orally reaches the epidermal skin within 24 hours and probably renders an individual with contagious ringworm noninfective within 24 to 48 hours. Topical dyes and imidazole derivatives applied to overt lesions will also prevent spread from treated lesions.

Ketoconazole, an orally administered imidazole, has also been used systemically to treat difficult ringworm infections. It has mostly been used when griseofulvin treatment has failed or the patient is unable to take griseofulvin. A topical form of this imidazole is now available.[8]

Outbreaks of tinea capitis or corporis require the identification and treatment of all infections.[9] In responding to these outbreaks, it is important to inspect all contacts of cases diagnosed initially; that includes family and intimate contacts, as well as their environment, to identify and eliminate all possible sources of infection. Identification of the causal dermatophyte species may be useful in directing the search for environmental and animal sources of infection. Some animals, especially kittens, may be inapparent carriers. The public, especially parents, needs to be educated as to the danger of acquiring infection from infected children as well as from dogs, kittens, and other animals.

Immunization against dermatophytoses has been explored with whole mycelium or crude extracts. It is unlikely, however, that effective vaccines for dermatophytoses will ever be developed for general use.

Hookworm Disease: Ancylostomiasis, Necatoriasis, Uncinariasis

L.K. Eveland

Hookworms cause one of the most important diseases of humans in tropical and subtropical climates throughout the world, exacerbating both human misery and economic loss, especially in areas where poverty and unsanitary living conditions prevail. Disease prevalence has decreased in areas such as the United States and Puerto Rico, where improvements in socioeconomic conditions have elevated living standards. Infection leads to an iron-deficiency anemia that further impairs nutrition, thus retarding growth and impairing learning and cognitive development.[1] Hookworms infect nearly one quarter of the world's people, with prevalence estimates between 700,000 and 900,000 per year and deaths between 50,000 and 60,000.[2] This is particularly significant because in endemic areas 60% of the hookworms are harbored by less than 10% of the people, which theoretically should facilitate control.[3] Although frank disease is usually not apparent in well-nourished persons, disease occurs, as a significant amount of protein is lost into the intestinal tract in the form of plasma or tissue protein.[3] Disease manifestations are insidious and have historically been confused with innate shiftlessness.

The Parasites. *Necator americanus* and *Ancylostoma duodenale* are small nematodes, approximately 9 to 13 mm long, with specialized mouthparts resembling teeth or cutting plates for "biting" into the intestinal mucosa. They are the only species that cause hookworm disease in humans, although larvae of zoonotic hookworms cause dermatitis when they migrate through human skin. *N. americanus* and *A. duodenale* differ in their morphology, life cycles, and biology, which has important implications for how they infect and survive in their mammalian hosts and for their control. *A. duodenale* is apparently not as well adapted to its host as *N. americanus.* It is relatively short lived but more pathogenic, as measured by the severity of gastrointestinal symptoms,[4] blood loss, anemia,[5] and its heightened protease profiles.[6] *A. duodenale* increases the probability of contacting its host by producing a greater number of eggs, synchronizing maximal egg output with the season most favorable for free-living development and having robust larvae capable of infecting orally or percutaneously.[7]

Where the two species are found together, their relative abundance varies geographically with host age, sex, and other factors. *N. americanus* coexists with *A. duodenale* in southern India, Burma, Malaysia, the Philippines, Indonesia, Micronesia, Polynesia, and Portuguese West Africa, although it is the predominant species in these areas. In coastal Peru and Chile *A. duodenale* predominates.

A. duodenale is also found in southern Europe, northern coastal Africa, northern India, north China, and Japan. It has been described in native Paraguayan Indians, in the hill tribes of Fukien, China, and in the aborigines of western Australia.[8]

The life cycles of the two species are similar but differ in several important ways that influence their epidemiology, pathogenesis, diagnosis, treatment, and control. The eggs, approximately 60 by 40 μm, are usually at the four- to eight-cell stage of development when they are passed in human feces. If they are deposited in suitable moist, shady, sandy soil, they develop and hatch in 1 or 2 days into first-stage rhabditiform larvae (0.25 to 0.30 mm long by 17 μm wide), which have characteristics that distinguish them from *Strongyloides stercoralis* larvae and free-living larvae such as those of *Rhabditis* species. The rhabditiform larvae grow for 2 or 3 days, feeding on bacteria and organic debris. They then molt into second stage rhabditoid larvae (0.5 to 0.6 mm long), which continue to feed for several days, and then into third stage filariform larvae, which have no mouth opening. The filariform larvae, which infect humans by penetrating the skin, may remain viable in the soil for several weeks under favorable conditions. Both hookworm species are carried to and through the right heart to the lungs, then up the respiratory tree and down the digestive tract into the small intestine, where after a final molt they attach to the mucosa of the jejunum and upper levels of the ileum and develop into sexually differentiated adults. The lung migration is essential for the development of *N. americanus* but not for *A. duodenale.* After the worms reach the intestine, eggs of *N. americanus* usually appear in the feces within 40 to 60 days. *A. duodenale* has a much more variable prepatent period, ranging from 43 to 105 days.[9]

A. duodenale larvae can infect by the oral route and develop into adults without lung passage[10] and probably can also infect by the transplacental route.[1] Although the evidence is indirect, the facts that *A. duodenale* infects nursing infants with no apparent exposure to other routes of infection and that in a number of endemic areas there is a predominance of *A. duodenale* in infants strongly argue for transmammary transmission.[3]

The prepatent period for *A. duodenale* is long because arrested larvae may persist for extended periods in deep tissues.

A. duodenale larvae sequester in the muscles of experimental animals,[11] and at least 28-day-old muscle larvae of *A. caninum* develop to adulthood when fed to dogs.[3] These observations indicate that meatborne *A. duodenale* infection of humans is possible through the ingestion of larvae in paratenic hosts, although no work has been done to explore the actual epidemiological significance of this means of transmission.[3] The duration of infections is highly variable; many worms are eliminated within a year, but records of longevity range from 4 to 20 years for *N. americanus* and 5 to 7 years for *A. duodenale.*[8]

Infection and Disease. The pathogenesis of hookworm disease begins when the larvae enter any portion of the skin with which they make contact, producing a stinging sensation of minor or moderate intensity, depending upon the number of larvae penetrating and the sensitivity of the host. Skin reactions vary from erythematous papules lasting 7 to 10 days to vesiculation and edema.[3] Secondary bacterial infections may also occur, especially if the itching lesions are abraded by scratching. This so-called "ground itch" or "dew itch" must be distinguished from the characteristic "cutaneous larva migrans (CLM)" caused by the zoonotic *Ancylostoma braziliense,* which it may sometimes resemble. CLM is characterized by tortuous inflammatory areas in the dermis associated with swelling, erythema, papular dermatitis, and pruritus. *N. americanus* sometimes migrates in the skin and produces a mild CLM, which is of shorter duration than that caused by *A. braziliense.*[8]

Although migrating hookworm larvae do not usually produce pulmonary symptoms, they do produce minute focal hemorrhages when they break out of pulmonary capillaries and may produce clinical pneumonitis in massive infections. Wakana disease, which has been described in Japan, sometimes results following the ingestion of *A. duodenale* larvae, penetration of the larvae into mucous membranes of the mouth and pharynx, and their migration to the lungs. The initial symptoms that occur shortly after the larvae are ingested are pharyngeal itching, hoarseness, salivation, nausea, and vomiting, followed by an illness of several days duration that includes coughing, dyspnea, wheezing, urticaria, nausea, and vomiting.[3] Infiltrations may be visible on chest x-ray films.[8] Because the disease can be produced by heat-killed organisms, it is presumed to be caused by an allergic reaction to the larvae.[12]

Although light infections are usually asymptomatic, acute, heavy hookworm infections can produce gastrointestinal symptoms similar to those of acute peptic ulcer, which include fatigue, nausea, vomiting, and burning and cramping abdominal pain. Blood eosinophilia occurs, and Charcot-Leyden crystals may be present in the feces. The acute disease occurs more frequently with *A. duodenale* than with *N. americanus.*

As the infection progresses, anemia resulting from chronic blood loss may be accompanied by a loss of appetite and congestive heart failure. Geophagia and pica may develop, with constipation resulting from the dietary change. The worms suck blood, but they actually utilize only 40% of the ingested erythrocytes that pass through their bodies.[13] However, they also spill a significant amount of blood by lacerating the mucosa during feeding.[13,14] Blood loss from mucosal damage increases disproportionately in heavy infections because the worms attach and reattach more frequently because of mating competition, especially early in the infection.[8] The worms also produce an anticoagulant that may enhance the blood loss.[15]

Classic hookworm disease is an iron-deficiency, microcytic, hypochromic anemia resulting directly from blood loss. Intestinal injury and changes in motility might contribute to disordered absorption of nutrients for the host, but hookworm patients usually are no more malnourished than uninfected subjects.[3]

In general, good nutrition consisting of iron, other minerals, and animal protein mitigates the disease associated with light to moderate hookworm infections, even though it does not affect the existing hookworm population or protect an individual from infection. In extremely heavy infections, disease cannot be ameliorated by diet alone. Although the disease is usually associated with heavy infections, it has long been a mystery why it occurs in some persons with only light infections while other persons with extremely heavy infections have no signs or symptoms. The answer appears to lie in the availability of dietary iron stores rather than diet per se,[13] because in hookworm endemic areas dietary intake of iron appears to be generally adequate.[3] It is likely that those more susceptible to disease cannot absorb sufficient iron for reasons unrelated to their hookworm infection, such as concurrent intestinal diseases.[16]

Remote organs may also be indirectly affected by hookworm infection. Thus, chronic anemia of hookworm disease may also be accompanied by increased pulmonary vital capacity, increased tolerance of tissue cells to anoxia, and lowered systolic pressure and peripheral blood flow. The heart may dilate and show increased collateral circulation of coronary arteries with an accompanying decreased risk of myocardial infarction.[8] Changes may occur in bone marrow because of blood loss; retroperitoneal lymph nodes can become enlarged secondary to antigenic stimulation; and the anemia and anoxia of hookworm disease are sometimes associated with fatty deterioration of the heart, liver, and kidneys.[3]

Infections that produce more than 5000 eggs per gram (EPG) of feces are considered heavy; 2000 to 5000 EPG, moderately heavy; 500 to 2000 EPG, moderately light; and less than 500 EPG, light. Light infections are usually not of clinical grade, but medium and heavy infections are often associated with significant anemia. Diagnosis is complicated in early infections because hookworm anemia may actually begin before eggs are detectable, when larval and immature hookworms first reach the mucosa and begin to cause blood loss.[1] Hookworm disease should be suspected in a person with a subnormal hemoglobin level, Charcot-Leyden crystals in the feces, and a history of exposure. Although heavy infections may be detected by direct fecal smears, in light infections (< 500 EPG of feces), concentration techniques are usually needed to demonstrate the eggs. Several excellent concentration methods are available, including zinc flotation and several modifications of formalin-ether and formalin-ethyl acetate techniques. Unless anemia is present or the intake of dietary iron is inadequate, light infections are usually not treated. Hookworm eggs may develop and hatch in fecal specimens stored for more than 24 hours at room temperature or above. It is then necessary to distinguish the rhabditiform larvae from those of free-living nematodes and *Strongyloides stercoralis.*

Epidemiology. The most favorable conditions for the development of hookworm larvae and completion of the life cycle include loose, moist, shady, sandy humus, promiscuous defecation or the use of improperly treated human feces (night soil) as fertilizer, and the opportunity for humans to come into contact with the soil. An important epidemiological factor appears to be the presence of dung beetles that thrive in such soil and bury human feces efficiently.[8] Rainfall is required to provide adequate moisture for the larvae to migrate, aggregate, and reach human skin on grass or other moist surfaces. Temperature is an important factor in determining which species of hookworm is found, because *A. duodenale* withstands colder temperatures than *N. americanus,* which conversely can tolerate much higher temperatures than *A. duodenale.* The infective larvae may remain viable in the soil for months during periods of drought or low temperatures.

White males are much more susceptible to infection than females or nonwhites, and it has been suggested that heavily infected persons are genetically predisposed to such levels of infection.[17] For epidemiological purposes the amount of hookworm disease in a community depends on both the prevalence and intensity of infection, as measured by egg output.[3] However, people who contribute large numbers of eggs to the environment are not necessarily those who are the greatest source of infection for others, because infective larvae show a high degree of aggregation in the soil.[18]

Prevention and Control. Theoretically, hookworm disease could be reduced by the sanitary disposal of human feces, wearing shoes and protective clothing, the use of ovicides or larvicides, vaccines, and adequate chemotherapy for mass therapy or individual use. However, the mere availability of properly constructed sanitary latrines does not assure their use, as local habits, customs, or beliefs regarding hygiene may be major obstacles.[3] It has been demonstrated that children, and to a lesser extent adults, fail to use sanitary facilities when present but prefer the convenience of defecating among bushes in backyards or nearby fields.[19] Shoes and protective clothing are not a reasonable expectation because they are expensive, difficult to clean, and can be extremely uncomfortable in hot weather. Health education should encourage people to defecate where free-living stages cannot develop or survive, such as on saline soils, open, dry, fallow land, or in flooded fields.[3]

At present no effective vaccines are available. Although there is little direct evidence that protective immunity to hookworm develops in humans, epidemiological evidence suggests the possibility. A cDNA clone encoding a specific antigenic protease may be a candidate immunogen in human beings.[3]

In general, only persons at highest risk for disease as determined by egg output and iron-deficiency anemia should be treated. Little benefit is gained from treating individuals with light infections in endemic areas, as reinfection commonly occurs in such foci. Persons who return from endemic areas to good sanitary conditions and adequate nutrition may not require treatment.[3]

Thiabendazole is larvicidal, and mebendazole is ovicidal and larvicidal. Albendazole kills both preintestinal and intestinal worms, but it is not known whether it affects arrested larvae of *A. duodenale.*[3] Bephenium hydroxynaphthoate is effective against *A. duodenale,* and also against *N. americanus* when combined with tetrachlorethylene, although the latter is difficult to obtain for human use in the United States. Tetrachlorethylene is effective when used alone in higher doses but should not be used if *Ascaris* worms are present. Pyrantel pamoate is useful against both species and is useful for combined infections with *Ascaris.*

The objective of control actions should be to lower the intensity of the infection, which will reduce morbidity and gradually disrupt transmission. To achieve this objective further research is needed in (1) development of species- and stage-specific diagnostic tests, (2) investigation of the consequences of arrested development of hookworms, (3) study of hookworm transmission in various regions in the context of varied cultural factors, (4) quantification of the effects of morbidity on individuals and communities, (5) investigation of the relationships between hookworm disease and human nutrition, (6) elucidation of the human host response to infection, and (7) the search for potential vaccines.[1]

Schistosomiasis

S.Y.Li Hsü

Schistosomiasis or bilharziasis, a chronic debilitating disease with significant morbidity and some mortality, affects more than 200 million people in the endemic area world-wide. It is one of the main occupational risks encountered in rural areas in developing countries and is second only to malaria in tropical and subtropical areas in socioeconomic and public health importance.[1] The disease is caused by blood flukes—the *Schistosoma. S. japonicum, S. mansoni,* and *S. haematobium* are the three species of importance for humans.

Biology and Life Cycles. The schistosome requires an intermediate and a definitive host to complete its life cycle. Asexual multiple reproduction takes place in the molluscan intermediate host and sexual reproduction in the definitive vertebrate host. The mature female measures from 7.2 to 26 mm in length and 0.25 to 0.5 mm in width, whereas the mature male measures from 6.5 to 20 mm in length and 0.5 to 1 mm in width. They remain in copula for their entire lifespan, an average of 5 to 8 years, but sometimes as long as 30 years. The main habitat of *S. japonicum* is the superior mesenteric vein but may extend farther in the vascular system; *S. mansoni,* the inferior mesenteric vein; and *S. haematobium,* the vesical and pelvic venous plexuses. The differences in their main habitat may be partially due to their different capacities for production of eggs. A preferred specific site would be necessary to facilitate distribution or evacuation of eggs to maintain their life cycles. The daily egg production of *S. japonicum* is 1500 to 3000, that of *S. mansoni* 300, and that of *S. haematobium* approximately 50. Eggs of *S. japonicum* are globular in shape, without spines; *S. mansoni,* oval with a lateral spine; and *S. haematobium,* oval with a terminal spine. The eggs are deposited in the venules of the intestine or urinary bladder, break through the submucosa and mucosa into the lumen, and are evacuated through the feces or urine. Free-swimming miracidia hatch from eggs in the water, penetrate the appropriate snail host, and develop into mother sporocysts, which produce multiple daughter sporocysts. Each of the daughter sporocysts produces a great number of cercariae. The fork-tailed cercariae propel themselves toward the surface of the water. When humans contact the infested water, cercariae penetrate the skin, lose their tails, and are transformed into schistosomula. They then enter a venule or lymphatic vessel and migrate to the right side of the heart, then to the lungs, and thence to the liver sinusoids, where they begin to mature. On reaching maturity they pair and migrate to their final habitats, where the eggs are released and the life cycle is repeated.

Distribution. Schistosomiasis is endemic in many tropical and subtropical countries. The distribution is dependent on the existence of the appropriate snail host and necessary environmental conditions. The intermediate snail host of *S. japonicum* is amphibious, *Oncomelania* spp.; of *S. mansoni* is aquatic, *Biomphalaria* spp. and *Tropicorbis* spp.; and of *S. haematobium* is aquatic, *Bulinus* spp., *Planorbatius metidjensis,* or the limpet, *Ferrisia tenuis. S. japonicum* is confined to the Far East, distributed in parts of China, Malaysia, Indonesia, the Philippines, and to a smaller extent, Japan.[2] Among the three species, *S. mansoni* has the most widespread distribution, ranging from the Arabian peninsula to South America and the Caribbean. *S. haematobium* is endemic in the Middle East and Africa. The important reservoir hosts for *S. japonicum* are mice, dogs, goats, rabbits, cattle, sheep, rats, pigs, horses, and buffalo.[3] In *S. mansoni* and *S. haematobium,* human infection is almost exclusively derived from human sources, although natural infection of *S. mansoni* has been found in monkeys and baboons and of *S. haematobium* has been found in monkeys, baboons, and chimpanzees.[2]

Treatment. Three drugs commonly used against schistosomiasis in humans are praziquantel, oxamniquine, and metrifonate. Praziquantel, a heterocyclic pyrazino-isoquinoline, is the drug of choice, effective against all species of schistosomes. No mutagenic, carcinogenic, embryotoxic, or teratogenic activity has been established. It is the drug with the least side effects for *S. japonicum* infections. Three doses of 20 mg/kg given at 4-hour intervals are recommended.[1,4] A single dose of praziquantel of 40 mg/kg is recommended for *S. mansoni* or *S. haematobium.*[1,4] In certain areas where *S. mansoni* or mixed infections are prevalent, a dose of 60 mg/kg may be required. The drug is well tolerated, since even advanced hepatosplenic schistosomiasis has been successfully treated without adverse side-effects.[5] Oxamniquine, a tetrahydroquinoline, is active only against *S. mansoni.* For the strain of South American origin, a single dose of 15 mg/kg is adequate for adults, and two doses of 10 mg/kg once daily are recommended for children.[1,4] For the strain of African origin a total dose of 30 to 60 mg/kg given over 2 to 3 consecutive days is required, dependent upon the specific geographic area. Metrifonate,[1,4] an organophosphorus ester, is active only against *S. haematobium.* Three doses of 7.5 mg to 10 mg/kg given at 2-week intervals are required.[1,4] Side effects of the above three drugs are transient and mild and include abdominal discomfort, diarrhea, headache, dizziness, and drowsiness. However, changes of electroencephalograms (EEG), electrokymograms, and hepatic enzyme have occasionally been observed with oxamniquine treatment.[4]

Diagnosis. Definite diagnosis is made by identifying characteristic eggs in the stool or urine sample, or by tissue biopsy. Samples taken at three different times should be examined carefully before a negative report is given. Concentration techniques should be employed for all urine and stool specimens. For detection of eggs in the stool, sedimentation and hatching methods are commonly used. The quantitative Kala (cellophane) thick fecal smear is used to evaluate intensity of infection.[6] It has become a standard diagnostic tool in epidemiology for international comparison of data.[1] The filtration technique is a good method for detecting eggs in urine and providing quantitative data on the intensity of infection. Samples are passed through polycarbonate[7] or polyamide fibers[8] by pumps or syringe. Eggs collected on the filters are then counted. If eggs cannot be found in a chronic symptomatic case, a rectal biopsy snip should be employed.[6] The tissue sample is pressed between two glass slides and examined by light microscopy.

When eggs cannot be demonstrated in the excreta, serology and skin testing may have to depend on determining positive cases in early infection such as Katayama disease, late chronic infection, or in ectopic schistosomiasis. Immunological tests are available but generally are nonspecific and cannot differentiate simple infection from those with complications. Indirect immunofluorescence (IFAT), enzyme-linked immunosorbent assay (ELISA), and the circumoral precipitin test (COPT) are commonly used. ELISA is particularly useful in epidemiological studies.[1] The ELISA test with egg antigen has been recently reported to be highly sensitive and specific in cases with hepatosplenomegaly.[9] In addition, radiological investigation and ultrasonography can provide valuable aids to diagnosis.[10]

Pathological and Clinical Manifestations. Most of the pathological changes and clinical manifestations of schistosomiasis result from the host's immunological response to schistosomula, adult worms, and especially the eggs. The severity of the disease depends on the species, strain, location of parasites, intensity and duration of infection, frequency of reinfection, and the host's reactivity. Mild infections without symptoms often occur. The course of infection may be divided into four progressive stages: invasion, maturation, established infection, and chronic infection with its attendant complications.

In the invasion stage, papular dermatitis may occur upon cercarial penetration of the skin of the sensitized host. Petechial hemorrhages, foci of eosinophilia, and leukocytic infiltration may be produced in the lung or in the liver when schistosomula migrate through the lungs and reach the liver. During this period, transitional symptoms of fever, malaise, cough and a generalized allergic reaction may appear. The syndromes are induced by secretions, excretions, and breakdown products of cercariae and schistosomula.[11]

Active schistosomiasis starts with worm maturation and the beginning of egg production. Severe cases of active schistosomiasis known as Katayama fever are not uncommon in *S. japonicum* or after heavy *S. mansoni* infection. Chills, fever, headache, dermatitis, eosinophilia, hepatosplenomegaly, generalized lymphadenopathy, and gastrointestinal discomfort are the common symptoms.[11] Recovery usually occurs several weeks later, but there are some fatalities. The syndromes probably result from strong host immune responses to large amounts of antigenic materials which are suddenly released from schistosome worms and eggs.[12]

In the established stage, intense egg deposition and excretion take place. Eggs are primarily responsible for the pathological changes. Eggs of *S. japonicum* and *S. mansoni* secrete proteolytic enzymes that erode the tissue, break through the intestinal wall, and cause diarrhea and blood in the stool. In a similar fashion, eggs of *S. haematobium* break through the bladder and cause dysuria, urinary frequency, and hematuria. Other eggs may be trapped at the original site or swept back into the bloodstream and distributed to the liver, spleen, or other ectopic foci, where they provoke an inflammatory tissue response and granuloma formation. This may cause thrombosis of vessels, formation of papillomas in the intestinal and bladder wall, or enlargement of the liver and spleen. The severity of disease is closely correlated with the schistosome's capacity for egg production and the location of the egg in the body. The eggs of *S. japonicum* and *S. mansoni* are primarily deposited in the mesenteric lymph nodes, the intestine, and also in the liver, causing both gastrointestinal and hepatosplenic schistosomiasis. Of the three species, *S. japonicum* has the highest capacity for egg production and widest egg distribution, resulting in severe and disseminated disease. In *S. mansoni* infection the rectum and colon are affected more than other parts of the gastrointestinal tract. The eggs of *S. haematobium* are deposited in the vesicle plexus, causing primarily vesicle schistosomiasis, with lesions in the urinary bladder, genitalia, and to a lesser extent in the colon.

The chronic stage with its attendant complication is generally observed only in heavy infection.[13,14] It develops gradually with an increase of granulomatous formation, fibrous proliferation, and vascular obliteration. Fibrosis induced by the granulomatous immunoreaction around the eggs is responsible for most of the pathological changes and clinical manifestations seen in this stage.

In intestinal schistosomiasis, fibrous sandy patches, polyps, thickening of the intestinal wall and adhesions of the thickened mesentery and omentum to the intestine may occur.[15,16] Complications include secondary bacterial infection and intestinal obstruction. In hepatosplenic schistosomiasis the liver gradually shrinks with increasing fibrosis. Symmers' pipe-stem fibrosis develops around the periportal tract.[17,18] Pylethrombophlebitis, with or without eggs, and vascular fibrotic lesions are commonly seen. Many small branches of portal veins are obstructed by egg emboli and associated fibrosis. Larger veins may be occasionally found to be occluded by granulomatous formation around disintegrated dead worms. These changes may result in blockage of portal blood flow, leading to presinusoidal hypertension, hepatosplenomegaly, portosystemic collateral circulation, ascites, and esophageal varices.[11,15,16]

Pulmonary schistosomiasis can be observed in all three species of schistosome infection. Eggs may be carried to the lungs because of occasional migration of worms into the vena caval or vertebrate venous systems or by a systemic collateral circulation developed in chronic cases of *S. japonicum* and *S. mansoni* infection.[2] This results in fibrosis of the pulmonary capillary bed and leads to obliterative arteriolitis, pulmonary hypertension, and in some cases, cor pulmonale with right-sided heart failure.[19]

In urinary schistosomiasis, fibrosis and calcification of the eggs in the urinary bladder may impair bladder function. Fibrosis of the neck of the bladder and opening of the ureter result in obstruction of urine flow and may lead to the development of hydroureter and hydronephrosis or even uremia. Chronic ulceration and irritation of the bladder epithelium lead to formation of polyps, which may in time undergo malignant changes.[20]

In cerebrospinal schistosomiasis, ectopic eggs may cause granuloma formation in the central nervous system, resulting in focal damage.[21] *S. japonicum* often involves the brain, manifested as jacksonian epilepsy.[21] *S. mansoni* and *S. haematobium* often affect the spinal cord, causing myelitis.[22]

Schistosomiasis Dermatitis. Schistosomiasis dermatitis, the "swimmer's itch,"[23] is caused by infection with the avian or mammalian schistosome. The penetration and the death of cercariae in the skin provoke consecutive dermal inflammatory reactions including both humoral-mediated immediate hypersensitivities and cell-mediated delayed hypersensitivity with manifestation of urticarial wheal, macule, and pruritus. These symptoms last about 1 week. The severity of the symptoms increases with the frequency of reinfection.

Control and Prevention. Control and prevention of schistosomiasis are among the most complex problems in public health. Success in control depends on having a well-organized program based on a profound understanding of the epidemiology of the disease, the biology, ecology, and distribution of the parasite intermediate snail-host, and the geographic characteristics of the environment. It is also important to have sound knowledge of local socioeconomic conditions, support from health authorities, and cooperation of the communities.

Molluscicidal application, environmental modification, biological competition, chemotherapy, sanitation, and education are fundamental measures for schistosomiasis control.[1] For the most successful program an integrated method should be used. The particular combination of measures must be determined by local conditions and available resources. There are two essential approaches in reaching the optimal level of control: one emphasizes an interruption of transmission by eradication of snail hosts, and the other emphasizes reduction of prevalence and morbidity in the human population through chemotherapy.[24]

In snail control, molluscicidal, environmental, and biological methods have been used. Molluscicides provide a rapid and effective means of reducing the snail population and decreasing disease transmission. A suitable molluscicide must be safe and nontoxic to mammals and aquatic organisms, stable in storage, and simple to apply. Niclosamide and certain other amide compounds are the best choices. Natural molluscicides of plant origin have also been used in some countries.[25,26] Application of molluscicides must be planned according to the focal and seasonal patterns of disease transmission.

Long-lasting effects in the reduction of snail populations can be achieved by environmental modifications, such as the installation of overhead sprinklers and trickle-type irrigation systems, modification of canal design, alteration of water level, or lining of canals with cement. In addition, simple methods such as weed control and draining of unused standing water can also decrease the snail population. Biological snail control methods are still in experimental stages, and none has reached large-scale field trials. Fish, insects, and molluscan competitors have been studied in sufficient detail to be considered for use as biological control agents.[27]

Chemotherapy plays a key role in schistosomiasis control. It not only decreases morbidity and prevalence of disease but also reduces transmission. The three drugs—praziquantel, metrifonate, and oxamniquine—are primarily for large-scale chemotherapy in a schistosomiasis control program.[1] Selection of a chemotherapeutic agent, correct dosage, and frequency and timing of administration, must be carefully determined. The scope of treatment depends on local prevalence and available resources. Ideally, all positive cases would be treated to achieve maximal reduction of disease transmission.

Sanitation and water supply are important issues in an integrated schistosomiasis control program. Provision of improved latrines may protect snail-bearing waters from contamination with infectious human wastes. Installation of safe water systems may curtail the domestic use of contaminated water. Thus, both transmission and prevalence can be decreased. With respect to using the night soil as fertilizer, it is necessary to store the soil long enough to kill the eggs or to disinfect it with ammonium nitrate before the material is spread on the fields.

Health education is an integral part of any successful schistosomiasis control program. Schistosomiasis is a human-made disease. It is necessary that people learn to protect themselves from contact with infested water, to avoid polluting water sources, and to understand the importance of early diagnosis and treatment so that they willingly change their behavior and actively participate in the community control program.

The elimination of schistosomiasis through multiple measures, with emphasis on interruption of transmission and snail eradication, has been used for the last 4 decades. It has been successful in certain countries such as Japan[2] and large parts of China[3] but has proved to be beyond the resources of many endemic areas.[1] A new program for schistosomiasis control, by reducing morbidity and prevalence of the disease implemented through a primary health care unit, has been recommended by the World Health Organization. This approach emphasizes chemotherapeutic treatment of the population in combination with auxiliary measures of molluscicide use and improvements in sanitation, water supply, and education.[1,24] Successful short-term control has been reportedly achieved with this program in some endemic areas.[28-32] However, reinfection generally occurs. Even a small residual egg output can sustain disease transmission if the snail population is not controlled. A continuing schedule of screening and retreatment is required. Once prevalence has been reduced to the targeted level, a maintenance program is necessary to sustain it. Furthermore, long-term side effects (if any) of receiving repeated drug treatment and the possibility of producing drug resistance need to be considered.

Indeed, schistosomiasis control is extremely difficult and requires a continuous, concerted effort with a long-term full commitment at both the national and local levels. To facilitate control of the disease, a vaccine which could be used as an auxiliary measure is clearly needed. Since the discovery in 1961 of the use of cercariae of the nonhuman strain of *S. japonicum* as an immunizing agent against a challenge infection of human strain in Rhesus monkeys,[33] great effort has been expended in the study of schistosome immunity and vaccine development. A highly irradiated schistosome organism live vaccine has been developed through investigation of laboratory attenuation of cercariae by exposure to radiation.[34,35] This live vaccine can induce a strong acquired resistance in the skin and causes no significant lesions in the lungs or liver.[36] The immune effector mechanisms against schistosomiasis in skin have been documented.[37-40] Field trials in animals have been carried out in China, where the snail is difficult to control, and cattle and water buffaloes are major reservoirs of infection. Acquired resistance after vaccination was found to be as high as 75%.[41] If this vaccine was in use as a control measure in cattle, it could decrease the transmission rate in humans. Human trials with this vaccine have not been attempted. In recent years, several protective immunogens have been isolated.[4] It is hoped that based upon the knowledge of the effector mechanism obtained from the live vaccine, a defined vaccine against schistosomiasis for human use may be achieved in the near future.[42-44]

Personal protective measures against the disease require avoidance of contact with cercariae-contaminated water used for bathing, wading, washing, swimming, working, and drinking. People who must work with fresh water can be partially protected from infection by repellants, rubber boots, gloves, clothes, and so on. Repellants containing dibutylphthalate and benzylbenzoate as principal agents with turpentine as the base have been used with success. Wrapping the feet with cloth or puttees smeared with powdered *Thea oleosa* fruits may protect an individual from cercariae for 8 hours.[25]

For preventing the spread of schistosomiasis to uninfected areas before any water source development schemes begin, a proper design and management practice, planned by a panel of experts including an epidemiologist, ecologist, biologist, engineer, and public health official should be developed. The entire population including the new migrants should be screened and treated. Furthermore, a preventive measure strategy should be adopted for regulating any existing impoundment, and the use of land around it.[1] Prevention of the spread of the disease is essential in schistosomiasis control.

Toxic Shock Syndrome

Arthur L. Reingold
Lauri E. Markowitz

Toxic shock syndrome (TSS) is an acute multisystem illness due to infection with *Staphylococcus aureus*. Although TSS has occurred in association with a wide variety of different kinds of *S. aureus* infections, most reported cases have occurred in previously healthy young women who were menstruating and using tampons at the time of onset of illness. TSS has been categorized into menstrual and nonmenstrual cases for epidemiological purposes, but the clinical picture, microbiology, and treatment are similar in these groups.

Clinical Findings. Symptoms of TSS include fever, chills, vomiting, myalgias, dizziness, and diarrhea. Typically, onset is abrupt. On physical examination, patients have fever, hypotension, and rash. The rash has been described as a diffuse, sunburnlike erythroderma of the face and trunk. Oropharyngeal erythema, conjunctival injection, vaginal hyperemia, and muscle tenderness are common findings, and vaginal ulceration and discharge may also be present. Desquamation usually occurs 1 to 3 weeks after the acute illness and can be generalized or localized to the face or palms and soles, particularly around nailbeds. In nonmenstrual cases associated with *S. aureus* surgical wound infections the wound frequently does not display local signs of infection such as redness, tenderness, or drainage. Laboratory findings in patients with TSS may include leukocytosis, lymphocytopenia, thrombocytopenia, abnormal liver and renal function tests, hypocalcemia, hypophosphatemia, sterile pyuria, and proteinuria. The case-fatality rate for TSS is in the range of 3% to 5%. When death occurs, it is usually due to respiratory failure or irreversible hypotension.

The diagnosis of TSS is based on clinical criteria because a sensitive and specific laboratory test does not yet exist. According to the revised case definition the criteria for a definite case include high fever, a characteristic rash, evidence of hypotension, and subsequent desquamation of the rash.[1] In addition, there must be evidence of involvement of at least three organ systems. If tests for other illness such as Rocky Mountain spotted fever, leptospirosis, or rubeola are performed, the results must be negative. Because the criteria for inclusion as a case are strict, confusion of TSS with diseases that resemble it is unlikely. Patients whose illnesses meet the current case definition are usually severely ill and generally require hospitalization. It is clear that a much wider spectrum of clinical presentations of TSS exists, however, and that milder cases occur; their identification and characterization await development of a diagnostic laboratory test.

History. TSS is believed to be the same clinical entity as staphylococcal scarlet fever, cases of which have been reported in the medical literature since 1927.[2] Todd and associates introduced the name TSS in 1978 when they reported a series of seven children, aged 8 to 17 years, with high fever, erythroderma, hypotension, and renal and hepatic abnormalities, associated with infection with phage group I *S. aureus*.[3] TSS rose from being a disease of relative obscurity to one of notoriety when, in late 1979 and early 1980, an increasing number of cases were reported and it was recognized that most of these cases were occurring in young menstruating women.

A number of epidemiological studies performed in 1980 and 1981 showed that the use of tampons was associated with an increased risk of developing menstrual TSS.[4-8] In addition, four studies showed that a particular brand of tampons, when compared with other tampons, was associated with the highest risk of developing tampon-associated menstrual TSS,[4-6,9] and one study showed that the risk of developing tampon-associated menstrual TSS was related to the absorbency and chemical composition of tampons.[6] As a result, in September 1980 the manufacturer of the tampon brand that was particularly implicated voluntarily withdrew this product from the market. Later studies suggested that the increased risk of menstrual TSS among tampon users persisted and was associated with higher absorbency tampons.[10-11] As a result, the manufacturers of other brands began altering the chemical composition and reducing the absorbency of the tampons they produced. The absorbency of currently available tampons is approximately half that of tampons sold in 1980 to 1981.[12] Although cases of TSS continue to occur (Fig. 14-4) and use of currently available tampons continues to be associated with an increased risk of TSS, the number of cases reported annually has dropped. In addition, evidence from studies employing active surveillance or case detection methods suggests that the incidence of hospitalization for TSS associated with menstruation has, in fact, dropped substantially since 1980.[12-13]

Epidemiology. As of September 1989, over 2900 cases of TSS meeting the strict criteria had been reported to the Centers for Disease Control (CDC) as having occurred in the United States. Overall, 78% have been associated with menstruation; 19% have not been associated with menstruation; and in 3% the menstrual status was unknown. Of the reported menstrual cases, 99% have occurred in tampon users, whereas only 60% to 70% of menstruating women in the United States use tampons. The percentage of reported cases not associated with menstruation has increased from 7% in 1980, to 19%, 28%, 36%, and 41% in 1981–82, 1983–84, 1985–86, and 1987–88, respectively. The incidence of menstrual TSS in 1980 was estimated to be approximately 5 to 10 cases per 100,000 menstruating women per year.[7] Studies from several areas in the United States suggest that the incidence of menstrual TSS currently is in the range of 1 to 1 1/2 cases per 100,000 menstruating women.[12,14] Patients with menstrual TSS have ranged from 11 to 60 years of age, but almost 60% have been between the ages of 15 and 24; 98% have been white.

Patients with TSS not associated with menstruation have ranged from less than 1 to 80 years of age. Although reported menstrual cases have been primarily in whites, the racial distribution of patients with nonmenstrual TSS more closely reflects the racial distribution of the U.S. population. Of the nonmenstrual cases, 35% have occurred in men and boys. When the postpartum and nonmenstrual vaginal cases are excluded, there is only a slight female predominance.

The largest proportion of nonmenstrual cases, about one third, have occurred in association with nonsurgical cutaneous and subcutaneous *S. aureus* infections, such as abscesses, furuncles, infected burns, and insect bites. In addition, TSS cases have occurred in postpartum women, associated with either vaginal infection, mastitis, or infection of cesarean-section site, and in postoperative patients, associated with *S. aureus* surgical wound infections. Nonmenstrual TSS also has occurred in association with *S. aureus* infections at various body sites, and cases have been reported to develop coincident with or following diaphragm and contraceptive sponge use.

In the United States, cases have occurred in all states. While a disproportionate percentage of the cases reported in 1980 and 1981 were from a small number of states (Wisconsin, Minnesota, Utah, Colorado, and California), it is unknown to what extent this pattern reflected true geographic differences in incidence as opposed to increased surveillance activity in these states. However, studies employing active surveillance or review of hospital discharge records suggest that regional variation in the incidence of TSS is not entirely due to differences in diagnosis and reporting of cases.[14-15] Cases outside the United States have occurred in Canada, Europe, Israel, South Africa, Australia, New Zealand, and Japan. Most of the cases reported from outside the United States also have occurred in young menstruating women who were using tampons.

Possible risk factors for menstrual TSS, other than factors related to tampon use, have been evaluated in several epidemiological studies. None of the other factors examined, including sexual activity, duration and quantity of menstrual flow, bathing or physical activity during menstruation, douching, or use of vaginal deodorants, were found to be associated with an increased risk of menstrual TSS. An early finding that use of oral contraceptives may decrease the risk of menstrual TSS could not be substantiated in a later study.[11]

Bacteriology and Pathogenesis. Much research has been directed at characterizing TSS-associated *S. aureus* strains. Most *S. aureus* strains isolated from TSS patients are phage group I, with phage types 29 and 52 predominating.[16]

Because the clinical features of TSS, particularly the lack of bacteremia in most cases, suggest a toxin-mediated mechanism, attempts have been made to identify one or more toxins responsible for TSS. Substantial evidence now exists that toxic shock syndrome toxin-1 (TSST-1), an extracellular protein produced by *S. aureus,* can produce many, if not all, the signs and symp-

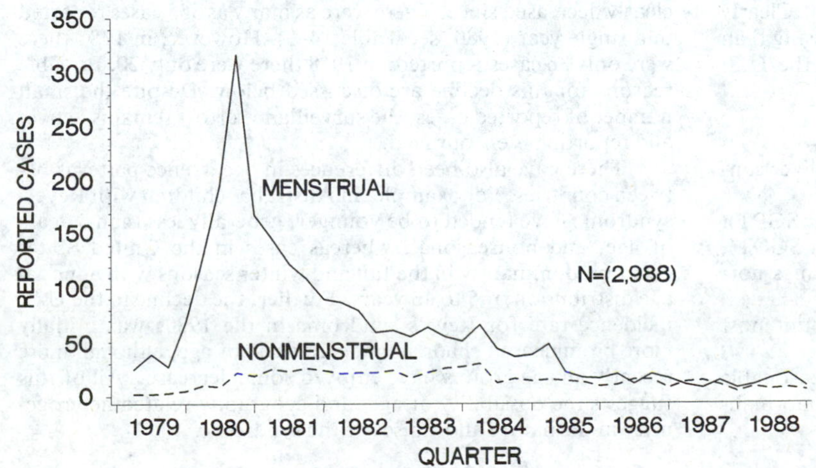

Figure 14-4. Toxic shock syndrome by quarter, United States, 1979 to 1988 (includes only cases meeting the CDC case definition).

toms of TSS. Of the many *S. aureus* strains from women with menstrual TSS studied, 90% to 100% make TSST-1, compared with only 10% to 30% of non-TSS associated strains.[17] Purified TSST-1 has been shown to have a variety of biological properties, many mediated by interleukin-1, and in vivo animal studies, have shown that it can produce a TSS-like illness in rabbits.[18-19] However, only 60% to 70% of *S. aureus* strains recovered from normally sterile sites in patients with nonmenstrual TSS make TSST-1, strongly suggesting that one or more other staphylococcal products can produce a similar or identical clinical illness.[20] Staphylococcal enterotoxin B has been proposed as the responsible toxin in many of these cases.[21]

In addition to characteristics of *S. aureus* strains, host factors and interactions between tampons and *S. aureus* have been studied. There is evidence that patients with TSS lack preexisting antibody to TSST-1, suggesting that host susceptibility may be important. In menstrual TSS the role of the materials used to manufacture tampons has been investigated both in the laboratory and in epidemiological studies. The epidemiological studies suggest that the chemical composition of tampons has an effect on the risk of developing menstrual TSS that is independent of the tampon's absorbency.[10] At the same time, laboratory studies have demonstrated that various tampons and their constituents have markedly different effects on the production of TSST-1 by *S. aureus* in vitro.[22] Some of these studies also suggest that binding of magnesium by tampons and resultant changes in available magnesium may play a role in regulating TSST-1 production.[23]

Therapy and Prevention. Therapy for TSS should be directed at correcting hemodynamic, electrolyte, and acid-base abnormalities. Correction of hypovolemia with intravenous fluids and, when necessary, maintenance of blood pressure with vasopressors are the mainstays of treatment. Supportive measures for complications such as renal failure or adult respiratory distress syndrome are also required in some cases. Antimicrobial therapy directed against *S. aureus,* such as a β-lactamase-resistant penicillin, cephalosporin, or vancomycin, is recommended. Although there is no evidence that antimicrobial therapy shortens or ameliorates the acute illness, there is evidence that antimicrobial therapy prevents recurrences. High-dose corticosteroids and calcium replacement may be of benefit in severe cases of TSS, although data supporting their use are largely anecdotal.

Although an assay that measures antibody to TSST-1 has been developed, its use in screening individuals for susceptibility to TSS cannot be recommended until it is known how well a given level of antibody correlates with protection against disease. Similarly, routine vaginal cultures in healthy women are of no benefit in determining who is at risk of developing TSS. It is hoped that ongoing epidemiological and laboratory research concerning the interaction between tampons and *S. aureus* will lead to the design of tampons that do not increase the risk of developing menstrual TSS. In the meantime, women who have had menstrual TSS should be advised to discontinue tampon use. Women who have not had TSS can minimize their already small risk of developing menstrual TSS by not using tampons.

Reye's Syndrome

Robert B. Wallace

What is now known as Reye's syndrome was first described in Australia in 1963,[1,2] and shortly thereafter a series of similar cases was published in the United States.[3] It is unclear whether cases occurred in prior eras. The syndrome was characterized by an acute encephalopathic clinical picture and fatty liver in children, often leading to death with major neurological and metabolic manifestations.[4] Epidemiological, clinical, and metabolic studies have added considerable information on the nature of the condition, but it remains a syndrome that is likely comprised of diverse causes and pathogenetic mechanisms.

Case Definition and Surveillance. Rates of occurrence of Reye's syndrome depend in part on the skill in clinical case recognition, the rigor of surveillance, and case definition. Clearly some definitions and criteria are much more encompassing than others. The epidemiological case definition used by the U.S. Centers for Disease Control[5] includes—

1. Acute noninflammatory encephalopathy with
   a. Microvascular fatty metamorphosis of the liver confirmed by biopsy or autopsy, or
   b. A serum alanine aminotransferase (ALT or SGPT), a serum aspartate aminotransferase (AST or SGOT), or a serum ammonia greater than three times normal.
2. If cerebrospinal fluid is obtained, leukocyte count must be $\leq 8/mm^3$.
3. In addition, there should be no other more reasonable explanations for the neurological or hepatic abnormalities.

Cases have been reported in the neonatal period and in adults, although most occur in infants and children. The syndrome has been clinically staged according to the level of consciousness and corresponding physical signs.[6]

Other definitions have been more specific,[7] but none will be wholly satisfactory until a "gold standard" for the diagnosis appears. Recent evidence suggests, for example, that at least some cases originally labeled as being the syndrome were associated with known inborn errors of metabolism.[7] Diagnosis rates may also vary according to the frequency of biopsy and autopsy, although the specificity of histopathological changes has been disputed. Continuous surveillance of Reye's syndrome began in 1976 in the United States, and the incidence of the syndrome has clearly decreased since. There were as many as 555 cases reported in a single year (1980, see Table 14–3). However, in 1987 there were only 36 cases reported; in 1988 there were only 20. Possible reasons for this decline are discussed below. Despite the small number of reported cases, the surveillance effort remains active, and reporting is encouraged.

There have also been differences in occurrence patterns between countries. For example, in Australia, children with Reye's syndrome have tended to be younger, generally less than 5 years of age, and nonseasonal, whereas cases in the United States occur predominantly in the fall and winter seasons with a modal age distribution of 5 to 15 years. Further, the decline in the U.S. incidence rate for Reye's syndrome in the 1980s was initially more prominent in children under 10 years of age, although more recently all age groups have enjoyed some decrease.[8] All of this suggests the possibility of age- and geography-related heterogeneity in the nature and causes of the syndrome.

TABLE 14-3. PREDOMINANT INFLUENZA STRAINS, REPORTED CASES OF REYE'S SYNDROME (RS) AND VARICELLA-ASSOCIATED RS, RS INCIDENCE, AND RS FATALITY RATE, UNITED STATES, 1974 AND 1977–1988[a]

Year[a]	Predominant Influenza Strains (Jan–May)	Total	Varicella-associated	Incidence of RS[b]	Case Fatality Rate (%)
1974	B	379	—	0.6	41
1977	B	454	73	0.7	42
1978	A(H3N2)	236	69	0.4	29
1979	A(H1N1)	389	113	0.6	32
1980	B	555	103	0.9	23
1981	A(H3N2)	297	77	0.5	30
1982	B	213	45	0.3	35
1983	A(H3N2)	198	28	0.3	31
1984	A(H1N1)+B	204	26	0.3	26
1985	A(H3N2)	93	15	0.2	31
1986	B	101	5	0.2	27
1987	A(H1N1)	36	7	0.1	29
1988	A(H3N2)	20	4	0.0	30

[a]Continuous RS surveillance began in December 1976. Data for 1988 are provisional. RS reporting year begins December 1 of previous year.
[b]Per 100,000 U.S. population <18 years of age (U.S. Bureau of the Census data).

Causes and Control of Reye's Syndrome. The causes of Reye's syndrome, including pathogenetic mechanisms, remain enigmatic. Sullivan-Bolyai and Corey have reviewed this area thoroughly.[9] Hypotheses include genetic predispositions, possibly related to selected inborn errors of metabolism, exposure to environmental toxins such as various chemicals, pesticides, and mycotoxins, and use of medications such as salicylates and antiemetics. Also, at least in the United States, most cases are preceded by an acute viral infection, usually beginning 7 to 10 days prior to syndrome onset. Instances of infection with many categories of viruses have been documented, but the two most prominent are varicella and influenza B. Table 14-3 shows that 5% to 30% of reported cases were varicella associated and explores the relation of case rates to the prevalent influenza strain.[6] The synergistic effect of a second or dual viral infection in causing the syndrome has been postulated. Other viruses have been the subject of speculation but have not yet been rigorously evaluated.

The 1980s were characterized by the epidemiological assessment as to whether salicylates, particularly aspirin, have a causal role in the syndrome. After some anecdotal reports and case-series, several case-control studies were performed in the United States. Although some of these were criticized on methodological grounds, in aggregate they suggested that the syndrome was at least in part related to the use of aspirin as treatment for the febrile illness preceding or during syndrome onset.[10] No evidence was found for acetaminophen or other medications. In fact, the decline in Reye's syndrome incidence noted above has been related to public education and the subsequent decline in the use of aspirin for febrile conditions in children.[11] However, aspirin does not likely explain all cases of the syndrome, and other forces, yet unidentified, may be at work. In other countries such as Australia, aspirin was not related to the syndrome, particularly in children under 5 years of age [12]; some of these cases are turning out to be other defined metabolic disorders.

Summary. Reye's syndrome appears to be an important and at least partially preventable entity, even if not fully characterized or etiologically explained. Continued surveillance is necessary to assess its public health impact, search for additional causes, and detect any important increases in incidence.

REFERENCES

Lyme Disease

1. Steere AC: Lyme Disease. N Engl J Med 321:586–596, 1989
2. Lyme disease and other spirochetal diseases. Rev Infect Dis, II S6:S1433–S1525, 1989
3. Anderson JF: Preventing Lyme disease. Rheum Dis Clin North Am 15:757–766, 1989

Dermatophytosis

1. Head ES, Henry JC, Macdonald EM: The cotton swab technique for the culture of dermatophyte infections—Its efficacy and merit. J Am Acad Dermatol 11:797–801, 1984
2. Ajello L: Geographic distribution and prevalence of the dermatophytes. Ann NY Acad Sci 89:30, 1960
3. English MP, Gibson MD: Studies in the epidemiology of tinea pedis. I. Tinea pedis in school children. II. Dermatophytes on the floors of swimming-baths. Br Med J: 1442–1448, 1959
4. English MP: The epidemiology of animal ringworm in man. Br J Dermatol 86 (suppl 8):78, 1972
5. Georg L: Epidemiology of the dermatophytes: Sources of infection, modes of transmission and endemicity. Ann NY Acad Sci 89:69, 1960
6. Mitchell PC, Clayton YM: Some observations on fungal infections in tropical climates. Proc R Soc Med 55:559–561, 1962
7. Allen AM, et al: Griseofulvin in the prevention of experimental human dermatophytosis. Arch Dermatol 108:233–236, 1973
8. Brown C, Caro I, Condry P, et al: Multicenter clinical evaluation of ketoconazole in the treatment of cutaneous fungal infections. Cutis 33:578–581, 1984
9. Grappel SF, Bishop CT, Blank F: Immunology of dermatophytes and dermatophytosis. Bacteriol Rev 38:222–250, June 1974

Hookworm Disease: Ancylostomiasis, Necatoriasis, Uncinariasis

1. Crompton DWT, McKean PG, Schad GA: Hookworm disease: current status and new directions. Parasitol Today 5:1–2, 1989
2. Warren, KS: Selective Primary Health Care and Parasitic Diseases. In McAdam KPWJ (ed): Frontiers of Infectious Diseases: New

Strategies in Parasitology. Edinburgh: Churchill Livingstone, 1989, pp 217–231
3. Schad GA, Banwell JG: Hookworms. In Warren KS, Mahmoud AAF (eds): Tropical and Geographic Medicine. New York: McGraw-Hill, 1990, pp 379–393
4. Chandler AC: Hookworm Disease: Its Distribution, Biology, Epidemiology, Pathology, Diagnosis, Treatment and Control. New York: Macmillan, 1929
5. Matsusaki G: Hookworm diseases and prevention. In Morishita K et al (eds): Progress of Medical Parasitology in Japan. Tokyo: Meguro Parasitological Museum 3:187–282, 1966
6. Pritchard DI, McKean PG, Schad GA: An immunological and biochemical comparison of hookworm species. Parasitol Today 6:154–156, 1990
7. Hoagland KE, Schad GA: *Necator americanus* and *Ancylostoma duodenale* life history parameters and epidemiological implications of two sympatric hookworms of humans. Exp Parasitol 44:36–49, 1978
8. Beaver PC, Jung RC, Cupp EW: Clinical Parasitology, 9 edt. Baltimore: Lea & Febiger, 1984, p 270
9. Komiya Y, Yasuraoka K: The biology of hookworms. In Morishita K, et al (eds): Progress of Medical Parasitology in Japan. Tokyo: Meguro Parasitological Museum 2:5–114, 1966
10. Okamoto K: An experimental study of the migration route and development of *Ancylostoma duodenale* in pups after oral infection. J Kyoto Pref Med Univ 70:145–152, 1961
11. Soh CT: The distribution and persistence of hookworm larvae in the tissues of mice in relation to species and to routes of inoculation. J Parasitol 44:515–519, 1958
12. Harada Y: Wakana disease and hookworm allergy. Yonago Acta Med 6:109–118, 1962
13. Roche M, Layrisse M: The nature and causes of "hookworm anemia." Am J Trop Med Hyg 15(6), part 2), 1966
14. Kalkofen UP: Intestinal trauma resulting from feeding activities of *Ancylostoma caninum.* Am J Trop Med Hyg 23:1046–1053, 1974
15. Carroll SM, Howse DJ, Grove DI: The anticoagulant effects of the hookworm, *Ancylostoma caninum.* Thromb Haemostas 51:222–227, 1984
16. Variyam EP, Banwell JG: Nutrition implications of hookworm infection. Rev Infect Dis 4:830–835, 1982
17. Behnke JM: Do hookworms elicit protective immunity in man? Parasitol Today 3:200–206, 1987
18. Hominick WM, Dean CG, Shad GA: Population biology of hookworms in west Bengal: Analysis of numbers of infective larvae recovered from damp pads applied to the soil surface at defaecation sites. Trans R Soc Trop Med Hyg 81:978–986, 1987
19. Kan S: Soil-transmitted helminthiases among inhabitants of an oil-palm plantation in West Malaysia. J Trop Med Hyg 92:263–269, 1989

Schistosomiasis

1. World Health Organization: The control of schistosomiasis. WHO Technical Report Series No. 728. Geneva: World Health Organization, 1985
2. Beaver PC, Jung RC, Cupp EW: Schistosomes of blood flukes. In Clinical Parasitology. 9 edt. Philadelphia: Lea & Febiger, 1984, pp 415–448
3. Mao SP, Shao BR: Schistosomiasis control in the People's Republic of China. Am J Trop Med Hyg 31:92–99, 1982
4. Abramowicz M (ed): Handbook of Antimicrobial Therapy. New Rochelle, NY: The Medical Letter, 1988
5. Coutinho A, Domingues AL: Specific treatment of advanced schistosomiasis liver disease in man: Favourable results. Mem Inst Oswaldo Cruz 82 (suppl 4):335–340, 1987
6. Jordan P: Diagnostic and laboratory techniques. In Jordan P, Webbe G (eds): Schistosomiasis, Epidemiology, Treatment and Control. London: Heinemann, 1982, pp 165–183
7. Peters PA, Mahmoud AAF, Warren KS, Ouma JH, Arap Siongkok TK: Field studies of rapid accurate means of quanitifying *Schistosoma haematobius* eggs in urine samples. Bull WHO 54(2):159–162, 1976
8. Mott KE: A reusable polyamide filter for diagnosis of *Schistosoma haematobius* infection by urine filtration. Bull Soc Pathol Exot 76:101–104, 1983
9. Khalil HM, Makled MK, el Sibae MM, et al: The immunodiagnosis of *Schistosoma mansoni* infection in the different clinicoparasitological stages. J Egypt Soc Parasitol 19(2):653–667, 1989
10. Davis A: Recent advances in schistosomiasis. Q J Med 226:95–110, 1986
11. Warren KS: The pathology, pathobiology and pathogenesis of schistosomiasis. Parasitology Sup Nature 273:609–612, 1978
12. Borot DL: Immunopathology of *Schistosoma mansoni* infection. Clin Microbiol Rev 2:250–269, 1989
13. Cook JA, Baker ST, Warren KS, et al: A controlled study of morbidity of schistosomiasis in St. Lucian school children, based on quantitive egg excretion. Am J Trop Med Hyg 23:625–633, 1974
14. Cheever AW: A quantitative post-mortum study of *Schistosomiasis mansoni* in man. Am J Trop Med Hyg 17:38–60, 1968
15. Warren KS: The pathology of schistosome infections. Helminth Abstr 42:529–633, 1973
16. Cheever AW, Andrade ZA: Pathological lesions associated with *Schistosoma mansoni* infection in man. Trans R Soc Trop Med Hyg 61:629–639, 1967
17. Symmers WSC: Note on a new form of liver cirrhosis due to the presence of ova of *Bilharzia haematobium.* J Pathol Bact 9:237–239, 1903
18. Lichlenberg V, Sadum F, Cheever EH, et al: Experimental infection with *Schistosoma japonicum* in chimpanzees: parasitologic clinical serologic and pathological observations. Am J Trop Med Hyg 20:850–893, 1971
19. Wunschmann D, Ribas E: [Chronic cor pulmonale due to granulomatous and obliterating pulmonary arteritis caused by schistosomiasis] Chronisches cor pulmonale durch granulomatose und obliterienrende pulmonale arteriitis dei schistosomiasis. Zentralbl Allg Pathol 135(3):241–247, 1989
20. Sharfi AR, Rayis AB: The continuing challenge of Bilharzial ureteric stricuture. Scand J Urol Nephrol 23(2):123–126, 1989
21. Scrimgeour EM, Gajdusek DC: Involvement of the Central Nervous System in *Schistosoma mansoni* and *Schistosoma haematobium* infection. Brain 108:1023–1038, 1985
22. Cohen J, Capildo R, Rose FC, Pallis C: Schistosomal myelopathy. Br Med J 1:1258, 1977
23. Hunter GW III: Schistosome cercarial dermatitis and other rare schistosomes that may infect man. In Marcial Rojas RA (ed): Pathology of Protozoal and Helminthic Disease. New York, NY: Robert E. Krieger, 1975, pp 450–468
24. World Health Organization: Epidemiology and control of schistosomiasis. WHO Technical Report Series No. 643. Geneva: World Health Organization, 1980
25. Hsü HF, Hsü SYL: Schistosomiasis in the Shanghai area. In Quinn JR (ed): China medicine as we saw it. DHEW Publication No. (NIH) 75-684, 1974, pp 345–363
26. Makanga B, Odyek O: Mollusc-killing agents from *Khaya grandifoliola.* Trop Med Parasitol 40:117–118, 1989
27. McCullough FS: Biological control of the snail intermediate hosts of human *Schistosoma* spp: A review of its present status and future prospects. Acta Trop 38:5–13, 1981
28. Gryseels B: The relevance of schistosomiasis for public health. Trop Med Parasitol 40(2):134–142, 1989
29. Janitschke K, Telher AA, Wachsmuth J, Jahia S: Prevalence and control of *Schistosoma haematobium* infections in the Amran subprovince of the Yemen Arab Republic. Trop Med Parasitol 40:181–184, 1989
30. Nassif S: A review of achievements of the national schistosomiasis control program in middle and upper Egypt areas. Mem Inst Oswaldo Cruz 82(suppl 4):83–87, 1987

31. Kloetzel K, de Azevedo, Vergetti AM: Repeated mass treatment of *Schistosomiasis mansoni:* Experience in hyperendemic areas of Brazil. II. Micro-level evaluation of results. Ann Trop Med Parasitol 82(4):367–376, 1988
32. Spencer HC, Ruiz-Tiben E, Mansour NS, Cline BL: Evaluation of UNICEF/Arab Republic of Egypt WHO schistosomiasis control project in Beheira Governorate. Am J Trop Med Hyg 42(5):441–448, 1990
33. Hsü SYL, Hsü HF: New approach to immunization against *Schistosoma japonicum.* Science 1961, pp 133:766
34. Hsü HF, Hsü SYL, Osborne JW: Immunization against *Schistosoma japonicum* in rhesus monkeys produced by irradiated cercariae. Nature 194:98–99, 1962
35. Hsü SYL, Hsü HF, Osborne JW: Immunization of rhesus monkeys against schistosome infection of cercariae exposed to high doses of X-radiation. Proc Soc Exp Biol Med 131:1146–1149, 1969
36. Li YL, Hsü SYL, Hsü HF, Osborne JW, Robinson H, Ohnishi Y: Autoradiographic study of the attrition of migrating schistosomula in the skin of mice. I. Mice immunized with highly X-irradiated *Schistosoma mansoni* cercariae. Proc CAMS and PUMC 4(3):153–156, 1989
37. Hsü SYL, Hsü HF, Penick GD, Hanson HO, Schilleer HJ, Cheng HF: Immunoglobulin E, mast cells and eosinophils in the skin of rhesus monkeys immunized with X-irradiated cercariae of *Schistosoma japonicum.* Int Arch Allergy Appl Immunol 59:383–393, 1979
38. Hsü SYL, Hsü HF, Penick GD, Lust GL, Osborne JW, Cheng HF: Mechanism of immunity to schistosomiasis: Histopathological study of lesions elicited in rhesus monkeys during immunizations and challenge with cercariae of *Schistosoma japonicum.* J Reticuloendoth Soc 18:167–185, 1975
39. Hsü SYL, Hsü HF: Further discussion on the new hypothesis for the mechanism of immunity to schistosome infection. Proc Int Conf Schistosomiasis, Cairo, Egypt, Oct 1975, 2:573–582, 1978
40. Hsü SYL, Hsü HF, Hanson HO: Immunoglobulins and complement in the skin of rhesus monkeys immunized with X-irradiated cercariae of *Schistosoma japonicum.* Z Parasitenkd 66:133–143, 1981
41. Hsü SYL, Xu ST, He YX, Shi FH, Shen W, Hsü HF, Osborne JW, Clarke WR: Vaccination of bovines against *Schistosomiasis japonica* with highly irradiated schistosomula in China. Am J Trop Med Hyg 33:891–898, 1984
42. Smithers SR: Parasiotology. Improving prospects for a schistosomiasis vaccome (News). Nature 323:205–206, 1987
43. Capron A, Dessaint TP, Capron M, et al: Immunity to schistosomes: Progress towards a vaccine. Science 238:1065–1072, 1987
44. Sher A, James SL, Correa-Oliveira R, Hieny S, Pearce E: Schistosome vaccines: Current progress and future prospects. Parasitology 98:S61–S68, 1989

Toxic Shock Syndrome

1. Reingold AL, et al: Toxic shock syndrome surveillance in the United States, 1980 to 1981. Ann Intern Med 96:875–880, 1982
2. Stevens FR: The occurrence of *Staphylococcus aureus* infection with a scarlatiniform rash. JAMA 88:1957–1958, 1927
3. Todd J, Fishaut M, Kapral F, Welch T: Toxic-shock syndrome associated with phage-group-I staphylococci. Lancet 2:1116–1118, 1978
4. Schlech WF, Shands KN, Reingold AL, et al: Risk factors for the development of toxic-shock syndrome: Association with a tampon brand. JAMA 248:834–839, 1982
5. Kehrberg MW, Latham RH, Haslam BT, et al: Risk factors for staphylococcal toxic-shock syndrome. Am J Epidemiol 114:873–879, 1981
6. Osterholm MT, Davis JP, Gibson RW, et al: Tri-state toxic-shock syndrome study: I. Epidemiologic findings. J Infect Dis 145:431–440, 1982
7. Davis JP, Chesney PJ, Wand PJ, LaVenture M, the Investigation and Laboratory Team: Toxic-shock syndrome: Epidemiologic features, recurrence, risk factors, and prevention. N Engl J Med 303:1429–1435, 1980
8. Shands KN, Schmid GP, Dan BB, et al: Toxic-shock syndrome in menstruating women: Its association with tampon use and *Staphylococcus aureus* and the clinical features in 52 cases. N Engl J Med 303:1436–1442, 1980
9. Helgerson SD, Foster LR: Toxic shock syndrome in Oregon: Epidemiologic findings. Ann Intern Med 96:909–911, 1982
10. Berkley SF, et al: The relationship of tampon characteristics to menstrual toxic shock syndrome. JAMA 258:917–920, 1987
11. Reingold AL, et al: Risk factors for menstrual toxic shock syndrome: Results of a multistate case-control study. Rev Infect Dis 11:S35–S42, 1989
12. Petitti DB, et al: Update through 1985 on the incidence of toxic shock syndrome among members of a prepaid health plan. Rev Infect Dis 11:S22–S27, 1989
13. Todd JK, et al: Toxic shock syndrome II. Estimated occurrence in Colorado as influenced by case ascertainment methods. Am J Epidemiol 122:857–867, 1985
14. Gaventa S, et al: Active surveillance for toxic shock syndrome in the United States, 1986. Rev Infect Dis 11:S28–S34, 1989
15. Markowitz LE, et al: Toxic shock syndrome: Evaluation of national surveillance data using a hospital discharge survey. JAMA 258:75–78, 1987
16. Altemeier WA, et al: *Staphylococcus aureus* associated with the toxic-shock syndrome: Phage typing and toxin capability testing. Ann Intern Med 96(Part 2):978–982, 1982
17. Schlievert PM, et al: Identification and characterization of an exotoxin from *Staphylococcus aureus* associated with toxic-shock syndrome. J Infect Dis 143:509–516, 1981
18. Parsonnet J: Mediators in the pathogenesis of toxic shock syndrome: overview. Rev Infect Dis 11:S263–S269, 1989
19. Melish ME, et al: Endotoxin is not an essential mediator in toxic shock syndrome. Rev Infect Dis 11:S219–S230, 1989
20. Garbe PL, et al: *Staphylococcus aureus* isolates from patients with nonmenstrual toxic shock syndrome: Evidence for additional toxins. JAMA 253:2538–2542, 1985
21. Schlievert PM: Staphylococcal enterotoxin B and toxic shock syndrome toxin-1 are significantly associated with non-menstrual TSS. Lancet 1:1149–1150, 1986
22. Lee AC, et al: Investigation by syringe method of effect of tampons on production in vitro of toxic shock syndrome toxin 1 by *Staphylococcus aureus.* J Clin Microbiol 25:87–90, 1987
23. Kass EH: Magnesium and the pathogenesis of toxic shock syndrome. Rev Infect Dis 11:S167–S175, 1989

Reye's Syndrome

1. Anderson RMcD: Encephalitis in childhood: pathologic aspects. Med J Aust 1:573–575, 1963
2. Reye RDK, Morgan G, Baral J: Encephalopathy and fatty degeneration of the viscera: A disease entity in childhood. Lancet 2:749–752, 1963
3. Johnson GM, Scurletis TD, Carroll NB: A study of sixteen fatal cases of encephalitis-like disease in North Carolina children. NC Med J 24:463–473, 1963
4. Trauner DA: Reye's syndrome. Curr Probl Pediatr 12:1–31, 1982
5. Centers for Disease Control: Follow-up on Reye Syndrome-United States. 1987 and 1988. MMWR 29:321–322, 1980
6. Centers for Disease Control: Reye Syndrome surveillance-United States, 1987 and 1988. MMWR 38:325–327, 1989
7. Gauthier M, Guay J, LaCroix J, Lortie A: Reye's syndrome. A reappraisal of diagnosis in 49 presumptive cases. Am J Dis Child 143:1181–1185, 1989

8. Barrett MJ, Hurwitz ES, Schonberger LS, Rogers MF: Changing epidemiology of Reye syndrome in the United States. Pediatrics 77: 598–602, 1986
9. Sullivan-Bolyai JZ, Corey L: Epidemiology of Reye syndrome. Epidemiol Rev 3:1–26, 1981
10. Hurwitz ES: Reye's syndrome. Epidemiol Rev 11:249–253, 1989
11. Arrowsmith JB, Kennedy DL, Kuritsky JN, Faich GA: National patterns of aspirin use and Reye syndrome reporting, United States, 1980 to 1985. Pediatrics 79:858–863, 1987
12. Orlowski JP, Campbell P, Goldstein S: Reye's syndrome: a case control study of medication use and associated viruses in Australia. Cleveland Clin Med J 57:323–329, 1990

SECTION THREE

Environmental Health

Edited by Arthur L. Frank

15

The Status of Environmental Health

Arthur L. Frank

The broad area of environmental health continues to be an important public health concern. Increasingly, barriers between workplace and ambient environment—pollution via the air, soil, or water—are coming down. Concerns range from the exposure of a single individual all the way to global concerns for "spaceship earth."

The field of environmental health, especially as practiced in workplace settings, combines routine clinical medicine, preventive measures, and curative health care. Routine clinical medicine includes preemployment examinations and workplace injury evaluation and also has elements of fitness-to-work characteristics in many settings. Preventive examinations at the workplace can include regular monitoring examinations for the effects of noxious exposures and workplace-related screening examinations for hypertension, hearing loss, and other afflictions, and in increasing numbers of settings, periodic examinations related to length of employment are being carried out. Also, with greater frequency, intervention programs with regard to smoking cessation, weight reduction, nutrition, stress reduction, and other preventable conditions are being incorporated into overall workplace health programs.

This section of the book reflects both the traditional and historical concerns of occupational and environmental health but continues to keep abreast of new and emerging problems and to reflect a better appreciation of the integrated role of a variety of health professions. New discussions on such problems as multiple chemical sensitivity and the role of industrial hygiene are examples of such new areas. Increasingly, one finds that workplace exposure may be well controlled but that contamination of surrounding air, soil, or water may threaten the health of those who live in the environment of an industrial facility.

A continuing serious problem in the area of occupational and environmental health is the insufficient number of trained personnel in the field. Clearly there are too few adequately trained occupational medicine physicians, and the number being graduated yearly in the United States, less than 100 per year, may not even be sufficient to replace those who leave the field, much less to allow for expansion. Primary care physicians receive too little training in occupational medicine, although they are the group that provides the greatest amount of occupational medicine in the United States. There also are too few trained ergonomicists and safety specialists, to cite two examples.

Significant administrative and judgmental issues continue to make work in these areas difficult. In the workplace there is for some the potential problem of conflicting interests between employer and employee, and the physician is at risk of losing his traditional role as a patient advocate. In reality there should be no loss of such a role, and it must be recognized that in a workplace setting often what is best for the worker is a prompt and healthful return to work, which meshes well with corporate interests. Nevertheless, there should never be any risk-taking that puts the well-being of workers in jeopardy. The ability of laboratory-based toxicologists to measure increasingly smaller amounts of potentially toxic materials and to translate such measurements into information regarding real or potential health effects is increasingly problematic. A basic question then arising is, "Does the mere presence of a material mean that harm will result?" The issue of individualized risk compared to the public's risk following low-levels of exposure is always present. Recognizing that we cannot expect to live in a risk-free environment, we must also quickly recognize that "acceptable" risk levels are not to be left solely to the judgment of physicians but are ultimately societal issues needing to be judged by a wider constituency. Although the individual risk following a particular exposure may be low, on a societal basis with thousands or even millions exposed, a different approach may need to be taken with regard to workplace or environmental protection. Political, social, economic, cultural, and other considerations must be evaluated alongside medical considerations.

The judgment of physicians with regard to individual patients is still central to the approach of clinical medicine. To practice occupational medicine in a good medical tradition requires obtaining a suitable environmental and occupational history. The effects of these exposures, be they at the workplace, at home, or elsewhere, may be felt minutes after exposure or not for decades. The interaction of a variety of factors, such as the use of alcohol and drugs or smoking, is relevant to the study of environmental exposures. Table 15-1 provides a format for obtaining the essential features of an environmental-occupational history.

This section reviews basic toxicological principles and examines exposure to significant dusts, metals, chemicals, and pesticides. Physical factors such as thermal extremes, noise, and ergonomic issues are discussed. Chapters dealing with more global issues, such as water, waste, and food, are followed by chapters on regulations, approach to special groups, preventive strategies, and the problems of housing and environmental warming. Although medical and scientific concerns are at the

TABLE 15-1. ENVIRONMENTAL AND OCCUPATIONAL EXPOSURE HISTORY

Current work: ____________________

How long at this job? ____________________

Description of work: ____________________

____

Any contact with dust, fumes, chemicals, radiation, noise, etc?
_______ Yes _______ No If yes, describe: ____________

____

Describe any adverse effects noted: ____________________

____

Are any fellow workers ill? _______ Yes _______ No
If yes, describe: ____________________

Do you use any protective equipment at work?
_______ Yes _______ No

Previous job history	*From*	*To*	*Exposures*
First regular job	______	______	________
Next job	______	______	________
Next job	______	______	________
Vacation or temporary job	______	______	________
Vacation or temporary job	______	______	________

Military service or related exposures: ____________________

____

Have you lived near an industrial facility or has a family member worked in a setting where hazardous materials have been brought home? _______ Yes _______ No
If yes, describe: ____________________

Hobby history: ____________________

Smoking history: ____________________

Alcohol and drug use history: ____________________

Comments: ____________________

heart of this material, the social context in which these problems are found, is also recognized.

While much is already known and new information constantly accumulates, many serious questions about environmental health remain unanswered. Let us hope that as we approach the next century, we will further clarify and illuminate these factors and deal with their solution.

I have been struck in recent years by the shifting of emphasis away from workplaces to environmental exposures and the infiltration of nontraditional clinical and preventive medicine practices into workplaces. A few institutional-specific examples will, perhaps, highlight this, but one suspects that this experience is more widely appreciated elsewhere as well. In a recent review of 21 cases of arsenic poisoning seen at our medical center, not one was traced to an occupational setting. They were all environmentally related, either by accidental or intentional ingestion, or resulted from malevolent intent. The only inquiries regarding gasoline exposure have been related to environmental aspects due to leaking storage tanks. While fairly routine inquiries regarding traditional occupational exposures persist, some of the problems of greatest concern that have come to my attention have involved environmental issues, either via air pollution or water pollution, and the number of inquiries regarding the broad area of environmental risk assessment is increasing.

In the traditional workplace, ergonomics, especially musculoskeletal problems, are a major area of concern at levels of interest not apparent 5 years ago. Increasingly, enlightened workplaces are seeking to add a whole array of preventive health services, and these may range from daily workplace exercises to periodic health examinations to screening examinations to health fairs for employees and their families. Implications with regard to the costs of health care are enormous, especially as connected with employment, and it should be noted that in recent years a significant number of work actions have been related to the specific issue of the costs of health care at the workplace.

16

Toxicology

Principles of Toxicology

Michael Gochfeld

Toxicology is the study of the harmful effects of chemicals, including drugs, on living organisms. This chapter focuses on conceptual issues rather than facts regarding specific toxic substances. The concepts relate to properties of toxic substances in general, how they enter and move through the body, and the pathophysiological effects they exert on various targets within the body that may ultimately lead to effects on health.

Oser[1] traces the history of toxicology to Paracelsus (1493–1541), who recognized that a substance that is physiologically ineffective at a very low dose might be toxic at a high dose and therapeutic at an intermediate dose. Toxicology developed under the combined impetus of a quest for therapeutic agents and concern over adulterated foods. In 1906 the United States enacted the Pure Food and Drug Act, which perhaps was stimulated more by works such as Upton Sinclair's *The Jungle*[2] than by toxicologists.[1]

The process by which a chemical achieves its effect can be characterized by the following chain: concentration of agent in an environmental medium or matrix, exposure of the host, entry into the body, internal distribution, dose-reaching target, and effect on target. Internal distribution and the dose reaching the target organ, tissue, or cell are constantly modified by binding of the chemical to carrier molecules, by metabolic activation (or inactivation), by storage in various tissues (e.g., fat), and ultimately by excretion.[3] These processes are demonstrated in Figure 16–1.

Each of these factors requires detailed investigation, and each has important implications for the dose of a chemical that reaches targets within the body and thus for the health effects of chemicals. Accordingly, this chapter deals with the classification of toxic chemicals, the manner in which exposure occurs and how it can be measured, the absorption and distribution of chemicals within the body, and finally, the kinds of toxic effects that are produced.

Table 16–1 indicates the factors that influence the uptake and toxicity of a material and the susceptibility of the host. Uptake varies by route of exposure and bioavailability. A given chemical may be readily absorbed from the lungs but may not be absorbed through the skin or intestinal tract.

BRANCHES OF TOXICOLOGY

Toxicology is a broad discipline embracing such medical disciplines as pathology, pharmacology, clinical toxicology, molecular biology, and biochemistry. Historically, toxicology was linked with pharmacology and focused extensive attention on the toxic effects of pharmaceuticals. Industrial toxicology emerged to investigate the toxic effects of raw materials, intermediate materials, and products and wastes produced by commerce. Recently, important linkages, such as the relationship of toxicology to behavior, genetics, and nutrition, have opened new research horizons. Toxicology is concerned with both lethal and sublethal effects, and indeed much recent investigation has focused on pathophysiological and behavioral changes not clearly identified as disease.

Uptake, metabolism, distribution, and excretion are major influences on toxic effects, and an extensive literature examining these factors has emerged. Recently, toxicology has gone beyond these influences to examine the mechanism by which toxic substances achieve their effects on the target organ, tissue, cell, or molecule. Indeed, molecular toxicology is clearly a new frontier in this evolving discipline[4] and is linked closely with molecular epidemiology, which examines the distribution in populations of physiological changes at the molecular level.

Toxicological data are a major basis for environmental risk assessments, which in turn are increasingly used by regulatory agencies to assess chemical hazards, determine priorities for hazardous waste site cleanups, establish governmental policies, and set levels of allowable exposure. Such risk assessments produce quantitative or qualitative estimates of the magnitude of risk associated with a particular dose or with exposure of a population to a particular chemical, physical, or biological agent.

TYPES OF STRESSORS

The stressors that potentially harm the body can be broadly classified as physical (noise, temperature, radiation), biological (infectious, immunological), chemical, and psychosocial. Toxicologists focus mainly on chemicals, both synthetic ones and those of natural biological origin, and to a lesser extent on physical agents such as radiation. Classes of stressors interact with one another. Thus radiation, infection, or psychological stress may modify the effects of toxic chemicals, and vice versa, and there is increasing attention to the effects of two or more chemicals administered together where synergistic or antagonistic effects may occur.

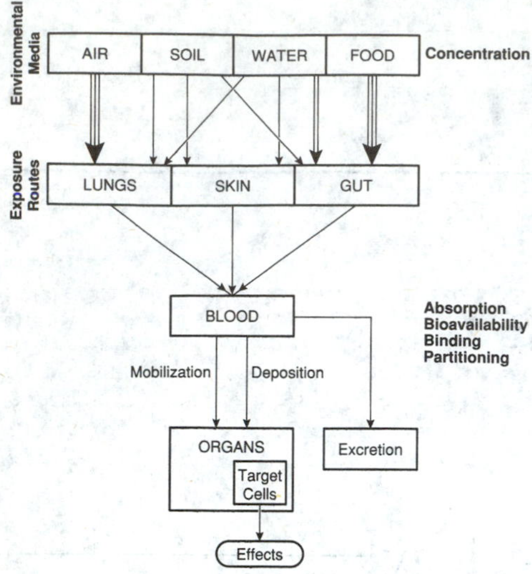

Figure 16–1. A multicompartment model of toxicant distribution.

DEFINITIONS

The following definitions will be helpful in understanding toxicology.

Bioavailability. the ability of a substance that enters the body to be liberated from its environmental matrix (water, tissue, soil) and to enter the circulation.

Intermediary metabolism. the metabolic change(s) that a chemical undergoes once it reaches the cells of the body. The liver is the primary site of intermediary metabolism. Harmful compounds can be made less harmful (detoxification), or benign compounds may be converted into a biologically harmful metabolite (metabolic activation).

Mechanism. the way in which the toxic substance acts on a cellular or subcellular level to disrupt the living organism. Some toxic agents are metabolic poisons; others disrupt cell membranes, interfere with chemical reactions, or bind to nucleic acids.

Susceptibility. the ability of a living thing to be harmed by an agent. Susceptibility is influenced by genotype, by age, and by environmental factors such as nutrition, prior exposure, and underlying state of health (e.g., immune status).

Threshold. the lowest dose of a chemical that has a detectable effect.

Toxic effect. damage to an organism measured in terms of a loss, reduction, or change of function; may be reported as a symptom or detected as a sign. Effects that are considered adverse in one person may be desirable or therapeutic in another.

TABLE 16–1. FACTORS THAT MODIFY TOXICITY

▪ Host	▪ Environment
Species, strain, genotype	Temperature
Age	Light: cycle, intensity, spectral distribution
Gender	Air: flow rate, ion content, humidity
Infectious/immunological history	**▪ Toxicant**
Behavioral stress history	Matrix/bioavailability
Activity level/fitness	Physical form
Nutritional status	Chemical form
Toxicant exposure history	

Toxicity. the intrinsic ability of a substance to harm living things. This varies from substances such as sodium chloride (a dose of 0.9% being isotonic and therapeutic) to some naturally occurring toxins such as aflatoxin B1 or botulinum toxin, which are toxic at levels well below 1 ppt.

Xenobiotic. a substance foreign to the body. Xenobiotics include all non-naturally occurring chemicals and many of biologic origin that do not occur in the target species. Although the term is usually used in the context of toxic chemicals, most pharmaceutical agents are xenobiotics.

CLASSIFICATION, OR TAXONOMY, OF TOXIC AGENTS

One can organize knowledge in toxicology in terms of chemical agents or types of effect. Thus chemicals can be classified on the basis of their structure, their source, their use, their mechanism of action, or their target organ. The lists below are not intended to be exhaustive.

Classification by Structure

Organic chemicals	Inorganic chemicals
Aromatics (e.g., phenols, methylbenzenes)	Anions
Polyaromatics (and chlorinated polyaromatics)	Cations
Aliphatic hydrocarbons (e.g., alkanes, alkenes)	Heavy metals
Chlorinated hydrocarbons	Metalloids (e.g., selenium)
Amines	
Nitriles	
Ethers, ketones, aldehydes, alcohols	

Classification by Source. Many plants and animals secrete chemicals designed to keep them from being eaten. Butterflies, such as the monarch, may incorporate plant alkaloids into their own tissues, rendering themselves inedible. Beetles may squirt cyanide compounds to deter predators. Plants that have once been partially eaten by herbivores may load increased levels of distasteful compounds in newly regenerated leaves. Similarly, many fungi may secrete chemicals that inhibit bacterial growth. A wide variety of these naturally occurring bioactive substances, or "toxins," have been adapted into some of our most familiar pharmaceuticals, such as antibiotics.

Natural or biological compounds, or "toxins"	Synthetics
Plants	Industrial reagents, byproducts or products
Bacteria	Pharmaceuticals
Invertebrates	
Vertebrates	

Classification by Use. Often in clinical toxicology the first thing one learns about a chemical exposure is the type of compound. Thus a would-be suicide may be brought in with "an overdose," or a worker may have been overcome while "using a solvent," or a homeowner may report that "some pesticide spray" has made him ill. The following are examples of common classes of materials that may have toxic effects:

Solvents	Pesticides	Pharmaceutical agents
Paints, dyes, coatings	Organochlorine	Detergents, cleansers
	Organophosphates	

Classification by Mechanism of Action. Much exciting research in modern toxicology focuses on the mechanism by which a bioactive substance interacts with and alters its targets to produce its unwanted effects.

Enzyme disruption	Macromolecular binding (e.g., DNA, protein)	Formation of free radicals and active oxygen
Enzyme induction	Cell membrane disruption	Sensitizers
Metabolic poisons	Competitive binding of active sites	Irritants

Classification by Target Organ. Toxins can act on any organ system in the body. The effects on these target organs are discussed in other chapters in this section. Standard toxicology textbooks (e.g., Klaasen et al., 1986) are organized by organ system, and several of the general readings deal with organ systems. The next discussion in this chapter deals specifically with neurobehavioral toxicology. The following is a list of toxins classified by the target organ:

Neurotoxin	Pulmonary toxin	Reproductive system toxin
Hematotoxin	Metabolic toxin	Genotoxin (including mutagens)
Nephrotoxin	Endocrine toxin	Carcinogen (including initiators and promoters)
Hepatotoxin	Dermatotoxin	Teratogens
Cardiotoxin		

The liver is of particular importance because many substances, particularly ingested xenobiotics, are transported directly to the liver. There they undergo metabolism, which may either detoxify or activate them. The liver may conjugate substances to facilitate their excretion in the urine or may actually secrete some substances into the bile. Liver cells are particularly vulnerable to toxins, and toxic hepatitis, often manifested by abnormalities in liver function, is a common occurrence.

CHEMICAL STRUCTURE AND TOXICOLOGY

Several chemical principles play important roles in toxicology. They influence how the chemical behaves in its environmental matrix, how it is absorbed into, metabolized, distributed through, and excreted from the body, and how it exerts its toxic effect.

Chemical Species. Although a rose may be a rose, a chemical may not always be what it appears to be. Thus toxicologists have demonstrated that slight modifications in a chemical may drastically alter its effect.[5] This is particularly true for certain metals which, in an organic complex, may have drastically different and more serious effects than in the elemental or ionic form. Examples include methylmercury and tributyl tin compared with inorganic mercury or tin compounds. Organic species have been incorporated into biocides such as fungicidal seed dressing and into marine paints to thwart the growth of barnacles.[6,7] A chemical variant of a metal is called a species. This term may also refer to the valence state; thus trivalent chromium and hexavalent chromium are species of chromium,[8] and because CrIII is an essential nutrient whereas CrVI is a potent lung carcinogen,[9] the difficulty of reliably speciating chromium (analyzing the concentrations of CrIII and CrVI in an environmental sample) impedes our ability to protect potentially exposed persons.

Isomers and Congeners. Isomeric structure may affect toxicity. Butane, a four-carbon chain, can appear as either normal (linear) butane or (branched) isobutane. Behavior in the body and toxicity may vary greatly among isomers and congeners. Thus different chlorinated dibenzodioxins vary more than a thousandfold in their toxicity.[10] Two isomers (e.g., *cis-* and *trans*-isomers) have the same chemical structure but a different atomic arrangement. Congeners have the same basic structure but different numbers of atoms. For instance, dichlorophenol and trichlorophenol are congeners, whereas 2,4-dichlorophenol and 2,5-dichlorophenol are isomers.

Structure-Activity Relationships. The converse of the variation in toxicity between isomers and congeners is the fact that chemicals that are structurally similar may have similar types of toxic effects on the body,[11] although the effects may be modulated in intensity by adjacent atoms. This forms the basis for much pharmaceutical research, the quest for agents that have a desired effect without undesired side effects. Understanding structure-activity relationships is important in toxicology because one can often infer the effects of a chemical by knowing the effects of related compounds. Thus many short-chain chlorinated hydrocarbons have a common general anesthesia effect, even though their potency varies with their structure. Similarly many metal ions are nephrotoxic, affecting the proximal kidney tubule,[12] and many hallucinogenic compounds share a common active group.

ACUTE AND CHRONIC TOXIC EFFECTS AND EXPOSURE

The terms "acute" and "chronic" can refer either to conditions of exposure or to the resultant health effects. A single "acute" exposure to a toxic chemical may be sufficient to induce health effects that in turn may be either acute (followed by recovery), subacute, or chronic. Chronic exposure may be followed by no adverse health effects (if the dose is low), by acute effects (which may occur when a sufficient dose is accumulated), or by chronic effects. In addition to having a long duration, chronic effects tend to be irreversible.

More specifically with respect to toxicological studies in animals, acute toxic effects can be defined as "the adverse effects occurring within a short time of . . . a single dose or multiple doses . . . within 24 hours," whereas subchronic toxicity is "the adverse effects occurring as a result of the repeated daily . . . dosing of a chemical . . . for part (< 10%) of the life span."[13] Chronic exposure refers to dosing of animals for more than 10% of their life span.[14]

CHEMICALS IN THE ENVIRONMENT

Environmental toxicology is generally concerned with chemicals in food, water, and air. In the broadest sense, however, the environment includes our home, community, and workplace, and our behavior greatly influences the microenvironment that we frequent and the exposures that we experience. It is customary to deal with the environment in terms of its specific medium: soil, water, air, and living organisms (biota). Each of these media has relevance to human exposure through routes such as ingestion, inhalation, and percutaneous absorption.

Chemicals in Soil. Soils have complex physical structures and compositions that vary greatly. Some are rich in organic material, and others are poor. Some are coarse grained and porous, others fine grained and impervious. The ionic charge of soil particles and pH properties influence the movement of chemicals through soils. Some toxic elements occur naturally in some soils. The minerals that are highly concentrated in most soils (e.g., calcium, silicon, aluminum, and iron) are fortunately relatively nontoxic. This is probably not an accident, because plants and animals coevolved with their environment and would have had to develop tolerances to elements with which they come in daily contact. As an example, in the nickel-rich soils of New Caledonia, the flora is tolerant of nickel.

Human activities have resulted in the deposition of many toxic substances in the soil. Such anthropogenic deposits arise because of mining and slag-dumping operations, the fallout of air pollutants, construction activities, and the discharge of industrial or agricultural wastes.

Once a chemical is deposited on soil, it may remain in place, may be washed away by water flowing over the surface, or may percolate down through the soil, usually aided by water. Liquid wastes move more quickly than solid ones, although oily wastes may move relatively slowly. Depending on a chemical's structure and charge, it may bind to soil particles, may remain in solution, or may form a complex with organic constituents.

Some chemicals may be readily leached from the upper layers of soil and carried down or away by water. Others may undergo biodegradation or photodegradation with the aid of microorganisms or sunlight. Some chemicals, for example, the chlorinated hydrocarbon pesticides and polychlorinated biphenyls (PCBs), tend to remain unchanged in the soil for many years. They are referred to as persistent chemicals.

Soil particles that form a fine dust can remain airborne and may be inhaled. Particles less than 5 μm in diameter are likely to reach the alveoli. Other particles may settle on food or water and be ingested. People may also ingest particles of soil that get on their fingers or under their nails or that are on the outer surfaces of vegetables. However, of much greater concern is the quantity of soil that preschool children may consume. Activities of toddlers brings them into close proximity with dirt. They crawl on it, get it on their hands, and transport it to their mouth. In addition, children with pica may deliberately eat dirt, particularly dirt that is rich in such minerals as lead.

Chemicals in Water. Environmental toxicologists are concerned with contamination of surface and ground water. Both of these can serve as water sources for communities. Many industrial and municipal wastes, both treated and untreated, are discharged directly into surface waters. Although the regulatory climate is changing with regard to water pollution, there are still numerous discharge permits that allow toxic chemicals to be piped into streams, lakes, rivers, canals, and the oceans. Solubility in water is the primary factor determining the behavior of chemicals in water. Many metal salts dissolve readily, whereas most larger organic molecules do not.

Drinking-water sources are regulated with regard to several pollutants. For example, the concentration of trihalomethanes (e.g., chloroform, dichlorobromomethane) cannot in total exceed 100 ppb in a water supply. (Refer to Chapter 35 on water.)

Chemicals in Air. Air pollution remains a major public health concern. Recent attention has focused on ozone because of photochemical oxidation. Probably the main substrate for excess ozone formation are oxides of nitrogen (the term for the family) emitted in automobile exhaust. Another substance of concern is sulfur dioxide, which forms an irritating acid mist. Both ozone and sulfur dioxide are irritating to the respiratory system.

Air pollution indoors has become a major concern since the fuel crisis of the early 1970s. Recently constructed office buildings tend to be relatively airtight, and fuel conservation programs greatly reduce the amount of fresh air (makeup air) added to air conditioning. It is substantially cheaper to recirculate cooled air (summer) or heated air (winter), rather than taking in outside air and paying to cool or heat it continuously. "Tight building syndrome" and "indoor air pollution" are rubrics applied to a variety of problems usually experienced in office buildings. Offending agents include carbon dioxide in elevated amounts, burning insulation in overheating air compressors, cigarette smoke, copier chemicals, ozone, fiberglass, and sulfuric acid. Episodes involving these substances frequently affect a large number of employees, who may notice an unusual smell and have a variety of nonspecific symptoms of irritation. Although some investigators have labeled these episodes as cases of mass psychogenic illness,[15] most studies have identified a correctable ventilation or contamination problem.

Many homes contain unsuspected air pollutants that are hazardous to health. Radon gas, a breakdown product from naturally occurring radioactive materials in soil, is a lung carcinogen. It occurs in many parts of the United States and may occur in relatively high concentrations in certain homes. A more common but less dreaded pollutant is nitrogen dioxide, which is formed by combustion in a gas cooking range. Elevated levels of this irritant can be measured in a kitchen while cooking is in progress. Children living in homes with gas ranges may have an excess of respiratory symptoms.[16]

Community exposure to airborne contaminants has become an issue of concern when solid waste incinerators or industrial facilities are planned. Attention is focused on a variety of pollutants that may be emitted from the stack. A variety of pollution control devices (such as bag house filters, scrubbers, and electrostatic precipitators) may be installed, but although they advertise 99.9999% efficiency, they never achieve 100% efficiency, allowing some pollutants to escape. It remains a major challenge for persons charged with risk assessment to determine where these contaminants fall, in what form they fall, and whether the amounts are sufficient to threaten health, ecosystems, or property.

Air is the major route of exposure for industrial workers. Many processes cause the emission of vapors, smokes, or mists that can be inhaled. Most of the standards regarding industrial exposure refer to airborne concentrations, above which inhalation could lead to adverse health effects.[17]

Food. Food may contain toxic chemicals from a variety of sources. Although regulations governing pesticide reentry (e.g., the minimum number of days between spraying and harvest) are designed to minimize residual pesticides in food, many vegetables still contain some pesticide residues. Some residues may be surface sprays that adhere to plant tissue, whereas others are systemic substances taken up through the roots and incorporated into the tissue. The uptake by plants of toxic chemicals from the soil has already been mentioned. Hormones and antibiotics used in promoting animal growth can also be detected in certain foods, as can food additives used to prolong shelf life or to enhance flavor, texture, or color. Some of these compounds have been demonstrated to have toxic effects in long-term investigations of low-level exposure. (See Chapters 24 and 34 on Pesticides and Food.)

Biological Amplification in the Food Chain. Among the phenomena that influence the movements of chemicals in the environment is the process of biological amplification. This phenomenon has been demonstrated in a variety of ecosystems and has implications for human exposure. Most examples of bioamplification concern lipophilic chemicals such as chlorinated hydrocarbons or organometallic compounds such as methylmercury. These substances may be present in water or soil at the level of parts per million. When taken up by planktonic organisms, they tend to concentrate in the lipids of these organisms and only a small fraction of the uptake is excreted. When the plankton are consumed by low-level predators such as fish larvae or shrimp, they, too, retain the lipophilic contaminant. These minute animals are then eaten by small fish, which are in turn eaten by larger ones, and the larger ones may then be consumed by birds or perhaps by humans. At each step up the food chain (what ecologists call trophic levels), the organism is in positive balance—that is, it takes in and sequesters more than it excretes, and incorporates an ever-increasing amount of contaminant in its fat until a steady state is reached where excretion balances intake. If the concentration factor is 10 for each level, then the plankton, swimming in water with a 1 ppm concentration, would contain 10 ppm, the fish larvae 100 ppm, the small fish 1000 ppm, and the large fish 10,000 ppm. This example leaves the hapless human consuming a huge dose of the amplified toxic material. A high lipid:water partition coefficient enhances bioamplification. However, some non-lipophilic materials may also undergo bioamplification if they concentrate in some other tissue (i.e., the thyroid) or bind to macromolecules.

Pharmaceuticals and Abused Substances. Pharmaceuticals and abused substances are grouped together because of the high concentrations of bioactive agents deliberately introduced into the body. In fact, many abused substances originally developed as pharmaceuticals (e.g., amphetamines, barbiturates, and narcotics) have profound toxic effects, quite apart from their addictive properties. By whatever route, and whether legal or illicit, these chemicals are used because of their high level of bioactivity. Even when the dosage used is in the therapeutic range, there may be undesired side effects that are actually manifestations of toxicity. These effects may occur in most users (e.g., the soporific effects of diphenhydramine) or rarely (e.g., anaphylaxis caused by penicillin). Certainly the most widespread toxic exposures involve the chronic inhalation of tobacco smoke by the smoker and the chronic consumption of ethanol.

EXPOSURE TO TOXIC SUBSTANCES

Understanding human exposure to toxic substances is the unique feature of environmental medicine. Traditional approaches such as taking a history remain important, but much more sophisticated approaches are required to understand exposure that takes place in the home, community, and workplace. Exposure may occur through air, through water, through food, and through dermal contact.

One can visualize several levels of exposure. The first level involves being in the vicinity of the offending agent (e.g., living in a community with an arsenic smelter). The next level of exposure concerns direct contact with the agent—breathing contaminated air, drinking affected water, or exposing the skin to direct contact with a toxic substance. The third level of exposure concerns the amount of contaminant that actually enters the body and remains. For example, if one breathes air containing benzene vapor or asbestos fibers, how much of the contaminant remains within the body and how much is exhaled? In the case of ingested material, how much is absorbed from the intestinal tract and how much is excreted? In the case of dermal contact, how much penetrates the skin? This level of exposure depends, for example, on the bioavailability of the substance, the intactness of the skin, and the function of the intestinal tract. The final level concerns the exposure of the target (cell, tissue, organ) to the contaminant; this exposure is also called the internal dose.[18]

Exposure to a specific substance is modified by the substance itself and by its bioavailability—for example, whether it is in a soluble or an insoluble form, whether it is volatile, whether there is a vehicle or carrier that promotes absorption into the body (or, conversely, whether it is bound to a matrix from which it cannot be released), and whether it is highly volatile. Exposure is also modified by the condition and behavior of the host—for example, whether the skin is intact, a dietary substance promotes or inhibits uptake, and whether the host is breathing rapidly (e.g., a jogger may be jogging on a crowded urban avenue).

Exposures can be measured by analyzing water, food, and air samples and various products for their concentration of particular substances. Recently the highly sophisticated field of exposure assessment has emerged; it combines chemical analysis, behavioral studies, and mathematical modeling to estimate the dose received by an individual.[18]

Although one usually thinks of ingestion in terms of food or water, there has been great concern over the amount of soil ingested by children. Because children who are very young are more vulnerable to toxic agents such as lead, and because children who are undernourished are both more vulnerable and more likely to eat soil (as a result of a condition known as pica), it has been feared that ingestion of soil may be an important route of contaminant ingestion by children. Various attempts have been made to estimate how much soil an actively playing child consumes in a day. Estimates of 1 g have been used (e.g., by the Environmental Protection Agency dioxin risk assessment), although the actual amount is probably closer to 0.1 g.[19] Ingested soil often contains organic and inorganic pollutants bound to small soil particles.

Exposure varies with the form or species of the pollutant. For example, organic mercury is primarily taken up by ingesting contaminated food items, whereas inorganic mercury can enter the body readily through the respiratory tract. Organic arsenic is ingested with seafood, whereas arsine, a gas, is inhaled.

Advances in instrumentation and analytical chemistry have supported great strides in direct measurement of environmental exposure. Laboratories that would formerly have yielded concentrations of "zero" or "nondetectable" now provide results at parts per trillion or less (e.g., femtograms per gram). Thus the so-called "vanishing zero"[20] is an indication of the ability to analyze smaller and smaller quantities of an agent. Unfortunately, the ability to deal environmentally and sociopolitically with exposures to toxic agents has not kept pace with technological improvements.

The discipline of industrial hygiene is particularly concerned with estimating and preventing exposure to workplace hazards.[21] For airborne hazards, industrial hygienists use a variety of pumps and collection media to capture pollutants in a known volume of air. These pollutants are then quantified and extrapolated in the laboratory to determine how much of the material a worker is exposed to in an 8-hour period. In the case of particulates, it is necessary to establish a size distribution to determine the portion that is of respirable size (usually less than 5 μm in diameter). Because exposures are not constant throughout the day, measurements must be made either several times during the day or during several 8-hour work shifts. Exposures are expressed in terms of a time-weighted average (TWA) corrected to an 8-hour exposure.[17] (See Environmental Risk Assessment, this chapter.)

Bioavailability. An important aspect of exposure is bioavailability.[22] How readily is a toxicant released from its environmental matrix? In the case of ethanol dissolved in water, there is virtually 100% uptake of the alcohol into the bloodstream. In the case of a metal bound to protein in food, the uptake may depend on the efficiency of protein digestion. In the case of substances bound to soil, bioavailability may vary greatly. Research on 2,3,7,8-tetrachlorodibenzo-*p*-dioxin (TCDD; "dioxin"), for example, has emphasized bioavailability. Gallo and colleagues[23] demonstrated that dioxin bound to soil in Newark, N.J., had a very low bioavailability, probably because of a high degree of organic compounds in the soil, whereas dioxin from the sandy soil at Times Beach, Mo., had a much higher bioavailability.

Bioavailability is also important for plants and consequently for humans who consume the plants. Certain pollutants in soil may be taken up by the plant and translocated to the leaves or fruits, which are subsequently harvested for human consumption. Depending on such factors as the chemical species, concentration, pH, and competing ions, the plant may take up a large amount of the pollutant or none at all. If the pollutant is taken up, it is likely to be translocated and subsequently consumed by humans.

FACTORS AFFECTING TOXICITY

Toxicokinetics and Pharmacodynamics. Toxicokinetics is the study of the distribution and differential concentration of a toxic substance and its metabolites throughout the body. It is based on the different rate constants of metabolic processes in different tissues under different circumstances and, for example, on different partitioning coefficients and binding properties. Different reactions are competitive, so the amount of material available for metabolism depends on the amount that has been sequestered in fat, bound to protein, or excreted in the urine.

The fate of every substance that enters the body depends on its absorption, transport, metabolism, storage, and excretion. Metabolism, for example, alters the binding properties and solubility of the original chemical and influences whether it will be stored or excreted. Dynamic equilibria exist for all these processes, and one may refer to Figure 16–1 for the various status changes that constitute the pharmacodynamics of a substance.

As an example of pharmacodynamics, Fick's law describes the passage of a xenobiotic across a membrane as proportional to the concentration gradient, the membrane surface area, and a compound-specific permeability coefficient. The latter, in turn, depends on the condition of the membrane and the lipid:aqueous partitioning of the compound. Two factors influencing the entry of chemicals into cells are the perfusion rate of the organ and the diffusion rate of the substance across the membrane. Excretion via urine, feces, exhaled air, or sweat is, in turn, determined by the relative solubility of the compound and its delivery to the kidneys, liver, lungs, or skin. In general, compounds that are water soluble or appropriately conjugated are excreted via urine, whereas lipid-soluble compounds are secreted via the bile into the intestine.

Metabolic Activation vs Detoxification. An important feature of metabolism is its ability to either reduce or enhance toxicity. Although it was formerly taught that the liver was the major site of detoxification of xenobiotics, it has recently been recognized that many toxic agents are inert until they reach the liver and are metabolically activated, usually through an oxidative reaction. This process results in more highly reactive intermediate compounds that can interfere with other metabolic reactions or "attack" membranes, organelles, or macromolecules.

Sequestration of Xenobiotics. The amount of a substance available to affect a target organ or for excretion depends on how much has been stored or bound. Sequestration of an agent in an organ need not be permanent. Stored substances may be slowly or quickly released from such relatively inactive depots as bone or fat. Lipophilic substances such as chlorinated hydrocarbons (dichlorodiphenyltrichloroethane [DDT], PCB, TCDD) and organometallic compounds are generally found in fatty tissues or in lipid components of cells and membranes. They may be released in large concentrations from fat during starvation or illness. Metal ions such as strontium and lead compete with calcium for deposition in bone, which therefore provides a long-term storage depot for these ions.

Routes of Excretion. Xenobiotics and their metabolites are excreted mainly through the urine and feces but also through the lungs, in sweat, and by the sloughing of skin and hair. Renal clearance is greatest for substances that are water soluble or that are conjugated into hydrophilic complexes. Fecal excretion usually occurs for substances that are lipophilic or that can be conjugated into lipophilic complexes. Enterohepatic cycles may exist to interfere with excretion. A substance that is lipophilic can be secreted into the intestine, from which it is immediately reabsorbed, redistributed to the liver, conjugated with bile, and returned to the gut.

Volatile compounds are excreted through the lungs. At any moment the concentration of these compounds in expired air depends on how much has just been inspired (but not absorbed) and on how much is released to the lungs from the bloodstream. Measurement of volatile compounds in expired air is gaining increasing utility as a means of monitoring exposure.

Short-chain chlorinated hydrocarbons are highly volatile, and whether consumed in water or inhaled, they are excreted via the lungs. Once they reach the liver, they are oxidatively metabolized into polar metabolites that are water soluble but no longer available from excretion in the air.

DOSE-RESPONSE CURVE

Although many toxicological studies simply regard the presence or absence of a particular effect (the quantal response), the hallmark of toxicology is the dose-response curve.[24] The reason is that a high dose of a substance usually has a greater effect than a low dose. In the dose-response curve (Fig. 16–2) the dose is indicated along the x-axis and the response along the y-axis. Most commonly the response is measured as the percentage of exposed animals that show a particular effect. The response could also reflect severity of effect in an individual subject. The typical dose-response curve has the sigmoid shape illustrated. It is a cumulative-percentage response curve.

It is customary to measure dose in terms of the amount of the agent divided by the body weight of the organism (e.g., milligrams of chemical per kilogram of body weight). In some cases (e.g., acute toxic effects or sensitization of the skin, eyes, or respiratory tree) the toxicant is not distributed throughout the

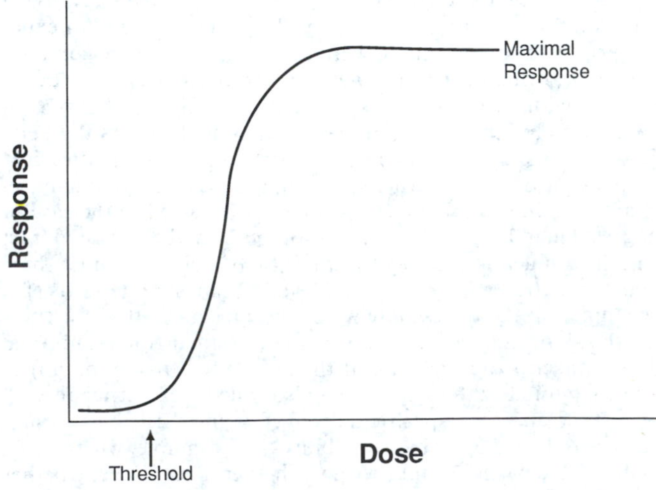

Figure 16–2. The dose-response curve.

body, and the dose per kilogram of body weight is therefore not a good predictor of effect. In such cases, different units must be used, such as concentration in a volume of air or on an area of skin.

In an interpretation of dose-response data from animal studies, it is necessary to know the species, strain, age, and sex of the test animals and the conditions of exposure, as well as the dose. Next, it is necessary to determine the endpoint. Endpoints include death, presence of a lesion (e.g., a tumor), number of lesions, and anatomical, biochemical, physiological, or behavioral changes. Thus if one were concerned with neurotoxic, nephrotoxic, and lethal characteristics of a particular chemical, one would draw three dose-response curves, graphing the severity of each effect against the dose. Thus difficulty in speech occurs at a much lower dose than did coma and death.

The common features of most dose-response curves are shown in Figure 16–2. Initially there is a flat portion, where an increase in dose produces no effect. This is the subthreshold phase. The threshold is the lowest dose that produces an observable effect. Beyond that point the curve tends to rise steeply and often enters a linear phase, where the increase in response is proportional to the increase in dose. Eventually a maximal response is reached and the curve flattens out. This usually means that all the exposed persons or at least all the susceptible persons have shown the effect. Various endpoints have been used to reflect toxicity. Traditionally toxicologists were interested in the LD_{50}, the lethal dose for 50% of the exposed animals. Various chemicals could be ranked in terms of their LD_{50}. In recent years a variety of other responses such as physiological and behavioral responses are defined, and one speaks of the response dose (RD_{50}) or the effective dose (ED_{50}).

Threshold. The threshold (see Fig. 16–2) is a familiar concept to physiologists and biochemists. A particular response may not occur at a very low dose or intensity of stimulus. Thresholds probably exist for most toxic exposures. Thus we can live normal lives even though we are exposed to myriad chemicals, albeit at extremely low (subthreshold) levels. Experience with radiation, however, indicated that even at very low doses there was a measurable (albeit very low) response; the threshold was either not measurable or very close to zero. This led to an understanding of a no-threshold approach to carcinogens.[25]

The concept of a threshold is a source of great controversy in the case of carcinogens,[26] in which, theoretically at least, a single molecule may be the critical molecule that induces a cancer transformation in a cell.[27] Some scientists believe that there must be a threshold for cancer as there is for other toxic reactions. Others argue, on theoretical grounds, that because no threshold (below which no cancer risk exists) has been demonstrated, there must not be a threshold. Perhaps the largest group of scientists are undecided about the no-threshold concept for carcinogens or believe that the concept may be valid for some but not all carcinogens. In light of the ongoing controversy, some governmental regulatory agencies have concluded that until greater certainty is achieved, it is prudent to act as though there is no threshold for carcinogens. Thus the application of a no-threshold approach to carcinogens can be viewed as a policy decision rather than a scientific decision.[28]

Particularly controversial is the Delaney Amendment to the Food, Drug and Cosmetic Act, which states that a known carcinogen cannot be added to food at any concentration. This act is based on the presumption that there is no threshold for a carcinogen below which ingestion is safe. However, the Delaney Amendment does not restrict the sale of food that contains naturally occurring substances or pesticide residues that may be carcinogens.

Latency. Latency is the time between a stimulus and a response or, in toxicology, the time between an exposure and an effect. In some cases (e.g., acute exposure to hydrogen sulfide) the effect is felt in seconds and the latency is therefore measured in seconds. In the case of asbestos-induced mesothelioma, a cancer of the lining of the chest or abdomen, the latency may be on the order of 40 years; that is, the cancer may not develop until 40 years after the first exposure occurred.[29]

If the latency is very short, as with acute effects, it is usually easy to establish a cause-effect relationship. When the latency is much longer, the cause may have been forgotten before the outcome is realized. Accordingly, only sophisticated epidemiological studies can identify cause-effect relationships with long latencies. In some cases there is a dose-response relationship with latency as the effect, because at higher doses latency is reduced.

SYNERGISM AND ANTAGONISM

When two chemicals are administered together or when a person is exposed to a mixture of chemicals, there may be various interactions, identified as follows: (1) independence or additivity: each substance produces its own effect appropriate for its dose; (2) synergism: the combined effect is greater than either substance would produce alone or additively (i.e., the effect is multiplicative); (3) antagonism: the combined effect is less than one would expect from either chemical administered alone. A classic example of synergism is the case of asbestos and smoking.[30] Synergism may occur when substance A enhances the effect of substance B, promotes its activation, or interferes with its degradation and excretion. Antagonism occurs when A interferes with the uptake of B, competes with it for metabolic enzymes or substrates, or enhances its degradation or excretion.

REVERSIBILITY

Because most people recover from most toxic exposures, it is clear that many toxic effects are reversible. Inhibition of a biochemical pathway may be reversed if a competing agent is introduced to bind up the xenobiotic. The death of a cell is not reversible, but in almost all organs the regeneration of new cells occurs to take over the role of the damaged cells. In the case of genetic damage to the nucleic acid molecules, sophisticated biochemical reactions called "DNA repair" mechanisms are brought into play and eliminate, in various ways, the damaged DNA. The mechanism(s) of DNA repair become less efficient with age, and this is believed to be one of the factors associated with the increased incidence of cancer in older people.

SUSCEPTIBILITY

Although it is well known that individual humans vary in their susceptibility to different stressors, and although some of the factors modifying susceptibility are well known, there is little research literature on this particular topic. In experimental animals, species, strain, gender, and age influence susceptibility. Indeed, some strains are bred for enhanced susceptibility to certain diseases. If a population of organisms is exposed to a fixed dose of a chemical, one can graph the responses with a histogram and determine the number of individuals with no response and of those with a low, medium, or high response. If a response is quantitative, a smoothed histogram can be drawn. This might show a normal or log-normal distribution, or it might vary greatly from normal. If only one gender is susceptible, the curve will be skewed. If both very young and very old animals are susceptible, the curve will be bimodal.

BIOLOGICAL EFFECTS

Pathologists recognize several categories or classes of pathogenic change in organisms, organs, tissues, and cells, including: (1) physical trauma, (2) chemical poisoning, (3) inflammation, (4) infection, (5) neoplasia, and (6) immune response. Recently attention has focused on subcellular and molecular targets of poisons. Toxicology is concerned with all these forms and levels of injury.

RECEPTORS

Advances in biochemistry include the recognition of receptors as an important part of toxic interactions. Although some toxic interactions take place in solution, toxicologists have increasingly recognized that toxic effects usually involve binding of the toxicant to some active receptor site on an enzyme or membrane. A familiar example is the binding of neuroinhibitory substances to the receptors on the postsynaptic membrane or the myoneural junction. Receptors are important components of normal cellular function and account for the remarkable specificity of many cell processes. Most familiar are the receptors on the postsynaptic membrane that initiate a nerve impulse when binding acetylcholine. It is now realized that many hormone effects are mediated by hormone-specific receptors in particular target tissues. Some toxic effects occur because a xenobiotic is capable of binding to a hormone receptor or a neuroreceptor and of interfering with the normal action of the endogenous chemical; for example, 2,3,7,8-TCDD binds to estrogen receptors.[31]

A normal feature of receptor models is that they are reversible, allowing the same biological function to be rapidly repeated. Toxic effects involving receptors often are much less reversible (e.g., the binding of carbon monoxide to hemoglobin, or the anticholinesterase effects of organophosphate pesticides). One result of this lesser reversibility is competitive inhibition between the xenobiotic and the endogenous compound.

MECHANISMS OF TOXICITY

Metabolic Poisons. Metabolic poisons are substances that disrupt metabolic pathways and are therefore competitive inhibitors. Binding to an enzyme and altering its tertiary structure or interfering with its active site is a common mechanism of toxicity.

Macromolecular Binding. Chemicals may bind to various macromolecules such as proteins, hemoglobin, and nucleic acids. The presence of DNA adducts may reflect genotoxic or carcinogenic properties, and the quest for these molecular markers of exposure is an important frontier in toxicological research.

Subcellular Poisons. Some substances act within cells to alter the structure or function of internal membranes such as endoplasmic reticulum or of organelles such as mitochondria. Many chemicals act on mitochondria, interfering with their energetic function and resulting in swelling and loss of detail on electron micrographs.

Cellular Poisons. Cellular poisons are substances that damage cells and cell membranes, causing necrosis or lysis. Membranes are functional as well as structural entities, and chemicals that interfere with membrane transport systems may have major consequences. Toxic agents may react with either the protein or lipid component of the membrane. Many naturally occurring toxins, for example, the hemolysins in certain plants and snake venoms, cause the lysis of cells. Some heavy metals act directly on the cell membrane, interfering with the sulfhydryl binding responsible for membrane integrity and altering membrane fluidity.[32]

Immunotoxins. Immunotoxins are substances that suppress the immune response. They may act on different components of the immune system. Some toxins affect γ-globulins. Some agents interfere with the production or function or life span of the T and B lymphocytes. T cells mature in the thymus and are the main factor in cell-mediated immunity. B cells control antibody-mediated or humoral immunity. T cells are classified on the basis of surface antigens, and it is now possible to quantify a variety of T cell populations and determine which functions have been inhibited. The initial site of action may be in the bone marrow or in the bloodstream. The synthesis of immunoglobulins by the liver may be altered. Substances known to interfere with the immune system include polyhalogenated aromatic compounds (e.g., 2,3,7,8-TCDD), metals (e.g., lead and cadmium), pesticides, and even air pollutants (e.g., NO_2, SO_2, tobacco smoke).

Sensitizers. Sensitizers are substances that act through the immune system to induce an increased immune response. They can be complete allergens or haptens. The main target organs are the skin itself and the respiratory system. Nickel and *Rhus* plants are common examples of skin sensitizers that cause contact dermatitis. Occupational asthmas reflect sensitization of the lung and airways to aerosols. A particular type of sensitization is the syndrome of so-called multiple chemical sensitivity, in which some individuals appear to develop multisystem responses to very low levels of chemicals and to have these effects generalized to chemicals other than those to which they were originally exposed. Numerous clinicians have encountered such individuals, and the identification of an immune mechanism that would account for symptoms is a controversial research area.[33]

Neuroendocrine Poisons. Many chemicals have very specific actions on components of the nervous and endocrine systems. These poisons may interfere with the synthesis or release of hormones or transmitters or may competitively or destructively block their action.

Mutagenic Substances. Some substances interact with genetic material, causing either point mutations, chromosomal damage, or interference with meiosis, mitosis, or cell division.

Substances With Reproductive System Effects. The processes of gametogenesis, fertilization, implantation, embryogenesis, organogenesis, and birth are complex and subject to many errors. Major errors incompatible with life generally result in spontaneous abortion, which can be viewed as a quality control procedure. Adverse reproductive consequences include failure to form gametes (e.g., azoospermia) and formation of abnormal gametes. Once gametes are formed, several factors may intervene to prevent the initiation of embryogenesis. There is concern that many synthetic chemicals, particularly those which bind to hormone receptors, may interfere with one or more of these steps. A notable case is dibromochloropropane (DBCP), a nematocide, which induced azoospermia in the men who manufactured and packaged it. Some of these men never recovered normal spermatogenesis after cessation of exposure. Lead also interferes with spermatogenesis. A long list of chemicals have been implicated in toxic effects on the male reproductive system (including interference with spermatogenesis, semen quality, erection, and libido). The list of chemicals affecting the female reproductive system includes cancer chemotherapeutic agents, other pharmaceuticals, metals, insecticides, and various industrial chemicals.[34]

Teratogenic Substances. Some substances interfere with the complex processes of morphogenesis. Depending on the stage of embryogenesis or fetogenesis, they may affect various organ systems, leading to embryonic death, major structural birth defects, slowed maturation, or even such postnatal problems as learning difficulties.[35] In general, exposure before implantation is likely to be lethal. Exposure during organogenesis may result in birth defects or embryonic death. Later in fetal life, intrauterine growth retardation or fetal death may occur, or functional changes that interfere with birth or postnatal development may occur. Approximately 3% of live-born infants have detectable congenital abnormalities; additional congenital defects may become apparent later in life. Some defects are genetic or chromosomal in origin, but some are due to chemical exposures (including drugs taken by the mother).

The recently recognized field of behavioral teratology involves study of some of these effects, such as the impact of lead exposure on psychomotor development and learning. The fetal alcohol syndrome reflects the specific toxic effects of ethanol ingested by the mother on the development and behavior of the newborn infant.

MICROSOMAL ENZYME INDUCTION

Because of the specificity of enzymes, the body cannot maintain a full supply of all the enzymes that may be needed for every situation. Accordingly, many substances induce the synthesis of the enzymes that will act on them, and within 12 to 24 hours the amount of enzyme present within a cell may increase by several orders of magnitude. Some enzyme systems are highly specific and act only on a single substrate, whereas others are nonspecific and catalyze classes of reactions on a wide range of substrates. The substrates vary in their potency at inducing enzymes. Enzyme induction plays an important role in metabolizing xenobiotics, either enhancing their toxicity or reducing it. However, the most important consequence of enzyme induction is sometimes the greatly accelerated metabolism of endogenous bioactive compounds. The cytochrome P-450 system is an example of an enzyme system that metabolizes a wide range of xenobiotics.

OXIDATIVE STRESS

Oxygen, in addition to its critical role in supporting cellular respiration and oxidation-reduction reactions throughout the body, plays a more sinister role in toxicity. Normally there is a balance between oxidative and antioxidant reactions. However, the oxidative reactions, so necessary for life, are now believed to play important roles in inflammation, aging, carcinogenesis, and toxicity.[36]

Toxicologists speak of reactive oxygen species, some of which are free radicals. Oxygen can receive an electron and form superoxide anion radicals, which can react with hydrogen to form hydrogen peroxide, which, in turn, reacts with free electrons and hydrogen ions to form water and a highly reactive hydroxide radical.

$$O-O + e^- \rightarrow O-O\cdot$$
$$O-O\cdot + e^- + H^+ \rightarrow H-O-O-H$$
$$H-O-O-H + e^- + H^+ \rightarrow H_2O + \cdot OH$$

In the course of these reactions the highly reactive free radicals, particularly the hydroxy radical, are available to attack macromolecules, initiating a variety of toxic effects. The superoxide anion radical is formed in many oxidation reactions in which oxygen acts as an electron receptor.

In response to the potential harm that these reactive oxygen species may cause, the body has evolved antioxidant defenses (see Sies[36] for a more detailed description). The defenses include water-soluble vitamin C and the lipid-soluble vitamins E and A. Superoxide dismutase, a metalloprotein, and glutathione-dependent peroxidases, in association with glutathione reductase, scavenge free radicals. One of the consequences of free radical formation is a reaction with lipids, including those in cell and organelle membranes, to form lipid peroxides, which in turn lead to cell damage and dysfunction.

CARCINOGENESIS: INITIATION AND PROMOTION

Cancer is not a single disease but includes a great many diseases that share a common property of uncontrolled cell proliferation. Normally cell proliferation proceeds in controlled fashion, ensuring an adequate number of new cells for any given physiologic task. Substances that cause cancer, carcinogens, have a variety of actions. It is customary to divide carcinogenesis into two stages, *initiation* and *promotion*. Initiation is the process by which the genetic material of the cell is altered, predisposing it to cancer.[37] Initiation is a process to which humans are exposed all their lives. The changes that constitute initiation may be reversed by repair mechanisms or may lie dormant, perhaps controlled by the immune system. Promotion is the process by which initiated cells are stimulated or allowed to become cancerous.[38]

An effect that is manifested in clinically apparent signs or symptoms is likely to be a significant health effect that requires prevention. There are, however, measurable effects, the significance of which is controversial. Is hyperplasia or hypertrophy under moderate stress a sign of healthy physiological adaptation, or is it pathological? A person with hemolysis adequately compensated by reticulocytosis will show no sign of illness.[39] Does this natural biologic adaptation put an unacceptable and eventually unhealthful strain on the body? Is there a limit to the body's ability to compensate for stress? Is a certain level of stress beneficial? Some writers have suggested that "hormesis," the beneficial effects of low levels of otherwise toxic substances, actually enhances the body's ability to confront stressors.[40]

Many articles have been written in this controversial area, and at present most of the opinion lies outside the realm of science. It can be said that organisms protected from stressors do not necessarily thrive (e.g., gnotobiotic individuals are susceptible to subsequent exposure to infectious agents). In the case of oxidant-induced hemolysis in a person with glucose-6-phosphate dehydrogenase deficiency, it is safe to say that controlling exposure to the oxidant is desirable. However, because the body's ability to compensate is sufficient, the "susceptible" person should not be discriminated against or denied employment simply because some hemolysis will occur initially.[39]

TARGET ORGANS

A traditional approach to describing the effects of toxic chemicals is to examine them in terms of the target organ system and the consequent pathophysiological effects. Chapters in standard toxicology textbooks (e.g., Klaasen et al., 1986) are devoted to each of these systems, and they will not be discussed here.

CLINICAL EVALUATION OF TOXICITY

Clinical evaluation of persons exposed to toxic chemicals involves a number of diagnostic approaches.

History. A detailed medical, social, environmental, and occupational history may provide evidence of certain health effects as well as relevant exposures. The occupational history (see Chapter 15) should include a detailed list of all employment (including moonlighting and parttime jobs and the employment of other household members).[41] For each job, one documents the kinds of activities performed, exposures experienced, and protective equipment available and used. The interviewer should obtain detailed information on how the patient actually performs a task and whether the patient associates symptoms with particular tasks, exposures, or time periods. Postshift versus preshift symptoms, and symptoms that recur on Monday morning or disappear on vacation, are clues to a work-related exposure. The interviewer should also elicit information on whether coworkers or spouses have similar symptoms.

Physical Examination. The examiner may detect certain effects related to chemical exposure. For maximal value the physical examination must be based on the history. Thus a history of tingling in the toes leads to a more intensive neurological and vascular examination of the extremities.

Laboratory Tests. Although laboratory tests are often included automatically in diagnostic studies, they tend to have a low yield. In the case of specific hematotoxins, one may see a reduction (or an increase) in circulating white blood cells, red blood cells, platelets, or reticulocytes. Specific tests are more likely to be productive if they are selected to correspond with known exposures (e.g., creatinine tests after nephrotoxin exposure or liver function tests after hepatotoxin exposure).

Liver Function Tests. Some tests, such as the alanine and aspartate aminotransferase tests, measure liver cell injury. These enzymes are normally present in the blood in small amounts but are released in larger amounts when the liver is damaged. Other tests may be true function tests. For example, the indocyanine green test, although long abandoned by clinicians, may be resurrected for the specific examination of patients exposed to hepatotoxins. This dye enters the liver cells and is conjugated into a water-soluble form that can be quickly excreted. If liver cells are not functioning, the dye remains in the bloodstream, and this failure to excrete the dye can be measured. Such tests are nonspecific—that is, they indicate damage but provide no clues as to cause.

Kidney Function Tests. Clinical tests for kidney disease are not sufficiently sensitive to detect early exposure to nephrotoxins.[42] A variety of new, although still somewhat esoteric, tests are being studied as ways of monitoring persons exposed to nephrotoxins. Lauwerys and Bernard[42] recommend monitoring of high-molecular-weight (e.g., albumin) and low-molecular-weight (e.g., β_2-microglobulin) proteins in urine.

Clinical Evaluation vs Surveillance. The clinical evaluation of some patients can become extremely involved and expensive. The same tests have often been used to monitor groups of healthy workers to determine excessive chemical exposure. However, care must be exercised in designing a medical surveillance protocol for workers, because tests designed to detect gross clinical illness are often insensitive and inappropriate for detecting subclinical changes in apparently healthy persons.

CAUSALITY: ENVIRONMENTAL CHEMICAL EXPOSURE AND HEALTH EFFECTS

In the laboratory, establishing a chemical exposure as the cause of an adverse effect on health depends on sound experimental design and careful attention to alternative hypotheses. It may or may not involve careful definition of the mechanism by which the effect is achieved. In the community, determination of cause and effect is much more difficult. Under these "natural" conditions, the hazardous substance is not always identified or may be present in mixtures, and the dose and the conditions and time frame of exposure are seldom known. It may also be difficult to ascertain who has been exposed. Often there is a bewildering array of symptoms and signs attributed, perhaps only tentatively, to the putative cause. Simply defining relevant health effects may be a costly and frustrating venture, and linking the effects to specific exposures may be impossible.[43]

Scientists and clinicians may not appreciate that the courts impose entirely different standards on establishing causation. Moreover, standards of causation differ under different bodies of law. Thus in some jurisdictions one may have to establish a "reasonable probability," whereas in others, causation must be "more likely than not" or one must be able to say that "without this event the outcome probably would not have occurred." In some circumstances one must establish an attributable risk—that is, one must determine how much of the outcome can be related to a particular exposure. In other cases the causation is assumed unless proved otherwise.[44] For example, the U.S. Congress required the Veterans Administration to give veterans "the benefit of the doubt" in cases involving herbicide exposure.

TOXICITY TESTING

Toxicologists employ a wide variety of systems and paradigms to test chemicals in order to predict their effects on human health or the environment. The factors that affect toxicity in humans (see Table 16–1) must be considered in designing the experiments. One must choose the appropriate animal model or in vitro test system. If animals are used, the genetic strain, gender, and age of the animal must be selected. The dosage schedule, including whether doses will be single or multiple, the duration of dosing, and appropriate dose levels, must be chosen. The route of administration should be relevant to natural conditions of exposure, the experiment should last long enough to fully encompass any effects that have a long latency, and naturally, appropriate control animals must be selected. In addition to these design features, an experiment must adhere to established good laboratory practice standards, which mandate how animals must be cared for and how data must be recorded. This provides for appropriate quality assurance methods.[13,14] Increasingly, however, a variety of in vitro test systems are replacing many studies traditionally done in animals.

ANIMAL WELFARE AND ANIMAL RIGHTS

Toxicologists have become increasingly attentive to the animal welfare and animal rights movements. Proponents of animal rights argue that animals have intrinsic rights which, in the extreme, should protect them from any and all use in experimental research. Animal "rights" are not guaranteed by either human or divine law; however, animal welfare is clearly an important issue. Experimental animals should be spared unnecessary stress, discomfort, or pain. Increasingly researchers have sought alternative models that do not require whole animals. At the same time, animal research has been redesigned to use fewer animals and to minimize pain. The National Science Foundation and the National Institutes of Health have recognized the importance of animal welfare not only from a humane perspective but because stressed animals may not provide an appropriate response in experimental situations. Accordingly researchers using animals must take into account animal care guidelines that stipulate the conditions under which animals must be kept and the availability of veterinary care. Research protocols must be reviewed by institutional animal care committees.

The conflict over animal welfare reaches its peak when primates are used. Primates are expensive to acquire and maintain, and most studies of primates can afford only a few animals, who often live under somewhat stressed conditions. In addition, because extrapolation from primates to humans is not always more appropriate than extrapolation from other animal models, most toxicology research does not involve primates.

REGULATING TOXIC EXPOSURES

The past two decades have seen emergence of a complex governmental framework to regulate toxic chemicals in the environment. Each agency has a distinct jurisdiction; unfortunately the regulations of one agency may not always be consistent with those of another. Among these agencies and programs are the Food and Drug Administration, the Occupational Health and Safety Administration, the Consumer Product Safety Commission, and the Environmental Protection Agency (see Chapter 34 on Regulation of Chemicals in the United States).

Neurobehavioral Toxicology

Michael Gochfeld
Nancy Fiedler
Joanna Burger

The nervous system is a prominent target organ for many poisons that can interfere with neuromuscular or synaptic transmission or with nerve conduction or that can cause degeneration of myelin sheaths, axons, glial cells, or neurons. Some toxic effects, such as the weakness produced by anticholinesterases or the peripheral neuropathy associated with lead poisoning, may be clinically apparent. Subclinical changes may be detected by neurophysiological techniques, whereas other, even more subtle changes may require new neurobehavioral testing approaches. The acute effects associated with anesthetics, such as lightheadedness, fainting, coma, and death, are dramatic manifestations of neurotoxicity. Increasingly, however, neurobehavioral toxicology has become concerned with chronic effects such as impaired learning, memory, vigilance, and depressed psychomotor performance. Neurobehavioral evaluations of exposed individuals or groups provide an opportunity to evaluate objectively the many nonspecific symptoms reported. For example, symptoms attributed to metal toxicity include weakness, dizziness, irritability, listlessness, anorexia, depression, anosmia and visual disturbances, disorientation, incoordination, ataxia and paralysis, insomnia or sleepiness, and finally psychiatric symptoms or personality changes.

In the past 15 years increasing attention has been paid to neurobehavioral toxicity, in recognition of the observation that subtle behavioral changes may occur at doses lower than those required to cause frankly pathological changes or clinical symptoms.[1–4] Neurobehavioral toxicology has built on the major advances in understanding behavior provided by ethologists and experimental psychologists. The pharmaceutical industry has contributed to the field's development through its quest for psychoactive drugs as well as its scrutiny of neurotoxic side effects. In 1973, the National Institute for Occupational Safety and Health convened the Behavioral Toxicology Workshop for Early Detection of Occupational Hazards,[2] which reviewed research findings on many substances in various organisms, charted future directions, and carefully considered the tools that could be applied to evaluating behavioral toxic effects.[1] Since that time the field has grown rapidly, and there are a variety of experimental paradigms and clinical approaches for detecting behavioral manifestations of neurotoxicity.[6,7] There have been extensive reviews of experimental and clinical findings[8,9] (see also General References in the Neurobehavioral Toxicology section of the references collected at the end of this chapter), and an entire journal, first published in 1979, is devoted to the field.[10]

Whereas evaluation of nervous system function was formerly the domain of the neurologist and electrophysiologist, a new dimension has been added with the advent of validated neurobehavioral test batteries. Because neurobehavioral toxins affect the higher levels of function and functional integration, often without apparent anatomical or physiological changes, they pose certain problems for the clinician. Thus neurobehavioral testing is a necessary component of evaluating neurotoxicity. However, because many of the neurobehavioral tests are new and remain to be validated, they are more useful for epidemiological studies of groups of people rather than for the clinical assessment of individuals. In this discussion we review the target components of the nervous system, the kinds of behavioral abnormalities seen, and some of the neurobehavioral tests currently used for evaluating such abnormalities. Only brief consideration is given to examples of neurotoxins.

TARGET COMPONENTS OF NERVOUS SYSTEM

In analyzing neurobehavioral and neurological effects of xenobiotics, one can subdivide the nervous system into various target components. The major anatomical divisions are as follows:

Autonomic nervous system

Parasympathetic nerves
Sympathetic nerves

Peripheral nervous system

Sensory receptors and integrators
Sensory nerves
Motor nerves

Central nervous system

Brain
- Cerebral cortex
- Cerebellum
- Basal ganglia
- Brain stem

Spinal cord

Recognized effects on the autonomic nervous system are primarily biochemical. Toxins structurally similar to neurotransmitters may act to enhance (agonist) or inhibit (antagonist) the normal function of either the parasympathetic or sympathetic system. The parasympathetic system is concerned with normal maintenance activities (e.g., peristalsis). A drug that inhibits this action (e.g., many antidiarrheal agents) may bring the peristaltic action to a standstill. Many widely used drugs have primary effects or side effects on the autonomic system.

Effects on the peripheral nervous system often result from chronic exposures. Peripheral neuropathies may occur when a xenobiotic kills nerve cells or destroys the axon. Myelinopathies involve the destruction of the myelin sheath, which plays an important role in rapid nerve conduction. Even subtle damage to the myelin can be detected by nerve conduction velocity studies. Axonopathies involve a dying back of the axon itself (e.g., that caused by n-hexane). These defects can be detected by neuropathologists. More elusive are pathological changes that affect associations among neurons in the brain. Improved histochemical approaches allow pathologists to detect changes in innervation (e.g., between two nuclei in the brain) and the localized destruction of specific types of nerve cells. Many neurobehavioral effects are due to agonistic or antagonistic actions on neurotransmission in the central nervous system. At the subcellular level, the differential impact of organic and inorganic lead on the microtubule assembly suggests an additional mechanism subject to disruption by certain toxins.

Peripheral neuropathies are important manifestations of a number of neurotoxic exposures, such as exposure to lead. Such neuropathies also occur in systemic diseases such as diabetes. Peripheral neuropathies may affect either sensory nerves or motor nerves or both. Usually it is the sensory nerve fibers that are most susceptible, as in the case of lead,[11] and the sense of touch, temperature sensitivity, and vibration sensation may be the first to go. Longer fibers tend to be more susceptible, and the neuropathies tend to appear in the feet before they appear in the hands.

Effects in the brain tend to be much more complex. The components of the nervous system as targets of neurotoxic compounds having already been examined, it is apparent that the most complex aspects of nervous system function cannot be tested by traditional electrophysiological or clinical means. Accordingly the field of neurobehavioral toxicology is emerging as an important and overlooked branch of toxicology. Our understanding of how the brain achieves the so-called higher functions (e.g., learning, memory, creativity, cognition) remains primitive. Ablation studies (opportunistic or deliberate) and computer analogy are examples of approaches to understanding brain function, and there is an extensive experimental and human psychology literature on brain functions; yet for most clinical purposes the brain remains a "black box." There is also a need for fusion among disciplines because, for example, the extensive literature on the neurobehavioral effects of alcohol and hallucinogens is seldom cited by researchers in occupational or environmental science.

SELECTED NEUROBEHAVIORAL TOXINS

This section briefly treats some of the types of neurobehavioral toxins. Specific neurotoxins are considered in detail in many of the texts listed in the General References, such as Spencer and Schaumburg, Klaasen et al., and Hartman. Many commonly occurring chemicals are neurotoxic. Table 16–2 indicates the variability in effects produced by some common neurotoxins. Virtually all solvents, whether aliphatic or aromatic, and whether chlorinated or not, have acute effects on the nervous system, many solvents sharing common anesthetic properties. Particularly on the basis of research in Scandinavia,[12–14] important chronic effects of solvent exposure also are apparent in both animals and workers. Nerve conduction remains altered for many years after cessation of solvent exposure, and memory and learning, mood, impulse control, and motivation are impaired.[15]

TABLE 16–2. EXAMPLE OF BEHAVIORAL IMPAIRMENTS ASSOCIATED WITH VARIOUS TOXIC SUBSTANCES

	Pb	As	Mn	Hg	CS_2	Solv	OPP
Acute psychosis			+		+		
Emotional lability			+	+	+		
Memory impairment	+	+	+		+		
Psychomotor	+			+	+	+	+
Neurasthenia	+	+	+	+		+	
Extrapyramidal			+		+		
Neuropathy	+	+					
Tremor			+	+	+		

Key: CS_2 = carbon disulfide; Solv = solvents; OPP = organophosphate pesticides.

The effects of styrene have been studied in several occupational groups,[16,17] and both specific changes (impaired reaction time) and more general mood alterations have been found. Carbon disulfide effects are manifested in almost all components of the central and peripheral nervous systems.[18] Evidence of peripheral neuropathy (paresthesia, numbness), cranial neuropathy, dementia (confusion), parkinsonism, acute psychosis, irritability, and memory loss have been attributed to this compound.[19,20] Carbon monoxide at relatively low levels (equivalent to carboxyhemoglobin $< 10\%$) impairs vigilance, tracking, and the ability to drive.[21,22]

Many metals, for example, lead, mercury, manganese, and arsenic, are also neurotoxic but tend to have discrete nervous system effects (Table 16–2). Lead has been the most extensively studied neurotoxic metal, and the literature documents effects on most aspects of neurobehavioral function.[23,24] The species of metal influences its impact. Thus organic tin compounds cause weakness and paralysis as well as central nervous system disturbances. Organic arsenic affects the optic nerve and retina, whereas inorganic arsenic produces polyneuritis and weakness. Tremors and, in severe cases, ataxia occur with either inorganic or organic mercury poisoning; however, organic mercury also produces visual field changes, whereas inorganic mercury produces personality disturbances characterized as "erethism." This syndrome involves irritability, labile temper, pathological shyness (avoidance of close friends), depression, loss of sleep, fatigue, and blushing. In some cases there is even a dose-response curve between the occurrence of symptoms and the concentration of mercury in urine.

A more esoteric compound is 1-methyl-4-phenyl-1,2,3,6-tetrahydropyridine (MPTP), a synthetic substance produced accidentally in the attempted synthesis of meperidine analogues by substance abusers. MPTP has a specific effect on the substantia nigra, leading to irreversible parkinsonian symptoms.[25]

These examples indicate the breadth of substances that affect neurobehavioral performance and the spectrum of effects. The reader should also consider the extensive literature on ethanol and hallucinogens, which have their primary effects on neurobehavioral performance.

ANIMAL MODELS IN NEUROBEHAVIORAL TOXICITY

In addition to clinical reports and epidemiological studies, animal research contributes significantly to our understanding of neurotoxicity and neurobehavioral changes. No animal model adequately mimics the complex neurobehavioral performance of humans, particularly in the intellectual domain. Although gorillas and chimpanzees appear to behave similarly to humans in some respects and are genetically very close to humans, our evolutionary divergence is particularly apparent in those functions that are the domain of the neurobehaviorist. Thus, although the neuropathologist and electrophysiologist would be able to assess the function of a gorilla or chimpanzee and translate it to humans, the clinical psychologist would be sorely challenged to evaluate behavior and psychodynamics and would revert to conditioning paradigms[26] regularly applied to "lower" primates and rodents. Although primate research is attractive, one must consider that the lineage of human evolution diverged from that of the New World and Old World monkeys many millions of years ago; hence it may be illusory to assume that monkeys, so widely favored in research, offer useful animal models for behavioral changes involving so-called higher functions. In addition to evolutionary considerations, primate research is extremely expensive, and many of the species used in research are threatened or endangered in the wild. Moreover, for wide-ranging, highly social species such as most primates, captivity may produce a chronic level of stress which itself interferes with all aspects of behavior. Finally, most laboratory studies of primate behavioral responses are based on samples of one to five individuals.

Many important advances in understanding brain function have been derived from studies in avian and rodent models. Rodent studies allow large sample sizes to be employed, whereas avian studies take advantage of the fact that, like humans, birds rely primarily on visual and acoustic rather than olfactory and tactile communication. Traditional animal research has provided useful paradigms for human neurobehavioral studies. The fact that a chemical produces the same effect on learning in a wide variety of animal species is important validation of its role in humans. Similarly, although our assessment of higher-level functions in humans relies on functions or responses that are uniquely human (reading, speech), the basic structural arrangement and function of the human nervous system do not differ from those of other vertebrates. Thus eye-limb coordination, cerebellar function, and even learning are common to all vertebrates, and even cognition may be identified in many so-called "lower" organisms.[27] In recognition of the important contribution of animal behavior studies to shaping our understanding of human behavior,[28] three pioneers of animal behavior research, Konrad Lorenz, Nikolaas Tinbergen, and Karl von Frisch were awarded the Nobel Prize in Biology and Medicine in 1973.

Animal experimentation also provides the opportunity to assess exposures and effects that cannot be studied in humans. Developing species-appropriate test batteries is an exciting challenge for behavioral toxicologists.[26,29,30] Animal studies have focused on discrimination of stimuli, learning deficits, disturbance of locomotion or balance, decreased performance of previously learned tasks, memory deficits, altered activity patterns, and changes in normal behavior patterns related to reproduction or maintenance. A wide variety of paradigms have been employed in the attempt to understand the effects of stress on the nervous system, and many of them can be applied to humans. In addition, some research has examined how the neurobehavioral effects of a toxic chemical or physical stressors can be exhibited in offspring of the exposed individual.

Learning Tasks. Experimental intervention allows specific probes of behavior and performance. Early testing employed Y mazes and other learned visual-discrimination tasks. Experiments with rats examined how toxins affect the speed of learning a maze after a reward or punishment was offered in one or the other arms of the maze.[31-33]

Conditioning Studies. In studies involving conditioning of psychomotor performance, animals are trained to perform tasks in response to certain stimuli. They are then exposed to a substance, and the disruption of performance is quantified.[26,34] With time, the behavioral tests have become more sophisticated and now include such paradigms as nonspatial and spatial delayed matching to a sample, serial position sequences, and multiple fixed-interval reinforcement tests in animals previously trained with operant conditioning.[26,35-38] These studies examined learned behavior and relied on the production of the desired behavior, followed by measurement of its sensitivity to environmental stimuli.[26] Alterations in visual performance can be useful endpoints in conditioned animals.[39] The great advantage of these methods is that they can detect subtle differences in the behavior of animals that otherwise appear normal; however, they do require experience in the operant conditioning techniques.

Naturalistic Studies. Naturalistic studies of behavior, conducted in the laboratory and in the field, observe behaviors that occur naturally in the organism's life-style (e.g., locomotion, balance, or predator defense).[29,40] In many of these studies the toxic agent, such as lead, interferes with learning or with retention of learning (i.e., the subsequent performance of learned tasks).

Under natural conditions, animals have somewhat predictable or stereotyped ways of behaving that can be quantified. Such behaviors may be directly relevant to survival and successful reproduction. Toxic substances that affect such behavior can have far-reaching effects on fitness. Some behaviors examined include the accuracy and pecking rate of pigeons,[41] activity rates in mice[42] or rats,[43] nest-site defense in falcons,[40] monkey behavior,[44] dove courtship sequences,[45] begging behavior and food manipulation in terns,[29] and web weaving in spiders.[46] In most of these studies the effect was clearly demonstrable by directly observing individual animals.

The advantage of the naturalistic behavioral studies is that the behaviors are important for fitness and have been shaped and perhaps optimized by evolution. Thus predator avoidance is a natural part of an animal's behavioral repertoire, whereas pushing a button may not be. Conversely, operant conditioning paradigms afford tighter control of experimental situations. Yet natural behaviors such as locomotion,[30] exploration, righting ability, depth perception, thermoregulation, aggression, avoidance,[47] learning, and parental recognition are all amenable to laboratory and field experimentation where variables can be controlled.[29,48] Laties and Cory-Slechta[49] caution that confounding factors may influence behavioral outcome in laboratory studies.

Although most neurotoxicology studies in animals examine the direct effect of exposure, some multigeneration studies have yielded important results,[50,51] showing that the children and even grandchildren of treated animals may manifest behavioral deficits. Exposure of one or both parents can affect behavior in offspring. If both parents are exposed, the impact is greater than if either one is exposed alone.[50]

It seems reasonable to conclude that animal behavioral models will continue to be useful for understanding many aspects of behavioral toxicology, for developing useful questions and approaches to clinical application, and for validating generalizations developed in humans. Conversely, for some of the higher functions, humans will remain the primary test subjects, and improved epidemiological studies employing both old and new psychometric approaches will be fruitful. These studies must be opportunistic, recognizing exposures that have already occurred, whereas the animal models will allow the use of controlled exposures and testing of new paradigms.

SYSTEMATIC ANALYSIS OF THE NERVOUS SYSTEM

Evolutionary selection has honed the vertebrate sensory systems to provide information about position, food, mates, and danger. The pathways from receptor to brain and the central integration required to process the information are highly complex and are vulnerable to damage from toxic agents.

Vision. Neuroophthalmologists, neurologists, and ophthalmologists examine the eyes and visual system for evidence of damage. Electrooculography can provide objective measures of eye muscle function. Visual evoked potentials are used in electroencephalographic techniques to measure brain-wave responses to light. Neurobehaviorists test such functions as visual perception and eye-hand coordination. Direct perceptual changes include loss of visual acuity, alteration of visual fields, and changes in color sensitivity and in flicker fusion. Valciukas and Singer[7,52] emphasized the value of complex perceptual tasks detected by embedded figures (Fig. 16–3). These different approaches thus evaluate the ability to direct the eyes, the receptive capability of the eye itself, and ultimately the ability of the brain to process and respond to information transmitted from the eye.

Hearing. The physician's physical examination includes the status of the ear canal and eardrum, and a relatively crude measurement of hearing and of bone versus air conduction. Audiometric examination of hearing is extremely commonplace, and although the equipment is not inexpensive, it is used in such high volume that examinations should be relatively inexpensive. In the presence of entirely normal hearing, however, performance of tasks involving auditory reaction time or auditory memory may be impaired. As with the eye, some tests evaluate the external receptor and others the response of the brain to sound. Persistent loud noise damages the sensory cells of the inner ear, which in effect are the interface between the hearing mechanism and the brain. Certain neurotoxic chemicals, for instance the antibiotics streptomycin and kanamycin, damage the auditory nerve pathway. More subtle changes in the ability to detect loudness, pitch, and timbre are the domain of the psychoacoustician, and in special cases can be evaluated as part of a neurobehavioral assessment.

Olfaction. Unlike virtually all other mammals, humans rely relatively little on olfaction to find their food or detect danger. Nonetheless, olfaction has been shown to influence human appetite and sexual development.[53] Unlike moths, which can locate a potential mate from a few molecules of a pheromone emitted a kilometer away, humans rely primarily on sight and sound for communication with mates. We are, however, capable of distinguishing the odor of our mates from that of other persons of the opposite sex. Loss of olfaction (hyposmia or anosmia) can be disabling because of its profound impact on taste and nutrition. However, objective evaluation of olfaction has been difficult. A recent University of Pennsylvania test battery offers substantial promise of changing that.[54] The olfactory battery is satisfactory for individual clinical evaluation but is generally still too expensive for large-scale screening.

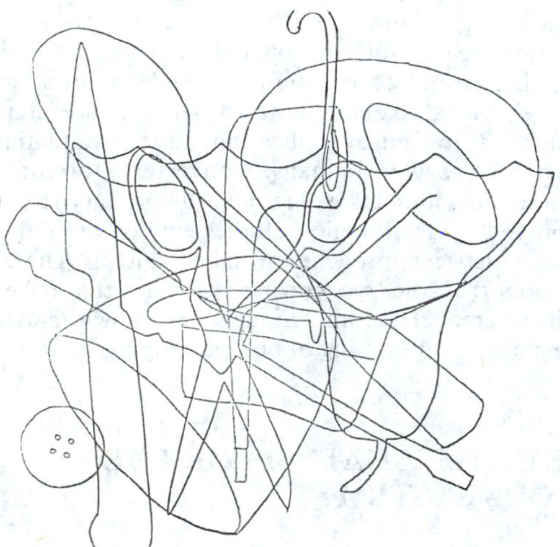

Figure 16–3. A plate from the Embedded Figures Test.

Taste. Although the food industry conducts extensive subjective research on taste, there is little objective literature on the impact of chemicals on taste sensitivity. Although many chemicals have a specific "taste," others seem to have an abnormal taste, such as the metallic taste that characterizes lead poisoning (but is not a lead taste) and the garliclike taste that occurs with selenium ingestion (but is not a selenium taste). There is a close linkage between olfaction and taste, although the peripheral receptors differ, and diminished olfactory sensitivity or discrimination will interfere with taste. Taste actually lends itself to objective study more readily than olfaction because one can control and determine the concentration of a substance in solution more easily than in air.

Touch. Physical examination of light touch and pain sensation and of temperature and two-point discrimination can be elaborate and time-consuming, but an experienced neurologist can detect subtle nervous system malfunction. Evaluation of touch is complex because in addition to skin receptors, there are receptors in underlying tissues and muscle. Other tests of sensory deficit include tests of the ability to detect numbers traced on the skin and of the ability to recognize the shape of objects. These tests are described in standard physical diagnosis textbooks.

Vibration. Vibratory sensation appears to be sensitive to peripheral nerve damage. Recent attempts to quantify vibratory sensation have had substantial success in several workplace settings.[55] A variety of devices have been developed for assessing vibratory sensation. Assessments generally consist of having the subject press a fingertip or other body part against the detector and indicate when a vibration is felt. The amplitude and frequency of the vibration can be adjusted, and the subject's reported threshold can be determined. The pressure applied by the patient potentially confounds the measurement, but the use of a forced-choice paradigm[55] somewhat compensates for this deficiency.

Temperature. Ability to discriminate slight changes in temperature is also affected by chemical exposure. Devices that provide objective control of temperature, in combination with a forced-choice paradigm, allow the clinician or researcher to evaluate this modality.[55]

Position Sense. The dorsal columns of the spinal cord carry information on position to the brain, and the sensorimotor system compensates by adjusting tone. Tests for sway and straight-line walking and the Romberg tests are traditional ways of measuring the performance of these tasks. In addition to testing position sense, these tests assess whether motor and vestibular functions are intact.

Motor Function. Neuromuscular function provides the organism with its main modes of manipulating its environment or manipulating itself within its environment. Motor deficits may be due to muscle disease, disorders of the motor cortex or pathways, changes in the reflex pathways controlling tone, or central disorders that interfere both with volition and with fine tuning and coordination of motor function.

A physical examination can detect muscle mass changes (particularly asymmetry) and physical weakness caused either by overall lack of well-being or by disease of the muscles or nervous system. Behavioral tests focus on the motor system as a manifestation of central function—for example, in terms of reaction time (see below), rapid alternating movements, and fine muscle control. Many compounds that produce acute intoxication (i.e., alcohol) affect sensorimotor function and cause alterations of gait and posture. Some neurotoxins affect motor nerves, which may lead to reduced strength, coordination, and fine muscle control. Loss of ability to perform previously learned motor sequences (i.e., apraxias) may be an indication of neurotoxic effects, and some of the animal paradigms appear directly analogous to this deficit.

Vestibular Function. The labyrinth and vestibular apparatus provides for maintenance of equilibrium and awareness of position. It senses the position of the eyes and head and reflexively controls tone in the limbs and body. Its function depends on the saccular and utricular macules, which sense linear acceleration of the head, and on the semicircular canals, which sense angular acceleration. Visual and proprioceptive impulses also feed this system. Disruption of either the sensory components or the central vestibular function can cause dizziness and vertigo. Certain toxins, such as ethanol, can have a specific impact on this system. A sway test is a gross procedure that evaluates the intactness of vestibular function as well as of proprioceptive input.

Basal Ganglia. The basal ganglia and cerebellum constitute the extrapyramidal motor system, often a target of toxic chemicals. The functional relationships of the basal ganglia to the striatum and cerebral cortex are described in standard texts. Damage to these ganglia or to the cortical-striatal-pallidal-thalamic-cortical loop is associated with a variety of disorders, including ataxias, tremors, akinesia or dyskinesia, athetosis, dystonia, and myoclonus. This system is characterized by the variety of neurotransmitters (e.g., γ-aminobutyric acid, dopamine) associated with particular functional components. Toxic damage by MPTP to the substantia nigra, for example, is known to produce parkinsonism.[25] Selected neurobehavioral tests of fine motor function may detect early damage to this system.

Cerebellar Function. The cerebellum, in conjunction with the cortex and the basal ganglia, refines motor function. Its role can be viewed as quality control. It contributes to balance, posture and tone, repetitive movement, coordination, and spatial location. Gross cerebellar dysfunction is manifested as a staggering gait, swaying or stumbling, ataxias involving movements of specific limbs in which the timing of contraction of antagonistic muscle groups is disrupted, and loss of controlled rapid alternating movements (dysdiadochokinesia).

Personality and Mood. A number of epidemiological studies indicate that overall personality changes may be important manifestations of neurobehavioral toxic effects. Erethism attributable to inorganic mercury (see above) is probably the classic example. Additional examples of general changes in mood and personality that do not necessarily reflect focal changes are mood changes associated with the use of solvents[56] and formaldehyde[57] and altered classroom behavior attributed to exposure to lead.[58]

DIAGNOSIS OF NEUROBEHAVIORAL DEFICITS

Complete neurobehavioral examination is an interdisciplinary endeavor requiring the participation of a physician, psychologist, and electrophysiologist. A complete examination includes an interview, a physical examination, and one or more neurobehavioral tests, supplemented where necessary by electrophysiological studies.

Interview. The interview provides the examiner with an important opportunity to observe the mood, affect, and behavior of the individual. It can be supplemented with a structured interview and mental status examination. The interview allows one to explore the contribution of "organic" and "psychological" changes and to detect anxiety, depression, and changes in intellectual function and other performance.

Physical Examination. The physician can observe posture and gait and can test cerebellar function, cranial nerve function, gross peripheral sensation, muscle strength and mass, and reflexes. Changes in some of the complex tasks, such as resisting sway and heel-to-toe walking or heel-to-shin, can be sensitive in detecting neurological deficits. Additional details on the neurological examination are provided in texts on neurology and clinical diagnosis.

Paper-and-Pencil Tests. These tests include a variety of questionnaires and other tests, many of them part of longstanding psychometric batteries (described below).

Specialized Apparatus. These include devices to measure visual and auditory reaction time and visual, auditory, olfactory, vibration, and temperature thresholds; block design tests; and devices for measurement of manual dexterity with pegboards.

Computerized Test Batteries. In the late 1970s, perhaps in response to the flexibility and popularity of electronic arcade games, researchers recognized the potential of computers to challenge the nervous system in repeatable, objective fashion and to score performance in real time. The emergence of neurobehavioral toxicology has coincided with the ascendancy of the microcomputer, and it is no surprise that some of the early developments in neurobehavioral testing have relied heavily on the computer.[6] Many traditional psychometric tests have been adapted for computer application. The advantages of the computer are (1) consistency of application, (2) reduced need for highly trained testers, and (3) automatic recording of data in real time. Disadvantages have been (1) logistical considerations such as unreliable hardware and software, and capital costs of purchasing several computers, (2) computer illiteracy of most target populations, (3) lack of motivation and stimulation usually provided by a live examiner and loss of opportunity to observe performance, and (4) lack of normative data.

Electrophysiological Studies. In addition to electroencephalography, electromyography, and nerve conduction studies, a variety of specific electrophysiological techniques, including electronystagraphy, electrooculography, and assessment of evoked potentials, have been employed clinically.

RATIONALE FOR NEUROBEHAVIORAL TESTING

In the presence of uncertainty, a major rationale for neurobehavioral testing is the assumption that subtle behavioral changes may be the most sensitive indicator of exposure to toxic substances.[4] Moreover, there is the increasing recognition that levels of exposure formerly thought safe or unlikely to produce adverse health effects are now known to have far-reaching consequences for important behavioral functions. Most evident among these consequences is the impact of low-level lead exposure on hyperactivity and intellectual development in children.[58,59]

Just as liver function tests can measure cell damage, conjugation, or metabolic ability, so neurobehavioral tests target distinct functions. These targeted functions include vigilance, time and accuracy of perception and task performance, simple and complex reaction times, visual-motor coordination, and intellectual function such as vocabulary and arithmetic skills, memory, learning, and associative functions.

PSYCHOMETRIC TESTS IN NEUROBEHAVIORAL EVALUATION

Although many gross changes can be detected during an interview and a mental status examination, psychometric tests are useful in extending the sensitivity of the examination by detecting and quantifying subclinical effects. Those psychometric tests with a long history of validation and a data base of normative data can be particularly useful. Newer tests, lacking such normative data, may be difficult to interpret on an individual basis but may be useful in large-scale screenings or epidemiological studies. Table 16–3 summarizes some commonly used tests, the function they assess, and their validation status.

The following is a discussion of the core functions that potentially need to be assessed if a patient is exposed to neurotoxins. The tests cited as illustrative of various functions are those which have normative data to allow interpretation of individual performance. Unlike making group comparisons for research purposes, assessing dysfunction in an individual is dependent on having a standard, either individual or group norms, against which individual performance can be compared. For example, if a patient's performance on a test of a particular function is markedly lower (e.g., two or more standard deviations below the mean) than that of comparable peers (e.g., those of similar age, sex, race, and socioeconomic status), the clinician may suspect deficits caused by exposure to a toxic substance. Confronted by a poor test performance, the clinician must ascertain that the standard of performance in use is reasonably comparable to the demographic profile. It is particularly necessary to be alert to cultural biases on these tests.

A number of investigators and clinicians have developed neurobehavioral test batteries.[60,61] In general, these batteries include tests of several basic functions necessary for higher-order cognitive functioning. Although the specific tests may differ, the basic functions tested are consistent. In an effort to standardize assessment of neurobehavioral function in the world community, and therefore to develop a coherent picture of how potential neurotoxins are affecting human health, the World Health Organization has recommended a core battery of tests. The functions to be assessed include psychomotor functions, cognitive nonverbal and verbal functions, memory and learning, perceptual speed, and mood.[62] A test can assess a particular function or more than one function. For example, reaction time is a basic skill that is also assessed on more complex tests. Thus a slowed reaction time will interfere with a patient's ability to complete more complex tests involving memory or construction of complex figures.[63]

TABLE 16–3. AVAILABILITY OF NORMATIVE DATA* FOR VARIOUS NEUROBEHAVIORAL TESTS

Test	Function
Visual Reaction Time	Psychomotor
Auditory Reaction Time	Psychomotor
Santa Ana	Psychomotor
Grooved Pegboard	Psychomotor
WAIS subtests	
Digit-Symbol	Perception/encoding
Digit Span, Auditory	Memory
Vocabulary and Comprehension	Cognitive verbal
Block Design	Cognitive nonverbal
California Verbal Learning Test	Cognitive verbal
Benton Retention Test	Memory
Embedded Figures Test	Perception profile of mood traits
SCL-90	Mood affect

Key: WAIS = Wisconsin Adult Intelligence Scale; SCL = Symptom Checklist.
*Validated on large normal and nonnormal populations.

Psychomotor Function. "Psychomotor function" refers to those tasks that require the integration of sensory-perceptual processes such as vision or hearing with motor responses. The tests used to assess this function have varying levels of complexity. For example, a test of simple reaction time in response to a visual or auditory cue provides the simplest method of assessing psychomotor function. The patient is instructed to press a button (motor response) as quickly as possible after the presentation of a visual stimulus such as a letter or an auditory stimulus such as a tone. The time between presentation of one stimulus and the next can be varied and can affect performance. At a more complex level, a patient may be asked to place pegs into holes (e.g., in a grooved pegboard) as quickly as possible.[64] Such a task requires more motor skill than a test of simple reaction time. Tests of psychomotor function (e.g., digit symbol) have consistently been the most sensitive indicators of cognitive deficits caused by neurotoxins.[65]

Perception. Tests of perceptual speed are generally timed tests that require sequencing of digits or numbers, or encoding of symbols. The tests are generally simple but require speed in working with symbols. The best known of such tests is the Digit Symbol subtest of the Wechsler Adult Intelligence Scale—Revised (WAIS-R).[66] This timed test requires the patient to identify symbols with their corresponding number according to a key chart that is in front of the patient. Although memory substantially aids performance, it is not necessary because the key is always present. Exposure to certain neurotoxins that interfere with performance will increase the time required. Because this task is somewhat more complicated than a simple reaction, it offers another level of assessment of the effects of neurotoxins on cognitive abilities. The Digit Symbol subtest in particular has been shown to be sensitive to the effects of neurotoxins.[9] The Embedded Figures Test[52] (Fig. 16–4) requires the subject to identify meaningful and familiar shapes from a complex drawing during a limited period.

Memory and Learning. Tests of memory and learning assess a patient's short-term memory by presenting stimuli (e.g., words, digits, pictures) visually or aurally and asking the patient either to recall or recognize these stimuli immediately or within a short period. The Digit Span subtest of the WAIS-R requires the patient to recite immediately an increasing string of digits presented aurally by an examiner.[66] On computer batteries this has been modified to provide a visual presentation of digits. There need be no concordance between performance on the aural and the visual Digit Span subtests. Similarly, the California Verbal Learning Test involves the presentation of a string of words that the patient is asked to recall.[67] Other memory tests (e.g., the Benton Retention Test[68]) involve the presentation of pictures of abstract drawings or actual objects and require that the subject recognize the picture from a set. Short-term memory loss is one of the most frequent clinical complaints of patients exposed to neurotoxins.[9] If a patient's performance on a short-term memory task is well below his general ability as assessed by a vocabulary test, then complaints of memory problems may be substantiated.

Overall Intellectual Ability. Tests of cognitive verbal ability are generally more familiar to the patient and include tests of vocabulary and comprehension (e.g., the WAIS-R[66]). These tests are generally regarded as most resistant to the effects of neurotoxins because they reflect abilities that are well rehearsed and long-standing.[63] Significant decline of a person's verbal abilities usually reflects serious or chronic damage. Such deficits can occur with significant head injury or stroke but generally not with exposure to neurotoxins unless the latter has occurred for a number of years at significant levels,[9] producing a well-defined dementia. Thus a patient's performance on a vocabulary test may be used, in the absence of information about premorbid function, as an estimate of premorbid ability. Relatively poor performance on tests of other functions such as memory or concentration may indicate deficits caused by neurotoxins.

Tests of cognitive nonverbal functions are generally more complex and reflect general ability. These tests integrate spatial perceptual skills with some form of motor response. Probably the best known of these tests is the Block Design subtest of the WAIS-R.[66] This test requires the patient to assemble blocks to replicate a two-dimensional picture of a design. Thus it requires perceptual and motor skills of a more complex nature than the simpler psychomotor tests described above.

Mood and Affect. Patients exposed to neurotoxins often complain also of mood changes. For example, patients report being depressed, anxious, and irritable. Although a number of instruments exist that can document these complaints and compare an individual patient with a normative group, the cause of these symptoms cannot be ascertained. That is, such symptoms may be secondary to other cognitive deficits or may be a primary effect of exposure to neurotoxins. The Profile of Mood States[69] and the Symptom Checklist-90[70] both document levels of mood disturbance. The factors to which these symptoms can be attributed require a clinical assessment of other potential agents or stressors or both in an individual patient's life that could be causing mood disturbance (e.g., divorce).

Vigilance. Vigilance is the general effective responsiveness of the central nervous system to external stimuli. The reticular formation in the mesencephalon is primarily responsible for influencing cortical arousal, and vigilance varies as a monotonic function of arousal. A variety of tests are used to assess vigilance; for example, in the proofreading test the patient is asked to find a certain number of errors during a fixed period. Other approaches include presenting a stimulus requiring a response in a long sequence of irrelevant stimuli.[22]

Temporal Properties of Performance. One of the most subtle measures of neurobehavioral deficits tests the slowing of function. Whereas peripheral neuropathies are characterized by the slowing of nerve impulse conduction, it is the slowing of central nervous system functions that is evaluated in neurobehavioral testing. Whether this can be thought of as an "increased resistance" in the central nervous system or the need for adaptation, wherein alternative pathways are sought for particular functions, is a subject for future research. It is not known whether cells die, interconnections shrink or wither, or biochemical communication is inhibited, but probably all of these mechanisms apply.

The simplest measure in the time domain is reaction time. Reaction time may be discordant depending on whether the signal is administered visually or acoustically (or for that matter via any other sensory modality). A classic substance that prolongs reaction time is ethanol. More subtle changes include a reduced number of answers or of right answers in timed tests or prolonged time to accomplish a fixed task. An example is the pegboard test, in which an individual must place as many pegs as possible into the appropriate holes in 1 minute.

BEHAVIORAL TERATOLOGY

The developing nervous system undergoes dramatic growth and expansion of function, not only before birth, but throughout the first decade of life. Anatomical changes such as increasing myelinization occur during the first years of life, and associations are formed that make possible complex motor patterns, fine-tuning of coordination, concept formation, pattern recognition, and more highly learned tasks such as speech and communication. For some tasks, such as the learning of language, there appear to be "critical periods" during which learning proceeds more rapidly and effectively. Animals or humans that are isolated from speakers during the critical period may find it difficult or impossible to learn speech at a later time. There may be critical periods for development of other functions as well.[29] As organisms mature, their locomotor ability, learning, and knowledge should increase appropriately for their age. There is increasing evidence that even low-level chemical exposure may have a profound impact on the orderly acquisition of nervous system function. The magnitude of such changes is not fully appreciated, and the field of behavioral teratology is in a rapid growth phase.

Probably the best documented behavioral teratogen is lead. At blood lead levels formerly thought innocuous (i.e., $<25\ \mu g/dl$), children may still show depressed intellectual development.[58,59] Elementary-school children with higher body burdens of lead were rated by their teachers as being more easily distracted, less persistent, less independent and organized, more hyperactive and impulsive, more easily frustrated, and showing poorer overall functioning, compared with children in the lower lead groups.[58] Needleman et al.[58] showed remarkable dose-response relationships between dentine-lead levels and poor ratings. Children with higher lead levels had poorer performance on verbal and digit span components of IQ tests.[58]

CONFOUNDERS OF BEHAVIORAL PERFORMANCE

Neurobehavioral evaluation requires the concentration and cooperation of the subject; yet these behaviors, too, may be diminished in a chemical-exposed individual. Interpretation of test results in the individual must take into account a variety of confounders which will be briefly mentioned below. Many of the confounders have a *global* effect, that is, they interfere with all aspects of performance rather than with performance on particular subtests. Subjects who have a high level of anxiety may find it difficult to concentrate on complex tasks, particularly on tests of vigilance. Lack of familiarity with the test context or with the expectations of the examiner, particularly if the testing is not conducted in one's first language, will certainly interfere with performance. Subjects who believe that they are being evaluated for poisoning may be hesitant about participating in so many "psychological" tests and may suggest that the examiners believe that their complaints are not "real."

Lack of sleep or drowsiness, a recent full meal, or recent use of drugs, alcohol, or tobacco may also have global effects on performance. Examiners should elicit subjective evaluations of wakefulness and should carefully observe the subject. A pretest questionnaire should determine the time at which alcohol, cigarettes, or specific medications were used. Unrelated illnesses may affect performance. Diabetes or other metabolic states may interfere with alertness. Dementia from other causes will complicate interpretation of test results. Many neurobehavioral functions decline steadily with age.[4,71]

Bias of Tests. Perhaps the most important problems are the inherent intellectual and cultural biases of many of the tests. Designed for white, English-speaking, middle-class patients, the tests may require major modifications before being given to less educated or non-English-speaking cohorts, much less to worker populations from distant cultures. However, the principles of neurobehavioral testing will certainly be cross-cultural, and the successes of studying the cultural impact of psychology and development should be viewed as a challenge for the coming decade.

Learning Curves. Learning poses an additional confounding problem in interpreting neurobehavioral tests. The first performance of an unfamiliar task may go slowly and haltingly. The second performance (either intellectual or psychomotor) should greatly improve because of previous experience. Third and fourth repetitions may also improve performance, but at some point maximal capability will have been reached and there will be little further improvement. This phenomenon is known as a learning curve (Fig. 16–4). Some tasks are more resistant to learning than others. Even on the same task, some individuals learn more than others. In addition, the interval between previous performance and current performance is important. There may be little learning if a long time has elapsed. Also the ability to learn may itself be impaired in the subject.

This phenomenon makes it particularly difficult to interpret neurobehavioral tests for individuals. There is both intertask and interindividual variation in the learning curve, which can profoundly influence performance. Persons unfamiliar with computers may take time to learn computer tasks and may show great "learning" improvement. Indeed, some computer test batteries provide practice sessions for all tests to reduce the impact of a learning curve.

When any testing regimen is planned, the learning curve must be taken into account. If time allows, repeated practice sessions may bring all subjects to the maximal performance plateau, so that test results can be compared among groups. However, logistical considerations for testing that is already time and labor intensive seem to preclude this approach.

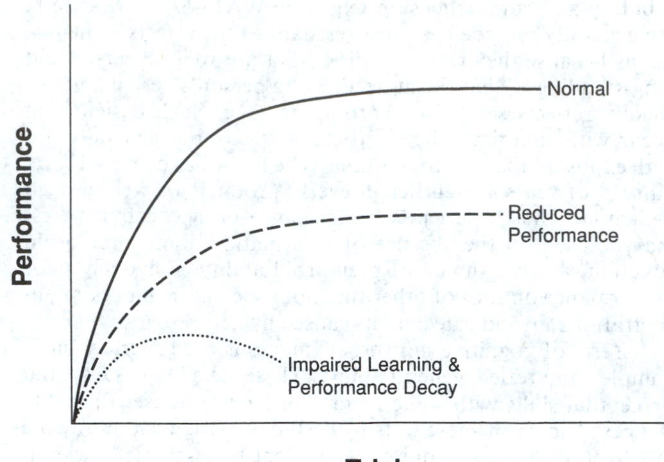

Figure 16–4. Example of a typical learning curve.

FUTURE DIRECTIONS

Building on the foundation of clinical psychology, behavioral toxicologists have assembled a variety of test approaches that yield important information about nervous system response to toxic chemicals. In many cases the mechanisms are uncertain and the pathological lesion is unrecognized. The lesions are likely to be biochemical rather than microanatomical, and the lesions presumably occur mainly in the brain. A neurotoxin may act on a discrete target such as the basal ganglia or may disrupt associations between different parts of the brain, interfering with intellectual functions such as cognition and memory. These all provide an active domain for research in a variety of disciplines using a variety of models.

Given the uncertainties, it is nonetheless apparent that deficits in function can be measured and validated. A major limiting factor, applicable to most clinical testing, is that without a baseline, subtle deviations from normal are difficult to evaluate. As the field of neurobehavioral testing matures and tests of an increasing number of "normal" persons are validated, greater certainty in evaluating subtle abnormalities may be achieved. Neurobehavioral assessment should complement neurophysiological and neurological assessment in the standard clinical evaluation of patients with nervous system symptoms.

Environmental Risk Assessment

Michael Gochfeld

Whereas causality between an exposure and an effect is often established in the case of one or more individuals, the process of risk assessment is concerned with groups. Risk assessment addresses the question of how much a risk will increase if a group of people are exposed to a certain amount of a hazardous substance or condition for a certain period. Major descriptions of the risk assessment process[1] and its role in policy[2] have been written. There is a rapidly growing literature on specific applications of risk assessment,[3,4] and an entire journal is devoted to the subject.[5] The social implications of the risk assessment process have been discussed by Lowrance[6] and by Imperato and Mitchell,[7] among others. Once a risk estimate has been calculated, it becomes a major problem to communicate the risk to responsible officials and potentially at-risk individuals, because the manner in which risk is perceived often bears little resemblance to the actual magnitude of risk.[8]

In its broadest sense,[9] environmental risk assessment covers a wide variety of natural hazards including earthquakes, floods, and hurricanes. However, this chapter will focus on the more narrow application to hazardous chemical and physical agents and their impact on human health.

There are several ways to apply environmental risk assessment to making policy decisions. One can assess risks associated with a variety of hazards (e.g., different types of hazardous waste sites) and use the findings to set priorities for remediation, starting first with those sites that pose the greatest risk to the greatest number of people. One can compare estimated risk with a level of so-called acceptable risk and decide whether to take action. One can treat the reduction of risk as a benefit and perform a cost-benefit analysis for any proposed solution, recognizing that benefit considered in terms of life or health is not easily compared with monetary costs. In another mode, one can contrast the risks of two or more alternative decisions (e.g., to clean or not to clean, or to ban or not to ban) and then choose the path with the lowest risk. This is called risk-risk balancing.

One common goal of environmental risk assessment is to establish an acceptable level of exposure to some continuing hazard and an appropriate regulatory approach or policy to protect the public from greater exposure.[10] However, what constitutes unacceptably high risk to one person (e.g., skydiving) may be a provocative challenge to another. The process of establishing *acceptable risk* involves decisions based on human and social values, not biomedical considerations. In the case of cancer risks, it has become traditional to state that exposure to a hazard is acceptable if the overall risk of cancer does not increase by more than one in a million exposed people. For example, if we accept for the sake of argument that approximately 25% of people die of cancer, an increase of one death per million, or of 10^{-6}, means that instead of 250,000 out of a million people dying of cancer, the number will be 250,001. Clearly this immeasurably small elevation of risk cannot be identified by any current or projected epidemiologic methods. Most epidemiologists are content if they can identify as real a 50% increase in risk.

ACCEPTABLE RISK

Before one determines whether a risk is acceptable, it is necessary to define an endpoint. Table 16–4 provides a spectrum of endpoints ranging from early death from cancer to emotional discomfort. There is a tendency to treat the first entries as the most consequential, and risk assessment has been preoccupied with cancer. Yet some people are indeed disabled by their emotional reactions to hazardous exposures.

Society must determine how safe it wants to be[11] and how much it is prepared to sacrifice for that level of security. Unfortunately, the persons who most often decide whether to invest in environmental safety are usually not those most at risk. Acceptable risk may be defined (e.g., by the Environmental Protection Agency [EPA]), as an excess lower than 10^{-6}; this means that the exposure level at which a population is estimated to have a 10^{-6} increase in risk is the cutoff point between acceptable and unacceptable.[6,7] Some persons argue that this level of risk is unrealistically low because most of the risks that people willingly face (e.g., driving an automobile, smoking a cigarette) are much higher. Indeed, the cancer risk of living in a home with 4 picocuries of radon per cubic meter is on the order of 10^{-2} or 10^{-3}, but many people choose not to test their homes or remediate the elevated level.[12]

TABLE 16–4. SPECTRUM OF ADVERSE CONSEQUENCES CONSIDERED BY RISK ASSESSORS*

- **Shortening of Life**
  Cancer vs other causes
- **Illness or Injury Leading to Disability**
  Acute vs chronic
  Permanent vs temporary disability
  Serious vs minor disability
- **Illness or Injury with Temporary Disability Followed by Recovery**
  Chronic vs acute
  Serious vs minor disability
- **Physical Discomfort without Disability**
- **Psychological Disorder with Behavioral Consequences**
  Posttraumatic stress disorder
  Anxiety reaction
  Stress reaction
  Chronic frustration and anger
- **Emotional Discomfort**

*Each of these categories is weighted by the number of persons involved.

RISK ASSESSMENT vs RISK MANAGEMENT

One of the historical problems with risk assessment is the confusion between analyzing a level of risk and controlling that risk. Early risk estimates were often modified by concerns over what it would take to manage the risk, and some policy makers considered risk management an integral part of risk assessment.[13] Accordingly the term *risk analysis* was introduced to refer to a value-free process of estimating risk, independent of any management or economic considerations. May[14] criticized the use of cost-benefit analysis in evaluating risk data in which a company blatantly chooses to accept and pay for a certain level of risk rather than reengineer a product to make it safer.

Risk assessment is used in applications for siting permits for hazardous facilities such as liquified natural gas depots, hazardous waste incinerators, and municipal solid waste incinerators. Because many risk assessments are broad estimates, and because of the controversies over the risk assessment process, many management applications of risk analyses may be premature. Nonetheless, risk analysis has played an important role in many governmental decisions on such matters as the management of dioxin-contaminated soil and the setting of safe drinking water standards. It is important to keep risk management and risk assessment separate.

ENVIRONMENTAL RISK ASSESSMENT PROCESS

The basic approach to environmental risk assessment is outlined below. For the most part, this process describes the risk assessment for carcinogens, which differs somewhat from risk assessment for noncarcinogens.[1]

Hazard Identification. The first step in risk assessment is to define the hazard and establish an endpoint. This means identifying a toxic substance or mixture and naming one or more endpoints (e.g., lung cancer, neurotoxic effects) that are of concern.

Hazard Assessment. Hazard assessment, sometimes called dose-response assessment, usually involves extensive review of the toxicological and epidemiological literature to ascertain whether dose-response curves can be constructed for the endpoints of concern, or whether specific thresholds have been determined. The goal is to construct a dose-response curve from the existing studies. The EPA Carcinogen Assessment Group has prepared cancer potency estimates for a number of common carcinogens.

Exposure Assessment. A critical and, until recently, an overlooked component of risk assessment is an estimate of exposure.[15] Although measurement of exposure is important, exposure assessment often involves mathematical models or projections of exposure under different scenarios. Exposure assessment must take into account the measured or estimated concentration of a substance in any or all environmental media (air, soil, water, food) and all applicable routes of exposure (inhalation, ingestion, the cutaneous route). This requires knowing how individuals behave: where they spend their time, what they eat, and how much they drink. It must incorporate estimates of bioavailability to provide a final estimate of the internal dose—the dose actually delivered to the target site.

Risk Characterization. Risk characterization (or analysis) involves a quantitative estimate of the exposure level that would result in a particular level of excess risk (greater than background risk level in a nonexposed population). In the case of cancer, one constructs a dose-response curve based on animal studies of cancer and performs a low-dose extrapolation to estimate the dose that would produce a particular excess in the mortality from cancer (usually a 10^{-6} increase). The data used may involve the presence of tumors, the number of tumors per animal, or the time to tumor development after initial dosing. A variety of biological models of carcinogenesis have been advocated, each leading to selection of different mathematical extrapolations. Among these are the linear no-threshold model,[16] the Armitage-Doll multistage model,[17] and the Moolgavkar-Vernon-Knudsen model[18]; the latter model emphasizes mutational events involved in initiation rather than promotion. No single model will explain all cancer-causing processes. Risk assessment texts provide details on the various mathematical models in use.[19,20] The linear nonthreshold model assumes that no threshold exists for a carcinogen.[16] The linearized multistage model is probably the most widely accepted and takes into account multistage models of carcinogenesis.[21] Other models, such as dose-distribution models, give higher estimates of dose and are considered less protective of the public health, although future research may validate their use for some substances. It is possible that where several models give similar estimates of risk for a substance, and one model gives a very divergent estimate of risk, one can safely rely on the evidence of the concordant estimates.

LOW-DOSE EXTRAPOLATION OF RISK

Toxicological research has usually been done at relatively high doses, often orders of magnitude greater than the doses encountered in the home, community, or workplace. Moreover, a single study usually involves only two or three different doses, plus the no-dose control. How can one ascertain the risk facing humans at a low dose from the outcome in animals exposed at a high dose? Depending on which biological model one believes is appropriate for a particular chemical, one selects from a variety of mathematical models, each purporting to describe a realistic biological concept. For example, if the risk assessor believes that the dose-response curve is linear and has no threshold (a common belief regarding carcinogens), one may employ the "linear no-threshold model." At the other end of the spectrum is the so-called probit model.

Risk analyses for noncancer endpoints use a variety of approaches based on the lowest dose known to produce an effect or on the highest dose known to produce no effect.[20] Ideally one would use data from epidemiological studies including the most sensitive human subpopulations, in which there has been a lifetime of adequate exposure by appropriate routes as well as a lifetime of follow-up (to ensure that events with long latency are not missed). This condition is virtually never met. One must rely either on incomplete epidemiological studies or more frequently on animal studies. Because most published animal studies were not designed for risk assessment, one must be selective. Studies with very short term exposure or with short-term follow-up are usually not incorporated into risk assessments.

NOEL and NOAEL. In toxicological studies the acronym NOEL refers to "no observable effect level," and the acronym NOAEL refers to "no observed adverse effect level." The NOAEL is the highest dose at which there is no biological or statistically significant adverse effect.

LOAEL. The acronym LOAEL refers to the "lowest observed adverse effect level." In some studies, even the lowest dose induced a significant effect. Rather than throw out such studies, there has been a tendency to use these data but to treat the LOAEL differently from a NOAEL. Because most toxicological data used in risk assessment were not collected with risk assessment in mind, one is often confronted with LOAELs rather than NOAELs.

Safety Factor. The safety factor (SF) is a margin of safety introduced into the regulatory process to account for uncertainties in the biomedical data base. Various SFs are introduced in a multiplicative manner. Thus we may use an SF of 10 in an extrapolation from animals to humans[20] and another 10 to protect the most sensitive persons. The composite SF of 100 is commonly used by regulatory agencies. If, however, the toxicological data base is inadequate, one may opt to introduce another factor of 10 for uncertainty, which leads to an SF of 1000. Moreover, if the only data available are LOAELs rather than NOAELs, or if synergism is suspected, then another SF of 10 may be incorporated. Although the choice of these values was arbitrary, subsequent data analyses have tended to support their utility.[20]

Making the Calculations. In using NOELs, NOAELs, and LOAELs, one selects the highest NOAEL or the lowest LOAEL reported in the literature as the starting point for calculations. One also makes certain assumptions about exposure. The standard human target is the 70 kg adult. However, if susceptible subpopulations include children, females, or ethnic groups, a more appropriate mass should be chosen. Exposure is assumed to occur during a 70-year life span, but in many cases involving childhood exposure a different critical period is selected.

The human acceptable dose can be calculated as follows:

$$\text{Dose} = \frac{\text{Concentration of agent in media} \cdot \text{Estimated intake of media}}{\text{Body weight} \cdot \text{Product of all SFs}}$$

Examples of applications of this approach with much additional detail are provided by Hallenbeck.[20]

Acceptable Daily Intake. The end result of a risk assessment is a determination of an acceptable, or "safe," level of exposure. The acceptable daily intake (ADI) is the amount of a substance to which a person can be exposed on a daily basis without suffering a deleterious effect. Most risk assessments have been done with cancer as the endpoint and have relied on a series of mathematical models believed to reflect appropriately the various biological models of carcinogenesis. Unfortunately the various models yield vastly different estimates, and the choice among them and the development of an ADI become political and economic, rather than scientific. For noncancer endpoints, the process, at least, is simpler.

Reference Dose. As part of a critical reevaluation of risk assessment for noncancer and nongenetic endpoints, the EPA established the concept of a reference dose. It uses safety factors, here called "uncertainty factors," or UFs and adds to these an additional modifying factor (MF) for "professional judgment."[22] The reference dose RfD is estimated from the following formula:

$$\text{RfD} = \text{NOAEL}/(\text{UF} \cdot \text{MF})$$

CANCER RISK ASSESSMENT

Much of the literature on risk assessment has been concerned with cancer. One reason is that community concerns about cancer caused by long-term low-level exposures were frequently encountered by the EPA and provided the main stimulus for risk assessment. The basic process of risk assessment begins with a review of the literature on toxicological studies of a particular chemical. Then one can analyze either the number of animals that developed cancer at each dosage level, the number of cancers per animal, or the time required to develop the tumor.

A variety of mathematical models have been used for low-dose extrapolation of cancer risks. In general the one-hit linear, no-threshold model produces the highest estimate of risk (or conversely the lowest allowable dose), whereas the logit and probit models are at the opposite end of the spectrum.[19] The one-hit model assumes a linear relationship between dose and outcome, with the slope of the line determined from the available studies. It assumes no threshold and is basically drawn from our understanding of radiation and cancer. Multistage models take into account our understanding of chemical carcinogenesis as a process involving initiation and promotion. Crump[21] proposed a linearized multistage model, now widely used.

INTERSPECIES EXTRAPOLATION

One of the controversial aspects of risk assessment is comparing effects among species. (See Huff and Rall discussion in Chapter 21, this text.) It is important to realize that such basic phenomena as the presence of enzymes and consequent metabolism vary not only among species but among strains of a species, between the sexes, and even with age. The response of experimental animals (or of human subjects) may vary with many factors. In some cases the fact that a toxic substance produces the same effect (e.g., bladder cancer or leukemia) in several species of animals makes one confident that interspecies extrapolation is valid. When a carcinogen produces cancer in many species, but in each species involves a different organ system, extrapolation is more uncertain. Finally, a substance may be a carcinogen in one species but not another.

A high correlation between a single chemical's estimated carcinogenic potency in animals and its potency in humans, based on both animal studies and human epidemiological studies, validates the use of animal toxicological data.[23] The basic problem is that one does not know whether humans are more or less susceptible to an agent than is the experimental animal used in a study. Incorporating a safety factor of 10 assumes that humans are no more than tenfold more sensitive. However, humans are just as likely to be less sensitive than more sensitive, and in many cases the degree of sensitivity is not known. Thus, in the case of 2,3,7,8-TCDD ("dioxin"), guinea pigs are approximately 1000 times more sensitive than rats, but it is not clear whether humans are more sensitive than guinea pigs or rats or even perhaps are less sensitive than either to specific effects.

INTERPRETING THE MODEL

Before selecting a model, one establishes a level of acceptable risk.[6,11] For example, one would calculate the dose of chemical that would increase the cancer risk by one case in a million. The mathematical model would allow extrapolation downward until that very low dose associated with one-in-a-million excess risk is reached.

If the linear nonthreshold model is used, the dose will be much lower than if the probit model is used. Environmentalists seeking to prevent any unnecessary exposure to carcinogens will tend to favor the model giving the lowest allowable dose, whereas an industrialist responsible for controlling exposures in and around the factory will feel more comfortable if a probit model is used, thus relaxing his or her burden somewhat. Unfortunately, much of the debate over which model to use has focused on the political consequences of the choice rather than on the scientific requirements—perhaps the inevitable result of the slow progress toward determining the biological basis for model selection for specific chemicals. The biological underpinnings are important to an understanding of the mechanisms by which toxic substances produce their effects at the molecular and cellular levels.

In addition to estimating a critical dose, one can calculate the 95% confidence limits around an estimate. To ensure protection of the public health, one reports the upper 95% confidence limit as the "upper bound" of the risk estimate. In addition, the EPA has established a science-policy decision of using a no-threshold model in cancer risk assessment.[16]

One compromise solution is the linearized multistage model.[21] This model takes into account the two-stage process of carcinogenesis, recognizing that a single hit may not be sufficient to cause a cancer. The dose estimated by the linearized multistage model is intermediate between the doses estimated by the other models. The EPA has also selected a "one-in-a-million excess risk," often indicated as a 10^{-6} excess risk, as the point at which it will make decisions to regulate exposures.

Several phenomena render a particular risk assessment more useful to policymakers. Where these phenomena are present, one's confidence in the outcome increases. Where they are absent, there is a clear need for additional research to provide a sounder scientific basis for the risk estimate.

Biological Plausibility. "Biological plausibility" means that the putative health effect in a study is already known to be caused by the agent under investigation.

Consistency. Consistency has been achieved if two or more studies yield comparable findings of excess risk (preferably in different test models).

Concordance. Concordance is present if the same endpoint (e.g., type of tumor) arises in more than one species, strain, or sex. Even more important, there is concordance if the type of pathologic change found in animal models is the same one found in humans (e.g., bladder cancer after exposure to certain organic dyes).

INDIVIDUAL vs COLLECTIVE RISK

The process of risk assessment is concerned with collective risks. Risk assessment does not impart information about individuals. Policymakers, likewise, are concerned with protecting groups from unacceptable exposures and risks. However, most decisions regarding risks are made at the individual level; even when a group is exposed, its members try to interpret and respond to the risk as individuals. Although risk is estimated for a group, the risk assessor realizes that the distribution of the risk estimate may mean that the risk is actually much lower or much higher than the estimate. In reality, whatever the true risk, each individual has behaviors that modify his own risk; thus individual risk may be much lower or much higher than group risk.

LIMITATIONS OF RISK ASSESSMENT

Although risk assessment is becoming increasingly important to policymakers, it is essential to understand its limitations. (1) For the most part, risk assessment has been and will continue to be based on published animal research. However, until recently, toxicological research on animals was not designed with quantitative risk assessment in mind; hence the choice of doses and of the number of animals used may have been appropriate for descriptive purposes but not for the low-dose extrapolations used in risk assessment. (2) Many of the endpoints of concern for humans have not been adequately studied in animal models. (3) The uncertainties inherent in extrapolating from animals to humans have engendered controversy. (4) Human epidemiological studies of adequate power are usually too sparse to contribute to risk assessment, resulting in the continued necessity of relying on animal models. (5) Human exposure data are often inadequate. (6) In cancer risk assessments there are dramatic differences depending on which mathematical model is used. (7) Risk estimates based on collective exposure are not easily translated into individual risk. (8) Finally, the continuing debate over what constitutes an acceptable level of risk often overrides biomedical risk estimates.

Although these concerns interfere with performance and application of risk assessments, the process has become increasingly robust and therefore serves useful functions in ordering priorities, comparing the risks of different solutions, and providing some data for the establishment of policy.

RISK PERCEPTION AND RISK COMMUNICATION

Some persons engage in extremely risky behavior on a regular basis as part of their job, and they may receive hazardous duty pay in recognition of this risk. Others engage in risks for recreational purposes or thrill. At the opposite pole of such risk-taking behavior are risk-aversive persons, who are usually perceived as timid. One might predict that a risk-taking individual, such as a skydiver or a mercenary soldier, would willingly undertake other risks such as smoking, driving without a seat belt, or living with radon or next to a hazardous waste dump, whereas risk-aversive individuals would take public transportation to a 9-to-5 job, frequently check their homes for radon, have their car undergo frequent safety inspections, and shun all activities or exposures that would enhance their risk of becoming ill or hurt.

However, risk perception is not that simple. Some persons who willingly take great risks in certain aspects of life fear having their drinking water contaminated even at immeasurably low levels. That individuals generally tend to overestimate negligible risks and underestimate severe ones is a source of frustration to risk managers and policymakers alike and has engendered the rapidly growing field of "risk perception" analysis.[24] Unfortunately, much of the energy of risk perception analysis has been aimed at a particular goal: how to convince people to accept a particular level of risk that is politically or economically expedient. Although the origin is not usually recognized, the field has its roots in the study of "marketing," which emerged in the 1950s and 1960s in an effort to understand factors motivating purchasing decisions. Although the risk perception literature rarely references its parent discipline, many common principles can be recognized. Nonetheless, important advances and generalizations have been developed by Covello et al.,[25] among others.

Lowrance[6] is credited with popularizing the understanding of risk perception and what constitutes acceptable risk. He examined a series of dichotomous factors that influence human perception of risk. Some of these are shown in Table 16–5.

The goal of risk perception research is to understand how people appreciate risks, how they make their risk-taking and risk-avoiding decisions, and how to bring their understanding of specific risks into congruence with the actual levels of risk. A correct understanding of risk levels will reduce anxiety caused by overestimating risk and may prevent significant exposure caused by underestimating risk. All too often, risk managers have the goal of reducing anxiety and encouraging people to accept exposures, particularly those which would be costly to mitigate. Examples of the need to enhance awareness and increase the response to underestimated exposures include the need to convince people to have their homes tested for radon, and their exposure mitigated if the radon level is high, and the need to support continued educational efforts to warn people about the hazards of smoking tobacco.

RISK COMPARISONS

Risk assessors often lament irrational public reaction to risks, not realizing that individuals must put risk into very personal contexts. It has become popular to present new risks in terms of familiar ones. Common reference points include the risk of driving so many miles in a car, the radiation risk of a transcontinental air flight, and the lung cancer risk from smoking a pack of cigarettes per day. A risk lower than these should presumably be acceptable. Yet individuals may rationally accept the necessary risk of transcontinental flight while shunning the perceived risk of having a communications tower constructed in their community. The concept of risk comparison thus makes more sense to the communicator than the communicatee. The dichotomies shown in Table 16–5 help us understand this apparent paradox.

MEDIA COVERAGE OF RISK

One often gains the impression that newspaper and television coverage exaggerates the hazards of everyday life, with stories that bear little relationship to the actual magnitude of the public health hazard.[26] Nonetheless, the media are an important source of hazard and risk information for many people and could therefore play a crucial role in providing a balanced perspective on risk. Although many toxicologists shun journalists for fear of being misquoted, there is a substantial basis for believing that environmental news coverage can be improved if communication among toxicologists, risk assessors, and reporters can be developed.[27]

FUTURE DIRECTIONS

Risk assessment procedures and applications continue to be refined. For cancer risk assessment, new studies will provide more refined low-dose extrapolations. Moreover, they will take into account the fact that cancer is not one disease but many and that

TABLE 16–5. RISK PERCEPTION DICHOTOMIES

Acceptable or Reduces Apparent Riskiness	Unacceptable or Increases Apparent Riskiness
Risk assumed voluntarily or self-imposed	Risk borne involuntarily or imposed by others
Adverse effect immediate	Outcome delayed
Alternatives not available, a necessity	Alternatives available, a luxury
Risk certain	Risk uncertain
Occupational exposure	Community exposure
Familiar hazard	Feared or "dreaded" hazard
Consequences reversible	Consequences irreversible
Some benefit gained from assuming risk	No apparent benefit to persons at risk
Hazard associated with perceived good	Someone else profits at "my expense"

Modified from Lowrance.[6]

a model appropriate for leukemia or angiosarcoma of the liver may not work for breast cancer or mesothelioma. Risk assessment continues to play an important role in regulatory agencies,[10,28,29] allowing them to establish priorities and facilitating decisions. As the shortcomings are realized, slavish devotion to risk assessment results can be avoided while the process continues to provide useful information. As the risk communication process improves, individuals may find it easier to translate a community-based risk assessment into a personal decision analysis, but regulators are unlikely ever to be completely satisfied with how the public perceives and responds to environmental risks.

REFERENCES

Principles of Toxicology

1. Oser BL: Toxicology then and now. Regulatory Toxicol Pharmacol 7:427–443, 1987
2. Sinclair U: The Jungle. New York: Viking, 1946 (originally published 1905)
3. Gibaldi M, Perrier D: Pharmacokinetics. New York: Marcel Dekker, 1982
4. Goldstein BD (chair), Subcommittee on Reproductive and Neurodevelopmental Toxicology: Biologic Markers in Reproductive Toxicity. Washington, D.C.: National Academy Press, 1989
5. Sipes IG, Gandolf AJ: Biotransformation of toxicants. In Klaasen CD, Amdur MO, Doull J (eds): Cassarett & Doull's Toxicology. 3rd edt. New York: Macmillan, 1986, pp 64–98
6. Agency for Toxic Substances and Disease Registry: Toxicological profile: Mercury. Atlanta: Centers for Disease Control, 1989
7. Laughlin RB Jr, Linden O: Fate and effects of organotin compounds. Ambio 14:88–94, 1985
8. Nieboer E, Jusys AA: Biologic chemistry of chromium. In Nriagu JO, Nieboer E (eds): Chromium in the Natural and Human Environments. New York: John Wiley & Sons, 1988, pp 21–80
9. Agency for Toxic Substances and Disease Registry: Toxicological profile: Chromium. Atlanta: Centers for Disease Control (USPHS,ATSDR/TP-88/10), 1989
10. Agency for Toxic Substances and Disease Registry: Toxicological profile for 2,3,7,8-tetrachlorodibenzo-*p*-dioxin: TCDD and dioxins. Atlanta: Centers for Disease Control, 1989
11. Enslein K: Estimation of toxicological endpoints by structure-activity relationships. Pharmacol Rev 36:131–135, 1984
12. Buchet J-P, Roels H, Bernard A, Lauwerys R: Assessment of renal function of workers exposed to inorganic lead, cadmium or mercury vapor. J Occup Med 22:741–750, 1980
13. Chan PK, O'Hara GP, Hayes AW: Principles and methods for acute and subchronic toxicity. In Hayes AW (ed): Principles and Methods of Toxicology. New York: Raven Press, 1982, pp 1–51
14. Stevens KP, Gallo MA: Practical considerations in the conduct of chronic toxicity studies. In Hayes AW (ed): Principles and Methods of Toxicology. New York: Raven Press, 1982, pp 53–77
15. Colligan MJ, Pennebaker J, Murphy L (eds): Mass Psychogenic Illness. Hillsdale, N.J.: Lawrence Erlbaum Assoc., 1982
16. Goldstein BD, Melia RJW, du V Florey C: Indoor nitrogen oxides. Bull NY Acad Med 58:873–882, 1981
17. American Conference of Governmental Industrial Hygienists: Threshold Limit Values and Biological Exposure Indices for 1989–1990, Cincinnati: ACGIH, 1988 [updated annually]
18. Lioy P: Total human exposure analysis: A multidisciplinary science for reducing human contact with contaminants. Environ Sci Technol 24:938–945, 1990
19. Exposure Assessment Group: Estimating Exposures to 2,3,7,8-TCDD. Washington, D.C.: U.S. Environmental Protection Agency, 1988 (EPA/600/6-88/005)
20. Zweig G: The vanishing zero: The evolution of pesticide analyses. Essays Toxicol 2:156–198, 1970
21. Plog B: Fundamentals of Industrial Hygiene. 3 edt. Chicago: National Safety Council, 1988
22. Rowland M, Tozer TN: Clinical Pharmacokinetics: Concepts and Applications. Philadelphia: Lea & Febiger, 1980
23. Umbreit TH, Hesse EJ, Gallo MA: Bioavailability of dioxin in soil from a 2,4,5,-T manufacturing site. Science 232:497–499, 1986
24. Tallarida RJ, Jacob LS: The Dose-Response Relation in Pharmacology. New York: Springer-Verlag, 1979
25. Lowrance WW: Of Acceptable Risk. Los Altos, Calif.: William Kaufmann, Inc., 1976
26. Cohrssen JJ, Covello VT: Risk analysis: A Guide to Principles and Methods for Analyzing Health and Environmental Risks. Washington, D.C.: U.S. Council on Environmental Quality, 1989
27. U.S. Environmental Protection Agency: Proposed guidelines for carcinogen risk assessment. Federal Register 49:46294–46301, 1984
28. National Research Council: Regulating Pesticides in Food: The Delaney Paradox. Washington, D.C.: National Academy Press, 1987
29. Selikoff IJ, Lee DHK: Asbestos and Disease. New York: Academic Press, 1978
30. Hammond EC, Selikoff IJ: Relation of cigarette-smoking to risk of death of asbestos-associated disease among insulation workers in the United States. In Bogovski (ed): Biological Effects of Asbestos. IARC Scientific Publication No. 8. Lyon, France: International Agency for Research on Cancer. 1973
31. Gallo MA, Esse EJ, MacDonald GJ, Umbreit TH: Interactive effects of estradiol and 2,3,7,8-tetrachloro-dibenzo-*p*-dioxin on hepatic cytochrome P-450 and mouse uterus. Toxicol Lett 32:123–132, 1986
32. Amoruso MA, Witz G, Goldstein BD: Alteration of erythrocyte membrane fluidity by heavy metal cations. Toxicol Industr Health 3:135–144, 1987
33. Cullen MR: The worker with multiple chemical sensitivities. State-of-the-Art Reviews in Occupational Medicine 2:655–662, 1987
34. Dixon RL, Hall JL: Reproductive Toxicology. In Hayes AW (ed): Principles and Methods of Toxicology. New York: Raven Press, 1982, pp 107–140
35. Needleman H, Gunnoe C, Leviton A, Reed R, Peresie H, Maher C, Barrett P: Deficits in psychologic and classroom performance of children with elevated dentine lead levels. N Engl J Med 300:689–695, 1979
36. Sies H: Oxidative Stress: Introductory Remarks. In Sies H (ed): Oxidative Stress. New York: Academic Press, 1985, pp 1–10
37. Report of the EPA Workshop on the Development of Risk Assessment Methodologies for Tumor Promoters. Washington, D.C.: Environmental Protection Agency, 1987 (EPA/600/9-87/013)
38. Armitage P: Multistage models of carcinogenesis. Environ Health Perspect 63:195–201, 1985
39. Amoruso MA, Ryer J, Easton D, Witz G, Goldstein BD: Estimation of risk of glucose-6-phosphate dehydrogenase–deficient red cells to ozone and nitrogen dioxide. J Occup Med 28:473–479, 1986
40. Luckey TD, Venugopal B, Hutcheson D: Heavy metal toxicity, safety and hormology. Environ Qual Safety (suppl 1). New York: Academic Press, 1975
41. Burger J, Gochfeld M: A hypothesis on the role of pheromones on age of menarche. Med Hypotheses 17:39–46, 1985
42. Lauwerys R, Bernard A: Preclinical detection of nephrotoxicity: Description of the tests and appraisal of their health significance. Toxicol Lett 46:13–30, 1989
43. Kimbrough RD: Determining exposure and biochemical effects in human population studies. Environ Health Persp 48:77–79, 1983
44. LaDou J (ed): Occupational Health Law: A Guide for Industry. New York: Marcel Dekker, 1981

General References

American Conference of Governmental Industrial Hygienists: Threshold Limit Values and Biological Exposure Indices 1990–1991. Cincinnati: ACGIH, 1990 (updated annually)

Baselt RC: Disposition of Toxic Drugs and Chemicals in Man. Davis, Calif.: Biomedical Publications, 1978

Berg GL (ed): Farm Chemicals Handbook. 72nd edt. Willoughby, Ohio: Meister Publishing CO., 1986

Gibson GG, Hubbard R, Parke DV (EDS): Immunotoxicology. New York: Academic Press, 1983

Haddad LM, Winchester JF: Clinical management of poisoning and drug overdose. Philadelphia: WB Saunders Co., 1983

Hayes AW: Principle and Methods of Toxicology. 2nd edt. New York: Raven Press, 1989

Hodgson E, Gutherie FE: Introduction to Biochemical Toxicology. New York: Elsevier, 1980

Hodgson E, Levi PE: A Textbook of Modern Toxicology. New York: Elsevier, 1987

Jakoby WB, Bend JR, Caldwell J (eds): Metabolic Basis of Detoxication. New York: Academic Press, 1982

Klaassen CD, Amdur MO, Doull J: Casarett and Doull's Toxicology. 3rd edt. New York: Macmillan, 1986

Lauwerys RR: Industrial Chemical Exposure: Guidelines for Biological Monitoring. Davis, Calif.: Biomedical Publications, 1983

Loomis TA: Essentials of Toxicology. 3rd edt. Philadelphia: Lea & Febiger, 1978

Ottoboni A: The Dose Makes the Poison. Berkeley, Calif.: Vincente Books, 1984

Sies H: Oxidative Stress. New York: Academic Press, 1985

U.S. Department of Health and Education: NIOSH Pocket Guide to Chemical Hazards. Cincinnati: National Institute for Occupational Safety and Health, 1983

Selected Organ Systems

Goldstein BD (Chair) and Subcommittee on Reproductive and Neurodevelopmental Toxicology: Biologic Markers in Reproductive Toxicity. Washington, D.C.: National Academy Press, 1989

Kimmel CA, Buelke-Sam J: Developmental Toxicology. New York: Raven Press, 1981

McLachlan JA, Pratt RM, Markert CL (eds): Developmental Toxicology: Mechanisms and Risk. Cold Spring Harbor, N.Y.: Cold Spring Harbor Laboratories, 1987

Marzulli FN, Maibach HI (eds): Dermato-toxicology. New York: Hemisphere, 1983

Porter GA: Nephrotoxic Mechanisms of Drugs and Environmental Toxins. New York: Plenum, 1982

Spencer PS, Schaumburg HH: Experimental and Clinical Neurotoxicology. Baltimore: Williams & Wilkins, 1980

Weening JJ: Mechanisms leading to toxin-induced impairment of renal function, with a focus on immunopathology. Toxicol Lett 46:205–226, 1989

Zimmerman HJ: Hepatotoxicity: The Adverse Effects of Drugs and Other Chemicals on the Liver. New York: Appleton-Century-Crofts, 1978

Neurobehavioral Toxicology

1. Weiss B: Tools for the assessment of behavioral toxicity. In Xinteras C, Johnson BL, de Groot I, (eds): Behavioral Toxicology: Early Detection of Occupational Hazards. Washington, D.C.: National Institute for Occupational Safety and Health, 1974, pp 444–449
2. Xinteras C, Johnson BL, de Groot I: Behavioral Toxicology: Early Detection of Occupational Hazards. Washington, DC: National Institute for Occupational Safety and Health, 1974
3. Zenick H, Reiter LW: Behavioral toxicology an emerging discipline. Research Triangle Park, N.C.: U.S. Environmental Protection Agency, 1977
4. Valciukas JA, Lilis R: Psychometric techniques in environmental research. Environ Res 21:275–297, 1980
5. Johnson BL, Anger WK: Behavioral toxicology. In Rom W (ed): Environmental and Occupational Medicine. Boston: Little, Brown & Co., 1983, pp 329–350
6. Baker EL, Letz R, Fidler A: A computer-administered neurobehavioral evaluation system for occupational and environmental epidemiology. J Occup Med 27:206–212, 1985
7. Valciukas JA, Singer RM: An embedded figures test in environmental and occupational neurotoxicology. Environ Res 28:183–198, 1982
8. Weiss B, Laties VG: Behavioral Pharmacology: The Current Status. New York: Alan R. Liss, 1985
9. Hartman DE: Neuropsychological Toxicology. New York: Pergamon Press, 1988
10. Neurobehavioral Toxicology. Journal published by ANKHO International Inc., Fayetteville, N.Y. (1st volume, 1979)
11. Singer R, Valciukas JA, Lilis R: Lead exposure and nerve conduction velocity: The differential time course of sensory and motor nerve effects. Neurotoxicology 4:193–202, 1983
12. Seppalainen AM: Neurophysiological findings among workers exposed to organic solvents. Scand J Work Enviorn Health 7(suppl 4):29–33, 1981
13. Lindstrom K, Martelin T: Personality and long-term exposure to organic solvents. Neurobehav Toxicol 2:89–100, 1980
14. Flodin U, Edling C, Axelson O: Clinical studies of psychoorganic syndromes among workers with exposure to solvents. Am J Industr Med 5:287–295, 1984
15. National Institute for Occupational Safety and Health: Organic solvent neurotoxicity. Curr Intell Bull 48:1–39, 1987
16. Cherry N, Waldron HA, Wells GG, Wilkinson RT, Wilson HK, Jones S: An investigation of the acute behavioural effects of styrene on factory workers. Br J Industr Med 37:234–240, 1980
17. Lindstrom K, Harkonen H, Hernberg S: Disturbances in psychological functions of workers occupationally exposed to styrene. Scand J Work Environ Health 3:129–139, 1976
18. Cavanaugh JV: Peripheral neuropathy caused by chemical agents. CRC Crit Rev Toxicol 2:365–376, 1980
19. Teisinger J: New advances in the toxicology of carbon dislufide. Am Industr Hyg Assoc J 35:55, 1974
20. Vigilani EC: Carbon disulfide poisoning in viscose rayon factories. Br J Industr Med 11:235, 1954
21. Laties VG, Merigan WH: Behavioral effects of carbon monoxide on animals and man. Ann Rev Pharmacol Toxicol 19:357–392, 1979
22. O'Hanlon JF: Preliminary studies of the effects of carbon monoxide on vigilance in man. In Weiss B, Laties VG (eds): Behavioral Toxicology. New York: Plenum, 1975, pp 61–75
23. Valciukas JA, Lilis R, Fischbein A, Selikoff IJ: Central nervous system dysfunction due to lead exposure. Science 201:465–467, 1978
24. Agency Toxic Substances and Disease Registry: The Nature and Extent of Lead Poisoning in Children in the United States: A Report to Congress. Washington, D.C.: U.S. Department of Health and Human Services, 1988
25. Langston JW, Ballard P, Tetrud JW, Irwin I: Chronic parkinsonism in humans due to a product of meperidine-analog synthesis. Science 219:979–980, 1983
26. Laties VG: How operant conditioning can contribute to behavioral toxicology. Environ Health Perspect 26:29–35, 1978
27. Griffin DR: The Question of Animal Awareness: Evolutionary Continuity of Mental Experience. New York: Rockefeller University Press, 1976
28. Lorenz K: On Aggression. New York: Harcourt, Brace & World, 1966
29. Burger J, Gochfeld M: Early postnatal lead exposure: behavioral effects in common tern chicks (*Sterna hirundo*). J Toxicol Environ Health 16:869–886, 1985
30. Reiter L: Use of activity measures in behavioral toxicology. Environ Health Perspect 26:9–20, 1978
31. Brown DR: Neonatal lead exposure in the rat: Decreased learning as a function of age and blood lead concentration. Toxicol Appl Pharmacol 32:628–637, 1975
32. Ogilvie DM. Sublethal effects of lead acetate on the Y-maze performance of albino mice (*Mus musculus* L.) Can J Zoology 55:771–775, 1977
33. Zenick H, Padich R, Tokarek T, Aragon P: Influence of prenatal

and postnatal lead exposure on discrimination learning in rats. Pharmacol Biochem Behav 8:347–350, 1978

34. Cory-Slechta DA, Weiss B, Cox C: Delayed behavioral toxicity of lead with increasing exposure concentration. Toxicol Appl Pharmacol 71:342–352, 1983
35. Rice DC, Gilbert SG, Willes RF: Neonatal low-level lead exposure in monkeys: locomotor activity, schedule-controlled behavior, and the effects of amphetamine. Toxicol Appl Pharmacol 51:503–513, 1979
36. Rice DC: Behavioral deficit (delayed matching to sample) in monkeys exposed from birth to low levels of lead. Toxciol Appl Pharmacol 75:337–345, 1984
37. Dietz DD, McMillan DE, Mushak P: Effects of chronic lead administration on acquisition and performance of serial position sequences by pigeons. Toxicol Appl Pharmacol 47:377–384, 1979
38. Laties VG, Evans HL: Methylmercury-induced changes in operant discrimination in the pigeon. J Pharmacol Exp Ther 214:620–628, 1980
39. Rice DC, Gilbert SG: Early chronic low-level methylmercury poisoning in monkeys impairs spatial vision. Science 206:759–771, 1982
40. Fox GA, Donald T: Organochlorine pollutants, nest-defense behavior and reproductive success in merlins. Condor 82:81–84, 1980
41. Evans KL, Garman RH, Laties VG: Neurotoxicity of methylmercury in the pigeon. Neurotoxicology 3:21–36, 1982
42. Silbergeld E, Goldberg A: A lead-induced behavioral disorder. Life Sciences 13:1275–1283, 1973
43. Sauerhoff M, Michaelson: Hyperactivity and brain catecholamines in lead-exposed developing rats. Science 182:1022–1024, 1973
44. Bushnell PJ, Bowman RE, Allen JR, Marlar RJ: Scotopic vision deficits in young monkeys exposed to lead. Science 195:333–335, 1977
45. McArthur MLB, Fox GA, Peakall DB, Philogene BJR: Ecological significance of behavioral and hormonal abnormalities in breeding ring doves fed an organochlorine chemical mixture. Arch Environ Contam Toxicol 12:343–353, 1983
46. Witt PN: Drugs alter web-building of spiders: A review and evaluation. Behav Sci 16:98–113, 1971
47. Barthalamus GT, Leander JD, McMillan DE, Mushak P, Krigman MR: Chronic effects of lead on schedule-controlled pigeon behavior. Toxicol Appl Pharmacol 42:271–284, 1977
48. Burger J, Gochfeld M: Lead and behavioral development: effects of varying dosage and schedule on survival and performance of young common terns (*Sterna hirundo*). J Toxicol Environ Health 24:173–182, 1988
49. Laties V, Cory-Slechta DA: Some problems in interpreting the behavioral effects of lead and methylmercury. Neurobehav Toxicol 1(suppl 1):129–135, 1979
50. Brady K, Herrera Y, Zenick H: Influence of parental lead exposure on subsequent learning ability of offspring. Pharmacol Biochem Behav 3:561–565, 1975
51. Dahlgren RB, Linder RL: Effects of dieldrin in penned pheasants through the third generation. J Wildlife Manage 39:320–330, 1974
52. Valciukas JA, Singer RM: An embedded figures test in environmental and occupational neurotoxicology. Environ Res 28:183–198, 1982
53. Burger J, Gochfeld M: A hypothesis on the role of pheromones on age of menarche. Med Hypotheses 17:39–46, 1985
54. Doty RL, Gregor T, Monroe C: Quantitative assessment of olfactory function in an industrial setting. J Occup Med 28:457–460, 1986
55. Bove F, Litwak MS, Arezzo JC, Baker EL: Quantitative sensory testing in occupational medicine. Semin Occup Med 1:185–188, 1986
56. Morrow LA, Ryan CM, Goldstein G, Hodgson MJ: A distinct pattern of personality disturbance following exposure to mixtures of organic solvents. J Occup Med 31:743–750, 1989
57. Kilburn KH, Seidman BC, Warshaw R: Neurobehavioral and respiratory symptoms of formaldehyde and xylene exposure in histology technicians. Arch Environ Health 40:229–233, 1985
58. Needleman H, Gunnoe C, Leviton A, Reed R, Peresie H, Maher C, Barrett P: Deficits in psychologic and classroom performance of children with elevated dentine lead levels. N Engl J Med 300:689–695, 1979
59. Lin-Fu JS: The evolution of childhood lead poisoning as a public health program. In Chisholm JJ, O'Hara DM (eds): Lead Absorption in Children: Management, Clinical and Environmental Aspects. Baltimore: Urban & Schwarzenberg, 1982, pp 1–10
60. Baker EL, Letz R: Solvent neurobehavioral testing in monitoring hazardous workplace exposures. J Occup Med 28:126–129, 1986
61. Hanninen H, Lindstrom K: Behavioral Test Battery for Toxicopsychological Studies. Helsinki: Institute of Occupational Health, 1979
62. World Health Organization: Organic Solvents and the Central Nervous System. Copenhagen: WHO, 1985 (Document 5)
63. Lezak M: Neuropsychological Assessment. New York: Oxford University Press, 1983
64. Matthews CG, Klove H: Instruction Manual for the Adult Neuropsychology Test Battery. Madison, Wis.: University of Wisconsin Medical School, 1964
65. Gamberale F: Use of behavioral performance tests in the assessment of solvent toxicity. Scand J Work Environ Health 11(suppl 1):65–74, 1985
66. Wechsler D: WAIS-R Manual. New York: The Psychological Corp., 1981
67. Delis D, Kramer J, Kaplan E, Ober B: California Verbal Learning Test Manual. New York: The Psychological Corp., 1987
68. Benton A: Visual Retention Test Manual. New York: The Psychological Corp., 1974
69. McNair D, Lorr M, Droppleman LF: Profile of Mood States: Manual. San Diego: Educational and Industrial Testing Service, 1981
70. Derogatis L: SCL-90-R Manual-II. Baltimore: Clinical Sociometric Research, 1983
71. Doty RL, Shaman Pl, Applebaum SL, Giberson R, Siksorski L, Rosenberg L: Smell identification ability: Changes with age. Science 226:1441–1443, 1984

General Readings

Anastasi A: Psychological Testing. New York: Macmillan, 1976.

Brown GG, Nison R: Exposure to polybrominated biphenyls: Some effects on personality and cognitive functioning. JAMA 242:523, 1979

Feldman RG, Ricks NL, Baker EL: Neuropsychological effects of industrial toxins: A review. Am J Industr Med 1:211–227, 1980

Gale A, Edwards JA (eds): Physiological Correlates of Human Behavior. New York: Academic Press, 1983 (3 vols.)

Hanninen H: Behavioral effects of occupational exposure to mercury and lead. Acta Neurol Scand 66:(suppl) 92:167, 1982

Hartman DE: Neuropsychological Toxicology. New York: Pergamon Press, 1988

Huber F, Markl H: Neuroethology and Behavioral Physiology. New York: Springer-Verlag New York. 1983

Jason KM, Kellogg CK: Behavioral neurotoxicity of lead. In Singhal RL, Thomas JA (eds): Lead Toxicity. Baltimore: Urban & Schwarzenberg, 1980, pp 241–271

Johnson BL: Prevention of Neurotoxic Illness in Working Populations. New York: John Wiley & Sons, 1987

LaDou J (ed): Occupational Health Law: A Guide for Industry. New York: Marcel Dekker, 1981

Lehner PN: Handbook of Ethological Methods. New York: Garland STPM Press, 1979

Olishifski JB (ed): Fundamentals of industrial hygiene. 2nd edt. Chicago: National Safety Council, 1979

Reiter L: An introduction to neurobehavioral toxicology. Environ Health Perspect 26:5–7, 1978

Reiter L: Use of activity measures in behavioral toxicology. Environ Health Perspect 26:9–20, 1978

Spencer PS, Schaumburg HH: Experimental and Clinical Neurotoxicology. Baltimore: Williams & Wilkins, 1980

Tinbergen N: The Study of Instinct. New York: Oxford University Press, 1974

Valciukas JA, Lilis R: Psychometric techniques in environmental research. Environ Res 21:275–297, 1980

Weiss B: Behavioral toxicology and environmental health science: Opportunity and challenge for psychology. Am Psychol 38:1174, 1983

Weiss B: Experimental implications of behavior as a criterion of toxicity. In Weiss B, Laties VG (eds): The Current Status. Behavioral Pharmacology. New York: Alan R. Liss, 1985

Weiss B: Behavior as a measure of adverse responses to environmental contaminants. Handbook Psychopharmacol 18:1–57, 1984

Xinteras C, Johnson BL, de Groot I: Behavioral Toxicology: Early Detection of Occupational Hazards. Washington, D.C.: U.S. Department of Health, Education, and Welfare, National Institute for Occupational Safety and Health, 1974 (publication No. DHEW (NIOSH) 74–126

Yerkes RM: The mental life of monkeys and apes: a study of ideational behavior. Behav Monogr 3:1–145, 1916

Yerkes RM: The mind of a gorilla: memory. Comp Psychol Monogr 5(2):1–91, 1928

Zbinden G, Cuomo V, Racagni G, Weiss B (eds): Application of Behavioral Pharmacology in Toxicology. New York: Raven Press, 1983

Zenick H, Reiter LW: Behavioral toxicology: An emerging discipline. Research Triangle Park, U.S. Environmental Protection Agency, N.C.: 1977

Environmental Risk Assessment

1. National Research Council: Risk Assessment in the Federal Government. Washington, D.C.: National Academy Press, 1983
2. U.S. Environmental Protection Agency: Risk assessment guidelines for carcinogenicity, mutagenicity, complex mistrues, suspect developmental toxicants, and estimating exposures. Federal Register 51:33992–34054, 1986
3. Derby SL, Keeney RL: Risk analysis: Understanding "how safe is safe enough." Risk Analysis 1:217–224, 1981
4. Lave LB: Quantitative Risk Assessment in Regulation. Washington, D.C.: Brookings Institution, 1982
5. Risk Analysis: An International Journal of the Society for Risk Analysis. New York: Plenum Press 1981 to present
6. Lowrance WW: Of Acceptable Risk. Los Altos, Calif.: William Kaufmann, 1976
7. Imperato PJ, Mitchell G: Acceptable Risks. New York: Viking, 1985
8. Kasperson RE, Renn O, Slovic P, Brown HS, Emel J, Goble R, Kasperson JX, Ratick S: The social amplification of risk: a conceptual framework. Risk Analysis 8:177–187, 1988
9. Whyte AV, Burton I: Environmental Risk Assessment. New York: John Wiley & Sons, 1980
10. Goldstein BD: Risk assessment/risk management is a three-step process: In defense of EPA's risk assessment guidelines. J Am Coll Toxicol 7:543–549, 1988
11. Fischoff B, Slovic P, Lichtenstein S, Read S, Combs B: How safe is safe enough? A psychometric study of attitudes towards technological risks and benefits. Policy Sciences 8:127–152, 1978
12. Sandman PM: Hazard Versus Outrage: The Case of Radon. New Brunswick, N.J.: Environmental Communication Research Program, 1988
13. Doderlein JM: Understanding risk management. Risk Analysis 3: 17–21, 1983
14. May WW: $s for lives: ethical considerations in the use of cost/benefit analysis by for-profit firms. Risk Analysis 2:35–46, 1982
15. Lioy P: Assessing total human exposure to contaminants. Environ Sci Technol 24:938–945, 1990
16. U.S. Environmental Protection Agency: Proposed guidelines for carcinogen risk assessment. Federal Register 49:46294–46301, 1984
17. Armitage P: Multistage models of carcinogenesis. Environ Health Perspect 63:195–201, 1985
18. Moolgavkar SH, Knudsen AG Jr: Mutation and cancer: A model for human carcinogenesis. J Natl Cancer Inst 66:1037–1052, 1981
19. Krewski D, Van Ryzin J: Dose response models for quantal response toxicity dates. In Csorgo M, Dawson D, Rao JNK, Saleh E (eds): Current Topics in Probability and Statistics. New York: Elsevier/North Holland, 1981
20. Hallenbeck WH: Quantitative evaluation of human and animal studies. In Hallenbeck WH, Cunningham KM (eds): Quantitative Risk Assessment for Environmental and Occupational Health. Chelsea, Mich.: Lewis, 1986, pp 43–60
21. Crump KS, Howe RB: The multistage model with a time-dependent dose pattern: Application to carcinogenic risk assessment. Risk Analysis 4:163–176, 1984
22. Barnes DG, Dourson M: Reference dose (Rfd): Description and use in health risk assessments. Regul Toxicol Pharmacol 8:471–486, 1988
23. Allen BC, Crump KS, Shipp AM: Correlation between carcinogenic potency of chemicals in animals and humans. Risk Analysis 8:531–544, 1988
24. Slovic P, Fischoff B, Lichtenstein S: Why study risk perception. Risk Analysis 2:83–94, 1982
25. Covello VT, Sandman P, Slovic P: Risk communication, risk statistics, and risk comparisons: A manual for plant managers. Washington, D.C.: Chemical Manufacturers Assoc., 1988
26. Greenberg MR, Sachsman DB, Sandman PM, Salomone KL: Network evening news coverage of environmental risk. Risk Analysis 9:119–126, 1987
27. Sandman P, Sachsman D, Greenberg M, Gochfeld M: Environmental Risk and the Press. New Brunswick, N.J., Transaction Books, 1987
28. National Research Council: Risk Assessment in the Federal Government. Washington, D.C.: National Academy Press, 1983
29. Environmental Protection Agency: Risk assessment guidelines for carcinogenicity, mutagenicity, complex mixtures, suspect developmental toxicants, and estimating exposures. Federal Register 51: 33992–34054, 1986

General Readings on Risk Assessment

Conway RA. Environmental Risk Analyses for Chemicals. New York: Van Nostrand, 1982

Hallenbeck WH, Cunningham KM: Quantitative Risk Assessment for Environmental and Occupational Health. Chelsea, Mich.: Lewis, 1986

Hoel DG, Merrill RA, Perera FP: Risk quantitation and regulatory policy. Banbury Reports 19:1–386, 1985

Kandel A, Avni E: Engineering risk and hazard assessment. Boca Raton, Fla.: CRC Press, 1988

Lave LB: Quantitative Risk Assessment in Regulation. Washington, D.C.: Brookings Institute, 1982

Long FA, Schweitzer GE: Risk Assessment at Hazardous Waste Sites. American Chemical Society Symposium, 1982, p 204

Lowrance WW: Of Acceptable Risk. Los Altos, Calif.: William Kaufmann, 1976

Oftedal P, Brogger A: Risk and Reason: Risk Assessment in Relation to Environmental Mutagens and Carcinogens. New York: Alan R. Liss, 1986

Saxena J: Hazard Assessment of Chemicals. Vols. 1 and 2. New York: Academic Press, 1983

Silbergeld E: Epidemiology versus risk assessment: Resolving some old controveries. Risk Analysis 8:555–558, 1988

Stara JF, Erdreich LS: Advances in health risk assessment for systemic toxicants and chemical mixtures: An international symposium. Toxicol Industr Health 1(4):1–364, 1985

Travis CC: Carcinogen Risk Assessment. New York: Plenum, 1988

Whyte AV, Burton I: Environmental Risk Assessment. New York: John Wiley & Sons, 1980

Selected Readings on Quantitative Risk Assessment

Allen BC, Crump KS, Shipp AM: Correlation between carcinogenic potency of chemicals in animals and humans. Risk Analysis 8:531–544, 1988

Altshuler B: Modeling of dose-response relationships. Environ Health Perspect 42:23–27, 1981

Andersen ME, Clewell HI, Gargas ML, Smith FA, Reitz RH: Physiologically based pharmacokinetics and the risk assessment process for methylene chloride. Toxicol Appl Pharmacol 87:185–205, 1987

Armitage P: Multistage models of carcinogenesis. Environ Health Perspect 63:195–201, 1985

Crump KS: A critical analysis of a dose-response assessment for TCDD. Food Chemical Toxicol 26:79–83, 1988

Knight FH: Risk, Uncertainty and Profit. New York: Harbor Torchbooks, 1921

Moolgavkar SH, Knudsen AG Jr: Mutation and cancer: A model for human carcinogenesis. J Natl Cancer Inst 66:1037–1052, 1981

National Academy of Science, Safe Drinking Water Committee: Drinking Water and Health. Vols. 6 and 10. Washington, D.C.: National Academy Press, 1986, 1987

Paustenbach DJ: The Risk Assessment of Environmental Hazards. New York: John Wiley & Sons, 1989

Tardiff RG, Rodricks JV: Toxic Substances and Human Risk: Principles of Data Interpretation. New York: Plenum, 1987

Van Ryzin J: Quantitative risk assessment. J Occup Med 22:321–326, 1980

Selected Readings on Risk Perception and Risk Communication

Covello VT, Sandman P, Slovic P: Risk Communication, Risk Statistics, and Risk Comparisons: A Manual for Plant Managers. Washington, D.C.: Chemical Manufacturers Assoc., 1988

Epple D, Slovic P: Taxonomic analysis of perceived risk: Modeling individual and group perceptions within homogeneous hazard domains. Risk Analysis 8:435–456, 1988

Fischoff B: How safe is safe enough? A psychometric study of attitudes towards technological risks and benefits. Policy Sciences 9:127–152, 1958

Freudenburg WR: Perceived risk, real risk: Social science and the art of probabilistic risk assessment. Science 242:44–49, 1988

Green CH, Brown RA: Through a glass darkly: Perceiving perceived risks to health and safety. Dundee, Scotland: University of Dundee School of Architecture, 1980

Johnson B, Covello V (eds): Social and Cultural Construction of Risk: Essays on Risk Selection and Perception. Boston: Reidel, 1987

Kahneman D, Slovic P, Tversky A: Judgement Under Uncertainty: Heuristics and Biases. New York: Cambridge University Press, 1982

Krimsky S, Plough A: Environmental Hazards. Dover, Mass.: Auburn House, 1988

Otway H, Wynne B: Risk communication: Paradigm and paradox. Risk Analysis 9:141–146, 1989

Sandman PM: Apathy versus hysteria: Public perception of risk. In Batra LR, Klassen W (eds): Public Perception of Biotechnology. Bethesda, Md.: Agricultural Research Institute, 1987, pp 219–231

Sandman P, Sachsman D, Greenberg M, Gochfeld M: Environmental Risk and the Press. New Brunswick, N.J.: Transaction Books, 1987

Short JF Jr: Social dimensions of risk: The need for a sociological paradigm and policy research. American Sociologist 22:167–172, 1987

Slovic P: Informing and educating the public about risk. Risk Analysis 6:403–415, 1986

Slovic P: Perception of risk. Science 236:28–290, 1987

Slovic P, Fischoff B, Lictenstein S: Facts versus fears: Understanding perceived risk. In Kahneman D, Slovic P, Tversky A (eds): Judgement Under Uncertainty: Heuristics and Biases. New York: Cambridge University Press, 1982

von Winterfeldt D, John RS, Borcherding K: Cognitive components of risk ratings. Risk Analysis 1:277–288, 1981

Selected Readings on Applications of Risk Assessment

Covello VT, Lave LB, Moghiss A, Uppuluri VRR (eds): Uncertainty in risk assessment, risk management and decision making. New York: Plenum, 1987

Denison RA, Silbergeld EK: Risks of municipal solid waste incineration: An environmental perspective. Risk Analysis 8:343–357, 1988

Ditz DW: Hazardous waste incineration at sea: EPA decision making on risk. Risk Analysis 8:499–508, 1988

Gough M: Science policy choices and the estimation of cancer risk associated with exposure to TCDD. Risk Analysis 8:337–342, 1988

Hance BJ, Chess C, Sandman P: Improving dialogue with communities. Trenton, N.J.: Department of Environmental Protection, 1988

Kroes R: Contribution of toxicology toward risk assessment of carcinogens. Arch Toxicol 60:224–228, 1987

Kunreuther H, Lathrop JW: Siting hazardous facilities: Lessons from LNG. Risk Analysis 1:289–302, 1981

Kunreuther H, Slovic P: Decision making in hazard and resource management. In Kates RW, Burton I (eds): Geography, Resources and Environment. Vol. 2. Chicago: University of Chicago Press, 1986, pp 153–187

Rodricks J, Taylor MR: Application of risk assessment to food safety decision making. Regul Toxicol Pharmacol 3:275–307, 1983

Rycroft TW, Regens JL, Dietz T: Incorporating risk assessment and benefit-cost analysis in environmental management. Risk Analysis 8:415–420, 1988

Sandman PM: Getting to maybe: Some communications aspects of hazardous waste facility siting. In Lake RW (ed): Resolving Locational Conflict. New Brunswick, N.J.: Environmental Community Research Program, 1987, Rutgers University, 1987, pp 324–344

Viscusi WK, Magat WA: Learning About Risk: Consumer and Worker Responses to Hazard Information. Cambridge, Mass.: Harvard University Press, 1987

17

Asbestos and Other Fibers

Kaye H. Kilburn

ASBESTOS

Asbestos-associated Diseases

Clinical Recognition of Asbestosis. Asbestosis is defined as a fibrotic disease of the lung from asbestos exposure that occurs after a suitable latent period. Pathologic changes consisting of cellular infiltrates and fibrosis surround small bronchioles, limit forced expiratory flow, and thereby impair pulmonary function. Asbestosis is diagnosed from chest radiographs by diffuse irregular opacities in the lung fields or by circumscribed or diffuse pleural thickening. These abnormalities are defined by international criteria.[1]

Asbestos exposure produces *no acute symptoms.* The pathological changes of fibrosis in lung or pleura are well advanced when recognition of *radiographic features* permits "early diagnosis" before *breathlessness on exertion* and *cough productive of phlegm* develop. Usually asbestosis has been incubating for years, frequently two decades or more from the first exposure; the time between exposure and manifestation is called the "latent" period. Asbestos and cigarette smoking are *synergistic* in impairing function and producing fibrosis and carcinoma.

History. Although man's first use of asbestos is lost in antiquity, it is mentioned by Plinius, who referred to asbestos as *immun vivum,* "durable linen." Charlemagne is supposed to have had an asbestos tablecloth that was cleaned after feasts by being tossed into the flames. The exceptional properties of asbestos fiber—resistance to combustion, durability, and resistance to friction—have made it useful for many types of insulation and heat protection in modern industrial society. H. Montague Murray,[2] a London physician, recognized a new disease in the badly scarred lungs of an asbestos worker, presumably in a textile factory, who died after a brief illness characterized by extreme breathlessness. Murray connected the workplace exposure to the scarring in testifying before an inquiry at the British Government Commission on Occupational Disability in 1907 and stated hopefully that with the recognition of the cause, he would predict few future cases. The singular finding was largely ignored until 1924, when Cooke[3] published a clear description of pulmonary fibrosis in a woman who had worked for 20 years in an asbestos textile factory. Although this report attracted some attention to the condition, the possibility that it was simply a manifestation of tuberculosis, the plague of those times, was the excuse largely to ignore the entity. Cooke[4] also introduced the name "pulmonary asbestosis" as a pneumoconiosis, one of the dust diseases named by Zenker 60 years earlier.

After further scattered reports of the exposure of individual workers, usually those in asbestos textile factories but sometimes insulators, to these woven asbestos products, an epidemiological investigation was conducted by Merewether and Price[5] into the condition of the workers in British asbestos textile factories. They systematically associated factory dust containing asbestos with asbestosis, which was recognized during life by radiographic findings that had been reported by Pancoast et al.[6] in 1918. The study by Merewether and Price demonstrated clear relationships, focusing in the card rooms, between levels of dust and prevalence of asbestosis. Studies of the workers' lungs in the fatal cases by Gloyne[7] showed the propensity of the lesions for membranous and respiratory bronchioles. Later in the 1930s there were two industrywide studies. One, undertaken for the Metropolitan Life Insurance Co. by Lanza et al.,[8] reported that two thirds of the x-ray films of 126 persons selected more or less at random from those with 3 or more years of employment had findings of asbestosis. In 1938, Dreessen et al.[9] studied 511 employees of asbestos textile factories in North Carolina. He found a low prevalence of abnormalities in the x-ray films, but the workers studied were largely newly hired hands with short-term exposure. It is important to note that when several dozen workers who had been discharged from these same factories were traced, x-ray films of many of them showed chest abnormalities characteristic of asbestosis.[10–12] Thus, with the publication of the Dreessen study and the associated reports, it was clear that asbestosis produces abnormalities in the chest x-ray film and shortness of breath.

In the 1930s, additional reports of insulators, boilermakers, and men in other trades who manufactured or used asbestos showed that they had abnormal x-ray films, shortness of breath and in some cases rales in the chest, clubbing of the digits, and cyanosis. However, World War II intervened before there was useful control of exposure; thus further intelligence about the pervasiveness and widespread nature of asbestosis was left to the 1960s and 1970s, when studies in the shipbuilding and construction trades showed how widespread were abnormal chest x-ray findings in workers exposed to asbestos. Large studies of asbestos miners and millers first pointed out that in men so exposed, airways obstruction and reductions in vital capacity and in dif-

TABLE 17-1. DEATHS AMONG 17,800 ASBESTOS INSULATION WORKERS IN THE UNITED STATES AND CANADA (JANUARY 1, 1967, TO DECEMBER 31, 1976)[a]

Underlying Cause of Death	Expected[b]	Observed		Ratio, Observed/Expected	
		(BE)	(DC)	(BE)	(DC)
Total deaths, all causes	1658.9	2271	2271	1.37	1.37
Total cancer, all sites	319.7	995	922	3.11	2.88
Cancer of lung	105.6	486	429	4.60	4.06
Pleural mesothelioma	c	63	25	—	—
Peritoneal mesothelioma	c	112	24	—	—
Mesothelioma, n.o.s.	c	0	55	—	—
Cancer of esophagus	7.1	18	18	2.53	2.53
Cancer of stomach	14.2	22	18	1.54	1.26
Cancer of colon-rectum	38.1	59	58	1.55	1.52
Cancer of larynx	4.7	11	9	2.34	1.91
Cancer of pharynx, buccal	10.1	21	16	2.08	1.59
Cancer of kidney	8.1	19	18	2.36	2.23
All other cancer	131.8	184	252	1.40	1.91
Noninfectious pulmonary diseases, total	59.0	212	188	3.59	3.19
Asbestosis	c	168	78	—	—
All other causes	1280.2	1064	1161	0.83	0.91

[a] Number of workers, 17,800; person-years of observation, 166,853.
[b] Expected deaths are based on white male age-specific U.S. death rates of the U.S. National Center for Health Statistics, 1967–1976.
[c] Rates are not available, but these have been rare causes of death in the general population.
BE = Best evidence, indicating number of deaths categorized after review of best available information (autopsy, surgical, clinical); DC = number of deaths as recorded from death certificate information only.

fusing capacity occurred before there were abnormalities in the chest x-ray film.[13]

Lung Cancer. Lung cancer was first associated with asbestos exposure in reports of individual patients in the 1930s. However, as with cancer caused by cigarette smoking, the full impact developed slowly. Merewether,[14] who was the first to conduct a population-based study, reported to the British Inspectorate of Factories in 1947 that 13.5% of the asbestos textile workers whom he had studied in 1931 had died of lung cancer within 16 years. Hueper[15] collected the experience of the 1930s and earlier and by 1942 concluded in his textbook that asbestos was one of the principal causes of lung cancer and was more important than arsenic or radium. However, it remained for Richard Doll,[16] in a well-designed study of a textile factory cohort, a defined population, to call attention to the long latency of cancer and to account for all causes of death for comparison. This report, published in 1955, provided convincing evidence of the association between occupational exposure to asbestos and lung cancer; the increase was tenfold above the expected incidence. New evidence continued to accrue with the report of Mancuso and Coulter,[17] which confirmed Doll's findings in the United States, and Selikoff[18] first reported a large excess of lung cancer among the users of asbestos, that is, insulators. The finding that the users were in danger vastly amplified the number of persons who could be expected to have an increased risk of lung cancer and raised the urgency of control. With the use of a 10-year prospective study of mortality rates in almost 18,000 insulators begun in 1967, Selikoff et al.,[19] by 1979, found excessive death rates not only for lung cancer, mesothelioma, and asbestosis but also for cancers of the gastrointestinal tract, larynx, oropharynx, and kidney (Table 17–1), and they measured interactions between cigarette smoking and asbestos in these cancers (Table 17–2). Age-standardized rates per 100,000 person-years are as follows: Individuals who neither worked with asbestos nor smoked cigarettes had a calculated death rate of 11.3; asbestos workers who did not smoke had a rate of 58.4. Smokers in general (not asbestos workers) showed a rate of 122.6, whereas those who had both types of exposure, cigarettes and asbestos, had a rate of 601.6.

Mesothelioma, a Twentieth-century Tumor. Klemperer and Rabin,[20] in 1931, described the features of this tumor, its rarity, and the characteristic spread on the pleural surface, and reasoned that the carcinogen responsible must be one that could penetrate to these inaccessible surfaces of the pleura and peritoneum. Reports of mesotheliomas in subjects exposed to asbestos

TABLE 17-2. AGE-STANDARDIZED LUNG DEATH RATES[a] FOR CIGARETTE SMOKING AND/OR OCCUPATIONAL EXPOSURE TO ASBESTOS DUST COMPARED WITH NO SMOKING AND NO OCCUPATIONAL EXPOSURE

Group	Exposure to Asbestos?	History Cigarette Smoking	Death Rate	Mortality Difference	Mortality Ratio
Control	No	No	11.3	0.0	1.00
Asbestos workers	Yes	No	58.4	+47.1	5.17
Control	No	Yes	122.6	+111.3	10.85
Asbestos workers	Yes	Yes	601.6	+590.3±	53.24

[a] Rate per 100,000 person-years standardized for age on the distribution of the person-years of 12,051 asbestos workers followed prospectively 1967–1976. Control subjects included 73,763 like men in a prospective study at the American Cancer Society for the same decade. Number of lung cancer deaths based on death certificate information.

were scattered throughout the 1940s and 1950s. Rarity was its principal property until Wagner et al.,[21] in 1960, reported 47 mesotheliomas in people who had been associated with the crocidolite works in South Africa 15 years earlier. Such a clear association between a rare tumor and a mineral species was unprecedented, but it was quickly corroborated by a number of other studies. Despite the lack of controls in the Wagner study, the germinal observations were confirmed statistically and by population-based data. Consequently the diagnosis of a mesothelioma now provokes a search for asbestos exposure that is seldom unfulfilled. Latent intervals of 30 to 40 years are characteristic. Many recent and current patients were exposed in U.S. shipyards during the development and support of a two-ocean navy and shipping during World War II.

Asbestos Minerals

Fibers and Fibrils. "Asbestos" is a convenient name given to naturally occurring fibrous minerals and includes commercial serpentine and amphibole fibers but excludes fibrous forms of other minerals such as wollastonite, brucite, gypsum, and calcite. Chrysotile, the serpentine asbestos, occurs in "cobs" about the size of a hand that are found in pockets often within platelike and nonfibrous silica deposits. The fibers are, in turn, composed of fibrils. The fibers can be seen with an optical microscope; the fibrils that compose them are of micrometer size, and therefore single fibrils isolated or in tissue are ordinarily visible only with an electron microscope. Fortunately there are crude associations among "dustiness" (the gravimetric measurement of the total airborne burden), the visible fibers recognized with the optical microscope (particularly with the help of phase-contrast or polarized light), and the concentrations of fibrils that are visible with the electron microscope. For industrial hygiene, the rough relationships between total dust measured gravimetrically from air samples and fibers visible with the light microscope have produced reasonable dose-response relationships in miners and millers of asbestos, asbestos textile workers, and workers producing asbestos (calcite) pipe. Estimates of maximal human exposure to fine fibers range widely from several hundred fibrils per cubic meter to several hundred millions of fibrils per cubic meter.

Sources. The commercially important asbestos fibers are chrysotile, amosite, and crocidolite. Chrysolite, or white asbestos, is mined mainly in Canada's Quebec Province and in the Ural mountains of the Soviet Union, but it is also found in commercial quantities in the United States, particularly in Arizona and California. In contrast to the single serpentine species, the amphiboles are represented by three major species of commercial importance. Crocidolite, or blue asbestos, is highly associated with mesothelioma. Amosite is called brown asbestos because of its content of iron; it was named for the Asbestos Mining Organization of South Africa. Anthophyllite is of little commercial importance except for deposits in Finland. Important for human exposure, although of less commercial importance, is actinolite, or fibrous tremolite, which contaminates minerals; examples include crocidolite and talc from many sources, particularly the deposits in the Gouverneur district of New York State.

In terms of numbers of human subjects exposed, mining and milling of asbestos is less important than is its use in thermal insulation and construction materials (Table 17-3). The contamination potential is large because of dispersal of the fibrils into the air of "massive containers" such as ships and of industrial facilities such as aluminum refineries, copper smelters, glass and fiberglass factories, paper mills, and powerhouses. Airborne fibrils spread to all workers, well beyond those whose hands contact asbestos products.

Uses of Asbestos in Industry and Construction. Asbestos has been widely used in industry and construction.[22] The general uses are in heat insulation, friction-resistant products, and construction. As heat insulation, asbestos cloth is used in blankets, gloves, suits, and boiler packing and is combined with magnesia in pipe insulation. Asbestos combined with portland cement, or blue mud, was widely used in free-form insulation around pipes and boilers (Fig. 17-1). Friction products include the obvious brake shoes and pads, clutch facing, and other woven products that must resist both friction and the heat generated thereby. In many senses the full tragedy of asbestos exposure has been borne by workers in the construction trades, where, for reasons not at all clear but including availability, cheapness, and binding properties, asbestos has been used widely, as thermal insulation in drywall, in spray ceilings, paint, floor tile, and ceiling tile, and as filler in a wide range of other products. Analogous to fine sand, as the inert material in paint, asbestos has been added to products whether or not it conferred useful properties.

Peak Use of Asbestos. The peak use of asbestos in the United States was probably in the early 1970s, although it can be seen in

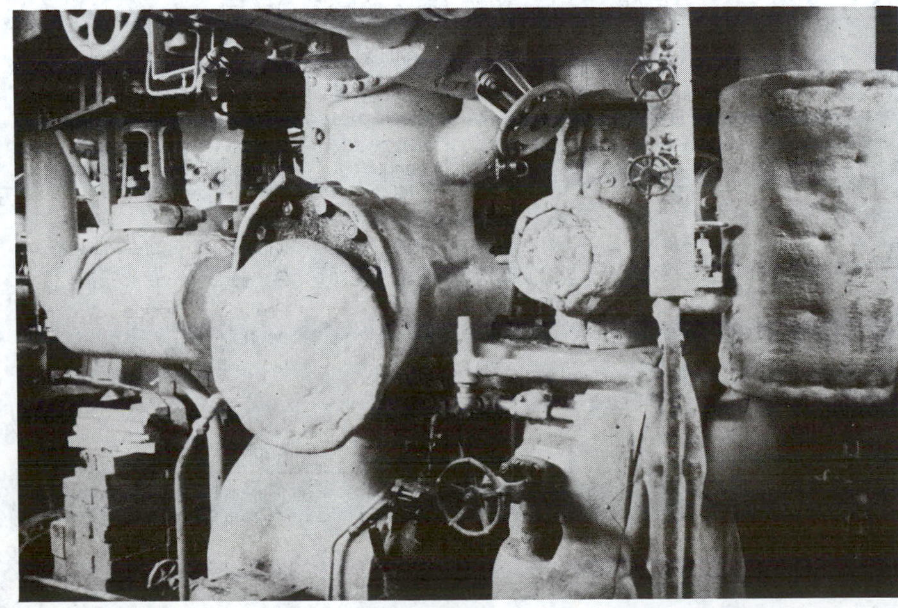

Figure 17-1. Asbestos insulation aboard ship. Asbestos repairs in engine rooms and similar areas carry the potential for asbestos exposure not only of shipyard workers[50] but also of engine room and other shipboard personnel.

TABLE 17-3. ASBESTOS-CONTAINING MATERIALS FOUND IN BUILDINGS

Subdivision	Generic Name	Asbestos (%)	Dates of Use	Binder/Sizing
Surfacing material	Sprayed or troweled on	1–95	1935–1970	Sodium silicate, portland cement, organic binders.
Preformed thermal insulating products	Batts, blocks, and pipe covering			
	85% magnesia	15	1926–1949	Magnesium carbonate
	Calcium silicate	6–8	1949–1971	Calcium silicate
Textiles	Cloth[a]			
	Blankets (fire)[a]	100	1910–present	None
	Felts	90–95	1920–present	Cotton/wool
	Blue stripe	80	1920–present	Cotton
	Red stripe	90	1920–present	Cotton
	Green stripe	95	1920–present	Cotton
	Sheets	50–95	1920–present	Cotton/wool
	Cord/rope/yarn[a]	80–100	1920–present	Cotton/wool
	Tubing	80–85	1920–present	Cotton/wool
	Tape/strip	90	1920–present	Cotton/wool
	Curtains[a] (theatre, welding)	60–65	1945–present	Cotton
Cementitious concretelike products	Extrusion panels	8	1965–1977	Portland cement
	Corrugated	20–45	1930–present	Portland cement
	Flat	40–50	1930–present	Portland cement
	Flexible	30–50	1930–present	Portland cement
	Flexible perforated	30–50	1930–present	Portland cement
	Laminated (outer surface)	35–50	1930–present	Portland cement
	Roof tiles	20–30	1930–present	Portland cement
	Clapboard and shingles:			
	Clapboard	12–15	1944–1945	Portland cement
	Siding shingles	12–14	Unknown–present	Portland cement
	Roofing shingles	20–32	Unknown–present	Portland cement
	Pipe	20–15	1935–present	Portland cement
Paper products	Corrugated			
	High temperature	90	1935–present	Sodium silicate
	Moderate temperature	35–70	1910–present	Starch
	Indented	98	1935–present	Cotton and organic binder
	Millboard	80–85	1925–present	Starch, lime, clay
Roofing felts	Smooth surface	10–15	1910–present	Asphalt
	Mineral surface	10–15	1910–present	Asphalt
	Shingles	1	1971–1974	Asphalt
	Pipeline	10	1920–present	Asphalt
Asbestos-containing compounds	Caulking putties	30	1930–present	Linseed oil
	Adhesive (cold applied)	5–25	1945–present	Asphalt
	Joint compound		1945–1975	Asphalt
	Roofing asphalt	5	Unknown–present	Asphalt
	Mastics	5–25	1920–present	Asphalt
	Asphalt tile cement	13–25	1959–present	Asphalt
	Roof putty	10–25	Unknown–present	Asphalt
	Plaster/stucco	2–10	Unknown–present	Portland cement
	Spackles	3–5	1930–1975	Starch, casein, synthetic resins
	Sealants, fire/water	50–55	1935–present	Caster oil or polyisobutylene
	Cement, insulation	20–100	1900–1973	Clay
	Cement, finishing	55	1920–1973	Clay
	Cement, magnesia	15	1926–1950	Magnesium carbonate
Asbestos ebony products		50	1930–present	Portland cement
Flooring tile and sheet goods	Vinyl/asbestos tile	21	1950–present	Poly(vinyl)chloride
	Asphalt/asbestos tile	26–33	1920–present	asphalt
	Sheet goods/resilient	30	1950–present	Dry oils
Wallcovering	Vinyl wallpaper	6–8	Unknown–present	—
Paints and coatings	Roof coating	4–7	1900–present	Asphalt
	Airtight	15	1940–present	Asphalt

Data modified from: Lory EE, Coin DC. February 1981. Management Procedure for Assessment of Friable Asbestos Insulating Material. Port Hueneme, Calif.: Civil Engineering Laboratory Naval Construction Battalion Center. The U.S. Navy prohibits the use of asbestos-containing materials when acceptable nonasbestos substitutes have been identified.

[a] Laboratory aprons, gloves, cord, rope, fire blankets, and curtains may be common in schools.

Figure 17–2 that yearly consumption was virtually level from 1950 through 1969, at more than 7000 metric tons. The profile is similar for the remainder of the developed nations of the world. Less is known about the Soviet Union, but from personal inspection, it is obvious that asbestos has been widely used in construction.

Patterns of Use. In response to a flood of asbestos litigation and regulation since the mid 1970s, patterns of use have changed, sometimes abruptly, in Western countries. Asbestos has been excluded from many consumer products, from building materials, and most recently from brakes and friction goods. Pioneering synthetic brake materials, Volvo Corporation, in Sweden, produced pads and shoes that although twice as expensive last three or four times as long as asbestos. Although we were sanguine about abolishing the use of asbestos, episodes remind us that all has not gone as well as hoped. For example, asbestos continued to be installed in New Jersey schools without warning labels well into the early 1980s, and in 1986 an inventory of a U.S. Navy warehouse for ship fittings disclosed 130 products containing asbestos. Many of these were gaskets and other relatively low-exposure items, but others included thermal insulation and blankets. Because the use of asbestos accompanied industrialization, particularly the intense industrialization of the twentieth century, a key question is, What is in store for the developing countries? It appears that economic determinants take precedence over health; for example, in Israel, asbestos pipe containing

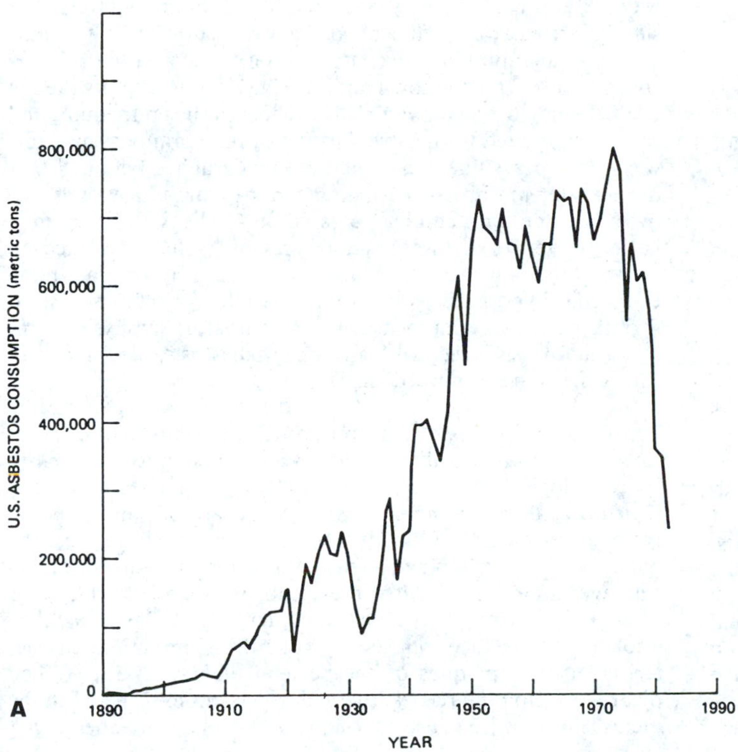

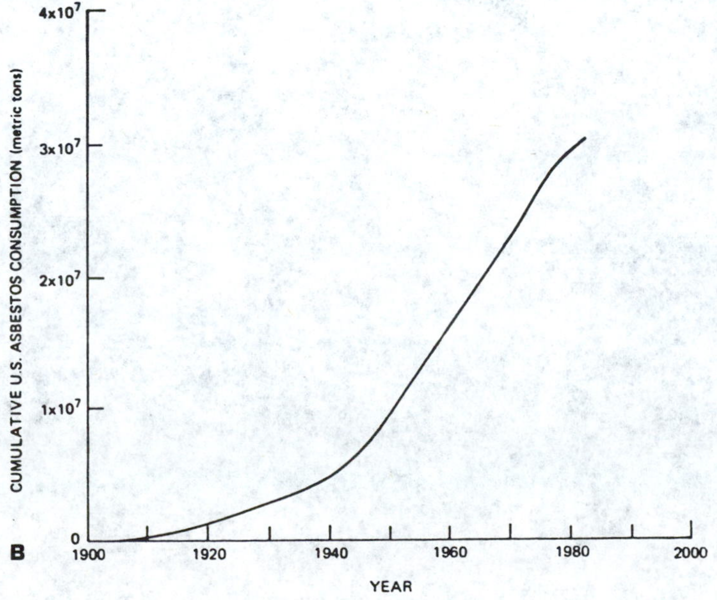

Figure 17–2. A. Annual U.S. consumption of asbestos from 1890 to 1982. **B.** Cumulative U.S. consumption of asbestos from 1905 to 1982, which exceeded 30 million metric tons. Based on data from U.S. Bureau of Mines, 1973, 1978, 1983.

crocidolite was manufactured through the decade of the 1970s, and asbestos continues in place in sugar mills and oil refineries in Mexico, Brazil, and China.

Removal of Asbestos. Fragmentation and degeneration, particularly caused by heat and vibration, increase the potential liberation of fibrils from asbestos, particularly when it is disturbed by renovation, removal, or repair.[23] Thus it appears that the highest doses for workers may be generated during removal of asbestos, particularly if attention is not given to wetting material down and restricting the area to properly suited personnel who are well trained in using air-supply respirators.[22] Under these conditions, if the asbestos is placed in plastic bags and buried, the hazard is minimized. However, much of the asbestos removal and renovation have been taking place without these safeguards, and levels of more than 100 fibers per millimeter have been measured during these activities.

BIOLOGICAL EFFECTS OF ASBESTOS

Molecular Effects. The in vitro properties of asbestos include effects over large surface areas of asbestos fibrils on the hemolysis of red blood cells. Chrysotile has been shown to mediate the uptake of exogenous DNA into monkey cells in such a way that the genes on the DNA are expressed.[24] Several cultured human cell lines show the toxic effects of chrysotile and amosite.[25–28] Pleural mesothelial cells showed marked proliferation.[26] Dose-response cytotoxic effects were found in a cultured line of macrophages, and amphiboles caused hyperplasia and squamous cell metaplasia.[27] In normal and transformed epithelial cell lines, chrysotile was more toxic than amosite in terms of cell numbers and of plasminogen activator assay results.[28]

Cellular Effects. Studies begun by Heppleston[29,30] and by Allison[31] and associates two decades ago showed the importance of signals generated by macrophages that have phagocytosed asbestos fibrils. In contrast, quartz is disturbingly lethal for cells. Macrophages that have phagocytosed asbestos fibrils are strongly implicated in the pathogenesis of fibrosis in animal models[32,33] and in the human lung, where asbestos causes both recruitment and proliferation.[34] Observations of cells in vitro and in permeable chambers implanted in the peritoneum of rats showed that macrophages produce peptides that stimulate fibroblasts to replicate and produce collagen. These peptides have been identified as fibronectin and other fibroblast-stimulating factors.[35,36] Asbestos is less cytotoxic and yet generates fibroblast-stimulating factors, including fibronectin, which may explain how asbestos simulates collagen production in the pathogenesis of asbestosis.[37]

Target Organ. Processing asbestos in the lung[38,39] evidently begins in airways, particularly the small airways where fibrils impinge. Short-term clearance depends on fiber size and type; chrysotile, for example, clears from guinea pig lungs faster than does amosite.[40] There are no studies of the acute response in the airways,[39] but the probable scenario is that the fibrils penetrate the epithelium by passing between the epithelial cells, cross the basement membrane, and probably lodge in the connective tissue, where macrophages are attracted. Macrophages on the airway surfaces may phagocytose some fibrils, but many fibrils are simply carried away on the mucociliary escalator. Others, apparently a small minority, are coated with iron-rich protein and become asbestos (ferruginous) bodies (Fig. 17–3). Certainly the site of thickening of the airway walls is beneath the epithelium, and cells are attracted to the alveolar side of membranous small airways. It appears likely, as suggested by Craighead et al.,[41] that the next step in fibrosis is bridging, via the lymphatic vessels, between the peribronchiolar scars, linking them together in a latticelike network. It was assumed previously that this linked-up network "shrank" the lung, that is, reduced its volume; however, this hypothesis is no longer tenable. Volumes lost to shrunken zones are compensated for by areas of emphysema. Interstitial fibrosis is seen with advanced asbestosis, particularly in subjects who have smoked cigarettes.

Transport of Fibrils. Transport of fibrils occurs to other sites, clearly to the regional lymphatic vessels and into the pleural space. A logical pleural pathogenesis by Hillerdal[42] suggests that the fibrils, absorbed in small airways and alveoli, move via the lymphatic vessels or within cells to the pleural surface, cross the pleural space, and impinge on the parietal pleura, where the macrophages are retained. Here they send signals to fibroblasts or perhaps also to mesothelial cells to undergo fibroblastic proliferation and to produce collagen.[43] Under this stimulation, characteristic hyaline plaques of the parietal pleura develop. When pleural effusion intercedes, there may be symphysis between the pleural layers, with dense adhesions. At this stage it appears that

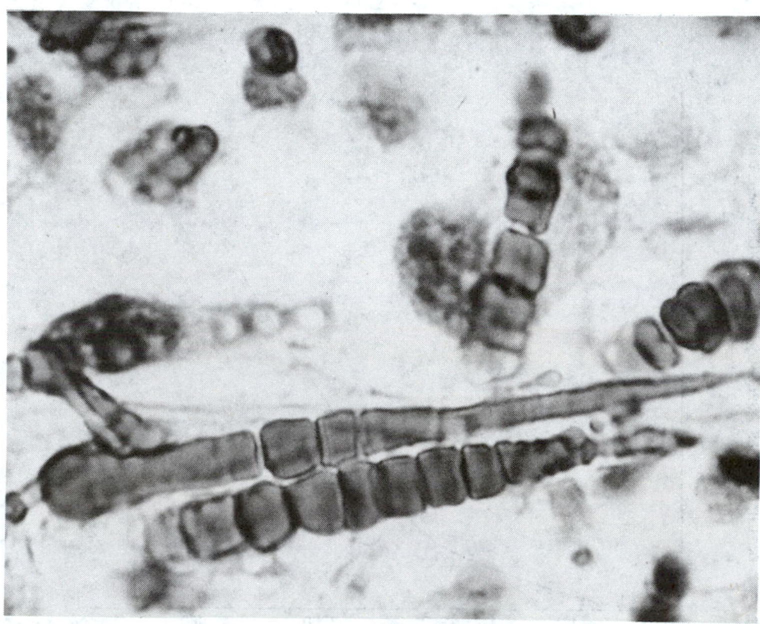

Figure 17–3. Asbestos (ferruginous) bodies in lung tissue consist of an asbestos core with an iron protein coat that make them appear tan or brown. (×600.)

in some instances fibrosis invades the lung from pleural surfaces via the perivenous lymphatics in a retrograde direction. Perhaps this occurs because pleural symphysis obliterates the pleural space so that it is no longer accessible as a sump for the fibrils, which have moved toward the peripheral portions of the lung. Fibrils remain in the perivenous lymphatics. Whatever the mechanism, such fibrous strands, as seen on cut surfaces of the lung or on high-resolution computer-augmented tomographs, are most dense at the pleura and attenuate progressively toward the hilum.

Immune Responses. Disturbances of the immune system, particularly the association of rheumatoid factor with asbestosis,[44,45] have posed several unresolved questions concerning, first, whether those subjects who develop rheumatoid factor are more susceptible to the clinical manifestations of disease after asbestos exposure, second, whether immune globulin synthesis is stimulated by asbestos, and third, whether such elevations enhance the development of asbestosis. Alterations in populations of lymphatic T cells have also been associated with asbestos exposure and with asbestosis.[45,46] However, the meaning of these observations is uncertain and poses questions similar to those regarding the role of immune globulins.

Summary. Macrophage products, exportable peptides that stimulate fibroblasts to proliferate and to produce collagen, have been observed in cell systems and diffusion chambers of plants and animals.[30,31] More recently, it has been clear that fibronectin and at least one other fibroblast-stimulating factor can be stimulated by asbestos in cells.[47-49] Implantation of asbestos and man-made fibers in the pleural space of experimental animals, and refinements of this technique with milling and sizing of the fibrils, led Stanton and Wrench[50] to propose that it was the physical properties—the diameters and lengths of the fibers or fibrils—that were responsible for neoplasia expressed as mesothelioma. Intracellular asbestos fibrils interfere with chromosome aggregation in mitosis, although whether this interference is linked to neoplasia is unclear.[24] It appears that physical, surface, and chemical properties of the fibrils may be important in cell proliferation, particularly to form tumors.

Human Exposure

Workers. After airborne asbestos fibrils are respired, they affect the small airways, or alveoli, of the human lung. Thus the important means of human exposure is the sharing of the air space into which asbestos, in pure form or as a component, has been dispersed. It is also clear that a textile factory, as in the first studied instances, or a ship, power station, factory, smelter, or refinery where there is heat conservation and protection, is a *container,* which increases the dose and enhances the possibilities of exposure by raising the concentration within the contiguous spaces without dissipation into the outdoors. Thus, when asbestos insulation was sprayed on the structural steel of high-rise buildings in New York City, sprayers were heavily exposed (Fig. 17-4) and asbestos was detected in ambient air as far away as Cape May, N.J. However, it is clear that the sprayers themselves, within the skeleton of the buildings, were at greatest risk. Asbestos spray insulation is a potent form of asbestos exposure. It is possible that, in mining and milling, moisture and non-asbestos rock bind fibers together and impair their discharge of fibrils into the air. In comparison, textile operations, in which the fibers are carded and spun, would produce maximal opportunity for the generation of fibrils into the workplace air, similar to the spraying of asbestos insulation. Obviously, partially bound asbestos-containing materials are less hazardous than those which are friable and which readily release fibers or allow for the generation of fibrils into the air. The use of compressed air to clear dust from brake drums represents a large-scale disturbance of very fine fibrils (Fig. 17-5), as does the removal of insu-

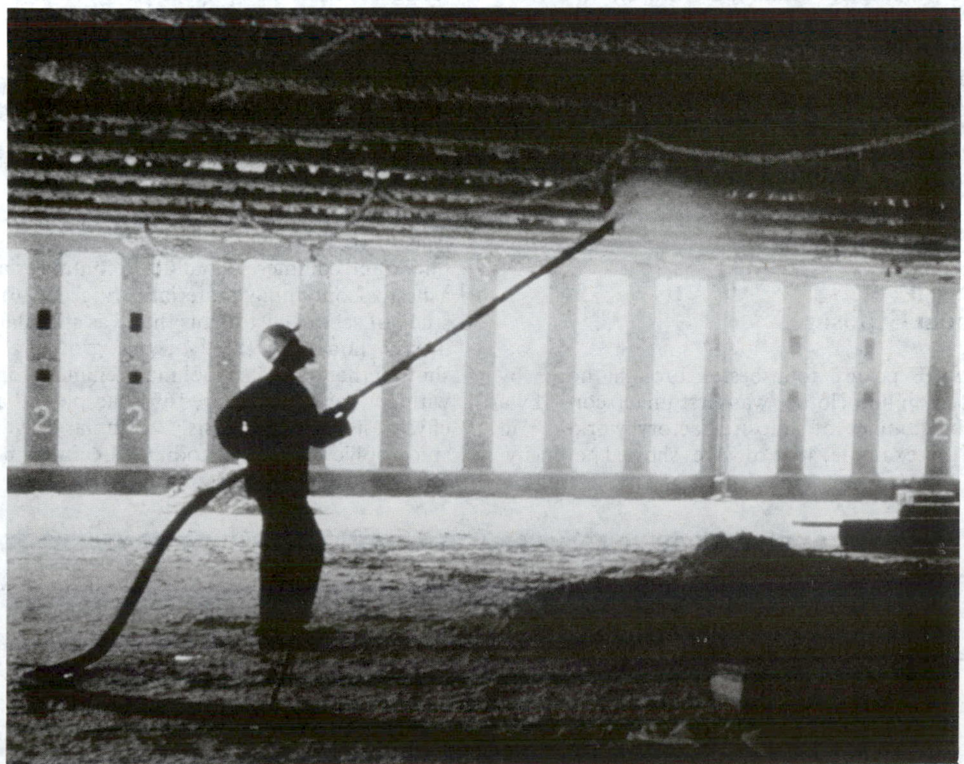

Figure 17-4. Insulator wearing a mask is spraying structural steel with asbestos insulation. His mask is inadequate personal protection. Other workers and the community were also exposed. This practice stopped in the 1970s.

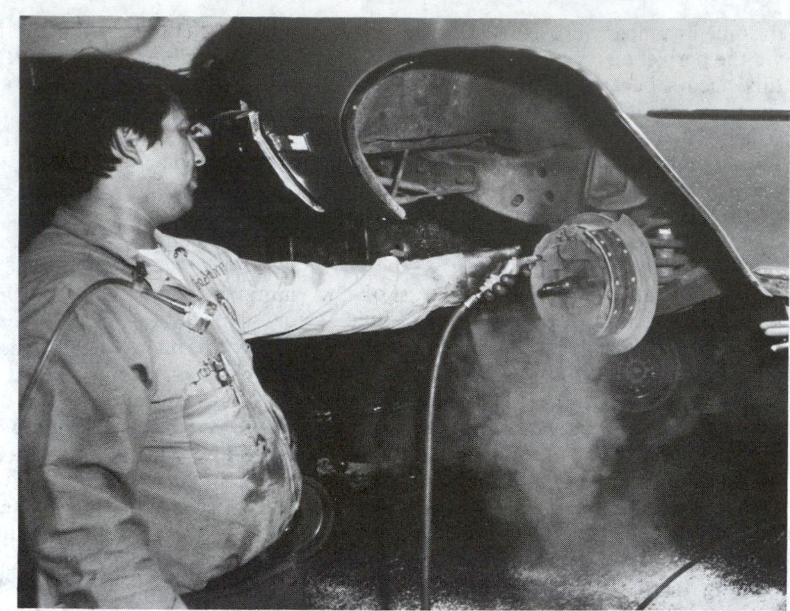

Figure 17–5. Removal of dust from brake drum and back plate using compressed air generates cloudy or fine fibers and dust.

lation that had cooked in place on boilers or steam lines. If one considers the prevalence of asbestosis as a reflection of cumulative exposures in trades in which workers use or are within the airspace of asbestos goods, it is clear that insulators, sheet metal workers, boilermakers, and pipefitters rank very high, whereas at the same construction sites, electricians, carpenters, laborers, workers, and mechanics have less exposure. Thus the prevalence of disease is less in the latter groups after 15 to 25 years.

Judged by the prevalence and severity of chest radiograph abnormalities, bystander tradesmen working in shipyards and, in particular, on board ship, have as much exposure as those who are installing or ripping out insulation.[51] Ships with perforated plates comprising decks and the hull as the outside container are ideal for maintaining fibrils in the air, similar to asbestos textile factories. Thus the important matter in taking a patient's history is to determine whether he is involved in a heat-conserving or heat-protecting operation, and whether asbestos is present and in what proximity to the subject. For example, asbestosis has been diagnosed in cafeteria and office workers employed in asbestos pipe plants where they had shared the airspace of a single structure with production workers for 15 or 20 years.

Secondary Human Exposure

Family Members. Exposure to asbestos brought home by workers on their person and clothes was first underscored by a classic study of the families of amosite factory workers[52] in Patterson, N.J. In this example, 48% of wives showed parenchymal or pleural evidence of asbestosis, 21% of daughters, and 42% of sons (Table 17–4). Shifting to a less intense work exposure, that of shipyards, another family study showed that 11.3% of wives, 2.1% of daughters, and 7.6% of sons, had signs of asbestosis (Table 17–5).[53] Although consumer electrical goods such as irons, hairdryers, and fans have contained asbestos, to this time there has been no evidence of disease resulting from exposure at the levels of fibrils released from electric irons, electric hairdryers, or even asbestos-containing artificial logs burned in fireplaces. However, this does not excuse continuance of such exposure, and the Consumer Products Safety Administration has been responsive in seeing that consumer goods are free of asbestos.

Schools and Other Buildings. The matter of passive bystander asbestos exposure in buildings containing asbestos as part of their heat insulation on steam pipes and boilers, as part of insulation ducts leading to the rooms, as material sprayed on ceilings and walls, or as construction materials has been the subject of contentious discussion, rule making, and litigation in the past decade.[54,55] Surveys by the U.S. Environmental Protection Agency (EPA) have estimated that 31,000 schools and 733,000 public and commercial buildings contain friable, easily crumbled asbestos-containing material[22] (Fig. 17–6). In a preliminary study of school custodians that was stimulated by the finding of mesotheliomas in three of this group, a Los Angeles study showed that of 205 school maintenance workers and custodians with 10 years on the job, 16% had pleural and 13% had parenchymal signs of asbestosis.[56] A similar prevalence was found in a study of New Jersey custodians (Levine S: personal communica-

TABLE 17–4. PREVALENCE OF RADIOGRAPHIC ABNORMALITIES AMONG HOUSEHOLD CONTACTS OF ASBESTOS FACTORY WORKERS

Relationship	Total Examined	Parenchymal Opacities	Pleural Abnormality	Parenchymal and/or Pleural	Mean Duration of Exposure
Wives	162	40 (25%)	58 (36%)	77 (48%)	2.2 ± 2.4 y
Daughters	224	15 (7%)	34 (15%)	46 (21%)[a]	2.4 ± 2.6 y
Sons	151	31 (21%)	47 (31%)	63 (42%)	2.3 ± 2.8 y
Siblings	81	15 (19%)	22 (27%)	30 (37%)	2.1 ± 2.1 y
Others	61	12 (21%)	17 (28%)	23 (38%)	3.6 ± 3.3 y
Total	679	129 (19%)	178 (26%)	239 (35%)	

[a] Prevalence of radiographical abnormalities significantly higher among sons than daughters. $\chi^2 = 19.6$, $P < 0.001$.

TABLE 17-5. PREVALENCE OF ASBESTOSIS OF LUNGS AND/OR PLEURA FOR SHIPYARD WORKERS AND FAMILY CONTACTS AND IN LONG BEACH AND MICHIGAN COMPARISON POPULATIONS

Groups	*n*	Percent with Asbestosis
Male shipyard workers	288	64.2
Female shipyard workers	71	21.1
Wives of shipyard workers	274	11.3
Sons of shipyard workers	79	7.6
Daughters of shipyard workers	140	2.1
Comparison population		
Long Beach census tract men	673	3.7
Long Beach census tract women	674	0.6
Michigan sample men	594	0.5
Michigan sample women	583	0.0

tion). In neither of these studies did data with certainty exclude from analysis custodians with prior exposure to asbestos, nor was it possible to ascertain which ones were working on the maintenance of boilers and of heat- and power-generating facilities. A study in Boston schools[57] showed that of 52 custodians, 40% had pleural markers of asbestosis and only 1 (1.9%) had pulmonary changes. These studies make the point that some maintenance and school custodial workers have asbestosis as a result of workplace exposure. The studies also raise the possibility that teachers and students sharing these air spaces may show signs as well, but neither teachers nor children have been studied. Such a study would best be done in teachers exposed to asbestos for at least 20 years; the prevalence of asbestos-induced changes on chest x-ray examination should be determined, and those with other sources of exposure to asbestos should be excluded from the study. One method applicable to the study of students would be to ask adults attending 20-year high school reunions to undergo chest x-ray examinations to ascertain whether they have an increased prevalence of asbestosis; those with occupational exposure, as determined by questionnaire, would of course be excluded from the study. Many schoolboards have removed asbestos from the schools; some have issued bonds for this purpose, and some have sued the suppliers of asbestos-containing products to recover the costs. In response to considerable pressure from consumer groups and legislatures, the EPA has recommended removal of such products when air levels of asbestos are 0.1 to 0.01 fiber per milliliter.[21] In a sense, asbestosis as a problem can be solved when a society is willing to make changes on the basis of the known harmfulness of asbestos, without waiting to assess morbidity and mortality rates in a particular instance of exposure.[53,54]

ASBESTOSIS

Diagnosis. The diagnosis of asbestosis requires, first, a history of exposure, usually occupational or as a bystander in a trade in which asbestos has been used. Second, a suitable period must have elapsed since the start of exposure, so that the usual incubation (latent) period for developing asbestosis has been completed. The third criterion is the presence of typical pulmonary or pleural abnormalities on the chest x-ray film. The latent period, at the levels of exposure prevalent in developed countries in the past 30 years, is at least 10 years, with progressively higher prevalences of asbestosis found at 20, 30, and 40 years. In most shipbuilding and construction trades, among workers who were virtually continuously exposed for 25 to 35 years, the prevalence of asbestosis, including pleural disease, is 25% to 35%. Pulmonary abnormalities are seen on a full-size posteroanterior chest radiograph as irregular opacities in the lower half of the lung fields near the lateral pleural surfaces. The radiographic technique used optimizes the visualization of vascular markings in peripheral lung fields.[1] Pleural signs are circumscribed or diffuse areas of pleural thickening, so-called hyaline plaques of the parietal pleura, which are seen best when located laterally or on the diaphragm but may also be located posteriorly or anteriorly and may be seen face on (en face), or in profile. Descriptions of the patterns of changes in chest radiographs as a result of asbestosis have been progressively enhanced and detailed by the International Labor Organization (ILO) working committees since 1919. The 1980 revision[1] included a set of standard radiographs with the major ILO categories portrayed (Fig. 17-7A to E). Pleural changes are described by their location, thickness, and extent (Fig. 17-7F). Use of the ILO classification scheme has improved communication between investigators in various countries. Although radiographic pulmonary or parenchymal signs of asbestosis are distinct from pleural signs, recent studies of several thousand exposed workers showed that the functional implications are similar: both impair expiratory flow and produce air trapping.[58-60] Furthermore, despite radiographic distinctions between circumscribed plaquelike and diffuse pleural thickening, there was no difference in physiological impairment except that greater impairment occurred when diffuse thickening surrounded the base of the lung.

Pathology. The pathological changes in asbestosis were first described by the British pathologist Roodhouse Gloyne[7] as cellular aggregates and cell proliferation around the small airways, the terminal and respiratory bronchioles. The primacy of this lesion was obscured in later descriptions of severe fibrosis extending throughout the lung, with dense aggregates of macrophages and asbestos bodies in the surviving alveoli. These observations led to characterization of asbestosis as an interstitial fibrosis. However, in the past decade, descriptions of the human pathological changes and considerable animal experimentation have refocused attention on the membranous and respiratory bronchioles as the focus of fibrosis (Fig. 17-8). Subsequent bridging extends between the bronchioles, creating a latticework; additional interstitial fibrosis may develop at a more advanced stage.[41] A possible second and more distinctive lesion probably involves the perivenous lymphatics and has been visualized on extended-scale computer-assisted tomograms of subjects with increased markings in the lung bases.[61,62] This lesion creates a distinct pattern on the extended-scale tomograms. Fibrosis is well visualized peripherally and attenuates as it extends toward the hilum. This is in contrast to ordinary vascular and bronchial markings, which attenuate toward the pleural surfaces. Accentuated secondary lobular septa occur at about 1 cm intervals along the lateral margins of the lung, where they are recognized as laddering on the chest radiograph.

A small percentage of asbestos-exposed subjects have their course complicated by pleural effusions. Healing of these effusions may obliterate the costophrenic angles and produce diffuse pleural scarring by a variant pathogenesis.[63,64]

Undoubtedly, fibrils migrate to the pleura from their locus of deposition in small airways or alveoli.[42] Whether they are translocated as free fibrils or within macrophages after phagocytosis is still unknown. In either case they must exit the lung to the pleural space and move with the lymph flow to the parietal pleural lymphatic vessels.[42] Here they apparently stimulate macrophages or stimulate the retention of the macrophages in the outer layers of the pleura and once again stimulate fibroblastic proliferation. Thus circumscribed thickening (plaques) is found in the lower two thirds of the lateral dorsal and ventral parietal pleura and in the dome of the diaphragm. Plaques are disks composed of dense hyalinized collagenous connective tissue up to several millimeters in thickness.

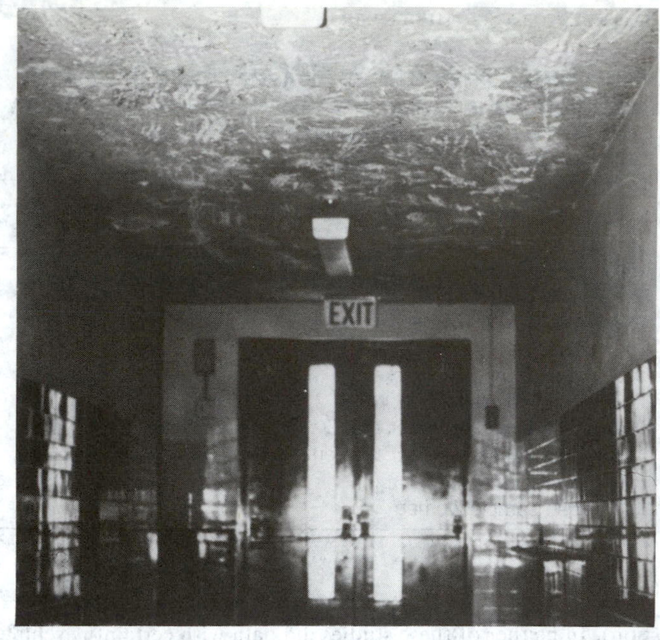

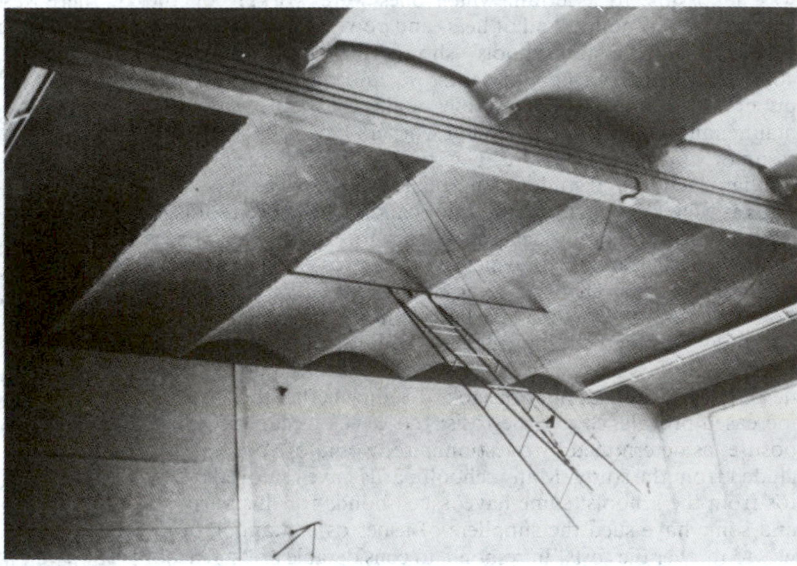

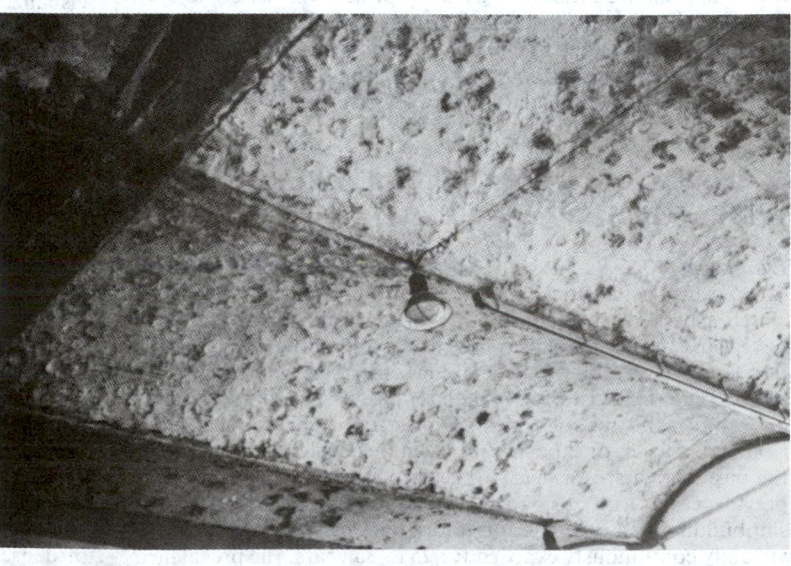

Figure 17–6. A. Asbestos-coated ceiling in a public hallway. **B.** Ceiling of a gymnasium in an elementary school (no basketball marks). **C.** Ceiling of a gymnasium in a high school showing evidence of damage from basketballs thrown by students. (**B.** *and* **C.** *used by permission from* Guidance for Controlling Asbestos-containing materials in Buildings. *Washington, D.C.: U.S. Environmental Protection Agency, June 1985 (EPA 560/5-85-024).*)

Clinical Features. During the past 50 years, other clinical features have been described in asbestosis. The principal symptom is shortness of breath on exertion; onset is insidious, and the symptom gradually worsens before either recognition of radiograph abnormalities in the lung or a diagnosis. Cough with phlegm production is common, and when it is present for a duration of 3 months in 2 succeeding years, chronic bronchitis is diagnosed. Bronchitis increases in prevalence as the duration of asbestos exposure passes 20 years, even in workers who have never smoked.

Physical examination of the chest reveals decreased breath sounds as the prime feature. Wheezing on forced expiration increases in frequency as the lesions on x-ray films become more profuse. Fine crepitant rales may be heard after the radiographic changes are moderately advanced (ILO category 2/2 and greater) but are rare earlier. Peripheral cyanosis and clubbing of the phalanges, although described in advanced asbestosis, are such uncommon signs that their presence should arouse suspicion of other causes. Asbestos "warts," which occur from inoculation of asbestos fibers through the skin, once common in insulators who handled asbestos daily, are now rarely seen.

Physiological Impairment. The principal pathological lesions caused by the presence of asbestos in the lungs involve the membranous and respiratory bronchioles. These lesions physically narrow these small airways and limit mid and terminal flow rates,[65,66] that is, obstruct expiratory air flow as the earliest physiological lesion in asbestosis.[13,58] Large numbers of workers have been studied to provide significant numbers of workers who were not exposed to cigarette smoke so that the effect of asbestos alone could be confirmed.[13,58] Thus it appears that the obstruction of the small airways occurs before the irregular opacities of asbestosis are visible on the posteroanterior chest film (Fig. 17–9A). It is also clear that this airflow limitation produces air trapping evidenced by an increase in the ratio of the residual volume (RV) to total lung capacity (total gas volume [TGV]) (RV/TGV ratio) and that it is this increase in residual volume which reduces vital capacity (Fig. 17–9B). This observation led to the concept that asbestosis is a restrictive lung disease similar to idiopathic pulmonary fibrosis. However, vital capacity is a reliable measure of restrictive disease, that is, loss of lung volume only in the *absence of obstruction.*[67] Using a reduced vital capacity to indicate restriction allowed an erroneous concept to creep into the understanding of the physiological picture of asbestosis in the absence of measurements of the total lung capacity that were not influenced by air trapping. In the presence of air trapping, gas dilution using helium or nitrogen is not a reliable method of measuring total lung capacity, as has been well demonstrated in patients with emphysema. Thus radiographic[68] or body plethysmographic methods must be used for accurate measurement of total lung capacity.[67] In the latter method, care must be taken to measure expiratory reserve volume carefully. When this is done, total lung capacity is generally slightly increased (about 10%) in asbestosis (Fig. 17–9C). Most of this increase is attributable to the effect of cigarette smoking; 85% of workers exposed to asbestos also smoked cigarettes for many years (Table 17–6).

The profusion of irregular opacities on the chest radiograph is used as the anatomical measure of severity of asbestosis, and key pulmonary function measurements are plotted against this anatomical score; progressive impairment of airflow and air trapping is seen with an increasing profusion of opacities on roentgenograms[59,60] (Fig. 17–9). Further limitation of expiratory flow from 25% to 75% of vital capacity, which indicates increased airways obstruction, increases air trapping, but the total lung capacity is maintained. As the ratio of forced expiratory volume in 1 second to vital capacity decreases progressively, air trapping, measured as the RV/TGV ratio, increases and the forced expiratory volume in 1 second and the vital capacity both decrease; lung volume, however, is maintained. In fact, in a study of 8000 workers, of whom 46 had severe asbestosis and ILO profusions of 2/3 and greater, none had reduced thoracic gas volume. Four additional subjects with apparent restrictive disease had had part or all of one lung removed because of lung cancer. In summary, "a small, tight lung" does not characterize asbestosis but, rather, is an airways obstructive disease in which total lung volume, the real measure of restrictive lung disease, actually increases by about 10% above predicted values because of cigarette smoking. It is also clear that gas transfer capacity—that is, the diffusing capacity for carbon monoxide, measured during a single breath-holding effort of 10 seconds—does not decrease until there is considerable air trapping and reduction in vital capacity; thus a decrease in gas transfer capacity is not an early detector of asbestosis impairment.

Cigarette Smoking Interaction. There is a profound interaction in men with asbestosis between cigarette smoking and an increasing profusion of irregular opacities (Table 17–6).[69] Cigarette smoking produces obstructive lesions of the small airways and causes emphysema by departitioning the distal portion of the lung. Because of these well-known effects of cigarette smoke on the lung airways, obstruction in asbestos workers was attributed to cigarette smoke. However, recent studies that have included large numbers of workers who have never smoked show that the physiological pattern of airways obstruction is characteristic of asbestosis alone.[13,58–60]

Not only is there a strong correlation between the profusion of irregular opacities and physiological impairment, but impairment can be measured in workers after 15 years of exposure in the absence of radiographic lesions. Airways obstruction also characterizes the physiological pattern in those workers who show only pleural signs of asbestosis, either circumscribed or diffuse.[70] This confirms the hypothesis, clearly stated a decade ago by Fridriksson et al.[71] and confirmed by a large number of physiological studies, that airways obstruction characterizes asbestotic pleural disease. Subjects with both pleural and parenchymal asbestosis have greater functional impairment than those with either pleural or pulmonary changes alone.

Pleural Effusions and Their Sequelae. The recognition that pleural effusions occur in subjects with asbestosis without other proximate causes was probably delayed until tuberculosis became rare in American workers. During the past two decades, there have been reports[63,64] of pleural effusions that last weeks to months, are without bacterial flora, stigmata of tuberculosis, or malignant cells, and have a benign course. However, such effusions may be antecedent to diffuse pleural thickening with adhesions between the visceral and parietal pleura and obliteration of costophrenic angles. Careful inquiry of workers with obliterated costophrenic angles and pleural thickening has found many with histories of pleural effusion. Follow-up of some reported subjects has been likewise confirmatory.[64] From these observations it is inferred that fibrosis, more dense in the periphery of the lung and attenuating toward the hilum, which is recognized with ex-

TABLE 17-6. PULMONARY PARENCHYMAL ASBESTOSIS OF PROFUSION 1/0 OR MORE (INTERNATIONAL LABOR ORGANIZATION CRITERIA IN 419 MIDWESTERN INSULATORS BY HISTORY OF CIGARETTE SMOKING

Smoking Category	Mean Age (Years)	Number with Asbestosis/ Number in Population	Percent	Risk Ratio
Nonsmokers	40	7/97	7.2	
Exsmokers	44	29/131	22.1	3.1
Current smokers	48.2	37/191	19.4	2.7

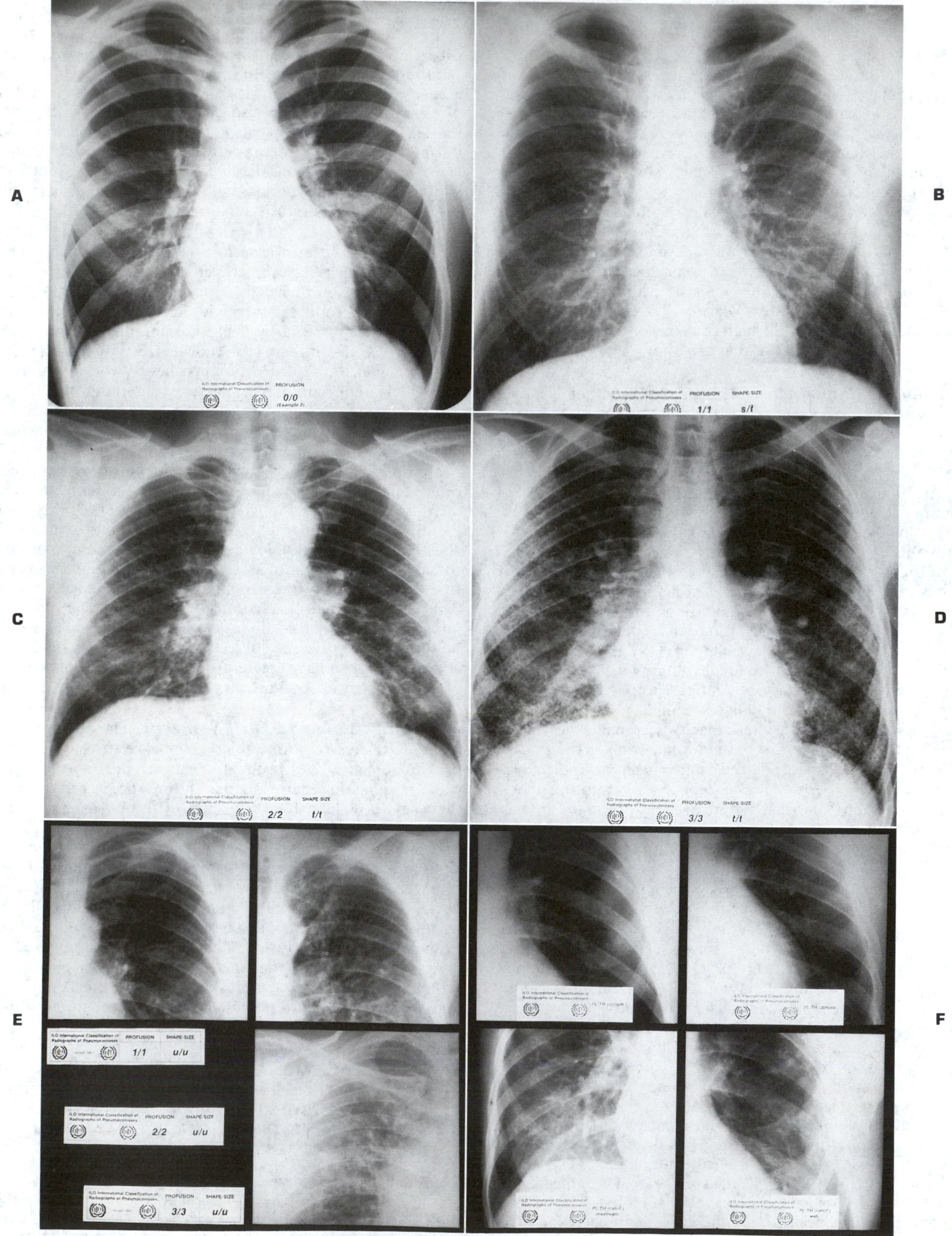

Figure 17–7. For legend see opposite page.

Figure 17–7. The International Labor Organization (ILO) classification for pneumoconiosis has provided criteria for asbestosis on chest x-ray films since 1959, using a scheme that originated in 1916. Classification is based on a standard 14 × 17 = inch posteroanterior radiograph of a technical quality that distinguishes details in the lungs. In 1980, copies of radiographs were supplied for normal, 0/0, and for the three major categories of profusion of opacities for each size: s, t, and u. 1/1-slight opacities, notable in outer lung regions; 2/2 = moderate opacities, partly obscuring pulmonary vessels; and 3/3 = opacities so profuse as to obscure the pulmonary vessels. **A** shows the standard films for opacities 3 to 10 mm in diameter (u/u). **F** shows circumscribed plaque (UL), diffuse pleural plaques (UR), calcified diaphragmatic plaque (LR), and calcified wall (LL).

Technical quality. With modern x-ray equipment, dedicated technicians can produce nearly ideal maximally inflated chest radiographs in all instances except morbid obesity, severe infirmity, or distortion of the chest cage or internal organs. The common correctable error is underinflation, which is recognized when the right side of the diaphragm is above the ninth intercostal space. Such films must be repeated after the subject is instructed in holding a deep breath. Films of high quality can be ensured if a qualified reader repeats suboptimal films before the subject leaves the x-ray unit.

The 12-point scale. The profusion of opacities was classified into one of four major categories by comparison with standard radiographs and a number, 0 to 3, written to the left of the slash. If during this rating the major category above or below was seriously considered as an alternative, this was recorded on the right side of the slash. thus, "2/1" represents a profusion of major category 2 but with category 1 having been seriously considered. Profusion without serious doubt, in the middle of the major category was recorded as 2/2. If the category above was seriously considered, profusion was recorded as 2/3.

ILO CLASSIFICATION OF CHEST RADIOGRAPHS FOR ASBESTOSIS

Small Opacities Irregular		Short (1971) Classification	1980 Extended Classification
Profusion		1, 2, 3	0/0, 0/1, 1/0, 1/1, 1/2, 2/1, 2/2, 2/3, 3/2, 3/3, 3/4
		1 = slight, 2 = moderate, 3 = advanced	
Type		s, t, u	s, t, u
		s = width to about 1.5 mm	
		t = width exceeding 1.5 mm and up to 3 mm	
		u = width exceeding 3 mm and up to 10 mm	
Extent		—	6 zones: right and left—upper, middle, and lower
Large opacities:	>10 mm		
Pleural thickening:			
Chest wall	▪ **Circumscribed** (plaques)		
	Face-on (en face)		Right, left
	Width (a, b, c)		
	Extent (1, 2, 3)		
	▪ **Diffuse**		
	Face on		
	Width (a, b, c)		
	Extent (1, 2, 3)		
	Diaphragm		Right, left
	Costophrenic angle obliteration		Right, left
	a = maximum width up to ≈ 5 mm		
	b = maximum width > ≈ 5 mm and up to ≈ 10 mm		
	c = maximum width > ≈ 10 mm		
	1 = total length up to one fourth (of the projection of the lateral chest wall)		
	2 = total length exceeding one fourth but not half of the projection of the lateral chest wall		
	3 = total length exceeding half of the projection of the lateral chest wall		

Additional symbols: classification of other abnormalities on the x-ray films.

ax	= coalescence of small pneumoconiotic opacities	fr	= fracture rib
bu	= bullae	hi	= enlargement of hilar or mediastinal lymph nodes
ca	= cancer of lung or pleura	ho	= honeycomb lung
cn	= calcification of small pneumoconiotic opacities	id	= ill-defined diaphragm
co	= abnormality of cardiac shape or size	ih	= ill-defined heart outline
cp	= cor pulmonale	kl	= septal (Kerley's) lines
cv	= cavity	od	= other significant abnormalities
di	= marked distortion of intrathoracic organs	pi	= pleural thickening
ef	= effusion	px	= pneumothorax
em	= definite emphysema	rp	= rheumatoid pneumoconiosis
es	= eggshell calcification of hilar or mediastinal lymph nodes	tb	= tuberculosis

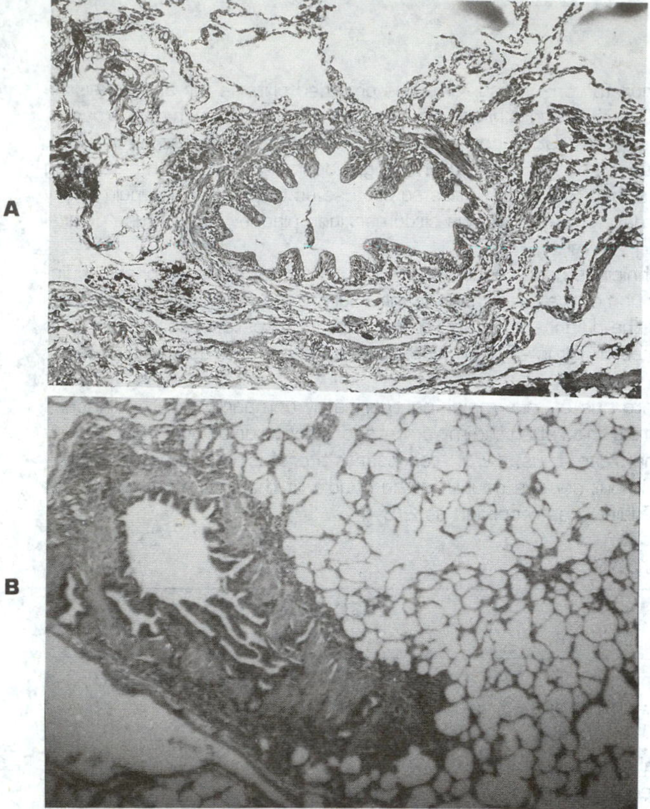

Figure 17-8 **A.** A normal terminal bronchiole (small airway) has thin walls beneath the epithelial layer and is near to alveoli. **B.** An abnormal terminal bronchiole is surrounded by a thick cuff of connective tissue.

tended-scale, computer-augmented tomography[61,62] (Fig. 17-10), may be due to asbestotic pleural effusions. It is clear that these workers have more functional impairment than others with pleural asbestos disease.[70] The logical inference that these workers are the ones with development of thick pleural encasement of the lungs, which on occasion has required surgical removal (decortication) for relief of lung trapping, is not yet confirmed.

Mesothelioma

The pleura and peritoneum are lined with mesothelial cells. These cells are derived from mesoderm and may develop into connective tissue cells or epithelial cells. Asbestos is translocated to mesothelial cells and initiates tumors that grow rapidly, have an excellent blood supply, thus rarely showing necrosis, and kill by interference with vital functions, although they frequently show microscopic metastases as well. By 1931, Klemperer and Rabin[20] had described the modern concept of mesothelioma. Tumors arise in response to asbestos fibers or fibrils that have either penetrated the lung to reach the pleural space or penetrated the bowel wall to reach the peritoneum. Mesotheliomas grow and spread rapidly and widely over the surfaces, displacing or engulfing vital organs rather than invading them (Fig. 17-11). In the peritoneum or pleura the bumpy growths are white or light yellow and vascular without necrosis. Histological sections show either a dense fibroblastic connective tissue, with stroma cells forming tubular structures resembling capillaries, or small vessels or glands, or a combination of these two distinct fibroblastic and epithelial types.[72] It is often difficult to distinguish the tumors from metastatic adenocarcinoma from lung, pancreas, colon, or stomach without ultrastructural and histochemical studies.[73]

Rare tumors such as these, when they occur even in small numbers, serve as sentinel or signal neoplasms strongly suggesting exposure to specific materials. Thus mesotheliomas indicate the presence of asbestos. Nasal sinus carcinomas connote exposure to nickel carbonyl or wood dust from certain tropical hardwood trees. Angiosarcoma of the liver in the United States suggests exposure to vinyl chloride monomer, but similar tumors of the liver occur in Africa after aflatoxin exposure. Historically, the first examples were probably the scrotal cancers in the chimney sweeps, which Percival Pott causally related to coal tar.

Overall, the incidence of mesothelioma varies between 1:1000 and 1:10,000 deaths or fewer, but in insulators who have been heavily exposed throughout their careers, 8% to 10% of deaths are attributable to mesothelioma. Instances of family exposure, that is, contamination of the home by asbestos brought into it by a worker in a shipyard or an asbestos factory, continue to add to the number of deaths, as do subjects who had exposures for only a year or so. The latency period is 35 to 40 years on average, although it may be as brief as 5 years, which means that the asbestos-exposed person is at risk throughout his lifetime. There is no relation to cigarette smoking, nor is there convincing evidence for a dose-response or an enhanced risk from intensive or prolonged exposure to asbestos. Amphiboles may be more potent than is chrysotile. Thus in the shipbuilding trades the incidence of mesothelioma is related to the number of workers at risk in all of the trades, whereas the prevalence of asbestosis is much higher in more heavily exposed workers such as pipe coverers, pipe fitters, and boilermakers.

That asbestos causes mesothelioma is unmistakable; however, experimental implanting of fibers of various types and sizes into the pleural space of rats and guinea pigs has shown that fibrous glass, rock wool, palygorskite, and brucite are all capable of causing mesothelioma.[50] In Turkey, erionite, a fibrous zeolite, has been associated with an extraordinary prevalence of mesotheliomas around Cappadocia.[74,75] Before zeolite can be accepted as a cause, however, it must be noted that fibrous tremolite has also been found in this area and is a contaminant of natural products used for building material. Thus fibrous tremolite, an amphibole, may be responsible for the mesotheliomas. The experiments of Stanton and Wrench,[50] cited previously, demonstrated that other mineral fibers and vitreous fibers produced mesotheliomas and sounded a note of caution against widespread adoption of these substitutes for asbestos. Carbon fibers, because of their size and shape, may share the potential for inducing mesothelioma. Furthermore, if they do so, then they and vitreous fibers may also produce pulmonary fibrosis.

Management of mesothelioma is discouraging to the patient and frustrating to the physician. Survival for 1 year after diagnosis is usual; rarely do patients live 5 years. Used alone, radiotherapy, chemotherapy, and surgery offer no advantage to the natural course. Debulking of the tumor surgically, if possible, and multidrug chemotherapy, with doxorubicin (adriamycin), cyclophosphamide, and *cis*-platinate, increase the after-diagnosis life span about 1 year. Because of invasion of nerves, pain relief is the major concern.

Lung Cancer

The major public health concern and principal cause of death from asbestosis in developed countries is lung cancer. In some groups of asbestos-exposed workers the lung cancer mortality rate is as high as one in five. The cocausality with cigarette smoking is clear, and the relative risk may be 50 to 100 times as high in the asbestos-exposed smoker as in the non-asbestos-exposed subject who has never smoked[19,76] (see Table 17-2). Because 65% to 85% of workers exposed to asbestos have smoked and about

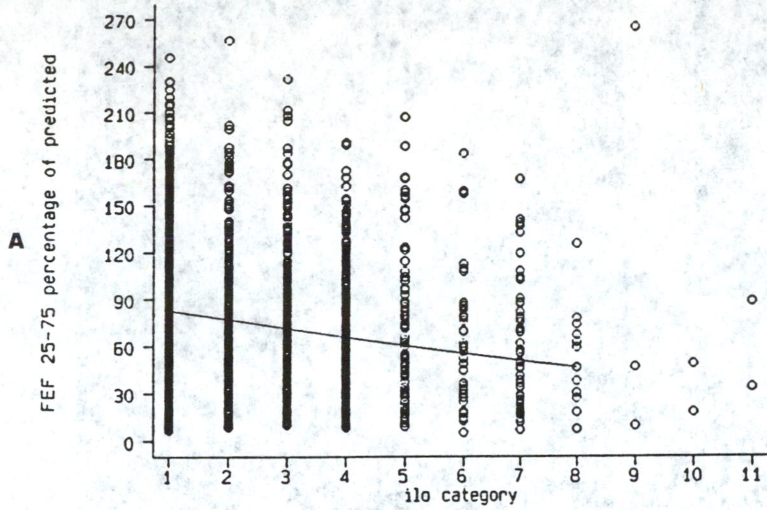

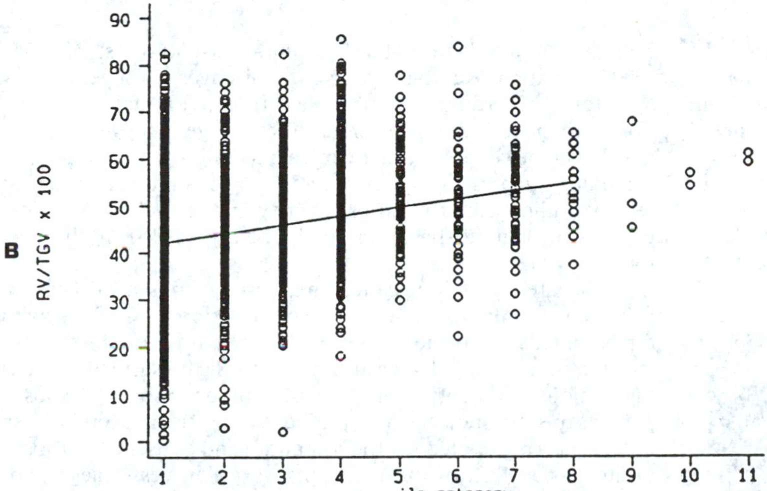

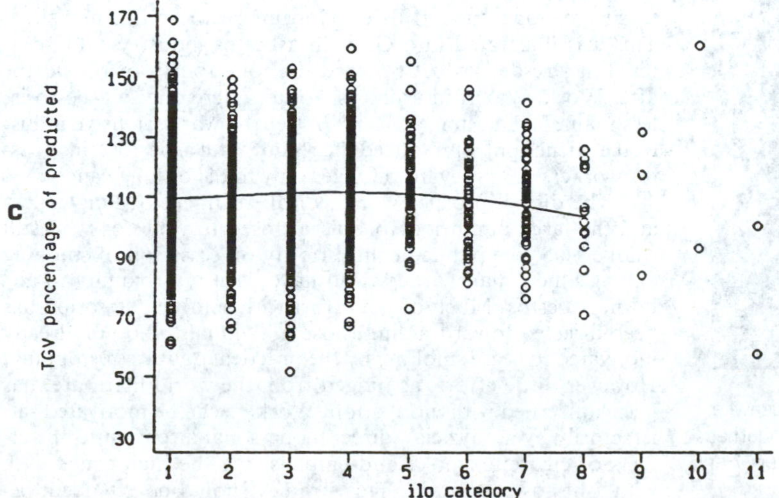

Figure 17-9. A. Forced expiratory flow [FEF_{25-75}] as percentage of the predicted flow at mid-expiratory phase, is plotted against the extent of asbestosis plotted as the profusion of irregular opacities on a chest radiograph by ILO category for 4572 asbestos-exposed workmen [1 = 0/0, 2 = 0/1, 3 = 1/0, 4 = 1/1, 5 = 1/2, 6 = 2/1, 7 = 2/2, 8 = 2/3, 9 = 3/2, 10 = 3/3, 11 = 3/+]. The regression line shows that flows decrease significantly with increasing severity of asbestosis. **B.** Ratio of residual volume to thoracic gas volume [*RV/TGV*], a measure of air trapping, is plotted against the profusion of irregular opacities on chest radiographs for the population of 4572. The regression line shows that air trapping increases significantly with increasing severity of asbestosis. **C.** Thoracic gas volume [*TGV*], as percentage of the predicted value, is plotted against the profusion of irregular opacities in this same population. The regression line shows an elevated volume with a tendency to decrease with greater severity of asbestosis.

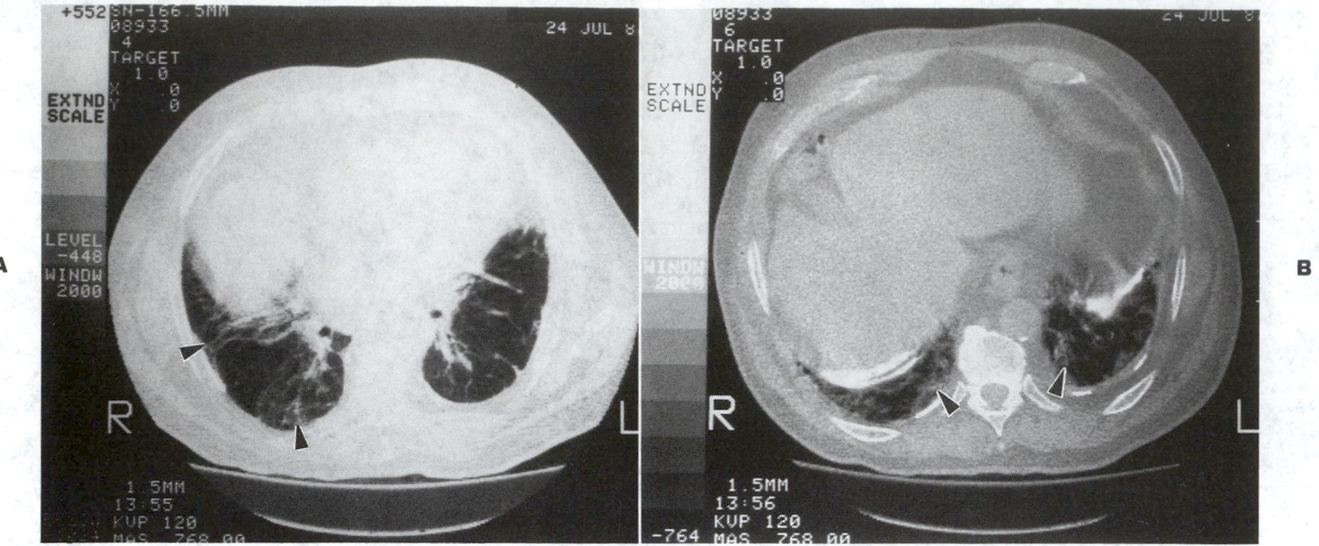

Figure 17-10. A. Extended-scale, computer-augmented scan shows pleura plaques (*white*) and networks of abnormal connective tissue (*arrows*) extended from mid-lung structures to the chest wall and to plaques on the right (*R*) side. **B.** Similar scan has gray-shaded area showing connective tissue.

50%, at this writing, continue to do so,[77] their excessive risk of lung cancer invites smoking cessation intervention. Although the smoking rate for males in the general population is now less than 30% and there is clear evidence that stopping smoking reduces the risk of cancer,[78] more than 60% of workers in surveyed occupational groups in the construction, shipbuilding, and metal trades continue to smoke. Thus there are workers with an extreme risk of cancer for whom there is only one practical approach: motivate them to discontinue smoking. Treatment of lung cancer has advanced but little in the past 30 years. Only 5% to 8% of patients survive 5 years after discovery of the cancer by symptoms or ordinary clinical detection. Although investigations with genetic markers and surface antigens suggest that we may be on the verge of earlier clinical recognition, the logistics of extending the present expensive and time-consuming methods to several million asbestos-exposed active and retired workers suggest that little immediate benefit can be expected from this avenue.

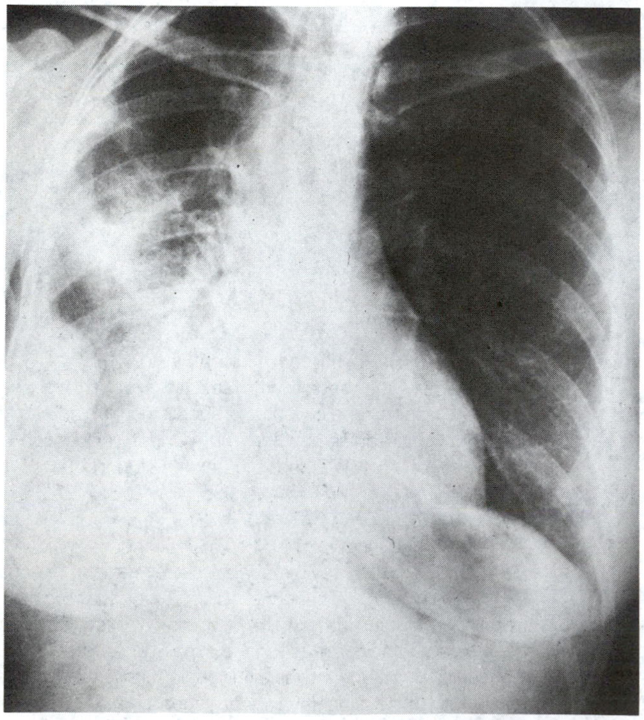

Figure 17-11. Pleural mesothelioma in a 35-year-old housewife. Her father, a shipyard employee, had brought dusty work clothes home from the shipyard to be cleaned. He died of lung cancer. Her mother died of pleural mesothelioma.

The latency for lung cancer in asbestos-exposed workers appears to be similar to that in non-asbestos-exposed workers, with a peak incidence in the early 60s.[19,76,79] Because of the demonstration of a rapidly decreasing risk with the cessation of smoking, serious and continuous efforts to induce asbestos-exposed persons to stop smoking are a public health priority. Similar risk reduction is postulated for the bystander and household-exposed groups, as well as for those persons who share lesser degrees of exposure in buildings containing asbestos. Although proof that the tumors are due to asbestos is at times difficult in the absence of radiographically demonstrated asbestosis, a recent study showed that almost all the lungs removed for cancer from asbestos-exposed individuals show microscopic fibrosis.[80] One lesson from history is clear: when asbestos exposure is sufficiently great that asbestosis is a principal cause of death, then the opportunity to survive long enough to develop lung cancer is diminished. This was illustrated in a German asbestos industry study centered in Dresden, which showed that one fourth of the deaths after World War II in asbestos workers were due to asbestosis; less than 3% had lung cancer.[81] After the war, extensive industrial hygiene controls reduced the risk of fatal asbestosis in asbestos workers, and they lived longer only to die of lung cancer.

The dismal prospect for medical treatment of lung cancer and the large number of people exposed to asbestos who still smoke place the public health priority on cessation of smoking among blue collar workers who have been in proximity to airborne asbestos. Much of the effort with smoking cessation has been directed toward aiding those individuals who are already motivated to cease smoking by the practical politics of stopping. However, little effort, as judged from the world literature, has been concerned with motivation. Workers can be motivated satisfactorily by a physician directing personal attention to the effects of cigarette smoke and emphasizing the high cancer risk with asbestos exposure.[77] This strategy should be extended, because in the United States and most of the developed world, the pattern during the past 20 years has been to reduce asbestos exposure progressively so that we now face a problem of dealing with a population of millions of people who were exposed in the previous era. Clearly their risk of lung cancer can be substantially reduced if they cease smoking and thereby improve public health and decrease medical and social costs.

Other Asbestos-related Neoplasms

Attribution of other neoplasms to asbestos is complex, meaning that large numbers of study subjects and a long time are required because many individuals in the study populations also smoke cigarettes, use alcohol, and are exposed to other occupational carcinogens. However, associations have been made between asbestos exposure and neoplasms of the pancreas and kidney, certain types of lymphoma, and neoplasms of the gastrointestinal tract, including the esophagus, mouth, and colon. The most extensive study, which serves to anchor the experience, is that of the heat and frost insulators, a cohort of 17,800 workers who have been studied by Selikoff et al.[19] since January 1967. In this group the ratio of observed to expected cancers of the esophagus, larynx, kidney, pharynx, and buccal mucosa was greater than 2, whereas the ratio for cancers of the stomach, colon, and rectum was greater than 1.5. Thus it appears that these common epithelial cancers are related to asbestos exposure, although the relationships of several are complex because of causal interaction with cigarette smoke and alcohol.

The mortality rate from asbestos disease is elevated 2.6 times the expected rate, and that due to lung cancer is 9.1 times the expected rate.[76] Of British workers certified by medical panels as having asbestosis on the basis of sufficient exposure and the presence of two of four conditions (radiological [pulmonary] abnormality, pulmonary functional impairment, basal rales, and finger clubbing), 39% died of lung cancer, 9% of mesothelioma, and 20% of asbestosis. Selikoff et al.,[19] studying all deaths in U.S. and Canadian insulators, found in the first 10 years an excess of deaths nearly 1.4 times the expected number, with deaths from cancer 3.11 times the expected number. Lung cancer accounted for 21.4% of deaths, mesothelioma 7.7%, and asbestosis 7.3%.

Societal Impact

Beginning slowly in the 1970s, workmen's compensation and tort litigation were both undertaken for workers with mesothelioma, lung cancer, and asbestosis who were either threatened by death or showed impairment of function. In part because of 50 different laws in the 50 states, there are no accurate figures on the numbers of plaintiffs who have successfully threaded their way through the legal maze of workers' compensation. This system was a social construct to avoid litigation and provide compensation without adversarial confrontation. It was focused on workplace injuries. The price for the plaintiff was to forgo other legal redress for injury or illness. In practice, obtaining workers' compensation may be more difficult than pursuing third-party litigation. Thus society, employing public assistance, disability compensation, Social Security payments, Medicare, and Medicaid, has borne those costs after the workers' resources have been exhausted.

In the mid-1970s, civil actions (torts) began to be filed against major asbestos suppliers and manufacturers on behalf of patients with asbestos disease. More than a decade of such litigation has made the use of asbestos expensive because insurance is difficult or impossible to buy. Juries awarded large sums to a small fraction of plaintiffs with asbestos disease, particularly those with fatal neoplasms. Smaller awards or settlements were made for pulmonary impairment along with asbestosis in the lungs. The associated (nonpulmonary) neoplasms and pleural asbestosis have fared less well, with smaller jury awards and less frequent settlements. The coresponsibility of cigarette smoking has not been accepted by the tobacco companies, nor has litigation succeeded against them for their contribution to the lung cancer death toll. In 1978 the U.S. Congress asked for an appraisal of workers' compensation programs for occupationally related lung disease, which included asbestosis, byssinosis, and black lung, as the prelude to an omnibus bill. However, no omnibus bill has been passed. Although on paper the situation remains perhaps worse than it was in 1978, society has responded through the courts. The bankruptcy proceedings of Johns Manville and several of the other asbestos firms affirm their loss of insurability and their large costs in fighting and settling asbestos cases. Meanwhile, installation and use of new asbestos have virtually ceased. More members of the exposed workforce know the hazards and hygiene of asbestos removal. Exposure has certainly decreased in developed countries. Currently the burden of asbestosis is on the individual who tries to obtain Social Security, county welfare, public assistance, disability compensation, or Medicare payments. The likelihood of obtaining such help apparently depends on luck.

Regulations to control exposure in the workplace were enacted in 1977; a temporary standard allowed workers to be employed in environments that contained up to 2 fibers per milliliter of air, or 2 million fibers per cubic meter.[82,83] The National Institute for Occupational Safety and Health has recommended to the Occupational Safety and Health Administration (OSHA), a 0.1 fiber per milliliter industrial exposure in the United States. Currently the level is at 0.2 fiber per milliliter. In view of the temporizing slowness of this approach, it is reassuring that the use of asbestos in the United States has steadily fallen since 1978, that it is or will be proscribed in most consumer products, that in California a home cannot be sold without an asbestos inspection and amelioration of the problem, and that there is a general sense of asbestos avoidance. New asbestos products are not being installed because of EPA rulings regarding most new construction. The EPA expanded its asbestos ban to most uses in July 1989[84] but provided for three phase-out stages over a period of 7 years, and brake blocks, pipe, and shingles are not affected until 1996. Only 10% of products were phased out in 1990; not until 1996 will 60% of products be affected—surely an example of "deliberate speed." Resolution of the problem will be slow because workers are still removing asbestos that was in place before the new regulations. Although in many jurisdictions removal is done with reasonable protection, including disposable suits and air-supply respirators, by specially trained workers, there are still some fly-by-night removal companies using laborers who do not even know the dangers of asbestos, let alone having had any instructions in its safe handling. Such avoidance of responsibility also characterized earlier eras in this industrial society. Such unconscionable disregard of human suffering underscores the need for tighter controls and genuine accountability. Criminal penalties may be needed. On the optimistic side, friction products such as brakes and clutch facings can be made free of asbestos materials, and although they cost more than the products replaced, early experience suggests that they need to be replaced less often. Asbestos use in the United States fell from 240,000 metric tons in 1984 to 85,000 metric tons in 1987.[84,85]

NATURAL NONASBESTOS AND MAN-MADE MINERAL FIBERS

Natural Nonasbestos Fibers

Nonasbestos fibers constitute a large collection of minerals; more than 150 minerals listed by the Mine Safety and Health Administration occur in fibrous form or may contain fibers. A fiber is an elongated polycrystalline unit whose form resembles cotton or animal hair. Some mineralogists define fibers as particles with an aspect ratio (length to diameter) equal to or greater than 10 to 1. "Asbestiform" denotes a type of silicate fiber that has a high tensile strength, extreme aspect ratio (i.e., high length/diameter ratio), flexibility, heat resistance, and aggregation of fibrils into bundles. Chrysotile is a good example. The Occupational Safety and Health Administration has defined asbestos fiber as being greater than 5 μm in length with an aspect ratio of 3 to 1 or greater.

The pulmonary toxicity of fibers is related to the dose delivered and to the dimensions and durability of the fiber. Fibers with long residence time because of high durability are more toxic than those with shorter residence times. Pleural or peritoneal injection of fibers such as amosite and crocidolite, chrysotile, anthophyllite, tremolite, attapulgite, erionite (zeolite), borosilicate glass, aluminum silicate glass, mineral wool, aluminum oxide, potassium titanate, silicon carbide, sodium aluminum carbonate, and wollastonite produces mesotheliomas.[1] It is clear that both in solution and in animal tissues, including lung tissue, the amphiboles have greater durability than does chrysotile.

There is considerable question concerning the toxicity of talc, a sheetlike silicate, because in the deposits usually found in North America it is contaminated by significant amounts of tremolite, anthophyllite, and quartz.[2] It appears that exposure to pure cosmetic talc, that is, talc with minimal fiber content, produces little or no toxic reactions. Thus it appears that the toxicity of talc is due to its fiber contamination, or perhaps to its silica content, if elevated.

Vermiculite, a family of hydrated magnesium-aluminum-iron silicates, is sheetlike. The mineral is expanded by heat after removal from the mines and used for insulation and for fillers in paint, plasters, rubber, and other materials. Once again, the health hazard from vermiculite seem to be related to its contamination with fibrous tremolite.[3]

Zeolites, a group of crystalline and hydrated aluminum silicate minerals, consist of extremely fine tubes of mordenite or erionite. The tubes are 10 to 20 μm in length and less than 1 to 3 μm in diameter. Naturally occurring deposits of zeolites are distributed worldwide, but adverse health effects have largely been investigated in the vicinity of Karain, Turkey, in the central Anatolia.[4,5] Although mesotheliomas, pleural thickening, and plaques were attributed to exposure to erionite, it appears that there is contamination of chrysotile and tremolite.[4] The implication of the Turkish experience is either that the samples of airborne fibers in Karain, with an average of less than 0.01 fiber per cubic meter and a peak level of 1.38 fibers per cubic meter, are significantly below the current standard for asbestos fibers and thus reflect an unrecognized hazard from low-level airborne fiber exposure or, alternatively, that low-level exposure to tremolite, in contrast to erionite, may be responsible for the adverse health effects.[2] Wollastonite is also found in sites scattered around the world. A study in Finland showed that workers from a limestone-wollastonite quarry had a high frequency of pleural thickening and pulmonary fibrosis. Fibrosis was observed in only 3% of a worker cohort in the United States, but reductions in expiratory airflow were related to dust levels.[6] Further studies of effects of erionite and wollastonite on human populations are essential before conclusions can be drawn, but these materials should be handled with caution.

Man-made Fibers

The physical characteristics of fibers made by humans, with slag, rock, glass, or ceramics used as starting material, vary greatly with the conditions of manufacture.[7] The same applies to the most recent species of fiber, carbon fiber. Carbon fibers are used in making sailboat masts and aircraft components (as in the Stealth bomber). The same considerations of dose, dimensions, and durability that apply to natural fibers also apply to the man-made filaments.[8] These products have a wide range of diameters. It is clear that little human respiratory hazard should be predicted for fibers with diameters greater than 10 μm because there is no way for these fibers to be split into fragments that are respirable. However, inspection of numerous samples of fibrous glass shows that the current commercial materials are highly heterogeneous, with some fibers having diameters of 1 μm. Both rotary spinning and flame attenuation produce fibers less than 1 μm (Fig. 17-12A and B). It is clear that, beginning with the work of Stanton and Wrench,[1] these fibers cause mesotheliomas and pleural scars in the animal pleura and peritoneum. Currently the National Institute for Occupational Safety and Health[9] recommends that fibrous glass exposure be limited to 3 fibers per cubic meter and that these fibers be less than 3.5 μm in diameter and equal to or greater than 10 μm in length. Rotary spinning, the process analogous to that for making cotton candy, requires less energy and is replacing flame attenuation for producing fine fibers. Because the thermal coefficient, a measure of insulating capacity, is increased as fiber diameters are reduced (Fig. 17-12C) where high thermal coefficients are needed with low weight, such as in aerospace applications, fine fiberglass is used preferentially. Fine fiberglass is also used in refrigerator doors and in insulation used in industrial construction and home building because it is mixed heterogeneously with larger fibers. This usage exposes production and construction workers to some respirable airborne fibers.

Effects of Nonrespirable Fibers

The effects of the nonrespirable fibers are largely due to mechanical irritation of the skin, such as itching, burning, and irritation of the conjunctivae and the nasal and pharyngeal passages.[10] Such irritation clears on removal from exposure and can be treated similarly to that from exposure to natural irritants such as peach fuzz or stinging nettle. Striking dermatographism may be seen in sensitive individuals and may preclude further exposure.

Effects of Respirable Fibers

There is much still to learn about the handling by animal cells of fine fibers, particularly the differential effects on cells when fibers are of different lengths. It is clear that longer fibers resist phagocytosis and give rise to ferruginous bodies after variable periods of residence. Moreover, shorter fibers are phagocytized and, after this process, release peptides that stimulate recruitment of cells for production of collagen and other fibers.[11] Animal experiments have consistently shown that intrapleural injection of fibers produces mesothelioma.[1] Inhalation, even for a long period in rodents[12-14] and in monkeys,[13] produces macrophage accumulations and granulomas containing fibrous glass but little fibrosis. In rats, plaques developed on the visceral pleura.[13]

Insulators using materials with a high thermocoefficient and low weight in fuselages of aircraft or space vehicles should be studied to learn whether these fine fibers cause adverse health effects. The practical problem is that many of these workers were previously exposed to asbestos used in these applications or in similar work. Furthermore, the manufacturing sites for fiberglass tend to be, or to have been in the recent past, rich in asbestos for heat conservation. Finally, the duration of human exposure in many of these facilities has been less than the 20 or 25 years, which is the "latent period" usually needed to produce effects of asbestos exposure. Therefore, although it is logical that the hazard from fine fiberglass is analogous to that from asbestos, this has not yet been demonstrated by human data.

Effects of fine fibers on human health have been predicted, by analogy to asbestos, and studied in sites of fiberglass production and use.[7] Unfortunately, the effective dose has seldom been measured in terms of respirable fibers; thus the studies that fail

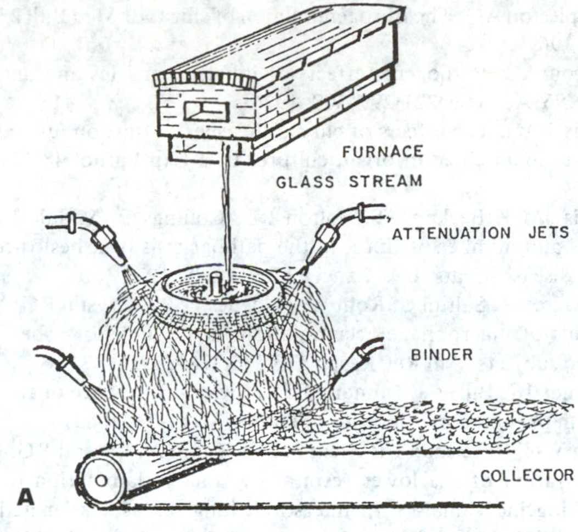

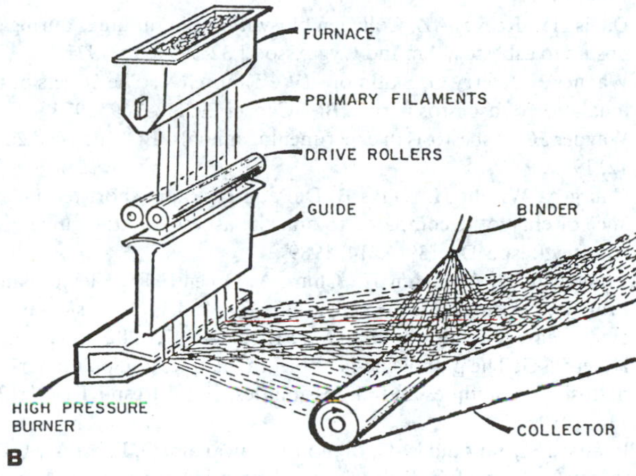

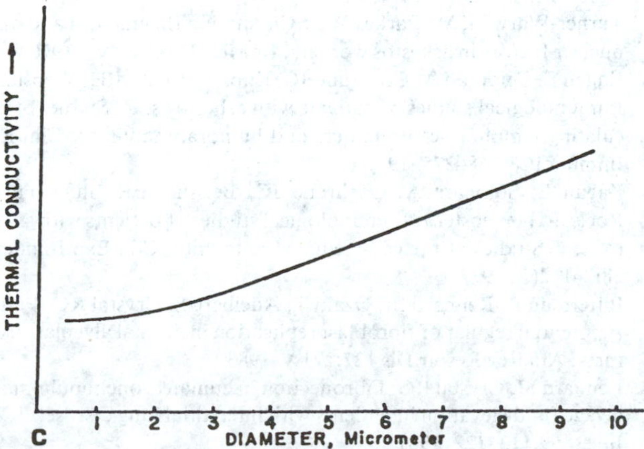

Figure 17-12. A. Rotary process of producing fine fiberglass utilizes both centrifugal force and air jets to attenuate the glass. Heterogeneous fiber diameters result. **B.** Flame attenuation provides heat and drive force to pull the fibers into smaller diameters. **C.** Insulating capacity, the reciprocal of thermal conductivity, is increased as fiber diameter is reduced.

to show health effects may be studies of materials that are largely nonrespirable.[15] As after asbestos exposure, symptoms may occur after a long latency period. Symptoms include the chronic effects of fibrotic disease, namely, shortness of breath, but there are no alerting, or acute, symptoms after exposure to submicronic particles.[16] Thus airway and eye irritation are associated with coarse but not fine fibers. Studies have shown chronic bronchitis and bronchiectasis with bloody sputum in workers in fibrous glass production.[16] Unfortunately, these studies were not carefully controlled for other exposures, particularly for cigarette smoking. Radiographic studies of workers at seven fibrous glass and mineral wool facilities have demonstrated that 10% had small radiographic opacities with a profusion of 0/1 to 1/1.[17] Physiological impairment has not been measured.[15,16]

Mortality rates for fibrous glass workers have been studied without regard to the respirability (size) of the fibers; generally there have been no excess deaths from malignant or nonmalignant respiratory disease.[18] One study that showed an increased mortality rate found that it was due to bronchiectasis and silicosis,[16] without a clearly demonstrable or plausible link to fibrous glass. Two large studies currently under analysis include a 17-plant study in the United States under the auspices of the Thermal Insulation Manufacturers Association and a 72-plant European study by the European Insulation Manufacturers Association. Both show that mortality rates differ from those of the control populations. Preliminary analyses of results have raised serious questions about the suitability of national vs regional vs area controls for tracking cancer mortality rates. The mortality rate question remains unsettled[19] because these problems are general, beyond merely understanding the effects of fiberglass. However, in societies whose members are highly contaminated by chemicals, suitable comparison groups are difficult to locate. Human mesotheliomas resulting from exposure to fiberglass have not been identified.

Public Health Considerations

Research. Because of the analogous dimensions, durability, and respirability of fine fibrous glass and other man-made fibers, there is a need for studies of health effects in a population that has been exposed for a suitable latent period, at least more than 20 years, and that has had *no exposure* to asbestos. Studies of such populations have not yet appeared but are needed so that the best alternatives to asbestos in many applications can be chosen. Meanwhile, the association of mesothelioma with silica filaments in sugar cane factory workers in India[20] raises the specter of an unusual "natural fiber" of plant origin mimicking asbestos exposure. A better history of exposure, examination of lung tissue, and analysis of its fiber content with scanning electron microscopy and energy-dispersive analysis will help answer such problems of competing etiology.

Control Measures. It seems ironic that we are witnessing widespread adoption of fibrous glass and, despite the lessons of 75 years, facing this adoption without the key information needed to determine the human health risks.[8,9] Clearly, determination of the health hazards of fine man-made fibers is a high priority before widespread use in the production and applications industries produces a problem for the next century that mimics the one we have experienced with asbestos. Meanwhile, it is prudent to regard materials that contain fibers of respirable dimension as needing the same precautions as does asbestos.[21]

REFERENCES

Asbestos

1. International Labour Office: U/C International Classification of Radiographs of Pneumoconiosis in Occupational Safety and Health Series. Geneva: International Labour Office, 1980

2. Murray HM: Report of the Departmental Committee on Compensation for Industrial Disease. London: HM Stationery Office, 1907
3. Cooke WE: Fibrosis of the lungs due to the inhalation of asbestos dust. Br Med J 2:147, 1924
4. Cooke WE: Pulmonary asbestosis. Br Med J 2:1024–1026, 1927
5. Merewether ERA, Price CV: Report on effects of asbestos dust on the lungs and dust suppression in the asbestos industry. London: HM Stationery Office, 1930
6. Pancoast HK, Miller TG, Landish HRM: A roentgenologic study of the effects of dust inhalation upon the lungs. Am J Roentgenol (N.S.) 5:129–138, 1918
7. Gloyne SR: The morbid anatomy and histology of asbestosis. Tubercule (London) 14:445–451, 493–497, 550–559, 1933
8. Lanza AJ, McConnell WJ, Fehnel JW: Effects of the inhalation of asbestos dust on the lungs of asbestos workers. Public Health Rep 50:1–48, 1935
9. Dreessen WC, Dallavalle JM, Edwards TI, et al: A study of asbestosis in the asbestos textile industry. Public Health Bull 241:1–147, 1938
10. Donnelly J: Pulmonary asbestosis: Incidence and prognosis. J Ind Hyg 18:222–228, 1936
11. Shull JR: Asbestosis: A roentgenologic review of 71 cases. Radiology 27:279–292, 1936
12. McPheeters SB: A survey of a group of employees exposed to asbestos dust. J Ind Hyg 18:229–239, 1936
13. Becklake MR, Fournier-Massey G, McDonald JC, Siemiatycki J, Rossiter CA: Lung function in relation to chest radiographic changes in Quebec asbestos workers. I. Methods, results and conclusions. Bull Physio Pathol Resp 6:637–659, 1970
14. Merewether ERA: Annual Report of the Chief Inspector of Factories. London: HM Stationery Office, 1947
15. Hueper WC: Occupational tumors and allied diseases. Springfield, Ill.: Charles C Thomas, Publisher, 1942
16. Doll R: Mortality from lung cancer in asbestos workers. Br J Ind Med 12:81–86, 1955
17. Mancuso TF, Coulter EJ: Methodology in industrial health studies: The cohort approach, with special reference to an asbestos company. Arch Environ Health 6:210–222, 1963
18. Selikoff IJ: Asbestos disease in the United States, 1918–1975. Rev Fr Mal Resp 4:7–24, 1976
19. Selikoff IJ, Hammond EC, Seidman H: Mortality experiences of insulation workers in the United States and Canada, 1943–1976. Ann NY Acad Sci 3301:91–116, 1979
20. Klemperer P, Rabin CB: Primary neoplasms of the pleura: A report of five cases. Arch Pathol 11:385–412, 1931
21. Wagner JC, Sleggs CA, Marchand P: Diffuse pleural mesothelioma and asbestos exposure in the North Western Cape Province. Br J Ind Med 17:260–271, 1960
22. Guidance for Controlling Asbestos-containing Materials in Buildings. Washington, D.C.: U.S. Environmental Protection Agency, June 1985 (EPA 560/5-85-024)
23. Spurny KR: On the release of asbestos fibers from weathered and corroded asbestos cement products. Environ Res 48:100–116, 1989
24. Appel JD, Fasy TM, Kohtz DS, Kohtz JD, Johnson EM: Asbestos fibers mediate transformation of monkey cells by exogenous plasmid DNA. Proc Natl Acad Sci (USA) 85:7670–7674, 1988
25. Mossman BT, Craighead JE, MacPherson BV: Asbestos-induced epithelial changes in organ cultures of hamster trachea: Inhibition by retinyl methyl ether. Science 207:311–313, 1980
26. Rajan KT, Wagner JC, Evans PH: The response of human pleura in organ culture to asbestos. Nature 238:346–347, 1972
27. Wade MJ, Lipsin LE, Tucker RW, Frank AL: Asbestos cytotoxicity in a long-term macrophage-like cell culture. Nature 264:444–446, 1976
28. Neugut AI, Eisenberg D, Silverstein M, Pulkribek P, Weinstein IB: Effects of asbestos epithelial cell lines. Environ Res 17:256–265, 1978
29. Heppleston AG: Silica and asbestos: Contrasts in tissue response. Ann NY Acad Sci 330:725–744, 1979
30. Heppleston AG: The fibrogenic action of silica. Br Med Bull 25:282–287, 1969
31. Allison AC: Pathogenic effects of inhaled particles and antigens. Ann NY Acad Sci 221:299–308, 1974
32. Davis JMG: The effects of chrysotile asbestos dust on lung macrophages maintained in organ culture. Br J Exp Pathol 48:379–385, 1967
33. Davis JMG, Beckett ST, Bolton RE, Collings P, Middleton AP: Mass and number of fibres in the pathogenesis of asbestos-related lung disease in rats. Br J Cancer 37:673–688, 1978
34. Spurzem JR, Saltini C, Rom W, Winchester RJ, Crystal RG: Mechanisms of macrophage accumulation in the lungs of asbestos-exposed subjects. Am Rev Respir Dis 136:276–280, 1987
35. Wagner JC, Burns J, Munday DE, McGee J: Presence of fibronection in pneumoconiotic lesions. Thorax 37:54–56, 1982
36. Rom WN, Bitterman PB, Rennard SI, Catin A, Crystal RG: Characterization of the lower respiratory tract inflammation of nonsmoking individuals with interstitial lung disease associated with chronic inhalation of inorganic dusts. Am Rev Respir Dis 136:1429–1434, 1987
37. Davis HV, Reeves AL: Collagen biosynthesis in rat lungs during exposure to asbestos. Am Ind Hyg Assoc J 32:599–602, 1971
38. Wagner JC, Berry G, Skidmore JW, Timbrell V: The effects of the inhalation of asbestos in rats. Br J Cancer 29:252–269, 1974
39. Wagner JC: Asbestosis in experimental animals. Br J Ind Med 20:1–12, 1963
40. Churg A, Wright JL, Gilks B, DePaoli L: Rapid short-term clearance of chrysotile compared to amosite asbestos in the guinea pig. Am Rev Respir Dis 139:A214, 1989
41. Craighead JE, Abraham JL, Churg A, Green FHY, Kleinerman J, Pratt PC, Seemayer TA, Vallyathan V, Weill H: Asbestos-associated disease. Arch Pathol Lab Med 106:544–597, 1982
42. Hillerdal G: The pathogenesis of pleural plaques and pulmonary asbestosis: Possibilities and impossibilities. Eur J Respir Dis 61:129–138, 1980
43. Rennard SI, Jaurand M-C, Bignon J, Kawanami O, Ferrans VJ, Davidson J, Crystal RG: Role of pleural mesothelial cells in the production of the submesothelial connective tissue matrix of lung. Am Rev Respir Dis 130:267–274, 1984
44. Turner-Warwick M, Parkes WR: Circulating rheumatoid and antinuclear factors in asbestos workers. Br Med J 3:492–495, 1970
45. Kagan E, Solomon A, Cochrane JC, Kuba P, Rocks PH, Webster I: Immunological studies of patients with asbestosis. II. Studies of circulating lymphoid cell numbers and humoral immunity. Clin Exp Immunol 28:268–275, 1977
46. Kagan E, Solomon A, Cochrane JC, Beissner EI, Gluckman J, Rocks PH, Webster I: Immunological studies of patients with asbestosis. I. Studies of the cell-mediated immunity. Clin Exp Immunol 28:261–267, 1977
47. Bitterman P, Rennard SI, Ozaki T, Adelberg S, Crystal RG: PGE_2: A potential regular of fibroblast replication in normal alveolar structures. Am Rev Respir Dis 127:271A, 1983
48. Rennard SI, Crystal RG: Fibronection in human bronchopulmonary lavage fluid elevation in patients with interstitial lung disease. J Clin Invest 69:113–122, 1981
49. Rennard SI, Bitterman PB, Crystal RG: Pathogenesis of granulomatous lung disease. IV. Mechanisms of fibrosis. Am Rev Respir Dis 30:492–496, 1984
50. Stanton MF, Wrench C: Mechanisms of mesothelioma induction with asbestos and fibrous glass. JNCI 48:797, 1972
51. Kilburn KH, Warshaw RH, Thornton JC: Asbestosis, pulmonary symptoms and functional impairment in shipyard workers. Chest 88:254–259, 1985
52. Anderson HA, Lilis R, Daum SM, Selikoff IJ: Asbestosis among household contacts of asbestos factory workers. Ann NY Acad Sci 330:387–399, 1979
53. Kilburn KH, Lilis R, Anderson HA, Boylen CT, Einstein HE, Johnson SJS, Warshaw RH: Asbestos disease in family contacts of shipyard workers. Am J Public Health 75:615–617, 1985

54. Nicholson WJ, Swoszowski EJ jr, Rohl AN, Todaro JD, Adams A: Asbestos contamination in United States schools from use of asbestos in surfacing materials. Ann NY Acad Sci 330:587–596, 1979
55. Sawyer RN, Swoszowski EJ Jr: Asbestos abatement in schools: Observations and experiences. Ann NY Acad Sci 330:765–775, 1979
56. Balmes JR, Warshaw R, Chong S, Kilburn KH: Effects of occupational exposure to asbestos containing materials in public schools. Am Rev Respir Dis 129:A174, 1984
57. Oliver LC, Sprunce NL, Green RE: Asbestos-related disease in public school custodians. Am Rev Respir Dis 139:A211, 1989
58. Kilburn KH, Warshaw RH, Einstein K, Bernstein J: Airway disease in non-smoking asbestos workers. Arch Environ Health 40:293–295, 1985
59. Kilburn KH, Warshaw RH: Correlation of pulmonary functional impairment with radiographic asbestosis (ILO category). Am Rev Respir Dis 139:A210, 1989
60. Kilburn KH, Warshaw RH: Evidence for airways obstruction with increasing profusion of irregular opacities in asbestos exposed workers. Chest, 1991 (In press)
61. Wollmer P, Jakobsson K, Albin M, Albrechtsson U, Brauer K, Eriksson L, Johnson B, Skerfving S, Tylen U: Measurement of lung density by x-ray computed tomography. Chest 91:865–869, 1987
62. Aberle DR, Gamsu G, Ray CS: High-resolution CT of benign asbestos-related disease: Clinical and radiographic correlation. Am J Radiol 151:883–891, 1988
63. Gaensler EA, Kaplan AI: Asbestos pleural effusion. Ann Intern Med 74:178–191, 1971
64. Epler GR, McLoud TC, Gaensler EA: Prevalence and incidence of benign asbestos pleural effusion in a working population. JAMA 247:617–622, 1982
65. Morris JF, Koski A, Johnson LC: Spirometric standards for healthy nonsmoking adults. Am Rev Respir Dis 103:57–67, 1971
66. Morris JF, Koski A, Breese JD: Normal values and evaluation of forced end-expiratory flow. Am Rev Respir Dis 111:755–762, 1975
67. Miller A: Pulmonary function tests in clinical and occupational lung disease. Orlando, Fla.: Grune & Stratton, 1986, pp 258–443
68. Harris TR, Pratt PC, Kilburn KH: Total lung capacity measured by roentgenograms. Am J Med 50:756–763, 1971
69. Kilburn KH, Lilis R, Anderson HA, Miller A, Warshaw RH: Interaction of asbestos, age and cigarette smoking in producing radiographic evidence of diffuse pulmonary fibrosis. Am J Med 80:377–381, 1986
70. Kilburn KH, Warshaw RH: Pulmonary functional consequences of pleural asbestos disease circumscribed and diffuse. Chest 98:965–972, 1990
71. Fridriksson HV, Hedenstrom H, Hillerdal G, Malmberg P: Increased lung stiffness in persons with pleural plaques. Eur J Respir Dis 62:412–424, 1981
72. Suzuki Y: Pathology of human malignant mesotheliomas. Semin Oncol 8:268–282, 1980
73. Suzuki Y, Churg J, Kannerstein M: Ultrastructure of human malignant mesothelioma. Am J Pathol 85:241–262, 1976
74. Baris YI, Sakin AA, Ozesmi M, Kerse I, Ozen E, Kolocan B, Altinors M, Ghoktepeli A: An outbreak of pleural mesothelioma and chronic fibrosing pleurisy in the village of Karain Urgup in Anatolia. Thorax 33:181–192, 1978
75. Lilis R: Fibrous zeolites and endemic mesothelioma in Cappadocia, Turkey. J Occup Med 23:548–558, 1981
76. Berry G: Mortality of workers certified by pneumoconiosis medical panels as having asbestosis. Br J Ind Med 38:130–137, 1981
77. Kilburn KH, Warshaw RH: Effects of individually motivated smoking cessation on male blue collar workers. Am J Public Health 80:1334–1337, 1990
78. Hammond EC, Selikoff IJ, Seidman H: Asbestos exposure, cigarette smoking and death rates. Ann NY Acad Sci 330:473–490, 1979
79. Selikoff IJ, Seidman H, Hammond EC: Mortality effects of cigarette smoking among amosite asbestos factory workers. J Natl Cancer Inst 65:507–513, 1980
80. Kipen HM, Lilis R, Suzuki Y, Valciukas JA, Selikoff IS: Pulmonary fibrosis in asbestos insulation workers with lung cancer: A radiological and histopathological evaluation. Br J Ind Med 44:96–100, 1987
81. Jacob G, Anspach M: Pulmonary neoplasia among Dresden asbestos workers. Ann NY Acad Sci 132:536–548, 1965
82. Peto J: Dose-response relationships for asbestos-related disease: Implications for hygiene standards. II. Mortality. Ann NY Acad Sci 330:195–203, 1979
83. Berry G, Lewinsohn HC: Dose-response relationships for asbestos-related disease: Implications for hygiene standards. I. Morbidity. Ann NY Acad Sci 330:184–194, 1979
84. EPA announces final regulation to ban new asbestos products. Washington, D.C.: U.S. Environmental Protection Agency, Office of Public Affairs (A107), 1989
85. EPA orders more bans on asbestos. Salt Lake Tribune, July 7, 1989

Nonasbestos Fibers Including Man-made Mineral Fibers

1. Stanton MF, Wrench C: Mechanisms of mesothelioma induction with asbestos and fibrous glass. JNCI 48:797–821, 1972
2. Lockey JE, Moatamed F: Health implications of non-asbestos fibers. In Gee B (ed): Occupational Lung Diseases. New York: Churchill Livingstone, 1984, pp 75–98
3. Hassell PA, Sluis-Cremer GK: X-ray findings, lung function and respiratory symptoms in black South African vermiculate workers. Am J Ind Med 15:21–29, 1989
4. Baris YI, Sahin AA, Ozesmi M, Kerse I, Ozen E, Kolacan B, Altimors M, Goktepeli A: An outbreak of pleural mesothelioma and chronic fibrosing pleurisy in the village of Karain Urgup in Anatolia. Thorax 33:181–192, 1978
5. Lilis R: Fibrous zeolites and endemic mesothelioma in Cappadocia, Turkey. J Occup Med 23:548–553, 1981
6. Hanke W, Sepulveda M-J, Watson A, Jankovic J: Respiratory morbidity in wollastonite workers. Br J Ind Med 41:474–479, 1984
7. Kilburn KH: Flame-attenuated fiberglass: Another asbestos? Am J Ind Med 3:121–125, 1982
8. Stanton MF: Fiber carcinogenesis: Is asbestos the only hazard? J Natl Cancer Inst 52:633–634, 1974
9. National Institute for Occupational Safety and Health: Criteria for a Recommended Standard Occupational Exposure to Fibrous Glass. U.S. Public Health Service, Department of Health, Education, and Welfare publication No. DHEW (NIOSH) 77–152, 1977
10. Bjornberg A: Glass fiber dermatitis. Am J Ind Med 8:395–400, 1985
11. Maroudas NG, O'Neill CH, Stanton MF: Fibroblast anchorage in carcinogenesis by fibres. Lancet 1:807–809, 1973
12. Gross P, Kaschak M, Tolker EB, Babyak MA, de Treville RTP: The pulmonary reaction to high concentrations of fibrous glass dust. Arch Environ Health 20:696–704, 1970
13. Mitchell RI, Donofrio DJ, Moorman WJ: Chronic inhalation toxicity of fibrous glass in rats and monkeys. J Am Coll Toxicol 5:545–574, 1986
14. Smith DM, Ortiz LW, Archuleta RF, Johnson NF: Long-term health effects in hamsters and rats exposed chronically to man-made vitreous fibres. Ann Occup Hyg 31:731–754, 1987
15. Enterline PE, Marsh GM, Esmen NA: Respiratory disease among workers exposed to man-made fibers. Am Rev Respir Dis 128:1–7, 1983
16. Bayliss DL, Dement JM, Wagoner JK, Blejer HP: Mortality patterns among fibrous glass production workers. Ann NY Acad Sci 271:324–335, 1976
17. Nasr AN, Ditchek T, Scholtens PA: The Prevalence of Radiographic Abnormalities in the Chests of Fiber Glass Workers: Occupational Exposure to Fibrous Glass. U.S. Department of Health, Education, and Welfare Publication No. USPHS NIOSH 76–151, 1976
18. Enterline PE, Marsh GM, Henderson V, Callahan C: Mortality up-

date of a cohort of U.S. man-made mineral fiber workers. Presented at the International Symposium on Man-made Mineral Fibers in the Working Environment, Copenhagen, October 29, 1986

19. Doll R: Overview and conclusions. Symposium on Man-made Mineral Fibers, Copenhagen, October 1986. Ann Occup Hyg 31:805–819, 1987

20. Das PB, Fletcher AG Jr, Deodhare SG: Mesothelioma in an agricultural community of India: A clinicopathological study. Aust NZ J Surg 46:218–226, 1976

21. Hallin N: Report on Mineral Wool Dust in Construction Sites. Stockholm, Sweden: Bygghalsan, The Construction Industry's Organization for Working Environment, Safety and Health, 1981

18

Coal Workers' Pneumoconiosis

James A. Merchant

Historical Perspective. Lung disease among underground coal miners has been a recognized occupational hazard since at least the mid-seventeenth century. Miners' black lung, now called coal workers' pneumoconiosis (CWP), was first documented among Scottish coal miners in 1836.[1] Although the disease was thought to be disappearing in Britain at the turn of this century, wider use of chest radiographs following World War I showed pneumoconiosis, similar to silicosis, among coal miners in South Wales. As a measure of public acceptance of this disease, British coal miners were first awarded compensation for silicosis under the Workmen's Compensation Act in 1931.

In marked contrast is the story of CWP in the United States. Appreciation of CWP as an occupational hazard and public health problem occurred at a much later date, as did legislation to deal with CWP and associated respiratory disease. The first systematic study of coal miners was conducted by the U.S. Public Health Service between 1928 and 1931 in the anthracite coal fields in eastern Pennsylvania.[2] Because of the relatively high silica content and similarity to silicosis, the term "anthracosilicosis" was used to describe the pneumoconiosis found among those miners. Among the entire population studied ($n = 2711$), 23% were found to be affected. The prevalence of pneumoconiosis also was found to be related to the number of years underground, particles per cubic meter, and free silica content. "Pulmonary infection" was more frequent among miners with higher dust exposure and greater than 15 years underground. Among miners over age 55, pulmonary tuberculosis was as much as 10 times more frequent than in the general population.

One reason for the relatively late recognition of CWP as a distinct disease entity in the United States was the early emphasis placed on the etiological role of silica in pneumoconiosis. The Hawk's Nest tragedy (1932 to 1934), in which more than 400 workers died of acute silicosis and tuberculosis after working on the tunnel at Gauley Bridge, West Virginia, reinforced the prevalent theory that silica content was the important etiological agent in pneumoconiosis.[3] Experimental research on pneumoconiosis at Saranac Lake, N.Y., focused heavily on silica and significantly influenced this area of investigation for a generation.[4] By 1934, British physicians were beginning to accept coal dust as an occupational exposure that could result in disability and death. In 1942, the Committee on Industrial Pulmonary Diseases of the Medical Research Council introduced the term "coal workers' pneumoconiosis."[5]

Little additional progress was made in the United States until 1954, when the Public Health Service published a bibliography of American and British reports on respiratory disease among coal miners.[6] Following this, studies by Levine and Hunter,[7] Lieben et al,[8] and Stoeckle et al[9] further documented the importance of coal workers' pneumoconiosis. At the direction of Congress, the Public Health Service began a comprehensive survey of the Appalachian coal fields in 1963. Of 2549 working miners and 1191 nonworking miners, 9% of the working and 18% of the nonworking miners were found to have radiographic evidence of pneumoconiosis.[10] This study, published in 1968, together with the disastrous November 20, 1968, Farmington, W. Va., mine explosion that killed 78 miners, triggered pressure from miners, their union (the United Mine Workers of America), and public health advocates, and led to passage of the Federal Coal Mine Health and Safety Act of 1969 (Public Law 91-173). This was the first American mining bill to recognize the importance of both health and safety hazards and provide a mandate for strong preventive measures.

Legislation. Although the Federal Coal Mine Health and Safety Act of 1969 was a landmark piece of legislation, it was by no means the first or last legislation to deal with occupational hazards of mining (Table 18–1). The 1969 act addressed several issues specifically and has in many respects served as a model for subsequent occupational safety and health legislation. The provisions included the following[11]:

- Mandatory health standards to be prescribed by the Secretary of Health and Human Services (HHS)
- Right of entry for inspection (Department of Interior) and investigation (HHS)
- Power to close mining operations, issue abatement orders, and penalize operators for noncompliance
- Provide a respirable dust standard of 3 mg/m^3 to be reduced to 2 mg/m^3 3 years after passage of the act
- Medical surveillance of underground coal miners through entry and periodic medical examinations
- Transfer of miners (transfer rights) with evidence of pneumoconiosis, without loss of pay (rate retention), to a low dust area (now < 1 mg/m^3)
- Autopsies on deceased miners, administered by the National Institute for Occupational Safety and Health (NIOSH) through the National Coal Workers' Autopsy Study

- Compensation for miners with total disability and for dependents of miners who die of the disease
- Research and training

The medical surveillance provisions of the act were implemented through specifications developed by the NIOSH Appalachian Laboratory for Occupational Safety and Health in August 1970. Since that date, more than 350,000 examinations have been performed.

Subsequently, Title IV of the 1969 act has been amended twice by Congress, each time liberalizing requirements that qualify miners for benefits and making coal operators responsible for providing trust funds to pay these benefits. In 1977, the entire 1969 act was revised and largely incorporated into a new, comprehensive mining law—the Federal Mine Safety and Health Amendments Act (Public Law 95-164)—which now also extends many of the provisions of the 1969 act to metal and nonmetal miners. Significant new responsibilities were given to the Department of Labor (Mine Safety and Health Administration) for establishing health standards and mine inspections and to HHS (NIOSH) for research and surveillance in noncoal mines.

Definition. CWP is a specific occupational lung disease arising from the prolonged inhalation of coal mine dust. Black lung is a generic term that has been used legislatively and popularly to mean any lung disease that may arise from coal mine employment; this has translated into pathologically defined CWP, and also obstructive airway disease among coal miners, for compensation purposes. CWP occurs in two forms: (1) simple CWP and (2) complicated CWP, or progressive massive fibrosis (PMF). The characteristic lesion of simple CWP is the coal macule, which is a focal collection of dust-laden macrophages at the division of the respiratory bronchioles together with associated focal emphysema.[12] Micro- and macronodules of simple CWP usually are smaller than 1 cm in diameter. Complicated CWP, or PMF, consists of solid, heavily pigmented masses averaging 2 cm in diameter, located commonly in the apical region of the lung and occurring on a background of simple CWP.

Environmental Exposures. It is important to realize that significant exposure to coal dust may occur not only in underground mines but also in strip and auger mining, in coal preparation plants, and in coal-handling operations. U.S. coal reserves are extensive, covering some 400,000 square miles across the country (Fig. 18–1). Coal in the United States may be classified by four ranks: lignite, sub-bituminous, bituminous, and anthracite. Anthracite deposits, which are mined on a limited basis only in northeastern Pennsylvania, are associated with higher exposures to respirable free silica and have been associated with higher rates of pneumoconiosis. The relative toxicity of bituminous coals, of which there are many grades, appears to vary. CWP occurs less frequently among western U.S. miners than among Appalachian miners. Lignite, which also is mined on a limited basis, has not been adequately studied epidemiologically.

Table 18–2 summarizes the industrial processes and jobs in which exposure to coal dust may occur among the estimated 200,000 workers at risk. Workers engaged in face work, drilling, and coal preparation often have the highest exposures to respirable coal dust and free silica and thus the highest rates of CWP.

Although the focus of this chapter is on CWP, other associated health effects, including emphysema, bronchitis, and pulmonary vascular and cardiac abnormalities, will be mentioned.

Pathophysiology. Simple CWP as pathologically defined consists, at a minimum, of the characteristic coal macule lesion(s).[12] These may occur as microscopic manifestations of CWP associated with little or no functional impairment. With greater dust deposition in the lung, micronodules (less than 7 mm in diame-

TABLE 18–1. COAL MINING HEALTH AND SAFETY LEGISLATION IN UNITED STATES

1865:	Bill is introduced to create Federal Mining Bureau. It is not passed.
1910:	Bureau of Mines is established but specifically denied right of inspection.
1941:	Bureau of Mines is granted authority to inspect, but it is not given authority to establish or enforce safety codes [Title I, Federal Coal Mine Safety Act].
1946:	Federal Mine Safety Code for Bituminous Coal and Lignite Mines is issued by the Director, Bureau of Mines [agreement between Secretary of the Interior and the United Mine Workers of America] and included in the 1946 [Krug-Lewis] UMWA Wage Agreement.
1947:	Congress requests coal mine operators and state agencies to report compliance with the Federal Mine Safety Code; 33% compliance is reported.
1952:	Title II of the Federal Coal Mine Safety Act is passed. All mines employing 15 or more persons underground must comply with the act. Enforcement is limited to issuing orders of withdrawal for imminent danger or for failure to abate violations within a reasonable time.
1966:	Amendments to 1952 law are passed. Mines employing under 15 employees are included under 1952 act; stronger regulatory powers are given to Bureau of Mines, such as the provision permitting the closing of a mine or section of a mine because of an unwarrantable failure to correct a dangerous condition.
1969:	Federal Coal Mine Health and Safety Act is passed. The hazards of pneumoconiosis are, for the first time, given prominence, in addition to those of accidents.
1972:	Black Lung Benefits Act of 1972 is passed. Several sections of the Title IV are amended, liberalizing the awarding of compensation benefits.
1977:	Federal Mine Safety and Health Act of 1977 is passed. It amends Coal Mine Health and Safety Act of 1969 largely by adding health and safety standard setting, inspections, and research provisions for metal and nonmetal miners, while leaving the 1969 act largely intact. This act also consolidates health and safety compliance activities for general industry [OSHA] and mining [MSHA] in the Department of Labor.
1977:	Black Lung Benefits Revenue Act of 1977 is passed. This provides for an excise tax on the sale of coal by the producer to establish trust funds to pay black lung benefits.
1977:	Black Lung Benefits Reform Act of 1977 is passed, to improve and further define provisions for awarding black lung benefits. Additionally, it establishes [a mandate] that a detailed study of occupational lung disease would be undertaken by the Department of Labor and NIOSH.

From Key MM, Kerr LE, Bundy M [eds]: Pulmonary Reactions to Coal Dust. New York: Academic Press, 1971, with permission.

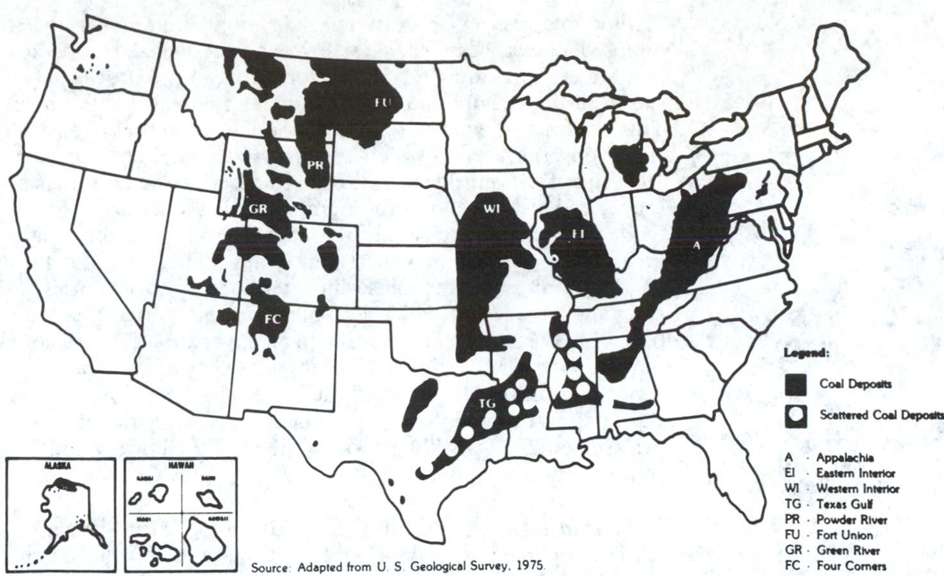

Figure 18-1. Coal deposits in United States.

ter) and nodules (larger than 8 mm but less than about 1 cm) are found, predominantly in the upper lung zones (Fig. 18-2). These nodules consist of collagen in addition to a preponderance of reticulin. With increased profusion of nodular lesions in the lung come greater functional abnormalities, but until marked, CWP often is not associated with significant respiratory symptoms or limiting impairment.

PMF invariably occurs on a background of simple CWP and its probability increases with the severity of simple CWP (Fig. 18-3).[13] PMF lesions usually occur in the posterior portion of the upper lobes and in the superior segment of the lower lobes. Unlike silicotic lesions, they cut easily and may have cavities containing inky fluid. The margins may be rounded or irregular, with fibrous strands extending into adjacent lung tissue.

Caplan's syndrome, consisting of pulmonary nodules associated with rheumatoid arthritis, occurs rarely in coal miners. The nodules, Caplan lesions, are similar to large (up to 5 cm) silicotic nodules on gross examination, usually have smooth borders and concentric internal laminations, and in contrast to PMF lesions, often have little dust contained with the lesion.[12]

Although other forms of emphysema occur in coal miners as they do in the general population, focal emphysema is integral to the coal macule (Fig. 18-2). Focal emphysema is associated with local loss of elastic fibers and alterations in capillary density. In PMF, particularly with the larger lesions, clinical, physiological, and pathological evidence of both chronic obstructive and restrictive lung disease is common. The panlobular, irregular, centrilobular, and bullous emphysema associated with these massive lesions is often extensive and destructive; it frequently results in marked pulmonary impairment.[12] Increasing pathological and physiological evidence has strengthened the view that coal mine dust exposure causes centrilobular emphysema.[14,40,41]

Chronic bronchitis, characterized pathologically by hypertrophy and hyperplasia of the bronchial mucous glands with an associated increase in the goblet cells of the small airways, occurs in association with CWP. Clinically defined as the chronic production of phlegm, chronic bronchitis is a frequent clinical finding among coal miners.[15] Only one vascular lesion is accepted as specific to CWP. This consists of muscular hypertrophy involving small pulmonary arteries as they traverse the coal macule. It is postulated that this lesion may contribute to alterations in perfusion, but this has not been demonstrated. In PMF, occluded and destroyed blood vessels are common and contribute to right

TABLE 18-2. OCCUPATIONAL EXPOSURES ASSOCIATED WITH CWP

Exposure	Industry or Occupation
Coal dust [lignite, sub-bituminous, bituminous, and anthracite]	Coal mine construction Strip and auger mining Underground mining, inspection Coal preparation Coal loading and transportation

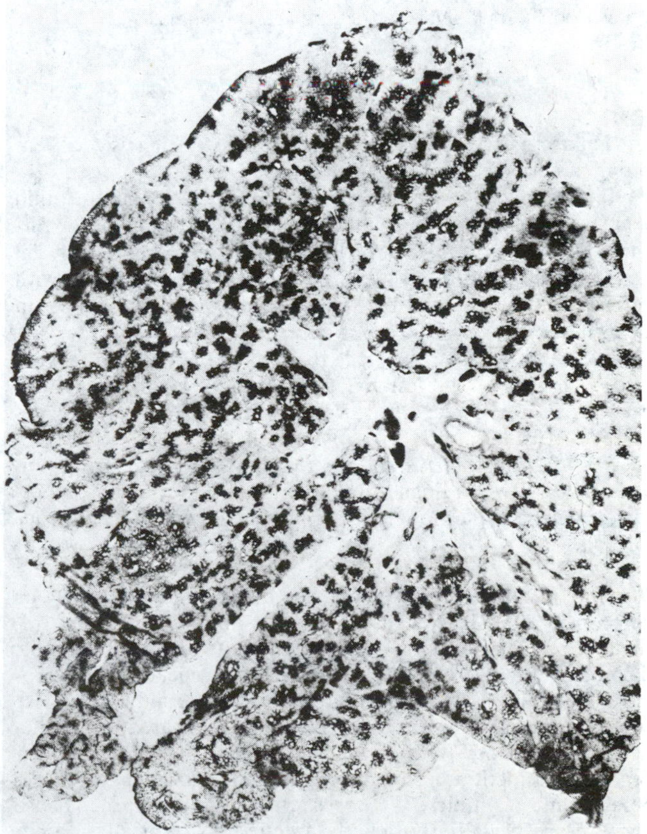

Figure 18-2. Whole lung section showing simple CWP with associated focal emphysema but otherwise preserved lung architecture.

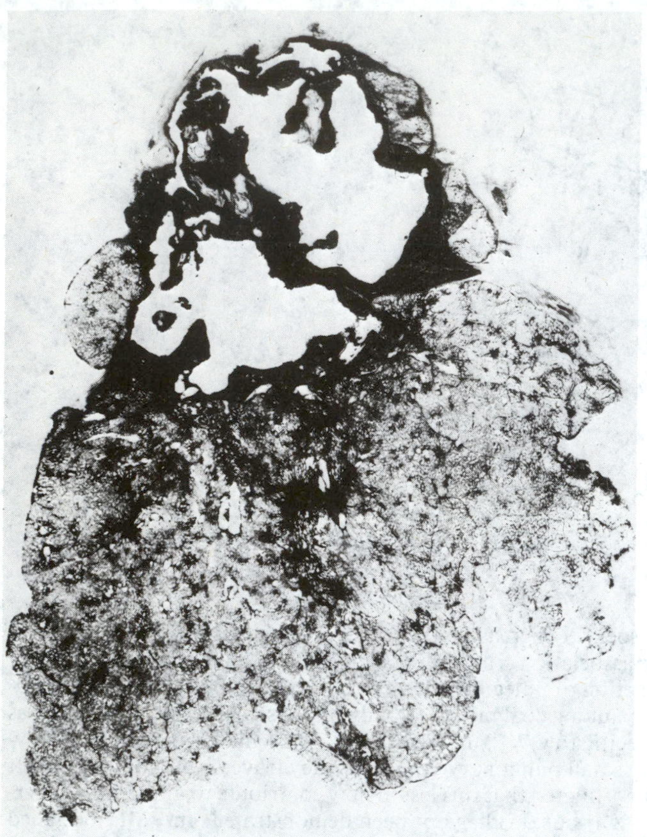

Figure 18-3. Whole lung section showing progressive massive fibrosis with cavitation involving the superior segments of the lung on a background of simple CWP and extensive emphysema.

ventricular hypertrophy or cor pulmonale, which is frequent among miners with severe CWP.[12]

Physiologically, miners with simple CWP have been found to have increased residual volumes, decreased maximal expiratory flow rates, reduction in Pa_{O_2}, increased alveolar arterial oxygen differences, and slight hyperventilation, especially with exercise.[16] These findings may be nonexistent or slight in those in the earliest stages of CWP, but become progressively more significant with increasing extent of disease. In PMF (again varying with the extent of the lesions), moderate-to-severe airway obstruction is manifested by markedly reduced flow rates, decreased diffusing capacity, perfusion defects, and reduced Pa_{O_2}, together with obstructive and restrictive mechanical changes in the lung.[16] These findings often are marked. Pulmonary hypertension with cor pulmonale is a frequent manifestation of advanced PMF.

Clinical Features. There are no pathognomonic signs or symptoms of CWP. In the early stages of CWP, workers frequently are asymptomatic and without functional impairment. Chronic cough and phlegm are, however, associated with prolonged inhalation of coal dust and with cigarette smoking. These symptoms per se also are not necessarily associated with functional impairment. With advanced simple CWP, shortness of breath and functional impairment become more common, yet some advanced simple CWP cases remain symptom free. Those with PMF, especially those with large lesions, typically present with cough, phlegm, shortness of breath, and signs of cor pulmonale.

The chest radiograph is a simple and relatively accurate method to assess CWP. Although it is known that unless superimposed, the earliest lesions of CWP are undetected by radiographic examination, the correlation between the profusion of CWP pathologically and radiographically is reasonably good. This has led to the development of a series of international classifications, the latest of which is the International Labor Office's 1980 classification; this can be used to describe the extent, size, shape, and distribution of radiographic opacities and also to describe pulmonary, cardiac, pleural, and other thoracic abnormalities that may appear on a chest radiograph.[17] This classification divides simple pneumoconiosis into four major subcategories (0, 1, 2, and 3), each of which is subdivided into three categories (i.e., 0/1, 1/1, and 1/2), resulting in an approximation to a continuous scale. PMF is divided into three categories (A, B, and C), depending on the diameter of the largest lesion. Although designed as an epidemiological instrument, this classification also has been adopted worldwide to describe CWP clinically and for compensation purposes.

Epidemiology. A great deal of epidemiological investigation has been directed toward the study of CWP and associated conditions. Early epidemiological studies established an association between coal mining, respiratory disease, and pulmonary infections. More recent studies have identified specific risk factors and health effects and have led to new hypotheses about yet-unexplained observations.

Mortality patterns among coal miners have been studied principally in Great Britain and the United States. These studies have generally shown increased standard mortality ratios (SMRs) for accidents, respiratory disease, respiratory tuberculosis, and stomach cancer.[18-21] Mortality rates by major radiographic category have shown minimal-to-moderate elevations in SMRs for all miners, no significant difference between those with category 0 and those with other categories of simple CWP, but significant differences between those with category 0 and those with complicated CWP.[22]

Of particular interest is the question of carcinogenesis. Among coal miners, widely divergent results have been reported in SMRs for lung cancer.[19,23] Among those with evidence of respiratory disease, low lung cancer mortality has suggested competing risks.[24] Two recent case control studies found no coal mine dust exposure–lung cancer risk, but did find the anticipated increase in lung cancer among smoking miners.[25] By contrast, stomach cancer mortality has been almost uniformly increased in coal mining cohorts in both Britain and the United States.[18,19,26] Ong and co-workers[27] have hypothesized, supported by laboratory mutagenesis data, that compounds in coal may undergo intragastric nitrosation or interaction with exogenous chemicals or both to form carcinogenic compounds that may with time cause stomach cancer. The most comprehensive retrospective cohort mortality study in the United States has been published by Rockette.[26] This report summarizes and largely supports earlier observations and serves as an excellent reference on coal miner mortality.

Morbidity studies of coal miners have concentrated on the association between radiographic evidence of CWP and dust exposure. Dust suppression effected after 1950 resulted in a downward shift in the prevalence of CWP among British miners. In 1959 the Institute of Occupational Medicine in Edinburgh, with the support of the National Coal Board, began a long-term cohort study of 26 collieries. This massive study has provided the most comprehensive available data on dose-response relationships. After 10 years of study, analysis of the respirable dust and radiographic findings provided clear dose-response relationships, which resulted in new dust standards in the United States and interim dust standards in Great Britain.[28] A subsequent study of 10 of the original collieries provided a longer follow-up and shifted the dose-response curve to the left, indicating a slight underestimation based on earlier data (Fig. 18-4).[29] As a part of this study, free silica content in respirable samples was assessed

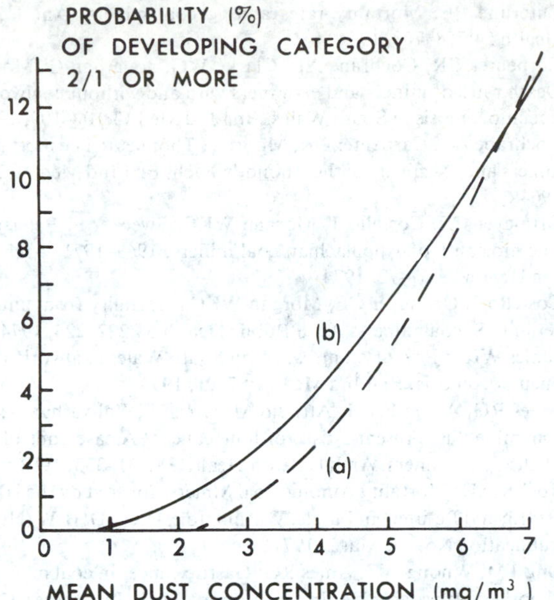

Figure 18-4. Lines [a] and [b] are estimates of probabilities of developing category 2 or 3 of simple pneumoconiosis over an approximately 35-year working life at the coalface, in relation to the mean dust concentration experienced during that period. [a] is based on 10 years of data, Interim Standards Study, Pneumoconiosis Field Research. [b] is update of [a], based on 20 years of data, Pneumoconiosis Field Research. *[From Hurley JF, et al: Simple Pneumoconiosis and Exposure to Respirable Dust: Relationships From Twenty-five Years' Research at Ten British Coal Mines. Institute of Occupational Medicine, Report No. TM/79/13.]*

and found not to influence pneumoconiosis risk, which did vary significantly and unaccountably between collieries. It was, however, found that a small number of miners with rapid progression had higher exposure to free silica. Recently available data from similar studies in the United States conducted by NIOSH are consistent with the British pneumoconiosis field research data[30,31] (Fig. 18-5).

Because of the strong association between PMF and respiratory impairment and increased mortality, the attack rate of PMF has been of particular interest. Miners with evidence of CWP by

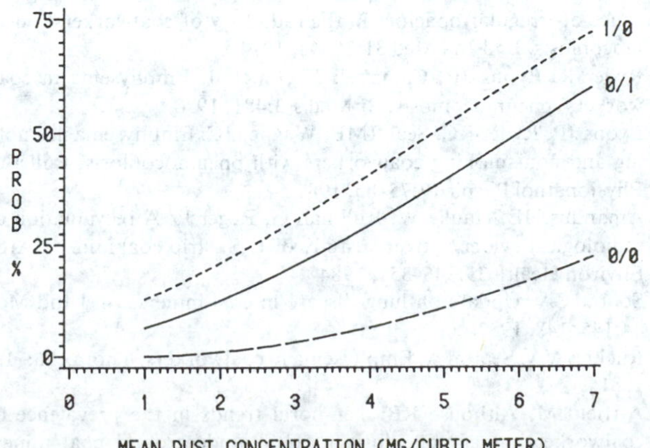

Figure 18-5. Ten-year predicted incidence and progression of CWP for various starting categories. *[From the Division of Respiratory Disease Studies/NIOSH.]*

radiograph have been found to have an increasing probability of developing PMF with increasing radiographic category of CWP.[28] The attack rate of PMF has been found to rise with increasing radiographic category of CWP and increased progression of CWP and among younger miners but not among those with pulmonary tuberculosis, as once suspected.[13,32] These studies are important because they serve as the basis for recommending removal of a miner with radiographic evidence of CWP from areas of high dust exposure.

While radiographic evidence of CWP has been the major focus of epidemiological research on CWP, recent attention has focused on the effect of coal dust exposure on obstructive airway disease (bronchitis and emphysema). Both of these diseases result in airway obstruction, frequently called chronic obstructive pulmonary disease (COPD). These diseases are known to be of multifactorial etiology. Cigarette smoking is widely accepted as a major risk factor in both bronchitis and emphysema. Although earlier studies questioned the association between coal dust exposure and bronchitis, more comprehensive reports support an association between bronchitis and dust exposure in addition to a smoking effect. Recent results from the NIOSH longitudinal study of U.S. coal miners confirm that coal mine dust exposure contributes significantly to an increased decline in FEV_1 over time but somewhat less than the average effect of smoking.[33-35] Evidence of CWP by radiograph does not appear to affect the prevalence of bronchitis, nor does smoking appear to influence the prevalence of CWP.[36] Although differences in spirometry between bronchitic and nonbronchitic miners have been observed, their significance has been questioned and awaits prospective evaluation.

Focal emphysema is associated with the coal macule as the characteristic lesion of CWP. More extensive, destructive, centriacinar emphysema is seen in a certain proportion of miners' lungs.[37] These miners usually are cigarette smokers and it is difficult in an individual case to determine the relative importance of coal mine dust and cigarette smoking in the pathogenesis of these lesions. A recent study of coal miners with pneumoconiosis suggests, however, that centrilobular emphysema may play a much more important role in coal miners' lung impairment than appreciated previously.[38]

Prevention. The key to preventing coal workers' pneumoconiosis is prevention of prolonged inhalation of significant concentrations of coal dust. This can be accomplished in two ways: (1) by the control of respirable coal mine dust through proper ventilation of mining operations or (2) by removal of miners with early evidence of CWP to low-dust jobs. Of these two, dust control clearly is more effective. These two provisions were mandated by Congress in the Federal Coal Mine Health and Safety Act of 1969 and have been implemented successfully in underground operations of the U.S. coal industry.

Since passage of the 1969 act, respirable dust levels have been reduced for most high-risk jobs to meet the 2.0 mg/m³ standard. Although the vast majority of mining sections are in compliance, certain operations such as long walls have proved difficult to adequately ventilate and have achieved only marginal dust control. Dust concentration in surface mines has averaged less than half that of underground mining; however, high exposure to coal dust and free silica may occur for those who drill, crush, and prepare coal for transport. Attention recently has been drawn to silicosis among drillers in the anthracite mines in eastern Pennsylvania.[39]

NIOSH CWP surveillance on U.S. miners after 3 years of employment and at 4- to 5-year intervals thereafter has documented decreases in radiographic prevalence of CWP from 17.7% in round 1 ending in 1974, to 5.4% in round 2, to 4.7% in round 3, and to 4.2% in round 4, which ended in 1986. The initial decrease in prevalence was the result of a substantial shift in the working population, with older miners leaving employment and new miners coming into employment between rounds, rather than any reduction in the rate of CWP among those with 20 or more years underground. The fourth round of surveillance began in 1983 and allowed assessment of 12 years of improved dust control.[42] Trends in CWP incidence suggest the dust standard is playing a protective role, but longer follow-up is necessary to assess the adequacy of the 2 mg/m^3 respirable dust standard.[30]

REFERENCES

1. Thomson W: On black expectoration and deposition of black matter in the lungs. Med Chir Tr 20:230, 1836
2. Sayers RR, Bloomfield JJ, Dallavalle JM, et al: Anthraco-Silicosis (Miners' Asthma): A Preliminary Report of a Study Made in the Anthracite Region of Pennsylvania. Spec. Bull. No. 41. Harrisburg, Penn.: Pennsylvania Department of Labor and Industry, 1934
3. Subcommittee of the Committee of Labor, House of Representatives: An Investigation Relating to Health Conditions of Workers Employed in Construction and Maintenance of Public Utilities. Washington, D.C.: 74th Congress, HJ Res. 449:2603, 1936
4. Pendergrass E: Personal communication
5. Medical Research Council of Great Britain: Chronic Pulmonary Diseases in South Wales Coalminers (1942, 1943). Medical Research Council of Great Britain, Spec. Rep. Ser. 243, 244
6. Doyle HN, Noehren TH: Pulmonary Fibrosis in Soft Coal Miners: An Annotated Bibliography on the Entity Recently Described as Soft Coal Pneumoconiosis. Washington, D.C.: U.S. Public Health Bibliography, Ser. 11, 1954
7. Levine MD, Hunter MB: Clinical study of pneumoconiosis of coal workers in Ohio River Valley. JAMA 163:1-9, 1957
8. Lieben J, Pendergrass E, McBride WW: Pneumoconiosis study in central Pennsylvania coal mines. I. Medical phase. J Occup Med 3:493-506, 1961
9. Stoeckle JD, Hardy HL, King WB, Nemiah JC: Respiratory disease in U.S. soft-coal miners: Clinical and etiological considerations. A study of 30 cases. J Chronic Dis 15:887-905, 1961
10. Lainhart WS, Felson B, Jacobson G, Pendergrass EP: Pneumoconiotic lesions in bituminous coal miners and metal miners. Arch Environ Health 16:207-210, 1968
11. Lee DHK: Historical aspects. In Key MM, Kerr LE, Bundy M (eds): Pulmonary Reactions to Coal Dust, 1953-1977. New York: Academic Press, 1971, p 9
12. Kleinerman J, Green F, Harley RA, et al: Pathology standards for coal workers' pneumoconiosis. Arch Pathol Lab Med 108:8, 1979
13. McLintock JL, Rae S, Jacobsen M: The attack rate of progressive massive fibrosis in British coal miners. In Walton WH (ed): Inhaled Particles III, Vol. 2. London: Unwin, 1971, pp 933-950
14. Worth G: Emphysema in coal workers. Am J Ind Med 6:401-403, 1984
15. Kibelstis JA, Morgan EJ, Reger R, et al: Prevalence of bronchitis and airways obstruction in American bituminous coal miners. Am Rev Respir Dis 108:886-893, 1973
16. Lapp NL, Seaton A: Pulmonary function. In Key MM, Kerr LE, Bundy M (eds): Pulmonary Reactions to Coal Dust. New York: Academic Press, 1953-1977, 1971
17. International Labor Office: International Classification of Radiographs of the Pneumoconioses. Geneva: ILO, 1979
18. Stocks P: On the death rates from cancer of the stomach and respiratory diseases in 1949-1953 among coal miners and other male residents in countries of England and Wales. Br J Cancer 16:592-598, 1962
19. Enterline PE: Mortality rates among coal miners. Am J Public Health 54:758-768, 1964
20. Carpenter GR, Cochrane AL, Clarke WG, Jonathan G, Moore F: Death rates of miners and ex-miners with and without coalworkers' pneumoconiosis in South Wales. Br J Ind Med 13:102-109, 1956
21. Cochrane AL, Carpenter GR, Moore F, Thomas J: The mortality of miners and ex-miners in the Rhondda Fach. Br J Ind Med 21:38-45, 1964
22. Ortmeyer CE, Costello J, Morgan WKC, Swecker S, Petersen M: The mortality of Appalachian coal miners, 1963-1971. Arch Environ Health 29:67-72, 1974
23. Costello J, Ortmeyer CE, Morgan WKC: Mortality from lung cancer in U.S. coal miners. Am J Public Health 64:222-224, 1974
24. James WRL: Primary lung cancer in South Wales coalworkers with pneumoconiosis. Br J Ind Med 12:87-91, 1955
25. Ames RG, Amandus H, Attfield M, Green F, Vallyathan V: Does coal mine dust present a risk for lung cancer? A case-control study of U.S. coal miners. Arch Environ Health 38:331-333, 1983
26. Rockette H: Mortality Among Coal Miners Covered by the UMWA Health and Retirement Funds. Washington, D.C.: DHEW (NIOSH) Publication No. 77, March 1977
27. Ong TM, Whong WZ, Ames RG: Gastric cancer in coal miners: An hypothesis of coal mine dust causation. Med Hypotheses 12:159-165, 1983
28. Jacobsen M, Rae S, Walton WH, Rogan JM: The relation between pneumoconiosis and dust exposure in British coal miners. In Walton WH (ed): Inhaled Particles III, Vol. 2. London: Unwin, 1971, pp 903-919
29. Hurley JF, Copland L, Dodgson J, Jacobsen M: Simple Pneumoconiosis and Exposure to Respirable Dust: Relationships from Twenty-Five Years' Research at Ten British Coal Mines. Report No. TM/79/13. Edinburgh: Institute of Occupational Medicine, 1979
30. Attfield M, Reger R, Glenn R: The incidence and progression of pneumoconiosis over nine years in U.S. coal mines: I. Principal findings. Am J Ind Med 6:407-415, 1984
31. Attfield M, Reger R, Glenn R: The incidence and progression of pneumoconiosis over nine years in U.S. coal mines: II. Relationship with dust exposure and other potential causative factors. Am J Ind Med 6:417-425, 1984
32. Cochrane AL, Moore F, Thomas J: The radiographic progression of progressive massive fibrosis. Tubercle 42:72-77, 1961
33. Hankinson JL, Reger RB, Morgan WKC: Maximal expiratory flows in coal miners. Am Rev Respr Dis 116:175-180, 1977
34. Rogan JM, Attfield MD, Jacobsen M, et al: Role of dust in the working environment in development of chronic bronchitis in British coal miners. Br J Ind Med 30:217-226, 1973
35. Attfield M: Longitudinal decline in FEV_1 in U.S. coal miners. Thorax, 40:132-137, 1985
36. Lyons JP, Ryder RC, Campbell H, Clarke WG, Gough J: Significance of irregular opacities in the radiology of coalworkers' pneumoconiosis. Br J Ind Med 31:36-44, 1974
37. Ryder R, Lyons JP, Campbell J, Gough J: Emphysema in coalworkers' pneumoconiosis. Br Med J 3:481, 1970
38. Lyons JP, Ryder RC, Seal RME, Wagner JC: Emphysema in smoking and non-smoking coalworkers with pneumoconiosis. Bull Eur Physiopathol Respir 17:75-85, 1981
39. Amandus HE, Hauke W, Kullman G, Reger R: A reevaluation of radiological evidence from a study of U.S. strip coal miners. Arch Environ Health 39:346-351, 1984
40. Soutar CA: Update on lung disease in coal miners. Br J Ind Med 44:145-148, 1987
41. Ruckley VA, Seaton A: Emphysema in coalworkers. Thorax 36:716, 1981
42. Attfield M, Althouse RB: Temporal trends in the prevalence of coalworkers' pneumoconiosis in U.S. underground coal miners based on surveillance data for the period 1970-1986. In press 1991

19

Silicosis

Ruth Lilis

Silicosis is a fibrotic lung disease produced by the inhalation of dust containing free crystalline silicon dioxide (SiO_2). Free silica and silicates represent a large part of the earth's crust. Silicon and oxygen are the two most important elements in the crust; about 27.7% of its composition is silicon, and 46.6% is oxygen. Free silica is the most widespread naturally occurring substance known to have a fibrogenic effect on the lungs. It occurs in crystalline and amorphous forms. The crystalline forms that are fibrogenic are quartz, tridymite, and cristobalite; cryptocrystalline forms (consisting of minute crystals) are flint, chert, opal, and chalcedony. There are numerous forms of amorphous silica.

At high temperatures (800° to 1000° C), quartz, the most common crystalline form of free silica, is converted into tridymite, and at even higher temperatures (1100° to 1400° C) it is transformed into cristobalite. Flint, chert, opal, chalcedony, and amorphous forms of free silica, including kaolin and diatomaceous earth, also are transformed into tridymite and cristobalite at these temperatures. This effect of high temperatures is of importance, since both tridymite and cristobalite are more potent than quartz in producing pulmonary fibrosis.

History. Silicosis undoubtedly originated in antiquity with the mining and processing of metals and building stone. Agricola, in his book *De Re Metallica* (1556), was probably the first to recognize the adverse effects of inhaled dust. He stated that dust entering miners' lungs caused ulcerated lungs and consumption. The disease was so lethal that some women had seven husbands in succession. The first monograph on miners' diseases, *Von der Bergsucht,* by Paracelsus in 1567, included a classic description of miners' phthisis. Distinctive pathological features were described first by van Diemerbroeck, who described how the lungs of stonecutters dying of "asthma" cut like masses of sand (*Anatomi Corporis Humani,* 1672). Bernardino Ramazzini included a description of diseases of stonemasons and miners in *De Morbis Artificium Diatriba* (1700). In England the disease (phthisis) was described in flint knappers, needlepointers, knife grinders, fork sharpeners, and cutters of sandstone. Holland (1843) found that 30 of 97 grinders in Sheffield had grinders' asthma (silicosis). John Scott Haldane (1923) described the cellular storage and retention of dust, including the long-term retention of silica, and recommended better ventilation of mines and factories. The distinction between tuberculosis and silicosis followed Koch's discovery of the tubercle bacillus in 1882. The earliest description of silicosis in the United States, in the nineteenth century, was of employees of a cutlery plant; the disease was then detected among miners, in some of whom it reached high incidence levels. Tunnel work also generated numerous cases of silicosis. The tunnel at Gauley Bridge in West Virginia, where many workers contracted both acute and chronic silicosis in the 1930s, attracted much public attention. This resulted in the initiation of dust suppression and respiratory protection methods, improved industrial hygiene, and the introduction of laws for compensation of silicosis victims.

Although the magnitude of the silicosis risk was gradually reduced in tunnel drilling and mining operations, significant silica exposure continued to occur in other industrial operations, such as foundries, the manufacture and use of silica flour, the production of detergent soaps with a high content of free silica, and sandblasting.

Work Exposures

Mines. The quartz content of the ores mined and the intensity of the exposure to the dusts determine the relative risks of working in the following situations: metal ore mines, especially gold, copper, tin, silver, nickel, tungsten, uranium, and platinum; coal mines (drilling through rock or work in areas with narrow seams); mines or quarries for silicates (talc, kaolin, bentonite, mica, clays, etc.), slate, graphite, and fluorspar and their processing; drilling for exploration; and crushing operations.

Quarries. Quarries of materials with high free crystalline silica content (quartz, sandstone, granite, slate, porphyry, etc.) and the processing of such materials place workers at risk for silicosis. Sandstone is almost pure silica; granite may have a variable silica content, 20% to 70%; and slate usually is approximately 40% silica. The cottage industry producing slate pencils in India has produced numerous cases of severe silicosis.[1]

Tunnels. Tunnel drilling and other excavations in rocks with high SiO_2 content may represent a severe hazard, especially since ventilation usually is poor. Among the earliest studies of silicosis in the United States were those of disease in subway and tunnel builders in New York City in the mid-1920s. Cases of silicosis also have been traced to the excavation of deep foundations in sandstone in Australia.

Stonemasonry. Stonemasons may be subjected to significant and seldom well-controlled silica exposure. Sandstone and granite are the most important materials.

Foundry Work. A significant risk of silica exposure is associated with the mixture of sand and clays used for molds; the temperature of the molten metal poured into the molds fuses some sand to the surface of the castings and converts some quartz into tridymite or even cristobalite. Sometimes the molds are dusted with powders of high free-silica content, which adds a significant risk. The separation of castings from molds and cores, by shaking or knocking or automatically on vibrating tables, generates dangerous concentrations of dust. Fettling, the process by which the remnants of molds are removed from the castings by various abrading and polishing techniques, carries a substantial risk.

Grinding. Grinding and polishing with sandstone or other abrasive materials of high silica content have been replaced largely by less hazardous procedures, since these methods have resulted in numerous severe cases of silicosis. Nevertheless, grinding with such synthetic materials as Carborundum does not totally eliminate the risk, since remnants of the silica-containing mold are a source of airborne silica dust. Crushed sand, sandstone, and quartzite have been used for metal polishes and sandpaper.

Sandblasting. Sandblasting, used, for example, in foundries, in construction work, especially for the polishing of metal surfaces before painting and for cleaning building stone, and in the etching of glass and plastics, is an extremely hazardous occupation with high levels of exposure to very fine particles. Steel shot, iron garnet, and Carborundum sometimes are used instead of sand, but this has not universally eliminated the risk because in some areas these materials are used in only a small proportion of sandblasting activities. Sandblasting of relatively small objects can be done in enclosed chambers operated from the outside. A hazardous exposure persists, however, for workers entering the sandblasting booths to remove the objects or clean the floors. Sandblasting in construction work or shipbuilding cannot be enclosed; hence adequate respiratory protection of all persons in the work area is essential. Sandblasting was banned in the United Kingdom in 1951 and in the European Economic Community in 1966 but is still widely used in the United States, where cases of rapidly progressing silicosis attributed to this type of exposure have been reported.[2]

Brick-making. Manufacture of refractory brick and other refractory products (especially the acid refractories) carries a high risk of silicosis. Quartzite, sandstone, sands, or grits with a high quartz content are crushed, milled, shaped, dried, and fired at high temperatures, and a proportion of quartz is converted to tridymite and cristobalite.

Bricklaying. Bricklaying and dismantling or repair of refractory bricks in ovens, furnaces, kilns, and boilers carry a high risk of silicosis, especially because of the cristobalite along with the quartz.

Pottery. The pottery industry may generate significant risks when the raw materials (mostly clays) contain free silica, even though use of powdered flint, which was a major source of silica in the pottery industry in Great Britain, has been discontinued. Glazes with variable contents of quartz also are used; firing at high temperatures (up to 1400° C) may create another source of significant silica exposure. In the United States, wollastonite, a calcium metasilicate, is used instead of flint, quartz, sand, and china clay, and therefore the health hazard in this industry is less than that reported in Great Britain in the past.

Glass. Glass industry workers, especially those grinding and polishing with fine quartz, and sandblasters of glass have considerable silica exposure.

Soaps. Manufacture of abrasive soaps containing fine sand (silica flour) has in the past been a cause of rapidly progressing silicosis, "abrasive soap pneumoconiosis."

Fillers. Fillers used in the paint, rubber, plastic, and paper manufacturing industries may include silica flour, a finely ground, highly toxic quartz. It is sometimes incorrectly labeled as amorphous silica.[3] Rapidly progressing silicosis has resulted from the production of silica flour in Australia[4] and the United States.[5]

Enamel. Vitreous enameling, using mixtures of pulverized materials with a quartz component and high temperatures, may present a significant risk; enamel spraying is particularly hazardous.

Diatomaceous Earth. Calcined diatomaceous earth carries a significant risk, since part of the amorphous silica is transformed through calcination into cristobalite and tridymite. It is used in filters, absorbents, and abrasives and may generate significant exposure and risk of silicosis.

Ceramic Fiber Insulation. Ceramic fiber insulation is being used increasingly as a refractory lining for heat-treating and preheating furnaces in the iron and steel industry. Recent studies have shown that the fibers undergo partial conversion to cristobalite when exposed to high temperatures.[6]

Occurrence. Accurate data on the occurrence of silicosis in various industries and in different parts of the world are difficult to obtain and hard to compare, in part because of different notification systems. Cross-sectional surveys of exposed populations, such as miners, indicate the prevalence of the disease. The attack rate or incidence of the disease is less well known. The incidence of silicosis undoubtedly increased in the majority of the industrialized countries until the 1950s. Methods of dust suppression and control that had been developed and applied mainly in large industrial facilities then led to a decrease in the incidence of silicosis. Dust control became more rigorous as the hazards were recognized, but smaller industries and new industrial processes continued to expose workers to dangerous levels of silica.

In industrialized countries with intensive mining, such as West Germany, silicosis is still one of the most important problems of occupational medicine; as many as 3500 new cases were diagnosed in 1960, and approximately 1500 deaths due to silicosis occurred annually in the 1960s—five times more than the total number of fatal work accidents. France reported a similar number of silicosis deaths in the 1960s.

In India, silicosis was diagnosed as soon as systematic examinations of miners were initiated in the 1950s and 1960s. In the Bihar mining area, 34% of those examined were found to have advanced silicosis. Similarly, in Japan a high prevalence of silicosis (63%) was found in some metal ore miners.

Much of the available information is based on compensation cases. Because the criteria for compensation differ in each country, only general impressions can be gained. In the United Kingdom, for example, 721 persons were awarded industrial injury compensation for silicosis in 1957; in 1969, only 162 new awards for silicosis were made. Mining, quarrying, and slate industries had not shown a significant downward trend, however.

In the United States, the incidence of silicosis has decreased in the Vermont granite quarries,[7] but metal mining is still an important cause of silicosis. A survey of more than 76% of the work force in 50 metal mines, conducted by the Public Health Service and the Bureau of Mines between 1958 and 1961, revealed a silicosis prevalence of 3.4%. In one third of cases, complicated silicosis was present. Prevalence was related to silica content of the rock, occupation, and length of exposure. Trasko[8] estimated the total number of silicosis cases in 20 states to be about 6000. Miners and foundry workers were each represented by more than 1600 cases, but the number of cases was probably underestimated. In a British study of foundry workers,[9] the prevalence of simple pneumoconiosis was 34% among fettlers and 14% in foundry floor workers. Similar data for the United States are not available.

In 1971, milling of bentonite (sodium montmorillonite) was

found to have produced severe silicosis in Wyoming[10]; a silicosis risk in this industry had not been suspected in the past.

In 1983, the National Institute of Occupational Safety and Health estimated that approximately 3.2 million workers in 238,000 plants in the United States were potentially exposed to crystalline silica.

Watts et al (1984)[11] analyzed respirable silica exposures in metal and nonmetal mines in the United States (41,502 samples taken in 1974 to 1981). Workers in sandstone, clay, shale, and various nonmetallic mineral mills had the highest exposures to silica dust. Crushing, grinding, sizing, and bagging operations and general labor had the highest exposures.

In 1984 the U.S. Mine Safety and Health Administration identified approximately 2400 work sites in coal mines where the level of 5% silica in respirable dust had been exceeded, representing the work environment of 15,000 to 20,000 coal miners (about 10% of U.S. coal miners). Floor and roof samples were found to contain 18% to 82% quartz; coal itself contained only 1% to 4%.[12] Continuous mining machines, cutting of roof, floor, and inclusion rock bands, and roof bolting operations were the major sources of silica exposure.

Mean quartz content of respirable dust was found to range from 4.2% to 14% in Belgium, 0.8% to 9.3% in Germany, 1.5% to 10.3% in Great Britain, 0.4% to 12.5% in the Soviet Union, and 2.1% to 12.7% in Bulgarian coal mines.[13]

The median silica content of respirable dust in 1743 personal air samples collected by the U.S. Occupational Safety and Health Administration in U.S. foundries from 1974 to 1981 ranged from 7.3% to 12.0%; during melting, 56.4% of the samples had more than 0.12 mg/m^3 respirable silica. Of 10,850 samples collected in iron and steel foundries, 23% had concentrations in excess of 0.20 mg/m^3 respirable silica.

Reports on a high (37%) prevalence of silicosis in workers in silica flour mills, with a significant proportion of cases developing massive fibrosis,[5] and reports of acute silicosis in sandblasters in the Louisiana Gulf area[14] point to the fact that silicosis continues to be an important occupational health risk, although the number of individuals affected probably has been reduced substantially.

Effects on Health. Classic silicosis is a chronic and slowly progressive disease. Acute silicosis and silico-proteinosis (alveolar lipoproteinosis-like silicosis) occur in epidemic outbreaks under circumstances of heavy silica exposure. Sandblasting, abrasive soap manufacture, tunnel drilling, and refractory brick manufacture have been the major sources of such outbreaks.

Dust concentration, particle size (in the 2 to 0.1 μm range, which penetrate respiratory bronchioles and alveoli), and duration of dust exposure define the hazard. Thus high concentrations of fine dust overburden the limited direct clearance capacity of the distal zones of the lung, and longer exposures increase the risk of developing silicosis.

The interactions of concentration, particle size, and duration of exposure are the main determinants of the attack rate, latency period, incidence, rate of progression, and outcome of the disease.

In industrial processes in which silica-containing materials are heated at temperatures exceeding 800° C so that transformation into tridymite and cristobalite occurs, the higher fibrogenic potency of these forms of SiO_2 results in a higher attack rate and more severe silicosis. In the superficial layers of refractory brick that have been repeatedly subject to contact with molten metal, cristobalite may reach a concentration of 94%. Fusicalcination of diatomaceous earth also results in high cristobalite concentrations (up to 35%).

Many theories have been proposed to explain the fibrogenic effect of silica. It had been generally accepted that silica particles were ingested by alveolar macrophages and that this eventually led to the death and disintegration of the cell. Among the contents released from dead macrophages a factor (or factors) that stimulates fibroblast function, synthesis of hydroxyproline, and thus collagen formation had been detected. Damaged macrophages were thought to attract other macrophages, which ingested the liberated silica particles and were injured in their turn; a reticular network appears, followed by collagen deposition, and eventually hyalinization of collagen occurs.

Recent studies in human subjects and on animal models have shown that alveolar macrophages that have engulfed silica particles maintain normal viability, including unaltered phagocytosis. These macrophages produce chemical mediators, such as interleukin-1, macrophage-derived growth factor, and fibronectin, which enhance the inflammatory process.[15]

In experimental studies and in an investigation of human subjects with silicosis, silica particles have been shown to initially produce an alveolitis, characterized by sustained increases in the total number of alveolar cells, including macrophages, lymphocytes, and neutrophils.

Biochemical analyses of bronchial lavage fluid have shown increased levels of lactate dehydrogenase, β-glucuronidase (markers of cytotoxicity), lecithin and phosphatidylglycerol (two components of lung surfactant), and glucosaminoglycans (major constituents of interstitial matrix).

In experimental silicosis models[16] the initial histopathological lesion, alveolitis, progressed to the characteristic nodular fibrosis of simple silicosis. Sustained increases in cellularity, enzyme release, and glycosaminoglycan were found by repeated bronchial lavage.

In a recent study using bronchial lavage in three groups of silica-exposed granite workers—(1) those without silicosis, (2) those with nodular silicosis, and (3) those with silicotic massive progressive fibrosis—proliferation of fibroblasts was increased in the lavage fluid of those with simple silicosis and in the group with complicated coalescent silicosis. In this last group, with massive progressive fibrosis, markers of fibrogenic activity, such as glucosaminoglycans, fibronectin, and procollagen 3, also were significantly increased.[16]

Interestingly, gallium scans and bronchial lavage have detected a subclinical alveolitis even in workers exposed to granite dust who have no radiologically detectable silicotic changes. This initial stage then progresses; macrophage-derived humoral factors enhance fibroblast growth, leading to fibrosis characteristic of silicosis. In complicated silicosis, markers of a high-intensity fibrotic process, fibronectin and procollagen 3, were found to be significantly increased.

Inhalation of crystalline silica particles produces a rapid increase in the rate of synthesis and deposition of lung collagen. Silica-induced fibrosis is unique among all the animal models and most human fibrotic lung disease thus far examined in that the excess collagen deposited in the lung contains normal ratios of the two major collagen types of the lung, types I and II; nevertheless it is biochemically different from normal lung collagen. The difference seems to be due to altered intermolecular cross-links; there is an increased hydroxylysine content of collagen. Dysfunctional cross-links are more likely to be derived from hydroxylysine. Hydroxylysine replaces lysine in the primary structure of a specific collagen α-chain to form the altered cross-links.

Another important property of crystalline silica is that it enhances the production of reactive oxygen metabolites by polymorphonuclear leukocytes. Antioxidant enzymes, such as superoxide dismutase and catalase, are inhibited.

Reactive oxygen metabolites have a deleterious effect on cellular and subcellular membranes. Lactate dehydrogenase (LDH), a cytoplasmic enzyme, the lysosomal enzyme β-*N*-acetylglucosaminidase (β-NAG), and β-glucuronidase are found in higher than normal concentrations in bronchial lavage fluid from these workers because of the damaging effect of crystalline silica on cellular and lysosomal membranes.

In the alveolar spaces of rats exposed to very high concentrations of quartz or cristobalite a material similar to that found in human alveolar lipoproteinosis together with a significant increase in the number of type II alveolar cells have been detected. Alkaline phosphatase is a marker for alveolar type II cells. This alveolar material is acellular and has a high phospholipid content, with osmophilic bodies similar to those present as inclusions in type II alveolar cells. Phosphatidylcholine and phosphatidylglycerol are components of the increased amounts of surfactant found in the alveolar spaces under such circumstances.

Thus it seems that two different types of reactions can occur as a result of the penetration of silica particles into alveolar spaces: triggering of a fibrogenic reaction by altered macrophages or production of excess phospholipids by type II alveolar cells. The rate at which silica particles accumulate in the alveoli is of great importance; exposure to high concentrations results in lipoproteinosis; exposure to relatively lower concentrations of silica, over longer periods of time, leads to the development of typical nodular fibrosis. Most silicosis cases are of the classic nodular type, characterized by the presence of collagenous and hyaline nodules.

The possibility that immunologic reactions are involved in the silicotic process has been considered repeatedly. The hypothesis that silica particles alter proteins and thus produce antigens that induce the production of autoantibodies has not been confirmed by immunofluorescence studies in experimental silicosis.

Increased prevalence of circulating antinuclear antibodies (ANA) has been reported in sandblasters with silicosis[17,18]; in some studies an increase in rheumatoid factor has also been reported although other studies have not confirmed this finding.[19] The role of such antibodies is unclear. It is thought that they may reflect the macrophage destruction due to silica and the release of cell contents.

Antibodies to lung connective tissue have been shown[20] to stimulate silica-exposed macrophages to release a factor that increases the production of collagen. Although the presence of human autoantibodies against denaturated collagen has been demonstrated in arthritis, lupus, and other chronic disorders associated with collagen breakdown, their role in the fibrogenic process of the pneumoconioses is not yet established.

Pathology. Silicotic nodules are readily felt in the lung and seen on the cut surface. Their size usually varies between 2 and 6 mm; they are hard, grayish, and more frequent in the apical and posterior parts of the lung. Sectioned nodules show a characteristic whorled pattern. The hilar lymph nodes most often are enlarged and also contain silicotic nodules.

Large fibrotic masses tend to be located mostly in the upper and posterior parts of the lungs; they are the result of coalescence of individual nodules when their profusion is high. Cavitation in large fibrotic masses can occur and most often is due to complicating tuberculous infection; cavitation due to ischemic necrosis is relatively rare in silicosis. Emphysema frequently is present when large fibrotic masses have developed. Enlargement of the right chambers of the heart and the pulmonary artery can be found in advanced silicosis.

In a classic example of nodular disease in gold miners, the quartz content of the lungs is 2.5 to 3 g of the total 7 to 10 g dust content; in foundry workers it is between 1 and 2 g with approximately 10 g total dust content. In contrast, in stellate or diffuse fibrosis in hematite miners, the total dust content may be 60 g with 3.5 g quartz, and in coal miners, 40 to 55 g with 1 to 1.5 g quartz.[21]

Silicotic nodules initially appear in the area of the respiratory bronchiole and around arterioles. The nodules consist of concentric layers of collagen; hyalinization of the collagen occurs with time and progresses from the center to the periphery of the nodule; reticulin fibers usually are present in the periphery. A cellular peripheral layer is characteristic of relatively early lesions; it consists mostly of fibroblasts and macrophages. Particles of silica can be found in the center of the nodules; polarized light is particularly useful to visualize the birefringent SiO_2 particles.

The alveoli around the silicotic nodule most often are normal, although scar emphysema occasionally can be observed; centrilobular emphysema is not a feature of silicosis.[22,23] Small pulmonary arterioles and venules are involved in the fibrotic process and often obliterated. With continuous exposure the silicotic nodules grow and new nodules appear. Progression may continue even after exposure has been discontinued, especially when the dust is characterized by high silica concentration and small particle size.

Coalescence of nodules occurs when the profusion of silicotic nodules has increased beyond a critical level. Dense hyalinized collagen masses develop in which individual nodules can still be identified, especially at the periphery. These lesions destroy the normal architecture of the lung; necrosis in the avascular center can occur even in the absence of tuberculous infection, although the latter is a frequent complication.

In rapidly developing silicosis, because of exposure to high concentrations of fine silica particles, the characteristic pathological features consist of the rapid development of numerous small nodules, together with areas of diffuse fibrosis and the rapid coalescence of nodules into large fibrotic masses.

Acute or hyperacute silicosis resembles idiopathic alveolar lipoproteinosis and has been associated with extremely high exposures to pure or almost pure free silica and very small particle sizes. The term *silico-lipoproteinosis* has been proposed for this condition.[24] Exposures in the manufacture of abrasive soap, quartz milling, the grinding of quartzite and sandstone to produce silica flour, and sandblasting with quartzite have been associated with silico-lipoproteinosis.

In this form of silicosis, the lungs are firm and edematous. A few silicotic nodules can be present; alveolar walls are infiltrated by mononuclear and plasma cells or thickened by fibrosis, and alveoli are filled with an eosinophilic PAS-positive lipid and proteinaceous fluid with numerous fine granules and desquamated cells. The latter are mostly type II alveolar cells, containing osmiophilic lamellar bodies. Diffuse interstitial pulmonary fibrosis is present, but silicotic nodules are rare or absent. These lesions have been reproduced in experimental animals exposed to inhalation of high concentrations of fine quartz particles.[25,26]

Proteinuria and renal failure have been associated with silica exposure from sandblasting or refractory bricks.[27,28] This appears to represent the effect of high levels of renal silicon dioxide crystals transferred to the kidney after pulmonary deposition.

Clinical Features. Classic nodular silicosis sometimes can be completely asymptomatic, although relatively numerous silicotic nodules can be present on the chest x-ray film. In most such cases, no abnormalities can be detected on physical examination. As the disease progresses, cough, sputum production, and dyspnea on exertion gradually develop in most cases. In some there is only a dry cough; in others small amounts of mucoid sputum are produced. An increased susceptibility to repeated respiratory infections develops in many patients and can result in larger amounts of mucopurulent sputum.

In the advanced stages of silicosis, distortion of the normal architecture of the bronchi develops, especially when coalescence into massive fibrosis has taken place. Rhonchi and wheezes can be detected in such cases and paroxysms of coughing can occur. Shortness of breath develops gradually as the disease progresses; initially it is limited to heavy exercise, but later it manifests itself with moderate or even minor efforts. Physical signs are practically absent in the initial stages of silicosis. With the development of massive fibrosis or of a major infectious complication such as tuberculosis, abnormalities on percussion and auscultation (rales, rhonchi, areas of reduced or increased resonance) and cyanosis can develop.

Cor pulmonale is the most frequent complication of silicosis in industrialized countries. Pulmonary hypertension, with a loud second pulmonic sound and corresponding electrocardiographic signs, can be detected; overt congestive heart failure with hepatomegaly and peripheral edema is less frequent and is thought to occur mainly in cases with significant associated emphysema or marked chronic bronchitis.

In patients with "acute" silicosis similar to idiopathic alveolar lipoproteinosis, symptoms develop rapidly over a period of several weeks or months; time from onset of exposure to first symptoms can vary from less than 1 year to a few years. Fatigue, cough, sputum production (mostly mucoid), chest pain of pleuritic type, rapidly progressive shortness of breath, weight loss, and rapid deterioration are characteristic for such cases. Shortness of breath at rest, cyanosis, and abnormalities on percussion and auscultation with presence of crepitations are noted frequently. The rapid and fatal course of the disease leads to death in hypoxic respiratory failure.[29]

Radiographic Findings. The radiographic changes in silicosis are essential for the diagnosis and classification of the disease, for the evaluation of its progression, and for the detection of important complications, such as tuberculosis, emphysema, and cor pulmonale. Nevertheless, it should be emphasized that pathological changes precede, often by several years, the appearance of the earliest radiographic changes, since to be detected on the standard posteroanterior chest film the pathological changes (silicotic nodules) have to reach a certain size, profusion, and radiological density. Because of this radiological latency period of silicosis, a normal chest x-ray film does not exclude the existence of the pathological process of silicosis in a person with significant exposure. Nevertheless, the disease seldom is symptomatic in this stage of radiological latency, with the notable exceptions of "acute silicosis," alveolar lipoproteinosis, and chronic bronchitis due to silica.

The earliest radiographic changes consist of fine linear-reticular opacities, often described as "lace-like" in the upper and middle lung fields and extending to the periphery. These linear-reticular opacities increase in thickness with time.

The most characteristic radiographic abnormalities are silicotic nodules (Fig. 19–1), which usually appear initially in the middle and upper right lung fields. The earliest discrete round opacities are small, with a diameter of 1 to 3 mm and of low radiopacity. The diameter of silicotic nodules increases with time, as does their profusion and radiopacity, and they become more visible in most of the lung fields, with the exception of the lower lateral areas. The International Labor Office's *Classification of Radiographs of Pneumoconioses* (1980) grades simple silicosis according to the profusion of the opacities, from 1/0 to 3/+, and to the size of most of the nodules, p for less than 1.5 mm, q for between 1.5 and 3 mm, and r for opacities with a diameter of more than 3 mm but less than 10 mm. The nodules often are seen against a background of a linear-reticular pattern.

As the number of rounded opacities increases, the profusion progresses, and eventually coalescence of nodules, initially in small limited areas in the upper lateral parts of the lung fields, becomes apparent. At this stage when coalescence into large opacities is suspected (and their size is relatively small, less than 5 cm in diameter), they are classified as Ax. This marks the point at which simple silicosis progresses to complicated silicosis.

As the large opacity becomes definite, it is classified according to size into category A (less than 5 cm), B (one or more opacities with a diameter of more than 5 cm but with a combined area

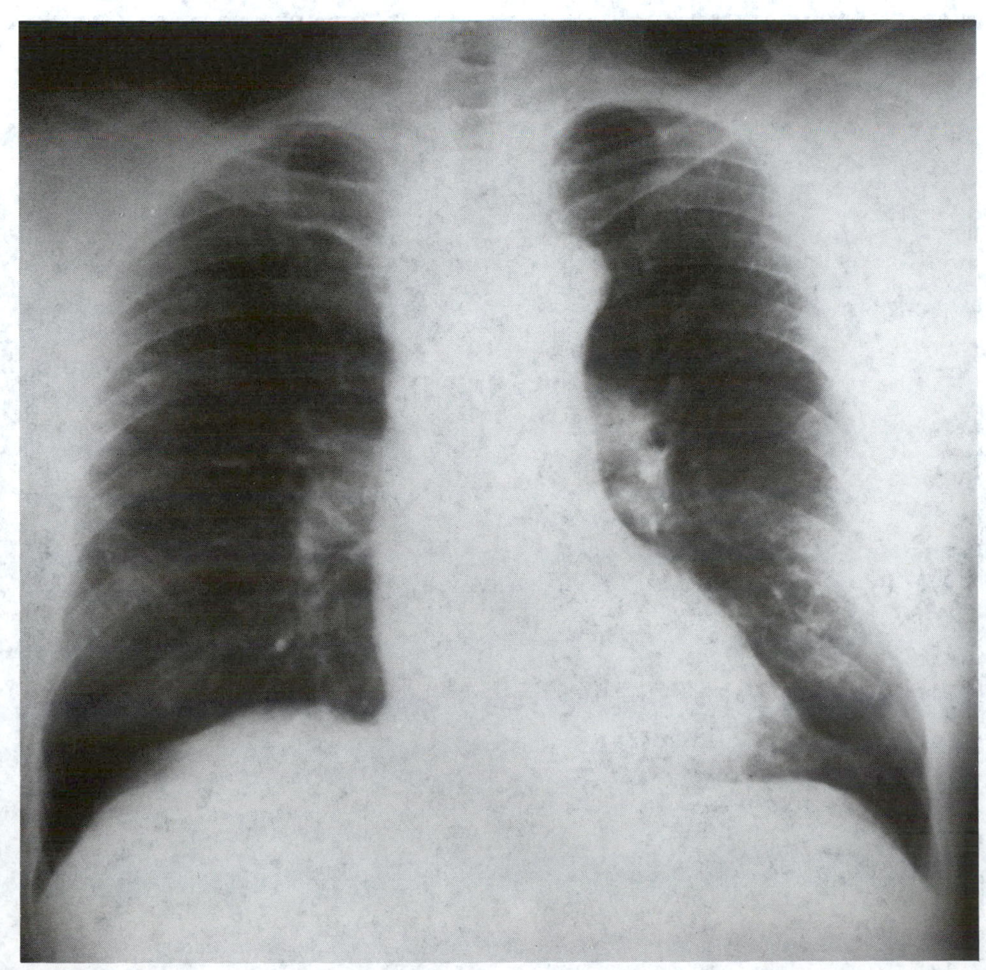

Figure 19–1. Simple silicosis. Small, rounded opacities (q-diameter, approximately 3 mm) in upper lung fields, bilaterally.

of less than the equivalent of the right upper zone), and C (one or more opacities whose combined area exceeds the equivalent of the right upper zone). The large opacities in silicosis usually are bilateral and most often located in the upper, but also in the middle, lung fields (Figs. 19–2 and 19–3). When the opacities are observed over time, contraction may be noted, and migration to the enlarged hilar opacities is not unusual. Distortion of the pulmonary and mediastinal structures is frequent in this stage, as are emphysematous changes, including bullae, in the rest of the lung. Hilar lymph node enlargement is observed quite consistently in silicosis; calcification of the periphery of the lymph nodes, "eggshell" calcification, may be present occasionally. Pleural adhesions also may be found; quite characteristic are the longitudinal pleural plicatures extending from the diaphragmatic pleura along the interlobal fissures.

In acute silicosis the radiological latency period, a few months to 2 years, is much shorter than in classic silicosis. The radiological abnormalities are different from those of classic (nodular) silicosis, a fact that may have contributed to the underestimation of the incidence of this form of silicosis. Early changes consist of a diffuse haziness of reticular, irregular opacities in the middle and lower lung fields. Rounded and linear opacities develop rapidly over the entire lung fields. Occasionally, very small opacities are the main feature. The hilar shadows are only moderately enlarged. Rapid coalescence and large opacities, sometimes involving an entire lobe, can be observed in some cases; in others the numerous small, rounded opacities do not coalesce, and death ensues rapidly.

Alveolar lipoproteinosis is characterized by diffuse, hazy infiltrates found most often in the lower lung fields, particularly above the diaphragm. Changes similar to those characteristic for pulmonary edema are present sometimes; in other cases, small, rounded opacities indicating alveolar filling can be observed.

Pulmonary Function. With classic silicosis the typical change in pulmonary function is a gradual reduction in lung volume, beginning with reduction in vital capacity. The functional changes are less than would be predicted from the radiographic evidence. Airway obstruction, however, often is present because chronic bronchitis frequently coexists, especially in foundry workers, brickworkers, hematite miners, and workers in user industries. The diffusing capacity is normal until relatively late in the course of the disease. Thus in classic silicosis there is a decrease in total lung capacity, vital capacity, and residual volume, with arterial blood oxygen tension normal or slightly decreased. A mixed pattern of restrictive and obstructive ventilatory dysfunction is found most often in advanced, complicated silicosis.

Imbalance of ventilation-perfusion occurs in the more advanced stages of the disease. Impairment of gas exchange and signs of cor pulmonale can develop. The coexistence of chronic bronchitis with airway obstruction results in reduced forced expiratory volume in 1 second (FEV_1), reduced flow at 25% to 75% of vital capacity, and in increased airway resistance. With severe obstruction arterial blood oxygen tension is reduced and carbon dioxide tension increased. Acute silicolipoproteinosis almost always causes marked restrictive dysfunction with reduced diffusing capacity and arterial desaturation.

Complications. The complications of silicosis include tuberculosis, cor pulmonale, and Caplan's syndrome.

Tuberculosis has been the most persistent problem over the past 150 years. There is no doubt that involvement of the lungs

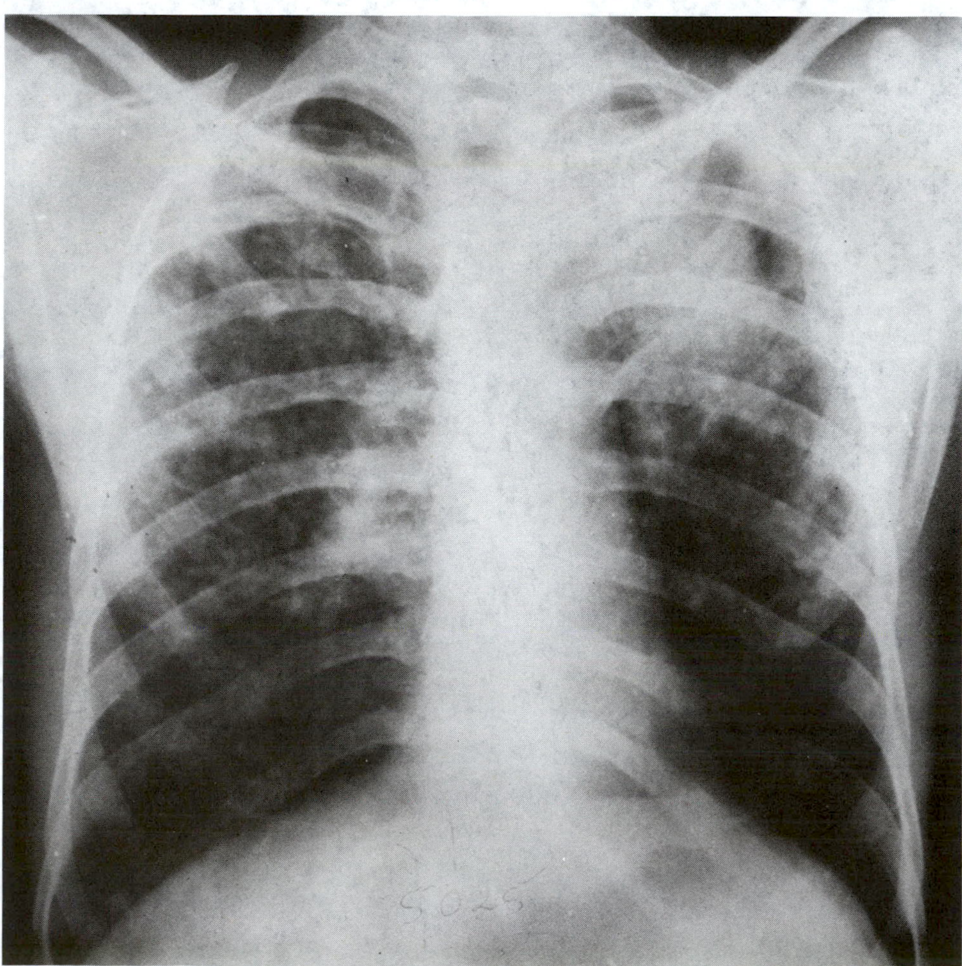

Figure 19–2. Small, rounded opacities (r-diameter, approximately 3 to 10 mm) predominantly in upper and middle lung fields; large opacity due to coalescence of nodules in left upper lung field (size B, according to International Classification of Radiographs of Pneumoconioses).

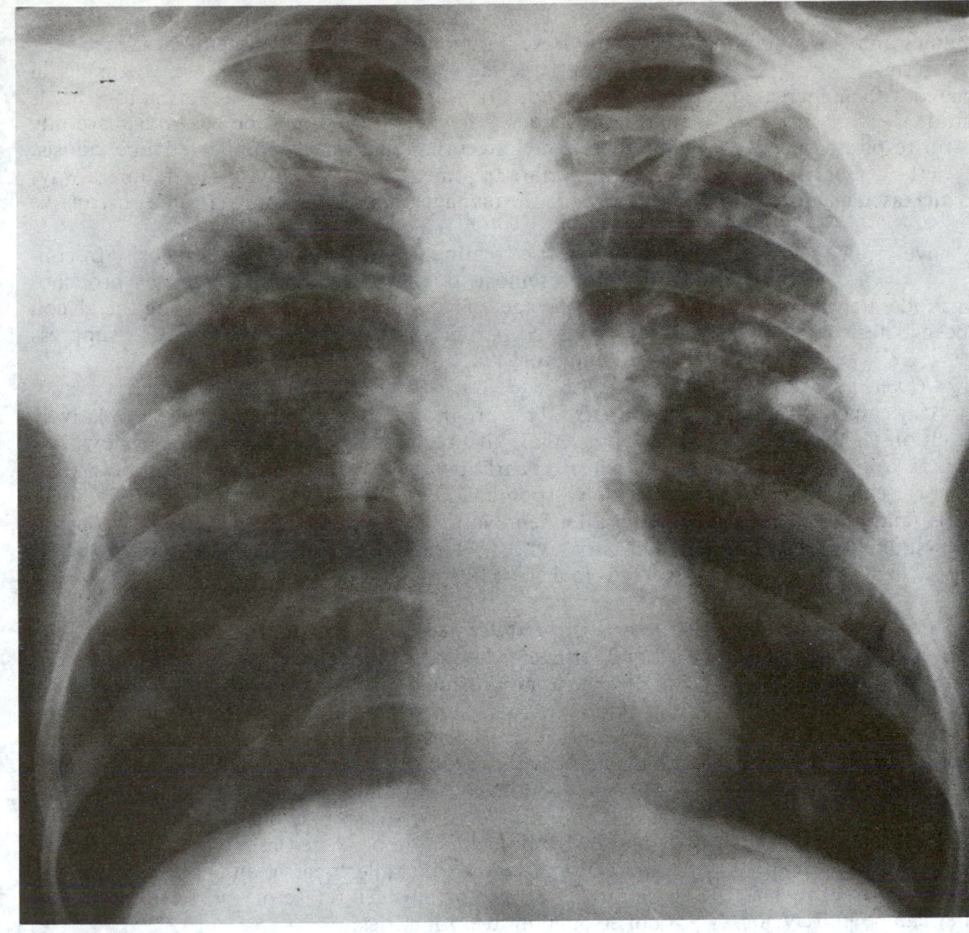

Figure 19–3. Rounded opacities (r/q) in upper and middle lung fields; bilateral multiple large opacities due to coalescence of nodules.

by silicosis increases the susceptibility for tuberculosis infection. In contrast, there is no added risk of tuberculosis after exposure to asbestos or other nonsilica dusts. Thus patients with silicosis in whom tuberculosis is suspected on the basis of a positive tuberculin test and a suggestive x-ray film should be treated with antituberculous chemotherapy because demonstration of mycobacteria by smear or culture is difficult in silicotuberculosis, and the disease sometimes advances rapidly.

Chronic bronchitis is not infrequent in some occupational groups exposed to silica dust, such as foundrymen.[9] Bronchitis due to acute or subacute infections of the distorted bronchi associated with advanced silicosis has been well characterized.

Emphysema is considered a side effect in the silicotic process. Small areas of scar emphysema can be found around nodules; coalescence of nodules into fibrotic masses often produces larger areas of emphysema, often bullous, mostly in the lower lung fields.

Cor pulmonale is a well-recognized complication of silicosis; the massive involvement of the pulmonary vasculature in the fibrotic process with obliteration of numerous arterioles eventually results in a marked increase in resistance and consequently in pulmonary artery pressure. Right ventricular heart failure with overt clinical signs is seen less frequently, although it is not unusual. In such cases death due to congestive heart failure can occur. In cases with coexistent emphysema and chronic bronchitis with marked airflow obstruction or complicating tuberculosis, right ventricular heart failure is encountered more frequently.

Progressive systemic sclerosis (scleroderma) has been reported by some investigators to be associated with silicosis with a frequency greater than would be expected in the population at large. It is not clear in these cases whether the association was merely due to coincidence.

Caplan's syndrome, the association between rheumatoid arthritis and silicosis, is rare. It is characterized by the appearance of large nodules (more than 1 cm in diameter) on a background of preexisting silicotic nodules. The larger nodules of Caplan's syndrome occasionally cavitate.

Renal lesions have been described in cases in which heavy occupational exposure to free silica has led to silico-lipoproteinosis. Glomerular and tubular lesions have been described. Proteinuria and hypertension were associated with these renal lesions.[22] The silica content of the kidney was found to be high in such cases.

In recent years the problem of a possible carcinogenic effect of silica has received considerable attention. Experimental studies on the possible carcinogenic effect of crystalline silica have been conducted on rats, mice, and hamsters, using various routes of administration: inhalation, intratracheal instillation, intrapleural, and intraperitoneal injection.

Findings from these studies were negative in mice and hamsters. In rats the incidence of adenocarcinoma of the lung and squamous cell carcinoma was significantly increased, and the intraperitoneal injections caused malignant lymphomas.

In a substantial mortality experience reported from Hamburg,[29] lung cancer occurred in 2.3% of 688 deaths from silicosis and in 3.99% of 212,887 control deaths in men over 20 years of age.

Epidemiological studies have been conducted on numerous silica-exposed groups, such as metal ore miners, coal miners, and workers in the granite and stone industry, the ceramics, glass, and related industries, foundries, and in persons diagnosed as having silicosis. There were methodologic difficulties with many of these studies; confounding by cigarette smoking and insufficient information on exposure to other carcinogens, such as radon (mostly in mining and quarrying operations), polycyclic aromatic hydrocarbons (mostly in foundries), and arsenic (in metal ore mining and possibly in the ceramics and glass industries), were the most important issues of concern.

Metal ore mining has not been associated with an increased incidence of respiratory cancer in some studies[30,31]; in other cohorts of metal ore miners, mortality rates for respiratory cancer were found to be 20% to 50% above levels in the general population.[32,33] In most studies of coal miners no increased incidence of lung cancer has been detected.

Studies of granite workers generally have yielded negative findings also.[34,35]

In the ceramics and pottery industry a moderately increased mortality from respiratory cancer has been detected in some studies.[36,37]

A number of recent reports on foundry workers have pointed to slightly to moderately increased respiratory cancer mortality.[38-40]

The International Agency for Research on Cancer monograph on the evaluation of the carcinogenic risk of silica (1987) concluded that "there is sufficient evidence for carcinogenicity of crystalline silica to experimental animals [and that] there is limited evidence for the carcinogenicity of crystalline silica to humans."[13]

Diagnosis. A history of exposure to free silica is important for the diagnosis of silicosis. A detailed work history is necessary, with appropriate attention to occupations held in the past, since the latency period for the appearance of characteristic chest x-ray abnormalities is often decades, especially with relatively low silica concentrations in the airborne dust.

The other essential element for a correct diagnosis of silicosis is a good quality chest x-ray film. Nodular silicosis is not difficult to recognize, although nodular opacities can be found in many other diseases. Enlarged hilar opacities are quite characteristic for silicosis. Pulmonary function tests are not particularly helpful in the diagnosis of silicosis since they can be entirely normal in the presence of well-developed nodular opacities. When abnormalities are present, they are most often of a mixed, obstructive-restrictive type, although cases with only restrictive or obstructive dysfunction also can be found.

The differential diagnosis has to exclude conditions such as sarcoidosis, miliary tuberculosis, carcinomatous lymphangitis, pulmonary hemosiderosis, rheumatoid lung, fibrosing alveolitis, alveolar microlithiasis, and histoplasmosis.

Massive fibrosis seldom presents difficulties in diagnosis, although early in its development, when a single large opacity is detected, differential diagnosis with lung cancer can be a problem. The presence of nodular opacities around the large opacity most often facilitates the correct diagnosis of silicosis with coalescent, massive fibrosis.

The diagnosis of tuberculosis in the presence of silicosis is difficult; this complication should always be considered, and frequent sputum cultures are indicated.

The diagnosis of acute silicosis is more difficult than that of classic nodular silicosis because the radiographic changes are less characteristic and the clinical course more rapid. Idiopathic alveolar proteinosis, acute allergic alveolitis, and tuberculosis have to be considered in the differential diagnosis. A careful occupational history with evidence of exposure to high silica dust levels is extremely important for the diagnosis of this form of silicosis.

Treatment. Although poly-2-vinyl-pyridine-1-oxide and polybetaine prevent silicosis in experimental animals, possibly by altering the surface charge on silica particles, the results of clinical trials have been unrewarding. Treatment of patients with silicosis by the inhalation of powdered aluminum was undertaken in the 1950s, but aluminum itself carries the risk of diffuse interstitial fibrosis. Thus neither of these forms of prophylactic treatment can be recommended.

There is no specific treatment for established silicosis; therapy of complications, such as bronchitis and pneumonitis, is important to prevent rapid deterioration of functional status.

Prompt treatment of silico-tuberculosis with regimens in which isoniazid, rifampin, and ethambutol are given together is most satisfactory. The treatment should be vigorous, carefully monitored, and longer than that for uncomplicated tuberculosis.

Appropriate treatment for congestive heart failure always has to include the management of coexisting chronic obstructive bronchitis.

No specific treatment is useful for acute silicosis. In contrast, lipoproteinosis due to silica can be treated by bronchopulmonary lavage, which may be helpful in clearing the alveoli of the deposited particles,[41] and by steroid therapy to suppress the inflammatory reaction.

Prognosis. The prognosis for nodular silicosis is relatively good, particularly if the progression of the disease is slow. For acute silicosis, early death is almost the rule. Lipoproteinosis may resolve spontaneously without treatment or may improve rapidly after removal of free silica from the lung by bronchopulmonary lavage. There is some evidence that lipoproteinosis proceeds to diffuse fibrosis if left untreated.[42]

Control and Prevention. The recognition of the silicosis hazard and stringent dust control engineering measures are essential. Frequent monitoring of airborne dust levels is needed to ensure a safe working environment. The effectiveness of dust control measures in preventing silicosis has been emphasized dramatically by the reduction in silicosis in Great Britain and the European Economic Community since sandblasting was outlawed. A special effort is necessary to avoid exposure to cristobalite and tridymite, which are produced in the calcining of silica within diatomaceous earth, fuller's earth, and particularly in the regrinding of broken or salvaged refractory brick, in the scaling of boilers, and in steel foundries.

Reduction of exposure to quartz above the threshold limit value of

$$\frac{10\ \mathrm{mg/m^3}}{\%\mathrm{SiO_2} + 2}$$

would reduce the silicosis attack rate considerably. The National Institute for Occupational Safety and Health has proposed a further reduction of the time-weighted average silica exposure to 50 $\mu g/m^3$. The effects of dust levels on other workers in the area must be considered because even if sandblasters or brick grinders are protected by appropriate respirators, workers in other trades within the same area may be affected. Failure to apply occupational standards to workplaces employing five or fewer workers also has resulted in cases of silicosis. In addition, it appears essential to regard silica in quantities of 5% or less within other rock, such as limestone, kaolin, gypsum, graphite, or portland cement, as important and capable of producing disease if total dust concentrations are as high as they often are in mining or other operations. The problem of silica exposure in foundries is well known and may require changes in technology to bring it under control. Personal respiratory protection is valuable when it is otherwise impossible to control environmental dust levels.

REFERENCES

1. Jain SM, Sepha GC, Khare KC, Dubey VS: Silicosis in slate pencil workers. Chest 71:423–426, 1977
2. Buechner HA, Ansari A: Acute silico-proteinosis, a new pathologic variant of acute silicosis in sandblasters, characterized by histologic features resembling alveolar proteinosis. Dis Chest 55:274–284, 1969
3. Banks DE, Morring KL, Boehlecke BE: Silicosis in the 1980's. Am Ind Hyg Assoc J 42(1):77–79, 1981

4. Zimmerman PV, Sinclair RA: Rapidly progressive fatal silicosis in a young man. Med J Aust 2:704–706, 1981
5. Banks DE, Morring KL, Boehlecke BE: Silicosis in silica flour workers. Am Rev Respir Dis 124:445–450, 1981
6. Gantner BA: Respiratory hazard from removal of ceramic fiber insulation from high temperature industrial furnaces. Am Ind Hyg Assoc J 47:530–534, 1986
7. Ashe HB, Bergstrom DE: Twenty six years' experience with dust control in the Vermont granite industry. Ind Med Surg 33:973–978, 1964
8. Trasko VM: Some facts on the prevalence of silicosis in the United States. Arch Ind Health 14:379–386, 1956
9. Lloyd-Davies TAL: Respiratory Disease in Foundry Men. London: HM Stationary Office, 1971
10. Phibbs BP, Sundin RE, Mitchell RS: Silicosis in Wyoming bentonite workers. Am Rev Respir Dis 103:1–17, 1971
11. Watts WF, Parker DR, Johnson RL, Jensen KL: Analysis of Data on Respirable Quartz Dust Samples Collected in Metal and Nonmetal Mines and Mills. Information Circular 8967. Washington D.C.: Bureau of Mines, U.S. Department of the Interior, 1984
12. Jankowski RA, Nesbit RE, Kissel FN: Concepts for controlling quartz dust exposure of coal mine workers. In Peng SS (ed): Coal Mine Dust Conference Proceedings. Cincinnati: American Conference of Governmental Industrial Hygienists, 1984, pp 126–136
13. Silica and some silicates. In Evaluation of the Carcinogenic Risk of Chemicals to Humans, vol. 42. International Agency for Research on Cancer, 1987, pp 39–143
14. Hughes JM, Jones RN, Gilson JC, et al: Determinants of progression in sandblasters' silicosis. In Walton WH (ed): Inhaled Particles V. Oxford: Pergamon Press, 1983, p 701
15. Davis GS: Pathogenesis of silicosis. Lung 164:139–154, 1986
16. Begin R, Masse S, Sebastian P, Martel M, Bosse J, Duois F, Geoffroy M, Labbe J: Sustained efficacy of aluminum to reduce quartz toxicity in the lung. Exp Lung Res 13:205–222, 1987
17. Jones RN, Turner-Warwick M, Ziskind M, Weill H: High prevalence of antinuclear antibodies in sandblaster silicosis. Am Rev Respir Dis 113:393–395, 1976
18. Turner-Warwick M, Cole P, Weill H, Jones RN, Ziskind M: Chemical fibrosis: The model of silica. Ann Rheum Dis 36(suppl):47–50, 1977
19. Warrell DA, Harrison BDW, Fawcett IW, et al: Silicosis among grindstone cutters in North Nigeria. Thorax 30:389–398, 1975
20. Lewis DM, Burrel R: Induction of fibrogenesis by lung antibody treated macrophages. Br J Ind Med 33:25–28, 1976
21. Nagelschmidt G: The relationship between lung dust and lung pathology in pneumoconiosis. Br J Ind Med 17:247–259, 1960
22. Gardner LV: Pathology of so-called acute silicosis. Am J Public Health 23:1240–1249, 1930
23. Heppleston AG: The fibrogenic action of silica. Br Med Bull 25:282–287, 1969
24. Parkes WR: Diseases due to free silica. In Occupational Lung Disorders. 2 edt. London: Butterworth, 1982, pp 134–174
25. Gross P, deTreville RTP: Alveolar proteinosis: Its experimental production in rodents. Arch Pathol 86:255–261, 1968
26. Heppleston AG: A typical reaction to inhaled silica. Nature 213: 199–200, 1967
27. Saldanha LF, Rosen VJ: Silicon nephropathy. Am J Med 59:95–103, 1975
28. Giles RD, Sturgill BC, Suratt PM, Bolton WK: Massive proteinuria and acute renal failure in a patient with acute silico-proteinosis. Am J Med 64:336–342, 1978
29. Ruttner JR, Heer HR: Silikose and Lungenkarzinom. Schweiz Med Wochenschr 99:245–249, 1969
30. Brown DP, Kalplan SD, Zumwalde RD, Kaplowitz M, Archer VE: Retrospective cohort mortality study of underground gold mine workers. In Goldsmith DF, Winn DM, Shy CM (eds): Silica, Silicosis, and Cancer. Controversy in Occupational Medicine. New York: Praeger, 1986, pp 335–350
31. Lawler AB, Mandel JS, Scuman LM, Lubin JH: Mortality study of Minnesota iron ore miners: Preliminary results. In Wagner WL, Rom WN, Merchant JA (eds): Health Issues Related to Metal and Nonmetallic Mining. Boston: Butterworths, 1983, pp 211–226
32. Muller J, Wheeler WC, Gentleman JF, Suranyi G, Kusiak RA: Study of Mortality of Ontario Miners, 1955–1977. Part I. Toronto: Ontario Ministry of Labour/Ontario Workers' Compensation Board/Atomic Energy Control Board of Canada, 1983
33. Costello J: Mortality of metal miners. A Retrospective Cohort and Case-Control Study. In Proceedings of an Environmental Health Conference, Park City, Utah, 6–9 April 1982. Morgantown, WV: National Institute of Occupational Safety and Health, 1982
34. Davis LK, Wegman DH, Monson RR, Froines J: Mortality experience of Vermont granite miners. Am J Ind Med 4:705–723, 1983
35. Costello J, Graham WGB: Vermont granite workers' mortality study. In Goldsmith DF, Winn DM, Shy CM (eds): Silica, Silicosis, and Cancer. Controversy in Occupational Medicine, New York: Praeger, 1986, pp 437–440
36. Thomas TL: A preliminary investigation of mortality among workers in the pottery industry. Int J Epidemiol 27:175–180, 1982
37. Forastiere F, Lagorio S, Michelozzi P, Cavariani F, Arca M, Borgia P, Perucci C, Axelson O: Silica, silicosis, and lung cancer among ceramic workers: A case-referent study. Am J Ind Med 10:363–370, 1986
38. Sherson D, Iversen E: Mortality among foundry workers in Denmark due to cancer and respiratory and cardiovascular disease. In Goldsmith DF, Winn DM, Shy CM (eds): Silica, Silicosis, and Cancer. Controversy in Occupational Medicine, New York: Praeger, 1986, pp 403–414
39. Fletcher AC: The mortality of foundry workers in the United Kingdom. In Goldsmith DF, Winn DM, Shy CM (eds): Silica, Silicosis, and Cancer. Controversy in Occupational Medicine, New York: Praeger, 1986, pp 385–401
40. Silverstein M, Maizlish N, Park R, Silverstein B, Brodsky L, Mirer F: Mortality among ferrous foundry workers. Am J Ind Med 10:27–43, 1986
41. Ramieriz RJ, Keiffer RE, Ball WC: Bronchopulmonary lavage in man. Ann Intern Med 63:819–828, 1965
42. Hudson AR, Halprine GM, Miller JA, Kilburn KH: Pulmonary interstitial fibrosis following alveolar proteinosis. Chest 65:700–702, 1974

20

Health Significance of Metals

Philippe Grandjean

The term *metal* has important meanings in physics and chemistry. In environmental medicine the term is interpreted slightly differently, so that arsenic and selenium are included with the metals. Nutritionists often refer to trace metals as those constituting less than 1 g of the human body, an arbitrary limit that would exclude iron. Although *toxic metals* is a term commonly applied to a specific group of metals, all metals have toxic effects if given in sufficient quantity. Frequently heavy metals (those with a gravity of 4 g/cm^3 and above) are considered the greatest health hazard. This belief is related to the observation that the toxicity of the metals tends to increase toward the right and downward in the periodic system. However, gravity as such is of little medical significance and would not account for the toxic potential of beryllium. Rather, the relative toxicity on a molar basis would seem to be related to the affinity to various ligands and the resulting biochemical activity. On the basis of such considerations, the metals may be separated into soft metals (class B), with a higher affinity for sulfur and nitrogen than toward oxygen, and hard metals (class A), in which the opposite is the case.[1]

Among the metals considered in this chapter, aluminum, barium, beryllium, magnesium, and lanthanides (rare earths) belong to the less toxic class A, and the other metals are either borderline or class B metals.

In contrast to organic compounds, which may be broken down by detoxification processes, metals always remain metals. However, some changes may occur because of oxidation and reduction, as with mercury vapor and chromate, and most metals are bound to organic compounds, notably proteins such as transferrin or metallothioneine. Some metals form rather stable organometal compounds with a covalent bond between carbon and the metal. Some organic compounds, such as tetra-alkyl lead, are dealkylated in the body. On the other hand, methylation in the liver is an important part of arsenic and selenium kinetics. These metabolic processes frequently result in changed toxic potentials.

When metal is present as airborne particles, retention in the airways is governed by physical principles related to the aerodynamic diameter of the particles. Some metal compounds are corrosive and exert their effects on the mucous membranes. Such is the case with osmium tetroxide and zinc chloride. In other situations, systemic effects, whether mediated by oral or respiratory intake, are most important and depend on the amount absorbed. Solubility of metal compounds then becomes significant. In the gut some interaction between metals may occur. Zinc and copper tend to mutually inhibit the absorption of each other. The same appears to be true for iron and cobalt, but the absorption of both is increased in iron deficiency. In addition, phosphate and other components may decrease the absorption because of the formation of insoluble compounds. The variability is illustrated by the fact that gastrointestinal absorption of lead sulfide is barely detectable, but a soluble compound ingested during a fasting period may result in a 50% absorption.

Exposure potentials have increased considerably because of the development of metallurgy and associated processes and the contamination from energy production. Workers, surroundings, and consumers may now be heavily exposed to chemical elements rare in the earth's crust. Air pollution with lead from human activities is more than 10 times greater than atmospheric emissions of lead from natural sources. The amounts of cadmium, zinc, and other metals in anthropogenic air pollution also are comparatively large. Table 20–1 shows an arbitrary grouping of some metals according to their abundance and the annual production rate. Although only major tendencies would appear from such crude grouping, the rarer metals seem to cause much less prevalent exposures than do the metals common in the earth's crust. However, production figures tend to increase, and a doubling is expected within a decade or two for several metals, in particular, aluminum, molybdenum, nickel, and rare earths.

The metals have all occurred in the biosphere since primeval times, although mostly in lower concentrations than today; some of the common metals actually were used in metabolic processes and became essential nutrients (Table 20–1). When the intake of essential metals is insufficient, signs of deficiency may develop. Many such cases have occurred as part of multiple nutrient deficiencies or as a result of long-term parenteral nutrition.

The increased metal exposure levels also have possible toxicological significance.[2] When toxicity is compared, the rare metals appear to be more toxic than the elements that are more common components of the earth's crust and the "natural" environment. In Table 20–1, the molar limits for occupational exposure have been used for classifying metals into three groups with different toxicities. LD_{50} values from animal experiments could have been used also and would yield almost the same results.

In preventive medicine the target organ is of special importance. The earliest effects of metal toxicity are said to originate from the target organ, sometimes referred to as the critical organ. As a consequence, if effects in the target organ can be

TABLE 20-1. NATURAL OCCURRENCE, PRODUCTION, AND HEALTH SIGNIFICANCE OF METALS AS INDICATED BY ARBITRARY GROUPING OF RELEVANT PARAMETERS

Abundance in Earth's Crust	Annual (1978) Production	Occupational Exposure Limit	Significance of Daily Oral Intake
▪ GROUP I			
Common ($>10^{-2}$ mol/kg)	Large ($>10^{11}$ mol/y)	High ($>10^{-4}$ mol/m^3)	Deficiency recorded
Al, Fe, Mg, Mn, Ti	Al, Cu, Fe, Mg, Mn, Zn	Al, Fe, Mg, Ti, Zn	Cr, Cu, Fe, Mg, Se, Zn
▪ GROUP II			
Medium (10^{-4}–10^{-2} mol/kg)	Medium (10^{9}–10^{11} mol/y)	Medium (10^{-6}–10^{-4} mol/m^3)	Unknown or no significance
Ba, Be, Co, Cr, Cu, Ni, V, Zn, Zr	Ba, Cr, Mo, Ni, Pb, Sb, Sn, Ti, Zr	As, Ba, Be, Cd, Co, Cr, Cu, Mn, Mo, Ni, Sb, Se, Sn, Ta, V, W, Zr, rare earths	Ag, Al, Be, Mn, Mo, Ni, Os, Pt, Sb, Sn, Ta, Te, Ti, Tl, V, W, Zr, rare earths
▪ GROUP III			
Rare ($<10^{-4}$ mol/kg)	Low ($<10^{9}$ mol/y)	Low ($<10^{-6}$ mol/m^3)	Environmental toxicity recorded
Ag, As, Cd, Hg, Mo, Os, Pb, Pt, Sb, Se, Sn, Ta, Te, Tl, U, W, rare earths	Ag, As, Be, Cd, Co, Hg, Os, Pt, Se, Ta, Te, Tl, U, V, W, rare earths	Ag, Hg, Os, Pb, Pt, Te, Tl, U	As, Ba, Cd, Co, Hg, Pb, U

Modified from data collected by Bergqvist.[2]

prevented, no other toxicity should be expected. However, prevention becomes somewhat more difficult when considering that the critical effect of respiratory exposure to chromate or nickel compounds is respiratory cancer; such stochastic effects may be totally prevented only if exposures are eliminated effectively. Other complex problems relate to the prevention of contact dermatitis in persons who have developed metal allergies; even oral intake of the offending metal has in some cases induced or worsened the hand eczema. Individual susceptibility therefore must be taken into account. In this regard interactions between metals are also important. Thus zinc supplements may prevent cadmium toxicity in experimental animals, and mercury and selenium seem to form a rather stable complex that has a low toxicity.

Acute, fulminant cases of poisoning rarely are difficult to diagnose, in part because of the immediate relation to the exposure. As preventive efforts become more efficient, the patterns of adverse effects change and in fact become more difficult to recognize. Most metals accumulate to some degree in the body, and storage depots or "slow compartments" may slowly release metals to the blood or may actually be the site of delayed toxicity. Insidious, delayed effects of chronic exposures often are hard for the clinician and patient to detect. In the absence of pathognomonic symptoms and a history of a recent hazardous exposure, an etiological diagnosis may be impossible to verify. If no causative explanation is found, specific preventive precautions are hard to suggest. Thus the partial success of prevention actually makes further preventive efforts more difficult.

The human body has a certain capacity to withstand potentially adverse effects of environmental exposures. Exposures to toxic metals may not necessarily result in apparent toxicity; low doses could conceivably cause a weakening of the body defenses, that is, a decrease in reserve capacity.[3] This effect may not be readily observable, but it could lead to increased susceptibility to subsequent exposures to other hazards. This interaction would be in accordance with the notion of multicausal disease. Although metals by such mechanisms may increase the risk of developing a range of diseases, their contribution will be difficult to document in individual cases.

The diagnosis of acute metal poisoning frequently has been supported by the detection of increased or toxic levels of the metal in blood or urine. Methods have now been further refined and become routine parameters for biological monitoring of metal exposures.[4] Recent developments have included more sensitive analyses and methods for in vivo detection of cadmium in kidney and liver, for measurement of lead levels in teeth, and for assessment of various biochemical abnormalities that indicate early biological effects of metal exposures. Biological monitoring is expected to become an important part of future preventive activities with regard to environmental and occupational metal exposures. However, because metals are ubiquitous and often disseminated through a multitude of pathways, the sources of human exposures must be known before a preventive strategy can be planned.[5]

In the following pages, individual metals are dealt with in alphabetical order. The general outline includes environmental occurrence, uses, and exposure sources; absorption and fate in the human organism; essential functions and toxic effects in humans; diagnosis; and preventive measures and limits applicable. References have been limited to a few key studies or reports. For more detailed information and reference to additional literature sources, some recent handbooks should be consulted.[6,7]

ALUMINUM

Exposures. Aluminum is the most common metal in the earth's crust. The most important aluminum ore is bauxite, but andalusite also is used. Aluminum is a light metal with a high resistance against corrosion and is used in light metal alloys, in particular with magnesium. Kitchenware, aluminum foil, and automobile bodies are important uses, and the aircraft industry is one of the major consumers. The most intense occupational exposures occur in the aluminum refineries, where the metal is produced by electrolysis of aluminum oxide dissolved in molten cryolite. Refinery and foundry workers, welders, and grinders working with aluminum or its alloys may be exposed to high levels of aluminum fumes or particles. Aluminum chloride is used in petroleum processing and in the rubber industry, and alkyl compounds are used as catalysts in the production of polyethylene. Other aluminum compounds also are widely used, notably for flocculation of drinking water and medical treatment of ulcers.

Aluminum compounds in soil are soluble at a pH below 5.5, and soft drinking water may contain 1 mg/L or more of aluminum flocculants. Water levels usually are below 10 μg/L. Dairy products and fish contain little aluminum, but meat products and vegetables may exhibit relatively high levels. The total daily intake through food and beverages usually is between 5 and 10 mg, but much higher intake levels have been recorded. Aluminum silicate is used as an anticaking agent, and milligram quantities frequently occur as part of the normal daily intake. Small amounts may be released from aluminum pots and pans at low pH levels, especially when rhubarb or other acid foods are heated. Much higher intakes originate from antacid therapeutics, and ulcer patients may ingest several grams of aluminum hydroxide every day.[8]

Aluminum is barely absorbed from the gastrointestinal tract, probably because sparingly soluble aluminum phosphate is formed. Patients who ingest aluminum-containing antacids appear to absorb about 0.1% of the amount ingested. In the presence of citrate, aluminum is much more readily absorbed. Inhaled fine aluminum dust can be retained in the alveoli with the potential for chronic effects. Although other organs do not retain aluminum for long periods, aluminum concentration in the lungs increases with advancing age. When released to the blood, aluminum appears to be effectively excreted, almost entirely in the urine.

Effects. Salts of aluminum are irritants because acid is liberated on hydrolysis. Thus conjunctivitis, eczema, and upper airway irritation may result from aerosol exposures; even local necrosis of the cornea has been recorded. Pulmonary changes have been described in persons with severe occupational exposure to bauxite fumes during World War II. This so-called shaver's disease probably was caused by the combined effects of quartz and aluminum dust. More recently exposures to fine aluminum oxide dust (probably about 50 mg/m^3) apparently have caused irregular opacities on chest x-ray films, and this simple pneumoconiosis has been named aluminum lung or aluminosis, although the pathogenesis is by no means clear.[9] The most frequent symptoms of aluminosis are dyspnea and dry cough. Early reports suggested that lung fibrosis occurred in cryolite workers, but more recent studies have suggested that the fibrogenicity of this aluminum ore is minimal. Unilateral pneumothorax has been seen more often than expected in workers exposed to aluminum dust. In the past, beneficial effects have been attributed to inhalation of fine aluminum powder as treatment against silicosis, but no adverse effects have been reported.

Aluminum exposure may cause some biochemical changes of limited or unknown relevance, but the most important toxic potential is related to its neurotoxicity. This problem has been studied in particular in patients undergoing dialysis.[10] Because of the limited ability of these patients to excrete aluminum in the urine, aluminum from the dialysis water and from aluminum hydroxide gels, which are taken to bind phosphate, accumulate in the body, in particular in the brain, which seems to be at least a partial cause of dialysis dementia. The early symptoms are speech impairment and dysphasia, followed by myoclonic movements, seizures, and progressive global dementia with prominent symptoms from the parietal lobe. This disease appears to be irreversible, and survival beyond a few years is uncommon.

In addition, aluminum seems to accumulate, although to much less an extent, in the brains of patients with presenile dementia of the Alzheimer type. This accumulation could be a phenomenon secondary to the disease development, since the possible causative role of aluminum has not yet been determined. However, one or two reports suggest that encephalopathy may develop as an apparent result of heavy occupational aluminum exposure. Thus aluminum is undoubtedly neurotoxic, but to what extent this is true in individual patients with normal kidney function still has to be clarified.[10]

Dialysis osteodystrophy is a complication in about 2% of patients undergoing long-term dialysis treatment. It causes sclerosis and osteoporosis, leading to skeletal pains and multiple fractures.[10] Dialysis osteodystrophy is closely associated with long-term aluminum accumulation, but the exact role of this metal in its pathogenesis is not yet known. Bone toxicity has been described in patients receiving long-term parenteral nutrition containing aluminum-contaminated casein hydrolysate.[11] Also, a few cases of osteomalacia have been described in patients who had ingested large doses of aluminum-containing antacid for extended periods.[8] A negative phosphate balance may be part of the explanation for osteomalacia in patients with normal kidney function. Animal experiments, however, have indicated that aluminum has a biochemical effect on bone formation that leads to a vitamin D–resistant osteomalacia.

Prevention. Serum aluminum levels are used extensively in the monitoring of patients undergoing dialysis treatment. Although high levels of aluminum may be estimated accurately by most laboratories, reference levels have decreased substantially during recent years, indicating an improved contamination control in the laboratories. Serum levels below 10 μg/L (0.37 μmol/L) usually are considered normal. Dialysis patients frequently have serum levels of 50 μg/L (1.85 μmol/L) and above, and the risk of adverse effects is much higher if the serum aluminum level exceeds 100 μg/L (3.7 μmol/L). Aluminum has a short biological half-life in the blood of persons with normal kidney function, thus rendering aluminum measurements in serum samples of limited value in occupational health practice. Urinary excretion of aluminum in healthy persons, however, may be a useful parameter in diagnosing short-term exposures,[12] but urinary levels up to 1 mg/L (37 μmol/L) may be found in patients ingesting aluminum-containing antacids.

Aluminum toxicity in dialysis patients may be prevented by using dialysis water with an aluminum concentration below 10 μg/L (0.37 μmol/L) after reverse osmosis or other effective treatment and by restriction of or possible substitution for oral aluminum-containing phosphate binders. In Western Europe about 200 people per million inhabitants currently need dialysis, and the number of patients increases by 8% to 10% per year. Thus this problem is of considerable importance. Solutions used for parenteral nutrition should be examined for aluminum contents, and low-level products should be preferred. Desferrioxamine has limited therapeutic use as an aluminum chelator.

The exposure limits recommended by the American Conference of Governmental Industrial Hygienists (ACGIH) are 10 mg/m^3 for aluminum metal and oxide, 5 mg/m^3 for aluminum pyropowders and welding fumes, and 2 mg/m^3 for soluble aluminum salts and (unstable) aluminum alkyls. Only the sparingly soluble forms of aluminum dust are considered inert dust. As a limit for urinary aluminum excretion at the end of a workday, 200 μg/L (7.4 μmol/L) has been recommended.

ANTIMONY

Antimony is used as an alloy with lead and other metals and for semiconductors and thermoelectric devices, and antimony compounds also are widely used, especially as pigments. Occupational antimony exposures occur in the mining and refining of the metal and in the production of pewter, solder, storage battery plates, and Babbitt metal. Exposure to antimony compounds has been reported from production of abrasives, textile dyeing, and handling of pigments and catalysts. Antimony-containing pharmaceuticals (antimony pentasulfide as cough medicine and tartar emetic or stibophen against leishmaniasis and schistosomiasis) are still in wide use in certain parts of the world.

The medical literature on antimony mainly deals with the use of organic compounds as therapeutic agents. Much less information is available on the significance of environmental and occupational exposures.[13] Antimony compounds have been ingested accidentally in a few cases when acid fruit juices dissolved the metal from enameled containers. The symptoms occurred almost immediately: abdominal pains with nausea and vomiting, which were of short duration. Several reports on health effects related to occupational antimony exposures are difficult to evaluate because arsenic may have occurred as a contaminant and been responsible for some of the caustic and irritant effects. Although cardiotoxicity has been documented as a side effect in antimony pharmaceuticals, only a few reports of electrocardiogram (ECG) changes related to occupational exposures have been published. More commonly, antimony compounds have given rise to irritation of the mucous membranes, irritant eczema, and even chemical burns and perforation of the nasal septum. In particular, antimony trioxide frequently causes the so-called antimony spots, that is, the small, intensely itchy erythematous papules that develop on exposed, moist skin in hot environments; they are fortunately of short duration. A simple, benign pneumoconiosis is related to antimony exposures, but free silica may have been a partial cause in some of the more serious cases reported.[9] A carcinogenic potential of antimony trioxide has been documented in rats; a relation to increased frequency of abortions has been reported in one study.

In the presence of strong acid, stibine (SbH_3) may be formed. Storage battery workers and metal etchers may be exposed to this hazard. This gas is toxic and causes severe hemolysis, shock, central nervous system (CNS) symptoms, and even death due to anuria.

Most antimony absorbed is excreted rather rapidly, Sb(V) mostly in the urine, and Sb(III) mostly through the gastrointestinal tract. A slow compartment seems to exist, and accumulation in lungs, liver, kidneys, thyroid, and adrenals has been indicated. Severe toxicity has not been documented at urine levels below 1 mg/L (8.2 μmol/L), but biological monitoring of antimony levels in blood and urine so far has been used only rarely. The limit for occupational antimony exposures is 0.5 mg/m^3; for stibine this level corresponds to 0.1 ppm. Antimony trioxide exposure is regarded as potentially carcinogenic.

ARSENIC

Exposures. Arsenic occurs widely in the environment. The earth's crust contains an average of 5 μg/g, frequently in association with other elements, such as copper, lead, and zinc. Seawater usually contains 6 to 30 μg/L, and some crustaceans may contain as much as 100 mg/kg, but most arsenic in seafood occurs as organic complexes. Other food items contain little arsenic, but well water may be severely contaminated, especially in certain parts of South America and Taiwan. Fowler's solution (sodium arsenite) was used in the past to treat leukemia, psoriasis, and other diseases. Although redundant in most countries, arsenic may still be used for therapeutic purposes in some parts of the world. Arsenic present in coal and oil shale may result in increasing environmental contamination by this element.

Occupational exposure to arsenic occurs in the following branches of industry: metal smelting, where arsenic occurs as a contaminant or by-product; production and use of various alloys, especially with lead and copper; production and use of pesticides (e.g., calcium and lead arsenate); production of opal glass; certain kinds of enameling; production of pharmaceuticals (e.g., salvarsan, used in the past for treatment of syphilis, and antiparasitic drugs such as carbarsone); production of paints and coatings, including antifouling compounds; leather tanning and the taxidermist industry; and the production, handling, and analysis of arsenic and arsenic compounds. When arsenic-containing ores are heated, arsenic trioxide (As_2O_3, white arsenic) is formed, and this compound constitutes the main product for the arsenic-consuming industry. Experimental studies suggest that As(III), as found in arsenic trioxide from smelter fumes, is more toxic than As(V), which occurs in arsenate compounds, such as wood treatment products. Arsine (AsH_3) is particularly toxic. However, little is known about the speciation of arsenic in occupational exposures.[14]

Easily soluble arsenic compounds may be absorbed rather efficiently through the respiratory and gastrointestinal tracts; absorption through the skin also has been documented. Following absorption, inorganic arsenic is first bound to the globin of erythrocyte hemoglobin. Subsequently, arsenic may be released, distributed within the body, and bound to sulfhydroxyl groups of enzymes, thus causing adverse biochemical effects. Some conversion of As(V) to As(III) may take place. Arsenobetaine, the arsenic analogue of betaine, appears to constitute the main proportion of arsenic contents of fish and crustacea. This compound is excreted in unchanged form in the urine relatively rapidly; arsenocholine from fish seems to be oxidized to arsenobetaine in the mammalian body. The kinetics and toxicological significance of other organoarsenic compounds are unknown. The biological half-life for inorganic arsenic in the blood is about 2 days, probably even less for arsenobetaine. After an acute exposure to inorganic arsenic the arsenic excretion in urine often is increased for more than a week. An additional, somewhat slower excretion occurs through hairs, nails, and skin cells. Both skin and lungs may constitute a "slow" arsenic compartment with a long biological half-time. Insufficient information is available concerning the specific kinetics of As(III) and As(V) in humans. However, arsenic should be regarded as a cumulative toxin that can cause chronic intoxications.

Effects. The acute intoxication is frequently an accident or suicide attempt in which arsenic trioxide or lead arsenate has been ingested. Fatal doses are usually 100 mg and above. The first symptoms occur from the gastrointestinal tract—that is, vomiting, colic, and diarrhea, followed by fever, cardiotoxicity, peripheral edema, and shock, which can lead to death within 12 to 48 hours. Patients who survive an acute intoxication usually exhibit anemia and leukopenia and may experience peripheral nervous damage 1 to 2 weeks later. Late effects include loss of hair and nail deformities. Recovery from peripheral neurotoxicity is slow and may take several months.[14,15]

Another kind of acute poisoning may occur after inhalation of the extremely toxic arsine (AsH_3), which smells like garlic.[16] This compound is formed when arsenic (frequently as an impurity) comes into contact with strong acid. Prolonged inhalation of 10 ppm or more of arsine is lethal. The patient first experiences dizziness, headache, pains in the stomach, arms, and legs, and subsequently hemolysis, icterus, and kidney damage, which may lead to death.

Under chronic exposure conditions the critical effect is usually a polyneuropathy of the sensorimotor type causing paresthesias in the extremities, muscle weakness, especially in the fingers, motor incoordination, and neuralgic pains. This peripheral neuropathy may be a late result of an acute exposure or the only lasting result of a long-term exposure to arsenic, although chronic skin symptoms often occur at the same time. A subclinical neuropathy, detectable by neurophysiological methods, has been described in relation to relatively low arsenic exposures.[17] Long-term exposure to inorganic arsenic compounds can cause chronic eczema, hyperpigmentation of the skin, and hyperkeratosis, especially on foot soles and palms. Development of skin cancer may be seen at a later time: squamous cell carcinomas, mostly at hyperkeratoses on the extremities, and basal cell carcinomas in any region. Vascular effects may be Raynaud's disease, acrocyanosis, and necroses ("blackfoot disease"). More rarely, arsenic exposure causes cardiotoxicity, liver enlargement with possible portal hypertension, and instances of angiosarcoma and toxic effects in the CNS, including decreased hearing. Chronic irritation of respiratory mucous membranes causes secretion, a hoarse voice, and cough. Repeated damage to the mucous membrane by white arsenic may cause defects in the nasal septum. Chronic irritation in the eyes may cause keratoconjunctivitis. Epidemiological evidence from studies of pesticide production workers, sprayers, smelter workers, residents near polluting industries, and patients treated with arsenicals convincingly indicates that respiratory exposure to arsenic results in an increased risk of lung cancer. In most studies the exposures were mixed, and the effects of As(III) and As(V) cannot be separated. Arsenic may act synergistically with tobacco smoke in causing lung cancer. Excess cancer rates in several organs also have been documented in persons exposed to drinking water severely contaminated with arsenic. Teratogenic effects have been reported in experimental animals.

Prevention. Biological monitoring of arsenic levels in blood is of limited interest because arsenic is cleared rapidly from the blood. Hair analysis has been used in forensic medicine, but the significance of external contamination excludes the use of this method in the surveillance of dust exposures in industry. Measurement of arsenic levels in urine may be used for the evaluation of current exposures because a major part, about 60% at steady state, of the absorbed arsenic is excreted in the urine. However, the somewhat variable proportion excreted by this route, the daily variations related to the short biological half-life, and the contribution of arsenic compounds from food items render urine tests for total arsenic useful only on a group basis. Excretion of more than 1 mg/L (13 μmol/L) can be used as an indication of arsenic intoxication. Normally the arsenic content in urine is below 100 μg/L (1.3 μmol/L), but levels of at least 200 μg/L (2.7 μmol/L) may be seen after a good seafood meal. Improved analytical methods have indicated that after a person has been exposed to inorganic arsenic compounds, the urinary arsenic will be up to 20% inorganic arsenic and up to 20% monomethylarsinate and that the remainder will be dimethylarsinate (cacodylate).[4] Background levels of these compounds would probably be below 20 μg/L (0.27 μmol/L) unless exposures from contaminated wells were prevalent. Seafood contains primarily stable organoarsenicals that do not influence urinary excretion of the above-mentioned compounds.

The limit for airborne arsenic and inorganic arsenic compounds is 0.2 mg/m^3. For arsine the airborne limit corresponds to 0.05 ppm. Arsenic trioxide production has been classified as a cancer risk. However, on the basis of the carcinogenic effects, the National Institute for Occupational Safety and Health (NIOSH) has recommended a limit of 0.002 mg/m^3 for all arsenic compounds; exposures below this limit would result in minor or undetectable increases of arsenic levels in urine. An expert group from the World Health Organization (WHO) and the Food and Agriculture Organization (FAO) of the United Nations has suggested a maximum allowable daily limit (MADL) for intake of inorganic arsenic of 0.002 mg/kg body weight.

BARIUM

Barium is the heaviest of the stable alkaline earths. The main ore is barite, which is mainly used in drilling muds. Small amounts are used in glass and ceramic glazes, paper coating, and pesticides and as a plastic stabilizer. Sparingly soluble barium salts cause negligible gastrointestinal absorption. Thus the use of barium sulfate as x-ray contrast material is generally safe. If absorbed, barium mainly accumulates in the skeleton. Inhalation of insoluble barium compounds has produced a benign pneumoconiosis, baritosis, which is reversible and causes minor, if any, symptoms.[9,18] Soluble barium salts cause potassium depletion in the blood and subsequently hypokalemia. In barium poisoning the first symptom is smooth muscle stimulation (vomiting, colic, diarrhea), followed by general muscle stimulation; in severe cases, paralysis develops. In the Szechwan province of China an endemic periodic, familial paralysis was traced to the table salt produced from a mine with a high barium content. The occupational exposure limit for soluble barium compounds is 0.5 mg/m^3.

BERYLLIUM

Beryllium, the fourth lightest element, is extracted from beryl ore. Most cases of beryllium-induced disease have been the result of exposures in connection with the production of fluorescent lamps.[19] The application of this metal is greatly expanding. Beryllium is used for coating of cathode ray tubes, for example, for radar equipment, in electrical or electronic instruments, and in nuclear reactors. Moreover, beryllium is used in many light metal alloys for the space and aircraft industry. Although adverse effects of beryllium are now seen infrequently, the increasing use of this metal could again result in a higher risk of inadvertent exposures.

Most beryllium salts are practically insoluble at neutral pH, and therefore absorption after oral intake is limited. Skin contact may result in sufficient penetration to cause an allergic dermatitis. Inhalation of beryllium dusts is the major hazard. Once absorbed, excretion is slow. Animal studies suggest that peak urinary beryllium excretion occurs 10 to 30 hours after inhalation exposure. An acute, severe exposure to airborne beryllium may inflame mucous membranes and cause a chemical pneumonia. After severe beryllium exposure the disease generally develops within a few days, becoming rapidly progressive and occasionally lethal.[9] Most patients survive the acute phase and recover within 12 months.

Berylliosis, a chronic disease syndrome, is different from the acute intoxication and is rather similar to sarcoidosis. The pulmonary granulomatosis can evolve following the acute phase after a long, but variable latency period. Berylliosis also can occur without a preceding acute episode, and the diagnosis may not be made until several years after cessation of exposure. The most frequent symptom is dyspnea on exertion. Paroxysmal coughing occurs, especially in the morning and on physical exertion. The chest x-ray film usually reveals a mixture of small, rounded, irregular opacities, and histological studies show interstitial cellular infiltration and granuloma formation. Pulmonary function tests show decreased diffusion, later followed by more generalized pulmonary impairment. Granulomas also may occur in the liver and other organs, but the Kveim test for sarcoidosis is negative. The lymphocyte blast transformation test is positive for beryllium, apparently even before development of symptoms and also during steroid treatment. The abnormal chest x-ray film does not necessarily reflect the severity of symptoms, but incapacitation due to poor pulmonary function may occur. The course of the disease is irregular with recurrences that result in a further progression. Steroid treatment is beneficial and may keep some patients free of symptoms for long periods, although no complete recovery has been recorded.[9]

The beryllium case registry at NIOSH recorded almost 900 cases between 1952 and 1982. As little as 45 μg of this metal inhaled in a matter of several minutes is sufficient to cause acute disease. Chronic disease cases have occurred in several household contacts. Exposures after 1970 have caused few cases.[19]

Experimental evidence confirms that beryllium may be a carcinogen. However, epidemiological studies have not shown with certainty that beryllium-exposed persons suffer lung cancer more frequently than expected.

Biological monitoring plays no role in the prevention of excess beryllium exposures. The limit for occupational beryllium exposure is 0.002 mg/m^3. NIOSH has recommended that the time-weighted exposure limit be decreased to 0.001 mg/m^3.

CADMIUM

Exposures. The earth's crust contains an average cadmium concentration of 0.55 μg/g, and small amounts of this metal are always found in food items. Of concern is the increasing concentration of cadmium deposited in agricultural soils by airborne cadmium particles and by phosphate fertilizers and sewage sludge used for fertilization. Cadmium is a relatively mobile metal in soils, and many crops retain relatively high cadmium levels. In particular, tobacco leaves are high in cadmium. The total daily intake of cadmium via food varies according to diet composition, but averages range from a low of 10 to more than 50 μg/d.[20]

The most important application of this metal is cadmium plating for corrosion treatment of metals, especially iron and steel.[21] Brazing is sometimes carried out with solders containing cadmium. Rechargeable nickel-cadmium batteries are used increasingly in modern electronic products. To a limited degree, cadmium also is used in certain copper alloys and in bearing metal. Cadmium rods are used in nuclear power plants. Cadmium sulfide and selenide are used as pigments in enamel, ceramics, glass, plastic, and leather. Many of these uses are now being restricted in certain countries to limit cadmium releases to the environment. Accordingly, the risk of occupational exposure to cadmium may be decreasing also. However, considerable cadmium exposure still may be a result of various work processes, such as welding or cutting of metals with cadmium-containing coatings, spray painting with cadmium pigments, or primary production of copper and zinc from cadmium-containing ores. Raw phosphate often contains significant amounts of cadmium, and exposures may occur during the production of phosphate fertilizers. This metal has a melting point of 320° C, and dangerous fumes are generated by comparatively low temperatures.

Animal experiments suggest that 10% to 40% of inhaled cadmium is absorbed, whereas 2% to 10% of oral intake is transferred to the bloodstream, the gastrointestinal absorption being higher in persons with iron deficiency. After absorption, cadmium is bound to albumin, and uptake by the liver induces synthesis of metallothionein. Cadmium then is chelated by this small protein, the complex being stored intracellularly in the liver from where it is slowly released to the blood and subsequently excreted through the kidney glomeruli; most is again reabsorbed by the tubulus cells, and an accumulation in the kidney cortex takes place. In general, about one half of the human body's burden of cadmium is located in liver and kidneys. The liver is the main storage organ for cadmium in the body, but the highest concentration eventually is reached in the kidneys. The biological half-life is at least 10 years, probably closer to 20 years, and cadmium therefore seems to accumulate in the body during the major part of a lifetime.[20]

Effects. Acute cadmium poisoning most frequently occurs after inhalation of cadmium fumes, for example, during the cutting of cadmium-plated steel with an oxyacetylene torch. Slowly developing symptoms can sometimes indicate that hazardous exposure is continuing. Generally the first symptoms appear a few hours after the exposure and may suggest metal fume fever, but a toxic pneumonitis then develops. In some cases of acute exposure, gastrointestinal effects develop in a day or so, and in such cases the symptoms are less severe and the prognosis is much better. However, recovery often is slow and may take months. The few literature reports suggest that such cases are rare.[20,21] Several years after acute cadmium pneumonitis, progressive pulmonary fibrosis has been observed.

Acute oral cadmium poisoning occurs, for example, when large amounts of the metal are released from solder materials in soft-drink machines or from ceramic glazes of kitchenware. As little as 20 mg of cadmium induces vomiting, and gastrointestinal absorption of toxic amounts causes salivation, nausea, headache, abdominal pains and cramps, and diarrhea. In severe cases, ulcerative gastroenteritis and constipation develop, and systemic toxicity may subsequently include effects on lungs, liver, and kidneys.

In long-term cadmium poisoning the metal accumulates in the body, where the kidneys are the target organ.[20] The toxic damage seems to occur mostly in the proximal tubules, but glomerular changes often appear at a later state and in some cases may even be the first indication of cadmium-induced nephropathy. The first sign of kidney dysfunction is usually an increased excretion of low-molecular proteins in the urine, notably β_2-microglobulin, retinol-binding protein, and albumin. Even after cessation of exposure, this proteinuria continues to worsen and is associated with an accelerated decrease in glomerular filtration rate.[22] In cases of glomerular dysfunction, larger proteins also occur in the urine. As tubular reabsorption further deteriorates, calcium, phosphorus, amino acids, and glucose are excreted in excess quantities. These changes may relate to an increased incidence of kidney stones in cadmium-exposed workers. In severe cases the kidney dysfunction results in changes of electrolyte and protein balance, and a long-lasting, severe loss of protein and minerals may lead to skeletal changes. Such effects were seen in Japan, where a large number of patients suffered osteomalacia with skeletal pains and pseudofractures, the so-called itai-itai disease, as a result of severe, environmental cadmium exposure in conjunction with nutritional deficiencies. A few cases of industrial origin have occurred in other countries.

Low-level environmental exposure to cadmium in women more than 60 years of age has been related to increased urinary excretion of total protein, amino acids, β_2-microglobulin, and albumin.[23] Thus the possibility exists that cadmium pollution in many industrialized areas could accelerate the age-related decline of renal function in populations without occupational exposure.

Some studies suggest that long-term inhalation of cadmium can lead to emphysema.[20] This disease also has been linked to cadmium retention in the lungs in smokers. Other effects of long-term cadmium exposure include mild anemia, anosmia, and abnormal liver function tests. Animal experiments suggest that cadmium may cause hypertension, but epidemiological data are inconclusive.

A recent experimental animal study has suggested that pulmonary exposure to cadmium oxide may cause lung cancer. Epidemiological evidence has suggested only a weak relation to cancer, in particular prostate cancer. Animal experiments suggest that this metal may be a teratogen.

Prevention. The cadmium concentration in the blood is an indication of the current exposure (during the last few months) and is used frequently for biological monitoring.[20] Levels below 1 μg/L (9 nmol/L) are seen in nonsmokers, but smokers often have levels up to 5 μg/L (44 nmol/L). For industrial exposures a previous limit for blood cadmium of 5 μg/100 ml will not protect against kidney damage under long-term exposure conditions. Preferably blood cadmium should not exceed 15 μg/L (0.13 μmol/L). Urinary excretion of cadmium is limited in the beginning, and it increases only under rather heavy, acute exposures. Higher urinary cadmium levels are found more frequently when the kidneys over a long period have accumulated rather large amounts of cadmium, which then starts to leak, and an upper normal level of 3 μg/L (27 nmol/L) is then exceeded.[20] When tubular and perhaps glomerular dysfunction develop, relatively large amounts of cadmium are then excreted in the urine, thus decreasing the kidney burden of the metal. Considerable evidence suggests that the threshold for development of nephrotoxicity may be exceeded when the cadmium concentration in the kidney cortex reaches about 200 μg/g, a level that would correspond to a urinary cadmium excretion of 10 μg/L (89 nmol/L) and a daily absorption of 10 to 15 μg over a lifetime. The level of

β_2-microglobulin or, preferably, retinol-binding protein may be assessed in urinary samples, but excess levels usually are caused by early or imminent kidney damage (i.e., when preventive efforts have failed).

ACGIH has accepted a limit of 50 $\mu g/m^3$, which also applies as a ceiling limit for cadmium fumes. This limit is in accordance with the conclusions drawn by a WHO expert group.[24] However, the carcinogenic potential would suggest that all exposures should be minimized. Many countries have adopted regulations concerning cadmium release from ceramic glazes and other materials that may leach cadmium to food and beverages. With regard to dietary intake of cadmium, a WHO/FAO expert group several years ago suggested a provisional tolerable weekly intake (PTWI) limit of 0.4 to 0.5 mg/wk. Since then, kidney function in the elderly has turned out to be more vulnerable than expected,[23] and lifelong cadmium accumulation from environmental exposures would seem eventually to cause adverse effects, perhaps even below the PTWI. Therefore a reevaluation may be expected. However, the current PTWI already seems to be exceeded by some population groups, and prevention of cadmium pollution from all sources appears to be a major environmental priority.

CHROMIUM

Exposures. The average chromium concentration in the earth's crust is 300 $\mu g/g$, and chromium most commonly occurs as trivalent compounds. Divalent compounds are rather unstable, and hexavalent chromates released to the environment are reduced to trivalent compounds in the presence of oxidizable substances. Only scattered information is available on environmental exposures to chromium. In general, daily intakes through food appear to average less than 50 μg. However, the chemical form of chromium present in food and drinking water is largely unknown.

Occupational exposures to chromium occur in several industries[25]: production of chromium and chromium compounds, stainless steel, and other metal alloys; chromium plating of metals; production of heat-resistant bricks with chromate additives; use of chromates as pigments and dichromates for tanning; welding of chromium-plated metals and chromium-containing alloys; development of photographic emulsions; and production and usage of wood preservatives. The main consumption of chromium is in the steel industry, and stainless steel usually contains between 8% and 18% chromium. In addition, chromate in cement results in considerable cutaneous exposures.

The gastrointestinal uptake of Cr(VI) is on the order of 3% or 4%, while the absorption of Cr(III) is less than 1%, but organic complexes of chromium may be absorbed more easily. The fate of inhaled chromium particles and the transfer within the body depend on the solubility of the compounds. The Cr(VI) ion readily passes through biological membranes, but the Cr(III) ion does not. Excretion is mainly in the urine.

Effects. Chromium is an essential trace metal (previously referred to as the glucose tolerance factor) for several species, including humans. Glucose intolerance, weight loss, and peripheral neuropathy in patients undergoing long-term intravenous nutrition may be cured by Cr(III) supplements. High-sugar diets, strenuous exercise, physical trauma, and infection may provoke a deficiency in persons with low chromium intake.[26] However, the public health consequences of widespread marginal intakes of this trace metal are unclear.

The toxicity of the various chromium compounds varies, partly in relation to the different solubilities. In general, hexavalent compounds are more easily soluble than the trivalent compounds. The chromate ion is strongly oxidizing. The major effects include corrosion of skin and mucous membranes, allergic responses, and carcinogenicity.[25,27] Trivalent chromium is less toxic, apparently because of the lower solubility and lower biological mobility. However, Cr(III) may be the ultimate toxin in relation to some of the effects related to Cr(VI) exposure.

Long-term inhalation of Cr(VI) compounds in chromium-plating workshops has in the past caused severe corrosion of the nasal mucous membrane, often with a resulting defect in the nasal septum. The ulcer is not painful, but bleeding and sneezing often occur. Irritation of airways, cornea, and conjunctiva also may result. Presently these effects are seen more rarely. Chromate may cause circumscribed ulcers (chrome holes) at the knuckles, nail roots, or other exposed skin areas. Even though they may be quite deep, they are almost painless. Healing often takes several weeks and leaves a depressed scar, but the ulcers apparently are not related to development of skin cancer.

Chromium is one of the best known allergens in the occupational environment, and chromate is frequently the most common cause of allergic contact dermatitis among males. Cement eczema is a common occupational disease in bricklayers, masons, and other workers in the building trades, and it is caused most often by chromate allergy. In some countries the addition of 0.4% ferrous sulfate to the cement is required by law because it effectively reduces the chromate to insoluble Cr(III) compounds. Many cases of chromium allergy also have been seen in tanners, furriers, and workers exposed to Cr(VI) compounds in photographic laboratories and in relation to wood treatment. Although Cr(VI) may be the primary sensitizer, subsequent allergic responses allegedly have been elicited by Cr(III) also. In a few cases chromate also has been identified as a cause of asthma, probably mediated by a type I allergic reaction. Chromite mining apparently has caused several cases of a benign pneumoconiosis.

Chromium is a well-documented human carcinogen,[28] and occupational exposures from the production of chromates, chromium pigments, and perhaps ferrochrome have caused an increased frequency of cancer in the respiratory tract. An increased occurrence of lung cancer in some groups of welders may be due to the content of insoluble chromates in welding fumes from stainless steel. Although trivalent chromium compounds may constitute the ultimate carcinogens, exposures to such compounds have not been shown in epidemiological studies to cause cancer.

Prevention. Biological monitoring of chromium levels in the urine is useful after an exposure to soluble, hexavalent chromium compounds. Renal excretion of chromium reflects three major compartments with a half-life of about 7 hours, 2 to 4 weeks, and 3 to 5 years. In persons without occupational exposures, urinary chromium excretion averages about 1 $\mu g/L$ (20 nmol/L). In long-term exposure to chromium trioxide an air level of 0.1 mg/m^3 corresponds to about 40 $\mu g/L$ (0.8 $\mu mol/L$) or 30 $\mu g/g$ creatinine (65 $\mu mol/g$); lower concentrations are seen with shorter lasting exposures. The erythrocytes tend to accumulate chromium from Cr(VI) exposures; the above-mentioned level of chromium trioxide exposures will result in average whole-blood concentrations of about 35 $\mu g/L$ (0.7 $\mu mol/L$). Exposure to trivalent compounds or sparingly soluble chromates will not result in detectable changes in body fluids available for biological monitoring.

The exposure limit for chromate ore processing and certain insoluble chromates is 0.05 mg/m^3, but for the metal and all other compounds the limit is 0.5 mg/m^3. NIOSH has considered monochromates and bichromates of hydrogen, lithium, sodium, potassium, rubidium, cesium, and ammonium, in addition to chromium acid anhydride, as noncarcinogenic forms of Cr(VI) for which an average exposure limit of 0.025 mg/m^3, with a ceiling limit of 0.05 mg/m^3 for any 15-minute period, is recommended. All other Cr(VI) compounds were regarded as carcinogenic, and a permissible exposure limit of 0.001 mg/m^3 has been suggested. Skin contact with Cr(VI) compounds should be avoided, and any skin contamination should be removed immediately with soap and water. This problem is even more important for patients with chromate allergy who may have to avoid contact with leather products and plastic articles with leachable chromate pigments. The sulfur on matches contains chromate also. On the other hand, chromium alloys release only insignificant amounts because of oxide formation in the surface layer. A daily dietary intake of 0.05 to 0.2 mg of chromium is considered safe and adequate for adults. Although daily chromium intake may be marginal in large population groups, the need for chromium supplements in healthy persons still is unclear.

COBALT

Cobalt is a rare element that comprises only about 0.001% of the earth's crust. Thus human exposures from natural sources are limited, and daily intake through food usually has been estimated at somewhat below 50 μg. Cobalt levels in drinking water usually are low and of little concern, and atmospheric levels frequently are undetectable.

Occupational exposures have become prevalent.[29] The most important use is in "hard metal," which consists of various metal carbides (mainly tungsten) cemented by a cobalt binder. Cobalt also has found considerable use in alloys to which it adds a high melting point, tensile strength, and resistance to corrosion. Cobalt compounds are used increasingly as catalysts, including desiccators in paints. Cobalt pigments are used in ceramic and glass products. The alloys are used extensively in the electrical, automobile, and aircraft industries, and cobalt also is used for electroplating.

Absorption in the gastrointestinal tract varies but probably averages about 25% for soluble compounds unless cobalt is ingested in the form of vitamin B_{12} and in iron deficiency, which increases the absorption of cobalt. Cobalt induces hematopoiesis and has a therapeutic application in patients with refractory anemia. Ingestion of excessive amounts of cobalt will induce vomiting and diarrhea.

Cobalt is an essential micronutrient and has important actions as an enzyme activator and as a component of vitamin B_{12}. Cobalt deficiency has not been documented in humans, but enzootic deficiency may be a problem in certain regions of the United States, Australia, Scotland, and other parts of the world. Thus cobalt is added to cattle feed and sometimes to fertilizers.

Respiratory exposure to cobalt dust may lead to airway irritation and asthma that may progress to chronic obstructive lung disease; exposure levels below 0.05 mg/m^3 seem to prevent the appearance of such cases.[29] Cobalt dust retained in the lungs is of additional health significance. Cemented carbide production workers may develop a pneumoconiosis called hard-metal lung, frequently following long-term exposures of more than 10 years; this disease most likely is due to the cobalt exposures. The first radiological signs of this diffuse, interstitial fibrosis usually are more prominent hilar regions and increased irregular and nodular opacities in the middle and lower lobes. The pathogenesis of cobalt-induced pulmonary disease is not known in detail, but some individual hypersensitivity may predispose patients to the pulmonary reactions.[9]

Cutaneous exposures to cobalt are common. Small concentrations of this metal are present in cement, and cobalt may contaminate cutting oils and leach from metal objects. Cobalt allergy is frequent but occurs mainly in combination with allergy to nickel or chromate. Hand eczemas in patients with such cross-reactions have a relatively poor prognosis.

Although the highest concentrations of cobalt are retained in the liver, no adverse effects have been documented in this organ. Cobalt is a goitrogen and induces thyroid hyperplasia. Cardiotoxicity is perhaps an important hazard.[30] An outbreak of cardiomyopathy, sometimes complicated by pericardial effusion, was reported in Quebec City 20 years ago. This disease occurred exclusively in beer drinkers, and subsequent investigations showed that the local brewery added cobalt sulfate to the beer. The same practice was discovered in Omaha, Neb., in Minneapolis, Minn., and in Brussels, Belgium, where similar epidemics occurred. The cardiomyopathy was highly lethal and could not be explained solely by the addition of about 1 mg of cobalt to each liter of beer; potentiating effects of other factors have been suggested. After the addition of cobalt was discontinued, the epidemics faded away. Moreover, several cases have been linked to industrial cobalt exposures.

Limited evidence from experimental studies suggests potential carcinogenicity. However, epidemiological data are difficult to evaluate because of concomitant exposures to nickel and arsenic.[31]

Biological monitoring may be of some use. The kinetics of cobalt in the organism show the existence of two fast compartments with half-lives of up to 2 days, but about 10% of absorbed cobalt is excreted much more slowly. Urinary cobalt excretion levels average less than 1 μg/L (0.017 μmol/L) unless the individual takes a mineral supplement. Following occupational exposures, urinary excretion levels may be 100 times higher, but the levels may change rapidly because of the short half-life. Thus more information may be obtained on the average long-term exposure by measuring the cobalt level in urine on a Monday morning after an exposure-free period.

Occupational exposures to cobalt metal fumes and dust should be limited as much as possible. Because of the increasing awareness concerning hard metal disease, a limit of 0.05 mg/m^3 for cobalt metal dust and fumes has been adopted by ACGIH.

COPPER

Copper is a widely used metal that has both beneficial and adverse health effects.[32] It is used in electrical equipment, in alloys, and in plumbing and heating. The daily intake through food averages about 2 mg or more. Copper is necessary for various metalloenzymes, but human copper deficiency has been documented only in extreme situations. Accidental intake of large amounts of this metal results in acute gastrointestinal symptoms. Copper sulfate has actually been used as an emetic but rarely now because of the potential absorption of toxic quantities of the metal. Systemic effects include hemolysis, icterus, anemia, and kidney and liver damage. Such effects have occurred primarily after suicidal ingestion of large amounts. Occupational exposures to copper fumes and fine dust may cause metal fume fever, and copper dust is a respiratory irritant. Several cases of "vineyard sprayer's lung" were described from the use of copper sulfate in an antimildew spray in Portugal; these reports may suggest that copper aerosols could act as a lung fibrogen. Patients with Wilson's disease (hepatolenticular fibrosis) accumulate copper in the liver related to insufficient formation of the copper-binding ceruloplasmin; these patients and the heterozygous carriers may be particularly sensitive to excess copper exposures. Increased susceptibility to copper also is seen in infants; long-lasting diarrhea and suspected cases of chemical hepatitis have been ascribed to copper from corroded water pipes.[33] Copper from kitchen utensils is the apparent cause of the Indian childhood cirrhosis syndrome. Biological monitoring of blood levels may be of interest. Excretion is mainly through the bile. Increased copper concentrations in serum (above 20 mg/L, i.e., 0.31 mmol/L) are seen in pregnant women, in relation to oral contraception, and in alcoholism. The impact of occupational exposures on serum and urine concentrations is poorly documented. The exposure limit for copper dusts or mists is 1 mg/m^3, and for copper fumes, 0.1 mg/m^3, although ACGIH has suggested 0.2 mg/m^3 for fumes. Copper is included in the list of essential minerals, with a recommended daily dietary intake of 2.3 mg for adults.

IRON

This common metal constitutes about 5% of the earth's crust. Iron is necessary for life but is toxic at excess exposures.[34] Iron deficiency is the most prevalent metal deficiency syndrome in humans, especially among women in the reproductive age group and certain groups of small children. Several nutrients interfere with iron absorption, but it is always increased in case of deficiency. Ingestion of iron supplements in considerable excess may cause acute gastrointestinal lesions followed by metabolic acidosis, toxic hepatitis, and shock. Chronic iron overload leads to hemosiderosis and liver cirrhosis. Foundry workers, grinders, and welders are exposed to considerable quantities of iron oxide fumes, which accumulate in the lungs and may result in siderosis, a benign and reversible pneumoconiosis. Detectable fibrosis seems to occur only when the exposures have included silica. However, the reticulonodular markings of siderosis on the chest x-ray film may be difficult to distinguish from the appearance of other diseases. Hematite miners have exhibited an excess incidence of lung cancer; although iron may not be the primary cause, an interaction between the iron dust and other factors, such as radon and asbestos, is possible. The exposure limit for iron oxide fumes is 5 mg/m^3 and is 1 mg/m^3 for soluble iron salts. Recommendations for daily iron intakes suggest that iron supplements are necessary for large population groups, but the supplement always should be stored in child-proof containers.

Iron pentacarbonyl may be formed when carbon monoxide comes in contact with iron at high partial pressures. This liquid is extremely toxic, and the inhaled vapor results almost immediately in headache, dyspnea, and dizziness. The symptoms then fade, only to return after several hours when pulmonary consolidation and cerebral edema are progressing. The ACGIH exposure limit is 0.1 ppm.

LEAD

Exposures. Lead occurs at a concentration of 12 μg/g in the earth's crust. The most important lead ore is galena (PbS), but several other minerals are used to a minor degree. Lead has a wide spectrum of applications that result in environmental dissemination and human exposures.[35] Metallic lead is used in various alloys, and several inorganic compounds have important uses. Almost 10% of the production is used for organolead compounds, tetraethyl lead, and tetramethyl lead, which are added to gasoline as octane boosters. These compounds are dealt with separately. The extensive use of lead has resulted in substantial redistributions in the biosphere, particularly as a result of the air pollution, which has reached a maximum of about 1000 tons a day, mainly emitted in the northern hemisphere. Calculations of natural lead exposures, supplemented by measurements of lead retention levels in archeological samples of bones and teeth, suggest that current lead exposure levels average almost 100 times more than typical exposure levels in premetallurgical times.[36] The daily oral intake of lead in America currently seems to average about 100 μg; levels below 30 μg have been found in some European countries. The major sources of lead contamination include gasoline additives, lead-based paint, lead-soldered food cans, ceramic glazes, and industrial pollution. Drinking water levels may be of particular concern in soft-water areas where lead pipes are used; the highest lead concentrations occur in the "first draw" water in the morning.

The melting point for lead is 327° C, and hazardous evaporation results when the temperature exceeds about 500° C. This fact is important where lead is melted or molded in factories and workshops. Various inorganic compounds are used as pigments and desiccators, for corrosion treatment and enameling, as additives to glass, and as stabilizers in polyvinyl chloride (PVC) plastic. Lead compounds used in ceramic glazes usually are fritted, that is, aggregated as larger particles by preheating.

Occupational lead exposure occurs in particular in the following processes: primary production of lead from lead ores; secondary lead production from used automobile batteries and scrap metal; production of batteries; welding and flame cutting of lead-containing or minimum-treated alloys; molding of lead-containing alloys in foundries; soldering with lead solder if the temperature is too high; production of, and spray painting with, paints containing lead pigments and desiccators; addition of lead stearate as stabilizer in PVC plastic; batch mixing with lead compounds for the production of crystal glass; and grinding and sandblasting of lead alloys and coatings. Several thousand workers in Finland and Denmark have been examined at several hundred factories and workshops, and the results of these screening studies suggest that the highest lead exposures occurred at lead smelters and battery plants. Occasionally, high exposures were found at battery repair shops, automobile radiator repair shops, pewter foundries, other lead alloy foundries, PVC-plastic production plants, crystal glassworks, ship-disassembly facilities, and scrap metal handling. High lead exposures also were documented in instructors from indoor shooting ranges, workers producing leaded panes, and in gunsmiths. Exposure may be considerable in small workshops with few employees and poor hygiene (Fig. 20–1).

Inorganic lead compounds are absorbed only to a minor degree in the gastrointestinal tract of adults, usually about 10% or slightly less, somewhat higher during fasting, somewhat lower when excess calcium, phosphate, and phytate are present. However, the immature gastrointestinal tract is relatively permeable to lead, and balance studies in small children have suggested that oral intake may result in absorption rates of 30% to 50%.

Almost all lead in the blood is bound to the erythrocytes, and the lead content of serum or plasma is so low that it cannot be measured reliably by conventional analytical methods. Measurements therefore refer to the lead content of whole blood (or erythrocytes). Because of the low solubility of lead phosphate, lead accumulates in calcified tissues. About 95% of the lead burden of an adult is located in the skeleton, with a long biological half-life related to the slow tissue remodeling rate. However, skeletal lead is more mobile in children. Much less lead is present in the soft tissues, and the half-life is generally about 2 months.

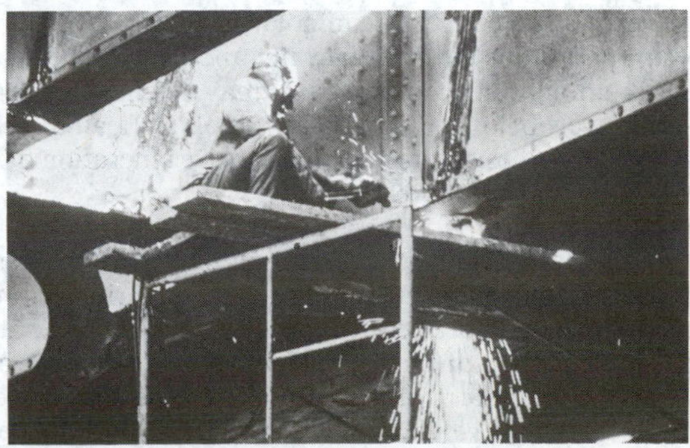

Figure 20–1. Burning through metal structures covered with lead-containing paint may generate high levels of lead in the working environment.

The brain probably constitutes an exception: lead passes only slowly through the blood-brain barrier, and the biological half-life seems to be more than a year. The placenta does not constitute a principal barrier to lead passage, and the fetus therefore is exposed to lead through the mother. Some lead is excreted into the gastrointestinal tract, but excretion is mainly in the urine. Only low concentrations of lead have been detected in human milk.

Effects. Lead has a great affinity to certain radicals and functional groups, such as $-SH$ and $-NH_2$. Lead is an important enzyme inhibitor. Of clinical importance are the chronic effects on blood cells and nervous system. In acute poisoning, gastrointestinal toxicity dominates, but encephalopathy may result in children. Kidney damage and other organ toxicity also may occur.[35]

Anemia is a typical symptom in classic lead poisoning.[35] Lead inhibits the Na-K-ATPase in the cell membranes of the erythrocytes, making them less stable and thereby shortening their life-span. An accumulation of bilirubin in the blood also is seen along with decreased haptoglobin. Of less importance quantitatively is the interference with hemoglobin synthesis, several steps of the heme formation being inhibited by lead. Most sensitive is the enzyme aminolevulinic acid dehydrase (ALAD), which is inhibited even at lead serum concentrations as low as 5 μg/dl (0.24 μmol/L). The ALAD activity correlates closely with the lead content in the blood. ALAD is useful for the examination of persons with relatively low lead exposures, but the analysis must take place within a few hours of sampling the blood. In severe occupational lead exposure the activity of this enzyme in the erythrocytes is extremely low.

Less sensitive to lead is the incorporation of ferrous ion into protoporphyrin IX to form heme. When this reaction is inhibited, zinc substitutes for iron, and the resulting zinc protoporphyrin (ZPP) binds instead of heme to the hemoglobin molecule, thereby rendering the hemoglobin unable to carry oxygen. The ZPP content of each erythrocyte reveals the lead exposure at the time the cell was formed. A blood sample contains erythrocytes that have been formed within the last 4 months or so, and the ZPP concentration in the blood therefore is an indication of the average lead exposure within this time interval. The measurement may be carried out in a few seconds with a portable fluorometer. In adult men the ZPP concentration increases significantly when the blood-lead concentration averages above 25 μg/dl (1.2 μmol/L). In women the threshold is somewhat lower because of their increased sensitivity related to lower iron stores in the body. In children the threshold for ZPP increase seems to be about 15 μg/dl (0.73 μmol/L). An increased amount of ZPP in the blood also can be caused by iron deficiency alone, but iron deficiency may, at the same time, make the patient more sensitive to the toxic effects of lead.

Other steps in the heme formation also can be affected. When the average lead serum level exceeds 40 μg/dl (1.9 μmol/L), excess excretion of δ-aminolevulinic acid (ALA), coproporphyrin, and other intermediary metabolites can be detected. Although hemoglobin concentrations may be entirely normal at blood lead levels below 60 μg/dl (2.9 μmol/L), lead toxicity affects the hematopoiesis; after a blood loss, regeneration of erythrocytes is significantly depressed.[3]

Lead affects both the central and the peripheral nervous systems.[35] In the past, acute toxic encephalopathy occurred in relation to severe lead exposure in certain occupations, but such cases now are rare. More recently, cases in adults have been related to consumption of moonshine whiskey distilled in old car radiators. Children are more susceptible to the central nervous system effects, and severe cases of encephalopathy with seizures still occur, sometimes as a result of ingestion of lead-containing paint flakes from peeling walls.

Research has shown insidious effects that produce a chronic toxic encephalopathy in adults. This syndrome in exposed workers has some similarity to the nonspecific effects seen in workers with long-term exposures to neurotoxic solvents.[37] Typically, the patient is taken to the physician or the hospital by the wife who is worried about his failing health and his unbearable irritability. Clinical examination and neuropsychological testing frequently show that attention, concentration, memory, and abstraction are affected. Cross-sectional studies have indicated that early effects, detectable by psychological tests, may develop when blood lead concentrations exceed 40 μg/dl (1.9 μmol/L) for extensive periods. One prospective study has shown impaired performance in men when a serum lead level of 30 μg/dl (1.5 μmol/L) was exceeded, as compared with the performance of a reference group.

Similarly, effects have been detected in children with elevated levels of lead in the blood in the absence of any past history of acute lead toxicity. The studies suggest that attention and vigilance are sensitive measures of lead toxicity, and decreased performance may be detected in lowered IQ tests. Several other factors may influence the performance of small children in such tests, and the contribution of lead to decreased functioning of children has raised considerable controversy. Most studies are difficult to interpret because of inaccurate retrospective exposure assessment, possible selection bias, and the significance of confounders and effect modifiers. When carefully evaluated, however, the studies in concert suggest that even low lead levels may contribute to decreased performance of children. The general impression is that levels only slightly above 10 μg/dl (0.49 μmol/L) very well could cause measurable deficits. For example, lead-associated dysfunctions were found in a group of Danish children, most of whom had blood lead concentrations below this level.[38] Prospective studies suggest that intrauterine lead exposure is even more serious because of the particular vulnerability of the fetus. Whether the effects are reversible is unclear. However, a follow-up study recently indicated that lead-related dysfunctions in the early school years are associated with a significantly reduced chance of a child's being admitted to high school several years later.[39] Thus the insidious changes seen on a relatively flat dose-response relationship may well have rather severe public health implications.

The adult patient with acute lead poisoning has a weak handshake and decreased function of the extensor muscles of the forearm ("lead palsy," Teleky's sign). Although such obvious effects are now seen rarely, a decreased nerve conduction velocity has been documented in several studies, and electromyography has shown fibrillations and a decreased number of motor units at maximal effort. Related subjective symptoms may include muscle weakness, fatigue, pains in the extremities, and sometimes even tremor.[37] The earliest detectable effects on nerve conduction velocity appear to occur when blood lead levels exceed 40 μg/dl (1.9 μmol/L), as suggested by one prospective study and several cross-sectional investigations. Children may be somewhat more sensitive to peripheral nervous system effects, the decrease in nerve conduction velocity perhaps starting at relatively small increases in blood lead.

Acute lead exposure may also impair kidney function, but this effect appears to be reversible. In chronic exposures, hyperuricemia and a decreased clearance of creatinine and urea have been seen, and a statistical association has been reported with hypertension and gout.[35]

Symptoms from the gastrointestinal tract include anorexia, dysphagia, constipation, and in some cases diarrhea and can be a result of chronic exposures as well as of acute intoxication. In severe poisoning, colicky pains occur, and the blood lead level is frequently above 150 μg/dl (7.3 μmol/L). Periodic colic may continue for a few days, and several such patients have been subjected to surgery for a suspected appendicitis or ulcer. The colic is due to cramps in the smooth muscles of the intestines. The same mechanism may contribute to the occasional finding of hypertension and to the typical lead pallor.[35]

Under chronic exposure conditions and bad oral hygiene the accumulation of lead sulfide can cause a formation of a blue-gray seam at the gingival edge, the so-called lead seam. This sign is rare.

Some studies have suggested that severe lead exposure may decrease life expectancy, in particular because of an increased incidence of stroke. A similar tendency also has been postulated in relation to kidney disease, and kidney cancer has been suggested by animal studies. Although lead may be a weak cancer promotor and may augment the development of other disease, current lead exposure levels probably would not cause a detectable increase in cause-specific mortality, although the influence on individual health could be considerable. Teratogenic effects are well documented, and some reports have indicated toxic effects on sperm.

The diagnosis of lead poisoning may be difficult because the effects are nonspecific. In an adult patient, however, the combination of colicky pains, anorexia, constipation, insomnia, and irritability, perhaps supplemented by a low-normal hemoglobin and an increased serum bilirubin, would suggest lead poisoning. In children, lead toxicity may be even more difficult to recognize, especially in insidious cases. Screening programs for lead exposure therefore are paramount, and a blood test should be performed in individual cases at the least suspicion.

Prevention. The current lead exposure of an individual is best reflected in the lead concentration of whole blood. Signs of acute intoxication in adults usually are related to levels above 80 μg/dl (3.9 μmol/L), but mild cases can be seen at 60 μg/dl (2.9 μmol/L). Prevention of adverse health effects requires that blood lead levels be maintained below 40 μg/dl (1.9 μmol/L). Furthermore, the Occupational Safety and Health Administration (OSHA) lead standard includes the provision that blood lead concentrations be kept below 30 μg/dl (1.5 μmol/L) in men and women workers who intend to have children. Long-term exposure may be evaluated by measuring the ZPP level in the blood, and this test can be used efficiently for screening purposes. Medical surveillance is required as an additional safeguard and must be made available to all employees exposed above the action level of 30 $\mu g/m^3$ for more than 30 days a year. Blood lead examination must be carried out at least every 6 months, and every 2 months if the blood lead level exceeds 40 μg/dl (1.9 μmol/L). The removal protection provision means that workers with a blood lead level above 50 μg/dl (2.4 μmol/L), or if otherwise indicated by the medical surveillance, should be removed (without losing pay or benefits) until the level has returned to 40 μg/dl or below. If the air lead level cannot be kept below 50 $\mu g/m^3$, engineering control measures must be initiated. Regular air monitoring is required if levels exceed the action limit of 30 $\mu g/m^3$. The standard also includes provision for employee information and respirator use.

In the screening program for childhood lead exposure the Centers for Disease Control distinguishes between several classes of risk according to the lead and protoporphyrin levels in the blood. The acceptable limit for safe lead levels in the blood has been 25 μg/dl (1.2 μmol/L). This limit is expected to be decreased so that it is in better agreement with current research results. A recent report from the Agency for Toxic Substances and Disease Registry (ATSDR)[40] concluded that in 1984 between 3 and 4 million children in the United States had blood lead concentrations above 15 μg/dl (0.72 μmol/L). In addition, about one-half million children are born each year with a blood lead level above 10 μg/dl (0.48 μmol/L). These estimates document that lead pollution is a major public health problem. Although of serious dimensions in the United States, even higher average blood lead concentrations have been reported from countries in Latin America and Eastern Europe, thus indicating the international scope of the problem.

A WHO/FAO expert group recommended some years ago that the weekly oral intake (PTWI) of lead should be below 3 mg. This limit may protect most adults against adverse effects of lead, but even when adjusting for the body weight, the limit will not protect children sufficiently. Thus a PTWI for total lead intake in children has been set at 25 μg/kg body weight. The limit for lead in drinking water is 50 μg/L, and some countries have adopted a slightly higher limit for lead contents of wine, which occasionally can contain milligram quantities in a bottle if the lead cap has been eroded. Also, specific limits may apply to ceramic glazes. The lead release is usually measured by means of a 5% dilute acetic acid test. The test is conducted during three 30-minute boiling periods. Exposures also are limited by setting standards for the lead content of paints. Efforts have been initiated in some parts of the United States to remove old, peeling lead paint as part of restoration of houses with a lead hazard; continuing cases of lead poisoning in children suggest that these efforts are insufficient.

Organolead Compounds

Organolead compounds have a covalent bond between lead and carbon, resulting in chemical and toxic properties that differ from those of inorganic lead.[41] Tetraethyl lead has been used since 1924, and tetramethyl lead since 1960, as octane boosters of gasoline. Although the formation of methylated lead compounds in aquatic sediments may be possible, pollution with organolead compounds in cities is entirely due to gasoline lead. Evaporation from the carburetor and gasoline tank is a problem of older automobiles, and filling stations also contribute substantial amounts of organolead vapors. In addition, uncombusted organolead compounds may be present in considerable quantities in the exhaust gases during cold starts. In some European cities, up to 10% of the lead levels in the air has been organic lead. In the United States the organolead contribution is less because of improved engine designs and the considerable decrease in the use of lead additives; at the present time a small part of total gasoline sales is of leaded gas.

Organolead compounds are produced at several facilities in the United States and Europe. Occupational exposures may occur during the production, transportation, and blending procedures with raw gasoline. Particularly hazardous procedures include the cleaning of large storage tanks, where the inside organolead levels have been extremely high and have caused a large number of fatal intoxications. Organolead compounds may pass through the skin but apparently only in minor quantities when diluted in gasoline.

Because of their lipid solubility, organolead compounds may pass through membranes, including the blood-brain barrier. In the body they are dealkylated to the trialkyl lead compounds responsible for the toxic actions. Symptoms of acute poisoning are sleepiness, dizziness, and fatigue, and at higher exposure levels, insomnia, hallucinations, and a toxic psychosis may ensue. The measurement of blood lead levels is of limited use, but lead excretion in the urine may provide important information. At organolead intoxications the lead content in the urine is usually 150 μg/L (7.3 μmol/L) or higher, sometimes appreciably higher. It is necessary therefore to keep the lead levels below 100 μg/L (4.9 μmol/L) and preferably much below this level.

The latency period may be a few hours in severe poisoning but up to a day or so in milder cases. Fatalities usually are not encountered until 1 to 2 days after the acute exposure; in less severe cases, improvement begins in less than 2 weeks. Chronic sequelae have been described but appear to be relatively minor. Similarly, symptoms of chronic intoxication are mild and may resemble the nonspecific symptoms of the prodromal period.

Gasoline sniffing has been reported in several ethnic groups in different parts of the world; most frequently, gasoline sniffers are teenagers from traditional societies under severe cultural and social pressures. A euphoric state with hallucinations results from inhalation of gasoline fumes, and subsequent effects including nausea, vomiting, agitation, and anxiety could be partly due to organolead toxicity. More likely, the ataxia, tremor, confusion, and other neurological symptoms seen in habitual gasoline sniffers are produced by organolead compounds.

The occupational exposure limit for tetraethyl lead is 0.075 mg/m^3, and for tetramethyl lead, 0.07 mg/m^3; the ACGIH limits are 0.1 and 0.15 mg/m^3, respectively. This situation may be somewhat difficult to understand, since inorganic lead, to which the organolead compounds are detoxified, has a lower exposure limit. Environmental pollution with organolead compounds will decrease as older car models are scrapped and the lead content of the leaded gasoline is decreased. Most cars in the United States are now equipped with catalytic converters and must use unleaded gasoline; the same is true in Japan. Other countries, in particular most of Western Europe, have introduced unleaded gasoline more recently; although unleaded gasoline is required only for new cars with converters, a lower tax on unleaded gasoline has spurred increased sales. However, organolead consumption is increasing in many developing countries.

MAGNESIUM

Magnesium, a light metal, is essential for life, but excess exposures may have adverse effects.[42] Magnesium is required as an activator for at least 300 enzymes, and a daily intake of 0.6 g for adults has been recommended. Deficiency may be caused by insufficient intake, decreased absorption, and increased loss; alcoholism, parenteral nutrition, certain drugs, and various diseases are the principal causes of magnesium deficiency. The observation of decreased serum magnesium after myocardial infarction has led to clinical trials using magnesium infusions for these patients; although its biochemical mechanisms still are incompletely known, magnesium supplements seem to protect against arrhythmias and the risk of infarction-related deaths.[43] Occupational exposures to magnesium oxide produce eye and upper airway irritation, and controlled exposure with magnesium oxide fumes has demonstrated that metal fume fever may be induced in humans. Magnesium metal slivers implanted in the skin cause a slow-healing burn with ulceration. About one half of the magnesium in the body is retained in the skeleton, and a similar amount is contained intracellularly, but only about 1% is found in the serum. However, measurements of serum and urine magnesium levels are frequently useful. The current standard for occupational magnesium oxide exposure is 10 mg/m^3. The daily requirement for this essential element in food is about 0.3 to 0.4 g.

MANGANESE

The earth's crust has an average manganese content of 1000 $\mu g/g$. Manganese has a wide range of applications. Ferromanganese is its main product; 90% of the ferromanganese produced is used in various metal alloys, including welding rods. Other applications include dry batteries (manganese dioxide) and pigments for the glass and ceramics industry. Methylcyclopentadenyl manganese tricarbonyl (MMT) is used as an octane-boosting additive to gasoline. Occupational exposures to manganese may occur in the primary production and in the various user industries, especially when manganese-containing alloys are welded. Daily intakes through food are usually about 3 to 5 mg but may vary considerably, depending on the intake of cereals and rice, which are high in manganese.[44] High levels in drinking water rarely become a matter of medical concern because low limits are enforced for technical reasons. Increasing use of MMT in gasoline could cause atmospheric manganese levels above 1 $\mu g/m^3$ in cities, and similar levels may be encountered near ferromanganese plants.

The gastrointestinal absorption of manganese appears to be below 5% of that ingested, although its absorption can be inhibited by iron and is higher in iron deficiency; a considerable excretion occurs through the bile, some of which is reabsorbed. Manganese is an essential element in metalloenzymes and as enzyme activator, but deficiency states are unlikely to occur under normal circumstances.[44]

Characteristically, manganese-related diseases appear to be rare. Two different pictures may emerge: pulmonary and neurological pathologies.[24,44] In acute respiratory exposure to manganese a chemical pneumonitis may develop with cough, phlegm, fever, and changes on the chest x-ray film. Also, manganese aerosols may cause metal fume fever (as described under Zinc). Manganese conceivably may decrease the resistance to pneumonia and other lung diseases. Thus in Norwegian studies made about 50 years ago an increased frequency of pneumonia was related to severe community exposure from a ferromanganese factory. Reports of industrial and neighborhood exposures confirmed this finding. The dose-response relationship is not at all clear, however, but pulmonary effects in workers are unlikely to occur at manganese exposures below 0.3 mg/m^3.

Manganism is a central nervous system disease with clinical manifestations similar to those of parkinsonism.[45] This chronic intoxication has been described primarily in miners and workers in ore processing plants. The onset is delayed and sometimes occurs after the exposure has ceased. The first symptoms are nonspecific, such as asthenia, fatigue, headache, irritability, and memory difficulties. The more characteristic signs then develop insidiously: stiff movements, hoarse and low voice, stiffened facial expression, muscular hypertonia, and tremor. At least partial recovery may be achieved by treatment with L-dopa. Recent studies have suggested that the early, nonspecific symptoms occur at an increased frequency in welders and other workers with increased exposures to manganese. Although these preliminary data are from a few cross-sectional studies in which other exposures could distort the findings, they may indicate that a subclinical stage of manganese neurotoxicity could be relatively prevalent.[24] Interestingly, the severe manganism appears to affect only a small proportion of the exposed persons, and individual vulnerability may therefore be of importance.

Biological monitoring for manganese is of some interest and needs further exploration. In the blood some of the manganese has a half-life of about 1 month. Urine analyses are not useful, except perhaps in the case of MMT exposure, but analysis of hair samples occasionally has been used for screening purposes.[44]

The limit for occupational exposures is 5 mg/m^3. However, because of the possible subclinical effects on the CNS, a WHO working group[24] has recently recommended a limit of 0.3 mg/m^3. Although few countries have adopted a limit this low, the exposure limits for manganese have tended to decrease. In the surveillance of workers exposed to manganese above the WHO recommendation, neurological tests could be considered so that the exposure can be stopped if early neurotoxic effects develop. Because of the beneficial effects of trace amounts of manganese, a daily intake of about 2.5 to 5.0 mg of this metal in the diet has been recommended.

MERCURY

Exposures. The toxicity of mercury has been known since antiquity, but therapeutic effects also were used in a variety of drugs. In particular, mercury became an important drug from the sixteenth century when syphilis patients were treated with mercurous chloride (calomel). Such treatments invariably caused numerous intoxications. Occupational mercury poisoning has been described vividly in the past, for example, by Ramazzini, who almost 300 years ago noted about mirror makers: "At Venice on the island called Murano where huge mirrors are made, you may see these workmen gazing with reluctance and scowling at the reflection of their own sufferings in their mirrors and cursing the trade they have adopted."

The earth's crust contains an average mercury concentration of 0.05 to 0.08 μg/g, but large variations occur. Natural evaporation of mercury is the chief source of atmospheric pollution with this metal. Cinnabar, or mercury sulfide, has been used since ancient times as a pigment and constitutes the most important mercury ore. Environmental exposures in mercurous zones, where cinnabar occurs, may be considerable. Fresh water contains mercury levels up to 0.2 μg/L, unless contaminated, and most mercury is present in the particle fraction. In seawater, mercury is more easily soluble as a chloride complex. The mercury eventually finds its way to the sediments, where it is bound as sulfides under anaerobic conditions. Some microorganisms in the sediments are able to methylate mercury, possibly as a detoxication process. Methylmercury accumulates in fish, particularly in fatty species. Most of the mercury present in fish is in the form of methylmercury, and the highest levels usually are present in freshwater fish and saltwater carnivores; because of demethylation, liver from seals and whales is high in inorganic mercury.[46]

Mercury is used for a variety of instruments, including thermometers, manometers, and electrical equipment. Mercury also is used for the production of fluorescent light tubes, as a catalyst in the chemical industry, including the production of chlorine, and in amalgams for dentistry. Mercury may evaporate at room temperature; the rate depends on the surface area, temperature, and ventilation. Thus increased amounts of mercury will evaporate if it is scattered on the floor as small droplets. The amount that evaporates at 40° C is four times the amount that evaporates at 20° C. At saturation the air at 20° C contains 15 mg/m^3, which is more than 100 times the occupational exposure limit.

Inorganic mercury compounds are used for the production of certain pharmaceuticals, including mercurous bromide, certain inorganic pesticides, antifouling agents for marine paints, and various other purposes, such as treatment of felt for hats.

Organomercury compounds contain a covalent bond between mercury and carbon, and the organic part of the molecule is often an alkyl group or an alkoxyalkyl group. The former compounds are more toxic because they are more easily absorbed and more slowly metabolized. Organomercury compounds are used as a fungicide on seed grain. Methylmercury was used extensively for this purpose in the past, until environmental effects were discovered, and now methoxymethylmercury is the compound preferred. The paper and pulp industry previously has used these compounds as antislime agents. Phenylmercury has been used as a fungicide in paint. The decomposition of phenylmercury on application may produce considerable mercury vapor.

The various uses of mercury and mercury compounds result in occupational exposures in a range of occupations. Also, the industrial use of mercury may lead to releases to the environment, in particular through sewage water. Local river systems and bays have been contaminated by chloralkaline plants, paper and pulp industries, and pesticide factories. Minamata Bay in Japan was severely contaminated by a factory that used methylmercury as a catalyst in the production of vinyl chloride.

Inhaled metallic mercury vapors are almost completely absorbed in the alveoli. Absorption of the metal in the gastrointestinal tract is negligible unless some is retained, for example, in diverticula or the appendix. Inorganic mercury compounds from aerosols may be absorbed through the lungs as well, and some absorption (about 5% to 10% for soluble compounds) also takes place in the gastrointestinal tract. A higher absorption rate has been demonstrated in newborn rats, but data on humans are lacking. The organomercury compounds also are absorbed when taken in by this route, methylmercury almost completely.[46]

In the blood, inorganic mercury is almost evenly distributed between plasma and erythrocytes, but about 90% of organomercury compounds are bound to the cells. Mercury vapor and methylmercury are lipophilic and may pass biological membranes, including the blood-brain barrier and placenta, depositing considerable amounts in the CNS and the fetus, respectively. The vapor dissolved in the blood and tissues is rapidly oxidized. Mercuric ions become bound to some extent to metallothionein and accumulate in the kidneys. Excretion is mainly through feces and urine, but significant amounts may be eliminated in perspiration. The presence of ethanol in the blood influences the equilibrium between dissolved mercury vapor and mercury ions. Thus after ethanol ingestion, mercury vapor may be detected in the expired air of persons with high levels of mercuric ions in their blood. When selenium is present in the blood, a complex is formed that has a longer half-life but decreased toxicity, as judged from animal experiments. Methylmercury is metabolized slowly in the liver; methylmercury excreted in the bile may be demethylated by intestinal microorganisms and is excreted partly as inorganic mercury in the feces.[46]

Effects. Acute mercury vapor poisoning causes severe airway irritation, chemical pneumonitis, and pulmonary edema. Tremor may indicate nervous system involvement, but pulmonary distress is usually the cause of death. Ingestion of inorganic compounds results in symptoms of gastrointestinal corrosion and irritation, such as vomiting, bloody diarrhea, and stomach pains. Shock and acute kidney dysfunction with uremia may ensue. The lethal dose is about 1 g. Cutaneous exposure to mercury compounds may result in local common allergens in patients with contact dermatitis.

Chronic intoxication may appear a few weeks after the onset of a mercury exposure. More commonly, the exposure has lasted for several months or years. The symptoms depend on the degree of exposure and the type of mercury in question. The symptoms may involve the oral cavity, the nervous system, and the kidneys.[24]

Severe exposure to inorganic mercury causes an inflammation of gingiva and oral mucosa, which become tender and bleed easily. Salivation is increased, most obviously so in subacute cases. Often the patient complains of a metallic taste in the mouth. Especially when oral hygiene is bad, a gray border is formed on the gingival edges. If the inflammation develops further, the teeth may loosen and the salivary glands swell. Nasal bleeding also may occur, and changes in taste and odor sensations have been reported.

Mercury may damage both the peripheral and the central nervous systems. In exposures to mercury vapor, the CNS is the critical organ. The classic triad of symptoms includes erethism, intention tremor, and the gingivitis described above. The fine intention tremor of fingers, eyelids, lips, and tongue may progress to spasms of arms and legs. A jerky micrographia is typical as well. Along with the tremor, disturbances in the autonomic nervous system may cause excess perspiration and flushing of the skin. Pains in arms and legs and paresthesias may be related to a toxic polyneuritis. The changes in the CNS have psychological effects known as erethism: restlessness, irritability, insomnia, concentration difficulties, decreased memory, and depression, sometimes in combination with shyness, unusual psychological vulnerability, anxiety, and total neglect concerning economic problems and daily needs. In some cases a toxic psychosis develops. Newer studies suggest that early stages of erethism may occur; Russian authors have dubbed this psychoasthenic-vegetative syndrome "micromercurialism." The main problem appears to be decreased memory; headache, dizziness, and irritability also are part of the picture.

Kidney damage may occur during exposure, but chronic

loads with inorganic mercury compounds also may cause proximal tubular damage, as indicated by an increased excretion of small proteins in the urine, for example, β_2-microglobulin, retinol-binding protein, and albumin. The mechanism for this effect is not known in detail, but a synergistic action between mercury and cadmium has not been demonstrated. Glomerular damage seems to be caused by an autoimmune reaction to mercury complexes in the basal membrane, and mercury-related cases of nephrotic syndrome have been traced to this pathogenesis.

A different syndrome, the so-called "pink-disease" or acrodynia, was diagnosed frequently in children treated with teething powders that contained calomel, until 30 years ago, when the cause was discovered and teething powders were phased out. It also was seen occasionally in children who had inhaled mercury vapor from broken thermometers. A recent case in Michigan was due to mercury vapor released from interior house paint containing phenylmercury fungicide. A generalized eruption develops, and the hands and feet show a characteristic scaly, reddish appearance. In addition, the children are irritable, sleep badly, fail to thrive, perspire profusely, and have photophobia.

Mercury from amalgam fillings has been associated with a range of nonspecific symptoms. Some mercury vapor is released from the fillings, particularly during chewing; analysis of mercury in brain and kidney from autopsies has suggested an increased retention in relation to amalgam fillings. Although perhaps resembling "micromercurialism," the symptoms are nonspecific and an epidemiological study failed to identify a relationship to amalgam fillings.[47] This observation does not exclude the possible existence of some form of individual susceptibility to the mercury. However, anecdotal evidence of reversal of symptoms due to removal of fillings is difficult to explain; the removal procedure results in a briefly increased exposure and the mercury already retained in the body will be eliminated only slowly. With the large number of persons with mercury fillings, this uncertainty is unfortunate. However, at least from an environmental viewpoint, the introduction of safer alternatives should be recommended.

Intoxications with alkoxyalkyl or aryl compounds are similar to intoxications with inorganic mercury compounds because these organomercurials are relatively unstable. Alkyl mercury compounds, such as methylmercury, produce a different syndrome.[46] The earliest symptoms are paresthesias in the fingers, tongue, and face, particularly around the mouth. Later on, disturbances occur in the motor functions, resulting in ataxia and dysphasia. The visual field is decreased, and in severe cases total blindness may result. Similarly, impaired hearing may progress to complete deafness. This syndrome is known from cases of methylmercury intoxication in Japan, Iraq, and other countries where methylmercury-treated grain has been used for baking. Children are more susceptible to the toxic effects of methylmercury than adults are, and congenital methylmercury poisoning may result in a cerebral palsy syndrome, even though the mother remains healthy or suffers only minor symptoms caused by the exposure. In various populations with a high consumption of large marine fish or marine mammals, methylmercury intakes may approach the levels that produced such serious disease in Japan and Iraq. However, no clear-cut cases of intoxication have been reported in these populations, and the possibility is that the methylmercury accumulated in natural food chains is associated with selenium, which has a protective effect against the toxic actions of the mercury.

The prognosis of milder poisoning with inorganic mercury is excellent, but some sequelae may remain after chronic exposures to mercury vapor, and methylmercury poisoning has a less optimistic prognosis.

Prevention. Biological monitoring is useful in the diagnosis of mercury exposure and in the control of occupational exposure levels. In the blood, inorganic mercury has a half-life of about 30 days, and methylmercury has a half-life about twice as long. Unfortunately, blood levels do not reflect mercury retained in the brain, where mercury after vapor inhalation has a half-life of several years. Urine levels usually are preferred as an indicator of occupational exposures. Long-term mercury vapor exposures should respect a time-weighted average limit of 25 $\mu g/m^3$ and a corresponding urinary mercury excretion limit of 50 $\mu g/L$ (0.25 $\mu mol/L$).[24] Induction of minimal tremor by mercury vapor has been reported at exposures above this level. With regard to methylmercury the earliest effects, such as paresthesias, appear to occur when blood concentrations are above 200 $\mu g/L$ (1 $\mu mol/L$), but a safety factor of 10 should be applied to take into account possible individual susceptibility and the increased vulnerability of the fetus. In populations without considerable consumption of marine food, blood mercury concentrations usually are below 5 $\mu g/L$ (0.025 $\mu mol/L$). Methylmercury is incorporated in hair, and hair analyses for mercury screening have proved useful and quite reliable as indicators of individual exposures during the preceding months. Methylmercury toxicity has been seen at hair levels above 50 $\mu g/g$ (0.25 $\mu mol/g$). At steady state the mercury content in 1 L of blood is about four times the content of 1 g of hair. Thus a limit of 10 $\mu g/g$ (0.05 $\mu mol/g$) hair to protect against fetal methylmercury toxicity corresponds to about 40 $\mu g/L$ (0.20 $\mu mol/L$) blood.

Preventive measures should include the limitation of mercury released from industrial operations into the environment. One of the important nonindustrial sources is in discarded batteries (for cameras and watches) and thermometers. Some countries have instituted a practice of collecting and recycling the mercury from such consumer products. If mercury is used for fungicidal treatment of grain, the grain should be dyed red to indicate that it is unsuitable for human consumption. Concentration limits have been proposed for various fish products, especially for tuna, swordfish, and shark. A level of 0.5 or 1.0 mg/kg frequently is used. However, eel, halibut, and freshwater fish frequently may contain more than 1 mg/kg, especially in areas with local pollution sources. A PTWI level has been recommended at 0.3 mg/wk, of which no more than 0.2 mg/wk may be methylmercury.

The current occupational exposure limits are 0.1 mg/m^3 for aryl and inorganic mercury compounds, 0.05 mg/m^3 for mercury vapor, and 0.01 mg/m^3 for alkyl compounds.

MOLYBDENUM

The largest deposit of molybdenite, the major molybdenum ore, is in Climax, Colo. Most of the molybdenum consumption is in alloys but various compounds also are used as catalysts and pigments. Considerable experimental evidence is available on the essential functions of molybdenum but little information has been gathered on the toxic potential.[48] The human intake of this metal appears to be below 0.5 mg/d unless substantial contamination occurs. Absorption of molybdenum in food may be about 25% to 50% in humans, and excretion is mainly through the urine; the biological half-life in the blood is probably only a few hours, although some molybdenum may be retained in the liver and other tissues for a longer time. Molybdenum serves as a constituent of three oxidases, including xanthine oxidase, but deficiency states have not been reported in humans. Molybdenum poisoning in livestock may produce "teart disease" with anemia, growth retardation, and bone abnormalities, especially if the copper intake is low. In humans the frequent occurrence of arthralgias in some Armenian villages has been linked to the high intake of molybdenum, possibly through abnormalities of uric acid metabolism. Increased serum ceruloplasmin and mildly elevated serum uric acid were reported in workers from a molybdenite roasting plant; nonspecific complaints included joint pains and back pain possibly related to the exposure.[49] Pulmonary fibrosis has been reported in experimental animals, and a few cases of pneumoconiosis have been seen in workers exposed to sparingly soluble forms of molybdenum. The current exposure limits are 5 mg/m^3 for soluble compounds. A dietary intake of 0.15 to 0.5 mg of this metal daily has been recommended for adults as safe and adequate.

NICKEL

Exposures. Although the earth's crust contains an average nickel concentration of 80 μg/g, ores of sufficient quality occur only at a few places, notably Sudbury, Ontario. Nickel is used particularly for alloys but also for surface treatment of metals, as a catalyst, in the electronics industry, and in the production of nickel-cadmium batteries. Nickel exposures occur in the production trades and the various user industries, for example, stainless steel welding. The nickel intake through food may average about 0.1 to 0.2 mg/d, but it varies considerably because high contents may be encountered in legumes, cereals, nuts, and chocolate. Nickel may leach to food and beverages from nickel-plated or nickel-containing kitchen utensils. Limited information is available on gastrointestinal absorption, which seems to be about 5%. Internal exposures also may result from implantation of orthopedic prostheses and from intravenous infusion of nickel-contaminated solutions.[50,51]

Effects. Nickel apparently has a limited acute toxicity in humans, including airway irritation, but the important adverse effects relate to allergic eczema and respiratory cancers. However, nickel carbonyl may cause acute pulmonary disease and systemic toxicity.[50]

Respiratory exposure to nickel compounds in nickel production plants increases the risk of nasal and respiratory cancers. Animal experiments have indicated that a range of nickel compounds may be carcinogenic under various administration regimens, but epidemiological studies have not demonstrated whether a hazard is related only to nickel compounds present in refineries or to all nickel compounds. An increased respiratory cancer risk has been seen in some welders, but the contribution by nickel in welding fumes has not been elucidated. Most respiratory cancers in refinery workers have been primary carcinoma of the lung, but nasal cancers may be 100 times as frequent as would be expected. A recent evaluation of the epidemiological data from the refineries has shown a high risk associated with exposures to soluble nickel, mainly nickel sulfate, in addition to the oxide and sulfide forms; depending on kinetic factors, all nickel may be carcinogenic.[28]

Nickel allergy is the most frequent cause of contact eczema in women. The development of allergy is provoked frequently by earrings, but metal buttons, bracelets, and watches are frequent causes also. More rarely, the primary allergy develops because of an occupational exposure. However, hand eczema often results as a consequence of exposures at work if nickel allergy already is present, as indicated, in the past, for example, by earlobe dermatitis. Some studies suggest that about 10% to 15% of women become allergic to nickel and that almost half of them at some point develop hand eczema, in some cases so severe that the patient has to stop working. A much smaller proportion of the male population appears to be allergic to nickel. Nickel allergy may be increasing in prevalence, and it most frequently develops during the teenage years.[51] Limited evidence suggests that hand eczema in a nickel-allergic patient may develop or progress as a result of increased nickel intake through food.[52] In addition, inhalation allergy has resulted in asthmatic symptoms in a few recorded cases, but these two types of allergy probably are not related.

Nickel carbonyl, $Ni(CO)_4$, is a liquid and can evaporate at room temperature. Nickel carbonyl is produced in the Mond refining process of nickel. In addition, it may be formed or used in other branches of industry, such as electronics, oil refining, and plastics. After an acute exposure, dyspnea, headache, dizziness, vomiting, and substernal and hypogastric pain may occur, followed by a virtually symptom-free interval of 12 to 36 hours. Severe pulmonary symptoms then develop, and physical examination suggests pneumonia. Cerebral toxicity and death may ensue within 3 to 10 days. Pulmonary cancer has been reported in animal experiments, but the epidemiological evidence is uncertain on this point.

Prevention. Exposure to soluble nickel compounds and nickel carbonyl, which is metabolized to form nickel ions and carbon monoxide, may be evaluated by analysis of nickel concentrations in plasma and urine. The biological half-life in the body and the release from particles retained in the lungs will depend on the solubility of the nickel compounds concerned. Nickel in the blood seems to be cleared relatively rapidly by the kidneys, and animal experiments suggest a half-life of a few days. Therefore limits for plasma levels must depend on the nickel speciation in the exposure. Nickel levels in plasma usually are below 2 μg/L (0.03 μmol/L) in persons without occupational exposures, at least when the analysis has been carried out by an experienced laboratory.

The ACGIH limits are 1 mg/m^3 for nickel metal, nickel sulfide roasting, fumes, and dust; 0.1 mg/m^3 for soluble compounds; and 0.05 ppm for nickel carbonyl. NIOSH has recommended that the permissible exposure limit for nickel be reduced to 0.015 mg/m^3 and for nickel carbonyl to 0.001 ppm.

Specific preventive measures apply with regard to nickel-induced contact dermatitis. Primary prevention would mean that nickel-containing or nickel-plated metals should not be used in products that come into contact with the skin. Unfortunately, current fashions and the usefulness of nickel in cheap alloys (including coinage metal) seem to strongly oppose such measures. At any rate, contact with such products should be limited, if not totally avoided, in patients who have already developed an allergy to nickel. Many dermatologists have experienced some success in advising their patients to refrain from eating beans, cereals, nuts, and chocolate and from using nickel-plated kitchen utensils. The degree of nickel leaching may be determined by Fisher's test (dimethylglyoxime and ammonium hydroxide), which enables the allergic patient to identify and discard objects that could provoke an outbreak of dermatitis.[51]

OSMIUM

Osmium, a hard metal, occurs as osmiridium (a natural alloy with iridium) and as an impurity of other metal ores. Environmental exposures have limited significance, but the information on kinetics in the human body is incomplete. Of main interest is osmium tetroxide (osmic acid), which is used for various laboratory purposes, mainly as a fixative for tissue sections. The highly volatile osmium tetroxide also may be formed by oxidation of the finely divided metal. Inhalation of osmium tetroxide causes immediate irritation of the mucous membranes with cough and shortness of breath. These symptoms may last for several hours after a short exposure. Osmium tetroxide also has corrosive effects on the eyes, as indicated by severe irritation and lacrimation. After these symptoms have ceased, the patient may see large halos around lights until the tissue damage has been completely repaired. Skin contact results in irritant dermatitis. Repeated respiratory exposures allegedly have caused headache, insomnia, chronic airway irritation, and gastrointestinal disturbance. The permissible limit for occupational exposures to osmium tetroxide is 0.002 mg/m.[3]

PLATINUM

Platinum is used in jewelry, in dentistry, and in chemical and electrical industries. Platinum compounds are used in electroplating and photography and as a catalyst in the petroleum and pharmaceutical industries. Exposures to hexachloroplatinic acid and platinum tetrachloride are most frequent. When inhaled, the platinum compounds may cause upper airway irritation with violent sneezing, dyspnea, wheezing, and even cyanosis. Platinum rhinorrhea and platinum asthma are more typical clinical pictures that fade away shortly after the worker has left work for the day. Skin contact produces a scaly erythema, sometimes urticaria, mostly on the hands and forearms. These allergic manifestations have been called platinosis. Long-term effects, such as lung fibrosis, are unlikely, but a worker with a past history of platinosis may not be able to work with platinum again without suffering a severe reaction to minute amounts of platinum salts in the atmosphere. Some platinum compounds, notably *cis*-diamino-dichloroplatinum (cisplatin), inhibit cell growth in tumors and therefore have been used as cytostatic agents in cancer therapy. With the extensive precautions for handling such drugs, exposures of hospital personnel should be minimal; for surveillance purposes, urinary excretion of platinum could be determined. Environmental exposures result from industrial emissions and from the use of catalytic converters on automobile exhaust systems. Platinum is used as a catalyst, and about 1 μg of the metal is lost per mile of driving. The limit for occupational exposures is 0.002 mg/m^3 for soluble platinum salts, and the ACGIH has adopted a limit of 1 mg/m^3 for platinum metal.

RARE EARTHS

The rare earths or lanthanides constitute a group of metals that includes lanthanum and 14 elements in the periodic system that follow it. They occur in monazite and several other common minerals. Most extensively used are cerium and lanthanum. Major uses include steel alloys, lighter flints, catalysts, and additives in glass manufacture. Misch metal is an unseparated mixture of rare earths and yttrium. It has been suggested that these metals will experience a rapidly increasing demand, particularly for production of alloys. Thus exposure potentials may change in the future. To date, few problems have been discovered as a result of occupational exposure. A small number of reports have described cases of benign pneumoconiosis related to rare earth exposures, and similar conditions have been produced in animal experiments. Subcutaneous implantation of some rare earths has caused granulomas. Gastrointestinal absorption is limited and possibly negligible. Experiments with laboratory animals have documented toxic effects on several organ systems, especially fatty liver degeneration, blocking of the reticuloendothelial system, and interference with calcium metabolism. Because of the pyrophoric effects, rare earths may cause thermal burns and eye injuries. Although the limited information available suggests that these metals belong among the relatively less toxic ones, their increasing use and the scarcity of data concerning them should inspire additional studies and considerable caution in the handling of rare earths. Yttrium, which often is dealt with as a rare earth, has an exposure limit of 1 mg/m^3.

SELENIUM

Selenium often is referred to as a metalloid that shares some chemical properties with sulfur. Selenium is usually a by-product of primary copper production. This element has found considerable use in semiconductor technology and other electronic applications, in photocopy machines, as pigments in paints and glass, as an ingredient in certain alloys, in antidandruff shampoos, and in several other applications. Perhaps the most intensive exposures occur in sulfide ore refineries, but harmful exposures also may result when selenium-containing rectifiers are overloaded or when scrap metal is melted. Environmental selenium exposure varies geographically, with average daily dietary intakes varying from below 10 μg in parts of China and New Zealand to a high of about 300 μg in Venezuela and 750 μg in other areas of China. Increased levels may be due to emissions from coal combustion and manufacturing industries, but geological factors are generally most important. Some plants concentrate selenium and may contain up to several thousand parts per million.

Until recently the physiological role and toxic properties of selenium have been a matter of serious concern with regard to domestic animals but are of much less concern in connection with human health. Acute poisoning (''blind staggers'') and chronic toxicity (''alkali disease'') have been known in livestock for about 50 years. Later, selenium deficiency was discovered as the cause of white muscle disease in ruminant animals, hepatosis diatetica in swine, and exudative diathesis in chickens. Although toxicity in humans has been known for a long time, beneficial effects are now being characterized.

Soluble selenium compounds are almost completely absorbed from the gastrointestinal tract. Absorption through the skin may occur as well. The selenium concentrations in serum and urine seem to reflect recent absorption. Part of the selenium in the body is associated with a glutathione peroxidase, and the activity of this enzyme is linked closely to selenium levels. Selenium compounds are metabolized in the liver, in part by reduction and methylation. Dimethylselenide is an intermediary metabolite that is exhaled when its formation at high selenium exposures exceeds the further formation of trimethylselenonium ions, which are excreted in the urine. The kinetics depend on the absorption level and on interfering substances, including arsenic, cadmium, and mercury.

Inhalation of selenium results in mucous membrane irritation, gastrointestinal symptoms, elevated body temperature, headache, and malaise. Garlicky breath from dimethylselenide frequently is present. This symptom was noted by the housekeeper of Berzelius, who discovered selenium. In fact most of the systemic toxicity may be due to the liberation of this metabolite from the liver. Selenium dioxide and oxichloride are strong irritants and may produce burns and pulmonary edema. Because selenium is assimilated in the body, the nail beds become tender, and deformed nails develop; skin, teeth, and hair may become red from precipitation of amorphous selenium. Hydrogen selenide, which is more toxic than hydrogen sulfide, is generated by a reaction of metal selenides with water or acids; immediate symptoms are related to its irritant properties and nervous system depression, but frank pulmonary edema may develop after several hours. Seleniferous food has been related to enamel dysplasias in children, brittle hair, abnormal nail growth, some nonspecific symptoms, and delayed prothrombin time.[53]

Selenium deficiency is becoming an important medical entity. Keshan disease, an endemic, juvenile cardiomyopathy in China, occurs in selenium-low areas; successful treatment of a large number of patients apparently has been achieved by selenium supplements. Low selenium intakes may predispose patients to the development of some forms of cancer and arteriosclerosis. In addition, clinical improvement has been recorded in other groups of patients, including some on parenteral nutrition and some with lipidoses of the CNS. However, much more information needs to be discovered in these areas before conclusions concerning minimal daily intakes can be made, although a daily intake of 0.05 to 0.2 mg currently is recommended. However, in Finland where the daily selenium intake was considered marginal, selenium was added to agricultural fertilizers; serum selenium concentrations now reflect daily intakes regarded as adequate. It is unclear whether possible supplements should be taken in the form of organic compounds, such as selenomethionine. These compounds steadily increase selenium concentration in the erythrocytes, but the effect on glutathione peroxidase levels off. The toxic potential of the compounds concerned also must be considered.

Limited experience has been gathered on monitoring occupational selenium exposures. Measurement of selenium in urine and hair appears promising, perhaps supplemented by analysis of exhaled air for the possible presence of dimethylselenide. Selenium toxicity has been recorded at blood selenium concentrations above 600 μg/L (7.6 μmol/L) and at daily urinary excretion levels above 600 μg (7.6 μmol). Selenium deficiency would be likely to develop at blood concentrations below 30 μg/L (0.38 μmol/L) and at urinary excretion levels below 3 μg/d (0.04 μmol/d). A physiological decrease in blood selenium levels occurs during pregnancy. The occupational exposure limit is 0.2 mg/m^3 for selenium and its inorganic compounds and is 0.05 ppm for selenium hexafluoride, an airway irritant.

SILVER

Conventional uses of silver, such as jewelry, silverware, and photographic emulsions, have been augmented by a range of other applications resulting from developments in coatings and alloy technology. Silver solder also is in use, although the adverse effects related to the cadmium content have necessitated a change of ingredients. Argyria is a bluish discoloration of the skin due to deposition of silver metal particles. A localized form is due to penetration of particles through the corneum, but generalized argyria is due to absorption of silver compounds into the body. Argyrosis of the respiratory tract has been diagnosed by bronchoscopy, but ocular argyrosis, especially as evidenced by conjunctival discoloration, may be more easily detected. These signs occur as a result of occupational exposures but also may be caused by oral or dermal pharmaceuticals containing silver; they appear to be relatively benign.[54] The current exposure limit is 0.01 mg/m^3 for silver metal and soluble silver compounds, but ACGIH has recommended a limit of 0.1 mg/m^3 for silver metal.

TANTALUM

Tantalum is used increasingly in alloys for electronic equipment and applications in the nuclear and aerospace industries. Additional uses include surgical prostheses and additives in glass manufacture. Few health problems have been attributed to occupational exposure to this metal. Animal experiments suggest that airway irritation and pneumonitis may result from inhalation of tantalum dusts, and sequelae in the form of emphysema, slight fibrosis, and epithelial hyperplasia have been recorded. The current occupational exposure limit is 5 mg/m^3.

TELLURIUM

Tellurium is similar to selenium and occurs as an impurity of various metal ores. It is used in various alloys and for rubber compounding. Tellurium causes garlicky breath at a lower exposure level than selenium does. Not surprisingly, some workers from an electronic company were referred to Dr. Harriet L. Hardy of the Massachusetts Institute of Technology with the chief complaint that their wives refused to kiss them. This symptom disappears about a week after cessation of selenium exposure but is longer lasting when caused by tellurium. In addition, tellurium also causes dry mouth and inhibits perspiration. The exposure limit is 0.1 mg/m^3, but for the irritant tellurium hexafluoride, it is 0.02 ppm or 0.2 mg/m^3.

THALLIUM

Thallium is a rare element in the biosphere and has been used by humans for only about 100 years. Early uses included thallium as a therapeutic agent against syphilis, dysentery, and other diseases, but the most important current application is as a rodenticide or insecticide. Thallium has important uses in various industrial processes, including the fabrication of phosphorescent pigments and glassware, and as a catalyst in organic synthesis. Environmental thallium pollution occurs near mines and refineries because zinc, cadmium and copper ores usually contain thallium. Most environmental effects have been due to extensive application of thallium rodenticides.

Thallium compounds are without taste and odor, and lethal doses may be less than 1 g. Absorption through the skin has led to several cases of intoxication, and gastrointestinal absorption is almost complete. Many poisonings have been related to the easy access in the past to thallium pesticides. The acute effects include nausea, vomiting, diarrhea, and possibly gastrointestinal bleeding within a few days, accompanied by a motor polyneuropathy with muscle weakness associated with mental disturbances, such as irritability, concentration difficulties, somnolence, and, in severe cases, delirium and convulsions. Hair loss (alopecia) occurs about 1 to 3 weeks after the acute exposure. Thus the characteristic triad, gastroenteritis, polyneuropathy, and hair loss, is seen only at a rather late stage of the intoxication. In survivors of severe poisoning, some nervous system damage may remain after recovery.

Inhalation of thallium-containing dust at work over longer time periods may be associated with vague symptoms of joint pains, anorexia, fatigue, and trembling, accompanied by partial hair loss and polyneuropathy. No specific treatment of thallium poisoning is available, although several chelators may have marginal effects, and prevention is therefore of utmost importance.

Excretion is mainly through the gastrointestinal tract and the kidney. Urine levels of thallium may remain high for several weeks, although plasma concentrations have decreased. A biological half-life of several days has been indicated by experiments on rodents, but longer half-lives in slow compartments may exist in humans. A slow excretion takes place through hair and nails, which may provide a profile of recent thallium levels in the body. The limit for occupational exposure to soluble thallium compounds is 0.1 mg/m^3.

TIN

Tin has been used for many centuries in brass and pewter and currently is also used in tin-plating, which consumes about half the total tin production, tinfoil, collapsible tubes, and pipes. Cans for food products often are plated with tin on the inner side, and leaching to acid contents may be considerable, especially if the can is left open for a few days. The dietary intake of tin is variable, although the range is mostly about 1 to 4 mg/d. A large number of organotin compounds are in use, for example, dioctyltin as a stabilizer in PVC, triorganotins as pesticides, in particular fungicides and antifouling agents, and various compounds as catalysts.[55]

Ingestion of 50 mg of tin causes vomiting, but only a small percentage of this is absorbed in the gastrointestinal tract. Organotin compounds are absorbed more easily, also through the skin, but detailed information on human exposures is unavailable. Tin may be an essential element in some species, perhaps including humans. Inhalation of tin dust is usually not a matter of major concern. However, an apparently benign pneumoconiosis, called stannosis, has been described in relation to considerable exposures to tin dust. On the x-ray film, stannosis appears as rounded opacities that are denser than the nodules in silicosis. This clinical picture may already be developed 3 to 5 years after the onset of exposure, but pulmonary function abnormalities are minor, if detectable at all.[9]

The organotin compounds, including dialkyl and trialkyl compounds, are strong skin irritants. The systemic toxicity in experimental animals has been studied in some detail; the neurotoxic potential is higher in trialkyltins than in dialkyltins, and it decreases with the length of the alkyl chains. Thymus degeneration and other immunotoxic effects have been induced by diorganotin compounds. More than 200 human cases of poisoning, half of them fatal, were described after the application of an ointment containing organotin compounds (diethyltin and triethyltin) against staphylococcal infections. The symptoms included headache, vomiting, dizziness, visual disturbances, convulsions, and paresis. Similar, but less severe, symptoms have been described in workers exposed to organotin compounds, including trimethyltin and triphenyltin.

The limit for occupational exposure to tin is 2 mg/m^3, and for organotin compounds, 0.1 mg/m^3. Biological monitoring seems to be of limited use, although urinary tin excretion may be worth studying more closely. In the preventive measures, eye protection and prevention of skin contact with organotin compounds should be included.

TITANIUM

The chief use for titanium is in titanium dioxide pigments. It is used in paints, paper coatings, pharmaceuticals, and bread flour, for example, because of its extreme whiteness and high index for refraction. Titanium tetrachloride may be encountered as an intermediate and as a catalyst; the carbide is a component of "hard metal," and titanium metal is alloyed with other metals. The daily intake, mainly through food, may be up to a few milligrams, depending on local paint sources and the content of titanium dioxide additives in food items such as bread and cheese. Occupational exposures mainly concern the metal and the dioxide, which appear to be generally nontoxic. Findings of obstructive lung disease, pulmonary fibrosis, and airway irritation in titanium-exposed workers could be due to exposures to other chemicals, and the contribution of titanium is yet to be determined. Titanium tetrachloride is a strong irritant because acid is liberated when it comes in contact with water, and pulmonary edema may result. Systemic toxicity is known from experimental toxicology but is probably of little importance in environmental health, since titanium is poorly absorbed from the gastrointestinal tract. Titanocene, an organotitanium compound, has been carcinogenic when injected into rodents. Also, titanium phosphate, a fibrous material, may possess important biological activities. The consumption of this metal is rapidly increasing, and additional studies of its health significance would be warranted. Titanium dioxide is regarded a nuisance dust with an exposure limit of 10 mg/m^3.

TUNGSTEN

Tungsten (or wolfram) is present in the environment in small quantities. Major exposures are associated with the primary production of tungsten and with the manufacture of tungsten carbide for hard metal products. Although a considerable fraction of soluble tungsten compounds are absorbed in the gut, urinary excretion is rapid. Systemic toxicity has been produced in laboratory animal experiments but appears to be of little relevance to human exposure situations. Pulmonary disease has been documented from the manufacture of cemented carbide tools, but the adverse effects probably are caused by cobalt, and any contribution from tungsten exposures is difficult to assess. The ACGIH limits are 1 mg/m^3 for tungsten and soluble compounds, and 5 mg/m^3 for insoluble compounds. NIOSH has recommended similar limits.

URANIUM

Uranium is radioactive and may cause serious chemical toxicity. Most natural uranium is uranium 238, which has a half-life of almost 5 billion years. It is extracted from ores that may contain less than 1% of the metal. Exposure to caustic uranium hexafluoride vapor may occur during the concentration process. Its main use is as fuel in nuclear power plants, but small amounts are used as pigments and catalysts. Gastrointestinal absorption varies with solubility, and human studies would suggest that perhaps 20% of uranium from food is absorbed. Tetravalent uranium is oxidized in the organism to hexavalent ions that are excreted through the glomeruli. At low pH, uranyl ions (UO_2^{2+}) will be reabsorbed in the tubules, where they may cause cell damage or necrosis. Increased excretion of albumin and catalase has been detected in such cases. This process may be prevented by infusion of sodium bicarbonate; regeneration seems to be possible, and the prognosis of nonlethal cases therefore is fairly good. Less soluble uranium compounds from respiratory exposures tend to accumulate in the lungs, making them the primary sites of retention. Such accumulation, especially if the uranium is enriched with ^{235}U, would tend to have effects associated with the α-radiation. However, the excess cancer risk in uranium miners seems to be mainly due to radon gas and radon daughters. Uranium sometimes may occur in drinking water, and such contamination has been linked to excess excretion of β_2-microglobulin in the urine as an indication of early tubule dysfunction. The standard for occupational exposure to uranium is 0.2 mg/m^3.

VANADIUM

At an average concentration of about 1.5 mg/g, vanadium is one of the more frequent metals in the earth's crust. Some minerals contain rather high concentrations of vanadium, but this metal is produced primarily from vanadium-containing iron ores. Vanadium often is used in various alloys, frequently in the form of ferrovanadium, which accounts for most vanadium consumption. Vanadium oxides are important catalysts in the inorganic and organic chemical industries, and other vanadium compounds are used in the electronics, ceramics, glass, and pigment industries. Occupational exposure to vanadium also may occur at primary production of other metals when the ores contain considerable amounts of vanadium; certain qualities of oil contain much vanadium, and unexpected exposures may occur when burners and filters are being serviced.[56]

The daily intake through food is frequently below 0.1 mg,

and gastrointestinal absorption may be less than 1%. Vanadium is an essential element for chickens and rats, but how essential it is to humans has not been determined. Environmental exposures have not been reported to cause significant toxicity, but the possible health significance of vanadium pollution from fly ash probably needs further study.

Pentavalent vanadium compounds are more toxic than tetravalent compounds are.[56] Vanadium pentoxide (V_2O_5) dust and fumes cause conjunctivitis, rhinitis, and other irritations of the mucous membranes and, in severe cases, dyspnea and chemical pneumonitis. Some workers become particularly sensitized, whereas others seem to adapt to it. Vanadium-induced cough may be particularly bothersome, since it lasts for several days; the mechanism is probably both bronchoconstriction and increased secretion of mucus. These changes are reversible in most cases, but chronic bronchitis has been recorded as an apparent long-lasting effect following long-term exposures. Animal studies have indicated that vanadium could induce systemic effects, such as fatty degeneration of liver and kidneys, polycythemia, and cardiotoxicity at high doses. In humans a lowering of serum cholesterol levels has been demonstrated, as well as a reduction of cystine in fingernails. After oral intake of vanadium the tongue may have a green coating.

Vanadium is efficiently excreted in the urine, and about one half the absorbed amount is excreted within the first 1 to 2 days, but the existence of a slower compartment with a half-life of about several weeks has been suggested. Analysis of urine samples for vanadium at the end of a workday may be useful to indicate the acute exposure levels, and levels below 30 μg/L (0.6 μmol/L) are believed to reflect safe exposures. The limit for occupational exposures to vanadium pentoxide is 0.05 mg/m^3.

ZINC

Zinc is a common and essential metal with a low toxic potential. Its concentration in the earth's crust is 40 mg/kg. This metal is added to bronze, brass, and various other alloys to add corrosion resistance, and it is used for galvanizing steel and other iron products. In the presence of carbon dioxide and humidity a surface film of alkaline zinc carbonate is formed, which protects against corrosion. Various zinc compounds are used in the chemical, ceramic, pigment, plastic, rubber, and fertilizer industries. Most frequently used are zinc oxide, carbonate, sulfate, chloride, and some organic compounds. The most significant occupational exposures occur during alloy founding, galvanizing, zinc smelting, and welding, especially of galvanized metals.[57]

The daily intake of zinc varies considerably. Seafood and meat are high in zinc. Also, soft drinking water may contain high concentrations of zinc leached from the water pipes. The average oral intake is several milligrams. The gastrointestinal absorption is difficult to evaluate because the major excretion route is through the gut. Also, the absorption of zinc may vary with the speciation and the presence of phytate, calcium, phosphate, and vitamin D. Under normal circumstances the absorption probably is about 25% to 50%, and under zinc deficiency the absorption may approach 100%.

Zinc is an essential metal, and more than 20 zinc-dependent enzymes have been identified. Zinc deficiency in children has resulted in endocrine disturbances with retarded growth and delayed puberty. This condition may be cured completely when zinc therapy is instituted. Acrodermatitis enterohepatica, a rare familial skin disease, has been found to be related to deficient zinc absorption. In addition, recent research has suggested that zinc supplements may be beneficial in certain dermatological conditions and in accelerating wound healing in surgical patients. Zinc also seems to somewhat protect against cadmium toxicity. However, in the occupational setting, the latter metal is a frequent impurity in zinc and may result in serious adverse effects.

Oral zinc poisoning has occurred in a few instances as a result of zinc release from galvanized food containers. Symptoms have included nausea, vomiting, stomach pains, and diarrhea.

Inhalation of high concentrations of zinc oxide may cause metal fume fever,[57] a condition that also may be caused by freshly formed oxides of several other metals, including copper, magnesium, manganese, and nickel. This condition also is referred to by other names, such as metal shakes or zinc chills. The metal oxide particles tend to aggregate after their formation and are unable to pass through to the lungs as easily; therefore only the freshly formed particles cause the disease. A few hours after the exposure, the first symptoms may be slight feeling of malaise, dry cough, sore throat, and a sweet, metallic taste in the mouth. An influenza-like syndrome develops 6 to 8 hours later, with chills, muscle pains, headache, and medium-grade fever, which is followed by sweating and recovery. Blood tests show leukocytosis, increased sedimentation rate, and lactate dehydrogenase. Depending on the extent of the exposure, the total attack usually lasts less than 24 hours, and the patient usually returns to work the next morning. Many workers have experienced repeated, almost weekly, spells of metal fume fever, and chronic damage could conceivably occur. However, this question is difficult to address, and none of the current evidence suggests that repeated attacks of metal fume fever leave sequelae. In fact the patient develops a temporary resistance after each spell, and metal fume fever therefore is seen mostly on Mondays, which accounts for the name, "Monday morning fever." The mechanism of metal fume fever is not yet known.

Zinc chloride is used extensively as a flux in soldering, and incautious work practices have caused spattering of caustic droplets. In contact with water, hydrochloric acid is liberated, and the result is painful burns. Zinc chloride also is used in smoke bombs, and inhalation of the fumes has had corrosive effects in the airways, with pulmonary edema and, in the survivors, bronchopneumonia.

Biological monitoring is yet of limited importance. The urine represents only a minor part of the total amount excreted. Decreased serum zinc concentrations may be attributed to pregnancy, alcoholism, or chronic disease, but increases are minimal in relation to occupational exposures.

Metal fume fever seems to be caused by zinc fume levels of 15 mg/m^3, but insufficient information is available on exposures below that level. The exposure limit for zinc oxide fumes is 5 mg/m^3. The standard for zinc chloride fumes is 1 mg/m^3; for other zinc exposures, the limit is 10 mg/m^3. With regard to the beneficial effects, recommended values for daily requirements are 15 mg for adults, 20 mg for pregnant women, and 25 mg for lactating women.

ZIRCONIUM

Zirconium has limited uses, the chief ones being in glass and ceramics production, shielding materials for nuclear power plants, and some alloys. The meager evidence contains no well-documented case of zirconium toxicity in industry. However, use of deodorants containing this metal has induced subcutaneous granulomas, possibly due to hypersensitivity. The exposure limit is 5 mg/m^3.

REFERENCES

1. Nieboer E, Richardson DHS: The replacement of the nondescript term "heavy metals" by a biological and chemically significant classification of metal ions. Environ Pollut 1(Series B):3–26, 1980

2. Bergqvist U: New Metals: A Study on the Use of and Exposure to Certain Metals and Their Compounds From a Toxicological Viewpoint. USIP Report 83-11. Stockholm: University of Stockholm, Institute of Theoretical Physics, 1983
3. Grandjean P, Jensen BM, Sandø SH, Jørgensen PJ, Antonsen S: Delayed blood regeneration in lead exposure: An effect on reserve capacity. Am J Public Health 79:1385–1388, 1989
4. Lauwerys R: Industrial Chemical Exposure: Guidelines for Biological Monitoring. Davis, Calif.: Biomedical Publications, 1983
5. Grandjean P: Monitoring of environmental exposures to toxic metals. In Brown SS, Savory J (eds): Chemical Toxicology and Clinical Chemistry of Metals. London: Academic Press, 1983, pp 99–112
6. Friberg L, Nordberg GF, Vouk VB (eds): Handbook on the Toxicology of Metals, Vol II. 2nd edt. Amsterdam: Elsevier, 1986
7. Clarkson TW, Friberg L, Norgberg GF, Sager PR (eds): Biological Monitoring of Toxic Metals. New York: Plenum, 1988
8. Spencer H, Lender M: Adverse effects of aluminum-containing antacids on mineral metabolism. Gastroenterology 76:603–606, 1979
9. Parkes WR: Occupational Lung Disorders. 2nd edt. London: Butterworth, 1982
10. Wills MR, Savory J: Aluminum poisoning: Dialysis encephalopathy, osteomalacia, and anaemia. Lancet 2:29–34, 1983
11. Ott SM, Maloney NA, Klein GL, Alfrey AC, Ament ME, Coburn JW, Sherrard DJ: Aluminum is associated with low bone formation in patients receiving chronic parenteral nutrition. Ann Intern Med 98:910–914, 1983
12. Sjögren B, Lundberg I, Lidums V: Aluminum in the blood and urine of industrially exposed workers. Br J Ind Med 40:301-304, 1983
13. Criteria for Recommended Standard: Occupational Exposure to Antimony. DHEW (NIOSH) Publication No. 78–216. Cincinnati: National Institute for Occupational Safety and Health, 1978
14. Criteria for a Recommended Standard: Occupational Exposure to Inorganic Arsenic. New Criteria 1975. DHEW (NIOSH) Publication No. 75-149. Cincinnati: National Institute for Occupational Safety and Health, 1975
15. World Health Organization: Arsenic. Environmental Health Criteria 18. Geneva: WHO, 1981
16. Arsine (Arsenic Hydride) Poisoning in the Workplace. Current Intelligence Bulletin No. 32, DHEW (NIOSH) Publication No. 79–142. Cincinnati: National Institute for Occupational Safety and Health, 1979
17. Feldman RG, Niles CA, Kelly-Hayes M, Sax DS, Dixon WJ, Thompson DJ, Landau E: Peripheral neuropathy in arsenic smelter workers. Neurology 29:939–944, 1979
18. Doig AT: Baritosis: A benign pneumoconiosis. Thorax 31:30–39, 1976
19. Hardy H: Beryllium disease: A clinical perspective. Environ Res 21:1-9, 1980
20. Lauwerys R: The Toxicology of Cadmium. Environment and Quality of Life Series, EUR 7649. Luxembourg, Belgium: Commission of the European Communities, 1982
21. Criteria for a Recommended Standard: Occupational Exposure to Cadmium. DHEW (NIOSH) Publication No. 76–192. Cincinnati: National Institute for Occupational Safety and Health, 1976
22. Roels HA, Lauwerys RR, Buchet JP, Bernard AM, Vos A, Oversteyns M: Health significance of cadmium induced renal dysfunction: a five year follow up. Br J Ind Med 46:755–764, 1989
23. Roels HA, Lauwerys RR, Buchet J-P, Bernard A: Environmental exposure to cadmium and renal function of aged women in three areas of Belgium. Environ Res 24:117–130, 1981
24. World Health Organization: Recommended Health-Based Limits in Occupational Exposure to Heavy Metals. Technical Report Series 647. Geneva: WHO, 1980
25. Criteria for a Recommended Standard: Occupational Exposure to Chromium (VI). DHEW (NIOSH) Publication no. 76–129. Cincinnati: National Institute for Occupational Safety and Health, 1976.
26. Anderson RA: Essentiality of chromium in humans. Sci Total Environ 86:75–81, 1989
27. Langård S (ed): Biological and Environmental Aspects of Chromium. Amsterdam: Elsevier, 1982
28. Chromium, Nickel and Welding Exposures. IARC Monographs on the Evaluation of the Carcinogenic Risk of Chemicals to Humans, Vol. 50. Lyon, France: International Agency for Research on Cancer, (in press)
29. Criteria for Controlling Occupational Exposure to Cobalt. DHHS (NIOSH) Publication No. 82–107. Cincinnati: National Institute for Occupational Safety and Health, 1982
30. Alexander CS: Cobalt-beer cardiomyopathy. Am J Med 53:395–417, 1972
31. Jensen AA, Tüchsen F: Cobalt exposure and cancer risk. CRC Crit Rev Toxicol (in press)
32. Committee on Medical and Biological Effects of Environmental Pollutants, National Research Council: Copper. Washington, D.C.: National Academy of Sciences, 1977
33. Müller-Höcker J, Meyer U, Wiebecke B, et al. Fatal copper storage disease of the liver in a German infant, resembling Indian childhood cirrhosis. Virchows Arch 411:379–385, 1987
34. Committee on Medical and Biological Effects of Environmental Pollutants, National Research Council: Iron. Baltimore: University Park Press, 1978
35. U.S. Environmental Protection Agency: Air Quality Criteria for Lead. Research Triangle Park, N.C.: U.S. EPA, 1986
36. Grandjean P: Ancient skeletons as silent witnesses of lead exposures in the past. CRC Crit Rev Toxicol 19:11–21, 1988
37. Cullen MR, Robins JM, Eskenazi B: Adult inorganic lead intoxication: Presentation of 31 new cases and a review of recent advances in the literature. Medicine 62:221–247, 1983
38. Hansen ON, Trillingsgaard A, Beese I, Lyngbye T, Grandjean P: A neuropsychological study of children with elevated dentine lead level: Assessment of the effect of lead in different socioeconomic groups. Neurotoxicol Teratol 11:205–213, 1989
39. Needleman HL, Schell A, Bellinger D, Leviton A, Allred EN: The long-term effects of exposure to low doses of lead in childhood. N Engl J Med 322:83–88, 1990
40. The Nature and Extent of Lead Poisoning in Children in the United States: A Report to Congress. Atlanta, Ga.: Agency for Toxic Substances and Disease Registry, 1988
41. Grandjean P (ed): Biological Effects of Organolead Compounds. Boca Raton, Fla.: CRC Press, 1984
42. Rude RK, Singer FR: Magnesium deficiency and excess. Ann Rev Med 32:245–259, 1981
43. Rasmussen HS, McNair P. Nørregaard P, Backer V, Lindeneg O, Balslev S. Intravenous magnesium infusion in acute myocardial infarction. Lancet 1:234–236, 1986
44. World Health Organization: Manganese. Environmental Health Criteria 17. Geneva: WHO, 1981
45. Mena I: Manganese. In Bronner F, Coburn JW (eds): Disorders of Mineral Metabolism, Vol. I. Trace Minerals. New York: Academic Press, 233–270, 1981
46. World Health Organization: Mercury. Environmental Health Criteria 1. Geneva: WHO, 1976
47. Ahlqwist M, Bengtsson C, Furunes B, Hollender L, Lapidus L: Number of amalgam tooth fillings in relation to subjectively experienced symptoms in a study of Swedish women. Community Dent Oral Epidemiol 16:227–231, 1988
48. Winston PW: Molybdenum. In Bronner F, Coburn JW (eds): Disorders of Mineral Metabolism, Vol. I. Trace Minerals. New York: Academic Press 295–315, 1981
49. Walravens PA, Moure-Eraso R, Solomons CC, Chapell WR, Bentley G: Biochemical abnormalities in workers exposed to molybdenum dust. Arch Envrion Health 34:302–307, 1979
50. Nickel in the Human Environment. IARC Scientific Publications No. 53. Lyon, France: International Agency for Research on Cancer, 1984
51. Menné T, Maibach H (eds). Nickel and the Skin. Boca Raton, Fla.: CRC Press, 1989
52. Nielsen GD, Jepsen LV, Jørgensen PJ, Grandjean P, Brandrup F: Nickel-sensitive patients with vesicular hand eczema: Oral challenge with a diet naturally high in nickel. Br J Dermatol (in press)

53. Yang G, Yin S, Zhou R, Gu L, Yan B, Liu Y, Liu Y: Studies of safe maximal daily dietary Se-intake in a seleniferous area in China. J Trace Elem Electrolytes Health Dis 3:123–130, 1989
54. Rosenman KD, Moss A, Kon S: Argyria: Clinical implications of exposure to silver nitrate and silver oxide. J Occup Med 21:430–435, 1979
55. World Health Organization: Tin and Organotin Compounds: A Preliminary Review. Environmental Health Criteria 15. Geneva: WHO, 1980
56. Criteria for a Recommended Standard: Occupational Exposure to Vanadium. DHEW (NIOSH) Publication No. 77-222. Cincinnati: National Institute for Occupational Safety and Health, 1977
57. Criteria for a Recommended Standard: Occupational Exposure to Zinc Oxide. DHEW (NIOSH) Publication No. 76-104. Cincinnati: National Institute for Occupational Safety and Health, 1975

21

Diseases Associated with Exposure to Chemical Substances

Organic Compounds

Ruth Lilis

ORGANIC SOLVENTS

Organic solvents comprise a large group of compounds (alcohols, ketones, ethers, esters, glycols, aldehydes, aliphatic and aromatic saturated and nonsaturated hydrocarbons, halogenated hydrocarbons, carbon disulfide, etc.) with a variety of chemical structures. Their common characteristic, related to their widespread use in many industrial processes, is the ability to dissolve and readily disperse fats, oils, waxes, paints, pigments, varnishes, rubber, and many other materials.[1,2]

Solvent exposure affects many persons outside industrial and occupational settings. The use of solvents in household products and in arts, crafts, and hobbies has significantly increased the population that may be affected by repeated exposure. Moreover, the deliberate inhalation of solvents as a form of addiction (''sniffing'') occurs, especially in younger population groups.

Some solvents are well known for their specific toxic effects on the liver, kidney, and bone marrow,[3] and a few organic solvents have specific toxicity for the nervous system. Carbon disulfide may induce a severe toxic encephalopathy with acute psychosis[3]; methyl alcohol may induce optic neuritis and atrophy; methyl chloride and methyl bromide may cause severe acute, even fatal, toxic encephalopathy. Exposures to n-hexane, methyl-n-butyl ketone,[4-6] and carbon disulfide have produced peripheral neuropathy.

Most organic solvents share some common nonspecific toxic effects, the most important of which are those on the central nervous system (CNS). The depressant narcotic effects of organic solvents have long been recognized; numerous members of this heterogeneous group of chemical compounds have been used as inhalation anesthetics (chloroform, ethyl ether, trichloroethylene, etc.).

The sequence of stages of anesthesia achieved with volatile solvents is of interest: the cerebral cortex is affected first; the lower centers of reflex activity in the brain stem and medulla oblongata, which control vital cardiovascular and respiratory functions, are the last to be depressed. This characteristic sequence makes it possible to use volatile anesthetic compounds for medical purposes. The earliest manifestations of the anesthetic effects of solvents are slight disturbances in psychomotor coordination. These may progress to more pronounced incoordination and, if exposure continues, through an excitation stage of longer or shorter duration, to loss of consciousness.

Occupational exposure to solvents may reproduce the entire sequence of medical anesthesia, up to loss of consciousness and even death through paralysis of vital cardiovascular and respiratory centers. While such severe cases of occupational solvent poisoning are relatively uncommon under normal conditions, they may occur with unexpected accidental overexposure.

The initial manifestations of CNS depression are frequent in workers handling solvents or mixtures of solvents in various industrial processes. A low boiling point, with generation of significant airborne concentrations of vapor, large surfaces from which evaporation may take place, lack of appropriate enclosure and/or exhaust ventilation systems, relatively high temperature of the work environment, and physical exercise implicit in the actual work performed (increasing the ventilatory volume per minute and thus the amount of solvent vapor absorbed) may all contribute to uptake of sufficient solvent to induce prenarcotic CNS symptoms.

Early prenarcotic effects are dizziness, nausea, headache, slight incoordination, paresthesia, increased perspiration, tachycardia, and hot flushes. These symptoms are mostly subjective and transitory, and their causal relationship with solvent exposure has therefore often been overlooked. The transitory nature of prenarcotic symptoms is due to the common characteristics of the metabolic model for solvents: once exposure ceases after the end of the work shift, the body burden of solvents is usually rapidly depleted, mostly eliminated through exhalation. The prenarcotic symptoms subside as the concentration of solvent in blood and in the CNS decreases.

With exposure to higher concentrations or with longer exposure, more marked incoordination and a subjective feeling of drunkenness may occur. The risk of accidents is increased, even with early prenarcotic symptoms and more so with more pronounced symptoms.

While acute overexposure of higher magnitude with loss of consciousness is generally accepted as a serious condition (with possible persistent after effects, including neurological deficit), the long-term effect of repeated episodes of slight prenarcotic symptoms has remained unexplored until relatively recently, although it had been recognized that such symptoms are an expression of functional changes in some cortical neurons.

It had been suspected for some time that repeated functional change may lead to permanent impairment of neuronal functions, and various possible mechanisms had been considered, including interference with cell membrane or neurotransmitter functions or even neuronal loss. Since no regeneration of neurons occurs, neuronal loss can result in permanent, irreversible neurological damage. The diffuse nature of such effects and the lack of major, well-localized neurological deficits have contributed to the relatively slow recognition of chronic, irreversible solvent-induced neurological impairment.

Repeated exposure to organic solvents may result in the gradual development of persistent symptoms, such as headache, tiredness, fatigue, irritability, memory impairment, diminished intellectual capacity, difficulty in concentration, emotional instability, depression, sleep disturbances, alcohol intolerance, loss of libido and/or potency. These symptoms, often reported by workers with repeated solvent exposure and mentioned in many studies on chronic effects of solvents, had received relatively little attention until recently, probably because of their nonspecific nature. Nevertheless, the term *toxic encephalosis* was proposed as early as 1947.[7] More recently, the term *psycho-organic syndrome* has been used for this cluster of symptoms related to long-term solvent exposure. Effects on the CNS, including the diencephalic centers of the autonomic system with their interrelationships with endocrine functions, are probably important components in the development of the syndrome.

Over the last several years, chronic neurotoxicity of solvents related to long-term exposure has received increasing attention. Research has been particularly active in the Scandinavian countries. Epidemiological studies of exposed workers and control groups have significantly contributed to recognition of the association between the psycho-organic syndrome and exposure to solvents; neurobehavioral and electrophysiologic methods, including electroencephalographic, visual evoked potential, and nystagmographic investigations, have added objective, quantitative measures for the assessment of CNS functions.

In case-control studies,[8,9] neuropsychiatric disease has been found to occur more frequently among solvent-exposed workers than in age-matched controls. In a large study performed in Denmark, in which solvent-exposed painters were compared with nonexposed bricklayers,[10] the painters had a relative risk of 3.5 for disability due to cryptogenic presenile dementia. With modern methods of investigation and brain imaging, including pneumoencephalography, computed tomographic (CT) scan, and cerebral blood flow studies, diffuse cerebral cortical atrophy has been demonstrated in cases of chronic solvent poisoning.[11-16]

Thus recent studies converge to indicate that long-term exposure to solvents may lead to chronic, irreversible brain damage. The clinical expression is that of intellectual impairment and decrements in performance, which can be detected by means of neurobehavioral testing; electroencephalographic abnormalities are frequent and characterized mostly by a diffuse low wave pattern. The underlying pathological changes are represented by cortical atrophy; these changes can be of different severity, with extreme cases of severe diffuse cerebral and cerebellar cortex atrophy in chronic poisoning due to solvent sniffing addiction.[13,17,18]

The axons and myelin sheaths may also be affected by organic solvents. This is well known for peripheral nerves, and peripheral neuropathy has been well documented with exposure to such solvents as carbon disulfide, methyl-*n*-butyl ketone and *n*-hexane. While specific CNS effects are known also to occur with carbon disulfide, little is known about the chronic CNS effects of the other solvents capable of producing peripheral neuropathy. Recent research has shown that solvents such as *n*-hexane and methyl-*n*-butyl ketone have an effect on both long and short axons and that axonal degeneration of fibers in the anterior and lateral columns of the spinal cord, cerebellar vermix, spinocerebellar tracts, optic tracts, and tracts in the hypothalamus can also occur.[6,19]

ALIPHATIC HYDROCARBONS

Aliphatic hydrocarbons are mostly derived from petroleum by distillation or cracking; their chemical structure is relatively simple, since they are linear carbon chains of various lengths with a certain number of hydrogen atoms attached. They are either saturated (alkanes or paraffins) or unsaturated (alkenes or olefins, with one or several double bonds) and alkynes or acetylenes, with one or more triple bonds.

The aliphatic hydrocarbons occur in mixtures that have numerous industrial uses: natural gas; heating fuel; jet fuel; gasoline; solvents for a variety of materials such as pigments, dyes, inks, pesticides, herbicides, resins, and plastic materials; in degreasing and cleaning; in the extraction of natural oils from seeds; and increasingly as raw material for the synthesis of numerous compounds in the chemical industry.

Compounds with a low number of carbon atoms are gases (methane, ethane, propane, butane). Compounds with a higher number of carbon atoms (up to eight) are highly volatile liquids at room temperature, whereas those with longer carbon chains have higher boiling temperatures and usually do not generate dangerous air concentrations. Compounds with more than 16 carbon atoms are solids. The only adverse effect attributed to the lower members of the group is the indirect one they might exert when present in high concentrations, displacing oxygen.

Toxic effects of *paraffins* (alkanes) are significant for the highly volatile liquid compounds from pentane through octane. These compounds are potent depressants of the CNS, and overexposure may result in deep anesthesia with loss of consciousness, convulsions, and death through inhibition of the respiratory center. Such high levels of exposure are infrequent under usual circumstances, but they may occur accidentally. Moderate irritation of mucous membranes of the airways and conjunctivae is a common but less severe effect; degreasing of the skin might contribute to dermatitis, with repeated contact. Aspiration of liquid mixtures of aliphatic hydrocarbons into the airways or accidental ingestion of such liquids usually results in chemical pneumonitis, often severe and necrotizing.

Chronic toxic effects of aliphatic hydrocarbons have been identified only rather recently. *N*-hexane has been shown to be one of the substances that may result in toxic peripheral neuropathy, affecting both the sensory and motor components of peripheral nerves, initially in the lower extremities but eventually, with longer exposure, also in the upper extremities. Paresthesia, numbness, and tingling progressing from distal to proximal, distal hypoesthesia (touch, pain), followed by muscle weakness due to motor deficit, with difficulty in walking and eventual muscular atrophy, and diminished or absent deep tendon reflexes, are the characteristic clinical findings. Electromyographic abnormalities indicating peripheral nerve lesions, including abnormal fibrillation pattern, and significant decrease in nerve conduction velocities (sensory and motor) are usually detected. Axonal degeneration and secondary demyelination have been found to be the underlying pathological abnormalities. Abnormalities in visual, auditory, and somatosensory evoked potentials have been reported after experimental *n*-hexane exposure; longer latencies and central conduction times were interpreted as reflecting neurotoxic effects at the level of the cerebrum, brain stem, and spinal cord.[20]

N-hexane peripheral neuropathy, first described by Japanese investigators[21] in 1969, has since been repeatedly reported from various European countries and the United States.[22] It has also been reproduced in animal experiments at concentrations as low as 250 ppm. Nevertheless, outbreaks of toxic peripheral neuropathy due to *n*-hexane have continued to be reported. Relatively recently such cases have occurred in press proofing workers in Taiwan, associated with exposure to a solvent mixture with a high (60%) *n*-hexane content. The outbreak of peripheral neuropathy cases had been preceded by a gradual change (to a high *n*-hexane content) in the solvent mixture used to clean rollers of press proofing machines.[23] Cases of *n*-hexane subacute, predominantly motor, peripheral neuropathy have also been reported in young adults and in children after several months of glue sniffing. Although functional improvement after discontinuation of toxic exposure has been reported, in some cases full recovery has not been observed, even after long term (16 years) follow-up.[24-26] More recently, experiments involving exposure of rats to high concentrations of *n*-hexane have revealed adverse effects on the seminiferous epithelium; repeated exposures resulted in severe, irreversible testicular lesions.[27] The main *n*-hexane metabolites are 2-hexanol and 2,5-hexanedione. In experiments on rats, 2-hexanol was found to be mostly excreted during exposure while 2,5-hexanedione was mainly excreted after the end of exposure. *N*-hexane accumulates in adipose tissue where it persists longer (estimated half-life, 64 hours); complete elimination from fat tissue after cessation of exposure has been estimated to require at least 10 days.[28]

The maximum concentration of 2,5-hexanedione in urine was delayed with higher exposure levels. Measurement of urinary 2,5-hexanedione levels has been proposed for the biological monitoring of workers exposed to *n*-hexane.[29] In humans chronically exposed to a mixture of hexane isomers with concentrations ranging from 10 ppm to 140 ppm, the urinary 2,5-hexanedione excretion ranged from 0.4 to 21.7 mg/L.[30] Urinary concentrations of 2,5-hexanedione in subjects not exposed to *n*-hexane or related hydrocarbons were found to range from 0.12 to 0.78 mg/L.[31] The urinary 2,5-hexanedione excretion reaches its highest level 4 to 7 hours after the end of exposure.[32] Biological monitoring to assess worker exposure to toxic chemicals has gained increasing recognition, especially for occupations characterized by highly variable exposure levels. The American Conference of Government Industrial Hygenists has recommended biological exposure indices (BEIs—levels of a biological indicator after an 8-hour exposure to the current threshold limit value) for a limited number of widely used chemicals; *n*-hexane is one of these.[33] 2,5-Hexanedione was found to be significantly correlated with a score of electroneuromyographic abnormalities. There is general agreement that, for practical purposes, the urinary concentrations of 2,5-hexanedione can predict the likelihood of subclinical peripheral neuropathy in persons exposed to *n*-hexane.[34] 4,5-Dihydroxy-2-hexanone as a metabolite of *n*-hexane has recently been identified in rats and in humans; it is excreted in amounts that at times exceed those of 2,5-hexanedione. It has been suggested that this metabolite indicates a route of detoxification.[35] While there is no definitive evidence that other aliphatic hydrocarbons, such as pentane, heptane, or octane, have similar effects, some case reports suggest an association.

Commercial hexane that had been used in industrial processes where workers had peripheral neuropathy was found to contain 2-methyl pentane, 3-methyl pentane, and methyl cyclopentane, in addition to *n*-hexane. The neurotoxicity of these compounds has been tested in rats, and significant effects on peripheral nerves of a similar type but of lesser magnitude than those of *n*-hexane were detected. The order of neurotoxicity was found to be *n*-hexane > methyl cyclopentane > 2-methyl pentane = 3-methyl pentane.[36]

Other solvent mixtures, such as one containing 80% pentane, 5% hexane, and 14% heptane, have produced cases of peripheral neuropathy in humans. White spirit mixtures containing more than 10% *n*-nonane have been shown by neurophysiological and morphological criteria, to produce axonopathy in rats after 6 weeks of daily exposure. Since the various members of the group are most often used in mixtures, a time-weighted average (TWA) of 100 ppm (350 mg/m^3) has been proposed.[3]

Peripheral neuropathy similar to that associated with hexane has been found to result from exposure to methyl *n*-butyl ketone. DiVincenzo et al[37] identified the metabolites of *n*-hexane and of methyl *n*-butyl ketone; the similarity of chemical structure between the metabolites of these two neurotoxic agents suggested the possibility of a common mechanism in the very similar peripheral neuropathy.

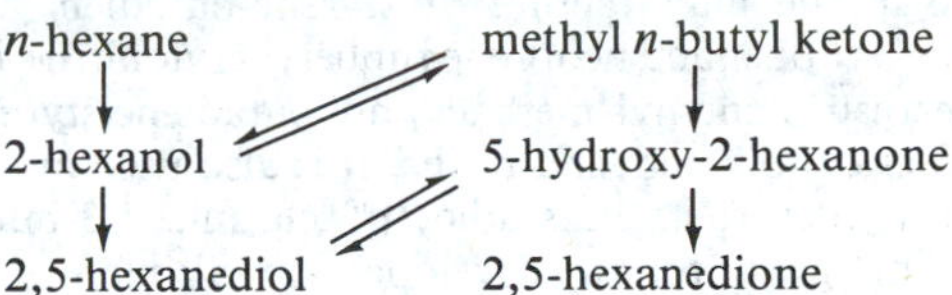

It is now well established that 2,5-hexanedione is the most toxic metabolite. The biochemical mechanism of 2,5-hexanedione neurotoxicity is related to its covalent binding to protein lysyl residues and cyclization to pyrroles. Pyrrole oxidation and subsequent protein cross-linking then lead to the accumulation of neurofilaments in axonal swellings, the histopathologic earmark of gamma-diketone peripheral neuropathy. Massive accumulation of neurofilaments has been shown to occur within the axoplasm of peripheral and some central nervous system fibers.[38]

Ethyl-*n*-butyl ketone (EBK, 3-heptanone) had not been reported until recently to produce toxic neuropathy. In a recent study, EBK administered in relatively high doses for 14 weeks by gavage produced a typical central peripheral distal axonopathy in rats, with giant axonal swelling and hyperplasia of neurofilaments. Methyl-ethyl ketone (MEK) potentiated the neurotoxicity of EBK and increased the urinary excretion of two neurotoxic gamma-diketones, 2,5-heptanedione and 2,5-hexanedione. The neurotoxicity of EBK seems to be due to its metabolites, 2,5-heptanedione and 2,5-hexanedione. MEK potentiates EBK neurotoxicity by inducing the metabolism of EBK to its neurotoxic metabolites.[39]

Commercial-grade methyl-heptyl ketone (MHK, 5-methyl-2-octanone) also produced toxic neuropathy in rats, clinically and morphologically identical to that resulting from *n*-hexane, methyl-*n*-butyl ketone (MBK), and 2,5-hexanedione. The MHK mixture was found by gas chromatography-mass spectrometry to contain 5-nonanone (12%), MBK (0.8%) and C_7—C_{10} ketones and alkanes (15%), besides 5-methyl-2-octanone. Purified 5-nonanone produced clinical neuropathy, whereas purified 5-methyl-2-octanone was not neurotoxic; given together with 5-nonanone, it potentiated the neurotoxic effect. In vivo conversion of 5-nonanone to 2,5-nonanedione was demonstrated.[40] The toxicity of 5-nonanone was shown to be enhanced by simultaneous exposure to MEK. This effect is attributed to the microsomal enzyme inducing properties of MEK.[41] The neurotoxicity of methyl-*n*-butyl ketone has been shown to be enhanced by other aliphatic monoketones, such as methyl-ethyl ketone, methyl-*n*-propyl ketone, methyl-*n*-amyl ketone, and methyl-*n*-hexyl ketone; the longer the carbon chain of the aliphatic monoketone, the stronger the potentiating effect on methyl-*n*-butyl ketone neurotoxicity seemed to be.[42]

Neuropathological studies have shown that the susceptibility of nerve fibers to these linear aliphatic hydrocarbons and ketones is proportional to fiber length and the diameter of the axon. Fibers in the peripheral and central nervous systems undergo axonal degeneration, with shorter and smaller fibers generally being affected later. The long ascending and descending tracts of the spinal cord, the spinocerebellar and the optic tracts, can be affected. Giant axonal swelling, axonal transport malfunction, and secondary demyelination are characteristic features of this central peripheral distal axonopathy.

The unsaturated *olefins* (with one or more double bonds),

such as ethylene, propylene, and butylene, and the diolefins, such as 1,3-butadiene and 2-methyl-1,3-butadiene, mainly obtained through cracking of crude oil, are of importance as raw materials for the manufacture of polymers, resins, plastic materials, and synthetic rubber. Their narcotic effect is more potent than that of the corresponding saturated linear hydrocarbons, and they have moderate irritant effects.

1,3-Butadiene, a colorless, flammable gas is a by-product of the manufacture of ethylene; it can also be produced by dehydrogenation of *n*-butane and *n*-butene. Major uses of 1,3-butadiene are in the manufacture of styrene-butadiene rubber, polybutadiene rubber and neoprene rubber, acrylonitrile-butadiene-styrene resins, methyl methacrylate-butadiene-styrene resins, and other copolymers and resins. It is also used in the production of rocket fuel. In studies of chronic 1,3-butadiene inhalation, malignant tumors developed at multiple sites in rats and mice, including mammary carcinomas and uterine sarcomas in rats and hemangiosarcomas, malignant lymphomas, and carcinomas of the lung in mice.[43] Other important effects were atrophy of the ovaries and testes. Ovarian lesions produced in mice exposed by inhalation to 1,3-butadiene included loss of follicles, atrophy, and tumors (predominantly benign, but also malignant granulosa cell tumors). Ovarian lesions have been detected for only 8 of 300 chemicals tested.[44] A macrocytic megaloblastic anemia, indicating bone marrow toxicity, was also found in inhalation experiments on mice.[45]

Epidemiological studies on occupational groups exposed to 1,3-butadiene in the manufacture of styrene-butadiene rubber were conducted. The results in some studies were inconclusive, most probably because of the relatively short period of observation from onset of exposure and the relatively small number of workers in the cohorts. The standardized mortality ratio for non-Hodgkin's lymphoma was found to be increased in a large cohort of employees at a butadiene-production facility. There were, nevertheless, no clear exposure group or latency period relationships.[46] 1,3-Butadiene is metabolized to 1,2-epoxy-3 butene. This metabolite has been shown to be carcinogenic in skin-painting experiments on mice. 1,3-Butadiene has been found to be mutagenic in in vitro tests on *Salmonella* and genotoxic to mouse bone marrow in vitro in the sister chromatid exchange test. Binding of carbon 14–labeled 1,3-butadiene to liver DNA was demonstrated in mice and rats.[47] The International Agency for Research on Cancer concluded in 1986 that the evidence of a carcinogenic effect of 1,3-butadiene in humans is inadequate but that there is sufficient evidence of carcinogenic potential in experimental animals to consider a carcinogenic risk in humans.[48]

The National Institute for Occupational Safety and Health has recommended that the present OSHA standard of 1000 ppm TWA for 1,3-butadiene be reexamined, since carcinogenic effects in rodents (mice) have been observed at exposure levels of 650 ppm. To minimize the carcinogenic risk for humans, it was recommended that exposures be reduced to the lowest possible level.

Isoprene (2-methyl-1,3-butadiene), a naturally occurring volatile compound and close chemical relative of 1,3-butadiene, has been recently studied in inhalation experiments on rats. A mutagenic metabolite, isoprene diepoxide, was tentatively identified in all tissues examined.[49]

The principal member of the series of aliphatic hydrocarbons with triple bonds—*alkynes*—is acetylene (HCCH), a gas at normal temperature. Acetylene is widely used for welding, brazing, metal buffing, metallizing, and other similar processes in metallurgy. It is also a very important raw material for the chemical synthesis of plastic materials, synthetic rubber, vinyl chloride, vinyl acetate, vinyl ether, acrylonitrile, acrylates, trichloroethylene, acetone, acetaldehyde, and many others.

While the narcotic effect of acetylene is relatively low and becomes manifest only at high concentrations (15%) not found under normal circumstances, the frequent presence of impurities in acetylene represents the major hazard. Phosphine is the most common impurity in acetylene, but arsine and hydrogen sulfide may also be present. The hazard is especially significant in acetylene-producing facilities or when acetylene is used in confined, poorly ventilated areas.

ALICYCLIC HYDROCARBONS

Alicyclic hydrocarbons are saturated (cycloalkanes, cycloparaffins, or naphthenes) or unsaturated cyclic hydrocarbons, with one or more double bonds (cycloalkenes or cycloolefins). The most important members of the group are cyclopropane, cyclopentane, methylcyclopentane, cyclohexane, methylcyclohexane, ethylcyclohexane, cyclohexene, cyclopentadiene, and cyclohexadiene. These compounds are present in crude oil and its distillation products.

Cyclopropane is used as an anesthetic. Most of the members of the group are used as solvents and, in the chemical industry, in the manufacture of a variety of other organic compounds, including adipic, maleic, and other organic acids; methylcyclohexane is a good solvent for cellulose ethers. Their toxic effects are similar to those of their linear counterparts, the aliphatic hydrocarbons, but they have more marked narcotic effects; the irritant effect on skin and mucosae is similar.

COMMERCIAL MIXTURES OF PETROLEUM SOLVENTS

Mixtures of hydrocarbons obtained through distillation and cracking of crude oil are gasoline, petroleum ether, rubber solvent, petroleum naphtha, mineral spirits, Stoddart solvent, kerosene, and jet fuels. These are all widely used commercial products.

The composition of these mixtures is variable: all contain aliphatic saturated and nonsaturated hydrocarbons, alicyclic saturated and nonsaturated hydrocarbons, and smaller amounts of aromatic hydrocarbons such as benzene, toluene, xylene, and polycyclic hydrocarbons; the proportion of these components varies. The boiling temperature varies from 30° to 60°C for petroleum ether to 175° to 325°C for kerosene; the hazard of overexposure is higher with the more volatile mixtures with lower boiling temperatures.

The toxic effects of these commercial mixtures of hydrocarbons are similar to those of the individual hydrocarbons: the higher the proportion of volatile hydrocarbons in the mixture, the greater the hazard of acute CNS depression, with possible loss of consciousness, coma, and death resulting from acute overexposure. Exposure to high concentrations, when not lethal, is usually followed by complete recovery. Nevertheless, irreversible brain damage may occur after prolonged coma. The underlying pathologic change is represented by focal microhemorrhages. The irritant effects on the respiratory and conjunctival mucosae are generally moderate.

Exposure to lower concentrations over longer periods is common; the potential effects of aromatic hydrocarbons, especially benzene, have to be considered under such circumstances. Bone marrow depression with resulting low red blood cell counts and leukopenia with neutropenia and/or low platelet counts can develop, and medical surveillance should include periodic blood counts for the early detection of such effects; cessation of exposure to mixtures containing aromatic hydrocarbons is necessary when such abnormalities occur. Long-term effects of benzene exposure include increased risk of leukemia; therefore exposure should be carefully monitored and controlled so that the recommended standard for benzene not be exceeded.

Chronic effects on the central and peripheral nervous systems with exposure to commercial mixtures of hydrocarbons have received more attention only in recent years. Since some of the common components of such mixtures have been shown to produce peripheral neuropathy and to induce similar degenerative changes of axons in the CNS, such effects might also result from exposure to mixtures of hydrocarbons. Long-term exposure to solvents, including commercial mixtures of hydrocarbons, has been associated, in some cases, with chronic, possibly irreversible CNS impairment. Such effects have been documented by clinical, electrophysiological, neurobehavioral, and brain-imaging techniques.

Accidental ingestion and aspiration of gasoline or the other mixtures of hydrocarbons can occur, mainly during siphoning, and result in severe chemical pneumonitis, with pulmonary edema, hemorrhage, and necrosis.

Gasoline and other hydrocarbon mixtures used as engine fuel have a variety of additives to enhance desired characteristics. Lead tetraethyl probably has the highest toxicity. Workers employed in the manufacture of this additive and in mixing it with gasoline have the highest risk of exposure, and their protection has to be extremely thorough. Ethylene dibromide (EDB) is another additive with important toxicological effects; recently it has received increased attention.

Skin irritation, related to the degreasing properties of these solvents, and consequent increased susceptibility to infections is frequent when there is repeated contact with such mixtures of hydrocarbons or with individual compounds. Chronic dermatitis is a common finding in exposed workers; protective equipment and appropriate work practices are essential in its prevention.

Prevention and Surveillance. Exposure to airborne aliphatic hydrocarbons should be controlled so as not to exceed a concentration of 350 mg/m^3 as a time-weighted average. This concentration is equivalent to 120 ppm pentane, 100 ppm hexane, and 85 ppm heptane. For the commercial mixtures, a similar TWA has been recommended, except for petroleum ether (the most volatile mixture) for which a TWA of 200 mg/m^3 is recommended.[3] Exposure to benzene should not exceed the recommended standard of 1 ppm (3.2 mg/m^3), given the marked myelotoxicity of benzene and the increased incidence of leukemia. There is a definite need to monitor for the presence and amount of aromatic hydrocarbons in mixtures of petroleum solvents.

Medical surveillance programs should aim at the early detection of such adverse effects as toxic peripheral neuropathy, chronic CNS dysfunction, hematological effects, and dermatitis. Since accidental overexposure may result in rapid loss of consciousness and death (CNS depression), adequate and prompt therapy for such cases is urgent. Education of employees and supervisory personnel concerning potential health hazards, safe working practices (including respirator use when necessary), and first-aid procedures is essential.

AROMATIC HYDROCARBONS

Aromatic hydrocarbons are characterized by a benzene ring in which the six carbon atoms are arranged as a hexagon, with a hydrogen atom attached to each carbon—C_6H_6. According to the number of benzene rings and their binding, the aromatic hydrocarbons are classified into three main groups:

1. Benzene and its derivatives: toluene, xylene, styrene, etc.
2. Polyphenyls: two or more noncondensed benzene rings—diphenyls, triphenyls
3. Polynuclear aromatic hydrocarbons: two or more condensed benzene rings—naphthalene, anthracene, phenanthrene, and the carcinogenic polycyclic hydrocarbons (benz[a]pyrene, methylcholanthrene, etc.)

Distillation of coal in the coking process was the original source of aromatic hydrocarbons; an increasing proportion is now derived from petroleum through distillation, dehydrogenation of cycloparaffins, and catalytic cyclization of paraffins.

Benzene

Benzene is a clear, colorless, volatile liquid with a characteristic odor; the relatively low boiling temperature (80° C) is related to the high volatility and the potential for rapidly increasing air concentrations.

Commercial-grade benzene contains variable amounts—up to 50%—of toluene, xylene, and other constituents that distill below 120° C. More important is the fact that commercial grades of other aromatic hydrocarbons, toluene and xylene, also contain significant proportions of benzene (up to 15% for toluene); this also applies to commercial mixtures of petroleum distillates, such as gasoline and aromatic petroleum naphthas, where the proportion of benzene may reach 16%. Therefore, benzene exposure is a more widespread problem than would be suggested by the number of employees categorized as handling benzene as such; many others exposed to mixtures of hydrocarbons or commercial grades of toluene and xylene may also be exposed to significant concentrations of benzene.

Exposure to benzene may occur in the distillation of coal in the coking process; in oil refineries; and in the chemical, pharmaceutical, and pesticides industries, where benzene is widely used as a raw material for the synthesis of products. Exposure may also occur with its numerous uses as a solvent, in paints, lacquers, and glues; in the linoleum industry; for adhesives; in the extraction of alkaloids; in degreasing of natural and synthetic fibers and of metal parts; in the application and impregnation of insulating material; in rotogravure printing; in the spray application of lacquers and paints; and in laboratory extractions and chromatographic separations. An important use of benzene in some parts of the world is as an additive in motor fuel, including gasoline. In Europe, gasolines have been found to contain up to 5% benzene; in the United States levels up to 2% have been reported. Environmental levels of benzene in areas with intense automotive traffic have been found to range from 1 to 100 ppb.[50] The largest amounts of benzene are used for the synthesis of other organic compounds, mostly in enclosed systems, where exposure is generally limited to equipment leakage, liquid transfer, and repair and maintenance operations. Exposures with the use of benzene as a solvent or solvent component present a more difficult problem, since enclosure of such processes and adequate control of airborne concentrations have not been easily achieved.

Production has continuously expanded, reaching 11 billion pounds in 1976. It is estimated that more than 2 million workers are exposed to benzene in the United States.[3] In recent years there has been increasing concern with respect to benzene in hazardous waste-disposal sites. Benzene has been found in almost one third of the 1177 National Priorities List hazardous waste sites. Other environmental sources of exposure include gasoline filling stations, vehicle exhaust fumes, underground gasoline storage tanks that leak, wastewater from industries that use benzene, and ground water next to landfills that contain benzene. Consumer products that contain benzene include glues, adhesives, some household cleaning products, paint strippers, some art supplies, and gasoline.[51]

Inhalation of the vapor is the main route of absorption; skin penetration is of minor significance. Benzene retention is highest in lipid-rich organs: in adipose tissue and bone marrow, benzene concentrations may reach a level 20 times higher than the blood concentration; its persistence in these tissues is also much longer. Elimination is through the respiratory route (45% to 70% of the amount inhaled); the rest is excreted as urinary metabolites. Benzene is metabolized in the liver by the mixed-function microsomal oxidases; the first intermediate in its biotransformation, benzene epoxide, is possibly the active substance responsible for the carcinogenic effect of benzene. The metabolites of benzene include phenol, catechol, hydroquinone, *p*-benzo-quinone, and *trans-trans*-mucondialdehyde. It has been shown that deoxyribonucleic acid (DNA) adducts (guanine nucleoside adducts) are formed by incubation of rabbit bone marrow with ^{14}C-labeled benzene; *p*-benzoquinone, phenol, hydroquinone, and 1,2,4-benzenetriol also form adducts with guanine.[52] Catechol and hydroquinone were found to be highly potent in inducing sister chromatid exchanges and delaying cell division; these effects were much more marked than those of benzene and phenol.[53]

Exposure to high airborne concentrations of benzene results in CNS depression with acute, nonspecific, narcotic effects; with very high exposure (thousands of ppm), loss of consciousness and depression of the respiratory center or myocardial sensitization to endogenous epinephrine with ventricular fibrillation may result in death. Recovery from acute benzene poisoning is usually complete if removal from exposure is prompt; in cases of prolonged coma (after longer exposure to high concentrations), diffuse or focal electroencephalographic (EEG) abnormalities have been observed for several months after recovery, together with such symptoms as dizziness, headache, fatigue, and sleep disturbances.

Chronic benzene poisoning is a more important risk, since it can occur with much lower exposure levels. It can develop insidiously over months or years, often without premonitory warning symptoms, and result in severe bone marrow depression. Benzene is a potent myelotoxic agent. Red blood cell, white blood cell, and platelet counts may initially increase, but more often anemia, leukopenia, and/or thrombocytopenia are found. The three cell lines are not necessarily affected to the same degree, and all possible combinations of hematological changes have been found in cases of chronic benzene poisoning. In some older reports, the earliest abnormalities have been described as reduction in the number of white blood cells (WBCs) and relative neutropenia; in later studies, lower than normal red blood cell (RBC) counts and macrocytosis with hyperchromic anemia have been found more often to be the initial hematologic abnormalities.[54,55] Thrombocytopenia has also been frequently reported.[56] The bone marrow may be hyperplastic or hypoplastic; in extreme cases, bone marrow failure with aplastic anemia may be seen.

Hematologic abnormalities detected in the peripheral blood do not always correlate with the pattern of bone marrow changes. Relatively minor deviations from normal in the blood count (RBCs, WBCs, or platelets) may coexist with marked bone marrow changes (hyperplastic or hypoplastic) and abnormalities are sometimes first found after cessation of exposure. Benzene-induced aplastic anemia can be fatal, with hemorrhage secondary to the marked thrombocytopenia and increased susceptibility to infections due to neutropenia. The number of reported cases of severe chronic benzene poisoning with aplastic anemia gradually decreased after World War II, because of better engineering controls, progressive reduction of the permissible exposure limits, and efforts to substitute less toxic solvents for benzene in numerous industrial processes. Suppression of cell growth and function in the lymphocytic line have also been shown to result from benzene exposure and to be correlated with the concentrations of benzene metabolites. The possibility that depressed immune system function might contribute to carcinogenesis has been raised.[57]

Leukemia secondary to benzene exposure has been repeatedly reported since the 1930s.[58,59] All types of leukemia have been found; myelogenous leukemia (chronic and acute) and erythroleukemia (Di Guglielmo's disease) apparently more frequently, but acute and chronic lymphocytic or lymphoblastic leukemia is represented as well. Malignant transformation of the bone marrow has been noted years after cessation of exposure, an added difficulty in the few epidemiological studies on long-term effects of benzene exposure. In Italy, with a large shoe-manufacturing industry, where benzene-based glues had been used for many years, at least 150 cases of benzene-related leukemia were known by 1976.[60] In Turkey more than 50 cases of aplastic anemia and 34 cases of leukemia have been reported from the shoe-manufacturing industry.[61] Epidemiological studies in the U.S. rubber industry[62] have indicated a more than threefold increase in leukemia deaths; occupations with known solvent exposure (benzene widely used in the past and still a contaminant of solvents used) showed a significantly higher leukemia mortality than other occupations. Lymphatic leukemia showed the highest excess mortality. Detailed examination of solvent-exposure histories in 15 cases of lymphocytic leukemia and 30 matched controls revealed that case subjects were 4.5 times as likely as controls to have had direct exposure to both benzene and other solvents.[63] Mean duration of benzene exposure was short, more than half of the cohort having been exposed for less than 1 year. The risk of leukemia was much higher in workers exposed 5 years or more (SMR of 2100). Four additional cases of leukemia occurred among employees not encompassed by the definition of the cohort.[64] In Japan the incidence of leukemia among Hiroshima and Nagasaki survivors was found to be significantly increased by occupational benzene exposure in the years subsequent to the bomb.[65]

Chromosomal aberrations in lymphocytes of benzene-exposed workers have been well documented[66,67]; they were shown to persist even years after cessation of toxic exposure. The "stable" aberrations are more persistent and have been considered to be the origin of leukemic clones. Cytogenetic effects of benzene have been reproduced in animal models. In rats exposed to 1000 and 100 ppm, a significant increase in the proportion of cells with chromosomal abnormalities was detected; exposure to 10 and 1 ppm resulted in elevated levels of cells with chromosomal abnormalities that showed evidence of being dose-related, although they were not statistically significant.[68] A significant increase in sister chromatid exchanges in bone marrow cells of mice exposed to 28 ppm benzene for 4 hours was also reported.[69] Recently toxic effects on reproductive organs have received increased attention. In subchronic inhalation studies, histopathological changes in the ovaries (characterized by bilateral cyst formation) and in the testes (atrophy and degenerative changes, including a decrease in the number of spermatozoa and an increase in abnormal sperm forms) have been reported.[70]

Experimental evidence of the carcinogenicity of benzene has been very limited in the past.[71] Recently several experimental studies have demonstrated carcinogenic effects of benzene in experimental animals; in addition to leukemias,[72,73] benzene has produced in rodents significant increases in the incidence of Zymbal gland carcinomas, cancer of the oral cavity, hepatocarcinomas, and possibly mammary carcinomas and lymphoreticular neoplasias.[74] In experimental studies on mice, in addition to a high increase in leukemias, a significant increase in lymphomas was found.[75] The National Toxicology Program has recently completed an oral administration experimental study in which malignant lymphoma and carcinomas in various organs, including skin, oral cavity, alveoli/bronchioli, and mammary gland, in mice, and carcinomas of the skin, oral cavity, and Zymbal gland in rats were found with significantly increased incidence. Thus NTP concluded that there was now clear evidence of carcinogenicity of benzene in rats and mice[76]; EPA has come to the same conclusion.[51]

The International Agency for Research on Cancer (IARC)

has recently updated its evaluation of benzene carcinogenicity (1988) and acknowledged the existence of limited evidence for chronic myeloid and chronic lymphocytic leukemia. In addition, it was noted that recent studies had suggested an increased risk of multiple myeloma,[77] while others indicate a dose-related increase in total lymphatic and hematopoietic neoplasms.

There is little information on developmental toxicity of benzene in humans. Case reports have documented that normal infants without chromosomal aberrations can be born to mothers with an increased number of chromosomal aberrations[78,79]; other investigators have reported increases in the frequency of sister chromatid exchanges and chromatid breaks in children of women exposed to benzene and other solvents during pregnancy. In animal experiments benzene has not been found to be teratogenic; a decrease in fetal weight and an increase in skeletal variants have been associated with maternal toxicity.

Prevention and Control. Prevention of benzene poisoning and of malignant transformation of the bone marrow is based on engineering control of exposure. The threshold limit value (TLV) for benzene has been repeatedly reduced in the last several decades.[2,3] In 1987 the Occupational Safety and Health Administration (OSHA) occupational exposure standard for benzene was revised to 1 ppm TWA, with a 5 ppm short-term exposure limit (STEL). The National Institute for Occupational Safety and Health (NIOSH) has recommended that the standard be revised to a TWA of 0.1 ppm, with a 15-minute ceiling value of 1 ppm.

Biological monitoring through measurements of urinary metabolites of benzene is useful as a complement to air sampling for the measurement of benzene concentrations.

Elevation in the total urinary phenols (normal range 20 to 30 mg/L) indicates excessive benzene exposure, and 50 mg/L should not be exceeded. The urinary inorganic/total sulfate ratio may also be monitored. Biological monitoring is recommended at least quarterly but should be more frequent when exposure levels are equal to or higher than the TWA. Current methods of biological monitoring lack sensitivity at levels corresponding to inhalation exposures below 10 ppm. A urinary phenol level of 75 mg/L was found to correspond to a TWA exposure to 10 ppm; in other studies the urinary phenol level corresponding to 10 ppm benzene was 45 to 50 mg/L. Preplacement and periodic examinations should include a history of exposure to other myelotoxic chemical or physical agents or medications and of other hematologic conditions. A complete blood count, a mean corpuscular volume determination, reticulocyte and platelet counts, and the urinary phenol test are basic laboratory tests. The frequency of these examinations and tests should be related to the level of exposure.[3] Possible neurological and dermatological effects should also be considered in comprehensive periodic examinations. Adequate respirators should be available and should be used when spills, leakage, or other incidents of higher exposure occur.

In recent years the possibility of excessive benzene ingestion from contaminated water has received increasing attention. Benzene concentrations in water have been found to range from 0.005 ppb (in the Gulf of Mexico) to 330 ppb in contaminated well water in New York, New Jersey, and Connecticut. In 1985 the Environmental Protection Agency (EPA) proposed a maximum contamination level (MCL) for benzene in drinking water at 0.005 mg/L; this standard was promulgated in 1987.[80]

Toluene

Toluene (methylbenzene, $C_6H_5CH_3$) is a clear, colorless liquid, with a higher boiling point (110° C) than benzene and therefore lower volatility. The production of toluene has increased markedly over the last several decades because of its use in numerous chemical synthesis processes, such as those of toluene diisocyanate, phenol, benzyl, and benzoyl derivatives, benzoic acid, toluene sulfonates, nitrotoluenes, vinyl toluene, and saccharin. Toluene is also used as a solvent, mostly for paints and coatings, and is often a component of mixtures of solvents. Technical grades of toluene contain benzene in variable proportions, reaching 25% in some products.

Hematological effects in workers exposed to toluene have been reported in the past.[1,2,81] Such effects were most probably due to the benzene content of toluene or to prior benzene exposure. Animal experiments indicate that pure toluene has no myelotoxic effects.[82] Toluene has been shown to induce microsomal cytochrome P-450 and mixed-function oxidases in the liver. Exposure to toluene concentrations higher than 100 ppm results in CNS depression, with prenarcotic symptoms and in moderate eye, throat, airway, and skin irritation. These effects are more pronounced with higher concentrations.

Numerous reports on toluene addiction (sniffing) have indicated that irreversible neurological effects are possible. Diffuse encephalopathy with dramatic acute manifestations, including hallucinations, convulsions, and coma, can occur.[83] Severe multifocal CNS damage[83–88] with impairment in cognitive, cerebellar, brain stem, auditory, and pyramidal tract function has been well documented in glue sniffers. Diffuse electroencephalographic abnormalities are usually present. Cerebral and cerebellar atrophy have been demonstrated by CT scans of the brain; brain stem atrophy has also been reported.[86] Progressive optic neuropathy and sensory hearing loss developed in some cases.[89] Peripheral neuropathy associated with severe CNS damage has been reported.[87]

Hepatotoxic and nephrotoxic effects have also been found in cases of toluene addiction; the possibility that other toxic agents might have contributed cannot be excluded. Sudden death in toluene sniffers has been reported and is thought to be due to arrhythmia secondary to myocardial sensitization to endogenous catecholamines,[90] a mechanism of sudden death similar to that reported with trichloroethylene and other halogenated hydrocarbons.

Adverse developmental effects in offspring of women who are solvent sniffers have been reported. These include CNS dysfunction, microcephaly, minor craniofacial and limb abnormalities,[91] and growth retardation.[92] Experimental results[93] confirm adverse developmental effects: skeletal abnormalities and low fetal weight were observed in several animal species (mice, rabbits). Adverse reproductive effects have not been detected in humans or in experimental studies.[94] Toluene has been found to be nonmutagenic and nongenotoxic. There are no indications, from human observations, that toluene has carcinogenic effects; long-term experimental studies on several animal species have been consistently negative.

Prevention and Control. The recommended TWA for toluene is 100 ppm. It is important to monitor the benzene content of technical grades of toluene and to control exposures so that the TWA of 1 ppm for benzene is not exceeded. Engineering controls, such as enclosure and exhaust ventilation, are essential for the prevention of excessive exposure; adequate respirators should be provided for unusual situations, when higher exposures might be expected.[3]

Biological monitoring of exposure can be achieved by measuring urinary hippuric acid, the main urinary metabolite of toluene. Excretion of hippuric acid in excess of 3 g/L indicates an exposure in excess of 100 ppm. A second important urinary metabolite of toluene is o-cresol[95]; as for hippuric acid, the excretion of o-cresol reaches its peak at the end of the exposure period (work shift). Interindividual differences in the pattern of toluene metabolism have been found, resulting in variable ratios between urinary hippuric acid and o-cresol. For these reasons, biological monitoring should include measurements of both urinary metabolites. Preemployment and periodic medical examinations should encompass possible neurological, hematological, hepatic, renal, and dermatological effects. Hematological tests, as indicated for benzene, have to be used because, as noted, variable amounts of benzene may enter commercial grades of toluene.

Potential environmental toluene exposure is currently also of concern.[94] The largest source of environmental toluene release is the production, transport, and use of gasoline, which contains 5% to 7% toluene by weight. Toluene in the atmosphere reacts with hydroxyl radicals; the half-time is about 13 hours. Toluene in soil or water volatilizes to air; the remaining amounts undergo microbial degradations. There is no tendency toward environmental buildup of toluene. Toluene is a very common contaminant in the vicinity of waste-disposal sites, where average concentrations in water have been found to be 7 to 20 μg/L and average concentrations in soil 70 μg/L. The EPA, in a 1988 survey, found toluene in groundwater, surface water, and soil at 29% of the hazardous waste sites tested. Toluene is not a widespread contaminant of drinking water; it was present in only about 1% of groundwater sources in concentrations lower than 2 ppb.

Xylene

Xylene (dimethylbenzene, $C_6H_4(CH_3)_2$) has three isomeric forms: *ortho-, meta-,* and *para*xylene. Commercial xylene is a mixture of these but may also contain benzene, ethylbenzene, toluene, and other impurities. With a boiling temperature of 144° C, xylene is less volatile than benzene and toluene. It is used as a solvent and as the starting material for the synthesis of xylidines, benzoic acid, phthalic anhydride, and phthalic and terephthalic acids and their esters. Other uses are in the manufacture of quartz crystal oscillators, epoxy resins, and pharmaceuticals. It is estimated that 140,000 workers are potentially exposed to xylene in the United States. As with toluene, early reports on adverse effects of xylene have to be evaluated in light of the frequent presence of considerable proportions of benzene in the mixture.[2,3]

Xylene has been shown to induce liver microsomal mixed-function oxidases and cytochrome P-450 in a dose-dependent manner.[96,97] The metabolism of *n*-hexane to its highly neurotoxic metabolite 2,5-hexanedione was shown to be markedly enhanced in rats pretreated with xylene.[97] Xylene also increases the metabolism of benzene and toluene. Thus, when present in mixtures with other solvents, xylene can increase the adverse effects of those compounds, which exert their toxicity mainly through more toxic metabolites.

Xylene was also found to facilitate the biotransformation of progesterone and 17 β-estradiol in pregnant rats by inducing hepatic microsomal mixed-function oxidases. Decreased blood levels of these hormones were thought to result in reduced weight of the fetuses.[98]

Acute effects of xylene exposure are depression of the CNS (prenarcotic and narcotic with high concentrations) and irritation of eyes, nose, throat, and skin. Liquid xylene is irritant to the skin, and repeated exposure may result in dermatitis. Hepatotoxic and nephrotoxic effects have been found in isolated cases of excessive exposure. Myelotoxic effects and hematologic changes have not been documented for pure xylene; the possibility of benzene admixture to technical-grade xylene has to be emphasized.

The TWA for xylene exposure is 100 ppm. The metabolites of *ortho-, meta-,* and *para*xylene are the corresponding methyl hippuric acids. A concentration of 2.05 g *m*-methyl hippuric acid was found to correspond to 100 ppm (TLV) exposure to *m*-xylene.[99] Prevention, control, and medical surveillance are similar to those indicated for toluene and benzene. Complete blood counts, urinalysis, and liver function tests should be part of the periodic medical examinations.

Styrene

Styrene (vinyl benzene, $C_6H_5CH=CH_2$), a colorless or yellowish liquid, is used in the manufacture of polystyrene (styrene is the monomer; at temperatures of 200° C, polymerization to polystyrene occurs) and of copolymers with 1,3-butadiene (butadiene-styrene rubber) and acrylonitrile (acrylonitrile-butadiene-styrene, ABS). The most important exposures to styrene occur when it is used as a solvent-reactant in the manufacture of polyester products in the reinforced plastics industry. TWA exposures can be as high as 150 to 300 ppm, with excursions into the 1000 to 1500 ppm range.[100]

The metabolic transformation of styrene is characterized by its conversion to styrene-7,8-oxide by the mixed function oxidases and cytochrome P-450 enzyme complex. Styrene-7,8-oxide is mutagenic in several prokaryotic and eukaryotic test systems. It has been shown to produce single-strand breaks in DNA of various organs in mice: kidney, liver, lung, testes, and brain.[101] Styrene-7,8-oxide is an alkylating agent and reacts mostly with deoxyguanosine, producing 7-alkylguanine, and with deoxycytidine, producing N-3-alkylcytosine. Chromosome aberrations and sister chromatid exchanges were reported to be significantly increased in several studies of styrene-exposed workers. Styrene-7,8-oxide is a potent carcinogen in rodents.

Mandelic acid and phenyl glyoxylic acid are the main urinary metabolites of styrene.

Styrene has an irritant effect on mucous membranes (eyes, nose, throat, airways) and skin. Inhalation of high concentrations may result in transitory CNS depression, with prenarcotic symptoms. Chronic neurotoxic effects have been reported with repeated exposure to relatively high levels in the boat-construction industry, mostly in Scandinavian countries, where styrene is widely used by brush application on large surfaces. Electroencephalographic changes, performance test abnormalities, and peripheral nerve conduction velocity changes have been reported.[102] There is no indication, from epidemiological studies, that styrene is carcinogenic.

Contact allergy to styrene has recently been reported.[103] Cross-reactivity on patch testing with 2-, 3-, and 4-vinyl toluene (methyl styrene) and with the metabolites styrene epoxide and 4-vinyl phenol was found to be present.

Prevention. In view of reports of persistent neurological effects with long-term exposure, the present federal standard for a styrene TWA of 100 ppm appears to be too high, and reduction has been suggested. The NIOSH has proposed a TWA of 50 ppm. Biological limits of exposure have been proposed corresponding to a TLV of 50 ppm styrene. At the end of the shift, urinary MA should not exceed 800 mg/g creatinine and the sum of MA + PGA should not be more than 1000 mg/g creatinine. In the morning, before the start of work, the values should not exceed 150 and 300 mg/g creatinine, respectively.[104] Preemployment and periodic medical examinations should assess neurological status, liver and kidney function, and hematological parameters.

HALOGENATED HYDROCARBONS

The compounds in this group result from the substitution of one or more hydrogen atoms of a simple hydrocarbon by halogens, most often chlorine. Simple chlorinated hydrocarbons are used in a wide variety of industrial processes. The majority are excellent solvents for oils, waxes, fats, rubber, pigments, paints, varnishes, etc. In the chemical industry these compounds are used for chlorination in the manufacture of such products as plastics, pesticides, and other complex halogenated compounds.[1,2] Most are nonflammable; some, such as carbon tetrachloride, have been used as fire extinguishers (this use has been stopped because of the high toxicity of carbon tetrachloride and the formation of highly irritant combustion products). The most widely used simple chlorinated hydrocarbons are as follows:

Monochloromethane (methyl chloride)	CH_3Cl
Dichloromethane (methylene chloride)	CH_2Cl_2
Trichloromethane (chloroform)	$CHCl_3$
Tetrachloromethane (carbon tetrachloride)	CCl_4
1,2-Dichloroethane (ethylene chloride)	CH_2ClCH_2Cl
1,1-Dichloroethane	$CHCl_2CH_3$
1,1,2-Trichloroethane	$CH_2ClCHCl_2$
1,1,1-Trichloroethane (methyl chloroform)	CH_3CCl_3
1,1,2,2-Tetrachloroethane	$CHCl_2CHCl_2$
Monochloroethylene (vinyl chloride)	$CHCl=CH_2$
1,2-Dichloroethylene (*cis* and *trans*)	$CHCl=CHCl$
Trichloroethylene	$CHCl=CCl_2$
Tetrachloroethylene	$CCl_2=CCl_2$

Many of the members of this series of compounds have a low boiling point and are highly volatile at room temperature; hazardous exposure levels may develop in a very short time. The application of heat is common in numerous industrial processes; air concentrations of halogenated hydrocarbons increase sharply under such circumstances.

Many industrial solvents are sold as mixtures. These may sometimes contain highly toxic products, and hazardous exposure may occur without the exposed person's knowledge of the specific chemical composition of the solvent mixture used. Toxic effects of halogenated hydrocarbons are multiple and potentially severe; the severity varies from compound to compound. Carbon tetrachloride has been generally accepted as the prototype for a hepatotoxic agent; other members of the group have similar or lesser hepatotoxicity.

The majority of the compounds have a narcotic effect on the central nervous system; in this respect they are more potent than the hydrocarbons from which they are derived. Some (chloroform, trichloroethylene) were used as anesthetics until their marked toxicity was recognized. Moderate irritation of mucous membranes (conjunctivae, upper and lower airways) is also a common effect of halogenated hydrocarbons.

With acute overexposure or repeated exposures of a lesser degree, toxic damage to the liver and kidney is common; the severity of these effects is largely dependent on the specific compound and on the level and pattern of exposure. Individual susceptibility may also contribute but is of lesser importance. Halogenated hydrocarbons may produce liver injury and centrilobular necrosis with or without steatosis. They also have marked nephrotoxicity; tubular cellular necrosis is the specific lesion that may lead to anuria and acute renal failure. Many of the fatalities due to acute overexposure to halogenated hydrocarbons have been attributed to this effect, although concomitant liver injury was always present.[1,2]

The toxicity of many halogenated solvents is associated with their biotransformation to reactive electrophilic metabolites, which can alkylate macromolecules and thus produce organ injury. The microsomal mixed function oxidases and cytochrome P-450 complex of enzymes are effective in the biotransformation of halogenated solvents. Chloroethanes (1,2-dichloroethane, 1,1,1-trichloroethane, and 1,1,2,2,-tetrachloroethane) have been shown to be also metabolized by hepatic nuclear cytochrome P-450; the metabolites are similar to those resulting from hepatic microsomal P-450, indicating similar pathways of metabolic transformation. It is suggested that the metabolism of 1,2-dichloroethane and 1,1,2,2-tetrachloroethane by nuclear cytochrome P-450 may in part mediate mutagenicity and carcinogenicity.[105]

Food deprivation, more specifically a low intake of carbohydrates, and alcohol consumption have been shown to enhance the metabolic transformation of the halogenated hydrocarbon solvents chloroform, carbon tetrachloride, 1,2-dichloroethane, 1,1-dichloroethylene, and trichloroethylene.[106,107]

Recently it has been proposed that the nephrotoxicity of some compounds in this group is due to metabolic transformation in the kidney of the glutathione conjugates into the corresponding cysteine conjugates. The cysteine conjugates may be directly nephrotoxic or they may be further transformed in the kidney by renal cysteine conjugate β-lyase into reactive alkenyl mercaptans.[108]

Another toxic effect, more recently identified, is related to the arrhythmogenic properties of halogenated hydrocarbons. These were first reported with chloroform and trichloroethylene used as anesthetics; they have also been found to occur with occupational exposure and, more recently, in persons addicted to the euphoric effects of short-term exposure (solvent sniffers).[3] Ventricular fibrillation secondary to myocardial sensitization to endogenous epinephrine and norepinephrine has been postulated as the mechanism underlying the arrhythmias and sudden deaths.

The hepatotoxicity of carbon tetrachloride has been studied extensively, both clinically and in various experimental models. The mechanisms of toxic liver injury, the underlying biochemical and enzymatic disruptions, and the corresponding ultrastructural changes have been progressively defined. The possible development of hepatic cirrhosis after repeated exposure to carbon tetrachloride has been reported.[109] An unusual type of fibrosis of the liver and spleen, including subcapsular fibrosis and the development of portal hypertension, has been found to be a potential effect of vinyl chloride exposure.[110]

Liver carcinogenicity has been documented for several compounds of this series. Hepatocellular carcinoma developing several years after acute carbon tetrachloride poisoning has been reported.[109,111] In other cases long-term exposure, even without overt acute toxicity, may lead to the same end result. In animal studies, carbon tetrachloride has proved a potent hepatocarcinogen.

Chloroform and trichloroethylene have been shown to be hepatocarcinogens in animals.[112] Human data are not available; no long-term epidemiological study has been reported, and the possibility exists that instances of hepatocellular carcinoma may have occurred in workers exposed to these substances without recognition of the etiological link between exposure and malignancy. That this is a possibility has been illustrated by the example of vinyl chloride. Hemangiosarcoma of the liver was identified as one of the possible effects of vinyl chloride exposure in 1974, and many cases have since been reported from various industrial countries. Some of these cases had occurred in prior years, but at that time the link between toxic exposure and malignancy had not been suggested. Only after the etiological association was established, both by the first human cases reported and by results of animal experiments,[113] was information on many other cases published. There are indications that vinyl chloride may induce hepatoma as well as hemangiosarcoma. Vinylidene chloride has also come under close scrutiny, since animal data seem to indicate a carcinogenic effect. Chemical enhancement of viral transformation of Syrian hamster embryo cells has been demonstrated for 1,1,1-trichloroethane, 1,2-dichloroethane, 1,1-dichloroethane, chloromethane, and vinyl chloride; other chlorinated methanes and ethanes did not show such an effect.[114,115]

Exposure to halogenated hydrocarbons and other volatile organic compounds in the general environment, from various sources including contaminated water and toxic waste–disposal sites, has received increasing attention during recent years. Methods have been developed to determine individual exposures with personal monitors to determine ambient air levels and special spirometers for the collection of expired air samples; gas chromatography—mass spectroscopy analysis—has permitted adequate detection and has clarified patterns of relationships between breathing zone concentrations and results of breath analysis. In a study on students in Texas and North Carolina, air has been found to be the major source of absorption, except for two trihalomethanes, chloroform and bromodichloromethane. Estimated total daily intake from air and water ranged from 0.3 to 12.6 mg, with 1,1,1-trichloroethane at the highest concentrations.[116] Monitoring of airborne levels of mutagens and suspected carcinogens, including linear and cyclic halogenated hydrocarbons, has been undertaken in many urban centers of the United States. Average concentration levels for halogenated hydrocarbons were in the 0 to 1 ppb range.[117] Similar efforts have been undertaken regarding the monitoring of water contamination with halogenated hydrocarbons. Rivers, lakes, and drinking water from various sources have been tested. Analytical methods have been developed for the detection of volatile organic compounds, including chlorinated hydrocarbons, in fish and shellfish.[118] Since the long-term effects of low-level exposure to halogenated hydrocarbon solvents, especially with regard to carcinogenicity and mutagenicity, are not known, it is necessary to monitor current exposures from all possible sources and to reduce such exposures to a minimum to protect the health of the general population.

Carbon Tetrachloride

The production of carbon tetrachloride in the United States has varied from 250 to 400 million kg in recent years. It is currently used mainly in the synthesis of dichlorofluoromethane (fluorocarbon 12) and trichlorofluoromethane (fluorocarbon 11); a small proportion is still applied as a fumigant and pesticide for certain crops (barley, corn, rice, rye, wheat) and for agricultural facilities, such as grain bins and granaries.

Airborne concentrations of carbon tetrachloride in the general environment have been found to vary from 0.05 to 18 ppb. In rural areas, levels of CCl_4 were lower, in the range of 80 to 120 ppt. The photodecomposition of tetrachloroethylene results in the formation of about 8% (by weight) carbon tetrachloride[119] and is thought to be possibly responsible for a significant proportion of atmospheric carbon tetrachloride. Available data on the amounts of CCl_4 released into the atmosphere have shown a considerable decrease between 1978 and 1983.[120]

Carbon tetrachloride has also been found in rivers, lakes, and drinking water. About 95% of all surface water supplies contain less than 0.5 μg/L; in drinking water, detectable levels ($>$0.2 μg/L) were present in 3% of 945 samples tested.[121]

The ability of the liver to metabolize foreign chemicals (as well as many endogenous biologically active substances such as hormones) may result in detoxification or, on the other hand, in the conversion of some chemicals into metabolites of higher toxicity. The toxicity of carbon tetrachloride (CCl_4) is enhanced by its metabolic transformation in the liver. Induction of mixed-function microsomal enzymes significantly increases CCl_4 toxicity, while inhibition of the enzymatic system decreases its toxicity.

Carbon tetrachloride can produce disruption of all elements of the hepatocyte-plasma membrane, endoplasmic reticulum, mitochondria, lysosomes, and nucleus. The resulting cellular destruction is reflected in zonal (centrilobular) necrosis, which can be accompanied by steatosis. The corresponding clinical manifestation is hepatocellular jaundice; in severe cases hepatic failure and death may occur. With lesser exposure, less extensive subclinical pathologic changes may result; nonspecific symptoms, such as fatigability, loss of appetite, and nausea, may be present without jaundice. Elevated serum enzymes (SGOT, SGPT, LDH), bilirubin and sometimes alkaline phosphatase, a rise in bromsulphalein retention, reduction of prothrombin, and increased urinary urobilin excretion may nevertheless be detected. Repeated toxic insults may lead to the development of postnecrotic cirrhosis.

The toxic effect of carbon tetrachloride is due to a metabolite, a free radical (CCl_3) that appears to produce peroxidation of the unsaturated lipids of cellular membranes. Metabolism of CCl_4 to the more toxic metabolite (free radical) is thought to occur in the endoplasmic reticulum. Cytochrome P-450 is destroyed in the process. As the metabolite accumulates, membranes of lysosomes and mitochondria are also injured, and necrosis results.

Individual variation in the response to CCl_4 is now better understood; previous mixed-function microsomal enzyme induction has been shown to enhance CCl_4 toxicity through enhanced metabolic transformation to the active intermediate free radical. Alcohols, ketones, and some other chemical compounds enhance carbon tetrachloride toxicity: ethanol, isopropyl alcohol, butanol, acetone, PCBs and PBBs, chlordecone and trichloroethylene have all been shown to potentiate CCl_4 toxicity, mostly by hepatic enzyme induction.[122] These observations are important for the assessment of potential toxicity of chemical mixtures, including those from waste-disposal sites, that could be or are found to contaminate drinking water. A recent outbreak of clinically overt carbon tetrachloride poisoning in a printing plant in Taiwan[123] was associated with the combined use of CCl_4 and isopropyl alcohol.

Irreversible (covalent) binding of carbon tetrachloride metabolites to hepatic macromolecules has been demonstrated with the use of radiolabeled carbon tetrachloride (C^{14} or Cl^{36}). Binding of radiolabeled CCl_4 to DNA has also been reported.[124] Experimental evidence of carcinogenicity in mice and rats has accumulated. Liver tumors, including hepatocellular carcinomas, developed in various strains of mice, and benign and malignant liver tumors developed in rats.[125]

Prevention and Control. The federal OSHA standard for a permissible exposure limit (PEL) for carbon tetrachloride exposure is 2 ppm. Replacement by less toxic substances, engineering controls, and enclosed processes are necessary. Respiratory protection should be available for emergency situations. Medical surveillance must include careful evaluation of liver and kidney function, central and peripheral nervous system function, and the skin. The World Health Organization has adopted a guideline for permissible CCl_4 concentration of 0.003 mg/L in drinking water.[126]

Chloroform

Chloroform is a colorless, very volatile liquid, with a boiling point of 61° C. Most of the more than 300 million pounds produced annually in the United States is used in the manufacture of fluorocarbons. Chloroform has also been used in cosmetics and numerous products of the pharmaceutical industry; the FDA banned these uses in 1976. Another application of chloroform has been as an insecticidal fumigant for certain crops, including corn, rice, and wheat. Chloroform residues have been detected in cereals for weeks after fumigation. They have also been found in food products, such as dairy produce, meat, oils and fats, fruits, and vegetables, in amounts ranging from 1 to more than 30 mg/kg.

The presence of chloroform in the water of rivers and lakes, in ground water, and in sewage treatment plant effluents has been documented at various locations. In drinking water, concentrations of 5 to 90 μg/L have been detected. Chlorination of water is thought to be responsible for the presence of chloroform in water (Chapter 35).

Chloroform has toxic effects similar to those of carbon tetrachloride, but fewer severe cases have been reported after industrial exposure. Chloroform undergoes metabolic transformation; one of the metabolites has been shown to be phosgene

($COCl_2$). Microsomal cytochrome P-450 is active in the metabolism of chloroform; induction of cytochrome P-450 results in increased chloroform hepatotoxicity.[127] Methyl-*n*-butyl ketone (MBK) and 2,5,-hexanedione, the common metabolite of MBK and *n*-hexane, have been shown to enhance chloroform hepatotoxicity by induction of cytochrome P-450.[128,129] Extensive covalent binding to liver and kidney proteins has been found after administration of ^{14}C-chloroform to mice; this was in direct relationship with the extent of hepatic centrilobular and renal proximal tubular necrosis.[130] The National Cancer Institute report on the carcinogenic effect of chloroform in animals (hepatocellular carcinomas in mice and renal tumors in rats) draws attention again to the lack of long-term epidemiologic observations. As with other carcinogens, industrial exposure must not exceed the limit of detection, and appropriate engineering methods must be used to protect the health of employees. The NIOSH recommended a ceiling of 2 ppm.[112] Environmental exposure of the general population to chloroform in water and food has also to be reduced to a minimum, given the fact that sufficient experimental evidence for the carcinogenicity of chloroform has accumulated.

Trichloroethylene

Trichloroethylene (TCE) is a colorless, volatile liquid with a boiling point of 87° C. Trichloroethylene was thought to be much less toxic than carbon tetrachloride and was used, to a large extent, to replace CCl_4 in many industrial processes. It is one of the most important chlorinated solvents. Its main applications are as a dry cleaning agent and a metal degreaser. In smaller amounts, it is used in extraction of fats and other natural products, in the manufacture of adhesives and industrial paints, and in the chemical industry, mainly in the production of fluorocarbons.

NIOSH estimated that 3.5 million workers in the United States are occupationally exposed to trichloroethylene; about 100,000 are exposed full time.[131]

Trichloroethylene is absorbed rapidly through the respiratory route, and only a relatively small fraction of the amount inhaled is eliminated unchanged in the exhaled air. The metabolic transformation of trichloroethylene has been shown to proceed through formation of a complex with cytochrome P-450; several pathways can then follow:

- Destruction of heme
- Formation of chloral, which can be reduced to trichloroethanol or oxidized to trichloroacetic acid
- Formation of trichloroethylene oxide, which then decomposes into carbon monoxide and glyoxylate
- Formation of metabolites that bind irreversibly to protein, RNA and DNA

The relative proportion of these four different metabolic pathways can vary. The levels of protein adducts, especially DNA adducts, vary from species to species. This may explain species differences reported in carcinogenicity bioassays.[132] In some experiments using radiolabeled ^{14}C-trichloroethylene in mice and rats, no direct evidence of formation of liver DNA adducts could be detected. Covalent binding to liver and kidney RNA and to DNA in kidney, testes, lung, pancreas, and spleen was found to be due to metabolic incorporation, particularly into guanine and adenine.[133,134]

In humans, most trichloroethylene is metabolized to trichloroacetic acid and trichloroethanol. The urinary excretion of these metabolites can be used for biologic monitoring of trichloroethylene exposure; trichloroethanol excretion reaches its peak 24 hours after exposure, while trichloroacetic acid reaches its highest urinary level 3 days after exposure. Trichloroethylene has been shown to inhibit δ-aminolevulinic acid dehydratase (ALA-D) in rats; an increased excretion of δ-aminolevulinic acid in urine was also found.[135]

Trichloroethylene has a depressant effect on the CNS; prenarcotic and narcotic symptoms can develop in rapid sequence with high concentrations of vapor. TCE is also an irritant to the skin, conjunctivae, and airways.

Hepatotoxicity and nephrotoxicity of trichloroethylene are much lower than those of carbon tetrachloride[136]; there are few reports of acute fatal toxic hepatitis[137] and only isolated reports of acute renal failure[138,139] due to TCE. Trichloroethylene was shown to enhance the hepatotoxicity of carbon tetrachloride, possibly potentiating lipid peroxidation.[140] Sudden deaths in young workers exposed to TCE have been reported repeatedly and have been attributed to ventricular fibrillation, through myocardial sensitization to increased levels of epinephrine.[90] Chronic effects on the central and peripheral nervous system have been described; hepatotoxicity with moderate, long-term exposure has not been found in humans.

Trichloroethylene has been reported to be a hepatocarcinogen in experimental animals. An increased incidence of hepatocellular carcinomas was found in mice, but this effect was not observed in rats.[125] Kidney adenocarcinomas, testicular Leydig cell tumors, and possibly leukemia were found to be significantly increased in some experimental studies in rats.[131] Exposure of rats to TCE has not been shown to result in teratogenic effects.[141] TCE exposure does not produce dominant lethal mutations in mice.[142] An increased proportion of morphologically abnormal spermatozoa was found in mice exposed to TCE by inhalation.[143]

Medical surveillance of populations currently exposed or exposed in the past is necessary, with special attention to long-term and potential carcinogenic effects, neurological effects, and liver and kidney function abnormalities.[112]

The present federal standard for a permissible level of occupational TCE exposure is 50 ppm. A lower exposure limit has been proposed in view of information on carcinogenicity in animals. Exposure of the general population to TCE has received increasing attention. In 1977 the FDA proposed a regulation prohibiting the use of TCE as a food additive; this included the use of TCE in extraction processes in the manufacture of decaffeinated coffee and of spice oleoresins.

Trichloroethylene has been found in at least 460 of 1179 hazardous waste sites on the National Priorities List.[131] Federal and state surveys have shown that between 9% and 34% of water supply sources in the United States are contaminated with TCE; the concentrations are, on the average, 1 to 2 ppb or less. Higher levels have been found in the vicinity of toxic waste–disposal sites; under such circumstances concentrations of several hundred up to 27,000 ppb have been detected.[131] In 1989 the EPA established a drinking water standard of 5 ppb.

Perchloroethylene

Perchloroethylene is used in the textile industry for dry cleaning, processing, and finishing. More than 70% of all dry-cleaning operations in the United States use perchloroethylene. Another important use is in metal cleaning and degreasing. Perchloroethylene is also a raw material for the synthesis of fluorocarbons.

Perchloroethylene (tetrachloroethylene) is similar in most respects to trichloroethylene. Its hepatotoxicity, initially thought to be very low, has been well documented,[144] with abnormal levels of liver enzymes after exposure and persistence of elevated urinary urobilinogen and serum bilirubin in asymptomatic persons.

An arrhythmogenic effect of perchloroethylene has also been well documented in humans; premature ventricular contractions in young adults were frequent with high blood levels of perchloroethylene and disappeared completely after removal from exposure.[145]

Deaths due to massive perchloroethylene overexposure continue to be reported,[146,147] especially from small dry cleaning establishments. In recent years experimental data on the underlying mechanisms of chronic neurotoxicity due to perchloroethylene have accumulated. Increases in the brain content of an astroglial protein (S-100) and of glutamine synthetase, a biomarker for astroglial hypertrophy, provide biochemical evidence of astroglial proliferation secondary to neuronal damage.[148,149] The metabolism of perchloroethylene is characterized by a cytochrome P-450 catalyzed oxidative reaction[150]; an epoxide intermediate has been postulated, but current technology has not yet allowed its isolation. For the biological monitoring of exposure to perchloroethylene, measurements of urinary trichloroacetic acid and blood levels of perchloroethylene can be used. A blood level of 1 mg/L found 16 hours after exposure corresponds to a TWA exposure of less than 50 ppm. Such an exposure was found to result in no adverse effects on the CNS, liver, or kidney. The excretion of urinary trichloroacetic acid is slow and therefore not very useful for biological monitoring.

In chronic inhalation studies[151] perchloroethylene increased the incidence of leukemia in rats and hepatocellular adenomas and carcinomas in mice. Epidemiological studies on workers exposed to perchloroethylene are considered inconclusive. The IARC and the EPA have classified perchloroethylene as a category 2B carcinogen. The NIOSH has designated perchloroethylene as a carcinogen and has recommended that occupational exposure be limited to the lowest feasible limit. In 1986 the American Conference of Government Industrial Hygienists recommended a TLV-TWA of 50 ppm.[152]

Mutagenicity tests with perchloroethylene have been negative. No increase in the rate of chromosomal aberrations or sister chromatid exchange was detected in workers occupationally exposed to perchloroethylene.[153]

Contamination of the general environment with perchloroethylene has been documented. Perchloroethylene may be formed in small amounts through chlorination of water. It has been found in drinking water in concentrations of 0.5 μg/L to 5 μg/L. In trace amounts, it has also been detected in foodstuffs. The EPA (1987) has recommended that perchloroethylene in drinking water not exceed 0.5 mg/L.[152]

Methyl Chloroform

Methyl chloroform (1,1,1-trichloroethane) has recently gained widespread use because of its relatively low toxicity.[154] It is mostly used as a dry-cleaning agent, vapor degreaser, and aerosol vehicle and in the manufacture of vinylidene chloride. Hepato- and nephrotoxicity are low, but narcotic effects and even fatal respiratory depression have been reported. Cardiac arrhythmias due to myocardial sensitization to epinephrine have sometimes led to fatal outcomes.

Methyl chloroform, rather than its metabolites, produces the arrhythmias; pretreatment of rabbits with phenobarbital resulted in lower blood levels of methyl chloroform and a decreased incidence of arrhythmias.[155]

Fatal cases of 1,1,1-trichloroethane poisoning continue to be reported. In one such case, symmetrical infarction of the lenticular nuclei and of the occipital cortex were found in a patient who survived an acute poisoning for 3 years without recovering consciousness.[156] Intentional inhalation of typewriter correction fluid has resulted in at least 27 deaths; 3 additional deaths were reported in 1988.[157] 1,1,1-Trichloroethane and trichloroethylene are the components of this commercial product. Decrease in the availability of toluene-based glues, because of measures to combat glue sniffing, has resulted in abuse of more accessible solvents, such as 1,1,1-trichloroethane, which was the cause of three fatal cases within a period of 6 months reported from Scotland.[158] In subchronic inhalation experiments 1,1,1-trichloroethane was shown to lead to a decrease in DNA concentration in several brain areas of Mongolian gerbils. These results were interpreted as indicating decreased cell density in sensitive brain areas.[159]

Technical-grade methyl chloroform was found often to contain vinylidene chloride; elimination of this contaminant seems desirable in view of its potential carcinogenic and mutagenic risk.[160]

Vinyl Trichloride

Vinyl trichloride (1,1,2-trichloroethane) is a more potent narcotic and is a potent hepatotoxic and nephrotoxic agent. In an experimental study[161] significant increases in hepatocellular carcinomas and adrenal pheochromocytomas were found in mice. No similar findings were detected in rats. DNA adduct formation in vivo was found to occur to a greater extent in mouse liver than in rat liver.[162] The IARC (1987) has classified 1,1,2-trichloroethane in group 3 (not classifiable as to its carcinogenicity in humans). The EPA (1988) has included 1,1,2-trichloroethane in category C (possible human carcinogen).[163] The permissible level for occupational exposure to 1,1,2-trichloroethane is 10 ppm.[164] The EPA (1987) has recommended that the concentration in drinking water not exceed 3 μg/L.[163]

Tetrachloroethane

Tetrachloroethane (1,1,2,2-tetrachloroethane) is the most toxic of the chlorinated hydrocarbons. It is an excellent solvent and has been widely used in the past in the airplane industry, from which numerous cases of severe and even fatal toxic liver injury have been reported. This has prompted its replacement by other, less toxic solvents in most industrial processes. Toxic liver damage due to tetrachloroethane is known to have been associated with the development of cirrhosis of the liver.

1,1,2,2-Tetrachloroethane has produced hepatocellular carcinomas in mice. In rats, no significant increase in hepatocellular carcinomas was found.[125] It has been recommended that occupational exposure to 1,1,2,2-tetrachloroethane not exceed 1 ppm.[165]

Vinyl Chloride

Vinyl chloride, an unsaturated, asymmetrical chlorinated hydrocarbon, has found widespread use in the production of the polymer polyvinyl chloride. Although its industrial use had expanded in the 1940s and 1950s, it was not until 1973 that its hepatotoxicity[166] and carcinogenicity[167] were recognized. The acute narcotic effects had long been known: some rather unusual chronic effects had been reported in the 1960s, their main feature being Raynaud's syndrome involving the fingers and hands, skin changes described as similar to those of scleroderma, and bone abnormalities with resorption and spontaneous fractures of the distal phalanges. This syndrome was reported under the name *vinyl chloride acroosteolysis.*[168]

In 1973 peculiar hepatosplenic changes were described in vinyl chloride–exposed workers in Germany.[166] Soon thereafter, the first cases of hemangiosarcoma of the liver were reported in workers of one vinyl chloride–polyvinyl chloride polymerization plant in the United States,[167] and the search for similar cases elsewhere led to the identification of some 90 such otherwise rare tumors in workers of this industry in many industrialized countries.

The nonmalignant pathological changes in the liver are characterized by activation of hepatocytes, smooth endoplasmic reticulum proliferation, activation of sinusoidal cells including lipocytes, nodular hyperplasia of hepatocytes and sinusoidal cells, dilation of sinusoidal spaces, networklike collagen transformation of the sinusoidal walls, moderate portal fibrosis, and subcapsular fibrosis.

Portal hypertension has been the prominent feature in some cases of nonmalignant vinyl chloride liver disease; esophageal varices and bleeding have occurred. Fatty degenerative changes in the hepatocytes and focal necrosis have sometimes been observed and are thought to be more pronounced in cases studied shortly after cessation of toxic exposure.

The dilation of sinusoidal spaces and the proliferative changes of sinusoidal cells are precursors of the malignant transformation and the appearance of angiosarcomas. While the pathological characteristics of hemangiosarcomas may differ, and several types (sinusoidal, papillar, cavernous, and anaplastic) have been described, the biological characteristics are similar, with rapid growth and a downhill clinical course. No effective therapeutic approach has been identified. Excess lung cancers, lymphomas, and brain tumors have also been reported in some epidemiological studies.[169] Random cases of hepatocellular carcinoma have been seen after vinyl chloride exposure, but the association is still not fully established. Hemangiosarcoma of the liver is a very rare tumor, and therefore the identification of vinyl chloride as the etiologic carcinogen was facilitated.

In experimental animals exposed to vinyl chloride, carcinomas of the liver (hepatomas) also occur; sometimes both hemangiosarcoma and hepatoma have been found in the same animal. Malignant tumors of kidney, lung, and brain have also been found with increased incidence. Vinyl chloride is a transplacental carcinogen in the rat.

Vinyl chloride is metabolically activated by liver microsomal enzymes to intermediates that bind covalently to proteins and nucleic acids.

The toxic active metabolite of vinyl chloride is, according to several groups of investigators, most probably the epoxide chloroethylene oxide:

```
Cl     H          Cl   O   H
 \    /             \ / \ /
  C = C  ---------->  C---C
 /    \             /     \
H      H           H       H
```

The electrophilic epoxide may react with cellular macromolecules, including nucleic acids; covalent and noncovalent binding occurs. The vinyl chloride epoxide metabolite appears to represent an optimal balance between stability that allows it to reach the DNA target and reactivity that leads to DNA binding and thus to the carcinogenic effect.[170] Proven sites of alkylation are adenine, cytosine, and guanine moieties of nucleic acids and sulfhydryl groups of protein. Covalent binding with hepatocellular proteins can lead to liver necrosis; it has been observed that after microsomal enzyme induction, high doses of vinyl chloride may result in acute necrosis of the liver. Binding to DNA is considered potentially important for mutagenicity and carcinogenicity. Under normal circumstances, altered DNA molecules are eliminated through physiological enzymatic systems. With defective function of repair mechanisms, cell populations modified by the toxic metabolite develop, with increasing metabolic autonomy and eventual malignant growth.

Active research on the metabolic transformations of vinyl chloride has also resulted in a better understanding of the metabolic transformations of other chlorinated hydrocarbons, identification of reactive intermediate products (epoxides), and structural reasons for higher or lower reactivity.

Tetrachloroethylene, 1,2-*trans*-dichloroethylene, and 1,2-*cis*-dichloroethylene have been found not to be mutagenic, while trichloroethylene, 1,1-dichloroethylene, and vinyl chloride are mutagenic.

The respective epoxides have been found to be symmetrical and relatively stable for the first group but asymmetrical, unstable, and highly reactive for the second.

```
                 Symmetrical                    Asymmetrical
             (relatively stable)                 (unstable)

                Cl   O   Cl                     Cl   O   H
                  \ / \ /                         \ / \ /
Tetra              C---C                Tri        C---C
                  /     \                         /     \
                Cl       Cl                     Cl       Cl

                H    O   H                      Cl   O   H
                  \ / \ /                         \ / \ /
Cis 1,2 di         C---C                1,1 di     C---C
                  /     \                         /     \
                Cl       Cl                     Cl       H

                H    O   Cl                     Cl   O   H
                  \ / \ /                         \ / \ /
Trans 1,2 di       C---C                Vinyl      C---C
                  /     \               chloride  /     \
                Cl       H                      H        H
```

Mutagenicity of vinyl chloride has been demonstrated in a variety of test systems.[171–173] Cytogenetic studies have indicated that vinyl chloride produces chromosomal aberrations.[174,175] The federal standard for exposure to vinyl chloride is 1 ppm for an 8-hour period; the ceiling of 5 ppm should never be exceeded for more than 15 minutes. Air-supplied respirators should be available and are required when exposure levels exceed these limits.

Vinyl Bromide

Production of vinyl bromide in the United States has expanded only very recently.[112] It is used in the chemical, plastic, rubber, and leather industries. Experimental studies have shown that vinyl bromide has produced angiosarcoma of the liver, lymph node angiosarcoma, lymphosarcoma, and bronchioloalveolar carcinoma in rats exposed to 50 and 25 ppm by inhalation. Mutagenicity of vinyl bromide has also been reported.[176] On the basis of these data, the NIOSH and OSHA jointly recommended that vinyl bromide be considered a potential carcinogen for humans and be controlled in a way similar to vinyl chloride, with a recommended exposure standard of 1 ppm.

Vinylidene Chloride

Vinylidene chloride (1,1-dichloroethylene), like other vinyl halides, is used mainly in the plastics industry; it is easily polymerized and copolymerized to form plastic materials and resins with valuable properties.

In experimental studies, vinylidene chloride has been found to be carcinogenic in rats and mice: angiosarcoma of the liver, adenocarcinoma of the kidney, and other malignant tumors have been produced in inhalation experiments with concentrations as low as 25 ppm.[177] A limited study of workers occupationally exposed to vinylidene chloride[178] did not demonstrate an excessively high cancer mortality; nevertheless, the possibility of a carcinogenic risk for humans exposed to vinylidene chloride cannot yet be excluded. Vinylidene chloride has been shown to be mutagenic in several assay systems.[179] Embryotoxicity and fetal malformations have been observed in rats and rabbits after inhalation exposure to maternally toxic concentrations. Vinylidene chloride has not been shown to produce chromosomal aberrations or sister chromatid exchanges. In some experiments, vinylidene chloride has induced unscheduled DNA synthesis in rat hepatocytes and has alkylated DNA and induced DNA repair in mouse liver and kidney; the validity of these results has been questioned. The IARC has concluded that no evaluation of the carcinogenic risk of vinylidene chloride in humans could be made.[180] The recommended exposure standard[82] for vinylidene chloride is 1 ppm.

Ethylene Dichloride

Ethylene dichloride (1,2-dichloroethane, $ClCH_2—CH_2Cl$) is a colorless liquid at room temperature; with a boiling temperature of 83.4° C, it is highly volatile. Ethylene dichloride has a rapidly increasing volume of annual production; approximately 10 to 13 billion pounds was manufactured in the United States in recent years. Most of it (approximately 75%) is used in the production of vinyl chloride; it has also found applications in the manufacture of trichloroethylene, perchloroethylene, vinylidene chloride, ethylene amines, and ethylene glycol. It is a frequent constituent of antiknock mixtures of leaded gasoline and a component of fumigant insecticides. Other uses are as an extractor solvent, as a dispersant for nylon, viscose rayon, styrene-butadiene rubber, and other plastics, as a degreasing agent, as a component of paint and varnish removers, and in adhesives, soaps, and scouring compounds.

The main route of absorption is by inhalation; absorption through the skin is also possible. Ethylene dichloride is metabolized by cytochrome P-450; chloroacetoaldehyde and chloroacetic acid are the resulting metabolites. Microsomal cytochrome P-450 and nuclear cytochrome P-450 have been shown to metabolize ethylene dichloride. The possibility that the metabolic transformation of ethylene dichloride by nuclear cytochrome P-450 may in part mediate its mutagenicity and carcinogenicity has been considered.[105] Covalent alkylation of DNA by ethylene dichloride has been demonstrated.[181]

Narcotic and irritant effects occur during or soon after acute overexposure; hepatotoxic and nephrotoxic effects become apparent several hours later and can be severe, with centrilobular hepatic necrosis, jaundice, or proximal renal convoluted tubular necrosis and anuria; fatalities with high exposure levels have been reported.[2,3] A hemorrhagic tendency in acute ethylene dichloride poisoning has also been reported; disseminated intravascular coagulopathy and hyperfibrinolysis have been found in several cases. Experiments on rats and mice fed ethylene dichloride in corn oil revealed a statistically significant excess of malignant and benign tumors.[112] Several experimental studies point to the importance of glutathione conjugation in the metabolic transformation of 1,2-dichloroethane.[182]

The metabolic pathways for 1,2-dichloroethane biotransformation are saturable; saturation occurs earlier after ingestion than after inhalation.[182] Such differences in metabolic transformation have been thought to explain differences in results of experimental carcinogenicity studies, positive after oral administration[183] but negative in inhalation experiments.[184] A statistically significant increase in sister chromatid exchanges was detected in bone marrow cells of mice after acute 1,2-dichloroethane exposure.[185]

Ethylene dichloride has been found to be mutagenic in a variety of bacterial systems.[186] It was also shown to significantly enhance the viral transformation of Syrian hamster embryo cells.[187] Testing for teratogenic effects and dominant lethal effects in mice was negative.[188]

Environmental surveys conducted by the EPA have detected 1,2-dichloroethane in groundwater sources in the vicinity of contaminated sites[189] in concentrations of about 175 ppb (geometric mean). In a survey of 14 river basins in heavily industrialized areas in the United States, 1,2-dichloroethane was present in 53% of more than 200 surface water samples. In drinking water the compound has been detected at concentrations ranging from 1 to 64 μg/L.[190] The OSHA permissible exposure limit for occupational exposure has been reduced to 1 ppm.[191] The maximum contaminant level (MCL) for drinking water has been regulated by the EPA[187] at 0.005 mg/L. The EPA has classified 1,2-dichloroethane for its carcinogenic potential in group 2B.

Ethylene Dibromide

Ethylene dibromide (1,2-dibromoethane, $BrCH_2CH_2Br$) (EDB) is a colorless liquid with a boiling point of 131° C. One of the most important uses is in antiknock compounds added to gasoline to prevent the deposition of lead on the engine cylinder. It has also been used as a fumigant for grains, fruit, and vegetables, as a soil fumigant, as a special solvent, and in organic synthesis.

EDB has an irritant effect on the skin, with possible development of erythema, blistering, and ulceration after prolonged contact. It is also a potent eye and respiratory mucosal irritant. Systemic effects include CNS depression; after accidental ingestion, hepatocellular necrosis and renal proximal tubular epithelium necrosis have been reported. Cases of fatal ethylene dibromide poisoning have been reported as late as 1984; exposure occurred while victims were working inside a tank that had contained ethylene dibromide residues.[192] In experimental studies, hepatotoxicity and nephrotoxicity have been found at exposure levels of 50 ppm in all animals tested (rats, guinea pigs, rabbits, and monkeys).

EDB has been shown to produce significant decreases in cytochrome P-450 levels in liver, kidney, testes, lung, and small intestine microsomes. Hepatic microsomal mixed-function oxidase activities decreased in parallel with the cytochrome P-450 content.[193]

EDB exerts a toxic effect on spermatogenesis in bulls, with oligospermia and degenerative changes in spermatozoa.[194] This adverse effect on spermatogenesis has also been found in rams and in rats.[195,196] Effects of ethylene dibromide on spermatogenesis have been studied in 46 men employed in papaya fumigation; the highest measured exposure was 262 ppb, and the geometric mean was 88 ppb. When compared with a nonexposed reference group, there were statistically significant decreases in sperm count, in percentage of viable and mobile sperm and in the proportion of sperm with specific morphologic abnormalities.[197]

Mutagenic effects of EDB have been detected in several test systems.

A teratogenic effect is suspected; in rats and mice an increased incidence of CNS and skeletal malformations was found to be related to ethylene dibromide exposure. The carcinogenicity of EDB has been well documented in several bioassays on rats and mice exposed through various routes, including inhalation of 10 and 40 ppm. An increased incidence of various malignant tumors occurred in one or both sexes of one or both species tested. Among these were tumors of the mammary gland and nasal cavity, alveolar bronchiolar carcinomas, hemangiosarcomas, and tumors of the adrenal cortex and kidney.[196,198,199]

An epidemiological study[3,200] of a relatively small group of EDB-exposed workers suggests an increase in total mortality and total deaths from malignant diseases in the population with higher exposure.

EDB is considered to be a bifunctional alkylating agent because of the two replaceable bromine atoms. It may form covalent bonds with cellular constituents; the reaction with DNA is thought to be especially important, with possible covalent cross-links between DNA strands. Irreversible binding of EDB to DNA and RNA has been demonstrated. A complex between reduced glutathione and ethylene dibromide seems to be implicated in the covalent binding of EDB to DNA; this is unusual in that glutathione seems to play a role in the bioactivation of the carcinogen, as opposed to its more typical detoxification reactions.[201]

Environmental exposure of the general population to EDB has recently received increased attention.

Several uses of EDB—as an antiknock additive in leaded gasoline, for soil fumigation, fumigation of citrus and other fruit to prevent insect infestation, and treatment of grain-milling equipment—have resulted in contamination of air, water, fruit, grain, and derived products.

EDB has been found in groundwater in areas where it had been extensively used for soil fumigation. In the air of major cities, levels of EDB ranging from 16 to 59 ppt have been detected. Citrus fruits that had been fumigated were found to contain amounts of EDB of several hundred parts per billion; in lychee fruit (imported to Japan from Taiwan) levels varying from 0.14 to 2.18 ppm were detected.[202] An important and rather widespread contamination problem is that of EDB residues in commercial flour; levels from 8 ppb to 4 ppm were detected. In some ready-to-eat food products levels up to 260 ppb were found.

In 1983 the Environmental Protection Agency (EPA) introduced regulations to discontinue the use of EDB for soil fumigation, grain fumigation, treatment of grain-milling equipment, and postharvest fruit fumigation.[203] In 1984 the EPA recommended guidelines for acceptable levels of the chemical in food for human consumption, based on samplings of grain stocks and packaged foods in markets. It was recommended that EDB concentrations in grain intended for human consumption not exceed 900 ppb; for flour the residue level should not be higher than 150 ppb, and for ready-to-eat products it should not be more than 30 ppb. These guidelines have been critically reviewed and requests for even lower acceptable levels have been made. The proposed OSHA TWA standard for ethylene dibromide exposure is 100 ppb. NIOSH has recommended 45 ppb.

Methyl Chloride and Methyl Bromide

Methyl chloride and methyl bromide are gases at normal temperatures. Methyl chloride (CH_3Cl) is used in the chemical industry as a chlorinating agent but mainly as a methylating agent; it is also used in oil refineries for the extraction of greases and resins, as a solvent in the synthetic rubber industry, and as an expanding agent in the production of polystyrene foam. In recent years methyl chloride has been used primarily in the production of methyl silicone polymers and resins and organic lead additives for gasoline.[204] Methyl bromide (CH_3Br) is used as a fumigant for soil, grain, warehouses, and ships. Other important uses are as a methylating agent, a herbicide, a fire-extinguishing agent, a degreaser, in the extraction of oils, and as a solvent in aniline dye manufacture. Currently most of the methyl bromide produced in the United States is used to manufacture pesticides.

Methyl chloride and methyl bromide are irritants; exposure to high concentrations may result in toxic pulmonary edema. They are potent depressants of the CNS; with high exposure, toxic encephalopathy with visual disturbances, tremor, delirium, convulsions, and coma may occur and may be fatal. Permanent neurological deficits have been reported after recovery from acute toxic encephalopathy caused by methyl chloride and methyl bromide. Hepatotoxic and nephrotoxic effects may also occur.

Fatal poisonings after accidental exposure to high concentrations of methyl bromide, used as a fumigant, continue to be reported.[205-207] Methyl chloride, methyl bromide, and methyl iodide are alkylating agents; all three are direct mutagens in in vitro tests. They are also carcinogenic in experimental models. Methyl chloride has produced a teratogenic effect (heart malformation) in offspring of pregnant mice exposed by inhalation.[208] Methyl chloride and methyl bromide have been shown to produce testicular degeneration.[209,210]

Recently the hemoglobin adduct methyl cysteine was proposed as a biological indicator of methyl bromide exposure.[211] The NIOSH recommends that methyl chloride and methyl bromide be considered as potential occupational carcinogens.[208] The IARC (1986) found the evidence of carcinogenicity in humans and animals inconclusive.[204] The 1987 TLV for methyl chloride is 50 ppm; for methyl bromide, it is 5 ppm.

Chloroprene

Chloroprene (2-chloro- 1,3-butadiene, $H_2C=CCl—CH=CH_2$) is a colorless, flammable liquid with a low boiling point of 59.4°C. The major use is as a monomer in the manufacture of synthetic rubber, neoprene, since it can polymerize spontaneously at room temperature. The annual neoprene production in the United States is approximately 400 million pounds.

Inhalation of vapor and skin absorption are the routes of absorption. Chloroprene is an irritant of skin and mucosae (eyes, respiratory tract); it is a potent CNS depressant and has definite liver and kidney toxicity. Hair loss has also been associated with chloroprene exposure.

There are very few epidemiological studies on long-term effects of chloroprene. An excess of lung cancer and skin cancer has been reported by Russian investigators; the mean age of chloroprene-exposed workers with cancer was significantly younger than that in other groups.[112,212] The methodological limitations of these studies preclude firm conclusions on the carcinogenicity of chloroprene. A cohort study of chloroprene production and polymerization workers[213] gave negative results with regard to lung cancer but raised the possibility of an increased incidence of gastrointestinal cancer and hematopoietic and lymphatic cancer. Methodological difficulties of this latter study make it impossible to reach definitive conclusions.

Experimental studies on the carcinogenicity of chloroprene have been assessed by the International Agency for Research on Cancer and found to be inconclusive.[214]

An immunosuppressive effect of chloroprene is suspected.[112] Chloroprene produces degenerative changes in male reproductive organs. Reproduction of male mice and rats was affected after inhalation of chloroprene in concentrations of 12 to 150 ppm.[215] Reduction in the number and mobility of sperm and testicular atrophy have been observed in rats after chloroprene exposure.[214] In experiments on rats and mice, it was also found to be embryotoxic.[112]

Chloroprene has been shown to be mutagenic in several test systems.[179,216,217] Chromosome aberrations have been reported in bone marrow cells of exposed rats. In several groups of chloroprene-exposed workers, an increased incidence of chromosome aberrations in peripheral blood lymphocytes was noted.[210]

Prevention. Occupational exposure to chloroprene should be limited to a maximum concentration of 1 ppm.[217] Protective equipment to exclude the possibility of skin absorption, safety goggles, and air-supplied respirators are necessary to minimize exposure. Medical surveillance must be aimed not only at detection of short-term toxic and irritant effects but also at long-term effects on the CNS, liver and kidney function, reproductive abnormalities, and cancer risk.

Fluorocarbons

Fluorocarbons are hydrocarbons with fluorine, often with additional chlorine or bromine substitution of hydrogen atoms in their molecules. Most of them are nonflammable gases, and some are liquids at room temperature. Contact with open flame or heated metallic objects results in decomposition products, some of which are highly irritant, especially with chlorofluorocarbons (hydrogen fluoride, hydrogen chloride, phosgene, chlorine).

The fluorocarbons are used as refrigerants (Freon is one of the most widely used trademarks), as aerosol propellants, in fire extinguishers, for degreasing of electronic equipment, in the production of polymers, and as expanding agents in the manufacture of plastic foam.

Exposure to fluorocarbons in chemical plant operations and production is generally low but highly variable; high exposures can occur in areas without proper ventilation, during tank farm operations, tank and drum filling, and cylinder packing and shipping. Exposure to fluorocarbons can also occur during manufacturing, servicing, or leakage of refrigeration equipment.

The use of fluorocarbons as solvents in the electrical and electronic industry can generate higher exposures, especially when open containers are used. Emissions of fluorocarbons from plastic foams, where they have been entrapped during foam blowing, is another source of exposure. Use of fluorocarbons in sterilization procedures for reusable medical equipment, mostly with ethylene oxide, does not usually generate major exposures.

Fluorocarbons, especially trichlorofluoromethane (FC 11), have been used in the administration of certain drugs by inhalation, mostly sympathomimetics and corticosteroids for the treatment of asthma.[161]

Fluorocarbons with the widest use are the following:

- Bromotrifluoromethane
- Dibromodifluoromethane
- Dichlorodifluoromethane
- Dichloromonofluoromethane
- Dichlorotetrafluoroethane
- Fluorotrichloromethane
- 1,1,1,2-Tetrachloro-2,2-difluoroethane
- 1,1,2,2-Tetrachloro-1,2-difluoroethane
- 1,1,2-Trichloro-1,2,2-trifluoroethane
- Bromochlorotrifluoroethane
- Chlorodifluoromethane
- Chloropentafluoroethane
- Chlorotrifluoroethylene
- Chlorotrifluoromethane
- Difluoroethylene
- Fluoroethylene
- Hexafluoropropylene
- Octafluorocyclobutane
- Tetrafluoroethylene

Irritative effects of fluorocarbons are mild; after exposure to decomposition products, such effects may be severe. A bronchoconstrictive effect after inhalation of fluorocarbons has been demonstrated to occur at concentrations higher than 1000 ppm.

Narcotic effects occur at high concentrations. Liver and kidney toxicity have been reported with fluoroalkenes, thought to be more toxic than fluoroalkanes. Fatalities have been reported after acute overexposure to high concentrations of fluorocarbons used as refrigerants; in some of these cases simultaneous exposure to methyl chloride or to phosgene (a decomposition product of fluorocarbons) made it difficult to assess the contribution of fluorocarbon exposure to the lethal outcome.

A significant increase in the number of deaths from bronchial asthma was observed in Great Britain and found to coincide in time with the introduction and use of bronchodilator aerosols with fluorocarbon propellants. After withdrawal of these products from over-the-counter sale, the number of deaths from bronchial asthma decreased significantly.[218] Numerous deaths due to inhalation of fluorocarbon FC 11 (trichlorofluoromethane) have occurred. Addiction to fluorocarbon propellants in bronchodilator aerosols has been reported.[219]

Experimental evidence from studies on various animal species, documenting the arrhythmogenic properties of fluorocarbons, has established that sudden deaths due to cardiac arrhythmias, most probably through a mechanism similar to that identified for many chlorinated hydrocarbons, can occur with exposure to fluorocarbons. This prompted a reassessment of the permissible exposure levels.

Mutagenicity tests were conducted on a series of fluorocarbons in two in vitro systems. Chlorodifluoromethane (FC 22), chlorofluoromethane (FC 31), chlorodifluoroethane (FC 142b), and trifluoroethane (FC 143a) gave positive results in one or two of the tests. Potential carcinogenicity was considered, and limited carcinogenicity bioassays have indicated that FC 31 and FC 133 were potent carcinogens.[220]

Fluorocarbons that are lighter than air accumulate at high altitudes, where they may interact with and degrade the ozone layer, leading to penetration to the earth's surface of greater amounts of ultraviolet light. The problem of the ozone layer depletion is thought to be more specifically related to the fully halogenated, nonhydrogenated fluorocarbons, which produce free radical reactions with ozone by photodissociation in the upper atmosphere. Regulatory action has been taken to eliminate the use of fluorocarbon aerosol products in the United States. Other aspects of fluorocarbon use are still under consideration.

ALCOHOLS AND GLYCOLS

Alcohols are characterized by the substitution of one hydrogen atom of hydrocarbons by a hydroxyl (—OH) group; glycols are compounds with two such hydroxyl groups. Both are used extensively as solvents. Under usual industrial exposure conditions, alcohols and glycols do not represent major acute health hazards, mostly because their volatility is much lower than that of most other solvents.

Cases of severe poisoning with methyl alcohol or ethylene glycol are usually caused by accidental ingestion. They have an irritative effect on mucous membranes; the narcotic effect is much less prominent than with the corresponding hydrocarbons or halogenated hydrocarbons.

Glycols are liquids with low volatility; the low vapor pressure prevents significant air concentrations, except when the compounds are heated or sprayed. Inhalation or skin contact does not usually result in absorption of toxic amounts; accidental ingestion accounts for the majority of poisoning cases. Glycols are used mainly as solvents and, because of their low freezing point, in antifreeze mixtures.

Methyl Alcohol

Methyl alcohol (methanol, wood alcohol, CH_3OH) is used in the chemical industry in the manufacture of formaldehyde, methacrylates, ethylene glycol, and a variety of other compounds such as plastics, celluloid, and photographic film.[2,3,153] It is also used as a solvent for lacquers, adhesives, industrial coatings, inks, and dyes and in paint and varnish removers. It is used in antifreeze mixtures, as an additive to gasoline, and as an antidetonant additive for aircraft fuel.

Methyl alcohol is a moderate irritant and depressant of the CNS. Systemic toxicity due to inhalation and skin absorption of methyl alcohol has been reported with very high exposure levels because of large amounts being handled in enclosed spaces. Accidental ingestion of methyl alcohol can be fatal; after a latency period of several hours (longer with smaller amounts), neurological abnormalities, visual disturbances, nausea, vomiting, abdominal pain, metabolic acidosis, and coma may occur in rapid sequence.

Toxic optic retrobulbar neuritis is a specific effect of methyl alcohol and may result in permanent blindness due to optic atrophy. Nephrotoxic effects and toxic pancreatitis have also been reported. Methyl alcohol is slowly metabolized to formaldehyde and formic acid; the extent to which these metabolites are responsible for the specific toxic effects has not been completely clarified.

Control of acidosis is very important in methyl alcohol poisoning, and intravenous bicarbonate has been beneficial. Since methanol is metabolized by alcohol dehydrogenase, and its metabolites were considered more toxic than methanol itself, ethanol was thought to be helpful through competition for the metabolizing enzyme. Hemodialysis has markedly improved the outlook in accidental methanol poisoning, as has the adequate management of metabolic acidosis.

Prevention. The federal standard for methanol exposure is 200 ppm.[3] Warning signs must be posted wherever methyl alcohol is stored or can be present in the working environment, with emphasis on the extreme danger of blindness if swallowed. Employees' education and training must be thorough. Medical surveillance with attention to visual, neurological, hepatic, and renal functions is necessary. Formic acid in urine and methyl alcohol in blood can be used for the assessment of excessive exposure.

Allyl Alcohol

Allyl alcohol ($H_2C=CHCH_2OH$) is a liquid with a boiling point of 96.0° C. It is used in the manufacture of allyl esters and of monomers for synthetic resins and plastics, in the synthesis of a variety of organic compounds, in the pharmaceutical industry, and as a herbicide and fungicide.

Absorption occurs through inhalation and percutaneous penetration. Allyl alcohol is a potent irritant for the eyes, the respiratory system, and the skin. Muscle pain underlying the site of skin absorption, lacrimation, photophobia, blurring of vision, and corneal lesions have been reported.[2] The marked irritant properties probably prevent greater exposure, which would result in liver and kidney toxicity, effects found in experimental animals but not reported in humans.

Prevention. The federal standard for permissible exposure limit to allyl alcohol is 2 ppm. Protective equipment is very important, given the possible skin absorption; the material of choice is neoprene.

Isopropyl Alcohol

Isopropyl alcohol ($CH_3CHOHCH_3$, isopropanol) is a colorless liquid with a boiling point of 82.3° C and high volatility. It is used in the production of acetone and isopropyl derivatives. Other important uses are as a solvent for oils, synthetic resins, plastics, perfumes, dyes, and nitrocellulose lacquers and in the extraction of sulfonic acid from petroleum products. Isopropyl alcohol has many applications in the pharmaceutical industry, in liniments, skin lotions, mouthwashes, cosmetics, rubbing alcohol, etc.

Isopropyl alcohol absorption takes place mainly by inhalation, although skin absorption is also possible. The irritant effects are slight; dermatitis has seldom been reported. Depressant (narcotic) effects have been observed in cases of accidental or intentional isopropyl alcohol ingestion. Coma and renal tubular degenerative changes have occasionally resulted in death. Acetone has been found in the exhaled air and in urine; isopropyl alcohol concentrations in blood can be measured.

In the early 1940s an unusual clustering of neoplasms of the respiratory tract—malignant tumors of the paranasal sinuses, lung, and larynx—was reported in an isopropyl alcohol manufacturing facility.[221] Similar observations have been reported by Hueper[222,223] and by Bittersohl.[224] It was thought that the carcinogenic compounds were associated with the "strong acid process" and especially with heavier hydrocarbon oils (tars) containing polyaromatic compounds.

In the more modern direct catalytic hydration (weak acid process) of propylene, the isopropyl oil seems to contain compounds with lower molecular weight, although the precise composition is not known. Attempts to identify the carcinogen(s) in experimental studies have not been successful,[3] and the question of a carcinogen present in the manufacture of isopropyl alcohol is still open.

Prevention. The federal standard for a permissible level of isopropyl alcohol exposure is at present 400 ppm.

Ethylene Chlorhydrin

Ethylene chlorhydrin (CH_2ClCH_2OH)—synonyms: glycol chlorohydrin, 2-chloroethanol, β-chloroethyl alcohol—is a very toxic compound.[2] It is used in the synthesis of ethylene glycol and ethylene oxide and in a variety of other reactions, especially when the hydroxyethyl group ($—CH_2CH_2OH$) has to be incorporated in molecules. Other uses are as a special solvent, for cellulose acetate and esters, resins, waxes, and for the separation of butadiene from hydrocarbon mixtures. Agricultural applications include seed treatment and application to accelerate the sprouting of potatoes.

Ethylene chlorhydrin is absorbed through inhalation and readily through the skin. It is irritant to the eyes, airways, and skin. Exposure to high concentrations may result in toxic pulmonary edema. Systemic effects are marked: depression of the CNS, hypotension, visual disturbances, delirium, coma and convulsions, hepatotoxic and nephrotoxic effects with nausea, vomiting, hematuria, and proteinuria. Death may occur as a result of pulmonary edema or cerebral edema. Even cases with slight or moderate initial symptoms may be fatal.

Prevention. The federal standard for the limit of permissible exposure is 5 ppm. The use of ethylene chlorhydrin other than in enclosed systems should be completely eliminated. Protective clothing should use materials impervious to this compound; rubber is readily penetrated and has to be excluded. Protective clothing must be changed regularly so that no deterioration will jeopardize its purpose.

Ethylene Glycol

Ethylene glycol ($OHCH_2CH_2OH$) is a viscous colorless liquid, used mainly in antifreeze and hydraulic fluids but also in the manufacture of glycol esters, resins, and other derivatives and as a solvent.

CNS depression, nausea, vomiting, abdominal pain, respiratory failure, and renal failure with oliguria, proteinuria, and oxalate crystals in the urinary sediment are manifestations of ethylene glycol poisoning.[2] Glycolic acid is the metabolite that is found in the highest concentrations in blood; serum and urine levels of glycolic acid correlate with clinical symptoms.[225] The active enzyme is alcohol dehydrogenase.[153] It is estimated that 50 deaths occur annually in the United States from accidental ingestion of ethylene glycol. Hemodialysis has been successfully used in the treatment of accidental ethylene glycol poisoning by ingestion.[226,227] The therapeutic use of 4-methyl pyrazole, an alcohol dehydrogenase inhibitor, was also recently recommended for the management of accidental or suicidal ethylene glycol poisoning.[228]

Prevention. No federal standard for ethylene glycol exposure has been established. The American Conference of Industrial Hygienists recommended a threshold limit value of 100 ppm. The most important preventive action is to alert employees to the extreme hazard of ingestion. Adequate respiratory protection should be provided wherever the compound is heated or sprayed.

Increasing use of glycols as deicing agents for aircraft and airfield runways has generated concern about surface water contamination that may result from runoff. Degradation of ethylene glycol in river water is complete within 3 to 7 days (depending on temperature); degradation of diethylene glycol is somewhat slower. At low temperatures (8°C or less), both glycols degrade at a minimal rate.[229]

Diethylene Glycol

Diethylene glycol is similar in its effects to ethylene glycol; its importance is mainly historical, since more than 100 deaths occurred in the United States when it was used in the manufacture of an elixir of sulfanilamide. Fatal cases were caused by renal proximal tubular necrosis and renal failure.[2]

ETHYLENE GLYCOL ETHERS AND DERIVATIVES

The most important alkyl glycol derivatives are ethylene glycol monoethyl ether, (ethoxyethanol, cellosolve) ($CH_3CH_2OCH_2CH_2OH$) and its acetate; ethylene glycol monomethyl ether (methoxyethanol, methyl cellosolve) ($CH_3OCH_2CH_2OH$) and its acetate; and ethylene glycol monobutyl ether (butoxyethanol, butyl cellosolve) ($CH_3CH_2CH_2CH_2OCH_2CH_2OH$).[2] These compounds are colorless liquids with wide applications as solvents for resins, lacquers, paints, varnishes, coatings (including epoxy resin coatings), dyes, inks, adhesives, and plastics. They are also used in hydraulic fluids, as anti-icing additives, in brake fluids, and in aviation fuels. Ethylene glycol monoethyl ether is used in the formulation of adhesives, detergents, pesticides, cosmetics, and pharmaceuticals.

Inhalation, transcutaneous absorption, and gastrointestinal absorption are all possible. These derivatives are irritants for the mucous membranes and skin. The acetates are more potent irritants. Corneal clouding, usually transitory, may occur. Acute overexposure may result in marked narcotic effects and encephalopathy; pulmonary edema and severe kidney and liver toxicity are also possible. At lower levels of exposure, CNS effects result in such symptoms as fatigue, headache, tremor, slurred speech, gait abnormalities, blurred vision, and personality changes.

Anemia is another possible effect; macrocytosis and immature forms of leukocytes can be found. Exposure to ethylene glycol monomethyl ether has also been associated with pancytopenia. In animal experiments, butyl cellosolve has been shown to produce hemolytic anemia; this has not been reported in humans.

Exposure to ethylene glycol monomethyl ether and to ethylene glycol monoethyl ether has been shown to result in adverse reproductive effects in mice, rats, and rabbits.[230] These effects include testicular atrophy, degenerative testicular changes,[231] abnormal sperm head morphology, and infertility in males. Exposure of pregnant animals resulted in increased rates of embryonic deaths and in various congenital malformations.[232,233] The acetate esters of ethylene glycol monomethyl ether and of ethylene glycol monoethyl ether have produced similar adverse male reproductive effects.

A cross-sectional study of 97 workers exposed to ethylene glycol monomethyl ether, with semen analysis in 15, did not reveal abnormalities other than a possibly smaller testicular size.[234] The occurrence of adverse male reproductive effects in humans cannot be excluded on the basis of this study.

Prevention. Federal standards for permissible exposure limits are ethylene glycol monoethyl ether, 200 ppm; ethylene glycol monoethyl ether acetate, 100 ppm; ethylene glycol monomethyl ether, 25 ppm; ethylene glycol monomethyl ether acetate, 25 ppm; and ethylene glycol monobutyl ether, 50 ppm.

The American Conference of Governmental Industrial Hygienists has recommended a TLV of 25 ppm for ethylene glycol monomethyl ether and 100 ppm for ethylene glycol monoethyl ether; this latter TLV was lowered in 1981 to 50 ppm. In 1982 it was proposed that the time-weighted average exposure limits for both these compounds and their acetates be reduced to 5 ppm in view of the testicular effects observed in recent animal studies.[230,235]

ORGANIC ACIDS, ANHYDRIDES, LACTONES, AND AMIDES

These compounds have numerous industrial applications. Their common clinical characteristic is an irritant effect on eyes, nose, throat, and the respiratory tract. Skin irritation can be severe, and some of the acids (formic, acetic, oxalic, and others) can produce chemical burns. Accidental eye penetration may result in severe corneal injury and consequent opacities. Toxic pulmonary edema can occur after acute overexposure to high concentrations.

Phthalic Anhydride

Phthalic anhydride ($C_6H_4(CO)_2O$) is a crystalline, needlelike white solid. It is used in the manufacture of benzoic and phthalic acids, as a plasticizer for vinyl resins, alkyd and polyester resins, in the production of diethyl and dimethyl phthalate, phenolphthalein, phthalamide, methyl aniline, and other compounds.

Phthalic anhydride as dust, fumes, or vapor is a potent irritant for the eyes, respiratory system, and skin; with prolonged skin contact, chemical burns are possible. Repeated exposure may result in chronic industrial bronchitis. Phthalic anhydride is also a potent sensitizing substance: occupational asthma can be severe and hypersensitivity pneumonitis has been reported. Skin sensitization may result in exzematiform dermatitis.

Prevention. The federal standard for phthalic anhydride is a TLV of 1 ppm. Enclosure of technological processes where phthalic anhydride is used and protective clothing, including gloves and goggles, are necessary; respiratory protection must be available. Periodic examinations should focus on possible sensitization and chronic effects, such as bronchitis and dermatitis.

Maleic Anhydride

Maleic anhydride (O CO CH = CO) is used mainly in the production of alkyd and polyester resins; it has also found applications for siccatives. Maleic anhydride can produce severe chemical burns of the skin and eyes. It is also a sensitizing substance and can lead to clinical manifestations similar to those described for phthalic anhydride. The 1987 TLV is 0.25 ppm.

Trimellitic Anhydride

Trimellitic anhydride (1,2,4-benzenetricarboxylic acid, cyclic 1,2-anhydride, $C_9H_4O_5$) is used as a curing agent for epoxy resins and other resins, in vinyl plasticizers, polyesters, dyes and pigments, paints and coatings, agricultural chemicals, surface-active compounds, pharmaceuticals, etc. Chemical pneumonitis has been reported after an epoxy resin containing trimellitic anhydride was sprayed on heated pipes.[236] Respiratory irritation after exposure to high concentrations of trimellitic anhydride was reported in workers engaged in the synthesis of this compound. It was also found that in some cases sensitization occurs after variable periods following onset of exposure (sometimes years); allergic rhinitis, occupational asthma, and hypersensitivity pneumonitis can be manifestations of sensitization.[237] Trimellitic anhydride as the etiologic agent in cases of sensitization was confirmed by inhalation challenge tests.[237a,238]

Prevention. The NIOSH recommended in 1978 that trimellitic anhydride be considered an extremely toxic agent, since it can produce severe irritation of the respiratory tract, including pulmonary edema and chemical pneumonitis; sensitization, with occupational asthma or hypersensitivity pneumonitis can occur at lower levels. Guidelines for engineering controls and protective equipment have been outlined by NIOSH.[3] The current OSHA TLV standard is 0.04 mg/m^3.

Beta-Propiolactone

Beta-propiolactone ($\underline{O\,CH_2\,CH_2\,C}=O$) is a colorless liquid with important applications in the synthesis of acrylate plastics; it is also used as a disinfectant and as a sterilizing agent against viruses. It is easily absorbed through the skin; inhalation is also important.

Beta-propiolactone is a very potent irritant. In animal experiments it has been found to produce hepatocellular necrosis, renal tubular necrosis, convulsions, and circulatory collapse. In several animal studies it has also been shown to be carcinogenic; skin cancer, hepatoma, and gastric cancer have been induced. Reports on systemic or carcinogenic effects in humans are not available.

Beta-propiolactone is included in the federal standard for carcinogens; no exposure should be allowed to occur. Protective equipment designed to prevent all skin contact or inhalation is necessary; this includes full-body protective clothing and full-face air-supplied respirators. Showers at the end of the shift are absolutely necessary. The 1987 TLV is 0.05 ppm.

N, N-Dimethylformamide

N, N-dimethylformamide, $HCON(CH_3)_2$, is a colorless liquid with a boiling point of 153° C. It is miscible with water and organic solvents at 25° C. It has excellent solvent properties for numerous organic compounds and is used in processes where solvents with low volatility are necessary. Its major applications are in the manufacture of synthetic fibers and resins, mainly polyacrylic fibers and butadiene. It is absorbed through inhalation and through the skin and is irritating to the eyes, mucous membranes, and skin.[2] Adverse effects of absorption include loss of appetite, nausea, vomiting, abdominal pain, hepatomegaly, and other indications of liver injury. Recently clusters of testicular germ cell tumors have been reported among airplane manufacturing employees and tannery workers.[239] An increased incidence of cancer (oropharyngeal and melanoma) was reported in a cohort of formamide-exposed workers.[240] In animal experiments nephrotoxicity has also been detected. The federal standard for a permissible exposure limit is 10 ppm (30 mg/m^3).

N, N'-Dimethylacetamide

N, N'-dimethylacetamide, ($CH_3CON(CH_3)_2$) is a colorless liquid that is easily absorbed through the skin. Inhalation is a less important route of absorption, since the volatility is low. *N, N'*-dimethylacetamide is used as a solvent in a variety of industrial processes.

Hepatotoxicity is the most severe adverse effect; hepatocellular degenerative changes and jaundice have been reported in exposed workers. Experimental studies have also indicated hepatotoxicity as the prominent effect in rats and dogs. With high exposure, depressant neurotoxic effects become evident. Dimethylacetamide has recently been shown, in experiments on rodents, to produce testicular changes in rabbits and rats. Its hepatotoxicity was comparable to and possibly higher than that of dimethyl formamide.[241]

The federal standard for a PEL is 10 ppm (35 mg/m^3). Protective equipment to exclude percutaneous absorption is necessary, as are eye and respiratory protection if high vapor concentrations are possible.

Acrylamide

Acrylamide ($CH_2=CH\ CO\ NH_2$) is a white crystalline material with a melting point of 84.5° C and a tendency to sublime; it is readily soluble in water and in some other common polar solvents. Large-scale production started in the early 1950s[242]; the major industrial applications are as a vinyl monomer in the production of high-molecular polymers such as polyacrylamides. These have many applications, including the clarification and treatment of municipal and industrial effluents and potable water; in the oil industry (for fracturing and flooding of oil-bearing strata); as flocculants in the production of ores, metals, and coal; as strengtheners in the paper industry; for textile treatment, etc. Although the pure polyacrylamide polymers are nontoxic, the problem of residual unreacted acrylamide exists, since up to 2% residual monomer is acceptable for some industrial applications. The Food and Drug Administration (FDA) has established a maximum 0.05% residual monomer level for polymers used in paper or cardboard in contact with food; similar levels are accepted for polymers used in clarification of potable water. Since acrylamide has cumulative toxic effects, it has been recommended that the general population not be exposed to daily levels in excess of 0.0005 mg/kg.

The initial indication of a marked neurotoxic effect of acrylamide came when a recently introduced acrylamide production method (from acrylonitrile) was first used in 1953; several workers experienced weakness in their extremities, with numbness and tingling, strongly suggestive of toxic peripheral neuropathy.[243] Cases of acrylamide neuropathy have since been reported from Japan, France, Canada,[244] and Great Britain.[245]

Acrylamide is readily absorbed through the skin, which is considered an important route of absorption. Respiratory absorption and ingestion of acrylamide are also important; severe cases of acrylamide poisoning have resulted from ingestion of contaminated water in Japan.

Acrylamide poisoning in occupationally exposed workers has occurred after relatively short periods of exposure (several months to a year). Erythema and peeling of skin, mainly in the palms but also on the soles, usually precede neurologic symptoms; excessive fatigue, weight loss, and somnolence are followed by a slowly progressive symmetrical peripheral neuropathy. The characteristic symptoms include muscle weakness, unsteadiness, paresthesia, signs of sympathetic nervous system involvement (cold, blue hands and feet, excessive sweating), impairment of superficial sensation (touch, pain, temperature) and position sense, diminished or absent deep tendon reflexes in legs and arms, and the presence of Romberg's sign. Considerable loss of muscle strength may occur, and muscular atrophy, usually starting with the small muscles of the hands, has been reported. This toxic neuropathy has a distal to proximal evolution; the earliest and most severe changes are in the distal segments of the lower and upper extremities, and progression occurs with involvement of more proximal segments ("stocking and glove" distribution). Signs indicating CNS involvement are somnolence, vertigo, ataxic gait, and occasionally slight organic mental syndrome. EEG abnormalities have also been described.

Sensory nerve conduction velocities have been found to be more affected than motor nerve conduction velocities; potentials with markedly prolonged distal latencies are described. Recovery after cessation of exposure is slow; it may take several months to 2 years. Experimental acrylamide neuropathy has been produced in all mammals studied; medium-to large-diameter fibers and long fibers are more susceptible to the primary giant axonal degeneration and secondary demyelination characteristic of acrylamide neuropathy. CNS pathology consists of degenerating fibers in the anterior and lateral columns of the spinal cord, gracile nucleus, cerebellar vermis,[246] spinocerebellar tracts, CNS optic nerve tracts, and tracts in the hypothalamus.

Changes in somatosensory evoked potentials have been found to be useful in the early detection of acrylamide neurotoxicity. They precede abnormalities of peripheral nerve conduction and behavioral signs of intoxication.[247] Deterioration of visual capacity, with an increased threshold for visual acuity and flicker fusion and prolonged latency in visual evoked potentials, was reported in monkeys. These abnormalities were detected before overt signs of toxicity became apparent.[248]

An underlying mechanism of acrylamide peripheral neuropathy has been found to be impaired retrograde transport of material from the more distal parts of the peripheral nerve. The buildup of retrogradely transported material has been shown to be dose-related. Changes in retrograde axonal transport are thought to play an initial and important role in the development of toxic axonopathies, possibly the primary biochemical event in acrylamide neuropathy.[249] Alterations in retrograde transport appear before detectable changes in peripheral nerve function.

Local disorganization of the smooth endoplasmic reticulum, forming a complex network of tubules intermingled with vesicles and mitochondria, is thought to be responsible for the focal stasis of fast-transported proteins. These seem to be the earliest changes detectable in axons damaged by acrylamide.[250]

Acrylamide has been reported to produce effects on neurotransmitter and neuropeptide levels in various areas of the brain. Elevated levels of 5-hydroxyindolacetic acid in all regions of the rat brain were interpreted as being the result of an increased serotonin turnover. Changes in the affinity and number of dopamine receptor sites have also been reported.[251] Elevated levels of some neuropeptides were detected mainly in the hypothalamus.[252] Significant decreases in plasma levels of testosterone and prolactin were found after repeated acrylamide administration.[252]

Experimental neurotoxicity studies of 14 acrylamide analogues were undertaken; 5 produced neuropathy. The order of neurotoxicity was acrylamide > N-isopropylacrylamide > N-methylacrylamide = methacrylamide > N-hydroxymethylacrylamide. All these compounds also produced testicular atrophy, with degenerative changes in the epithelial cells of seminiferous tubules. Acrylamide produces chromosomal aberrations in mouse bone marrow cells. The micronucleus test was also positive.[253] Recent oncogenicity studies on rats treated with acrylamide in drinking water for 2 years have been positive for a number of tumors (central nervous system, thyroid, mammary gland, uterus in females, and scrotal mesothelioma in males).[254]

In a mortality study involving a cohort of 371 employees exposed to acrylamide, an excess in total cancer deaths was due to excess in digestive and respiratory cancer in a subgroup that had had previous exposure to organic dyes.[255]

Control and Prevention. Engineering designs that prevent the escape of both vapor and dust into the environment are necessary; enclosure, exhaust ventilation, and automated systems must be used to minimize exposure. Prevention of skin and eye contact is especially important in handling of aqueous solutions, and closed systems are to be preferred.

The present recommended TWA for acrylamide exposure is 0.3 mg/m^3. Skin exposure has to be carefully avoided by the use of appropriate protective clothing and work practices. Showers and eyewash fountains should be available for immediate use if contamination occurs. Preemployment and periodic medical examinations with special attention to skin, eyes, and nervous system are necessary. It is essential that employees be warned of the potential health hazards and the importance of personal hygiene and careful work practices. Frequent inspection of fingers and hands by medical or paramedical personnel is useful in detecting peeling of skin, which usually precedes clinical neuropathy.

ALDEHYDES

Aldehydes are aliphatic or aromatic compounds with the general structure:

$$\mathrm{R{-}\overset{\displaystyle O}{\overset{\|}{C}}{-}H}$$

The aldehydes are highly reactive substances and are used extensively throughout the chemical industry. Formaldehyde is a gas that is readily soluble in water; the other aldehydes are liquids.

The common characteristic of aldehydes is their strong irritative effect on the skin, eyes, and respiratory system. Acute overexposure may result in toxic pulmonary edema. Sensitization to aldehydes is possible, and allergic dermatitis and occupational asthma can occur.

Formaldehyde

Formaldehyde (HCHO) is a colorless gas with a strong odor, which is readily soluble in water; the commercial solutions may contain up to 15% methanol to prevent polymerization. It has numerous industrial applications in the manufacture of textiles, cellulose esters, dyes, inks, latex, phenol, urea, melamine, pentaerythrol, hexamethylenetetramine, thiourea, resins, and explosives and as a fungicide, disinfectant, and preservative. More than half of formaldehyde is used in the United States in the manufacture of plastics and resins: urea-formaldehyde resins, phenolic, polyacetal, and melamine resins. Among the many other uses is in the manufacture of 4,4′-methylene dianiline and 4,4′-methylene diphenyl diisocyanate. Some relatively small-volume uses of formaldehyde are in agriculture, for seed treatment and as a soil disinfectant, in cosmetics, deodorants, in photography, and in histopathology.

Formaldehyde has been found to be a relatively common contaminant of indoor air; it originates in urea-formaldehyde resins used in the production of particle board or in urea-formaldehyde foam used for insulation. Such insulation has been applied in the United States in approximately 500,000 houses during the period 1975 to 1980. Concentrations of formaldehyde in residential indoor air have varied from 0.01 to 31.7 ppm.[256]

Significant concentrations of formaldehyde have been found in industrial effluents, mainly from the production of urea-, melamine-and phenol-formaldehyde resins, and also from users of such resins (e.g., plywood manufacturers). In water, formaldehyde undergoes rapid degradation and therefore does not represent a major source of absorption. Formaldehyde is also readily degraded in soil. Bioaccumulation does not occur.

Other sources of formaldehyde exposure for the general population are from cigarette smoke (37 to 73 μg/per cigarette) and from small amounts in food, especially after the use of hexamethylenetetramine as a food additive.

Formaldehyde resins applied to permanent-press textiles can emit formaldehyde when stored. Fingernail hardeners containing formaldehyde are a relatively recent addition to the potential sources of formaldehyde exposure.

Absorption occurs through inhalation. Skin and eye contact may result in chemical burns. Acute overexposure to very high concentrations may result in pulmonary edema. Sensitization resulting in allergic dermatitis is not uncommon; occupational asthma is also possible.

Formaldehyde carcinogenicity assays have recently revealed that exposure inhalation to concentrations of 14.3 ppm resulted in a significantly increased incidence of squamous cell carcinomas in rats of both sexes.[257] In mice only a very small number of squamous cell carcinomas (two) developed; the incidence was not statistically significant. Dysplasia and squamous metaplasia of the respiratory epithelium, rhinitis, and atrophy of the olfactory epithelium were observed in mice; similar lesions were seen in rats, and goblet cell hyperplasia, squamous atypia, and papillary hyperplasia were also found. A recent 2-year experimental study on rats investigated the effects of formaldehyde in drinking water. Although pathologic changes in the gastric mucosa were found in the high-dose rats, no gastric tumors or tumors at other sites were detected.[258]

Mortality studies on human populations exposed to formaldehyde only are rare. A study of pathologists and laboratory technicians in Great Britain was negative.[259] Among morticians practicing embalming[260] in New York State, an excess of skin cancer, kidney cancer, and brain cancer was found, although the small numbers preclude definitive conclusions. There were no cancers of the nose or nasal sinuses and no excess of respiratory cancer. A cohort study of 2490 employees in a chemical plant manufacturing and using formaldehyde was also conducted. An elevated proportional mortality for digestive tract cancer in white males was found; the small numbers make it difficult to draw conclusions. No deaths from cancers of the nose or nasal sinuses had occurred. The duration of employment was relatively short. The studies had a very limited power to detect excess mortality from nasal cancer.[256] In a large retrospective cohort mortality study of more than 11,000 workers exposed to formaldehyde in the garment industry, significant excess mortality from cancer of the buccal cavity and connective tissue were found. The incidence of such cancers as leukemia and lymphoma was higher than expected without reaching the level of statistical significance.[261]

Formaldehyde is mutagenic to bacteria, yeast, and *Drosophila* but not in other systems, including mammalian cells in culture. Formaldehyde is metabolized to carbon dioxide and formate. Studies using ^{14}C-formaldehyde have demonstrated the presence of ^{14}C-labeled cellular macromolecules.[262] Formaldehyde has been reported to react with nucleic acids[263] and to induce DNA-protein cross-links.[264] Sister chromatid exchanges in lymphocytes of formaldehyde-exposed anatomy students showed a small but statistically significant increase when compared with preexposure findings in the same persons.[265]

The federal standard for formaldehyde is 1 ppm (1.2 mg/m^3). Engineering controls are essential to control exposure. Protective equipment to prevent skin contact, adequate respirators for situations in which higher exposure could result, proper work practices, and continuous education programs for employees are necessary. The Environmental Protection Agency and the Occupational Health and Safety Administration, in their consideration of available epidemiological and toxicological studies, now regard formaldehyde as a possible human carcinogen, although the evidence in humans is limited and controversial.[266]

Acrolein

Acrolein ($H_2C=CHCHO$), a clear liquid, is used in the production of plastics, plasticizers, acrylates, synthetic fibers, and methionine; it is produced when oils and fats containing glycerol are heated. It is one of the strongest irritants. Skin burns and severe irritation of eyes and respiratory tract, including toxic pulmonary edema, are possible.

Recently, acrolein was shown to be embryotoxic and teratogenic in rats, after intraamniotic administration[267]; similar effects were reported for chick embryos. Acrolein is genotoxic and causes DNA single-strand breaks and DNA cross-links in human bronchial epithelial cells.[268] Acrolein has been shown to form cyclic deoxyguanosine adducts when it reacts with DNA in vitro and in *Salmonella typhimurium* cultures.[269]

The federal standard for a permissible exposure limit for acrolein is 0.1 ppm.

Other widely used aldehydes are acetaldehyde and furfural. They have irritant effects but are less potent in this respect than formaldehyde and acrolein.

ESTERS

Esters are organic compounds that result from the substitution of a hydrogen atom of an acid (organic or inorganic) with an organic group. They constitute a very large group of substances with a variety of industrial uses in plastics and resins, as solvents, and in the pharmaceutical, surface coating, textile, and food-processing industries.

Narcotic CNS effects and irritative effects (especially with the halogenated esters such as ethyl chloroformate, ethyl chloroacetate, and the corresponding bromo- and iodo- compounds) are common to most esters. Sensitization has been reported with some of the aliphatic monocarboxylic halogenated esters. Some of the esters of inorganic acids have specific, potentially severe toxicity. For a discussion of phosphate esters, see Pesticides, Chapter 24.

Dimethylsulfate

Dimethylsulfate, $(CH_3)_2SO_4$, is an oily fluid. It is used mainly for its methylating capacity; another use is as a solvent in the separation of mineral oils. Absorption is mainly through inhalation, but skin penetration is also possible.

Toxic effects are complex and severe; many fatalities have occurred. After a latency period of several hours, the irritant effects on the skin, eyes, and respiratory system become manifest; toxic pulmonary edema is not unusual. Vesication of the skin and ulceration can occur. Eye irritation usually results in conjunctivitis, keratitis, photophobia, palpebral edema, and blepharospasm. Irritation of the upper airways may also be severe, with dysphagia and sometimes edema of the glottis. Dyspnea, cough, and shallow breathing are the signs of toxic pulmonary edema. If the patient survives this critical period, 48 hours later the signs and symptoms of hepatocellular necrosis and renal tubular necrosis may become manifest.

At very high levels of exposure, neurotoxic effects are prominent, with somnolence, delirium, convulsions, temporary blindness, and coma.

Dimethylsulfate is an alkylating agent. In experimental studies on rats it has been shown to be carcinogenic. Prenatal exposure has also produced tumors of the nervous system in offspring. The IARC has concluded that there is sufficient evidence of dimethyl sulfate carcinogenicity in animals and that it has to be assumed to be a potential human carcinogen.[270] In inhalation experiments on rodents, embryotoxic and teratogenic effects have also been observed.[271]

The federal standard for a permissible level of dimethylsulfate exposure is 0.1 ppm.

Diethylsulfate, methylchlorosulfonate, ethylchlorosulfonate, and methyl-*p*-toluene sulfonate have effects similar to those of dimethyl sulfate, and the same extreme precautions in their handling are necessary. The skin, eyes, and respiratory tract should be protected continuously when there may be exposure to dimethylsulfate or the other esters that have similar effects. Contaminated areas should be entered only by trained personnel with impervious protective clothing and air-supplied respirators.[2]

KETONES

The chemical characteristic of this series of compounds known as ketones is the presence of the carbonyl group. Their general structure is

$$R-\underset{\underset{O}{\|}}{C}-R'$$

Ketones are excellent solvents for oils, fats, collodion, cellulose acetate, nitrocellulose, cellulose esters, epoxy resins, pigments, dyes, natural and synthetic resins (especially vinyl polymers and copolymers), and acrylic coatings. They are also used in the manufacture of paints, lacquers, and varnishes and in the celluloid, rubber, artificial leather, synthetic rubber, lubricating oil, and explosives industries. Other uses are in metal cleaning, rapidly drying inks, airplane dopes, as paint removers and dewaxers, and in hydraulic fluids.

The most important members of the ketone group, because of extensive use, are as follows:

- Acetone CH_3COCH_3
- Methyl-ethyl-ketone $CH_3COCH_2CH_3$
- Methyl-*n*-propyl ketone $CH_3(CH_2)_2COCH_3$
- Methyl-*n*-butyl ketone $CH_3CO(CH_2)_3CH_3$
- Methyl isobutyl ketone $CH_3COCH_2CH(CH_3)_2$
- Methyl-*n*-amyl ketone $CH_3CO(CH_2)_4CH_3$
- Methyl isoamyl ketone $CH_3CO(CH_2)_2CH(CH_3)_2$
- Diisobutyl ketone $(CH_3)_2CHCH_2COCH_2\ CH(CH_3)_2$
- Cyclohexane $C_6H_{10}O$
- Mesityl oxide $CH_3COCH = C(CH_3)_2$
- Isophorone(3,5,5-trimethyl-2-cyclohexen-1-one)
- $C_{10}H_{14}O$

Methyl isobutyl ketone is used in the recovery of uranium from fission products. It has also found applications as a vehicle for herbicides, such as 2,4,5-T, and insecticides. Many of the ketones are valuable raw materials or intermediates in the chemical synthesis of other compounds. For example, approximately 90% of the 2 billion pounds of acetone produced each year is used by the chemical industry for the production of methacetylates and higher ketones.

The major route of absorption is through inhalation of vapor; with some of the ketones, such as methyl-ethyl ketone (MEK) and methyl-butyl ketone (MBK), skin absorption may contribute significantly to the total amount absorbed if work practices allow for extensive contact (immersion of hands, washing with the solvents).

All the ketones are moderate mucous membrane irritants (eyes and upper airways); at higher concentrations CNS depression with prenarcotic symptoms progressing to narcosis may occur.

A specific neurotoxic effect of MBK, peripheral neuropathy, was reported in 1975[272] in workers exposed in the plastic coatings industry. In 1976 similar cases were identified among spray painters.[273] Cases of peripheral neuropathy were also found in furniture finishers exposed to MnBK and in workers employed in a dewaxing unit in a refinery, where the exposure was reported to be to MEK.

The toxic sensorimotor peripheral neuropathy caused by MnBK exposure is very similar to that caused by other neurotoxic substances such as acrylamide and *n*-hexane. Typically, sensory dysfunctions (touch, pain, temperature, vibration, and position) are the initial changes, affecting the hands and feet. Distal sensory neuropathy can be the only finding in some affected persons; in more severe cases motor impairment (muscle weakness, diminished or abolished deep tendon reflexes) in the distal parts of the lower and then the upper extremities becomes manifest. With progression, and in more severe cases, both the sensory and motor deficits may also affect the more proximal segments of the extremities; muscle wasting may be present in severe cases. Electromyographic abnormalities and slowing of nerve conduction velocity can be detected in the vast majority of cases; these electrophysiological abnormalities are useful for early detection, since they most often precede clinical manifestations. The clinical course is protracted, and cessation of toxic exposure does not result in recovery in all cases; progressive dysfunction was observed to occur for several months after exposure had been eliminated.

Animal experiments have demonstrated that exposure to methyl-*n*-butyl ketone (MnBK) results in peripheral neuropathy in all tested species; moreover, mixed exposure to MEK and MnBK (in a 5:1 ratio) resulted in a more rapid development of peripheral neuropathy in rats than exposure to MnBK alone, indicating a potentiating effect of MEK.[274] These experimental data are of importance for human exposure, since mixtures of solvents are often used.

MnBK produces primary axonal degeneration, with marked increase in the number of neurofilaments, reduction of neurotubules, axonal swelling, and secondary thinning of the myelin sheath. Spencer and Schaumberg[275] have identified similar changes in certain tracts of the CNS, the distal regions of long ascending and descending pathways in the spinal cord and medulla oblongata, and preterminal and terminal axons in the gray matter. For this reason, they have proposed central-peripheral distal axonopathy as a more appropriate term for this type of neurotoxic effect. The "dying back" axonal disease therefore seems not to be limited to the peripheral nerves but to be quite widespread in the CNS. Recovery from peripheral neuropathy is slow; it is thought that recovery of similar lesions within the CNS is unlikely to occur and might result in permanent deficit, such as ataxia or spasticity.[275]

The predominant metabolite of MnBK identified by DiVincenzo et al[37] is 2,5-hexanedione. A similar type of giant axonal neuropathy was reproduced in animals exposed to this metabolite. 2,5-Hexanedione is also the main metabolite of *n*-hexane, another solvent with marked similar neurotoxicity. Other metabolites of MnBK are 5-hydroxy-2-hexanone, 2-hexanol and 2,5-hexanediol; all have been shown to produce typical giant axonal neuropathy in experiments on rats.[3] The transformation of MnBK to its toxic metabolites is mediated by the liver mixed-function oxidase system.[37] MEK potentiates the neurotoxicity of MnBK by induction of the microsomal mixed-function enzyme system.

It is generally accepted that 2,5-hexanedione, the gamma-diketone metabolite of MnBK, has the most marked neurotoxic effect of all MnBK metabolites. Another ketone, ethyl-*n*-butyl ketone (EnBK, 3-heptanone) has also been reported to produce typical central-peripheral distal axonopathy in rats. MEK potentiated EnBK neurotoxicity; the excretion of two neurotoxic γ-diketones—2,5-heptanedione and 2,5-hexanedione—was increased.[39]

Technical-grade methyl-heptyl ketone (MHK) was also found to produce toxic neuropathy in rats; the effect was shown to be due to 5-nonanone. Metabolic studies have demonstrated the conversion of 5-nonanone to 2,5-nonanedione, MnBK, and 2,5-hexanedione.[40] Other γ-diketones—2,5-heptanedione and 3,6-octanedione—have also produced neuropathy.[19]

Nephrotoxic (degenerative changes in proximal convoluted tubular cells) and hepatotoxic effects have been detected in experimental exposure of several animal species to the following ketones: isophorone (at 50 ppm), mesityl oxide (at 100 ppm), mesityl isobutyl ketone (at 100 ppm), cyclohexanone (at 190 ppm), and diisobutylketone (at 250 ppm).

Prevention. Appropriate engineering, mainly enclosure and exhaust ventilation, and adequate work practices preventing spillage and vapor generation are essential to maintain exposure to ketones below the exposure limits. Adequate respiratory protection is recommended for situations in which excessive concentrations are possible (maintenance and repair, emergencies, installation of engineering controls, etc.). Appropriate protective clothing is necessary, and skin contact must be avoided.

All ketones are flammable or combustible, and employees should be informed of this risk as well as of the specific health hazards. Warning signs in the work areas and on vessels and special educational programs for employees, especially new employees, are necessary as part of a comprehensive prevention program.

The NIOSH recommends that occupational exposure to ketones be controlled so that the TWA concentration does not exceed the following exposure limits:

MnBK	1 ppm
Isophorone	4 ppm

Mesithyl oxide	10 ppm
Cyclohexanone	25 ppm
Diisobutyl ketone	25 ppm
Methyl isobutyl ketone	50 ppm
Methyl isoamyl ketone	50 ppm
Methyl *n*-amyl ketone	100 ppm
Methyl *n*-propyl ketone	150 ppm
MEK	200 ppm
Acetone	250 ppm

The marked neurotoxicity of at least one member of this group (MnBK), the slow recovery in cases of distal axonal degeneration, and the possibility that irreversible damage may occur, possibly also in the central nervous system, indicate the need for appropriate protection and medical surveillance.[3] The experimental evidence of nephrotoxic and hepatotoxic effects in animal studies and the lack of information on such potential effects in humans are to be taken into consideration in the comprehensive approach to prevention, medical surveillance, and record keeping. Neurophysiological methods—electromyography and nerve conduction velocity measurements—are indicated wherever MnBK, mixtures of MEK and MnBK, or other neurotoxic ketones are used. Liver-function tests and indicators of renal function should be included in the periodic medical examination along with the physical examination and medical history.

ETHERS

Ethers are organic compounds characterized by the presence of a —C—O—C—group. They are volatile liquids, used as solvents and in the chemical industry in the manufacture of a variety of compounds. Some of the halogenated ethers are potent carcinogens (see Halogenated Ethers.) While all ethers have irritant and narcotic properties, dioxane ($O—CH_2—CH_2—O—CH_2—CH_2$) has marked specific toxicity.

Diethylene Dioxide (Dioxane)

Dioxane is a colorless liquid with a boiling temperature of 101.5° C. It has applications as a solvent similar to those indicated for the ethylene glycol ethers; it is also a good solvent for rubber, cellulose acetate and other cellulose derivatives, and polyvinyl polymers. Dioxane has been used in the preparation of histologic slides as a dehydrating agent.

Absorption is mainly through inhalation but also through the skin. Dioxane is slightly narcotic and moderately irritant. The major toxic effect is kidney injury, with acute renal failure due to tubular necrosis; in some cases, renal cortical necrosis was reported. Centrilobular hepatocellular necrosis is also possible. Dioxane was recently tested in an in vitro cell transformation assay and was found to be very active.[276] Dioxane has been shown to be carcinogenic (by oral administration) in rats and guinea pigs.[277]

Prevention. The federal standard for the permissible exposure limit is 100 ppm; because of the high toxicity, the ACGIH recommended 50 ppm. Protective equipment, appropriate work practices, and medical surveillance are similar to those indicated for the ethylene glycol ethers.

Carbon Disulfide

Carbon disulfide (CS_2) is a colorless, very volatile liquid (boiling temperature, 46° C). It is used in the production of viscose rayon and cellophane.[3] Another important application is in the manufacture of carbon tetrachloride. Other uses are in the manufacture of neoprene cement and rubber accelerators, the fumigation of grain, various extraction processes, as a solvent for sulfur, iodine, bromine, phosphorus, and selenium, in paints, varnishes, paint and varnish removers, and in rocket fuel. Absorption is mainly through inhalation; skin absorption has been demonstrated but is practically negligible.

After inhalation at least 40% to 50% of carbon disulfide is retained, while 10% to 30% is exhaled; less than 1% is excreted unchanged in the urine.

Oxidative metabolic transformation of carbon disulfide is mediated by microsomal mixed-function oxidase enzymes.[278] The monoxygenated intermediate is carbonyl sulfide (COS); the end product of this metabolic pathway is CO_2, with generation of atomic sulfur. Atomic sulfur is able to form covalent bonds.

Carbon disulfide is a very volatile liquid, and high airborne vapor concentrations can easily occur; under such circumstances, specific toxic effects on the central nervous system are prominent and may result in severe acute or subacute encephalopathy. The clinical symptoms includes headache, dizziness, fatigue, excitement, depression, memory deficit, indifference, apathy, delusions, hallucinations, suicidal tendencies, delirium, acute mania, and coma. The outcome may be fatal; in less severe cases, incomplete recovery may occur with persistent psychiatric symptoms, indicating irreversible CNS damage. Many such severe cases of carbon disulfide poisoning have occurred in the past, during the second half of the nineteenth century in the rubber industry in France and Germany; as early as 1892 the first cases in the rubber industry were reported from the United States. Acute mania often led to admission to hospitals for the insane. With the rapid development of the viscose rayon industry, cases of carbon disulfide poisoning became more frequent, and Alice Hamilton repeatedly called attention to this health hazard in the rubber and rayon viscose industries.[279,280] In 1938 an extensive survey of the industry was published by the Pennsylvania Department of Labor and Industry.[281] The first exposure standard for carbon disulfide in the United States was adopted in 1941.[282] As late as 1946, cases of carbon disulfide psychosis were reported as still being admitted to state institutions for the mentally ill,[2] often without any mention of carbon disulfide as the etiological agent. Chronic effects of carbon disulfide exposure were recognized later, when the massive overexposures leading to acute psychotic effects had been largely eliminated.

Peripheral neuropathy of the sensorimotor type, initially involving the lower extremities but often also the upper extremities, with distal to proximal progression, can lead in severe forms to marked sensory loss, muscle atrophy, and diminished or abolished deep tendon reflexes. CNS effects can also often be detected in cases of toxic carbon disulfide peripheral neuropathy; fatigue, headache, irritability, somnolence, memory deficit, and changes in personality are the most frequent symptoms.[2,283] Optic neuritis has often been reported. Constriction of visual fields has been found in less severe cases.

Electromyographic changes and reduced nerve conduction velocity have been useful in the early detection of carbon disulfide peripheral neuropathy.[283,284] Behavioral performance tests have been successfully applied for the early detection of CNS impairment.[285]

With the recognition of carbon disulfide peripheral neuropathy, efforts to further reduce the exposure limits were made. As the incidence of carbon disulfide peripheral neuropathy decreased, previously unsuspected cardiovascular effects of long-term carbon disulfide exposure, even at lower levels, became apparent. Initially cerebrovascular changes, with clinical syndromes including pyramidal, extrapyramidal, and pseudobulbar manifestations, were reported with markedly increased incidence and at relatively young ages in workers exposed to carbon disulfide.[286] A significant increase in deaths due to coronary heart disease was documented[287,288] in workers with long-term carbon disulfide exposure at relatively low levels, and this led to the lowering of the TLV to 10 ppm in Finland in 1972.

A higher prevalence of hypertension and higher cholesterol and lipoprotein levels have also been found in workers exposed to carbon disulfide and most probably contribute to the higher incidence of atherosclerotic cerebral, coronary, and renal disease. A high prevalence of retinal microaneurysms was found in Japanese and Yugoslavian workers exposed to carbon disulfide; retinal microangiopathy was more frequent with longer carbon disulfide exposure.[289]

Adverse effects of carbon disulfide exposure on reproductive function and more specifically on spermatogenesis have been reported in exposed workers, with significantly lower sperm counts and more abnormal spermatozoa than in nonexposed subjects.[290] This toxic effect on spermatogenesis was confirmed in experiments on rats, where marked degenerative changes in the seminiferous tubules and degenerative changes in the Leydig cells, with almost complete disappearance of spermatogonia, were found.

Carbon disulfide has a high affinity for nucleophilic groups, such as sulfhydryl, amino, and hydroxy. It binds with amino groups of amino acids and proteins and forms thiocarbamates; these tend to undergo cyclic transformation, and the resulting thiazolidines have been shown to chelate zinc and copper (and possibly other trace metals), essential for the normal function of many important enzymes. The high affinity for sulfhydryl groups can also result in interference with enzymatic activities.

Effects of carbon disulfide on catecholamine metabolism have been reported. The concentration of norepinephrine in the brain decreased in rats exposed to carbon disulfide, while dopamine levels increased in both the brain and the adrenal glands. The possibility that carbon disulfide might interfere with the conversion of dopamine to norepinephrine has been considered; the converting enzyme dopamine-β-hydroxylase contains copper, and the copper-chelating effect of carbon disulfide probably results in its inhibition.[291]

Carbon disulfide interference with vitamin B_6 metabolism has also been considered as a possible mechanism contributing to its neurotoxicity. Carbon disulfide reacts with pyridoxamine in vitro, with formation of a salt of pyridoxamine dithiocarbonic acid.

Carbon disulfide has been shown to produce a loss of cytochrome P-450[292] and to affect liver microsomal enzymes. This effect is thought to be related to the highly reactive sulfur (resulting from the oxidative desulfuration of carbon disulfide), which binds covalently to microsomal proteins.

Carbon disulfide peripheral neuropathy is characterized by axonal degeneration, with multifocal paranodal and internodal areas of swelling, accumulation of neurofilaments, abnormal mitochondria, and eventually thinning and retraction of myelin sheaths.[293]

Such axonal degeneration has been detected also in the central nervous system, mostly in long-fiber tracts. Thus carbon disulfide neuropathy is of the type described as central peripheral distal axonopathy, very similar to those produced by *n*-hexane and methyl-*n*-butyl ketone. Covalent binding of the highly reactive sulfur to enzymes and proteins essential for the normal function of axonal transport is thought to be the mechanism of axonal degeneration leading to carbon disulfide peripheral neuropathy.

Approximately 70% to 90% of absorbed carbon disulfide is metabolized. Several metabolites are excreted in the urine. Among these, thiocarbamide and mercaptothiazolinone have been identified.[294,295]

The urinary metabolites of carbon disulfide have been found to catalyze the iodine-azide reaction (i.e., the reduction of iodine by sodium azide). The speed of the reaction is accelerated in the presence of carbon disulfide metabolites, and this is indicated by the time necessary for the disappearance of the iodine color. A useful biological monitoring test has been developed[296] from these observations; departures from normal are found with exposures exceeding 16 ppm. It has been recommended that workers with an abnormal iodone-azide test reaction at the end of a shift, in whom there is no recovery overnight, should be removed (temporarily) from carbon disulfide exposure.

Prevention. The present federal standard for a permissible level of carbon disulfide exposure is 10 ppm. Prevention of exposure should rely on engineering controls, and mostly on enclosed processes and exhaust ventilation. When unexpected overexposure can occur, appropriate[3] respiratory protection must be available and used. Skin contact should be avoided, and protective equipment should be provided; adequate shower facilities and strict personal hygiene practices are necessary. Worker education on health hazards of carbon disulfide exposure and the importance of adequate work practices and personal hygiene must be part of a comprehensive preventive medicine program. Medical surveillance should encompass neurologic (behavioral and neurophysiological), cardiovascular (electrocardiogram and ophthalmoscopic examination), renal function, and reproductive function assessment. The iodine-azide test is useful for biological monitoring; it is an integrative index of daily exposure.

AROMATIC NITRO- AND AMINO- COMPOUNDS

Aromatic nitro-and amino- compounds make up a large group of substances characterized by the substitution of one or more hydrogen atoms of the benzene ring by the nitro- ($—NO_2$) or amino-($—NH_2$) radicals; some of the compounds have halogens (mainly chlorine and bromine) or alkyl radicals (CH_3, C_2H_5, etc.). Substances of this group have numerous industrial uses in the manufacture of dyes, pharmaceuticals, rubber additives (antioxidants and accelerators), explosives, plastic materials, synthetic resins, insecticides, and fungicides. New industrial uses are continuously found in the chemical synthesis of new products.[2] The physical properties of the aromatic nitro-and amino- compounds influence the dimension of the hazards they may generate. Some are solid, and some are fluids with low volatility; most are readily absorbed through the skin, and dangerous toxic levels can easily be reached in persons thus exposed.

A common toxic effect of most of these compounds is the production of methemoglobin and thus interference with normal oxygen transport to the tissues. This effect is thought to result not through a direct action of the chemical on hemoglobin but through the effect of intermediate metabolic products, such as paraaminophenol, phenylhydroxyl-1-amine, and nitrosobenzene. The microsomal mixed-function oxydases system is directly involved in these metabolic transformations.

Methemoglobin (Met Hgb) results from the oxidation of bivalent Fe^{+2} in hemoglobin to trivalent Fe^{+3}. Methemoglobin is a ferrihemoglobin (Hgb $Fe^{+3}OH$) as opposed to hemoglobin, which is a ferrohemoglobin. Methemoglobin cannot serve in oxygen transport, since oxygen is bound (as —OH) in a strong bond and cannot easily be detached. The transformation of hemoglobin into methemoglobin is reversible; reducing agents, such as methylene blue, favor the reconversion. In humans methemoglobin is normally present in low concentrations, not exceeding 0.5 g/100 ml whole blood. An equilibrium exists between hemoglobin and methemoglobin, the latter being continuously reduced by intracellular mechanisms in which a methemoglobin reductase-diaphorase has a central place.

The production of methemoglobin after exposure to and absorption of nitro- and amino-aromatic compounds results in hypoxia, especially when higher concentrations of Met Hgb (in excess of 20% to 25% of total Hgb) are reached. The most prominent and distinctive symptom is cyanosis (apparent when Met

Hgb exceeds 1.5 g/100 ml); most of the other symptoms and signs are due to the effects of hypoxia on the central nervous and cardiovascular systems. With high levels of methemoglobinemia, coma, arrhythmias, and death may occur. After cessation of exposure, recovery is usually uneventful, taking place in a matter of hours or days, depending on the specific compound. Methemoglobinemia develops more rapidly with aromatic amines, such as aniline, than with nitro- aromatic compounds; with the latter, the reconversion of methemoglobin into hemoglobin is slower (several days).

While the methemoglobin-forming effect is of an acute type, several significant chronic toxic effects have resulted from exposure to some of the members of this group. Liver toxicity, with hepatocellular necrosis, can be prominent, especially for polynitro-aromatic derivatives. Aplastic anemia is another severe effect, sometimes associated with the hepatotoxic effect, especially with trinitrotoluene.

The major nitro- and amino-aromatic compounds are as follows:

Aniline	$C_6H_5NH_2$
Nitrobenzene	$C_6H_5NO_2$
Dinitrobenzene	$C_6H_4(NO_2)_2$
Trinitrobenzene	$C_6H_3(NO_2)_3$
Dinitrotoluene	$C_6H_3\ CH_3\ (NO_2)_2$
Trinitrotoluene	$C_6H_2\ CH_3\ (NO_2)_3$
Nitrophenol	$C_6H_4\ OH\ NO_2$
Dinitrophenol	$C_6H_3\ OH\ (NO_2)_2$
Tetranitromethylaniline (tetryl)	$C_6H_2(NO_2)_3\ N(CH_3)\ NO_2$
Toluylenediamine	$C_6H_3\ CH_3\ (NH_2)_2$
Xylidine	$C_6H_3\ (CH_3)_2\ NH_2$
Phenylenediamine	$C_6H_4(NH_2)_2$
4,4′-Diaminodiphenyl methane (methylene dianiline)	$NH_2(C_4H_4)\ CH_2\ (C_4H_4)NH_2$

Diazo-positive metabolites (DPM) have been proposed as biological indicators of aromatic nitro- and amino- compound absorption, including that of trinitrotoluene.[297]

Nitrobenzene

Nitrobenzene, easily absorbed through the skin and the respiratory route, is known to have resulted in numerous cases of industrial poisoning. Its toxicity is higher than that of aniline, and liver and kidney damage are not unusual, although most often these are transitory. Anemia of moderate degree and Heinz bodies in the red blood cells may also be found.

Dinitrobenzene

Dinitrobenzene, especially the meta- isomer, is more toxic than both aniline and nitrobenzene. Liver injury, sometimes severe, may even result in hepatocellular necrosis.

Dinitrotoluene

Dinitrotoluene is another compound that may produce toxic hepatitis.

Trinitrotoluene

Trinitrotoluene (TNT) has produced thousands of cases of industrial poisoning. The first reported cases occurred during World War I, and several hundred fatalities were reported from the ammunition industry in Great Britain and the United States. During World War II, there were another several hundred cases and a smaller number of fatalities in both countries.[2]

Absorption takes place through the skin and also through the respiratory and gastrointestinal routes.

Functional disturbances of the gastrointestinal, central nervous, and cardiovascular systems, and skin irritation or eczematous lesions may precede the development and clinical manifestations of toxic liver injury or aplastic anemia. Abdominal pain, loss of appetite, nausea, and hepatomegaly may be the first indications of toxic hepatitis. Clinically recognizable jaundice can be preceded by moderate elevations in bilirubin levels and a decrease in total plasma protein levels.

According to available records, toxic hepatitis developed in approximately 1 of 500 workers exposed, but the fatality rate was around 30% and higher in some reported series. High urinary coproporphyrin levels are a feature of TNT-induced toxic hepatitis. Acute liver failure may develop rapidly and may be fatal. Massive subacute hepatocellular necrosis has been found in fatal cases. A chronic, protracted course with development of cirrhosis was observed in other cases. Postnecrotic cirrhosis becoming clinically evident as long as 10 years after apparent recovery from TNT-induced acute toxic hepatitis has also been reported.

The number of nonfatal cases of TNT poisoning during World War II is unknown, since only fatalities due to hepatocellular necrosis or to aplastic anemia were reported. It is almost certain that many cases of toxic hepatitis were never diagnosed during exposure, and the number of such cases eventually resulting in chronic liver disease—postnecrotic cirrhosis—is unknown. Acute hemolytic anemia has been reported after TNT exposure of workers with glucose-6-phosphate dehydrogenase deficiency.[298] Early equatorial cataracts were described in workers exposed to TNT.[299,300]

Urinary metabolites of trinitrotoluene are 4-aminodinitrotoluene and 2-aminodinitrotoluene[301]; they can be used for biological monitoring of exposed workers. Complete blood counts, bilirubin, prothrombin, liver enzyme (SGOT, SGPT, etc.) levels, and urinary coproporphyrins have been recommended in the medical surveillance of exposed workers.

Toluylenediamine

Toluylenediamine can produce severe toxic liver damage, with massive hepatic necrosis.

Xylidine

Xylidine has been shown to produce severe toxic hepatitis; postnecrotic cirrhosis has developed in experimental animals.

4,4′-Diaminodiphenylmethane

More than 200 million pounds of 4,4′-diaminodiphenylmethane are manufactured each year in the United States. It is widely used in the production of isocyanates and polyisocyanates,[112] which are the basis for polyurethane foams. Other uses are as an epoxy hardener, as a curing agent for neoprene in the rubber industry, and as a raw material in the production of nylon and polyamideimide resins.

4,4′-Diaminodiphenylmethane was the cause of an epidemic outbreak (84 cases) of toxic hepatitis with jaundice in Epping, England, in 1965 (an episode since known as "Epping jaundice"). The accidental spillage of the chemical from a plastic container and contamination of flour used for bread was the cause of this epidemic.[302] Both the contaminated bread and the pure aromatic amine produced similar lesions in mice.

In 1974 the first industrial outbreak of 13 cases of toxic hepatitis[303] caused by 4,4′-diaminodiphenylmethane (methylene dianiline, MDA) was reported. The aromatic amine had been used as an epoxy resin hardener for the manufacture of insulating material. The pattern of illness was similar to that described for the Epping epidemic, with abrupt onset, epigastric or right upper quadrant pain, fever, and jaundice. The duration of the illness ranged from 1 to 7 weeks. Skin absorption had been important in some of the cases.

Another small outbreak of methylene dianiline poisoning occurred when 6 of approximately 300 men who applied epoxy resins as a surface coat for concrete walls at the construction site of a nuclear power electric generating plant contracted toxic hepatitis 2 days to 2 weeks after starting work. The clinical picture was similar to the cases previously described. Methylene dianiline has been shown to produce hepatocellular necrosis in all animals tested, although there are species differences. Cirrhosis has developed in rats and dogs in several experimental series.[304]

MDA exhibits all the characteristics of a direct or predictable hepatotoxin, such as dose dependency, short latent period, and effect on animal models. Nephrotoxicity has also been demonstrated in animal experiments. In recent years 4,4-diaminodiphenylmethane has been the etiologic agent of an increasing number of cases of contact allergies.[305]

Limited data suggest that workers in the textile, dye, and rubber industries experience a higher incidence of gallbladder and biliary tract cancer than control groups.[3] In view of the very large number of chemicals used, however, direct association with MDA has not been established. Long-term observations on workers uniquely exposed to chemicals of this group are almost nonexistent, and therefore no firm conclusions can be drawn.

In a chronic feeding experiment on rats and mice, MDA was found to produce thyroid carcinoma, hepatocellular carcinoma, lymphomas, and pheochromocytomas. The NIOSH recommended that MDA be considered a potential human carcinogen and that exposures be controlled to the lowest feasible limit.[306] The IARC concluded that there is sufficient evidence for carcinogenic effect of 4,4-methylenedianiline in experimental animals to consider a carcinogenic risk to humans.[307]

Dinitrochlorobenzenes

Dinitrochlorobenzenes are strong skin sensitizers.[2]

Paraphenylenediamine and Paraaminophenol

Paraphenylenediamine and paraaminophenol are dye intermediates and are used mostly in the fur industry. They are potent skin and respiratory sensitizers. Severe occupational asthma is not unusual in exposed workers.[2] Paraphenylenediamine was shown to induce sister chromatid exchanges in ovary cells of Chinese hamsters.[308]

4,4′-Methylene-Bis-Ortho-Chloroaniline

4,4′-Methylene-bis-ortho-chloroaniline (MOCA) is used mainly in the production of solid elastomeric parts, as a curing agent for epoxy resins, and in the manufacture of polyurethane foam. Absorption through inhalation and skin contact is possible. In rats, liver and lung cancer have followed the feeding of MOCA. MOCA is included in the federal standard for carcinogens; all contact must be avoided.

Tetranitromethylaniline (Tetryl)

Tetryl is a yellow solid used in explosives and as a chemical indicator.[2] It can be absorbed through inhalation and skin absorption. It is a potent irritant and sensitizer; allergic dermatitis can be extensive and severe. Anemia with hypoplastic bone marrow has occurred. In animal experiments, hepatotoxic and nephrotoxic effects have been detected.

Prevention and Control. Adequate protective clothing and strict personal hygiene with careful cleaning of the entire body, including hair and scalp, are essential to minimize skin absorption, which is particularly hazardous with this group of substances. Clean work clothes should be supplied at the beginning of every shift. Soiled protective equipment must be immediately discarded. Adequate shower facilities and a mandatory shower at the end of the shift, as well as immediately after accidental spillage, are necessary. Respirators must be available for unexpected accidental overexposure.

Medical surveillance should comprise dermatological examination and hematological, liver, and kidney function evaluation. Workers must be informed of the health hazards and educated and trained to use appropriate work practices and first-aid procedures for emergency situations.

ALIPHATIC AMINES

Aliphatic and alicyclic amines are derivatives of ammonia (NH_3) in which one atom (primary amine) or more hydrogen atoms (secondary or tertiary amines) are substituted by alkyl, alicyclic, or alkanol radicals (ethanolamines). They have a characteristic fishlike odor; most are gases or volatile liquids. They are widely used in industry; one of the most important applications is as "hardeners" (cross-linking agents) and catalysts for epoxy resins. Other uses are in the manufacture of pharmaceutical products, dyes, rubber, pesticides, fungicides, herbicides, emulsifying agents, and corrosion inhibitors.

The amines form strongly alkaline solutions that can be very irritating to the skin and mucosae. Chemical burns of the skin can occur. Skin sensitization and allergic dermatitis have been reported.[2] Some of the amines can produce bronchospasm, and cases of amine asthma have been documented.[2] Corneal lesions may result from accidental contact with liquid amines or solutions of amines.

Prevention. Appropriate engineering controls, protective clothing, and eye protection (goggles), air-supplied respirators when concentrations exceeding the federal standard for exposure limits (from 3 to 10 ppm for various amines) are expected, and training programs for employees are necessary to prevent adverse effects due to exposure to these compounds.

ORGANIC NITROSO-COMPOUNDS

The organic nitroso-compounds comprise nitrosamines and nitrosamides, in which the nitroso-groups (—N=O) are attached to nitrogen atoms

$$O{=}N{-}N\begin{matrix}\diagup R_1 \\ \diagdown R_2\end{matrix}$$

and C-nitroso-compounds in which the nitroso-groups are attached to carbon atoms. Nitrosamines are readily formed by the reaction of secondary amines with nitrous acid (nitrite in an acid medium).

A large number of *N*-nitroso-compounds are known; several examples of dialkyl, heterocyclic, and aryl alkylnitrosamines with marked toxic activity are shown above, together with two *N*-nitrosamides, *N*-nitrosomethyl urea, and *N*-nitro-*N*′nitro-*N*-methyl guanidine. The nitrosamines are more unstable in an alkaline medium, yielding the corresponding dialkanes; they are extensively used in synthetic organic chemistry for alkylating reactions.

Toxicological interest in the *N*-nitroso-compounds was first

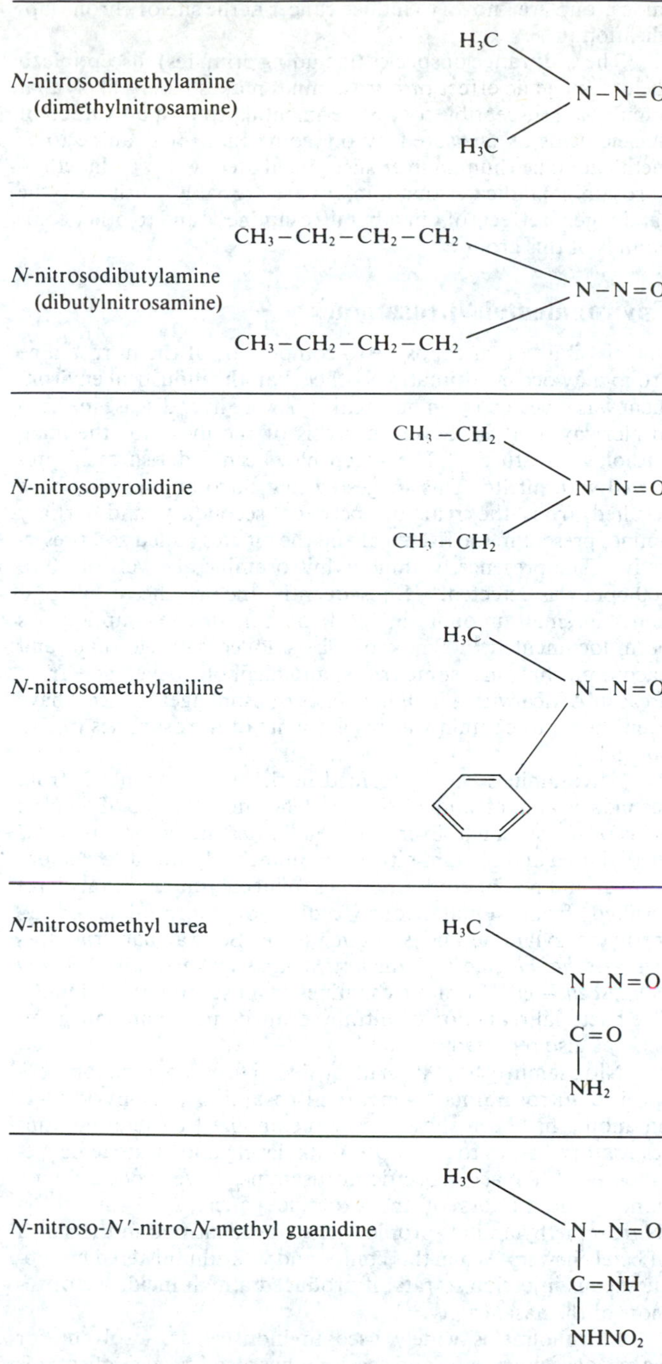

aroused in 1954, when Barnes and Magee[309] reported on the hepatotoxicity of dimethylnitrosamine. This compound had recently been introduced into a laboratory as a solvent, and two cases of clinically overt liver damage were etiologically linked to it. A search of the literature at that time revealed only a single short report of the toxic properties of dimethylnitrosamine (DMN). Hamilton and Hardy had reported in 1949 that the use of DMN in an automobile factory had been followed by illness in some of the exposed workers. Experiments on dogs showed DMN to be capable of producing severe liver injury.

As a solvent, DMN is highly toxic and dangerous to handle, although its volatility is relatively low. The absence of a specific odor or irritant properties may favor the absorption of toxic amounts without any warning; contamination of skin and clothes may pass unnoticed.

Information on the industrial uses of nitrosamines is incomplete. A relatively large patent literature indicates many potential applications. The manufacture of rubber, dyes, lubricating oils, explosives, insecticides and fungicides, the electrical industry, and the industrial applications of hydrazine chemistry appear to be the main uses for nitrosamines.

The use of DMN as an intermediate in the manufacture of 1,1-dimethylhydrazine is well known. *N*-nitrosodiphenylamine is used in the rubber industry as a vulcanizing retarder, and dinitrosopentamethylene-tetramine is used as a blowing agent in the production of microcellular rubber.

Experiments conducted by Barnes and Magee[309] indicated that DMN readily produced severe liver injury in rats, rabbits, mice, guinea pigs, and dogs. Centrilobular and midzonal necrosis, depletion of glycogen and fat deposition, and dilation of sinusoidal spaces were the prominent changes in the acute stage. Hemorrhagic peritoneal exudate and bleeding into the lumen of the gut were striking features; such changes are not encountered in liver injury caused by carbon tetrachloride, phosphorus, or beryllium. Repeated doses were found to result in fibrosis of the liver. These experimental observations pointed to the conclusion that DMN, shown to produce severe liver injury in a variety of experimental animals, had been the etiological agent in the development of cirrhosis of the liver in the two laboratory technicians handling the solvent.

In 1956 Magee and Barnes[310] reported on the hepatocarcinogenicity of DMN. The metabolic degradation of DMN in the liver was shown by Heath[311] to proceed through enzymatic oxidative demethylation; the resulting monomethyl nitrosamine is then decomposed, and diazomethane was thought by Magee to be the alkylating agent with carcinogenic potential.

In 1962 Magee and Farber,[312] by administering ^{14}C DMN to rats, were able to demonstrate the methylation of nucleic acids in the liver, especially at the N7 site of guanidine. Thus an alteration of the genetic information in the hepatocyte was detected and was considered the basis for the carcinogenic effect. This was the first experimental proof of such a molecular alteration of DNA by a carcinogen.

The discovery of the role of drug-metabolizing microsomal enzymes in the biotransformation of DMN into a carcinogen opened an important field of investigation. Similar pathways were found to be effective for another compound of this group, diethyl nitrosamine.[313]

Several consecutive activation reactions were postulated, the first step being the enzymatic C-hydroxylation. The —C hydroxylases are present not only in the microsomal fraction of the liver but also in other organs and tissues. Druckrey and coworkers[313] undertook a systematic and thorough experimental testing program of a variety of *N*-nitroso-compounds. They were able to demonstrate that the acute hepatotoxic effect was also caused by the alkylating intermediate metabolites. In agreement with Magee and Farber,[312] they concluded that the acute toxicity is due to alkylation of proteins and enzymes, while the carcinogenic effect is related to the alkylation of nucleic acids. Several fundamentally important observations were also made:

1. A carcinogenic effect of a single dose of some of these compounds was demonstrated (tumors developed after various latency periods), and the kidney, liver, esophagus, stomach, and CNS were the main organs in which the primary tumors were detected.
2. The site of the primary malignant tumor was found to be, for certain compounds, in a clear relationship with the administered dose.
3. DMN was shown to be a more potent carcinogen than diethylnitrosamine.
4. The transplacental carcinogenicity of DMN was demonstrated; hepatocarcinogenicity was detected in offspring of treated pregnant rats.

5. Di-*n*-butyl-nitrosamine induced hepatocellular carcinoma and cirrhosis of the liver when administered orally in relatively high amounts. With the gradual decrease of the dose, fewer hepatocellular carcinomas and more cancers of the esophagus and the urinary bladder were found. Diamylnitrosamine resulted in hepatocellular carcinoma when given in high doses. Subcutaneous injections resulted in squamous cell and alveolar cell carcinoma of the lung, in addition to relatively few hepatocellular carcinomas. This finding was thought to be important since it indicated that lung cancer can develop not only after inhalation of carcinogens but also as a result of absorption of carcinogens through other routes.

Cyclic *N*-nitroso compounds (*N*-nitroso -pyrrolidine, -morpholine, -carbethoxypyperazine) were also found to produce hepatocellular carcinomas. Heterocyclic nitrosamines (*N*-nitrosoazetidine, *N*-nitrosohexamethyleneimine, *N*-nitrosomorpholine, *N*-nitroso-pyrrolidine, and *N*-nitrosopiperidine) result in characteristic hepatic centrilobular necrosis; they have also been shown to produce a high incidence of tumors of the liver and other organs.[314]

In an experimental model, pancreatic cancer developed in Syrian hamsters after subcutaneous administration of three nitrosamines, including *N*-nitro-2,6-dimethylmorpholine.[315] *Ras*-oncogene activation was investigated in bladder tumors of male rats given *N*-butyl-*N*-(4-hydroxybutyl) nitrosamine. Enhanced expression of *p* 21 was detected in all tumors.[316]

DMN was shown to induce, besides typical centrilobular necrosis, veno-occlusive lesions in the liver in animals followed for longer periods after a high, nearly lethal dose. Prolonged administration[317] of relatively low doses of dimethylnitrosamine (100, 50, and 25 ppm in the diet) resulted in gross, nodular cirrhosis of the liver; with the lower doses, longer survival of the animals was achieved, and several malignant liver-cell-type tumors occurred.

The dialkylnitrosamines, stable compounds, are decomposed by enzymatic action only and result in cell damage after having undergone an enzymatic activation process in organs that have adequate enzymatic systems. The toxic, mutagenic, teratogenic, and carcinogenic effects of nitroso-compounds all depend on this biologic activation by enzymatic reactions. Inhibition of hepatic microsomal enzymatic systems by a protein-deficient diet has been shown to result in a decrease in dimethylnitrosamine toxicity, confirming that the hepatotoxic effect is dependent on microsomal enzymatic activation.

The predominant effect of the dialkylnitrosamines is liver injury, the characteristic lesion being a hemorrhagic type of centrilobular necrosis. This specificity of action is related to the fact that these compounds require metabolic transformation–activation for their toxic effect. The enzymatic systems effective for these metabolic transformations are present in highest amounts in the microsomal fraction of the liver but also in the kidney, lung, and esophagus. Species differences have been documented; these metabolic differences parallel differences in the main site of effects—toxic, carcinogenic, or both.

In contrast to the relative chemical stability of nitrosamines, the nitrosamides show varying degrees of instability. Many of these compounds yield diazoalkanes when treated with alkali, and they are extensively used in the synthetic chemical industry.

The nitrosamides differ in their effects from the nitrosamines; they have a local irritation effect at the site of administration; some have marked local cytopathic action, sometimes resulting in severe tissue necrosis. *N*-methyl-*N*-nitrosomethane causes severe necrotic lesions of the gastric mucosa and also periportal liver necrosis. In addition to their local action, some of the nitrosamides have a radiomimetic effect on organs with rapid cell turnover, with the bone marrow, lymphoid tissue, and small intestine being injured most. Several substances of the nitrosamide group are known to induce cancer at the site of chronic application.

The wide range of species (including primates) susceptible to the carcinogenic effect of nitrosamines makes it very likely that humans are susceptible too. Experimental proof of alkylation of nucleic acids as measured by the conversion of guanine to 7-methylguanine (human liver slices incubated with ^{14}C dimethylnitrosamine) indicates that humans are probably sensitive to the carcinogenic effects of dimethylnitrosamine[318] and to other compounds of this group.

Environmental Nitrosamines

The possibility that exposure to compounds of the nitrosamine group may occur in situations other than the industrial environment was revealed by an outbreak of severe liver disease in sheep in Norway in 1960. Severe necrosis of the liver was the main pathologic feature.[319] The sheep had been fed fish meal preserved with nitrite. This suggested that nitrosamines may have resulted from the reaction between secondary and tertiary amines present in the fish meal and the nitrites added as a preservative. The presence of dimethylnitrosamine at levels of 30 to 100 ppm was detected.[320] Subsequently, the presence of nitrosamines in small amounts in food for human consumption has been documented.[320] Smoked fish, smoked sausage, ham and bacon, mushrooms, some fruits, and alcoholic beverages (from areas in Africa with a high incidence of esophageal cancer) have been shown to contain various amounts of nitrosamines (0.5 to 40 μg/kg).

Nitrosamines can be formed in the human stomach from secondary amines and nitrites.[321] The methylation of nucleic acids of the stomach, liver, and small intestine in rats given ^{14}C methyl urea and sodium nitrite simultaneously was also demonstrated, and malignant liver and esophageal tumors in rats have resulted from simultaneous feeding of morpholine or *N*-methylbenzylamine and sodium nitrite. Several bacterial species—*Escherichia coli, E. dispar, Proteus vulgaris,* and *Serratia marcescens*—can form nitrosamines from secondary amines.[322] The bacterial reduction of nitrate to nitrite in the human stomach was also reported in 1969.[323]

Nitrosamines have been identified in tobacco. One tobacco-specific nitrosamine, 4-(methylnitrosamino)-1-(3-pyridyl)-1-butanone, has been shown to be metabolized by fetal hamster respiratory tissues to form DNA-alkylating and clastogenic metabolites.[324] Tobacco-specific nitrosamines have produced lung tumors and tumors of the exocrine pancreas in rats.[325] *N*-(Nitrosomethylamino) propionitrile was identified in the saliva of betel chewers. When this compound was administered by subcutaneous injection to rats, it produced a high incidence of tumors of the nasal cavity.[326]

Morpholine is widely used in industry as a solvent for waxes, dyes, pigments, and casein; it has also found applications in the rubber industry.

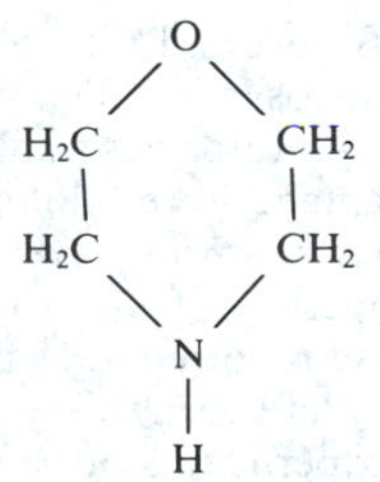

```
         O
       /   \
   H2C       CH2
    |         |
   H2C       CH2
       \   /
         N
         |
         H
```

As an anticorrosive agent and as an emulsifier (after reaction with fatty acids), morpholine is used in the manufacture of cleaning products. Long considered a relatively nontoxic substance, morpholine was also used in the food industry, in the coating of fresh fruit and vegetables (fatty acid salts of morpholine), and for anticorrosive treatment of metals (including those to be used in the food industry). Industrial occupational exposure and household exposure are therefore quite frequent. Absorption of morpholine through the oral route may, in the presence of nitrites from alimentary sources, result in the production of hazardous gastric levels of nitrosamine. In the rubber industry, efforts have been made to replace amino-compounds that can generate *N*-nitrosamines in accelerators with "safe" amino components. Derivatives of the dithiocarbamate and sulfenemide class were synthesized and found to be suitable for industrial application.[327]

The organic *N*-nitroso-compounds are characterized by marked acute liver toxicity; chronic absorption of smaller amounts has been shown to result in cirrhosis in experimental animals. Initial reports of human cases of postnecrotic cirrhosis, however, have not been followed by other reports on human effects. Suitable epidemiological data are not yet available on the real incidence of toxic liver damage, cirrhosis of the liver, hepatocellular carcinoma, and other malignant tumors in industrially exposed populations.

More recently, the presence of nitrosamines in cutting oils was reported.[1] The formation of nitrosamines had been suspected, since nitrites and aliphatic amines are known constituents of some cutting fluids. Concentrations of nitrosamines up to 3% have been found in randomly selected cutting oils; metal machining operators using cutting oils may therefore be significantly exposed to nitrosamines. Semisynthetic cutting oils and the synthetic cutting fluids most often contain amines as a soluble base and nitrites as additives. NIOSH estimated that almost 800,000 persons are occupationally exposed in the manufacture and use of cutting fluids, and issued guidelines for industrial hygiene practices in an effort to minimize skin and respiratory exposure.

Laboratory research conducted over the last 20 years has identified the organic nitroso-compounds as some of the most potent carcinogens, mutagens, and teratogens for a variety of animal species. The possibility of nitrosamine formation from nitrites (or nitrates) and secondary or tertiary amines in the stomach and the possibility of a similar effect attributable to microorganisms normally present in the gut and frequently in the urinary tract suggest a potential hazard for the population at large.

EPOXY COMPOUNDS

Epoxy compounds are cyclic ethers characterized by the presence of an epoxide ring.

```
     O
    / \
 -C---C-
  |   |
```

These ethers, with an oxygen attached to two adjacent carbons, readily react with amino, hydroxyl, and carboxyl groups and also with inorganic acids to form relatively stable compounds. The epoxide group is very reactive and can form covalent bonds with biologically important molecules.

Industrial applications have expanded rapidly in the manufacture of epoxy resins, plasticizers, surface-active agents, solvents, etc.

Most epoxy resins are prepared by reacting epichlorhydrin with a polyhydroxy compound, most frequently bisphenol A, in the presence of a curing agent (cross-linking agents—"hardeners," mainly polyamines or anhydrides of polybasic acids, such as phthalic anhydride). Catalysts include polyamides and tertiary amines; diluents such as glycidyl ethers, styrene, styrene oxide or other epoxides are sometimes used to achieve lower viscosity of uncured epoxy resin systems.

Epoxy compounds can adversely affect the skin, the mucosae, the airways, and the lungs; some have hepatotoxic and neurotoxic effects. Most epoxy compounds are very potent irritants (eyes, airways, skin), and they can produce pulmonary edema. Skin lesions can be due to the irritant effect or to sensitization. Respiratory sensitization can also occur. Carcinogenic effects in experimental models have been demonstrated for several epoxy compounds.

Epichlorhydrin

Epichlorhydrin (1-chloro-2,3,-epoxypropane, $CH_2OCH\text{-}CH_2Cl$) is a colorless liquid with a boiling point of 116.4° C. The most important uses are for the manufacture of epoxy resins, surface-active agents, insecticides and other agricultural chemicals, coatings, adhesives, plasticizers, glycidyl ethers, cellulose esters and ethers, paints, varnishes, and lacquers.[2,3]

Absorption through inhalation and skin is of practical importance. Epichlorhydrin is a strong irritant of the eyes, respiratory tract, and skin. Skin contact may result in dermatitis, occasionally with marked erythema and blistering. Skin sensitization with allergic dermatitis has also been reported. Severe systemic effects have been reported in a few cases of human overexposure: these included nausea, vomiting, dyspnea, abdominal pain, hepatomegaly, jaundice, and abnormal liver function tests.

In experimental studies, nephrotoxic effects have been found; an adverse effect on liver mixed-function microsomal enzymes has also been reported.[328] In experiments on rats, epiochlorhydrin was found to significantly decrease the content in cytochrome P-450 of microsomes isolated from the liver, kidney, testes, lung, and small intestine mucosa.[329]

In experimental studies on rats, it was found that the incidence of squamous cell nasal carcinoma was significantly higher than in control animals. A previous experimental study[330] had also indicated a carcinogenic effect of epichlorhydrin. Limited epidemiological data have produced equivocal results. The carcinogenic risk to humans cannot be considered as having been fully assessed because of insufficient follow-up periods and relatively small cohorts. The IARC has concluded that there is sufficient evidence of carcinogenicity in animals but as yet inadequate evidence in humans.[331]

Chromosomal aberrations have been found in exposed workers.[332] Several experimental studies suggest that interference with male reproductive function can result from epichlorhydrin exposure. In rats, epichlorhydrin was found to produce progressive testicular atrophy, reduction of sperm concentration, and an increase in the number of morphologically abnormal spermatozoa.[333] Testicular function was studied in 128 epichlorhydrin-exposed workers in two plants, and the results were compared to those in a control group of 90 chemical plant workers unexposed to agents known to affect spermatogenesis; no significant differences were detected.[334] Epichlorhydrin did not produce teratogenic effects in rats, rabbits,[335] or mice.[336]

Epichlorhydrin is considered a bifunctional alkylating agent; it reacts with nucleophilic molecules by forming covalent bonds; cross-linking bonds may also be formed. These chemical characteristics are believed to be of importance for their carcinogenic, mutagenic, and reproductive effects.

Prevention. The recommended standard[3] for exposure to epichlorhydrin is 2 mg/m^3 (0.5 ppm), with a ceiling of 19 mg/m^3 (5 ppm) not to exceed 15 minutes. In 1978, when data on a potential carcinogenic effect in humans became available, additional emphasis was given to the importance of minimizing occupational exposure to epichlorhydrin by engineering and work-practice controls.

Ethylene Oxide

Ethylene oxide (1,2-epoxyethane, H_2COCH_2), is a colorless gas used in the organic synthesis of ethylene glycol and glycol derivatives, ethanolamines, acrylontrile, polyester fibers, and film and surface-active agents; it has been used as a pesticide fumigant and for sterilization of surgical equipment. Ethylene oxide is highly reactive and potentially explosive; it is relatively stable in aqueous solutions or when diluted with halogenated hydrocarbons or carbon dioxide.

Ethylene oxide is a high-volume production chemical; production capacity in the United States was 6.1 billion pounds a year in 1981. Exposure to ethylene oxide is very limited in chemical plants, where it is produced and used for intermediates, mostly in closed systems. Maintenance and repair work, sampling, loading and unloading, and accidental leaks can generate exposure.

Although only a small proportion of ethylene oxide is used in health care and medical equipment manufacturing industries, and even less for sterilization of equipment in medical care facilities, NIOSH has estimated[337] that more than 75,000 employees in sterilization areas have been exposed; concentrations as high as hundreds of parts per million were found on occasion, mostly in the vicinity of malfunctioning or inadequate equipment.

Absorption occurs through inhalation. Ethylene oxide is a strong irritant, especially in aqueous solutions. Severe dermatitis and even chemical burns, marked eye irritation, and toxic pulmonary edema have occurred with high concentrations. Allergic dermatitis may develop. With high levels of exposure, CNS depressions with drowsiness, headaches, and even loss of consciousness have occurred. A number of cases of sensory motor peripheral neuropathy have recently been reported in personnel performing sterilization with ethylene oxide.[338] Removal from exposure resulted in gradual improvement over several months. The distal axonal degenerative changes have been reproduced in rats exposed to 500 ppm for 13 weeks.[339]

Ethylene oxide has been shown to be mutagenic in several assay systems.[337] Covalent binding to DNA has been demonstrated.[340,341] Chromosomal aberrations and sister chromatid exchange have been found to occur with significantly increased frequency in workers exposed to ethylene oxide[337] at concentrations not exceeding a time-weighted average of 50 ppm (but with occasional excursions to 75 ppm).

Adverse reproductive effects (reduced numbers of pups per litter, fewer implantation sites, and a reduced ratio of fetuses to number of implantation sites) were observed in rats exposed to 100 ppm ethylene oxide. An increased proportion of congenital malformations (mostly skeletal) was also reported. Women hospital employees exposed to ethylene oxide were found to have a higher incidence of miscarriages than a comparison group.[342]

In 1981 the NIOSH recommended that ethylene oxide be regarded in the workplace as a potential carcinogen and that appropriate controls be used to reduce exposure. This recommendation was based on the results of a carcinogenicity assay, clearly indicating that ethylene oxide can produce malignant tumors in experimental animals.[337] In a chronic inhalation study, mononuclear cell leukemias and peritoneal mesotheliomas were found to be significantly increased in ethylene oxide exposed rats; both were dose-related and occurred at concentrations of 33 ppm.

A mortality study of workers in a Swedish ethylene oxide plant[343] showed an increased incidence of total cancer deaths, with leukemia and stomach cancer accounting for most of these excess cancer deaths. Other chemical exposures (including some well-known carcinogens) had also been possible in that plant. An excess of leukemia was also found in another plant in which 50% ethylene oxide and 50% methyl formate were used for sterilization of hospital equipment.[344] The small number of observed deaths and the complex chemical exposures[343] do not allow definitive conclusions regarding the human evidence of ethylene oxide carcinogenicity, although it is entirely consistent with the experimental data. The current (1987) TLV for ethylene oxide is 1 ppm.

Glycidyl Ethers

Glycidyl ethers are characterized by the group:

$$-C-O-CH_2-\overset{\overbrace{\quad O \quad}}{CH-CH_2}$$

Their most important use is for epoxy resins; diglycidyl ether of bisphenol A is one of the basic ingredients used to react with epichlorhydrin.[82] Glycidyl ethers are also used as diluents, to reduce the viscosity of uncured epoxy resins systems. These find applications in protective coatings, bonding materials, reinforced plastics, etc. The NIOSH estimates that about 1 million workers are exposed to epoxy resins; it is difficult to reach an accurate estimate of the number exposed to glycidyl ethers, but it is probably around 100,000 workers.

Glycidyl ethers are irritants for the skin and mucosae; dermatitis and sensitization have been reported. In experimental studies, an adverse effect on spermatogenesis and testicular atrophy have been the result of glycidyl ether exposure of several species (rats, mice, rabbits) to concentrations as low as 2 to 3 ppm. A potent effect on lymphoid tissue, including atrophy of the thymus and of lymph nodes, low white blood cell counts, or bone marrow toxicity have also been reported in rats, rabbits, and dogs. Information on immunosuppressive or myelotoxic effects in humans is not available, and the possibility that such effects have not been detected in the past cannot be excluded. The present federal standard for permissible exposure limits are listed below[112];

Allyl glycidyl ether	5 ppm
n-Butyl glycidyl ether	25 ppm
Diglycidyl ether	0.1 ppm
Isopropyl glycidyl ether	50 ppm
Phenyl glycidyl ether	1 ppm

Relevance to Humans of Carcinogenesis Results from Laboratory Animal Toxicology Studies

James Huff
David P. Rall

Basic and applied research using laboratory animals is fundamental for the discovery of new drugs and other beneficial chemical substances. Likewise, toxicological characterization of chemicals remains essential to the identification of any potential hazards that these agents may impose on public health.

Clinical and epidemiological studies, which frequently involve the observation and evaluation of human experience with exposure to possibly hazardous agents, obviously offer the most direct means of assessing the human health risks associated with such exposures.[1] In the case of chronic diseases such as cancer, however, the long time interval or latency period that often exists between the initial exposure to the hazardous agent of interest and the onset of clinically recognizable disease may mean that there will not yet be sufficient human experience with the agent to determine its full toxicological potential. In other instances an agent may have been present in the human environment long enough for its toxicological effects to be apparent, but lack of adequate historical exposure data on persons whose initial exposures occurred one or more decades in the past may inhibit the use of available epidemiological information in the quantitative estimation of potential health risks.[2-7] As a result, data generated from laboratory experiments will often form the primary basis for the identification and evaluation of possible human health risks.[8-11]

The adequacy of experimental data for identifying potential health risks and, in particular, for estimating their probable magnitude has been the subject of scientific question and debate. Laboratory animals can and do differ from humans in a number of respects that may affect responses to hazardous exposures.[1,12] For example, humans are much larger than the typical experimental animal, have significantly longer life spans, frequently suffer from one or more concomitant diseases, may be subject to an exposure regimen for the agent of interest that is markedly different from that of their laboratory counterpart, may process (i.e., metabolize, store, excrete) that agent in question in a different manner,[13,14] and, as a species, are much more genetically heterogeneous than most experimental animals. Nevertheless, experimental evidence to date certainly suggests that there are more physiologic, biochemical, and metabolic similarities between laboratory animals and humans than there are differences. These similarities increase the probability that results observed in a laboratory setting will predict similar results for humans.[15,16]

Today, for example, ill patients need not fear that they will suffer some unknown toxic side effect from a new drug, because laboratory animals are used as scientifically valid surrogates for humans in the development of new and safe pharmaceuticals. This can be done because of the remarkable similarities among animal species. Considerable basic research has provided the knowledge that the biological processes controlling life at the molecular, cellular, tissue, organ, and system levels hold striking parallels from one mammalian species to another. As Weiss and Laties[17] have elucidated: "Evolution is what saves us from chaos. . . . Differences among various forms of life are much less striking than similarities. Arguments that assert a sharp discontinuity between man and other living creatures in the fundamental mechanisms of behavior are asserting one of biology's least likely possibilities."

Chemicals and Adverse Health Effects. Certain human diseases have been traced to exposure to environmental and occupational chemicals; several select examples follow[10,18]:

- Lung cancer to asbestos,[19-23] arsenic,[24] bischloromethyl ether,[25] aluminum production,[18] iron and steel founding,[18,26] and others
- Liver hemangiosarcoma to vinyl chloride[27]
- Mesothelioma to asbestos[20,28]
- Leukemia to benzene[18,29-33] and chlorambucil[18,34]
- Male sterility to chlordecone (kepone)[35] and dibromochloropropane[36]
- Neurologic disease to chlordecone,[37] methylmercury,[38] lead,[39] methyl-butyl ketone,[40] and *N*-methyl-4-phenyl-1,2,3,6-tetrahydropyridine[41]
- Chronic renal disease to phenacetin and acetaminophen[42]

Control of unnecessary or excessive exposures is a key element of preventive medicine. The evidence that links a chemical to a disease is critical for the regulatory agencies that must make decisions to control chemicals,[43] but it is also important to the physician and the health care worker who need to diagnose a disease that may be caused by a chemical or who may advise a patient to take personal actions to avoid exposure. In essence, preventing human exposure to such hazardous chemicals prevents the associated human diseases.

The key role of the environmental health scientist is to identify chemicals that are toxic so that public health will be protected by subsequent reduction or elimination of exposures to essential chemicals (e.g., vinyl chloride) or by discontinuation of the use of a chemical that may be unnecessary (e.g., colors and dyes) or easily replaced (e.g., fumigants).[44] The apparently ideal and certainly the most convincing manner of establishing effects of a chemical on humans is through the study of proven human disease (that is, the conduct of well-designed epidemiological studies on exposed human populations compared with unexposed or "control" populations).

Epidemiology. Both the prospective and retrospective epidemiological approaches have shortcomings, however, and for several reasons cannot be used to predict or assure safety. Often exposed and unexposed populations or cohorts need to be large, and yet frequently this is not the case; thus the sensitivity (or power) of epidemiological studies is typically weak. Epidemiology alone cannot identify or predict the effects a material will have until after humans have been exposed and perhaps fallen ill, become moribund, or died. Likewise, if exposure has been ubiquitous, it may not be possible to assess the effects of a material because there is no unexposed or adequate control group. Morbidity statistics obtained before extensive use of a relatively new material can sometimes be useful, but when latent periods are variable and usually of long duration, and times of introduction and removal of materials overlap, historical data on chronic effects are typically unsatisfactory. It is usually difficult to determine or to calculate concentration or duration of past human exposures and to identify small changes in common effects that may be important if the population is large. Finally, interactions usually cannot be controlled and multiple exposures are sure to occur. Despite these shortcomings and the observational nature of epidemiology, it appears that reasonable criteria have been developed and accepted for the qualitative establishment of causality in a study[45]; quantitative assessment is a less certain process.[46,47] For negative epidemiological evidence, interpretation and confident validation become even more difficult because proving a study showing no evidence of any association must be approached with extreme care.[48]

Superimposed on the recognized assumptions, strengths, and weaknesses of the epidemiological process is the need for a more dispassionate and disinterested approach.[49] For instance, Peto[49] has characterized the politics of cancer as having been dominated on both sides by exaggeration and self-interest.

Human and Animal Concordance. These comments are not meant to suggest that human epidemiology is not useful and important but only to stress that in the absence of adequate human data primary reliance must be placed on the use of laboratory animals to determine the toxic effects of hazardous chemicals for extrapolation to humans.[1] There is, however, the continuing scientific debate regarding the suitability of laboratory animals as surrogates for humans. Both theoretical consideration and accumulated experience indicate that it is appropriate to evaluate in laboratory animals chemicals to which humans are or will be exposed and to use these experimental results to predict in general terms what is likely to occur in human populations.[50] Essential to this premise is the knowledge, derived from considerable basic research, that biological processes of molecular, cellular, tissue, and organ functions that control life are strikingly similar from one mammalian species to another. Such processes as sodium and potassium transport and ion regulation, energy metabolism, and DNA replication vary little in the aggregate as one moves along the phylogenetic ladder. The classic work on the transmission of neural impulses in the squid axon is directly relevant to humans. Extensive renal function studies in fish, rodents, and dogs set the basis for our current understanding of renal function and the treatment of hypertension in humans. Also, the processes of cell replication and development of cancer are analogous in all mammalian species.

Many scientists who are expert in the care, feeding, and understanding of rodents and their response to carcinogens and noncarcinogens appear reluctant to apply their knowledge to predict what may happen when humans are exposed to these chemicals. This is, perhaps, understandable. Scientists are taught to follow the long-honored process from the initial idea, formulate and propose a hypothesis, then design and execute an experiment or series of experiments that can rigorously test that hypothesis. Only then does the scientist publicly explain to other scientists the nature of the hypothesis and the results of the experiment, usually at specialized meetings or in subject-oriented journals. In projecting the results of carcinogenicity studies from laboratory animals to predict what may logically happen to humans, the scientist might consider that the opportunity to test the "idea" or hypothesis has been denied. The idea or hypothesis is, of course, the prediction that a chemical will or will not produce some estimated probability of adverse effects or cancers in humans given a certain level of exposure for a certain period or interval of time.

The laboratory scientist, accustomed to being able to close the circle from hypothesis, to test, to acceptance or rejection, to new hypothesis generation, is uncomfortable when lawyers, economists, journalists, and politicians take the hypothesis and use it in a system in which the circle cannot be closed and in which the answer often cannot be known with certainty. In fact, in most basic research areas the "circle" is rarely closed; the usual course of events leads to other questions that need answering.

Nonetheless, there are instances in which the circle has been closed—in which, irrespective of the sequence of events, carcinogenicity data are available from laboratory animals and from human exposure. These data coming from the human experience are among the most precious possessed by the biomedical community because the human suffering involved in their acquisition could have been prevented or reduced and because the possibility of further human suffering can be prevented or ameliorated by using these findings in an intelligent and expeditious manner.

Properly studied examples in which laboratory animals and human populations have been exposed to the same carcinogenic chemicals offer an opportunity to answer this important question: Do the biological responses to a particular chemical observed in laboratory animals predict similar responses in humans? The answer can be illustrated best by describing international efforts dealing with chemical carcinogenesis.

Chemicals and Cancer. Since 1971 the International Agency for Research on Cancer (IARC), a part of the World Health Organization (WHO), has been evaluating the epidemiological and experimental evidence of carcinogenicity of chemicals, industrial processes, and occupations. Included in the 53 volumes of the IARC *Monographs on the Evaluation of Carcinogenic Risks to Humans* published through 1991 are evaluations or reevaluations on close to 750 chemicals, groups of chemicals, industrial processes, occupational exposures, or cultural habits.[10,18,51-54] Of these 850 agents, data on humans were available for only about 25% (or approximately 216 agents).[10,51-53,55] The IARC has thus far identified 56 agents recognized and accepted widely as being linked unequivocally to human cancers; these divide logically into five categories (Table 21-1): eight single chemicals, 10 groups (or mixtures) of chemicals, 17 individual or combination pharmaceuticals, 12 industrial processes or occupations, and seven environmental or cultural-life-style risk factors.[10,56,57] Tomatis et al.[10] have identified four other environmental risk factors as causally associated with human cancers—hepatitis B virus, human T-cell leukemia virus, ionizing radiation, and ultraviolet radiation—and another five risk factors for which an association with the occurrence of human cancer has been observed although a causal relation has not been fully established—*Clonorchis sinensis, Schistosomia haematobium, Opisthorchis viverrini,* Epstein-Barr virus, and papillomavirus. Thus a total of 61 agents are known to cause cancer in humans.

All the single-entity or groups of chemicals known to cause cancer in humans (Table 21-1) are also carcinogenic in experimental models; moreover, in each case there is a concordant target organ in both humans and in at least one of the animal species studied.[10,15,18,52,53,55] (Available experimental data on talc containing asbestiform fibers is considered inadequate.)

Pharmaceuticals listed in Table 21-1 have comparative concordance on 14 of the 17: methyl-CCNU (leukemogen in humans) has been evaluated in only one study in rats, where lung is a suspected target organ; for MOPP and treosulfan (both induce leukemia in humans) there are either inadequate data or no data at all. Of the 12 processes or occupations shown in Table 21-1, none have been evaluated properly in whole-animal laboratory experiments. Other than using sentinel animals or catching and examining native stock, the design and conduct of mimic experiments on these processes are not logically or logistically possible. The seven "life-style" agents grouped in Table 21-1 have good complementation among species; however, neither alcoholic beverages nor smokeless tobacco has been studied adequately in experimental animals.

Therefore, of the 56 known human carcinogens, 44 have been or could be studied in long-term experiments on laboratory rodents; the 12 processes cannot. All 39 human carcinogens that have undergone adequate experimental studies have been shown to cause cancer in animals and exhibit concordance for tumor sites.[10,53] Of the five that may appear to show a lack of agreement, three (methyl-CCNU, MOPP, talc with asbestiform fibers) are considered to have been studied inadequately and two (alcoholic beverages and treosulfan) have yet to be evaluated in animals.

Further, the IARC identified an additional 41 chemicals, groups of chemicals, or industrial processes that are *probably* carcinogenic to humans (Table 21-2)[10,18]; 16 have limited evidence of carcinogenicity in humans, whereas the other 25 were placed in this category largely on the basis of sufficient evidence

TABLE 21-1. THE FIVE CATEGORIES OF AGENTS LINKED UNEQUIVOCALLY TO HUMAN CANCERS[a]

▪ SINGLE CHEMICALS

1. 4-Aminobiphenyl
2. Benzene
3. Benzidine
4. Bis(chloromethyl)ether (technical grade)
5. Chloromethyl methyl ether (technical grade)
6. Mustard gas (sulfur mustard)
7. 2-Naphthylamine
8. Vinyl chloride

▪ GROUPS (OR MIXTURES) OF CHEMICALS

1. Arsenic and arsenic compounds[b]
2. Asbestos
3. Chromium (VI) compounds[b]
4. Coal-tars
5. Coal-tar pitches
6. Mineral oils, untreated, and mildly treated
7. Nickel and nickel compounds[b]
8. Shale oils
9. Soots
10. Talc containing asbestiform fibres

▪ INDIVIDUAL OR COMBINATION PHARMACEUTICALS

1. Analgesic mixtures containing phenacetin
2. Azathioprine
3. *N,N*-Bis(2-chloroethyl)-2-naphthylamine (chlornaphazine)
4. 1,4-Butanediol dimethanesulfonate (myleran)
5. Chlorambucil
6. 1-(2-Chloroethyl)-3-(4-methylcyclohexyl)-1-nitrosourea (methyl-CCNU)
7. Ciclosporin
8. Cyclophosphamide
9. Diethylstilbestrol
10. Estrogen-replacement therapy
11. Estrogens, nonsteroidal[b]
12. Estrogens, steroidal[b]
13. Melphalan
14. 8-Methoxypsoralen (methoxsalen) plus UV radiation
15. MOPP[c] and other combined chemotherapeutics including alkylating agents
16. Oral contraceptives, combined[d]
17. Oral contraceptives, sequential[d]
18. Thiotepa
19. Treosulfan

▪ INDUSTRIAL PROCESSES OR OCCUPATIONS[b]

1. Aluminum production
2. Auramine (manufacture of)
3. Boot and shoe manufacture and repair
4. Coal gasification
5. Coke production
6. Furniture/cabinet making
7. Hematite underground mining, with exposure to radon
8. Iron and steel founding
9. Isopropyl alcohol manufacture using the strong-acid process
10. Magenta (manufacture of)
11. Painters (occupational exposure as)
12. Rubber industry

▪ ENVIRONMENTAL AND CULTURAL RISK FACTORS[e]

1. Aflatoxins
2. Alcoholic beverages
3. Betel quid with tobacco
4. Erionite
5. Radon and its decay products
6. Tobacco products, smokeless (chewing tobacco, oral snuff)
7. Tobacco smoke

[a] Adapted from Tomatis et al., 1989; IARC Monographs on the Evaluation of Carcinogenic Risks to Humans, Volumes 1–53, 1972–1991; and IARC Supplement 7, 1987.
[b] The evaluation of carcinogenicity to humans applies to the group of chemicals as a whole and not necessarily to all individual chemicals within the group.
[c] Procarbazine, nitrogen mustard, vincristine, and prednisone.
[d] There is also conclusive evidence that these agents protect against cancer of the ovary and endometrium.
[e] An additional four human carcinogens have been identified by Tomatis et al, 1989: hepatitis B virus, human T-cell leukemia virus, ionizing radiation, and ultraviolet radiation.

from studies in laboratory animals. Another 180 agents have been designated as *possibly* carcinogenic to humans; eight of these had limited evidence in humans (Table 21-2).

Complementary to the IARC effort and in response to the U.S. Congress, the National Toxicology Program (established in 1978) publishes an *Annual Report on Carcinogens*[58] that contains a series of monographs on substances that "are known to be carcinogenic to humans or that may reasonably be anticipated to be carcinogenic." In the fifth *Annual Report,* for example, there were 22 substances, groups of substances, or technological processes designated as being carcinogenic to humans and 140

TABLE 21-2. AGENTS CONSIDERED *PROBABLE* OR *POSSIBLE* CARCINOGENIC RISKS TO HUMANS[a]

▪ *PROBABLE:* THOSE HAVING *LIMITED EVIDENCE OF CARCINOGENICITY* IN HUMANS AND *SUFFICIENT EVIDENCE* IN EXPERIMENTAL ANIMALS

1. Acrylonitrile
2. Androgenic (anabolic) steroids (testosterone)
3. Beryllium and beryllium compounds[b]
4. Bischloroethyl nitrosourea (BCNU)
5. Cadmium and cadmium compounds[b]
6. Chloramphenicol (inadequate in animals)
7. p-Chloro-o-toluidine and its strong-acid salts
8. Creosotes[b]
9. Diesel engine exhaust[b]
10. Diethyl sulfate
11. Ethylene oxide
12. Formaldehyde
13. Nitrogen mustard
14. Phenacetin
15. Polychlorinated biphenyls[b]
16. Silica, crystalline

▪ *PROBABLE:* THOSE HAVING *SUFFICIENT EVIDENCE OF CARCINOGENICITY* IN EXPERIMENTAL ANIMALS[c]

1. Adriamycin
2. Benz[a]anthracene
3. Benzidine-based dyes[b]
4. Benzo[a]pyrene
5. 1-(2-Chloroethyl)-3-cyclohexyl-1-nitrosourea (CCNU)
6. Chlorozotocin
7. Cisplatin
8. Dibenz[a,h]anthracene
9. Dimethylcarbamoyl chloride
10. Dimethyl sulfate
11. Epichlorohydrin
12. Ethylene dibromide
13. *N*-Ethyl-*N*-nitrosourea
14. 5-Methoxypsoralen
15. 4,4′-Methylene bis (2-chloroaniline) (MOCA)
16. *N*-Methyl-*N*′-nitro-*N*-nitrosoguanidine (MNNG)
17. *N*-Methyl-*N*-nitrosourea
18. *N*-Nitrosodiethylamine
19. *N*-Nitrosodimethylamine
20. Procarbazine hydrochloride
21. Propylene oxide
22. Styrene oxide
23. Tris(1-aziridinyl)phosphine sulfide (thiotepa)
24. Tris(2,3-dibromopropyl phosphate)
25. Vinyl bromide

▪ *POSSIBLE:* THOSE HAVING *LIMITED EVIDENCE OF CARCINOGENICITY* IN HUMANS[d]

1. Carpentry and joinery[e]
2. Chlorophenols[b]
3. Chlorophenoxy herbicides[b]
4. Dimethylformamide
5. Rock wool
6. Slag wool
7. Textile manufacturing industry[c]

[a] Adapted from Tomatis et al., 1989; IARC Monographs on the Evaluation of Carcinogenic Risks to Humans, Volumes 1–53, 1972–1991; and IARC Supplement 7, 1987.
[b] The evaluation of carcinogenicity to humans applies to the group of chemicals as a whole and not necessarily to all individual chemicals within the group.
[c] Evidence in humans considered inadequate or absent.
[d] These eight agents exhibit *limited* or *inadequate* evidence in experimental animals.
[e] Occupation or manufacturing process.

that may reasonably be anticipated as being carcinogenic to humans.[58] (A summary copy may be obtained from the National Toxicology Program, P.O. Box 12233, Research Triangle Park, NC 27709, U.S.A.)

Chemical Carcinogenesis. Clearly, the accumulated experience in the field of carcinogenesis supports the concept that cancer development is a multistep process and that multiple genetic changes are required before a normal cell becomes fully neoplastic.[59,60] Likewise, studies of human tumors suggest that the multistep paradigm, together with similar genetic events, is involved in the development of cancer in humans and that the carcinogenic process is virtually indistinguishable among mammals (e.g., laboratory rodents and humans). The foregoing, plus the knowledge that all chemicals known to induce cancer in humans that have been studied under adequate experimental protocols also cause cancer in laboratory animals, leads most prudent investigators to the persuasive speculation that the obverse would similarly hold true: chemicals shown unequivocally to induce cancer in laboratory animals should be considered capable of causing cancer in humans. Nonetheless, this biologic conundrum of scientific debate will surely continue.

Yet, as more and more advancements are made in molecular carcinogenesis, the mechanisms of cancer induction within the mammalian domain will allow us to shed more light on the major objectives of using animals as predictive surrogates for humans. In basic cellular functions, *ras* genes are likely to play a fundamental role based on their high degree of conservation throughout eukaryotic evolution; using the H-*ras* gene as a particular example, the human and rat protein sequence is identical.[61]

These proto-oncogenes are cellular genes that are expressed during normal growth and development processes. These proto-oncogenes can be activated to become cancer-causing oncogenes by point mutations or by gross DNA rearrangement (chromosomal translocation or gene amplification).[62] These lesions are especially revealing for chemicals that are apparently nonmutagenic and yet cause point mutations in chemically (furan and furfural) exposed B6C3F1 mice.[63] Distinct oncogene activation in spontaneous versus chemically induced[64,65] and in benign versus malignant neoplasms[64,66,67] greatly enhances the use of molecular events in the risk-assessment process. Moreover, loss of specific regulatory functions (i.e., tumor-suppressor genes) represents an important feature in neoplastic transformation.[68-70] This further permits us to come closer to the public health objective of preventing (or reducing) chemically induced and chemically associated cancers in humans.[71-74]

In addition, a majority of the human carcinogens have been studied as a class for genetic toxicity.[75,76] The IARC group 1 chemicals and groups of chemicals[18,77] were evaluated for genetic toxicity on the basis of their ability to mutate *Salmonella* or induce chromosome aberrations or micronuclei in rodent bone marrow. Results confirmed that hormones, metals, and asbestos fibers, though not well tested, are usually not genotoxic in these two test systems.[76,78] The 21 organic chemicals (Table 21-1; tobacco smoke and smokeless tobacco) were positive in rodent bone marrow and, except for benzene, were positive in *Salmonella* as well.

Moreover, for several chemicals, now recognized and documented as human carcinogens, the evidence was first obtained from experiments in laboratory animals: 4-aminobiphenyl, bis (chloromethyl) ether, diethylstilbestrol, mephalan, 8-methoxypsoralen plus ultraviolet radiation, mustard gas, and vinyl chloride.[1,79,80] With some of these chemicals the first notice of tumor induction in experimental animals indicated that tumors did not occur in the same organs that later appeared to be the targets in humans.[79,81] However, in all cases there is at least one tumor site in common for humans and experimental animals for the recognized human carcinogens.[10]

Suspected Chemical Carcinogens. Because epidemiological data are often absent, public health decisions must continue to be based largely on animal data. Historically, this logical concept has served the public well as preventive medicine. Thus, while we hope that subsequent epidemiological studies on the recognized animal chemical carcinogens do not identify causal associations with human cancer, these chemical carcinogenesis findings in laboratory animals frequently, if not almost always, constitute the primary basis for identifying and predicting potential human health hazards.[1,9,71,72,74] Yet several other chemicals identified first as causing cancer in laboratory animals are beginning to show some associations with human cancers. For instance, 1,3-butadiene, a potent rodent carcinogen,[82-84] appears to be causally associated with the development of lymphatic and hematopoietic cancers in humans.[85,86] In a nested case-control study of the styrene-butadiene rubber industry (*note:* the rubber industry as a whole is considered a human carcinogen[87]), Matanoski et al.[88] found that leukemia cases were associated with exposure specifically to butadiene (odds ratio = 9.4; 95% confidence interval = 2.1-22.9).

Certain other chemicals with strong animal data and limited human evidence (see Table 21-2) seem to be prime candidates for further evaluation as potential human carcinogens: 1,3-butadiene and leukemia (as mentioned above); hair dye use and leukemia/lymphoma,[89,90] drinking water and urinary bladder cancer,[91] sulfuric acid mist and other acid mists and lung cancer,[92] dimethylformamide and testicular cancer,[93-96] ethylene oxide and leukemia,[97-99] ethylene dibromide and lymphoma,[100-101] formaldehyde and lung cancer,[102-108] acrylonitrile and lung cancer[18,109-112] and prostate cancer,[111,113] methylene chloride and liver cancer,[114-116] and 4-chloro-*o*-toluidine and urinary bladder cancer.[117] Others that have varying degrees of positive evidence of an association with human cancers are given in Table 21-2.[10,18,51] As stated by Doll[118,119] the final number of proven occupational carcinogens may eventually be quite large.

Regarding causes of cancer in humans, Doll and Peto[120] argued that the causes of 97% of human cancers can be explainable, with a large proportion (10% to 70%; best estimate, 35%) due to "diet." Using the most relevant and common sites of human cancer, Schmahl et al.[121] estimate that only one third of the cancers (in the Federal Republic of Germany) can be assigned etiologically to exogenous carcinogenic agents or to life-style. These latter authors stress that indirect primary prevention, based on the probable summation of subcarcinogenic effects of single carcinogens identified from animal experiments, may lead to a reduction in carcinogen-induced cancers, even if the effects of a particular carcinogenic compound cannot be determined precisely. Regarding the influence of diet, Schmahl et al.[121] agree with Byers and Graham,[122] who indicate that the relationship between dietary factors and cancer risks has not revealed a single unequivocal conclusion of causality.

Pesticides and Qualitative Risk Evaluation. The use of pesticides evaluated for carcinogenicity in long-term studies in rodents will serve as a means to illustrate the spectrum of results for a large and typical class of chemicals.[123] Of the nearly 400 chemicals so far studied by the National Cancer Institute (the first 200 studies during 1976–1981) and by the National Toxicology Program (the latter 200 chemicals for the years 1982–1991),[9,67,124] 63 are considered to be pesticides.[123] From this group, 26 (41%) were considered positive for carcinogenicity (Table 21-3) in *at least one* of the four experiments performed on rodents (generally male and female Fischer rats and male and female B6C3F1 mice) and 37 (59%) were judged to exhibit no or equivocal evidence of carcinogenicity (Table 21-3).

To place these results in some comparative perspective, one measure of "qualitative potency" could depend on the number of positive responses among the four experiments that are usually performed on each chemical; another empirical value comes from the number and similarity of positive target tissues, organs, and systems. Because all long-term studies on important chemicals are designed and conducted with the highest exposure concentrations that will not markedly jeopardize the well-being of the rodents or diminish their average life span, with the exception of sequela due to carcinogenic responses,[9,125,126] these experiments can be considered as having a generic exposure value of "one," or unit equivalency, and can be treated as comparable regardless of the actual exposure concentrations. Doing this signals 12 chemicals that cause cancers in both species; 6 of these 12 chemicals were carcinogenic in each of the four experiments, whereas the other 6 were carcinogenic in three of four experiments. Three chemicals were each studied twice, with the gavage route of exposure and subsequently with the inhalation route. In all cases the chemicals exhibited carcinogenic responses, regardless of route, albeit the target tissues were different for one and similar for the others: for DBCP the primary site by gavage was the forestomach (in female rats an increase in mammary gland tumors was seen also); by inhalation exposure to DBCP, the target organs were nasal cavities, lung, and tongue.[127] EDB by oral intubation induced neoplasms in the forestomach and at distant sites as well (circulatory system, liver, and lung); lesions observed in the inhalation study included the nasal cavity, lung, circulatory system, and mammary gland.[128] In both feed studies with nitrofen the major target site was the liver in mice. As with most chemicals studied for carcinogenicity, these were nominated and selected because of a priori suggestion that they might be carcinogenic.[9,67] Unfortunately, in the case of pesticides at least (and most other chemicals that are dubbed potentially carcinogenic), the prospective speculation based often on structure-activity-relationships, short-term test results, and toxicology information has not proved to be particularly useful or predictive. These indices are most valuable for classes of chemicals (e.g., benzidine-based dyes, anthraquinones, epoxides, nitrosamines), although minor structural changes in two closely related *p*-phenylenediamine dyes (a methyl versus an ethanol moiety) imparts major differences in carcinogenic responses.[129]

If this qualitative agreement is accepted, the next question concerns quantitative aspects of the broad area of risk assessment. There are at least two aspects to this: (1) What will be (or is) the exposure level in the human population? Clearly, the answers are needed, and fortunately it is usually a straightforward task to obtain current or recent past estimates. Nonetheless, there are significant difficulties in obtaining accurate exposure estimates based on historical reconstruction.[47] (2) What is the quantitative relationship between the amount of a carcinogen that causes cancer in laboratory animals and in the human population? This is particularly difficult. Dose-response data can be easily, if expensively, obtained from metabolic and kinetic experiments on laboratory animals. Except for pharmaceuticals, however, similar data are rare in human populations, but they are of unusual value.

Dose-Response Quantitation. The first systematic attempt to estimate and compare dose-response relationships comes from the U.S. National Academy of Sciences–National Research Council panel report on pest control.[130] For the few carcinogens for which data are available to make comparisons, the total induced incidence in humans and the intensity of exposure are not well documented, and the duration and conditions of exposure in humans and laboratory animals are usually not comparable. Nevertheless, to bring together some of the data and to encourage more adequate comparative studies, the panel reviewed and evaluated the available information for six human carcinogens—aflatoxin, benzidine, chlornaphazine, cigarette smoke, diethylstilbestrol (DES), and vinyl chloride—for which human exposure and induced cancer incidence can be at least roughly estimated, since those carcinogens are already known to affect humans. Of course, this could introduce a bias exaggerating the sensitivity of humans relative to laboratory animal systems. Other factors may introduce an opposite bias. For two carcinogens, DES and vinyl chloride, human observations are for considerably less than a full lifetime, so that the reported incidence may be a serious underestimation of the eventual total. Also, these two compounds and aflatoxin are known as human carcinogens because they are associated with types of cancer that otherwise occur uncommonly in the unexposed population. If these carcinogens also induce more common types of cancer, even at much higher frequency, this could go undetected, again giving rise to an underestimate of their overall carcinogenicity to humans. The limited conclusion reached by the panel follows:

> If the data from the most sensitive published test on animals are used to predict life-time human incidence on a dose per body weight basis, the result seems approximately correct for benzidine, chlornaphazine, and cigarette smoking. For aflatoxin, the predicted human incidence is about ten times greater than estimated from existing epidemiologic studies; for vinyl chloride it is about 500 times higher. For DES, the human incidence predicted from the result of a single dose administered to newborn female mice is about 50 times higher than that estimated from studies of adenocarcinomas in daughters of women given DES during pregnancy. Thus, as a working hypothesis, in the absence of countervailing evidence for the specific agent in question, it appears reasonable to assume that the life-time cancer incidence induced by chronic exposure in man can be approximated by the life-time incidence induced by similar exposure in laboratory animals at the same total dose per body weight. [See Table 21–4.]

Similar results have been reported by Crouch and Wilson.[131] Earlier Meselson and Russell[132] evaluated and compared the mutagenic and carcinogenic potency of 14 chemicals representing a variety of structures; these authors concluded that the carcinogenic potency for humans may be roughly equal to that in rodents, if the carcinogenic potencies are expressed in terms of the average normal life spans. Later comparisons by Piegorsch and Hoel[133] showed a significant correlation between mutagenic and carcinogenic potencies, but the observed scatter was considered too large for the overall result to be predictive. Using mammalian data, Shipp et al.[134] found significantly high correlations between quantitative estimates of risk made from animal data and those made from human data,[134] lending further support for the use of animals for protecting human health.

From data available so far, therefore, it appears that chemicals that are carcinogenic in laboratory animals are likely to be carcinogenic in human populations and that, if appropriate studies can be performed, there is qualitative predictability. Also, there is evidence that there can be a quantitative relationship between the amount of a chemical that is carcinogenic in laboratory animals and that which is carcinogenic in human populations.[134] The standard two-sex, two-species lifetime toxicity study in environmental animals—beginning at weaning, ending at death, usually with mice and rats, using multiple dose levels of the chemical being evaluated—can provide worthwhile information on the kinds of toxic effects caused by the chemical (qualitative toxicity) and the doses or concentrations needed to produce these toxic effects (quantitative toxicity). These long-term experiments are the standard assay to determine whether a chemical can cause cancer and one that gives useful information as to effects on certain organ systems (liver, endocrine systems, etc.).[11,135] These long-term studies are relatively weak for predicting effects on reproductive capacity, prenatal and postnatal growth and development, and certain neurobehavioral functions and on identification of chemicals that damage genetic information transfer (mutagens). Further, these chemical carcinogenesis

TABLE 21-3. LONG-TERM CHEMICAL CARCINOGENICITY RESULTS FOR AGRICHEMICALS IN FOUR SEX-SPECIES EXPERIMENTAL GROUPS STUDIED BY THE NATIONAL CANCER INSTITUTE OR BY THE NATIONAL TOXICOLOGY PROGRAM

Chemical Name	TR No.	Route	Carcinogenicity Results			
			MR	FR	MM	FM
▪ CARCINOGENIC RESPONSE IN AT LEAST 1 OF THE 4 GROUPS						
Aldrin	021	Feed	E	E	P	N
Captan	015	Feed	N	N	P	P
Chloramben	025	Feed	N	N	E	P
Chlordane	008	Feed	N	N	P	P
Chlorobenzilate	075	Feed	E	E	P	P
3-Chloro-2-methylpropene	300	Gav	CE	CE	CE	CE
Chlorothalonil	041	Feed	P	P	N	N
Daminozide	083	Feed	N	P	E	N
1,2-Dibromo-3-chloropropane	028	Gav	P	P	P	P
(DBCP)	206	Inh	P	P	P	P
1,2-Dibromoethane (EDB)	086	Gav	P	P	P	P
	210	Inh	P	P	P	P
1,4-Dichlorobenzene	319	Gav	CE	NE	CE	CE
1,2-Dichloropropane	263	Gav	NE	EE	SE	SE
1,3-Dichloropropene (Telone II)	269	Gav	CE	SE	IS	CE
Dichlorvos	342	Gav	SE	EE	SE	CE
Dicofol	090	Feed	N	N	P	N
Ethylene oxide	326	Inh			CE	CE
Heptachlor	009	Feed	N	E	P	P
Mirex	313	Feed	CE	CE		
Monuron	266	Feed	CE	NE	NE	NE
Nitrofen	184	Feed	N	N	P	P
	026	Feed	IS	P	P	P
Piperonyl sulfoxide	124	Feed	N	N	P	N
Sulfallate	115	Feed	P	P	P	P
Tetrachlorovinphos	033	Feed	N	P	P	P
Toxaphene	037	Feed	E	E	P	P
2,4,6-Trichlorophenol	155	Feed	P	N	P	P
Trifluralin	034	Feed	N	N	N	P
▪ NO DISTINCT CARCINOGENIC RESPONSES IN ANY OF THE GROUPS						
Aldicarb	136	Feed	N	N	N	N
Anilazine	104	Feed	N	N	N	N
Azinphosmethyl	069	Feed	E	N	N	N
Calcium cyanamide	163	Feed	N	N	N	N
2-Chloroethyltrimethylammonium chloride	158	Feed	N	N	N	N
Chloropicrin	065	Gav	IS	IS	N	N
Clonitralid	091	Feed	N	E	IS	N
Coumaphos	096	Feed	N	N	N	N
Diazinon	137	Feed	N	N	N	N
Dichlorvos	010	Feed	N	N	N	N
Dieldrin	021	Feed	N	N	E	N
	022	Feed	N	N		
1,2-Dichlorobenzene	255	Gav	N	N	N	N
Dichlorodiphenyldichloroethane (TDE)	131	Feed	E	N	N	N
Dichlorodiphenyltrichloroethane (DDT)	131	Feed	N	N	N	N
Di(*p*-ethylphenyl) dichloroethane (DDD)	156	Feed	N	N	N	E
Dimethoate	004	Feed	N	N	N	N
Dioxathion	125	Feed	N	N	N	N
Endosulfan	062	Feed	IS	N	IS	N
Endrin	012	Feed	N	N	N	N
Fenthion	103	Feed	N	N	E	N
Fluometuron	195	Feed	N	N	E	N
Lindane	014	Feed	N	N	N	N
Malaoxon	135	Feed	N	N	N	N
Malathion	024	Feed	N	N	N	N
	192	Feed	N	N		
Methoxychlor	035	Feed	N	N	N	N
Methyl parathion	157	Feed	N	N	N	N
Mexacarbate	147	Feed	N	N	N	N

TABLE 21-3. LONG-TERM CHEMICAL CARCINOGENICITY RESULTS FOR AGRICHEMICALS IN FOUR SEX-SPECIES EXPERIMENTAL GROUPS STUDIED BY THE NATIONAL CANCER INSTITUTE OR BY THE NATIONAL TOXICOLOGY PROGRAM (Continued)

			Carcinogenicity Results			
Chemical Name	**TR No.**	**Route**	**MR**	**FR**	**MM**	**FM**
Parathion	070	Feed	E	E	N	N
Pentachloronitrobenzene	061	Feed	N	N	N	N
	325	Feed			NE	NE
o-Phenylphenol	301	Skin			NE	NE
Phosphamidon	016	Feed	E	E	N	N
Photodieldrin	017	Feed	N	N	N	N
Picloram	023	Feed	N	E	N	N
Piperonyl butoxide	120	Feed	N	N	N	N
Rotenone	320	Feed	EE	NE	NE	NE
2,3,5,6-Tetrachloro-4-nitroanisole	114	Feed	N	N	N	N
Triphenyltin hydroxide	139	Feed	N	N	N	N

TR = NTP Technical Report; Gav= Gavage; Inh = Inhalation; MR = Male rats; FR = Female rats; MM = Male mice; FM = Female mice
For experiments evaluated by the NCI or the NTP prior to June 1983, results are reported as "positive" [P], "negative" [N], "equivocal" [E], or "inadequate" [IS]. In June 1983 the NTP adopted the use of "categories of evidence": two of the five categories correspond to positive results ["clear evidence" [CE] and "some evidence" [SE] of carcinogenicity], one is for uncertain findings ["equivocal evidence" [EE]], one is for negative studies ["no evidence" [NE]], and one is for studies that cannot be evaluated because of major flaws ["inadequate studies" [IS]].

studies are expensive. One study costs hundreds of thousands of dollars, takes at least 5 years to design, conduct, complete, and evaluate, and requires hundreds of hours of professional time as well as considerable laboratory space and equipment. Realistically, it is not reasonable or logical to evaluate, one by one in this rigorous experimental way, the more than 40,000 to 60,000 chemicals already introduced for commercial use. Current world capacity for such carcinogenesis studies is limited to about 200 new chemicals each year.[136]

Many of these problems would be alleviated if relatively simple short-term tests were available, at least for screening, so that the more extensive whole-animal lifetime studies could be reserved for detailed information on chemicals for which there is already good evidence of toxicity. In vitro test systems, such as those in which the chemical is incubated with specially constructed strains of *Salmonella* involving reverse mutations, are rapid, relatively inexpensive, and about 50% to 90% effective in identifying known carcinogens.[137] Tennant et al.[138] evaluated four widely used in vitro genetic toxicity assays for their ability to predict the carcinogenicity of selected chemicals in rodents. These assays were mutagenesis in *Salmonella* and mouse lymphoma cells and chromosome aberrations and sister chromatid exchanges in Chinese hamster ovary cells. Seventy-three chemicals evaluated in 2-year carcinogenicity studies conducted by the National Cancer Institute and the National Toxicology Program were used in this evaluation. Results from the four in vitro assays did not show significant differences in individual concordance with the rodent carcinogenicity results; the concordance of each assay was approximately 60%. Within the limits of this study there was no evidence of complementarity among the four assays, and no battery of tests constructed from these assays improved substantially on the overall performance of the *Salmonella* assay. The in vitro assays, which represented a range of three cell types and four end points, did show substantial agreement among themselves, indicating that chemicals positive in one in vitro assay tended to be positive in the other in vitro assays. Still further work may be needed to clarify reasons for negative results and for validation of positive data.

TABLE 21-4. PREDICTED HUMAN INCIDENCE OF CANCER BASED ON MOST SENSITIVE ANIMAL SPECIES

Compound	Human Incidence
Benzidine	Same
Chlornaphazine	Same
Cigarette smoke	Same
Alfatoxin B[1]	10 times greater
DES	50 times greater
Vinyl chloride	500 times greater than existing epidemiological studies would suggest

From NAS/NRC Environmental Studies Board, 1975, with permission.[130]

A feature of animal studies that is somewhat controversial and not always understood is the need to employ high concentrations of the agent being evaluated. This need emerges from at least three requirements: (1) that the number of experimental animals must be kept within reasonable limits, (2) that it be possible to estimate relatively low cancer incidences in terms of a human population (e.g., 1 per 100,000), and (3) because these same studies are also designed to characterize long-term toxic effects of chemicals in these animals, the exposure concentrations must be high enough to elicit some toxicity, albeit without unduly compromising health or life span (effects, incidentally, that are rarely associated with neoplasia induction by some indirect mechanism.)[139] For several chemicals the exposure concentrations used in the 2-year studies in rodents are the same or less than those to which humans are exposed (e.g., benzene,[32] 1,3-butadiene,[84] and methylene chloride).[140]

Other studies also reinforce the general concept that laboratory animals and humans respond similarly to chemical exposure. In an experimental analysis of the short-term toxicity of more than 20 cancer chemotherapeutic agents in laboratory animals and humans, it was shown that the toxic doses were highly correlated if expressed on a dose per kilogram of body weight basis and almost identical if expressed as dose per body weight to the two-thirds power.[141] This would suggest that humans may be up to ten times more sensitive than the typical small laboratory animal if the comparison is made on the basis of dose per kilogram of body weight.

Other features might argue for greater human sensitivity. Smaller animals tend to metabolize and excrete foreign organic chemicals more rapidly than do larger mammals; therefore, higher body burdens develop in humans over the years than develop in mice and rats in a 2-year experimental period. For example, the biological half-life of 2,3,7,8-tetrachlorodibenzo-*p*-dioxin in humans is about 7 years whereas in rodents the half-life was much shorter—31 days in rats and 11 days in mice and hamsters—even as a proportion of life span.[142] Because chemically induced cancer is viewed as originating in one or a few cells, it is relevant that a human has hundreds of times more susceptible cells than does a mouse or a rat. A latent period intervenes between the original carcinogenic stimulus and the eventual manifestation of cancer. The cells of small animals "turn over" or replicate themselves at perhaps twice the rate of cells in larger mammals such as humans, and latent periods are longer in large animals. The human life span, however, is about 30 to 35 times that of the mouse or rat, and this may make humans more susceptible.

In summary, it appears likely that the natural or synthetic compounds that are carcinogenic in animal models will likewise be carcinogenic in humans. These models, using adequate laboratory animal experimental results, may also yield estimates of risk. There are, however, numerous constraints on the capacity of animal model systems to serve as the primary or only tools for evaluating potential adverse health effects from the large number of chemicals in commercial use today or the abundance and diversity of complex chemical mixtures.[143] Short-term or medium-term in vivo bioassays[144] and in vitro systems using prokaryotic and eukaryotic cells hold promise as tools for the primary screening of potentially toxic chemicals.

The aim of toxicology has always been the prevention of injury; this remains the guiding principle. The emphasis on prevention and on finding means of choosing less hazardous ways of working with chemicals, including the development of appropriate regulations and controls,[43] should receive even more emphasis in the next decade.[50]

Polychlorinated Biphenyls (PCBs)

Alf Fischbein

Polychlorinated biphenyls (PCBs) are a group of complex synthetic organic chemicals that belong to the class of chlorinated aromatic hydrocarbons. Because of their useful chemical characteristics, such as chemical and thermal stability, they have been widely used in industry. Their excellent dielectric or nonconductor (insulating) properties have rendered them very useful as components of dielectric fluid in transformers, capacitors, and other electrical equipment. Thus PCBs are present in these items in conjunction with other chemicals used for the same purpose, including chlorinated benzenes and epoxy compounds. PCBs have also been used as additives to paints and surface coatings, inks, and adhesives. Other uses include components in fluid in hydraulic systems, such as those present in metal presses, elevators, and forklifts, in heat exchangers, and for microencapsulation of dyes in carbonless copying paper. PCBs have also been used in immersion oil for microscopic analysis. Although most of the principal uses have been in fairly enclosed systems, some uses have made possible more direct entry of these chemicals into the environment.

PCBs have attracted much public health concern; media attention to this group of chemicals is common, especially in connection with accidental spills and the detection of PCBs at toxic waste sites or in waterways and in association with fires involving transformers and other equipment containing PCBs. It is the only group of chemicals in the United States that is specifically controlled by an act of Congress, reflecting the policy of the authorities to control their spread in the environment.[1] Well-documented chronic health effects in humans as a result of environmental or occupational exposures to PCBs have not been reported.[2] However, because of their chemical stability and low degree of biodegradation, they are very persistent in certain sectors of the environment. Their ubiquity in the human environment has resulted in the accumulation of these substances in biota and human tissues.

The manufacturing of PCBs, which began in the 1920s, was discontinued in the United States in 1977, and their use has been very much restricted to enclosed systems. The regulatory framework concerning PCBs, in an attempt to dispose of these chemicals and to minimize the possibility of PCBs reentering the human environment, is extensive in the United States.[3–6] The National Institute for Occupational Safety and Health recommends an occupational exposure limit to all PCBs of 1.0 $\mu g/m^3$, determined as a time-weighted average (TWA) concentration for up to a 10-hour workday, or a 40-hour workweek. The Occupational Safety and Health Administration's permissible occupational exposure limits are 0.5 mg/m^3 for mixtures with 54% chlorine content and 1 mg/m^3 for 42% chlorine mixtures for an 8-hour workday. It is estimated that more than 750 million pounds of PCBs are distributed throughout the United States in more than 900 million items of equipment. Certain occupational groups may, therefore, continue to be at risk of possible exposure, including utility workers handling transformers and capacitors, electricians, appliance service workers, and workers involved in decontaminations after hazardous spills.[7–9]

When the risk to humans of exposure to PCBs is being evaluated, consideration must be given to other chemically related compounds that are present in most environments where PCBs are found.

Recent accidents, especially fires involving transformers containing PCBs and other chlorinated compounds, have focused attention on potential health effects to fire fighters and emergency crew workers. It is essential to note in this context that heating or pyrolysis of materials containing PCBs and chlorinated benzenes can, under some circumstances, generate the chemically related and toxic polychlorinated dibenzofurans (PCDFs) and polychlorinated dibenzodioxins (PCDDs), respectively.[10,11] The degree to which these chemicals are causally related to health effects attributed to situations in which PCBs are present in the exposure source is unclear. It appears, however, that PCDFs, often referred to as "contaminants," have played a major role in causing some of the clinical signs and symptoms reported in connection with two major outbreaks of accidental poisonings in Japan and in Taiwan. In those episodes, to be described in greater detail below, persons were accidentally exposed by ingesting rice oil that had become contaminated with heat exchange fluid initially thought to contain PCBs but subsequently found to contain both PCDFs and other polychlorinated compounds such as polychlorinated quaterphenyls (PCQs). These were also identified in the blood of patients who had consumed the contaminated oil.[12] It is likely that exposure to these chemicals will become of even greater health concern in the future, especially among occupational groups engaged in firefighting and cleanup operations.

Chemistry and General Toxicity. PCBs are produced by the chlorination of biphenyl hydrocarbons at elevated temperatures in the presence of anhydrous chlorine and a catalyst, such as iron or ferric chloride. The chlorination results in a biphenyl nucleus in which multiple chlorine atoms are substituted on either or both aromatic rings. Substitution of ring positions by chlorine ranges from dichloroisomers (two substitutions) to decachloro derivatives (ten substitutions). Commercial PCB mixtures contain several congeners and comprise 209 known individual isomers.

PCBs appear as colorless crystals when isolated in pure form. Most commercial products are liquids. Their solubility in water is low, ranging from 0.007 to 5.9 mg/L for the most commonly occurring isomers. On the other hand, they are soluble in oils and organic solvents.[13]

PCBs were manufactured in the United States under the trade name Aroclor. Most of these commercial mixtures are numerically described according to their chlorine content; for example, Aroclor 1254 and Aroclor 1260 refer to 54% and 60% chlorine content, respectively. The degree of chlorination and specific isomerism have been shown to be related to biological activity and environmental persistence. Likewise, higher chlorinated PCBs tend to be less readily metabolized than PCB mixtures with lower chlorine content. PCBs are lipophilic compounds and accumulate readily in adipose tissue. They have low acute toxicity, and it is the potential risk of chronic or delayed effects that is of public health concern.

Environmental Contamination. During the course of widescale industrial manufacturing of PCBs from the 1920s to the early 1970s, there were ample possibilities for PCBs to enter the human environment, since no restrictions existed regarding either their use or their disposal. It was not until 1966 that PCBs were identified as a major environmental pollutant. This was determined after a survey of wildlife and vegetation in the archipelago of Stockholm, Sweden, had provided evidence of the presence of PCBs in many tissue and plant samples.[14] Similar findings were subsequently made by analysis of samples taken from areas remote from industrial activity, and scientists throughout the world detected PCBs in several locations soon thereafter.[15] There is no evidence suggesting that PCBs are formed in the environment from natural sources; thus their presence in the environment is a reflection of contamination associated with man-made production and long-term industrial use of PCBs. Despite recent regulations concerning their use and disposal, there are still significant reservoirs of PCBs in the environment that constitute a potential source of exposure to humans in the future.

The principal sources of PCBs that contribute to the environmental contamination include industrial and municipal effluents and paper recycling. The latter is related to the use of PCBs in carbonless copy paper and subsequent contamination and migration to food products from packing materials. Incineration of paper and other PCB-containing products under conditions that do not destroy PCBs is another potential source of exposure. Release of PCBs into soil, primarily from disposal sites, is also considered to be a source of potential future exposure; it is uncertain whether such exposure is associated with increased absorption among persons in communities located in the vicinity of waste sites.[16]

Accumulation of PCBs in freshwater biota has been of particular concern, since fish can be a major source of PCB exposure to humans via the food chain. Surveys of various water sources in the United States have revealed that some fish from waters known to have been contaminated with PCBs from industrial wastes in the past exceeded the Food and Drug Administration tolerance level of 2 mg/kg. Such water sources include Lake Michigan, the Fox River in Wisconsin, and the Hudson River in New York State.

Because of the ubiquity of PCBs in the environment and potential magnification through the food chain, PCBs are present in most humans. In the United States, serum PCB levels ranging from 0 to 20 ppb are frequently found among persons of the general population without a history of any specific occupational or environmental source of exposure. Polychlorinated biphenyls have also been detected in human breast milk. Significant correlation between consumption of fish from waters contaminated with PCBs and serum levels of PCBs have been reported.[17]

Experimental Laboratory Studies. The toxicity of PCBs has been evaluated extensively in numerous experimental animal studies. A wide spectrum of toxic effects on the skin, liver, lipid metabolism, and the immune, endocrine and reproductive systems have been reported.[18,19]

One of the principal biochemical effects of PCBs is their ability to induce microsomal enzymes in the liver. Two types of enzyme inducers are known. One group increases cytochrome P-450 content associated with increases in benzo(a)pyrene hydroxylase and ethylmorphine dimethylase activities. A second group of inducers, which include polycyclic hydrocarbons, stimulates the formation of cytochrome P-448 and increases hydroxylation. PCBs induce both cytochrome P-450 and cytochrome P-448 systems in rats.[20] Since several endogenous and exogenous compounds are metabolized by these enzyme systems, an increased metabolism of these compounds can be expected. Thus, PCBs have been shown to affect the metabolism of testosterone, progesterone, and estrogen by their ability to induce liver microsomal enzymes.

The induction of these enzyme systems has the potential for assisting in detoxification of other exogenous substances. However, certain chemicals become more toxic after having undergone metabolic activation, by the P-450 and P-448 systems, to toxic intermediates. The significance of these biochemical effects for human health is unknown.

Dermatological abnormalities are frequent findings in PCB-exposed animals; the pilosebaceous unit of the skin appears to be the most commonly affected organ. Acneiform lesions are considered typical sequelae of exposure to PCBs and related substances in laboratory studies. Enlargement of the meibomian glands and swelling of the upper eyelids are also manifestations associated with experimental animal PCB poisoning.[20]

Certain types of PCB have been found to produce hepatomas and hepatocellular carcinomas in mice and rats.[21,22] Similar to what applies for many other toxic effects, a wide range of differences have been noted between various species in their biological responses to PCBs.[23] In terms of risk assessment, it is therefore a complicated task to determine which animal model is the most appropriate predictor of the carcinogenic risk for man of long-term exposure.

Human Health Effects. Despite the widespread industrial use of PCBs since the 1930s, it was not until 1966 that PCBs were first recognized as a major environmental pollutant, as mentioned above.[14] Reports causing initial concern about adverse effects of excessive exposure to chlorinated naphthalenes, PCBs, and related substances began to occur in the 1930s and 1940s.[24-26] These reports described multiple skin lesions characterized by chloracne and, occasionally, systemic health effects among workers who either manufactured these chemicals or used products containing mixtures of them. In one investigation, reporting effects of contact with an insulation material known as Halowax, the attack rate of skin symptoms ("cable rash") was very high. An association was made between clinical findings and the handling of the insulation material. The material contained a mixture of chlorinated substances, known to be capable of causing the observed skin abnormalities. Halowax contained chlorinated naphthalenes as the principal ingredient, a known cause of chloracne and liver dysfunction, and had a biphenyl compound as a minor ingredient.

In most instances, in which adverse effects have been attributed to exposure to PCBs, concomitant exposure to other halogenated hydrocarbons, including polychlorinated naphthalenes, styrene chloride, and polychlorinated dibenzofurans, has occurred. A report from 1954 described chloracne among workers with exposure to an Aroclor compound in a heat exchanger system. Whether contaminants were present in the heated oil was not reported.[27]

The difficulty in attributing adverse health effects in humans to "pure" exposure to PCBs has been a continuous scientific problem and has complicated the assessment of public health risk and the identification of health effects associated with various types of exposure to PCBs. This is particularly illustrated by the two major epidemic outbreaks of diseases initially thought to be caused by the accidental consumption of food items contaminated by PCBs but later found to have been associated with more complex exposures.[28] This became known only after the analytical methods for the determination of these chemicals had been satisfactorily developed.

Yusho and Yu-cheng. During the summer of 1968 a large number of patients in a certain area of Japan sought medical attention because of a variety of skin symptoms.[29,30] Characteristic signs, diagnosed as chloracne, were present in the majority of affected persons; the clinical hallmarks of chloracne, such as comedones, pustules, and straw-colored cysts, were observed. Other abnormalities noted on the skin and mucous membranes included hyperpigmentation, swelling of the eyelids, eye discharge (caused by hypersecretion of the meibomian glands), and hyperemia of the conjunctiva. Approximately 80% of the first group of patients evaluated manifested skin symptoms. Skin abnormalities, particularly dark brown pigmentation and facial edema, were also noted among newborn infants; they were also found to exhibit low birthweight, pigmented nails, and dental abnormalities.[29-31]

Epidemiological investigation demonstrated that affected persons had consumed food prepared in a certain rice cooking oil, which had been produced or distributed on two consecutive days from a company. It was estimated initially from an analysis of the chlorine contents of the oil that the PCB concentration was approximately 2000 to 3000 ppm. When subsequent, improved analytical methods were applied, it became evident that other chlorinated compounds must have been present in the oil as well, since the PCB concentration was determined to be approximately 1000 ppm in a sample of the original oil. The other chlorinated compounds found in the oil included polychlorinated quaterphenyls (PCQs) and polychlorinated dibenzofurans (PCDFs). Among the latter group of chemicals, more than 40 different isomers were identified.[28]

The clinical findings made in the affected persons in Japan became known as "PCB poisoning" or "yusho" (in Japanese literally "oil disease"). Clinical observations similar to those made in patients with yusho were reported in connection with a second outbreak of intoxication that occurred in Taiwan in 1979. The oil consumed in that incident contained 100 ppm PCBs and 0.1 ppm PCDFs. The clinical syndrome appearing as a result of this episode was named yu-cheng (in Chinese literally "oil disease").[30,31]

In addition to the dermatological abnormalities mentioned above, effects in other organ systems were noted in both epidemics. Abnormal liver function test results were reported in some of the severely affected persons. One of the more prominent clinical-biochemistry findings in patients with both yusho and yu-cheng was elevated serum levels of triglycerides. Neurophysiological examinations revealed predominantly sensory neuropathy, although abnormal test results of measurement of motor nerve conduction velocity have also been reported, particularly in patients with yu-cheng. Nonspecific general symptoms included excessive fatigue, anorexia, and weight loss. Effects on the respiratory and immune systems were also reported.[32]

Transplacental exposure and possibly exposure through breast milk that occurred in connection with the intoxication in Taiwan is likely to have resulted in signs of poisoning among children born to exposed mothers. In addition to skin and mucous membrane abnormalities, developmental effects were also noted.[33] These observations represent an unusual description of effects in offspring associated with this type of exposure.

A carcinogenic effect from the exposure experienced by survivors of the yusho and yu-cheng episodes have not been established with certainty; future epidemiological surveillance of exposed persons after a sufficient latency period is necessary to assess this in detail.

There appears to be a fairly general consensus that the contaminants—i.e., polychlorinated dibenzofurans (PCDFs), polychlorinated quaterphenyls (PCQs), and perhaps others—have been substantial contributing factors in the development of the clinical and biochemical effects observed in yusho and yu-cheng. This has been suggested by the results of chemical analyses of both the oils and tissue samples of various organs from affected persons. Although widely known as "PCB poisonings," the epidemic incidents in Japan and in Taiwan should be considered in the light of the more recent findings, which associate the observed effects with exposure to the mixture of halogenated hydrocarbons.[28,34]

Occupational Exposure to PCBs and Their Contaminants. In contrast to the often severe clinical manifestations noted in patients with yusho and yu-cheng, investigations of occupationally overexposed workers have not demonstrated clinical abnormalities of similar intensity. Except for the early reports mentioned above, describing skin and liver abnormalities in workers with histories of exposure to mixtures of other chlorinated compounds (e.g., chlorinated naphthalenes) and PCBs, overt clinical findings have been rare in more recent investigations.

Abnormal liver function tests and various dermatological abnormalities, including some cases suggestive of chloracne, have been reported.[35] However, the majority of studies have not identified clinically noticeable effects in workers, despite their long-term exposure and their having high serum levels of PCBs, in many instances higher than those found in the patients with either yusho or yu-cheng. Thus, the presence of a high serum concentration of PCBs (i.e., even several times those typically found in the general population) is usually not associated with clinical abnormalities in workers' populations.[36]

Significant correlations between serum levels of PCBs and some of the commonly performed liver function tests have been reported. Although correlations reach statistical significance in many studies, the results of liver function tests have mostly been within the normal range as compared with nonexposed workers.[37-41]

Other clinical-biochemistry parameters, such as plasma triglyceride levels, have also been found to be significantly correlated with serum levels of PCBs in some investigations.[42] It is unclear whether there is a direct cause-effect relationship between serum lipids and PCBs or whether this observation is a consequence of the lipophilic properties of PCBs. Thus a positive association between PCBs and serum lipids could be related to the increased solubility of PCBs in serum with higher lipid concentrations.[43,44]

Other health consequences attributed to PCBs and their contaminants, such as adverse reproductive effects, immunosuppression, respiratory symptoms, neurological abnormalities, and effects on the endocrine system that were described among patients with yusho and yu-cheng, have not been well documented in occupationally exposed subjects. Dose-response relationships have been poorly defined in studies of human populations.

Mortality studies have been conducted on a few occupationally exposed groups. One investigation addressed the mortality among employees potentially exposed to PCBs during a 10-year period in a refinery plant, and excess mortality due to melanoma and cancer of the pancreas was reported. Exposure to several chemicals other than PCBs was present during many years, and the population was small. Association with PCBs is questionable.[45]

Additional studies of workers employed in capacitor manufacturing have likewise provided limited information.[46] The number of deaths is small in general, and meaningful interpretations are often difficult to make. However, excess deaths due to cancer of the digestive system were found in two studies, but the risk with regard to specific organs has not been determined.[47] Deaths due to cancer of the liver, the gallbladder, and the biliary tract are of particular interest in one of the studies.[48] Other investigations have not demonstrated similar mortality patterns and have been inconclusive.[49]

Mortality studies of occupationally exposed populations have not demonstrated conclusive evidence that exposure to PCBs increases the risk of cancer. Further epidemiological surveillance and updating of ongoing investigations are necessary for more definitive evaluation of this matter.[19,50]

Low-level Environmental Exposure. Health effects of levels of exposure commonly encountered in the general environment and associated with serum concentrations of PCBs considered to be within acceptable range (0 to 20 ppb total PCBs) have not been reported. Association between blood pressure and serum levels of PCBs was reported in one study of a community population in the southern United States.[51] Other concomitant exposures and significant associations with blood pressure were also recognized in that study. A follow-up study addressing the issue of an association between blood pressure and exposures experienced by patients with yusho did not find a similar relationship.[52] The information derived from more recent investigations on occupationally exposed populations indicates that clinically observable adverse health effects are rare, even among workers with significantly elevated serum levels of PCBs.

There appears to be a discrepancy between both the acute and chronic effects noted in yusho and yu-cheng patients on the one hand and the general absence of clinical abnormalities among occupationally exposed groups on the other. It appears that extrapolations cannot be made from the unique episodes in the Far East to effects from either occupational or environmental exposures. The complexity of the nature of exposures in any "PCB-related" incident, such as exposure to pyrolytic components of PCB-containing materials, makes it difficult to relate health effects, whether symptoms or clinical signs, to "pure" PCBs.

Because of the awareness of the ubiquitous presence of PCBs in the environment, concern is often expressed by persons or groups about potential adverse health effects of various types of exposure to materials containing PCBs. Typical situations include brief contact with contaminated soil (e.g., from a leaking transformer or similar equipment) or being present in the vicinity of an ongoing accidental fire involving electrical instruments containing dielectric fluids. Evidence of significantly increased absorption of PCBs or adverse clinical effects from these chemicals has rarely been reported to occur under such exposure circumstances; in the future, more attention is likely to be called to the potential for exposure to the chlorinated compounds generated during combustion of materials containing PCBs and related substances.

Disposal and Destruction. The disposal of PCBs is strictly regulated. The Toxic Substances Control Act has prescribed specific regulations for the disposal of PCBs. Among the types of disposal methods approved by the U.S. Environmental Protection Agency are landfill disposal, high-temperature incineration, and chemical dechlorination. The different disposal methods are aimed at the destruction of specific items and wastes containing PCBs. For example, nonliquid PCB-containing materials are most frequently disposed of in landfills, while the disposal of free fluids is not permitted in a landfill unless the fluid contains 500 ppm PCBs prior to dilution. For liquids with PCBs at a concentration of or exceeding 500 ppm, incineration is the preferred method of disposal.[1] To avoid the formation of PCDFs and PCDDs, incineration has to take place at very high temperature, in the range of 1500° C.[53]

Dechlorination and other chemical modification are the techniques most often applied to PCBs in mineral oil. Some of these methods make recycling of the purified mineral oil possible for reuse in transformers. Degradation of PCBs also occurs in nature by bacterial action.[54] Major efforts are currently being made throughout the world to dispose of PCBs and related chemicals, and international coordination appears to be desirable.[55]

Exposure Tests and Clinical Evaluation. Clinical evaluation of persons is usually confined to those with previous employment in environments where there has been a potential for exposure to PCBs and related substances. Maintenance personnel in industrial facilities where transformers and similar electrical equipment are still in use constitute another group frequently undergoing examination.

Several laboratories throughout the United States perform analysis of PCBs in serum. The serum concentration of PCBs is a good indicator of exposure and absorption, which primarily occurs via the lungs or through the skin. As mentioned, elevated serum levels of PCBs are sometimes present in symptom-free persons with a history of excessive exposure. The levels measured in an individual or a group of workers are best evaluated in comparison with those found in nonoccupationally exposed normal controls. There are great variations in laboratory techniques, and the same laboratory should perform the analyses in sequential measurements. Routine measurement of PCDFs and other contaminants is usually not widely performed by clinical biochemistry laboratories; determination of PCDF levels usually must be performed by specialized research laboratories. The identification of these compounds in serum and adipose tissue is likely to be of greater interest in the future. This is because of potential exposure among certain occupational groups, such as fire fighters and workers who are engaged in decontamination in connection with accidental fires involving equipment containing chlorinated substances that frequently accompany PCBs in electrical insulation materials.

Clinical examination should focus on examination of the skin, with attention to the presence of comedones, papules, pustules, and straw-colored cysts consistent with chloracne. The location of acne lesions associated with chlorinated substances differs from that seen in acne vulgaris (youth acne), but the diagnosis must often be made by an experienced occupational dermatologist. The occurrence of typical chloracne after occupational exposure to pure or not heated PCBs is rare.

Liver function tests are usually part of a routine medical examination. Despite the nonspecific and insensitive nature of such clinical biochemistry tests (γ-GTP, AST [SGOT], ALT [SGPT], alkaline phosphatase, and bilirubin), they are frequently used both for screening purposes and in the evaluation of individual patients. History of alcohol and drug use should be considered when the results of liver function tests are evaluated. The usefulness of these tests is usually increased when the individual worker serves as his or her own control in serial tests that are performed in relation to certain exposure situations.

Measurements of serum cholesterol and triglyceride levels are useful procedures in general health maintenance and may be of additional significance among persons with a history of significant exposure to PCBs. Fractionation of serum lipids into high- and low-density lipoproteins has also been suggested in evaluation of occupationally exposed groups. It is uncertain whether associations between serum lipids and serum or plasma levels of PCBs are a reflection of the solubility of PCBs in lipids or whether there is a direct cause-effect relationship between these two variables.

Evaluation of the endocrine system and the nervous system (neurophysiological studies) and testing of immune status can hardly be considered part of a routine battery of laboratory tests in the evaluation of PCB-exposed workers and must be performed in accordance with presenting symptoms and the clinical judgment of the individual examiner. Although abnormalities in these organ systems were reported in yusho and yu-cheng, these are usually not associated with a history of occupational or environmental exposure to PCBs.

Polybrominated Biphenyls (PBBs)

Alf Fischbein
J. George Bekesi
Peter Tsang

Polybrominated biphenyls (PBBs), which have a chemical structure similar to that of polychlorinated biphenyls (PCBs), are mixtures of brominated biphenyls produced industrially by perbromination of the biphenyl ring. Their principal use has been as fire retardants in thermoplastic resins, lacquers, and polyurethane foam. Like other halogenated hydrocarbons, PBBs are lipophilic and they are resistant to chemical and metabolic degradation. While there is potential for accumulation of these compounds in biota and along the food chain, the use of PBBs has been relatively limited and worldwide environmental contamination by PBBs similar to that related to PCBs has not occurred. However, a unique accidental exposure situation involving PBBs took place in the state of Michigan in 1974. This unfortunate episode has necessitated studies of a wide spectrum of toxic effects in both exposed animals and humans. Unprecedented longitudinal immunological investigations of exposed populations has provided a basis of biochemical markers of exposure for future epidemiological surveillance.

PBB Exposure in the State of Michigan. Health effects of exposure to PBBs were essentially unknown before a major outbreak of PBB poisoning occurred in the state of Michigan in 1974, when some 1000 kg of a commercial preparation containing PBBs was inadvertently substituted for a dairy cattle feed supplement (i.e., magnesium oxide).[1] The contaminating agent was a mixture of brominated biphenyls consisting primarily of penta-, hexa-, and octabromo biphenyls. It is estimated that the PBB concentration in the contaminated feed supplement was between 4000 and 13,500 ppm. Small amounts of brominated naphthalene and brominated methylfuran were also reported to be present in mixture.[2]

Initially this outbreak was epizootic. It was estimated that cattle on approximately 25 farms had consumed as much as 200 g of PBBs per head. Because of widespread contamination of livestock, the episode subsequently had implications for human health and resulted in extensive investigations of these chemicals and their potential acute and chronic health effects on residents in Michigan.

Adverse effects of PBBs were first described in lactating cows in 1974 and included anorexia, weight loss, decrease in milk production, abnormal hoof growth, hyperkeratosis, alopecia, and severe infections of the joints.[3] In numerous cases, cachexia and death followed within a few months after ingestion of the PBB-containing compound. Subsequently, more than 500 dairy and poultry farms were quarantined during 1974. Some 30,000 head of cattle, 1.5 million chickens, and 5 million eggs died or were destroyed. Despite these quarantine actions, it became evident that exposure to PBBs among the general population of Michigan was widespread. In some persons who had consumed products from their own highly contaminated farms the exposure was especially high, up to 10 g. In a study of postmortem specimens from a series of autopsies from the Grand Rapids area in Michigan, which was considered one of the high-exposure regions, PBBs were detected in 192 of 196 samples 10 years after the accident. The chemicals were primarily distributed in perirenal adipose tissue, adrenals, and thymus.[4] Ninety-six percent of farmers with a history of potentially high exposure had detectable levels of PBBs (i.e., more than 0.5 ppm) in their serum and persons living on or consuming products from quarantined farms had significantly higher PBB levels than those living on nonquarantined farms. Furthermore, it was estimated that the elimination half-time of PBBs in adipose tissue is at least 7.8 years and that PBBs are likely to persist in tissues of contaminated persons throughout their lifetime.[5,6]

Animal Experimental Data. Early toxicological data derived from animal experiments indicated that PBBs are fat-soluble substances and that they are stored in the thymus, liver, brain, and adipose tissues, where they persist for long periods. Polybrominated biphenyls have also been shown to pass through the placenta and are excreted in milk.[7] A wide spectrum of toxic effects on the liver, thyroid, thymus, and lymph nodes were described; these included intrahepatic bile duct hyperplasia, thyroid gland hyperplasia, and the induction of hypocellular lymph nodes with a depleted T-cell–dependent area.[8] Significant thymic atrophy and chronic injury to the lymphatic tissues were also described as components of the "toxic PBB syndrome."

A tumor-promoting property has also been reported for PBBs. They were found to induce hepatocellular carcinomas in rats[9] and tracheal papillomas in hamsters.[10] The mechanism of their tumor-promoting capacity remains obscure. According to one theory, PBBs may inhibit cell-to-cell communications, either directly or indirectly, through necrosis-induced compensatory hyperplasia.[11] Iron may cause a marked synergistic increase in their carcinogenicity,[12] whereas vitamin A may have some inhibitory effect.[13] Moreover, PBBs have been demonstrated to induce DNA synthesis as well as expression of cytochrome P-450 genes in the small intestinal mucosa of rats.[14]

Health Effects. Concomitant with the rapid generation of animal toxicological data concerning PBBs, investigations about potential health effects were undertaken. According to one study, a high prevalence of clinical symptoms was reported in Michigan dairy farmers and members of their families. Four major categories of symptoms were recognized: neurological, musculoskeletal, dermatological, and gastrointestinal. The neurological symptoms were the most prominent and included headaches, dizziness, irritability, decreased capacity for physical and intellectual work, and memory impairment. The musculoskeletal symptoms consisted of arthritis-like abnormalities with pain and swelling of joints, joint deformity in some cases, and various degrees of impaired movement. Knees and ankles were mostly affected. Affected individuals often reported multiple symptoms from several organ systems. The neurological and musculoskeletal symptoms, however, were the most prevalent. Thus the presence of a "human toxic PBB syndrome" was suggested.[15]

PBB-Induced Immune Dysfunction. The clinical studies were accompanied by investigations of the potential immunotoxic effects by PBBs in Michigan dairy farmers and other residents in the state. The interest in studying the immunobiological aspects of PBB exposure was stimulated by the observed effects of PBBs on the thymus and lymphoid tissues in affected cattle and in animal experiments. That the immune system was a potential target organ for PBB-related toxicity was also suggested by the observations of a higher concentration of the most abundant hexa-isomers (HBB) on the surface membrane of white blood cells of Michigan dairy farm residents as compared to erythrocytes and plasma components.[16]

Initial studies[17,18] included 332 adult dairy farmers from Michigan, 156 persons from the general population of the state, and 29 chemical plant workers who had been engaged in the manufacture of PBBs. Significant deviation from normal in both percentage and absolute number of T lymphocytes was observed in the PBB-exposed farmers and chemical workers with a reduction of T cells and an increase in null cells (i.e., lymphocytes without detectable surface markers). In contrast, the markers for monocytes, determined by peroxidase staining or latex ingestion, did not differ from the controls.

However, both direct occupational and indirect exposure to PBBs resulted in various degrees of abnormalities in cell-mediated immunity (CMI) according to our own observations. In vivo CMI was measured by the delayed cutaneous hypersensitivity response to PPD, mumps, *Candida*, Varidase, and dermatophytin. Whereas 43 of 46 tested persons of a control group responded to at least one recall antigen, 18% of the Michigan dairy farmers were completely anergic to each of the recall antigens. The functional integrity of peripheral blood lymphocytes of PBB-exposed persons was also assessed by evaluation of lymphoblastogenesis with T cell mitogen (phytohemagglutinin, PHA), T cell-dependent B cell mitogen (pokeweed mitogen, PWM), and T cell–independent B cell antigen (SAC, streptococcus aureus). Marked decreases were observed in lymphocyte responses to T cell–specific mitogens as well as in the proliferative T lymphocyte responses in the mixed lymphocyte culture reaction. Although the number of B lymphocytes was well preserved among the exposed persons, a functional anomaly reflected by a decreased response to the B cell mitogen was observed. The latter effect could represent either a defect in the B cell per se or some alteration in the ratio between helper T cells and the suppressor T cell subpopulation.

Effects on the humoral immune system have also been observed and associated with PBB exposure. A dose-response relationship was suggested by the observation that the farm residents with the highest exposure to PBBs exhibited elevated levels of IgG, IgM, and IgA, increased levels of C3, and reduced concentrations of C4. Associations between cellular abnormalities, such as polyclonal hypergammaglobulinemia, reduced T cell population, and dysfunction and increase in number of null cells, and heightened in vivo response to recall antigens as well as neurological and musculoskeletal symptoms was also suggested.

Despite such observations, no apparent relationship between serum or adipose levels of PBBs and clinical symptoms or immune dysfunction was detected. However, family clustering of the observed abnormalities independent of sex and age was noted, suggesting the importance of the common dietary source rather than genetic predisposition.

An opportunity was given in 1981 and 1983 for long-term follow-up of farm residents originally examined in 1976 and a control group of dairy farmers from another state.[19,20] This made it possible to determine whether the immunological abnormalities originally observed were reversible or persistent. The follow-up examination provided results similar to those obtained in 1976, with high correlations between the two examinations for both T cell and B cell functions ($r = 0.87$ and $r = 0.85$, respectively). In a large number of persons a decreased response to T cell mitogen was accompanied by a corresponding decrease in the number of T lymphocytes.

The persistence of immunological abnormalities and the long half-life of PBBs in human tissues warrant long-term epidemiological surveillance of the exposed populations. A carcinogenic effect of PBBs in humans has not been demonstrated conclusively; it must be recognized, however, that the observation period from the time of initial exposure is relatively short for any conclusive evidence to have been obtained, if the latency period for PBB-related carcinogenic effects follows the pattern that is characteristic for many occupational and environmental exposures. Future epidemiological surveillance is necessary.

There are also indications that PBBs are transmitted to nursing infants via mother's milk.[21] A recent investigation of 285 serum samples from 4-year-old children in Michigan demonstrated that PBBs were detected in 13% to 21% of the samples.[22] Fetal toxicity has been shown to accompany maternal toxicity in experimental animals. Observed effects have included increased hepatic weight, decreased body weight gain during gestation, and delayed ossification.[23] Lower survival rates from birth to weaning and increased mortality rate after 2 years, including the development of hepatocellular carcinomas, have also been reported in offspring of rats fed PBBs during pregnancy.[24]

Evaluation of PBB-related effects in developing children have not yet been performed on a large-scale basis, but this matter also requires future epidemiological surveillance.

REFERENCES

Organic Compounds

1. Browning E: Toxicity and Metabolism of Industrial Solvents. Amsterdam: Elsevier, 1965
2. Finkel AJ: Hamilton and Hardy's Industrial Toxicology, 4 edt. Boston: John Wright, 1983
3. U.S. Department of Health, Education, and Welfare, Public Health Service, CDC, NIOSH: Criteria for a Recommended Standard—Occupational Exposure to: Trichloroethylene, 1978; Benzene, 1974; Carbon Tetrachloride, 1976; Carbon Disulfide, 1977; Alkanes (C5-C8), 1977; Refined Petroleum Solvents, 1977; Ketones, 1978; Toluene, 1973; Xylene, 1975; Trichloroethylene, 1978; Chloroform, 1974; Epichlorhydrin, 1976; Ethylene Dichloride (1,2, dichloroethane), 1978 (revised); Ethylene Dichloride (1,2 dichloroethane), 1976; Ethylene Dibromide, 1977; Methyl Alcohol, 1976; Isopropyl Alcohol, 1976; Acrylamide, 1976; Formaldehyde, 1977. Washington, D.C.: Government Printing Office
4. Cavanagh JB: Peripheral neuropathy caused by chemical agents. CRC Crit Rev Toxicol 2:365–417, 1973
5. Spencer PS, Schaumburg HH: A review of acrylamide neurotoxicity. II. Experimental animal neurotoxicity and pathologic mechanisms. Can J Neurol Sci, August 1974, pp 152–169
6. Spencer PS, Schaumburg HH: Experimental neuropathy produced by 2,5-hexanedione—a major metabolite of the neurotoxic industrial solvent methyl n-butyl ketone. J Neurol Neurosurg Psychiatry 38(8):771–775, 1975
7. Borbely F: Erkennung und Behandlung der organischen Losungs-

mittel-vergiftungen. Bern: Medizinischer Verlag Hans Huber, 1947

8. Axelson O, Hane M, Hogstedt C: A case referent study on neuropsychiatric disorders among workers exposed to solvents. Scand J Work Environ Health 2:14–20, 1976
9. Olsen J, Sabroe S: A case-reference study of neuropsychiatric disorders among workers exposed to solvents in the Danish wood and furniture industry. Scand J Soc Med 16:44–49, 1980
10. Mikkelson S: A cohort study of disability pension and death among painters with special regard to disabling presenile dementia as an occupational disease. Scand J Soc Med 16:34–43, 1980
11. Juntunen J, Hupli V, Hernberg S, Luisto M: Neurological picture of organic solvent poisoning in industry: a retrospective clinical study of 37 patients. Int Arch Occup Environ Health 46(3):219–231, 1980
12. Elofsson S-A, Gamberale F, Hindmarsh T, et al: Exposure to organic solvents: a cross-sectional epidemiologic investigation on occupationally exposed car and industrial spray painters with special reference to the nervous system. Scand J Work Environ Health 6:239–273, 1980
13. Escobar A, Aruffo C: Chronic thinner intoxication: clinico-pathologic report of a human case. J Neurol Neurosurg Psychiatry 43(11):986–994, 1980
14. Arlien-Sborg P, Bruhn P, Gyldensted C, Melgaard B: Chronic painters' syndrome: chronic toxic encephalopathy in house painters. Acta Neurol Scand 60(3):149–156, 1979
15. Arlien-Sborg P, Bruhn P, Christensen EL, Gyldensted C, Damgaard M: Chronic painters' disease: a follow-up study of 26 former house painters with occupational toxic encephalopathy. Ugeskr Laeger 143(46):3069–3074, 1981
16. Arlien-Sborg P, Henriksen L, Gade A, Gyldensted C, Paulson OB: Cerebral blood flow in chronic toxic encephalopathy in house painters exposed to organic solvents. Acta Neurol Scand 66(1):34–41, 1982
17. Sasa M, Igarashi S, Miyazaki T, et al: Equilibrium disorders with diffuse brain atrophy in long-term toluene sniffing. Arch Otorhinolaryngol 221(3):163–169, 1978
18. King MD, Day RE, Oliver JS, Lush M, Watson J: Solvent encephalopathy. Br Med J Clin Res 283(6292):663–665, 1981
19. Spencer PS, Schaumberg HH (eds): Experimental and Clinical Neurotoxicology. Baltimore: Williams & Wilkins, 1980
20. Chang YC: Neurotoxic effects of n-hexane on the human central nervous system: evoked potential abnormalities in n-hexane polyneuropathy. J Neurol Neurosurg Psychiatry 50(3):269–74, 1987
21. Yamamura Y: N-hexane polyneuropathy. Folia Psychiatr Neurol Jpn 23:45–57, 1969
22. Herskowitz A, Ishii N, Schaumburg H: N-hexane neuropathy—a syndrome occurring as a result of industrial exposure. N Engl J Med 285:82–85, 1971
23. Wang J-D, Chang Y-C, Kao K-P, Huang C-C, Lin C-C, Yeh W-Y: An outbreak of n-hexane induced polyneuropathy among press proofing workers in Tapai. Am J Ind Med 10(2):111–118, 1986
24. Kurihara K, Kita K, Hattori T, Hirayama K: N-hexane polyneuropathy due to sniffing bond G10: clinical and electron microscope findings. Brain Nerve (Tokyo) 38(11):1011–1017, 1986
25. Hall D MB, Ramsey J, Schwartz MS, Dookun D: Neuropathy in a petrol sniffer. Arch Dis Child 61(9):900–901, 1986
26. Oryshkevich RS, Wilcox R, Jhee WH: Polyneuropathy due to glue exposure: case report and 16-year follow-up. Arch Phys Med Rehabil 67(11):827–828, 1986
27. De Martino C, Malorni W, Amantini MC, Barcellona PS, Frontali N: Effects of respiratory treatment with n-hexane on rat testis morphology. I. A light microscopic study. Exp Mol Pathol 46(2):199–216, 1987
28. Perbellini L, Mozzo P, Brugnone F, Zedde A: Physiologico-mathematical model for studying human exposure to organic solvents: kinetics of blood/tissue n-hexane concentrations and of 2,5-hexanedione in urine. Br J Ind Med 43(11):760–768, 1986
29. Iwata M, Takeuchi Y, Hisanaga N, Ono Y: Changes of n-hexane metabolites in urine of rats exposed to various concentrations of n-hexane and to its mixture with toluene or methyl n-butyl ketone. Int Arch Occup Environ Health 53(1):1–8, 1983
30. Perbellini L, Amantini MC, Brugnone F, Frontali N: Urinary excretion of n-hexane metabolites: a comparative study in rat, rabbit and monkey. Arch Toxicol 50(3–4):203–215, 1982
31. Fedtke N, Bolt HM: Detection of 2,5-hexanedione in the urine of persons not exposed to n-hexane. Int Arch Occup Environ Health 57(2):143–148, 1986
32. Ahonen I, Schimberg RW: 2,5-Hexanedione excretion after occupational exposure to n-hexane. Br J Ind Med 45(2):133–136, 1988
33. Lowry LK: Biological exposure index as a complement to the TLV. J Occup Med 28(8):578–582, 1986
34. Governa M, Calisti R, Coppa G, Tagliavento G, Colombi A, Troni W: Urinary excretion of 2,5-hexanedione and peripheral polyneuropathies in workers exposed to hexane. J Toxic Environ Health 20(3):219–228, 1987
35. Fedtke N, Bolt HM: The relevance of 4,5-dihydroxy-2-hexanone in the excretion kinetics of n-hexane metabolites in rat and man. Arch Toxicol 61(2):131–137, 1987
36. Takeuchi Y, Ono Y, Hisanaga N: An experimental study on the combined effects of n-hexane and toluene on the peripheral nerve of the rat. Br J Ind Med 38(1):14–19, 1981
37. DiVincenzo GD, Kaplan CJ, Dedinas J: Characterization of the metabolites of methyl n-butyl ketone, methyl iso-butyl ketone, methyl ethyl ketone in guinea pigs and their clearance. Toxicol Appl Pharmacol 36:511–522, 1976
38. DeCaprio AP: Molecular mechanisms of diketone neurotoxicity. Chem Biol Interact 54(3):257–270, 1985
39. O'Donoghue JL, Krasavage WJ, DiVincenzo GD, Katz GV: Further studies on ketone neurotoxicity and interactions. Toxicol Appl Pharmacol 72(2):201–209, 1984
40. O'Donoghue JL, Krasavage WJ, DiVincenzo GD, Ziegler PA: Commercial grade methyl heptyl ketone (5-methyl-2-octonone) neurotoxicity: contribution of 5-nonanone. Toxicol Appl Pharmacol 62(6):307–316, 1982
41. Shifman MA, Graham DG, Priest JW, Bouldin TW: The neurotoxicity of 5-nonanone: preliminary report. Toxicol Lett 8(4–5):283–288, 1981
42. Misumi J, Nagano M: Experimental study on the enhancement of the neurotoxicity of methyl n-butyl ketone by non-neurotoxic aliphatic monoketones. Br J Ind Med 42(3):155–161, 1985
43. U.S. Dept. of Health and Human Services, Public Health Service, Centers for Disease Control, National Institute for Occupational Safety and Health: NIOSH Current Intelligence Bulletin 41: 1,3-Butadiene. Washington, D.C.: NIOSH, Feb. 9, 1984
44. Maronpot RR: Ovarian toxicity and carcinogenicity in eight recent national toxicology program studies. Environ Health Perspect 73:125–130, 1987
45. Irons RD, Smith CN, Stillman WS, Shah RS, Steinhagen WH, Leiderman: Macrocytic-megaloblastic anemia in male NIH Swiss mice following repeated exposure to 1,3-butadiene. Toxicol Appl Pharmacol 85(3):450–455, 1986
46. Downs TD, Crane MM, Kim KW: Mortality among workers at a butadiene facility. Am J Ind Med 12(3):311–329, 1987
47. deMeester C: Genotoxic properties of 1,3-butadiene. Mutat Res 195(1–4):273–281, 1988
48. IARC Monographs on the Evaluation of the Carcinogenic Risk of Chemicals to Humans. Vol 39. Some Chemicals Used in Plastics and Elastomers. Lyon, France: International Agency for Research on Cancer, 1986, pp 155–179
49. Dahl AR, Birnbaum LS, Bond JA, Gervasi PG, Henederson RF: The fate of isoprene inhaled by rats: comparison to butadiene. Toxicol Appl Pharmacol 89(2):237–248, 1987
50. Sandmeyer EE: Aromatic hydrocarbons. In Clayton GD, Clayton FE (eds): Patty's Industrial Hygiene and Toxicology, 3 edt rev. Vol. 2B. New York: John Wiley, 1981
51. Toxicological Profile for Benzene. Agency for Toxic Substances and Disease Registry, U.S. Public Health Service, 1989
52. Rushmore T, Snyder R, Kalf G: Covalent binding of benzene and

its metabolites to DNA in rabbit bone marrow mitochondria in vitro. Chem Biol Interact 49(1–2):133–154, 1984

53. Morimoto K, Wolff S: Increase in sister chromatid exchanges and perturbations of cell division kinetics in human lymphocytes by benzene metabolites. Cancer Res 40(4):1189–1193, 1980
54. Greenburg L: Benzol poisoning as an industrial hazard. VII. Results of medical examination and clinical tests made to discover early signs of benzol poisoning in exposed workers. Public Health Rep 41:1526–1539, 1926
55. Greenburg L, Mayers MR, Goldwater L, Smith AR: Benzene (benzol) poisoning in the rotogravure printing industry in New York City. J Ind Hyg Toxicol 21:295–420, 1939
56. Savilahti M: More than 100 cases of benzene poisoning in a shoe factory. Arch Gewerbepathol Gewerbehyg 15:147–157, 1956
57. Cronkite EP, Inoue T, Carsten AL, Miller ME, Bullis JE, Drew RT: Effects of benzene inhalation on murine pluripotent stem cells. J Toxicol Environ Health 9:411–421, 1982
58. Vigliani EC, Saita G: Benzene and leukemia. N Engl J Med 271: 872–876, 1964
59. DeGowin RL: Benzene exposure and aplastic anemia followed by leukemia 15 years later. JAMA 185:748, 1963
60. Vigliani EC: Leukemia associated with benzene exposure. Ann NY Acad Sci 271:143–151, 1976
61. Aksoy M, Erdem S, Dincol G: Types of leukemia in chronic benzene poisoning: a study in thirty-four patients. Acta Haematol 55:65–72, 1976
62. McMichael AJ, Spirtas R, Kupper LL, Gamble JE: Solvent exposure and leukemia among rubber workers: an epidemiologic study. J Occup Med 17:234–239, 1975
63. Arp EW Jr, Wolff PH, Checkoway H: Lymphocytic leukemia and exposures to benzene and other solvents in the rubber industry. J Occup Med 25(8):598–602, 1983
64. Rinsky RA, Young RJ, Smith AB: Leukemia in benzene workers. Am J Ind Med 2(3):217–245, 1981
65. Ishimaru T, Okada H, Tomiyasu T, et al: Occupational factors in the epidemiology of leukemia in Hiroshima and Nagasaki. Am J Epidemiol 93:157–165, 1971
66. Tough IM, Smith PG, Court-Brown WM, Harnden DG: Chromosome studies on workers exposed to atmospheric benzene. Eur J Cancer 6:49–55, 1970
67. Forni A, Cappellini A, Pacifico E, Vigliani EC: Chromosome changes and their evolution in subjects with past exposure to benzene. Arch Environ Health 23:285–391, 1971
68. Styles J, Richardson CR: Cytogenetic effects of benzene: dosimetric studies on rats exposed to benzene vapour. Mutat Res 135(3): 203–209, 1984
69. Tice RR, Vogt TF, Costa DL: Cytogenetic effects of inhaled benzene in murine bone marrow. In Genotoxic Effects of Airborne Agents. Environ Sci Res 25:257–275, 1982
70. Ward CO, Kuna RA, Snyder NK, Alsaker RD, Coate WB, Craig PH: Subchronic inhalation toxicity of benzene in rats and mice. Am J Ind Med 7:457–473, 1985
71. Lignac GEO: Benzene leukemia in humans and in white mice. Krankheitsforsch 9:403–453, 1932
72. Goldstein BD, Snyder CA, Laskin S, et al: Myelogenous leukemia in rodents inhaling benzene. Toxicol Lett 13(3–4):169–173, 1982
73. Snyder CA, Goldstein BD, Sellakumar AR, Albert RE: Evidence for hematotoxicity and tumorigenesis in rats exposed to 100 ppm benzene. Am J Ind Med 5(6):429–434, 1984
74. Maltoni C, Conti B, Cotti G: Benzene: a multipotential carcinogen; results of long-term bioassays performed at the Bologna Institute of Oncology. Am J Ind Med 4(5):589–630, 1983
75. Cronkite EP: Benzene hematotoxicity and leukemogenesis. Blood Cells 12:129–137, 1986
76. NTP: Toxicology and carcinogenesis studies of benzene. Research Triangle Park, NC: National Toxicology Program, 1986
77. Rinsky RA, Alexander B, Smith MD, et al: Benzene and leukemia: an epidemiological risk assessment. N Engl J Med 316:1044–1050, 1987
78. Forni AM, Capellini A, Pacifico E, Vigliani EC: Chromosome changes and their evolution in subjects with past exposure to benzene. Arch Environ Health 23:385–391, 1971
79. Messerschmitt J: Bone-marrow aplasias during pregnancy. Nouv Rev Fr Hematol 12:115–28, 1972
80. EPA (Environmental Protection Agency): Health advisory for benzene. Washington, DC: Office of Drinking Water, 1985
81. Capellini A, Alessio L: The urinary excretion of hippuric acid in workers exposed to toluene. Med Lav 62:196–201, 1971
82. Gerarde HW: Toxicological studies on hydrocarbons. II. A comparative study of the effects of benzene and certain mono-n-alkylbenzenes on hemopoiesis and bone marrow metabolism in rats. AMA Arch Ind Health 13:468–474, 1956
83. King MD, Day RE, Oliver JS, Lush M, Watson JM: Solvent encephalopathy. Br Med J Clin Res 283(6292):663–665, 1981
84. Knox JW, Nelson JR: Permanent encephalopathy from toluene inhalation. N Engl J Med 275:1494–1496, 1966
85. Fornazzari L, Wilkonson DA, Kapur BM, Carlen PL: Cerebellar, cortical and functional impairment in toluene abusers. Acta Neurol Scand 67(6):319–329, 1983
86. Lazar RG, Ho SU, Melen O, Daghestani AN: Multifocal central nervous system damage caused by toluene abuse. Neurology 33(10):1337–1340, 1983
87. Streicher HA, Gabow PA, Moss AH, Kano D, Kaehny WD: Syndromes of toluene sniffing in adults. Ann Intern Med 94(6):758–762, 1981
88. Malm G, Lying-Tunell O: Cerebellar dysfunction related to toluene sniffing. Acta Neurol Scand 62(3):188–190, 1980
89. Ehyai A, Freeman FR: Progressive optic neuropathy and sensorineural hearing loss due to chronic glue sniffing. J Neurol Neurosurg Psychiatry 46(4):349–351, 1983
90. Reinhardt DF, Azar A, Maxfield ME, Smith PE, Mullin LS: Cardiac arrhythmias and aerosol "sniffing." Arch Environ Health 22:265, 1971
91. Hersh JH, Podruch PE, Rogers G, et al: Toluene embryopathy. J Pediatr 106:922–927, 1985
92. Goodwin TM: Toluene abuse and renal tubular acidosis in pregnancy. Obstet Gynecol 71:715–718, 1988
93. Courtney KD, Andrews JE, Springer J, et al: A perinatal study of toluene in CD-1 mice. Fundam Appl Toxicol 6:145–154, 1986
94. Toxicological Profile for Toluene. Agency for Toxic Substances and Disease Registry, U.S. Public Health Service, 1989
95. Hasegawa K, Shiojima S, Koizumi A, Ikeda M: Hippuric acid and o-creosol in the urine of workers exposed to toluene. Int Arch Occup Environ Health 52(3):197–208, 1983
96. Toftgard R: Effects of xylene exposure on the metabolism of antipyrine in vitro and in vivo in the rat. Toxicology 28(1–2):117–131, 1983
97. Toftgard R, Halpert J, Gustafsson JA: Xylene induces a cytochrome P-450 isozyme in rat liver similar to the major isozyme induced by phenobarbital. Mol Pharmacol 23(1):265–271, 1983
98. Unguary G, Varga B, Horvath E, Tatrai E, Folly G: Study on the role of maternal sex steroid production and metabolism in the embryotoxicity of para-xylene. Toxicology 19(3):263–268, 1981
99. Ogata M, Taguchi T: Quantitative analysis of urinary glycine conjugates by high performance liquid chromatography: excretion of hippuric acid and methyl hippuric acids in the urine of subjects exposed to vapours of toluene and xylene. Int Arch Occup Environ Health 58(2):121–129, 1986
100. Criteria for a Recommended Standard . . . Occupational Exposure to Styrene. U.S. Department of Health and Human Services, Public Health Service, Centers for Disease Control, National Institute for Occupational Safety and Health, 1983
101. Solveig-Walles SA, Orsen I: Single-strand breaks in DNA of various organs of mice induced by styrene and styrene oxide. Cancer Lett 21(1):9–15, 1983
102. Harkonen H, Lindstrom K, Seppäläinen AM, et al: Exposure-response relationship between styrene exposure and central nervous functions. Scand J Work Environ Health 4:53–59, 1978

103. Sjoborg S, Fregert S, Trullson L: Contact allergy to styrene and related chemicals. Contact Dermatitis 10(2):94–96, 1984
104. Droz PO, Guillemin MP: Human styrene exposure. V. Development of a model for biological monitoring. Int Arch Occup Environ Health 53(1):19–36, 1983
105. Casciola LA, Ivanetich KM: Metabolism of chloroethanes by rat liver nuclear cytochrome P-450. Carcinogenesis 5(5):543–548, 1984
106. Sato A, Nakajima T: Dietary and ethanol-induced alteration of metabolism and toxicity of organic solvents. In Abstract Book, International Conference on Organic Solvent Toxicity, Stockholm, Oct. 15–17, 1984, p 16
107. Nakajima T, Koyama Y, Sato A: Dietary modification of metabolism and toxicity of chemical substances, with special reference to carbohydrate. Biochem Pharmacol 31(6):1006–1011, 1982
108. Anders MW, Jakobson I: Biotransformation of halogenated solvents. In Abstract Book, International Conference on Organic Solvent Toxicity. Stockholm, Oct. 15–17, 1984, p 7
109. Johnstone RT: Occupational Medicine and Industrial Hygiene. St. Louis: CV Mosby, 1948
110. Popper H, Thomas LB, Telles NC, et al: Development of hepatic angiosarcoma in man induced by vinyl chloride, thorotrast, and arsenic. Am J Pathol 92:349–376, 1978
111. Tracey JP, Sherlock P: Hepatoma following carbon tetrachloride poisoning. NY State J Med 68:2202–2204, 1968
112. U.S. Department of Health, Education and Welfare, Public Health Service: CDC, NIOSH, Current Intelligence Bulletin. Bull. 2, Trichloroethylene, June 6, 1975; Trichloroethylene, February 28, 1978; Bull. 28, Vinyl Halides Carcinogenicity, September 21, 1978; Bull. 25, Ethylene Dichloride, April 19, 1978; Bull. 1, Chloroprene, January 20, 1975; Bull. 9, Chloroform, March 15, 1976; Bull. 21, Trimellitic Anhydride (TMA), February 3, 1978; Bull. 8, 4,4-Diaminodiphenyl-methane (DDM) January 30, 1976; Bull. 15, Nitrosamines in Cutting Fluids, October 6, 1976; Bull. 30, Epichlorhydrin, October 12, 1978. Washington, D.C.: GPO
113. Maltoni C: Predictive value of carcinogenesis bioassays. Ann NY Acad Sci 271:431–447, 1976
114. Hatch GG, Mamay PD, Ayer ML, Castro BC, Nesnow S: Methods for detecting gaseous and volatile carcinogens using cell transformation assays. Environ Sci Res, Genotoxic Eff Airborne Agents 25:75–90, 1982
115. Hatch GG, Mamay PD, Ayer ML, Castro BC, Nesnow S: Chemical enhancement of viral transformation in Syrian hamster embryo cells by gaseous and volatile chlorinated methanes and ethanes. Cancer Res 43(5):1945–1950, 1983
116. Wallace L, Zweidinger R, Erikson M, et al: Monitoring individual exposure: measurements of volatile organic compounds in breathing zone air, drinking water, and exhaled breath. Environ Int 8(1–6):269–282, 1982
117. Singh HB, Salas LJ, Stiles RE: Distribution of selected gaseous organic mutagens and suspect carcinogens in ambient air. Environ Sci Technol 16(12):872–880, 1982
118. Reinert KH, Hunter GV, Savatino T: Dynamic heated headspace analysis of volatile organic compounds present in fish tissue samples. J Agric Food Chem 31(5):1057–1060, 1983
119. Singh BH, Lillian D, Appleby A, Lobban L: Atmospheric formation of carbon tetrachloride from tetrachloroethylene. Environ Lett 10:253–256, 1975
120. Toxicological Profile for Carbon Tetrachloride. Agency for Toxic Substances and Disease Registry, U.S. Public Health Service, 1989
121. Letkiewicz F, Johnston P, Macaluso C, et al: Carbon tetrachloride; occurrence in drinking water, food and air. Washington, D.C.: U.S. Environmental Protection Agency, Office of Drinking Water, 1983
122. Pessayre D, Colbert B, Descatoire V, et al: Hepatotoxicity of trichloroethylene-carbon tetrachloride mixtures in rats. Gastroenterology 83:761–772, 1982
123. Deng JF, Wang JD, Shih TS, et al: Outbreak of carbon tetrachloride poisoning in a color printing factory related to the use of isopropyl alcohol and air conditioning systems in Taiwan. Am J Ind Med 12:11–19, 1987
124. Días Gómez MI, Castro JA: Covalent binding of carbon tetrachloride metabolites to liver nuclear DNA, proteins, and lipids. Abstract No. 223. Toxicol Appl Pharmacol 45:315, 1970
125. Monographs on the Evaluation of the Carcinogenic Risk of Chemicals to Humans. Vol. 20. Some Halogenated Hydrocarbons. Lyon, France: International Association of Research on Cancer, 1979
126. WHO: Guidelines for drinking water quality. Volume 1. Recommendations. Geneva: World Health Organization, 1984
127. Jernigan JD, Harbison RD: Role of biotransformation in the potentiation of halocarbon hepatotoxicity by 2,5-hexanedione. J Toxicol Environ Health 9(5–6):761–781, 1982
128. Branchflower RR, Schulick RD, George JW, Pohl LR: Comparison of the effects of methyl-n-butyl ketone and phenobarbital on rat liver cytochrome P-450 and the metabolism of chloroform to phosgene. Toxicol Appl Pharmacol 71(3):414–421, 1983
129. Jernigan JD, Pounds JG, Harbison RD: Potentiation of chlorinated hydrocarbon toxicity by 2,5-hexanedione in primary cultures of adult rat hepatocytes. Fundam Appl Toxicol 3(1):22–26, 1983
130. Ilett KF, Reid WD, Sipes IJ, Krishna G: Chloroform toxicity in mice: correlation of renal and hepatic necrosis with covalent binding of metabolites to tissue macromolecules. Exp Mol Pathol 19:215–229, 1973
131. Toxicological Profile for Trichloroethylene. Agency for Toxic Substances and Disease Registry, U.S. Public Health Service, 1989
132. Miller RE, Guengerich FP: Metabolism of trichloroethylene in isolated hepatocytes, microsomes, and reconstituted enzyme systems containing cytochrome P-450. Cancer Res 43(3):1145–1152, 1983
133. Bergman K: Interactions of trichloroethylene with DNA in vitro and with RNA and DNA of various mouse tissues in vivo. Arch Toxicol 54(3):181–193, 1983
134. Parchman LG, Magee PN: Metabolism of ^{14}C trichloroethylene to $^{14}CO_2$ and interaction of a metabolite with liver DNA in rats and mice. J Toxicol Environ Health 9(5–6):797–813, 1982
135. Koizumi A, Fujita H, Sadamoto T, et al: Inhibition of delta-aminolevulinic acid dehydratase by trichloroethylene. Toxicology 30(2):93–102, 1984
136. Lachnit V, Brichta G: Trichloroethylene and liver damage. Zentralbl Arbeitsmed 8:56–62, 1958
137. James WRL: Fatal addiction to trichloroethylene. Br J Ind Med 20:47–49, 1963
138. Kleinfeld M, Tabershaw IR: Trichloroethylene toxicity—report of five fatal cases. Arch Ind Hyg Occup Med 10:134–141, 1954
139. Gutch CF, Tomhave WG, Stevens SC: Acute renal failure due to inhalation of trichloroethylene. Ann Intern Med 63:128–134, 1965
140. Pessayre D, Cobert B, Descatoire V, et al: Hepatotoxicity of trichloroethylene-carbon tetrachloride mixtures in rats: a possible consequence of the potentiation by trichloroethylene of carbon tetrachloride-induced lipid peroxidation and liver lesions. Gastroenterology 83(4):761–772, 1982
141. Healy TE, Poole TR, Hopper A: Rat fetal development and maternal exposure to trichloroethylene 100 ppm. Br J Anaesth 54(3):337–341, 1982
142. Slacik-Erben R, Roll R, Franke G, Uehleke H: Trichloroethylene vapours do not produce dominant lethal mutations in male mice. Arch Toxicol 45(1):37–41, 1980
143. Land PC, Owen EL, Linde HW: Morphologic changes in mouse spermatozoa after exposure to inhalation anesthetics during early spermatogenesis. Anesthesiology 54(1):53–56, 1981
144. Stewart RD: Acute tetrachloroethylene intoxication. JAMA 208:1490, 1969
145. Abedin Z, Cook RC, Milberg RM: Cardiac toxicity of perchloroethylene (a dry-cleaning agent). South Med J 73(8):1081–1083, 1980
146. Lukaszewski T: Acute tetrachloroethylene fatality. Clin Toxicol 15(4):411–415, 1979
147. Levine B, Fierro MF, Goza SW, Valentour C: A tetrachloroethylene fatality. J Forensic Sci 26:206–209 (cited in EPA 1985a), 1981
148. Rosengren LE, Kjellstrand P, Haglid KG: Tetrachloroethylene:

levels of DNA and S-100 in the gerbil CNS after chronic exposure. Neurobehav Toxicol Teratol 8(2):201–206, 1986
149. Briving C, Jacobson I, Hamberger A, Kjellstrand P, Haglid KG, Rosengren LE: Chronic effects of perchloroethylene and trichloroethylene on the gerbil brain amino acids and glutathione. Neurotoxicologist 7(1):101–108, 1986
150. Buben JA, O'Flaherty EJ: Delineation of the role of metabolism in the hepatotoxicity of trichloroethylene and perchloroethylene: a dose-effect study. Toxicol Appl Pharmacol 78(1):105–122, 1985
151. NTP (National Toxicology Program): Toxicology and carcinogenesis tetrachloroethylene (perchloroethylene) (CAS No. 127-18-4) in F344/N rats and B6C3F1 mice (inhalation studies). Natl Toxicol Program Tech Rep Ser 311, 1986
152. Toxicological Profile for Tetrachloroethylene. U.S. Department of Health and Human Services, Public Health Service, Agency for Toxic Substances and Disease Registry, 1990
153. Ikeda M, Koizumi A, Watanabe T, Endo A, Sato K: Cytogenetic and cytokinetic investigations on lymphocytes from workers occupationally exposed to tetrachloroethylene. Toxicol Lett 5(3–4):251–256, 1980
154. Stewart RD: Methyl chloroform intoxication: diagnosis and treatment. JAMA 215:1789, 1971
155. Carlson GP: Effect of alterations in drug metabolism on epinephrine-induced cardiac arrhythmias in rabbits exposed to methyl chloroform. Toxicol Lett 9(4):307–313, 1981
156. Gresham GA, Treip CS: Fatal poisoning by 1,1,1-trichloroethane after prolonged survival. Forensic Sci Int 23(2–3):249–253, 1983
157. Troutman WG: Additional deaths associated with the intentional inhalation of typewriter correction fluid. Vet Hum Toxicol 30(2): 130–132, 1988
158. Macdougall IC, Isles C, Oliver JS, Clark JC, Spilg WG: Fatal outcome following inhalation of Tipp-Ex. Scott Med J 32(2):55, 1987
159. Karlsson JE, Rosengren LE, Kjellstrand P, Haglid KG: Effects of low-dose inhalation of three chlorinated aliphatic organic solvents on deoxyribonucleic acid in gerbil brain. Scand J Work Environ Health 13(5):453–458, 1987
160. Henschler D, Reichert D, Metzler M: Identification of potential carcinogens in technical grade 1,1,1-trichloroethane. Int Arch Occup Environ Health 47(3):263–268, 1980
161. National Cancer Institute: Bioassay of 1,1,2-trichloroethane for possible carcinogenicity. Report. ISS DHEW/PUB/NIH-78-1324. NCI-CG-tr. PB-283337. 1978
162. Mazzullo M, Colacci A, Grilli S, et al: 1,1,2-Trichloroethane: evidence of genotoxicity from short-term tests. Jpn J Cancer Res 77:532–539, 1986
163. Toxicological Profile for 1,1,2-Trichloroethane. Agency for Toxic Substances and Disease Registry, U.S. Public Health Service, 1989
164. OSHA: Air contaminants: Final rule. U.S. Department of Labor. Occupational Safety and Health Administration. 29 CFR 1910.1000. Federal Register 54(12):2332–2960, 1989
165. National Institute for Occupational Safety and Health: Recommendations for a workplace exposure to 1,1,2,2-tetrachloroethane. Occup Saf Health Rep 3:1271–1278, 1977
166. Marsteller HJ, Lelbach WK, Muller R, Gedigk P: Unusual splenomegalic liver disease as evidenced by peritoneoscopy and guided liver biopsy among polyvinyl chloride production workers. Ann NY Acad Sci 246:95–134, 1975
167. Creech JL Jr, Johnson MN: Angiosarcoma of liver in the manufacture of polyvinyl chloride. J Occup Med 16:150, 1974
168. Wilson RH, McCormick WE, Tatum CF, Creech JL: Occupational acroosteolysis: report of 31 cases. JAMA 201:577, 1967
169. Waxweiler RJ, Stringer W, Wagoner JK, Jones J: Neoplastic risk among workers exposed to vinyl chloride. Ann NY Acad Sci 271:40, 1976
170. Bolt HM: Metabolism of genotoxic agents: halogenated compounds. Monitoring human exposure to carcinogenic and mutagenic agents, proceedings of a joint symposium held in Espo, Finland, 12–15 December, 1983, IARC Scientific Publication No. 59, pp 63–71, 1984
171. Garro AJ, Guttenpaln JB, Milvy P: Vinyl chloride dependent mutagenesis: effects of liver extracts and free radicals. Mutat Res 38(2):81–88, 1976
172. Greim H, Bonse G, Radwan Z, et al: Mutagenicity in vitro and potential carcinogenicity of chlorinated ethylenes as a function of metabolic oxirane formation. Biochem Pharmacol 24:2013–2017, 1975
173. Henschler D, Bonse G, Greim H: Carcinogenic potential of chlorinated ethylenes—tentative molecular rules. INSERM 52:171–175, 1976
174. Heath CW Jr, Dumont CR, Gamble J, Waxweiler RJ: Chromosomal damage in men occupationally exposed to vinyl chloride monomer and other chemicals. Environ Res 14:68–72, 1977
175. Purchase IFH, Richardson CR, Anderson D: Chromosomal and dominant lethal effects of vinyl chloride. Lancet 2:410–411, 1975
176. Bartsch H, Malaveille C, Barbin A, et al: Alkylating and mutagenic metabolites of halogenated olefins produced by human and animal tissues. Proc Am Assoc Cancer Res 17:17, 1976
177. Maltoni C: Recent findings on the carcinogenicity of chlorinated olefins. Environ Health Perspect 21:1–5, 1977
178. Ott MG, Fishbeck WA, Townsend JC, Schneider EJ: A health study of employees exposed to vinylidene chloride. J Occup Med 18:735–738, 1976
179. Bartsch H, Malaveille C, Montesano R, Tomatis L: Tissue mediated mutagenicity of vinylidene chloride and 2-chlorobutadiene in *Salmonella typhimurium*. Nature 255:641–643, 1975
180. IARC Monographs on the Evaluation of the Carcinogenic Risk of Chemicals to Humans. Vol. 39. Some Chemicals Used in Plastics and Elastomers. Lyon, France: International Agency for Research on Cancer, 1986, pp 195–226
181. Reitz RH, Fox TR, Ramsey JC, et al: Pharmacokinetics and macromolecular interactions of ethylene dichloride in rats after inhalation or gavage. Toxicol Appl Pharmacol 62(6):190–204, 1982
182. Reitz RH, Fox TR, Ramsey JC, et al: Pharmacokinetics and macromolecular interactions of ethylene dichloride in rats after inhalation or gavage. Toxicol Appl Pharmacol 62(6):190–204, 1982
183. National Cancer Institute: Bioassay of technical grade 1,2-dichloroethane for possible carcinogenicity. Bethesda, MD: National Cancer Institute, Division of Cancer Cause and Prevention, Carcinogenesis Testing Program. NCI-CG-TR 55, 1978
184. Maltoni C, Valgimigli L, Scarnato C: Long-term carcinogenic bioassays on ethylene dichloride administered by inhalation to rats and mice. In: Ames BN, Infante P, Reitz R (ed): Ethylene Dichloride: A Potential Health Risk? Banburry Report No. 5. Cold Spring Harbor, NY: Cold Spring Harbor Laboratory, 3–33, 1980
185. Giri AK, Hee S Sq: In vivo sister chromatid exchange induced by 1,2-dichloroethane on bone marrow cells of mice. Environ Mol Mutagen 12(3):331–334, 1988
186. Moriya M, Ohta T, Watanabe K, et al: Further mutagenicity studies on pesticides in bacterial reversion assay systems. Mutat Res 116(3–4):185–216, 1983
187. Hatch GG, Mamay PD, Ayer ML, Castro BC, Nesnow S: Chemical enhancement of viral transformation in Syrian hamster cells by gaseous and volatile chlorinated methanes and ethanes. Cancer Res 43(5):1945–1950, 1983
188. Lane BW, Riddle BL, Borzelleca JF: Effects of 1,2-dichloroethane and 1,1,1-trichloroethane in drinking water on reproduction and development in mice. Toxicol Appl Pharmacol 63(3):409–421, 1982
189. EPA. Health assessment document for 1,2-dichloroethane: final report. Washington, D.C.: Office of Health and Environmental Assessment, U.S. Environmental Protection Agency, EPA 600/8-84-006F, 1985
190. Toxicological Profile for 1,2-Dichloroethane. Agency for Toxic Substances and Disease Registry, U.S. Public Health Service, 1989
191. OSHA. Occupational Safety and Health Administration. U.S. Department of Labor. Federal Register 12(12):2937, 1989
192. Letz GA, Pond SM, Osterloh JD, Wade RL, Becker CE: Two fatalities after acute occupational exposure to ethylene dibromide, JAMA 252(17):2428–31, 1984

193. Moody DE, Clawson GA, Woo CH, Smuckler EA: Cellular distribution of cytochrome P-450 loss in rats of different ages treated with alkyl halides. Toxicol Appl Pharmacol 66(2):278–289, 1982
194. Amir D: Individual and age differences in the spermicidal effect of ethylene dibromide in bulls. J Reprod Fertil 44:561–565, 1975
195. Amir D, Gledhill BL, Garner DL, Nicolle JC, Tadmor A: Spermiogenic, epididymal and spermatozoal damage induced by a peritesticular injection of ethylene dibromide to rams. Anim Reprod Sci 6(1):35–50, 1983
196. Wong LCK, Winston JM, Hong CB, Plotnick H: Carcinogenicity and toxicity of 1,2-dibromoethane in the rat. Toxicol Appl Pharmacol 63(2):155–165, 1982
197. Ratcliffe JM, Schrader SM, Steenland K, Clapp DE, Turner T, Hornung RW: Semen quality in papaya workers with long term exposure to ethylene dibromide. Br J Ind Med 44(5):317–326, 1987
198. Olson WA, Habermann RT, Weisburgen EK, et al: Induction of stomach cancer in rats and mice by halogenated aliphatic fumigants. J Natl Cancer Inst 51:1993–1995, 1973
199. Carcinogenesis Bioassay of 1,2-dibromoethane (CAS No. 106-93-4) in F344 Rats and B6C3F1 Mice (inhalation study). NIH Publ. Iss. NIH-82-1766, 1982
200. Ott MG, Scharnweber HC, Langner RR: The mortality experience of 161 employees exposed to ethylene dibromide in two production units. Report submitted to NIOSH by the Dow Chemical Co., Midland, Mich., March 1977
201. Ozawa N, Guengerich FP: Evidence for formation of an S-(2-(N7-guanyl)ethyl)glutathione adduct in glutathione-mediated binding of the carcinogen 1,2-dibromoethane to DNA. Proc Natl Acad Sci USA 80(17):5266–5270, 1983
202. Sekita H, Takeda M, Uchiyama M: Analysis of pesticide residues in foods: 33. Determination of ethylene dibromide residues in litchi (lychee) fruits imported from Formosa. Eisei Shikenjo Hokoku 99:130–132, 1981
203. Ethylene dibromide: Decision and emergency order suspending registrations of pesticide products containing EDB. Federal Register, Feb. 6, 1984, part II
204. Halogenated Hydrocarbons: IARC monographs on the evaluation of the carcinogenic risk of chemicals to humans. Vol. 41. Lyon, France: International Agency for Research on Cancer, 1986, pp 161–186
205. Chavez CT, Hepler RS, Straatsma BR: Methyl bromide optic atrophy. Am J Ophthalmol 99(6):715–719, 1985
206. Behrens RH, Dukes DCD: Fatal methyl bromide poisoning. Br J Ind Med 43(8):561–562, 1986
207. Ishizu S, Kato N, Morinobu S, Nagao N, Yamano Y, Ito I: Cases of severe methyl bromide poisoning in persons residing above a warehouse. Jpn J Ind Health 30(1):54–60, 1988
208. NIOSH. Current Intelligence Bulletin 43. Monohalomethanes. Pub. No. 84–117, p. 22. Washington, D.C.: U.S. Government Printing Office, Sept. 27, 1984
209. Hamm TE, Raynor TH, Phelps MC, Auman CD, Adams WT, Proctor JE, Wolkowski-Tyl R: Reproduction in Fischer-344 rats exposed to methyl chloride by inhalation for two generations. Fundam Appl Toxicol 5(3):568–577, 1985
210. Eustis SL, Haber SB, Drew RT, Yang R SH: Toxicology and pathology of methyl bromide in F-344 rats and B6C3F1 mice following repeated inhalation exposure. Fundam Appl Toxicol 11(4):594–610, 1988
211. Iwasaki K: Determination of S-methylcysteine in mouse hemoglobin following exposure to methyl bromide. Ind Health 26(3):187–190, 1988
212. Khachatryan EA: The occurrence of lung cancer among people working with chloroprene. Probl Oncol 18:85, 1972
213. Pell S: Mortality of workers exposed to chloroprene. J Occup Med 20:21–29, 1978
214. IARC Monographs on the Evaluation of the Carcinogenic Risk of Chemicals to Humans: Vol. 19. Some Monomers, Plastics and Synthetic Elastomers, and Acrolein. Lyon, France: International Association of Research on Cancer, 1979
215. Von Oettingen WF, Hueper WC, Deichmann-Grubler W, Wiley FH: 2-Chlorobutadiene (chloroprene): its toxicity and pathology and the mechanism of its action. J Ind Hyg Toxicol 18:240–270, 1936
216. Vogel E: Mutagenicity of carcinogens in Drosophila as function of genotype-controlled metabolism. In deSerres FJ, Fouts JR, Bend JR, Philpot RM (eds): In Vitro Metabolic Activation in Mutagenesis Testing. Amsterdam: Elsevier, 1976, pp 63–79
217. National Institute for Occupational Safety and Health: Criteria for a recommended standard occupational exposure to chloroprene. DHEW (NIOSH) Publ. No. 77-210. Washington, D.C.: U.S. Government Printing Office, 1977
218. Clayton GD, Clayton FE (eds): Patty's Industrial Hygiene and Toxicology, 3 edt rev. Vol. 2B. Toxicology. New York: John Wiley, 1981
219. Brennon PD: Addiction to aerosol treatment. Br Med J 287:1877, 1983
220. Longstaff E, Robinson M, Bradbrook C, Styles JA, Purchase IF: Genotoxicity and carcinogenicity of fluorocarbons: assessment by short-term in vitro tests and chronic exposure in rats. Toxicol Appl Pharmacol 72(1):15–31, 1984
221. Weill CS, Smyth HR Jr, Nale TW: Quest for a suspected industrial carcinogen. Arch Ind Hyg Occup Med 5:535–547, 1952
222. Hueper WC: Occupational and Environmental Cancers of the Respiratory System. New York: Springer-Verlag, 1966, pp 8–9, 22, 104–107
223. Hueper WC: A Quest into the Environmental Causes of Cancer of the Lung. Public Health Monogr No. 36. U.S. Department of HEW, Public Health Service. Washington, D.C.: U.S. Government Printing Office, 1955, p 38
224. Bittersohl G: Carcinogenic effect of isopropyl oil. Arch Geschwulstforsch 43:250–253, 1974
225. Hewlett TP, McMartin KE, Lauro AJ, Ragan FA Jr: Ethylene glycol poisoning: the value of glycolic acid determinations for diagnosis and treatment. J Toxicol Clin Toxicol 24(5):389–402, 1986
226. Younossi-Hartenstein A, Roth B, Iffland R, Sticht G: Short term hemodialysis for ethylene glycol poisoning. J Pediatr 109:731–732, 1986
227. Jacobsen D, Hewlett TP, Webb R, Brown ST, McMartin KE, et al: Ethylene glycol intoxication: evaluation of kinetics and crystalluria. Am J Med 84:145–152, 1988
228. Baud FJ, Galliot M, Astier A, Bien DV, Bismuth C, et al: Treatment of ethylene glycol poisoning with intravenous 4-methylpyrazole. N Engl J Med 319:97–100, 1988
229. Evans W, David EJ. Biodegradation of mono-, di-, and triethylene glycols in river waters under controlled laboratory conditions. Water Res 8(2):97–100, 1974
230. U.S. Dept of Health and Human Services, PHS, Centers for Disease Control: NIOSH Current Intelligence Bulletin No. 39: Glycol Ethers 2-Methoxyethanol and 2-Ethoxyethanol. Washington, D.C.: U.S. Government Printing Office, 1983
231. Miller ER, Ayres JA, Young JT, McKenna MJ: Ethylene glycol monomethyl ether. I. Subchronic vapor inhalation study in rats and rabbits. Fundam Appl Toxicol 3(1):49–54, 1983
232. Nagano K, Nakayama E, Dobayashi H, et al: Embryotoxic effects of ethylene glycol monomethyl ether on mice. Toxicology 20(4): 335–344, 1981
233. McGregor DB, Willins MJ, McDonald P, et al: Genetic effects of 2-methoxyethanol and bis(2-methoxyethyl) ether. Toxicol Appl Pharmacol 70(2):303–316, 1983
234. Cook RR, Bodner KM, Kolesar RC, et al: A cross-sectional study of ethylene glycol monomethyl ether process employees. Arch Environ Health 37(6):346–351, 1982
235. American Conference of Governmental Industrial Hygienists: Supplemental Documentation for 1982. Cincinnati, Ohio, 1982
236. Rice DL, Jenkins DE, Gray JM, Greenberg SD: Chemical pneumonitis secondary to inhalation of epoxy pipe coating. Arch Environ Health 32:173–178, 1977
237. Zeiss CR, Pattersin R, Pruzansky JJ, et al: Trimellitic anhydride-induced airway syndromes: Chemical and immunologic studies. J Allergy Clin Immunol 60:96–103, 1977

237a. Leach CL, Hatoum NS, Ratajczak HV, Zeiss CR, Garvin PJ: Evidence of immunologic control of lung injury induced by trimellitic anhydride. Am Rev Respir Dis 137(1):186–190, 1988
238. Fawcett DW, Taylor AJ, Pepys J: Asthma due to inhaled chemical agents—epoxy resin systems containing phthalic acid anhydride, trimellitic acid anhydride and triethylene tetramine. Clin Allergy 7:14, 1977
239. Ducatman AM, Conwill DE, Crawl J: Germ cell tumors of the testicles among aircraft repairmen. J Urol 136(4):834–836, 1986
240. Chen JL, Fayerweather WE, Pell S: Cancer incidence of workers exposed to dimethylformamide and/or acrylonitrile. J Occup Med 30(10):813–818, 1988
241. Kennedy GL Jr, Sherman H: Acute and subchronic toxicity of dimethylformamide and dimethylacetamide following various routes of administration. Drug Chem Toxicol 9(2):147–170, 1986
242. Spencer PS, Schaumburg HH: A review of acrylamide neurotoxicity. I. Properties, uses and human exposure. Can J Neurol Sci 1:143–150, 1974
243. Fassett DW: Organic acids, anhydrides, lactones, acid halides and amides, thioacids. In Patty FA (ed): Industrial Hygiene and Toxicology. Vol. 2. Toxicology. New York: Interscience, 1963, pp 1832–1835
244. Auld RB, Bedwell SF: Peripheral neuropathy with sympathetic overactivity from industrial contact with acrylamide. Can Med Assoc J 96:652–654, 1967
245. Fullerton PM: Acrylamide toxicity in man. Electroencephalogr Clin Neurophysiol 28:426, 1970
246. Ghetti B, Wisniewski HM, Cook RD, Schaumburg HH: Changes in the CNS after acute and chronic acrylamide intoxication. Am J Pathol 70:78, 1973
247. Arezzo JC, Schaumburg HH, Vaughan HG Jr, Spencer PS, Barna J: Hind limb somatosensory evoked potentials in the monkey: the effects of distal axonopathy. Ann Neurol 12(1):24–32, 1982
248. Merigan WH, Barkdoll E, Maurissen JPJ: Acrylamide-induced visual impairment in primates. Toxicol Appl Pharmacol 62(6): 342–345, 1982
249. Jakobsen J, Brimijoin S, Sidenius P: Axonal transport in neuropathy. Muscle Nerve 6(2):164–166, 1983
250. Chretien M, Patey G, Souyri F, Droz B: Acrylamide-induced neuropathy and impairment of axonal transport of proteins. 2. Abnormal accumulations of smooth endoplasmic reticulum as sites of focal retention of fast transported proteins: electron microscope radioautographic study. Brain Res 205(1):15–28, 1981
251. Agrawal AK, Squibb RE: Effects of acrylamide given during gestation on dopamine receptor binding in rat pups. Toxicol Lett 7:233–238, 1981
252. Ali SF, Hong J-S, Wilson WE, Uphouse LL, Bondy SC: Effect of acrylamide on neurotransmitter metabolism and neuropeptide levels in several brain regions and upon circulating hormones. Arch Toxicol 52(1):35, 1983
253. Adler ID, Ingwersen I, Kliesch U, el Tarras A: Clastogenic effects of acrylamide in mouse bone marrow cells. Mutat Res 206(3):379–385, 1988
254. Johnson KA, Gorzinski SJ, Bodner KM, Campbell RA, Wolf CH, Friedman MA, Mast RW: Chronic toxicity and oncogenicity study on acrylamide incorporated in the drinking water of Fischer 344 rats. Toxicol Appl Pharmacol 85(2):154–168, 1986
255. Sobel W, Bond GG, Parsons TW, Brenner FE: Acrylamide cohort mortality study. Br J Ind Med 43(11):785–788, 1986
256. IARC Monographs on the Evaluation of the Carcinogenic Risk of Chemicals to Humans. Vol. 29. Some Industrial Chemicals and Dyestuffs: Formaldehyde. Lyon, France: International Association of Research on Cancer, 1982
257. U.S. Dept. of Health and Human Services. Public Health Service. Centers for Disease Control: NIOSH Current Intelligence Bulletin 34. Formaldehyde: Evidence of Carcinogenicity. Washington, D.C.: U.S. Government Printing Office, 1981
258. Til HP, Woutersen RA, Feron VJ, Hollanders VH, Falke HE, Clary JJ: Two-year drinking water study of formaldehyde in rats. Food Chem Toxicol 27(2):77–87, 1989
259. Harrington JM, Shannon HS: Mortality study of pathologists and medical laboratory technicians. Br Med J 2:329–332, 1975
260. Walrath J, Fraumeni JR Jr: Proportionate mortality among New York embalmers. In Gibson JE (ed): Formaldehyde Toxicity. Washington, D.C.: Hemisphere Publishing Corp., 1983, pp 227–236
261. Stayner LT, Elliott L, Blade L, Keenlyside R, Halperin W: A retrospective cohort mortality study of workers exposed to formaldehyde in the garment industry. Am J Ind Med 13(6):667–681, 1988
262. Pruett JJ, Scheuenstuhl H, Michaeli D: The incorporation and localization of aldehydes (highly reactive cigarette smoke components) into cellular fractions of cultured human lung cells. Arch Environ Health 35:15–20, 1980
263. Chaw YFM, Crane LE, Lange P, Shapiro R: Isolation and identification of cross-links from formaldehyde-treated nucleic acids. Biochemistry 19:5525–5531, 1980
264. Thomas JO: Chemically induced DNA-protein cross-links. In Smith KC (ed): Carcinogenesis and Radiation Biology. New York: Plenum, 1976, pp 193–205
265. Yager JW, Cohn KL, Spear RC, Fisher JM, Morse L: Sister chromatid exchanges in lymphocytes of anatomy students exposed to formaldehyde-embalming solution. Mutat Res 174(2):135–139, 1986
266. Formaldehyde. Council on Scientific Affairs. JAMA 261(8):1183–1187, 1989
267. Slott VL, Hales BF: Teratogenicity and embryolethality of acrolein and structurally related compounds in rats. Teratology 32(1):65–72, 1985
268. Grafstrom RC, Dypbukt JM, Willey JC, Sundqvist K, Edman C, Atzori L, Harris CC: Pathobiological effects of acrolein in cultured human bronchial epithelial cells. Cancer Res 48(7):1717–1721, 1988
269. Foiles PG, Akerkar SA, Chung FL: Application of an immunoassay for cyclic acrolein deoxyguanosine adducts to assess their formation in DNA of *Salmonella typhimurium* under conditions of mutation induction by acrolein. Carcinogenesis 10(1):87–90, 1989
270. IARC Monographs on the Evaluation of the Carcinogenic Risks of Chemicals to Humans. Lyon, France: International Agency for Research on Cancer, 1982, Supply 4, pp 119–120
271. Environmental Health Criteria 48, Dimethyl Sulfate, Geneva: World Health Organization, 1985, p 55
272. Allen N, Mendell JR, Billmaier DJ, et al: Toxic polyneuropathy due to methyl n-butyl ketone. Arch Neurol 32:209–218, 1975
273. Malloy JS: MBK neuropathy among spray painters. JAMA 235:1455–1457, 1976
274. Saida K, Mendell JR, Weiss HS: Peripheral nerve changes induced by methyl n-butyl ketone and potentiation by methyl ethyl ketone. J Neuropathol Exp Neurol 35:207–225, 1976
275. Spencer PS, Schaumburg HH: Ultrastructural studies of the dying-back process. IV. Differential vulnerability of PNS and CNS fibers in experimental central-peripheral distal axonopathies. J Neuropathol Exp Neurol 36:300–320, 1977
276. Sheu CW, Moreland FM, Lee JK, Dunkel VC: In vitro BALB/3T3 cell transformation assay of nonoxynol-9 and 1,4-dioxane. Environ Mol Mutagen 11(1):41–48, 1988
277. IARC Monographs on the Evaluation of Carcinogenic Risk of Chemicals to Man. Vol. 11. Cadmium, Nickel, Some Epoxides, Miscellaneous Industrial Chemicals and General Considerations on Volatile Anaesthetics. Lyon, France: International Agency for Research on Cancer, 1976, pp 247–253
278. Dalvy RA, Neal RA: Metabolism in vivo of carbon disulfide to carbonyl sulfide and carbon dioxide in the rat. Biochem Pharmacol 27:1608, 1978
279. Hamilton A: Industrial Poisons Used in the Rubber Industry. Bulletin No. 179. Washington, D.C.: U.S. Department of Labor, Bureau of Labor Statistics, 1915, pp 5–64
280. Hamilton A: The making of artificial silk in the United States and some of the dangers attending it. In U.S. Department of Labor, Division of Labor Standards: Discussion of Industrial Accidents and Diseases. Bulletin No. 10, Washington, D.C.: U.S. Government Printing Office, 1937, pp 151–160

281. Harrisburg, Pennsylvania, Department of Labor and Industry, Occupational Disease Prevention Division: Survey of Carbon Disulphide and Hydrogen Sulphide Hazards in the Viscose Rayon Industry. Bulletin No. 46. Washington, D.C.: U.S. Government Printing Office, 1938
282. American Standards Association: Allowable Concentrations of Carbon Disulfide. ASA Z37.3-1941. New York: ASA, 1941
283. Lilis R: Behavioral effects of occupational carbon disulfide exposure. In Xintaras C, Johnson BL, de Groot I (eds): Behavioral Toxicology, Early Detection of Occupational Hazards. Washington, D.C.: U.S. Dept. of HEW, Public Health Service, Centers for Disease Control, National Institute for Occupational Safety and Health, 1974, pp 51–59
284. Seppäläinen AM, Tolonen MT: Neurotoxicity of long-term exposure to carbon disulfide in the viscose rayon industry—a neurophysiological study. Work Environ Health 11:145–153, 1974
285. Hänninen H: Psychological picture of manifest and latent carbon disulfide poisoning. Br J Ind Med 28:374–381, 1971
286. Vigliani EC: Carbon disulphide poisoning in viscose rayon factories. Br J Ind Med 11:235–244, 1954
287. Tiller JR, Schilling RSF, Morris JN: Occupational toxic factor in mortality from coronary heart disease. Br Med J 4:407–411, 1968
288. Nurminen M: Survival experience of a cohort of carbon disulphide exposed workers from an eight-year prospective follow-up period. Int J Epidemiol 5:179–185, 1976
289. Goto S, Hotta R: The medical and hygienic prevention of carbon disulfide poisoning in Japan. In Brieger H, Teisinger J (eds): Toxicology of Carbon Disulphide. Amsterdam: Excerpta Medica Foundation, 1967, pp 219–230
290. Lancranjan I: Alterations of spermatic liquid in patients chronically poisoned by carbon disulphide. Med Lav 63:29–33, 1972
291. Magos L, Jarvis JAE: The effects of carbon disulfide exposure on brain catecholamines in rats. Br J Pharmacol 39:26, 1970
292. DeMatteis F: Covalent binding of sulfur to microsomes and loss of cytochrome P-450 during the oxidative desulfurization of several chemicals. Mol Pharmacol 10:849, 1974
293. Juntunen J, Linnoila I, Haltia M: Histochemical and electron microscopic observations on the myoneural functions of rats with carbon disulfide-induced polyneuropathy. Scand J Work Environ Health 3:36, 1977
294. Pergal M, Vukojevic N, Cirin-Popov N: Carbon disulfide metabolites excreted in the urine of exposed workers. I. Isolation and identification of 2-mercapto-2-thiazolinone-5. Arch Environ Health 25:38, 1972
295. Pergal M, Vukojevic N, Djuric D: II. Isolation and identification of thiocarbamide. Arch Environ Health 25:42, 1972
296. Djuric D, Surducki N, Berkes I: Iodine-azide test on urine of persons exposed to carbon disulfide. Br J Ind Med 22:321–323, 1965
297. Ahlborg G Jr, Ulander A, Bergstrom B, Oliv A: Diazo-positive metabolites in urine from workers exposed to aromatic nitroamino compounds. Int Arch Occup Environ Health 60(1):51–54, 1988
298. Fenakel G: Acute hemolysis due to trinitrotoluene in glucose-6-phosphate dehydrogenase deficiency. Harefuah 109(7–8):188–189, 215, 1985
299. Harkonen H, Karki M, Lahti A, Savolainen H: Early equatorial cataracts in workers exposed to trinitrotoluene. Am J Ophthalmol 95(6):807–810, 1983
300. Hathaway JA: Subclinical effects of trinitrotoluene: a review of epidemiology studies. In Rickett DE (ed): Toxicity of Nitroaromatic Compounds. New York: Hemisphere Publishing Corp, 1985, pp 255–274
301. Ahlborg G Jr, Einisto P, Sorsa M: Mutagenic activity and metabolites in the urine of workers exposed to trinitrotoluene (TNT). Br J Ind Med 45(5):353–358, 1988
302. Kopelman H, Robertson MH, Sanders PG, Ash I: The Epping jaundice. Br Med J 1:514, 1966
303. McGill DB, Motto JD: An industrial outbreak of toxic hepatitis due to methylenedianiline. N Engl J Med 291(6):278–282, 1974
304. Schoental R: Carcinogenic and chronic effects of 4,4′-diaminodiphenylmethane, an epoxy resin hardener. Nature 219: 1162–1163, 1968
305. Gailhofer G, Ludvan M: Change in the allergen spectrum in contact eczema 1975–1984. Derm Beruf Umwelt 35(1):12–6, 1987
306. Current Intelligence Bulletin 47, 4,4-methylenedianiline (MDA), Publication No. 86–115. Cincinnati, Ohio: NIOSH, U.S. Department of Health and Human Services, 1986
307. IARC Monographs on the Evaluation of the Carcinogenic Risk of Chemicals to Humans. Vol. 39. Some Chemicals Used in Plastics and Elastomers. Lyon, France: International Agency for Research on Cancer, 1986, pp 347–365
308. Lee H, Perng L-Y, Shiow S-J, Chou M-Y, Chou M-C, Lin J-Y: Induction of sister chromatid exchange in cultured Chinese hamster cells by short-term treatment with hair dye components. J Chin Biochem Soc 15(1):34–38, 1986
309. Barnes JM, Magee PN: Some toxic properties of dimethylnitrosamine. Br J Ind Med 11:167, 1954
310. Magee PN, Barnes JM: Carcinogenic nitroso compounds. Adv Cancer Res 10:163, 1956
311. Heath DF: The decomposition and toxicity of dialkylnitrosamines. Biochem J 85:72, 1962
312. Magee PN, Farber E: Toxic liver injury and carcinogenesis: methylation of rat-liver nucleic acids by dimethylnitrosamine in vivo. Biochem J 83:114, 1962
313. Druckrey H, Preussman R, Ivankovic S, Schmahl D: Organotrope carcinogene Wirkungen bei 65 verschiedenen *N*-Nitroso-Verbindungen an BD-Ratten. Z Krebsforsch 69:103–201, 1967
314. Goodal CM, Lijinsky W, Tomatis L: Tumorigenicity of *N*-nitroso-hexa-methyleneimine. Cancer Res 28:1217, 1968
315. Kokkinakis DM, Scarpelli DG: Carcinogenicity of *N*-nitroso (2-hydroxypropyl) (2-oxopropyl) amine, *N*-nitrosobis (2-hyroxypropyl) amine and *cis*-*N*-nitroso-2,6-dimethylmorpholine administered continuously in the Syrian hamster, and the effect of dietary protein on *N*-nitroso (2-hydroxypropyl) (2-oxopropyl) amine carcinogenesis. Carcinogenesis 10(4):699–704, 1989
316. Fujita J, Ohuchi N, Ito N, Reynolds SH, Yoshida O, Nakayama H, Kitamura Y: Activation of H-*ras* oncogene in rat bladder tumors induced by *N*-butyl-*N*-(4-hydroxybutyl) nitrosamine. J Natl Cancer Inst 80(1):37–43, 1988
317. LePage RN, Christie GS: Induction of liver tumors in the rabbit by feeding dimethylnitrosamine. Br J Cancer 23:125, 1969
318. Montesano R, Magee PN: Metabolism of dimethylnitrosamine by human liver slices in vitro. Nature 228:173, 1970
319. Sakshaug H, Sognen E, Hansen MA, Koppang N: Dimethylnitrosamine: its hepatotoxic effect in sheep and its occurrence in toxic batches of herring meal. Nature 206:1261, 1965
320. Ender F, Ceh L: Occurrence of nitrosamines in foodstuffs for human and animal consumption. Food Cosmet Toxicol 6:569, 1968
321. Sander J: Kann Nitrit in der Menschlichen Nahrung Ursache einer Krebsentstehung durch Nitrosaminbildung sein? Arch Hyg Bakt 151:22, 1967
322. Sander J: Nitrosaminsynthese durch Bakterien. Hoppe Seylers Z Physiol Chem 349:429, 1968
323. Sander J, Seif F: Bakterielle Reduktion von Nitrit im Magen des Menschen als Ursache einer Nitrosamin-Bildung. Arzneimittelforsch 19:1091, 1969
324. Joshi PA, Schuller HM, Rossignol G, Castonguay A: In vitro morphological changes induced by 4-(methylnitrosamino)-1-(3-pyridyl)-1-(butanone) in fetal hamster respiratory tract tissue. Cancer Lett 44(3):173–8, 1989
325. Rivenson A, Hoffman BBT D Prokopczyk B, Amin S, Hecht SS: Induction of lung and exocrine pancreas tumors in F344 rats by tobacco-specific and Areca-derived N-nitrosamines. Cancer Res 48(23):6912–7, 1988
326. Prokopczyk B, Brunnemann KD, Bertinato P, Hoffman D: The role of N-(nitrosomethylamino) propionitrile in betel-quid carcinogenesis. IARC Sci Publ 84:470–473, 1987
327. Wacker CD, Spiegelhalder B, Borzsonyi M, Brune G, Preussmann

R: Prevention of exposure to N-nitrosamines in the rubber industry: new vulcanization accelerators based on "safe" amines. IARC Sci Publ 84:370–374, 1987

328. Lawrence WH, Malik M, Turner JE, Autian J: Toxicity profile of epichlorhydrin. J Pharm Sci 61:1712–1717, 1972
329. Moody DE, Clawson GA, Woo CH, Smuckler EA: Cellular distribution of cytochrome P-450 loss in rats of different ages treated with alkyl halides. Toxicol Appl Pharmacol 66(2):278–289, 1982
330. Van Duuren BB, Godschmidt BM, Katz C, Seidman I, Paul JS: Carcinogenic activity of alkylating agents. J Natl Cancer Inst 53:695–700, 1974
331. IARC Monographs on the Evaluation of the Carcinogenic Risk of Chemicals to Humans. Lyon, France: International Agency for Research on Cancer, 1982, Suppl 4, pp 122–124
332. Kucerova M, Zurkov VS, Polvkova Z, Ivanova JE: Mutagenic effect of epichlorhydrin. II. Analysis of chromosomal aberrations in lymphocytes of persons occupationally exposed to epichlorhydrin. Mutat Res 48:355–360, 1977
333. Kluwe WM, Gupta BN, Lamb JC IV: The comparative effects of 1,2-dibromo-3-chloropropane and its metabolites, 3-chloro-1,2-propane oxide (epichlorhydrin), 3-chloro-1,2-propanediol(a-chlorohydrin), and oxalic acid, on the urogenital system of male rats. Toxicol Appl Pharmacol 70(1):67–86, 1983
334. Milby TH, Whorton MD, Stubbs HA, et al: Testicular function among epichlorhydrin workers. Br J Ind Med 38(4):372–377, 1981
335. John JA, Gusohow TS, Ayres JA, et al: Teratologic evaluation of inhaled epichlorhydrin and alkyl chloride in rats and rabbits. Fundam Appl Toxicol 3(5):437–442, 1983
336. Marks TA, Gerling FS, Staples RE: Teratogenic evaluation of epichlorhydrin in the mouse and rat and glycidol in the mouse. J Toxicol Environ Health 9(1):87–96, 1982
337. U.S. Department of Health and Human Services, Public Health Service, Centers for Disease Control: NIOSH Current Intelligence Bulletin No. 35. Ethylene Oxide (ETO). Washington, D.C.: U.S. Government Printing Office, 1981
338. Finelli P, et al: Ethylene oxide-induced polyneuropathy: a clinical and electrophysiologic study. Arch Neurol 40:419–421, 1983
339. Ohnishi A, et al: Ethylene oxide induces central peripheral distal axonal degeneration of the lumbar primary neurones in rats. Br J Ind Med 42:373–379, 1985
340. Sulovska K, Lindgren DR, Erikkson G, Ehrenberg L: The mutagenic effect of low concentrations of ethylene oxide in air. Hereditas 62:264, 1969
341. Ehrenberg L, Hiesche KD, Osterman-Golkar, Wennberg I: Evaluation of genetic risks of alkylating agents: tissue doses in the mouse from air contaminated with ethylene oxide. Mutat Res 24:83–103, 1974
342. Hemminki K, et al: Spontaneous abortion in hospital staff engaged in sterilizing instruments with chemical agents. Br Med J 285:1461–1463, 1982
343. Hogstedt C, Rohlen BS, Berndtsson O, Axelson O, Ehrenberg L: A cohort study of mortality and cancer incidence in ethylene oxide production workers. Br J Ind Med 36:276–280, 1979
344. Hogstedt C, Malmquist N, Wadman B: Leukemia in workers exposed to ethylene oxide. JAMA 241:1132–1133, 1979

Relevance to Humans of Carcinogenesis Results from Laboratory Animal Toxicology Studies

1. Rall DP, Hogan MD, Huff JE, Schwetz BA, Tennant RW: Alternatives to using human experience in assessing health risks. Ann Rev Public Health 8:355–385, 1987
2. Hoel DG, Merrill RA, Perera FP (eds): Risk Quantitation and Regulatory Policy. Banbury Report 19. New York: Cold Spring Harbor Laboratory, 1985, pp 1–368
3. NRC Commission on Life Sciences (1983): Risk Assessment in the Federal Government: Managing the Process. Washington, D.C.: National Academy Press, 1983, pp 1–191
4. DHHS Task Force on Health Risk Assessment: Determining Risks to Health: Federal Policy and Practice. Dover, Mass.: Auburn House Publishing Co, 1986, pp 1–410
5. Rothman KJ: Modern Epidemiology. Boston: Little, Brown & Co, 1986, pp 1–358
6. Fraumeni JF Jr, Hoover RN, Devesa SS, Kinlen LJ: Epidemiology of cancer. In DeVita VT Jr, Hellman S, Rosenberg SA (eds): Cancer: Principles and Practice of Oncology. Vol. 1. 1989, pp 196–235
7. Tyler CW Jr, Last JM: Epidemiology. Chapter 2, this text.
8. International Agency for Research on Cancer (IARC): Reports on long-term and short-term assays for carcinogens: a critical appraisal. Report 1. Long-term assays for carcinogenicity in animals. IARC Sci Publ 83:14–83, 1986
9. Huff JE, McConnell EE, Haseman JK, et al: Carcinogenesis studies: results of 398 experiments on 104 chemicals from the U.S. National Toxicology Program. Ann NY Acad Sci 534:1–30, 1988
10. Tomatis L, Aitio A, Wilbourn J, Shuker L: Human carcinogens so far identified. Jpn J Cancer Res 80:795–807, 1989
11. Lijinsky W: In vivo testing for carcinogenicity. In Cooper CS, Grover PL (eds): Handbook of Experimental Pharmacology. Vol. 94/I. Berlin: Springer-Verlag, 1990, pp 179–209
12. Rall DP: Species differences in carcinogenesis testing. In Origins of Human Cancer. New York: Cold Spring Harbor Laboratory, 1977, pp 1383–1390
13. NRC/NAS: Pharmacokinetics in Risk Assessment: Drinking Water and Health. Vol. 8. Washington, D.C.: National Academy Press, 1987, pp 1–475
14. Hoel DG, Kaplan NL, Anderson MW: Implication of nonlinear kinetics on risk estimation in carcinogenesis. Science 219:1032–1037, 1983
15. Rall DP: Laboratory animal toxicity and carcinogenesis testing: underlying concepts, advantages and constraints. Ann NY Acad Sci 534:78–83, 1988
16. Hogan MD, Hoel DG: Extrapolation to man. In Hayes AW (ed): Principles and Methods of Toxicology, 2 edt. New York: Raven Press, 1989, pp 879–891
17. Weiss B, Laties VG: Comparative pharmacology of drugs affecting behavior. Fed Proc 26:1146–1156, 1987
18. IARC Monographs on the Evaluation of Carcinogenic Risks to Humans: Overall Evaluations of Carcinogenicity: An Updating of IARC Monographs. Lyon, France: International Agency for Research on Cancer, 1987, Vols 1 to 42, suppl 7
19. Doll R: Mortality from lung cancer in asbestos workers. Br J Ind Med 12:81–86, 1955
20. Kilburn KH: Asbestos and other fibers. Chapter 17, this text.
21. Saracci R: Asbestos and lung cancer: an analysis of the epidemiological evidence on the asbestos-smoking interaction. Int J Cancer 20:323–331, 1977
22. EPA Airborne Asbestos Health Assessment Update. Research Triangle Park, NC: U.S. Environmental Protection Agency, 1986, pp 1–198
23. IPCS International Programme on Chemical Safety: Environmental Health Criteria 53: Asbestos and Other Natural Mineral Fibres. Geneva: WHO, 1986, p 194
24. Lee AM, Fraumeni JF: Arsenic and respiratory cancer in man—an occupational study. J Natl Cancer Inst 42:1045–1052, 1969
25. Figueroa WG, Raszkowski R, Weiss W.: Lung cancer in chloromethyl methyl ether workers. N Engl J Med 288:1096–1097, 1973
26. IARC Monographs on the Evaluation of the Carcinogenic Risk of Chemicals to Humans: Polynuclear Aromatic Compounds. Part 3. Industrial Exposures in Aluminum Production, Coal Gasification, Coke Production, and Iron and Steel Founding. Lyon, France: International Agency for Research on Cancer, 1984, pp 133–190
27. Creech JL, Johnson MN: Angiosarcoma of liver in the manufacture of polyvinyl chloride. J Occup Med 16:150–158, 1974
28. Wagner JC, Sleggs CA, Morehand P: Diffuse pleural mesothelioma and asbestos exposure in the North Western Cape Province. Br J Ind Med 17:260–271, 1960
29. IARC Monographs on the Evaluation of the Carcinogenic Risk of

Chemicals to Humans: Some Industrial Chemicals and Dyestuffs. IARC Monographs, Vol 29. Lyon, France: International Agency for Research on Cancer, 1982, pp 93–148
30. Bailer AJ, Hoel DG: Metabolite-based internal doses used in a risk assessment of benzene. Environ Health Perspect 82:177–184, 1989
31. Lucier GW, Hood GER (eds): Symposium on benzene metabolism, toxicity and carcinogenesis. Environ Health Perspect 82:1–349, 1989
32. Huff JE, Hasemen JK, DeMarini DM, et al: Multiple-site carcinogenicity of benzene in Fischer 344 rats and B6C3F1 mice. Environ Health Perspect 82:125–163, 1989
33. Nicholson WJ, Landrigan PJ: Quantitative assessment of lives lost due to delay in the regulation of occupational exposure to benzene. Environ Health Perspect 82:185–188, 1989
34. IARC Monographs on the Evaluation of the Carcinogenic Risk of Chemicals to Humans: Some Antineoplastic and Immunosuppressive Agents. Vol 26. Chlorambucil. Lyon, France: International Agency for Research on Cancer, 1981, pp 115–136
35. Cannon SB, Veazey JM, Jackson RS, et al: Epidemic Kepone poisoning in chemical workers. Am J Epidemiol 107:529, 1978
36. Whorton D, Krauss RM, Marshall S, Milby TH: Infertility in male pesticide workers. Lancet 2:1259–1261, 1977
37. Taylor JF, Selhorst JB, Houff S, Martinez J: Chlordecone intoxication in man. Neurology (Minneap) 28:626, 1978
38. Bakir F, Damluji L, Amin-Zaki M, et al: Methylmercury poisoning in Iraq: an interuniversity report. Science 181:230–241, 1973
39. Needleman HL, Gunnae C, Leviton A, et al: Deficits in psychologic and classroom performance of children with elevated dentine lead levels. N Engl J Med 300:689–695, 1979
40. Allen N: Toxic polyneuropathy due to methyl-n-butyl ketone. Arch Neurol 32:209, 1975
41. Burns RS, Church CC, Markey SP, et al: A primate model of parkinsonism: selective destruction of dopaminergic neurons in the parts compacta of the substantia nigra by N-methyl-4-phenyl-1,2,3,6-tetrahydropyridine. Proc Natl Acad Sci 80:4546–4550, 1983
42. Sandler DP, Smith JC, Weinberg CR, et al: Analgesic use and chronic renal disease. N Engl J Med 320:1236–1271, 1989
43. Bingham E, Meader WV: Governmental regulation of environmental hazards in the 1990s. Annu Rev Public Health 11:419–434, 1990
44. Yang RSH, Huff JE, Boorman GA, et al: Chronic toxicology and carcinogenesis studies of telone II by gavage in Fischer-344 rats and B6C3F1 mice. J Toxicol Environ Health 18:377–392, 1986
45. Johnson BL, Turturro A, Freni SC, Hogan MD, Huff JE: Risk assessment and risk management of toxic substances: A report to the Secretary, DHHS, 1985, pp 336–386
46. Hoel DG: The impact of occupational exposure patterns on quantitative risk estimation. In Banbury Report 19: Risk Quantitation and Regulatory Policy. New York: Cold Spring Harbor Laboratory, 1985, pp 105–118
47. Hoel DG, Landrigan PJ: Comprehensive evaluation of human data. In Tardiff RG, Rodricks JV (eds): Toxic Substances and Human Risk. New York: Plenum, 1987, pp 121–130
48. Doll R, Wald NJ (eds): Interpretation of negative epidemiological evidence for carcinogenicity: Proceedings of a Symposium, Oxford, Lyon: IARC Sci Publ 65: 1–232, 1985
49. Peto R: Distorting the epidemiology of cancer: the need for a more balanced overview. Nature 284:297–300, 1980
50. Nelson N: Toxics and public health in the 1990s. Annu Rev Public Health 11:29–37, 1990
51. IARC Monographs on the Evaluation of Carcinogenic Risks to Humans. Lyon, France: International Agency for Research on Cancer. 1972–1990, Vols 1–48
52. Vainio H, Kemminki K, Wilbourn J: Data on the carcinogenicity of chemicals in the IARC Monographs programme. Carcinogenesis 6:1653–1665, 1985
53. Wilbourn J, Haroun L, Heseltine E, et al: Response of experimental animals to human carcinogens: an analysis based upon the IARC Monographs programme. Carcinogenesis 7:1853–1863, 1986
54. Tomatis L: Environmental cancer risk factors: a review. Acta Oncol 27:465–472, 1988
55. IARC Biennial Report. Lyon, France: International Agency for Research on Cancer 1988–1989, pp 1–246
56. Tomatis L, Agthe C, Bartsch H, et al: Evaluation of the carcinogenicity of chemicals: a review of the monograph program of the International Agency for Research on Cancer (1971–1977). Cancer Res 38(4):877–885, 1978
57. Merletti F, Heseltine E, Saracci R, et al: Target organs for carcinogenicity of chemicals and industrial exposures in humans: a review of results in the IARC Monographs on the Evaluation of Carcinogenic Risk of Chemicals to Humans. Cancer Res 44:2244–2250, 1984
58. Department of Health and Human Services, National Toxicology Program (NTP) Fifth Annual Report on Carcinogens. Research Triangle Park, N.C.: 1989, pp 1–746
59. Barrett JC: A multistep model for neoplastic development: role of genetic and epigenetic changes. In Barrett JC (ed): Mechanisms of Environmental Carcinogenesis. Vol 2. Boca Raton, Fla: CRC Press, 1987, pp 117–126
60. Boyd JA, Barrett JC: Genetic and cellular basis of multistep carcinogenesis. Pharmacol Ther 46:469–486, 1990
61. Barbacid M: *ras* Genes. Ann Rev Biochem 56:779–827, 1987
62. Anderson MW, Maronpot RR, Reynolds SH: Role of oncogenes in chemical carcinogenesis: extrapolation from rodents to humans. In Bartsch H, Hemminki K, O'Neill IK (eds): Methods for Detecting DNA Damaging Agents in Humans: Applications in Cancer Epidemiology and Prevention. IARC Sci Publ 89:477–485, 1988
63. Reynolds SH, Stowers SJ, Patterson RM, et al: Activated oncogenes in B6C3F1 mouse liver tumors: implications for risk assessment. Science 237:1309–1316, 1987
64. Reynolds SH, Stowers SJ, Patterson RM, et al: Oncogene activation of spontaneous and chemically induced rodent tumors: implications for risk analysis. Environ Health Perspect 78:175–177, 1988
65. Reynolds SH, Stowers SJ, Maronpot RR, et al: Detection and identification of activated oncogenes in spontaneously occurring benign and malignant hepatocellular tumors of the B6C3F1 mouse. Proc Natl Acad Sci USA 83:33–37, 1986
66. Wiseman RW, Stowers SJ, Miller EC, et al: Activating mutations of the C-Ha-ras protooncogene in chemically induced hepatomas of the male B6C3F1 mouse. Proc Natl Acad Sci USA 83:5825–5829, 1986
67. Huff JE, Eustis SL, Haseman JK: Occurrence and relevance of chemically induced benign neoplasms in long-term carcinogenicity studies. Cancer Metastasis Rev 8:1–21, 1989
68. Barrett JC, Oshimura M, Koi M: Role of oncogenes and tumor suppressor genes in a multistep model of carcinogenesis. In zur Hausen H, Schlehofer JR (eds): Critical Molecular Determinants of Carcinogenesis. Vol 39. Austin: University of Texas Press, 1987, pp 45–56
69. Barrett JC, Wiseman RW: Relevance of cellular and molecular mechanisms of multistep carcinogenesis to risk assessment. In Byrd DM III, Wilson JD (eds): Inferring Carcinogenic Effects in One Species With Data From a Different Species. New York: Telford Press (in press)
70. Weinberg RA: Oncogenes, antioncogenes, and the molecular bases of multistep carcinogenesis. Cancer Res 49:3713–3721, 1989
71. Office of Science and Technology (OSTP): Chemical carcinogens: a review of the science and its associated principles. Federal Register, pp 10371–10442, 1985
72. Office of Science and Technology (OSTP): Chemical carcinogenes: a review of the science and its associated principles. Environ Health Perspect 67:201–232, 1986
73. Office of Technology Assessment (OTA): Assessment of Technologies for Determining Cancer Risks from the Environment. Washington, D.C.: OTA, 1981, pp 1–240
74. Office of Technology Assessment (OTA): Identifying and Regulating Carcinogens: Background Paper. Washington, D.C.: Government Printing Office, 1987, pp 1–251
75. Shelby MD: The genetic toxicity of human carcinogens and its implications. Mutat Res 204:3–15, 1988
76. Shelby MD, Zeiger E: Activity of human carcinogens in the *Salmo-*

nella and rodent bone-marrow cytogenetics tests. Mutat Res 234: 257–261, 1990

77. IARC Monographs on the Evaluation of Carcinogenic Risks to Humans: Genetic and Related Effects: An Updating of Selected IARC Monographs from Volumes 1 to 42. Suppl 6, Lyon, France: International Agency for Research on Cancer, 1987, pp 727
78. Bartsch H, Malaveille C: Prevalence of genotoxic chemicals among animal and human carcinogens evaluated in the IARC Monograph series. Cell Biol Toxicol 5(2):115–127, 1989
79. Tomatis L: The predictive value of rodent carcinogenicity tests in the evaluation of human risks. Ann Rev Pharmacol Toxicol 19: 511–530, 1979
80. IARC Monographs programme preamble. IARC Monogr Eval Carcinog Risks Hum 48:13–31, 1990
81. Tomatis L: The value of long-term testing for the implication of primary prevention. In origins of human cancer. New York: Cold Spring Harbor Laboratory, 1977, pp 1339–1357
82. Huff JE, Melnick RL, Solleveld A, et al: Multiple organ carcinogenicity of 1,3-butadiene in B6C3F1 mice after 60 weeks of inhalation exposure. Science 227:548–549, 1985
83. Melnick RL, Huff JE, Bird M, Aquavella JF: Toxicology, carcinogenesis, and human health aspects of 1-3,butadiene: symposium overview. Environ Health Perspect 86:3–5, 1990
84. Melnick RL, Huff J, Chou BJ, Miller RA: Carcinogenicity of 1,3-butadiene in C57B1/6 and C3HF1 mice at low exposure concentrations. Cancer Res 50:6592–6599, 1990
85. Divine BJ: An update on mortality among workers at a 1,3-butadiene facility—preliminary results. Environ Health Perspect 86:119–128, 1990
86. Matanoski GM, Santos-Burgoa C, Schwartz L: Mortality of a cohort of workers in the styrene-butadiene polymer manufacturing industry (1943–1982). Environ Health Perspect 86:107–117, 1990
87. IARC Monographs on the Evaluation of the Carcinogenic Risk of Chemicals to Humans. Vol 28. The Rubber Industry. Lyon, France: International Agency for Research on Cancer, 1982, pp 1–486
88. Matanoski GM, Santos-Burgoa C, Zeger SL, Schwartz L: Epidemiologic data related to health effects of 1,3-butadiene. In Bates DV, Dungworth DL, Lee PN, et al (eds): ILSI Monographs: Assessment of Inhalation Hazards: Integration and Extrapolation Using Diverse Data. New York: Springer-Verlag, 1989, pp 201–214
89. Cantor KP, Blair A, Everett G, et al: Hair dye use and risk of leukemia and lymphoma. Am J Public Health 78:570–571, 1988
90. IARC Monographs on the Evaluation of the Carcinogenic Risk of Chemicals to Humans. Vol 27. Some Aromatic Amines, Anthraquinones and Nitroso Compounds, and Inorganic Fluorides Used in Drinking-water and Dental Preparations: Appendix 1 Epidemiological evidence relating to the possible carcinogenic effects of hair dyes in hairdressers and users of hair dyes. Lyon, France: International Agency for Research on Cancer, 1982, pp 307–318
91. Cantor KP, Hoover R, Hartge P, et al: Bladder cancer, drinking water source, and tap water consumption: a case-control study. J Natl Cancer Inst 79:1269–1279, 1987
92. Beaumont JJ, Leveton J, Knox K, et al: Lung cancer mortality in workers exposed to sulfuric acid mist and other acid mists. J Natl Cancer Inst 79:911–921, 1987
93. Levin SM, Baker DB, Landrigan PJ, Monaghan SV: Testicular cancer in leather tanners exposed to dimethylformamide. Lancet 2:1153, 1987
94. Ducatman AM, Conwill DE, Crawl J: Germ cell tumors of the testicle among aircraft repairmen. J Urol 136:834–836, 1986
95. Ducatman AM: Dimethylformamide, metal dyes, and testicular cancer. Lancet 1:911, 1989
96. Testicular cancer in leather workers—Fulton County, New York. MMWR 38:105–106, 111–114, 1989
97. Hogstedt C, Aringer L, Gustavsson A: Epidemiologic support for ethylene oxide as a cancer-causing agent. JAMA 255:1575–1578, 1986
98. Hogstedt LC: Epidemiological studies on ethylene oxide and cancer: an updating. In Bartsch H, Hemminki K, O'Neill IK (eds): Methods for Detecting DNA Damaging Agents in Humans: Applications in Cancer Epidemiology and Prevention. IARC Sci Publ 89:265–270, 1988
99. Hertz-Picciotto I, Neutra RR, Collins JF: Ethylene oxide and leukemia. JAMA 257:2290, 1987
100. Hertz-Picciotto I, Gravitz N, Neutra R: How do cancer risks predicted from animal bioassays compare with the epidemiologic evidence? The case of ethylene dibromide. Risk Anal 8:205–213, 1988
101. Alavanja MC, Rush GA, Stewart P, Blair A: Proportionate mortality study of workers in the grain industry. J Natl Cancer Inst 78:247–252, 1987
102. Blair A, Stewart PA, Hoover RN, Fraumeni JF Jr: Cancers of the nasopharynx and oropharynx and formaldehyde exposure. J Natl Cancer Inst 78:191–193, 1987
103. Blair A, Stewart PA, Hoover RN: Mortality from lung cancer among workers employed in formaldehyde industries. Am J Ind Med 17:683–699, 1990
104. Stayner LT: Human studies of formaldehyde exposure and cancers of the respiratory tract. In Feron VJ, Bosland MC (eds): Nasal Carcinogenesis in Rodents: Relevance to Human Health Risk. Proceedings of the TNO-CIVO/NYU Nose Symposium, Veldhoven, Netherlands, 1988, pp 98–109
105. AMA Council on Scientific Affairs: Formaldehyde. JAMA 261: 1183–1187, 1989
106. IPCS International Programme on Chemical Safety: Environmental Health Criteria 89: Formaldehyde. Geneva: World Health Organization, 1989, pp 1–219
107. Soffritti M, Maltoni C, Maffei F, Biagi R: Formaldehyde: an experimental multipotential carcinogen. Toxicol Ind Health 5:699–730, 1989
108. Sterling TD, Weinkam JJ: Reanalysis of lung cancer mortality in a National Cancer Institute study on "mortality among industrial workers exposed to formaldehyde." Exp Pathol 37:128–132, 1989
109. Delzell E, Monson RR: Mortality among rubber workers. VI. Men with exposure to acrylonitrile. J Occup Med 24:767–769, 1982
110. Koerselman W, van der Graaf M: Acrylonitrile: a suspected human carcinogen. Int Arch Occup Environ Health 54:317–324, 1984
111. O'Berg MT, Chen JL, Walrath J, Pell S: Epidemiologic study of workers exposed to acrylonitrile: an update. J Occup Med 27:835–840, 1985
112. Theiss AM, Frentzel-Beyme R, Link R, Wild H: Mortality study of chemical workers in different plants with exposure to acrylonitrile (Ger.). Zentralbl Arbeitsmed 30:259–267, 1980
113. Chen JL, Walrath J, O'Bert MT, Burke CA, Pell S: Cancer incidence and mortality among workers exposed to acrylonitrile. Am J Ind Med 11:157–163, 1987
114. Hearne FT, Grose F, Pifer JW, Friendlander BR, Raleigh RL: Methylene chloride mortality study: dose-response characterization and animal model comparison. J Occup Med 29:217–228, 1987
115. Hearne FT, Pifer JW, Crose F, Katz GV: Authors reply to letter to the editor. J Occup Med 30:478–481, 1988
116. Mirer FE, Silverstein M, Park R: Methylene chloride and cancer of the pancreas. J Occup Med 130:475–476, 1988
117. Stasik MJ: Carcinomas of the urinary bladder in a 4-chloro-o-toluidine cohort. Int Arch Occup Environ Health 60:21–24, 1988
118. Doll R: Occupational cancer: problems in interpreting human evidence. Ann Occup Hyg 28:291–305, 1984
119. Doll R: Occupational cancer: a hazard for epidemiologists. Int J Epidemiol 14:22–31, 1985
120. Doll R, Peto R: The causes of cancer. Oxford Medical Publications, Oxford University Press, 1981, p 112, J Natl Cancer Inst 66: 1197–1308, 1981
121. Schmahl D, Preussmann R, Berger MR: Causes of cancer—an alternative view to Doll and Peto (1981). Klin Wochenschr 67:1169–1173, 1989
122. Byers T, Graham S: The epidemiology of diet and cancer. Adv Cancer Res 41:1–61, 1984
123. Yang RSH, Huff J, Germolec DR, et al: Biological issues in extrapolation. In Ragsdale NN, Menzer RE (eds): ACS Symposium Series 414: Carcinogenicity and Pesticides: Principles, Issues, and Rela-

tionships. Washington, D.C.: American Chemical Society, 1989, pp 142-163

124. Haseman JK, Huff JE, Zeiger E, McConnell EE: Comparative results of 327 chemical carcinogenicity studies. Environ Health Perspect 74:229-235, 1987
125. Huff JE, Moore JA: Carcinogenesis studies design and experimental data interpretation/evaluation at the National Toxicology Program. In Jarvisalo J, Pfaffli P, Vainio H (eds): Industrial Hazards of Plastics and Synthetic Elastomers. New York: Alan R. Liss, 1984, pp 43-64
126. McConnell EE: The maximum tolerated dose: the debate. J Am Coll Toxicol 8:1115-1120, 1989
127. Huff JE: 1,2-Dibromo-3-chloropropane. Environ Health Perspect 47:365-369, 1983
128. Huff JE: 1,2-Dibromoethane (ethylene dibromide). Environ Health Perspect 47:359-363, 1983
129. Kari FW, Mennear JH, Farnel D, Thompson RB, Huff JE: Comparative carcinogenicity of two structurally similar phenylenediamine dyes (HC Blue No. 1 and HC Blue No. 2) in F344/N rats and $B6C3F_1$ mice. Toxicology 56:155-165, 1989
130. NAS/NRC Environmental Studies Board (1975): Contemporary Pest Control Practices and Prospects: The Report of the Executive Committee. 1. Pest Control: An Assessment of Present and Alternative Technologies. Washington, D.C.: NAS, 1975, pp 66-83
131. Crouch E, Wilson R: Interspecies comparison of carcinogenic potency. J Toxicol Environ Health 5:1095-1118, 1979
132. Meselson M, Russell K: Comparisons of carcinogenic and mutagenic potency. In Hiatt HH, Watson JD, Winsten JA (eds): Origins of Human Cancer: Book C: Human Risk Assessment. New York: Cold Spring Harbor Laboratory, 1977, pp 1473-1481
133. Piegorsch WW, Hoel DG: Exploring relationships between mutagenic and carcinogenic potencies. Mutat Res 196:161-175, 1988
134. Shipp AM, Crump KS, Allen BC: Correlation between carcinogenic potency of chemicals in animals and humans. Comments Toxicology 2:289-303, 1988
135. Lijinsky W: Commentary: importance of animal experiments in carcinogenesis research. Environ Mol Mutagen 11:307-314, 1988
136. IARC Information Bulletin on the Survey of Chemicals Being Tested for Carcinogenicity. Publication No. 13. Lyon, France: International Agency for Research on Cancer, 1988, p 403
137. Ames B, McCann J, Yamasaki E: Methods for detecting carcinogens and mutagens with the *Salmonella* mammalian microsome mutagenicity test. Mutat Res 31:347-364, 1975
138. Tennant RW, Margolin BH, Shelby MD, et al: Prediction of chemical carcinogenicity in rodents from in vitro genetic toxicity assays. Science 236:933-941, 1987
139. Hoel DG, Haseman JK, Hogan MD, Huff J, McConnell EE: The impact of toxicity on carcinogenicity studies: implications for risk assessment. Carcinogenesis 9:2045-2052, 1988
140. Mennear JH, McConnell EE, Huff JE, Renne RA, Giddens E: Inhalation toxicology and carcinogenesis studies of methylene chloride (dichloromethane) in F344/N rats and $B6C3F_1$ mice. Ann NY Acad Sci 534:343-351, 1988
141. Freireich EJ, Gehan EA, Rall DP, Schmidt LH, Skipper HE: Quantitative comparison of toxicity of anticancer agents in mouse, rat, hamster, dog, monkey, and man. Cancer Chemother Rep 50:219-244, 1966
142. Zeise L, Huff JE, Salmon AG, Hooper NK: Human risks from 2,3,7,8-tetrachlorodibenzo-*p*-dioxin and hexachlorodibenzo-*p*-dioxins. Environmental and Occupational Cancer. Scientific Update. Adv Mod Environ Toxicol 17:293-342, 1990
143. Rall DP: Carcinogens in our environment. In Vainio H, Sorsa M, McMichael AJ (eds): Complex Mixtures and Cancer Risk. IARC Sci Publ 104:233-239, 1990
144. Ward JM, Ito N: Development of new medium-term bioassays for carcinogens. Cancer Res 48:5051-5054, 1988

General References

Ames BN, Gold LS: Too many carcinogens: Mitogenesis increases mutagenesis. Science 249:970-971, 1990

Baserga R: The cell cycle: Myths and realities. Cancer Res 50:6769-6771, 1990

Chhabra RS, Huff JE, Schwetz BS, Selkirk J: An overview of prechronic and chronic toxicity/carcinogenicity experimental study designs and criteria used by the National Toxicology Program. Environ Health Perspect 86:313-321, 1990

Cohen SM, Ellwein LB: Cell proliferation in carcinogenesis. Science 249:1007-1011, 1990

Davis DL, Hoel, D (eds): Trends in cancer mortality in industrial countries: Ann NY Acad Sci 609:1-347, 1990

Dubach UC, Rosner B, Strumer MD: An epidemiologic study of analgesic drugs: Effects of phenacetin and salicylate on mortality and cardiovascular morbidity (1968 to 1987). N Engl J Med 324:155-160, 1991

DHHS/NTP: Fifth Annual Report on Carcinogens. Research Triangle Park, N.C.: National Toxicology Program. 1989, 745 pages

Eustis SL: The sequential development of cancer: A morphological perspective. Toxicol Lett 49:267-281, 1989

Hakama M, Beral V, Cullen JW, Parkin DM (eds): Evaluating Effectiveness of Primary Prevention of Cancer. IARC Scientific Publications No. 103. Lyon, France: International Agency for Research on Cancer. 1990, 206 pages

Haseman JK: Use of statistical decision rules for evaluating laboratory animal carcinogenicity studies. Fund Appl Toxicol 14:637-648, 1990

Haseman JK, Huff JE: Arguments that discredit animal studies lack scientific support. Chem Engin News 69:49-51, 1991

Haseman JK, Huff JE, Rao GN, Eustis SL: Sources of variability in rodent carcinogenicity studies. Fund Appl Toxicol 12:793-804, 1989

Huff JE: Chemical toxicity and chemical carcinogenesis. Is there a causal connection? In Use of Mechanistic Data to Evaluate the Carcinogenicity of Chemicals to Humans. IARC Sci. Pub. Lyon, France: International Agency for Research on Cancer. 1991 (in press)

Huff JE: Long-term chemical carcinogenesis studies: Strategy, results, and relevance to public health. Scand J Work Environ Health 1991 (in press)

Huff JE: Classification of chemical carcinogens: Levels of evidence of carcinogenicity developed and used by the National Toxicology Program (1983-1990). Scand J Work Environ Health 1991 (in press)

Huff JE: Merit and value of using experimental findings in the risk assessment process. Scand J Work Environ Health 1991 (in press)

Huff JE, Haseman JK: Long-term chemical carcinogenesis experiments for identifying potential human cancer hazards. Collective data base of the National Cancer Institute and National Toxicology Program (1976-1991). Environ Health Perspect 1991 (in press)

Huff JE, Haseman JK, Rall DP: Scientific concepts, value, and significance of chemical carcinogenesis studies. Ann Rev Pharmacol Toxicol 31:621-652, 1991

Huff JE, Cirvello J, Haseman JK, Bucher JR: Chemicals associated with site-specific neoplasia in 1394 long-term carcinogenesis experiments in laboratory rodents. Environ Health Perspect 1991 (in press)

Huff JE, Hoel DG: Hazard identification. Perspective and overview on the concepts and value of the initial phase in the risk assessment process of cancer and human health. Scand J Work Environ Health 1991 (in press)

IARC Monographs on the Evaluation of Carcinogenic Risks to Humans: Preamble. Lyon, France: International Agency for Research on Cancer. 1990, 415 pages

Melnick RL: Does chemically induced cell proliferation predict liver carcinogenesis? Cancer Res 1991. Submitted for publication

Melnick RL, Huff JE: 1,3-Butadiene: Toxicity and carcinogenicity in laboratory animals and in humans. Rev Environ Contam Toxicol 1991 (in press)

Muir C: Epidemiology, basic science, and the prevention of cancer: Implications for the future. Cancer Res 50:6441-6448, 1990

Parkin DM, Laara E, Muir CS: Estimates of the worldwide frequency of sixteen major cancers in 1980. Int J Cancer 41:184-197, 1988

Preston-Martin S, Pike MC, Ross RK, Jones, Henderson BE: Increased cell division as a cause of human cancer. Cancer Res 50: 7415-7421, 1990

Rao GN, Huff JE: Refinement of long-term toxicity and carcinogenesis studies. Fund Appl Toxicol 15:33-43, 1990

Steenland K, Stayner L, Greife A, Halperin W, Hayes R, Horning R, Nowlin S: Mortality among workers exposed to ethylene oxide. N Engl J Med 324:402–407, 1991

Stolley PD: The risks of phenacetin use (editorial). N Engl J Med 324:191–193, 1991

Tomatis L, Aitio A, Day NE, Heseltine E, Kaldor J, Miller AB, Parkin DM, Riboli E: Cancer: Causes, Occurrence and Control. IARC Scientific Publications No. 100. Lyon, France: International Agency for Research on Cancer. 1990, 352 pages

Vainio H: Classification of chemical carcinogens: Categories of evidence of carcinogenicity developed and used by the International Agency for Research on Cancer 1972–1991. Scand J Work Environ Health 1991 (in press)

Vainio H, Coleman M, Wilbourn J: Carcinogenicity evaluations and ongoing studies: The IARC databases. Environ Health Perspect 1991 (in press)

Walker AM, Cohen AJ, Loughlin JE, Rothman KJ, DeFonso LR: Mortality from cancer of the colon or rectum among workers exposed to ethyl acrylate and methyl methacrylate. Scand. J. Environ. Health 17:7–19, 1991

Ward E, Carpenter A, Markowitz S, Roberts D, Halperin W: Excess number of bladder cancers in workers exposed to ortho-toluidine and aniline. J Natl Cancer Inst 83:501–506, 1991

Weinstein IB: The origins of human cancer: Molecular mechanisms of carcinogenesis and their implications for cancer prevention and treatment--twenty-seventh G. H. A. Clowes Memorial Award Lecture. Cancer Res 48:4135–4143, 1988

Weinstein IB: Mitogenesis is only one factor in carcinogenesis. Science 251:387–388, 1991

Polychlorinated Biphenyls (PCBs)

1. Woodyard JP, King JJ: PCB Management Under TSCA. The Hazardous Waste Management Handbook Series. New York: Executive Enterprises Co., Inc. 1989
2. Kimbrough RD: Human health effects of polychlorinated biphenyls (PCBs) and polybrominated biphenyls (PBBs). Ann Rev Pharmacol Toxicol 27:87–111, 1987
3. Requiring EPA to prescribe marking and disposal regulations for PCBs by July 1, 1977. Federal Register 42:26563–26577, May 24, 1977
4. Regulations concerning storage, transport and use of PCBs after July 2, 1979. Federal Register 44:31514, May 31, 1979
5. Environmental Protection Agency: Polychlorinated biphenyls (PCBs); manufacturing, processing, distribution in commerce and use prohibition; use in closed and controlled waste manufacturing processes. Federal Register 47(204):46980–46996, 1982
6. Polychlorinated biphenyls spill cleanup policy. Federal Register 52(63):10688, April 2, 1987
7. Letz G: The toxicology of PCBs—an overview for clinicians. West J Med 138:534–540, 1983
8. Nadeau RJ, Allen HL, Prince RG: Hazard assessment and criteria development methodology applied at PCB incidents. In Government Institutes, Inc.: Hazardous Material Spills. Proceedings, April 19–22, 1982, Milwaukee, Wisconsin. Rockville, Md: Government Institutes, Inc., 1982
9. Moseley CL, Geraci CL, Burg J: Polychlorinated biphenyl exposure in transformer maintenance operations. Am Ind Hyg Assoc J 43: 170–174, 1982
10. Buser HR, Busshardt HR, Rappe C: Formation of polychlorinated dibenzofurans (PCDFs) from the pyrolysis of PCBs. Chemosphere 1:109–119, 1978
11. Hutzinger O, Blumich MJ, von den Berg M, Olie K: Sources and fate of PCDDs and PCDFs: an overview. Chemosphere 14:581–600, 1985
12. Kashimoto T, Miyata H, Shigehiko F, Kunita N, Ohi G, Tung TC: PCBs, PCQs and PCDFs in blood of yusho and yu-cheng patients. Environ Health Perspect 59:73–78, 1985
13. Waid JS (ed): PCBs and the environment. Vol 1. Boca Raton, Fla: CRC Press, 1987
14. Jensen S: The PCB story. Ambio 1:123–131, 1972
15. Risebrough RW, Reiche P, Peakall DB, Herman SG, Kirven MN: Polychlorinated biphenyls in the global ecosystem. Nature 220: 1098–1102, 1968
16. Stehr-Green PA, Burse VW, Welty E: Human exposure to polychlorinated biphenyls at toxic waste sites: investigations in the United States. Arch Environ Health 43:6:420–424, 1988
17. Schwartz PM, Jacobson SW, Fein G, Jacobson JL, Price HA: Lake Michigan fish consumption as a source of polychlorinated biphenyls in human cord serum, maternal serum and milk. Am J Public Health 73:293–296, 1983
18. Toxicological profile for selected PCBs (aroclor-1260, -1254, -1248, -1232, -1221 and -1016). Agency for Toxic Substances and Disease Registry (ATSDR). U.S. Public Health Service. ATSDR/TP-88/21, June 1989
19. Alvares AP, Bickers DR, Kappas A: Polychlorinated biphenyls: new type of inducer of cytochrome P-448 in the liver. Proc Natl Acad Sci USA 70:1321–1325, 1973
20. Allen JR: Response of the non-human primate to PCB exposure. Fed Proc 34:1965–1979, 1975
21. Kimbrough RD, Linder RE: Induction of adenofibrosis and hepatomas of the liver in Balb/cd mice by polychlorinated biphenyls (Aroclor 1254). J Natl Cancer Inst 53:547–552, 1974
22. Kimbrough RD, Squire R, Linder RE, et al: Induction of liver tumors in Sherman strain female rats by polychlorinated biphenyl (Aroclor 1260). J Natl Cancer Inst 55:1453–1459, 1975
23. McConnell EE: Comparative toxicity of PCBs and related compounds in various species of animals. Environ Health Perspect 60:29–33, 1985
24. Jones JW, Alden HS: An acneform dermatergosis. Arch Dermatol Syphilol 33:1022–1034, 1936
25. Schwartz L: An outbreak of halowax acne (''cable rash'') among electricians. JAMA 122:158–161, 1943
26. Good CM, Pensky N: Halowax acne (''cable rash''): a cutaneous eruption in marine electricians due to certain chlorinated naphthalenes and diphenyls. Arch Dermatol Syphilol 48:251–257, 1943
27. Meigs JW, Albom JJ, Siyali DS: Chloracne from an unusual exposure to Arochlor. JAMA 154:1417–1418, 1954
28. Kuratsune M: Yusho. In Kimbrough RD (ed): Halogenated Biphenyls, Terphenyls, Naphthalenes, Dibenzodioxins and Related Products. Amsterdam: Elsevier/North Holland Biomedical Press, 1980, pp 287–302
29. Higuchi K (ed): PCB Poisoning and Pollution. New York: Academic Press, 1976
30. PCB Poisoning in Japan and Taiwan. In Kuratsune M, Shapiro RE (eds): Progress in Clinical and Biological Research, Vol. 137. New York: Alan R. Liss, 1984
31. Environmental Health Perspectives, U.S. Department of Health and Human Services, National Institute of Environmental Health Sciences, vol. 59, February 1985
32. Nakanishi Y, Shigematsu N, Kurita Y, Matsuba K, Kanegae H, Ishimaru S, Kawazoe Y: Respiratory involvement and immune status in yusho patients. Environ Health Perspect 59:31–36, 1985
33. Rogan WJ, Gladen BC, Hung KL, Koong SL, Shih LY, Taylor JS, Wu YC, Yang D, Regan NB, Hsu CC: Congenital poisoning by polychlorinated biphenyls and their contaminants in Taiwan. Science 241:334–336, 1988
34. Rappe C, Buser HR, Kuroki Y, Masuda Y: Identification of polychlorinated dibenzofurans (PCDFs) retained in patients with yusho. Chemosphere 4:259–266, 1979
35. Maroni M, Colombi A, Arbosti G, Cantoni S, Foa V: Occupational exposure to polychlorinated biphenyls in electrical workers. II. Health effects. Br J Ind Med 38:55–60, 1981
36. Acquavella JF, Hanis NM, Nicolich MJ, Phillips SC: Assessment of clinical, metabolic, dietary and occupational correlations with serum polychlorinated biphenyl levels among employees at an electrical capacitor manufacturing plant. J Occup Med 28:1177–1180, 1986
37. Ouw HK, Simpson GR, Siyali DS: Use and health effects of Aroclor 1242, a polychlorinated biphenyl in an electrical industry. Arch Environ Health 31:189–194, 1976

38. Fischbein A, Wolff MS, Lilis R, Thornton J, Selikoff IJ: Clinical findings among PCB-exposed capacitor manufacturing workers. Ann NY Acad Sci 320:703–715, 1979
39. Chase KH, Wong O, Thomas D, Stal BW, Berney BW, Simon RK: Clinical and metabolic abnormalities associated with occupational exposure to polychlorinated biphenyls. J Occup Med 24:109–114, 1982
40. Emmett EA, Maroni M, Schmith JM, Levin B, Jefferys J: Studies of transformer repair workers exposed to PCBs. I. Study design, PCB concentrations, questionnaire and clinical examination results. Am J Ind Med 13:415–427, 1988
41. Kimbrough RD: Occupational exposure. In Kimbrough RD (ed): Halogenated Biphenyls, Terphenyls, Naphthalenes, Dibenzodioxins and Related Products. Amsterdam: Elsevier/North Holland Biomedical Press, 1980, pp 373–397
42. Smith AB, Schloemer J, Lowry LK, Smallwood AW, Ligo RN, Tanaka S, Stringer W, Jones M, Hervin R, Glueck CJ: Metabolic and health consequences of occupational exposure to polychlorinated biphenyls. Br J Ind Med 39:361–369, 1982
43. Brown JF Jr: Polychlorinated biphenyl (PCB) partitioning between adipose tissue and serum. Bull Environ Contam Toxicol 33:277–280, 1984
44. Lawton RW, Ross MR, Feingold J, Brown JF Jr: Effects of PCB exposure on biochemical and hematological findings in capacitor workers. Environ Health Perspect 60:165–184, 1985
45. Bahn AK, Rosenwaike I, Herrman N, Grover P, Stellman J, O'leary K: Melanoma after exposure to PCB. N Engl J Med 295:450, 1976
46. Brown DP, Jones M: Mortality and industrial hygiene study of workers exposed to polychlorinated biphenyls. Arch Environ Health 36:120–129, 1981
47. Bertazzi PA, Ribolidi L, Pesatori A, Radice L, Zochetti C: Cancer mortality of capacity manufacturing workers. Am J Indust Med 11:165–176, 1987
48. Brown DP: Mortality of workers exposed to polychlorinated biphenyls—an update. Arch Environ Health 42:333–339, 1987
49. Gustavsson P, Hogstedt C, Rappe C: Short-term mortality and cancer incidence in capacitor manufacturing workers exposed to polychlorinated biphenyls (PCBs). Am J Ind Med 10:341–344, 1986
50. International Agency for Research on Cancer (IARC): Polychlorinated biphenyls and polybrominated biphenyls. IARC Monogr Eval Carcinog Risk Chem Hum 18:3–124, 1978
51. Kreiss K, Zack MM, Kimbrough RD, Needham LL, Smrek AL, Jones BT: Association of blood pressure and polychlorinated biphenyls, JAMA 245:2505–2509, 1981
52. Akagi K, Okumura M: Association of blood pressure and PCB level in yusho patients. Environ Health Perspect 59:37–39, 1985
53. Piver WT, Lindstrom FT: Waste disposal technologies for polychlorinated biphenyls. Environ Health Perspect 59:163–177, 1985
54. Furukawa K: Microbial degradation of polychlorinated biphenyls (PCBs). In Chakrabarty A.M. (ed): Biodegradation and detoxification of environmental pollutants. Boca Raton, Fla: CRC Press, 1982, pp 33–37
55. Jones GRN: Polychlorinated biphenyls: where do we stand now? Lancet 2 (Sept. 30):791–794, 1989

Polybrominated Biphenyls (PBBs)

1. Carter LT: Michigan's PBB incident: chemical mix-up leads to disaster. Science 192:240–243, 1976
2. Kay K: Polybrominated biphenyls (PBB) environmental contamination in Michigan, 1973–1976. Environ Res 13:74–93, 1977
3. Jackson TF, Halbert FL: A toxic substance associated with the feeding of polybrominated biphenyls-contaminated concentrate to dairy cattle. J Am Vet Med Assoc 165:437–439, 1974
4. Miceli JN, Nolan DC, Marks B, Hariharan M: Persistence of polybrominated biphenyls (PBB) in human post-mortem tissue. Environ Health Perspect 60:399–403, 1985
5. Wolff MS, Aubrey B, Camper F, Haymes N: Relation of DDE and PBB serum levels in farm residents, consumers, and Michigan Chemical Corporation employees. Environ Health Perspect 23:177–181, 1978
6. Wolff MS, Anderson HA, Selikoff IJ: Human tissue burdens of halogenated aromatic chemicals in Michigan. JAMA 247:2112–2116, 1982
7. Gutenmann WH, Lisk DJ: Tissue storage and excretion in milk of polybrominated biphenyls in ruminants. J Agric Food Chem 23:1005–1007, 1975
8. Farber T, Kasza L, Giovetti A, et al: Effect of polybrominated biphenyls (Firemaster BP) on the immunologic system of the beagle dog. Toxicol Appl Pharmacol 45:343–344, 1978
9. Tsushimoto G, Trosko JE, Chang CC, Aust SD: Inhibition of metabolic cooperation in Chinese hamster V79 cells in culture by various polybrominated biphenyl (PBB) congeners. Carcinogenesis 3:181–186, 1982
10. Wasito L, Sleight SD: Promoting effect of polybrominated biphenyls on tracheal papillomas in Syrian golden hamsters. J Toxicol Environ Health 27:173–187, 1989
11. Evans MG, el-Fouly MH, Trosko JE, Sleight SD: Anchored cell analysis/sorting coupled with the scrape-loading/dye transfer technique to quantify inhibition of gap-junctional intercellular communication in WB-F344 cells by 2,2′, 4,4′, 5,5′ - hexabromobiphenyl. J Toxicol Environ Hlth 24:261–271, 1988
12. Smith AG, Francis JE, Carthew P: Iron as a synergist for hepatocellular carcinoma induced by polychlorinated biphenyls in Ah responsive C57BL/10ScSn mice. Carcinogenesis 11:437–444, 1990
13. Rezabek MS, Sleight SD, Jensen RK, Aust SD: Effects of dietary retinyl acetate on the promotion of hepatic enzyme-altered foci by polybrominated biphenyls in initiated rats. Food Chem Toxicol 27:539–544, 1989
14. Traber PG, Chianale J, Florence R, Kim K, Wojcik E, Gumucio JJ: Expression of cytochrome P450b and P450e genes in small intestinal mucosa of rats following treatment with phenobarbital, polyhalogenated biphenyls, and organochlorine pesticides. J Biol Chem 263:9449–9455, 1988
15. Anderson HA, Lilis R, Selikoff IJ, et al: Unanticipated prevalence of symptoms among dairy farmers in Michigan and Wisconsin. Environ Health Perspect 23:217–266, 1978
16. Roboz J, Suzuki RK, Bekesi JG, et al: Mass spectral identification and quantification of polybrominated biphenyl in blood compartments of exposed Michigan chemical workers. J Environ Pathol Toxicol 3:363–378, 1979
17. Bekesi JG, Holland JF, Anderson HA, et al: Lymphocyte function of Michigan dairy farmers exposed to polybrominated biphenyls. Science 199:1207–1209, 1978
18. Bekesi JG, Roboz JP, Solomon S, et al: Altered immune function in Michigan residents exposed to polybrominated biphenyls. In Gibson GG, Hubbard R, Parke DV (eds): Immunotoxicology. New York: Academic Press, 1983, pp 181–191
19. Bekesi JG, Roboz J, Fischbein A, Mason P: Immunotoxicology: environmental contamination by polybrominated biphenyls and immune dysfunction among residents of the state of Michigan. Cancer Detect Prev 1(suppl):29–37, 1987
20. Bekesi JG, Roboz J, Fischbein A, Roboz JP, Solomon S, Greaves J: Immunological, biochemical and clinical consequences of exposure to polybrominated biphenyls. In Dean JH, Luster MI, Munson AE, Amos H, (eds): Immunotoxicology and Immunopharmacology: New York: Raven Press, 1985, 393–405
21. Brilliant LB, Van Amburg GA, Isbister J, Humphrey H, Wilcox K, Eyster J, et al: Breast-milk monitoring to measure Michigan's contamination with polybrominated biphenyls. Lancet 2:643–646, 1978
22. Jacobson JL, Humphrey HE, Jacobson SW, Schantz SL, Mullin MD, Welch R: Determinants of polychlorinated biphenyls (PCBs), polybrominated biphenyls (PBBs) and dichlorodiphenyl trichloroethane (DDT) levels in the sera of young children. Am J Public Health 79:1401–1404, 1989
23. Breslin WJ, Kirk HD, Zimmer MA: Teratogenic evaluation of a polybromodiphenyl oxide mixture in New Zealand white rabbits following oral exposure. Fundam Appl Toxicol 12:151–157, 1989
24. Groce DF, Kimbrough RD: Stunted growth, increased mortality, and liver tumors in offspring of polybrominated biphenyl (PBB) dosed Sherman rats. J Toxicol Environ Health 14:695–706, 1984

22

Multiple Chemical Sensitivities

Mark R. Cullen

During the 1980s a curious clinical syndrome emerged in occupational and environmental health practice: an apparent intolerance to low levels of manufactured chemicals. Although it still lacks a widely agreed on definition or designation, the disorder idiosyncratically occurs in individuals who have experienced a single or recurring episodes of a typical chemical intoxication or injury such as solvent or pesticide poisoning. Subsequently, an expansive array of divergent environmental contaminants in air, food, or water may elicit respiratory, gastrointestinal (GI), dermal, and central nervous system (CNS) symptoms at doses far below those typically producing toxic reactions. Although the affected organs show no objective signs of impairment, patients' suffering may be extreme, causing considerable dysfunction and disability.

Although such reactions to chemicals are doubtless not new, it appears that multiple chemical sensitivities (or MCS, as the syndrome is now most frequently called) is occurring and presenting to medical attention far more commonly than in the past. Although little is known about its epidemiology (see below), it has become prevalent enough to have attracted its own group of specialists—clinical ecologists or environmental physicians—and substantial public controversy. Unfortunately, despite widespread debate over who should treat patients with the disorder and who should pay for it, little compelling research has yet emerged to resolve virtually any important scientific questions; the cause and pathogenesis, as well as strategies for treatment and prevention of MCS, remain entirely unknown. This state of affairs notwithstanding, MCS is clearly occurring and causing significant morbidity in the workforce and general populations and requires constructive scientific investigation.

Definition and Diagnosis. Although, as noted, there is not yet a consensus on one definition of MCS, certain salient features allow its differentiation from other well-characterized entities:

1. Symptoms begin after a more typical occupational or environmental disease, such as an intoxication or chemical insult. This "initiating" problem may have been one episode, such as accidental smoke inhalation, or repeated episodes, as in daily solvent intoxication. Often this event or events were mild and self-limited and may blur almost imperceptibly into the syndrome that follows.
2. Symptoms, initially often similar to those of the initiating illness, begin to occur after reexposure to lower levels of the same or related compounds.
3. Generalization of symptoms occurs such that multiple organ–system complaints are involved. Invariably these include symptoms referrable to the CNS, such as fatigue, confusion, and headache.
4. Generalization of precipitants occurs such that low levels of chemically diverse agents can elicit the responses, often at levels orders of magnitude below accepted threshold limit values (TLVs) or guidelines.
5. Work-up of complaints fails to reveal impairment of organs that would explain the pattern or intensity of complaints.
6. Frank psychosis or systemic illness that might explain the multiorgan symptoms is absent.

Although not every patient will fit this description precisely, it is important to consider each point before "labeling" patients with MCS or including them in any study population. Each criterion serves to rule out other disorders with which MCS may be confused: typical somatization disorder, classic sensitization to environmental antigens (e.g., occupational asthma), pathological sequelae of organ system damage (e.g., reactive airways dysfunction syndrome after a toxic inhalation), or a masquerading systemic disease (e.g., cancer with paraneoplastic phenomena). On the other hand, it is important to recognize that MCS is not a diagnosis of exclusion, nor should exhaustive and therapeutically disruptive (see below) tests be required in most cases. Even though many variations will be encountered, MCS has a quite unmistakable character that should allow prompt recognition in most cases.

In practice, the most difficult diagnostic problems with MCS fall into two categories. The first occurs with patients early in their course in whom it is often challenging to separate MCS from the more classic occupational or environmental health problem that generally precedes it. For example, patients who have experienced untoward reactions around organic solvents may find their reactions are persisting even when they have been removed from high-exposure areas or after these exposures have been properly abated; clinicians may assume that high exposures still exist and direct their attention to that, an admirable but unhelpful error. This is especially troublesome in the office setting, where MCS may be seen as a complication of typical sick building syndrome (see below). Whereas the typical office worker will respond quite promptly to steps that improve indoor air quality, the patient who has acquired MCS typically will continue to experience symptoms despite the far lower exposures involved. Again, continued attempts to improve the air quality may frustrate patient and employer alike.

Later in the disorder, confusion often is created by patients' reactions to chronic illness. The MCS patient who has been symptomatic for many months is often depressed and anxious, as are most medical patients with new chronic diseases to which they have not adapted. This may lead to a focus exclusively on psychiatric aspects, of which the chemically stimulated symptoms are viewed as part. Without questioning the importance or recognizing and treating these complications of MCS, nor the possibility that MCS itself has psychological origins, the underlying pattern of MCS must be recognized if appropriate management is to proceed.

Pathogenesis. It is not known what sequence of events causes some individuals to progress from a self-limited episode or episodes of occupational or environmental disease to potentially disabling symptomatic responses to very low levels of ubiquitous chemicals. Several theories have been offered, as described below.

The clinical ecologists and their adherents attribute the illness to immune dysfunction caused by excessive cumulative burden of xenobiotic material in susceptible hosts. Factors that enhance susceptibility in this theory include relative or absolute nutritional deficiencies (e.g., vitamins, antioxidants, essential fatty acids), the presence of subclinical infections such as candidal or other yeasts, and other life stresses.[1,2] In this view, the role of the "initiating" illness is important only insofar as it may contribute heavily to environmental overload, which is the cornerstone of the theory.

A less radical view, but one still based on immune dysfunction, is that MCS represents an amplification of traditional allergic phenomena due to neural or other sensory inputs.[3,4] According to this theory, underlying atopic manifestations may be elicited and modified by a range of chemicals, not directly triggering the classic cascades but interacting with them. Proponents cite the generally low upper respiratory tract irritation thresholds of hay fever sufferers and the known effects of irritants and odors on airway smooth muscle in asthmatics as perhaps better characterized examples of these phenomena.

Critics of clinical ecology have invoked a primarily psychological view of MCS, characterizing it in the spectrum of somatoform illness.[5] Variations of this view include the concept that MCS is a variant of classic posttraumatic stress disorder[6] or a conditioned response to an unpleasant environmental experience.[7] In these views, the initiating illness plays an obviously more central role in the pathogenesis of the disorder. Host factors may also be important, especially, for example, the predisposition to somaticize.

Less well developed positions have been profferred, suggesting that MCS may represent an unusual biological sequela of the initial injury.[8] As such, the disorder may be mediated by diverse mechanisms related to neurotoxicity (e.g., when the initiating illness is due to solvents or pesticides), injury to the respiratory tract (e.g., after an acute inhalational episode), or, less commonly, other organ system effects. In this view, MCS is seen as a final common pathway of divergent disease mechanisms.

Unfortunately, despite considerable literature on the subject, especially by the clinical ecologist group, little compelling clinical or experimental science has been published to prompt enthusiasm for any of these views or to refute them. Virtually no investigator has rigorously defined the population on which various tests have been performed nor carefully controlled these tests against an appropriately matched group of referent subjects. Neither subjects of research nor observers have generally been blinded to clinical status or research hypotheses. In the end, almost all existing data must be characterized as anecdotal.[9]

Most unfortunate of all, the legitimate debate over the etiological basis of the disorder has been heavily clouded by dogma. Since major economic decisions may hinge on the terms in which a case or cases generally are viewed (e.g., patient benefit entitlements, physician reimbursement acceptance), many physicians' strong views of the illness have inhibited scientific progress as well as patient care. It is essential to an understanding of MCS that the above theories are extant and often well known to patients, who often have very strong views themselves. As such, MCS differs markedly from other environmentally related disorders, such as massive fibrosis in miners, in which uncertainty about pathogenesis has not interfered with efforts to study the problem or manage its victims.

Epidemiology. Given the absence of a clear case definition, it is not surprising that detailed knowledge about the occurrence of MCS is lacking. Although estimates of its prevalence in the population range as high as 1% to 2%, the scientific basis of these remains obscure.[10] Almost all available data derive from anecdotal reports of practitioners who have treated patients with the disorder.

Despite the limitations of the data base, some general observations merit mention. Compared with other chronic occupational disorders, MCS appears to occur more commonly in somewhat younger workers (especially those in the fourth and fifth decades) and among those of higher socioeconomic status. Economically disadvantaged and nonwhite individuals seem underrepresented in most reports, although this may be an artifact of differential access, disease perception, or diagnostic bias. Women seem to be more frequently affected than men. Importantly, epidemiological evidence strongly suggests host idiosyncrasy as a factor, since clusters of cases rarely occur even after outbreaks of acute occupational or environmental disease that predispose.

In addition to these demographic features, some insights may be gleaned about the settings in which the illness occurs. Although many develop after nonoccupational exposures, for instance, in cars and homes, several groups of chemicals appear to account overwhelmingly for the majority of initiating events—organic solvents, pesticides, and respiratory irritants. Although this may be a function of the broad usage of these materials in our workplaces and general environment, they appear to be overrepresented in the histories of MCS patients. The other special setting in which many cases occur is in the so-called tight building, with victims of the typical "sick building syndrome" occasionally evolving into classic MCS pictures. Although the two illnesses share many symptoms in common, their epidemiological features readily distinguish them. "Sick building syndrome" typically affects most individuals sharing a common ("sick") environment and responds characteristically to environmental improvement; MCS occurs in isolation and does not abruptly respond to quantitative modifications of the environment.

A final issue of considerable interest is whether MCS is, in fact, a truly new disorder or whether it has only recently come to attention because of widespread interest in the environment as a source of human disease. Views on this are split, largely along the same lines as opinion regarding the pathogenesis of the disorder. Those who suspect a primarily biological role for environmental agents, including the clinical ecologists, would argue that MCS is uniquely a twentieth-century disease with rapidly rising incidence because of increased chemical contamination of the environment.[1,2] Contrarily, those who invoke primarily psychological mechanisms have argued that only the societal context of the disease is in any sense new. According to this view, the social perception of the environment as a hostile agent has resulted in the evolution of new symbolic content to the age-old problem of psychosomatic disease, changing the perception of patient and physician but not the fundamental disease mechanism.[11]

Natural History. Although MCS has yet to be subjected to careful clinical study sufficient to delineate its course or outcome, anecdotal experience with large numbers of patients has shed some preliminary light on this issue, which may be important in appropriate management. Based on this information, the general pattern of illness appears to be one of initial progression as the process of generalization evolves, followed by cyclical periods of gradual improvements and exacerbations. Although the patient generally perceives these cycles to be related to environmental alterations or treatment trials, the pattern seems to have some life of its own as well, although the basis for it is far from clear.

Two important corollaries follow from this observation. First, other than during the early stages in which the process emerges, there is little evidence to suggest that the disease is in any sense progressive.[12] Patients do not tend to deteriorate from year to year, nor have obvious complications such as infections or organ system failure resulted. There is no evidence of mortality from MCS, although virtually every patient becomes convinced that progression and death are inevitable, based on the profound change in perception of health that the disorder engenders.

Even though this observation may provide the basis for a sanguine prognosis and reassurance, it has been equally clear from described clinical experience that true remission of symptoms is also highly improbable. Various good outcomes have been described, but these are invariably based on improved patient function and sense of well-being. The underlying tendency to react adversely to chemical exposures continues, although symptoms may become sufficiently tolerable to allow return to a near-normal life style.

In sum, MCS appears to be a disorder with well-defined upper and lower bounds in outcome. Neither limit has been confirmed by large, well-characterized series, but it is probably not premature to include this assumption in planning treatment and assisting in vocational rehabilitation.

Clinical Management. Little is known about treatment of patients with MCS. Although a vast array of modalities have been proposed and tried, none has been subjected to the usual scientific standards to determine efficacy. As with other aspects, theories of treatment follow closely the theories of pathogenesis. Clinical ecologists, convinced that MCS represents immune dysfunction caused by excessive body burden of xenobiotics, focus much of their attention on reducing burden by strict avoidance of chemicals[1,2]; some have advocated extreme steps resulting in complete alterations in patient life style. This approach is often accompanied by efforts to determine "specific" sensitivities by various forms of skin and blood testing—none as yet validated by acceptable standards—and using therapies akin to desensitization to induce "tolerance." Coupled with this are a variety of strategies to bolster underlying immunity with dietary supplementation, eradication of "infections" (e.g., *Candida*), and other metabolic supports. A most radical approach involves efforts to eliminate toxins from the body by chelation or accelerated turnover of fat (where some presumed causal agents are stored).

Those inclined to a more psychological view of the disorder have explored alternative approaches consistent with their theories. Supportive individual or group therapies and more classic behavioral methods have been described.[13] However, as with the more biological theories, the efficacy of these approaches remains conjectural.

Although none of these modalities is likely to be directly dangerous, limitations to present knowledge suggest that they are best reserved for settings in which well-controlled trials are being undertaken. In the meantime, certain treatment principles, discussed below, can be justified based on present knowledge and experience.

Taking steps to limit, to the extent possible, the search for the mysterious "cause" of the disease is an important first aspect of treatment. Many patients will have had considerable work-up by the time MCS is considered and will equate, not totally irrationally, extensive testing with extensive pathologic findings. Uncertainty feeds this cycle, as well as patients' common underlying fear that they have been irrevocably poisoned.

Whatever the clinician's theoretical proclivity, he or she must ensure that the patient understands the existing knowledge and uncertainty about MCS, including specifically that its cause is unknown. The patient must be reassured that the possibility of a psychological basis does not make the illness less real, less serious, or less worthy of treatment. Further reassurance that the disease will not lead to death is also valuable, coupled with caution that total cure is unrealistic.

Steps to remove patients from the most obviously offensive aspects of their environment are almost always necessary, especially if a patient still lives or works in the same environment where the initiating illness occurred. Although radical avoidance is probably counterproductive, given the goal of improving function, protection from daily misery is important in establishing the strong therapeutic relationship that the patient needs. In general, this means a vocational change, which will require attention to sufficient benefits to make this option viable for the patient. For cases due to an occupational illness, however mild, workers' compensation may be available; most jurisdictions will compensate for MCS if it can be demonstrated to be a complication of some disorder that is more easily understood as work related.

Having established this foundation of support, the goal of all subsequent therapy should be to develop improved function. Obviously psychological problems, for instance, adjustment difficulties, anxiety, or depression, should be treated, as should coexistent pathologic findings such as usual allergic manifestations. Unfortunately, since these patients do not tolerate chemicals readily, nonpharmacological approaches may be necessary. Beyond these measures, patients need direction, counseling, and reassurance to begin the challenging process of adjusting to an illness that they do not understand and for which there is no established treatment. To the extent consistent with tolerable symptoms, patients should be encouraged to expand the range of their activities (including work) and should be discouraged from passivity, dependence, or resignation, which intermittently recur throughout the course of the illness. No evidence suggests that an unpleasant exposure carries more risk than short-term provocation of symptoms.

Although it is appropriate to provide patients with all available factual information about MCS, many patients will get desperate and may try available alternative treatment modalities, sometimes several at once or in sequence. It is probably not reasonable to resist such efforts or to undermine a therapeutic relationship on this account but rather to hold steadily to a single coherent perspective, treating the "treatment" as yet another troublesome aspect of a troublesome condition.

Prevention. Primary prevention cannot be seriously considered, given present knowledge of pathogenesis of the disorder or the host factors that render certain individuals susceptible to it. At this time, the most reasonable approach is to reduce the opportunities in the workplace and ambient environment for the kinds of acute exposures that appear to precipitate MCS in some hosts, especially solvents and pesticides. Better ventilation in offices would probably be helpful as well.

Secondary prevention appears to offer some greater control opportunity, although no intervention has been studied. Because psychological factors may play a role in victims of environmental mishaps, careful, early management of such individuals seems advisable, even if the prognosis from a biological perspective is good. For example, patients seen in clinics or emergency rooms after acute illnesses should have their reactions to the events explored and should probably receive very close follow-up examination if they express undue fears of long-term effects or recurrence. Equally important, efforts must be made on behalf of such patients to ensure that preventable recurrences do not occur, since recurrences may be an important pathway leading to MCS by whichever mechanism—biological or psychological—is truly responsible.

REFERENCES

1. Bell IR: Clinical Ecology. Colinas, Calif.: Common Knowledge Press, 1982
2. Levin AS, Byers VS: Environmental illness: A disorder of immune regulation. Occup Med 2:669–682, 1987
3. Adkinson NF: Environmental influences on the immune system and allergic reactions. Environ Health Perspec 20:97, 1977
4. Muranaka M, Suzuki S, Koizuni K, et al: Adjuvant activity of diesel exhaust particles for the production of IgE antibodies in mice. J Allerg Clin Immunol 77:616, 1986
5. Brodsky CM: Psychological factors contributing to somatoform diseases attributed to the workplace. The case of intoxication. J Occup Med 25:459–464, 1983
6. Schottenfeld RS, Cullen MR: Occupation-induced post-traumatic stress disorder. Am J Psychol 142:198–202, 1985
7. Bolle-Wilson K, Wilson RJ, Bleecker ML: Conditioning of physical symptoms after neurotoxic exposure. J Occup Med 30:684–686, 1988
8. Bach B, Molhave L, Pederson OF: Human reactions during controlled exposures to low concentrations of organic gases and vapors known as normal indoor air pollutants. In Berglund B, Lindvall T, Sundell J (eds): Indoor Air: Proceedings of the Third International Conference on Indoor Air Quality and Climate, vol. 3. Stockholm: Swedish Council for Building Research, 1984, pp. 397–402
9. Cullen MR: Multiple chemical sensitivities: Summary and directions for future investigations. Occup Med 2:801–804, 1987
10. Mooser SB: The epidemiology of multiple chemical sensitivities. Occup Med 2:663–668, 1987
11. Brodsky CM: Multiple chemical sensitivities and other "environmental illnesses": A psychiatrist's view. Occup Med 2:695–704, 1987
12. Terr AL: Environmental illness: A chemical review of 50 cases. Arch Intern Med 146:145–149, 1986
13. Lewis BM: Workers with multiple chemical sensitivities: Psychosocial interventions. Occup Med 2:791–800, 1987

23

Pulmonary Responses to Gases and Particles

Kaye H. Kilburn

This chapter defines the functional zones of the human lung, describes responses to occupationally polluted air, reviews the adverse health effects caused by environmental air pollution, and considers indoor air pollution.

FUNCTIONAL ZONES OF HUMAN LUNG

The lung has two regions: the conducting airways and the gas-exchanging alveolar zone. In the former, a mucociliary escalator removes deposited particles. The alveolar zone, which includes alveolarized respiratory bronchioles and alveolar ducts, lacks this ability[1] (Fig. 23-1). The two zones have vastly different defences, and thus their susceptibilities to damage differ. For example, water-soluble gases such as sulfur dioxide and ammonia absorb to proximal conducting airways, while relatively insoluble ozone and nitrogen dioxide damage the non-mucous-covered alveolar zone (Table 23-1). The airways selectively filter particles from the nose to the alveolar ducts. Thus, large particles (50 μm in diameter) lodge in the nose or pharynx, but particles must be under 10 μm (and usually below 5 μm) to reach the alveolar zone.[2] Fungal spores with diameters of 17 to 20 μm affect only proximal conducting airways (Fig. 23-2), while the 1 μm diameter spores of *Micropolyspora faeni* affect alveoli as well (Fig. 23-3). As a first approximation, reactions to particles can be predicted from their size, which is best defined by the mean median diameter, and from solubility in water. Where fibers and fibrils lodge is predicted from aerodynamic diameter, not from length.

OCCUPATIONALLY POLLUTED AIR

Acute Alveolar Reactions

Asphyxiant Gases. Asphyxiant gases, which include carbon dioxide, carbon monoxide, hydrogen cyanide, hydrogen sulfide, methane, and the fluorocarbons, essentially displace oxygen from alveoli and cause death. Their properties, exposure sources, toxicity, and applicable standards for occupational exposure in the United States are listed in Table 23-1. Carbon dioxide stimulates respiration at concentrations under 10% but depresses breathing at higher concentrations and is anesthetic. The occupational hazard generally occurs in men going into poorly ventilated chambers, often underground. For example, carbon dioxide, methane, and hydrogen sulfide are generated from manure collected from cattle feeding lots or from sewage and in wells, pits, silos, holds of ships, or abandoned mine shafts. Workers entering these areas collapse after a few breaths. Tragically, the first attempted rescuer often dies of asphyxiation before it is realized that the exposure is lethal.

Arc welding is a particular hazard in small compartments, since it does not require oxygen but burns organic material with oxygen to produce carbon monoxide; if ventilation is restricted, lethal quantities of carbon monoxide may accumulate in the compartment. Methane, as coal damp, is an asphyxiant and an explosion hazard for miners. Community contamination with hydrogen sulfide has occurred from coal seams in Gillette, Wyo., from evaporative (salt crystallization) chemistry in Trona, Calif., and from hydrocarbon petroleum refining in Ponca City, Okla., and Nipoma, Calif. However, the most serious incident of this type was the Bhopal, India, disaster of 1984. Methyl isocyanate (used in manufacturing the insecticide carbaryl [Sevin]) escaped from a 21-ton liquid storage tank, killing over 2300 people and injuring more than 30,000.

Hydrogen sulfide inhalation produced nausea, headache, shortness of breath, sleep disturbances, and throat and eye irritation at concentrations of 0.003 to 11 mg/m^3 during a series of intermittent air pollution episodes over a 2-month period. Hydrogen sulfide at concentrations of about 150 ppm quickly paralyzes the sense of smell, so that victims may be unaware of danger. Instantaneous death has occurred at levels of 1400 mg/m^3 (1000 ppm) to 17,000 mg/m^3 (12,000 ppm). As the level of hydrogen sulfide increases in the ambient environment, symptoms vary from headache, loss of appetite, burning eyes, and dizziness at low concentrations, to low blood pressure, arm cramps, and unconsciousness at moderate concentrations, to pulmonary edema, coma, and death at higher concentrations. The recommended occupational standard for carbon dioxide is 0.5%, but for carbon monoxide it is 50 ppm for an 8-hour workday, with a single exposure to 200 ppm considered dangerous for chronic as well as acute impairment of the central nervous system (CNS). Since hydrogen sulfide is highly toxic even at low concentrations, the Occupational Safety and Health Administration (OSHA) has not set a time-weighted average for an 8-hour day. Instead, 20 ppm has been set as a maximum 15-minute exposure.

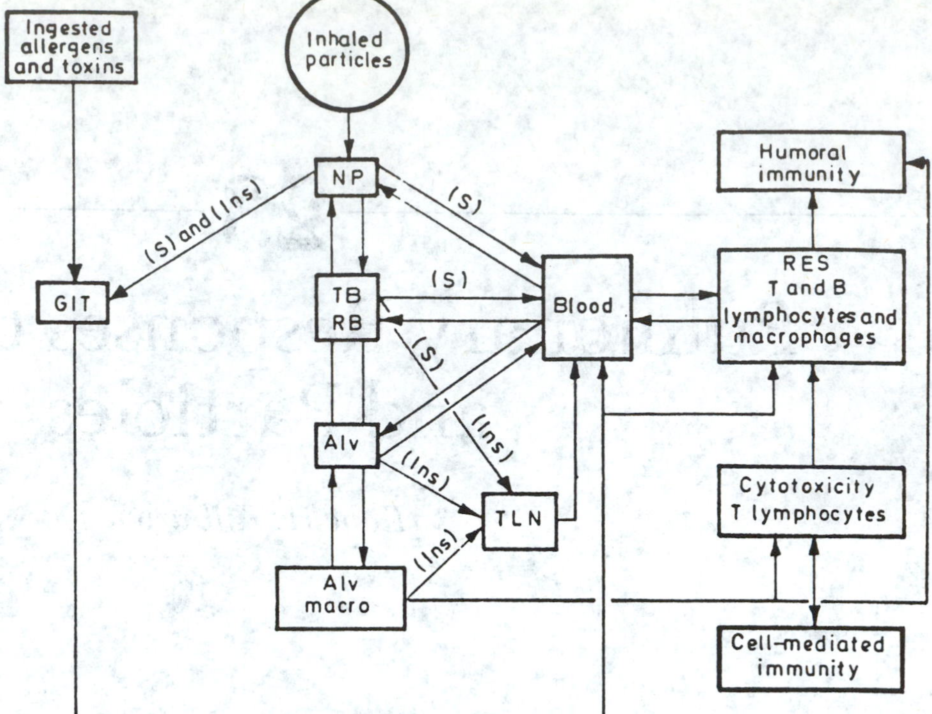

Figure 23-1. Diagram showing the possible fates and influence of inhaled aerosols and ingested materials. Alv., alveolus; Alv. macro, alveolar macrophages; GIT, gastrointestinal tract; Ins, insoluble particles; NP, nasopharynx; RB, red blood cell; RES, reticulo-endothelial system; S, soluble particles; TB, terminal bronchioles; TLN thoracic lymph nodes. *[Adapted from Kilburn, 1968,[1] by courtesy of the Editor of American Review of Respiratory Diseases]*

TABLE 23-1. PROPERTIES, SOURCES, AND TOXICITY OF COMMON GASES

Name	Formula	Color and Odor	Sources of Exposure	Health Effects: Acute	Health Effects: Chronic	OSHA (TWA)[a] (ppm)	IDLH[b] (ppm)
▪ ASPHYXIANT GASES							
Carbon dioxide	CO_2	c, ol	M, We, FC	A, H, D, Ch		5,000	50,000
Carbon monoxide	CO	c, ol	CS, T, FC	A, H, Cv, Co		50	1,500
Carbon disulfide	CS_2	c, so	CM	H, D	Np	20	500
Hydrogen sulfide	H_2S	c, re	Ae, D, Ng, P	A, Pe, D, H, Co	Np	(20) ceiling	300
Methane	CH_4	c, ol, f	Ng, D	A			
▪ OXIDANT GASES							
Ozone	O_3	c, po	S, EA, W, AC	T, Pe, Mm, Tp	AO	0.1	10
Nitrogen oxides	NO	rb, po	W	T, Mm, Pe, Tp		25	100
	NO_2 (N_2O_4)	rb, po	CS, W, FC	Ch	AO	5	50
▪ IRRITANT GASES							
Sulfur dioxide	SO_2	c, po	P	T, Mm, Tp, Pe, Ch		5	100
Ammonia	NH_3	c, po	Ae, Af, Cm	A, Pe, Mm, Tp, T, Ch		50	500
Formaldehyde	HCHO	c, po, p	CS, CM	T, Mm, Ch, Tp	AO, Ca		
Acetaldehyde	CH_3CHO	c, po, p	CS, CM	T, Mm, Ch, Tp	AO	2	100
Acrolein		c, po, p	CS, CM	T, Mm, Ch, Tp	AO	0.1	5
Chlorine		gy, po	CM	Pe, Mm, Ch, T, H, D, L	AO	1	25
Bromine		rb, po	CM	Pe	AO	1	10
Fluorine		y, po	CM	Pe	AO	0.1	25
Hydrogen fluoride	HF	c, po	CM	Pe, T, Mm, B	AO	3	20
Hydrogen bromide	HB_r	c, po	CM	Pe, T, Mm, B	AO	3	50
Hydrogen chloride	HCL	c, po	CM	Pe, T, Mm, B	AO	5	100
Phosgene	$COCl_2$	c ol-po	CM	Pe, T, Mm, Ch Tp, B	AO	0.1	2
Carbon tetrachloride	CCl_4	c, so		H, D, Pe	L, Np	10	300
Chloroform	$CHCl_3$	c, so	CM	H, D, Pe, Co	L, Np	50	1,000
Vinyl chloride	$CH_2{=}CHCL$	c, so, p	CM	H, D, Mm	Ca, AOL, Np	1	5
Vinylidene chloride	$CH_2{=}CCl_2$	c, so, p	CM	B, Mm	Ca	10	50

Color and Odor: c, colorless; f, flammable; gy, green, yellow; o, odorless; p, polymerizes; po, pungent; rb, red-brown; re, rotten eggs; so, sweet.
Sources: AC, aircrew; Ae, animal excreta; Af, agrifertilizer; CM, chemical manufacture; CS, cigarette smoke; D, dumps; EA, electric arcs; FC, fuel combustion; M, mining; Ng, natural gas; P, petroleum drilling, refining; S, stratosphere; T, tunnels; W, welding; We, Wells.
Health Effects: A, asphyxiant; AO airways obstruction; AOL, acroosteolysis; B, burns skin; Ca, cancer; Ch, cough; Co, coma; Cv, depresses heart rate; D, dizziness; H, headache; L, liver; Mm, mucous membrane irritation; Np, neuropsychological toxin; Pe, pulmonary edema; T, tearing; Tp, tracheal pain.
[a] TWA, time weighted average.
[b] IDLH, level of immediate danger to life or health.

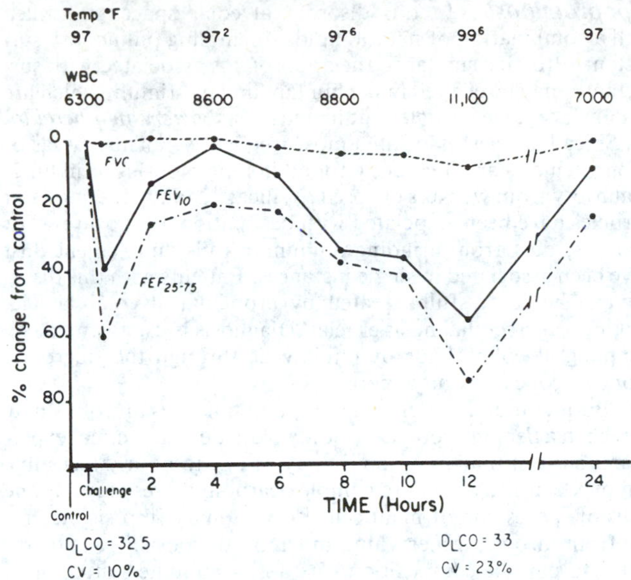

Figure 23-2. Effects of exposure to aspergilli.

Oxidant Gases. A potent oxidizing agent, ozone is a bluish pungent gas generated by electrical storms, arcs, and ultraviolet light. Ozone and nitrogen oxides are important in environmental air pollution. At high altitudes the ozone shield protects against solar radiation. Excess ozone is found on board high-flying, long-distance aircraft, particularly over the North Pole, if adequate adsorption is absent. Exposure to ozone, nitrogen dioxide, and other oxidant gases is found mainly in welding, near electric generation, and in the chemical industry (Table 23-1). Nitrogen dioxide has a pungent odor most remarkable in fuming nitric acid, silos containing alfalfa, and manufacture of feeds, fertilizers, and explosions. Although ozone and nitrogen dioxide irritate mucous membranes and the eyes, they exert their effects in the distal zone of the lung, the respiratory bronchioles and alveoli ducts. These gases enter alveolar epithelial cells, produce swelling, and secondarily affect the capillary endothelial cells. The thin alveolar membranes are then rendered permeable to plasma fluids and proteins, which leads to pulmonary edema after exposure to large concentrations. Exposure to nitrogen oxides, principally nitrogen dioxide generated in silos by silage, in animal feed processing, and in nitrocellulose film fires in movie theaters, caused subacute necrotizing bronchiolitis in survivors of acute pulmonary edema. Sulfur dioxide may also cause alveolar edema but is extremely irritating; unless doses are unbearably high, the nose and upper airways absorb enough to reduce the amount reaching the alveoli.

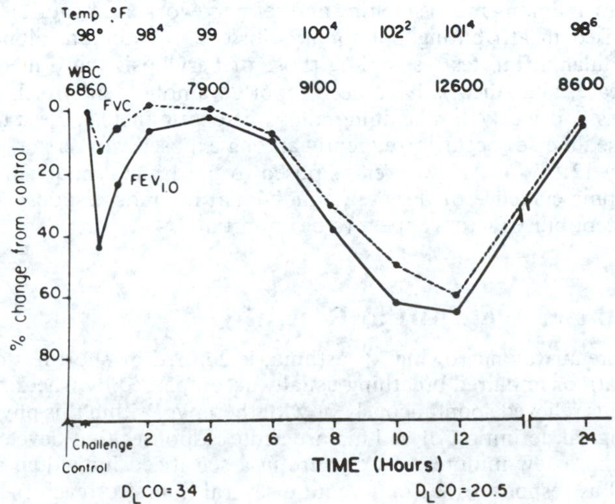

Figure 23-3. Effects of exposure to thermophiles.

Irritant Gases. The irritant gases include several halogens, fluorine, bromine, and chlorine, hydrochloric acid, hydrogen fluoride, phosgene (a poison gas used in World War I), sulfur dioxide, ammonia, and dimethyl sulfate. Vanadium pentoxide, osmium, and platinum as finally divided fumes act like gases. The sources are generally industrial processing, although inadvertent production may occur. In addition, bromine and chlorine are injected to sterilize municipal water supplies, so that large amounts of concentrated gas are stored in heavily populated cities. One of the desulfurization processes for petroleum uses vanadium pentoxide as a catalyst for hydrogen sulfide, and although portions of this are regenerated, workplace and environmental exposures have occurred. When ammonia is injected into soil as liquid ammonia for agricultural or industrial purposes, workers may inhale large quantities.

Although these gases are classified as irritants, in large quantities they damage alveolar lining cells and capillary endothelial cells, causing alveolotoxic pulmonary edema. They may also severely damage the epithelial surface of airways. The mechanism is pulmonary edema from destruction of both alveolar epithelial cells and the capillary endothelium, such that the fluid and protein that the lymphatic system cannot remove overflow into alveoli. The fluid moves up into the terminal bronchioles and hence into the conducting airways, to be heard as rales on examination.

Particles. Particles causing alveolar edema include small fungal spores such as *M. faeni,* bacterial endotoxins, and metal fumes (particles), particularly vanadium pentoxide, osmium, platinum cadmium, and cobalt. Particles may be generated from vegetable crops used as food, fiber, or forage, as aerosols from sewage or animal fertilizer, or from petroleum desulfurization in large enough amounts that acute inhalation produces pulmonary edema. Onset may range from minutes to hours.

Mixtures. Mixtures created by combustion of fuel, such as diesel exhaust in mines and welding fumes, particularly in compartments with limited ventilation, may reach edemagenic levels due to concentrations of ozone, nitrogen dioxide, formaldehyde, and acrolein. Again, if combustion or arcing takes place in a limited air space without adequate ventilation, pulmonary edema or acute airways obstruction is likely.

Therapy. Afflicted individuals require oxygen delivered under positive pressure by mask. This restores for oxygenation alveoli blocked by foaming of edema fluid and rapidly improves systemic oxygenation. Morphine (which is a respiratory depressant), diuretics, fluid restriction, or adrenal corticosteroids are secondary measures. Speed is crucial. If breathing is impaired or the patient is unconscious, intubation and artificial ventilation may be required.

Control. Control and surveillance include avoiding areas where harmful gases may collect. Personnel must don self-contained breathing apparatus or air supply respirators before entering such areas and work in such areas only with adequate provision for air exchange. All rescuers of afflicted individuals should wear an individual air or oxygen supply or enter with a means by which they can be retrieved safely by a fellow worker if needed.

Appropriate and specific rules should be devised and posted for personnel.

Prevention. Opportunities for gas leakage and accumulation should be minimized by industrial hygiene surveillance; the above advice postulates that every effort has been made to minimize leakage and maximize avoidance.

Chronic Alveolar Disease

Extrinsic allergic alveolitis, lipoproteinosis, and granulomatous alveolitis are disorders of the alveolar cells or alveolar spaces that are caused by inhalation of chemically active particles. They are described briefly below.

Nongranulomatous Alveolitis, Allergic Pneumonitis. The original description of extrinsic allergic alveolitis, or farmer's lung, implicated inhalation of fungal spores and vegetable material from hay or grain dust,[3] which recruited cells to alveoli. Some exposed farmers developed shortness of breath, and frequently precipitating antibodies to crude preparations of fungi were found in their serum. However, antibodies were also found in asymptomatic farmers. Farmer's lung occurred in areas where animal feeds were stored wet, with the consequent enhanced generation of fungal spores. Classic descriptions came from Northwest England,[4] Scotland,[5] and the North-Central U.S. dairy states.[6] Both the size of the spores, under 7 μm to be respirable but under 3 μm to reach alveoli, and their solubility influence the disorder. Their toxins, including endotoxins, are important in the pathogenesis of farmer's lung, and hypersensitivity may be responsible for part of the pathological picture. Whether this is type IV allergy or also type III is not clear. Initial high-dose exposure to spores frequently produces both airway narrowing and acute pulmonary edema (see Fig. 23-3).[7] Hospitalization with oxygen therapy has been required. After repeated exposure and development of precipitating antibodies, many cells may be recruited into alveoli. This pneumonitis can be lethal with repeated heavy exposure. On the other hand, the reaction may clear completely during absence from exposure. Adrenal corticosteroids frequently help resolve the acute phase but do not affect the chronic fibrotic stage.

Berylliosis. Beryllium, a dense, corrosion-resistant metal, produces fulminant chemical pneumonia when inhaled as a soluble salt in large doses. Inhalation of fumes or fine particles leads to chronic granulomatous alveolitis. Originally beryllium disease was interpreted as an accelerated sarcoidosis.[8] First recognized in workers making phosphores for fluorescent lamps, berylliosis is recognized pathologically by noncaseating granuloma with giant cells and the absence of necrosis. Specific helper-inducer T cells accumulate in the lung, leading to its identification as a hypersensitivity disease.[9] Insidious shortness of breath was accompanied by characteristic x-ray changes, which led to hospitalization in a tuberculosis sanitarium. Patients with accelerated sarcoidosis were brought to the attention of Dr. Harriet Hardy, who isolated the cause as beryllium from 42 materials used at work by the original patients.[8] Subsequently, the problem was recognized in workers from other electrical factories using beryllium nitrate phosphores. Some of the patients with advanced disease died. Those with less advanced berylliosis gradually improved but were left with residual interstitial fibrosis.[10] Because beryllium is irreplacable in nuclear reactors and in exotic alloys for spacecraft, exposure to beryllium fumes continues to be a problem for both engineers and skilled workers. Beryllium must be handled in a protective enclosure.

Lipoproteinosis. In this disorder alveolar spaces are filled with a combination of neutral lipids resembling pulmonary surfactant. Proteins similar to the apoproteins associated with surfactant[11] may be elicited in the human lung by stimuli, which are usually inorganic particles but include *Myobacterium tuberculosis*. Silica has been associated most frequently.[12] Thus, areas of lipoproteinosis are frequently found in lung biopsies or in lungs at autopsy from workers exposed to silica.[13] Many other types of particles have been associated with occupational exposures. For example, dust from grinding aluminum rails and cement dust have been associated in single instances. Patients with this disorder can be successfully treated by bronchial alveolar lavage, making a correct diagnosis crucial. Diagnosis is usually made by sampling alveolar fluids by minilavage through the fiberoptic bronchoscope or by lung biopsy.

Both granulomatous and nongranulomatous alveolitis may be seen in a person exposed to moldy plant debris. Animal experiments suggest that granulomas may be due to poorly digestible complex chitins, which are complex carbohydrates forming the walls of spores and of plant cells.[14] Pulmonary fibrosis may result from chronic farmer's lung and lipoproteinosis.[15] Whether it is due to particle composition, the host's immune status, or to other factors is unknown.

Fibrosis. Chronic interstitial fibrosis has been observed after exposure to hard metal (tungsten carbide), silicon carbide, rare earths, copper (as sulfate in vineyard sprayer's lung), aluminum, beryllium, and cadmium. As mentioned above, in berylliosis, fibrosis follows the granulomatous sarcoidlike response. Aluminum has been associated with fibrosis in workers making powdered aluminum for paints.[16] It is an infrequent disease that still requires separation from asbestosis and silicosis because of these confounding exposures in aluminum refineries.

With hard metal there is less doubt about specificity.[17] To make hard metal, powdered tungsten and carbon are fluxed with cobalt. Animals exposed to cobalt alone show the same lesions seen in workers, namely, proliferation of alveolar and airway cells.[18] One similarity to the beryllium reaction is that removing the worker from exposure leads to prompt improvement; reexposure causes exacerbation. Its similarity to farmer's lung or alveolar lipoproteinosis suggests that lung lavage may be helpful. Adrenal corticosteroids help reverse the airways obstruction. Cadmium has the unusual distinction of producing both pulmonary edema (acute respiratory distress syndrome), particularly when fumes are generated from silver soldering, and pulmonary fibrosis, which is fine and nonnodular in cadmium refinery workers.[19] Because of the frequency of asbestos exposure and asbestosis among metal smelting and refinery workers,[20] caution is advised in attributing pulmonary fibrosis to cadmium alone. Nodular infiltrates resembling those of berylliosis, hard metal disease, and silicosis have been reported among dental technicians and workers machining alloys of exotic metals. Because these illnesses occur infrequently among exposed workers (e.g., only 12.8% of 425 workers exposed to hard metal had radiographic evidence of disease),[21] individual immune response or susceptibility factors appear to be important.

Asthma, Acute Airway Reactivity

Acute airway narrowing, or asthma, is defined by shortness of breath or impaired breathing usually accompanied by wheezing that is relieved spontaneously or with therapy. Within this physiological definition of asthma are acute responses that develop within a few minutes of exposure in a sensitized individual as well as responses that may require several hours to reach their peak after exposure, as with cotton dust.[22]

Prevalence. The prevalence of occupational asthma has been estimated for only a few situations. Although the total number of workers at risk is known in the United States using data compiled by the National Institute of Occupational Safety and Health, the prevalence of asthma is known only within wide limits for portions of this population. For example, in 1973 the prevalence of byssinosis varied from 5% to 60% among the 700,000 U.S. textile workers. Estimates of disability from byssinosis were as high as 35,000 workers, although most of these individuals had already retired from the workforce. Based on the shift of cotton carding, spinning, and weaving to developing countries, world exposure to cotton dust may be 10 times the U.S. estimate.[23] Although in the United States effective dust control in textile mills mandated by National Occupational Safety and Health Standards[24] has reduced the prevalence of byssinosis to 5% or less, no dust controls exist in many countries.

Because the processing of common materials, for example, cereal grains and flour, maximizes opportunities for exposure, farmers, grain handlers, millers, and bakers probably constitute the largest group with reactive airways disease in the world.[25–27] Fortunately, exposures that produce the highest prevalence of airways reactivity, such as exposure to diisocyanates and cotton dust, have been controlled in the United States or the amounts used reduced.[28] An estimated 8 million workers in the world are exposed to welding gases and fumes. Such exposure produces symptoms but practically no acute airway response and relatively mild impairment of function. This is detectable 10 or 11 years after beginning exposure and is greater in cigarette smokers.[29]

Diagnosis. Acute or reactive airway response is recognized by an increased resistance to expiratory flow from either contraction of airway smooth muscle or swelling of airway walls. Tightness in the chest, shortness of breath, and wheezing develop quickly or insidiously. Nonproductive cough occurs with increasing frequency, but as mucus secretion is stimulated, the cough becomes productive. Generalized wheezing is heard low and posterior as the lung empties during forced expiration. Alternatively, scattered localized wheezing may be heard. The chest x-ray film is usually negative, but any abnormalities are most often due to preexisting disease. The exception is occasional hyperinflation with increased radiolucency and even a low and flattened diaphragm, suggesting emphysema. A second exception is accentuated venous markings and a prominent minor lung fissure, suggesting pulmonary edema. Symptoms occur within a few hours of beginning work, are more frequent on Monday or the first day back after a holiday, and gradually increase during the work shift.[22] The diagnosis is confirmed by finding decreases in expiratory flow when comparing measurements at the middle or end of the shift with those made before entry to the workplace. The workplace is convenient to find cross-shift decrements, but if specific agent testing is needed a laboratory exposure may be required.[3,7] Workers' exposure must be long enough to simulate workplace conditions. With management's cooperation, exposures can be measured during the work shift and dose-response curves constructed.

Mechanisms. Acute airway responses may be nociceptive, inflammatory, or immune. The reactive segment of a work force includes but is not limited to atopic individuals, those with IgE antibodies. In the instance of toluene diisocyanate (TDI), which has been well studied, reactivity to low doses does not appear to correlate with atopic status.[30] Etiologies of many workplace exposures are imperfectly understood because cotton dust, grain dust, flour, coal dust, and foundry dust are complex mixtures. Only a few chemical agents can be singled out as specific causes. Included are metal fumes from zinc, copper, magnesium, aluminum, osmium, and platinum. Clearly endotoxin from gram-negative bacteria and possibly from fungi is an important one. Many organic, naturally occurring food, fodder, and fiber plant products are enriched with endotoxin. Endotoxin concentrations increase with senescence of plants and thus are maximal at harvest time, as with cotton.

Causal Agents. To cover comprehensively the occupational exposures of importance is an encyclopedic job. However, Table 23-2 provides an index of the categories of materials and types of reactions. Causative agents are logically grouped so the reader can add new materials and reactions to them.

Control, Surveillance, and Prevention. The first principle of control and prevention is to reduce exposure for all workers by improved industrial hygiene. This has been demonstrated in the control of byssinosis (cotton dust disease) in the United States. Since 1973, dust has gradually been reduced in cotton textile mills. Abatement was so successful that after 15 years there was debate on whether byssinosis had existed. However, it continues to be a problem in the waste cotton industry[31] and in developing countries[32] lacking adequate engineering controls. The second principle of control and prevention is to remove reactive individuals from exposure. Reactively is judged from symptoms or objectively from impaired function. Often individuals who react sharply to inhaled agents select themselves out of work. Because removing impaired workers from cotton textile mills did not improve their function, at least in the short term, it appears that byssinosis is a disease for which surveillance should be longitudinal as well as across the acute shift exposure so that workers whose function deteriorates at an accelerated rate can be removed from exposure before they have suffered enough impairment to interfere with their ability to work. This can be determined after measurements at 6- and 12-month intervals after the baseline measurement. Annual and semiannual surveillance by pulmonary function testing was mandated by the cotton dust standards invoked by OSHA in 1978[24] under the 1970 Health and Safety Act.

Chronic Airway Disease: Chronic Bronchitis

Definition. Chronic bronchitis is defined by the presence of phlegm or sputum production for more than 3 months of 2 succeeding years. Cough is generally the presenting symptom. It is probably the most common respiratory disease in the world.[33]

Effects of Cigarette Smoking. The prevalence of chronic bronchitis is related mainly to the widespread smoking of cigarettes, a plague of this century largely since World War I. Although the habit is on the wane in the United States, it appears to be entrenched in Europe and to have taken developing nations by storm, where the peak prevalence of cigarette smoking may not yet have been reached. Certainly there is no evidence that quitting has become the more accepted social behavior, as it has in the United States. Chronic bronchitis has such a high prevalence in cigarette smokers, particularly 20 years or more after they start smoking, that it often takes careful analysis to find occupational chronic bronchitis. This is because blue collar workers are more frequently cigarette smokers than the average population.[34]

Occupational effects can be assessed most securely by studying large populations of individuals who have never smoked.[35] Alternately, effects of cigarette smoking and occupational exposure can be partitioned by adjusting predicted function values

TABLE 23-2. PARTICLES AFFECTING HUMAN LUNGS: CLASSES AND EXAMPLES

Source	Persons Affected	Airways	Alveoli	Reference
▪ BACTERIA				
Aerobacter cloaceae *Phialophora* species	Air conditioner, humidifier workers		+	Friend JAR: Lancet 1:297, 1977
Escherichia coli endotoxin	Textile workers (mill fever)	+	+	Pernis B, et al: Br J Ind Med 18:120, 1961
Pseudomonas sp	Sewer workers	+	+	Rylander R: Schweiz Med Wochenschr 107:182, 1977
▪ FUNGI				
Aspergillus sp *Micropolyspora faeni*	Farmers	+		Emanuel DA, et al: Am J Med 37:392, 1964
Aspergillus clavatus	Malt workers	+		Channell S, et al: Q J Med 38:351, 1969
Cladosporium sp	Combine operators	+	+	Darke CS, et al: Thorax 31: 294–302, 1976
Verticillium sp *Alternaria* sp *Micropolyspora faeni*	Mushroom workers	+	+	Lockey SD: Ann Allergy 33:282, 1974
Penicillium casei	Cheese washers	+		Minnig H, deWeck AL: Schweiz Med Wochenschr 102:1205, 1972
Penicillium frequentans	Cork workers (suberosis)	+		Arila R, Villar TG: Lancet 1:620, 1968
Thermoactinomyces (vulgaris) sacchari	Sugar cane workers (bagassosis)	+	+	Seabury J, et al: Proc Soc Exp Biol Med 129:351, 1968
▪ AMEBA				
Acanthamoeba castellani *Acanthamoeba polyphaga* *Naegleria gruberi*	Air conditioning, humidifier workers	+	+	Edwards JH, et al: Nature 264:438, 1976
▪ VEGETABLE ORIGIN				
Barley dust	Farmers	+		McCarthy PE, et al: Br J Ind Med 42:106–110, 1985
Carbon black	Production workers	+		Crosbie WA: Arch Environ Health 41:346–353, 1986
Castor bean (ricin)	Oil mill workers	+		Panzani R: Int Arch Allergy 11:224–236, 1957
Cinnamon	Cinnamon workers	+		Uragada CG: Br J Ind Med 41:224–227, 1984
Coffee bean	Roasters	+		Freedman SD, et al: Nature 192:241, 1961 Van Toorn DW: Thorax 25: 399–405, 1970
Cotton, hemp, flax jute, kapok	Textile workers	+		Roach SA, Schilling RSF: Br J In Med 17:1, 1960 Jamison JP, et al: Br J Ind Med 43:809–813 1986 Buck MG, et al: Br J Ind Med 43:220–226, 1986
Flour dust	Millers	+		Tse KS, et al: Arch Environ Health 27:74, 1973
Grain dust	Farmers	+		Warren P, et al: J Allergy Clin Immunol 53:139, 1974 Awad el Karim MA, et al: Arch Environ Health 41: 297–301, 1986
Gum arabic, gum	Printers	+		Gelfand, HH: J Allergy 14:208, 1954
Papain	Preparation workers		+	Flindt MLH: Lancet 1:430, 1978
Proteolytic enzymes—*Bacillus subtilis* (subtilisin, alcalase)	Detergent workers		+	Pepys J, et al: Lancet 1:1181, 1969

TABLE 23-2. PARTICLES AFFECTING HUMAN LUNGS: CLASSES AND EXAMPLES (Continued)

Source	Persons Affected	Airways	Alveoli	Reference
▪ VEGETABLE ORIGIN (cont'd)				
Soft paper	Paper mill workers	+		Enarson DA, et al: Arch Environ Health 39:325–330, 1984
				Thoren K, et al: Br J Ind Med 46:192–195, 1989
Tamarind seed powder	Weavers	+		Murray R, et al: Br J Ind Med 14:105, 1957
Tea	Tea workers	+		Zuskin ES, Kuric Z: Br J Ind Med 41:88–93, 1984
Tobacco dust	Cigarette, cheroot factory	+		Viegi G, et al: Br J Ind Med 43:802–808, 1986
				Huuskonen MS, et al: Br J Ind Med 41:77–83, 1984
Wood dust	Those who work with Canadian red cedar, South African box-wood, rosewood (*Dalbergia* sp)	+		Chan-Yeung M, et al: Am Rev Respir Dis 108:1094–1102, 1973
				Carosso A, et al: Br J Ind Med 44:53–56, 1987
				Vedal S, et al: Arch Environ Health 41:179–183, 1986
	Furniture workers		+	Gerhardsson MR, et al: Br J Ind Med 42:403–405, 1985
▪ ANIMAL ORIGIN				
Ascaris lumbricoides	Zoologists	+		Hansen K: Occupational Allergy. Springfield, Ill.: Charles C Thomas, 1958
Ascidiacea	Oyster culture	+		Nakashima T: Hiroshima J Med Sci 18:141, 1969
Dander	Farmers, fur workers, grooms	+		Squire JR: Clin Sci 9:127, 1950
Egg protein	Turkey and chicken farmers	+		Smith AB, et al: Am J Ind Med 12:205–218, 1987
Feathers	Poultry workers	+		Boyer RS, et al: Am Rev Resp Dis 109:630–635, 1974
Furs	Furriers			Zuskin E, et al: Am J Ind Med 14: 189–196, 1988
Insect chitin (*Sitophilus granarius*)	Flour	+		Lunn JA, Hughes DTD: Br J Ind Med 24:158, 1967
Mayfly	Outdoorsmen	+		Figley KD: J Allergy 11:376, 1940
Screwfly	Screw-worm controllers	+		Gibbons HL, et al: Arch Environ Health 10:424–430, 1965
King crab	Processors	+		Orford RR, Wilson JT: Am J Ind Med 7:155–169, 1985
Pancreatic enzymes	Preparation workers	+	+	Colten HR, et al: N Engl J Med 292:1050–1053, 1975
				Flood DFS, et al: Br J Ind Med 42:43–50, 1985
Rat serum and urine	Laboratory workers	+	+	Taylor AN, et al: Lancet 2:847, 1977
				Agrup G, et al: Br J Ind Med 43:192–198, 1986
Swine confinement	Farm workers	+		Donham KJ: Am J Ind Med 5:367–375, 1984
▪ CHEMICALS				
▪ Inorganic				
Beryllium	Metal workers		+	Saltini C, et al: N Engl J Med 320:1103–1109, 1989
Calcium hydroxidetricalium silicate	Cement workers	+		Eid AH, El-Sewefy AZ: J Egypt Med Assoc 52:400, 1969
Chromium	Casters	+		Dodson VN, Rosenblatt EC: J Occup Med 8:326, 1966
Copper sulfate and lime	Vineyard sprayers		+	Pimental JC, Marques F: Thorax 24:678–688, 1969

(*continued*)

TABLE 23-2. PARTICLES AFFECTING HUMAN LUNGS: CLASSES AND EXAMPLES (Continued)

Source	Persons Affected	Airways	Alveoli	Reference
▪ **CHEMICALS** (cont'd)				
▪ **Inorganic** (cont'd)				
Hard metal	Sintering and finishing workers	+	+	Meyer-Bisch C, et al: Br J Ind Med 46:302–309, 1989
Vanadium pentoxide	Refinery workers	+		Zenz C, et al: Arch Environ Health 5:542, 1962
Nickel sulfate	Platers	+		McConnell LH, et al: Ann Intern Med 78:888, 1973
Platinum chloroplatinate	Photographers	+		Pepys J, et al: Clin Allergy 2:391, 1972
Titanium chloride	Pigment workers		+	Redline S, et al: Br J Ind Med 43:652–656, 1986
Titanium oxide	Paint factory			Oleru UG: Am J Ind Med 12:173–180, 1987
Tungsten carbide (cobalt); hard metal	Hard metal workers	+	+	Coates EO, Watson JHL: Ann Intern Med 75:709, 1971
Zinc, copper, magnesium fumes	Welders, bronze workers (metal fume fever)	+		Gleason RP: Am Ind Hyg Assoc J 29:461, 1968
Iron, chromium, nickel (oxides)	Welders	+		Kilburn KH: Am J Indust Med 87:62–69, 1989
▪ **Organic**				
Aminoethyl ethanolamine	Solderers			McCann JK: Lancet 1:445, 1964
Ayodicarbonemide	Plastic injection molders	+		Whitehead LW, et al: Am J Ind Med 11:83–92, 1987
Chlorinated biphenyls	Transformer manufacturers		+	Shigematsu N, et al: PCB's Environ Res 1978
Colophony (pine resin)	Solderers	+		Fawcett IW, et al: Clin Allergy 6(4):577, 1976
Diazonium salts	Chemical workers	+		Perry KMA: Occupational Lung Disease. In Perry KMA, Sellers TH (eds): Chest Diseases. London: Butterworth Publishers, 1963, p 518
Diisocyanates—toluene, diphenylmethane	Production workers, foundry workers	+		Brugsch HG, Elkins HG: N Engl J Med 268:353–357, 1963 Zammit-Tabona M, et al: Am Rev Respir Dis 128:226–230, 1983
Formaldehyde (Permapress, urethane foam)	Histology technicians, office workers	+		Popa V, et al: Dis Chest 56:395, 1969; Alexandersson R, et al: Arch Environ Health 43:222, 1988
Paraphenylenediamine	Solderers	+		Perry KMA: Occupational lung diseases. In Perry KMA, Sellers TH (eds): Chest Diseases. London: Butterworth Publishers, 1963, p. 518; Dally KA, et al: Arch Environ Health 36:277–284, 1981
Paraquat	Sprayers	+	+	Bainova A, et al: Khig-i zdravespazane 15:25, 1972
Penicillin, ampicillin	Production workers, nurses	+		Davies RJ, et al: Clin Allergy 4:227, 1974
Parathion	Sprayers	+		Ganelin RS, et al: JAMA 188:108, 1964
Piperazine	Chemists	+		Pepys J: Clin Allergy 2:189, 1972
Polymer fumes (polytetrafluoroethylene)	Teflon manufacturers, users	+	+	Harris DK: Lancet 2:1008, 1951 Lewis CE, Kirby GR: JAMA 191:103, 1965
Polyvinyl chloride	Fabrication workers	+		Ernst P, et al: Am J Ind Med 14:273–279, 1988

TABLE 23-2. PARTICLES AFFECTING HUMAN LUNGS: CLASSES AND EXAMPLES (Continued)

Source	Persons Affected	Airways	Alveoli	Reference
▪ **SYNTHETIC FIBERS**				
Nylon, polyesters, dacron	Textile workers		+	Pimental JC, et al: Thorax 30:204, 1975
Rubber (neoprene)	Injection press operators	+		Thomas RJ, et al: Am J Ind Med 9:551–559, 1986
Tetralzene	Detonators	+		Burge SB, et al: Thorax 39:470, 1984
Vinyl chloride (phosgene, hydrogen chloride)	Meat wrappers (asthma)	+		Sokol WN, et al: JAMA 226:639, 1973
	Firefighters		+	Dyer RE, Esch VH: JAMA 235:393, 1976
	Polymerization plant workers		+	Arnard A, et al: Thorax 33:19, 1978

for expiratory flows for duration of smoking using standard regression coefficients.[36] Similarly, accelerated functional deterioration or increased prevalence of symptoms across years of occupational exposure after adjusting for the cumulative effects of smoking may show the effects of occupational exposure. Based on interactive effects of cigarette smoking with occupational dusts and fumes and with atmospheric air pollution in many studies, if the age decrement for forced expiratory volume (FEV_1) in a person who has never smoked exceeds 21 to 25 ml/y, this represents an unusual decrement. Cigarette smoking alone in men increases the age-associated decrement by 9 ml/y, an almost 40% increase. Women show no such effect, probably because they smoke fewer cigarettes daily. Thus in groups of men decrements in FEV_1 of greater than 30 ml/y would be attributable to occupational or environmental exposures. Airborne particle burdens increase decrements with age.

Occupational Exposures. Many dusts of occupational exposure, including those containing silica, coal, asbestos, and cotton (including flax and hemp) dust, and exposures during coking, foundry work, welding, and papermaking increase the prevalence or lower the age of appearance of chronic bronchitis. Although it is clear that high exposures to silica and asbestos produce pneumoconiosis, lower doses cause airways obstruction. Symptoms and later airways obstruction from cotton and other vegetable dusts have been well studied since recognition more than a century ago.[37] In the 1960s studies in British textile mills (using American-grown cotton), the severity of this Monday-morning asthma (byssinosis) and of shortness of breath and tightness in the chest were correlated with concentrations of respirable cotton dust.[38] Similarly, exposure to welding gases and fumes has been associated with accelerated reductions in expiratory flows.[29] It is noteworthy that the trades of shipbuilding and construction work, so frequently associated with asbestosis and to a lesser extent with silicosis, are also strongly correlated with chronic bronchitis, as are coal mining[39,40] and work in foundries.[41] The common thread is inhalation of respirable particles with inflammation stimulated by one or more chemically active species contained or adsorbed. Clinical signs are cough with mucus production due to goblet cell hyperplasia in small airways and to hyperplasia of mucous glands in large bronchi and exertional dyspnea due to small airways obstruction.[42]

Inhalation of 200 to 400 ppm of sulfur dioxide by rats or guinea pigs produces a useful model of chronic bronchitis. However, the levels exceed, by two orders of magnitude, levels found in usual smelting or metal roasting operations to which workers are exposed or by three magnitudes the most ambient air pollution exposures. However, human exposures are almost always accompanied by quantities of respirable particles. Similarly, exposure to chlorine, fluorine, bromine, phosgene, and vapors of hydrogen fluoride and hydrogen chloride produce bronchitic reactions, but because exposure is seldom continuous, these pulses of damage tend to produce cycles of injury and repair rather than chronic bronchitis.

Gases are adsorbed on particles in many occupational exposures. Examples include welding, metal roasting, and smelting operations, as well as in foundries or situations where compressed air jets are used for cleaning. Gas molecules adsorbed on particles deposit in small airways.[2] This deposition is studied in animal models with gases and pure carbon. Carbon, by itself an innocuous particle, adsorbs gas molecules and creates a nidus of damage because the particle is difficult to remove and the adsorbed gas molecules leach into cells.[43] Perhaps the best example is the adsorption of ozone, nitrogen dioxide, and hydrocarbons on respirable particles[35] in Los Angeles, Mexico City, Athens, and other cities where large amounts of fossil fuel are combusted with limited atmospheric exchanges because of mountains, prevailing winds, and weather conditions.

The prevalence of occupational chronic bronchitis has declined in the postindustrial era in the United States, Great Britain, and Northern Europe. Byssinosis and chronic bronchitis from cotton dust have been on the wane since the early 1970s.[44,45] A similar decline in prevalence in workers in foundries, coke ovens, welding, and other dusty trades is attributed to better awareness of the health hazards and improved air hygiene often dictated by economic or processing imperatives.[39,41,46]

Natural History. The natural history of chronic bronchitis in urban dwellers has been investigated since the early nineteenth century.[47] Chronic inhalation of polluted air stimulates mucus production, recognized by cough and phlegm, which define chronic bronchitis epidemiologically.[48] Chronic bronchitis identified by the symptoms of cough and sputum was studied in over 1000 English civil servants and transport workers over a decade.[48,49] Approximately the same proportion were symptomatic at the end of the decade as at the beginning, although some individuals had left and others had entered the symptomatic group over the interval.[49]

Clearly, the prevalence of chronic bronchitis increases with age in both females and males. The male predominance may be entirely due to cigarette smoking. The latent period before deterioration of expiratory airflow may be long if chronic bronchitis begins in childhood or early adulthood but short if it begins in late middle age.[49,50]

Chronic bronchitis has another course, that with an abrupt onset of bronchitis, which is not associated with cigarette smoking or occupational exposure.[50] It is more common in women and is generally preceeded by a viral or chemical respiratory illness, after which there is chronic phlegm production and more rapid than expected airflow limitation with deterioration of pulmonary function. When shortness of breath accompanies the cardinal symptoms, airflow limitation is generally present, and the yearly decrements in function are usually twice as large as predicted. For many individuals who smoke and have had an insidious onset of shortness of breath, expiratory airflow declines more steeply after age 50.[49]

Epidemiology. Since the early 1960s atmospheric air pollution has been recognized as an important cause of chronic bronchitis.[51] Studies in Groningen, The Netherlands,[52] Cracow, Poland,[53] and London[49] firmly established that episodic severe pollution increased mortality and that chronic levels of atmospheric air pollution were associated with increased prevalence and morbidity from chronic bronchitis. Mortality from asthma and chronic bronchitis fell in Japan when sulfur dioxide air pollution decreased.[54] In 1986, restudy of Italian schoolchildren showed that previously reduced expiratory flows rose to levels of controls when air pollution decreased.[55]

Control Measures. Control measures for chronic bronchitis depend on avoiding exposure—to cigarette smoke, to contaminated respirable particles in coal mines, smelters, and foundries, and to air pollution from fossil fuel combustion. Socioeconomic level is also important, since as the standard of living rises, the prevalence of chronic bronchitis falls. Control ultimately depends on improving the population's general health and curtailing its exposure to respirable particles.

Surveillance. Effects of a personal, occupational, or atmospheric air pollution control program are best assessed by surveying symptoms and pulmonary functional performance of a random sample of the affected population. Most essential data—the prevalence of chronic bronchitis and measurement of expiratory airflow—are easily obtained and can be appraised frequently. Measures that decrease exposure should reduce the prevalence of cough and phlegm and the rate of deterioration of expiratory airflow.

Prevention. The prevention of chronic bronchitis essentially centers on avoiding generation of respirable particles into the human air supply. Cigarette smoking cannot be condoned. Air filtration helps if particle generation is not avoidable, as in cotton textile mills. Socioeconomic measures include cleaner combustion of fossil fuels, reduction of human crowding, provisions for central heating, and improvements in the standard of living. Patients with acute bronchitis should receive broad-spectrum antibiotics in an attempt to reduce chronic bronchitis of abrupt onset.

Neoplastic Disease of Airways

Lung cancer from occupational exposure to uranium, asbestos, chromate pigments, and arsenic was described before the worldwide epidemic of lung cancer from cigarette smoking. Unfortunately, early reports often failed to mention cigarette smoking, so that secure attribution of cause was delayed until large studies had sufficient numbers of individuals who had never smoked. Certainly with asbestosis, there is firm data on which to establish the causal linkage of asbestos to lung cancer without smoking. The histological types of cancer are those seen in the general population, including adenocarcinoma, squamous cell, undifferentiated, and small- or oat cell carcinoma. One sentinel disorder has been described—small-cell carcinoma after exposure to chloromethyl ethers.

The association of lung cancer with exposure to polycyclic aromatic hydrocarbons in coke oven workers and roofers has been clearly established and follows Percival Pott's attribution of the scrotal skin cancers in chimney sweeps to coal tar in London, 200 years ago. Similarly, the occupational exposures to radon, radium, and uranium in mining and metalworking cause lung cancers. A recent example is uranium-mining Navaho Indians on the Colorado Plateau, who, despite a low prevalence of smoking and a low consumption of cigarettes among those who smoke, had a tenfold increase (observed and expected) in lung cancer.[56] Sentinel nasal sinus cancers and excessive lung cancers have resulted from exposure to the nickel refining in calcination of impure nickel and copper sulfide to nickel oxide or in the carbonyl process.

Lung cancer may be caused by other exposures to nickel, to chromium, and to arsenic but the data are less convincing than the foregoing examples.[57] Thus, another agent or agents may be responsible for the cancer mortality from lung cancer in smelter workers. That this additional factor may be asbestos was suggested in recent studies of copper smelter workers and aluminum refinery workers, whose prevalences of asbestosis were between 8% and 25% using the International Labor Organization (ILO) criteria for x-ray diagnosis.[20]

It appears that the common denominator for the higher pulmonary disease prevalence and lung cancer mortality among metal smelter workers may be asbestos. In these work sites asbestos has been used for heat insulation, for patching of calciners, retorts, and roasters, and for heat protection for personnel. In a way reminiscent of the studies before the contribution of cigarette smoking was recognized, it appears that the contribution of asbestos must be taken into account before attributing cancer or irregular opacities in the lung to the useful metals.

ENVIRONMENTAL AIR POLLUTION

History. The famous fogs along the Thames in the City of London chronicled by Sir Arthur Conan Doyle in the Sherlock Holmes stories 100 years ago underscored a problem first noted in the early seventeenth century, at the beginning of the Industrial Revolution. In fact, John Evelyn described the conditions in 1621. That this type of exposure could produce death was first recognized in the Meuse Valley of Belgium during a thermal inversion in December 1930.[51] Sixty people died. In Denora, Pa., a town of about 14,000 people along the Monongahela River with steel mills, coke ovens, a zinc production plant, and a chemical plant manufacturing sulfuric acid, a continuous temperature inversion created a particularly malignant fog that caused many illnesses and 20 deaths in October 1948. Deaths occurred the third day after onset. In December 1952, a particularly vicious episode produced excessive mortality in London among infants, young children, and elderly persons with cardiorespiratory disease. High values reported were 4.5 mg/m^3 for smoke and 3.75 mg/m^3 for sulfur dioxide. A 1953 episode in New York City called further attention to this twentieth-century plague. Other episodes described in Tokyo, Yokohama, New Orleans, and Los Angeles led to investigation of the health effects of environmental air pollution in the 1960s and early 1970s.

A singular air pollution episode swept across the Northern hemisphere between November 27 and December 10, 1962. Excessive respiratory symptoms were observed in Washington, D.C., New York City, Cincinnati, and Philadelphia. London, England, had 700 excess deaths due to high sulfur dioxide levels, and in Rotterdam, The Netherlands, sickness, absenteeism, and increased hospital admissions occurred, with a fivefold increase in sulfur oxides. Hamburg, W. Germany, reported increase of sulfur dioxide and dust and increased heart disease mortality; in Osaka, Japan, 60 excess deaths were linked to high pollution levels.

Currently, several cities stand out as worst cases of air pollution. Mexico City, with extreme levels of pollution and an altitude of 7000 feet in an enclosed valley with over 20 million people, is the world's capital of air pollution. Athens, located like Los Angeles with a mountain backdrop to prevailing westerly winds, has experienced such serious pollution as to jeopardize some of its monuments of antiquity. Adverse health effects from air pollution have been observed in Saõ Paulo and Cubatao, Brazil, which have many diesel vehicles, a heavy petrochemical industry, and fertilizer plants. Brazil is experimenting with methyl alcohol as fuel for internal combustion engines. As more developing countries industrialize, the lessons that should have been learned from Denora, London, and New York are ignored.

Sources. The major source of modern environmental air pollution is combustion of fossil fuels.[58] During this century oil (gasoline)-based transportation has become the predominant contributor, a shift from coal for space heating and industrial production. In fact, the internal combustion automobile engine is now the major source of both particles and gases, including hydrocarbons. The interaction of atmospheric gases with hydrocarbons under sunlight (photocatalysis) produces ozone and nitrogen dioxide. Adding these to the direct products of combustion in air produces the irritating acrid smoke and smog, a word coined to describe the mixture of smoke and fog. Thus, the horizon of many cities shows a burnished copper glow from nitrogen oxides. The smog in Los Angeles has remained practically static for 30 years; efforts to ameliorate the problem have simply kept pace with the additional population and its motor vehicle exhaust.[59,60]

In certain areas, such as the Northeastern United States, industrial processing, coking, steel production, paper mills, and oil refineries contribute their selective and somewhat specific flavor to the problem.[61] In occupational exposures, the particles are of respirable size and gases adsorb on them. Flyash, from the combustion of coal in power stations, from space heating, and in industry, consists of fused glass spheres with adsorbed metals and acidic gases.[62] Adsorbed chemicals increase particle toxicity and determine the zones of injury in the lung.

Waste incineration has increased the burden in the air, and greater population has nearly exhausted available canyons and open spaces for land fills for garbage around major cities. Although it appears that selective incineration under properly controlled conditions may help solve the solid waste problem, it increases the burden of particles and gases in the atmosphere unless carefully controlled. Moreover, nature may be responsible for freak episodes of air pollution. In 1986, release of carbon dioxide from Lake Nyos in West Africa killed 1700 people as they slept, and already the lake may be partly recharged.[63]

Regulated Pollutants. Since 1970 in the United States, carbon monoxide, hydrocarbons, sulfur dioxide, nitrogen oxides, and ozones have been regulated by the Environmental Protection Agency (EPA). In various urban areas, ozone and oxidant concentrations have been defined above which occupants are alerted to limit physical activity. Although the respirable particles, particularly flyash, hydrocarbons, and coated carbon particles from diesel engines, provide the principal components that make the visible pollution, recently considerable attention has focused on acids and chlorofluorocarbons.

Chlorofluorocarbons manufactured as refrigerants and also used to power convenience aerosols have been identified as the specific chemicals that liberate chlorine into the stratosphere, where it combines with ozone to reduce the ultraviolet shield.[64,65] The combination of loss of the ozone shield and increase in carbon dioxide from combustion of fuel and destruction of tropical rain forests, among other causes, has increased atmospheric carbon dioxide, leading to global warming, the so-called greenhouse effect.[66] This constitutes an entirely different but potentially very serious complication of environmental air pollution. Northern Europeans, particularly in Sweden, Norway, and the city of Cologne, W. Germany, have been greatly concerned with the problem of acid rain, which is precipitation of large amounts of acid from acidic gases combined with water.[67] The acidity of these solutions has been sufficient to etch limestone buildings and to acidify lakes and reservoirs, killing aquatic life and changing natural habitats. Ozone loss (which increases the risk of cancer[68]), acid rain, and global warming are likely to produce future human health problems.

Modifiers. The effects of particles and gases in the atmosphere are lessened by wind and rain dilution and made worse by thermal inversion. Studies in Tokyo showed that the heat worked with ozone to produce respiratory symptoms in schoolchildren.[69] There have been enough spontaneous experiments to show that stopping automotive transportation in a city such as New York, for a day or two, is sufficient to ameliorate problems from rising levels of air pollutants. Thus, it appears obvious that a solution to transportation in urban areas would greatly relieve air pollution. Because combustion of diesel fuel and gasoline in automobiles and trucks is the major problem, it appears that designing cleaner engines is fundamental to improving air quality. Alternate fuels emphasizing methanol and ethanol alone or mixed with gasoline may be important and are included in the EPA plans for clearer air for the United States in the next decade. Almost 20 years of retrofit (regressive) engineering, the installation of catalytic converters, has been less satisfactory. Although it has kept levels of air pollution from increasing in Los Angeles, it is unclear whether this technology would help in Mexico City, Athens, or São Paulo.

Effects. Toxicity is determined by particle size, adsorption, and respiratory deposition profiles.[70] Respirable particles are those capable of depositing beyond the ciliated conducting airways of the human lung.[1] The effects of air pollution can be classified as symptoms, impaired pulmonary function, respiratory diseases, and mortality. Acute symptoms, including eye irritation, nasal congestion, and chest tightness, appear to be due to the oxidant gases, aldehydes, and hydrocarbons largely in the gaseous phase, including peroxyacetyl nitrate.[71] In the most sensitive 7% to 10% of the population, exposure to these same gases may limit expiratory air flow, with wheezing and cough. Symptoms increase with exercise and are usually relieved within a few hours of removal from exposure.

Large studies of European populations exposed to air pollution have shown that airways obstruction varied on days of greater or lesser levels of sulfur dioxide and particles.[52–55] However, the question of reversibility is unanswered. Whether or how quickly airflow limitation is relieved by removal from exposure has not been tested. Meanwhile, to assume that the situation resembles that of cigarette smoking, in that airways obstruction is irreversible, is justified.

The prevalence of chronic bronchitis in the exposed population is one of the most reliable indicators of exposure to the gases and particles of atmospheric air pollution.[71] A number of classic studies—Grotingen, The Netherlands; Cracow, Poland; London; Tokyo; and Los Angeles—have shown that prevalence of chronic bronchitis rises with level and duration of air pollution.[72] Obviously, this is best studied in individuals who have never smoked and in children. The production of enough mucus to necessitate coughing for its removal appears to be essentially a protective mechanism for the respiratory tract. Both clinical and experimental data show goblet cell metaplasia in small airways[42] and goblet cell and mucous gland hyperplasia in larger conducting airways. This latter finding is the consistent pathological accompaniment of chronic bronchitis in autopsies from exposed populations.[73]

Deaths from the air pollution disasters, and from current levels of air pollution, have largely occurred in infants who have died of pneumonia and in adults with cardiorespiratory disease, particularly chronic bronchitis and emphysema. Those with precarious respiratory function are highly susceptible to additional insult and by analogy constitute, in the picturesque lumberjack terms, "standing dead timber," susceptible to the "strong wind" provided by a prolonged period of increased air pollution.

Other results of severe air pollution include the retardation of children's mental development from airborne lead,[74] which constituted the principal reason for first regulating lead tetraethyl and similar additives and finally removing them from gasoline and motor fuel in the United States during the 1970s. The clear inverse relationship between lead and population intelligence is being experienced once again, this time in Mexico City.[75]

INDOOR AIR POLLUTION

Living Agents. Illness associated with exposure indoors has been observed repeatedly[76,77] and reviewed at length.[78,79] Episodes such as in Pontiac, Mich., have stimulated investigations into bacterial and fungal contamination with some fruitful results. For example, Legionnaires' disease was discovered from an investigation of illnesses occurring at a convention of the American Legion at the Bellvue Stratford Hotel in Philadelphia. Its etiology was a bacterium since named *Legionella pneumophila.*[80] Episodes of the tight building syndrome became more frequent with the energy crisis of 1973. These many investigations failed to find a bacterial or fungal source and engendered a search for chemical contamination.

Sources of Chemicals. Indoor air receives gases, vapors, and some particles generated by the activities therein (Table 23-3). Their concentrations reflect the amounts generated or released in the volume, the number of air exchanges, and the purity of make-up air. Thus, human effluents, chiefly carbon dioxide and mercaptans, combine with products of space heating and cooking, cigarette smoke, and contributions from air-conditioning systems. Added to these are outgassing of building construction, adhesive, and decorating materials to make a potent witches' brew. If the building has a sufficient number of air exchanges, the concentration gradient may be reversed and the building atmosphere made hospitable. On the other hand, reducing the air exchanges to conserve heat or cold can lead to build-up of noxious odors, vapors, and gases. Location of air intakes, types of filtration, and refrigeration and heating systems all contribute to the quality of indoor air.

Formaldehyde. Because many building materials are bonded with resins that use formaldehyde, this gas, which also is a constituent of cigarette smoke and is used in permanent press fabrics, has been consistently found in indoor air.[81] Most studies have found major contamination from cigarette smoking. Thus, prohibition of smoking indoors makes air more pleasant. Cooking, particularly with natural gas, generates nitrogen oxides that rival formaldehyde in their capacity to irritate.

Asbestos. During the late 1970s and early 1980s, concern for release of asbestos from construction materials into indoor air stimulated measurement of fiber levels.[82] Generally these have been well below occupational levels, usually between 0.01 and 0.0001 fiber per milliliter. However, during repair or renovation of heating systems, with maximal conservation of air, levels may reach 0.2 to 1.0 fiber per milliliter. The experience with asbestos

TABLE 23-3. SELECTED GUIDELINES FOR AIR CONTAMINANTS OF INDOOR ORIGIN[a]

Contaminant[b]	Concentration	Exposure Time	Comments
Acetone—O	—	—	—
Ammonia—O	—	—	—
Asbestos	—	—	Known human carcinogen; best available control technology
Benzene—O	—	—	Known human carcinogen; best available control technology
Carbon dioxide	4.5 g/m^3	Continuous	—
Chlordane—O	5 μg/m^3	Continuous	—
Chlorine	—	—	—
Cresol—O	—	—	—
Dichloromethane—O	—	—	—
Formaldehyde—O	120 μg/m^3	Continuous	W. German and Dutch guidelines
Hydrocarbons, aliphatic—O	—	—	—
Hydrocarbons, aromatic—O	—	—	—
Mercury	—	—	—
Ozone—O	100 μg/m^3	Continuous	—
Phenol—O	—	—	—
Radon	0.01 working level	Annual average	Background 0.002–0.004 working level
Tetrachloroethylene—O	—	—	—
Trichloroethane—O	—	—	—
Turpentine—O	—	—	—
Vinyl chloride—O	—	—	Known human carcinogen; best available control technology

[a] Reprinted with permission from American National Standards Institute/American Society of Heating, Refrigeration, Air-Conditioning Engineers: Standard 62-1981—Ventilation for Acceptable Indoor Air Quality. New York: The Society, 1981, 48 pp which states: "If the air is thought to contain any contaminant not listed [in various tables], guidance on acceptable exposure . . . should be obtained by reference to the standards of the Occupational Safety and Health Administration. For application to the general population the concentration of these contaminants should not exceed 1/10 of the limits which are used in industry. . . . In some cases, this procedure may result in unreasonable limits. Expert consultation may then be required." "These substances are ones for which indoor exposure standards are not yet available."

[b] Contaminants marked "O" have odors at concentrations sometimes found in indoor air. The tabulated concentrations do not necessarily result in odorless conditions.

has raised concerns about fibrous glass, which has been widely used in insulation. Even less is known of its possible effects on health.

Freon and Chlorofluorocarbons. The leakage of freon, a refrigerants used in air-conditioning systems, is particularly noxious because phosgene is generated at ignition points such as electric arcs, burning cigarettes, and open flames. This problem was first identified aboard nuclear submarines, which remained submerged for long periods. Paint was demonstrated to be the most potent contributor to indoor pollution on board these vessels. Regulations now prohibit painting less than 30 days before putting to sea.

Radon. Another concern indoors is radon and daughter products, which may concentrate in indoor air due to building location (e.g., the granite deposits of Reading Prong in Pennsylvania, New York, and New Jersey) or be released from concrete and other building materials.[83] As with asbestos, the human health hazard of large exposures to radon and daughter products is well known from the miners of Schneeberg, Germany, and Jacymov, Czechoslovakia. The long-term health impact of low doses of radon products from basements, particularly from building materials or the substrata of rock, is poorly demonstrated.[84] Decisions of this type are difficult both for individuals and from a public health perspective, and thus both legislation and rulemaking have wavered in the breezes of indecision.

In summary, living organisms do cause disease in buildings spread by heating and air-conditioning systems. It is unknown if materials such as trichloroethylene, which appears in culinary water that is dispersed into the air by showering and other water use, make chronic exposure dangerous. Such low-level exposure appears to produce harmful effects after 20 or 25 years.[72]

Effects

Symptoms. The major ill effects from indoor exposure begin several minutes to several hours after exposure and disappear in a few hours or overnight after individuals exit the building. They recur on reentry. Symptoms include fatigue, feeling of exhaustion, headache, and sometimes anorexia, nausea, lack of concentration, and lightheadedness. As occupants talk about their problems, irritability and recent memory loss may be noted along with the irritation of eyes and throat. Attempts to demonstrate physiological changes are beset by difficulties in measuring slight changes and interpreting the findings. This has led to concerns over possible mass hysteria, or "crowd syndrome." The methods for proving these diagnoses are frequently poorly grounded. Despite trials and errors and a rather large literature, there is as yet no standard investigational method for these problems. However, the following are suggested.

Investigation. Use a standard inventory of symptoms and obtain information on as many occupants of a structure as possible. Affective disorder inventories such as the profile of mood states are useful. This information should be accompanied by mapping of affected and unaffected subjects' work areas and their locations in the building. Air sampling should aim at recognizing groups such as aldehydes, solvents, mercaptans, oxidant gases, chlorofluorocarbons (freons), and carbon monoxide. The decision to use physiological tests for pulmonary or neurological function should be made after reviewing the exposure and the symptom inventories.

Control and Prevention. Provision for adequate air exchange with entrainment of fresh air not contaminated by motor vehicle exhaust or effluents from surrounding industrial activities is the most prudent control and preventive method. Source removal of contaminated air should be applied to welding, painting, and similar operations. Internal filtration of air is sometimes useful in removing particles. It works in textile mills and metal machining operations but is rarely useful in indoor pollution, where total particle burdens are rarely more than 0.2 mg or 0.3 mg/m^3. On high-altitude aircraft, activated charcoal absorbers for ozone are workable, as they are on submarines. However, the cost of these, compared with air exchanges, is prohibitively high for buildings. Freon, formaldehyde, solvents, and asbestos should be controlled to as low doses as possible in the indoor environment. These concerns will develop and compromises be made as pushed by the nation's need to conserve energy.

REFERENCES

1. Kilburn KH: A hypothesis for pulmonary clearance and its implications. Am Rev Resp Dis 98:449–463, 1968
2. Kilburn KH: Particles causing lung disease. Environ Health Perspect 55:97–109, 1984
3. Pepys J: Hypersensitivity disease of the lungs due to fungi and organic dusts. In Kolos A (ed): Monograph in Allergy, Vol. 4. New York: Karger, 1969, pp 1–147
4. Morgan DC, Smyth JT, Lister RW, et al: Chest symptoms in farming communities with special reference to farmer's lung. Br J Ind Med 32:228–234, 1975
5. Grant IWB, Blyth W, Wardrop VE, et al: Prevalence of farmer's lung in Scotland: A pilot survey. Br Med J 1:530–534, 1972
6. Roberts RC, Wenzel FJ, Emanuel DA: Precipitating antibodies in a midwest diary farming population toward the antigens associated with farmer's lung disease. J Allergy Clin Immunol 57:518–524, 1976
7. Schlueter DP: Response of the lung to inhaled antigens. Am J Med 57:476–492, 1974
8. Hardy HL, Tabershaw IR: Delayed chemical pneumonitis in workers exposed to beryllium compounds. J Ind Hyg Toxicol 28:197–211, 1946
9. Saltini C, Winestock K, Kirby M, Pinkston P, Crystal RG: Maintenance of alveolitis in patients with chronic beryllium disease by beryllium-specific helper T cells. N Engl J Med 320:1103–1109, 1989
10. Hardy HL: Beryllium poisoning—lessons in control of man-made disease. N Engl J Med 273:1188–1199, 1965
11. Passero MA, Tye RW, Kilburn KH, Lynn WS: Isolation characterization of two glycoproteins from patients with alveolar proteinosis. Proc Natl Acad Sci (USA) 70:973–976, 1973
12. Davidson JM, MacLeod WM: Pulmonary alveolar proteinosis. Br J Dis Chest 63:13–28, 1969
13. Heppleston AG, Wright NA, Stewart JA: Experimental alveolar lipo-proteinosis following the inhalation of silica. J Pathol 101:293–307, 1970
14. Smetana HF, Tandon HG, Viswanataan R, Venkitasubrunarian TA, Chandrasekhary S, Randhawa HS: Experimental bagasse disease of the lung. Lab Invest 11:868–884, 1962
15. Seal RME, Hapke EJ, Thomas GO, Meck JC, Hayes M: The pathology of the acute and chronic stages of farmer's lung. Thorax 23:469–489, 1968
16. Mitchell J, Mann GB, Molyneux M, Lane RE: Pulmonary fibrosis in workers exposed to finely powdered aluminum. Br J Ind Med 18:10–20, 1961
17. Coates EO, Watson JHL: Diffuse interstitial lung disease in tungsten carbide workers. Ann Intern Med 75:709–716, 1971
18. Schepers GWEH: The biological action of particulate cobalt metal. AMA Arch Ind Health 12:127–133, 1955
19. Smith TJ, Petty TL, Reading JC, Lakshminarayans: Pulmonary effects of chronic exposure to airborne cadmium. Am Rev Respir Dis 114:161–169, 1976
20. Kilburn KH: Re-examination of longitudinal studies of workers. Arch Environ Health 44:132–133, 1989

21. Meyer-Bisch C, Pham QT, Mur JM, Massin N, Moulin JJ, Teculescu D, Carton B, Pierre F, Baruthio F: Respiratory hazards in hard-metal workers: A cross sectional study. Br J Ind Med 46:302–309, 1989
22. Merchant JA, Lumsden JC, Kilburn KH, et al: Dose response studies in cotton textile workers. J Occup Med 15:222–230, 1973
23. WHO Environmental Health Criteria Programme: Environmental health criteria for vegetable dusts. Draft prepared by Professor A. Bouhuys, Yale University School of Medicine, New Haven, Conn, 1979
24. Department of Labor: Occupational Safety and Health Administration: Occupational exposure to cotton dust, Part III. Federal Register, June 23, 1978
25. Bongers P, Houthuijs D, Remijn B, Brouwer R, Biersteker K: Lung function and respiratory symptoms in pig farmers. Br J Ind Med 44:819–823, 1987
26. Manfreda J, Cheang M, Warren CPW: Chronic respiratory disorders related to farming and exposure to grain dust in rural adult community. Am J Ind Med 15:7–19, 1989
27. Anto JM, Sunyer J, Rodriguez-Roisin R, Suarez-Cervera M, Vazquez L: Community outbreaks of asthma associated with inhalation of soybean dust. N Engl J Med 320:1097–1102, 1989
28. Musk AW, Peters JM, Wegman DH: Isocyantes and respiratory disease: Current status. Am J Ind Med 13:331–349, 1988
29. Kilburn KH, Warshaw RH: Pulmonary function impairment from years of arc welding. Am J Med 87:62–69, 1989
30. Diem JE, Jones RN, Hendrich DJ, et al: Five-year longitudinal study of workers employed in a new toluene diisocyanate manufacturing plant. Am Rev Respir Dis 126:420–428, 1982
31. Engelberg AL, Piacitelli GM, Petersen M, Zey J, Piccirillo R, Morey PR, Carlson ML, Merchant JA: Medical and industrial hygiene characterization of the cotton waste utilization industry. Am J Ind Med 7:93–108, 1985
32. Pei-lian L, Christiani DC, Ting-ting Y, Nai-yi S, Zhi-Chu G, He-lian D, Wei-de Z, Jun-Wei H, Mu-Zhen L: The study of byssinosis in China: A comprehensive report. Am J Ind Med 12:743–753, 1987
33. Ciba Guest Symposium: Terminology, definitions and classification of chronic pulmonary emphysema and related conditions. Thorax 14:286, 1959
34. Kilburn KH, Warshaw RH: Effects of individually motivating smoking cessation on male blue collar workers. Am J Public Health 80:1334–1337, 1990
35. Hodgkin JE, Abbey DE, Euler GL, Magie AR: COPD prevalence in non-smokers in high and low photochemical air pollution areas. Chest 86:830–838, 1984
36. Miller A, Thornton JC, Warshaw RH, Bernstein J, Selikoff IJ, Teirstein AS: Mean and instantaneous expiratory flows, FVC and FEV_1: Prediction equations from a probability sample of Michigan, a large industrial state. Bull Eur Physiopathol Respir 22:589–597, 1986
37. Schilling RSF, Hughes JPW, Dingwall-Fordyce I, Gilson JC: An epidemiological study of byssinosis among Lancashire cotton workers. Br J Ind Med 12:217–226, 1955
38. McKerrow CB, McDermott M, Gilson JC, Schilling RSF: Respiratory function during the day in cotton workers: A study in byssinosis. Br J Ind Med 15:75–83, 1958
39. Lowe CR, Khosla T: Chronic bronchitis in ex-coal miners working in the steel industry. Br J Ind Med 29:45–49, 1972
40. Sluis-Cremer GK, Walters LG, Sichel HS: Ventilatory function in relation to mining experience and smoking in a random sample of miners and non-miners in a Witwatersrand Town. Br J Ind Med 24:13–25, 1967
41. Davies TAL: A survey of respiratory disease in foundrymen. London: HM Stationery Office, 1971
42. Karpick RJ, Pratt PC, Asmundsson T, Kilburn KH: Pathological findings in respiratory failure. Ann Intern Med 72:189–197, 1970
43. Boren HG, Lake S: Carbon as a carrier mechanism for irritant gases. Arch Environ Health 8:119–124, 1964
44. Merchant JA, Lumsden JC, Kilburn KH, et al: An industrial study of the biological effects of cotton dust and cigarette smoke exposure. J Occup Med 15:212–221, 1973
45. Kilburn KH: Byssinosis 1981. Am J Ind Med 2:81–88, 1981
46. Higgins ITT, Cochrane AL, Gilson JC, Wood CH: Population studies of chronic respiratory disease. Br J Ind Med 16:255–268, 1959
47. Oswald NC, Harold JT, Martin WJ: Clinical pattern of chronic bronchitis. Lancet 2:639–643, 1953
48. Fletcher CM: Chronic bronchitis, its prevalence, nature and pathogenesis. Am Rev Respir Dis 80:483–494, 1959
49. Fletcher CM, Peto R, Tinker C, Speizer FE: The Natural history of chronic bronchitis and emphysema. Oxford: Oxford University Press, 1976
50. Gregory J: A study of 340 cases of chronic bronchitis. Arch Environ Health 22:428–439, 1971
51. Goldsmith JR: Effects of air pollution on human health. In Stern AC (ed): Air Polution, 2 ed. New York: Academic Press, 1968, pp 547–615
52. Van der Lende R, Kok T, Peset R, Quanjer Ph.H, Schouten JP, Orie NGM: Longterm exposure to air pollution and decline in VC and FEV_1. Chest 80:23S–26S, 1981
53. Kryzyanowski M, Jedrychowski W, Wysocki M: Factors associated with the change in ventilatory function and the development of chronic obstructive pulmonary disease in the 13 year follow-up of the Cracow study. Am Rev Respir Dis 134:1011–1090, 1986
54. Imai M, Yoshida K, Kitabtake M: Mortality from asthma and chronic bronchitis associated with changes in sulfur oxides air pollution. Arch Environ Health 41:29–35, 1986
55. Arossa W, Pinaci SS, Bugiani M, Natale P, Bucca C, de Candussio G: Changes in lung function of children after an air pollution decrease. Arch Environ Health 42:170–174, 1987
56. Samet JM, Kutvirb DM, Waxweiler RJ, Kay CR: Uranium mining and lung cancer in Navajo men. N Engl J Med 310:1481–1484, 1984
57. Sunderman FW Jr: Recent progress in nickel carcinogenesis. Toxicol Environ Chem 8:235–252, 1984
58. Comar CL, Nelson N: Health effects of fossil fuel combustion products: Report of a workshop. Environ Health Perspect 12:149–170, 1975
59. Health and Welfare Effects Staff Report: Ambient air quality standard for ozone. Sacramento, Calif.: Research Division Air Resources Board, 1987
60. South Coast Air Quality Management District: Seasonal and diurnal variation in air quality in California's south coast air basin. El Monte, Calif., 1987
61. Rahn KA, Lowenthal DH: Pollution aerosol in the Northeast: Northeastern-Midwestern contributions. Science 228:275–284, 1985
62. Fisher GL, Chang DPY, Brummer M: Fly ash collected from electrostatic precipitators: Microcrystalline structures and the mystery of the spheres. Science 192:553–555, 1976
63. Kerr RA: Nyos, the Killer Lake, may be coming back. Science 244:1541–1542, 1989
64. Hively W: How bleak is the outlook for ozone? American Sci 77: 219–224, 1989
65. Rowland SF: Chlorofluorocarbons and the depletion of stratosphericozone. American Sci 77:36–45, 1989
66. Houghton RA, Woodwell GM: Global climate change. Scientific American 260:36–44, 1989
67. La Bastille A: Acid rain—how great a menace? National Geographic 160:652–680, 1981
68. Jones RR: Ozone depletion and cancer risk. Lancet 2:443–446, 1987
69. Kagawa J, Toyama T, Nakaza M: Pulmonary function test in children exposed to air pollution. In Finkel AJ, Duel WC (eds): Clinical Implications of Air Pollution Research. Acton, Mass.: Publishing Sciences Group, 1976
70. Natusch FS, Wallace JR: Urban aerosol toxicity: The influence of particle size. Science 186:695–699, 1974
71. World Health Organization Regional Office for Europe, Copenhagen: Air quality guidelines for Europe. WHO Regional Publications, European series, No. 23, 1987
72. National Research Council: Epidemiology and air pollution. Washington, D.C.: National Academy Press, 1985

73. Reid L: Measurement of the bronchial mucous gland layer: A diagnostic yardstick in chronic bronchitis. Thorax 15:132–141, 1960
74. Needleman HL, Gunnoe C, Leviton A, Reed R, Peresie H, Maher C, Barrett P. Deficits in psychologic and classroom performance of children with elevated dentine lead levels. N Engl J Med 300:689–695, 1979
75. Grove N: Air—an atmosphere of uncertainty. National Geographic 171:502–537, 1987
76. Arnow PM, Fink JN, Schlueter DP, Barboriak JJ, Mallison G, Said SI, Martin S, Unger GF, Scanlan GT, Kurup VP: Early detection of hypersensitivity pneumonitis in office workers. Am J Med 64:236–242, 1978
77. Hodgson MJ, Morey PR, Attfied M, Sorenson W, Fink JN, Rhodes WW, Visvesvara GS: Pulmonary disease associated with cafeteria flooding. Arch Environ Health 40:96–101, 1985
78. National Academy Press: Indoor Pollutants. Washington, D.C.: The Press, 1981
79. Spengler JD, Sexton K: Indoor air pollution: A public health perspective. Science 221:9–17, 1983
80. Morey PR: Microbial agents associated with building HVAC systems. Presented at The California Council–American Institute of Architects' National Symposium on Indoor Pollution: The Architect's Response. San Francisco, Nov. 9, 1984
81. Konopinski VJ: Formaldehyde in office and commercial environments. Am Ind Hyg Assoc J 44:205–208, 1983
82. Board on Toxicology and Environmental Health Hazards, Commission on Life Sciences, National Research Council: Asbestiform fibers: Nonoccupational health risks. Washington, D.C.: National Academy Press, 1984
83. Archer VE: Association of lung cancer mortality with Precambrian granite. Arch Environ Health 42:87–91, 1987
84. Stebbings JH, Dignam JJ: Contamination of individuals by radon daughters: A preliminary study. Arch Environ Health 43:149–154, 1988

24
Pesticides

Marion Moses

HISTORY

Pesticides are among the few toxic substances deliberately added to our environment. They are, by definition, toxic and biocidal, since their purpose is to kill or harm living things. Pesticides are ubiquitous global contaminants found in air, rain, snow, soil, groundwater, surface water, fog, even the arctic ice pack. All living creatures tested throughout the world are contaminated with pesticides—birds, fish, wildlife, domestic animals, livestock, and human beings, including newborn babies.

The Federal Insecticide Fungicide and Rodenticide Act (FIFRA) defines pesticides as "economic poisons . . . substances intended for preventing, destroying, repelling or mitigating any . . . form of life declared to be pests."

Pesticide use dates back to ancient times with the use of sulfur and arsenic. Use of botanicals such as nicotine (tobacco extract) began in the sixteenth century, and pyrethrum (from chrysanthemums) in the nineteenth century. In the United States, widespread use of copper-arsenic compounds, such as Paris green against the Colorado potato beetle, began in the 1860s. Use of other metallic compounds containing mercury and lead soon followed.

Widespread use of synthetic chemicals in pest control began in the middle to late 1940s. In 1939, Swiss chemist Paul Mueller discovered the insecticidal properties of dichlorodiphenyl trichloroethane (DDT), marketed in 1942. German scientists experimenting with nerve gas during World War II synthesized the organophosphorus insecticide parathion, marketed in 1943. Marketing of the phenoxy herbicides 2,4-D and 2,4,5-T also began in the early 1940s.

The use of DDT dust on allied troops in Italy averted a typhus epidemic in 1942. This made World War II the first war in history in which more soldiers died of their wounds than of disease. DDT and related chlorinated hydrocarbon insecticides and parathion and related organophosphate insecticides became major pest control agents in the 1950s and 1960s. They were extensively used in agriculture in the developed countries and in malaria and other vector control in developing countries.

The first serious challenge to the use of toxic synthetic pesticides was the book *Silent Spring,* by the biologist Rachel Carson, published in 1962. Carson indicted DDT and related chlorinated hydrocarbon insecticides, documenting environmental persistence, bioaccumulation in the fatty tissue of humans and animals, severe toxic effects on nontarget species, especially birds and fish, and potentially devastating ecological and human health effects. A presidential commission was set up to investigate Carson's charges. In 1970 the authority for pesticide regulation and administration of FIFRA was transferred from the U.S. Department of Agriculture to the newly formed Environmental Protection Agency (EPA). In 1972, FIFRA was amended with provisions for protection of human health and the environment from toxic pesticides.

In 1939 there were 32 pesticide products registered with the U.S. Department of Agriculture. In 1987 there were 1200 active-ingredient pesticide chemicals formulated into 37,000 commercial products registered with the EPA. The EPA estimates there are 30 major basic producers of pesticides in the United States, 100 smaller producers, 3300 companies that formulate the finished product, 29,000 pesticide distributors and dealers, and 40,000 commercial pest control firms.[1]

CLASSIFICATION

The term *pesticide* is generic and applies to all chemicals used in pest control. Pesticides are classified according to the type of pest they are active against: insecticides (ants, aphids, beetles, bugs, caterpillars, cockroaches, mosquitoes, moths, termites), herbicides (weeds, grasses, algae), fungicides (mildew, molds, rot, plant diseases), acaricides (mites, ticks), rodenticides (rats, gophers, ground squirrels), pisicides (fish), avicides (birds), molluscicides (snails, slugs), and nematicides (nematodes or nonsegmented soil worms).

Other chemicals the EPA regulates as pesticides are classified by function: defoliants (cause leaves to fall off), desiccants (dry out plants), disinfectants (destroy or inactivate bacteria, other microbes), repellents (primarily of insects, birds), attractants (pheromones, lures, baits), chemosterilants (sterilize insects), growth regulators (stimulate or retard growth of insects or plants).

Pesticide classification is also by chemical type: organophosphates, N-methyl carbamates, chlorinated hydrocarbons, bisdithiocarbamates, organotins, botanicals, arsenicals, phenoxyaliphatic acids, pyrethroids, phenol derivatives, and microbials. Fumigant is a classification based on physical state (gas).

USE

In 1985, total world pesticide use was more than 6 billion pounds, according to World Health Organization (WHO) estimates.[2] These figures do not include wood preservatives and disinfectants. Pesticide use doubled every 10 years between 1945 and 1985.

The United States, which is the world's largest user, accounts for 20% of the total. In 1987 the EPA estimated the United States used 1 billion pounds of conventional pesticides, 1 billion pounds of wood preservatives, and 400 million pounds of disinfectants, with a total expenditure of $7 billion.[2] The second largest user of pesticides is Brazil.

Pesticides are broadly classified into agricultural and nonagricultural use. Primary nonagricultural uses are for wood preservation, public health, maintenance of right-of-way, structural, industrial, and home and garden.

Agricultural Use

Agriculture uses 75% of all the pesticides in the United States (excluding wood preservatives and disinfectants). In 1987 the U.S. EPA estimated 814 million pounds of pesticides were used in agriculture: 505 million pounds of herbicides (62%), 179 million pounds of insecticides (22%), and 70 million pounds of fungicides (9%).[1] About 75% of use is for three crops—corn, soybeans, and cotton.

Pesticide use in food, fiber, and field crops in the United States has changed significantly over the past 2 decades. There has been a decrease in use of insecticides and a marked increase in use of herbicides, which now account for two thirds of all agricultural pesticide use. Most chlorinated hydrocarbon pesticides are banned or severely restricted in the United States, including DDT, aldrin, endrin, dieldrin, chlordane, heptachlor, lindane, toxaphene, and hexachlorobenzene (see Table 24-4). Methoxychlor and endosulfan are nonpersistent chlorinated hydrocarbons widely used on food crops.

Because of the restriction and banning of most chlorinated hydrocarbons in agriculture, there has been an increase in the use of the more acutely toxic organophosphate and N-methyl carbamate insecticides as replacements. Widely used organophosphates include parathion, azinphosmethyl (Guthion), mevinphos (Phosdrin), methamidophos (Monitor, Tamaron), diazinon (Spectracide), chlorpyrifos (Lorsban), and dichlorvos (DDVP). Widely used N-methyl carbamates include aldicarb (Temik), methomyl (Lannate, Nudrin), carbaryl (Sevin), and carbofuran (Furadan).

The most widely used herbicides include: alachlor (Lasso), atrazine, 2,4-D, glyphosate (Roundup), paraquat (Gramoxone), simazine, and trifluralin (Treflan).

Current pesticide use in Canada and Western Europe is similar to that in the United States. Use patterns in other parts of the world, particularly Latin America, the Asia-Pacific region, and Africa, are similar to U.S. use in the 1950s, with insecticides accounting for 60% to 80% of use and herbicides for about 10% to 15%. Use of DDT, aldrin/dieldrin, toxaphene, BHC (benzene hexachloride), lindane, and hexachlorobenzene is widespread in agriculture and in public health in many developing countries.

Brazil, Mexico, Argentina, and Columbia account for about 90% of pesticide use in Latin America. China is the largest consumer in the Asia-Pacific region, followed by India, South Korea, and Indonesia. Sudan and Egypt are major users in Africa.

Nonagricultural Use

Wood Preservatives. The EPA estimates that annual nonagricultural use of pesticides in the U.S. is about 1.5 billion pounds, of which 1 billion pounds is for wood preservation. Of this amount, 950 million pounds is for a single chemical use—creosote on railroad ties. Pentachlorophenol is used for preservation of utility poles, dock pilings, and lumber for construction purposes. The pulp and paper products industry uses large amounts of slimicides.

Structural Pest Control. Structural pest control by commercial firms is a major nonagricultural use. It includes treatment of office buildings, schools, hotels, hospitals, theaters, supermarkets, department stores, restaurants, sports facilities, food storage facilities, aircraft, and homes for a wide variety of pests—mainly ants, cockroaches, fleas, termites, and rodents. A 1982 survey found that 30% of private households had used the services of a pest control firm in the previous year. Chlordane for termite control was the predominant home use pesticide before its banning in 1989 and was used in more than 30 million homes in the United States.

The Texas Pest Control Association estimates that every year there are 8 to 10 million commercial extermination jobs in homes, businesses, restaurants, schools, and other buildings. The 200,000 termite treatments done each year in Texas account for 20% of all termite jobs in the United States. The Structural Pest Control Board estimated that Texas consumers spend more than $1 billion each year for pest control services.

Lawn Care and Turf Management. Use of insecticides, fungicides, and herbicides is extensive in lawn treatment, golf courses, and other turf management. Commercial treatment of home lawns is increasing because of aggressive marketing by chemical lawn treatment companies. The lawn care industry estimates it services 6 to 7 million residential lawns annually. Golf courses are also intensively chemically managed. Use of methyl bromide and other fumigants is extensive and increasing in such turf management.

State and Local Government. Municipal, county, and state government agencies use large amounts of pesticides. A major use is herbicides for maintenance of right-of-way on highways, railroad beds, power transmission lines, and park and recreation areas. Other uses include mosquito and rodent control and treatment of drinking water supplies.

Federal Government. The federal government is also a major user of pesticides. The Department of Defense used large amounts of defoliants for forest and crop destruction during the war in Vietnam. The most widely used was a 50/50 mixture of the phenoxy herbicides 2,4-D and 2,4,5-T, known as Agent Orange. The Drug Enforcement Administration (DEA) authorizes the use of defoliants and herbicides, including paraquat and 2,4-D, in drug eradication programs on federally owned land. The U.S. Agency for International Development assists Mexico and other Latin American countries in spraying herbicides on marijuana and coca plants.

Industrial Use. Pesticides, primarily fungicides, are used as mildewcides, preservatives, and antifoulants in paints, glues, pastes, metalworking fluids and in fabrics used for tents, tarpaulins, sails, tennis nets, and exercise mats. Carpets and upholstery are treated with insecticides for protection from insects and moths. Pesticides are used in a wide variety of consumer products, including cosmetics, shampoos, soaps, household disinfectants, cardboard and other food packaging materials, and in many paper products. Water for industrial purposes and in cooling towers is treated to prevent growth of weeds, algae, fungi, and bacteria. Canals, ditches, reservoirs, and other water channels are similarly treated.

Over-the-Counter. About 65 million pounds of pesticides are sold directly to the public as aerosols, foggers, pest strips, baits, pet products, and lawn and garden chemicals. C.H. Kline Company estimated total nationwide sales of home and garden pesticides were $1.9 billion in 1984, which was double 1980 sales and quadruple 1975 figures. With few exceptions, most of the pesticides in home and garden products are different formulations of agricultural pesticides. Home use pesticides include the herbicides 2,4-D, glyphosate (Roundup) and simazine; the insecticides diazinon (Spectracide), chlorpyrifos (Dursban), carbaryl (Sevin), dichlorvos (DDVP), methoxychlor, malathion, pyrethrins, pyrethroids, and propoxur (Baygon); and the fungicides maneb, captan, benomyl, and chlorothalonil (Daconil, Bravo).

Public Health. On a worldwide basis the chief public health use of pesticides is in malaria control. The ambitious program begun by the World Health Organization (WHO) in 1955 to eradicate malaria is a failure. The primary reason is the increasing resistance of the mosquito vector to insecticides. In several areas of the world the *Anopheles* mosquito is resistant to *all* insecticides, and there is a resurgence of deaths from malaria. Other important uses are for the vectors of filariasis, onchocerciasis, schistosomiasis, and trypanosomiasis. WHO estimates that the 100 million pounds of pesticides used for public health programs in developing countries in 1980 account for 10% of pesticide use.[2] In the United States, public health uses are primarily for mosquito and rodent control and treatment of drinking water.

Regulation. The EPA lacks much of the exposure data it needs to perform accurate and reliable risk assessments for exposure of the general public to nonagricultural pesticides. Nonagricultural use of pesticides is unregulated, and there are no good data on the amount and consequences of unrestricted homeowner and other use. A Government Accounting Office (GAO) investigation in 1986 determined that "the pesticide industry sometimes make safety claims that the EPA considers to be false or misleading." The GAO also noted that consumers who apply pesticides around their homes or hire professional applicators are not told that the pesticides have not been tested for chronic health effects by current standards.[3]

EXPOSURE TO PESTICIDES

Those with the greatest exposure to pesticides are workers who handle the concentrated technical formulations. They include pesticide formulation workers; farmers, agricultural, and other workers who mix and apply pesticides; structural pest control operators (exterminators); and lawn, golf course, and turf maintenance workers. Exposures are generally much lower in pesticide manufacturing workers, since batch processing requires almost no direct contact.

Field workers who cultivate and harvest crops are exposed to pesticide residues on leaf surfaces, on the crop itself, in the soil, or in the duff (decaying plant and organic material that collects under vines and trees). These workers are also exposed to overspray from crop dusting aircraft and drift from ground rig applications, especially airblast sprayers in groves and orchards.

Nonoccupational exposures to bystanders and community residents from drift are increasing as residential housing developers build adjacent to agricultural groves, orchards, and fields. Significant concentrations of pesticides can drift a mile or more from the site of initial application, depending on droplet size and wind conditions; lower concentrations can drift many miles. Off-gassing from fields where fumigants such as methyl bromide have been injected into the soil is also a potential source of exposure to community residents. In California, off-gassing from a gladiola field required evacuation of a community.[4]

Pesticides are readily absorbed through the skin, the respiratory tract (inhalation), and the gastrointestinal tract (ingestion). The eye also readily absorbs pesticides and can be a significant route of exposure in splashes and spills. The chief route of occupational exposure to pesticides is the skin and not, as commonly believed, the respiratory system. Fumigants, which are in the form of gases, are a notable exception, which accounts in part for their greater toxicity. However, the skin is a route of absorption for them as well. Pesticides can persist on the skin for many months after exposure.[5] The respiratory tract can be an important route of absorption for the general public from over-the-counter products in the form of aerosols, foggers, smoke bombs, and pest strips.

The rate of absorption of pesticides into the body is product specific and depends on the properties of the active-ingredient pesticide and the inert ingredients in a particular formulation.

Basic types of pesticide formulations include *dusts,* a mix of the dry pesticide ingredient with finely ground clay, talc, or volcanic ash; *granules,* a mix of the active ingredient with clay or sand particles much larger than dusts; *wettable powders,* a distribution of the pesticide in dry, powderlike particles for mixture with water before application; *emulsifiable concentrate,* a liquid containing the technical material, an organic solvent, an emulsifier, spreader, and sticker (the solvent dissolves the pesticide, and the emulsifier allows it to be mixed with water); *flowables,* a special type of liquid formulation containing finely ground solid particles of pesticide suspended in liquid; *seed treatments,* which are similar to wettable powders but in which the particles are more finely ground so a coating adheres to the seed; *drenches,* a slurry or strong solution of a systemic pesticide for soaking roots of seedling plants or cuttings; and *baits,* a mixture of the pesticide with palatable grains, pastes, or other food attractive to the pest.

The formulated product thus may contain the active-ingredient pesticide diluted with water, oil, solvents, adjuvants, spreaders, stickers, and a variety of other "inert" ingredients. Typical solvents are light aromatics such as xylene; chlorinated organics such as 1,1,1-trichloroethane; and mineral spirits.

Inert does not mean the ingredient is not chemically or biologically reactive, only that it is not active as a pesticide. Often the "inert" ingredients are more toxic than the pesticide itself or pose a more significant potential chronic health hazard. Over-the-counter aerosol pesticide products may contain carcinogenic solvents such as trichloroethylene and methylene chloride as "inert" ingredients.

Because of trade secret provisions in the FIFRA law it is almost impossible to find out what inert ingredients are in a pesticide product. Material Safety Data Sheets provide information on the active ingredient only and usually only on acute toxicity. In cases of poisoning, the effects may be from the active ingredient pesticide, the "inert" ingredient, or a combination of the two.

TOXICOLOGY

Organophosphate Pesticides

Organophosphate pesticides are similar to nerve gases and exert their toxic effect by inhibition of the nervous system enzyme acetylcholinesterase (cholinesterase). Cholinesterase breaks down the neurotransmitter acetylcholine at synaptic sites and is critical in the transmission of nerve impulses. The signs and symptoms of organophosphate poisoning are due to the subsequent build-up of acetylcholine at synaptic sites in muscles, glands, autonomic ganglia, and the brain.

There are two types of enzymes capable of hydrolyzing choline esters in humans. "True" cholinesterase is found in red blood cells (RBC), and pseudocholinesterase is found in plasma.

Both RBC and plasma cholinesterase activity may be decreased in liver and other diseases, but the decrease is small compared with the degree of inhibition by organophosphate pesticides.

Decreased activity of cholinesterase in the blood is a biological indicator of poisoning by organophosphates. Testing RBC and plasma cholinesterase activity levels is therefore an excellent tool for diagnosing organophosphate pesticide poisoning and for monitoring worker exposure. A 10% to 40% reduction in activity usually results in latent poisoning without clinical manifestations. A 50% to 60% reduction results in mild poisoning. A reduction of 70% to 80% results in moderate poisoning, and 90% reduction in activity results in severe poisoning that may be fatal without treatment.

The rate of reduction in activity of cholinesterase greatly affects the development of signs and symptoms. A rapid reduction over a few minutes or hours can produce marked signs and symptoms. A gradual drop of the same magnitude over a period of days or weeks may cause only minimal signs and symptoms. In an occupational exposure setting a reduction of enzyme activity 25% or more from a preexposure or "baseline" level is evidence of excess absorption and indication for removal of the worker from any additional exposure.

Atropine, which blocks the effect of acetylcholine, is the antidote for organophosphate pesticide poisoning. Pralidoxime (2-PAM), if given within 24 to 48 hours of exposure, can reactivate cholinesterase and restore function of the enzyme. After this time "aging" of the enzyme-pesticide complex occurs, and it is refractory to reactivation.

Organophosphate pesticides and one in particular, parathion, are responsible for most of the occupational poisonings and deaths in the United States and throughout the world. Other highly toxic pesticides in this chemical class are mevinphos (Phosdrin), methamidophos (Monitor, Tamaron), and azinphosmethyl (Guthion).

Symptoms of poisoning occur soon after exposure, usually within 4 to 12 hours. Fatigue, headache, dizziness, nausea, vomiting, chest tightness, excess sweating, salivation, abdominal pain, and diarrhea are signs and symptoms of mild poisoning. In moderate poisoning the victim usually cannot walk, has generalized weakness, difficulty in talking, muscular fasciculations, and miosis, besides the symptoms mentioned above. In severe poisoning the victim is usually unconscious with marked miosis, flaccid paralysis, respiratory difficulty, increased bronchial secretions, and cyanosis. Pulmonary edema may be present, and convulsions can occur. Death from respiratory paralysis may occur without treatment.

Central nervous system effects also occur, such as restlessness, anxiety, tremulousness, dizziness, insomnia, excessive dreaming, nightmares, slurring of speech, confusion, difficulty in concentrating, and, with severe exposure, convulsions and coma.

The organophosphates are readily metabolized by the body, and with early and proper treatment most occupationally poisoned workers will recover. In cases of accidental or suicidal ingestion, recovery depends on the amount ingested and the interval before emergency treatment and resuscitation. Recovery appears to be complete. However, recent studies suggest there may be long-term neurobehavioral effects after recovery from acute poisoning.[6] The potential chronic effects of long-term, low-level exposures have not been studied. Delayed neurotoxicity due to organophosphates is discussed below under Chronic Health Effects.

N-Methyl Carbamates

The N-methyl carbamate pesticides are similar to the organophosphates in their acute toxic effects and like them are inhibitors of the enzyme cholinesterase. However the inhibition of the enzyme is readily reversible, and symptoms appear earlier. Workers are thus more likely to remove themselves from exposure. Except for an aldicarb (Temik)-related tractor accident death of a young farm worker,[7] no occupational deaths have been reported from these compounds in the United States.

Tests of RBC and plasma cholinesterase are less useful in poisoning with the N-methyl carbamate pesticides. Unlike the irreversible phosphorylation of the enzyme by the organophosphates, carbamylation is readily reversible and can occur in vitro during transport of the specimen to the laboratory.

The antidote for N-methyl carbamate poisoning is atropine. Unless there is exposure to an organophosphate pesticide as well, use of 2-PAM is not recommended, since it is usually unnecessary and may be harmful. The use of 2-PAM is contraindicated in poisoning with carbaryl (Sevin).[8]

Widely used toxic N-methyl carbamates include aldicarb (Temik), methomyl (Lannate), carbofuran (Furadan), and oxamyl (Vydate). Methyl isocyanate (MIC), the chemical that caused thousands of poisonings and deaths in Bhopal, India, in 1984, is an intermediate in the manufacture of N-methyl carbamate insecticides.

Chlorinated Hydrocarbons

The exact mechanism of toxicity of the chlorinated hydrocarbon pesticides, which include DDT, aldrin, endrin, dieldrin, toxaphene, lindane, chlordane and heptachlor, is not known. They are central nervous system stimulants and in toxic doses cause anxiety, tremor, hyperexcitability, and generalized seizures, which can result in death. Convulsions or abnormal electroencephalograms (EEG) have been found in workers manufacturing aldrin, dieldrin, and endrin or applying dieldrin as a spray. Some of these workers showed no overt signs or symptoms of clinical toxicity. The EEG abnormalities in some cases persisted long after exposure ceased. Toxic hepatitis, cholestatic jaundice, and a wide range of abnormalities in liver function have occasionally been reported in the occupationally exposed.

In general most of the chlorinated hydrocarbons are of lower acute toxicity than the organophosphates and N-methyl carbamates. Chlorinated hydrocarbon pesticides are highly lipophilic and biodegrade slowly, with long half lives. Their metabolites are persistent and ubiquitous contaminants of human fatty tissues and breast milk. The most commonly found pesticides or metabolites are DDE, dieldrin, transnonachlor, oxychlordane, heptachlor expoxide, beta-BHC, and hexachlorobenzene.

One of the most serious outbreaks of poisoning from a chlorinated hydrocarbon pesticide in the United States occurred between March 1974 and July 1975 in Hopewell, Virginia, in a plant manufacturing and formulating the insecticide chlordecone (Kepone). More than half the workers were severely poisoned, with clinical manifestations of nervousness, apprehension, tremor, head bobbing, opsoclonus, ataxia, and visual and speech disturbances. Weight loss, pleuritic chest pain, and arthralgia were also reported. The most severely affected worker developed a toxic psychosis with active hallucinosis. Unlike poisonings with other chlorinated hydrocarbons, generalized seizures did not occur. Further examination of the workers revealed abnormalities in nerve conduction velocity, and sperm abnormalities with oligospermia and decreased motility. Chlordecone levels were as high as 32 ppm in the blood, 91 ppm in the fat, and 173 ppm in the liver of affected workers; 94% of the family contacts of the workers had detectable levels in their blood.[9]

In July 1975 the plant was closed by the Virginia State Department of Health. EPA canceled the registration of chlordecone in 1976. Mirex, a compound chemically similar to Kepone and which degrades to Kepone, was previously widely used for fire ant control in the southeastern United States.

One of the most serious outbreaks of poisoning from a chlorinated hydrocarbon pesticide outside the United States occurred in Turkey from 1956 to 1959. Seed wheat for planting, treated with the fungicide hexachlorobenzene, was sold for food in several villages. More than 3000 cases of acquired porphyria cutanea tarda were reported, with a mortality rate of about 10%. The largest number of deaths was in infants who nursed from mothers who had porphyria or who had eaten bread made from the contaminated wheat.

Those affected manifested blistering and epidermal lysis of the skin with poor healing, often complicated by suppuration leading to arthritis and osteomyelitis, particularly of the fingers. Also present were hyperpigmentation, hypertrichosis, weight loss, hepatomegaly, thyroid and lymph node abnormalities, and increased excretion of porphyrins in the urine.[10] Turkey banned hexachlorobenzene in 1959. The United States still allows its use for seed treatment.

Hexachlorobenzene is a contaminant of the herbicide Dacthal and the fungicide chlorothalonil (Bravo, Daconil). It is a widespread environmental contaminant as a by-product of perchlorethylene manufacture. Hexachlorobenzene is a ubiquitous contaminant of human breast milk.

Phenolic and Cresolic Pesticides

All these pesticides, which include pentachlorophenol (Penta, PCP), dinoseb (DNBP, dinotro [-phenol]), DNOC (4,6-dinitro-ortho-o-cresol), and dinocap, are highly toxic. They exert their effects by the uncoupling of oxidative phosphorylation, resulting in interference with cellular respiration and a severe hypermetabolic state. Clinical manifestations include anorexia, flushing, severe thirst, weakness, marked sweating, and severe hyperthermia, which can progress to coma and death. Profuse diaphoresis distinguishes this type of poisoning from heat stroke, with which it may be confused. Aspirin is contraindicated in the treatment of hyperthermia from poisoning with these compounds. All are toxic to the liver, kidneys, and nervous system. They are readily absorbed by all routes of exposure, especially the skin. Ambient weather conditions of high temperature and humidity enhance the toxicity of these chemicals. Many occupationally related deaths have occurred from these compounds. In 1983 a young farm worker in Texas died after 3 days of applying dinoseb to cotton while using a leaking backpack sprayer.

Dinoseb, DNOC, and related compounds are widely used in agriculture as herbicides and insecticides. They stain the skin yellow on contact. Diffuse yellowing of the skin and the sclerae (jaundice) is a sign of hepatotoxicity and indicates serious poisoning. The EPA emergency suspended most uses of dinoseb in 1986 and banned it in 1989. It is still manufactured in the United States for export.

The primary use of pentachlorophenol is as a wood preservative for utility poles, dock pilings, and construction lumber. Sodium pentachlorophenate is used in water for industrial processes to prevent growth of weeds, algae, fungi, and bacteria and as a molluscicide. There are reports of occupational deaths from its use as a wood preservative and as a molluscicide in agriculture and of deaths in infants in a newborn nursery where it was used in washing of diapers. There are also reports of illness related to its volatilization from treated wood surfaces, especially in log cabins. The main effects were eye and mucosal irritation, but there was also serious damage to the eye, with diminution of vision or blindness.

Dibenzodioxins and dibenzofurans contaminate technical pentachlorophenol. Chloracne may be seen in workers exposed to these contaminants.

Phenoxyaliphatic Acid Herbicides

2,4-D (2,4-dichlorophenoxy acetic acid), 2,4-DP (2,4-dichlorophenoxy proprionic acid), 2,4-DB (2,4-dichlorophenoxy butyric acid), MCPA (2-methyl-4-chlorophenoxy acetic acid), MCPP, and dicamba (2-methyl-3,6-dichlorobenzoic acid) are widely used herbicides in the United States. There are hundreds of different formulations for use in agriculture, maintenance of right-of-way, turf management, and lawn and garden use. The EPA suspended the registration of 2,4,5-T (2,4,5-trichlorophenoxy acetic acid) and silvex (2,4,5-trichlorophenoxy proprionic acid) in 1979, which were banned in 1989.

The acute oral and dermal mammalian toxicity of these compounds is relatively low, and they are readily metabolized and excreted. However, they can be contaminated with dioxins, which are toxic contaminants in products and intermediates made from chlorinated phenols. There are 75 different isomers of dioxin, of which 2,3,7,8-tetrachlorodibenzo-p-dioxin (TCDD), which contaminates 2,4,5-T and silvex, is the most toxic. 2,3,7,8-TCDD is carcinogenic and teratogenic in animals at very low doses.

The toxic effects of 2,3,7,8-TCDD in humans are known from episodes of illness in workers heavily exposed during explosions, accidents, and the manufacture of 2,4,5-T, and the 2,4,5-trichlorophenol from which it is made. Consistently reported signs and symptoms include hyperirritability, sleep disturbances, insomnia or hypersomnia, loss of vigor and drive, decreased libido, and in some cases, impotence. Effects on the liver range from abnormalities in liver enzymes to toxic hepatitis and elevated lipids. Psychiatric manifestations were frequent and often severe. The most severely affected workers developed sensory-motor peripheral neuropathy. Porphyria cutanea tarda, an acquired defect in metabolism of porphyrins by the liver, has also been reported.

Chloracne, a skin disease characterized by comedones, cysts, pustules, and inflammatory skin changes, is the most commonly reported effect of exposure to 2,3,7,8-TCDD. It generally occurs within 4 to 6 weeks of exposure and can persist for as long as 30 years after cessation of exposure. Most children who developed chloracne after environmental exposure to 2,3,7,8-TCDD from an explosion at a factory in Italy in 1976 had recovered completely 10 years later.

Controversy has surrounded the use of Agent Orange, a 50/50 mixture of 2,4,5-T and 2,4-D, used by the U.S. military as a defoliant in Vietnam from 1962 to 1969. Chronic long-term health effects in Vietnam veterans and birth defects in their children have been alleged. Studies by the Centers for Disease Control in Atlanta and the Australian government have found no increased risk for Vietnam veterans to father children with birth defects. Preliminary findings from studies of air force pilots who flew the spray missions in Vietnam (Ranch Hands) reveal no major clinical problems specifically related to 2,4,5-T exposure. Ground troops have not been adequately studied.

Bipyridyl Herbicides

Paraquat (Gramoxone) is one of the most widely used herbicides in the world. It is also the most toxic and has been responsible for thousands of deaths. Diquat, a related compound, is mainly used for aquatic weed control and is less toxic than paraquat.

Paraquat is an epithelial toxin and a powerful irritant that can cause severe injury to the eyes, skin, nose, and throat, resulting in ulceration, epistaxis, and severe dystrophy or complete loss of the fingernails. High mortality is associated with the ingestion, accidental or suicidal, of paraquat. Acute poisoning causes damage to the liver, kidney, and myocardium. These effects, though severe, are reversible, and in most cases the patient will recover from renal and hepatic failure only to die of asphyxiation due to a relentlessly progressive pulmonary fibrosis. Death may occur in hours or 1 to 3 or more weeks after ingestion, depending on the dose and treatment. Dermal exposure to paraquat can cause fatal pulmonary fibrosis, and deaths have been reported in farmers, a landscape maintenance worker, and from application to the skin for treatment of lice and scabies.

Paraquat's mechanism of toxicity is likely due to reaction with molecular oxygen to form a superoxide ion with resulting lipid peroxidation. There is no antidote to paraquat poisoning, and most patients who absorb or ingest an amount sufficient to cause severe organ toxicity do not survive.

Fumigants

Fumigants are highly toxic and the most acutely hazardous to workers of any pesticide compounds. Most are alkylating agents, mutagens, carcinogens, neurotoxic, and hepatotoxic. They are responsible for many occupational deaths, especially methyl bromide. Because they are in the form of a gas, they are readily absorbed through the lungs and rapidly distributed throughout the body. The central nervous system, lungs, liver, and kidneys can be severely affected. Pulmonary edema can occur and is a frequent cause of death. Severe neurotoxic and behavioral effects, including toxic psychosis, can result from poisoning with methyl bromide. Such mental and behavioral changes can occur after acute overexposures or from low-level chronic exposure and can be progressive and irreversible.[11]

Commonly used structural fumigants are methyl bromide and sulfuryl fluoride. Commonly used soil fumigants are methyl bromide and dichloropropane-dichloropropene (D-D, Telone II). Methyl bromide is odorless at low concentrations and contains the "tear gas" Chloropicrin as a warning agent. Aluminum phosphide is used in shipping of grains and methyl bromide in fumigation of a wide variety of commodities such as spices, nuts, and fruits. The soil fumigants dibromochloropropane (DBCP) and ethylene dibromide (EDB) were banned in 1979 and 1984, respectively. See below for discussion of chronic effects of DBCP on the reproductive system.

Insect Repellents

N,N-diethyl-m-toluamide (Deet, Off) first marketed in 1954, is a widely used insect repellent. It is applied directly to the skin and is effective against mosquitoes, ticks, fleas, gnats, biting flies, and chiggers. Its use has been increasing, especially in children, because of public concerns regarding ticks that carry Lyme disease. It is extensively used by the military for troops in the field.

Deet is neurotoxic and can cause death if ingested. Systemic toxicity can also be caused by absorption through the skin, and fatalities have been reported in infants and children after repeated dermal exposure or exposure to high concentrations. The clinical picture is one of toxic encephalopathy, with slurring of speech, tremor, convulsions, and coma. It has been recommended that all high strength (more than 75%) formulations be withdrawn from the market.[12]

ACUTE EFFECTS

Poisoning and Death

Acute health effects of pesticides range from irritant effects on the eye and upper respiratory tract, to contact dermatitis, to systemic poisoning, which can lead to death.

The WHO estimates that the total number of acute unintentional poisonings annually throughout the world is between 3.5 to 5 million cases, of which 3 million are severe poisonings, resulting in 20,000 deaths. They estimate that intentional poisonings number 2 million, with 200,000 resulting in death (suicide). They further estimate another million cases of chronic effects.[2]

The number of pesticide poisonings in the U.S. is not known, but estimates are that there are 300,000 agricultural worker pesticide poisonings each year.[13] In California, the only state that requires and enforces mandatory reporting by physicians of occupational pesticide-related illness, doctors reported 1211 cases in 1986. Most of the cases were in agricultural workers. Since many affected workers never see a doctor or are not properly diagnosed, these numbers are underestimates.[14]

There are several reasons for the underreporting of pesticide-related occupational disease. In mild and moderate poisoning the signs and symptoms are nonspecific and may be confused with common illnesses such as gastroenteritis, upper respiratory disease, and other flulike illness. Workers often do not know or suspect that their signs and symptoms may be due to pesticide exposure. Doctors often do not know how to recognize early mild forms of pesticide poisoning and do not take even a minimal occupational history. There may be strong dysincentives to report illness, by both the employer and the worker. The employer does not want his insurance premium to increase or to disrupt the harvest of a highly perishable crop, or his workers may not be covered by workers' compensation. The workers must maximize income and cannot afford to take time off from work. Also many workers justifiably fear the loss of their job if they complain, or ask to be sent to a doctor.

A study of emergency room visits and hospitalizations for pesticide-related illness in Nebraska in 1984 found an annual incidence of 1.35 cases per 10,000 population.[15] An EPA study of hospital admissions for pesticide poisoning estimated an annual rate of 8.2 per 100,000 hospital admissions for pesticide poisoning. Of 192 deaths, 120 (66%) were intentional, 48 (25%) were nonoccupational, and 24 (12.5%) were occupational.[16] A death certificate study reported 52 pesticide related deaths in 1974, with 30% being in children less than 10 years old. Pesticide storage in soft drink bottles and other inappropriate containers in the reach of children is a major cause of morbidity and mortality.

Of 1,368,748 human exposure cases reported by 64 poison control centers throughout the U.S. in 1988, 56,674 (4.1%) were due to pesticides. Organophosphates and carbamates, alone or in combination, accounted for 33% of the cases; rodenticides for 19%; herbicides for 8%, and chlorinated hydrocarbons for 7%. Of the 545 fatalities, 20 (3.7%) were from pesticides; 15 were suicides, 3 were accidents, and 2 were unknown. Organophosphates, alone or in combination, were responsible for 9 of the deaths, and herbicides (2,4-D, diquat and paraquat) for 5.[17]

Developing countries account for 25% of pesticide use, but 50% of acute poisonings and 75% of deaths. Most of the occupational poisonings and deaths are from highly toxic organophosphates such as parathion and methamidophos (Monitor).

However, pesticides thought to be "safe" can cause severe poisoning and death. In 1975, five deaths and 2800 poisonings occurred in Pakistan during the spraying of malathion for malaria control.[18] Malathion is one of the least toxic organophosphates, and there were no reports of occupational poisonings and deaths before this incident. The contaminant isomalathion, a toxic isomerization product found in one of the formulations, was responsible for the deaths. WHO has now changed the specifications so that this toxic contaminant must be below a certain percentage for malathion used in malaria control.

The number of pesticide deaths from suicide is increasing, especially among the poor in developing countries. In one study the percentage of pesticide-related deaths that were suicides was 60% in the Philippines, 73% in Sri Lanka, and 90% in Trinidad-Tobago.[19] In Sri Lanka most of the suicides are from ingestion of paraquat. Paraquat is also responsible for about 1300 deaths a year from suicide in Japan, despite reformulation in a gelatinous form difficult to swallow and addition of a stench agent and an emetic.

Effects on Skin

Workers in agriculture are at four times greater risk of skin disease than workers in other industries. Most pesticide-related skin problems are primary irritant or contact dermatitis. Propargite (Omite), sulfur, glyphosate (Roundup), captan (Orthocide), methyl bromide, creosote, triadimefon (Bayleton), and cryolite exposures are the most frequently reported causes of contact dermatitis in California agricultural workers. The "inert" ingredients in a pesticide may be responsible for or contribute to the dermatitis, especially organic solvents and petroleum distillates.

Pesticides also can be sensitizers, that is, cause allergic contact dermatitis. Some workers can be permanently disabled, since they cannot tolerate even minute exposures to the pesticide. Sunlight can aggravate the dermatitis, adding to the disability. Pesticides known to cause allergic contact dermatitis include alachlor (Lasso), benomyl (Benlate), Botran, captan, captafol (Difolatan), folpet, dazomet, anilazine (Dyrene), maneb, Mancozeb, Zineb, thiram, naled (Dibrom), PCNB (pentachloronitrobenzene), propachlor, pyrethrums, and pyrethroids. It is often difficult to determine if the allergic contact dermatitis is from pesticides exposure or from the crop itself. Patch testing is necessary to identify the allergen and confirm the diagnosis.[20]

Other Acute Effects

People with debilitating medical conditions affecting the respiratory or cardiovascular system may be more susceptible to adverse effects from pesticide exposure at levels tolerated by those not affected. Those with asthma or severe allergies may be at higher risk as well.

CHRONIC HEALTH EFFECTS

Chronic effects of concern in pesticide-exposed populations include cancer, birth defects, neurotoxicity (including neurobehavioral deficits and neuropsychological changes), and adverse effects on reproduction and fertility. Chronic effects may occur with no prior indication of acute health effects. Most workers have chronic exposure to low-levels of many different pesticides (and "inert" ingredients) over a working lifetime. The extent and magnitude of chronic health problems from occupational and environmental exposure to pesticides is not known because appropriate studies have not been done.

Cancer

Recent epidemiological studies show increased risk of cancer in humans occupationally and environmentally exposed to pesticides. There are reports of statistically significantly increased risk for non-Hodgkin's lymphoma, leukemia, multiple myeloma, liver cancer, testicular cancer, brain cancer, and lung cancer, in U.S. farmers, agricultural workers, pest control operators, and pesticide manufacturing workers. There are reports of increased risks in similar pesticide-exposed populations for non-Hodgkin's lymphoma in New Zealand and Sweden; multiple myeloma in Australia, Finland, and New Zealand; testicular cancer in England, Wales, and Sweden; liver cancer in Sweden; brain cancer in Italy, and lung cancer in East Germany.[21]

In the early 1970s, several case reports suggested a possible association between pesticide exposure and neuroblastoma and colorectal cancer in children. Studies show household pesticide use by the parents is a risk factor for children with primary brain cancer or acute lymphocytic leukemia.[21]

Sterility

In 1977, several men working in the pesticide formulation division of a California chemical company noticed they had not recently fathered children. Sperm tests showed them to be either azoospermic (complete absence of sperm) or oligospermic, with sperm counts of less than 20 million. The fumigant 1,2-dibromo-3-chloropropane (DBCP), used in agriculture as a nematicide, was responsible. Two of the sterile workers had not had any exposure to DBCP for 9 and 13 years, respectively, and both had fathered children before their exposure to the pesticide. A follow-up 8 years later found that while some had recovered, in others the damage to their testes was permanent.[22] Studies of other workers exposed to DBCP or a similar pesticide, ethylene dibromide (EDB), also showed lowered sperm counts and impaired fertility.

DBCP is the most frequently found contaminant of groundwater in California. Thousands of drinking water wells in agricultural counties where soil injection was extensive are heavily contaminated and can no longer be used. The EPA banned DBCP in 1979, except for use on pineapple in Hawaii. Only after extensive contamination of the Maui aquifer did the EPA totally ban it in 1989. DBCP is still leaching into groundwater in California, 10 years after all use stopped because of its long life in soil and continual downward movement into the aquifers. EDB, which replaced DBCP in 1979, was banned in 1984. It is also a widespread contaminant of groundwater, particularly in the state of Florida, which relies on aquifers for more than 90% of its water. Both DBCP and EDB are potent animal carcinogens.

Birth Defects

Birth defects, which are the leading cause of infant mortality and a major cause of infant morbidity in the United States, are relatively rare, occurring in 3% to 7% of all births. In one of the few studies of farm workers, of all births in a California County Hospital, infants of agricultural workers had a high prevalence of limb-reduction defects. A larger follow-up study showed an association between residence in agricultural counties and limb-reduction defects.[23] There are occasional case reports of birth defects associated with occupational exposure to pesticides during the first trimester. Recently a pregnant woman working in cauliflower oversprayed with Metasystox-R, a known animal teratogen, delivered a chromosomally normal child with multiple severe defects who died 2 weeks later.

Studies in Arkansas, New Zealand, and Hungary of parental environmental or occupational exposures to the phenoxy herbicides 2,4,5-T and 2,4-D found no association between exposure to these herbicides and major structural defects.

Vietnam veterans have also raised concerns about their exposure to Agent Orange. Two well-conducted case-control studies by the Centers for Disease Control in Atlanta and by the Australian government found no relationship between service in Vietnam and fathering a child with a birth defect.

The failure to find a high rate of birth defects associated with pesticide exposures may be due to the embryotoxicity or fetotoxicity of the pesticide.[24] The embryo or fetus may be poisoned in utero and spontaneously aborted early in the pregnancy. A U.S. study of maternal occupation and fetal death found farm worker women to be at increased risk for spontaneous abortion.[25] A study in India found increased rates of spontaneous abortion, stillbirth, and sterility in vineyard workers.[26]

Chronic Neurotoxic Effects

Pesticide-induced Delayed Neuropathy. Certain organophosphate pesticides can cause delayed neuropathy involving long and large diameter fibers in the spinal cord and peripheral nervous system. Demyelination results in muscle weakness that may progress to paralysis, with the lower extremities usually more severely affected than the upper. Onset is usually 2 to 4 weeks after the acute exposure. Organophosphates known to cause delayed neuropathy in hens (the experimental animal used for testing) include EPN, trichlorfon (Dipterex), dichlorvos (DDVP), DEF, isofenphos (Oftanol), and leptophos (Phosvel).

Pesticide-induced delayed neuropathy is thought to be the cause of severe neurological disease in 12 workers at a pesticide plant in Texas that manufactured leptophos for export. Four employees were diagnosed with multiple sclerosis, two with psychiatric disorders, and three with encephalitis. The National Institute for Occupational Safety and Health (NIOSH) determined that the neuropathy was work related.[27] Leptophos used in cotton production caused paralysis and death in thousands of water buffalo in Egypt.

Two case reports of suicidal ingestion of organophosphates suggest that humans may be more susceptible to pesticide-induced delayed neuropathy than the hen. Chlorpyrifos (Dursban, Lorsban) may be implicated in such delayed neuropathy in a 20-year-old man who suicidally ingested chlorpyrifos.[28] Chlorpyrifos is coming into increasingly wider use in over-the-counter insecticides, pet collars, and for termite and cockroach infestations and in lawn and garden products. Unlike other organophosphates, chlorpyrifos has a long residual action and is stored in fatty tissue.

Neurobehavioral and Neuropsychological Effects. Several early case reports document that organophosphate pesticides can cause profound mental and psychological changes. In a study using mental patients as research subjects, administration of a small amount of pesticide resulted in an apparently permanent exacerbation of acute psychosis in a previously stable patient. There are several other case reports of mental illness or severe psychological disturbances in pesticides applicators, as well as behavioral changes such as anxiety, difficulties in concentration, memory deficits, and other subtle effects.[29]

Few follow-up studies are available in persons poisoned by pesticides to determine if any long-term or delayed effects were present. One such study examined 117 of 235 individuals 3 years after occupational poisoning by organophosphate pesticides, mainly parathion and Phosdrin. Thirty-three still had complaints 3 years later; in 10 of these individuals in whom the central nervous system was involved, the complaint was mainly of visual disturbances. No major psychiatric or neurological sequelae were found.[30] A recent study investigated neuropsychological status of 100 persons poisoned by organophosphate pesticides (mainly parathion), an average of 9 years before, compared with nonpoisoned controls. The poisoned subjects had significant differences in measures of memory, abstraction, and mood. Twice as many had scores consistent with cerebral damage or dysfunction, and personality scores showed greater distress and complaints of disability.[6]

The fumigant methyl bromide can cause toxic psychosis and irreversible neurological and neurobehavioral sequelae after recovery from acute poisoning or from chronic overexposure.[11] Chlordecone (Kepone) can cause toxic psychosis with active hallucinosis.[9]

Other Neurological Disease. The street drug MPTP (1-methyl-4-phenyl-1,2,3,6-tetrahydropyridine) is known to induce Parkinson's disease in drug abusers.[31] Methyl phenylpyridine (MPP), a toxic metabolite of MPTP, is similar in structure to the herbicide paraquat. Case reports of Parkinson's disease in pesticide applicators and a higher prevalence of the disease in agricultural areas of Quebec with high pesticide use led to consideration of pesticides as a possible risk factor for the disease.[32]

CARCINOGENICITY AND TERATOGENICITY

The EPA classifies pesticides into five categories depending on the weight of the evidence for cancer in humans:

A. Human carcinogen
B. Probable human carcinogen
  B1. Sufficient evidence of carcinogenicity from animal studies with limited evidence from epidemiologic studies
  B2. Sufficient evidence of carcinogenicity from animal studies with inadequate or no epidemiologic data
C. Possible human carcinogen. Limited evidence of carcinogenicity in the absence of human data
D. Not classifiable as to human carcinogenicity. Inadequate or no human and animal data for carcinogenicity
E. Evidence of noncarcinogenicity for humans. No evidence of carcinogenicity in at least two animal species in adequate studies, based on available evidence, and does not mean is not a carcinogen under any circumstances

The EPA classifies arsenic as A and cadmium as B1. Pesticides in the B2 classification (probable human carcinogens) include the *insecticides* amdro, chlordane/heptachlor, chlordimeform, DDT/DDE/DDD, dichlorvos (DDVP, Vapona), dieldrin, propoxur (Baygon); the *fungicides* captafol (Difolatan), captan, chlorothalonil (Daconil, Bravo), folpet, hexachlorobenzene, maneb/Mancozeb/Zineb (based on contamination with ethylene thiourea, ETU); the *fumigants* dibromochloropropane (DBCP), ethylene dibromide (EDB), and dichloropropane/dichloropropene (D-D, Telone II); the *herbicides* acetochlor, aciflurofen, alachlor (Lasso), amitrole, oxadizaon (Ronstar); and the *plant growth regulator,* daminozide (Alar).[33]

Widely used pesticides that the EPA classifies as teratogens include the *fungicides* benomyl, captafol, folpet, hexachlorobenzene, Mancozeb, maneb, tributyltin oxide, triphenyltin fluoride, and triphenyltin acetate; the *herbicides* acrolein (Aqualin), bentazon (Basagran), cyanazine (Bladex), bromoxynil, 2,4-D, dinocap, dinoseb, diquat, fluazifop-butyl (Fusilade), nitrofen (TOK), picloram, sodium arsenite, 2,4,5-T, and trifulralin; the *insecticides* avermectin, chlordimeform, endosulfan, ethion, phosmet (Imidan), methyl parathion, mirex, and trichlorfon.[34]

REGULATION AND CONTROLS

Legislation. The Federal Insecticide Act of 1910 was primarily a labelling law to control adulteration. It was repealed by the Federal Insecticide Fungicide and Rodenticide Act (FIFRA) of 1947. FIFRA was administered by the U.S. Department of Agriculture (USDA) until 1970, when control passed to the Environmental Protection Agency. Most pesticides on the market were approved by the USDA in the 1940s through the 1960s, without the chronic toxicity testing required by the current law. In 1972 the U.S. Congress passed extensive amendments to FIFRA, including requirements that all pesticides be "reregistered" by 1975 to meet current health and safety standards. The testing required falls into nine areas: oncogenicity or carcinogenicity, chronic toxicity, reproductive toxicity, teratogenicity, gene mutation, chromosomal aberrations, DNA damage, and delayed neurotoxicity.

As of 1986, only one pesticide active ingredient, of the 1200 registered, has met all current reregistration standards.[34] The weakest part of FIFRA is the enforcement of these scientific requirements. In 1988 Congress amended FIFRA to requiring reregistration of all pesticides currently on the market by 1997. The registrants (producers) must provide the missing scientific data (called "data gaps") or face loss of registration of the pesticide.

All pesticides must be registered with the EPA before they can be sold. Registration is contingent upon submission by the registrant (manufacturer) of scientific evidence that when used as directed, the pesticide will effectively control the indicated pest(s); that it will not injure humans, crops, livestock, wildlife,

TABLE 24-1. ENVIRONMENTAL PROTECTION AGENCY TOXICITY CATEGORIES FOR PESTICIDES

	Toxicity Class and Signal Word Required on Label	Median Lethal Dose[a] in Rats				
		Oral (mg/kg)	Dermal (mg/kg)	Respiratory (mg/L)	Eye	Skin
I	Highly toxic **Danger**	< 50	< 200	< 0.2	Corneal opacity; irreversible in 7 d	Corrosive
II	Moderately toxic **Warning**	50–500	200–2,000	0.2–2	Corneal opacity; reversible in 7 d	Severe irritation at 72 h
III	Minimally toxic **Caution**	500–5,000	2,000–20,000	2–20	Irritation; reversible in 7 d	Moderate irritation at 72 h
IV	Practically nontoxic **Caution**	> 5,000	> 20,000	> 20	No irritation	Mild irritation

[a]The median lethal dose is the amount of the chemical that will kill 50% of the animals exposed to it. The lower the median lethal dose, the more hazardous the chemical.

or the environment; and that it will not result in illegal residues in food and feed.

All pesticides are classified as either general or restricted use. Restricted use pesticides must be applied by a state-certified applicator or under the supervision of a certified applicator. The states vary enormously in the quality of their education and training programs for pesticide applicators. Usually one person on each farm or ranch is certified, most often a supervisor or foreman. In actual practice, most work is done by persons "under the supervision of a certified applicator," and most workers applying restricted use pesticides are not certified. Many are not even minimally trained and cannot read the labels or do not understand them.[35]

Enforcement. The EPA delegates administration and enforcement of FIFRA to the states through working agreements. In most states, enforcement authority is in the state department of agriculture. The pesticide label is the keystone of FIFRA enforcement, and any use inconsistent with the label is illegal. The label must contain brand name, chemical name, percentage active ingredient(s) and inert ingredient(s); directions for use; pests it is effective against; crops, animals, or sites to be treated; dosage, time, and method of application; reentry interval; preharvest interval; protective clothing and equipment required for application; first aid and emergency treatment; name and address of the manufacturer; and toxicity category.

All pesticides are classified into four toxicity categories depending on the median lethal dose (LD_{50}). The EPA regulates pesticides on the basis of these categories, which must be on the pesticide label. Toxicity category I pesticides are the most toxic, and toxicity category IV the least. Table 24–1 describes these categories in more detail. The WHO also classifies pesticides by acute toxic hazard. The WHO recommendations, which differ from the EPA, are shown in Table 24–2.

Other federal agencies with responsibilities for enforcement of pesticide regulations include the Food and Drug Administration (FDA), the Department of Agriculture (USDA), and the Federal Trade Commission (FTC). The EPA sets the maximum legal residues of pesticides (called tolerances) allowed to be on food at the time of retail sale but does not enforce them. The FDA is responsible for enforcement of tolerances in fruits, vegetables, grains, feed, and fiber. The USDA is responsible for enforcement of tolerances in meat, poultry, and fish. The FTC protects consumers against false and deceptive advertising claims by pesticide distributors and professional applicators; the commission has brought only three actions in the past 10 years.

Worker Protection. Workers who manufacture or formulate pesticides are covered under the provisions of the Occupational Safety and Health Act (OSHA). Pesticide applicators and agricultural workers are covered by FIFRA; thus the majority of workers exposed to pesticides are under the jurisdiction of the EPA.

Federal EPA worker safety standards are minimal, and those that do exist are weak. The EPA has proposed stronger worker safety standards under section 170 of FIFRA, which may be finalized in 1990. These regulations will cover workers in nurseries, greenhouses, and forestry, as well as agricultural workers in horticulture and field crops.

One of the few worker protection standards that applies to field workers are re-entry intervals. These intervals are quarantine periods after a pesticide has been sprayed before workers are permitted to enter the field for cultivation or harvest activities. If a specific interval is not on the label, then fields may be re-entered "when sprays have dried, and dusts have settled."

The State of California has set its own re-entry intervals, and they are much more stringent than those set by the EPA. Table 24–3 lists the reentry intervals for selected pesticides in California and nationally.

TABLE 24-2. WHO RECOMMENDED CLASSIFICATION OF PESTICIDES BY HAZARD

Hazard Class		Median Lethal Dose[a] in Rats			
		Oral		Dermal	
		Solids (mg/kg)	Liquids (mg/kg)	Solids (mg/kg)	Liquids (mg/kg)
IA	Extremely hazardous	≤ 5	≤ 20	≤ 10	≤ 40
IB	Highly hazardous	5–50	20–200	10–100	40–400
II	Moderately hazardous	50–500	200–2,000	100–1,000	400–4,000
III	Slightly hazardous	> 500	> 2,000	> 1,000	> 4,000

[a]The median lethal dose is the amount of the chemical that will kill 50% of the animals exposed to it. The lower the median lethal dose, the more hazardous the chemical.

TABLE 24-3. REENTRY INTERVALS IN DAYS FOR SELECTED PESTICIDES, CALIFORNIA DEPARTMENT OF FOOD AND AGRICULTURE AND EPA, 1988

	CALIFORNIA						EPA
Pesticide	***Apples***	***Citrus***	***Corn***	***Grapes***	***Peaches***	***Other***	***All Crops***
All toxicity category I pesticides[a]	1	1	1	1	1	1	–
Aldicarb [Temik]	1	1	1	1	1	1	1
Anilazine [Dyrene]	2	2	2	2	2	2	–
Carbofuran	–	–	14	–	–	–	2
Chlorpyrifos [Lorsban]	–	2	–	–	–	–	4
Diazinon	–	5	–	5	5	–	–
Dioxathion	–	30	–	30	30	–	1
Disulfoton	2	2	2	2	2	2	1
Endosulfan	2	2	2	2	2	2	2
Ethion	2	30	2	14	14	2	1
Guthion	14	30	–	21	14	14	1
Methidathion	2	30,40[b]	2	2	2	2	1
Methomyl [Lannate]	2	2	2	7	2	–	2
Methyl parathion	14	14	14	14	21	14	1
Mevinphos [Phosdrin]	2	4	2	4	4	2	2
Monitor	2	2	2	2	2	2	1
Monocrotophos	2	2	2	2	2	2	1
Parathion [ethyl]	14	30,45,60,90[c]	14	21	21	14	2
Phorate [Thimet]	2	2	7	2	2	2	1
Phosalone [Zolone]	–	7	–	35[d]	1	1	1
Propargite [Omite]	–	14	–	14	–	–	7
Propargite [Omite CR]	–	42[e]	–	–	–	–	–

[a] In California, all toxicity category I pesticides have a 1 day reentry interval.
[b] Depending on the concentration used.
[c] Depending on the concentration used and the time of year applied.
[d] No longer registered for use on grapes in California due to several reentry poisonings.
[e] No longer registered for use on citrus in California due to severe reentry poisonings.

TABLE 24-4. PESTICIDES BANNED, SUSPENDED, OR SEVERELY RESTRICTED IN THE UNITED STATES

Pesticide	Action	Year
Aldrin	All uses cancelled except termite control	1974
BHC	All uses cancelled	1978
Chlordane	Cancellation for most uses, except termite control	1978
	All uses cancelled	1988
Chlordimeform	Registration voluntarily withdrawn	1989
DBCP	All uses cancelled except on pineapple in Hawaii	1979
	Use on pineapple cancelled	1985
DDT	All agricultural use cancelled	1972
	Use only for public health emergencies	
Diazinon	Use on golf courses and sod farms cancelled	1986
Dieldrin	Cancellation of most uses	1974
Dinoseb	Emergency suspended and registration cancelled	1986
EDB	All uses cancelled	1984
Endrin	Voluntary cancellation	1985
EPN	Use as mosquito larvacide cancelled	1983
Heptachlor	All uses cancelled except seed treatment	1978
	Seed treatment cancelled	1989
Lindane	Indoor smoke fumigation use cancelled	1986
Mirex	All uses cancelled except on pineapple in Hawaii	1977
Nitrofen [TOK]	Voluntary cancellation	1983
2,4,5-T/silvex	Emergency suspension of registration	1979
	All uses cancelled	1985
Toxaphene	All uses cancelled except sheep and cattle dip and on bananas and pineapple in Puerto Rico and The Virgin Islands	1982

Banned, Suspended, and Severely Restricted Pesticides. Table 24–4 lists selected pesticides that have been banned, suspended or severely restricted for use in the United States. Many pesticides that are banned or severely restricted in the U.S., Canada, and Western Europe, are widely used in developing countries. About one third of the pesticides banned in the United States are still manufactured for export. The most recent examples are dinoseb (banned in 1986) and daminozide (Alar) (banned in 1989).

The Pesticide Action Network (PAN), a coalition of over 300 nongovernment organizations from 50 countries, has called for the worldwide ban of a group of pesticides called "the dirty dozen." These pesticides are aldicarb (Temik), chlordane/heptachlor, chlordimeform, DBCP/EDB, DDT, aldrin/dieldrin/endrin, BHC/lindane, paraquat, parathion (methyl and ethyl), pentachlorophenol, and 2,4,5-T. Table 24–4 lists which of these pesticides are banned in the United States.

An executive order signed in 1979 requires agencies such as the Agency for International Development to file environmental impact statements before beginning projects in foreign countries. Another executive order requires the United States to inform developing countries if an exported pesticide is banned in the United States and to obtain official approval before it can be exported.

REFERENCES

1. U.S. Environmental Protection Agency: Pesticide Industry Sales and Usage, 1987 Market Estimates. Washington, D.C.: EPA, Office of Pesticide Programs, November 1988
2. World Health Organization: Public Health Impact of Pesticides Used in Agriculture. Report of a WHO/UNEP Working Group. Geneva: WHO, 1989
3. U.S. General Accounting Office: Nonagricultural Pesticides, Risks and Regulation. GAO/RCED-86-97. Washington, D.C.: GAO, April 1986
4. Goldman LR, Mengle D, Epstein DM: Acute symptoms in persons residing near a field treated with the soil fumigants methyl bromide and chloropicrin. West J Med 147:95–98, 1987
5. Kazen C, Bloomer A, Welch R, et al: Persistence of pesticides on the hands of some occupationally exposed people. Arch Environ Health 29:315–318, 1974
6. Savage EP, Keefe TJ, Mounce LM, et al: Chronic neurological sequelae of acute organophosphate poisoning. Arch Environ Health 43:38–45, 1988
7. Lee MH, Randsell JF: A farmworker death due to pesticide toxicity: A case report. J Toxicol Environ Health 14:239–246, 1984
8. Morgan DP: Recognition and management of pesticide poisonings, 4 edt. EPA-540/9-88-001, Washington, D.C.: U.S. Environmental Protection Agency, March 1989
9. Taylor JR, Selhorst JB, Houff SA, et al: Chlordecone intoxication in man. I. Clinical Observations. Neurology 28:626–630, 1978
10. Cripps DJ, Goemen A, Peters HA: Porphyria turcica, twenty years after hexachlorobenzene intoxication. Arch Dermatol 116:46–50, 1980
11. Hine CH: Methyl bromide poisoning. J Occup Med 11:1–10, 1969
12. Editorial: Are insect repellants safe? Lancet 2:610–611, 1988
13. Wasserstrom RF, Wiles R: Field duty: U.S. farmworkers and pesticide safety. Washington, D.C.: World Resources Institute, July 1985
14. California Department of Health Services: Pesticides: Health aspects of exposure and issues surrounding their use. Continuing Education Seminar for Health Personnel Course Syllabus and Manual. Berkeley, Calif.: Hazard Evaluation Section, June 1988
15. Rettig BA, Klein DK, Sniezek JE: The incidence of hospitalizations and emergency room visits resulting from exposure to chemicals used in agriculture. Neb Med J 7:215–219, 1987
16. U.S. Environmental Protection Agency: National Study of Hospital Admitted Pesticide Poisonings. Washington, D.C.: Office of Pesticide Programs. EPA, April 1976
17. Litovitz TL, Schlmitz BF, Holm KC: 1988 annual report of the American Association of Poison Control Centers National Data Collection System. Am J Emerg Med 7:495–545, 1989
18. Baker EL Jr, Zack M, Miles JW, et al: Epidemic malathion poisoning in Pakistan malaria workers. Lancet 1:31–34, 1978
19. Davies JE, Lee JA: Changing profiles in human health effects of pesticides. In Greenhalgh R, Roberts TR (eds): Pesticide Science and Biotechnology. London: Blackwell Scientific Publications, 1987, pp 533–538
20. Adams RM: Occupational Skin Disease. New York: Grune & Stratton, 1983
21. Moses M: Cancer in humans and potential occupational and environmental exposure to pesticides. Abstracts of selected epidemiological studies and case reports. Am Assoc Occup Health Nurse J 37:131–136, 1989
22. Eaton M, Schenker M, Whorton D, et al: Seven-year follow-up of workers exposed to 1,2-dibromo-3-chloropropane. J Occup Med 28:1145–1150, 1986
23. Schwartz DA, LoGerfo JP: Congenital limb reduction defects in the agricultural setting. Am J Public Health 78:654–657, 1988
24. Schardein JL: Chemically Induced Birth Defects. New York: Marcel Deckker, 1985
25. Vaughn TL, Daling JR, Starzyk PM: Fetal death and maternal occupation: An analysis of birth records in the State of Washington. J Occup Med 26:676–678, 1984
26. Rita P, Reddy PP, Reddy SV: Monitoring of workers occupationally exposed to pesticides in grape gardens of Andhra Pradesh. Environ Res 44:1–5, 1987
27. Xintaras C, Burg JR, Tanaka S, et al: Occupational exposure to Leptophos and other chemicals. NIOSH pub. no. 78-136, Washington, D.C.: U.S. Government Printing Office, 1978
28. Lotti M, Moretto A, Zoppellari R, et al: Inhibition of lymphocytic neuropathy target esterase predicts the development of organophosphate-induced delayed polyneuropathy. Arch Toxicol 59:176–179, 1986
29. Sharp DS, Eskenazi B, Harrison R, et al: Delayed health hazards of pesticide exposure. Ann Rev Public Health 7:441–471, 1986
30. Tabershaw IR, Cooper WC: Sequelae of acute organophosphate poisoning. J Occup Med 8:5–20, 1966
31. Kopin IJ: MPTP: An industrial chemical and contaminant of illicit narcotics stimulates a new era in research on Parkinson's disease. Environ Health Perspect 75:45–51, 1987
32. Rajput AH, Uitti RJ, Stern W, et al: Geography, drinking water chemistry, pesticides and herbicides and the etiology of Parkinson's disease. Can J Neurol Sci 14:414–418, 1987
33. Moses M: Pesticide-related health problems and farmworkers. AAOHN J 37:115–130, 1989
34. U.S. General Accounting Office: Pesticides, EPA's Formidable Task to Assess and Egulate Their Risks. BAO/RCED-86-125. Washington, D.C.: GAO, April 1986
35. Moses M: A field survey of pesticide-related working conditions in four locations in the U.S. and Canada. Monitoring the international code of conduct on the distribution and use of pesticides in North America. Pesticide Education and Action Project, San Francisco, Calif., 1988

25

Illness Due to Thermal Extremes

Edwin M. Kilbourne

THERMOREGULATION

As a homeothermic ("warm-blooded") species, humans must maintain a relatively constant deep body (core) temperature. The temperatures of more superficial body parts can vary but only within limits. Substantial deviations from "normal" body temperatures can result in adverse effects that range in severity from minor annoyance to life-threatening illness.

The principal physical processes affecting thermoregulation are heat production by metabolism, heat loss by evaporation, and heat loss or gain by conduction, convection, and radiation.[1] Metabolic heat is generated from the myriad biochemical reactions that maintain life and must be dissipated constantly. Evaporative heat loss occurs as moisture on body surfaces and in the respiratory tract is transformed from liquid to gas.

By conduction, heat may be gained from, or lost to, solid objects in contact with the body. Whether heat is gained or lost depends on whether the object in question is hotter or colder than the body surface with which it is in contact.

Although conduction also is involved in the transfer of heat between the body and fluids (gases and liquids), such heat transfer usually is termed "convection" because of the substantial role played by the flow of fluid medium (e.g., air or water) over body surfaces in facilitating heat transfer. The distinction between convection and pure conduction is illustrated particularly well by the common case of a person surrounded by air. Absolutely still air has extremely low thermal conductivity (only 6.1×10^{-5} calories s^{-1} cm^{-1} $°C^{-1}$).[2] Nevertheless, convective heat loss to cold air can be very substantial in high winds at low temperatures.

When applied to heat, the term "radiation" refers to the low frequency (infrared) electromagnetic radiation emitted by all objects at a temperature greater than 0° Kelvin (absolute zero). The greater the temperature of an object, the more radiation it emits. When these electromagnetic waves strike an object that is not transparent to them and from which they are not reflected, the object is warmed. The energy is then reemitted by the warmed object. The net effect of this radiation back and forth is that objects in close proximity tend toward the same temperature, and this process occurs even if the objects are in a vacuum. The biological importance of infrared radiation is that thermal comfort and equilibrium depend not only on the ambient air temperature (which must be measured in the shade to limit the effect of solar radiation) but also on the temperature of surrounding objects. For instance, if a wall of a room is warmed by the sun, that wall will tend to warm a person in the room, whether or not the air temperature is affected.

HEAT-RELATED ILLNESS

Heat Stress

Heat stress may result from alteration of any of the physical processes involved in the transfer of heat to or from the body. A runner in a long-distance race or a soldier on strenuous military maneuvers may suffer heat stress as a result of increased metabolic heat production caused by physical activity. A steelworker may experience heat stress because of the radiant heat emitted from a furnace at the workplace. At a hazardous waste site, a worker who must wear a heavy, impermeable suit may develop heat stress as the air in the suit becomes humid (decreasing evaporative cooling) and warm (limiting heat loss by convection).

During an urban summer heat wave, several factors may combine to exacerbate heat stress. The pavement and concrete buildings absorb radiant solar heat, which they emit during the night, a time that would otherwise be one of respite from heat. Evaporative cooling may be limited by high summer humidity. Convective cooling can be decreased by tall buildings that block the movement of air.[3]

People seek relief from heat stress by altering one or more of the processes by which the body gains or loses heat. They may rest (lowering metabolic heat production), move to the shade (avoiding radiant solar heat), sit in front of a fan (increasing convective and evaporative heat losses), or swim (facilitating heat loss by conduction/convection through water).

The acute physiological response to heat stress includes perspiration and peripheral vasodilation. Perspiration increases cutaneous moisture, allowing greater evaporative cooling. Peripheral vasodilation tends to reroute blood flow, enhancing transmission of heat from the body's core to its periphery.[4,5]

With continuing exposure to heat stress, a process of physiological adaptation takes place. Although maximal adaptation may take weeks, significant acclimatization occurs within a few days of the first exposure. Acclimatization results in increased sweating, and the salt content of sweat is greatly reduced. After acclimatization, exercise in the heat elicits less of an increase in heat rate and in core and skin temperatures.[6,7]

Indexes of Heat Stress. In most circumstances four environmental variables (dry-bulb air temperature, humidity, air speed, and radiant heat energy) summarize the effect of the physical processes affecting thermal homeostasis.[8,9] Ambient (dry-bulb) air temperature gives an indication of the ease with which the body can discharge metabolic heat into the air by means of convection. However, air temperature alone is an unsatisfactory indicator of the amount of heat stress a person may suffer. High humidity limits evaporative cooling, and for any given temperature, heat stress increases as humidity rises. On the other hand, air of a given temperature usually feels cooler as it moves faster (unless ambient temperature is high), since air movement generally facilitates both evaporative and convective heat losses. Finally, increased radiant heat energy adds to heat stress independent of ambient temperature, humidity, and air movement.

Several heat indexes have been developed that attempt to express the net contribution of some or all of these four variables as a single number reflecting their combined thermal effect on a human being. One of the earliest such indexes is known as "effective temperature" (ET), an empirical scale based on the subjective reports of the thermal sensations of volunteers placed in a wide variety of conditions of temperature, humidity, and air movement.[10] On the basis of their responses, a nomogram was developed from which one can read the ET corresponding to a specific set of values of dry-bulb temperature, wet-bulb temperature (a measure of humidity), and airspeed. In its original version, the ET of any such combination is equal to the dry-bulb temperature of still, saturated air that would produce the same subjective thermal effect.

A modification of this scheme, the corrected effective temperature, substitutes globe thermometer temperature for dry-bulb temperature. The globe thermometer is a dry-bulb thermometer with the bulb located at the center of a 6-inch diameter, thin, copper sphere, the outside of which is painted matte black. The globe thermometer is affected by radiant heat in addition to dry-bulb temperature and wind speed. The corrected effective temperature scheme thus yields a single number for the net effect of a particular set of conditions of temperature, humidity, air movement, and radiant heat energy.

Although the original ET index was developed in 1923, physiologists and engineers still use it as a standard for measuring thermal comfort. However, because of concern that the original ET scale is too sensitive to the effect of humidity at low temperatures and not sensitive enough to humidity at high temperatures, a reformulated version of ET has been published.[11,12]

The wet-bulb globe temperature (WBGT) is a heat stress index calculated as the weighted average of wet-bulb, globe, and dry-bulb thermometer temperatures:

$$\text{Outdoors: } WBGT = 0.7T_{wb} + 0.2T_g + 0.1\,T_{db}$$
$$\text{Indoors: } WBGT = 0.7T_{wb} + 0.3T_g$$

where T_{wb} is the temperature read by a naturally convected wet-bulb thermometer, T_g is the globe thermometer temperature, and T_{db} is the dry-bulb temperature. The WBGT thus reflects all four of the major environmental variables affecting heat stress. Its formulas were chosen to yield values close to those of the ET for the same conditions.[13] The WBGT has been used to assess the danger of heatstroke or heat exhaustion occurring in persons exercising in hot environments. Curtailing certain types of activities when the WBGT is high decreases the incidence of serious heat-related illness among military recruits.[14] Current standards and recommendations for limiting heat stress in the workplace generally are expressed in terms of WBGT, although a person's degree of acclimatization, the energy expenditure required, and the amount of time spent performing the stressful task often are factored in also.[15] Thus no single WBGT value can be used as a heat exposure limit for all occupational situations.

The "Botsball" (BB) or wet globe thermometer, developed by Botsford, consists of a thermal probe within a black sphere 6 cm in diameter, the surface of which is covered with black cloth kept wet by water in a reservoir. Like WBGT, the BB is affected by ambient temperature, humidity, wind speed, and radiant heat. However, the BB is smaller and lighter than the equipment required to take WBGT readings and has a shorter stabilization time. Thus it is easier to take a Botsball measurement than a WBGT measurement in an employee's personal work space. This ease of use is its principal advantage over WBGT. The following is the approximate numerical relationship in degrees Celsius of BB to WBGT[16]:

$$WBGT = (1.01 \times BB) + 2.6$$

Steadman's scheme of apparent temperature (AT) is favored currently by meteorologists and climatologists as a measure of the heat stress associated with a given set of meteorological conditions (Table 25–1). Unlike effective temperature, which was derived empirically, AT is the product of mathematical modeling based on principles of physics and physiology. The AT for a given set of conditions of temperature, humidity, airspeed, and radiant heat energy is equal to the dry-bulb temperature with the same predicted thermal impact on an adult walking in calm air of "moderate" humidity with surrounding objects at the same temperature as ambient air (no "extra" radiation).[17]

There are other heat stress indexes, and no attempt is made here to present an exhaustive list. The subject has been reviewed by Lee.[13] Any index that attempts to predict heat stress solely from environmental data is limited. Such indexes necessarily make assumptions regarding metabolic heat production, clothing, and body shape and size. Thus at best these indexes are approximations. In addition, data needed to calculate some indexes are difficult to obtain. For example, globe thermometer readings may not be easily available.

Heatstroke

The most serious illness caused by elevated temperature is heatstroke. In heatstroke the core body temperature is elevated to greater than 105° F (40.6° C), and temperature elevations to 110° F (43.3° C) or higher are not uncommon. Mental status is altered; lethargy proceeds to confusion, stupor, and finally unconsciousness. Classically, sweating is said to be absent or diminished, but many victims of clear-cut heatstroke perspire profusely. The outcome often is fatal, even when patients are brought quickly to medical attention; death/case ratios of 40% or more have been reported.[18–22]

Initial treatment is directed toward the rapid lowering of body temperature. A patient can be cooled with an ice water bath, ice massage, or specialized evaporative cooling procedures. Rectal temperature should be monitored continuously, both to monitor the efficacy of hypothermic treatment and to guard against the development of clinically significant hypothermia, which can occur if cooling is continued too long. In general, intensive hypothermic treatment should be discontinued when the rectal temperature is brought down to about 102° F (38.9° C).

Further treatment is supportive and directed toward the many potential complications of hyperthermia. Hypovolemia, hypokalemia or hyperkalemia, rhabdomyolysis, hypocalcemia, and bleeding diathesis may require intensive, supportive treatment. If the clinical circumstances suggest a concomitant infection, empirical antibiotic therapy may be indicated. Recovery

TABLE 25-1. APPARENT TEMPERATURE IN °C SHOWING EFFECT OF HUMIDITY AT HIGHER TEMPERATURE (WIND AND RADIATION COMPONENTS NOT SHOWN)

Dry-Bulb Temperature (°C)	Relative Humidity (%)										
	0	**10**	**20**	**30**	**40**	**50**	**60**	**70**	**80**	**90**	**100**
20	17.1	17.5	17.9	18.4	18.8	19.2	19.6	20.0	20.4	20.8	21.2
22	19.1	19.6	20.1	20.6	21.1	21.5	22.0	22.4	22.8	23.2	23.5
24	21.3	21.9	22.4	22.9	23.3	23.8	24.2	24.6	25.2	25.8	26.4
26	23.6	24.2	24.7	25.1	25.6	26.1	26.7	27.3	28.0	28.9	29.8
28	25.4	25.9	26.5	27.1	27.8	28.6	29.4	30.4	31.7	32.8	34.3
30	27.1	27.7	28.4	29.2	30.1	31.1	32.3	33.7	35.3	37.2	39.6
32	28.7	29.5	30.4	31.4	32.8	34.0	35.7	37.6	40.1	43.0	
34	30.3	31.3	32.5	33.8	35.0	37.4	39.6	42.7	46.0		
36	31.9	33.1	34.6	35.5	37.3	40.0	43.0	48.3			
38	33.4	35.0	36.8	39.0	41.8	45.3	49.7				
	Relative Humidity (%)										
	0	**5**	**10**	**15**	**20**	**25**	**30**	**35**	**40**	**45**	**50**
40	35.0	35.9	36.9	38.0	39.2	40.6	42.0	43.9	45.8	48.2	50.6
42	36.6	37.4	38.2	39.6	40.9	42.9	45.0	46.7	48.6		
44	38.1	39.4	40.8	42.4	44.4	46.5	49.0	51.8	54.1		
46	39.7	41.2	43.0	45.0	47.4	50.1	53.3				
48	41.2	43.1	44.5	46.8	49.6	52.8					
50	42.8	45.0	47.5	50.5	54.0	58.1					

From Steadman RG: A universal scale of apparent temperature. J Climate Appl Meteorol 23:1674–1687, 1984

may be rapid or slow, depending on the severity of the insult. Maximal recovery may not occur for a period of days or weeks, and there may be permanent neurological residua.[18,22]

Heat Exhaustion

Unlike heatstroke, heat exhaustion is not principally a failure of thermoregulation. It is a milder illness than heatstroke and is caused primarily by the unbalanced or inadequate replacement of water and salts lost in perspiration due to thermal stress. In contrast to heatstroke, which may develop in a matter of minutes or hours, heat exhaustion typically occurs after several days of high temperatures. Body temperature may be normal or moderately elevated, but it is uncommon for it to exceed 102° F (38.9° C). The symptoms, primarily dizziness, weakness, and fatigue, are those of circulatory distress. Heat exhaustion often is severe enough to require hospitalization, especially of elderly patients. Treatment is supportive and directed toward normalizing fluid and electrolyte balance. Although generally rapid, the speed of recovery depends on the extent of the underlying fluid and electrolyte imbalances.[21,22]

Heat Syncope and Heat Cramps

Heat syncope and heat cramps occur principally in persons exercising in the heat. Heat syncope is a transient fall in blood pressure with an associated loss of consciousness. Consciousness generally returns promptly in the recumbent posture. The disorder is thought to arise from circulatory instability due to cutaneous vasodilation in response to heat stress. Prevention is accomplished by avoiding strenuous exercise in the heat, unless one is well trained and acclimatized.[23]

Heat cramps are muscle cramps, particularly in the legs, that occur during or shortly after exercise in a hot environment. They are thought to result from transient fluid and electrolyte abnormalities. Heat cramps decrease in frequency with athletic training and acclimatization to hot weather. They may be treated by increasing salt intake.[21]

Effects of Heat on Reproduction

Among men, frequent or prolonged exposure to heat can result in elevated intrascrotal temperatures, causing a substantial decrease in sperm count.[24] Occupational exposure to heat has been associated with delayed conception.[25] A decrease in brain weight and other adverse neurological effects have been observed in the offspring of female mice made hyperthermic during pregnancy.[26] In humans, maternal hyperthermia has been implicated in the genesis of neural tube defects.[27,28]

Epidemiology

In an average summer in the United States, about 200 persons die with death certificate diagnoses of heat-related illness.[29] If there is a heat wave, however, that number may increase greatly. During the summer of 1980 when a major heat wave affected large portions of the central and southern United States, more than 1700 deaths were attributed to heat.[30] Geographic analysis indicates that such deaths are not uniformly distributed within the population at risk. Rather, they tend to cluster in certain "high-risk" areas.[31]

The health effects of heat waves have been evaluated at specific locations. In July 1980, in St. Louis and Kansas City, Mo., deaths from all causes were, respectively, 57% and 65% greater than expected. Nevertheless, physicians attributed only 40% and 67% of the excess deaths to the heat.[32] This pattern (recognized heat-related deaths accounting for only a fraction of the increased mortality noted during heat waves) has been observed several times by different investigators. In general, recognized heat-related deaths comprise up to 50% of the heat wave mortality increase.[33]

Diagnoses of death due to cerebrovascular and cardiovascular diseases often account for a large part of the remainder of the increase.[34,35] Such findings are of particular interest, because some studies indicate that heat stress may induce some degree of blood hypercoagulability.[36,37] Heat stress therefore may favor the development of thrombi and emboli and may cause an increase in fatal strokes and myocardial infarctions.

The increase in mortality during heat waves is paralleled by an increase in nonspecific measures of morbidity. During hot weather the numbers of hospital admissions and emergency room visits increase.[32,38]

Excess mortality due to heat waves occurs primarily in urban areas. Suburban and rural areas are at far less risk.[32,38] The urban predominance of adverse health consequences of the heat may be explained in part by the phenomenon of the urban "heat island."[3] The masses of stone, brick, concrete, asphalt, and cement that are typical of modern urban architecture absorb much of the sun's radiant energy, functioning as heat reservoirs and reradiating that heat during nights that would otherwise be cooler. In many urban areas there are few trees to provide shading. In addition, tall buildings may effectively decrease wind velocity, decreasing in turn the cooling convective and evaporative effects of moving air. Other factors contributing to the severity of heat-related health effects in cities include the relative poverty of some urban areas.[32,38] Poor people are less able to afford cooling devices such as air conditioners and the energy needed to run them.

Impact on Elderly. The elderly are at particularly high risk of severe, heat-related health effects. Except for infancy and early childhood, the risk of death due to heat increases throughout life as a function of age (Fig. 25-1). During the 1980 heat wave in the United States, 64% of those who died as a result of the heat were at least 65 years old; 72% were at least 60 years old.[30] In St. Louis and Kansas City, Mo., during the same period, about 71% of heatstroke cases occurred in persons aged 65 and over, despite the fact that this group constituted only about 15% of the population.[32] A similar predominance of elderly casualties during other heat waves has been noted.[39]

The predisposition to heat-related illness among the elderly may be explained in part by impaired physiological responses to heat stress. Vasodilation in response to heat requires increased cardiac output, but persons older than 65 are less likely to have the ability to increase cardiac output and decrease systemic vascular resistance during hot weather.[40] Moreover, the body temperature at which perspiring begins increases with increasing age.[41] The elderly are more likely to have underlying diseases or to be taking medications (major tranquilizers and anticholinergics) that have been reported to increase the risk of heatstroke.[42–45] Finally, elderly persons do not perceive differences in temperature as well as younger persons. This attribute may render an older person less able to effectively regulate his or her thermal environment.[46]

Other Factors Affecting Risk. Infants and young children are also at increased risk from the heat, although their death rates due to heat are lower than those of the elderly. Healthy babies kept in a hot area have been found to run temperatures as high as 103° F, and mild fever-causing illnesses of babies may develop into frank heatstroke as a result of heat stress.[47] In children, sensitivity to heat is greatest in those less than 1 year old. The 5- to 9-year-old age group has the lowest mortality rate by age for the United States (Fig. 25-1). The risk of both fatal and nonfatal heatstroke is increased in infants and young children.[48] Children with congenital abnormalities of the central nervous system and with diarrheal illnesses appear to be particularly vulnerable.[47,48] Parents may contribute to risk by failing to give enough hypotonic fluid during the heat and dressing or covering the child too warmly.[48,49]

In the United States, death rates due to heat generally are higher in males than in females. This trend is most evident among young adults and is much less evident at the extremes of age (Table 25-2). The reasons for the apparent increased risk for males are not known, but differences between the sexes in patterns of thermal exposure may be maximal during young adult life and may be the causal factor.

During urban heat waves the rate of heatstroke is disproportionately high in poor neighborhoods. In the United States the association of the black race with relatively low socioeconomic status may well explain the disproportionately high heatstroke rates of blacks in this country.[32,38] No biologically based vulnerability of any particular race has been shown.

Chronic illnesses resulting in loss of the ability to care for oneself or in a bedfast or relatively immobile life-style are more frequent in heatstroke cases than in controls. No specific chronic disease is known to be as effective a predictor of heatstroke as this more general characterization.[42]

Persons with a history of prior heatstroke have been shown to maintain thermal homeostasis in a hot environment less well than comparable volunteers who have never suffered heatstroke.[50] Whether heatstroke causes damage to the body's ability to regulate its temperature or thermoregulative abnormalities antedate the first heatstroke is not known. Nevertheless, persons with a history of heatstroke should be considered at increased risk of a recurrence.

Obesity is an important factor affecting heat tolerance. Obese subjects exercising in a hot environment show a greater increase in rectal temperature and heart rate than do lean subjects.[51,52] The insulating effect of subcutaneous fat impedes the transfer of metabolic heat from core to surface. Soldiers in the U.S. army who died of heatstroke during basic training in World War II were more likely to be obese than their peers were.[53] Nevertheless, obesity may not have an important influence on the rate of heatstroke in the elderly, largely sedentary population that is at greatest risk during a heat wave.[42]

Persons affected by other, less common conditions also may tolerate the heat poorly. These conditions include congenital ab-

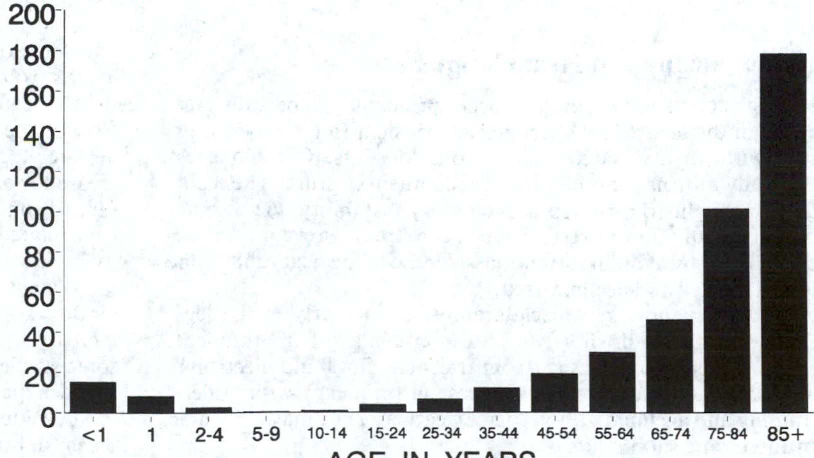

Figure 25-1. Rates of death per 10 million population per year attributed to heat (International Classification of Diseases, Eighth and Ninth Revisions, Code E900) by age, United States, 1975–1985.

TABLE 25-2. U.S. RATES OF DEATH PER 10 MILLION POPULATON PER YEAR DUE TO HEAT AND COLD (1975–1985) BY SEX AND AGE WITH RATE RATIOS

	Heat (ICD E900[a])			Cold (ICD E901[a])		
Age (y)	Male	Female	RR[b]	Male	Female	RR[b]
<1	15.6	14.7	1.1	12.6	6.3	2.0
1	8.7	8.0	1.1	2.7	2.3	1.2
2–4	2.6	2.7	1.0	2.2	1.2	1.8
5–9	0.9	0.2	4.5	1.2	0.4	3.0
10–14	1.2	0.6	2.0	3.9	0.6	6.5
15–24	6.7	1.1	6.1	16.0	3.3	4.9
25–34	10.8	2.4	4.5	19.4	4.5	4.3
35–44	19.8	4.8	4.1	37.4	6.9	5.4
45–54	29.8	9.6	3.1	69.6	16.2	4.3
55–64	41.3	20.3	2.0	105.7	22.8	4.6
65–74	58.5	37.4	1.6	144.1	37.5	3.8
75–84	108.8	96.9	1.1	273.0	101.5	2.7
85+	200.1	168.0	1.2	465.5	226.9	2.1

[a] International Classification of Diseases code for cause of death.
[b] Rate ratio (male/female).

sence of sweat glands and scleroderma with diffuse cutaneous involvement. In both conditions, perspiration is markedly diminished, resulting in impaired thermoregulation in a hot environment.[54,55]

Some drugs predispose the patient to heatstroke. Neuroleptic drugs (e.g., phenothiazines, butyrophenones, and thioxanthenes) in particular have been strongly implicated.[43,45] Phenothiazine-treated animals survive in a hot environment for shorter periods than controls, and heatstroke occurs with increased frequency in patients taking these drugs.[42,56] Neuroleptics appear to impair thermoregulatory function in both directions, sensitizing to cold and heat.[56]

Anticholinergics have decreased heat tolerance in laboratory tests of human volunteers. Persons treated with anticholinergics while exposed to heat had a decrease or cessation of perspiring and a rise in rectal temperature.[44] Many commonly used prescription drugs (e.g., tricyclic antidepressants, some antiparkinsonian agents) and nonprescription drugs (e.g., antihistamines, sleeping pills) have prominent anticholinergic effects; in one study the use of such drugs was more common in heatstroke victims than in controls.[42] The likely mechanism of action appears to be inhibition of perspiration.

Certain stimulant and antidepressant drugs taken in combination or in overdose quantities may induce the syndrome of heatstroke. Severe hyperthermia has been reported to result from an overdose of amphetamine, amphetamine taken with a monoamine oxidase inhibitor, and a tricyclic taken in combination with a monoamine oxidase inhibitor.[57–59]

Global Warming

Although predictions regarding climate change remain the subject of intense controversy, a number of expert climatology investigators anticipate a substantial increase in global temperature over the next several decades. Such predictions are based on the current and anticipated future accumulation of atmospheric gases that tend to retain solar energy as heat in the vicinity of the earth ("greenhouse effect"). Average global temperatures are predicted to rise by 2° to 6° C (3.6° to 10.8° F) during the next century.[60] Although an increase of this magnitude may not sound threatening, it is close to the change in average global temperature since the Ice Age extreme 18,000 years ago.[60,61]

Even small changes in average temperature can potentially translate into substantial numbers of deaths and cases of severe illness. For example, the areally weighted average summer (June through August) temperatures of about 74° F (23.3° C) for the state of Missouri in 1979, 1982, and 1985 were associated with few reported heat-related deaths. The average temperature of the summer of 1980, when some 300 heat-related deaths were reported in the state, was higher by only about 6° F (3.3° C) (Fig. 25-2). Figure 25-2 also illustrates the close correlation of average summer temperature with the number of heat-related deaths reported.

Other health consequences, in addition to those caused by direct exposure of human beings to the heat, probably will result from any significant global warming that occurs. This complex subject has been reviewed elsewhere.[61] (See Chapter 39.)

Of course, many factors may intervene to reduce the heat-related morbidity and mortality that might otherwise result from a gradual increase in average temperatures. Such factors include human physiological acclimatization to the warming trend, changes in behavior or building construction to reduce heat exposure, and mitigation of climate change itself through a reduction in the emission of greenhouse gases or by other means. Nevertheless, the potential health threat posed by global warming should be recognized. Further scientific research and thoughtful formulation and implementation of policy will be required to adequately address the complex issues involved. (See also Chapter 39.)

Prevention

In most parts of the United States, heat waves severe enough to threaten health do not occur every year. Several relatively mild summers may intervene between extensive heat waves. The erratic occurrence of heat waves hinders prevention planning. It is administratively difficult to plan for adequate resources to be available if needed but not wasted if not needed.

Programs to prevent heat-related illness should concentrate on measures whose efficacy is supported by empirical data. Many heatstroke prevention efforts for the community at large have been based on the distribution of electric fans to persons at risk. Nevertheless, a study of the 1980 heat wave in Missouri did not show a significant protective effect of fans.[42] Examination of some of the indexes of heat stress shows them to be consistent with this finding. As dry-bulb temperature increases, wind speed causes an increasingly smaller decrement in AT until finally at dry-bulb temperatures above about 36° C (96.8° F), the AT actually increases with increasing wind speed. ET similarly increases with increasing wind speed at high temperatures. Other physiologic experimentation has confirmed the inability of increasing air movement to increase heat tolerance at high temperatures.[62] Fans thus appear unlikely to offer protection from heat under the conditions of very high ambient temperature at which

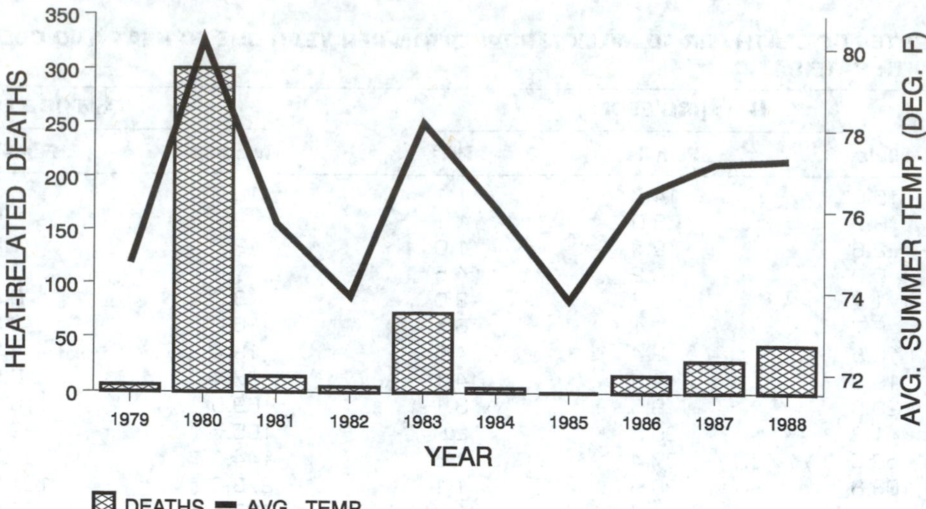

Figure 25-2. Heat-related deaths and areally weighted average summer (June through August) temperatures, Missouri, 1979–1988. *(Adapted from Centers for Disease Control. Heat-related deaths—Missouri, 1979–1988. MMWR 38:437, 1989.)*

heat-related health effects are most likely to occur. Moreover, since heat stress indexes suggest that fan use actually might be harmful under certain conditions, the distribution of free fans during heat waves as a relief measure probably should be abandoned.

Air conditioning, on the other hand, effectively prevents heatstroke. In one study 24-hour air conditioning led to a 98% decrease in fatal heatstroke. In addition, simply spending more time in air-conditioned places (regardless of whether there was a home air conditioner) was associated with a fourfold reduction in heatstroke.[42] Thus setting up air-conditioned heat wave shelters may be an effective means of preventing heatstroke. Even if such shelters cannot be provided, elderly and other persons at high risk can be encouraged to spend a few hours each day at some public air-conditioned place, such as a movie theater or shopping mall.

Heatstroke is an occupational risk for an estimated 6 million Americans who work in ''hot'' industries (e.g., foundries, glassworks, and mines). To prevent heat-related illness among the occupationally exposed, the U.S. National Institute for Occupational Safety and Health (NIOSH) recommends acclimatizing new workers and those returning from leave, arranging frequent rest periods in a cool environment, scheduling hot operations for the coolest part of the day, making drinking water readily available, conducting preemployment and periodic medical examinations, and instructing workers and supervisors about preventive measures and early recognition of heat-related illnesses.[15]

COLD-RELATED ILLNESS

Seasonal Trends in Mortality

In the United States there is a marked seasonal trend in overall mortality (Fig. 25-3). The death rate is greatest in midwinter and lowest in the late summer. This pattern of mortality also occurs in other countries in the temperate zones of both the northern and southern hemispheres, although the mortality curves of the two hemispheres are 6 months out of phase.[1]

The tendency for death to occur in the winter is most marked in the elderly and becomes increasingly prominent with age. For persons aged 45 or younger, however, the pattern is reversed: the death rate is lowest in the winter and greatest in the summer.[63]

The extent of seasonal variation in mortality in the United States varies greatly by cause of death. The death rates for diseases of the heart, cerebrovascular disease, pneumonia, influenza, and chronic obstructive pulmonary disease show substantial increases in the winter. On the other hand, the occurrence of death due to malignant neoplasms remains virtually constant throughout the year.[63,64]

Some of the seasonal winter increase in deaths due to chronic diseases such as stroke and myocardial infarction may reflect seasonal changes in underlying risk factors for vascular diseases. For example, it is well documented that blood pressure in humans is seasonal and is higher in the winter.[65] Cold stress can physiologically potentiate the coagulation of blood, possibly contributing to the winter excess of deaths due to stroke and ischemic heart disease.[66] In addition, many types of exercise are practiced seasonally, with sedentary periods tending to occur in winter.[67]

The winter death increase cannot be attributed entirely to the direct effect of cold exposure. The increase occurs even in states noted for their relatively mild winter climates (e.g., Florida and Hawaii) and is of approximately the same order of magnitude as in colder states (e.g., Minnesota and Montana).[63] Low winter humidity may contribute to the winter death excess, since it favors the transmission of certain infectious agents, notably influenza.[68] In addition, winter increases in deaths caused by certain unintentional injuries may reflect seasonal increases in certain behaviors. For example, deaths due to fire are more common in the winter, perhaps a result of the use of fireplaces and heating devices. Finally, the peaks and valleys in the U.S. death rate have not always come in midwinter and late summer, respectively, as they usually do now. In the early part of this century the peak was usually in February or March and the nadir in June.[64] This change in seasonal pattern is further evidence that temperature is not necessarily the most important determinant of the seasonal aspect of mortality.

Cold Stress and Its Indexes

The two most important adaptive physiological responses to the cold are vasoconstriction and shivering. Peripheral vasoconstriction causes a rerouting of some blood away from cutaneous and other superficial vascular beds toward deeper tissues in which the blood's heat is less easily lost. In addition, blood is rerouted from the superficial veins of the limbs to the venae comitantes of the major arteries. Such rerouting activates a ''countercurrent'' mechanism by which arterial blood warms venous blood before the venous blood returns to the core. Conversely, venous blood

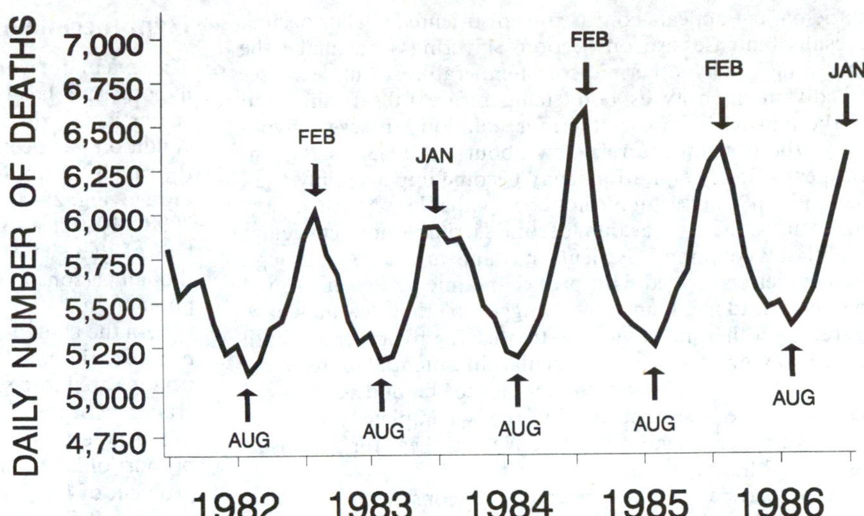

Figure 25-3. Mean daily number of U.S. deaths from all causes by month, United States, January 1982–January 1987.

cools arterial blood so that it gives up less heat when it reaches the periphery. The result is a fall in the temperature of superficial body parts in defense of core temperature. Thus the difference between skin and core temperatures is an approximate measure of the efficacy of vasoconstriction.[1,69]

Humidity and radiant heat energy tend to be less important in the evaluation of cold environments than of hot. Thus the popular "wind chill" index of Siple expresses the intensity of cooling expected from a cold environment as a function of ambient temperature and wind speed:

$$H = (10.45 + 10s^{1/2} - s)(33 - t)$$

where H is the wind chill expressed in kcal m^{-2} h^{-1}, s is the wind speed in m s^{-1}, and t is the ambient temperature in degrees Celsius.[70] The value of H permits comparison of the cooling effect of various temperature and wind speed combinations. The subjective thermal perception associated with any given value of H is influenced greatly by one's level of activity and the type and amount of clothing worn.

Often the wind chill effect is described in terms of a wind chill equivalent temperature. This is the temperature that would produce the same intensity of cooling as the temperature-wind speed combination under consideration if the wind speed were some arbitrarily chosen reference value.[71] A wind chill equivalent temperature can be calculated from a modification of the Siple formula:

$$t_{eq} = 33 - \frac{(10.45 + 10s^{1/2} - s)(33 - t)}{(10.45 + 10s_{ref}^{\ 1/2} - s_{ref})}$$

where t_{eq} and t are the wind chill equivalent and ambient temperatures in degrees Celsius, and s and s_{ref} are the actual and reference wind speeds in m s^{-1}. Wind-chill equivalent temperatures in degrees Fahrenheit for a reference wind speed of 4 mph (1.79 m s^{-1}) are listed in Table 25-3.

The wind chill formula of Siple has been criticized as being too sensitive to changes in wind speed when wind speed is low and not sensitive enough to changes in wind speed at higher velocities.[71] The formula clearly is only an approximation, since for any temperature, H, the wind chill, is maximal at winds of 25 m s^{-1} (56 mph) and decreases as wind speed goes even higher, a physical impossibility.

Hypothermia

The term "hypothermia" refers to either the unintentional or purposeful lowering of core body temperature. Hypothermia has been induced purposefully to decrease oxygen consumption during surgical procedures. Unintentional hypothermia may occur as a result of overexposure to cold and is a problem of considerable public health importance. It is the only type of hypothermia considered further herein.

By general agreement hypothermia is said to be clinically significant when core temperature falls to 95° F (35° C) or lower. As body temperature drops, consciousness becomes clouded,

TABLE 25-3. WIND CHILL EQUIVALENT TEMPERATURES IN DEGREES FAHRENHEIT FOR REFERENCE WIND SPEED OF 4 MILES PER HOUR

	Actual Wind Speed (mph)						
Temperature	**4**	**5**	**10**	**20**	**30**	**40**	**50**
40	40	37	28	18	13	10	9
35	35	32	22	11	5	2	1
30	30	27	16	4	−2	−6	−7
25	25	22	10	−3	−10	−14	−15
20	20	16	4	−10	−18	−22	−23
15	15	11	−3	−18	−25	−29	−31
10	10	6	−9	−25	−33	−37	−39
5	5	1	−15	−32	−41	−45	−47
0	0	−5	−21	−39	−48	−53	−55
−5	−5	−10	−27	−46	−56	−61	−63
−10	−10	−15	−33	−53	−64	−69	−71
−15	−15	−20	−40	−60	−71	−77	−79
−20	−20	−26	−46	−67	−79	−85	−87

and the patient appears confused or disoriented. Pallor occurs, the result of intense vasoconstriction. Shivering is maximal in the higher range of hypothermic core temperatures, but decreases markedly in intensity as body temperature falls further and hypothermia itself impairs thermoregulation. In severe hypothermia (body temperature below about 86° F [30° C]), consciousness is lost, respirations may become imperceptibly shallow, and the pulse may not be palpable. At such low temperatures, the myocardium becomes irritable and ventricular fibrillation is common.[72] Patients may appear dead even though they may yet be revived with proper treatment. Persons found apparently dead in circumstances suggesting that they may have suffered hypothermia should be treated for hypothermia until death can be confirmed.[73] In particular the potential for recovery of cold-water drowning victims should not be underestimated, since there have been reports of virtually complete recovery in patients who were without an effective heartbeat for periods as long as 2 1/2 hours.[74]

Hypothermia occurs both as a direct consequence of overexposure to the cold (primary hypothermia) and as the apparent result of thermoregulatory failure due principally to other severe illness (e.g., sepsis, myocardial infarction, central nervous system damage, metabolic derangements), although cold exposure may contribute to such secondary hypothermia. Primary hypothermia has a better prognosis than hypothermia that occurs as a result of concomitant illness.[75] Death is more likely in patients who present with particularly low body temperatures.[76]

The question of the best method(s) for rewarming hypothermic patients remains controversial, and treatment varies considerably among different clinicians.[76] Regardless of the method of rewarming used, all but mild hypothermia cases require intensive medical care, especially treatment directed toward supporting circulation and respiration, correcting electrolyte and acid-base disturbances, and optimizing intravascular volume. Hypoglycemia should be considered and corrected if present. In addition, the patient must be treated for any predisposing medical condition.[77,78]

Local Tissue Injury

Local tissue injury as a result of exposure to cold may be seen in hypothermia cases but often occurs independently from it. Frostbite, the actual freezing of tissue, primarily affects acral body parts (e.g., distal extremities, ears, and nose) and can occur over a period of minutes to hours in severe cold. Frostbite often lessens tissue viability to the point that amputation may be required. Such injuries may be frequent during a spell of unusually cold weather.[79]

Hypothermia in the Elderly

The extent to which indoor cold causes clinically significant hypothermia has been increasingly appreciated in recent years. In particular, the special vulnerability of elderly persons to this condition has been recognized. After the first few years of life the rate of death due to the cold increases steadily with advancing age (Fig. 25-4). In the United States, there are approximately 700 to 1000 deaths due to cold exposure each year. More than half of these cases occur in persons aged 60 years or older, although persons in this age group comprise less than 16% of the population.[80,81]

In the United States the annual number of deaths due to exposure to the cold has increased in recent years.[82] Because elderly persons are more susceptible to hypothermia, the increasing average age of the U.S. population may account for at least some of the increase. Since hypothermia deaths typically involve a disproportionate number of persons without a fixed address,[83] the problem of homelessness in the United States may be an additional contributing factor.

The extent of hypothermia morbidity is difficult to measure. A national wintertime survey conducted in Great Britain of 1020 persons aged 65 and over showed that relatively few (0.58%) persons surveyed had hypothermic morning deep-body temperatures (≤35° C) and that none had hypothermic evening temperatures. Nevertheless a substantial number (10%) had near-hypothermic temperatures (≤35.5° C but >35° C).[84] In contrast, 3.6% of 467 patients more than 65 years old admitted to London hospitals in late winter and early spring were hypothermic.[85] The fact that hypothermia is relatively common among elderly persons admitted to hospitals, although it is virtually absent in the community, has been interpreted as showing that most elderly Britons with hypothermia are hospitalized quickly.

The apparent cold sensitivity of the elderly may be the result of physiological factors. Collins and associates[86] found that a high proportion of persons aged 65 and older failed to develop physiologically significant vasoconstriction in response to a controlled cold environment and that the proportion of such persons increased with the age of the cohort examined. These elderly subjects with abnormal vasoconstriction tended to have relatively low core temperatures. The basal metabolic rate declines substantially with age, requiring elderly people to battle cold stress from a relatively low level of basal thermogenesis.[87] Shivering, a mechanism by which metabolic thermogenesis can be increased, may be impaired in some older persons.[88] Voluntary muscular activity also releases heat, but the elderly are more prone than others to debilitating chronic illnesses that limit mobility. Metabolic heat produced through the oxidation of brown fat is less

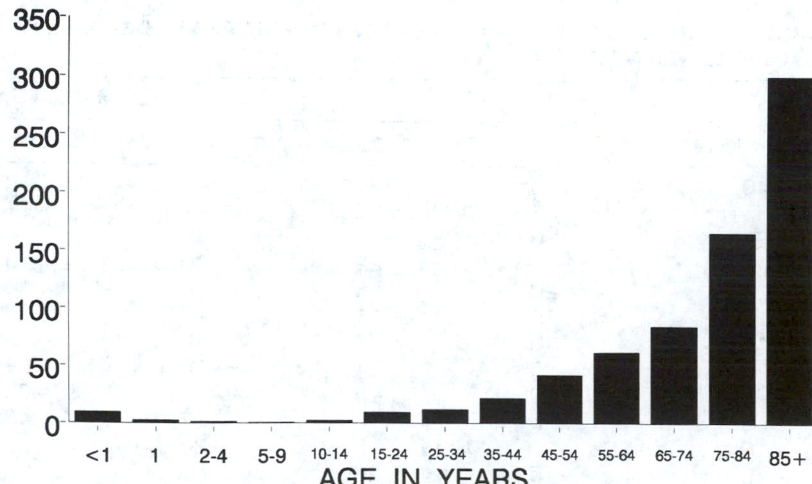

Figure 25-4. Rates of death per 10 million population per year attributed to cold (International Classification of Diseases, Eighth and Ninth Revisions, Code E901) by age, United States, 1975-1985.

available to the elderly, in whom this type of adipose tissue is less abundant than in children and younger adults.[89]

Elderly persons do not appear to perceive cold as well as younger persons and may voluntarily set thermostats to relatively low temperatures.[46,90] In addition, the rising cost of energy in recent years, together with the relative poverty of some elderly people, may discourage them from setting their thermostats high enough to maintain comfortable warmth.

Drugs Predisposing to Hypothermia

Ethanol ingestion is an important predisposing factor for hypothermia. The great majority of patients in many hypothermia case series are middle-aged alcoholic men.[83,91] Ethanol produces vasodilation, interfering with the peripheral vasoconstriction that is an important physiological defense against the cold.[69] Although ethanol-containing beverages are sometimes taken in cold surroundings for the subjective sense of warmth they produce, this practice is dangerous. Ethanol also indirectly predisposes one to hypothermia by inhibiting hepatic gluconeogenesis and thus producing hypoglycemia in carbohydrate-depleted persons (e.g., many chronic alcoholics). Ethanol-induced hypoglycemia clearly has been shown to produce hypothermia in healthy volunteers.[92]

Treatment with the neuroleptic drugs (phenothiazines, butyrophenones, and thioxanthenes) also predisposes the patient to hypothermia. Chlorpromazine, the prototypical drug of this group, has been used to induce hypothermia pharmacologically.[1,93] Chlorpromazine suppresses shivering, probably by a central mechanism, and causes vasodilation.[56] The hypothermic action of drugs of this class becomes more pronounced with decreasing ambient temperature.[94]

Other Risk Factors

Infants under 1 year of age have a higher rate of death due to cold than older children have (Fig. 25-4). Neonates, especially premature or small-for-gestational-age babies, are at particularly high risk. Although the mechanisms for maintaining thermal homeostasis (vasoconstriction and thermogenesis by shivering) are present at birth, they seem to function less effectively than in older children. Infants have a relatively large ratio of heat-losing surface/heat-generating volume, and the layer of insulating subcutaneous fat is relatively thin. Perhaps most important, babies are unable to control their own environment. They are totally dependent on others to keep them warm, and if sufficient warmth is not provided, hypothermia results.[69]

Hypothermia in infants can be a substantial public health problem in areas with severe winter weather. During December and January of the winters of 1961–1962 and 1962–1963, 110 severely hypothermic (temperature $< 90°$ F, 32.2° C) babies were admitted to hospitals in Glasgow, Scotland. Mortality in this group was 46%.[95] Hypothermia, however, is not restricted to cold climates. In tropical climates, hypothermia among babies and young children also can be a problem in winter. Children and infants suffering from protein-calorie malnutrition are particularly susceptible.[96]

In older children and young adults, lethal hypothermia is relatively infrequent (Fig. 25-4). However, persons in this age group are still susceptible to an overwhelming cold stress. Unintentional immersion in very cold water can lead rapidly to hypothermia.[97] Cold and wet weather may be especially dangerous, because the insulating properties of clothing are markedly reduced by moisture.[98]

The rate of death due to cold is greater in males than in females in all age groups (Table 25-2). Behavioral differences resulting in increased frequency of exposure to cold may account for the particularly great relative risk of males during the teenage years through late middle age, but such differences do not fully explain the apparent difference between the sexes in susceptibility.

Hypothermia is common among elderly persons with hypothyroidism. Persons with myxedema (severe hypothyroidism) may be hypothermic with no unusual cold stress. A low level of thyroid hormone results in a low rate of metabolic heat production, leading to hypothermia.[99]

Prevention

Hypothermia is best prevented by limiting the cold stress of susceptible populations. Thus programs that help the elderly poor to receive financial assistance in paying heating bills may be helpful. Both government agencies and utility companies have been involved in establishing programs that either provide direct financial aid toward the payment of elderly people's energy bills or allow deferred payments. Awareness of the problem of neonatal hypothermia by pediatricians and communication of this concern to new parents may help prevent hypothermia in infants.

Children and young adults who are at low risk from the cold nevertheless should take appropriate precautions when they venture into a cold environment. The clothing chosen should provide sufficient insulation, and care should be taken that it does not get wet. In particular, one should guard against the possibility of immersion in cold water.

REFERENCES

1. Collins KJ: Hypothermia: The Facts. New York: Oxford University Press, 1983
2. Weast RC (ed): CRC Handbook of Chemistry and Physics. Boca Raton, Fla.: CRC Press, 1981
3. Clarke JF: Some effects of the urban structure on heat mortality. Environ Res 5:93–104, 1972
4. Rowell LB: Human adjustments and adaptations to heat stress. Where and how? In Folinsbee LJ, Wagner JA, Borgia JF, et al (eds): Environmental Heat Stress: Individual Human Adaptations. New York: Academic Press, 1978, pp 3–27
5. Nadel ER, Roberts MF, Wenger CB: Thermoregulatory adaptations to heat and exercise: Comparative responses of men and women. In Folinsbee LJ, Wagner JA, Borgia JF, et al (eds): Environmental Heat Stress: Individual Human Adaptations. New York: Academic Press, 1978, pp 29–38
6. Bonner RM, Harrison MH, Hall CJ, Edwards RJ: Effect of heat acclimatization on intravascular responses to acute heat stress in man. J Appl Physiol 41:708–713, 1976
7. Wyndham CH, Rogers GG, Senay LC, Mitchell D: Acclimatization in a hot, humid environment: Cardiovascular adjustments. J Appl Physiol 40:779–785, 1976
8. Steadman RG: The assessment of sultriness. Part I: A temperature-humidity index based on human physiology and clothing science. J Appl Meteorol 18:861–873, 1979
9. Steadman RG: The assessment of sultriness. Part II: Effects of wind, extra radiation, and barometric pressure on apparent temperature. J Appl Meteorol 18:874–885, 1979
10. Yaglou CP: Temperature, humidity, and air movement in industries: The effective temperature index. J Ind Hyg 9:297–309, 1927
11. American Society of Heating, Refrigerating, and Air Conditioning Engineers (ASHRAE): Handbook of Fundamentals. Atlanta: ASHRAE, 1981
12. American Society of Heating, Refrigerating, and Air Conditioning Engineers (ASHRAE): 1989 ASHRAE Handbook: Fundamentals (I-P ed). Atlanta: ASHRAE, 1989
13. Lee DHK: Seventy-five years of searching for a heat index. Environ Res 22:331–356, 1980

14. Minard D, Belding HS, Kingston JR: Prevention of heat casualties. JAMA 1655:1813–1818, 1957
15. National Institute for Occupational Safety and Health: Criteria for a Recommended Standard: Occupational Exposure to Hot Environments. Revised Criteria 1986. Washington, D.C.: U.S. Government Printing Office, 1986
16. Beshir MY, Ramsey JD, Burford CL: Threshold values for the Botsball: A field study of occupational heat. Ergonomics 25:247–254, 1982
17. Steadman RG: A universal scale of apparent temperature. J Climate Appl Meteorol 23:1674–1687, 1984
18. Hart GR, Anderson RJ, Crumpler CP, et al: Epidemic classical heat stroke: Clinical characteristics and course of 28 patients. Medicine 61:189–197, 1982
19. Gauss H, Meyer KA: Heat stroke: Report of one hundred and fifty-eight cases from Cook County Hospital, Chicago. Am J Med Sci 154:554–564, 1917
20. Ferris EB Jr, Blankenhorn MA, Robinson HW, Cullen GE: Heatstroke: Clinical and chemical observations on 44 cases. J Clin Invest 17:249–262, 1938
21. Knochel JP: Environmental heat illness: An eclectic review. Arch Intern Med 133:841–864, 1974
22. Knochel JP: Heat stroke and related heat stress disorders. Dis Mon 35:301–377, 1989
23. National Institute for Occupational Safety and Health: Criteria for a Recommended Standard: Occupational Exposure to Hot Environments. Washington, D.C.: U.S. Department of HEW, 1972
24. Levine RJ: Male fertility in hot environments [Letter]. JAMA 252:3250–3251, 1984
25. Rachootin P, Olsen J: The risk of infertility and delayed conception associated with exposures in the Danish workplace. J Occup Med 25:394–402, 1983
26. Shiota K, Kayamura T: Effects of prenatal heat stress on postnatal growth, behavior and learning capacity in mice. Biol Neonate 56:6–14, 1989
27. Miller P, Smith DW, Shepard TH: Maternal hyperthermia as a possible cause of anencephaly. Lancet 1:519–521, 1978
28. Layde PM, Edmonds LD, Erickson JD: Maternal fever and neural tube defects. Teratology 21:105–108, 1980
29. Centers for Disease Control: Heatstroke: United States, 1980. MMWR 30:277–279, 1981
30. 1980 Mortality Computer Tape. Hyattsville, Maryland: National Center for Health Statistics.
31. Martinez BF, Annest JL, Kilbourne EM, Kirk ML, Lui K-J, Smith SM: Geographic distribution of heat-related deaths among elderly persons. Use of county-level dot maps for injury surveillance and epidemiologic research. JAMA 262:2246–2250, 1989
32. Jones TS, Liang AP, Kilbourne EM, et al: Morbidity and mortality associated with the July 1980 heat wave in St. Louis and Kansas City, Missouri. JAMA 247:3327–3331, 1982
33. Ellis FP: Heat illness. Trans R Soc Trop Med Hyg 70:402–425, 1976
34. Schuman SH, Anderson CP, Olicer JT: Epidemiology of successive heat waves in Michigan in 1962 and 1963. JAMA 189:733–738, 1964
35. Schuman SH: Patterns of urban heat wave deaths and implications for prevention: Data from New York and St. Louis during July, 1966. Environ Res 5:59–75, 1972
36. Keatinge WR, Coleshaw SRK, Easton JC, Cotter F, Mattock MB, Chelliah R: Increased platelet and red cell counts, blood viscosity, and plasma cholesterol levels during heat stress, and mortality from coronary and cerebral thrombosis. Am J Med 81:795–800, 1986
37. Strother SV, Bull JMC, Branham SA: Activation of coagulation during therapeutic whole body hyperthermia. Thromb Res 43:353–360, 1986
38. Applegate WB, Runyan JW Jr, et al: Analysis of the 1980 heat wave in Memphis. J Geriatr Soc 29:337–342, 1981
39. Austin MG, Berry JW: Observations on one hundred cases of heatstroke. JAMA 161:1525–1529, 1956
40. Sprung CL: Hemodynamic alterations of heat stroke in the elderly. Chest 75:362–366, 1979
41. Crowe JP, Moore RE: Physiological and behavioral responses of aged men to passive heating. J Physiol 236:43P–45P, 1973
42. Kilbourne EM, Choi K, Jones TS, et al: Risk factors for heatstroke. A case-control study. JAMA 247:3332–3336, 1982
43. Wise TN: Heatstroke in three chronic schizophrenics: Case reports and clinical considerations. Compr Psychiatry 14:263–267, 1973
44. Littman RE: Heat sensitivity due to autonomic drugs. JAMA 149: 635–636, 1952
45. Adams BE, Manoguerra AS, Lilja GP, Long RS, Ruiz E: Heatstroke: Associated with medications having anticholinergic effects. Minn Med 60:103–106, 1977
46. Collins KJ, Exton-Smith AN, Dore C: Urban hypothermia: Preferred temperature and thermal perception in old age. Br Med J 282:175–177, 1981
47. Cardullo HM: Sustained summer heat and fever in infants. J Pediatr 35:24–42, 1949
48. Danks DM, Webb DW, Allen J: Heat illness in infants and young children. A study of 47 cases. Br Med J 2:287–293, 1962
49. Bacon C, Scott D, Jones P: Heatstroke in well-wrapped infants. Lancet 1:422–425, 1979
50. Shapiro Y, Magazanik A, Udassin R, et al: Heat intolerance in former heatstroke patients. Ann Intern Med 90:913–916, 1979
51. Bar-Or O, Lundegren HM, Buskirk ER: Heat tolerance of exercising obese and lean women. J Appl Physiol 26:403–409, 1969
52. Haymes EM, McCormick RJ, Buskirk ER: Heat tolerance of exercising lean and obese prepubertal boys. J Appl Physiol 39:457–461, 1975
53. Schickele E: Environment and fatal heat stroke: An analysis of 157 cases occurring in the army in the U.S. during World War II. Milit Surgeon 98:235–256, 1947
54. MacQuaide DHG: Congenital absence of sweat glands. Lancet 2:531–532, 1944
55. Buchwald I: Scleroderma with fatal heat stroke. JAMA 201:270–271, 1967
56. Kollias J, Ballard RW: The influence of chlorpromazine on physical and chemical mechanisms of temperature regulation in the rat. J Pharmacol Exp Ther 145:373–381, 1964
57. Ginsberg MD, Hertzman M, Schmidt-Nowara WW: Amphetamine intoxication with coagulopathy, hyperthermia, and reversible renal failure. Ann Intern Med 73:81–85, 1970
58. Stanley B, Pal NR: Fatal hyperpyrexia with phenelzine and imipramine. Br Med J 2:10–11, 1964
59. Lewis E: Hyperpyrexia with antidepressant drugs. Br Med J 1:1671–1672, 1965
60. Schneider SH: The greenhouse effect: Science and policy. Science 243:771–781, 1989
61. Leaf A: Potential health effects of global climatic and environmental changes. N Engl J Med 321:1577–1583, 1989
62. Kamon E, Avellini B: Wind speed limits to work under hot environments for clothed men. J Appl Physiol 46:340–345, 1979
63. Feinlieb M: Statement of Manning Feinleib. In Deadly Cold: Health Hazards due to Cold Weather. Washington, D.C.: U.S. Government Printing Office, 1984, pp 85–125
64. Rosenwaike I: Seasonal variation of deaths in the United States, 1951–1960. J Am Stat Assoc 61:706–719, 1966
65. Giaconi S, Ghione S, Palombo C, Genovesi-Ebert A, Marabotti C, Fommei E, Donato L: Seasonal influences on blood pressure in high normal to mild hypertensive range. Hypertension 14:22–27, 1989
66. Keatinge WR, Coleshaw SRK, Cotter F, Mattock M, Murphy M, Chelliah R: Increases in platelet and red cell counts, blood viscosity and arterial pressure during mild surface cooling: Factors in mortality from coronary and cerebral thrombosis in winter. Br Med J 289:1405–1408, 1984
67. Dannenberg AL, Keller JB, Wilson PWF, Castelli WP: Leisure time physical activity in the Framingham offspring study. Am J Epidemiol 129:76–88, 1989
68. Schulman JL, Kilbourne ED: Experimental transmission of influenza virus in mice: II. Some factors affecting incidence of transmitted infection. J Exp Med 118:267–275, 1963

69. Maclean D, Emslie-Smith D: Accidental Hypothermia. Oxford: Blackwell Scientific Publications, 1977
70. Siple PA, Passel CF: Measurement of dry atmospheric cooling in subfreezing temperatures. Proc Am Philos Soc 89:177–199, 1945
71. Steadman RG: Indices of wind chill of clothed persons. J Appl Meteorol 10:674–683, 1971
72. MacGregor DC, Armour JA, Goldman BS, Bigelow WG: The effects of ether, ethanol, propanol, and butanol on tolerance to deep hypothermia. Experimental and clinical observation. Dis Chest 50:523–529, 1966
73. Althaus U, Aeberhard P, Schupback P, Nachblur BH, Muhlemann W: Management of profound accidental hypothermia with cardiorespiratory arrest. Ann Surg 195:492–495, 1982
74. Young RSK, Zaineratis EL, Dooling EC: Neurological outcome in cold water drowning. JAMA 244:1233–1235, 1980
75. Miller JW, Danzl DF, Thomas DM: Urban accidental hypothermia: 135 cases. Ann Emerg Med 9:456–460, 1980
76. Danzl DF, Pozos RS, Auerbach PS, et al: Multicenter hypothermia survey. Ann Emerg Med 16:1042–1055, 1987
77. Anonymous: Treatment of hypothermia. Med Lett Drugs Ther 28:123–124, 1986
78. Laub GW, Banaszak D, Kupferschmid J, Magovern GJ, Young JC: Percutaneous cardiopulmonary bypass for the treatment of hypothermic circulatory collapse. Ann Thorac Surg 47:608–611, 1989
79. Bishop HM, Collin J, Wood RFM, Morris PJ: Frostbite in Oxfordshire: The impact of a severe winter on an unprepared civilian population. Injury 15:379–380, 1984
80. Mortality Tapes from 1968–1980. Hyattsville, Md: National Center for Health Statistics.
81. 1980 Census. Washington, D.C.: U.S. Bureau of the Census.
82. Centers for Disease Control: Hypothermia prevention. MMWR 37:780–782, 1988
83. Centers for Disease Control: Exposure-related hypothermia deaths—District of Columbia, 1972–1982. MMWR 31:669–671, 1982
84. Fox RH, Woodward PM, Exton-Smith AN, et al: Body temperatures in the elderly: A national study of physiological, social, and environmental conditions. Br Med J 1:200–206, 1973
85. Goldman A, Exton-Smith AN, Francis G, O'Brien A: A pilot study of low body temperatures in old people admitted to hospital. J R Coll Physicians Lond 11:291–306, 1977
86. Collins KJ, Dore C, Exton-Smith AN, et al: Accidental hypothermia and impaired temperature homeostasis in the elderly. Br Med J 1:353–356, 1977
87. Shock NW, Watkin DM, Yiengst MJ, et al: Age differences in the water content of the body as related to basal oxygen consumption in males. J Gerontol 18:1–8, 1963
88. Collins KJ, Easton JC, Exton-Smith AN: Shivering thermogenesis and vasomotor responses with convective cooling in the elderly. J Physiol 320:76P, 1981
89. Heat J: The distribution of brown adipose tissue in the human. J Anat 112:35–39, 1972
90. Watts AJ: Hypothermia in the aged: A study of the role of cold-sensitivity. Environ Res 5:119–126, 1971
91. Weyman AE, Greenbaum DM, Grace WJ: Accidental hypothermia in an alcoholic population. Am J Med 56:13–21, 1974
92. Haight JSJ, Keatinge WR: Failure of thermoregulation in the cold during hypoglycemia induced by exercise and ethanol. J Physiol 229:87–97, 1973
93. Courvoisier S, Fournel J, Ducrot R, Kolsky M, Koetschet P: Proprietes pharmacodynamiques du chlorhydrate de chloro-3 (dimethylamino-3′ propyl)-10 phenothiazine (4.560 R.P.). Arch Int Pharmacodyn Ther 92:305–361, 1953
94. Higgins EA, Iampietro PF, Adams T, Holmes DD: Effects of a tranquilizer on body temperature. Proc Soc Exp Biol Med 115:1017–1019, 1964
95. Arneil GC, Kerr MM: Severe hypothermia in Glasgow infants in winter. Lancet 2:756–759, 1963
96. Cutting WAM, Samuel GA: Hypothermia in a tropical winter climate. Indian Pediatr 8:752–757, 1971
97. Bullard RW, Rapp GM: Problems of body heat loss in water immersion. Aerospace Med 41:1269–1277, 1970
98. Pugh LGC: Clothing insulation and accidental hypothermia in youth. Nature 209:1281–1286, 1966
99. Forester CF: Coma in myxedema. Arch Intern Med 111(6):100–109, 1963

26

Ionizing Radiation

Vladimir Dvorak

Naturally occurring ionizing radiation of cosmic and terrestrial origin has been part of the environment throughout the evolution of life. Additional exposures have been added to this natural radiation background during the century, becoming an important concern of public health. However, centuries before the radioactivity was discovered, lung disease was seen in miners from Central European mines; the disease eventually was recognized as lung cancer caused by exposure to high concentrations of radon decay products in poorly ventilated mines.

The discovery of x-rays at the end of the nineteenth century prompted vigorous pursuit to use ionizing radiation as a tool in diagnostic and therapeutic medicine and in research and industry. Severe health consequences of overexposure to x-rays and cases of radium poisoning of dial painters have contributed to the intensive research on adverse health effects and to the development of radiation protection on an international basis. Indeed, the International Commission for Radiological Protection (ICRP) was established as early as 1928.

With the onset of military use of nuclear energy, followed by the promotion of its peaceful applications and the widespread use of sources of ionizing radiation, concerns were raised as to the potential genetic and somatic risks of population exposure. Long-term epidemiological studies and the vast experimental data reviewed periodically by national and international bodies serve as the basis of the system of radiation dose limitation.

TYPES OF IONIZING RADIATION: QUANTITIES AND UNITS

Ionizing radiation includes electromagnetic radiation, such as gamma rays or x-rays, and particulate radiation of different mass and charge, such as helium nuclei (alpha particles), electrons (beta particles), protons, or neutrons. Both types are present in a natural radiation background and in man-made radiation (sources of which are devices such as x-ray tubes or nuclear reactions). Disintegration of radioactive nuclides, naturally occurring or produced artificially, is called radioactivity.

The activity of a radioactive material is the number of nuclear disintegrations per unit of time. The unit of activity is a becquerel (Bq); 1 Bq = 1 disintegration per second. Formerly, the unit of activity was curie (Ci), which is 3.7 10^{10} disintegrations per second, corresponding with approximately 1g of radium 226.

The absorbed dose of radiation is the energy imparted per unit mass of the irradiated material. The unit of absorbed dose is joule per kilogram, for which the special name gray (Gy) is used.

The same absorbed dose, expressed in Gy, caused by different types of radiation can have different degrees of biological effect. The relative biological effectiveness (RBE) is used in radiobiology, the reference radiation being x-rays or gamma rays. For the purposes of radiation protection, a quantity called the dose equivalent is used. The dose equivalent is a product of the absorbed dose (in Gy) and a quality factor Q. The quality factor is a function of the capability of each type of radiation to produce ionizations along its path, expressed as the linear energy transfer (LET). The ICRP recommends the values, for example, $Q = 1$ for x-rays, gamma rays, and beta particles; $Q = 20$ for alpha particles. The x-rays and the beta and gamma radiation have the ionizations sparsely distributed along the track and therefore are considered low-LET radiations. Alpha particles and other densely ionizing radiations can produce hundreds or thousands times more ionizations per unit length—hence high-LET radiations. The unit of the dose equivalent is the sievert (Sv). The relationship between the currently used International System of Units (SI) and the older units still found in recent literature, together with the quantity exposure, are given in Table 26–1.

ICRP[1] recommended in 1977 that a weighted sum of the radiation dose equivalents in the most radiosensitive organs and tissues should be the basis for radiation protection assessments. This weighted sum is called the effective dose equivalent. The unit is the same as for the dose equivalent, the sievert. The effective dose equivalent is determined using the ICRP organ weighting factors given in Table 26–2.[2]

EFFECTS

DNA is considered the most important target for cell killing caused by ionizing radiation. DNA may be damaged either by ionizations occurring in the DNA itself (direct effect) or by radicals, particularly by the OH radical, produced in the immediate vicinity of DNA by interaction of radiation with water molecules (indirect effect). The DNA damage includes single- and double-

TABLE 26-1. UNITS[a]

Quantity	SI Unit	Conventional Unit (Symbol and Value in SI Units)
Exposure	No special name [C kg^{-1}]	1 roentgen [R] = 2.58×10^{-4} C kg^{-1}
Absorbed dose	1 gray [Gy] = 1 J kg^{-1}	1 rad [rad] = 0.01 Gy
Dose equivalent	1 sievert [Sv][b] = 1 J kg^{-1}	1 rem [rem][b] = 0.01 Sv

[a]Where the abbreviations C, kg, and J in the table stand for coulomb, kilogram, and joule, respectively.
[b]The magnitude of the dose equivalent in sievert or rem depends on the LET of the radiation.
From NCRP, 1989.[6]

strand breaks, the latter being produced more aptly by high-LET radiation than by low-LET radiation; correspondingly, lower ability for repair has been implicated for high-LET radiation. The high-LET radiation has been found to be more effective than low-LET radiation in cell culture experiments concerning inactivation, mutation, and cell transformation. Experimental evidence indicates that for the low-LET radiation the effectiveness of a given dose decreases with decreasing dose rate. This dose-rate effect is due to such factors as the repair of sublethal damage, redistribution of the cells within the mitotic cycle, and the compensatory cellular proliferation. At the cellular level, irradiation can result in cell death or lead to changes that may be compatible with subsequent cellular division. Depletion of cells at the tissue level can lead to early changes, such as the acute radiation syndrome, in which tissue sensitivity is a determinant of clinical response to different dose levels, or local tissue reaction, such as radiation dermatitis. The changes that do not lead to cell death can be the initial step in the subsequent development of delayed somatic effects, particularly tumor induction, or genetic effects in the case of gonadal exposure.

Early Effects of High Doses of Radiation

Data from radiation accidents, the atomic bombings in Nagasaki and Hiroshima, and from radiation therapy have been reviewed recently,[3] including available information from the 1986 Chernobyl accident. Symptoms, therapy, and outcomes, with respect to different dose ranges of whole-body irradiation by low-LET, high dose rate in man, are given in Table 26-3. Early prodromal response, mediated through the autonomic nervous system, consists of gastrointestinal reactions (anorexia, nausea, vomiting, intestinal cramps, diarrhea) and neuromuscular signs (fatigue, apathy, sweating, headache, and hypotension) and may occur from hours to 2 days after irradiation. Time between exposure and onset of prodromal signs depends on dose; the dose that induces vomiting in 50% of individuals is about 2 Gy. Doses above 50 Gy result in death from cerebrovascular injury, called neurological syndrome, in 2 days. Doses between about 10 and 50 Gy lead to the gastrointestinal syndrome, deaths occurring mostly between days 6 and 9. The intestinal mucosa damage and marrow failure determine the clinical findings. Doses from about 1 Gy up to several grays result in bone marrow syndrome. The lymphocyte count is the earliest sensitive indicator of radiation injury in blood, the counts being reduced to about 50% of normal within the first 48 hours after doses of 1 to 2 Gy.

As part of the acute radiation syndrome or in the case of nonhomogeneous irradiation, other tissues may be affected; for example, radiation dermatitis may be caused by a broad range of doses from about 1.5 Gy up, depending on the area irradiated and the type of radiation (with higher photon energies, maximum dose may be to the dermis because of the dose build-up). Permanent sterility in men requires more than 6 Gy; at lower doses, temporary sterility occurs. Higher sensitivity has been found after fractionated irradiation than after an acute dose, because the most sensitive differentiating forms of spermatogonia are present at a low proportion at any given time. In women, permanent sterility occurs after doses in the range of about 4 to 10 Gy; older women are more susceptible because the number of follicles decreases with age.

Prenatal Irradiation

Knowledge of the effects of prenatal human irradiation is based mainly on long-term epidemiological studies of persons exposed in utero in Hiroshima and Nagasaki. During the first years, microcephaly, often combined with mental retardation, and growth retardation were reported in a broad range of estimated values. Later on, more subtle impairments have been studied; a

TABLE 26-2. RECOMMENDED VALUES OF THE WEIGHTING FACTORS, w_T, FOR CALCULATING EFFECTIVE DOSE EQUIVALENT AND THE RISK COEFFICIENTS FROM WHICH THEY WERE DERIVED [a]

Tissue (T)	Risk Coefficient	w_T
Gonads	40×10^{-4} Sv^{-1} [40×10^{-6} rem^{-1}]	0.25
Breast	25×10^{-4} Sv^{-1} [25×10^{-6} rem^{-1}]	0.15
Red bone marrow	20×10^{-4} Sv^{-1} [20×10^{-6} rem^{-1}]	0.12
Lung	20×10^{-4} Sv^{-1} [20×10^{-6} rem^{-1}]	0.12
Thyroid	5×10^{-4} Sv^{-1} [5×10^{-6} rem^{-1}]	0.03
Bone surfaces	5×10^{-4} Sv^{-1} [5×10^{-6} rem^{-1}]	0.03
Remainder[b]	50×10^{-4} Sv^{-1} [50×10^{-6} rem^{-1}]	0.30
Total[c]	165×10^{-4} Sv^{-1} [165×10^{-6} rem^{-1}]	1.00

[a]Values from ICRP, 1977.[1]
[b]A w_T of 0.06 is to be assigned to each of the five remainder tissues receiving the highest dose equivalents and the other remainder tissues are to be neglected. (When the gastrointestinal tract is irradiated, the stomach, small intestine, upper large intestine and lower large intestine are to be treated as four separate organs and each may therefore be included in the five remainder tissues depending on the magnitude of the dose equivalent they receive when compared to the dose equivalent received by other remainder tissues and organs.)
[c]The total for somatic risk alone is 125×10^{-4} Sv^{-1} [125×10^{-6} rem^{-1}], which for radiation protection purposes is often rounded to a nominal value of 1×10^{-2} Sv^{-1} [1×10^{-4} rem]. Genetic risk is 40×10^{-4} Sv^{-1} [40×10^{-6} rem^{-1}].
From NCRP, 1987.[2]

TABLE 26–3. TOTAL-BODY IRRADIATION IN MAN: SCHEMATIC CLASSIFICATION OF DOSE RANGES: SYMPTOMS, THERAPY, AND OUTCOME

	Prodromal Symptoms		Clinical Characteristics			Therapy, Clinical Course, and Outcome				
									If Injury Is Fatal	
Acute Dose (Gy)	**Incidence (%)**	**Latency**	**Syndrome or Organ Involved**	**Characteristic Symptoms**	**Critical Period After Exposure**	**Therapy**	**Prognosis**	**Lethality (%)**	**Death Within**	**Usual Cause of Death**
>50	100	Minutes	Neurological syndrome	Cramps, tremor, ataxia, lethargy, impaired vision, coma	1–48 h	Symptomatic	Hopeless	100	1–48 h	Cerebral edema
10–15	100	0.5 h	Intestinal syndrome	Diarrhea, fever, electrolytic imbalance	3–14 d	Palliative	Very poor	90–100	2 wk	Enterocolitis shock
5–10	100	0.5–1 h	Bone marrow syndrome	Thrombopenia, leukopenia, hemorrhage, infections, epilation	2–6 wk	Bone marrow transplantation, transfusions of leukocytes and platelets, optimal care (isolation, antibiotics, fluids)	Uncertain, depending on success of therapy	0–90	Weeks	Infections or hemorrhage or both
2–5	50–90	1–2 h	Bone marrow syndrome	Thrombopenia, leukopenia, hemorrhage, infections, epilation	2–6 wk	Transfusions of leukocytes and platelets, optimal care (isolation, antibiotics, fluids), bone marrow transplantation	Uncertain, depending on success of therapy	0–90	Weeks	Infections or hemorrhage or both
1–2	0–50	>3 h	Bone marrow	Mild leukopenia and thrombopenia	2–6 wk	Symptomatic	Excellent	0–10	Months	Infections or hemorrhage or both

From UNSCEAR, 1988.[3]

recent reevaluation[4,5] has brought quantitative evidence concerning brain damage by irradiation, particularly between 8 and 15 weeks following fertilization (Table 26–4). Pathogenetically, neuronal death, impairment of the migration of neurons to the cortical zone, and faulty synaptogenesis could play a role in the occurrence of mental retardation. The authors have stressed the limited nature of the data. With all their reservations it is an important finding that for mental retardation, plausible interpretations either could not prove the existence of a, thus far, presumed threshold value of dose or would lead to identification of a threshold, the 95% lower boundary of which would appear to be in the range of 0.12 to 0.23 Gy. The other two developmental periods under study have not changed previous knowledge substantially: the probability of radiation-related mental retardation is lower for the period 16 to 25 weeks after conception, and no exposure-related mental retardation has been found in the first 8 weeks.

Cancer risk with respect to exposure in utero also has been studied for decades. In the Hiroshima and Nagasaki study, those persons exposed to prenatal irradiation have demonstrated no excess risk of leukemia, and until recently no radiation-related risk for solid cancers has been seen either. However, evaluation of data on prenatal exposure for the period from 1950 through 1984[5] showed an increased risk of malignant solid tumors. The limited evidence is consistent with the fact that early postnatal irradiation has shown carcinogenic risk also but only many years after exposure. The site-specific solid tumors observed in both groups have been the same, that is, bladder, breast, colon, ovary, stomach, and thyroid.

About 30 years ago, epidemiological studies of children exposed to x-irradiation in utero were initiated, and an association of childhood cancer has been shown; however, methodological difficulties, such as those related to the relevance of the reasons for the diagnostic use of x-ray examinations, have not allowed for definitive conclusions that would be widely accepted. From a practical point of view, progress in the reduction of prenatal irradiation including the introduction of ultrasonography have contributed to reduction of prenatal exposures.

Cancer

Carcinogenesis is the main delayed somatic effect of ionizing radiation. Tumors induced by irradiation are indistinguishable from those originating from other causes. Epidemiological studies are the principal source of information for cancer risk determination. The subjects of the studies include atomic bomb survivors, population groups with higher exposures incurred in the past because of the then allowed higher occupational or medical exposures (external or internal), and groups of persons subjected to accidental irradiation.

Several factors influence the probability that an irradiated individual will develop cancer and in which tissue it will develop. First is the radiation dose with its temporal and spatial distribution and radiation quality. Host factors include age at exposure, tissue susceptibility, gender, and genetic characteristics. Other factors, particularly environmental, may affect susceptibility of the host or interact with radiation, for example, smoking, dietary habits, or chemical exposure.

Age at exposure is an important factor; tissue susceptibility may be expected to relate to the proliferative activity of cells, which is reflected in recent findings of excess cancer in atomic bombing survivors exposed prenatally or in the first years of life, and in data showing decreased susceptibility with increasing age. Generally the excess cases, particularly those of solid tumors, occur at those stages in life in which cancer prevalence increases in nonirradiated populations. The sex ratio for persons with radiation-induced tumors is similar to that for nonexposed persons with the same tumors. Differences in latency are considerable; leukemia, except for chronic lymphatic leukemia, is a prominent radiation-induced cancer, with latency at least 2 to 4 years after exposure and peak occurrence at about 10 years; most of the cases occur within 30 years after irradiation. Solid tumors show longer latency, often decades after exposure. Radiation-induced cancer has been found in many tissues. To the long recognized cancers, such as tumors of the breast, thyroid, and lung, more are being added with longer follow-up periods of the principal groups studied; the recent additions are tumors of the colon and ovary and multiple myeloma. Excess cases also have been seen after internal contamination, for example, osteogenic sarcomas in persons contaminated with radium 226 or after repeated injections of radium 224. Some tumors, such as chronic lymphatic leukemia, squamous cell carcinoma of the cervix, and Hodgkin's disease, have not been found to be induced by ionizing radiation. In some studies the general patterns of tumor occurrence have not been observed: no excess leukemia cases following pelvic irradiation for cancer of the cervix or following prenatally exposed persons in Hiroshima and Nagasaki have been reported; tumors in patients subjected to irradiation for ankylosing spondylitis appear to be less frequent than expected after approximately 20 years from time of exposure.

The shape of the dose-response relationship continues to be the single most important problem for assessing cancer risk. The data suitable for quantitative evaluation of cancer occurrence after irradiation are in the range of about 0.5 to 1.5 Gy in atomic bombing survivors. Higher values may affect the quantitative assessment by recently recognized higher mortality from all diseases except neoplasms at dose levels from about 2 Gy and above.[5] For levels below this range the determination of risk is based on limited human data, animal experiments, research of mechanisms of carcinogenesis, and development of models.

The high incidence of cancer deaths from other causes makes it increasingly more difficult to determine statistically excess cases caused by radiation with decreasing doses (the calcu-

TABLE 26-4. EFFECT ON DEVELOPING BRAIN OF EXPOSURE TO IONIZING RADIATION IN WEEKS 8–15 FOLLOWING FERTILIZATION

Effect	Risk at 1 Gy	Comments
Severe mental retardation	Increased 50-fold	Risk rises from 0.8% at 0 Gy to 44% at 1 Gy.
Intelligence test score	Decreased 24–33 pts.[a]	This is a decline of about two standard deviations.
School performance	Decreased 1.0–1.3 pts.[b]	This is a fall from the class 50 percentile to the lowest 10 percentile.
Seizures, unprovoked	Increased 20-fold	Risk rises from 0.9% at 0 Gy to 20% at 1 Gy.

[a] Note these values do not represent the upper and lower confidence limits, but the range of central estimates based on samples, including and excluding persons known to be mentally retarded.

[b] Again this is not the confidence interval, but the range of central estimates seen over the four grades in school that have been studied.

From Schull, 1990.[5]

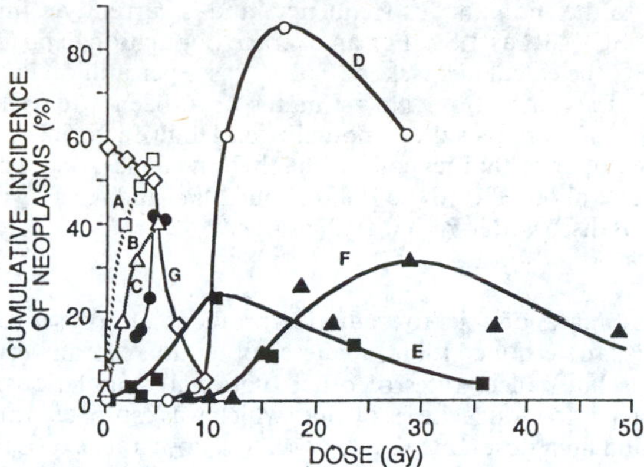

Figure 26–1. Dose-incidence curves for different neoplasms in animals exposed to external radiation: [A] myeloid leukemia in x-irradiated mice [▫] [Upton *et al*, 1958]; [B] mammary gland tumors at 12 months in gamma-irradiated rats [△] [Shellabarger *et al*, 1969]; [C] thymic lymphoma in x-irradiated mice [●] [Kaplan and Brown, 1952]; [D] kidney tumors in x-irradiated rats [○] [Maldague, 1969]; [E] skin tumors in alpha-irradiated rats [percentage incidence × 10] [▪] [Burns *et al*, 1968]; [F] skin tumors in electron-irradiated rats [percentage incidence × 10] [▲] [Burns *et al*, 1968]; [G] reticulum cell sarcoma in x-irradiated mice [◇] [Metalli *et al*, 1974]; [H] lung adenomas in neutron-irradiated mice [*] [Ullrich *et al*, 1976]. *[Modified from UNSCEAR, 1972. From Upton, 1984].*

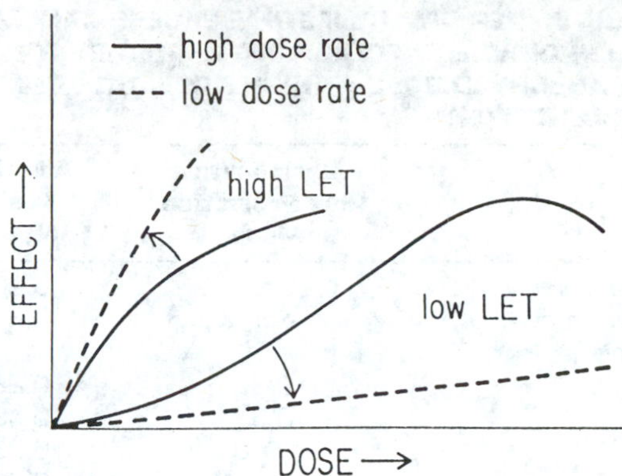

Figure 26–2. Schematic dose-response curves for incidence of tumors in relation to dose and dose rate of high-LET and low-LET radiation. *[From Upton, 1984; see also Thomson et al, 1982; Sinclair, 1983.]*

lated lifetime risk of fatal cancer for doses below 100 mSv is a fraction of a percent).

Animal experiments have provided an array of dose-response relationships (Fig. 26–1).[6] The lower incidence at high dose levels in some cases might be interpreted as being due to cell killing. Radiobiological concepts based on rapid progress of cellular research are themselves contributing to an understanding of carcinogenesis as a multistage process in which the initiation may be caused by ionizing radiation. A simplified concept of relationship between dose and dose-rate of high-LET and low-LET radiation with respect to tumor incidence is given in Figure 26–2.[6]

Several models of dose-response relationship are given in Figure 26-3.[7] International and national bodies periodically have been evaluating empirical data and theoretical concepts with respect to these models. At this time for different tumors the dose-response relationship may be approximated by one or more of the models. Thus the quantitative risk assessment depends heavily on the preferred model used. The BEIR V Committee's preferred risk model is a linear function of dose; thus a risk can be calculated even for low doses below the range of observation. The Committee acknowledges the departure from linearity cannot be excluded at low doses with resulting increase or decrease of risk and that there may be a threshold in the

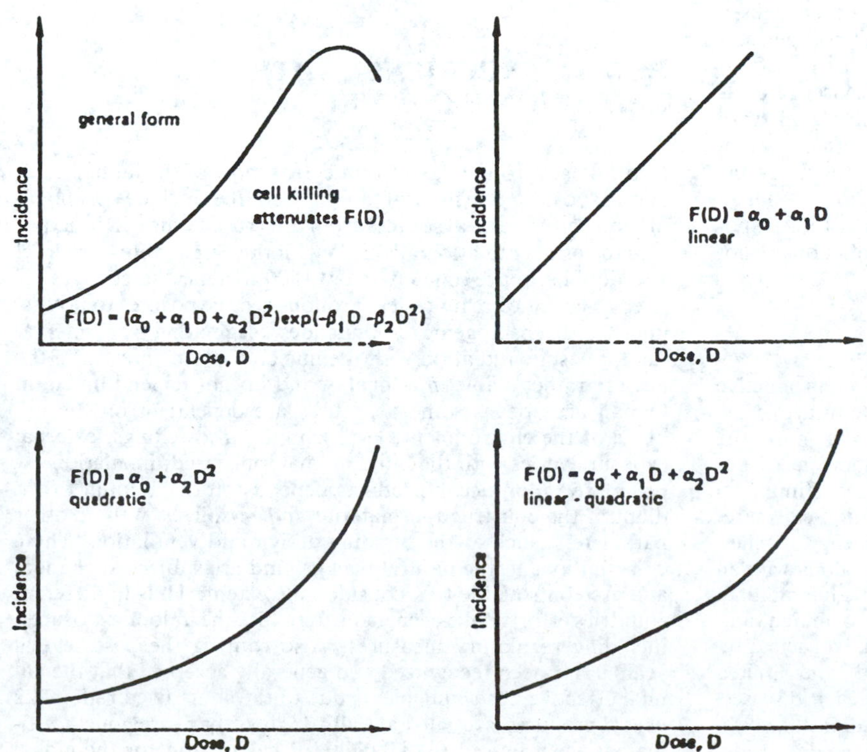

Figure 26–3. Dose-response curves for four different mathematical models relating cancer incidence to radiation dose. *[From BEIR III Report, NAS/NRC, 1980.[7]]*

TABLE 26-5. PER CAPUT LIFETIME EXCESS CANCER DEATHS PROBABILITY FOLLOWING EXPOSURE TO 1 Gy ORGAN ABSORBED DOSE AT HIGH DOSE RATE OF LOW-LET RADIATION (%)[a]

	Multiplicative Risk Projection Model	Additive Risk Projection Model
Red bone marrow	0.97	0.93
All cancers except leukemia	6.1	3.6
Bladder	0.39	0.23
Breast[b]	0.6	0.43
Colon	0.79	0.29
Lung	1.5	0.59
Multiple myeloma	0.22	0.09
Ovary[b]	0.31	0.26
Esophagus	0.34	0.16
Stomach	1.3	0.86
Remainder	1.1	1.0
Total	7.1	4.5

[a] Based on the population of Japan using an average age risk coefficient.
[b] Value has to be divided by 2 to calculate the total and other organ risks.
From UNSCEAR, 1988.[3]

millisievert range. Therefore the possibility that there may be no risk from exposure comparable to those from external natural background variation cannot be ruled out. With all the caveats and further qualifications discussed in extenso by the United Nations Scientific Committee on the Effects of Ionizing Radiation (UNSCEAR)[3] and the Biological Effects of Ionizing Radiations (BEIR) V Committee of the National Research Council,[8] the UNSCEAR estimates are given in Table 26–5; UNSCEAR restricted its estimate of cancer risk to a Japanese population with an exposure of 1 Sv, high-rate low-LET radiation. It should be noted that the reevaluation of the dosimetry of atomic bomb survivors, adopted in 1986 as the DS86 dosimetry system, has led to a lower estimated contribution of neutron dose and changes in gamma dose estimates as compared to the dose estimates used from 1965 to 1986. The result was an increase of risk per unit dose gamma and much less valid estimates of the effects of human exposure to neutrons. No increase in the cancer rate has been demonstrated in population groups living in regions with high natural gamma radiation background (often several millisieverts annually), such as those in Brazil, India, or the People's Republic of China, where monazite sands contain high concentrations of natural radionuclides. Studies at these exposure levels could indicate if risks from low level radiation are not underestimated.

Genetic Effects

Ionizing radiation damages the genetic material in reproductive cells, and the resulting mutations are transmitted to future generations. The genetic effects have been studied from the time of the *Drosophila* experiments in the 1920s. The development of nuclear energy and widespread use of radiation sources stimulated efforts to evaluate genetic risk of human population exposure. For the evaluation, knowledge of the normal frequency of genetically related diseases in the population is needed, along with an estimate of the risk of radiation dose. At this time human data are not sufficient for estimates of genetic risk due to human radiation exposure; therefore extensive experimental data sets, predominantly from mice and primates, are used, and limited human data are considered. Frequency of mendelian diseases, dominants, and x-linked and chromosome aberrations has been estimated to be between 1% and 2%. The doubling dose is defined as that dose required to induce the number of mutations equal to the spontaneous frequency, and is currently estimated by UNSCEAR[3] as 1 Sv. For an average population exposure of 0.01 Sv, the calculated risk is 10 to 20 cases per million liveborn in the first generation. No estimates have been attempted by UNSCEAR for congenital anomalies and multifactorial diseases because of uncertainties concerning their incidence, once considered to be about 3%, in the 1980s about 10%, and recently above 50%, as discussed in recent evaluations.[8,9]

• • •

Estimates of risks for radiation protection purposes require that risks determined for a Japanese population be transferred to the baseline cancer rates of other (national) populations. The next step is to reduce the risk value, which was estimated for high dose and high dose-rate to low dose, low dose-rate exposure.

Estimates of the value of this dose-rate effectiveness factor (DREF) are for low-LET radiation between 2 and 10. Currently, ICRP is considering the use of a value of 2 for the factor it calls dose and dose rates effectiveness factor (DDREF).[10]

For radiation protection purposes, the ICRP and regulatory bodies in many countries recognize the deterministic (nonstochastic) effects for which a threshold value may be identified, for example, acute postirradiation syndrome and the stochastic effects (such as cancer or genetic effects) for which a threshold value may not exist. In the ICRP system of dose limitation, limits are set to prevent the occurrence of the deterministic effects and, for the stochastic effects, to limit the risk to acceptable levels. To reduce exposure further, the ALARA concept (doses to be kept *a*s *l*ow *a*s *r*easonably *a*chievable) has been applied. In practice, most of the workers have exposures at about 10% of the limit (currently 50 mSv annually) or lower. Therefore, after years of the legal limit being 50 mSv in many countries, the lower value of 20 mSv annually expected to be proposed by the ICRP should be attainable.

According to the IRPA recommendations, practices using ionizing radiation should be justified, and dose reduction below dose limits should be achieved through the process of optimization.

HUMAN EXPERIENCE WITH RADIATION EXPOSURE

Natural background has accounted for most of the human radiation exposure. The natural radiation sources include cosmic radiation and terrestrial sources from the crust of the earth. Exposure to cosmic radiation increases with the height above sea level and doubles approximately every 1500 meters; the changes related to latitude are much less pronounced. Exposures to potassium 40 or to cosmogenic radionuclides, originating from interaction of cosmic radiation with the nuclei of atoms present in the air, are rather stable in a locality and do not depend much on human activities. Some exposures are dependent on the use made of the environment. For example, in dwellings, external exposure varies with the building materials used; inhalation exposure to radon decay products depends on the amount of radium in the construction material and in soil, as well as other parameters, such as the building design and ventilation. These contributions to the natural background are subject to changes and are controllable to a considerable extent. Thus in different countries efforts have been made to reduce the indoor exposures, including regulatory measures. Also, during the past several years it has been recognized and generally accepted that the annual effective dose equivalents due to the short-lived radon 222 decay products are substantially higher than previously estimated; according to the UNSCEAR calculation for the global population, approximately half the annual effective dose equiv-

TABLE 26-6. SUMMARY OF ESTIMATES OF EFFECTIVE DOSE EQUIVALENT

Source of Practice	Present Annual Individual Doses (mSv): Per Caput (World Population)	Present Annual Individual Doses (mSv): Typical (Exposed Individuals)	Collective Dose Commitments: Million Man Sv	Collective Dose Commitments: Equivalent Years of Background
▪ ANNUAL			**▪ PER YEAR OF PRACTICE**	
Natural background	2.4	1-5	11	1
Medical exposures (diagnostic)	0.4-1	0.1-10	2-5	0.2-0.5
Occupational exposure	0.002	0.5-5	0.01	0.001
Nuclear power production	0.0002	0.001-0.1	0.001 (0.03)[a]	0.0001 (0.004)[a]
▪ SINGLE			**▪ PER TOTAL PRACTICE**	
All test explosions together	0.1	0.01	5 (26)[a]	0.5 (2.4)[a]
Nuclear accidents			0.6[b]	

[a] The additional long-term collective dose commitments from radon and carbon-14 for nuclear power production and carbon-14 for test explosions are given in parentheses.
[b] Chernobyl.
From UNSCEAR, 1988.[3]

alent is caused by radon (Table 26-6). The annual effective dose equivalent estimated for the United States (NCRP 1987) is given in Figure 26-4.

Radon

Radon and its short-lived decay products can cause bronchogenic carcinoma in uranium miners at exposures of about 100 WLM; data from Ontario suggest that it can be caused by even lower exposures: about 50 WLM or below. The units used for miners' exposure are the working level (WL), defined as any combination of short-lived radon daughters in 1 L of air that will result in the emission of 1.3×10^5 MeV of potential alpha energy, and WLM, defined as exposure to 1 WL for a working month of 170 hours. The relationship between WL and activity depends on the ratio of decay products of radon in the air. In homes, 1 WL corresponds to radon concentrations of about 200 pCi/L.

Radon and its decay products are present in outdoor air and in structures; their concentration can vary considerably. A low percentage of dwellings may have concentrations similar or even higher than those in uranium mines. Therefore concerns have risen that exposure to radon decay products in dwellings also may cause lung cancer in the general population. The U.S. Environmental Protection Agency (EPA) has estimated that 5000 to 20,000 lung cancers per year may be caused by environmental exposure to radon in dwellings in the United States alone. The EPA recommends that remedial action be taken in dwellings with radon concentrations of 4 pCi/L or more. Most of the homes have lower concentrations. A review of different models of radon-related lung cancer[11] illustrates an uncertainty of quantitative risk estimates at lower levels of exposure; the transfer of risk coefficients from miners to the general population is difficult because of different parameters of air quality, time distribution of dose, and different biological characteristics of the subjects. In many countries, preventive measures have been implemented in newly constructed dwellings, and efforts to identify older dwellings with higher levels are underway. More than 20 epidemiological studies of general population groups have been initiated; the problems with interpretation of preliminary results recently have been reviewed.[12]

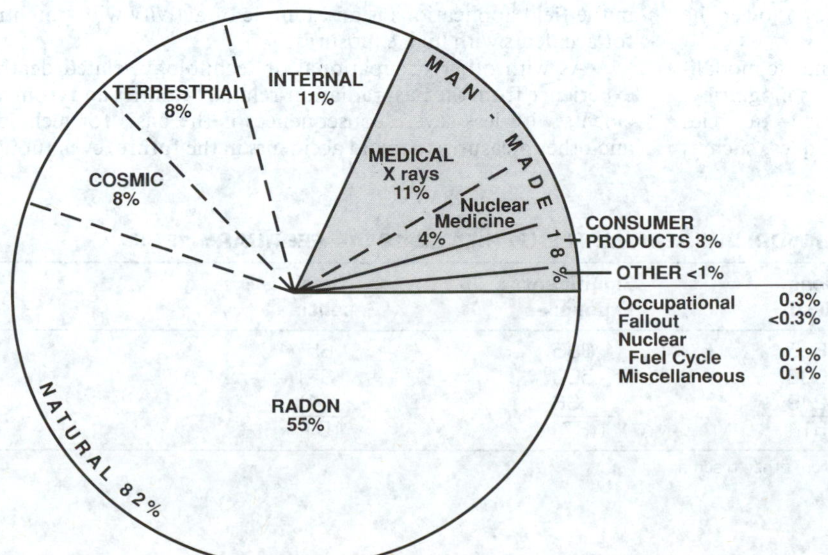

Figure 26-4. Percentage contribution of various radiation sources to total average effective dose equivalent in U.S. population. *(From NCRP, 1987.[13])*

Data from miners indicate that there is a synergistic effect when exposure to radon decay products is combined with cigarette smoking. Therefore educational efforts acknowledging this are prudent.

Medical Radiation

Medical radiation has a unique position among uses of ionizing radiation, because direct benefit to those exposed is intended. To evaluate exposures, information on frequency of examinations and on absorbed dose per examination is needed. These data are available from developed countries, less so from many other countries, and no data are available for about half of the world's population. Availability of radiodiagnosis in different countries can be assessed by population per x-ray machine. In some countries the index is less than 2000 people per x-ray machine; in other countries it is several hundred thousand people per machine. In many developing countries, one to two thirds of the x-ray machines are out of order.[3]

The total frequencies of diagnostic x-ray examinations in countries in which one physician is available for less than 1000 population are in the range of 450 to 1300 examinations per 1000 population. In some countries 15 to 20 examinations per 1000 population are performed annually. Mass chest x-ray examination campaigns in some countries increase the frequencies.

Of the total number of diagnostic x-ray examinations in industrialized countries, chest examinations account for about 30%, examinations of the extremities, of the abdomen, and of the digestive tract account for 18% to 20%. In countries with lower availability of examinations there is an increase of chest examinations expressed as a percentage of the total.

Absorbed dose per examination has been reduced because of improvements in diagnostic instrumentation over the last 2 decades. However, considering the expenses to replace equipment that may otherwise be kept operational for many years, reduction of doses per examination accompanied by improved diagnostic information is a continuous process. It has long been recognized that with the same equipment, great differences in patient doses per examination are realized, depending on how the personnel use it. The importance of personnel qualifications, training, and attitude in lowering the doses cannot be overemphasized. This applies to reduction of unnecessary somatic doses but even more to gonadal doses. The necessary precautions are of the utmost importance when infants and children are examined. As important as the change from photofluorography to chest radiography and improvements in collimation or gonadal shielding have been, there are various other ways to lower the patient doses.

Also, the ever-increasing availability of diagnostic modalities, such as computed tomography, ultrasound, sonography, and magnetic resonance imaging, is influencing the frequencies of x-ray examinations. Some interventional techniques, such as percutaneous transluminal coronary angioplasty, require prolonged fluoroscopy times with higher skin-absorbed doses in a wide range up to 0.5 Sv per one stenosis dilated. In mammography the absorbed dose per examination has been reduced considerably over the past years, enabling its extensive use.

Frequencies of nuclear medicine examinations in vivo are much lower than those of x-ray examinations. In industrialized countries, the annual frequencies are one to two orders of magnitude lower than those of x-ray examinations. Absorbed dose per examination has been reduced by the development of the nuclear diagnostic systems but even more by the introduction of radionuclides with short half-lives, such as technetium 99m. Reduction of dose from nuclear medicine examinations is also a long-term endeavor because of costs of the systems and new radiopharmaceuticals.

Estimates of doses were attempted for the world population.[3] The per caput annual effective dose equivalent from diagnostic x-ray procedures may be in the range 0.4 to 1.0 mSv, as compared to the estimated value of 2.4 mSv from natural sources. Exposure from dental or diagnostic nuclear medicine examinations is much lower. Medical irradiation is the largest man-made source contributing to the worldwide population radiation dose.

Accidents and Incidents

In the early years of exploration of x-rays and radium many pioneers had localized or total body exposures because of lack of preventive measures. More than 300 deaths were thought to have been caused by the exposures. The toll led to the introduction of ever-improving radiation protection. By the time of the onset of World War II the basic principles of radiation protection against external exposure and internal contamination were in use.

Major radiation accidents from 1944 to February 1989 were reviewed by Lushbaugh et al.[14] The authors have analyzed available information from the United States and from other countries worldwide. Altogether, 101 fatalities were reported during the period (Table 26–7). The authors pointed out that not all of them were due to radiation tissue damage. Analysis of the 305 accidents contained in the Radiation Accident Registry (Table 26–7) distinguished three more frequently occurring groups of accidents related to criticality, radiation-emitting devices, and radioisotopes. After 1980, only two criticality accidents occurred: in Argentina in a research reactor in 1984 and in Chernobyl in 1986. Accidents due to loss of control over the sealed sources dominate the reported incidents. Industrial radiography in the field applications is an example of activity with potential for accidents with high exposures.

As with other occupational or technology-related deaths, experience from the past radiation-related fatalities and from accidents with less severe consequences is the basis for technical and other measures to avoid accidents in the future, even though

TABLE 26–7. MAJOR RADIATION ACCIDENTS WORLDWIDE HUMAN EXPERIENCE 1944—FEBRUARY 1989

Number of Accidents	Persons Involved	Significant Exposures	Total Fatalities[a]
303	5,865	1,335	65
[1	116,500	500[b]	32]
{1	249	36	4}
305	122,614	1,871	101

[a] Includes deaths due to acute radiation effects and deaths from other trauma.
[b] USDOE/NRC accident dose criteria.
[]—Chernobyl data.
{}—Goiania, Brazil, Data.
Adapted from DOE—REAC/TS Radiation Accident Registries.

the radiation-related fatality rates are lower than in many other industries. It is one of the goals of radiation protection to achieve and maintain occupational exposures at levels associated with risks in industries considered safe.

The Chernobyl accident occurred in the Soviet Union in 1986, causing extensive contamination of the local area and resulting in contamination in Europe and the northern hemisphere. According to the report of the United Nations Scientific Committee on the Effects of Atomic Radiation issued in 1988, from the point of view of individual risk the radiological impact of the accident was apparently negligible outside the affected area within the Soviet Union, either because the contamination levels were low or because preventive measures, particularly the ban on consumption of contaminated foodstuffs, prevented high exposure.[3] The large extent of regions contaminated by this type of accident was unanticipated. The deposition pattern and subsequent transfer of radionuclides to food and the resulting human exposure, external and internal, were inhomogeneous. Iodine 131, cesium 134, and cesium 137 contributed most significantly to the exposure. According to information from the Soviet authorities, the reactor accident occurred in the course of a low-power engineering test, during which safety systems had been switched off. The uncontrollable instabilities that developed caused explosions and fire, which damaged the reactor and allowed radioactive gases and particles to be released into the environment. The fire was extinguished and the reactor core sealed off by the tenth day after the accident. The fatalities occurred among the reactor personnel and the fire fighters. Two persons died immediately; others were radiation-related deaths. Radiation doses to the local population were below levels causing immediate effects, and the residents were evacuated from a 30 km exclusion zone. Agricultural activities were halted, and further evaluation of the environmental contamination (as well as decontamination activities) has been started.

The UNSCEAR calculations of the first-year committed effective dose equivalents in 34 countries are given in Figure 26–5. The 1-year value of effective dose equivalent from natural sources is 2.4 mSv.[3]

Nuclear Power

By the end of 1989, nuclear energy accounted for 16% of the world's electricity. The 426 reactors operating in 26 countries had an installed capacity of more than 300 gigawatts (GW). The so-called nuclear fuel cycle includes mining and milling of uranium ores, enrichment of the isotopic content of uranium 235 for most reactor types and fabrication of fuel elements, production of energy in thermal reactors, reprocessing of the spent fuel, disposal of radioactive waste, and transportation of nuclear materials throughout the specialized facilities.

The concentrations of radionuclides in effluents are usually low, and estimates of exposures are based on measurements of releases and models of transfer of radionuclides through the environment, rather than on monitoring members of the population, which is either infeasible or impracticable. The contribution from this source to the population exposure is given in Table 26–6 and in Figure 26–4.

• • •

Radiation protection has developed from using basic principles of protection against external irradiation in occupational settings—shielding, distance, time, and training—to a system of dose limitation encompassing almost all human activities connected with radiation exposure. However, because for some effects it has not been possible to define a threshold dose below which there is no health risk and because exposures currently experienced by population groups are at the levels for which evidence of excess disease is not available, assumptions must be made concerning the risk. The public's perception of risk varies for different sources. For example, although there is a general acceptance of exposures connected with medical uses of ionizing

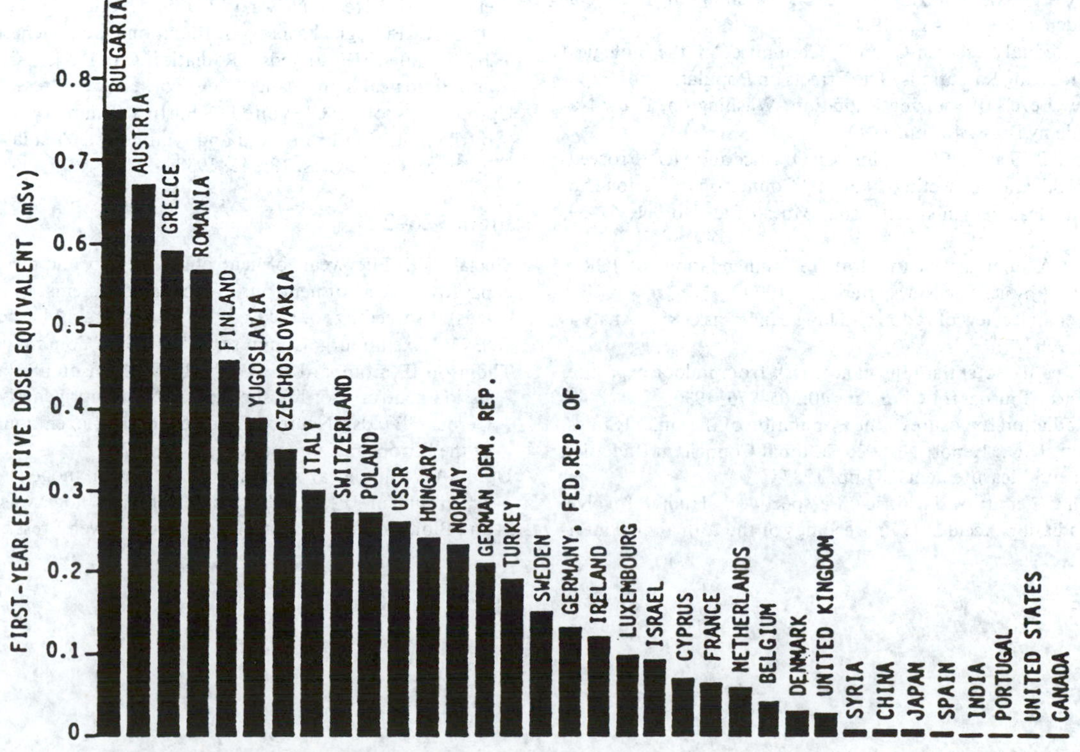

Figure 26–5. Country average first-year committed effective dose equivalent from the Chernobyl accident. (From UNSCEAR, 1988.[3])

radiation, the perceived risk often is higher for other applications, for example, low-level radioactive waste sites.

Opponents of nuclear power are concerned because of problems with waste disposal and the potential for an accident that could lead to exposures of members of the population. These concerns influence energy policy in many countries.

From the public health perspective the knowledge of ionizing radiation is more profound than that of many other environmental factors. The radiation protection measures, with emphasis on radiation accident prevention, have been sufficient to prevent undue health risks in most situations. The potential use of nuclear weapons is in another category together with other means of mass destruction.

REFERENCES

1. Recommendations of the International Commission on Radiological Protection. ICRP Publication 26. Oxford: Pergamon Press. 80 pp. 1977.
2. Recommendations on Limits for Exposure to Ionizing Radiation. Washington, D.C.: Report No. 91, National Council on Radiation Protection and Measurements. 72 pp. 1987
3. United Nations Scientific Committee on the Effects of Ionizing Radiation (UNSCEAR): Sources, Effects and Risks of Ionizing Radiation. 647 pp. New York: United Nations, 1988
4. Dunn K et al: Prenatal exposure to ionizing radiation and subsequent developments of seizures. Am J Epidemiol 131:114–123, 1990
5. Schull WJ: The Status of Somatic Risk Estimation. Proceedings of the 25th annual meeting, National Council on Radiation Protection and Measurements. Bethesda, Md.: Proc. No. 11, 27–42, 1990
6. Comparative Carcinogenicity of Ionizing Radiation and Chemicals. Washington, D.C.: Report No. 96, National Council on Radiation Protection and Measurements. 179 pp. 1989
7. BEIR III: National Research Council, Committee on the Biological Effects of Ionizing Radiations. The Effects on Populations of Exposure to Low Levels of Ionizing Radiation. Washington, D.C.: National Academy Press. 524 pp. 1980
8. BEIR V: National Research Council, Committee on the Biological Effects of Ionizing Radiations. The Effects on Populations of Exposure to Low Levels of Ionizing Radiation. Washington, D.C.: National Academy Press. 421 pp. 1990
9. Abrahamson S: Genetic Risk Estimates: Of Mice and Men. Proceedings of the 25th annual meeting, National Council on Radiation Protection and Measurements. Bethesda, Md.: Proc. No. 11, 61–69, 1990
10. Clarke RH: A summary of the draft recommendations of ICRP, 1990. Health Physics Soc Newsletter 28:9, 1990
11. Samet JM et al: Review of radon and lung cancer risk. Risk Analysis 10:65–75, 1990
12. Harley NH et al: Potential lung cancer risk from indoor exposure. Ca—A Cancer Journal for Clinicians 40:265–275, 1990
13. Ionizing Radiation Exposure of the Population of the United States. Washington, D.C.: Report No. 93, National Council on Radiation Protection and Measurements. 87 pp. 1987
14. Lushbaugh CC et al: An Historical Perspective of Human Involvement in Radiation Accidents. Proceedings of the 25th annual meeting, National Council on Radiation Protection and Measurements. Bethesda, Md.: Proc. No. 11, 171–186, 1990

General References

BEIR IV: National Research Council, Committee on the Biological Effects of Ionizing Radiations. Health Risks of Radon and Other Internally Disposited Alpha-Emmitters. Washington, D.C.: National Academy Press. 602 pp. 1988

Eisenbud M: Environmental Radioactivity, 3 edt. Orlando, Fla.: Academic Press, 1987

Recommendations of the International Commission on Radiological Protection. ICRP Publication 60. Oxford: Pergamon Press. 215 pp (approx).

Figure 26–1

Burns F, Albert RE, Heimback RD: RBE for skin tumors and hair follicle damage in the rat following irradiation with alpha particles and electrons. Radiat Res 36:225, 1968

Kaplan HS, Brown MB: A quantitative dose response study of lymphoid-tumor development in irradiated C57 black mice. J Natl Cancer Inst 13:185, 1952

Maldague P: Comparative study of experimentally induced cancer of the kidney in mice and rats with x-rays. In Radiation-induced Cancer, IAEA STI/PUB/228. Vienna: International Atomic Energy Agency, 1969, p 439

Metalli P, p, Covelli V, DiPaola M, Silini G: Dose incidence data for mouse reticulum cell sarcoma. Radiat Res 59:21, 1974

Shellabarger CJ, Bond VP, Cronkite EP, Aponte GE: Relationship of dose to total-body ^{60}Co radiation to incidence of mammary neoplasia in female rats. In Radiation-induced Cancer, IAEA/STI/PUB/228. Vienna: International Atomic Energy Agency, 1969, p 161

Ullrich RL, Jernigan MC, Cosgrove GE, Satterfield LC, Bowles ND, Storer JB: The influence of dose and dose rate on the incidence of neoplastic disease in RFM mice after neutron irradiation. Radiat Res 68:115, 1976

United Nations Scientific Committee on the Effects of Ionizing Radiation (UNSCEAR): Ionizing Radiation: Levels and Effects. Vol. I: Levels. Vol. II: Effects. New York: United Nations, 1972

Upton AC: Biological aspects of radiation carcinogenesis. In Boice JD, Jr, Fraumeni JF, Jr (eds): Radiation Carcinogenesis: Epidemiology and Biological Significance. New York: Raven Press, 1984, p 9

Upton AC, Wolff AC, Wolfe FF, Furth J, Kimball AW: A comparison of the induction of myeloid and lymphoid leukemias in X-irradiated RF mice. Cancer Res, 18:842, 1958

Figure 26–2

Sinclair WK: Fifty years of neutrons in biology and medicine: The comparative effects of neutrons in biological systems. In Booz J, Ebert H (eds): Proceedings of the Eighth Symposium in Microdosimetry. EUR 8395. Luxembourg: Commission European Communities, 1983, p 1

Thomson JF, Lombard LS, Grahn D, Williamson FS, Fritz TF: RBE of fission neutrons for life shortening and tumorigenesis. In Broerse JJ, Gerber GB (eds): Neutron Carcinogenesis. Luxembourg: Commission of the European Communities, 1982, p 75

Upton AC: Biological aspects of radiation carcinogenesis. In Boice JD, Jr, Fraumeni JF, Jr (eds): Radiation Carcinogenesis: Epidemiology and Biological Significance. New York: Raven Press, 1984, p 9

27

Nonionizing Radiation

Arthur L. Frank
Louis Slesin

The term *nonionizing radiation* refers to several forms of electromagnetic radiation of wavelengths longer than those of ionizing radiation. As wavelength elongates, the energy value of electromagnetic radiation decreases, so all nonionizing forms of radiation have less energy than cosmic, gamma, and x-radiation have. In order of increasing wavelength, nonionizing radiation includes ultraviolet (UV) radiation, visible light, infrared radiation, microwave radiation, and radiofrequency radiation. The latter two are often treated as a single category. The energy, frequency, and wavelength range for electromagnetic forces are shown in Table 27-1. All forms of electromagnetic radiation have the same velocity of 3×10^{10}cm/s in a vacuum.

Radiation is emitted continuously from the sun over a wide range; the solar spectrum reaching earth ranges from 290 nm in the ultraviolet range to more than 2000 nm in the infrared range with a maximum intensity at about 480 nm in the visible range. The radiation from the sun is modified as it passes through the earth's atmosphere. Ozone, which is found in the upper atmosphere, absorbs the highest energy ultraviolet radiation. Infrared radiation is absorbed by water vapor, and other wavelengths are altered by passage through smoke, dust, and gas molecules.

Any object above absolute zero temperature emits radiation, much of it as infrared radiation. At low temperatures, only long wavelength radiation is emitted, but as the temperature of the object increases, shorter wavelength radiation is emitted. Heated metal gives off a red glow; if heating continues, the metal becomes "white hot" as energy throughout the whole visible spectrum is given off. Heated gases may give off wavelengths in the ultraviolet, visible, or infrared regions. Ultraviolet radiation is given off with the use of extremely high temperature welding equipment such as carbon or electric arcs.

The biological effect of radiation exposure depends on the type and duration of exposure and on the amount of absorption by the organism. The carcinogenic and other effects of ionizing radiation are discussed in Chapter 26. Various types of ionizing radiation will be considered separately.

ULTRAVIOLET RADIATION

The sun is the major source of ultraviolet radiation. There are some man-made sources such as electric arc lights, welding arcs, plasma jets, and special ultraviolet bulbs. The amount of ultraviolet radiation reaching the earth from the sun varies with season, time of day, latitude, altitude, and specific atmospheric conditions. Intensity is greatest at midday and is greater in summer than in winter. In a summer month, about as much ultraviolet radiation reaches the earth's surface as in the entire period from autumn to spring equinoxes. Total ultraviolet exposure is greater on a cloudy day due to reflection, and snow reflects about 75% of ultraviolet radiation. Therefore, sunburn may be more severe on a cloudy than a clear day and may be especially severe in those spending a great deal of time on snow. Window glass and light clothing filter out ultraviolet radiation efficiently.

There is a wide range of potential occupational exposures[1,2] to ultraviolet radiation in both outdoor work and industrial settings (Table 27-2).

Biological Effects. Since ultraviolet radiation has little penetrating power, the organs that are affected are primarily the skin and the eyes. Ultraviolet radiation is strongly absorbed by nucleic acids and proteins, and the effects in man are largely chemical rather than thermal. Mutations resulting from ultraviolet exposure occur in organisms such as plants and flies but not in man, because of the low penetration.

Short-term effects on man include acute changes in the skin. These are of four types: (1) darkening of pigment, (2) erythema (sunburn), (3) increase in pigmentation (tanning), and (4) changes in cell growth. Ultraviolet radiation does not penetrate through the subcutaneous tissue. The corneum, or outermost layer of skin, which is about 0.03 mm thick, absorbs the shortest wavelength ultraviolet radiation. The longer the wavelength, the deeper the radiation penetrates; the longest ultraviolet radiation passes through the corneum and corium into the malpighian layer. The darkening of preformed pigment occurs immediately and is particularly noted at wavelengths between 300 and 400 nm. The erythema (sunburn) does not begin for at least one-half hour, and there are several peaks within the ultraviolet spectrum with variable times of maximum effect, ranging from 12 hours for radiation at 254 nm to 48 hours for radiation at 297 nm. Darker skin has a protective effect, and estimates for the darkest skin shades suggest a twofold to tenfold threshold value for erythema production. Subsequent exposure reduces the threshold value for erythema production. The increase in pigmentation (tanning) results from a migration of melanin pigment into more superficial skin cells and also from an increased production of melanin pigment. Ultraviolet radiation works as a catalyst to ox-

TABLE 27-1. ENERGY, FREQUENCY, AND WAVELENGTH RANGE FOR ELECTROMAGNETIC FORCES

Type of Radiation	Energy Range	Frequency Range	Wavelength Range
Ionizing (includes cosmic, gamma, and x-ray)	>12.4 eV	>3000 THz	<100 nm
Ultraviolet	6.2–3.1 eV	1500–750 THz	200–400 nm
Visible	3.1–1.8 eV	750–429 THz	400–700 nm
Violet			400–424
Blue			424–491
Green			491–575
Yellow			575–585
Orange			585–647
Red			647–700
Infrared	1.8 eV–1.2 meV	429 THz–300 GHz	700 nm–1 mm
Microwave	1.2 meV–1.2 μeV	300 GHz–300 MHz	1 mm–1 m
Radiofrequency	1.2 μeV–1.2 neV	300 MHz–300 kHz	1 m–1 km

Adapted from NIOSH Technical Report—Ionizing Radiation, Washington, D.C.: NIOSH Publication No. 78-142, 1978.

idize tyrosine to dihydroxyphenol 1-alanine, which is a precursor of melanin. Changes in skin cell growth follow exposure to ultraviolet radiation. First, there occurs a cessation of cell growth followed after 24 hours by an increase in cell division. At this time there is an intra- and intercellular edema that thickens the skin. Eventually there is shedding of cells by scaling. Severe reactions can be seen with blistering, desquamation, or even ulceration of the skin.

Ultraviolet radiation also causes acute effects on tissues of the eye. Exposure can lead to keratitis, inflammation of the cornea, and conjunctivitis. The keratitis may develop after a latent period of several hours and returns to normal in a few days. Since the cornea possesses a large number of nerve endings, even a small amount of inflammation can be painful. The effect in the eye is independent of skin color, and there appears to be no development of protection of the eye with repeated exposures.

Long-term effects of ultraviolet exposure include an increase in the rate of aging of skin with degeneration of skin tissue and a decrease in elasticity. Late effects of ultraviolet on the eye include the development of cataracts. The most serious chronic effect of ultraviolet exposure is skin cancer.

More than 90% of skin cancers occur on parts of the body exposed to sunlight. Approximately 40% of all cancers in the United States are skin cancers, and in general they are the most common malignancy in light-skinned populations. Rates for skin cancer vary from less than 2 cases per 100,000 in dark-skinned populations to more than 100 per 100,000 in South African whites and Australians.[3] The incidence of skin cancer on a worldwide basis correlates with decreasing latitude. Skin cancer occurs in great excess in those with outdoor occupations such as agricultural, forestry, and marine workers. Most skin cancers in man are of epithelial cell origin; most commonly noted are basal cell carcinomas followed in frequency by squamous cell carcinomas.

Some individuals, for example, those with xeroderma pigmentosum, have particular sensitivity to ultraviolet radiation and are at increased risk for developing disease on exposure. Photosensitivity reactions occur after exposure to a variety of chemicals and drugs, including dyes, phenothiazines, sulfonamides, and sulfonylureas.

Ultraviolet radiation has an important role in the prevention of rickets. Vitamin D is produced by the action of ultraviolet radiation on 7-dehydrocholesterol or related steroidal compounds.

TABLE 27-2. OCCUPATIONAL EXPOSURE TO ULTRAVIOLET RADIATION

Aircraft workers	Glassblowers
Barbers	Metal casting inspectors
Bath attendants	Oil field workers
Construction workers	Railroad track workers
Drug makers	Ranchers
Electricians	Seamen
Farmers	Steel mill workers
Fishermen	Tobacco irradiators
Food irradiators	Vitamin D makers
Foundry workers	Welders

Protection. Protective measures include administrative controls, equipment design, and personal protection. Administrative actions include education and instruction of individuals who will be exposed, posting of notices, limiting access in the workplace, and regulation of exposure time. Equipment design includes placement of ultraviolet sources within suitable housing and the use of appropriate glass shields. Personal protection includes the use of shields, goggles, and appropriate clothing. Polyvinyl chloride can be used for gloves, and the use of barrier creams is also possible. Exposure during recreation, such as winter sports and sunbathing, should be done in moderation, especially by fair-skinned persons.

Recommended Values for Protection Against Ultraviolet Radiation. Based on regulations adopted from the American Conference of Governmental and Industrial Hygienists in 1976, the federal limits in the United States are as follows:

1. For the near ultraviolet spectral region (320 to 400 nm), total irradiance incident upon the unprotected skin or eye should not exceed 1 mW/cm^2 for periods greater than 10^3 seconds (approximately 16 minutes) and for exposure times less than 10^3 seconds should not exceed 1 J/cm^2.
2. For the actinic ultraviolet spectral region (200 to 315 nm), radiant exposure incident upon the unprotected skin or eye should not exceed the values given in Table 27-3 within an 8-hour period.

3. To determine the effective irradiance of a broadband source weighted against the peak of the spectral effectiveness curve (270 nm), the following weighting formula should be used:

$$E_{eff} = \Sigma E_\lambda S_\lambda \Delta_\lambda$$

where

E_{eff} = effective irradiance relative a E_λ
E_λ = monochromatic source at 270 nm spectral irradiance in $W/cm^2/nm$
S_λ = relative spectral effectiveness (unitless)
Δ_λ = band width in nanometers

4. Permissible exposure time in seconds for exposure to actinic ultraviolet radiation incident upon the unprotected skin or eye may be computed by dividing 0.003 J/cm by E_{eh} in W/cm^2. The exposure time may also be determined using Table 27–4, which provides exposure times corresponding to effective irradiances in $\mu W/cm^2$.

TABLE 27–4. THRESHOLD LIMIT VALUES FOR ULTRAVIOLET RADIATION

Duration of Exposure per Day	Effective Irradiance, E_{eff} ($\mu W/cm^2$)
8 h	0.1
4 h	0.2
2 h	0.4
1 h	0.8
30 min	1.7
15 min	3.3
10 min	5.0
5 min	10.0
1 min	50.0
30 s	100.0
10 s	300.0
1 s	3000.0
0.5 s	6000.0
0.1 s	30,000.0

VISIBLE LIGHT

Visible light[4,5] is radiation with a wavelength between 400 and 700 nm. The sun is the major source of visible light, but it can also be produced by heating tungsten or other filaments and by electrical discharge in a gas such as mercury or neon. Any ultraviolet radiation given off is largely absorbed by the glass enclosing the bulb.

The abnormal biological effects of visible radiation are generally not serious. A flash of light will bleach visual pigments, causing "spots" in the visual field. Intense visible light, such as one may experience by staring directly into the sun for extended periods, may cause coagulation of the retina, and the scotoma that results may be permanent. Snow blindness results from overexposure to sunlight and is characterized by conjunctivitis and keratitis accompanied by photophobia. Use of appropriate lenses will protect against the above effects.

Of potentially greater seriousness are injuries caused by lasers. Laser stands for *l*ight *a*mplification of *s*timulated *e*mission of *r*adiation. Lasers are used in industry, communications, surveying, construction, medicine, and electronics. There are many types of laser apparatus, but all are characterized by their ability to produce an intense, monochromatic, coherent beam in which all waves are parallel and all are in phase. There are three types of lasers: (1) continuous, (2) pulsed, and (3) Q-switched, which are pulsed, but the beam is turned on and off at a rapid rate to produce a beam with higher peak power of shorter duration than the pulsed variety.

TABLE 27–3. THRESHOLD LIMIT VALUES (TLV) FOR ULTRAVIOLET RADIATION

Wavelength (nm)	TLV (mJ/cm^2)	Relative Spectral Effectiveness (S_λ)
200	100.0	0.03
210	40.0	0.075
220	25.0	0.12
230	16.0	0.19
240	10.0	0.30
250	7.0	0.43
254	6.0	0.5
260	4.6	0.65
270	3.0	1.0
280	3.4	0.88
290	4.7	0.64
300	10.0	0.30
305	50.0	0.06
310	200.0	0.015
315	1000.0	0.003

Because the laser is a light beam, it follows all the laws of optics and can be manipulated like other light beams. When focused on a spot, a laser can produce enormous heat for drilling and related purposes.

Burns may occur with exposure to lasers, either to the skin or to the eye, if the laser beam hits the retina. This can cause blindness. Lasers also emit ultraviolet radiation, which can cause corneal damage, and infrared radiation, which can cause opacification of the lens.

Threshold values have been proposed for a wide variety of laser equipment.

ILLUMINATION

Units for Expressing Amount of Light. The amount of visible radiation (light) emitted by a luminous object, such as an electric light bulb, is measured in terms of candle power, based on a standard international candle. The amount of illumination that falls on a surface from a light source is expressed in terms of foot-candles. One foot-candle of illumination is the intensity of illumination at any point on a surface 1 foot away from a light source of 1 candle power. The illumination falling on a surface varies inversely as the square of the distance from the light source. The total amount of light that falls on 1 square foot of surface, all points of which are 1 foot from a light source of 1 standard candle, is called 1 lumen, lumen being the term used to measure light flux. The brightness of the light source or of an object reflecting light is usually expressed in terms of foot-lamberts or candles per square inch. One foot-lambert is equivalent to 1 lumen emitted per square foot of the light source. One candle per square inch is the candle power emitted per square inch of light source and is equivalent to 452 foot-lamberts.

General Principles of Illumination

Intensity of Illumination. Sufficient illumination is essential for visual acuity, maximum speed of seeing, prevention of eye fatigue and eye strain, and thus for efficient work and prevention of accidents. Definite proof that poor illumination leads to permanent eye injury is lacking, but the character of the illumination may affect psychological reactions. Most authorities agree that high levels of illumination, except under such unusual circumstances as direct viewing of the sun, do not produce harmful effects on the eye. The human eye is adapted for vision outdoors where foot-candle levels may range from 1000 in the shade to 10,000 in the sun.

Standards of illumination usually are set in terms of the amount of illumination that falls on the work area. Since vision depends on the light reaching the eye, however, the important consideration is not the amount of illumination on the desk or workbench but the amount of light reflected to the eye. For example, if there are 50 foot-candles of illumination falling on a white object, which reflects about 80% of the visible light, then 40 foot-candles of illumination are reflected toward the eye. If the same amount of light falls on a dark object, which reflects 20% of the light, only 10 foot-candles of illumination are reflected to the eye. Hence it is necessary to specify different standards of illumination for different circumstances, depending on the amount of light reflected from each work area.

Authorities differ on the amount of illumination essential for vision. Visual acuity and speed of vision increase markedly with an increase in illumination up to about 10 foot-candles, and then increase more slowly up to about 20 foot-candles. The rate of improvement with higher levels of illumination appears to be low. These data are based on visual tasks where the background had a reflection factor of 80% and where there was optimum contrast in color (black letters on a white background). Hence 15 to 20 foot-candles can be accepted as a bare minimum level of illumination for vision under the most optimum conditions. When the reflection factor is reduced, as in work on dark colors or when the contrast in color between the object and its background is reduced, higher levels of illumination are necessary for good visual acuity and speed of vision. Higher levels are required also for continuous eye work and for fine work, that is, when the size of the object is very small. Persons with poor vision or eye defects require more illumination than those with normal eyesight. Generally it is recommended that when the contrast in color and brightness between the object and the immediate background is good and when the object being viewed is the size of normal print, the lighting for continuous eye work should supply a minimum of 30 foot-candles on the object. Where poor contrasts exist or the size of the object is small, the minimum illumination requirement should be set at 50 foot-candles. Higher levels are necessary under certain conditions, such as in printing and typesetting, for finer work, or when working on black objects. In 1965, the American National Standards Institute (ANSI) in cooperation with the Illuminating Engineering Society published an American Standard Practice for Industrial Lighting, including a list of the current recommended practice foot-candles in service applicable to many types of industrial operations. More recently, the Illuminating Engineers and some other authorities have recommended much higher levels of illumination, but the 1965 standards were reconfirmed in 1970 by the American National Standards Institute and adopted by the United States Department of Labor as the standards to be used under the 1971 Occupational Safety and Health Act.

Brightness and Glare. The amount of light reaching the eye from a light source or by reflection from an object is commonly designated as the brightness of the source or object and is usually expressed in foot-lamberts. Although the eye can adapt to very high levels of brightness, such as daylight outdoors, it cannot tolerate great contrasts in brightness between the central field of vision and the surrounding area. Such contrasts interfere with vision and may produce an uncomfortable sensation. In viewing an object against its surroundings, the visual acuity is greatest when the surrounding area has the same brightness as the central field of vision. The brightness of this central field should never be less than that of the surroundings. On the other hand, the brightness contrast between the central field of vision (subtending an angle of 1 minute at the eye) and the immediate surroundings (assuming the latter to be an area that subtends an angle of 60 degrees) should not exceed a ratio of 10:1. Brightness ratios smaller than 5:1, even 3:1, are more desirable for continuous work. Contrasts in brightness within an angle of 30 degrees are especially uncomfortable. Greater contrasts in brightness can be tolerated between the central and peripheral fields of vision, but even here the contrasts in brightness should not be great. For example, the brightness of the ceiling should not be more than 10 times greater than that of the task area. To avoid contrasts in brightness, good general illumination, rather than only local lighting on the work, must be provided throughout the entire area.

Brightness contrasts are produced also when bright light sources are in the field of view. If the eye is adapted to a high level of illumination and the contrast is not great, a bright light in the field of vision does not produce discomfort, for example, when viewing an automobile headlight during daylight; if the eye is not adapted to bright light or if the contrast in brightness between the light and the surroundings is great, as an automobile headlight at night, an uncomfortable glare sensation is produced. The degree of the glare sensation depends on the distance of the eye from the light source, the brightness of the light source in relation to that of its surroundings, and the position of the light source in the field of vision in relation to that of the object on which the eye is focused. Excessive reflection from shiny surfaces, so-called reflected glare, produces an uncomfortable sensation and may completely obliterate the outline of an object. These localized bright spots, whether they be due to unprotected light sources or to reflected glare, markedly reduce critical vision. The effect of glare on vision increases sharply in older age groups; bare light bulbs should never be permitted in the field of vision.

Differences in Illumination. Great differences in illumination between one work space and another or between a work area and a hallway are dangerous if people are required to move from one space to the other. When passing from a brightly lighted area to one with a low level of illumination, the visual acuity is markedly decreased until dark adaptation has occurred. Although some adaptation occurs fairly rapidly, it requires at least one-half hour for adequate readjustment of vision to dim light. The greater the light adaptation, the slower the dark adaptation that follows. During the readjustment period, the ability of the eye to see clearly is so reduced that the danger of accidents is increased. It is because of this physiological fact that relatively high levels of illumination are recommended for stairs, hallways, storage rooms, and so forth. Adaptation requires only a few minutes when passing from a dimly lighted space to one at a high level of illumination.

When the level of illumination falls below 0.1 millilambert, vision becomes a function of the rods in the retina rather than the cones. Since the rods are not sensitive to red light but the cones are, dark adaptation may be produced in bright light by wearing red glasses that protect the rods but allow cone vision. Excessive exposure to ultraviolet radiation causes a decrease in dark adaptation.

Color of Light and Surroundings and Surface Finish. A contrast in color between the object and its immediate background is important; the more definite the color contrast, the greater the visual acuity and speed of vision. The value of color contrast is due partly to the dissimilarity in color and partly to differences in the amount of light reflected by the different colors. Recognition of an object becomes most difficult when a black object is viewed against a black background. Here, differences in texture and shadows are necessary for vision. Higher levels of illumination are required where the color contrast is reduced.

The color quality of the light from the common illuminants has little or no effect on visual discrimination. Hence it is not very important, except where a particular color is essential for the work, so long as sufficient light reaches the eye.

The color and finish of the walls, ceiling, furniture, and machinery are of great importance in illumination because the amount of light reflected is determined chiefly by the color. For example, light gray reflects 75% of the visible light, whereas light blue reflects only 55%. Dark blue reflects 8%, and black cloth 1%. In areas where good visual functioning is required, it is recommended that the colors of the surroundings be selected so that the following percentages of reflection are obtained: from ceilings 75% to 85%; from walls 50% to 60%; from school desks 35% to 50%; from office desks 30% to 35%; from machines 20% to 30%; and from floors 15% to 30%. To obtain good diffusion of light and to avoid glare spots, a flat finish is recommended. All polished specular surfaces should be eliminated. The light should be uniformly distributed and harsh shadows avoided. Multiple or contrasting colors often are used for accident prevention, for example, to indicate moving parts of machines, edges of steps, steam lines, and other dangerous objects.

Recommendations: Artificial and Natural Lighting

Artificial Illumination. It is evident from the above discussion that a basic amount of general illumination must be supplied to all areas of a room to prevent great contrasts in brightness. Local or supplemental lighting, in addition to general lighting, is necessary when very high levels of illumination are required, when illumination is needed in specific areas not accessible to general lighting, where the light must come from a particular angle, where hand readjustments are needed, where shadows are required, for the prevention of reflected glare, and in various other circumstances. Supplementary lighting sources should be arranged so that other persons in the vicinity are not exposed to excessively bright spots of light. Local lighting without general illumination is undesirable for the reasons discussed above.

Lighting fixtures fall into four types:

1. Totally indirect units give diffuse illumination with no shadows or glare, but they are uneconomical and accumulate dirt. Good reflection from the ceiling is necessary, but excessive brightness of the ceiling must be avoided.
2. Direct units are economical but cause shadows, produce glare, and give spot rather than diffuse illumination. They are used chiefly with high ceilings or for local lighting.
3. Semiindirect units are satisfactory when equipped with diffusers, when ceiling reflection is adequate, and when they are properly placed to avoid too much brightness in the field of view.
4. Large units having a lower candle power per square inch, for example, long tabular fluorescent lights give less concentrated lighting than round tungsten-filament bulbs, which have a higher brightness per unit area (Table 27-5). Large units with moderate brightness also may cause discomfort if placed directly in the field of view, however.

Exposed bulbs should never be allowed within the visual field. When fluorescent bulbs are used on alternating current, two bulbs must be used together and arranged so as to prevent the cycle flicker or stroboscopic effect. All lighting units become less efficient with time, chiefly because of the accumulation of dirt; continuous maintenance is necessary.

Natural Illumination. Daylight, if properly arranged, may be a very effective source of good illumination in a room. Much more difficulty is encountered in designing for daylighting than for artificial lighting, however. The amount of daylight reaching a room varies with the location and orientation of the building, with the presence of surrounding buildings, and with the time of day, season, weather, and degree of atmospheric pollution. Furthermore, whereas artificial lighting can be evenly spaced throughout a room and directed as desired, daylight is available only from certain areas, and its distribution is more difficult to control. Because of these variable factors, only a few general recommendations for providing daylight illumination can be given.

Windows facing south give maximum heat in cold climates but considerable glare; those facing north are advised for buildings in warm climates. The glass area should be at least 20% of the floor area of the room. The tops of the windows should be as near the ceiling as possible, since the higher the windows, the more effectively the light reaches the opposite side of the room. An increase in the height of a window produces a much greater increase in illumination than a proportional increase in the width. The width of the room should not be more than approximately twice the distance from the floor to the top of the window when windows are only on one side of the room because of the rapid decrease in illumination across the room. Too often the illumination near a window is excessively bright while the illumination in another part of the room is below the minimum required for good vision. Windows on two sides of the room are desirable, but where windows are only on one side of a room, the glass area should extend the full length of the room if possible. It

TABLE 27-5. BRIGHTNESS OF NATURAL AND ARTIFICIAL LIGHT SOURCES

Light Source	Brightness	
	Foot-lamberts	***Candles per Square Inch***
Sun as observed at earth's surface	450,000,000	1,000,000.0
Full moon, clear sky	1,500	3.3
1000 W type H-6 mercury lamp	104,000,000	230,000.0
400 W type H-1 mercury lamp	443,000	980.0
Brightest spot on bulb of:		
500 W tungsten-filament lamp	131,000	290.0
100 W tungsten-filament lamp	58,800	130.0
40 W tungsten-filament lamp	24,800	55.0
30 W fluorescent, 1-inch tube [white]	2,400	5.3
40 W white fluorescent, 1 1/2 in tube	1,750	3.9
100 W white fluorescent, 2 1/8 in tube	2,180	4.8

From Taylor: Illum Engin 37:19, 1947, with permission.

is recommended that windows should not be in the field of view for normal working conditions. The size and position of monitors and skylights also must be related to the size of the building. Since direct sunlight often produces excessive brightness, it is necessary to provide some means of sunlight control, such as venetian blinds, shades, louvres, outside projectors, and glass block. For maximum reflection and diffusion the interiors of rooms should be painted in light colors. Where feasible, the outside walls of neighboring buildings situated opposite the windows can be painted a light color to increase the light reflected to the room. Supplementary artificial lighting is necessary for use when the daylight is reduced by clouds or sunset.

A complete discussion of recommended practices for daylighting in schools, factories, offices, and homes has been published by the Committee on Daylighting of the Illuminating Engineering Society.

INFRARED RADIATION

Infrared radiation, of longer wavelength than visible light, ranges in wavelength from 700 nm to 1 mm. All objects above absolute zero radiate some infrared radiation. Objects of higher temperature radiate to objects of lower temperature; the sensation of a hot stove results from this. Infrared radiation is the most important part of the spectrum for the production of heat.

Infrared radiation causes dilation of the capillary bed of the skin and if strong enough can cause a burn. Infrared radiation can cause damage to the eye and is a cause of cataract development among glassblowers and others. Occupations exposed to infrared radiation are listed in Table 27-6.

EXTREMELY LOW FREQUENCY ELECTROMAGNETIC FIELDS

Extremely low frequency (ELF) radiation refers to the 0 to 300 Hz frequency band. Distribution lines, transmission lines, and substations, which operate at 60 Hz in the United States and at 50 Hz in Europe, are the most common sources of ELF EMF exposures. Electronic office equipment, such as video display terminals, copiers, and laser printers, and home appliances, such as electric blankets, also emit ELF fields.

Although scientists have been investigating the health effects of ELF EMFs for decades, much of the work has focused on electric fields. It was only in the mid-1980s that their attention turned to magnetic fields. In the 1990s most magnetic field studies are on the biological consequences of magnetic field exposures.

A draft EPA report released in June 1990 stated that epidemiological studies of ELF exposures and leukemia, lymphoma, and cancers of the nervous system among children and workers "show a consistent pattern of response that suggests, but does not prove, a causal link."[6] The epidemiological studies, when combined with cellular studies, support the hypothesis that ELF EMFs act as a cancer promoter. Indeed, in May 1989 the congressional Office of Technology Assessment (OTA) concluded that even relatively weak ELF fields can cause biological changes and that, although the implications remain unclear, "there are legitimate reasons for concern."[7]

TABLE 27-6 OCCUPATIONAL EXPOSURE TO INFRARED RADIATION

Bakers	Foundry workers
Blacksmiths	Glass workers
Chemists	Solderers
Cooks	Steel mill workers
Electricians	Welders

Epidemiological Studies: Residential and Occupational. In 1979, Wertheimer and Leeper[8] first identified a link between childhood cancer and ELF exposures. The study was repeated under the auspices of the New York Power Line Project by a team headed by Savitz,[9] who essentially replicated the original findings: children who lived near high-current distribution lines had higher risks of brain tumors and leukemia. The scientists who oversaw the New York project concluded that if the association between EMFs and cancer was causal, "10–15% of all childhood cancer are attributable to magnetic fields." The Wertheimer-Leeper and Savitz studies suggest that a possible threshold for cancer risks is 2.3 to 3.0 milligauss (mG). Studies of adults exposed to magnetic fields at home are inconclusive. (These magnetic field levels are very small; the Earth's magnetic field is on the order of 500 mG. There is one key difference, however: the Earth's field is essentially static, and an ELF magnetic field is constantly oscillating.)

Wertheimer and Leeper[10–12] also have shown that EMF exposures, from electric blankets and ceiling cable heating systems, can lead to developmental delays and miscarriages. Savitz et al.[13] also have shown that the children of mothers who used electric blankets during pregnancy had significantly higher risks of brain tumors and leukemia.

In a series of studies in the United Kingdom, Perry[14] has shown that those exposed to ELF radiation are more likely to suffer from depression and to commit suicide.

Interestingly, the increased risk of cancer and depression may stem from the same cause: the effects of EMFs on the pineal gland. EMFs, like visible light, can suppress the pineal gland's production of melatonin, which can inhibit carcinogenesis.

There have been more than 30 studies indicating a positive association between cancer, particularly leukemia and brain tumors, and on-the-job EMF exposures. Most use job categories as the index of exposure. The strongest link has been observed with brain tumors.

One of the most interesting and potentially most troubling is the possible link between EMF exposure and breast cancer. Two articles presented at scientific meetings in 1989[15] and 1990[16] have documented an increased risk of male breast cancer among telephone linemen. A number of researchers are encouraging investigations to determine whether female breast cancer also is associated with EMF exposure.

There are now more than 22 studies under way worldwide examining the link between EMF exposures and cancer; 12 are residential studies, and 10 are occupational studies. Unlike earlier efforts most of these use both direct and indirect measurements of EMF levels. Results will appear throughout the early part of the decade of the 1990s.

Cellular and Animal Studies. Although an increasing number of epidemiological studies point to a link between ELF radiation and cancer, it is still not clear how these fields interact with biological systems. A considerable body of evidence has emerged pointing to the cell membrane as the primary site of interaction between ELF fields and the cell. This includes studies that focus on the movement of calcium ions in brain tissue (Adey,[17] Bawin and Adey,[18] and Blackman et al.[19]) and interference with DNA synthesis and RNA transcription (Goodman and Henderson[20] and Liboff et al.[21]).

Of particular relevance to cancer are the studies by Byus et al.[22] showing increased ornithine decarboxylase (ODC) activity in cells exposed to EMFs; ODC activity is elevated in all rapidly growing cells, including cancer cells. The study of Phillips et al.[23] indicates that tumor cells proliferate at a much faster rate when exposed to EMFs and also are more resistant to attack by the immune system.

Standards and Regulations. There is little consistency among the various magnetic field guidelines and standards currently proposed by state governments and international agencies. In 1989, the International Radiation Protection Association adopted interim limits for ELF magnetic field public exposures.[24] These limits are not based on the cancer risk because "this association is not proven" and because "present data do not provide any basis for health risk assessment useful in the development of exposure limits."

In the United States, only Florida has adopted magnetic field limits: 150 to 250 mG at the edge of new transmission line right-of-ways. New York has adopted an interim limit of 200 mG for new high-voltage lines. These standards are not based on health effects, rather on what is technologically achievable. In 1990, New Jersey suggested that it would adopt an "as low as reasonably achievable (ALARA) approach to public EMF exposures."

As of 1991 there are no federal ELF exposure guidelines.

Litigation. A number of suits have been filed against utilities alleging that power lines either pose unacceptable health hazards or cause a reduction in property values because of fear of hazards. Among the major recent cases are the following:

In 1986 the Klein Independent School District won an award against Houston Lighting & Power for building a power line on the school property. The jury concluded that there are potential health effects associated with exposures to power line EMFs. In addition to damages of $104,275 the court also awarded the school district $25 million in punitive damages, which was later overturned. The utility eventually rerouted the line at its own expense.

In 1988 approximately 60 New York landowners sued the New York Power Authority for $66.5 million in damages, claiming that the 345 kV Marcy-South power line had created a "cancer corridor" that destroyed the market value of their property. In September 1989 the judge ruled against the health effects argument but awarded the first landowner approximately $95,000 for "indirect damages." The utility appealed the award, and the landowners filed a counterappeal, reopening the health effects arguments.

In June 1989 a Florida judge ruled that children attending a Boca Raton elementary school may not play in the school yard bordering on high-voltage lines. The suit was brought by three parents who sought unsuccessfully to close the school because of potential EMF hazards.

At least one suit is in progress alleging that EMFs from a power line caused the brain cancer death of a young man in Houston.

Funding. The major sponsor of ELF biological effects research in the United States is the Electric Power Research Institute (EPRI), which is supported by utilities around the country. In 1989, EPRI's budget for ELF bioeffects research was $6 million. The U.S. Department of Energy is the next largest sponsor with a fiscal year 1991 ELF budget on the order of $3 million.

VIDEO DISPLAY TERMINALS

There are some 30 million video display terminals (VDTs) in U.S. offices plus millions more in American homes. The long-term health consequences of VDT work are unclear, although the data suggest that workers can suffer debilitating repetition strain injuries (RSIs) and chronic stress. More controversial and less well documented are risks due to the weak EMFs from VDTs, which have been linked to miscarriages, birth defects, and, by analogy to power line EMFs, to cancer.

As early as 1981, the National Institute for Occupational Safety and Health (NIOSH) reported high rates of RSIs, musculoskeletal disorders, and job stress among VDT operators. NIOSH recommended what has since become commonly accepted: an environment designed for VDT work and frequent rest breaks. Since then, numerous surveys and studies have shown a higher rate of these health complaints among VDT workers compared with non-VDT workers. For instance, in 1989, NIOSH reported that RSIs accounted for 39% of all occupational illnesses reported to the Occupational Safety and Health Administration (OSHA) in 1987—up from 28% in 1984. Although these statistics include RSIs among *all* workers, the trend also is clearly discernible among VDT workers.

The increasing use of computer monitoring of worker productivity is aggravating the already high level of stress among VDT workers. Monitoring cancer can include counting the number of keystrokes per unit of time, tracking the frequency and length of rest breaks, and listening to operators' telephone conversations.

Complaints of eyestrain, neck strain, backaches, and other discomfort can be overcome to some extent with ergonomically correct furniture and training on how to use it. In 1988, a voluntary standard was adopted by the Human Factors Society, which prescribes in great detail the desired environment for VDT work, including specifications for computer furniture, lighting, keyboards, and displays.[25]

With the exception of eyestrain, there appear to be few short-term effects on vision. One 1988 report from the VDT eye clinic at the University of California, Berkeley, however, indicated that VDT workers had more trouble focusing. Full-scale studies are needed to investigate these findings. The long-term picture is much more uncertain because of the almost total lack of research. Ophthalmologists also report that those with uncorrected refractive errors can be hit especially hard by VDT work; most experts agree that eye examinations should be required for all VDT workers.

In dry climates, especially Scandinavia, there have been persistent reports of skin rashes among VDT workers. Research in this area is continuing, and those involved disagree over whether rashes actually are linked to VDT work.

The question of whether EMFs from VDTs cause pregnancy problems or even cancer remains unresolved, at least partially because of the limited number of epidemiological and laboratory studies. The deflection coils that move the electron beam within the VDT's cathode ray tube generate two types of EMFs: very low frequency and extremely low frequency. Very low frequency EMFs have been linked to pregnancy problems, whereas extremely low frequency EMFs have been associated with miscarriages, cancer, and immune dysfunction.

Concerns over pregnancy risks among VDT users first surfaced with anecdotal reports of "clusters" of miscarriages and birth defects among the offspring of office workers. At first the possibility that adverse pregnancy effects could be linked to VDT work was discounted, as was the more specific concern that the EMFs of the VDTs might be directly involved. In 1982, Leal, working in Delgado's laboratory in Madrid, reported that extremely weak, pulsed EMFs could damage developing chick embryos. This finding was later confirmed by an international research effort, the "Henhouse Project." Swedish researchers then extended the Leal studies by using EMFs designed to mimic those emitted by VDTs. In a series of experiments, two different laboratories reported that the EMFs from the VDTs were indeed biologically active, causing birth defects in one study and miscarriages in another study using a different strain of mice. Recent studies have shown that the risk is greatest during the earliest stages of pregnancy, a finding that calls into question avoidance strategies, such as alternative work policies now offered in many workplaces.

In 1988, Goldhaber and coworkers[26] at Kaiser Permanente in Oakland, Calif., published an epidemiological study that appeared to support the concerns raised by the cluster reports. They found that women who used VDTs for more than 20 hours a week during the first trimester of pregnancy had twice as many miscarriages as non-VDT workers. Goldhaber's study was unable to identify the factors responsible for the increase. Among the possibilities listed were stress, ergonomics, EMFs, and of course chance. Other studies also have found a statistically significant link between VDT work and miscarriage, although these findings often have been attributed to recall bias—the tendency for women who have miscarried to report more VDT use than was actually the case—or confounding factors, such as stress or smoking. A more definitive answer to the pregnancy risk question will emerge with the completion of the first large-scale *prospective* study now being conducted at Mount Sinai Medical Center in New York City. In addition, NIOSH reported the results of its own epidemiological study early in 1991 and found no effect of VDT use.[27]

Because EMFs from VDTs decay quickly with distance, some experts are recommending that VDT users keep an arm's length from the terminal and make sure they do not sit within 3 to 4 feet of a neighbor's terminal, especially the side or the back of VDTs where the EMFs are highest.

Office workers also should be made aware that copying machines and laser printers emit strong levels of EMF radiation, although these also decay rapidly with distance.

RADIOFREQUENCY AND MICROWAVE RADIATION

Radiofrequency and microwave (RF-MW) radiation refers to electromagnetic radiation in the frequency band between 3 MHz and 300 GHz. RF-MW radiation has a wide range of applications: most commonly, radio and television broadcasting, cellular telephone transmitters, radar, satellite communications, industrial heating (including MW ovens), point-to-point communication relay links, medical diathermy, and hyperthermia for cancer treatment.

RF-MW biological effects depend on the number of different factors: power density (usually expressed in milliwatts per square centimeter [mW/cm^2]), frequency, waveform, and orientation in the field.

For many years the general consensus was that tissue heating at high intensities was the only biological effect of RF-MW radiation exposure. Over the past decade, however, many experts have come to believe that RF-MW radiation can have nonthermal biological effects as well, including cancer promotion, changes in endocrine gland functions and in the blood-brain barrier, and cataract formation.

The specific absorption rate (SAR) is the unit of measurement most often used to define the amount of energy a biological system absorbs from RF-MW radiation, especially for thermal effects. SARs are measured in units of watts per kilogram (W/kg). For humans an SAR of 4 W/kg is approximately equivalent to a power density of 10 mW/cm^2 at frequencies of 30 to 300 MHz.

There have been very few studies of the long-term effects of low-level, nonthermal exposures to RF-MW radiation. The vast majority of studies have addressed only the acute hazards. The original version of a draft EPA report on the carcinogenicity of EMFs recommended that RF-MW radiation be designated as Class C: possible human carcinogen. The designation was removed from the draft report before its June 1990 release.[28]

Biological Effects. In the mid-1980s, after a detailed literature review, EPA issued a report concluding that significant biological effects occur at SARs of approximately 1 W/kg—four times lower than the threshold level cited in the ANSI safety guidelines (see below). EPA's conclusion was based on research that showed effects at 1 W/kg on endocrine gland function, blood chemistry, hematology, and immunology.

Acute high-level exposures to RF-MW radiation can cause persistent health problems, including memory loss. For example, there was a report in 1988 of a military pilot who accidentally stood in front of a functioning MW fighter radar system for approximately 5 minutes. The next morning the pilot found a small, painful lump on the back of his neck that continued to grow. During the next few weeks the pilot noticed problems with his short-term memory. His memory lapses persisted for a number of months.

Laboratory and Animal Experiments. One of the earliest studies to identify nonthermal RF-MW biological effects was by Prausnitz and Susskind[29] who exposed mice to pulsed 9.27 GHz MW radiation at a level of 100 mW/cm^2 and found an indication of leukemia. Their study was never replicated.

In 1982, Szmigielski et al.[30] published a landmark study of MW cancer promotion, which showed that 2450 MHz (in the MW range) can act as a cocarcinogen with benzo-a-pyrene.

Researchers at the Johns Hopkins Applied Physics Laboratory found that pulsed 2.45 GHz MWs can affect the endothelial layer of the cornea in primates at average power levels of 5 mW/cm^2. Their research, like many other studies, indicates that pulsed radiation is more biologically potent than continuous-wave radiation.

A single acute exposure of the eye to high-intensity RF-MW radiation (100 mW/cm^2), if applied for a sufficient time, can lead to cataract formation in some experimental animals. Some experts, notably Zaret, believe that the threshold for cataract formation is much lower.

The only chronic animal study of RF-MW exposures ever undertaken, by Guy and coworkers at the University of Washington School of Medicine in Seattle, indicated that pulsed 2450 MHz radiation caused a statistically significant increase in malignant tumors among rats. The rats in the Guy study were exposed to an SAR of 0.4 W/kg, precisely the SAR level specified by ANSI as safe (see below). No single type of tumor predominated, although there were indications of an effect on the endocrine system.

In 1990, a study by Cleary and colleagues[31] showed that brain tumor cells continued to proliferate at an abnormally high rate 5 days after a 2-hour RF-MW exposure at levels of 5 or 25 W/kg.

Epidemiological Studies. One of the first studies to link cancer to RF-MW exposures in a human population was a 1985 study by Szmigielski showing a tripling of the incidence of cancer among military personnel exposed to RF-MW radiation compared with unexposed servicemen. For blood-forming organs and lymphatic tissues the rates were nearly seven times those expected. Szmigielski currently is in the midst of a prospective study of military personnel; preliminary results support the results of the retrospective study.

In 1987 the Hawaii Department of Health found that Honolulu residents living near radio and television towers had a significantly higher incidence of cancer than those living elsewhere in the city.

In general there have been extremely few epidemiological studies of RF-MW-exposed populations.

Funding. In the United States the military historically has been the predominant sponsor of RF-MW health effects research. As of 1990, essentially all ongoing research is being funded by the U.S. Air Force and the U.S. Army.

RF-MW Safety Standards. There are no enforceable federal standards to protect the public or workers from RF-MW radiation. The 1982 ANSI standard of 1 mW/cm^2 at body resonant frequencies (30 to 300 MHz) has become the de facto national RF-MW health guide in the United States. At lower frequencies the standard increases to 100 mW/cm^2 for the 300 kHz to 3 MHz band and increases to 5 mW/cm^2 at 1500 MHz. ANSI used a safety factor of 10 to arrive at its exposure limit of 1 mW/cm^2, based on an SAR of 0.4 W/kg. A committee is at work at revising the standard; it is expected in 1991.

In 1986 the National Council on Radiation Protection and Measurements (NCRP), a group chartered by the U.S. Congress, recommended an occupational standard essentially identical to ANSI's but advised that the maximum exposure for the general population should be one-fifth the occupational levels.

In 1988, EPA abandoned its multiyear project of setting a federal standard for RF-MW exposures; the agency had originally decided to set a 100 μW/cm^2 standard but did not go forward in the face of political opposition.

The Occupational Safety and Health Administration (OSHA) has a voluntary exposure guideline of 10 mW/cm^2. This standard is based on the 1966 ANSI standard.

Exposure standards in Eastern Europe and the Soviet Union are significantly lower than those in the United States. In the Soviet Union the occupational exposure standard is 100 μW/cm^2, and 10 μW/cm^2 above 300 MHz for the general public.

Litigation. Most RF-MW health effects and product liability suits are settled out of court for undisclosed amounts. The following cases are two of the largest electromagnetic field (EMF) settlements ever made public.

In 1989, Antionette Yannon, the widow of a New York Telephone Company radio technician, settled a 1976 product liability suit against RCA Corporation for $250,000. Yannon claimed that RCA was responsible for the wrongful death of her husband Samuel at the age of 62 because of long-term MW exposure. Samuel Yannon worked on MW relay equipment for 15 years on top of the Empire State Building in New York City. In his last months, Samuel Yannon lost almost all sight, memory, speech, and motor coordination and was diagnosed as suffering from chronic brain syndrome with psychotic overtones due to biological brain changes resulting from prolonged exposure to shortwave radiation.

In 1990 the Boeing Company agreed to pay Robert Strom, a former electromagnetic pulse (EMP) technician, more than $500,000 to settle his claim that he and other Boeing EMP workers were used as human research subjects without their knowledge or consent. Strom alleged that he contracted leukemia at the age of 45 from occupational exposure to EMP radiation. From 1983 to 1985, Strom tested the effects of EMP on electrical and electronic components of the MX "Peacekeeper" missile. (EMP is a type of nonionizing radiation emitted in a nuclear detonation; in the 1980s the U.S. military and its contractors embarked on an ambitious program requiring testing to protect electronic equipment from EMP radiation.)

A number of veterans have won out-of-court settlements for cataracts resulting from exposure to radar and communication equipment.

REFERENCES

1. Hughes D: Hazards of Occupational Exposure to Ultraviolet Radiation. Occupational Hygiene Monograph No. 1. Leeds, England: University of Leeds Industrial Services, 1978
2. Occupational Exposure to Ultraviolet Radiation: NIOSH Criteria Document. Washington, D.C.: U.S. Department of HEW, NIOSH Publication No. 73-11009, 1973, p 108
3. Urbach F: Geographic distribution of skin cancer. J Surg Oncol 3: 219–234, 1971
4. American National Standards Institute: Practice of Industrial Lighting A 11.1, 1965 (reaffirmed 1970). Practice for Office Lighting A 132.1, 1966. Guide for School Lighting A 23.1, 1962 (reaffirmed 1970). New York: The Institute
5. Illuminating Engineering Society, Committee on Daylighting: Recommended Practice of Daylighting. Baltimore: The Society, 1950
6. Environmental Protection Agency: Evaluation of the Potential Carcinogenuity of Electromagnetic Fields. Workshop Review Draft, No. EPA/600/6-9/005A. Washington, D.C.: The Agency, 1990
7. Office of Technology Assessment: Biologic Effects of Power Frequency Electric and Magnetic Fields—Background Paper, No. OTA-BP-E-53. Washington, D.C., 1989
8. Wertheimer N, Leeper E: Electrical wiring configurations and childhood cancer. Am J Epidemiol 109:273–284, 1979
9. Savitz D et al: Case control study of childhood cancer and exposure to 60 Hz magnetic fields. Am J Epidemiol 128:21–38, 1988
10. Wertheimer N, Leeper E: Adult cancer related to electrical wires near the home. Int J Epidemiol 11:345–355, 1982
11. Wertheimer N, Leeper E: Possible effects of electric blankets and heated waterbeds on fetal development. Bioelectromagnetics 7:13–22, 1986
12. Wertheimer N, Leeper E: Fetal loss associated with two seasonal sources of electromagnetic field exposure. Am J Epidemiol 129:220–224, 1989
13. Savitz D, John E, Kleckner R: Magnetic field exposure from electric appliances and childhood cancer. Am J Epidemiol 131:763–773, 1990
14. Perry S: Power frequency magnetic fields: depressive illness and myocardial infarction. Public Health 102:11–18, 1988
15. Matanoski G, Elliott E, Breysse P: Cancer incidence in New York telephone workers [Abstract]. Annual Department of Energy-Electric Power Research Institute Contractors Review, 1989
16. Demers P et al: Occupational exposure to electromagnetic radiation and breast cancer in males [Abstract]. Am J Epidemiol 132:775–776, 1990
17. Adey WR: Joint actions of environmental non-ionizing electromagnetic fields and chemical pollution in cancer promotion. Environ Health Perspect 86:297–305, 1990
18. Bawin SM, Adey WR: Sensitivity of calcium binding in cerebral tissue to weak environmental electric fields oscillating at low frequency. Proc Natl Acad Sci USA 76:1999–2003, 1976
19. Blackman C et al: Effects of ELF (1-120 Hz) and modulated (50 Hz) RF fields on the efflux of calcium ions from brain tissue in vitro. Bioelectromagnetics 6:1–11, 1985
20. Goodman R, Henderson A: Exposure of salivary gland cells to low-frequency electromagnetic fields alters polypeptide synthesis. Proc Natl Acad Sci USA 85:3928–3932, 1988
21. Liboff AR et al: Effects of electromagnetic stimuli in bone and bone cells in vitro: Inhibition of responses to parathyroid hormone by low-energy, low frequency fields. Proc Natl Acad Sci USA 79:4180–4184, 1982
22. Byus C, Pieper S, Adey WR: The effects of low energy 60 Hz environmental electromagnetic fields upon the growth-related enzyme ornithine decarboxylase. Carcinogenesis 8:1385–1389, 1987
23. Phillips J, Winters W, Rutledge L: In vitro exposure to electromagnetic fields: Changes in tumour cell properties. Int J Radiat Biol 49:463–469, 1986
24. International Radiation Protection Association: Interim guidelines on limits of exposure to 50/60 Hz electric and magnetic fields. Health Phys 58:113–122, 1990
25. Human Factors Society: American National Standard for human factors engineering of visual display terminal workstations. (ANSI/HFS 100-1988), 1988
26. Goldhaber M, Polen M, Hiatt R: The risks of miscarriage and birth

defects among women who use VDTs during pregnancy. Am J Ind Med 13:695–706, 1988

27. Schnorr TM, Grajewski BA, Hornung RW, et al: Video display terminals and the risk of spontaneous abortion. N Engl J Med 324(11): 727–733, 1991
28. Environmental Protection Agency: Evaluation of the Potential Carcinogenicity of Electromagnetic Fields. Workshop Review Draft No. EPA/600/6-90/00SA, Washington D.C., 1990
29. Prausnitz S, Susskind C: Effects of chronic microwave irradiation on mice. IRE Trans Bio-Med Electronics 9:104–108, 1962
30. Szmigielski S et al: Accelerated development of spontaneous and benzopyrene-induced skin cancer in mice exposed to 2450 MHz microwave radiation. Bioelectromagnetics 3:179–192, 1982
31. Cleary S, Liu L-M, Merchant R: Glioma proliferation modulated in vitro by isothermal radiofrequency radiation exposure. Radiat Res 121:38–45, 1990

General References

Ahlbom A: A review of the epidemiologic literatures on magnetic fields and cancer. Scand J Work Environ Health 14:337–343, 1988

Archimbaud E et al: Acute myologenous leukemia following exposure to microwaves. Br J Haematol 73:272–273, 1989

Becker RO, Selden G: The Body Electric. New York: William Morrow, 1985

Brown HD, Chattopadhyay SK: Electromagnetic field exposure and cancer. Cancer Biochem Biophys 9:295–342, 1988

Grandjean E: Ergonomics in Computerized Offices. Philadelphia: Taylor & Francis, 1987

National Council on Radiation Protection and Measurements: Biological Effects and Exposure Criteria for Electromagnetic Fields. Bethesda, Md.: NCRP, 1986

National Institute of Child Health and Development: Proceedings of the NICHD Workshop on the Reproductive Effects of VDT Use. Reprod Toxicol 4:39–69, 1990

Salzinger K et al: Altered operant behavior of adult rats after perinatal exposure to a 60 Hz electromagnetic field. Bioelectromagnetics 11:105–116, 1990

Savitz D, Calle E: Leukemia and occupational exposure to electromagnetic fields: Review of epidemiologic surveys. J Occup Med 29:47–51, 1987

Speers M, Dobbins J, Miller V: Occupational exposures and brain cancer: A preliminary study of East Texas residents. Am J Ind Med 13:629–639, 1988

Thomas T et al: Brain tumor mortality risk among men with electrical and electronics jobs: A case-control study. Natl Conser Dist 79:233–238, 1987

Wilson B, Stevens R, Anderson L: Extremely Low Frequency Electromagnetic Fields: The Question of Cancer. Columbus, Ohio: Battelle Press, 1990

28

Noise as a Health Hazard

Aage R. Møller

Noise can be hazardous to health chiefly in two ways: (1) it can damage the ear, and (2) it can influence a number of other bodily functions. In addition, the permanent or temporary decrease in hearing acuity from noise exposure may make speech communication difficult. Noise can also mask warning signals. Thus, it poses a risk to safety and therefore a risk to the general health of workers.

Because the potential to cause damage to the ear is the most apparent and best-known health risk of noise, it will be discussed first. The other effects of noise will be discussed later in the chapter.

EFFECT OF NOISE ON HEARING

Noise is commonly used to describe sounds that are unwanted or unpleasant, in contrast to sounds such as music or speech. Several textbooks, in fact, define noise as sound that is discordant and nonperiodic, probably because such sound often has unpleasant qualities. The potential of noise to damage hearing, however, is entirely related to such physical properties as its intensity, the length of time over which subjects are exposed to it, and its time pattern and is not related to whether the sound is pleasant or not. It would therefore be more appropriate to use the general term *sound* in discussing the hazards to hearing. However, we will use *noise* to describe sound that may be damaging to the ear because this word has traditionally had negative connotations and thus will be identified more readily with health hazards.

Noises of intensity and duration sufficient to cause hearing impairment are usually associated with industry. However, since it is solely the physical characteristics of the sound that determine its potential for causing hearing loss, the origin of the sound by itself has no influence on the degree of risk it presents for hearing damage. Thus, sounds to which people are exposed during recreational activities may pose as great a hazard to hearing as noise associated with work activities (including military activities, where gunshot noise in particular poses a high degree of risk).

Individual variation in susceptibility to noise is great, and probably factors that are not yet known affect an individual's risk of noise-induced hearing loss. Thus, only the degree of risk (probability) for acquiring a hearing loss can be predicted on the basis of our present knowledge about how the physical characteristics of noise and time of exposure to noise affect hearing. The risk of noise-induced hearing loss is in proportion to the intensity and duration of the noise, with the risk of injuring one's hearing increasing with the length of exposure. The character of the noise—continuous or transient (such as gunshots)—also plays a role. Thus, different types of noise pose different degrees of risk of hearing loss, even though the overall intensity of the noises is the same; impulsive sounds such as gunshots generally pose a greater risk than continuous noise.[1] The spectral composition of the noise and the pattern of exposure (constant intensity vs fluctuating intensity or noise interspersed with intervals of relative silence) are also important factors that affect the degree of risk of hearing loss.

The first effect of exposing an ear to noise of a certain intensity for a certain period of time is a reduction in hearing (elevated auditory threshold). This reduction in hearing is greatest immediately after the exposure and decreases gradually. If the noise has not been too loud or the exposure too long, hearing will gradually return to its original level, a type of hearing loss known as a temporary threshold shift (TTS). If the noise is louder than a certain value or the exposure time is longer than a certain time, then the hearing threshold never returns to its original value, causing a permanent threshold shift (PTS). The time course of the change in hearing threshold is illustrated schematically in Figure 28-1.

While a TTS probably results from temporarily impaired function of the sensory cells in the inner ear, a PTS is associated with irreversible damage to these cells. This damage can be seen when the cells are examined histologically under high-power magnification. An example of such damage is illustrated in Figure 28-2, which shows a scanning electron micrograph of the sensory cells (hair cells) in the inner ear of a monkey before and after exposure to gunshot noise. Hearing in persons with damaged hair cells cannot be restored. Noise exposure may also damage neural structures in the auditory nervous system, but the exact nature and extent of this damage is poorly understood.

As has been noted, the intensity and the duration of exposure to noise primarily determine the degree of permanent hearing damage caused by the noise, and the hazard to hearing increases as the intensity and length of exposure increase. The distribution of a noise's energy over the frequency spectrum is also important: low-frequency sounds are considered to be less damaging than high-frequency sounds of the same physical in-

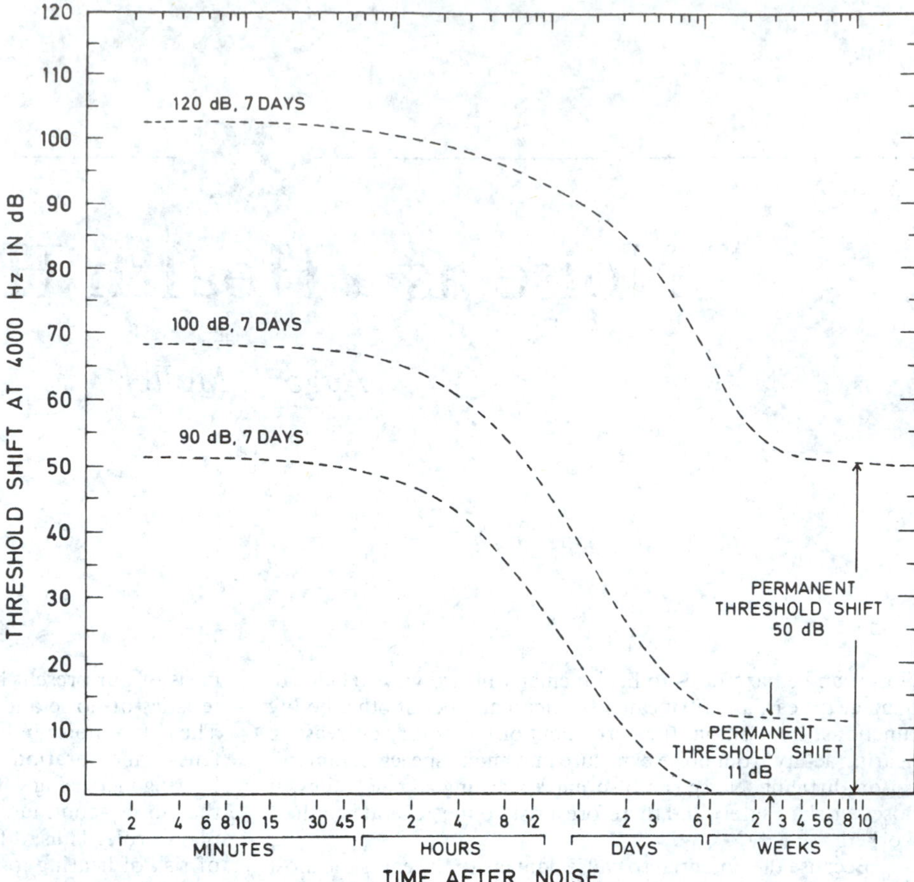

Figure 28-1. Schematic diagram illustrating how noise can affect hearing. The graph shows the hearing loss (threshold shift) at 4000 Hz a certain time (horizontal axis) after noise exposure. Noise with an intensity below a certain value is expected to give rise to a temporary threshold shift (*90 dB, 7 days curve*), while a louder noise (*100 dB, 7 days*) results in a permanent threshold shift. A very intense noise (*120 dB, 7 days*) gives rise to a considerable permanent shift in threshold. *(Adapted from Miller J: J Acoust Soc Am 56:3, 1974, with permission.)*

tensity. Another parameter of noise important in determining its potential to cause hearing loss is whether it is continuous or impulsive in nature; impulsive noise is more likely to cause hearing loss than is continuous noise of the same intensity and spectrum.

Because there is great individual variation in susceptibility to noise-induced hearing loss, people who are exposed to exactly the same noise for exactly the same period of time may not suffer the same degree of hearing loss. Some people can tolerate high-intensity noise for a lifetime and not suffer any substantial degree of hearing loss, but other people may acquire a substantial hearing loss from exposure to much less intense noise. Attempts have been made to estimate an individual's susceptibility to PTS

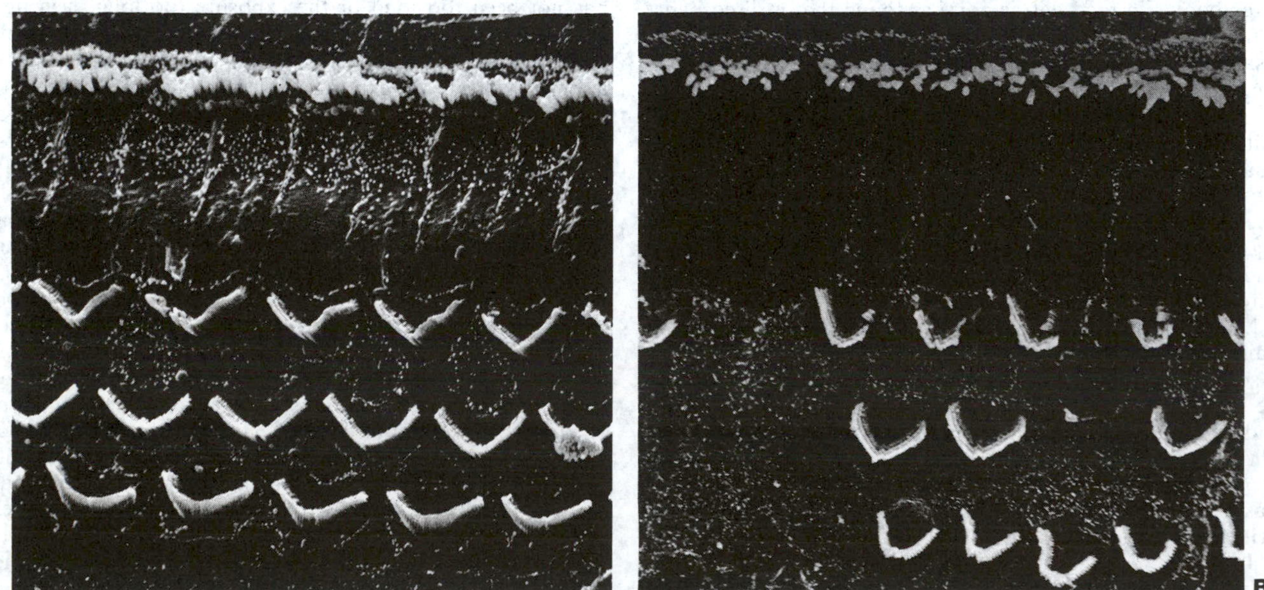

Figure 28-2. Scanning electron micrographs of sensory cells (hair cells) from a small segment of the basilar membrane of a monkey. **A.** Normal hair cells. **B.** Hair cells after noise exposure (gunshots). *(Courtesy Professor Hans Engstrom, Uppsala, Sweden.)*

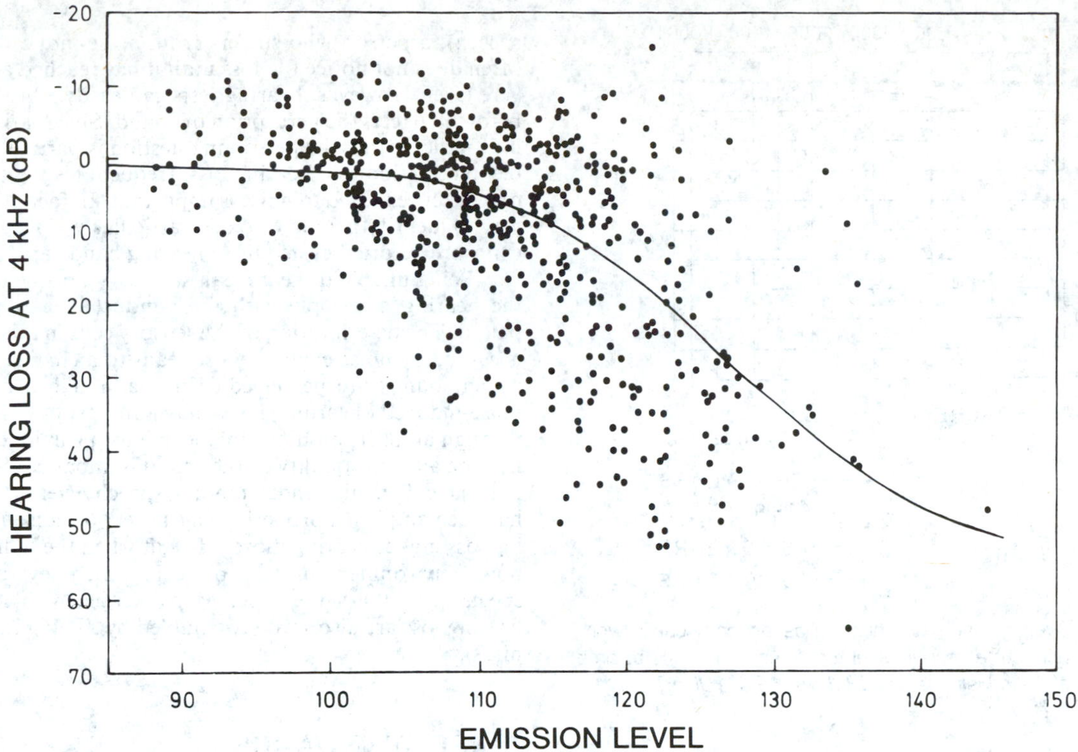

Figure 28–3. Threshold shift (hearing loss) at 4 kHz as a function of the total amount of noise exposure (emission value). Each point represents an individual person, and the solid lines are the mean values of the threshold shifts. The emission value is L_{eq} + 10 log (*T*), where L_{eq} represents the sound level (measured with A-weighting) that is exceeded during 2% of the exposure time *T* (in months). For example, exposure to 85-dB noise during 20 years of work corresponds to 85 + 10 log (20 × 12) = 85 + 10 log 240 = 85 + 24 = 109. The threshold shift given is the threshold shift measured minus the threshold shift assumed to be normal considering the age of the person (everyone experiences some hearing loss as part of the normal process of aging, which is called presbycusis). For continuous noise, L_{eq} deviates only slightly from the A-weighted sound intensity, but for noise that contains transient or intermittent noises (i.e., noises that vary considerably in intensity), the difference between these two values is great. The graph thus shows that the *average* hearing loss as a result of exposure to continuous noise with a sound intensity of 85 dB(A) for 20 years is less than 5 dB at 4 kHz, but that a number of people experience a 30-dB to 40-dB threshold shift. *(From Burns W and Robinson DW: Hearing and Noise in Industry. London, HMSO, 1970.)*

by the degree of TTS evidenced on exposure to a test sound that is not loud enough to cause permanent hearing loss. However, the results of these attempts have been rather discouraging, and it seems that there is no correlation between susceptibility to PTS and the degree of TTS in any individual person. At the present time the only way to determine such individual susceptibility is to test at frequent intervals the hearing of workers exposed to loud noise.

However, the distribution of susceptibility to PTS in a large population is relatively well known. Figure 28–3 shows hearing losses at 4 kHz for a number of people as a function of the noise emission level.[2] This measure combines the two characteristics of noise (duration and intensity) assumed to be of the greatest importance in defining its potential for harm but does not take into account the nature of the noise (time pattern or spectrum).

Although we do not yet know which factors determine susceptibility to noise, recent studies in animals have pointed toward some factors that may predispose a subject to noise-induced hearing loss. For example, studies in rats that were genetically predisposed to high blood pressure showed that these rats acquired a higher degree of hearing loss from noise exposure than did normal rats when both groups were exposed to noise for their entire lifetimes.[3,4] Although these findings have not been duplicated in humans, the results of some human studies support a relationship between high blood pressure and hearing loss from noise exposure[5] (see also p. 529). Alterations in cochlear blood flow may also affect susceptibility to noise.[6] More recent animal studies have disclosed that activation of a particular neural circuit in the brainstem (the olivocochlear bundle) may protect the ear from noise-induced hearing loss.[7] The results of these recent studies underline the complexity of the way noise affects and gives rise to hearing loss; they also shed some light on several unexplained effects of the exposure pattern and nature of the noise in producing noise-induced hearing loss. Research along these lines is likely to provide knowledge that may lead within the foreseeable future to the development of more efficient ways to assess an individual's susceptibility to noise-induced hearing loss.

NATURE OF NOISE-INDUCED HEARING LOSS

Hearing loss is measured in decibels* relative to a normative average hearing threshold. Such baseline thresholds are obtained

**dB, the abbreviation for decibel, is a logarithmic measure, used here as a measure of sound pressure. One decibel is one tenth of a logarithmic unit (a ratio of 1:10). The reason for using a logarithmic measure of sound pressure to measure hearing threshold is that the subjective sensation of sound intensity is* approximately *related to the logarithm of the sound pressure.*

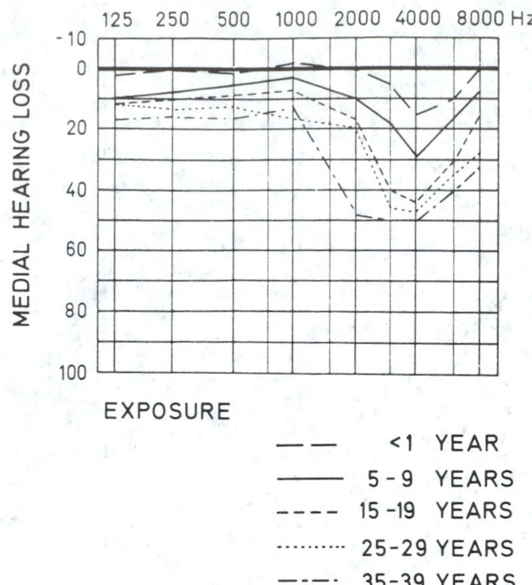

Figure 28-4. Average estimated hearing losses for industrial workers exposed to noise of a certain level for different lengths of time. *[From Taylor et al: J Acoust Soc Am 38:113–120, 1965.]*

by measuring the hearing thresholds of young people who have had no known exposure to noise. However, slightly different standards for "normal" hearing are used in different parts of the world (American National Standard Institute [ANSI] in the United States[8]; International Organization for Standardization [ISO] in Europe[9]), which may need to be taken into account when the risk of noise-induced hearing loss is evaluated. The difference between the hearing threshold of an individual and the "standard" hearing threshold is known as the hearing level (HL) and is measured in decibels. When the HL is plotted on the vertical axis as a function of the frequency tested, the resulting graph is known as an audiogram. Usually, the hearing thresholds are determined only in the frequency range of 125 to 8000 Hz (8 kHz), despite the fact that a person with normal hearing can hear sounds in the frequency range of 18 to 20,000 Hz.

Examples of estimated hearing loss taken from data obtained in a study of workers in the weaving industry are shown in Figure 28–4 as "predicted" audiograms. The individual curves on this audiogram represent different durations of noise exposure in years. As seen, the estimated hearing loss is greatest in a restricted frequency range around 4 kHz, but with continuing exposure the frequency range of hearing loss widens and the magnitude of the loss increases. These results obtained in weavers are typical for those exposed to noise in various manufacturing industries where the noise tends to be of a broad spectrum and continuous in nature. Although many hypotheses have been presented, we do not know why the greatest hearing loss resulting from exposure to the broadband noise that is common in industries occurs around 4 kHz. We do know, however, that the frequency distribution of hearing loss depends to some extent on the spectrum of the noise. When the hearing-damaging effect of a noise with a narrow spectrum (i.e., its energy is limited to a narrow range of frequencies) is studied, the hearing loss usually is greatest over a frequency range slightly above (about ½ octave) the range at which the noise has its highest energy. However, the precise relationship between the spectrum of a noise and the distribution of hearing loss it can cause is not fully known.

Since hearing loss induced by industrial noise usually first affects the hearing threshold at frequencies around 4000 Hz (and thus above the 300- to 3000-Hz range essential for perception of speech), a person who suffers from noise-induced hearing loss often does not notice the loss until it has reached a relatively severe level. However, hearing tests can easily reveal hearing loss before it affects the perception of sound. Since early hearing loss may indicate that the person in question is particularly susceptible to noise-induced hearing loss, frequent testing of the hearing of workers exposed to noise is important. In fact, it is a powerful way to identify people who are particularly susceptible to noise exposure before they acquire a hearing handicap.

Being unable to hear weak sounds is not the only way that the hearing of people with noise-induced hearing loss is impaired. The deterioration of the sensory cells in the inner ear that is caused by noise exposure also leads to a change in the way in which sounds are perceived. Thus, although a person with a noise-induced hearing loss may understand some sounds through amplification (asking people to speak louder or using a hearing aid), the quality of the sound is impaired. Such a person may have difficulty understanding speech, even when the sound has been amplified properly. This aspect of noise-induced hearing loss makes hearing more difficult when the individual is in a noisy environment or in a place in which several people are speaking at the same time. Many people with noise-induced hearing loss are also severely troubled by ringing in the ears (tinnitus).

NOISE STANDARDS

To reduce the risk of noise-induced hearing loss, a number of recommendations of acceptable noise levels have been established and appear in the form of noise standards. Different countries have adopted slightly different standards, and the ways in which the standards are enforced also differ. All presently accepted standards use a single-value measure of noise level and the duration of the exposure to calculate the risk the noise represents for causing permanent noise-induced hearing loss. Some of these standards include correction factors regarding the nature of the sound, for instance, impulsive vs continuous sounds.

Establishing Noise Standards and Damage Risk Criteria. The maximal noise level and duration accepted in most industrial countries is either 85 or 90 dB(A),* for 8 hours a day, 5 days a week. In Europe the 85-dB(A) level is more common, whereas in the United States 90 dB(A) is the level stated by the Occupational Safety and Health Administration (OSHA), although certain measures have to be taken if workers are exposed to noise levels above 85 dB(A) (for a review of noise standards see Suter[10]).

Individual variation in susceptibility to noise-induced hearing loss makes it impossible to predict what hearing loss an individual will acquire when he or she is exposed to a certain noise. Therefore, at best the standards merely predict the percentage of people in a population with normal hearing who will acquire less than a certain specified (acceptable) hearing loss when exposed to noise no louder than a certain value. When evaluating the so-called noise standards it is important to keep this in mind.[11,12] Noise standards are thus based on the fact that a certain percentage of a normal-hearing population will acquire a permanent hearing loss (threshold elevation) greater than a certain value averaged over certain frequencies. The "allowed" hearing loss and the frequencies at which it is measured vary among standards and have been modified at intervals.

**The (A) after dB indicates that the noise spectrum has been weighted to place less emphasis on low frequencies than on high frequencies because low-frequency sounds generally pose less risk for causing hearing loss than high-frequency sounds.*

There has been a tendency to adjust these criteria downwards to allow for less permanent hearing loss. In the beginning of the era in which efforts were made to reduce (or prevent) noise-induced hearing loss, the *acceptable hearing loss* was defined as the level of hearing loss at which an individual begins to experience difficulty in understanding everyday speech in a quiet environment. This definition was based on the American Academy of Ophthalmology and Otolaryngology (AAOO) guidelines for evaluation of hearing impairment,[13] which state that the ability to understand normal everyday speech at a distance of about 1.5 m (5 ft) does not noticeably deteriorate as long as the hearing loss does not exceed an average value of 25 dB at frequencies 500, 1000, and 2000 Hz. On the basis of this, an average hearing loss of 25 dB at frequencies of 500, 1000, and 2000 Hz was taken to be the hearing loss that resulted in a just-noticeable handicap. This level of hearing loss was originally designated in the United States as the level of handicap at which a worker was entitled to receive workman's compensation for loss of earning power (it is puzzling that this degree of hearing loss was later designated as acceptable).

More recently, some controversy about what constitutes a hearing impairment has emerged. The AAOO had focused on average hearing loss at 500, 1000, and 2000 Hz,[14] but the National Institute for Occupational Safety and Health (NIOSH) criteria document[15] states that the ability to hear sounds at 25 dB below normal at 500, 1000, and 2000 Hz is not sufficient to assure that speech will be understood under normal conditions, even though this hearing threshold might be adequate under the optimal conditions in which speech reception is usually tested for audiological purposes. It has therefore been advocated that the average hearing loss at 1000, 2000, and 3000 Hz be used as a basis for evaluating the effects of noise exposure, instead of at 500, 1000, and 2000 Hz. However, to date this definition has not won general acceptance.

The Environmental Protection Agency (EPA) recommended to OSHA that 25 dB average hearing loss at 1000, 2000, and 4000 Hz be accepted as the standard for when difficulties in understanding normal speech begin.[16] The justification for excluding the hearing level at 500 Hz from calculations of hearing handicaps due to noise exposure is that hearing loss at 500 Hz is more often the result of factors other than noise exposure, such as middle ear disease. The inclusion of the hearing level at 3000 Hz in a composite describing the ability to understand normal speech seems justified because hearing at 3000 Hz is important for speech perception.

It has also been suggested that the average hearing level of 25 dB be replaced by 22 dB, while keeping the same frequencies defined by the EPA (1000, 2000, and 4000 Hz).[17] The reasoning behind this suggestion was endorsed by the AAOO, which, however, maintained that a "low fence" of 25 dB was acceptable.[18] In general, these changes in how measured pure tone thresholds should be weighted to obtain a single number to best define a hearing handicap that affects speech communication have led to a more realistic way of describing the handicap of hearing loss.

Only hearing loss induced by noise has been discussed as imposing a handicap. However, the total acceptable hearing loss is that induced by noise plus whatever is assumed to be the result of other causes such as age (presbycusis). Presbycusis also varies greatly among individuals. Nevertheless, it is the total hearing loss that determines the degree of handicap. So although noise-induced hearing loss may not be at a level regarded to be a handicap according to the noise standard, older persons may suffer a level of hearing loss that can be handicapping, despite not having been exposed to noise that exceeded the standard.

Present Noise Standards. In the United States, legislation that covers noise includes the Federal Aviation Act of 1958, the 1969 Amendment of the Walsh-Healy Public Contracts Act, the Occupational Safety and Health Act of 1970, the Noise Control Act of 1972, and the Mine Safety and Health Act of 1978. These acts require certain agencies to regulate noise.

In Europe, legislation in various countries on industrial noise limitations has largely been guided by recommendations made by the ISO. These recommendations have generally set an upper limit of acceptable noise exposure at 85 dB(A) for 8 hours a day, 5 days per week, but in the United States 90 dB(A) has been the standard.

The ISO recommendation is based on the probabilities of acquiring a hearing loss of 25 dB, averaged for 500, 1000, and 2000 Hz, with exposure to noises of different intensities for variable lengths of time. According to ISO recommendations,[9] as much as 10% of a population with initially normal hearing will acquire a hearing loss of 25 dB or more, averaged over frequencies 500, 1000, and 2000 Hz, after 40 years of exposure to noise at a level of 85 dB(A). For a 90 dB(A) noise level, those experiencing hearing loss increases to 21%. These values are based on studies of workers in the weaving industry, and research indicates that the number of people with noise-induced hearing losses may be higher in other industries. However, the risk of hearing impairment doubles when the daily average noise exposure of 85 dB(A) increases to 90 dB(A), regardless of which data are used (see Suter[10]). Many European countries have chosen 85 dB(A) as the upper limit of acceptable noise exposure for 8 hours.

Recently, proposals have been put forward to lower the standard in the United States from 90 dB(A) to 85 dB(A).[19] Accordingly, a recent OSHA hearing conservation amendment states that a noise monitoring program is mandatory in environments where the daily average noise level is 85 dB(A) or higher.[20] The monitoring program must be so designed that it identifies people who are exposed to noise levels of 85 dB(A) (8-hour weighted average) or more. If people are exposed to noise levels of 90 dB(A) or higher for 8 hours per day, measures must be taken to reduce the noise; and if these measures do not result in a reduction of the noise level to at least 90 dB(A) or lower, workers must participate in a hearing conservation program and employers must make available to workers personal hearing protection devices (ear protectors) and conduct hearing tests at specified intervals during employment. If a hearing loss of 10 dB average over frequencies 2000, 3000, and 4000 Hz is detected, the person must be referred for further evaluation, and action must be taken to avoid further deterioration of hearing.

As early as 1972, NIOSH, in its criteria document,[15] recommended that the 90 dB(A) permissible exposure limit be lowered to 85 dB(A). This recommendation also included suggestions about audiometrical testing, use of hearing protectors, notification of workers, and how records should be kept. Only some of these suggestions were accepted by the U.S. Secretary of Labor, however, and the permissible exposure limit still remains at 90 dB(A), although audiometrical testing and certain other hearing conservation measures are now required when workers are exposed to noise above 85 dB(A). It has been advocated that noise standards be modified to reduce the number of people who acquire a hearing loss that can be regarded as a social handicap. The maximal tolerable noise level for an 8-hour exposure is around 75 dB(A) if significant noise-induced hearing loss is to be eliminated.[21] One of the main obstacles in adopting a lower noise level such as the proposed 85 dB(A) was economic concerns: the cost of having all workplaces comply with such regulations was considered prohibitive. However, a much less expensive alternative, having all *new* equipment comply with regulations, was not even considered.

In the United States the EPA has regulated exposure to noise for the general population, deciding that no more than 5 dB hearing loss can be allowed at 4000 Hz as a result of environmental noise.[22]

The fact that present noise standards are based on a simplified measure of noise, dB(A), adds to the uncertainty in predicting the risk of acquiring a hearing loss through exposure to a certain noise. As discussed earlier, this single-valued dB(A) measure does not contain any information about the spectrum of the noise, nor does it include any information about whether the noise contains sharp transient sounds or sounds with other characteristics important in hearing loss (see p. 523).

Relationship Between Noise Level and Exposure Time. A conversion factor must be established to estimate the acceptable noise level when the exposure to noise is less than 8 hours per day. Again the conversion factor differs throughout the world. Thus, in Europe a 3-dB doubling factor is commonly used to estimate how high a noise level is acceptable when the exposure time to the noise is less than 8 hours per day, but a 5-dB doubling factor is used in the United States. A 3-dB doubling factor implies that a reduction of the exposure time by a factor of 2 is equivalent to a reduction in the noise level by 3 dB. That is, when the exposure time is reduced from 8 hours per day to 4 hours per day, this rule assumes that a sound level 3 dB higher would be acceptable. Or if the exposure time to noise is 2 hours per day, a sound level 6 dB higher can be accepted, and so on. This rule reflects the equal energy principle, which assumes that the total energy of the noise determines the risk for permanent hearing loss. However, using a 5-dB doubling factor means that every time the exposure time is reduced by a factor of 2, the noise level can be increased by 5 dB without increasing the risk of hearing loss. This implies that exposure to a noise for less than 8 hours per day decreases the risk more than the equal energy principle implies and, therefore, that a higher total energy can be tolerated when the exposure time to noise is reduced.

The noise standard presently in effect in the United States (29 CFR 1910.95) states that the maximum time-weighted exposure level acceptable is 90 dB(A) for 8 hours with a 5-dB trading relation (doubling factor) between exposure time and intensity: this trading relation means that although the maximum acceptable noise level for 8 hours is 90 dB(A), the maximum for half the time (4 hours) is 5 dB more (95 dB(A)). This noise level for this time is considered to be as hazardous as a 2-hour exposure to 100 dB(A), a 1-hour exposure to 105 dB(A), a 30-minute exposure to 110 dB(A), and a 15-minute exposure to 115 dB(A).

Using a fixed doubling factor implies that a worker should be equally safe from acquiring a hearing loss when exposed to noises of the same total sound energy, independent of whether the noises are presented as short-duration high-level noises or long-duration low-level noises. The value of the doubling factor for which this is true is, however, in dispute. The results of recent research indicate that a doubling factor of 5 dB may be adequate for relatively low noise levels but that a smaller doubling factor (3 dB, i.e., equal energy) more correctly reflects the hazards presented by noise of a high level.

The validity of the equal energy principle has been questioned because animal experiments have shown that hearing loss progresses more rapidly than predicted in response to loud, short-duration sounds. Thus, it seems that a doubling factor of less than 3 dB should be applied when the noise level is above a certain value. In the United States, standards have been tightened accordingly by stating that no worker should be exposed to continuous noise above 115 dB(A) or impulsive noise above 140 dB(A), thus setting a ceiling for acceptable combination of noise intensity and exposure time.

Because the level of noise exposure usually varies during a work day, noise exposure is often described by its *equivalent level* (L_{eq}), which is defined as the level of a noise that has the same *average* energy as the noise measured during a work day. The equivalent level is measured by summing the total noise energy to which a person is exposed and dividing it by the duration of exposure. The calculation of this equivalent level assumes that the equal energy principle discussed above is valid.

MEASUREMENT OF NOISE

Measurements of sound levels are usually made at a location where people work. However, several factors are thereby left in doubt. One is the effect of the head and pinna on the sound that actually reaches the ear. These two structures amplify sounds within a rather narrow range of frequencies (between 2 and 5 kHz) by as much as 10 to 15 dB. If the noise contains much energy in that range, the level of sound that actually reaches the ear may be as much as 10 to 15 dB higher than the actual reading on a sound level meter placed in the person's location when the person is not present.

Particular measurement problems also arise when the noise is impulsive in nature. Since the ear requires 100 ms to integrate a sound to perceive its loudness, noise level meters in earlier times integrated sound over about 100 ms to provide a reading that was in accordance with the perceived loudness of the sound. This integration time is appropriate when the level of the sound is measured to assess its ability to annoy the hearer. However, when noise levels are measured for the purpose of assessing the risk they pose to hearing, a much shorter integration time should be used because the cochlea integrates sound energy over 2 to 3 ms. Since presently available sound level meters (so-called impulse sound level meters) have an integration time of 35 ms, they underestimate the peak intensities of impulsive sounds and thus the potential of such sounds to affect the cochlea (see Bruel[23]).

Another important factor of sound measurement is the variation in noise level at different locations. Usually, a person does not maintain one work position but walks around, making the average exposure difficult to estimate. Noise dosimeters have been developed to improve the accuracy of measurements of noise exposure. These devices, worn by the person whose noise exposure is to be measured, register the sound level near the ear or sometimes at other locations on the body and integrate the energy over an entire working day. Noise dosimeters thus function similarly to radiation monitors.

PREVENTION OF NOISE-INDUCED HEARING LOSS

Naturally, the preferred method for preventing noise-induced hearing loss is to reduce the noise in a workplace below levels associated with significant risk to the people who work there. This method has often been disputed because of its serious economic implications; however, when noise restrictions are implemented on new equipment only, the economic consequences are small. Although rebuilding old machinery for the purpose of reducing noise can be costly, in the construction of new machinery state-of-the-art engineering can reduce noise without excessive economic consequences. As an example, over a decade ago a new, fast papermaking machine with a noise level of 85 dB(A) was constructed using known technology to replace old machinery with a noise level of more than 110 dB(A).[24] In fact, the noise level did not exceed 82 dB(A) in many workplaces in which this new equipment was installed, and the total cost of reducing noise was only 1.1% of the total cost of the plant.

When old equipment is to be converted, it may cost less than $1000 per worker to comply with 90 dB(A) standards and about $1600 per worker to comply with 85 dB(A) standards (see Bruce,[25] Table 4, page 609; see also Suter[10]). Undeniably, the cost of noise reduction in several industries is greater than in the example given, but it is equally obvious that in many branches of industry the cost is less, and there may even be cases in which the cost would be negligible. For this reason, setting a noise standard at a certain dB(A) value may in some cases be counterproductive because it provides no initiative to reduce the noise level below the standard, even when substantial reductions in noise level, beyond that necessary to meet the standard, could be achieved at minimal cost and improve worker comfort and productivity immeasurably.

It has been claimed that the problem of noise-induced hearing loss can be solved by personal protection devices (ear defenders). However, wearing ear protectors for long periods may be hot and inconvenient, and they impair speech communication even beyond the impairment caused by the noisy environment. In addition, ear protectors make it more difficult for people to hear alarm signals or other acoustical signs of danger.

Nevertheless, there are times when ear protectors are appropriate. Two types are in common use: earmuffs, which are attached to a helmet or headband, and earplugs. Earmuffs can be removed more easily than earplugs and are therefore better suited for intermittent use, for example, when people are walking in and out of noisy areas (such as airports), whereas earplugs are most practical for people who spend long periods of time in noisy environments. The sound attenuation of different types of earplugs and earmuffs depends not only on the type of device but also on how well it fits the individual person. Even results of laboratory testing where more ideal situations can be achieved show great variability. When the sound attenuation of various protective devices is measured in the laboratory, earmuffs attenuate sound more than earplugs do.[26] However, when hearing loss is assessed in people using these two types of ear protectors, earmuffs are usually shown to be less efficient than earplugs, even though earmuffs attenuate sound more.[26,27] This discrepancy may be due to the way sound attenuation is measured, or possibly since earmuffs are easier to remove, they may not always be worn when indicated.[27] In addition, earmuffs tend to lose some of their sound attenuating power over time, thus they become less efficient in reducing noise-induced hearing loss. Earplugs may also offer more efficient protection to some individuals but less to others because earplugs must fit into the ear canal, the size of which varies widely in people. The sound attenuating power of earmuffs is less dependent on the anatomy of the wearer.[28]

These problems were studied recently in shipyards, where there is often a combination of intense, relatively continuous noise and superimposed impulsive noise, thus presenting an extreme hazard to hearing.[29] When workers were divided into two groups according to the intensity of the noise to which they were exposed, those in the low-intensity noise group suffered more hearing loss than did those in the high-intensity noise group. This surprising result is likely related to the workers' differing habits of wearing ear protectors: many more workers exposed to high-intensity noise than low-intensity noise wore ear protectors. In fact, because the number of workers in the high-intensity noise group who did not wear ear protectors was so low, no analysis could be made in this group of the relative benefit of wearing ear protectors, but in the low-intensity noise group, 1.73 times more workers who did not wear protectors suffered hearing loss than did those who wore protectors.[27]

If the noise level to which people are exposed cannot be reduced below harmful levels, then measuring hearing loss at frequent intervals becomes an important part of a hearing conservation program, and it is the only known method of identifying people who are especially susceptible to noise-induced hearing loss. Since a hearing loss usually begins in the high-frequency range, above the frequencies used for everyday speech, it may not be noticed at first by the sufferer. However, such a hearing loss can easily be detected using ordinary pure tone audiometry. Persons who show such deterioration of hearing at high frequencies may be made aware that they are beginning to acquire a noise-induced hearing loss. The progress of hearing deterioration can usually be halted by moving to a less noisy environment, thus preventing the hearing loss from reaching levels at which it becomes a social handicap. Modern hearing conservation programs focus on identifying persons who risk acquiring such a hearing loss so that they can take steps to avoid a handicap. Many more people could no doubt be spared such a decline in the quality of their lives if more would take these simple precautions.

EFFECTS OF NOISE ON OTHER BODILY FUNCTIONS

The effects of noise on bodily functions other than hearing are poorly understood. Noise exposure has been reported to cause an increase in blood pressure and alterations in other important bodily functions such as changes (usually increases) in the secretion of pituitary hormones.[30] However, more experimental evidence needs to be gathered to determine what the exact effects are and to distinguish between acute and long-term effects of noise on these functions.

Alterations in the body's immune reactions and an increase in sensitivity to epinephrine and norepinephrine of the vascular system have been reported.[31] Although it is known that the acute effect of noise on autonomic reactions increases as noise intensity is increased, the effect of the time pattern of noise on this response is less well understood than is its effect on hearing.[30] We know little about the ability of noise to alter excretion of pituitary hormones over extended periods of time.[21]

It has been known for a long time that workers in noisy industries have a higher incidence of peripheral circulatory problems and heart problems than do those who are not exposed to such high levels of noise.[32] However, because many other adverse factors besides noise exist in industrial environments, it has been difficult to identify the results of noise exposure alone.

The effect of noise on blood pressure perhaps has been most thoroughly studied but has not been fully elucidated. During acute exposure to noise, blood pressure usually increases. The effect of noise on this bodily function is assumed to be mediated by the autonomic nervous system. Some reports[33] have shown that prolonged exposure to noise had a lasting effect on blood pressure in monkeys. In other studies[3] no effect was found on the normal increase in blood pressure with age that occurs in rats with normal blood pressure at birth nor in animals with hereditary high blood pressure (spontaneously hypertensive rats) when such rats were exposed to noise for their entire lives.[3,34,35] (Unexpectedly, however, the spontaneously hypertensive rats developed considerably greater degrees of hearing loss from exposure to noise than did rats without this hereditary predisposition to high blood pressure.[3,34])

Some retrospective studies (e.g., Jonsson and Hansson[5]) of the effects of exposure to noise on the blood pressures of industrial workers found that workers who were exposed to industrial noise had higher systolic and diastolic blood pressures, but other studies (e.g., Sanden and Axelsson[36]) found no relationship between noise-induced hearing loss and blood pressure in shipyard workers. However, shipyard workers who had the highest degrees of noise-induced hearing loss had the greatest increases in heart rate during work, although the increases were not correlated with noise level.[36] Again, there is no evidence that such an increase in heart rate has any long-term effects. If the results of the above-mentioned experiments in spontaneously hypertensive rats[3,4,34] can be applied to humans, then the results of the study of hypertension reported by Jonsson and Hansson[5] may have to be reevaluated: by using hearing loss as the criterion for degree of noise exposure, they may have inadvertently selected workers who were predisposed to hearing loss because of their hypertension and not vice versa, as was intended.

SOUNDS ABOVE AND BELOW AUDIBLE FREQUENCY RANGE (ULTRASOUND AND INFRASOUND)

Sounds not audible to humans because their frequencies are outside our audible range are known as ultrasounds and infrasounds. The range of hearing in humans is usually given as 16 to 20,000 Hz in young people. The high-frequency limit usually shifts downward with age: at 50 years it averages 10,000 Hz, although there is great individual variation. While the high-frequency limit is well defined (the hearing threshold rises abruptly when that frequency is exceeded), threshold increases much more gradually at the lower end of the frequency scale, and sounds with frequencies below 10 Hz may be audible if they are intense. There is no evidence to indicate that exposure to sounds that are not audible can damage the ear.

Ultrasounds are heavily attenuated when transmitted in air and therefore decrease rapidly in intensity with distance from the source. Although very high intensities of ultrasound can kill furred animals such as mice, rats, and guinea pigs because of the buildup of heat by sound absorption in the fur, such an effect could not occur in humans because bare skin cannot absorb enough energy to cause damage.

Exposure to low-frequency sounds (infrasounds) of high intensity has lately been reported to cause various diffuse symptoms such as headache, nausea, and fatigue. Although few controlled studies have been conducted, it is possible that exposure to such sounds may have some effect on general bodily functions. The results of some recent experiments indicate that infrasounds may *decrease* blood pressure, possibly through stimulation of the vestibular part of the inner ear. However, there is no evidence that such sounds can be hazardous to hearing.

REFERENCES

1. Price GR, Kim HN, Lim DJ, Dunn D: Hazard from weapons impulses: Histological and electrophysiological evidence. J Acoust Soc Am 85:1245–1254, 1989
2. Burns W, Robinson DW: Hearing and Noise in Industry. London, Her Majesty's Stationery Office, 1970, p 241
3. Borg E, Møller AR: Noise and blood pressure: Effects of lifelong exposure in the rat. Acta Physiol Scand (Stockh) 103:340–342, 1978
4. Borg E: Noise, hearing, and hypertension. Scand Audiol (Stockh) 10:125–126, 1981*a*
5. Jonsson A, Hansson L: Prolonged exposure to a stressful stimulus (noise) as a cause of raised blood pressure in man. Lancet 1:86–87, 1977
6. Axelsson A, Borg E, Hornstrand C: Noise effects on the cochlear vasculature in normotensive and spontaneously hypertensive rats. Acta Otolaryngol (Stockh) 96:215–225, 1983
7. Rajan R, Johnstone BM: Contralateral cochlear destruction mediates protection from monaural loud sound exposures through the crossed olivocochlear bundle. Hear Res 39:263–278, 1989
8. American National Standard Institute (ANSI) Standard for Audiometrics, S3.6, 1969
9. International Organization for Standardization (ISO): Assessment of Occupational Noise Exposure for Hearing Conservation Purposes. (Recommendation R1999) 1971
10. Suter AH: The development of federal noise standards and damage risk criteria. In Lipscomb DM (ed): Hearing Conservation in Industry, Schools, and the Military. London: Taylor & Francis Publishing Co., 1988, pp 45–66
11. Kryter KD: Impairment to hearing from exposure to noise. J Acoust Soc Am 53:1211–1234, 1973
12. Møller AR: Noise as a health hazard. Ambio 4:6–13, 1975
13. American Academy of Ophthalmology and Otolaryngology (AAOO), Committee on Conservative of Hearing: Guide for Evaluation of Hearing Impairment, 1959
14. American Academy of Ophthalmology and Otolaryngology (AAOO): Guide for Conservation of Hearing in Noise (rev. ed). Rochester, Minnesota: Trans Am Acad Ophthalmol Otolaryngol (suppl), 1973
15. National Institute for Occupational Safety and Health (NIOSH) Criteria for a Recommended Standard: Occupational Exposure to Noise. Publication No. HSM 73-11001, 1972
16. Environmental Protection Agency (EPA): Testimony of Alvin F. Meyer, Jr. at the public hearings on proposed standards for occupational exposure to noise (submitted to U.S. Department of Labor, Occupational Safety and Health Administration as Exhibit 57 in docket OSH-011), 1973
17. Suter AH: The ability of mildly hearing impaired individuals to discriminate speech in noise. Washington, D.C.: U.S. Environmental Protection Agency (EPA #550/9–78–100) and U.S. Air Force (#AMRL-TR-78-4) reports, 1978
18. American Academy of Ophthalmology and Otolaryngology (AAOO), Committee on Hearing and Equilibrium, and the American Council of Otolaryngology, Committee on Medical Aspects of Noise: Guide for evaluation of hearing handicap. JAMA 241:2055–2059, 1979
19. Suter A: Essentials of noise regulations. Otolaryngol Clin North Am 21(3):551–562, 1979
20. Occupational Safety and Health Administration (OSHA): Occupational Noise Exposure: Hearing Conservation Amendment, Final Rule. Federal Register 48:9738–9785, 1983
21. Kryter KD: Extra auditory effects of noise. In Henderson D, Hamernik RP, Dosaujh DS, Mills JHM (eds): Effects of Noise on Hearing. New York: Raven Press, 1976, pp 531–546
22. Environmental Protection Agency (EPA), Office of Noise Abatement and Control Information on Levels of Environmental Noise: Requisite to Protect Public Health and Welfare with Adequate Margin of Safety. Washington, D.C.: Environmental Protection Agency (EPA #550/9–74–004), 1974
23. Bruel PV: Noise: Do We Measure It Correctly? Naerum, Denmark: Bruel and Kjaer, 1975, p 40
24. Møller AR: Noise as a health hazard. Scand J Work Environ Health 3:73–79, 1977*a*
25. Bruce RD: The economic impact of noise control. In Cantell RW (ed): Symposium on Noise: Its Effects and Control. The Otolaryngologic Clinics of North America. Philadelphia: W.B. Saunders Co., 1979, pp 601–607
26. Erlandsson B, Hakanson H, Ivarsson A, Nilsson P: The difference in protection efficiency between earplugs and earmuffs. Scand Audiol (Stockh) 9:215–221, 1980
27. Nilsson R, Lindgren F: The effect of long term use of hearing protectors in industrial noise. Scand Audiol (Stockh) (suppl) 12:204–211, 1980
28. Edwards RG, Hauser WP, Moiseev NA, Broderson AB, Green WW: Effectiveness of earplugs as worn in the workplace. Sound Vib 12:12–20, 1978
29. Nilsson R, Liden G, Sanden A: Noise exposure and hearing impairment in the shipbuilding industry. Scand Audiol (Stockh) 6:59–68, 1977
30. Welch BL, Welch AS: Physiological Effects of Noise. New York: Plenum Press, 1970
31. Osguthorpe JD, Mills JH: Non-auditory effects of low-frequency

noise exposure in humans. Otolaryngol Head Neck Surg 90:367–370, 1982

32. Adrinkin AA: Influence of sound stimulation on the development of hypertension. Clinical and experimental results. Cor Vasa (Prague) 3:285–293, 1961
33. Peterson EA, Augenstein JS, Travis DC, et al: Noise raises blood pressure without impairing auditory sensitivity. Science 211:1450–1452, 1981
34. Borg E: Physiological and pathogenic effects of sound. Acta Otolaryngol (Stockh) (suppl) 381:1–68, 1981*b*
35. Borg E: Noise-induced hearing loss in normotensive and spontaneously hypertensive rats. Hear Res 8:117–130, 1982
36. Sanden A, Axelsson A: Comparison of cardiovascular responses in noise-resistant and noise-sensitive workers. Acta Otolaryngol (Stockh) (suppl) 377:75–100, 1981

General References

Burns W, Robinson DW (eds): Hearing and Noise in Industry. London: Her Majesty's Stationery Office, 1970

Hamernik RP, Henderson D, Salvi R (eds): New Perspectives on Noise-Induced Hearing Loss. New York: Raven Press, 1982

Kryter KD: The Effects of Noise on Man, 2 edt. New York: Academic Press, 1985

Lipscomb DM (ed): Hearing Conservation in Industry, Schools, and the Military. Boston: Little, Brown & Company, 1988

Pickles JO: Physiology of the Ear, 2 edt. New York: Academic Press, 1988

Salvi RJ, Henderson D, Hamernik RP, Colletti V: Basic and Applied Aspects on Noise-Induced Hearing Loss. New York: Plenum Press, 1985

29
Ergonomics

W. Monroe Keyserling
Thomas J. Armstrong

Ergonomics is the study of humans at work and the evaluation of the stresses that occur in the work environment and the ability of people to cope with these stresses. The goal of ergonomics is to design facilities (e.g., factories and offices), furniture, equipment, tools, and job demands to be compatible with human dimensions, capabilities, and expectations, and thus reduce stress. All work, regardless of its nature, places both physical and mental stresses on the worker. As long as these stresses are kept within reasonable limits, work performance will be satisfactory and the worker's health and well-being will be maintained. However, if stresses are excessive, undesirable outcomes may occur in the form of errors, accidents, injuries, and a decrement in health.

Ergonomics is a multidisciplinary science with four major areas of specialization:

1. *Human factors engineering* (sometimes called engineering psychology) is concerned with the information processing requirements of work. Major applications include designing displays (e.g., gauges, warning buzzers, signs, instructions) and controls to enhance performance and minimize the likelihood of error.[1-3]
2. *Anthropometry* is concerned with the measurement and statistical characterization of body size. Anthropometric data provide important information to the designers of clothing, furniture, machines, and tools.[4]
3. *Occupational biomechanics* is concerned with the mechanical properties of human tissue, particularly the response of tissue to mechanical stress. A major focus of occupational biomechanics is the prevention of overexertion disorders of the low back and upper extremities.[5]
4. *Work physiology* is concerned with the responses of the cardiovascular system, pulmonary system, and skeletal muscles to the metabolic demands of work. This discipline is concerned with the prevention of whole body and localized fatigue.[6]

The primary emphasis of this chapter is the prevention of overexertion injuries and syndromes that result from physical stressors in the work environment. The following are typical examples:

- A farm worker experiences pain in the lower back that is attributed to the awkward stooping posture required to harvest vegetables.
- A firefighter experiences fatigue and heat exhaustion because of the excessive heat and the intense physical exercise and heavy impermeable protective clothing required.
- A nurse's aide suffers a back strain when transferring a patient from a hospital bed to a wheelchair.
- A poultry worker develops numbness and tingling in the hand and fingers because of the repetitive hand motions associated with dismembering chickens.

These health problems are not the result of accidents. (An *accident* is defined as an unanticipated, sudden, and discrete event that has an undesired outcome such as property damage, injury, or death.[7]) Instead, they can be generally classified as overexertion or overuse disorders and conditions caused by performing regular and predictable work requirements of the job.

Anthropometry, biomechanics, and work physiology are the ergonomic disciplines most relevant to the development of programs for ameliorating overexertion injuries. Applications of these disciplines are presented in the following discussions. Additional information pertaining to human factors engineering can be found in the references.[1-3]

ANTHROPOMETRY

Anthropometry is concerned with measuring the size of the human body and using this information to design facilities, equipment, tools, and personal protective equipment (e.g., gloves and respirators) to accommodate the physical dimensions of the user.

As illustrated in Figure 29-1, most anthropometric design problems are not trivial because of the large variation in body dimensions within a typical work population. In this example a designer must specify the height of an overhead conveyor used to transport parts between two areas of a plant. If the conveyor is too high, short workers would not be able to load or unload parts without elevating the shoulder to an extended reach posture. On the other hand, if the conveyor is too low, tall workers could sustain head injuries from collisions with hung parts.

If it is decided that the primary goal is to avoid head injuries to tall workers, the designer must provide sufficient overhead clearance to accommodate 95% of the U.S. male population by positioning the conveyor so that the lowest point of the hung

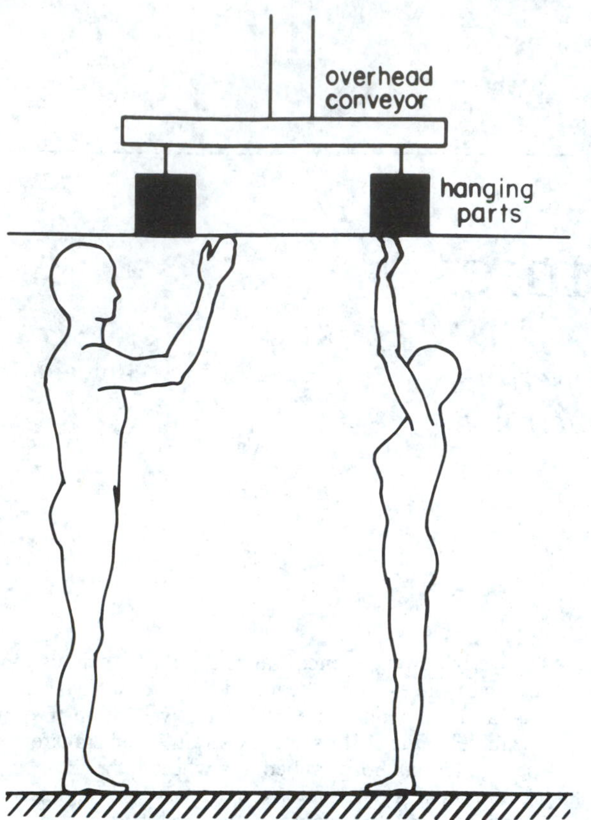

Figure 29-1. For safety reasons an overhead conveyor should be higher than the stature of a tall worker [ninety-fifth percentile male illustrated]. This can create a difficult reach for a short worker [fifth percentile female illustrated].

parts is 189.4 cm (74.6 in) above the floor. (NOTE: This dimension is computed using nude stature data for a ninety-fifth percentile male from Table 29-1 and adding 2.5 cm [1 in] as an adjustment for shoes.[8,9]) With this design a short worker (a fifth percentile female is illustrated) can reach the parts only by raising the shoulder into an elevated, awkward position, which may cause fatigue or musculoskeletal injury.[10] In this situation there is no simple solution that will simultaneously satisfy the needs of persons who are exceptionally tall or exceptionally short.

In anthropometry the characterization of body size must consider the large variations in dimensions from person to person and from population to population. Consequently, statistical methods are used to analyze body dimensions, and the results are typically reported as means and standard deviations for various body segments.[4] Extensive tables of these statistics are available in reference texts.[3,4,8,9] By assuming that dimensions follow the "normal" or "log-normal" distribution, statistical procedures can be used to compute dimensions for various percentiles of the population of interest. Table 29-1 presents a summary of useful body dimensions for anthropometric applications.

Characterization of body size is further complicated by a lack of consistency in a person's body dimensions (i.e., it is not necessarily true that a tall person will have both long legs and a long torso). Statistical procedures have been developed that can be used to predict one body dimension based on another.[4] Although many of these procedures are quite complex, a relatively simple procedure developed by Drillis and Contini[11] can be used to estimate link lengths based on a person's stature. The method uses the following formula:

$$\text{Link length} = K \times \text{Stature} \qquad (1)$$

where K is a coefficient obtained from Figure 29-2 that corresponds to the dimension of interest. Stature data from Table 29-1 and coefficients from Figure 29-2 can be used to estimate the average limb size for a given stature.

Example: Estimate the average knee height of a fifth percentile U.S. female.
Solution: First, find the stature of a fifth percentile female:

Fifth percentile female stature = 151.1 cm. (from Table 29-1)

Next, find K for knee height:

$$K_{\text{knee}} = 0.285 \text{ (from Fig. 29-2)}$$

Finally, substitute these values into Eq. (1):

$$\begin{aligned} \text{Knee height} &= 0.285 \times 151.1 \text{ cm} \\ \text{Knee height} &= 43 \text{ cm} \\ \text{Knee height (with shoes)} &= 43 \text{ cm} + 2.5 \text{ cm} \\ &= 45.5 \text{ cm (18 in)} \end{aligned}$$

Link-length data can also be used to estimate reach limits. Reach limits are important for determining where objects should be positioned so that they can be grasped without excessive body

TABLE 29-1. BODY DIMENSIONS FOR 5TH, 50TH, AND 95TH PERCENTILES OF U.S. CIVILIAN POPULATION

	U.S. Civilian Females (percentile)			U.S. Civilian Males (percentile)		
Dimension	**5th**	**50th**	**95th**	**5th**	**50th**	**95th**
Stature [cm]	151.1	161.5	172.2	163.6	175.3	186.9
Floor-knee	43.1	46.0	49.1	46.6	50.0	53.3
Floor-hip	80.1	85.6	91.3	86.7	92.9	99.1
Floor-elbow	95.2	101.7	108.5	103.1	110.4	117.7
Floor-shoulder	123.6	132.1	140.9	133.8	143.4	152.9
Floor-eye	141.4	151.2	161.2	153.1	164.1	174.9
Floor-finger	57.0	60.9	64.9	61.7	66.1	70.5
Floor-wrist	73.3	78.3	83.5	79.3	85.0	90.6
Center-shoulder	19.5	20.8	22.2	21.1	22.6	24.1
Shoulder-elbow	28.1	30.0	32.0	30.4	32.6	34.8
Elbow-wrist	22.1	23.6	25.1	23.9	25.6	27.3
Wrist-finger	16.3	17.4	18.6	17.7	18.9	20.2
Foot length	23.0	24.5	26.2	24.9	26.6	28.4
Foot breadth	8.5	9.0	9.6	9.2	9.8	10.5

Stature from NASA [8] and link lengths from Drillis and Contini.[11] See Figure 29-2 for definition of links.

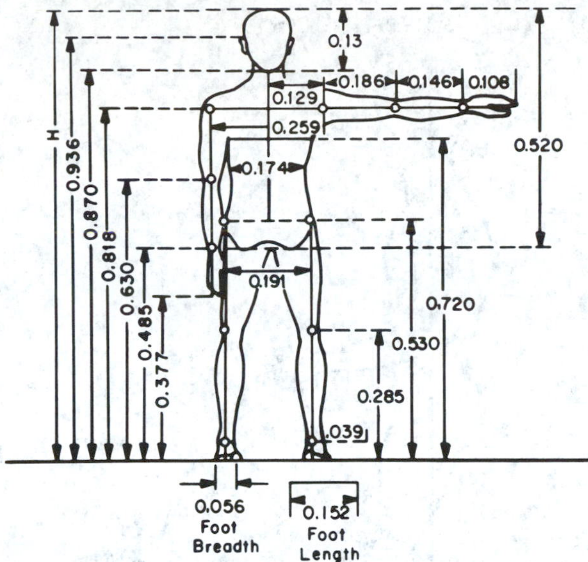

Figure 29-2. Link lengths of body segments expressed as a proportion of stature. *[From Drillis and Contini.[11]]*

motion or awkward postures. The following example demonstrates the use of link-length data to compute reach limits in the sagittal plane.

Example: Estimate the average sagittal reach limit for a fifth percentile U.S. female standing in an erect posture.
Solution: The reach limits are determined by the location of the shoulder and the length of the upper extremity measured from the shoulder to the fingertip. These dimensions are available from the link-length constants in Figure 29-2 and the U.S. female stature data in Table 29-1. First, use the Drillis and Contini method to locate the position of the shoulder:

Stature = 151.1 cm (from Table 29-1)
Shoulder height = 0.818 × 151.1 = 123.6 cm
Shoulder height (with shoes) = 123.6 cm + 2.5 cm = 126.1 cm

Next, compute the length of the arm from the shoulder to the fingertip:

Upper arm length = 0.186 ×151.1 cm = 28.1 cm
Forearm length = 0.146 ×151.1 cm = 22.1 cm
Hand length = 0.108 ×151.1 cm = 16.3 cm
Total length = Upper arm + Forearm + Hand = 66.5 cm

The average reach limits for the fifth percentile U.S. female can be estimated by drawing a 66.5 cm radius arc about a point 126.1 cm above the floor as illustrated in Figure 29-3A. Workers who are larger than the fifth percentile female (i.e., most of the working population) would have a greater reach envelope because of their longer link lengths.

Caution should be exercised when reach data are used. Excessive fatigue and soft tissue injury can result from repeated reaches to the limits of the reach envelope.[11] As a general rule, repetitive reaching should be limited to about one half the envelope. As shown in the following example, link length data can be used with postural constraints to describe a reduced reach envelope:

Example: Estimate the sagittal reach envelope of a fifth percentile U.S. female if shoulder flexion is limited to 30 degrees and if the hand remains below shoulder height.
Solution: See Figure 29-3B. The reach envelope can be estimated by first rotating the entire arm (i.e., upper arm, forearm, and hand) to a shoulder forward flexion angle of 30 degrees (i.e., 60 degrees below the horizontal). Up to this point the reach envelope is identical to the envelope shown in Figure 29-3A. Since additional shoulder flexion is prohibited by the constraints of the problem, the remaining portion of the reach envelope is determined by rotating the forearm and hand about the elbow. Finally, the maximum vertical reach is limited to 126.1 cm to keep the hand below shoulder height.

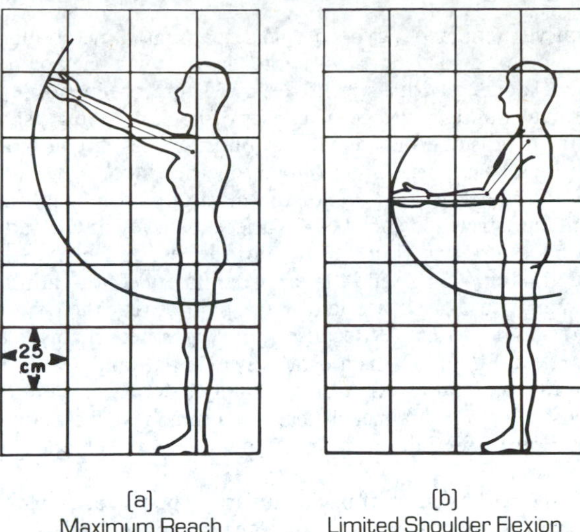

[a]
Maximum Reach

[b]
Limited Shoulder Flexion

Figure 29-3. [a] Sagittal plane reach limits of a 5th percentile female with the arm fully extended and no restrictions on shoulder elevation. [b] Reach limits with the shoulder restricted to 30 degrees forward flexion.

In the following discussion on biomechanics, several examples are presented that illustrate how awkward postures can contribute to the onset of musculoskeletal and nerve disorders. Body posture is frequently determined by the physical dimensions of a work station and the location and orientation of equipment and tools. Anthropometric methods such as the reach envelope prediction method presented in Figure 29-3 can be used during the design of work stations to avoid situations that require awkward working postures.

OCCUPATIONAL BIOMECHANICS

Biomechanics is the subdiscipline of ergonomics concerned with the mechanical properties of human tissue, particularly the resistance of tissue to mechanical stresses. Many mechanical stresses in the environment can cause *overt* injuries (e.g., a concussion when a worker is struck in the head by a dropped object). In most cases, overt injury hazards are readily recognized and can be controlled through safety engineering techniques such as machine guarding and personal protective equipment.[7] Other stresses in the environment are more subtle and can cause *cumulative* injuries and disorders. These stresses may be external (e.g., a vibrating tool that causes white finger syndrome) or internal (e.g., tension in a tendon when the attached muscle contracts). Hazards that cause cumulative injuries are frequently difficult to recognize because the health effects are not necessarily temporally correlated to exposure. Although injuries and disorders caused by cumulative stress occur in all parts of the body, the back and the upper extremities are the most commonly affected areas.

LOWER BACK PAIN

Lower back pain is a nonspecific condition that refers to complaints of acute or chronic pain and discomfort in or near the lumbosacral spine, which can be caused by inflammatory, degenerative, neoplastic, gynecological, traumatic, metabolic, and other types of disorders.[12] Most episodes of lower back pain cannot be associated with a specific lesion. Therefore in most epidemiological studies the specific causes of back pain (e.g., sprains and strains, disc herniation, facet abnormalities) are not identified since all categories are grouped together.[13]

Lower back pain is one of the most common health problems in industrialized societies. In a recent survey of U.S. adults, lower back pain was found in 14% of the respondents.[14] Studies in Scandinavia have found that approximately 80% of adults experience at least one episode of back pain during their working years (ages 18 to 65).[15] Because many episodes of lower back pain are disabling, it is the most costly occupational health problem in the United States. Approximately 2% of workers experience disabling back pain each year, resulting in workers compensation costs of $16 billion for medical services and compensation for lost time.[12]

Because the causes of back pain are so poorly understood, it is difficult to specify a treatment plan. In most episodes, people with back pain are able to cope with the problem without seeking medical treatment. Most disabling episodes resolve themselves within a 2-week period with only conservative treatment (bedrest and aspirin). Isometric abdominal exercises have also been shown to be effective as part of a conservative management strategy. Surgery should not be considered during the first 3 months unless indicated by a specific diagnosis.[16]

The following occupational risk factors are associated with the development of back pain:

1. *Forceful exertions during manual materials handling,* such as lifting, pushing, or pulling of heavy loads[17–19]
2. *Awkward trunk postures,* such as flexion, lateral bending, axial twisting, or prolonged sitting[20,21]
3. *Whole body vibration,* usually transmitted through a vibrating seat or platform[22]
4. *Repetitive or prolonged exposure* to any of the above risk factors[23]

Truck drivers experience back pain more than any other occupational group does.[23] Many truck drivers load and unload their own rigs; this activity often requires heavy lifting, sometimes combined with awkward posture (e.g., trunk flexion when they bend down to grasp an object on the floor of the trailer). Truck drivers also spend a considerable part of their workday seated and are exposed to high levels of whole-body vibration because many vehicle and seat suspension systems do not adequately isolate the driver from roadway bumps and shocks.

Other occupations at high risk for back pain include nurses and nurses aides, garbage collectors, warehouse workers, and mechanics.[24] All these occupations require heavy lifting and associated materials-handling tasks.

Lifting. Because of the hazards associated with manual lifting, the National Institute for Occupational Safety and Health (NIOSH) has issued a technical report entitled *Work Practices Guide for Manual Lifting.*[18] This document discusses the various risk factors associated with lifting and describes procedures for evaluating and classifying manual tasks to keep metabolic and L5/S1 disk compressive loads within acceptable limits.

To use the NIOSH guide, it is necessary to measure six task variables:

1. Object weight (*L*): measured in kilograms.
2. Horizontal location (*H*): the location of the object's center of gravity measured in the sagittal plane midway between the ankles. (To simplify measurements the body centerline is assumed to be the midpoint of the line joining the ankles, as illustrated in Figure 29–4.) This is measured in centimeters.

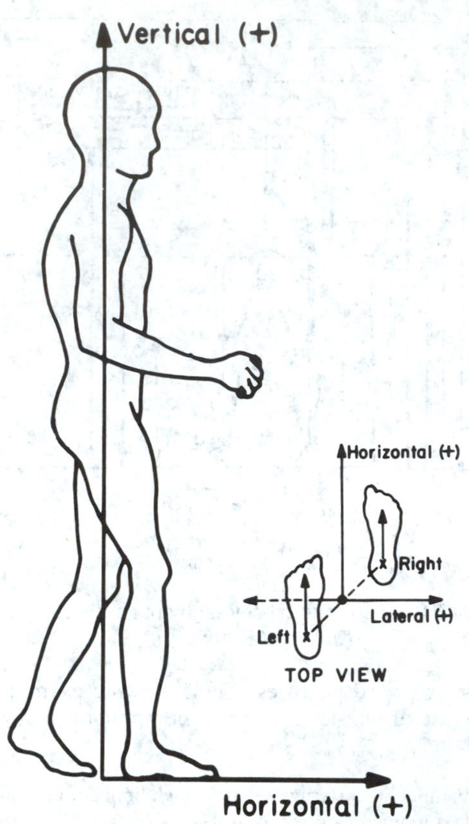

Figure 29–4. Horizontal and vertical locations of the hands when using the NIOSH Work Practices Guide for Manual Lifting. *[From NIOSH.[18]]*

3. Vertical location (*V*): the location of the hands at the origin of the lift, measured vertically from the floor or working surface in centimeters. See Figure 29–4.
4. Lift distance (*D*): the vertical displacement of the object (origin to destination) over the course of the lift, measured in centimeters.
5. Frequency of lifting (*F*): the number of lifts per minute, averaged over the time that manual lifting is performed.
6. Duration of lifting: classified as *occasional* if lifting activities can be performed in less than 1 hour or *continuous* if the duration of lifting exceeds 1 hour.

These variables are substituted into an equation (discussed below), which is used to compute an *acceptable lift* (AL) and a *maximum permissible lift* (MPL). After the AL and the MPL are computed, the job can be classified into one of three risk categories:

1. *Acceptable:* If the weight of the lifted object is less than the AL, the job is classified as acceptable. This means that most members of the U.S. workforce could perform the job with only a nominal risk of injury.
2. *Administrative controls required:* If the weight of the object falls between the AL and MPL, the job is assigned to this category, which means that some members of the workforce would have difficulty performing the lift (because of limited strength) or would be at increased risk of injury. Action must be taken to protect these individuals, such as redesigning the job so that it would fall into the "acceptable" category or implementing administrative procedures such as employee selection or training.

3. *Hazardous:* If the lifted object weighs more than the MPL, the job is classified as hazardous. This means that most members of the workforce would be at a substantial risk of injury if they were required to perform this job. The only acceptable approach to resolving this situation is job redesign to eliminate lifting stresses or reducing these stresses to acceptable levels.

The acceptable lift is computed using the following formula:

$$AL = 40\,kg \times HF \times VF \times DF \times FF \qquad (2)$$

where

HF is the *horizontal factor* computed as $(15/H)$, where H is the horizontal location (defined above). In general, H is never less than 15 cm because of body interference or greater than 80 cm because of reach limitations.
VF is the *vertical factor* computed as $[1 - (.004 \times |V - 75|)]$, where V is the vertical location (defined above). In general, V is never less than 0 (floor level) or greater than 175 cm (the reach limit for most people).
DF is the *distance factor* computed as $[0.7 + (7.5/D)]$, where D is the lift distance (defined above). The DF is never greater than 1.0. If the computed DF is greater than 1, it should be set to 1.0.
FF is the *frequency factor* defined as $[1 - (F/M)]$, where F is the frequency of lifting (defined above) and M is the maximum frequency that can be sustained. Values for M are presented in Table 29-2. For lifts that occur less than once every 5 minutes, the FF should be set to 1.0.

Once the acceptable lift (AL) has been determined, the maximum permissible lift (MPL) is computed using the following formula:

$$MPL = 3 \times AL \qquad (3)$$

For additional information on measurements and computations, including examples, refer to reference 18.

The most effective way for reducing back injuries and disorders associated with manual lifting is to implement engineering controls (e.g., changes in equipment, work station layout, work methods) to reduce exposure to the risk factors discussed above. Possible approaches are briefly outlined below:

1. Can the weight of an object be reduced? For example, is it possible to put fewer parts in a tote pan or to resize bags containing bulk materials such as powdered chemicals?
2. If the weight of the load cannot be reduced, can a mechanical assist (e.g., hoist, conveyor, articulating arm) be provided to reduce the forces exerted by workers?
3. Can low reaches be eliminated by delivering objects to the worker at knee height or above? Can a lift table be installed to allow the worker to pick up objects without trunk flexion?
4. Can horizontal reach distances be reduced by eliminating or relocating barriers that prevent workers from getting as close to the object as safely as possible before they start the lift? Forward reaches should be easily accomplished with only the arms and should require no trunk flexion.

TABLE 29-2. MAXIMUM LIFTING FREQUENCY (*M*) WITH THE *NIOSH WORK PRACTICES GUIDE FOR MANUAL LIFTING*[18]

	Vertical Location (V) of Lift	
Work Duration	**(>75 cm)**	**(<75 cm)**
Less than 60 min	18	15
60–480 min	15	12

5. Can a rotation schedule be developed that allows workers to alternate between jobs with heavy lifting requirements and jobs with insignificant lifting requirements? This reduces the cumulative exposure to lifting stresses.

If engineering changes do not bring the job within the acceptable zone defined by NIOSH, administrative controls should be implemented. One technique currently available to evaluate a person's ability to perform strenuous work is strength testing. Several studies have shown that strength tests that accurately simulate a job can be used to achieve an effective job-employee match and to reduce back injuries.[25,26] Strength testing and other administrative procedures should not be used, however, unless it has been proved that engineering controls are not feasible.

Awkward Posture. Frequently, workers complain of musculoskeletal pains and disorders that can be attributed to the uncomfortable or unnatural postures required by their jobs. Often these problems are caused by work station designs improperly matched to the size of the worker or to the task he or she is required to perform.

Awkward trunk posture during work activities can be caused by poor work station layout. The neutral position of the trunk occurs when it is in a vertical upright position with no axial twisting. Trunk flexion (forward bending in the sagittal plane) can usually be attributed to one of two causes: (1) reaching down to grasp an object lower than the level of the hands when a person is standing erect with the arms hanging in a relaxed vertical position or (2) reaching forward to grasp an object that is too far in front of the body. Lateral bending (in the frontal plane) and axial twisting are usually associated with reaching for objects either to the side of or behind a worker's body. Laboratory and field studies have shown that these nonneutral postures are associated with local muscle fatigue and excessive rates of back pain.[18,27–29] A good way to prevent awkward trunk postures is to locate all items that must be touched or grasped within the reach limits shown in Figure 29–3B.

Because working posture is a function of an individual's anthropometry, a work station layout that is good for one person may not be appropriate for workers who are considerably larger or smaller. For this reason, adjustability should be incorporated into the work station wherever possible.

Seated Work. Because of the rapid growth of service and information industries and technological advances in manufacturing methods, an increasing number of workers are spending a major fraction of their workday in a seated posture. Sitting provides many ergonomic benefits, such as a reduction in the amount of body weight borne by the tissues of the feet and lower extremities, a reduction in whole-body energy expenditure because of decreased muscle activity, and stabilization of the body for tasks that require precise manual dexterity. The primary disadvantage of sitting is increased stress on the spine.[5]

Clinical and epidemiological studies have shown that prolonged sitting is associated with increased rates of lower back pain.[20,30] A possible explanation is that when a person moves from a standing to a sitting posture, the pelvis rotates backward, flattening the normal lordotic curve of the lower spine.[31,32] This flattening compresses the anterior portion of the disc, increases intradiscal pressure, and places tension on the exterior portion of the disc, on the apophyseal joint ligaments, and on the erector spinae muscles.[33,34] These stresses affect the supply of nutrients to the disc and surrounding tissue and may be related to the development of back disorders.

Spinal stresses associated with sitting are affected by the design of the chair. An important design consideration is the angle between the backrest and the seat pan. As this angle is increased, pelvic rotation and lumbar flattening is reduced.[28] This can be accomplished by tilting the seat pan forward to create a sit-stand

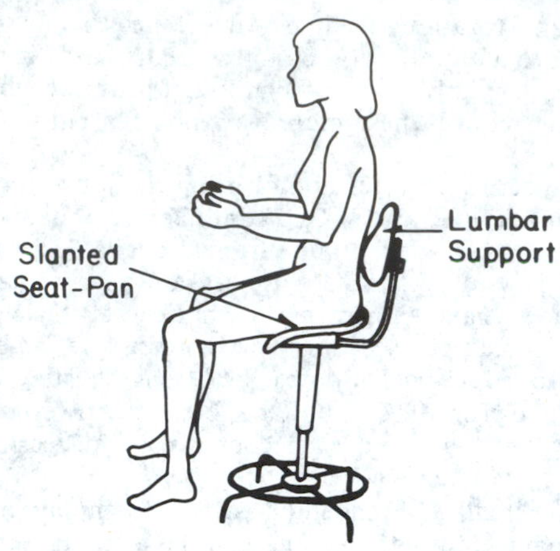

Figure 29-5. Work chair with a forward sloping seatpan and a backrest lumbar support. *[From Yu C, Keyserling WM: Appl Ergonomics 20:17–25, 1989.]*

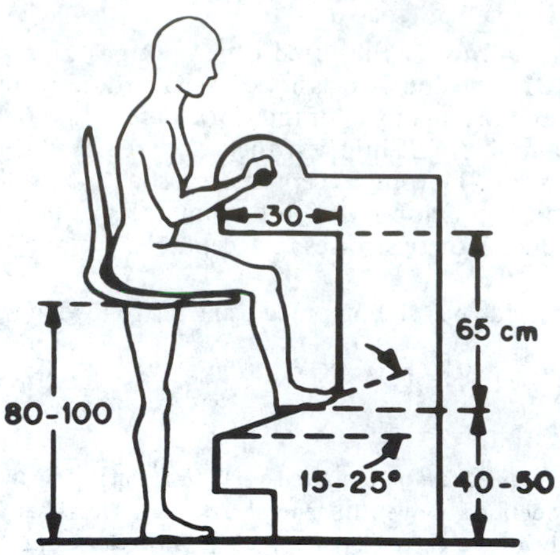

Figure 29-6. Example of a workbench and seat configuration that permits a worker to alternate between standing and sitting. *[From Grandjean E: Fitting the Task to the Man—An Ergonomic Approach. London: Taylor and Francis, 1980.]*

posture as illustrated in Figure 29–5 or by rotating the backrest in a rearward direction from the vertical. Jobs that require the worker to lean forward while sitting (e.g., sewing, many bench assembly tasks, microscope work) should have forward-slanting seat pans. A recent field study of full-time sewing machine operators found that comfort was enhanced and fatigue reduced by tilting the seat pan to slant forward at an angle 15 degrees below the horizontal.[35] Furthermore, laboratory experiments have demonstrated that intradiscal pressures can be reduced up to 50% by increasing the included angle between the seatpan and backrest from 90 to 110 degrees.[28] Adding a lumbar support to the backrest also reduces intradiscal pressure.[28]

The height and shape of the seatpan are also important considerations in chair design. If the seat is too high, the worker's feet dangle, causing pressure on the underside of the thigh. This can interfere with circulation and cause swelling in the feet and lower legs. If the seat is too low, the thighs do not make good contact with the seat pan, and an excessive amount of body weight will be borne by the ischial tuberosities and surrounding tissue. This may cause considerable discomfort, particularly if the person is sitting on an unpadded seat or is sitting for a prolonged period. To accommodate the range of body sizes found in the working population, it is suggested that seat height be adjustable between 38 and 53 cm, measured from the floor to the front of the seatpan.[36] This adjustment should be easy to perform and not require any special tools. Ease of adjustment is particularly important if the chair is used by more than one person (e.g., where the same work station is used by both day-shift and night-shift workers).

Where feasible, the seat and the associated work area should be designed to avoid prolonged static postures.[37] This concept is shown in Figure 29–6. At this work station the seat and work bench are designed to allow the user to alternate between standing and sitting postures at will. (NOTE: the dimensions in Figure 29–6 show the ranges of adjustability required to accommodate the various body sizes found in the population.)

Another method for preventing prolonged sitting is to modify the job description to include occasional tasks that must be performed away from the primary work station. This allows the worker to periodically stand up and walk during the shift.

In the selection or design of a work seat it is important to match the characteristics of the chair to the requirements of the job. For example, workers who must periodically reach behind or to the side of the body typically prefer seat pans that swivel, and workers who perform precision assembly tasks prefer stable seat pans.[38]

CUMULATIVE TRAUMA DISORDERS OF UPPER LIMB

Cumulative trauma disorders is a term used to refer to a family of chronic muscle, tendon, and nerve-related disorders caused, precipitated, or aggravated by repeated or sustained exertions of the upper limb.[39–41] Although these disorders can occur anywhere in the body, the upper limb is one of the most common sites. Examples of these disorders include myalgia, tendinitis, bursitis, and carpal tunnel syndrome. These disorders may cause significant pain, impairment, and disability, but they often go unreported out of ignorance or fear. These disorders also may be episodic and poorly localized, making it difficult to distinguish them from normal fatigue or to determine exactly when and where they occur.

One of the earliest references to these disorders is that of Bernardino Ramazzini,[42] who in 1713 attributed "diseases reaped by certain workers" to "violent and irregular motions and unnatural postures." Gray[43] in 1893 described "washerwomen's sprain," which is commonly referred to as de Quervain's disease or tendinitis of the extrinsic abductor and extensor muscles of the thumb near the radial styloid process.[44]

Morbidity. Insurance claims for tendinitis were recorded in the early twentieth century. For example, Zollinger[45] reported 929 cases of crepitant tenosynovitis attributed to repeated strain from Swiss insurance records in 1927. More recently, Jensen et al.[46] reported that 6% of workers' compensation reports from 26 states were related to inflammation or irritation of the joints, tendons, muscles, or nerves.

Occupational activities often are cited as a cause of these problems in clinical case series from both industrial and nonindustrial clinics. For example, Pozner[47] reported a sudden outbreak of acute tenosynovitis in soldiers assigned to agricultural work in 1942. In a 1947 report of six cases of median nerve compression in the carpal tunnel, Brain et al.[48] concluded, "There can be little doubt that occupation is a causal factor." Hymovich and Lindholm[49] reported 66 disorders associated with repetitive motion in an electronics assembly firm, which was a rate of 6.6 cases per 100 workers per year. More recently, Masear et al.[50] reported an unusually high incidence, 14.8%, of carpal tunnel syndrome among workers at a meat processing plant versus less than 1% in the general population. Similar clinical findings have been reported by other investigators.

Since the passage of the 1970 Occupational Safety and Health Act (OSHA),[51] employers are required to maintain a record of all cumulative trauma disorders or "disorders associated with repeated trauma. Examples include: . . . synovitis, tenosynovitis, and bursitis; Raynaud's phenomenon; and other conditions due to repeated motion, vibration, and pressure."[52]

The U.S. Department of Labor uses such records for determining if employers are in compliance with the general duty clause of OSHA, which requires that "Each employer shall furnish to each of his employees employment and a place of employment which are free from recognized hazards that are likely to cause death or serious physical harm to his employees."[51]

Employers are expected to monitor the incidence of cumulative trauma disorders and intervene when new cases and high-incidence jobs are identified.

Although workers' compensation reports, clinical case reports, and OSHA records show that many workers are afflicted with cumulative trauma disorders, these records probably underestimate the actual number. A study by Fine et al.[53] of two automobile assembly plants found that personal absences and plant medical visits outnumbered OSHA and compensation records by as much as 100 to 1.

In summary, the overall incidence and severity of various cumulative trauma disorders in the United States are not yet available. The available data, however, suggest that despite significant underreporting, these disorders are still a major cause of impairment and work disability.

Risk Factors. A review of the possible causes of upper extremity cumulative trauma disorders and the arguments for and against each are beyond the scope of this chapter. Instead, the discussion will focus on how the available information can be used in applied studies for control of cumulative trauma disorders. Risk factors can be classified as occupational or nonoccupational; the relative contribution of each risk factor appears to vary significantly from one situation to another. For example, carpal tunnel syndrome has been reported as a side effect of oral contraceptives in groups of childbearing women.[54] In a study of cumulative trauma disorders and worker and work factors, however, repetitive and forceful exertions were found to be the most significant causes of carpal tunnel syndrome, whereas oral contraceptive use was not a significant finding.[55] In yet another study, vibrating tools and gynecological surgery were significant factors.[56] All possible factors should be considered in each individual case and work setting.

Individual Risk Factors. Commonly cited individual risk factors include age, female gender, acute trauma, rheumatoid arthritis, diabetes mellitus, hormonal factors, wrist size or shape, and vitamin deficiency.[57] These factors should be evaluated as possible causes in each case or work situation. It has not yet been shown that worker selection based on the presence or absence of personal factors results in a significant reduction in the incidence of cumulative trauma disorders in the work place. Attempts to use these factors for worker selection or screening should be regarded as experimental and must include appropriate safeguards of individual risks and rights. It may be advisable to monitor workers with recognized personal risk factors and to even counsel these people in regard to the potential risks.

Occupational Risk Factors. The following occupational risk factors are commonly cited[2,57–59]:

- Repetitive or sustained exertions
- Forceful exertions
- Certain wrist postures
  Ulnar deviation of the wrist
  Wrist flexion or hyperextension
  Forearm and shoulder postures
  Extreme reaching
- Localized mechanical stresses
- Low temperatures
- Vibration

These factors are not unique to one particular industry, occupation, or job but can be found to varying degrees in all jobs and can thus be referred to as "generic" factors or ergonomic stresses. In some cases it is possible to measure these factors on ratio scales, but since continuous dose-response models have not yet been developed, these measurements should be regarded as nominal and ordinal.[60] This makes it possible to identify the least and most stressful jobs in terms of generic risk factors. These rankings can be used to select job designs that minimize ergonomic stress. Combining ergonomic job analysis with health surveillance should make it possible to identify affected workers and to perfect interventions to minimize risk of upper limb disorders. A schematic of this process for the control of cumulative trauma disorders is shown in Figure 29–7.

Surveillance. Health surveillance may include both passive and active forms. Passive surveillance includes the monitoring of medical visits, insurance claims, and OSHA logs.[53,59–61] Evidence cited previously suggests that the fidelity of passive surveillance may be highly variable from one situation to another. If the accuracy of the passive data in a given situation is doubted, it should be verified by active surveillance.[59,62–65] Active surveillance includes health interviews and physical examinations. Active surveillance can be viewed as analogous to monitoring the biological burden of environmental contaminants.

Sample passive surveillance data from an instrument assembly company are illustrated in Table 29–3. This plant, employing 114 production workers and 581 office workers, experienced 18 upper limb cumulative trauma disorders in a 6-month period. Each of these cases was investigated for possible personal and work-related causes when initially reported. In addition, case totals by department were tabulated. After 6 months, two manufacturing departments, assembly areas II and V, emerged with the largest number of cases. Further analysis of these data by incidence rate indicates that the risk of cumulative trauma disorders is much greater in area II than in area V.

Relative risk and attributable risk statistics provide insight into how much the risk is increased by factors associated with a given area and how many cases might be prevented by a completely effective control program.[59,61,66] The ideal comparison

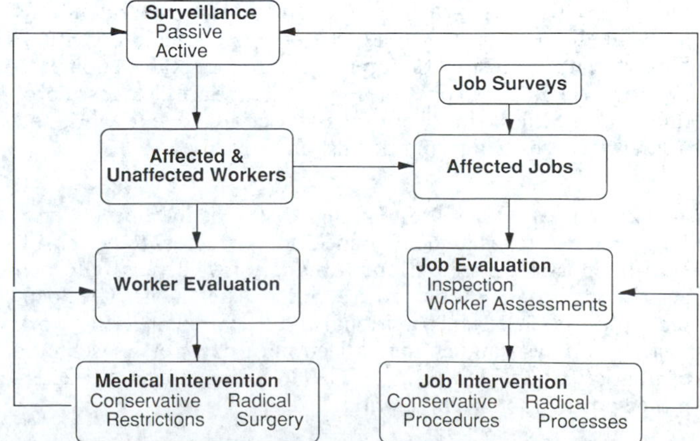

Figure 29–7. A comprehensive program for control of cumulative trauma disorders includes surveillance, job analysis, medical and work interventions and evaluation of interventions.

TABLE 29-3. CUMULATIVE TRAUMA CASE REPORTS FOR 6-MONTH PERIOD AT INSTRUMENT ENGINEERING AND MANUFACTURING PLANT

Dept.	Population	Cases	Incidence[a]	Rel.[b] Risk	Attrib.[c] Risk
1	13	0	0.0	**	**
2	12	4	66.7	44.5	65.2
3	23	0	0.0	**	**
4	23	1	8.7	5.8	7.2
5	39	4	20.5	13.7	19.0
6	4	1	50.0	33.3	48.5
Total	114	10	17.5	11.7	16.0
▪ **KEYING**					
<4 h/d	133	1	1.5	1.0	0.0
4–6 h/d	253	2	1.6	1.1	0.1
>6 h/d	195	5	5.1	3.4	3.6
Total keying	581	8	2.8		

[a] Cases per 100 workers per year.
[b] Relative risk with respect to keying <4 h/d.
[c] Attributable risk with respect to keying <4 h/d.

department is a large, stable age-and gender-matched population that does not perform handwork so that the incidence of upper limb disorders can be fully attributed to nonwork factors. It is difficult to find a large group of workers who do not perform any handwork. Therefore the comparison population should be the one with minimal exposure to generic risk factors. In the example shown in Table 29-3 the 133 persons who perform keying for less than 4 hours a day are the best comparison population. With these measures, area II has the highest relative and attributable risks, but area V also is elevated and merits attention. Although the relative risk and attributable risk are zero for some departments, it should not be concluded that the long-term incidence rate is zero. Even for a relatively high incidence rate of 10 cases per 100 workers per year, the expected number of cases in assembly areas I and III would be 0.65 and 1.15 cases during this 6-month period. The absence of cases in these departments is not outside of the range of normal statistical variation. Therefore continued surveillance is warranted.

Formal statistical procedures are available for these analyses, but they often are limited by statistical power and available sample sizes.[66] For example, a case control study designed to have an 80% chance of finding a difference between one population with a 10% incidence rate and a second population with a 20% incidence rate with a 5% chance of a type I error would require 196 persons in each group.[66] In addition, several months are generally required to assess the effects of the intervention. Unfortunately, most work populations are not stable enough to rigorously evaluate all possible factors. There are changes in production schedules, turnover in the work force due to work and nonwork causes, plant shut downs, and so on.

Job Analysis. Once cases and high-risk jobs have been identified, the next step is to identify specific risk factors to be considered for possible intervention. Job analysis is divided into two activities: documentation and ergonomic assessment. The documentation is based on traditional industrial engineering work methods analysis and entails collection of data for a systematic evaluation of the job.[41,59,67,68] The following items are determined during job documentation:

Objective. why the job is performed.

Standard. the production quantity and quality expectations.

Staffing. the number of persons performing the job.

Method. the steps required to perform each task.

Work station layout. blueprints or a sketch of the work place with dimensions that can be used to determine reach distances.

Materials. parts and substances used in the production process.

Tools. devices used to accomplish the work objective.

Environment. where the work is performed and surrounding conditions.

Ergonomic Assessment. The ergonomic assessment entails characterization of stresses that may contribute to a cumulative trauma disorder. This discussion will focus on identification and measurement of stresses at nominal and ordinal levels.

Repeated and Sustained Exertions. The number of exertions per hour or shift can be estimated from the work standard and methods analysis. Rankings of stress should be adjusted upward if workers have difficulty keeping up with an assembly line, making production quotas, or meeting deadlines. Rankings should be adjusted downward if workers frequently can pause briefly while waiting for equipment or materials.

Forceful Exertions. Forces can be identified by inspecting the work methods for steps that involve resisting gravity, finishing surfaces (e.g., grinding, polishing, or trimming), or reaction forces (using a manual or powered tool to tighten a screw or nut). Force requirements of each step may be rank ordered based on the following:

- The magnitude of weight, resistance, and reaction forces
- Friction
- Balance (well-balanced tools require lower exertions than poorly balanced tools)
- Posture (pinch grips require more exertion than power grips do)
- Pace
- Gloves

Jobs that require workers to get, hold, or use a heavy object should be ranked as more forceful than ones that require workers to get, hold, or use a light part in the same way. The ranking may be adjusted upward if objects or glove surfaces are slippery or if objects are poorly balanced or supported with the ends of the fingers. Rankings also should be increased for rapid moves or if stiff or bulky gloves are used.

Posture Stresses. Stressful postures can be identified by inspecting work elements for steps that involve repeated or sustained maximum reach, elevation of the elbows, reaching behind the torso, full elbow flexion, full forearm rotation, wrist deviation (side to side), wrist flexion, full wrist extension, or a pinch grip (Fig. 29-8). Posture analysis may be performed by directly observing the job or by observing videotapes played back in slow motion.[58,69] Also, it often is possible to predict posture on the basis of the work station design and tool specifications.[57,58] Posture stress rankings should be increased as deviation from neutral positions, duration, and frequency increase.

Localized Mechanical Stresses. Stresses can be identified by inspecting work methods for steps that involve contact of the body with external objects. Edges of the external objects that are hard, sharp, or otherwise unsuitable for supporting the body should be documented. Rankings should be adjusted upward for hard and sharp contact surfaces and for high contact forces.

Low Temperature. Exposure to low temperatures can be identified by inspecting work methods for steps that result in exposure to cold air, tools, or materials. Rankings may be based on tem-

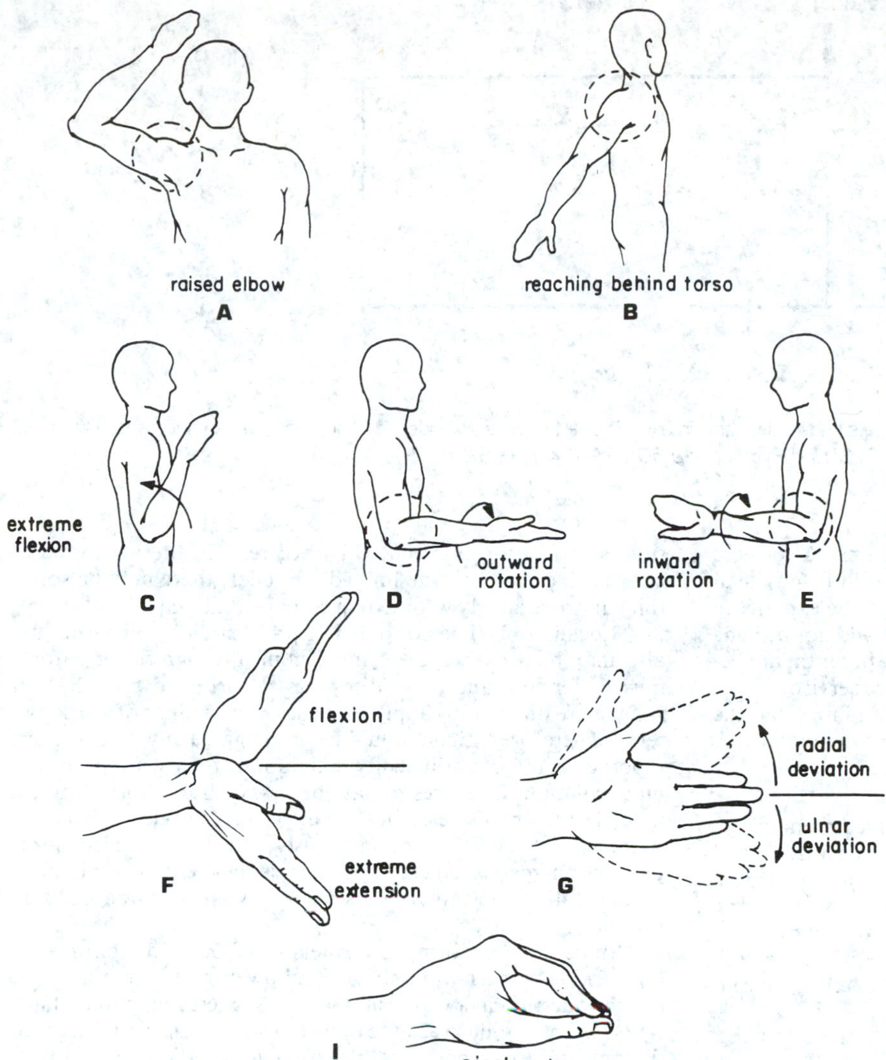

Figure 29-8. Stressful postures for prolonged or repeated exertions. *[From Armstrong TJ. In Corlett N, Wilson J, Manenica I (eds): The Ergonomics of Working Postures. London: Taylor and Francis, 1986.]*

perature but should be adjusted for thermal conductivity and protective equipment. It may also be necessary to adjust rankings for clothing since finger skin temperature is affected by the body core temperature.

Vibration Exposure. Vibration exposure can be identified by inspecting the work methods for steps that involve the use of stationary or hand-held power tools, impact tools, or controls connected to vibrating equipment. Instrumentation is available for quantitative vibration measurements. In the absence of proper instrumentation, rankings may be based on the duration or frequency of contact with vibrating objects. For example, a grinding or buffing job would probably be rated higher in terms of vibration stress than an assembly job that requires periodic use of a power wrench.

Assessment of ergonomic stresses may be supplemented by worker interviews. Interviews should be carefully designed to avoid suggesting to workers how they should feel. Also it is important that all workers be asked the same question. One way of doing this is through the use of surveys in which workers rate discomfort or perceived exertion.[70-72] An example of a survey in which a visual analogue scale was used to assess the weights used in an automobile trim shop is shown in Figure 29-9.[73] These data show a significant increase in ratings toward "too heavy" as the tool mass increases above 2 kg. It cannot be said that workers will not develop a cumulative trauma disorder if they use tools that weigh less than 2 kg, but in the absence of better data, worker ratings may be used as a design or selection benchmark. Designing lifting tasks to match acceptable levels of perceived exertion has been reported to reduce the risk of back disorders from overexertion.[74-76] While this has not been shown for upper limb disorders, it is a tenable hypothesis.

Intervention. Work elements ranked high in terms of ergonomic stresses should be redesigned to minimize those stresses. Possible strategies may focus on the redesign or modification of methods, tools, work stations, and production processes. Worker training may also be considered, but most ergonomic stresses are determined by the work requirements and cannot be reduced through training. Worker training has not been shown to be an effective way of reducing risk of cumulative trauma disorders. Details of ergonomic interventions to reduce generic stresses have been described elsewhere.[41,59,77,78]

Evaluation of Control Measures. There are as yet no specification standards for acceptable ergonomic stresses. Therefore it is necessary to evaluate interventions to ascertain their effectiveness. Evaluation may be accomplished through reanalysis of the job, measurement of localized discomfort or exertion, and ongoing surveillance of health data.

Management of Restricted Workers. It is unrealistic to expect to prevent all cumulative trauma disorders in the work place. The causes of these multifactorial problems are not yet un-

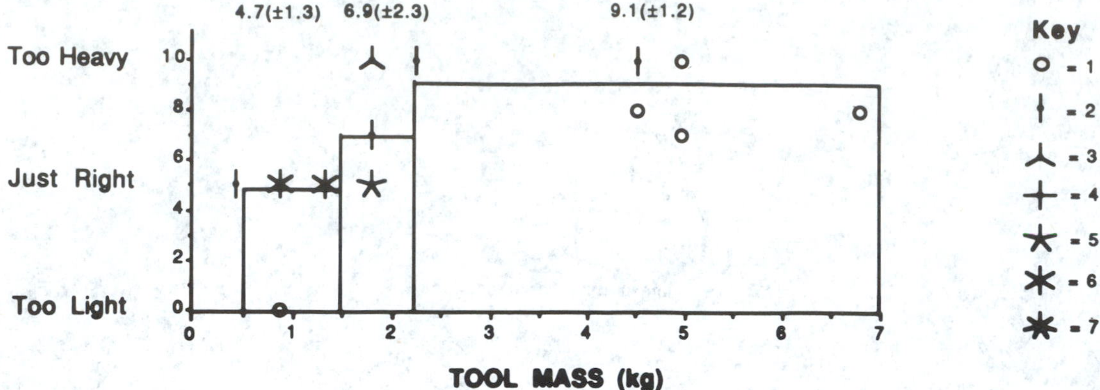

Figure 29-9. Ratings of 33 tools by 23 workers show that tools in excess of 2 kg were considered "too heavy" in an automobile trim shop. *(From Armstrong TJ, Punnett L, Ketner P: Am Ind Hyg Assoc J 50:639–645, 1989.)*

derstood well enough to design jobs with zero risk. Also there probably will continue to be some cases because of individual risk factors. It is necessary to provide for people who experience these impairments of the upper limb so that they do not become long-term disability cases. The details of such a program are beyond the scope of this chapter. The worker, supervisor, engineer, and physician must cooperate to determine what the worker can do and to find or modify jobs to accommodate any limitations.[79-81]

The Ergonomics Team. Control of cumulative trauma disorders involves health professionals, supervisors, engineers, and workers. Thus an ergonomics program is best managed by a team comprised of persons from each of these areas.[59,79,82] The team should meet regularly to review health data and new and old cases, set goals, recommend allocation of resources to control ergonomic stresses, and review the progress of ergonomic interventions.

WORK PHYSIOLOGY

Fatigue. Basmajian and Deluca[83] describe fatigue as a process that results in physiological, psychological, and mechanical alterations that if carried too far will result in failure to maintain desired work performance. Fatigue can be divided into "local" and "whole-body" categories. Localized fatigue is a process that occurs in the affected tissues. For example, holding a suitcase fatigues the muscles, tendons, and ligaments of the upper limb. If the suitcase is heavy enough or is held long enough, the person holding it will experience pain and trembling and will ultimately let go. Whole-body fatigue refers to processes that occur in many tissues at once. For example, shoveling challenges not only the muscles, tendons, and ligaments of the upper limb but also the tissues of the lower limbs and back and the cardiopulmonary system. If the scoops are heavy enough or if the task is performed long enough, the person shoveling will experience pain in one or more areas and elevated heart and ventilation rates. Ultimately the shoveler will slow down or stop.

Localized Fatigue. Localized fatigue can be distinguished from other effects in that it is completely reversible and in that the time required for development and recovery is generally less than 24 hours. Also, there is a direct cause and effect relationship between the work activity and the symptoms. Altering the work activity will generally provide prompt relief. For example, a seated operator usually gets relief from stretching, changing seat position, standing up, or from a night of rest. If altering the work activity does not provide immediate relief, there may be something more seriously wrong than so-called fatigue.

Localized fatigue not only is a problem in its own right but also may be a harbinger of more clinically significant chronic muscle, tendon, and nerve disorders.[10,84] Predictive models for fatigue are difficult to apply because of variability of work patterns. Therefore fatigue should be investigated any time workers report discomfort or difficulty maintaining their work pace. The most common measures of fatigue assess discomfort patterns, perceived exertion, electrical changes in muscle activity, or tremor.[37,83,84] This discussion focuses primarily on discomfort patterns and perceived exertion because they require minimal instrumentation and should be useful to anyone with nominal clinical skills.

In its simplest form, assessment of effort or discomfort entails asking workers how they feel; however, it is important to ask the question in a way that does not suggest they should hurt. It also is important to ask the question so that the actual areas of discomfort can be identified. Several scales and procedures have been suggested and used for this purpose. One such scale is the Borg scale, on which ten verbal anchor points are arranged in a geometric progression on a 14-point scale.[70] Borg showed that this scale of perceived exertion had a high correlation with heart rate in persons exercising on a treadmill. The 14-point scale corresponded to the change in heart rates from 50 to 190 beats per minute. Borg later adjusted this scale from 0 to 10 points as shown in Table 29-4.

Another way to query a worker is with a visual analogue scale. Visual analogue scales are lines with verbal anchor points at various locations.[71,72,84] The subjects place a check at the location on the line that corresponds to the level of their perceived discomfort or effort (Table 29-4). Studies by Harms-Ringdahl[84] found subject ratings of elbow pain using the 10-point Borg scale and a visual analogue scale agreed favorably. As a practical matter, the visual analogue scale may be the easiest to use in work settings, where subjects do not have time to read and contemplate all the verbal anchor points.

Another method of assessing localized fatigue was described by Corlett and Bishop[85] in an intervention study of localized fatigue among spot welders. These investigators introduced the use of a "body part discomfort diagram," a silhouette of the body divided into 12 sectors. Subjects were first asked to indicate their overall feeling by drawing a mark on a seven-point visual analogue scale. Next they were asked to identify areas of discomfort on the "body part discomfort diagram." Finally they were asked to rank the areas of discomfort. In this way it was possible to identify consistent areas of worker discomfort that corre-

TABLE 29-4. BORG AND VISUAL ANALOGUE SCALES USED TO MEASURE PERCEIVED EXERTION AND DISCOMFORT

▪ **BORG SCALE[70]**

0	Nothing at all
0.5	Very, very weak (just noticeable)
1	Very weak
2	Fairly weak
3	Moderate
4	Somewhat strong
5	Strong
6	
7	Very strong
8	
9	
10	Very, very strong (almost maximal) Maximal

▪ **VISUAL ANALOGUE SCALE[71]**

|____|

Very Uncomfortable Work — Very comfortable Work

From Borg[70] and Price et al.[71]

sponded to the design of spot welding machines. That information was used to redesign the spot welders, and the process was then repeated to evaluate the redesigned spot welders.

There is some controversy about the analysis of these data as categorical data with nonparametric statistics versus continuous data with parametric statistics. Borg[70] described these data as "categorical with analogue properties." Price[71] argued that visual analogue scales could be treated as ratio scales. Nonparametric methods of analysis (e.g., Spearman's rank correlation and Wilcoxon sign rank tests) are the most conservative way of analyzing rating data, but parametric analysis (e.g., analysis of variance and regression analysis) is most convenient.[86]

Electromyography entails the use of electrodes, preamplifiers, amplifiers, rectifiers, frequency analyzers, and recorders to measure electrical responses of muscles to work.[83,87] Needle electrodes often are used in laboratory studies to examine individual muscles, whereas surface electrodes are most commonly used in field studies to examine groups of muscles. Objectivity and insensitivity to subject attitude are advantages of electromyography. Another advantage can be the specificity of the measurement to a single muscle or group of muscles. This specificity can be a disadvantage if the major site of fatigue is in the connective tissue. Requirements for specialized equipment and trained technicians are disadvantages of electromyography.

Fatigue may also be assessed by comparing work loads and times with published endurance curves.[88] The ability to evaluate proposed job designs from descriptions of work rates and loads before actual implementation is a significant advantage of this approach. Work loads generally are expressed as a fraction or percentage of total strength. Thus for a given weight the relative work load for a weak subject is greater than that for a strong subject. Because of difficulty in determining the population strength and in characterizing jobs as a discrete sequence of forces, these methods cannot be applied with a great deal of precision. A final disadvantage is that work endurance may not be a suitable end point, since workers will inevitably experience unacceptable pain before reaching exhaustion.[27,83]

Whole-body Fatigue. Whole-body work occurs when multiple muscles repeatedly contract and relax in conjunction with the performance of a task. Common examples include walking, climbing stairs, and moving materials from one location to another (carrying, shoveling, pushing). Whole-body fatigue occurs when the metabolic demands of working muscles throughout the body exceed the capacity of the cardiovascular and pulmonary systems to deliver oxygen and glucose to working muscles and to remove products of metabolism. Common symptoms include shortness of breath and feelings of general weakness. These symptoms increase with the intensity and duration of work activities.

The metabolic demands of a job can be expressed in terms of the rate of energy expenditure (common units include kilocalories per minute and British thermal units [BTUs] per minute). Endurance limits for whole-body work are generally predicted as a fraction or percentage of a person's physical work capacity (PWC).[18,89-91] PWC is frequently measured in units of kilocalories or BTUs per minute determined during a graded exercise test in a clinic.[92,93] PWC varies within the working population. Factors that determine PWC include age, sex, weight, heredity, and physical fitness. Tables of PWC for various populations have been published elsewhere.[18,90,92-94] Variability within the population is an important consideration in evaluating stress; a job that is relatively easy for a person with high PWC can be extremely fatiguing for a person with low capacity.

The literature on work capacity and duration was reviewed by a NIOSH-sponsored committee when they were developing the *Work Practices Guide for Manual Lifting*.[18] This group concluded that a person can work at an intensity equal to his or her PWC for only short periods (4 minutes or less). As the duration of work increases, the intensity must be adjusted downward. If a task is performed continuously for an hour, the average energy expenditure rate should not exceed 50% of PWC. For a typical 8-hour work shift the average rate should not exceed 33% of PWC.[90,91,93] In establishing energy expenditure criteria for jobs that require repetitive lifting, the NIOSH committee recommended that the energy expenditure rate should not exceed 6.5 kcal/min for occasional, short-duration lifting tasks (1 hour or less).[18] For continuous, 8-hour lifting activities the rate should not exceed 3.5 kcal/min.

To assess the potential for whole-body fatigue, it is necessary to measure or estimate the energy expenditure rate of a job. This is usually done in one of three ways:

1. Indirect calorimetry: Energy expenditure rates can be estimated by measuring oxygen uptake.[93] This technique requires that the workers being studied wear a face mask or mouth piece and special equipment for recording ventilation rates and differences in oxygen content between inspired and expired air.
2. Table look-up: An alternative to indirect calorimetry is extrapolation from another job. This is a common practice of industrial engineers for estimating fatigue allowances, of heating and cooling engineers for assessing thermal burdens, and of medical personnel for planning cardiac rehabilitation.[89,92,95]
3. Elemental analysis of work tasks: The energy requirements of a job can be estimated from an elemental task analysis.[96] Traditional industrial engineering analysis is used to break the job down into work elements, and the energy increment of each element is estimated by using empirical equations. The increments for each task are added to the resting metabolic rate.

Whole-body fatigue can be controlled through good job design. Energy expenditure requirements can be reduced by designing the workplace to minimize unnecessary movements (e.g., walking, stooping, squatting, or climbing) and providing mechanical assists such as hoists and conveyors for moving heavy materials. If these approaches are not feasible, it may be necessary to provide rest allowances to prevent excessive fatigue.[89]

SUMMARY

Many worker health and safety problems can be attributed to failure to anticipate the capacity and behavior of the entire work population. Accidents, back and upper limb disorders, and localized and whole-body fatigue are all too common examples of these problems. Ergonomics is the application of epidemiology, anthropometry, biomechanics, physiology, psychology, and engineering to the evaluation and design of work for preventing injury and illness while maximizing productivity. Ergonomics is not yet an exact science; therefore all interventions should include appropriate evaluations to ascertain their effectiveness.

REFERENCES

1. Sanders MS, McCormick EJ: Human Factors in Engineering and Design, 6 edt. New York: McGraw-Hill, 1987
2. VanCott HP, Kincade RG (eds): Human Engineering Guide to Equipment Design. Washington DC: US Government Printing Office, 1972
3. Kantowitz BH, Sorkin RD: Human Factors: Understanding People—System Relationships. New York: John Wiley & Sons, 1983
4. Roebuck JA, Kroemer KHE, Thomson WG: Engineering Anthropometry Methods. New York: John Wiley & Sons, 1975
5. Chaffin DB, Andersson GBJ: Occupational Biomechanics. New York: John Wiley & Sons, 1984
6. Astrand P, Rodahl K: Textbook of Work Physiology, 2 edt. New York: McGraw-Hill, 1977
7. Keyserling WM: Occupational safety: prevention of accidents and overt trauma. In Levy BS, Wegman DH (eds): Occupational Health—Recognizing and Preventing Work-related Disease, 2 edt. Boston: Little, Brown, 1988, pp 105–120
8. NASA: Anthropometric Source Book, Vol 1: Anthropometry for Designers. Washington, D.C.: National Aeronautics and Space Administration (Ref. Pub. 1024), 1978
9. Pheasant S: Bodyspace—Anthropometry, Ergonomics, and Design. London: Taylor and Francis, 1986
10. Hagberg M: Local shoulder muscular strain—symptoms and disorders. J Human Ergol 11:99–108, 1982
11. Drillis R, Contini R: Body Segment Parameters. Report No. 1166-03 (Office of Vocational Rehabilitation, Dept. of HEW). New York: NYU School of Engineering and Science, 1966
12. Snook SH: The cost of back pain in industry. Spine: State Art Rev 2:1–5, 1987
13. Kelsey JL, Hochberg MC: Epidemiology of musculoskeletal disorders. Ann Rev Public Health 9:379–401, 1988
14. Holbrook TL, Grazier K, Kelsey JL, Stauffer RN: The Frequency of Occurrence, Impact and Cost of Selected Musculoskeletal Conditions in the United States. Chicago: American Academy of Orthopedic Surgeons, 1984
15. Berquist-Ullman M, Larsson U: Acute low back pain in industry. Acta Orthop Scand (Stockholm) (suppl 170), 1977
16. Waddell G: A new clinical model for the treatment of low back pain. Spine 12:632–644, 1987
17. Snook SH: Approaches to the control of back pain in industry: job design, job placement and education/training. Spine: State Art Rev 2:45–59, 1987
18. NIOSH: Work Practices Guide for Manual Lifting. Cincinnati: National Institute for Occupational Safety and Health (Pub No. 81-122), 1981
19. Bigos SJ, Spengler DM, Martin NA, Zeh J, Fisher L, Nachemson A, Wang MH: Back injuries in industry—a retrospective study. Part II: injury factors. Spine 11:246–251, 1986
20. Magora A: Investigation of the relation between low back pain and occupation. Indus Med Surg 41:5–9, 1972
21. Keyserling WM, Punnett L, Fine LJ: Trunk posture and back pain: identification and control of occupational risk factors. Appl Indus Hyg 3:87–92, 1988
22. Frymoyer JW, Pope MH, Clements JH, Wilder DG, MacPherson B, Ashikaga T: Risk factors in low back pain. J Bone Joint Surg [Am] 65:213–218, 1983
23. Kelsey JL, Hardy RJ: Driving motor vehicles as a risk factor for acute herniated lumbar intervertebral disc. Am J Epidemiol 102:63–73, 1988
24. Klein BP, Jensen RC, Sanderson LM: Assessment of workers' compensation claims for back sprains or strains. J Occup Med 26:443–448, 1984
25. Chaffin DB, Herrin GD, Keyserling WM: Pre-employment strength testing—An updated position. J Occup Med 20:403–408, 1978
26. Keyserling WM, Herrin GD, Chaffin DB: Isometric strength testing as a means of controlling medical incidents on strenuous jobs. J Occup Med 22:332–336, 1980
27. Chaffin DB: Localized muscle fatigue—Definition and measurement. J Occup Med 15:346–354, 1978
28. Andersson GBJ, Ortengren R, Herberts F: Quantitative electromyographic studies of back muscle activity related to posture and loading. Orthop Clin North Am 8:85–96, 1977
29. Snook SH: The design of manual handling tasks. Ergonomics 21:963–985, 1978
30. Andersson GBJ: Epidemiologic aspects of low back pain in industry. Spine 6:53–60, 1981
31. Keegan JJ: Alterations of lumbar curve related to posture and sitting. J Bone Joint Surg [Am] 35:589–603, 1953
32. Andersson GBJ, Ortengren R, Nachemson A, Elfstrom S: The influence of backrest inclination and lumbar support on lumbar lordosis. Spine 4:52–58, 1979
33. Adams MA, Hutton WC, Scott JRR: The resistance to flexion of the lumbar intervertebral joint. Spine 5:245–253, 1980
34. Holm S, Nachemson A: Variation in nutrition of the canine intervertebral disc induced by motion. Spine 8:866–874, 1983
35. Yu C, Keyserling WM: Evaluation of a new work seat for industrial sewing operations: Results of three field studies. Appl Ergonomics 20:17–25, 1989
36. Andersson GBJ, Ortengren R, Nachemson A, Elfstrom G: Lumbar disc pressure and myoelectric back muscle activity during sitting. Studies on an experimental chair. Scand J Rehab Med 3:104–114, 1974
37. Grandjean E: Fitting the Task to the Man—An Ergonomic Approach. London: Taylor & Francis, 1980
38. Yu C, Keyserling WM, Chaffin DB: Development of a Workseat for industrial sewing operations: Results of a laboratory study. Ergonomics 31:1765–1786, 1988
39. Hershenson A: Cumulative injury: A national problem. J Occup Med 21(10):674–676, 1979
40. WHO: Identification and control of work-related diseases, Report of a WHO Expert Committee, WHO Technical Report Series 714, p 9, Geneva: WHO 1985
41. Armstrong TJ: Ergonomics and cumulative trauma disorders of the hand and wrist. In Hunter JM, Schneider LH, Mackin EJ, Callahan AD: Rehabilitation of the Hand, Surgery and Therapy. St. Louis: The C.V. Mosby Co., 1990, pp 1175–1191
42. Ramazzini B: Treatis on the disease of workers, 1713. Translated by WC Wright, 1940, New York: Hafner Publ Co., 1964
43. Gray H: Anatomy, Descriptive and Surgical, 13 edt. 1893, p 491. See Muckart RD: Stenosing tendovaginitis of abductor pollicis longus and extensor pollicis brevis at the radial styloid (de Quervain's Disease). Clin Orthop 33:201–208, 1964
44. de Quervain F: Ueber Eine Form von Chronischer Tendovaginitis. Correspondenz-Blatt Schweizer Aerzte 25:389–394, 1895
45. Zollinger F: A few remarks on the question of tubercular tendovaginitis and bursitis after an accident. Arch Orthop Unfallchirurgie 24:456–467, 1927
46. Jensen R, Klein B, Sanderson L: Motion-related wrist disorders traced to industries, occupational groups. Monthly Labor Rev 106(9):13–16, 1983

47. Pozner H: A report on series of cases of simple acute tenosynovitis. J R Army Med Corps 78:142–142, 1942
48. Brain W, Wright A, Wilkinson M: Spontaneous compression of both median nerves in the carpal tunnel. Lancet 1:277–282, 1947
49. Hymovich L, Lindholm M: Hand, wrist, and forearm injuries: The result of repetitive motion. J Occup Med 8(11):573–577, 1966
50. Masear R, Hayes J, Hyde A: An industrial cause of carpal tunnel syndrome. J Hand Surg 11A:222–227, 1986
51. Occupational Safety and Health Act, Public Law 91-596, Section 5a, 1970
52. OSHA: Recordkeeping Requirements under the Occupational Safety and Health Act of 1970, OSHA No. 200, U.S. Dept. of Labor, Occupational Safety and Health Administration, 1978
53. Fine LJ, Silverstein BA, Armstrong TJ, Anderson CA, Sugano DS: The detection of cumulative trauma disorders of the upper extremities in the workplace. J Occup Med 28:675–678, 1986
54. Sabour M, Fadel H: The carpal tunnel syndrome, a new complication ascribed to the pill. Am J Obstet Gynecol 107:1265–1267, 1970
55. Silverstein BA, Fine LJ, Armstrong TJ: Occupational factors and carpal tunnel syndrome. Am J Ind Med 11:343–358, 1987
56. Cannon LJ, Bernacki EJ, Walter SP: Personal and occupational factors associated with carpal tunnel syndrome. J Occup Med 23:255–258, 1981
57. Armstrong TJ, Silverstein BA: Upper-extremity pain in the workplace—role of usage in causality. In Clinical Concepts in Regional Musculoskeletal Illness. New York: Grune & Stratton, 1987
58. Armstrong TJ: Upper extremity posture: Definition, measurement and control. In Corlett N, Wilson J, Manenica I (eds). The Ergonomics of Working Postures. London: Taylor and Francis, 1986, pp 59–73
59. Putz-Anderson V: Cumulative Trauma Disorders, A Manual for Musculoskeletal Diseases of the Upper Limbs. New York: Taylor and Francis, 1988
60. Kleinbaum DG, Kupper LL, Morgenstern H: Epidemiological Research—Principles and Quantitative Methods. Belmont, Calif.: Lifetime Learning Publications, 1982
61. Wegman DH, Eisen EA: Epidemiology. In Levy BS, Wegman DH (eds): Occupational Health, Recognizing and Preventing Work-related Disease. Boston: Little, Brown, 1988, pp 55–73
62. Waris P, Kuorinka I, Kurppa K: Epidemiologic screening of occupational neck and upper limb disorders. Scand J Work Environ Health 5(suppl 3):25–38, 1979
63. Armstrong TJ, Fine L, Silverstein B: Occupational risk factors of cumulative trauma disorders of the hand and wrist, a final report. Contract No. 200-82-2507, National Institute for Occupational Safety and Health, Cincinnati: December 1985
64. Fine LJ, Silverstein BS: Work-related disorders of the neck and upper extremity. In Levy BS, Wegman DH (eds): Occupational Health, Recognizing and Preventing Work-related Disease. Boston: Little, Brown, 1988, pp 358–370
65. Matte T, Baker E, Honchar P: The selection and definition of targeted work-related conditions for surveillance under SENSOR. Am J Pub Health 79(suppl.):21–25
66. Hennekens CH, Buring JB: In Mayrent S.L. (ed): Epidemiology in Medicine. Boston: Little, Brown, 1987, pp 260-264
67. Barnes R: Motion and Time Study, Design and Measurement of Work. New York: John Wiley and Sons, 1980
68. Niebel B: Motion and Time Study. Homewood, Ill.: Richard D. Irwin, 1986
69. Armstrong TJ, Foulke J, Joseph B, Goldstein S: An investigation of cumulative trauma disorders in a poultry processing plant. Am Ind Hyg Assoc J 43:103–116, 1982
70. Borg GAV: Psychophysical bases of perceived exertion. Med Sci Sports Exerc 14:377–381, 1982
71. Price DD, McGrath PA, Rafil A, Buckingham B: The validation of visual analogue scales as ratio scale measures for chronic and experimental pain. Pain 17:45–56, 1983
72. Scott J, Huskisson EC: Graphic representation of pain. Pain 2:175–184, 1976
73. Armstrong TJ, Punnett L, Ketner P: Subjective worker assessments of hand tools used in automobile assembly. Am Ind Hyg Assoc J 50:639–645, 1989
74. Snook SH, Campanelli RA, Hart JW: A study of three preventive approaches to low back injury. J Occup Med 20:478–481, 1978
75. Liles DH, Deivanayagam S, Ayoub MM, Mahajan P: A job severity index for the evaluation and control of lifting injury. Hum Factors 26:683–693, 1984
76. Herrin GD, Jaraiedi M, Anderson CK: Prediction of overexertion injuries using biomechanical and psychophysical models. Am Ind Hyg Assoc J 47:322–330, 1986
77. Human Factors Section, Eastman Kodak: Ergonomics for People at Work. Belmount, Calif.: Belmount Learning Publications, 1983
78. Armstrong T, Radwin R, Hansen D, Kennedy K: Repetitive trauma disorders: Job evaluation and design. Hum Factors 28:325–336, 1986
79. McKenzie F, Storment J, Van Hook P, Armstrong T: A program for control of repetitive trauma disorders associated with hand tool operations in a telecommunications manufacturing facility. Am Ind Hyg Assoc J 46:674–678, 1985
80. Bruening LA, Beaulieu D: The return to work phase for the patient with cumulative trauma. In Hunter JM, Schneider LH, Mackin EJ, Callahan AD (eds): Rehabilitation of the Hand, Surgery and Therapy. St. Louis: The C.V. Mosby Co., 1990, pp 1192–1196
81. Berlin S: On-site evaluation of the industrial worker. In Hunter JM, Schneider LH, Mackin EJ, Callahan AD (eds): Rehabilitation of the Hand, Surgery and Therapy. St. Louis: The C.V. Mosby Co., 1990, pp 1214–1217
82. Joseph B: Analysis of a program for control of cumulative trauma disorders in the auto industry. In Ergonomic Interventions to Prevent Musculoskeletal Injuries in Industry. Chelsea: Lewis Publishers, 1987, pp 133–150
83. Basmajian JV, Deluca CJ: Muscles Alive—Their Functions Revealed by Electromyography, 5 edt. Baltimore: Williams & Wilkins, 1985
84. Harms-Ringdahl K: On assessment of shoulder exercise and load-elicited pain in the cervical spine—biomechanical analysis of load-EMG-methodological studies of pain provoked by extreme position. Scand J Rehab Med (suppl. 14), 1986
85. Corlett EN, Bishop RP: The ergonomics of spot welders. Appl Ergonomics 9:23–32, 1978
86. Freund JE, Walpol RE: Mathematical Statistics. 3 edt. Englewood Cliffs, N.J.: Prentice-Hall, 1980
87. Habes D: Muscle activity of the low-back associated with repetitive leaning tasks in industry. Appl Ergonomics 15:297–301, 1984
88. Rohmert W: Problems in determining rest allowances. Part I: Use of modern methods to evaluate stress and strain in static muscular work. Appl Ergonomics 4:91–95, 1973
89. Karger D, Hancock W: Advanced Work Measurement. New York: Industrial Press, 1982
90. Bonjer FH: Actual energy expenditure in relation to the physical working capacity. Ergonomics 5:29–31, 1962
91. Bink B: The physical working capacity in relation to working time and age. Ergonomics 5:25–38, 1962
92. The Exercise Standards Book. Dallas: American Heart Association, 1979
93. Kamon E, Ayoub M: Ergonomics guide to assessment of physical work capacity. Am Ind Hyg Assoc J (Suppl, June):1–9, 1976
94. Murrell KFH: Human performance in industry. New York: Reinhold, 1965, p 376
95. ASHRAE Handbook 1990 Fundamentals. Atlanta: American Society of Heating, Refrigerating and Air-Conditioning Engineers, 1990
96. Garg A, Chaffin DB, Herrin GD: Prediction of metabolic rates for manual materials handling jobs. Am Ind Hyg Assoc J 39:661–674, 1978

30

Industrial Hygiene

Sanford W. Horstman

Industrial hygiene is the science of protecting human health through control of the work environment. This discipline arose out of the realizations that humans are greatly influenced by their work environment and that many of the illnesses that were being observed from industry are not only controllable but, in fact, can be eliminated in many cases.

Historically, the term "industrial hygiene" arose out of the English health and sanitation movement, or hygiene and sanitation movement, active in Great Britain in the early 1800s. The term "hygiene" is traceable to the goddess Hygeia, the greek mythological goddess of health, and thus the health and hygiene movement was a movement to promote health and healthful sanitary environmental conditions. By extension, this concept was applied to work in the industrial environment, and from this came the title "industrial hygienist."

Industrial hygiene in the United States traces its earliest development to the work of Alice Hamilton, who during the first and second decades of the twentieth century presented substantiated evidence of relationships between illness and exposure to toxins. In addition, she proposed a variety of concrete solutions to these problems. Much of her work was published in her autobiography, *Exploring the Dangerous Trades* (1943, Little, Brown), which highlights her work in the lead industries during the early parts of this century. As a result of the increasing focus on the relationship between employment and accidents and illness, public awareness became more widespread, and legislation was proposed and passed. In 1908, the federal government passed a compensation act for certain civil employees, and in 1911, the first state compensation laws were passed. The American Conference of Governmental Industrial Hygienist (ACGIH) was formed in 1938, representing a large and diverse group of individuals focused on protection of workers. In 1939, the American Industrial Hygiene Association was formed, and publication of a journal in the area of industrial hygiene and industrial hygiene control began shortly thereafter. The impact of the second World War and the immediate postwar period provided some impetus for the incorporation of industrial hygiene concepts in the private sector. Increased federal legislation addressing the environment called for research, training, and, in the 1960s, regulation. This development of regulation by the federal government, along with the continued development of the worker's compensation system, which was essentially complete by 1948 in all states in the United States, set the stage for the landmark Occupational Safety and Health Act (OSHAct).

The Occupational Safety and Health Administration (OSHA) became official on April 28, 1971, the effective date of the OSHAct. This organization was created in the Department of Labor to discharge the responsibilities assigned under the Act. The Act gives the Secretary of Labor a number of powers, including the authority (1) to promulgate, modify, and revoke safety and health standards, (2) to conduct inspections and investigations, (3) to issue citations and to propose penalties, (4) to require employers to keep records of safety and health data, (5) to petition the courts to restrain imminent danger situations, and (6) to approve or reject state plans for programs under the Act. The authority includes the right of access to the records of other federal agencies and a shared responsibility with other federal agency heads for the adequacy of programs in the organizations reporting to them.

The Act authorizes the Secretary to have the Department of Labor conduct training of personnel involved in the performance of duties related to their responsibilities under the Act and, in consultation with the U.S. Department of Health and Human Services (DHHS), to provide training and education to employers and employees. The Secretary and his designees are authorized to consult with employers, employees, and organizations regarding prevention of injuries and illnesses. The Secretary, after consultation with the Secretary of the DHHS, may grant funds to the states for identification of program needs and plan development, experiments, demonstrations, and administration and operation of programs. In conjunction with the Secretary of the DHHS, the Secretary of Labor is charged with developing and maintaining a statistics program for occupational safety and health.

Health standards are promulgated under the OSHAct by the Labor Department, with technical advice from the National Institute for Occupational Safety and Health (NIOSH), an agency of the DHHS.

The Labor Department regulations dealing with OSHA are published in Title 29 of the Code of Federal Regulations (CFR) as

29 CFR Part 1910	General Industry Standards
29 CFR Part 1915	Maritime Standards
29 CFR Part 1926	Construction Standards

NIOSH was established within the Department of Health, Education, and Welfare (now the DHHS) under the provision of

Public Law 91-596, the OSHAct. Administratively, NIOSH is located within DHHS's Centers for Disease Control of the Public Health Service. NIOSH is the principal federal agency engaged in research to eliminate on-the-job hazards to the health and safety of American workers. NIOSH responsibilities include identification of occupational safety and health hazards and recommendation of changes of the regulations limiting them. It also has obligations for training occupational health personnel.

NIOSH studies include not only the effects of exposure to hazardous substances used in the workplace but also the psychological, motivational, and behavioral factors involved in occupational safety and health. Much of the institute's research centers on specific hazards, such as asbestos and other fibers, beryllium, coal tar pitch, volatiles, silica, noise, and stress.

At the NIOSH Appalachian Laboratory for Occupational Safety and Health (ALOSH), research has focused on coal workers' pneumoconiosis (black lung disease) and other occupational respiratory diseases. Also located at the facility is the NIOSH Testing Certification Branch, which evaluates and certifies the performance of workers' personal safety equipment.

Under the authority of the OSHAct, NIOSH conducts research for new occupational safety and health standards. Its recommended standards are transmitted to the Department of Labor, which has the responsibility for development, promulgation, and enforcement of the standards.

NIOSH has a training grant program to develop baccalaureate and graduate programs in colleges and universities, and it offers a spectrum of short-term training courses for upgrading the knowledge and skills of present occupational health practitioners.

Workplace investigations are conducted also in a health hazard evaluation program, under which NIOSH responds to requests from employers and employee representatives to investigate a workplace, collect environmental samples, make toxicity determinations, and provide medical examinations for workers. The results of these investigations, including recommendations for work practices, personal protective equipment, and engineering controls, are reported back to company or plant management, employee representatives, and OSHA.

A third agency that plays an important role in the practice of industrial hygiene is the Environmental Protection Agency (EPA). In 1976, Congress enacted the Toxic Substances Control Act (TSCA), PL 94-469. The Act provides the EPA with the authority to require testing of chemical substances entering the environment and to regulate them when necessary. The regulatory actions include toxicity testing and environmental monitoring. This authority supplements and closes the loop of already existing hazardous substances laws in the EPA and other federal agencies. In 1976, Congress also enacted the Resource Conservation and Recovery Act (RCRA), PL 94-580, and put into place a universal hazardous waste management program applying not only to federal agencies but also to the private sector. RCRA greatly expanded the federal government's role in solid waste disposal management, with emphasis on hazardous waste disposal. Since 1980, general waste management requirements of RCRA have included proper notification and recording of hazardous waste activities, along with adequate packing, labeling, and manifesting of wastes for shipment. An RCRA permit is required for storage, treatment, or disposal of hazardous waste on-site or off-site. Standards for treatment, storage, and disposal (TSD) facilities include rigorous facility management plans, preparedness and prevention of emergencies and releases, contingency plans, operating records and reports, groundwater protection for land disposal facilities, and closure and postclosure plans with financial responsibility assurance.

The new RCRA requirements, following the amendments of 1984, make TSD facilities responsible for assessing human exposure to current and past waste management operations and for corrective action to remedy releases of hazardous constituents into the environment.

The RCRA regulations also require worker training, development of safe handling procedures, and emergency response measures. Documentation of training is required, and inspectors may require a review of the documentation.

In 1980, Congress enacted the Comprehensive Environmental Response, Compensation, and Liability Act (CERCLA), PL 96-510. This act established the Superfund program to handle emergencies at uncontrolled waste sites, to clean the sites, and to deal with related problems. In 1986, CERCLA was reauthorized by Congress to provide additional funding and additional provisions. The new authorities and programs in this reauthorization, which are of considerable interest to the industrial hygienist, include underground storage tanks, emergency planning, risk assessment, community right-to-know, research, development, demonstrations, and training.

The reauthorization amendment to CERCLA also established a comprehensive federal program to promote various research, development, demonstration, and training activities, including

1. Techniques for detecting, assessing, and evaluating health effects of hazardous substances
2. Methods to assess human health risks
3. Methods and technologies to detect hazardous substances and to reduce volume and toxicity

With the passage of the OSHAct, the establishment of NIOSH, and the strengthening of environmental laws under the EPA, the development of industrial hygiene accelerated rapidly. This has given rise to an era in which there is greater focus not only on the occupation but also on control and evaluation of the impact of industries on the environment and the ecosystem as a whole.

Within the United States, three organizations have had a strong influence on the continued development of industrial hygiene as a profession. These organizations are the American Conference of Governmental Industrial Hygiene (ACGIH), the American Industrial Hygiene Association (AIHA), and the American Board of Industrial Hygienists (ABIH).

The American Conference of Governmental Industrial Hygienists (ACGIH) is an organization devoted to the administrative and technical aspects of worker health protection. The ACGIH was organized in 1938 and, as the name suggests, was composed of industrial hygienists employed by the federal government and was formed as a medium for the exchange of ideas and experiences as well as the promotion of standards and techniques in industrial health. Since its inception, the ACGIH has contributed substantially to the development and improvement of official industrial health services to industry and labor. At the present time, the ACGIH has an international membership drawn from professional and technical personnel in governmental agencies or educational institutions engaged in occupational health activities. ACGIH is known for its many publications, which address important professional issues and applications. Three of the most widely used publications emanate from ACGIH technical committees: *Threshold Limit Values and Biological Exposure Indices, Air Sampling Instruments,* and *Industrial Ventilation—A Manual of Recommended Practice.*

ACGIH was a founding member of the International Occupational Hygiene Association (IOHA). Established in 1987, the IOHA has 13 members, representing 10 different countries. Objectives of the IOHA include (1) promotion and development of occupational hygiene throughout the world, (2) promotion of the exchange of occupational hygiene information among organizations and individuals, (3) encouragement to further develop occupational hygiene at a professional level, and (4) maintenance and promotion of a high standard of ethical practice in occupational hygiene. Although the IOHA is still in the organizing stage, its potential influence as an international society of teachers, researchers, and practitioners of occupational hygiene (industrial hygiene in the United States and some other countries) is great.

The American Industrial Hygiene Association (AIHA) is a nonprofit professional society for persons practicing industrial hygiene in industry, government, labor, academic institutions, and independent organizations. Nearly 11,000 professionals currently are affiliated with AIHA. Of these, over 7300 are members of the national AIHA association, and the rest are members of local AIHA sections. Membership is drawn from the United States, Canada, and 43 other countries.

The AIHA was established in 1939 by a group of industrial hygienists in response to the need for an association devoted exclusively to industrial hygiene. AIHA is a national professional society of persons engaged in protecting the health and well-being of workers and the general public through scientific application of knowledge about chemical, engineering, physical, biological, or medical principles to minimize environmental stress and to prevent occupational disease.

The AIHA's purpose is to promote recognition, evaluation, and control of environmental stresses arising in or from the workplace or its products and to encourage increased knowledge of industrial and environmental health by bringing together specialists in this professional field.

The American Board of Industrial Hygiene (ABIH) was established in 1959 to improve the practice and educational standards of the profession of industrial hygiene. The ABIH issues three categories of certificates awarded on successful completion of written qualifying examinations. The first certifies that the individual has the required education, experience, and professional ability in the comprehensive practice of industrial hygiene (CIH). The second certifies as to education, experience, and professional ability of the individual in the application and practice of a specialized aspect of industrial hygiene. The specialized aspects are designated by the following words: acoustical, air pollution, chemical, engineering, or radiological (CIH). The third is the Industrial Hygienist in Training (IHIT) certification, which refers to individuals who are permitted to take the core examination after receiving an appropriate bachelor's degree or after completion of a graduate degree in industrial hygiene. After 5 years of professional level industrial hygiene experience, the same individuals are eligible to take the comprehensive examination, either in the comprehensive practice of industrial hygiene or in an individual specialty area, such as engineering control or chemistry of industrial hygiene. A fourth category, the Occupational Health and Safety Technologists (OHST) designation, is a joint certification with the Board of Certified Safety Professionals (BCSP). The OHST examination procedure is administered by the BCSP.

Each applicant for a certificate must meet certain minimum eligibility requirements and must pass the two-part examination. The first part, the core examination, covers general aspects of industrial hygiene to the degree that, in the opinion of the Board, should be familiar to the candidate. The second part of the examination consists of different sets of questions for each category of certificate to be issued. Those seeking certification in the comprehensive practice of industrial hygiene will be given detailed questions covering the comprehensive aspects. Those seeking certification in a specialized aspect will be required to provide answers to questions largely pertinent to, but not confined to, that particular specialty.

The ABIH also administers a certification maintenance program for CIHs. The purpose of the certification maintenance program is to ensure that CIHs continue to develop and enhance their professional skills throughout their careers. Persons certified in either comprehensive practice or one specialty aspect become members of the American Academy of Industrial Hygiene and their names are published in the annual roster of the Academy. The names of IHITs also are published in the Academy roster.

In the international arena, the work of the International Labor Organization (ILO) and its sister agency at the United Nations, the larger World Health Organization (WHO), including the International Agency for Research on Cancer (IARC), has had important influences on industrial hygiene practice, particularly outside the United States.

The ILO was founded in Geneva in 1919 as an autonomous part of the League of Nations, becoming, in 1946, the first specialized agency associated with the United Nations. Whereas its early efforts focused mainly on labor standards and human rights in the workplace, issues of occupational safety and health have been of increasing importance since the 1930s.

Industrial hygiene, as it is currently practiced, has been defined by the ABIH as that science and art devoted to the anticipation, recognition, evaluation, and control of those environmental factors or stresses arising in or from the workplace that may cause sickness, impaired health or well-being, or significant discomfort and inefficiency among workers or among citizens of the community. Thus, an industrial hygienist, according to this definition, would be a person who has professional degrees and training in the areas of engineering, chemistry, physics, medicine, or related biological sciences who by virtue of special studies and training has acquired competence.

In the recognition of health hazards within a particular industry, the practitioner of industrial hygiene brings to this task elements of toxicology, physiology, and an understanding of industrial chemistry. Increasingly, the focus is placed on anticipation of occurrence of hazards early in the development of an industrial process. Thus, one can plan for potential problems before construction or implementation of a particular process. For existing processes, the industrial hygienist is responsible for recognition and identification of potential health hazards in the workplace, as well as the estimation of existing exposures to health hazards as a part of that recognition.

The second area of focus of industrial hygiene is in the evaluation of health hazards after their recognition. In this aspect of his or her work, the industrial hygienist normally will sample and observe the working environment. This will include measurements of the chemical and physical parameters (e.g., heat, noise, ventilation) of the workplace. Where existing engineering or work practice controls are in place, careful evaluation of the performance and efficiency of these controls is necessary. In addition, the industrial hygienist may analyze biological and environmental samples and interpret the results of these samples in terms of existing health standards or known effects. Where there are no standards or existing base of information, the practitioner will evaluate the results on the basis of previous studies or by analogies to known hazards and, where these comparisons are difficult, by the exercise of prudent judgment until sufficient evidence regarding the potential for health hazard is documented.

After the recognition and evaluation of problems, the industrial hygienist focuses on the control of workplace health hazards, which involves the elements of education, administration, and engineering. One of the earliest goals after evaluation and recognition is to convince management and members of the work force of the value of control, since inevitably such controls cost money and will have some effect on the work practices of the work force. After this initial step, administration controls should be designed and instituted, followed by design of an evaluation of engineering control systems. Since ventilation frequently is an important consideration in control of exposures, the industrial hygienist must have a working knowledge of this important factor. If no practicable engineering or administrative control is possible, the industrial hygienist should specify, implement, and evaluate a program for personal protective equipment use by the work force. The use of personal protective equipment normally is considered less desirable in the long run than eliminating or totally controlling exposure of the worker by engineering controls.

The ABIH has examined the domains of practice of industrial hygienists and has used these to design their certification examinations. An abbreviated version of the domain of practice is included in Table 30–1, which shows the types of considerations under each of the various headings that industrial hygienists are expected to perform. Certainly, the role of industrial hygienist in industry and government today has expanded well beyond the traditional role as the practitioner has moved into broader areas of environmental and occupational concern. The industrial hygienist frequently is involved in estimating the environmental impact of a product or a process and frequently works in conjunction with experts in air and water to limit the problems created by various processes. The industrial hygienist often is involved in emergency planning as required by SARA Title III and is a key figure in planning the emergency response plans in the event of an accident. In a more prospective role, the industrial hygienist is increasingly becoming involved in studies involving epidemiologists and occupational physicians in the attempt to monitor potential developing problems in industry or in the environment. In an effort to establish retrospectively historical exposure data, industrial hygienists frequently work closely with epidemiologists and use their knowledge of historical processes and exposures that existed during those processes to assist in establishing probable exposures of the study population.

In large industry settings, the industrial hygienist often works as a member of a multidisciplinary team. One example is an occupational health program involving multiple disciplines, including occupational medicine, occupational health nursing, industrial hygiene, safety, and perhaps health physics. These health professionals who are members of management not only must work closely with each other but also must have an effective relationship with other management members. This is especially true when working with the human resources or labor relations areas. Such a program not only affects the worker but also can influence personnel and labor relations favorably in such areas as workers' compensation, sickness and absence policies, and group insurance.

Industrial hygienists often work closely with the occupational physician, particularly when relating observed symptoms to exposure and the use of biomonitoring techniques to estimate exposure. The use of biomonitoring techniques is increasing rapidly and is a useful parallel documentation process to the conventional air monitoring techniques used previously.

Increasingly, industrial hygienists in industry are finding themselves directly responsible for aspects of environmental protection activities, including hazardous waste, emergency planning, community right-to-know, and general air pollution emission control. In governmental roles, industrial hygienists are charged with evaluation of these programs from a regulatory point of view. The industrial hygienist in the manufacturing industry frequently works closely with the design engineer and design laboratories, beginning as early as the basic laboratory investigation or pilot plant stage of product development. This involvement is a cost-effective way of ensuring that a safe and healthful workplace will be maintained while new products are being introduced and that if problems develop, prompt action can be taken for their elimination or control.

The industrial hygienist may be involved as a consumer complaint investigator or provide technical service to the users of a particular product. This becomes more relevant as the concept of third-party liability makes an increasing impact on the profession. Prompt problem-solving intervention for the consumer end of the manufacturing process is an effective way to avoid large-scale problems.

The profession of industrial hygiene has changed and expanded over the years. The introduction of new technologies can be expected to broaden it even further as new demands and opportunities in the control and prevention of occupational and environmental disease manifest themselves. This will bring changes in requirements for the education and background of individuals who will enter the industrial hygiene profession.

TABLE 30–1. DOMAIN OF PRACTICE

Recognizer of health stressors
- Foresee health stressor in plants and operations
- Identify potential workplace health stressors
- Recognize existing exposures to health stressors
- Set priorities by recording, organizing, and analyzing data

Evaluator of health stressors
- Develop data collection plan
- Obtain samples and make observations of environmental factors
- Analyze biological and environmental specimens
- Analyze and interpret results of observations

Controller of health stressors
- Educate people about health and environmental stressors
- Prescribe appropriate personal protective equipment (PPE)
- Design and prescribe engineering controls
- Design and prescribe administrative measures
- Communicate recommendations to appropriate people
- Verify efficiency of control measures

Manager of industrial hygiene programs
- Develop, implement, and evaluate the industrial hygiene program

Ethics
- Standards of ethical and professional conduct

31

Surveillance, Monitoring, and Screening in Occupational Health

Diana L. Ordin

Disease surveillance, a powerful public health tool, is the systematic collection, analysis, and interpretation of health data in order to detect, control, and prevent health problems.

Surveillance has long been used in the battle to control communicable disease. Because of inherent methodological and political difficulties, surveillance of occupational disease and injury in the United States has trailed far behind communicable disease surveillance and far behind programs in other countries.[1] During the past 15 years, however, major efforts have been made by occupational safety and health professionals in various settings to use surveillance in their battle against this important and preventable public health problem.

COMPONENTS OF SURVEILLANCE

Surveillance for occupational disease and injury has three basic components.[1]

1. The detection and enumeration of occupationally related morbidity and mortality. Identification and counting are the essential first steps for evaluating the extent of the problem and the efficacy of control measures. This component encompasses detection of well-recognized occupational disease and previously unrecognized adverse health effects related to work. It also may involve detection of conditions likely to result in disease or injury, such as elevated air levels of toxic agents in the workplace.
2. Data evaluation and interpretation to characterize trends and identify new patterns or clusters of disease and injury.
3. Intervention to decrease the incidence or severity of occupational disease and injury identified in data collection and analysis. The scope of intervention strategies is broad, encompassing education of workers, employers, and health care providers, broad-based screening efforts to detect additional disease cases, recommendations for changes in workplace design or use of personal protective equipment, additional toxicological or epidemiological studies, and adoption of new health and safety regulations.

Surveillance activities are undertaken by various types of organizations, including federal and state agencies, large companies and unions, and occupational medicine clinics. These surveillance efforts extend beyond the strict epidemiological definition of surveillance (see Chapter 2) to encompass other traditional public and occupational health activities, including

- Medical screening: Testing to diagnose disease in individuals at an early and, hopefully, reversible stage
- Medical monitoring: The routine measurement of health indices, with analysis and interpretation of the data
- Biological monitoring: The sampling of body tissue for toxic agents, their metabolites, or other physiological indicators of exposure
- Exposure monitoring: Involving air measurements of chemicals to which workers are exposed

What makes occupational health surveillance distinct from each of these individual activities is that, in surveillance, information from various sources is integrated and interpreted. The ultimate purpose is not merely to find cases or assess air measurements or obtain mortality statistics but rather to see what that information tells us about the causes, occurrence, patterns, trends, and means to prevent occupational disease and injury.

Epidemiological Surveillance

Epidemiological surveillance is the macroscopic surveillance perspective, carried out primarily by public health agencies on a statewide or nationwide basis. These efforts seek to identify and quantify illness, injury, or excessive exposure and monitor trends in their occurrence across different industry types, over time, and between geographic areas.

In the 1980s the National Institute for Occupational Safety and Health (NIOSH) (see Chapter 33) and several state health departments launched major efforts to improve the epidemiological surveillance of occupational diseases and injuries. These efforts have focused on NIOSH's list of 10 leading work-related diseases and injuries (Table 31-1).

Case Counting and Data Evaluation. Various sources of data are being explored for their use in quantifying occupational illness and injury in the United States. These data include

TABLE 31-1. NIOSH LIST OF 10 LEADING WORK-RELATED DISEASES AND INJURIES IN UNITED STATES[a]

1. Occupational lung diseases: Asbestosis, byssinosis, silicosis, coal workers' pneumoconiosis, lung cancer, occupational asthma
2. Muscoloskeletal injuries: Disorders of the back, trunk, upper extremity, neck, lower extremity; traumatically induced Raynaud's phenomenon
3. Occupational cancers (other than lung): Leukemia, mesothelioma, cancers of the bladder, nose, and liver
4. Severe occupational traumatic injuries: Amputations, fractures, eye loss, lacerations, and traumatic deaths
5. Cardiovascular diseases: Hypertension, coronary artery disease, acute myocardial infarction
6. Disorders of reproduction: Infertility, spontaneous abortion, teratogenesis
7. Neurotoxic disorders: Peripheral neuropathy, toxic encephalitis, psychoses, extreme personality changes (exposure-related)
8. Noise-induced loss of hearing
9. Dermatological conditions: Dermatoses, burns (scaldings), chemical burns, contusions (abrasions)
10. Psychological disorders: Neuroses, personality disorders, alcoholism, drug dependency

[a] Three criteria were used to develop the list: frequency of occurrence of the disease or injury, its severity in the individual case, and its amenability to prevention. The conditions listed under each category are to be viewed as selected examples, not comprehensive definitions of the category.
From MMWR 32(2):24, 1983.

workers' compensation claims, health insurance statistics, Occupational Safety and Health Administration (OSHA) (see Chapter 2) records, hospital discharge information, disease registries, birth and death certificates, laboratory reporting of abnormal results (e.g., heavy metal blood and urine tests), national health surveys, information obtained annually from employers by the Bureau of Labor Statistics, and physician reporting of occupational disease. Physician reporting of some occupational illnesses is now required in at least 32 states and the District of Columbia.[2]

Each of these databases has strengths and weaknesses,[3] and identifying and strengthening the most useful data sources are an important priority of NIOSH and state health departments.

Intervention. Current occupational health surveillance efforts by public health agencies usually include a response component. Intervention activities have included

- Medical screening of co-workers of affected individuals
- Comprehensive evaluation of workplaces where health effects have been detected
- Development of educational programs and consultative services for primary care physicians who need assistance in identifying and managing occupational disease
- Drafting of new regulations
- Recommendations and educational outreach for workers, unions, and management

The case counting and data evaluation tools then are used to ascertain the effectiveness of these interventions.

Medical Surveillance in the Workplace

In workplace-based medical surveillance, the three basic surveillance components of disease and injury detection, data evaluation and interpretation, and intervention are focused on the hazards and potential hazards of a particular workplace, company, or group of workers. Thus, a prerequisite to the development of such programs is careful identification and characterization of these hazards.

Methods for identifying and characterizing hazards may include review of plant inventory and processes, review of the material safety data sheets (MSDS), which must be provided by chemical manufacturers and suppliers, walkthrough investigations, discussions with employees, and air monitoring. Consultation with safety experts, industrial hygienists, ergonomists, and engineers can facilitate identification of the workplace hazards. Ideally, exposure to these hazards can be prevented or minimized through the primary preventive measures of engineering controls (such as ventilation or isolation), product substitution, protective equipment, and good work practices. But because current strategies for primary prevention often are inadequate and never are failsafe, medical surveillance programs are warranted.

Screening for Known Effects of Exposure. Most workplace-based medical surveillance programs consist largely of medical screening for previously undiagnosed disease or for adverse physiological effects caused or influenced by workplace exposures.

Screening is aimed at secondary prevention—the early detection of recognized adverse health effects. The detection of these adverse effects in a workplace population indicates that primary preventive measures must be instituted, modified, or enforced.

Screening Principles. Population-based disease screening has long been acknowledged as a powerful public health strategy, and the principles governing selection of health problems appropriate for community screening have been articulated (see Chapter 2). Most of these criteria are equally appropriate in screening for the adverse effects of workplace exposures. However, screening in the occupational setting has several unique features, and a set of principles for such screening has been proposed by Halperin et al.[4]

Perhaps the most important of these amended principles concerns the detection of disease at a subclinical or treatable stage. Community disease screening is recommended to be undertaken only when the disease is treatable or can be diagnosed at a discernible latent or early symptomatic stage. In occupational disease screening, however, detection of a disease or other adverse effect in an individual worker raises the possibility that a potentially widespread problem exists in that workplace. Thus, such detection could result in prevention of the effect in similarly exposed workers and is justifiable even if there is no available treatment for the affected individual.

Another traditional screening principle requiring modification in the occupational setting is the cost–benefit consideration. For community screening, this involves balancing the cost of case finding against the benefits to be derived from a similar expenditure on other aspects of community medical care. Thus, cost and simplicity of the screening test are key factors in population-based screening efforts. In the industrial setting, however, screening cost is not the only factor to be considered. Some screening tests are required by federal law. Concern for employee health on moral and ethical grounds, requests for screening programs by concerned and increasingly knowledgeable employees, and potential long-term financial benefit through reduction of litigation, insurance, and workers' compensation costs are additional motivating factors. The relative benefits of expenditure on screening tests vs new machinery or machinery redesign also may be taken into consideration. Thus, screening tests for occupational disease do not necessarily need to be simple or inexpensive.

Selecting a Screening Test. Depending on the agent, any combination of four approaches may be used in screening for known adverse effects of exposures.

1. Diagnosis of overt disease, as in the use of chest x-rays to detect silicosis in sandblasters or spirometry to diagnose byssinosis in cotton workers
2. Examination for physical signs, such as nasal perforation in chromium workers or gynecomastia in males working with synthetic estrogens
3. Questionnaires to elicit symptoms, such as headaches in solvent-exposed workers or painful blanching of fingers (Raynaud's phenomenon) in workers exposed to vibration
4. Laboratory testing to identify pathophysiological and biochemical abnormalities signifying preclinical adverse effects, such as the use of nerve conduction studies to detect early peripheral neuropathy in workers exposed to carbon disulfide, liver function tests to detect early hepatotoxicity in chlorinated hydrocarbon exposure, and blood cell examinations to detect early hematotoxicity in benzene exposure

The selection of appropriate screening tests for exposed workers requires identification of specific workplace hazards, literature review to delineate the potential adverse health effects of those hazards, evaluation of what, if any, screening tests are useful for identifying those health effects, and determination of which workers should undergo screening with what frequency. There is a growing body of literature dealing with such testing and excellent summary material is available.[5,6]

In surveillance for previously unidentified adverse health effects, there often is information available to help focus the search. Monitoring may be undertaken for adverse effects detected in animal studies but not yet detected or investigated in human populations. Adverse effects known to be caused by agents with structural similarities to the agent under consideration may be sought. Damage to organ systems previously demonstrated to be especially vulnerable to toxins, such as kidney, liver, lung, nervous system, and reproductive system, should be evaluated in the exposed population.

All programs should be reevaluated periodically in light of the rapidly advancing identification and evaluation of new screening tests, environmental and biological monitoring assays, potential risk factors, and exposure-related health effects.

OSHA Screening Requirements. Most employer-sponsored workplace screening efforts are limited to those required by OSHA. These regulations require medical examinations for 24 occupational exposures as well as a medical evaluation for respirator use (Table 31-2). OSHA uses the term "surveillance" in referring to these examinations, but, in fact, they are screening programs.

The screening requirements in many of the OSHA standards generally are acknowledged to be outdated. In particular, the effectiveness of annual chest x-rays and sputum cytology in screening for lung cancer in all workers exposed to certain lung carcinogens (e.g., coke oven emissions and arsenic), irrespective of the amount and duration of exposure, is widely questioned. Performing a nonspecific physical examination for workers exposed to agents for which a specific human cancer site has not yet been identified (e.g., 2-acetylaminofluorene, 4-aminodiphenyl, 3,3′-dichlorobenzidine, 4-dimethylaminozobenzene) also is recognized to be an ineffective screening tool.

Although OSHA officials state that the agency is still enforcing these screening requirements,[7] OSHA is now considering new regulatory activity that would greatly expand federally mandated screening efforts as well as enable the screening requirements to better keep pace with the ever-expanding body of knowledge in this area. Approaches under consideration include "prescriptive requirements for specific chemicals," "broader requirements for chemicals that have similar health effects," and "allowing medical professionals to decide when and what test would be useful."[8]

Ambient and Biological Monitoring. In a well-designed workplace occupational health program, ambient monitoring—the measurement of levels of known toxic agents in workplace air and other media—is undertaken to ascertain the effectiveness of primary preventive measures (such as engineering controls) and to determine whether potentially hazardous worker exposure is taking place.

Although ambient monitoring is a necessary constituent of primary prevention, the measured airborne concentration of a chemical agent does not necessarily correlate with the quantity actually absorbed by exposed workers. Unless the monitoring is continuous (which is seldom the case), dangerous surges in ambient levels may be missed. In addition, considerable interindividual variation exists in personal hygiene habits and work practices (such as handwashing, use of protective equipment, smoking on the worksite), as well as dermal, pulmonary, and gastrointestinal absorption rates. Each of these factors could lead to potentially toxic body burdens of a workplace agent despite acceptable ambient measurements.

The use of personal protective equipment, such as respirators or special clothes or gloves, may decrease a worker's absorption of toxic workplace agents. This equipment is often so uncomfortable and inconvenient, however, that workers simply do not wear it. The use of this equipment occasionally may be medically contraindicated for those with respiratory or cardiovascular problems. In addition, no protective device is failsafe.

Thus, even with allegedly safe workplace air levels and approved safety equipment, an individual worker's absorption of and consequent internal exposure to potentially harmful amounts of toxic agent cannot be excluded. To circumvent this problem, biological monitoring is used in the workplace as an important tool in medical surveillance. Such monitoring is designed to measure chemical agents and their metabolites or early, nonpathological indicators of internal exposure in the tissues of exposed individuals to determine whether and how much absorption has taken place. Since the aim of biological monitoring is to detect biochemical evidence of absorption before any adverse effect has occurred, it is essentially a means for primary prevention.

Examples of biological monitoring currently undertaken in occupational settings include determination of blood lead levels, measurement of solvent concentrations in expired air, measurement of heavy metals and solvent metabolites in urine, and analysis of red blood cell cholinesterase in workers exposed to anticholinesterase pesticides.

It is important to note that the mere existence of analytical tools to quantify an agent or metabolite in human tissue does not necessarily signify that such measurement is appropriate for biological monitoring.[9] For an assay to be useful, sufficient toxicological information must be available on the human absorption and metabolic fate of the agent. The correlation between measured levels and health effects, or availability of population norms or preexposure data for comparison purposes, and some notion of the intra-and interindividual variability in such measurements also should be known. When information is available, biological monitoring can complement environmental monitoring in ensuring that worker exposure levels are acceptable and can provide a more accurate estimate of health risk.

Other Data Useful in Surveillance of Exposed Workers. In addition to medical screening tests, ambient monitoring, and biological monitoring, other data may be useful for surveillance of exposed workers. Workplace accident and illness records, company medical insurance data, workers' compensation claims, absenteeism data, retiree death certificates, and the results from other components of a workplace employee health

TABLE 31–2. MEDICAL SCREENING PROVISIONS IN OSHA STANDARDS

Agent/Worker Group	Primary Adverse Health Effects To Be Detected by Screening	Examination Interval[a]	Examination Contents[a]
2-Acetylaminofluorene	Cancer (site unspecified)	Annual	Hx, PE
Acrylonitrile	CNS effects, dermatitis, lung cancer, GI cancer	Annual	Hx, PE, CXR, fecal blood[b]
4-Aminodiphenyl	Cancer (side unspecified)	Annual	Hx, PE
Arsenic, inorganic	Skin lesions (including cancer), lung cancer, nasal septal perforation	Annual or semiannual[b]	Hx, PE, CXR, sputum cytology[b]
Asbestos	Pulmonary disease, lung and GI cancer, mesothelioma	Annual	Hx, questionnaire,[c] PE, CXR,[b] PFTs
Benzene	Hematological disease, including aplastic anemia and leukemia	Annual	Hx, CBC, PFTs
Benzidine	Cancer (site unspecified)	Annual	Hx, PE
bis-Chloromethyl ether	Cancer (site unspecified)	Annual	Hx, PE
Coke oven emissions	Lung cancer, kidney cancer, skin cancer	Annual or semiannual[b]	Hx, PE, CXR, PFTs, U/A, sputum and urine cytology[b]
Cotton dust	Byssinosis	Biennial, annual, or semiannual[d]	Hx, questionnaire, PFTs
1,2-Dibromo 3-chloropropane	Male and female germ cell toxicity, cancer (site unspecified)	Annual	Hx, PE, reproductive tests[e]
3,3′-Dichlorobenzidine	Cancer (site unspecified)	Annual	Hx, PE
4-Dimethylaminoazobenzene	Cancer (site unspecified)	Annual	Hx, PE
Ethylene oxide	Leukemia, dermatitis, reproductive toxicity, neurological toxicity, pulmonary toxicity	Annual	Hx, PE, CBC, reproductive tests[e]
Ethyleneimine	Cancer (site unspecified)	Annual	Hx, PE
Formaldehyde	Mucous membrane irritation, skin and pulmonary sensitization	Annual	Questionnaire,[c] PE, PFTs
Lead	Hematological effects, renal disease, reproductive toxicity, neurological disease	Exam: at least annual[f]; biomonitoring: at least semiannual[f]	Hx, PE, CBC, U/A, BUN, Cr, biomonitoring[f]
Methyl chloromethyl ether	Cancer (site unspecified)	Annual	HX, PE
α-Naphthylamine	Cancer (site unspecified)	Annual	Hx, PE
β-Naphthylamine	Cancer (site unspecified)	Annual	Hx, PE
4-Nitrobiphenyl	Cancer (site unspecified)	Annual	Hx, PE
N-Nitrosodimethylamine	Cancer (site unspecified)	Annual	Hx, PE
Noise	Hearing loss	Annual	Audiometry
β-Propiolactone	Cancer (site unspecified)	Annual	Hx, PE
Vinyl chloride	Hepatic disease, hepatic cancer	Annual or semiannual[b]	Hx, PE, LFTs
Employees using respirators	Conditions causing inability to wear respirator	"Periodically"[g]	[g,h]
Hazmat workers	[h]	Annual	Hx, PE[h]
Laboratory workers	[h]	[h]	[h]

Hx, medical, work, family history; PE, physical examination; CXR, chest x-ray; LFTs, routine serum liver function test; CBC, complete blood count, or other routine hematological test; U/A, urinalysis; PFTs, pulmonary function tests (spirometry only), BUN, serum blood urea nitrogen; Cr, serum creatinine; CNS, central nervous system; GI, gastrointestinal.

[a] All standards require preplacement and termination as well as periodic examinations. For most standards, additional examinations are mandated in emergency situations, for symptomatic employees, or at the discretion of the examining physician.

[b] Frequency determined by age of employee, years of exposure, or both.

[c] Questionnaire provided in appendix to standard.

[d] Frequency determined by exposure level and PFT results.

[e] If requested by physician or employee.

[f] Examination and biomonitoring frequency determined by previous blood lead levels and symptomatology.

[g] The formaldehyde standard requires annual PFTs for respirator users; the benzene standard requires PFTs every 3 years.

[h] Testing to be determined by physician.

From U.S. Department of Labor, Occupational Safety and Health Administration, Washington, DC: General Industry OSHA Safety and Health Standards (29 CFR 1910), 1988. Hazardous Waste Operations and Emergency Response (29 CFR 1910.120), 1989. Occupational Exposures to Hazardous Chemicals in Laboratories (29 CFR 1910.1450), 1990.

program may prove useful in identifying adverse health effects related to work.

Data Analysis, Interpretation, and Intervention. As in epidemiological surveillance, periodic analysis of aggregate data for evidence of known toxicity, unanticipated adverse health effects, and evidence of a correlation between exposure and adverse health effects is an essential part of workplace medical surveillance. Subtle group changes ascertainable only by statistical evaluation may provide early indication of a problem.

For screening tests, abnormal aggregate results may occur either as a change in the mean test result in the exposed group or as an increase in the number of exposed individuals with abnormal results. A positive correlation between adverse screening results and exposure (as determined by environmental or biological monitoring or by rougher approximations of exposure, such as work location) helps corroborate an etiological relationship between the exposure and the abnormal findings. Consideration of other possible reasons for the abnormal results, such as confounding factors or statistical artifact, is appropriate, but the first response always should be the prompt evaluation of workplace conditions and other workers to determine the need for immediate preventive or remedial action.

Possible intervention measures in response to a suspect or proven health hazard identified through medical surveillance include further medical or industrial hygiene evaluation, job or process modification, engineering controls, work practice controls, use of protective equipment, and education programs.

PROBLEMS IN OCCUPATIONAL DISEASE AND INJURY

Both epidemiological and workplace-based medical surveillance efforts are fraught with some inherent difficulties.

Lack of Data on Adverse Health Effects. Despite the considerable literature on adverse effects of workplace exposures, the vast majority of the nearly 10 million chemicals potentially used in U.S. workplaces[10] have never been studied for their potential effects on human health. Animal toxicological data can offer an approximation of human health risk but often are unavailable or inapplicable for several reasons.

First, until very recently, no toxicological testing was required before the introduction of a chemical into the general environment or the workplace, and thus there was little incentive for investment in such testing. United States regulatory agencies, such as the Food and Drug Administration, Environmental Protection Agency, and Consumer Products Safety Commission, have published testing guidelines, some of them in fact requirements, for pharmaceuticals, food additives, pesticides, and household substances. Relatively few workplace agents are covered by these regulations, however, and testing now required does not evaluate their safety for humans under conditions of workplace exposure.

Second, workers generally are exposed to mixtures of chemicals both inside and outside the workplace, and such mixtures rarely undergo testing. Third, chemical intermediates present in the workplace but not in the final products do not require evaluation under current regulations.

Finally, the utility of toxicological testing is limited by the inherent problem of extrapolating animal data to conditions of human exposure. Not only are mice and other laboratory animals different from men and women, but also the exposure routes and extreme exposure conditions of most traditional toxicological tests are seldom analogous to those encountered by humans in the workplace. Thus, although laboratory toxicology data often can provide information useful in protecting employees from the adverse effects of their workplace exposures, they by no means provide all necessary information.

The study of adverse effects of exposures in human populations can provide information more directly applicable to the workplace setting. However, epidemiological study of exposed workers is usually complex and costly. Many of the adverse health effects, such as cancer, pulmonary diseases, and neurological deficits, have long latency periods as well as relatively high background incidence levels in the general population. Thus, large study groups and extended follow-up periods are required. Additional problems may include inadequacy of available medical and employment records, poor or nonexistent exposure data, and employer reluctance to acknowledge the need for such studies. Because of these difficulties, relatively few agents have been studied systematically in human populations, and these investigations have been undertaken only after an occupational disease problem has been suspected.

Thus, historically, most adverse health effects have been discovered through epidemics of disease in exposed workers. In most of these epidemics, the connection between occupation and disease has been made only because so great a number of workers were affected (as with silicosis in miners) or because the disease was so rare in the general population (as with angiosarcoma of the liver in vinyl chloride exposure and mesothelioma in asbestos exposure) that recognition of the occupational connection was unavoidable.

Difficulty in Ascribing Adverse Health Effects to Workplace Exposures. Even when the association between a chemical exposure and a disease or adverse health effect is clearly documented in the scientific literature, it may be difficult to establish an etiological relationship in an individual.

The end points used in occupational health screening, such as abnormal liver function tests, headaches, or lung cancer, are usually clinically indistinguishable from identical findings caused by other factors. For example, an employee's lung cancer may be causally related to arsenic exposure at work, radon exposure at home, cigarette smoking, or (most probably) a combination of the three. An employee working with trichloroethylene may have elevated hepatic enzyme levels secondary to the workplace exposure, alcohol use, or medication. Thus, a careful and complete history of occupational and nonoccupational exposures is required for appropriate diagnosis and treatment.

Defining what is abnormal for an individual may itself be difficult, since there is such a broad range of normal values for most laboratory tests. For example, an individual whose usual hematocrit is 50% can lose as much as one fifth of his or her red blood cell mass and still be within a laboratory's normal range. This problem can be minimized if each individual serves as his or her own control by using preexposure baseline data obtained at the time of hire.

Defining what is abnormal for aggregate data also may be problematic. The workforce often is demographically different from the general population and usually is healthier (the so-called healthy worker effect). This means that the use of population-based norms for data analysis may be misleading. In practice, the most reliable comparison data are preexposure information from the workers under surveillance or results from an unexposed but otherwise similar employee group.

In both worker-based and epidemiological surveillance, the systematic search for a possible relationship between workplace exposures and morbidity and mortality is bound to yield statistically significant relationships due to confounding factors or chance. Further investigation often is necessary before definitive conclusions may be drawn. Although it is desirable to avoid undue alarm through precipitate announcement of tentative data, positive findings must not be ignored. Further evaluation of workplace exposures and work practices, close clinical follow-up of workers at possible risk, and preliminary dissemination of the information to affected employees, scientific colleagues, and government agencies should be undertaken promptly.

Inadequate Physician Training. The average U.S. physician receives only 4 hours of training in occupational medicine during medical school.[11] Although the number of residencies and fellowships in occupational medicine expanded greatly during the 1980s, instruction in occupational and environmental medicine is still woefully lacking in most primary care residencies where the physicians likely to see the initial signs, symptoms, diseases, and injuries related to workplace exposures are being trained.

The lack of physician knowledge about occupational medicine leads to underdiagnosis of work-related diseases and, to a lesser extent, injuries. This underdiagnosis has a marked effect on epidemiological surveillance, which primarily uses existing morbidity and mortality data to identify and track occupational disease and injury.

Theoretically, lack of physician education should affect work-based surveillance programs to a lesser degree, since such programs are designed specifically to identify occupational disease and injury. The lack of training, however, may also characterize the company physician responsible for the design and implementation of workplace medical programs, so the need for appropriate surveillance may not be recognized, or an inadequate program may be instituted.

Strategies to address this problem have been outlined in a recent report by the Institute of Medicine,[12] and the 1990s should see implementation of some of these recommendations on national, state, and local levels. New occupational medicine textbooks aimed at primary care clinicians[13] and the recent publication of general articles on occupational medicine in major journals read by the primary care community[14] should help in addressing this problem. Health provider education also is included in most NIOSH-sponsored surveillance activities.

Difficult Interventions. Even when occupational diseases and injuries are readily identifiable and known to be reducible, the interventions required to achieve reduction are often arduous and expensive.

For the primary care physician, whose recognition of occupational disease is key to epidemiological surveillance efforts as well as to patient health, there are major disincentives for diagnosis and appropriate management of occupational disease and injury. These include the vast amount of time and effort involved in obtaining exposure and toxicological information and dealing with the workers' compensation system and OSHA and physician concern over jeopardizing patient livelihood. The Institute of Medicine report suggests various methods for removing these disincentives.[12]

Political and economic factors impede the enactment of new government regulations and programs. Implementation of recommendations for workplace modifications or medical screening programs may be costly and thus may encounter employer opposition. Designing and implementing effective educational strategies for workers, employers, and health care providers is notoriously difficult.

THE FUTURE OF SURVEILLANCE ACTIVITIES

Despite the complexities of conducting occupational disease and injury surveillance and screening, the 1980s saw impressive developments in this area in the United States. These include

- Escalating surveillance activities by NIOSH and state health departments
- OSHA's efforts to develop a standard for workplace medical surveillance
- Increasing worker and employer awareness of occupational health issues, resulting in part from OSHA's Hazard Communication Standard[15]
- Attention to this issue by various national institutions, such as the Institute of Medicine,[12] National Research Council,[16] and the U.S. Congress[17]
- Increased recognition of occupational medicine's importance by medical specialty boards, such as the American Board of Internal Medicine and the American Board of Family Medicine, and professional organizations, such as the American Medical Association
- The establishment of some state-funded occupational health clinics (e.g., New York, Connecticut)
- An increase in the number of occupational medicine residencies and fellowships
- The availability of some private and federal grant monies to nurture medical school training in this area

Hopefully, these trends will continue into the 1990s, augmented by increased OSHA standard-setting and enforcement and by the continuing activism of occupational health and safety professionals, health care providers, and concerned workers and employers.

RELATIONSHIP OF MEDICAL SURVEILLANCE TO OTHER ASPECTS OF WORKPLACE OCCUPATIONAL HEALTH PROGRAM

Workplace medical surveillance can serve to enhance other aspects of a comprehensive occupational health program. In turn, several of the traditional components of an employee health service can be used for surveillance purposes.

Comprehensive information on the components of an occupational health program and how to set up such a program is readily available.[18] The following discussion is focused on the relationship of some of these components to occupational disease and injury surveillance.

Preplacement Examinations. The purpose of preplacement examinations is to ensure appropriate job placement by matching the physical requirements and hazards of the job to the medical capabilities of a job candidate. The examination should be designed to assess whether an employee is likely to be able to carry out the job duties without harm to self or others.

It has long been recognized that medical problems unrelated to employment can affect a worker's ability to perform safely his or her job responsibilities. Examples include back injuries, which may limit heavy lifting, cardiovascular disease, which can decrease exercise and heat tolerance, and pulmonary disease, which can affect work capacity as well as ability to wear respiratory protective equipment.

As is the case in most areas of medicine, the medical history, in this case coupled with knowledge of the exposures and physical requirements of the job, usually provides sufficient information to determine fitness for duty. For example, someone with chronic knee problems is unlikely to tolerate work involving constant climbing on ladders or roofs, someone with coronary artery disease is unlikely to tolerate the metabolic load of firefighting, and an insulin-dependent diabetic with frequent hypoglycemic episodes would probably be a danger to self and others operating moving equipment, such as a crane or forklift.

Beyond commonsense use of the medical history, few tests have demonstrated predictive value in this setting, and some of the most frequently used tests have been shown to have little predictive value. For example, spinal x-rays are still widely used in industry to exclude those with radiological abnormalities such as spondylolisthesis and spondylosis, which, it is presumed, predispose to back injuries on the job. Yet studies have shown that x-ray abnormalities per se do not correlate well with subsequent lost-time back injury.[19] Chest x-rays and pulmonary function tests are performed routinely to determine an applicant's ability to wear respiratory protective equipment, yet there are no validated criteria for using these tests to determine fitness for respirator use.[20]

Discussion with personal physicians, work capacity evaluation by physical or occupational therapists, with testing under conditions simulating the physical requirements of the job, and exercise testing, with personal protective equipment as appropriate, to assess job performance capability may provide more objective data when fitness-for-duty status is unclear based on the medical history and physical examination.

In the context of occupational surveillance, the preplacement examination acquires additional use by serving as a baseline medical assessment of an employee before workplace exposure.

Discrimination Issues in the Preplacement Examination. Besides potentially affecting fitness-for-duty, preexisting disease and risk factors may render a worker more vulnerable to the toxic effects of workplace chemicals. Such factors include exposures outside the workplace (e.g., in second jobs or through environmental contamination), lifestyle habits (e.g., cigarette smoking and alcohol use), and possibly age, sex, nutritional status, and genetic makeup.

Examples of those who might be at increased risk of suffering adverse effects from workplace exposures include atopic individuals, who may be more susceptible to the dermatological irritant effects of industrial agents, or employees with impaired renal function, who may tend to accumulate agents and metabolites normally metabolized or excreted by the kidney.

The use of cigarettes, alcohol, and prescription or nonprescription drugs can in themselves lead to serious medical problems, and these agents also may influence the metabolism and excretion of workplace agents so as to increase their toxic potential. Exposures at second jobs or through general environmental contamination may increase the workplace risk either additively or synergistically.

There is increasing debate about the effects of age, sex, nutritional status, and genetic makeup on susceptibility to the adverse effects of workplace exposures. Few definitive examples of such effects are available, other than the increased gastrointestinal absorption of lead in children and the increased risk of ultraviolet skin damage, including skin cancer, in Caucasians. The growing interest in and concern over this issue emanate not only from its scientific merit but also from its potential role in legitimizing age, sex, ethnic, and racial discrimination. The possible use of genetic tests (such as assays for hemoglobin abnormalities or enzyme deficiencies) to identify and exclude potential employees who might be hypersusceptible to the adverse effects of workplace toxins exemplifies the problem, since some of these traits are more prevalent among certain ethnic groups. At present, there is no scientific basis for the use of such tests in a workplace medical program except in the context of a rigorous study protocol with appropriate informed consent.

Detection of nonoccupational factors or diseases that might render a worker more vulnerable to the toxic effects of a workplace exposure merits several possible actions. Counseling and lifestyle modification programs may be used to combat substance abuse and to aid in control of medical problems, such as hypertension and cardiovascular disease. Appropriate job modifications may obviate the problem. Positive findings should lead to exclusion of a worker from a particular job only as a last resort.

The 1990 Americans with Disabilities Act, which forbids the use of medical testing by employers unless the results provide information about the person's ability to perform job-related functions and also bans medical testing of applicants until a job offer is made, should help ensure that such tests are not abused.

Injury and Illness Treatment. Evaluation and treatment of work-related and, at some worksites, nonwork-related illness and injury may be included in an occupational health program. The benefit to the employer and employee of including illness and injury treatment in an occupational health program depends largely on the sophistication of management on occupational health and safety issues, the competence and professionalism of the occupational health personnel, and the status of labor–management relations at the worksite.

In the ideal situation, ongoing involvement of the occupational health team in evaluation and treatment of work-related medical problems will help ensure appropriate treatment, will result in better surveillance of work-related health problems, and will lead to evaluation of the workplace to prevent recurrence of the illness or injury in the affected employee or development of the illness or injury in other employees.

Return-to-Work Examinations. Because many physicians lack expertise in occupational medicine, employees may be sent back to work after personal or work-related illness or injury without knowledgeable evaluation of their ability to perform their jobs without harm to themselves or others.

In a state-of-the-art occupational health program, return-to-work examinations are performed after prolonged medical absence (e.g., longer than 2 weeks) to ensure employees' fitness for duty or outline appropriate work restrictions. If the employee is considered to be unfit for his or her usual work, plans are made with the treating physician for appropriate treatment, rehabilitation, or both. The purpose of these examinations is to prevent exacerbation or recurrence of the illness or injury in the affected employee and to protect other workers.

These examinations also serve an important surveillance function, enabling occupational health personnel to be continually aware of unusual illness or injury patterns that merit investigation for possible work-relatedness.

Periodic Fitness-for-Duty Examinations. Periodic examinations of employees to determine their continued fitness for work are performed for many jobs where the nature of the work demands constant assurance of medical capability. For some jobs, these examinations are required, and their contents are specified by federal regulatory agencies. Examples include bus and truck drivers, covered by the Department of Transportation (DOT), and pilots, covered by the Federal Aviation Agency (FAA).

Workers who wear respiratory protection in the course of their job duties are required by OSHA to be medically cleared to use this equipment. The examination contents and frequency are not at this time mandated in the regulation, but recommended approaches have been published.[20]

For some jobs, such as heavy equipment operation or work involving climbing to great heights, the desirability of periodic fitness-for-duty evaluation is obvious. Because the aim of these examinations is similar to those required of truck and bus drivers (i.e., to screen for conditions that could cause sudden loss of consciousness or otherwise impair the employee's ability to safely perform the job without harm to self and others), the DOT examination protocol often is used.

For the purpose of integrating a surveillance program into an existing clinical framework, surveillance examinations may be conducted concurrently with fitness-for-duty examinations, since the content of the two examinations may have considerable overlap.

Health Promotion. Workplace health promotion, designed to maintain or improve the overall health of employees through risk factor identification and modification and early disease detection, has greatly proliferated in the past decade. Reasons for these expanded efforts include increased national emphasis on wellness and disease prevention and employer efforts to decrease employee absenteeism and health care costs.

Health promotion activities, with their emphasis on prevention, offer a forum for reiterating the importance of prevention of occupational disease and injury. Despite the obvious desirability of general wellness for employees, it is important for the occupational health team to maintain its primary focus on detection and prevention of work-related injury and illness and to remind both management and workers continually of their occupational health and safety responsibilities.

Drug Testing. Preemployment, random, and for-cause testing of employees' blood, urine, or both for evidence of alcohol or illegal drug use has become a popular practice in industry, as well as a contentious legal and ethical issue for management, workers, and workplace health and safety professionals.

One of the often-stated purposes of employee drug testing is to decrease work-related accident rates. Although there have been claims that drug testing has indeed accomplished this, well-controlled studies evaluating the effectiveness of drug testing are not generally available. A review article addressing this question and most of the other myriad issues surrounding workplace drug testing has been published recently.[21]

REFERENCES

1. Landrigan P: Improving the surveillance of occupational disease. Am J Public Health 79(12):1601, 1989
2. Freund E, Seligman PJ, Chorba TL, et al: Mandatory reporting of occupational diseases by clinicians. MMWR 39(RR-9):19, 1990
3. Baker EL, Melius JM, Millar JD: Surveillance of occupational illness and injury in the United States: Current perspectives and future directions. J Public Health Policy 9(2):198, 1988
4. Halperin WE, Ratcliffe J, Frazier TM, et al: Medical screening in the workplace: Proposed principles. J Occup Med 28(8):547, 1986
5. NIOSH/OSHA Occupational Health Guidelines for Chemical Hazards. DHHS (NIOSH) Publications Nos. 81-123, 88-118, 89-104.
6. Rempel D (ed): Medical surveillance in the workplace. State Art Rev Occup Med 5(3), 1990
7. Yodaiken RE: Director, Office of Occupational Medicine, OSHA. Personal communication, 7/6/90
8. Medical surveillance programs for employees. Occup Safety Health Rep 20(13):643, 1990
9. Lauwerys RR: Industrial Chemical Exposure: Guidelines for Biological Monitoring. Davis, CA: Biomedical Publications, 1983
10. American Chemical Society 1989 Annual Report
11. Levy BS: The teaching of occupational health in U.S. medical schools: Five-year follow-up of an initial survey. Am J Public Health 75(1):79, 1985
12. Institute of Medicine: Role of the Primary Care Physician in Occupational and Environmental Medicine. Washington, DC: National Academy Press, 1988
13. Rosenstock L, Cullen MR: Clinical Occupational Medicine. Philadelphia: W.B. Saunders, 1986, 1991
14. Cullen MR, Cherniack MG, Rosenstock L: Occupational medicine. JAMA 322(9):594-601, 322(10):675-683, 1990
15. Hazard Communication (29 CFR 1910.1200). General Industry OSHA Safety and Health Standards, U.S. Department of Labor, Occupational Safety and Health Administration, Washington, DC, 1988
16. National Research Council: Counting Injuries and Illnesses in the Workplace. Washington, DC: National Academy Press, 1987
17. U.S. Congress, Committee on Government Operations: Occupational Illness Data Collection: Fragmented, Unreliable and Seventy Years Behind Communicable Disease Surveillance. Washington, DC: U.S. Government Printing Office, 1984
18. Felton JS: Occupational Medical Management. Boston: Little, Brown, 1990
19. Himmelstein J, Andersson BJ: Low back pain: Risk evaluation and preplacement screening. State Art Rev Occup Med 3(2):255, 1988
20. Harber P: The evaluation of pulmonary fitness and risk. State Art Rev Occup Med 3(2):285, 1988
21. Osterloh J: Drug testing in the workplace. State Art Rev Occup Med 5(3):517, 1990

32

Special Working Groups

Workers with Disabilities

Harriet L. Rubenstein

The employment of people with disabilities raises challenging medical, social, legal, and ethical issues. Employers traditionally have viewed people with disabilities as unemployable, citing as potential problems the negative attitudes of customers and nondisabled co-workers, the inability of disabled workers to meet production and quality standards, the costs of removing architectural barriers, providing special equipment, and making necessary job modifications, and an inevitable increase in health, disability, and liability insurance costs. In a 1987 survey of over 900 corporate managers conducted by Louis Harris for the International Center for the Disabled (ICD), 66% of those whose company had not hired a disabled person in the preceding 3 years cited a lack of qualified applicants as an important reason. Only 10% of top management displayed strong optimism toward disabled people as a potential source of employees, and most managers thought their company was already doing enough to employ the disabled and should not make greater efforts in this area.[1]

Consequently, in 1985, two thirds of working age adults with work disabilities were not in the labor force; that is, they were neither employed nor actively seeking work, at a large financial cost to society. That same year, the federal government spent $62 billion on subsidies, medical care, and other programs for disabled persons, of which 93% went to support out-of-work individuals with disabilities.[2] Ironically, a 1986 ICD survey of working-age disabled Americans revealed that two thirds of those not in the labor force would like to have a job.[3] In the same survey, disabled adults who were not working at all or not working full-time reported a number of barriers to their integration into the workforce, set out in Table 32–1. Although limitations in activity and the need for care, the two most frequently cited barriers, are difficult for policymakers to address, additional survey results suggest that many disabled adults may be unaware of available rehabilitation and medical services.[3] Interestingly, although 70% of disabled adults receiving benefits reported that they would lose some benefits if they started working full-time, only 18% of unemployed or underemployed disabled adults cited fear of a loss of benefits as an important reason for their employment status.[3] Many of the other reported obstacles are more amenable to change through employer education, worker training, and public policies targeted to the employment-related needs of the disabled.

A combination of demographic, social, political, and economic factors, however, is improving employment prospects for the disabled. Over the past decade, the number of young entrants to the job market has dropped, as the last of the baby boom generation completed their schooling. At the same time, the economy is growing, with employment expected to increase 19% by the year 2000.[4] Facing a shortage of qualified job applicants, employers in many parts of the country must consider new recruitment strategies, and both older and disabled job seekers stand to benefit. Legal requirements, particularly those of the federal 1973 Rehabilitation Act and similar state laws, have provided the disabled with some protection from employment discrimination and forced many employers to make "reasonable accommodations" to the needs of qualified disabled job applicants. Passage of the 1990 Americans with Disabilities Act, prohibiting employment discrimination against any qualified individual with a disability because of that disability, will compel more employers to reevaluate their hiring practices. (Publ. No. 101–336, 104 Stat. 327 [1990].)

Changes in the U.S. economy also are improving employment opportunities for people with disabilities. During the next decade, most growth in the economy will continue to occur in wage and salary jobs in the services industry, where jobs are more suitable than ever for the disabled.[4] Moreover, high technology equipment and software that perform tasks that certain disabilities preclude—for example, scanners that "read," light pens that "type," and speech synthesizers—are increasingly making disability irrelevant at the workplace.

Skyrocketing disability-related costs are providing another incentive for employment of the disabled. According to the ICD managers survey, over two thirds of employers believe they have a responsibility to rehabilitate their employees who become disabled, and an equally large majority believe it is more cost-effective to rehabilitate disabled employees and return them to work than to pay them disability benefits and replace them.[1]

Moreover, studies indicate that employers who hire or retain workers with disabilities are highly satisfied with their performance.[1,5] The overwhelming majority of managers polled in the ICD survey gave disabled employees a good or excellent rating on overall job performance. They reported that disabled employees perform on a par with or above their nondisabled counterparts with respect to their willingness to work hard, reliability, attendance and punctuality, productivity, desire for promotion, and leadership ability.[1] Another study reported that disabled employees work safely and may even be more careful than their nondisabled colleagues.[5]

As employers respond to these social, legal, and economic pressures, health professionals will be called on increasingly by

TABLE 32-1. REASONS WHY DISABLED ADULTS ARE NOT WORKING AT ALL OR NOT WORKING FULL-TIME

Reason	% Citing as Important Reason
Disability severely limits activity	78
Need for medical treatment/therapy	52
Employer attitudes toward disability	47
Full-time work is unavailable or cannot be found in line of work	40
Lack of necessary skills, education, or training	38
Lack of transportation to and from work or housing near work	28
Need for special equipment or devices	23
Loss of benefits or insurance payments	18
Childcare or other family responsibilities	15

From Harris et al., 1986.[3]

policymakers, employers, advocates for the disabled, and others to help in the design and implementation of programs and policies aimed at integrating people with disabilities into the workforce.

Demographic Profile

A discussion of disability should begin by distinguishing between "impairment" and "disability." Impairment is an alteration of health status that can be described in purely medical terms. Usually, a physician makes a determination of impairment. Disability is an alteration of a person's capacity to meet personal, social, or occupational demands as a result of a medical impairment. Disability determinations generally are made by someone other than a physician using physician-generated information on impairment.[6] Two persons with the same impairment may have different disabilities depending on their age, living situation, education, work experience, skills, and psychological and other factors. The distinction between disability and impairment becomes most significant in the context of disability evaluations conducted for purposes of determining an individual's eligibility for public or private disability insurance benefits, workers' compensation, or similar program. This is discussed more fully below.

Statistics on the prevalence of disability in the U.S. population vary according to the definition of "disabled" and the content, design, and methodology of the survey. This section focuses on work disability, that is, limitations in the amount or type of work that an individual can perform as a result of a medical impairment. Estimates derived from the 1983–1985 National Health Interview Survey place the prevalence of work disability at 11.5% of the U.S. working-age population.[7] The 1988 Bureau of the Census Current Population Survey (CPS) estimated that 8.6% of 16 to 64 year olds, or approximately 13.4 million adults, are work disabled.[8] CPS data, although acknowledged underestimates, provide valuable information on the labor force activity and earnings of persons with a work disability.

The population of noninstitutionalized 16 to 64-year-old disabled adults divides itself into three relatively equal segments: 31.3% are in the labor force, 42% receive Social Security, Supplemental Security Income, or some other retirement or disability income because of their disability, and 26.7% are neither on payrolls nor on aid rolls.[9] The distribution of disabled adults among these three categories varies markedly by sex. Approximately 44% of disabled men compared to 25% of disabled women are in the labor force, probably in large part a function of cultural pressures regarding appropriate sex roles.[9] Research evidence suggests, however, that employment contributes to higher perceived health status among disabled women, and policies and programs, such as job retraining, must focus on enabling disabled women to participate in the labor force in greater numbers.[10]

Age, schooling, income, and race all correlate highly with work disability status (Table 32–2).[8] The likelihood of having a work disability is strongly related to age, with persons 55 to 64 years old nearly four times as likely as persons 25 to 34 years old to be work disabled. The relationship between work disability status and years of school completed also is strong. Persons who have completed less than 8 years of school have a disability rate that is more than triple that of high school graduates and eight times that of college graduates. The inverse relationship between work disability and formal education remains significant even when controlling for age. Suggested explanations for this relationship include, on the one hand, the negative impact of disability on a person's ability to attend school and, on the other hand, the association between low levels of schooling and two potential risk factors for disability: poverty and employment in physically demanding jobs.[8]

Income also exhibits an inverse relationship to work disability, with 21.9% of working-age adults in poverty having a work disability compared with only 5.6% of those with an income of at least twice the poverty threshold.[8]

Finally, race correlates with work disability, with blacks having a much higher likelihood than either whites or Hispanics of being work disabled.[8]

Of those disabled adults who are in the labor force, approximately two thirds are in the prime working years, ages 25 to 54. Disabled adults in the labor force are better educated and enjoy markedly higher incomes than the general population of disabled adults.[9] Table 32–3 depicts the labor force activity of working-

TABLE 32-2. PERCENT OF PERSONS 16 TO 64 YEARS OLD WITH A WORK DISABILITY, BY SELECTED CHARACTERISTICS: 1988

Characteristics	Both Sexes	Males	Females
Total	8.6	8.7	8.4
▪ AGE (YEARS)			
16–24	3.8	4.1	3.6
25–34	5.6	5.9	5.6
35–44	7.1	7.7	6.5
45–54	10.3	10.3	10.2
55–64	22.3	22.4	22.2
▪ YEARS OF SCHOOL COMPLETED[a]			
Less than 8 years	29.7	29.1	30.2
8	24.6	23.9	25.2
9–11	17.7	17.5	17.9
12	8.8	9.3	8.4
13–15	7.5	8.4	6.7
16 or more	3.8	3.8	3.8
▪ INCOME/POVERTY RATIO			
Less than 1.00	21.9	24.4	20.3
1.00–1.24	17.8	19.0	16.8
1.25–1.49	13.4	13.4	13.4
1.50–1.99	11.3	12.8	9.9
2.00 and over	5.6	5.8	5.3
▪ RACE AND HISPANIC ORIGIN[b]			
White	7.9	8.2	7.7
Black	13.7	13.7	13.8
Hispanic origin	8.2	8.4	7.9

[a] Universe is persons 25 to 64 years old.
[b] Persons of Hispanic origin may be of any race.
From Labor Force Status and Other Characteristics of Persons with a Work Disability, 1989.[8]

TABLE 32-3. LABOR FORCE STATUS BY WORK DISABILITY STATUS, NONINSTITUTIONALIZED PERSONS 16–64 YEARS: 1988

	With a Work Disability (%)			With No Work Disability (%)		
	Male	**Female**	**Total**	**Male**	**Female**	**Total**
In labor force	35.7	27.5	31.6	88.9	69.5	78.9
Employed full-time	(23.4)	(13.1)	(18.2)	(74.8)	(47.1)	(60.6)
Unemployed	(5.1)	(3.9)	(4.9)	(5.5)	(3.6)	(4.6)
Not in labor force	64.3	72.5	68.4	11.1	30.5	21.1
Total	100.0	100.0	100.0	100.0	100.0	100.0

Adapted from Labor Force Status and Other Characteristics of Persons with a Work Disability, 1989.[8]

age men and women by work disability status in 1988. Workers with disabilities are distributed throughout all occupation groups in both the public and private sectors and as self-employed workers.

Accommodating the Worker with Disabilities

Legal Requirements. Numerous federal and state laws prohibit discrimination in employment on the basis of "handicap." At the federal level, the principal statute has been the Rehabilitation Act of 1973.[11] For purposes of the Act, a handicapped individual is any person who either has a physical or mental impairment that substantially limits one or more major life activities or has a record of such an impairment or is regarded as having such an impairment. Section 501 prohibits employment discrimination on the basis of handicap by the federal government. Section 503 requires that employers with federal contracts in excess of $2500 take affirmative action to employ and promote qualified handicapped individuals. Section 504 prohibits private employers who receive federal financial assistance from discriminating against "otherwise qualified individuals with handicaps." An estimated three million firms, approximately half the businesses in the country, may be covered by the Act.[12] The Americans with Disabilities Act of 1990 (the ADA) becomes effective in July 1992 and by 1994 will cover all private sector employers with 15 or more employees. The ADA strengthens and expands current federal law. In addition, virtually every state has enacted laws prohibiting discrimination in public and private employment on the basis of handicap. These laws usually have wider coverage than the federal statute but vary markedly as to employers covered, protected handicapping conditions, and available remedies.

Neither the federal nor state laws require an employer to hire, promote, or retain every disabled person for every job. Rather, the employer can establish job qualifications and then make employment decisions based on the individual's ability to perform the essential duties of the job. Most antidiscrimination statutes require that the job qualifications established by the employer be job-related and consistent with business necessity and the safe performance of the job. Judicial interpretations of federal and state laws emphasize the necessity for an individualized determination of an applicant's or an employee's ability to perform a job. Categorical rejection of an individual based on the type of impairment or the nature of the medical condition, without consideration of specific limitations in relation to specific job requirements, most likely will be found violative of these employment discrimination statutes.

If a handicapped person cannot perform the essential functions of a job, both federal and state laws require employers to make "reasonable accommodation" for the physical and mental limitations of the applicant or employee unless the accommodation would impose an "undue hardship" on the conduct of the employer's business. Although what is "reasonable" must be determined on a case-by-case basis, regulations implementing the federal Rehabilitation Act provide some general guidance. According to these regulations, reasonable accommodation may include making workplace facilities readily accessible to and usable by handicapped persons, job restructuring, part-time or modified work schedules, acquisition or modification of equipment or devices, the provision of readers or interpreters, and other similar actions.[13] These regulations also set forth the following factors to be considered in the determination of "undue hardship": the overall size of the employer's operation with respect to number of employees, number and type of facilities, and size of budget, the type of business operation, including composition and structure of the workforce, and the nature and cost of the accommodation needed.[14] Determination of undue hardship also must be made on a case-by-case basis, balancing the benefits to the disabled individual and society against the burdens to the employer.

Job Analysis. Conducting a job analysis is the first step in a rational assessment of any individual's ability to perform the essential requirements of a job and a prerequisite to job accommodation determinations. Mistaken assumptions as to the skills required and hazards posed by a particular job or the type or extent of an individual's limitations can result in discrimination against persons with disabilities and in poor employment decisions generally. A written job analysis systematically identifies the following components of a job: the specific tasks involved, the frequency of their performance and their importance to successful job completion, the specific worker experience, knowledge, skills, and behaviors required, the tools and equipment used, time and motion requirements, and the prevailing working conditions, including physical, chemical, and psychological hazards.

A thorough job analysis begins with a review of existing job descriptions and training manuals. Discussions with supervisors and direct observations and interviews of incumbent workers should follow, with a completed draft of the job analysis submitted to supervisors and incumbent workers for validation and final ranking of job duties. Input from physicians, occupational health nurses, safety managers, industrial hygienists, ergonomists, and other professionals may be needed. Data available under the federal OSHA Hazard Communication Standard and Medical Access regulation and state and local right-to-know laws can facilitate development of an accurate depiction of working conditions. Determining the actual level of worker exposure to particular hazards will require environmental monitoring as well as evaluation of the effectiveness of ventilation systems, respirators, or other protective measures being used.

Using the job analysis, an employer can develop a profile of the skills, characteristics, and experience that are required for successful job performance. This profile will be useful in decisions involving the hiring, training, compensation, promotion, and retention of all workers, both disabled and nondisabled. The job analysis is particularly useful when determining what, if any, modifications can be made to a job in order to accommodate people with disabilities. Performing the job analysis may uncover working conditions that should be changed to protect the health and safety of all workers and of the surrounding community.

Analogous to the job analysis, an evaluation of the individual applicant or employee must be performed to determine his or her suitability for the job and any accommodations that may be needed. Evaluation should be made of the individual's technical or professional qualifications, physical and mental functioning, and personal attributes, such as assertiveness, organizational skills, and independence. The role of the clinician in these evaluations is discussed more fully below.

Job Accommodation. With a thorough job analysis in hand, an employer can more readily identify those areas in which adjustments and adaptations can be made to enable an individual with a functional limitation to be hired or promoted or to return to work after an illness or injury. The range of potential modifications is as varied as the functional limitations needing accommodation. Many modifications will protect the health and safety and enhance the productivity of all workers. Still others, such as ramps, will benefit the employer by also accommodating the needs of older or disabled customers or those with small children.

Wheelchair users need ramps, easily opened doors, and space for their chairs entering and exiting as well as within work areas. Often, simply raising an ordinary desk or worktable is sufficient to allow the wheelchair-bound user to work comfortably. Specially designed and mechanically adjustable workstations also are available. The limited range of reach of wheelchair users and others with upper body strength and extension problems may be simply and inexpensively accommodated by moving equipment or devices from one side of a work area to the other. In addition, a variety of devices are available to extend a person's reach and grasp.

Lift assist devices, such as hydraulic tailgates and scissor lifts, can accommodate the worker with a back disorder or a history of cardiovascular disease and can prevent injuries when made available to all workers.

Many individuals with severe strength and motion limitations, such as those caused by quadriplegia or cerebral palsy, can operate telephones, computers, and even manufacturing equipment with the installation of switches that can be operated with one's mouth or a headstick or by rolling a wheelchair across a strip on the floor.

People with visual impairments can be accommodated by raised lettering or Braille symbols on signs and elevator buttons. Enlarged print and electronic readers with speech or braille output enable the visually impaired to read printed material and access computers.

Accommodations for hearing-impaired workers include amplification of existing telephone equipment or installation of telephone devices for the deaf (TDD) and use of vibration techniques or activation of light sources to provide greater awareness of surrounding activities.

Workers with severe allergies to particular chemicals may require installation of ventilation systems in the work area or substitution of the offending agent with a safer alternative. These modifications will protect the health of all potentially exposed workers.

Mentally retarded workers or those with a history of mental illness often can be accommodated very inexpensively. Extra training, dissection of complex tasks into simpler components, and sensitive supervision may be all that is necessary to ensure comprehension and productivity.

Flexible scheduling of arrival, departure, lunch and break times, and part-time or seasonal employment may enable workers with disabilities to work around their special transportation needs or their treatment or therapy schedules.

Job restructuring and modification and reassignment and recombination of tasks can allow disabled workers to perform that portion of a job that is unaffected by their impairments. Where workers are represented by a labor union, the collective bargaining agreement will need to be consulted before these changes can be made. ICD survey results indicate that despite allegations to the contrary, the overwhelming majority of employers have not encountered resistance from labor unions when making job modifications or reassignments that would allow a newly disabled employee to return to work.[1]

Determining what job accommodation is necessary should begin with input from the disabled individual, who can offer constructive advice as to what adjustments need to be made. Agencies dealing with specific disabilities, such as State Commissions for the Blind and Visually Impaired, state and local rehabilitation agencies, Governors' Committees on Employment of Persons with Disabilities, and occupational therapy departments at local rehabilitation hospitals, are good resources for assistance in providing appropriate accommodation. Often, some of the state agencies can help pay for more expensive types of equipment. The Job Accommodation Network (JAN) is a national information and consultation service whose mission is to assist employers and rehabilitation professionals with the hiring, retention, and advancement of persons with disabilities through job accommodation. JAN's services are available to all employers, without charge.

Most building design modifications have emphasized solutions that permit people with disabilities to gain access to a building or facility. Little attention has been paid to providing safe egress for the disabled during time of emergency, and more research into innovative evacuation technologies is sorely needed. In the meantime, disabled workers and their employers will need to rely on more traditional techniques. Strict compliance with building and fire codes, installation and maintenance of all recommended safety features, and scrupulous adherence to safe work practices will promote safety for all building occupants, including those with disabilities. Early detection systems, two-way communication methods, and safe areas of refuge—compartments within a building where people can await the arrival of rescue personnel—facilitate the safe evacuation of both disabled and nondisabled occupants.

As with other job modifications, disabled workers must be included in the evacuation planning process, since they are in the best position to identify the assistance they would need. Possible modifications include visual or other sensory alarm systems to supplement traditional audio signal systems for the hearing impaired, tactile maps along with traditional evacuation maps for the visually impaired, and evacuation chairs for transportation of disabled persons down stairs. Disabled employees must be included in all evacuation drills to ensure that appropriate and sufficient accommodations have been made.

In most cases, the cost of accommodating people with disabilities in the workplace is modest. In the ICD survey of managers, three fourths of respondents reported that the average cost of employing a disabled person is about the same as the cost of employing a nondisabled person in the same job. The large majority of managers in companies that have made accommodations reported that the cost of making these accommodations has not been expensive.[1] Another study of job accommodation in over 900 firms found that approximately one half of the accommodations cost nothing, and another 18% cost less than \$100.[15]

Vocational Rehabilitation. Currently, two separate vocational rehabilitation systems operate in the United States, one public sector, and one private sector, each having different objectives, serving clients with different types of disabilities, and providing a different mix of services.

Public sector vocational rehabilitation operates as a federal–state partnership aimed at maximizing the vocational potential of disabled individuals. Once evaluated, a disabled client is prescribed an appropriate rehabilitation regimen that may include restorative surgery, on-the-job training, or formal education. Ideally, on completion of the program, the participant is placed in competitive employment. Public agency clients usually have little or no vocational experience and limited labor market skills.

Over the past decade, private sector vocational rehabilitation agencies have emerged, primarily to serve the needs of employers and their workers' compensation insurance carriers, concerned over the skyrocketing cost of work-related disability. The mission of the private sector agencies is to return disabled persons to work at their predisability level of earnings as quickly as possible by whatever means are appropriate. In contrast to public service agencies, which emphasize training and formal schooling programs, private agencies rely on placement services and job site modifications.

Studies of public sector vocational rehabilitation programs generally have found that the benefits to the individual and to society outweigh the costs.[16] Few data are available on the cost-effectiveness of the private sector programs. On the other hand, the ICD survey reported that the majority of disabled persons who had participated in a vocational rehabilitation program found that it provided little or no help to them in securing employment. In light of employer reports that a major obstacle to employing the disabled is the lack of qualified applicants, it appears that the provision of potentially valuable vocational rehabilitation services is desperately in need of reexamination and revision.

Role of the Clinician

The clinician most commonly confronts the issue of work disability in two contexts: when performing medical evaluations of workers applying for disability benefits and when performing worker fitness and risk evaluations as part of preplacement medical examinations of new hires or as part of return-to-work examinations of employees who recently have suffered an illness or injury.

Disability Evaluations. There are three major compensation systems in the United States to which people can turn for financial support when they can no longer work because of an illness or injury: Social Security Disability Insurance (SSDI) and Supplemental Security Income (SSI), workers' compensation, and private disability insurance plans. The three programs differ in their definition of disability, their legal and medical eligibility criteria, and their schedule of benefits. Workers' compensation program requirements and benefit levels even differ from state to state. Furthermore, the nature and scope of the physician's role vary among each of these systems and often are confusing to the patient, the physician, the employer, and even program administrators. For example, SSDI and SSI require the treating physician to determine only the applicant's degree of medical impairment. The determination of ability to work rests with an administrative body. Under most private disability insurance plans, however, the treating physician determines both impairment and ability to work. These complex and often conflicting systems can be frustrating for individuals with disabilities and for their physicians.

The disability evaluation process may require a clinician to assume any one or more of three very different and potentially conflicting roles: patient advocate and counselor, source of information for the determining agency, and adjudicator and certifier of impairment or disability.[17]

As advocate and counselor, the physician should advise the patient with a work incapacity of the availability, advantages, and potential pitfalls of the various compensation programs. Physicians treating patients with work disability need to be sensitive to the complex psychological, social, and economic impacts of disability on patients and their families. Referrals to psychologists, social workers, and rehabilitation specialists may be as significant as those to medical specialists. Where appropriate, physicians should encourage and assist patients with disabilities to return to the workforce. With the patient's consent, the physician can work with the employer to identify and design necessary accommodations.

Once a patient has applied for benefits, the physician will likely be asked to provide medical records and other documentation of impairment. The physician should respond promptly, with only that information relevant to the patient's specific disability determination. For example, information regarding a patient's diabetes would be irrelevant to a workers' compensation claim based on a low back injury. In all cases, a signed request for release of information must first be obtained from the patient.

An employer or insurance company request for a treating physician to evaluate a patient's impairment places that physician in the role of adjudicator. In this role, the physician faces the greatest potential for conflict with the patient, who may feel betrayed by the physician's adherence to legal requirement that appear unfair to the patient. In all cases, physicians need to state explicitly to their patients which role they are assuming and the potential conflicts that may arise. More thorough discussions of the physician's role in disability evaluation appear elsewhere.[17,18]

Selection Screening. Motivated by the dramatic increase in health insurance, workers' compensation, and related benefit costs, growing numbers of employers have turned to selection screening—the use of medical criteria in the selection and maintenance of a workforce—to identify healthier workers and thereby contain costs.[19] Preplacement and return to work examinations are two popular examples of selection screenings, the purposes of which are to determine current fitness for work and to evaluate the risk of future illness and injury.

Fitness-for-work evaluations require the clinician to assess an applicant's or employee's current health in order to determine whether the individual is medically capable of performing the essential tasks of the job under consideration. If not, the clinician must then determine what accommodations or modifications in the workplace or the job might enable the individual to perform that job. The clinician performing a fitness-for-work evaluation must be totally familiar with the specific job demands, the work environment, and the potential for modifications. A thorough job analysis helps to ensure the relevance of the fitness-for-work evaluation. The significant medical uncertainty that permeates these evaluations suggests that accommodation and job trial are preferable over outright exclusion of potentially impaired individuals.[20]

Risk evaluations attempt to predict whether currently capable individuals are at increased risk of illness or injury in relation to performance of the proposed job because of such factors as current health conditions, past medical or work histories, genetic makeup, environmental exposures, or behavioral patterns. If a determination of increased risk is made, potential job modifications or personal risk factor modifications that might reduce the risk must be considered. Again, the uncertainty of these determinations makes accommodation, employee education and counseling, and job trial preferable to restrictive hiring and placement schemes.[20]

Worker fitness and risk evaluations raise numerous medical, legal, and ethical dilemmas for the clinician. In most instances, few data exist to support a determination of whether, and to what extent, a particular characteristic is, in fact, a risk factor for a specific adverse outcome or the likelihood of a specific outcome given the identified risk factor and the anticipated job demands or exposures. Questions arise as to whether individuals at increased risk for work-related injury or illness should be permitted to assume that risk, provided that their employment does not endanger co-workers or the public. Clinicians may be under pressure from employers to reveal specific medical diagnoses and other information concerning an applicant or employee. A thorough discussion of these dilemmas is beyond the scope of this chapter. Detailed analyses are available elsewhere.[19,21]

Conclusion

Despite the proscriptions and requirements of federal and state statutes, 25% of working-age disabled adults report that they have experienced employment discrimination because of their disability.[3] Advocates for the rights of the disabled worked hard for passage of the ADA, which prohibits discrimination against the disabled in employment, in the provision of public services, notably transportation, in telecommunications, and in public accommodations and services. Implementation and enforcement of the ADA are essential to the integration of people with disabilities into the mainstream of American life.

Public health professionals can promote and facilitate the employment of people with disabilities by educating employers, employees, colleagues, policymakers, and the public about the work abilities of the disabled and by dispelling those myths and stereotypes that foster the social and economic isolation of individuals with disabilities.

Migrant and Seasonal Farmworkers

Harriet L. Rubenstein

Harsh social, economic, and political conditions combine to make migrant and seasonal farmworkers probably the most at-risk of American workers. These same factors render the traditional analyses of occupational health status inadequate to the task of describing the impact of hazardous working conditions on the health of farmworkers.

Over the last decade, agriculture has ranked consistently among the three most hazardous U.S. industries, and in 1987, agricultural workers ranked first in the rate of work-related fatalities and disabling injuries. Their death rate of 49 per 100,000 workers was above that of 38 and 35 per 100,000 for mining and construction, respectively, and well above the 10 per 100,000 for all industries combined. Their disabling injury rate of 50 per 1000 exceeded the 37 and 30 per 1000 for mining and construction and 16 per 1000 for all industries combined.[1] In addition to safety hazards, poor sanitation, infectious agents, pesticides, and excessive heat jeopardize the health of farmworkers. Tragically, economic necessity for migrant families dictates that children often must work and play in the fields alongside their parents, exposed to an array of potentially life-threatening health and safety hazards.

Poverty, along with social, cultural, linguistic, and geographic isolation, impedes the ability of migrant and seasonal farmworkers to obtain adequate housing, nutrition, health care, education, and social services. Inadequate housing, often provided by the employer and situated in close proximity to the fields, reproduces and exacerbates occupational exposures.

Federal and state laws that protect most workers from dangerous or oppressive working conditions totally or partially exclude farmworkers. The National Labor Relations Act, which provides legal protection for the unionization and collective bargaining activities of most workers, does not cover farmworkers. Consequently, a mere 2.5% of U.S. agricultural wage and salary workers enjoy union representation, compared to 14.5% of private nonagricultural workers and 42.5% of government employees.[2] Unions generally are credited with securing improved conditions for workers both legislatively and contractually, and the low rate of unionization among farmworkers contributes to their harsh working conditions and meager wages and benefits.

The workers' compensation laws in nearly half of the states exclude farmworkers, who then cannot receive payments for lost wages and related medical expenses when they suffer work-related disabilities. The federal Occupational Safety and Health Act (OSHAct), which regulates workplace exposures to hazardous conditions, excludes farms with fewer than 11 employees from its oversight. Consequently, the majority of farmworkers do not enjoy OSHA protection. The child labor proscriptions of the federal Fair Labor Standards Act allow children to toil in the fields at a younger age than in most other workplaces. Farmworkers do not enjoy the full protection of the Act's minimum wage and overtime provisions, nor do they have full rights under the federal Social Security Act, and they are often the victims of employer nonreporting and fraud.[8]

Demographic Profile

By virtue of their mobility, geographic and linguistic isolation, seasonal employment, and, for many, their undocumented status, migrant and seasonal farmworkers defy accurate census and demographic description. Enumeration difficulties are compounded by definitional differences—whether nonmigratory seasonal workers, undocumented foreign workers, and accompanying dependents are included—and by the conflicting political agendas of the government agencies and farmworker advocacy organizations doing the counting. Generally, seasonal farmworkers are distinguished from migrants in that the former live and harvest crops in their own communities, whereas the latter travel various distances to find employment. Because many workers shift back and forth between seasonal and migrant status, depending on political, economic, weather, and other conditions, this distinction becomes artificial. Our inability to count accurately the farmworker population is significant because underestimations translate into reduced funding for desperately needed health, education, legal, and other service programs targeted to these groups.

Estimates of the number of seasonal and migrant farmworkers and their dependents range upward from 1.3 million, but a comprehensive analysis of data from various sources places the number at 5 million.[4] The racial composition of the migrant workforce has evolved in recent years, with a marked increase in the proportion of migrants from Cuba, Haiti, and other Caribbean islands. A recent survey estimated that 71% of migrant farmworkers are Hispanic, 16% are black, and 11% are white. Two thirds are male, and most are young. Not surprisingly, over half of migrant farmworkers have not completed high school, and almost one third have an eighth grade education or less.[5] The Minimum Wage Study Commission reported in June 1981 that half of migrant farmworkers surveyed earned at or below the federal minimum wage or within 25 cents above it.[6] The average annual income from farm and nonfarmwork for the head of the household was $3418 in 1986.[5] Fringe benefits, such as sick leave and vacation pay, are virtually unheard of, except under a few negotiated contracts. Consequently, when farmworkers are sick and cannot work, they do not eat either. Because most are paid on a piecework basis rather than an hourly rate, any injury or illness that interferes with eye-hand coordination, such as "mild" pesticide poisoning, acts directly to depress wages.[4]

The movement of migrant farmworkers from their home bases upstream to their various work sites crosses more than 41 states in complex patterns. Most migrants follow one of three main paths—or streams—Atlantic, Pacific, and midcontinent. The Atlantic stream originates in the citrus groves of Florida, moves up through Appalachia and into New England, harvesting apples, cranberries, mushrooms, and tobacco. The midcontinent stream originates in Texas and travels through the Central Plains to Wisconsin and Ohio. The Pacific stream, originating in southern California, flows up the west coast.

U.S. Agricultural Production

Increasing consolidation and mechanization, along with intensive chemical usage, have characterized U.S. agricultural production over the last 50 years. Farms have become both fewer and larger, with 14.5% of the farms with the highest income controlling 51.4% of the cropland.[7] Mechanization has had a dual impact on farmworkers' health and well-being. With the mechanization of many hazardous hand labor processes has come a decrease in the rate of some occupational injuries. On the other hand, mechanization has contributed to unemployment and often has required changes in production methods, such as increased use of herbicides, that have an adverse impact on worker health.[8]

Migrant and seasonal farmworkers are concentrated in labor-intensive crops, primarily fruits and vegetables, where hand cultivation and harvesting are still necessary. Sixty-five percent of hired farmworkers on farms employing more than 10 workers are involved in the production of vegetables, fruits, nuts, tobacco, and sugar. Harvesting operations, which involve contact with foliage during high pesticide application periods, employ more than 50% of seasonal workers. Crop cultivation employs 27% of seasonal workers, and more than one third of these workers cultivate cotton, a crop with a very high rate of pesticide applications.[8]

Approximately 1.08 billion pounds of pesticides were used in the United States in 1984, 79% of these in agriculture.[9] Pesticides are chemicals or biological agents used to destroy or control unwanted plants, insects, fungi, rodents, bacteria, and other pests. Some persist in the environment over long periods of time and accumulate in human, animal, and plant tissue. Pesticide formulators combine one or more active ingredients—compounds targeted to control a specific pest—with a number of inert ingredients designed to make the pesticide more effective or usable. Although inert ingredients have no intended pesticidal effect and are inactive against the target species, they may have adverse health effects and include such highly toxic substances as formaldehyde and dioxane.

The pattern of pesticide use has evolved significantly over the past 30 years. The environmentally persistent organochlorine pesticides, popular in the 1950s, were replaced by the less persistent but more acutely toxic organophosphate and carbamate compounds, and later by the pyrethroids and other compounds. From 1966 to 1980, herbicide use doubled as farmers replaced mechanical cultivation with chemical weed control. Herbicides now account for two thirds of the total poundage by active ingredient of all pesticides used in the United States. During the same time period, insecticide use rate has been halved, and fungicide use has decreased substantially.[8] The significance of fungicide use, however, outstrips the volume of its use because many fungicides, applied to fruits and vegetables, are carcinogenic, teratogenic, or both[10] (see Chapter 24).

General Health Status

Serious deficiencies in sanitation, housing, education, nutrition, and access to health care operating synergistically with hazardous occupational exposures, notably to pesticides and communicable diseases, create a bleak health status picture for the farmworker population.

A survey of active Colorado migrant workers found that 50.5% identified their health as fair or poor compared to 6.1% of the general U.S. population.[11]

A review of farmworker health data from migrant health centers and community surveys found that dermatitis, injuries, respiratory problems, musculoskeletal ailments, eye problems, gastrointestinal problems, and diabetes were the most frequently reported health problems. Additionally, surveys indicated that the majority of migrant and seasonal farmworkers and their families seek medical attention for acute ailments rather than for preventive services or the management of chronic ailments.[3] One survey compared the most frequent diagnoses of the upstream migrant health centers with those of the home base centers. Gastroenteritis and parasitic infections were common diagnoses for the upstream clinics but not for those downstream, a finding consistent with the effects of substandard migrant labor camps and unsanitary field conditions. The percentage of upstream clinics reporting dermatitis as one of the most frequent reasons for patient visits was twice that of downstream sites, consistent with the increased exposure to pesticides and plant material that occurs during the active work season.[12]

The distinction between the living and working conditions of migrants is blurred. When upstream, many migrants live in housing units supplied by the employer and often located adjacent to the fields where they work. The quality of housing provided is variable, ranging from relatively comfortable dwellings to converted chicken coops lacking indoor plumbing, electricity, ventilation, regular garbage removal, and a fresh water supply. These conditions foster the harboring and transmission of infectious diseases. Workers housed in units adjacent to pesticide-sprayed fields are subject to pesticide drift or even to direct spray. Some migrants are forced to live out in the open, sleeping and eating in the fields in which they toil. For these workers, the occupational hazards described below are ever present.

Language barriers and lack of education often make it difficult or impossible for farmworkers to protect themselves from crew leader abuses or to read and understand pesticide warning labels and posted signs.

Ironically, hunger and malnutrition are rampant among those who replenish our produce shelves. Migrant farmworkers are among the three population groups most vulnerable to malnutrition,[13] which contributes to poor dental health, obesity, cardiovascular disease, diabetes, and anemia. Nutritional deficiencies also increase the toxicity of many pesticides.[8]

A number of studies document nutritional deficiencies among migrant farmworker families. A screening of 327 children of Mexican-American migrants between the ages of 2 months and 7 years found that 16.5% of those screened were anemic.[14] A survey of migrant farmworkers in Colorado classified 12% of women as anemic and found that one third of eligible migrant women were not enrolled in the federal Women, Infants, and Children (WIC) supplemental food program.[3] A chronic disease screening of migrant and seasonal farmworkers in Utah and North Dakota found 12% of Utah migrants and 21% of North Dakota migrants to have decreased hematocrit.[3] A survey of Colorado migrant workers found that 43% of families and 67.8% of solo males had difficulty getting good food while away from home. The lack of money, transportation, refrigeration, and cooking facilities helps explain this finding. Forty percent of families and 58% of solo males reported running out of money to buy food during the previous year.[11]

Poor housing and malnutrition combined with the recent influx of immigrants has led to an increase in tuberculosis among farmworkers. A recent survey of all reported cases of tuberculosis in 29 states found that farmworkers are six times more likely to develop the disease than the general population of employed persons.[15]

Despite their exceptional needs, migrant and seasonal farmworkers face a number of obstacles to receiving adequate and necessary health care, and various aspects of medical care use by these workers are low.[16]

The federal Office of Migrant Health operates 122 health centers located in 40 states and Puerto Rico and serving over 400 geographic areas. Even these centers have had limited impact. In fiscal 1985, they provided health care to only 17% of the nation's migrant and seasonal farmworkers and their dependents.[17]

Financial barriers to care include lack of money or health insurance and unfamiliarity with free or sliding scale services. Because migrants usually work a 6-day week, the inability or unwillingness of health care providers to offer evening hours and the lack of sick leave benefits means workers must forfeit wages to receive care. As many as 32.2% of migrant health centers responding to a survey reported operating only during weekdays between 8 AM and 5 PM.[12] The tendency of most agricultural areas to be medically underserved and the lack of transportation from the fields or labor camps also impede access. Cultural and linguistic barriers between immigrant farmworkers and health care providers discourage these workers from seeking care and discourage providers from reaching out to this community. For undocumented workers, fear of detection and deportation by immigration authorities is a significant deterrent to their pursuit of health care and other services. When migrant families finally do use the health care system, they often must leave the area before they can receive all the necessary follow-up care. Providers should bear this in mind when designing and offering services to this population.

Work-related Health Problems

Pesticide-related Illnesses. The primary route of farmworker exposure to most pesticides is through dermal absorption. Inhalation and ingestion are secondary avenues of exposure. Fieldworkers who cultivate and harvest crops are exposed to pesticide residues on foliage, on the crops themselves, and in the dusty soil and decaying organic material that collects in the fields. Aerial and ground pesticide application exposes workers through direct spray and through drift of pesticides sprayed on adjacent fields. In a survey of Colorado migrants, one third reported that, at some time, pesticides had been applied to an area while they were working it, and 13% reported having pesticides spilled or sprayed on them at some time in the past.[11] In a survey of southern Florida farmworkers, nearly one half of the respondents reported having been directly sprayed on at least one occasion while working.[18]

Deficiencies in sanitation in the fields and in nearby labor camps exacerbate pesticide exposures. Pesticide residues contaminate irrigation water that may be used for drinking, cooking, and bathing. The increasing use of chemigation, putting pesticides in the irrigation water, underscores this problem. The lack of adequate toilet and handwashing facilities in the fields means that workers may eat and smoke with pesticide-contaminated hands, may use pesticide-contaminated leaves or twigs as a substitute for toilet paper, and may contaminate the genital area after elimination because they are unable to wash their hands.

The Federal Insecticide, Fungicide and Rodenticide Act (FIFRA), authorizes the Environmental Protection Agency (EPA) to regulate the manufacture, distribution, and use of pesticides. Key provisions of the Act include product registration and labeling. As of 1984, EPA had registered approximately 50,000 pesticide products formulated from about 600 active and 1200 inert ingredients. Most pesticides have not been fully tested and evaluated, however, in accordance with current testing requirements aimed at determining a pesticide's potential for causing cancer, reproductive disorders, birth defects, and other chronic health problems. In addition, FIFRA's trade secret provisions severely handicap EPA's ability to evaluate the hazards posed by inert ingredients. The EPA currently is reregistering all pesticides. Estimates are that this process will extend into the twenty-first century.[9]

EPA also regulates farmworkers' exposure to pesticides in the fields, making them the only workers whose occupational exposure to toxic substances is not regulated by OSHA. Currently, reentry intervals—time periods that must elapse between pesticide application and worker entry into a treated field—are the primary method of preventing acute poisonings arising out of contact with pesticide residues. EPA has established specific reentry intervals for only a few pesticides. For the rest, fields may be reentered legally, but not necessarily safely, "when dusts have settled and sprays have dried."[19]

Reentry intervals have severe limitations. They do not even claim to protect workers from the carcinogenic and other chronic effects of pesticide exposure. In addition, a number of studies and case reports demonstrate their inadequacy in preventing acute effects.[3,20] In one case, an outbreak of dermatitis cases among orange pickers was linked to their exposure to a pesticide whose formulation had been modified by the addition of a new inert ingredient intended to prevent leaf burns. The inert ingredient also extended the degradation period of the active ingredient, a known potential skin and eye irritant. Regulators did not adjust the reentry or preharvest intervals accordingly, and as a result, 114 of 198 exposed workers suffered dermatitis of varying severity. A smaller number suffered eye irritation, with some requiring medical treatment.[20]

Other traditional measures to prevent toxic exposures, such as protective clothing and frequent washing of exposed skin, are unrealistic and ineffective. Growers often fail to supply protective clothing, and workers are loathe to wear the hot, cumbersome gear. The lack of handwashing facilities in the fields prevents timely removal of residues.

Adequate data on the extent and magnitude of pesticide-related and other occupational morbidity and mortality among farmworkers are unavailable for several reasons. Access barriers described earlier discourage farmworkers from seeking care for work-related illnesses. Lack of training in occupational medicine impedes physician recognition and diagnosis of these illnesses. Pesticide poisonings, for example, often are mistaken for flu and gastroenteritis. Moreover, nearly one third of migrant health centers responding to a survey admitted that they do not routinely screen patients regarding their occupational or environmental exposures.[12] Workers' compensation benefits often are unavailable or unknown to farmworkers. Additionally, there is no national surveillance system to track pesticide or other work-related illnesses.

In California, the only state to mandate physician reporting of pesticide-related illnesses, physicians report only an estimated 1% to 2% of residue-related illnesses.[21] Using California statistics and extrapolating this data to the national farmworker labor force yields an estimated 313,300 cases of pesticide-related illness annually.[8]

Acute health effects of mild pesticide exposure include increased salivation, tearing, blurred vision, diarrhea, slowed heart rate, weakness, headaches, and listlessness. Severe exposure may cause difficulty in breathing, respiratory failure, paralysis, convulsions, coma, and death. The organophosphate and carbamate pesticides, which inhibit the action of the enzyme cholinesterase, are the most toxic and have been responsible for the great majority of systemic poisonings and deaths in agricultural workers.[10]

Little is known about the magnitude of pesticide-related chronic health effects, and additional research is needed. A number of pesticides can cause allergic contact dermatitis, a chronic debilitating skin condition that can lead to permanent disability, since even minute exposure to the pesticide can be intolerable. Many commonly used pesticides are known or suspected animal carcinogens. Studies have shown pesticide-exposed workers to be at increased risk for malignant lymphoma, multiple myeloma, and cancer of the gastrointestinal tract, lung, testes, and brain.[10] Studies and case reports have associated pesticides with birth defects, sterility, and spontaneous abortion.[10] Organophosphate pesticides have been associated also with neurological and behavioral abnormalities, including ataxia, tremors, vertigo, drowsiness, anxiety, confusion, defective memory, convulsions, and coma.[3,10]

Effects of Inadequate Sanitation. The basic public health principle that poor sanitation increases the prevalence of disease has been well understood and universally accepted for over 100 years. Nevertheless, U.S. migrant and seasonal farmworkers have lived and worked under conditions analogous to those faced by third world populations.

In 1984, only an estimated 22% to 45% of farms provided workers with toilets, handwashing facilities, and potable water in the fields, either voluntarily or in compliance with state law.[22] After farmworker advocates waged a 15-year battle to win their constituents the same basic sanitation protection afforded to all other workers in this country, OSHA issued a federal field sanitation standard in 1987. The standard requires agricultural employers who hire 11 or more workers to provide them with free drinking water, toilets, and wash water in the fields.[22] The standard protects between 15%[23] and 36%[22] of U.S. field hand laborers. The few existing state-mandated field sanitation regulations are rarely adequate, often violated, and poorly enforced and, therefore, do little to improve conditions.[22]

The lack of adequate sanitation facilities contributes to farmworkers' increased risk of communicable diseases, heat stress, urinary tract infections, and pesticide-related illnesses. Working in hot environments, farmworkers who minimize their fluid intake in an effort to limit the need to urinate, risk dehydration and heat stress. Evidence indicates that migrant workers' relative risk of developing a heat-related illness is over four times that of the general working population.[24] Farmworkers, especially women, who try to retain their urine, risk developing urinary tract infections. The rate of these infections among migrant workers is estimated at 3.5 times that of the general population.[24] Those who urinate and defecate in the fields contaminate the water in irrigation pipes and ditches and expose co-workers to such communicable diseases as dysentery, hepatitis, typhoid fever, and parasitic infections. Estimates place the rate of parasitic infection among migrants at 20 times that of the general population and the rate of bacterial gastrointestinal infection at 11 times that of the general population.[24] A chart audit for fecal-related symptoms conducted in a Utah clinic serving both migrant farmworkers and an urban poor population found that the migrants, who lacked field sanitation facilities, displayed a clinic use rate for diarrhea that was 20 times higher than that of the urban poor. Similar findings applied to other enteric disease symptoms.[25] The impact of sanitary deficiencies on pesticide-related illness has already been discussed.

Dermatitis. A number of data sources point to dermatitis as the foremost work-related health problem in agriculture.[3] Farmworkers face nearly four times the risk of developing skin disease as workers in other industries.[24] Pesticides and allergenic plants and crops are the primary culprits. Their effects are exacerbated by constant exposure to the sun, sweat, chapped or abraded skin, and the lack of appropriate protective gear and adequate handwashing facilities. Patch testing generally is necessary to determine whether a rash is chemical or plant related.

Musculoskeletal Problems. Farmworkers face many of the hazards traditionally associated with musculoskeletal problems, including lifting and carrying heavy loads, fast-paced work necessitated by the piece rate wage system, and awkward work positions. For example, the short-handled hoe, *el cortito,* requires the worker to labor in a doubled-over position and is linked with development of back strain and other ailments. Significantly, the ban on its use in California is associated with a 34% decrease in the rate of sprain and strain injuries among relevant California farmworkers.[26] No national ban on its use has been issued.

Injuries. Farmworkers suffer a wide variety of injuries, including acute pesticide poisonings, fractures in falls from ladders, strains from heavy lifting, eye injuries from chemicals and debris ejected by machinery, cuts and lacerations from knives and machetes, and a host of crush, contusion, fracture, and amputation injuries associated with heavy equipment use. Piece work, heat stress, the effects of mild pesticide exposure, long hours, and awkward working positions contribute to the risk of injury. Often, large distances separate the fields from the nearest health care facility and frustrate the receipt of prompt and appropriate treatment.

Recommendations

The secondary legal status of this country's migrant and seasonal farmworkers lies at the heart of their political, social, and economic plight. Changes in labor, health and safety, and social welfare legislation are necessary to provide this population with equal protection.

Farmworker advocates have called for the creation of a national clearinghouse and resource center on farmworker health.[3] Funding for research on farmworker occupational hazards and their effects is desperately needed, as is a national surveillance system to monitor work-related illnesses and injuries.

Farmworkers need to receive culturally and linguistically appropriate worker education materials that explain on-the-job hazards and appropriate preventive measures.

Clinicians practicing in areas where migrant and seasonal farmworkers live and work cannot serve this population effectively without a clear picture of their living and working conditions and an understanding of the relationship between these conditions and their patients' health and well-being. This is particularly significant for clinicians who treat migrants when they are downstream and who, therefore, may have difficulty appreciating the significance of upstream conditions. Clinicians need training in the importance and methods of taking a thorough occupational and environmental history and in recognition, diagnosis, and treatment of pesticide and other work-related illnesses and injuries.

It is useful to remember that the pesticide and sanitation-related hazards that compromise the health of exposed farmworkers also contaminate produce and groundwater and, thereby, have a negative impact on the health of consumers and surrounding communities.[27] Community and environmental activists and concerned consumers, working in concert with farmworker advocates, can be a powerful force for changing the policies and practices of both government regulators and growers.

Minority Workers

Harriet L. Rubenstein

Racial and ethnic discrimination in wages and working conditions is a longstanding tradition in the American workplace. Historically, each new wave of immigrants worked the dirtiest, heaviest, and most dangerous jobs until, a generation or two later, a new immigrant group arrived to replace them. Discriminatory hiring and other employment practices, however, have prevented blacks, Hispanics, Asian Pacific Islanders, and Native Americans from scaling the job ladder as successfully as other immigrant groups. Despite remedial legislation, a disparity in job placement between minority and white workers persists. Most available information applies to black workers, but the issues discussed are applicable to other minorities as well.

Another disparity is the burden of morbidity and mortality borne by blacks and other minorities as compared with the white population. Based on key indicators, the health of blacks and other minority Americans lags 20 to 30 years behind that of whites.[1] The premise underlying this section is that the disproportionate representation of blacks in America's more hazardous industries and occupations places them at increased risk for occupational disease and injury and contributes to their diminished health status relative to the white population.

General Health Status

The nation's 28.1 million blacks constitute 12% of the population and are this country's largest minority group. In 1984, the median family income of blacks was $15,430, 56% of that of whites. The proportion of black Americans below the poverty level was 33.8%, nearly triple the 11.5% of whites. Twenty percent of blacks report having no regular source of medical care compared to 13% of whites.[2] Blacks assess their own health status less favorably than whites do theirs. In 1987, 42.1% of whites rated their own health as excellent compared to 29.5% of blacks, and 8.5% of whites rated their own health as fair or poor compared to 16.7% of blacks.[3] Objective measures support these subjective assessments.

In 1983, the life expectancy of black males was 65 years, 7 years less than that of white males, and the life expectancy of black females, at 74 years, trailed that of white females by 5 years. Black American infant mortality rate runs twice as high as that of whites.[2]

The death rate from all causes for blacks is 1.5 times that for whites. Table 32–4 lists the six causes of death that, taken together, account for roughly 80% of these excess deaths and the percent contribution of each. Although heart disease and stroke account for nearly one third of the excess deaths, the death rates from these two causes are declining. From 1968 to 1982, the stroke mortality rate of blacks dropped 51% and their coronary heart disease mortality rate declined 42%.[1] Improvements in hypertension control have contributed to this trend.

The picture for blacks becomes grimmer when we look at trends in cancer incidence and mortality, both in absolute numbers and relative to whites. Between 1974 and 1983, the incidence of cancer at all sites increased 18.4% among black males, more than double the 7.8% increase among white males. For black females, the 3.9% increase was more than five times the 0.7% increase among white females.[2] Between 1950 and 1985, cancer mortality rates for all sites for black males increased 84%, nearly quadruple the 22% increase in white males. During this same period, black males suffered a 400% increase in mortality from cancer of the respiratory system compared to a 169% increase for white males.[4]

Although smoking bears substantial blame for cancer incidence and mortality, particularly for lung cancer,[5] an examination of smoking patterns among blacks suggests that other risk factors must play a significant role as well. One study analyzing data from the 1970 and 1979–1980 National Health Interview Surveys compared smoking-related risk factors for lung cancer in black vs white males. Proportionally more black than white males were "never smokers" and fewer were "ever smokers," although more blacks were "current" and fewer were "former" smokers than whites. Black smokers smoked approximately 65% of the number of cigarettes smoked by their white counterparts, and blacks reported almost consistently that they started to smoke at an older age than whites. The authors concluded that blacks have fewer smoking-related lung cancer risk factors than whites and ascribed the racial differential in lung cancer incidence and mortality to differences in workplace exposures.[6]

A National Cancer Institute study analyzing changing patterns of lung cancer mortality between 1950 and 1975 underscores the need to look beyond smoking for an explanation of the greater incidence of lung cancer among blacks relative to whites. Cohort analysis drawn from National Center for Health Statistics data revealed that the age-specific lung cancer mortality rates of nonwhites were only two-thirds those of whites for males born in the late 1800s, resembled those of whites for males born around 1900, and surpassed by 50% those of white males born around 1915. The authors concluded that racial differences in smoking patterns and in the quality of lung cancer diagnosis and reporting could not adequately explain the higher rates of lung cancer among nonwhites, particularly nonwhite males aged 45 to 64 years. Instead, the authors suggested workplace exposures as a likely culprit.[7]

In fact, the sharp rise in black Americans' cancer-related morbidity and mortality since 1950 is consistent with both the historical and current patterns of black employment in American industry and the 15 to 40 year latency period for occupational cancers.

TABLE 32–4. AVERAGE ANNUAL TOTAL AND EXCESS DEATHS IN BLACKS: SELECTED CAUSES OF MORTALITY, UNITED STATES, 1979–1981

	Excess Deaths Males and Females Cumulative to Age 70	
Causes of Excess Death	***Number***	**%**
Heart disease and stroke	18,181	30.8
Homicide and accidents	10,909	18.5
Cancer	8,118	13.8
Infant mortality	6,178	10.5
Cirrhosis	2,154	3.7
Diabetes	1,850	3.1
Subtotal	47,390	80.4
All other causes	11,552	19.6
Total excess deaths	58,942	100.0
Total deaths, all causes	138,635	
Ratio of excess deaths to total deaths		42.5%
Percent contribution of six causes to excess death		80.4%

From Report of the Secretary's Task Force on Black and Minority Health, Vol I: Executive Summary, U.S. Department of Health and Human Services, August 1985.

Black Employment Patterns

The outbreak of World War I triggered a migration of southern black field hands, tenant farmers, and sharecroppers to the highly industrialized urban centers of the North. Aggressive recruitment campaigns, launched by northern businessmen facing both expanding markets for munitions and other war-related goods and a dwindling labor pool, lured southern blacks living under difficult political, social, and economic conditions. During the next 45 years, 4.5 million blacks would travel northward in pursuit of more promising living and working conditions. However, employers typically assigned black Americans to the hot, dirty, backbreaking, unskilled, low-paying, and generally least desirable jobs that were believed to best suit black workers. On average, more than 8 of every 10 black men worked as unskilled laborers in foundries, building trades, meatpacking companies, on the railroads, or as servants, porters, janitors, cooks, and cleaners. Many of these jobs exposed black workers to carcinogens and other hazards for as many as 60 hours a week. A relative few obtained work in semiskilled or skilled occupations. The majority of black women worked as domestic servants or in service-related jobs.[8] World War II sparked a second wave of northern migration, with 1.6 million blacks, nearly one sixth of the total southern black population, migrating north and west in search of new jobs. The exodus continued through the 1950s and, at a slightly slower pace, during the 1960s as well.[9]

Favorable economic conditions and passage of the Civil Rights Act of 1964 allowed blacks to make substantial headway in employment during the 1960s. Three recessions between 1970 and 1980, however, dampened job opportunities and slowed occupational mobility considerably. Despite some inroads into white collar jobs during this period, black males in 1980 were twice as likely as white males to occupy laborer jobs and only half as likely to be employed in professional or technical occupations.[10]

As evidenced by the private sector employment data in Table 32–5, blacks in 1987 continue to be overrepresented in most blue collar occupations, where they are generally more apt to face work-related hazards, and are underrepresented in most white collar occupations.[11] A survey of federal and state labor officials revealed that Hispanics and Asians are heavily overrepresented in sweatshops, defined as workplaces violating both safety or health and wage or child labor laws.[12]

TABLE 32-5. BLACK WORKERS AS A PERCENTAGE OF VARIOUS OCCUPATIONS

Occupation	% Black Workers	
Total private sector employment	12.5	
Total white collar	8.8	
Officials and managers		4.9
Professionals		4.7
Technicians		9.6
Sales workers		10.3
Office and clerical workers		13.6
Total blue collar	15.2	
Craft workers		9.3
Operators		17.2
Laborers		19.5
Service workers		25.1

From U.S. Equal Employment Opportunity, EEO-1, 1987.[11]

Relationship Between Minority Employment and Health

The absence of essential occupational disease surveillance data severely hampers efforts to determine the relationship between the health status and the occupational status of black and other minority workers. No data sources exist that include information both on the health and safety hazards and exposures of particular jobs and on the racial or ethnic composition of workers in those jobs. Moreover, occupational injury and illness incidence data are not reported by race or ethnicity and are not broken down into the same or comparable occupational categories as are data on racial distribution among occupations.

Nevertheless, a number of studies, piecing together data from various sources, have estimated the rate of excess work-related morbidity and mortality suffered by black workers. Using 1975 OSHA death and lost workday injury and illness data and Equal Employment Opportunity Commission employment figures, one study estimated that blacks face a 37% greater risk than whites of sustaining a work-related illness or injury and a 24% greater risk of dying from work-related causes.[13] A follow-up study, using similar data from 1984–1985, found that black workers' excess risk of job-related injury and illness had diminished to 23%.[14]

In studies integrating census, occupational injury and illness, and other data, Robinson has attempted to quantify the excess risk of work-related morbidity faced by minority workers.[15-17] One study determined that the average black worker is in an occupation 37% to 52% more likely to produce a serious accident or illness than that of the average white worker. Because this disparity held strong even after controlling for differences in education and on-the-job experience, Robinson concluded that black workers with education and experience comparable to whites will nevertheless find themselves in substantially more dangerous occupations.[15]

In a later study, Robinson examined trends in the excess risk of occupational injuries faced by blacks relative to whites between 1968 and 1986. He found that the racial risk differential for disabling occupational injuries declined 50% among men, from a ratio of 1.78 in 1968 to 1.60 in 1977 and then to 1.41 in 1986. The trend among women was substantially less encouraging for blacks. The overall risk differential increased 20%, so that by 1986, black women faced nearly the same injury risk as white men. Robinson attributes this divergence to the rise in injury rates in those industries and occupations where black women are concentrated.[16]

In the only study to separate the experience of Hispanic workers from that of non-Hispanic whites, Robinson found that California's Hispanic and black workers are each exposed to higher risks of occupational injury and acute illness than are non-Hispanic white workers, even after controlling for education and work experience.[17]

Epidemiological Evidence

Most epidemiological studies of occupational disease fail to examine and report on the incidence or causes of job-related health problems among black or other minority workers. Nevertheless, results of a few studies suggest, or in some instances actually illustrate, an association between disparate employment practices and the diminished health status of black and other minority workers.

The U.S. Public Health Service conducted one of the earliest studies suggesting an association between excess morbidity and mortality in blacks and job placement patterns. The study uncovered an unusually high incidence of respiratory cancer and nasal septum perforation among chromate workers and found that black workers suffered significantly greater excess morbidity and mortality than did whites. These excesses could not be explained by differences in smoking patterns. Although white workers tended to have worked in the industry longer than blacks, the percentage of black workers employed in the dry ends of the plant, where exposure to carcinogenic chromium compounds was greatest, was over 2.5 times that of white workers.[18]

The most comprehensive and compelling series of studies examined the long-term mortality experience of steelworkers employed in 1953 in the steel mill coke plants, where coal is transformed into metallurgical coke for use in the blast furnace. Initial study results disclosed that mortality from respiratory cancer for men employed in the coke plant was twice that observed generally among steelworkers and that all of this differential was due to a threefold excess in black workers.[19] Further study determined that this excess lung cancer mortality was limited to men employed at the coke ovens, where exposure to such carcinogens as benzo(a)pyrene is greatest. These men were found to have a risk of lung cancer 2.5 to 3 times greater than that predicted. The greatest part of this excess was attributable to an almost sevenfold excess risk of lung cancer in men working for 5 years or longer on the tops of the ovens, where concentrations of carcinogenic emissions are highest. A critical finding was that the apparent differential in respiratory cancer rates between black and white coke plant workers was a function of the overrepresentation of blacks in jobs requiring full-time work at the topside of the ovens. In fact, whereas only 2.1% of white coke oven workers worked full-time topside for at least 5 years, 10.7% of black workers were so employed. When both type and duration of exposure were accounted for, the relative risks of lung cancer for white and black coke oven workers were of about the same magnitude.[20]

A pulmonary function survey of 6631 textile mill employees found that 58% of the workers with symptoms of byssinosis, or brown lung disease, worked in the high dust areas of opening, picking, and carding, which employed only 10.1% of the total workforce. Further analysis demonstrated a positive association between byssinosis and length of employment. Discrimination had kept blacks out of the mills up until 1960. Consequently, only 17% of blacks had worked there more than 10 years. Nevertheless, the prevalence of byssinosis among black males was 53% greater than among white males, and although blacks made up 34% of the study population, they comprised 41% of the byssinosis cases. Part of the explanation for this pattern lay in the disproportionate assignment of blacks to the three dustiest departments. Opening, picking, and carding employed 6% of white mill workers but 18% of black mill workers, and 54% of workers in these areas were black.[21]

A study of rubber workers looked for relationships between mortality excesses in male rubber workers between 1964 and 1973 and specific jobs held within the industry between 1940 and 1960. With regard to cancer, the strongest associations tended to be with work areas at the front end of the production line, especially the compounding and mixing area, where the likelihood of contact with early reaction by-products was high. Compounding and mixing workers showed an elevated risk of mortality from stomach, lung, prostate, bladder, lymphatic, and hematopoietic cancers and lymphatic leukemia. The authors noted that only 3% of white workers as compared with 27% of black workers had worked in the compounding and mixing areas for at least 5 years.[22]

A proportional mortality ratio study of construction equipment and diesel engine manufacturing plant workers exposed to solvents, cutting oils, and metal fumes and dusts reported a significant excess of pancreatic cancer and non-Hodgkin's lymphomas in blacks with 20 or more years of service. Acknowledging limitations in the study, including absence of work histories, the authors nevertheless suggested that their findings might be relevant to the already described marked increase in cancer mortality in black males.[23]

Another study examined the hospital inpatient records of burn victims and found the incidence of work-related burns for black males to be double that of white males and for black females to be triple that of white females. The authors proposed that this disparity might reflect differences in exposure to high-risk situations for burn injury, associated with differential work opportunities between blacks and whites.[24]

A standardized proportional mortality study of deaths among auto repair and auto body shop workers uncovered a threefold excess in lymphopoietic cancer, particularly multiple myeloma, in black workers. Once again, the absence of good work histories made any correlation with on-the-job exposures impossible.[25]

Unemployment and Disemployment

Discriminatory employment practices have placed blacks at increased risk for work-related morbidity and mortality, and high rates of unemployment in the black community and the threat of disemployment operate together to exacerbate this problem.

In 1988, 11.7% of black workers were unemployed, 2.5 times the rate of white workers.[26] Such a high rate of unemployment has a chilling effect on the willingness of black workers to refuse or complain about a hazardous job. If an employer is either unwilling or unable to make modifications to reduce or eliminate a hazardous condition, the affected worker is forced to choose between continued exposure and disemployment. "Disemployment" is defined as job loss due to the need for removal from a hazardous exposure in order to prevent continuation or worsening of an occupational illness or injury.[27] Although all workers potentially face this choice, minority workers and those who are older, unskilled, or undocumented or have disabilities face added difficulties securing a new job. These workers may find the immediate threat of disemployment, and its concomitant loss of health insurance, more compelling than the potential threat of an occupational illness, particularly one with a long latency period.

Summary

Activities targeted to eliminating the disparate health status of blacks and other minorities relative to whites must address the role occupational exposures play in creating this inequality. The work of Robinson and of others demonstrates that race discrimination is an enduring characteristic of the American workplace, with blacks and other minorities more likely to face on-the-job hazards than their white counterparts with comparable education and experience. Eliminating racial inequality in working conditions is, therefore, a prerequisite to eradicating racial inequality in health status measures. Creative and aggressive implementation and enforcement of labor and civil rights legislation appears to be necessary to bring about change.

Regardless of the success of these efforts, public health professionals can advocate for and participate in more modest but nevertheless useful measures, many of which will accrue to the benefit of all workers. Health care providers serving the minority community and minority-intensive industries are in the best position to recognize work-related disease in their patients and to alert and initiate follow-up activities with affected workers, unions, employers, government agencies, and occupational health professionals. Primary care providers need to receive education in occupational health, both in training programs and as part of postgraduate continuing education. Minority workers themselves need culturally and linguistically appropriate educational materials and training programs that will help them to identify workplace hazards and to use the resources available for reducing these hazards.

Work-related injury and illness statistics and occupational disease surveillance data should include information on race and ethnic background to help identify patterns of morbidity and mortality among minority workers. Epidemiological studies of particular industries or occupations need to develop race-specific data on both workplace exposures and rates of excess morbidity.

Health and social service professionals can play a critical advocacy role on behalf of minority workers attempting to improve their working conditions or to secure workers' compensation or other benefits.

Efforts to improve the working conditions of minority workers should not overshadow the need to ameliorate those of all workers. For black and other minority workers to secure the right to suffer occupational illness and injury at the same rate as white workers would be a hollow victory.

Women Workers

Harriet L. Rubenstein

The occupational health problems of women workers merit special attention for several interrelated reasons. First, the historic and ongoing segregation of women into occupational categories demands that attention be paid to the hazards accompanying "women's work" (see Table 32–6). Although sex discrimination in employment often masquerades as protection of the weaker sex, the reality is that women's work—from housework to nursing to electronics assembly—poses an array of threats to the health, safety, and well-being of women. Recent studies of the Canadian fish-processing[1] and poultry[2] industries are challenging the conventional wisdom that female-intensive jobs are somehow protective of women's health or that women are more susceptible than men to workplace hazards. Few studies have examined and relatively little is known about the impact of occupational exposures on women's health, particularly the chronic low-level exposures that characterize the clerical and service occupations to which women have largely been relegated. Consequently, many of the health hazards women workers face go unrecognized, the misconception of safe women's work is perpetuated, and opportunities for both prevention and compensation are missed.

In addition, the health of working women demands special attention because women in the labor force continue to shoulder the bulk of housework and caregiver responsibilities. These multiple and perhaps conflicting roles qualitatively affect women's work experience and its impact on their health. Finally, women's unique physical role in reproduction gives rise to both legitimate and misguided health concerns in the workplace that require careful scrutiny.

Profile of Women in the Labor Force

The past 40 years have witnessed a startling shift in the primary work setting of U.S. women, from unpaid labor in the home to paid labor outside the home. In 1987, 56% of women over the age of 16, nearly 54 million women, participated in the labor force, up from 31.8%, less than 17 million women, in 1947.[3] Women in 1987 accounted for 44.8% of the civilian labor force[4] and will be the major source of new entrants through the end of the century, accounting for 63% of the net labor force growth up to that time.[5]

Economic necessity brings most women to the workplace.

TABLE 32–6. POTENTIAL HAZARDS AND THEIR EFFECTS IN SELECTED FEMALE-INTENSIVE OCCUPATIONS

Occupation	Hazards	Possible Health Effects
Household workers[a]	Cleaning agents	Dermatitis, mucous membrane and respiratory irritation
	Infectious agents	Rubella, varicella, influenza
	Heavy lifting	Musculoskeletal injuries
	Job insecurity	Stress
Clerical workers	Ergonomic hazards	Musculoskeletal fatigue, stress
	VDTs	Eye strain, musculoskeletal fatigue, stress
	Indoor air pollution (e.g., microbes, volatile organic compounds)	Eye mucous membrane and respiratory irritation, headaches, fatigue
Healthcare workers[a]	Infectious agents	Hepatitis B, AIDS, tuberculosis, etc.
	Ethylene oxide	Suspect carcinogen and mutagen, reproductive hazard
	Lifting patients, equipment	Musculoskeletal injuries
	Ionizing radiation	Carcinogenesis, mutagenesis
	Slippery floors	Muscoloskeletal injuries
Clothing/textile workers[a]	Cotton dust	Byssinosis
	Dyes, fabric treatment	Dermatitis, respiratory irritation, carcinogenesis
	Noise	Hearing loss
	Piecework	Stress, injuries
Retail sales workers	Prolonged standing	Varicose veins, low back strain
	Indoor air pollution	Eye, mucous membrane and respiratory irritation, headaches, fatigue
Hairdressers and cosmetologists[a]	Hair dyes, solvents, aerosol propellants	Dermatitis, respiratory and mucous membrane irritation, central nervous system depression

[a] Occupation characterized by poverty of significant fractions of full-time female workers.[7]

Sixty percent of women in the labor force are either single, divorced, widowed, or separated or have husbands earning less than $15,000 a year.[4] Ironically, job segregation and outright wage discrimination leave year-round full-time women workers with a median income of $16,843, only 65% of that of men.[4] Despite the media attention paid to the movement of women into nontraditional jobs, women remain concentrated in a few, low-wage job "ghettos" (Tables 32–7 and 32–8). Fifty-eight percent of all working women are employed in either clerical, service, or sales occupations, where the median annual earnings are $4500, $8100, and $9100, respectively, below the national average for all occupations.[6] In fact, a large number of employed women work full-time and still live at or below the poverty level. Black and unmarried women are especially hard hit. Seventy-one percent of the occupations held by black unmarried women are ones in which at least 13% of the workers are impoverished.[7] Many of the occupations characterized by impoverishment and poverty among full-time women workers also are characterized by exposure to known or suspected carcinogens and other hazards (Table 32–6).

Aside from occupational segregation, wage discrimination depresses women's earnings substantially below those of their male counterparts (Table 32–9). One implication of this earnings differential is that most employed women are less able than most men to protect their health through spending on nutrition, housing, and recreation and to purchase health insurance and health services.

Married women and women with children are significantly increasing their participation in the workforce. In 1987, 56% of married women were active members of the labor force, up from 40% in 1972.[4] Today, 56% of women with preschool-age children are working, nearly a fivefold increase since 1950.[8] In fact, married women with children under age 2 comprise the fastest growing segment of the workforce.[8] In 1988, almost 11 million families were headed by women, compared to 1.5 million in 1950. Contrary to popular myth, nearly 88% of these women are in the workforce. Nevertheless, families maintained by women have a poverty rate more than three times that of all families.[8]

Traditional women's jobs also are those with low rates of unionization. In 1988, 15% of working women, as opposed to 22.5% of working men, were represented by unions.[9] The lack of union protection contributes to the gender wage gap, limits women's ability to improve their working conditions, and fosters job insecurity, all of which factor into the job-related stress experienced by working women.

TABLE 32–7. SELECTED OCCUPATIONS WITH HIGH PERCENTAGE OF WOMEN WORKERS, 1988 ANNUAL AVERAGES

Occupation	% Women
Secretaries	99.1
Dental assistants	98.7
Prekindergarten and kindergarten teachers	98.2
Dental hygienists	97.6
Childcare workers	97.3
Licensed practical nurses	96.0
Teacher's aides	95.9
Cleaners and servants	95.6
Registered nurses	94.6
Typists	94.5
Bank tellers	91.0
Eligibility clerks, social welfare	90.3
Billing clerks	90.2
Hairdressers and cosmetologists	89.5
Electrical and electronic equipment assemblers	70.0

From Employment and Earnings 36(1), U.S. Department of Labor, Bureau of Labor Statistics, January 1989, pp 183–188.

TABLE 32–8. PERCENT DISTRIBUTION OF WOMEN WORKERS BY OCCUPATIONAL CATEGORY, MAY 1989

Occupation	% of Working Women
Administrative support (including clerical)	27.5
Service	17.4
Professional specialty	14.9
Sales occupations	13.2
Executive, administrative, and managerial	11.3
Operators, fabricators, and laborers	9.1
Technicians and related support	3.4
Precision production, craft and repair	2.1
Farming, forestry, fishing	1.2
Total	100.0

From Employment and Earnings, U.S. Department of Labor, Bureau of Labor Statistics, June 1989, p 46.

Stress

Stress is a ubiquitous occupational hazard associated in varying degrees with all types of work and affecting both women and men. Stress may contribute to the development of heart and cerebrovascular disease, hypertension, peptic ulcer and inflammatory bowel disease, and musculoskeletal problems. Evidence suggests that stress alters immune function and may facilitate the development of cancer. Anxiety, depression, neuroses, and alcohol and drug problems all are associated with stress.[10]

Employed women confront a variety of job-related stressors. Hazardous working conditions have both a direct effect on health (Table 32–6) and an indirect effect through the subjective distress they engender. Multiple roles, particular job characteristics, sexual harassment, and the threat of work-related violence are some of the significant sources of occupational stress for working women.

Health Effects of Multiple Roles. Despite women's increasing role in the workforce, their traditional family responsibilities persist. Employed women, regardless of marital status, still assume nearly all the responsibility for housework, household management, child care, and care of older and disabled family members.[11] The hours required to run a home and the time required at the worksite add up to an average 80-hour work week for women compared to a 50-hour work week for men.[12]

The conventional wisdom has predicted that women's entry into the workforce and their exposure to the job stressors for-

TABLE 32–9. MEDIAN WEEKLY EARNINGS OF FULL-TIME WAGE AND SALARY WORKERS FOR SELECTED OCCUPATIONS, ANNUAL AVERAGES 1986

Occupation	Median Weekly Earnings		Female Earnings as % of Male Earnings
	Male	*Female*	
Financial managers	$703	$458	65
Physician	$728	$505	69
Cashiers	$209	$174	83
Information clerk	$347	$250	72
Janitors and cleaners	$261	$207	79
Supervisors, production	$495	$297	60
Electrical and electronic equipment assemblers	$305	$255	84

From Current Population Survey, U.S. Department of Labor, Bureau of Labor Statistics, 1986 Annual Averages.

merly the province of men, compounded by the stress of multiple role burdens, would compromise the health status of employed women. The underlying implicit assumptions—that the role of housewife is women's natural state and that housework provides a safe haven from physical hazards and stressors—are acknowledged increasingly as unfounded. We now know that housework exposes women to a variety of chemical and other hazards (Table 32-6) and that the roles of wife and mother have their own attendant risks.

Research evidence on the health effects of women's employment suggests that, overall, gainfully employed women enjoy better health than housewives, based on both subjective and objective health status indicators.[13-15] The relative contribution to this health status differential made by the healthy worker effect—the self-selection of healthy women into the labor force and of women in poor health out of the labor force—remains unresolved.[14,16]

The San Antonio Heart Study examined the relationship between women's employment status and the presence of cardiovascular risk factors and found highly significant differences favoring employed women over homemakers in levels of high density lipoprotein (HDL) cholesterol, ratio of HDL cholesterol to total cholesterol, and triglycerides. This protective effect of employment was more pronounced for women in professional, managerial, sales, and clerical occupations than for those in blue collar jobs.[15] Other studies have determined that women's mortality risk has not been affected negatively by employment.[17,18] In fact, in one study, employed, married women with a child in the home had the lowest risk of mortality.[18]

The Framingham Heart Study called attention to the potential increased risk for coronary heart disease faced by women clerical workers who ever had married and had raised children.[19] This finding has not reappeared in subsequent studies,[19,20] and one study found that women clerical workers in the United States have the best health profile of all occupational categories.[20]

Mounting evidence suggests that employment acts as both a potential buffer against stress and a potential source of stress for working women. The findings of one study indicate that the social support and integration gained through work are salient aspects of employment that contribute to the health status advantage enjoyed by employed women.[13] Alternatively, another study found that satisfaction with life situations correlated more closely with health than did employment in and of itself.[21]

Whether multiple roles per se jeopardize women's health is only the threshold question. The evidence that the benefits of employment may outweigh its risks should not obscure what those risks are and the important health differentials that may be related to the types and qualities of roles occupied by working women.

In particular, attention must be paid to the demands that child and dependent care responsibilities place on working women. With 65% of all women with children under age 18 working outside the home[8] and no comprehensive national child care policy, the search for quality, affordable child care haunts most working mothers. Child care arrangements require continuous attention and remain a source of stress for working mothers until the children leave home. Child care is a family's fourth largest expense, after housing, food, and taxes. For some mothers who want to work, the cost of child care precludes their joining the labor force. A lack of affordable child care prevents an estimated 60% of mothers receiving public assistance from participating in education and training programs.[22]

The federal government has been slow to respond to the increasing demand for child and other dependent care, and initiatives in this area have been limited primarily to tax credits. Moreover, between 1977 and 1986, direct federal outlays for child care programs, which benefited mainly poor and low-income families, declined nearly 25%.[22] A small percentage of employers are providing some kind of child care assistance, including information and referral services, various forms of financial assistance, and on-site care. Child care also is becoming an important organizing tool and bargaining issue for labor unions, some of which have established child care information and referral networks or won contract language providing for flex-time and alternative work schedules or on-site centers.

The need for maternity leave presents a related stressor for many working women. The United States is the only industrialized nation that does not provide directly for maternity benefits through federal legislation. The Pregnancy Discrimination Act of 1978 (the Act) amended Title VII of the Civil Rights Act of 1964 to prohibit discrimination with respect to compensation, terms, conditions, and privileges of employment on the basis of "pregnancy, childbirth, or related medical conditions." The Act makes it illegal for an employer to fire or refuse to hire or promote a woman because of pregnancy. In addition, the Act requires employers of 15 or more employees to provide workers unable to work because of pregnancy, childbirth, or related medical conditions the same health or temporary disability insurance, sick leave, seniority credits, and reinstatement privileges that are provided to workers temporarily disabled from other nonwork-connected causes. Although the law prohibits pregnancy-related employment discrimination, it does not require employers to provide special benefits for pregnant workers, such as unpaid or paid leave with reinstatement, or to institute new programs.

Some states have placed an affirmative duty on employers. A few mandate maternity disability insurance. Others require employers to grant pregnant women short-term, unpaid disability leave with reinstatement. Still others require employers to provide either parent with unpaid leave with reinstatement to care for a newborn or newly adopted child. Those women who are not covered by any policy often must use a combination of sick days, vacation days, or leave without pay during this period. This patchwork of protection is inadequate, and national legislation is needed to address this problem.

Job Characteristics. Female-intensive occupations exhibit many of the job characteristics associated with work-related stress. For example, clerical and assembly work are characterized by a lack of control over work pace and methods, repetitious and monotonous tasks, time pressures, narrow job content, piece rate wage system, and electronic monitoring. Women in nursing, teaching, and social service occupations experience stress from the overwhelming demands created by their responsibility for the welfare of others and the stark contrast between role expectations and reality.

Women also experience stress from having to prove themselves to co-workers and supervisors. In one study of business school graduates, 83% of women respondents compared with 53% of men reported that they always or often felt that they had to be the best at all they did.[11] This can be an especially dangerous problem for women in nontraditional jobs, such as the construction trades, where women may feel pressured to attempt unsafe work as a way of proving their abilities and establishing credibility with their male peers.

Sexual Harassment. Sexual harassment on the job affects between 36% and 88% of working women in both traditional and nontraditional jobs.[23] Any unwanted verbal or physical advance, ranging from sexual comments and innuendos to pressure for sexual favors accompanied by outright or subtle job threats to physical assault, qualifies as sexual harassment. Noncompliant women or those who report their harasser's actions often face retaliation, including mandatory overtime, excessive scrutiny of job performance, public ridicule, sabotage of their work product, and denial or alteration of safety equipment. In the extreme, sexual harassment leads to loss of job, promotion, or training and other benefits. In addition to economic effects, sexual harassment also is associated with psychological trauma and stress-related physical symptoms, such as nausea, headache, depression, and drastic weight change. In one survey, 25% of women reporting unwanted sexual advances sought medical or psychological help in connection with the experience.[23]

Sexual harassment may be a violation of Title VII of the Civil Rights Act and of state fair employment practice laws. Clinicians should advise women in these situations to seek help from their union and co-workers, local women's organizations, the Equal Employment Opportunity Commission, and relevant state or local agencies.

Threat of Violence. Little attention has been paid to violence as an occupational hazard or to personal insecurity as a work-related stressor for employed women. For example, nurses and aides working in psychiatric hospitals confront violent patients on a daily basis, and social service workers often are victimized by frustrated clients. A study of fatal occupational injuries among Texas women revealed that homicides accounted for 53% of work-related fatalities. The highest workplace homicide rates were found among women workers in gasoline service stations, food, bakery, and dairy stores, and eating and drinking establishments.[24] A study of sexual assault of women at work in Ohio and in Memphis, Tennessee, found female convenience food store clerks and cashiers to be at substantially increased risk for rape.[25]

Inadequate security systems and insufficient staffing contribute to personal insecurity for employed women. This area deserves further study and demands development of creative preventive strategies.

Health professionals may be called on by employers and unions to assist in the establishment of workplace stress management programs. Programs that focus on helping women to develop coping skills and to use relaxation techniques may be helpful, but only in the short term. Long-term effective stress management requires that both employers and employees look beyond individual strategies to the social and economic context of women's work and to the organizational stressors in the workplace. Employers should be encouraged to look for and rectify job segregation, sexual harassment, and stress-producing job characteristics where they exist in their workplaces and to implement innovative support programs for working women. For example, from 1987 to 1988, the proportion of workplaces offering flexible work hours increased nearly fourfold, from 11% to 43%.[8] More advances such as this are needed.

Clinicians should be alert to job stress as an etiological agent in both the physical and mental health problems of their patients. Workers' compensation claims for stress-related disorders are difficult but not impossible to win, and their number is growing. Clinicians should take every opportunity to support their patients' efforts to rectify stressful working conditions.

Finally, health professionals and their organizations can involve themselves in supporting public policy initiatives that will reduce work-related stress, such as child care or parental leave legislation.

Ergonomic Issues

Although ergonomic problems beset both men and women workers (see Chapters 15 and 29), women are particularly at risk because most tools, workstations, and personal protective equipment are designed to fit "the average male" and because so many women are concentrated in jobs where they are confined to a desk or other often poorly designed workstation for much of the day, performing machine-paced, repetitive tasks.

Carpal tunnel syndrome (CTS), a disabling hand disorder resulting from nerve compression inside the wrist, is one of several cumulative trauma, or repetitive strain, disorders associated with hand-intensive, and female-intensive jobs, such as garment worker, cash register operator, poultry deboner and video display terminal (VDT) operator. Although a number of nonoccupational factors have been reported to be associated with CTS, research evidence demonstrates that CTS is strongly associated with high force–highly repetitive work.[26]

In one study, over 25% of 600 VDT operators at a single facility were diagnosed with CTS or pre-CTS as a result of the repetitive motion required by work at an improperly located keyboard.[27] By the early 1990s, two thirds of American office workers, most of them women, will use VDTs.[8] CTS is only one of several ergonomic-related health problems reported by VDT operators. Fatigue, headache, visual disturbances, backstrain, and other musculoskeletal disorders all have been reported by VDT users and are associated with poor workstation and equipment design, improper lighting, and stressful job demands. Results of a study of adverse reproductive outcomes, potentially associated with VDT use, suggest that significantly elevated miscarriage rates among clerical workers using VDTs for more than 20 hours per week actually may be related to the onerous and stressful working conditions associated with much of data entry and other full-time clerical VDT work.[28]

A fundamental tenet of ergonomics is that the job should be modified to fit the worker, not the worker to fit the job. Adherence to this principle requires that equipment manufacturers and employers consider the physical and mental health implications of workplace, equipment, and job design and bear in mind the variability in size, strength, and other characteristics among all workers. In the case of VDTs, the National Institute for Occupational Safety and Health has made specific recommendations aimed at preventing ergonomic-related health problems.[29]

Obtaining proper-fitting personal protective equipment (PPE) is another ergonomics-related challenge encountered by women working in both female-intensive and nontraditional jobs. A 1980 survey of 154 manufacturers and suppliers found that for most categories of PPE, fewer than half of all companies surveyed provided items with women's sizing.[30] Improperly fitting PPE increases women's exposure to workplace hazards and detrimentally affects their health and safety.

Reproductive Hazards

Myths and misinformation permeate medical and lay decision-making concerning occupational hazards to reproduction. Many physicians and employers appear to rely more on cultural beliefs than on scientific data when deciding whether, and to what degree, pregnancy has an impact on a woman's ability to perform various job tasks. Research and regulatory priorities and workplace policies virtually disregard the male role in procreation, the vulnerability of the male reproductive system to toxic agents, and the potential for adverse reproductive outcomes outside of pregnancy. Consequently, women are both underprotected and overprotected from workplace reproductive hazards while the reproductive health of men and the health of the fetus remain in jeopardy.

A reproductive health hazard is any agent that causes reproductive impairment in adults or developmental impairment or death in an embryo/fetus or child. Potential adverse reproductive outcomes include male and female infertility, decreased libido, altered menses, early fetal loss, spontaneous abortion, prematurity or low birthweight, birth defects, abnormal growth and development, difficulties with lactation, and childhood cancer as a manifestation of transplacental carcinogenesis.

Despite extremely limited surveillance of reproductive dysfunction in the U.S. population, some estimates of the magnitude of the problem exist. An estimated 8.4% of couples are "unintentionally" infertile, between 30% and 75% of pregnancies end in spontaneous abortion, nearly 7% of infants born are of low birthweight, and 7% have detectable birth defects.[31]

The degree to which occupational exposures contribute to

this burden of reproductive impairment is unknown. Few of the thousands of substances used commonly in the workplace have been evaluated for their reproductive effects and even fewer for their potential adverse impact on and through the male reproductive system. Those studies that have been conducted are fraught with methodological weaknesses that frustrate efforts to link particular exposures with particular negative reproductive outcomes.[32] Nevertheless, the significance of workplace exposures lies not in their numerical impact but in the fact that these exposures are potentially preventable.

Human and animal studies have identified at least 500 known or suspected reproductive hazards found in the workplace, a few of which are listed in Table 32–10. OSHA has regulated only four agents—ionizing radiation, lead, dibromochloropropane, and ethylene oxide—on the basis of their potential to cause reproductive dysfunction.

Studies have implicated both paternal and maternal exposures, occurring before and after as well as during pregnancy, in the genesis of adverse pregnancy outcomes. Some toxins may affect the fetus adversely even though exposure predates conception. Exposure to physical or chemical mutagens can damage the germ cells of either parent and result in spontaneous abortion of the conceptus or birth defects in the offspring arising from the damaged cells. Maternal exposures before conception also can affect fetal development if the toxin persists in the mother's body. For example, the storage of PCBs in fat cells and lead in bone exists in a steady state with the blood so that the fetus can be exposed to these body stores through the maternal circulation.[33]

TABLE 32–10. SELECTED KNOWN AND SUSPECTED REPRODUCTIVE HAZARDS AND THEIR EFFECTS

Agent	Parental Exposure	Effect
Inorganic lead	Maternal	Menstrual disorders Decreased fertility Spontaneous abortion Behavioral/developmental disabilities Breast milk contamination
	Paternal	Decreased fertility Prematurity Spontaneous abortion Perinatal mortality
Dibromochloropropane (DBCP)	Paternal	Decreased fertility
Ethylene oxide	Maternal	Spontaneous abortion Mutagenesis
Infectious agents (rubella, cytomegalovirus, hepatitis B, varicella)	Maternal	Birth defects
Heat	Paternal	Decreased fertility
Carbaryl (insecticide)	Maternal	Birth defects
	Paternal	Decreased fertility
Organic solvents	Maternal	Menstrual disorders Spontaneous abortions Toxemia of pregnany Birth defects
	Paternal	Decreased fertility Spontaneous abortions Birth defects
Anesthetic agents	Maternal	Spontaneous abortions Birth defects
	Paternal	Birth defects
Ionizing radiation	Maternal	Infertility Reproductive disorders in offspring Cancer in offspring Birth defects
	Paternal	Decreased libido Infertility Mutagenesis

During pregnancy, the timing of an exposure is a significant determinant of its effect. Exposures occurring during the first 3 weeks of embryonic life are most likely to result in severe damage to or death of the embryo. Exposures during weeks 4 through 9 of gestation, when most organogenesis is occurring, are most likely to induce classic birth defects. Subsequent exposures may cause postnatal growth or functional abnormalities or damage to the central nervous, immune, or endocrine system that continues to develop throughout gestation. An agent may be harmful to the embryo or fetus but have no effect on the mother.

Postnatal parental exposures also can affect the growth and development of the offspring. Contaminated work clothes brought into the home by either parent can expose the child to asbestos, lead, or other hazards. Breast milk can be contaminated by workplace toxins, such as PCBs, lead, and mercury, which may then be transmitted to the nursing child.

A number of studies have examined the effects of various physical and mental stressors in the workplace on pregnancy and the fetus, with mixed and often conflicting results.[34–37] One study found that the birthweights of full-term infants were progressively lower when the mothers continued work outside the home during the third trimester of pregnancy. The growth retardation was most severe when mothers had jobs requiring standing, continued working until near term, were hypertensive, or had children to care for at home. Third trimester employment, however, did not seem to shorten the length of gestation regardless of postural requirements.[24] Another study found a positive relationship between prematurity and "occupational fatigue," the elements of which included standing 3 or more hours a day, working on an industrial machine requiring effort, working at tasks requiring little attention, and working in a humid, noisy environment. Shift work, night work, and work extending beyond 8 hours a day, 5 days, or 40 hours a week also were associated with prematurity.[35]

A study of hospital workers found that the rate of preterm delivery was significantly higher for women whose jobs involved at least two or three of the following working conditions: long periods of standing, carrying heavy loads (other than lifting patients), and heavy cleaning involving the washing of floors and windows.[26]

Another study compared pregnancy outcomes of employed women and housewives by looking at Apgar score, birthweight, incidence of fetal distress, and prolonged gestational age and rates of prematurity, perinatal death, and malformation. The authors concluded that there was little evidence that working during pregnancy is in itself a risk factor for adverse pregnancy outcome.[37]

The postural and exertional requirements of some jobs, for example, nursing or retail sales, may necessitate modification of work activity at some point during pregnancy. The American Medical Association Council on Scientific Affairs has published guidelines that set out the various stages in gestation through which healthy women with normal uncomplicated pregnancies should be able to perform specific tasks without undue difficulty or risk to the pregnancy. Table 32–11 sets out these guidelines.

In general, a pregnant woman should be able to continue employment until the onset of labor.[38] The determination of whether she can work a particular job and what, if any, modifications are necessary should be made by the woman and her health care provider on a case by case basis, considering the

TABLE 32-11. GUIDELINES FOR CONTINUATION OF VARIOUS LEVELS OF WORK DURING PREGNANCY

Job Function	Week of Gestation	Job Function	Week of Gestation
Secretarial and light clerical	40	Climbing	
Professional and managerial	40	Vertical ladders and poles	
Sitting with light tasks		Repetitive	
Prolonged [>4 h]	40	[>4 times/8-h shift]	20
Intermittent	40	Intermittent	
Standing		[<4 times/8-h shift]	28
Prolonged [>4 h]	24	Stairs	
Intermittent		Repetitive	
[>30 min/h]	32	[>4 times/8-h shift]	28
[<30 min/h]	40	Intermittent	
Stooping and bending below knee level		[<4 times/8-h shift]	40
Repetitive		Lifting	
[>10 times/h]	20	Repetitive	
Intermittent		>23 kg	20
[<10 >2 times/h]	28	<23 >11 kg	24
[<2 times/h]	40	<11 kg	40
		Intermittent	
		>23 kg	30
		<14 >11 kg	40
		>11 kg	40

From Goldhaber et al.[28]

postural, exertional, and other requirements of the job, the potential workplace exposures and their effects, the woman's general physical condition and health status, and her pregnancy experience.[33] Guidelines exist to assist the clinician's decision-making.[39]

A clinician should obtain a thorough occupational history from both partners at the first prenatal visit as well as when evaluating infertility, spontaneous abortion, or other adverse reproductive outcomes.

Some employers, under the guise of protecting the fetus from hazardous exposures, have developed policies that exclude women from certain jobs or otherwise restrict their activities in the workplace. These fetal protection policies or exclusionary policies are highly suspect. Most are directed solely at women despite the potential for paternal exposures to jeopardize the health of the fetus. These policies also ignore the potential for reproductive hazards to endanger the health of other organ systems as well. For example, known or suspected mutagens also have been implicated in carcinogenesis.

One study of the reproductive health policies and practices of nearly 200 Massachusetts chemical and electronics companies revealed a lack of awareness of and attention to reproductive hazards in the workplace.[40] Only 60% of 105 firms reporting the use of at least one of four known reproductive hazards—lead, mercury, ionizing radiation, and glycol ethers—included information on reproductive risks in their worker health and safety training. The survey also found that corporate exclusionary and transfer practices often were unrelated to current scientific knowledge about the effects of particular agents on reproduction or the categories of workers actually at risk. Although 20% of respondents had instituted some form of exclusionary policy, in all but one instance, these policies were aimed solely at women, and by far the greatest number of restrictions were placed on pregnant women, despite the presence in the workplace of agents harmful to the male reproductive system as well.

Some employers offer voluntary transfer policies that maintain the wages and benefits of workers at risk, ideally defined as men and women who are trying to conceive. Although laudable, these policies are of limited applicability, since most small firms lack the requisite flexibility and economic stability to support such practices.

Long-term solutions to the problem of reproductive hazards must begin with education of workers, employers, clinicians, and policymakers. Reproductive health should no longer be identified exclusively with a healthy pregnancy or maternal exposures. Reproductive hazards, like other hazards, should be either eliminated or controlled through the use of engineering controls, work practices, and other traditional hazard control methods.

Child Labor

Susan H. Pollack
Harriet L. Rubenstein
Philip J. Landrigan

Child labor is defined as employment of children less than 18 years of age. It is a common phenomenon in American society, and over the past 5 years, the number of employed children has been increasing steadily. According to provisional data from the U.S. Department of Labor, more than 4 million children in the United States were legally employed in 1988. These child workers include the urban high school student working in a fast food establishment, the suburban 11-year-old delivering newspapers, and the rural child working on a neighbor's farm. Despite the existence of federal and state statutes that regulate the hours and safety conditions under which minors may work, illegal child labor persists in the United States.[1] Detected violations of child labor laws have increased from 9200 in 1983 to more than 22,500 in 1989.[2] Four-year-olds "help out" in factory sweatshops, passing fabric between their mothers' sewing machines to increase the speed of piecework. Fourteen-year-olds work on dangerous and legally prohibited machinery in belt and garment factories, bakeries, and butcher shops. Children do industrial homework on school nights, and they pick vegetables in fields still wet with pesticides.

A combination of economic and social factors is responsible for the increasing prevalence of child labor. Demographic and technological changes have created labor shortages in some regions of the country, particularly the Northeast, and projected population declines and worker shortages suggest that this impetus to employ children will intensify in the years ahead. Despite a relatively strong economy, 20% of American children live below the poverty line today, substantially more than did two decades ago. For these children, financial need presents a compelling reason to seek employment. Unstable world conditions, particularly war and poverty in Central America, have led increasing numbers of illegal immigrants to enter the United States. These immigrants, especially children without parents, are highly vulnerable to exploitation in the workplace because of their overwhelming need for income and their fear of discovery by immigration officials. Finally, officially sanctioned relaxation in enforcement of federal child labor law over the past 8 years has undermined its historic intent and effectiveness.[3]

Historical Perspective

Child labor has a long history. In the Middle Ages, children worked in agriculture and as apprentices to artisans.[4] In Colonial America, children who helped out on their own farms and households commonly were hired out to perform similar tasks for neighbors, a practice that has continued in rural areas almost without change. Under these conditions, proximity to family and social relationships provided some degree of protection for the child worker.[5]

Child labor underwent major expansion and restructuring during the eighteenth century as a consequence of the industrial revolution's need for large numbers of workers. Most mill owners preferred to hire children rather than adults because child workers were cheaper, more tractable, and as labor unions developed, less likely to strike.[6] Families sent children as young as 11, especially girls, to work in the mills, where the wages they could earn far exceeded the income of their parents at home on rural farms. These young girls often were victims of sexual exploitation outside of the workplace in addition to exploitation inside the factories, where they commonly labored for 12 or more hours a day, 6 days a week.[7] Depiction of the horrors of child labor in the literature[8,9] and art of the eighteenth and nineteenth centuries sparked great popular revulsion against the worst abuses, but the practice nevertheless continued.

In Britain, concern over the plight of working children stimulated passage of the first legislation protecting the health of all workers.[4,6] The 1802 Health and Morals of Apprentices Act fixed the maximum number of hours of work for apprentices, forbade night work, and ordered the walls of factories to be washed twice each year and workrooms to be ventilated. In the United States, concerns about working children led to the enactment of compulsory education laws in the eighteenth and nineteenth centuries. For example, an 1874 New York State law mandated schooling for all 8 to 14-year-old children and proscribed work on school days.[6]

Despite federal and state legislation, child labor continued to be a major problem during the first third of the twentieth century, largely because of inadequate enforcement of existing statutes. The need for enforcement was demonstrated tragically by the death of 146 women and children in the 1911 Triangle Shirtwaist fire in New York City, only 8 years after the passage of landmark child labor and fire protection legislation.[10]

Between 1916 and 1930, Congress enacted three major pieces of child labor legislation, but the U.S. Supreme Court invalidated all three. Finally, in 1938, Congress passed the Fair Labor Standards Act (FLSA), which remains the major federal legislation governing child labor today. Major reductions in child labor occurred during the 40 years after passage of the FLSA. Although provisions of the Act helped to produce this decrease, automation, structural shifts in the American industrial economy, reductions in family size, and restrictive immigration policies all contributed to the declining use of child laborers.

After World War II, widespread emphasis on the personal and societal value of education and a generally strong economy combined to further decrease the prevalence of child labor in most sectors of the economy. The major exception was in agricultural employment, which was exempted from many of the provisions of the FLSA. Consequently, the employment of children in agriculture remained common and is to the present time relatively underregulated.

Fair Labor Standards Act and Work Permit System

Under the Fair Labor Standards Act, no child under the age of 16 years may work during school hours, and a ceiling is set on the number of hours of employment permissible for each school day and each school week. Employment in any hazardous nonagricultural occupation is prohibited for anyone less than 18 years old. Thus, no one under age 18 may work in mining, logging, brick and tile manufacture, roofing, or excavating, or as a helper on a vehicle or on power-driven machinery. Work with meat-processing machinery, delicatessen slicers, and supermarket boxcrushers is specifically prohibited. In agriculture, where the restrictions are much less stringent, hazardous work is prohibited only until age 16, and all work on family farms is totally exempted. According to the law, however, no child under age 16 working on a nonfamily farm is allowed to drive a tractor with an engine over 20 horsepower or to handle or apply pesticides and herbicides.[11]

Although the FLSA provides a broad framework for the regulation of child labor, most administration of the law occurs on a state level, largely through the work permit system. Work permits are issued to children by state and local school systems. This authority was placed within the schools to allow for discretion in the issuance and rescission of a work permit based on a student's academic performance. In reality, however, most school systems, overwhelmed by more pressing responsibilities, virtually never exercise their discretionary authority. Administration of the FLSA in most states also suffers from a lack of centralized data collection on the number or types of work permits issued or the industries in which children are employed. Thus, in most states, only meager information is available on the number and ages of employed children or on the nature of their employment.

Illegal Child Labor

Despite the FLSA, illegal employment of children continues to occur in all industrial sectors and often exists under sweatshop conditions.[12–14] A sweatshop is defined as any establishment that routinely and repeatedly violates wage, hour, or child labor laws and the laws protecting occupational safety and health.[15] Traditionally, these shops have been considered fringe establishments, such as those in the garment and meat-packing industries. Increasingly, however, restaurants and grocery stores, not typically considered to be sweatshops, also are satisfying the definition.

In an effort to quantify the magnitude of illegal child labor in the absence of readily available national statistics, the General Accounting Office (GAO) surveyed the directors of state labor departments in 1987.[15] The GAO found that in Chicago, half of the approximately 5000 restaurants met the criteria for sweatshops and that about 25,000 workers were employed in such establishments. In New Orleans, 25% of the 100 apparel firms (employing 5000 workers) were estimated to be sweatshops. In Los Angeles and New York, anywhere from 500 to 2000 or more sweatshops were thought to exist. The problem is not confined to large urban areas. In 1987, several high school students employed by a chain restaurant in a small West Virginia town quit after having tried unsuccessfully to negotiate with the manager to stop keeping them past midnight on school nights.[16]

Benefits and Risks

Parents, employers, vocational counselors, and working children cite numerous potential advantages of employment.[17] Work can foster the development of discipline, teamwork, and a sense of responsibility in the working child. It can encourage the unfolding of new skills and provide an opportunity to sample different vocations. An employer provides a role model for working youth and may evolve into a mentor. Work historically has offered youth economic opportunity, and it provides money that can be used for a college education, to help feed the family, for travel, or for personal extras not otherwise available. In recent years, as the number of American children living below the poverty line has increased and as available college financial assistance for those in the middle class has dwindled, these economic opportunities have assumed great importance. Finally, work offers youth a sense of personal worth for a job well done.

Employment of children does, however, present potential risks to the intellectual, moral, and emotional development of the working child. Additionally, work may pose risks to a child's physical health and safety.

One of the principal hazards of child labor is that it can interfere with school performance, mortgaging the child's educational and financial future for today's short-term economic gain. Employed children risk having inadequate time for school homework and increased fatigue on school days. Teachers of children in areas where preholiday employment is common or industrial homework is escalating have noted declines in the academic performance of previously adequate students.[17,18] These children fall asleep at their desks and have difficulty in learning. Even if they maintain their academic performance, working children may be unable to participate as actively in afterschool activities and sports as their nonworking peers. Adequate rest and time to play are necessary for children to develop, grow, and learn.

Child labor may affect childhood development adversely by encouraging antisocial behavior or by interfering with the formation of moral judgment,[19] particularly if the employer's values, morals, or work habits are not those society would wish to inculcate in young workers. When an employer hires children without working papers, pays them "off the books," illegally keeps them at work after midnight, or asks them to work on dangerous and legally prohibited machinery, the employer sends socially inappropriate messages to the child about the relative importance of abiding by the law.

The second major risk of child labor is that hazardous working conditions threaten the physical safety and health of working children. Injury is the leading cause of death for children above age 1 year in the United States. Approximately 10,000 children die from injuries each year.[20] In 1990, we still do not have a reliable nationwide system for collection of data on work-related fatalities or injuries suffered by minors, and most major publications discussing the epidemiology of childhood injury fail to consider work as a causal or contributing factor.[21,22] Nevertheless, the limited data available characterizing the risks of work-related injury and illness faced by working children suggest that a significant public health problem exists. Injuries to working children are noted on hospital records and in workers' compensation awards. A 1985 study reviewing adolescent injury-related emergency room visits in Massachusetts found that 24% of the visits with an identified site of injury had occurred on the job.[23]

The GAO has developed a partial picture of youth fatalities and injuries in the workplace using data from state workers' compensation programs and OSHA citation information.[2] Based on workers' compensation reports from 33 states, at least 48 minors were killed and 128,000 others were injured on the job in 1987 and 1988. Injuries generally involved strains, sprains, cuts, punctures, dislocations, and lacerations. In California, nearly half of all injuries occurred in the retail trade industry, and about one third of all injuries occurred in restaurants and food stores.

During fiscal years 1987 and 1988, the OSHA reported conducting 59 inspections of workplaces where workers under age 19 had died.[2] These deaths most often were a result of fractures, electrocutions, and asphyxiations. Of the 59 inspections, 48 (81%) resulted in citations of the employer for violating safety or health requirements.

An analysis of workers' compensation claims reported to the Supplementary Data System of the Bureau of Labor Statistics in 1980 examined injuries occurring in persons under age 18.[24] A total of 23,823 workers' compensation claims for this age group were reported in the 24 participating states during that year. Approximately 10% of claims were for children under age 16. The rates of injury in 16 and 17-year-olds were equivalent to 12.6 per 100 full-time male workers and 6.6 per 100 full-time female workers. Serious injuries included fractures, dislocations, and amputations. Machines and vehicles accounted for over 14% of claims, despite being proscribed for child work under the FLSA. Approximately one half of the claims were from workers in the retail trade industry. Another 21% of claims were from service industry workers. In nine states without a minimum number of days of disability as a prerequisite to workers' compensation, rates of injury were 11.5 and 9.4 per 100 full-time 16 and 17-year-old workers in trade and service industries, respectively. Comparable rates of injury for workers of all ages reported in this survey were 7.4 and 5.2 per 100 full-time workers in these two industries.

A review of New York State Workers' Compensation records for 1980 through 1987 found that more than 1100 awards every year were made to children under age 18 for work-related injury.[25] More than 40% of these injuries involved some degree of permanent disability. Although older children accounted for more of the injuries, younger children incurred more serious and disabling injuries. Children under age 15 received 99 of the 1333 awards in 1986, a representative year.

Even less is known about the incidence and severity of work-related illness in children, although children are known to experience a variety of toxic exposures at work. These exposures include formaldehyde and dyes in the garment industry, solvents in paint shops, organophosphate pesticides in agriculture and lawn care, asbestos in building abatement projects, and benzene in gasoline service stations. Given the range and potential toxicity of these exposures, it is quite possible that some as yet undefined fraction of adolescent asthma, leukemia,[26] and other chronic disease is related to toxic exposures to children in the workplace. Almost no work has been done to explore the possibility that differences in metabolism, respiratory rates, and body surface area may make young workers more susceptible to toxic agents than their adult counterparts. Also ignored is the possible increased risk for diseases of long latency faced by young workers because of their additional years of potential exposure compared to adult workers.

Hazard of Injury

Urban Child Labor. There are no recent epidemiological studies of the health hazards associated with urban child labor. The available information comes, therefore, from case reports and from evaluation of the types of employment available to urban children.

Garment industry sweatshop work appears to be an increasingly common and hazardous source of employment for urban children.[27] Children who work in shops where pleating is done may suffer burns, since the process involves high temperature fixation of the fabric. Exposure to solvents and dyes in poorly ventilated leather shops poses long-term neurological hazards. Large cutting blades and industrial leather punches create amputation and crush hazards. High-speed sewing machines can rapidly sew a child's finger or hand.

Fire hazards in urban sweatshops are created by blocked exit doors and accumulation of combustible materials. Electrocution hazards result from overloaded electrical supplies, workstations located close to exposed wire, and bare fuse boxes. These same conditions are known to have contributed to the deaths of 146 women and children in the 1911 Triangle Shirtwaist fire in New York City.[10] The large number of fire code violations being discovered today by the Garment Industry Task Force Inspectors of the New York State Department of Labor[28] suggests that workers, including children, are at very high risk of dying of fire if these conditions are not alleviated.

Stocking shelves and working at the cash register of grocery stores is legal work for children aged 14 and older, and urban grocery stores rely heavily on a young workforce. Although there is no literature concerning repetitive motion injuries among child cashiers, such injuries, including carpal tunnel syndrome, are known to pose problems for adult cashiers. The usual configuration of stock in big-city markets, where space is at a premium and items are stacked to a much greater vertical height than in other locales, poses risks both of ladder falls and of injuries from falling objects. Lacerations may be caused by cardboard boxes and by the knives used to open them. Although children are prohibited by law from operating the machines that are used to crush or bale these boxes, an 11-year old boy in the Bronx, New York, was killed in December 1988, when he became entangled in a boxcrusher.

Delicatessen and bakery slicers both have been shown to be sources of serious injury among teenage workers, although their use is legally prohibited for children under 18 years old. In the early 1980s, a teenage boy in New York City was brought to the emergency room with an amputated arm. He said he had been "helping out" in a butcher shop. A few months later, another teenage boy was brought to the same emergency room with his arm amputated after "helping out" in the same shop.[29] In 1988, a 17-year-old girl in New York City amputated several fingers when a bakery dough slicer came down on her hand.[30]

The fast food industry is one of the largest employers of youth in the United States today. Minor lacerations and burns are common hazards in these establishments. There is also a risk of electrocution, although this risk may have been lessened by changes mandated subsequent to the 1987 death by electrocution of a teenage worker in a hamburger restaurant. The cause of the boy's electrocution was a power outlet on a wet floor in an improperly grounded building.[31] Workers in fast food restaurants may have excessive microwave exposure, since heavy use of the microwave equipment tends to damage the seals of food ovens. In an effort to hasten the efficiency of food delivery, safety power cutoffs on microwave cookers may be circumvented.[32] The extent of occupational exposure to microwaves has not been quantified, nor is the risk fully quantified, but concern exists over the possibility that exposure to microwaves in repeated high doses may cause eye damage, with subsequent cataract formation.

Suburban and Small Town Child Labor. Children in small towns have a wide variety of job opportunities: delivering newspapers or pizzas, caring for lawns, working in gas stations, working in restaurants and fast food establishments, working at sales jobs in retail stores, and stocking shelves and working the registers in supermarkets. These jobs present potential exposure to diverse safety and health hazards.

Lawn care is associated with mower-related injuries, including amputation of fingers and toes as well as eye injuries caused by flying rocks propelled by mower blades. Exposures to pesticides and herbicides also may occur. Newspaper delivery is associated with motor vehicle injuries to children on bicycles and on foot. Employment of teenagers in gas stations may be associated with airborne and dermal exposure to benzene, a carcinogenic solvent contained in unleaded gasoline. The delivery of pizzas and other hot food items has proven to be extremely hazardous to working children, particularly when unrealistic delivery deadlines encourage reckless and dangerous driving by young and often inexperienced motor vehicle operators.[33,34]

Rural Child Labor. Rural children work primarily in agriculture and face the same health and safety hazards as adult agricultural workers, including lacerations, amputations, and crush injuries from farm machinery, blunt trauma from large animals, motor vehicle accidents involving farm vehicles on public roads, suffocation on grain elevators and silos, and exposure to pesticides. Small physical size, inadequate training, and age-inappropriate task assignment may superimpose additional risks on young workers. Although the numbers of children working in agriculture are not as large as in other sectors, the potential hazards, especially those involving machinery and large animals, coupled with the historical lack of regulation of agriculture, create an important problem. Agriculture has come to surpass mining as the most dangerous occupation in the United States, accounting in 1980 for 61 fatalities per 100,000 workers.[35] Perhaps for this reason, much of the scanty literature available on work-related injury and illness in children focuses on agricultural employment.

Rivara compiled a picture of childhood farm-related morbidity and mortality in 1985.[36] He found that nearly 300 children and adolescents die each year from farm injuries, and 23,500 suffer nonfatal trauma. The rate for 15- to 19-year-old boys is double that of young children and 26-fold higher than for girls. More than half (52.5%) of those children fatally injured on farms die without ever reaching a physician, an additional 19.1% die in transit to a hospital, and only 7.4% live long enough to receive inpatient care. The most common cause of fatal and nonfatal injury is farm machinery. Tractors accounted for one half of these machinery-related deaths, followed by farm wagons, combines, and forklifts. A study of Wisconsin farm tractor fatalities between 1971 and 1975 revealed that 29% of the fatalities occurred to male farm residents under the age of 19.[37]

Cogbill et al. reviewed the cases of 105 farm trauma patients 19 years old or younger admitted to a Wisconsin Level II trauma referral center.[38] They found a bimodal age distribution, with peaks at ages 4 and 14 years. All 13- to 18-year-olds were working at the time of their injury. Six of the teenagers were critically injured.

Swanson et al. also noted a bimodal peak of childhood farm injuries, in which the adolescent peak is accounted for by working children.[39] A review of 88 cases of injury in rural adolescents found that 29 were definitely working at the time of injury, and another 20 may have been working. Older children were involved in accidents with tractors more than twice as often as younger children. Power takeoffs (rotating drive shafts that transfer power from a tractor to a piece of attached farm machinery) were a second important cause of injury.

The FLSA requires that all 14 and 15-year-olds hired as farm employees must have completed a safety education course before operating machinery. These regulations do not apply, however, to children working on their family farms. Furthermore, this safety requirement is not being met even on farms where it is required by law. In 1984, a 16-year-old New York boy died while working on a neighbor's farm when the machine he was unloading caught and pulled him in, leaving him torn and crushed. He had been working since age 11 but had no work permit and no tractor permit.[17] Although both a license and an inspected and registered car are required to drive on public roads, a farm vehicle need not have a certificate of inspection and can be driven by anyone, including a child with no license.

A 1989 article by Broste et al. from the Marshfield Clinic in Wisconsin describes hearing loss among high school farm students.[40] The article is of historical as well as medical note, since it represents perhaps the only report of occupational illness in adolescents. Audiometric examinations of 872 vocational agriculture students were conducted over a 3-year period. Students who were actively involved in farm work had increased prevalence of high frequency, early noise-induced hearing loss as compared to their peers who were not actively involved in farm work. The authors suggest that education and provision of hearing protection would be appropriate preventive measures, since students using hearing protection had a lower prevalence of hearing loss. The authors conclude that farm teenagers may be at increasing risk for hearing loss and other occupational illnesses as economic pressures compel them to take additional responsibility for farm operations formerly performed by hired help or by their parents, who are now forced to work off the farm to supplement family income.

International Child Labor. Child labor is a serious problem beyond the borders of the United States.[41-44] According to the International Labour Organization (ILO), at least 200 million children worldwide under the age of 14 are employed. In some countries, children constitute 15% to 25% of the total workforce. Children are employed as rug weavers in the middle East, underground tin miners in South America, metal workers, fireworks makers, textile weavers, and glass blowers. Injuries, illnesses, and disability are common among working children worldwide.

Child labor is associated in virtually all countries—both industrialized and developing—with poverty, inadequate educational opportunities, and failure to enforce existing laws and standards. Particularly severe abuses have been documented in so-called free enterprise zones, industrial areas established in many countries in which relaxation has been permitted in the enforcement of labor and environmental laws.

Options for Prevention

A variety of preventive strategies will need to be undertaken to reduce the illness and injury associated with both legal and illegal child labor.

Enforcement. Relaxation in the enforcement of federal regulations protecting child workers, along with a decrease in the number of inspectors and, consequently, a decrease in the number of inspections, has contributed to the current resurgence of child labor abuses in the United States. Strong enforcement of existing legislation and regulations is necessary to protect the health and safety of working children and to encourage legitimate employers whose businesses are financially endangered by those who hire children under illegal working conditions.

Education. Working children and their parents, employers, and school authorities, as well as physicians and other health care providers, need to be educated about the hazards associated with child labor and the relevant legal proscriptions. Education of child workers should attempt to temper their usual enthusiasm and lack of fear of industrial hazards. School authorities exercising their responsibilities under the work permit system and health care providers performing physical examinations of job applicants under age 18 years have a unique opportunity to ensure that minors are not working in prohibited occupations or in other unproscribed yet hazardous situations. Health care providers, particularly emergency room staff, need to remember that work can be a cause of injury and illness in childhood. The importance of an occupational history cannot be overemphasized. Finally, the business community must be educated on the hazards of child labor and reminded of their responsibilities under the law.

Surveillance. One of the major impediments to defining and resolving the problem of child labor in the United States is the lack of up-to-date descriptive data on the size and demographic characteristics of the population of working children. Data on the incidence of work-related injuries and illnesses in children are limited and fragmented. Federal and state governments need to develop mechanisms for collecting these data more efficiently and for accessing data sets that are potentially useful, but currently only minimally available, such as information on work permits issued by local school boards. Furthermore, federal and state agencies should institute active surveillance of occupational injuries and illnesses in minors, using workers' compensation claims, hospital visits, and other sources to identify occupational sentinel health events for follow-up and preventive intervention. Active surveillance and epidemiological studies of work-related injury and illness in minors also will facilitate evaluation of the effectiveness of current laws and may suggest possible modifications, such as additions to the list of proscribed occupations.

REFERENCES

Workers with Disabilities

1. Harris L, and Associates: The ICD Survey II: Employing Disabled Americans. New York, March 1987
2. The President's Committee on Employment of the Handicapped: Out of the Job Market: A National Crisis, Washington, DC, 1987, p 1
3. Harris L, and Associates: The ICD Survey of Disabled Americans: Bringing Disabled Americans into the Mainstream. New York, March 1986
4. Report of the Secretary of Labor: Labor Market Shortages. January 1989, p 2
5. E.I. duPont de Nemours and Company: Equal to the Task. Wilmington, DE, 1982
6. Committee on Mental and Physical Impairment, American Medical Association: Guides to the Evaluation of Permanent Impairment, 2 edt. Chicago: AMA, 1984
7. LaPlante MP: Data on disability from the National Health Interview Survey, 1983–85. Corte Madera, CA: InfoUse, 1988
8. Labor Force Status and Other Characteristics of Persons With a Work Disability: 1981 to 1988. Current Population Reports, Series P 23, No 160. U.S. Department of Commerce, Bureau of the Census, July 1989
9. Bowe F: Disabled in 1985: A Portrait of American Adults. Hot Springs, Arkansas Research and Training Center in Vocational Rehabilitation, 1986
10. Kutner NG: Women with disabling health conditions: The significance of employment. Women Health 9(4):21–31, 1984
11. United States Code, title 29, sec. 701–796
12. Rothstein MA: Legal considerations in worker fitness evaluations. In Himmelstein JS, Pransky GS (eds): Worker Fitness and Risk Evaluations. State Art Rev Occup Med. Philadelphia: Hanley & Belfus, April–June 1988, chap 4
13. 45 Code of Federal Regulations Part 84.12(b)
14. 45 Code of Federal Regulations Part 84.12(c)
15. O'Bryant T: Facts about hiring people with disabilities. Worklife—A Publication on Employment and People with Disabilities. 1(3):8–10, 1988

16. Dean DH: Costs and benefits of vocational rehabilitation: An employer's perspective. Employment Relations Today 15(2):141–147, 1988
17. Carey TS, Hadler NM: The role of the primary physician in disability determination for Social Security Insurance and workers' compensation. Ann Intern Med 104:706–710, 1986
18. Himmelstein J, Pransky GS: Work incapacity, impairment and disability evaluation. In Levy BS, Wegman DH (eds): Occupational Health: Recognizing and Preventing Work-Related Disease, 2 edt. Boston: Little, Brown and Co, 1988, Chap 12
19. Rothstein MA: Medical Screening and the Employee Health Cost Crisis, Washington, DC: Bureau of National Affairs, 1989
20. Pransky GS, Frumkin H, Himmelstein JS: Decision-making in worker fitness and risk evaluation. In Himmelstein JS, Pransky GS (eds): Worker Fitness and Risk Evaluations. State Art Rev Occup Med. Philadelphia: Hanley & Belfus, April–June 1988, chap 2
21. Derr PG: Ethical considerations in fitness and risk evaluations. In Himmelstein JS, Pransky GS (eds): Worker Fitness and Risk Evaluations, State Art Rev Occup Med Philadelphia: Hanley & Belfus, April–June 1988, chap 3

Migrant and Seasonal Farmworkers

1. National Safety Council: Accident Facts, 1988 edt
2. U.S. Department of Commerce, Bureau of the Census: Statistical Abstract of the United States. 1989
3. Wilk VA: The Occupational Health of Migrant and Seasonal Farmworkers in the United States. Washington, DC: Farmworker Justice Fund, 1986
4. Lillesand D, Dravitz L, McClellan J: An Estimate of the Number of Migrant and Seasonal Farmworkers in the United States and the Commonwealth of Puerto Rico. Washington, DC: Legal Services Corporation, 1977
5. Association of Farmworker Opportunity Programs: Partnerships: Helping Migrant Farmworkers Help Themselves. Washington, DC, 1988
6. Report of the Minimum Wage Study Commission. Washington, DC: U.S. Government Printing Office, 1981
7. U.S. Department of Agriculture: Agricultural Statistics. Washington, DC: U.S. Government Printing Office, 1988
8. Coye MJ: The health effects of agricultural production: I. The health of agricultural workers. J Public Health Policy 6(3):349–370, 1985
9. U.S. General Accounting Office: Pesticides: EPA's Formidable Task to Assess and Regulate Their Risks. Washington, DC: GAO/RCED-86-125, 1986
10. Moses M: Pesticide-related health problems and farmworkers. Am Assoc Occup Health Nurses J 37(3):115–130, 1989
11. Littlefield C, Stout CL: A survey of Colorado's migrant farmworkers: Access to health care. Int Migration Rev 21(3):688–707, 1987
12. Hicks W: Migrant health: An analysis. Primary Care Focus July/Aug: 6–23, 1982
13. Schaefer AE: Nutritional needs of special populations at risk. Ann NY Acad Sci 300:419–427, 1977
14. Smith G, DeAngelis C, Hanser J: The health status of a subgroup of migrant American children. Clin Pediatr 19(5):900–903, 1978
15. Goldsmith MF: As farmworkers help keep America healthy, illness may be their harvest. JAMA 261(22):3207–3213, 1989
16. Walker GM Jr: Utilization of health care: The Laredo migrant experience. Am J Public Health 69(7):667–672, 1979
17. Wilk VA: The Occupational Health of Migrant and Seasonal Farmworkers in the United States Progress Report. Washington, DC: Farmworker Justice Fund, 1988
18. Florida Rural Legal Services: Danger in the field: The myth of pesticide safety. 1980
19. Worker Protection Standards for Agricultural Pesticides (40 CFR 170) Fed Reg 39:16890, 1974
20. Saunders LD, Ames RG, Knaak JB, et al: Outbreak of Omite-CR-induced dermatitis among orange pickers in Tulare County, California. J Occup Med 29(5):409–413, 1987
21. Kahn E: Pesticide-related illness in California farmworkers. J Occup Med 18(1):693–696, 1976
22. Field Sanitation: Final Rule (29 CFR 1928). Fed Reg 52:16050, 1987
23. Migrant Legal Action Program Inc., Farmworker Justice Fund Inc.: Post hearing proposed findings of fact and conclusions of law. Docket No. H-308, U.S. Department of Labor, Occupational Safety and Health Administration. In the matter of: Proposed Farmworker Field Sanitation Standard. August 30, 1984
24. Ortiz JS: Composite summary and analysis of hearing held by the Department of Labor, Occupational Health and Safety Administration on field sanitation for migrant farm workers. Docket No. H-308. October 21, 1985
25. Arbab DM, Weidner BL: Infectious diseases and field water supply and sanitation among migrant farm workers. Am J Public Health 76(6):694–695, 1986
26. Whiting WB: Occupational illness and injuries of California agricultural workers. J Occup Med 17(3):177–181, 1975
27. Coye MJ: The health effects of agricultural production: II. The health of the community. J Public Health Policy 7(3):340–354, 1986

Minority Workers

1. U.S. Department of Health and Human Services: Report of the Secretary's Task Force on Black and Minority Health, Vol 1: Executive Summary. August 1985
2. The Office of Disease Prevention and Health Promotion, U.S. Public Health Service: Disease Prevention/Health Promotion: The Facts, Palo Alto, CA: Bell Publishing Co, 1988
3. National Center for Health Statistics: Health, United States, 1988. DHHS Pub. No. (PHS) 89-1232, Public Health Service. Washington, DC: U.S. Government Printing Office, March 1989
4. National Center for Health Statistics: Health, United States, 1987. DHHS Pub. No. (PHS) 88-1232, Public Health Service. Washington, DC: U.S. Government Printing Office, March 1988
5. Centers for Disease Control. The Surgeon General's 1989 report on reducing the health consequences of smoking: 25 years of progress (executive summary). MMWR 38(suppl S-2), 1989
6. Sterling TD, Weinkam JJ: Comparison of smoking-related risk factors among black and white males. Am J Ind Med 15:319–333, 1989
7. Blot WJ, Fraumeni JF Jr: Changing patterns of lung cancer in the United States. Am J Epidemiol 115(5):664–673, 1982
8. Crew SR: The great migration of Afro-Americans, 1915–40. Monthly Labor Rev 110(3):34–36, 1987
9. Mancuso TT, Sterling TD: Lung cancer among black and white migrants in the U.S. Etiologic considerations. J Natl Med Assoc 67(2):106–111, 1975
10. Westcott DN: Blacks in the 1970's: Did they scale the job ladder? Monthly Labor Rev 105(6):29–38, 1982
11. U.S. Equal Employment Opportunity Commission: 1987 EEO-1 Employment Analysis Report. Unpublished material
12. U.S. General Accounting Office: "Sweatshops" in the U.S.: Opinions on their extent and possible enforcement options. GAO/HRD-88-130BR. August 1988
13. Kotelchuck D: Occupational injuries and illness among black workers. Health/PAC Bulletin 81–82(April):33–34, 1979
14. Campbell AB: Analysis of occupational injuries and illnesses among black workers (1984). Unpublished thesis. Hunter College, CUNY, New York, 1987
15. Robinson JC: Racial inequality and the probability of occupation-related injury or illness. Milbank Mem Fund Q/Health Soc 62(4):567–590, 1984
16. Robinson JC: Trends in racial inequality and exposure to work-related hazards, 1968–1986. Am Assoc Occup Health Nurses J 37(2):56–63, 1989
17. Robinson JC: Exposure to occupational hazards among Hispanics, blacks, and non-Hispanic whites in California. Am J Public Health 79(5):629–630, 1989

18. Gagager WM, cited by Davis M, Rowland A: Occupational Disease Among Black Workers: An Annotated Bibliography. Berkeley, CA: Labor Occupational Health Program, 1980
19. Lloyd JW, Lundin FE Jr, Redmond CK, et al: Long-term mortality study of steelworkers. IV. Mortality by work area. J Occup Med 12(5):151–157, 1970
20. Redmond CK, Ciocco A, Lloyd JW, et al: Long-term mortality study of steelworkers. VI. Mortality from malignant neoplasms among coke oven workers. J Occup Med 14(8):621–629, 1972
21. Martin CF, Higgins JE: Byssinosis and other respiratory ailments. A survey of 6,631 cotton textile employees. J Occup Med 18(7):455–462, 1976
22. McMichael AJ, Spirtas R, Gamble JF, et al: Mortality among rubber workers: Relationship to specific jobs. J Occup Med 18(3):178–185, 1976
23. Mallin K, Berkeley L, Young Q: A proportional mortality ratio study of workers in a construction equipment and diesel engine manufacturing plant. Am J Ind Med 10:127–141, 1986
24. Rossignol AM, Locke JA, Boyle CM, et al: Epidemiology of work-related burn injuries in Massachusetts requiring hospitalization. J Trauma 26(12):1097–1101, 1986
25. Park R, Silverstein M, Maizlish N, et al: Mortality among workers in auto repair and auto body shops. NIOSH Contract No. 210-81-5104. September 1986
26. U.S. Department of Labor, Bureau of Labor Statistics: Employment in perspective: Minority workers. Report 764. Fourth quarter 1988
27. Friedman-Jimenez G: Occupational disease among minority workers. A common and preventable public health problem. Am Assoc Occup Health Nurses J 37(2):64–70, 1989

Women Workers

1. Messing K, Reveret J-P: Are women in female jobs for their health? A study of working conditions and health effects in the fish-processing industry in Quebec. Int J Health Serv 13(4):635–648, 1983
2. Mergler D, Brabant C, Vezina N, et al: The weaker sex? Men in women's working conditions report similar health symptoms. J Occup Med 29(5):417–421, 1987
3. Labor Force Statistics Derived From the Current Population Survey, 1948–87. Bulletin 2307. U.S. Department of Labor, Bureau of Labor Statistics, August 1988, p 567
4. Twenty Facts on Women Workers. Fact Sheet No. 88-2. U.S. Department of Labor, Women's Bureau, 1988
5. Facts on U.S. Working Women: Women and Workforce 2000. Fact Sheet No. 88-1. U.S. Department of Labor, Women's Bureau, January 1988
6. Labor Market Problems of Older Workers. Report of the Secretary of Labor, January 1989, p 38
7. Stellman JM: The working environment of the working poor: An analysis based on workers' compensation claims, census data and known risk factors. Women Health 12(3/4):83–101, 1987
8. 9 to 5, National Association of Working Women: 9 to 5 Profile of Working Women. Cleveland, Ohio: 9 to 5, March, 1989
9. U.S. Department of Labor, Bureau of Labor Statistics: Employment and Earnings. January 1989, p 225
10. Baker DB: Occupational stress. In Levy BS, Wegman DH (eds): Occupational Health: Recognizing and Preventing Work-Related Disease, 2 edt. Boston: Little, Brown and Co, 1988, chap 20
11. Zappert LT, Weinstein HM: Sex differences in the impact of work on physical and psychological health. Am J Psychiatry 142(10): 1174–1178, 1985
12. Report of the Public Health Service Task Force on Women's Health Issues. Public Health Rep 100(1):73–106, 1985
13. Hibbard JH, Pope CR: Employment status, employment characteristics, and women's health. Women Health 10(1):59–77, 1985
14. Froberg D, Gjerdingen D, Preston M: Multiple roles and women's mental and physical health: What have we learned? Women Health 11(2):79–96, 1986
15. Hazuda HP, Haffner SM, Stern MP, et al: Employment status and women's protection against coronary heart disease. Am J Epidemiol 123(4):623–640, 1986
16. Waldron I, Herold J, Dunn D, et al: Reciprocal effects of health and labor force participation among women: Evidence from two longitudinal studies. J Occup Med 24(2):126–132, 1982
17. Passannante MR, Nathanson CA: Women in the labor force: Are sex mortality differentials changing? J Occup Med 29(1):21–28, 1987
18. Kotler P, Wingard DL: The effect of occupational, marital and parental roles on mortality: The Alemeda County Study. Am J Public Health 79(5):607–612, 1989
19. Haynes SG, Feinleib M: Women, work and coronary heart disease: Prospective findings from the Framingham Heart Study. Am J Public Health 70(2):133–141, 1980
20. Verbrugge L: Physical health of clerical workers in the U.S., Framingham, and Detroit. Women Health 9(1):17–41, 1984
21. Jougla E, Bouvier-Colle MH, Maguin P, et al: Health and employment of a female population in an urban area. Int J Epidemiol 12(1):67–76, 1983
22. Women, Work and Child Care. Washington, DC: National Commission on Working Women of Wider Opportunities for Women, 1989
23. Crull P: Sexual harassment and women's health. In Chavkin W (ed): Double Exposure: Women's Health Hazards on the Job and at Home. New York: Monthly Review Press, 1984, Chap 5
24. Davis H, Honchar PA, Suarez L: Fatal occupational injuries of women, Texas 1975–84. Am J Public Health 77(12):1524–1528, 1987
25. Seligman PJ, Newman SC, Timbrook CL, et al: Sexual assault of women at work. Am J Ind Med 12:445–450, 1987
26. Silverstein BA, Fine LJ, Armstrong J: Occupational factors and carpal tunnel syndrome. Am J Ind Med 11:343–358, 1987
27. Additional repetitive motion problems found by communication workers, BNA told. Occup Safety Health Reporter 17(34):1341–1342, 1988
28. Goldhaber MK, Polen MR, Hiatt RA: The risk of miscarriage and birth defects among women who use visual display terminals during pregnancy. Am J Ind Med 13:695–706, 1988
29. Morbidity and Mortality Weekly Reports: Working with video display terminals: A preliminary health rise evaluation. MMWR 29(25):307–308, 1980
30. Murphy DC, Henefin MS, Stellman JM: Personal protective equipment for women: Results of a manufacturers' and suppliers' survey. Transactions of the forty-third annual conference of governmental industrial hygienists 1981, 62–72
31. U.S. Congress, Office of Technology Assessment: Reproductive Health Hazards in the Workplace. Washington, DC: U.S. Government Printing Office, OTA-BA-266, December 1985
32. Rosenberg MJ, Feldblum PJ, Marshall EG: Occupational influences on reproduction: A review of recent literature. J Occup Med 29(7): 584–591, 1987
33. Welch LS: Decisionmaking about reproductive hazards. Semin Occup Med 1(2):97–106, 1986
34. Naeye RL, Peters BS: Working during pregnancy: Effects on the fetus. Pediatrics 69(6):724–727, 1982
35. Mamelle N, Laumon B, Lazar P: Prematurity and occupational activity during pregnancy. Am J Epidemiol 119(3):309–322, 1984
36. Saurel-Cubizolles MJ, Kaminski M, Llado-Arkhipoff, et al: Pregnancy and its outcome among hospital personnel according to occupation and working conditions. J Epidemiol Commun Health 39:129–134, 1985
37. Marbury MC, Linn S, Monson RR, et al: Work and pregnancy. J Occup Med 26(6):415–421, 1984
38. Council on Scientific Affairs: Effects of pregnancy on work performance. JAMA 251(15):1995–1997, 1984
39. U.S. Department of Health, Education and Welfare, National Institute for Occupational Safety and Health: Guidelines on Pregnancy and Work. DHEW (NIOSH) Publication No. 78-118, 1977
40. Daniels C, Paul M, Rosofsky R: Family, Work & Health, Boston: Department of Public Health, 1988

Child Labor

1. Corbin T: Child labor law survey of teenagers. Albany: New York State Department of Labor, Division of Research and Statistics, Working Paper No. 5, Sept 1988
2. U.S. General Accounting Office: "Sweatshops" and child labor violations: A growing problem in the United States. W. Gainer before the Capitol Hill Forum on the Exploitation of Children in the Workplace, Nov 21, 1989
3. Landrigan PJ: The hazards to children of industrial homework. Testimony before the U.S. Dept of Labor. New York, March 29, 1989
4. Hunter D: The Diseases of Occupations, 5 edt. London: The English Universities Press, Ltd, 1974
5. Postol T: Child labor in the United States: Its growth and abolition. Am Educator 13(2):30–31, 1989
6. Trattner WI: Crusade for the Children: A History of the National Child Labor Committee and Child Labor Reform in America. Chicago: Quadrangle Books, 1970
7. Rosner J: Emmeline. New York: Pocket Books, 1980
8. Dickens C: Hard Times. London, 1854
9. Trollope A: The Life and Adventures of Michael Armstrong, the Factory Boy. London: Colburn, 1840
10. Werthheimer BM. "We Were There"—The Story of Working Women in America. New York: Pantheon Books, 1977
11. National Child Labor Committee: Child Labor and Related Law Compendium. Excerpt from Dorianne Beyer. New York, 1986
12. Bagli CV: Child labor and sweatshops—Growing problems in the city. Observer, October 3, 1988
13. Bagli CV: Some "hard workers" in garment district are just 12 or 14. NY Observer, January 9, 1989
14. Powell M: Babes in toil-land: Child labor and the city's sweatshops. NY Newsday, January 8, 1989
15. U.S. General Accounting Office: Sweatshops in the U.S.—Opinions on their Extent and Possible Enforcement Actions. Washington, DC: August 1988 (Publ. No. GAO/HRD-88-130 BR)
16. West Virginia high school student: 1987 personal communication to Susan H. Pollack
17. New York State Department of Labor: Hearings on Child Labor Law Review. Albany, Buffalo, Manhattan, Hauppauge, L.I., and Syracuse, 1988
18. Schiffley Embroidery Cases: Personal communication from Dorothy Come (retired United States Department of Labor) to Susan H. Pollack
19. Cohen S: Social and Personality Development in Childhood. New York: MacMillan, 1976, pp 163–186
20. Waller AE, Baker SP, Szocka A: Childhood injury deaths: National analysis and geographical variations. Am J Public Health 79(3):310–315, 1989
21. Centers for Disease Control: Prevention of Injuries to Children and Youth: A Selected Bibliography. Atlanta: Center for Environmental Health and Center for Health Promotion and Education, CDC, 1987
22. Baker SP: Childhood injuries: The community approach to prevention. J Public Health Policy 2:35–246, 1981
23. Anderka M, Gallagher SS, Azzara CA: Adolescent work-related injuries. Presented at American Public Health Association Meeting, Washington DC, November 1985
24. Schober SE, Handke JL, Halperin WE, et al: Work-related injuries in minors. Am J Ind Med 14(5):585–595, 1988
25. Pollack SH, Belville R, Landrigan P, et al: Epidemiologic studies in the health hazards of child labor. In preparation.
26. Rinsky RA, Smith AB, Hornung R, et al: Benzene and leukemia—An epidemiologic risk assessment. N Engl J Med 316:104–1050, 1987
27. Pollack S: Personal observations on visits to the garment industry sweatshops in New York City in conjunction with the New York State Department of Labor Apparel Industry Task Force, 1988–1989
28. McDaid H: Personal communication to Susan H. Pollack, 1989
29. Drucker E: Comments on proposed revision of legislation on child labor. Testimony submitted to the Sub-Committee on Labor Standards, Committee on Education and Labor, U.S. House of Representatives. New York: Montefiore Medical Center, Department of Social Medicine, September 1982
30. Scott G: Teenager's fingers severed in Queens bakery accident. NY Newsday, September 29, 1988
31. Division of Safety Research, National Institute for Occupational Safety and Health: FACE program, January 22, 1988
32. Gilman C: Personal communication to Susan H. Pollack, 1989
33. Kelly M: A deadly delivery program. Boston Globe, July 19, 1989
34. Kinney J, National Safe Workplace Institute: Personal communication to Susan H. Pollack, 1989
35. Wilkerson I: Farms, deadliest workplace, taking the lives of children. NY Times, September 16, 1988, p 1
36. Rivara FP: Fatal and nonfatal farm injuries to children and adolescents in the United States. Pediatrics 76:567–573, 1985
37. Karlson T, Noren J: Farm tractor fatalities: The failure of voluntary safety standards. Am J Public Health 69(2):146–149, 1979
38. Cogbill TH, Busch HM, Stiers GR: Farm accidents in children. Pediatrics 76(4):562–566, 1985
39. Swanson JA, Sachs MI, Dahlgren KA, Tinguely SJ: Accidental farm injuries in children. Am J Dis Child 141:1276–1279, 1987
40. Broste SK, Hansen DA, Strand RL, Steuland DT: Hearing loss among high school farm students. Am J Public Health 79(5):619–622, 1989
41. Albright J, Kunstel M, McKay R: Stolen childhood, a global report on the exploitation of children. Atlanta: Cox Newspaper Enterprises, June 21–26, 1987
42. Anti-Slavery Society: Child Labour Series. Birmingham (England): Third World Publications, 1978–1981
43. Waldron HA: Danger: Children at work. Br J Ind Med 45:73–74, 1988
44. World Health Organization Study Group: Children at Work: Special Health Risks. (Technical Report Series 756) Geneva: WHO, 1987

33

Occupational Safety and Health Standards

Eula Bingham

Until 1970, there was almost total reliance on state and local governments and market forces to improve working conditions related to occupational injuries, death, and disease. For more than 50 years, state governments had attempted to inspect workplaces and to advise employers about hazards. Few of these programs, however, had adequate enforcement authority to compel abatement of dangerous conditions. In some states, no attempt was made by government to change workplace conditions, either by enforcement or by persuasion. Variations in state legislation resulted in comprehensive, strong regulation in some states (e.g., California and Michigan) and nonexistent regulation in others (e.g., Texas). The doctrine of states' rights and a tradition of state regulation in the area of labor standards protected this status quo.

A second traditional approach was to trust private sector mechanisms to provide worker protection. Workers' compensation insurance carriers made some attempt to improve workplace safety for economic reasons. Many carriers provide consultative service to their clients and charge lower rates to large companies that are successful in reducing injuries. Unfortunately, insurance companies' consultative resources are limited and are not available to all who might need them. Whereas it may be possible to increase economic incentives to large firms by basing their premium rates on accident experience, it is not possible to provide this same incentive to small firms that have too few employees to record a statistically significant accident experience.

These economic incentives are inadequate where health problems are concerned because occupational diseases are not often diagnosed as workplace related. Occupational diseases often have complex origins. Many years may elapse between exposure and the appearance of symptoms, making physicians and compensation boards reluctant to attribute the symptoms to time spent with specific employers or to exposure to particular working conditions. Even today, estimates of the number of occupational diseases compensated range between 1% and 10%.

A third approach evolved to cope with occupational safety and health problems. Industry-based organizations filled the vacuum by producing guidelines for safe work practices for various types of industrial equipment and processes and for "acceptable" exposure limits to certain harmful substances. These consensus standards were adopted by the Occupational Safety and Health Administration (OSHA) in 1972 as federal standards.

Thus, a long series of private, voluntary efforts and a slowly evolving pattern of government initiatives (e.g., against federal contractors who violated standards) tested a variety of approaches to improving safety and health. These experiences served as the basis for broad federal legislation. Since legislators had a record of approaches that had not worked, it became clear that voluntary compliance approaches and consensus guidelines would have to be backed by a technically experienced federal enforcement staff and that inadequate state safety and health efforts would have to be reshaped to meet national standards of effectiveness. The economic realities of the marketplace had overwhelmed voluntary efforts, and the weak incentives of workers' compensation programs and of the states appeared unable to act effectively because of a need to compete among themselves for industry and jobs.

The Occupational Safety and Health Act (OSHAct) was signed into law in 1970. It featured a strong standards-setting authority vested in the Secretary of Labor. The standards-setting process was open to labor, industry, and public inputs at all stages. The word "standard" connotes uniformity, consensus, and regulatory power. OSHA standards are an attempt, through the federal government's regulatory powers, to set a minimum level of protection for workers against specific hazards and to achieve that level through enforcement, education, and persuasion.

Sections 6 and 3(8) of the OSHAct govern the standards-setting process. They contain three major schemes under which standards can be promulgated: (1) a short-lived authority for adoption of existing consensus standards, (2) development and promulgation of new or amended standards, and (3) promulgation of temporary emergency standards.

CONSENSUS STANDARDS

At the time the OSHAct was passed, a large body of so-called consensus standards was already in existence, developed as guidelines by such groups as the American National Standards Institute (ANSI), the National Fire Prevention Association (NFPA), and the American Conference of Governmental Industrial Hygienists (ACGIH). The guidelines represented industry's agreement on certain reasonable exposures, work practices, and equipment specifications. In order to establish as rapidly as possible a body of occupational safety and health rules already familiar to employers, Congress required adoption of these guidelines but recognized that many were seriously out of date. The legislative history of the Act emphasized that any standards would need constantly to be improved and replaced and that new comprehensive standards were especially needed in the occupational health area.

Many of the consensus standards contained provisions that were irrelevant to safety and health (e.g., several pages of specifications for the wood to be used in ladders). The standards were adopted wholesale, however, without significant deletions, in the interest of speed. Competing priorities made it impossible to evaluate and amend the body of standards within the 2-year deadline allowed by Congress.

Thus, OSHA began with initial standards derived from previous industry use, which had these key weaknesses.

1. They were unduly complex.
2. They were often obsolete. One standard, for example, prohibited the use of ice in drinking water, a rule that dated from a time when ice was cut from contaminated rivers.
3. The consensus standards were guidelines. They were not designed for enforcement and the adjudicatory process. Provisions that should have been advisory became inflexible law.
4. They reflected industry consensus as to acceptable practice and were not necessarily designed for the greatest protection to workers.
5. Some standards were related only tangentially to the safety or health of workers, for example, the requirement for coat hooks in toilet stalls.

In 1978, OSHA removed the most inappropriate of these rules from the books. At that time, 1110 standards provisions were proposed for deletion. After participation by labor and the business community, 927 finally were eliminated. Further improvements have included an updated fire protection standard (1978).

PERMANENT STANDARDS

Section 6(b) of the Act outlines the nine-step process for setting permanent safety or health standards.

1. *Decision to initiate standards development project.* The Secretary of Labor may begin the process on the basis of recommendations from the National Institute of Occupational Safety and Health, petitions of private parties, research findings from any source, accident and injury data, congressional input, or court decisions, with interested parties given time to prepare testimony and to estimate the impact that regulations might have.
2. *Drafting the proposal.* Including economic and environmental impact statements to fulfill the requirements of the National Environmental Policy Act of 1969. Economic studies determine whether regulatory analysis will be required.
3. *Advisory committee.* Composed of representatives of labor and industry, the safety and health professions, and recognized experts from government or the academic world.
4. *Revision and review.* By technical experts and attorneys. Where appropriate, review by other agencies also occurs.
5. Federal Register *publication.* The public is invited to comment.
6. *Informal hearings.* To allow further public comment.
7. *Staff analysis of records.* Major issues requiring policy decisions are defined and presented to the assistant secretary. Alternate approaches, if appropriate, are presented.
8. *Final standard.* The staff develops a proposed final standard based on the record of rule making and submits the proposal for internal reviews.
9. *Final publication.* The completed final standard is published in its entirety in the *Federal Register.* A petition for review of the standard may be filed in a federal circuit court of appeals.

This process is only an outline. The length of time between steps may stretch for months or years. At times, proposals are abandoned after first hearings or public comment, and the decision to proceed with a rule making is reevaluated. If appropriate, an entirely new proposal is developed.

TEMPORARY EMERGENCY STANDARDS

The OSHAct requires that the Secretary of Labor "shall provide . . . for an emergency temporary standard to take immediate effect upon publication in the *Federal Register* if employees are exposed to grave danger from exposure to substances or agents determined to be toxic or physically harmful or from new hazards." These standards are promulgated without the extensive public participation characteristic of permanent standards. The Act requires that they be replaced with a permanent standard within 6 months. Emergency temporary standards may be used as a "proposed standard" in the permanent standards proceedings.

CONTENTS OF OSHA STANDARDS

OSHA standards are written to control risks even if exposure continues throughout a person's working life. The effectiveness of the technology available for controlling exposures and the characteristics of the hazard in the particular workplace determine how compliance with the standard will be achieved.

The standards are variable in several areas. The technical content necessarily differs according to the hazard being regulated, although it is possible to group related problems in a single standard. A specification approach or a performance approach may be employed, or the two approaches may be combined.

Specification Standards. Specification standards tell precisely what protection an employer must provide. This approach has been used most often in developing safety standards. The advantage of specification standards is that they tell the employer exactly what must be provided to "be in compliance." The disadvantage of the specification standards is that they tend to be inflexible and may restrict an employer's efforts to provide equivalent protection using alternative—and sometimes more satisfactory—methods. In such instances, employers may be granted a variance by OSHA.

Performance Standards. The trend in OSHA regulation is toward performance standards that set exposures but leave the means of compliance largely to the decision of the employer. This greater degree of flexibility allows the employer to consider alternative methods and equipment and choose those most suited to the particular technology. Performance standards, however, do not give the employer carte blanche to substitute less effective means of protection (such as personal protective equipment) for engineering controls of dangerous emissions or other hazards.

Health standards generally are addressed by way of the performance, rather than the specification, approach. Although many large corporations prefer performance standards in both the safety and health areas, it is advantageous, at least for small employers, to have an acceptable specific method of compliance included in the appendix of a performance standard.

THRESHOLD LIMIT VALUES, PERMISSIBLE EXPOSURE LIMITS, AND ACTION LEVELS

Older occupational health standards (still used in many countries) were based on threshold limit values (TLVs) developed by the ACGIH. In this system, maximum exposures usually were set based on the level of a contaminant known to produce acute effects, allowing some margin for safety and considering what was readily achievable by employers. Unfortunately, such limits do not protect against long-term or subclinical effects on the body, such as changes in blood chemistry, liver function, or the reaction time of the central nervous system. In addition, these values were derived mainly for healthy, young adult, white males, not for the broader makeup of working populations and were not designed to address the problem of carcinogens.

Permissible exposure limits (PELs) are used in the newer OSHA health standards. The lead standard, for example, contains a PEL of 50 μg of lead per cubic meter of air, averaged over an 8-hour period. PELs are based on consideration of the health effects of hazardous substances.

MEDICAL REMOVAL PROTECTION

Medical removal protection (MRP) is a protective, preventive health mechanism complementing the medical surveillance portion of some OSHA standards. The lead standard, for example, calls for temporary removal for medical purposes of any worker having an elevated blood lead level. During the period of removal, the employer must maintain the worker's earnings, seniority, and other employment rights and benefits as though the worker had not been removed.

Medical removal protection is essential. Without it, the major cost of health hazards falls directly on the worker and the worker's family in the event of illness, death, or lost wages. Without a requirement for the protection of workers' wages and job rights, removal could easily take the form of transfer to a lower-paying job, temporary layoff, or termination. A worker who participates in the medical surveillance program might risk losing his or her livelihood. The alternative has sometimes been to resist participation and thereby lose the protection that surveillance offers.

An interesting leveraging effect of MRP is its role as an economic incentive for employers to comply with the OSHA standards. For example, employers who do not comply with the lead standard will have a greater number of removals and thus will have higher labor costs over a long period, whereas employers who invest in the control technology will experience savings from lowered removal costs.

COMPLIANCE

To comply with the PELs, employers first conduct an industrial hygiene survey, including environmental sampling. This process identifies contaminants, their sources, and the severity of exposure. The employer then devises methods to reduce exposure to permissible levels. Methods commonly employed by industrial hygienists to control exposures fall into three basic categories: engineering controls, work practice controls (including administrative controls), and personal protective equipment.

Engineering controls employ mechanical means or process redesign to reduce exposure. The contaminant may be eliminated, contained, diverted, diluted, or collected at the source. Examples of this type of control include process isolation or enclosure, such as is used in uranium fuel processing. Employee isolation and machine and process enclosure also are used to protect workers from excessive fumes or noise. Closed material-handling systems, product substitution, and exhaust ventilation are commonly employed.

Work practice controls rely on employees to perform certain activities in a carefully specified manner so that exposures are reduced or eliminated. For example, employers may instruct workers to keep lids on containers, to clean spills immediately, or to observe specific, required hygiene practices. Such work practices are often required to complement engineering controls. This is particularly true in cases where engineering controls cannot provide complete compliance with the standard. Noise hazards often are controlled by a combination of engineering steps and work practices limiting the amount of time workers are exposed to excessive noise levels.

Personal protective equipment (PPE) controls exposure by isolating the employee from the emission source. Respirators are a common type of PPE, used when protection from an inhaled contaminant is required. PPE is used to supplement engineering controls and work practices. Often overlooked is the great importance of personal hygiene, which includes the use of protective clothing to provide barriers to both the worker and the worker's family, provision for shower facilities, and cleaning of protective clothing so that contaminants are not transferred to others.

Engineering control is the best method for effective and reliable control of worker exposure to many substances. It acts at the source of the emission and eliminates or reduces employee exposure without reliance on self-protective action by the employee. Work practices also act on the source of the emission but rely on employee behavior, which requires supervision, motivation, and education for effectiveness. Although PPE provides a cheaper alternative to engineering controls, it does so at the expense of safety and reliability. The equipment does not eliminate the source of the exposure, often fails to provide the degree of protection required (or fails to provide it with certainty in all cases), and may create additional hazards by interfering with vision, hearing, and mobility.

Individual differences in employees also affect the acceptability of PPE. Some employees develop infections from ear-protection devices and respirator facepieces, and some who have impaired breathing cannot use respirators safely or comfortably. Additionally, PPE is made in standard sizes and facial configurations that may not properly fit female workers and unusually large or small workers.

SETTING STANDARDS PRIORITIES

OSHA should progress from a reactive, priority-setting system to one with an information-based approach. Highest priority must be given to hazards that cause irreversible adverse health effects. For example, OSHA's cancer policy could be modified to increase the speed with which the particular carcinogens are regulated, with priorities shaped according to the population of the workers exposed, current exposure levels, and the potency of a substance. Consideration should be given to the ways in which these substances are used in actual operations and to the likelihood of substantial accidental exposures.

These same criteria can be applied to other health hazards. In the safety standards area, a parallel process must occur, which should include guidance in the establishment of standards for reducing deaths due to inappropriately designed lock-out procedures, for reducing musculoskeletal injuries, and for controlling the development of stress-related diseases associated with newer technologies. Recommendations from the National Institute of Occupational Safety and Health (NIOSH), public petitions, court decisions, and new research findings also will shape priorities for standards development.

For both safety and health standards, OSHA must judge whether scientific and technical evidence is sufficient to demonstrate the need for a new or revised regulation and to support the development of a standard that will withstand court challenges. Consideration must be given to the feasibility of implementing technological changes in affected industries.

REGULATORY COSTS ANALYSES

Critics of occupational safety and health standards encourage the use of theoretical economic models based on cost-benefit analysis. Common sense indicates that the numbers of workers exposed, the severity of hazards, and the technological feasibility must be considered in setting standards. These factors should be explicit in OSHA's priority-setting processes. Precise costs and benefits, however, cannot be measured.

The costs of standards compliance can be estimated with some precision. New equipment, engineering modifications, and work practices have readily measurable costs. Industry, however, sometimes overestimates these costs by several magnitudes in their testimony against standards. Actual costs for vinyl chloride standards compliance turned out to be but a fraction of those indicated in public testimony. More recently, even with the thoroughly worked and reworked estimates of the costs to comply with the cotton dust standard, it appears that costs were overestimated by the government and industry both.

The benefits of regulation, however, are more difficult to calculate. One cannot count all accidents that were avoided as one can number the accidents and injuries that actually occurred. One cannot identify precisely the health benefits that will accrue in 10, 20, or 30 years from current reduced exposures to toxic substances or carcinogens. The data for prediction do not exist, and causality mechanisms in occupational disease are too complex to be defined with the same certainty as the costs of a new ventilating system.

The largest problem with cost-benefit analysis, however, is not lack of information. It is the impossibility of weighing lives spared against the dollar costs for prevention. Workers are coming to realize that hazardous pay differentials are in fact based on a dangerously false assumption that lives can be valued and, in effect, prorated on a cash basis. Public debate over regulatory costs, fortunately, has begun to clarify this issue and to uncover the hidden social costs of failure to regulate out of deference to faulty labor market mechanisms. These hidden social costs include not only loss of life and health of workers but also increased incidence of illness and death among families of workers exposed to some substances, such as lead and asbestos, and disruption of family and community life due to death and disability of workers and to local environmental effects of industrial contaminants. This relationship was seen clearly in the Kepone disaster in Hopewell, Virginia, and the ensuing long battles over compensating workers with asbestos-related diseases.

OTHER CONSIDERATIONS

Particularly important for the NIOSH and the OSHA is participation in international occupational health and safety forums to achieve full awareness of available research and enforcement experience, including those of the Commission of the European Communities, the International Labour Organization, the World Health Organization, and many foreign national governments. It is critical that the United States share information internationally and encourage other nations to adopt effective health and safety standards. Without comparable standards in other countries, U.S. industries can choose to export hazardous processes, such as asbestos milling or pesticide formulation. This is doubly unacceptable because it not only exposes foreign workers to hazardous conditions but also would tend to export jobs along with the hazards.

CONCLUSION

Standards alone will not guarantee healthful, safe working conditions. Inspections to determine whether there is compliance, along with citations and penalties when compliance is inadequate, are necessary. Training and education of workers and employers are required. Government cannot provide direct, constant enforcement of employee protection. This effort must be assisted by employer and employee participation.

Workers' rights to a safe and healthful workplace are facilitated in part by the existence of employer standards, by federal and state enforcement activities, but most of all by the workers' own knowledge and vigilance. The OSHAct recognizes this fact. It reinforces the workers' rights, with guarantees against reprisals by employers, to make complaints and to obtain abatement for their efforts to clean their work environment. Whether improvements come from voluntary employer action, from direct enforcement, or from labor-management negotiations, health and safety standards are essential to define the necessary levels of protection and the acceptable means of attaining them.

34

Food and Dairy Sanitation

Joseph F. Frank
Harold M. Barnhart

Sanitation is the control of factors in the environment that affect public health. Before the twentieth century, sanitation centered on the home and the immediate environment. Sanitary practices were applied with little understanding of the basic principles of sanitation, resulting in a lack of effectiveness. Industrialization, urbanization, and changes in work and social habits have broadened the scope of activities that can affect an individual's health and well-being, especially in regard to food, its preparation, and its consumption. Today, individuals in developed countries particularly have little control over the production and processing of the food they consume; the responsibility for food protection lies mainly with food processors, food service personnel, and regulatory agencies. Individuals do have control, however, over food handling in the home, where most foodborne illness, if we include unreported cases, probably originates.

Protection of the public from foodborne hazards involves maintenance of sanitary control over harvesting or slaughter, processing, preserving, distribution, storage, and preparation of food for institutional or home consumption. Sanitary control of the food processing and food service industry would be impossible without laws that authorize sanitary regulations and standards. After passage of the Food, Drug, and Cosmetic Act (FDCA) in 1938, the United States began to monitor food sanitation relative to interstate commerce. Since then, the act has been amended numerous times to keep pace with technological advances and new practices. Sanitation control is less effective in many less-developed countries. The World Health Organization (WHO) helps these countries set and monitor sanitation standards. The purpose of sanitary control is the same throughout the world—to prevent illnesses resulting from the consumption of unsafe foods.

The objectives of food sanitation are not only to protect the public health but also to reduce economic and nutritional losses from microbial and chemical degradation. The maintenance of aesthetic quality is also considered an objective of sanitation practices in developed countries. Food processing and preparation procedures are designed to attain these objectives, with effective sanitation programs functioning as an essential safeguard. In the past, regulators have been criticized for overemphasizing inspection criteria relating to noncritical factors such as physical facilities and appearances as opposed to critical points such as time-temperature relationships. This criticism has become less relevant as principles of the hazard analysis critical control point (HACCP) system have become understood and implemented by both industry and government sanitarians.

Sanitary control of food processing and food service in developed countries is in general successfully implemented; however, in many less-developed countries procuring an adequate supply of safe and nutritious food is a major problem. In these countries concern for sanitation may not be great, physical facilities are often poor, and lower aesthetic standards often prevail. Less-developed countries rely on the Food and Agriculture Organization (FAO)/WHO Codex Alimentarius Commission for guidelines on international food standards.[1] As food supply increases and living standards are raised, developing countries usually pay increased attention to food sanitation.

Reducing risk of foodborne illness involves identifying major hazards associated with a particular food and then utilizing the appropriate control mechanisms to reduce the risk associated with these hazards. Statistics on foodborne illness are required to accomplish this analysis. In the 1920s the U.S. Public Health Service began publishing annual summaries of milkborne diseases reported by individual states. Today the Centers for Disease Control (CDC) publishes the *Morbidity and Mortality Weekly Report* (*MMWR*) as well as annual summaries of surveillance programs for foodborne and waterborne disease. Canada established its national foodborne disease reporting system in 1973, and Health and Welfare Canada has issued annual summaries since 1976, many of which are published in the *Journal of Food Protection*. WHO's surveillance program of foodborne disease in Europe has operated since 1981.[2] A list of common foodborne disease agents is given in Table 34–1.

Among the difficulties in obtaining reliable judgments on hazards and risks of foodborne illness are the incompleteness of the data due to unreported cases, an inability to always obtain samples of suspect food for laboratory analysis, and an inability to interview or identify victims. Consequently, much foodborne illness goes unreported, and hazards may go unidentified or underestimated. In the United States, 47% (1983–1987) and in Canada 55% (1979–1983) of the outbreaks in which a vehicle was determined were situations where food was mishandled in a food service establishment.[3-8] A vehicle was either unknown or unspecified in 29.6% and 29.8% of the outbreaks in the United States and Canada respectively. Between 1983 and 1987, in 40.9% of the reported outbreaks in the United States where the vehicle was identified the food was eaten at a food service establishment or other mass-gathering events (Table 34–2). In Canada from 1979 to 1983, 43.3% of outbreaks where the vehicle was confirmed occurred in a food service establishment, school, or institution. Only 16.8% of foodborne outbreaks in Canada

TABLE 34-1. FOODBORNE DISEASES BY ETIOLOGY

Bacterial:	*Salmonella* (numerous serotypes)
	Staphylococcus aureus
	Clostridium perfringens
	Campylobacter jejuni
	Clostridium botulinum
	Bacillus cereus
	Listeria monocytogenes
	Vibrio parahaemolyticus
	Yersinia enterocolitica
	Shigella
	Vibrio cholerae
	Streptococcus groups A, D
	Escherichia coli
	Brucella
Parasitic:	*Trichinella spiralis*
	Giardia lamblia
Viral:	Hepatitis A
Chemical:	Ciguatoxin
	Heavy metals
	Mushroom poisoning
	Scombrotoxin

(1979–1983) and 5.5% in the United States (1974–1979) were a result of mishandling at the food processing plant. Because of the rapid and widespread distribution of processed foods, however, these outbreaks often place large numbers of individuals at risk before the implicated food can be recalled.

The etiology of foodborne disease is strikingly similar in developed countries. Differences in the numbers of outbreaks and cases reported for each country are in part due to varying effectiveness of the reporting systems. Data from the CDC show that bacterial agents are the overwhelming cause of foodborne illness. Between 1983 and 1987, 66.0% of the outbreaks and 90% of the confirmed cases in the United States were bacterial illnesses (Table 34-3). A similar pattern is evident in Europe and Canada. The etiological agents most often responsible for foodborne disease in the United States have consistently been identified as *Salmonella* species, *Staphylococcus aureus,* and *Clostridium perfringens,* which are similarly reported in Canada and European countries. *Salmonella* is the most frequently confirmed causative agent, although others have emerged as important foodborne disease agents. England, Wales, and Ireland reported in 1984 that *Campylobacter* accounted for more reported gastrointestinal infections than *Salmonella.*[9] WHO reports that for the years 1979 to 1986, a global increase in *Salmonella* cases is apparent. An increase in cases in 56% of the reporting European countries is thought to be related to consumption of poultry and eggs.[10]

COMMON FOODBORNE DISEASES

Foodborne Intoxications

Botulism. The great majority of incidents of botulism have been associated with home-canned vegetables and fruits; they comprise only 3% of the outbreaks in the United States. Vegetables and fruits are most often implicated in the United States, whereas in the Soviet Union, Canada, and Japan most reported outbreaks were associated with fish or fish products.

Staphylococcal Intoxication. Staphylococcal intoxication is one of the leading causes of foodborne disease. Although staphylococcal intoxication is less frequently reported as a foodborne illness than salmonellosis, it probably causes more illness than surveillance data indicate.

The severity of staphylococcal intoxication depends on the amount of enterotoxin ingested. The enterotoxins responsible for foodborne illness are stable; even boiling for 30 minutes does not completely destroy their toxicity.

Foods Implicated. Any food that provides a good growth medium for staphylococci can be involved in an outbreak of staphylococcal intoxication; meats including ham, pork, beef, chicken, and turkey are usually implicated. Milk and milk products, baked goods such as cream-filled pastries, and mixed salads are occasionally implicated. The most common vehicle is pork, particularly ham that has been prepared whole and is difficult to cool

TABLE 34-2. INCIDENTS WHERE FOOD WAS EATEN

Where Acquired	Home	Delicatessen/ Cafeteria/ Restaurant	School	Picnic	Church	Camp	Unknown Other	Total
▪ **U.S.**[a]:								
1983	61	50	12	5	7	2	50	187
1984	45	61	8	5	3	1	62	185
1985	82	61	7	7	10	1	52	220
1986	62	54	10	0	2	1	52	181
1987	32	54	3	4	0	4	39	136
% of total	(31.0%)	(30.8%)	(4.4%)	(2.3%)	(2.4%)	(1.0%)	(28.1%)	909
▪ **CANADA**[b]:								
1979	110	301	28	—[c]	—	—	287	726
1980	120	293	24	—	—	—	229	666
1981	87	194	20	—	—	—	217	518
1982	137	328	51	—	—	—	330	846
1983	243	331	27	—	—	—	272	873
1984	243	404	35	—	—	—	382	1064
% of total	(20.0%)	(39.4%)	(3.9%)				(36.6%)	4,693

[a] From annual summaries, CDC Foodborne Disease Outbreaks, 1983–1987.
[b] From Todd ECD, 1985, 1987, 1988, 1989.[5–8]
[c] Not reported.

TABLE 34-3. CONFIRMED TOTALS: FOODBORNE DISEASE OUTBREAKS BY ETIOLOGY

	Bacterial		Chemical		Parasitic		Viral	
	Outbreaks (%)	Cases (%)	Outbreaks (%)	Cases (%)	Outbreaks (%)	Cases (%)	Outbreaks (%)	Cases (%)
1983	67.9	89.6	24.1	3.3	2.1	0.1	5.9	7.0
1984	69.2	89.7	22.7	2.6	5.9	0.7	2.2	7.4
1985	65.0	96.3	26.4	1.7	4.1	0.2	4.5	1.8
1986	66.7	83.6	26.5	3.7	4.4	1.2	3.3	11.5
1987	61.0	92.5	28.7	1.6	2.9	0.2	7.4	5.7
Average	66.0	90.3	25.7	2.6	3.9	0.5	4.7	6.7

rapidly and thoroughly reheat. Hams are frequently served at social functions.

Foodborne Infections

Salmonellosis. Salmonellosis can be caused by any one of the *Salmonella* species because all are pathogenic to man. Reporting of salmonellosis is probably as extensive as reporting of any other etiological agent, particularly since 1963, when the national *Salmonella* Surveillance Program was established in the United States.

Foods Implicated. Because animals are the natural reservoir for *Salmonella,* foods of animal origin are most often implicated in outbreaks of foodborne salmonellosis. Poultry, meat, and eggs are primary sources of *Salmonella* in food service operations. Between 1963 and 1975, poultry accounted for 21%, meat 15%, and eggs 11%, for a total of 47% of the vehicles responsible for disease transmission.[11] From 1985 to 1987 there seems to be a resurgence of egg-associated salmonellosis in the United States. Seventy-seven percent of outbreaks in the northeastern states with identified food vehicles were associated with eggs or foods that contained eggs.[12]

C. perfringens Infection. The first reported gastroenteritis caused by foods containing large numbers of *C. perfringens* occurred in the 1890s. Not until 1946 did experiments on human volunteers with cultures and filtrates of *C. perfringens* produce symptoms of gastroenteritis. Recognition of *C. perfringens* as a foodborne pathogen has steadily increased since then, especially after Hobbs et al[13] described outbreaks associated with *C. perfringens* in Great Britain. The disease is caused by enterotoxin-producing strains of *C. perfringens.*

Foods Implicated. Meats and meat products prepared for food service are frequently involved in outbreaks of *C. perfringens.* Implicated items have included turkey, chicken, soups and gravies, meat pies, pork, beef, veal, and mutton. It is almost impossible to prevent contamination of raw meats with *C. perfringens.* It is present in cooked as well as uncooked foods. The survival and growth of the organism requires anaerobic conditions, which are present in a large beef roast or turkey. The numbers of contaminating organisms are not usually high; however, it is not uncommon for caterers, restaurants, or institutions to cook meats and poultry a day before serving. The items are then stored overnight, handled, sliced, reheated, and served. This delay in serving provides ample opportunity for the organism to multiply to numbers sufficient to cause an outbreak.

Other Foodborne Diseases

Campylobacteriosis. *Campylobacter jejuni* is now considered by many the most frequent cause of bacterial diarrhea in the United States.[14] *C. jejuni* is more commonly associated with diarrheal disease in humans than are other *Campylobacter* species. Many reservoirs of *C. jejuni* exist. It can be isolated from swine, cattle, sheep, rodents, chickens, turkeys, and other fowl. Cats, dogs, and other household pets are commonly infected. The disease appears to be transmitted by the fecal-oral route through contaminated food and water or direct contact with fecal material from infected people or animals. Livestock carcasses in slaughterhouses are often positive for *C. jejuni,* which indicates the presence of the pathogen in food marketing channels. The CDC has only recently begun to report the incidence of confirmed outbreaks of campylobacteriosis in its Foodborne Disease Surveillance summary. In 1980 five outbreaks were confirmed; since that year, reports have identified 3 to 13 outbreaks annually. Most proven outbreaks of campylobacteriosis have involved raw milk or contaminated water; yet surveys consistently implicate poultry as the source of most cases. The difficulty in detecting *Campylobacter* results in the current incomplete understanding of its association with foods and the food service situation.

Listeriosis. *Listeria monocytogenes* has only recently become established as a cause of foodborne illness. The outbreaks that have occurred since 1981 have implicated several foods as vehicles, but dairy products have received the most attention because of several serious outbreaks.[15-17] The incidence of listeriosis in humans is low compared to that of other leading causes of foodborne illness; however, its mortality rate ranges from 20% to about 50% in individual cases or outbreaks.[18] Clinical manifestations in adults include meningitis, meningoencephalitis, or septicemia. These symptoms may be preceded by typical gastroenteritis symptoms. Listeriosis may include neonatal sepsis or meningitis and puerperal sepsis, which occurs during pregnancy and may result in perinatal sepsis and stillbirth of the fetus.[19]

Foods Implicated. The diversity of foods that may transmit listeriosis to humans is still being studied. Poultry and meats are likely carriers because the organism can be readily isolated from the animals. A U.S. survey showed that 43%, 48%, and 70% of pork sausage, poultry, and ground beef, respectively, contained *L. monocytogenes.*[20] Vegetables including lettuce, celery, and tomatoes have also been implicated,[21] although a Canadian study found tomatoes, celery, lettuce, radishes, and pasteurized milk to be free of *L. monocytogenes,* while 20%, 56.3%, and 86.4% of fermented sausages, chicken legs, and ground meats, respectively, were positive.[22] *L. monocytogenes* competes with other microflora and proliferates at refrigeration temperatures. Its presence in a food should be considered a significant potential health risk.

Yersiniosis. Yersiniosis, the disease caused by *Yersinia enterocolitica,* has caused health problems throughout the world. The enterocolitis mimics acute appendicitis. Important reservoirs of *Y. enterocolitica* include swine, cattle, chickens, and dogs. Leistner et al.[23] found the organism to be present in fecal samples and meat from chicken, beef, and pork. Its presence in various foods has been reported by Lee.[24] In a survey of raw milk, 48% of the samples analyzed were positive for the organism.[25] Outbreaks of the illness have been reported more frequently in Europe and Japan than have been reported in the United States. Numerous outbreaks have also been reported in Scandinavian countries. It is of some concern to the food industry because it grows at recommended refrigeration temperatures; however, its full significance as a foodborne pathogen has not yet been determined.

Vibriosis. The disease caused by *Vibrio parahaemolyticus* is generally associated with seafood, since it is commonly found in a marine environment, especially in coastal and estuarine water. It is the most important foodborne agent in Japan and may be responsible for more than 70% of the cases reported there since the 1960s. *V. parahaemolyticus* has been isolated from fish, oysters, shrimp, and crabs. Outbreaks show seasonal variation, with a peak during summer and fall. The disease seems to be transmitted exclusively as a foodborne illness. Infected food handlers have not been identified as a source of the organism, although cooked seafood has been contaminated by raw seafood, food contact surfaces, or contaminated hands. In addition, *Vibrio vulnificus* is of great concern because it may not be detected using standard shellfish quality indicators.[26] Its role as a foodborne pathogen is not fully understood. *V. parahaemolyticus* has rarely been isolated from patients in the United States. The CDC has reported only 11 confirmed cases in its last 5-year summary. Additional epidemiology of *V. parahaemolyticus* is presented by Blake et al.[27]

Bacillus cereus Intoxication. *Bacillus cereus* gastroenteritis has been known since the 1950s when reports from Europe suggested that the organism could be a foodborne pathogen. Outbreaks have been reported in Europe, the U.S.S.R., and Canada. Various foods including rice, spices, meats, soups, sausage, and puddings have been implicated, depending on whether it is a diarrheal or an emetic toxin-producing strain involved. No *B. cereus* outbreak was reported in the United States until 1966. Sixteen outbreaks were reported to the CDC from 1984 to 1987.

ADMINISTRATION OF FOOD SANITATION

International Food Standards

The FAO of the United Nations and WHO created the Codex Alimentarius Commission to implement a food standards program. The Joint FAO/WHO Food Standards Program was created to protect the health of consumers and ensure fair practices in world food trade, to promote coordination of food standards activities of international organizations, to formulate food standards, and to publish accepted standards in the Codex Alimentarius.[28] These standards are classified as Codex Commodity Standards (applicable to specific food commodities), Codex General Standards (applicable to various commodities), and Codex Maximum Limits for Pesticide Residues. Acceptance and implementation of these standards is up to individual governments, but accepted standards must apply equally to imported and domestically produced foods. The following types of acceptances are permitted:

1. *Full Acceptance.* The country ensures that foods that do not comply with the standard will not be distributed within its jurisdiction. Distribution of products that comply with the standard and are safe for consumption will not be hindered.
2. *Target Acceptance.* The country intends to accept the standard after a stated number of years but until then will not hinder the distribution of products that do not conform to the standard and are safe for consumption.
3. *Acceptance with Specified Deviations.* The standard is accepted with specifically stated deviations.
4. *Limited Acceptance.* This applies to pesticide residue limits only. The country concerned will not hinder the importation of food that complies with the pesticide limit and will not use the Codex Maximum Limit to impose a more stringent standard on imported foods than is applied domestically.

The International Dairy Federation (IDF) was formed to promote uniformity of standards for dairy products and to provide an international forum for the exchange of scientific and technical information. The organization has over 98 groups of experts, many of which review scientific data relating to possible standards, encourage research when information is lacking, and ultimately propose and review standards. The IDF works closely with the Codex Alimentarius Commission in developing standards for dairy product sanitation and safety.

Food and Drug Administration

The Food and Drug Administration (FDA) is the federal agency responsible for administering provisions of the FDCA of 1938, whose objectives include ensuring that foods are wholesome, safe to eat, and produced under sanitary conditions. Important modifications to the FDCA include the Pesticide Chemicals Amendment, the Food Additive Amendment, and the Color Additive Amendment. The FDA also administers other food-related federal statutes such as the Fair Packaging and Labeling Act (1966), the Public Health Service Act (1944), the Import Milk Act (1927), and certain provisions of the Federal Meat Inspection Act (1967), the Poultry Products Inspection Act (1957), and the Egg Products Inspection Act (1970). The last three acts are administered in conjunction with the U.S. Department of Agriculture (USDA). Food items containing over 2% poultry or 3% meat are regulated by the USDA.

Provisions of the amended FDCA relating to food safety require the FDA to act (1) if a food contains substances harmful to human health, (2) if food additives that are not approved for safety are used, (3) if a food contains pesticide residues in excess of tolerances established by the Environmental Protection Agency, (4) if a food is prepared or stored under unsanitary conditions, (5) if a food contains filth or is decomposed, (6) if colors that are not approved for safety are added to food, (7) if the food container or package contains substances that may be unsafe, and (8) if the food is from a diseased animal or an animal that died from a cause other than slaughter.

In addition to its public health objectives, the FDA is also responsible for ensuring fair packaging and labeling and for protecting the public from adulteration for economic gain. Generally, the FDA has jurisdiction only over food products in interstate commerce and the manufacturers of these products. State governments have jurisdiction over products produced and sold solely within their states.

Food Additives. The Food Additives Amendment to the FDCA regulates both incidental and intentional food additives. Additives in common use at the time the amendment was passed (1958) were exempt from regulation and classified as "generally recognized as safe" (GRAS). Substances on this list include common spices and seasonings, various acids such as citric and lactic, vegetable gums, and chemicals such as sodium bicarbonate. The GRAS list of several hundred food additives is presently under review by the FDA, with substances found to be of questionable safety being removed from the list. Non-GRAS substances can be approved as food additives, but the organization wishing to use the substance must first demonstrate to the FDA that the substance is safe. Such testing is time consuming and expensive, since animal feeding studies, and in some cases human tests, are required.

The Food Additives Amendment also contains the Delaney Clause, which prohibits approval as a food additive of any substance that has been found to cause cancer in animals or humans or that has been shown to be carcinogenic by any other appropriate test. The clause is controversial because animal feeding tests usually involve feeding large amounts of the test substance. Requiring such tests is based on the reasoning that there is no proven level below which carcinogens exhibit no effect; consequently a substance shown to be carcinogenic at high levels will also be carcinogenic at low levels. Although some might question this reasoning, it is impossible to prove the absence of an effect at low doses.[29] The Delaney Clause has also been criticized for not permitting a risk-benefit analysis of a food additive. In the case of saccharin the public preferred to assume the risk of consuming a substance that does not meet the requirements of the Delaney Clause rather than do without the additive's benefits.

U.S. Department of Agriculture

The USDA is responsible for inspection, grading, and certification of all agricultural products. Many of the product grading programs are voluntary, although a USDA grade often facilitates marketing of a commodity. Mandatory inspection of animals for slaughter, slaughtering conditions, and meat processing facilities is required by the Wholesome Meat Act (1967) and the Wholesome Poultry Act (1968). These acts provide that all red meat and meat products and all poultry products, whether in interstate or intrastate commerce or imported, must be processed under federal standards. Inspection of meats in intrastate commerce can be administered by states that have developed programs equivalent to those of the USDA. The original federal Meat Inspection Act was passed in 1906 partially as a result of the publication of Upton Sinclair's novel *The Jungle*. The original Poultry Inspection Act was not passed until 1957. Both acts only apply to meat and poultry products in interstate commerce.

Inspection Procedures. Animals are inspected prior to slaughter, and those with communicable diseases or an unhealthy appearance are rejected for human consumption. Carcasses and organs are also inspected for signs of disease and atypical appearance. Individual organs, parts of carcasses, or whole carcasses can be condemned. Only gross pathology is detectable during the postmortem inspection; for example, pork containing trichinae could pass. Poultry is inspected under procedures similar to those for meat.

The Egg Products Inspection Act (1970) authorizes mandatory inspection of eggs and egg products. Egg products include liquid, frozen, or dried whites, yolks, or whole eggs. The entire egg processing operation is inspected continuously, from the selection of the shell egg for breaking to the packing and storage of the final product. Inspectors can classify certain eggs as being for "restricted" use. Restricted classification include "dirty," "checks" (cracked but not leaking), "leakers," "incubator rejectors," and "unsuitable for human consumption." "Dirty" eggs and "checks" are segregated for further processing. All other "restricted" eggs are destroyed.

Administration of Milk Sanitation

In the late nineteenth century milk was recognized as an important disease vector, especially in rapidly growing cities where milk delivery by individual producers was no longer feasible and milk delivered in bulk by milk trains could cause massive outbreaks of disease. In an attempt to protect the public health and prevent the sale of willfully adulterated milk, city governments passed ordinances requiring permits for the delivery of milk into their jurisdictions. These milk ordinances set conditions under which permits were granted and revoked. The legality of these ordinances has been upheld by the courts.

As the dairy processing industry grew, the multiplicity of milk ordinances severely hindered efficient marketing and distribution of milk. To encourage uniformity in regulations, the U.S. Public Health Service developed a model milk ordinance in 1924. The recommendations of this ordinance, which has become known as the Pasteurized Grade A Milk Ordinance (PMO) and which was revised in 1978,[30] have been widely accepted by state, county, and municipal regulatory agencies. The provisions of the PMO are enforced through inspection of production, transportation, and processing facilities and the testing of raw and pasteurized product. Enforcement is either at the local or state level.

The PMO is designed to accomplish three goals: (1) to provide a milk supply that is free of health hazards; (2) to provide a pure product unadulterated by water, pesticides, filth, or other contaminants; and (3) to provide a product produced under the most sanitary conditions practicable. To accomplish these goals, the ordinance addresses all phases of milk production and processing, including animal health, the design, construction materials, and maintenance of facilities and equipment, milking procedures, equipment cleaning and sanitation, environmental sanitation and water supply, storage and transportation facilities, and refrigeration and pasteurization requirements, including acceptable time-temperature treatments and equipment design and operation. Temperature, microbiological, and chemical standards are included for raw and pasteurized milk and milk products (Table 34–4).

After obtaining a Grade A license, producers and processors are inspected at regular intervals, and product samples are tested to assure continued compliance. The license can be revoked if three of the last five samples tested do not meet chemical, bacteriological, or temperature standards or if violations documented by the inspector are not corrected.

Although the widespread adoption of the PMO provides uniformity of regulations between states, enforcement must also be uniform if milk is to move freely throughout the country. To facilitate interstate milk shipment, the FDA supervises the Inter-

TABLE 34–4. CHEMICAL, MICROBIOLOGICAL, AND TEMPERATURE STANDARDS FOR GRADE A MILK

▪ RAW MILK FOR PASTEURIZATION	
Temperature	Cooled to 7° C or less within 2 h after milking, provided that the blend temperature after subsequent milkings does not exceed 10° C
Bacterial limits	Individual producer milk not to exceed 100,000/ml prior to commingling with other producer milk
Antibiotics	No detectable inhibitory zone using the *Bacillus stearothermophilus* disc assay
Somatic cells	Individual producer milk not to exceed 1,000,000/ml
▪ PASTEURIZED MILK AND MILK PRODUCTS	
Temperature	Cooled to 7° C or less and maintained thereat
Bacterial limits	20,000/ml (except for cultured products)
Coliform	10/ml—bulk milk transport tank shipments shall not exceed 100/ml
Phosphatase	Less than 1 g/ml by Scharer Rapid Method or equivalent
Antibiotics	No detectable zone

state Milk Shippers Agreement. This voluntary program requires the receiving agency to accept the inspection and enforcement procedures of the shipper's locality if they are similar to or exceed those of the PMO; this decreases duplication of inspection.[31] FDA inspectors periodically check state milk control programs to ensure compliance with PMO recommendations. The FDA also evaluates laboratories licensed by states for testing of milk designated for interstate shipment. Laboratory equipment and testing procedures are evaluated for compliance with official procedures. Reproducibility of testing between laboratories is evaluated using split samples.

Nearly all fluid milk sold at retail is designated Grade A Pasteurized, indicating it was produced and processed under the provisions of the PMO. In most states, milk produced for manufacturing purposes does not need to meet Grade A standards. Such milk is usually designated as Manufacturing Grade. Recommendations for the sanitary control of Manufacturing Grade milk were first published by the USDA in 1963.[32] These have been adopted by many states. Dairy product manufacturers wishing to market USDA graded products or ship products across state lines must submit to inspection by that agency. Consequently, there is an increasing degree of uniformity in the sanitary control of Manufacturing Grade milk.

SANITARY CONTROL OF FOOD PRODUCTION AND DISTRIBUTION

The major objective of sanitary control of food production is to produce food stuffs free of biological or chemical substances that may be injurious to health. Attaining this objective requires maintaining control over fertilization, irrigation, pests, harvesting, animal health, raw product transportation, and storage. The degree of sanitary control mandated by governmental agencies should correspond to the public health risks inherent in the production of each food commodity. For this reason, some food production enterprises such as dairying are closely controlled through frequent inspections and sample analysis, whereas others such as crop production are subject to minimal regulatory control. Some foods such as milk, eggs, and meat cannot be produced without substantial risk of contamination with pathogenic microorganisms. With these foods we rely on processing, preservation or cooking, and frequent and thorough sanitary monitoring to maintain their safety.

Crop Production

Sanitary control of crop production begins with the selection of seed varieties and continues through growing, harvesting, and storage. Sanitary control during all these stages not only ensures that the food marketed is safe but also results in improved appearance, nutritional value, and shelf life.

Variety Selection. Selection of disease and insect resistant plant varieties is of prime importance in the production of safe plant foods. Using such varieties may not eliminate the need for pesticide applications, but it may allow for reduced application. Selection of varieties suitable for the growing climate can help reduce heat- or drought-induced stress, which weakens the plant's resistance to disease and insect damage, thus increasing risk to public health (see following section on pesticide application).

Fertilization. Both chemical fertilizers and sewage sludge can be sources of toxic metal contamination. Sewage sludge contains a variety of metals in relatively high and variable concentrations. Some metals such as copper and nickel accumulate in the soil but are not taken up by plants.[33] Boron does not accumulate in soil to the same extent, but excessive levels can lead to crop poisoning. The accumulation of cadmium, lead, and mercury in soils treated with sewage sludge poses a potential health hazard. Pathogenic microorganisms, pesticides, and industrial chemicals can also be found in sewage sludge. The FDA has set acceptable limits for cadmium, lead, and polychlorinated biphenyls (PCBs) in sludge for fertilizer use. In addition the use of sewage sludge on soils for growing plants usually consumed fresh has been prohibited.[34] Swedish and Australian researchers have reported that chemical fertilizers may contain more cadmium than sewage sludge. Soil acidity resulting from acid rain may increase uptake of cadmium in plants.[33] Fertilizers derived from animal manure and animal processing waste may carry various pathogenic microorganisms, especially viruses and bacteria.[35,36]

Irrigation. The use of untreated sewage or contaminated water for crop irrigation can result in contamination of food crops with pathogens. Green leafy vegetables are at special risk. Application of sewage effluent using drip irrigation can be accomplished without increased public health risk.[37]

Pesticide Application. The major hazard associated with the use of pesticides is posed by exposure during application rather than during food consumption. The organophosphorous and carbamate pesticides most often used are highly toxic but rapidly degrade in the environment. Recommended application procedures must be followed so that pesticide concentrations in the harvested crop will be at acceptable levels. Pest control before harvest can be just as important as pest control after harvest. For example, insect damage to corn before harvest can lead to growth of toxigenic mold in the kernels.[38]

Harvest. Harvest should be timed so that the proper degree of ripening has taken place. Overripe fruit is easily damaged, and damaged areas provide an opportunity for microbial growth, including toxigenic molds.[39] Contamination of crops with pathogens can occur if harvesting is done by hand, so field workers should have use of hygienic toilet facilities.

Storage. Fruits and vegetables must be stored at proper temperature and relative humidity to preserve freshness and to inhibit tissue deterioration resulting from enzymatic or microbial activity. Grains should be harvested when they are free of excess moisture. They are often dried before storage and then must be protected from moisture to prevent mold growth. Toxigenic molds are commonly isolated from stored grains. Storage facilities must be designed to protect grain from rodent infestation. Treatment of stored grains or flours with insecticides may also be necessary. Since insecticides such as ethylene dibromide are no longer permitted for food application, irradiation has become an acceptable alternative for insect control in grain products (see discussion of food preservation).

Animal Production

The primary focus of sanitation in animal production is on the control of zoonoses. Since meat is often marketed without undergoing treatment to inactivate microorganisms, it can become a source of pathogenic and food poisoning microorganisms in the food preparation environment. Zoonoses also constitute an occupational hazard for meat handlers. Since edible animal tissues often become contaminated with fecal material, zoonoses transmissible to humans through both animal tissue and feces must be controlled. Some animal infections transmissible to humans include helminthic parasites, brucellosis, trichinosis, toxoplasmosis, salmonellosis, campylobacteriosis, yersiniosis, *Escherichia coli* gastroenteritis, and listeriosis.

Methods used to control zoonoses during animal production include vaccination, identification and destruction or treatment of ill animals, and quarantining of herds when necessary. In some cases eliminating the pathogen from the feed source is required for effective control; examples include trichinosis in swine and salmonellosis in poultry. Transportation and holding of animals before slaughter should take place in clean facilities and should involve a minimum of stress to the animal, since animals often contract disease during this stage of production. For a zoonoses control program to be effective, veterinarians must inspect live animals before slaughter for signs of infection.

Seafood Procurement and Processing

Fish. The sanitary objectives of primary concern to the fishing industry are (1) minimizing bacterial contamination of the product and (2) handling and processing fish in such a way that growth of endogenous and exogenous bacteria and activity of endogenous enzymes are minimized. Fish are particularly susceptible to microbial spoilage and enzymatic decomposition; consequently, sanitary conditions during harvesting and processing and either frozen storage or storage on ice are required. Sources of exogenous bacterial contamination include ship surfaces, ice (usually contaminated after delivery to the ship), bilge water, and the fishermen themselves. The sanitary inspection of fishing boats and ships is useful for controlling these problems. On the dock, unsanitary unloading and exposure to flies and bird droppings must be prevented. During filleting, contamination with fish feces and the quality of the rinse water are of concern. Fish caught in unpolluted water are seldom contaminated with human pathogens; however, *V. parahaemolyticus* can be found on fish from unpolluted shallow coastal or estuarine waters,[40] and *Clostridium botulinum* type E is often found in the gut of fish taken from certain areas. Common intoxications associated with consumption of fish include histamine poisoning resulting from the growth of histamine-producing bacteria, and ciguatera poisoning resulting from ingestion of fish that have fed on toxic algae.[41]

Shellfish. Sanitary procurement of shellfish such as oysters, clams, and mussels is of special concern because the whole animal, including the gastrointestinal tract, is consumed raw or partially cooked. In addition, bacteria, chemical contaminants, viruses, and fine particulate matter are concentrated in shellfish when they feed. As a result, the sanitary quality of shellfish is related to the quality of the estuarine waters in which they have been harvested. Shellfish should not be harvested from waters contaminated with wastewater where wastewater treatment is inadequate or unreliable. Shellfish growing areas are surveyed for safety by the U.S. Public Health Service. Only those waters not subject to sewage contamination and having coliform counts of under 70 organisms per 100 ml are approved for harvesting. Shellfish transferred from marginally polluted areas to unpolluted waters and left at least 14 days will purify themselves.

Although the transmission of typhoid fever by shellfish is no longer of major concern in most parts of the world, concern over the transmission of viral hepatitis and *V. vulnificus* septicemia has increased. Current standards for shellfish harvesting appear to be adequate in assuring a safe product[42]; however, unauthorized harvesting and illegal sale is a problem.

Milk Production

Since the development of the fluid milk industry in the early twentieth century, public health officials have recognized the potential of milk for large-scale transmission of disease. As late as 1923, there were 15 outbreaks and 423 cases of milkborne typhoid fever reported in the United States.[43] Since then, improvements in herd health and standardized pasteurization methods have made milk a relatively safe food. Even so, recent outbreaks of salmonellosis and listeriosis have focused attention on improving sanitary control over milk processing. Even though milk is pasteurized, maintenance of sanitary quality during production and transportation to the processing facility is important in reducing the possibility of contamination of the pasteurized product by pathogens and in increasing flavor quality and shelf life. Sanitary control of milk production depends on maintaining herd health, using wholesome feeds, and preventing the entrance and growth of microorganisms in the milk. Pasteurization of milk inactivates pathogens but will not reduce levels of microbial toxins, antibiotics, chemical adulterants, or off-flavors.

Dairy Cow Health. The use of mechanical milking equipment and sanitary milking practices has reduced the opportunity for contamination of milk through human contact to such an extent that milk production personnel using modern milking facilities are no longer considered an important source of pathogenic contaminants. The cow itself, however, is a major source of pathogenic and toxigenic bacteria. Consequently, maintenance of herd health is an important aspect of sanitary milk production. Unfortunately, even healthy animals can transmit disease through their milk.[44] Milkborne diseases of contemporary importance include salmonellosis, campylobacteriosis, listeriosis, staphylococcal food poisoning, brucellosis, and yersiniosis.[45] With the possible exception of yersiniosis, infected animals are a major source of causative organisms for these illnesses. On the other hand, diseases associated with consumption of manufactured dairy products are most often the result of contamination from equipment, water, and human handlers after the milk has been pasteurized. Disease risks associated with consumption of raw milk are much greater than those associated with consumption of pasteurized products.[46]

Salmonellosis. Although milk and dairy products are not the major vehicle for salmonellosis in the United States, milkborne salmonellosis is common in regions where raw milk is consumed.[45] The *Salmonella* species chiefly associated with cattle and raw milk is *Salmonella dublin,* although *Salmonella typhimurium* is also prevalent in the United States.[44] *S. dublin* can cause a long-term carrier state in cattle, which can then shed the organism in their feces, infecting the milking environment, other animals, and the milk during the milking process. Some dairy cattle have been found to shed *S. dublin* into milk through the mammary gland. This is a chronic asymptomatic condition.[44]

Eliminating *Salmonella* species from dairy cattle herds is difficult and presently uneconomical. Common sources of the organism are birds and rodents, feed, animal wastes, and other cattle. Animal wastes are often held in lagoons and then used to irrigate crops. *Salmonella* species can survive this process and recontaminate the herd. Since dairy cattle are housed in relatively open environments, it is difficult to eliminate contamination from outside sources. The trend toward maintaining larger herds in less space increases the opportunity for infection to pass among cows. Currier[44] concluded, "We do not have the ability to eradicate *Salmonella* infection from a dairy herd or preclude their reintroduction." *Salmonella* species are isolated from about 5% of dairy herd milk.[45]

Campylobacteriosis. Milkborne campylobacteriosis is associated almost exclusively with the consumption of raw milk. The causative organism is usually *C. jejuni.* Large outbreaks have occurred in Great Britain, including one that involved 2500 children.[47] Several outbreaks have occurred in the United States.[45] Many milkborne outbreaks involve small children and are thus particularly serious. Typical outbreaks result when school children tour dairy farms and sample raw milk. A more unusual outbreak occurred when raw milk was served to a group of 233 persons, and 80 persons became ill.[48] *Campylobacter* species are difficult to isolate from raw milk because they are usually present in very low numbers. In surveys of raw milk in which sensitive detection methods were used (less than 1 organism per ml), from 1% to 2% of individual farm milk was found contaminated.[49,50] Low levels of *Campylobacter* survive in raw milk[50] and do represent a health hazard.[51] Diagnosing campylobacteriosis in dairy cattle is difficult because the organisms are not easily isolated and because of the presence of asymptomatic carriers. Since *Campylobacter* reservoirs are farm animals such as cattle, pigs, and chickens, as well as humans and wild birds, it is unlikely that the infection of cattle with this organism can be prevented in the present farm environment.

Brucellosis. Approximately 10% of reported cases of brucellosis are associated with the consumption of dairy products.[52] The products most often implicated are raw milk and cheese made from raw milk. The popularity of raw goat's milk cheese, especially that brought into the United States from Mexico, is a significant portion of the foodborne brucellosis problem.[45] Implicated dairy foods processed in the United States are usually traced to dairy cattle infected with either *Brucella abortus* or *Brucella suis* if the cattle have had contact with swine.[46] The porcine strain is more virulent to humans than the bovine strain. Many cases of brucellosis in humans may have been transmitted by cattle infected with *B. suis.*[53] Brucellosis in cattle is called Bang's disease, or infectious abortion. The organism localizes in the uterus of pregnant animals and mammary glands of lactating animals, with the result that it is shed into the milk. Brucellosis in cattle is controlled through the removal and slaughter of infected animals. Calf immunization is also considered effective. Herd infections are detected by means of a ring test that examines milk for antibodies.

North American and European countries have undertaken extensive government-supported programs to eradicate brucellosis from dairy animals. Although total eradication has not been achieved, these programs have been successful in decreasing incidence of the disease in animals and humans. In the United States, 27% of dairy herds had at least "suspicious" ring test results in 1952, but only 0.27% of dairy herds were positive in 1970. In 1977, eight states were brucellosis free, and only infectious rates in Texas, Louisiana, Mississippi, and Florida exceeded 10 herds per 1000.[54] Since various animals may act as reservoirs for *B. abortus,* eradication of this organism in domestic cattle may not be possible in regions of the world where cattle cannot be segregated from such sources.[55]

Yersiniosis. In recent years milk has been implicated as a vehicle in outbreaks of yersiniosis. The organism involved is usually *Y. enterocolitica,* although one case of illness from *Yersinia pseudotuberculosis* associated with raw goat's milk was reported.[56] Outbreaks of yersiniosis have been associated with both raw and pasteurized milk.[57,58] *Y. enterocolitica* is commonly found in raw milk, although nearly all isolates are "environmental" nonpathogenic strains.[25] Both the milking animal and the environment are considered possible sources for contamination of raw milk. Sources on the farm include water, birds, and farm animals.[59] Pasteurized milk can be contaminated from environmental sources within the processing plant,[60] although these contaminants are generally nonpathogenic types. *Y. enterocolitica* can grow in milk held at 3°C.[61] The organism survives in inadequately cleaned and sanitized equipment, which can result in contamination of pasteurized product. Swine are the major on-farm reservoir of *Y. enterocolitica* strains pathogenic for humans. In one outbreak that may have involved several thousand people, pasteurized milk was probably contaminated by milk crates that had been returned from a swine farm. Mud trapped on the bottoms of the crates was not removed by the dairy plant's cleaning procedure.[62] Stacking of the filled crates resulted in the contamination of milk carton tops.

Listeriosis. Only recently has *L. monocytogenes* been implicated in dairy product–associated illness. *L. monocytogenes* can infect the mammary gland of the cow and be excreted into the milk. Hayes and associates[63] isolated the organism from 12% of raw milk samples. The organism is psychrotrophic and can grow on moist surfaces in processing plants, resulting in postprocess contamination.[64] There have been recent outbreaks of milkborne and cheeseborne listeriosis.[65,66] The mortality rate in these outbreaks was about 30%.

Staphylococcal Food Poisoning. If raw milk is not rapidly chilled, staphylococci can grow and produce enterotoxin.[67] Staphylococcal food poisoning associated with fluid milk is rare in the United States because raw milk is cooled rapidly and stored cold until pasteurization. Staphylococci in raw milk are often associated with clinical or subclinical mastitis, although apparently healthy animals may also excrete the organisms.[67]

Mastitis. Mastitis is an inflammation of the mammary gland usually associated with microbial infection. Approximately 50% of the cows in the United States have mastitis, usually in a subclinical form.[68] Subclinical mastitis is detected by measuring the somatic cell concentration in the milk. Somatic cell counts greater than 500,000/ml are generally considered an indication of the disease. Individual producer milk (milk from one herd) is considered unsuitable for Grade A classification if the somatic cell count exceeds 1,000,000/ml (Table 34–4). Mastitis in dairy cows is usually caused by either *Streptococcus agalactiae* or *S. aureus. S. agalactiae* is an obligate parasite of the cow's mammary gland and poses no hazard to public health. However, the secretion of *S. aureus* into milk may pose a hazard if temperatures suitable for growth are encountered (see previous discussion). Coliform bacteria and nonagalactiae streptococci are occasionally associated with mastitis but pose no known health threat. Other less common causes of mastitis are *L. monocytogenes* and various species of *Pasteurella* including *P. multocida* and *P. haemolytica. Pasteurella* species most often associated with mastitis are considered opportunistic pathogens for humans.[46]

The public health hazard associated with mastitis is slight, at least when milk is pasteurized. The contamination of milk with antibiotics used for the treatment of mastitis is of concern. This problem is discussed under Incidental Adulterants.

Safety of Raw Milk. Mandatory pasteurization and sanitation procedures have made milk one of the safest foods available. Several states, however, still allow the sale of raw milk, usually "certified" raw milk. The "certified" designation indicates that the milk was produced under stringent sanitary guidelines and meets the strict microbiological standards of the American Association of Medical Milk Commissions, Inc. (AAMMC).[69] In the nineteenth century when the AAMMC was formed, there was a need for safer milk because modern pasteurization procedures had not yet been developed and milkborne disease was widespread. Certification of milk was instituted to provide a safer product for infants and persons in poor health. At the time it was initiated, certification was beneficial to the public health. Current evidence, however, shows that the "certified" trademark is no longer indicative of a safer product.[44,45] Between 1971 and 1975, for instance, 35 of 113 cases of salmonellosis from *S. dublin* reported in California were associated with consumption of raw milk from one certified dairy, even though this dairy produces only 0.05% of California's fluid milk.[70] Campylobacteriosis has also been associated with the consumption of certified raw milk produced in Georgia and California.[45] It is apparent that raw milk can still be a vehicle for disease transmission even though it has very low coliform and total aerobic bacteria populations. Production of raw milk free of *Salmonella* species or *Campylobacter* species is difficult (see previous discussion).

Infections associated with the consumption of raw milk may not always take the form of acute outbreaks typical of food poisoning[44] because contamination is usually intermittent and at very low levels. Unfortunately, the persons most likely to be infected under these circumstances are infants, the very old, and the infirm—the same persons for whom some physicians prescribe the consumption of raw milk and who may be led to drink raw milk because of its purported healthful properties. It is ironic the "certified" label, which was developed to improve public health, is now increasing health risks for the segment of population that it was designed to protect. Of 74 persons who became ill with salmonellosis between 1971 and 1974 after consumption of raw milk in California, 50% had an underlying debilitating condition, 75% were hospitalized, and 20% died.[71]

Although infants and adults who have trouble digesting pasteurized milk are often advised to consume raw milk, raw milk cannot be considered more digestible than the pasteurized equivalent. The mechanisms of milk intolerance—hypersensitivity to bovine proteins, lactose intolerance, and a toxic heat labile protein—are not exacerbated by pasteurization.[72]

Sanitary Milking Procedures. Producing milk of high sanitary quality requires clean cows, milking machines that are properly sanitized and maintained, a clean milking environment, and rapid cooling of the milk. The milking environment and milking procedures recommended for production of fluid milk are described in the PMO.[30]

The milking environment includes the cow yard, the milking parlor, and milk house. This environment must be designed and maintained to minimize opportunities for contamination of the milk. The cow yard is the area outside the milking parlor where cows are held before milking. The yard should be landscaped to minimize standing water, and manure should be regularly removed. Modern milking parlors are designed to reduce the labor and time required to milk large herds. They should be constructed so that they can be easily cleaned. Feed storage should be in dust-tight containers. There should be sufficient air circulation to prevent condensation. Milking parlors often include stalls for automatic washing of udders before milking.

The milk house or room is to be used only for the cooling and storage of milk and the washing, sanitizing, and storing of utensils and containers used during milking. The milk room is usually constructed so that there is no direct opening between it and the milk parlor or any other animal holding facility. It should be kept free of insects and rodents and constructed so that it is easily cleaned.

Another important aspect of a sanitary milking environment involves proper toilet facilities with disposal of waste in such a manner that it does not contaminate groundwater. An adequate sanitary water supply is also required for proper cleaning and rinsing of animals, equipment, and utensils.

In addition to a clean environment, specific milking procedures described in the PMO must be followed to ensure sanitary milk production. To prevent contamination with abnormal milk or milk containing antibiotics, all cows with symptoms of mastitis and those undergoing antibiotic treatments of any kind should be milked last or with separate equipment. This milk must be segregated to prevent the spread of infection and the contamination of milk-handling utensils. Cows ready for milking should be clean—especially their udders, flanks, bellies, and tails. Just before milking, the cows' udders and teats should be cleaned, sanitized, and dried with single-use paper towels. This preparative cleaning not only lowers the concentration of bacteria in the milk but also helps control the spread of mastitis. The cows can then be milked with well-maintained, cleaned, and sanitized milking equipment. Cleaning and sanitizing procedures are discussed in a following section.

In modern dairies, milk is pumped directly from the milking machines to the cooling and storage tank. The milk should be cooled to 7°C within 2 hours after milking. Since the milk is usually picked up every other day, more than one milking will be collected before the tank is emptied. When warm fresh milk is added to cold milk in the tank, the blend temperature should not exceed 10°C. Farm holding tanks often do not have sufficient refrigeration capacity to achieve this rate of cooling.[73]

Transportation and Handling of Raw Milk. There are various systems for delivering milk from the farm to the processing plant. In many countries, the farmer delivers milk in cans once or twice a day to a central receiving station where it is cooled and delivered to the processing plant by tank truck. Milk producers located near the processing plant deliver their milk directly to the plant. If milk is not cooled on the farm, it should be transported to the receiving station or processing plant immediately after each milking.

In the United States and other milk producing areas where large dairy herds predominate, farm storage (bulk) tanks with refrigeration are common. This milk is usually picked up by tank truck every other day. When a tank truck is used to collect milk at the farm, judgments concerning the acceptability of the milk must be made before loading because the milk is mixed (commingled) with milk from other farms. If a single producer's milk has high bacteria levels, off-flavors, or antibiotic contamination or is otherwise adulterated, it will adulterate the whole truckload. For this reason, the milk of each producer must be monitored for sanitary compliance on a regular basis. Samples for microbiological and chemical analyses, including tests for microbial inhibitors, aerobic bacteria, somatic cells, and added water, are taken from each farm storage tank. A milk sample from the truck is also tested when it arrives at the receiving station or processing plant. If the milk is acceptable, it is unloaded into large storage tanks, where additional mixing takes place. A major concern associated with the modern bulk milk handling system is the possibility that milk from one producer containing a toxin or pathogen will result in tens of thousands of pounds of contaminated milk. The rarity of disease outbreaks associated with fluid milk can be ascribed to the effectiveness of pasteurization procedures and enforcement of the PMO.

Incidental Chemical Adulterants

Incidental chemical adulterants are (1) environmental contaminants or industrial chemicals that accidentally find their way into food and (2) chemicals such as pesticides and antibiotics used in the production of food that may be at unacceptable levels as a result of improper use. As various incidents of food contaminated with heavy metals or aromatic halogenated hydrocarbons have demonstrated, incidental chemical adulterants can cause severe and widespread public health hazards. This section concentrates on the control of acute episodes of contamination rather than the control of chronic low-level contamination, which is usually beyond the control of food sanitarians. Probably 80% or more of incidental chemical residues in food animals occur through feed contamination or feed additives.[74]

Heavy Metals. Mercury and lead are the heavy metals of greatest concern as food adulterants; cadmium, tin, zinc, and arsenic pose a lesser threat to public health. These substances find their way into food through their release into the environment by industry, through the application of sewage sludge on crops, and through the use of metal-containing food storage containers. The release of mercury-containing industrial waste into waterways is a public health hazard, and this practice is now banned. In the environment, mercury compounds are methylated and concentrated by environmental flora. Metallic or mercuric mercury compounds are not considered hazardous; however, alkyl mercury is highly toxic. Alkyl mercury is concentrated in the food chain to such an extent that fish from contaminated waters will be toxic to humans. In Japan, consumption of fish contaminated with methyl mercury has caused birth defects and poisoning.[33] The fish contained up to 29 mg/kg of methyl mercury, with human consumption as high as 30 μg/d. The mercury in alkyl mercury compounds used as seed protectants is ingested by birds and causes severe illness when the seeds are consumed by humans.[75] This seed treatment is not legal in the United States.

Lead is prevalent in the environment and the food supply and slowly accumulates in the human body. The effects of chronic low-level exposure to lead include intellectual impairment (see Chapter 20). Subclinical poisoning characterized by decreased heme biosynthesis may cause anemia.[33] Lead can contaminate foods in several ways, including from naturally occurring concentrations of lead present in soil and water. Additional environmental contamination results from the use of leaded gasoline, water runoff from mining operations, and pollution from lead smelting. More direct contamination of food is associated with the use of lead-containing pesticides and tin cans. Of these sources, the use of tin cans may be the most pervasive. The FDA estimates that 13% to 14% of the lead in the average diet has leached into canned food from lead-containing solder on tin cans.[76] Leaching of lead is affected by the type of food and its pH, the amount of lead in the solder, and the type of protective coatings inside the can. Since decreasing amounts of lead are being used in can solder, canned food should contain less lead in the future. Lead-containing glazes on earthenware dishes originating in underdeveloped countries are particularly hazardous.[77]

Food prepared or stored in galvanized containers has been implicated as a cause of metal poisoning.[78] Tin poisoning from food packaged in tin cans occurs occasionally when fruit or fruit juice cans lack a complete lacquer coating. Levels of tin in such products range from 100 to 365 ppm.[79]

Mining operations can cause contamination of water supplies with cadmium and arsenic. Cadmium poisoning has been caused by consumption of rice grown in contaminated water.[80] Cadmium levels in the rice were as high as 0.69 ppm, whereas the normal background level is less than 0.2 ppm. Use of sewage sludge on fields may be an important cause of elevated cadmium levels in vegetables and meat.[80]

Aromatic Halogenated Hydrocarbons. PCBs and polybrominated biphenyls (PBBs) have contaminated foods at levels that may be hazardous. Since these substances are persistent in the environment, their use and disposal is now severely limited. They are strongly lipophilic and consequently accumulate in animal fat and milk. PCBs have found their way into food through leakage into soil and water from landfills where various electrical devices were deposited and from food packaging materials made from recycled contaminated paper. Since 1971, chronic exposure to PCBs has decreased because of a ban on their production and governmental control over their disposal. Danger from their accidental use and illegal disposal still exists, however. In Montana, PCBs from a damaged transformer contaminated animal meal; this resulted in the contamination of millions of pounds of animal feed and food.[81]

A fire retardant containing PBBs was accidentally used in formulating animal feeds in Michigan. This accident resulted in the destruction of about 30,000 cattle and over 1 million fowl. The total cost of the contamination was estimated at $215 million. Circumstances leading to the accident are summarized by Kay.[82] Levels of PBBs found in milk were as high as 595 ppm, in poultry meat as high as 4600 ppm, in eggs up to 59 ppm, and in cattle tissue as high as 27,000 ppm.

Pesticides. Chemical pesticides include insecticides, fungicides, herbicides, and rodenticides. Only insecticides are discussed here because they have been most often associated with foodborne hazards. Commonly used insecticides include chlorinated hydrocarbons, organophosphates, and carbamates. Acute foodborne poisoning associated with pesticides is usually a result of accidental spillage on a raw product such as flour or grain or improper application before harvest. Regulatory aspects of pesticide use are discussed by Petersen and Chaisson.[83]

Chlorinated hydrocarbon insecticides including DDT, chlordane, heptachlor, and lindane were widely used until the mid-1960s. Their use is now restricted because of their persistence in the environment, their tendency to accumulate in living organisms, and the potential danger of chronic toxicity to humans and animals. Acute poisoning from chlorinated hydrocarbon insecticides is rare.

Organophosphorus and carbamate insecticides have high toxicity and are more often associated with cases of acute food poisoning. These insecticides are widely used and rapidly degrade in the environment. A large outbreak of carbamate (aldicarb) food poisoning associated with contaminated melons has been reported.[84] Aldicarb is not legally approved for use on melons. (See Chapter 24.)

Antibiotic Residues. About $50 million worth of meat and milk are discarded annually because of antibiotic contamination. Meat contamination can result from the common practice of incorporating low levels of antibiotics such as chlortetracycline and oxytetracycline in poultry, swine, and cattle feeds to stimulate growth. Although residues are seldom found in commercial meats, there is concern that animals will develop antibiotic-resistant microflora in their digestive tracts and that this resistance might be transferred to human pathogens.[85]

In the ongoing battle against bovine mastitis, dairy cows are being treated with higher doses of a greater variety of antibiotics. Antibiotics given to cattle by almost any route (oral, intravenous, intramuscular, intramammary) can contaminate the milk. Milk from treated cows usually must be discarded for 72 hours after treatment to ensure an uncontaminated product. Antibiotics used for mastitis therapy include penicillin, streptomycin, neomycin, and polymyxin.[86] The dairy industry supports the education of milk producers in the prevention of antibiotic contamination because bacterial cultures used in the manufacture of products such as cheese and yogurt will be inhibited by low-level antibiotic contamination. The industry spends about $20 million per year in its efforts to keep antibiotics out of milk.[86] A survey of nonfat dry milk by the USDA found 63 antibiotic-positive samples out of 2265 tested (2.8%).[87]

Antibiotic residues in foods present public health risks. Individuals with antibiotic-mediated hypersensitivity, especially those sensitized by therapeutic applications, are at greatest risk.[88] In one case, consumption of 1 L of penicillin-contaminated milk per day (4000 units per day) caused a reaction.[89] In addition, attempts to manufacture cheese with antibiotic-contaminated milk can provide an opportunity for growth of pathogenic or toxigenic microorganisms because of delayed acid production.[90] Further health concerns involve the selection for resistant microorganisms in food and in the gut of persons who might regularly consume antibiotic-contaminated food. There is no evidence that the antibiotic-resistant microflora of raw milk is associated with antibiotic contamination.[91]

Growth Hormones. Synthetic growth hormones such as diethylstilbesterol (DES) are able to increase the rate and efficiency of weight gain in beef cattle by 10% to 15%. When used as a feed additive, synthetic hormones leave no detectable residue in the meat tissue, but they may be found in part-per-billion amounts in the liver. These organ meat residues will disappear rapidly after withdrawal of the animal from the feed because they are rapidly metabolized and excreted. DES is banned for use as a feed additive on the basis of its being a carcinogen, but other synthetic hormones are allowed.

Mycotoxins. Mycotoxins are toxic metabolites of molds that contaminate food either when mold grows on the food during storage or when foods are derived from animals fed contaminated feed. The most important mycotoxins affecting human health are aflatoxins, which are considered the most potent naturally occurring carcinogens known. Other mycotoxins include sterigmatocystin, ochratoxin, patulin, and trichothecenes.[92] Molds capable of producing mycotoxins include species of *Penicillium, Aspergillus,* and *Fusarium.*

Aflatoxins have been found in various foods and feeds, including grains, oilseeds, peanuts, pistachios, and dairy products. For some foods such as peanuts and pistachios, which are difficult to harvest free of aflatoxin, the FDA has set contamination limits at 20 ppb.[93] These foods may contain aflatoxin B-1, the most carcinogenic of the group. Milk products can be contaminated with aflatoxin M-1, a metabolite of B-1, which is only one hundredth as carcinogenic but just as toxic. Milk is contaminated with aflatoxin when cows are given contaminated feed. Feed becomes contaminated when weather conditions permit mold growth before harvest or when grains are not sufficiently dried for storage. About 1% of the aflatoxin B-1 in dairy cattle feed ends up in milk as M-1.[38] Acute poisoning from aflatoxins is rare. However, aflatoxin in milk is of special concern because milk is a major food for infants and children and the rapidly growing young are considered most susceptible to induction of carcinogenesis.[94]

FOOD PLANT SANITATION

From the perspective of food sanitation, the objective of a food processing plant is to convert raw food of good quality into a shelf-stable product, without degradation of the food or exposure of it to filth or potentially harmful microbial or chemical contaminants. Accomplishing this objective requires concern for sanitation when choosing a plant site, designing equipment, and operating the plant. An operational plant should maintain a sanitation program that ensures that the food is stored and processed in a sanitary environment. If a food processing plant lacks effective sanitation, high-quality raw foods can easily be converted into contaminated, spoiled, or hazardous products.

Plant Design

The food processing plant structure should provide a barrier to animal vectors and environmental contaminants such as dust and water. Since the plant structure may not always be a perfect sanitary barrier, some thought should be given to plant location. A food processing plant should not be located close to sources of airborne or waterborne chemical or microbial contaminants. There should be a plentiful supply of treated or readily purified water. The plant surroundings should be landscaped to ensure good drainage and maintained to provide dust and animal vector control. Processing-plant waste should be disposed of or treated so that air and water quality are not jeopardized.

A processing plant should be designed to provide separate rooms for receiving raw product, processing and packaging, dry storage, and finished product storage. The flow of materials through the plant should be controlled to avoid contamination of processed products with raw products, returned product, or dust from dry storage areas. Airflow between rooms should also be controlled to prevent processing and packaging areas from being contaminated by the "dirtier" areas of the plant. Microorganisms such as *Salmonella, Listeria,* molds, and bacterial endospores can be spread by air currents. Special precautions should be taken to maintain uncontaminated air in the processing-packaging area. A common solution is to maintain a positive pressure of filtered air in critical rooms.

The floors, walls, and ceiling of processing plant rooms should be designed for easy cleaning and avoidance of condensate formation. Although these surfaces do not come in contact with food, they, as well as piping and floor drains, can increase the level of microbial contaminants in the processing environment. Cleanliness of these areas is of crucial importance in the control of *L. monocytogenes,* which grows on damp surfaces[95] including floor and sink drains, pipes, walls, and floors. It is very difficult to avoid condensate formation in most food processing facilities, making cleanliness of these surfaces the major means of control over microbial growth. Additional preventive measures include reducing relative humidity in high-risk areas and insulating cold pipes and equipment. Floor drains are an important source of airborne microorganisms during water and waste drainage.[96] Standard drain designs make it difficult to prevent this contamination.

The heating-ventilation-air conditioning (HVAC) system in a food plant can also be a source of contamination. To ensure that particulate and microbial contaminants are removed, circulating air must pass through a suitable filtration system. Regular maintenance and monitoring of the HVAC system is crucial for sanitary operation.[97]

Sanitary Equipment Design

Food processing equipment should not be a source of chemical or microbial contamination and should be easy to clean and sanitize. Achieving this objective requires proper selection of construction materials, use of proper construction techniques, and a design in which ease of cleaning and providing an effective barrier to environmental contamination are given high priority. Construction materials should be smooth, nonabsorbent, and corrosion resistant. Stainless steel is considered the best all-purpose construction material for food-handling equipment. Equipment should be constructed so that food contact surfaces are manufactured from one piece of material or have as few seams and joints as possible. If welds are required, they should be smooth, flush with the surroundings, and corrosion resistant. Internal corners and angles of food contact surfaces must be rounded to facilitate cleaning. Rotating shafts must have a close-fitting, easily cleaned seal. Tank openings should have raised edges, to prevent contamination with liquids. To be easily cleaned, equipment must either be suitable for clean-in-place (CIP) systems or be readily dissembled by hand.

Guidelines for the design of milk-handling and processing equipment have been developed through the combined efforts of three agencies: the U.S. Public Health Service, the International Association of Milk, Food and Environmental Sanitarians, and the Milk Industry Foundation. These guidelines, known as 3-A (three agency) standards, have provided uniformity in the sanitary design of dairy equipment. These standards are published in the *Journal of Dairy and Food Sanitation* (before 1985, see *Journal of Food Protection*). General standards for the sanitary design of food handling equipment have been developed by the National Sanitation Foundation (NSF Building, Ann Arbor, MI 48105). NSF standards are especially applicable to food service equipment.

Equipment Cleaning

Principles of Cleaning. The removal of soil from equipment surfaces is necessary both to eliminate food for microbial growth and to achieve effective destruction of microorganisms during chemical sanitation. Adequate cleaning occurs when a cleaning agent (detergent) and water are applied to a surface with enough energy to remove the soil. The required energy can be supplied in the form of mild heat and physical force, as is the case with hand cleaning using a brush, or in the form of higher temperatures combined with turbulent flow of the cleaning solution, as is the case with CIP systems.

Most recommended cleaning procedures involve four steps: prerinse, cleaning, postrinse, and drying. The prerinse removes gross amounts of food or soil that remain on the surface so that the cleaning power of the detergent can be maximized. The temperature of the water should be warm enough to melt fat so that it can be removed; however, the water temperature must not be so hot that it "cooks" protein onto the surface. The recommended prerinse water temperature for removing milk solids is 39° to 46°C. Water temperature is also critical for the cleaning step. Very hot water (70° to 77° C) and strong cleaning agents are required for CIP or circulation cleaning. Temperatures and cleaning agents used in hand cleaning are limited by human tolerance and safety. In the postrinse step, all detergent and dissolved or emulsified soil are removed from the equipment surface. Hot water is normally used so that soil does not redeposit on the equipment. In some cases, acidified water is used in a postrinse to prevent mineral deposits from forming. The final step in cleaning is draining and drying. Pipelines and tanks should be designed so that they drain thoroughly. It is undesirable to have pools of rinse water remaining in or on equipment, as this can provide moisture for microbial growth. If an acid rinse is used, equipment surfaces will be left at a low pH (4.0 to 5.0), which offers additional antimicrobial effects.

Types of Soil. The selection of a cleaning agent depends to a large extent on the nature of soil to be removed and the mineral content of the available water. Food residues that are high in protein or fat require specific cleaning agents. Dried-on or baked-on soil is more difficult to remove and requires special cleaning procedures. In addition to food constituents, the soil may consist of dust, lubricants, microorganisms, and mineral deposits. The isolation of *L. monocytogenes* from conveyer belt lubricant has increased attention in the cleaning of lubricated areas.[64]

Water Quality. Minerals in water can reduce the efficiency of cleaning compounds and increase the formation of insoluble mineral films. Cleaning compounds intended for use with hard water contain chemical precipitants or chelating agents for removing calcium and magnesium. Water for cleaning is often softened by using ion exchange to avoid the expense of chemical softeners added to the cleaning compound. Rinsing with hard water under alkaline conditions will result in the formation of a mineral film. Since most cleaning compounds are alkaline in reaction, the film will not be removed by subsequent cleaning and will continue to accumulate, forming what is known as waterstone or milkstone. These deposits appear as a white film on dry stainless steel. Mineral deposits can usually be removed by using an acidic cleaning agent. Rinsing with acidified water prevents their formation and therefore is generally recommended in dairy and other food processing plants.

Cleaning Agents. Cleaning compounds usually consist of several cleaning agents because a single agent seldom has all the functional properties necessary for effective soil removal. A good cleaning compound will function in four steps[98]: (1) wetting and penetrating to bring the detergent solution into intimate contact with the soil; (2) displacing soil from the equipment surface by saponifying fat, peptonizing proteins, and dissolving minerals; (3) dispersing soil in the cleaning solution by dispersion, deflocculation, or emulsification; and (4) preventing redeposition of the dispersed soil onto the clean surface through good rinsing properties.

Food industry cleaning compounds are based on either acid or alkaline cleaning agents with added sequesterants and wetting agents. Most commonly used cleaning compounds are alkaline based. Caustic soda (sodium hydroxide) is effective in removing protein and fat deposits. It is not safe for use in manual cleaning but is used in CIP and circulation systems. Sodium carbonate (soda ash) and mixtures of sodium carbonate and sodium bicarbonate (sesquicarbonate) are alkalis often used for manual cleaning. The cleaning ability of alkali compounds is enhanced by the addition of hypochlorite. Chlorinated alkalis are the most commonly used cleaning compounds for CIP systems. Acid cleaners, usually containing weak acids such as phosphoric, are used for removing mineral deposits. The most common sequesterants used in cleaning compounds are the polyphosphates, especially sodium hexametaphosphate and sodium tetrametaphosphate. Amounts required depend on the hardness of the water. Wetting agents or surfactants function by lowering the surface tension of the solution, increasing its ability to penetrate soil. They also act as emulsifying agents. Sulfonated alcohols and alkyl aryl sulfonates are commonly used surfactants.

Cleaning Systems. Although cleaning solutions can be applied either manually or through recirculation, recirculation (CIP) systems are usually preferred because they reduce human error and allow the use of higher temperatures and stronger cleaning agents. Modern CIP systems are microprocessor controlled to minimize chemical and energy use while maintaining temperature and flow control.

Sanitizing Equipment

Sanitizing is the process of inactivating microorganisms on equipment surfaces. Sanitizing does not usually sterilize the surface but should inactivate all pathogenic microorganisms and most other vegetative cells. Chemicals, heat, and radiation can all be used as sanitizing agents. For sanitizing agents to be effective, surfaces must be clean, since food and mineral residues protect microbial cells from physical and chemical inactivation. To minimize recontamination, all food contact surfaces should be sanitized immediately before use.

Chemical Sanitizers. Numerous chemical sanitizing agents are available for food industry use. The major types are chlorine, iodine, quaternary ammonium, and acid-anionic compounds (Fig. 34–1).

Chlorine Compounds. These compounds release chlorine into water, with subsequent formation of hypochlorous acid. Commonly used inorganic compounds include sodium and calcium hypochlorite. Sodium hypochlorite is the preferred inorganic chlorine sanitizer because it is economical, soluble, and effective in hard water. It inactivates vegetative cells, microbial spores, and viruses. The minimum treatment with hypochlorite for effective sanitation is at least 1 minute of exposure to 50 ppm available chlorine at 24° C. Lower temperatures and alkaline solutions require longer exposure times. Since free chlorine reacts indiscriminately with organic matter, additional chlorine must be added to compensate. If the surface is clean, concentrations of 150 to 200 ppm hypochlorite will provide sufficient available chloride. Hypochlorite corrodes stainless steel if exposure is excessive (greater than 3 to 4 minutes or concentrations greater than 500 ppm), and it is irritating to the skin. Organic chlorides such as Chloramine T (Fig. 34–1) are less irritating and less corrosive. Organic chlorides release chlorine at a slower rate than inorganic chlorides but are not as stable or soluble. Longer exposure times are required. Most chlorine compounds exhibit greatest effectiveness in neutral or slightly acidic solutions; however, acidic hypochlorite solutions are very corrosive.

Iodine Compounds. Sanitizers that contain iodine are normally used in the form of an iodophore, that is, iodine bound to a nonionic surfactant in an acidic solution. When mixed with water, the iodophore releases free iodine. An iodophore solution has an amber color that can be used to judge its strength. Iodophores must be used at pH 6.0 or lower to obtain adequate release of free iodine, and they must not be heated above 49° C because the iodine will sublimate, resulting in a health hazard. Iodine is less corrosive and irritating than chlorine, but iodine is also less effective than chlorine against spores and viruses. Iodine com-

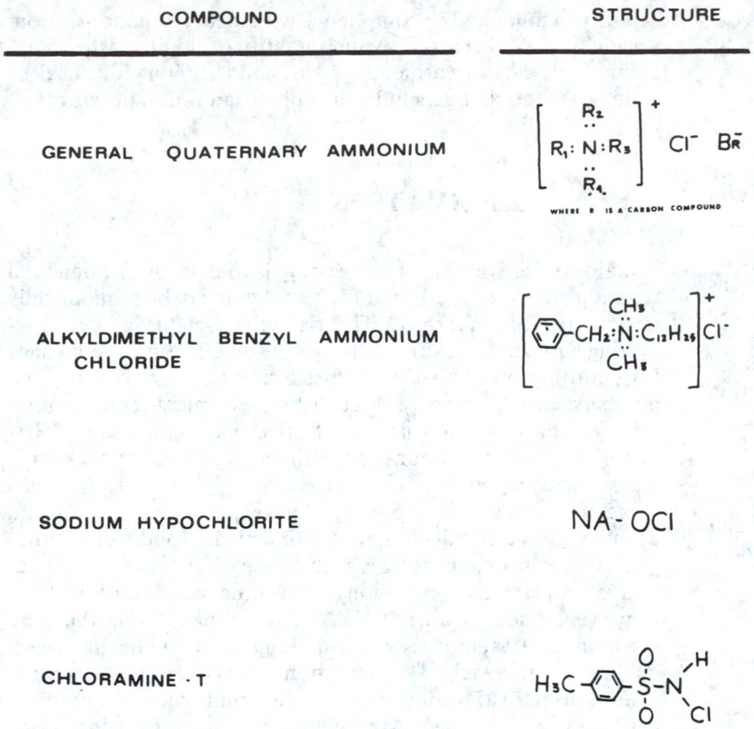

COMPOUND	STRUCTURE
GENERAL QUATERNARY AMMONIUM	$[R_1:\ddot{N}:R_3\text{ with }R_2, R_4]^+$ Cl^- Br^- (WHERE R IS A CARBON COMPOUND)
ALKYLDIMETHYL BENZYL AMMONIUM CHLORIDE	$[C_6H_5\text{-}CH_2:\ddot{N}(CH_3)_2:C_{12}H_{25}]^+ Cl^-$
SODIUM HYPOCHLORITE	NA-OCl
CHLORAMINE-T	$H_3C\text{-}C_6H_4\text{-}S(=O)_2\text{-}N(H)Cl$

Figure 34–1. Chemical structure of some common sanitizing agents.

pounds are more likely to produce off-flavors in certain foods, especially dairy products. The careless use of iodine sanitizers can result in undesirable levels of iodine in the food supply, although cattle feed supplements are the major source of iodine in milk.[99]

Quaternary Ammonium Compounds. Quaternary ammonium compounds (QACs) are cationic wetting agents with bactericidal activity. Their chemical structure consists of a chlorine or bromine salt of ammonia, with the hydrogens substituted with *n*-alkyl, benzyl, methyl, or ethyl groups (Fig. 34–1). QACs are active over a wide pH range and can be used at high temperatures. They are also noncorrosive and nonirritating. A major disadvantage in using them is a reduction in activity caused by calcium or magnesium in the water. With chelation of minerals, a solution of 200 ppm is effective if exposure is for 30 seconds. These compounds are generally less bactericidal than chlorine or iodine sanitizers, but they do have higher residual activity. They are often used for sanitation of food and nonfood contact surfaces. They must be used with care in cultured-product plants because their residual activity will inhibit growth of lactic starter cultures.

Acid Wetting Agents. Acid wetting agents are mixtures of bactericidal organic acids, anionic or nonionic wetting agents, and phosphoric acid. Sanitizing effectiveness is dependent on the low pH (2.0 to 2.5) maintained by the phosphoric acid. Acid wetting agents are noncorrosive and effective in hard water, but they have slower bactericidal action than the previously discussed chemical sanitizers. They have both cleaning and sanitizing ability and can be used to accomplish both tasks in one step. Their sanitizing effectiveness is lowered if excess soil is present.

Heat Sanitizing. Moist heat is an effective sanitizing agent when used on clean equipment. Normal practice is to circulate hot water (93° C) for 5 to 30 minutes.[68] Minimum treatments using steam are 76.7° C for 15 minutes, 93.3° C for 5 minutes, or 1-minute exposure to a steam jet. Minimum treatments using water at 93.3° C are 5 minutes for equipment and 2 minutes for dishes and utensils. Heat sanitation is often not economical in a food processing plant because of heating and cooling costs. Dairy farms and other small-scale food handling operations may find heat sanitation appropriate.

Radiation Sanitizing. Ultraviolet (UV) radiation can be used to sanitize air, nonporous surfaces, and water. A contact time of at least 2 minutes is required for effectiveness. UV radiation is used to sanitize water used as a food ingredient and water for washing and cooling foods. UV lights are also used in packaging areas to reduce airborne microflora.

Cleanliness and Health of Personnel

An important aspect of sanitation in both food processing and food service establishments is the cleanliness and health of personnel. This topic is discussed in detail under Food Service Sanitation. Modern food processing facilities are designed so that direct contact between personnel and the food product is avoided as much as possible. Manual food handling can not always be eliminated, especially during some packaging operations. Whenever there is a reasonable possibility of contact between food and a food handler, precautions must be taken. These precautions are outlined in the Good Manufacturing Practices published by the FDA.[100] Good health, clean hands, and clean clothing are required. Also precautions should be taken to keep personnel from inadvertently contaminating food with foreign substances such as hair, jewelry, and tobacco. Control of employee traffic through critical areas of the processing plant is useful in avoiding the spread of microorganisms.

Plant Sanitation Programs

Every food processing plant should have an effective program designed to assure the sanitary handling and processing of products and ingredients. The program should be managed by an appropriately trained person who reports directly to the top management of the organization. The cooperation and support of management is necessary for a sanitation program to be effective. Management is legally responsible for sanitary conditions at the organization's food processing plants, even if authority has been delegated. A food plant sanitation program at minimum should include in-plant inspections, employee training and education, insect and rodent control, monitoring of water supply, and sanitary waste disposal.

In-Plant Inspections. In-plant inspections should be designed to ensure that the processing plant is complying with state and federal regulations. In food processing plants where good sanitation is critical for extending shelf life, in-plant inspections should be more rigorous than required by regulatory authorities. Inspections may be wholly visual or may include microbiological, compositional, or filth analysis of product samples. Inspections are best if they are conducted at irregular intervals and hours so that realistic appraisals of actual operating conditions are obtained. The inspector should use a form containing all the critical points to be observed. When inspections involve the collection and analysis of food samples, company standards must be developed to indicate when corrective action is needed. Such standards should usually be well within the limits set by regulatory agencies. In some cases, microbiological standards not required by regulations will be useful for maintaining high quality and long shelf life of the product. The HACCP system should be used to determine sampling points, frequency of sampling, and types of analyses (see subsequent section on HACCP).

Important aspects of a sanitation program that can be controlled through inspections are (1) checking the precision of instruments and charts used for determining and recording time-temperature treatments, (2) determination of the adequacy of cleaning/sanitizing procedures, (3) adequacy of pest control procedures, (4) adequacy of housekeeping practices throughout the plant, (5) adequacy of personnel cleanliness and training, and (6) adequacy of chemical storage and container labeling procedures. Employee facilities such as washrooms and lunchrooms should be inspected for cleanliness. A common sanitary hazard in food processing plants is disorder and clutter, which makes proper cleaning difficult and provides hiding places for pests.

Rodent and Insect Control. Rodents and insects contaminate food through chewing, depositing urine and feces, and leaving behind filth such as insect parts and rodent hairs. Rodents and insects have the ability to spread pathogenic microorganisms. Prevention or management of animal infestation often requires the services of pest control professionals. Effective control measures include eliminating breeding and hiding areas in the plant vicinity, erecting physical barriers to prevent entrance into the plant, maintaining clean orderly premises, and using pesticides and traps when necessary.

Employee Training and Education. Employee education is the basis of all effective sanitation programs, since sanitation depends on the day-to-day work habits and hygiene of employees. Employees should be taught how to perform their jobs in a sanitary manner and the importance of sanitation to public health and product quality. The plant inspection often offers an excellent opportunity for employee education. Inspections also call the attention of management to areas where additional education and training are needed.

Water Quality. There are two ways in which water quality has an impact on food plant sanitation. First, the water supply can be a source of pathogenic or food spoilage microorganisms. The presence of coliform bacteria is used as an indicator of fecal contamination, since it is not practical to analyze directly for pathogens. Second, the mineral content of water can adversely affect cleaning and sanitizing procedures. Consequently, periodic monitoring of the water supply for coliform bacteria and hardness is usually included in food sanitation programs.

Waste Treatment. Most food processing plants produce large amounts of liquid or solid waste, which must be disposed of in a sanitary manner and in compliance with local regulations. Monitoring of the concentration and quantity of liquid waste, maintenance of waste treatment systems, and sanitary disposal of solid waste should be included in a plant sanitation program.

FOOD PRESERVATION

A major objective of food processing is to delay nutritional and organoleptic deterioration of food so that it can be economically transported and marketed. This objective is achieved by (1) retarding autodecomposition through the inactivation of enzymes, (2) retarding microbial-induced deterioration by reducing cell numbers and growth, (3) retarding chemical deterioration through anaerobic and light-protective packaging, and (4) lessening damage from animal pests through protective packaging and storage procedures.

Some forms of food preservation such as pasteurization and canning are specifically designed to inactivate foodborne pathogens, whereas other processes such as dehydration and refrigeration rely on effective sanitation and eventual cooking of the food to prevent disease transmittal. A gross breakdown in the food preservation system does not usually have public health consequences because lack of preservation most often results in rapid deterioration of the commodity to the point where it cannot be marketed or consumed. Marginally effective processing, however, can have severe public health consequences if spoilage organisms are killed but pathogens survive. For example, low-acid canned foods can be given a marginal heat treatment that preserves the food organoleptically but allows survival and subsequent growth of *C. botulinum*.

The food processing objective of delaying or preventing microbial spoilage also results in protecting the public health because measures that are used to limit the presence and growth of spoilage microorganisms also limit the presence and growth of pathogens and toxin producers. Some pathogens such as *Salmonella* species and *L. monocytogenes* remain relatively unaffected by preservation methods such as dehydration, refrigeration, and freezing. Consequently, when relying on these preservation methods, precautions must be taken to prevent entry of pathogens into the food product. This is especially important for foods such as nonfat dried milk and salad vegetables that might not be cooked before consumption.

Pasteurization

Pasteurization is a mild heat treatment (under 100° C) designed to inactivate pathogens and heat-sensitive spoilage microorganisms while minimizing changes in organoleptic quality. Foods high in acid, alcohol, or sugar (such as juices, fruit preserves, and beer) are pasteurized mainly to increase shelf life. Pasteurization of milk and eggs is designed to eliminate pathogens, although a longer shelf life is also obtained.

Both milk and shelled eggs must be pasteurized before entering interstate commerce because of the high risk of disease transmission associated with the raw products. Minimum acceptable time-temperature treatments are based on the destruction of *Coxiella burnetii* in milk and *Salmonella* species in eggs. Pasteurization of eggs involves a minimal heat treatment because of the susceptibility of egg white to coagulation. The recommended treatment of 56.7° C for 3 1/2 minutes for egg white will result in a 1000-fold to 10,000-fold decrease in viable salmonellae.[101] Normal contamination is usually less than one organism per gram, so there is a substantial safety factor in this recommendation. Chemical additives such as metal salts and polyphosphates and pH adjustment can be used to increase heat sensitivity of the salmonellae and reduce the severity of the required heat treatment. Additives are necessary to restore the whipping properties of the egg white after pasteurization.[102]

Milk Pasteurization. The two most widely used methods for pasteurizing fluid milk products are the low-temperature-long-time (LTLT), or holding, method and the high-temperature-short-time (HTST), or continuous, method. The minimum LTLT treatment for milk is 63° C for 30 minutes. This treatment is used when small quantities of product are to be pasteurized. The minimum HTST treatment is 72° C for 15 seconds. This treatment is usually accomplished using a continuous flow plate heat exchanger, which includes a heating section where warm milk is heated to pasteurization temperature, a holding tube in which heated milk is kept for the required time, a regenerative section in which the cold raw milk is warmed by the hot pasteurized milk, and a cooling section where the warm pasteurized milk from the regenerative section is cooled to 4° C or lower (Fig. 34–2).

Other parts that are essential for legal operation of an HTST system are a flow diversion valve, a float control tank, and a timing pump (Figs. 34–2 and 34–3). The flow diversion valve is a temperature-controlled three-way valve installed at the outlet of the holding tube. If milk flowing through this valve is at or above pasteurization temperature, it flows through the valve to the regenerative section for cooling. If the fluid is below pasteurization temperature, it is automatically diverted to the float control tank for repasteurization. The float control tank utilizes a float valve to maintain raw milk at a constant supply level and thus provides consistent fluid pressure to the system. A positive displacement timing pump provides constant flow through the system. Flow rate is critical, since the length of the holding tube is set to provide the required holding time at a specific flow rate. Continuous monitoring and recording of holding tube temperature is required for all milk pasteurization systems.

HTST systems have proven effective in inactivating pathogens in fluid milk products with minimal changes in flavor and nutritional value. Even relatively heat resistant pathogens such as *L. monocytogenes* are inactivated by the treatment.[103] Pasteurized milk is occasionally implicated as a vehicle for foodborne illness. The source of *S. typhimurium* in a large milk-associated outbreak in Illinois was never determined.[104] In an earlier outbreak, the implicated pasteurized milk contained the same strain of *S. typhimurium* as the raw milk.[105] Whether contamination resulted from inadequate heat processing or recontamination could not be determined. In an outbreak of listeriosis associated with milk the contaminating strain was also isolated from raw milk, but no processing deficiencies were observed.[66] *L. monocytogenes* has been recovered from pasteurized ice cream products, but it is believed to occur as a result of postpasteurization contamination.[64]

Blanching

Blanching is a mild heat treatment applied to fruits and vegetables prior to preservation by freezing, drying, or canning. Hot water or steam are used as heating media. Blanching before drying or freezing inactivates tissue enzymes that would cause flavor, color, and nutritional deterioration during storage. Unwanted changes in texture caused by blanching of fruits can be avoided by using chemical inactivation of enzymes, antioxidants, or sugar syrups to prevent oxidation. Blanching prior to canning is not necessary to inactivate enzymes, but it removes dissolved gases and wilts tissue to facilitate packing. Blanching can reduce microbial content by as much as 99%.[106] Blanching is not a reliable method for eliminating pathogens from food.

Canning

Canning is a method of preserving foods by heating in hermetically sealed cans or pouches so that all pathogenic and toxin-forming organisms and all organisms capable of growing in the food at room temperature are inactivated. Canned foods are "commercially sterile" in the sense that there may be a small number of heat-resistant viable spores in the product that do not germinate and grow under normal storage conditions. Canned foods are classified as acid (pH < 4.6) and low acid (pH > 4.6). Canning processes for low-acid foods are of public health concern because spores of *C. botulinum* can germinate and grow in these foods. Low-acid foods such as beans, corn, beets, tuna, salmon, mushrooms, and pot pies are known to be naturally contaminated with spores of *C. botulinum*. Although *C. botuli-*

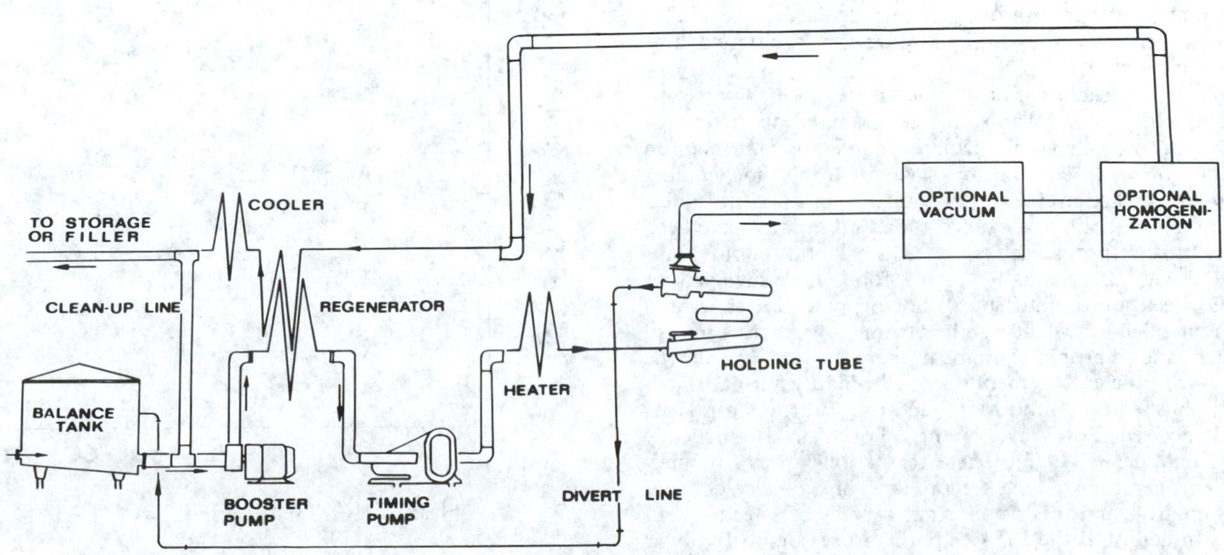

Figure 34-2. Diagram of a high-temperature–short-time milk pasteurization system.

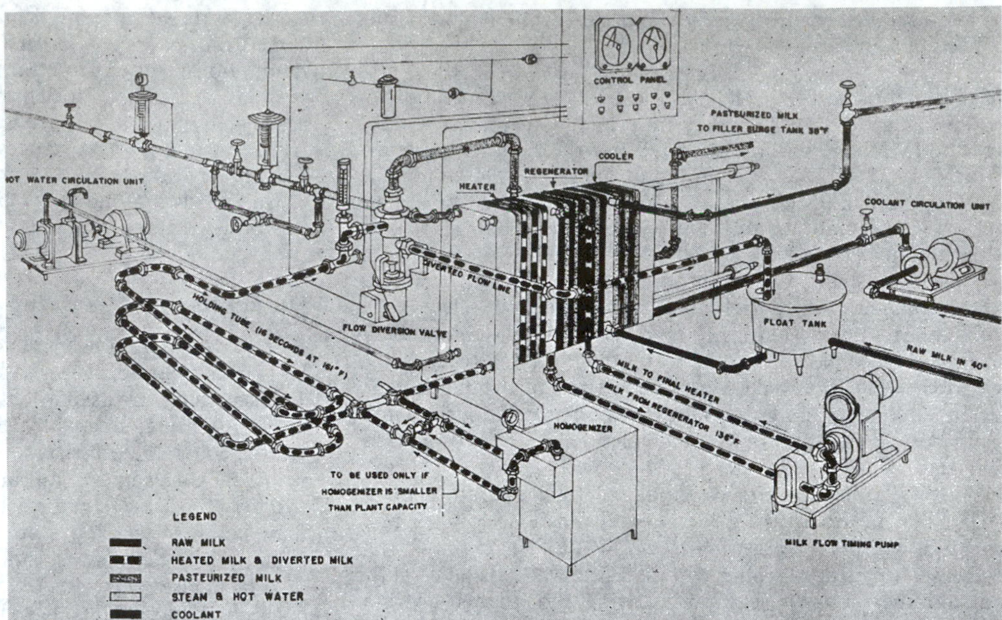

Figure 34-3. Schematic flow through HTST pasteurization equipment. *[Courtesy Delaval Separation Co., Poughkeepsie, New York.]*

num is a gas producer, cans may become toxic without noticeable swelling or off-flavor development.[107]

The critical points of the canning process are the heat treatment and the can seal. The heat treatment for low-acid foods must be severe enough to inactivate all spores of *C. botulinum.* Heat destruction of bacteria and their spores follows a logarithmic death curve (Fig. 34-4). This means that if 1 minute of exposure at a given temperature destroys 90% of a bacterial population, the next minute will destroy 90% of the remaining population, and so on. The "D" value (decimal reduction time) is defined as the time in minutes required to reduce a bacterial population by 90% at a given temperature. Commercial canners use a 12 D heat treatment based on the heat resistance of either *C. botulinum* or a more heat-resistant spoilage organism such as *Clostridium sporogenes* (PA 3679) or *Bacillus stearothermophilus* (FS 1518). If the product contained 1 million *C. botulinum* spores per can before processing (an unusually high number), the 12 D treatment would decrease the population to one viable spore in 1 million cans (a 12 log reduction). Heat processes are calculated for specific products in specific containers. Any change in product composition, pH, particle size, filling weight, or container size and shape may require that a different heat treatment be used.

Even if the heat treatment is adequate, faulty can seams may negate the process by allowing recontamination. After processing, canned foods are immediately cooled by immersion in cold water. Since the can develops vacuum at this time, cooling water will be sucked in if there are faulty seams. Cases of botulism from consumption of canned tuna and salmon have been attributed to postprocess leakage.[108] Other botulism outbreaks associated with commercially canned foods have involved vichyssoise (leek and potato soup), hot pepper, beef stew, and mushrooms. These incidents resulted from faulty process control equipment and improper equipment operation. As a result, the FDA initiated the enforcement of Good Manufacturing Practices, as published in "Good Manufacturing Practices for Thermally Processed Low-Acid Canned Foods in Hermetically Sealed Containers" (1973). These regulations specify requirements for operator training, record keeping, quality control, process control, and other important aspects of effective processing. In addition, the FDA requires processors to file their heat treatments and to report any spoilage or processing abnormalities that could have a negative impact on public health.

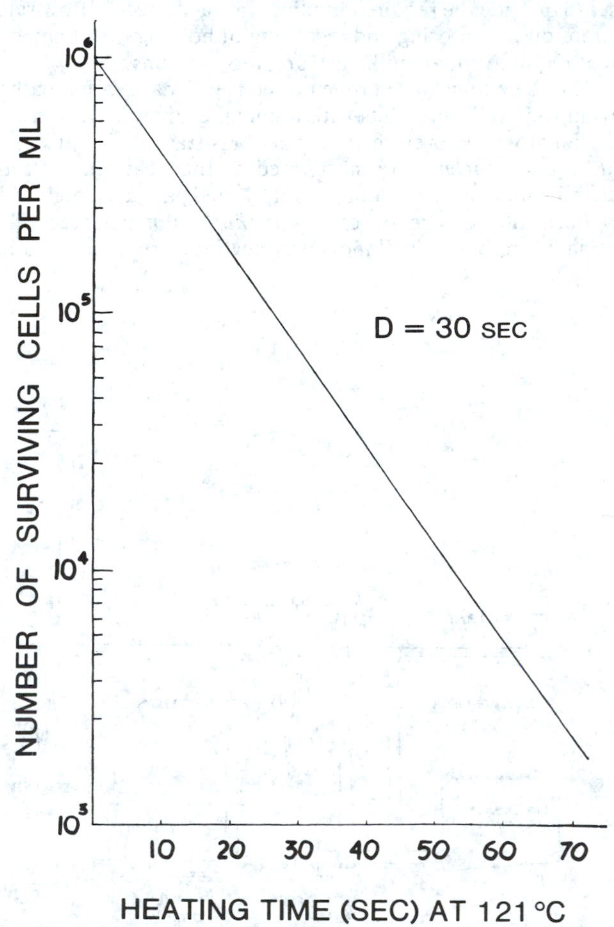

Figure 34-4. Typical heat inactivation curve for a bacterial population.

Botulism outbreaks involving commercial foods receive much media attention and are important because of the potential involvement of a large number of consumers. Since 1899, however, 72% of botulism outbreaks have been traced to home processed foods and only 9% to commercially processed foods.[109]

More food products are being heat processed in bulk by continuous flow sterilization and then aseptically packaged in cans, cartons, or pouches. This type of processing often results in improved quality over traditional canning because a less severe heat process is required. Milk can be processed in this manner by utilizing temperatures of about 140° C and holding times of only a few seconds. Commercially sterile, aseptically packaged foods require stringent processing and quality control to prevent underprocessing or posttreatment contamination. No health hazard has been associated with these foods.

Refrigeration

Maintaining foods at temperatures below 15° C without freezing delays deterioration and involves minimal damage to the food; however, this delay may be only a few days to a few weeks. Fruits and vegetables are still "alive" after harvest. Refrigeration slows tissue metabolism in these foods and thus maintains nutritional value, the living tissue's natural resistance to microbial spoilage, and the organoleptic qualities associated with freshness. The refrigeration of animal carcasses slows anaerobic respiration of the muscle tissue and results in improved tenderness and juiciness. Refrigeration of fresh meats is especially important for delaying microbial spoilage and autodegradation. Physiologically inactive foods such as milk and fresh juices are refrigerated to delay microbial spoilage and oxidative deterioration. The safety of refrigerated foods that are consumed fresh is assured only by preventing contamination with pathogenic organisms from harvest to retail.

Home refrigerators are usually set at 4° to 7° C. Psychrotrophic (cold-tolerant) bacteria will grow in food held at these temperatures, leading to spoilage. Most refrigerated food spoilage problems are caused by aerobic, gram-negative organisms, unless the food is stored under low oxygen conditions as with modified atmosphere packaging. Only a few foodborne pathogens will grow at refrigeration temperatures. These include *L. monocytogenes, Y. enterocolitica,* and *C. botulinum* type E. The potential for growth of these organisms in precooked and minimally processed refrigerated foods is currently of concern to regulatory and industry food microbiologists.[110]

Freezing

Freezing foods to below −10° C results in complete inhibition of microbial growth. The freezing process itself usually results in a decrease in microbial numbers, although the extent of this effect is highly variable. The rate of freezing and thawing has a major influence on microbial survival because most inactivation occurs between −1° and −5° C.[106] At temperatures maintained during frozen storage (−15° to −20° C), inactivation of pathogenic bacteria is slow; consequently, one cannot rely on freezing to eliminate bacterial pathogens from foods. Freezing can produce sublethal injury of bacteria, with the result that it is possible to underestimate numbers when conventional microbiological enumeration techniques are used. Sublethally injured pathogens can recover and regain their pathogenicity when growth conditions become favorable.[111] Since freezing has a negligible effect on survival of spores, outgrowth of *C. botulinum* can occur if thawed foods are mishandled. Microbial toxins present in foods are not significantly affected by frozen storage.

Freezing can be used to eliminate animal parasites including protozoa, cestodes, and nematodes from foods. Frozen storage times and temperatures have been determined for eliminating *Toxoplasma gondii,* larvae of *Trichinella spiralis,* and cysts of *Taenia saginata* from foods.[112] Holding times are generally in the range of 1 to 20 days at −10° to −20° C. Pork to be used in uncooked, cured sausages can be frozen at −15° C or lower for 20 days or more to achieve the destruction of *T. spiralis.*

Dehydration

Many foods including milk, eggs, fruits, and vegetables are sometimes preserved by dehydration. Weight and volume reduction through water removal is economically beneficial when high-moisture foods must be stored or transported or when a long shelf life is required. Although dehydration will inactivate many food pathogens, salmonellae, listeriae, and staphylococci can be expected to survive in stored dried foods. Staphylococcal enterotoxin also survives the drying process, even though the cells that produced the toxin may be inactivated.[113] The dehydrated foods most often associated with disease outbreaks are milk and egg products, since they are often rehydrated and consumed without further heat treatment. Ungutted dried fish have recently been implicated in an international outbreak of type E botulism.[114]

The modern method of drying milk produces a superior product by subjecting the milk to a minimal amount of heat through spray drying and then preparing a powder for reconstitution as "instant" milk by remoistening and redrying. But this process provides greater opportunity for the survival and growth of salmonellae and staphylococci than does the old drum drying process. Instances of staphylococcal food poisoning from dried milk have resulted from holding concentrated milk at temperatures that permit microbial growth with resultant toxin formation before dehydration.[45,115] Contamination of milk with *Salmonella* species can occur at various points after preheating (pasteurization). Air contamination can be a major problem since large volumes of air are used during spray drying. Dust and milk powder contaminated by rodents, birds, and insects can become airborne sources of *Salmonella* species. Improperly maintained or ineffective air filters may not remove these contaminants.[90] Milk solids may accumulate in the "instantizing" chamber, where enough moisture exists to support bacterial growth. Contamination of milk powder with *Salmonella* species can be prevented through pasteurization, holding concentrated milk at 65° C or above, preventing buildup of milk residue on product contact surfaces, effective filtration of drying air, and protecting the dried product from moisture.[45] The USDA detected *Salmonella* contamination in up to 1.9% of product samples tested between 1970 and 1978.[116] Outbreaks of salmonellosis traced to powdered milk consumption were reported in 1966 and 1979.[45]

Nondairy Food Fermentations

Bread, pickles, certain sausages, wine, and beer are all produced by fermentation. In these foods the microbial conversion of sugar into either acids or ethanol and carbon dioxide is essential in converting the raw product to the traditional food. In foods such as pickles, fermented sausages, sauerkraut, wine, and beer the fermentation process also acts as a preservative. With the exception of some fermented sausages, foodborne illness is not a problem with these foods because of the high acid or alcohol content of the products.

Manufacture of dry and semidry sausages of the salami or cervelat type involves an incubation period in which a lactic acid fermentation lowers the pH of the meat to 4.2 to 5.0.[117] Naturally occurring lactobacilli or added *Pediococcus cerevisiae* are responsible for the fermentation. If fermentation conditions are not adequately controlled and the pH is not promptly lowered, staphylococci may grow on the sausage surface. This was apparently the case in a 1979 outbreak of staphylococcal food poisoning. The safety of fermented sausages is difficult to evaluate, since staphylococci may die off during the typical 1-month to 20-month curing period and leave the enterotoxin behind at random locations on the sausage surface.[118]

Dairy Fermentations

The manufacture of cultured dairy products typically involves addition of multiple cultures of lactic acid bacteria to pasteurized milk or cream. Lactose in the milk is converted to lactic acid and—depending on the particular culture—other acids and low molecular weight compounds. The ability of dairy industry starter cultures to inactivate and inhibit growth of pathogenic bacteria varies with culture strain, inoculation level, and incubation temperature. Inhibitory effects of lactic acid bacteria result not only from lactic acid production but also from production of acetic and formic acid, hydrogen peroxide, and antibiotics.[119] Cultured milk and cream products such as yogurt, buttermilk, and sour cream offer little opportunity for pathogen survival because of their low pH (4.0 to 4.7).

In contrast to cultured milks, cheese products have been implicated in various outbreaks of foodborne disease. If cheese is made from raw milk, pathogens present in the milk are trapped in the curd. They may multiply during manufacture and survive in the finished product. USDA regulations state that raw milk cheese must be held at least 60 days before sale to provide for sufficient pathogen inactivation. However, this holding time does not ensure a product free of microbial toxins or viable pathogens.[90] Consumption of raw milk cheese has resulted in cases of brucellosis, salmonellosis, and staphylococcal food poisoning. A recent outbreak of listeriosis resulted when cheese sold as made from pasteurized milk was actually manufactured in part from raw milk.[65] This outbreak resulted in over 100 fatalities. After a thorough review of the literature, Keough[90] concluded that even after 120 days of storage there is an unjustifiable risk involved in the consumption of raw milk cheese.

Cheese made from pasteurized milk is occasionally involved in disease outbreaks as a result of faulty pasteurization or, more commonly, recontamination during manufacture, curing, or packaging. Antibiotic or bacteriophage contamination of milk often results in slow acid production by the starter culture, providing an opportunity for growth and toxin production by staphylococci.[67] When acid production is delayed by washing curd during manufacture of certain varieties, the cheese is susceptible to coliform growth.[120] In one survey of soft and semisoft cheeses, 17% were found to contain over 10,000 fecal coliforms per gram.[121] The pH of surface-ripened cheeses such as Brie and Limburger can increase to such an extent during ripening that foodborne pathogens can grow.[122] The potential hazard was revealed by an outbreak of enteropathogenic *E. coli* illness associated with imported Camembert cheese.[123] In this case, polluted water was probably the source of contamination. In recent years there have been several recalls of imported surface-ripened cheeses because of contamination with *L. monocytogenes,* although no outbreaks were reported. An outbreak of salmonellosis associated with Cheddar cheese was notable for its widespread occurrence and for the very low numbers of salmonellae found in the cheese.[124] The high fat and protein content of cheese appear to protect the organisms from destruction in the digestive tract, resulting in an infective dose as low as 100 organisms.

Chemical Preservatives

Chemical preservatives are added to foods to prevent microbial or chemical deterioration. Common preservatives include organic and inorganic acids, antioxidants, and chelating agents. Sugar and salt are the most common chemical preservatives. Sugar, usually in the form of sucrose or corn syrup (glucose), inhibits microbial growth by reducing available water and oxidation by acting as a barrier to oxygen. Salt also preserves foods by binding free water. A single chemical is seldom used as the sole method of preservation. Pickles are preserved through the combined effects of salt, acid, and refrigeration or pasteurization. Sausages can be preserved through the combined effects of salt, sugar, nitrite, and refrigeration. The combined effect of multiple preservatives utilizes what is known as the hurdle concept.[125] Each preservative treatment acts as a hurdle that organisms must clear to grow. Even if one hurdle is not sufficient for preservation, additional hurdles can be utilized to prevent growth and provide a safe food. This concept is of particular importance in its application to refrigerated foods because pathogens such as *L. monocytogenes* and *Y. enterocolitica* can grow in most foods if refrigeration is the only preservative.

Concern about the health effects of various chemical preservatives has led to the reformulation of some foods to decrease the use of certain preservatives. Levels of salt and sugar have been reduced in many foods, and nitrite has been reduced or eliminated in many cured meats. Care must be taken that a reduction in the use of "undesirable" chemical preservatives does not lead to an increased risk of foodborne illness. The controversy over eliminating nitrates and nitrites provides a good example of this problem. Nitrites and the nitrosamine compounds formed from nitrite when food is heated have been found to be mutagenic and carcinogenic. Product reformulation has led to the near elimination of nitrosamine formation in all cured meats except bacon, which when fried may contain less than 10 ppb.[126] Restricting the use of nitrites, however, could have increased the risk of botulism because nitrite is the major inhibitor of *C. botulinum* growth in cured meats. Combinations of other botulinum inhibitors such as ascorbic acid, sorbic acid, sodium hypophosphite, and lactic cultures are used as compensation for reduced nitrite levels to provide for a safe product.[127]

Sodium and potassium salts of sulfite, bisulfite, and metabisulfite are used in the food industry as enzyme and microbial inhibitors. Sulfite residues in foods have caused respiratory distress in asthmatics and gastrointestinal upset and other symptoms in sensitive individuals.[128,129] Consequently the use of sulfiting agents throughout the food industry and by restaurants has been severely restricted. Ascorbic and citric acids are good substitutes for sulfites for some uses such as maintaining freshness of cut vegetables in food service salad bars.

Chemical preservatives intentionally added to foods either are classified as food additives whose use is restricted by the FDCA, or are classified by the FDA as GRAS substances whose use is restricted by FDA-published Good Manufacturing Practices.

Irradiation

Ionizing radiation can destroy spoilage and pathogenic organisms in foods without causing adverse organoleptic or nutritional changes.[130] Since only a small rise in temperature occurs during the process, quality characteristics of the raw unprocessed food are retained. Mild irradiation treatments can be used as a form of pasteurization to improve shelf life and inactivate pathogens and parasites. This low-dose treatment is called "radurization" if food spoilage bacteria are the primary target or "radicidation" if a specific pathogen is the major target. High-dosage irradiation for producing "commercial sterility" is not in common use.

Irradiation at doses for pasteurization-type treatments (under 1 mrad) produces virtually no organoleptically detectable changes in the food.[131] A major criticism of irradiation food processing is that the chemical products resulting from the treatment may be toxic; however, a joint FAO-IAEA-WHO report[132] addressing this issue concluded that any food irradiated with an average dose of 1 mrad or less is wholesome and should be approved for human consumption without the need for additional toxicological testing. Commercially feasible applications using this dosage include control of sprouting in potatoes and onions, control of insect infestation in rice, wheat, and other grains, prolonging the shelf life and reducing pathogen contamination of fresh fish and poultry, delaying ripening and controlling insect damage in fruits, and the destruction of *Trichinella* and *Salmonella* in fresh meat.

Irradiation of poultry, wheat, wheat flour, potatoes, spices, natural flavorings, and dehydrated seasonings is approved by the FDA. Irradiation is considered by regulatory agencies to be a food additive rather than a processing treatment. Consequently, each application must meet stringent criteria for safety as outlined in food additive regulations. This approach greatly increases the expense of obtaining regulatory approval. In addition, public acceptance of irradiated foods presents an important barrier to their use. People may believe such foods to be radioactive or otherwise unsafe. Irradiation of foods has been studied for over 40 years. The process has been found to pose no threat to human health, to pose no special microbiological problems, and to produce foods of high nutritional quality.[130,133] Irradiation of foods may actually prove beneficial to public health by allowing decreased use of pesticides and fumigants of questionable toxicity such as the now-banned ethylene dibromide that was used to treat grains, cereals, and fruits.

FOOD SERVICE SANITATION

Sanitation measures applied to food service must be dynamic enough to stay abreast of the changing processes and equipment in food service if public health problems are to be minimized. The continued occurrence of foodborne illnesses is due in part to changes in the food service industry but also to changes in the public's life-style and eating habits. These changes have resulted in a more diversified food service industry, including fast-food service, delicatessens, and other carryout operations, cafeterias, and complete service restaurants. The increased mobility of a growing population, women in the work force and school-aged children away from the home results in more meals eaten out and a growing number of food service establishments. This increases the potential for greater numbers of foodborne illness outbreaks. In spite of this increased risk the number of outbreaks reported nationally is undoubtedly much lower than actually occurs.[134] The symptoms of foodborne intoxications or foodborne infections may be severe but are usually transient in nature. Consequently the victim fails to have his condition diagnosed, contributing to the underreporting of foodborne diseases.

Sanitation in food processing, preparation, and service plays an integral part in the control of foodborne disease agents.[135] A thorough understanding of basic sanitation principles and the epidemiological characteristics of the important foodborne disease agents is essential if measures to prevent foodborne illness are to be successful.

Plan Review

State and local ordinances include requirements for plan reviews of food service establishments. This requirement is intended as a safeguard to ensure that all aspects of sanitation are addressed in the construction or remodeling of a structure. Plan reviews provide the regulator with a layout, arrangement, and construction materials of all work areas in a facility. The location, type, size, and installation information of all fixed equipment should be supplied and approved by the health authority before any work is done. Once approved, the establishment in question must be constructed or converted according to the approved plans and specifications. Similar recommendations appear in the Food Service Sanitation Manual published by the Department of Health and Human Services.[136]

Personnel Training

Since employees are one of the major sources of contamination in food service, the health and personal hygiene of employees is of paramount importance in a sanitation program designed to protect food against contamination. An employee showing little or no outward sign of an illness may still transmit a disease agent. Therefore, any employee who is affected with a respiratory infection, or who has an infected wound or lesion, or who is infected with any disease that may be communicable through food should not be working in any capacity in food service if this could result in food contamination or contamination of food contact surfaces.[136] The recommendation appears in one form or another in most states' regulations for food service.

It is the responsibility of food service managers and supervisors to see that no employee infected with any communicable disease works in an area where food might be contaminated (or other employees infected) and that they are not allowed to return until the communicable period for the disease has passed. This judgment may be difficult to make because an infected worker may not show signs of illness. Therefore, it is essential that food handlers be adequately educated and conscious about the consequences of poor judgment in this regard. Employees can be motivated through education to realize that strict sanitation standards should prevail over other considerations. They must have an appreciation of the relationship of good personal hygiene to the total food sanitation effort. It is the responsibility of managers and supervisors to instill in workers a health consciousness and an understanding of the basics of good health and healthful practices.

In 1971 the National Conference on Food Protection recommended that knowledge of safe food handling practices should be disseminated to all food handlers and especially management personnel. The FDA developed such a program with several states; its objectives were to (1) increase significantly the level of consumer food protection by having certified management personnel, (2) promote a more cooperative effort between the regulatory agency and the food service industry in meeting sanitation requirements, (3) conduct a series of food service training courses to certify those persons competent in food protection, and (4) see that this training resulted in reciprocity between regulatory agencies and within the food service industry. The FDA then recommended uniform, national food service sanitation training.

The FDA developed uniform subject matter and recommended minimum instruction time for management training courses (15 contact hours). Training covers food, food protection methods, and foodborne diseases; facilities, sanitation, water and waste disposal, cleaning and sanitizing, nonfood supplies, and physical facilities; foodhandlers, personal hygiene, food handling practices, and operational problems; and management, motivation, personnel training, and self-inspection techniques. Certification is for a period of 5 years.

By 1983 a large number of manager training programs had been conducted in the United States. Thirty-one states offered one or more manager training programs that met the uniform, national recommended criteria. Training was sponsored by government organizations (local, state, and federal), industry organizations, and academic institutions.[137] Nineteen states reported no training programs. Reciprocity with other training programs varied from state to state, and mandatory manager certification varied with the particular jurisdiction. In 1985 the FDA began offering a certification examination for food service managers. A recent survey indicated that 3 states have statewide mandatory certification programs, 17 have voluntary programs, and 20 states now have local jurisdictions with certification programs.[138] Longree[139] presents an excellent volume on manager-employee responsibilities in food service training and sanitation.

Personal Hygiene

The food handler is the ultimate source of health consciousness. It is imperative that employees observe strict habits of personal hygiene while they work and whenever their work activities are interrupted. When the food handler temporarily leaves work, he must thoroughly wash his hands with soap and water before returning. This should be done after eating, drinking, smoking, or using the toilet. If the person sneezes or coughs, the nose and mouth should be covered to prevent direct contamination of foods or food contact surfaces. Specific regulations state that employees shall thoroughly wash their hands and the exposed portions of their arms with soap and warm water before starting work, during work as often as necessary to keep them clean, and after smoking, eating, drinking, or using the toilet. To achieve this, toilet facilities must be adequate in number and properly located and maintained. They should be located to permit convenient use by all employees in food preparation areas and utensil-washing areas. The lavatories should be accessible to employees at all times, located in or immediately adjacent to rest rooms, and adequately supplied with soap, towels or a hand dryer, and wastebaskets. Sinks used for food preparation or for washing equipment or utensils should not be used for hand washing. The lavatories and all related fixtures should be clean and in good repair. Employees shall keep their fingernails clean and trimmed because these can also contaminate food.[136]

Employees working in and individuals entering a food service area must use hair and beard restraints. Hair has been shown to be an excellent harborage for microorganisms, so precautions must be taken to avoid having hair fall into the food. Employees should always keep their hair clean and neat as well.

The clothing of food service employees can be important in the prevention of food contamination. The outer garments of all employees should be neat and reasonably clean. Most regulations do not specifically require special clothing to be worn while engaged in food service; however, it is often preferable to wearing street clothing. If special clothing is required, then facilities to store both work and street clothing should be available in dressing rooms separate from toilet facilities and kept clean and sanitary like all other food related areas. It is undesirable to allow workers to wear work clothing home because this may be another source of contamination.

Food Supplies

A variety of national and international as well as state and local agencies are concerned with providing a wholesome food supply for the food service industry. Under the jurisdiction of the United Nations are WHO, the FAO, and the United Nations International Children's Emergency Fund (UNICEF). Although these are not regulatory agencies, they coordinate global health activities ranging from disseminating research information to supporting nutrition, child and infant health, control of communicable disease, and development of food and agriculture programs.

In the United States several agencies are involved directly or indirectly in protecting the food supply and in regulating food sanitation. Within the FDA is the Division of Retail Food Protection, which assists the food service industry in providing safe, wholesome food to the consuming public. This division publishes the "Food Service Sanitation Manual." The FDA also develops national sanitation standards for retail food operations, monitors all foods shipped interstate, and has jurisdiction over food sanitation and related sanitary conditions of all interstate public systems such as airlines, ships, and trains.

The USDA by authority of the meat, poultry products, and egg products inspection acts protects the food supply to food service establishments.[140] The section in this chapter on administration of food sanitation provides additional information on these and other agencies.

State and local authorities are responsible for the daily monitoring of food supplies in food service operations. Their regulations are usually patterned after, and are at least as stringent as, federal standards. State food service regulations are enforced by a variety of agencies.

All food service regulations set criteria for conditions or commodities such as

1. Food shall be in sound condition, free from spoilage, filth, or other contamination, and safe for human consumption.
2. Food shall be obtained from sources that comply with all laws relating to food processing and shall have no information on the label that is false or misleading.
3. The use of food in hermetically sealed containers that was not prepared in a food processing establishment is prohibited.
4. Fluid milk and milk products used or served shall be pasteurized and shall meet the Grade A quality standards as established by law.
5. All baking products shall have been prepared in permitted food service establishments or in an approved food processing establishment.
6. Fresh and frozen shucked shell fish (oysters, clams, or mussels) shall be packed in nonreturnable packages identified with the name and address of the original shell stock processor, shucker-packer, or repacker and with the interstate certification number issued according to law.
7. Only clean whole eggs, with shell intact and without cracks or checks, pasteurized liquid frozen or dry eggs, pasteurized dry egg products, or commercially prepared and packaged hard-boiled, peeled eggs may be used.

These criteria state that food generally, and especially that from potentially hazardous foods, be obtained from sources considered satisfactory. The CDC reports for the years 1978 through 1981 indicate that about 4% of reported outbreaks were associated with food from unapproved sources.

Water Supplies

Nonpotable water can be a vehicle for disease transmission. If unsafe water is used, it can contaminate food, equipment, utensils, and the employees' hands. The use of nonpotable water in a food service establishment is therefore prohibited. During 1984–1985 the CDC reported several incidences of water-related disease outbreaks where the location of the outbreak was a restaurant. These outbreaks were associated with contaminated ice or ground water sources such as wells or springs.[3]

Enough potable water for the needs of the food service establishment must be supplied, under pressure, at the required temperatures for all equipment that uses water and at appropriate temperatures at all fixtures. Water and ice should be provided from approved sources and properly handled, transported, and dispersed to protect the consumer and employee. Hot and cold water is necessary for the proper sanitizing and washing of surfaces, equipment, and utensils and for adequate employee hand washing. Occasionally bottled water must be brought in to a food service establishment. Bottled and packaged potable water must be from an approved source and handled and stored in such a way to protect it from contamination. Bottled water must be dispersed from the original container to avoid contamination. Ice, whether made on premises or transported from some other source, must be made from potable water if it is to be used for human consumption.

Equipment and Utensils

The surfaces of all multi-use equipment and utensils, work areas, and even dining areas must be effectively cleaned and sanitized to minimize the possibility of contamination of foods and thereby transmission of disease to consumers or employees. Therefore, the materials from which equipment and surfaces are constructed, their design and fabrication, where and how they are installed to facilitate cleaning are of great importance. Maintaining these surfaces and equipment in a good state of repair is also imperative in an effective food service sanitation program.

The NSF in Ann Arbor, Michigan, a noncommercial, nonprofit organization, has provided leadership and guidance in the construction, design, and installation of food service equipment.[141] It sponsors research and education programs to establish and disseminate information about standards for equipment and services relating to the food service industry. NSF also brings together regulatory agencies, business and industry, and the consuming public to address concerns about standards for equipment, products, procedures, and services.

NSF recommendations and most food service regulations will contain a statement that multiuse equipment and utensils shall be constructed and repaired with materials that are smooth, corrosion resistant, nontoxic, stable, and nonabsorbent under use conditions and shall not impart an odor, color, or taste or contribute to the adulteration of food. Materials that easily corrode under normal use, chip, crack, or dent may either impart toxic substances to food or provide harborages for microorganisms, especially if the material cannot be adequately cleaned using recommended procedures. Nonfood contact surfaces must be smooth and of corrosion resistant material, or rendered corrosion resistant, or painted. Nonfood contact surfaces may be of lesser concern but should be noncracking, nonchipping, and so on, so that materials will not inadvertently get into food. The use of wood as a food contact surface is discouraged because it will absorb and hold water, easily cut or chip, is difficult to clean and sanitize effectively, and can harbor large numbers of microorganisms. Plastics that under normal use are resistant to scratching, scoring, chipping, decomposition, and distortion and that allow for cleaning and sanitizing are permitted for repeated use.

Design and fabrication considerations for food service equipment stress ease of cleaning, maintenance, and service. Food contact surfaces of equipment should be smooth, free of open seams and internal corners, and easily cleanable. Equipment and surfaces should be accessible without being disassembled, disassembled without use of tools, or easily disassembled with simple tools. Equipment cleaned-in-place should be designed so that all food contact surfaces will be cleaned using the circulating cleaning system, and the system should be self-draining or easily emptied. A discussion of cleaning agents and sanitizers is given under Food Processing in this chapter.

Food service equipment should be located to prevent contamination of food and food contact surfaces and to permit thorough cleaning of the equipment and adjacent surfaces. Equipment should not be exposed to unprotected sewer lines or water lines or located near stairwells. Portable equipment on tables or counters should have clearance between the counter and equipment, which will facilitate cleaning of the equipment and adjacent areas. Floor-mounted equipment should be sealed to the floor or installed on a platform elevated 6 inches for ease of cleaning of the equipment and all adjacent units and walls. Proper installation and location of equipment can reduce the potential for food contamination but may not completely eliminate hazards. CDC reports that for the years 1983 to 1987 approximately 12% of the reported foodborne disease outbreaks were thought to have contaminated equipment as a contributing factor.

Food contact surfaces can be a source of contamination. Surfaces are readily contaminated with *Salmonella, C. perfringens,* and *S. aureus* if they are present. Sanitation of saws, slicing machines, knives, and other contact surfaces is extremely important. Foods of animal origin, which have not been previously processed, should be handled and prepared separately from other foods. The preparation area and equipment should be thoroughly cleaned and sanitized to avoid cross-contamination.

These and other aspects of equipment or utensil sanitation can play an important role in the transmission of disease. Difficult to clean equipment will likely lead to a buildup of food residue, which harbors organisms and also attracts rodents and insects. NSF and FDA recommendations should be thoroughly considered when equipment for food service is being selected.

Food Preparation and Storage

A review of research literature and CDC reports of confirmed foodborne disease outbreaks indicates that unsafe time-temperature relationships are the single most important contributing factor in these episodes. These abuses occur in the transport, storage, preparation, cooking, service, or postcooking storage of foods. The FDA recommendation for the preparation and holding of potentially hazardous food is

> At all times, including while being stored, prepared, displayed, served, or transported, food shall be protected from potential contamination, including dust, insects, rodents, unclean equipment and utensils, unnecessary handling, coughs and sneezes, flooding, drainage, and overhead leakage or overhead drippage from condensation. The temperature of potentially hazardous food shall be 45° F or below or 140° F or above at all times, except as otherwise provided in the ordinance.[136]

Bacteria grow best at or near their optimum temperature for growth. When food is mishandled, it is usually kept at a temperature close to this optimum temperature and long enough to support microbial growth. This handling or storage temperature under certain circumstances may project into the FDA recommended "safe temperature" range and still allow hazardous organisms to survive and even multiply. Bryan[142] has completed several studies on time-temperature relationships in preparation of food for service. Table 34-5 gives the conditions identified as factors contributing to the occurrence of outbreaks of foodborne disease resulting from mishandled foods in the United States. These data indicate that factors most likely to lead to an outbreak include unsafe time-temperature conditions during cooling, cooking, hot holding, and reheating, as well as preparing food a day or more ahead of serving time (coupled with inadequate storage practices). Time-temperature abuses oc-

TABLE 34-5. FACTORS CONTRIBUTING TO CONFIRMED U.S. OUTBREAKS OF FOODBORNE DISEASE RESULTING FROM MISHANDLED FOOD (1983–1987)

Contributing Factors[a]	%
Improper holding temperatures	57.9
Inadequate cooking	25.0
Poor personal hygiene	30.5
Contaminated equipment	23.4
Food from unsafe source	14.7
Other factors	19.5

[a] Factors reported in 47.5% of all confirmed outbreaks.
(From annual summaries, CDC Foodbourne Disease Outbreaks, 1983–1987.)

curred as factors in 82.9% of the confirmed outbreaks in which contributing factors were reported.

Cooking Temperatures

Bryan and McKinley[143] studied roast beef preparation practices in food service establishments for the likelihood of contamination. They evaluated the possibilities of survival or growth of organisms during each stage of operation. Workers' hands were a source of *S. aureus,* samples of raw beef contained both *C. perfringens* and *S. aureus,* and dried beef-jus mix was a source of *C. perfringens.* There were many opportunities for microbial contamination during food service operations. These included handling of raw beef, checking doneness during cooking, carving of meat, trimming, boning, wrapping, and rewrapping. Their data indicated that geometric centers of roasts seldom reached time-temperature values lethal to vegetative foodborne disease bacteria. They determined that vegetative foodborne pathogens could survive in 76% of the geometric centers and on 5% of the surfaces of beef during cooking and that survival of these organisms could occur in 36% of the geometric centers and on 11% of the surfaces of the cooked beef during postoven temperature rise periods.

Three common methods of cooking foods for food service, especially entrees, are the conventional oven, microwave oven, and some forms of slower cooking, including steam-jacketed kettles. Conventional ovens are the most commonly used, and in institutional food preparation, cooking kettles are used to prepare larger quantities. More recently the use of microwave cooking has introduced reduced overall cooking time, brought about energy savings, reduced manpower requirements, and reduced food preparation space. The survival of foodborne disease bacteria in food cooked by these methods as well as by the slow cookers used in many homes has been studied.[144] Data indicated that conventional oven and slow cooking methods resulted in greater cumulative lethal time-temperature effects than did microwave cooking because of the slower heating involved. Microwave heating of nonfluids was quite irregular, while the conventional oven was intermediate and the slow cooking methods most uniform. Postoven temperature rise produced continued decreases in viable cell numbers except for *Streptococcus faecalis,* which increased slightly during holding periods after microwave cooking. Significant temperature differences were demonstrated within meat loaves cooked by different methods, especially microwave. This has important implications because of reheating practices employed in food service.

The FDA recommends that "Potentially hazardous foods requiring cooking shall be cooked to heat all parts of the food to a temperature of at least 140° F." However, U.S. consumer taste preference has dictated that beef is seldom cooked to internal temperatures that would inactivate foodborne pathogens. The required minimum cooking temperature caused significant problems for processors of cooked roast beef and cooked beef because they could not produce a product that possessed the rare beef color that satisfied consumers. Independent laboratories developed alternative roasting procedures that produced a quality, safe product having the desired color. The USDA accepted these alternative cooking time-temperatures, and they appear in the Federal Register 1978.[145]

Surveillance data indicate that meat and poultry and meat-containing entrees are major vehicles in foodborne disease outbreaks. How these items are cooked in food service must be scrutinized. More research should be done to identify factors that play an important role in this phase of food service.

Handling and Cold Storage

How food is handled after cooking is important to its safety. The most important factor contributing to foodborne disease outbreaks is inadequate cooling practices. Unacceptable cooling practices include storing foods in large containers or otherwise in bulk in refrigerators, leaving foods at room temperature for several hours, storing foods in refrigerators at temperatures above recommended levels, unrefrigerated transport of foods in trucks or automobiles, and storage of foods in ovens that are turned off.[146] Inadequate cooling has also been found to be the most frequently identified factor contributing to outbreaks in Canada and in England.

Cooked foods are cooled to prevent growth of microorganisms. Most common foodborne disease organisms will grow very slowly or not at all at temperatures at or below 7° C. Food should be cooled rapidly, which is not possible unless the temperature of the refrigeration unit is much lower than 7° C. FDA recommendations state that "Potentially hazardous food requiring refrigeration after preparation shall be cooled to an internal temperature of 45° F (7° C) or below. Potentially hazardous foods of large quantities shall be rapidly cooled utilizing such methods as shallow pans, agitation, quick chilling or water circulation external to the food container so that the cooling period shall not exceed 4 hours." Bryan and McKinley[143] found that during cooling of cooked roasts 83% of geometric centers of roasts and 79% of surfaces of roasts were kept at incubation temperatures long enough to permit the growth of mesophilic bacteria including *C. perfringens.* The time that food was stored within the 7° to 60° C range frequently exceeded 4 hours and was usually more than 8 hours. When roasts were stored refrigerated in covered pans, both the centers and surfaces cooled very slowly.

Several types of food services such as airline catering establishments, schools, or institutions may require or contract for food preparation off site. Low temperature storage during transport from one site to another is important.[147] Holding foods that should be refrigerated at temperatures above 7° C for a long time may permit the growth of foodborne disease bacteria.

Reheating and Hot Storage of Foods

All hot foods must be maintained at a minimum temperature of 60° C. Cooked foods are often stored on steam tables, under infrared lamps, or in hot air ovens before being served. This practice is appropriate if adequate internal temperatures are maintained, if a uniform temperature is maintained throughout the holding device, and if no power fluctuation or failure occurs during storage. Because food may be held within the incubation range for pathogenic bacteria because of poor operation or design, hot holding can be one of the most hazardous practices in food service. Foods should be cooked to 60° C before being placed in a hot holding device and served reheated, or chilled and adequately reheated if the temperature falls below 55° C.[148]

In a study of cook and chill food service systems, Sawyer and associates[149] evaluated reheating of foods by conduction, convection, and microwave radiation. They found that the internal end temperature of beef loaf did not meet FDA recommendations (> 74° C) for reheated products in 83% of situations observed. Temperature variability of reheated food at its point of service demonstrated a potential for foodborne illness in hospital food service and possibly other food service situations. The practice of hot holding freshly cooked or refrigerated and reheated foods, especially meats, should be avoided if storage extends several hours. Reheated foods should be checked for adequate internal serving temperatures.

Equipment and Utensil Cleaning and Sanitizing

The purpose of cleaning and sanitizing is to inactivate microorganisms and to remove residual soil from equipment surfaces. It is impractical to remove all soil and contaminants, so by definition a sanitizer is an agent that reduces the microbial contaminants on a cleaned surface to safe levels, as determined by public health requirements.

Effective sanitation in food preparation and in food service begins with good management and depends on management to maintain high standards. Effective cleaning and sanitizing involves many factors, including the use of proper detergent, proper sanitizer, and water at appropriate temperatures. Other important factors include those discussed previously such as appropriate materials and design of food service equipment and its proper location and installation.

Dishwashing Machines and Manual Cleaning

Food service regulations contain minimum standards for the cleaning and sanitizing of equipment and utensils by both manual and mechanical means. The objective of cleaning by either method is to remove soil and prevent the accumulation of food residue, which may harbor pathogenic bacteria or toxins. Local and state food regulations generally follow FDA recommendations.[150] Manual cleaning systems should include a sink with not fewer than three compartments for hot detergent washing, rinsing, and sanitizing. Work areas must be provided for adequate precleaning, scraping, or soaking of equipment and utensils. The food contact surfaces of all equipment and utensils should be sanitized using specific procedures, including immersion for at least 30 seconds in water at 77° C, immersion for 1 minute in 50 ppm available chlorine at 24° C, or immersion for 1 minute in 12.5 ppm available iodine (pH 5.0) at 24° C. Other sanitizing agents are permitted as discussed previously in this chapter.

Mechanical cleaning and sanitizing may be done using spray-type or immersion dishwashing machines. Mechanical cleaning must provide adequate water pressure for washing and rinsing. Two types of machines are available: those using hot water for sanitizing and those using chemicals for sanitizing. Hot water sanitizing machines must provide wash water of 60° to 74° C and final rinse water of 74° to 82° C, depending on the design of the machine. Chemical sanitizing machines must provide wash water of at least 49° C, sanitizing rinse water of 24° C, and chemical sanitizer equivalent to the effect of 50 ppm available chlorine as hypochlorite at 24° C for 1 minute. All manual or mechanical cleaning and sanitizing systems need to be kept clean daily and in good repair. The choice of using hot water or chemical sanitizer systems is made based on several considerations including initial cost, operating costs, and ease of operation. The effectiveness of either system is also dependent on design.[151]

FDA has published recommendations for the frequency of cleaning tableware, kitchenware, and food contact surfaces that are to be washed, rinsed, and sanitized after each use. Equipment used on a continuous basis throughout the day for potentially hazardous foods and food contact surfaces of grills, griddles, and similar cooking devices should be cleaned and sanitized at regular intervals. Nonfood contact surfaces should be cleaned as often as necessary to keep equipment free of dust, dirt, and food particles.

Garbage Disposal

A food service establishment generates solid waste ranging from waste unusable food to waste paper and other types of rubbish including boxes and various packaging containers. The proper handling and disposal of this waste is critical to a good sanitation program. Improper disposal is a problem because (1) it causes odors; (2) garbage and refuse is attractive to insects and rodents, providing food and harborage; (3) it can be a source of bacterial contamination of food, utensils, equipment, and food contact surfaces; and (4) it can be a nuisance, making cleaning and sanitation difficult.

Food service regulations largely refer to the storage of garbage in durable, easily cleanable, insect-and rodent-proof containers that do not leak. There should be a sufficient number of containers to hold all garbage, and the containers should be thoroughly cleaned inside and out so that no food, equipment, or food preparation areas are contaminated. Containers stored outside the establishment including dumpsters, compactors, and compactor systems should be easily cleanable, kept covered at all times, and cleaned frequently to minimize insect and rodent attraction. The handling of garbage and other refuse should be done in a manner that avoids any possible contamination of food, equipment, utensils, and hands, prevents attraction of insects and rodents, does not create a nuisance with odor, and is not a hindrance to housekeeping, cleaning, and sanitizing.

Insects and Rodents

Infestation of a food service establishment by insects and rodents is prohibited because they are capable of transmitting diseases to humans through contamination of food and food contact surfaces. Therefore, their control is essential and must be directed first to the prevention of their entry into an establishment. Once insects or rodents gain entrance to an establishment the control program is directed towards eradication methods. Food service regulations are directed toward preventing conditions that attract and provide harborage and prevention of their entry into structures through cracks, crevices, doors, windows, skylights, or other points of entry.

Effective insect and rodent control programs should be carried out by certified professionals. Local health officials should be consulted for approval of methods used for eradication. In all cases, eradication methods should be used that will pose no danger of chemical contamination of food, utensils, and equipment. Information on rodentborne disease control through rodent stoppage is available through the CDC.[152]

Airline Food Service Sanitation

The current trend in civil aviation is for aircraft to be built for greater passenger carrying capacity, with greater speed and range. Consequently a greater number of meals are served to more passengers who are confined for longer periods of time. This trend coupled with increases in international travel to all parts of the globe including areas of poor sanitation has placed a strain on airline food service, water supplies, and waste disposal. More frequent travel into these regions has made sanitation an integral part of all airline and airport operations. The basic principles of sanitation do not change; however, their application becomes more important.

The Inflight Food Service Association, Inc. (IFSA) is a coordinating or consulting agency that assists all commercial airlines in establishing sound sanitation programs and promotes a self-inspection program by the airlines and airline caterers. Its "Airline Catering Sanitation Guide" was used as the foundation for this effort.[153] IFSA's current airline food service personnel training program is focused on HACCP principles and includes manager certification.

Food prepared for consumption on the ground is usually prepared on the premises, a short time before being served, and usually on demand. Airline caterers are burdened with menus many times prepared off premises, many hours before the meal is served, and often hundreds of miles away. Therefore, particular attention must be paid to all aspects of food protection and procedures of operation. Food purchasing, receiving, storage, preparation, holding, delivery, and final service on board the aircraft must be closely monitored. The IFSA recommends that all canned goods and staples be obtained from acceptable food processing plants, that paper goods be received adequately protected, and that all perishable food items including meats, poultry, dairy products, and eggs be from approved sources.

Likewise, bakery products, fruits, and vegetables must meet standards set by the USDA.

Aircraft meals are prepared in kitchens that are either operated by catering concerns, supervised by airline personnel, or directly controlled by the airline itself. Direct control is the best method of ensuring appropriate standards for food quality. Criteria for food preparation facilities have been discussed previously. The same criteria that apply to any totally ground-based food service operation apply to aircraft food service, from physical facilities to standards for food and water supplies, cleaning and sanitation of equipment and utensils, and protection against infestation. Time-temperature combinations for refrigerated, frozen, or hot food storage are critical.

Unique problems arise with the packaging of food, equipment, and utensils for service on board the aircraft and with the transport system from the catering kitchens to the aircraft. Within this food service system, basic food protection assumes even greater significance in the prevention of foodborne illness. Complete meals are often prepared as a tray assembly and stored until heated just prior to service to the passenger. Cold foods are stored refrigerated. Hot foods may be containerized, placed in preheated containers at 60° C while in the kitchen, and held at an appropriate temperature during transport to the aircraft. Containers meant for transport or holding of both hot and cold foods must be inspected regularly. They must be free of defects, which could impair proper temperature control. The proper cold or hot temperature must be maintained at all times. Frozen foods must be quickly cooled to a storage temperature of −18° C to minimize moisture loss. Blast freezers are usually used, and a vapor-proof cover to all meal trays is used to help reduce water loss. These foods should remain frozen until thawed for service.

All vehicles used to transport food should be fabricated of an approved material. This includes the doors, walls, ceilings, and floors. If kitchens are located some distance from the airport, vehicles should be refrigerated. This is especially critical in tropical areas. After food and equipment is loaded aboard the aircraft, these same vehicles are often used to remove dirty equipment, waste, and surplus food; therefore, vehicle sanitation is very important. They should be cleaned and sanitized daily.

The galleys of aircraft vary with the size and type of aircraft. They provide facilities for storage of cold, hot, or reheated meals (Fig. 34–5). Dairy products and cold food items are stored at < 7° C. These units might operate at higher temperatures, so cold meals should be served early in the flight. Hot meals on short flights should be stored in heat retaining ovens and served early in a flight. Hot meals served later in a flight are usually refrigerated or frozen and reheated in conventional or microwave ovens.

Microwave ovens provide the unique capacity of thawing and heating frozen meals in a very short period of time. Hot meals can be stored frozen and reheated in a matter of seconds. This capacity avoids the hazard of relatively long storage in heat retaining ovens, which might produce conditions favorable for the growth of pathogenic bacteria. Additional safety is provided if hot meals are always served soon after take-off.

Aircraft galleys should be constructed of materials and designed to facilitate cleaning and sanitation. Adequate solid waste receptacles should be provided, and all used utensils and equipment, food waste, and surplus food should be removed and replaced with fresh meals and equipment for each flight. Solid waste should not be off-loaded in the same transport vehicle used to load fresh equipment and food into the aircraft. The crew should observe the aircraft for indications of infestation. The presence of insects usually indicates a food source. Measures should be taken to ensure their elimination.

Flight attendants serving food to passengers should observe the same food handling and sanitary practices as in any ground-based food service operation. Attention to personal hygiene is essential. Attendants must have clean hands, clean clothes, and handle food and utensils in a sanitary manner. Eating utensils should be prepackaged.

The flight crew is usually required to eat different meals if they are consumed a few hours before a flight. Likewise, if a meal or meals is to be consumed in flight, it is essential that the pilot and copilot be given different menus from different food sources. This is an absolute safety measure to protect against the possibility of a foodborne illness. Dire problems could result should the entire crew become ill during a flight. Flight kitchen personnel and flight attendants must be made aware of this precaution.

A survey of food preparation practices of several airline ca-

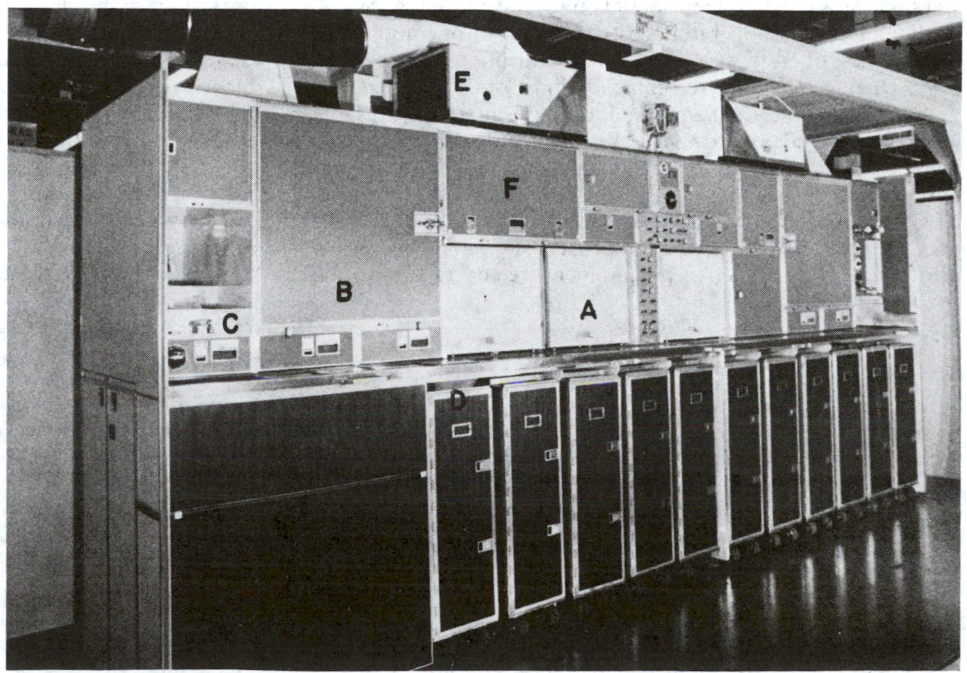

Figure 34–5. Aircraft galley. *A.* Conventional ovens (3). *B.* Refrigerator-freezers (2). *C.* Water supply. *D.* Meal carts (11). *E.* Air chillers for meal carts. *F.* Miscellaneous storage.

terers indicated that generally safe foods are provided. However, had some of the foods been contaminated, pathogens would have survived cooking and reheating and multiplied excessively during meal storage.[147] Indeed, outbreaks of foodborne illnesses do occasionally affect airline passengers and crew. Airline-associated incidences occur infrequently, largely because of the short-haul nature of most flights. If the incubation period of the illness exceeds a flight's duration, the passengers will have proceeded to their destinations, and any epidemiological follow-up is lost. On long flights staphylococcal intoxication has been reported on numerous occasions. Also, cases of *V. parahaemolyticus* gastroenteritis, salmonellosis, shigellosis, and noncholera vibrio gastroenteritis have been reported.

The CDC reported an outbreak in February 1975 in which almost 200 passengers and crew aboard a flight from Tokyo to Paris experienced vomiting, diarrhea, and abdominal cramps on stopping in Copenhagen.[154] Ham served on board had been prepared by a food handler with an infected lesion. The ham was held at room temperature 6 hours during preparation, held 14 hours at 10° C as a part of the tray assembly, and held 8 hours on board the aircraft at room temperature before being heated and served. Enterotoxin positive *S. aureus* of identical phage type was isolated from the cook's lesion, patient feces, vomitus, and leftover ham samples.

Staphylococcal intoxication has often been implicated in airline foodborne illness in part because of its short incubation period, but other foodborne illnesses have also caused problems. In 1976 passengers to Australia succumbed to *V. parahaemolyticus* gastroenteritis after consuming prawns prepared in Asia. In another incident, typhoid was contracted by six passengers traveling to Australia. Water taken aboard in an Asian country was implicated as the source of the infection.

The FDA found an increasing number of regulation deficiencies while inspecting over 2000 commercial flights from 1983 to 1985. In 1983, only 1% of airplanes monitored had food improperly prepared or stored, while in 1985 this number was 6%. The problem seems to be an airline catering problem, not an airline problem. A major outbreak of salmonellosis occurred in 1984 that affected an estimated 2700 passengers flying to the United States on 29 flights. One hundred eighty-six cases on these flights to 11 cities were confirmed.

In 1985 an outbreak of illness among cruise ship passengers involved 29 individuals of which 23 had flown to the embarkation port aboard two flights of the same commercial airline. Data indicated a relationship between the airline and the cruise ship aboard which the illness occurred. A snack of a pork and cheese sandwich was served aboard both flights, which were catered by the same facility. Interviewed passengers from both flights indicated consumption of the sandwich was significantly associated with illness. Passengers indicated the sandwich was cold, had no taste, or tasted "funny." While this outbreak occurred aboard a cruise vessel, its cause originated with food from a commercial airline. This episode emphasizes the complexity of today's public transportation network and the importance of immediate and complete follow-up in data collection in these events.[155]

Outbreaks aboard aircraft usually arise from food being held at improper temperatures after preparation and while on board the airplane. Unfortunately, airline food service has problems associated with the transport system, limiting space and weight restrictions, facilities for storage, reheating, or cooling. It is especially important that flight crews be given adequate training in basic food sanitation and be knowledgeable of the basic epidemiology of foodborne illnesses. A WHO publication by Bailey[156] thoroughly reviews health considerations of global air travel and application of measures for sanitary control at airports and aboard aircraft. Also available is a handbook on airline sanitation from the U.S. Public Health Service.[157]

Cruise Ship Sanitation

Shipboard food sanitation and food service, in contrast to aircraft catering, more nearly parallels food service in ground-based operations. Most cruise vessels serve luxurious meals, including many cold items over the duration of a cruise, usually lasting 1 to 2 weeks. In ocean-going vessels the space allocated to storage of raw materials is adequate; the space provided for refrigerated storage is often limited, especially aboard older vessels, resulting in improper storage of both cooked and some raw foods. These conditions combined with inadequate cooking can result in conditions conducive to foodborne illness outbreaks. Conditions for cooking and preparing meals are also less than ideal because of space constraints. Inspections have indicated that poor personal hygiene and lack of supervision and training of food handlers are deficiencies on vessels on which outbreaks have occurred. Early data from shipboard outbreaks reported to the CDC in the 1960s and 1970s implicated a variety of vehicles, including water and a number of foods, especially seafood cocktails, shrimp, and lobster.[158]

The U.S. Public Health Service instituted a Vessel Sanitation Program (VSP) in 1975. The VSP established a surveillance system that requires the captain of any cruise ship that docks in the United States to report by radio 24 hours before arrival the number of passengers who consulted the ship's physician for diarrhea. The CDC is notified if > 3% of the passengers are reported as having diarrhea during the cruise. In addition to surveillance for diarrheal illness on cruise ships, the VSP includes periodic unannounced sanitation inspections of cruise ships by the CDC.

The CDC has maintained a computerized list of ship captain's reports of diarrheal disease on cruises terminating at U.S. ports for 15 years. By definition, a diarrheal illness is the occurrence in a 24-hour period of three or more loose stools or of a greater than normal (for the person) amount of loose stools. Recent tabulated data excluded cruises with fewer than 100 passengers, cruises less than 3 or more than 15 days long, and cruises to Alaska, since they do not terminate in the contiguous 48 states. Captains on 97.7% of all cruises reported diarrheal illness in fewer than 10 passengers and in less than 3% of passengers for 98.8% of all cruises. These reports compared closely with ship physician's reports and had a specificity of 99.5% in identifying ships on which > 3% of passengers had diarrhea.[159]

Conditions aboard vessels are unique and may play an important role in food sanitation. The establishment of the VSP brought about the program's Operations Manual, which provides recommendations for all food protection measures, including food and water quality, food preparation, safe disposal of wastes, and deinfestation methods.[160]

An ocean-going vessel provides an opportunity in some cases for crew or passengers to obtain seafood by fishing from the deck. Operations guidelines stress that all food must be from sources that comply with all laws relating to food and food handling.

A possible source of contamination is nonpotable water (seawater), which may be utilized in other areas or operations on board ship. All saltwater taps, except for fire hydrants, must be removed from all food service, storage, and preparation areas. Only potable water is to be used for deck washing in these areas. In all instances, the potable water system is not to be subjected to contamination through cross-connections to nonpotable water or through backsiphonage. All potable water hose, caps, fittings, and connections must be clearly marked and stored as such and not mixed with those used for nonpotable water supplies.

Potable water should be chlorinated or brominated to at least 2.0 ppm at the time of bunkering. Batch halogenation of bunkered water is not recommended. Any distillation plant that supplies water to the potable water system should not be operated in polluted or harbor areas. Unfortunately, it may be difficult to know when seawater is polluted.

Space is limited aboard a ship, yet relatively long-term food storage is necessary because all meals are prepared on board. Factors unique to vessel configuration or construction must be considered. Drainage lines that carry liquid waste should not pass directly overhead or horizontally through areas where food is stored, handled, prepared, or served. The garbage and refuse storage room should be constructed so as to be easily cleaned and of ample size and located so as to prevent contamination in food preparation and storage areas.

Like land-based food service, a variety of causes have been identified for outbreaks occurring aboard vessels. In 1979 an outbreak of gastroenteritis was reported to the CDC in which 32% of the ship's 1149 passengers were suffering from a diarrheal illness. This was followed the next week by a second outbreak aboard the same vessel. Diarrhea was reported to the ship's physician by 26 of 1160 passengers and 18 of 540 crew, and many more passengers complained of gastrointestinal illness. Stool cultures revealed *Salmonella heidelberg* isolated from 17 of 21 ill passengers and 4 of 6 well passengers. More than 60 of 269 food handlers were positive for *Salmonella* group B at the time of the report. Multiple deficiencies in sanitation were identified, particularly in food handling and preparation. The same *Salmonella* serotype was cultured from 7 of 35 food samples. Turkey and macaroni salad from an evening buffet were originally implicated, and several other items were subsequently found to be contaminated.[161]

Two outbreaks occurred on two consecutive cruises of a commercial vessel in 1986. First, 392 passengers and 30 crew developed gastroenteritis, which peaked on the fifth and sixth day of the cruise. On the next voyage a second outbreak occurred in which 321 passengers and 48 crew developed gastroenteritis. A sanitation inspection revealed problems associated with water chlorination, food contamination, and food preparation and holding. Numerous deficiencies were identified related to food and water sanitation. The sanitation inspection scores were 18 and 16 out of a possible 100 points, respectively. No bacterial pathogen was identified with either episode; however, a rise in antibodies to Norwalk virus was demonstrated in some ill crew and passengers from the first voyage.[162]

Of 22,767 cruises during the period 1975 to 1985, excluding certain trips of longer duration or having fewer than 100 passengers, as described above, 0.6% or 98 of the remaining 17,322 cruises reported that > 3% of passengers had consulted the ship's physician for a diarrheal illness. The proportion of those occurring in the period 1980 to 1985 decreased, with only 34 cruises so identified during this period. Forty-nine outbreaks were investigated, with 45 considered to be shipboard outbreaks. The major bacterial pathogens were *V. parahaemolyticus* and *E. coli*. Norwalk or Norwalk-like virus was implicated in 6 outbreaks, and for 24 outbreaks the pathogen was unknown.[159]

Food and waterborne disease aboard cruise ships occurs for various reasons, including storage or handling of foods at temperatures where pathogens readily grow, cross-contamination of cooked and raw foods, poor personal hygiene by food handlers, and the improper use of nonpotable water in food preparation areas. Inadequate training of food handlers may be an important factor. Ocean-going vessels share all of the food sanitation problems associated with land-based food service, in addition to some that are unique to their environment. Of course, their sanitation standards must be no less rigorous.

Hazard Analysis Critical Control Point

HACCP is a quality-assurance program, a preventive system of control, in which a series of actions are identified that should be taken to ensure food safety for all processed or prepared foods.[163] These actions include (1) detecting hazards and assessing their severity and probability of occurrence, (2) identifying critical processing or handling control points, (3) establishing criteria for control and putting control measures into effect, (4) monitoring the critical control points, and (5) taking immediate action to correct problems whenever the results of monitoring indicate that the criteria are not met. All the human elements that could influence the safety of foods processed or served in an establishment should be considered. Bauman,[164] in an early, basic discussion of HACCP, defined these concepts for food processing; however, they are applied equally well in food service. Bryan[165] has discussed the practices and processes that lead to the outbreak of foodborne disease in homes, in food service operations, and in food processing plants. All of these factors should be included in a HACCP system approach to evaluating any operation or facility.

Discussions with managers and food handlers can determine the method by which foods are received, stored, reconstituted or thawed, handled during preparation, cooked, handled after cooking, held hot, cooled, reheated, and served. When these data are combined with the methods of cleaning equipment and hygienic practices of workers, a routine flow diagram for foods through the operation can be constructed. The flow diagram should show time-temperature combinations, survival and growth of microorganisms, and a designation of potential points for contamination. Time-temperature combinations of heat processes and storage practices can be identified to help understand the hazards. A diagram should show all pertinent information for preparation steps, processing, and equipment used. Critical control points should be identified, and measures for prevention and control specified. Such a diagram need only be done once for each potentially hazardous food at each establishment, unless there are changes in the process, food equipment, or personnel, then only the modifications need be identified.

Critical control points in food processing and food service include time-temperature controls, sanitation techniques, and the quality of raw material. An operations step where control is critical should be monitorable, have controllable conditions, be monitored before or during operation, have established control criteria, and be a condition of moderate to high risk, and when criteria are not met, appropriate action is taken.[163] These critical control points can be monitored by sampling raw materials and product from each step in preparation or processing, as well as swabs of food contact surfaces.

The concept of HACCP has been applied to the monitoring of a variety of different food service systems.[166,167] Its use is not limited to conventional food service or food processing operations and may be applied to situations ranging from street vendors to Third-World home environments.[168,169] The HACCP approach may be focused on the control of a specific foodborne pathogen as in the International Commission of Microbiological Specifications for Foods (ICMSF) recommendations for the control of salmonellosis in developing countries.[170] Using the HACCP approach, Bryan and Bartleson[171] found that foods cooked in Mexican-style restaurants usually reached temperatures that would inactivate vegetative pathogenic bacteria. Cooking temperatures were adequate; however, cooling practices for foods was noted to be a problem. During reheating, products often failed to reach a minimum of 165° F. The process of adding sauces after steaming of rice lowers the pH, but cooling and reheating seem to be critical control points for beans, rice, and ground meat used in this type of food service facility. Bryan[172] has discussed the application of HACCP principles in a variety of food preparation systems including several different ethnic foods.

HACCP procedures can identify those elements that are known to cause outbreaks of foodborne disease in food processing and food service operations. An excellent volume giving an overview of the application of the HACCP system to ensure microbiological safety and quality of foods was recently published by ICMSF.[173] For HACCP to succeed, however, control measures must be properly administered and utilized, and critical control points must be monitored. Having properly accomplished this, a more successful food protection program is possible. Bryan[174] has summarized the significant factors in HACCP monitoring for food service operations. Many of these factors also apply to food processing operations. They include the following.

1. Appraise incoming foods as to source, brand, appearance, history of processing, quality, pH, a_w, type and damage of packaging, and type of quantity of contaminants.
2. Appraise methods of storing raw, frozen, chilled, and dry foods to determine situations that facilitate contamination or promote microbial growth.
3. Appraise situations that could permit contamination during handling of raw products, during reconstitution of dehydrated foods, during thawing of frozen foods, and during preparation of foods to be served without subsequent heating.
4. Measure time-temperature exposure of foods during cooking to determine whether pathogens could survive.
5. Appraise situations that could permit cooked foods to become contaminated during handling.
6. Measure time-temperature exposures of cooked foods during hot holding to determine whether pathogens could survive or bacteria could multiply.
7. Measure time-temperature exposure of foods during room temperature or refrigerated storage to determine whether bacteria could multiply.
8. Measure time-temperature exposure of foods during reheating to determine whether any pathogens could survive.
9. Appraise situations that facilitate contamination of foods while they are either being served or packaged for carryout orders.
10. Appraise cleaning procedures to determine whether pathogens are removed from equipment and utensils.
11. Appraise understanding of supervisors and workers about foodborne disease hazards and their prevention and supervision and training provided by management.
12. Determine the conditions (including pH, a_w, microbiological quality) of food at all stages of preparation, at the time of serving, and of any leftovers.

REFERENCES

1. Kermode G: Food Standards for the World. World Health Organization, 1983, pp 11–13
2. Institute of Veterinary Medicine-Robert von Ostertag-Institute: WHO Surveillance Programme for Control of Foodborne Infections and Intoxications in Europe, 2nd Report. Berlin (West), The Institute, 1983
3. Centers for Disease Control: Foodborne Disease Outbreaks, Waterborne Disease Outbreaks. Surveillance Summaries (5-Year). Atlanta: CDC, 1990
4. Bryan FL: Prevention of foodborne diseases in foodservice establishments. J Environ Health 41:198–206, 1979
5. Todd ECD: Foodborne and waterborne disease in Canada—1979 annual summary. J Food Prot 48:1071–1078, 1985
6. Todd ECD: Foodborne and waterborne disease in Canada—1981 annual summary. J Food Prot 50:982–991, 1987
7. Todd ECD: Foodborne and waterborne disease in Canada—1982 annual summary. J Food Prot 51:56–65, 1988
8. Todd ECD: Foodborne and waterborne disease in Canada—1984 annual summary. J Food Prot 52:503–511, 1989
9. Institute of Veterinary Medicine-Robert von Ostertag-Institute: WHO Surveillance Programme for Control of Foodborne Infections and Intoxications in Europe, #6 Newsletter, 1984
10. Institute of Veterinary Medicine-Robert von Ostertag-Institute: WHO Surveillance Programme for Control of Foodborne Infections and Intoxications in Europe, #24 Newsletter, 1990
11. Cohen ML, Balke PA: Trends in foodborne salmonellosis outbreaks, 1963–1975. J Food Prot 40:798–800, 1977
12. St. Louis ME, Morse DL, Potter ME, DeMelfi TM, Guzewich JJ, Tauxe RV, Blake PA: The emergence of grade A eggs as a major source of *Salmonella enteritidis* infections. JAMA 259:2102–2107, 1988
13. Hobbs BC, Smith ME, Oakley CL, et al: *Clostridium welchii* food poisoning. J Hyg (London) 51:75–101, 1953
14. Blaser MJ, Berkowitz ID, LaForce FM, Cravens J, Reller LB, Wen-Lan LouWang: Campylobacter enteritis: Clinical and epidemiological features. Ann Intern Med 91:179–185, 1979
15. McLauchlin J: *Listeria monocytogenes:* Recent advances in the taxonomy and epidemiology of listeriosis in humans. J Appl Bacteriol 63:1–11, 1987
16. Fleming DW, Cochi SL, MacDonald KL, Brondum J, Hayes PS, Plikaytis BD, Holmes MB, Audurier A, Broome CV, Reingold AL: Pasteurized milk as a vehicle of infection in an outbreak of listeriosis. New Engl J Med 312:404–407, 1985
17. James SM, Fannin SL, Agee BA, Gall B, Parker E, Vogt J, Run G, Williams J, Lieb L, Prendergast T, Werner SB, Chin J: Listeriosis outbreak associated with Mexican-style cheese—California. MMWR 34:357, 1985
18. Boucher M, Yonekura ML: Perinatal listeriosis (early onset): Correlation of antenatal manifestations and neonatal outcome. Obstet Gynecol 68:593–597, 1986
19. Seeliger HPR, Finger H: Listeriosis. In Remington JS, Klein JO (eds): Infectious Diseases of the Fetus and Newborn Infant. Philadelphia: W.B. Saunders, 1976, p 33
20. Lee WH, McClain D: Personal communication. Beltsville, Maryland: Food Safety and Inspection Service, U.S.D.A., 1987
21. Ho JL, Shands KN, Friedland P, Eckind P, Fraser DW: An outbreak of type 4b *Listeria monocytogenes* infection involving patients from eight Boston hospitals. Arch Intern Med 146:520–521, 1986
22. Farber JM, Sanders GW, Johnston MA: A survey of various foods for the presence of *Listeria* species. J Food Prot 52:456–458, 1989
23. Leistner L, Hechelmann H, Kashiwazaki M, Albertz R: Nachweis von *Yersinia enterocolitica* in faeces und fleisch von schweinen, rindern und geflugel. Fleischcwirtschatf 55:1599–1602, 1975
24. Lee WH: An assessment of *Yersinia enterocolitica* and its presence in foods. J Food Prot 40:486–489, 1977
25. McManus C, Lanier JM: *Salmonella, Campylobacter jejuni* and *Yersinia enterocolitica* in raw milk. J Food Prot 50:51–55, 1987
26. Tacket CO, Brenner F, Blake PA: Clinical features and an epidemiological study of *Vibrio vulnificus* infections. J Infect Dis 149:558–561, 1984
27. Blake PA, Weaver RE, Hollis DG: Diseases of humans (other than cholera) caused by vibrios. Ann Rev Microbiol 34:341–367, 1980
28. Codex Alimentarius Commission: Procedural Manual. Italy: FAO/WHO, 1981
29. Doull J: Food safety and toxicology. In Roberts HR (ed): Food Safety. New York: John Wiley, 1981, pp 295–316
30. Public Health Service/Food and Drug Administration: Pasteurized Milk Ordinance. Washington, D.C.: U.S. Government Printing Office, Publication No. 229, 1978
31. Townsend L: Why are Grade A surveys necessary? J Food Prot 43:73–75, 1980
32. United States Department of Agriculture: Requirements for milk for manufacturing purposes and its production and processing. Fed Reg 37:7046–7066, 1972
33. Reilly C: Metal Contamination of Food. London: Applied Science Publishers, 1980
34. Jelinek CF, Braude GL: Management of sludge use on land. J Food Prot 41:476–480, 1978
35. Dazzo F, Smith P, Hubbell D: The influence of manure slurry irriga-

tion on the survival of fecal organisms in Scranton fine sand. J Environ Quality 2:470–473, 1973

36. Duboise SM, Moore BE, Sorber CA, Sagik BP: Viruses in soil systems. Crit Rev Microbiol 7:245–285, 1979
37. Sadovski AY, Fattal B, Goldberg D: Microbial contamination of vegetables irrigated with sewage effluent by the drip method. J Food Prot 41:336–340, 1978
38. Marth EH: Aflatoxin in milk, cheese and other dairy products. Proceedings of the 1st Biennial Marschall International Cheese Conference. Madison, Wisconsin: Marschall Dairy Ingredients Division, Miles Laboratories, 1978, pp 241–248
39. Harrison MA: Presence and stability of patulin in apple products: A review. J Food Safety 9:147–153, 1989
40. Hackney CR, Dicharry A: Seafood-borne bacterial pathogens of marine origin. Food Technol 42(3):104–109, 1988
41. Taylor S: Marine toxins of microbial origin. Food Technol 42(3):94–98, 1988
42. Clem JD: Microbiological considerations in the handling and processing of molluskan shellfish. In Chichester CO, Graham HD (eds): Microbial Safety of Fishery Products. New York: Academic Press, 1973, pp 53–58
43. United States Public Health Service: Summary of Milkborne Disease Outbreaks Reported by State and Local Health Authorities as Having Occurred in the United States. 1923–1946. Washington, D.C.: U.S. Public Health Service, 1948
44. Currier RW: Raw milk and human gastrointestinal disease: Problems resulting from legalized sale of certified raw milk. J Public Health Policy 2:226–234, 1981
45. Bryan FL: Epidemiology of milk-borne diseases. J Food Prot 46: 637–649, 1983
46. Snyder IS, Johnson W, Zottola EA: Significant pathogens in dairy products. In Marth EH (ed): Standard Methods for the Examination of Dairy Products, 14 edt. Washington, D.C.: American Public Health Association, 1978, pp 11–32
47. Jones PH, Willis AT, Robinson DA, et al: *Campylobacter enteritis* associated with the consumption of free school milk. J Hyg 87:155–170, 1981
48. Todd ECD: Foodborne and waterborne disease in Canada—1983 annual summary. J Food Prot 52:436–442
49. Lovett J, Grancis DW, Hunt JM: Isolation of *Campylobacter jejuni* from raw milk. Appl Environ Microbiol 46:459–462, 1983
50. Doyle MP, Roman DJ: Prevalence and survival of *Campylobacter jejuni* in unpasteurized milk. Appl Environ Microbiol 44:1154–1158, 1982
51. Robinson DA: Infective dose of *Campylobacter jejuni* in milk. Br Med J 282:1584, 1981
52. Centers for Disease Control: *Brucella* Surveillance Annual Summary. Atlanta: CDC, 1972–1979
53. Beattie CP, Rice RM: Undulant fever due to *Brucella* of the porcine type—*Brucella suis.* JAMA 102:1670–1674, 1934
54. Johnson BG: Progress of Cooperative State-Federal Brucellosis Eradication Program. Washington, D.C.: United States Animal Health Association, 1977
55. Thimm BM: Brucellosis. New York: Springer-Verlag, 1982
56. Prober CG, Tune B, Hoder L: *Yersinia pseudotuberculosis* septicemia. Am J Dis Child 133:623–624, 1979
57. Black RE, Jackson RJ, Tsai T, et al: Epidemic *Yersinia enterocolitica* infection due to contaminated chocolate milk. N Engl J Med 298:76–79, 1978
58. de Grace M, Laurin MF, Belanger C, et al: *Yersinia enterocolitica* gastroenteritis outbreak—Montreal. Can Dis Week Rep 2(11):41, 1976
59. Toma S, Lafleur L: Survey on the incidence of *Yersinia enterocolitica* infection in Canada. Appl Microbiol 28:469–473, 1974
60. Hughes D: Repeated isolation of *Yersinia enterocolitica* from pasteurized milk in a holding vat at a dairy factory. J Appl Bacteriol 48:383–385, 1980
61. Amin MK, Draughon FA: Growth characteristics of *Yersinia enterocolitica* in pasteurized skim milk. J Food Prot 50:849–852, 1987
62. Aulisio CC, Lanier JM, Chappel MA: *Yersinia enterocolitica* 0:13 associated with outbreaks in three southern states. J Food Prot 45:1263, 1982
63. Hayes PS, Feeley JC, Graves LM, et al.: Isolation of *Listeria monocytogenes* from raw milk. Appl Environ Microbiol 51:438–440, 1985
64. FDA/MIF/IICA: Recommended guidelines for controlling environmental contamination in dairy plants. Dairy Food Sanitat 8:52–56, 1988
65. Centers for Disease Control: Listeriosis outbreak associated with Mexican-style cheese—California. MMWR 34:357–359, 1985
66. Fleming DW, Cochi SL, MacDonald KL, et al: Pasteurized milk as a vehicle for infection in an outbreak of listeriosis. New Engl J Med 308:404–407, 1985
67. Minor TE, Marth EH: Staphylococci and Their Significance in Foods. New York: Elsevier, 1976
68. Campbell JR, Marshall RT: The Science of Providing Milk for Man. New York: McGraw-Hill, 1975
69. American Association of Medical Milk Commissions: Methods and Standards for the Production of Certified Milk. Alpharetta, Georgia: The Association, 1976
70. Werner SB, Humphrey GL, Kamei I: Association between raw milk and human *Salmonella dublin* infection. Br Med J 1:238–241, 1979
71. Kamei I, Mahoney L, Sachs RR, et al: Human *Salmonella dublin* infections associated with the consumption of certified raw milk—California. MMWR 23:175, 1979
72. Sandine WE, Daly M: Milk intolerance. J Food Prot 5:437, 1979
73. Oz HH, Farnsworth RJ: Laboratory simulation of fluctuating temperature of farm bulk tank milk. J Food Prot 48:303–305, 1985
74. Biehl ML, Buck WB: Chemical contaminants: Their metabolism and their residues. J Food Prot 50:1058–1073, 1989
75. World Health Organization: Conference on intoxication due to alkylmercury-treated seed. Bulletin WHO Suppl 1, 1976
76. Food and Drug Administration. Fed Reg 44:51233, 1979
77. Harris RW, Elsea WR: Ceramic glaze as a source of lead poisoning. JAMA 202:544–546, 1967
78. Anon: Heavy metal poisoning at a high school's home economics "food" class. J Food Prot 49:77, 1986
79. Todd ECD: Foodborne and waterborne disease in Canada—1980 annual summary. J Food Prot 50:150–160, 1987
80. Munro IC, Charbonneau SM: Environmental contaminants. In Roberts HR (ed): Food Safety. New York: John Wiley, 1981, pp 141–180
81. Centers for Disease Control: Follow-up on polychlorinated biphenyls exposure—Idaho, Montana. MMWR 28:559–560, 1979
82. Kay K: Polybrominated biphenyls (PBB) environmental contamination in Michigan, 1973–1976. Environ Res 13:74–94, 1977
83. Petersen B, Chaisson C: Pesticides and residues in food. Food Technol 42(7):59–64, 1988
84. Centers for Disease Control: Aldicarb food poisoning from contaminated melons—California. MMWR 35:254–258, 1986
85. Siddique IH: Antibiotic residues in foods. In The Safety of Foods. Westport, Connecticut: AVI Publishing, 1968, pp 358–359
86. Barnard SE: Antibiotic detection programs. J Food Prot 45:1178, 1982 (abst)
87. Meister HE: Surveillance of milk products for penicillin as done by the dairy division of the U.S. Department of Agriculture. J Food Prot 38:621–623, 1975
88. Olson JC Jr, Sanders AC: Penicillin in milk and milk products: Some regulatory and public health considerations. J Food Prot 38:630–633, 1975
89. Vickers HR, Bagratuni L, Alexander S: Dermatitis caused by penicillin in milk. Lancet 1:358, 1958
90. Keogh BP: Reviews of the progress of dairy science. Section B. The survival of pathogens in cheese and milk powder. J Dairy Res 38:91–111, 1971
91. Hankin L, Lacy GH, Stephens GR, Dillman WF: Antibiotic-resistant bacteria in raw milk and ability of some to transfer antibiotic resistance to *Escherichia coli.* J Food Prot 42:950–953, 1979

92. Bullerman LB, Buchanan RL: Mycotoxins other than aflatoxins—Their relationships to food safety. Introduction. J Food Prot 44:701, 707, 1981
93. Labuza TP: Regulation of mycotoxins in foods. J Food Prot 46:260–265, 1983
94. Stoloff L: Aflatoxin M in perspective. J Food Prot 43:226–230, 1980
95. Gabis D, Faust RE: Controlling microbial growth in food processing environments. Food Technol 42(12):81–83, 1988
96. Heldman DR, Seiberling DA: Environmental sanitation. In Harper JW, Hall CW (eds): Dairy Technology and Engineering. Westport, Connecticut: AVI Publishing, 1976, pp 272–321
97. Kang YJ, Frank JF: Biological aerosols: A review of airborne contamination and its measurement in dairy processing plants. J Food Prot 52:512–524, 1989
98. Harper WJ: Sanitation in dairy food plants. In Guthrie RK (ed): Food Sanitation. Westport, Connecticut: AVI Publishing, 1972, pp 130–160
99. Bruhn JC, Franke AA, Bushnell RB, et al: Sources and content of iodine in California milk and dairy products. J Food Prot 46:41–46, 1983
100. Food and Drug Administration: Current Good Manufacturing Practice in Manufacturing, Processing, Packing, or Holding Human Food. Part 110, Title 21, Code of Federal Regulations, 1969
101. Elliot RP, Hobbs BC: Eggs and egg products. In Microbial Ecology of Foods, Vol. II. New York: Academic Press, 1980, pp 521–556
102. Kline L, Sugihara TF, Bean ML, Ijichi K: Heat pasteurization of raw liquid egg white. Food Technol 19:1709–1718, 1965
103. Doyle MP: Effect of environmental and processing conditions on *Listeria monocytogenes*. Food Technol 42(4):169–171, 1988
104. Centers for Disease Control: Update: Milk-borne salmonellosis—Illinois. MMWR 34:215–216, 1985
105. Centers for Disease Control: *Salmonella gastroenteritis* associated with milk—Arizona. MMWR 28:117, 119–120, 1979
106. Jay JM: Modern food microbiology. New York: Van Nostrand Reinhold, 1986
107. Townsend CT, Yee L, Mercer WA: Inhibition of the growth of *Clostridium botulinum* by acidification. Food Res 19:536–548, 1954
108. Hersom AC, Hulland ED: Canned Foods. New York: Churchill Livingstone, 1980
109. Centers for Disease Control: Botulism in the United States, 1899–1977. Atlanta: U.S. Public Health Service, 1979
110. Lechowich RV: Microbiological challenges of refrigerated foods. Food Technol 42(12):84–89, 1988
111. Hurst A: Injury and its effect on survival. In International Commission on Microbial Specifications for Foods: Microbial Ecology of Foods. Vol. I. New York: Academic Press, 1980, pp 205–214
112. Olson JC Jr, Nottingham PM: Temperature. In International Commission on Microbiological Specifications for Foods: Microbial Ecology of Foods. Vol. I. New York: Academic Press, 1980, pp 1–37
113. Bergdoll MS: Staphyloenterotoxins in dried foods. In The Microbiology of Dried Foods. New York: International Association of Microbiological Societies, 1969, pp 225–240
114. Centers for Disease Control: International outbreak of Type E botulism associated with ungutted, salted whitefish. MMWR 36:812–813, 1987
115. Minor TE, Marth EH: *Staphylococcus aureus* and staphylococcal food intoxications. A review. III. Staphylococci in dairy foods. J Milk Food Technol 35:77–82, 1972
116. Centers for Disease Control: Salmonellosis associated with consumption of nonfat powdered milk—Oregon. MMWR 28:129–130, 1979
117. Pederson CS: Microbiology of Food Fermentations. Westport, Connecticut: AVI Publishing, 1971
118. Centers for Disease Control: Staphylococcal food poisoning associated with Genoa and hard salami—United States. MMWR 28:179–180, 1979
119. Babel FJ: Antibiosis by lactic culture bacteria. J Dairy Sci 60:815–821, 1977
120. Frank JF, Marth EH, Olson NF: Behavior of enteropathogenic *Escherichia coli* during manufacture and ripening of brick cheese. J Food Prot 41:111–115, 1978
121. Frank JF, Marth EH: Survey of soft and semisoft cheese for presence of fecal coliforms and serotypes of enteropathogenic *Escherichia coli*. J Food Prot 41:198–200, 1978
122. Frank JF, Marth EH, Olson NF: Survival of enteropathogenic and non-pathogenic *Escherichia coli* during manufacture of Camembert cheese. J Food Prot 40:835–842, 1977
123. Marier R, Wells JG, Swanson RC, Callahan W: An outbreak of enteropathogenic *Escherichia coli* foodborne disease traced to imported French cheese. Lancet 2:1376–1378, 1973
124. Fontaine RE, Cohen ML, Martin WT, Vernon TM: Epidemic salmonellosis from Cheddar cheese. Surveillance and prevention. Am J Epidemiol 111:242–253, 1980
125. Scott VN: Interaction of factors to control microbial spoilage of refrigerated foods. J Food Prot 52:431–435, 1989
126. Nitrite Safety Council: A survey of nitrosamines in sausages and dry-cured meat products. Food Technol 34:45–53, 1980
127. Hotchkiss JH, Cassens RG: Nitrate, nitrite, and nitroso compounds in foods. Food Technol 41(4):127–134, 1987
128. Schwartz HJ: Sensitivity to ingested metabisulfite: Variations in clinical presentation. J Allergy Clin Immunol 71:487–489, 1983
129. Stevenson DD, Simon RA: Sensitivity to ingested metabisulfites in asthmatic subjects. J Allergy Clin Immunol 68:26, 1981
130. Skala JH, McGown EL, Waring PP: Wholesomeness of irradiated foods. J Food Prot 50:150–160, 1987
131. Ingram M, Roberts TA: Ionizing irradiation. In Microbial Ecology of Foods. Vol. I. New York: Academic Press, 1980, pp 46–67
132. WHO: Wholesomeness of Irradiated Food. World Health Organization Technical Report Series, No. 659. Geneva: WHO, 1981
133. Institute of Food Technologists: Radiation preservation of foods. Food Technol 37:55–60, 1983
134. Hauschild AHW, Bryan FL: Estimate of cases of food and waterborne illness in Canada and the United States. J Food Prot 43:435–440, 1980
135. Longree K: Quantity Food Sanitation, 3 edt. New York: John Wiley, 1980
136. Food and Drug Administration Food Service Sanitation Manual DHEW Publication No. (FDA) 78-2081. Washington, D.C.: U.S. Government Printing Office, 1976
137. Food and Drug Administration: A Registry of Manager Training and Certification Programs in Food Protection. Washington, D.C.: Department of Health and Human Services, 1983
138. Speer SC, Kane BE Jr: Certification of food service managers: A survey of current opinion. J Food Prot 53:269–274, 1990
139. Longree K, Baker GG: Sanitary Techniques in Foodservice, 2 edt. New York: John Wiley, 1982
140. U.S. Department of Agriculture: Meat and Poultry Inspection Regulations (with revisions). Washington, D.C.: U.S. Printing Office, 1986
141. National Sanitation Foundation: Food Service Equipment Standards (Current revision date for each of the 21 independent food standards). Ann Arbor, Michigan: National Sanitation Foundation
142. Bryan FL: Prevention of foodborne diseases in foodservice establishments. J Environ Health 41:198–206, 1979
143. Bryan FL, McKinley TW: Hazard analysis and control of roast beef preparation in foodservice establishments. J Food Prot 42:4–18, 1979
144. Fruin JT, Guthertz LS: Survival of bacteria in food cooked by microwave oven, conventional oven, and slow cookers. J Food Prot 45:695–698, 1982
145. Federal Register. Washington, D.C.: U.S. Department of Agriculture #30793, 1978

146. Bryan FL: Factors that contribute to outbreaks of foodborne disease. J Food Prot 41:816–827, 1978
147. Bryan FL, Seabolt KA, Peterson RW, Roberts LM: Time-temperature observations of food and equipment in airline catering operations. J Food Prot 41:80–92, 1978
148. Bryan FL: Hazard analysis of foodservice operations. Food Technol 35:78–87, 1981
149. Sawyer CA, Naidu YM, Thompson S: Cook/chill foodservice systems: Microbiological quality and endpoint temperature of beef loaf, peas and potatoes after reheating by conduction, convection and microwave radiation. J Food Prot 46:1036–1043, 1983
150. Georgia Department of Human Resources: Rules and Regulations for Food Service Chapter 290-6-14. Atlanta: Georgia Department of Human Resources, 1985
151. Deoring RD: Comparison of low temperature and conventional dishwasher systems. Proceedings for the Society for the Advancement of Food Service Research, November, 1980
152. Centers for Disease Control: Rodent-borne Disease Control through Rodent Stoppage, 1977. DHEW Publication No. (CDC) 77-8343. Atlanta: CDC, 1977
153. Inflight Food Services Association, Inc.: Airline Catering Sanitation Guide, 1976
154. Centers for Disease Control: MMWR 24:57–59, 1975
155. Centers for Disease Control: MMWR 35:383–384, 1986
156. Bailey J: Guide to Hygiene and Sanitation in Aviation. Geneva: WHO, 1977
157. U.S. Public Health Service: Handbook on Sanitation of Airlines. DHEW Publication No. 308. Washington, D.C.: U.S. Government Printing Office, 1964
158. Merson MH, Hughes JM, Lawrence DN, et al: Food and waterborne disease outbreaks on passenger cruise vessels and aircraft. J Milk Food Technol 39:285–288, 1976
159. Addiss DG, Yashuk JC, Clapp DE, Blake PA: Outbreaks of diarrheal illness on passenger cruise ships, 1975–1985. Proceedings Annual Meeting APHA, New Orleans, 1987
160. U.S. Department of Health and Human Services: Vessel Sanitation Program Operations Manual. Atlanta: CDC, 1989
161. Centers for Disease Control: MMWR 28:145–146, 1979
162. Centers for Disease Control: MMWR 35:383–384, 1986
163. Bryan FL: Hazard Analysis Critical Control Point (HACCP) Concept. Dairy Food Environ Sanit 10:416–418, 1990
164. Bauman HE: The HACCP concept and microbiological hazard categories. Food Technol 28:30–34, 1974
165. Bryan FL: Risks of practices, procedures and processes that lead to outbreaks of foodborne diseases. J Food Prot 5:663–673, 1988
166. Bryan FL, Sugi M, Miyashiro L, et al: Hazard analysis of duck in Chinese restaurants. J Food Prot 45:445–449, 1982
167. El-Sherbeeny MR, Saddik MF, Aly ES, Bryan FL: Microbiological profile and storage temperatures of Egyptian rice dishes. Intern J Food Microbiol 2:355–364, 1985
168. Bryan FL, Silvia C, Michanie SC, Alverez P, Paniagwa A: Critical control points of street-vended foods in the Dominican Republic. J Food Prot 51:373–383, 1988
169. Bryan FL, Michanie SC, Vizcarra MM, Obdulia NS, Taboada D, Fernandez NM, Requejo EG, Munoz BP: Hazard analyses of food prepared by inhabitants near lake Titicaca in the Peruvian Sierra. J Food Prot 51:412–418, 1988
170. Simonsen B, Bryan FL, Christian JHB, Roberts TA, Tompkin RB, Silliker JH: Prevention and control of food-borne salmonellosis through application of hazard analysis critical control point (HACCP). Intern J Food Microbiol 4:227–247, 1987
171. Bryan FL, Bartleson CA: Mexican-style foodservice operations: Hazard analyses, critical control points and monitoring. J Food Prot 48:509–524, 1985
172. Bryan FL: Safety of ethnic foods through application of the hazard analysis critical control point approach. Dairy Food Sanit 8:654–660, 1988
173. International Commission on Microbiological Specifications for Foods (ICMSF) of the International Union of Microbiological Societies: Microorganisms in Foods: Application of the hazard analysis critical control point (HACCP) system to ensure microbiological safety and quality. Boston: Blackwell Scientific Publications, 1988
174. Bryan FL: Hazard analysis critical control point approach: Epidemiologic rationale and application to food service operations. J Environ Health 44:7–14, 1981

35

Water Quality Management

Daniel A. Okun

Water is a necessity and an amenity. Wholesome and abundant, it supports and enriches life. Unwholesome or scarce, it is a threat to health and to life itself. This chapter concerns the adequacy and quality of water in the service of people.

The amount of water in the world is fixed, some 1500 million km^3 in all. Only about 0.2% of this is fresh water, readily available for use. Fresh waters run to the sea and become saline, but evaporation of water from the seas and precipitation on land, the hydrologic cycle, restores these fresh waters continuously so that the quantity of fresh water is relatively fixed.

Early settlements were located near water, and the water resources were then ample for all purposes, although history does describe instances in which communities disappeared because declining water supplies resulted from local changes in climate. The present water crisis has arisen from population growth and urbanization, which puts pressure on the fixed sources of fresh water available locally. These pressures have resulted in insufficient quantity and deterioration in quality of water to the extent that a continuously increasing investment must be committed to providing water and maintaining its quality. The problems with water generally arise from the concentration of people and their activities in settlements. This chapter is devoted primarily to the provision of a safe and adequate water supply and the sanitary removal of wastewaters from communities.

USES OF WATER

The uses of water in a community are many, and the requirements in quantity and quality are varied. Conventionally, it has been convenient and economical to provide a single water supply sufficient in quantity to serve all uses and suitable in quality to meet drinking requirements, even though only a small fraction of the total water supply is actually used for drinking.

The uses of water include (1) drinking and culinary purposes; (2) personal cleanliness, including bathing and laundering; (3) household cleanliness; (4) heating and air conditioning; (5) urban irrigation; (6) cleaning streets; (7) recreational purposes, including swimming pools and the watering of playing fields; (8) amenity purposes, such as public fountains and ornamental ponds; (9) power production from hydropower and steam power; (10) commercial and industrial purposes, including industrial process waters and cooling; (11) fire protection; and (12) carrying away wastes from all manner of establishments.

The quantities required for each use vary substantially. In a typical American community, the average per capita consumption is about 600 L per day, allocated approximately as shown in Tables 35–1 and 35–2. These are average annual figures. In summer, the daily demand may be 50% greater, mainly because of increased urban irrigation. In Asia and Africa, per capita consumption may be only 50 L per day.

WATER SYSTEMS

To serve these uses, communities require sources of water, transmission pumps and mains, treatment plants, and distribution systems for delivering water to each user (Fig. 35–1). Transmission systems and treatment plants should be designed for the maximum day, which occurs generally in summer and is about 150% of the average demand. The distribution system should meet the peak demand during the day, which may be 150% to 300% of the maximum day demand, being larger for smaller communities where the peak is determined by requirements for fire protection. Concomitant are a sewerage system for collecting the wastewaters from each user in the community and treatment facilities for rendering the wastewaters suitable for disposal or reuse. Some 80% of the population of the United States in more than 60,000 communities is served by water supply and sewerage systems. The remaining population, not always in rural areas, is served by individual wells and wastewater-disposal systems, generally septic tanks and tile fields for percolation of the septic tank effluents.

PROPERTIES OF WATER

Water is a unique substance. "Pure" water is a clear, colorless, tasteless, and odorless fluid. It is a strong solvent, and in nature it washes gases from the atmosphere, dissolves minerals and

This chapter is based on chapters prepared for earlier editions by the late Prof. Gordon M. Fair of Harvard University. I am indebted to Professors Mark D. Sobsey and James E. Watson, Jr., of the University of North Carolina at Chapel Hill for their contributions relating to microbiology and radiological standards, respectively.

TABLE 35-1. ALLOCATION OF WATER USED IN U.S. COMMUNITIES

Use	(%)
Residential	40
Commercial	15
Industrial	25
Public	5
Unaccounted for	15
Total	100

TABLE 35-2. ALLOCATION OF INTERIOR RESIDENTIAL WATER USE

Use	(%)
Drinking and cooking	5
Bathing	30
Toilet flushing	40
Laundry	15
Dishwashing	5
Miscellaneous	5
Total	100

Depending upon the nature of the residence and the climate, exterior residential use, primarily for lawn watering, may range from 5% to more than 150% of interior use, averaging about 75%.

humic substances from the soil through which it flows, and carries substantial quantities of silt as it flows. Many of the uses to which water is put further affect its quality. Accordingly, water is seldom useful without some kind of treatment. In addition, microorganisms find their way into waters and, depending on circumstances, may prosper or die. Some of these microorganisms are beneficial or at least not harmful. Others may be pathogenic. Many scourges of mankind have been waterborne, and the potential for spread of enteric disease is always present.

At normal atmospheric pressure, water freezes at 0° C and boils at 100° C. Because it has its greatest density at 4° C, ice floats on the surface, keeping bodies of water from freezing solid, an important phenomenon that keeps aquatic creatures alive and permits lakes and reservoirs to serve as sources of water even at subfreezing temperatures. The specific heat of water is high, resulting in the ameliorating effects of large water bodies on climate and temperature. The surface tension of water is also high, resulting in the concentration of many contaminants on its surface in monomolecular layers.

Water is an important constituent of living matter, constituting about 70% of the weight of the human body. It is a medium for transferring nutrients and waste materials as well as maintaining thermostability through heat transfer and evaporation. The water intake of an adult varies from 2 to 2.5 L per day, about half of which is lost through the skin and lungs and the other half in feces and urine. It is this latter half that needs to be managed properly if adequate sanitation is to be maintained and the spread of disease avoided. Water management involves protecting water supplies for people from damage by people.

SOURCES OF WATER

Water may be abstracted for use from any one of a number of points in its movement through the hydrological cycle shown in Figure 35-2. The specific source to be developed for any community depends on the quantity and quality of the source and its case of development.

The *safe yield* of the source must be sufficient to serve the

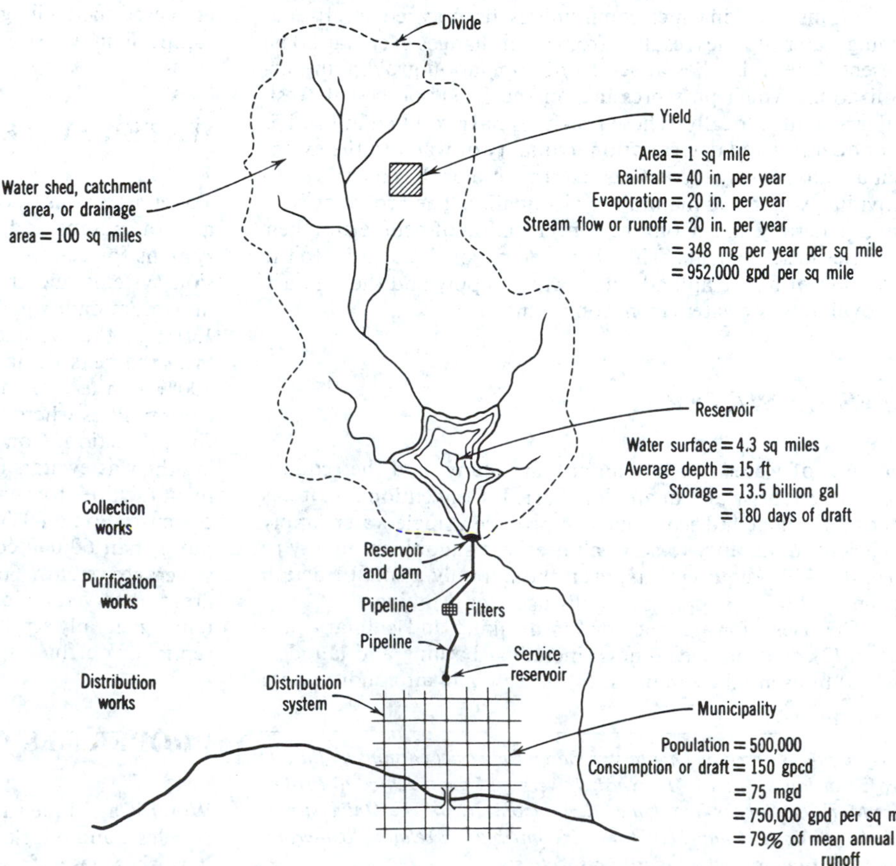

Figure 35-1. Rainfall, run-off, storage, and draft in the development of surface water supplies. *(From Fair GM et al, 1971, with permission.[1])*

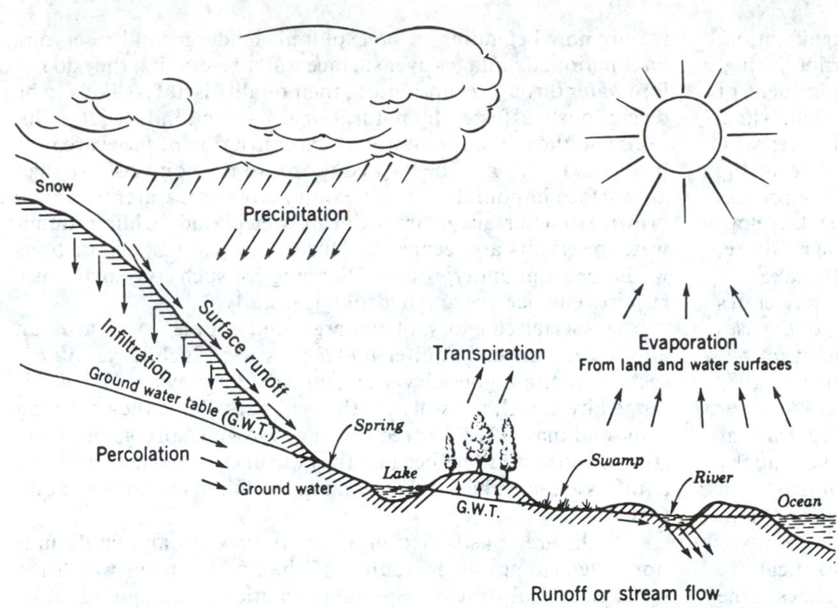

Figure 35-2. The water cycle. *[From Fair GM et al, 1971, with permission.[1]]*

population expected at the end of the design period, which may be 10 to 50 years in the future. The safe yield is generally defined as the yield that is adequate 95% of the years, or 19 out of 20 years on the average. Where reliability of supply is important, such as in industrial areas, the safe yield may be taken as that available 99% of the years. Where seasonal storage is not available, the yield must be adequate to meet the maximum day demand. With seasonal storage, it need only meet the average annual demand.

The role of the engineer is in the selection of the most suitable source from the various options available. The most common sources of water are listed below.[1]

Rainwater. Rainwater is the source of all fresh water. It may be collected directly from roofs and other prepared catchments and stored in cisterns. Because catchment areas for the direct capture of rainwater are necessarily limited in size, such supplies are useful only for individual households or small communities. Households in the Southwest are examples of the former, and paved catchments in Gibraltar are examples of the latter. The quality of rainwater is generally good, being free of minerals, but it may be contaminated by gases and particles it washes out of the atmosphere and by the accumulation of dust and other debris on the catchments. For example, gaseous sulfur and nitrogen oxides are emitted from power plants that use fossil fuels. These gases react with atmospheric water, forming dilute solutions of sulfuric and nitric acids. The precipitation of these acids ("acid rain") has begun to have serious impacts on surface water quality and on the biota that depend upon water.

Surface Water. The earliest sources of water for large communities were rivers and lakes, which readily afforded the quantity needed. The large drainage areas required for such run-of-river or lake supplies inevitably subject them to activities, such as urban and industrial development, that result in quality degradation. Water supplies for Philadelphia, Cincinnati, and New Orleans are typical of run-of-river supplies. Such supplies have historically been the source of waterborne epidemics (e.g., in the nineteenth century) and still pose disease hazards in situations where treatment is inadequate, as in the developing countries of Asia, Africa, and Latin America. The development of filtration and disinfection of water by chlorination at about the turn of the century rendered such waters free of pathogenic organisms and suitable for community supplies. Since the onset of the chemical revolution beginning in the mid-twentieth century, waters obtained from large watersheds, such as those of the Ohio and Mississippi rivers, inevitably contain numerous synthetic organic chemicals used in cities, in industry, and on the farm, some of which have been identified as being carcinogenic, mutagenic, teratogenic, or otherwise toxic. These chemicals are not easily removed in wastewater or water treatment or in the environment during passage downstream, so that use of such sources is once again brought into question. It was the identification of many synthetic organic chemicals in the lower Mississippi River that provided the impetus for the passage of the Safe Drinking Water Act (PL 93-523) in 1974. The groundwork for this act had been laid by the Community Water Supply Survey conducted by the Public Health Service (PHS) in 1969,[2] which indicated that many public water supplies, particularly those serving small communities, were not providing adequate service and were not in a position to meet the requirements of the 1962 PHS Drinking Water Standards.

A safer option is the use of smaller watersheds, which do not have naturally sustained flows during all periods of the year but, by the storage of wet-weather flows in impounding reservoirs, can provide substantial quantities of water for use during dry periods. Such small watersheds are generally found in upland areas and are often free of the major urban and industrial development that results in the chemical pollution that is now a growing concern.

Boston, New York, and San Francisco are examples of cities that have developed upstream sources. The quality of these upstream sources has often been so high that up to now the only treatment required is disinfection. Pressure for development of such heretofore protected watersheds is now threatening to degrade them, and special efforts will be required in the future to identify such protected watersheds and preserve them.

Natural and man-made lakes may improve or degrade waters drawn from their watersheds. Storage in a lake provides opportunities for coagulation and sedimentation of colloidal and suspended solids that are tributary to the lake. Some measure of disinfection is accomplished by exposure to sunlight, provided there is time for biochemical stabilization of organic matter and for die-away of microorganisms. Furthermore, storage in a lake or reservoir attenuates high levels of contaminants that may result from rainstorms or accidents on the watershed, such as spills from tankers.

On the other hand, storage in lakes or reservoirs may degrade water quality through eutrophication, biomagnification, and thermal stratification. Eutrophication, or overnourishing, of a water body occurs naturally as a result of the influent of nutrient materials, particularly phosphorus and nitrogen, which support the growth of algae. In a standing body of water with adequate sunlight, these nutrients tend to accumulate in the algae. As the algae settle, the lake tends slowly to fill, a process that naturally might take a considerable length of time. Development on a watershed, particularly urbanization and agriculture, adds significantly to sediment and nutrient input to the lake; the former reduces the capacity of lakes, and the latter accelerates the process of eutrophication to the point where many of the uses of the lake are adversely affected. The increasing concentrations of algae are difficult to remove in water treatment, and they often impart unpleasant taste and odors to the water. Another impact of storage is the bioaccumulation of small concentrations of chemicals and other contaminants that are taken up by aquatic life in the lake. These may affect the quality of fish taken from the lake and may also increase the levels of these contaminants beyond what they would be in a flowing river.

Lake quality is further affected by thermal stratification. During the summer, the warmer, lighter water accumulates in the upper layers of the lake. The density difference is sufficient to interfere with mixing, thereby preventing the lower layers of the lake from obtaining atmospheric oxygen. Organic matter reduces the dissolved oxygen in the lower levels of the lake, often resulting in anaerobic conditions with the accumulation of hydrogen sulfide, carbon dioxide and, because of the increasing acidity under such circumstances, increasing solution of such metals as iron and manganese. Thus such waters, which may otherwise have been satisfactory for water supply, become exceedingly troublesome. Microorganisms tend to accumulate at the thermocline, the zone of rapidly changing temperature and density that separates the upper and lower layers. Management of water quality requires an understanding of the chemical, biological, and hydrological phenomena that occur in such waters.

Groundwater. Groundwaters are recharged by percolation of rainwater and runoff through the ground. Groundwater is abstracted by means of natural springs, wells, or infiltration galleries (horizontal wells). Groundwaters tend to be more highly mineralized than surface waters because of the solution of minerals as they percolate through the ground. They are, however, generally of higher sanitary quality as they are not nearly so subject to pollution as surface sources, and passage of the water through the soil serves to improve their bacteriological quality. Groundwater pollution, particularly from toxic waste discharges and leaching of landfills has become a major problem, however, and considerable care is required to protect such sources. Once a groundwater aquifer is contaminated with chemicals, many years may be required for it to be cleansed, if cleansing is indeed possible.

Yields of groundwaters are a function of the volume and size of soil interstices. In general, it is far more difficult to determine the yields of groundwater sources than of surface water sources. Such determinations depend on extensive hydrogeological exploration, including the construction of test wells and the conduct of pumping tests. Accordingly, groundwaters have not generally been as fully exploited as they might be and have been used primarily for smaller communities. On the other hand, some groundwater supplies have been overpumped, or "mined," where withdrawals have exceeded recharge. This has resulted in a steady lowering of the elevation of the water surface underground, the *water table,* diminishing the amount that can be abstracted and increasing the cost of pumping. Such excessive abstractions have also resulted in subsidence of the ground above, threatening structures and increasing the potential for flooding.

The use of groundwaters in conjunction with surface waters is only now beginning to be explored. Underground reservoirs have major advantages over surface water reservoirs: they do not lose water through evaporation; their quality is not so likely to be deleteriously affected by natural or urban and industrial pollution; and they do not require the expropriation of large areas of land. Also, they may be located nearer to the points of use than are surface impoundments. In conjunctive use, water would be drawn from surface sources during wet periods while groundwater reservoirs are recharged. During dry periods, abstractions would be from underground. Planning for such conjunctive use requires engineering and hydrological study.

A special category of underground source is the artesian aquifer, a confined aquifer under pressure. Such an aquifer is recharged at a higher elevation some distance away. When it is tapped by a well, the water in the well rises above the confining layer and may often be free flowing. Flowing springs originate from artesian aquifers because they are under pressure. Artesian aquifers are less likely to be contaminated than unconfined aquifers.

Wells are constructed in a variety of ways and configurations, depending on the nature of the aquifer from which the water is to be abstracted. Special precautions are required, however, to assure that wells are protected from surface water runoff by being encased properly, with the casing extending above ground surface.

After construction, wells must be disinfected before being tested for water quality. Sampling of water from a well is, however, pointless if the *sanitary survey* indicates that the well is not protected from contamination by surface runoff. A sample taken during a dry period may show good quality, but the water will inevitably be contaminated by surface runoff if the well is not adequately protected.

Ocean and Brackish Waters. These are unsuitable for water supply but, in conditions of dire necessity, fresh water can be obtained from them by one of several desalination processes. The most appropriate method for desalination of seawater is thermal distillation. Distillation is widely used in oil-rich areas where water is extremely limited, such as the Middle East and the West Indies. With brackish waters, where the salt content is less than 10% that of seawater, reverse osmosis or electrodialysis may be used. All methods of desalination are energy intensive. With the relative increase in the cost of energy as compared with other costs, desalination is not likely to be a feasible option for community water supplies except in situations where a high investment in providing water can be justified, such as for tourism or for industrial, military, or political purposes.

Water Reclamation and Reuse. Far more attractive than desalination in water-short areas is the reclamation of wastewaters for reuse for nonpotable purposes.[3] As a substantial portion of community water supply is required for urban irrigation and other nonpotable uses, water reuse is becoming increasingly attractive in communities where water resources are limited. Impetus for water reuse has also resulted from the increasingly rigorous requirements for wastewater treatment, which lead to production of an effluent of too high a quality at too high a cost for it to be discarded.

Early reuse developed from wastewater disposal by irrigation, a practice widely followed in Europe for more than a century. In the United States, early water reuse was exemplified by the utilization of the effluent from the Baltimore wastewater treatment facilities for the Bethlehem Steel Sparrow's Point plant in the 1930s.

The modern approach to water reuse is the development of distribution systems for nonpotable waters for a variety of purposes, including urban irrigation, residential, and industrial use. Such dual distribution systems were pioneered in Colorado Springs, Colorado; Pomona and Irvine, California; and St. Petersburg, Florida. In these instances, the nonpotable distribution systems carry secondary wastewater effluent additionally treated by coagulation, filtration, and disinfection, processes used for treatment of potable waters drawn from polluted sources. Inadvertent ingestion of water from such a nonpotable system would not be a source of waterborne disease. The main difference between the potable and nonpotable waters would be that the nonpotable waters, having as their source the wastewaters of a community, would not be free of the chemicals that are inevitably present in such wastewaters and that are not removed in wastewater or water supply treatment, but that are hazardous if ingested over a long period of time.

In 1958 the United Nations Economic and Social Council stated, "No higher quality water, unless there is a surplus of it, should be used for a purpose that can tolerate a lower grade."[4] This policy is beginning to be adopted in water-short areas of the United States. In Florida, for example, where consumptive use permits are required for all abstractions of water, the policy is that a permit will not be issued if a lower-quality water can be used and is available. Nonpotable reuse is becoming so widely adopted that the American Water Works Association has published a *Manual on Dual Distribution Systems,*[5] and some 14 states have adopted regulations for water reclamation and reuse.

Selection of Sources. A community and its engineers facing the need to provide a community's water supply must recognize that each situation is unique. Topography, climate, the availability of untapped water resources, population density, land use, and myriad other characteristics help differentiate one situation from another; none is precisely like that of any other community. The guiding principle in the selection of the source is provided in the National Interim Primary Drinking Water Regulations promulgated by the U.S. Environmental Protection Agency (EPA) in 1976:

> Production of water that poses no threat to the consumer's health depends on continuous protection. Because of human frailties associated with protection, priority should be given to the selection of the *purest source.* Polluted sources should not be used unless other sources are economically unavailable, and then only when personnel, equipment, and operating procedures can be depended on to purify and otherwise continuously protect the drinking water supply.[6] [Emphasis added.]

Earlier drinking water standards established by the U.S. Public Health Service expressed similar sentiments. Because the primary concern with water quality had been transmission of waterborne infectious disease, and because conventional filtration and disinfection with chlorine had assured protection against such disease, many cities throughout the United States opted for run-of-river supplies that were conveniently available, even though they did not constitute the "purest" source. The relatively new threat to health arising from the "chemical revolution," with the creation of many new long-lasting synthetic organic chemicals, has given new meaning to the concern for selecting the purest source, particularly because methods of monitoring for many of these chemicals are not yet available. Given options in the selection of sources, prudence dictates a search for the purest source. This might mean development of groundwaters or upstream sources free of urban and industrial pollution. Where these are not adequate in quantity to provide all the water required in a community, consideration is being given to dual systems, using the protected source for potable purposes and polluted sources or reclaimed wastewaters for nonpotable purposes.

Protection of Sources. Where high-quality sources of water supply are available, whether surface or underground, they are subject to despoilation from development on the watershed or recharge areas. Only in rare instances is the land on the watershed or recharge area under the control of the water purveyor; these areas are generally the responsibility of the local authorities, that have planning jurisdiction. Even where the water purveyor owns the land or the local authority that has dominion over the land is served by the water supply, the pressure of development can lead to degradation of the water supply.

In a landmark case, water companies in Connecticut sought to sell off portions of their wholly owned protected watersheds for development. After considerable study, legislation was enacted that forbade the sale of watershed lands for development. In response to a suit against the State of Connecticut by the water companies, the U.S. District Court upheld the State:

> . . . the obvious purpose of the legislation is the protection of the health and welfare of the State's inhabitants . . . watershed properties are critical to water purity . . . the State is ensuring the ability of the water companies to provide pure water to its customers.[7]

More generally, local authorities have planning jurisdiction over watershed lands and recharge areas, and they must work closely with the water purveyor in developing land use strategies that would protect the integrity of the water supplies. Such strategies would include regulations specifying maximum densities, limits for impervious areas, setbacks from the banks of streams and reservoirs, permissible activities, etc.[8,9] The promulgation and enforcement of such regulations require great courage and leadership on the part of elected and appointed officials because they sharply curtail the opportunities for financial profit from development.

While the greatest attention is generally given to the numerical limits for specific contaminants, far more attention is being given to the "sanitary survey," which can assure a high quality of water in the first place, and its adequate handling and distribution to the user. The regulations state:

> Knowledge of physical defects or of the existence of other health hazards in the water supply system is evidence of a deficiency in protection of the water supply. Even though water quality analyses have indicated that the quality requirements have been met, the deficiencies must be corrected before the supply can be considered safe.[6]

Obvious deficiencies include pollution of the source, inadequate treatment, cross-connections with sources of contamination, inadequate capacity resulting in low pressure, and inadequate operation of the facilities, including inadequate disinfection and failure to provide standby facilities in the event of power or other equipment failure.

In contention is whether or not the discharge of a pollutant upstream of the water intake is a deficiency. While many laws exist directed to the prevention of the discharge of toxic substances into the environment in general and water bodies in particular, implementation of these laws is uncertain at best. Little assurance can be given that a water supply drawn from a source that drains large urban and industrial areas will, in fact, be free of potentially harmful chemicals. The best course is to avoid discharging wastes above water supply intakes and to avoid installing intakes below waste discharges.

POTABLE WATER QUALITY

In the United States, protection of the public health was initially a responsibility of the states, with federal initiatives only where interstate activities were concerned. The U.S. Public Health Service Drinking Water Standards were first adopted in 1914 to protect the health of the traveling public. These standards were often adopted by individual states and came to be applicable to water supplies generally. Initially, because of their limited application, primary emphasis was on physical and bacterial parameters, the first to assure esthetic quality and the second to prevent the transmission of waterborne disease. These standards were updated periodically. In 1962, the standards were extensively revised to include chemicals and radioactivity for the first time. The only chemicals for which limits were established were heavy metals. Recognition of the problem of synthetic organic chemicals surfaced with the establishment of an upper limit for carbon chloroform extract (CCE). This served as a comprehensive, gross surrogate for synthetic organic chemicals, although it could not distinguish between those chemicals that are innocuous and those harmful to health. These standards required systems that have adequate capacity to meet peak demands without development of low pressures or other health hazards, that the quality be assessed at the free-flowing outlet of the consumer, and that the facilities be under the responsible charge of personnel whose qualifications are acceptable to the regulatory agency.

It was not until passage of the Safe Drinking Water Act (SDWA) in 1974 that public water supply systems in the United States came under the federal aegis. Under this law, the National Interim Primary Drinking Water Regulations were established and maximum contaminant levels (MCLs) were set. They are summarized in Table 35-3.[6] Contaminants not directly related to safety but only to esthetic quality are titled secondary drinking water standards and SMCLs are summarized in Table 35-4. For the first time, six synthetic organic chemicals, all well-known biocides, were included. However, no measure of total synthetic organic chemical concentration was called for. The 70,000 chemicals now in commercial production and the thousand or so introduced each year, many of which reach water sources, were ignored.

The SDWA mandated that the National Academy of Sciences (National Research Council) conduct studies on the health effects associated with contaminants found in drinking water. A series of nine reports has been published under the title *Drinking Water and Health*.[10] The first, published in 1977, is a 939-page compendium of health effects associated with microbiological, radioactive, particulate, inorganic, and organic chemical contaminants found in drinking water, including risk assessments for cancer resulting from exposure to chemical contaminants in drinking water. The others, published through 1989, add information on chlorination and disinfection byproducts in water, toxicology, epidemiological risks, risk assessments on additional chemicals, and suggested no-adverse-response levels (SNARLs) for acute and chronic exposures to chemicals in drinking water, and pharmacokinetics.

In 1981, an MCL was added for trihalomethanes (THMs), including chloroform, formed by the reaction of chlorine used for disinfection with water containing organics. An interesting aspect of the THM standard was that it was not to apply to communities of less than 10,000 population because the technology involved in meeting and monitoring for the standard was believed to be beyond the resources of such small communities, which make up more than 95% of community water supplies in the United States.

Troubled by the slow pace of establishment of new MCLs, the Congress enacted amendments to the Safe Drinking Water Act in 1986, which represented a quantum increase in requirements for the regulation of the quality of drinking water. The principal revision was that new contaminants are to be added to the regulations in a timely fashion, with a total of 83 by 1989 and at least 25 new contaminants every 3 years thereafter. In addition, MCL goals (MCLGs) are to be established for each contaminant at a level at which no known adverse effects on health would occur and that allows an adequate margin of safety. For known carcinogens, MCLGs are set at zero. The MCL is to be as

TABLE 35-3. NATIONAL INTERIM PRIMARY DRINKING WATER REGULATIONS (MCL)

Contaminant	MCL
Inorganic Chemicals	
Arsenic	0.05 (mg/L)
Barium	1
Cadmium	0.010
Chromium	0.05
Fluoride	1.4–2.4*
Lead	0.05*
Mercury	0.002
Nitrate (as N)	10
Selenium	0.01
Silver	0.05
Organic chemicals	
Chlorinated hydrocarbons	
Endrin	0.0002
Lindane	0.004*
Methoxychlor	0.1*
Toxaphene	0.005*
Chlorophenoxys	
2,4-D	0.1*
2,4,5-T. Silvex	0.01*
Trihalomethanes	0.100*
Turbidity	1 unit
Microbiologic contaminants	1 coliform bacterium per 100 ml as the arithmetic mean of all samples per month
Radioactivity	
Combined radium 226 and radium 228	5 pCi/L
Gross alpha particle activity (including radium 226 but excluding radon and uranium)	15 pCi/L
Average annual concentration of beta particle and photon radioactivity not to produce annual dose equivalent greater than	4 mrem per year
Tritium	20,000 pCi/L
Strontium 90	8 pCi/L

* Subject to early revision;consult the *Federal Register* or EPA for up-to-date regulations.
From the Environmental Protection Agency, 1976.

TABLE 35-4. INTERIM NATIONAL SECONDARY DRINKING WATER REGULATIONS (SECONDARY MAXIMUM CONTAMINANT LEVELS)

Contaminant	SMCL
Chloride	250 mg/L
Color	15 color units
Copper	1 mg/L
Corrosivity	Noncorrosive
Foaming agents	0.5 mg/L
Hydrogen sulfide	0.5 mg/L
Iron	0.3 mg/L
Manganese	0.05 mg/L
Odor	3 threshold odor number
pH	6.5–8.5
Sulfate	250 mg/L
TDS	500 mg/L
Zinc	5 mg/L

TABLE 35-5. VOLATILE ORGANIC CHEMICAL ADDITIONS TO PRIMARY DRINKING WATER REGULATIONS IN TABLE 35-3

Contaminant	MCL (mg/L)	MCLG (mg/L)
Benzene	0.005	zero
Carbon tetrachloride	0.005	zero
p-Dichlorobenzene	0.075	0.075
1,2-Dichloroethane	0.005	zero
1,1-Dichloroethylene	0.007	0.007
1,1,1-Trichloroethane	0.20	0.20
Trichloroethylene	0.005	zero
Vinyl chloride	0.002	zero

close to the MCLG as is feasible. The promulgation of these MCLs and MCLGs is behind schedule.

Only the contaminants listed in Table 35-5, all volatile organic chemicals, had been added by 1989. Tables 35-6 and 35-7 list other contaminants that have been proposed for regulation, while Table 35-8 contains a priority list of contaminants that may be considered for inclusion in the regulations in the future. In addition, the EPA listed 29 chemicals that must be monitored by the states if their waters are vulnerable and another 84 proposed for monitoring at the discretion of the states. Table 35-9 lists possible additions to the list of secondary MCLs. Regulation of these contaminants is to become effective in 1991, 1992, and 1993, but the actual dates may be somewhat later. However, their identification does provide early warning for water purveyors as they plan for future investments. A major problem for water purveyors and local regulatory authorities is that the new regulations are published piecemeal, as they are approved, in the *Federal Register* and no single publication that codifies all the regulations is available 14 years after the Interim Regulations[6] were published.

Other regulations mandated by the 1986 Amendments to the SDWA include:

- The establishment of the best available technology (BAT) to meet the MCLs and MCLGs promulgated.
- Prohibition of the use of lead materials in water supply systems or in plumbing used to convey drinking water, with a requirement for public notice where lead is present and/or where the water is sufficiently corrosive to cause leaching of lead.
- Regulations for the protection of groundwater sources.
- Regulations specifying criteria under which filtration will be required for surface water sources, including quality of the source, vulnerability of the watershed to pollution, and protection offered by watershed management practices.

Among the criteria established to avoid filtration are the following:

- Fecal coliform ≤ 20/100 ml or total coliform ≤ 100/100 ml 90% of the time.
- Turbidity ≤ 5 NTU immediately before disinfection.
- Maintenance of a watershed control program that minimizes the potential for contamination by *Giardia lamblia* and viruses.
- Performance of an annual sanitary survey.

TABLE 35-6. PROPOSED REGULATIONS FOR SYNTHETIC ORGANIC CHEMICALS

SOC	Proposed MCL (mg/L)	Proposed MCLG (mg/L)
Acrylamide	treatment technique	zero
Alachlor	0.002	zero
Aldicarb	0.01	0.01
Aldicarb sulfone	0.04	0.04
Aldicarb sulfoxide	0.01	0.01
Atrazine	0.003	0.003
Carbofuran	0.04	0.04
Chlordane	0.002	zero
2,4-D*	0.07	0.07
Dibromochloropropane (DBCP)	0.0002	zero
o-Dichlorobenzene	0.6	0.6
cis-1,2-Dichloroethylene	0.07	0.07
trans-1,2-Dichloroethylene	0.1	0.1
1,2-Dichloropropane	0.005	zero
Epichlorohydrin	treatment technique	zero
Ethylbenzene	0.7	0.7
Ethylene dibromide (EDB)	0.00005	zero
Heptachlor	0.0004	zero
Heptachlor epoxide	0.0002	zero
Lindane*	0.0002	0.0002
Methoxychlor*	0.4	0.4
Monochlorobenzene	0.1	0.1
PCBs (as decachlorobiphenyls)	0.0005	zero
Pentachlorophenol	0.2	0.2
Styrene	0.005	zero/0.1
Tetrachloroethylene	0.005	zero
Toluene	2.0	2.0
Toxaphene*	0.005	zero
2,4,5-TP (Silvex)*	0.05	0.05
Xylene	10	10

* Proposed change in MCLs in Interim Regulations, as shown in Table 35-3.

TABLE 35-7. CONTAMINANTS BEING CONSIDERED FOR MCLs AND MCLGs BY EPA (IN ADDITION TO THOSE CURRENTLY REGULATED AS SHOWN IN TABLES 35-3 AND 35-5)

▪ MICROBIAL	
Giardia lamblia	Plate count
Viruses	*Legionella*
▪ VOLATILE ORGANIC CHEMICALS	
Chlorobenzene	trans-1,2-Dichloroethylene
cis-1,2,-Dichloroethylene	Tetrachloroethylene
Methylene chloride	Trichlorobenzene(s)
▪ SYNTHETIC ORGANIC CHEMICALS	
Aldicarb	PCBs (polychlorinated biphenyls)
Aldicarb sulfoxide	Atrazine
Aldicarb sulfone	Phthalates
Chlordane	Acrylamide
Dalapon	DBCP (dibromochloropropane)
Diquat	1,2-Dichloropropane
Endothall	Pentachlorophenol
Ethylbenzene	Picloram
Glyphosate	Dinoseb
Heptachlor	Alachlor
Heptachlor epoxide	EDB (ethylene dibromide)
Carbofuran	Epichlorohydrin
1,1,2-Trichlorethane	Stylene
Vydate	Toluene
Simazine	Xylene
Stylene	Adipates
PAHs (polynuclear aromatic hydrocarbons)	Hexachlorocyclopentadiene
	2,3,7,8-TCDD (dioxin)
▪ INORGANIC CHEMICALS	
Antimony	Nitrite
Asbestos	Thallium
Sulfate	Beryllium
Copper	Cyanide
Nickel	
▪ RADIOLOGICAL CONTAMINANTS	
Natural Uranium	Radon

- Contiguous monitoring of disinfectant residual and maintenance of no less than 0.2 mg/L in the distribution system.

Altogether, regulations for the assurance of safe water are expected to be in continuous flux for the foreseeable future.

CHEMICAL CONTAMINANTS

Maximum contaminant levels in drinking waters have been set for eight metals, nitrates, fluorides, and six organic chemicals plus trihalomethanes (THMs), as shown in Table 35-3. In arriving at MCLs, the total environmental exposure of humans to the specific toxin is considered. An attempt is made to set lifetime limits at the lowest practical level in order to minimize the amount of toxicant carried by water, particularly when other sources such as food or air are known to represent the major exposure. The toxicological basis for each of the limits is provided in the appendix of the Drinking Water Regulations and in the *Federal Register* from time to time as new contaminants are proposed for regulation.[6] Limits are not given for every toxicant or undesirable contaminant that might be in the public water supply, as scientific data are not available for many of the chemicals of concern. Also, the analytic burden for assessing the presence and concentration of all the chemicals of concern would be inordinately great. As it is, the determination of these chemicals requires experienced analysts and sophisticated instrumentation. Most larger water supply laboratories are equipped with atomic

TABLE 35-8. PRIORITY CONTAMINANTS THAT MAY REQUIRE ESTABLISHMENT OF MCLs AND MCLGs

▪ POSSIBLE SUBSTITUTES FOR CONTAMINANTS IN TABLE 35-7	
Aluminum	Sodium
Dibromomethane	Vanadium
Molybdenum	Zinc
Silver	
▪ DISINFECTANTS AND THEIR BY-PRODUCTS	
Ammonia	Chloropicrin
Bromochloroacetonitrile	Cyanogen chloride
Bromodichloromethane	Dibromoacetonitrile
Bromoform	Dibromochloromethane
Chloramines	Dichloroacetonitrile
Chlorates	Halogenated acids, alcohols, aldehydes, ketones, and other nitriles
Chlorine	Hypochlorite ion
Chlorine dioxide	Ozone byproducts
Chlorite	
Chloroform	
▪ OTHER ORGANIC COMPOUNDS	
Bromobenzene	2,2-Dichloropropane
Bromomethane	2,4-Dinitrotoluene
Chloromethane	ETU
o-Chlorotoluene	Isophorone
p-Chlorotoluene	Metolachlor
Cyanazine	Metribuzin
Dicamba	2,4,5-T
1,1-Dichloroethane	1,1,1,2-Tetrachloroethane
1,1-Dichloropropene	1,1,2,2-Tetrachloroethane
1,3-Dichloropropane	1,2,5-Trichloropropane
1,3-Dichloropropene	Trifluralin
▪ OTHER SUBSTANCES REPORTED AT HIGH CONCENTRATIONS	
Boron	*Cryptosporidium*
Strontium	

TABLE 35-9. CONTAMINANTS BEING CONSIDERED BY EPA FOR ADDITION TO THE LIST OF SECONDARY MCLs IN TABLE 35-4

Contaminant	SMCL (mg/L)
Aluminum	0.05
o-Dichlorobenzene	0.01
p-Dichlorobenzene	0.005
Ethylbenzene	0.03
Pentachlorophenol	0.03
Silver	0.09
Styrene	0.01
Toluene	0.04
Xylene	0.02

absorption spectrophotometers for determination of the metals. The gas chromatograph mass spectrometers required for determination of the synthetic organics are many times more costly, however, and fewer laboratories are equipped for these determinations. Utilities with the more protected sources will have fewer monitoring problems.

Heavy Metals. Among the classes of contaminants, the MCLs for the heavy metals appear to rest on the firmest basis; however, the data on the health effects of many individual metals are not adequate and the significance of combinations of contaminants has not been addressed. The MCLs for several metals, such as chromium and arsenic, are being reevaluated, and even so ubiquitous a metal as aluminum, which is used as a coagulant in water treatment, is being examined for possible neurological significance. (See Chapter 20.)

Of all the heavy metals, lead is of greatest concern. The heaviest concentrations of lead in water supplies result from the use of lead service piping. Waters remaining in lead pipes overnight, particularly soft waters, dissolve considerable lead. Lead is no longer authorized for piping, and existing lead-containing services should be gradually replaced. Meanwhile, customers with lead service pipes should allow the first flush of water each day to be wasted. Lead also originates from developments on watersheds, its load being a function of the length of streets in the area. The evidence is strong that even very low concentrations of lead are neurologically damaging to children, so that a reduction in the MCL for lead is expected in the next regulations. Also, an MCL and an MCLG of 1.3 mg/L for copper is being proposed.

Synthetic Organic Chemicals. Some 1000 specific synthetic organic chemicals (SOCs), at nanogram to microgram per liter concentrations, have been identified in drinking water supplies in the United States. These compounds result from industrial and municipal discharges, urban road runoff, and reaction of chlorine in water treatment with natural organics.

The 1986 SDWA Amendments represented a major step toward addressing SOCs. As shown in Tables 35–5 to 35–8 and in the requirements for monitoring by the states, hundreds of new SOCs will be brought under regulatory purview. While this will require a major change in commitment for water purveyors and regulators alike, determination of the principal impact of SOCs on health remains intractable; the MCLs and MCLGs are based on anticipated exposures to individual contaminants and the significance of exposures to combinations of these contaminations is still to be determined.

The problem of the synthetic organic chemicals that originate from industrial and municipal discharges and urban runoff is far less tractable because of their vast number, their highly variable concentrations, and the uncertainty as to their presence.

Most of the organic chemicals identified in drinking water have not yet been examined for their health effects, and the National Research Council indicates that only about 10% of the organic chemicals in water have been identified. Where effects have been established, these are generally based on animal studies on individual contaminants, and there is uncertainty as to the actual risk posed to humans who ingest very low concentrations of combinations of contaminants over an extended period of time. Such epidemiological studies as have been made are far from definitive. The National Research Council studies[10] offer ample evidence of the uncertainties involved in establishing acceptable levels of trace contaminants. What can be stated with certainty is that the situation with regard to acceptable levels of synthetic organic chemicals in drinking water is constantly changing and will undergo continuous reassessment.

Accordingly, the most prudent approach lies in selecting sources of water that are free of urban and industrial pollution. Although this does not guarantee that they would not be subject to airborne contaminants and runoff from the land, these contaminants may be more readily identified and managed.

Chlorine Reaction Products. The problem of chlorine reaction products, and other disinfectant reaction products as well, is also troublesome. The MCL for THMs, 0.100 mg/L, had been established as an expedient, rather than on the same health-risk basis as for other contaminants, one additional death per 1 million population over 70 years' exposure. This MCL is expected to be lowered to 0.025 or 0.050 mg/L, which will still allow it at higher risk than other contaminants. Another chlorine reaction product, 3-chloro-4-(dichloromethyl)-5-hydroxy-2(5H)-furanone (labeled MX), has been found in drinking waters drawn from surface waters. Although present only at nanogram levels, its high mutagenicity (more than 1 millionfold greater than the THMs) makes MX potentially a far more serious reaction product than THMs, accounting for an estimated 15% to 60% of the total mutagenicity of chlorinated waters. One problem with MX is that it is nonvolatile and therefore is not easily measured.

The epidemiological significance of chlorine reaction products was established in a case control study by the National Cancer Institute.[11] Through examination of some 8000 persons, including 2805 with bladder cancer, a significantly higher cancer risk was found for people who drank chlorinated surface tap water for at least 40 years than for people who drank unchlorinated groundwater. Those who drank the most chlorinated water had twice the risk as the lowest tap water users. Among nonsmokers, the relative risk for more than 60 years' exposure was 3.1 as compared with nonsmokers using unchlorinated water. From these data, it was inferred that 12% of bladder cancer in the study population was caused by the chlorinated surface water.

Nitrates. A temporary blood disorder, methemoglobinemia, has occurred in infants after ingestion of well waters containing nitrates in concentrations greater than 10 mg/L of nitrogen. Some 2000 cases of this disease have been reported in North America and Europe, with a 7% to 8% mortality rate. The disease results from the conversion in the gastrointestinal tract of innocuous nitrates to nitrites, which then convert hemoglobin to methemoglobin (which cannot transport oxygen), resulting in suffocation. Nitrites in water do not themselves pose a problem because they are unstable and are not present in sufficient concentrations to be troublesome. The disease has not been associated with ingestion of high-nitrate surface waters, although the reasons for this have not yet been established.

Since only infants are at risk and then only for a few months, a convenient solution where the public water supply cannot easily conform with the standards is to provide bottled water for infants during this brief period of risk.

Consumers of water supply systems that contain excessive nitrates or, for that matter, exceed any of the maximum contaminant levels established in the primary drinking water regulations must be informed by the purveyor through the media and by direct notification.

Fluorides. Fluoride is a normal constituent of all diets and is an essential nutrient. When the concentration is optimum, no ill effects result and the caries rate in children is 60% to 65% below the rates in communities with little or no fluorides in their water supplies. Excessive fluorides in drinking water supplies produce unsightly dental fluorosis, which increases with increasing fluoride concentration. The optimal fluoride level in drinking water differs from place to place, varying with amounts of fluorides in food and with climatic conditions, because the amount of water and therefore the amount of fluoride ingested by children is influenced by temperature (Chapter 62). In the interim primary regulations the optimum fluoride content varied from 0.7 to 1.2 mg/L with MCLs of 1.4 to 2.4 mg/L, with the higher values at temperatures below 12° C and the lower values at temperatures above 26.3° C. Currently the MCL for fluorides is 4 mg/L.

Some water supplies in the United States, particularly in the Southwest, contain fluorides naturally at or near the optimum level and have achieved the benefits of fluorides without intervention. Many communities throughout the country with water supplies containing less than the optimum level of fluorides have provided fluoride supplementation, although the decision to adopt fluoridation has not been without controversy. Communities with excessively high fluoride levels tend to reduce the concentrations by partial defluoridation, by changing the water source, or by adding a low-fluoride water to attain the optimum. The health effects of fluoridation have been studied intensively, and no side effects have been associated with optimum levels of fluoride in water. Although there is no scientific basis for considering added fluorides any different from naturally occurring fluorides, the issue continues to be examined.

Asbestos. While it has long been recognized that workers exposed to asbestos through inhalation may have marked increases in rates of lung cancer and pleural and peritoneal mesothelioma, and regulations to limit inhalation exposures to asbestos have been promulgated, asbestos is not mentioned in the Drinking Water Regulations.[6] Volume 1 of *Drinking Water and Health* suggests, however, that the possibility of long-delayed effects of the ingestion of asbestos through drinking water cannot be ignored and Volume 5, published 6 years later, concludes that an excess of gastrointestinal (GI) tract cancers is associated with occupational exposure to asbestos.[10] Although animal asbestos-ingestion studies have not produced convincing evidence of GI tumors, epidemiological studies did lead to the conclusion that ingestion of asbestos in drinking water increases the risk of cancer. Assuming a daily consumption of 2 L of water, a concentration of 110,000 fibers, as measured by transmission electronic microscopy (TEM), per liter may lead to one additional GI tract cancer per 100,000 persons exposed over a 70-year lifetime.

An MCL for asbestos is being considered (Table 35-7). In the meantime, the possibility of the presence of asbestos should be considered in the evaluation and selection of water sources and treatment. More than 20% of 365 cities surveyed in the United States had water containing more than 1 million TEM fibers per liter and more than 10% had more than 10 million fibers per liter. Much of this asbestos originates on watersheds and can be removed by filtration. Some, however, is attributed to the use of asbestos-cement pipes, but its significance is yet to be established.

Radionuclides. Radioactivity in public water supplies may be naturally occurring or man-made. Radium 226, among the more important of the naturally occurring radionuclides, is found in groundwaters as a result of geological conditions. Man-made radioactivity, on the other hand, finds its way into surface waters as a result of fallout from weapons testing and releases from nuclear power plants and users of radioactive materials.[12]

The establishment of limits for radioactivity suffers from the same uncertainties as those inherent in establishment of limits for synthetic organic chemicals, i.e., the assumptions that there is no threshold below which any dose is considered to be harmless and that health effects are proportional to the dose. Attempts are made, in establishing limits, to weigh the cost of achieving certain levels, both in uses of radioactivity forgone and in water supply decisions, as against the expected risks and benefits in reduced radiation exposures to the population.[13]

Some hint of the order of magnitude of the allowable concentrations can be ascertained by comparing the maximum contaminant levels permitted in the standards with dose levels established by the Federal Radiation Council.[4] The annual dose of man-made radionuclides, beta and photon emitters, via the drinking water route is limited to 4 mrem per year by the EPA as compared with 170 mrem specified by the Federal Radiation Council from all sources except radiation received for medical purposes and that due to natural background. An exposure of 4 mrem per year corresponds to a lifetime cancer risk increase of 0.025% in exposed groups.

In the case of natural radioactivity, primarily Radium 226 and Radium 228, the allowance for drinking water amounts to half the recommended daily intake via all routes.

The maximum contaminant level for gross alpha particle activity, 15 picocuries (pCi) per liter, is based on the conservative assumption that, if the radium concentration is 5 pCi/L, which is its limit, and the balance of the alpha particle activity is due to the most radiotoxic alpha particle-emitting chain, the total dose to bone would be equivalent to less than 6 pCi/L of Radium 226.

Because its control is less tractable, the natural radium contamination in drinking water is often of more concern than man-made radioactivity, particularly because it affects the small water supplies that draw from groundwaters. Some concentrations as large as 50 pCi/L have been reported, and some 500 community water supply systems deliver water that exceeds the standard. If other sources of water cannot be found, the radium can be removed by ion exchange, although this increases the concentration of sodium and may be of concern to that portion of the population requiring low-sodium diets.

Radon, a daughter product of radium, is a naturally occurring radionuclide in groundwater. Surveys indicate that about 70% of groundwater supplies have detectable radon, but only about 10% exceed 1000 pCi/L and, of these, fewer than 1% occur in communities of more than 500 people.[14] An MCL for radon is being considered, possibly between 500 and 1000 pCi/L. Aeration is an effective and simple method for removing radon from community water supplies. Granular activated carbon filters may be used for adsorption of radon for private supplies serving individual households, but the buildup of radioactivity on the GAC may present problems. Accordingly, while radon is not likely to pose a problem for larger community supplies, it may be a problem for individual or very small supplies.

Secondary Maximum Contaminant Levels. There are no direct health consequences from exceeding the levels shown in Tables 35-4 and 35-9. Effects are primarily of esthetic or economic concern. Waters high in hydrogen sulfide, iron, manganese, color, or odor may, even if satisfactory from a health standpoint, encourage a user to seek another less offensive source, which may not be safe. Corrosive action resulting from low pH and low alkalinity may have significant economic consequences as well as discoloring the water and imparting stains to clothing and fixtures. The significance of corrosivity on lead concentrations is discussed on p. 625.

Hardness in water is due primarily to the carbonate and sulfate salts of calcium and magnesium. More soap is required for bathing and laundering with hard water than with soft water. While no limit is specified for hardness or the constituents associated with hardness, many water supplies have incorporated softening to reduce the economic burden on customers who would otherwise be required to use excessive amounts of soap. With the development of synthetic detergents, which contain softening agents, hardness poses much less of a problem and softening may not be economically justified. Furthermore, epidemiological studies have suggested that there is an inverse relationship between the hardness of water and the cardiovascular disease mortality rate. While these studies are not conclusive, and there is not yet a basis for adding hardness to water supplies or for selecting a source based on higher hardness, there does appear to be less justification today for softening public water supplies. Individual large consumers, such as laundries, may find softening of their own supplies advisable.

Sulfates in drinking water are cathartic. The laxative dose for Epsom salt ($MgSO_4 \cdot 7H_2O$) is about 2 g. This dose would be obtained by ingesting 2 liters of water containing 390 mg/L of sulfate. This laxative effect of waters high in sulfates is more pronounced in occasional users, as those who ingest such waters continuously apparently become acclimated. A safeguard is that waters containing sulfate salts in concentrations that may have laxative properties also impart a slight taste that is noticeable to the occasional user if not to the chronic user. Hence there is considered to be no serious health consequence from the presence of high levels of sulfates in water.

Sodium is ingested as sodium chloride, table salt, in fairly liberal quantities, ranging from 4 to 24 g per day and averaging 10 g per day for American males. This represents a sodium intake of 1600 to 9600 mg per day. Intakes at these levels are considered to have no adverse effect on normal persons. Consequently, the sodium ion concentration in water supplies is of little consequence to the normal person. A sodium survey of 2100 public water supplies in 1963 indicated that 95% of the samples contained a sodium ion concentration under 250 mg/L, with almost 50% under 20 mg/L. At a 2 L intake per day, the 250 mg/L concentration would represent only a small portion of the total salt intake. Sodium levels are important, however, in the control of several disease conditions, including congestive heart failure and hypertension, which affect some 25 million Americans. A restricted sodium intake is recommended for these people. Water supplies with high concentrations of sodium might well furnish their entire daily allowance, permitting no salt ingestion with food. Although there is now no limit on sodium, water purveyors who furnish waters high in sodium should advise physicians in their service areas of the concentrations they can expect.

Softening of water, particularly by ion exchange, adds significant concentrations of sodium, which would be of consequence to that portion of the population on low-sodium diets. The use of home softeners, which are all based on ion exchange, adds substantial concentrations of sodium to water delivered in the home, concentrations of which consumers may not be aware. This constitutes another argument for a policy requiring water quality problems to be addressed centrally rather than in individual homes, where the costs for treatment are substantially higher and where the impacts on quality are uncertain.

Analytical Methods of Analysis. Methods of analysis for water quality, published in *Standard Methods for the Examination of Water and Wastewater*[15] by the American Public Health Association and other organizations, are updated every 5 years. These are being improved continually, with better methods replacing older technologies and with new methods for contaminants that are only recently being considered for regulation. These newer methods appear in the journals, but those being introduced before publication in *Standard Methods* are published in *The Federal Register*.

MICROBIOLOGICAL QUALITY

Five categories of pathogens are found in water: bacteria, viruses, protozoa, worms, and fungi. The principal bacterial waterborne diseases are typhoid, cholera, and shigellosis (bacillary dysentery), all of which attacked the industrialized countries of the world in the mid-nineteenth century and are still major causes of morbidity and mortality in Asia, Africa, and Latin America.

The coliform determination that has been used as a measure of fecal contamination since the early twentieth century is valuable, not because the coliform organisms are pathogenic but because they are always present in the normal intestinal tract of humans and other warm-blooded animals and are found in great numbers in fecal wastes. Thus, while their presence may not signify that a water is a health hazard, their absence provides reasonable evidence of bacteriologically safe water.

Some bacteria included in the total coliform group have wide distribution in the environment but are not evident in all fecal discharges. Other coliforms may be found in fecal discharges but usually in smaller numbers than *Escherichia coli,* the predominant coliform in humans and other warm-blooded animals. Various coliforms have different survival times in the environment, and an assessment of the presence of these different species may indicate the nature of the water contamination. In waters recently contaminated by fecal discharges, however, the fecal coliform organisms are present in larger numbers and the fecal coliform count is a useful test to affirm the presence of fecal pollution.

Nevertheless, the presence of any type of coliform organism in treated water suggests either inadequate treatment or contamination of the treated water. Coliform bacteria, whether fecal or nonfecal, should not be present in significant numbers in any potable water supply.

Unfortunately, coliform determinations are somewhat tedious and time consuming, despite recent simplifications of the methods and modifications that produce results within 24 hours. By the time the results of the bacterial analyses are in hand, the water sampled will already have been ingested. For quality-control purposes, the frequent determination of turbidity levels and disinfectant residuals, which can be on-line in real time, are now used for quality control in addition to periodic coliform determinations. The product of the disinfectant residual concentration (C) and the time of contact (T), or CT in milligrams per liter-minutes, to achieve a specified degree of inactivation of a target pathogen in water at a given pH and temperature, is becoming the basis for disinfection regulations in the United States. For example, in the current regulations for drinking water derived from surface sources, the target organism for disinfectant CT values is the protozoan cyst *Giardia lamblia.* Table 35–10 indicates CT values for selected temperatures, pHs, and disinfectants based on *Giardia lamblia,* the most resistant. The additional 2-log inactivation required by the regulations is expected to be achieved by filtration before disinfection. For drinking water derived from surface sources, filtration is recommended before disinfection to reduce turbidity in order to better remove pathogens and also to reduce disinfection requirements.

TABLE 35–10. CT* VALUES FOR 1-LOG INACTIVATION OF *GIARDIA LAMBLIA*†[20]

		Temperature °C			
	pH	**0.5**	**5**	**10**	**15**
Free chlorine‡	6	49	35	26	19
	7	70	50	37	28
	8	101	72	54	36
	9	146	146	78	59
Ozone		0.97	0.63	0.48	0.32
Chlorine Dioxide		2.1	8.4	7.4	6.3
Chloramines, preformed		1270	730	620	500

*C = concentration of disinfectant (mg/L); T = contact time (minutes)
†Prefiltration removes about 2 logs of *Giardia lamblia.*
‡Based on free chlorine of 2 mg/L; varies somewhat with other concentrations.

Turbidity interferes with the effectiveness of disinfection, and many pathogens and indicator organisms in water are associated with the particulate matter comprising turbidity. For this reason, a turbidity standard is included in the primary drinking water regulations. The standard has been modified from the 5 units in the 1962 standards and the 1 unit in the 1976 regulations by relating the turbidity limit of drinking water produced from surface sources to the options for filtration. Filtered water supplies must achieve a turbidity of < 1 unit, although turbidity up to 5 units is allowed in exceptional cases for unfiltered or slow sand-filtered waters. The requirement in the 1989 regulations for filtration (and associated pretreatment, such as coagulation and flocculation) as well as disinfection of drinking water produced from surface sources is intended to adequately control contamination by *Giardia lamblia* as well as enteric viruses, bacteria, and turbidity.

Viruses of human origin have been identified as causative agents of waterborne disease. The viruses of concern include the enteroviruses (hepatitis A virus, polioviruses, coxsackieviruses, and echoviruses), rotaviruses, reoviruses, adenoviruses and the Norwalk-type gastroenteritis viruses ("small, round viruses" or SRVs). In all, more than 100 different human enteric viruses are recognized, and new ones continue to be discovered. Numerous outbreaks of hepatitis A and Norwalk gastroenteritis, a few outbreaks of rotavirus gastroenteritis, and possibly some of poliomyelitis have been identified as waterborne, some from waters that were ostensibly treated to satisfactory standards, although this is not yet well established.

However, there is no MCL standard for viruses in the regulations because virology techniques have not yet been perfected to the point where they can be used for the routine monitoring of water quality required for regulation. As viruses in substantial numbers are expected to be present where polluted sources are used or where wastewater reclamation is practiced, technology-based standards designed to control viruses continue to be the basis for regulations until a reliable viral indicator system is developed or the procedures for enteric virus examination become simple, reliable, and rapid.

In untreated wastewaters and fecal material some 50,000 to 100,000 coliform organisms can be expected per virus unit, although this ratio can be substantially different during virus disease outbreaks. Viruses survive longer in natural waters and are more resistant to treatment processes than coliforms, however, and the ratio for a treated water may be substantially lower.

The role of waterborne viruses in the spread of disease is still to be adequately quantified. There is a hypothesis that polluted waters that are inadequately treated, but that meet present drinking water standards, may in fact contain low levels of human viruses that might cause subclinical infections and illness in susceptible persons. This, in turn, might result in spread of the virus by person-to-person contact. Epidemiological studies of waterborne viral disease, other than during epidemics, are difficult to mount, and it may be many years before the relationship between viral contamination of water and health can be established.

Protozoan infections, particularly amebic dysentery, are estimated to affect up to 10% of the U.S. population. Because of the small number of cysts excreted and their ready removal in nature and in treatment, relatively massive pollution is required for the initiation of waterborne outbreaks of amebic dysentery.

Giardiasis, caused by a flagellated protozoa, *Giardia lamblia,* has emerged as one of the most important waterborne infectious diseases in the United States, with 92 outbreaks causing nearly 25,000 cases from 1978 to 1986, more than for any other waterborne disease of known etiology.[16] Most outbreaks have been attributed to the ingestion of surface waters without adequate treatment. Because of their ability to survive for long periods in natural waters, waterborne giardiasis may be a problem where *Giardia* is endemic in wild animal populations. Apparently, meeting coliform standards without effective coagulation and filtration in addition to chlorination does not assure the destruction of *Giardia* cysts. This has become another reason for recommending filtration of all surface waters.

Another protozoan now recognized as being responsible for waterborne disease is *Cryptosporidium,* a coccidian protozoan that is fecally excreted and present in polluted water as a highly resistant, relatively small (3 to 6 μm diameter) oocyst. The natural history of this agent is similar to that of *Giardia lamblia.* A recent outbreak in Great Britain indicates that conventional treatment may be inadequate to prevent waterborne outbreaks by this agent if the source water is heavily contaminated.[17] The outbreak serves to emphasize the importance of protecting source waters from excessive fecal contamination by animal as well as human sources.

Worm infections generally result from unsanitary disposal of fecal material and, as they are not a function of the distribution of water, are not generally addressed through water treatment. Worm infections are caused by pollution of the soil on which people, particularly children, walk barefoot (hookworm) or by irrigation or fertilization with wastewaters or fecal material of vegetables that are eaten raw. The most important of the worm infections is schistosomiasis. While water supply has been shown to reduce schistosomiasis by making available proper bathing and laundering facilities, which reduce exposure to polluted waters, in general the control of schistosomiasis requires the sanitary disposal of human wastes and the control of the snail hosts. While schistosomiasis does not occur in the United States, the snail hosts and larvae of schistosomes that cause swimmer's itch do occur in some parts of the country, where they are transported from one body of water to another by infected waterfowl.

Bacteriological Examination of Drinking Waters. Determination of coliform organisms in drinking waters is routinely required by the purveyor, the regulatory agency, or both. Because the number of coliform organisms in drinking water is small and the organisms are not necessarily randomly distributed, the 1989 coliform MCL is based on the frequency of positive 100 ml samples collected over time. No more than 5.0% of the samples collected per month can be positive for coliform, and if fewer than 40 samples are collected monthly, no more than 1 can be positive for coliform. The number of samples required each month is based on the size of the population served by the water supply, with larger service populations requiring larger numbers of samples. A coliform-positive sample requires the collection of repeat samples for coliform analysis within 24 hours of obtaining positive results. Furthermore, cultures from coliform-positive samples must be further analyzed for fecal coliforms or *E. coli,* that, if positive, are considered to represent a serious violation requiring notification of the state agency and further investigative and corrective actions.

Four alternative tests can be used for coliform analysis of water, but the total sample size must be 100 ml in all cases. The basis of all tests is to detect aerobic or facultative anaerobic, Gram-negative, rod-shaped, non-spore-forming bacteria that ferment lactose with the production of acid and gas within 24 to 48 hours of incubation at 35° C. The multiple-tube fermentation technique is done by adding 10 ml portions of the sample to 10 separate tubes of lactose-containing medium (or 20 ml portions to five separate tubes of medium). Positive (growth plus gas production) tubes after 48 hours of incubation at 35° C are transferred to confirmatory medium, and, if any are positive, the sample is confirmed positive for coliforms. The membrane filter test (MFT) is done by filtering a 100 ml sample through a membrane filter that retains the bacteria. The membrane is placed on the surface of coliform medium in a petri dish and incubated for 24 hours at 35° C. If coliforms are present, they will produce characteristic-appearing colonies on the surface of the membrane that can be readily counted with the unaided eye or under a low-power microscope. The presence-absence (P-A) coliform test is done by using a single 100 ml sample. Growth with the production of acid or acid plus gas is presumptively positive, and these cultures are transferred as in the MFT test for confirmation. Another coliform test that can be performed with multiple tubes or a single P-A container uses a non-lactose-containing medium in which coliforms are detected because they grow by 24 hours at 35° C on a minimal medium containing the substrate ortho-nitrophenyl-galactoside (ONPG). Growth causes hydrolysis of this substrate and acid production, which is detected by a dye in the medium that changes color when acidified.

Microbiology of Recreational Waters. Until 1986 the bacteriological quality of bathing waters recommended by the EPA was based on a fecal coliform level not exceeding a log mean of 200/100 ml over a 30-day period.[16] This criterion, which was used by some 95% of the states and territories of the United States, was first proposed in 1968 and was based on only the sketchiest of epidemiological data. Furthermore, it provides regulatory officials with a "go–no go" number of doubtful validity.

From 1972 to 1982 the EPA engaged in a long-term recreational water quality research program that examined the relationship between water quality and swimming-associated acute infectious disease, first in marine bathing areas[17] and then in fresh water bathing areas.[18,19] In both types of water a linear relationship was found between *E. coli* and enterococci density and swimming-associated gastrointestinal symptoms rates, such as shown in Figure 35–3. Fecal coliforms did not exhibit such a relationship.

Measurable health effects were associated with enterococcus or *E. coli* densities in seawater as low as 10/100 ml via a route in which 10 to 50 ml of water is ingested. At equivalent indicator densities, the health effects were approximately one-third as great as in fresh water.

The best use of these relationships is in the selection of acceptable risks, followed by estimates of relevant bacterial densities and their translation into effluent guidelines for degree of wastewater treatment and location of outfalls. Much more information is needed, however, particularly with regard to die-away of both indicators and pathogens and identification of the pathogens responsible for gastrointestinal illness.

EPA produced guidelines in 1986 recommending that the states adopt the enterococcus criterion for marine waters and either the enterococcus or *E. coli* criterion for fresh waters. While the states were left to select appropriate bacterial densities, the EPA recommended a geometric mean of about 35/100 ml for both waters, corresponding to a geometric mean of 200/ml fecal coliform.[20]

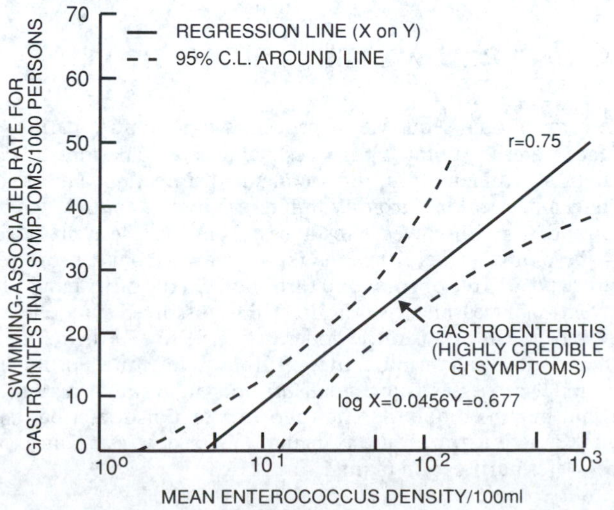

Figure 35–3. Recommended health effects criterion for marine recreation waters. *[From Cabelli VJ, 1983.[18]]*

Water Standards as Applied in Developing Countries. High infant mortality rates in developing countries, often more than tenfold greater than in industrialized countries, are attributed in good part to inadequate water supply and sanitation. That some 1.5 billion people are estimated to lack reasonable access to safe water led the United Nations, on November 10, 1980, to inaugurate the International Drinking Water Supply and Sanitation Decade (1981 to 1990). An excellent reference, *Water and Human Health,* on the relationship between water and disease in developing countries was prepared by McJunkin.[21]

Considerable controversy has arisen concerning the standards to be applied to community water supplies in developing countries. It has been argued that the availability of water for household use and personal cleanliness may be more important than the quality of that water. The cost of assuring quality such as is required in the United States and other industrialized countries may be so great as to militate against the installation of any water supply facilities at all. Thus there is pressure to relax drinking water standards in developing countries. On the other hand, bacterial standards must necessarily be a function of the incidence of bacterial disease. The success of water-sanitation programs in the United States in the twentieth century has resulted in the virtual disappearance of waterborne typhoid and cholera. Consequently, U.S. bacterial standards could be relaxed considerably without much likelihood of any increase in waterborne disease. On the other hand, in countries where typhoid and cholera are endemic and periodically epidemic, if water is not to be a vehicle for the spread of the diseases the bacterial standards may have to be somewhat more stringent. Health status, water use habits, and economic circumstances should all help determine the standards that are most appropriate.[22]

Chemical standards may be of less importance in the developing countries because these chemicals are not likely to be present in large numbers or concentration and chronic disease resulting from long-term exposure to low concentrations of SOCs is not likely to be a problem in the face of high rates of enteric disease.

The World Health Organization (WHO) had adopted separate drinking water standards for Europe and the developing countries of Asia, Africa, and Latin America. Recognizing that these standards were used primarily as guides to countries for establishing their own standards, WHO has published *Guidelines for Drinking Water Quality.*[23] It considers all health effects issues but also the practical application of the guidelines to developing countries. The guidelines comprise three volumes: Volume 1 includes recommended values for all contaminants, including SOCs, together with guidelines for their application and attainment; Volume 2 provides the health effects criteria on which Volume 1 is based; and Volume 3, "Drinking Water Quality Surveillance for Small Community Supplies" contains guidelines for developing countries, emphasizing microbiological rather than chemical problems.

However, the introduction of oral rehydration therapy (ORT), a relatively new and simple ministration that averts many child deaths from diarrhea, has diverted attention from water supply and sanitation (WS&S). The principal attractiveness of ORT is its apparent low cost per diarrheal death averted as compared with WS&S. However, WS&S provides many more benefits that are essential to sustaining the lives saved by ORT and vital to maintaining and enhancing the lives of both children and adults.[24] WS&S *prevents* diarrhea, and many other diseases as well, releases women from the heavy and time-consuming burden of carrying water from distant possibly contaminated sources, and improves the quality of life in the community. WS&S is a long-term investment in preventive health, while ORT is a response to an immediate life-threatening situation. The costs are not high, and, without WS&S and hygiene education, ORT programs are not likely to improve child health status.

TREATMENT OF WATER AND WASTEWATER

The treatment of waters to make them suitable for subsequent use requires physical, chemical, and biological processes.[1] These processes may take place in nature. Where natural processes cannot assure a desired quality, these processes need to be engineered in water treatment plants.[25-27]

Engineering processes are increasingly necessary, in part because the contamination that impairs the quality of water is increasingly man-made and resistant to nature's purification process and in part because of growth of population and its activity in the face of fixed natural resources. The unit processes used in water treatment are listed in the following. Those used for purifying water for drinking are described below, while those used for treating wastewater are described beginning on p 638.

Distillation. Evaporation and condensation maintain the hydrologic cycle. Engineered distillation is used for desalination and for other applications where special water quality may be needed. Distillation produces the purest water of any of the processes listed, with only volatile organics persisting.

Gas Exchange. Oxygen is added to waters, and dissolved gases such as carbon dioxide and hydrogen sulfide are removed. This helps in reducing taste and odors and may also assist in the oxidation of iron and manganese, making them more easily removable. Aeration is an important natural process, helping to restore water quality in polluted rivers and other bodies of water. It is also used in water purification and wastewater treatment.

Coagulation. Colloidal and suspended particles are brought together to form large *flocs* that settle more easily. This occurs in nature in lakes and other bodies of water, but it is an important process in water purification and is aided by the addition of coagulants such as alum (aluminum sulfate) or synthetic polymers. The floc is then removed by sedimentation, filtration, or both.

Flocculation. In nature, mixing is induced by the velocity of flow in rivers or by wind-, thermal-, or density-induced currents in lakes. This mixing causes interparticle contact. In treatment plants, flocculation is engineered and aids, with the process of coagulation, in the formation of large-floc particles that are more easily removed.

Sedimentation. Under the action of gravity, particulates, including bacteria, settle to the bottom. Because the settling velocities of these small particles are low, turbulence or swift currents interfere with sedimentation so that the process is effective only in slow-moving bodies of water such as lakes. In engineered works, special tanks that minimize extraneous currents are used, encouraging the settling of the smallest and most dense particles. Coagulation assists in sedimentation.

Filtration. Water passes through granular media, and fine particulates are removed by adhesion to the grains and by sedimentation in the pore spaces. Removal of particles by filtration is not accomplished by straining, as the particles removed are generally much smaller than the spaces between the grains of the medium. In some instances, biological growth on the filter helps with the removal of particles and assists with biochemical degradation of the adsorbed organic matter. Natural filtration occurs as water percolates through the soil.

Adsorption. While some adsorption takes place in filtration, often special media designed to adsorb contaminants may be used. Activated carbon, both in granular form as filters and in powdered form as an additive to water, is used to adsorb taste and odors and a wide variety of organic chemicals.

Ion Exchange. Resins, both natural and synthetic, are used to remove specific ions. The most common are zeolites used for removing calcium and magnesium, two hardness-producing ions, and replacing them with sodium.

Disinfection. A wide variety of disinfection procedures is available for the destruction of microorganisms that may cause disease. Sterilization is not intended or necessary. The most common disinfection procedure is chlorination.

• • •

A wide variety of other unit processes is available for specific purposes, such as treatment to help prevent corrosion and processes for the handling of the solids (sludge) that accumulate in treatment. The handling and disposal of sludge is a difficult problem, particularly at wastewater treatment plants where the sludge is often noxious and can constitute a health hazard. Other processes may be required for the removal of specific substances such as ammonia, phosphorus, radioactivity, or specific contaminants. In general, one or more of the unit processes mentioned will be used.

Where the aim is a potable water, the selection of the treatment processes is dependent on the quality of the water source. For example, groundwaters may require only aeration and disinfection, while heavily polluted surface waters may require all the processes. Community wastewaters, except for the presence of industrial wastewater discharges, tend to be much the same, and the treatment processes are selected to provide an effluent that protects the receiving water and the subsequent uses to which that water may be put. If the effluent is to be discharged into an ocean, fewer processes are likely to be required than if the effluent is intended for discharge into a small, fragile stream or for reuse for nonpotable purposes. The full use of natural purification processes and the selection and sizing of these units is involved in process design, which precedes the engineering design of the treatment facility.

ENGINEERED WATER PURIFICATION

The conventional sequence of processes for the purification of surface water for potable purposes includes flocculation and coagulation, sedimentation, filtration, and disinfection. This treatment removes color, turbidity, microorganisms, colloidal particles, and some dissolved substances. Some of these processes may be omitted where the waters are drawn from a protected source and are free of color and turbidity. On the other hand, the conventional treatment is not directed to dissolved synthetic organic chemicals and is only moderately effective in the removal of heavy metals and radioactivity. If these constitute a problem, additional processes, such as adsorption on granular activated carbon, may be required. The following sections describe, and Figure 35–4 illustrates, the principal unit processes required in most water purification plants.

Coagulation. The processes described here include chemical addition, rapid mixing, and flocculation. The purpose is to remove finely divided suspended material, colloidal material, microorganisms, and to some extent dissolved substances, particu-

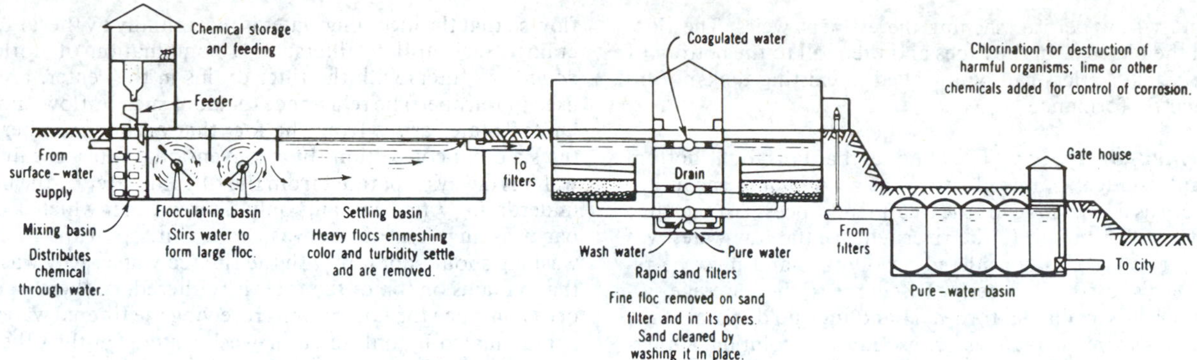

Figure 35-4. Typical water treatment plant profile. *(From Fair GM et al, 1971, with permission.[1])*

larly those of larger molecular size, by bringing them together into flocs sufficiently large to be removed by sedimentation, filtration, or both. The raw water may be highly colored and free of turbidity or turbid and free of color. The particles responsible for the color and turbidity are not discernible to the naked eye. After coagulation, however, the individual floc particles are easily observed, being on the order of 1 to 2 mm in diameter.

The principal coagulants are alum, aluminum sulfate ($Al_2(SO_4)_3 \cdot 14H_2O$) available in solid or liquid form, and ferric salts such as ferric sulfate. These aluminum and iron salts, on solution, form trivalent aluminum and ferric ions. These ions react with alkalinity, which may be naturally present or, if not, may be provided through the addition of lime or soda ash.

$$Al_2(SO_4)_3 + 6HCO_3^- = 3SO_4^{--} + 2Al(OH)_3 + 6CO_2$$

The addition of these coagulants reduces the pH of the water. Since optimum coagulation is a function of pH, coagulation may require pH adjustment.

While the aluminum hydroxide is essentially insoluble and forms a loosely bound gelatinous structure, which might appear to be the basis for the floc formation, the process is one in which the trivalent ions interact with the materials in the water to reduce the forces of repulsion among them, allowing them to come together in larger and larger aggregates, which then grow by accretion. As natural colloids are largely negatively charged, the positive ions are effective in neutralizing and allowing their coagulation.

Where large amounts of coagulants are required, the pH is reduced, tending to make the water somewhat more corrosive. The use of natural or synthetic polymers can reduce coagulant requirements some tenfold. The proper amount of coagulant and polymer and the optimum pH are determined by jar tests or by pilot plant studies prior to the design of the facility. Jar tests are then run routinely as a guide to the adjustment of chemical dosages with changing temperature and quality of the raw water.

Chemical feeding equipment selection is based on the needed chemical, the required precision of feeding, and the variety of dosages necessitated by changing quality, which is generally gradual, or the changing flow, which may be sudden and frequent.

After the chemicals are added to the water, it is customary to provide rapid mixing equipment to be certain that the chemicals are distributed uniformly in the water. Turbine or propeller mixers are commonly used, although if the water is to be pumped, the chemical may be added on the suction side of the pump using the pump as the mixer. Hydraulic mixing may be used. Pipes themselves can be used if there are sufficient bends to assure the necessary turbulence, or stators may be inserted in a pipe. The time required for rapid mixing is on the order of seconds.

The coagulation process is aided by flocculation produced in special tanks, where mechanical paddles or diffused air stirs the water gently, promoting the conjunction of suspended particles. The resulting large flocs then settle easily. Where sufficient head is available, the flocculation can take place in baffled tanks. This method is suited to developing countries, where the use of imported mechanical equipment is to be minimized. Generally, the more flexible power-driven mechanical devices are used in industrialized countries. The parameter of concern in the design of such tanks is the velocity gradient, the velocity variation across an element of water. In practice, the velocities in flocculation tanks vary from about 1 m/s at the entrance to the tanks, decreasing to about 0.2 m/s near the outlet, with a retention time of 30 minutes. Specific requirements vary with different raw waters and variations in temperature, so that the flocculator is designed to accommodate the worst situation, which generally occurs in winter.

Sedimentation. The effluent from the flocculation tanks with large but variable-sized flocs is led into sedimentation tanks, where the flocs are encouraged to settle. The detention time, again depending on the water to be treated, varies from about 2 to 6 hours. The required capacity is divided into two or more units to permit one unit to be out of service without requiring shutdown of the plant. Commonly, these tanks are rectangular in plan and about 4 to 5 m deep. Where the rate of accumulation of floc at the bottom of the tanks is expected to be too great to be easily removed manually, mechanical sludge collectors may be installed. Where the sludge can be stored at the bottom of the tank for several months without creating problems in treatment, and removed manually, mechanical sludge collectors can be dispensed with, saving the cost of equipment and maintenance.

Another useful configuration, particularly where space is at a premium, is the upward flow or sludge blanket clarifier, in which the water after flocculation moves up through a floc blanket, which is suspended in the tank by the upward velocity. The impurities are removed in the blanket, and the effluent is clear. These upward-flow units were initially developed for softening, but their economies have encouraged their use in conventional treatment as well. A compact arrangement for the upflow unit in combination with the flocculator is in concentric tanks, the flocculator in the center and sedimentation on the outside. Unless first-class supervision of operation can be assured, however, the conventional horizontal-flow sedimentation tank is preferred because it is far less subject to upset.

An improvement in the efficiency of these sedimentation tanks can be obtained by increasing the area on which the floc can settle. Initially, this was done by installing intermediate bottoms in horizontal-flow tanks. A more effective approach is the installation of a series of sloping plates or tubes installed in the top of the sedimentation tank through which the floc-bearing waters must flow before reaching the effluent weirs. The flocs settle on the plates or in the tubes and then fall to the bottom of the tank. Such settlers can be installed in existing tanks to improve their performance.

Management of Sludge. The material that falls to the bottom of the tank, sludge, is now identified as a *residual* to encourage its recovery as a byproduct of the treatment process. At one time this sludge was returned to the river whence the raw water was drawn, but today it is considered a pollutant and must be reclaimed or disposed of properly. Discharge to the sewerage system, if a sewer is available, for final handling and disposal at the wastewater treatment plant is an expeditious solution. Otherwise, transport by truck to a landfill or other acceptable place for disposal may be required. In such instances, dewatering of the sludge is appropriate to reduce the cost of transportation. For this purpose, sand drying beds, vacuum filtration, filter presses, or centrifuges, all processes similar to those used for handling sludges in wastewater-treatment plants (see p. 644), may be used. Where alum and/or lime is used in the water-treatment process, their recovery may be economical.

Filtration. Floc particles that escape the sedimentation tank are removed in filters. The conventional filter is about 1 m in depth and is made up of sand grains varying in size from 0.5 to 1.0 mm. The granular material rests on a bed of graded gravel or on a specially designed underdrain system made of porous plates or false bottoms of various types with small orifices to assure uniform backwashing. As water passes down through the filter beds, the floc settles in the interstices or is adsorbed onto the surface of the sand grains. When the amount of floc accumulated in the filter is sufficiently great to impede the flow of water by increasing the head loss to 2 to 3 m, the filter is backwashed, using filtered water sometimes accompanied by air. A filter run may last some 48 hours, and the filter washing takes about 10 minutes. Some 3% to 5% of the filtered water is required for backwashing, and the dirtied backwash water can be retained and returned to the plant influent. The cleansing of the filter is accomplished by expanding the sand bed with water introduced into the bottom of the filter. On completion of the wash, the sand settles back into place with the finest particles at the top and the coarsest at the bottom. This configuration of particles limits the effectiveness of the filter, as the top layer tends to remove most of the floc particles and the remainder of the depth of the filter goes unused. One approach now widely accepted to help alleviate this situation is the use of dual media or even multimedia filters, where granular materials of different specific gravity are used. Most common is the dual media filter, where coarser anthracite grains with a specific gravity of about 1.5 rest on top of a silica sand with a specific gravity of 2.65. In backwashing such a filter, the larger grains of the lighter anthracite always remain on the top of the filter, permitting the full depth of the bed to be more effectively used.

The rate of application to the filters ranges from 4 to 10 m/h, depending on the quality of the water. The engineer selects the sizes and loadings of the pretreatment and filter units to minimize the overall cost. Where the raw waters are of high quality and coagulation and sedimentation are not required, as is the case when water is drawn from upland reservoirs with low turbidity and color, direct filtration is used with the addition of a very small amount of coagulant and coagulant aids. Such direct filtration is widely practiced in the treatment of water for swimming pools and for many industrial uses.

Inasmuch as filters are periodically taken out of service for washing, there must be multiple units. Also, because of the many valves and other fittings required in each filter, there is a limit to their size, so that larger water-treatment plants may have many separate filter units.

A preferred mode for operating sand filters would be upflow so that the incoming water is met initially by the largest sand grains. Such upflow filters, or a combination of upflow and downflow filters with the filter drains in the center, are widely used in Europe. The reluctance to adopt such upflow units in the United States arises from the fact that an upflow filter constitutes a cross-connection. In a conventional filter, the unfiltered water is always separated from the filtered water by the bed. The underdrain system contains only filtered water which is used for backwashing. The dirtied wash water on top of the filters after washing should not mix with the filtered water. Any wash water that remains on top of the filter is refiltered, so there is never an occasion when the underdrains receiving the filtered water can be contaminated by unfiltered or wash water. On the other hand, the purified effluent from upflow filters occupies the same space above the filters as is occupied by the wash water during washing and contamination of the filtered water is quite possible. In many European plants, where filters are used primarily to remove iron and manganese from groundwaters and there is no bacterial contamination, such cross-connections are of little consequence. Also, in reclamation of wastewaters where the production of potable water is not intended, upflow filters may be used.

The earliest filters, introduced in the middle of the nineteenth century for use without pretreatment by coagulation and sedimentation, were slow sand filters. The rate of application to the slow sand filter is on the order of 0.15 m/h, requiring an area about 50 times greater than conventional filters. The slow sand filter operates by the creation on its top layer of a film of material removed from the water, including microorganisms, called a *schmutzdecke*. It is this living filter that removes color, turbidity, and bacteria. The top layer is easily clogged, however, and the top 3 to 5 cm of sand is removed periodically for washing. Immediately after removal of the *schmutzdecke,* the performance of the filter may be somewhat poorer, but it is quickly restored. Several cleanings take place before the washed sand is restored to the filter. Slow sand filters have much to commend them in small communities and in developing countries, because they require a minimum of mechanical equipment and much less skilled supervision than conventional rapid sand filters. In fact, slow sand filters are used exclusively in treating the water from the rivers Thames and Lee for the city of London. Many cities in Europe that draw from polluted sources use slow sand filters. To permit somewhat greater loads on slow sand filters, it is customary to precede the slow sand filtration with pretreatment by rapid sand filters or microstrainers, drums made of finely woven steel mesh that remove algae and other large particles, permitting the slow sand filters to operate for longer periods between cleanings. Chemical coagulants are not used.

Diatomaceous earth filters are used for industrial water supplies and many specialized applications. The water to be filtered is mixed with diatomaceous earth and forced through a porous septum in a pressure shell, forming a filtering layer several millimeters thick on the surface of the septum. When the filter is clogged, the flow is reversed, the diatomaceous earth is dislodged and washed away, and a new cycle of operation is initiated. Filters of considerable capacity can be provided in a small space, so such units are particularly suitable for mobile installations, swimming pools, and many industrial water supplies. However, they are not well suited for handling coagulated waters as they clog quickly. More important, the small thickness of diatomaceous earth does not provide the security against breakthroughs of unfiltered water that is provided by the meter depth of sand in conventional filters. Hence, they have not been widely adopted in municipal practice.

Communities with hard water, generally groundwater, often use filters containing ion-exchange resins for softening. For treatment plants drawing upon highly polluted sources, granular activated carbon filters to adsorb chemicals are being introduced.

Such filter units, identified as "point-of-use" treatment devices, have been introduced for home use for attachment to the household supply or even to a single faucet. These units have enjoyed some vogue because of the commercial exploitation of uncertainties with regard to the public supplies. They are costly, however, and of doubtful value. They may operate properly initially, but if the media are not replaced or recharged at regular intervals, they begin to do more harm than good. These filters are of no value in removing bacteria and often actually result in an increase in the bacterial content of water because of the growth of bacteria within the filter itself. The home unit for water softening is much less necessary today with the availability of synthetic detergents. If home softening is desired, the water softener is best attached to the household hot water tank and the washing machines, rather than softening the entire supply.

Home remedies are uncertain and costly, and they can be afforded by only the relatively well-to-do segment of the population. The growing use of household filters and bottled water, a sign that the public has lost faith in the quality of the water supply, should stimulate corrective action by water purveyors and regulatory agencies.

Disinfection. Disinfection with chlorine has been the single most important process for assuring the bacteriological safety of potable water supplies. Waterborne epidemics have virtually disappeared in the industrialized countries of the world. Such waterborne outbreaks as have occurred have generally been traced to failures in chlorination.

To be used in water treatment, water disinfectants must possess the following properties:

1. They must destroy bacteria, viruses, and amebic cysts in water within a reasonable time despite all variations in water temperature, composition, and concentration of contaminants.
2. They must not be toxic to humans and domestic animals, unpalatable, or otherwise objectionable.
3. They must be reasonable in cost and safe and easy to store, transport, handle, and apply.
4. Their residual concentration in the treated water must be easily, and preferably automatically, determinable.
5. They must be sufficiently persistent so that the disappearance of the residual would be a warning of recontamination.

As it is not feasible to continuously monitor bacteriological or virological quality of water and to have the results before the water is distributed to the consumer, the ability to detect a residual concentration of a known bactericidal disinfectant (C) after exposure for a certain time (T) at a certain pH and temperature is the key quality-control test. Table 35–10 shows CT values for various conditions and disinfectants.

The use of chlorine or one of its derivatives meets these requirements most economically; however, other methods of disinfection are sought for two reasons: (1) chlorine added to some waters imparts an undesirable taste and odor, particularly where phenol is present, and (2) the reaction of chlorine with organic matter, even where these organics are not themselves of health significance, has resulted in the formation of a wide range of reaction products. One group of these, trihalomethanes, including chloroform, has been shown to cause cancer in animals. The problems created by the use of chlorine have been exacerbated because chlorine is a useful oxidant that can remove taste and odors economically and which, when added at the beginning of a treatment process, facilitates subsequent treatment by reducing the concentration of microorganisms that can cause difficulty in sedimentation tanks and filters. Because of the wide use of prechlorination, particularly with waters drawn from polluted sources such as the Mississippi and Ohio rivers, many water supplies do not meet the standard for trihalomethanes of 100 μg/L. This problem is readily addressed by the use of better sources of water or by adequate treatment before the disinfecting dose of chlorine is added. Humic organics, phenols, and other precursors of the trihalomethanes should be removed before the addition of chlorine. This requires abandoning the process of prechlorination. While the removal of natural organics through coagulation, sedimentation, and filtration can be readily accomplished, the removal of synthetic organic chemicals in polluted waters is more difficult.

The adoption of substitutes for chlorine must be initiated with great care. Other disinfectants may themselves produce compounds of which far less is known than of the trihalomethanes. Also, some of the other methods of disinfection, such as chloramination, do not provide the same level of microbiological safety as chlorine. Nevertheless, knowledge of all methods of disinfection might help reveal a combination that provides the required safety while minimizing the undesirable side effects. For example, the use of another method for disinfection, such as those described below with chlorine added primarily to assure bacterial safety by providing the water with a measurable chlorine residual, may be suitable.

A wide range of other methods of disinfection, including the use of strong oxidants, is available. Boiling water will disinfect it, but this is suitable only as an emergency measure for individual consumers. It is not a reasonable community approach.

While sunlight is a natural disinfectant, irradiation by ultraviolet light is an engineered process that can be tailored to the need. A mercury vapor arc lamp emitting invisible light of 25 to 37Å units applied to a water free of light-absorbing substances, particularly suspended matter that will protect microorganisms against the light, is a useful method of disinfection. There is no way of continuously monitoring the effectiveness of the process, however, and therefore it has not yet found application in municipal potable water supply practice in the United States, although it is used in the Soviet Union.

Silver ions are bactericidal at concentrations as low as 15 μg/L, but the action is quite slow. Larger concentrations that speed up the process are unacceptable because of possible side effects from the silver. Furthermore, silver ions are neither viricidal nor cysticidal in appropriate concentrations, and silver is expensive. Nevertheless, silver-coated sand may be appropriate for specialized installations. Copper ions are strongly algicidal, and copper sulfate is often used for algae control in lakes and reservoirs. However, copper is not bactericidal.

Pathogenic bacteria do not survive in highly acid or alkaline waters, below 3 or above 11 pH. Where the treatment process brings the water to these pH levels, as might be the case through the use of lime, some disinfection benefits accrue. Otherwise, the use of acids or alkalis as disinfectants is not feasible.

Oxidizing Chemicals. Oxidizing chemicals include the halogens (chlorine, bromine, iodine), ozone, and other oxidants, such as potassium permanganate and hydrogen peroxide. Potassium permanganate has found wide use as a replacement for chlorine for taste and odor control, but it is not as effective as a disinfectant. Ozone is useful for destroying odors and color and is also an effective if expensive disinfectant, but it suffers from the fact that it leaves no residual suitable for monitoring. Among the halogens, gaseous chlorine and a wide variety of chlorine compounds are economically most useful. Bromine and iodine have been employed on a limited scale for the disinfection of swimming pool waters as well as in tablets for disinfecting small quantities of drinking water in the field.

Ozone. Ozone is produced on site by the corona discharge of high-voltage electricity into dry air or oxygen. Ozone is corrosive and toxic, and strong concentrations in the atmosphere, from its photochemical genesis in conjunction with hydrocarbon vapors from automobile exhaust, are responsible for oxidant smogs that are eye, throat, and lung irritants. In the vicinity of a plant using ozone, its effect can often be seen on vegetation. Nevertheless, ozone is used effectively and efficiently as an oxidant, a deodorant, a decolorant, and a disinfectant in both drinking water and wastewaters. Because the production of ozone is expensive and energy-intensive, and because ozone residuals disappear rapidly from water and are not available for quality control, ozone is used for special applications and not as a general replacement for chlorine. The combination of ozone for pretreatment while providing some disinfection, to be followed by chlorination, has become a popular sequence in Europe and is beginning to be used in the United States to reduce the level of THMs in finished water. Intensive research into the characteristics, biocidal efficiency, and reaction products of ozone is being undertaken, although it is not expected that it will replace chlorine entirely because it leaves no residual.

Chlorine. Chlorinated lime (CaClOCl) was the first chlorine disinfectant used for public water supplies. It is a hygroscopic white powder that readily absorbs both moisture and carbon dioxide from the air with the loss of chlorine. Because it is unstable, it was rapidly replaced by hypochlorites. This was shortly followed by elemental chlorine (Cl_2), produced by the electrolysis of brine, in liquid form for storage and transmission in steel cylinders. Liquid chlorine is still by far the most common form of chlorine to be used for water supply and wastewater disinfection. Calcium hypochlorite ($Ca(OCl)_2$) is stable and is used for small installations. It is easily stored in solid form in small containers, and 1% to 3% solutions can be made up as needed. Sodium hypochlorite solution (NaOCl) is also used for small installations and increasingly for large installations where the transportation of liquid chlorine is considered too hazardous because of the danger of leakage. Chlorine is heavier than air and is extremely toxic, so that all handling and dosing of liquid and gaseous chlorine must be done with care. Chlorine dioxide (ClO_2) is used in special instances, particularly where tastes and odors may be a problem. It is produced directly in water by the reaction of elemental chlorine with sodium chlorite ($NaClO_2$).

The on-site generation of hypochlorite by electrolysis of brine may be appropriate for communities in isolated locations where power is available but the delivery of chlorine may be difficult.

When chlorine or its derivatives are added to water in the absence of ammonia or organic nitrogen, hypochlorous acid (HOCl), hypochlorite ion (OCl^-), or both are formed, with the distribution between the two depending on pH. These are referred to in practice as free available chlorine. When ammonia or organic nitrogen is present, monochloramine (NH_2Cl_2), dichloramine ($NHCl_2$), and nitrogen trichloride (NCl_3) may be formed, the distribution among the species again being a function of pH. Generally, the first two of these prevail and are referred to as chloramines or combined available chlorine. Because the disinfecting power of each of these varies widely, the chemistry of chlorination must be fully understood so that the chlorine may be used effectively and disinfection assured.

Although the purpose of adding chlorine is to destroy microorganisms, most of the substances in water that react with the chlorine are inert organic materials, both natural and manmade, as well as other reducing substances. To the extent that the organic matter and other chemicals that cause chlorine demand can be removed from water by treatment before the addition of chlorine, both the required addition of chlorine and the formation of chlorinated organic compounds will be reduced.

When chlorine is added to water, it is hydrolized immediately and completely, according to the following reaction:

$$Cl_2 + H_2O \rightleftarrows HOCl + H^+ + Cl^-$$

Hypochlorous acid ionizes in part into H^+ and OCl^-. At pH below 5, the chlorine exists almost entirely as HOCl and above pH 10 as OCl^-. Between these two pHs, the percent of chlorine added as HOCl at 20° C is

$$\frac{100}{1 + 2.5 \times 10^{pH} / 10^8}$$

At pH 7, 80% of the chlorine is in the form of HOCl. The distribution is important because HOCl has a much higher killing power than OCl^-. Figure 35–5 indicates that at pH 10 some 50-fold greater chlorine residuals are required for a 99% kill of *E. coli* in 30 minutes at 2° to 5° C, as compared with requirements at pH 7.

When ammonia or its salts are present in chlorinated water, chloramines are formed. Monochloramine is formed in the pH range of 6 to 8, while dichloramine predominates at lower pH values. The chloramines appear as part of the residual chlorine, but as they are considerably less effective disinfecting agents than hypochlorous acid, it is important to differentiate them in analysis. To assure adequate disinfection, a free residual must be formed; this requires the addition of more than enough chlorine to react with all the ammonia and organic compounds present. The great advantage of obtaining free available chlorine is that most tastes and odors that can be oxidized by chlorine are destroyed, and rigorous disinfection, even to the inactivation of viruses, can be assured as long as the proper combination of chlorine residual concentration, pH, time of contact, and temperature are observed.

While hypochlorites can be added with solution feeders much as any other chemical solutions are added in water treatment, special equipment is required for adding elemental chlorine. Chlorine is transported in liquid form in steel cylinders, but chlorine gas also exists within the cylinder, and it is the gas that is drawn off for solution in a water stream, feeding into the water to be treated. For large rates of use, particularly in wastewater treatments where the amounts of chlorine used are substantially greater than in water supply disinfection, the chlorine may be withdrawn from the steel tank as a liquid and vaporized in special evaporation equipment. The solubility of chlorine gas in water is about 7300 mg/L at 20° C at one atmosphere. Below 9.5° C, chlorine combines with water to form chlorine hydrate, chlorine ice, which may obstruct feeding equipment. Therefore it is important that chlorine feeding equipment and the water that may come in contact with the gas be kept above this temperature.

Because chlorine is highly toxic, it must be handled with

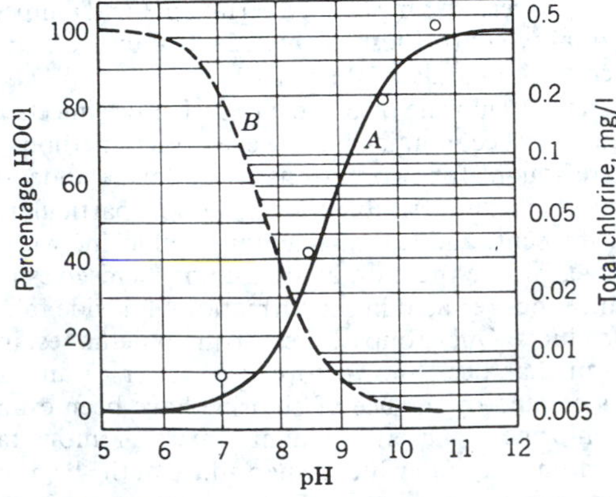

Figure 35–5. Observed concentration of free available chlorine required for 99% kill of *E. coli* in 30 min at 2 to 5°C (curve A and right-hand scale) and percentage of HOCl in the total chlorine (curve B and left-hand scale). *(From Fair GM et al, 1971, with permission.[1])*

great care and under adequate safeguards. Its odor threshold is about 3.5 ppm by volume. Concentrations of 30 ppm or more induce coughing, and exposures for 30 minutes to concentrations of 40 to 60 ppm are dangerous, with 1000 ppm being rapidly fatal. Because chlorine gas is heavier than air, it concentrates in tunnels and lower levels of buildings at the water treatment plants. Therefore, special facilities are provided for handling chlorine, with separate entrances to feeding and weighing rooms, adequate automatic ventilation, and safety equipment including appropriate gas masks stored nearby.

Inasmuch as chlorine is the most important safeguard for microbiological safety, no breakdown in chlorine feeding can be tolerated. Thus, units must be adequate in size and be duplicated so that failure of any single unit would not interfere with continuous chlorination. An ample number of filled cylinders must be available, with at least two cylinders on line at all times so that an empty cylinder can be replaced without interfering with chlorination. Most chlorinators operate under vacuum to prevent leakage of chlorine gas. The vacuum is created by the feed water being pumped under pressure through a venturi throat in the feeder. The pressure of water required for this feed water line must be substantially greater than the water pressure in the line being fed. Accordingly, separate pumps are required. Failure of these pumps because of a power failure would mean the cessation of chlorination. Therefore, suitable alarms with provision for standby power can help assure continuous operation.

Portable chlorinators that operate off the pressure in the cylinders may be used for emergency chlorination or for chlorination of water mains, wells, tanks, and reservoirs in the field.

After the chlorine is added, sufficient contact time, which depends on the particular water but is generally on the order of 30 minutes, must be provided. The product of the concentration, *C,* and time of contact, *T,* the *CT,* is the operating parameter (see Table 35-10). In water treatment plants, this can be done in a clear well at the plant. In wastewater treatment plants, on the other hand, special chlorine contact chambers are constructed. It may be that sufficient treated water transmission mains exist to provide adequate contact time before the first customer is reached even at highest flows. This would make a contact chamber necessary; however, it is then necessary to be able to sample for chlorine residual at a point at least 30 minutes flow distant from the point of addition.

Chlorination is now routinely automated to permit automatic variation of dosage to account for variations in flow and chlorine demand and to maintain a constant chlorine residual. The chlorine dosages and residuals are recorded, and it is common to maintain an alarm to give warning of any departure from the required chlorine residual.

Corrosion Inhibition. The treated water may be more corrosive because of the addition of coagulants and chlorine, both of which reduce pH. Also many natural waters are quite soft and corrosive. To avoid corrosion of pipelines, hot water heaters, and plumbing fittings, it is general practice to reduce the corrosivity of the water. This is done either by adding sufficient alkalinity and raising the pH to render the water noncorrosive or by adding a hexametaphosphate sequestering agent, which tends to form a light coating in the pipes and mitigates the effect of any corrosion that might occur. Corrosion control is also important to minimize lead concentrations in water where lead is present in household water plumbing.

Adsorption. Depending on the source of water, a treatment plant may use one or more of the processes described. None of these processes, however, are directed against the SOCs present in waters that drain urban and industrial areas, although some removal of these organics can be expected when powdered activated carbon is used for taste and odor control. The organics in water were initially characterized by passing the water sample through activated carbon filters on which the organics are adsorbed and then dissolving these organics with chloroform. The 1962 U.S. Public Health Service Drinking Water Standards had a limit for this carbon chloroform extract of 0.2 mg/L. It was recognized that many of the organics adsorbed on the filter were of no health concern, and that many organics that might be of health concern were not adsorbed at all. The use of GAC filters for treating water drawn from polluted sources is now being introduced in an attempt to remove some, if not all, of these refractory organic chemicals. At the time of this writing, many pilot plants have been built but there is little experience with the long-term use of these GAC filters full scale. They have limited capacity, require recharging, and may release contaminants into the finished water. In time, the larger cities that draw from polluted sources, such as the lower Delaware, Hudson, Ohio, and Mississippi rivers, are likely to incorporate GAC filters into their treatment. This represents a small proportion of the total water supplies in the country. Smaller supplies that draw from polluted sources will be constrained in their adoption of GAC filters because of their inadequate operating and monitoring capabilities. One beneficial effect of requiring such additional treatment may be that water purveyors now drawing on polluted sources will examine other options. For example, Vicksburg, Mississippi, which had been drawing its water supply from the Mississippi River prior to passage of the SDWA, switched to groundwater. This possibility does exist for other cities and may be more attractive than trying to monitor for and remove the myriad SOCs present in these rivers. Also, the cost of installation and operation of GAC filters, together with the cost of monitoring, may make higher-quality sources a more attractive option.

WATER DISTRIBUTION

A water supply system, including the treatment plant, is designed to meet the average demand on the maximum day. Use, however, varies from hour to hour and may reach a peak during a fire. Accordingly, the distribution system, which includes the high lift pumps that deliver the treated water to the system, the transmission mains for the treated water, the piping in the streets that serves the individual houses, hydrants on the system for firefighting, and service reservoirs, must be based on peak demand requirements. Each customer is served by a connection to the main in the street generally through a meter. In order to assure continuity of service, pumps are selected so that, in the event any single pump is down for repairs, the remaining pumps can handle the requirements. Also, it is customary to provide standby power, generally through diesel engines. Distribution system piping, most commonly cement-lined ductile cast iron pipe, is 6 inches and larger in diameter. This minimum size is required for fire protection. The pipe network is designed with sufficient interconnections so that in the event of any pipe break, the service, including water for fire protection, can be provided via other routes. The system is designed to maintain a minimum pressure of 20 psi (about 280 kg/cm^2) during peak flows to permit service to be maintained at least to the second floor of homes without creating a backdraft that might pollute the supply. Higher buildings need to be served by their own pumping stations. Elevated service reservoirs are used to help maintain these pressures by storing water for peak hours, firefighting, or an emergency.

The introduction of dual water supply systems, potable and nonpotable, requires that the two systems be kept physically separate and easily distinguishable. This is accomplished by using different materials and colors for the pipe and hydrants and different-shaped valve boxes.[5]

The operation and maintenance of the distribution system

so that it may perform in an emergency is an obligation of the water supply authority. It is to the credit of the water industry in the United States that power failures occur with considerably greater frequency than failure of water services.

WASTEWATER COLLECTION AND DISPOSAL

In common with other living organisms, humans discharge to the environment waste substances that, in turn, reenergize the endless cycle of nature. With urbanization and industrialization, waste products have increased in volume and in kind, and their impact on the environment has intensified.

Human wastes are discussed under two headings: so-called night soil and wastewaters. Each exerts its influence on specific environmental resources; night soil principally on the soil, water-carried wastes principally on water, but both in some degree on the atmosphere and in some places or in some ways on soil and water together. Some of the effects on the environment have, in turn, reacted on our health and general well-being.

Night Soil. The expression *night soil* is used to describe human body wastes, excreta, or excrement, or the combination of feces and urine voided by humans. The term itself derives from the practice of carting away accumulations of human ordure at night. Night soil is one of several components of urban refuse in parts of the developing world. In industrialized countries, except in parts of Japan, night soil no longer exists as such, because excreta are flushed away by water into the sewerage system.

The disposal of night soil is a problem of economy, convenience, general cleanliness, and personal hygiene. The danger of exposure to infectious diseases is proportional to the concentration of the causative agents which tends to be high in countries that do not yet have sewerage systems. The unsightliness of excrement does not injure the public health, and neither do the odors disseminated by decomposing urine and feces. Yet they are offensive to the senses and interfere with the enjoyment of an otherwise attractive environment. From this standpoint alone, their elimination is important.

Night soil is the source of a wide variety of GI infections. Its safe disposal has important public health implications, and it is understandable why this has become a concern of official health agencies even though needed operations are commonly left to other departments of local government.

Composition and Quantities. The two components of night soil—feces and urine—vary much in amount (but only slightly in composition) with the diet and age distribution of the general population and the consumption of water and other liquids. Fecal matter contains food residues, the remains of bile and intestinal secretions, cellular substances from the alimentary tract, and bacterial cells in large numbers. The per capita amount of fecal matter excreted daily is estimated at about 90 g for well-fed people, ranging up to an average of 150 g for adult males. It becomes lower, more or less in proportion to body weight, in populations that are not so fully nourished.

On the basis of wet solids, fecal matter contains about 1% nitrogen, much the same relative amount of phosphoric acid, and approximately one fourth that weight of potash. The number of coliform organisms alone is well in excess of 100×10^9, and there is a wide variety of other bacteria in fecal discharges. Bacterial cells, indeed, make up about one fourth of the weight of feces.

The infective danger of human feces is illustrated by the isolation of more than 100×10^9 *Salmonella typhosa* from some carriers of typhoid fever bacilli, in the millions of cysts of *Entamoeba histolytica* from carriers of amebic dysentery, and of similar numbers of virus units of poliomyelitis in the stools of those infected with this virus. Infectious hepatitis is the most important, if the least understood, of the viral diseases transmitted from the feces of infected persons. The eggs of intestinal parasites vary in number with the degree of infection, but the per capita figures do not come anywhere near the magnitudes of bacterial pathogens. Of particular importance in certain tropical parts of the world is the discharge in feces of the eggs of the blood fluke that causes schistosomiasis.

The principal components of urine are water, urea, and mineral ash. The weight of urine excreted is about 1000 g per capita daily, running up to 1500 g in adult males. Compared with fecal matter, however, urine is richer in fertilizing elements; daily per capita production of nitrogen is almost ten times as great, of phosphoric acid perhaps two times, and of potash about eight times. It follows that urine constitutes the most agriculturally valuable part of human excreta. At the same time, urine is normally sterile and, in fact, destroys bacteria in fecal matter with which it is left in contact for any length of time. It is quite salty because of a daily per capita excretion of 5 to 9 g of chlorides.

As chemical fertilizers have become economical in industrial parts of the world, the use of human excreta has been abandoned with mounting zeal and in clear opposition to established folkways. It is doubtful that education in hygiene and esthetics could have done as much in so short a time. With increasing cost of chemical fertilizers, primarily because of the high energy costs involved in their manufacture, interest in using human wastes for fertilizer is being revived.

The circulation of enteric pathogens in the environment is a function of many things, including the prevalence of the causative agents through cases and carriers, the rate of survival of the excreted organisms in different environments and climates, the nature of the vehicle of infection, and the minimum infective dose with due consideration of immunological factors. Operating in favor of control are low incidence, rapid die-off, warm climates (except for the production of insects that may serve as vectors of disease), and protection of possible vehicles of infection, such as drinking water, natural ice, shellfish, bathing waters, and the soil, including foods raised upon it.

Collection and Disposal. In some parts of the world—or regionally in some countries—night soil is disposed of on site; in others it is collected and emptied into a sewerage system or dumped into an open water course or treated by itself or jointly with wastewater. On-site disposal is often primitive. A clump of bushes or trees satisfies the urge for privacy for defecation, and excreta are scattered over the ground in disregard of religious injunctions such as the Mosaic law of burial (Deuteronomy 23:12, 13).

Most common in on-site disposal is the privy, which provides privacy but may neglect sanitation. Four common types of privy are shown in Figure 35–6.

Privies that are not properly built or well maintained may constitute as much of a hazard as their absence. The vault and pail privies require regular and frequent emptying, which has worked satisfactorily when well-managed in villages and the unsewered outskirts of sewered communities. Poorly operated, these systems can be a nuisance and a threat to health.

Because it is successful in operation and low in cost, the earth pit privy has found wide use in rural areas. The pit is usually shallow enough to lie above groundwater, yet deep enough to be shunned by flies because of its darkness and large enough to hold its accumulation for a year or two. A concrete slab floor includes either a riser with self-closing seat or an opening and foot rests, and a screened vent that prevents moisture from condensing on the underside of seat and lid.

The danger of contaminating groundwater supplies must be clearly recognized for deep pit privies. No arbitrary rules can be laid down for the minimum safe distance of any privy from a

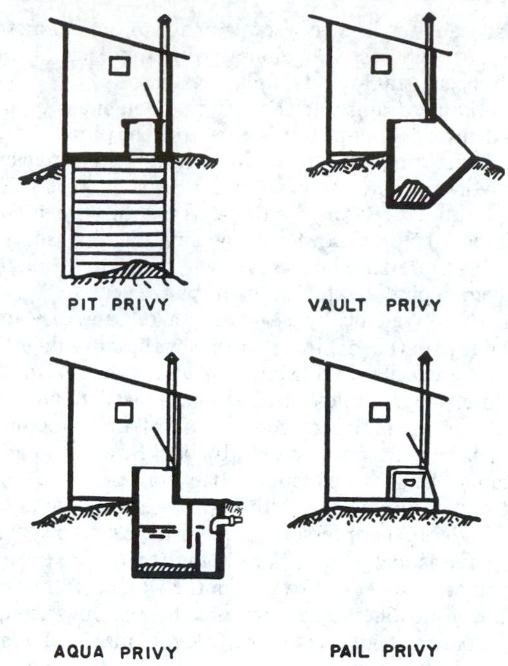

Figure 35-6. Types of privies.

well. Everything depends on the height and direction of groundwater flow and the nature of the soil. In sand, a distance of 50 feet or more should intervene for safety. No safe distance can be prescribed where the privy is in a limestone or similar aquifer from which drinking water is drawn. Pollution of groundwater can be prevented by using watertight concrete vaults, which must be cleaned out at suitable intervals.

For vacation or other homes in isolated areas, electric toilets that incinerate the fecal material are available. For aircraft, pleasure boats, and similar situations, recirculating chemical toilets are used, with provision made for their emptying into sewerage systems or treatment facilities.

The sanitary privy can be the instrument for materially reducing the incidence of intestinal diseases, particularly in developing countries. It cannot, however, be considered a satisfactory method of excreta disposal in densely populated villages or congested urban slums.

Water Pollution. Household wastes from kitchen, bathroom, and laundry are conveniently flushed away by water as domestic wastewater, and manufacturing wastes are discarded as industrial wastewaters. The system of underground pipes and appurtenances into which wastewaters are poured is called the sewerage system.

Cities built sewers initially to protect their streets and low-lying areas from inundation by flooding rainstorms—not to carry away human body wastes. The sewers were stormwater drains, not sanitary sewers. The *cloaca maxima,* which drained the Roman Forum to the Tiber, is such a sewer and continues in service to this day. Water carriage of wastes of human activity did not come into purposeful use until the nineteenth century. Then, under the impact of the Industrial Revolution, the explosive growth of urban communities placed so sudden and heavy a burden on existing waste storage and vehicular transport for its removal that stormwater drains were pressed into service for domestic wastes, creating a combined sewerage system. When summers grew hot and waste loads great, however, the streams into which the sewers emptied began "to seethe and ferment under a burning sun," because the oxygenating capacity of their waters had been surpassed. One remedy was the construction of intercepting sewers along the banks of larger bodies of water. These conduits were made big enough to transport the dry weather flow and deliver it beyond the town to points of possible disposal without nuisance. Stormwaters had to be spilled, together with their share of municipal wastes, into the otherwise protected waters. This weakness of the combined system of sewerage is as yet unresolved in the older cities of the United States. Separate systems of sewerage did not come in significant use until the beginning of the twentieth century, when the treatment of wastewater was introduced. Today they are the system of choice. The reasons for this are patent: protection of water courses within the community against pollution and treatment of all the wastewaters unaffected by rainwater.

Understandably, the need for reducing the burden of waste matters imposed upon the waters in streams was established first in densely settled industrial communities. Depending on the capacity of the waters to receive the wastes and stabilize them without nuisance, removal progressed from the separation of gross, generally settleable, pollutional constituents (primary treatment); to the separation of fine or dissolved, generally nonsettleable, pollutional components by biological treatment (secondary treatment); and ultimately to the removal of the small concentrations of specific classes of residual pollutants (tertiary treatment).

The disposal of water-carried domestic and industrial wastes involves collection through plumbing systems of the wastes in houses and other buildings, followed either by on-site disposal of these wastes or their delivery to the public sewer; collection of the wastes emptied into public sewers; treatment of the communal and industrial wastewaters; and their ultimate disposal onto land or into receiving waters.

Modern wastewater treatment in the United States began in the 1920s and for a half-century was devoted to protecting the best uses of the waters into which the wastewaters were discharged. The classes of uses were as follows:

A. Drinking water, and protection of shellfish laying beds
B. Bathing waters
C. Aquatic life
D. Industrial and agricultural water supply
E. Navigation and disposal of wastewaters without nuisance

Standards were established for each of these classes, and the treatment required was then established to maintain these standards. For example, class A and B waters for drinking and bathing have rigorous bacterial standards, which are not applicable to waters for other purposes. Treatment facilities discharging to class A and B waters were required to provide bacterial removal. Dissolved oxygen levels did not need to be so high in waters used for industry or agriculture as in waters for aquatic life. Accordingly, the treatment to remove biochemical oxygen demand needed to be greater when discharges were to class C waters, intended for protecting aquatic life, than when they were to class D waters.

These standards were the responsibility of the individual states. Some states were more rigorous in their implementation of standards than others. Accordingly, some streams were allowed to become highly polluted and unfit for any use. The environmental movement originating in the 1960s addressed this problem, leading to passage of Public Law 92-500, the Federal Water Pollution Control Act Amendments of 1972, which, with its 1977 amendments, is called the Clean Water Act. Among the goals of this act were that water quality in the nation's waters provide for the protection and propagation of fish, shellfish, and wildlife and provide for recreation in and on the waters, all to be achieved by 1983. This eliminated classifications D and E. Another national goal stated in the act was that the discharge of pollutants into navigable waters be eliminated by 1985, a goal that was recognized by professionals as being unattainable and that has since come to be recognized by all as unfeasible. The environmental movement focused far more on the quality of the aquatic environment (i.e., fishable and swimmable) than on public health, and little in PL 92-500 was directed to preservation of receiving waters for potable water supplies. In the United States, the greatest threat to the public health from pollution of water sources is from the nondegradable SOCs. Not even tertiary treatment of wastewaters addresses these chemicals; nor are waters routinely monitored for them. In some instances, fish have been found to contain dangerously high levels of chemicals discharged from industries upstream, and proscriptions against the eating of these fish have been established by health authorities. Similar concern has not yet been expressed by public agencies about drinking waters drawn from streams in which these contaminated fish swim. With the growing concern about the relationship between drinking water and health, however, more attention is now being devoted to this problem. Meanwhile, the arbitrary separation, both in legislation and administration, of water pollution control and drinking water protection militates against a comprehensive attack on this issue.

One important provision of the Clean Water Act is the requirement for National Pollution Discharge Elimination System (NPDES) permits for all sewered, so-called point-source, discharges. The permits list the conditions that have to be met by the dischargers, and together they afford a useful tool for wastewater management. The problems of nonpoint-source wastewaters, such as urban and agricultural runoff, however, remain less tractable, although a permit system is being considered for urban runoff, initially targeted at communities of 100,000 population or more.

Drainage of Buildings. The plumbing system of dwellings and other buildings is the terminus of water supply and the beginning of wastewater disposal. As shown in Figure 35-7, the central components of house drainage systems are a vertical stack and a connecting, nearly horizontal house drain leading to the house sewer that leads to the street sewer or to an on-site method of disposal. For tightness, all piping, with the exception of the house sewer, is metallic or rigid plastic.

Each fixture drains into the system through a trap in which a sealing depth of water prevents air within the piping from seeping into the building. Usually malodorous, this air may at times contain toxic and flammable contaminants. Fixture traps also keep out vermin. Accordingly, the seals of traps are intended to remain intact. To prevent their being siphoned by aspiration or blown by back-pressure because of water rushing through them or past them in pipes or stacks, the traps are vented.

Important hygienically is the proper relating of water supply to drainage in the manifold fixtures within dwellings, hotels, hospitals, mercantile establishments, and industrial buildings. For full safety, water inlets must discharge well above the high-water mark of the fixture to keep its waters from being sucked or forced back into the water system by backflow. If an adequate air gap cannot be provided, special backflow preventers must be installed in the supply pipe. Although water supply systems are normally under higher pressure than drainage systems, pressures are reduced drastically at times of high draft—e.g., during fires or when pipes break. The pressure in the water system may then drop below atmospheric pressure and the resulting negative (in relation to barometric) pressure differential may pull dangerous pollutants into the system.

Drainage of Towns. Sewerage systems, whether separate or combined, are in a sense vascular systems of underground conduits that collect the spent water of the community for treatment and disposal.[28] Sewers begin in the high-lying parts of the town, point progressively downhill, and increase in size as they take in more and more wastewaters from larger and larger tributary areas. In the United States, street sewers are at least 8 inches in diameter, and house sewers at least 6 inches. Sanitary and combined sewers are laid deep enough to drain the lowest fixtures in the properties they serve. However, when basements are very deep, as in tall buildings, their wastewaters are lifted into the street sewer by

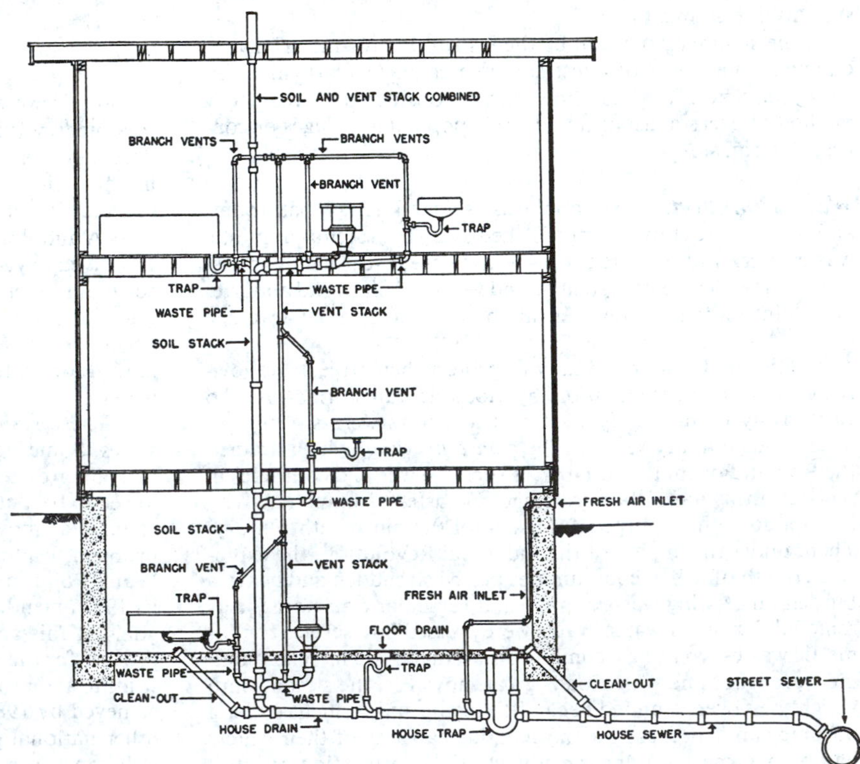

Figure 35-7. House plumbing system.

pumps or ejectors. Sewers are generally of vitrified tile or concrete, with joints of premolded rubber or plastic to maintain watertightness.

The slopes on which sewers are laid are set more or less by existing street grades. If the town is flat, sewers must still be laid on minimum grade, becoming quite deep, and pumping stations must lift the wastewater back to minimum depth, making for a costly system. Alternative systems, using vacuum or pressure sewers to avoid the need for laying sewers to grade, have application in special situations.

For inspection and cleaning, manholes are generally built into the system at changes in grade and direction and also at intermediate points in long, straight runs.

Rainwater enters combined or storm sewers through street inlets with catch basins necessary for combined sewerage systems. The outlets of catch basins to their sewers are trapped to contain the air in the sewer and to keep sand and gravel out of it. Street inlets in separate storm systems are left untrapped.

Quantity and Composition of Wastewater. During dry weather, the volume of wastewater[1] is about 70% of water used. The flow fluctuates by the day, the week, and the season. Maximum rates are as much as 200% greater than the daily average. Some industrial uses introduce still greater differences. In wet weather and for some time after, groundwater adds to flow, depending upon the tightness of the sewers and the wetness of the ground.

Intercepting sewers for combined systems are designed to carry as much water as can be economically and technologically justified. Where rains are steady and gentle (in England, for example), interceptors are designed for up to six times the dry weather flow, because spills are then rare. Where most storms are intense and of short duration, as they are in the United States, the frequency and volume of stormwater overflow is not altered much by oversizing the interceptors to carry more than the peak dry weather flow.

Wastewater shares the fundamental quality of the water supply but is debased by the waste load imposed upon it, by influx of groundwater, and in combined sewers by varying quantities of rainwater and street wash. The longer it flows or stands, the more its constituents disintegrate; fecal matter and paper become unrecognizable as such; bacteria and other saprophytes multiply enormously; and the respiration of living organisms and incidental biochemical changes reduce the oxygen originally dissolved in the water, so that fresh sewage becomes first stale and then anaerobic or septic. Wastewater is obnoxious to the senses when it putrefies; it is dangerous to health when it contains pathogenic microorganisms.

Figure 35–8 shows the normal concentration and physical state of the impurities in wastewater of moderate strength from a water supply that is not highly mineralized. The components are chosen to identify in a comprehensive manner how much of the load of solids carried in sewage is capable of settling out, how much is colloidal and in solution and can therefore be removed only by chemical or biological precipitation, and how much is likely to be decomposed, degraded, or putrefied because it is organic.

In general, wastewater is analyzed for the purpose of ascertaining or predicting its effects on bodies of water into which it is to be discharged and for evaluating the performance of treatment processes. The test for biochemical oxygen demand (BOD) is worthy of special mention. This test measures the oxygen requirements of bacteria and other organisms as they feed upon and bring about the decomposition of organic matter. These requirements are important because they decree whether the receiving body of water remains aerobic (oxygen present) or anaerobic (oxygen exhausted). Hence, the BOD test is a measure of the putrescible load placed on treatment works and on bodies of water into which treatment plants empty.

In the United States, the per capita contribution of 5-day, 20° C BOD to domestic wastewater averages 54 g, of which 42 g is in suspension, 19 g is settleable from suspension, and 12 g is dissolved. This compares with a per capita contribution of 250 g of solids, of which 90 g are suspended, 54 g are settleable, and 160 g are dissolved. Industrial wastes may add to these amounts appreciably. Their relative strength is conveniently expressed in terms of the number of people who would exert an equivalent BOD load. Especially high BODs are added to municipal wastewater by breweries, canneries, distilleries, packinghouses, milk plants, tanneries, and textile mills.

Industrial Wastewaters. Because BOD characterizes only organic wastes typical of human discharges, where industrial wastes are present, the chemical oxygen demand (COD) or the total organic carbon (TOC) determination may be useful. Where industrial organics or heavy metals are suspected, these too must be monitored in wastewater streams and treatment plant effluents, particularly where wastes are discharged into waters to be used for drinking or that provide the environment for edible fish.

Many industrial wastewaters interfere with treatment processes by imposing heavy loads on the plants or by impairing biological treatment because of toxic components in the wastewaters. Accordingly, industries may be required to pretreat their wastes before being permitted to discharge them to a municipal sewerage system. In addition, they are often required to reimburse the municipality for handling these wastewaters, generally in accordance with their volume and strength.

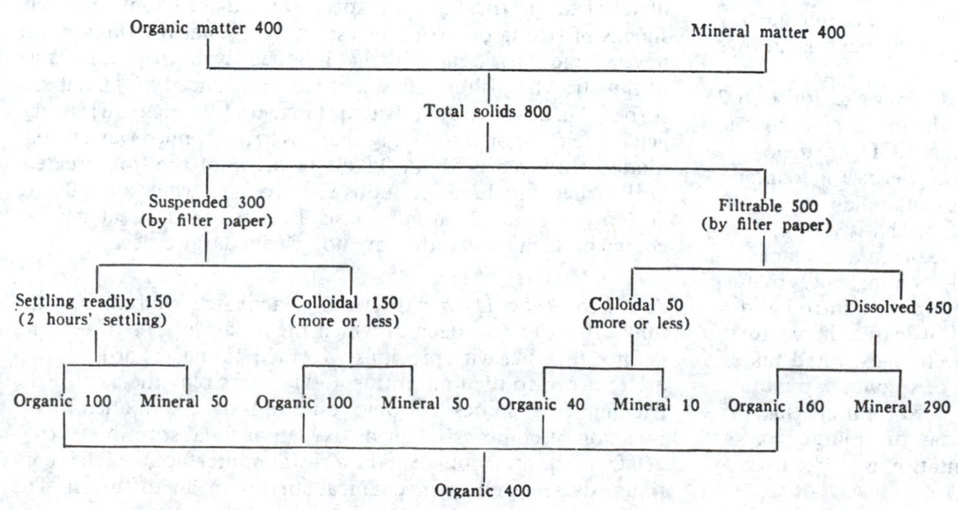

Figure 35-8. Concentration and physical state of solids in wastewater of moderate strength. Numbers are parts per million or milligrams per liter. They are generalized approximations; considerable departures from them might be expected.

In addition, many industrial wastewaters are discharged directly into receiving waters, thereby requiring NPDES permits under the Clean Water Act. These wastewaters contain myriads of contaminants of all types. Two approaches have been taken together to address this problem. The first is based on technology, the requirement for the use of the best available technology economically achievable, with guidelines established by EPA for each of the 21 industrial categories. The second is based on monitoring polluting chemical compounds; initially 65 compounds and classes of compounds were identified, which could include thousands of individual pollutants. This was refined to a list of 129 so-called "priority pollutants." Establishing standards for these, as well as monitoring procedures, is a formidable and expensive task, so it can be expected that they will need to be addressed on a selective basis. For example, the establishment of an MCL for a particular compound in drinking water would strongly suggest consideration of including it among those to be regulated in effluents that discharge to waters that are drawn upon for potable supplies.

Wastewater Treatment. With few exceptions, water purification and wastewater treatment processes are alike in concept and in kind.[1] They differ only in the amounts of pollutants they must remove and in the degree of purification they must accomplish.

The key operations in wastewater treatment plants are directed to the separation of the imposed load from the carrying water. The unloaded solids constitute sewage sludge or, in the current vernacular, residuals. The desired phase separation or mass transfer of removable solids is set in motion in a number of different ways that include physical, chemical, and biological unit operations. Moreover, since wastewater is rich in nutrients, it is understandable that air or oxygen must be introduced into some treatment processes if the wastes are to be kept fresh and odorless. This, too, is a form of mass transfer—in this case as aeration or gas transfer, accompanied coincidentally by a sweeping out of gases and odors of decomposition. By contrast, anaerobic conditions may favor the degradation of putrescible matter in the dewatering and stabilization of sewage sludge.

The common unit operations and their useful combinations are as follows:

Preliminary Treatment. Screens or comminutors are often placed at the influent of treatment plants to remove or macerate rags and other large objects that may interfere with subsequent treatment units. Similarly, grit chambers remove heavy sand and grit that may be troublesome in the plant, if not in a receiving stream.

Sedimentation. The workhorse of wastewater treatment plants is the settling tank. In it, settleable solids are removed by sedimentation. These are similar to sedimentation tanks in water treatment except that, because the settled sludge can become quickly putrescible, mechanical sludge-removal equipment is always provided.

Primary sedimentation tanks hold the sewage for 1 to 2 hours. During this time, 50% to 70% of the influent suspended solids, including 30% to 50% of the influent BOD, are deposited on the tank bottom. The sludge is bulky because it contains about 95% water and is putrescible because its solids are volatile (organic) to the extent of about 72% on a dry basis.

Intermediate and secondary or final sedimentation tanks remove the flocs or sludges formed in biologically treated wastewaters. When wastewater treatment was first introduced, a recognized goal was the introduction of at least primary treatment in all the industrialized countries. In the United States, Public Law 92-500 mandates a minimum of secondary treatment (i.e., biological treatment), although the need for more than primary treatment for discharges to the ocean or to large rivers is questioned. In general, primary sedimentation is a precursor to biological treatment.

Chemical Coagulation and Flocculation. This is similar to water treatment, although the amounts of aluminum and iron salts required may range as high as 100 mg/L. Reductions as high as 80% to 90% in suspended solids and 70% to 80% in BOD are obtained. The sludges from chemical treatment are generally more troublesome than primary treatment sludges.

Biological Treatment. Biological treatment units are designed to encourage a high rate of growth and activity of scavenging microorganisms. The physical result is twofold: (1) conversion of finely divided, colloidal, and dissolved organic matter into settleable cell substance by biosynthesis and (2) reduction of the energy level of much of the remaining organic matter by bioanalysis, degradation, or oxidation. The wastes must not be toxic to bacteria and other microorganisms. As already mentioned, secondary or biological treatment is the minimum treatment to be provided by U.S. communities, with but few exceptions. This treatment removes about 85% of the BOD, resulting in an effluent BOD of about 30 mg/L.

Two uniquely biological treatment operations have continued in wide service over the years: trickling filtration and activated sludge aeration. Flow sheets for treatment works that include, respectively, high-rate trickling filters and activated-sludge units are shown in Figure 35–9. A third treatment approach finding favor today is the rotating biological contactor, which provides for the establishment of biological growths on a fixed medium while not requiring the large areas necessary for trickling filters.

Trickling Filters. Structurally, trickling filters are beds of stone or plastic media 1 to 4 m deep. The beds have extensive surfaces to which microorganisms adhere as zoogleal slimes or biomasses that are supplied (1) with nutrients by the wastes trickling over them from top to bottom and (2) with oxygen by air sweeping up or down of its own accord through the filter bed.

The wastewaters are distributed over the circular filters from arms rotating over the bed, propelled—in much the same way as an ordinary lawn sprinkler—by their own jets issuing horizontally from rows of nozzles.

The filter effluent is collected by a system of underdrains large enough to carry the flows from the bed and to transmit enough air to the zoogleal slimes to keep the operation aerobic. The biomass that builds up in the filter is kept in balance by sloughing into the filter effluent for capture in the secondary settling tank. The effluent of modern filters is normally recycled for dilution of influent and greater efficiency. For strong wastes or high loadings, two or more units may be placed in series.

Trickling filters can produce effluents containing, after sedimentation, less than 20 mg of BOD and suspended solids per liter. Their performance is not greatly affected by transient shocks of strong or toxic wastes, implying that the filter slimes have a large reserve capacity that is not easily destroyed. Because of this, trickling filters are sometimes introduced as "shock absorbers" in advance of activated sludge units, which are less rugged in their response to taxing changes in the applied wastewater. Sludge produced is about 0.05% to 0.1% of the flow treated. Ordinarily, this sludge contains 92% to 95% water and 60% to 70% organic matter on a dry basis. Because of the great area occupied by such plants, they are not used in large cities.

Activated Sludge Units. Structurally, activated sludge units are tanks 10 to 15 feet deep in which the wastewater is mixed and aerated together with previously formed biomasses or flocs that are returned to the tank influent. The flocs play the part of the trickling-filter slimes. Aerobic conditions are maintained by the injection of compressed air or oxygen or by absorption of oxygen from the atmosphere at the air–water interface, which is continuously renewed by mechanical stirring or air diffusion. The

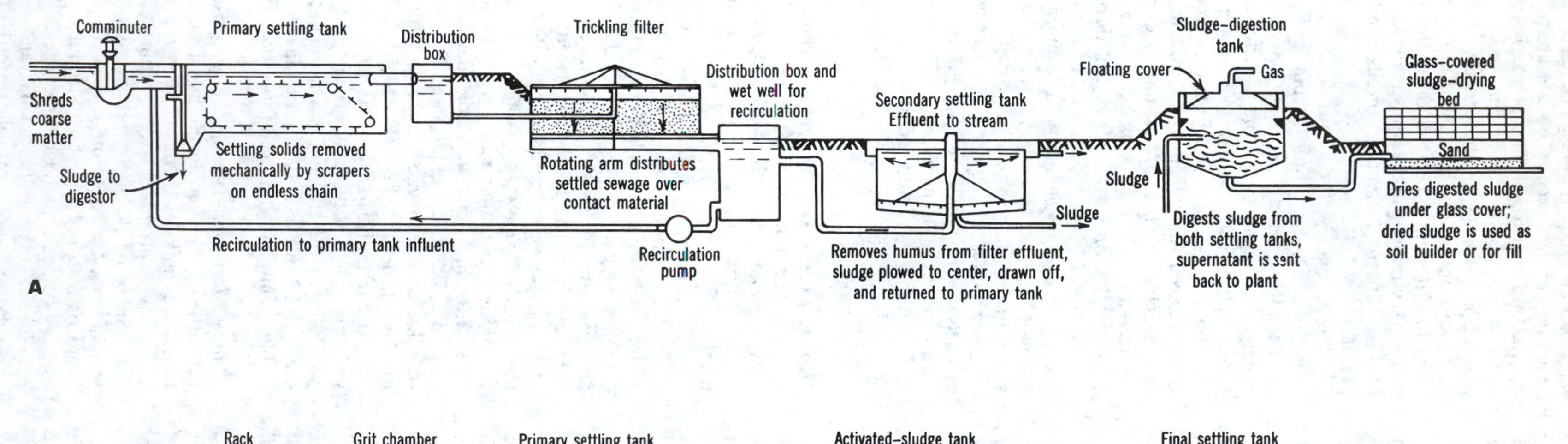

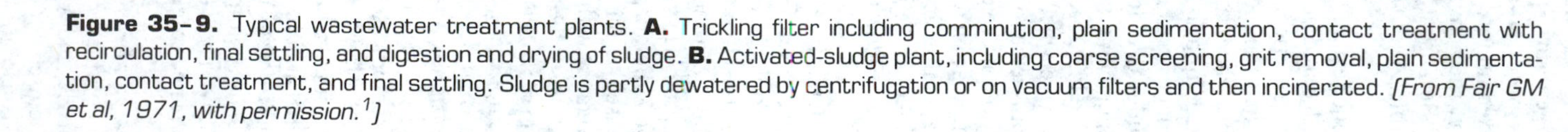

Figure 35-9. Typical wastewater treatment plants. **A.** Trickling filter including comminution, plain sedimentation, contact treatment with recirculation, final settling, and digestion and drying of sludge. **B.** Activated-sludge plant, including coarse screening, grit removal, plain sedimentation, contact treatment, and final settling. Sludge is partly dewatered by centrifugation or on vacuum filters and then incinerated. *[From Fair GM et al, 1971, with permission.[1]]*

flocculant solids, the activated sludge, are then removed in final settling tanks.

The biomass that builds up in the aeration unit is maintained by returning a useful amount of sludge to the process from the final settling tank. Therefore, recycling is built into the activated sludge process. Transfer of organic matter to the zooglean flocs by adsorption and its stabilization and oxidation take several hours. Sludge return in the vicinity of 25% by volume of incoming sewage produces about 2500 mg of suspended solids per liter of the mixed liquor.

Because it is watery, the activated sludge wasted from the process is large in bulk. Because it consists principally of living cells, it is highly putrescible. About 0.5% of the flow is wasted as sludge.

Modern activated sludge plants are flexible, making it possible to vary returned sludge and air in quantities and ways that meet changing needs and experience. Three variants of the conventional process serve as examples. In *modified aeration,* the period of aeration is shortened, and the concentration of suspended solids in the mixed liquor is reduced. Less air is required, but the degree of treatment is reduced. In *step aeration* or *step loading,* the returned sludge is added to a fraction of the inflowing sewage, the remainder being introduced at equal distances along the path of the mixed liquor. The returning sludge renews its activity without being overwhelmed. In *complete mixing,* the influent is introduced transverse to the flow. This avoids "shock loading" of the sludge even more effectively than step loading. Sludge may be kept in circulation within the aeration unit until it is no longer degradable, a practice favored in small plants or when the organic substances in the wastes being treated are completely soluble. Milk-processing wastes are of this kind.

Stabilization Ponds. A system of stabilization ponds is like a river wound up in one spot. The ponds are constructed in porous or tight soil as rude basins about 1 m deep. They expose large surfaces to air and light. Putrescible wastewaters are held in them for several weeks. During this time, settleable solids sink to the bottom, and organic matter decomposes. Under favorable climatic conditions, carbon dioxide, nitrogen, phosphorus, and other nutrients are released to the water during decomposition and stimulate profuse algal growths. During daylight hours, oxygen is produced by photosynthesis and helps keep the ponds aerobic. At night, carbon dioxide is lost to the atmosphere. Seepage and evaporation are not great.

Except in winter at high latitudes, when they are covered with ice, properly dimensioned ponds remain aerobic, and both BOD and coliforms are reduced to acceptable levels. Climatic and operational factors enter into the performance of stabilization ponds so greatly that allowable loadings cannot be set with certitude. Depending on circumstances, winter loadings may be no more than 20, summer loadings as high as 400 persons per 1000 m^2. The green alga *Chlorella* is a common bloom. Its small spherical cells are not easily separated from the effluent, but the incentive remains to convert waste nutrients into useful algal proteins that can be harvested safely and economically as animal feeds.

Because of their large area, stabilization ponds are introduced only where waste volumes are not too large and land is not too costly. Odors may arise, and treatment sites must be selected with care. The ponds themselves are simple to construct and are particularly suitable in developing countries.

Tertiary Treatment. In many instances, secondary treatment is insufficient to maintain water quality in receiving streams and lakes, and tertiary treatment is required. When tertiary treatment involves physical-chemical treatment, it is characterized as advanced waste treatment (AWT). Often the tertiary treatment is required to remove additional BOD, which can be accomplished by adding a second stage of biological treatment or by carrying the process to nitrification, which oxidizes the oxygen-demanding ammonia, relieving oxygen pressures on receiving streams. Other tertiary treatment processes are for the removal of phosphorus and/or nitrogen. Phosphorus is generally removed chemically, while nitrogen can be removed biologically or by ammonia stripping, a gas exchange process. It should not be necessary to remove both phosphorus and nitrogen. These are nutrients that stimulate eutrophication, or fertilization, in lakes and other still or slow-moving bodies of water. Generally, one or the other of these nutrients is limiting, and its removal may control eutrophication.

Unfortunately, these nutrients originate also in nonpoint sources, such as from runoff from fertilized urban and agricultural lands, which are more difficult to control. Removal of phosphorus and nitrogen from wastewaters may then not be sufficient to effect any improvement in receiving waters.

Where wastewater reclamation is intended, filtration may be introduced for polishing the effluent, increasing its clarity, and reducing the chlorine demand for disinfection. In some special instances, the filter may be activated carbon to reduce the color and the concentration of synthetic organics.

As the efficiency of removal of pollutants is increased, the cost of removing each additional unit of pollution increases exponentially. After secondary treatment achieves 85% removal, an additional 10% removal may cost much more than removal of the first 40%. Going from 97% to 99% removal may cost as much as the entire effort of going from zero to 97%. Moreover, the operation and energy costs are exceedingly high. Accordingly, authorities should demonstrate ample justification in public benefits, including public health, before selecting treatment levels.

Disinfection of Wastewaters. Chlorine is the principal disinfectant, with contact times of at least 15 minutes at maximum flow rates, and residuals of 0.2 to 1.0 mg/L. For 99.9% reduction of coliform organisms, chlorine dosages range from 5 to 25 mg/L.

Chlorination is called for only where effluents are to be discharged into waters used for shellfish growing, drinking, or bathing. Chlorination of effluents may create three problems: (1) chloramines are formed, which may be toxic to aquatic life; (2) in reaction with organics, chlorinated hydrocarbons of potential health significance may be formed; and (3) beneficial microorganisms, as well as pathogens, are destroyed, thereby reducing the ability of the receiving water to biochemically stabilize the organic matter remaining. In contrast with the United States, where EPA had initially mandated chlorination for every effluent, no effluents are chlorinated in Great Britain, even where they discharge into waters to be used for drinking. Disinfection of effluents needs to be evaluated carefully in each instance.

An alternative to chlorination of effluents is the use of ultraviolet light, which eliminates the impact on aquatic life and the possibility of the creation of chlorinated hydrocarbons. To be successful, however, UV requires an effluent of consistently low turbidity, implying the need for tertiary filtration.

Sludge Management. Sludge comprises the settled solids removed from the flow during its passage through primary sedimentation tanks with or without the benefit of coagulating chemicals, or after biological treatment. Sludge accumulates the lion's share of the living organisms that find their way into wastewaters. Sludge teems with predators such as the ciliated protozoa that feed upon bacteria and thereby accelerate the dieaway of bacterial pathogens. Sludge drying deprives the organisms of moisture needed for survival.

Fresh primary-tank solids are the most dangerous, solids from biological treatment units less so, solids that have been subjected to biological decomposition still less, and air-dried solids the least. Heat-dried solids are microbiologically safe. The period of survival of enteric viruses in sludge is still unknown; for enteric bacteria, such as the typhoid bacillus, it is reported as about 1 week. Viable cysts of *E. histolytica* have been isolated from sludge held for 10 days at 30° C, and viable hookworm eggs after 41 days. For sludge held 6 months, a 10% survival of *Ascaris* eggs was noted; but when pulverized sludge was heated to 103° C for 3 minutes, all eggs were destroyed.

Treatment. Generally speaking, sludge is of little value and is disposed of in the cheapest possible way. In normal circumstances, however, it is neither feasible nor economical to get rid of the large volumes of sludge generated without dewatering it, destroying its organic (putrescible) constituents, or both. Why it pays to reduce the water content of sludge is exemplified by the fact that reducing the moisture content of sludge from 98% (2% solids) to 96% (4% solids) doubles the proportion of solid matter and in consequence halves the volume of sludge to be handled. Dewatering and destruction of organic matter are indeed the primary objectives of sludge treatment. The wide range of options for the handling of sludges is illustrated in Figure 35–10.

Sludge Digestion. Sludge is an abundant source of food for saprophytic bacteria and other organisms. Different groups of living things use different types of nutrients originally contained in the sludge or produced in the course of decomposition. As the nutritive elements are used up, the sludge becomes stable and, in its final state of degradation, inoffensive to sight and smell. The sludge is then well digested. The end products of digestion are gases, liquids, and residues of mineral and conservative organic substances. Losses by gasification and liquefaction, destruction of water-binding colloids, and physical compaction of solids reduce the bulk of the sludge and prepare it for dewatering.

Organic solids digest under both aerobic and anaerobic conditions. They do so in nature in swamps and river deposits. In the preparation of sludge for land disposal, however, it is simpler and more economical to digest the solids anaerobically. The principal gas released during aerobic decomposition is carbon dioxide; during anaerobic digestion it is combustible methane (65% to 80% by volume). The potential heat energy of the methane is a prime factor in the economy of anaerobic sludge digestion. The gas may be burned under a boiler or in a gas engine. The power released as heat and mechanical energy is put to use for the heating of buildings and digestion units, air compression, pumping, and minor laboratory purposes. On a per capita basis, the normal daily volume of gas generated is about 0.03 m^3 from primary settling tanks and nearly the same amount again from biological treatment units. Ground garbage and some organic industrial wastes increase the gas yield appreciably. The fuel value of the gas is about 24,000 kilojoules (BTU's) per cubic meter, more than that of most synthetic illuminating gases.

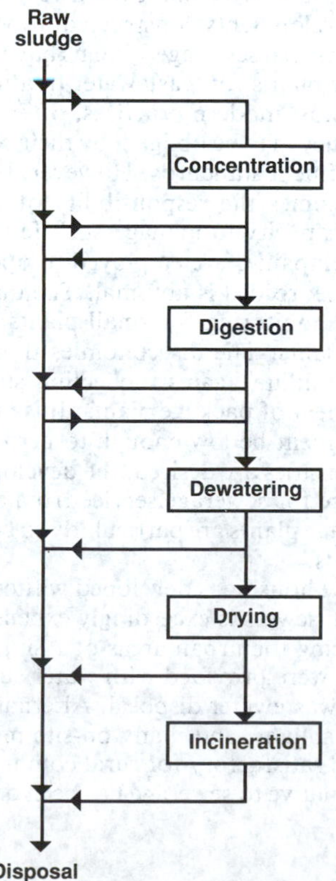

Figure 35–10. Flow diagram for the handling of wastewater treatment plant sludges, with arrows indicating possible flow paths. *(From Okun DA, Ponghis G, 1975.[29])*

Anaerobic sludge digestion units are heated, covered, insulated tanks in which the sludge is stored until it is dense, essentially odorless, and readily dewatered. The temperature of the sludge mass is kept at an optimal operating value—normally about 35° C. In modern, high-rate installations, digestion is promoted by stirring as well as by heating. Digestion tank capacity requirements range from 0.07 m^3 per capita for sludge from primary treatment up to twice that for all the sludge from an activated sludge plant.

Where sludge treatment is by mechanical dewatering and heat-drying or incineration, sludge digestion is not necessary; where it is practiced, capacities may be much less than indicated above because digestion need not be complete. The destruction of organic matter at high temperatures and pressures by wet combustion is finding some application.

Sludge Drying. For small works, the cheapest and therefore the most common method of dewatering sludge is drying it in the open air. To this purpose, digested sludge is run or pumped onto beds of sand and gravel or other suitable porous material. Part of the sludge moisture evaporates at its surface, and part seeps through the supporting bed into underdrains. Drying times vary with climate and character of sludge. The required area is about 0.1 m^2 per capita for well-digested primary sludge and twice that amount for biological sludges. When sludge has lost enough moisture to become a spadable cake, it is removed from the drying beds for final disposal.

In works of moderate and large size, it pays to dewater sludge mechanically.

Sludge Disposal. Some seacoast towns pump wet sludge to sea; others load partially dewatered sludge onto vessels or scows and carry it out to dumping grounds at sea. This practice is being reevaluated.

Dewatered sludge is a suitable material for disposal in a properly designed landfill by itself or in combination with municipal refuse. Wet sludge can provide useful moisture, humus, and nutrients for composting operations. The use of sludge as a fertilizer may be warranted as a measure of nitrogen and phosphorus conservation and soil building. To this purpose, some municipalities are able to dispose of wet sludge, or sludge cake, to farmers. Tank trucks with fixed nozzles that plow and discharge the liquid sludge into the soil have become popular. In general, only commercially dry (heat-dried to less than 10% moisture) activated sludge has been found sufficiently marketable in the United States—for use on lawns and golf greens—to meet the expense of dewatering and heating.

Because of the low cost and the convenience of chemical fertilizers, however, the production of heat-dried sludge for sale is seldom economically rewarding. This may change, though, as rising energy costs increase the costs of chemical fertilizers. In the few instances where heat-dried activated sludge is marketed, as from Milwaukee, the capital investment in the facilities has already been paid off and further capital investment is not warranted. Where suitable sites for sludge disposal are not economically available, the sludge must be incinerated, leaving only the ash for disposal. In some communities, incineration of sludge with municipal refuse has been found feasible.

The ultimate disposal of wastewater sludges, particularly when they may contain pathogens, heavy metals, and synthetic organic chemicals, has raised many questions. All of the methods of disposal, whether by discharge to sea, application to agricultural land, burying in landfills, composting, or incineration have come under attack. The EPA has been wrestling with this problem since passage of the 1977 Clean Water Act Amendments, and final regulations are to be promulgated in 1991. The regulations involve contaminant limits for heavy metals and organics in the sludges, in milligrams per kilogram, and loading rates, in kilograms per hectare, for various land applications, as well as technology, monitoring, and reporting requirements. Ultimate disposal will likely be by land application and landfills for communities that have such land available to them and, for larger cities, incineration. With land applications, a major concern is the potential for impact on water supplies.

Wastewater Disposal. Outfall sewers are used to discharge the treated wastewater into the receiving body of water. If outfalls are to be effective, they must be designed and situated to disperse the effluent quickly and thoroughly throughout the receiving water. In streams, this is not difficult; in lakes, tidal estuaries, and the ocean it is not simple. Outfall locations must be chosen with an eye to waterworks intakes, shellfish layings, bathing beaches, and recreational areas. This calls for the study of water movements of all kinds: normal currents, wind-induced and tidal movements, and eddy diffusion created by differences in the density of the sewage and the receiving water. Density is a function of water temperature and the concentration of dissolved solids, or salinity.

Wastewaters are generally warmer and lighter than the water into which they are discharged. Emptied into a receiving body of water near its surface—especially the brackish waters of tidal estuaries—the wastewater rides on top of the diluting water, does not mix appreciably, and tends to form a slick, noticeable for many miles. Nevertheless, the temperature-density equilibria are so delicate that every situation and season must be handled individually. Under some conditions, for example, subsurface discharge of wastewaters into a deep fresh-water lake may build up a large mass of undispersed wastes around the outfall. Otherwise, subsurface and submarine outfalls are widely used. The lighter liquid rises like a smoke plume through the receiving body of water, and there is good dispersion. This is stepped up further by discharging the wastes through a number of outlets spaced so as not to interfere with one another.

The purification accomplished in streams can be improved by engineering works that either supply water for dilution during periods of low flow, lengthen the time of downstream passage of the receiving water, or introduce air into the flowing water, either directly by injection or indirectly by agitation. In low-water regulation, water is released from upland reservoirs in the same or neighboring catchment areas, or water is pumped back or recycled from the more voluminous flows of lower river reaches or other water courses. Times of travel and self-purification are normally lengthened by impoundages within the polluted stretches of the stream. The reservoirs are not made so deep that they stratify and undergo eutrophication. Compressed air has been introduced with some success into critical reaches of polluted streams from stationary compressors and piping or from floating, occasionally self-propelled, barges.

A somewhat unusual example of controlled dilution of wastewaters is the construction of fish ponds in which effluent is mixed with clean river water to create an ecosystem favorable for the cultivation of fish and the raising of ducks. Large crops of organisms that serve as food for fish and ducks are raised in the aquatic meadows of these ponds. Both impoundages and fish ponds are variations on stabilization ponds that receive raw or treated wastes without the benefit of diluting waters.

On-Site Disposal of Domestic Wastewaters. Where running water has been introduced into kitchens, bathrooms, laundries, and outbuildings of farms and fringe-area houses but there is no public sewerage, the wastewaters must be disposed of on site. Usually, this is done through septic tanks or cesspools, which involve simple settling and subsurface leaching. For success, the amount of sewage cannot be large in relation to the leaching area, and the soil must be porous. Where the volume of wastewater is high or the soil is tight, more sophisticated and costly treatment methods patterned after municipal processes must be introduced. Of special concern is the contamination, both chemical and biological, of nearby wells. Septic tanks derive their name from the septic or anaerobic condition created by the decomposition of the settling solids or accumulating sewage sludges. All septic tanks must be emptied of accumulated sludge from time to time. Septage is generally disposed of to community wastewater treatment plants.

The ability of soil to absorb settled sewage is explored by digging test holes, filling them with water, and clocking the time required for the water to drop a given distance in the stratum in which leaching is to take place.

Septic tanks and tile fields may be suitable for truly rural areas, but they have been adopted by builders for housing developments where they inevitably cause trouble, generally because the tile fields become clogged and the septic tanks overflow, creating a local health hazard. Even where soil conditions are suitable, septic tanks and tile fields should not be used unless at least about 4000 m^2 (1 acre) is available per dwelling unit.

Housing developments constructed in periurban areas not accessible to municipal sewerage systems have led to the proliferation of package plants for wastewater treatment. These plants do conform to most modern practices, often providing tertiary treatment, and they may be obliged, by their NPDES permits, to meet exacting effluent standards. However, their operation and maintenance becomes the responsibility of the home owners, who have little capacity to manage such facilities. Even where private utility companies are employed to operate these plants, their performance record is abysmal. The quality of personnel and the cost of monitoring for small plants are little different than for large plants. The diseconomies that accompany such small facilities militate against collecting sufficient funds for proper management of package plants. It is preferable that densities of development be low enough to permit septic tanks or, where greater densities are desired, the development must be obligated to arrange for sewerage service from a nearby large municipality. Package plants are particularly to be avoided on water supply watersheds.

Where dense housing is developed without sewers, retrofitting an area with sewers is exceedingly expensive. This is a serious problem facing the urban areas of Asia, Africa, and Latin America, which were provided with water supplies but no adequate means of wastewater disposal. Alternatives to costly sewerage are being sought, and many on-site methods of disposal have been found satisfactory for rural communities, but to date no suitable alternative to sewerage has been developed for urban areas.

Wastewater Reclamation (see p. 622). Wastewaters are a water resource, and their reclamation for reuse serves both to conserve limited quantities of fresh water and to reduce the load of pollution on receiving bodies of water. The following purposes have been served by wastewater reclamation.[3]

1. Irrigation, both agricultural and urban
2. Industrial use, both process and cooling
3. Recreation, through establishment of lakes and ponds
4. Nonpotable residential and commercial use, including toilet flushing.

Reclamation for potable purposes is not recommended, as sound drinking water practice requires that priority should be given to the purest source. Treatment and monitoring technology are not adequate to assure safety where wastewaters are to be used directly for potable purposes.

Reclamation for irrigation and land disposal of wastewaters are different. Irrigation is the beneficial use of wastewaters for growing crops or lawns. Land disposal is a method of wastewater disposal where harvesting of crops is incidental. Many of the constraints and benefits are the same.

Land disposal may be useful in smaller communities where ample land is available and the soil conditions are appropriate. Where the nutrients in wastewaters would be troublesome if discharged to a body of water, on land they constitute an important plus, particularly as chemical fertilizers become more costly. Land disposal provides a method for removing the nutrients in the soil, to be picked up by harvested crops.

Each situation is unique, permitting certain rates of application and requiring specific treatment. Because the wastewaters are produced year-round, but cannot be applied to the land during periods of heavy rainfall or freezing, seasonal storage is required. Soil scientists can make useful contributions to resolution of these problems.

Where wastewaters are to be reused, the treatment needs to be tailored to the specific reuse, with more intensive treatment and more stringent standards as the uses become of greater public health concern. The California Department of Health has prepared *Wastewater Reclamation Criteria,* which guide in the regulation of many hundreds of reclamation projects in the state. The highest degree of treatment is for nonpotable distribution systems, which include urban irrigation, toilet flushing, industry, etc., as well as spray irrigation of food crops and nonrestricted recreational impoundments (i.e., those that permit body contact). On the basis of the Pomona Study, an appropriate quality would appear to be produced by secondary wastewater treatment followed by coagulation, direct filtration, and disinfection with chlorine.

Essential to such reclamation are reliability of operation of the treatment facilities and continuous monitoring of effluent quality with a capacity to automatically reject effluent that does not meet the bacterial, turbidity, and chlorine residual standards.[30]

ORGANIZATION FOR WATER QUALITY MANAGEMENT

Human ecology is distinguished from the ecology of other biological systems by our ability to reason, inquire, and invent. As a result, we have developed the means for adjusting the environment to ourselves. This is a never ending task, as development continues to interfere with the environment, often creating new hazards to health. We must continue efforts to protect ourselves against disease processes that have environmental causes. Among other things, this requires the collaboration of persons with many different skills.

Engineers have long been members of public agencies that have as one of their responsibilities the initiation, approval, and control of public works related in one way or another to human health and well-being. In England, the start was made through the promotion of the "sanitary idea," which found expression in the sanitation of growing industrial towns. In the United States, it was begun at the state level for the protection of the purity of inland waters and continued at the federal level for the safety of interstate travelers and the protection of interstate waters. At the international level, water sanitation has been promoted by international treaty; examples are the control of oil pollution of international waters in the seas and oceans of the world and the maintenance of acceptable standards of water quality in international bodies of fresh water such as the Rhine, the Rio Grande, and the chain of lakes and rivers along the boundary between the United States and Canada.

At another level, municipal, county, or regional authorities are generally responsible for the provision and operation of water supply and wastewater treatment facilities. Regulation through monitoring of water quality, review of plans for treatment works, and data from their operations is the responsibility of state agencies. At one time, this responsibility almost always rested with the state health agency, but gradually separate pollution control agencies were established. At the federal level, the EPA administers the national water supply and water pollution control programs.

Because the waters of the earth know no political boundaries—although they often become international and interstate borders by political choice—some countries have found it expedient to establish national water authorities.

As revealed by the PHS Community Water Supply Survey,[2] one of the problems with the quality of water service arises from the excessive fragmentation of the water supply industry. More than half the water supply systems in the United States serve fewer than 1000 people. The same is true for sewerage and wastewater disposal. Such small systems cannot afford the quality of design and operation of complex facilities that large communities can, and yet the needs are much the same. Moreover, smaller communities are in competition with each other for limited water resources, and they lose the advantages of the economies and efficiencies of scale.

One clear solution is the regionalization of water management, which has been approached in a revolutionary way by England and Wales with the creation of ten regional water authorities based on hydrological boundaries.[31] Each authority owns, operates, and finances all the facilities for water supply, wastewater collection and disposal, and water-based recreation. The success of this approach is revealed by the fact that more than 99% of the population is served by public water supplies and by the way in which England met the 1975–1976 drought, the most severe in a millennium. While the integrated approach to water management was abandoned in 1989 by privatization of the water supply, sewerage, and wastewater disposal functions of the authorities, this regional approach can be studied with profit, and elements of it adopted, by all who are responsible for water quality management. Whatever form of organization is adopted, its ultimate task is to manage water resources in the service of people while protecting their health and the quality of the environment.

REFERENCES

1. Fair GM, Geyer JC, Okun DA: Elements of Water Supply and Wastewater Disposal. New York: John Wiley, 1971
2. Community Water Supply Survey, U.S. Public Health Service, 1969. Summarized in McCabe LJ, et al: Study of community water supply systems. J Am Water Works Assoc 62:670, 1970
3. Camp, Dresser & McKee, Inc: Guidelines for Water Reuse. Environmental Protection Agency, 600/8-80-036, 1980

4. United Nations Economic and Social Council: Water for Industrial Use, Report No. E-3058 ST/ECA/50, 1958
5. American Water Works Association: Manual on Dual Distribution Systems, No. M24, Denver: AWWA, 1983
6. Environmental Protection Agency: National Interim Primary Drinking Water Regulations, 1976
7. U.S. District Court, District of Connecticut: Bridgeport Hydraulic Co. et al. *v.* The Council on Water Company Lands of the State of Connecticut et al, Civil No. B-75-212, December 1977
8. University of North Carolina: Protecting Drinking Water Supplies Through Watershed Management: A Guidebook for Devising Local Programs. Chapel Hill, North Carolina: Center for Urban and Regional Studies, 1982
9. Burby RJ, Okun DA: Land use planning and health. Annu Rev Public Health 4:47–67, 1983
10. National Research Council: Drinking Water and Health. Washington, D.C.: National Academy Press, Vol. 1, 1977; Vols. 2 and 3, 1980; Vol. 4, 1982; Vol. 5, 1983; Vol. 6, 1986; Vols. 7 and 8, 1987; Vol. 9, 1989
11. Cantor KP, Hoover R, et al: Bladder cancer, drinking water source, and tap water consumption: a case-control study. J Natl Cancer Inst 19(6):1269–1279, 1987
12. Cothern CR: Radioactivity in Drinking Water. Washington, D.C.: Environmental Protection Agency, EPA 570/9 81 002, 1981
13. National Academy of Sciences—National Research Council: The Effects on Populations of Exposure to Low Levels of Ionizing Radiation. Washington, D.C.: GPO, 1972
14. Longtin JP: Radon, Radium and Uranium Occurrence in Drinking Water from Groundwater Sources. Proceedings of National Conference of American Water Works Association, June 1987. Denver: The Association
15. Standard Methods for the Examination of Water and Wastewater: American Public Health Association, American Water Works Association, Water Pollution Control Federation, 16 edt. Denver: The Association, 1989
16. Craun GF: Surface water supplies and health. J Am Water Works Assoc 80:40, 1988
17. Cabeth VJ: Health Effects Criteria for Marine Recreational Waters. Washington, D.C.: Environmental Protection Agency, EPA-600/1-80-031, August 1983
18. Colbourne JS: Thames Water Authority's Experience with *Cryptosporidium,* Proceedings of 1989 Water Technology Conference American Water Works Association, Denver 1990
19. Dufour AP: Health Effects Criteria for Fresh Recreational Waters. Washington, D.C.: Environmental Protection Agency, EPA-600/1-84-004, August 1984
20. Environmental Protection Agency, Federal Register, Part II 40 CFR, Parts 141 and 142, June 29, 1989
21. McJunkin FE: Water and Human Health. Washington, D.C.: U.S. Agency for International Development, July 1982
22. Thomas HA Jr: The animal farm. J Am Water Works Assoc 56: 1087, 1964
23. World Health Organization: Guidelines for Drinking Water Quality, 3 Volumes, Geneva, 1984
24. Okun DA: The value of water supply and sanitation development: An assessment. Am J Public Health 78:1463, 1988
25. American Water Works Association: Water Quality and Treatment. New York: McGraw-Hill, 1971
26. American Society of Civil Engineers, American Water Works Association, Conference of State Sanitary Engineers: Water Treatment Plant Design. Denver: American Water Works Association, 1989
27. Water Pollution Control Federation and American Society of Civil Engineers: Wastewater Treatment Plant Design. New York: American Society of Civil Engineers, 1977
28. Water Pollution Control Federation and American Society of Civil Engineers: Design and Construction of Sanitary and Storm Sewers. Alexandria, Va.: The Federation, 1969
29. Okun DA, Ponghis G: Community Wastewater Collection and Disposal. Geneva: World Health Organization, 1975
30. California Department of Health Services: Wastewater Reclamation Criteria. California Administrative Code, Title 22, Division 4, 1978
31. Okun DA: Regionalization of Water Management: A Revolution in England and Wales. Essex, England: Applied Science Publishers, 1977

36

Solid and Radioactive Waste Disposal

Solid Waste Disposal

Masaru Tanaka
Hiroshi Takatsuki
Yoshinori Itokawa

QUANTITY AND QUALITY OF SOLID WASTE

Solid wastes are classified into general waste and industrial waste, according to the generating source.

Although there are some statistics available regarding details of waste quantity and waste quality in individual countries, neither statistical object items nor the degree of statistical accuracy have been standardized. In spite of this, integrated data in relation of solid waste quantity in the world have been shown to give scope to the problem of worldwide solid waste generation.

Table 36–1 shows a comparison of solid waste quantity among a group of advanced industrial countries where large amounts of solid waste are generated.

Quantities of industrial waste, such as factory waste or sewage sludge generated and discharged by industrial activities, are generally from two times to some tens of times greater than the quantity of general waste generated and discharged from municipal activity, such as household, commercial, and business waste.

It is difficult to explain each individual item of various types of industrial waste, since differing waste items need different disposal systems. On the contrary, in view of public health considerations, one is more interested in disposal of municipal solid waste than of industrial waste.

Table 36–2 shows a comparison of quantity, physical composition, and method of disposal of municipal solid waste in various countries. It is difficult to obtain a mean value of the relative data from the statistics available from Asian countries; instead, individual city data are compiled in Table 36–2.

The definition of municipal solid waste differs a bit among individual cities. In general, however, municipal solid waste includes household, commercial, business, and public street waste. In some countries, municipal solid waste includes industrial waste and construction waste, because the definition of municipal solid waste includes all the waste generated and discharged by municipal activities. On the other hand, household waste comprises those items generated and discharged from individual activities and subject to periodic collection.

Individual amounts of household waste vary among countries, although the mean value of all the Western Europe type of advanced industrial countries is approximately 700 to 800 g per capita per day, while that of industrial waste is approximately 1200 to 1500 g per capita per day.

Municipal solid waste disposal methods vary between countries. Landfill disposal is the dominant method in many countries, including the United States and the United Kingdom, but incineration is the dominant method in Switzerland and Japan. Material recovery from municipal solid waste, including composting, represents a large portion of the disposal methods used in some countries.

Regarding the content and constitution of municipal solid waste, there may be various measurement and classification methods in many countries. However, the outline or the feature data can be obtained. For example, the fact that municipal waste includes twigs and weeds in the United States indicates that there is much backyard material in household waste. The ratio of plastic material contained in municipal solid waste is more than 10% in Japan and Switzerland, whereas the ratio in other countries is less than 7%.

The ratio of incombustible materials in municipal solid waste is high in Asian countries, and it may indicate the influence of ashes generated from coal or charcoal used for fuels and heating.

COLLECTION AND TRANSPORTATION

As part of solid waste management, collection and transportation are important. Particularly with regard to municipal solid waste management in general, it is said that approximately 70% of the total cost will go to expenditures for waste collection and transportation.

Figure 36–1 shows the expenditure ratio of municipal solid waste management in Tokyo, Japan, for example. It indicates that 70% of the whole management cost goes to expenditure for waste collection and transportation, more specifically 40% for waste collection and 30% for waste transportation.

Collection and transportation expenses amount to such a

TABLE 36-1. COMPARISON OF SOLID WASTE GENERATION IN VARIOUS COUNTRIES (UNIT: 1,000 TONS PER YEAR)

	General Waste[a] (1)	Industrial Waste[b] (2)	Agricultural and Forestry Waste (3)	Mine and Construction Waste (4)	Overall Industrial Waste (5) = (2) + (3) (4)	Quantity of all Waste[c] (6) = (1) + (5)	Year of Survey
Japan	41,530	166,071	62,702	83,498	312,271	353,801	1985
(Quantity of final disposal*)	16,048				91,000	107,048	
United States	148,000	7,615,100	Unknown	3,526,500 -5,040,500		11,300,000	1987 Report
(Quantity of final disposal*)		392,580					
United Kingdom	18,000[d]	91,700	250,000	75,000	416,700	434,700	
Italy	13,960	30,500	Unknown	4,400	34,900	48,860	1977
Austria	1,630	728[e]				2,358[e]	1984
Holland	4,100	14,570	500	57,000 -67,000	72,070 -82,070	76,170 -86,170	
Canada	25,354[f]	60,500	40,000	600,000	700,500	725,854	
Switzerland	2,500	565.7	Unknown	3,000[g]	3,565.7	6,065.7	
Sweden	2,500	5,850	65,000 [(3) + (4)]		70,850	73,350	
Spain	10,600						1984
Denmark			Unknown	1.6		3,435	1987
Hungary	2,700	14,326	22,991[h]	7,820	45,137		1980
France	17,800	150,000	568,000	Unknown	718,000	735,000	1984
Poland							
Portugal	2,000						
West Germany	23,100					36,512[e] [(1) + (2)]	1979, 1983
Norway	1,900[i]	2,120					

* Final disposal is considered to be "landfill."
[a] Those categorized as municipal and household waste, even though they can be classified into household, commercial, business, etc. in view of the source.
[b] In the case of sewage sludge, incineration residue, etc. are aggregated, the values have been added.
[c] In some cases, quantity of agricultural and mine residue waste have not been added.
[d] Total quantity of general waste due to business waste category is 1,400 × 1,000 tons per year.
[e] Unknown if quantity of in-company recovered waste has been added.
[f] Total quantity of general waste due to household waste category is 12,677 × 1,000 tons per year.
[g] Quantity of commercial waste discharged from small businesses has been added.
[h] Since the rate of the inquiry sheet recovery was low, the actual quantity can be estimated as follows: (30,000 to 35,000 × 1,000 tons per year). Resource recovery rate is more than 90%.
[i] Total quantity of general waste due to household is 800 × 1,000 tons per year.

large percentage because of labor costs. In waste management only 2 to 3 tons of urban waste may be collected and hauled from an urban collection route by a collector vehicle, which needs at least a driver and a collection crew of two or three members. In some countries one still sees a common type of truck with an open bed although from a good public health standpoint, it is desirable to use a compartment type of collection vehicle to preclude scatter of waste, stench, seepage, and so forth. There are various types of compartmental collection vehicles, and all are designed to use a compaction mechanism to achieve effective transportation. Figure 36–2 shows the cross section of a typical compartment-type waste-collection vehicle that uses hydraulic compaction press device.

There are various kinds of public garbage cans. Many countries employ containers of the bucket type made of plastic or metal, but standard-size plastic bags are employed for common use in Japan to achieve an effective waste-collection system.

Frequency of waste collection is different, depending on waste quantity and local conditions. It is desirable to make collections at least once a week in view of flies' regular hatching time period. In some settings, such as restaurants, it is common practice to provide daily collection service from midnight through early morning.

In recent years many cities have been using source-separation collection systems. There are various kinds of source separation, such as separation of combustibles and non-combustibles and resource-recoverable waste and hazardous waste.

A number of experiments have been conducted in several countries in an effort to achieve rational management of waste collection and transportation. Some countries have been successful in utilizing a pipe instead of traditional vehicles for waste collection and hauling in order to save labor costs. In reality, it seems difficult to adopt this practical pipeline collection system except in special areas, such as high-density population zones with severe traffic problems. There is a pressing need to achieve an effective vehicle collection and hauling system using large collector vehicles together with development of improved hauling systems with a network of transfer stations. In any case, the collection and transportation system is one of the most important factors, not only in terms of the total social and economic system but also as a close contact point between the municipal environmental administration and the area's inhabitants.

INCINERATION

A basic principle of waste disposal is recovery of usable materials from waste and reuse of generated solid waste as much as possible. One also wishes to stabilize the waste, minimize hazardous elements, and then carry out sanitary disposal of the residue.

Among the various methods of waste disposal, the incineration method has progressed rapidly in recent years in Japan and some European countries. The level of waste quantity reduction

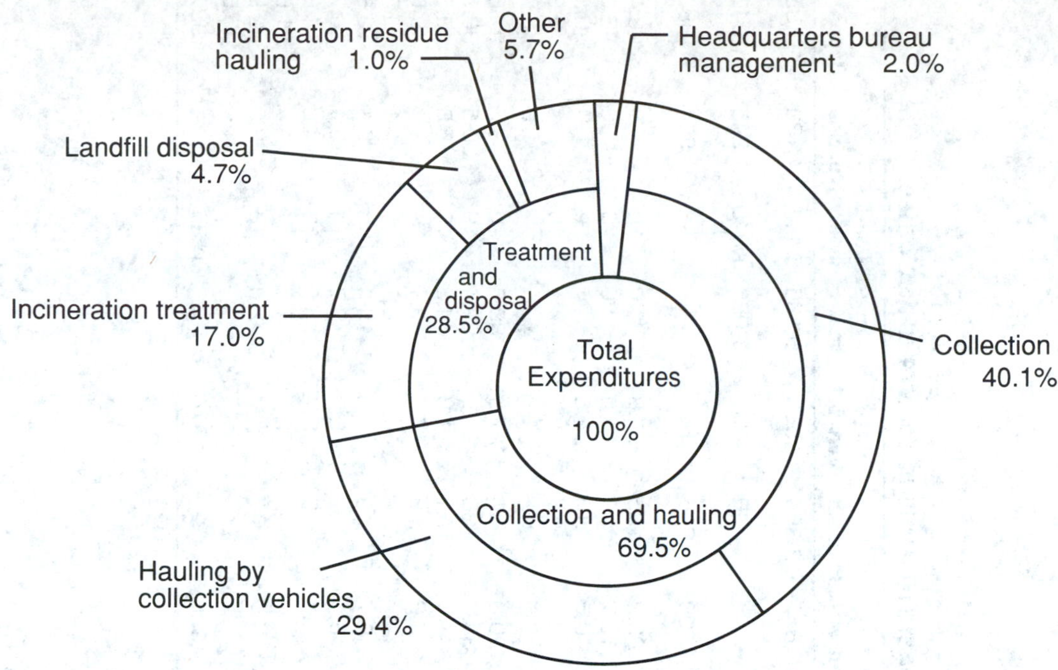

Figure 36-1. Breakdown of waste management expenses [Tokyo Metropolis, 1987].

is as large as 1/15 to 1/20. Incineration is highly valued for its ability to stabilize and eliminate hazardous material. It turns perishable organic material into inorganic matter and kills pathogenic organisms through high ambient temperature conditions. According to the three principles of quantity reduction, stabilization, and harmlessness, the incineration method accompanied by a prompt disposal procedure is highly valued in cities with heavy population density, where it is difficult to secure enough landfill space for waste disposal.

The basic principle of incineration is to burn things at high temperature, causing oxidation. When organic materials, such as paper, fresh garbage, and plastics, are subjected to combustion, all the material becomes inorganic in its transformation to CO_2 and H_2O. Many organic materials would finally becomes CO_2 and H_2O after passage of long periods of time, allowing for decomposition of bacteria. However, the particular feature of the incineration method is that it takes advantage of the instantaneous oxidation effect of the combustion reaction. Furthermore, since the combustion reaction generates calorific energy at the time of the oxidation, the ambient temperature becomes higher during the reaction process and kills pathogenic bacteria, insect nits, and other organisms that adhere to waste, as well as decomposing stench elements generated with waste putrefaction. The incombustible residue becomes ash, which is stabilized inorganic matter, and is discharged from the incinerator.

Waste incinerators are classified into two types: the stoker combustion type and the fluidized bed type. They are also classified into two types of operation: the batch-combustion method (intermittent supply method) (Fig. 36-3) and the continuous-combustion method (Fig. 36-4).

With the stoker type of incinerator, waste is placed on a cast-iron grill and fresh air is supplied through the grill to burn waste. With the fluidized bed type, incineration material such as sand is placed within a cylindrical type of incinerator and then waste is taken and placed on the sand. Next, fresh air is supplied from the bottom section to make the sand operate under fluidized conditions (Fig. 36-5). The number of incinerators of the fluidized bed type in practical use has been rapidly increasing in recent years. However, most of them are of small size, and experience in the use of large equipment is still rare.

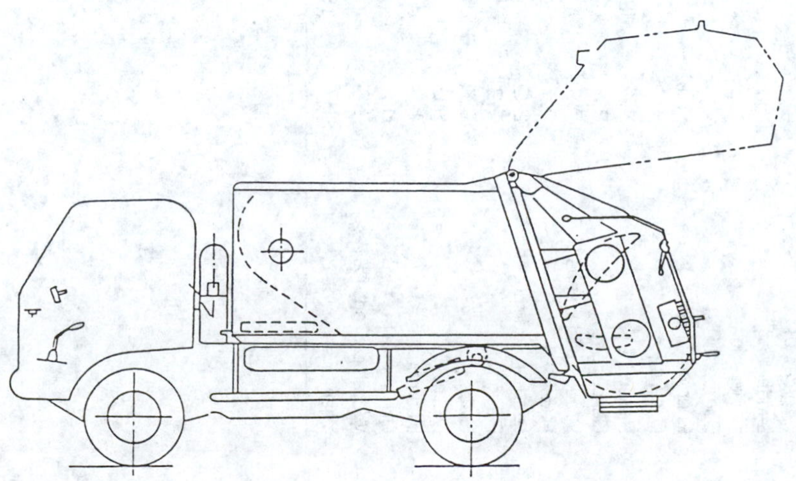

Figure 36-2. Compartment type of waste-collection vehicle with a waste compaction press.

TABLE 36-2. QUANTITY, PHYSICAL COMPOSITION, AND DISPOSAL METHOD OF MUNICIPAL SOLID WASTE IN VARIOUS COUNTRIES AND CITIES

Country	U.S.A.	West Germany	Italy	U.K.	France	Spain	Canada	Holland	Hungary	Sweden	Austria	Switzer-land	Den-mark	Norway	Japan
Population (unit: 1,000)	227,000	61,000	56,244	55,836	54,330	39,000	25,354	13,850	10,657	8,399	7,566	6,485	5,111	4,180	122,185
Municipal waste (g/cap•d)	1,605	1,460		1,585		745	1,370	1,444		1,468	781	1,056	1,840	1,245	1,040
Household waste (g/cap•d)			680	814	970			811	700	815	594			524	863
Landfill (%)	85	65	73.5	88	34.4	81.3	95.7	45	86.3	35	59.8	20	18	65	23.4
Incineration (%)	5	32	24	11	35.9	4.5	4		10.7	55	16.3	80	70	23	72.6
Compost (%)		3	2		8.0	14.2			0.5	10	24.0		2	4 }	0.1
Recovery (%)	10		0.5	1			0.3						10	}	3.9
Others (%)					8.9				2.5					8 }	
Paper (%)	37.1	20.0	22.3	33.9	28		38.9	24.0	20.0	40	27.2	30.6	29	33.5	27.6
Garbage (%)	8.1	42.3	42.1	23.4	25		30.6 }		34.7	30	22.5	29.4	19	30.5	36.9
Woods and weeds (%)	17.9	2.3					6.7 }	51.0		1	1.8	4.3	12	5.3	2.6
Fiber (%)	2.1 }			4.1	3		3.6 }	2.2	5.3	3	7.9	3.1		3.1	3.6
Leather and rubber (%)	2.5 }	7.6						1.1				0.7		1.1	0.7
Plastic (%)	7.2 }		7.2	4.2	5		4.9	6.5	5.7	9	6.0	13.4	5	5.1	12.6
Glass (%)	9.7	11.6	7.1	14.4	8		6.5	6.7	6.1	7	6.0	8.7	4	5.1	6.7
Metal (%)	9.6	3.9	3.0	7.1	7		6.2	2.8	4.4	3	8.4	5.9	13	4.0	4.8
Incombustible (%)	1.8	11.5		7.1	15		2.5	2.1 }	23.8		15.1	1.5		1.4	1.6
Others (%)	0.1	0.8	18.3	5.8			0.3	3.6 }		7		2.4	13	2.9	2.9
Water content (%)	23		44.2				26.5								45.0
Year of survey	1987	1980	1980	1980			1977		1986		1974		1985		1987

TABLE 36-2. QUANTITY, PHYSICAL COMPOSTION, AND DISPOSAL METHOD OF MUNICIPAL SOLID WASTE IN VARIOUS COUNTRIES AND CITIES (Continued)

City (Country)	Peking (China)	Seoul (Korea)	Bangkok (Thailand)	Bombay (India)	Tokyo (Ward) (Japan)	Nagoya (Japan)	Kyoto (Japan)	Sapporo (Japan)
Population (unit: 1,000)	9,880	10,287	5,609	8,243	8,341	2,148	1,473	1,618
Municipal waste (g/cap•d)	993	2,800	879	382	1,571	1,151	1,200	1,695
Household waste (g/cap•d)					1,148	873	641	808
Landfill (%)	100	99.6	91.9	100	40	20	3	37
Incineration (%)	0	0.4	0	0	59	79	96	63
Compost (%)	0	0	8.1	0				
Recovery (%)					1	1	1	0
Others (%)								
Paper (%)	7.8	14.4	13.9	10	37.3	20.9	26.9	25.2
Garbage (%)	29.2	25.9	36.5	20	24.1	37.1	39.8	46.6
Wood and weeds (%)	2.6	2.1	14.9	20	5.0	2.5	1.3	1.7
Fiber (%)					3.8	4.0	4.1	2.4
Leather and rubber (%)					0.4	0.9	0.7	
Plastic (%)	2.8	6.1	11.0	2	11.0	12.8	13.9	12.5
Glass (%)	2.4	5.9	2.0	0.2	7.7	7.2	5.6	7.1
Metal (%)	1.1		1.8	0.2	6.3	5.5	3.8	3.7
Incombustible (%)	49.6	45.6	19.5	41.6	0.8	2.6	1.9	0.8
Others (%)	4.5		0.4	6	3.6	6.6	2.0	
Water content (%)	36.4	27.9	59.1	40	36.7		44.5	50.1
Year of survey								

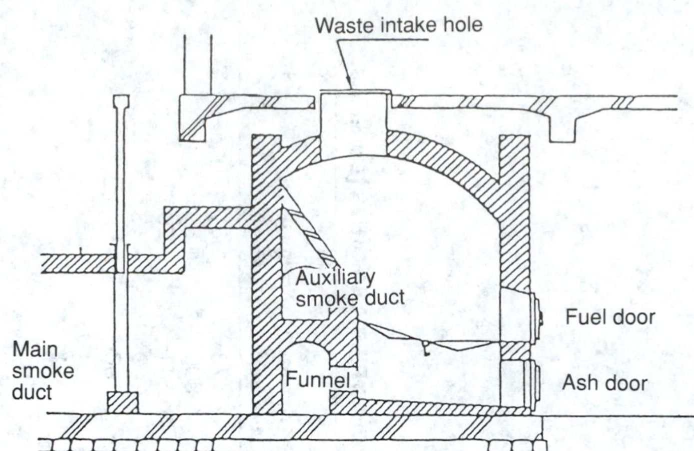

Figure 36-3. Example of fixed-bed stoker batch-combustion type of waste incinerator.

With the batch-combustion method, waste is intermittently fed into the incinerator for combustion. When a quantity of the unburned portion of the waste contained within the incinerator reaches a certain level, the next batch is dumped into the incinerator. With this method the waste is kept burning at the same position in the incinerator. This is called a fixed-grade type of incinerator. It is not suitable for bulky waste combustion.

In big cities the stoker-type continuous-combustion incinerators are generally used. The waste collected and hauled by vehicles from collection stations is unloaded into the pit. The pit capacity is usually approximately two to three times the daily disposal capacity of the incinerator. Next the waste is picked up in a large bucket on a crane installed at the upward portion of the pit and placed into the intake hole (hopper) of the incinerator. The hopper is an entrance for incoming waste, and it is always filled with waste to preclude flow-out and flow-in of surplus air. The waste is placed within the hopper and then gradually slides down into the stoker grade, being pulled by its own weight, and is slowly conveyed for burning in the presence of fresh air supplied from the downward section of the incinerator. The slope angle of the inclined stoker is approximately 30 degrees, and it functions as a conveyer floor. It will take 1 to 2 hours for the

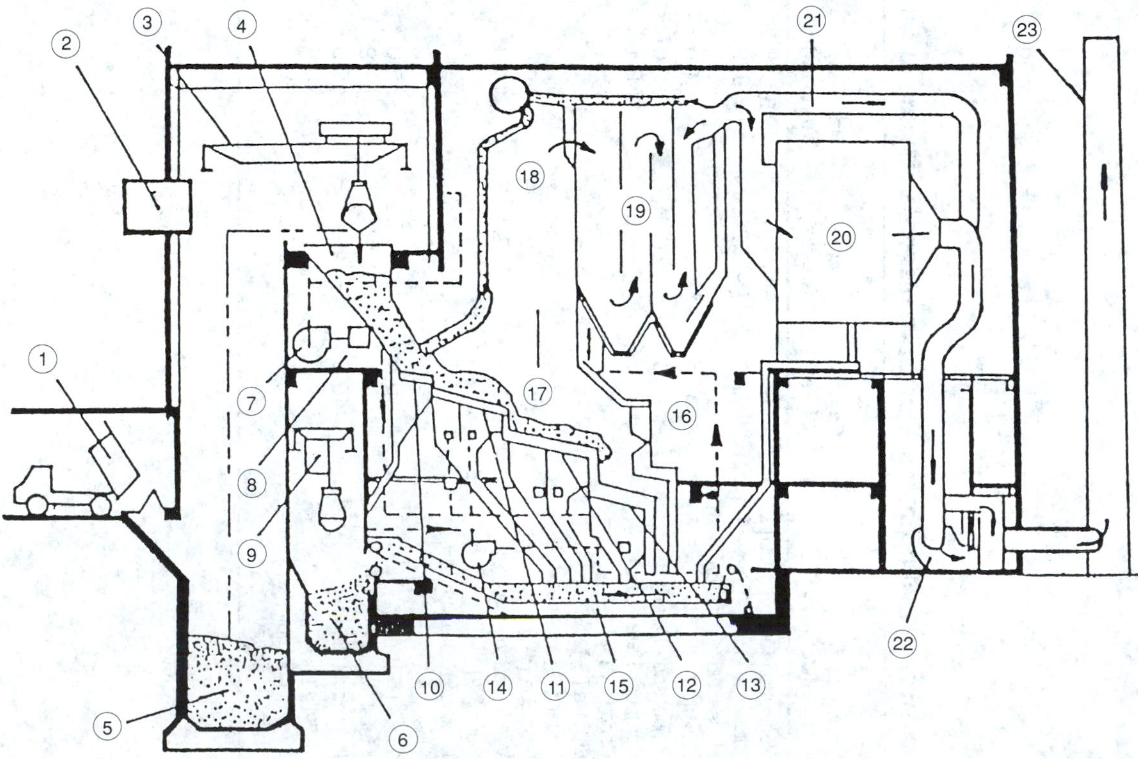

1, Waste collector/hauling vehicle. *2*, Crane operator room. *3*, Waste supplier crane. *4*, Waste hopper. *5*, Waste pit. *6*, Ash pit. *7*, Burner air compressor. *8*, Steam type air pre-heater. *9*, Ash pick-out crane. *10*, Waste supplier. *11*, Dry Stoker. *12*, Burner stoker. *13*, After burner stoker. *14*, Furnace thermostat air compressor. *15*, Ash cooling equipment. *16*, Auxiliary burner. *17*, First combustion chamber. *18*, Second combustion chamber. *19*, Waste heat boiler. *20*, ESP collector. *21*, ESP bypass. *22*, Induction ventilator. *23*, Chimney.

Figure 36-4. Example of representative facility of continuous-combustion type of incinerator.

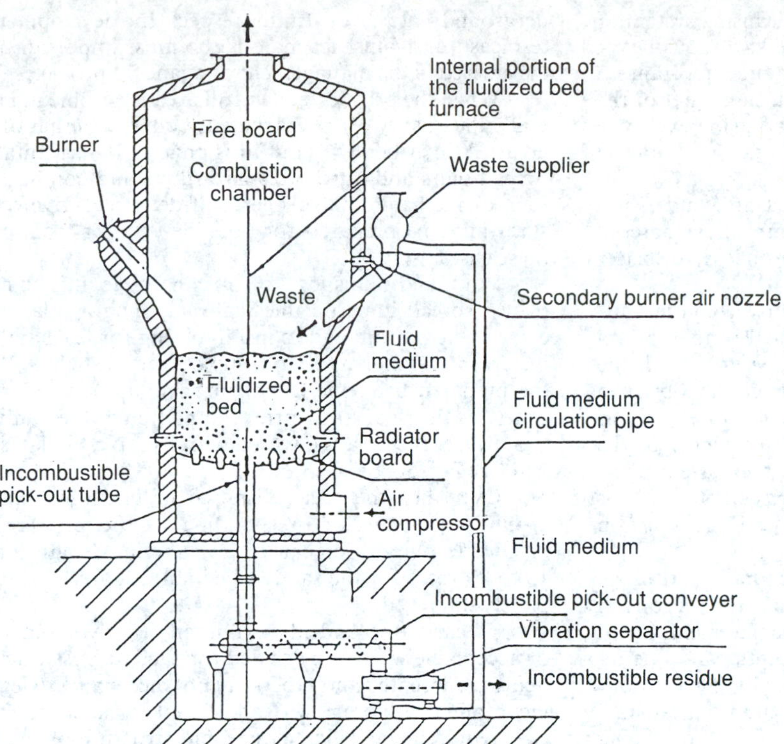

Figure 36-5. Fluidized bed type of incinerator.

burning waste on the stoker to move from the starting position to the ending position. The ash remaining after combustion, the residue, is allowed to soak into the quenching bath to extinguish and then is further conveyed toward the outside of the incinerator for collection. At the same time the combustion gases pass through the combustion chamber toward the boiler tube for cooling or are subjected to a cold water spray for cooling and then are transported to the electrostatic precipitator or a multicyclone for dust collection. With sophisticated incinerators, the combustion gas is further transported to the hazardous gas eliminator to remove various kinds of hazardous gas, such as hydrogen chloride, and is finally exhausted from the chimney. The temperature within the incinerator is stabilized to keep it constant at approximately 900° C at the exit portion of the combustion chamber. Also, pressure of the internal section of the incinerator is stabilized to keep it negative in order to prevent leakage of combustion gas through the gap space of the incinerator during operation. Waste-disposal capacity of this continuous-combustion type of incinerator is, in general, approximately 200 to 300 tons a day.

Regulations regarding the content of the exhaust gas varies by country (Table 36-3). Black smoke is eliminated with the use of multicyclone or electrostatic precipitators in the dry system, while venturi scrubbers are used in the wet system. With waste incinerators, sulfuric acid gas (SO_2) is a minor problem, since sulfur content is low in the case of municipal solid waste.

The chief problem gas is hydrogen chloride (HCl). In municipal solid waste, the quantity of plastic waste is high and plastics contain chlorides in such forms as vinyl chloride and others. When incinerated, this causes generation of high-density HCl gas contained in the combustion gas of the waste incinerator. Two types of countermeasure against the HCl gas have been employed in accordance with the exhaust gas regulation: (1) the dry type of system using a lime spray system and (2) the wet type of cleansing system using a caustic soda solution (sodium hydroxide) or a caustic potash solution (potassium hydroxide). The wet system should be employed to suppress exhaust HCl gas density at less than 20 ppm.

Oxides of nitrogen are generated by nitrogen content contained in the waste, and the density in the exhaust gas may reach 200 to 300 ppm. To suppress it to levels less than 100 ppm, various means must be applied in the incineration procedures.

Regarding concerns about dioxin, a number of countries, including Sweden, have enforced strict regulations. Other countries, however, have not taken strict countermeasures while awaiting the results of current active research.

TABLE 36-3. COMPARISON OF WORLDWIDE EXHAUST GAS REGULATIONS

Country	Dust (mg/m^3)	HCl (mg/m^3)	Hg (mg/m^3)	Cd (mg/m^3)	HF (mg/m^3)	TCDD (mg/m^3)	SOx (mg/m^3)	NOx (mg/m^3)
Japan (O_2 12%)	100–200	700						
Sweden (CO_2 12%)	20	100	0.03	—	—	0.1		
West Germany (O_2 10%)	<10	<10	0.10	0.1	<1	—	<50	<300
Denmark (O_2 10%)	40	100	0.1	0.1	2	1.0		
Switzerland (O_2 11%)	50	30	0.10	0.2	5	—		

HF = hydrofluoric acid; NOx = oxides of nitrogen; SOx = oxides of sulfur; TCDD = dioxin.

NOTE: West Germany's exhaust gas regulation stipulated the following other than those shown in the table: With regard to all the heavy metals (As, Pb, Co, Cr, Cu, Mn, V, Sn, Sb) in total <1.0 mg/m^3, all organic material <10 mg/m^3, CO <50 mg/m^3.

The previously mentioned wet type of cleansing system or electrostatic precipitator is able to collect the hazardous heavy metals, such as mercury, cadmium, etc. The more important remaining problem is how to dispose of the cleansing water or the fly ash that remains in the dust collector. Chelating ion-exchange resin is used for mercury, and coagulation and precipitation methods are used for other heavy metals.

Performance of waste incinerators is measured and evaluated by ignition loss or by the quantity of combustible material in the residue. In other words, the less the ignition loss, the better the incinerator completes waste combustion.

In Japan present regulations stipulate for the continuous-combustion type of incinerator that less than 7% to 10% remains, corresponding to the size of the incinerator. With the large incinerator used in recent years, caloric energy obtained from the waste combustion process is used to generate steam to assist with electric power generation, hot water supply to the community, and so forth. At present, some of the waste incinerators have an electric power generation capacity of 5000 kW or more. Sterilization of pathogenic bacteria caused by combustion is an appreciated public health measure.

Since incineration-related technology has improved in recent years, it appears to have practical future applications in major cities around the world. In spite of the achievements noted above, however, there may be different perceptions by the inhabitants of surrounding communities, especially if hazardous materials are to be loaded in the incinerator, and if no satisfactory countermeasure are presented to the community regarding generation of hazardous materials, such as dioxin.

LANDFILL

The most commonly used method of waste disposal throughout the world is landfill disposal. Although the term sounds like a simple and outdated waste disposal method, it is still effective. Since ancient days, it has seemed best and the most natural method to bury organic waste matter, turning it back into the ground, where it serves as an excellent ground conditioner. With landfill disposal, waste disintegrates gradually, undergoing the decomposition process by mild reactions mediated by bacteria in the ground over a long period of time.

While in some highly populated cities where there is great competition for uses of land, incineration disposal methods may be preferred because of the rapidity with which decomposition takes place, the landfill disposal method continues to be an important and necessary method for municipal waste disposal and will continue to be so in the future. Even with more municipal waste being disposed of by incineration methods, the remaining material, such as fly ash, bottom ash, and incombustibles, will have to be finally disposed of in landfill disposal sites. Moreover, the landfill disposal method is reevaluated for its inherent advantage in view of need of separation processing of hazardous waste from the surrounding environment and for future land-reclamation planning. Economics must be considered with regard to the use of land for landfill purposes or other uses, as well as consideration of environmental factors.

There are two classifications of landfill: (1) inland landfill and (2) ocean landfill. This is a location-based classification, and there are other classification methods as well. For example, there is the classification based on water content, such as dry-type landfill and wet-type landfill. Also, one can classify by type of leachate; then the classification should be based on the difference between aerobic and anaerobic conditions. There are large differences between bacteria affecting decomposition conditions in aerobic landfill areas compared to anaerobic landfill areas. These differences greatly influence the quality and content of the leachate. If the leachate contains high levels of organic material, it may cause water pollution when it flows into rivers or into underground water beds. In this respect, the development of countermeasures against leachate is the most important issue to be considered in the management of a landfill project.

When the prospected landfill area is aerobic in nature, generally the quality of the leachate is better than that of anaerobic areas. Also, when the landfill is anaerobic fermentation sometimes occurs and introduces hazardous and combustible gases, such as methane or hydrogen sulfide. Preventive countermeasures must be prepared for possible disaster from eruption of these gases.

With landfill disposal of fresh garbage, it is common practice to spread impermeable material, such as plastic sheets or clay, at the bottom and to install piping for leachate, next placing crushed stone on top to complete the waste bed. When using the prepared bed, one layers garbage and soil on top of each other. At the final stage, after completion of the sandwich piling procedure, the area is covered with soil to a thickness of 1.5 to 2 m (see Fig. 36–6).

Over time the waste disposed of underground will cause ground subsidence, corresponding to the process of underground decomposition caused by bacteria. Usually it takes from 10 to 20 years for the sandwiched landfill area to become completely stabilized.

To carry out landfill work in an orderly manner, the types of acceptable waste are decided for each disposal facility. Some items are accepted and others are not, according to legal requirements and regulations, with additional consideration of site-specific requirements, such as size and structure of the facility. A system to check waste at the acceptance gate should be established. Furthermore, it is absolutely necessary to establish a monitoring system to check surrounding environmental conditions not only during but also after completion of the waste-disposal operation.

Experience teaches that problems happen more frequently when management of the landfill is transferred to another party. It is necessary to firmly establish and to operate the monitoring system before, during, and after the actual waste disposal in the landfill site.

RESOURCE RECOVERY AND RECYCLING

Following are the three methods for material recovery and recycling:

1. Resource recovery without property conversion of the recovered material. In this type of waste recycling recovered wastes are used. Such re-used refuse includes (a) ferrous metal or aluminum cans, transformed into raw material for remanufacture, and (b) glass bottles which are cleansed, sterilized, and reused as new.
2. Resource recycling with conversion of the recovered material. In this type of waste recycling, recovered wastes are used after conversion processing. It utilizes material such as (a) kitchen garbage or excessive sludge to prepare compost and (b) incinerator residue and slag to be used for road construction material and so forth.
3. Resource recycling with energy recovery. In this type of waste recycling, combustible and nonhazardous wastes are fed into an incinerator and the obtained calorific resource is either transmitted to a boiler installed next to the combustion zone and converted into thermal electromotive energy or used to obtain fuel produced by high-temperature pyrolysis treatment of plastic material.

Among the three methods the first reuses waste material before generation of waste and the other two reuse generated waste in the treatment and disposal process.

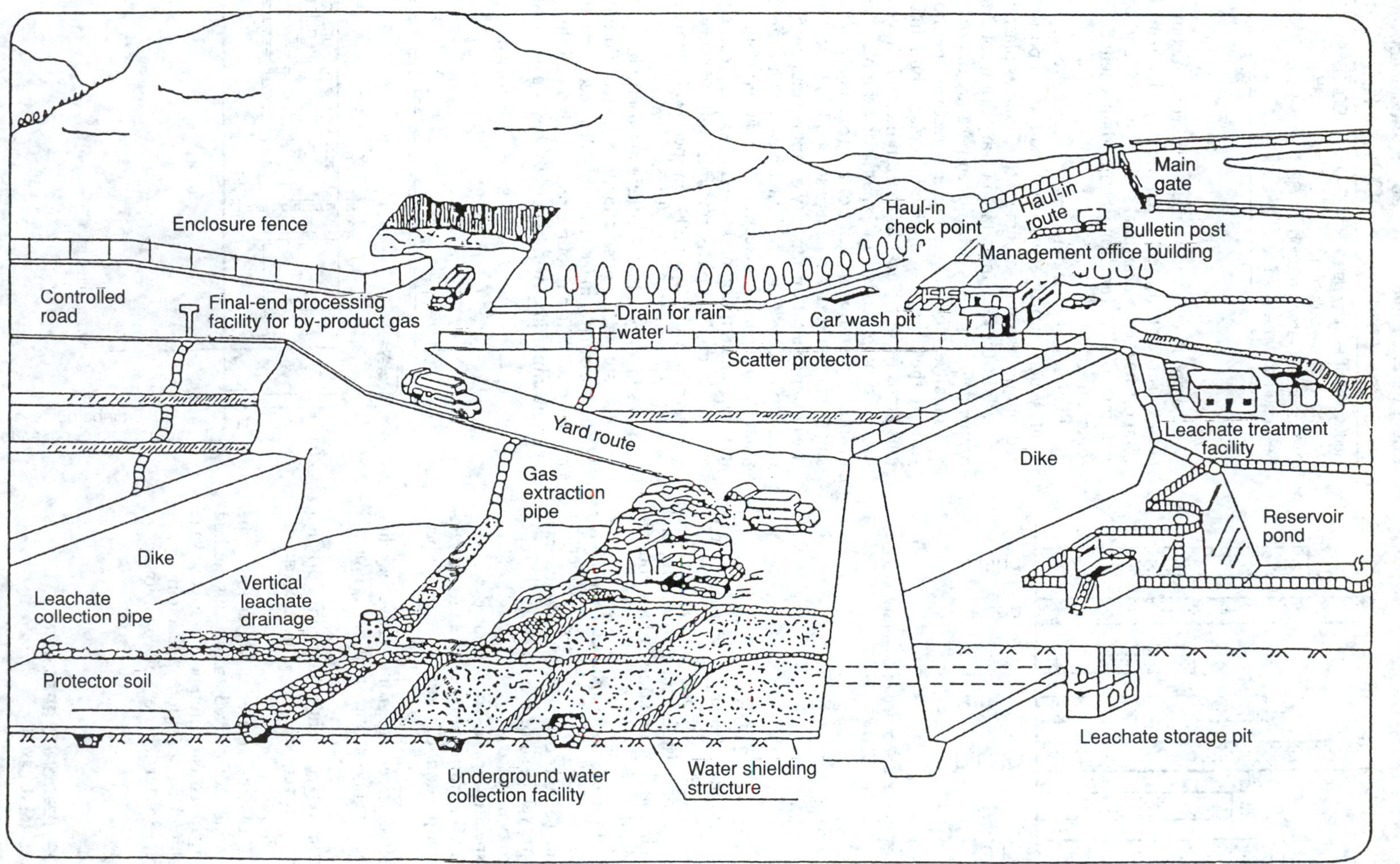

Figure 36-6. Concept of a landfill facility for household waste disposal.

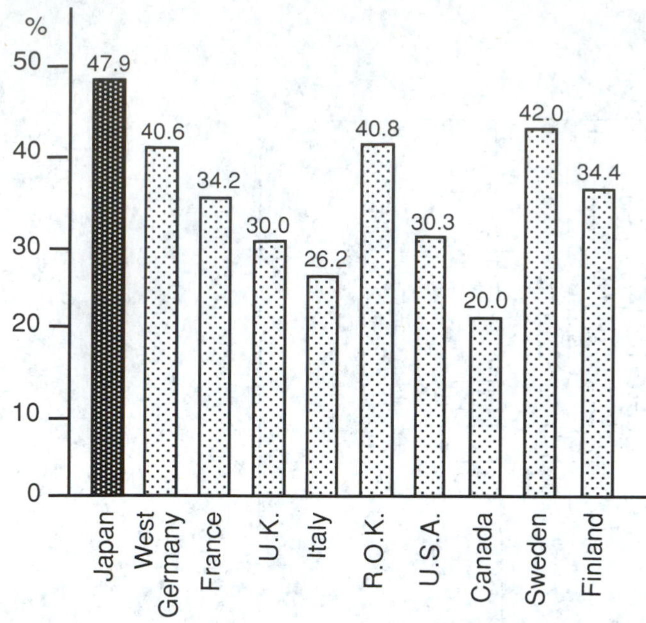

Figure 36-7. Ratio of wastepaper recovery of the individual countries.

Waste-recycling methods 1 and 2 above are associated with efficient waste quantity reduction and energy saving. However, to achieve excellent results from these, it is necessary to develop an effective all-in-one system of waste sorting, collection, and reutilization. Cooperation in source separation by local community inhabitants is also helpful.

Figure 36–7 shows the ratio of wastepaper recovery in individual countries at the present time, and there are considerable differences among individual countries. It is useful to encourage and promote wastepaper recycling since it is said that 1 ton of wastepaper is equivalent to twenty trees.

Table 36–4 shows specified ratios of resource recovery within Japan. All the recycling ratios are observed to be relatively high. However, major portions of the waste have not been fully reutilized.

Table 36–5 lists expected percentages for effective recycling of various materials, with energy savings and environmental protection factors.

Although the key factor is effective minimization of original waste generation, resource recovery and recycling are also important aspects of waste disposal.

Regarding recycling of the material-conversion type (method 2), composting has already proved useful. This method produces compost from organic waste (municipal waste, sewage sludge, etc.), using aerobic decomposition reaction by agrobacteria, and then finds reuse as fertilizer or soil conditioner.

TABLE 36-4. RATIOS OF RESOURCE RECOVERY FOR CANS AND BOTTLES IN JAPAN

• Aluminum cans	: The ratio of recovery is 41.7% (1988)
• Steel cans	: The ratio of recovery is 40.2% (1988)
• Glass bottles	: The ratio of container usage is 47.6% (1989)

TABLE 36-5. EFFECT ON NATURAL RESOURCE AND ENVIRONMENT PROTECTION BY RECYCLING

Effect on Environment Protection	Paper (%)	Aluminum (%)	Iron (%)	Glass (%)
Reduction of energy use	23–74	90–97	47–74	4–32
Reduction of air pollution	74	95	85	20
Reduction of water pollution	35	97	76	—
Reduction of water use	58	—	40	50

Composting is widely used in European countries, but it is not as prevalent in the United States and Japan. Even though compost has some drawbacks, such as odor and contained foreign material, it functions better than chemical fertilizer for some soil conditions.

Figure 36–8 is a diagram of a typical compost-processing plant. When municipal waste is used for composting, it is shredded and undesirable foreign matter, such as plastic and glass, is separated. It is then mixed in a rotary drum for 2 to 3 days at a proper degree of moisture and temperature to produce compost.

Finally, one can assess energy-recovery methods. In recent years, at the large waste-incinerator plants built in big cities, various kinds of waste heat utilization methods have already been shown to be practical. In Japan, for example, there are waste incinerators with a capacity of approximately 600 tons per day and the attached steam generation boilers have a potential electric power generation capacity of approximately 5,000 kW. This makes possible the use of boiler steam as a heat source for regional heating and for electric power generation, both to supply in-plant consumption and to sell as excess electric power. However, such application is possible only for large incineration plants with a capacity of 200 tons per day or more and the rated calorific value of 1,500 kcal/kg or more.

In summary, although there are useful and efficient methods of waste management and although techniques are available to maximize material use, there is still a need for better municipal management. Such resource recovery and recycling will have increasing importance with regard to the global environment.

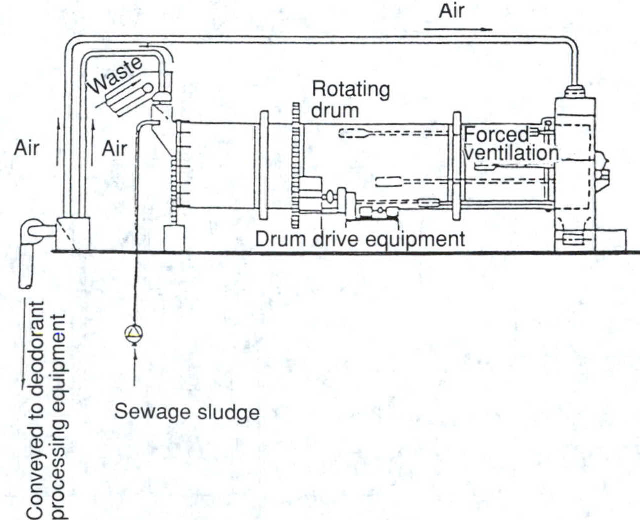

Figure 36-8. Block diagram of a rotary drum type of compost-processing facility.

Radioactive Waste Disposal

Vladimir Dvorak

Radioactive wastes originating from peaceful uses of nuclear energy are conventionally classified, according to both their physical and chemical properties and their origin, into two broad categories: low-level and high-level wastes. Another recognized categorization has three levels—low, intermediate, and high.

Low-level Radioactive Wastes. There are three classes of low-level radioactive wastes, with progressively more stringent requirements for packaging and disposal practices to provide reasonable assurance that exposures of the public, should they occur, present a small fraction of the current dose limits.

The class A wastes consist of slightly contaminated trash (e.g., from laboratories) and must meet the requirement to decay to harmless levels during the 100 years of planned institutional control. This also applies to the class B wastes, which must be packaged in containers that will retain their integrity for at least 300 years. The containers for class C wastes must also retain their integrity for 300 years and are placed at greater depth or behind concrete barriers that will retain their integrity for at least 500 years so as to minimize the possibility of inadvertent intrusion. The sites selected must enable quantification of hydrogeological features and must be designed and operated so that movement of radionuclides is minimized and can be described quantitatively. Further technical requirements include solidification of liquid wastes or their packaging in material capable of absorbing twice the volume of the liquid waste. Legal requirements deal with ownership of land (state or federal) and with assurance of continuity of institutional control.[1,2]

The requirements reflect the relative risk of different classes of wastes, which is related to the physical and chemical properties of radionuclides and their compounds. The radionuclides with short half-lives that are used in nuclear medicine can be stored long enough to decay to negligible activities, provided that proper storage is assured. In the case of trace amounts of radionuclides with longer half-lives, such as tritium, carbon 14, or sulfur 35 in aqueous solutions, release into the sewer system may be permitted. For biological samples, e.g. from experimental work, incineration may be an option when legally permitted and after exposure evaluation.[3,5]

The physical forms, volumes, and activities of low-level radioactive waste reflect the diversity of waste generators as indicated in a recent study in New York State[4] (Tables 36–4 and 36–5). During the last decade the total yearly volumes and activities decreased. The reductions were due to the use of waste compaction, incineration, storage for decay of radionuclides with short half-lives, and changes in operations and radionuclides used by the waste operators. Wilkerson et al.[5] reviewed the problems and solutions concerning radioactive waste in biomedical and academic institutions.

TABLE 36–6. GENERATORS OF DIFFERENT TYPES OF LOW-LEVEL RADIOACTIVE WASTES

- **Academia**
  - Absorbed liquids
  - Animal carcasses
  - Compacted trash
  - Institutional laboratory waste
- **Industry**
  - Absorbed liquids
  - Compacted trash
  - Depleted uranium
  - Sealed sources
- **Medical Facilities**
  - Absorbed liquids
  - Compacted trash
  - Institutional laboratory waste
  - Sealed sources
- **Utilities**
  - Contaminated plant hardware
  - Dry compressible waste
  - Evaporator bottoms
  - Filter sludges
  - Irradiated components
  - Spent resins
- **Government**
  - Absorbed liquids
  - Compacted trash
  - Contaminated plant hardware

Adapted from Maile H D: Bull NY Acad Med 65:439, 1989.

TABLE 36–7. RADIOACTIVITY AND VOLUME OF SHIPPED DISPOSAL MATERIAL

	Radioactivity (%)	Volume (%)
Academia	0.3	4.4
Industry	55.2	8.8
Medical facilities	0.4	24.1
Utilities	44.1	60.4

NOTE: Government contributed less than 0.1% to the radioactivity and about 1.8% to the volume of the materials shipped.
Adapted from Maile H D: Bull NY Acad Med 65:439, 1989.

The disposal facilities range from simple trenches, which may be about 10 m deep, 25 m wide, and 100 to 200 m in length, to engineered disposal facilities, such as concrete structures containing conditioned wastes and capped with water-resistant materials.[6] Groundwater contamination is the most important exposure pathway; therefore, evaluation of potential contamination for the periods hundreds of years after closure is required. Exposures from currently operated disposal facilities account for a small fraction of annual limits.

In the United States, selection of the disposal sites and construction of the disposal facilities by individual states or groups of states called compounds has often been slowed because of controversial stances on safety issues by the parties involved.[1,7]

High-level Radioactive Waste. The high-level waste includes spent fuel from nuclear power plants, radioactive liquids and solids from reprocessing of spent fuel, and other highly radioactive materials.

The spent fuel elements are placed on site in the cooling fuel storage pool to reduce their radioactivity and temperature. After about 6 months, the fuel elements can be transferred to a reprocessing plant, enabling recovery of fissile material. Some percentage of the world's yearly spent fuel is being reprocessed commercially in the United Kingdom and France. Generally, the spent fuel is stored at nuclear power plant sites. Proposals for the permanent disposal of high-level radioactive wastes, such as geologic isolation in mined cavities or solidification and disposal at the nuclear plant site, have been explored. Because the high-level wastes are being kept on site, population exposures from this source have not been evaluated.

REFERENCES

1. Eisenbud M: Management strategies for low-level radioactive waste disposal. Bull NY Acad Med 65:451–460, 1989
2. Eisenbud M: Environmental Radioactivity. 3 edt. Orlando, Fla.: Academic Press, 1987
3. Hamrick PE, Wall BE, Simon SL: Incineration and monitoring of low-level S-35 wastes at a biological research institution. Health Physics 57:191–194, 1989

4. Mailie HD: Low level radioactive waste: sources, content, and significance. Bull NY Acad Med 65:439–450, 1989
5. Wilkerson A, Klein RC, Party E, Gershey EL: Low-level radioactive waste from U.S. biomedical and academic institutions: policies, strategies, and solutions. Annu Rev Public Health 10:299–317, 1989
6. United Nations Scientific Committee on the Effects of Ionizing Radiation (UNSCEAR). Sources, Effects and Risks of Ionizing Radiation. New York: United Nations, 1988
7. Covello VT: Communicating information about the health risks of radioactive waste: a review of obstacles to public understanding. Bull NY Acad Med 65, 467–482, 1989

37

Aerospace Medicine

Roy L. DeHart

DEFINITION AND HISTORY

Aerospace medicine is "that specialty of medical practice within preventive medicine that focuses on the health of a population group defined by the operating aircrews and passengers of air and space vehicles, together with the support personnel who are required to operate them."[1] The practice of aerospace medicine tends to reverse the usual order of traditional or curative medicine. Normally the physician is treating abnormal physiology (illness) in a normal (terrestrial) environment. The physician concerned with the care of the aviator or astronaut most frequently deals with a normal (perhaps supernormal) individual in an abnormal (aeronautical) environment. This unusual aeronautical environment was first explored by a young scientist and physician, Pilatre de Rozier. The exploration took place in one of the large Montgolfier balloons on November 21, 1783, in Paris when, accompanied by a passenger, he ascended in free flight to a height of 85 m. Unfortunately, some 2 years later this first aeronaut also became the first victim of this unforgiving aeronautical environment when he fell from an altitude of 1000 m following the explosion of a compound hydrogen and hot air balloon.

In this same year another physician, an American named Jeffries, persuaded a Frenchman named Blanchard to allow him to join a proposed flight to cross the English Channel in order to make scientific observations. Jeffries took with him on the flight scientific instruments to measure the environment and vacuum flasks for collecting air samples. From the beginning, scientific inquiry, particularly that related to man's adaptation to the aeronautical environment, has been a motivation equal to the excitement and passion of flight.

Since its earliest beginnings, flight has required man to adapt to or to protect himself from multiple environmental stressors. Progress in flight has required continuing improvement in man's adaptation or in the devices that he uses for protection. Such progress has always been marked by the sacrifices made by those who push the envelope of aeronautical and astronautical activity. On December 17, 1903, on a windswept beach in Kitty Hawk, North Carolina, the Wright brothers succeeded in accomplishing sustained powered flight for 12 seconds over a distance of 40 m. In less than 15 years, thousands of these powered flying machines swarmed over the battlefields of the "Great War." During this rapid expansion of military aviation the seed of aviation medicine sprouted, took root, and grew.

Aviation Medicine. Early in World War I the value of the airplane for use in combat was established. It proved to be a valuable observation platform and an armed combat vehicle that could carry war beyond the trench lines. As frequently occurs with technology, military motivation stimulated the rapid development of higher performance aircraft and their production in great numbers. Large numbers of aviators were needed to fly the aircraft, and soldiers were selected to enter flight training with little more regard for their physical attributes or capabilities than that used to select any infantryman. Soon the unforgiving environment of aeronautics became evident with the soaring accident rates and the accompanying high mortality. Initially, far more aviators were dying in training than in combat. One of the solutions to successfully reducing this aircraft accident carnage was the development of medical standards for the selection of aviators and training a cadre of physicians to understand the aeronautical environment and its unique demands on human physiology. From its beginning the orientation of this discipline of medicine has been and is prevention of injury and illness and maintenance of health.

During the interwar period advances in aeronautical technology continued, and enhanced personal protection equipment permitted the aviator to optimize the new improvements in speed, altitude, and lift. The aircraft became a commercial carrier, hauling freight, mail, and passengers. Concern for human limitations in the aeronautical environment now extended beyond the crew to passengers. Pressurized cabins were developed to protect both the aviator and the passenger from cold, hypoxia, and hypobarics. This period saw a consolidation and institutionalization of aviation medicine in the United States. Many flight surgeons trained in World War I helped in forming airline medical departments. In 1929 the Aviation Medical Association was formed by some of these same physicians. Physical standards were developed by the government for aviators in general aviation.

Military aviation played an important role in the hostilities of World War II. Again there was rapid expansion of technology, the aircraft industry, flight personnel, and in medical personnel with orientation and training in aviation medicine. Although aircraft continued to fly higher and faster, the first concern of the physician supporting the aircrew was one of preventive medicine through the selection of individuals with physical attributes compatible with flight and the health maintenance of aircrews to enhance their ability to perform in the hostile aeronautical environment.

Space Medicine. The department of space medicine was officially established at the United States Air Force School of Aerospace Medicine under the directorship of Dr. Hubertus Strughold on February 9, 1949.[2] One of Dr. Strughold's early contributions to the field was the establishment of space equivalent altitudes. This represented the altitudes where, for all practical purposes, space equivalency was achieved either because of consideration of human physiology or aeronautical factors of the aircraft. Unlike the historical developments in aviation, extensive investigations into man's ability to adapt to the environment of space flight were undertaken. Stringent physical standards were adopted for potential astronauts in order to reduce, to the lowest possible degree, potential adverse health effects of space flight. The principles of clinical preventive medicine were at the forefront in this selection process and in the health maintenance program for America's astronauts.

The first manned flight in space, circumnavigating the globe, was performed by Soviet cosmonaut Yuri Gagarin on April 12, 1961. In February 1962 American astronauts joined the Soviets with the successful orbital flight of John Glenn.

Biomedical oversight for the United States' space program is headquartered at the National Aeronautics and Space Administration's facility at the Johnson Space Center, Houston, Texas. Following successful lunar flights and space laboratory missions, the United States entered into a nearly routine operation with the space transportation system or "shuttle." Medical planning is well under way toward the continuing human habitation of an orbiting space station.

The Specialty of Aerospace Medicine. Shortly after World War II the Aero Medical Association initiated activities for the establishment of a training program for medical specialists in the field of aviation medicine. In 1953 the American Board of Preventive Medicine (ABPM) approved the decision to authorize certification in aviation medicine. The first group of physicians was certified in the specialty that same year. As of 1990, approximately 1000 physicians have been certified in the specialty.

Recently the ABPM initiated the development of a Certificate of Added Competency in Undersea Medicine. This is of interest to aerospace medicine as it is related to the hyperbaric environment, an environment used to treat dysbarism or aviator's bends.

With the advent of space flight, both the association and the specialty changed names to appropriately reflect their activities in both the aeronautical and astronautical environments. The name of the specialty was officially changed by the ABPM to aerospace medicine.

TRAINING AND EDUCATION

Few physicians have the opportunity to gain experience in aerospace medicine until their postgraduate years. Typically, physicians will be introduced to the specialty via one of two routes. Those practitioners with an interest in aviation may turn to the Federal Aviation Administration (FAA) for orientation and training as an aviation medical examiner (AME) to support general aviation. Each year the FAA conducts postgraduate educational courses for new physicians who are becoming AMEs and refresher training for established AMEs. The second route is via the military, where the three services conduct their own training programs for flight surgeons. Historically, most physicians who have entered the field of aerospace medicine have done so via the military route. These courses are basically introductory and focus on the clinical preventive medical aspects of evaluation and care of the aviator.

Residency Programs. Aerospace medicine is one of the smallest specialty training programs in the United States, both with regard to training sites and number of residents. Its program is similar in structure to other training programs in preventive medicine. Two programs are under the Department of Defense (DOD) sponsorship. The Air Force program is headquartered at the United States Air Force School of Aerospace Medicine, San Antonio, Texas, and the Navy program is managed at the Naval Aerospace Medical Institute, Pensacola, Florida. The only civilian program is housed at Wright State University, College of Medicine, Dayton, Ohio. Fewer than 50 residents are in training at any one time, with 25 to 30 candidates sitting for the specialty board examination annually.

THE AEROSPACE ENVIRONMENT

The characteristic that distinguishes aerospace medicine from other medical fields is the complex environment in which flight takes place. Stressors that impinge on humans in this unique environment, either singularly or in combination, include reduced availability of oxygen, reduced atmospheric pressure, thermal extremes, brief and sustained acceleration fields, ionizing radiation, and null gravity fields. For men and women to perform successfully in this potentially hazardous environment, the principles of preventive medicine apply in the selection, health maintenance, and engineering protection of aircrew.

The Biosphere. The chemical and physical properties of the atmosphere vary with the attained altitude. Although the properties are frequently described in terms of altitude, it must be appreciated that the atmosphere is dynamic in that specific characteristics are altered by season, the earth's rotation, and latitudes. For practical purposes the components and their relative percentage of the atmosphere remain relatively constant up to an altitude of approximately 90 km. The major constituents of the atmosphere are nitrogen (78%) and oxygen (21%). The remaining 1% of the atmosphere consists of argon, carbon dioxide, helium, krypton, xenon, hydrogen, and methane. The actual percentages of these constituents vary with the water content of the atmosphere, which is altitude-dependent. As one ascends, the air becomes dryer.

Regardless of the altitude within the aeronautical frame of reference, the percentage of oxygen available to an individual at sea level is basically the same as that found at 90 km. The difference is that the partial pressure of oxygen is much reduced at altitude. Consequently the physiological availability of oxygen is likewise reduced.

One constituent of the atmosphere has received considerable attention in recent years because of concern for potential adverse health effects should it be reduced. Ozone is produced in the upper atmosphere by the photodissociation of molecular oxygen. Ozone attains maximum density at an altitude of approximately 22 km but is present in measurable concentrations from 10 to 35 km. Reduction in the ozone concentration would increase the level of ultraviolet radiation reaching the earth's surface. (See Chapter 39.)

At sea level the column of air creates an atmospheric pressure of 760 mm Hg, 760 torr or 1013.2 millibars. As one ascends in altitude, there is less of a column of air and thus less air pressure; however, this relationship is not linear: the density of the air decreases exponentially. Consequently, at a height of 5.5 km the air density is one half that found at sea level, and at 11 km the density is one quarter. In practice the actual heights are somewhat greater because of the effects of temperature.

Although we usually consider the border for space to begin at 200 km or higher, the biological or physiological equivalent of space, as defined over 30 years ago by Strughold, is much lower. To protect an individual at an altitude of 20 km, it is necessary to provide essentially the same engineering solutions for such parameters as respiration and pressure as if the individual were already at space altitude. Consequently a number of space equivalent altitudes for various parameters to support human life are far lower than the 200 km used to define the physical environment of space.

Oxygen Systems. Hypoxia, which may have any one of several causes, has devastating effects on normal physiological function. In aviation, one is faced with the potential for hypoxia resulting from a deficiency in alveolar oxygen exchange. This oxygen deficiency is due to a reduction in the oxygen partial pressure in inspired air, which occurs at altitude because of reduced oxygen in the ambient air. The alveolar partial pressure of oxygen is the most critical factor in this problem. In aviation, two factors must be considered in understanding hypoxia at altitude.

Not only may the partial pressure of oxygen be low, for example, the available oxygen is reduced by half in the ambient air at 6 km, but the ambient pressure may be insufficient to permit gas exchange at the alveoli. Considering that water vapor at normal body temperature is 47 mm Hg and the residual alveolar carbon dioxide pressure is 40 mm Hg, then for any air exchange to occur in the lung, the ambient pressure must exceed 87 mm Hg. Even if the aviator is breathing 100% oxygen, if the ambient pressure of that oxygen is no higher than 87 mm Hg, it would be impossible to overcome the gas pressures already present at the alveoli and thus provide oxygen.

Hypoxia is particularly dangerous because its signs and symptoms produce little discomfort and no pain. Between 2000 and 3000 m the subtle symptoms may produce deficiencies in night vision and some drowsiness. Unfortunately, intellectual impairment can be an early manifestation of hypoxia, thus compromising the ability of an individual to behave rationally. Thinking is slow and calculations are difficult. Both memory and judgment are faulty, and reaction time is delayed. This condition can be rapidly treated by administering oxygen at altitudes between 3000 and 10,000 m and adding positive pressure oxygen up to 14,000 m or by enclosing the individual in a pressurized system with available oxygen at altitudes out to space.

To avoid discomfort and potential hazard in flying at altitude, the most logical solution is to carry your terrestrial environment with you. Although it is not the usual case, the same principle applies for many aircraft systems, particularly passenger-carrying aircraft. The body of the aircraft becomes a pressure vessel in which the air pressure and oxygen availability are similar to that at sea level. For a number of practical reasons, such as passenger comfort and avoiding clinical hypoxia for most passengers, and the additional cost of maintaining a sea level environment, the actual cabin altitude for most commercial aircraft is set at approximately 2500 m. Although passengers will note some pressure changes in the ears or sinuses, the change is gradual and rarely causes pain or discomfort. In most cases the passenger is not even aware of these pressure changes. The altitude is set so that most passengers are able to fly without experiencing any hypoxic symptoms. Occasionally, passengers with a compromised pulmonary or cardiovascular system may require supplemental oxygen, since their reserve is inadequate to compensate for the relatively small changes in oxygen partial pressure.

In the absence of a pressurized cabin the aviator may be forced to adapt by wearing a self-contained pressure system. Although the public is most familiar with "space suits" from television reporting, similar suits have been used for nearly a half century by military aviators flying high-altitude missions.

Provided the ambient pressure is adequate, supplemental oxygen systems permit high altitude flying and provide a safety factor for passengers on commercial airliners. Most systems employ an oxygen storage system of either pressurized gas or liquid oxygen. The source of oxygen is then connected through a regulator or metering device to an oxygen mask worn by the user. Another less commonly used oxygen storage system uses solid chemicals which, when activated, release oxygen. Two devices have been developed recently to provide on-board oxygen generation systems. The fuel-cell concept has been developed for space flight and is basically an electrolysis system freeing oxygen from water. A second system uses the reversible absorption properties of fluomine for oxygen. In this technology, pressurized air is forced over a fluomine bed, and the pressure is then reduced, allowing the absorbed oxygen to be released. Other techniques have included the molecular sieve device, which is used to filter oxygen from air; a similar technology employs a permeable membrane that passes oxygen preferentially to other constituents of the atmosphere.

Biodynamics. The first powered flight aviation death occurred in the United States when an army lieutenant sustained fatal injuries while flying with Orville Wright. Since that initial accident, there has been an ever-increasing sophistication in the science of aircraft accident prevention and aircrew and passenger protection.

Acceleration occurs whenever the velocity of an object changes. This change may occur either in direction or in magnitude. For convenience, transitory and sustained accelerations in aerospace applications are expressed in terms of "G." G is defined as the magnitude of acceleration when the velocity change approximates 9.8 m/s^2. Transitory acceleration is of such a short duration that the body does not reach a steady-state status. Protection from transitory acceleration has generally centered around two technologies: the development of restraint devices, such as lap belts and shoulder harnesses, and the design of crew space to reduce the possibility of contact.

Accident protection technology has been employed in the design of the airframe to absorb energy and improvements in the seat structure to reduce mechanical failure.

Primarily in military aviation, escape systems have been designed that often impart a new acceleration field. Ejection seats and capsules are designed to carry the occupant free of the aircraft envelope even on the ground at zero speed or in adverse conditions during uncontrolled descent. These new components of acceleration are specifically designed to remain within human tolerance.

During World War I, fighter pilots began reporting visual changes when they engaged in a pull-out or during aerial combat. Research work using a human centrifuge demonstrated, in 1935, the effects of blackout during sustained acceleration. Sustained acceleration is achieved when the body has sufficient time to reach equilibrium with the effects of the acceleration. In this context, G has been used to reflect a ratio of weight. Consequently, a pilot flying a maneuver in an aircraft in which he sustains 4 G would likewise experience an increase in body weight from 175 to 700 pounds. In such an acceleration a flight helmet with equipment weighing 10 pounds becomes a mass of 40 pounds. As any mass exposed to such a field will experience a proportionate increase in weight, this has dynamic effects on the body's hydrostatic column and thus on cardiovascular function. For example, the hydrostatic column from the heart to the eye in a normal terrestrial environment is 30 cm; when exposed to a plus 6 G acceleration environment, it becomes 180 cm. In this example the body's blood pressure would be unable to overcome the hydrostatic pressure, and blood flow to the level of the eyes would cease.

Because of the hydrostatic pressure of the eyeball, a pilot will experience blackout wherein vision is lost but consciousness is maintained. When tested on a centrifuge using a standard protocol, the typical aviator, relaxed and without any protective devices, experienced blackout between 4 and 5.5 G. The same aviator, when allowed to strain to increase blood pressure, was able to increase his tolerance 0.5 G to 1.5 additional G. Two critical factors impact the degree of tolerance: the rate of onset of the acceleration and its duration.

Further protection is available using mechanical devices such as an anti-G suit. The suit is basically a lower torso device with bladders to press on the abdomen, thighs, and calves. These bladders inflate when a sensor is stimulated by acceleration. Such devices increase the G tolerance by 2 G. Research performed nearly 2 decades ago demonstrated that an anti-G suit properly worn during performance of a straining maneuver can increase G tolerance from approximately 4 G to about 9 G. Other mechanisms used to enhance acceleration tolerance for pilots have included body positioning to orient the long axis of the body more perpendicular to the acceleration vector. Positive pressure breathing is also shown to be helpful in increasing tolerance as it increases intrathoracic pressure.

The biomechanical force environments in aerospace systems can be enormous, with generation of severe noise and vibration. Human exposure to these forces may affect performance and contribute to adverse health outcomes. Prevention is the key to proper management of these stressors.

Vibration is a series of oscillations of velocity that involve displacement and acceleration. The frequency of these vibrations is described in terms of the numbers of complete cycles of motion taking place in 1 second. Amplitude of vibration is defined as the maximum displacement about a position of rest. The vibration field may be generated by mechanical devices, such as engines, or from aerodynamically induced mechanisms. Mechanical transmission of vibration to the body usually occurs in the frequency range below 100 Hz. Each major body segment and internal organ system has its own frequency to which it is most susceptible. For example, the thoracoabdominal viscera are most susceptible to vibration in the 2 to 12 Hz range. Excessive vibration and noise can have adverse effects on motor performance, vision, and communications.

Spatial Disorientation. The complex neurosensory system that we terrestrials use to maintain our orientation in the three-dimensional plane of our normal existence is inadequate for the three-dimensional dynamic environment of aerospace.

The vision sensory system is by far the most important modality for providing us input to maintain spatial orientation. Visual information processing, however, is acted on by the vestibular system and, to some degree, by proprioception and motion.

Vestibular function in maintaining spatial orientation is not as clearly defined or evident as vision. Once we are deprived of visual cues, the vestibular system becomes a major source of orientation cues in our normal environment. The visual-vestibular interface is important in the fine-tuning of our spatial orientation activities. However, an individual with a nonfunctional vestibular system is able to perform well as long as visual cues are adequate.

In the environment of flight the aviator is exposed to far more complex motion inputs than the physiological system is designed to process. Not infrequently, visual cues may be in conflict with apparent motion and velocity cues processed by the vestibular system. These conflicting cues may lead to severe spatial disorientation or induce episodes of motion sickness. In flight the visual system may be subjected to various illusions, which may cause the pilot to assume a position in free space that is inaccurate. At night or in inclement weather the pilot may not have any external visual cues.

The phenomenon of autokinesis, the apparent motion of a single point of light due to the searching movement of the eyes, although not unique to the aviation environment, is most often perceived in flight. The phenomenon occurs during night flight when the pilot is tracking a single light, such as another aircraft, against the black background of the sky. Within approximately 10 to 15 seconds of visual fixation upon the light the observer will perceive an apparent motion of up to 20 degrees per second. Although the exact mechanism is unknown, the phenomenon is thought to be caused by small movements of the eye, which result in the apparent oscillation of the object being observed.

Vestibular illusions are often more severe and may produce a fatal outcome. These illusions are generally produced by velocity changes that generate input from the semicircular ducts and otolith organs.

Disorientation accidents in military aircraft account for approximately 18% of fatal mishaps. Measures that may be employed to prevent these accidents include modifying flight procedures to reduce the opportunity for disorientation; improving the ease of interpretation of information presented by flight instruments; increasing proficiency in instrument flying, which will permit the pilot to overcome false sensory input; and educating the pilot regarding his or her own physiological frailty and the need for dependence on and acceptance of flight instrument information.

Space. The transition from the terrestrial to the space environment is not a well-demarcated line but rather a continuum that varies with altitude depending upon the parameter discussed. Manned flight and near-earth orbit at altitudes in excess of 240 km require a self-contained vehicle sealed from the near vacuum of space. At this altitude the air density is so low that there is no practical method for compressing the gases to supply both pressure and oxygen to the craft's inhabitants. Although the sun's radiation may heat the vehicle, occupants must be protected from the extreme cold of the ambient environment. While in orbital flight the astronaut will experience a nearly gravity-free or weightless environment. This occurs when the gravitational force vector is counter-balanced by the centrifugal force imparted to the vehicle as it travels tangential to the earth's surface. Long-term exposure to this near-null gravity environment has important biomedical ramifications that as yet are not fully defined.

The earth's atmosphere serves as an insulator to shield us from many of the potential dangers of space radiation. Once a person is in space, this protection is no longer available, and ionizing radiation must be a concern. Three types of radiation present hazards: primary cosmic radiations, geomagnetically trapped radiation (also known as the Van Allen belts), and radiation produced by solar flares. The environment of space is similar in many ways to the aeronautical environment; however, the duration of exposure is much more prolonged in space, and null-gravity is essentially unique.

OPERATIONAL AEROSPACE MEDICINE

The physician practicing aerospace medicine as a clinical specialty must be not only an astute clinician in the office setting but also a practitioner able to grasp the nuance of the environment of flight. One flight surgeon when asked what he did was heard to reply, "I operate on airplanes." This sarcastic response was an attempt at humor. However, the response was not far off the mark if one gives "operating" a broader definition than surgery. The physician may well be an operator while flying.

The stressors impinging on aircrew vary with the type of flight vehicle, whether a single-seat private plane or a multicrew space habitat. Consequently the physician serving as an AME or flight surgeon (FS) must be cognizant of the aircrew's flight environment. For ease of discussion these operational flight environments are defined as civil aviation, military aviation, and space operations.

Civil Aviation. This category of flight operations includes commercial aviation and private or recreational flying. Airlines represent an international industry with over 8000 aircraft worldwide transporting nearly 800 million passengers over 900 billion air miles per year. With the deregulation of the airline industry in the United States, air taxi and air commuter operations have grown to fill the vacuum left when airlines pulled out of small airport terminals. Most large corporations in the United States either own or lease aircraft for business purposes. Other commercial activities include air ambulance service, flight training, aerial application, air cargo, and the new growth industry of commercial parcel delivery.

In the United States there are approximately 450,000 general aviation private pilots flying 220,000 recreational aircrafts. Another 150,000 hold commercial pilot certificates.

The magnitude of preventive medicine intervention by the aerospace physician takes on added meaning when one realizes that all U.S. licensed aviators are required to have an initial medical examination prior to issuance of their license and periodic assessments as long as they continue to fly. To examine these 600,000 aviators, the FAA has designated 7,000 physicians as AMEs. These physicians have undergone special training conducted under the auspices of the FAA; they may have had experience as military flight surgeons and frequently are private pilots themselves. The examination is performed to a rigorous protocol, and detailed physical standards have been promulgated.

The periodicity and sophistication of the examination is dictated in part by the class of the license exercised by the aviator. The airline captain must meet a more stringent standard, more frequently, than is required of the private pilot. In all cases the medical examination is reviewed by medical personnel at the FAA's Civil Aeromedical Institute (CAMI). Approximately 2000 medical examinations are received each business day by the office. This represents one of the largest longitudinal medical data bases in the country; unfortunately, resources to use the tools of epidemiology for fully studying this wealth of data have not been available. Another employment category required to meet flight medical standards is air traffic controller. These 12,000 federal employees stationed throughout the United States must meet, as a minimum, the physical standards required of private pilots, and just as with pilots, these examinations are repeated periodically.

CAMI also has responsibility for conducting research to address issues of health and safety for flight deck and cabin crew as well as for the private aviator and passengers. Toward this goal the institute has conducted research and recommended standards on emergency aircraft lighting, egress systems, restraint systems, breathing equipment, emergency breathing devices, and flotation systems.

Military Aviation. One would expect that the Air Force has the largest number of military aircraft. Although the numbers vary from year to year, this may not be the proper conclusion in view of the large number of Army fixed and rotary wing aircraft. The fewer number of available aircraft to the Navy and Marines in no way diminishes the aeromedical support required.

The Air Force has by far the widest range of aeronautical activities. Low and slow describes some Air Force missions, while others are truly into the fringes of space. Current fighter aircraft are capable of readily exceeding the physiological tolerance of the pilot with rapid onset, high G. The response of fighter aircraft is so fast that controls are now electronic rather than hydraulic or mechanical. Large transport aircraft are capable of nearly endless flight with air-to-air refueling. With rest facilities and multiple crew, the aircraft can simply keep on flying; the only restriction is the crew rest requirements of its human operators. For over 2 decades it has been predicted that aeronautical design will take aircraft performance beyond the performance of the pilot. That time has arrived as aeronautical engineers are forced to curtail performance characteristics because the human operator would fail.

Army aviation medicine has for some years concentrated on unique facets of rotary wing operations and pilot adaptability. In past years, helicopter crashes that were survivable in terms of impact force frequently ended in fire and death of the occupants. With intense research and redesign this hazard has been significantly reduced. The military necessity of helicopter operations in adverse weather conditions and at night have created human factor challenges that have only in part been successfully addressed by technology.

The unique challenge for naval aviation medicine is related to aircraft carrier operations. Not only is the flight surgeon responsible for health maintenance of the flight crews but also for maintaining health surveillance for the 5000 men on board the carrier. The word "independent" has been used to describe a prominent characteristic of this medical service. The flight surgeon is the public health officer for this isolated community and oversees all aspects of hygiene, epidemiological surveillance, health maintenance, and medical disaster preparedness aboard ship.

The Navy has just celebrated the fiftieth anniversary of the Thousand Aviator Program,[3] one of the first large cohort, longitudinal health surveillance programs undertaken in the United States. More than 1000 aviators and aviation cadets were examined using psychological and physiological assessment procedures. This ongoing study has reviewed cardiovascular status, overall morbidity and mortality rates, and the effects of the aviation experience on the overall health of the individual.

In addition to the stress of prolonged periods at sea and the unique flying environment of carrier operations, the Navy and its operation of high performance aircraft share with the other services many of the challenges of extreme physiological stress.

Space Operations. The United States' manned space program has enjoyed successes; unfortunately, it has also experienced several disasters that continue to remind one that space operations are neither routine nor free from potential catastrophic failures. The Soviet Union likewise has experienced success and disaster in space.

As experience has accumulated with man-days in space and monitoring of increasing numbers of astronauts in the space environment, medical concerns have focused on the physiological effects of null gravity. Based on our current experience for short duration flights, the biomedical challenges include space adaptation syndrome (space motion sickness), cardiovascular deconditioning, loss of red cell mass, and bone mineral loss. For shuttle operations the first two concerns are primary. Space adaptation syndrome has been experienced by up to one third of the shuttle crew. This syndrome occurs in the early segments of orbital flight and may adversely affect early mission performance.

Fluid shift and deconditioning effects occur even during the relatively short duration of the shuttle orbital missions. Performance during orbit does not appear to be compromised, but with the increasing G upon reentry, performance decrements are possible.

As preparations proceed for a continuous habitat in space, the remaining biomedical challenges will become important. The Soviet Union has successfully maintained cosmonauts in orbit for over a year. Biomedical data obtained from those individuals are awaiting publication.

The space station operation introduces additional challenges for maintaining astronauts on long duration missions. The environmental control systems must be able to maintain potable water and uncontaminated air reliably for long periods. Microbe overgrowth must be prevented. Food and sanitation issues need to be addressed with resupply providing only one solution. Health maintenance surveillance and emergency medical treatment will require attention. Crew work-rest cycles and psychological considerations remain challenges, as do biologically efficient extravehicular activities. In the summer of 1989, on the occasion of the twentieth anniversary of the Apollo manned landing, President George Bush proposed several goals for space operations to be achieved over the next several decades. These goals include a successful manned space station, establishment of a manned lunar base, and Mars exploration. These goals grip the imagination and challenge the aerospace medical specialist.

PERSONNEL, PASSENGERS, AND PATIENTS

In general the people most involved in the aerospace industry are flight crews, cabin personnel, and ground staff; passengers, who represent the chief revenue source for commercial aviation; and patients, who may be transported either by an airline or air ambulance service.

Personnel. American flag carrier airlines are responsible for the direct employment of approximately 460,000 workers including 51,000 flight deck and 77,000 cabin crew members. The remaining employees make up the maintenance teams, counter servicing and baggage personnel, and those engaged in administration and management. The preventive health surveillance and medical monitoring of these individuals are provided via a variety of health service mechanisms. A number of the larger airlines maintain modern, sophisticated medical departments providing both occupational and aviation medicine services to the workforce. Other airlines have elected to keep only a minimal medical presence in-house and to contract for or otherwise provide services to employees. Smaller airlines have found it successful to hire the periodic services of an aeromedical consultant and to contract out health services. Less common is contracting all health services without the benefit of corporate medical oversight.

Airlines providing comprehensive aviation medical services will provide many, if not all, of the services detailed in Table 37–1.

Many of the activities for either flight crew or ground personnel are clinical preventive medicine services. The sophistication of the preemployment examination depends on the job description of the future employee. In part, because of the enormous training investment in pilots, airlines try to select pilots who are free of active disease, who have few precursors to chronic illness, and who do not exhibit high-risk life-style behavior.

Prior to the promulgation of the regulation dealing with urine drug screening by the Department of Transportation, many airlines had already initiated such a policy. Recognizing their obligation to public safety, airline companies began by the mid-1980s to implement a drug-free work policy. From the perspective of public health and preventive medicine, two components of this policy are essential—education and treatment. Broad-based educational programs were initiated for all employees, including flight personnel, maintenance crews, and management. Individuals who recognized their own drug dependency were encouraged to step forward and receive treatment and support. Management then worked with employee representatives to establish guidelines and rules for implementing a drug abuse protection program. Most airlines established a drug screening component to their preemployment processing. Drug testing for cause was also implemented; however, fewer airlines established a no-notice urine drug screening program. These programs continue to evolve, and both legislation and litigation will clearly modify the process.

Approximately 2 decades ago, airlines in association with the Airline Pilots Association and with cooperation from the FAA, initiated a model alcoholic rehabilitation program. With few exceptions it had been the FAA policy to revoke the medical certificate of airline pilots who had alcoholism. Such a practice was devastating, requiring counseling, support, and treatment for those whose licenses were revoked. Once identified as an alcoholic, the pilot, even though he may have been seeking help, lost his livelihood. The new program encouraged self-identification since treatment was now available and because if it was successful, the pilot would be able to return to the cockpit. This program involved supervisors, peers, medical personnel, FAA supervision, and, perhaps most importantly, close affiliation with Alcoholics Anonymous. Hundreds of pilots have been successful in these recovery programs and have returned to the cockpit. This program provides an excellent model for industry in general and clearly recognizes the importance of continuing support to the recovering alcoholic.

Although many pilots earn their livelihood in commercial aviation, most aviators in the United States are private pilots who fly for recreation or business. Whether the aircraft is a wide-bodied, multiengine, commercial passenger airliner, a high-performance jet fighter, or a single-engine private aircraft, the aviation environment and its potential adverse effects on human physiology remain. Although the level to which stress is imposed on the aviator is determined in large measure by the flight profile of the aircraft, all aviators are exposed to some adverse environmental factors associated with flight. Prevention or amelioration of adverse effects resulting from the flight environment continues to be a key component of the practice of aerospace medicine. Flight personnel whose health and well-being may be compromised by illness or by self-imposed stress compromise their performance as aviators and thus have a potential adverse effect on flight safety.

Illness and Disease. Aviation is among those few avocations or vocations where the incapacitation of the operator could have dire effects. Once airborne, the aircraft is dependent on the pilot to safely complete the flight. Although there are many assists to the aviator both in the aircraft and on the ground, the number of aircraft capable of fully automated flight is small. Consequently, public safety dictates that the potential for pilot incapacitation be minimized.

There are many physical afflictions an aviator may have without undue risk to flight safety. However, certain medical conditions are currently considered incompatible with safe flight. The clinical skills of the aerospace medicine specialist are most tested in diagnosing occult disease and determining the risk such a condition may impose on flight safety and the aviation activities of the aviator.

Unexplained loss of consciousness or epilepsy are examples of conditions that may create an unacceptable risk to the pilot and to the public. Diabetes mellitus requiring medication and exertional angina are other examples where the risk to public safety may take precedence over the individual pilot's desire to continue flying. *Clinical Aviation Medicine* addresses most common afflictions and their aeromedical implications.[4]

Therapeutic Medications. Physicians write more than 1.5 billion prescriptions for therapeutic medications each year in the United States. An even greater number of over-the-counter medications are purchased annually. With this degree of drug ingestion

TABLE 37–1. AIRLINE AVIATION MEDICAL SERVICES

Preemployment medical examination	Employee assistance program
Drug abuse testing	Acute care
Psychological profile or personality inventory	Emergency response service
Physiological training	Periodic medical assessment
Wellness or health maintenance program	Job-related illness or injury monitoring
	Return to work assessment

among the U.S. population, it is most probable that medication is being taken by a substantial percentage of aviators. Both therapeutic effects and adverse side effects may create situations that adversely affect flight performance. One of the most common side effects of medications is drowsiness or loss of concentration. A pilot on a long, uneventful flight must be vigilant in order to fight boredom and inattention. He or she may also be experiencing mild hypoxia. If one adds to this scenario the side effects of medication, the results could be tragic. Most studies have shown that adverse effects of medications are enhanced by the flight environment. Recognizing that pilots may be unaware of some of the common adverse effects of medication, Mohler published a guide written in layman's terms specifically addressing this issue for pilots.[5]

The DOD, because it supervises the health care of its pilots, simply removes the aviator from flight duty until completion of the therapeutic regimen. For long-term or chronic disease requiring therapy, such as mild hypertension, limited prescription medications are available, provided a prior trial has demonstrated that the pilot experiences no adverse side effects. In the civilian sector, such control of health care is essentially nonexistent. This is true even for commercial airlines that may attempt to monitor the health status of their pilots. Consequently both the physician providing treatment and the pilot taking medication must be educated to the potential dangers of adverse side effects in flight.

Nontherapeutic Drugs. The two most commonly used drugs in this category are cigarettes and alcohol. Although the incidence of alcohol-related aircraft accidents has fallen in response to an extensive educational effort on the part of the FAA, alcohol continues to be associated with approximately 15% of all aircraft accidents. Alcohol and altitude are synergistic, both in the effects upon the central nervous system and in regard to slowing metabolic clearance rates. Ground-based simulation and actual in-flight performance have demonstrated that blood alcohol levels as low as 0.04% (40 mg/dl) adversely compromise flight performance.

Habitual cigarette smokers commonly have blood carbon monoxide levels in excess of 5%. This represents a reduction in the blood oxygen level equal to that of a nonsmoker at an altitude of 2200 m. Consequently the aviator who smokes is placing his body physiologically at a higher altitude than indicated and thus compromises altitude tolerance.

Work-Rest Cycles. Numerous factors in the aerospace environment enhance the onset of fatigue. One of the more significant of these factors is the erratic schedule many aviators maintain while flying. Weather remains the greatest cause for flight schedule disruption in private, business, or commercial aviation. Although larger, more expensive aircraft are now equipped with electronic measures to reduce the impact of weather on flight schedules, problems remain. There are regulatory controls, work rules, and common sense methods in place to reduce inadvertent or intentional fatigue factors. Although a pilot may fly only the prescribed number of hours over a particular time period, there is no assurance that there was either the opportunity or ability to obtain adequate rest in the interval.

The excitement of a new place, insomnia in a strange bed, circadian rhythm asynchrony, and work-related anxiety may contribute to restless sleep and inadequate rest. Then a new workday begins, which may in fact be in the middle of the pilot's biological night. Such circumstances are not infrequent and do lead to both acute and chronic fatigue for aircrew members.

For the private pilot, time schedules are frequently self-imposed, which initially may have been realistic but become severely disrupted with the passage of a storm front. Nevertheless the individual attempts to reach the next destination, ignoring the length of time without rest and the manifestations of fatigue. Fatigue is rarely cited as the primary cause of an aircraft accident; however, it often appears as a contributing factor.

Aging. For a number of years, the FAA has had in place the Age 60 Rule. This rule directs that air transport pilots flying for commercial airlines may not serve as pilots beyond age 60 years. This is not a medical regulation but one promulgated through operations. There is no such age limitation for other categories of flying. All others, regardless of age, may continue aviation activities as pilots as long as a current medical certificate is maintained and other evaluation requirements of the license are met.

The Age 60 Rule had its origin some years ago before sophisticated medical diagnostic techniques were available and predated the advanced simulators, which are now able to measure subtle performance decrements. It was recognized that the risk for sudden incapacitation in flight increased with age, particularly cerebral vascular accidents and heart attacks. The wisdom at the time said such a rule was necessary to reduce the potential for such events by controlling the population at risk. Although the rule is currently being sustained in the courts, considerable epidemiological evidence is being put forward in an attempt to overturn what some have described as age discrimination.

Passengers. Commercial airlines have both an obligation and a commitment to provide safe, reliable, and comfortable service to their passengers. In general this is the experience of millions of passengers flying each year. Table 37-2 provides comparative accident data for road, rail, and air travel. Travel by domestic airlines remains one of the safest forms of transportation.

Safety. Many of the safety features in modern commercial aircraft go unrecognized by the passengers. The number of emergency exits are specified to assure rapid evacuation in case of an emergency. Both airline seats and seat belts are designed to sustain considerable impact force in order to protect and restrain the passenger. Other than the preflight demonstration, few passengers have seen the emergency oxygen masks, which are available at every seat location in aircraft flying at substantial altitudes. Emergency lighting has been designed to provide illumination in case of power failure and floor level track lighting leading to the emergency evacuation routes has been installed recently. The most important safety feature is not equipment but the cabin attendant. Although most passengers look to these individuals to make the flight more comfortable by providing service and assistance, the cabin attendant's primary purpose is to provide safety instructions and help to passengers in case of emergencies.

Scheduled domestic aircraft are equipped with an expanded first-aid kit, which provides basic equipment and medication for inflight medical emergencies, provided a practitioner is on

TABLE 37-2. COMPARATIVE ACCIDENT DATA FOR ROAD, RAIL, AND AIRLINE TRAVEL 1971-1987

	Passenger Fatalities Per 100 Million Passenger-Miles			
Year	***Automobiles and Taxis***	***Buses***	***Passenger Trains***	***Domestic Scheduled Aircraft***
1971	1.90	0.19	0.24	0.15
1975	1.40	0.15	0.08	0.08
1980	1.32	0.15	0.04	0.01
1985	0.96	0.04	0.03	0.07
1987	0.92	0.03	0.13	0.07

From The National Safety Council: Accident Facts. Washington, D.C: U.S. Government Printing Office, 1988.

board. The actual number of in-flight medical incidents per year is relatively small; one such incident occurs per 10 million passenger-miles flown. In the domestic setting, an airline would divert to the nearest appropriate field should a medical emergency occur. Such diversions occur approximately once per 2 million passengers carried or one per 3 billion passenger-miles flown. Table 37–3 lists examples of the kind of passenger injury and illness experienced by major air carriers for 1 year.[6]

Circadian Asynchronization ["Jet Lag"]. Transmeridian flights commonly are disruptive to the passenger's awake-sleep cycle. There is considerable individual sensitivity to disruption of the normal body rhythm. Time shifts of 3 to 4 hours often will alter the body's homeostasis. The recovery time is dependent not only on the number of time zones crossed but also on the direction of flight. Body cycle disruptions occurring after crossing six or more time zones appear to be relatively persistent when one is flying east, lasting upward of 11 days; symptoms from flying west persist for no more than 1 or 2 days. Measures recommended to reduce the impact of this circadian asynchronization include adjusting daily activities several days before the flight, changing meals to the new time, eating light meals, avoiding alcohol, and using hypnotics during and following the flight, as well as allowing specific rest periods on arrival at the destination.

Patients. There are few absolute contraindications to transporting patients by air. Patients who suffer from dysbarism, acute myocardial infarction, pneumothorax, or air embolism can be moved with relative safety provided appropriate precautions are taken and preparations made. Assuming that maximum effort has been made to stabilize the patient, the question should be asked, "Are the benefits of air transportation real, and do they justify the clinical risks and financial costs?" The DOD has the greatest experience with transporting seriously ill and injured patients. The Army Air Force proved the benefit of aeromedical evacuation by fixed-wing aircraft in World War II. The Viet Nam War provided the laboratory for developing the technology for patient transport by helicopter.

The military aeromedical evacuation system employing the McDonnell-Douglas C-9A represents the nation's main resource for fixed-wing medical transport. The U.S. Army's Military Assistance and Safety and Traffic (MAST) helicopter units established the nation's first major network of rotary wing medical evacuation capabilities.

Commercial air ambulance services are available in all large communities in the United States. To date, there are no federally mandated air ambulance standards, and consequently the quality of service varies over a wide spectrum. Recognizing the potential problem, the industry itself has developed standards to enhance the service to the patient through improved training of personnel and placement of specialized equipment aboard the aircraft. Most visible is the medical center helicopter used to transfer critically ill and injured patients and neonates to tertiary medical facilities.

The environment of flight, such as vibration, noise, and pressure changes, has dictated the modification of standard life-support equipment. Many aircraft used in patient transfer routinely carry this specialized equipment. Two additions are flight-certified incubators for neonatal transport and respirators.

Medical conditions requiring particular insight into the physiology and environment of flight are air embolism and pressure change–induced decompression sickness, or dysbarism. In the transfer of such patients it is imperative that pressure changes routinely experienced in flight be avoided. Some aircraft, such as the Hercules C-130, can be overpressurized to maintain the cabin below sea level pressure provided they fly at a relatively low altitude.

Optimal treatment of decompression sickness requires transfer of the patient to a hyperbaric environment. Much of the physiology of altitude or hypobarics has parallels with elevated pressure. The clinical procedures first developed to manage dysbarism have been adopted as an adjunct in the treatment of other medical afflictions. Hyperbaric oxygen administered in a pressure chamber has proven helpful in treatment of carbon monoxide poisoning, air embolism, clostridia infection, and refractory osteomyelitis. Questions remain on the efficiency of hyperbaric oxygen treatment in some of these examples because of the lack of adequate control studies.

Airline companies are frequently called on to make special provisions for the transfer of ill or injured patients in the normal cabin environment of an airliner. Provided such a transfer does not represent a hazard to other passengers, stretchers are available that extend over three airline seats. The patient must be accompanied by at least one attendant. The expense is significant because of the block of seats required by the stretcher apparatus.

Prevention is the hallmark of aeromedical support to personnel, passengers, and patients: prevention of disease and risk behaviors that might compromise the longitudinal health of aircrew personnel; prevention of injury or death to passengers through safety design of aircraft and safe airline operations; and prevention of further complications to the air-transported patient through planning, training, and equipping aeromedical transportation systems.

TABLE 37–3. PASSENGER INJURY AND ILLNESS EXPERIENCE FOR 1 YEAR

Injury or Illness	Number
▪ **Type of Injury**	
Contusions or sprains	238
Inside aircraft	118
On steps	91
In terminal	10
Struck by objects	11
Struck by seat belt buckle	8
Burns	29
Spilled food	25
Exploding matches	3
Fuel in eyes	1
Lacerations	13
Dental injury	4
Ear injury	3
Total	287
▪ **Type of Illness**	
Cardiovascular	124
Respiratory	87
Neuropsychiatric (including 25 cases of air sickness)	55
Gastrointestinal	28
Eye, ear, nose, and throat	26
Other (diabetes, dermatologic, orthopedic)	22
Total	342

COMMUNITY AND INTERNATIONAL HEALTH

Aerospace flight operations have the potential for disrupting the environment and serving as a mechanism for the introduction of disease. Within the United States, regulations have helped reduce the impact of flight operations on the environment. The potential for disease transmission has been reduced with the implementation of international sanitary regulations and other control mechanisms.

Disease Transmission. The spread of epidemics by movement of populations has been well-documented throughout history. In days past an infected individual traveling by land or sea usually became symptomatic, and thus the disease was apparent before the person reached his or her destination. With today's high-speed jet traffic it is not only possible but also likely that an individual infected with a communicable disease could be asymptomatic yet incubating the disease at the time of arrival at the destination. Today it is possible to fly to nearly any destination on the globe with 24 hours. Lathrop and Wolfe[7] implicate the aircraft in the spread of cholera, penicillin-resistant gonorrhea, influenza, rubella, and Lassa fever. Shilts, in *And The Band Played On,* describes how a flight attendant, with his ability to move rapidly from city to city, may have served as a vector of the human immunodeficiency virus.[8]

Recognizing the potential importance of the aircraft as a mechanism to spread disease and vectors, the first sanitary convention for aerial navigation convened in 1933. The convention's focus was curtailment of the spread of yellow fever, including limiting the distribution of the mosquito vector *Aedes aegypti.* This convention eventually became the World Health Organization (WHO) Committee on Hygiene and Sanitation in Aviation. International airlines are required to comply with the International Health Regulations published by WHO, which primarily address the following:

1. Promulgation of the application of epidemiological principles
2. Enhancement of sanitation at international airports
3. Reduction or elimination of factors contributing to the spread of disease
4. Elimination of disease vector transportation
5. Enhancement of epidemiological techniques to halt the introduction or establishment of a foreign disease

To accomplish these tasks, WHO provides assistance in implementing the necessary strategies. The following specific requirements have been established to allow a nation to designate "sanitary airports":

1. An organized and properly equipped medical service
2. A system for the care and transport of individuals suspected of having a regulated disease
3. A system for disinsection and disinfection and methods to control vectors and rodents
4. Access to a biological laboratory
5. An on-site facility for yellow fever vaccination

Vector Control. Disinfection procedures vary from airline to airline. The principal objective of these procedures is to kill mosquitos and other insect vectors of disease. At one time it was common when one was flying to or from tropical areas to have cabin attendants pass through the aircraft with activated aerosol cans spraying insecticide. Another procedure, which was less obvious, was to disseminate an insecticide vapor from several fixed stations in the aircraft. Current regulations permit residual treatment of the aircraft with permethrin. A common practice was the "blocks-away" disinsection technique, in which insecticide would be introduced into the passenger cabin immediately after the aircraft was closed and was taxiing to take off. An alternative method was to use aerosol insecticide prior to arrival at the destination airport. In any case, to be effective, it is necessary that insecticides be used before off-loading passengers, cargo, and luggage. It is becoming more common for live animal cargo to be transported by air. The issues of disease and vectors must be addressed with such cargo.

Large pieces of expensive equipment are also being transported by air. When the equipment has been used in the field, it is extremely difficult to assure that all fomite contamination has been removed prior to air transportation to another country. Washing and steam cleaning of the exterior of such equipment has become regular practice. The use of some form of pesticide is commonly required before the equipment is allowed to be unloaded after it has crossed international borders.

Airline Community Health. A commercial airliner, whether traveling domestic or international routes, provides a partially closed, self-contained environment. Air is brought on board, filtered, condensed, warmed, and if necessary, neutralized for irritants such as ozone and oxides of nitrogen. Potable water must be available as well as beverages safe for human consumption. The catering service must provide food items, which frequently include both preprepared meals and other items requiring some degree of preparation. Provisions must be made for the generation of solid and hazardous waste. Toilet facilities must be provided that require retention tanks to hold sewage until servicing can be provided on the ground. Arrangements for the collection of trash and sewage and its proper disposal on arrival must be made. These details may prove relatively simple in the domestic environment but may become extremely complex with international flights. In some international situations, all food products must be incinerated at the destination airport to ensure no introduction of a plant or animal disease.

THE ENVIRONMENT

Noise. One of the more noticeable features of aerospace operations is noise. The Department of Transportation estimates that approximately 3% of the U.S. population, 7 million persons, have been exposed to a potentially hazardous level of aircraft noise. The Environmental Protection Agency (EPA) is authorized under the Noise Pollution and Abatement Act (1970) and the Noise Control Act (1972) to institute noise control abatement procedures around airports. The FAA has also been assigned responsibilities to reduce environmental noise. Regulatory requirements set goals and timelines for airport operators to submit and comply with noise compatibility programs.

Since the implementation of these laws, efforts have been undertaken by airframe manufacturers to control aircraft noise at its source. Numerous design changes have been made in engines primarily to reduce noise. Airports may require specific landing and departure patterns including engine power adjustments to comply with abatement controls. Some airports have found it necessary to curtail nighttime operations to satisfy objections by the community surrounding the airport. All levels of government have taken an active role in assuring the compatibility of land use around airfields, both with regard to safety and noise control.

Sonic Booms. A sonic boom is generated when an aircraft exceeds the speed of sound and produces an advancing shockwave, which as it passes an observer is heard as a boom or thunderlike sound. With the exception of the British-French Concord supersonic transport (SST), sonic booms are produced primarily by military aircraft flying at supersonic speeds. The general community response to sonic booms has remained negative. Thus commercial SST operations have been limited to over-water flights, and high-speed military operations are limited to narrow corridors with low population densities.

Anticipating the development of the SST, both in this country and in Europe, numerous studies were conducted in the

United States. Although actual complaints were few and of no serious consequence, stories continued to abound regarding sonic boom–generated snow avalanches, depressed egg production, disrupted mink farming, and adversely affected livestock production. In response to communities with preconceived perceptions of adverse effects, the FAA has prohibited civil aircraft flights at supersonic speeds over United States territory.

The "Greenhouse Effect" and Ozone Depletion. Aerospace operations contribute to approximately 1% of the nation's total emissions of hydrocarbons, oxides of nitrogen, and carbon monoxide. In certain areas such as Atlanta and Chicago where aircraft operations are intense, emission levels have increased to approximately 3% of the average level. Under the Clean Air Act, airlines have markedly reduced the practice of inflight fuel dumping. Economics have also dictated a change in this policy. The principal environmental problem of the fuel is its contribution to photochemical pollution. The formation of the condensation trail, or con-trail, consists of the emissions of the aircraft's engines condensing and freezing in the cold ambient temperature of altitude. It has been suggested that heavy jet traffic may cause weather changes in areas surrounding major airport hubs.

Ozone depletion is receiving an appropriate international response. In the 1970s there was much concern that oxides of nitrogen would serve as catalysts for ozone depletion at the high altitudes of the SST flights. It was estimated that an SST fleet of 100 aircraft would decrease the ozone layer by 10%. This concern played an important role in the decision by this country to withdraw from the SST commercial competition. With additional research and a better understanding of the high altitude atmospheric chemical relationship the fears of ozone depletion from this source were shown to be exaggerated.

THE FUTURE

As we approach the twenty-first century, all projections point to more people flying higher and faster. The technology of aerospace systems will continue to improve, and the degree of automation of both air and space craft will continue to increase. Large numbers of men and women will be required to maintain and operate the expanding fleet of aerospace vehicles. New exotic materials will be introduced by the aerospace industry, requiring special medical surveillance programs to ensure the safety and health of those working with these new substances.

The challenges to public health and the environment will continue. With the continued expansion of international commerce via rapid air and space transport, the potential for transporting disease, vectors, and fomites will continue. Increasing air traffic in finite, three-dimensional space will result in some compromise to environmental factors. Airports will continue to expand, challenging community aesthetics and introducing social and environmental concerns.

With all of the opportunities and challenges of the future, aerospace medicine will continue to have an important niche in the ecology of health services.

REFERENCES

1. Directory of Graduate Medical Education Programs. Chicago: American Medical Association, 1989
2. Peyton G: Fifty years of aerospace medicine. Washington, D.C.: U.S. Government Printing Office, 1967
3. Caudill RP: Naval aviation medicine. In DeHart RL (ed): Fundamentals of Aerospace Medicine. Philadelphia: Lea and Febiger, 1985
4. Rayman RB: Clinical Aviation Medicine, 2 edt. Philadelphia: Lea and Febiger, 1989
5. Mohler SR: Medication and Flying: A Pilot's Guide. Boston: Boston Publishing Co, 1982
6. DeHart RL, Gullett CC: Aviation medical support to airlines. In DeHart RL (ed): Fundamentals of Aerospace Medicine. Philadelphia: Lea and Febiger, 1985
7. Lathrop GD, Wolfe WH: Role of aircraft in the transmission of disease. In DeHart RL (ed): Fundamentals of Aerospace Medicine. Philadelphia: Lea and Febiger, 1985
8. Shilts R: And the Band Played On. New York: St. Martin's Press, 1987

General References

DeHart RL (ed): Fundamentals of Aerospace Medicine. Philadelphia: Lea and Febiger, 1985

Ernsting J, King PF (eds): Aviation Medicine, 2 edt. London: Butterworth, 1988

Hawkins FH: Human Factors in Flight. London: Grover Technical Press, 1987

Nicogossian AE, Huntoon CL, Pool SL (eds): Space Physiology and Medicine, 2 edt. Philadelphia: Lea and Febiger, 1989

38

Housing and Health

John M. Last

All humans need shelter: protection against the elements, somewhere to store food and prepare meals, and a secure place to raise offspring. The effects of housing conditions on health have been known since antiquity. Deplorable living conditions in urban slums became a political issue in the nineteenth century when vivid descriptions by journalists, novelists, and social reformers aroused public opinion. Osler's *Principles and Practice of Medicine* (1892) and Rosenau's *Preventive Medicine and Hygiene* (1913) noted the association between overcrowding and common serious diseases such as tuberculosis and rheumatic fever.

OVERVIEW OF HOUSING CONDITIONS IN THE WORLD

Housing conditions have greatly improved in the affluent industrial nations throughout the second half of the twentieth century, but more than two thirds of the households in the world are in developing countries, the great majority of them in rural areas; the most prevalent indoor environment in the world is the same now as throughout history—huts in rural communities.[1] But this is changing. Urbanization is rapidly transforming the distribution of populations in the developing world, where the proportion living in urban areas rose from less than 25% to over 33% between 1970 and 1985; by 2025, if present trends continue, the proportion living in urban areas in the developing world is expected to exceed 50%,[2] and in the world as a whole the urban population will comprise 65% or more. Many cities will be very large (see Table 70–2, Chapter 70).

Many of these new urban dwellers have terrible living conditions. In the last 20 years there has been a great increase in the numbers of people living in periurban slums in developing countries. They often lack sanitation, clean water supplies, access to health care, and other basic services such as elementary education. The proportion of people in such circumstances ranges between 20% and over 80% in most cities throughout Africa, Latin America, and South, South-east and South-west Asia. The plight of children is especially deplorable; infant mortality rates exceed 100 in many places.[3] Children are often abandoned by parents who cannot provide for them and must fend for themselves from ages as young as 5 or 6 years; many turn to crime and child prostitution to survive.

These shanty-towns and periurban slums endanger the health and security of many millions in Latin America, Africa, and many parts of Asia. Accurate numbers are impossible to obtain because the missing services include enumeration by census-takers and because situations change so rapidly, but in Mexico City, Lima, Santiago, Rio De Janeiro, São Paulo, and Bogota, well over half the total population live in the periurban slums.[3] In the mid-1980s, there were as many as 30 million periurban slum-dwellers in these six cities alone. Others are even worse off: worldwide, an estimated 100 million people are entirely homeless, living on the streets without possessions, often from infancy onward. Although this is a problem mainly in developing countries, homeless people have increased in numbers in the most affluent industrial nations in the last decade, often forced out of their homes by hard economic times. Public health departments in large cities such as New York and London have been obliged to spend increasing proportions of their budgets on emergency shelter for growing numbers of homeless destitute families.

Increasing numbers, an estimated 15 million in 1989, live in refugee communities[4] in Africa and the Middle and Far East where housing conditions are equally deplorable, sometimes worse than in periurban slums. Refugee communities may have health services, but these are seldom adequate; supplies and continuity of services are often precarious; the safety and security of the inhabitants is often threatened by hostilities, and their long-term prospects for a better life are poor.

Industrially developed nations are experiencing other challenging new health problems related to housing conditions. Rising land values and the need to provide cheap housing for expanding populations have led to proliferation of high-rise, high-density apartment housing. Publicly supported housing projects economize by restricting living space and providing few amenities. This kind of dwelling creates new sets of problems: emotional tensions attributable to living too close to the neighbors, inadequate play areas for children, poor services, and defective elevators and communal washing machines. Only a small minority of people, predominantly the educated professional classes (such as many readers of this book), enjoy comfortable, aesthetically pleasing, healthy living conditions.

INDOOR ENVIRONMENT

Indoor climate and indoor air pollution, biological exposure factors, and various physical hazards encountered inside the home are encompassed by the term *indoor environment*.

The indoor climate may be the same as that out of doors, or it may be modified by heating, cooling, or adjustment of humidity levels, and often in sealed modern buildings, by all of these.

Physical Hazards. Physical hazards in the indoor environment include toxic gases, respirable suspended particulates, asbestos fibers, ionizing radiation, notably radon and "daughters," nonionizing radiation, and tobacco smoke.

Indoor air may be contaminated with dusts, fumes, pollen, and microorganisms. The principal indoor air pollutants in industrially developed nations are summarized in Table 38–1. Many of these pollutants are harmful to health. Some occur mainly in sealed office buildings, and others, such as tobacco smoke, in private dwellings.

In developing countries, indoor air pollution with products of biomass fuel combustion is a pervasive problem (Table 38–2). The fumes from cooking fires include high concentrations of respiratory irritants that cause chronic obstructive pulmonary disease (COPD) and that sometimes contain carcinogens too. Premature death from COPD is common among women who from their childhood have spent many hours every day close to primitive cooking stoves, inhaling large quantities of toxic fumes.[5]

The toxic gases specified in Table 38–1 come from many sources. Formaldehyde is emitted as an off-gas from particle board, carpet adhesives, and urea formaldehyde foam insulation; it is a respiratory and conjunctival irritant and sometimes causes asthma. It is not emitted in sufficient concentrations to constitute a significant cancer risk. Although rats exposed to formaldehyde do demonstrate increased incidence of nasopharyngeal cancer, there is only weak evidence of elevated cancer incidence or mortality rates even among persons occupationally exposed to far higher concentrations than occur in domestic settings. Nonetheless, ureaformaldehyde foam insulation has been banned in many jurisdictions on the basis of the evidence for carcinogenicity in rats. Gases and vapors from volatile solvents, such as cleaning fluids, have diverse origins. There is a wide range of other pollutants, such as many organic substances, oxides of nitrogen, sulfur, and carbon, ozone, benzene, and terpines.[6] All such toxic substances can be troublesome, especially in sealed air-conditioned buildings and most of all when the air is recirculated to conserve energy used to heat or cool the building. In combination with fluorescent lighting, these gases and suspended particulate matter can produce an irritating photochemical smog that may cause chronic conjunctivitis and nasal congestion.

Imperfect ventilation can become a serious hazard if it leads to accumulation or recirculation of highly toxic gas such as carbon monoxide; this is especially likely when coal or coke is used as cooking or heating fuel in cold weather and vents to the outside are closed to conserve heat.

Asbestos was used for many years as a fire retardant and insulating substance in both domestic and commercial buildings. Its dangers to health have led to restriction or banning of its use and to expensive renovations aimed at removing it (see Chapter 17). Fibrous glass insulation may present hazards similar to those of asbestos but less severe.

Ionizing radiation, in particular radon and "daughters," can be a health hazard, especially if houses are sealed and air recirculated, in which case there is greater opportunity for higher concentrations to accumulate. Sources of radon include trace amounts of radioactive material incorporated in cement used to construct basements. Radon can also be emitted from soil or rocks in the environment where the houses are built.

Nonionizing radiation, notably extremely low frequency electromagnetic radiation (ELF), has attracted much attention since the observation of cancer incidence at higher rates than expected among children living close to high voltage power lines.[7] No convincing relationship has been demonstrated between childhood cancer and exposure to ELF from domestic appliances, with the possible exception of electric blankets.[8] Microwave ovens and television screens are safe. The nature of the relationship, if any, between ELF and cancer remains controversial, however.

Tobacco smoke is often the greatest health hazard attributable to physical factors in the indoor environment. Infants and children are significantly more prone to respiratory infections,

TABLE 38–1. SOURCES AND POSSIBLE CONCENTRATIONS OF INDOOR POLLUTANTS

Pollutant	Sources	Range of Concentrations
Respirable particles	Tobacco smoke Stoves Aerosol sprays	0.05–0.7 mg/m^3
Carbon monoxide	Combustion equipment Stoves, gas heaters	1–115 mg/m^3
Nitrogen dioxide	Gas cookers Cigarettes	0.05–1.0 mg/m^3
Sulfur dioxide	Coal combustion	0.02–1.0 mg/m^3
Carbon dioxide	Combustion Respiration	600–9000 mg/m^3
Formaldehyde	Particle board Carpet adhesives Insulation	0.06–2.0 mg/m^3
Other organic vapors [benzene, toluene, etc.]	Solvents, adhesives, resin products, aerosol sprays	0.01–0.1 mg/m^3
Ozone	Electric arcing, UV light sources	0.02–0.4 mg/m^3
Radon and "daughters"	Building materials	10–3000 Bq/m^3
Asbestos	Insulation, fireproofing	1 + fiber/cm^3
Mineral fibers	Appliances	100–10,000/m^3

NOTE: Tobacco smoke, benzene, radon and daughters, asbestos, and possibly formaldehyde are carcinogens; most others on this list are respiratory, or conjunctival irritants. Carbon dioxide is an asphyxiant, carbon monoxide is a lethal poison.

TABLE 38-2. INDOOR AIR POLLUTION FROM BIOMASS FUEL COMBUSTION IN DEVELOPING COUNTRIES

	SPM (mg/m^3)	BaP (mg/m^3)	CO (mg/m^3)	NO_2 (μg/m^3)	Other
Nigeria, Lagos	—	—	1076	15,168	SO_2, 38 ppm Benzene, 86 ppm
Papua New Guinea	0.84	—	35.5	—	HCHO, 1.2 ppm
Kenya Highlands	4.0	145	—	—	BaH, 224 μg/m^3 Phenols, 1.0 μg/m^3 Acetic acid, 4.6 μg/m^3
India, Ahmedabad					
Cattle dung	16.0	8250	—	144	SO_2, 242 μg/m^3
Dung and wood	21.1	9320	—	326	SO_2, 269 μg/m^3
India, Gujarat	2.7–10	2220–6070			
Monsoon	56.6	19300			

BaP = benz-a-pyrene; SPM = suspended particulate matter.
Data from de Koning et al., 1985, and WHO: *Air Quality Guidelines*. Regional Reports series 23. Copenhagen: WHO, 1987.

and nonsmoking spouses are more prone to chronic respiratory illnesses and to tobacco-related respiratory cancer when living in the same house as a habitual cigarette smoker. Cigarette smoking is a hazard in another way as well: about 20% to 25% of deaths in domestic fires are a result of smoking.

Biological Hazards. Biological hazards in the indoor environment include many varieties of pathogenic microorganisms. *Mycobacterium tuberculosis* survives for long periods in dark and dusty corners. *Legionella* lives in air conditioners, water-cooled air conditioning systems, stagnant water pipes, and shower stalls, for example. Mites that live on mattresses, cushions, and infrequently swept floors cause asthma, as may many organic dusts and pollens. Many other infections, especially those spread by the fecal-oral route, occur most often when homes are dirty, verminous, or rat infested. Food storage and cooking facilities should be kept scrupulously clean at all times because many varieties of disease-carrying vermin are attracted by filth and because food scraps can be an excellent culture medium for many pathogens that cause food poisoning or other diseases.

Socioeconomic Conditions. Socioeconomic conditions are related to the quality of housing in many ways, some already alluded to. Crowding always tends to be greater among the poor than among the rich; this increases risks of transmitting communicable diseases and often imposes additional emotional stress that probably contributes to domestic violence. Street accidents involving children are more common in poor than in wealthy neighborhoods because the children often have no other place than the street to play. Poor people generally live in poorly equipped and maintained homes, adding to the risk of domestic accidents ranging from falls down poorly lit stairwells to electrocution. Lead poisoning is a particular hazard for children in dilapidated houses where they are likely to ingest dried out flakes of lead-based paint. Emissions from factory smelter stacks contribute to environmental lead and other toxic metal contamination, also more often present in poor than in well-to-do neighborhoods, because the former are more often located in or close to heavily industrialized areas.

HOUSING CONDITIONS AND MENTAL HEALTH

Many descriptive studies by social epidemiologists and psychiatrists have demonstrated a consistent association between mental disorders and urban living conditions.[9] There is also a close relationship between mental health and social class.[10] Those who cannot cope with the competitive pressures of industrial and commercial civilization because they suffer from such disorders as schizophrenia, alcoholism, or mental retardation and have inadequate family and social support systems drift downward to the lowest depths of the slums or become homeless street people. There are estimated to be between 500,000 and 2 million homeless mentally ill persons in the United States.[11] Schizophrenia and alcoholism have maximum prevalence in slums and skid row districts, and depression, manifested by attempted and accomplished suicide, is clustered in neighborhoods where a high proportion of the people live in single-room rented apartments.[12] Behavior disorders such as adolescent delinquency, vandalism, and underachievement at school have high prevalence in dormitory suburbs occupied mainly by low-paid workers, where recreational facilities for young people are often inadequate and schools are often of inferior quality. Bad housing does not cause these problems; they are usually symptoms of more complex social pathology. A different set of factors contribute to the syndrome called "suburban neurosis," which occurs among women who remain housebound for much of the time while their husbands are at work and their children are at school[13]; this condition has been alleviated by television, which by bringing faces and voices into the house relieves loneliness.

HOUSING STANDARDS

Public health workers are directly concerned about the quality of housing because of the many ways it can affect health. Local health officials have special powers to intervene when health is threatened by inadequate housing conditions. A handbook frequently revised by the Centers for Disease Control and the American Public Health Association, *Housing and Health; APHA-CDC Recommended Minimum Housing Standards,*[14] sets out specific details on basic equipment and facilities, fire safety, lighting, ventilation, thermal requirements, sanitation, space requirements (occupancy standards), and the special requirements for rooming houses. This valuable reference spells out general guidelines that can be used by local authorities as the basis for regulations, but there are no universal legally enforcible standards until local jurisdictions introduce them. *Health Principles of Housing,*[15] a WHO manual, gives guidance on a wide range of behavioral factors that can influence health in relation to housing conditions, for example, by providing guidelines on ways to reduce psychological and social stresses by ensuring privacy and comfort and on the housing needs of populations at special risk such as pregnant women, the handicapped, and the elderly infirm. Both these booklets should be part of the library of every local health officer.

STATISTICAL INDICATORS OF HOUSING CONDITIONS

Health planning requires every kind of information pertinent to community health, including statistics on housing conditions. Useful information is routinely collected at the decennial census on density of occupancy (persons per bedroom), cooking and refrigerating facilities, and sanitary conditions. Perusal of tables showing these and other housing statistics enables health planners to identify neighborhoods at high risk of diseases associated with crowding and poor sanitation.

Census tables also enable health planners to identify less obtrusive health hazards, such as proportions of elderly persons living alone, whether in small apartments or multiple-room dwellings that perhaps were once the family home before all the others in the family moved away or died, leaving an elderly person as sole resident. Once such neighborhoods are identified, public health nurses and other community health workers can more easily locate the individuals at risk, who may need but have not yet asked for help.

In addition to census tables, there are other useful sources of information on neighborhoods with a high incidence of social pathology. Fire departments record false alarms and fires deliberately lit; police departments record details of vandalism and calls to settle domestic disturbances, and schools record absenteeism and truancy. All can be analyzed by area, thus pin-pointing high-risk neighborhoods; this method has been used as part of a program aimed at improving the chances of getting a good start in life for children from disadvantaged homes. There is a high correlation between these indicators of social pathology in a neighborhood, such as a high-rise, high-density apartment complex for low-income families, and the incidence of emotional disturbances and similar behavioral upsets among young and teenaged children.[16]

HEALTHY COMMUNITIES AND HEALTHY CITIES

As part of the initiative for "Health for all by the year 2000" that followed resolutions passed at the World Health Assembly in 1977,[17] health planners in many nations, notably in the European Region of WHO, began active planning for health promotion (to be distinguished from disease prevention). Health promotion (see Chapter 1) requires action by many individuals and groups not usually identified with care of the sick or prevention of disease. The definition of health promotion, "the process of enabling people to increase control over and improve their health," implies that people may often have to take action aimed at improving their living conditions. The Healthy Cities movement is a coordinated program involving community health workers, local elected officials in urban affairs, and a wide variety of community groups who collectively seek to upgrade living conditions. Initially, some of the participating cities were relatively healthy places to live (e.g., Toronto, Canada) while others, (e.g., Liverpool, England) were not. The Healthy Cities initiative emphasizes activities that could be expected to enhance good health, such as provision of improved recreational facilities, services for children and their mothers (including basic education for the mothers as well as the children), and aggressive action to eradicate urban wasteland, industrial pollution, toxic dump sites, and other forms of urban blight.[18] From modest beginnings the Healthy Cities movement has spread all over the world, and in some places has extended beyond cities to embrace rural communities.[19] Since the environment in which people live, grow, work, and play so manifestly influences their health and happiness, the Healthy Cities initiative is potentially among the most valuable means at our disposal to make this environment healthful.

SPECIAL HOUSING NEEDS

Elderly and handicapped people require accommodation that has been adapted to enable easier access (ramps, handrails, wide doors to permit passage of wheelchairs), to facilitate storage and preparation of food (low-placed cupboards and stoves with front-fitted switches, which are inadvisable in homes where there are small children), and with special equipment for bathing and toileting (strong handrails, wheelchair access). Special accommodation of this type is often segregated, which tends to set the occupants apart in an urban ghetto for the elderly and handicapped. Integrated special housing is preferable, as examples in Denmark, Sweden, and the United Kingdom have demonstrated; in this setting, elderly, infirm, and younger handicapped persons live among healthy families, which many of them prefer and which helps to accustom healthy people to making allowances for their less fortunate fellow-citizens.

CONCLUSION

This is a brief summary of a complex and diverse field. The essential requirements of the domestic environment have been stressed, along with some of the obvious adverse effects of unsatisfactory housing.

The home should provide more than mere shelter and a safe place to raise children. It should be the setting in which the family lives and grows together, where bonds of affection and mutual trust are formed and strengthened, where socialization into the prevailing culture and intellectual stimulation are occurring, and where privacy is available when it is wanted and needed. Doxiadis[20] coined the term *ekistics,* meaning the science of human settlements, to encompass the many interactive factors that make living space compatible with good physical, mental, emotional, and social health and well-being. The arrangement of dwelling units, their relationship to the natural and to the manmade environment, and their interior structure and function all play a part in creating a housing environment conducive to good health. Many less easily described and unmeasurable factors, such as the innumerable ways that people can interact, also contribute to the ambience of the living space. These intangible factors would receive more attention in a better world than this if we were really intent on applying all possible means to the end of promoting and preserving the public's health.

REFERENCES

1. de Koning HW, Smith KR, Last JM: Biomass fuel combustion and health. Bull WHO 63:11–26, 1985
2. Tabibzadeh I, Rossi-Espagnet A, Maxwell R: Spotlight on the cities; Improving urban health in the developing world. Geneva: WHO, 1989
3. Urbanization and its implications for child health. Geneva: WHO and UN Environmental Programme, 1988

4. World Health Organization: Global Estimates, 1990. Geneva: WHO/HST, 1990
5. Last JM: Biomass fuels. In Environmental Determinants of Health Associated with the Production, Distribution and Use of Energy. Geneva: WHO, 1991
6. Indoor air quality: organic pollutants. WHO Regional Office for Europe, Euro Reports and Studies No. 111, 1987
7. Wertheimer N, Leeper E: Electrical wiring configurations and childhood cancer. Am J Epidemiol, 109:273–284, 1979
8. Savitz D, John EM, Kleckner RC: Magnetic field exposure from electric appliances and childhood cancer. Am J Epidemiol 131:763–773, 1990
9. Srole L, Langner TS, Michael ST, et al: Mental Health in the Metropolis: the Mid-town Manhattan Study. New York: McGraw-Hill, 1962
10. Dohrenwend BP, Dohrenwend BS: Social status and psychological disorder: a causal inquiry. New York: Wiley, 1969
11. American Psychiatric Association Report on the Homeless Mentally Ill. Washington D.C.: The Association, 1984
12. Hare EH: Mental illness and social conditions in Bristol. J Ment Sci 102:349–357, 1956
13. Hare EH, Shaw GK: Mental health on a new housing estate. Oxford: Oxford University Press, 1965
14. Wood EW: Housing and Health: APHA-CDC Recommended Minimum Housing Standards. Washington DC: APHA, 1986
15. Health Principles of Housing. Geneva: WHO, 1989
16. Offord DR, Barrette PA, Last JM: A comparison of school performance, emotional adjustment and skill development of poor and middle-class children. Can J Public Health 76:157–163, 1985
17. Resolution 30.43, World Health Assembly. Geneva: WHO, 1977
18. Kickbusch I (ed): WHO Healthy Cities Project: WHO Healthy Cities Papers 1–5. Copenhagen: FADL Publishers for WHO, 1988–1989. The five papers published so far are (1) Promoting health in the urban context (1988), (2) Five-year planning framework (1988), (3) A guide to assessing healthy cities (1988), (4) The new public health in an urban context (1989), and (5) Good planets are hard to find (1989)
19. Lacombe R: Villes et villages en sante: l'experience Quebecoise. Can J Public Health 80:3–5, 1989
20. Doxiadis CA: Action for Human Settlements. New York: Norton, 1977

39

Global Environment, Health, and Health Services

John M. Last

This chapter considers greenhouse gases and global temperature, ozone depletion and ultraviolet irradiation, acid precipitation, environmental pollution, aspects of population dynamics that relate to these environmental changes, and the effects of these phenomena on health[1-3] and health services.[4] Though some of what follows is speculative, it is based on the judgment of many atmospheric physicists, biologists, and ecologists. The majority view among these experts is that the environment of our planet is changing in ways that could have serious consequences for human health. All people need to behave in ways that will minimize further harm. Public health workers should prepare to face new challenges that will arise as the global environment changes in the next few decades.

GREENHOUSE GASES, AMBIENT TEMPERATURE, CLIMATE, AND WEATHER

Svante Arrhenius pointed out in 1896 that the earth and its mantle of atmosphere behave like a greenhouse.[5] In 1937, G.T. Trewartha used the term "greenhouse effect" to describe how atmospheric gases in the troposphere stabilize the earth's temperature. These gases permit the passage of visible and ultraviolet (UV) radiation from the sun, which warms the earth's surface but blocks the escape back into space of reflected infrared (IR) radiation. This has been known and understood for a long time, but only in the 1980s did we begin to appreciate its ominous implications. The greenhouse effect maintains the biosphere within a temperature range that sustains life. Without the greenhouse effect, almost all the radiant heat from the sun would be reflected back into space, and the surface temperature would be many degrees below freezing. (The surface temperature falls if solar radiation is blocked by dust in the stratosphere, as has happened sometimes after massive volcanic eruptions; the same thing could follow occlusion by smoke and dust after multiple nuclear bomb explosions, the hypothetical phenomenon called "nuclear winter."[6])

Atmospheric physicists are concerned about the rising concentration of greenhouse gases and have predicted that the temperature of the biosphere will rise as a result.[7] The responsible gases are carbon dioxide, oxides of nitrogen, methane, chlorofluorocarbons (CFCs), ozone, and miscellaneous others. All are due to human activity—exhaust emissions from internal combustion engines and coal-burning electric power generators, and various industrial processes. Methane also comes from agricultural and other sources such as rotting vegetation.

Since accurate recording began, the concentration of these gases in the troposphere has accelerated sharply, mainly because of the enormous increase in the scale of combustion of fossil fuels[8] (Fig. 39–1). Accumulating greenhouse gases are beginning to raise global temperature—an estimated 0.5° to 1° C from 1880 to 1990, more rapidly in the last 10 years than in earlier periods (Fig. 39–2).

A temperature rise of up to 3° to 4° C in the next 50 to 100 years has been predicted; this is greater and faster than at any time in the last 140,000 years and could overwhelm the capacity of many species to adapt. A change of this magnitude would affect local, regional, and global ecosystems, sea levels and ocean currents, prevailing winds, fresh water supplies, agriculture, forests, fisheries, industry, transport, urban planning, demographics, and human health. Some effects are mutually reinforcing, so a small additional change in an existing trend could have massive consequences, in accordance with the mathematics of catastrophe theory.[9] There are far-reaching economic and political consequences and security implications.

Changes in the configuration of jet streams, prevailing winds, and ocean currents could alter the distribution of rainfall in many regions, making some wetter, others drier. The American Midwest is expected to get drier, drastically reducing grain production.

Some of these changes are probably already in progress. Six of the ten hottest summers since record keeping began occurred in the 1980s; the summer of 1988 not only was unusually hot but also was a bad season for grain crops throughout the world, leading to a drastic reduction in world grain reserves from about 100 to about 55 days.[10] Grain reserves continued to decline in the next two seasons.

As grasslands and prairies get hotter, they dry out and become even hotter, and the self-correcting effects of vegetation on microclimates is lost. This is one of several feedback loops that accentuate climate change. Temperate zone warming induces a decline in soil moisture that impairs grain production. Moreover, some grain crops, for example, corn and rice, germinate only within a narrow temperature range and would fail in a sustained series of excessively hot growing seasons.

Food crops may be affected in other ways. An unpredictable effect of climate change is altered habitat for pests such as

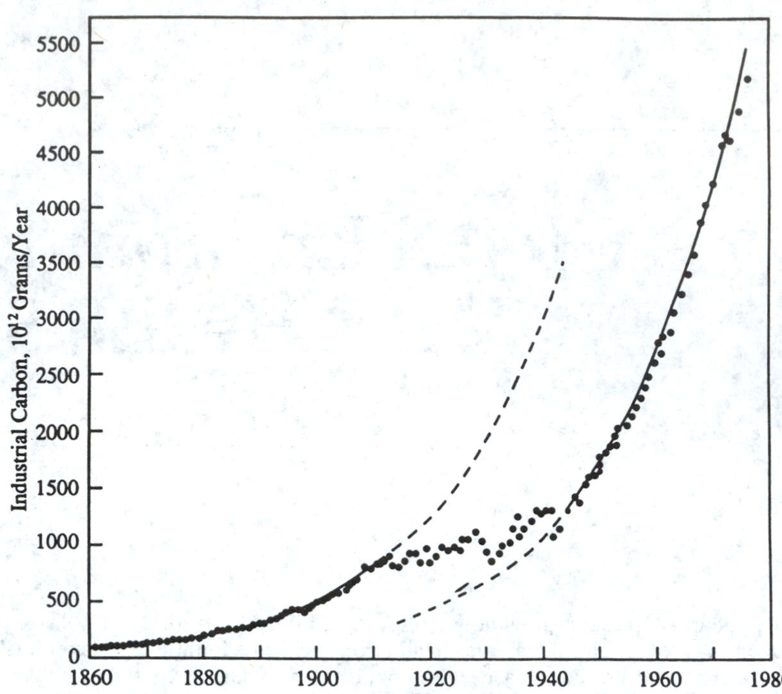

Figure 39-1. Industrial carbon dioxide production since the late nineteenth century; the rate has been exponential, with minor perturbations due to world wars and depressions. [*From Abrahamson DE (ed): The Challenge of Global Warming. Washington, D.C.: Island Press, 1989.*]

insects, fungus, and microorganisms that cause blight and other diseases of grain, fruits, and vegetables such as potatoes.

Changes in the composition of vegetation on large land masses lead to and are accentuated by wider temperature swings. Many species of trees in temperate zone forests cannot survive at ambient temperatures exceeding even by only a few degrees those that prevail now.

Forests are disappearing because of human depredation. In the tropics, primeval rain forests are being slash-burned to clear land for agriculture or are being cut to gather hardwood trees. In temperate zones such as the high-rainfall regions of the Pacific slopes of North America, forests have been subjected to clear-cut logging. Slash-burning of tropical rain forests contributes to the atmospheric burden of carbon dioxide and is causing the loss of many species of plants and animals, as well as reducing the amount of vegetation available to metabolize carbon dioxide, further aggravating the atmospheric carbon dioxide buildup.

In high latitudes the warming could thaw permafrost, releasing long-frozen rotting vegetation in arctic bogs and ponds. This would lead to emission of large amounts of methane, adding yet more to the burden of atmospheric greenhouse gases.

Because oceanic upwelling and thermal air currents are destabilized by global warming, violent weather disturbances such as hurricanes are likely to become more frequent; the relatively predictable pattern of tropical cyclones may already be changing, if recent unprecedented storms in Europe are an indication.

An important consequence of global warming is sea-level rise due to thermal expansion of the sea water mass and to melting of ice caps. The likely extent of polar and alpine ice melt is difficult to predict. In a worst-case scenario the entire Antarctic ice shelf would break away and melt, causing a sea-level rise of 5 to 7 m; most experts consider this unlikely; a conservative estimate is a sea-level rise of 1 to 1.5 m in the next 50 to 100 years. This would be enough to submerge coastal wetlands and disrupt their ecosystems. This process may be aggravated by other factors. For example, the annual monsoon floods in Bangladesh are

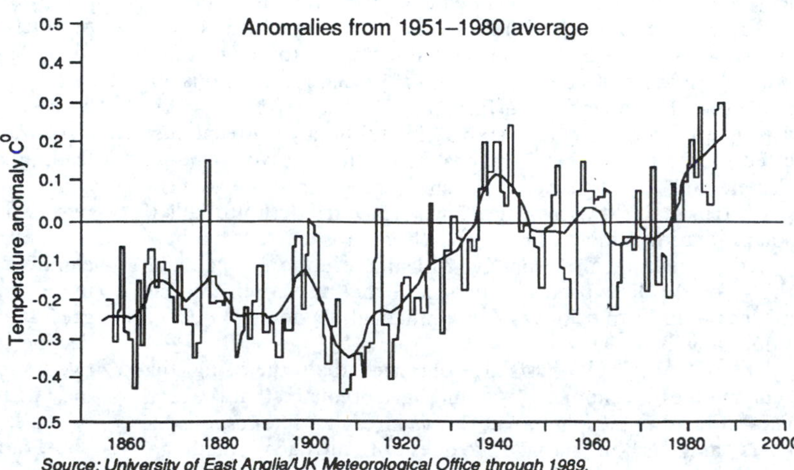

Figure 39-2. Annual average surface temperature of the earth 1856 to 1989. [*From The Globe and Mail, Toronto.*]

made worse by deforestation of the Himalayas, leading to a deluge of run-off rains in contrast to more gentle water-level rise when vegetation impeded the flow.

Many of the world's important fishing grounds are dependent on ecosystems involving coastal wetlands and the diverse flora and fauna they support, so coastal flooding would contribute to depletion of fish stocks. In some areas, for example, the Grand Banks off Newfoundland, fish catches are already falling sharply because of overfishing in past years. In many places, fish once plentiful at the surface are now found only at great depths. Drift-net fishing accelerates depletion, indiscriminately taking everything that lives in the sea. Ecological disasters such as massive oil spills increase the danger to fishing grounds.

All the above phenomena add up to a serious threat to food security. There could be severe food shortages, perhaps worldwide famines by early in the twenty-first century.

A sea level rise of 1 to 1.5 m would drown many coastal communities: most of Bangladesh and the Netherlands, and unless protective dikes are built, parts of many large cities—London, New York, Washington, Miami, Tokyo, Shanghai, Calcutta, Jakarta, Singapore, Lagos, Copenhagen, and Leningrad, to name a few—but there are many more. Sea level rise therefore will greatly increase the numbers of "ecological refugees" (discussed later).

Fresh water supplies are threatened by salination of coastal estuaries. Potable fresh water resources may decline not only because of this but also because sea water infiltrates subterranean water tables, as in many parts of Florida where porous limestone readily permits passage of salt water. Another cause of fresh water shortage is depletion of fossil water and artesian basins; for example, the water table below the southern United States is being withdrawn more rapidly than it can be replenished. Elsewhere, depletion of artesian water is causing subsidence, which leads to seasonal floods, as in Bangkok and Venice.[11] Moreover, water supplies are often polluted with toxic waste, constituents of domestic refuse, human excreta, or all of these.

Global warming will change the distribution of vegetation. The capability of grain crops and trees to "migrate" from hot to cooler zones is debatable.[12] As forest canopies recede from temperate zones, they are replaced by cultivated land or pasture (grassland or savannah); the distribution of noxious weeds, including many allergens, also shifts, and so will the myriad species of insects whose habitats are related to specific varieties of vegetation. Areas now devoted to grain crops will become drier, desertified; topsoil is lost in dust storms.

The distribution of insect vectors of disease will change: as the temperate zones get warmer, they will become more hospitable to ticks and hematophagous insects such as anophelene and culicine mosquitoes; consequently many arthropodborne diseases are likely to extend over a wider range.

Over the next 50 years the average annual number of very hot days is expected to double in the temperate zone cities of the world. The "heat island" phenomenon that makes cities warmer than surrounding rural areas will lead to longer and more severe heat waves than we are accustomed to now. This will strain utilities and essential services such as fire departments. Heat waves increase the demand for air conditioning, but unless solar energy is used, extra consumption of fossil fuels makes matters worse by adding further to the burden of greenhouse gases.

OZONE DEPLETION AND ULTRAVIOLET IRRADIATION

The stratospheric ozone layer is located at an altitude of 12 to 24 km. This layer provides protection against the harmful biological effects of UV irradiation. There are three wavelengths of UV radiation. The longest and least dangerous is UV-A (320 to 400 nm), the shortest and most dangerous is UV-C (200 to 290 nm); this is blocked by stratospheric nitrogen oxides and ozone. The midband UV-B radiation, 290 to 320 nm, penetrates in greater amounts when stratospheric ozone is attenuated. UV-B causes DNA damage proportional to the amount of exposure.

In the early 1970s an expert panel of the National Academy of Sciences examined the threat to the stratospheric ozone layer presented by lighter-than-air chemicals capable of destroying ozone by converting its molecules into oxygen. The principal chemicals discussed at that time were oxides of nitrogen, emitted as exhaust gases by high-flying supersonic jet aircraft, and CFCs. The panel recommended limiting the production of CFCs, which are used as propellants in spray-cans, aerating agents, refrigerants, and solvents, and advised the US government not to develop supersonic passenger jet aircraft because of the destructive effects of their exhaust gases on the ozone layer.[13,14]

The stratospheric ozone layer has been under observation since the first satellites were launched into orbit in the 1950s. It was observed to be thinning over Antarctica in 1984–1985. Repeated observations have confirmed the attenuation and charted its progress. Between 1956 and 1976, the first 20 years of observations from space, the ozone layer was stable; since then its thickness over Antarctica has declined by a third or more. Attenuation has also been observed in the northern hemisphere. In 1990 the southern hemisphere attenuation was the most widespread yet, extending over the inhabited areas of southern Australia and Argentina. On average worldwide the stratospheric ozone layer has declined by 4% in the last 12 years.[15] The period of observation is short, and the natural history of the ozone layer is imperfectly understood; we know little about how ozone is produced from oxygen molecules, how it circulates, or how it is degraded again into oxygen. The attenuation could be part of a natural cycle of fluctuation, but it is following a pattern that accords with predictions based on the atmospheric buildup and physical chemistry of CFCs.

Stratospheric ozone depletion must not be confused with tropospheric ozone accumulation; ozone is a toxic greenhouse gas in the troposphere, but a vital protective layer against potentially lethal UV-B irradiation in the stratosphere.

The human health effects of increased ultraviolet (UV-B) irradiation due to ozone depletion, described later, are less important than adverse effects on single-celled and small organisms, notably plankton in surface layers of the oceans—the beginning of many important food chains. Many species of pollen and nitrogen-forming soil bacteria may also be at risk, although it is difficult to say when such effects may begin or what will be their consequences. The implications for evolution of a large increase in UV-B irradiation (i.e., the mutagenic effects) are unpredictable but are unlikely to be desirable. Of course UV radiation also contributes to global warming.

ACID PRECIPITATION

Acid precipitation is due mainly to the solution of sulfur dioxide in water vapor to produce sulfuric acid. Sulfur dioxide is the principal polluting gas emitted from combustion of coal, especially soft coal. Other gases that produce acid precipitants include oxides of carbon (carbonic acid) and nitrogen (nitric acid). They are usually emitted high into the atmosphere from tall chimney stacks and travel far on the wind, often across international borders. Downwind from heavily industrialized areas, the rain sometimes has a pH of 4.0 or even lower.

The effects of acid precipitation are primarily ecological. Although some adverse human health effects have been demonstrated, the associations are weak and inconsistent, for example, between acid fog and chronic respiratory disease[16] and between acid haze and certain varieties of cancer.[17] Acid precipitation has serious effects on delicate aquatic ecosystems and also on some species of plants and trees, causing severe damage to the growing ends of many trees. Some alpine trees are rapidly killed by acid mist or cloud, leading to deforestation and soil erosion. The effects of acidifying chemicals, that is, oxides of sulfur, ozone, chlorine, and nitrogen oxides, are synergistic. Indirectly, acid precipitation adversely affects human health if essential food chains are disrupted. Other indirect health effects may follow changes in trace element concentrations. Economic consequences are serious: for instance, maple trees and the lucrative maple sugar industry face extinction in eastern Canada and the northeastern United States.

ENVIRONMENTAL POLLUTION

Water, soil and food throughout the world are contaminated by heavy metals, for example, organic mercury compounds, lead, and cadmium, by organic chemical compounds such as PCBs and dioxins, and by radioactive waste products.

Environmental mercury contamination has several causes. It is mainly due to the presence of trace amounts of mercury in emissions from coal-burning electric power stations. This has led to worldwide fallout of mercury in rainfall, amounting to about 6×10^9 g/y.[18] Mercury enters marine ecosystems and is concentrated in food chains that end with fish (or fish-eating birds and humans). Acid precipitation accelerates the chemical changes. The environmental burden of toxic organic compounds of mercury has increased by two orders of magnitude since the beginning of the industrial revolution, a fact verified by assay of sea birds' plumage obtained from museum specimens. Some ecologists have suggested that women in the reproductive years should not eat fish more often than once or twice weekly because of accumulation of the body burden, which puts the early developing fetus at risk. Mercury passes across the placenta and can cause Minamata disease (See Chapter 20).

Environmental lead contamination is a serious problem in many industrial areas because of the presence of lead in fallout from smelter stacks and in leaded gasoline. Low-level lead intoxication causes mild mental retardation (see Chapter 20). In some urban industrial areas elevated lead levels (measured in dentine from primary teeth) and a statistically significant associated reduction in IQ have been observed among high proportions of elementary age school children.[19]

Many organic chemicals, notably PCBs and dioxins, have become widespread in the environment; those that are passed through food chains because they resemble enzymes in chemical structure or because they are fat soluble have been disseminated worldwide, even in the high Arctic. Their biological effects remain controversial, although in laboratory animals and in some human exposures there is evidence that PCBs and dioxins are teratogenic, mutagenic, and carcinogenic.

Chemical pollution of underground aquifers and of rivers and lakes has occurred in many parts of the world, often leading to public outrage. Evidence of adverse effects on health, however, remains elusive. Chemical waste dumps in Niagara Falls, New York, attracted notoriety in the early 1970s when persons living near the Love Canal dump site became ill; there were some deaths from leukemia and cancer, although a cause-effect relationship could not be established.[20] In 1975, Canadian wildlife biologists studied an epidemic of reproductive failure (embryonic death, failure to hatch, gross deformities of chicks) among herring-gull and other marine bird colonies on Lake Ontario. This was associated with extremely high concentrations of dioxins and PCBs in the birds' livers and egg yolks; the source was a toxic spill into the Niagara River about 1970.[21-23] No firm evidence of adverse human reproductive outcomes has been demonstrated, but gross malformations of marine birds and high rates of hatching failure have been consistently observed ever since. Chemical contamination of aquifers and wells is suspected as the cause of several cancer and leukemia clusters; but in all such instances the epidemiological and toxicological evidence is weak. The same is true of several examples of environmental contamination with radioactive waste, as at Sellafield in England, where the evidence has repeatedly been reviewed but proof of harm to human health has been difficult to establish.[24] Only massive disasters such as Chernobyl are unequivocally harmful to human health.

Radioactive waste products from nuclear power stations and nuclear weapons production have become a serious disposal problem in many countries. It has been customary to dispose of nuclear waste with extremely long half-lives by burying it, for example, in abandoned mine shafts. This short-term solution fails to recognize that some nuclear waste will remain radioactive for periods measurable in units of time more customary among geologists than human biologists.

DEMOGRAPHIC CHANGES RELATED TO GLOBAL ENVIRONMENTAL CHANGES

Ultimately the cause of almost all these problems is that there are so many people on earth, consuming so much energy and producing so much waste. The growth rate of human populations has been exponential for several generations (Fig. 39–3). The cost of this spectacular reproductive success has been the loss of many wilderness areas and extinction of an increasing number of species of other living creatures that competed against humans or human agricultural and industrial development for a share of the same finite resources of space, land, water, and nourishment. This human swarming has also been accompanied by industrial development with exponential increases in fossil fuel combustion. The problems are aggravated by the perception that resources are limitless and by haphazard and often irresponsible disposal of industrial waste.

The sincerely held beliefs of many millions of adherents to several of the world's religions, and in many nations the prevailing political philosophy, are impediments to limiting human reproductive exuberance. The biological cost of unrestrained family size, that is, extinction of other species, has not been considered in religious beliefs and political programs that proscribe effective contraception.

As resources have been depleted in some parts of the world, the people who previously lived in these places have had to leave when their environment could no longer sustain them. In the past the main reason for movement of "ecological refugees," especially in Africa, has been desertification; sea level rise could soon become another cause of population movement. There are increasing numbers of ecological refugees in many developing countries, notably in expanding periurban slums in Latin America and parts of Africa and Asia. Ecological refugees are also beginning to alter the sociodemographic composition of developed nations in Western Europe and North America.[25]

Mass migrations are a public health problem: people carry their diseases with them and are at risk of other diseases at their destination. When their cultural, linguistic, or ethnic backgrounds differ from those of the host nation, there are often barriers to provision of health care. Sometimes immigrants become members of an underclass that has little contact with health services. Additional problems arise from competition for jobs and from cultural clashes between immigrants and established residents. These can strain the fabric of health care and other services. Family disruption can also be a complication.

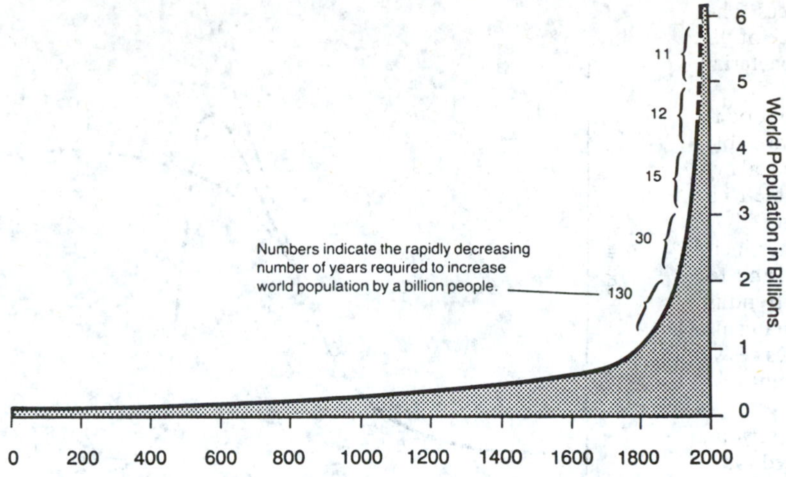

Figure 39-3. Population growth rates since antiquity; the period required for increase by each successive billion has been getting progressively shorter.

THREATS TO SECURITY

Competition for diminishing resources is a potential and often an actual cause of conflict among and within nations. Many localized wars in the last 40 years fall into this category, although most are attributed to ideological, religious, or ethnic differences. As we enter the 1990s, regional and local conflicts remain widespread. It is easy to imagine a world in which peace, order, and good government are replaced by fragmentation into anarchic warring communities. The only goal of all such communities would be to survive; aspirations to improve the human condition would be an impossible luxury.

No matter what the underlying causes may be, all wars disrupt civil order, including provision of health care, and also disrupt food supplies. Conflicts where food supplies are already scarce are bound to aggravate the scarcity.

POLITICAL IMPLICATIONS

There has never been a greater need for long-term vision and planning by leaders of every nation. The United Nations (UN) agencies and organizations concerned about the environment, such as the United Nations Environmental Programme and the World Meteorological Organization, have demonstrated their capability for collaborative efforts, but these organizations lack political power. When irrefutable facts demonstrate that the situation has become urgent, as happened in the mid-1980s with stratospheric ozone depletion, some nations collaborated in signing the Montreal Protocol that called for sharp reductions in CFC production and use worldwide. However, there are no powers to enforce compliance, and many nations either have not signed the Montreal Protocol or intend to ignore it. In November 1990 at a meeting in Geneva, heads of all nations but one agreed to reduce carbon emissions as a step toward control of the greenhouse effect. The exception was the United States, which is responsible for about 25% of global carbon emissions; the reason for the US noncompliance was the economic disruption it would cause.

HEALTH EFFECTS OF GLOBAL ENVIRONMENTAL CHANGES

It is difficult to measure some of the environmental changes discussed above. There is controversy about some predictions, disagreement over interpretation of empirical observations, and argument about whether or when global warming, climate change, altered habitats, and sea level rise will begin.[26] There are large error factors in models that attempt to predict future climate and weather. It is also most difficult to relate the measurements and models to effects on human health.

Causal relationships, credibility, and public acceptance of the evidence are difficult enough to establish even when we have straightforward causes and effects like cigarette smoking and lung cancer. Existing effects, if any, of the global environmental changes discussed here have not included obvious evidence of damage to human health. We have no indicators of adverse health effects, let alone adequate methods of relating these effects to environmental causes. Moreover some predicted health effects are indirect and remote—mass starvation following crop failure for instance, although if this occurs, it will be too late to take steps to prevent its underlying causes.

Some probable effects of global environmental change on human health have already been suggested. We can expect a rise in prevalence of diseases and premature deaths related to heat stress; this primarily affects the very young, the very old, and persons with chronic respiratory and cardiovascular diseases. Prolonged hot weather also appears to aggravate tendencies toward violent and antisocial behavior, leading to more episodes of domestic violence as well as riots and other forms of civil disturbance which could become another public health problem.

Increased atmospheric pollution, dust, and greater quantities of atmospheric allergens lead to higher incidence and prevalence of allergic respiratory diseases. Chronic respiratory diseases associated with acid precipitation and with rising concentrations of atmospheric dusts and pollens also will become more prevalent.

The range of some vector-borne diseases is likely to extend more widely into temperate zones now free of these diseases. These diseases include malaria, arthropodborne virus and rickettsial diseases such as viral hemorrhagic fevers, dengue, viral encephalitides, tickborne diseases such as typhus and Lyme disease, and perhaps bubonic plague. The range of bats that carry rabies is also likely to extend more widely.[27] We have effective vaccines and other preventive and therapeutic measures against some but not others on this list.

Drinking water and many staple foods are increasingly threatened with contamination by toxic chemicals, which have caused environmental disasters such as the reproductive failure among marine birds on the Great Lakes in the mid-1970s and the bizarre diseases that afflicted both cattle and humans after contamination of a batch of cattle feed with polybrominated biphenyls (PBBs) in Michigan in 1974[28] (see Chapter 21).

Many sewage treatment plants would be inundated by a quite modest sea level rise, as they are now by flash floods after heavy rainstorms, causing deterioration of sanitary services. The consequence would be increased incidence and prevalence of diarrheal diseases, including parasitic infections as well as bacterial and viral infections of the gastrointestinal tract.

Long-term low-level chemical pollution of water and food is frustratingly difficult to study: there have been innumerable complaints and investigations, but only rarely is unequivocal evidence found of adverse human health effects attributable to a particular toxic substance in the environment. See Chapter 21.

Increased levels of UV irradiation will lead to higher incidence rates of melanotic and nonmelanotic skin cancer and to higher incidence of cataract. There is evidence that this trend is already established.[29,30] Impaired immune defense mechanisms are a further consequence of UV irradiation; this reduces resistance to infection and increases susceptibility to malignant disease.

Disrupted crops and other food supplies may well be serious enough to cause episodes of localized, perhaps generalized famine. This effect of global climate change presents the greatest threat to the greatest numbers of people. Even without this, populations in many parts of the world are likely to experience chronic undernutrition, with consequent impaired resistance to infections of all kinds. Since the 1970s there have been repeated small-scale famines in parts of Africa; these are but harbingers of what we might expect to occur on a much larger scale soon. Together or separately, these factors greatly increase the risk of severe and widespread epidemics, for example, of influenza.

The combination of all these processes could be enough to alter the direction of the exponential growth rate of the human population. Much of our thinking about the future, from economic forecasts to plans for care of the elderly and future industrial expansion, has been based on assumptions that the rate of growth of populations will continue on its present course well into the twenty-first century; the United Nations Statistical Office forecasts a world population of 14 billion before the growth curve levels off.[31] No serious demographic or economic forecasts have been based on alternative assumptions, for instance, on the possibility that the human population growth curve might behave like that of other biological organisms in a closed, finite system.[32] We are, of course, living in a closed and finite system, the biosphere. Like a bacterial colony in a culture medium, we are susceptible to depletion of nutriments and to poisoning by our own waste products. The growth curve of the human population could go into reverse: the exponential growth phase might be succeeded by a phase of precipitous decline (Fig. 39–4). Such a possibility was among the scenarios produced 20 years ago by the Club of Rome.[33] It accords with catastrophe theory and with empirical observations of closed biological systems. An extreme scenario suggests extinction of the human species, but a more likely possibility is rapid decline, perhaps by two or three orders of magnitude.

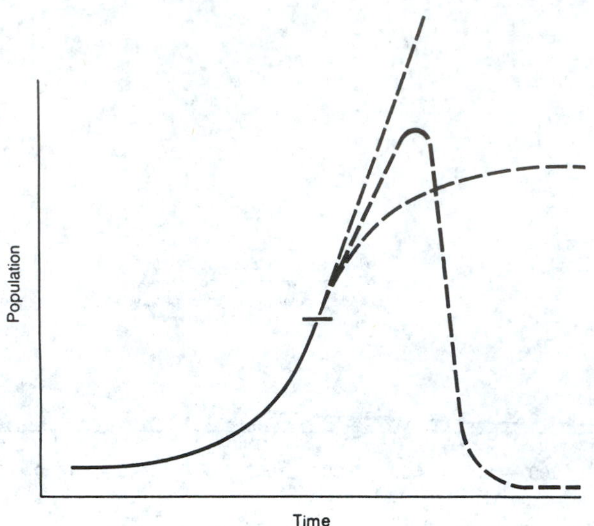

Figure 39–4. Possible outcomes of population growth; exponential growth cannot continue indefinitely and must eventually be followed by a phase of leveling off or decline.

IMPLICATIONS FOR THE FUTURE OF HEALTH CARE SYSTEMS

Instabilities of economic and political systems disrupt the provision of personal and public health services. The kind of instabilities likely to accompany the changes described here could lead to the collapse of organized health services in many parts of the world. In an era of scarcity of food, water, money, and other resources and of the threat to survival suggested above, priorities must be reassessed. Our present health care system is strongly oriented toward tertiary care, is extravagant, and gets more costly for progressively diminishing returns with every passing year.

We expend huge sums on high-technology care, mainly of the irretrievably ill; estimates of the distribution of individual life-time health care expenditure suggest that 60% or more of lifetime expenses for medical care are incurred in the last six months of life. We have other priorities in the wrong places.

We put too much emphasis on "curative" measures (which are often only palliative) and not enough on preserving and protecting health. This is part of the value system of our culture, epitomized in many ways, for instance, in our pursuit of remedies for obesity. Obesity and other diseases due to overeating disappear rapidly in an era of scarcity.

Instead of our preoccupation with ways to prolong individual lives (on average by only a few months[34]), we should become concerned about the survival of communities. The child survival strategies developed by the United Nations Childrens Fund (UNICEF) have proven efficacious in many developing nations,[35] but without effective family planning programs, enhancing child survival makes matters worse by leading to greater population pressures.[36] Promoting literacy of women in the reproductive years is an essential part of family planning programs.

Many health services are inadequately equipped to cope with heat emergencies: we may soon need facilities to manage large numbers of cases of heat exhaustion and heat stroke; upgrading these facilities has high priority. Health services are often inadequately equipped also to cope with the medical and public health emergencies associated with natural disasters such as extensive floods that follow severe rainstorms. The emergencies include management of large numbers of people suddenly rendered homeless and vulnerable to infections, such as gastrointestinal infections that increase in incidence because sewage treatment plants have been flooded. Booster doses of immunizing agents are another high priority for people after natural disasters.

Other public health measures will become more important than they have been in the past. Environmental monitoring of water and food, public health nutrition (national food policies), and immunization programs will have to be given higher priority, as will people-management techniques, for example, to cope with refugees.

Most important are family planning programs and policies. Ultimately the problems we face are due to overpopulation. The world needs nothing so much as a few generations of single-child families. If this could be accomplished, instead of the human and mathematical catastrophe of precipitous decline in numbers, we would experience a leveling-off of population and stabilizing of the global environmental situation. To achieve this would require an unprecedented effort and unanimity of purpose worldwide.

CONCLUSION: WHAT CAN WE DO?

Not merely humanity but all life on earth is facing the most serious ecological crisis since the last ice age, perhaps the most serious since the cataclysmic upheaval that led to the extinction of dinosaurs 65 million years ago. By any standards this is a public health problem of enormous dimensions. How can we address this problem? Can we extricate ourselves from the predicament that confronts us?

Addressing and solving public health problems requires all the following: knowledge about the nature and causes of the problem, technical capability to solve the problem, a sense of values that the problem matters, and the political will to mobilize the necessary resources to deal with the problem.

A report of the United Nations World Commission on the Environment and Development, *Our Common Future,*[37] contained clear statements on three of these four essential requirements for dealing with the problem and sensibly addressed the fourth, the question of political will. However, with rare exceptions, leaders of nations, of industry and commerce, and ordinary people everywhere have ignored this important report. Few pay attention to serious reviews of the global situation and steps we should be taking to control it, even when the reports are commercially published and widely marketed, as are the annual reports of the Worldwatch Institute.[38]

Like earlier volumes in the series, the 1990 Report of the Worldwatch Institute[39] argues cogently for "sustainable development" with many suggestions for greater use of solar power and human muscle power, as well as increased efforts at cleaning the environment—the air, the water, the land. These ideas are stated in the form of a code of environmental conduct in *Environment and Health,*[40] a document produced after a conference of representatives from countries of the European Region of WHO in December 1989. This document sets out clearly the elements of public policy that will be needed to transform the environmental status of European nations. The economic and political implications of this charter are, however, likely to impede necessary effective steps to implement it.

The relentlessly increasing numbers of humanity and their demands for development, economic equity, and security make many such suggestions seem impractical. The Worldwatch Institute also makes a strong case for converting world economies from warlike to peaceful activities, a case strengthened by the striking political realignments that took place in the second half of 1989. Yet despite these political changes, many wars continue unabated in developing countries, and the nations of the world continue to spend far more on military than socially useful activities such as education and health enhancement.[41]

The Challenges. We know quite a lot about the nature and causes of global environmental change. It is impossible not to be awestruck by its complexity, its connection to the technical, economic, and sociopolitical basis of civilized life. It is impossible not to be intimidated by the implications for virtually every aspect of civilized life of attempting to retard, let alone to halt or reverse, the responsible industrial activities.

Increased concern demonstrated by frequent mass media discussions, the growth of "green" political parties, declining popularity of "disposable" consumer goods and environmentally unfriendly packaging and the like have had little impact on the pace at which our planet is deteriorating. Small cars that consume less gasoline than the larger models of the 1950s and 1960s still consume gasoline and still are often occupied by just one person when they clog the freeways during rush hours. In the industrial nations the average person produces well over a ton of nonrecyclable garbage every year. In these and many other ways most people demonstrate their indifference to our predicament. There is an element of denial in this attitude, akin to the dying man's denial that he has an incurable disease or to the adolescent's belief that death is a remote event that will not be hastened by taking risks.

The difficult challenges are further compounded by great differences in values between the industrially developed and the developing nations; in the former, concern exists and is growing greater, and there is some motivation to begin conserving resources; but in developing nations that are beginning to industrialize, there is much resistance and resentment among political and industrial leaders when environmental scientists suggest that industrial development must be slowed or stopped.

Possible Responses. One response that has high priority is to develop international networks of concerned health professionals, for which an excellent model exists. A loose-knit but cohesive medical organization, International Physicians for the Prevention of Nuclear War (IPPNW), successfully brought to widespread public knowledge the medical consequences of a large-scale nuclear conflict and in that way did much to force many national leaders, especially those in the two super powers, to confront the reality of their warlike posturing. The efforts of IPPNW were crowned with the award of the Nobel Peace Prize. What is needed now is a similar coalition of health workers all over the world, aimed at bringing to greater public notice the health consequences of the deteriorating global environment. Although most individuals and national leaders seem relatively indifferent to the environmental deterioration that is so evident to all, the dangers to their own and their children's health might motivate them to take action, if these dangers were effectively and dramatically drawn to their attention. One way to do this would be to develop and publicize plans to deal with the environmental catastrophes that can be predicted with reasonable reliability as consequences of the trends now evident in the global environment. If it were widely perceived that health professionals as a social institution collectively take this threat seriously, there is some prospect that other important groups in society might also take it seriously enough to do something about it.

In addition, planning to cope with these catastrophes is urgently needed for its own sake. Almost certainly there will be climatic catastrophes, for which at present we are ill-prepared.

If all industrial uses of fossil fuels and CFCs stopped today, the atmosphere would continue to deteriorate for decades. It would take many years and cost trillions of dollars for us to convert to solar and other nonpolluting energy sources. Fossil fuel–based industry is not going to stop today, or tomorrow. We can expect greenhouse gases to continue accumulating. Global warming is inevitable. Our best hope is to begin preparing for its widespread consequences. For those of us in the health professions, this means preparing to shift priorities away from high-technology tertiary care services, which will become increasingly irrelevant, and concentrating on expanding and improving all aspects of public health services.

REFERENCES

1. Leaf A: Potential health effects of global climatic and environmental changes. N Engl J Med 321:1577–1583, 1989
2. McCally M, Cassel CK: Medical responsibility and global environmental change. Ann Intern Med 113:467–473, 1990
3. Potential health effects of climatic change. Geneva: World Health Organization, WHO/PEP/90.10, 1990

4. Last JM: A vision of health in the 21st century: Medical response to the greenhouse effect. Can Med Assoc J 140:1277–1279, 1989
5. Arrhenius S: On the influence of carbonic acid in the air upon the temperature on the ground. Philosophical Magazine 41:237–276, 1896
6. Turco RP, et al: Nuclear winter: Global consequences of multiple nuclear explosions. Science 222:1283–1292, 1983
7. Schneider SH: Climate modeling. Sci Am 256(5):72–80, 1987
8. Schneider SH: The greenhouse effect: Science and policy. Science 243:771–781, 1989
9. Woodcock A, Davis M: Catastrophe Theory. New York: Dutton, 1978
10. Brown LR: Feeding six billion. Worldwatch 2(5):32–40, 1989
11. la Riviere JWM: Threats to the world's water. Sci Am 261:80–94, 1989
12. Roberts L: How fast can trees migrate? Science 243:735–737, 1989
13. Climatic Impact Committee, National Academy of Sciences: Environmental Impact of Stratospheric Flight: Biological and Climatic Effects of Aircraft Emissions in the Stratosphere. Washington D.C.: National Academy of Sciences, 1975
14. Panel on Stratospheric Chemistry and Transport, Committee on Impacts of Stratospheric Change, National Academy of Sciences: Stratospheric Ozone Depletion by Halocarbons: Chemistry and Transport. Washington D.C.: National Academy of Sciences, 1979
15. Stolarsky RS: The Antarctic ozone hole. Sci Am 258:30–36, 1988, and presentation at NIEHS Conference on Global Atmospheric Change and Health. Raleigh, N.C., November 1989
16. Shy CM, Goldsmith JR, Hackney JD, et al: Health effects of air pollution. Am Thoracic Soc News 4:22–63, 1978
17. Gorham ED, Garland CF, Garland FC: Acid haze air pollution and breast and colon cancer mortality in 20 Canadian cities. Can J Public Health 80:96–100, 1989
18. Fitzgerald W: Mercury and methyl mercury in the environment: Present and future concerns. Paper presented at NIEHS Conference on Global Atmospheric Change and Health. Raleigh, N.C., November 1989
19. Mushak P, Davis JM, Crocetti AF, Grant LD: Prenatal and postnatal effects of low-level lead exposure: Integrated summary of a report to the US Congress on childhood lead poisoning. Env Res 50:11–36, 1989
20. Committee on Response Strategies to Unusual Chemical Hazards, Board of Toxicology and Environmental Health Hazards: Proceedings of Workshop on Plans for Clinical and Epidemiological Followup after Area-wide Chemical Contamination. Washington D.C.: National Academy of Sciences, 1982
21. Peakall DB, Fox GA, Gilman AP, et al: Reproductive success of herring gulls as an indicator of Great Lakes water quality. In Afghan BK, Mackay D (eds): Hydrocarbons in the aquatic environment. New York: Plenum, 1980, pp 337–344
22. Gilman AP, Peakall DB, Hallett DJ, Fox GA, Norstrom RJ: Herring gulls (*Larus argentatus*) as monitors of contamination in the Great Lakes. In Animals as Monitors of Environmental Pollutants. Washington D.C.: National Academy of Sciences, 1979, pp 280–289
23. Fox GA, Last JM: Unpublished data, 1980–1982
24. Black D, Adelstein AM, Berry RJ, et al: Investigation of the possible increased incidence of cancer in West Cumbria: A report of the independent advisory group. London: Her Majesty's Stationery Office, 1984
25. Charting Canada's Future: A Report of the Demographic Review. Ottawa: Health and Welfare Canada, 1989
26. Global Change. Science 245:449, 1990
27. Shope R: Global warming and public health. Health Environ Digest 4(9):1–4, 1990
28. Anderson HA, Lilis R, Selikoff IJ, et al: Unanticipated prevalence of symptoms among dairy farmers in Michigan and Wisconsin. Environ Health Perspect 23:217–226, 1978
29. Lee JAH: Melanoma and exposure to sunlight. Epidemiol Rev 4:110–136, 1982
30. Sunlight, ultraviolet radiation and the skin. NIH Consensus Conference Statement, Vol. 7 No. 8, May 8–10, 1989
31. UN Department of International Economic and Social Affairs: World Population Trends and Policies. New York: UN Statistical Office, 1983
32. Andrewartha HG, Birch LC: The distribution and abundance of animals. Chicago: University of Chicago Press, 1954, Part IV, pp 557–665; Williamson M: Island Populations. Oxford: Oxford University Press, 1981
33. Meadows DH, Meadows DL, Randers J, Behrens WW: The Limits to Growth: A Report for the Club of Rome's Project on the Predicament of Mankind. New York: Potomac Associates, Universe Books, 1972
34. McKinlay JB, McKinlay SM, Beaglehole R: Influence of medical care on mortality and morbidity. Int J Health Services 19:181–208, 1989
35. Grant JM: The State of the World's Children (annual reports of UNICEF). New York: Oxford University Press
36. King M: Health is a sustainable state. Lancet 336:664–667, 1990
37. United Nations World Commission on Environment and Development: Our Common Future (the Brundtland Report). Oxford and New York: Oxford University Press, 1987
38. Brown LR, Durning A, Flavin C, et al: State of the World 1989 (Annual Report of the Worldwatch Institute). New York: Norton, 1989
39. Brown LR, Durning A, Flavin C, et al: State of the World 1990. New York: Norton, 1990
40. Environment and Health: The European Charter and Commentary. Copenhagen: WHO European Regional Office, Regional Office Publications, No. 35, 1990
41. Sivard RL, Brauer A, Roemer MI: World Military and Social Expenditures. Washington D.C.: World Priorities, Inc, 1989

SECTION FOUR

Behavioral Factors Affecting Health

Edited by Jonathan E. Fielding

40

Social Determinants of Disease

S. Leonard Syme

The prevention of disease is a major goal of public health programs. In developing and implementing prevention programs, environmental factors are increasingly recognized as important components. In part, this recognition is based on the fact that many diseases of concern involve large numbers of people and that it is more cost-effective to prevent such diseases at an environmental level than at a "one-to-one" individual level. A concern for environmental factors also has developed because of the difficulty in getting individuals to change their behaviors; in many cases it is more efficient to change the environment than to encourage individuals, one at a time, to change their behaviors. Yet a third reason for the increasing interest in environmental factors is the fact that the distribution of many diseases remains relatively constant over time even though individuals come and go from the population; this constancy of rate suggests that there is something about the environment that elicits a characteristic rate of disease in different population groups.

This chapter is concerned with the influence on health of social factors in the environment. This limited focus is not meant to suggest that the social environment stands alone in its relationship to health and disease. The term *environment* is a general one describing many different conditions and influences under which any person or thing lives or develops. This term has been used to describe many phenomena, including the air we breathe, the water we drink, the geographic regions and buildings in which we live, the groups to which we belong, and the climatic conditions we experience.[1] Although one can distinguish between the man-made environment, the natural environment, and the social and cultural environment, none of these aspects exists independently of the others: the environment is the result of the continuing interaction between natural and human-made components, social processes, and the relationships between individuals and groups. In spite of these interconnections, it often is useful to closely examine specific components of the whole.

RATIONALE FOR ENVIRONMENTAL APPROACH TO DISEASE PREVENTION

Magnitude of Disease Problem

The first reason for the consideration of environmental factors in efforts to prevent disease is based on the sheer magnitude of many of the diseases with which we are concerned (including coronary heart disease, cancer of various sites, arthritis, mental illness, diabetes, and stroke). Consider coronary heart disease, a disease of substantial prevalence in all of the developed nations of the world. In the United States, approximately 6 million people have atherosclerotic disease.[2] If a permanent, 100% effective cure with no relapses were available for this disease, treatment would require 28% of available physician time during that year.

The relatively high cost of this program in terms of physician time would be acceptable except that enormous numbers of new people would continue to develop heart disease for the first time, since the treatment program would not deal with people "at risk" for heart disease. If these at-risk people were included, the expanded program would require 91% of available physician time. Even the higher cost of this activity might be considered acceptable since it could achieve a permanent and completely effective cure for a major disease. It must be noted, however, that although the program would virtually exhaust all available physician resources, it would not solve the problem because it would not deal with those forces in society that brought about the problem in the first place: about 1% of healthy people over the age of 30 in the United States (about 1,130,000 people) are expected to become at risk for the first time each year because they (1) start smoking, (2) become overweight, or (3) develop elevated levels of a risk factor.

Although a one-to-one approach to diseases of great prevalence clearly is of value to patients, families, and friends, it does little to alter the distribution of disease in the population because new people develop disease even as sick people are cured. Thus an individual approach exhausts substantial medical care resources but does little to address the environmental factors that have initiated the problem. In this circumstance an environmental approach to prevention clearly is more efficient.

Difficulties in Changing Behavior

A second reason for the consideration of environmental factors in disease prevention is that the prevention of so many diseases requires that people change their behaviors. To prevent disease we increasingly ask people to begin to do things they have not done previously, to stop doing things they have been doing for years, and to do more of some things and less of others. This behavioral approach to disease prevention contrasts with programs that attempt to do something *to* people. Although some diseases and conditions can be treated best by injection, surgery, or other nonbehavioral manipulations, most chronic diseases cannot. Chronic diseases and conditions such as cancer, diseases

The assistance of Diane Helmer, PhD, in the preparation of this chapter is gratefully acknowledged.

of the cardiovascular system, cirrhosis, and chronic respiratory diseases are associated to a greater or lesser degree with particular behaviors and hopefully can be prevented or treated by behavior change.[3,4]

Of course, it is one thing to identify a risk behavior and another thing to ensure that people will actually change that behavior. It is of little value to identify a hazardous behavior if people will not change it. Although there certainly are examples of successful programs to change behavior, the evidence suggests that behavior change is a difficult and complex challenge.[5] Although many different factors need to be considered in helping people change their behavior, one factor rarely considered is that of the environment. It is difficult to expect that people will easily change their behavior when many forces in the social, cultural, and physical environments conspire against such change.[6–8] If successful behavior change programs are to be developed to prevent diseases, more attention must be given not only to the behavior and risk profiles of individuals but also to the environmental context within which people live. Community-based programs directed at cigarette smoking already are underway in Richmond, California, and in a nationwide study involving 11 paired communities.[9]

Patterning of Disease Rates

The third reason for considering environmental factors in disease prevention programs is that groups often have a characteristic pattern of disease over time even though individuals come and go from these groups. If groups have different rates over time, there may be something about the group that either promotes or discourages disease among individuals in those groups. A considerable amount of research has been done in hopes of identifying such environmental factors so that interventions might be developed to prevent or control disease.

The search for causes in the environment is especially important because we have not been completely successful in pinpointing the causes of disease using conventional, individually oriented epidemiology models. This limited success can be illustrated by referring once again to the case of coronary heart disease. Several collaborative long-term community studies in the United States of several thousand middle-aged people have shown that high serum cholesterol, high blood pressure, and cigarette smoking are important risk factors for the development of coronary heart disease.[10] After adjusting for age, men with all three of these risk factors had more than six times the chance of developing a first major coronary attack than did men with none of the risk factors; the relative risks for people having one or two of these risk factors compared to men with none are 2.4 and 4.5, respectively.[11]

On the other hand, as Marmot and Winkelstein have shown,[12] only 14% of people with all three of these risk factors actually had coronary heart disease during 10 years of observation in these community studies; 86% did not have a coronary event. Of people with one or two risk factors, only 5% and 9%, respectively, had an event in the 10-year period of study. Thus, even though these three risk factors clearly are associated with an increased relative risk of disease, few people with the risk factors actually developed disease. Looked at another way, of all the people who developed coronary heart disease in these community studies over the 10-year follow-up period, only 17% had all three risk factors, and only 58% had two or more risk factors. Therefore many people develop coronary heart disease for reasons not entirely explainable by these three risk factors. Although this observation should not de-emphasize the importance of the three established risk factors, it does suggest that other factors also may be involved in the etiological process.

That environmental factors might be involved in the etiology of a broad range of diseases has been forcefully suggested both by McKeown[13] and by McKinlay and McKinlay.[14] These scholars have concluded that the dramatic decline since 1900 in overall mortality in both Britain and the United States cannot be explained by the introduction and use of medical interventions. Indeed, many medical measures against disease (both chemotherapeutic and prophylactic) were introduced several decades after a marked decline in mortality from those diseases already had taken place. McKinlay and McKinlay cite five diseases that in their view did benefit from medical intervention: influenza, pneumonia, diphtheria, whooping cough, and poliomyelitis. They note, however, that even if the decline in these diseases was totally attributable to medical measures, at best their decline accounts for only 3.5% of the total decline in mortality. In assessing these statistics, McKeown has argued that most of the decline in mortality since the second half of the nineteenth century was primarily due to improvements in hygiene and to rising standards of living, especially improved nutrition.

This emphasis on the importance of environmental factors in the etiology and control of diseases has a long history, especially in reference to the study of infectious diseases.[15] In spite of this long-standing concern with the environment, most work on the prevention, treatment, and control of noninfectious diseases has focused, in one way or another, on the individual. As a consequence, although we may refer to the importance of an environmental perspective for noninfectious diseases, we have very little specific and precise information about how the environment affects the incidence, severity, and persistence of these diseases and even less information about how they can be prevented by environmental interventions. This problem can be illustrated by reference to three factors that exhibit characteristic and well-recognized disease patterns but for which explanations remain unclear: socioeconomic status, marital status, and gender.

Socioeconomic Status. One of the most persistent disease patterns observed in public health research is that people in the lowest socioeconomic groups have the highest rates of morbidity and mortality. The consistency of this finding dates from the twelfth century.[16] Further, this differential has been observed throughout the world, regardless of whether the dominant causes of death and disability were attributed to infectious or noninfectious conditions and regardless of the specific methods used to assess socioeconomic status.[17]

In a massive nationwide survey of mortality in the United States, Kitagawa and Hauser[18] found that mortality rates varied dramatically among socioeconomic groups for both men and women, whether socioeconomic status was studied in relation to education, income, or occupation: the lower the socioeconomic level, the higher the death rate. In addition, Kitagawa and Hauser found that those in lower socioeconomic groups had higher death rates for every cause of death except, among women, cancer of the breast and motor vehicle accidents (Table 40–1). Higher rates of morbidity also have been observed among those in lower socioeconomic groups. These higher morbidity rates include virtually every disease as well as mental illnesses and conditions such as schizophrenia, depression, unhappiness, worry, anxiety, and hopelessness.[17,19]

In spite of the fact that socioeconomic status is such a well-recognized and important risk factor for disease, we know little of the reasons for its importance. There are at least two explanations for this. One is that socioeconomic status is so powerful a risk factor that we almost always statistically control for its influence in research so that we can study other factors of interest. If we did not do this, the effect of socioeconomic status would overwhelm everything else under study. In consequence, socioeconomic status rarely is studied as a phenomenon in its own right. The second explanation is more subtle: we tend to study risk factors that we think we can do something about, and socioeconomic status seems not readily amenable to intervention. As we have noted, however, it turns out not to be as easy as we thought to get people to change their diet, stop smoking, or in

TABLE 40–1. PERCENTAGE DIFFERENCE IN MORTALITY RATIO BETWEEN HIGHEST AND LOWEST EDUCATION LEVELS, BY CAUSE OF DEATH, FOR WHITES 25 TO 63 YEARS, UNITED STATES, 1960[a]

	Percentage Difference in Mortality Ratio			
Cause of Death	**White Males**		**White Females**	
Tuberculosis	776		b	
Malignant neoplasms	31		23	
Stomach		123		b
Intestine, rectum		21		66
Lung, bronchus, trachea		93		37
Breast		b		−22
Uterus		b		109
Other neoplasms		5		12
Diabetes	45		332	
Cardiovascular-renal diseases	33		109	
Vascular lesions of CNS		27		103
Rheumatic fever		24		26
Arteriosclerotic disease		25		139
Hypertension		79		158
Other cardiovascular diseases		71		72
Influenza, pneumonia	159		b	
Cirrhosis of liver	2		16	
All accidents	127		24	
Motor vehicle accidents		84		−4
Other accidents		163		
Suicide	74			
Other causes of death	100		48	

[a] Adapted from Kitagawa and Hauser, 1973.[18] Mortality ratios for nonwhites are not shown because of insufficient data. In this table, the percentage differential in mortality ratio is computed by dividing the *difference* in ratios by the ratio at the lowest education level. Any given percentage figure in the table may be read as the percentage by which the ratio at the lowest education level is *higher* than the ratio at the highest education level.

[b] Insufficient data to calculate ratios.

other ways to change their behavior. Further, it is inappropriate to conclude that we cannot intervene in regard to socioeconomic status without first knowing its essential ingredients. If the important ingredient in socioeconomic status is income, interventions may indeed be difficult. On the other hand, if the important ingredient is education or a way of looking at the world, there may be things we can do. In any case, without an understanding of the components involved in socioeconomic status, it seems unwise to decide ahead of time that interventions are impossible.

One way of studying this problem is to focus on socioeconomic status in some detail. Marmot and his colleagues[20] have done research on British civil servants that provides an opportunity to study socioeconomic status carefully. British civil servants in the highest grade (administrators) have the lowest rate of coronary heart disease, and those in the lowest grade (mainly unskilled manual workers) have rates 4 times as high (Fig. 40-1). After such coronary heart disease risk factors as high serum cholesterol, cigarette smoking, high blood pressure, insufficient physical activity, glucose intolerance, and lack of social support, had been taken into account, the rate of those at the bottom was reduced to 3 times as high. However, about 60% of the difference in coronary heart disease rates among civil service grades remained unexplained after this adjustment. More interesting is the fact that workers in professional and executive jobs (grade 2) and in clerical jobs (grade 3) have coronary heart disease rates 2 and 3.2 times as high as administrators. This finding poses a challenge. Although it is reasonably simple to come up with possible explanations for the fact that those at the bottom have higher rates than those at the top, these explanations do not account for the fact that those close to the top have higher rates of disease than those at the top. Factors such as inadequate medical

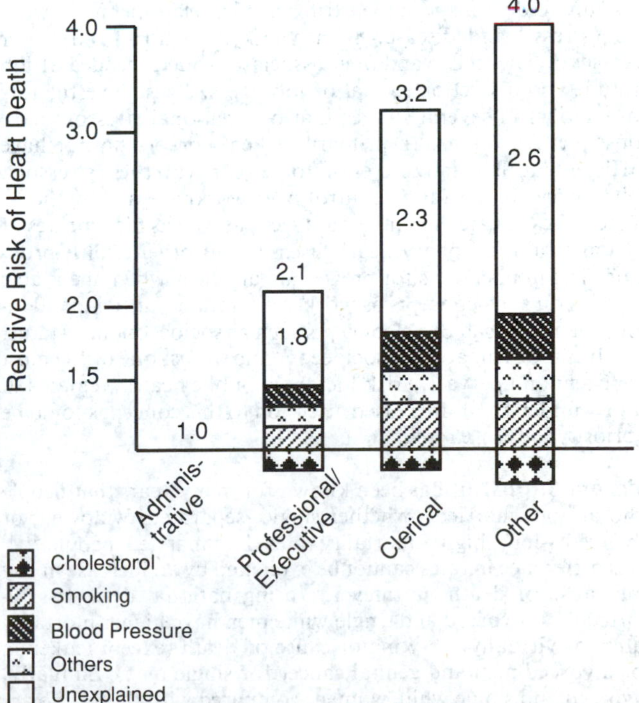

Figure 40–1. Relative risk of coronary heart disease death by civil service rank—Male Civil Service Workers, London, England. Number at top of column: Unadjusted relative risk. Number in column: Adjusted relative risk. *[Adapted from Marmot MG et al, 1978.[20]]*

care, unemployment, low income, racial factors, poor nutrition, poor housing, and poor education may account for higher rates of disease among those in class 5, but they do not explain why professionals and executives in the British civil service have rates twice as high as administrators.

This gradient of disease is not unique to British civil servants. It has been observed in a wide variety of populations in many different countries, and it is not confined to a single disease entity or age group.[19,21] The gradient has been observed for many body systems, including the digestive, genitourinary, respiratory, circulatory, nervous, blood, and endocrine systems. It has been observed also for most malignancies, congenital anomalies, infectious and parasitic diseases, accidents, poisoning and violence, perinatal mortality, diabetes, and musculoskeletal impairments.

It is difficult to explain why those one or two steps from the top have higher rates of disease than those at the top and especially to explain why this gradient exists for so many diseases in so many different geographic locations. One hypothesis involves the concept of "control of destiny." It could be postulated, for example, that the lower one is in the socioeconomic status hierarchy, the less control one has over the factors that affect life and living circumstance.

This hypothesis is general, and it does not specify whether control involves money, power, information, prestige, experience, or something else. Over the years many social scientists have studied many concepts related to the idea of "control of destiny" and it may be of value to look for common denominators in that body of work. The list of such concepts includes mastery,[22] self-efficacy,[23,24] locus of control,[25,26] learned helplessness,[27] the ability to control,[28,29] predictability,[30] desire for control,[31] sense of control,[32-34] powerlessness,[35] hardiness,[36] and competence.[37] If these ideas, or something like them, are supported by research evidence, an avenue for intervention might become available that is more precise and understandable than simply suggesting that we change "socioeconomic status."[38]

Research on job stress already is supporting the usefulness of this approach. For many years researchers have tried unsuccessfully to demonstrate the existence of a relationship between "job stress" and disease. Such a link was shown only after Karasek,[39] Theorell,[40] and their associates added the idea of job latitude and discretion to that of job stress. These investigators have shown in several studies that occupational stressors have consequences for health primarily when workers do not have sufficient latitude and discretion for coping with these stressors. When workers have little control over workpace and methods, higher rates of catecholamines are seen, as well as higher rates of mental strain, coronary heart disease, and other health problems. The implications for prevention are clear when one is able to focus on such concepts as worker discretion, latitude, and involvement, instead of on concepts such as socioeconomic status.

It is unfortunate that socioeconomic status, one of the most persistent and pervasive risk factors in public health, remains so poorly understood. Increased attention to this concept should be a priority in future research.

Marital Status. It has been known for many years that people who are not married—whether single, separated, widowed, or divorced—have higher mortality rates than married people.[41-43] This difference in rates cannot be explained by an increase in any one cause of death. Ortmeyer,[42] using national data, has reported that divorced and single white men have higher mortality rates for virtually every major cause of death (except leukemia for divorced men and genital cancer for single men). Similarly, divorced and single white women, compared with those who are married, have higher death rates for almost all causes of death.

In an effort to account for the fact that single, widowed, and divorced persons have more disease than married persons, Weiss[44] compared these groups in terms of a variety of disease risk factors. Using data from the U.S. Health Examination Survey, he studied a sample of 6672 adults with and without coronary heart disease and found that adjustment for such risk factors as high serum cholesterol, high systolic and diastolic blood pressures, and obesity did not diminish the differences observed for marital status.

Considerable attention is now being given to this issue, especially to the effect of different types of work on women in various marital circumstances and the way in which these relationships are affected by variations in socioeconomic status. At present, however, the effect of marital status on health remains largely unexplained.

Gender. One of the most well-established facts among students of health and disease is that men have higher mortality rates than women.[45] In 1980, men in the United States had an age-adjusted death rate 80% higher than women, and, as would be expected, men's life expectancy is about 7.5 years less than women. This excess of male deaths occurs at every age and for every major cause for which comparison is possible. The largest male excess occurs for suicide and homicide (age-adjusted ratios of 3.33 and 3.86, respectively) and the lowest for diabetes (age-adjusted ratio of 1.02). These patterns generally are similar in all the developed nations of the world. Further, since 1900 the differential in mortality between the sexes has been increasing.

Wingard[46,47] has examined two proposed explanations for this differential: a biological explanation stating that women are biologically more "fit" than men and a social or life-style explanation purporting that men behave in ways more damaging to health. After a detailed review of such possible life-style explanations as marriage, parenthood, employment, hard-driving behavior, cigarette smoking, and physical activity, she concluded that none of these, singly or together, eliminated the sex differential in mortality. In fact, in one study multivariate adjustments for all known risk factors actually increased the sex differential. Once again then a major factor known to influence rates of disease remains largely unexplained.

These examples of patterned consistency of disease rates among socioeconomic, marital, and gender groups emphasize the importance of environmental factors in the study of disease etiology; they also illustrate how little is known about these major issues.

SOCIAL FACTORS AND THE INCIDENCE OF DISEASE

The first modern argument for the inclusion of social factors in environmental studies of disease etiology was that offered by Emile Durkheim in his classic research on suicide. Durkheim's book *Le Suicide* was published in France in 1897 but was not translated into English until 1951.[48] This work is among the first examples of the systematic and organized use of the statistical method to further the sociocultural investigation of disease. Durkheim noted that although suicide is one of the most individualistic acts imaginable, it can be understood only in terms of the social setting within which it takes place. At the time Durkheim wrote, it was known that suicide varied among different groups and times. Suicide rates were higher for Protestants than for Catholics, higher for the unmarried than for the married, higher for soldiers than for civilians, higher for noncommissioned officers than for enlisted men, higher in times of peace than in times of war and revolution, and higher in times of both prosperity and recession than in times of economic stability.

Durkheim acknowledged that there were many different reasons for committing suicide (e.g., economic problems, sickness, personal failure); he pointed out, however, that suicide rates differ among social groups and that such differences persist over time and cultural setting, even though individuals may come and go and even though individual problems may vary within the groups. To explain this difference in group rates, Durkheim argued, one must refer to social factors. He reasoned that if different groups have different suicide rates, there must be something about the social organization of the groups that encourages or deters individuals from suicide. Durkheim's research led him to conclude that the major factor affecting suicide rates was the degree of social integration of groups. He suggested that the extent to which the individual was integrated into group life determined whether he would be motivated to commit suicide. This emphasis on the importance of social ties is a theme that also emerges from current research. Aside from Durkheim's substantive contribution regarding suicide, however, is the important epidemiological observation that systematic, patterned differences in disease rates among groups must be explainable in group terms. This idea continues to be the major rationale for research on social factors in disease etiology.

During the last 30 years, research evidence has accumulated regarding the role of several social factors in disease etiology. Although most of this work has been done in reference to coronary heart disease, other diseases also have been studied. From this work several themes can be identified that are supported by a relatively large body of consistent empirical evidence.

Mobility and Disease

Much early research on social factors was concerned with the impact of various types of mobility on the occurrence of disease. Two early studies on this topic showed that persons who changed jobs or residences had higher rates of disease.[49,50] Later studies confirmed these findings not only for people who moved from jobs and homes but also for people who moved from one life circumstance to another. Higher rates of disease have been noted among southern rural workers who moved to industrial jobs[51] and among college-trained monks from lower class origins.[52] In a follow-up study conducted in Evans County, Georgia, between 1960-1969, Kaplan and associates[53] found twice the incidence of coronary heart disease among lower status persons who moved upward in social status during the period studied as compared to those who remained at the same level, again adjusting for the effect of other known risk factors.

Shekelle and his colleagues[54] studied the incidence of coronary heart disease over a 5-year period among 1472 men aged 42 to 57 years. They found that inconsistencies in social status (e.g., wife with more education than husband) assessed at the beginning of the study were associated with a subsequent increased risk of coronary heart disease: men with four or five inconsistencies had six times the risk of coronary heart disease as compared to men with no inconsistencies. These findings were not explained by the effects of such other risk factors as serum cholesterol, blood pressure, blood glucose, educational status, relative weight, or cigarette smoking.

Many other studies and reviews have reported an increased rate of disease in mobile persons,[55-60] but several studies have failed to confirm these findings. For example, Hinkle et al.[61] and Williams[62] found no relationship between occupational advancement and coronary heart disease among employees of industrial firms. As Lehman[63] and Kaplan et al.[53] have pointed out, however, industrial firms may not be appropriate settings for the study of social mobility because of the truncated status distributions that exist in such cases. Haynes et al.[64] recently studied various types of mobility in the community setting of Framingham, Massachusetts, and reported no statistically significant associations between coronary heart disease and occupational mobility, educational mobility, or status incongruity for the overall sample of men and women in various age groups.

A major test of the mobility hypothesis was undertaken in a study of Japanese migrants to the United States.[65] Japanese men were studied in Japan, Hawaii, and California using comparable study methods. A gradient in coronary heart disease morbidity[66] and mortality[67] was observed in this group; the lowest rates were in Japan, the highest in California, and the intermediate rates were in Hawaii. This gradient was not explained by differences in these populations regarding serum cholesterol, diet, blood pressure, or cigarette smoking. Thus the principal coronary heart disease risk factors did not account for most of the increase in coronary heart disease rates among the Japanese migrants. However, in a special study of Japanese living in California,[68] two subpopulations were observed. One subpopulation, migrants who had adopted Western life-styles and were considered "acculturated," had coronary heart disease rates 2.5 to 5 times higher than the second group, who had retained traditional Japanese ways (Fig. 40-2). In this study acculturation was assessed

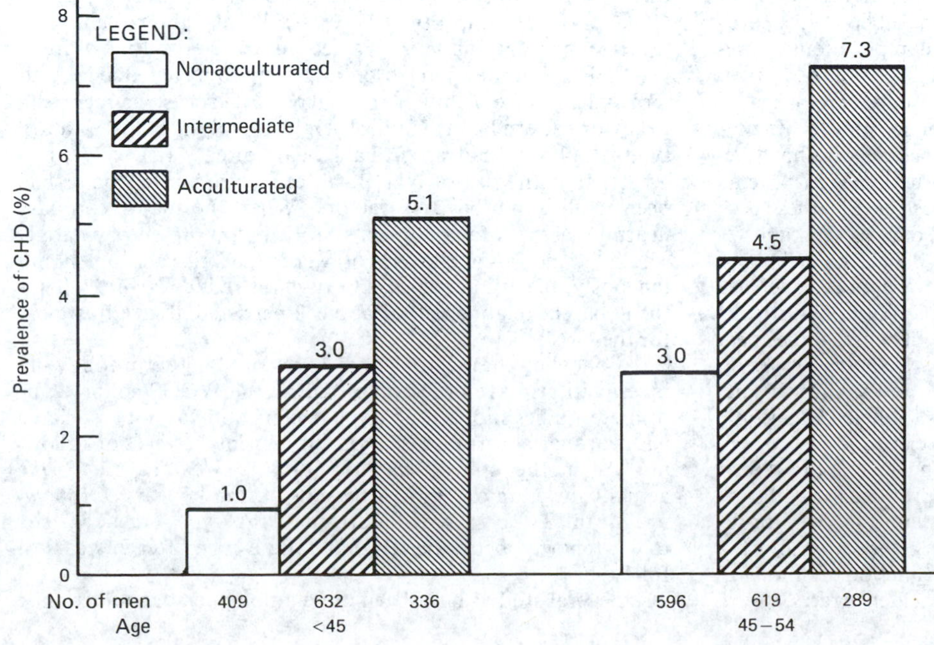

Figure 40-2. Acculturation and coronary heart disease among Japanese Americans living in California. *[Adapted from Marmot MG, Syme SL, 1976.[68]]*

in reference to the subjects' association with Japanese friends and the Japanese community, both in childhood and adulthood. Findings from this study suggest that mobility per se does not increase coronary heart disease rates since those migrants who retained Japanese life-styles exhibited rates similar to those of Japanese living in Japan.

The ways in which mobility affects the incidence of disease are not clear. Few data are available on the subject of whether disease risks increase because of (1) the changes necessitated by mobility, (2) the situation to which the mobile person moves, or (3) characteristics predisposing certain persons to become mobile. The Japanese data suggest that mobility by itself is not a major factor. However, Tyroler and Cassel[69] found that change can influence disease rates even when individuals remain in place. These investigators studied the trend of mortality rates among residents of rural counties in North Carolina as some of these counties became urbanized. They found that coronary heart disease mortality rates increased among the residents of those counties that had experienced the most urbanization. Two possible explanations—differences in diagnostic custom with increasing urbanization and selective migration—were shown to be unlikely. One interpretation is that rates of disease can increase when social change occurs, even though people stay put.

Clearly, the links between mobility and disease are complex and require further study. Nonetheless, it seems reasonable to conclude that mobility somehow is involved in disease etiology. The majority of studies suggest a consistent increase of disease rate associated with occupational, geographic, intergenerational, and situational mobility. Although none of these studies is without flaw, the overall pattern of findings is impressive because many different investigators working independently have come up with similar findings in spite of using different approaches and methods in different population groups.

Life Events

Closely related to research on mobility is the work attempting to establish a link between stressful life events and disease. In 1967, Holmes and Rahe[70] developed the Social Readjustment Rating Scale to record such life events as change in residence, injury, job changes, death of loved ones, and birth of children. Over the years various suggestions have been offered to refine this scale and increase its usefulness.[71] From use of the scale in one form or another, a relatively large body of data has developed suggesting an association between a wide variety of life events and a broad array of disease outcomes, including eczema, tuberculosis, coronary heart disease, childhood illnesses, and complications of pregnancy. However, much of this research has been retrospective: persons who already have experienced an illness are asked to identify stressful life events within a year or so prior to their illness. This weakens the evidence because people who have become ill often attempt retrospective reconstruction of past events to explain their current situation, and it is possible that these people would be more likely than healthy persons to recall and report life events to account for their state of ill health.

Prospective studies showing that life events can increase rates of illness have been reported by Parens et al.,[72] Thurlow,[73] and Spilken and Jacobs.[74] However, most of these studies deal with the incidence of relatively minor diseases (such as upper respiratory infections, gastrointestinal upset, and skin problems) among people who have come to physicians for help. The people studied in these investigations generally have been willing to seek help for conditions that clearly allow personal discretion. It may be that those motivated to report life event problems also may be more motivated to seek medical aid for such minor health problems. Thus these prospective data showing a relationship between life events and illness may be more a function of illness-reporting than of true differences in disease incidence rates.

These methodological problems are not involved in bereavement studies such as that conducted by Parkes et al.[75] In that research the investigators followed 4486 widowers, 55 years of age and older, for 9 years after the deaths of their wives. Of these men, 213 died during the first 6 months of bereavement, a rate 40% higher than would have been expected for married men of the same age. After the first 6 months the mortality rate gradually fell to that of married men and remained at that lower level. Similar findings have been reported by Jacobs and Ostfeld,[76] Maddison and Viola,[77] and Rees and Lutkins.[78] Jacobs and Ostfeld[76] conclude that the attributable risk of death for persons losing a spouse may be as high as 50%.

Many of these studies on bereavement have been criticized for methodological shortcomings. However, most of these criticisms have been addressed in a major, comprehensive, and well-controlled study by Helsing and associates[79] in Washington County, Maryland. In this 10-year retrospective cohort study the investigators found that bereavement carried an increased mortality risk for men, but not for women. The excess risk among men persisted even after account had been taken of such factors as age, education, age at first marriage, cigarette smoking, church attendance, and socioeconomic status. Further, and unlike other investigators, Helsing and associates found the increased mortality risk among widowers to persist throughout the 10-year study period (and not just for 6 months or so).

It is clear that the relationship between life events and disease is not simple or clear cut. It seems reasonable to think that the occurrence of life events must be mediated by personality, perception, previous experiences, social context, and coping styles.

Behavior Pattern

Of all the research on ways people cope with stressful life events, probably most attention has been focused on "type A" behavior. This behavior pattern is said to be exhibited by persons engaged in a relatively chronic and excessive struggle to obtain an unlimited number of things from the environment in the shortest time or against the opposing efforts of other persons or things.[80]

For almost 30 years, Friedman, Rosenman, Jenkins, Brand, and others have published a series of articles showing an increased rate of coronary heart disease among men characterized by this behavior pattern. The most compelling evidence from this group was based on the study of 3524 men in the Western Collaborative Group Study (WCGS).[81] This study was a prospective investigation and involved an 8 1/2-year follow-up. It was found that men judged on interview to have behavior pattern A had twice as much coronary heart disease as men with behavior pattern B. In a multiple logistic analysis of these data,[82] type A subjects had a coronary heart disease risk 2.37 times greater than the risk of type B subjects before adjustments had been made for other risk factors. When the major coronary heart disease risk factors (age, systolic blood pressure, cigarette smoking, and serum cholesterol) were taken into account simultaneously, the estimated relative risk was reduced to 1.97. Thus the apparent relative risk of about 2 persisted after adjustment for these risk factors.

Following these initial studies, several long-term follow-up investigations have been completed on the WCGS cohort. One of these studies showed that type A behavior was not associated with coronary heart disease mortality during 22 years of follow-up.[83] In another study it was found that case fatality rates were actually lower among type A persons during 15 years of follow-up.[84] A third study of this cohort found that type A men, aged 61 to 81, reported better health than type B men after 22 years of follow-up.[85]

Several studies have been done among persons undergoing

coronary angiography. Angiograms have the advantage of yielding a direct, quantitative assessment of the extent of disease, but persons undergoing angiography are not necessarily representative of the general population, and results from studies of such patients therefore might lead to biased findings. The results from studies using angiographic patients are mixed: some studies show a relationship between type A behavior and degree of atherosclerosis,[86-90] but others do not.[91-94] Dimsdale and colleagues[92] have suggested that these inconsistent results may in fact be a reflection of the different ways that people are selected for angiography in different communities.

Other studies on type A behavior have used community samples. Results from the large community study of Framingham, Massachusetts, using a set of self-administered questions similar to those used in the WCGS, are generally consistent with results from that study[95]: type A behavior was significantly associated with the incidence of coronary heart disease among men and women in the 45 to 64 age group but not among older age groups. A study in Belgium and France[96] on 3200 men, using another questionnaire similar to the interview used in WCGS, also found that type A behavior was significantly associated with the incidence of coronary heart disease after a follow-up period of 4.5 to 8 years.

Negative evidence regarding type A behavior comes from the Multiple Risk Factor Intervention Trial[97] (MRFIT) and the Aspirin Myocardial Infarction Study[98] (AMIS). Data from MRFIT showed that type A behavior, assessed in ways closely similar to the method used in the WCGS, was unrelated to the incidence of coronary heart disease among 3110 men at high risk to develop the disease. Similarly, data from AMIS showed that type A men who survived a first myocardial infarction were at no greater risk of a second infarction than type B men who also had survived a first infarction. It is not yet clear how seriously to regard these negative reports since in both cases only men at high risk to develop disease were studied. On the other hand, both studies were conducted carefully in large populations, and in both cases the identification of type A behavior did not demonstrate even modest predictive power.

One of the ways to evaluate the importance of a suspected risk factor is to determine whether the incidence of disease is reduced after the risk factor is removed. A major intervention project to alter type A behavior recently has been completed with interesting results. In this study[99] 862 postmyocardial infarction patients received general cardiological counseling, but an experimental group consisting of 592 patients also received counseling to reduce type A behavior. After 3 years of follow-up, patients in the experimental group experienced coronary heart disease only half as often as those in the control group (7.2% vs 13% incidence, respectively). The significance of this finding will be better evaluated after additional experience accumulates in other intervention studies.[100]

These mixed findings from research on type A behavior have led to a new generation of research focused on particular components of the behavior patterns, rather than on the global phenomenon. Most component research has been directed to "hostility." Assessing hostility from the type A-structured interview, positive relationships with coronary heart disease have been observed in prospective[101] and angiographic studies.[94,102] With the Cook-Medley Hostility Inventory, positive correlations have been found between hostility and coronary heart disease in two other prospective studies[103,104] and in one angiographic study.[105] Recently, however, Helmer and colleagues[106] failed to confirm this association in a study of men and women undergoing angiographic procedures.

Other components being studied include antagonism and resentment,[107] time urgency,[108] anger,[109,110] need for control,[111] self-involvement,[112] self-esteem,[113] and hardiness.[114] The complexities involved in this research are formidable,[115] and it will be of interest to observe continuing developments in this important field.

Social Support

Another approach to the study of coping resources involves social support networks. One of the first studies of this factor was undertaken in 1972 by Nuckolls et al.[116] Complications of pregnancy and delivery were studied in 107 white, married primiparae of similar age and social class, all of whom gave birth in the same medical facility. Women reported on life changes both before and during pregnancies and on the presence or absence of social supports. Women with frequent life changes before or during pregnancy had no more complications than those with few life changes. However, among women who experienced frequent life changes and who *also* reported poor social support, 90% had one or more complications of pregnancy. Although this study was conducted in a small population, it generated interesting findings that also were consistent with the observations made by Durkheim in 1897 regarding the importance of supportive interpersonal relations for health and well-being.

The concept of social support subsequently was studied in a much larger community sample in Alameda County, California.[117] In that study an increased mortality rate was observed in persons previously identified as having fewer friends and social relationships. This study was conducted among a random sample of 6928 adults whose mortality experiences were monitored for 9 years after the baseline interview. Social ties were assessed in terms of marital status, contact with friends and relatives, church membership, and organizational affiliations. Persons with more social ties had lower mortality rates than those with fewer ties, and this relationship existed in all age groups and for both sexes. Although the relative risk associated with social networks was slightly reduced after considering relative weight, cigarette smoking, alcohol consumption, physical activity, health practices, and health status at baseline, those with weak networks still had mortality rates 2 to 3 times higher than those with strong ties (Fig. 40-3).

Since the Alameda County study, several other studies have been done to test the social support hypothesis. The results from this research are generally, but not completely, supportive of the findings from California. In Tecumseh, Michigan, House and his colleagues[118] studied 2754 men and women who had originally been interviewed and medically examined in 1967 to 1969. The mortality experience of this group was followed until 1978–1979. Using a measure of social networks similar but not identical to that used in Alameda County, these investigators found basically the same relationship between networks and mortality as in Alameda County for men but not for women (again, after adjusting for such factors as age, smoking, alcohol consumption, education, employment status, occupation, height and weight, and several measures of health status as determined at the baseline examination).

In Evans County, Georgia, Schoenbach et al[119] attempted to replicate the Alameda County results in a study of 2059 men and women followed from 1967–1969 to 1980. Using a measure of social networks generally comparable to that used in Alameda County and in Tecumseh, these investigators found that two network measures were only modestly related to this outcome. In all comparisons, however, the influence of networks on mortality was weaker than that observed in Alameda County.

In their study of 7639 Japanese American men living in Hawaii, Reed and his colleagues[120] found an inverse relationship between coronary heart disease and social support in a prevalence design but failed to confirm that observation in a study of incidence. In a follow-up on these men from 1965–1968 through 1978, no significant association was observed between social networks and various measures of coronary heart disease. On the

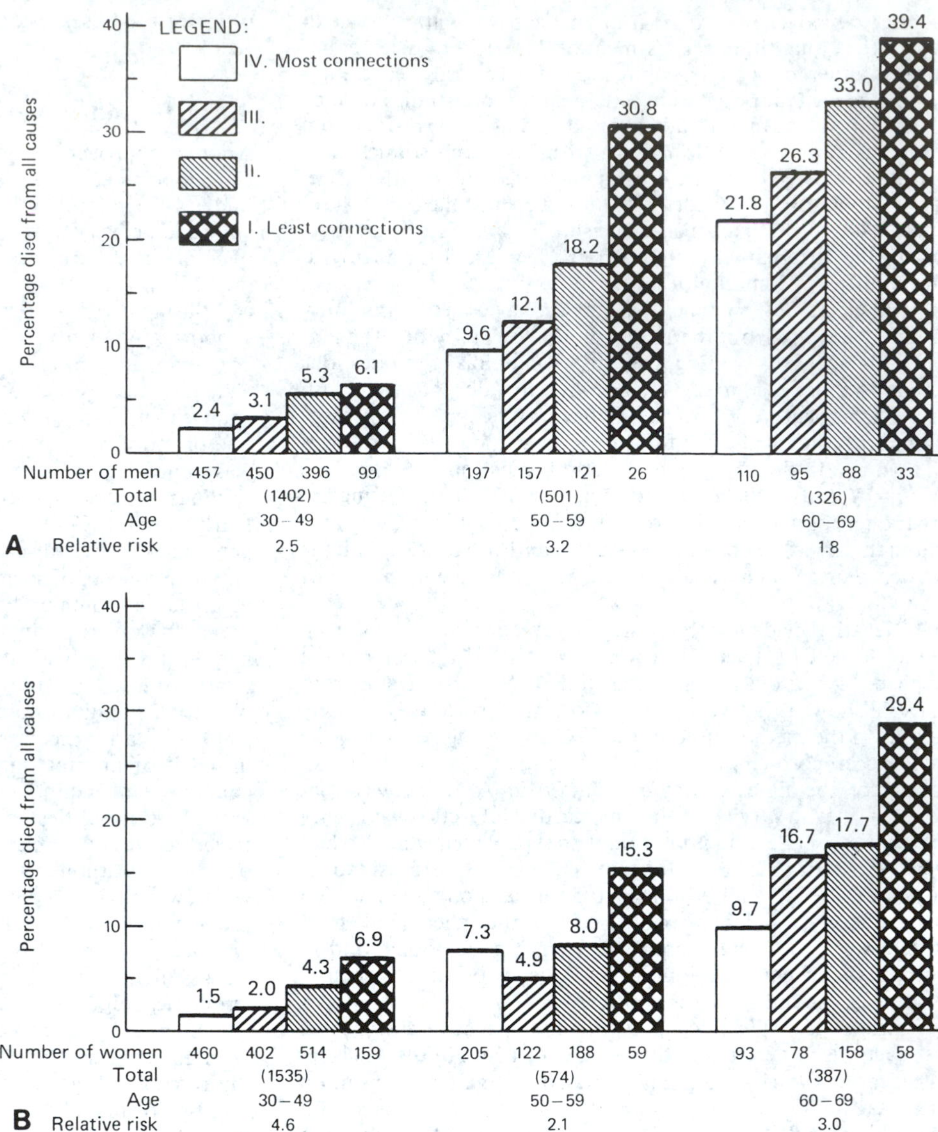

Figure 40-3. Social ties and 9-year mortality in Alameda County, California. **A.** Men. **B.** Women. *(From Berkman L, Syme SL, 1979.[117])*

other hand, results from a study in Durham County, North Carolina,[121] of 331 men and women over 65 years of age showed a strong relationship between social networks and mortality during a 30-month follow-up period (after account had been taken of age, race, sex, economic resources, physical health, activities of daily living, stressful life events, smoking, and several psychological traits).

In a recent study of social support and social networks in eastern Finland, Kaplan and his colleagues[122] found a strong association between networks and mortality from all causes of death. This study involved a representative sample of 13,301 men and women followed for 5 years. After adjustments for age, serum cholesterol, blood pressure, smoking, obesity, education, residence, health status, and family history, the most isolated men had an all-cause death rate twice as high as those most socially connected. The odds ratios for death from cardiovascular and ischemic heart diseases were 1.6 and 1.7, respectively. In striking contrast to these findings for men, no increase in mortality rate associated with social connections was seen for women.

As is evident from this brief account, several large studies have shown that weak social ties are associated with an increased risk of disease, but results from Michigan and Georgia are only partially consistent with this conclusion, and those from Hawaii are not supportive. Several reviews[123-125] have critically assessed this literature and concluded that something of importance is going on, but the precise ingredients of this "something" are not yet clear. One possible explanation for the inconsistent pattern of findings may be that a few simple questions about relationships (e.g., about marriage, clubs, and number of friends) may be enough to separate those with ties from those without ties in a large urban area like Alameda County, but they are not precise enough in smaller, more rural communities.[118] Thus it may be that more sensitive, detailed, and culturally appropriate questions about relationships may be necessary in small towns like Tecumseh, Michigan, in rural areas like Evans County, Georgia, and in close-knit groups such as Japanese American men in Hawaii. The research now underway on this issue will, it is to be hoped, clarify this interesting point.

Another important dimension in research on social support is the effort to define it more precisely. Research has focused on such aspects as number of friends, number of close friends, frequency of seeing people, and satisfaction with the quantity and quality of relationships. In one approach to the study of this issue, Seeman and Syme[126] compared the relative importance of several different social support and network components in a study of men and women undergoing coronary angiography. In assessing the predictive power of these various components, the most powerful one to emerge was the instrumental dimension.

Compared to other definitions of social support, less coronary atherosclerosis was seen among people who could count on specific people to help them when they needed specific kinds of help (e.g., to borrow money, help with household repairs, advice on problems). Further work will be necessary to better define the importance of various dimensions of social networks and social support for health and well-being.

TOWARD A MORE APPROPRIATE SOCIAL EPIDEMIOLOGY

Although several social factors have been identified in this chapter as increasing risk to disease, some of the evidence presented is conflicting and contradictory. Possible explanations for this inconsistency are that (1) investigators have used different research designs in different populations, (2) they have defined concepts differently, and (3) they have used crude, imprecise, and noncomparable assessment tools. These are problems typical of many new research fields, and they tend to be resolved in time as research experience accumulates. Nevertheless, in view of these design and measurement problems, it is especially interesting to note that research on social factors has yielded such a consistent pattern of findings.

There are at least two other possible explanations for this uneven pattern of research findings. One is that we have been using an inappropriate disease classification system that yields misleading and incomplete findings. The other possible explanation is that we have for the most part been studying disease in adults when a more useful strategy would have been to study the early years of life.

Use of Appropriate Disease Classification Scheme

The possibility that social epidemiology may be using an inappropriate disease classification scheme was powerfully suggested by John Cassel. In an influential article written in 1976,[127] Cassel noted that a wide variety of disease outcomes was associated with similar circumstances. For example, he cited the remarkably similar set of risk factors that characterize people who develop tuberculosis or schizophrenia, people who become alcoholics, and those who are victims of multiple accidents or commit suicide. Cassel also noted that this phenomenon generally had escaped comment. To explain this he suggested that investigators usually are "concerned with only one clinical entity, so that features common to multiple disease manifestations have tended to be overlooked."

When researchers focus on a clinical entity, they are consciously or unconsciously adopting a clinical classification scheme that may be useful in clinical settings but that may not be as useful in studies of disease etiology. The clinician uses a classification scheme that has proved useful in the treatment of diseases and in making prognostic estimates for such diseases. However, when epidemiologists observe that several different clinical entities have one risk factor in common, it is not unreasonable to consider a new disease classification that unifies these disparate clinical entities based on the features they have in common.

This is not a new idea. For many years infectious disease epidemiologists have grouped together different clinical entities based on their similarities in modes of transmission. Thus different clinical conditions have been grouped together according to whether they are waterborne, airborne, vectorborne, or foodborne. These environmental classifications may not be of direct value in the treatment of sick people, but they certainly are of value in identifying those aspects of the environment to which interventions can be directed. A comparable set of environmental categories for noninfectious diseases does not exist. The reasons for this are not clear, but it may be that diseases such as coronary heart disease, cancer, and arthritis often are viewed as being diseases "of the individual" and not as diseases influenced by environmental factors. As we have seen, the fact that so many diseases exhibit patterned consistencies in populations suggests that there may indeed be environmental factors associated with the occurrence of these diseases.

An illustration of this environmental perspective is provided by a research project currently underway among bus drivers in San Francisco.[128] Several previous studies have noted that bus drivers have a higher prevalence of hypertension as well as of diseases of the gastrointestinal tract and the musculoskeletal system as compared with workers in other occupations. These results have been obtained from studies of different transit systems, under different conditions, and in several countries.[129-134] Based on these findings, it has been suggested that certain aspects of the occupation of bus drivers may create an increased risk of disease for workers in that occupation.

From a clinical viewpoint it is of value to identify drivers with disease in order to treat them. It also would be of value to teach drivers about better posture, more healthful eating habits, and alternative ways of dealing with job stress. However, from an environmental perspective, it would perhaps be more useful to identify those aspects of the job itself that might be changed to prevent diseases by identifying characteristics of the job that are associated with increased disease risk.

In this study of drivers, their exposure to noise, vibration, and carbon monoxide fumes is being monitored, but particular attention is being paid to the social environment of the driver.[135] For example, in preliminary studies of drivers the "tyranny of the schedule" has been forcefully brought to attention. Drivers must keep to a specific schedule, but in almost every instance this schedule is arranged without realistic reference to actual road conditions and in fact cannot be met. If this and other characteristics of the job that are associated with disease can be identified, it may be possible to introduce interventions, not merely among bus drivers, but directly on those environmental factors associated with the job. For example, it may be that by changing the way in which schedules are arranged, the bus company will be able to earn more money than it loses because of lower rates of absenteeism, sickness, accidents, and, in particular, turnover of employees.

In the case of bus drivers a clinical focus either on hypertension, gastrointestinal diseases, or musculoskeletal disorders clearly is useful. However, from environmental and preventive perspectives, it might be more useful to group together these different diseases and conditions associated with a common work exposure so that they can be studied as related phenomena. If this is not done, the circumstances they share will not likely be appreciated.

In spite of the usefulness of looking at groups of diseases in this way, almost all research on noninfectious disease is directed more or less exclusively toward one or another clinical entity. Although this is understandable (not only because of the enormous influence of the clinical tradition but also because funding for research is so firmly focused on well-established and recognized clinical entities), it has serious consequences. One consequence is that the power of our research is compromised: if a risk factor is associated with several diseases and if we study it with reference to only one disease, its more general importance is not likely to be appreciated and in fact may be missed entirely. The concept of social support provides an illustration of this problem. As noted previously, the absence of social support is moderately related to an increased risk of coronary heart disease, complications of pregnancy and delivery, suicide, and several other diseases and conditions. It also is associated with an increased rate of all-cause mortality. If we could study all of the disease consequences associated with inadequate social support, we might develop a much clearer understanding of its importance for disease etiology. Indeed, by studying social support in relation to only one disease, we may be missing what is most important about the concept.

Let us pursue this example one step further. The fact that those with weak social supports have higher rates of many different diseases and conditions is not immediately plausible biologically. Two models come to mind to account for this observation. One model is that the concept of social support includes many diverse elements and that each of these elements separately influences the likelihood of different diseases. This often is the explanation offered to account for the higher rate of so many diseases associated with cigarette smoking. The second model is that social support affects bodily defenses to such an extent that with weak supports, people are more vulnerable to a wide range of disease agents.[136-144] In this case the presence of specific viruses, bacteria, or air pollutants would not result in disease unless the person was vulnerable to them. For this reason the presence of weak social support would predict whether people would get sick but not what disease they would get. This latter model is attractive because it would account for the fact that several psychosocial factors are related to many different diseases (involving many organ systems) and that most well-recognized, disease-specific risk factors are only modestly predictive of those diseases.

The use of the concept of social support in this way is of course merely illustrative. A whole new area of research is now emerging showing the link between a wide range of psychosocial factors and immunologic function. This area, referred to as psychoneuroimmunology, is growing rapidly and promises to expand our understanding in this important but little understood field.[145] One of the central debates in this work is whether the relationship between a psychosocial variable such as anger or hardiness and a specific disease should be studied, or whether it is more appropriate to study a generalized bodily response.[146-147] Over time the results of this debate will provide information useful not only for studies of disease etiology but for intervention programs also.

Study of Appropriate Age Groups

It is disappointing that after almost 40 years of epidemiological research on noninfectious diseases, we are not further along in our understanding of their risk factors. We have only an imperfect knowledge of psychosocial risk factors, but our knowledge of other risk factors is limited also. In addition, even when we have identified risk factors, we have had substantial difficulty in getting people to change behavior to lower that risk. Part of the explanation for this state of affairs is that we are dealing with complex issues that are difficult to define and measure. Part of the difficulty also is that our most powerful research method, the experiment, is difficult to use in human populations. Both of these explanations are reasonable. But another aspect of the problem may be that we typically study adults when we ought to be studying infants and children.

The rationale for this view is that many of the risk factors studied in adults have their origins in childhood and "track" into adult years. Children with high blood pressure tend more often to be hypertensive as adults.[148-149] Obese children tend more often to become obese adults.[150] The same pattern exists for serum cholesterol values, height, and respiratory function.[151-152] The importance of socioeconomic status for disease occurrence in adults was documented previously; Kaplan and Salonen[153] have shown that childhood socioeconomic status is a more powerful predictor of heart disease in adults than adult socioeconomic status is.

One of the most intriguing findings comes from a follow-up study of children involved in an early education program. This study reported a 22-year follow-up of low income children, 3 and 4 years of age, from Ypsilanti, Michigan.[154] These children had been assigned randomly either to a program offering special education before enrollment in regular school or to no program. As shown in Table 40–2, children who had 1 or 2 years of early education were more likely than those in the control group to complete high school and be employed; they were less likely to have been arrested, to have been on public assistance, and, for girls, to have had a teenage pregnancy. Since these children were assigned at random to the program, these reported differences probably are attributable to the program itself and not to such other factors as motivated parents or differences in baseline intellectual level. It is interesting that 1 or 2 years of exposure to an early education program would, at age 19, make such a difference in living circumstances.

It is hardly original to suggest that experiences in early life are important for later life. In spite of the fact that this relationship is well known, it is difficult to find solid research evidence demonstrating this phenomenon. Many pediatricians and child development experts believe that early experiences are important but base their view on personal experience and intuition. It is not surprising that they have so little data to rely on because it is difficult to conduct follow-up research covering 40 or 50 years. Nevertheless, if one could review the data already available in many long-term data sets, it might be possible to document more precisely how much tracking really occurs and with what strength. If certain physical or psychological traits do track, are we doomed as adults? What other factors modify the impact of early experiences?[155] One interesting study of high-risk children in Kauai, Hawaii,[156] for example, suggests that subsequent life events can buffer or ameliorate earlier experiences and that childhood "high risk" status can in fact be modified.

If it could be established more clearly that certain risk factors are initiated early in life, it might be more appropriate to initiate interventions at that time instead of many years later. Although this might make intuitive sense, it is difficult to shift the financial and organizational resources necessary to do this without a sound body of research evidence to support it. In any case, given our difficulty in making sense of risk factors in the adult years and of developing effective intervention programs, it may be useful now to at least explore this issue as a practical and reasonable alternative.

In summary, a more appropriate social epidemiology would take advantage of current discrepancies and inconsistencies in the research evidence by developing better research methods and instruments, by thinking about more appropriate disease classification systems, by exploring more precisely the ways in which

TABLE 40-2. EFFECTS OF PRESCHOOL THROUGH AGE 19—PERRY PRESCHOOL STUDY[a]

Outcome	No. Responding	Preschool Group	No Preschool	*P*
Employed	121	59%	32%	0.032
High school graduation	121	67%	49%	0.034
College or vocational training or both	121	38%	21%	0.029
Ever detained/arrested	121	31%	51%	0.022
Females: Teen pregnancies per 100	49	64	117	0.084

[a] Adapted from Berrueta-Clement, 1984.[154]

psychosocial factors affect immune function, and by considering more systematically the possibility that what happens early in life may hold an important key to understanding what happens later in life.

ENVIRONMENTAL INTERVENTIONS

This chapter has been concerned primarily with the prevention of disease. It has been argued that although disease prevention can and should be encouraged as we work with both healthy and sick individuals, more attention now must be given to an environmental approach to prevention. Environmental approaches have a long history in public health and have been of great importance in the control of infectious diseases. They have been much less prominent with reference to noninfectious diseases. There are many reasons for this, but one important factor may be our reluctance to encourage environmental interventions for fear they may preempt individual freedom and choice by limiting options and by allowing the few to dictate to the many. In fact, environmental interventions can be seen in precisely the opposite way—as increasing freedom of choice and options. For example, teenagers can hardly be considered free agents when the tobacco industry places enormous pressure on them to smoke. Providing structural alternatives to teenagers would give them more options for making choices than are now possible. Similarly, when a food market has a wide selection of unhealthful foods prominently and attractively displayed at cheap prices (while healthy foods are more expensive and hidden on the bottom shelf), the consumer hardly has a full range of options equally available. The environmental pressures now in place often favor unhealthful interests; introduction of healthful environmental changes can be seen as redressing the balance by providing people with greater freedom of choice among a broader range of alternatives.

The importance of social factors in the etiology of many diseases is becoming increasingly clear. The evidence for some factors is weak; for others it is still unclear. Nevertheless, it is impressive that an increasingly large body of consistent findings is being generated in spite of these major methodological problems. We may not be ready at present to use the data emerging from this research in public health programs, but it is clear that we will need to use them soon because today most serious diseases are greatly influenced by the social environment. For these reasons interventions in the social environment clearly are necessary, and continued research on social factors therefore must become an important priority in both public health planning and program development.

REFERENCES

1. Lindheim R, Syme SL: Environments, people and health. Annu Rev Public Health 4:335–359, 1983
2. U.S. Department of HHS: Disease Prevention/Health Promotion: The Facts. Palo Alto, Calif.: Bull Publishing, 1988
3. Hamburg D: In Elliot GR, Parron DL (eds): Health and Behavior: Frontiers of Research in the Biobehavioral Sciences. Washington, D.C.: National Academy of Science Press, 1982
4. Lalonde M: A New Perspective on the Health of Canadians: A Working Document. Ottawa: Information Canada, 1974
5. Syme SL: Strategies for health promotion. Prev Med 15:492–507, 1986
6. Leventhal H, Cleary PD: The smoking problem: A review of the research and theory in behavioral risk modification. Psychol Bull 88:370–405, 1980
7. Dekker E: Youth culture and influences on the smoking behavior of young people. In Smoking and Health. Proceedings of the Third World Conference. Washington, D.C.: U.S. Department of HEW, Public Health Service, 381–392, 1975
8. Syme SL, Alcalay R: Control of cigarette smoking from a social perspective. Annu Rev Public Health 3:179–199, 1982
9. National Cancer Institute: Community Intervention Trial for Smoking Cessation. Bethesda, M.D.: NCI, 1988
10. Pooling Project Research Group: Relationship of blood pressure, serum cholesterol, smoking habit, relative weight and ECG abnormalities to incidence of major coronary events: Final report of the Pooling Project. J Chronic Dis (Special Issue) 31:201–306, 1978
11. Inter-Society Commission for Heart Disease Resources: Primary prevention of the atherosclerotic diseases. Circulation 42:A55–A95, 1970
12. Marmot M, Winkelstein W Jr: Epidemiologic observations on intervention trials for prevention of coronary heart disease. Am J Epidemiol 101:177–181, 1975
13. McKeown T: The Role of Medicine: Dream, Mirage or Nemesis. London: Nuffield Provincial Hospitals Trust, 1976
14. McKinlay JB, McKinlay SM: The questionable contribution of medical measures to the decline of mortality in the United States in the twentieth century. Health Soc Summer:405–428, 1977
15. Rosen G: From Medical Policy to Social Medicine: Essays on the History of Health Care. New York: Science History Publications, 1974
16. Antonovsky A: Social class, life expectancy and overall mortality. Milbank Mem Fund Q 45:31–73, 1967
17. Syme SL, Berkman LF: Social class, susceptibility and sickness. Am J Epidemiol 104:1–8, 1976
18. Kitagawa EM, Hauser PM: Differential Mortality in the United States. Cambridge, Mass.: Harvard University Press, 1973
19. Haan MN, Kaplan GA, Syme SL: Socioeconomic status and health: Old observations and new thoughts. In Bunker JP, Gomby DF, Kehrer BH (eds): Pathways to Health: The Role of Social Factors. Palo Alto, Calif.: H.J. Kaiser Family Foundation, 1989
20. Marmot MG, Rose G, Shipley M, Hamilton PJS: Employment grade and coronary heart disease in British civil servants. J Epidemiol Community Health 3:244–249, 1978
21. Susser MW, Watson W, Hopper K: Sociology in Medicine. New York: Oxford University Press, 1985
22. Pearlin LI, Menaghan EG, Leibeerman MA, Mullan JT: The stress process. J Health Soc Behav 22:337–356, 1981
23. Bandura A: Self-efficacy mechanisms in human agency. Am Psychol 37:122–147, 1982
24. O'Leary A: Self-efficacy and health. Behav Res Ther 23:437–451, 1985
25. Rotter JB: Some problems and misconceptions related to the construct of internal versus external reinforcement. J Consult Clin Psychol 43:56–67, 1975
26. Wallston KA, Wallston BS: Who is responsible for your health? The construct of health locus of control. In Sanders GS, Suls J (eds): Social Psychology of Health and Illness. Hillsdale, N.J.: Erlbaum, 1982
27. Seligman MEP: Helplessness: On Depression, Development, and Death. San Francisco: Freeman, 1975
28. Glass DC, Singer JE: Urban Stress: Experiments on Noise and Social Stressors. New York: Academic Press, 1972
29. Sherrod DR: Crowding, perceived control, and behavioral aftereffects. J Appl Soc Psychol 4:171–186, 1974
30. Cohen S: Aftereffects of stress on human performance and social behavior. Psychol Bull 88:82–108, 1980
31. Burger J: Desire for control and achievement-related behaviors. J Pers Soc Psychol 48:1520–1533, 1985
32. Langer EJ: The Psychology of Control. Beverly Hills, Calif.: Sage, 1983
33. Rodin J: Aging and health: Effects of the sense of control. Science 233:1271–1276, 1986
34. Schulz R: Effects of control and predictability on the physical and

psychological well-being of the institutionalized aged. J Pers Soc Psychol 33:563–573, 1976
35. Bauman KE, Udry JR: Powerlessness and regularity of contraception in an urban Negro male sample: A research note. J Marriage Fam 34:112–114, 1972
36. Kobasa SC: The hardy personality: Toward a social psychology of stress and health. In Sanders GS, Suls J (eds): Social Psychology of Health and Illness. Hillsdale, N.J.: Erlbaum, 1982
37. Libassi MF, Maluccio A: Competence-centered social work: Prevention in action. J Primary Prev 6:168–180, 1986
38. Syme SL: Control and health: A personal perspective. In Steptoe A, Appels A (eds): Stress, Personal Control and Health. New York: John Wiley, 1989
39. Karasek R, Baker D, Marxer F, Ahlbom A, Theorell T: Job decision latitude, job demands, and cardiovascular disease: A prospective study of Swedish men. Am J Public Health 71:694–705, 1981
40. Theorell T, Alfreddson L, Knox S, Persk A, Svensson J, Waller D: On the interplay between socioeconomic factors, personality and work environment in the pathogenesis of cardiovascular disease. Scand J Work Environ Health 10:373–380, 1984
41. Carter H, Glick PC: Marriage and Divorce: A Social and Economic Study. Cambridge, Mass.: Harvard University Press, 1970
42. Ortmeyer CF: Variations in mortality, morbidity, and health care by marital status. In Erhardt LL, Berlin VE (eds): Mortality and Morbidity in the United States. Cambridge, Mass.: Harvard University Press, 1974, pp 159–188
43. Thiel HG, Parker D, Bruce T: Stress factors and the risk of myocardial infarction. Psychol Res 17:43–57, 1973
44. Weiss NS: Marital status and risk factors for coronary heart disease: The United States Health Examination Survey of Adults. Br J Prev Soc Med 27:41–43, 1973
45. Wingard DL: The sex differential in morbidity, mortality, and lifestyle. Annu Rev Public Health 5:433–458, 1984
46. Wingard DL: The sex differential in mortality rates: Demographic and behavioral factors. Am J Epidemiol 115:205–216, 1982
47. Wingard DL, Suarex L, Barrett-Connor E: The sex differential in mortality from all causes and ischemic heart disease. Am J Epidemiol 117:165–172, 1983
48. Durkheim E: Suicide: A Study in Sociology. Simpson G (ed and trans). Glencoe, Ill.: Free Press, 1951
49. Syme SL, Hyman MM, Enterline PE: Some social and cultural factors associated with the occurrence of coronary heart disease. J Chronic Dis 17:277–289, 1964
50. Syme SL, Borhani MO, Buechley RW: Cultural mobility and coronary heart disease in an urban area. Am J Epidemiol 82:334–346, 1965
51. Cassel J, Tyroler HA: Epidemiological studies of cultural change: I. Health status and recency of industrialization. Arch Environ Health 3:25–33, 1961
52. Caffrey B: A multivariate analysis of sociopsychological factors in monks with myocardial infarctions. Am J Public Health 60:452–458, 1970
53. Kaplan BH, Cassel JC, Tyroler HA, Cornoni JC, Kleinbaum DG, Hames CG: Occupational mobility and coronary heart disease. Arch Intern Med 128:938–942, 1971
54. Shekelle RB, Ostfeld AM, Paul O: Social status and incidence of coronary heart disease. J Chronic Dis 22:381–394, 1969
55. Bruhn JG, Chandler B, Miller MC, Wolf S, Lynn TN: Social aspects of coronary heart disease in two adjacent ethnically different communities. Am J Public Health 56:1493–1506, 1966
56. Bakker CB, Levinson RM: Determinants of angina pectoris. Psychosom Med 29:621–633, 1967
57. Smith R: Factors involving sociocultural incongruity and change: A review of empirical findings. Milbank Mem Fund Q 45:23–37, 1967
58. Marks RU: Factors involving social and demographic characteristics: A review of empirical findings. Milbank Mem Fund Q 45:51–108, 1967
59. Jenkins CD: Psychologic and social precursors of coronary disease. N Engl J Med 284:244–255, 307–317, 1971
60. House JS, Jackman MF: Occupational stress and health. In Ahmed PI, Coelho GV (eds): Towards a New Definition of Health. New York: Plenum, 1979
61. Hinkle LE, Whitney LH, Lehman EW, Dunn J, Benjamin B, King R, Plakum A, Flehinger B: Occupational, educational and coronary heart disease. Science 151:238–246, 1968
62. Williams CA: The relationship of occupational change to blood pressure, serum cholesterol and specific overt behavior patterns [doctoral dissertation]. University of North Carolina at Chapel Hill, 1968
63. Lehman EW: Social class and coronary heart disease: A sociological assessment of the medical literature. J Chronic Dis 20:381–391, 1967
64. Haynes SG, Levine S, Scotch M, Feinleib M, Kannel WB: The relationship of psychosocial factors to coronary heart disease in the Framingham Study. II. Prevalence of coronary heart disease. Am J Epidemiol 107:384–402, 1978
65. Syme SL, Marmot MG, Kagan A, Kato H, Rhoads G: Epidemiologic studies of coronary heart disease and stroke in Japanese men living in Japan, Hawaii and California: Introduction. Am J Epidemiol 102:477–480, 1975
66. Marmot MG, Syme SL, Kagan A, Kato H, Cohen JB, Belsky J: Epidemiological studies of coronary heart disease and stroke in Japanese men living in Japan, Hawaii and California: Prevalence of coronary and hypertensive heart disease and associated risk factors. Am J Epidemiol 102:514–525, 1975
67. Worth RM, Kato H, Rhoads G, Kagan A, Syme SL: Epidemiology studies of coronary heart disease and stroke in Japanese men living in Japan, Hawaii and California: Mortality. Am J Epidemiol 102:481–490, 1975
68. Marmot MG, Syme SL: Acculturation and coronary heart disease in Japanese-Americans. Am J Epidemiol 204:225–247, 1976
69. Tyroler HA, Cassel J: Health consequences of culture change: II. Effect of urbanization on coronary heart mortality in rural residents. J Chronic Dis 17:167–177, 1964
70. Holmes TH, Rahe RH: The Social Readjustment Rating Scale. J Psychosom Res 11:213–218, 1967
71. Dohrenwend BS, Dohrenwend BP: Stressful Life Events: Their Nature and Effects. New York: Wiley-Interscience, 1974
72. Parens H, McConville BJ, Kaplan SM: Prediction of frequency of illness from the response to separation: A preliminary study and replication attempt. Psychosom Med 28:162–176, 1966
73. Thurlow HJ: Illness in relation to life situation and sick-role tendency. J Psychosom Res 15:73–88, 1971
74. Spilken AZ, Jacobs MA: Prediction of illness behavior from measures of life crisis, manifest distress, and maladaptive coping. J Psychosom Res 33:251–264, 1971
75. Parkes CM, Benjamin B, Fitzgerald RG: Broken heart: A statistical study of increased mortality among widowers. Br Med J 1:740–743, 1969
76. Jacobs S, Ostfeld A: An epidemiological review of the mortality of bereavement. Psychosom Med 39:344–357, 1977
77. Maddison D, Viola A: The health of widows in the year following bereavement. J Psychosom Res 12:297–306, 1968
78. Rees WD, Lutkins SJ: Mortality of bereavement. Br Med J 4:13–16, 1967
79. Helsing K, Szklo M, Comstock G: Factors associated with mortality after widowhood. Am J Public Health 71:802–809, 1981
80. Dembroski TM (ed): Proceedings of the Forum on Coronary-Prone Behavior. DHEW Publication No. NIH 78-1451. Washington, D.C.: U.S. Government Printing Office, 1977
81. Rosenman RH, Brand RJ, Jenkins CD, Friedman M, Straus R, Wurm M: Coronary heart disease in the Western Collaborative Group Study: Final follow-up experience of 8½ years. JAMA 233:872–877, 1975
82. Brand RJ: Coronary prone behavior as an independent risk factor for coronary heart disease. In Dembroski TM, Weiss SM, Shields

JL, Haynes SG, Feinleib M (eds): Coronary-Prone Behavior. New York: Springer-Verlag, 1978
83. Ragland DR, Brand RJ: Coronary heart disease mortality in the Western Collaborative Group Study: Follow-up experience of 22 years. Am J Epidemiol 127:462–475, 1988
84. Ragland DR, Brand RJ: Type A behavior and mortality from coronary heart disease. N Engl J Med 318:65–69, 1988
85. Shoham-Yakubovich I, Ragland DR, Brand RJ, Syme SL: Type A behavior pattern and health status after 22 years of follow-up in the Western Collaborative Group Study. Am J Epidemiol 128:579–588, 1988
86. Review Panel on Coronary-Prone Behavior and Coronary Heart Disease: Coronary-prone behavior and coronary heart disease: A critical review. Circulation 63:1199–1215, 1981
87. Blumenthal JA, Williams R, Kong Y, et al: Type A behavior and angiographically documented coronary disease. Circulation 58:634–639, 1978
88. Frank KA, Meller SS, Kornfield DS, et al: Type A behavior and coronary heart disease: Angiographic confirmation. JAMA 240:761–763, 1978
89. Williams RB, Haney TL, Lee KL, et al: Type A behavior, hostility, and coronary atherosclerosis. Psychosom Med 42:539–549, 1980
90. Zyzanski SJ, Jenkins CD, Ryan T, et al: Psychological correlates of coronary angiographic findings. Arch Intern Med 136:1234–1237, 1976
91. Dimsdale JE, Hackett TP, Hutter AM, et al: Type A personality and extent of coronary atherosclerosis. Am J Cardiol 42:583–586, 1978
92. Dimsdale JE, Hackett TP, Hutter AM, Block PC, Catanzano D, White PJ: Type A behavior and angiographic findings. J Psychosom Res 23:273–276, 1979
93. Dembroski TM, MacDougall JM, Williams RD: Components of Type A, hostility and anger: Relationships to angiographic findings. Psychosom Med 47:219–233, 1985
94. MacDougall JM, Dembroski TM, Dimsdale JE: Components of Type A, hostility and anger: Further relationships to angiographic findings. J Health Psychol 4:137–152, 1985
95. Haynes SG, Feinleib M, Kannel WB: The relationship of psychosocial factors to coronary heart disease in the Framingham Study: III. Eight-year incidence of coronary heart disease. Am J Epidemiol 3:37–58, 1980
96. French-Belgian Collaborative Group: Ischemic heart disease and psychological patterns: Prevalence and incidence studies in Belgium and France. Adv Cardiol 29:25–31, 1982
97. Shekelle RB, Hulley SB, Neaton JD, Billings JH, Borhani NO, Gerace TA, Jacobs DR, Lasser NL, Mittlemark MB, Stamler J: The MRFIT behavior pattern study: II: Type A behavior and incidence of coronary heart disease. Am J Epidemiol 122:559–570, 1985
98. Aspirin Myocardial Infarction Study Research Group: A randomized, controlled trial of aspirin in persons recovered from myocardial infarction. JAMA 243:661–668, 1980
99. Friedman M, Thoresen CE, Gill JJ, Powell LH, Ulmer D, Thompson L, Price VA, Rabin DD, Breall WS, Dixon T, Levy R, Bourg E: Alteration of Type A behavior and reduction in cardiac recurrences in postmyocardial infarction patients. Am Heart J 108:237–248, 1984
100. Friedman M, Thoresen CE, Gill JJ, Ulmer D, Powell LH, Price VA, Brown B, Thompson L, Rabin D, Breall WS, Bough E, Levy R, Dixon T: Alteration of type A behavior and its effects upon cardiac recurrences in postmyocardial infarction subjects: Summary results of the Recurrent Coronary Prevention Project. Am Heart J 112:653–665, 1986
101. Matthews KA, Glass DC, Rosenman RH: Competitive drive, pattern A, and coronary heart disease: A further analysis of some data from the Western Collaborative Group Study. J Chronic Dis 30:489–498, 1977
102. Dembroski TM, MacDougall JM, Williams RD: Components of Type A, hostility and anger: Relationship to angiographic findings. Psychsom Med 47:219–233, 1985
103. Shekelle RB, Gale M, Ostfeld AM: Hostility, risk of coronary heart disease and mortality. Psychosom Med 45:109–114, 1983
104. Barefoot JC, Dahlstrom WG, Williams RB: Hostility, CHD incidence and total mortality: A 25 year follow-up study of 255 physicians. Psychosom Med 45:59–63, 1983
105. Williams RB, Haney TL, Lee KL: Type A behavior, hostility, and coronary atherosclerosis. Psychosom Med 42:539–549, 1980
106. Helmer DH, Ragland DR, Syme SL: Hostility and coronary artery disease. Am J Epidemiol 133:112–122, 1991
107. Hecker MH, Chesney MA, Black GW: Coronary-prone behavior in the Western Group Collaborative Study. Psychosom Med 50:153–164, 1988
108. Kanner AD, Coyne JC, Schaefer C, et al: Comparison of two modes of stress management: Daily hassles and uplifts vs. major life events. J Behav Med 4:1–38, 1981
109. Kahn HA, Medalie JH, Newfeld HN, et al: The incidence of hypertension and associated factors: The Israeli Ischemic Heart Disease Study. Am Heart J 84:171–182, 1972
110. Haynes SG, Feinleib M, Kannel WB: The relationship of psychosocial factors to coronary heart disease in the Framingham study: Eight-year incidence of coronary heart disease. Am J Epidemiol 111:37–58, 1980
111. Glass DC: Behavior Patterns, Stress and Coronary Disease. Hillsdale, N.J.: Erlbaum, 1977
112. Scherwitz L, Berton K, Leventhal H: Type A behavior, self-involvement, and cardiovascular response. Psychosom Med 40:593–609, 1978
113. Matthews KA: Psychological perspectives on the Type A behavior pattern. Psychol Bull 91:293–323, 1982
114. Kobasa SC, Maddi SR, Kahn S: Hardiness and health: A prospective study. J Pers Soc Psychol 42:168–177, 1982
115. Matthews KA, Haynes SG: Type A behavior and coronary disease risk: Update and critical evaluation. Am J Epidemiol 123:923–960, 1986
116. Nuckolls KB, Cassel J, Kaplan BH: Psychosocial assets, life crises, and the prognosis of pregnancy. Am J Epidemiol 95:431–441, 1972
117. Berkman LF, Syme SL: Social networks, host resistance, and mortality: A nine year follow-up study of Alameda County residents. Am J Epidemiol 109:186–204, 1979
118. House JS, Robbins C, Metzner HL: The association of social relationships and activities with mortality: Prospective evidence from the Tecumseh Health Study. Am J Epidemiol 116:123–140, 1982
119. Schoenbach VJ, Kaplan BH, Fredman L, Kleinbaum DG: Social ties and mortality in Evans County, Georgia. Am J Epidemiol 123:577–591, 1986
120. Reed D, McGee D, Yano K, Feibleib M: Social networks and coronary heart disease among Japanese men in Hawaii. Am J Epidemiol 117:384–396, 1983
121. Blazer D: Social support and mortality in an elderly community population. Am J Epidemiol 115:684–694, 1982
122. Kaplan GA, Salonen JT, Cohen RD, Brand RJ, Syme SL, Puska P: Social connections and mortality from all causes and cardiovascular disease: Prospective evidence from Eastern Finland. Am J Epidemiol 128:370–380, 1988
123. Broadhead WE, Kaplan BH, James SA, Wagner EH, Schoenbach VJ, Grimson R, Heyden S, Tibblin G, Gehlbach SH: The epidemiologic evidence for a relationship between social support and health. Am J Epidemiol 117:521–537, 1983
124. Cohen S, Syme SL (eds): Social Support and Health. New York: Academic Press, 1985
125. House JS, Landis KR, Umberson D: Social relationships and health. Science 241:540–545, 1988
126. Seeman TE, Syme SL: Social networks and coronary artery disease: A comparison of the structure and function of social relations as predictors of disease. Psychosom Med 49:341–354, 1987
127. Cassel J: The contribution of the social environment to host resistance. Am J Epidemiol 104:107–123, 1976
128. Ragland DR, Winkelby MA, Schwalbe J, Holman BL, Morse L,

Syme SL, Fisher JM: Prevalence of hypertension in bus drivers. Int J Epidemiol 16:208–214, 1987

129. Morris JN, Kagen A, Pattison DC, Gardner MJ, Raffle PAB: Incidence and prediction of ischaemic heart disease in London busmen. Lancet 553, Sept. 10, 1966
130. Netterstrom B, Laursen P: Incidence and prevalence of ischaemic heart disease among urban bus drivers in Copenhagen. Institute of Social Medicine, University of Copenhagen, Denmark. Scand J Soc Med 2:75–79, 1981
131. Berlinguer G: Maladies and Industrial Health of Public Transportation Workers. Italian Institute of Social Medicine, 1962
132. Pikus VG, Taranikkova VA: Hypertension disease in drivers of passenger motor transport. Ter Arkh 47:135, 1975
133. Garke C: Health and Health Risks Among City Bus Drivers in West Berlin. Institute for Social Medicine and Epidemiology of the Ministry of Health, 1980
134. Winkelby MA, Ragland DR, Fisher JM, Syme SL: Excess risk of sickness and disease in bus drivers: A review and synthesis of epidemiologic studies. Int J Epidemiol 17:124–134, 1988
135. Winkelby MA, Ragland DR, Syme SL: Self-reported stressors and hypertension: Evidence of an inverse association. Am J Epidemiol 127:124–134, 1988
136. Bartrop RW, Lockhurst E, Lazarus L, Kiloh HG, Penny R: Depressed lymphocyte function after bereavement. Lancet:834–836, 1977
137. Jackson GG, Dowling HF, Anderson TO, Riff L, Saporta J, Turek M: Susceptibility and immunity to common upper respiratory viral infection—The common cold. Ann Intern Med 53:719–738, 1960
138. Jemmott JB III, Borysenko JZ, Borysenko M, McClelland DC, Chapman R, Meyer D, Benson H: Academic stress, power motivation, and decrease in salivary secretory immunoglobulin and secretion rate. Lancet:1400–1402, 1983
139. Kiecolt-Glaser JK, Garner W, Speisher C, Penn GM, Holliday J, Glaser R: Psychosocial modifiers of immuno-competence in medical students. Psychosom Med 46:7–14, 1984
140. Schleifer SJ, Keller SE, Camerino M, Thornton JC, Stein M: Suppression of lymphocyte stimulation following bereavement. JAMA 250:374–377, 1984
141. Totman RG, Kiff J: Life stress and susceptibility to colds. In Oborne DJ, Gruneberg MM, Eiser JR (eds): Research in Psychology and Medicine. New York: Academic Press, 1979, pp 141–149
142. Sklar LS, Anisman H: Stress and coping factors influence tumor growth. Science 205:513–515, 1979
143. Visitainer MA, Volpicelli JR, Seligman MEP: Tumor rejection in rats after inescapable shock. Science 216:437–439, 1982
144. Laudenslager ML, Ryan SM, Drugan RC, Hyson RL, Maier SF: Coping and immunosuppression: Inescapable but not escapable shock suppresses lymphocyte proliferation. Science 221:568–571, 1983
145. Ader R (ed): Psychoneuroimmunology. New York: Academic Press, 1981
146. Syme SL: Control and health: An epidemiologic perspective. In Schaie KW, Rodin J, Schooler C (eds): Self-Directedness: Cause and Effects Throughout the Life Course. Hillsdale, N.J.: Erlbaum, 1990, pp 213–229
147. Cohen S: Control and the epidemiology of physical health: Where do we go from here? In Schaie KW, Rodin J, Schooler C (eds): Self-Directedness: Cause and Effects Throughout the Life Course. Hillsdale, N.J.: Erlbaum, 1990, pp 231–240
148. Kuller LH, Crook M, Almes MJ: Dormont High School (Pittsburgh, PA) blood pressure study. Hypertension 2(suppl I):109–116, 1980
149. Rosner B, Hennekens CH, Kass EH, Miall WE: Age-specific correlation analysis of longitudinal blood pressure data. Am J Epidemiol 106:306–313, 1977
150. Clarke WR, Woolson RF, Lauer RM: Changes in ponderosity and blood pressure in childhood: The Muscatine Study. Am J Epidemiol 124:195–206, 1986
151. Venters MH: Family life and cardiovascular risk: Implications for the prevention of chronic disease. Soc Sci Med 22:1067–1074, 1986
152. Samet JM, Tager IB, Speizer FE: The relationship between respiratory illness in childhood and chronic air-flow obstruction in adulthood. Am Rev Respir Dis 127:508–523, 1983
153. Kaplan GA, Salonen JT: Socioeconomic conditions in childhood are associated with ischaemic heart disease during middle age. Br Med J 301:1121–1123, 1990
154. Berrueta-Clement JR, Schweinhart LJ, Barnett WS, Epstein AS, Weikart DP: Changed Lives: The Effects of the Perry Preschool Program on Youths Through Age 19. Ypsilanti, Mich.: High/Scope Press, 1984
155. Richmond JB, Beardslee WR: Resiliency: Research and practical implications for pediatricians. Dev Behav Pediatr 9:157–163, 1988
156. Werner E: High-risk children in young adulthood: A longitudinal study from birth to 32 years. Am J Orthopsychiatry 59:72–81, 1989

General References

Kaplan HB (ed): Psychosocial Stress: Trends in Theory and Research. New York: Academic Press, 1983

Gentry WD (ed): Handbook of Behavioral Medicine. New York: Guilford Press, 1985

Cohen S, Syme SL (eds): Social Support and Health. New York: Academic Press, 1985

Hamburg D, Elliot GR, Parron DL (eds): Health and Behavior: Frontiers of Research in the Biobehavioral Sciences. Washington, D.C.: National Academy of Sciences Press, 1982

Antonovsky A: Health, Stress, and Coping. San Francisco: Jossey-Bass, 1979

Susser MW, Watson W, Hopper K: Sociology in Medicine. New York: Oxford University Press, 1985

41

Health Behaviors and Health Promotion

Dennis D. Tolsma
Jeffrey P. Koplan

In 1979 the opening sentence of *Healthy People,* the Surgeon General's Report on Health Promotion and Disease Prevention, stated flatly, "The health of the American people has never been better."[1] By any reasonable measure of health status, the statement was a fair assessment of the public's health. Yet, as the Report was quick to note, a renewed commitment to prevention was a central challenge, one in which major emphasis would need to focus on new and emerging health risks—risks that to a significant extent arise from personal behavior choice.

This is the case not only in the United States and other industrialized nations but also increasingly in the developing world as well. Although communicable disease remains a significant health problem, such modern ("Western") dilemmas as smoking, substance abuse, injury risks, and even overweight and lack of exercise plague the peoples of many parts of the world. Behavior plays a prominent role in these new plagues and is influenced by many factors, including cross-cultural communications of unprecedented global breadth and speed.

ROLE OF BEHAVIORS IN HEALTH

A multitude of factors influence health: personal factors, such as genetic, physiological, psychological, and demographic variables; environmental factors, such as hazards encountered in work, community, home, and recreation; and societal factors, such as cultural and socioeconomic variables. Nevertheless, behavioral risks have become increasingly visible as underlying causes of preventable morbidity and premature death. This was documented in a series of analyses undertaken for "Closing the Gap," a health policy consultation sponsored by the Carter Center of Emory University. The consultants undertook to measure the generic (underlying) risk factors that contribute most to 14 leading causes of morbidity and mortality. Based on the findings of these analyses, a panel of experts identified alcohol, tobacco, injury, and unintended pregnancy as the highest priority precursors. (Three other precursors that ranked nearly as high were overnutrition, including obesity and high serum cholesterol levels, handguns, and dental problems.) To the final list were added two generic health problems: gaps in primary care and mental health issues (violence, depression, and substance abuse).[2] Clearly, these priority precursors are either behavior choices or risk factors in which behavioral choice plays a major role.

A few illustrations from the analyses show the range of behavioral risks that influence health. The analysis of diabetes mellitus indicated that "prevention of obesity may reduce the incidence of type II diabetes by one half and gestational diabetes by as much as one third."[3] It is also estimated that if all the 1 million diabetics who continue to smoke were to stop, the incidence of peripheral vascular disease could be reduced by 30%.[3]

The analysis of cancer reviewed a broad array of attributable risks for cancers of various sites. Table 41–1 illustrates the health impacts of smoking, diet, and alcohol on major cancers. Overall, 24% of deaths, 21% of life-years lost before age 65, 21% of hospital days, and 16% of direct medical care costs were attributable to these behavior-related precursors.[4]

The Closing the Gap analysis of cardiovascular disease calculated population-attributable risk fractions for major risk factors of cardiovascular disease.[5] For premature death (defined as potential years of life lost before age 65), smoking was estimated to cause 30% of life-years lost. Similarly, 18% of life-years lost because of cardiovascular disease was attributed to high blood pressure and 9% to elevated cholesterol. These three variables accounted for more than half of each measured health burden of cardiovascular disease (Table 41–2).

The equations used did not permit separate estimates for lack of exercise as a risk factor. A recent meta-analysis of studies of exercise and heart disease concludes that lack of exercise is causally related to increased risk of heart disease, and that the relative risk of this factor is the same order of magnitude as those of moderate smoking and elevated cholesterol.[6] Nonpharmacological measures, that is, nonsmoking and protective behavioral choices in exercise, diet, and weight loss, can reduce the health impact of cardiovascular disease substantially.[7–9]

A summary analysis, combining the findings of the 14 individual Closing the Gap analyses, suggests that "approximately two thirds of deaths in the United States are attributable to a preventable precursor."[10] Six precursors—tobacco, alcohol, injury risks, high blood pressure, overnutrition, and gaps in primary prevention—accounted for three fourths of the preventable health impact. Tobacco was the strongest precursor for deaths, life-years lost, and hospital days. Four precursors that were strongly related to personal health behavior—tobacco, high blood pressure, overnutrition, and alcohol—accounted for approximately 1 million preventable deaths, nearly 4 million potential years lost, and 45.5 million days of hospital care.[10]

Population-based trials commonly examine cause-specific

TABLE 41–1. HEALTH IMPACT OF MAJOR CANCERS ATTRIBUTABLE TO SELECTED RISK FACTORS, UNITED STATES, 1980

Cancer Site	Risk Factor	Number of Deaths	Number of Years Lost (to age 65)	Number of Hospital Days (100,000s)	Cost (millions)
Lung	Smoking	67,140	253,667	2,548	$1,212
Colorectal	Diet	11,444	27,546	645	260
Breast	Diet	7,504	43,454	449	253
Cervix	Smoking	1,320	9,431	136	43
Pancreas	Smoking	5,931	15,866	135	63
Bladder	Smoking	4,347	4,513	153	131
Larynx	Smoking	2,552	9,235	198	178
	Alcohol	583	2,108	45	41
Percentage of all cancers		24	21		16

Adapted from Rothenberg et al.[4]

death rates as the outcome in question. Lack of change in total mortality, even when cause-specific reductions occur, has been interpreted as evidence that risk reduction interventions may be less efficacious than claimed.[11] However, others argue that overall mortality rates are not the best measure for success of health promotion programs. "The primary purpose of most health promotion activities in developed countries is to improve the quality of life, to 'compress' morbidity, and to extend *active* life expectancy."[12]

From a public health perspective, precursors of disease are of interest if they are causal and modifiable. Although behavioral risk factors meet both conditions, health promotion more suitably focuses on population prevalence rather than on the status of a single individual for two reasons. First, individuals can enter and leave exposure categories and vary the "dosage," which they do frequently and over significant periods of time before the consequence becomes clinically visible. Second, it is difficult to link a behavior choice by any given individual to his or her subsequent health status despite clear, sometimes dramatically increased, relative risks associated with the behavior. Indeed, for most people health behavior is like a lottery in reverse: it is the minority that loses rather than wins.[13]

Nevertheless, accumulated evidence indicates that health behavior choices, far from being refractory, deeply ingrained human characteristics, are modifiable and sometimes change at a pace that equates to rapid social change. Nutrition is a complex issue; dietary preferences are rooted in childhood determinants of eating behavior and influenced by family and cultural values. Nevertheless, the American public in the 1970s made substantial reductions in consumption of saturated fats. Per capita consumption of red meats, whole milk, and similar sources of fat has continued to decrease, although fat continues to represent too large a share of the typical American diet.[14]

Injury prevention practices also have been changing. Now more than half of all infants ride in cars in a certified car seat rather than in a parent's arms.[15] Moreover, after years of public education culminating in the passage of state laws requiring seat belt use, the prevalence of seat belt use has shown significant percentage increases.[16] There is increasing societal agreement that drunk driving is unacceptable behavior, and driving while drunk seems to be declining. Between 1982 and 1987 the proportion of intoxicated drivers in fatal crashes dropped from 30% to 25%.[17]

Another striking example of population behavior change in public health is the 25-year decline in cigarette smoking. From 1965 to 1987, the overall prevalence of smoking dropped from 40% to 29%; for men the drop was almost 20 points, from 50.2% to 31.7%.[18] Clearly, despite the addictive potency of tobacco, millions of individuals quit smoking, millions more were deterred from starting, and the population prevalence of a major hazardous behavior changed in a significant way.

Not all parts of society adopt or maintain healthful behaviors at the same rate, and some of the most vulnerable social groups typically lag behind. Again, smoking provides an object lesson. Although overall rates of smoking have declined among both men and women, the rate of decline has been lower for women, particularly for young women, with obvious consequences both for the health of these women and their infants.[19] There is a higher prevalence of smoking in persons in racial and ethnic minorities, and these smokers quit less often than those in nonminority groups.[18]

Socioeconomic variables are important factors influencing both the adoption of health practices and the success of intervention strategies. The association of poverty with mortality and illness has been clear for a long time. Survival rates have been shown to vary, over an 18-year follow-up, directly with class of family income: the lower the income, the lower the survival rate.[20] Studies have identified at least 23 health problems that are more frequent at lower socioeconomic levels in the United States.[21]

Formal educational attainment appears to have a particularly strong association with personal behavior choices. At virtually every level, from "no high school" through "graduate de-

TABLE 41–2. HEALTH IMPACT OF CARDIOVASCULAR DISEASE ATTRIBUTABLE TO SELECTED RISK FACTORS, UNITED STATES, 1980

Risk Factor	Number of Deaths	Number of Years Lost (to age 65)	Number of Cases (est.) (1000s)	Direct Costs (millions)
Smoking	162,564	534,870	3,891	$4,509
High blood pressure	295,162	319,499	3,536	6,289
Serum cholesterol	101,766	159,333	4,791	7,655

Adapted from White et al.[5]

gree,'' for both men and women, the less education people have, the greater the likelihood that they are current smokers (Fig. 41-1).[22] This inverse pattern has been observed consistently in both the United States and Canada for cigarette smoking, lack of physical activity, lack of seat belt use, and in safety practices (e.g., not having a smoke detector in the home).[23] (The opposite pattern has been noted for alcohol use and for driving after excessive alcohol use.)

THE CONCEPT OF HEALTH PROMOTION

The fundamental importance of personal health behaviors as a determinant of health has been acknowledged as early as human thought about health and its care has been recorded. For contemporary health promotion, the Canadian document known popularly as the Lalonde Report was a landmark.[24] It introduced the ''health field concept'' as a framework for analysis of public health problems. By looking at health in terms of four fields, human biology, life-style, environment, and health care organization, this approach accomplished several things. First, it shifted consideration of the causes of sickness and death to an understanding of the contributions made by each of the fields and thus to the potential for prevention that each embodies. Second, examination of the health fields facilitated identification of intervention strategies available to realize the prevention opportunities. Finally, the report's publication and wide distribution as a public policy document elevated life-style issues and, by extension, the field of health promotion to the level of health care organization issues, despite the vast disparity in resource expenditures among the health fields. Subsequent analyses using the health field approach attributed as much as half of all premature deaths to life-styles.[25,26]

In the United States this was elaborated by two federal policy documents that received wide distribution and visibility. The first, Healthy People, the Surgeon General's Report on Health Promotion and Disease Prevention, firmly established prevention as a key strategy of national health policy and made health promotion a prominent element of the prevention strategy.[1] The report grouped strategy elements into three basic categories: (1) health promotion directed at population groups, (2) health protection directed at population groups, and (3) personal preventive health services.

A companion document, *Promoting Health/Preventing Disease: Objectives for the Nation,* followed the same conceptual framework in setting prevention objectives for 1990.[27] Of the 226 objectives, 78 were presented under the rubric ''health promotion.'' As many as 30 others, presented under the rubrics ''health protection'' and ''preventive health services,'' addressed either consequences of health behaviors or personal and professional education. Thus nearly half the national prevention objectives bear relevantly on health promotion. The widespread adoption of these 1990 objectives as a framework for public health action has given additional impetus to health promotion activities.[28]

In spite of the evident growth of health promotion programs in the decade since these documents appeared, an accepted definition of health promotion has been elusive. *Healthy People* did not explicitly define the term but suggested its aim is ''the development of community and individual measures which can help [people] to develop lifestyles that can maintain and enhance the state of well-being.''[1] In both the Lalonde Report and *Healthy People* the focus on health behavior is an *etiological* one: a focus on causal linkages to health outcomes.

These and other health promotion definitions acknowledge that behavior choices are influenced by many external factors and discuss the need for parallel strategies to reinforce, through community and societal actions, behavior choices that promote health. In another type of definition, the focus is on *intervention processes.* Green's widely cited definition of health promotion carefully incorporates both individual and societal measures: health promotion is ''any combination of health education and related organizational, economic and political interventions designed to facilitate behavioral and environmental changes conducive to health.''[29]

For some the focus on individual behavior as an etiologic agent and on strategies whose impact is measured in reduction of health-risking behaviors carries ethical and philosophical dilemmas.[30-32] A commonly cited concern is that ''the intensifying focus on individual behavior [seems] nothing short of an ideological effort to divert attention from the social and environmental causes of disease and death.''[33]

From this perspective, health promotion is better defined from a systems change, or *socioecological,* viewpoint. One such definition, developed by the European Regional Office of the World Health Organization (WHO) and issued under the title Ottawa Charter for Health Promotion, states, ''Health promotion is the process of enabling people to increase control over, and to improve, their health.''[34] In this concept the function of health promotion is to ''advocate for health,'' to ''enable people to achieve their fullest health potential,'' and to ''mediate between differing interests in society for the pursuit of health.''[34] At this end of the definitional spectrum, virtually all the focus is on modification of political and social systems, and modest at-

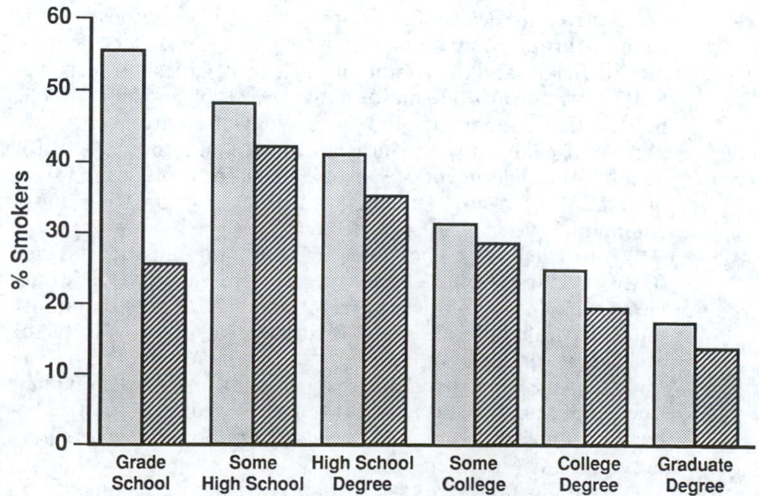

Figure 41-1. The inverse relationship of adult smoking prevalence and educational attainment. *Dotted bars* represent white men; *slashed bars,* white women. Age adjusted for smokers aged 25 years or older. *[From Remington P et al: JAMA 253:2975, 1985.[22]]*

tention is paid either to behavioral outcomes or to public health and health educational intervention strategies. An additional weakness of this conceptualization of health promotion is the explicit incorporation of such public health disciplines as environmental health, pollution control, and occupational safety and health under the purview of health promotion. Such an aggregative definition seems to obscure rather than clarify health promotion as a public health strategy.

Other definitions approach health promotion as a positive concept of human capacity, not a negative assignment of blame. One defines health promotion in reference to a positive concept of health, strengthening the reserves for, and reducing the risks to, health.[35] Another argues that a public health approach to health promotion includes actions in support of both personal and community responses, that is, individual and collective citizen involvement in defining priority health promotion needs and stimulating community efforts to address them.[36]

We believe that the definition of health promotion proposed by Green remains a serviceable framework for public health action.[29] The attainment of health promotion objectives is appropriately measured by changes in population prevalence of behavioral risk factors, community changes, and health status and quality of life improvements that may reasonably be expected on the basis of scientific knowledge.

For readers responsible for designing, managing, or allocating resources to health promotion programs or setting health promotion priorities, a technical report prepared by an ad hoc work group of the American Public Health Association extends this framework in the form of Criteria for the Development of Health Promotion and Education Programs.[37] These criteria, intended as guidelines for establishing the feasibility and appropriateness of health promotion programs in a variety of settings, are summarized in Table 41-3. Each of these criteria is supplemented by a series of issues or questions that illuminate the central characteristics of health promotion programs.

STRATEGIES AND SETTINGS

Interventions designed to reduce behavioral risk factors and their consequences logically lead to consideration of settings in which they can appropriately, economically, and effectively be mounted.[37] There is general agreement that community, school, work site, and health care settings are most appropriate for health promotion activities.

TABLE 41-3. CRITERIA FOR THE DEVELOPMENT OF HEALTH PROMOTION AND EDUCATION PROGRAMS

1. A health promotion program should address one or more risk factors which are carefully defined, measurable, modifiable, and prevalent among the members of a chosen group, factors which constitute a threat to the health status and the quality of life of target group members.
2. A health promotion program should reflect a consideration of the special characteristics, needs, and preferences of its target group[s].
3. Health promotion programs should include interventions which will clearly and effectively reduce a targeted risk factor and are appropriate for a particular setting.
4. A health promotion program should identify and implement interventions which make optimum use of available resources.
5. From the outset, a health promotion program should be organized, planned, and implemented in such a way that its operation and effects can be evaluated.

From American Public Health Association Technical Report: Criteria for the development of health promotion and education programs. Am J Public Health 77[1] 89–92, 1987[37]

Community-based Health Promotion

In community health in general, and even more so in health promotion, many community institutions and resources are essential partners. A central and critical partner is the public health department. The role health departments play in health promotion derives from their core functions in public health. A report of the Institute of Medicine on the future of public health identifies the core functions as *assessment, policy development,* and *assurance.*[38] Assessment includes systematically collecting, analyzing, and making available information on community health status and needs. Policy development includes leadership in developing public health policies that are based on scientific knowledge and community need. Assurance is the responsibility to ensure that public health needs are met by encouraging actions by other public or private entities, by requiring action through regulation, or by providing services directly. In the case of health promotion, all three of these core functions contribute directly to behavioral risk reduction.

An extensive community health promotion program called PATCH—Planned Approach to Community Health—was launched in 1982 as a collaboration between state and local health departments and the Centers for Disease Control. Some 12 states and more than 40 communities are involved. Although the program draws substantially from the experience of North Karelia and similar U.S. studies,[39] it differs in that it is not an intervention trial. The health department partners work with community residents and institutions to define local priorities, set measurable objectives, collect community data, and undertake health promotion programs. Use of locally specific data, including a community behavioral risk factor survey, vital statistics, and opinion leader interviews, is a key element for assuring that PATCH objectives and strategies will be supported by the community.[40] PATCH programs typically have generated several dollars in additional support for every $1 initially received in financial assistance. This planned approach also has been successful in gaining intersectorial cooperation, for example, in school health education, highway safety, and work site smoking policies.[41]

Another community-based model being demonstrated both in North America and Europe emerged from a 1984 Toronto workshop, Healthy Toronto 2000.[42] Known as Healthy Cities or Healthy Communities, this concept was subsequently launched in a number of Canadian cities, followed by a WHO-sponsored European project and by projects in the United States sponsored by Indiana University and the California Health Department. The Canadian model, which is premised on a socioecological perspective on health behaviors, seeks to accomplish social changes through cooperative efforts of political leaders, government officials, and the community. Healthy Cities' projects typically work toward five major aims: (1) establishment of public policies that support health, (2) creation of environments supportive of health, (3) encouragement of community action for health, (4) development of personal skills for health, and (5) reorientation of health services toward health promotion and a community-based health services system.[42]

A problem often encountered at the community level is lack of a systematic way to choose targets and select proven strategies. One solution to this may be found in a series of community intervention handbooks, each focused on a specific risk factor and a defined target population.[43–45] Each handbook follows the same sequence of steps: diagnosis, intervention, and action plan. The handbooks provide a guide for understanding a specified behavior, estimating community needs and resources, and organizing community interventions.[46]

An important private-sector initiative has been launched by the Kaiser Family Foundation in association with other philanthropic groups. Plans include expending up to $40 million, over 10 years, to support community health promotion efforts, along with regional technical resource centers on which communities can draw to plan and evaluate their efforts.[47] A particular priority of this initiative is health promotion programs targeted to the needs of minority groups.

Racial and ethnic minorities experience more than 58,000 excess deaths from chronic diseases when compared to the more favorable mortality rates of nonminority populations, and many of these are attributable to behavioral risk factors.[48] Thus responsible and responsive programs are needed to address the health promotion concerns of minorities in a culturally sensitive fashion.[37,49]

One example of such programs is a physical exercise program for members of the Zuni tribe. Evaluation results indicate quantitative improvements in both weight and diabetes control.[50] In another program, residents of a black Atlanta neighborhood designed and implemented the Community Health Assessment and Promotion Project (CHAPP). Community concern about high blood pressure led to support for a weight loss and exercise program. Results of the intervention included a significant loss of weight compared with a control population. Perhaps because of a concerted effort to develop culturally appropriate strategies, this community-guided intervention was able to avoid one of the difficulties of many minority health promotion programs: falloff in participation rates.[51]

Broad participation is a vital ingredient of successful community health promotion programs.[52,53] A number of important intervention trials, particularly in cardiovascular disease, have drawn on both behavioral theory and community organization research to incorporate community health promotion strategies in their approaches, for example, the North Karelia, Finland, Project,[54] the Stanford Five Cities Project,[55] and the Pawtucket Heart Health Program.[56] Community organization skills and principles reinforce the efforts of health promotion practitioners in disseminating health information, motivating decisions to adopt healthful behaviors, providing opportunities to change behavior, and maintaining such changes.[57]

It is evident from health promotion definitions and community organization principles that behavior is determined by multiple influences and that the community is a particularly apt setting to address these interventions at several levels. A model of behavioral determinants has been proposed, using theoretical frameworks to array determinants into five groups:

1. *Interpersonal factors:* Characteristics of the individual such as knowledge, attitudes, behavior, self-concept, and skills (includes the developmental history of the individual)
2. *Interpersonal processes and primary groups.* Formal and informal social network and social support systems, including the family, work group, and friendship networks
3. *Institutional factors:* Social institutions with organizational characteristics and formal (and informal) rules and regulations for operation
4. *Community factors:* Relationships among organizations, institutions, and informal networks within defined boundaries
5. *Public policy:* Local, state, and national laws and policies[58]

Researchers from the University of Texas Health Science Center, on the basis of their work in a number of intervention projects, have proposed a multilevel intervention model that conceptualizes interventions as directed toward three levels: individuals, organizations, and governments.[59] Figure 41-2 illustrates how a community-based health promotion program can

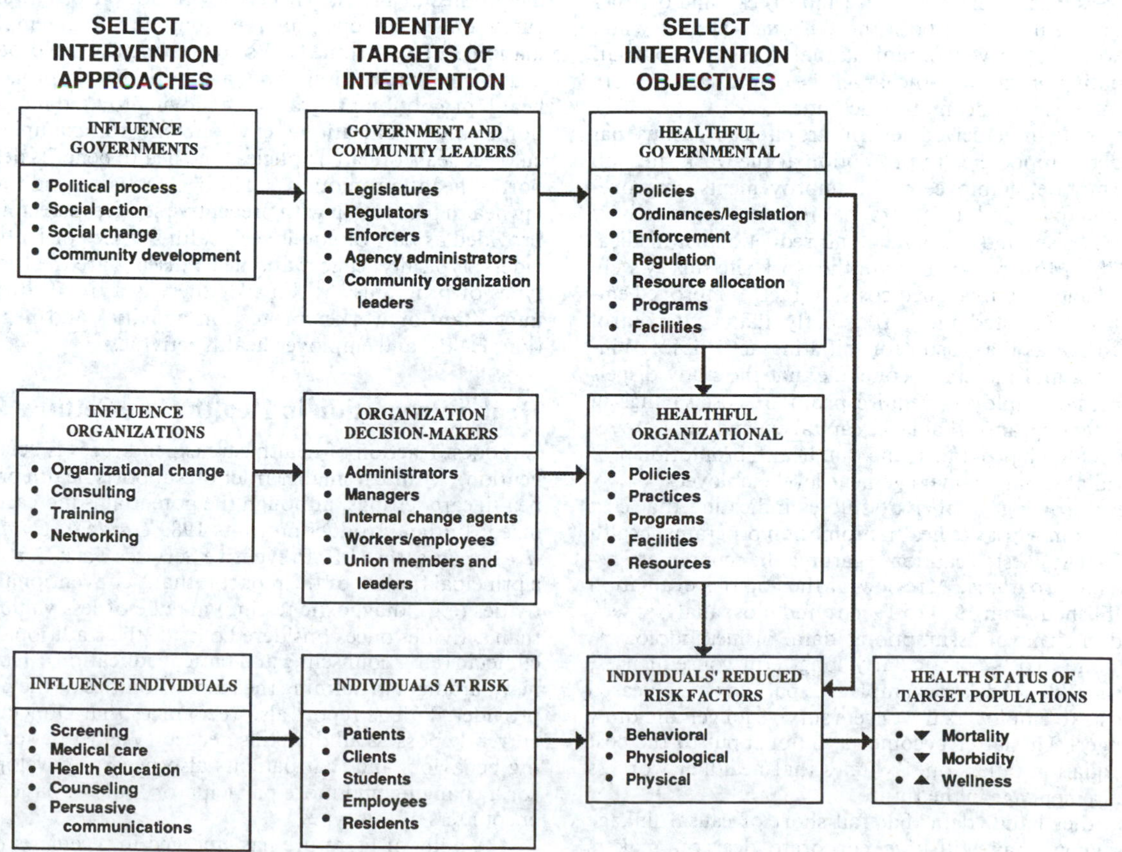

Figure 41-2. A model of the multiple levels of intervention targets available to health promotion programs. *[Reprinted from Simons-Morton DG et al. Family & Community Health, vol. 11, no. 2, p. 29, with permission of Aspen Publishers, Inc., © 1988.]*

address health behaviors and health status outcome through actions at each level of intervention.

Numerous examples of successful projects have been described that document success in community organization, community change, and behavioral change.[60] The PATCH, Zuni, and CHAPP projects described above are illustrative of such interventions, as is the San Francisco-based Tenderloin Senior Organizing Project. This 10-year-old program has helped inner-city elderly residents solve a number of problems through actions at the municipal, neighborhood, and individual levels.[61] Moreover, transferring "ownership" to a broader base may be essential to long-term survival. A recent case study of a project that terminated when its federal funding ended demonstrates that intervention effectiveness does not automatically lead to long-term institutionalization, an ultimate mark of program success.[62]

Work Site-based Health Promotion

Interest in health promotion and health education programs conducted in the work setting has been steadily increasing, and business leaders view these programs as consistent with employee health and good business.[63] This growth seems unlikely to abate. A survey of the nation's largest corporations, the *Fortune* 500 list, to which half responded, suggests that two thirds of these corporations have health promotion programs. Many of these are slated for expansion, and one third of the corporations without programs indicated that they plan to initiate them.[64]

More than half of American workers are employed at work sites with 50 or more employees. The National Survey of Worksite Health Promotion Activities documents the nature and extent of health promotion activities in work sites of this size.[65] The survey indicates that two out of three of these work sites now offer at least one health promotion activity. The most commonly offered activities are smoking control, health risk assessment, back care, stress management, exercise and fitness, and off-the-job accident prevention.[64] In both the *Fortune* 500 survey and the broader work site survey, organizational size is an important factor in initiating programs—the larger the employer, the more likely it is to offer health promotion activities.

A wide variety of perceived benefits are cited as reasons that business leaders support health promotion at the work site: job satisfaction, morale, employee health improvements, improvements in productivity and in factors that influence productivity (such as absenteeism and turnover), and reductions in medical care costs.[63,66,67] Most respondents in the work site survey were satisfied that benefits outweighed costs; in fact, "improved employee health" was cited more frequently than "to control health care costs" as the reason for initiating activities.[66] Windom, McGinnis, and Fielding[68] conclude that the study dispels three myths: that employers require proof of cost savings in order to initiate programs, that large capital expenditures are required to launch such programs, and that health promotion programs are available only to management-level employees.

Despite a growing number of studies indicating that cost savings result from work site health promotion programs, health economists have suggested caution regarding the economic benefits of work site programs. A review of the copious evaluation literature published from 1974 to 1986 found most analyses seriously flawed in terms of assumptions, data, or methodology.[69] Certain economic costs, particularly long-term consequences, often were not addressed, for example, the paradox of increased long-term costs to employers if workers survive longer and draw pensions longer. The latter becomes a major input to the cost side of the equation unless one assumes that healthier workers will defer retirement age in the future.[70]

On the other hand, data that fall short of causal linkage with cost savings may still give corporate decision makers enough confidence in the positive benefits of the program to warrant the investment.[71] Given the practical limits to research in the work setting, the lack of sound evidence of cost savings does not mean that there are none, but rather reflects the need for careful reading and additional evaluation.[71]

Among the better known programs nationally are the Live for Life program of Johnson & Johnson, the AT&T Total Life Concept program, the Employee Health Promotion program of the Group Health Cooperative of Puget Sound, and the Blue Cross–Blue Shield of Indiana program.[72] The Johnson & Johnson program was evaluated recently in terms of cost and care utilization; controls experienced significantly greater per capita hospital costs incurred under the employee health benefits program.[73] School faculty and staff in Oregon also have been the focus of work site health promotion. Benefits of such programs may include not only health benefits, such as improved attitudes toward personal health, with carryover to student attitudes, but also perceived academic benefits, such as improved quality of instruction.[74]

Increasingly, workplace health promotion programs are being targeted to individuals at highest risk or groups who have not been well reached in the past, for example, blue-collar employees[75] and women.[76] Some programs also extend the work site program to a larger community of dependents[77] and retirees.[78] Although much of the focus on workplace health promotion has been on employer-sponsored programs, labor unions historically have been involved in health promotion also and are increasingly initiating programs as benefits to their members.[79] The likelihood of a particular workplace health promotion innovation being adopted probably is influenced by the interlocking network of interests of employers, employees, and health promotion providers.[80]

Several trends appear to be emerging that affect work site health promotion. First, employee assistance programs (EAPs) traditionally have focused on providing assessment, short-term counseling, and referral to employees with substance abuse and mental health problems; health promotion programs have focused on educational interventions aimed at employee populations.[81] Today some EAPs are moving toward broad-scale education and prevention, from a case-finding approach. Second, health promotion programs are moving toward increased attention to the organizational environment, for example, corporate culture, health-related policies, and health benefits design in support of health promotion.[82] Third, there is a trend towards linking health promotion with preventive services screening activities provided as part of employee health services or by outside providers; typically, cancer and heart disease are the focus of these types of programs.[83,84] Finally, there is a trend toward greater integration of worker protection activities and health promotion, EAPs, and employee health activities.[83,85]

Health Promotion in Health Care Settings

A modest fraction of health care expenditures is devoted to prevention.[86] A much smaller fraction supports health promotion in health care settings, although the potential is increasingly recognized. In the introduction to its 1989 *Guide to Clinical Preventive Services,* the U.S. Preventive Services Task Force states that a principal finding of the report is that "conventional clinical activities (e.g., diagnostic testing) may be of less value to patients than activities once considered outside the traditional role of the clinician (e.g., counseling and patient education). This suggests a new paradigm in defining the responsibilities of the primary care provider."[87] The report also recognizes that clinicians may not currently possess all the skills needed to assist patients in changing behaviors and that patients also need to develop new skills for a changing and more participatory role in patient-physician encounters of this type.

A body of literature has emerged in recent years regarding successful strategies for medical personnel to counsel patients and help accomplish behavior change. Some of this focuses on specific risk factors, such as smoking[19,88] and exercise.[7,89] Others address counseling approaches, such as patient-physician counseling[90] and reinforcement by office staff.[91] Many publications report that patient counseling and education can be carried out successfully and integrated into clinical settings.[92-95]

Hospitals also have found new roles in health promotion. The number of hospitals providing patient education services has increased steadily since the mid-1970s. In 1987, more than 87% of reporting hospitals indicated to the American Hospital Association (AHA) that they offer patient education on an inpatient basis and almost 73% offer this service to outpatients.[96] One of the first conditions for which hospitals typically began to provide patient education was diabetes, and detailed patient education standards have been set for this.[97] Currently many different subjects are covered, ranging from high blood pressure control to chronic disease management to adherence by elderly patients to prescribed medication regimens.[96]

In addition, the AHA surveys reported that more than 70% of hospitals offer one or more community health promotion programs. Between 1984 and 1987, rapid growth occurred in such areas as work site health promotion programs, employee assistance programs, industrial or occupational health services, and fitness facilities. The latter category more than doubled during that period, from 240 to 629 hospitals.[96-98]

Hospitals embark on health promotion programs for various reasons. One hospital administrator sees changing market conditions as forcing hospitals to assume new roles in their communities. Health promotion has become an attractive business option, with potential for opening new markets, generating new sources of revenue, and identifying asymptomatic individuals in need of services.[99] Community health promotion and other services such as screening and detection, often offered free, also enhance the public image of health care institutions.[100,101] However, respondents to the 1987 AHA survey ranked "quality of care" and "community service" first and second as possible rationales for hospital health promotion, ahead of "public relations," "referral source," and "revenue source."[96]

Health maintenance organizations (HMOs), because they are reimbursed by a fixed capitation fee, have incentives to prevent ill health and would therefore seem a likely provider of health promotion services to their members. However, of 203 HMOs reporting, more than 50 had no wellness activities. Possibly, relatively rapid turnover of membership and the time lapse between some health promotion activities and prevented health outcome make the economic benefits seem less attractive to HMOs. The most commonly cited benefit of HMO-sponsored wellness activities was "helping to retain current members by demonstrating the commitment of the HMO to keeping members healthy."[102] Other HMO rationales for investment in health promotion may be marketing to new members and altering the mix of subscribers by attracting younger, healthier persons interested in health promotion.

Many health professionals, in addition to medical and dental practitioners, are able to provide health promotion services. Among these are nurses,[103] occupational therapists,[104] certified nurse midwives, certified physician assistants, registered dental hygienists, registered dietitians,[105] and other allied health professionals.[106]

A number of studies of health promotion provided in a health care setting have documented positive behavioral, health care utilization, and health outcome results, for example, reduced diabetic hospitalizations through a patient education and support system[107] and a simple self-help education program in an HMO that reduced physician visits for upper respiratory illness.[108] A controlled clinical trial in which smoking cessation services were incorporated in prenatal care reported significant reductions in maternal smoking and increases in birth weight for the study group as compared with the control group.[109] In a hospital-based hypertension trial, inner-city black women in the study group that received education and support services demonstrated behavior changes and reduced blood pressure and experienced a 50% reduction in mortality at 5-year follow-up as compared with a control group.[110]

These findings suggest that physicians and other health workers in hospital, clinic, HMO, and physician office settings can effectively provide health promotion services. A number of personal health behaviors affect, and can be influenced by, the health care system, for example, seeking appropriate health care and preventive services, adopting or maintaining protective health practices, adhering to preventive and therapeutic regimens, and keeping appointments.[36,111,112]

The barrier is not a lack of availability of preventive technologies.[113] Rather, such issues as education and attitudes of providers, motivation and expectation of patients, and aspects of health care organization such as access and reimbursement impede successful incorporation of health promotion in health care settings.[105,111,114-117] The health system is a long way from accomplishing its potential in health promotion.[118]

School-Based Health Promotion

Childhood and adolescent development includes the establishment of attitudes and behaviors that directly and indirectly influence the future health of those involved. Early behavior choices directly influence the current health status of young people, for example, sexuality,[119] drug use,[120] drinking, and driving.[121] Lifelong maintenance of protective health behaviors (e.g., nonsmoking[18] and regular aerobic exercise[7]) contributes to both quantity and quality of life.[122]

The 1987 National Adolescent School Health Survey was the first such national survey since the 1960s to measure several critical adolescent behavioral risks and the adolescents' perceptions of the risks.[121] A random sample of eighth- and tenth-grade students reported engaging in behaviors that increase health risks. For example, 56% of the students reported they had not worn a seat belt on their most recent trip. About 25% of boys and 42% of girls indicated that they had seriously considered suicide at some point in their lives. Among eighth graders, 51% said they had tried smoking tobacco, 77% said they had used alcohol, and 15% said they had tried marijuana. Significant majorities of respondents had correct perceptions of sexual risk factors for human immunodeficiency virus (HIV) infection, and smaller majorities understood sexually transmitted disease signs; however, a significant fraction of the respondents were unsure or had incorrect perceptions. Widely varying percentages reported having received instruction in school, depending on the health topic surveyed (Fig. 41-3). The area for which health education was reported most frequently was the effects of tobacco, alcohol, and drugs.[121]

Since 48 million children and youth attend school daily, it is apparent that schools have great potential to promote health. School health education is viewed both domestically and internationally as an essential part of education and of school health more generally.[123,124] Although many states have general policies encouraging school health education, only 27 have specific requirements for high school graduation.[125] The nation's health objectives for the year 2000 establish measurable targets both for high school graduation rate (90%) and for the proportion of schools (75%) providing quality school health education.[126] The American School Health Association has developed an agenda for the nation's schools outlining activities involved in achieving the Objectives for the Nation.[127]

School health joins the interests and skills of two major institutions of our society: education and public health. In concept, school health has been viewed, since the early 1900s, as including three basic elements: school health education, school health services, and school health environment.[128] More recently, in line with the evolution of health promotion, the concept of school health has broadened to include efforts that ad-

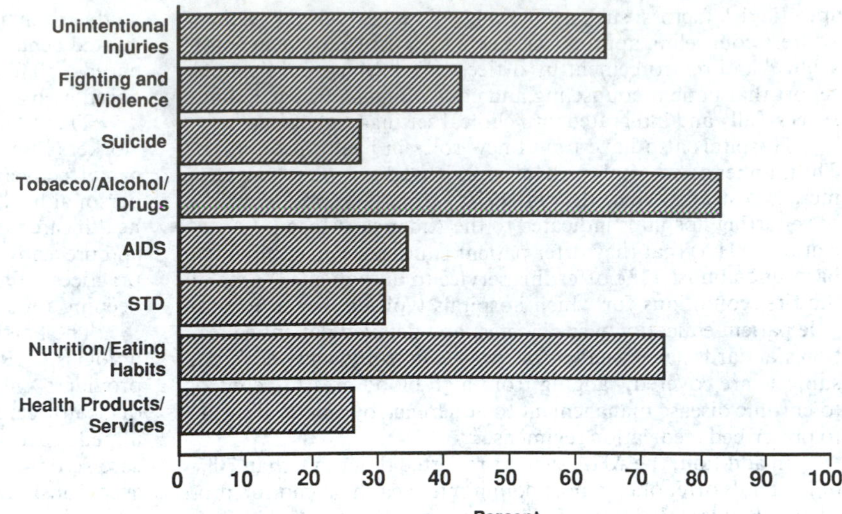

Figure 41-3. Percent of high school students reporting that they had received instruction in school in these indicated health promotion topics, 1987 Adolescent School Health Survey.

dress short- and long-term outcomes comprehensively (Fig. 41-4).[128,129]

The work of school counselors and school psychologists increasingly includes broader based interventions in support of the physical and emotional health of students. Emotional problems of young people likely to spill over into the educational setting range from psychopathologies (e.g., suicide attempts) to problem behaviors (e.g., delinquency) to health-compromising behavior (e.g., anorexia).[130] The role of the school psychologist need not be limited to psychopathology; it can also provide behavioral science guidance to develop school health programming to promote healthful behavior choices.[131]

School food services provide 27 million lunches and 3 million breakfasts daily; formats, menus, and innovations adopted in this important part of public education can either reinforce or undermine nutritional health promotion.[132] Strategies to help students learn about nutrition can be augmented by strategies aimed at organizational changes that support these learning experiences, for example, vending machine policies and school lunch menus in line with nutritional guidelines.[133]

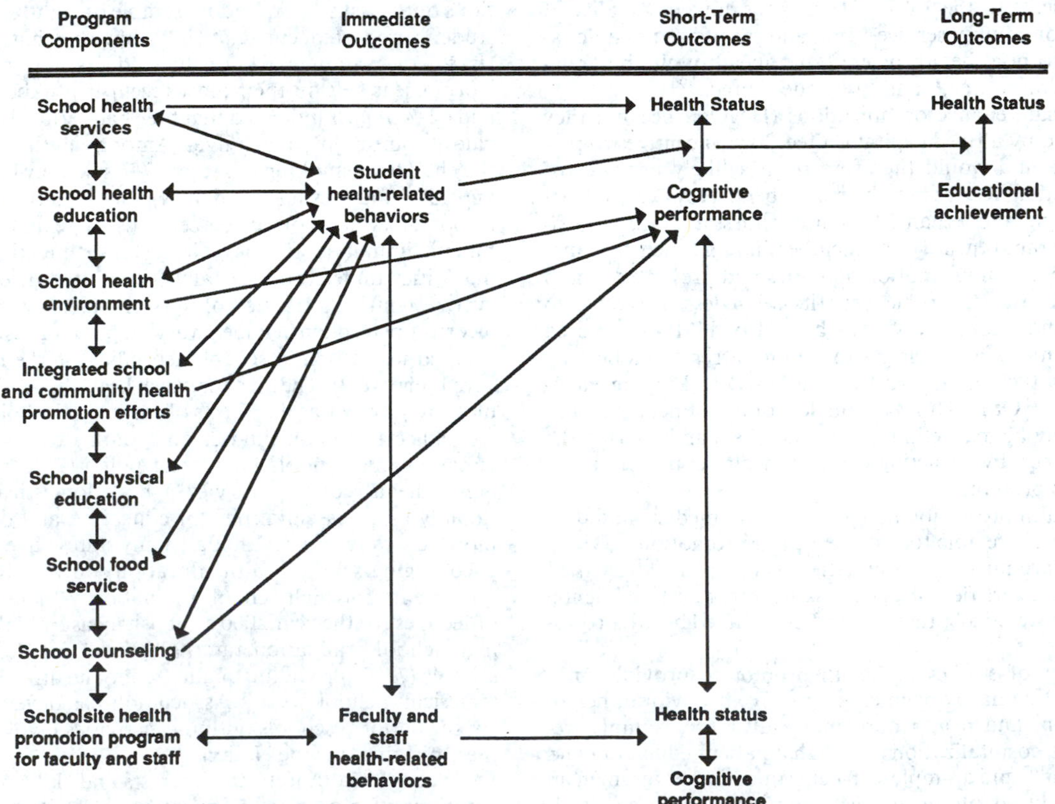

Figure 41-4. Comprehensive school health—a model of the relationships of eight components with behavioral and educational outcomes. *[From Allensworth DD, Kolbe LJ: The comprehensive school health program: Exploring an expanded concept. Reprinted with permission from Journal of School Health 57[10]:410, December 1987. Copyright 1987. American School Health Association, P.O. Box 708, Kent, OH 44240.]*

Physical education in schools is a vital element of health promotion. Unfortunately, a games-oriented approach to physical education, emphasizing sports skills and motor development, tends to be the norm in American schools, although a health-oriented approach is beginning to gain acceptance.[134] The findings of two National Children and Youth Fitness Studies do not offer encouragement regarding the exercise levels of American children.[135,136] A recent study found that only 6.1% of the time spent on various activities during elementary school physical education was devoted to aerobic physical activity.[137] None of the 1990 prevention objectives relating to physical activity for children is likely to be met when the data are fully analyzed.[137]

Ample data exist to show that well-conceived, well-executed school health education, carried out with fidelity to the curricula and with appropriately trained teachers, can increase health knowledge, attitudes, and behaviors. In a major controlled study of fifth- and sixth-grade children in four curricula, educationally significant improvements were observed at 3-year follow-up.[139] As expected, it was relatively easy to produce knowledge gains with a few hours of instruction, but these curricula also accomplished positive changes in health behavior and health attitudes, with maximum impact reached at about 50 hours—the optimum "dose" of this "intervention."[139]

A number of school health education curricula have become well established, including Growing Health,[140] the Teenage Health Teaching Modules Program for Teachers and Students,[141] and Know Your Body.[142] In a randomized trial of Growing Healthy, smoking behavior in a study group receiving fifth- and sixth-grade units of the curriculum was compared with that of control groups who did not receive the instruction. Growing Healthy is a comprehensive curriculum for kindergarten through seventh grade; tobacco is addressed within a broader health behavior framework. Although little difference was observed in smoking rates in fifth and sixth grades, at follow-up in the seventh grade the smoking rate in the study group was 37% lower than in the control group.[143] If all U.S. students received an equally effective school health education experience, an estimated 146,000 fewer seventh-grade students would be smokers each year than if none had this experience (Fig. 41-5).[143]

Teenage pregnancy is a serious U.S. problem; most pregnancies among women under 20 years of age are unintended. Starting in 1982, a "School and Community Program for Sexual Risk Reduction among Teens" was begun in a South Carolina county. The intervention was a combination of specific educational messages and skills and broad community involvement, including parents, teachers, representatives of churches, and community leaders. Compared with three control counties, which experienced net increases in the estimated pregnancy rate among females aged 14 to 17, the study population reduced its pregnancy rate by 54%.[144] A case study has documented the intervention strategy and methods used.[145]

These and other data argue for a comprehensive approach to school health education in preference to one-time or single-subject approaches.[128] A comprehensive approach is one that is planned and sequential, and introduces concepts and materials at developmentally appropriate points in the child's growth. Moreover, the term *comprehensive* means more than including all appropriate topics or all grades from kindergarten to twelfth grade, although both are features of a sound approach. In particular, comprehensive school health curricula should provide opportunities to develop needed skills and qualities, for example, decision-making and communication skills, resistance to persuasion, and a sense of self-efficacy and self-esteem. The growing support for this approach is illustrated by the current expansion of HIV education in schools. Integrating HIV content into a comprehensive program of school health is strongly endorsed by the Centers for Disease Control,[119] the Presidential Commission on the Epidemic of HIV Infection,[146] and leading educational organizations.[147,148]

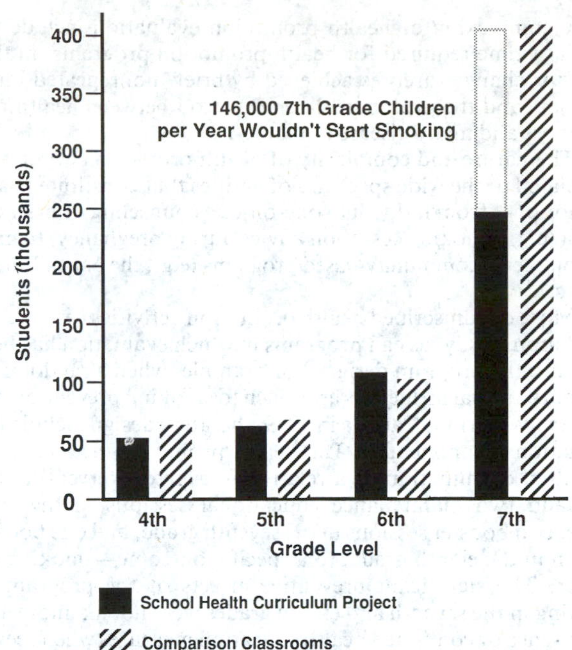

Figure 41-5. Estimated reduction in numbers of children smoking that would result from nationwide exposure to comprehensive school health education. *[From Christenson GM Gold RS, Katz M, Kreuter MW: Preface. Journal of School Health 55[8]:296, October 1985. Copyright 1985. American School Health Association, P.O. Box 708, Kent, OH 44240.]*

EVALUATION

The Office of Technology Assessment of the U.S. Congress defines medical technologies as the drugs, devices, and medical and surgical procedures used in medical care and the organizational and supportive systems within which such care is provided.[149] As such we should consider health promotion activities to be preventive medical technologies and as suitable for assessment or evaluation as organ transplantation, magnetic resonance imaging (MRI) scans, or zidovudine. Health promotion has particular features that make its evaluation sometimes different and often more difficult to perform than diagnostic or therapeutic technologies. Nevertheless, it is possible to apply similar concepts of efficacy, effectiveness, and cost-effectiveness in evaluating health promotion activities.[150]

Efficacy is used to refer to a program, activity, or technology being assessed under optimal conditions. Similar assessment done under field conditions is referred to as effectiveness. Most health promotion programs are studied after they are in place. As in diagnostic or therapeutic technologies, preventive technologies do not always establish their efficacy before becoming operational. Thus effectiveness studies require assessments of a program's inherent value and how it is implemented, how available it is, and its level of acceptance.

The evaluation of health promotion programs is complicated by the multitude of activities undertaken to achieve an impact on a given health target, such as coronary heart disease. These may include mass media education, use of community leaders and groups, population-based risk factor screening and education, adult education class, school-based education, health professional education, and community-wide risk factor education campaigns.[151] Thus evaluation involves assessing the ultimate impact on disease rates but also the individual effectiveness of each component of the program. Other factors contributing to the complexion of health promotion evaluation include the length of time required for health promotion programs, in that behavior change rarely is achieved by brief, nonrepeated interventions, and the prolonged latency period between health risk behaviors and many disease outcomes.

The nature and complexity of health promotion evaluation are related to the wide spectrum of entities that constitute health promotion—from individual one-on-one counseling of brief duration (e.g., smoking cessation advice during pregnancy) to massive long-term community-based programs (e.g., the North Karelia Project).[152]

More circumscribed health promotion activities can be evaluated more easily, as can programs in which evaluation has been built into the program design. For example, when a randomized trial of the social influences approach to smoking prevention was begun in Waterloo, Canada in 1979, the study design included an evaluation component.[153] The health promotion activity itself permitted examination of a relatively discrete intervention (six core and two maintenance educational sessions in the sixth grade, two booster sessions in the seventh grade, and one booster session in the eighth grade) to a specific outcome—smoking behavior. The significant preventive effects of the program on smoking in the seventh and eighth grades were not maintained in the absence of continued health education measures when reevaluated at the end of the twelfth grade.[154]

Similarly, when a legislative act mandating motorcycle helmet usage is enacted, one might expect motorcycle collision-related skull and spinal injuries and deaths to decline rapidly.[155] Thus the evaluation of such legislation as a health promotion technology should permit study of health outcomes in a relatively short time frame and also conclusions to be drawn of causal inference.

More complex health promotion programs, such as community-based comprehensive cardiovascular disease control programs, are much more complicated to evaluate.[156] Significant differences, such as a 5.6% decrease in serum cholesterol in the intervention area of North Karelia vs a 1.6% decrease in a reference area over the first 5 years of the program, may disappear when evaluations are repeated over longer time intervals, often because of larger secular trends.[152,157] Even in such large-scale heart disease control projects, different approaches, such as high-risk vs community-based strategies, can be considered as alternative technologies and evaluated as such.[158] Reviews of evaluations of community heart disease control programs,[159] tobacco control efforts,[160] injury prevention and control activities,[161] and school-based health programs[162] are being prepared for publication.

There is increasing interest in evaluating health technologies, including health promotion programs, not only in regard to their effectiveness (Do they work?) but also for their cost-effectiveness (How much do we spend to gain some finite measure of positive health outcome?).

The cost effectiveness of health promotion measures is influenced by several methodological considerations and the nature of health promotion itself. First, there is often a delay between instituting a health promotion activity and realization of the health effect. The longer this delay, the more program costs rise and the more health benefits decrease. The process of "discounting" contributes to this relationship. Discounting is a process for computing how much a dollar, payable in the future, is worth today.[163] The present value of a future dollar depends on the number of years in the future it is obtained and on the annual rate at which it is discounted, the "discount rate." Present dollars and health benefits are valued more than future ones. If a discount rate of 5% is used, then future health benefits (e.g., quality-adjusted life-years saved) and future cost-savings are decreased in value at the rate of 5% per year between intervention and outcome. Thus, within a few years, each additional year of life saved is valued at only a fraction of an undiscounted year (and similarly with dollars saved). Whether screening for hypertension, promoting smoking cessation, or encouraging exercise regimens, when the benefits to be evaluated are, respectively, the prevention of stroke, lung cancer, or coronary heart disease (events not expected to occur for another 15 to 30 years), the methodological requirements of discounting diminish benefits and magnify costs.

Another issue in conducting these analyses involves how we value the elderly and the concept of productivity.[164] Costs in cost-effectiveness analysis can be considered as direct and indirect. Direct costs are those associated with medical care, both acute and chronic. Indirect costs are those that represent lost income, either acutely at the time of illness or more long-term because of disability or death. Indirect costs can contribute greatly to the total sums tallied in an economic analysis. For persons unemployed or retired, dollars saved by preventing future illness usually would include only direct costs. In addition, in a narrow unidimensional perspective, mortality in members who did not belong to the work force could be seen as a net societal economic gain. This is a complex issue and involves our valuing the elderly in our society for far more than their current economic contribution, our understanding that the elderly "paid for" the benefits they receive after retirement during their working years, and our making health policy decisions on considerations beyond the economic aspects, such as ethical, social, and legal considerations.

Another factor that influences cost-effectiveness analysis of health promotion is the question of who pays the costs and who reaps the benefits. Although from a societal perspective a given program may be seen as "cost-effective" (a relative term that requires comparison to some standard or competing technology), it may not be cost-effective to the person or organization incurring the costs. This factor can be seen in settings such as HMOs, where an investment may be made for a health promotion program for a young population, many of whom may be obtaining medical care (or enjoying the benefits of averted illness) in later years with other providers.

There is a growing literature on the economics of health promotion activities. A cost-effectiveness study of the hypertension control program in the North Karelia Project shows a cost under $6000 (at 10% discount rate) per quality-adjusted life-year gained, a ratio that compares favorably with most therapeutic interventions applied after the appearance of hypertensive heart disease.[165] In a larger economic analysis of the North Karelia Project the authors conclude, that "On narrow economic grounds the project generated benefits in excess of costs even over the first 5 years of the project when some but not all of the benefits of the preventive programme started to emerge."[166]

When management alternatives for coronary heart disease were compared (standardized for a 55-year-old man using 1985 dollars), cost-effectiveness in dollars per year of life saved (YOLS) ranged from $4500/YOLS for smoking cessation programs to $17,800/YOLS for cholesterol level reduction using oat bran to $95,000/YOLS for coronary artery bypass graft surgery (three vessel disease, ejection fraction greater than 50%).[167]

Behavioral interventions for non-insulin-dependent diabetes mellitus, such as exercise and weight reduction, have been shown to have a cost-utility ratio of $10,870 per well-year saved, which compares favorably with many other clinical care interventions.[168]

SUMMARY

For many of the major causes of illness, disability, and death in the United States today, individual behavior is a principal factor.

Similarly, human behavior can be a critical factor in promoting health. Thus behavior choices influence our likelihood of being infected with HIV, suffering or surviving an injury, and having coronary heat disease, lung cancer, or cirrhosis. Choices we make in diet, use of alcohol or tobacco, sexual behavior, and driving behavior contribute to how "healthy" we are and will be.

Health promotion, both for individuals and communities, seeks to maximize health, both through influencing people to make appropriate behavior choices and through creating an environmental context that encourages these choices. Health promotion takes place in a wide variety of settings, from the streets (information from billboards or wall posters) to one's home (information from the print and the electronic media). Community, school, work site, and health care settings are important focuses for health promotion activities.

In addition, health promotion varies in scope, from individual counseling to large community-based programs. Many of these health promotion activities have been demonstrated to be effective and, as such, have contributed to the increasingly longer and healthier lives members of our society enjoy today.

REFERENCES

1. Healthy People: The Surgeon General's Report on Health Promotion and Disease Prevention. Washington, D.C.: U.S. Department of HEW Publication No. 79-55071, 1979
2. Foege WH, Amler RW: Introduction and methods. In Amler RW, Dull HB (eds): Closing the Gap: The Burden of Unnecessary Illness. Am J Prev Med 3(suppl 5):3–6, 1987
3. Hermann WH, Teutsch SM, Geiss LS: Diabetes mellitus. In Amler RW, Dull HB (eds): Closing the Gap: The Burden of Unnecessary Illness. Am J Prev Med 3(suppl 5):72–82, 1987
4. Rothenberg R, Nasca P, Mikl J, et al: Cancer. In Amler RW, Dull HB (eds): Closing the Gap: The Burden of Unnecessary Illness. Am J Prev Med 3(suppl 5):30–42, 1987
5. White CC, Tolsma DD, Haynes SG, McGee D Jr: Cardiovascular disease. In Amler RW, Dull HB (eds): Closing the Gap: The Burden of Unnecessary Illness. Am J Prev Med 3(suppl 5):43–54, 1987
6. Powell KE, Thompson PD, Casperson CJ, Kendrick JS: Physical activity and the incidence of coronary heart disease. Annu Rev Public Health 8:253–287, 1987
7. Harris SS, Casperson CJ, DeFriese GH, Estes EH Jr: Physical activity counseling for health adults as a primary preventive intervention in the clinical setting. JAMA 261:3590–3598, 1989
8. National High Blood Pressure Coordinating Committee: 1984 Report. Arch Intern Med 144:1045–1057, 1984
9. Consensus Conference: Lowering blood cholesterol to prevent heart disease. JAMA 253:2080–2086, 1985
10. Amler RW, Eddins DL: Cross-sectional analysis: Precursors of premature death in the United States. In Amler RW, Dull HB (eds): Closing the Gap: The Burden of Unnecessary Illness. Am J Prev Med 3(suppl 5):181–187, 1987
11. McCormick J, Skrabanek P: Coronary heart disease is not preventable by population interventions. Lancet 2:839–841, 1988
12. Fries JF, Green LW, Levine S: Health promotion and the compression of morbidity. Lancet 1:481–483, 1989
13. Beauchamp DE: Public health is social justice. Inquiry 13:3–14, 1976
14. The Surgeon General's Report on Nutrition and Health. Washington, D.C.: U.S. Department of HHS Publication No. (PHS) 88-50210. Government Printing Office, 1986
15. The 1990 Health Objectives for the Nation: A Midcourse Review. Washington, D.C.: U.S. Department of HHS, Government Printing Office, 1986
16. Comparison of observed and self-reported seat belt use rates—United States. MMWR 37:549–551, 1988
17. Fell JC, Nash CE: Intoxicated Drivers and Pedestrians on U.S. Public Roads: Collision Losses and Changes in the 1980's. Research Notes. Washington, D.C.: U.S. Department of Transportation, National Highway Safety Administration, 1989
18. Reducing the Health Consequences of Smoking: 25 Years of Progress. A Report of the Surgeon General. Atlanta: U.S. Department of HHS Publication No. (CDC) 89-8411, Centers for Disease Control, 1989
19. Mason JO, Tolsma DD, Peterson HB, Hogue CJR: Health promotion for women: Reduction of smoking in primary care settings. Clin Obstet Gynecol 31:989–1002, 1988
20. Berkman LF, Breslow L: Health and Ways of Living: The Alameda County Study. New York: Oxford University Press, 1983
21. Kaplan GA, Haan MN, Syme SL, et al: Socioeconomic status and health. In Amler RW, Dull HB (eds): Closing the Gap: The Burden of Unnecessary Illness. Am J Prev Med 3(suppl 5):125–129, 1987
22. Remington PR, Foreman MR, Gentry EM, et al: Current smoking trends in the United States. The 1981-83 behavioral risk factor surveys. JAMA 253:2975, 1985
23. Stephens T, Schoenborn CA: Health Habits in the US and Canada. NCHS Vital and Health Statistics, Series 5, No. 3. Hyattsville, Md.: U.S. Department of HHS Publication No. (PHS) 88-1429, 1988
24. Lalonde M: A New Perspective on the Health of Canadians. Ottawa: Information Canada, 1974
25. Dever GEA: An epidemiologic model for health policy analysis. Soc Indicators Res 2:453–466, 1977
26. The Leading Causes of Death in the United States. Atlanta: Centers for Disease Control, 1977
27. Promoting Health/Preventing Disease: Objectives for the Nation. Washington, D.C.: U.S. Department of HHS, Government Printing Office, 1980
28. Office of Disease Prevention and Health Promotion: A Review of State Activities Related to the Public Health Service's Health Promotion and Disease Prevention Objectives for the Nation. Washington, D.C.: ODPHP Monograph Series, Mar 1986
29. Green LW: National policy in the promotion of health. Int J Health Educ 22(3):161–168, 1979
30. Becker MH: The tyranny of health promotion. Public Health Rev 14:15–25, 1986
31. Levin L: Every silver lining has a cloud: The limits of health promotion. Soc Policy 18(1):57–60, 1987
32. Milio N: Promoting health promotion: Health or hype. Community Health Stud 10:427–437, 1986
33. Bayer R, Moreno JD: Health promotion: Ethical and social dilemmas of government policy. Health Aff 5(2):72–84, 1986
34. Ottawa Charter for Health Promotion. Ottawa: World Health Organization, European Regional Office, 1986
35. Breslow L: Health status measurement in the evaluation of health promotion. Med Care 27(suppl 3):S205–S216, 1989
36. Mason JO, Tolsma DD: Personal health promotion. In Holbrook JH (ed): Disease Prevention and Health Promotion: A Handbook for Physicians. New York, Praeger, 1986, pp 1–10
37. APHA Technical Report: Criteria for the development of health promotion and education programs. Am J Public Health 77(1):89–92, 1987
38. Institute of Medicine: The Future of Public Health. Washington, D.C.: Academy Press, 1988
39. Puska P: Involving people and community—keynote address. Proceedings of the XIII World Conference on Health Education, 1988. Houston: University of Texas Health Science Center, 1989
40. Kreuter MW: Involving people and community—response. Proceedings of the XIII World Conference on Health Education, 1988. Houston: University of Texas Health Science Center, 1989
41. Fuchs JA: Planning for community health promotion: A rural example. Health Values 12(6):3–8, 1988
42. Hancock T: Healthy cities: The Canadian project. Health Promotion 26(1):2–4, 1987
43. Smoking Control Among Women: Community Intervention Handbook. Atlanta: Centers for Disease Control, 1987
44. Promoting Physical Activity Among Adults: Community Intervention Handbook. Atlanta: Centers for Disease Control, 1988

45. Simons-Morton BG, Brink SG, Parcel GS, et al: Preventing acute alcohol-related health problems among adolescents and young adults. Atlanta: Centers for Disease Control, 1990
46. Brink SG, Simons-Morton DG, Parcel GS, Tiernan KM: Community intervention handbooks for comprehensive health promotion programming. Fam Community Health 11(1):28–35, 1988
47. Henry J. Kaiser Family Foundation: Health Promotion Resource Center, Stanford Center for Research in Disease Prevention. Palo Alto, Calif.: Health Promotion Resource Center, n.d.
48. Report of the Secretary's Task Force on Black and Minority Health, Vol. 1. U.S. Department of HHS, Government Printing Office, 1985
49. Pasick R: Health Promotion for Minorities in California. Berkeley, Calif.: University of California, Northern California Cancer Center, 1987
50. Heath GW, Leonard BE, Wilson RH, et al: Community-based exercise intervention—the Zuni diabetes project. Diabetes Care 10:579–583, 1987
51. Curry R: Mobilizing a Minority Community to Reduce Risk Factors for Cardiovascular Disease: An Exercise-Nutrition Handbook. Atlanta, Emory University School of Medicine and the Centers for Disease Control, 1989
52. Cook AL, Goeppinger J, Brink SE, Price LJ, et al: A reexamination of community participation in health: Lessons from three community health projects. Fam Community Health 11(2):1–13, 1988
53. Labonte R: Community health promotion strategies. Health Promotion 26:5–10, 32, 1987
54. McAlister A, Puska P, Salonen JT, et al: Theory and action for health promotion: Illustrations from the North Karelia Project. Am J Public Health 72(1):43–50, 1982
55. Farquhar J: The Stanford Five City Project: An overview. In Matarazzo J, Miller N, Weiss S, et al (eds): Behavioral Health. A Handbook of Health Enhancement and Disease Prevention. New York: John Wiley & Sons, 1984
56. Elder JP, McGraw SA, Abrams DA, et al: Organizational and community approaches to community-wide prevention of heart disease: The first two years of the Pawtucket Heart Health Program. Prev Med 15:107–115, 1986
57. Wakefield MA, Wilson DH: Community organization for health promotion. Community Health Stud 10:444–451, 1986
58. McLeroy KR, Bibeau D, Steckler A, Glanz K: An ecological perspective on health promotion programs. Health Educ Q 15:351–377, 1988
59. Simons-Morton DG, Simons-Morton BG, Parcel GS, Bunker JF: Influencing personal and environmental conditions for community health: A multilevel intervention model family and community health. J Fam Community Health 11(2):25–35, 1988
60. The Secretary's Community Health Promotion Awards: 1988. Atlanta: Centers for Disease Control, 1988
61. Minkler M: Health education, health promotion, and the open society: An historical perspective. Health Educ Q 16(1):17–30, 1989
62. Goodman RM, Steckler AB: The life and death of a health promotion program: An institutionalization case study. Int Q Community Health Educ 8(1):5–21, 1987–1988
63. Pearson CE: Health promotion and health education: The emerging role of the private sector. Hygie 7(2):20–22, 1988
64. Hollander RB, Lengermann JJ: Corporate characteristics and worksite health promotion programs: Survey findings from Fortune 500 companies. Soc Sci Med 26:491–501, 1988
65. Fielding JF, Piserchia PV: Frequency of worksite health promotion activities. Am J Public Health 79(1):16–20, 1989
66. Christenson GM, Kiefhaber A: The national survey of worksite health promotion activities. Am Assoc Occup Health Nurses 36:262–265, 1988
67. Sciacca JP: The worksite is the best place for health promotion. Personnel J 66(11):42–49, 1987
68. Windom RE, McGinnis M, Fielding JE: Examining worksite health promotion. Business Health 4(9):36–37, 1987
69. Warner KE, Wickizer TM, Wolfe RA, et al: Economic implications of workplace health promotion programs: Review of the literature. J Occup Med 30(2):106–112, 1988
70. Kristien MM: How much can business expect to profit from smoking cessation? Prev Med 12:358–381, 1983
71. Fielding JE: The proof of the health promotion pudding is . . . [Editorial]. J Occup Med 30(2):113–115, 1988
72. Opatz JP: Health Promotion Evaluation: Measuring the Organizational Impact. Stevens Point, Wis.: National Wellness Institute, Apr 1987, p 141
73. Bly JL, Jones RC, Richardson JE: Impact of worksite health promotion on health care costs and utilization: Evaluation of Johnson & Johnson's Live for Life program. JAMA 256:3235–3240, 1986
74. Blair SN, Tritsch L, Kutsch S: Worksite health promotion for school faculty and staff. J Sch Health 57:469–473, 1987
75. Kaiser J: Still on the sidelines: Health promotion has missed the mark with blue-collar workers. Health Action Managers 2(3):5–10, 1988
76. McDaniel SA: Women, work and health: Some challenges to health promotion. Can J Public Health 78(5):S9–S13, 1987
77. Vass M, Gatlin E, Walsh-Allis G: Health promotion should address the special needs of employee dependents. Business Health 5(8):53, 1988
78. Bezold C, Carlson RJ, Peck JC: The Future of Health and Work. Dover, Mass.: Auburn House, 1986
79. Kaiser J, Behrens R: Health Promotion and the Labor Union Movement. Washington, D.C.: Washington Business Group on Health (WBGH Worksite Wellness Series), Jul 1986, p 28
80. Orlandi MA: The diffusion and adoption of worksite health promotion innovations: An analysis of barriers. Prev Med 15:522–536, 1986
81. Ware BG: Workplace health promotion: Issues for the future. HealthLink 3(1):3–4, 1987
82. Roman PM, Blum TC: Formal intervention in employee health: Comparisons of the nature and structure of employee assistance programs and health promotion programs. Soc Sci Med 26:503–514, 1988
83. Eriksen MP: Cancer prevention in workplace health promotion. Am Assoc Occup Health Nurs J 36:266–270, 1988
84. Carpenter RA: The evaluation of a low-cost worksite health promotion program. Am Assoc Occup Health Nurs J 36:276–281, 1988
85. Jordan-Marsh M, Vojtecky MA, Marsh DD: Workplace health promotion/protection: Correlates of integrative activities. J Occup Med 29:353–356, 1987
86. McGinnis JM: National priorities in disease prevention. Issues Sci Tech 5(2):46–52, 1988
87. U.S. Preventive Services Task Force: Guide to Clinical Preventive Services. Baltimore: Williams & Wilkins, 1989, pp LIX–LXII
88. Kottke TE, Battista RN, DeFriese GH, et al: Attributes of successful smoking cessation interventions in clinical practice: A meta-analysis of 42 controlled trials. JAMA 259:2882–2889, 1988
89. Simons-Morton BG, Pate RP, Simons-Morton DG: Prescribing physical activity to prevent disease. Postgrad Med 83:165–176, 1988
90. Roter DL, Hall JA, Katz NR: Patient-physician communication. A descriptive summary of the literature. Patient Educ Counseling 12:99–119, 1988
91. Vogt HB, Kapp C: Patient education in primary care practice. Postgrad Med 81:273–278, 1987
92. Green LW: How physicians can improve patients' participation and maintenance in self-care. West J Med 147:346–349, 1987
93. Mullen PD, Green LW, Persinger G: Clinical trials of patient education for chronic conditions: A comparative analysis of intervention types. Prev Med 14:753–781, 1985
94. Bartlett EE: Introduction: Eight principles from patient education research. Prev Med 14:667–669, 1985
95. Fried RA, Iverson DC, Nagle JP: The Clinician's Health Promotion Handbook. Denver: Mercy Medical Center, 1985, pp 9–21

96. American Hospital Association: Census of Hospital-Based Health Promotion Programs: 1987. Chicago: The Association, 1988, p 73
97. National Diabetes Advisory Board: National Standards for Diabetes Patient Education Programs. Bethesda, Md.: The Board, 1983
98. American Hospital Association: Hospital-Based Health Promotion Programs: Report and Analysis of the 1984 Survey. Chicago: The Association, 1985
99. Howerton RB Jr: Health promotion: An administrator's perspective. Fitness Business Oct 1987, pp 45–47
100. Warner KE: Cost savings: Is there a better argument for health promotion. Promoting Health 5(1):4–5, 1984
101. McBrien M: Health promotion: Education or marketing strategy? Nurs Success Today 3(5):16–17, 1986
102. Bernton CT: What is the future for health promotion in HMO's?: Results of a national survey of 340 members of AMCRA. Am J Health Promotion 1(4):24–27, 1987
103. Murphy MM: Why won't they shape up? Resistance to the promotion of health. Can J Public Health 73:427–430, 1982
104. Jaffe E: The role of occupational therapy in disease prevention and health promotion. Am J Occup Ther 40:749–752, 1986
105. Holcomb JD, Mullen PD, Fasser CE, et al: Health behaviors and beliefs of four allied health professions regarding health promotion and disease prevention. J Allied Health 14:373–385, 1985
106. McTernan EJ, Rice NC: An overview of the role of allied health professionals in the health promotion and disease prevention movement. J Allied Health 15:289–292, 1986
107. Miller LV, Goldstein J: More efficient care of diabetic patients in a country hospital setting. N Engl J Med 286:1388–1391, 1972
108. Zapka J: Self care for colds: A cost-effective alternative to upper respiratory infection management. Am J Public Health 69:814–816, 1979
109. Sexton MJ, Hebel JR: A clinical trial of change in maternal smoking and its effect on low birth weight. JAMA 251:911–915, 1984
110. Morisky DE, Levine DM, Green LW, et al: Five-year blood pressure control and mortality following health education for hypertensive patients. Am J Public Health 73:672–677, 1983
111. McGinnis JM, Hamburg MA: Opportunities for health promotion and disease prevention in the clinical setting. West J Med 149:468–474, 1988
112. Byham LD, Vickery CE: Compliance and health promotion. Health Values 12(4):5–12, 1988
113. Wynder EL, Orlandi MA: Editorial. Prev Med 16(1):131–133, 1987
114. Orlandi MA: Promoting health and preventing disease in health care settings: An analysis of barriers. Prev Med 16(1):119–130, 1987
115. Price JH, Desmond SM, Losh DP, Krol RA: Family practice physicians' perceptions and practices regarding health promotion for the elderly. Am J Prev Med 4(5):274–281, 1988
116. Freeman SH: Health promotion talk in family practice encounters. Soc Sci Med 25:961–966, 1987
117. Horowitz MM, Byrd JC, Gruchow HW: Attitudes of faculty members, residents, students, and community physicians towards health promotion. J Med Educ 62:931–934, 1987
118. Blum A: Medical activism. In Taylor RB, Ureda JR, Denham JW (eds): Health Promotion: Principles and Clinical Applications. Norwalk, Conn.: Appleton-Century-Crofts, 1982, pp 373–391
119. Guidelines for effective school health education to prevent the spread of AIDS. MMWR 37(suppl 2):1–14, 1988
120. Johnson LD, O'Malley PM, Bachman JG: National Trends in Drug Use and Related Factors among American High School Students and Young Adults, 1975–1986. Rockville, Md.: National Institute on Drug Abuse, 1987
121. Results From the National Adolescent Student Health Survey. MMWR 38(9):147–150, 1988
122. Fries JF: Aging, natural death, and the compression of morbidity. N Engl J Med 303(3):130–135, 1980
123. Lohrman DK, Gold RS, Jubb WH: Social health education: A foundation for school health programs. J Sch Health 57:420–425, 1987
124. International Union for Health Education: Policy statement on education of the school age child. Hygie 6(3):5–6, 1987
125. School Health in America: An Assessment of State Policies to Protect and Improve the Health of Students, 4 edt. Kent, Ohio: American School Health Association, 1988
126. U.S. Department of Health and Human Services, Public Health Service: Healthy People 2000: National Health Promotion and Disease Prevention Objectives. Full Report with Commentary. Washington, D.C.: Government Printing Office. USDHHS Publication No. 91-50212, 1990
127. Allensworth DD, Wolford CA: Schools as agents for achieving the 1990 health objectives for the nation. Health Educ Q 15:3–15, 1988
128. Allensworth DD, Kolbe LJ: The comprehensive school health program: Exploring an expanded concept. J Sch Health 57:409, 1987
129. Kolbe LJ: Increasing the impact of school health promotion programs: Emerging research perspectives. Health Educ 17(5):47–52, 1986
130. Perry C: Health promotion at school: Expanding the potential for prevention. Sch Psychol Rev 13(2):141–149, 1984
131. Thomas A: School psychologist: An integral member of the school health team. J Sch Health 57:465–468, 1987
132. Frank GC, Vaden A, Martin J: School health promotion: Child nutrition programs. J Sch Health 57:451–460, 1987
133. Parcel GS, Simons-Morton BG, O'Hara NM, et al: School promotion of healthful diet and physical activity: Impact on learning outcomes and self-reported behavior. Health Educ Q 16:181–199, 1989
134. Pate RR, Corbon CB, Simons-Morton BG, Ross JG: Physical education and its role in school health promotion. J Sch Health 57:445–450, 1987
135. Ross JG, Gilbert GG: The National Children and Youth Fitness Study. J Physical Educ Recreation Dance 56(1):45–50, 1985
136. Ross JG, Pate RR: The National Children and Youth Fitness Study. II. A summary of findings. J Physical Educ Recreation Dance 58(1):51–56, 1987
137. Parcel GS, Simons-Morton BG, O'Hara M, et al: School promotion of healthful diet and exercise behavior: An integration of organizational change and social learning theory interventions. J Sch Health 57:150–156, 1987
138. Progress toward achieving the 1990 national objectives for physical fitness and exercise. MMWR 38:449–453, 1989
139. Connell DB, Turner RR, Mason EF: Summary of findings of the school of health education evaluation. J Sch Health 55:316, 1985
140. Growing Healthy. New York: National Center for Health Education, 1986
141. Health Is Basic: Teenage Health Teaching Module Program for Teachers and Students. Newton, Mass.: Education Development Center, 1983
142. Know Your Body. New York: American Health Foundation, n.d.
143. Christenson GM, Gold RS, Katz M, Kreuter MW: Preface to results of the school health education evaluation. J Sch Health 55:295, 1985
144. Vincent ML, Clearie AF, Schluchter MD: Reducing adolescent pregnancy through school and community-based education. JAMA 257:3382–3386, 1987
145. Reducing Adolescent Pregnancy Through School/Community Educational Interventions. A South Carolina Case Study. Atlanta: Centers for Disease Control, 1988
146. Report of the Presidential Commission on the Human Immunodeficiency Virus Epidemic. Washington, D.C.: Government Printing Office, 1988
147. Fraser K, Mitchell P: Effective AIDS Education: A Policymaker's Guide. Alexandria, Va.: National Association of State Boards of Education, 1988
148. National School Boards Association: Reducing the Risk: A School Leader's Guide to AIDS Education. Leadership Reports, vol. 2. Alexandria, Va.: The Association, 1988
149. U.S. Congress Office of Technology Assessment: Assessing the Efficacy and Safety of Medical Technologies. U.S. Government Printing Office, Stock No. 052-003-00593-0, September 1978

150. Flay BR: Efficacy and effectiveness trials (and other phases of research) in the development of health promotion programs. Prev Med 15:451–474, 1986
151. Mittelmark MB, Luepker RV, Jacobs DR, et al: Community-wide prevention of cardiovascular disease: Education strategies of the Minnesota Heart Health Program. Prev Med 15:1–17, 1986
152. Puska P, Nissinen A, Tuomilehto J, et al: The community-based strategy to prevent coronary heart disease. Conclusions from the ten years of the North Karelia project. Annu Rev Public Health 6:147–159, 1985
153. Flay BR, Ryan KB, Best JA, et al: Are social psychological smoking prevention programs effective? The Waterloo Study. Behav Med 8:37–59, 1985
154. Flay BR, Koepke D, Thomason SJ, et al: Six-year follow-up of the first Waterloo School smoking prevention trial. Am J Public Health 10:1371–1376, 1989
155. Evans L, Frick MC: Helmet effectiveness in preventing motorcycle driver and passenger fatalities. Accid Analy Prev 20:447–458, 1988
156. Jacobs DR, Luepker RV, Mittelmark MB, et al: Community-wide prevention strategies: Evaluation design of the Minnesota Heart Health Program. J Chronic Dis 39:775–788, 1986
157. Pietinen P, Nissinen A, Vartiainen E, et al: Dietary changes in the North Karelia project (1972-1982). Prev Med 17:183–193, 1988
158. Kottke TE, Puska P, Salonen JT, et al: Projected effects of high-risk versus population-based strategy in coronary heart disease. Am J Epidemiol 121:697–704, 1985
159. Vartiainen E, Heath G, Ford E: Assessing population-based programs to reduce blood cholesterol level and saturated fats. Int J Technology Assessment Health Care (publication pending)
160. MacVie J, Davis R: Assessing community interventions in reduction of tobacco use. Int J Technology Assessment Health Care (publication pending)
161. Chorba TL: Assessing technologies for preventing injuries in motor-vehicle crashes. Int J Technology Assessment Health Care (publication pending)
162. Dwyer T, Viney R, Jones M: Assessing school health education programs. Int J Technology Assessment Health Care (publication pending)
163. Weinstein MC, Fineberg HV: Clinical Decision Analysis. Philadelphia: WB Saunders, 1980
164. Avorn J: Benefit and cost analysis in geriatric care. Turning age discrimination into health policy. N Engl J Med 310:1294–1300, 1984
165. Nissinen A, Tuomilehto J, Kottke TE, Puska P: Cost effectiveness of the North Karelia Hypertension Program, 1972-1977. Med Care 24:767–780, 1986
166. Engleman SR, Forbes JF: Economic aspects of health education. Soc Sci Med 22:443–458, 1986
167. Kinosian BP, Eisenberg JM: Cutting into cholesterol: Cost-effective alternatives for treating hypercholesterolemia. JAMA 259:2249–2254, 1988
168. Kaplan RM, Atkins CJ, Wilson DK: The cost-utility of diet and exercise interventions in non-insulin-dependent diabetes mellitus. Health Promotion 2:331–340, 1988

42

Smoking: Health Effects and Control

Jonathan E. Fielding

> Tobacco drieth the brain, dimmeth the sight, vitiateth the smell, hurteth the stomach, destroyeth the concoction, disturbeth the humours and spirits, corrupteth the breath, induceth a trembling of the limbs, exsiccateth the windpipe, lungs, and liver, annoyeth the milt, scorcheth the heart, and causeth the blood to be adjusted.
>
> Tobias Venner
> *Via recta ad vitam Longam, 1638*

> This very night I am going to *leave off tobacco!* Surely there must be some other world in which this unconquerable purpose shall be realized.
>
> Charles Lamb, 1815

The custom of smoking dried tobacco leaves spread from America to the rest of the world after European colonization began in the sixteenth century. Given the deleterious effects of tobacco on cardiovascular, respiratory, and other body systems, coupled with its addictive properties and widespread use, it is perhaps the most dangerous of all psychoactive drugs. Its effects are soothing and tranquilizing, and under appropriate circumstances there is also a stimulant action. Physiological and psychological dependence occur, and there are severe withdrawal symptoms, a craving for tobacco, that makes this among the most refractory of all addictions.

Nicotine is the psychoactive compound in tobacco. However, smokers continue to smoke for several reasons. Some smoke for enjoyment or social reinforcement, and some to alleviate stress. Many young people perceive smoking as an attribute of maturity or sexual desirability. Pharmacological factors interact with stimuli in the social environment—social reinforcers—so that after many thousands of repetitions of inhaling tobacco fumes, confirmed smokers are inseparable from their cigarettes. Tolerance, the need for increasing amounts to achieve the same physiological response, develops to some but not all effects of nicotine. Heavy smokers who abruptly cease smoking experience a withdrawal syndrome of irritability, aggressiveness, hostility, depression, and difficulty in concentrating. These symptoms may last several days or even weeks and are accompanied by electroencephalographic changes. Many smokers who have such symptoms relapse if they try to quit.

OVERALL TOLL OF SMOKING

Excess Mortality. Cigarette smoking has been identified in the U.S. Surgeon General's reports since 1964 as the single most significant source of preventable morbidity and premature death. The estimated annual excess mortality from cigarette smoking in the United States exceeds 390,000, more than the total number of American lives lost in all wars during the twentieth century.[1]

Coronary heart disease (CHD), cancer, and various respiratory diseases account for the majority of excess mortality related to cigarette smoking.[1–4] It is estimated that of the 512,000 annual deaths from CHD, 115,000 (23%) are attributable to smoking.[1,5] Furthermore, 138,000 (29%) of the 477,000 cancer deaths in 1985 were attributable to smoking. Lung cancer caused 135,000 deaths in 1987 (28% of all cancers) and 79% of these deaths were attributed to smoking.[1,5] Other cancers strongly associated with smoking are those of the oral cavity, esophagus, larynx, and bladder; an association has also been demonstrated for cancers of the pancreas, kidney, and cervix.[1,3] Chronic obstructive pulmonary diseases (COPD), such as chronic bronchitis and emphysema, account annually for another 57,000 smoking-related deaths.[1,4]

Combining results from thousands of studies shows that smokers average a tenfold increased risk of acquiring lung cancer, a twofold increased risk of having a myocardial infarction, and a sixfold increased risk of acquiring COPD in comparison with nonsmokers.[6]

It has been estimated that an average of 5.5 minutes of life is lost for each cigarette smoked—about the time taken to smoke it. This estimate is based on an average reduction in life expectancy for cigarette smokers of 5 to 8 years. For a 25-year-old man smoking 1 pack per day (20 cigarettes), the reduction averages 4.6 years; for a man of the same age smoking 2 packs per day (40 cigarettes), 8.3 years of expected life are lost. Smoking-caused reduction in life expectancy is also affected by the age of smoking initiation. A person who begins smoking at the age of 15 years has an average of 8 years of reduced longevity, and one starting after 25 years of age faces an average 4-year reduction.[6]

Some analyses of differential mortality rates between genders suggest that a major cause of the differences after the age of 30 years is related to cigarette smoking prevalence. Increases in life expectancy differences between the two sexes since 1930 are largely attributable to cigarette smoking.[7] Although this appraisal probably overstates the contribution of smoking in gender longevity, smoking is responsible for at least part of the more than 7-year discrepancy between the sexes in the United States.

Economic Costs. The annual economic toll of smoking can be divided into direct and indirect costs. The U.S. Department of Health and Human Services estimated that the total direct health care cost associated with smoking in 1985 was $34 billion. The total indirect loss attributable to smoking because of lost productivity and earnings as a result of excess morbidity, disability, and premature death was estimated at $18 billion annually.[8] These figures translate into an annual per capita social cost of approximately $221 directly attributable to smoking,[8] with each nonsmoker shouldering an economic burden of providing medical care for smoking-induced illness that exceeds $110 (1990 dollars), paid primarily through taxes and health insurance premiums.[9]

Part of the cost of smoking is due to cigarette-caused fires, although this cost was not included in the calculations cited above. Smoking material related fires are the primary cause for all structural fires and all civilian fire deaths. Data from the National Fire Data Center show that 7 percent of all fires in residential occupancies result from smoking. Each year more than $320 million in property losses result from fires in residential and public mercantile occupancies caused by cigarettes, pipes, and cigars. Smoking results in fires that claim more than 1400 lives and injure another 3500 people annually.[10] Overall, smoking results in more than a quarter of all fire-caused mortality and accounts for close to $500 million in other losses.[10] Smoking materials were the cause of 5 percent of fires on national forest lands in 1979 through 1988, with a average yearly loss of 11,570 acres.[11]

CARDIOVASCULAR DISEASE

Coronary Heart Disease. CHD is related to several risk factors, one of which is tobacco use. Of the various disease manifestations associated with tobacco use, CHD is the leading cause of excess death and disability in the United States. In 1987 more than 45% of the 2,123,323 deaths in the United States were due to diseases of the circulatory system. Of cardiovascular deaths, 53%, or 412,138, were due to CHD, and 23% of the total CHD deaths were attributable to cigarette smoking.[1] On the basis of data from a very large recent U.S. study, smoking is estimated to cause 45% and 41%, respectively, of all CHD deaths of males and females less than 65 years of age, with 21% and 12% being the corresponding percentages for men and women 65 years of age and older.[1] On the basis of results from a variety of sources, a reasonable estimate is that 30% to 40% of all CHD deaths are attributable to smoking.

Evidence from both cohort and case-control studies support the statement in the 1983 Surgeon General's report that "cigarette smoking should be considered the most important of the known modifiable risk factors for coronary heart disease in the United States."[2] In early investigations, cigarette smoking, along with several other characteristics, was observed to be strongly associated with CHD. On the basis of this observation, 10 cohort studies were set up to determine the nature and degree of CHD risk attributable to smoking. These studies, accounting for more than 20 million person-years of observation, each revealed a higher incidence of myocardial infarction (MI) and death from CHD in cigarette smokers than in nonsmokers. This set of studies also demonstrated that whether in the United States, Canada, the United Kingdom, Scandinavia, or Japan, smokers as a group have excess CHD mortality that is approximately 70% greater than that of nonsmokers (Table 42–1).[2]

The National Cooperative Pooling Project used "pooled" data from five previous large cohort studies to examine more closely the effects of smoking on men aged 40 to 59 years. The pooled data (Table 42–2) showed that in those who smoked a pack of cigarettes or more per day at the time of their initial examination, the risk of having a first major coronary event was 2.5 times as great as in nonsmokers. The risk was greatest in heavy smokers (more than 1 pack a day), and the relative risk for smokers compared with nonsmokers tended to increase with age, up to 50 to 54 years of age, as shown in Table 42–2, with a dose-response relationship. After that age the relative risk decreased. This paradox is due to the rapid increase of CHD incidence with age (without cigarette smoking).[12]

Although most investigations of smoking-related risk of CHD have used male subjects predominantly, a study using all female subjects has reported that women smokers less than age 50 years who smoke a pack of cigarettes or more a day have twice the risk of having a nonfatal MI, compared with nonsmokers of the same age.[13] In a recent large study of female nurses, about half of the coronary events were attributable to smoking.[14] Other studies, both in the United States and abroad, have demonstrated consistently that female smokers who follow smoking patterns similar to those of male smokers have a similar increased risk of death from CHD, in comparison with nonsmokers.[2]

Further, results from cohort studies clearly demonstrate that the risk of death from CHD among both male and female smokers is increased by early smoking initiation (Table 42–3), number of cigarettes smoked per day, and depth of smoke inhalation. Male and female smokers have an increased relative risk of sudden cardiac death that is two to four times greater than that of nonsmokers. This risk is greater among young men and appears to be related to the number of cigarettes smoked per day.[15,16]

Smoking also appears to increase the risk of angina pectoris. After 24 years of follow-up, smokers in the Framingham Study had a slightly higher incidence of angina in all age groups compared with nonsmokers. Among smokers in the youngest age group (30 to 40 years of age), however, the incidence of angina pectoris was more than double that among nonsmokers (Fig. 42–1).[17] Smokers with angina pectoris have a higher rate of angina attacks than do nonsmokers with this symptom.[18,19]

Although smoking, hypertension, and hypercholesterolemia confer approximately the same average increase in the risk of CHD in various populations, smoking in combination with other CHD risk factors appears to have a synergistic effect on CHD mortality. With none of the other risk factors present, the annual CHD mortality rate is 54 per 1000 for smokers and 23 per 1000 for nonsmokers. If the three risk factors were acting in a purely additive fashion, the expected average CHD mortality rate for people with all three risks would be 116 per 1000; however, the actual rate is 189 per 1000.[2] A similar effect has been demonstrated in female smokers using oral contraceptives, who have an approximate tenfold increase in CHD mortality compared with women who neither smoked nor used oral contracep-

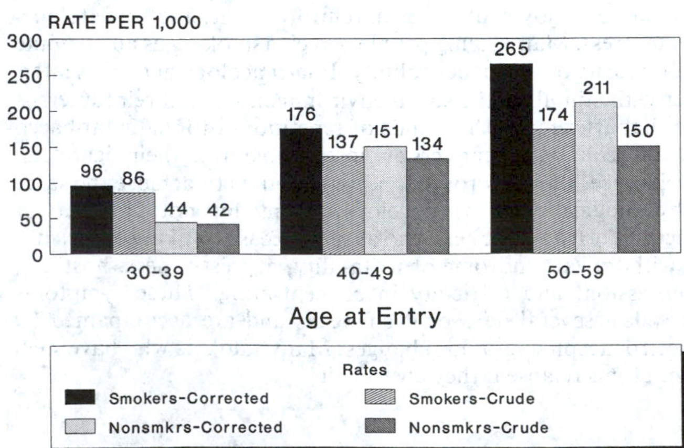

Figure 42-1. Twenty-four-year incidence of angina pectoris in men, by cigarette smoking status. *[From the U.S. Department of Health and Human Services, 1985.[2]]*

TABLE 42-1. CORONARY HEART DISEASE MORTALITY RATIOS BY AMOUNT SMOKED: RESULTS OF NINE COHORT STUDIES

Sex	Study	No. of Cigarettes per Day	Ratio
Males	U.S. veterans	Nonsmoker	1.00
		1-9	1.24
		10-20	1.24
		21-39	1.76
		40 or more	1.94
	American Cancer Society, 9-state study	Nonsmoker	1.00
		1-9	1.29
		10-20	1.89
		21-40	2.15
		41 or more	2.41
	Japanese in 29 health districts	Nonsmoker	1.00
		1-9	1.29
		15-24	1.59
		25-49	2.11
		50 or more	2.82
	American Cancer Society, 25-state study	Nonsmoker	1.00
		1-19	1.90
		20 or more	2.55
	Canadian veterans	Nonsmoker	1.00
		1-9	1.55
		10-20	1.58
		21 or more	1.78
	British physicians	Nonsmoker	1.00
		1-14	1.47
		15-24	1.58
		25 or more	1.92
	Swedish probability study	Nonsmoker	1.00
		1-7	1.50
		8-15	1.70
		16 or more	2.20
	California occupations	Nonsmoker	1.00
		About 1/2 pack	1.39
		About 1 pack	1.67
		About 1 1/2 packs	1.74
	Swiss physicians	Nonsmoker	1.00
		1-10	1.33
		10-19	1.42
		29-34	1.77
		35 or more	2.18
Females	British physicians	Nonsmoker	1.00
		1-14	0.96
		15-24	2.20
		25 or more	2.12
	Swedish probability study	Nonsmoker	1.00
		1-7	1.20
		8-15	1.60
		16 or more	3.00

From the U.S. Department of Health and Human Services, 1983.[2]

tives.[20] Diabetes confers an increased risk of CHD that is further increased if the women smoke.[21] Cigarette smoking also significantly increases CHD risk in those with familial hyperlipoproteinemia or hypercholesterolemia or both.[22,23]

Data from the cohort studies (Table 42-4) show that pipe and cigar smokers generally have a substantially lower risk of a major coronary event and subsequent CHD than do cigarette smokers. The risk of CHD-related death for pipe and cigar smokers, however, is still in the range of 1.02 to 1.40 compared with that for nonsmokers, with deeper smoke inhalation increasing the risk.[2] Among pipe and cigar smokers, former cigarette smokers tend to inhale and to have much higher venous-blood carboxyhemoglobin levels than do those who have never smoked cigarettes, and they are likely to be at higher risk for CHD.[24]

The positive effect of smoking cessation on both primary and secondary prevention of CHD has been extensively studied and validated. The 1990 Surgeon General's report evaluated this research and concluded that the risk of primary CHD is reduced by more than half by the end of the first year of cessation, followed by a gradual decline to the risk for that of a person who

TABLE 42-2. AVERAGE ANNUAL RISK (PER 1000 MAN-YEARS) OF FIRST MAJOR CORONARY EVENT BY SMOKING PATTERN AND AGE

	Age at Risk (Year)				
Smoking Pattern	**40–44**	**45–49**	**50–54**	**55–59**	**60–64**
All	3.1	6.4	8.0	12.6	19.9
Nonsmokers	[1.5]	3.0	3.6	7.3	15.5
Never smoked	[1.9]	[0.7]	[2.5]	8.7	11.4
Past smoker	[0.9]	5.5	4.3	6.1	15.5
<1/2 Pack per day	[1.7]	[4.7]	[5.9]	[6.4]	[7.5]
Cigar and pipe only	[2.1]	[2.2]	[2.1]	12.1	19.5
Cigarette smokers					
About 1/2 pack per day	[3.1]	[5.0]	[6.2]	15.5	24.3
About 1 pack per day	3.9	8.4	10.3	13.8	22.0
>1 Pack per day	4.9	12.2	17.4	22.5	26.8
Risk ratio					
>1 Pack per day vs nonsmokers		4.1	4.8	3.1	1.7

[ ] Based on fewer than 10 first events.
From the U.S. Department of Health and Human Services, 1983.[2]

TABLE 42-3. CORONARY HEART DISEASE MORTALITY RATIOS BY AGE AT START OF SMOKING (COHORT STUDIES)

			Smoker Mortality Ratio by Age (Year) of Initiation			
Study	**Age (Year)**	**Nonsmoker Ratio**	**≤14**	**15–19**	**20–24**	**≥25**
U.S. veterans	55–64	1.00	1.96	1.84	1.65	1.56
	65–74	1.00	2.03	1.66	1.54	1.55
American Cancer Society, 25-state study						
Males	45–54	1.00	3.47	3.11		2.37
	55–64	1.00	2.08	1.99		1.70
	65–74	1.00	1.54	1.62		1.17
Females	45–54	1.00	—	2.03		2.00
	55–64	1.00	—	1.64		1.74
	65–74	1.00	—	—		1.36

From the U.S. Department of Health and Human Services, 1983.[2]

TABLE 42-4. CORONARY HEART DISEASE MORTALITY RATIOS FOR MALE CIGARETTE, PIPE, CIGAR, AND MIXED PIPE AND CIGAR SMOKERS (COHORT STUDIES)

	Mortality Ratios				
Study	***Nonsmoker***	***Cigarette Smoker***	***Pipe Smoker***	***Cigar Smoker***	***Mixed Pipe and Cigar Smoker***
U.S. Veterans[a]	1.00	1.58	1.02	1.12	
American Cancer Society, 9-state study	1.00	1.70	—	1.28	
Swedish	1.00	1.70	1.40		
American Cancer Society, 25-state study[b]	1.00	1.90–2.55	1.08		
British physicians	1.00	1.62			1.03

[a] Smoker groups are "pure" smokers only.
[b] Ages 55 to 84 only.
From the U.S. Department of Health and Human Services, 1983.[2]

has never smoked. Among persons with diagnosed CHD, cessation is also effective in reducing the risk of a second CHD episode.[8] Similar findings have been reported for female ex-smokers.[25]

Peripheral Arterial Occlusive Disease. The most powerful risk factor predisposing persons to atherosclerotic peripheral arterial occlusive disease is cigarette smoking.[26] Cigarette smoking has been shown to be directly related to lower extremity atherosclerotic disease of both large and small arteries.[27] Smoking cessation can significantly reduce the risk of peripheral arterial disease for persons with diabetes.[28] Smoking prevalence is high among victims of aortoiliac (98%) and femoropopliteal (91%) disease.[29] Severe intermittent claudication is more frequent among nondiabetic smokers who consumed 15 cigarettes or more per day than among nonsmokers and lighter smokers.[30]

One epidemiological study found that in smokers consuming less than one pack of cigarettes per day, the relative risk of acquiring peripheral arterial occlusive disease was 11.53, compared with that in nonsmokers, and the relative risk in those who smoked more than one pack per day was 15.56 compared with that in nonsmokers. The relative risk of peripheral vascular disease in ex-smokers 1 to 5 years after cessation of smoking was 1.70, although for periods of cessation greater than 5 years the risk approached that in nonsmokers.[31] Limited studies of smokeless tobacco use have not demonstrated a high incidence of peripheral vascular disease in users. An elevated risk of peripheral vascular disease is not evident in cigar or pipe smokers.[2]

An autopsy study of atherosclerotic plaque in smokers found that the complexity and extent of plaque in the abdominal aorta increased with the number of cigarettes smoked. This study provides a rationale for the findings of several cohort studies that smokers have a twofold to threefold increase in abdominal aortic aneurysm mortality compared with nonsmokers.[2]

Cerebrovascular Disease. Both ischemic and hemorrhagic cerebrovascular diseases are major causes of death in the United States and together accounted for approximately 150,000 (7%) of all deaths in the United States in 1989. Each year there are more than 400,000 new events.[2] The Framingham Study estimated that the chances of suffering a stroke before the age of 70 years are 1 in 20, with incidence doubling each successive decade after the age of 45 years.[17] Although stroke deaths have declined substantially during the past two decades, the striking increase with age and the contribution of smoking remain constant.

Smoking has been well demonstrated as a causal factor in stroke.[32] The majority of cohort and case-control studies have shown smoker/nonsmoker stroke ratios ranging from 1.2 to 4.7,[2,33] and some of these studies have shown positive dose-response relationships. Smoking-related relative risk for subarachnoid hemorrhage may exceed those for other types of stroke. Cessation rapidly reduces risk, probably by more than 50% within 2 years.[32–34]

Female smokers who use oral contraceptives have been reported to be at increased risk of stroke, especially subarachnoid hemorrhage and thromboembolic events. In one case-control study of female smokers not using oral contraceptives, the relative risk for these events was 5.7 times greater than that for a nonsmoker, and for a female smoker and oral contraceptive user the relative risk increased to 21.9.[35] The risk increment associated with smoking, for both MI and stroke, is multiplicative in women older than 35 years of age who also use oral contraceptives.[36]

Chronic cigarette smoking in the absence of other risk factors appears to increase the risk of stroke by decreasing cerebral blood flow, probably by enhancing cerebral arteriosclerosis. In smokers with other risk factors, cerebral blood flow is reduced in an additive manner in comparison with that in nonsmokers with similar risk factors.[37]

Mechanisms of Cardiovascular Disease Development Related to Smoking. The mechanisms by which smoking contributes to the development and clinical manifestation of cardiovascular disease are not yet well understood. The systemic hemodynamic response to smoking includes increases in blood pressure, heart rate, cardiac output, myocardial contractile force, and velocity of contraction, with gradual return to baseline levels approximately 15 minutes after smoking.[13,38] These acute physiological effects are thought to result from nicotine stimulation of sympathetic ganglia, affecting the release of norepinephrine.[39] Another component of cigarette smoke, carbon monoxide, significantly reduces the oxygen-carrying capacity of normal hemoglobin by binding to it in an irreversible fashion. As a result, carboxyhemoglobin levels rise, oxygen binding affinity is diminished, and availability of oxygen for cellular aerobic metabolism is reduced.[40] The net result of the combined actions of nicotine and carbon monoxide on the cardiovascular system is an increased demand for myocardial oxygen in the presence of a limited supply, a set of conditions that could potentially precipitate myocardial ischemia.[41] Smoke products may also directly cause coronary artery spasm and increase platelet adhesiveness and aggregation.[42]

In addition to hemodynamic effects, smoking directly contributes to the development of atherosclerotic plaque in the coronary arteries by mechanisms that may include elevation of total serum cholesterol levels and reduction of high-density lipoprotein levels, abnormal synthesis of thromboxane A_2 and prostacyclin, and endothelial injury.[43,44]

CANCER

Lung Cancer. In the United States and other affluent industrial nations, carcinoma of the lung accounts for more deaths than any other cancer. Lung cancer mortality in the United States has risen sharply, from 18,300 in 1950 to 61,800 in 1969, 98,400 in 1979, and an estimated 142,000 in 1989.[5,45] Lung cancer now accounts for 35% of cancer deaths and 6% of all deaths in the United States. Eighty-three percent of lung cancer deaths are directly attributable to smoking, making smoking the leading cause of cancer deaths in the United States.[3,45]

Ninety percent of malignant lung tumors belong to four major cell types: squamous cell, small cell, large cell, and adenocarcinoma. Together these are commonly designated bronchogenic carcinoma. Of these cell types that account for the largest number of lung cancers, adenocarcinoma (35%) and small cell carcinoma (25%) have the strongest relationship to smoking and are usually found in persons with a smoking history of more than one pack per day for 10 years. Both types of tumors generally demonstrate a propensity to metastasize early and widely. Once symptomatic and unresectable, lung cancer has a 5-year survival rate of 5% to 10%; this rate, despite new therapies, has not changed significantly during the past 30 years.[46]

The rise in lung cancer rates in male smokers preceded that of female smokers. In 1964 the male/female ratio of death rates from lung cancer was 6:7. Whereas the incidence rate in males appears to have peaked in the 1980s, the rate for females has grown rapidly, by as much as 7% per year. Current lung cancer rates for women approximate male rates of three decades ago, and the male/female ratio has declined to about 2:1.[1] Lung cancer is replacing breast cancer as the leading cause of cancer death among American women.[47] In 1989 it is estimated that 93,000 men and 49,000 women died of lung cancer.[45]

Although the 1964 Surgeon General's report was the first official U.S. statement on the relationship of smoking and lung cancer, case-control studies in the 1940s and cohort studies in the 1950s had shown a clear association between smoking and lung cancer. The publication most influential in drawing medical attention to this relationship was the preliminary results from a 1956 cohort study of 40,000 British physicians older than 35 years of age, which showed that the age-adjusted death rate for lung cancer increased from 7 per 100,000 for nonsmokers to 166 per 100,000 for heavy smokers.[48]

Other cohort studies in various parts of the world further demonstrated the consistency, specificity, strength, coherence, and temporal nature of the association between smoking and lung cancer. Table 42-5 provides an outline of the lung cancer mortality ratios for smokers and nonsmokers from eight cohort studies used to establish this association. Overall, the subjects of these studies represent 17.5 million person-years of experience in five different parts of the world.[3] Although the mortality ratios vary among studies, smoker mortality rates for lung cancer ranged from 2 to 14 times those of nonsmokers. Strength of association was further enhanced by the dose-response relationship clearly illustrated by Table 42-5 and Figure 42-2. Data in Table 42-5 demonstrate the gradient of increasing risk of death from lung cancer as the number of cigarettes smoked per day increases. Increased consumption of cigarettes per day, whether filter or nonfiltered, results in an increased relative risk for both male and female smokers.[49]

Data from four large cohort studies confirm a direct relation between number of years of smoking and lung cancer mortality (Table 42-6). Lung cancer incidence appears to increase with the square of the amount smoked daily, but with the duration of smoking raised to a power of 4 or 5.[50] Smoking mechanics also affects lung cancer mortality: the degree of inhalation varies directly with smoking-associated mortality.[3] However, even smokers who report slight inhalation or none have a relative risk of cancer as much as eightfold and ninefold that for nonsmokers.[51] Both case-control and cohort studies have demonstrated some reduction in lung cancer risk in smokers who switched from nonfilter to filter cigarettes.[1] For those who have always smoked filter cigarettes, the risk of lung cancer may be reduced as much as one half compared with that for lifelong nonfilter smokers.[52,53]

For persons who stop cigarette smoking, the lung cancer mortality decrease is related to the smoking history (dose, duration, type of cigarette, and depth of inhalation) as well as the number of years since cessation. Risk reduction is gradual, and after 10 years the risk may still be 30% to 50% of the risk for continuing smokers (Table 42-7).[8]

Several cohort studies have reported an increased risk of

TABLE 42-5. LUNG CANCER MORTALITY RATIOS FOR MEN AND WOMEN, BY CURRENT NUMBER OF CIGARETTES SMOKED PER DAY (COHORT STUDIES)

	Men		Women	
Population	***Cigarettes Smoked/Day***	***Mortality Ratios***	***Cigarettes Smoked/Day***	***Mortality Ratios***
American Cancer Society, 25-state study	Nonsmoker	1.00	Nonsmoker	1.00
	1–9	4.62	1–9	1.30
	10–19	8.62	10–19	2.40
	20–39	14.69	20–39	4.90
	40+	18.71	40+	7.50
British physicians study	Nonsmoker	1.00	Nonsmoker	1.00
	1–14	7.80	1–14	1.28
	15–24	12.70	15–24	6.41
	25+	25.10	25+	29.71
Swedish study	Nonsmoker	1.00	Nonsmoker	1.00
	1–7	2.30	1–7	1.80
	8–15	8.80	8–15	11.30
	16+	13.70	16+	—
Japanese study all ages	Nonsmoker	1.00	Nonsmoker	1.00
	1–19	3.49	<20	1.90
	20–39	5.69	20–29	4.20
	40+	6.45		
U.S. veterans study	Nonsmoker	1.00		
	1–9	3.89		
	10–20	9.63		
	21–39	16.70		
	≥40	23.70		
American Cancer Society, 9-state study	Nonsmoker	1.00		
	1–9	8.00		
	10–20	10.50		
	20+	23.40		
Canadian veterans	Nonsmoker	1.00		
	1–9	9.50		
	10–20	15.80		
	20+	17.30		
California males in 9 occupations	Nonsmoker	1.00		
	About 1/2 pk	3.72		
	About 1 pk	9.05		
	About 1 1/2 pk	9.56		

From the U.S. Department of Health and Human Services, 1982.[3]

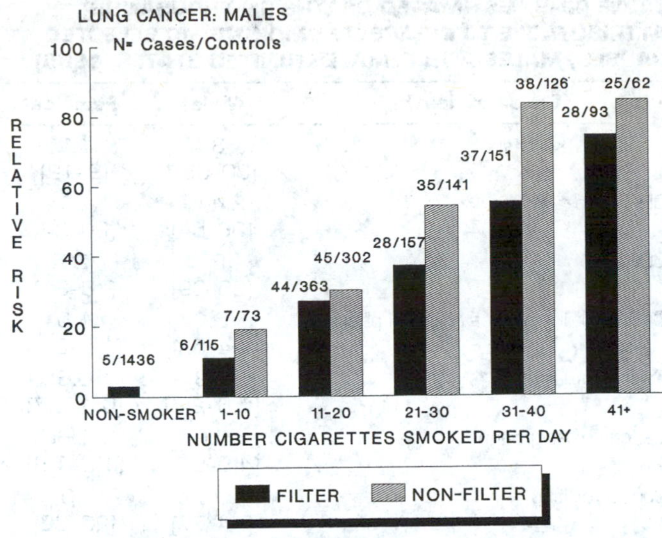

Figure 42-2. Relative risk of lung cancer for males by number of cigarettes smoked per day and long-term use of filter [F] or nonfilter [NF] cigarettes. *[From the U.S. Department of Health and Human Services, 1982.[3]]*

TABLE 42-6. LUNG CANCER MORTALITY RATIOS FOR MALES, BY AGE AT START OF SMOKING (COHORT STUDIES)

Study	Age (Year) at Start of Smoking	Mortality Ratios
American Cancer Society, 25-state study	Nonsmoker	1.00
	25+	4.08
	20–24	10.08
	15–19	19.69
	<15	16.77
Japanese study	Nonsmoker	1.00
	25+	2.87
	20–24	3.85
	<20	4.44
U.S. veterans	Nonsmoker	1.00
	25+	5.20
	20–24	9.50
	15–19	14.40
	<15	18.70
Swedish study	Nonsmoker	1.00
	19+	6.5
	17–18	9.8
	<16	6.4

From the U.S. Department of Health and Human Services, 1982.[3]

lung cancer among those who smoke pipes, cigars, or both. In general, the risk of lung cancer is much less for pipe and cigar smokers than for cigarette smokers, but greater than for nonsmokers.[3] Among pipe and cigar smokers, lung cancer death rates also exhibit dose-response relationships to smoking, as seen in Table 42-8.

In Denmark and the Netherlands, where the style of smoking pipes and cigars involves deeper inhalation than is generally practiced in the United States, rates of lung cancer for pipe and cigar smokers approach those for cigarette smokers. This suggests that condensates of cigar and pipe smoke have a carcinogenic activity similar to cigarette condensate, but the degree of

TABLE 42-7. LUNG CANCER MORTALITY RATIOS IN EX-CIGARETTE SMOKERS BY NUMBER OF YEARS SINCE STOPPED SMOKING

Study	Years Since Stopped Smoking	Mortality Ratio	
British physicians	1–4	16.0	
	5–9	5.9	
	10–14	5.3	
	15+	2.0	
	Current smokers	14.0	
U.S. veterans[a]	1–4	18.83	
	5–9	7.73	
	10–14	4.71	
	15–19	4.81	
	20+	2.10	
	Current smokers	11.28	
Japanese males	1–4	4.65	
	5–9	2.50	
	10+	1.35	
	Current smokers	3.76	
		Number of cigarettes smoked per day	
		1–19	*20+*
American Cancer Society, 25-state study (males 50–69)	<1	7.20	29.13
	1–4	4.60	12.00
	5–9	1.00	7.20
	10+	0.40	1.06
	Current smokers	6.47	13.67

[a] Includes data only for ex-cigarette smokers who stopped for other than physicians' orders.
From the U.S. Department of Health and Human Services, 1982.[3]

TABLE 42-8. LUNG CANCER MORTALITY RATIOS FOR CIGAR AND PIPE SMOKERS BY AMOUNT SMOKED

Smoking Type	Mortality Ratio	No. of Deaths
Nonsmoker	1.00	78
Cigar smokers		
<5 Cigars per day	1.14	12
5-8 Cigars per day	2.64	12
>8 Cigars per day	2.07	2
Pipe smokers		
<5 Pipefuls per day	0.77	2
5-19 Pipefuls per day	2.20	12
>19 Pipefuls per day	2.47	3
Cigar and pipe		
≤8 Cigars, ≤19 pipefuls	1.62	18
>8 Cigars, >19 pipefuls	2.19	2

From the U.S. Department of Health and Human Services, 1982.[3]

TABLE 42-9. ESTIMATED DEATHS (IN THOUSANDS) ATTRIBUTABLE TO CIGARETTE SMOKING: 10 SELECTED CAUSES, MALES AND FEMALES (UNITED STATES, 1985)

Cause of death	Males	Females
CHD, age <65 yr	34 (30–38)[a]	11 (9–12)
CHD, age ≥65 yr	44 (36–54)	26 (20–34)
COPD	37 (35–39)	20 (18–21)
Cancer of lip, oral cavity, and pharynx	5.1 (4.4–5.4)	1.6 (1.2–2.0)
Cancer of larynx	2.3 (1.6–2.7)	0.6 (0.4–0.7)
Cancer of esophagus	5.0 (4.0–5.7)	1.6 (1.3–1.9)
Cancer of lung	76 (74–77)	30 (20–32)
Cancer of pancreas	3.3 (2.1–5.0)	3.4 (2.8–5.1)
Cancer of bladder	3.1 (2.1–4.2)	1.1 (0.6–1.9)
Cancer of kidney	2.6 (1.8–3.5)	0.4 (0.1–1.5)
Cerebrovascular disease, age <65 yr	5.5 (3.9–7.0)	5.2 (4.3–6.2)
Cerebrovascular disease, age >65 yr	12 (8–17)	4.8 (1.9–11.4)
Ten causes	231 (220–242)	106 (98–115)

[a] Numbers in parentheses are 95% confidence intervals.
From the U.S. Department of Health and Human Services, 1989.[1]

exposure to susceptible organs is affected by the depth of inhalation.[3]

Although research during the past 25 years has led to a greatly expanded knowledge of the major factors contributing to the toxicity and carcinogenicity of cigarette smoke, the mechanisms responsible for lung tumor initiation from tobacco smoke constituents are complex and remain largely hypothetical.[3]

Oral, Laryngeal, and Esophageal Cancer. Large numbers of cohort and case-control studies from many countries show that smoking is an important risk factor for each of these three cancers. Also characteristic of the risk relationships for these cancers is the similarity of mortality ratios for smokers regardless of whether they smoke cigarettes, pipes, or cigars.[1] The estimated deaths attributable to smoking for each of these cancers are shown in Table 42–9; Table 42–10 displays attributable risk. Most cases in both sexes for each of these three cancers are attributable to smoking, with strong dose-response relationships at each of these sites. For all these sites, excess risk decreases with cessation, approximating the rate of a lifetime nonsmoker within 15 to 20 years. Alcohol appears to play a synergistic role with smoking for each of these cancers. In one study of oral cancer risk, for nonsmokers who consumed 7 ounces or more of alcohol per week the relative risk of death from oral cancer was 2.5 compared with that for nondrinkers. Those who consumed the same amount of alcohol and smoked one-half pack of cigarettes or less per day had approximately double the risk, but the relative risk rose to 24 if the smoker consumed 1 pack or more per day.[54]

Bladder and Renal Cancer. As seen in Tables 42–9 and 42–10, about 50% of bladder cancer cases in men and 40% in women are attributable to smoking, accounting for more than 4000 deaths per year. Relative risks for bladder cancer are 2 to 3, with a clear dose-response relationship and reduction in excess risk to near the level of a lifetime nonsmoker in about 15 years.[55,56]

Corresponding risks attributable to smoking and corresponding numbers of annual deaths are shown in Tables 42–9 and 42–10 for renal cancer. Relative risks from a variety of studies have ranged from 1 to 5, with most studies displaying a clear dose-response relationship.[1]

Pancreatic Cancer. In both men and women, smoking increases the risk of pancreatic cancer. Relative risks range from 2 to 3 in most studies, with dose-response relationships frequently, but not always, observed.[57] Attributable risk and annual smoking-related mortality rates are shown in Tables 42–9 and 42–10, respectively. The U.S. Veterans Study noted a 1.5 relative risk for pancreatic cancer among cigar, but not pipe, smokers.[3]

Stomach Cancer. Recent cohort and case-control studies have established that smoking consistently increases risk of cancer of the stomach, but to a limited degree, with an average relative risk of about 1.5 and a dose-response curve based on number of cigarettes smoked.[1]

Cervical Cancer. At least 15 epidemiological studies have consistently shown an increased risk of cervical cancer in cigarette smokers[58–60] after adjustment for other known causal factors such as early and frequent coitus, multiple sex partners, early pregnancy, and presence of sexually transmitted diseases. Relative risks have varied considerably but are probably below 2 for the average woman smoker. Recent findings of nicotine and cotinine in the cervical mucus of cigarette smokers[61] and of mutagenic mucus in the cervix of smokers[62] provide physical evidence supporting a causal relationship.

OTHER SMOKING-RELATED DISEASES

Chronic Obstructive Pulmonary Disease

An estimated 71,000 Americans died of COPD in 1986; 82% of these deaths were attributable to smoking. Rates increased with age and were 1.8 times higher in males than females and 2.8 times higher in white than in black people.[63] That the COPD mortality rate increased by 33% from 1979 to 1986 while smok-

TABLE 42-10. ESTIMATED ATTRIBUTABLE RISKS FOR 10 SELECTED CAUSES OF DEATH IN MALE AND FEMALE CIGARETTE SMOKERS (UNITED STATES, 1985)

Cause of death	Males (%)	Females (%)
CHD, age <65 yr	45 [40–50][a]	41 [34–48]
CHD, age ≥65 yr	21 [17–26]	12 [9–15]
COPD	84 [78–88]	79 [73–83]
Cancer of lip, oral cavity, and pharynx	92 [79–97]	61 [45–76]
Cancer of larynx	81 [57–93]	87 [56–97]
Cancer of esophagus	78 [62–89]	75 [57–87]
Cancer of lung	90 [88–92]	79 [75–82]
Cancer of pancreas	29 [18–43]	34 [25–44]
Cancer of bladder	47 [31–63]	37 [18–61]
Cancer of kidney	48 [32–64]	12 [3–43]
Cerebrovascular disease, age <65 yr	51 [36–65]	55 [45–65]
Cerebrovascular disease, age >65 yr	24 [16–35]	6 [2–14]

[a] Numbers in parentheses are 95% confidence intervals.
From the U.S. Department of Health and Human Services, 1989.[1]

ing prevalence decreased supports the observation of the long latency period between smoking exposure and COPD death. Data from both case-control and cohort studies consistently demonstrate a uniform increase in mortality for COPD among cigarette smokers compared with nonsmokers, with mortality ratios of 2.2 to 24.7 for one-pack-a-day cigarette smokers (Table 42-11). The reported relative risk of COPD for heavier smokers compared with nonsmokers is in the range of 30.[4] Dose-response relationships have been consistently observed, with the risk of death from COPD influenced not only by the number of cigarettes smoked per day but also by the depth of smoke inhalation and by the age at smoking initiation.[64,65]

The pathogenesis of COPD extends over the entire period of smoking history. Abnormal lung function (especially expiratory airflow) occurs as early as 2 years after smoking initiation.[66,67] Smokers as a group have a more rapid decline in forced expiratory volume at 1 second (FEV_1) with age than that observed in nonsmokers,[4] and the aggregate loss correlates well with cumulative pack-years of consumption of cigarettes.[68] Decline in lung function begins with inflammation in the small airways, although symptoms of such inflammation are not always a reliable indicator of smokers who will subsequently have symptomatic COPD. However, those smokers with a fast annual decline in FEV_1 appear to constitute a high-risk group for COPD development.[4,69]

Recent studies have identified the likely mechanism by which cigarette smoking induces COPD as an imbalance of levels of lower respiratory tract proteases and their inhibitors.[4] It is hypothesized that smoking results in an increased number of neutrophils in association with inflammation. They, in turn, secrete elastase, which can degrade elastin, a structural element of lung tissue.[70] Oxidizing agents in smoke reduce the activity of α_1-antiproteinase (α_1-antitrypsin), which normally blocks elastase activity.[70,71] Increased elastase activity eventually breaks down the alveolar walls,[4,72,73] causing emphysema.[72,73]

One of the first common symptoms of smoking-related respiratory problems is "smokers cough," which is associated with excess secretion of mucus.[4] On average, the prevalence of cough and phlegm increases threefold among male smokers and twofold among female smokers.[4] Smokers with cough and phlegm have reduced pulmonary function and are at increased risk for symptomatic COPD.[4,74]

Several large cohort studies have found that pipe and cigar smokers have an approximate twofold increase in COPD mortality compared with nonsmokers, but the case fatality rate for these groups of smokers is lower than for cigarette smokers.[4] After smoking cessation the rate of reduction of COPD excess risk is determined by prior smoking status (duration and daily consumption pattern) and number of years since cessation. In the U.S. Veterans Study, the mortality ratio for current smokers was about 12, and was reduced to 10 among ex-smokers 10 years after cessation. After more than 20 years, the mortality rate was still twice that of nonsmokers.[75] Persons with destructive changes can often stabilize after cessation but do not regain lost lung function.[4]

Gastrointestinal Disease. Smoking contributes to the development of symptomatic gastroesophageal reflux by lowering esophageal sphincter pressure and decreasing the competence of the esophagogastric barrier to reflux.[76] Nicotine decreases pyloric sphincter pressure, permitting increased reflux of duodenal contents into the stomach, including bile salts, exocrine pancreatic enzymes, and phospholipids, all of which can injure gastric mucosa.[1,77]

Smokers of both genders have a high prevalence of peptic ulcer disease, with a clear dose-response relationship based on amount smoked per day. Relative risks for prevalence of peptic ulcers and for duodenal ulcer mortality are in the range of 1.5 to 2.5 for smokers vs nonsmokers.[6] With or without cimetidine, duodenal ulcers heal more slowly in smokers.[78–81] Smoking cessation probably reduces the incidence of peptic ulcers and is an important component of peptic ulcer disease treatment.[1]

Diseases of the Mouth. Epidemiological studies from several countries have shown that cigarette smokers have more periodontal disease than nonsmokers, suggesting a possible causal role for cigarette smoking in the development of periodontal disease.[6,82,83] One large case-control study found that smokers have poorer periodontal status than ex-smokers, who in turn have poorer periodontal status than people who have never smoked. A strong association was noted between both the duration of smoking and cumulative consumption and the level of periodontal disease.[84] Among adult users of smokeless tobacco or snuff, the risk of oral disease has been well documented, and changes in the hard and soft tissues of the mouth (including gum recession and leukoplakia), discoloration of teeth, decreased ability to taste and smell, and advanced periodontal destruction have been reported.[85–87] One study of smokeless tobacco users in a high school population reported that 48 of these teenage users (averaging 1.7 years of smokeless tobacco use) had soft tissue lesions or periodontal inflammation or both, or erosion of dental hard tissues.[88]

HEALTH RISKS OF PASSIVE SMOKING

Constituents of Passive Smoke. Evidence of an adverse health effect of passive smoking is increasing. Involuntary smoking occurs when nonsmokers are exposed to the tobacco smoke exhaled by smokers in an enclosed environment.[89] Tobacco

TABLE 42-11. COPD MORTALITY RATES FOR MEN AND WOMEN BY NUMBER OF CIGARETTES SMOKED PER DAY (COHORT STUDIES)

	Men		Women		
Study	Cigarettes per Day	Mortality Ratios	Cigarettes per Day	Mortality Ratios	COPD Disease Classification
British physicians	Nonsmoker	1.00	Nonsmoker	1.00	Chronic bronchitis, emphysema, or both
	1–14	17.00	1–14	10.50	
	15–24	26.00	15–24	28.50	
	25+	38.00	25+	32.00	
U.S. veterans	Nonsmoker	1.00			Chronic bronchitis
	1–9	3.63			
	10–20	4.51			
	21–39	4.57			
	40+	8.31			
	Nonsmoker	1.00			Emphysema
	1–9	5.33			
	10–19	14.04			
	21–39	17.04			
	40+	25.34			
	Nonsmoker	1.00			Chronic bronchitis, and emphysema
	1–9	4.84			
	10–19	11.23			
	21–39	17.45			
	40+	21.98			
Canadian veterans	Nonsmoker	1.00			Chronic bronchitis
	1–9	7.02			
	10–20	13.65			
	21+	14.63			
	Nonsmoker	1.00			Emphysema
	1–9	4.81			
	10–20	6.12			
	21+	6.93			
Japanese	Nonsmoker	1.00	Nonsmoker	1.00	Emphysema
	<100,000[a]	0.51	<100,000	2.28	
	<200,000	2.57	<200,000	3.14	
	>300,000	1.93	>300,000	10.93	
California men in various occupations	Nonsmoker	1.00[b]			Emphysema
	About 1/2 pack	8.18			
	About 1 pack	11.80			
	About 1 1/2 pack	20.86			
American Cancer Society, 9-state study	Nonsmoker	1.00			All pulmonary diseases other than cancer[c]
	1–9	1.67			
	10–20	3.00			
	20+	3.64			

[a] Data for the Japanese study are for lifetime exposure by total number of cigarettes consumed.
[b] Nonsmokers in the California occupations study also include smokers of pipes and cigars.
[c] Pneumonia, influenza, tuberculosis, asthma, bronchitis, lung abscess, and so on.
From the U.S. Department of Health and Human Services, 1984.[4]

smoke in the environment is derived from two sources: (1) mainstream smoke emerging into the environment after being drawn through the cigarette, filtered by the smoker's lungs, and then exhaled, and (2) sidestream smoke arising from the burning end of the cigarette and entering directly into the environment. The two types of smoke share similar components, including oxides of nitrogen, nicotine, carbon monoxide, and various carcinogens and cocarcinogens. However, undiluted sidestream smoke has a higher pH, smaller particles, and higher concentrations of carbon monoxide and of many carcinogens.[90,91] Sidestream smoke contains a higher concentration of potentially dangerous gas-phase constituents and accounts for about 85% of the smoke in a room with smokers. However, because of dilution, nonsmokers are exposed to smaller doses of the products of tobacco combustion than active smokers.

Considerable work to develop sensitive and specific markers of exposure to passive smoking has identified cotinine[92–99] and, to a lesser extent, nicotine[100–106] as the best short-term markers for epidemiological studies. There is a strong dose-response correlation between urinary cotinine levels and self-reported exposure to tobacco smoke.[94–96]

Passive Smoking and Children's Health. Urinary cotinine concentrations in infants and young children correlate with the number of smokers reported in the home[93,98,100] and the number of cigarettes smoked by the mother during the prior 24 hours.[99]

Between 1974 and 1987, four prospective and nine case-control studies examined the possible effects of exposure to parental tobacco smoke on the frequency and severity of acute respiratory illness in children. Although a number of different research designs were used, the results have demonstrated a consistent increase in the frequency of both upper and lower respiratory tract problems among young children of smoking parents compared with the children of parents who do not smoke.[107-119] Pneumonia, bronchitis, bronchiolitis, and tracheitis, both as mild illnesses and for illnesses requiring hospitalization, have all been shown to increase significantly in children whose parents smoke. A dose-response curve has been observed for number of smoking parents and for level of maternal smoking, with one study estimating that an increase in the mother's smoking of five cigarettes per day results in an annual increase of 2.5 to 3.5 incidents of lower respiratory tract illness per 100 children at risk.[111,112] A French study correlated a higher incidence of tonsillectomy and adenoidectomy, as indexes of repeated respiratory infections, with parental smoking.[120] Other studies have demonstrated significant associations between parental smoking and an excess incidence of chronic middle-ear effusions and related ear infections.[121-125] Most of the observed effects are limited to the first year or two of life, although residual effects later in life cannot be ruled out.

A substantial number of cross-sectional studies also support an increased prevalence of chronic respiratory symptoms in children of smokers. Significant associations have been found between parental smoking and chronic wheeze, cough, and phlegm, although not all correlations in each study achieved statistical significance.[115,126-132] Overall, existing studies suggest that an excess prevalence of 30% to 80% of chronic respiratory disease symptoms in children of smokers, with effects observed throughout childhood.

Whether parental smoking leads to a decline in lung function in exposed children is a question that has so far defied clear-cut answers. During the decade ending in 1987, a total of 17 cross-sectional studies in the United States, China, and Italy assessed the physiological effects of exposure to environmental tobacco smoke on children's lung function. Results are divided almost equally between studies that found associations and those which did not.[115,129,131-135] Data suggesting a positive association have emerged from three ongoing longitudinal studies.[117,127,136-139] In general, younger children appear more strongly affected than older ones, with reductions in a standard measure of function such as FEV_1 by 1% to 5%, and with maternal smoking the strongest explanatory variable. Whether these small reductions predispose a child to the development of lung disease later in life is unknown.

Passive Smoking and Adults. Among healthy adults, the most common complaints after exposure to passive smoking are eye irritation (69%), headache (33%), nasal symptoms (33%), and cough (33%).[140] Exposure to tobacco smoke both precipitates and aggravates allergic attacks in some individuals with respiratory allergies and exacerbates other symptoms associated with allergies such as eye irritation, nasal symptoms, headaches, cough, wheezing, sore throat, and hoarseness.[90,140]

Passive Smoking and Lung Cancer. In 1985 three major bodies were independently convened to consider the evidence for health impacts of passive smoking. These three bodies, the U.S. Public Health Service, the National Research Council, and the Interagency Task Force on Environmental Cancer, Heart, and Lung Disease, reached a consensus that a substantial number of lung cancer deaths among nonsmokers can be attributed to involuntary smoking.[90,91,141] The National Research Council's review estimated the true relative risks (relative to subjects not exposed to smoking in the environment) for nonexposed nonsmokers married to smokers and for nonexposed nonsmokers married to nonsmokers as 1.41 to 1.87 and 1.09 to 1.45, respectively.[91] These estimates mean that between 2500 and 8400 of the approximately 12,200 annual lung cancer deaths in the United States not caused by smoking are attributable to environmental tobacco smoke.[91]

At least three prospective studies and 15 case-control studies have been published on this subject, with most investigators assessing exposure on the basis of nonsmokers' reporting that they were living with a smoker. The studies are reviewed in detail in the 1986 Surgeon General's report[90] and the 1986 publication of the National Academy of Sciences.[91] Each of the three prospective studies[142-144] reported a slightly higher risk of lung cancer in nonsmokers married to smokers, with reported relative risks of 1.18 to 2.25 and a weighted risk/ratio value of 1.44 (95% confidence intervals of 1.20 to 1.72).[90,91,145] An increased risk of lung cancer was found in nonsmokers married to smokers in 10 of the 15 case-control studies, with increases in 6 of the 10 studies reaching statistical significance. The odds ratios weighted average for these studies was 1.24 (95% confidence interval 1.04 to 1.50).

Although methodological problems limit interpretation of results of some of these studies, a wide body of evidence points to the likelihood of a causal effect of the involuntary inhalation of tobacco smoke on the risk of lung cancer in nonsmokers. While awaiting more definitive studies, individuals, employers, and those charged with developing public policy would be prudent to consider tobacco smoke a threat to the health of nonsmokers on the basis of current evidence of an association between environmental tobacco smoke and lung cancer.[146]

Passive Smoking and Other Diseases. The effect of passive smoking on chronic respiratory symptoms in adult nonsmokers has been the subject of very limited investigation. Although study results vary greatly, it appears that nonsmokers exposed to passive smoking may have a mild to moderate reduction in FEV_1, forced mid-expiratory flow, and forced end-expiratory flow.[2,146-163] Whether these reductions translate into overt health problems in otherwise healthy individuals or even in those with preexisting respiratory problems remains unknown.

At least five studies have examined the association between heart disease and exposure to tobacco smoke in nonsmokers.[144,152,161-163] Four have observed an association,[152,161-163] of which two have shown statistical significance.[161,163] However, a combination of methodological problems in most studies and small observed effect sizes do not yet permit any conclusion about causality. The National Research Council estimated that the relative risk of CHD in exposed nonsmokers would be approximately 1.02, an increase very difficult to detect or estimate.[91]

In Utero Effects of Maternal Smoking. The effects on the fetus of exposure to maternal smoke in utero have been extensively studied.[25] It is well documented that infants born to women who smoke during pregnancy weigh an average of 200 g less than those born to nonsmokers.[164] The incidence of low birth weight ($\leq$2500 g) in infants born to mothers who smoke is twice that in infants born to nonsmokers.[165] The relationship between maternal smoking and low birth weight is dose dependent and independent of other factors known to influence birth weight, including race, parity, maternal size, socioeconomic status, gender of child, and gestational age.[25]

In the offspring of smokers, low birth weight is primarily due not to a smoking-related reduction in the duration of gestation[6] but to direct retardation of fetal growth marked by decreases in body length and in head, chest, and shoulder circumference.[166] In 1985 the Centers for Disease Control defined the fetal tobacco syndrome as follows: (1) the mother smoked five or more cigarettes a day throughout the pregnancy; (2) the mother had no evidence of hypertension during pregnancy, specifically no preeclampsia and documentation of normal blood pressure at least once after the first trimester; (3) the newborn infant had symmetrical growth retardation at term, 37 weeks, defined as birth weight less than 2500g and a ponderal index (weight in grams divided by length) greater than 2.32; and (4) there is no obvious cause of intrauterine growth retardation, such as congenital malformation or infection.[1] Although fetal growth is diminished among maternal smokers, placenta/birth-weight ratios are larger in comparison with maternal nonsmokers,[167] probably because of the larger placental surface necessary to provide adequate fetal oxygenation in smokers. Smoking increases the level of carboxyhemoglobin in both maternal and fetal blood, with subsequent reduction in oxygen binding capacity and the pressure at which oxygen is delivered to fetal tissues, resulting in fetal hypoxia.[168] Smoking also increases the risk of maternal bleeding, including bleeding caused by abruptio placentae, during pregnancy.[169]

Maternal smoking is associated with higher fetal, neonatal, and infant mortality.[1] One large study showed adjusted infant mortality rates of 15.1 per 1000 for white nonsmokers and 23.3 for white women who smoked more than one pack per day. Comparable infant mortality rates for black women were 26.0 and 39.9, respectively.[170] Maternal smoking increases the risk of spontaneous abortion.[171] All the effects cited above demonstrate a dose-response relationship. The few studies that have examined the long-term consequences of maternal smoking in offspring suggest that there may be a slight increase in the incidence of mental retardation, cerebral palsy, epilepsy, hyperactivity, a shortened attention span, lower test scores, and electroencephalographic abnormalities.[172-174] However, these studies are limited by small numbers and infrequency of events of interest, making any conclusion premature.

TRENDS IN CIGARETTE USE

Prevalence of Cigarette Consumption Among Adults and Teenagers. Annual per capita consumption of cigarettes reached a peak of 4345 in 1963, a year before the first Surgeon General's report, and, except for an increase from 1971 through 1973, has steadily declined to an estimated 3121 in 1988 (Fig. 42–3). Overall numbers of cigarettes sold in the United States declined from 640 billion in 1981 to 574 billion in 1987.[175]

Since 1964, smoking in the United States has decreased yearly by an average of 0.5%. In the 1987 National Health Interview Survey, 28.8% of adults (persons 18 years of age and older) were reported to be current smokers. Rates for men were higher (31.2%) than for women (26.5%). For both sexes, smoking prevalence was highest in the 25- to 44-year age group (33.2%), followed closely by those 45 to 64 years of age (30.9%) and those 18 to 24 years of age (27.1%). Americans aged 65 to 74 years continued to smoke at a lower but still substantial rate (19%), with some decline after age 75 years (8.9%) (Table 42–12).[176]

Although the decreases in smoking prevalence are encouraging, analysis of the 1985 National Health Interview Survey revealed disturbing differences by age, gender, race, education, and socioeconomic status. These analyses examined overall prevalence, as well as rates of initiation and cessation.

Among men, the trend in smoking prevalence has been downward, both for white and black populations. The 1974 prevalence was higher among black men (40.6% vs 32.1% for white men), but their rate of decrease through 1985 was greater (−1.15% vs −0.87% per year). Although fewer women than men smoked, the rate of decrease among women was substantially less than that of men. For black women the decrease was −0.26% per year, whereas for white women it was slightly higher, −0.32% per year.[177]

During the period from 1974 to 1985, among ever smokers who had quit, fewer women (39.8%) than men (45.8%) were quitting and fewer black persons, both men (32.9%) and women (29.7%), had quit compared with white men (49%) and white women (43.3%). More disturbing were rates of smoking initiation, which were higher for women (34.6%) than men (33.4%). Overall the prevalence of initiation was higher among white (32.3%) than black (27.9%) persons, with fewer black men (27.5%) initiating smoking than white men (31.6%) and only slightly fewer black women (32.6%) than white women (33.1%).[177]

Formal educational attainment exhibited a striking association with smoking prevalence, initiation, and cessation rates. Among persons with a college education, 18.4% smoked vs 34.4% among high school graduates. Of college graduates, 57.1% have quit compared with 40.1% of high school graduates. The greatest educational disparity is in initiation rates. For those with a high school diploma or less, the initiation rate was 45.3%, whereas for those with some college education it was 16.4%. Less educated men and women initiated smoking at about the same rate (45.7% vs 44.4%), but women with some college education initiated smoking at a greater rate than comparable men (19.7% vs 12.4%).[178]

Persons who were unemployed, blue collar workers, per-

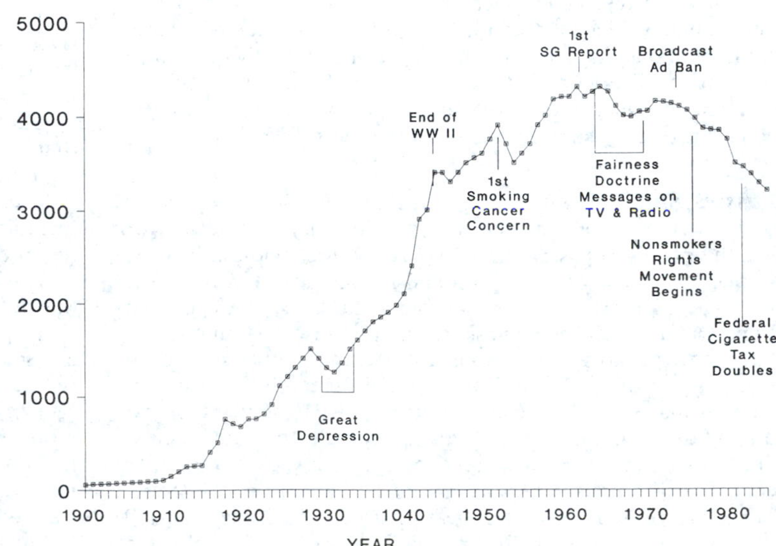

Figure 42–3. Adult per capita cigarette consumption and major smoking-and-health events. *[Adapted from Warner, 1985.[277]]*

TABLE 42-12. PERCENTAGE OF ADULTS WHO SMOKE CIGARETTES, BY SEX AND AGE (UNITED STATES, 1987)

Age (yr)	Men	Women	Total
18–24	28.1	26.1	27.1
25–44	35.6	30.8	33.2
45–64	33.5	28.6	30.9
65–74	20.2	18.0	19.0
≥75	11.3	7.5	8.9
Total[a]	31.2	26.5	28.8

[a] Ninety-five percent confidence intervals: men, 30.4 to 32.0; women, 25.8 to 27.2; total, 28.3 to 29.3.
From the Morbidity and Mortality Weekly Report, 1989.[176]

sons who were widowed, separated, or divorced, and those below the poverty level were more likely to have ever smoked or to be current smokers and to be heavy smokers (15 or more cigarettes a day).[179]

Daily smoking among high school seniors decreased from 27% in 1975 to 19% in 1987, whereas never smokers increased from 26% to 33% during that period (Table 42-13).[180] The 1987 National Student Health Survey found that 16% of eighth graders and 26% of tenth graders reported that they were current smokers. More than 50% of eighth graders had tried smoking, as had 63% of tenth-grade students.[181]

The Changing Cigarette. In the early 1950s, when smoking was first associated with lung cancer, a majority of Americans smoked unfiltered (plain) high-tar cigarettes, with average tar content greater than 35 mg per cigarette. Beginning in the 1960s, filters were introduced to reduce the amount of harmful substances reaching a smoker's lungs. Although early versions proved to be inefficient in lowering tar delivery, health concerns led to further changes in filter design and cigarette composition to reduce the amounts of tar and nicotine, at least as measured by standard smoking machines used to determine levels of these substances for labeling and advertising.

Tar is a complex mixture of compounds, including a number of identifiable carcinogens and cocarcinogens, and nicotine is generally accepted as the principal constituent responsible for a smoker's pharmacological response.[6] Between 1954 and 1975, the average tar content of a cigarette in the United States declined 50%, from 38 to 19 mg; by 1985 the average tar content was between 12.7 and 13 mg per cigarette. During the period from 1954 to 1985, average nicotine content was reduced from 2.3 to 0.9 mg.[182–184] The progression from high-tar, to unfiltered high-tar, to filtered middle-tar, and to filtered low-tar cigarettes has also been observed in Western European countries, including Germany, Switzerland, the United Kingdom, and France.[185]

TABLE 42-13. SMOKING STATUS (%) OF HIGH SCHOOL SENIORS (UNITED STATES, 1975–1987)

Year	Daily Smokers	Less Than Daily Smokers	Previous Smokers, Not in Last Month	Never Smokers
1975	27	10	37	26
1976	29	10	36	25
1977	29	10	38	24
1978	28	9	38	25
1979	26	9	40	26
1980	21	9	41	29
1981	20	9	42	29
1982	21	9	40	30
1983	20	9	41	29
1984	18	11	41	30
1985	19	11	39	31
1986	18	11	38	32
1987	19	11	38	33

From the Department of Health and Human Services, 1989.[1]

"Safe" and "less hazardous" low-tar and low-nicotine cigarettes, since their introduction to the U.S. cigarette market in the late 1960s and early 1970s, have had rapid increases in market share, from 2% in 1971 and 17% in 1976 to more than 60% in 1981[183–185] but declined to 54% in 1985 and 1986, indicating a return to a fuller-flavored cigarette.[176] In addition, the ultra-low-tar brands, since their introduction in the late 1970s, have captured 22.3% of the low-tar market.[185] (Low-tar cigarettes are defined as having <15 mg of tar per cigarette and ultra-low-tar brands as having up to 10 mg of tar per cigarette.) Similar patterns of consumption of low-tar cigarettes also occurred in Canada during this period.[186] The significant growth of the low-tar-cigarette market in the last decade is attributable to increased public awareness that cigarette smoking, particularly exposure to tar and nicotine, is detrimental to health.

Because of the widespread acceptance of cigarettes lower in tar and nicotine content, several cohort studies were conducted to ascertain the health consequences associated with reductions in cigarette tar and nicotine yields. One study followed more than 1 million people for 12 years and reported that those persons who smoked low-tar and low-nicotine brands (at that time defined as cigarettes having 17.6 to 25.8 mg tar per cigarette) had a 9% lower overall mortality rate than smokers of high-tar and high-nicotine cigarettes (defined as cigarettes having 25.8 to 35.7 mg tar per cigarette).[187] Results from the same study indicated that smokers of low-tar brands had a 26% reduction in lung cancer mortality rates compared with smokers of high-tar brands. Despite these reductions, lung cancer mortality and overall mortality among smokers of low-tar cigarettes were much greater than those of nonsmokers.[188]

With respect to heart disease, one cohort study reported a significant reduction (20%) in CHD mortality among low-tar cigarette smokers, but recent evidence from the Framingham Study suggests that smokers of low-tar, low-nicotine cigarettes and of filter cigarettes do not have a lower CHD incidence than smokers of high-tar, unfiltered brands.[187,189] This latter finding has been corroborated in later case-control studies, one of which reported the relative risk for nonfatal myocardial infarction among young men (30 to 54 years of age) smoking low-tar cigarettes to be 2.8 times that among nonsmokers.[190]

Evidence is unavailable on the relative risks of developing COPD from the smoking of low-tar, low-nicotine cigarettes. It appears, however, that the prevalence of cough and phlegm may be reduced slightly among smokers of these cigarettes.[4]

One study found that while ultra-low-yield cigarettes delivered much less exposure to tar, nicotine, and carbon monoxide than high- or low-yield cigarettes, the exposure was still substantial.[191] However, other studies have found that plasma nicotine and alveolar carbon monoxide levels in smokers using various low-tar brands correlated poorly with reported brand yields.[192–195] These findings imply that smokers may possibly compensate for reduced yields by altering their smoking methods, so the amount of tar and nicotine they receive may actually bear little relation to published yields, which are based on machine smoking under standardized conditions.

It is reported that changes in smoking methods are related to smokers' self-regulation of their blood-nicotine level[195] and that higher yields of nicotine can be obtained by alternating the frequency and depth of inhalation[196] or by mechanically compressing filter tips and blocking air channels with the lips or fingers.[1,197] (Air channels are four small holes at the periphery of a special filter, designed to allow inhalation of air to dilute toxic cigarette yields with each puff.) As a result of these practices, tar yields can be increased by 51%, nicotine by 69%, and carbon monoxide by 147% over their published yields.[194] A common but apt suggestion is that smoking machine parameters and methods used by the U.S. Federal Trade Commission to determine cigarette yields be updated to approximate more closely the patterns of human smoking behavior.

Smokeless Tobacco. Smokeless tobacco, as both chewing tobacco and snuff, contains tobacco leaves plus sweeteners, flavoring, and various scents. Chewing tobacco may be in the form of strands, cakes, or shreds and is either chewed or placed in the oral vestibule. Snuff, which is marketed in a small, round can, or "tin," is supplied dry or moist and is held ("dipped") between the gingiva and the lip or cheek. While the smoking of tobacco has declined, the use of smokeless tobacco has changed little during the past 20 years. The National Institute on Drug Abuse National Household Survey found that, in 1985, the prevalence of "ever use" among men and women 21 years of age or older was 19% and 3%, respectively.[198] Prevalence tends to be lower in the Northeast and higher in the South.[198] Long-term smokeless tobacco use increases the risk of periodontal disease and may increase the risk of oral cancer.[199] It may also predispose those who try it to become smokers of tobacco. Starting in 1986, smokeless tobacco products and advertisements were required by federal law to carry warning labels about the health hazards of use.

SMOKING CONTROL MEASURES

Smoking Cessation. Reduced prevalence of smoking suggests, and many national surveys confirm, that millions of smokers have stopped smoking and a substantial proportion of them have remained abstinent for many years. More than 90% of smokers wish to stop, and the majority of smokers have tried to do so one or more times.[200] Of those who have achieved long-term abstinence, the vast majority have stopped without the help of any formal programs, materials, or clinical interventions.[200] The stimuli for cessation differ substantially among individual smokers. Among stimuli reported by ex-smokers as contributing to their cessation and abstinence are health problems, such as emphysema or a myocardial infarction; strong family pressures, both from spouses and children; peer pressure from friends and co-workers; cost of cigarettes, especially for lower-income individuals; fear of potential adverse effects on personal health or on the health of children, or the likelihood of their starting to smoke; and concern for cleanliness and social acceptance.[1,200,201] In general, the greater the number of reasons a person has for stopping and the greater the number of cessation attempts, the greater will be the likelihood of long-term abstinence.

Smoking Cessation Classes. Smoking cessation programs have grown considerably in number, in the variety of their approaches, duration, and effectiveness. Most organized programs involve groups of 8 to 15 smokers led in a structured program by an experienced group leader who is often a psychologist or health educator. These programs share a reliance on behavioral techniques to augment the participant's skill in resisting the urge to smoke. Frequently, programs incorporate sensitization (e.g., aversion therapy) or desensitization (stimulus control) procedures to eliminate the urge to smoke and to control smoking as a response to environmental stimuli, such as drinking coffee or confronting a stressful situation.

Another frequently employed technique is contracting, by which the smoker gives money to a person or program; the money is returned only if smoking cessation and subsequent abstinence for an agreed-on period are accomplished. This is sometimes supplemented by having program participants make a public announcement of the date on which they will stop smoking. This approach is used in an attempt to increase commitment and take advantage of the participants' desire not to fail in the eyes of friends and co-workers. Self-monitoring, in which the time, place, and circumstances of each smoke are recorded, has also been used to sensitize smokers to personal smoking cues and to their limited control over their smoking habit.[1,202]

Group smoking-cessation programs may include only a few classes or as many as 15 sessions, but all organized programs continue through some period after the termination date to assist members as they go through the withdrawal process and deal with the craving to resume smoking. The two most common program models are the 1-week program, with sessions on 5 consecutive days, sometimes followed by one or two meetings during subsequent weeks, and programs of 2 to 4 weeks' duration in which cessation is scheduled to occur during the second or third week.

Success rates vary greatly. Major influencing variables include the nature of the program, program content, the instructor, the setting (e.g., clinical vs work site), entry cost, and degree of motivation. In most programs, initial termination rates are high, in the range of 70% to 90%, among persons who finish the program, but recidivism is also high; 6- and 12-month cessation rates are in the range of 10% to 40%.[203] Special classes to prevent relapse have recently been developed in the hope of increasing long-term abstinence rates.

In 1984, nicotine gum was introduced as an adjunct to other cessation activities, and 1987 sales of this product exceeded $60 million. Studies suggest that in conjunction with behavior-based cessation programs, it can sometimes lead to overall improvements in abstinence rates.[204,205]

The peer pressure and competitive spirit inherent at many work sites lend themselves to the use of contests. This approach has been reported to increase both effectiveness and cost-effectiveness of work-site risk-reduction programs targeted at risks such as smoking and obesity.[1]

Although persons who cease smoking because of participation in one organized program are usually a minority, those with sufficient motivation to attempt stopping once are likely to try again despite temporary failure, and some succeed on subsequent attempts. Therefore the traditional cross-sectional studies of smoking cessation probably reveal a much lower percentage of successful cessation than would cohort analyses of smokers studied for a period of several years.[206] Less encouraging is the evidence, from the Multiple Risk Factor Intervention Trial (MRFIT) and other longitudinal risk-reduction intervention studies, that recidivism can still occur after many years of abstinence.[207]

A new delivery vehicle for smoking cessation programs is the computer program, with formats and techniques similar to those of instructor-led group courses but with some instructional modules tailored to the specific demographic variables and the smoking history and pattern of the participant. The programs were initially developed for use with minicomputer and mainframe systems; new versions have emerged for use with microcomputers, such as the increasingly common personal computers. Effectiveness of computer-assisted courses has not yet been reported.

Clinical Interventions. Health professionals have had rapidly declining smoking rates. Data from 1985 showed that 16.7% of physicians and 14.1% of dentists were current smokers,[208] whereas only 9% of American Medical Association members surveyed in 1987 were smokers.[209] Smoking remained, in 1985, much more prevalent among nurses (23.4%).[208] Although most health professionals agree that the elimination of smoking is an essential part of health promotion, many underestimate their ability to be effective in promoting smoking cessation to their smoking patients. A survey of primary-care physicians in Massachusetts found that 90% routinely asked patients about smoking and that 58% were prepared to counsel patients about smoking.

Yet, only 3% expressed confidence about the success of their efforts.[210] Given that 70% or more (38 million) of the nation's 54 million adult smokers visit a physician at least once a year, however, even if only 5% to 10% of them followed their physician's advice to stop smoking, the impact would be considerable.[1] To emphasize the importance of counseling to prevent tobacco use, the U.S. Preventive Services Task Force recommended the following in 1989:

> Tobacco cessation counseling should be offered on a regular basis to all patients who smoke cigarettes, pipes, or cigars, and to those who use smokeless tobacco. The prescription of nicotine gum may be an appropriate adjunct for some patients. Adolescents and young adults who do not currently use tobacco products should be advised not to start.[211]

Special Community Intervention Programs. Controlled community intervention studies that focus on smoking cessation are still relatively scarce. Nevertheless, community trials for cardiovascular disease prevention in which cigarette smoking is a risk factor are providing promising results.

The best known of these studies is the Stanford Three-Community Study, involving three small communities (population approximately 20,000 each) nonrandomly assigned to control, media-only, and media and face-to-face study groups. Included in the study were annual thiocyanate measurements taken during a 4-year period to determine each participant's smoking status and 3-year smoking trends for each of the three groups. As Figure 42–4 clearly illustrates, smoking prevalence decreased markedly among the group receiving media and face-to-face intervention, whereas the other intervention group showed an initial decline that leveled after the first year of media intervention.[212] A follow-up study found some attrition in the intense-intervention group but reported that 32% of those who stopped smoking had sustained cessation after the study.[213]

In a similar study of three communities in Australia (the North Coast Study), the media and community programs group (which included physician-intervention programs in stress management and physical fitness) had a 6% to 15% smoking decrease, whereas the media-only group achieved an estimated 6% to 11% reduction. The control group had a slight decrease of 1% to 5% in smoking prevalence.[214]

Because of a number of methodological problems that exist with large-scale controlled community-intervention studies,[1] they cannot be accepted as conclusive tests of the effectiveness of community smoking-control programs, but they do provide a promising illustration and evaluation of what can be achieved through broad intervention designed to reduce smoking along with other cardiovascular risk factors.

Government and Private Sector Measures. Smokers and nonsmokers are increasingly separated in everyday activities. By the end of 1987, smoking restrictions had been passed by 42 states and the District of Columbia, with restrictions common in public transportation facilities (36 states), hospitals (34 states), schools (32 states), elevators (39 states), government buildings (31 states), and recreational facilities (30 states).[215-218] By 1989, more than 350 communities in the United States had passed laws restricting smoking in public places, a fourfold increase during a 3-year period.[219,220] Nonsmoking rental cars, sections of hotels and motels reserved for nonsmokers, and a few nonsmoking airlines provide a constant reinforcement that smokers are different and that many people wish to reduce their exposure to smoke at every possible opportunity.[221] In 1990, smoking was banned on all U.S. domestic flights of less than 6 hours' duration.

In addition, insurance companies are increasingly recognizing the overall impact of smoking on premature death and illness. For example, the Task Force on Smoker/Nonsmoker Mortality of the Society of Actuaries of America used the collective experience of five life insurance companies in developing a set of smoker-nonsmoker mortality ratios for men, varying by age. Smoker-nonsmoker ratios were determined to be 1.50 at the age of 25 years, increasing to a peak of 2.5 at the age of 45 years and decreasing thereafter with increasing age. Results of this and other studies have prompted almost all major life insurance underwriters (more than 200 companies) to offer premium discounts ranging from 10% to 30% for policy holders who have never smoked or have stopped for at least 12 months.[222] However, as of 1985, only about 15% of companies offering health and disability insurance provided nonsmoker discounts.[223] The trend in nonsmokers' discounts is slowly extending to fire, home owner, and automobile insurance policies; Farmers Insurance Group reports offering a 10% to 25% discount to drivers who have never smoked or have not smoked for at least 2 years.[221]

Since the U.S. Surgeon General's first Report on Smoking and Health in 1964, public and private health agencies have engaged in a broad variety of activities designed to reduce the incidence and prevalence of smoking. Although the impact of any single such effort is difficult to establish, growing evidence suggests a collective demonstrable effect, particularly on the prevalence of smokers. After comparing actual per capita consumption of cigarettes after 1964 with that projected on the basis of pre-1964 trends, one study concluded that the 1964 report led to an immediate transitory decrease of 4% to 5% in annual per ca-

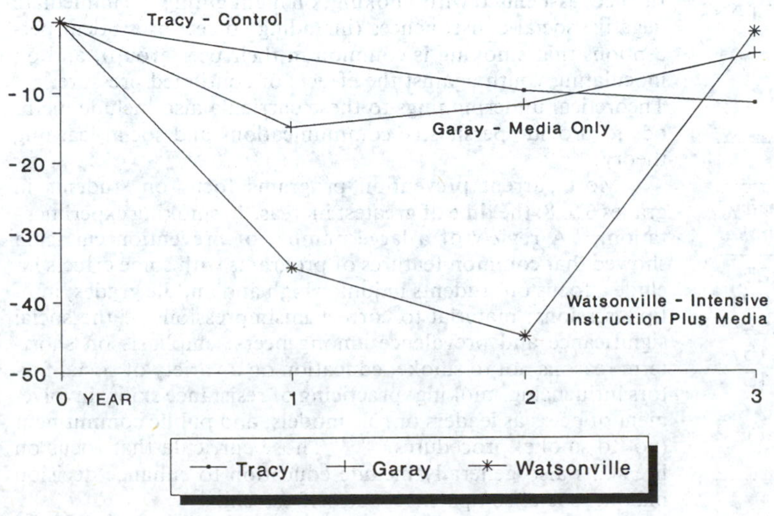

Figure 42–4. Comparison of cessation rates among smokers in communities subjected to varied intensities of education [Stanford Three-Community Study]. *[From the U.S. Department of Health and Human Services, 1984.[2]]*

pita consumption and that the cumulative effects of publicity and other public policies led to an actual smoking prevalence in 1978 of 40% lower than predicted.[224] This reduction below predicted levels translates into the avoidance of more than 200,000 premature smoking-related deaths between 1964 and 1978.[225] Such analyses must be interpreted cautiously because they rely heavily on assumptions of what would have occurred in the absence of antismoking campaigns.

One mechanism available to influence the consumption of tobacco is the taxation of cigarettes and other tobacco products. In the year ending June 30, 1987, the federal government received $4.8 billion (gross) from the 16 cents per pack tax. However, federal tax as a percentage of retail price declined from 30.3% in 1964 to 13.7% in 1987,[226] as did the percentage of state and federal revenues from cigarette taxes. At midyear 1988, state excise taxes ranged from 2 cents per pack in North Carolina to 38 cents in Minnesota, with an average state tax of 18.2 cents per pack. In addition, 40 states and the District of Columbia imposed general sales taxes as of 1987. By the same year, 27 states taxed smokeless tobacco, as did the federal government, but only at the rate of 8 cents per pound.[227] A California initiative petition to increase cigarette taxes by 25 cents per pack passed in 1988 despite an estimated $20 million campaign by the tobacco lobby to defeat it; as a result, California is collecting an additional $600 million per year from the sale of cigarettes.

Taxation increases price, which in turn reduces consumption. A large body of literature has developed regarding the demand-based price elasticity of cigarettes. Table 42–14 provides one set of estimates of the effects of price increases on both smoking prevalence and the quantity of cigarettes purchased by persons continuing to smoke.[228-231] Data for adults suggest that a 10% price increase leads to a 2.6% decline in the number of smokers and a 1% reduction in cigarette purchases among continuing smokers. By contrast, adolescent smoking appears much more affected by price changes: a 14% decrease in percentage of smokers is associated with a 10% price increase.[228,232]

Advertising and Promotion. Tobacco companies maintain that none of their advertising or promotions are intended to appeal to teenagers or preteen children. However, the nature of the activities promoted, often popular musical events and sporting events, as well as the effort in advertisements to associate smoking with maturity, glamour, and self-confidence, indicates a strong appeal to youth. In addition, cigarette companies give away free cigarettes to young people at rock concerts. As the prevalence of smoking in men and in white Americans declines, tobacco company marketing efforts have targeted women and minorities. In 1990, after the Secretary of the Department of Health and Human Services, Dr. Louis Sullivan, denounced R. J. Reynolds for "slick and sinister advertising" and for "promoting a culture of cancer," the company abruptly decided to cancel the launch of Uptown, their new cigarette aimed at blacks.[233] Only a month later, the same company was reported to be preparing to introduce a new cigarette aimed at "virile females," young, poorly educated, blue collar women.[234] These examples suggest that new tobacco product introductions aimed at young and minority populations are likely to be aggressively attacked as exploitative.

TABLE 42–14. ESTIMATES OF THE PRICE ELASTICITY OF DEMAND FOR CIGARETTES

Age group (ys)	Elasticities: Total	Participation	Quantity per Smoker
12–17	−1.40	−1.20	−0.25
20–25	−0.89	−0.74	−0.20
26–35	−0.47	−0.44	−0.04
36–74	−0.45	−0.15	−0.15
All adults (20–74)	−0.42	−0.26	−0.10
All ages (12–74)	−0.47	−0.31	−0.11

From the U.S. Department of Health and Human Services.[1]

Restrictions on tobacco advertising are likely to increase in the United States, following the pattern well established in many other countries. Canada passed legislation in 1988 to ban all tobacco advertising in newspapers and magazines published in Canada, as well as all point-of-sale advertising and promotion. In Europe a number of countries have enacted similar restriction or restrictions on the use of graphics in tobacco advertising, and it is likely that the European Economic Community will begin to address restrictions that would apply to all member nations.

Bans on advertising would most affect outdoor media, of which 1985 cigarette advertising expenditures accounted for 22.3% of the total.[235] In the same year, cigarette advertising accounted for 7.1% of magazine advertising and 0.8% of newspaper advertising revenues.

An important experiment to determine the effect of smoking counteradvertising began in California in 1990. During an 18-month period $28 million will be spend on such advertising as mandated by an initiative on smoking control passed in 1988. If it is successful in reducing smoking prevalence, it is likely that many other states will consider similar initiatives.

Smoking Prevention. Smoking prevention can be accomplished by a number of mechanisms: changes in public attitudes toward smoking acceptability, restrictions that limit supply to youth, high prices to reduce product affordability, and specific educational programs designed to reduce acquisition of the smoking habit. Since the mid-1960s, increasing attention has been given to developing valid theoretical models of smoking initiation and related prevention programs. The 1989 Surgeon General's report summarizes three approaches: (1) media-based prevention programs and resources, (2) smoking prevention as part of a multicomponent school health education curriculum, and (3) psychosocial approaches of social influence and generic life skills curricula.[1]

The newer curricula are distinctly different from their predecessors, which concentrated on exposing the evils of smoking, especially the long-term health effects. Evidence that knowledge of these effects did not translate into reduced smoking led to focusing on susceptibility of youth to peer pressure in the development of health behaviors.[236] Recent curricula share emphases on helping children understand and effectively cope with social influences associated with smoking, on highlighting the immediate negative social consequences (including correcting student perceptions that smoking is common in their peer group), and on inoculating youth against the effects of continued pressure.[1,237] Theoretical underpinnings to these curricula also include methods to provide persuasive communications and social learning theory.[238,239]

Most current prevention programs focus on students in grades 6 to 8, the time of greatest increase in smoking experimentation.[240] A review of a large number of prevention curricula showed that common features of programs with some effects include a focus on students in junior high and middle grades; multiple sessions; material to correct misimpressions of the social significance and prevalence among peers; emphasis on short-term reasons not to smoke; education on a variety of social factors influencing smoking; practicing of resistance skills; involvement of peers as leaders or role models; and public commitment (not to smoke) procedures.[240,241] Those curricula that focus on life skills also generally include education to enhance decision making, social competence, and self-esteem.[242]

A number of these curricula, when applied in the context of well-designed research studies, have been shown to delay the assumption of initial smoking experimentation and development of a smoking habit, although the effect size differs widely among programs.[241,243,244] What is less clear is effectiveness of the same curricula in a more widely disseminated group of schools and teachers. Training of teachers is undoubtedly a critical variable in the degree of success achieved. Also awaited are more longitudinal studies to assess whether the delay in smoking translates into lower prevalence throughout young adult life. If smoking is a gateway behavior to other drug use, evaluating the effect on reducing the age-specific incidence of other drug use behaviors merits priority attention.

Media-based prevention efforts may serve as effective complements to curricula-based programs but alone do not appear to have the desired effects on youth.[245]

An additional mechanism to reduce smoking behavior among youth is to increase the price of tobacco products. Teenagers appear to be more sensitive to price increases than adults, perhaps because the latter group are on average both more addicted and more affluent. One analysis of the cigarette excise tax concludes that an increase in the federal cigarette excise tax would encourage an additional 3.5 million Americans to forgo smoking, including more than 800,000 teenagers and almost 2 million young adults aged 20 to 35 years.[246] Any increase in real price can be expected to have similar effects. Preliminary information from California suggests that in the year after the state cigarette tax was raised by 25 cents a pack, the sale of cigarettes declined at least 10%.

A final approach to discouraging smoking among youth is the establishment of strong smoking policies in schools. According to an American Lung Association survey in 1985, 95% of school districts had a written policy or regulation on tobacco smoking in schools. Of survey respondents, 17% totally banned smoking (i.e., no smoking was allowed by anyone on school premises or at school functions). The proportion of districts prohibiting smoking by faculty, staff, or administrators, or a combination thereof, in school buildings increased from 11% in 1986 to 24% in 1988.[247] Growth of such policies not only directly discourages smoking by youth but increases the likelihood that their role models, some of whom are teachers, will be nonsmokers.

Smoking and the Workplace. Smoking is very costly to employers. For example, Control Data Corporation reports that when employee data were trichotomized into risk categories based on smoking behavior, the excess claims cost for the high-risk group over the low-risk group was 118%.[248] Control Data Corporation, Johnson & Johnson, and other companies report that smokers have significantly higher rates of absenteeism.[248-250] Best conservative estimates of the excess costs of employing a smoker are $450 to $1200/y (1990 dollars).[250,251]

Although the percentage of employees who smoke has gradually decreased, certain subpopulations, including those with limited formal education and those in craft, service, and some types of manufacturing jobs, retain rates that are much higher than average.

In the first National Survey of Worksite Health Promotion Activities, 35.6% of private firms with 50 or more employees reported some smoking cessation activities, with the lowest prevalence by industry (18.6%), in a category that includes construction, fishing, and mining, and the highest in the service industry (42%). Frequency rose from 18.5% at work sites with fewer than 100 employees to 57.6% at work sites with 750 or more employees.[252]

Work-site smoking-cessation programs may be provided on or off site, may be run by outside or in-house personnel, and may be an isolated activity or integrated into a comprehensive employee health promotion program. Company incentives for participation have included (1) full or partial payment of the program fee for the employee through direct payment to the vendor or tuition reimbursement to the employee, (2) refund of the program fee if the employee stops smoking by a predetermined milestone date, such as 6 months or 12 months after the program, and (3) contests for employees who are successful at stopping smoking, with small or large prizes awarded to all who stop, to some selected by a lottery, or to all in this group. Some employers provide the additional incentive of time released from work to attend smoking cessation classes. Literature reviews on results suggest that well conceived and executed programs can help a minority of participating employees to achieve long-term abstinence, but design and methodological limitations of many studies preclude a judgment on an expected cessation rate for most work-site programs. Approaches that appear to enhance program success include strong management support; good employer-employee relations; time released from work to participate; contribution by employees of at least a token amount of program cost; and choice of type of cessation program. Incentives, competition, and public feedback on progress appear to have less influence on program results.[253,254] One comprehensive work-site health promotion program that included smoking cessation, Live for Life (LFL), reported a verified decline among the *entire* work-site population of 22.6% for 2 years; at comparison work sites, the reduction in health-profile-only groups was 17.4%. In the LFL companies, 32% of high-risk smokers quit vs 12.9% in the health-profile-only companies.[249]

Workplace smoking policies, originally implemented primarily for safety reasons, have been adopted increasingly because of health concerns about the effects of passive smoking[146,255] In the National Survey of Worksite Health Promotion Activities, more than 76% of work sites with smoking cessation activities had a smoking policy in effect. The major reasons cited for adopting smoking policies were to protect the health of nonsmoking employees (39.1%) and to comply with regulations (38.2%).[256] As of 1987, 63% of personnel managers surveyed in companies with 1000 or more employees reported having smoking policies, compared with 52% in smaller companies.[215] Ironically, industries with a high potential for respiratory hazards (manufacturing, processing) and high prevalence of smoking employees are the least likely to have smoking policies.[215] Completely smoke-free work sites are the exception but growing rapidly in number. In 1987 the Bureau of National Affairs reported 79 places of business that were entirely smoke free, although many large and small workplaces have subsequently become smoke free.[215]

More than 90% of hospitals have a smoking policy, and bans are becoming more common, although as of 1986 not implemented in more than about 10% of hospitals.[257,258] Government work sites are increasingly covered by smoking policies, varying from a complete ban adopted by the U.S. Department of Health and Human Services in 1988 to policies restricting smoking in common areas such as conference rooms, elevators, and libraries. A major Department of Defense initiative to reduce smoking has included policies to create an environment that discourages smoking.[259] Laws in at least 31 states restrict smoking at public work sites, and other states have restricted smoking by administrative actions of the executive branch.

TOBACCO ECONOMICS

In 1989 consumers in the United States spent more than $41 billion on tobacco products, equal to 1.1% of all personal disposable income.[260] The industry indirectly accounts for about 2 million jobs, or 2.5% of all U.S. private sector employment.[9,261] The industry is highly concentrated, with only six major tobacco producers in the United States and with tobacco growing concentrated in six southern states. Of the 2.85 billion pounds of tobacco produced by domestic growers, 65% is used in domestic cigarette production and 35% is exported.[175] In monetary value, domestic tobacco exports account for 3.8% of all U.S. exports.[260]

In large part because of a price support control program first introduced in the 1930s, both the number of producers and the quantity produced are regulated through a complex system of quotas. As a result, the price of tobacco is maintained at artificially high levels, discouraging farmers from identifying alternative crops for their land. In 1989 the estimated gross income for tobacco was $3505 per acre, compared with corn ($262.73) and soybeans ($178.85).[260] In addition to price supports, tobacco farmers have benefited from the Drought Assistance Act of 1988. In fiscal year 1988, combined costs of loss of loan interest, administration of the price subsidy ($1.44 per pound in 1987[261]), and government regulation and supervision of tobacco exceeded $850 million.[262]

INTERNATIONAL PERSPECTIVE ON SMOKING

Smoking is a major preventable cause of death in most of the world. Although generalizations are difficult among industrialized nations, smoking prevalence is usually higher in men than in women, particularly in Japan. Prevalence is dropping for men while remaining constant or even increasing in women. In most European countries, Australia, and New Zealand, smoking prevalence is at U.S. levels or slightly higher (Table 42-15).[263] Significant public and private sector support exists for vigorous antismoking measures, particularly in the Scandinavian nations, New Zealand, and Australia. Under the aegis of the World Health Organization (WHO) Regional Committee for Europe, 32 participating countries agreed in 1988 to cooperate to combat smoking.[264] Partial or complete bans on tobacco advertising are becoming more common. Mandated health warnings, prevention activities in schools, and restriction of smoking in public and some private establishments are growing in frequency. Norway and Sweden have announced the objective of creating a smoke-free society within the next 10 to 20 years.[265,266]

TABLE 42-15. SMOKING PREVALENCE IN SELECTED COUNTRIES

	Smoking Prevalence			
Country	***Male***	***Female***	***M + F***	**Date of Survey**
Australia	37	30		1983
Bangladesh	70	20		1984
Bolivia	84	61	73	1986
Canada	31	28		1981
China	62	8	30	
Denmark	49	38	43	1987
Egypt	33	2	16	1981
France	49	26	37	1982
Germany (FDR)	44	29	36	1984
Hong Kong	33	4	19	1984
India	52	3		1984
Japan	66	14		1984
Korea	69	7	32	1981
Kuwait	52	12		
Malaysia	41	4	21	1984
Mexico	47	44	45	1984
Nigeria	53	3		
Poland	63	29		1983
Sweden	26	30	28	1986
Turkey	50	50		
United States	30	24	27	1987
United Kingdom	36	32		1984
Soviet Union	48	11	27	
Venezuela	69	67	68	1984
Yugoslavia	57	10		
Zambia	39	7	24	1983

From the World Health Organization, 1988.[263]

Consumption of tobacco products, primarily cigarettes, is growing in developing countries at an average rate of 2% per annum, double the rate of increase in the developed countries.[267] WHO estimates that more than half of the male population in developing countries smoke, compared with 5% of the women.[268]

Before the middle of this century, very few developing countries either produced tobacco or had significant consumption of manufactured cigarettes. In the late 1950s, cigarette manufacturers, sensing a shrinking domestic market because of the growing controversy surrounding smoking and lung cancer, sought to establish new markets in the Third World. These countries, with more than half of the world's population, who may be unaware of the health problems associated with smoking, represented a huge, potentially untapped resource for tobacco cultivation and cigarette manufacture, and marketing. More than 100 developing countries are involved in the growth, development, and processing of tobacco and its related products. The majority are poor and lack the resources to grow or import sufficient quantities of food for their populations; yet they divert agricultural land that could be utilized for growing staple crops, such as sorghum and maize, to tobacco cultivation. One explanation for this growth of a deadly industry is that the governments have been eager to emulate the practices of their more successful and wealthy neighbors in the industrialized world. In addition, they may perceive tobacco production as (1) a relatively simple mechanism for raising substantial revenue from taxation of tobacco products, (2) an easy way to generate foreign exchange necessary to buy commodities from abroad and to improve their balance of trade, and (3) a significant source of rural employment and wage production.[269]

China is a good example of the size and scope of the smoking problem because it is the largest producer and consumer of cigarettes in the world.[270] An estimated 300 million Chinese smoke, and one expert predicts that of all children less than 20 years of age in China today, 50 million will eventually die of diseases related to smoking.[271]

Economic data from tobacco-producing developing countries generally bear out the perceived value of this industry. For example, in 1980 the Nigerian Tobacco Company had gross revenues of $143 million, of which $51.5 million went to the government in the form of excise tax import duties and company taxes (compared with $25 million in 1965).[272] In India, tobacco accounted for approximately $1 billion in excise taxes and another $300 million in foreign exchange in 1981.[273] In Malaysia, of the nearly $460 million generated by cigarette sales, $120 million was retained by the government in various forms of taxes.[274] The short-run economic advantages of tobacco growth and consumption come at a high real cost. Most obvious are the direct, well-documented health problems associated with cigarette smoking. Moreover, other indirect effects of tobacco production include destruction of agricultural lands and forests and improper use of insecticides by rural farmers.

According to United Nations sources, the deforestation problem in many developing countries may soon become a "poor man's energy crisis."[275] This problem is traceable in large part to the need for wood to fuel fires that flue-cure many varieties of tobacco at high temperatures for about a week. Tobacco farmers in Third World countries, most of whom are dependent on wood as their sole source of energy, use approximately 2 hectares of trees for each ton of tobacco cured, equivalent to 2 trees for every 300 cigarettes, or 15 packs of cigarettes, produced.[276] A direct result of deforestation is soil erosion, which in hilly rural areas may lead to silt-filled rivers and dams during the rainy season and denuded croplands during growing seasons. In addition, because tobacco grows well in sandy soils and many developing countries are located in semiarid lands bordering deserts, tobacco is often grown on agricultural fringe land bordering deserts. As trees in nearby forests are cut down to provide fuel for the curing process, desertification is accelerated and farmers are forced to move into other, less arid regions, where cultivation of tobacco displaces staple food crops, leading to lost food production.[275]

Further, the lack of adequate education among rural area tobacco farmers regarding proper use of modern insecticides often leads to indiscriminate dispersal of the products in lakes and rivers. The resultant pollution endangers water sources of rural villagers and surrounding wildlife. Failure to use gloves and protective garments designed to limit exposure to toxic chemicals in insecticides also places rural tobacco farmers at an increased long-term risk of occupationally related diseases such as skin, lung, and bladder cancer.[276]

The major health consequences associated with smoking (e.g., cancer, heart disease, emphysema, COPD), which are well established in developed countries, are becoming increasingly prevalent in the developing world. For example, in China, the incidence of lung cancer increased more than sixfold during the period from 1970 to 1980, the delayed consequence of previous large cigarette consumption.[277] Similar disease patterns are appearing in Nigeria, with great increases in lung cancer and emphysema, which were rare 20 to 30 years before.[272] In India and Malaysia, a much higher incidence of smoking-related disease is being observed.[273,274]

In spite of increasing mortality from tobacco-related disease, the prevalence of smoking in the Third World is rising and major governmental efforts to control smoking and educate people about its health effects are rare. Although several developing countries have followed the examples of smoking-control legislation initiated in various industrialized countries, the majority of Third World governments ignore or give very limited acknowledgment to smoking and health issues while continuing to support tobacco production and to count on tobacco tax revenues.

There are disturbing parallels between the advertising and promotion techniques used to sell cigarette smoking in the United States and other developed countries in the late 1910s and throughout the 1920s and the efforts in the 1980s to promote smoking as a pleasurable status symbol in Third World countries. There is also a tragic difference. In the 1920s, neither producer, consumer, nor government knew of the direct adverse health effects of tobacco. Today, the scientific evidence is incontrovertible, and yet the developed countries, through their silence, trade, and foreign policies, implicitly encourage the growth of the tobacco industry in these countries. A legitimate question for all health professionals and public health leaders, particularly in developed countries, is whether we have an obligation to be active in warning developing countries about the high human cost of tacitly or explicitly encouraging smoking and tobacco cultivation. Among the recommendations for smoking control that developed countries could offer on the basis of our experience are the following:

1. Prohibit or severely limit advertisements of tobacco products.
2. Discourage, through economic means, adoption of cultivation of tobacco in lieu of staple crops.
3. Impose a heavy tax on all tobacco products.
4. Place warning labels on cigarette packets that are meaningful to the user population and rotate these messages frequently.
5. Use antitobacco advertising, particularly targeted at youth, to associate nonuse with high status, intelligence, popularity with peers, and other social attributes valued in that culture.
6. Restrict smoking in all public and private facilities where the public is aggregated (e.g., restaurants, movie houses, sport matches).
7. Develop explicit objectives for smoking control and a system of tracking progress toward meeting these objectives.

Powerful economic forces will continue to militate against a smoking control policy in developing countries. Only a concerted effort, including attaching conditions to economic aid by countries that are major contributors to the World Health Organization (WHO), the International Monetary Fund, the Food and Agriculture Organization (FAO), and the World Bank, is likely to be effective in helping Third World nations assign a high priority to smoking prevention and reduction.

CHALLENGES IN SMOKING CONTROL

Lessons from the considerable progress achieved in smoking control during the past 25 years can serve to confront remaining challenges successfully. Despite considerable progress, smoking remains the largest cause of preventable death in the United States and most of the industrialized world.

The growth of new knowledge about adverse health effects of smoking has been substantial. Public education campaigns have helped to translate scientific knowledge into improved public awareness of some smoking-caused problems, such as lung cancer, COPD, and cardiovascular disease, but awareness of other smoking-caused cancers and in utero effects is still limited. Passive smoking is increasingly appreciated as a health problem. From 1974 to 1989 the percentage of U.S. adults who believed that smoking is hazardous to nonsmokers' health increased from 46% to 81%.[1]

Public information efforts in support of smoking control have also benefited from the insatiable public desire for health information, which is reflected in a logarithmic growth in television health programming, routine coverage of health issues as part of broadcast news, and expanded health coverage and columns in newspapers and general interest magazines.

As public awareness of smoking-related diseases has given way to smokers' concerns that their habit is likely to adversely affect their health, more and more smokers have tried to quit, many successfully. Market responses to consumer concerns have included the filter cigarette, substantial reductions in average tar and nicotine content, and advertising copy implying that reductions in their components would decrease the health risk of cigarettes.

Overall, smokers in the United States are becoming socially isolated, especially in higher-income and well-educated groups, and sensitive to the concerns of the nonsmokers with whom they interact. Tobacco companies continue to spend large amounts of money to advertise and promote cigarettes, $931 million and $1450 million, respectively, in 1986.[278,279] Although the effects of these activities on overall cigarette consumption are difficult to assess, they are likely to make continuing smokers more comfortable with their addiction and less motivated to attempt cessation, while increasing recidivism by providing omnipresent clues that smoking is fun and relaxing and contributes to conviviality.

The inverse correlation between the percentage of health articles discussing smoking and cigarette advertising revenues as a percentage of total advertising revenue[280,281] suggests that the presence of cigarette advertising affects editorial decisions. As of 1990, one of the three major broadcasters, Columbia Broadcasting System, was controlled by the owners of a large tobacco company.

Limited experience with cigarette counteradvertising in broadcast media in the late 1960s strongly suggests that it can depress consumption, even in the presence of severalfold greater brand-specific pro-cigarette advertising. It is probable that reinitiation of counteradvertising through the mass media would significantly reduce per capita consumption of cigarettes. The impact of a broad-based ban on smoking advertising is more difficult to predict, but lack of reinforcement for smoking could lead to increased cessation attempts and higher long-term cessation rates.

From 1970 to 1986 the percentage of cigarette advertising and expenditures allocated to promotion increased from 12.8% to 60.9%.[280-282] Many of the promotional dollars sponsor sports events, such as skiing and tennis, that are associated with being healthy, being fit, and being outdoors. The subliminal message is that smoking contributes to health and fitness. Other tobacco company promotional money goes to blockbuster exhibitions at leading art museums, promoting the association of smoking with culture, sophistication, and artistic achievement. Perhaps sports figures asked to participate in events sponsored by cigarette companies could band together and decline these invitations. Alternatively, sports and entertainment stars might be willing to participate in counteradvertising, decrying the use of cigarette promotion money to create incorrect associations about the social and health aspects of smoking and emphasizing their own nonsmoking status.

Of all targets of opportunity, continuing the process of changing in social norms offers the greatest promise. Already, nonsmoking is an accepted norm in many socially defined groups in the United States. Rapid growth of community, state, and federal legislation and administrative actions limiting or banning smoking in places of public assembly, coupled with growing and increasingly stringent public and private employer restrictions on workplace smoking, should further limit smoking opportunities and increase the benefits of cessation to the individual. Public health agencies and preventive medicine practitioners can help accelerate social pressure not to smoke by supporting enactment of strict clean indoor air legislation and particularly enforcement, which is often lax.

Economic incentives can significantly affect cigarette consumption. Lower-income Americans, overrepresented among current smokers, may be especially sensitive to price increases in tobacco products. Although the addiction to nicotine may blunt the price elasticity of demand compared with other consumer products, data from the United States and other countries demonstrate that consumption decreases with escalating real prices. The recent enactment of an increase of 25 cents a pack in cigarette taxes in California will provide an excellent opportunity to better understand the price elasticity of different sociodemographic groups. The success of the California initiative process against the tobacco lobby could embolden other states to consider similar actions.

As the 80% of current smokers who want to quit attempt cessation, both public and private health organizations should be prepared to assist them. Referral to programs prescreened for their effectiveness should be encouraged. Physicians and other health care professionals should invariably take a smoking history and provide counseling on the benefits of quitting and encourage patients to continue to try regardless of failed past efforts. A smoking cessation prescription should be provided, perhaps including nicotine gum. Health professionals should provide positive reinforcement of the individual's ability to quit and encouragement to associate with nonsmokers.

Psychosocial prevention programs have demonstrated the ability to delay age-specific smoking initiation in students in grades 6 to 10. These curricula deserve broad dissemination and modification to target the highest-risk groups, including students from the lower socioeconomic backgrounds and those most likely to drop out of school. However, the impact of these curricula is likely to be limited unless they are coupled with mass media efforts that make smoking appear unattractive, socially unpopular, and sexually unappealing. Since tobacco use appears to be a common entry point for risk of other drug use, communications should stress that tobacco is a very addictive drug and can lead to use of drugs with even more immediate serious health risks.

America is groping for its role in dealing with international health threats to which it is a major contributor, such as global warming and acid rain. Exportation of tobacco and the role that American-based tobacco companies play in promoting use of their tobacco products in Third World countries, almost all having a real increase in per capita cigarette consumption, deserve to be viewed as exportation of a serious health threat to the citizens of countries we claim to want to help. As consumption declines in the United States, it is appropriate that the same government that is giving financial aid and excess foodstuffs to developing countries consider the appropriateness of permitting exportation of a substance that is addictive and that will become an even more important cause of preventable death as average longevity increases.

REFERENCES

1. Reducing the Health Consequences of Smoking: 25 Years of Progress. A Report of the Surgeon General. Washington, D.C.: U.S. Department of Health and Human Services, Public Health Service, Centers for Disease Control, Center for Chronic Disease Prevention and Health Promotion, Office on Smoking and Health, DHHS Publication No. (CDC) 89-8411, 1989
2. The Health Consequences of Smoking: Cardiovascular Disease. A Report of the Surgeon General. Washington, D.C.: U.S. Department of Health and Human Services, Public Health Service, Office on Smoking and Health, DHHS Publication No. (PHS) 84-50204, 1983
3. The Health Consequences of Smoking: Cancer. A Report of the Surgeon General. Washington, D.C.: U.S. Department of Health and Human Services, Public Health Service, Office on Smoking and Health, DHHS Publication No. (PHS) 82-50179, 1982
4. The Health Consequences of Smoking: Chronic Obstructive Lung Disease. A Report of the Surgeon General. Washington, D.C.: U.S. Department of Health and Human Services, Public Health Service, Office on Smoking and Health, DHHS Publication No. (PHS) 84-50205, 1984
5. Advance report of final mortality statistics, 1987. Monthly Vital Statistics Report 38(5,suppl), 1989. Washington, D.C.: U.S. Department of Health and Human Services, Public Health Service, Centers for Disease Control, National Center for Health Statistics
6. Smoking and Health: A Report of the Surgeon General. Washington, D.C.: U.S. Department of Health, Education and Welfare, Public Health Service, Office of the Assistant Secretary for Health, Office on Smoking and Health, DHEW Publication No. (PHS) 79-50066, 1979
7. Miller GH, Gerstein DR: The life expectancy of non-smoking males and females. Public Health Rep 98:343–349, 1983
8. Smoking and Health: A National Status Report, 2 edt. A Report to Congress. Washington, D.C.: U.S. Department of Health and Human Services, Public Health Service, Centers for Disease Control, Center for Chronic Disease Prevention and Health Promotion, Office of Smoking and Health, DHHS Publication No. (CDC) 87-8396 (revised 02/90), 1987
9. Warner KE: The economics of smoking: Dollars and sense. NY State J Med 83:1273–1274, 1983
10. National Fire Data Center, U.S. Fire Administration: Unpublished data, 1990

11. Fire and Aviation Management, U.S. Department of Agriculture Forest Service: Unpublished data, 1990
12. Pooling Project Research Group: Relationship of blood pressure, serum cholesterol, smoking habit, relative weight, and ECG abnormalities to incidence of major coronary events: Final report of the Pooling Project. J Chronic Dis 31:201–306, 1978
13. Rosenberg L, Miller DR, Kaufman DW, et al: Myocardial infarction in women under 50 years of age. JAMA 250:2801–2806, 1983
14. Willett WC, Green A, Stampfer MJ, et al: Relative and absolute excess risks of coronary heart disease among women who smoke cigarettes. N Engl J Med 317:1303–1309, 1987
15. Kannel WB, Thomas HE Jr: Sudden coronary death: The Framingham Study. Ann NY Acad Sci 382:3–21, 1982
16. Kuller L, Cooper M, Perper J: Epidemiology of sudden death. Arch Intern Med 129:714–719, 1972
17. Dawber TR: The Framingham Study: The Epidemiology of Atherosclerotic Disease. Cambridge, Massachusetts: Harvard University Press, 1980
18. Anderson EW, Andelman RJ, Strauch JM, et al: Effect of low-level carbon monoxide exposure on onset and duration of angina pectoris. Ann Intern Med 79:46–50, 1973
19. Wald N, Idle M, Smith PG, Bailey A: Carboxyhaemoglobin levels in smokers of filter and plain cigarettes. Lancet 2(8003):110–112, 1977
20. Shapiro S, Rosenberg L, Slone D, et al: Oral contraceptive use in relation to myocardial infarction. Lancet 1(8119):743–747, 1979
21. Suarez L, Barrett-Connor E: Interaction between cigarette smoking and diabetes mellitus in the prediction of death attributed to cardiovascular disease. Am J Epidemiol 120:670–675, 1984
22. Williams RR, Hasstedt SJ, Wilson DE, et al: Evidence that the men with familial hypercholesterolemia can avoid early coronary death: An analysis of 77 gene carriers in four Utah pedigrees. JAMA 255:219–224, 1986
23. Miettinen TA, Gylling H: Mortality and cholesterol metabolism in familial hypercholesterolemia: Long-term follow-up of 96 patients. Arteriosclerosis 8:163–167, 1988
24. Castleden CM, Cole PV: Inhalation of tobacco smoke by pipe and cigar smokers. Lancet 2(819):21–23, 1973
25. The Health Consequences of Smoking for Women. A Report of the Surgeon General. Washington, D.C.: U.S. Department of Health and Human Services, Public Health Service, Office of the Assistant Secretary for Health, Office on Smoking and Health, 1980
26. Kannel WB, Shurtloff D: The Framingham Study: Cigarettes and the development of intermittent claudication. Geriatrics 28:61–68, 1972
27. Criqui MH, Fronek A, Klauber MR, et al: Peripheral arterial disease in large vessels is epidemiologically distinct from small vessel disease [Abstract]. CVD Epidemiology Newsletter 37:67, 1985
28. Lithner F: Is tobacco of importance for the development and progression of diabetic vascular complications? Acta Med Scand 687(suppl):33–36, 1983
29. Tomatis LA, Fierens EE, Verbrugge GP: Evaluation of surgical risk in peripheral vascular disease by coronary arteriography. Surgery 71:429–435, 1972
30. Weinroth LA, Hertzstein J: Relation of tobacco smoking to arteriosclerosis obliterans in diabetes mellitus. JAMA 131:205–209, 1946
31. Weiss NS: Cigarette smoking and arteriosclerosis obliterans: An epidemiologic approach. Am J Epidemiol 95:17–25, 1972
32. Wolf PA, D'Agostino RB, Kannel WB, et al: Cigarette smoking as a risk factor for stroke: The Framingham Study. JAMA 259:1025–1029, 1988
33. Colditz GA, Bonita R, Stampfer MJ, et al: Cigarette smoking and risk of stroke in middle-aged women. N Engl J Med 318:937–941, 1988
34. Abbott RD, Yin Y, Reed DM, Yano K: Risk of stroke in male cigarette smokers. N Engl J Med 315:717–720, 1986
35. Petitti DB, Wingerd J: Use of oral contraceptives, cigarette smoking, and risk of subarachnoid hemorrhage. Lancet 2(8083):234–236, 1978
36. Stadel BV: Oral contraceptives and cardiovascular disease. Part 2. N Engl J Med 305:672–677, 1981
37. Rogers RL, Meyer JS, Shaw TG, et al: Cigarette smoking decreases cerebral blood flow suggesting increased risk for stroke. JAMA 250:2794–2800, 1983
38. Klein LW, Gorlin R: The systemic and coronary hemodynamic response to cigarette smoking. NY State J Med 83:1264–1265, 1983
39. Cryer P, Haymond M, Santiago J, Shah S: Norepinephrine and epinephrine release and adrenergic mediation of smoking-associated hemodynamic and metabolic events. N Engl J Med 295:573–577, 1976
40. Aronow WS, Rokow SN: Carboxyhemoglobin caused by smoking nonnicotine cigarettes: Effects in angina pectoris. Circulation 44:782–788, 1971
41. Kien GA, Sherrod T: Action of nicotine and smoking on coronary circulation and myocardial oxygen utilization. Ann NY Acad Sci 90:161–173, 1960
42. Fitzgerald GA, Oates JA, Nowak J: Cigarette smoking and hemostatic function. Am Heart J 115:267–271, 1988
43. Weitz JI, Crowley KA, Landman SL, et al: Increased neutrophil elastase activity in cigarette smokers. Ann Intern Med 107:680–682, 1987
44. Nowak J, Murray JJ, Oates JA, Fitzgerald GA: Biochemical evidence of a chronic abnormality in platelet and vascular function in healthy individuals who smoke cigarettes. Circulation 76:6–14, 1987
45. Cancer Facts and Figures—1989. New York: American Cancer Society, 1989
46. Jett JR, Cortese DA, Fontana RS: Lung cancer: Current concepts and prospects. Cancer 33:74–86, 1983
47. Cancer Facts and Figures—1988. New York: American Cancer Society, 1988
48. Doll R, Hill AB: Lung cancer and other causes of death in relation to smoking: A second report on the mortality of British doctors. Br Med J 2:1071–1081, 1956
49. Wynder EL, Stellman SD: Impact of long-term filter cigarette usage on lung and larynx cancer risk: A case-control study. JNCI 62:471–477, 1979
50. Doll R, Peto R: Cigarette smoking and bronchial carcinoma: Dose and time relationships among regular smokers and lifelong nonsmokers. J Epidemiol Commun Health 32:303–313 1978
51. Hammond EC: Smoking in relation to the death rates of one million men and women. In: Haenszel W (ed): Epidemiological Approaches to the Study of Cancer and Other Chronic Diseases. National Cancer Institute Monograph No. 19. Washington, D.C.: U.S. Department of Health, Education, and Welfare, Public Health Service, 1966, pp 127–204
52. Lubin JH, Blot WJ, Berrino F, et al: Patterns of lung cancer risk according to type of cigarette smoked. Int J Cancer 33:569–576, 1984
53. Lubin JH, Blot WJ, Berrino F, et al: Modifying risk of developing lung cancer by changing habits of cigarette smoking. Br Med J 288:1953–1956, 1984
54. Wynder EL, Mushinski MH, Spivak JC: Tobacco and alcohol consumption in relation to the development of multiple primary cancers. Cancer 40:1872–1878, 1977
55. McLaughlin JK, Mandel JS, Blot WJ, et al: A population-based case-control study of renal cell carcinoma. JNCI 72:275–284, 1984
56. Zahm SH, Hartge P, Hoover R: The National Bladder Cancer Study: Employment in the chemical industry. JNCI 79:217–222, 1987
57. Gordis L, Gold EB: Epidemiology of pancreatic cancer. World J Surg 8:808–821, 1984
58. Winkelstein W Jr, Shillitoe EJ, Brand R, Johnson KK: Further comments on cancer of the uterine cervix, smoking, and herpesvirus infection. Am J Epidemiol 119:1–8, 1984
59. Baron JA, Byers T, Greenberg ER, et al: Cigarette smoking in

women with cancers of the breast and reproductive organs. JNCI 77:677–680, 1986
60. Brinton LA, Schairer C, Haenszel W, et al: Cigarette smoking and invasive cervical cancer. JAMA 255:3265–3269, 1986
61. Sasson IM, Haley NJ, Hoffmann D, et al: Cigarette smoking and neoplasia of the uterine cervix: Smoke constituents in cervical mucus. N Engl J Med 312:315–316, 1985
62. Holly EA, Petrakis NL, Friend NF, et al: Mutagenic mucus in the cervix of smokers. JNCI 76:983–986, 1986
63. Vital statistics of the United States, 1986, Vol. 11. Mortality, Part A. DHHS Publication No. (PHS) 88-1122. Hyattsville, Maryland: National Center for Health Statistics, U.S. Department of Health and Human Services, Public Health Service, 1988, p 105
64. Dean G, Lee PN, Todd GF, Wicker AJ: Report on a second retrospective mortality study in North-east England. Part I. Factors related to mortality from lung cancer, bronchitis, heart disease and stroke in Cleveland County, with a particular emphasis on the relative risks associated with smoking filter and plain cigarettes. Research Paper No. 14. London: Tobacco Research Council, 1977
65. Hirayama T: Smoking and cancer in Japan: A prospective study on cancer epidemiology based on census population in Japan: Results of 13 years follow-up. In Tominaga S, Aoki K (eds): The UICC Smoking Control Workshop. Japan: The University of Nagoya Press, 1981, pp 2–8
66. Beck GJ, Doyle CA, Schachter EN: Smoking and lung function. Am Rev Respir Dis 123:149–155, 1981
67. Niewoehner DE, Kleinerman J, Rice B: Pathologic changes in the peripheral airways of young cigarette smokers. N Engl J Med 291:755–758, 1974
68. Dockery DW, Speizer FE, Ferris BG Jr, et al: Cumulative and reversible effects of lifetime smoking on simple tests of lung function in adults. Am Rev Respir Dis 137:286–292, 1988
69. Buist AS, Burrows B, Eriksson S, et al: The natural history of air flow obstruction in PiZ emphysema. Am Rev Respir Dis 127:435–445, 1983
70. Janoff A, Raju L, Dearing R: Levels of elastase activity in bronchoalveolar lavage fluids of healthy smokers and nonsmokers. Am Rev Respir Dis 127:540–544, 1983
71. Gadek JE, Fells GA, Zimmerman RL, et al: The anti-elastases of the human alveolar structures: Implications for the protease-antiprotease theory of emphysema. J Clin Invest 68:889–898, 1981
72. Lonkey SA, McCurren J: Neutrophil enzymes in the lung: Regulation of neutrophil elastase. Am Rev Respir Dis 127:59, 1983
73. Janoff A, Carp H, Laurent P, Raju L: The role of oxidative processes in emphysema. Am Rev Respir Dis 127:531–538, 1983
74. Burrows B, Knudson RJ, Cline MG, Lebowitz MD: Quantitative relationships between cigarette smoking and ventilatory function. Am Rev Respir Dis 115:195–205, 1977
75. Rogot E, Murray JL: Smoking and causes of death among U.S. veterans: 16 years of observation. Public Health Rep 95:213, 1980
76. Dennish GW, Castell DO: Inhibitory effect of smoking on the lower esophageal sphincter. N Engl J Med 284:1136–1137, 1971
77. Kivilaakso E, Fromm D, Silen W: Effect of bile salts and related compounds on isolated esophageal mucosa. Surgery 87:280–285, 1980
78. Piper DW, Shinners J, Grieg M, Thomas J, Waller SL: Effect of ulcer healing on the prognosis of chronic gastric ulcer. Gut 19:419–424, 1978
79. Korman MG, Hansky J, Eaves ER, Schmidt FT: Influence of cigarette smoking on healing and relapse in duodenal ulcer disease. Gastroenterology 85:871–874, 1983
80. Sontag S, Graham DY, Belsito A, et al: Cimetidine, cigarette smoking, and recurrence of duodenal ulcer. N Engl J Med 311:689–693, 1984
81. Lane MR, Lee SP: Recurrence of duodenal ulcer after medical treatment. Lancet 1:1147–1149, 1988
82. Bastiaan RJ, Waite IM: Effects of tobacco smoking on plaque development and gingivitis. J Periodontol 49:48, 1978
83. Sheiham A: Periodontal disease and oral cleanliness in tobacco smokers. J Periodontol 42:259–263, 1971
84. Ismail AI, Burt BA, Eklund SA: Epidemiologic patterns of smoker and periodontal disease in the United States. J Am Dent Assoc 106:617–621, 1983
85. Christen AG, Swanson BZ, Glover ED, Henderson AH: Smokeless tobacco: The folklore and social history of snuffing, sneezing, dipping, and chewing. J Am Dent Assoc 105:821–829, 1982
86. Christen AG, Armstrong WR, McDaniel RK: Intraoral leukoplakia, abrasion, periodontal breakdown, and tooth loss in a snuff dipper. J Am Dent Assoc 98:584–586, 1979
87. NIH Consensus Development Panel: National Institutes of Health consensus statement: Health implications of smokeless tobacco use. Biomed Pharmacother 42:93–98, 1988
88. Greer RO, Poulson TS: Oral tissue alterations associated with the use of smokeless tobacco by teenagers. Oral Surg Oral Med Oral Pathol 56:275–284, 1983
89. Weiss ST: Passive smoking and lung cancer: What is the risk? Am Rev Respir Dis 133:1–3, 1986
90. The Health Consequences of Involuntary Smoking: A Report of the Surgeon General. Washington, D.C.: U.S. Department of Health and Human Services, Public Health Service, Centers for Disease Control, DHHS Publication No. (CDC) 87-8398, 1986
91. National Research Council, Committee on Passive Smoking: Environmental tobacco smoke: Measuring exposures and assessing health effects. Washington, D.C.: National Academy Press, 1986
92. Benowitz NL, Kuyt F, Jacob P III, Jones RT, Osman AL: Cotinine disposition and effects. Clin Pharmacol Ther 34:604–611, 1983
93. Coultas DB, Howard CA, Peake GT, Skipper BJ, Samet JM: Salivary cotinine levels and involuntary tobacco smoke exposure in children and adults in New Mexico. Am Rev Respir Dis, 136:305–309, 1987
94. Wald NJ, Boreham J, Bailey A, et al: Urinary cotinine as marker of breathing other people's tobacco smoke. Lancet 1:230–231, 1984
95. Wald N, Ritchie C: Validation of studies on lung cancer in nonsmokers married to smokers. Lancet 1:1067, 1984
96. Foliart D, Benowitz NL, Becker CE: Passive absorption of nicotine in airline flight attendants. N Engl J Med 308:1105, 1983
97. Matsukura S, Taminato T, Kitano N, et al: Effects of environmental tobacco smoke on urinary cotinine excretion in nonsmokers: Evidence for passive smoking. N Engl J Med 311:828–832, 1984
98. Jarvis MJ, Russell MAH, Feyerabend C, et al: Passive exposure to tobacco smoke: Saliva cotinine concentrations in a representative population sample of non-smoking schoolchildren. Br Med J 291:927–929, 1985
99. Greenberg RA, Haley NJ, Etzel RA, Loda FA: Measuring the exposure of infants to tobacco smoke: Nicotine and cotinine in urine and saliva. N Engl J Med 310:1075–1078, 1984
100. Hoffmann D, Haley NJ, Adams JD, Brunnemann KD: Tobacco sidestream smoke: Uptake by nonsmokers. Prev Med 13:608–617, 1984
101. Russell MA, Feyerabend C: Blood and urinary nicotine in nonsmokers. Lancet 1:179–181, 1976
102. Feyerabend C, Ings RM, Russell MA: Nicotine pharmacokinetics and its application to intake from smoking. Br J Clin Pharmacol 19:239–247, 1985
103. Feyerabend C, Higenbottam T, Russell MA: Nicotine concentrations in urine and saliva of smokers and non-smokers. Br Med J 284:1002–1004, 1982
104. Benowitz NL, Jacob P III: Daily intake of nicotine during cigarette smoking. Clin Pharmacol Ther 35:499–504, 1984
105. Russell MA, West RJ, Jarvis MJ: Intravenous nicotine stimulation of passive smoking to estimate dosage to exposed non-smokers. Br J Addict 80:201–206, 1985
106. Jarvis M, Tunstall-Pedoe H, Feyerabend C, Vesey C, Salloojee Y: Biochemical markers of smoke absorption and self-reported exposure to passive smoking. J Epidemiol Community Health 35:335–339, 1984

107. Harlap S, Davies AM: Infant admissions to hospital and maternal smoking. Lancet 1:529–532, 1974
108. Colley JR, Holland WW, Corkhill RT: Influence of passive smoking and parental phlegm on pneumonia and bronchitis in early childhood. Lancet 2:1031–1034, 1974
109. Leeder SR, Corkhill RT, Irwig LM, Holland WW, Colley JR: Influence of family factors on the incidence of lower respiratory illness during the first year of life. Br J Prev Soc Med 30:203–212, 1976
110. Leeder SR, Corkhill RT, Irwig LM, Holland WW: Influence of family factors on asthma and wheezing during the first five years of life. Br J Prev Soc Med 30:213–218, 1976
111. Fergusson DM, Horwood LJ, Shannon FT, Taylor B: Parental smoking and lower respiratory illness in the first three years of life. J Epidemiol Community Health 35:180–184, 1981
112. Fergusson DM, Horwood LJ: Parental smoking and respiratory illness during early childhood: A six-year longitudinal study. Pediatr Pulmonol 1:99–106, 1985
113. Rantakallio P: Relationship of maternal smoking to morbidity and mortality of the child up to the age of five. Acta Paediatr Scand 67:621–631, 1978
114. Schenker MB, Samet JM, Speizer FE: Risk factors for childhood respiratory disease: The effect of host factors and home environmental exposures. Am Rev Respir Dis 128:1038–1043, 1983
115. Ekwo EE, Weinberger MM, Lachenbruch PA, Huntley WH: Relationship of parental smoking and gas cooking to respiratory disease in children. Chest 84:662–668, 1983
116. Pedreira FA, Guandolo VL, Feroli EJ, Mella GW, Weiss LP: Involuntary smoking and incidence of respiratory illness during the first year of life. Pediatrics 75:594–597, 1985
117. Ware JH, Dockery DW, Spiro A III, Speizer FE, Ferris BG Jr: Passive smoking, gas cooking, and respiratory health of children living in six cities. Am Rev Respir Dis 129:366–374, 1984
118. Fleming DW, Cochi SL, Hightower AW, Broome CV: Childhood upper respiratory tract infections: To what degree is incidence affected by day-care attendance? Pediatrics 79:55–60, 1987
119. Evans D, Levison MJ, Feldman H, et al: The impact of passive smoking on emergency room visits of urban children with asthma. Am Rev Respir Dis 135:567–572, 1987
120. Said G, Zalokar J, Lellouch J, Patois E: Paternal smoking related to adenoidectomy and tonsillectomy in children. J Epidemiol Community Health 32:97–101, 1978
121. Black N: The aetiology of glue ear: A case-control study. Int J Pediatr Otorhinolaryngol 9:121–133, 1985
122. Stahlberg MR, Ruuskanen O, Virolainen E: Risk factors for recurrent otitis media. Pediatr Infect Dis 5:30–32, 1986
123. Pukander J, Luotonen J, Timonen M, Karma P: Risk factors affecting the occurrence of acute otitis media among 2-to 3-year old urban children. Acta Otolaryngol (Stockh) 100:260–265, 1985
124. Kraemer MJ, Richardson MA, Weiss NS, et al: Risk factors for persistent middle-ear effusions: Otitis media, catarrh, cigarette smoke exposure, and atopy. JAMA 249:1022–1025, 1983
125. Iversen M, Birch L, Lundqvist GR, Elbrond O: Middle ear effusion in children and the indoor environment: An epidemiological study. Arch Environ Health 40:74–79, 1985
126. Charlton A: Children's coughs related to parental smoking. Br Med J 288:1647–1649, 1984
127. Burchfiel CM, Higgins MW, Keller JB, et al: Passive smoking in childhood: Respiratory conditions and pulmonary function in Tecumseh, Michigan. Am Rev Respir Dis 133:966–973, 1986
128. Weiss ST, Tager I, Speizer FE, Rosner B: Persistent wheeze: Its relation to respiratory illness, cigarette smoking, and level of pulmonary function in a population sample of children. Am Rev Respir Dis 122:697–707, 1980
129. Lebowitz MD, Burrows B: Respiratory symptoms related to smoking habits of family adults. Chest 69:48–50, 1976
130. Bland M, Bewley BR, Polland V, Banks MH: Effects of children's and parents' smoking on respiratory symptoms. Arch Dis Child 53:100–105, 1978
131. Dodge R: The effects of indoor pollution on Arizona children. Arch Environ Health 37:151–155, 1982
132. Kasuga H, Hasebe A, Osaka F, Matsuki H: Respiratory symptoms in school children and the role of passive smoking. Tokai J Exp Clin Med 4:101–104, 1979
133. Chen Y, Li WX: The effect of passive smoking on children's pulmonary function in Shanghai. Am J Public Health 76:515–518, 1986
134. Hasselblad V, Humble CG, Graham MG, Anderson HS: Indoor environmental determinants of lung function in children. Am Rev Respir Dis 123:479–485, 1981
135. Spinaci S, Arossa W, Burgiani M, et al: The effects of air pollution on the respiratory health of children: A cross-sectional study. Pediatr Pulmonol 1:262–266, 1985
136. Tager IB, Weiss ST, Munoz A, Rosner B, Speizer FE: Longitudinal study of the effects of maternal smoking on pulmonary function in children. N Engl J Med 309:699–703, 1983
137. Ferris BG Jr, Ware JH, Berkey CS, et al: Effects of passive smoking on the health of children. Environ Health Perspect 62:289–295, 1985
138. Berkey CS, Ware JH, Dockery DW, Ferris BG, Speizer FE: Indoor air pollution and pulmonary function growth in preadolescent children. Am J Epidemiol 123:250–260, 1986
139. Lebowitz MD, Holberg CJ, Knudson RJ, Burrows B: Longitudinal study of pulmonary function development in childhood, adolescence, and early adulthood. Am Rev Respir Dis 136:69–75, 1987
140. Speer F: Tobacco and the nonsmoker: A study of subjective symptoms. Arch Environ Health 16:443–446, 1968
141. Report of Interagency Task Force on Environmental Cancer, Heart and Lung Disease. Bethesda, Md., 1985
142. Hirayama T: Non-smoking wives of heavy smokers have a higher risk of lung cancer: A study from Japan. Br Med J 282:183–185, 1981
143. Garfinkel L: Time trends in lung cancer mortality among nonsmokers and a note on passive smoking. JNCI 66:1061–1066, 1981
144. Gillis CR, Hole DJ, Hawthorne VM, Boyle P: The effect of environmental tobacco smoke in two urban communities in the west of Scotland. Eur J Respir Dis (Suppl) 133:121–126, 1984
145. Wald NJ, Nanchahal K, Thompson SG, Cuckle HS: Does breathing other people's tobacco smoke cause lung cancer? Br Med J 293:1217–1222, 1986
146. Fielding JE, Phenow KJ: Health effects of involuntary smoking. N Engl J Med 319:1452–1460, 1988
147. Schilling RS, Letai AD, Hui SL, et al: Lung function, respiratory disease, and smoking in families. Am J Epidemiol 106:274–283, 1977
148. Schenker MB, Samet JM, Speizer FE: Effect of cigarette tar content and smoking habits on respiratory symptoms in women. Am Rev Respir Dis 125:684–690, 1982
149. White JR, Froeb HF: Small-airways dysfunction in nonsmokers chronically exposed to tobacco smoke. N Engl J Med 302:720–723, 1980
150. Kauffmann F, Tessier JF, Oriol P: Adult passive smoking in the home environment: A risk factor for chronic airflow limitation. Am J Epidemiol 117:269–280, 1983
151. Brunekreff B, Fischer P, Remijn B, et al: Indoor air pollution and its effect on pulmonary function of adult non-smoking women. III. Passive smoking and pulmonary function. Int J Epidemiol 14:227–230, 1985
152. Svendsen K, Kuller LH, Martin MJ, Ockene JK: Effects of passive smoking in the Multiple Risk Factor Intervention Trial. Am J Epidemiol 126:783–795, 1987
153. Kauffmann F, Dockery DW, Speizer FE, Ferris BG Jr: Respiratory symptoms and lung function in women with passive and active smoking [Abstract]. Am Rev Respir Dis 133:A157, 1986
154. Comstock GW, Meyer MB, Helsing KJ, Tockman MS: Respiratory effects of household exposures to tobacco smoke and gas cooking. Am Rev Respir Dis 124:143–148, 1981

155. Kentner M, Triebig G, Weltle D: The influence of passive smoking on pulmonary function: A study of 1,351 office workers. Prev Med 13:656–669, 1984
156. Jones JR, Higgins IT, Higgins MW, Keller JB: Effects of cooking fuels on lung function in nonsmoking women. Arch Environ Health 38:219–222, 1983
157. Weiss ST, Tager IB, Schenker M, Speizer FE: The health effects of involuntary smoking. Am Rev Respir Dis 128:933–942, 1983
158. Dahms TE, Bolin JF, Slavin RG: Passive smoking: Effects on bronchial asthma. Chest 80:530–534, 1981
159. Shepard RJ, Collins R, Silverman F: "Passive" exposure of asthmatic subjects to cigarette smoke. Environ Res 20:392–402, 1979
160. Wiedemann HP, Mahler DA, Loke J, et al: Acute effects of passive smoking on lung function and airway reactivity in asthmatic subjects. Chest 89:180–185, 1986
161. Hirayama T: Passive smoking: A new target of epidemiology. Tokai J Exp Clin Med 10:287–293, 1985
162. Garland C, Barett-Connor E, Suarez L, Criqui MH, Wingard DL: Effects of passive smoking on ischemic heart disease mortality of nonsmokers: A prospective study. Am J Epidemiol 121:645–650, 1985
163. Helsing KJ, Sandler DP, Comstock GW, Chee E: Heart disease mortality in nonsmokers living with smokers. Am J Epidemiol 127:915–922, 1988
164. Comstock GW, Shah FK, Meyer MB, Abbey H: Low birth weight and neonatal mortality rate related to maternal smoking on socioeconomic status. Am J Obstet Gynecol 111:53–59, 1971
165. Meyer MB, Jonas BS, Tonascia JA: Perinatal events associated with maternal smoking during pregnancy. Am J Epidemiol 103:464–476, 1976
166. Davies DP, Gray OP, Ellwood PC, Abernethy M: Cigarette smoking in pregnancy: Associations with maternal weight gain and fetal growth. Lancet 1:385–387, 1976
167. Wingerd J, Christianson R, Lovitt WV, Schoden EJ: Placental ratio in white and black women: Relation to smoking and anemia. Am J Obstet Gynecol 124:671–675, 1976
168. Christianson RE: Gross differences observed in the placentas of smokers and nonsmokers. Am J Epidemiol 110:178–187, 1979
169. Naeye RL, Harkness WL, Utts J: Abruptio placentae and perinatal death: A prospective study. Am J Obstet Gynecol 128:740–746, 1977
170. Kleinman JC, Pierre MB Jr, Madans JH, Land JH, Schramm WF: The effects of maternal smoking on fetal and infant mortality. Am J Epidemiol 127:274–282, 1988
171. Stein Z, Kline J, Levin B, Susser M, Warburton D: Epidemiologic studies of environmental exposures in human reproduction. In: Berg GG, Maillie HD (eds): Measurement of Risks. New York: Plenum Press, 1981, pp 163–183
172. Rantakallio P, Koiranen M: Neurological handicaps among children whose mothers smoked during pregnancy. Prev Med 16:597–606, 1987
173. Naeye RL, Peters EC: Mental development of children whose mothers smoked during pregnancy. Obstet Gynecol 64:601–607, 1984
174. Dunn HG, McBurney AK, Ingram S, Hunter CM: Maternal cigarette smoking during pregnancy and the child's subsequent development. II. Neurological and intellectual maturation to the age of 6 1/2 years. Can J Public Health 68:43–50, 1977
175. Tobacco: Situation and Outlook Report. Washington, D.C.: U.S. Department of Agriculture, Commodity Economics Division, Economic Research Service, USDA Publication No. TS-204, Sept 1988
176. Tobacco use by adults—United States, 1987. MMWR 38:685–687, 1989
177. Fiore MC, Novotny TE, Pierce JP, et al: Trends in cigarette smoking in the United States: The changing influence of gender and race. JAMA 261:49–55, 1989
178. Pierce JP, Fiore MC, Novotny TE, Hatziandreu EJ, Davis RM: Trends in cigarette smoking in the United States: Educational differences are increasing. JAMA 261:56–60, 1989
179. Novotny TE, Warner KE, Kendrick JS, Remington PL: Smoking by blacks and whites: Socioeconomic and demographic differences. Am J Public Health 78:1187–1189, 1989
180. Johnston LD, O'Malley PM, Bachman JG: National Trends in Drug Use and Related Factors Among High School Students and Young Adults, 1975–1986. Washington, D.C.: U.S. Department of Health and Human Services, Public Health Service, Alcohol, Drug Abuse, and Mental Health Administration, National Institute on Drug Abuse, DHHS Publication No. (ADM) 87-1535, 1987
181. Results from the National Adolescent Student Health Survey. MMWR 38:147–150, 1989
182. The Health Consequences of Smoking: The Changing Cigarette. A Report of the Surgeon General. Washington, D.C.: U.S. Department of Health and Human Services, Public Health Service, Office of the Assistant Secretary for Health, Office on Smoking and Health, DHHS Publication No. 81-50156, 1981
183. Report of "Tar," Nicotine, and Carbon Monoxide of the Smoke of 207 Varieties of Domestic Cigarettes. Washington, D.C.: Federal Trade Commission, 1985
184. Rickert WS: "Less hazardous" cigarettes: Fact or fiction? NY State J Med 83:1269–1272, 1983
185. Cigarette Report: Low Tar in Command. Tobacco International, April 1, 1983, pp 68–69
186. Rickert WS, Robinson JC: Yields of selected toxic agents in the smoke of Canadian cigarettes, 1969 and 1978: A decade of change? Prev Med 10:353–363, 1981
187. Lee PM, Garfinkel L: Mortality and type of cigarette smoked. J Epidemiol Community Health 35:16–22, 1981
188. Hammond EC, Garfinkel L, Seidman H, Lee EA: Tar and nicotine content of cigarette smoke in relation to death rates. Environ Res 12:263–274, 1976
189. Castelli WP, Dawber TR, Feinlab M, et al: The filter cigarette and coronary heart disease: The Framingham Study. Lancet 2:109–113, 1981
190. Kaufman DW, Helmrich SP, Rosenberg L, et al: Nicotine and carbon monoxide content of cigarette smoke and the risk of myocardial infarction in young men. N Engl J Med 308:407–413, 1983
191. Benowitz NL, Jacob P III, Yu L, et al: Reduced tar, nicotine, and carbon monoxide exposure while smoking ultralow—but not low—yield cigarettes. JAMA 256:241–246, 1986
192. Ebert RV, McNabb ME, McCusker KT, Snow SL: Amount of nicotine and carbon monoxide inhaled by smokers of low-tar, low-nicotine cigarettes. JAMA 250:2840–2842, 1983
193. Benowitz NL, Hall SM, Herning RI, et al: Smokers of low-yield cigarettes do not consume less nicotine. N Engl J Med 309:139–142, 1983
194. Hoffman D, Adams JD, Haley NJ: Reported cigarette smoke values: A closer look. Am J Public Health 73:1050–1053, 1983
195. Herning RI, Jones RT, Benowitz NC, Mines AH: How a cigarette is smoked determines blood nicotine levels. Clin Pharmacol Ther 33:84–90, 1983
196. Sutton SR, Russell MAH, Iyer R, et al: Relationship between cigarette yields, puffing patterns and smoke intake: Evidence for tar compensation. Br Med J 285:600–603, 1982
197. Kozlowski LT, Frecker RC, Khouw V, Pope MA: The misuse of "less hazardous" cigarettes and detection: Hole-blocking of ventilated filters. Am J Public Health 70:1202–1203, 1980
198. Rouse BA: Epidemiology of smokeless tobacco use: A national study. NCI Monogr 8:29–33, 1989
199. The Health Consequences of Using Smokeless Tobacco: A Report of the Advisory Committee to the Surgeon General. Washington, D.C.: U.S. Department of Health and Human Services, Public Health Service, National Institutes of Health, DHHS Publication No. (NIH) 86-2874, 1986
200. Healthy People: The Surgeon General's Report on Health Promotion and Disease Prevention. Rockville, Maryland: U.S. Public Health Service, 1979
201. Schwartz JL: Myths and realities of smoking cessation. NY State J Med 83:1355–1357, 1983

202. Leventhal H, Cleary PD: The smoking problem: A review of the research and theory in behavioral risk modification. Psychol Bull 88:370–405, 1980
203. Schwartz JL: Review and Evaluation of Smoking Cessation Methods: United States and Canada, 1978–1985. Washington, D.C.: U.S. Department of Health and Human Services, Public Health Service, National Institutes of Health, NIH Publication No 87-2940, April 1987
204. The Health Consequences of Smoking: Nicotine Addiction. A Report of the Surgeon General, 1988. Washington, D.C.: U.S. Department of Health and Human Services, Public Health Service, Centers for Disease Control, Center for Health Promotion and Education, Office on Smoking and Health, DHHS Publication No. (CDC) 88-8406, 1988
205. Tonnesen P, Hansen M, Helsted J, et al: Effect of nicotine chewing gum in combination with group counseling on the cessation of smoking. N Engl J Med 318:15–18, 1988
206. Stachnik T, Stoffelmayr B: Worksite smoking cessation programs: A potential for national impact. Am J Public Health 73:1395–1396, 1983
207. Ockene JK, Hymowitz N, Sexton M, Brotke SK: Comparison of patterns of smoking behavior change among smokers in the Multiple Risk Factor Intervention Trial (MRFIT). Prev Med 11:621–638, 1982
208. Garfinkle L, Stellman SD: Cigarette smoking among physicians, dentists, and nurses. CA 36:2–8, 1986
209. Harvey L, Shubat S: Physician Opinion on Health Care Issues, 1987 [Unpublished data]. Chicago: American Medical Association, 1987
210. Wechsler H, Levine S, Idelson RK, et al: The physician's role in health promotion: A survey of primary-care practitioners. N Engl J Med 308:97–100, 1983
211. U.S. Preventive Services Task Force: Counseling to prevent tobacco use. In Guide to Clinical Preventive Services. Baltimore: Williams & Wilkins, 1989
212. Farquhar JW, Wood PD, Breitrose H, et al: Community education for cardiovascular health. Lancet 1(8023):1192–1195, 1977
213. Meyer AJ, Nash JD, McAlister AL, et al: Skills training in a cardiovascular health education campaign. J Consult Clin Psychol 48:129–142, 1980
214. Egger G, Fitzgerald W, Frape G, et al: Result of a large-scale media antismoking campaign in Australia: North Coast "Quit for Life" Programme. Br Med J 286:1125–1128, 1983
215. Where There's Smoke: Problems and Policies Concerning Smoking in the Workplace, 2 edt. Washington, D.C.: Bureau of National Affairs, 1987
216. State Legislated Actions on Clean Air, Cigarette Excise Tax, and Sale of Cigarettes to Minors. Washington, D.C.: Tobacco-Free Young America Project, Oct 1987
217. State Regulations Limiting Smoking on School Property. Washington, D.C.: Tobacco-Free America Project, June 1988
218. State Legislated Actions on Tobacco Issues. Washington, D.C.: Tobacco-Free America Project, Oct 1988
219. Matrix of Local Smoking Ordinances. Berkeley, California: Americans for Nonsmokers' Rights, Aug 1988
220. The Health Consequences of Involuntary Smoking: A Report of the Surgeon General. Washington, D.C.: U.S. Department of Health and Human Services, Public Health Service, Centers for Disease Control, DHHS Publication No. (CDC) 87-8398, 1986
221. "Non-smoking, please": A money-saving proposition [News Features]. NY State J Med 83:1361–1363, 1983
222. Warner KE, Murt HA: Economic incentives for health. Ann Rev Public Health 5:107–133, 1984
223. National Association of Insurance Commissioners: Life and Health Actuarial (Ex5) Task Force results of field test of the Smoker/Nonsmoker Experience Exhibit. NAIC Proceedings 1987 2:687–705, 1987
224. Warner KE: Cigarette smoking in the 1970s: The impact of the antismoking campaign on consumption. Science 211:729–731, 1981
225. Warner KE, Murt HA: Premature deaths avoided by the antismoking campaign. Am J Public Health 73:572–577, 1983
226. Statistical Abstract of the United States 1988. Washington, D.C.: U.S. Bureau of the Census, U.S. Department of Commerce, 1988
227. Tobacco Institute: Monthly state cigarette tax report. Cigarette Tax Data, June 1988
228. Lewit EM, Coate D: The potential for using excise taxes to reduce smoking. J Health Economics 1:121–145, 1982
229. Lewit EM, Coate D, Grossman M: The effects of government regulation on teenage smoking. J Law Econ 24:545–569, 1981
230. Lewit EM: Regulatory and legislative initiatives. In: Proceedings of the Pennsylvania Consensus Conference on Tobacco and Health Priorities. Pennsylvania Cancer Plan, Pennsylvania Department of Health, Pennsylvania Interagency Council on Tobacco and Health, Statewide Health Coordinating Council, Oct 1985
231. Lewit EM: Unpublished data, 1987
232. Grossman M, Coate D, Lewit E, Shakotko RA: Economics and Other Factors in Youth Smoking. New York: National Bureau of Economic Research, Dec 1983
233. Ramirez A: Reynolds, after protests, cancels cigarette aimed at black smokers. The New York Times, Jan 20, 1990
234. Freedman AM, McCarthy MJ: New smoke from RJR under fire. The Wall Street Journal, Feb 20, 1990
235. Davis RM: Current trends in cigarette advertising and marketing. N Engl J Med 316:725–732, 1987
236. Flay BR, D'Avernas JR, Best JA, Kersell MW, Ryan KB: Cigarette smoking: Why young people do it and ways of preventing it. In: McGrath P, Firestone P (eds): Pediatric and Adolescent Behavioral Medicine, Vol. 10. New York: Springer Publishing, 1983, pp 132–183
237. McAlister AL, Percy C, MacCoby N: Adolescent smoking: Onset and prevention. Pediatrics 63:650–658, 1979
238. Flay BR, Ditecco D, Schlegal RP: Mass media in health promotion. Health Educ Q 7:127–143, 1980
239. Bandura A: Social Learning Theory. Englewood Cliffs, New Jersey: Prentice-Hall, 1977
240. Flay BR: Psychosocial approaches to smoking prevention: A review of findings. Health Psychol 4:449–488, 1985
241. Flay BR: What we know about the social influences approach to smoking prevention: Review and recommendations. In: Bell CS, Battjes R (eds): Prevention Research: Deterring Drug Abuse Among Children and Adolescents. NIDA Research Monograph 63. Washington, D.C.: U.S. Department of Health and Human Services, Public Health Service, Alcohol, Drug Abuse and Mental Health Administration, National Institute on Drug Abuse, DHHS Publication No. (ADM) 85-1334, 1985, pp 67–112
242. Botvin GJ, Wills TA: Personal and social skills training: Cognitive-behavior approaches to substance abuse prevention. In: Bell CS, Battjes R (eds): Prevention Research: Deterring Drug Abuse Among Children and Adolescents. NIDA Research Monograph 63. Washington, D.C.: U.S. Department of Health and Human Services, Public Health Service, Alcohol, Drug Abuse, and Mental Health Administration, National Institute on Drug Abuse, DHHS Publication No. (ADM) 85-1134, 1985, pp 8–49
243. Best JA, Thomson SJ, Santi SM, Smith EA, Brown KS: Preventing cigarette smoking among schoolchildren. Ann Rev Public Health 9:161–201, 1988
244. Biglan A, Ary DV: Methodological issues in research on smoking prevention. In: Bell CS, Battjes R (eds): Prevention Research: Deterring Drug Abuse Among Children and Adolescents. NIDA Research Monograph 63. Washington, D.C.: U.S. Department of Health and Human Services, Public Health Service, Alcohol, Drug Abuse, and Mental Health Administration, National Institute on Drug Abuse, DHHS Publication No. (ADM) 85-1134, 1985, pp 170–195
245. Flay BR: Mass media linkages with school-based programs for drug abuse prevention. J School Health 56:402–406, 1986
246. Warner KE: Smoking and health implications of a change in the federal cigarette excise tax. JAMA 225:1028–1032, 1986

247. School policies and programs on smoking and health—United States, 1988. MMWR 38:202–203, 1989
248. Brink SD: Health Risks and Behavior: The Impact on Medical Costs. Milwaukee: Milliman & Robertson, Inc., 1987
249. Shipley RH, Orleans CT, Wilbur CS, et al: Effect of the Johnson & Johnson Live for Life Program on employee smoking. Prev Med 17:25–34, 1988
250. Kristein MM: How much can business expect to profit from smoking cessation? Prev Med 12:358–381, 1983
251. Fielding JE: Effectiveness of employee health improvement programs. J Occup Med 24:907–916, 1982
252. Fielding JE, Piserchia PV: Frequency of worksite health promotion activities. Am J Public Health 79:16–20, 1989
253. Hallett R: Smoking intervention in the workplace: Review and recommendations. Prev Med 15:213–231, 1986
254. Klesges RC, Glasgow RE: Smoking modification in the worksite. In: Cataldo MF, Coates TJ (eds): Health and Industry: A Behavioral Medicine Perspective. New York: John Wiley & Sons, 1986
255. Walsh DC, McDougall V: Current policies regarding smoking in the workplace. Am J Indust Med 13:181–190, 1988
256. Fielding JE: Worksite health promotion survey: Smoking control activities. Prev Med 19:402–413, 1990
257. Holland RP: National Hospital Tobacco Smoking Policy Survey. Lancaster County: American Lung Association of Lancaster County and the Pennsylvania Academy of Family Physicians, 1988
258. Public Policy Opinion Poll: How Do Executives' Behavior and Views Match the Colleges' Public Statement. Chicago: American College of Healthcare Executives, Division of Research and Public Policy, Feb 1988
259. U.S. Department of Defense: Directive 1010.10 Health Promotion, March 1986
260. U.S. Department of Agriculture: Unpublished data, 1990
261. Tobacco Institute: Unpublished data, 1990
262. Tobacco Use in America Conference. Washington, D.C.: American Medical Association Public Affairs Group, 1989
263. Masironi R, Rothwell K: Tendance et effets du tabagisme dans le monde. World Health Statistics Quarterly 41:228–241, 1988
264. WHO Regional Committee for Europe: A Common Front Against AIDS and Tobacco. Press release, Sept 1987
265. Hauknes A, Bjartveit K: Norway: A pioneer effort to curb smoking [Letter to the Editor]. NY State J Med 83:1341–1342, 1983
266. Smoking control in Sweden. NY State J Med 85:404, 1985
267. Mackay J: Letter from Hong Kong: Battlefield for the tobacco war. JAMA 261:28–29, 1989
268. Smoking control strategies in developing countries. WHO Technical Report (series 695), 1983
269. Muller M: Preventing tomorrow's epidemic: The control of smoking and tobacco production in developing countries. NY State J Med 83:1304–1309, 1983
270. Tobacco: World Tobacco Situation, FT-11-86. Washington, D.C.: U.S. Department of Agriculture, 1986
271. Peto R: Future mortality from tobacco in China. Read before the Shanghai Symposium on Smoking and Health, Shanghai, China, November 14–16, 1987
272. Femi-Pearse D: Aspects of smoking in developing countries of Africa. NY State J Med 83:1312–1313, 1983
273. Nath UR: India's shame: A war on smallpox, but a welcome for cigarettes. NY State J Med 83:1320–1321, 1983
274. Teoth SK: Smoking in Malaysia: Promotion and control. NY State J Med 83:1317–1319, 1983
275. Whelam EM: A smoking gun: How the tobacco industry gets away with murder. Philadelphia: George F. Stickley Co., 1984, pp 166–176
276. Madeley J: The environmental impact of tobacco production in developing countries. NY State J Med 83:1310–1311, 1983
277. Sidel R, Sidel VW: The Health of China. Boston: Beacon Press, 1982
278. Warner KE: Selling Smoke: Cigarette Advertising and Public Health. Washington, D.C.: American Public Health Association, Oct 1986
279. Report to Congress Pursuant to the Federal Cigarette Labeling and Advertising Act. Washington, D.C.: Federal Trade Commission, May 1988
280. Dale KC: ACSH survey: Which magazines report the hazards of smoking? ACSH News and Views 3:1,8–10, 1982
281. White L, Whelan EM: How well do American magazines cover the health hazards of smoking? The 1986 survey. ACSH New and Views 7:1,7–11, 1986
282. Warner KE: Cigarette advertising and media coverage of smoking and health. N Engl J Med 312:384–388, 1985

43

Alcohol-related Health Problems

James G. Rankin
Mary Jane Ashley

The consumption of alcohol (ethyl alcohol, ethanol) is important to public health because it contributes to the etiology, course, and outcome of numerous acute and chronic physical, psychological, and behavioral problems[1] (Table 43–1). Although these alcohol-related problems are more frequent in people who are labeled "heavy drinkers," "alcohol abusers," "alcoholics," or "alcohol dependent," acute alcohol intoxication or relatively low levels of chronic alcohol consumption can produce serious adverse effects in individuals who otherwise fit within the social norms of alcohol use.[2,3] Furthermore, although heavy users of alcohol contribute disproportionately to the incidence of alcohol-related problems, the moderately drinking segment of the population, a much larger group, contributes the greater proportion of the problems.[4] Therefore, effective strategies to prevent alcohol-related problems must focus on drinkers generally and not just on the minority who use alcohol in large quantities.

GENERAL MECHANISMS OF ALCOHOL-RELATED DYSFUNCTION AND DAMAGE

A general schema of the mechanisms involved in alcohol-related tissue injury is provided in Figure 43–1. Tissue in this context refers to either a single type of cell or a single organ. Besides having direct toxic effects on target tissue, alcohol also may act indirectly through a variety of mechanisms. Other alcohol-associated behaviors involving tobacco, illicit drugs, and other drugs and chemicals, as well as non-alcohol-related disease processes, may contribute as cofactors to the development, course, and outcome of alcohol-induced primary damage. In addition, alcohol may act as a factor influencing the development, course, and outcome of coincidental diseases.

Much of the tissue damage that occurs in association with alcohol use has been attributed, at least in part, to direct toxic effects, for example, alcoholic hepatitis, cardiomyopathy, and neuronal degeneration. The effects on the nervous system are of greatest importance in the development of various alcohol-related problems associated with acute intoxication and withdrawal from alcohol, as well as alcohol dependence.[5,6] Acute effects are particularly important in circumstances under which drinkers may injure themselves or others.[7]

Alcohol also may act indirectly through the production of metabolic disturbances, endocrine changes,[8] impaired responses to infection,[9] aggravation of obstructive sleep apnea,[10] and displacement of dietary nutrients or impairment of their absorption or use,[11] as well as through the effects of diseases caused by alcohol.

Obstructive sleep apnea, a complication of alcohol use that occurs as a result of acute intoxication, is potentially important as a direct cause of morbidity and mortality.[10] It may contribute also to the course and outcome of other alcohol- as well as non-alcohol-related diseases. This disturbance and its precipitation and aggravation by alcohol have been recognized only recently.[12–15]

When an alcohol-related health problem does occur, its course and outcome may be influenced by whether or not the affected individual continues to be exposed to alcohol and alcohol-related hazards. Furthermore, course and outcome may be influenced by whether or not he or she seeks, has access to, receives, and adheres to effective treatment, not only for the complications of alcohol use but also for the drinking behavior itself.

A summary of the etiological significance of alcohol and associated variables that contribute to the excess mortality of heavy drinkers is provided in Table 43–2.

MORBIDITY AND MORTALITY

The important health problems related to alcohol use are alcohol dependence, injury, and debilitating or lethal diseases of the gastrointestinal, nervous, cardiovascular, and respiratory systems. Also important is a range of adverse pregnancy outcomes and fetal abnormalities caused by the embryotoxic and teratogenic effects of alcohol. The most common medical problems in alcohol-dependent and heavy drinking men, in terms of decreasing lifetime incidence, are trauma, acute alcoholic liver disease, peptic ulceration, chronic obstructive lung disease, pneumonia, hypertension, gastritis, epileptiform disorders, acute brain syndromes, peripheral neuritis, ischemic heart disease and cirrhosis[16] (Table 43–3). This pattern of lifetime morbidity contrasts greatly with the ranking in terms of excess mortality, namely, cardiovascular disease, suicide, accidents, cirrhosis, malignant neoplasms, pneumonia, and cerebrovascular disease.[17] These differences in patterns of morbidity and mortality are related to the lethality of the conditions, the risk of this population dying from these disorders compared with the community-at-large,[18] and the frequency of the conditions in the general adult population. The three most common causes of excess mortality, cardiovascular

TABLE 43-1. A SUMMARY OF ALCOHOL-RELATED PHYSICAL, PSYCHOLOGICAL, AND BEHAVIORAL PROBLEMS

- **Psychological and behavioral**
  Acute alcohol intoxication
  Acute alcohol poisoning
  Hangovers
  Blackouts
  Alcohol dependence
- **Acute alcohol withdrawal syndromes and alcoholic psychoses**
  Acute alcohol withdrawal syndrome
  Delirium tremens
  Acute auditory hallucinosis
  Depression
  Attempted suicide
  Suicide
- **Neurological**
  Subclinical neuropsychological impairment
  Epilepsy
  Peripheral neuropathy
  Cerebral atrophy
  Cerebellar atrophy
  Wernicke-Korsakoff syndrome
  Traumatic head injury
  Death from cerebrovascular disease
- **Gastrointestinal**
  Oropharyngeal carcinoma
  Acute esophageal dysfunction
  Mallory-Weiss syndrome
  Esophageal varices
  Esophageal carcinoma
  Erosive gastritis
  Acute gastroduodenal ulceration
  Atrophic gastritis
  Gastric carcinoma
  Disturbed small bowel motility
  Intestinal malabsorption
  Large bowel carcinoma
  Subclinical pancreatic dysfunction
  Chronic pancreatitis
  Pancreatic carcinoma
  Fatty liver
  Alcoholic hepatitis
  Cirrhosis
  Hepatocellular carcinoma
- **Cardiovascular**
  Cardiac arrhythmias
  Alcoholic cardiomyopathy
  Cardiac beriberi
  Hypertension
  Death from ischemic heart disease
- **Respiratory**
  Obstructive sleep apnea
  Chronic obstructive lung disease
  Pneumonia
  Lung abscess
  Pulmonary tuberculosis
  Laryngeal carcinoma
  Carcinoma of the lung
- **Endocrine–Metabolic**
  Hypoglycemia
  Hyperglycemia
  Diabetes
  Gout
  Lactic acidosis
  Derangements of mineral metabolism
- **Reproductive**
  Depressed testicular function
  Depressed ovarian function
  Carcinoma of the breast
- **Musculoskeletal**
  Acute and chronic myopathy
  Ischemic necrosis of the head of femur
  Osteoporosis
- **Hematological**
  Anemia
  Impaired leukocyte response to infection
  Thrombocytopenia
- **Traumatic injuries**
- **Ethanol–drug interactions**
- **Nutritional deficiencies**
- **Pregnancy outcome and developmental disorders**
  Spontaneous abortion
  Perinatal mortality
  Low birth weight
  Impaired development (physical, behavioral, intellectual)
  Congenital birth defects
  Fetal alcohol syndrome
  Pseudo-Cushing's syndrome in breast-fed infants
  Alcohol withdrawal in newborn

disease, suicide, and accidents, occur as *acute problems,* associated with sudden and usually unexpected death, whereas cirrhosis of the liver is the main *chronic* physical health *problem* in terms of incapacity and excess mortality.

HAZARDOUS DRINKING AND THE CONCEPT OF "SAFE" DRINKING

Hazardous Drinking

The term "hazardous drinking" has been used to describe levels of alcohol consumption that expose the drinker to a high risk of physical complications.[2] Under certain circumstances, relatively low levels of consumption on isolated occasions may result in damage to the individual drinker. There is evidence as well that levels of consumption far below those found in people diagnosed as alcohol-dependent are linked with increased risks of adverse health consequences.[4,19] A special case involves the survival and normal development of the fetus of the drinking pregnant woman.[20] In this instance, some authorities would assert that there is no safe level of consumption, or that it may be impossible to define such a level.[21] As information grows on how alcohol is hazardous to health, we find ourselves less secure in defining what is safe.[2,3] Rather, alcohol use involves a continuum of risk, defined by host and environmental factors as well as by the levels of alcohol consumption.

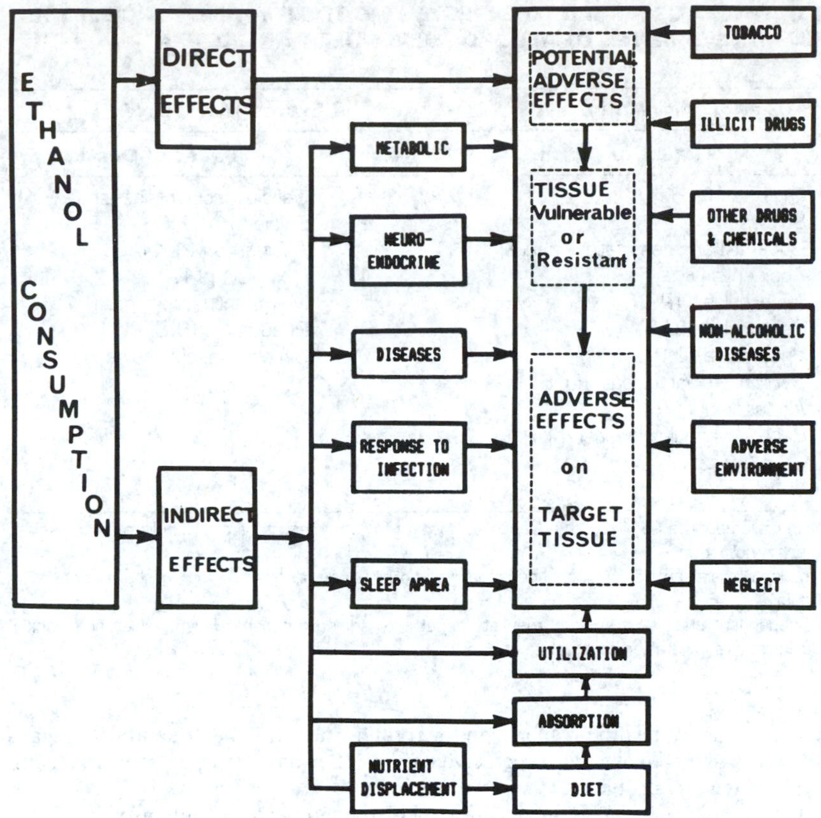

Figure 43–1. Schematic representation of the general mechanisms involved in the development of alcohol-related tissue injury.

"Safe" (Low-Risk) Drinking

Based on the concept of a continuum of risk, some organizations have proposed guidelines for "safe" (low-risk) drinking, which include both the characteristics and circumstances of the drinker as well as levels of consumption.[22–29]

One example of "safe" drinking guidelines is contained in the report of the Australian National Health and Medical Research Council (NHMRC), "Is there a safe level of daily consumption of alcohol for men and women? Recommendations regarding responsible drinking behavior," in which it is recommended that:

> responsible drinking be considered as the consumption of the least amount of alcohol that will meet an individual's personal and social needs and in any case:

TABLE 43-2. ETIOLOGICAL SIGNIFICANCE OF ALCOHOL AND ASSOCIATED VARIABLES IN THE EXCESS MORTALITY OF CHRONIC HEAVY DRINKERS

Cause of Death	Effects of Alcohol	Heavy Tobacco Smoking	Emotional Problems	Poor Food Habits	Other Personal Neglect	Increased Environmental Hazards
Tuberculosis		X		X	X	X
Carcinoma						
Mouth	XX	XX				
Larynx	XX	XX				
Pharynx	XX	XX				
Esophagus	XX	XX				
Liver	X					XX
Lung	X	XX				
Alcoholic cardiomyopathy	XX					
Other cardiovascular disease	XX	XX		X	X	
Pneumonia	XX	XX			XX	XX
Peptic ulcers	XX	X		X	X	
Liver cirrhosis						
Alcoholic	XX			X		
Nonalcoholic	X					XX
Suicide	XX		XX			
Accidents	XX	XX	X		X	X

X = probably indicated; XX = clearly indicated. Where a space is left blank, either the factor is probably of no significance or its role, if any, is unknown.
Modified from Popham et al, 1984.[18]

TABLE 43-3. RANKING OF LIFETIME INCIDENCE, RATIO OF OBSERVED TO EXPECTED MORTALITY, AND PERCENTAGE OF EXCESS MORTALITY FOR SELECTED CAUSES IN MALE SAMPLES OF ALCOHOL-DEPENDENT AND OTHER HAZARDOUS DRINKERS

Lifetime Incidence (%)[a]		Mortality Ratio[b]		Excess Mortality (%)[c]	
Rank	**Disease**	**Rank**	**Cause of Death**	**Rank**	**Cause of Death**
1	Trauma (81.9)[a]	1	Cirrhosis (7.6)[b]	1	Cardiovascular disease (21.4)[c]
2	Acute alcoholic liver disease (49.9)	2	Suicide (4.4)	2	Suicide (14.7)
3	Peptic ulcer (22.8)	3	Upper GI and respiratory cancer (4.1)	3	Accidents (11.1)
4	Obstructive lung disease (19.0)	4	Accidents (3.5)	4	Cirrhosis (11.0)
5	Pneumonia (16.8)	5	Tuberculosis (2.8)	5	Malignant neoplasms (11.8)
6	Hypertension (12.4)	6	Peptic ulcer (2.8)	6	Pneumonia (8.8)
7	Gastritis (11.5)	7	Pneumonia (2.3)	7	Cerebrovascular disease (5)
8	Epileptic disorders (10.9)	8	Cardiovascular disease (1.8)		
9	Acute brain syndromes (7.7)	9	All cancer (1.7)		
10	Peripheral neuritis (7.1)	10	Cerebrovascular disease (1.2)		
11	Ischemic heart disease (8.1)				
12	Cirrhosis (6.4)				

[a] Based on lifetime incidence of certain diseases and complications in male patients admitted to a Canadian hospital for the treatment of alcoholism. From Ashley et al.[16] The percentage, in brackets, is shown after each disease or complication.
[b] Based on analyses of ratios of observed to expected mortality by cause in male samples of alcohol-dependent and other heavy drinkers. From Popham et al.[18] The median mortality ratio, in brackets, is shown after each cause of death.
[c] Based on analyses of percentages of excess mortality in alcohol-dependent and heavy drinking men attributable to selected causes. From Ashley and Rankin, 1980.[17] The median percentage value for excess mortality, in brackets, is shown after each cause of death.

(a) that men should not exceed 4 units or 40 grams of absolute alcohol per day on a regular basis, or 28 units per week; that 4–6 units per day or 28–42 units per week be considered as hazardous and that greater than 6 units per day or 42 units per week be regarded as harmful;

(b) that women should not exceed 2 units or 20 grams of absolute alcohol per day on a regular basis, or 14 units per week; that 2–4 units per day or 14–28 units per week be considered as hazardous and that greater than 4 units per day or 28 units per week be regarded as harmful because of the biological differences between men and women;

(c) that abstinence be promoted as highly desirable during pregnancy;

(d) that persons who intend to drive, operate machinery or undertake activities in hazardous or potentially hazardous situations should not drink;

(e) that in any given situation it is difficult to say that there is an absolute safe level of consumption and thus in situations of any doubt people should not drink.[27]

In this report, a unit or standard drink was equivalent to 8 to 10 g of alcohol compared with Canada and the United States, where one unit or standard drink contains approximately 13.6 g of alcohol.

In essence, no level of alcohol consumption will always be safe for all individuals under all conditions. Rather, increasing levels of consumption hold a progressively increasing risk of causing either acute or chronic damage. Moreover, the level at which risk occurs and its significance are influenced by a combination of personal and environmental factors that render the individual more or less vulnerable to damage from alcohol.

ESTIMATING THE PUBLIC HEALTH IMPORTANCE OF ALCOHOL-RELATED PROBLEMS

In alcohol-consuming nations the public health importance of alcohol-related health problems usually is considered by each country to be significant.[30] There are differences, however, from country to country, concerning the impact of alcohol-related health problems on the total burden of ill health and with regard to what are perceived to be the major alcohol-related health problems.

The impact of alcohol-related health problems is felt, both directly and indirectly, by many different groups, those with alcohol-related health problems, their families, other individuals or groups who may suffer injury or loss due to the use of alcohol by others, those who provide services for the prevention and treatment of alcohol-related problems, and the community-at-large. Many of the effects are tangible but immeasurable, such as the pain and suffering experienced by the alcohol-damaged individual and his or her family. However, other manifestations of alcohol-related problems are suitable for empirical study, for example, the incidence and prevalence of alcohol-related health problems, the costs of health and social services attributable to these problems, the number of people who are disabled or die from alcohol-related problems, and the economic costs of illness, disability, and death.

Although it may be possible to make reasonably good estimates for specific aspects of mortality and morbidity, especially those components that are deemed to be directly related to alcohol, for example, the burden of alcoholic psychoses in specialized institutions, such directly related consequences are only a small part of the total problem. This is illustrated in a report on alcohol-related deaths in Canada in 1980 (Table 43–4). Of the almost 18,000 such deaths (10.5% of all deaths), the vast majority (88%) were classified as indirectly related; that is, they were due to accidents, cancers, and circulatory and respiratory diseases to which alcohol was a contributing factor.[31] This problem is further exemplified by U.S. studies in which only about 3% of recorded deaths were officially attributable to alcohol, 1.9% were attributable to an alcohol-related condition, and the remaining 1.2% had an alcohol-related condition listed along with the specified cause of death.[32] These figures compare with estimates that alcohol-dependence is responsible for 1 in 10 deaths in the United States.[33]

Despite such shortcomings in available statistics, there is no doubt about the serious toll of morbidity and mortality that alcohol use exacts from alcohol-consuming societies, such as the United States and Canada, countries ranking as moderate consuming nations. Selected indicators of the public health impact of alcohol use in Canada (Table 43–4)[31,34] illustrate this clearly.

TABLE 43-4. SELECTED INDICATORS OF THE PUBLIC HEALTH IMPACT OF ALCOHOL USE IN CANADA

Indicator	Year	Selected Findings		
Population 15 years and over drinking 14+ drinks per week[34]	1978–1979	Overall 12%	Males 19.4% Females 4.8%	
		Age group 20–24	Males 31.0% Females 8.1%	
Alcohol-dependent persons[31]	1980	600,000 persons; 1 in 19 [5.3% of] current drinkers		
Current drinkers 15 years and older with alcohol-associated problem[31]	1978–1979	Tension or disagreement with family or friends		6.1%
		Problems with health		2.3%
		Difficulty with driving		1.5%
		Injury to self or other		1.3%
		Trouble with the law		1.3%
		Trouble with school or work		1.2%
Current drinkers 15 years and over with at least one alcohol-associated problem[31]	1978–1979	Overall 9.7%	Males 12.4% Females 6.1%	
Alcohol-related deaths[31]	1980	17,974 [10.5%] of all deaths Directly related deaths: 2,110[a] Indirectly related deaths: 15,864[b]		

[a] Deaths due to alcohol-related cirrhosis, alcohol dependency syndrome, the nondependent abuse of alcohol, alcoholic psychoses, and accidental poisoning by alcohol.
[b] Deaths due to motor vehicle accidents, falls, fires, drownings, homicides, suicides [5554 in 1980], as well as circulatory and respiratory diseases and certain types of cancer [e.g., oral, esophageal, and laryngeal] totaling 10,310 in 1980.

In the period of these studies, 1979–1980, of Canadians 15 years and over, at least 12% regularly were consuming enough alcohol to be at increased risk of health consequences, 5% of current drinkers were alcohol-dependent, and almost 10% experienced at least one alcohol-related problem. More than 1 in 10 deaths were alcohol-related. In an earlier study of premature deaths and potential years of life lost in Canada in 1974, it was concluded that no other risk factor was responsible for more premature mortality than either smoking or hazardous drinking.[35] Although there is evidence that, since that period of study and in association with a plateauing and modest fall in alcohol consumption, there has been a significant decline in various indicators of alcohol-related health problems in Canada,[36,37] the adverse health consequences of drinking remain a major health problem. Furthermore, tobacco and alcohol continue to rate first and second as risk factors responsible for premature mortality.

One approach to quantifying the effects of alcohol-related health problems is to express them in monetary terms. Such an approach is useful because it provides an estimate of the relative distribution of the costs, for example, across organ systems or various health and social services, as well as a measure of total costs. Thus, these figures can be used to compare the costs of alcohol-related problems with other health problems as a basis for focusing the attention of the community or making policy decisions regarding the funding of prevention, treatment, and research.

An example of an economic approach to measuring the magnitude of alcohol-related problems is contained in Table 43–5, which provides an estimate of the costs of alcohol-related problems in the United States in 1983.[38,39] First, notice that the total cost is large, $116.875 billion. Of this amount, 89.0% was attributable to core costs, including losses in productivity associated with disability and death (76.2%) and costs incurred in the treatment and care of people with alcohol-related health problems (12.8%). Total alcohol-related health costs ranked a close second to heart and vascular disease, as the prime health cause of economic loss and were well ahead of cancer and respiratory disease. In this analysis, other related costs covered nonhealth alcohol-related costs attributable to motor vehicle crashes and fires, highway safety and the fire protection, and the criminal justice and social welfare systems. The costs of alcohol-related problems were equal to 3.54% of the gross national product, and the direct costs for health services were equal to 4.22% of the total costs of health services. Although these figures are large, very likely they are underestimates of the true economic costs of alcohol-related problems.

TRENDS IN ALCOHOL PRODUCTION AND CONSUMPTION

International and intranational variations in per capita consumption appear to be related to economic development, genetic influences, cultural heritage, traditions of temperance, and religious laws of abstinence. Among the eight geographic areas of the world, the highest median values of per capita consumption are found in Australasia (Australia and New Zealand), North America (Canada and the United States), and Europe,[40] the most economically developed regions. These regions share similar cultural heritages and have a long history of acceptance and use of alcohol. Much lower median values characterize the regions of Central and South America, the remainder of Oceania (excluding Australia and New Zealand), areas undergoing economic development, and Africa and Asia, where the effects of delayed economic development and traditions of temperance and prohibition are reflected. The last two regions have substantial numbers of countries in which the majority of the population is Moslem.[40,41] Islam has a strong prohibition on the use of alcohol.[42]

Since the end of World War II, there has been a general world trend of increased production and consumption of alcohol. Major absolute increases in per capita consumption were observed in Europe, North America, Australia, and New Zealand. The countries with the greatest increases were the German Democratic Republic (758%) and the Federal German Republic (272%) (Table 43–6).[43] The median percentage change for the 24 nations between 1950 and 1985 was an increase of between 70% and 82%. Italy had an increase of only 2%, and France had a fall of 23%. Most of the observed increases took place in the period 1950–1976, during which there were rises in all counties except France. During the period 1976–1980, the average annual increases were relatively minor and occurred in 14 countries, with no increase in 3 and small decreases in 7.[30,31] From 1980 and 1985, there were modest increases in 5 countries, no increases in 3, and declines in 16.

TABLE 43-5. ESTIMATED COSTS OF ALCOHOL-RELATED PROBLEMS IN THE UNITED STATES IN 1983

		$Billion	%
▪ **Core costs**			
Direct	Treatment	13.457	
	Health support services	1.549	
	Subtotal	15.006	12.8
Indirect	Mortality	18.151	
	Reduced productivity	65.582	
	Lost employment	5.323	
	Subtotal	89.056	76.2
Total core costs		104.062	89.0
▪ **Other related costs**			
Direct	Motor vehicle crashes	2.697	
	Crime	2.631	
	Social welfare administration	0.049	
	Other	3.673	
	Subtotal	9.050	7.8
Indirect	Victims of crime	0.194	
	Incarceration	2.979	
	Motor vehicle crashes	0.590	
	Subtotal	3,763	3.2
Total other related costs		12.813	11.0
▪ **Total costs**		116.875	100.0

Gross national product in 1983: $3305.0 billion; costs of alcohol-related problems: 3.54% of GNP.
Total costs of health services in 1983: $355.4 billion; cost of direct services for alcohol-related problems: 4.22% of total costs of health services.
Adapted from U.S. Department of Health and Human Services, 1987,[38] and Statistical Abstracts of the United States, 1985.[39]

Between 1960 and 1970, beer consumption rose on average 256% in Asia, 188% in Africa, 49% in North America, and between 30% and 72% in the rest of the world. During the same period, wine consumption increased 277% in the USSR, 139% in Asia, 133% in Oceania, 115% in Central America, and 74% in North America, and distilled spirits consumption rose 98% in Europe, 75% in Central America, 67% in Africa, 59% in South America, 51% in Asia, and 2% in North America. Overall, world consumption of alcoholic beverages increased 61% during this period. Between 1950 and 1980, the per capita consumption of alcohol increased 74% in the United States and 107% in Canada.[44]

Information on per capita consumption in 1978, 1980, and 1984 for the United States and for the 50 states and District of Columbia is provided in Table 43–7.[38,45] The highest per capita consumption, in liters of alcohol for the population aged 14 years and older, was in the District of Columbia (20.2), and the lowest was in Utah (5.8). The median value for all 51 regions was 10.0 liters. In general, the period 1978–1980 was one in which the progressive rise in alcohol consumption observed since 1935 peaked. There has been a constant downward trend since 1981. It has been noted that the decrease in the years 1981 through 1983 was the first time since Prohibition that consumption declined for 3 consecutive years.[38] This decline was observed in all states except Alaska, Delaware, Connecticut, Texas, and Virginia, where there were modest rises, and Kansas, where there was a plateauing. Two of the 25 regions above the median had areas that were legally dry compared with 13 of 25 regions below the median.

A number of explanations can be given for the plateauing and decline in consumption observed in recent years. These include changes in the characteristics of alcohol-consuming populations, responses to economic factors, and, finally, public-health oriented influences, including the possible impact of recent efforts by governments and other agencies to deal with alcohol problems and the growing awareness and concern among the general public about alcohol use and its associated problems.[46]

The decline in alcohol consumption in France was almost certainly, in part, due to national measures to reduce consumption because of concern about the health-related outcomes associated with the highest national per capita consumption.[47,48] However, the international trend that has been common to most, if not all, nations and that would seem the most logical explanation for the plateauing and decline of alcohol consumption internationally has been the economic recession in the 1970s[47] and ongoing financial circumstances that have either increased the relative prices of alcoholic beverages or decreased disposable incomes.

A FRAMEWORK FOR PREVENTION

Fundamental difficulties pervade attempts to prevent alcohol-related problems. These difficulties include the perceptions of those defining the problems, geographical and temporal variations in levels and patterns of consumption, the identification, range, and nature of the problems that occur in relation to consumption, and our understanding of the mechanisms that link these problems with alcohol consumption.

Basic to the definition and prevention of these problems are individual and group perceptions and experiences. Those whose objectives are concerned with promoting the production, distribution, and sales of alcoholic beverages naturally will view increases in these areas as desirable. On the other hand, those concerned with countering the adverse social, economic, and medical consequences usually consider increases in alcohol consumption as undesirable. A similar view would be held by others, who, for moral and religious reasons, define any use of alcohol as unacceptable.

The nature and scope of what is communicated to the com-

TABLE 43-6. PER CAPITA CONSUMPTION OF ALCOHOLIC BEVERAGES AS LITERS OF ABSOLUTE ETHANOL IN 24 COUNTRIES, TOTAL POPULATION, 1950, 1960, 1976, 1980, AND 1985, WITH TOTAL AND AVERAGE ANNUAL PERCENTAGE CHANGES

	Per Capita Consumption: Liters 100% Ethanol					% Change				
						Annual Average				Total
Country[a]	1950	1960	1976	1980	1985	1950–1960	1960–1976	1976–1980	1980–1985	1950–1985
1. France	17.2	17.3	16.5	14.8	13.3	+0.1	−0.3	−3	−2	−23
2. Portugal	—	10.9	14.1	11.0	13.1	—	+2	−5	+4	+20[b]
3. Spain	—	8.5	14.0	14.1	11.8	—	+4	0	−3	+38[b]
4. Italy	9.2	12.2	12.7	13.0	11.6	+3	+0.3	+0.6	−2	+2
5. Hungary	4.8	6.2	10.7	11.5	11.5	+3	+5	+3	0	+140
6. Switzerland	7.9	9.8	10.3	10.5	11.2	+2	+0.3	+0.4	+1	42
7. Federal German Republic	2.9	6.9	12.5	12.7	10.8	+14	+5	+0.4	−3	+272
8. Belgium	6.3	6.4	10.2	10.8	10.5	+2	+0.3	+0.4	−0.5	+67
9. German Democratic Republic	1.2	4.6	8.3	9.7	10.3	+28	+5	+4	+1	+758
10. Austria	5.0	8.7	11.2	11.0	9.9	+7	+2	−1	−2	+98
11. Denmark	3.6	4.2	9.2	9.2	9.9	+2	+7	0	+2	+175
12. Australia	6.1	6.5	9.6	9.8	9.4	+0.7	+3	+0.5	−0.8	+54
13. New Zealand	5.4	6.5	9.3	9.7	9.2	+2	+3	+1	−1	+70
14. Czechoslovakia	4.0	5.6	9.2	9.6	9.1	+4	+4	+1	−1	+128
15. Netherlands	2.1	2.6	8.3	8.8	8.5	+2	+14	+2	−0.7	+305
16. United States	5.0	4.8	8.1	8.7	8.0	−0.4	+4	+5	−2	+60
17. Canada	4.4	4.8	8.6	9.1	8.0	+0.9	+5	+1	−2	+82
18. Yugoslavia	—	4.7	8.9[c]	7.4	7.7	—	+6	−4	+0.8	+64[b]
19. United Kingdom	4.9	5.1	8.4	7.1	7.1	+0.4	+4	−4	0	+45
20. Poland	3.0	3.8	8.2	8.7	7.0	+3	+7	+2	−4	+133
21. Finland	1.7	1.8	6.4	6.4	6.5	−0.6	+16	0	+0.3	+282
22. Ireland	3.3	3.4	8.7	7.5	6.2	+0.3	+10	−3	−3	+88
23. Sweden	3.6	3.7	5.9	5.7	5.2	+0.3	+4	−0.8	−2	+44
24. Norway	2.2	2.5	4.3	4.6	4.2	+1	+5	+2	−2	+91

Percentage values of 1 or more are given to the nearest whole number and values of less than 1 to the nearest first decimal place.
[a] Ranked in order of 1985 consumption.
[b] 1960–1985.
[c] 1976.
From Moser, 1980,[30] for 1950–1976 statistics: Health and Welfare Canada, 1984,[31] for 1980 statistics; Produktschap voor Gedistilleerde Dranken, 1986,[44] for 1985 statistics.

munity-at-large and to those who set social and economic policies form the basis for attempts to resolve the problems that are so defined. The perception of this information by these groups, however, is predetermined, in part, by their own understanding of alcohol, its use, and its beneficial and adverse consequences.

Concepts, Theories, and Models of Alcohol Use and Alcohol-related Problems

Although it is clear that the pharmacological effects of alcohol, the personal characteristics of drinkers, and the environment within which drinking takes place all contribute to the development of drinking patterns and alcohol-related problems, no global model encompassing all of these influences has so far been developed and accepted. On the other hand, theories abound.[49]

Four main views on and of alcohol and alcohol-related problems underlie current community attitudes, beliefs, and approaches to prevention. These are moralistic and religious concepts, the disease concept, the integration model, and the availability (public health) model.

Moral and Religious Concepts. Some religious groups define any use of alcohol as sinful. Under Islamic law the drinking of any intoxicant is a criminal offence[42] punishable by 80 lashes.[50] Total abstinence from alcohol also has had strong associations with nonconformist Christian denominations.

The Total Abstinence Movement. The initial, public health-oriented Temperance Movement appeared in England, North America, and Australia in the early 1800s. This movement was eclipsed by the Total Abstinence Movement, which was concerned with the avoidance of sin and the maintenance of morals. The movement's leaders advocated temperance (abstinence) because they believed that alcohol could be a problem for anyone who drank and was the main cause of human suffering.[51,52] In Europe, North America, Australia, and New Zealand the Abstinence Movement provided the political force that was responsible for the enactment of a series of laws invoking either prohibition or severe restrictions on the conditions governing the sale and consumption of alcoholic beverages.[51,52] However, these laws failed to achieve their moral objectives.

With a shift in community values from cultural conservatism to cultural modernism the Total Abstinence Movement's influence was eclipsed by proalcohol forces.[53] Laws governing alcohol availability and abuse were abolished or eased. The commonly held view of Prohibition in the United States is that it was a failure, but there are major limitations to this view, since

TABLE 43-7. APPARENT CONSUMPTION OF ALCOHOLIC BEVERAGES IN THE UNITED STATES IN 1978, 1980, AND 1984 IN LITERS OF ETHANOL PER CAPITA AGED 14 YEARS AND OLDER BY STATE[a]

1984 Rank	State	Consumption (liters)			1984 Rank	State	Consumption (Liters)		
		1978	1980	1984			1978	1980	1984
1	District of Columbia	21.7	20.5	20.2	27	Oregon	11.0	10.7	10.0
2	Nevada	26.7	22.0	19.6	28	Michigan	10.7	10.0	9.8
3	New Hampshire	21.4	21.8	18.6	29	Maine	10.4	10.1	9.7
4	Alaska	14.1	14.2	14.6	30	North Dakota	10.6	10.7	9.7
5	California	13.5	12.8	12.1	31	Virginia (D = 3.3)	9.1	9.0	9.7
6	Wisconsin	12.9	13.1	12.1	32	South Carolina	10.1	9.3	9.5
7	Delaware	11.5	11.8	12.0	33	Georgia (D = 22.5)	9.7	8.9	9.4
8	Florida (D = 1.4)[b]	12.9	12.2	11.8	34	Idaho	10.2	9.8	9.2
9	Vermont	14.0	12.5	11.8	35	Nebraska (D = 0.1)	10.0	10.0	9.1
10	Colorado	13.4	12.7	11.7	36	South Dakota (D = 1.5)	9.4	9.7	8.8
11	Arizona	12.9	11.5	11.7	37	Missouri	9.0	9.2	8.6
12	Massachusetts	11.9	12.1	11.5	38	Ohio	8.6	8.8	8.6
13	Hawaii	12.7	12.5	11.2	39	Pennsylvania	9.0	9.0	8.5
14	Montana	12.1	12.2	11.2	40	Indiana	8.3	8.4	8.3
15	Rhode Island	12.0	11.9	11.1	41	North Carolina (D = 4.3)	8.4	8.3	8.1
16	Wyoming	13.3	12.9	10.8	42	Iowa	8.7	8.5	7.9
17	Maryland	11.9	11.7	10.8	43	Mississippi (D = 28.5)	8.5	7.9	7.8
18	New Jersey	10.6	10.7	10.7	44	Kansas (D = 2.0)	7.4	7.4	7.4
19	Texas (D = 10.0)	10.7	10.6	10.7	45	Tennessee (D = 27.2)	7.6	7.3	7.4
20	Connecticut	10.4	10.2	10.6	46	Oklahoma	8.0	7.4	7.2
21	Illinois	11.2	11.4	10.5	47	Alabama (D = 26.6)	7.7	7.0	7.2
22	New Mexico	11.5	11.3	10.4	48	Kentucky (D = 43.6)	7.3	7.2	7.0
23	Washington	11.8	11.8	10.2	49	Arkansas (D = 10.3)	7.0	6.9	6.7
24	Minnesota	10.5	10.8	10.1	50	West Virginia (D = 2.1)	7.2	6.9	6.4
25	New York	10.8	11.0	10.1	51	Utah	6.7	6.5	5.8
26	Louisiana (D = 1.4)	10.4	10.3	10.0					
United States 10.0									

[a]The District of Columbia has been referred to as a state for the purposes of this analysis.
[b]D indicates a state with legally dry areas, the number indicating the percentage of the state population living in dry area(s).
Of the 25 states with a per capita consumption above the national average, only 2 had dry areas. Of the 26 states with a per capita consumption below the national average, 13 had dry areas.
From Hyman et al, 1980,[46] and U.S. Department of Health and Human Services, 1987.[38]

during Prohibition, health and social problems associated with alcohol use certainly were reduced dramatically.[2,54]

The Disease Concept. In the period after Prohibition the Alcoholism Movement emerged with an alternative view of alcohol-related problems and their origins.[55] The focus of concern shifted from alcohol use generally in communities to the small proportion of those communities who drank to excess. The central thrust of the Alcoholism Movement was to explain why only a small proportion of the drinking population drank too much and, as a consequence, developed alcohol-related problems. This shift in focus was consistent with the general view of the community that, for most people, alcohol was not a problem.

The Alcoholism Movement has promoted the concept that alcoholism is a disease, that is, a biological condition for which those who are afflicted are not responsible and which leads to an inability to control the use of alcohol.[56] Corollaries of this view are that most problems of alcohol use are caused by those who suffer from alcoholism and that the vast majority of the community can drink with impunity.[55]

Currently this model has the widest community acceptance.[46] Not surprisingly, it is also the concept of alcohol-related problems promoted by the alcohol beverage industry[57] and others whose interests lie in promoting alcohol use.

In this context it is important to reflect on current general attitudes to psychoactive substances, including alcohol. Alcohol is unique among these substances in that its use for self-administered intoxication has become widely accepted. In the case of alcohol the focus has shifted from a bad substance, alcohol (Abstinence Movement), to bad users, or alcoholics (Alcoholism Movement). For other substances, particularly illicit drugs, the predominant community view is still that problems are caused in normal people by bad substances.

Genetic Theories of Alcoholism. Closely related to the disease concept are genetic theories of alcoholism. It has long been recognized that a familial history of alcohol-related problems is common. Despite this recognition there is still major disagreement on the degree to which such familial patterns are genetically or environmentally determined.

Studies of twins[58] and adoptees[59] have produced evidence for the importance of genetic factors. Indeed, as a result of the adoptees study it has been proposed that there are two types of alcoholism, mileau-limited alcoholism, which requires the presence of environmental factors for alcoholism to develop, and male-limited alcoholism, which does not.[59] Furthermore, there is evidence of a biochemical difference between individuals with these two types of alcoholism.[60]

Attractive as this hypothesis may be, a recent intensive review of the research literature on genetic inheritance of alcoholism concluded that no valid conclusions can be reached because of flaws in research to date.[61] However, it does seem likely that studies will confirm ultimately that both inherited and environmental factors are important in the development of alcohol dependence.

The Integration Hypothesis and Responsible Drinking. The integration hypothesis proposed that alcohol-related problems were the result of failure to integrate alcohol use into the everyday functions of that society. Major wine-producing countries, such as France, were held up as positive models of societies in which the integration of alcohol use had prevented the development of alcoholism.[62]

This hypothesis led to the introduction of responsible drinking as a concept for preventing alcohol-related problems. (The meaning of the term "responsible" in this context is different from that used in the context of the Australian NHMRC statement on "safe" drinking quoted earlier.[27]) If people could be taught to drink responsibly and if their drinking were integrated into the social fabric of everyday behaviors, fewer people would become alcoholic.[63] This hypothesis has served as the rationale for legislative changes since World War II, which eased or removed restrictions governing the availability and use of alcohol. Those who promoted, supported, or acted on this hypothesis either ignored or were unaware of the major health consequences linked to high levels of alcohol consumption in those countries considered to be models of integrated, responsible drinking, namely, France, Italy, Portugal, and Spain.

The Availability Theory. The availability theory is the framework adopted for the preventive strategies outlined in this chapter. These public health strategies concerned with the prevention of alcohol-related problems recognize that (1) alcohol is a risk factor for many health-related outcomes, (2) the magnitude of alcohol-related health problems in a population has a direct relationship to per capita consumption, and (3) preventive strategies must include among their key objectives a reduction in the per capita consumption of alcohol.[30,64]

This theory encompasses two principles. First, it is to be expected that a change in overall alcohol consumption in a population will be accompanied by a change in the same direction in the proportion of heavy users. Second, since heavy use of alcohol increases the probability of physical and social damage, it is to be expected that the average consumption usually will be closely related to the prevalence of such damage in the population. Therefore, measures expected to affect overall consumption usually will affect the prevalence of alcohol-related problems and hence should be of central concern in any prevention program.[57]

Since the late 1960s, particularly as a result of seminal research by Ledermann,[65,66] Terris,[67] de Lint and Schmidt,[68] Mäkellä,[69] and Skög,[70] the attention of those concerned with public health aspects of alcohol has shifted from individuals suffering from alcoholism with alcohol-related problems to the general overall consumption of alcohol in drinking communities, factors affecting this consumption, and the relationship between various levels of consumption and the development of alcohol-related disease and injury among drinkers as a whole. This shift in focus has been prompted not only by new research findings but also by concerns about the many inconsistencies and weaknesses in blaming alcoholic individuals for all or most alcohol-related problems.[54]

A substantial body of evidence now supports the view that increases in overall or per capita consumption are associated with higher rates of heavy drinking and, consequently, with increased frequencies of alcohol-related health problems.[2,54,66–68,71,72]

Per Capita Consumption and Alcohol-related Health Problems. Epidemiological research on alcohol-related health problems is substantially consistent with the availability model. Studies of relationships between per capita alcohol consumption and alcohol-related morbidity and mortality have focused on cirrhosis, where a strong positive correlation has been established.[74] Per capita consumption also has been correlated positively with total mortality in men,[66] international variations in deaths from diabetes mellitus,[75] deaths from alcohol-related disease,[76] alcoholism death rates,[77] and hospital admissions for alcohol dependence, alcoholic psychosis, liver cirrhosis, pancreatitis,[78] Wernicke's encephalopathy, and Korsakoff's psychosis.[79]

Implications of the Availability Model. Measures that lead to increases in per capita consumption in a population will result in greater proportions of the population drinking at levels associated with health risks and developing alcohol-related problems. Measures that reduce per capita consumption will result in decreases in these problems. Some of these effects may be seen almost immediately, whereas others may be evident only in the long term. Although the ultimate impact of control measures based on this model may be assessed in terms of the overall rate of alcohol-related health problems, their primary purpose is to reduce the incidence of these problems in the population.[80] Thus, such measures fall squarely into the realm of primary prevention.

This macroavailability (public health) model has not yet gained public acceptance.[46] Furthermore, since the model proposes that a reduction in alcohol-related problems is dependent on measures that would reduce the per capita consumption of alcohol, it is not surprising that the model has met with strong opposition. Presupposing that such a model were effectively promoted, it likely would take 20 to 30 years before it gained widespread acceptance.[46]

Barriers to the Prevention of Alcohol-related Problems

The Alcohol Beverage Industry. An appreciation of the nature, size, organization, resources, and practices of the alcohol beverage industry is essential in understanding the central factors influencing alcohol consumption and the development and implementation of effective prevention strategies. This industry is concerned primarily with the production, marketing, and sale of a very profitable commodity. The industry is committed to maximizing sales in existing markets and to developing new markets or market segments. The industry does not acknowledge that alcohol is a problem in its own right; alcoholics are held to be the cause of alcohol-related problems.[57] Furthermore, promotional activities are purported only to serve objectives related to beverage or brand preference and not to have any effect on consumption,[73] a claim similar to that of the tobacco industry.[81] This view is difficult to accept, given the widespread belief that similar promotional activities for nondependence-producing commodities are capable of developing new markets and expanding sales within existing markets.[46]

Central to the development and growth of the alcohol beverage industry in this century has been the emerging and constantly increasing dominance of the industry by transnational corporations. By the mid-1960s, a handful of giant corporations had achieved market dominance with regard to beer and distilled spirits in most counties. This consolidation within an ever decreasing number of corporations has continued since then. Today, these corporations are characterized by their immense size, global operations, diversification (4 of the 27 were among the top 20 food companies, and 5 were part of larger tobacco-based corporations), and vertical integration of operations relevant to the alcohol field (growth of raw materials, beverage production, packaging, transportation, marketing, distribution and sales[82]).

Two major mechanisms are used by these corporations to promote global sales of alcoholic beverages, namely, subsidization of the alcohol sector by the nonalcohol sectors of their operations and the use of existing, extensive, international networks for other products to distribute alcoholic beverages.[82] Nowhere has the impact of conglomerization of the alcohol industry been so conspicuous as in the extensive links developed recently between four of the seven transnational tobacco conglomerates that dominate world cigarette markets and alcohol corporations. As producers and distributors of one dependence-producing commodity, tobacco, they have brought their well-tested expertise to the other socially available, dependence-producing substance, alcohol.[82]

Clearly, transnational corporate structures and marketing strategies have contributed in a major way and will continue to contribute to the global availability and consumption of alcoholic beverages and, therefore to the global magnitude of alcohol-related problems. Effective prevention strategies to reduce alcohol consumption and its attendant problems will need to be pursued as assiduously and forcefully as are the efforts of the alcohol beverage industry and will require adequate resources and community and political support if they are to achieve lasting benefit. In this respect, two cardinal factors affecting per capita consumption of alcohol are attitudes to alcohol use and accessibility. As preventive strategies are developed and promoted, it is to be expected that the alcohol beverage industry will continue to pursue ways to counter them, for example, by influencing legislators through financial donations and lobbyists, forging links with other industries, influencing nongovernmental groups, punishing groups that oppose industry interests, organizing drinkers, funding research and researchers, and improving its image.[82]

Governments. The introduction of effective prevention strategies, of which the most basic one would be to increase the general understanding of the availability (public health) model, requires the involvement and support of governments and their agencies. With some exceptions, there is little evidence that policymakers in government are likely to make sustained attempts to promote this model. These policymakers are influenced largely by the prevailing community belief system and are lobbied intensively by interests opposed to the model. Further, they depend on current levels of consumption to maintain government revenues. If alcohol consumption increases, they stand to gain, at least in the short term, by additions to the public purse. The multiplicity of societal views and forces is evidenced in inconsistencies in governmental policies on the prevention of alcohol-related problems and in opposing policies within government, for example, in departments responsible for health and social services vs business and economic interests.[1] It is alleged that such conflicts have resulted in suppression of a government report[84] and in the cancellation of a World Health Organization project when data favoring control policies were presented.[85]

The setting of program objectives is complicated by differences in levels of alcohol consumption and related problems within and between countries, within and between states, and within and between communities. Differences in political orientation and organization, religion, social and economic circumstances, and other factors can lead to differing perceptions of the nature of and solutions to alcohol-related problems. These differences also are important with regard to the commitment of a nation or a community to the prevention of such problems. Successful application of effective strategies requires perseverance over the long term, a condition difficult to attain in many nations where periodic changes in leadership, philosophy, and objectives can be expected.[1]

Community Attitudes. We have referred to the multiplicity of views and forces that influence community attitudes to alcohol and its use. The major attitudinal influences promoting low levels of consumption have been moral and religious. These influences are reflected in low levels of per capita consumption in nations or states where moral or religious views aligned with abstinence exert a major effect, for example, Moslem nations and the state of Utah in the United States. In other areas, alcohol generally is accepted as a safe beverage for everyday use, although surviving fragments of restrictive legislation may still be in place from the Total Abstinence era, with some community groups still favoring their retention. Within such alcohol-consuming communities, the predominant pattern is one of abstinence and low levels of consumption.

There is no evidence, however, that this low consumption pattern is based on attitudes of moderation. After all, in alcohol-consuming nations, the evidence is that the population enjoys its use of alcohol, sees alcohol problems as only occurring in people who are alcohol-dependent, and, generally, will increase its levels of alcohol consumption within the legal and economic limits that are in force.[1] If there are possibilities of drinking more, the population seems likely to do so. Social pressures promoting drinking are such that a society may be prepared to modify isolated drinking-related behaviors, such as drinking and driving, in order to avoid specific alcohol-related problems while maintaining general drinking levels and behaviors.[1]

There is evidence of an increasing understanding of and support by communities and nongovernmental organizations for public health approaches to the prevention of alcohol-related problems. For example, Mosher and Jernigan[83] have pointed in the United States to

> The emergence of a growing consensus among health, non-profit, educational, and church agencies and organizations (which) is reflected in recent opinion polls. . . . Alcohol policy reforms, such as increases in alcohol taxes, health warning labels, restrictions on alcohol availability and alcohol advertising, receive strong public support. Support for alcohol taxes is perhaps the most surprising, since most other types of tax increases (except on tobacco) are strongly opposed.[83]

STRATEGIES FOR PREVENTION

Recognition of the relationships among per capita alcohol consumption, rates of heavy use, and the incidence of alcohol-related health problems has focused attention on primary prevention strategies aimed at the drinking population, generally with the principal objective of reducing per capita alcohol consumption. These strategies comprise two groups (Table 43–8). The first, health protection measures, are those that governments, other agencies, and industry can implement to reduce per capita consumption, essentially through the imposition of barriers to curtail consumer–product interaction, thus protecting people from harm.[86] The second group, health promotion measures, encourage healthy lifestyles in individuals and communities.[86] The two approaches are complementary and interactive, and it is unlikely that one would be effective without the other.[87–89] Preventive health services, a third group of measures aimed at the early detection of and effective intervention in hazardous drinking and its consequences, provide a backup, secondary prevention strategy.

Health Protection Measures

The health protection measures that might be considered include legislative and regulatory controls on the price of beverages, numbers, types, and locations of outlets, hours and days of sale, drinking age, alcohol content of beverages, other aspects of the alcohol production and distribution systems, and the service environment. Critical reviews suggest that measures addressing the economic and physical accessibility of alcohol are among the most effective.[2,30,38,46,47,54,73,83,90–96]

Public Awareness and Health Protection Measures. The adoption of health protection measures by a population will depend, at least in part, on its understanding of the rationale and need for such controls and the benefits to be realized. Therefore,

TABLE 43-8. CLASSIFICATION[a] OF PREVENTIVE MEASURES FOR ALCOHOL-RELATED PROBLEMS

	Health Protection	Health Promotion	Preventive Health Services
▪ **Definition**	Measures that can be used by government and other agencies, as well as by industry, to protect people from harm	Activities that individuals and communities can use to promote healthy lifestyles	Key preventive services that can be delivered to individuals by health providers
▪ **Specific objectives re alcohol problems**	To control accessibility to alcohol through economic, physical, legal, environmental, and other measures	To promote healthy lifestyles, including less harmful alcohol use	To detect harmful drinking and its consequences early and to intervene effectively
▪ **Examples of measures**	Economic Price controls Differential taxation Tax law Physical Times of sale Numbers/rates of outlets Types/locations of outlets Distribution systems Other Legal Drinking age Other Environmental Server intervention	Information and education Public education programs Health warning labels Targeted promotion Specific populations Specific problems Less hazardous drinking Beverage substitution Low alcohol content beverages Curtailment of negative lifestyle influences Advertizing and marketing Media portrayals	Early detection Effective intervention

[a]Based on categories defined in The Surgeon General's Report on Health Promotion and Disease Prevention, 1979.[87]

the implementation of these measures should be preceded and accompanied by social marketing designed to prepare the ground for consultation with policymakers, the media, and the public and to convince communities and their leaders of the legitimate role of public health considerations in the alcohol control debate.[97] These efforts would include educational programs to increase public awareness of the personal hazards of alcohol use, its adverse economic and other consequences for the community and for individuals, and the potential individual and public health benefits that would result from effective controls.[46,91] Appropriate methods and media should be employed to identify, inform, and involve the wide range of persons and groups in the community, including government, that have a stake in health protection measures.[72,86,92,97–99] Attention should be directed to the development of policies applicable and appropriate to the needs of local communities,[98] as well as broad national policies, and to the development of a capacity to respond quickly to unanticipated opportunities for policy initiatives.[97]

The Alcohol Beverage Industry and Health Protection Measures. The alcohol beverage industry has consistently and vigorously opposed the implementation of effective health protection measures, which, by their nature, are counter to its objectives. Therefore, it is essential that an overall preventive strategy include initiatives to overcome the barriers imposed by that industry.[85] Mosher and Jernigan,[83] in identifying areas where alcohol policy advocates can seek to overcome these barriers, suggest that they should take advantage of divisions that exist within the alcohol industry, form new coalitions with alcohol retailers in order to develop effective server intervention programs, use the threat of legal liability for damage associated with alcohol use, promote the establishment of regulations governing the sale and use of alcoholic beverages, develop organized, educated, and active constituencies at the local level, and use local organizations as the basis for developing broad coalitions at regional and national levels.

Economic Accessibility

Price Controls. Numerous studies, reviews, and reports have examined the use of price control via taxation in reducing alcohol consumption and alcohol-related problems. The accumulated evidence indicates that price control could be effective and, in some instances, powerful, both in relation to other measures and in combination with them.[2,38,46,47,54,73,88,90,91,94,96,100–103] According to Cook[104,105] and Cook and Tauchen,[106] doubling the federal tax on liquor in the United States would reduce the cirrhosis mortality rate by at least 20%. An effect on automobile fatalities also was postulated.[104] Holder and Blose[102] used a system dynamics model to study the effect of four prevention strategies—raising the retail price of all alcoholic beverages by 25% once, indexing the price of alcoholic beverages to the consumer price index (CPI) each year, raising the minimum drinking age to 21 years, and reducing high-risk alcohol consumption through state-of-the-art public education—on alcohol-related family disruptions and alcohol-related work problems, against a background of business as usual in three counties of the United States. Although both outcome measures were modestly sensitive to one-time changes in price, the largest effect was obtained by instituting a community education effort concurrently with indexing the prices of alcoholic beverages to the CPI. From an analysis of the price of beer and spirits, other economic and sociodemographic factors, and various regulatory control variables, Ornstein[107] concluded that price was the most important policy tool available to regulators in the United States. A similar conclusion arose from a study of the effects of various regulatory measures on the consumption of distilled spirits in the United States over a 25-year period.[108] Levy and Sheflin,[109] using methods intended to overcome the problem of beverage substitution when price control is not directed at all beverages, estimated that the price elasticity for total alcohol consumption, although less than 1 (implying that demand is inelastic), was large enough for price policies to be effective in reducing alcohol consumption. Others,[110–115] however, have been more guarded in their support for price manipulation as a control measure, pointing out the methodological limitations in econometric analyses, the modest or conflicting implications of some findings, and the possible role of countervailing forces.

In a study of individual drinkers, Kendell and colleagues[116,117] found that overall consumption and associated adverse effects fell 18% and 16%, respectively, among 463 "regular drinkers" in the Lothian region of Scotland when prices were increased via the excise duty. Heavy and dependent drinkers reduced their consumption at least as much as light and moderate drinkers, with fewer adverse effects as a result. Clinical data also show that alcohol-dependent persons reduce their alcohol consumption as a function of beverage costs.[118,119] Further, in an experimental study of price reductions during afternoon happy hours, Babor and associates[120] found that such reductions significantly increased alcohol consumption by both casual and heavy drinkers. With the reinstatement of standard prices, drinking in both groups returned to previous levels. These findings and others[88,90,105,106] seriously challenge the previously held view that a reduction in overall consumption does not affect consumption by the heaviest drinkers. Further, liver cirrhosis mortality rates, which are considered the most accurate indicator of the prevalence of heavy drinking, respond directly and rather quickly to major restrictions on availability, including economic ones, that produce declines in per capita consumption.[2,54,105] Indeed, the recent levelling off and decrease in cirrhosis mortality rates in Canada[31] and the United States[121] may be, in part, the result of current economic conditions affecting the price of alcohol relative to personal disposable income[47] and, consequently, the consumption of all drinkers, including heavy drinkers.

Price elasticities of alcoholic beverages vary among themselves, across time, and among countries.[2] In the United States, as in Canada and the United Kingdom, beer tends to be relatively price inelastic.[54,122,123] However, this general inelasticity does not hold in certain age groups. Grossman and colleagues[124–127] estimated the effects on young people of increases in alcoholic beverage prices with regard to alcohol use and motor vehicle mortality. They showed that for beer, the alcoholic beverage of preference in the young, the price elasticity was considerably higher than that usually reported, a 10 cent increase in the price of a package of six 12-once cans resulting in an 11% decrease in the number of youths drinking beer and a 15% decrease in the number of youthful heavy beer drinkers (three to five drinks per day).[124] Further, they predicted that a national policy simultaneously taxing the alcohol in beer and distilled spirits at the same rates and offsetting the erosion in the real beer tax since 1951 would reduce the number of youths 16 to 21 years old who drink beer frequently (four to seven times a week, about 11% of youths) and fairly frequently (one to three times a week, about 28% of all youths) by 32% and 24%, respectively.[124,125] Additional analyses showed dramatic effects of excise tax policies on motor vehicle accidents in youths.[125–127] In a multivariate analysis, it was estimated that a policy that fixed the federal beer tax in real terms since 1951 would have reduced the number of motor vehicle fatalities in youths ages 18 to 20 in the period 1975–1981 by 15%, and a policy that taxed the alcohol in beer at the same rate as the alcohol in liquor would have lowered fatalities by 21%. A combination of the two policies would have caused a 54% decline in the number of youths killed. In contrast, the enactment of a uniform drinking age of 21 years in all states would have reduced such fatalities by 8%, with considerable additional costs in enforcement. Since the principal objective of price control in the public health context is primary prevention, that is, a reduction in the incidence (new cases) of alcohol-related problems,[90] a differentially higher price sensitivity among young drinkers for beer is an especially important finding.

Price control via taxation has been recommended repeatedly as a strategy for stabilizing or reducing per capita consumption and, thereby, preventing alcohol-related health problems.[57,103,128,129] In the United States, recent public opinion polls indicate clear majority support for excise tax increases on alcohol for public health purposes.[103] However, federal excise taxes on distilled spirits, wine, and beer remained constant in nominal terms (current dollar value) between November 1, 1951, and the end of fiscal year 1985.[125] In 1985, the federal excise tax on distilled spirits was raised slightly (as a deficit reduction measure), but federal tax rates on beer and wine were not changed. Thus, the real price of alcoholic beverages has actually declined in recent years, such that between 1960 and 1980 the real price of liquor declined 48%, beer 27%, and wine 20%.[104] A similar situation has been documented in Ontario, Canada, where a taxation policy that would maintain a reasonably constant relationship between the price of alcohol and the consumer price index has been a key element in a long proposed, but unimplemented prevention strategy.[57]

Differential Taxation. Few data support differential taxation among the various beverages, since equally harmful public health effects result from their use.[30,54,73,88,90] More importantly, however, a taxation policy based on the absolute alcohol content of beverages, that is, equal taxation for equal alcohol content, could be used to favor differentially the consumption of low alcohol beverages, such as low alcohol beer.[73] Such a differential should be effected by increasing the price of regular strength beverages rather than by reducing the current price of low alcohol beverages.[2]

Tax Law. Recently, the role of tax law as a potential tool for the prevention of alcohol-related problems has been examined.[130,131] Current tax law in the United States supports the economic availability of alcohol in several ways. For example, taxpayers are permitted to deduct the cost of alcoholic beverages purchased for "ordinary and necessary business purposes." These deductions represented a $4 billion federal subsidy in support of alcohol consumption in 1979.[130] Federal law also permits a variety of tax deductions in connection with alcoholic beverage production and marketing.[130,131] These economic incentives favoring accessibility are an important consideration in a comprehensive approach to the prevention of alcohol-related problems via tax policy.

Physical Availability. The relationship between the physical availability of alcohol and alcohol consumption and related problems is multifaceted and complex. It is difficult to show the effect of small changes and to untangle the effects of changes in physical availability that take place simultaneously with others, either nonspecific changes (e.g., in the general economy) or specific changes (e.g., in the economic and legal accessibility of alcohol). It is not surprising, therefore, that the evidence concerning the effectiveness of limitations on physical accessibility is mixed.[2,30,46,54,73,92,94,132,133] Taken together, there is considerable evidence that controls on physical availability can alleviate alcohol-related problems and that the consumption of both heavy and moderate drinkers can be reduced.[92]

Prohibition is successful in reducing consumption and attendant health risks.[2,30,54,94] Such a situation prevails in some countries today.[94] With the institution of Prohibition in the United States earlier in this century, cirrhosis mortality rates fell dramatically and remained well below their former levels during the earlier years and to a considerable extent even in the later years, indicative of greatly decreased consumption.[54] On repeal of Prohibition and the subsequent increase in the availability of alcohol, consumption rose, and cirrhosis mortality rates gradually increased toward previous levels. Similar trends have been observed in the face of other severe limitations on availability, for example, in Paris during the two World Wars[2,71] and during some strikes and periods of rationing.[30,46,92,94] Under such conditions, the consumption of both heavy and moderate drinkers is reduced.[46,73,92,94]

Similarly, sudden, marked relaxations in the availability of alcohol are associated with increases in overall consumption, heavy drinking, and alcohol-related problems. The Finnish experience, which included a very marked increase in overall consumption in connection with liberalizing legislation that led to an extensive and rapid increase in outlets in previously dry areas, has been detailed[134] and summarized[91,94] elsewhere.

The effectiveness of less severe restrictions of physical accessibility on consumption is not as clear.[30,46,73,92,94,132,133] Indeed, some aspects have not been studied adequately.[30,94,132,133] Recent appraisals, however, do suggest that various aspects of physical accessibility are associated with alcohol consumption and alcohol-related problems in general populations.[92,94,132,133] Further, specific types of availability may have effects that are specific to certain problems, and in some instances, a control measure may alleviate one alcohol-related problem while exacerbating another.[21,132,133,135-137a] For example, Colon[137] found that restrictions on on-premise availability may reduce cirrhosis mortality rates, whereas Colon and Cutter[137] reported that such curtailment simultaneously may increase highway fatalities. These findings suggest that when on-premise outlets are fewer (and more geographically spread out), overall consumption may be decreased with a beneficial effect on cirrhosis mortality, but the chances of drinking and driving are greater, with adverse effects on motor vehicle accidents.[138]

Hoadley and colleagues[108] showed that state regulatory measures, excluding price, had an impact on per capita consumption of distilled spirits. In a multivariate analysis of data from the continental U.S. states over a 25-year period to 1980, bans on liquor by the drink, dry areas in a state, state monopolies on sale requiring visits to state stores, and a lower density of outlets all had negative impacts on consumption, but hours and days of sale did not. Neuman and Rabow[139] found that effortless, efficient physical availability explained a small but significant amount of the variance in individual consumption when normative factors were controlled statistically. They noted observations made by the beverage industry that grocery store availability increases sales, especially to women. They concluded that the effect of physical availability is best investigated at the local level, possibly in neighborhoods.

The complexity of evaluating changes in physical availability and developing appropriate public policy is illustrated in a study of the effects on liver cirrhosis and traffic accident mortality of changes in the rate and proportional distribution of types of alcohol outlets in Western Australia in comparison with a control state, Queensland.[140] During the after period, Western Australia had a 16.0% increase in the rates of licensed hotels, taverns, and stores in comparison to the control state but a 17.4% decrease in the rate of licensed clubs, restaurants, and other premises. These changes were associated with significant increases in male (+24.3%) and female (+29.3%) liver cirrhosis mortality but a significant decrease in male driver and motorcyclist mortality (−22.1%). The author attributed the increase in liver cirrhosis mortality relative to the control state to an increase in overall alcohol consumption, resulting from changes in the numbers and types of outlets in Western Australia. Similarly, he attributed the decrease in motor vehicle accident mortality to a decrease in the probability of drinking and driving as a result of either having more on-premise outlets (related inversely in a previous study[21] to motor vehicle accident mortality) or selling more alcohol in packaged form that would be more likely to be consumed at home or both. These different outcomes for two major health effects imply that a public health policy on availability should aim not only to reduce overall alcohol consumption, thereby reducing health effects that are related to total consumption (e.g., cirrhosis of the liver) but also to restrict consumption to locations and circumstances minimizing the probability of adverse effects arising primarily from the immediate effects of alcohol consumption (e.g., those from drinking and driving).

Times of Sale. Studies of days and hours of sale of alcoholic beverages provide some evidence of effects on patterns of consumption,[30,54,73,132,141] specific alcohol-related problems,[142-145] and problem drinking.[146] An attempt was made in Australia to reduce motor vehicle accidents associated with a 6 PM closing time for hotels by extending the time to 10 PM, on the premise that this would reduce the pressure to drink. The number of accidents was not reduced, but the peak accident time was shifted from 6 to 7 PM to 10 to 11 PM.[141] More recently, Smith[142] examined the effect on traffic accidents of introducing flexible hotel trading hours in Tasmania, Australia. Hotels stayed open for approximately the same duration each day but closed during uneconomical hours and remained open later than the previous 10:00 PM closing time. He found a significant increase of 10.8% in the number of accidents occurring from 10:00 PM to 6:00 AM, while there was no change in the accidents occurring before 10:00 PM. The additional accidents occurred after midnight. A study by Smith[143] of the effect of introducing Sunday drinking hours in Perth, Australia, suggested detrimental effects on traffic safety. A significant increase in the number of Sunday traffic casualty and reported property damage accidents followed the introduction of Sunday alcohol sales in Brisbane, Australia, an effect closely related in time to sales times.[144] Further, early opening may facilitate problem drinking.[145] In contrast, Olsson and Wikstrom[146] showed that the experimental Saturday closing of liquor retail stores in Sweden resulted in a small decrease in sales of alcohol and beneficial effects on detentions for drunkenness, other public order disturbances, assaults indoors and outdoors (including those in places of amusement and entertainment), and domestic disturbances.

Evaluations of the impact of the 1976 liberalization of Scotland's liquor licensing laws, which allowed bars to remain open for an extra hour in the evenings, permitted some all day licenses, and allowed public houses to open on Sunday, have yielded mixed results. Duffy and Plant[147] found no effect on mortality from liver cirrhosis, total alcohol-related mortality, or psychiatric hospital admissions for alcohol dependence, confirming earlier reports of little impact.[94] However, Northridge and colleagues,[148] in an uncontrolled study, presented evidence suggesting the possibility of a relationship between these liberalizations and admissions for self-poisoning associated with alcohol use.

Numbers and Rates of Outlets. Restrictions on the number and per capita rate of outlets in a community have been one of the most frequently used control measures related to alcohol accessibility.[54] Evidence concerning the impact of outlet frequency is mixed.[46,132] Some studies show a positive relationship between outlet frequency and consumption, others show no relationship, and a few show a negative relationship.[46,149] Also, the relationship between the rates of on- and off-premise availability and consumption may be different.[133,137]

The rate of change of outlet frequency is important.[30,46,94] In Scandinavia, marked increases in overall consumption followed the establishment of multiple outlets in what previously were largely dry areas.[46,134] Natural experiments of short-term restrictions on physical accessibility, for example, during strikes in beverage industries, suggest a minor effect on overall consumption, with a shift in consumption to beverages that are still available.[46] However, studies of strikes by alcohol monopoly employees in Finland and Sweden showed that even though alcoholic beverages were still available in on-premise locations, drinking was reduced in both moderate and heavy drinkers.[30,46,92,94]

Rabow and Watts[135] used multiple regression techniques to examine the relationship between general on- and off-premise accessibility and alcohol-related health and social problems in 51 California counties. Both on- and off-premise general outlets were positively related to cirrhosis mortality. The final regression model, however, did not predict cirrhosis mortality better than the initial model, which included only sociodemographic variables. In a subsequent study[136] of 213 California communities in which sociodemographic factors were controlled, general on- and off-premise availability both predicted cirrhosis mortality, whereas general off-premise availability and specific types of on-premise availability predicted public drunkenness. These and other recent findings[150-154] suggest that outlet rates are related to alcohol-related problems. Rush and colleagues,[153] in a study of alcohol availability, alcohol consumption, and alcohol-related damage in the 49 counties of Ontario, Canada, found robust statistical evidence that government policies restricting retail availability, as indicated by the rate of both off- and on-premise outlets per 1000 adults, will reduce per capita alcohol consumption and, in turn, will reduce the level of alcohol-related mortality and morbidity in the general population. This relationship was maintained when socioeconomic status, urbanism, and unemployment were incorporated into the statistical model.[154]

Types, Characteristics, and Locations of Outlets. Rabow and Watts[135,136] differentiated among five types of on-premise and two types of off-premise outlets with regard to effects on three types of alcohol-related arrest and cirrhosis mortality. When sociodemographic variables were controlled, beer bars were the best predictors of public drunkenness arrests and arrests for felony and misdemeanor drunk driving, but they were minimally correlated with cirrhosis mortality. This suggests that different types of outlets have effects that are alcohol problem-specific. Further, these effects, depending on local circumstances, may not influence all alcohol-related problems in the same direction, as shown in studies of outlet types and density in relation to highway safety and cirrhosis of the liver.[21,135,140]

The on-premise consumption of distilled spirits by the individual drink is widely permitted, but not ubiquitous, in the United States. In multiple regression analyses, Hoadley and associates[108] showed that the consumption of distilled spirits was lower in the absence of liquor-by-the-drink. Blose and Holder[155,156] found that the introduction of this serving practice in certain North Carolina counties was associated with statistically significant increases of 6% to 7.4% in total distilled spirits sales and of 16 to 24% in both the number of police-reported alcohol-related accidents and single vehicle accidents among male drivers 21 years of age and older, whereas no change was found in these accidents in counties not allowing this type of availability. Further, they documented substantial and diverse changes in the on-premise availability of distilled spirits resulting from the implementation of liquor-by-the-drink and pointed out difficulties in assessing the impact of specific changes in availability on overall availability, total consumption, and health and social outcomes.[157]

With regard to characteristics of on-premise outlets, different regulatory approaches have been attempted. Some have involved making drinking places more attractive to render drinking "more civilized," the idea being that such changes would give rise to fewer problems. Others have taken an opposite approach by making drinking in public places less attractive. These approaches have not been assessed carefully.[30,54] Single[95,158] has reviewed the small but growing body of literature based on tavern studies that has identified situational determinants of heavy or problem-related drinking, including the physical environment of the drinking setting. More studies are needed of the effects of television, games, music, physical design, and other manipulable factors of the drinking setting.[95]

Some evaluations of permitting sales in supermarkets and other stores selling various commodities have been attempted.[94] The effect seems to be dependent on local tradition and the suddenness of change.[30,94,139] Regression analyses on per capita wine consumption in four states of the United States indicated significant increases in wine consumption in two states where regulatory changes permitted the sale of wine in grocery stores where it had not been allowed before (and at somewhat lower prices than found in state-controlled stores) and in one of two states in which the regulatory changes permitted an increased selection of wines. The increases were additions to total consumption of alcohol, rather than substitutions for beer and spirits.[159] Smart,[160] however, was unable to detect an impact on consumption of selling wine in grocery stores in Quebec. Reasons postulated for the lack of impact included depressed economic conditions, the relative unpopularity of wine compared to other beverages, and the long-term trend toward lower alcohol consumption throughout Canada.

Smart[161] also studied purchases in two nearby liquor stores in Toronto, Canada, one self-service and the other clerk-service. The self-service store had more customers, who bought more and reported drinking more frequently in greater amounts and more on impulse. Beer and wine sales in minimarts (gasoline stations having a limited supply of groceries) have become a concern in some parts of the United States, particularly with regard to drinking and driving. There is a relationship between where people buy alcohol and where they drink it. Purchases from liquor stores, convenience stores, and minimarts more often result in public drinking and drinking in cars than do purchases from supermarkets.[162] Data from one minimart chain showed that 70% of those purchasing alcohol also purchased gasoline and that 40% of beer sales were single cans, suggesting immediate consumption.[162] Access to free alcohol on airplanes may be another matter of concern, particularly in relation to driving on flight arrival.[163] Drinking under special permits (such as at weddings, private receptions, and parties) is a neglected aspect of alcohol availability.[164] In Canada, these permits are issued for many different occasions and are most common in the provinces with the highest per capita consumption.

Distribution Systems. In some countries, control and distribution systems have been implemented with the specific goal of minimizing the harmful effects of alcohol, the Finnish State Alcohol Monopoly being one example.[30,165] This organization closely monitors alcohol consumption and alcohol-related problems, reports annually to Parliament, and, if necessary, proposes legislative amendments, particularly regulatory measures on availability and price. Most state monopolies, however, are established to stimulate production with the aim of increasing state revenue. Popham and colleagues,[54] in a review of research on the two different systems of control in the United States, a state monopoly and a licensed free-enterprise system, found no statistically significant differences in mean alcohol consumption or liver cirrhosis mortality rates. The authors stressed the limitations in these analyses. Recent analyses do suggest that the consumption of distilled beverages[108,166] and the incidence of alcoholism[166] are lower in those states of the United States in which monopolies controlling the distribution of distilled spirits are in place. Popham and associates[54] suggested that where a monopoly is comprehensive and the objective is control, as in Finland, rather than the generation of revenue, a beneficial effect on consumption and alcohol-related problems may result. Room[167] has drawn attention to the recent trend in the United States toward the dismantling of state monopolies, urging public health activists to take advantage of the prevention opportunities offered by these monopolies before it is too late to defend them.

Other Measures. Limitations on production, including raw materials, the commercial processing system, and home production, have been proposed and, in some instances, implemented.[30] Although limitations have been proposed for health reasons, most are for revenue or other purposes. Likewise, controls on importation are imposed largely to maintain trade balances, except in countries where prohibition is enforced.[30] According to Moser,[30] no country has been willing to reduce exportation of alcoholic beverages in order to prevent a rise in consumption in the recipient country. Measures for counteracting the disadvantages of reducing production sometimes have been implemented.[30]

Presumably for prevention purposes, a few states have imposed restrictions on the amounts of alcohol purchasable at any one time.[30] Other countries have adopted various rationing systems, with some effects on alcohol consumption and alcohol-related problems.[30] Usually, these measures have been abandoned, since they came to be largely circumvented or ignored.[46] However, the abolition in 1955 of a rationing system in place in Sweden since 1920 has been linked to a redistribution of alcohol consumption and a marked increase in the male liver cirrhosis mortality rate.[168]

Legal Accessibility

Legal Drinking Age. Age limitations represent a legal barrier to alcohol. Most countries have age restrictions on its purchase or consumption or both.[30] Although the data are neither unflawed nor entirely consistent, there is much evidence that the lower the drinking age, the higher the consumption of alcohol[30,125,169-172] and the incidence of alcohol-related problems, particularly among teenagers.[30,73,94,169,170,173,174]

Data from Ontario, Canada, provide one example of the effects of lowering the legal drinking age on both alcohol consumption and related problems. In 1971, the age was lowered from 21 to 18 years, the new age of majority. This was followed by increases in alcohol-related traffic accidents in teenagers and other indications of a marked increase of alcohol consumption and related problems, such as admissions for treatment and detoxification, virtually absent before, and reports of high school students drinking during lunch and being intoxicated in class.[73,169] As a result, public sentiment, which had previously supported a lowering in the drinking age, shifted in favor of raising it again, and in 1979, it was changed to 19 years, the rationale being that this would remove legal drinking from the high school population. A study conducted 2 months later suggested a minimal positive effect on the drinking behaviors of nonregular drinkers and on school-reported drinking behaviors but not on the drinking behavior of regular young drinkers (drinking episodes once a week or more).[175] That the effect was small was expected, as it was felt that too short a time had elapsed for a major impact. Longer-term data on driver alcohol-related accidents, as reported by the police, showed that the rate of alcohol involvement among all drivers declined 20% between 1979 and 1985. This decline was 36% in the youngest driver age group, 16 to 19 years. Thus, the raising of the drinking age was associated with a disproportionately sharper decline in alcohol-related driver accidents among teenagers.[176]

Similar effects of lowering and raising the drinking age on both alcohol consumption and related problems, especially motor vehicle accidents, have been reported in the United States[94,125,170-172,174,177-185] and elsewhere.[173] Age limitations also affect the occurrence of first alcohol use, which is usually several years younger than the legal drinking age. The lower the drinking age, the earlier first alcohol use occurs.[73]

Raising the drinking age in Massachusetts from 18 to 20 was associated with a minimal effect on drinking behavior and vehicular accidents.[179,180] There was a significant reduction in nonfatal crashes in 16- and 17-year-olds compared with the control area (New York) but no decline in single vehicle nighttime fatal crashes or in overall fatal crashes.[179] Nighttime single vehicle fatal accidents declined more in Massachusetts than in New York in the 18 to 19-year age group.[180] In New York,[171] a change in the alcohol purchase age from 18 to 19 years was followed by a decline in alcohol purchasing and consumption by the affected age group that was maintained over a 3-year follow-up.[184] In Tennessee, the implementation of a law denying alcohol to persons 19 through 20 caused a sudden dramatic decline in drunk driving in the affected age group that lasted for the study period of 2 years. In contrast, increased penalties for driving under the influence of alcohol, introduced 2 years before the legal drinking age change, had no effect.[185]

A study of the effect of raising the drinking age on fatal crashes in 10 states indicated a significant decrease in the ratio of single vehicle nighttime fatalities per 1000 licensed drivers in the age group affected by the change, whereas no significant change in the ratio was found among drivers in the comparison group aged 25 to 29 years. Further, the before–after changes in ratios for drivers in the affected age group were significantly greater than the corresponding changes in the comparison group. The single vehicle nighttime fatal crash involvement rate of drivers affected by the law change decreased an average of 21% in the 10 states.[181] Further analyses of data from 26 states confirmed these findings[182] and suggested a sustained effect. A 6-year follow-up study of the effect of the increase in the legal drinking age from 18 to 21 in Michigan also showed a sustained beneficial effect.[186]

In a comprehensive review of the impact of raising the minimum drinking age on traffic crashes involving young people in the age group directly effected by the changed law, the U.S. General Accounting Office concluded that significant reductions (ranging from 5% to 28% in four multistate studies) occurred in almost every instance.[103] It was noted that results from multiple studies using many methods are rarely so consistent. Further, the results appeared to be sustained, and two studies also found a decrease in the self-reported incidence of drinking and driving among young people directly affected by the raised legal minimum drinking age.

In 1982, the U.S. National Transportation Safety Board and the Presidential Commission on Drunk Driving recommended that all states raise the minimum drinking age to 21.[170] Federal legislation enacted in July 1984 provided for the withholding of a portion of federal highway grants from states not implementing a minimum age of 21 by October 1, 1986. By the deadline, most states had complied,[176] and by the end of 1988, all 50 states had raised the legal age for purchasing or consuming alcohol to 21 years.[187] A nationwide survey conducted in May 1985 showed that a clear majority of both parents of teenagers and other adults supported a minimum alcohol purchase age of 21, irrespective of residence in a state already having this restriction.[188]

The potential impact of legislation raising the legal drinking age goes beyond the drinking–driving problem.[170] The increase in the legal alcohol purchase age in New York from 18 to 19 years was associated with significant decreases in all drinking levels, including heavy drinking, among 17 and 18 year olds. Such changes in consumption could result in decreases in other alcohol-related problems, such as nonvehicular accidents, suicide, vandalism, delinquent behaviors and crime, and school problems.[185] However, a study of undergraduate students in 56 colleges and universities throughout the United States revealed few changes in collegiate drinking patterns attributable to the nationwide increase in the minimum age for alcohol purchase. Of 17 problems related to drinking, all but 5 remained stable over three time periods surveyed between 1982–1983 to 1987–1988. However, three problems related to drinking and driving showed a pattern of steady decline.[189]

Other Legal Restrictions. The access of other groups to alcohol has been limited legally, including that of persons who appear to be drunk (e.g., all states of the United States; Ontario, Canada), persons on public relief and mental patients (Switzerland), alcohol-dependent persons (some Swiss cantons), and, in Sweden until 1978, persons registered by a temperance board for alcohol abuse, persons found guilty of the illicit sale of alcohol, or persons sentenced, more than once in the last 12 months, for drunkenness, insober drinking, or drunken driving.[30,176] The effectiveness of such regulations has not been studied.[30]

Environmental Accessibility

Server Intervention. In North America, interest in the preventive potential of environmental barriers to accessibility is widespread, and initiatives are underway in many settings and jurisdictions.[83,190,191] "Server intervention," or, more appropriately, "responsible beverage service,"[192] refers to a broad set of strategies for creating more effective social, physical, and legal drinking environments for reducing both the risk of intoxication and the risk that intoxicated patrons will harm themselves and others.[87,193-196] The concept incorporates a comprehensive approach to the drinking context with the aim of decreasing environmental inducements toward unsafe drinking, especially, but not exclusively, with regard to drinking and driving. It encompasses three basic components, namely, server training, the legal context, and the drinking environment, bringing together a network of elements focusing on servers (commercial or social), managers and owners of commercial alcohol outlets, criminal statutes, dram shop liability, alcoholic beverage control statutes and regulations, alternative transportation (public or private), the interior and exterior design of drinking settings, and outlet location.[87,194,196] Policy and program elements have been specified.[197,198] A multidisciplinary research agenda for the specific strategies has been outlined,[87,195] and difficulties in evaluation are being recognized and addressed.[190-192,199]

In a review of evidence on the effectiveness of selected aspects of server intervention Saltz[192] concluded that, at least in the short term, there does seem to be an opportunity to reduce the risk of intoxication or the level of intoxication among patrons of licensed establishments. For example, the risk of intoxication was cut in half in the male patrons of a Navy club in which an extensive program was implemented.[200] Russ and Geller[201,202] found that trained servers initiated more server interventions than did untrained personnel and that the blood alcohol concentrations reached by patrons served by them was lower. In a Canadian study,[190,192,199] it was found that a training program increased the knowledge of servers with respect to alcohol, its effects, and how to deal with problems. Further, trained servers were found to have positive attitudes toward intervention, and they responded more appropriately when confronted with problematic and inappropriate behavior by patrons. Additional reports, cited by Saltz,[192] provided limited evidence of the effectiveness of techniques of effective alcohol management (TEAM) in sports facilities and of a short training program for servers and managers in selected establishments.

Although selected aspects of server training have been implemented and evaluated—with encouraging results—the systematic development and assessment of comprehensive community-based programs is rare.[192] Delewski and Saltz[191] have provided a preliminary assessment of one such program in California. With regard to the legal environment, The Model Alcoholic Beverage Retail Licensee Liability (Dram Shop) Act of 1985 has been prepared[203] and enacted in several states,[83,204] and server training programs are now mandatory in several jurisdictions.[83,190]

The widespread adoption of effective, comprehensive programs could have a significant impact on mortality and morbidity from drinking and driving. O'Donnell[205] showed that about half of intoxicated drivers involved in motor vehicle crashes came from licensed establishments, especially bars. In addition, such programs could have considerable structural and symbolic importance in reshaping regulatory functions and public attitudes toward the prevention of alcohol-related problems generally.[206,207]

Health Promotion Measures

The other major group of primary prevention measures aimed at reducing per capita consumption are those that promote less harmful alcohol use by individuals and communities.[86] These measures include active and passive education interventions, programs targeted at specific populations and problems, the direct facilitation and encouragement of less hazardous drinking, and the curtailment of negative lifestyle influences.

Information and Education

Public Education Programs. Although public education programs can affect public knowledge and attitudes, at least to some extent, and may be useful in bringing about an understanding of and support for alcohol control measures, convincing evidence that such programs result in behavior change leading to a reduction in per capita consumption is lacking.[30,33,38,46,94,96,208-211] Rootman[210] concluded, like others before[30,33,46,94,208,209] and after[38,96,211] him, that evidence for the effectiveness of public education programs in controlling alcohol consumption and preventing alcohol problems is equivocal. Although some studies suggest that these programs can affect alcohol consumption, most do not support this conclusion. The limitations of the data underlying this conclusion have been stressed repeatedly.[30,33,38,46,94,96,208-211] Since public education is the only preventive measure in the health-related alcohol control program in many countries, the need for well-designed and carefully evaluated experimental programs is evident.

Mass media campaigns can stimulate interest both in the prevention of alcohol-related health problems and in community-wide organization and development toward this end.[33] The media also are influential in setting public agendas—the press is more influential with opinion leaders and television with the general public.[46] Realistic goals for mass media interventions may not include changing health behavior.[210] Flay and Sobel[211] noted that the chief weaknesses in mass media campaigns are the failure to even reach the audience, the heavy reliance on information and fear messages, and the failure to target messages to identifiable audiences. They concluded that the most effective use of mass media programs is in combination with complementary elements, such as school programs, that include interpersonal communication. Although some media campaigns, in particular those that are sustained over a long period of time, focused on a specific behavior, and integrated with other approaches, may be effective,[210] overall these campaigns may be best suited for reinforcing existing attitudes and social norms.[96]

Health Warning Labels. Health warning labels on containers, in advertisements, and at the point of service or purchase comprise a passive approach intended to influence knowledge, attitudes, and behavior, one repeatedly recommended. In 1979, an attempt to legislate a general warning label failed to pass the U.S. Congress.[212] In the early 1980s, several local jurisdictions in the United States passed ordinances requiring the display, wherever alcoholic beverages are sold, of warning posters linking alcohol consumption during pregnancy to birth defects.[212] In New York City, the first (1983) jurisdiction to require such postings, evidence of the effectiveness of posters in increasing unaided awareness of the alcohol–birth defects link was found in both men and women.[213]

Support for health warning labels is widespread. In a Gallup poll conducted in 1986, 79% of Americans favored educational labeling on containers.[214] In a June 1987 report to the U.S. Congress, the literature on the effects of health warning labels was reviewed with three conclusions: health warning labels can have an impact on the consumer if they take account of factors that influence consumer response to warning labels, health warning labels can have an impact on the consumer if they are designed effectively, and studies of the impact of health warning labels in real world situations have concluded that the labels have an impact on consumer behavior.[215] In 1988, the Alcoholic Beverage Labeling Act was enacted. Rules and regulations implementing this act require the following warning on the labels of all containers of alcoholic beverages bottled on and after November 18, 1989, for sale or distribution in the United States: *Government Warning: (1) According to the Surgeon General, women should not drink alcoholic beverages during pregnancy because of the risk of birth defects. (2) Consumption of alcoholic beverages impairs your ability to drive a car or operate machinery, and may cause health problems.*[216]

This health warning is only a beginning. The American Public Health Association has called on the federal government to increase the effectiveness of alcohol warning labels by developing easily readable and rotating warnings that additionally include information on the risk of alcohol poisoning, cancer, addiction, and other long-term health problems. As well, it supports state and local laws and regulations requiring health and safety warning posters at locations where alcoholic beverages are sold.[217] The Safe Water and Toxic Enforcement Act of 1986 (Proposition 65) approved by California voters is an example of a state initiative requiring clear and reasonable warning to consumers regarding exposures to chemicals that can cause cancer or reproductive harm. This act subsequently enabled the posting and display of warning notices and signs in bars, restaurants, and off-premise retail settings about birth defects resulting from alcohol use in pregnancy.[218]

Targeted Health Promotion Programs

Specific Populations. Programs to promote less hazardous alcohol use have been aimed at specific population subgroups, notably the elderly, minorities, and subsets of women, youth, and the children of alcoholics.[30,33,38,219] Some elderly persons do become heavy drinkers, sometimes in conjunction with loss or loneliness resulting from retirement or the death of a spouse.[33,220-222] Proposed preventive approaches to reactive or situational drinking include interventions to strengthen coping mechanisms and improve socialization and interaction with peers, for example, self-help groups, as well as a greater emphasis on preretirement planning.[33,220,221] Attention has been drawn to gender issues in the primary prevention of alcohol problems.[223,224] Programs specifically targeted at women have been developed, but most have lacked adequate evaluation components,[224] and most have been targeted at drinking during pregnancy.[225] Some prevention programs have been aimed at ethnic and racial minorities; few have been adequately evaluated.[33,226-231] Although current data indicate that harmful alcohol use patterns in some racial groups can be attributed, at least partly, to sociocultural factors, uncertainty remains as to the role of genetic factors.[33,38] The recent recognition of the high risk of alcoholism among the children of alcoholics has precipitated prevention initiatives aimed at this population group. These require evaluation.[219]

Numerous education programs are aimed at subsets of youth and, as well, at groups of adults who interact with young people and are in a position to influence their drinking.[33,38,96] Significant increases in knowledge often are observed, as, in a few cases, are changes in attitudes toward alcohol or toward self and others, especially when attitude change has been an explicit goal and when instruction by peers and group discussion were part of the instructional method.[33,232] In some programs, notably those using peer leaders,[233] modest decrements in actual drinking have been found.[33] Generally, however, the impact of programs on alcohol consumption has been limited at best or uncertain.[38,96,232] Frequently, the evaluation has been imprecise or flawed.[33,38,96]

Given the multiple factors posited as playing roles in behavior change, it is not surprising that educational programs based exclusively or primarily on the transfer of factual information have limited effect on alcohol use. It is disappointing, however, that more comprehensive educational approaches have been similarly unsuccessful. An example is "Here's Looking at You," a model alcohol education curriculum employing a values clarification and decision-making approach.[38] Designed to enhance knowledge and self-esteem, instill appropriate attitudes, and teach decision-making skills necessary for youth to make responsible decisions about the use of alcohol, this curriculum, when implemented approximately as intended, was ineffective in achieving its goals.[234] A recent analysis suggests that the variables addressed in it make such a small independent contribution to alcohol consumption that even a highly successful classroom program would be unlikely to do much to prevent alcohol use or abuse by youth.[235]

Programs employing social influences approaches appear more promising. Project SMART tested the relative effectiveness of a program based on this approach (incorporating elements of peer pressure resistance training, correction of normative expectations, inoculation against mass media messages, information about parental and other adult influences, peer leadership, and other related components) against a drug-specific program based on values clarification and decision making (containing elements on the enhancement of self-esteem and self-image, stress management, values clarification, decision making, and goal setting) and a control situation.[236] In seventh grade students, the social influences approach was successful in delaying the onset of drug use, including alcohol use, whereas students receiving the other approach had significantly more alcohol use than did control students in the final posttests carried out about a year after the study began. Other studies, however, suggest that although specific program approaches may have specific effects on knowledge, attitudes and, possibly, behavior, program content is only one of several variables that may affect the outcome of prevention programs for schoolchildren.[237-239]

Recently, the initial effects of a comprehensive, community-based program for preventing drug abuse in youth have been reported.[240] In the Midwestern Prevention Project, 22,550 sixth and seventh grade adolescents in the Kansas City metropolitan area received the school-based drug education program component, with parental involvement in homework and mass media programming. The prevalence of cigarette smoking, alcohol use, and marijuana use were all significantly lower at the 1-year follow-up in the intervention condition relative to a delayed intervention condition (Indianapolis), indicating a slowing in drug use onset. Preliminary results of the 2-year follow-up suggest maintenance of the program effect over time. However, in a subsequent analysis of statistical issues in the evaluation of this project, it was pointed out that sampling variation was a plausible explanation for the intervention effect observed for alcohol use at 1 year.[241] Programs employing multiple community approaches may prove to be more successful than school-based programs in preventing adolescent alcohol use, but additional evidence of effectiveness is required.

In 1988, 97% of college campuses in the United States had some sort of education or prevention program, 77% had a special task force that focused on alcohol education and prevention, and 87% reported an increase since 1979 in educational programming efforts, including student workshops, discussion groups, speakers, alcohol and other drug awareness weeks, and media campaigns.[242] In a review of 14 programs with strong evaluation designs, Goodstadt and Caleekal-John[243] concluded that college programs are effective, particularly those that include field or laboratory experiences and occur over an extended period. However, Moskowitz[96] challenged this positive assessment, noting that selection bias may have accounted for the effects. In Ontario, Canada, the evaluation of a campus alcohol policies and education program (CAPE), although promising, has highlighted an array of implementation, maintenance, and evaluation difficulties.[244]

Specific Problems. Programs designed to encourage less hazardous drinking have been targeted at particular alcohol-related health problems. Programs for preventing damage to the fetus are one example. The best documented program is the Fetal Alcohol Syndrome Demonstration Program at the University of Washington in Seattle.[20,33] Although this comprehensive program was successful in increasing the number of women who became abstinent during pregnancy, it was less successful in reaching pregnant women drinking at higher levels associated with clear risks to the fetus. The need for more intensive strategies in high-risk pregnant women was further evident in results of interviews of different samples of pregnant women living in Seattle in 1974–1975 and 1980–1981.[245] In the interim, the study population was exposed to public media and education programs, coupled with a vigorous program of professional education. Although the proportion of women drinking during pregnancy decreased during this interval, the proportion drinking at least 1 ounce of absolute alcohol per day before pregnancy recognition was relatively unchanged, suggesting that problem-specific programs should be targeted to high-risk groups.

Drinking and driving programs are another example of education–information targeted to a specific alcohol-related problem. In a recent comprehensive review of school-based programs for the prevention of drinking and driving, it was concluded that programs based on accurate information, nonthreatening attempts to change attitudes, and behavioral peer intervention techniques consistently demonstrate knowledge gains and, in some cases, appropriate changes in attitudes and self-reported behavior immediately after the intervention, but these effects often dissipate with time. Their impact on actual drinking–driving behavior has not been examined, and although they hold promise, a number of development, implementation, and evaluation issues remain to be addressed.[246,247]

Two Canadian mass media campaigns on drinking and driving have been reviewed in the context of an evaluation of drinking–driving countermeasures.[248] These were well-designed programs with few of the methodological shortcomings common to many other studies. Both evaluated impacts on traffic safety, knowledge, and attitudes. Both campaigns were successful in conveying information to the public and producing short-term impacts on impaired driving. Attitudinal changes, however, were inconsistent, and the long-term impact was not determined in either study. The authors concluded that public education–information programs may educate the public and may have short-term impacts on impaired driving, but clear-cut evidence of reduced traffic accidents is still lacking. Atkin,[249] in drawing a similar conclusion, pointed out that the effectiveness of mass media campaigns will depend on how well they target specific audience segments and specific behavior changes, take into account the target audience's baseline knowledge, beliefs, attitudes, and values, determine which cognitive and affective orientations need to be made more or less salient, enhance personal efficacy and performance skills, use appropriate communication channels, and carry out preliminary component evaluation and pretesting research.

As well, mass media campaigns are more likely to be successful as part of a multifaceted intervention rather than as a stand-alone program.[250] In one community education program to reduce impaired driving, drink calculators were disseminated to customers of bars and licensed beverage outlets, bartenders and counter clerks were trained to demonstrate the use of the calculators, and demonstrations were presented in television spots.[251,252] Program components were evaluated in three matched communities, one receiving the multifaceted program, one receiving the TV spots only, and one serving as a control. After 6 months of intervention, a roadside survey of nighttime drivers indicated fewer drivers with blood alcohol concentrations above 0.05% in the community exposed to the multifaceted approach compared to the TV only and control communities.

With respect to drinking and driving (and other alcohol-related problems), it must be emphasized that the role of education goes well beyond the objective of changing personal alcohol use and safety behaviors. It includes the objectives of changing social norms and enhancing the actions of decision makers in addressing environmental influences on personal behavior and in enacting health protection measures.[250]

Less Hazardous Drinking. Another approach to preventing alcohol-related problems is to encourage new patterns of less hazardous drinking in place of traditional, more harmful ones. Opponents of this approach argue that such new drinking patterns develop in addition to, rather than in place of, existing patterns, resulting in increases in overall consumption.[253]

Beverage Substitution. A long-standing popular view is that beer is a beverage of moderation, alcohol-related problems being attributable mainly to the use of distilled spirits.[54,129] This view is promoted by the brewers and vigorously opposed by the distillers. If this view is valid, one approach to the prevention of alcohol-related problems would be to encourage the substitution of beverages of moderation for those deemed to be more hazardous. The beverage substitution approach, however, has been challenged.[253] There is little justification for promoting one beverage over another. With minor exceptions, all appear equally hazardous. It is the total amount of alcohol consumed rather than the specific beverage vehicle that determines most adverse health outcomes.[54,90,254–256] As well, this approach lacks empirical justification. Past attempts to change drinking patterns consistently have failed. Single[253] cited the striking situation in Finland after institution of a policy favoring the consumption of beer. Although beer consumption increased, it was not at the expense of hard liquor, the use of which continued to increase.[134,253] De Lint[254] concluded that the promotion of new drinking practices does not undermine traditional drinking patterns, with the net result that alcohol consumption is increased. On the other hand, restrictions on traditional drinking practices, for example, during strikes or as the result of price increases, do result in beverage substitution[47,253] without an increase in overall consumption.[253]

Low Alcohol Content Beverages. A variation on the beverage substitution approach is to encourage the use of low alcohol content beverages in place of traditional, regular strength ones. When a low alcohol content beer was marketed in Ontario, Canada, most use was substitutive.[257] However, the situations in which alcoholic beverages were used increased, with a concomitant increase in the use of beer in some persons' drinking practices. The most serious consequence from the public health viewpoint may be the expansion of some drinking repertoires in vulnerable areas, such as drinking with meals.[257] Mäkelä and associates[47] noted that product differentiation may recruit new consumers by breaking down cultural barriers that insulate certain groups from drinking. Youth and women appear to be more likely to accept new types of light and mixed drinks, but once they start to drink, they may switch to more traditional beverages. With the recruitment of new drinkers and drinkers to new drinking occasions, overall consumption will increase. On the other hand, the recruitment of drinkers of traditional, regular strength beverages to low alcohol content beverages might reduce overall consumption, with beneficial public health effects.

Skog[258] investigated the effect of introducing a new light beer in Norway. The introduction was moderately supported by advertising. Point estimates of consumption suggested substitution, but the effect was not statistically significant, and the shift was too small to be of public health importance. In Sweden, however, legislation removing medium strong beer from ordinary shops and replacing it with lower alcohol content beer has been credited with a substantial fall in the sale of alcohol. It may have been one of the factors contributing to sizable declines in mortality from and inpatient care for certain alcohol-related problems, including liver cirrhosis and pancreatitis.[259]

Whether or not less hazardous drinking patterns would result from a legislated lowering of the alcohol content of all beverages (thereby actually curtailing physical accessibility via a health protection measure) is not known,[73] but this approach is feasible.[260] Some drinkers might adjust their volume of consumption upward to compensate for the reduction of alcohol content.[73] That most drinkers would do so, however, seems unlikely, particularly if the usual packaging and service units for off- and on-premise purchase remained unchanged. Further, in an experimental situation, light beer is not readily discriminated from regular beer.[261–263] An alternative approach would be to decrease the size of traditional packaging and service units while leaving alcohol content unchanged.

A price policy (via taxation) favoring low alcohol content beverages could result in preferential shifts toward these beverages.[73] In introducing differential pricing, the cost of regular strength beverages should be increased relative to low alcohol content beverages, for which prevailing prices should be maintained.[46] Maintenance of a price structure that clearly favors the consumption of nonalcoholic beverages also is important. In parts of the United States, beer can be obtained at equal or less cost than soft drinks, an unheard of situation 20 years ago.[129] Such regulatory changes would be in keeping with changing public attitudes and practices in North America. The pubic is now less tolerant of heavy drinking, and beverage preferences are shifting to lower alcohol content beverages.[176,264]

Curtailment of Negative Lifestyle Influences. Whereas the alcohol beverage industry vigorously argues that its promotional efforts are intended only to affect the brand preferences of adult consumers, a consideration of actual practices indicates much broader objectives. These activities are designed to increase or at least maintain consumption by augmenting the variety of drinking practices and encouraging their diffusion, recruit new drinkers, increase or maintain the consumption of established drinkers, and favorably alter perceptions of the role of alcohol in society, particularly among the young, minorities, women, and other expansible markets.[46,73,257,265–268] Such activities undermine promotion of less hazardous alcohol use.

Advertising and Marketing. Whether alcohol beverage advertising per se increases overall consumption is controversial.[38,249,269] Some econometric data suggest a statistically significant, but small, positive relationship between advertising and consumption.[122,270] In analyses controlling for other variables, Strickland[271] found a small, statistically significant association between advertising and alcohol consumption in young Americans, and Franke and Wilcox[272] found that total advertising expenditure in the United States was significantly but weakly related to the consumption of wine and spirits. Schweitzer and associates[152] suggested that a ban on advertising in the United States would lead to a shift in consumption from beer to distilled spirits, which would be accompanied by a small decrease in total alcohol consumption. Other econometric studies, however, have shown no effect of advertising on total alcohol sales or beverage classes.[269] Smart[269] has stressed the limitations of most econometric studies, in particular their inability to examine the effects of advertising on groups targeted by the industry, such as youth, women, and minorities, and the limited range of advertising expenditures considered. Experimental studies of individual drinkers have shown that distilled spirits[273] and wine advertisements[274] may encourage drinking. Other investigations of the relationship between advertising and consumption, both at the population[275] and individual[276,277] levels, have failed to find important associations.

Since evidence on the potential effect of restrictions on alcohol advertising per se is equivocal[73,94,269,278,279] and unraveling the effects poses many logistic and methodological problems,[38,249,269] decisions to restrict advertising may need to be made on other than scientific grounds.[277–280] Advertising represents only one part of the marketing and promotional efforts of the alcohol industry that must be considered in determining an appropriate health promotion strategy.[73,265,281] Mosher[83,265] has described the total marketing concept employed by the industry to exploit the commercial beverage market. Intense promotional campaigns are but one of several strategies, including availability, price differentials, and product diversification, that comprise total marketing, an approach that places alcohol in its various forms in competition with all other beverages, including tap water.

Studies of the perceptions of Scottish children and adolescents refute the contention of the alcohol industry that advertisements are targeted only at persons who have attained the legal drinking age and provide evidence that advertising reinforces underage drinking[282,283] Alcohol advertising contributes to the social normative beliefs of adolescents regarding the acceptability of alcohol and to positive feelings toward drinking.[284] A nationwide survey of 1200 Americans, ages 12 to 22, found that alcohol advertising contributes to certain forms of problem drinking, specifically excessive drinking and drinking in dangerous contexts.[285] The targeting of U.S. college students for alcohol promotion, especially beer promotion, has been documented.[286] An expert panel has recommended that alcohol promotion and advertising be eliminated on college campuses where a high proportion of the audience is under the legal drinking age (now 21 years in all states).[287]

Media Portrayals. A pervasive form of alcohol promotion occurs through the portrayal of alcohol use on television[280,288–290] and in feature films.[291] Breed and de Foe[289] have documented the increased use of alcohol and alcohol-related acts in television situation comedies and dramas from 1950 to 1982 in the United States, noting that alcohol use in much television programming is a significant distortion of real life. For example, alcohol is the preferred beverage of characters, whereas in real life it ranks below water, soft drinks, coffee, and tea. They suggest that if modeling and social learning theories are borne out and if television stars continue their rate of drinking, increases in alcohol consumption and alcohol-related problems could occur. Wallack and colleagues,[290] in a study of prime time television programs in the fall of 1984, estimated that a regular viewer likely would see more that 20 drinking acts per evening. Many of these acts portray alcohol use in a glamorous context. Further, it is implied that alcohol is to be taken for granted, that its use is routine and even necessary, that most people drink, and that drinking is part of everyday life. Although the effects of these portrayals on viewers' actual consumption is not clear,[291] there is some evidence that the attitudes of children to alcohol may be influenced adversely.[292,293] Several approaches have been suggested,[294,295] including cooperative consultation to redress the distorted picture of alcohol use on television, with the goal of educating media personnel to make informed decisions about alcohol material without damaging entertainment value.

Preventive Health Services

Preventive health services comprise the third group of prevention strategies (Table 43–8). Unlike primary prevention strategies aimed at reducing per capita consumption with a resulting decrease in the incidence of heavy drinking and related problems, these services are secondary prevention measures aimed at the early detection of and effective intervention in heavy drinking, thus preventing its consequences. Inherently, secondary prevention is a less attractive approach. Nonetheless, it is a useful backup strategy when primary prevention is not possible. Given the failure of many communities to introduce effective primary prevention, a focus on preventive health services is appropriate.

Early Detection. Recent studies have shown that early identification of heavy drinkers is possible in several ways.[44,296,297] Much attention has been directed to the use of laboratory tests,[44,296–300] although a higher diagnostic accuracy of brief questionnaires, such as the Michigan Alcohol Screening Test (MAST) and the CAGE, has been demonstrated.[44,301,302] Their use in the assessment of high-risk individuals, such as hospital inpatients and primary care outpatients, has been shown to improve detection of problem drinkers in comparison to usual physician detection rates,[303,304] and their use is feasible in community settings as well.[305] Skinner and associates[306] showed that a brief, 5-item trauma scale is of value in the detection of excessive drinking and recommended its use, along with laboratory tests and a brief questionnaire. Cyr and Wartman[307] showed that two questions in the MAST ("Have you ever had a drinking problem?" and "When was your last drink?") are highly sensitive (91.5%) in combination. They recommended their inclusion as routine items in the medical history. A 10-item screening instrument has been developed by the World Health Organization incorporating questions on the amount and frequency of drinking, on dependence on alcohol and, on alcohol-related problems.[308] A disguised clinical screening procedure combining two history questions, five clinical examination items, and one laboratory test, has been developed.[308]

Skinner and associates[309–311] have identified a constellation of early indicators of alcohol abuse, including psychosocial factors, laboratory indicators, and clinical signs and symptoms. The more abnormalities found among these factors, the higher the likelihood of alcohol abuse. Of 108 clinical signs, medical history items, and laboratory tests, 17 clinical signs and 13 medical history items formed a highly diagnostic instrument, the Alcohol Clinical Index, suitable for use in clinical settings.[312] A probability of alcohol abuse exceeding 0.90 was found if four or more clinical items or four or more medical history items from the index were present. These results suggest that simple, noninvasive, immediate feedback clinical measures provide high diagnostic accuracy.

Effective Intervention. Recent evidence strongly suggests that brief interventions in the early stages of heavy drinking are both feasible and effective.[44] Edwards and colleagues,[313] in a controlled clinical trial of intensive inpatient–outpatient treatment vs brief advice for alcoholism, found the latter to be more effective in nondependent alcohol abusers after 2 years of follow-up,[314] whereas physically dependent patients achieved better results with more intensive treatment. In a randomized controlled trial of general practitioner intervention in patients with excessive alcohol consumption, Wallace and associates[315] showed that advice on reducing alcohol consumption was effective. If the results of their study were applied to the United Kingdom, intervention by general practitioners in the first year could reduce to moderate levels the alcohol consumption of some 250,000 men and 67,500 women who currently drink to excess. Other studies have shown the effectiveness of brief intervention in socially stable, healthy, problem drinkers who do not have a high degree of alcohol dependence and whose histories of problem drinking are short.[316–320] A careful assessment of alcohol dependence in detected heavy drinkers underpins the determination of the appropriateness of brief intervention.[311]

The degree of alcohol dependence also is crucial in determining whether the treatment goal should be moderation (i.e., controlled drinking) or abstinence.[44,311,321] Moderation appears to be a realistic alternative in problem drinkers who are not heavily alcohol dependent, as is often the case in the early-stage heavy drinkers.[44,48,311,317,322,323] It may be a more acceptable treatment goal, particularly in environments where alcohol use is especially diffuse[50] and among young drinkers, who may perceive the costs of abstinence to outweigh the risks from continued drinking.[311,324]

A five-step early intervention and treatment strategy for use in clinical practice settings has been developed,[311] along with self-help manuals[44] and procedures for teaching moderate drinking and abstinence.[325] Evaluations of brief interventions conducted as part of a general health screening project,[299] among problem drinkers in a general hospital,[326,327] in community referral centers for referred problem drinkers,[48,328] and in a family practice setting[329] are promising. This approach may be applicable beyond the clinical setting, for example, in the workplace, with considerable potential for public health impact.[33,48]

Skinner[330] has discussed the reasons why early detection and effective intervention strategies deserve major emphasis. To summarize: most heavy drinkers do not seek treatment for their alcohol problems, socially stable persons at early stages of problem drinking have a better prognosis, health professionals in primary care settings are in an excellent position to identify problem drinkers, and brief intervention by health professionals can be effective in reducing heavy alcohol use. Skinner cited reasons why early detection and effective intervention are not occurring, namely, widespread pessimism among health professionals about being able to intervene effectively, confusion regarding responsibility for confronting alcohol problems, uncertainly about the target population, lack of appreciation of what are appropriate interventions, and deficiencies in the practical skills and techniques to carry them out. He suggested that a simple basic strategy[330] for secondary prevention be adopted, that training materials and opportunities be readily available and incorporated into core education programs, and that strenuous efforts be made to convince key people in the health professions to give early detection and effective intervention a high priority.

THE PRIMACY OF PREVENTION

The need for public policy that takes into account the enormous toll of adverse health consequences arising from alcohol use is urgent. The general liberalization of alcohol control policies in North America and worldwide over the last three decades, accompanied by expanded production and vigorous promotion, has resulted in widespread, substantial increases in alcohol consumption and related problems. In developing healthy public policy, a reconciliation of economic, social, and political interests with the health aspects of alcohol use must be achieved. This will be a major undertaking. However, an environment conducive to such policy development is emerging in the United States with the leadership of organizations such as the National Association for Public Health Policy.

The usual response of governments to alcohol-related health problems has been to increase treatment services, leaving unaddressed the root cause: conflicting public policies. This approach implies unlimited resources for health care expenditures, certainly an unrealistic tenet in the current fiscal climate. Of necessity, a shift toward the implementation of effective preventive strategies will occur. Research conducted over the last three decades has provided a solid basis for the identification of such strategies. It is noteworthy that for the first time a reduction in alcohol consumption (to 2 gallons per person age 14 and older per year from a baseline of 2.54 gallons per person age 14 and older in 1987) has been recommended as a health objective for the United States by the year 2000.[331]

REFERENCES

1. Rankin JG, Ashley MJ: Alcohol-related problems and their prevention. In Last JM (ed): Maxcy-Rosenau Public Health and Preventive Medicine, 12 edt. Norwalk, Conn.: Appleton-Century-Crofts, 1986, pp 1039–1073
2. Bruun K, Edwards G, Lumio M, et al: Alcohol Control Policies in Public Health Perspective. The Finnish Foundation for Alcohol

Studies, Vol 25, Helsinki: The Finnish Foundation for Alcohol Studies, 1975

3. Popham RE, Schmidt W: The biomedical definition of safe alcohol consumption: A crucial issue for the researcher and the drinker. Br J Addict 73:233–235, 1978
4. Kreitman N: Alcohol consumption and the prevention paradox. Br J Addict 81:353–363, 1986
5. Kalant H: Effects of ethanol on the nervous system. In Tremolieres T (ed): International Encyclopedia of Pharmacology and Therapeutics, Vol 1, Section 20, Alcohol and Derivatives. Oxford: Permagon, 1970
6. Gross MM: Psychobiological contributions to the alcohol dependence syndrome: A selective review of recent research. In Edwards G, Gross MM, Keller M, et al (eds): Alcohol Related Disabilities. Geneva, World Health Organization, 1977, pp 107–131
7. Borkenstein RF, Crowther RF, Shumate RP, et al: The Role of the Drinking Driver in Traffic Accidents. Bloomington, Ind.: Department of Police Administration, Indiana University, 1964
8. Lieber CS: Medical disorders of alcoholism. Pathogenesis and treatment. In Smith LH Jr (ed): Major Problems in Internal Medicine, Vol 22. Philadelphia: WB Saunders, 1982
9. Lindenbaum J: Metabolic effects of alcohol on the blood and bone marrow. In Lieber CS (ed): Metabolic Aspects of Alcoholism. Baltimore: University Park Press, 1977, pp 215–247
10. Remmers JE: Obstructive sleep apnea. A common disorder exacerbated by alcohol. Am Rev Respir Dis 130:153–155, 1984
11. Rankin JG: Alcohol—A specific toxin or nutrient displacer. In Hawkens WW (ed): Drug-Nutrient Interrelationships: Nutrition & Pharmacology—An Interphase of Disciplines, Miles Symposium III. Hamilton, Ontario, McMaster University, 1974, pp 71–87
12. Taasan VC, Block AJ, Boysen PG, et al: Alcohol increases sleep apnea and oxygen desaturation in asymptomatic men. Am J Med 71:240–245, 1981
13. Issa FQ, Sullivan CE: Alcohol, snoring and sleep apnea. J Neurol Neurosurg Psychiatry 45:353–359, 1983
14. Bonora M, Shields GI, Knuth SL, et al: Selective depression by ethanol of upper airway respiratory activity in cats. Am Rev Respir Dis 130:156–161, 1984
15. Krol RC, Knuth SL, Bartlett D Jr: Selective reduction of genioglossal muscle activity by alcohol in normal human subjects. Am Rev Respir Dis 129:247–250, 1984
16. Ashley MJ, Olin JS, le Riche WH, et al: The physical disease characteristics of inpatient alcoholics. J Stud Alcohol 42:1–14, 1981
17. Ashley MJ, Rankin JG: Hazardous alcohol consumption and diseases of the circulatory system. J Stud Alcohol 41:1040–1070, 1980
18. Popham RE, Schmidt W, Israelstam S: Heavy alcohol consumption and physical health problems. A review of the epidemiologic evidence. In Smart RG, Cappell HD, Glaser FB, et al (eds): Research Advances in Alcohol and Drug Problems, Vol 8. New York: Plenum Press, 1984, pp 149–182
19. Péquignot G, Tuyns A: Rations d'alcool consommées "declarées" et risques pathologiques. In In INSERM. Paris: INSERM, 1975, pp 1–15
20. Streissguth AP, Clarren SK, Jones KL. Natural history of the fetal alcohol syndrome. Lancet 2:85–92, 1985
21. Little RE, Streissguth AP: Effects of alcohol on the fetus: Impact and prevention. Can Med Assoc J 125:159–164, 1981
22. Addiction Research Foundation: Know the Score. Toronto: Addiction Research Foundation, 1979
23. Health Education Council: That's the Limit. London: Health Education Council, 1986
24. Royal College of General Practitioners: Alcohol—A Balanced View. London: Royal College of General Practitioners, 1986
25. Royal College of Psychiatrists: Alcohol Our Favourite Drug. London: Tavistock, 1986
26. Alcohol Concern: The Drinking Revolution. Building a Campaign for Safer Drinking. London: Alcohol Concern, 1987
27. Pols RG, Hawks DV: Is there a safe level of daily consumption of alcohol for men and women? Recommendations regarding responsible drinking behavior. Technical Report for the National Health and Medical Research Council, Health Care Committee. Canberra: Australian Government Publishing Service, 1987
28. Royal College of Physicians: A Great and Growing Evil: The Medical Consequences of Alcohol Abuse. London: Tavistock, 1987
29. US Department of Health and Human Services: The Surgeon General's Report on Nutrition and Health. Summary and Recommendations. DHHS (PHS) Publication No. 88-50211. Washington, DC: US Government Printing Office, 1988
30. Moser J: Prevention of Alcohol-related Problems: An International Review of Preventive Measures, Policies, and Programmes. Published on behalf of the World Health Organization by the Alcoholism and Drug Addiction Research Foundation, Toronto, 1980
31. Health and Welfare Canada: Alcohol in Canada. A National Perspective, 2 edt, rev. Ottawa: Health and Welfare Canada, 1984
32. Van Natta P, Malin H, Bertolucci D, et al: The influence of alcohol abuse as a hidden contributor to mortality. Alcohol 2:535–539, 1985
33. US Department of Health and Human Services: Fifth Special Report to the US Congress on Alcohol and Health from the Secretary of Health and Human Services. DHHS Publication No. (ADM) 84-1291, Washington DC: US Government Printing Office, 1983
34. Ableson J, Paddon P, Strohmenger C: Perspectives on health. Statistics Canada, Catalogue 82-540. Ottawa: Occasional, 1983
35. Ouellet BL, Romeder J-M, Lance J-M: Premature mortality attributable to smoking and hazardous drinking in Canada. Am J Epidemiol 109:451–463, 1979
36. Smart RG, Mann RE: Large decreases in alcohol-related problems following a slight reduction in alcohol consumption in Ontario 1975–83. Br J Addict 82:285–291, 1987
37. Mann RE, Smart RG, Anglin L: Reductions in liver cirrhosis mortality in Canada: Demographic differences and possible explanations. Alcoholism Clin Exp Res 12:1–8, 1988
38. US Department of Health and Human Services: Sixth Special Report to the US Congress on Alcohol and Health from the Secretary of Health and Human Services. DHHS Publication No. (ADM) 87-1519, Rockville, MD: US Government Printing Office, 1987
39. US Bureau of the Census: Statistical Abstract of the United States, 106 edt. Washington, DC: US Bureau of the Census, 1985
40. Addiction Research Foundation: Statistics on Alcohol and Drug Use in Canada and Other Countries. Toronto: Addiction Research Foundation, 1982
41. Encyclopedia Britannica, 15 edt. Chicago: Encyclopaedia Britannica, 1977, Macropaedia, Vol 9, p 937
42. Baasher T: The use of drugs in the Islamic world. Br J Addict 76:233–243, 1981
43. Produktschap voor Gedistilleerde Dranken: How many alcoholic beverages are being consumed throughout the world. Schiedam, Nederland: Produktschap voor Gedistilleerde Dranken, 1986
44. Babor TF, Ritson EB, Hodgson RJ: Alcohol-related problems in the primary health care setting: A review of early intervention strategies. Br J Addict 81:23–46, 1986
45. Hyman MH, Zimmermann MA, Gurioli C, et al: Drinkers, Drinking and Alcohol-related Mortality and Hospitalizations. A Statistical Compendium, 1980 edt. New Brunswick, NJ: Center for Alcohol Studies, Rutgers University, 1980
46. Addiction Research Foundation: Alcohol, Public Education and Social Policy. Report of the Task Force on Public Education and Social Policy. Toronto: Addiction Research Foundation, 1981
47. Mäkelä K, Room R, Single E, et al: Alcohol, Society, and the State I: A Comparative Study of Alcohol Control. Toronto: Addiction Research Foundation, 1981
48. Babor TF, Treffardier M, Weill J, et al: Early detection and secondary prevention of alcoholism in France. J Stud Alcohol 44:600–616, 1983
49. Chaudron CD, Wilkinson DA: In Chaudron CD, Wilkinson DA (eds): Theories on Alcoholism. Toronto: Addiction Research Foundation, 1988
50. Coulson NJ: Islamic law. In Encyclopedia Britannica, 15 edt. Syd-

ney: Encyclopaedia Britannica, 1977, Macropaedia, Vol 9, pp 938–943

51. Harrison B: Drink and the Victorians. The Temperance Question in England 1815–1872. London: Faber & Faber, 1971
52. Levine HG: The discovery of addiction. Changing conceptions of habitual drunkenness in America. J Stud Alcohol 39:143–174, 1978
53. Gusfield J: Symbolic Crusade: Status Politics and the American Temperance Movement. Urbana, Ill.: University of Illinois Press, 6:140, 1963
54. Popham RE, Schmidt W, de Lint J: The effects of legal restraint on drinking. In Kissin B, Begleiter H (eds): The Biology of Alcoholism, Vol 4. Social Aspects of Alcoholism. New York: Plenum Press, 1976, pp 579–625
55. Beauchamp DE: Beyond Alcoholism. Alcohol and Public Health Policy. Philadelphia: Temple University Press, 1980
56. Alcoholics Anonymous: Alcoholics Anonymous, 3 edt. New York: Alcoholics Anonymous World Services, 1976
57. Schmidt W, Popham RE: Alcohol Problems and Their Prevention. A Public Health Perspective. Toronto: Addiction Research Foundation, 1980
58. Goodwin DW: Is Alcoholism Hereditary? New York: Oxford University Press, 1976
59. Cloninger CR, Bohman M, Sigvardsson S: Inheritance of alcohol abuse. Arch Gen Psychiatry 38:861–868, 1981
60. von Knorring A-L, Bohman M, von Knorring L, et al: Platelet monoamine oxidase as a biological marker in subgroups of alcoholism. Acta Psychiatr Scand 72:51–58, 1985
61. Lester D: Genetic theory—An assessment of the heritability of alcoholism. In Chaudron DC, Wilkinson DA (eds): Theories on Alcoholism. Toronto: Addiction Research Foundation, 1988, pp 1–28
62. Ullman AD: Sociocultural backgrounds conducive to alcoholism. Ann Am Acad Polit Sci 315:48–55, 1958
63. Chafetz M: Alcoholism prevention and reality. Q J Stud Alcohol 28:345–348, 1967
64. Single E: The availability theory of alcohol-related problems. In Chaudron DC, Wilkinson DA (eds): Theories on Alcoholism. Toronto: Addiction Research Foundation, 1988, pp 325–352
65. Ledermann S: Alcool, alcoolisme, alcoolisation. v.1. Données scientifique de caractère physiologique, economique et social, Vol. 1. Institut National d'Etudes Démographiques, Travaux et Documents, Cahier. No.29. Paris: Presses Universitaires de France, 1956
66. Ledermann S: Alcool, Alcoolisme, Alcoolization: Mortalité, Morbitité, Accidents du Travail. Institut National d'Etudes Démographiques, Travaux et Documents, Cahier. No 41. Paris: Presses Universitaires de France, 1964
67. Terris M: Epidemiology of cirrhosis of the liver. Am J Public Health 57:2076–2088, 1967
68. de Lint J, Schmidt W: The distribution of alcohol consumption in Ontario. Q J Stud Alcohol 29:968–973, 1968
69. Mäkelä K: Concentration of alcohol consumption. Scand Studies Ciminol 3:77–88, 1971
70. Skög O-J: Alkoholonsumets fordeling i befolkningen (The distribution of alcohol consumption in the population). Oslo: Natl Instit Alcohol Res, 1971
71. Schmidt W: Cirrhosis and alcohol consumption: An epidemiologic perspective. In Edwards G, Grant M. (eds): Alcoholism: New Knowledge New Responses. London: Croom Helm, 1977, pp 15–47
72. Schmidt W, Popham RE: An approach to the control of alcohol consumption. In Rutledge B, Fulton EK (eds): International Collaboration: Problems and Opportunities. Toronto: Addiction Research Foundation of Ontario, 1977, pp 155–164
73. Single E: International perspectives on alcohol as a public health issue. J Public Health Policy 5:238–256, 1984
74. Schmidt W: The epidemiology of cirrhosis of the liver: A statistical analysis of mortality data with special reference to Canada. In Fisher MM, Rankin JG (eds): Alcohol and the Liver. New York: Plenum Press, 1976, pp 1–26
75. Keilman PA: Alcohol consumption and diabetes mellitus mortality in different countries. Am J Public Health 73:1316–1317, 1983
76. La Vecchia C, Decarli A, Mezzanotte G, et al: Mortality from alcohol-related disease in Italy. J Epidemiol Community Health 40: 257–261, 1986
77. Imaizumi Y: Alcoholism mortality rate in Japan. Alcohol Alcoholism 21:159–162, 1986
78. Poikolainen K: Increasing alcohol consumption correlated with hospital admission rates. Br J Addict 78:305–309, 1983
79. Truswell AS, Apeagyei F: Incidence of Wernicke's encephalopathy and Korsakoff's psychosis in Sydney. Unpublished paper presented at a symposium, Alcohol, Nutrition and the Nervous System, Coppleston Postgraduate Medical Institute, University of Sydney, March 18, 1981
80. de Lint J, Schmidt W: Consumption averages and alcoholism prevalence: A brief overview of epidemiological investigations. Br J Addict 66:97–107, 1971
81. Warner KE: Selling Smoke, Cigarette Advertising and Public Health. Washington DC: Am Public Health Assoc, 1986
82. Cavanagh J, Clairmonte F: Alcoholic beverages: Dimensions of corporate power. In Cavanagh J, Clairmonte F, Room R (eds): The World Alcohol Industry with Special Reference to Australia, New Zealand and the Pacific Islands. Sydney: University of Sydney, 1985, pp 1–101
83. Mosher JF, Jernigan DH: New directions in alcohol policy. Annu Rev Public Health 10:245–279, 1989
84. Bruun K: Alcohol Policies in the United Kingdom. Stockholm: Sociologiska Inst.: Stockholm University, 1979, 53 pp
85. McBride RM, Mosher JF: Public health implications of the international alcohol industry: Issues raised by a World Health Organization project: Br J Addict 80:141–147, 1983
86. US Department of Health, Education, and Welfare: Healthy People, Surgeon General's Report on Health Promotion and Disease Prevention. Public Health Service, DEW(PHS) Publication No. 79-55071. Washington, DC: US Government Printing Office, 1979
87. Mosher JF: A new direction in alcohol policy: comprehensive server intervention. In Gerstein DR (ed): Toward the Prevention of Alcohol Problems: Government, Business, and Community Action. Section 4. Engaging the Business Sector. Washington DC: National Academy Press, 1984, pp 57–67
88. Moore MH, Gerstein DR: Alcohol and Public Policy: Beyond the Shadow of Prohibition. Washington, DC: National Academy Press, 1981, p 116
89. Simpson R: Health promotion: The relevance of policy and educational components. In Giesbrecht N, Cox AE (eds): Prevention: Alcohol and the Environment. Issues, Constituencies, and Strategies. Toronto: Addiction Research Foundation, 1986, pp 3–19
90. Popham RE, Schmidt W, de Lint J: The prevention of alcoholism: Epidemiological studies of the effects of government control measures. Br J Addict 70:125–44, 1975
91. Wodak AD, de Burgh SPH: Alcohol control policies. Aust Alcohol Drug Rev 2:68–75, 1983
92. Room R: Alcohol control and public health. Annu Rev Public Health 5:293–317, 1984
93. Gerstein DR (ed): Toward the Prevention of Alcohol Problems: Government, Business, and Community Action. Washington, DC: National Academy Press, 1984
94. Farrell S: Review of National Policy Measures to Prevent Alcohol-related Problems. Geneva: World Health Organization, 1985
95. Single E: The availability of alcohol: Prior research and future directions. Aust Drug Alcohol Rev 7:273–284, 1988
96. Moskowitz JM: The primary prevention of alcohol problems: A critical review of the research literature. J Stud Alcohol 50:54–88, 1989
97. Murray GG, Douglas RR: Social marketing in the alcohol policy arena. Br J Addict 83:505–511, 1988
98. Anderson P: Health authority policies for the prevention of alcohol problems. Br J Addict 84:203–209, 1989

99. Harrison L, Tether P: Data note 13. Alcohol policy and the British government bureaucracy. Br J Addict 83:451–460, 1988
100. Grant M, Plant M, Williams A (eds): Economics and Alcohol: Consumption and Controls. London: Croom Helm, 1983
101. Rush B, Steinberg M, Brook R: The relationship among alcohol availability, alcohol consumption and alcohol-related damage in the Province of Ontario and the State of Michigan 1955–1982. Adv Alcohol Substance Abuse 5:33–44, 1986
102. Holder HD, Blose JO: Reduction of community alcohol problems: Computer simulation experiments in three counties. J Stud Alcohol 48:124–135, 1987
103. Wagenaar AC, Farrell S: Alcohol beverage control policies: Their role in preventing alcohol-impaired driving. In Surgeon General's Workshop on Drunk Driving. Background Papers, Washington DC, December 14–16, 1988. US Department of Health and Human Services, Public Health Service. Rockville, MD: Office of the Surgeon General, 1989
104. Cook PJ: The effect of liquor taxes on drinking, cirrhosis and auto accidents. In Moore MH, Gerstein DR (eds): Alcohol and Public Policy: Beyond the Shadow of Prohibition. Washington, DC: National Academy, 1981
105. Cook PJ: Alcohol taxes as a public health measure. Br J Addict 77:245–250, 1982
106. Cook PJ, Tauchen G: The effect of liquor taxes on heavy drinking. Bell J Econ 13:379–390, 1982
107. Ornstein SI: A survey of findings on the economic and regulatory determinants of the demand for alcoholic beverages. Substance Alcohol Actions Misuse 5:39–44, 1984
108. Hoadley JF, Fuchs BC, Holder HD: The effect of alcohol beverage restrictions on consumption: A 25-year longitudinal analysis. Am J Drug Alcohol Abuse 10:375–401, 1984
109. Levy D, Sheflin N: New evidence on controlling alcohol use through price. J Stud Alcohol 44:929–937, 1983
110. Davies P: The relationship between taxation, price and alcohol consumption in the countries of Europe. In Grant M, Plant M, Williams A (eds): Economics and Alcohol: Consumption and Controls. London: Croom Helm, 1983
111. Maynard A: Modeling alcohol consumption and abuse: The powers and pitfalls of economic techniques. In Grant M, Plant M, Williams A (eds): Economics and Alcohol: Consumption and Controls. London: Croom Helm, 1983
112. Walsh BM: The economics of alcohol taxation. In Grant M, Plant M, Williams A (eds): Economics and Alcohol: Consumption and Controls. Croom Helm, 1983
113. McGuinness T: The demand for beer, spirits and wine in the UK, 1956–79. In Grant M, Plant M, Williams A (eds): Economics and Alcohol: Consumption and Control. London: Croom Helm, 1983
114. Heien D, Pompelli G: Stress, ethnic and distribution factors in a dichotomous response model of alcohol abuse. J Stud Alcohol 48:450–455, 1987
115. Walsh BM: Do excise taxes save lives? The Irish experience with alcohol taxation. Accid Anal Prev 19:433–448, 1987
116. Kendell RE, de Roumanie M, Ritson EB: Effect of economic changes on Scottish drinking habits, 1978–82. Br J Addict 78:365–379, 1983
117. Kendell RE, de Roumanie M, Ritson EB: Influence of an increase in excise duty on alcohol consumption and its adverse effects. Br Med J 287:809–811, 1983
118. Bigelow G, Liebson I: Cost factors controlling alcohol drinking. Psychol Record 22:305–314, 1972
119. Mello NK: Behavioural studies of alcoholism. In Kissin B, Begleiter H (eds): The Biology of Alcoholism, Vol 3. Physiology and Behaviour. New York: Plenum, 1972
120. Babor TF, Mendelson, JH, Greenberg I, et al: Experimental analysis of the "happy hour." Effects of purchase price on alcohol consumption. Psychopharmacology 58:35–41, 1978
121. Grant BF, Zobeck TS, Chan Ng M-J: Liver cirrhosis mortality in the United States, 1971–1985. Surveillance Report No. 8. Alcohol Epidemiologic Data System, Division of Biometry and Epidemiology, National Institute on Alcohol Abuse and Alcoholism, US Department of Health and Human Services, Public Health Service, Alcohol, Drug Abuse, and Mental Health Administration, June 1988
122. Duffy M: The influence of prices, consumer incomes and advertising upon the demand for alcoholic drink in the United Kingdom. Br J Alcohol Alcoholism 16:200–208, 1981
123. Ornstein SI: Control of alcohol consumption through price increases. J Stud Alcohol 41:807–818, 1980
124. Grossman M, Coate D, Arluck GM: Price sensitivity of alcoholic beverages in the United States. In Holder HD (ed): Control Issues in Alcohol Abuse Prevention: Strategies for Communities. Greenwich, Conn.: JAI Press, 1987
125. Coate D, Grossman M: Change in alcoholic beverage prices and legal drinking ages: Effects on youth alcohol use and motor vehicle mortality. Alcohol Health World Fall:22–25, 59, 1987
126. Saffer H, Grossman M: Beer taxes, the legal drinking age, and youth motor vehicle fatalities. J Legal Stud 16:351–374, 1987
127. Saffer H, Grossman M: Drinking age laws and highway mortality rates: Cause and effect. Econ Inquiry 25:403–418, 1987
128. Mosher JF, Beauchamp DE: Justifying alcohol taxes to public officials. J Public Health Policy 4:422–439, 1983
129. Vernberg WB: Alcohol Tax Reform. Proposed Position Paper. American Public Health Association. The Nation's Health August 1986
130. Mosher JF: Federal tax law and public health policy: The case of alcohol-related tax expenditures. J Public Health Policy 3:260–283, 1982
131. Mosher JF: Government policies concerning alcohol taxation: Beyond the excise tax debate. In Grant M, Plant M, Williams A (eds): Economics and Alcohol: Consumption and Controls. London: Croom Helm, 1983
132. Smith DI: Effectiveness of restrictions on availability as a means of reducing the use and abuse of alcohol. Aust Alcohol Drug Rev 2:84–90, 1983
133. MacDonald S, Whitehead P: Availability of outlets and consumption of alcoholic beverages. J Drug Issues 13:477–486, 1983
134. Makela K, Osterberg E, Sulkunen P: Drink in Finland: Increasing alcohol availability in a monopoly state. In Single E, Morgan P, de Lint J (eds): Alcohol, Society and the State. 2. The Social History of Control Policy in Seven Countries. Toronto: Addiction Research Foundation, 1981
135. Rabow J, Watts RK: Alcohol availability, alcoholic beverage sales and alcohol-related problems. J Stud Alcohol 43:767–801, 1982
136. Watts RK, Rabow J: Alcohol availability and alcohol-related problems in 213 California cities. Alcoholism Clin Exp Res 7:47–58, 1983
137. Colon I: Alcohol availability and cirrhosis mortality rates by gender and race. Am J Public Health 71:1325–1328, 1981
137a. Colon I, Cutter HSG: The relationship of beer consumption and state alcohol and motor vehicle policies to fatal accidents. J Safety Research 14:83–89, 1983.
138. Smart RG, Docherty D: Effects of the introduction of on-premise drinking on alcohol-related accidents and impaired driving. J Stud Alcohol 37:683–686, 1976
139. Neuman C, Rabow J: Drinkers' use of physical availability of alcohol: Buying habits and consumption level. Int J Addict 20:1663–1673, 1985–86
140. Smith DI: Effect on liver cirrhosis and traffic accident mortality of changing the number and type of alcohol outlets in Western Australia. Alcoholism Clin Exp Res 13:190–195, 1989
141. Raymond A: Ten o'clock closing—The effect of the change in hotel bar closing time on road accidents in the metropolitan area of Victoria. Aust Road Res 3:3–17, 1969
142. Smith DI: Effect on traffic accidents of introducing flexible hotel trading hours in Tasmania, Australia. Br J Addict 83:219–222, 1988
143. Smith DI: Effect on traffic accidents of introducing Sunday alcohol sales in Brisbane, Australia. Int J Addict 23:1091–1099, 1988

144. Smith DI: Impact on traffic safety of the introduction of Sunday alcohol sales in Perth, Western Australia. J Stud Alcohol 39:1302–1303, 1978
145. Smith DI: Comparison of patrons of hotels with early opening and standard hours. Int J Addict 21:155–163, 1986
146. Olsson O, Wikstrom P-O H: Effects of the experimental Saturday closing of liquor retail stores in Sweden. Contemp Drug Problems 11:325–353, 1982
147. Duffy JC, Plant MA: Scotland's liquor licensing changes: An assessment. Br Med J 292:36–39, 1986
148. Northridge DB, McMurray J, Lawson AAH: Association between liberalisation of Scotland's liquor licensing laws and admissions for self poisoning in West Fife. Br Med J 293:1466–1468, 1986
149. Dull RT, Giacopassi DJ: An assessment of the effects of alcohol ordinances on selected behaviours and conditions. J Drug Issues 16:511–521, 1986
150. Parker DA, Wolz MW, Harford TC: The prevention of alcoholism: An empirical report on the effects of outlet availability. Alcoholism Clin Exp Res 2:339–343, 1978
151. Harford TC, Parker DA, Pautler C, et al: Relationship between the number of on-premise outlets and alcoholism. J Stud Alcohol 40:1053–1057, 1979
152. Schweitzer SO, Intriligator MD, Salehi H: Alcoholism: An economic model of its causes and its control. In Grant M, Plant M, Williams A (eds): Economics and Alcohol: Consumption and Controls. London: Croom Helm, 1983
153. Rush BR, Gliksman L, Brook R: Alcohol availability, alcohol consumption, and alcohol-related damage. I. The distribution of consumption model. J Stud Alcohol 47:1–10, 1986
154. Gliksman L, Rush BR: Alcohol availability, alcohol consumption and alcohol-related damage. II. The role of sociodemographic factors. J Stud Alcohol 47:11–18, 1986
155. Blose JO, Holder HD: Liquor-by-the-drink and alcohol-related traffic crashes: A natural experiment using time-series analysis. J Stud Alcohol 48:52–60, 1987
156. Holder HD, Blose JO: Impact of changes in distilled spirits availability on apparent consumption: A time series analysis of liquor-by-the-drink. Br J Addict 82:623–631
157. Blose JO, Holder HD: Public availability of distilled spirits: Structural and reported consumption changes associated with liquor-by-the-drink. J Stud Alcohol 48:371–379, 1987
158. Single E: The control of public drinking: The impact of the environment on alcohol problems. In Holder HD (ed): Control Issues in Alcohol Abuse Prevention. Strategies for States and Communities. Advances in Substance Abuse, Supplement 1. Greenwich, Conn.: JAI, 1987
159. MacDonald S: The impact of increased availability of wine in grocery stores on consumption: Four case histories. Br J Addict 81:381–387, 1986
160. Smart RG: The impact of consumption on selling wine in grocery stores. Alcohol Alcoholism 21:233–236, 1986
161. Smart RG: Comparison of purchasing in self-service and clerk-service liquor stores. J Stud Alcohol 35:1397–1401, 1974
162. Ryan BE, Segars L: Mini-marts and maxi-problems. The relationship between purchase and consumption levels. Alcohol Health Res World Fall:26–29, 1987
163. Swann DR: Free-alcohol policy on airplanes. Can Med Assoc J 139:1051, 1988
164. Smart RG: Drinking under special occasion permits: A neglected aspect of alcohol control measures. J Stud Alcohol 49:196–199, 1988
165. Kortteinen T: State monopoly systems and alcohol prevention in developing countries: Report on a collaborative international study. Br J Addict 84:413–425, 1989
166. Spellman WE, Jorgenson MR: Liquor control and consumption. J Stud Alcohol 44:194–197, 1983
167. Room R: Alcohol monopolies in the US: Challenges and opportunities. J Public Health Policy 8:509–530, 1987
168. Norstrom T: The abolition of the Swedish alcohol rationing system: Effects on consumption distribution and cirrhosis mortality. Br J Addict 82:633–641, 1987
169. Smart RG, Goodstadt MS: Effects of reducing the legal alcohol-purchasing age on drinking and drinking problems. A review of empirical studies. J Stud Alcohol 38:1313–1323, 1977
170. Vingilis ER, DeGenova K: Youth and the forbidden fruit: Experiences with changes in the legal drinking age in North America. J Criminal Justice 12:161–172, 1984
171. Williams TP, Lillis RP: Changes in alcohol consumption by 18-year-olds following an increase in New York State's purchase age to 19. J Stud Alcohol 47:290–296, 1986
172. Engs RC, Hanson DJ: Age-specific alcohol prohibition and college students drinking problems. Psychol Rep 59:979–984, 1986
173. Smith DI, Burvill PW: Effect on juvenile crime of lowering the drinking age in three Australian states. Br J Addict 82:181–188, 1986
174. Cook PJ, Tauchen G: The effect of minimum drinking age legislation on youthful auto fatalities, 1970–1977. J Legal Stud 13:169–190, 1984
175. Vingilis E, Smart RG: Effects of raising the legal drinking age in Ontario. Br J Addict 76:415–424, 1981
176. Offer S: Report of the Advisory Committee on Liquor Regulation. Submitted to the Minister of Consumer and Commercial Relations, Province of Ontario, Canada, Toronto, February 1987, p 63
177. Wagenaar AC: Preventing highway crashes by raising the legal minimum age for drinking: An empirical confirmation. J Safety Res 13:57–71, 1982
178. Williams AF, Zador PL, Harris SS, et al: The effect of raising the legal minimum drinking age on involvement in fatal crashes. J Legal Stud 12:169–179, 1983
179. Smith RA, Hingson RW, Morelock S, et al: Legislation raising the legal drinking age in Massachusetts from 18 to 20: Effect on 16 and 17 year-olds. J Stud Alcohol 45:534–539, 1984
180. Hingson RW, Scotch N, Mangione T, et al: Impact of legislation raising the legal drinking age in Massachusetts from 18 to 20. Am J Public Health 73:163–170, 1983
181. Hoskin AF, Yalung-Mathews D, Carraro BA: Effect of raising the legal minimum drinking age on fatal crashes in 10 states. J Safety Res 17:117–121, 1986
182. DuMouchel W, Williams AF, Zador P: Raising the alcohol purchase age: Its effects on fatal motor vehicle crashes in 26 states. Washington, DC: Insurance Institute for Highway Safety, 1985, 23 pp
183. MacKinnon DP, Woodward JA: The impact of raising the minimum drinking age on driver fatalities. Int J Addict 21:1331–38, 1986
184. Williams TP, Lillis RP: Long-term changes in reported alcohol purchasing and consumption following an increase in New York's purchase age to 19. Br J Addict 83:209–217, 1988
185. Decker MD, Graitcer PL, Schaffner W: Reduction in motor vehicle fatalities associated with an increase in the minimum drinking age. JAMA 260:3604–3610, 1988
186. Wagenaar AC: Preventing highway crashes by raising the legal minimum age for drinking: The Michigan experience 6 years later. J Safety Res 17:101–109, 1986
187. Sternberg K: Alcohol consumer must be 21 years old in all states: Concerns remain about drunk driving. JAMA 260:2479–2480, 1988
188. Williams AF, Lund AK: Adults' views of laws that limit teenagers' driving and access to alcohol. J Public Health Policy 7:190–197, 1986
189. Engs RC, Hanson DJ: University students' drinking patterns and problems: Examining the effects of raising the purchase age. Public Health Rep 103:667–673, 1988
190. Single E: Paths ahead for server intervention in Canada. In Giesbrecht N, Conley P, Denniston R, et al (eds): Research, Action and the Community: Experiences in the Prevention of Alcohol and Other Drug Problems. Rockville, MD: Office for Substance Abuse Prevention, 1990, pp 239–246

191. Saltz RF, Delewski C: Experiences with community-based server intervention programs in California. In Giesbrecht N, Conley P, Denniston R, et al (eds): Research, Action and the Community: Experiences in the Prevention of Alcohol and Other Drug Problems. Rockville, MD: Office for Substance Abuse Prevention, 1990, pp 82–89
192. Saltz RF: Server intervention and responsible beverage service programs. In Surgeon General's Workshop on Drunk Driving. Background Papers, Washington, DC, December 14–16, 1988. US Department of Health and Human Services, Public Health Service. Rockville, MD: Office of the Surgeon General, 1989
193. Mosher JF, Wallack LM: The DUI project. Contemporary Drug Problems 8:193–206, 1979
194. Mosher JF: Server intervention: A new approach for preventing drinking and driving. Acid Anal Prev 15:483–497, 1983
195. Mosher JF: The impact of legal provisions on barroom behaviour: Toward an alcohol-problems prevention policy. Alcohol 1:205–211, 1984
196. Mosher JF: Server intervention: A guide to implementing local and state programs. In Holder HD (ed): Advances in Substance Abuse: Behavioral and Biological Research. Supplement 1. Control Issues in Alcohol Abuse Prevention: Strategies for States and Communities. Greenwich, CT: JAI, 1987
197. Saltz RF: Server intervention: Conceptual overview and current developments. Alcohol Drugs Driving 1:1–13, 1985
198. Saltz RF: Server intervention. Will it work? Alcohol Health Res World 10:12–19, 35, 1986
199. Gliksman L: Evaluating server training: In Giesbrecht N, Conley P, Denniston R, et al (eds): Research, Action and the Community: Experiences in the Prevention of Alcohol and Other Drug Problems. Rockville, MD: Office for Substance Abuse Prevention, 1990, pp 90–94
200. Saltz RF: The roles of bars and restaurants in preventing alcohol-impaired driving: An evaluation of server intervention. Evaluation Health Professions 10:5–27, 1987
201. Geller ES, Russ NW, Delphos WA: Does server intervention training make a difference? An empirical field evaluation. Alcohol Health Res World Summer:64–69, 1987
202. Russ NW, Geller ES: Training bar personnel to prevent drunken driving: A field evaluation. Am J Public Health 77:952–954, 1987
203. Mosher JF, Colman VJ: The Model Dram Shop Act of 1985. Alcohol Health Res World 10:4–11,35, 1986
204. Mosher JF: Dram Shop update. Bull Alcohol Policy 5:5, 1987
205. O'Donnell M: Research on drinking locations of alcohol-impaired drivers: Implications for prevention policies. J Public Health Policy 6:510–525, 1985
206. Bonnie RJ: Regulating conditions of alcohol availability: Possible effects on highway safety. J Stud Alcohol Suppl 10:129–143, 1985
207. Peters JE: Beyond server training. An examination of future issues. Alcohol Health Res World 10:24–27,35, 1986
208. Hochheimer JL: Reducing alcohol abuse: A critical review of education strategies. In Moore MH, Gerstein DR (eds): Alcohol and Public Policy: Beyond the Shadow of Prohibition. Washington, DC: National Academy, 1981
209. Moore MH, Gerstein DR: Shaping drinking practices directly. In Moore MH, Gerstein DR (eds): Alcohol and Public Policy: Beyond the Shadow of Prohibition. Washington, DC: National Academy, 1981
210. Rootman I: Using health promotion to reduce alcohol problems. In Grant M (ed): Alcohol Policies. Copenhagen: World Health Organization, 1985
211. Flay B, Sobel J: The role of mass media in preventing adolescent substance abuse. In Glynn TJ, Leukefeld CG, Ludford JP (eds): Preventing Adolescent Drug Abuse: Intervention Strategies. NIDA Research Monograph No 47. DHEW Pub No. (ADM)83-1280. Washington, DC:US Government Printing Office, 1983
212. Blume SB: Warning labels and warning signs: The battle continues across the Atlantic. Br J Addict 82:5–6, 1987
213. Prugh T: Point-of-purchase health warning notices. Alcohol Health Res World 10:36, 1986
214. Gallup G Jr: Public backs strong measures to fight alcohol, drug abuse. New York: Gallup Poll, December 18, 1986
215. US Department of Health and Human Services: Review of the Research Literature on the Effects of Health Warning Labels. A Report to the United States Congress. Washington, DC: Department of Health and Human Services, June 1987
216. US Department of the Treasury, Bureau of Alcohol, Tobacco and Firearms: Implementation of the Alcoholic Beverage Labelling Act of 1988 (Pub.L. 100-690); Health Warning Statement. Federal Register 54:7160–7164, 1989
217. American Public Health Association: Policy Statement 8812:Alcohol Warning Labels and Posters. Am J Public Health 79:357–358, 1989
218. Mosher JF (ed): California update. Bull Alcohol Policy 7:10, 1988
219. Blane HT: Prevention issues with children of alcoholics. Br J Addict 83:793–798, 1988
220. Williams M: Alcohol and the elderly: An overview. Alcohol Health Res World 8:3–9, 52, 1984
221. Brody JA: Aging and alcohol abuse. J Am Geriatr Soc 30:123–126, 1982
222. US Department of Health and Human Services, Public Health Service, Alcohol, Drug Abuse, and Mental Health Administration, National Institute on Alcohol Abuse and Alcoholism: Alcohol and Aging. Alcohol Alert, No.2. Rockville, Md., 1988
223. Morrissey ER: Of women, by women, or for women? Selected issues in the primary prevention of drinking problems. In Women and Alcohol: Health-Related Issues. National Institute on Alcohol Abuse and Alcoholism. Research Monograph-16. DHHS Publication No. (ADM) 86-1139. Rockville, Md: US Department of Health and Human Services, 1986
224. Ferrence RG: Prevention of alcohol problems in women. In Wilsnack S, Beckman L (eds): Alcohol Problems in Women. New York: Guilford Press, 1984
225. Blume SB: Women and alcohol. A review. JAMA 256:1467–1470, 1986
226. Watts TD, Wright R: Prevention of alcohol abuse among black Americans. An interview with TD Watts and Roosevelt Wright Jr. Minorities. Alcohol Health Res World 11:40,41,65, 1986–87
227. Dawkins MP: Alcoholism prevention and black youth. J Drug Issues 18:15–20, 1988
228. Galan FJ: Alcoholism prevention and Hispanic youth. J Drug Issues 18:49–58, 1988
229. Globetti G: Alcohol education programs and minority youth. J Drug Issues 18:115–129, 1988
230. Rhoades ER, Mason RD, Eddy P, et al: The Indian Health Service approach to alcoholism among American Indians and Alaska Natives. Public Health Reports 103:621–627, 1988
231. Edwards ED, Edwards ME: Alcoholism prevention/treatment and native American youth: A community approach. J Drug Issues 18:103–114, 1988
232. Bangert-Drowns RL: The effects of school-based substance abuse education—A metaanalysis. J Drug Educ 18:243–264, 1988
233. Perry C, Grant M: Comparing peer-led to teacher-led youth alcohol education in four countries. Alcohol Health Res World 12:322–326, 1988
234. Hopkins RH, Mauss AL, Kearney KA, et al: Comprehensive evaluation of a model alcohol education curriculum. J Stud Alcohol 49:38–50, 1988
235. Mauss AL, Hopkins RH, Weisheit RA, et al: The problematic prospects for prevention in the classroom: Should alcohol education programs be expected to reduce drinking by youth? J Stud Alcohol 40:51–61, 1988
236. Hansen WB, Johnson CA, Flay BR, et al: Affective and social influences approaches to the prevention of multiple substance abuse among seventh grade students: Results from Project SMART. Prev Med 17:135–154, 1988
237. Hansen WB, Graham JW, Wolkenstein BH, et al: Differential im-

pact of three alcohol prevention curricula on hypothesized mediating variables. J Drug Educ 18:143–153, 1988
238. Hansen WB, Malotte CK, Fielding JE: Tobacco and alcohol prevention: Preliminary results of a four-year study. Adolesc Psychiatry 14:556–575, 1987
239. Hansen WB, Malotte CK, Fielding JE: Evaluation of a tobacco and alcohol abuse prevention curriculum for adolescents. Health Educ Q 15:93–114, 1988
240. Pentz MA, Dwyer JH, MacKinnon DP, et al: A multicommunity trial for primary prevention of adolescent drug abuse. Effects on drug use prevalence. JAMA 261:3259–3266, 1989
241. Dwyer JH, MacKinnon DP, Pentz MA, et al: Estimating intervention effects in longitudinal studies. Am J Epidemiol 130:781–95, 1989
242. Anderson DS, Gadaleto A: Highlights of the 1988 College Alcohol Survey. Prevention Pipeline 2:15–16, 1989
243. Goodstadt MS, Caleekal-John A: Alcohol education programs for university students: A review of their effectiveness. Int J Addict 19:721–41, 1984
244. Gliksman L: Campus alcohol policies and education program (CAPE): practical consideration in a research evaluation. In Geisbrecht N, Conley P, Denniston R, et al (eds): Research, Action, and the Community: Experiences in the Prevention of Alcohol and Drug Problems. Rockville, Md.: Office for Substance Abuse Prevention, 1990, pp 75-81
245. Streissguth AP, Darby BL, Barr HM, et al: Comparison of drinking and smoking patterns during pregnancy over a six-year interval. Am J Obstet Gynecol 145:716–724, 1983
246. Mann RE, Vingilis ER, Leigh G, et al: School-based programmes for the prevention of drinking and driving: Issues and results. Accid Anal Prev 18:325–337, 1986
247. Mann RE, Vingilis ER, Stewart K: Programs to change individual behavior: Education and rehabilitation in the prevention of drinking and driving. In Laurence MD, Snortum JR, Zimring FE (eds): The Social Control of Drinking and Driving. Chicago: University of Chicago Press, 1988
248. Liban CB, Vingilis E, Blefgen H: The Canadian drinking–driving countermeasure experience. Accid Anal Prev 19:159–181, 1987
249. Atkin CK: Mass communication effects on drinking and driving. In Surgeon General's Workshop on Drunk Driving. Background Papers, Washington, DC, December 14–16, 1988. US Department of Health and Human Services, Public Health Service. Rockville, Md.: Office of the Surgeon General, 1989
250. Simons-Morton BG, Simons-Morton DG: Controlling injuries due to drinking and driving: The context and functions of education. In Surgeon General's Workshop on Drunk Driving. Background Papers, Washington, DC, December 14–16, 1988. US Department of Health and Human Services, Public Health Service. Rockville, Md.: Office of the Surgeon General, 1989
251. Worden JK, Flynn BS, Merrill DG, et al: Preventing alcohol-impaired driving through community self-regulation training. Am J Public Health 79:287–290, 1989
252. Graitcer PL: Evaluation of community interventions to reduce drunken driving. Am J Public Health 79:271, 1989
253. Single E: The "substitution hypothesis" reconsidered; a research note concerning the Ontario beer strikes in 1958 and 1968. J Stud Alcohol 40:485–491, 1979
254. de Lint J: Critical examination of data bearing on the type of alcoholic beverage consumed in relation to health and other effects. Br J Addict 72:189–197, 1977
255. Tuyns AJ, Esteve J, Pequignot G: Ethanol is cirrhogenic, whatever the beverage. Br J Addict 79:389–393, 1984
256. Feinman L, Lieber CS: Toxicity of ethanol and other components of alcoholic beverages. Alcoholism Clin Exp Res 12:2–6, 1988
257. Whitehead PC, Szandorowska B: Introduction of low alcohol content beer. A test of the addition-substitution hypothesis. J Stud Alcohol 38:2157–2164, 1977
258. Skog O-J: The effect of introducing a new light beer in Norway: Substitution or addition? Br J Addict 83:665–668, 1988
259. Romelsjo A: Decline in alcohol-related in-patient care and mortality in Stockholm County. Br J Addict 82:653–663, 1987
260. Whitehead PC: The prevention of alcoholism: Divergences and convergences of two approaches. Addictive Dis 1:431–443, 1975
261. Cox WM, Klinger E: Discriminability of regular, light and alcoholic and nonalcoholic near beer. J Stud Alcohol 44:494–498, 1983
262. McLaughlin K: An investigation of the ability of young male and female social drinkers to discriminate between regular, calorie reduced and low alcohol beer. Br J Addict 83:183–187, 1988
263. Russ NW, Geller ES: Exploring low alcohol beer consumption among college students: Implications for drunk driving. J Alcohol Drug Educ 3:1–5, 1988
264. Time Magazine (US ed): Blithe spirits for the sober set. Economics and Business. New York: Time Inc. August 18, 1986, pp 43,46
265. Mosher JF: Alcohol policy and the nation's youth. J Public Health Policy 6:295–299, 1985
266. Hacker GA, Collins R, Jacobson M: Marketing Booze to Blacks. Washington, DC: Center for Science in the Public Interest, 1987
267. Jernigan D: Alcohol and tobacco outdoor advertising in minority communities. Proposed policy statement. American Public Health Association. The Nation's Health, September 1989, pp 21–22
268. Mosher JF (ed): She can have it all: Alcohol promotion targets women. Bull Alcohol Policy 6:5,8, 1987
269. Smart RG: Does alcohol advertising affect overall consumption? A review of empirical studies. J Stud Alcohol 49:314–323, 1988
270. McGuinness AJ: An econometric analysis of retail demand for alcoholic beverages in the UK, 1956–1975. J Indust Econ 29:85–109, 1980
271. Strickland DE: Advertising exposure, alcohol consumption and misuse of alcohol. In Grant M, Plant M, Williams A (eds): Economics and Alcohol: Consumption and Controls. London: Croom Helm, 1983
272. Franke G, Wilcox G: Alcoholic beverage advertising and consumption in the United States, 1964–1984. J Advertising 16:22–30, 1987
273. McCarty D, Ewing JA: Alcohol consumption while viewing alcoholic beverage advertising. Int J Addict 18:1011–1018, 1983
274. Kohn PM, Smart RG: Wine, women, suspiciousness and advertising. J Stud Alcohol 48:161–168, 1987
275. Ogborne AC, Smart RG: Will restrictions on alcohol advertising reduce alcohol consumption? Br J Addict 75:293–296, 1980
276. Kohn PM, Smart RG: Impact of television advertising on alcohol consumption: An experiment. J Stud Alcohol 45:295–301, 1984
277. Kohn PM, Smart RG, Ogborne AC: Effects of two kinds of alcohol advertising on subsequent consumption. J Advertis 13:34–48, 1984
278. van Iwaarden T: Advertising, alcohol consumption and policy alternatives. In Grant M, Plant M, Williams A (eds): Economics and Alcohol: Consumption and Controls. London: Croom Helm, 1983
279. van Iwaarden MJ: Public health aspects of the marketing of alcoholic drinks. In Grant M (ed): Alcohol Policies. Copenhagen: World Health Organization Regional Publications, European Series No 18. 1985
280. Wallack L: Television programming, advertising, and the prevention of alcohol-related problems. Alcohol and the mass media. In Gerstein DR (ed): Toward the Prevention of Alcohol Problems: Government, Business, and Community Action. Washington, DC: National Acad Press, 1984
281. Wallack L: Alcohol advertising reassessed: The public health perspective. In Grant M, Plant M, Williams A (eds): Economics and Alcohol: Consumption and Controls. London: Croom Helm, 1983
282. Aitken PP, Leathar DS, Scott AC: Ten- to sixteen-year-olds' perceptions of advertisements for alcoholic drinks. Alcohol Alcoholism 23:491–500, 1988
283. Aitken PP, Eadie DR, Leathar DS, et al: Television advertisements for alcoholic drinks do reinforce under-age drinking. Br J Addict 83:1399–1419, 1988
284. Lieberman LR, Orlandi MA: Alcohol advertising and adolescent drinking. Alcohol Health Res World Fall: 30–33,43, 1987

285. Atkins CK, Neuendorf K, McDermott S: Role of alcohol advertising in excessive and hazardous drinking. J Drug Educ 13:313–325, 1983
286. Mills KC: Beverage promotion and alcohol-abuse prevention on the college campus. In Holder HD (ed): Control Issue in Alcohol Abuse Prevention: Strategies for States and Communities. Advances in Substance Abuse: Behavioural and Biological Research. Suppl 1:289–298, 1987
287. Denniston R: Advertising and marketing. Panel B. In US Department of Health and Human Services, Public Health Service, Surgeon General's Workshop on Drunk Driving. Proceedings, December 14–16, 1988. Washington, DC: Office of the Surgeon General, 1989
288. Greenberg BS: Smoking, drugging, and drinking in top rated TV series. J Drug Educ 11:227–234, 1981
289. Breed W, de Foe JR: Drinking and smoking on television, 1950–1982. J Public Health Policy 5:257–270, 1984
290. Wallack L, Breed W, Cruz J: Alcohol on prime-time television. J Stud Alcohol 48:33–38, 1987
291. Mosher JF: Alcohol and tobacco industry product placement in feature films. Proposed policy statement. American Public Health Association. The Nation's Health, September 1989, p 21
292. Sobell LC, Sobell MB, Riley DM, et al: Effect of television programming and advertising on alcohol consumption in normal drinkers. J Stud Alcohol 47:333–340, 1986
293. Futch EJ: Influence of televised alcohol consumption on children's social problem solving. Dissertation Abstracts International 45:1283-B, 1984
294. Kotch JB, Coulter ML, Lipsitz A: Does televised drinking influence children's attitudes toward alcohol? Addict Behav 11:67–70, 1986
295. Breed W, de Foe JR: Effecting media change: The role of cooperative consultation on alcohol topics. J Communications 32:88–99, 1982
296. Chang NC, Chao HM (eds): Early Identification of Alcohol Abuse. Research Monograph No. 17. US Department of Health and Human Services, DHHS Publication No (ADM) 85-1258. Rockville, Md.: National Institute on Alcohol Abuse and Alcoholism, 1985
297. Allen JP, Eckardt MJ, Wallen J: Screening for alcoholism: Techniques and Issues. Public Health Reports 103:586–692, 1988
298. Sanchez-Craig M, Annis HM: Gamma-glutamyl transpeptidase and high-density lipoproteins cholesteral in male problem drinkers: Advantages of a composite index for predicting alcohol consumption. Alcoholism Clin Exp Res 5:540–544, 1981
299. Kristenson H, Hood B: The impact of alcohol on health in the general population: A review with particular reference to experience in Malmo. Br J Addict 79:139–145, 1984
300. Storey EL, Anderson GJ, Mack U, et al: Desialylated transferrin as a serological marker of chronic excessive alcohol ingestion. Lancet 1:1292–1294, 1987
301. Bernadt MW, Mumford J, Taylor C, et al: Comparison of questionnaire and laboratory tests in the detection of excessive drinking and alcoholism. Lancet 1:325–328, 1982
302. Bush B, Shaw S, Cleary P, et al: Screening for alcohol abuse using the CAGE questionnaire. Am J Med 82:231–235, 1987
303. Moore RD, Bone LR, Geller G, et al: Prevalence, detection, and treatment of alcoholism in hospitalized patients. JAMA 261:403–407, 1989
304. Cleary PD, Miller M, Bush BT, et al: Prevalence and recognition of alcohol abuse in a primary care population. Am J Med 85:466–471, 1988
305. Spencer J, Bartu A, Harrison-Stewart A: Observations on community screening for alcohol problems: A pilot project to assess the feasibility of identifying heavy drinkers in a community setting. Alcohol Alcoholism 22:65–69, 1987
306. Skinner HA, Holt S, Schuller R, et al: Identification of alcohol abuse using laboratory tests and a history of trauma. Ann Intern Med 101:847–851, 1984
307. Cyr MG, Wartman SA: The effectiveness of routine screening questions in the detection of alcoholism. JAMA 259:51–54, 1988
308. Saunders JB, Aasland OG: WHO Collaborative Project on identification and treatment of persons with harmful alcohol consumption. Report of Phase 1. Development of a Screening Instrument. Geneva: World Health Organization, 1987
309. Skinner HA, Holt S, Israel Y: Early identification of alcohol abuse: 1. Critical issues and psychosocial indicators for a composite index. Can Med Assoc J 124:1141–1152, 1981
310. Holt S, Skinner HA, Israel Y: Early identification of alcohol abuse: 2: Clinical and laboratory indicators. Can Med Assoc J 124:1279–1295, 1981
311. Skinner HA, Holt S: Early intervention for alcohol problems. J R Coll Gen Pract 33:787–791, 1983
312. Skinner HA, Holt S, Sheu WJ, et al: Clinical versus laboratory detection of alcohol abuse: The alcohol clinical index. Br Med J 292:1703–1708, 1986
313. Edwards G, Orford J, Egert S, et al: Alcoholism: A controlled trial of "treatment" and "advice." J Stud Alcohol 38:1004–1031, 1977
314. Orford J, Oppenheimer E, Edwards G: Abstinence or control: The outcome for excessive drinkers two years after consultation. Behav Res Ther 14:397–416, 1976
315. Wallace P, Cutler S, Haines A: Randomized controlled trial of general practitioner intervention in patients with excessive alcohol consumption. Br Med J 297:663–668, 1988
316. Sanchez-Craig M, Leigh G, Spivek K, et al: Superior outcome of females over males after brief treatment for the reduction of heavy drinking. Br J Addict 84:395–404, 1989
317. Sanchez-Craig M, Annis HM, Bornet AR, et al: Random assignment to abstinence and controlled drinking: Evaluation of a cognitive-behavioural program for problem drinkers. J Consult Clin Psychol 52:390–403, 1984
318. Skutle A, Berg G: Training in controlled drinking for early-stage problem drinkers. Br J Addict 82:493–501, 1987
319. Zweben A, Pearlman S, Li S: A comparison of brief advice and conjoint therapy in the treatment of alcohol abuse: The results of the marital systems study. Br J Addict 83:899–916, 1988
320. Sannibale C: Differential effect of a set of brief interventions on the functioning of a group of "early-stage" problem drinkers. Aust Drug Alcohol Rev 7:147–155, 1988
321. Stockwell T: Can severely dependent drinkers learn controlled drinking? Summing up the debate. Br J Addict 83:149–152, 1988
322. Alden LE: Behavioural self-management controlled-drinking strategies in a context of secondary prevention. J Consult Clin Psychol 56:280–286, 1988
323. Taylor JR, Helzer JE, Robins LN: Moderate drinking in ex-alcoholics: Recent studies. J Stud Alcohol 47:115–121, 1986
324. Rush BR, Ogborne AC: Acceptibility of nonabstinence treatment goals among alcoholism treatment programs. J Stud Alcohol 47:146–150, 1986
325. Sanchez-Craig M: A Therapist's Manual for Secondary Prevention of Alcohol Problems. Procedures for Teaching Moderate Drinking and Abstinence. Toronto: Addiction Research Foundation, 1984
326. Chick J, Lloyd G, Crombie E: Counselling problem drinkers in medical wards: A controlled study. Br Med J 290:965–967, 1985
327. Elvy GA, Wells JE, Baird KA: Attempted referral as intervention for problem drinking in the general hospital. Br J Addict 83:83–89, 1988
328. Chick J: Secondary prevention of alcoholism and the Centres D'Hygiene Alimentaire. Br J Addict 79:221–225, 1984
329. McIntosh M, Sanchez-Craig M: Moderate drinking: An alternative treatment goal for early-stage problem drinking. Can Med Assoc J 131:873–876, 1984
330. Skinner HA: Early detection of alcohol and drug problems—Why? Aust Drug Alcohol Rev 6:293–301, 1987
331. US Department of Health and Human Services, Public Health Service: Healthy People 2000: National Health Promotion and Disease Prevention Objectives. Full Report with Commentary. Washington, DC: Government Printing Office.USDHHS Publication No. 91-50212, 1990

44

Prevention of Drug Abuse

C. Roberts Schuster
M. Marlyne Kilbey

In Western society we would like to believe that the only factor limiting an individual's ability to enjoy a healthy life is that set by one's genes. However, abuse of psychoactive drugs is a major threat to the realization of that birthright.

HEALTH AND COST IMPACT

The cost of drug abuse may be measured in adverse health effects reflected in expenditures for treatment of drug abuse and associated disorders as well as premature mortality and morbidity of persons abusing drugs. Related costs arise from lost productivity, crime, apprehension and incarceration, and rehabilitative social welfare programs. Adolescents are the only segment of our population that has not experienced improved health over the past 30 years.[1] In large part, this results from their disproportionate representation among the drug-abusing segment of our population. Homicides, suicide, and accidents account for over 77% of adolescent deaths, and drug abuse is implicated in over half of these deaths.[1]

In 1983, the economic impact of drug abuse was $60 billion.[2] Allowing for inflation, but not including the costs of AIDS-related disorders, the National Institute on Drug Abuse estimated that in 1988 drug abuse cost the nation approximately $75 billion, with roughly $52 billion in direct care costs and $23 billion in associated costs. A new dimension of the cost of drug abuse comes from recent data establishing a link between intravenous drug use and seropositivity for the human immunodeficiency virus (HIV). As of March 1989, the Centers for Disease Control estimated that the yearly cost of treating the 24,406 intravenous drug-abusing AIDS patients is in excess of $1.2 billion. Between 61,000 and 398,000 intravenous drug abusers in the United States are estimated to be infected with HIV.[3] The potential yearly cost of treating these persons for AIDS is a staggering $20 billion.

Much of the economic cost of drug abuse comes from crime (cost of losses to nondrug-abusing citizens and lost productivity of persons incarcerated, for example). A 1984 study[2] estimates these costs at 12.6% of the total economic burden for drug abuse, whereas crime-associated costs represent less than 3% of the costs of alcohol abuse and less than 2% of the costs of mental disorders. Clearly, improved efforts to prevent drug abuse would result in significant health improvement and economic savings.

DEFINITIONS

The term "psychoactive drug" refers to the various classes of exogenous substances that affect the central nervous system, inducing responses that generally are recognized subjectively as calming, energizing, or pleasurable. Legal restrictions on manufacture, production, or both of psychoactive substances vary from being nonexistent to being highly structured, and possession, use, or both of psychoactive substances can be legal (e.g., caffeine) or illegal (e.g., cocaine). Control of the availability of psychoactive substances is a fundamental approach to substance abuse prevention.[4]

One way the availability of psychoactive substances is controlled in the United States is through regulation under Title II of the Comprehensive Drug Abuse Prevention and Control Act of 1970, generally referred to as the Controlled Substances Act (CSA).[5] The act establishes five schedules of decreasing control from schedule I through V. It regulates possession and distribution of drugs and establishes penalties for individuals who violate the regulations. Schedule assignment is made on the basis of the drug's potential for abuse, current medical use, and safety, as well as the psychological and physiological dependence-producing properties of the drug. Table 44–1 lists five major types of drugs based on their pharmacological actions and shows their scheduling under the CSA, trade names of common drugs in the class, important medical uses, and certain physical and psychological dependence characteristics.

PHARMACOLOGY OF DRUGS OF ABUSE

For controlled substances, drug abuse may be defined as any use in a nonprescribed manner, and for noncontrolled substances, drug abuse may be thought of as any use in ways disapproved by society. For example, any use whatsoever of LSD constitutes abuse, whereas use of tobacco and alcohol by minors or excessive use of alcohol by adults may be termed abuse. Clearly, the definition of drug abuse is dependent on culture and historical period.[6–7] Drug dependence is defined as "a state of psychic or physical dependence, or both, on a drug, arising in a person following administration of that drug on a periodic or continuous basis."[8] Psychoactive substance abuse disorders involving excessive, compulsive, or detrimental use of drugs are conceptualized as mental disorders.[9]

TABLE 44-1. CONTROLLED SUBSTANCES—USES AND EFFECTS

Drugs/ CSA Schedules	Trade or Other Names	Medical Uses	Dependence		Tolerance	Duration (Hours)	Usual Methods of Administration	Possible Effects	Effects of Overdose	Withdrawal Syndrome
			Physical	Psychological						
▪ **Narcotics**										
Opium II III V	Dover's Powder, Paregoric Parepectolin	Analgesic, antidiarrheal	High	High	Yes	3–6	Oral, smoked	Euphoria, drowsiness, respiratory depression, constricted pupils, nausea	Slow and shallow breathing, clammy skin, convulsions, coma, possible death	Water eyes, runny nose, yawning, loss of appetite, irritability, tremors, panic, cramps, nausea, chills and sweating
Morphine II III	Morphine, MS-Contin, Roxanol, Roxanol-SR	Analgesic, antitussive	High	High	Yes	3–6	Oral, smoked, injected			
Codeine II III V	Tylenol w/Codeine, Empirin w/Codeine Robitussan A-C, Fiorinal w/Codeine	Analgesic, antitussive	Moderate	Moderate	Yes	3–6	Oral, injected			
Heroin I	Diacetylmorphine, Horse, Smack	None	High	High	Yes	3–6	Injected, sniffed, smoked			
Hydromorphone II	Dilaudid	Analgesic	High	High	Yes	3–6	Oral, injected			
Meperidine (Pethidine) II	Demerol, Mepergan	Analgesic	High	High	Yes	3–6	Oral, injected			
Methadone II	Dolophine, Methadone, Methadose	Analgesic	High	High–low	Yes	12–24	Oral, injected			
Other narcotics I II III IV V	Numorphan, Percodan, Percocet, Tylox, Tussionex, Fentanyl, Darvon, Lomotil, Talwin[b]	Analgesic, antidiarrheal, antitussive	High–low	High–low	Yes	Variable	Oral, injected			

▪ **Depressants**										
Chloral Hydrate IV	Noctec	Hypnotic	Moderate	Moderate	Yes	5–8	Oral	Slurred speech, disorientation, drunken behavior without odor of alcohol	Shallow respiration, clammy skin, dilated pupils, weak and rapid pulse, coma, possible death	Anxiety, insomnia, tremors, delirium, convulsions, possible death
Barbiturates II III IV	Amytal, Butisol, Fiorinal, Lotusate, Nembutal, Seconal, Tuinal, Phenobarbital	Anesthetic, anticonvulsant, sedative, hypnotic, veterinary euthanasia agent	High—moderate	High–moderate	Yes	1–16	Oral			
Benzodiazepines IV	Ativan, Dalmane, Diazepam, Librium, Xanax, Serax, Valium Tranxexe, Verstran, Versed, Halcion, Paxipam, Restoril	Antianxiety, anticonvulsant, sedative, hypnotic	Low	Low	Yes	4–8	Oral			
Methaqualone I	Quaalude	Sedative, hypnotic	High	High	Yes	4–8	Oral			
Glutethimide III	Doriden	Sedative, hypnotic	High	Moderate	Yes	4–8	Oral			
Other depressants III IV	Equanil, Miltown, Noludar, Placidyl, Valmid	Antianxiety, sedative, hypnotic	Moderate	Moderate	Yes	4–8	Oral			
▪ **Stimulants**										
Cocaine[a] II	Coke, Flake, Snow, Crack	Local anesthetic	Possible	High	Yes	1–2	Sniffed, smoked, injected	Increased alertness excitation, euphoria, increased pulse rate and blood pressure, insomnia, loss of appetite	Agitation, increase in body temperature, hallucinations, convulsions, possible death	Apathy, long periods of sleep, irritability, depression, disorientation
Amphetamines II	Biphetamine, Delcobese, Desoxyn, Dexedrine, Obetrol	Attention deficit disorders, narcolepsy, weight control	Possible	High	Yes	2–4	Oral, injected			
Phenmetrazine II	Preludin	Weight control	Possible	High	Yes	2–4	Oral, injected			
Methylphenidate II	Ritalin	Attention deficit disorders, narcolepsy	Possible	Moderate	Yes	2–4	Oral, injected			
Other stimulants III IV	Adipex, Cylert, Didrex, Ionamin, Melfiat, Plegine, Sanorex, Tenuate, Tepanil, Prelu-2	Weight control	Possible	High	Yes	2–4	Oral, injected			

(continued)

TABLE 44-1. CONTROLLED SUBSTANCES—USES AND EFFECTS (Continued)

Drugs/ CSA Schedules	Trade or Other Names	Medical Uses	Dependence		Tolerance	Duration (Hours)	Usual Methods of Administration	Possible Effects	Effects of Overdose	Withdrawal Syndrome
			Physical	Psychological						
▪ **Hallucinogens**										
LSD I	Acid, Microdot	None	None	Unknown	Yes	8–12	Oral	Illusions and hallucinations, poor perception of time and distance	Longer, more intense "trip" episodes, psychosis, possible death	Withdrawal syndrome not reported
Mescaline and peyote I	Mexc, Buttons, Cactus	None	None	Unknown	Yes	8–12	Oral			
Amphetamine variants I	2,5-DMA, PMA, STP, MDA, MDMA, TMA, DOM, DOB	None	Unknown	Unknown	Yes	Variable	Oral, injected			
Phencyclidine II	PCP, Angel Dust, Hog	None	Unknown	High	Yes	Days	Smoked, oral, injected			
Phencyclidine analogs I	PCE, PCPy, TCP	None	Unknown	High	Yes	Days	Smoked, oral, injected			
Other hallucinogens I	Bufotenine, Ibogaine, DMT, DET, Psilocybin, Psilocyn	None	None	Unknown	Possible	Variable	Smoked, oral, injected, sniffed			
▪ **Cannabis**										
Marijuana I	Pot, Acapulco Gold, Grass, Reefer, Sinsemilla, Thai Sticks	None	Unknown	Moderate	Yes	2–4	Smoked, oral	Euphoria, relaxed inhibitions, increased appetite, disoriented behavior	Fatigue, paranoia, possible psychosis	Insomnia, hyperactivity, and decreased appetite occasionally reported
Tetrahydrocannabinol I II	THC, Marinol	Cancer chemotherapy antinauseant	Unknown	Moderate	Yes	2–4	Smoked, oral			
Hashish I	Hash	None	Unknown	Moderate	Yes	2–4	Smoked, oral			
Hashish oil I	Hash oil	None	Unknown	Moderate	Yes	2–4	Smoked, oral			

[a] Designated a narcotic under the CSA.
[b] Not designated a narcotic under the CSA.

An understanding of the pharmacological properties of drugs is essential in the design of prevention efforts. Three processes are important in the development of drug abuse: (1) physical dependence, conceptualized as "an adaptive state that manifests itself by intense physical disturbances when the administration of a drug is suspended,"[8] (2) psychological dependence, conceptualized as a condition in which there is "a feeling of satisfaction and a psychic drive that requires periodic or continuous administration of the drug to produce pleasure or to avoid discomfort,"[8] and (3) tolerance, conceptualized as the need for increasingly higher doses of a drug to recapture the original effect of a dose.[10] All three of these processes reflect the pharmacological characteristics of a drug, individual characteristics of the person using them, and environmental characteristics particular to the setting(s) in which the drug is used. Much past and current research is designed to gain a better understanding of the processes themselves, the ways in which they interact, and their contribution to drug abuse. It should be noted, however, that drug abuse may exist in the absence of any or all of these processes. Adolescents' initial use of marijuana, for example, often is a response to peer pressure.

On initial use of a psychoactive drug, an individual is exposed to the reinforcing or pleasurable characteristics of the drug. The reinforcing–reward characteristic is an important factor in the initiation and maintenance of drug abuse. The more reinforcing the drug is, the more likely it is to be abused. This characteristic, termed the abuse liability of a drug, can be assessed in animal self-administration models. Work over the past 20 years has shown a strong correlation between the drugs that animals will self-administer and those that humans abuse.[11,12] With knowledge of its abuse liability, a drug can be scheduled in a manner to minimize its availability. Availability of a drug is seen as one of the principal determinants of the number of people who will try a drug and possibly go on to use it in a regular or compulsive fashion.[13,14] However, evaluation of abuse liability, although diagnostic of potential abuse, is not foolproof. For example, hallucinogens, such as mescaline, are not self-administered by animals[15] but are abused by humans. Nevertheless, knowledge of the general pharmacology and abuse liability of substances and the control of their distribution and use are useful steps in curtailing the amount of drug abuse that occurs. Both the basic research that establishes a drug's characteristics and the assignment of a drug to a schedule are an essential aspect of drug abuse prevention activities.

Narcotics. Narcotics (Table 44-1) include drugs ranging from heroin, which has no accepted medical use in the United States, to such drugs as morphine and meperidine, which are used commonly for their analgesic or antitussive properties. This class of drugs is widely abused. The degree of abuse depends on many factors, including the relative potency of the available formulations of the drug and economic and social factors.

Drugs listed under narcotics in Table 44-1 have opiumlike or morphinelike properties. These properties are shared with naturally occurring neuroactive peptides, for example, enkephalins and endorphins, which are active at certain brain sites[16] and coexist with norepinephrine, serotonin and other transmitters.[17] Narcotic drugs appear to be active in brain systems, mediating positive affective moods, and to mimic neuropeptides that may have evolved to guarantee that such essential acts as eating and sexual intercourse are repeated, thus increasing the probability of survival of the individual and the species.

Opium, the prototypical opioid, first extracted from the poppy plant, has been known to humanity since ancient times. Its medical analgesic uses were well established by the mid-sixteenth century, and opium smoking for purely subjective effects was an established practice in the Orient by the eighteenth century.[18] The structure of morphine, an alkaloid of opium, has been known since 1925, and synthetic derivatives are made by relatively simple modifications of morphine or thebaine, another alkaloid of opium. The effects of opioids are diverse, depending on many factors, and include altered endocrine and autonomic nervous system functions, changes in mood and pain perception, decreased gastrointestinal motility, drowsiness, nausea, respiratory depression, and vomiting.

Several types of brain receptors for opioid drugs have been identified, with morphinelike drugs appearing to have a preference for one subtype, the mu receptor. The site and mechanism of action of opioids are a focus of much current work by neuropharmacologists and other neuroscientists.[18,19]

Development of tolerance, dependence, and withdrawal to narcotics has been documented. It should be emphasized that tolerance and dependence reflect changes in drug disposition and pharmacodynamics but, in addition, are the result of an interactive process involving pharmacological characteristics of the drug, the individual's biology and behavior, and the individual's response to the setting. This principle is made clear in experiments in which the lethality of heroin has been shown to increase radically when rodents in a novel setting are given a heroin dose that they had tolerated previously in a familiar setting.[20] Tolerance to the many effects of a drug does not develop uniformly. For example, differentially greater tolerance to the euphorigenic effects of heroin with respect to its respiratory depressive characteristics may underlie at least some of the deaths associated with heroin overdoses.

Depressants. These include the drugs listed in Table 44-1 and alcohol, which is covered in Chapter 43. In general, the drugs shown under this heading share sedative and hypnotic properties and are used medically to produce drowsiness, sleep, and muscle relaxation and to prevent convulsions. The effects of these drugs are dose dependent, progressing from relaxation to sedation through hypnosis to stupor. In addition, barbiturates have anesthetic properties. In the 1950s, benzodiazepines were developed with high anxiolytic and low central nervous system depressant properties. This permitted relief of anxiety symptoms without suppression of cognitive, attention, or motor functions. Drugs listed as depressants have complex effects. Harvey[21] reviews their pharmacological properties. The relative degree of tolerance and dependence to these drugs varies from the benzodiazepines, assigned to schedule IV, to the barbiturates, which are associated with moderate to high abuse liability and are assigned to schedule II. Tolerance for and dependence on the various drugs of this class generalize within the class and across classes to some opiates and alcohol, thus showing cross-tolerance and cross-dependence. Since alcohol often is not recognized as a depressant drug in our society, its use with sedative–hypnotic drugs results in stupor and death more frequently than might be the case were alcohol's depressant characteristics more fully appreciated.[22]

Stimulants. Stimulant drugs generally are classified as excitatory in recognition of their main effect on the central nervous system. At low doses, stimulants are associated with feelings of increased alertness, euphoria, vigor, motor activity, and appetite suppression. At high doses, they cause convulsions. Changes in thought have been characterized on a continuum from hypervigilant through suspicion to paranoia. Amphetamine and cocaine-induced psychoses are described in chronic abusers.[23-25] Paranoid ideation generally is reported in persons with histories of chronic stimulant abuse, but transient psychotic symptoms have been reported with initial use of high doses,[26] and instances of psychoses associated with use of medically prescribed doses have been reported.[27] With repeated use, tolerance to some drug effects occurs, for example, euphoria and appetite suppression, whereas for other effects, for example, motor activity, stereotypy, and possibly paranoia, sensitization, an increased response to the drug, occurs.[28] Discontinuation of cocaine use results in symptoms characterized by three phases: crash, withdrawal, and extinction.[29] Thorough discussions of the general pharmacology of amphetamine and other sympathomimetic amines, including the various receptor systems at which they act, are available,[19,30] as is a comprehensive review of cocaine's behavioral pharmacology relevant to issues of abuse.[31]

Hallucinogens. Hallucinogens are the only category of abused drugs for which there is no accepted medical use. These drugs share an ability to distort perception and induce delusions, hallucinations, illusions, and profound alterations of mood. Mescaline and psilocin-containing plants have been used ceremonially for centuries, and LSD was synthesized by Hoffman in 1925. Under certain conditions, drugs from a variety of classes, in addition to those listed as hallucinogens in Table 44–1, show hallucinogenic properties. Because of similarities between experiences of persons ingesting hallucinogens and those of mentally ill persons and persons reporting profound religious experiences, these drugs also are termed psychotomimetics or psychedelics.

Hallucinogens can be classified as indolealkylamines, phenylethylamines, or phenylisopropylamines on the basis of their structure and pharmacology. As is true for other psychoactive substances, differential tolerance to the various effects can be demonstrated. For example, tolerance to the subjective effects of hallucinogens is greater than that seen for cardiovascular effects. Considerable cross-tolerance exists among drugs in this category. Drugs listed as phencyclidine-type hallucinogens are relatively new, and their potential for tolerance and dependence is not fully understood. Symptoms of physical dependence after abrupt withdrawal of phencyclidine have been described,[32] but similar reports for LSD do not exist. Jaffe[10] has discussed the pharmacology of hallucinogens in relation to their abuse.

Cannabis. Cannabis is obtained from the flowering top of the hemp plant. More than 60 cannabinoids have been isolated from the hemp plant, and 1-delta-9-tetrahydrocannabinol (delta-9-THC) has been identified as the isomer responsible for most of the characteristic effects of this category of drugs.[33] Cannabis affects cognition, memory, mood, motor coordination, self-perception, and sense of time and, under some conditions, produces feelings of relaxation and well-being. Tolerance is clearly seen after high doses and sustained use, and differential tolerance to the various effects and cross-tolerance occur to some hallucinogens.[34] Withdrawal symptoms characterized by irritability, restlessness, nervousness, decreased appetite, weight loss, and insomnia as well as delusions, paranoid ideation, and hallucinations have been reported.[10] Cannabis affects the cardiovascular system, increases heart rate, and differentially alters standing and supine blood pressure. Disruption of performance[35] and withdrawal symptoms[36] have been noted after discontinued use of delta-9-THC. A fuller discussion of the pharmacology of cannabis relative to its abuse is provided by Jaffe.[10]

EPIDEMIOLOGY

An understanding of the extent, nature, and duration of use and abuse of psychoactive drugs is a necessary prerequisite for developing effective and efficient drug abuse prevention and treatment programs. Three valuable sources of data are the National Household Survey on Drug Use, the Monitoring the Future Study, and the five-site Epidemiological Catchment Area (ECA) Program. The first two surveys are sponsored by the National Institute on Drug Abuse (NIDA) and the latter by the National Institute of Mental Health (NIMH).

Household Survey. The National Household Survey is based on responses to a detailed mail-in questionnaire plus face-to-face interviews of a large national probability sample of people 12 years of age or older.[37,38] The survey covers use of marijuana, cocaine, inhalants, hallucinogens, PCP, heroin, nonmedical use of four classes of psychotherapeutic drugs (stimulants, sedatives, tranquilizers, and analgesics), cigarettes and smokeless tobacco, and alcohol. Additional information gathered includes sex, race or ethnicity, density of population, region of residence, educational attainment, and employment. Use is documented for the past month, past year, and the respondent's lifetime. The 1985 survey interviewed 8038 persons, of whom 80.6% were white, 10.7% black, and 6.5% Hispanic. As shown in Table 44–2, approximately 37% of the population had used some illicit drug over their lifetime, and approximately 11% had used an illicit drug in the past month. Marijuana was the single most commonly used illicit drug, but use of multiple illicit drugs was even more common when lifetime experience was considered.

Reports of lifetime use differed by age. The lifetime use of

TABLE 44–2. PERCENT REPORTING USE OF MARIJUANA, NONMEDICAL USE OF ANY PSYCHOTHERAPEUTIC, AND OTHER ILLICIT DRUGS BY AGE GROUP IN LIFETIME AND PAST MONTH: 1985[a]

	Age Group (Years)				
	12–17	*18–25*	*26–34*	*35+*	**Total**
▪ Lifetime					
Use of any illicit drug (%)	29.5	64.3	62.2	20.4	36.8
Used					
Marijuana only (%)	10.6	26.0	25.0	7.2	14.2
Nonmedical psychotherapeutics only (%)	2.6	2.3	2.5	3.9	3.2
"More" illicit drugs[b] (%)	16.3	36.0	34.6	9.3	19.4
▪ Use Within the Past Month					
Use of any illicit drug (%)	13.9	24.1	20.0	3.4	11.2
Used					
Only marijuana (%)	7.8	11.9	9.1	1.2	5.3
Only nonmedical psychotherapeutics (%)	0.6	1.3	1.8	1.3	1.3
"More" illicit drugs[b] (%)	5.4	10.9	9.1	0.9	4.7

[a] Due to rounding, column percents may not total 100.0.
[b] The term "More" means that the respondent's use was not restricted to only marijuana or only the nonmedical use of psychotherapeutics.
From National Institute on Drug Abuse, 1985.[37]

marijuana and hashish was highest in 1985 for those aged 18 to 25 (60.3%) in comparison to those aged 26 to 34 (58.5%), 35+ (15.9%), and 12 to 17 (23.6%). Marijuana use peaked in 1979 and decreased in 1982 and 1985 for all ages except the 12 to 17-year-old group, where a nonsignificant increase from 11.5% (1982) to 12.0% (1985) was seen. Of special interest was the statistically significant decrease in past month use of marijuana (27.4% in 1982 to 21.8% in 1985) in 18 to 25 year olds who reported the highest lifetime use (Table 44–2). Almost twice as many males as females reported marijuana use in the past month (12.3% vs 6.8%), although at younger ages the difference was not as great (13.3% vs 10.6% at ages 12–17). Blacks reported more current marijuana use than whites or Hispanics (13.1 vs 9.1 vs 7.4%), but the age, sex, use pattern was complex. See Table 24 in NIDA, reference 37. In general, Table 24 shows that for the youngest age group (12–17), all males and white females reported more current use (between 10.9% and 13.7%) than black (5.5%) or Hispanic females (7.0%). As age increases, black males in increasingly higher percentages reported use, so that for persons 35 or over, 11.2% of black males reported use, with reports of current use for the other race and sex groups varying between 1.2% (Hispanic females) and 2.6% (Hispanic males). Since these data are not longitudinal, this pattern could reflect either of two situations. One is that black males continue use of marijuana at ages when other groups have stopped. The other is that black males discontinue drug use at the same rate as other groups, but older black males come from a proportionally larger group who began marijuana use some years ago.

Marijuana use in the past month was greatest in the unemployed (21.5%) compared to those employed full-time (11.7%) or part-time (10.25%). For people 18 or older, marijuana use was also higher in those having some college education (11.3%) than it was in college graduates (8.9%), high school graduates (9.9%), or those who did not graduate from high school (6.4%).

Cocaine use was less frequent than marijuana use, but 11.6% of those surveyed reported having tried it, 6.3% used it in the past year, and 2.9% used it in the past month. In the 1985 survey, route of use of cocaine was surveyed for the first time; 45.9% of the 12- to 17-year-old users reported having used freebase cocaine. This has serious implications for future prevention efforts, considering the increased availability of crack cocaine since 1985.

The National Household Survey also inquires about some of the consequences of drug use, and a large number of the persons sampled report concerns about their drug use. Of those who used marijuana 11 or more times in their lifetime, 37.2% report having tried to cut down their use, and 13.1% report they are dependent on the drug; 5.2% report having experienced withdrawal symptoms. See Table 73 in NIDA, reference 37. Among those who have used cocaine 11 or more times, 31.2% report having tried to cut down, 9.1% report dependence and 6.7% report withdrawal symptoms. See Table 74 in NIDA, reference 37. These data suggest that a significant percentage of the population is concerned about their drug use, and additional studies are needed to determine the ways in which these concerns are related to patterns of drug abuse or attempts to modify drug abuse behaviors.

Although the percent of the sample reporting use of some drugs may appear small, the total numbers of persons involved is not trivial. For example, the population estimated to have used cocaine 12 or more times in the past year in 1985 was slightly over 3.3 million persons, representing 1.6% of the white and 2.2% of the black population.

Monitoring the Future. The Monitoring the Future Study annually surveys 125 to 135 public and private high schools selected to provide a cross-section of the contiguous United States. Approximately 17,000 seniors complete the pencil and paper survey, and a representative sample of 2400 of them are followed in ensuing years. A review of the 1975–1987 data outlines the study design and procedures and presents an overview of key findings.[39] The survey covers 18 types of drugs for use at three periods: lifetime, annual, and past month (Table 44–3).

As in the Household Survey, marijuana was the most fre-

TABLE 44–3. 30-DAY PREVALENCE OF USE OF 18 TYPES OF DRUGS BY SUBGROUPS, CLASS OF 1987

	Marijuana	Inhalants[a]	Amyl/Butyl Nitrites	Hallucinogens	LSD	PCP	Cocaine[b]	Crack[b]	Other Cocaine[b]	Heroin	Other Opiates	Stimulants[c] (adjusted)	Sedatives	Barbiturates	Methaqualone	Tranquilizers	Alcohol	Cigarettes
All seniors	21.0[d]	2.8	1.3	2.5	1.8	0.6	4.3	1.5	4.1	0.2	1.8	5.2	1.7	1.4	0.6	2.0	66.4	29.4
Sex																		
Male	23.1	3.4	2.0	3.1	2.5	0.9	4.9	1.7	3.9	0.3	2.0	5.0	2.0	1.7	0.9	2.0	69.9	27.0
Female	18.6	2.2	0.7	1.8	1.1	0.4	3.7	1.1	4.0	0.1	1.7	5.2	1.3	1.1	0.3	2.0	63.1	31.4
College plans																		
None or <4 y	25.1	4.0	2.4	2.8	2.0	1.3	5.3	1.7	3.5	0.2	2.5	7.2	2.4	1.9	0.9	2.4	68.6	39.7
Complete 4 y	18.5	2.2	0.8	2.1	1.5	0.3	3.6	1.1	3.4	0.2	1.5	4.0	1.2	1.0	0.4	1.7	65.7	24.3
Region																		
Northeast	25.3	2.9	0.7	3.5	2.3	0.2	5.4	1.5	5.4	0.2	2.1	5.1	1.7	1.6	0.6	2.6	69.1	34.1
North Central	21.1	3.8	1.5	2.5	1.7	0.6	3.0	1.4	2.7	0.2	1.9	5.8	1.5	1.3	0.7	1.6	70.7	31.7
South	17.3	2.4	1.3	1.9	1.6	0.6	2.9	0.8	2.8	0.1	1.4	4.5	1.9	1.5	0.5	2.2	60.7	26.6
West	22.3	1.9	1.8	2.3	1.5	1.1	7.4	2.7	6.8	0.3	2.3	5.4	1.4	1.2	0.6	1.5	66.7	26.6
Population density																		
Large SMSA	23.1	2.0	1.0	3.3	2.1	0.6	5.7	2.0	5.9	0.1	1.9	5.2	1.6	1.3	0.5	2.2	66.3	29.3
Other SMSA	21.3	2.9	0.9	2.3	1.8	0.3	4.1	1.1	3.6	0.2	1.7	4.7	1.6	1.4	0.6	2.1	66.9	28.2
Non-SMSA	18.2	3.3	2.4	2.0	1.4	1.2	3.4	1.7	3.4	0.3	2.0	6.0	1.8	1.6	0.7	1.6	65.5	31.8

SMSA = Standard metropolitan statistical area.
[a] Unjustified for known underreporting of certain drugs.
[b] Cocaine data based on five questionnaire forms; crack data based on two questionnaire forms; and other cocaine data based on one questionnaire form.
[c] Based on the data from the revised question, which attempts to exclude the inappropriate reporting of nonprescription stimulants.
[d] Entries are percentages.

quently used illicit drug. The percentage reporting marijuana use (21%) approached that reporting cigarette use (29.4%). Of the 50.2% of high school seniors who reported any lifetime use of marijuana, over two thirds (34.6%) began use between seventh and tenth grades. See Table 15 in Johnston et al., reference 39.

Trends in lifetime prevalence for drug use show declines over the past 10 years. The year in which use peaked varied from 1979 for marijuana to 1985 for cocaine. Inhalant use is an exception to this pattern, with the lifetime prevalence fluctuating between 17% and 20% since its use was first measured in 1979. See Table 8 in Johnston et al., reference 39.

Between 1975 and 1978, an almost twofold increase in daily use of marijuana was reported such that in 1978, 10.7% of high school seniors were in this category. By 1987, reports of daily use had dropped to 3.3%, well below the 6% level reported in 1975. Noncontinuation, defined as the percentage of previous users of a specific drug who did not use it in the year before the survey, has been relatively stable for most drugs but has increased for marijuana from 16% in 1979 to 27.7% in 1987. Noncontinuation rates for more experienced users (10 or more times in their lifetime) are much lower than for less experienced users (fewer than 10 times in their lifetime). For example, in 1987, the noncontinuance rate for marijuana was 9.2% for the more experienced group compared to 27.7% for the less experienced group. For cocaine, noncontinuance rates were 7.6% for the more experienced group compared to 32.2% for the less experienced group.

Johnston and colleagues[39] associate decline in drug use with an increased perception of its adverse effects and peer disapproval of use. They report that the percentage who perceive smoking marijuana regularly as being a "great risk" has increased from less than 40% in 1978 to over 70% in 1987, and the percentage who disapprove of smoking marijuana regularly increased from 67.5% to 89.2% over the same period. See Fig. 21 and Table 17 in Johnston et al., reference 39. During the period in which reports of drug use have declined and beliefs of adverse consequences and social disapproval of use have increased, the perceived availability of drugs has either remained stable (marijuana) or increased (amphetamine and cocaine). See Fig. 27a in Johnston et al., reference 39.

The 30-day prevalence of marijuana use reported by Johnston and associates[39] is similar to the Household Survey finding that 21.8% of the 18 to 25-year group used marijuana in the past 30 days. This indicates that self-report data are reliable over these surveys. The question of validity of self-reports is, of course, crucial to an understanding of these survey data. An excellent overview of this issue is presented by Rouse and colleagues.[40] Large variations exist in drug use patterns within specific subgroups and from one local community to another. It is desirable to supplement national surveys with local surveys. Good discussions and examples of this point and other methodological considerations are available.[40,41] Beauvais and Oetting[42] emphasize that surveys of local drug use patterns must be completed in order for effective prevention programs to be tailored to the local community's needs.

Epidemiological Catchment Area (ECA) Studies. The ECA studies have provided population estimates of the numbers of people who can be classified as having a drug abuse or drug dependency disorder. Regier and associates[43] used the NIMH Diagnostic Interview Schedule, based on DSM-III, to identify the prevalence of drug abuse and drug dependency disorder in the five ECA catchment areas for persons aged 18 and older. Lifetime and 6-month prevalence rates for drug abuse/drug dependency disorder were 5.9% and 2.0%, respectively. The 1-month prevalence rate was 1.3%, with over twice as many men as women affected, 1.9% vs 0.7%. Drug abuse and drug dependency disorder predominantly affected persons under 25 years of age, with a rate of 4.8% for males aged 18 to 24. Prevalence rates for mental disorders, including drug abuse, in the 18 to 30-year-old group has been addressed specifically in the five-site ECA sample.[44] In this study, a 6-month prevalence rate of drug abuse/drug dependency disorder of 2.0% was found, with the median age of onset of 18. Early onset of anxiety or depression did not increase risk of alcohol abuse, but it approximately doubled the risk of drug abuse.[44]

Lower prevalence rates for drug abuse/drug dependency disorders in Mexican Americans compared to non-Hispanic whites have been reported for a Los Angeles ECA sample 18 years of age or older.[45] These data indicate that 6-month prevalence rates of drug abuse/drug dependency disorders are 2.8% for Mexican American men and 0.6% for Mexican American women vs 5.2% and 2.0% for non-Hispanic white men and women, respectively.

In summary, the epidemiological data establish that drug abuse in varying degrees of severity affects a sizable proportion of the general population, thus adding emphasis to the need for prevention efforts. They also reveal differential rates and patterns of use, suggesting that not all persons are equally at risk for drug abuse. Information on correlates of drug use suggest that variables associated with drug use include age, sex, race or ethnicity, employment, education, perception of adverse effects of drugs, and peer attitudes. In addition, epidemiological reports on noncontinuation of drug use indicate that the probability of stopping drug use is inversely related to the frequency of drug use.

ETIOLOGY

An understanding of the causal factors that give rise to the initiation and maintenance of drug abuse is fundamental to the development of prevention and treatment strategies. Substance abuse and substance abuse disorders are considered to result from complex interactions of biological, sociological, and psychological factors. A detailed discussion of the current major theoretical positions and the investigations they generate is beyond the scope of this chapter. However, since discussion of prevention activities is facilitated by an understanding of their relation to etiological models of drug abuse, a brief discussion is warranted.

Behavioral Genetics Studies. Behavioral genetics provides the framework for one line of etiological investigations. These studies use two experimental designs to look at the relationships among genetic factors, environmental factors, and an outcome behavior. The twin design compares identical twins and fraternal twins for similarity on a behavioral end point. The adopted-away design compares children adopted away at birth or shortly thereafter with those raised by their natural parents when both kind of parents either do or do not have the behavioral end point (e.g., alcoholism). Heritability, a statistical description of the portion of the variability in the behavior that can be ascribed to genetic factors, can be determined by both approaches. These designs can clarify the contribution of genetic and environmental factors to behavioral outcomes that have been shown to be familial—that is, their occurrence differs across families historically as has been shown for alcoholism.[46] Intelligence, personality, temperament, and psychopathology have been shown to be influenced by genetic factors using these experimental designs.

Nevertheless, it would appear that few complex behaviors are under the control of a single gene. A recent review of this work concluded that "genetic effects on behavior are polygenic and probabilistic, not single gene and deterministic" and that "genetic influence on individual differences in behavioral development is usually significant and often substantial" but "nongenetic factors are responsible for more than half of the variance for most complex behaviors."[47]

Behavioral Genetics of Alcoholism. (See Chapter 60.) Cadoret and colleagues[48] reviewed twin studies that indicated a greater concordance for alcoholism in monozygotic twins than in dizygotic twins. However, the 40% to 50% discordance in alcoholism seen in monozygotic twins suggests a strong influence of environmental factors in the development of alcoholism. Adopted-away studies of alcoholism have clearly established that sons of alcoholic mothers or fathers are at risk for increased rates of alcoholism, 23% vs 10% in the general population.[49] For daughters, a biological mother with alcoholism significantly increased the rate of alcoholism (10.3%). Rates (3.5%) for women with an alcoholic biological father were not significantly higher that those (2.8%) found in women whose biological parents were not alcoholic.[50] Cloninger and coworkers have been leaders in this field and note "an important general principle in genetic epidemiology is that disorders as prevalent as alcoholism have complex patterns of development involving the interaction of many genetic and environmental influences."[51] Genetic predisposition toward alcoholism is moderated by two types of factors, those that increase and those that decrease risk.[52–55] The identification of these factors and the ways in which they interact with any inherited factors are important to our understanding of alcoholism.

Behavioral Genetics of Substance Abuse [Drug Abuse or Alcoholism, Individually or in Combination]. Tarter[56] has theorized that temperament and its expression in personality constitute an important diathesis that, under certain developmental and environmental conditions, leads to drug abuse as well as alcoholism, a proposition that should be submitted to empirical investigation. However, few studies directly address this hypothesis. Work on the behavioral genetics of abuse of illicit drugs either by themselves or in combination with alcohol has been neglected. For example, there appears to be only one study focusing on drug abuse in adopted-away children,[57] and twin studies have focused on either alcohol[49–55] or nicotine.[58]

Cadoret and colleagues[57] identified possible or definite drug abuse in 25.2% of male and 7.0% of female adoptees, and many of these people used multiple drugs, including alcohol. Information on alcohol abuse, but not drug abuse, was available for the biological parents. Thus, it was possible to trace the intergenerational occurrence of alcoholism but not drug abuse. In this study, genetic influence on drug abuse in adoptees appeared to follow two possible routes: (1) antisocial behavior in biological relatives was associated with antisocial behavior in adoptees, which, in turn, was associated with drug abuse, and (2) alcoholism in the biological parents was associated with drug abuse in the adoptees in the absence of antisocial behavior. This latter route suggests that a predisposition for generalized substance abuse may be inherited. Characteristics of adoptive parents that increased the risk for drug abuse were divorce and parental psychiatric problems.

Familial Transmission Studies. Studies of the occurrence of drug abuse within families allow one to determine if there is a higher probability for drug abuse across successive generations in some family lines than in others. Although this design does not allow separation of environmental and biological factors, positive findings can be further explored through twin or adopted-away studies. One study that can be considered in this framework examined alcohol abuse in the parents of opiate addicts who were not alcoholic (422 persons) and opiate addicts (216 persons) who were also alcoholics.[59] Mothers of alcoholic addicts had significantly higher rates of alcoholism (9.7%) than did the mothers of nonalcoholic addicts (3.8%). Fathers of alcoholic addicts showed a nonstatistically significant increase in their rate of alcoholism (20.4%) over that of the fathers of nonalcoholic addicts (16%). These data provide partial support for familial clustering of alcoholism by showing that mothers of alcoholic addicts were more likely to be alcoholic than mothers of nonalcoholic addicts.

Four other studies have looked at opioid dependence and alcoholism in relatives of opioid-dependent probands.[60–63] Maddux and Desmond[63] reviewed the earlier studies and concluded that they support the clustering of opioid dependence, but not alcoholism, within families of addict probands. In this regard, the data support other work[62] suggesting that alcoholism tended to cluster in families of alcoholics and opioid abuse in families of opioid abusers and the possibility that vulnerability to abuse of a specific drug is transmitted genetically.

Maddux and Desmond[63] also looked at opioid dependence and alcoholism in the parents and siblings of 235 opioid-dependent persons whose use of alcohol also was evaluated. These opioid abusers had a 56% lifetime prevalence of alcoholism, which is elevated over the 24% lifetime prevalence for males estimated by the ECA. These data support other evidence of increased risk of codependency in this population. The alcoholism rate for fathers of these opioid abusers (33.2%) exceeded the ECA projections, whereas those for their mothers (4.3%), brothers (9.9%), and sisters (1.3%) did not. Siblings' rate of opioid dependence (16.6% for brothers and 2.2% for sisters) was greater than the estimated lifetime prevalence of 0.9% in the general population, whereas parental rate of opioid dependence (0.4% for fathers and zero for mothers) was not. The authors conclude that their study demonstrates familial clustering for opioid abuse but argue that this is not equivalent to familial transmission of susceptibility to abuse of a specific drug. In Maddux and Desmond's opinion, if familial transmission is operating, it consists of a generalized predisposition to either alcoholism or opioid dependence, with the principal substance of abuse being influenced by availability and peer influences. On balance, the Maddux and Desmond data fail to support the earlier studies or the hypothesis of a genetic vulnerability to abuse of a specific drug put forth by Hill and colleagues.[62]

Studies of the intergenerational patterns of addictive behavior could be designed using three different groups: alcoholics, drug abusers, and persons having both conditions, to look at the presence in different generations of alcoholism in combination with or independent of drug abuse. This design would provide information about whether or not susceptibility to abuse of a specific drug or a general risk for substance abuse is inherited.

Codependency and Comorbidity. Two factors that complicate consideration of the etiology of drug abuse are the presence of polydrug abuse (codependency) and the coexistence of drug abuse and a psychological disorder (comorbidity). In a recent review of 75 studies that evaluated the coexistence of alcoholism, drug abuse, or antisocial personality, these three conditions were found to be highly associated.[64] Of the 44 studies that examined the relationship between alcoholism and drug abuse, 80% described positive associations. Positive associations also were reported for 76% of the studies examining antisocial personality and drug abuse relationships and for 79% of the studies investigating antisocial personality and alcoholism relationships. Another study found increased alcoholism in opiate addicts—35% vs approximately 15% in the local community in which the study was carried out—and 54% of the addicts were diagnosed as having a major depressive disorder, whereas 27% were found to have an antisocial personality disorder.[59]

Little is known about the natural history of codependency and comorbidity in drug abusers. The ECA data indicate that developmentally, anxiety disorders precede drug abuse disorder, which, in turn, precedes alcohol disorders and major depressive episodes.[44] The lifetime prevalence of anxiety disorder is 14.6%, and the median age of onset is 15. Lifetime prevalence of drug abuse is 5.9%, and the median age at onset is 19. Lifetime prevalence for major depressive episode is 5.8%, and the median age at onset is 24. Drug abuse and either anxiety disorder or major depressive episode occurs in 4.6% of 18 to 30 year olds, and approximately 80% of multiple disorders have their onset before age 20. In 54.3% of individuals with multiple disorders, anxiety disorder precedes drug abuse, as do major depressive episodes in 19.6% of these individuals. For the remaining 26.1%, drug abuse precedes anxiety disorder or major depressive disorder. This information reinforces the idea that drug abuse prevention efforts should be tailored for young people. It also suggests that young people who are identified as having anxiety problems may need prevention programs especially formulated for their needs in order to avoid drug abuse. Finally, they remind us that drug abuse treatment programs need to address the needs of young persons, especially those who have co-occurence of drug abuse and anxiety.

Risk Factor Studies. Over the past 10 years, a number of risk factors, in addition to those discussed previously, have been identified as facilitating the initiation or augmentation of drug abuse in adolescents and young adults. The following risk factors have been identified relatively consistently[65-84]:

Parents' drug use[65-67]	Parents' educational level68
Family strife[67,69]	Peer drug use[70,71]
Early alcohol use[67,72]	Sensation seeking[73,74]
Low socioeconomic status[84]	Deviance[67,75,76]
Poor school grades[77,78]	Low self-esteem[67,79]
Depression[67,80]	Aggression[81,82]
Age[83]	

Two factors that are associated with declines in drug use in young adults are employment and marriage.[81,85]

In order to understand the progression of drug use from its initiation to the point where it becomes habitual or a drug abuse or drug dependency disorder develops, many factors have been evaluated to determine if their presence can be causally linked to continued drug use, drug abuse/drug dependency disorder, other psychological disorders, and criminal behavior. Kandel and coworkers outlined developmental periods of risk for drug abuse, progression patterns, and predictors of progression.[83,86,87] Data derived from a longitudinal sample of New York high school students, who were first interviewed in the tenth or eleventh year of school and again 9 years later, indicated that 90% of use began by age 18 for alcohol, by age 19 for cigarettes, and by age 20 for marijuana. Most use of other illicit drugs, except cocaine, was initiated before age 21. A progression from alcohol or cigarettes to marijuana and, subsequently, to other illicit drugs or to prescription drugs was identified that described the pattern of drug abuse involvement for most of the sample. Peers' use of marijuana was identified as an important factor for marijuana initiation. Current use of marijuana or prescription psychoactive drugs was strongly related to initiation of use of other illicit drugs. Initiation of prescription psychoactive drug use was related to multiple factors, including current or former use of illicit drugs, depression symptoms, maternal use of psychoactive drugs, and dropping out of school. Persistence of illicit drug use in young adulthood was related to the same factors that predict initiation in adolescence: peer use, delinquency, and unconventionality.[88] Kandel and coworkers identified important age effects in the initiation, escalation, and persistence of drug abuse. The age effects must be considered in conjunction with the period and cohort trends in drug use,[89] since the modal pattern of drug abuse across age may be subject to cultural influence. In addition, the modal pattern of drug abuse combines many subpopulations with differential risks of drug abuse. Identification of the parameters that separate these subgroups is critical if prevention programs are to be targeted to the needs of the specific groups.

Other work has found a highly significant linear relation between number of risk factors and extent of drug use in a high school population.[67,90] In a group of 994 adolescents, 8% used marijuana daily. Of these, 56% had 7 or more risk factors, and only 1% had zero risk factors.

Oetting and coworkers[70,91,92] have proposed that the peer cluster, which they define as the small intimate group who share beliefs and values, mediates the influence of other psychosocial variables on drug abuse. Furthermore, peer cluster effects are robust across various ethnic groups, whereas the importance of other variables, notably the mediating influence of anger and self-esteem, appears to vary from culture to culture in the direction and strength of their influence on drug abuse.[93]

The various studies of the etiology of drug abuse clearly indicate that primary prevention efforts should be targeted for certain populations distinguished on the basis of demographic or personal characteristics or both, especially those identified in the epidemiological studies reviewed earlier. In addition, since the probability of drug abuse may be related linearly to the number of risk factors present, intensity and content of prevention programs should be improved by tailoring them to both the extent and type of risk factors found in the population to whom the program is being delivered.

PREVENTION

Bukoski[94] has provided an overview of various models of drug abuse prevention, including public health, communicable disease, and risk factor models. In Bukoski's view, prior research supports the use of a combination of prevention strategies based on the level of the individual's psychosocial development and the extent of his or her drug use. In this model, termed comprehensive prevention, various prevention strategies are focused at four levels: individual, family, peer group, and community. An extensive review of primary drug abuse prevention activity is beyond the scope of this chapter. To provide a brief overview of primary prevention, we discuss a previous comprehensive review[95] and two meta-analyses describing earlier prevention programs.[96,97]

Review of Earlier Studies. Schaps and colleagues[95] studied 127 prevention programs operating between 1968 and 1977 to determine their effect on drug use and attitudes toward drug use. These programs used prevention strategies designed to provide specific information or skills relating to drug use consequences, changing attitudes, emotions, or behaviors, peer group processes, parenting, organizational processes, and other activities. In addition, many programs used peers in counseling, tutoring, or teaching. Almost half the programs offered more than one activity. Thus, a fivefold classification was used to categorize the combined program content: information, affective, information plus affective, counseling, and other. Duration, scope, and persistence of program delivery were determined to provide a measure of program intensity. Outcome measures yielded little evidence of an influence of the programs on drug use behaviors or attitudes. Many of these studies employed very weak outcome measures, however, that may have been unable to detect an effect. For example, Schaps rated only 20% of the studies as having a strong research design, with another 21% rated as acceptable. Among the best controlled studies were nine prevention programs that used peer or affective strategies alone or in combination with other strategies. Significant reductions in drug use behaviors were found in eight of these programs.

Meta-analysis of Earlier Studies. The utility of using peers to influence, teach, counsel, and facilitate the delivery of primary prevention programs to groups of young people was borne out in a meta-analysis[96] that compared outcome measures in 143 programs employing five major program modalities: (1) knowledge only, (2) affective only, (3) peer programs incorporating refusal skills or social and life skills, (4) knowledge plus affective, or (5) alternative programs dealing with activities or competence. Compared to other modalities, peer programs had significantly more influence on all outcome measures of alcohol, cigarette, and illicit drug use. Tobler[96] pointed out that use of peers facilitates positive outcomes in programs designed for the average student, but that programs using alternative strategies delivered with high intensity proved to be useful with special populations, including minority ethnic groups, adolescents with poor school performance, and those who already were using drugs.

Bangert-Drowns[97] also examined the relative strength of various models of prevention in 33 school-based alcohol and drug abuse prevention programs using meta-analyis techniques. He reported that all programs recorded positive changes in knowledge and attitudes about drug abuse. Use of peers in teaching roles appeared somewhat stronger than the other models in terms of the positive changes in knowledge and attitude. However, none of the models was associated with a significant decrease in drug use.

These evaluations of prevention programs, carried out over the past 15 to 20 years, indicate that the programs reviewed generally resulted in changes in drug abuse attitudes and knowledge but did not reliably result in changes in drug abuse behaviors. Comprehensive reviews[94,98–101] of issues of process, outcome, and impact research as they relate to drug abuse prevention suggest that there is a critical need for evaluation of process variables in order to determine which prevention program strategies work with whom and under what circumstances.

Antidrug Abuse Media Campaigns. Several lines of current work are converging to demonstrate that drug prevention can be marketed in much the same manner that other products are marketed. The Partnership for a Drug Free America is a coalition of national associations working in advertising that came together in a voluntary effort to change attitudes toward drugs through media campaigns. The National Institute on Drug Abuse staff has provided expert advice to the coalition to assure that the content of the campaigns adequately represents the potential adverse effects of drug use. The campaign's goals are to decrease acceptance of drug use, increase social disapproval of use, increase awareness of risks, increase parent–child communications about drug issues, and decrease demand for drugs.

Outcome research on the project is designed to track attitudes toward drug abuse and their relationship to reported drug use in a sample approximating the national audience. Black[102] found that the use of marijuana and cocaine was established by age 13 in approximately 10% of the population. Many children aged 9 to 12 reported being approached to buy drugs (16%) and that social pressures exist that promote drug use. For example, 39% find it hard to refuse friends who offer drugs, and 37% think drug users are popular.

Predictors of vulnerability in the 9 to 12-year-old group were older siblings' influence, peer influence, and beliefs about adverse effects. Age of first use and peer use are the strongest predictors of the extent of drug use in teenagers. Black children appear especially vulnerable to drug promotion. More black children aged 9 to 12 reported being approached to buy or use drugs than white children (27% vs 13%), and more black children reported that it was easy to buy or use drugs than white children (39% vs 16% for marijuana and 11% vs 6% for cocaine). More black than white adults also reported that drugs are easily accessible (44% vs 27% for marijuana, 34% vs 17% for cocaine, and 31% vs 14% for crack). These results serve to emphasize the importance of targeting prevention activities for those at risk, including the very young (age 8–12) and black children and adults.

Between 1987 and 1988, negative attitudes toward drug use increased in children, teenagers, and young adults. Increased negativity of attitudes toward drug use was more pronounced in those markets having high media exposure of the antidrug abuse materials in comparison with the rest of the country. Although teenage audiences were the hardest to influence, in communities with high exposure of the media materials, teens showed 8% to 20% increases in their negative view of drug use, whereas teenagers in the rest of the country showed 5% to 6% negativity shifts. Statistically significant declines in cocaine use were reported by college students in the communities where attitude changes were the greatest. The results of the first 2 years of this project suggest that accurate information packaged skillfully by advertising experts can be a powerful factor in changing drug abuse attitudes and drug use in targeted groups.

The trend of decreasing rates of drug use documented by Johnston and coworkers on the basis of data gathered in the Monitoring the Future studies[103–107] has been related to the increased perception of the risk of drug use and increased disapproval of drug use. Extensive statistical analyses indicated that although lifestyle factors account for some of the decrease in drug use, by far the most significant predictors are the perception of risk and attitude of disapproval factors. Thus, questions relating to the most efficient ways to produce these changes have taken on added importance.

One successful program has built on the research showing that sensation seeking is an important determinant of drug use, with junior and senior high school students who are high sensation seekers being two to seven times more likely to initiate use of an illicit drug than low sensation seekers. Donohew and colleagues[108] have manipulated the content of experimental public service announcements to elicit strong or weak sensory, affective, and arousal responses. Messages about a drug abuse hot line service were delivered to adolescents who differed in their levels of sensation seeking, and the recipients' intention to follow up by calling the hot line was measured. As predicted, intention to call the hot line was greatest when the sensation value of the message matched the sensation-seeking characteristics of the recipient. An interaction between sensation value of the message and drug use history was found, and intention to call the hot line was highest for drug users given the high sensation message and for nonusers given the low sensation message. This work promises to identify optimal methods of presenting material to individuals who vary in terms of their preferred level of sensory input and their drug experience and, thus, improve the efficiency of antidrug abuse public service campaigns.

Drug Abuse Resistance Skills Training. Much contemporary drug abuse prevention research is focused on providing young people with skills to resist peer and media forces that promote use of cigarettes and alcohol. Although use of these drugs is legal for adults, it should be remembered that their purchase is illegal for youngsters, and thus, use of cigarettes and alcohol can be considered abuse in a young population. Research on resistance skills training developed from studies conducted by Evans and coworkers[98–100] based on social learning theory, information processing theory, and developmental principles. Evans and coworkers developed films using same-age peers to deliver brief (less than 10 minutes) smoking cessation messages. Discussion and other materials were designed to reinforce the content of the films. Measures of knowledge, attitudes, intentions, and use were recorded as well as an objective, saliva-based measure of smoking. The 10 weeks postprogram measures showed that the rate of smoking initiation in the nonsmokers who had participated in either of two forms of the prevention program (8.6% and 10%) was approximately half the rate of the control group (18.3%).

Flay[109] reviewed four generations of work on social inoculation–peer resistance techniques in which the content of the material presented is closely linked to substance use behavioral end points. The Evans work described is termed "first generation." Fourth generation studies are described as large-scale field trials with numerous classrooms assigned to each intervention. In these studies, participation in the prevention program was clearly related to noninitiation of smoking that did not erode over a 2-year period.[110-112] When children who had never smoked before the intervention (early in sixth grade) were surveyed at the end of eighth grade, 60% of the children who had taken part in the prevention program had not initiated smoking compared to 47% of the children in the control program. Furthermore, children who were at high risk for smoking, as defined by having parents, siblings, and friends who smoked, appeared to benefit most from the intervention. High-risk children, who had not smoked before the intervention, were retested at the end of eighth grade. Sixty-seven percent of the high-risk children who were in the prevention program still had not initiated smoking, whereas only 22% of the high-risk control group remained nonsmokers.

In addition to pointing out specific research design and analysis issues, the work on drug abuse resistance skills training suggests that prevention can be enhanced by the development of objective, noninvasive measures of use. This point was demonstrated clearly by Evans and associates,[100] who found that presentation of a short film demonstrating that nicotine could be detected in saliva improved the accuracy of smoking self-reports. This procedure of convincing people that an objective measure of truthfulness of self-reports is available to the researcher is known as the "bogus pipeline" procedure, and it has become a standard feature of much smoking research. The improved validity and reliability associated with it strongly suggest that the development of relatively innocuous methods of testing for the presence of illicit drugs would strengthen drug abuse prevention research by allowing the bogus pipeline procedure to be used to enhance the validity of self-reports of drug use.

Cognitive–Behavioral Skills Training. Review of nine recent studies using the same basic social learning–persuasive communication theoretical framework as those reviewed by Flay[109] but concentrating on transmitting more general skills indicates that his model is an effective way of preventing drug abuse.[113] Although the nine studies shared some intervention strategies, others were unique to specific programs. Thus, the programs could be designated by their unique intervention elements, such as social assertiveness skills training,[114] cognitive–behavioral skills training,[115] decision skills training,[116] and life training skills.[117] All nine studies showed positive outcomes on one or more measures of smoking, and three reported significant effects on alcohol or marijuana use. The magnitude of the effects was "relatively large" demonstrating "that generic skills approaches to substance abuse prevention can produce about a 50% reduction in the incidence of substance use behavior."[113]

Comprehensive Model of Prevention. In addition to the issues, raised above, prevention research has adopted a goal of developing theoretically based, multimodal interventions that can be disseminated on a community-wide basis without the loss of impact and at a reasonable cost. One program that promises to meet these criteria has been developed by Pentz and associates.[118] This program includes mass media programming, school-based training of drug use resistance skills, parent involvement and education, community organization, and health policy components. The research project consists of a quasi-experimental design to be introduced sequentially to the entire adolescent population of 15 Kansas City metropolitan area communities and replication with a randomized experimental design in Indianapolis.

In the first 2 years of the study, 22,500 children enrolled in the sixth or seventh grade in 42 Kansas City area schools were surveyed. Base rates of drug use were essentially equal between prevention and control classrooms. The 1-year follow-up prevalence rates of cigarette, marijuana, and alcohol use was significantly lower for children enrolled in schools with prevention programs (17% vs 24% for cigarette, 7% vs 10% for marijuana, and 11% vs 16% for alcohol for the prevention and control groups, respectively). Future development of this model should provide guidelines to communities for providing cost-efficient, effective prevention measures to school-age children, who comprise one of the largest populations at risk for drug abuse.

The measure of drug use that has been most affected by school- and community-based prevention programs appears to be the onset of tobacco, marijuana, and alcohol use. Programs that are successful in delaying or preventing these behaviors in most children may not be sufficient to meet the needs of students whose risk of drug abuse is increased over that of the typical adolescent. In an examination of drug use in Native American youth and other minority groups, Oetting and coworkers[93,119] find that although drug use is dropping in these groups, it is only decreasing for those youths who are at little-to-moderate risk, with the behavior of youth at high risk remaining essentially unchanged.

Future work must address the specific needs of subpopulations. Likewise, future work will need to design early intervention programs for children with specific risks for drug abuse and employ long-term follow-up measures to determine the effect of the interventions on substance abuse. For example, Kellam and coworkers have initiated a prevention program with aggressive early elementary aged children who are at risk for drug abuse as teenagers.[120] This work and similarly designed studies will determine whether delaying the onset of smoking influences the onset of use of other drugs and whether or not nonuse of these substances during preteen and teenage years protects high-risk persons from abuse of drugs at later stages of life.

Once drug use is begun, frequency of use is an important variable in predicting whether or not it will be continued. Kandel and associates studied persons, identified at age 15 or 16 as having used illicit drugs at least 10 times, for their drug use at ages 24 or 25. Continuance rates of 80% for marijuana and 75% for other illicit drugs were found for men, and for women these rates were 71% for marijuana and 59% for other illicit drugs.[81] Thus, these data indicate that a large number of persons, particularly males, are likely to continue drug use. The household survey data indicate that people who use drugs are concerned about it. Taken together, these studies indicate a need for research on the transition from light to heavier drug use and the development of intervention programs targeted at people who are already abusing drugs but in whom the drug use pattern has not become so severe as to warrant a diagnosis of drug abuse/drug dependence disorder. Furthermore, the data suggest that intervention programs sensitive to the needs of and pressures on males in low socioeconomic groups, in which racial and ethnic minorities are overrepresented, would seem to be especially needed given the picture of continuation, and perhaps escalation, of drug use in this group.

Finally, much work remains to be done on the questions of codependency among the various forms of drug abuse and comorbidity with other mental disorders in order to determine to what degree prevention of drug abuse must be conceptualized as an activity independent of other mental health prevention activities.

TREATMENT OF DRUG ABUSE

The major goal of treatment is to eliminate or reduce drug use among drug abusers and drug-dependent persons who seek treatment or are referred for treatment and to prevent their relapse to drug use after treatment. Psychoactive substance use disorders[9] are characterized by maladaptive behavioral changes associated with more or less regular use of the substance or irregular use in amounts that impair functioning. Classification of psychoactive substance abuse disorders has undergone continual revision and refinement over the past 30 years and reflects the growth of empirical knowledge about the behavioral pharmacology of abused drugs and clinical experience with populations who abuse them. Psychoactive substance use disorders have been defined for 10 categories of drugs: alcohol, amphetamine, cannabis, cocaine, hallucinogen, inhalant, nicotine, opioid, phencyclidine, and sedative, hypnotic, or anxiolytic. In general, two subcategories exist for each disorder: dependence and abuse. In addition, polydrug dependence and abuse of other unspecified psychoactive substances is recognized. It is estimated that approximately 3 million Americans have psychoactive substance abuse disorders.

Most of the 37 million persons who indicated use of illicit drugs in the 1985 NIDA Household Survey do not use amounts of drug or suffer consequences of use that would cause them to be labeled as drug abusers or diagnosed as having psychoactive substance use disorders. There is no evidence that most of these people required assistance, beyond the kind of information that is widely available, to cease using illicit drugs. Another sizable group of persons whose abuse of illicit drugs becomes a problem find the help they need to change their behavior in self-help groups, such as the 12-step programs, or through personal resources, such as family, friends, and church. A small portion of the people who initiate use of an illicit psychoactive substance, who nonetheless comprise a large number of people, go on to use drugs in ways that are troublesome to them and their families and find that they are unable to initiate or maintain the behavior changes necessary to become drug free without the aid of a treatment program.

Over the past 30 years, treatment programs designed to provide services to drug abusers have been established by federal, state, and local governments. Two types of treatment exist, psychosocial and pharmacological, and they often are used in combination. There are three main modalities of treatment, detoxification, methadone maintenance, and drug free programs, which are provided generally in three settings, hospital inpatient, residential, and outpatient. Private, nonprofit, or for profit, facilities also are available, which usually are residential, inpatient programs that treat clients who pay for the service directly or through health insurance. In 1985, a year in which the Household Survey estimated that 37 million persons engaged in illicit or nonmedical use of drugs and in which we can presume that approximately 3 million persons were suffering from drug abuse disorders, about 0.5 million persons entered publicly funded treatment programs.[121] It is probably safe to say that many people who need treatment for drug abuse are not receiving it.

The National Drug and Alcoholism Treatment Unit Survey (NDATUS) conducted by NIDA is a voluntary survey of various aspects of treatment provided by private and public treatment facilities. In 1987, 6866 facilities reported providing treatment for alcoholism, drug abuse, or both. In a 12-month period (October 1987–October, 1988), 834,077 drug abuse clients were treated at 4880 facilities. Detoxification services were provided for 4.1% of the clients, methadone maintenance for 31.4%, and drug free treatment for 64.5%. The bulk of the clients were seen in outpatient settings (85.6%), with 10.4% in residential facilities and the remaining 4.1% in hospital inpatient settings. Males comprised 67.2% of the clients. Whites were 57.5%, blacks were 24.8%, and Hispanics were 15.9% of the total. People under 18 years of age comprised 15.4% of the clients, and 69.6% were between 21 and 44 years of age. Only 8.3% of the clients were 45 years of age or older.

Treatment Evaluation. Two large-scale treatment evaluation programs have been carried out from the early 1970s to the present. They have established that drug abuse treatment is successful in reducing illicit drug use and in improving the functioning of clients.

Drug Abuse Reporting Program (DARP). This was the first nationally based evaluation of the effectiveness of drug abuse treatment. This study obtained data from clients entering detoxification, methadone maintenance, residential, or drug free treatment between 1969 and 1973 and at periods thereafter for up to 12 years. DARP included 44,000 clients from 52 programs, and the findings were reported in detail.[122–124] Hubbard and colleagues[125] concluded that these studies provided convincing evidence of drug abuse treatment effectiveness in reducing drug use and criminal activity associated with drug use. The length of time spent in treatment was the variable most predicitive of success in treatment, and the modalities of treatment did not have different success rates. The DARP study clearly identified the chronic nature of drug abuse, since approximately 8 of 10 clients who were included in the 12-year follow-up study had reentered treatment at some time.

Treatment Outcome Prospective Study (TOPS). TOPS evaluated treatment received between 1979 and 1981.[125] The study used a longitudinal, prospective cohort research design. Approximately 10,000 clients who entered 37 urban treatment programs representing three modalities of treatment—methadone maintenance, residential, and outpatient drug free—were interviewed at intake, at 3-month intervals during treatment, and at 3 months and 1, 2, 3, and 5 years posttreatment. Not all former patients were selected at each follow-up period, but between 70% and 80% of the large number of clients designated were interviewed at each data collection point. TOPS patients are considered to be representative of the national treatment population.[126,127] Patient characteristics differed across the three treatment modalities in terms of previous treatment history for drug abuse, alcohol abuse, or mental illness, as well as in terms of referral to treatment through the criminal justice system. The length of time clients spent in treatment varied by type of program, with methadone clients averaging 38.4 weeks, residential clients 21.3 weeks, and outpatient drug free clients 14.6 weeks. Dropout rates for clients in the first month were 41.2% for outpatient drug free, 32.1% for residential, and 19.1% for methadone programs. However, half the clients who stayed in outpatient drug free and methadone programs 3 months or more completed treatment, as did 38% of those who remained in residential programs for this length of time. Clients in all programs were predominantly young, poorly educated men.

The most important predictor of success in treatment was length of time in the program, with 6 to 12 months of treatment being necessary to produce positive outcomes on drug use variables. One-year abstinence rates and improvement rates for clients in all three types of programs were similar for heroin, cocaine, and nonmedical use of psychoactive drugs. Between 40% and 50% of all clients remained abstinent at 1 year, and 70% to 80% showed improvement at 1 year in comparison to their pretreatment pattern of use. Marijuana use proved resistant to treatment, however. Between 55% and 65% of those clients who remained in treatment for 3 or more months used marijuana regularly in the year before entering treatment. At 1, 2, 3, and 5 years posttreatment, between 30% and 45% of these clients continued its regular use. Marijuana use was particularly persistent in young male clients. Heavy drinking in the year before entering treatment was characteristic of approximately one fourth of the methadone clients and one third of the clients in residential and outpatient drug free programs. Three to five years later, heavy drinking had decreased by 6% to 8%.

Duration of treatment also predicted success on other parameters. Clients who stayed in outpatient drug free treatment for at least 6 months or in residential treatment for at least 1 year were approximately twice as likely to be employed full-time in the year after treatment as were those whose stays were shorter. Methadone clients who completed treatment or remained in long-term treatment were 50% more likely to be employed full-time than methadone clients who dropped out of treatment. Suicidal indicators in clients treated for more than 3 months decreased by one third to one half in the 3- to 5-year posttreatment period compared with the year before entering treatment.

A study[128] confirmed the importance of time in treatment for positive outcomes but found sharp differences between programs in the percentage of methadone clients who used cocaine (16.3%) and heroin (24.4%) while in treatment. In the six programs studied, the percentage of clients who continued drug use while in treatment varied by a factor of 11 for heroin and of 8 for cocaine. The authors related continued use to program deficiencies, low methadone maintenance dosage, and length of time in program.

In the year before entering treatment, 33.3% of the methadone and outpatient drug free clients and 60% of the residential clients in the TOPS study had committed one or more predatory crimes, that is, aggravated assault, robbery, burglary, theft, auto theft, forgery or embezzlement, and sale of stolen property. At 3- to 5-years posttreatment, less than 10% of the residential treatment clients were engaged in any predatory crime. Rates of predatory crime involvement also were decreased by approximately 18% for clients of the methadone programs and by 20% for residential program clients. Length of time in treatment was associated with significantly decreased predatory crime for clients in all three types of programs. Harwood and colleagues[2] maintain that the costs of treatment are offset by the savings to society from the decreased amount of crime committed by these clients during and after treatment.

Reentry to treatment was very characteristic of the clients included in TOPS. Within a year of terminating the course of treatment that had brought them into contact with TOPS, almost one third had returned to treatment, with the average interval for returning being 3 months. Methadone program clients were more likely than clients of other programs to reenter treatment. This pattern, of course, emphasizes the chronic nature of drug abuse problems seen in persons dependent on licit[129] as well as illicit drugs.

In summary, the TOPS data conclusively show that for those who stay in treatment for reasonable lengths of time, the process leads to decreased drug use for most drugs, decreased predatory crime and suicidal intention, and improvement on a number of other variables associated with productive lives and that these benefits do not erode over a considerable period after treatment is concluded. On the other hand, it is obvious that not all clients who enter treatment programs become abstinent during that particular course of treatment and that a large number of people who terminate a course of treatment return for additional treatment. These data indicate that drug abusers require multiple periods of treatment, and future work needs to clarify how many courses of treatment are required by the population of drug abusers to enable the majority of them to lead drug-free lives.

Treatment Research. The information from the two large studies on the usefulness of treatment points to several problems that are the focus of much basic research on treatment processes. One major question concerns the nature of relapse—Why does a person who becomes free of drugs revert to their use? What constitutes psychological dependence? Are there ways to maximize the probability that a person will remain free of drug use? Much of the work in this field examines the contributions of learned factors in drug dependence.

Several investigators have concentrated on the role of environmental cues in relapse to drug use,[130,131] showing that when confronted with cues associated with drug use, abstinent drug abusers exhibit conditioned craving and withdrawal. These responses can be reduced by exposing the addict repeatedly to the conditioned stimuli in the absence of drug, that is, in an extinction procedure.[132,133] Childress and coworkers[134] have designed treatments for methadone outpatients, detoxifying methadone inpatients, abstinent opioid users, and abstinent cocaine users. Stimuli associated with an individual's specific craving and withdrawal responses are identified and extinguished, enabling the client to encounter these stimuli in the environment without discomfort or the desire to use drugs. This approach promises to decrease relapse in clients. For example, these investigators presented preliminary data on treatment of craving in clients being treated for cocaine abuse. Cue exposure in combination with psychotherapy proved better than other treatments in retaining the clients in treatment and decreasing the likelihood that their urine samples would be found to contain cocaine.

In order to improve treatment,[135] operant conditioning processes have been investigated to evaluate the role of the subjective effects of drugs, the ways in which drug-taking behaviors are reinforced, the role of verbal behavior, such as instructions, and the function of responses that are incompatible with drug abuse. In one study,[136] for example, methadone clients were permitted to take home their medication provided their urine tests did not show evidence of abuse of drugs. Under these conditions, illicit drug use was decreased.

Medication Development. Another line of ongoing research aimed at improving treatment of drug abusers focuses on developing medications that may be useful in blocking the reinforcing effects of drugs, in alleviating the craving for drugs once the person becomes drug free, or in lessening the adverse effects of drug withdrawal. Methadone has been available for use in opiate-dependent persons in treatment since the 1960s, and, as discussed above, methadone treatment is successful in reducing drug use and, improving other areas of functioning. Since 1984, naltrexone, an opiate antagonist that blocks the euphoric effects of heroin, has been available for treatment. Its use has been limited, however, and additional research is needed to evaluate the circumstances under which it will be useful.[137] Two drugs still being investigated that promise to be helpful are LAAM, a long-acting methadone-type drug, and buprenorphine, a methadone-type drug with less euphoriant and dependence-producing characteristics.[138,139] In addition, medications are needed that will block cocaine's euphoric properties as well as reduce cocaine craving. Initial work has indicated that desipramine treatment assists clients to abstain from cocaine use better than lithium or a placebo[140] and that flupenthixol decanoate administration helped retain crack addicts in treatment.[141] The National Institute on Drug Abuse recently has established medication development as a research priority, and it is hoped that this action will lead to the development of medications that will enable clinicians to treat those drug abusers who are not helped by current methods.

Aftercare. In the same way that increasing skills decreases the initiation of drug use (see Prevention discussion), the acquisition of skills helps former drug abusers to prevent relapse to drug use once treatment is completed. One current research program employs four modules—recovery training, self-help meetings, weekend and holiday recreational and social activities, and a network of senior ex-addicts—to specifically address factors that are related to relapse. The program is provided in an outpatient group setting for a 26-week period after discharge from a primary treatment program. The significant reduction in relapse to illicit opiates and increase in the percentage of persons holding jobs reported for the clients in this program[142] emphasize the high priority that should be given to aftercare in planning treatment programs.

CONCLUSION

Recent research on the epidemiology and etiology of drug abuse, as well as its prevention and treatment, has been presented. Epidemiological studies have provided information on the extent and pattern of drug abuse in the United States, and within the general population a trend of decreasing use of illicit drugs is clearly established. These trends are thought to reflect the improved methods for delivering primary prevention programs that have evolved over the past 20 years. There is a clear need to continue these programs and the research that leads to their improvement so that the recent gains are not lost and so that additional gains may be realized.

There are indications that drug abuse is continuing and may, in fact, be increasing in certain groups, notably the impoverished, residents of inner cities, and ethnic and racial minorities. In addition to these demographic risk factors, numerous other risk factors have been identified that suggest the need to tailor prevention, intervention, and treatment program to specific groups in the future.

In contrast to the opinion held by many people that treatment for drug abuse is futile, outcome studies demonstrate that treatment of drug abuse is useful in reducing abuse of drugs, drug-related antisocial behavior, and other adverse consequences of drug use. However, the high proportion of persons who drop out of treatment demonstrates the need for improved methods of treatment, including pharmacological methods of treating cocaine abuse or improving treatment of opiate abusers. Finally, the high relapse rate for drug abuse suggests the need for the design and delivery of intensive aftercare programs for persons who successfully complete drug abuse treatment.

REFERENCES

1. Blum R: Contemporary threats to adolescent health in the United States. JAMA 257:3390–3395, 1987
2. Harwood HJ, Napolitano DM, Kristiansen PL, Collins JJ: Economic Costs to Society of Alcohol and Drug Abuse and Mental Illness: 1980. Research Triangle Institute, Research Triangle, NC, report 2734/00-01FR to Alcohol, Drug Abuse and Mental Health Administration, Office of Program Planning and Coordination, Rockville, MD, 1984
3. Hahn RA, Onorato IM, Jones TS, Dougherty J: Prevalence of HIV infection among intravenous drug users in the United States. JAMA 261:2677–2684, 1989
4. Ashley MJ, Rankin JG: A public health approach to the prevention of alcohol-related health problems. Ann Rev Public Health 9:233–271, 1988
5. Fitzgerald PE (ed): Drugs of Abuse. US Department of Justice, Drug Enforcement Administration. Washington, DC: US Govt Printing Office, 1988
6. Falk JL, Feingold DA: Environmental and cultural factors in the behavioral action of drugs. In Meltzer HY (ed): Psychopharmacology: The Third Generation of Progress. New York: Raven Press, 1987, pp 1503–1510
7. Brecher EM: Licit and Illicit Drugs: The Consumers Union Report on Narcotics, Stimulants, Depressants, Inhalants, Hallucinogens and Marijuana—Including Caffeine, Nicotine and Alcohol. Boston: Little, Brown, 1972
8. Eddy NB, Halbach H, Isbell H, Seevers MH: Drug dependence: Its significance and characteristics. Bull WHO 32:721–733, 1965
9. American Psychiatric Association: Diagnostic and Statistical Manual of Mental Disorders. Washington, DC: American Psychiatric Association, 1987
10. Jaffe JH: Drug addiction and drug use. In Gilman AG, Goodman LS, Rall TW, Murad F (eds): The Pharmacological Basis of Therapeutics. New York: Macmillan, 1985, pp 532–581
11. Johanson CE, Balster RL: A summary of the results of a drug self-administration study using substitution procedures in rhesus monkeys. Bull Narc 30:43–54, 1978
12. Johanson CE, Schuster CR: Animal models of drug-self administration. In Mello NK (ed): Advances in Substance Abuse: Behavioral and Biological Research, Vol II. Greenwich, Conn.: JAI Press, 1981, pp 219–297
13. Cohen S: Coca paste and freebase: New fashions in cocaine use. Drug Abuse Alcohol News 9, 1980
14. Robins LN: The interaction of setting and predisposition in explaining novel behavior: Drug initiations before, in, and after Vietnam. In Kandel DB (ed): Longitudinal Research on Drug Use. Washington, DC: Hemisphere, 1978, pp 179–196
15. Deneau G, Yanagita T, Seevers MH: Self-administration of psychoactive substances by the monkey: A measure of psychological dependence. Psychopharmacologia 16:30–48, 1969
16. Hughes J, Smith TW, Kosterlitz HW, et al: Identification of two related pentapeptides from the brain with potent opiate agonist activity. Nature 258:577, 1975
17. Cooper JR, Bloom FE, Roth RH: The Biochemical Basis of Neuropharmacology. New York: Oxford University Press, 1986
18. Jaffe JH, Martin WR: Opioid analgesics and antagonists. In Gilman AG, Goodman LS, Rall TW, Murad F (eds): The Pharmacological Basis of Therapeutics. New York: Macmillan, 1985, pp 491–531
19. Koob GF, Bloom FE: Cellular and molecular mechanisms of drug dependence. Science 242:715–723, 1988
20. Siegel S, MacRae J: Environmental specificity of tolerance. Trends NeruoSci 7:140–142, 1984
21. Harvey SC: Hypnotics and sedatives. In Gilman AG, Goodman LS, Rall TW, Murad F (eds): The Pharmacological Basis of Therapeutics. New York: Macmillan, 1985, pp 229–371
22. Sellers EM, Busto U: Benzodiazepines and ethanol: Assessment of the effects and consequences of psychotropic drug interactions. J Clin Psychopharmacol 2:249–262, 1982
23. Ellinwood EH Jr: Amphetamine psychosis. I. Description of the individuals and process. J Nerv Ment Dis 144:273–283, 1967
24. Gawin FH, Ellinwood EH: Cocaine and other stimulants: Actions, abuse and treatment. N Engl J Med 318:1173–1182, 1988
25. Manschreck TC, Allen DF, Neville M: Freebase psychosis: Cases from a Bahamian epidemic of cocaine abuse. Comp Psychiatry 28:555–564, 1987
26. Jeri FR, Sanchez CC, del Pozo T, et al: Further experience with the syndromes produced by coca paste smoking. Bull Narc 30:1–11, 1978
27. Lesko LM, Fischman MW, Javaid JI, Davis JM: Iatrogenous cocaine psychosis. N Engl J Med 307:1153, 1982
28. Kilbey MM, Ellinwood EH Jr: Reverse tolerance to stimulant-induced behavior. Life Sci 20:1063–1076, 1977
29. Gawin FH, Kleber HD: Abstinence symptomatology and psychiatric diagnosis in cocaine abusers. Arch Gen Psychiatry 43:107–113, 1986
30. Weiner N: Norepinephrine, epinephrine, and the sympathomimetic amines. In Gilman AG, Goodman LS, Rall TW, Murad F (eds): The Pharmacological Basis of Therapeutics. New York: Macmillan, 1985, pp 145–180
31. Johanson CE, Fischman MW: The pharmacology of cocaine related to its abuse. Pharm Rev 41:3–52, 1989
32. Balster RL, Wessinger WD: Central nervous system depressant effects of phencyclidine. In Kamenka JM, Domino EF, Geneste P: Phencyclidine and Related Arylcyclohexylamines: Present and Future Applications. Ann Arbor, Mich.: NPP Books, 1983, pp 291–309
33. Mechoulam R: Marihuana chemistry. Science 168:1159–1166, 1970
34. Harris LS, Dewey WL, Razdan RK: Cannabis: Its chemistry, pharmacology, and toxicology. In Martin WR (ed): Drug Addiction II:

Amphetamine, Psychotogen, and Marihuana Dependence, Vol. 45. Handbuch der Experimentellen Pharmakologie. Berlin: Springer-Verlag, 1977, pp 371–429

35. Beardsley PM, Balster RL, Harris LS: Dependence on tetrahydrocannabinol in rhesus monkeys. J Pharmacol Exp Ther 239:311–319, 1986
36. Jones RT: Cannabis tolerance and dependence. In Fehr KO, Kalant H (eds): Cannabis and Health Hazards. Toronto: Addiction Research Foundation, 1983, pp 617–689
37. NIDA: National Household Survey on Drug Abuse: Main Findings 1985. National Institute on Drug Abuse, DHHS Publication No (ADM)88-1586. Washington, DC: US Govt Printing Office, 1988
38. NIDA: National Household Survey on Drug Abuse: Population Estimates. National Institute on Drug Abuse, DHHS Publication No (ADM)87-1539. Washington, DC: US Govt Printing Office, 1987
39. Johnston LD, O'Malley PM, Bachman JG: Illicit Drug Use, Smoking, and Drinking by America's High School Students, College Students, and Young Adults. DHHS Publication No (ADM)89-1602. Washington, DC: US Govt Printing Office, 1989
40. Rouse BA, Kozel NJ, Richards LG (eds): Self-report Methods of Estimating Drug Use: Meeting Current Challenges to Validity. NIDA Research Monograph No 57, (ADM)85-1402. Washington, DC: US Govt Printing Office, 1985
41. Murray DM, Perry CL, O'Connell C, Schmid L: Seventh-grade cigarette, alcohol, and marijuana use: Distribution in a north central U.S. metropolitan population. Int J Addict 22:357–376, 1987
42. Beauvais F, Oetting ER: Adolescent drug use: Findings of national and local surveys. J Consult Clin Psychol 58(4):385–394, 1990
43. Regier DA, Boyd JH, Burke JD, et al: One-month prevalence of mental disorders in the United States. Arch Gen Psychiatry 45:977–986, 1988
44. Christie KA, Burke JD Jr, Regier DA, et al: Epidemiologic evidence for early onset of mental disorders and higher risk of drug abuse in young adults. Am J Psychiatry 145:971–975, 1988
45. Burnam MA, Hough RL, Escobar JI, et al: Six-month prevalence of specific psychiatric disorders among Mexican Americans and non-Hispanic whites in Los Angeles. Arch Gen Psychiatry 44:687–694, 1987
46. Cotton NS: The familial incidence of alcoholism: A review. J Stud Alcoholism 40:89–116, 1979
47. Plomin R: Environment and genes: Determinants of behavior. Am Psychol 44:105–111, 1989
48. Cadoret RJ, Cain CA, Grove WM: Development of alcoholism in adoptees raised apart from alcoholic biologic relatives. Arch Gen Psychiatry 37:561–563, 1980
49. Bohman M, Cloninger R, Sigvardsson S, von Knorring AL: The genetics of alcoholisms and related disorders. J Psychiatr Res 21:447–452, 1987
50. Bohman M, Sigvardsson S, Cloninger CR: Maternal inheritance of alcohol abuse: Cross fostering analysis of adopted women. Arch Gen Psychiatry 38:965–969, 1981
51. Cloninger CR, Sigvardsson S, von Knorring AL, Bohman M: The Swedish studies of the adopted children of alcoholics: A reply to Littrell. J Stud Alcohol 49:500–509, 1988
52. Cloninger CR, Bohman M, Sigvardsson S: Inheritance of alcohol abuse: Cross-fostering analysis of adopted men. Arch Gen Psychiatry 38:861–868, 1981
53. Cloninger CR, Bohman M, Sigvardsson S, von Knorring AL: Psychopathology in adopted-out children of alcoholics. The Stockholm adoption study. Rec Devel Alcoholism 3:37–51, 1985
54. Wolin S, Bennett L, Noonan D: Family rituals and the recurrence of alcoholism over generations. Am J Psychiatry 136:589–593, 1979
55. Wolin S, Bennett L, Noonan D, Teitelbaum M: Disrupted family rituals: A factor in the intergenerational transmission of alcoholism. J Stud Alcohol 41:199–214, 1980
56. Tarter RE: Are there inherited behavioral traits that predispose to substance abuse? J Consul Clin Psychol 56:189–196, 1988
57. Cadoret RJ, Troughton E, O'Gorman TW, Heywood E: An adoption study of genetic and environmental factors in drug abuse. Arch Gen Psychiatry 43:1131–1136, 1986
58. Hughes JR: Genetics of smoking: A brief review. Beh Ther 17:335–345, 1986
59. Kosten TR, Rounsaville BJ, Kleber HD: Parental alcoholism in opioid addicts. J Nerv Ment Dis 173:461–469, 1985
60. Ellinwood EH, Smith WG, Vaillant GE: Narcotic addiction in males and females: A comparison. Int J Addict 1:33–55, 1966
61. O'Donnell JA: Narcotic Addicts in Kentucky. National Institute on Drug Abuse, DHHS Publication No 1881. Washington, DC: US Govt Printing Office, 1969
62. Hill SY, Cloninger CR, Ayre FR: Independent familial transmission of alcoholism and opiate abuse. Alcoholism Clin Exp Res 1:335–342, 1977
63. Maddux JF, Desmond DF: Family and environment in the choice of opioid dependence or alcoholism. Am J Alcohol Abuse 15:117–134, 1989
64. Grande TP, Wolf AW, Schubert DSP, et al: Associations among alcoholism, drug abuse and antisocial personality: A review of the literature. Psychol Report 55:455–474, 1984
65. Kandel DB: Adolescent marijuana use: Role of parents and peers. Science 181:1067–1070, 1973
66. Newcomb MD, Huba GJ, Bentler PM: Mother's influence on the drug use of their children: Confirmatory tests of direct modeling and mediational theories. Dev Psychol 19:714–726, 1983
67. Newcomb MD, Maddahian E, Bentler PM: Risk factors for drug use among adolescents: Concurrent and longitudinal analyses. Am J Public Health 76:525–531, 1986
68. Robinston TN, Killen JD, Taylor CB, et al: Perspectives on adolescent substance use: A defined population study. JAMA 258:2072–2076, 1987
69. Pandina RJ, Schuele J: Psychosocial correlates of adolescent alcohol and drug use. J Stud Alcohol 44:950–973, 1983
70. Oetting ER, Beauvais F: Peer cluster theory: Drugs and the adolescent. J Counsel Dev 65:17–22, 1986
71. Huba GJ, Wingard JA, Bentler PM: Beginning adolescent drug use and peer and adult interaction patterns. J Consult Clin Psychol 47:265–276, 1976
72. Tennant FS, Detels R, Clark V: Some childhood antecedents of drug and alcohol abuse. Am J Epidemiol 102:377–384, 1975
73. Huba GJ, Newcomb MD, Bentler PM: Comparison of canonical correlation and interbattery factor analysis on sensation seeking and drug use domains. Appl Psychol Meas 5:291–306, 1981
74. Segal B, Huba GJ, Singer JL: Prediction of college drug use from personality and inner experience. Int J Addict 15:849–867, 1980
75. Jessor R, Jessor SL: Problem Behavior and Psychosocial Development. New York: Academic Press, 1977
76. Jessor R, Jessor SL: Theory testing in longitudinal research on marijuana use. In Kandel DB (ed): Longitudinal Research on Drug Use: Empirical Findings and Methodological Issues. Washington, DC: Hemisphere, 1978, pp 41–71
77. Gossett JT, Lewis JM, Phillips VA: Psychological characteristics of adolescent drug users and abstainers: Some implications for prevention education. Bull Menninger Clin 36:425–435, 1972
78. Mills CJ, Noyes HL: Patterns and correlates of initial and subsequent drug use among adolescents. J Consult Clin Psychol 52:231–243, 1984
79. Kaplan HB: Increase in self-rejection as an antecedent of deviant responses. J Youth Adolesc 4:438–458, 1975
80. Aneshensel CS, Huba GJ: Depression, alcohol use, and smoking over one year: A four-wave longitudinal causal model. J Abnorm Psychol 92:134–150, 1983
81. Kandel DB, Simcha-Fagan O, Davies M: Risk factors for delinquency and illicit drug use from adolescence to young adulthood. J Drug Issues 16:67–90, 1986
82. Kellam SG, Brown CH, Rubin BR, Ensminger ME: Paths leading to teenage psychiatric symptoms and substance use: Developmental epidemiological studies in Woodlawn. In Guze SB, Earls FJ, Bar-

rett JE (eds): Childhood Psychopathology and Development. New York: Raven Press, 1983, pp 17–51
83. Kandel DB, Logan JA: Patterns of drug use from adolescence to young adulthood: I Periods of risk for initiation, continued use, and discontinuation. Am J Public Health 74:660–666, 1984
84. Auslander G: Social networks and the functional health status of the poor. J Community Health 13:197–209, 1988
85. Bachman JG, O'Malley PM, Johnston LD: Drug use among young adults: The impacts of role status and social environments. J Pers Soc Psychol 47:629–645, 1984
86. Yamaguchi K, Kandel DB: Patterns of drug use from adolescence to young adulthood: II Sequence of progression. Am J Public Health 74:668–672, 1984
87. Yamaguchi K, Kandel DB: Patterns of drug use from adolescence to young adulthood: III Predictors progression. Am J Public Health 74:673–681, 1984
88. Kandel DB, Raveis VH: Cessation of illicit drug use in young adulthood. Arch Gen Psychiatry 46:109–116, 1989
89. O'Malley PM, Bachman JG, Johnston LD: Period, age and cohort effects on substance use among American youth. Am J Public Health 74:682–688, 1984
90. Bry BH, McKeon P, Pandina RJ: Extent of drug use as a function of number of risk factors. J Abnorm Psychol 91:173–279, 1982
91. Oetting ER, Beauvais F: Peer cluster theory, socialization characteristics and adolescent drug use: A path analysis. J Counsel Psychol 34:205–213, 1987
92. Swaim RC, Oetting ER, Edwards RW, Beauvais F: Links from emotional distress to adolescent drug use: A path model. J Consult Clin Psychol 57:227–231, 1989
93. Oetting ER, Swaim RC, Edwards RW, Beauvais F: Indian and Anglo adolescent alcohol use and emotional distress: Path models. Am J Alcohol Drug Abuse 15:153–172, 1989
94. Bukoski WJ: A definition of drug abuse prevention research. In Donohew L, Sipher HE, Bukoski WJ (eds): Persuasive Communication and Drug Abuse Prevention. Hillsdale, NJ: Lawrence Erlbaum Associates, 1991, pp 3–19
95. Schaps E, DiBartolo R, Moskowitz J, et al: A review of 127 drug abuse prevention program evaluations. J Drug Issues 11:17–43, 1981
96. Tobler NS: Meta-analysis of 143 adolescent drug prevention programs: Quantitative outcome results of program participants compared to a control or comparison group. J Drug Issues 16:537–567, 1986
97. Bangert-Drowns RL: The effects of school-based substance abuse education—A meta-analysis. J Drug Educ 18:243–264, 1988
98. Evans RI: How can health lifestyles in adolescents be modified? Some implications from a smoking prevention program. In Routh DK (ed): Handbook of Pediatric Psychology. New York: Guilford Press, 1988, pp 321–331
99. Evans RI, Dratt LM, Raines BE, Rosenberg SS: Social influences on smoking initiation: Importance of distinguishing descriptive versus mediating process variables. J Appl Soc Psychol 18:925–943, 1988
100. Evans RI, Handon WB, Mittelmark MB: Increasing the validity of self-reports of smoking behavior in children. J Appl Psychol 62:521–523, 1977
101. Best A, Thompson SJ, Santi SM, et al: Preventing cigarette smoking among school children. In Breslow L, Fielding JE, Lave LB (eds): Annu Rev Public Health 9:161–201, 1988
102. Black GS: The attitudinal basis of drug use—1987 and changing attitudes toward drug use—1988. In Donohew L, Sipher HE, Bukoski WJ (ed): Persuasive Communication and Drug Abuse Prevention. Hillsdale, NJ: Lawrence Erlbaum Associates, 1991, pp 157–191
103. Johnston LD: A review and analysis of recent changes in marijuana use by American young people. In Marijuana: The National Impact on Education. New York: The American Council on Marijuana, 1982, pp 8–13
104. Johnston LD, Bachman JG, O'Malley PM: Highlights from Student Drug Use in America, 1975–1980. DHHS Publication No (ADM)81-1066. Washington, DC: US Govt Printing Office, 1981
105. Bachman JG, Johnston LD, O'Malley PM, Humphrey RH: Explaining the recent decline in marijuana use: Differentiating the effects of perceived risks, disapproval and general lifestyle factors. J Health Soc Behav 29:92–112, 1988
106. Bachman JG, Johnston LD, O'Malley PM: Explaining the Recent Decline in Cocaine Use Among Young Adults: Further Evidence that Perceived Risks and Disapproval Lead to Reduced Drug Use. Ann Arbor, MI: Institute for Social Research, 1989
107. Bachman JG, Johnston LD, O'Malley PM: How changes in drug use are linked to perceived risks and disapproval: Evidence from national studies that youth and young adults respond to information about the consequences of drug use. In Donohew L, Sipher HE, Bukoski WJ (eds): Persuasive Communication and Drug Abuse Prevention. Hillsdale, NJ: Lawrence Erlbaum Associates, 1991, pp 133–155
108. Donohew L, Palmgreen P, Lorch E: Sensation seeking and targeting of anti-drug PSAs. In Donohew L, Sipher HE, Bukowski WJ (eds): Persuasive Communication and Drug Abuse Prevention. Hillsdale, NJ: Lawrence Erlbaum Associates, 1991, pp 209–226
109. Flay BR: What we know about the social influences approach to smoking prevention: Review and recommendations. In Bell CS, Battjes R (ed): Prevention Research: Deterring Drug Abuse Among Children and Adolescents. DHHS Publication No (ADM)86-1334. Washington, DC: US Govt Printing Office, 1986, pp 67–111
110. Best JA, Flay BR, Towson SMJ, et al: Smoking prevention and the concept of risk. J Appl Soc Psychol 14:257–273, 1984
111. Flay BR, d'Avernas JR, Best JA, et al: Cigarette smoking: Why young people do it and ways of preventing it. In McGrath P, Firestone P (eds): Pediatric and Adolescent Behavioral Medicine. New York: Springer, 1983, pp 132–183
112. Flay BR, Ryan KB, Best JA, et al: Are social psychological smoking prevention programs effective? The Waterloo study. J Behav Med 8:37–59, 1985
113. Botvin GJ, Wills TA: Personal and social skills training: Cognitive-behavioral approaches to substance abuse prevention. In Bell CS, Battjes R (eds): Prevention Research: Deterring Drug Abuse Among Children and Adolescents. DHHS Publication No (ADM)86-1334. Washington, DC: US Govt Printing Office, 1986, pp 8–49
114. Pentz MA: Prevention of adolescent substance abuse through social skills. In Glynn TJ, Leukefeld CG, Ludford JP (eds): Preventing Adolescent Drug Abuse: Intervention Strategies. DHHS No (ADM)83-1280, 1983, pp 195–232
115. Schinke SP, Gilchrist LD: Primary prevention of tobacco smoking. J School Health 53:416–419, 1983
116. Wills TA: Stress, coping, and tobacco and alcohol use in early adolescence. In Shiffmans S, Wills TA (eds): Coping and Substance Use. Orlando, FL: Academic Press, 1985, pp 67–94
117. Botvin GJ, Tortu S: Preventing adolescent substance abuse through life skills training. In Price RH, Cowen EL, Lorion RP, Ramos-McKay J (eds): 14 Ounces of Prevention. Washington, DC: American Psychological Association, 1988, pp 98–100
118. Pentz MA, Dwyer JH, MacKinnon DP, et al: A multicommunity trial for primary prevention of adolescent drug use: Effects on drug use prevalence. JAMA 261:3259–3266, 1989
119. Beauvais F, Oetting ER, Wolf W, Edwards RW: American Indian youth and drugs: 1975–87. A continuing problem. Am J Public Health 79:634–636, 1989
120. Kellam SG, Anthony JC, Brown CH, et al: Prevention research on early risk behaviors: A cross-cultural study. In Schmidt MH, Remschmidt H (eds): Needs and Prospects of Child and Adolescent Psychiatry. Gottingen: Verlag-Hans Huber, 1989
121. Butynski W, Canova D: An Analysis of State Alcohol and Drug Abuse: Profile Data. Washington, DC: National Association of State Alcohol and Drug Abuse Directors, 1988
122. Sells SB (ed): Effectiveness of Drug Abuse Treatment, Vols 1, 2. Cambridge, Mass.: Ballinger, 1974
123. Sells SB, Simpson DD (eds): Effectiveness of Drug Abuse Treatment, Vols 3–5. Cambridge, Mass.: Ballinger, 1976

124. Simpson DD, Joe GW, Lehman WEK, Sells SB: Addiction careers: Etiology, treatment, and 12-year follow-up outcomes. J Drug Issues 16:107–121, 1986
125. Hubbard RL, Marsden ME, Rachal JV, et al: Drug Abuse Treatment: A National Study of Effectiveness. Chapel Hill, NC: The University of North Carolina Press, 1989
126. Allison M, Hubbard RL, Rachal JV: Treatment Process in Methadone, Residential and Outpatient Drug Free Programs. DHHS Publication No (ADM)85-1411, 1985
127. Hubbard RL, Bray RM, Cavanaugh ER, et al: Drug Abuse Treatment Client Characteristics and Pretreatment Behavior in 1979-1981 TOPS Admission Cohorts. DHHS Publication No (ADM)86-1453, 1986
128. Ball JC, Ross A, Jaffe JH: Cocaine and heroin use by methadone maintenance patients. Paper presented to 51st Annual Scientific Meeting of The Committee on Problems of Drug Dependence, Inc, 1989
129. Cohen S, Lichtenstein E, Prochaska JO, et al: Debunking myths about self-quitting. Am Psychol 44:1355–1365, 1989
130. Siegel S: Drug anticipation and the treatment of dependence. In Ray BA (ed.): Learning Factors in Substance Abuse. DHHS Publication No (ADM)88-1576, 1988, pp 1–24
131. O'Brien CP, Childress AR, McLellan AT, et al: Types of conditioning found in drug-dependent humans. In Ray BA (ed): Learning Factors in Substance Abuse. DHHS Publication No (ADM)88-1576). Washington, DC: US Govt Printing Office 1988, pp 44–61
132. Childress AR, McLellan AT, Ehrman R, O'Brien CP: Classically conditioned responses in opioid and cocaine dependence: A role in relapse? In Ray BA (ed): Learning Factors in Substance Abuse. DHHS Publication No (ADM)88-1576. Washington, DC: US Govt Printing Office, 1988, pp 25–43
133. Childress AR, McLellan AT, O'Brien CP: Nature and incidence of conditioned responses in a methadone population: A comparison of laboratory, clinic and naturalistic setting. In Harris L (ed.): Problems of Drug Dependence, 1985: Proceedings of the 47th Annual Scientific Meeting, The Committee on Problems of Drug Dependence, Inc. DHHS Publication No (ADM)86-1448. Washington, DC: US Govt Printing Office, 1986, pp 366–372
134. Childress AR, Ehrman R, McLellan AT, O'Brien CP: Reduction in cocaine craving and arousal through repeated exposure to drug-related "reminder" cues. Paper presented to 51st Annual Scientific Meetings of The Committee on Problems of Drug Dependence, Inc, 1989
135. Bickel WK, Kelly TH: The relationship of stimulus control to the treatment of substance abuse. In Ray BA (ed): Learning Factors in Substance Abuse. DHHS Publication No (ADM)88-1576. Washington, DC: US Govt Printing Office, 1988, pp 122–140
136. Higgins ST, Stitzer ML, Bigelow GE, Liebson IA: Contingent methadone delivery: Effects on illicit opiate use. Drug Alcohol Depend 17:311–322, 1986
137. Kleber HD, Topazian M, Gaspari J, et al: Clonidine and naltrexone in outpatient treatment of heroin withdrawal. Am J Drug Alcohol Abuse 13:1–17, 1987
138. Bickel WK, Stitzer ML, Bigelow GE, et al: A clinical trial of buprenorphine: Comparison with methadone in detoxification of heroin addicts. Clin Pharmacol Ther 43:72–78, 1988
139. Bickel WK, Stitzer ML, Bigelow GE, et al: Buprenorphine: Dose-related blockage of opioid challenge effects in opioid dependent humans. J Pharmacol Exp Ther 247:47–53, 1988
140. Gawin FH, Kleber HD, Byck R, et al: Desipramine facilitation of initial cocaine abstinence. Arch Gen Psychiatry 46:117–121, 1989
141. Gawin FH, Allen D, Humblestone MB: Outpatient treatment of "crack" cocaine smoking with flupenthixol decanoate. A preliminary report. Arch Gen Psychiatry 46:322–326, 1989
142. McAuliffe WE, Ch'ien JMN: Recovery training and self-help: A relapse-prevention program for treated opiate addicts. J Substance Abuse Treat 3:9–20, 1986

45

Prevention and Health Education

Lawrence W. Green

Biomedical and behavioral sciences have complicated the messages and methods of health education. No longer is the task simply one of informing and admonishing people about discrete actions they could take to protect themselves against single organisms or vectors of infectious diseases. Supplanting the germ theory with multicausal explanations of chronic and degenerative diseases has meant replacing proscriptions with probabilities and single actions with lifelong behavioral development and lifestyle change. Demographic and living conditions, at least in western countries, have shifted the emphasis of health education from survival and security to performance and productivity, from physical prowess to physical fitness, from mental hygiene to mental efficiency, from healthy people to healthful environments and policies.

Despite these shifts in the objectives of health education within the context of health promotion for the population at large, large segments of the population have yet to achieve the full benefit of the first epidemiological revolution. Poor people continue to suffer premature death and preventable morbidity from infectious diseases, nutritional imbalances, unsafe work and residential environments, limited access to health care, and inadequate knowledge and organization in their communities. Public health and preventive medicine carry a frontline responsibility to reach these underserved segments of the population with a more basic health education in the context of organizational, economic, and environmental supports for behavior and conditions of living conducive to health.

These perspectives on the meaning of health and on the demand for behavioral and environmental interventions have called traditional health education into question as being too narrow in concept and too soft in method. I review how recent advances in the science and art of health education have been applied in practical ways within medical and other settings for prevention and public health. Even where the goals are too ambitious for health education alone, as with health promotion for complex lifestyle changes in individuals and communities, health education remains an indispensable and primary component of organizational, economic, and environmental interventions designed to channel, support, or restrain behavior.

DEFINITIONS

The terms health education, patient education, self-care education, school health education, and health promotion are distinguished from each other as follows.[1]

Health education is any combination of learning experiences designed to predispose, enable, and reinforce voluntary adaptations of individual or collective behavior conducive to health.[2]

Patient education is initiated by medical care personnel to strengthen the motivation and ability of patients to adhere to prescribed medical or self-care regimens, including preparation for hospitalization, surgery, and rehabilitation.

Self-care education is designed to predispose, enable, and reinforce individuals (not necessarily patients) or groups in diagnosing, managing, and monitoring their own health care needs. It differs from health education only in the sense that it refers more specifically to the judgments and actions for which people traditionally have depended on professionals.[3]

School health education is initiated and directed by personnel in preschool, school, or college to develop the motivation and skills required by students to cope with challenges to health and to build the foundation of knowledge required to comprehend the further health learning scheduled for their future. This definition is intended to narrow the range of behavioral and health objectives for which schools are accountable and to emphasize outcomes to which schools will be most responsive.[4]

Similar definitions can be framed for other setting-specific, disease-specific, or behavior-specific enterprises, such as occupational health education, nutrition education, physical education, cancer education, diabetes education, or dental health education. Each may be seen as a subset of health education or of school health education, depending on the setting, function, or target population.

Health promotion is any combination of educational, organizational, economic, and environmental supports for behavior and conditions of living conducive to health. Health promotion thus goes beyond health education when the behavior in question is beyond the control of the individual or group at risk. Health promotion is a component of public health and preventive medicine. The U.S. national strategy in disease prevention and health promotion, for example, includes three components: health promotion directed at behavioral causes of health, health protection directed at environmental causes, and preventive health services directed at the organization of medical resources and services.[5] Health education is a subset or strategy within each of these but is the primary and dominant strategy in health promotion (Fig. 45–1).

Programs, activities, and methods that may be characterized as educational have vague boundaries. Most health education activities are embedded in other programs, and many are not identified as health education. Indeed, persons responsible

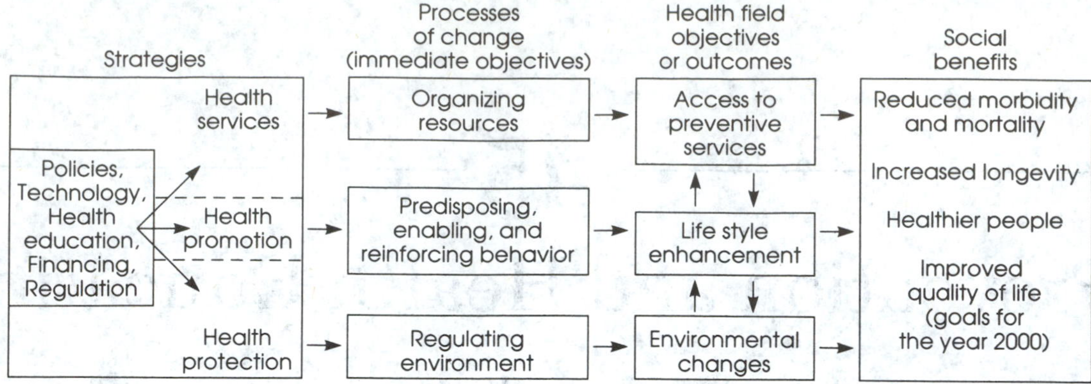

Figure 45–1. Functional relationships of health education strategies to immediate and long-term goals of health services, health promotion, and health protection.

for programs or studies sometimes disavow any association with health education in an attempt to distinguish their efforts as more innovative, modern, technological, behavioristic, client-centered, or scientific than they perceive health education to be. Alternative labeling occurs even when the methods employed clearly derive their approaches from education, educational psychology, educational technology, or health education itself.[6] Variations on self-care education, for example, have been referred to variously as "cognitive assessment and intervention procedures for relapse prevention,"[7] "self-monitoring . . . to provide feedback . . . in helping individuals assume more responsibility for their own care,"[8] and "helping people maximize their abilities to self-regulate [to] promote maintenance of behavior changes despite fluctuations in the physical and social environment."[9]

The alternative labels used for health education programs and activities reveal the scope and diversity of educational applications in areas concerned with health.

Motivation. The term "motivation" refers to that which drives behaviors from within the individual, not to something done to the person to influence behavior. Interventions can appeal to or reward people's motives, not motivate them.[10] This term has been used incorrectly in some programs to refer to the activities generally included in health education and to incentive schemes designed to appeal more directly to economic motives for behavioral change.[11]

Behavior Modification. Like motivation, the term "behavior modification" has expanded from its original applications by behaviorist psychologists to refer to a wider range of educational and political strategies for which the priority objectives are changes in behavior.[12] Most of the cognitive and training components of behavior modification, including self-monitoring, are essentially educational.

Health Counseling. This term and its variants (e.g., genetic counseling, diet counseling, patient counseling) represent an approach to voluntary change in health behavior. Most counseling methods of education have theoretical and philosophical roots in ego psychology, which is at extreme variance with behaviorism. Counseling is outside the scope of health education when it is more psychotherapeutic than informational in its method and content. Studies of doctor–patient interaction suggest a variety of purposes and tasks served by the reciprocal exchange of a counseling session besides educational purposes.[13]

Communications. The effects of communications on behaviors are studied in every sphere of human endeavor. Their applications in relation to health behaviors are usually within the scope of health education programming, except when they are used to advertise or promote products or causes that are inconsistent with the health needs of consumers.[14]

The foregoing examples of alternative labels used for health education activities illustrate what various programs may have in common and how they differ. Figure 45–2 provides an incomplete representation of these methods and techniques in relation to health education, suggesting aspects or applications of each that do not qualify as educational. The defining characteristic of health education is the voluntary participation of individuals in determining their own health practices. This is not merely a philosophical tenet. The durability of cognitive and behavioral changes is proportional to the degree of active rather than passive participation of the learner.[15]

Practical and legal reasons have led government and voluntary agencies to adhere to this usage of health education to avoid public resistance or reaction to programs that might be perceived as propaganda or as being manipulative, coercive, politically or commercially directed, threatening, or paternalistic.[16]

Other forms of health education that define its scope are community organization, community development, policy advocacy, in-service training, consultation, group work, computer-assisted instruction (CAI), other teaching machines and audiovisual methods, bibliotherapy, patient teaching, health fairs, exhibits, libraries, conferences, and social marketing.

These definitions are consistent with those applied in national planning for disease prevention and health promotion in several countries in recent years and with the philosophical and professional tenets of health education as commonly practiced worldwide in community, medical, occupational, and school settings. Health promotion is seen as the broader enterprise of creating a supportive environment for behaviors conducive to health. Health promotion must necessarily include health education but may require more structural, financial, technological, and even coercive interventions (e.g., regulatory or tax penalty laws) to influence behavior when it is deemed that such behavior threatens the health of others—as with reckless driving, irresponsible alcohol or drug abuse, marketing of harmful food products to young children, or smoking in crowded public places.[17]

Health education is more specifically limited to that range of behavior that is voluntary, self-directed, and relatively self-controlled. To the extent that the health outcomes to which health education may be addressed are not entirely controlled by behavior, health education may require the additional supports of medical services and resources and environmental controls over toxic and infectious agents, as suggested by the national disease prevention and health promotion strategy outlined in Figure 45-1. Even where organizational, economic, or environmental supports for behavior or health outcomes are paramount, health

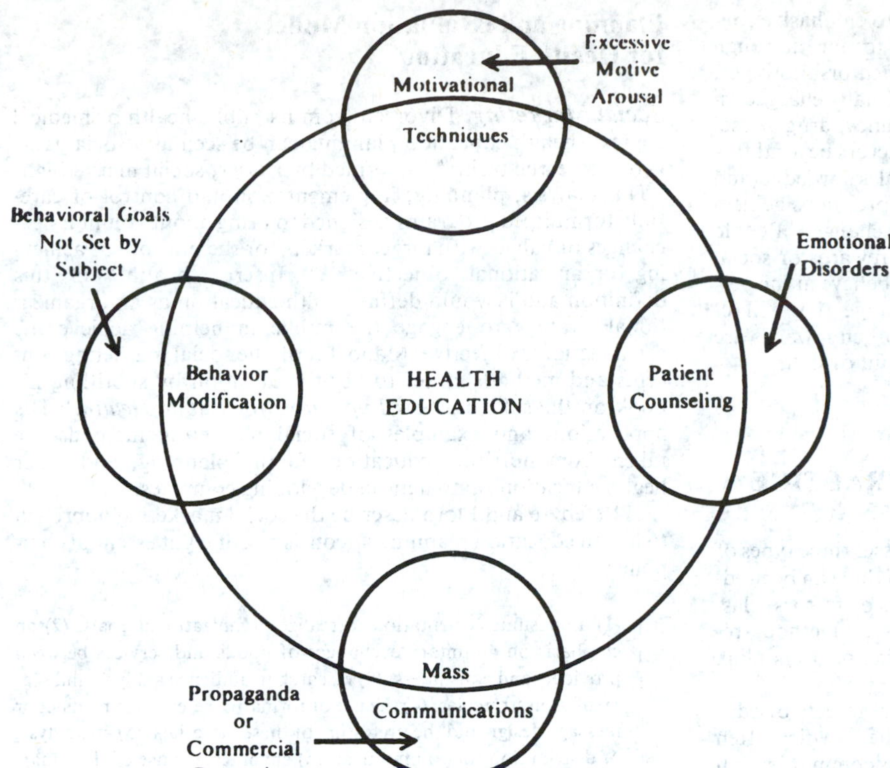

Figure 45-2. Examples of overlapping technologies for changing health-related behavior, showing the aspects of the technologies that fall outside the definition of health education.

education helps to gain the cooperation of political and administrative decision makers, directors and staffs of agencies dispensing services or resources, and the voting public.

Health education occurs through the mass media and in various settings: worksites (occupational health and safety, employee health promotion), medical (patient education, health education in primary care settings and hospitals), community agencies (voluntary health organizations, health fairs, health promotion events), and schools.

Patient education represents health education centered in medical care settings, but not necessarily limited to clinics or hospitals, to the patients themselves or to diagnosed health problems. It may include education to prevent the onset of symptoms, and it may be directed at family members.[18]

Because classrooms are the primary locus of school health education and because children or adolescents are the major target groups, the methods of school health education are largely pedagogical, and concentration is on the health and behavioral problems of children and youth. The other distinguishing characteristic of school health education is its limited responsibility for behavioral and health outcomes.

> It is taken as a task of school health education . . . that children at each age or grade should be helped to master those health maintenance skills necessary to cope with potential threats to their health in the coming age or grade, and those additional foundation skills necessary to benefit from the instructions next year in relation to the potential health problems of the year after that.[19]

THE CHANGING CIRCUMSTANCES OF HEALTH EDUCATION

In the earliest practice of health education, the health outcomes of primary concern were injuries and infectious diseases. The behavior required of children, youth, and adults was largely assumed to be in the sphere of personal safety or hygienic practices. Such practices were equated with good manners and moral development. By associating personal hygiene with socially acceptable behavior, a causal link was implied between personal responsibility for social good and the communicable nature of diseases spread by contact, or between behaving recklessly and endangering public safety.[20]

As the infectious diseases gave way to chronic, degenerative, developmental, and violent causes of death and disability, and as the overall death, disease, and disability rates of most nations declined, contagion no longer served as the underlying rationale for health education. Proper health behavior no longer can be prescribed entirely on the basis of the common good or family welfare. Unhealthful behavior must be proscribed in relation to increasingly personal, distant, and improbable or seemingly inevitable morbid events in the future. In contrast with the past, current generations are told that virtually every substance they consume and every pleasure they seek has some chance of harming them. In short, probabilities have replaced precept, data have replaced dictum, decision-making skills have replaced definitions of proper health conduct. The behavioral sciences have influenced understanding of the forces affecting behavior so that health educators today are expected to design their programs with traditional attention to knowledge, attitudes, and skills but also with methods and materials that take into account the circumstances that enable behavior to occur and that provide for rewards that will reinforce the desired behavior.[21] Attention to circumstances is understood to be especially important in health promotion, where the behaviors of increasing concern are heavily embedded in lifestyle and social learning. Dietary patterns, for example, will not yield to simplistic lesson plans that drill patients on food groups,[22] nor will smoking be prevented simply by increasing the percentage of students who know it may cause cancer.[23]

These shifts in the problems and patterns of health education have broadened the assumptions concerning cause-and-effect relationships between intervention and potential health benefits. Some educators and evaluators continue to emphasize content in health education and content mastery in testing, although the content itself has changed. Most health educators, however, have come to grips with the value-laden and socially charged issues of lifestyle changes, AIDS, teenage pregnancy, drug abuse, and smoking by placing greater emphasis on factors beyond factual knowledge. Bending too far from factual knowledge and understanding, however, has resulted in some programs achieving expedient change at the expense of durable change.[24] People will make token changes in response to token rewards or social influence, but unless they also understand and believe in the personally relevant reasons for maintaining the change, they will return to their former behavior as soon as the token rewards are withdrawn or the socially influential person is out of sight.[25]

NEW SCOPE OF THEORY AND PRACTICE

The modern practice of health education addresses three types of factors that may influence health behaviors and that can be modified by educational intervention. The three sets of factors, classified according to the types of interventions or methods required to modify them, are predisposing factors, enabling factors, and reinforcing factors.

Predisposing factors include the traditional targets of education, including knowledge, attitudes, and beliefs, which often change in response to one-way didactic and mass communication methods. The new variables in this category include values and perceptions, which require more interactive communication in order to clarify and adjust inconsistencies in values and misperceptions of reality. The defining characteristic of predisposing factors is their motivational force before the decision to take a given health action.[26]

Enabling factors may call for some community health education, family education, or staff education and organizational development within the primary care setting, worksite, or school to assure that the resources needed by patients, employees, or students to carry out the prescribed actions are accessible. The accessibility of resources or facilities in the community or the institution must concern those who recommend health practices that are blocked by circumstances. When the forces required to change these circumstances or to mobilize the needed resources go beyond education, strategies within the broader enterprises called health promotion, health services, or health protection are called into play.[27]

Reinforcing factors are becoming more prevalent in health education where the assumed causes of the behavior are largely social, such as peer influence. These factors may include token rewards (e.g., certificate of achievement) or tangible rewards (e.g., money) for successful trials or test performances, but more significant reinforcing factors are those associated with social learning.[28] One of the most fruitful lines of theory and research in recent health education efforts directed at the problems of smoking, drug abuse, and adolescent sexuality has been with concepts of *inoculation* against peer pressure: children are reinforced for demonstrating skills in declining or resisting the offer of a cigarette or pressure to engage in sexual activity, against their better judgment.

The most effective health education programs combine learning experiences directed at all three sets of factors influencing behavior, based on an educational diagnosis of the predominant variables in each category. A behavior that is highly motivated and reinforced will be frustrated if it is not also enabled. A motivated and enabled behavior that meets with social punishment or ridicule rather than reinforcement will not persist. Any review of contemporary research can be organized around the three sets of factors influencing health behavior.

Planning and Evaluation Models for Health Education

Social Marketing. Divorced from its public health or medical context, health education planning can be seen as a social marketing research task.[29] As defined by Kotler, social marketing is "The analysis, planning, implementation and control of carefully formulated programs designed to bring about voluntary exchanges of values with target markets for the purpose of achieving organizational objectives."[30] Insert "health" in this definition and it would define health education as an organizational strategy to engage the public in helping achieve the organization's objective. Manoff took the social marketing concepts and methods closer to health education by subtitling his book on the subject, *New Imperative for Public Health.*[31] His applications and examples of social marketing methods are taken from nutrition education, family planning, and other health education campaigns in developing countries.

Lefebvre and Flora describe the social marketing approach to health education planning as consisting of eight essential components:

> (1) a consumer orientation to realize organizational goals, (2) an emphasis on voluntary exchanges of goods and services between providers and consumers, (3) research in audience analysis and segmentation strategies, (4) the use of formative research in product or message design and the pretesting of these materials, (5) an analysis of distribution (or communication) channels, (6) use of the "marketing mix"—that is, utilizing and blending product, price, place, and promotion characteristics in intervention planning and implementation, (7) a process tracking system with both integrative and control functions, and (8) a management process that involves problem analysis, planning, implementation, and feedback functions.[32]

The PRECEDE Model. An alternative framework for health education planning has evolved from the specific application of social marketing, epidemiology, health psychology, medical sociology, and administrative sciences in the assessment of needs in the target population. The steps in this model can be traced from the causal chain of determinants and consequences implied in health education, as shown in Figure 45-3.[33] This represents a more focused application of the policy model in Figure 45-1. The diagnostic planning process begins with an analysis of the end points or ultimate outcomes as expressed by the population or individuals in terms of their quality of life or social problems. It then works back through the causal chain to the health determinants of the social problem. Once the health problems are identified, the model continues with an analysis of the behavioral determinants of each health problem. As with each preceding step, critical selection of the behaviors that are most important and potentially changeable must eliminate from further analysis those factors that fail to meet both criteria, or else the process becomes too cumbersome.

The next step is to identify the factors determining the behaviors previously identified. Finally, the administrative diagnosis identifies the educational resources and interventions that can be deployed to initiate the process of change in predisposing, enabling, and reinforcing behavior conducive to health.

The PRECEDE framework helped in the formulation of targeted and focused health education programs where earlier programs had been diffuse and inefficiently scattered over too many objects and processes of change. The acronym stands for *predisposing, reinforcing, and enabling constructs in educational diagnosis and evaluation.* It was intended to emphasize the repeated etiological search for what precedes the problem at hand. It borrows from the medical concept that accurate diagnosis must precede treatment. Too many health education pro-

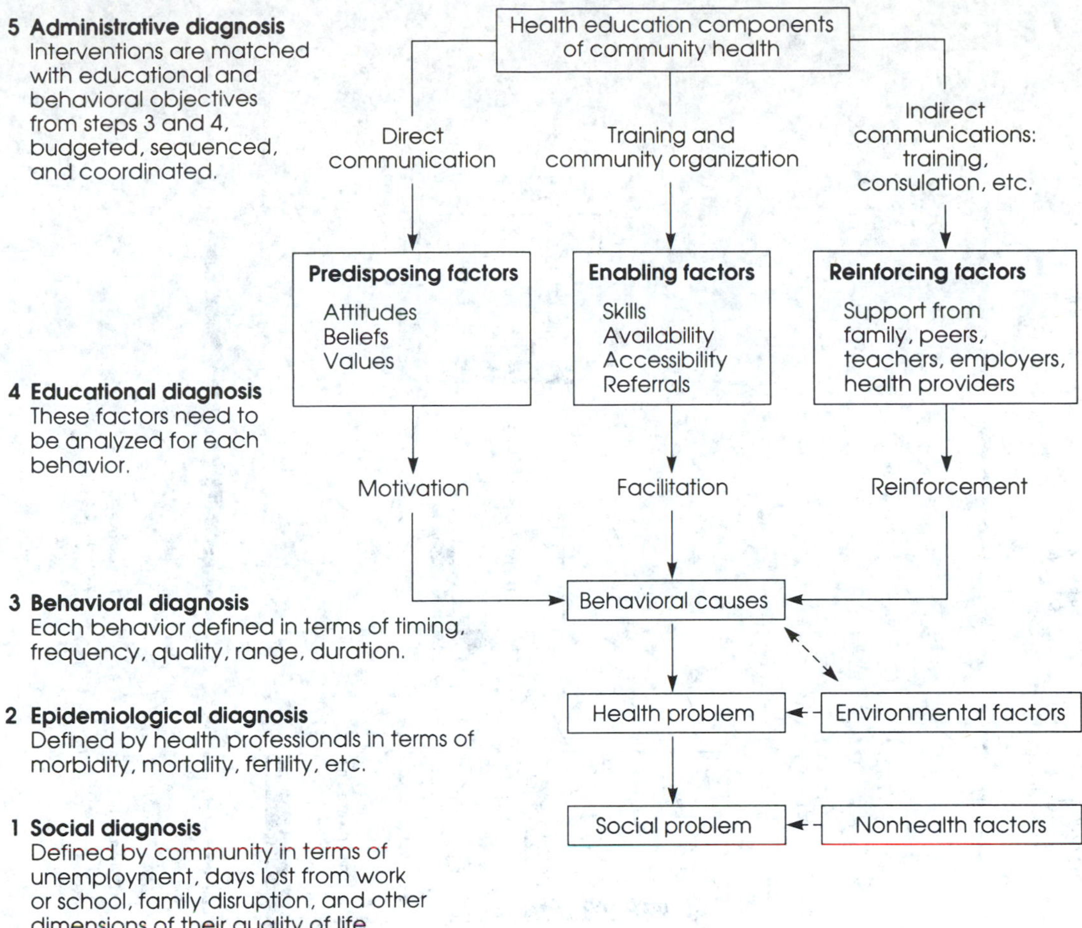

Figure 45-3. The five steps preceding the development of a specific plan of health education, related to the determinants of each level of outcome in a hierarchy of objectives for health programs, referred to as the PRECEDE framework.

grams had been conceived out of simplistic and undocumented assumptions about the causes of the problems they sought to change.

Critics of the PRECEDE framework pointed out that it left environmental determinants of health dangling in a residual category, implying that the responsibility for health should fall entirely on the people whose behavior was errant, regardless of their environmental circumstances. The framework also left the political, regulatory, and organizational context for implementation of programs to the imagination of the user. These concerns became increasingly important during the 1980s as the new policies in health promotion provided opportunities for health education to be teamed with more regulatory and organizational interventions, such as smoking ordinances and company arrangements for release time or facilities for employee participation in health programs. Such policies, regulations, and organizational arrangements supplement the educational interventions directed at enabling factors and environmental barriers to change.

With the health promotion movement, PRECEDE has evolved an additional set of appendages and steps in the planning and evaluation process referred to as PROCEED, for *policy, regulatory, and organizational constructs in educational and environmental development*. PROCEED, as seen in Figure 45-4, continues where PRECEDE leaves off, but with implementation rather than planning as the focus.

Social Learning Model. Of the three sets of factors—predisposing, enabling, and reinforcing—those that reinforce (reward or punish) health behavior are likely to be the most influential in relation to the development of complex behavior that must be maintained. Reinforcing factors determine whether a behavior that is motivated and enabled will occur or persist once it has been contemplated or tried. Depending on the social models demonstrating the behavior and the quality of feedback received in response to the behavior, the pattern of behavior will be more or less likely to develop and persist. Social learning theory has elaborated the reinforcing factors important to health education by showing how they can occur before the behavior has been enacted. These include efficacy expectations (Can I do it?) and outcome expectations (What benefit will it bring me?).[34] The theory also emphasizes vicarious learning and self-reinforcement as ways in which individuals can learn without necessarily receiving direct, external rewards.[35]

Patient education in primary care settings is ideally suited to offering some reinforcement for healthful behavior, but the most important sources of reinforcement are beyond the control of clinical personnel. These sources include the family, mass media, and peer influences, in that order of dominance for children. Peer influences, however, increase with age and eventually surpass the family in social influence on adolescents and young adults.[36] With advancing age, organizational, economic, and environmental factors play an increasing role in enabling and reinforcing health behavior.

If family influence, mass media, and peer pressure are beyond the direct control of the primary care setting and the school, perhaps the most promising contribution these institutional centers for health education may make is to prepare children and adults to recognize and to be able to resist mass media and peer pressures to adopt unhealthful practices. This approach

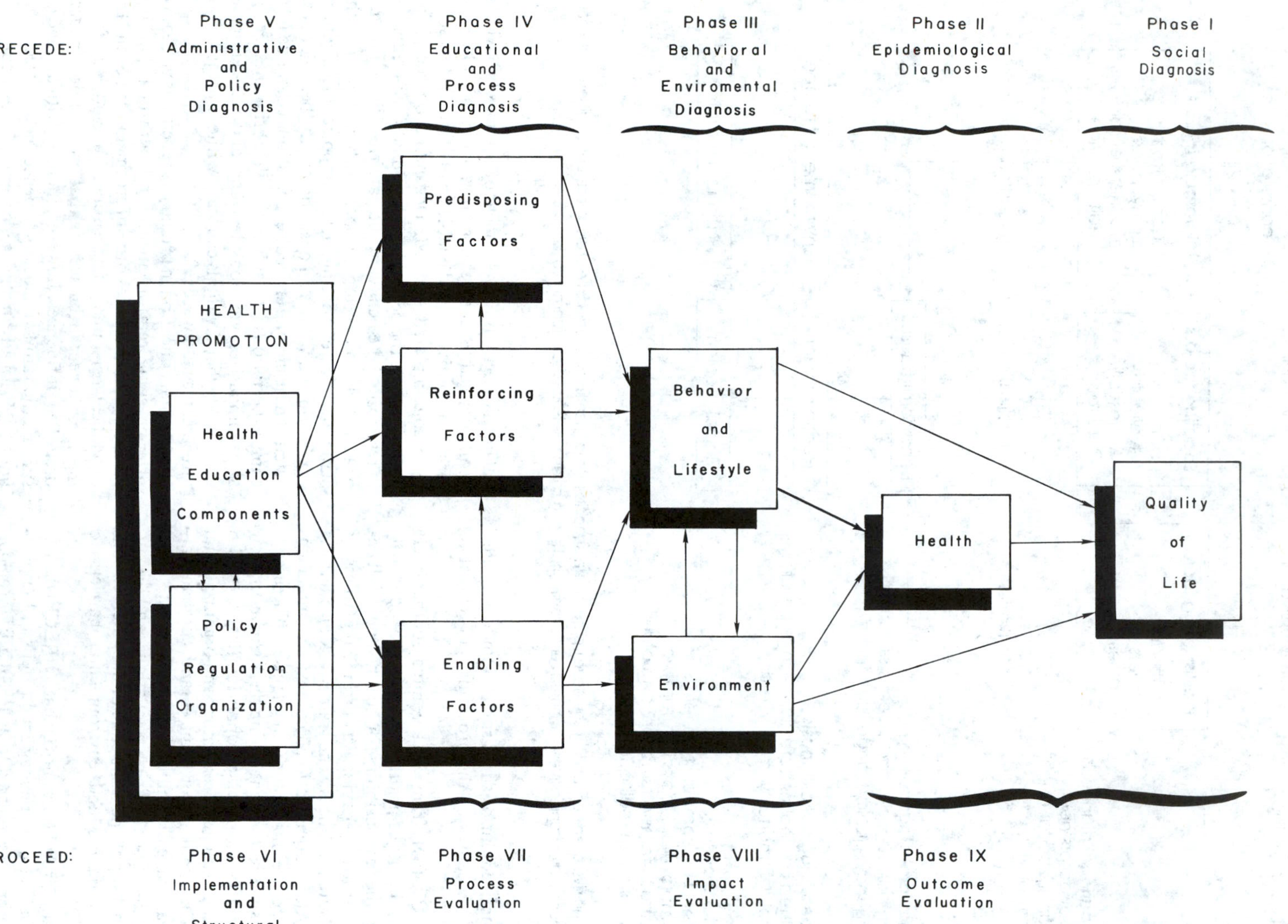

Figure 45-4. Phases of PRECEDE and PROCEED models for health education and health promotion.

has yielded impressive results in the delay of onset of smoking, alcohol, and drug use in children and adolescents.[37]

In summary, the evidence strongly supports the employment of methods in health education that help people resist peer pressure for unhealthful behavior and that take other social influences into account, especially those of family and the mass media. The appropriate level of parental involvement, however, is in dispute. It appears to be most effective to involve parents while the children are young, but some authorities emphasize the need for children to learn independent, adult-free decision making about health matters at younger ages.[38]

SELF-CARE EDUCATION IN MEDICAL SETTINGS

The most immediate and compelling opportunities for health education to influence behavioral risk factors are with patients in medical care settings. The evidence for effective interventions is stronger from randomized trials in this arena than from others. Especially well documented are studies in preoperative counseling to improve postoperative outcomes[39] and in patient education to reduce drug errors[40] and quit smoking.[41]

When possible, patients need to play a major role in the maintenance and management of their own health and disease. The increasing prevalence of chronic and degenerative disease, the increasing costs of medical care, and the increasing importance of patient behavior as a determinant of health outcomes all have forced growing attention on self-care education as an inescapable component of secondary prevention.[42]

The controversies center not on whether to allow self-care but on how to support it. How can the physician, for example, organize a medical practice that turns responsibility over to patients for a larger role in their own care without abrogating the physician's function? How can a medical practice devote sufficient resources to self-care education to be effective without stretching its resources so thin that medical procedures are compromised? How can the transfer to patients of responsibility for their own care provide for the necessary monitoring and surveillance of responsible medical care and secondary prevention?

The Role of the Clinical Setting. Conceding that self-care education is necessary still leaves open to debate whether health care workers in clinical settings should assume responsibility for it. Some have argued that self-care education belongs outside the medical sector, that nonmedical agencies can provide it at lower cost, with fewer conflicts of interest, and at less sacrifice to frank medical services. This argument is most credible with regard to the concerns of primary prevention or health promotion where the temptation to medicalize life-style issues draws the health care worker into some complex social, economic, and ethical arenas. How far should the physician or nurse go, for example, in pressing patients to stop smoking or to change eating habits that are highly interwoven with family, occupational, or ethnic ties? Should physicians extend the scope of their practice to intervene effectively on alcohol consumption, stress management, and physical fitness?

These questions cause some clinicians to hedge in the enthusiasm of their advice to patients and some patients to avoid a physician who advocates changes in health-related behavior without considering other dimensions of their life circumstances.[43]

Some of these issues apply also to nonmedical settings, but the costs relative to the risks and benefits can be lowered by educating people in groups, thus reducing overhead costs and unit costs of educational personnel, media, and facilities. Locating these educational functions outside the clinical practice of medicine also conserves the expensive time of the physician for more strictly medical problems, including the supervision of self-care in secondary prevention. Just as the hospital is not an ideal setting for the efficient and cost-effective provision of primary medical care, the primary care setting is less than ideal for the continuing supervision and education of most people (not to say patients) in their struggle with habits of daily living related to primary prevention.[44]

The clinical setting, nevertheless, is an ideal place to offer habituated patients a number of positive reinforcements, such as some initial encouragement, a medical rationale to help them perceive the benefits of behavioral change, the credibility of medical expertise and familiarity with their history, suggestions for strategies of behavioral change that fit their medical and economic circumstances, an authoritative referral for outside help, and periodic support of their progress with the habit on subsequent medical encounters. Physicians also can stimulate social support for their patients by asking family members to come in with the patients for health education or, better still, by treating the family as a unit. Physicians can in this way use their position in the community to coordinate life-style modification with agencies better equipped than they are to offer some types of health education and social support economically and effectively.[45]

In secondary prevention, on the other hand, the task is to respond early and effectively to signs or symptoms. Self-care education then does represent a larger opportunity for an effective and economical role for the clinical setting. The research on this aspect of patient education indicates that it holds the potential for large savings in unnecessary medical care costs, emergency room visits, hospitalization, absenteeism, disability days, and premature deaths and for improved quality of life for patients with chronic conditions.[46] It also may have the side benefits of reducing malpractice suits and broken appointments and of increasing patient satisfaction.[47] These and other benefits are achieved by enhancing patient understanding and participation in the development of the treatment or maintenance regimen and enhancing adherence to the prescribed regimen.[48]

The costs and possible tradeoffs of increased self-care education in primary care include the time and opportunity costs of the physician and other personnel that might have been devoted to more lucrative medical activities, the production or purchase costs of educational materials, the increased independence of patients, who make less frequent office visits, and the potential risks of mismanagement in less competent patients. The control of these costs and potential risks are discussed in the following paragraphs.

Implementation of Patient Education. A barrier to implementing self-care education in primary care may be the fear that it will become a bottomless pit of counseling on an array of psychological and social problems. The best way to overcome this barrier is to classify the major problems and needs of patients into categories that are broad enough to allow an initial triage of patients into a few educational treatment categories for each disease or self-care task. This will help to control the array. To control the sense of a bottomless pit, a stepped approach to each triage group is needed. These two strategies, applied in sequence, can limit the costs and can maximize the benefits of self-care education.

One approach to triage is to identify which source of support for the prescribed behavior is lacking. This educational diagnosis sorts patients into one of three groups where (1) personal motivation is lacking, (2) there is motivation, but a self-care skill or other resource is lacking, or (3) personal motivation and skill are both present, but there is little or no support for patients at home, school, or work. As seen in Figure 45–5, this classification yields a hierarchy of three categories of patients for whom qualitatively different educational objectives and methods can be

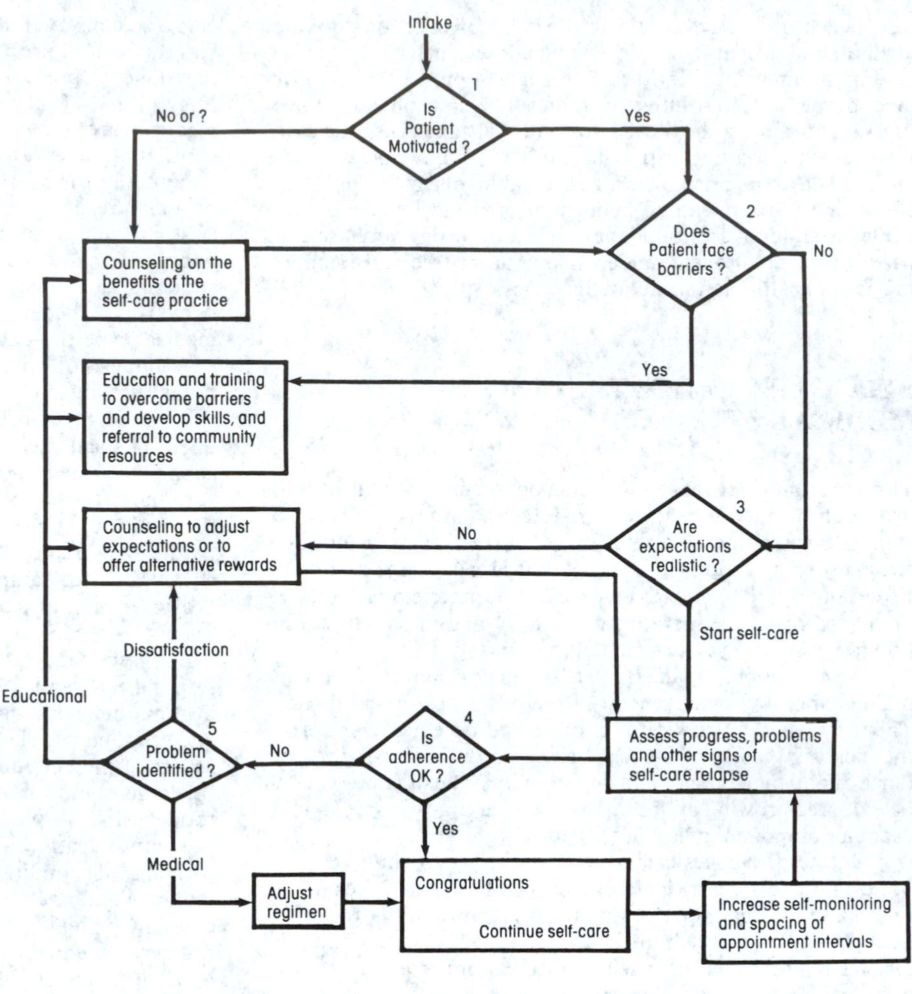

Figure 45-5. Algorithm for the triage and stepped approach to self-care education for patients in clinical settings.

drawn from the growing accumulation of health education literature organized around predisposing, enabling, and reinforcing factors.[49]

For the first category of patients, education in the form of direct communication can be designed to alter the predisposing beliefs, attitudes, and perceptions. Counseling the patients on three health beliefs in particular can be expected to provide the best motivational foundation to predispose them to take a more active role in self-care: (1) the belief that they are susceptible to the consequences of not following the prescribed regimen of self-care, (2) the belief that the consequences might be severe, and (3) the belief that the benefits of the recommended self-care methods outweigh the costs and inconvenience.[50]

The second group of patients faces the enabling factors of skill or resources as their primary barrier to self-care practice. These patients are motivated, but they will be frustrated if they are expected to carry out complicated or expensive self-care procedures without specific forms of help. The essential ingredients in the health care worker's initial responsibility to these patients are basic instruction and training to build the necessary skills, combined with an appropriate payment plan or a referral to a specific community source of equipment or supplies.[51]

The third group of patients has predisposing and enabling factors already in place, but their continuing practice of the recommended behavior is threatened by one or more social or environmental factors in the home or workplace. These factors will punish the patients for self-care, making the immediate social costs and inconvenience of the behavior outweigh the more distant medical rewards. The best educational antidote for patients in this group is to invite family members, with the permission of the patients, to discuss ways in which they can support the patients in following the self-care regimen. An alternative (for this group and others) is to form patient groups that meet periodically with or without invited partners to exchange self-care experiences and to provide mutual support and reinforcement. This, of course, is more economical and also provides the third category of patients a substitute form of social reinforcement for self-care when the home or work environment cannot be altered.

Physicians can be most helpful in referring patients to community organizations and resources, such as self-help groups, weight-control programs, voluntary agencies, and health education centers. These resources can provide the additional education, training, facilities, and social support necessary to predispose, enable, or reinforce the self-care practice. Return appointments to see patients after the referral can provide a responsible means of assuring that the needed help is being received in a form consistent with the medical indications for the recommended self-care. A follow-up appointment provides the patient with an additional incentive to pursue the referral and to act on the recommended self-care practices. It also identifies the strengths and weaknesses of community organizations in providing medically sound self-care education and support. The physician then can participate more effectively as a professional member of the community in correcting deficiencies in health education resources and services.

Monitoring Patient Education. Follow-up appointments are the standard method to verify the diagnosis, to evaluate progress of the treatment, and to correct any deficiencies in the treatment. The same principle applies in self-care, but it needs to be put in an operational form that takes into account the greater complexity and duration of the usual self-care regimen in secondary prevention (e.g., hypertension medications, weight control, sodium intake). A stepped-care approach is recommended for the systematic transfer of responsibility to patients and for the responsible monitoring of self-care practices.

The stepped-care approach proceeds from the triage method outlined in the previous section, moving the patients in group 1 to group 2 and from group 2 to group 3. Once patients are receiving the necessary environmental and social support for the recommended self-care practice, the next step can be to wean them from dependency on health professional supervision of the self-care practice. This can be accomplished with a minimum of risk only if patients learn to observe the same primary signals that physicians and other health professionals use in detecting an irregularity in the results of self-care (e.g., blood pressure readings in hypertensive patients, blood sugar readings in diabetic patients).

The means and the ends in self-care are as much self-monitoring as they are self-treatment. For example, educating hypertensive patients to take their own blood pressure readings at home or at work makes it possible to transfer not only the perfunctory aspects of following a rigid self-treatment regimen but also the evaluative function of monitoring and recording changes in the resulting blood pressure. The self-monitoring function can become a major source of reinforcement of proper self-treatment, so that two forms of self-care behavior are strengthened and become mutually reinforcing in a continuous feedback loop. This can make patients less dependent on the physician for evaluation as well as less dependent on family and friends for social reinforcement of self-care practices.

The ultimate step in a stepped-care program of self-care education establishes a truly collaborative relationship between the health care professional and the patient for treatment and monitoring. The health care professional assesses the quality of patient self-care and reduces the frequency of office visits according to the validation of patient self-assessments. Office visits may be more frequent if patients have multiple risk factors or medical, social, and economic complications. Some fail-safe signals should be included in the protocol for patient self-monitoring to ensure that patients call in response to some symptoms. Periodic mailing of self-monitoring records and a tickler file in the office can assure patients that they are not forgotten by the physician.

In general, the procedure for initiating stepped care would be to assign most patients to group 2 for skill training unless they obviously are unmotivated or already are skilled in self-treatment. Those who show little interest or motivation for self-treatment would be assigned to group 1 for education on the three health beliefs. Those who have the necessary resources to carry out the regimen can be advanced to group 3.

Even without standardized instruments for educational triage, the health care professional can make reasonable assessments and assignments by asking patients such questions as: What do you know about your illness? Do you have any specific fears or concerns about it? How serious do you think it is? What are your goals for the treatment of your condition? What are your feelings about the prescribed therapeutic regimen? Can you describe how you are going to go about your self-treatment? Do you expect to have any problems with family, friends, or employers in carrying out these procedures?

To provide for the additional education needed for self-monitoring, it will be most efficient to build it into the same three phases of predisposing, enabling, and reinforcing education as suggested in Figure 45–5. In summary, two conditions assure that the benefits of self-care education in clinical settings will outweigh the costs. If the behavior in question is related to a diagnosed medical condition rather than to a general health habit embedded in the lifestyle of patients and if the predisposing and enabling barriers for patients are not so great as to render them ineffective in trying to carrying out the recommended self-care practices, the physician can play a valuable role.

Even in primary prevention, the health care workers in clinical settings can encourage patients, present data on the expected benefits of behavioral change, explore the costs of attempting to change behavior, offer strategies for minimizing these costs, refer patients to community resources and programs, and follow-up with reinforcement for any progress the patients have made at the time of subsequent office visits.

HEALTH EDUCATION IN SCHOOL SETTINGS

Schools have been the object of much attention in health education and preventive health services, but there appears to be some disappointment with the outcomes. The disappointments stem largely from expectations that these programs and services should have given us more spectacular gains in health outcomes (i.e., morbidity and mortality reductions). In contrast to expectations, the 15- to 24-year age group, representing the immediate fruits of school health programs and services, is the only age group in the United States to have experienced an increased death rate in recent decades.[52] In addition, teenage pregnancies and sexually transmitted diseases have increased, and injuries from automobile crashes and violence remain highest in this age range.

The health services as we know them today cannot be expected to have prevented these problems, any more than school health education alone could have prevented them. A renewed partnership of health services with community social and educational agencies and private organizations would emphasize a different set of outcomes than those of primary importance to the health services. These mutually beneficial outcomes would be more in line with educational models than with those of medicine and public health.[53]

Public Health Models of Health Education Applied to Schools. Most health programs have had only marginal utility in schools because their end points (health outcomes) do not address the primary function of schools, namely, education. School health services and curricula have been supported or hosted by the educational establishment only to the extent that the health outcomes (or health problems prevented) were believed to have enhanced the educational mission of the schools.[54]

Within public health, health education has required more complex and difficult-to-test models because of the necessary linkages of cognitive, environmental, and behavioral variables, each of which is variously and sometimes tenuously related to the others and to health outcomes. A generic health education model is one that contains, by definition, a combination of interventions designed to predispose, enable, and reinforce voluntary adaptations of behavior conducive to health.

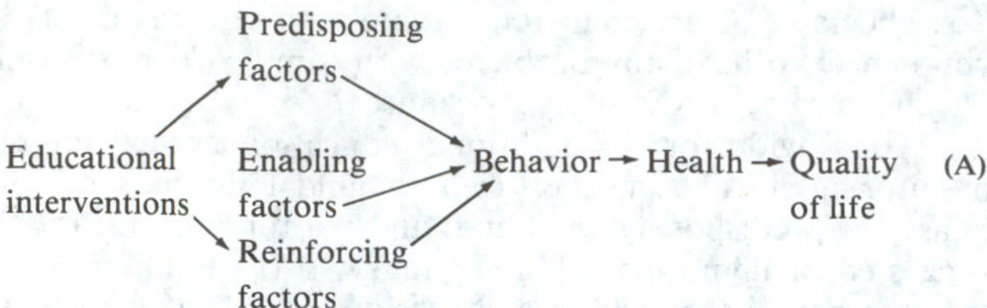

School Health Education Models. An impressive record of school health education impact on health behavior has accumulated in the past few years.[55] The most thoroughly documented is with improvements in knowledge, attitudes, and skills assumed to be important in the subsequent development of health behavior. In this hierarchy and sequencing of effects, an implicit model is imposed on, rather than inherent in, school health education.

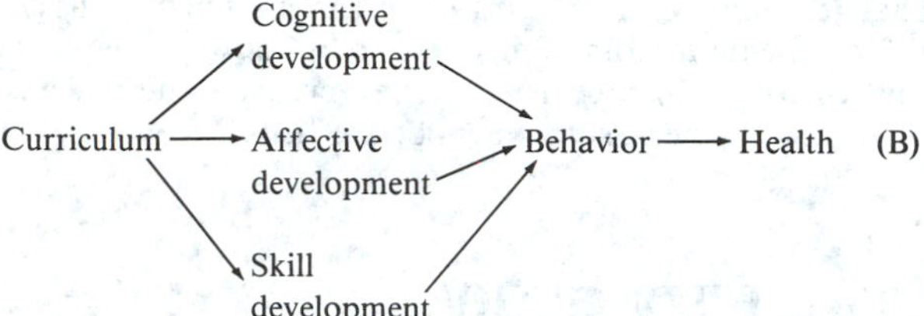

This model, derivative of the public health education model (A), places ultimate importance on health outcomes and the behaviors necessary to achieve them. The problem is that schools are neither medical institutions nor public health agencies and have never adopted the same mission and goals. School health educators have worked valiantly to live up to the expectations of their public health education colleagues, but they have been fighting an uphill battle within the education sector in recent years with the back-to-basics movement. The schools simply cannot be held accountable for solutions to all the ills of society, and the line is now being drawn more severely between the primary educational mission of the schools and the functions that other agencies would like them to serve.[56]

The Comprehensive School Health Program Model. One solution to this recognition that the classroom alone cannot be expected to accomplish behavioral and health outcomes was to return to a basic model of school health programs, one that was not derivative of public health education but rather of education in general. The generic model of school health promotion combines health teaching with school and community health services and interventions in the school and community environment to produce that level of health outcomes necessary to assure that students can perform effectively in school and achieve academically. The two significant departures of this model from the preceding models are (1) the combination of education with school and community services and environmental interventions to promote health and (2) the emphasis on health as a means to educational ends as well as an end in itself.

The comprehensive school health program model would approximate the following:

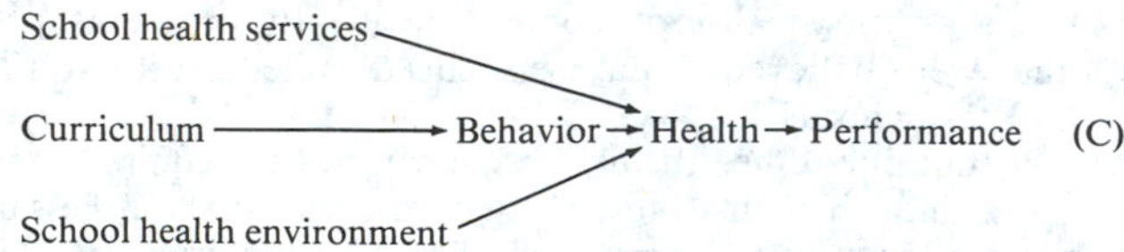

Schools are not obliged to justify their attention to performance and achievement in terms of their contribution to health, just as senior citizen centers are not obliged to justify their recreational programs in terms of their contribution to health. Yet both contribute to health and, therefore, could be construed as health services.

As portrayed in the foregoing review of models and assumptions, the major difference between those derived from the health fields (biomedical, public health, biobehavioral, and public health education) and those derived from education (e.g., the comprehensive school health model) is their respective placement of health as an ultimate outcome or as an instrumental outcome. Part of the disagreement in this lies in the missions of the two sectors, health and education. With the increasing complexity of etiologies and causal pathways for specific diseases and health problems, the health establishment seems ready to entertain more complex and time-lapsed models of intervention as related to health outcomes. The growing interest in disease prevention and health promotion attests to this. At the same time, the schools and their constituencies are demanding greater time on task and improved achievement scores of their students. The convergence of these trends suggests a new rationale for health education in schools in which behavioral and performance variables are targeted for the short-term outcomes:

Intervention → Lifestyle → Performance → Achievement (D)

The educational establishment will be more or less persuaded to adopt this model depending on the strength of evidence documenting the association between lifestyle and performance as measured in educational terms. A previous review assessed such evidence for children in four areas of lifestyle: sleep, exercise, diet, and stress.[57] The corresponding evidence for alcohol and drug abuse has been reviewed thoroughly elsewhere,[58] and the influence of such abuse on performance in school is hardly in doubt.

To maintain the interest and possible support of the health establishment, this model needs to be extended to show its potential contribution to health outcomes. The main argument affirming the relevance of this model to health is the pervasive and inescapable correlation between educational attainment and health.[59] The connection of educational attainment to health is explained most logically in behavioral terms, although genetic and economic factors undeniably enter into both the educational attainment and the health behavior of children and their parents. The empirical evidence supporting the causal link between educational attainment and health behavior is consistent but tenuous, in that it is not experimental. Similarly, the link between health behaviors and long-term health outcomes is widely documented and accepted but nearly impossible to establish experimentally.

With these caveats in mind, the following model would seem to place health education (curriculum) most appropriately within the context of schools:

School health services ↘
Health curriculum → Life-style → Performance → Achievement → Health (E)
School environment ↗

This, of course, is highly simplified, leaving out the exogenous influences of other aspects of the curriculum on performance, factors other than performance on achievement, and factors outside the school, including coordinated community health services and community health promotion efforts, on all the outcomes. The purpose of this model is simply to specify the essential elements linking school health education and related interventions with health outcomes in a causal chain that recognizes and gives primacy to the educational outcomes, which are the main, if not the sole, concern of the schools.

HEALTH PROMOTION IN THE COMMUNITY

The comprehensive school health model shown in (C) approximates at the school level what has come to be associated with health promotion at the community and national level in two ways. First, the combination of health education with organizational and environmental services and resources in support of health behavior, in both the school health model and in the health promotion model, relieves some of the unrealistic expectation of health education alone to accomplish behavioral and health outcomes. Second, the recognition that health is not necessarily an end in itself but may serve other values and social goals or quality-of-life concerns is in keeping with the positive concepts of health as "physical, mental, and social well-being" inherent in the earliest approaches to health education in the World Health Organization[60] and in the more recent formulations of policy in health promotion.[61]

This instrumentality of health is reflected in the resolution of the World Health Assembly of 1977: "The main social target of Governments and WHO in the coming decades should be the attainment by all the citizens of the world, by the year 2000, of a level of health that will permit them to lead a socially and economically productive life." Where the WHO, the Surgeon General, and private industries initiating worksite health promotion programs speak of productivity, the schools speak of performance and academic achievement. Where the school health models speaks of combining education with school health services and interventions in the school environment, national policy combines health promotion with health services and health protection, as reflected in Figure 45–1.

One other revelation that the health promotion movement has forced on health professionals is that there are more immediate benefits to be appreciated from lifestyle modification than most of them would normally count as health outcomes. Some would not be counted because they are too subjective, such as "feeling good," and "feeling more energetic." Others would not be counted because they are considered to have more to do with cosmetics, economics, or social norms than with objectively defined health. These include such outcomes of "healthier" lifestyle as weight control, agility, endurance, concentration, efficiency of movement, muscle tone, and independence or performance in activities of daily living.[62]

Together, these and related intangibles make up a large part of the quality-of-life or social concerns that were considered a consequence of health in the public health education model (A). They were given prominence there because public health education begins "where the people are" as a matter of principle or philosophy and because educational research, especially on adult populations,[63] has demonstrated that the commitment of people to the goals of a program increases the probability of their participation, cooperation, or behavioral response to a program.[64] Recognizing that the priority concerns of a population are seldom expressed in terms of health, public health education typically has worked to show people how health can contribute to their quality-of-life or social concerns.

LARGE-SCALE CAMPAIGNS AND COMMUNITY PROGRAMS

What distinguishes large-scale programs in health education and health promotion besides being bigger than their counterparts at the clinical, school, or worksite levels? Is there a qualitative difference in community or multicommunity programs from their component interventions in medical and other institutional settings, or do they merely represent the sum of these parts? Besides coordination of the pieces, what makes community programs run? Other than the additive effects of small-scale programs, what makes large-scale programs more or less effective?

These questions are at the heart of a public health approach to health education and health promotion. They defy simplistic answers that would merely distinguish community approaches from institutionally based programs in terms of magnitude, scope, or volume. There is something more than critical mass that holds such community or multicommunity programs together over time. They are more than medical models writ large, more than pedagogic methods transferred to the media, more than a step up the bureaucratic ladder from town to county or from province to nation.

Community or large-scale programs, even within large institutions, require a shift in perspective and employment of a distinct set of analytical and programmatic tools from those used with patients, clients, or customers. The differences reflect a blend of the distinctions between clinical and epidemiological methods of analysis, between strictly psychological and social-psychological theories, between counseling and mass media methods of communication, and between intraorganizational and interorganizational levels of intervention and management.

Three Generalizations and Propositions. Implications to be drawn from the experience and data on large-scale health education programs are as follows:

1. Large-scale health education and health promotion efforts require, above all, more planning and coordination than small-scale programs. More participants in the planning and execution means more meetings and telephone calls to achieve consensus, more letters and documents to convey concepts and procedures to more varied actors. The complexities grow exponentially with each additional organization or community added to the roster of participants, at least up to a point where added organizations or communities can be matched or clustered according to their similarities. Typically, such a point is not reached until many dissimilar organizations or communities have been accumulated. In short, a truly orchestrated large-scale program—as distinct from numerous replications of a small-scale program—requires additional planning and coordination for each unique unit added, multiplied by (not merely added to) the number of variations in prior units added.

2. As the number of units (organizations, communities) reaches a point where newcomers are more and more likely to be similar to some previous comers, large-scale programs begin to realize an economy of scale, which means that for each newcomer, the job of planning and coordination gets easier because it is more and more likely to be repetitious. The cost in time, effort, and resources per unit of production or service goes down as the number of organizations and people reached goes up. Some programs never reach their threshold level because their initial planning, production of materials, or coordination failed in the early stages to satisfy early participants, establish a reputation, and assure the diffusion of the program.

3. Diffusion of a new program depends both on satisfying the early adopters and on timing and placing interventions strategically according to stages in the natural history of the diffusion process. The natural history of the diffusion process as applied to organizations follows a logistic curve similar to the diffusion of innovations or ideas in populations.[65] Theories associated with the curve can describe and explain three important features of the diffusion process: **(a)** It helps us understand the characteristics and distribution of individuals or organizations according to their relative time of adoption as identified by their place in the diffusion curve. **(b)** A second understanding we gain concerns the lag time between awareness and adoption and how this lag time differs between early adopters and late adopters. **(c)** The third implication of diffusion theory is an understanding of the forces pushing the diffusion process forward and the forces holding it back, at each stage.

The Classification and Distribution of Adopters. Figure 45-6A shows the normal distribution of adoption over time, with the curve divided into standard deviations from the theoretical midpoint of the program or diffusion process. This curve has a vertical axis of numbers of new people or organizations adopting an idea or program at a given point in time. It is, therefore, an incidence curve, in epidemiological terms. The same phenomena and numbers can be expressed as a prevalence curve showing, as in Figure 45-6B, the cumulative number who have adopted up to a point in time. Here the same people who were adopting within one of the standard deviation categories of the incidence curve can be located and labeled on a segment of the cumulative S-shaped prevalence curve in Figure 45-6B.

Few, if any, government-sponsored programs could honestly claim to have entered at time zero on the adoption curve to which they sought to contribute. Usually they enter at a later stage. It is no criticism of government to say that in economies with free enterprise and extensive communication and marketing networks, the innovators and early adopters, and often the early majority, have been skimmed, like cream off milk, by commercial interests by the time government is called on to take action. Indeed, the relative deprivation of those who could not avail themselves of privately sponsored programs or services is often the impetus for government initiative in health. The previous adoption by the affluent and the middle majority causes an innovation related to health to be perceived more and more as a benefit, first negotiated in collective bargaining, then demanded as a right. Whether in the interest of equity or in the interest of health as a right, government agencies undertake large-scale programs in public health when previously acceptable circumstances have been redefined in the public's perception as unacceptable. As Sir Geoffrey Vickers said, "The history of public health might well be written as a record of successive redefinings of the unaccept-

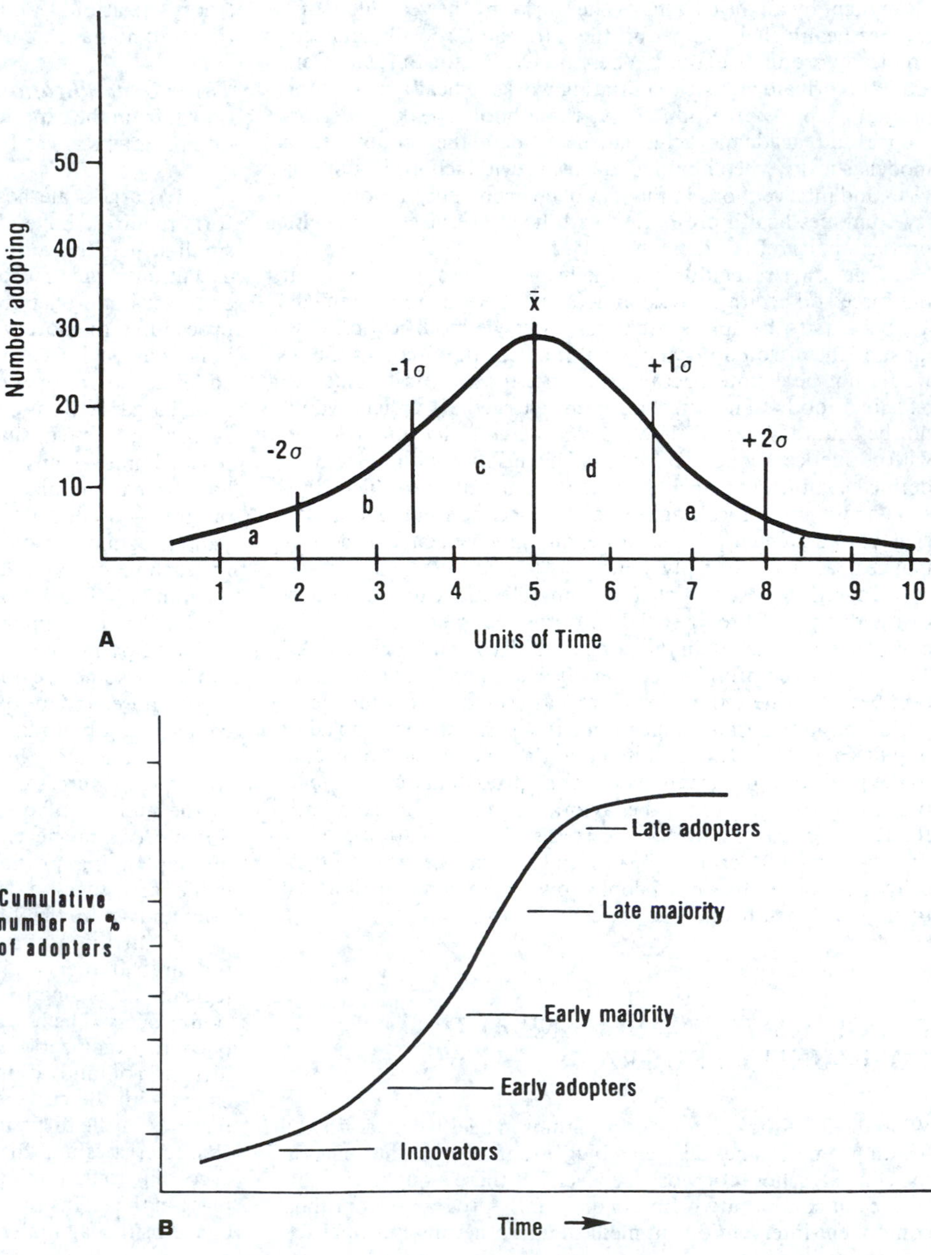

Figure 45-6. A. The incidence of adoption over time. **B.** The prevalence of adoption over time.

able.'' Health education has a large role in affecting the public's perception of acceptable and unacceptable conditions.

The late point of entry on the diffusion curve has several implications for public health campaigns. Some of these distinguish such government programs from large-scale commercial marketing efforts. Much has been said in the professional literature in recent years about the need to apply marketing principles and strategies in public health. The implicit criticism that public health has failed where commercial marketing has succeeded oversimplifies the task public health faces by equating a percentage point commercial gain in the early-adopter phase with a percentage point health behavior gain in the late-adopter phase.

The first implication of the point of entry on the diffusion curve has to do with the classification and distribution of people or organizations according to their order of adoption. Innovators and early adopters typically are more affluent and keyed in to national media. They are cosmopolitans who know the most about health and can afford the most in private purchase of health care products and services and least need some of the health products and services they buy. They are the upscale market of Madison Avenue in New York or of Bay Street in Toronto or of the Zona Rosa of Mexico City. They are the social models for the majority. Mass media alone can suffice in reaching them.

The early and late majorities attend less to national media and more to local media, and they respond less to media in general than to interpersonal influence. This is why most large-scale programs have put so much emphasis on involving the local media and organizational channels of communication rather than depending on network broadcasts or national publications. This middle majority is the primary target group of those public health programs addressing problems for which everybody is at some risk, such as food sanitation, fitness, stress, nutrition, and injury-control programs. All these relate to socially and culturally conditioned behaviors embedded in a complex web of lifestyle. This fact, in addition to the characteristics of people in this phase of the diffusion process, makes organizational and institutional channels essential to the health promotion and social modeling strategies required to support changes in their behavior. Media alone no longer suffice.

Finally, the late adopters and hard-to-reach are even more likely to be the primary targets of public health campaigns, especially in preventive health services, such as hypertension, immunization, maternal and child health, family planning, and occupational health and safety. The people and organizations in these late-adopter categories typically are disadvantaged in economic or status terms and are more isolated or alienated socially, and they tend to be suspicious of organizations, including government agencies, purporting to help them. Their use of media is more exclusively for entertainment, and their membership in organizations or coalitions is sporadic and limited in comparison with the earlier adopters. Reaching these people and organizations requires more expensive and labor-intensive forms of community organization, communication, and outreach. The payoff often is greater because of their high risk, but the cost per unit of service effectively delivered is necessarily higher.

The Gap between Exposure and Adoption. The second implication of the point at which health education programs enter the diffusion curve is the delay between intervention and results. For commercial marketing directed at innovators, early adopters, and the early majority, the lapses between awareness and interest, between interest and trial, and between trial and adoption or rejection are brief. As illustrated in Figure 45–7, the time elapsed in the decision and adoption stages represented by gaps e, f, and g at the early stages tends, on the average, to be shorter than the corresponding gaps a, b, and c for later adopters. Following these theoretical curves up the scale to the latest group to become aware of the innovation or program, the horizontal lines one might draw to connect the awareness curve with the adoption curve might be infinitely long on the time scale. It falls to public health education to overcome or offset this natural history of diffusion and adoption at this end of the curve.

To accomplish a percentage point increment in adoption at the public health end of the diffusion curve requires a great deal more effort and expense, as well as time, than an equal increment in the commercial marketing segments of the curve. This can be seen at a theoretical level just by contrasting the slope of the curve at the early-adopter stage, where the rate of adoption is increasing, with the slope at the late-adopter segments, where the rate of adoption is declining. This disparity in the boost of natural diffusion rates at the two ends of the time scale for a product, program, or service makes the simple comparisons of percentage points gained by commercial marketing and by public health campaigns manifestly unequal.

The Forces Operating on the Diffusion Curve. Figure 45–8 illustrates how a variety of forces stimulate or retard the rate of growth of adopters in a population. These forces need to be taken into account in large-scale programs as advantages to be exploited or barriers to be overcome. Most of these may be seen as inevitable natural forces, but even those that cannot be changed might be hastened or delayed in their impact. The nature of the services offered or the design of the program might be modified strategically to accommodate the forces impinging on the diffusion process at various points in time.

At the very least, communication channels and health education messages need to be adapted to the forces operating variously at successive stages of large-scale programs. Recognizing that many of the forces pushing or inhibiting the diffusion and adoption process are not strictly cognitive or motivational,

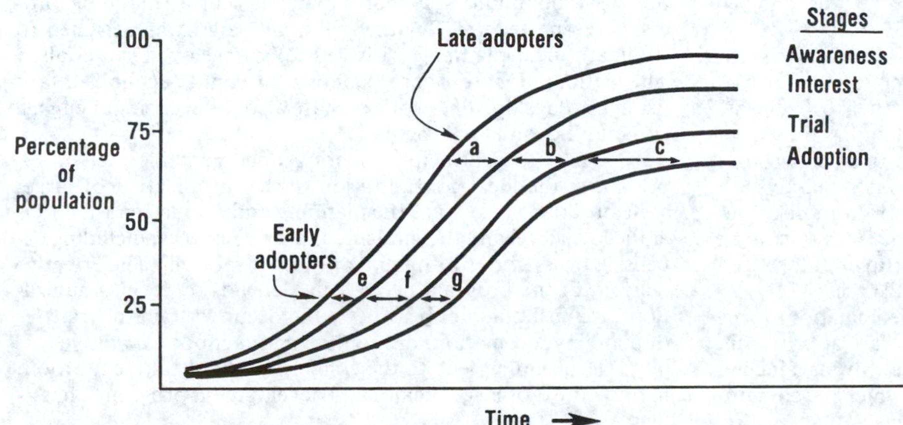

Figure 45–7. Differential time gaps between the stages of adoption for early adopters and late adopters. *[From Green L, McAlister A: Macro-intervention to support health behavior: Some theoretical perspectives and practical reflections. Health Educ Q 11[3]:323–339, 1984.]*

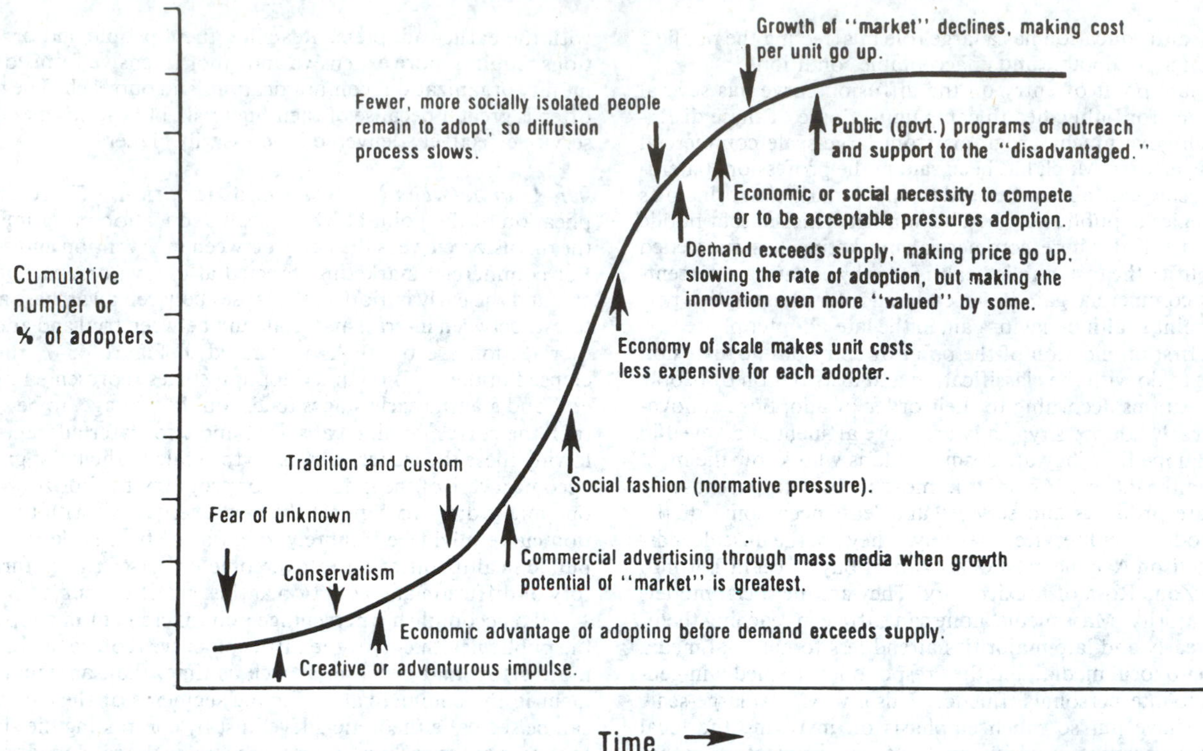

Figure 45–8. Examples of forces pushing the diffusion and adoption process up and those holding the process back at slower phases. *(From Green L, McAlister A: Macro-intervention to support health behavior: Some theoretical perspectives and practical reflections. Health Educ Q 11(3):323–339, 1984.)*

health promotion programs seek to mobilize organizational, economic, and environmental supports for the behavior advocated.

Examples of these strategies complementing the communications in the large-scale programs in the United States are the health styles, high blood pressure, and alcohol campaigns of recent years. Particular attention has been given to mobilization of community organizations and the channeling of communications through worksites and other settings where interpersonal influence could complement the formal communications of the media. The "Friends Can Be Good Medicine" campaign in California made the reduction of social isolation both a means and an end in itself. By encouraging the contact of people with their social support networks, the mental health goals of the program were served, and the diffusion process was facilitated.[66]

CENTRALIZATION vs DECENTRALIZATION

One thing that does not differ between large-scale and small-scale programs is the importance of the principle of participation. Involving people actively in identifying their own needs, setting their own priorities and goals, and planning their own programs of change applies equally at the individual, classroom, community, and national levels. The paradox for large-scale programs is that they require a degree of centralization of authority and responsibility almost by definition. Does this mean that large-scale programs should be avoided in favor of localized planning, implementation, and evaluation in all cases?

This policy question has stalemated implementation of the World Health Organization's primary health care approach in many countries where centralized planning is deeply ingrained in their systems. It also has limited the degree to which the community-based cardiovascular risk-reduction programs, such as those managed by the Stanford University and University of Minnesota research teams, have been able to achieve a truly community-based initiative and follow-through.

Decentralization has occurred most commonly in the implementation of large-scale programs, not in their planning or evaluation. This has given the concept of community participation a bad reputation in some circles as a form of exploitation, cooptation, or cheap labor for central agencies.

Asking communities and organizations to implement programs planned elsewhere and evaluated on someone else's terms might gain some followers, but usually with a limited commitment to the goals and methods of the programs. We have seen some of the national programs in the United States struggle with the problem in different ways. The National High Blood Pressure Education Program, for example, addressed it by convening numerous groups of representatives from far-flung organizations or communities to participate in central planning processes.[67] The federal Health Styles campaign was designed to stimulate local planning with centrally developed materials.[68] The National Institute for Alcohol Abuse and Alcoholism taps its highly developed network of state alcohol agencies to engage communities and local media.[69]

As a general principle, if not a documentable fact, it appears that the ideal configuration of decentralization of large-scale programs is to place the planning and evaluation functions at the local level and the implementation resources, including expensive productions of media, at the central level. The effective delivery of the program necessarily depends on local organizations, but it should not be expected to occur without the transfer of planning, evaluation, or monitoring functions as well.

All this might lead to the conclusion that health education, in the context of larger health and development programs, has as its primary function the arousal of individuals and communities to assess their own needs, set their own priorities, and to plan and evaluate their own programs.

SUMMARY

The mass media alone will not be effective unless organizational, economic, and environmental changes enable, and interpersonal communications reinforce, the behavioral change objectives. Systematic plans for organizing the community to support behavioral objectives need to be developed in coordination with the planned use of mass communication. The mass media can be powerful influences in society. In the complex process of social change for health promotion, however, the mass media represent only one of the numerous sectors that must be activated.

Theories of social psychology can be applied explicitly to enhance program effectiveness, but the same theories also lead to the conclusion that mass media are not likely to have much effect at the stage of diffusion in which these effects become public health issues unless they are reinforced and supported by families, peer groups, and other formal and informal community systems. Work with the mass media always must be coordinated with activities involving other important organizations and institutions.[70] Excessive dependence on mass media can be harmful to the social growth of individuals. In efforts to reach social objectives, overreliance on mass media similarly may retard the development of communities and of the less centralized systems of interpersonal communication and support that are needed for community self-reliance.

In the final analysis, it is not a question of how community forces can be mobilized in support of media or centralized objectives. It is a question of how the mass media can be used and supported by central agencies most appropriately and effectively in pursuit of community objectives. Large-scale programs still need to be seen as community-based programs. National and state objectives and resources still need to be adapted and tailored to communities and from there down to institutions, organizations, neighborhoods, families, and individuals.

REFERENCES

1. Green LW: Community Health, 6 edt. St. Louis: Mosby, 1990
2. Green LW, Kreuter MW, Deeds KB, Partridge KB: Health Education Planning: A Diagnostic Approach. Palo Alto, Calif.: Mayfield Publishing Co., 1980
3. Lewis FM: The concept of control: A typology and health-related variables. In Ward W (ed): Advances in Health Education and Promotion, Vol 2, Greenwich, Conn.: JAI Press, 1987
4. Kolbe LJ, Green LW, Foreyt J, et al: Appropriate functions of health education in schools. In Krasnagor N, Arasteh J, Cataldo M (eds): Child Health Behavior. New York: John Wiley, 1985
5. Healthy People: Surgeon General's Report on Health Promotion and Disease Prevention. Washington, D.C.: Government Printing Office, 1979
6. Green LW: Health education models. In Matarazzo JD et al (eds): Behavioral Health: A Handbook of Health Enhancement and Disease Prevention. New York: John Wiley, 1984
7. Marlatt GA: Cognitive assessment and intervention procedures for relapse prevention. In Marlatt GA, Gordon JR (eds): Relapse Prevention. New York: Guilford Press, 1985
8. Holli BB: Using behavior modification in nutrition counseling. J Am Diet Assoc 88:1530, 1988
9. Kirschenbaum DS: Self-regulatory failure: A review with clinical implications. Clin Psychol Rev 7:77–104, 1987
10. Rosenstock IM, Strecher VJ, Becker MH: Social learning theory and the health belief model. Health Educ Q 15:175–183, 1988
11. Kayman S: Applying theory from social psychology and cognitive behavioral psychology to dietary behavior change and assessment. J Am Diet Assoc 89:191–192, 1989
12. Mahoney MJ: Cognitive Behavior Modification. New York: Ballinger, 1977
13. Roter DL, Hall JA: Studies of doctor–patient interaction. Annu Rev Public Health 10:163–180, 1989
14. Faden RR: Ethical issues in government-sponsored public health campaigns. Health Educ Q 14:27–37, 1987
15. Green LW: The theory of participation: A qualitative analysis of its expression in national and international health policies. In Ward W (ed): Advances in Health Education and Promotion, Vol 1. Greenwich, Conn.: JAI Press, 1986
16. Green LW: Program Planning and Evaluation Guide for Lung Associations. New York: American Lung Association, 1987
17. Green LW, Raeburn J: Health promotion: What is it? What will it become? Health Promotion 3:151–159, 1988
18. Mullen PD: Health promotion and patient education benefits for employees. Annu Rev Public Health 9:305–332, 1988
19. Green LW, Heit P, Iverson D, et al: The school health curriculum project: Its theory, practice and measurement experience. Health Educ Q 17:14–34, 1980
20. Wikler D: Who should be blamed for being sick? Health Educ Q 14:11–25, 1987
21. Minkler M: Health education, health promotion and the open society: An historical perspective. Health Educ Q 16:17–30, 1989
22. Mayer JA, Dubbert PM, Elder JP: Promoting nutrition at the point of choice: A review. Health Educ Q 16:31–43, 1989
23. Flay BR: Social psychological approaches to smoking prevention: Review and recommendations. In Ward W (ed): Advances in Health Education and Promotion, Vol 2. Greenwich, Conn.: JAI Press, 1987
24. Green LW, Wilson AW, Lovato C: What changes can health promotion achieve and how long will these changes last? Prev Med 15:508–521, 1986
25. Green LW: The trade-offs between the expediency of health promotion and the durability of health education. In Maes S, et al (eds): Topics in Health Psychology. New York: John Wiley, 1988
26. Rodin J, Salovey P: Health psychology. Annu Rev Psychol 40:533–579, 1989
27. Steckler A, et al: Policy advocacy: Three emerging roles for health education. In Ward W (ed): Advances in Health Education and Promotion, Vol 2. Greenwich, Conn.: JAI Press, 1987
28. Best JA, Thompson SJ, Santi SM, et al: Preventing cigarette smoking among school children. Annu Rev Public Health 9:161–201, 1988
29. De Pietro R: A marketing research approach to health education planning. In Ward W, Simonds SK, Mullen PD, et al (eds): Advances in Health Education and Promotion. Greenwich, Conn.: JAI Press, 1987
30. Kotler P: Marketing for nonprofit organizations, 2 edt. Englewood Cliffs, NJ: Prentice-Hall, 1982
31. Manoff RK: Social Marketing: New Imperative for Public Health. New York: Praeger, 1985
32. Lefebvre RC, Flora JA: Social marketing and public health intervention. Health Educ Q 15:299–315, 1988
33. Green LW, Kreuter MW: Health Promotion Planning: An Educational and Environmental Approach. Palo Alto: Mayfield Publishing Co., 1991
34. Becker MH, Rosenstock IM: Comparing social learning theory and the health belief model. In Ward W (ed): Advances in Health Education and Promotion, Vol. 2. Greenwich, Conn.: JAI Press, 1987
35. Clark NM: Social learning theory in current health education practice. In Ward W (ed): Advances in Health Education and Promotion, Vol 2. Greenwich, CT: JAI Press, 1987
36. Israel BA, Rounds KA: Social networks and social support: A syn-

thesis for health educators. In Ward W (ed): Advances in Health Education and Promotion, Vol 2. Greenwich, Conn.: JAI Press, 1987
37. McAlister AL: The development and prevention of substance abuse: An introduction to research and policy. In Coates TJ, Peterson AC, Perry C (eds): Promoting Adolescent Health: A Dialog on Research and Practice. New York: Academic, 1982
38. Cohen RY, Felix MRJ, Brownell KD: The role of parents and older peers in school-based cardiovascular prevention programs: Implications for program development. Health Educ Q 16:245–253, 1989
39. Devine EC, Cook TD: A meta-analytic analysis of effects of psychoeducational interventions on length of postsurgical hospital stay. Nurs Res 32:267–274, 1983
40. Mullen PD, Green LW, Persinger G: Clinical trials of patient education for chronic conditions: A comparative meta-analysis of intervention types. Prev Med 14:753–781, 1985
41. Kottke TE, Battista RN, DeFriese G, et al: Attributes of successful smoking cessation interventions in medical practice. JAMA 259:2883–2889, 1988
42. Vickery DM, Kalmer H, Lowry D, et al: Effect of self-care education program on medical visits. JAMA 250:2952–2956, 1983
43. Lewis CE: Disease prevention and health promotion practices of primary care physicians in the United States. In Battista RN, Lawrence RS (eds): Implementing Preventive Services. New York: Oxford University Press, for Am J Prev Med 4(4)(suppl), 1987
44. Green LW: Some challenges to health services research on children and the elderly. Health Serv Res 19:793–815, 1985
45. Hatcher ME, Green LW, Levine DM, et al: Validation of a decision model for triaging hypertensive patients to alternate health education interventions. Soc Sci Med 22:813–819, 1986
46. Kernaghan SG, Giloth BE: Tracking the impact of health promotion on organizations: A key to program survival. Chicago: American Hospital Association, 1988
47. Green LW: Toward cost-benefit evaluations of health education: Some concepts, methods and examples. Health Educ Monogr 2(suppl):34–64, 1974
48. Mullen PD, Zapka JG: Assessing the quality of health promotion and patient education programs. HMO Pract 3:98–103, 1989
49. Green LW: What physicians can do to increase participation and maintenance of patients in self-care. West J Med 147:346–349, 1987
50. Janz NK, Becker MH: The health belief model: A decade later. Health Educ Q 11:1–47, 1984
51. Eriksen MP: The role of organizations in cancer prevention: Communities, worksites, schools, and hospitals. Cancer Bull 40:349–354, 1988
52. Fingerhut LA, Kleinman JC: Mortality among children and youth. Am J Public Health 79:899–901, 1989
53. Kolbe LJ: Indicators for planning and monitoring school health programs. In Kar SB (ed): Health Promotion Indicators and Actions. New York: Springer, 1989
54. Green LW: Bridging the gap between community health and school health. Am J Public Health 78:1149, 1988
55. Rundall TG, Bruvold WH: A meta-analysis of school-based smoking and alcohol use prevention programs. Health Educ Q 15:317–334, 1988
56. Kolbe LJ: What can we expect from school health education? J Sch Health 52:145–150, 1982
57. Kolbe LJ, Green LW, Foreyt J, et al: Appropriate functions of health education in schools. In Krasnagor N, Arasteh J, Cataldo M (eds): Child Health Behavior. New York: John Wiley, 1985
58. Perry CL (ed): Special issue on community programs for drug abuse prevention. J Sch Health 56:357–418, 1986
59. Green LW, Simons-Morton D: Education and life-style determinants of health and disease. In Holland WW, Detels R, Knox G (eds): Oxford Textbook of Public Health, 2 edt. London: Oxford University Press, 1991
60. World Health Organization: Expert Committee on Health Education of the Public. Geneva: WHO Tech Rep Series No 89, 1954
61. Green LW: Theory of participation: A qualitative analysis of its expression in national and international policies. In Ward W (ed): Advances in Health Education and Promotion, Vol 1. Greenwich, Conn.: JAI Press, 1986
62. Green LW: Research agenda: Building a consensus on research questions. Am J Health Promotion 1:70–72, 1986
63. Nyswander D: Education for health: Some principles and their application. Calif Health 14:65–70, 1956
64. Green LW, Raeburn J: Health promotion: What is it? What will it become? Health Promotion 3:151–159, 1988
65. Green LW, Gottlieb NH, Parcel GS: Diffusion theory extended and applied. In Ward W (ed): Advances in Health Education and Promotion, Vol 3. Greenwich, Conn.: JAI Press, 1989
66. Hersey JC, Kilbanoff LS, Lam DJ, Taylor RL: Promoting social support: The impact of California's "Friends Can be Good Medicine" campaign. Health Educ Q 11:293–311, 1984
67. Roccella EJ, Ward GW: The national high blood pressure education program: A description of its utility as a generic program model. Health Educ Q 11:225–242, 1984
68. Davis M, Iverson D: An overview and analysis of the Health Styles campaign. Health Educ Q 11:253–272, 1984
69. Maloney SK, Hersey JC: Getting messages on the air: Findings from the 1982 Alcohol Abuse Prevention Campaign. Health Educ Q 11:273–292, 1984
70. Flora JA, Maibach EW, Maccoby N: The role of media across four levels of health promotion intervention. Annu Rev Public Health 10:181–201, 1989

SECTION FIVE

Noncommunicable and Chronic Disabling Conditions

Edited by Elizabeth Barrett-Connor

46
Prevention of Chronic Illness

Robert B. Wallace
George D. Everett

Modern preventive practice not only removes barriers to good health but also positively promotes health. Prevention should be practiced by everyone in every setting: home, school, workplace, health care institutions, and recreational sites. The term *prevention* has varied connotations. It may indicate public policy, a philosophy, clinical or administrative skills, a research orientation, or public or personal care programs. This chapter considers the natural history and occurrence of chronic illness in populations and introduces the concepts of disease screening and the elements of sound preventive programs. The prevention of specific conditions of public health import are then considered in the remaining chapters of this section.

NATURAL HISTORY

Generalizations about chronic illnesses and their natural histories do not come easily. There are many gaps in knowledge of causes, pathogenesis, physiological and functional impact, and clinical trajectories, making understanding and development of preventive strategies complex and challenging. Several examples of inadequate knowledge of diseases and conditions that deters preventive strategies exist.

Some "chronic" illnesses are due to either infections directly, such as AIDS, or to the sequelae of infections, such as hearing loss after measles or influenza. Thus, as more chronic conditions are identified as having infectious causes, their prevention may employ methods commonly considered only for infectious agents.

Diseases such as atherosclerosis often have origins in childhood or young adulthood; thus, managing of risk factors in the clinically asymptomatic middle-aged adult may actually be *secondary,* not primary, prevention. This may also be true of certain cancers in which the pathogenic processes begin early, even when clinical disease is late. For example, breast cancer risk is related to age-at-menarche, although it is generally a disease of older women. One general implication is that preventive interventions labeled as primary but which are really secondary may be worthwhile maintaining even after the onset of overt clinical illness.

Conventional notions of chronic disease do not usually consider age-related physiological and anatomical changes with substantial health and functional perturbations. For example, age-related loss of muscle or brain cells may lead to important clinical problems, yet don't fit into conventional disease classifications. Giving disease names to such anatomical decrements and their functional consequences does not improve knowledge. However, it is possible that some portion of these decrements are preventable, as well as subject to rehabilitation, and these "conditions," whose progression is not necessarily inevitable, should be so evaluated.

A similar situation that has not been adequately studied involves the groups of symptoms and syndromes that affect health but are often not formalized as diseases. Examples include pain syndromes such as low back pain, itching and dry skin, and memory changes with age. In many instances these are poorly understood despite their health impact, and hence little attention is paid to prevention.

Diseases and conditions cluster in individuals for several reasons, including the multiple diseases caused by single exposures (e.g., tobacco) and the multiple organ abnormalities associated with single conditions (e.g., hypertension). These may be further combined with the multiple functional decrements of aging, so-called comorbidity.[1] Having multiple conditions and dysfunctions, with their various medical therapies, may change the natural history of each. For example, some antihypertensive medications may alter blood lipid levels in a manner favorable to atherogenesis. The altered natural history of comorbid conditions needs considerable study, with an emphasis on the value of preventive interventions. One consequence of prevention of multiple conditions is the need for integrating multiple risk factor interventions.[2]

OCCURRENCE

Central to preventive practice and policy is the definition of health and disease. Although no universally accepted definitions exist, they must be clearly specified operationally for measurement of population health status. As noted in the section above, most welcome are definitions that go beyond death and anatomical disruption to include clinical signs and symptoms, functional status and capacity, the nature of the physical and social environment, subjective well-being, and risk status. Using this framework, the occurrence and burden of chronic illness can be more fully understood and approached.

TABLE 46–1. DEATH RATES (PER 100,000) FOR LEADING CAUSES OF DEATH, UNITED STATES (1900 AND 1987)

1900				1987			
Rank and Cause of Death	***Rate***	***(%)***		***Rank and Cause of Death***	***Rate***	***(%)***	
1. Pneumonia and influenza	202.2	11.8		1. Diseases of the heart	312.4	35.8	
2. Tuberculosis (all forms)	194.4	11.3		2. Malignant neoplasms (cancer)	195.9	22.5	
3. Diarrhea, enteritis, ulceration of intestine	142.7	8.3		3. Cerebrovascular accidents	61.6	7.1	
4. Diseases of the heart	137.4	8.0		4. Accidents and adverse effects	39.0	4.5	
5. Intracranial lesions of vascular origin	106.9	6.2		5. Chronic obstructive pulmonary disease	32.2	3.7	
6. Nephritis	81.0	4.7		6. Pneumonia/influenza	28.4	3.3	
7. All accidents	72.3	4.2		7. Diabetes mellitus	15.8	1.8	
8. Malignant neoplasms (cancer)	64.0	3.7		8. Suicide	12.7	1.5	
9. Certain diseases of early infancy	62.2	3.6		9. Chronic liver disease	10.8	1.2	
10. Diphtheria	40.3	2.3		10. Atherosclerosis	9.2	1.1	

From National Center for Health Statistics: Monthly Vital Statistics Report 38(5).

Characterizing health and disease is also related to issues of taxonomy and nomenclature. While not reviewed here, those taxonomies that employ multidimensional descriptors, such as etiology, anatomy, physiology, functional impact, and prognosis, will provide a fuller understanding of the natural history, impact, and preventability. The following is a review of some approaches to ascertaining the occurrence of chronic disease in populations.

Mortality. Throughout the twentieth century there has been a marked decline in mortality rates in Western countries, particularly for infants and children but more recently for middle-aged adults and older persons as well. With this has been a dramatic shift in the distribution of causes of death from infections to cardiovascular diseases and cancers, with the persisting role of trauma. The leading causes of death in 1900 and 1987 in the United States are shown in Table 46–1. This transition reflects in part great strides in infection control, the emergence of chronic conditions associated with increased longevity, and improved surveillance and diagnosis of chronic diseases. However, as noted above, it is still possible that some "chronic" illnesses have infectious causes.

Chronic disease mortality in populations has been expressed in ways other than ranks or rates, such as years of life lost in a standard population prior to age 65 years. With such a representation, accidents, cancer, and suicides become relatively prominent. However, it has been argued that this method ignores ages over 65 years, where most chronic conditions and deaths occur and where many useful years of life still exist. Although mortality rates tell us about the occurrence and something of the causes of death, they often tell us little about the natural history of health, morbidity, dysfunction, and health services consumption during life, even when considering all information available on death certificates. Thus, other methods are obviously indicated.

Morbidity. Another approach to characterizing chronic illness in populations is to determine the rates for various discrete diseases, conditions, and syndromes. Unlike mortality data, morbidity surveys are often not available for many geographical areas. For the United States, the most complete data come from the surveys by the National Center for Health Statistics. An example from the ongoing Health Interview Survey is shown in Table 46–2 for skin and musculoskeletal conditions. Such findings could rarely be derived from death certificates, and while in some ways they more accurately reflect population health status for preventive considerations, there are shortcomings. For example, such rates depend in part on access to medical care and appropriate diagnostic labeling. Of themselves, they do not reflect disease severity, functional impact on the patient or rate of progression, and often neglect related mental and social issues. Symptoms and ill-defined clinical syndromes are usually underrepresented. Also, patterns of comorbidity are often not presented or even conceptualized.

Functional Status. To obviate some of these problems in presenting health status as morbidity alone, community surveys are now more frequently measuring health and disease in terms of the ability to perform basic physical and social functions.[3] An example of the population rates for requiring assistance with basic physical activities is shown in Table 46–3. Function status measures may be reported by survey respondents or proxies or may be directly measured by testing procedures. Thus, there are now population distributions available for physiological measures such as pulmonary function, blood hormone levels, grip strength, and cognitive testing. These data enhance the ability to assess preventive activities aimed at minimizing dysfunction and serve to summarize the cumulative impact of multiple conditions on the individual. While there are methodological issues related to the accuracy and interpretation of these variables and surveys tend to focus on the lower range of function, these data are critical for evaluating health maintenance and promotion programs.

Other Measures. Several additional approaches have been used in population surveys to enhance information available for preventive purposes. More work is being done in community sur-

TABLE 46–2. PREVALENCE OF SELECTED CHRONIC SKIN AND MUSCULOSKELETAL CONDITIONS REPORTED IN THE HEALTH INTERVIEW SURVEY, UNITED STATES (1988)

Chronic Condition	Prevalence per 1000 Persons
Skin	
Sebaceous skin cyst	6.1
Trouble with acne	18.8
Dermatitis	37.5
Trouble with dry (itching) skin	19.9
Musculoskeletal System	
Arthritis	129.9
Bone spur or tendonitis	10.2
Trouble with bunions	10.9
Trouble with corns and calluses	18.8

From National Center for Health Statistics: Vital and Health Statistics, Series 10, No. 173.

TABLE 46-3. AGE-STANDARDIZED HEALTH STATUS MEASURES, UNITED STATES (1988)

▪ Restricted Activity due to Acute and Chronic Conditions (per person per year)	
All restricted-activity days	14.4
Bed days	6.2
Work-loss days[a]	5.3
School-loss days[b]	4.9
▪ Limitation in Activity due to Chronic Conditions (percent of persons)	
All persons limited in activity	13.4
Persons limited in major activity	9.3
▪ Respondent-assessed Health Status (percent distribution)	
All health statuses[c]	100.0
Excellent	39.5
Very Good	27.8
Good	23.0
Fair	7.1
Poor	2.6

[a] For currently employed persons 18 years of age and older.
[b] For youths 5 to 17 years of age.
[c] Excludes a small number with unknown health status.
NOTE: Detailed tables show the 1988 estimates by age, sex, race, family income, geographic region, and place of residence.

veillance for mental illness, and "quality-of-life" measures are receiving more prominence.[4] Regular surveys of population hygienic behaviors and risk factor status, proximate to many chronic illnesses, are now routinely conducted. There is still considerable room for research on improved health status measures and related survey methods.

SCREENING FOR EARLY AND ASYMPTOMATIC CONDITIONS

One major activity in the prevention armamentarium is screening. The purpose of screening is to detect individuals with risk factors that predispose to disease development or with asymptomatic (latent) diseases that can be effectively treated. In general, screening is applied to a population of individuals with a low probability of the factors or diseases in question relative to individuals with symptoms of the condition.

There are several criteria that aid in selecting and applying an appropriate screening test.[5] (1) The disease should be common enough to warrant a search for its risk factors or latent stages because screening for excessively rare diseases may result in unacceptable cost-benefit ratios. (2) The morbidity or mortality of the untreated condition must be substantial. (3) An effective therapy must exist and should be more beneficial when applied to the presymptomatic rather than to the symptomatic stage. (4) The screening test should be acceptable to the population and suitable for routine application.

Even with rigid application of these screening criteria, major pitfalls may cause an erroneous assessment of a screening program's value. An example is *lead time,* the interval between presymptomatic disease detection by a screening test and symptom onset. If the natural history of a disease is variable or not thoroughly understood during the presymptomatic and symptomatic stages, a screening test may identify a presymptomatic condition earlier and increase the interval to overt morbidity but not change the ultimate outcome. *Length bias* occurs when there is a correlation between the duration of disease latency and the natural history of the symptomatic phase. If the mild form of a disease has a longer latency and is hence more easily found on screening than are more severe forms of disease, the screening test may appear falsely beneficial. These pitfalls can be fully resolved only through controlled trials of a screening procedure with long-term follow-up, as in the 18-year follow-up of the Health Insurance Plan clinical trial of mammography for detecting breast cancer.[6]

Selection and interpretation of screening tests require a combination of subjective and objective criteria. Objective criteria include operating characteristics, predictive value, and cost-effectiveness of the tests, which are tempered by subjective evaluations of individual and public acceptability and financing.

The operating characteristics of a test are its sensitivity and specificity. These characteristics apply to laboratory test data as well as other information collected from the medical history and physical examination. *Sensitivity* is the proportional detection of individuals with the disease of interest in the tested population, expressed as follows:

$$\text{Sensitivity (\%)} = \frac{\text{True positives}}{\text{True positives} + \text{False negatives}} \times 100$$

True positives are individuals with the disease and whose test result is positive. False negatives are individuals whose test result is negative despite having the disease. *Specificity* is the proportional detection of individuals without the disease of interest, expressed as follows:

$$\text{Specificity (\%)} = \frac{\text{True negatives}}{\text{True negatives} + \text{False positives}} \times 100$$

True negatives are individuals without the disease and whose test result is negative. False positives have a positive test result but do not have the disease. Sensitivity is limited by the proportion of cases missed by the test (false negatives) and specificity is limited by the proportion of noncases found to be positive (false positives). Ideally, a test would have a 100% sensitivity and specificity. No test has yet achieved this. Unfortunately, sensitivity and specificity are often inversely related. This relationship has been expressed as the receiver operating characteristic (ROC)[7] of a numerically continuous test result. The ROC allows optimal specification of test sensitivity and specificity, as shown in Figure 46–1. The sensitivity, or true-positive ratio, is displayed along the ordinate, and the specificity, or false-positive ratio, is exhibited on the abscissa. As the sensitivity increases, so does the false-positive ratio in most instances. When a ROC has been established for a test, any one of several sensitivity and specificity combinations may be evaluated for suitability in test application and contrasted with potential alternate tests.

Sensitivity and specificity values from the literature are most applicable to populations and test conditions similar to those under which the values were established. Further generalization or extrapolation of these values can be misleading.

Whereas the operating characteristics of a test are of major help in selecting a screening test, the predictive value of a test is a major aid in interpretation of a result. The *predictive value* of a *positive test* is the proportion of all individuals with positive tests who have the disease and is expressed as follows:

$$\text{Positive predictive value (\%)} = \frac{\text{True positives}}{\text{True positives} + \text{False positives}} \times 100$$

The predictive value of a negative test is the proportion of all individuals with negative tests who are nondiseased. This is expressed as follows:

$$\text{Negative predictive value (\%)} = \frac{\text{True negatives}}{\text{True negatives} + \text{False negatives}} \times 100$$

Predictive values are dependent on both the operating characteristics and the prevalence of the disease in the target population.

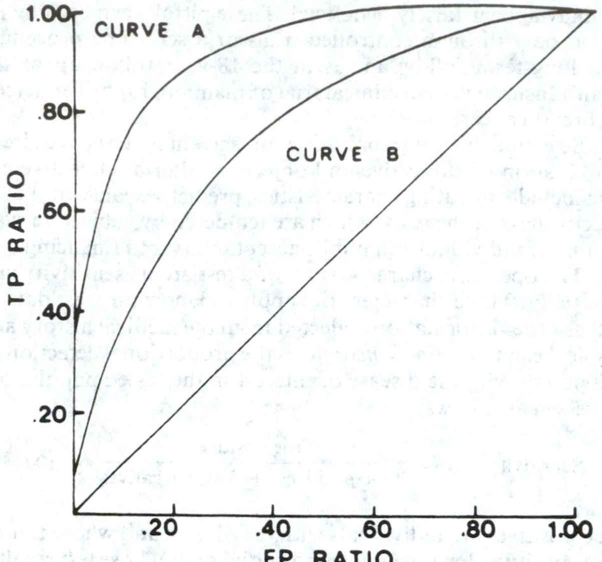

Figure 46-1. Hypothetical receiver operating characteristic (ROC) curve. The ordinate is the true-positive ratio and the abscissa is the false-positive ratio. Curve A demonstrates a greater true-positive ratio at all points along the abscissa than does curve B. For each point along curves A and B, the false-positive increases directly with the true-positive ratio. *(From Radiology 123:614, 1977, with permission.)*

For any given set of operating characteristics, the positive predictive value is directly related to prevalence, and the negative predictive value is inversely related to prevalence. Therefore, in screening situations where the prevalence is relatively low, the operating characteristics must be very high to avoid low positive predictive values. In most screening situations for serious fatal conditions, such as cancer, the test or test sequence offering the highest sensitivity ordinarily will be preferred. This has the effect of finding as many cases as possible but may correspondingly increase the number of false positives. The effect of sensitivity, specificity, and prevalence on predictive values has been demonstrated.[8]

Cost-effectiveness is especially important in screening programs because of the number of asymptomatic individuals who must be evaluated for the relatively small number of diseased cases. Formal cost-effectiveness analysis[9] should be undertaken before program initiation. The program's value must include an assessment of all costs and a realistic appraisal of effectiveness. Positive predictive values are usually well below 50% for most initial screening situations, so that secondary diagnostic evaluation is nearly always required to eliminate false positives, adding substantially to program cost. The exhaustive review of screening programs undertaken by the Canadian Task Force[10,11] includes recommendations weighted in part by consideration of cost-effectiveness.

Public screening, or mass screening, has inherent advantages from the standpoint of efficiency. The tests and procedures can be standardized and administered more cheaply than they can in other settings, generally without the need for direct physician supervision. For instance, in a large study evaluating breast cancer screening, the cost of the mammograms was clearly lower than what would be achievable in the individual clinical setting. To enjoy the efficiency of mass screening, such programs must be carefully organized and managed. Recipients of both normal and abnormal test results must be considered. Those with abnormal test results must have a properly organized follow-up evaluation protocol, and those with normal results should be informed of the predictive value of a normal test to avoid false reassurance. Even with the inherent efficiency of mass screening, most such programs must still be focused on high-risk populations to maximize program utility.

Screening programs may not be applied only to large asymptomatic populations but also should be applied in a clinical context, with screening performed on healthy subjects or those with unrelated medical problems. Comprehensive clinical screening with routine physical examinations or laboratory tests, or both, remains controversial, but several sound categorical screening and prevention programs have been proposed.[10-13] In the past, screening recommendations have been proposed for people being admitted to the hospital; these recommendations heavily emphasized multiphase laboratory tests. It now appears that these procedures have limited utility and high cost primarily because of numerous false-positive tests and irrelevant findings and should be discarded in favor of diagnostic and therapeutic activities directed at the clinical problems.[14-16]

GUIDELINES FOR EFFECTIVE PREVENTIVE PROGRAMS

Even with sufficient community survey information and program planning, additional guidelines exist that should help produce effective prevention programs. The following are not exhaustive but represent minimum guidelines:

1. *Programs must be based on scientific evidence.* Preventive programs must be based on adequate scientific evidence of their efficacy. Randomized trials should be conducted whenever possible to prove their worth, applying the same rigorous criteria that are used to determine clinical practices. For example, randomized community trials have been performed for vaccine evaluation and breast cancer screening but never for cytological screening of uterine cervical cancer. Such trials may be expensive but not in relation to the potential waste of inadequately tested interventions. Preventive programs often compete financially with personal care provision, non-health-related public programs, and even other preventive programs. In the long term, only proven programs will be maintained as competing priorities arise. Periodic redocumentation of program efficacy seems essential, including the adverse effects of such programs and their impact on health and illness rates other than those for which programs are targeted. Because many preventive practices have important economic consequences, their ultimate defense may be their scientific validity, and recent reviews of preventive maneuvers emphasize this.[10,17]

2. *Prevention programs should be supported by effective data systems.* Effective prevention often requires accurate determination of who has and who has not received a certain preventive service within a defined population. This promotes efficient planning, organization, administration, and evaluation. Most important, it allows resource allocation toward those most in need. Appropriate systems for maintaining these data can be useful in community-based programs but have special application in promoting preventive activities within clinical practice. Especially now with the use of automated systems, one can document demographic profiles and other indicators of high risk, maintain disease registers, monitor the receipt of preventive services, and facilitate merging these services with ongoing clinical activities. Requirements for a preventive medicine record system have been suggested.[18]

3. *Programs should be flexible.* As with all programs aimed at large numbers of people, there should be suitable administrative flexibility to reach as many people as possible. This may be reflected by variation in location of programs, hours, language of application, simplicity of instructions, mode of program pro-

vision, programmatic goals, and target population factors. Tailoring of programs to the needs, attitudes, and circumstances of potential recipients should enhance program success. Flexibility in amalgamating a preventive program with other clinical or community activities may improve acceptance and decrease costs, even if its individual identity is submerged. Public and individual acceptance is crucial to a particular program's success and also to the success of future programs.

4. *Programs must be sensitive to ethical issues.* There are several ethical dimensions to be considered in the design and conduct of preventive programs (see Chapter 75). The ethical issues of research in prevention are mainly those common to all human research. Community research, however, may entail acquiring personal information without consent, which requires considerable special care in data handling.

There are issues of ethics and values in presenting preventive recommendations to the public. Historically, many hygienic recommendations and reforms have been related to various moral or religious movements.[19] Some recommendations may inadvertently take on a moralistic or sermonizing tone not appreciated by all. Recommended practices may be contrary to some values or may seem overly paternalistic. Recommendations for public behavior raise issues of personal autonomy vs the common good. Life-style admonitions may sometimes imply that society is absolved of preventive responsibilities and that the onus of disease occurrence disproportionately lies with the individual, a process called "blaming the victim."[20] In some instances, health promotion may serve as a superficial banner for underlying political or entrepreneurial goals.

There are ethical issues relevant to the professional provision of personal preventive services. Any untoward risks of preventive maneuvers should be explained in advance, and iatrogenic problems clearly documented. In particular, screening programs offer special ethical concerns. A program may confer a false sense of security following a negative result. A positive screening result may unnecessarily stigmatize an individual, a process known as labeling. The social and emotional impact of either a negative or a positive test on a screenee should always be considered.

5. *Programs should be targeted to the recipients most in need.* Because preventive programs are generally costly, their untoward effects either are not entirely known or require minimization, and their impact on different risk groups is varied: some programs should be targeted to those persons who will derive the most benefit. Such targeting may be done on the basis of demographic, geographical, occupational, or other features indicating increased or excessive risk of a disease or condition. Sometimes identification of high-risk groups is difficult, but epidemiological data can often assist in pointing to those most vulnerable. On occasion, some family or population groups may be targeted solely because of previously elevated disease rates or prior incident conditions, since there is evidence that such events cluster.[21]

6. *Programs should muster a variety of community resources.* In general, there are many community resources available to assist in the design and provision of preventive programs. Involving a wide variety of public and private, voluntary and official, and professional and nonprofessional groups may not only improve program acceptance but also may avoid active or passive opposition from groups perceiving a political, social, or economic threat from the program.

7. *Effective prevention requires legislative action and social policy decisions.* Those promoting prevention must participate in the formulation of policy at the social, organizational, and legislative levels. Within the health care system, policy must dictate a structure that funds and provides preventive services. At the legislative level, there should be adequate provision for prevention research, services, and professional training. Many general legislative programs have direct or indirect preventive implications, such as environmental control, housing, road construction, or education. Governmental policy toward income equalization and military expenditure may have the most fundamental preventive implications for all. For those promoting preventive policies, the most difficult issue may be assigning priorities to the various programs in times of restricted resources.

8. *Programs should be continuous.* Most preventive programs of value must be conducted on a continuous basis. Freedom from a disease after a screening procedure usually does not mean that the condition will not arise in the future. Education programs should provide periodic reinforcement, as personal preventive behaviors may not always persist. Programs will be more effective as they become institutionalized into clinical or public health practice. When appropriate, however, certain programs should be curtailed or eliminated when no longer needed, such as when an infectious agent has been eradicated.

There are still many unanswered questions in prevention and many problems in search of valid solutions. Issues remain even when preventive practices seem firmly established. For example, how much of an intervention or behavior is optimal, both for an individual and for the community? What is the synergy of a preventive practice with other preventive activities? What is the net effect of the preventive practice on morbidity and mortality? Preventive practice should be continuously modernized to incorporate new findings in biology, clinical medicine, behavioral science, and public health. The remaining chapters in this section provide the scientific basis and practical recommendations for prevention of major chronic conditions in Western society.

REFERENCES

1. Guralnik JM, LaCroix AZ, Everett DF, Kovar MG: Aging in the eighties: The prevalence of comorbidity and its association with disability. Advanced Data from Vital and Health Statistics, No. 170. Hyattsville, Maryland: National Center for Health Statistics, 1989
2. Office of Disease Prevention and Health Promotion: Integration of risk factor intervention. U.S. Department of Health and Human Services, Public Health Service, November, 1986
3. Fillenbaum G: Assessment of health and functional status: An international comparison. In Kane RL, Evans JG, MacFadyen D (eds): Improving the Health of Older People: A World View. Oxford: Oxford University Press, 1990
4. See entire edition of J Chronic Dis 40(6), 1987
5. Wilson JMG, Jungner G: Principles and practice of screening for disease. Pub Health Pap No. 34. Geneva: WHO, 1968
6. Chu KC, Smart CR, Tarone RE: Analysis of breast cancer mortality and stage distribution by age for the Health Insurance Plan clinical trial. J Natl Cancer Inst 80:1125–1132, 1988
7. Greiner PF, Mayewski RJ, Mushlin AI, Greenland P: Selection and interpretation of diagnostic tests and procedures. Ann Intern Med 94(2):553, 1981
8. Galen RS, Gambino SR: Beyond Normality: The Predictive Value and Efficiency of Medical Diagnosis. New York: John Wiley, 1975
9. Weinstein MC, Stason WB: Foundations of cost-effectiveness analysis for health and medical practices. N Engl J Med 296:716, 1977
10. Canadian Task Force on the Periodic Health Examination: The periodic health examination. Can Med Assoc J 121:1193, 1979
11. Canadian Task Force on the Periodic Health Examination: The periodic health examination: 2. 1984 Update. Can Med Assoc J 130: 1278–1285, 1984
12. Breslow L, Somers AR: The lifetime health monitoring program: A practical approach to preventive medicine. N Engl J Med 296:601, 1977
13. Medical Practice Committee, American College of Physicians: Periodic health examination: A guide for designing individualized pre-

ventive health care in the asymptomatic patient. Ann Intern Med 95:729, 1981

14. Whitehead TP, Wotton IDP: Biochemical profiles for hospital patients. Lancet 2:1439, 1974
15. Korvin CC, Pearce RH, Stanley J: Admissions screening: Clinical benefits. Ann Intern Med 83:197, 1975
16. Burbridge TC, Edwards F, Edwards RG, Atkinson M: Evaluation of benefits of screening tests done immediately on admission to hospital. Clin Chem 22:968, 1976
17. U.S. Preventive Services Task Force: Guide to Clinical Preventive Services: An Assessment of the Effectiveness of 169 Interventions. Baltimore: Williams & Wilkins, 1989
18. Gray M, Fowler GH: Preventive Medicine in General Practice. Oxford: Oxford University Press, 1983
19. Whorton JC: Crusaders for Fitness—A History of American Health Reformers. Princeton, New Jersey: Princeton University Press, 1982
20. Ryan W: Blaming the Victim. New York: Vintage Books, 1971
21. Starfield B, Katz H, Gabriel A, et al: Morbidity in childhood—A longitudinal view. N Engl J Med 310:824, 1984

47
Cancer

David B. Thomas

Neoplasms are diseases characterized by abnormal proliferation of cells. If the proliferating cells do not invade surrounding tissues, the resultant tumor is benign; if they do invade, the tumor is malignant. Some benign neoplasms may be fatal, for example, histologically benign brain tumors that grow and displace normal brain tissue in the confined space of the skull and hepatocellular adenomas that rupture and cause bleeding into the peritoneal cavity. Some benign tumors such as intestinal polyps have a malignant potential. The term *cancer* usually implies a malignant tumor (malignancy) but refers also to brain tumors and some other benign neoplasms.

DESCRIPTIVE EPIDEMIOLOGY

Classification. Cancers are classified according to their organ or tissue of origin (site or topography code) and histological features (morphology code). A number of classification schemes have been developed, the most recent and widely used of which appears in Chapter 2 of the International Classification of Diseases, Tenth Revision (ICD-10), which is largely a topography code,[1] and the International Classification of Diseases for Oncology (ICD-O), which contains an expanded version of the topography code in ICD-10 as well as a detailed morphology code.[2]

SOURCES OF INCIDENCE AND MORTALITY RATES

Mortality rates are calculated from death certificate records and population census data. Mortality rates from various countries have been compiled periodically.[3] Cancer mortality rates for the United States are published by the National Cancer Institute (NCI).[4–6]

Population-based tumor registries, which have been established in many countries, provide information on incidence rates. These have been compiled in "Cancer in Five Continents,"[7] which is published periodically by the International Agency for Research on Cancer (IARC). The best source of cancer incidence rates for the United States is the Surveillance, Epidemiology, and End Results (SEER) program of the NCI, which supports a network of 10 population-based cancer registries throughout the country. Results from this program have been published by the NCI.[4,6] Both incidence and mortality statistics for the United States are summarized for the lay public and published annually by the American Cancer Society.[8]

Magnitude of the Cancer Problem. In the aggregate, cancer is second only to heart disease as a cause of death in the United States and accounts for about 22% of all deaths. Approximately 170 deaths from cancer occur per 100,000 people per year, compared to about 261 per 100,000 from heart disease, 51 per 100,000 from stroke, and 36 per 100,000 from accidents.[9] Based on U.S. mortality and incidence rates for 1973 to 1977, the lifetime probabilities of developing and dying from cancer have been estimated to be 30.8% and 15.1% respectively.[4] In economic terms, cancer is by far the most important health problem in the United States.[10]

Relative Importance of Specific Neoplasms. Age-adjusted incidence, mortality, and 5-year survival rates in men and women in the United States are shown in Table 47–1.[6] The five most common cancers in men are those of the lung, prostate, colon, bladder, and rectum; and the five cancers causing the most deaths per capita are those of the lung, prostate, colon, pancreas, and stomach. In women, breast cancer is by far the most common neoplasm, followed by cancers of the lung, colon, corpus uteri, and ovary. However, because the relative survival of women with breast cancer is higher than that of women with lung cancer, lung cancer and breast cancer are equally important causes of death; and mortality rates of lung cancer have actually exceeded those for breast cancer in recent years in many parts of the United States. The other cancers that are among the most important causes of death in American women are those of the colon, pancreas, and ovary.

Another way to judge the importance of a malignancy is by the number of years of life lost due to its occurrence in a population. This measure reflects the incidence of the cancer, the fatality rate in those who develop it, and the age at which the cancer tends to occur. This measure gives more weight to childhood cancers than mortality rates, and because of its economic implications, it can be of value in setting priorities for research and prevention. In order of estimated years of life lost, the 10 most important cancers in the United States are those of the lung, breast, colon and rectum, blood (leukemia), pancreas, lymphoid tissue (non-Hodgkin's lymphoma), prostate, brain, ovary, and stomach.[11]

TABLE 47-1. AVERAGE ANNUAL AGE-ADJUSTED (1970 STANDARD) INCIDENCE AND MORTALITY RATES (1982–1986) AND 5-YEAR RELATIVE SURVIVAL RATES (1980–1985 CASES) BY PRIMARY SITE AND SEX, ALL RACES, ALL SEER AREAS COMBINED (EXCEPT PUERTO RICO AND NEW JERSEY)

	Rates (per 100,000)				5-Year Relative Survival (%)	
	Incidence		Mortality			
Site	Male	Female	Male	Female	Male	Female
Buccal cavity and pharynx	17.2	6.6	5.2	2.0	49.7	54.4
Digestive system	99.3	65.9	55.0	34.3	35.9	40.5
Colon	42.0	32.4	20.5	15.0	54.7	54.8
Rectum and rectosigmoid	18.8	11.4	4.0	2.3	50.3	53.9
Pancreas	11.2	8.3	10.3	7.6	2.8	3.1
Stomach	12.3	5.5	8.4	3.8	15.5	19.1
Esophagus	6.1	1.9	5.5	1.6	6.6	9.3
Respiratory system	95.2	36.9	69.3	26.0	17.1	18.5
Lung and bronchus	84.2	34.4	66.1	25.2	11.6	15.5
Larynx	8.5	1.6	2.4	0.5	66.5	66.4
Bones and joints	1.0	0.7	0.6	0.3	48.5	55.8
Soft tissues (incuding heart)	2.5	1.8	1.2	1.1	61.0	60.7
Skin (excluding basal and squamous cell carcinoma)	14.1	9.1	3.9	1.7	68.3	86.5
Melanomas	10.8	8.3	2.7	1.4	75.3	86.5
Breast	0.8	97.3	0.2	27.3	81.6	75.4
Female genital system	—	47.9	—	15.3	—	65.8
Cervix uteri (invasive only)	—	8.8	—	2.7	—	66.0
Corpus uteri	—	22.3	—	2.1	—	81.9
Ovary	—	13.5	—	7.8	—	38.6
Male genital system	90.1	—	24.2	—	73.5	—
Prostate gland	85.1	—	23.7	—	72.1	—
Testis	4.0	—	0.7	—	91.2	—
Urinary system	41.0	13.1	10.8	3.9	70.9	64.6
Urinary bladder	28.9	7.5	6.1	1.7	78.1	73.5
Kidney and renal pelvis	10.9	5.1	4.6	2.0	52.8	52.4
Eye and orbit	0.8	0.6	0.1	0.1	73.8	78.9
Brain and nervous system	7.0	4.9	5.0	3.4	23.0	25.2
Endocrine system	3.1	6.3	0.7	0.7	81.0	92.1
Thyroid	2.5	5.9	0.3	0.4	90.7	94.8
Lymphomas	17.6	12.5	8.0	5.3	54.8	57.3
Non-Hodgkin's	14.3	10.1	7.1	4.8	48.4	52.1
Hodgkin's	3.2	2.3	0.9	0.5	74.2	76.3
Multiple myeloma	5.0	3.4	3.4	2.3	24.7	27.9
Leukemias	13.2	7.6	8.6	4.9	33.2	33.4
All sites	420.2	323.4	210.4	138.0	44.2	55.2

Data from NCI.[6]

The incidence rates of all cancers vary among the regions of the world, and the cancers of most importance in developing countries are different from those in developed countries such as the United States. In order of frequency of occurrence, the 10 most common cancers in developing countries are cancers of the cervix uteri, mouth and pharynx, esophagus, breast, lung, liver, colon and rectum, and the lymphomas and leukemias.[12]

Age. Cancers most probably arise from undifferentiated stem cells that are capable of mitotic division and differentiation. In adults, most cancers are carcinomas that arise from basal epithelial cells of ectodermal or endodermal origin. In children, most cancers are of mesodermal origin and consist largely of leukemias and lymphomas that arise from hematopoietic and lymphoid stem cells and sarcomas that probably develop from undifferentiated cells of embryonal origin.

Incidence rates for the most common childhood cancers in the United States are shown in Table 47–2.[13] The mortality rates for even the most frequent cancers in children are many times lower than the rates of comparable tumors for all ages (Table 47–1), which largely reflect rates in adults.

With some notable exceptions (e.g., cancers of the female breast and uterine cervix) there is an exponential increase in incidence rates with age for most adult malignancies. The median ages at which cancer was diagnosed from 1973 to 1977 was 66.9 for men and 63.5 for women,[4] and most cancers develop in the sixth, seventh, and eighth decades of life.

Sex. Most major cancers of nonsexual sites occur more frequently in men than women, exceptions being carcinomas of the thyroid, gallbladder, and extrahepatic bile ducts. Smoking-related cancers, described in detail subsequently, occur more frequently in men, at least in part because of their earlier and greater exposure to tobacco smoke. Some other cancers, such as carcinoma of the bladder and mesotheliomas, are more frequent in men, at least in part because of their greater occupational exposure to various chemical carcinogens and asbestos, respectively. Other cancers that occur more frequently in men include

TABLE 47-2. AVERAGE ANNUAL AGE ADJUSTED[a] INCIDENCE RATES PER MILLION (1973–1982) BY TYPE OF NEOPLASM AND SEX IN WHITES, NINE SEER AREAS COMBINED

	Rates per Million	
Type of Neoplasm	***Male***	***Female***
Leukemias	47.8	39.5
Acute lymphocytic	35.9	29.7
Lymphomas	20.3	11.5
Non-Hodgkin's	6.9	2.8
Hodgkin's	6.5	5.9
Brain and spinal	26.4	23.3
Astrocytoma	12.3	12.2
Medulloblastoma	6.9	4.4
Neuroblastoma	12.6	12.3
Wilm's tumor	7.9	10.0
Liver	2.1	1.1
Bone	5.4	5.6
Soft tissue sarcoma	9.0	8.2
Gonadal and germ cell	4.3	4.1
Epithelial neoplasm	3.2	5.8
All types	143.9	126.9

[a]Adjusted to standard world population under age 15: populations of 2400, 9600, 10,000, and 9000 for the age groups < 1, 1 to 4, 5 to 9, and 10 to 14, respectively.
Data from NCI.[13]

the lymphomas and leukemias, malignant melanomas, sarcomas of bone, and carcinomas of the nasopharynx, stomach, kidney, pancreas, colon, rectum, parotid gland, and liver. The reasons for the excess of these cancers in men are unknown. Women could either be constitutionally less susceptible to these neoplasms or less exposed to whatever (largely unknown) environmental factors contribute to their development.

Race and Geography. The frequency of occurrence of many cancers varies among racial groups residing in the same country. This variation could be due to either genetic differences among the races or to factors related to their distinct cultural patterns, social behavior, or economic status. Within individual races, rates of all cancers also vary considerably from one geographical region to another; and migrants from one country to another, or their descendants, tend to eventually develop most cancers at rates more similar to the native populations of their country of adoption than at rates similar to those in their country of origin. These observations imply that environmental factors play a large role in the etiology of most cancers.

In the United States, blacks have higher overall mortality rates of cancer than any other racial group,[14] and this observation has received much publicity and attention in recent years. Some of the increased mortality is due to poorer survival from some types of cancers,[15] most probably a result of delayed diagnosis and treatment. The incidence rates of some cancers are also higher in blacks than in other races. These include many of the smoking-related cancers (lung, pancreas) as well as those that have been related to both alcohol and tobacco use (mouth, esophagus, and larynx); liver cancer, which has been related to alcoholic cirrhosis; and cervical cancer, which is probably caused by a sexually transmitted agent. Black men in the United States have the highest rate of prostate cancer in the world. The explanation for this is unknown.

Some cancers appear to be related to a "Western" life-style. These include cancers that occur at lower rates in Chinese, Japanese, Latin Americans, and native North Americans than in U.S. whites[16]: cancers of the colon and rectum, which may be related to diets rich in animal products; cancers of the prostate, ovary, corpus uteri, breast, and testis, which have to some extent also been related to high consumption of meats and fats as well as to endocrinological and reproductive factors; cancers related to smoking and other chemical exposures, such as those of lung, larynx, bladder, and possibly kidney and pancreas; and Hodgkin's disease, which has been hypothesized to be due to a common infectious agent that, like polio viruses, causes clinically overt disease with a frequency directly related to the age of the person at the time of the initial infection. Other cancers occur more frequently in the nonwhite population than in the white population of the United States. These include stomach cancer, possibly related to use of preserved foods; esophageal and liver cancers, which may in part be caused by the production of carcinogens (nitrosamines and aflatoxins) in foods contaminated by bacteria or fungi; and cancers of the nasopharynx, liver, and cervix uteri, possibly caused by the Epstein-Barr virus (EBV), hepatitis B virus (HBV), and herpes simplex virus type 2 (HSV-2) or a papillomavirus, respectively.

Time Trends. Figure 47–1 shows trends in mortality rates for various cancers in the United States from 1930 to 1985.[8] The striking increase in rates of lung cancer is largely due to cigarette smoking. The reason for the marked decline in rates of stomach cancer is unknown but may be related to changes in dietary habits, with consumption of less preserved and more fresh and frozen foods. Mortality rates of uterine cancer largely reflect deaths caused by cancer of the cervix because invasive neoplasms arising from that site have a considerably poorer prognosis than do endometrial cancers. The decline in mortality from uterine cancer is probably due to a combination of three factors: a decrease in the number of women who still have a uterus because of an increase in rates of hysterectomies for nonneoplastic conditions, an increase in cytological screening, and a true decline (until recently) in the incidence of new cases. Following the change in sexual practices within the last three decades, there has recently been an increase in incidence and mortality rates of cervical cancer in several Western countries. The decline in liver cancer rates is, at least in part, due to improvements over time in diagnosis, with fewer individuals with cancers of other sites that have metastasized to the liver erroneously being diagnosed as having primary liver cancer. There has been either no change or only gradual and sometimes erratic changes over time in the mortality rates of such common cancers as those of the colon, rectum, pancreas, breast, and prostate and the leukemias. This indicates that the principal environmental determinants of these cancers are likely to be temporally stable factors that are well-ingrained in the social and cultural environment. The unremarkable changes in mortality over time also indicate that there has been little or no improvement in survival from many of the major cancers in the past several decades.

Temporal trends in mortality from cancer in children are much more encouraging. From 1950 to 1980, mortality rates declined 50% for leukemia, 32% for non-Hodgkin's lymphoma, 80% for Hodgkin's disease, 50% for sarcomas of bone, 18% for kidney cancer (largely Wilms' tumor), and 31% for all other cancers.[17] There has been little change in the incidence of these neoplasms in children, and these reductions in mortality are due to prolonged survival resulting from improved therapy.

Goals for the Year 2000. In 1984 the NCI set a goal to halve the cancer mortality rate by the year 2000.[18] This goal is a theoretical possibility because if the incidence rate of each cancer in the United States were reduced to equal the lowest rate observed for the same cancer in the world, then the overall cancer burden in the country would be reduced by about 80%. Part of the reduction was to be caused by reducing the prevalence of smoking to 16%. If this goal had been achieved by 1990, overall cancer mortality would have been reduced by 15% by the year 2000, but

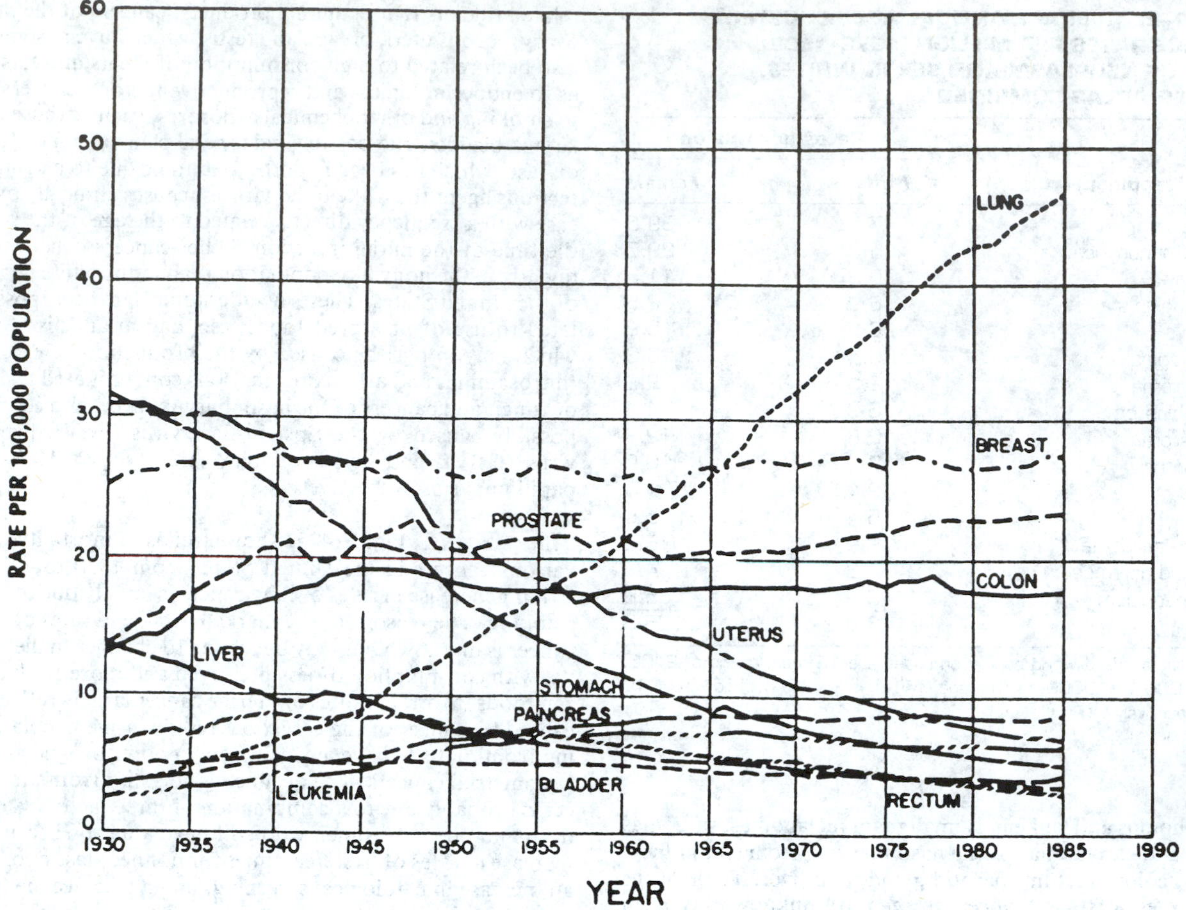

Figure 47–1. Cancer Death Rates by Site in the United States from 1930 to 1985. The population is age standarized based on the 1970 U.S. census. Rates are for both sexes combined, except rates for breast and uterine cancer are for females only and prostate cancer for males only. *[Data from U.S. National Center for Health Statistics and U.S. Bureau of the Census.]*

this did not occur. If this goal is reached by 2000, the reduction in mortality by then will be 8%. Eight percent of the cancer mortality reduction was to be caused by lowering the average fat intake to 30% of total calories and increasing the fiber intake to 20 to 30 g per day; but as of 1986 there had been no appreciable changes in fat or fiber consumption.[19] A 3% reduction in cancer mortality was to be achieved by more widespread screening for breast cancer (annual mammography coupled with physical examination of 80% of the 50- to 70-year-old women) and for cervical cancer (reaching 90% of women 20 to 39 years old and 80% of women 40 to 70 years old every 3 years). If trends seen up to 1986 in the amount of screening for breast and cervical cancers continue, these goals will not be met.[19] The remaining reduction in cancer mortality was to be achieved by more widespread state-of-the-art treatment. Estimates of the expected resulting reduction in cancer mortality vary from 10% to 26%, depending on the assumptions made about future changes in therapy. Some changes in both survival and the proportion of patients who receive appropriate therapy have occurred, but if the trends documented up to 1986 continue unchanged, the estimated 26% reduction in cancer mortality will not be realized.[19]

Although the goal of a 50% reduction in cancer mortality has been criticized as being overly ambitious and unrealistic, it continues to be of value in providing a focal point for the activities of basic and clinical scientists, epidemiologists, health planners and administrators, and community cancer control specialists.

ETIOLOGY AND PRIMARY PREVENTION

Criteria for Causality. Primary cancer prevention is prevention of the initial development of a neoplasm or its precursor. This can be accomplished only if one or more causes of the neoplasm are known and is achieved by reducing or preventing exposure to the causative agent. An agent is considered a cause if reducing or removing a population's exposure to it would result in a decrease in the amount of disease occurring in that population.

To determine whether an agent is a cause of a particular disease in humans, information from all relevant studies must be assessed critically. In making such an assessment, evidence for causality is strengthened if the criteria listed in Chapter 2 are met. Additional criteria include evidence that risk is decreased following a reduction in exposure and that the disease associated with the substance has unusual features (such as a specific histological type).

Attempts to determine whether an agent is carcinogenic in humans must often be made without information on all of these criteria. Yet, assessment of whatever evidence is available must frequently be made. Investigators must examine existing evidence to identify additional questions that should be addressed by further studies, physicians must assess available evidence to be able to give their patients adequate advice, and public officials must assess the evidence to determine needs for laws and regulations to limit exposure. Each must weigh the evidence for a causal relationship and consider the consequences of falsely implicating a substance as being carcinogenic when it is not and of failing to identify as carcinogenic a substance that is. All must also be willing to alter their opinions as results of additional investigations become available. Errors of judgment can be minimized by a clear understanding of basic epidemiological principles and by careful examination of available evidence using the above referenced criteria for assessing causality.

General Etiological Considerations. The series of cellular events that connect an undifferentiated stem cell and a malignant tumor cell are unknown. One current two-stage theory of carcinogenesis is that during division a stem cell produces an intermediate cell with altered genetic material as one of its daughter cells and during a subsequent division this intermediate cell in turn gives rise to a tumor cell with additionally altered DNA. The tumor cell then replicates to eventually form a tumor. Other multistage theories have been proposed, but this two-stage theory contains most of their important features. A mathematical model has been developed that shows the two-stage process to be compatible with the known epidemiological features of many of the important adult and childhood malignancies.[20]

This theory of carcinogenesis provides a logical explanation for the observation that multiple factors alter the risk of any neoplasm. These factors may represent tumor initiators, promoters, or inhibitors. Initiators are agents that cause the genetic damage to the stem or intermediate cells. Ionizing radiation, various chemicals, and (at least in animals) certain viruses most probably act as initiators. The nature of the genetic damage caused by initiators is unknown. One current school of thought is that initiators cause rearrangements in the DNA that result in increased expression or derepression of normal genes, known as oncogenes, that were perhaps operative in embryonic life.[21,22]

Promoters act to enhance the rate of growth and number of stem and intermediate cells that are the targets for initiators and to enhance the growth of tumor cells. Estrogens that enhance the proliferation of the endometrium probably act as promoters for endometrial cancer. Factors that alter immune mechanisms may also enhance tumor development, perhaps by reducing immunological destruction of transformed cells or tumor viruses.

There are a number of different mechanisms by which inhibitors of tumor development might act. They could, for example, reduce epithelial absorption of carcinogens, inhibit the enzymatic conversion of noncarcinogenic substances to active initiators or promoters, enhance the metabolic destruction of carcinogenic agents, promote DNA repair, or reduce the number of stem and intermediate cells susceptible to the carcinogenic effects of initiators by causing cell differentiation or destruction.

Although the mechanisms of action of many of the risk factors that have been identified for human cancers are unknown, these epidemiologically observed factors undoubtedly represent various initiating, promoting, and inhibiting agents. Human cancers are probably the end result of the cumulative effects of many of these agents. This explains why multiple risk factors are observed for all cancers and why only a small proportion of individuals who are exposed to most known carcinogens develop cancer.

Truly independent risk factors (i.e., those that are not surrogates for the same underlying cause) may alter the risk of cancer independently, synergistically, or antagonistically, depending on their modes of action (i.e., whether they represent initiators, promoters, or inhibitors).

It must be emphasized, however, that a risk factor can represent a cause in the public health sense, as defined previously, whether or not its precise mode of action is known. For example, the exact mechanism by which tobacco smoke increases a smoker's risk of lung cancer is unknown. Some evidence suggests that it acts as an initiator, and some points to a promoting action. In fact, tobacco smoke may act as both. For the purpose of primary prevention, however, the mechanism of action is unimportant. Cessation of smoking will prevent lung cancer, and that is what we need to know to take preventive action.

The latent period between exposure to a cancer risk factor and the development of a neoplasm also is dependent in part on the mechanism by which the factor operates. In general, long latent periods are associated with initiators, and shorter ones follow exposure to promoters. For example, mesotheliomas follow exposure to asbestos and breast cancers follow radiation to the chest usually only decades after exposure; yet, endometrial cancers can occur within 2 years of exposure to exogenous estrogens. Reticulum cell sarcomas have developed within just months of exposure to immunosuppressive drugs in persons with renal transplants.

There are many known causes of various cancers, and many risk factors that provide clues for further etiological research. These are described below. The best source of additional information is Reference 23.

Tobacco. Smoking and associated cancer risks are discussed in Chapter 42. Use of tobacco is responsible for the development of more neoplasms than are all other known causes of cancer combined. Table 47-3 shows relative risks of cancers at nine sites in cigarette smokers as estimated from eight cohort studies conducted in six countries.[24] The estimates shown are for individuals who have ever smoked; relative risks for heavy smokers of long duration are higher. Compared to nonsmokers, risk in the average cigarette smoker is increased approximately tenfold for lung cancer, eightfold for laryngeal cancer, fourfold for neoplasms of the mouth and pharynx, threefold for esophageal cancer, and twofold for cancers of the bladder, renal pelvis, ureter, and pancreas. Lesser increments in risk of neoplasms of the renal paryenchyma and stomach may also occur. Case-control studies conducted during the past decade also have shown a possible association between smoking and cancer of the uterine cervix, although this may be a spurious observation because of incomplete control for the confounding effects of sexual behavior, which may differ in smokers and nonsmokers.

Risks of a variety of neoplasms are also increased in users of other forms of tobacco. Compared to nonsmokers, risk in pipe and cigar smokers is approximately doubled for lung cancer, increased fourfold for cancer of the larynx, and doubled or tripled for neoplasms of the esophagus, oral cavity, and pharynx. Pipe smoking approximately triples one's risk of lip cancer, and chewing tobacco or using snuff results in a fourfold increase in the risk of oral cancer.[25]

Many of these estimates are based on studies of individuals

TABLE 47-3. RELATIVE RISKS OF NINE CANCERS IN CIGARETTE SMOKERS

	Relative Risks	
Cancer Site	***Range in Eight Cohort Studies***	***"Best" Estimate***
Lung	3.6–15.9	10.0
Larynx	6.1–13.6	8.0
Buccal cavity	1.0–13.0	4.0
Pharynx	2.8–12.5	4.0
Esophagus	0.7– 6.6	3.0
Bladder	1.0– 6.0	2.0
Pancreas[a]	1.6– 3.1	2.0
Kidney[a]	1.1– 1.5	1.5
Stomach[a]	0.8– 2.3	1.5

[a] Association with cigarette smoking is not firmly established.

who smoked cigarettes that were popular decades ago. Relative risks in comparable smokers of the newer filter and low-tar products are lower but still appreciable. Furthermore, the number of puffs per cigarette and the number of cigarettes smoked per hour are inversely proportional to the amount of nicotine in the tobacco. Low levels of nicotine therefore result in an increased exposure to carcinogens in tobacco smoke. There is no safe cigarette.

Side-stream smoke contains some carcinogens in higher concentration than mainstream smoke, and evidence is accumulating that nonsmokers exposed to tobacco smoke by their association with smokers may also be at increased risk of lung cancer. The best estimate to date is that risk is increased by about 30% in nonsmoking members of households with a resident smoker.[26]

In men in the United States, use of tobacco is responsible for about 90% of all lung cancer, 75% of all neoplasms of the mouth, pharynx, larynx, and esophagus, about 50% of the bladder cancers, and probably 40% of the cases of pancreatic cancer. For women, these proportions are about 75% of the lung cancers, 40% of neoplasms of the mouth, pharynx, larynx, and esophagus, 30% of the bladder cancers, and 25% of the cancers of the pancreas. About 35% of all cancer in U.S. males, 12% of all cancers in females, and 30% of all cancer deaths in both sexes combined can be attributed to use of tobacco. Passive smoking may account for much of the lung cancer not due to smoking or industrial exposures.

Population-attributable risks such as these are dependent on the proportion of people in the population who use tobacco, the relative risk of the particular cancer in users of tobacco, and the presence of other causes of the cancers of interest in the population. Estimates of population-attributable risks thus vary among populations, and the above values for the United States are different from values for other parts of the world.

Alcohol. The risk of several human neoplasms is clearly associated with alcohol consumption.[27,28] Hepatocellular carcinomas develop at an unusually high rate in alcoholics with macronodular cirrhosis. Risk is probably enhanced as a result of the rapid regeneration of liver cells in such individuals, although the exact mechanisms are not understood.

With the exception of the liver, risk is definitely increased only in those tissues that come in direct contact with the undigested alcohol. Risk is thus increased for carcinomas of the mouth (buccal cavity and pharynx), esophagus, and supraglottic larynx[29] but not, for example, of the lung, pancreas, or bladder. Results of studies of alcohol and cancers of the stomach and lower alimentary tract have been inconsistent but generally not supportive of a causal association.

Esophageal, oral, and laryngeal cancers are all related to smoking, and most studies show the effect of smoking on the risk of these tumors to be greater in drinkers than in nondrinkers. Alcohol thus appears to potentiate the carcinogenic effect of tobacco smoke. It is unclear whether alcohol increases the risk of these cancers in the absence of tobacco usage. Results of most studies suggest that it does, although so few heavy drinkers are nonsmokers that data from existing investigations are insufficient to provide a definitive answer. It is reasonable to assume, however, that because alcohol potentiates the effect of carcinogens in tobacco smoke, it is likely also to potentiate carcinogens from other sources.

It has been estimated that in U.S. men, alcohol consumption contributes to nearly half of the deaths due to oral and laryngeal cancers, 75% of the esophageal cancer deaths, and 30% of the fatal liver cancers.[30] Approximately 4% of all male cancer deaths and 2% of all female cancer deaths can be attributed to alcohol use. With the exception of liver cancer, most alcohol-related neoplasms develop as a result of smoking as well as drinking, and cessation of smoking would have nearly the same impact on the occurrence of these neoplasms as would cessation of drinking. (See also Chapter 43.)

Industrial Exposures. In 1987 an ad hoc committee of experts was assembled under the auspices of the International Agency for Research on Cancer in Lyon, France, to review published evidence for carcinogenicity in humans of 628 suspect chemicals and industrial processes.[31] The available evidence was considered sufficient to classify 50 of these as definitely carcinogenic for humans. Of the others, 37 were classified as probably carcinogenic for humans, and 159 were considered possibly carcinogenic. All but one of the remaining 382 were judged as not classifiable for their human carcinogenicity because of insufficient information, and one was classified as probably not carcinogenic to humans. Of the 50 substances and industrial processes classified as definitely carcinogenic for humans, 18 are specific industrial exposures. They are shown in the upper portion of Table 47–4, along with the neoplasms most strongly and consistently associated with them in human studies. Eleven others, shown in the lower portion of the table, are industrial processes. The specific carcinogens responsible for the enhanced risks in workers exposed to these processes are unknown.

TABLE 47–4. OCCUPATIONAL CAUSES OF CANCER

Specific Exposures	Site or Tumor Type
▪ **Specific Exposures**	
4-Aminobiphenyl	Bladder
Arsenic and arsenic compounds	Lung, skin
Asbestos	Lung, mesothelioma
Benzene	Leukemia
Benzidine	Bladder
Bis (chloromethyl) ether and chloromethyl methyl ether	Lung
Chromium compounds, hexavalent	Lung
Coal tar pitches	Skin, lung, bladder
Coal tars	Skin
Erionite	Mesothelioma
Mineral oils, untreated and mildly treated	Skin
Mustard gas (sulphur mustard)	Lung, larynx
2-Naphthylamine	Bladder
Nickel and nickel compounds	Sinonasal, lung
Shale oils	Skin
Soots	Skin, lung
Talc containing asbestiform fibers	Lung
Vinyl chloride	Liver, lung, brain, leukemia, lymphoma
▪ **Industrial Process**	
Aluminum production	Lung, bladder, lymphosarcomas and reticulosarcomas
Manufacture of auramine	Bladder
Boot and shoe manufacture and repair	Nasal, bladder
Coal gasification	Lung, bladder, skin
Coke production	Lung, bladder, skin
Furniture and cabinet making	Nasal
Hematite mining, underground, with exposure to radon	Lung
Iron and steel founding	Lung
Isopropyl alcohol manufacture, strong acid process	Sinonasal
Manufacture of magenta	Bladder
Rubber industry	Bladder, leukemia, lymphoma

The evidence that the agents shown in Table 47–4 are carcinogenic in humans comes from studies of relatively high exposure in the workplace. Exposures to most of these agents outside the workplace are sufficiently rare or at such low levels as to be of little importance. Exposures to arsenic, vinyl chloride, and particularly asbestos outside an industrial setting, however, are causes for concern.

There has been considerable controversy in recent years about the proportion of cancers that are attributable to known occupational exposures. Although estimates of over one third have been published, those estimates in the range of 5% are more generally accepted for the United States.[32]

Drugs. The ad hoc committee mentioned above also classified a number of drugs as definitely carcinogenic for humans. A variety of alkylating agents have been shown to cause acute nonlymphocytic leukemia, and some have also been implicated as causes of bladder carcinomas; squamous cell carcinomas of the skin have developed in patients with mycosis fungoides and psoriasis who were treated with topical nitrogen mustard. Other drugs that are likely causes of skin cancer include arsenic compounds (Fowler's solution) used systemically and topically, tar ointments, and methoxsalen used with ultraviolet light to treat psoriasis. The analgesic phenacetin has been strongly implicated as a cause of carcinomas of the renal pelvis and bladder.

Drugs are undoubtedly not an important cause of cancer. They account for less than 1% of the neoplasms in the United States. Furthermore, except for phenacetin, most of the known leukemogenic and carcinogenic drugs are used to treat conditions that are sufficiently life threatening to warrant accepting the associated risk of subsequent neoplasia. Nonetheless, the identification of drugs that cause cancer is of obvious importance to the practicing oncologist; the problem of drug-induced neoplasia will probably become greater in the future as more patients survive for longer periods of time and as more potentially carcinogenic and leukemogenic drugs come into use. The practicing physician should be aware of the known risks of subsequent neoplasia in patients receiving various chemotherapeutic agents and give support to formal epidemiological efforts to monitor new and existing drugs for their potential long-term carcinogenic effects.

Ionizing Radiation. A large number of epidemiological studies have clearly shown that ionizing radiation has caused a variety of human neoplasms.[33,34] These studies have largely involved following up individuals exposed to moderate or high doses from nuclear explosions, medical treatments, and occupational sources. Exposures have been both external and internal and have included X rays, gamma rays, neutrons, alpha particles, and beta particles.

Studies of individuals who have received total body radiation from external sources have shown that some organs are more susceptible to the carcinogenic effects of radiation than others, either because of their superficial location or because their cells are more radiosensitive. Among the atomic bomb survivors in Japan, there were large increases in rates of carcinomas of the anatomically exposed thyroid and mammary glands and of leukemias arising from the highly susceptible cells of the bone marrow; lesser increases in rates of lymphomas and carcinomas of the stomach, esophagus, and bladder were observed; and risks of cancer at other sites were either not altered or the increases were too small to measure with certainty. Risk of leukemia was also increased in early radiologists who took few precautions to reduce their general exposure to radiation and probably also in individuals exposed in utero to X rays from pelvimetry.

External sources of radiation directed at specific sites have resulted in a variety of neoplasms. Breast cancer was induced in women treated with X rays for a variety of benign breast conditions and in women who received multiple fluoroscopies of the chest in conjunction with pneumothorax treatment of tuberculosis. Individuals treated with X rays for ankylosing spondylitis have had increased rates of leukemia and lung cancer and, like the atomic bomb survivors, lesser increases in rates of lymphomas and cancers of the stomach and esophagus. Children treated with X rays for tinea capitis and enlarged thymus have developed leukemia and neoplasms of the salivary and thyroid glands. Those treated for an enlarged thymus have also had an increased risk of leukemia, and those with tinea capitis developed more brain tumors than expected.

Internal exposures to radiation have likewise resulted in increased risks of cancer at specific sites. Inhalation of radioactive dusts has contributed to the increased rates of lung cancer in the atomic bomb survivors and resulted in elevated rates of uranium and other radioactive substances in miners. Radium inadvertently swallowed by radium-dial watch painters and administered for treatment of ankylosing spondylitis was concentrated in osseous tissues and caused high rates of bone cancers. Individuals exposed to iodine 131 (^{131}I) in fallout from a hydrogen bomb test subsequently had increased rates of thyroid cancer. The radiopaque contrast material Thorotrast that was used to x-ray the liver has resulted in hepatic cancers as well as leukemias and lung carcinomas. Women receiving cervical radium implants and other forms of pelvic radiation for a variety of gynecological conditions have had increased rates of cancers of the colon, rectum, and possibly small bowel as well as leukemia.

The results of most studies show a linear increase in risk of neoplasms with the amount of radiation received over a wide range of observed doses, with a possible decrease in the slope of the dose-response curve at very high levels of exposure (perhaps due to cell killing). These observations are based primarily on studies of individuals who received from 10s to 100s of rads. Doses commonly received today are orders of magnitude lower, and it is uncertain whether the dose-response curve should be linearly extrapolated to these low levels to provide an estimate of the associated risk (Chapter 26). There may be a threshold level below which radiation does not induce neoplasms, perhaps because mechanisms of DNA repair are adequate. If so, linear extrapolation would yield estimates of risk to low levels of radiation that are too high. Conversely, chronic exposure to low levels of radiation might be more carcinogenic, rad for rad, than acute exposure at a higher dose. If so, linear extrapolations would underestimate the risk of low doses. Since there is little evidence for the latter possibility, most authorities believe that it is reasonable, as well as prudent, to assume a linear, nonthreshold dose-response curve.

Approximately half of all ionizing radiation received by individuals in the United States comes from natural background sources. These include cosmic rays, naturally occurring elements in the earth such as uranium, thorium, and radium, and emissions within the body from such isotopes as potassium 40 and carbon 14. These sources deliver about 80 mrems of ionizing radiation per year to a person living at sea level. Background doses received may be approximately doubled in individuals living in high altitudes or where concentrations of radium in the ground are unusually high. Radium decays to a radioactive gas, radon 222, which can seep into houses and accumulate under conditions of poor ventilation. Radon 222 is likely the cause of lung cancer in uranium miners, and whether the lower doses found in some homes also cause lung cancer is the subject of several ongoing investigations.[35] Approximately 43% of all ionizing radiation is received from medical sources, largely from diagnostic radiographs. These result in an annual exposure of about 92 mrems per year for the average U.S. citizen. Most other exposures are from mining and processing radioactive ores (2% to 3%), fallout from nuclear weapons (2% to 4%), and such consumer products as television sets and smoke detectors (1% to 4%).

The average person living at sea level in the United States

thus receives about 180 mrems of ionizing radiation per year. This is roughly equivalent to that received during an upper or lower gastrointestinal (GI) series, whereas only about 10 mrems are received from x-raying the chest.

Based on a linear, nonthreshold dose-response model, it has been estimated that approximately 1% of all cancer in the United States may be attributable to radiation from other than background sources. This estimate is, of course, too high if a threshold exists. Because most of the preventable radiation-induced neoplasms result from medical exposures, the responsibility for preventing them rests primarily with members of the medical profession. Political efforts to reduce the likelihood of environmental contamination from nuclear power plants and nuclear weapons would also obviously reduce the risk of radiation-induced neoplasms. (See also Chapter 26.)

Nonionizing Radiation. Sunlight is definitely a cause of squamous and basal cell carcinomas of the skin, as evidenced by the observations that these tumors tend to occur on exposed parts of the body, risk increases with the amount of sun exposure, and incidence rates are greater in light-skinned people than they are in dark-skinned individuals.[36,37]

The relationship of malignant melanomas of the skin to sunlight is more complicated.[38,39] Incidence rates are highest in low altitudes with sunny climates and in individuals with little natural skin pigmentation. Unlike other skin cancers, rates are not increased in individuals who regularly work outside, and although there is some tendency for these tumors to occur on exposed parts of the body, many do not. The results of some studies suggest that episodic exposures to the sun increase risk, and an investigation of migrants to Australia provided evidence that exposure at an early age may be of particular importance.[40] Incidence rates of melanomas of the skin have been increasing in recent years. The reason for this is unknown but may be related, at least in part, to destruction of the ozone layer in the upper atmosphere.

Because nonmelanotic skin cancers are common and largely attributable to sun exposure, sunlight accounts for approximately 10% of all neoplasms. It accounts for only about 2% of cancer deaths, however, both because these neoplasms are infrequently fatal and because the more fatal melanomas are related less strongly to sun exposure. All individuals, but particularly those with light skin who burn easily, should be encouraged to avoid excessive direct exposure to intense sunlight and to use sunshades and sunscreens.

Exogenous Sex Hormones. Diethylstilbestrol (DES) was used in the 1940s and 1950s to treat between one-half and five million women in the United States for threatened abortion. Approximately 80% of the female offspring who were exposed to DES while in utero have been found to have glandular epithelium resembling that of the endometrium, and presumably of Mullerian origin, in the vagina or cervix. A small portion of women with this condition, which is called adenosis, have developed clear cell adenocarcinomas of the vagina or (less frequently) the cervix when in their teens or twenties.[41] Fortunately, the risk of carcinoma is small, about 1/100,000 exposed women by the age of 34 years. This represents a small proportion of total cancers but a high proportion of neoplasms in this age group, including virtually all vaginal cancers. Women exposed in utero to DES with vaginal or cervical adenosis should be followed carefully for the development of clear cell carcinoma. Boys exposed in utero to DES are at increased risk of cryptorchidism, which is a risk factor for testicular cancer; and several studies have implicated prenatal DES exposure as a rare cause of testicular cancer.

These neoplasms represent the first documented instances of transplacental carcinogenesis in humans. This experience, along with that of leukemia in children following in utero exposure to radiation from pelvimetry, emphasizes the vulnerability of the growing fetus and the importance of minimizing in utero exposures to any suspected mutagens or carcinogens.

In some countries, DES is used as a "morning after" pill to prevent pregnancy. It has also been used to treat menopausal symptoms. Care must be exercised not to give DES inadvertently for these or other purposes to women who may be pregnant.

In considering the effects of exogenous female sex hormones on the risk of neoplasms in the women who take them, it is useful to categorize these substances according to their net estrogenic or progestogenic pharmacological effect. At one end of the spectrum are the pure progestational agents such as depomedroxyprogesterone acetate (DMPA), which is used as a long-acting injectable contraceptive in many countries (but not in the United States) and to treat malignant and benign proliferative disorders of the endometrium. The so-called minipills, which have been used in some parts of the world, are also progestogens. At the other end of the spectrum are the pure estrogen preparations. The most common of these are the conjugated "natural" estrogens (e.g., Premarin), used largely to treat or prevent symptoms and conditions associated with the menopause, and the nonsteroidal synthetic estrogen DES mentioned previously. Between these two ends of the estrogen-progestogen spectrum are the previously used sequential oral contraceptives, which contained only an estrogen in pills taken for 2 weeks of a cycle and which had a net estrogenic effect, and the commonly used combined oral contraceptives with an estrogen and a progestogen in each pill and therefore a net pharmacological effect more progestational than the sequential pills.

Risk of endometrial cancer is increased in women who have received estrogens for menopausal conditions and other reasons and in women who took sequential oral contraceptives.[42] On the other hand, risk is decreased in users of combined oral contraceptives.[43] One would therefore expect the pure progestational agents to be protective. The limited evidence available suggests that this is true. It has been advocated that a progestogen also be taken, either continuously with the estrogen or cyclically for a specified number of days each month, to reduce the risk of endometrial cancer in users of estrogens. The experience with sequential oral contraceptives suggests that cyclical treatment with a progestogen may not totally eliminate the carcinogenic effect of estrogens on the endometrium. Studies of this problem are currently being conducted.

Studies to determine whether risk of benign breast disease is altered in women who have ever taken menopausal estrogens have yielded inconsistent results, but two investigations have shown risk of fibrocystic disease to be increased in long-term users and in women exposed to high doses.[44] Combined oral contraceptives have been consistently shown to decrease risks of both fibrocystic disease and fibroadenomas (the two main types of benign breast tumors),[44] and this protective effect has been related to the progestogen content of the formulation used.

Although high doses of estrogens given to induce breast development have caused breast cancer in male transvestites, the results of three studies of women given high doses of DES for threatened abortion and of three other studies of women given more modest doses have yielded equivocal and inconsistent results.[45] Results from studies of breast cancer in relation to estrogens given at menopause are also inconclusive, with no consistent enhancement of risk observed among studies in women who ever used these products, in long-term users, or in users long after initial exposure. Risk has also not consistently been enhanced in users with or without various other risk factors for breast cancer, although some studies suggest that estrogens may reduce the protective effect of a premenopausal oophorectomy.[45] Multiple studies have consistently shown no increase in risk of breast cancer in women who have ever used combined oral contraceptives.[44] Some studies have shown risk to be enhanced in young women who used these products at an early age, before the birth of their first child, or in other subgroups of women, but other studies have not. The reasons for these discrepant findings are unknown, and this issue is under further investigation. Studies of breast cancer in relation to DMPA have likewise yielded inconsistent findings.[46,47]

Use of estrogens for menopausal indications has not consistently been shown to alter risk of ovarian cancers. Oral contraceptives clearly reduce the risk of epithelial ovarian cancer.[43] Risk in women who have ever used combined oral contraceptives is about 60% that of nonusers, and the risk decreases with duration of use. Studies to determine the effect of progestational agents on risk of ovarian cancer have not been completed.

Studies of cervical cancer and estrogens have not been conducted. Results of studies of combined oral contraceptives and cervical neoplasia are inclusive. Use of these products has been most consistently associated with invasive cervical cancer; results for carcinomas in situ are more variable.[43] One or more venereally transmitted agents undoubtedly contribute to the development of cervical cancer. Sexually promiscuous women are therefore at increased risk. In some cultures promiscuous women also have been those most likely to use oral contraceptives. Under such circumstances, one could observe a spurious association between use of oral contraceptives and cervical cancer unless variables related to sexual behavior are taken into account. Information on such variables is difficult to obtain accurately, and in many studies the confounding effect of sexual behavior has not been adequately considered. This may be an explanation for the inconsistent results of studies of carcinoma in situ in relation to oral contraceptive use. The somewhat more consistent findings for invasive disease may be due to incomplete control of the confounding effects of sexual activity or be spurious for other reasons. Alternatively, these results and an earlier observation[48] that oral contraceptives were associated with progression of cervical intraepithelial lesions may indicate that oral contraceptives promote the development of invasive disease. This issue is the topic of additional studies. There are also ongoing studies of progestogens and cervical cancer.

Combined oral contraceptives have clearly been shown to cause benign hepatic cell adenomas and focal nodular hyperplasia. These are highly vascular tumors that can rupture, bleed into the peritoneal cavity, and cause death. Fortunately, they are a rare complication of oral contraceptive use, occurring at a rate of less than 3 per 100,000 women years in women under 30 years of age.[49]

Four small case-control studies conducted in Britain and the United States have shown that primary liver carcinomas are rare complications of oral contraceptive use.[43,50] Some of these studies and a multinational study conducted largely in developing countries[51] provided evidence that this adverse effect is not mediated by enhancing the influence of other factors such as hepatitis B on risk.

There have been case reports of hepatomas developing in men who were treated with the androgen oxymetholone for various anemias and other medical conditions and in a body builder who took androgens. These reports probably represent a causal association, but formal epidemiological studies of this probable relationship have not been conducted.

Both case-control and cohort studies have failed to confirm earlier reports that risk of malignant melanoma is increased by use of oral contraceptives.[43] Isolated reports of associations between oral contraceptives and pituitary adenomas, choriocarcinomas, and thyroid tumors have also appeared, but these observations have not been convincingly confirmed by epidemiological investigations.[43]

The proportion of cancers caused by exogenous hormones is unknown. Rates of endometrial cancer have declined since the mid-1970s following a reduction in the use of estrogens that resulted from the discovery that estrogens caused carcinomas of the endometrium. Few estrogen-related breast cancers will occur with these changes in estrogen usage unless the addition of progestogens to replacement therapy regimens adversely affects risk of breast cancers. The protective effect of oral contraceptives against benign breast diseases, and cancers of the ovary and endometrium, undoubtedly outweigh the increased risk of liver tumors. Unless oral contraceptives are ultimately shown to increase risks of breast, cervical, or other cancers, it seems reasonable to conclude that they prevent more neoplasms than they cause.

Infectious Agents. Both DNA and RNA viruses have been shown to cause a variety of neoplasms in animals. The DNA viruses that have been most strongly linked to cancers in humans include EBV, HBV, HSV-2, and the papilloma viruses.

EBV has been strongly related to African Burkitt's lymphoma and nasopharyngeal carcinomas.[52] Almost 100% of the persons with these diseases have antibodies against EBV, compared to much lower percentages in unaffected persons, and antibody titers are higher in the cases. Also, a cohort study clearly showed EBV infection to precede the development of African Burkitt's lymphomas. In addition, the EBV genome has been demonstrated in tumor cells from most African Burkitt's lymphomas and virtually all nasopharyngeal carcinomas. EBV has been shown to induce lymphomas in several species of New World monkeys and to transform both human and other primate B-lymphocytes in vitro. Only a small proportion of individuals infected with EBV develop either of these neoplasms, however, and the worldwide distributions of the two malignancies are different. Therefore, either EBV is not a cause of these malignancies or, more probably, other factors must also be operative in conjunction with EBV for these tumors to develop. Chronic malaria, and the resultant immunosuppression or antigenic stimulation, may play a role in African Burkitt's lymphoma. Cofactors for nasopharyngeal carcinoma are unknown but may include human leukocyte antigen (HLA) type, other nasopharyngeal diseases, chemical exposures (e.g., the smoke from cooking fires), and dietary factors such as salted fish. EBV is not a necessary factor for Burkitt's lymphoma because only 15% to 25% of the cases outside Africa have evidence of prior EBV infection.

EBV may also contribute to the development of Hodgkin's disease.[53] It is known to cause infectious mononucleosis, and persons with this disease have a twofold to threefold increase in risk of Hodgkin's disease. Compared to controls, cases of Hodgkin's disease more frequently have antibodies against EBV and higher antibody titers. However, only 30% to 40% of the Hodgkin's disease cases have anti-EBV antibodies, and the EBV genome has not been demonstrated in tumor cells.

Although rare in the United States, hepatocellular carcinoma (hepatoma) is the most common cancer in some places, including parts of Africa and China. There is strong evidence that HBV is one cause of this disease.[54] The disease appears to develop in individuals who become chronic carriers of the hepatitis B surface antigen (HB_sAg). The prevalence of HB_sAg carrier state in the world correlates well with the incidence of hepatomas, and within both high- and low-risk areas the prevalence of HB_sAg is much higher in cases than in controls. One cohort study has shown that the antigenemia precedes development of the tumor. Determinants of the chronic HB_sAg carrier state are not fully understood. In high-risk areas, transmission to the child from the mother at or soon after birth, before immune competence is fully developed, appears to result in the child becoming a carrier. In adults, factors causing immunosuppression may play a role. It is uncertain whether the virus directly causes hepatomas or whether chronic antigenemia eventually causes chronic hepatitis and liver cirrhosis, which in turn leads to the development of hepatomas, perhaps in the presence of other carcinogens such as aflatoxins.

The epidemiological features of cervical cancer strongly suggest that one or more sexually transmitted agents play an etiological role in the development of this neoplasm. Virtually all sexually transmitted organisms have been hypothesized at one time or another to be the etiological agent, but no firm evidence exists at this time. During the 1970s and 1980s, HSV-2 was the subject of considerable research.[55] Most case-control studies showed cases to more frequently have antibodies against HSV-2 than controls, and early cohort studies showed higher rates of early neoplastic cervical lesions in women with than without evidence of HSV-2 infection. Other evidence for an etiological role for this virus includes the demonstration of antibodies against HSV-2–induced nonviron tumor antigens in higher proportions of cases than of controls, the presence of these antigens in some cells from cervical carcinomas, and induction of both in vitro cell transformations and cervical neoplasms in mice by inactivated HSV-2. However, HSV-2 DNA has not consistently been demonstrated in cervical cancer cells, and recent case-control and cohort studies have failed to confirm the serological results from earlier studies.

In the past 5 years the focus of attention has shifted to various types of human papilloma viruses (HPV).[56] Using a variety of DNA-DNA molecular hybridization techniques, evidence of HPV viral DNA has been demonstrated in high proportions of cervical cancers and in much lower proportions of non-neoplastic cervical tissues. DNA from types 16 and 18 are found most commonly in in situ and invasive cervical cancers, and types 6 and 11 are most frequently demonstrated in less severe interepithelial lesions. Also, the viral DNA in the carcinomas tends to be found integrated into the cellular genome, but that in the milder lesions is usually episomal. Types 16 and 18 have also been demonstrated in several cell lines derived from cervical carcinomas. Although these observations strongly suggest that certain types of HPV may be a cause of cervical cancer, conclusive evidence is lacking. Several formal epidemiological studies of this possible etiological relationship are currently in progress. One current hypothesis under consideration is that the papilloma virus acts as a tumor promoter by causing rapid proliferation of cells that in the presence of other carcinogens (including HSV-2) leads to the development of carcinomas.[57] Biological plausibility is supported by the observations that laryngeal carcinomas developed from papillomas of viral origin that were treated with X rays, and the skin lesions of epidermodysplasia verruciformis, which are caused by a papillomavirus, tend to undergo malignant transformation primarily in the presence of sunlight.

Papillomaviruses are also under investigation as causal factors in the development of carcinomas of the vulva and of the anus in both homosexual men and women who practice anal intercourse.

Certain RNA viruses have long been known to cause neoplasms in various animals; an example is the feline leukemia virus (which also causes immunosuppression in cats).

Individuals with acquired immunodeficiency syndrome (AIDS), caused by infection by the human immunodeficiency virus (HIV), an RNA virus, are at greatly increased risk of Kaposi's sarcoma and also have considerably higher rates of non-Hodgkin's lymphomas. (See also Chapter 6.) Many of the latter are extranodal, often involving the brain. Reports of other tumors occurring in AIDS patients, including Hodgkin's lymphomas and hepatomas, may not represent causal relationships. The human T-cell leukemia viruses (HTLV-1 and HTLV-2), have been strongly implicated as causes of T-cell leukemias, particularly in some areas of Japan and the Caribbean that are endemic for these viruses, but these agents probably are of little current importance in the United States.

Estimates of the proportion of cancers in the United States that are caused by viruses depend on which cancers are included in the list of neoplasms for which sufficient evidence for a viral etiology exists. The nasopharyngeal carcinomas and Burkitt's lymphomas that have evidence of prior EBV infection, and the proportion of hepatomas that are HB_sAg positive, represent about 0.25% of all neoplasms in U.S. citizens. Adding the cervical cancer cases will account for another 3% of the cancer cases in the United States. If, in addition, 30% of the Hodgkin's disease cases are included, another 0.3% is added for a total of about 3.5%. The T-cell leukemias and the Kaposi's sarcomas and B-cell lymphomas in persons with AIDS also constitute a small proportion of all malignancies in the United States, although their contribution to the total cancer burden will rise in the future as the number of AIDS-related cancer increases.

There are no proven methods of preventing these neoplasms, but prospects for prevention by means of vaccines against the suspected viral causes are promising. An inactivated HBV vaccine was shown to prevent the development of the chronic HB_sAg carrier state in infants born to mothers who were carriers,[58] and a trial of an inactivated HSV-2 vaccine is being conducted. Efforts are under way to develop vaccines against EBV and HIV. Barrier methods of contraception may reduce rates of transmission of sexually transmitted agents and could theoretically help prevent cervical and AIDS-related cancers.

Infectious agents other than viruses probably are of little importance as causes of cancer in the United States and other developed countries. In tropical areas, bladder cancer has been related to infection with *Schistosoma hematobium* and the liver fluke *Clonorchis sinensis* may be a cause of hepatic angiosarcomas.

Nutrition. Reasons for the large international differences in the incidence of most cancers are unknown. They are not due to differences among countries in the frequency of any of the known causes of cancer mentioned previously. Studies of rates in migrants have clearly shown that they are largely due to variation in environmental factors, not in genetic predisposition or susceptibility to carcinogens. Correlational studies have been conducted to identify factors that vary among countries in accordance with variations in the rates of various cancers. These have shown a variety of dietary components to be related to a number of different neoplasms. To investigate these associations further, many case-control studies have been conducted, several cohort studies have been initiated in populations whose members have variable dietary habits (e.g., vegetarian and nonvegetarian Seventh Day Adventists and Japanese with varying amounts of Western food in their diets), a variety of laboratory investigations to elucidate possible mechanisms for observed epidemiological findings have been performed, and randomized trials of dietary supplements or modifications have been started or planned.

Epidemiological studies of diet and cancer are difficult for a variety of reasons. One common problem in all epidemiological approaches is that many individual dietary constituents are highly correlated. For example, diets that are poor in animal protein are also likely to be poor in animal fat and high in carbohydrates and fiber. Under such circumstances, it is difficult to determine which of the interrelated dietary constituents (if any) is responsible for observed variations in risk. Another difficulty is that diet many years prior to the development of a neoplasm may be of the greatest etiological relevance. Such information is difficult (although not impossible) to obtain in case-control studies. Cohort studies can theoretically overcome this problem but must use large numbers and must be continued for decades and hence require large commitments of time and money. Partly because of these methodological problems, it cannot be stated with certainty that any cancer is caused by any specific dietary component or deficiency. Much work in the field of nutrition and cancer is now being done, however, and results strongly suggest that dietary factors contribute to the etiology of a variety of neoplasms. Some of the more likely mechanisms are briefly summarized in the following paragraphs.

Food items may be contaminated by preformed carcinogens. Aflatoxins produced by fungi that can grow in grains and other crops in warm moist climates have been linked to liver cancers in some parts of the world. In China, mutagens have been detected in fermented pancakes and vegetable gruels, and these have been related to both esophageal cancer in humans and neoplasms of the gullet in chickens; and nasopharyngeal carcinomas have been related to consumption of salted fish and fermented food during infancy. Also, some reports have linked coffee, especially decaffeinated products, to bladder cancer, with chemicals used in the decaffeination process hypothesized to account for this possible association.

Food additives may be carcinogenic. Although the evidence is weak, artificial sweeteners in high doses may increase the risk of bladder cancer.

Carcinogens may be formed in the body by bacteria. Nitrites may be ingested in small amounts with preserved meats and fish or formed in larger quantities from dietary nitrates, either spontaneously before being eaten or in the presence of bacteria in the body; and carcinogenic *N*-nitroso compounds may then be produced from ingested amines and nitrites by bacteria in the stomach of people with atrophic gastritis, in the bladder of individuals with urinary tract infection, or in the normal colon and mouth, to produce cancers of the stomach, bladder, colon, and esophagus, respectively.

Smoked and cured foods, as well as charcoal-broiled meats and some fruits and vegetables from contaminated areas, may contain carcinogenic polycyclic aromatic hydrocarbons.

A high-fat diet may increase bile production and produce an environment in the large bowel conducive to the growth of bacteria capable of forming carcinogens, and perhaps steroid hormones, from bile salts. Production of such substance provides one plausible explanation for the observed associations between a high-fat diet and cancers of the colon, breast, and prostate.

Overnutrition, leading to obesity, has been associated with endometrial and postmenopausal breast cancers. A possible mechanism is tumor promotion by excess endogenous estrogens. In postmenopausal women, estrogens are derived from androgens produced by the adrenal gland. This reaction takes place in adipose tissue and is enhanced in obese women. Also, early menarche is a risk factor for breast cancer, and late menopause is a risk factor for both breast and endometrial cancers; and both of these factors have been directly or indirectly related to overnutrition.

Fibers in diet may increase the bulk of the bowel contents and dilute intraluminal carcinogens. They may also enhance transit time through the gut. Both mechanisms would reduce contact of the colonic mucosa with carcinogens and explain the inverse association between dietary fiber and the risk of colon cancer.

Dietary constituents may also protect against cancer. Diets high in fresh fruits and raw vegetables have been associated with decreased risks of carcinomas of virtually all sites within the gastrointestinal and respiratory systems, the uterine cervix, and (less consistently) other tissues. Retinol (preformed vitamin A) has also been associated with reduced risks of some epithelial cancers. The occurrence of many of the potentially protective micronutrients are highly correlated in human diets, making it difficult to determine which micronutrients are most strongly associated with reduced risks. For these reasons, the specific substances in fruits and vegetables responsible for the apparent protective effects have not been conclusively identified. It is likely that different micronutrients operate at different sites, and a variety of protective mechanisms have been suggested. For example, the reduced risks of stomach and esophageal carcinomas may be due to inhibition by vitamin C of *N*-nitroso compound formation; vegetables of the Brassicaceae family have been hypothesized to induce activity of mixed-function oxidases, which may detoxify ingested carcinogens responsible for colon cancer development; and vitamins C and E and β-carotene quench free radicals that can cause DNA damage and initiate carcinogenesis. β-Carotene has quite consistently been associated with a reduced risk of lung and other respiratory tract cancers, and randomized trials of supplemental β-carotene and synthetic retinols are being conducted in humans to determine whether such neoplasms can be prevented by these substances.

Although existing evidence is insufficient to implicate definitely any specific dietary constituent as a causative or protective factor in humans, the bulk of current knowledge suggests the elements of a prudent diet.[59,60] Compared to the average Western diet, a prudent diet would be lower in meats and animal fats and higher in fresh fruits, vegetables, and fiber. Citrus fruits with high levels of vitamin C and vegetables of the Brassicacae family and those rich in β-carotene would be of particular importance. Smoked, charred, or cured meats and artificial sweeteners would be avoided or used in moderation, as would alcoholic beverages. Caloric intake would be optimized to avoid obesity. This diet would do no harm, probably reduce the risk of cancers, and be compatible with diets advocated to reduce risks of cardiovascular and cerebrovascular diseases.

Reproductive Factors. Single women and, more specifically, nulliparous women, are at increased risk of cancers of the ovary, endometrium, and breast. The mechanisms involved are not understood but undoubtedly differ among the three cancers. Risk of ovarian and endometrial cancers decreases with the number of pregnancies, whereas pregnancies beyond the first have a lesser protective effective against breast cancer risk. Risk of breast cancer increases strongly with age at birth of first full-term child, but risks of ovarian and endometrial cancer probably do not.

Mechanisms for these associations are not fully understood but undoubtedly involve endogenous pituitary and ovarian hormones. The development of ovarian (epithelial) tumors is probably promoted by gonadotropin stimulation and reduced by suppression of gonadotropins during pregnancy. Nulliparous women may, on the average, be less fertile than parous women, have more anovulatory menstrual cycles, and hence more constant production of estrogens without cyclical progesterone each month. This relative excess of estrogens could promote endometrial tumor development. Several mechanisms for the relationship of breast cancer to age at birth of first child have been proposed, but none appears adequate. Studies of the endocrinological events associated with childbearing and other endocrinological studies in women at varying risks of cancers of endocrine target organs have been conducted, and others are in progress, to attempt to explain more fully the mechanisms by which factors related to childbearing alter risk.

The observed association of age at birth of first child with breast cancer, at least theoretically, suggests a mean of primary prevention. Women who have their first child before age 20 have approximately one third the risk of women whose first child is born when they are over 35. Other factors must obviously be considered when a woman decides to have a child, and it would be inappropriate to advise a woman to become pregnant at an early age solely to reduce her future risk of breast cancer. Women should be informed of the strong protective effect of an early first birth, however, so that this effect, along with other factors, can be considered when decisions to have children are made.

Genetic Factors. Comparisons of incidence rates among countries and in migrants have shown that environmental factors contribute to the development of a high proportion of cancers. "Environmental" is used, however, in the broadest sense simply to mean "not primarily genetically predetermined." This is not to imply that genetic factors do not also play an important role in the genesis of many, or even all, tumors. Some individuals exposed to known carcinogens develop cancer, and others with apparently identical exposure do not. This may well be due to differences in genetic susceptibility to carcinogens.

Some common cancers have been shown to aggregate in families. Carcinomas of the breast and prostate, for example, occur more commonly in the relatives of afflicted than unafflicted individuals. This could be due either to common genes or to similarities in environment, however, and no clear Mendelian mode of inheritance is evident for either of these tumors.

Some cancers do, however, tend to be associated with specific genetic traits. Malignant melanomas occur predominantly in light-skinned individuals with blond or red hair and blue eyes; stomach cancers occur more frequently in persons with type A blood; and risk of nasopharyngeal carcinoma is associated with certain histocompatibility antigens (directly with HLA-2 and inversely with SIN-2). There are also some rare, genetically determined conditions with which an increased risk of a specific cancer is clearly associated. Examples include familial polyposis and cancer of the colon, xeroderma pigmentosum and skin cancers, and Fanconi's and Bloom's syndromes and leukemia. In addition, there are some cancers that appear to be, in part, genetically inherited[20]; the chromosomal locations of genes for retinoblastoma and Wilms' tumor have been identified. One current line of inquiry is the study of genetically determined variations in the activity of various enzymes that may be involved in the metabolism of various environmental carcinogens.

In another current method of investigation, attempts are being made to link the occurrence of cancers in family members with a genetic marker. An example of this is an observation that in 11 high-risk families, breast cancer was found to segregate as an autosomal dominant with the enzyme glutamate-pyruvate transaminase.[61] This suggests that, in these families, the "breast cancer allele" is chromosomally linked to the locus for the enzyme. However, this linkage was not observed in other groups studied and may not be of relevance for the genesis of breast cancer. Linkage analysis is nonetheless a useful method for genetic studies of cancer that is likely to provide additional etiological clues in the future.

Considerable theoretical work in recent years has involved the development of mathematical models to explain hereditary and nonhereditary cancers in terms of somatic and germ cell mutations and the kinetics of stem cell growth.[20]

Summary of Known Causes and Preventive Measures. Table 47-5 summarizes estimates of the proportion of new cancer cases and cancer deaths in the United States that are most likely due to various causes. The actual percentages shown are obviously rough approximations only, but they serve to indicate where preventive efforts should be directed to achieve the greatest reduction in incident cases. Efforts to reduce all forms of tobacco use should receive the highest priority. Elimination of all tobacco products would, in time, prevent three times as many cancer deaths as the elimination of all other known causes of cancer combined.

TABLE 47-5. PERCENTAGE OF U.S. CANCER CASES AND DEATHS MOST PROBABLY ATTRIBUTED TO VARIOUS FACTORS

	New Cases		Total Cancer Deaths
	Male	**Female**	
Tobacco	30	10	30
Alcohol/tobacco	5	2	3
Occupation	5	2	4
Drugs	<1	<1	<1
Ionizing radiation[a]	1	1	1
Sunlight	10	10	2
Exogenous hormones	0	?	<1
Life-style[b]	35	55	50

[a] Excluding background radiation.
[b] Includes factors related to diet, reproduction, sexual behavior, and possible infectious agents.

A second important point demonstrated in Table 47-5 is that over one third of the cancers in men and over one half of those in women are most likely related to currently unidentified or unproven factors to which people are subjected as a result of their style of living. These include infectious agents and factors related to diet, reproduction, and sexual behavior. Prospects seem bright for ultimately preventing cancers by altering these life-style factors.

There is already much that can be done to prevent cancer. The following is a summary of actions that can be taken:

1. Urge all users of tobacco to stop using this substance in any form, and encourage all nonusers not to start (especially the young).
2. Advise use of alcohol in moderation, if at all, especially by smokers and ex-smokers.
3. Support efforts to reduce exposures to known carcinogens in the workplace.
4. Support efforts to identify and reduce exposures outside the workplace to known carcinogens, such as arsenic, vinyl chloride, and asbestos.
5. Avoid unnecessary use of drugs that are known or suspected to be carcinogenic.
6. Use diagnostic radiographs prudently.
7. Urge individuals to avoid excess exposure to sunlight, especially if they are light skinned and easily sunburned.
8. When estrogens are prescribed, use the lowest dose necessary to achieve the therapeutic objective.
9. Avoid giving estrogens to pregnant women.
10. Caution women that sexual promiscuity enhances their risk of cervical cancer. Suggest use of barrier contraceptives to reduce risk of infection.
11. Caution men that homosexual behavior is associated with anal cancer and AIDS, which can lead to Kaposi's sarcoma and other malignancies. Suggest use of condoms.
12. Suggest a diet lower in fats and meats and higher in fresh fruits, vegetables, and fiber than the average American diet is.
13. Urge obese individuals to lose weight and others not to become overweight.
14. Apprise women of the protective effect against breast cancer of an early first full-term pregnancy.

SCREENING AND SECONDARY PREVENTION

Secondary prevention is the prevention of progression of a disease to a fatal outcome by means of early detection followed by definitive treatment. Screening is one component of early detection, which in turn is one aspect of secondary prevention. Secondary prevention against a cancer can only be achieved if there is a stage of that cancer that is amenable to cure and if there is a means of detecting the cancer at that stage.

Planning a Screening Program. A number of factors must be considered before initiating a screening program[62,63]:

1. *The sensitivity and specificity of the tests or procedures used for screening:* The number of diseased people that will be missed (false negatives) increases as the sensitivity of the test decreases, and the number of well people that will erroneously be considered possibly diseased

(false positives) increases as the specificity of the test decreases. (See also Chapters 2 and 46.)

2. *The target population:* Individuals at highest risk for the disease should be identified, and special efforts should be made to screen such persons. For example, Table 47-6 shows the characteristics of women at high risk of cervical and breast cancer; obviously screening programs for breast and cervical cancer should be aimed at different women.
3. *The prevalence of the disease in the target population:* For any test of given sensitivity and specificity, numbers of false-positive and false-negative test results are functions of the prevalence of the disease in the target population. More false-negative tests result if the disease is common, and of particular importance in screening for cancers, more false-positive tests occur if the disease is rare.
4. *The predictive value of a positive test:* This is the proportion of individuals with a positive test who actually have the disease. This proportion declines only slightly as test sensitivity decreases but declines markedly as test specificity declines. In addition, the predictive value of a positive test declines as the prevalence of the disease diminishes. For example, if we have a test of high sensitivity (e.g., 95%) and high specificity (e.g., 98%) and if the prevalence of the cancer in the target population is 1 per 1000, then only 4.6% of the individuals with a positive test will actually be found to have the disease on further evaluation. The rest will have a false-positive test.
5. *The consequences of false-positive tests:* A false-positive test is a false alarm. The consequences of this for the individual, the medical care system, and the screening program must be considered. How much inconvenience or psychological trauma will the erroneously screened individual have to bear? Are there sufficient facilities and personnel to provide the necessary diagnostic tests to determine who actually has the disease? What are the costs of these services and who will pay them? Do physicians want to have referred to them large numbers of healthy people for diagnostic evaluation? Will possible adverse reactions to the screening program by those falsely screened positive or by their physicians have a negative impact on the screening program itself?
6. *Consequences of a false-negative test:* A false-negative test gives the person screened a false sense of security, and the neoplasm may then progress to a noncurable stage and kill the patient. This could have medical-legal implications, particularly if a more sensitive test could have been used. One missed case can result in unfavorable publicity that can have an adverse impact on the screening program.
7. *Applicability of the test:* Can the test be administered to the people in the target population? Are special equipment or special resources needed (e.g., electrical power, water, a mobile van, transportation for the potential screenees)? Can the test be administered rapidly?
8. *Acceptability of the test:* Having made the test available to people in the target population, will the people agree to be screened? What kind of publicity should be given? Are there esthetic or cultural barriers (e.g., aversion to testing feces for occult blood or having a pelvic examination)? Is the cost to those being screened acceptably low?
9. *Adverse consequences of the test:* Is there a possibility that the test will do harm? This issue had originally been a great concern in using mammography to screen for breast cancer. The breast is a radiosensitive organ, high doses of ionizing radiation are known to cause breast cancer, and early mammographic techniques resulted in considerable levels of exposure. This controversy had an adverse impact on breast cancer screening programs, with many women fearing mammography. Similar problems should be anticipated with any future radiographic screening techniques.
10. *The evaluability of the program:* Public and private resources are all too often spent on service programs that are never evaluated, and program evaluators are all too often called on to assist in program evaluation after a project is fully underway, or even completed. The time to begin program evaluation is when the program is being planned.

TABLE 47-6. CERVICAL AND BREAST CANCER

Characteristics of Women at High Risk	Target Populations for Screening Programs
▪ Cervical Cancer	
Ages 25-60 Low socioeconomic status Nonwhite	Some minority groups
Prison inmates Prostitutes	Prisons, brothels
Infectious diseases: Syphilis Gonorrhea *Trichomonas vaginalis* HPV HSV-2	Venereal disease clinics Persons with positive serologic test for syphilis
Unmarried mothers	Obstetric clinics
Induced abortions	Abortion facilities
Other indices of sexual promiscuity: Broken marriages Extramarital relations Multiple partners	Selected cultural groups
Early age at first intercourse	Selected cultural groups
Cervical squamous dysplasia	Women with dysplasia
▪ Breast Cancer	
Age over 40 High SES White Single Nulliparous Nuns Late age at birth of first child	Affluent neighborhoods Professional women
?Obesity	
Family history of breast cancer	Mothers, daughers, and sisters of cases
Benign breast disease	Women with prior benign breast lesions
Previous breast cancer	Women with prior breast cancer
Ionizing radiation	Women with radiation of the chest

Evaluation of Methods of Secondary Prevention. The aim of secondary prevention is the prevention of fatal outcome. This implies that a method of secondary prevention of a disease should reduce mortality from that disease, and reduction in mortality should be the measure used to evaluate the method. This is not always done. Two other forms of evaluation have commonly been used, both of which can give misleading results.

One of these is the comparison of cases detected at screening with cases detected by other means, with respect to their stage at diagnosis. It is certainly not surprising that those detected at screening tend to be at a less advanced stage. This does not tell whether the early detection altered the course of the disease, however. This method of evaluation is based on the assumptions that early lesions have the same natural history as symptomatic lesions and that treatment of early lesions alters the course of the disease. Neither assumption is necessarily correct. For example, not all carcinomas in situ of the uterine cervix progress to invasive disease, and individuals with early lung cancer detected at screening with chest radiographs do not have a more favorable prognosis than do persons with lung cancer diagnosed later after development of symptoms.

The other misleading method of evaluating secondary prevention is the comparison of survival rates, or time to death, in cases detected at screening and cases detected by other means. There are two problems with this method. One is that the time from diagnosis to death may be longer for individuals who have been screened, not because their death is postponed but only because their disease is diagnosed earlier. This is referred to as lead time. The other problem is known as length bias sampling and results from the fact that neoplasms grow at varying rates; at any point in time (when screening is performed) more tumors will be progressing slowly than are progressing rapidly. Therefore, compared to symptomatic cases, a higher proportion of tumors detected at screening will be slow growing, so the patient's survival from time of detection will tend to be longer, even if early detection does not result in a prolongation of time-to-death.

Because of the problems of lead time and length bias sampling, there is no way of knowing from a comparison of survival rates or times from diagnosis to death whether a secondary prevention program results in a prolongation of life. This can only be done by comparing risks of dying (or risks of advanced disease as a surrogate for mortality) in screened and unscreened individuals.

Individuals who volunteer to be screened may differ from those who do not with respect to factors related to risk of death, and these factors must be taken into consideration when comparing mortality rates in screened and unscreened persons. This can be done in two ways. It is preferable to conduct a randomized trial of the secondary prevention method to be evaluated. The other method is to control statistically for differences between the screened and unscreened during data analysis.

The best example of a randomized trial of a procedure for secondary prevention is the study of mammography conducted among members of the Health Insurance Plan (HIP) in New York.[64] In 1963, approximately 62,000 women between the ages of 40 and 64 were randomly allocated to one of two groups. Approximately half were offered a series of four annual screenings by mammography and breast palpation (the experimental group). The other half served as a control group and received their usual medical care. Not all women in the experimental group agreed to participate. To eliminate a possible bias due to the remainder being volunteers, the mortality rate from breast cancer in the entire experimental group was compared to the breast cancer mortality rate in the control group. Inclusion of those not screened in the experimental group gave a conservative estimate of the impact of the program on breast cancer mortality that represented a combined evaluation of the efficacy and the acceptability of the screening procedures. After 5 years of follow-up, in women 50 to 60 years old there was over a 50% reduction in mortality from breast cancer; and breast cancer mortality was reduced by one third in older women. Although there was no beneficial effect on breast cancer mortality in women under 50 years old after 5 years, follow-up for 18 years showed a reduction in mortality from breast cancer in these women also. This observation serves to demonstrate the importance of long-term follow-up in studies of secondary prevention.

Once a screening technique is accepted as being useful, regardless of the evidence for its usefulness, a randomized trial becomes ethically questionable and operationally impossible. Other less satisfactory methods of evaluation then must be used. This is exemplified by the Pap smear for early detection of cervical cancer. When this technique was first introduced, it was greeted with such enthusiasm that suggestions for a randomized trial were not taken. The need to evaluate this procedure subsequently became evident, but by then it was too late for a randomized trial. As a result, a large number of less satisfactory epidemiological studies have been conducted to attempt to measure the effectiveness of the Pap smear.[65] Fortunately, in this instance most studies provide evidence that use of the Pap smear does reduce mortality from cervical cancer. Correlational studies have shown that mortality rates from cervical cancer in many populations have declined following the introduction of screening programs, that the magnitude of the decline is correlated with the amount of screening, and that the decline within some of the populations was greatest in those racial and age groups that received the most screening. Case-control studies of women with invasive cervical cancer have shown that, compared to normal controls, fewer of the cases had prior Pap smears. A cohort study showed, after controlling for socioeconomic differences between women who enrolled in a screening program and women who did not, that there was a decline in cervical cancer mortality rates in the screened women compared to an increase in rates in those not screened. None of these methods to evaluate the Pap smear are as satisfactory as a randomized trial would have been, although in the aggregate they do provide strong evidence that the procedure reduces mortality.

The HIP study was a pioneer effort and has served as a model for the evaluation of a number of subsequently developed methods of early detection. Results from these more recent trials are either preliminary or not yet available. Screening procedures that are developed in the future should be subjected to similar randomized trials.

Current Status of Secondary Prevention of Selected Cancers. A variety of techniques has been developed for the early detection of neoplasms. Unfortunately, few have been rigorously evaluated, and some that have do not show great promise.

By the time a lung tumor is radiographically visible, it is usually inoperable. Preliminary results of a randomized trial of sputum cytology in smokers show no reduction in mortality in those screened.[66]

Studies in industrial settings of urinary cytology for bladder cancer have not yielded encouraging results, and cytology for oral cancer has not been evaluated adequately.

Barium swallow and radiography have been used in Japan to detect early stomach cancer. Survival has been found to be better in those detected at screening than in other cases, and mortality rates from stomach cancer decreased in those screened but not in the general population. No randomized trial has been completed, however.

Several methods to screen for colorectal cancer by measuring occult blood in stool have been developed, and randomized trials are being conducted. Preliminary results do not show a reduction in colorectal cancer mortality due to screening, and the predictive value of a positive test is very low (many false positives).

Self-examination for breast and testicular tumors and for skin cancers has been advocated but not subjected to rigorous evaluation. Because of the low prevalence of testicular tumors, programs to teach men testicular self-examination are not likely to prevent many deaths. Randomized trials of breast self-examination are currently being conducted.

With the exception of the HIP study, which evaluated a combination of mammography and breast palpation, physical examinations by physicians or trained auxiliary personnel to detect early cancer have not been rigorously evaluated. These include digital rectal examination for rectal and prostate cancer and sigmoidoscopy for colorectal cancer.

α-Fetoprotein (AFP) blood levels have been used to screen for primary hepatocellular carcinoma in individuals serologically positive for HB_sAg in areas where hepatitis B is endemic and liver cancer highly prevalent. A study from China showed improved survival in asymptomatic persons with small tumors detected by this method, but studies to determine whether it reduces mortality from liver cancer have not been completed.

Cancers of the breast and cervix are the only neoplasms that have been shown beyond reasonable doubt to be amenable to secondary prevention. There are, however, some unresolved issues regarding screening for these conditions. In 1989, results from studies of the secondary prevention of breast cancer were reviewed, and the existing recommendations by various organizations for mammographic screening were summarized.[67] It is generally believed that this type of screening is beneficial for women over age 50 and should be performed annually. Although evidence is now accumulating that mammographic screening is also beneficial for women under age 50, the magnitude of this effect may be smaller than for older women. Also, the cost per life saved is greater in younger women because the prevalence of breast cancer is much lower than in older women. Trials are being conducted to further evaluate the efficacy and efficiency of mammographic screening in women of various ages.

Results of a critical review of cytological screening for cervical cancer were published in 1986.[68,69] By combining data from 10 screening programs in eight countries, it was shown that two negative cytological smears were more effective than one in reducing mortality from cervical cancer (presumably because of a reduction in false-negative diagnoses) and that the protective effect did not decline until 3 years after a second negative smear. Based on these findings, it is generally believed that screening for cervical cancer every 3 years is sufficient, after a woman has had two normal smears. Some women, however, do develop invasive disease soon after an apparently normal smear, and studies are needed to determine what proportion of such events are a result of prior false-negative smears and how many (if any) represent a rapidly progressing form of the disease.

Part of the proposed strategy to achieve the NCI goal of reducing the mortality from cancer by 50% by the year 2000 includes intensified efforts to achieve more widespread use of breast and cervical cancer screening. Results of ongoing investigations will be of importance in developing appropriate strategies for maximizing the benefits of these intensified efforts.

REFERENCES

Classification Schemes

1. The International Classification of Diseases and Related Health Problems, 10th Revision. Geneva: World Health Organization, 1991 (in press)
2. World Health Organization: International Classification of Diseases for Oncology, 2 edt. Geneva: WHO, 1990

Cancer Statistics

3. Kurihara M, Aoki K, Tominaga S (eds): Cancer Mortality Statistics in the World. Nagoya, Japan: The University of Nagoya Press, 1984
4. Surveillance, Epidemiology, and End Results: Incidence and Mortality Data, 1973–77. National Cancer Institute Monograph 57, NIH Publication No. 81-2330. Bethesda, Maryland: National Cancer Institute, 1981
5. Cancer Mortality in the United States: 1950–1977. National Cancer Institute Monograph 59, NIH Publication No. 82-2435. Bethesda, Maryland: National Cancer Institute, 1982
6. Cancer Statistics Review 1973–1986. NIH Publication No. 89-2789, Bethesda, Maryland: National Cancer Institute, 1989
7. Muir C, Waterhouse J, Mack T, Powell J, Whelan S (eds): Cancer Incidence in Five Continents, Vol. V. IARC Scientific Publications No. 88, Lyon, France: International Agency for Research on Cancer, 1987
8. American Cancer Society: Cancer Facts and Figures. New York: American Cancer Society, 1989
9. Silverberg E, Lubera J: Cancer Statistics, 1989. New York: American Cancer Society, 1989
10. Hartunian NS, Smart CN, Thompson MC: The incidence and economic costs of cancers, motor vehicle injuries, coronary heart disease, and stroke: A comparative analysis. Am J Public Health 70:1249–1260, 1980
11. Horm JW, Sonik EJ: Person-years of life lost due to cancer in the United States, 1970 and 1984. Am J Public Health 79:1490–1493, 1989
12. Parkin DM, Laara E, Muir C: Estimates of the worldwide frequency of sixteen major cancers in 1980. Int J Cancer 41:184–197, 1988
13. Austin DF, Flannery J, Greenberg R, et al: The SEER Program, 1973–82. In Parkin DM, Stiller CA, Draper GJ, et al (eds): International Incidence of Childhood Cancer, IACR Scientific Publications No. 87, Lyon, France: International Agency for Research on Cancer, 1988, pp 101–107
14. Myers MH, Hankey BF: Cancer Patient Survival Experience. Trends in Survival 1960–63 to 1970–73. Comparison of Survival for Black and White Patients. U.S. Department of Health and Human Services, NIH Publication No. 80-2138. Washington, D.C.: U.S. Government Printing Office, 1980
15. Cancer Among Blacks and Other Minorities: Statistical Profiles. NIH Publication No. 86-2785. Bethesda, Maryland: National Cancer Institute, 1986
16. Thomas DB: Epidemiologic studies of cancer in minority groups in the western United States. Natl Cancer Inst Monogr 53:103–113, 1979
17. Miller RW, McKay FW: Decline in U.S. childhood cancer mortality, 1950 through 1980. JAMA 251:1567–1570, 1984
18. Greenwald P, Sondik EJ: Cancer Control Objectives for the Nation: 1985–2000. NIH Publication No. 86-2880. Washington, D.C.: U.S. Government Printing Office, 1986
19. The Cancer Letter, Vol. 16, No. 1, 1990
20. Moolgavkar SH, Knudson HG: Mutation and cancer: A model for human carcinogenesis. J Natl Cancer Inst 66:1037–1052, 1981
21. Hamlyn P, Sikora K: Oncogenes. Lancet, 2:326–330, 1983
22. Robertson M: Oncogenes and the origins of human cancer. Br Med J 286:81–82, 1983
23. Schottenfeld D, Fraumeni JF Jr (eds): Cancer Epidemiology and Prevention. Philadelphia: W.B. Saunders, 1991 (in press)
24. Office on Smoking and Health: The Health Consequences of Smoking: Cancer. A Report of the Surgeon General. U.S. Department of Health and Human Services. Washington, D.C.: U.S. Government Printing Office, 1982
25. The Health Consequences of Using Smokeless Tobacco. A Report of the Advisory Committee to the Surgeon General. NIH Publication No. 86-2874. Bethesda, Maryland: National Cancer Institute, 1986
26. Blott WJ, Fraumeni JF Jr: Passive smoking and lung cancer. J Natl Cancer Inst 77:993–1000, 1986
27. Schottenfeld D: Alcohol as a co-factor in the etiology of cancer. Cancer 43:1462–1466, 1979
28. Tamburro CH, Lee H: Primary hepatic cancer in alcoholics. Clin Gastroenterol 10:457–477, 1981
29. Thomas DB: Sinonasal, nasopharyngeal, oral, pharyngeal, laryngeal, and esophageal cancers: Epidemiology and opportunities for primary prevention. In Chretien PB, Johns MF, Shedd DP, et al (eds): Head and Neck Cancer, Vol. 1. Philadelphia and Toronto: BC Decker Inc., 1985, pp 585–591
30. Rothman KJ: The proportion of cancer attributable to alcohol consumption. Prev Med 9:174–179, 1980

31. International Agency for Research on Cancer: IARC Monographs on the Evaluation of the Carcinogenic Risks of Chemicals to Humans. Overall Evaluation of Carcinogenicity: An Updating of IARC Monographs Volumes 1 to 42. IARC Monographs Supplement 7. Lyon, France: IARC, 1987
32. Higginson J: Proportion of cancers due to occupation. Prev Med 9:180–188, 1980
33. Jablon S, Bailar JC III: The contribution of ionizing radiation to cancer mortality in the United States. Prev Med 9:219–226, 1980
34. Upton AC: The biological effects of low-level ioning radiation. Sci Am 246:41–49, 1982
35. Samet JM: Radon and lung cancer. J Natl Cancer Inst 81:745–757, 1989
36. Scotto J, Fears TR, Fraumeni JF Jr: Incidence of Non-melanotic Skin Cancer in the United States. U.S. Department of Health and Human Services, NIH Publication No. 83-2433. Washington, D.C.: U.S. Government Printing Office, 1983
37. Fears TR, Scotto J, Schneiderman MA: Skin cancer, melanoma, and sunlight. Am J Public Health 66:461–464, 1976
38. McGovern VJ: Epidemiological aspects of melanoma: A review. Pathology 9:233–241, 1977
39. Lee JAH: Epidemiology of malignant melanoma: 10 years' progress. In Mackie RM (ed): Pigment Cell Cancers. Basel: Karger, 1983, pp 1–21
40. Holman CDJ, Armstrong BK, Heenan PJ, et al: The causes of malignant melanoma: Results from the West Australian Lions Melanoma Research Project. Recent Results Cancer Res 102:18–37, 1986
41. Herbst AL, Ulfelder H, Poskanzer DC: Adenocarcinoma of the vagina: Association of maternal stilbestrol therapy with tumor appearance in young women. N Engl J Med 284:878–881, 1971
42. Weiss NS: Epidemiology of endometrial cancer. In Lilienfeld AM (ed): Reviews in Cancer Epidemiology, Vol. 2. New York: Elsevier, 1983
43. Prentice RL, Thomas DB: On the epidemiology of oral contraceptives and disease. Adv Cancer Res 49:285–401, 1987
44. Thomas DB: The breast. In Michal F (ed): Safety Requirements for Steroid Contraceptives. Cambridge and New York: Cambridge University Press, 1989, pp 38–68
45. Thomas DB: Steroid hormones and medications that alter cancer risks. Cancer 62:1755–1767, 1988
46. World Health Organization: Facts about injectable contraceptives: Memorandum from a WHO meeting. Bull WHO 60:199–210, 1982
47. Paul C, Skegg DCG, Spears GFS: Depo-medroxyprogesterone (depo-provera) and risk of breast cancer. Br Med J 299:759–762, 1989
48. Stern E, Forsyth AB, Youkeles L, et al: Steroid contraceptive use and cervical dysplasia: Increased risk of progression. Science 190:1460–1462, 1977
49. Barrows GH, Christopherson WM: Human liver tumors in relation to steroidal usage. Environ Health Perspect 50:201–208, 1983
50. Palmer RJ, Rosenberg L, Kaufman DW, et al: Oral contraceptive use and liver cancer. Am J Epidemiol 130:878–882, 1989
51. The WHO Collaborative Study of Neoplasia and Steroid Contraceptives: Combined oral contraceptives and liver cancer. Int J Cancer 43:254–259, 1989
52. Evans A: Viruses. In Schottenfeld D, Fraumeni JF Jr (eds): Cancer Epidemiology and Prevention. Philadelphia: W.B. Saunders, 1982, pp 364–390
53. Gutensohn N, Cole P: Epidemiology of Hodgkin's disease. Semin Oncology 7:92–102, 1980
54. Arthur MJP, Hall AJ, Wright R: Hepatitis B, hepatocellular carcinoma, and strategies for prevention. Lancet 1:607–610, 1984
55. Melnick JL, Rawls WE, Adam E: Cervical cancer. In Evans AS (ed): Viral Infections of Humans: Epidemiology and Control, 3 edt. New York: Plenum Medical Book Co., 1989, pp 687–711
56. Koutsky LA, Galloway DA, Holmes HK: Epidemiology of genital human papillomavirus infection. Epidemiol Rev 10:122–163, 1988
57. ZurHausen H: Human genital cancer: Synergism between two virus infections or synergism between a virus infection and initiating events. Lancet 2:1370–1372, 1982
58. Beasley RP, Lee GC, Roan CH, et al: Prevention of perinatally transmitted hepatitis B virus infections with hepatitis B immune globulin and hepatitis B vaccine. Lancet 2:1099–1102, 1983
59. Graham S: Toward a dietary prevention of cancer. Epidemiol Rev 5:38–50, 1983
60. Palmer S: Diet, nutrition, and cancer: The future of dietary policy. Cancer Res (suppl) 43:2509s–2524s, 1983
61. King MC, Go RCP, Elston RC, et al: Allele increasing susceptibility to human breast cancer may be linked to the glutamate-pyruvate transaminase locus. Science 208:406–408, 1980
62. Lilienfeld AM: Some limitations and problems of screening for cancer. Cancer 33(suppl):1720–1724, 1974
63. Cole P, Morrison AS: Basic issues in population screening for cancer. J Natl Cancer Inst 64:1263–1272, 1980
64. Shapiro S: Statistical evidence for mass screening for breast cancer and some remaining issues. Cancer Detect Prev 1:347–363, 1976
65. Guzick DS: Efficacy of screening for cervical cancer: A review. Am J Public Health 68:125–134, 1978
66. Levin ML, Tockman MS, Frost JK, et al: Lung cancer mortality in males screened by chest x-ray and cytologic sputum examination: A preliminary report. Recent Results Cancer Res 82:138–146, 1982
67. Council on Scientific Affairs: Mammographic screening in asymptomatic women ages 40 years and older. JAMA 261:2535–2542, 1989
68. Hakama M, Miller AB, Day NE: Screening for Cancer of the Uterine Cervix. IARC Scientific Publication No. 76. Lyon, France: International Agency for Research on Cancer, 1986
69. IARC Working Group on Evaluation of Cervical Cancer Screening Programmes: Screening for squamous cervical cancer: Duration of low risk after negative results of cervical cytology and its implication for screening policies. Br Med J 293:659–664, 1986

48

Heart Disease

Henry Blackburn
Russell Luepker

Cardiovascular diseases (CVD) are important public health concerns around the world, particularly coronary or ischemic heart disease (CHD), hypertensive heart disease, and rheumatic heart disease. CHD remains the leading cause of adult death in industrial societies, although its incidence differs widely and the mortality ascribed to it is changing dramatically (Figs. 48–1 and 48–2). While deaths from CHD are rising in many populations, they are falling in others. The decline of age-adjusted U.S. deaths ascribed to CHD continues through 1986, for men and women, white and nonwhite (Fig. 48–3). Although causes of the decline are not precisely established, much is now known about U.S. trends in out-of-hospital deaths, in-hospital case fatality, and longer term survival after myocardial infarction.[1] Parallel to the CHD mortality trends are improvements in medical diagnosis and treatment, in population levels of risk factors, and in lifestyle.[2] Nevertheless, the critical explanatory data, including incidence trends from representative populations, are few. This deficiency, along with the difficulty of measuring change in diagnostic custom and in severity of CHD, or of its precursor, atherosclerosis, leaves considerable uncertainty about the causes of the mortality trends. Systematic surveillance is now in place in many countries to improve the future detection, prediction, and explanation of trends in CVD rates.[1–4]

Deaths ascribed to hypertensive heart disease have diminished over recent decades in many industrialized countries.[5] In West Africa, Latin America, and the Orient, however, the high prevalence still found in hospitals and clinics indicates the continued worldwide importance of hypertension.

Rheumatic fever and rheumatic valvular heart disease remain public health concerns in many developing countries and are still seen among disadvantaged peoples in affluent nations. On the other hand, syphilitic heart disease, a world-wide scourge until the 1940s, is now rare. Cardiomyopathies, often of unknown or infectious origin, constitute a common cause of heart disease in many regions, including Africa and Latin America. Finally, congenital heart disease continues to contribute to the heart disease burden among youth and adults of all countries.

The worldwide potential for primary prevention of most CVD is established by several salient facts: (1) the large population differences in CVD incidence and death rates; CVD is rare in many countries; (2) dynamic national trends in CVD deaths, both upward and downward; (3) rapid changes in CVD risk among migrant populations; (4) the identification of modifiable risk characteristics for CVD among and within populations; and (5) the generally positive results of preventive trials. There is much evidence that the risk of whole populations, as opposed to individual risk, is predominantly determined by mass sociocultural characteristics, which are in turn subject to change and to public policy.

CORONARY HEART DISEASE

CHD remains the leading cause of adult deaths in many industrial societies. Much knowledge about its causes and prevention has been derived from all research methods, including clinicopathological observations, laboratory-experimental studies, population studies, and clinical trials. The evidence of causation from all these disciplines is largely congruent. As a result, several ubiquitous cultural characteristics described below are now established as powerful influences on population risk of CHD. These influences and risk factors appear to be safely modifiable, for individuals and for entire populations.[1,6–9]

The sum of evidence suggests that there is widespread human susceptibility to atherosclerosis and, consequently, that CHD is maximally exhibited when the environment is unfavorable. These ubiquitous susceptibilities, exposures, and behaviors lead eventually to the mass precursors of CHD found among so many people in high-incidence societies. The rationale and the potential for preventive practice, as well as for public policy in prevention, are based on several well-established relationships: between risk factor levels and CHD, between health behaviors and risk factor levels, and between culture and mass behaviors.

Epidemiology

We summarize here what we consider to be the salient epidemiological observations about CHD:

- Population comparisons show large differences in CHD incidence and mortality rates (Fig. 48–1) and in the extent of its underlying vascular disease, atherosclerosis.
- Population differences in the mean levels and distributions of CHD risk characteristics (particular blood lipoprotein levels) are strongly correlated ecologically with population differences in CHD rates.
- Within populations, several risk characteristics (blood cholesterol and blood pressure levels and smoking habits)

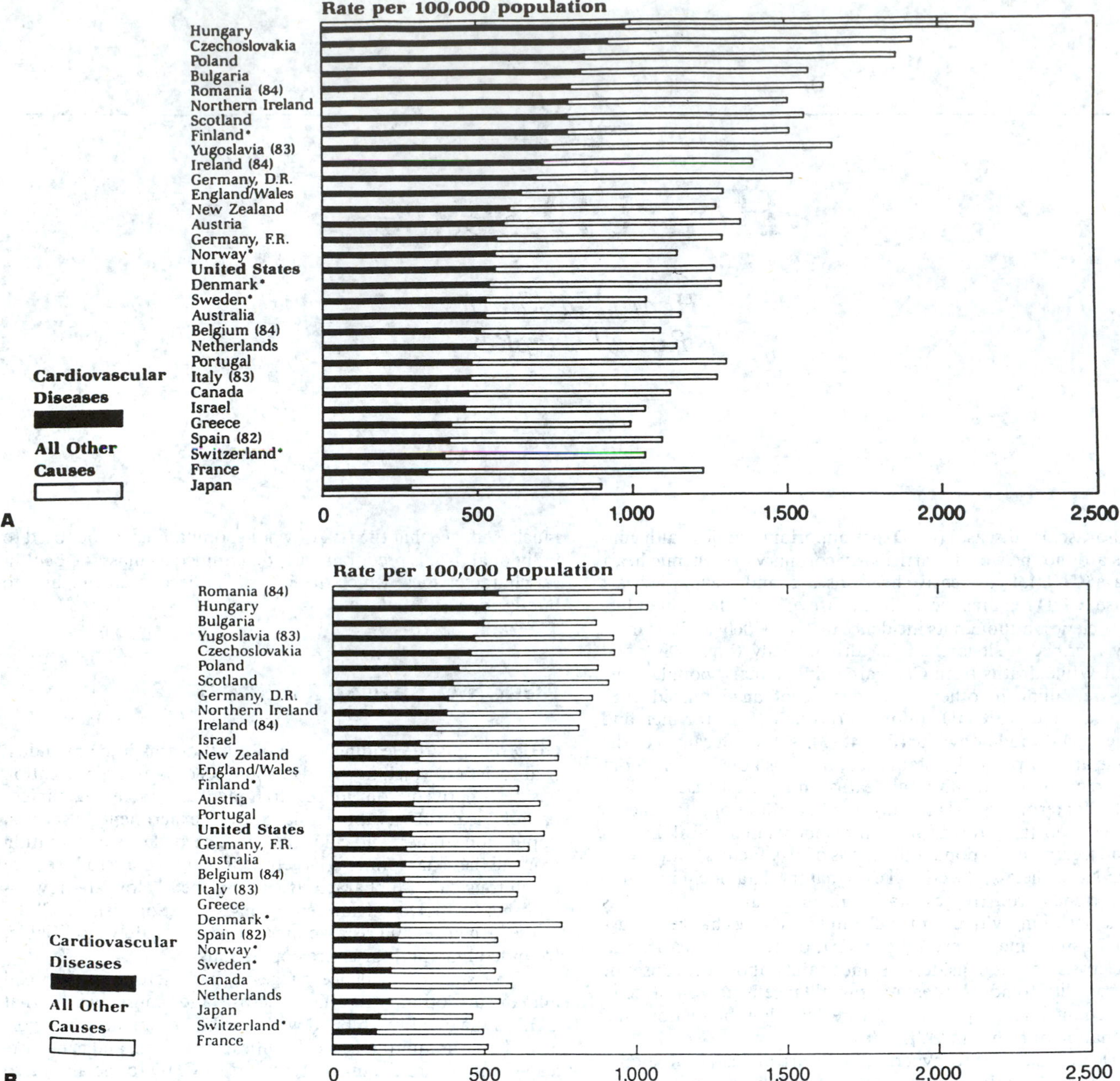

Figure 48–1. Death rate for all causes and cardiovascular diseases in men (**A**) and women (**B**) 35 to 74 years of age in selected countries, 1985. Note: ICD/9 390-459 for cardiovascular disease except as noted. Rates are adjusted to the European standard population. ICD/8 390-458 for cardiovascular disease. *(From World Health Organization.)*

are strongly and continuously related to future individual risk of a CHD event.

- Population differences in average levels of CHD risk characteristics are already apparent in youth. Individual values of children tend to "track" into adult years.
- CHD risk characteristics and incidence in migrants rapidly approach levels of the adopted culture.
- Trends in CHD mortality rates, both upward and downward, occur over relatively short periods of 5 to 10 years. These trends tend to be associated with changes in medical care and case-fatality rates as well as with trends in incidence and in population distributions of risk characteristics.
- The recent decrease in age-adjusted CHD mortality rates in the United States is shared by men and women, by whites and nonwhites, and by younger and older age groups (Fig. 48–4).
- The decrease in age-adjusted CHD mortality rates in the United States is associated with an even greater decrease in death rates from stroke and from all CVD. Moreover, in the last decades there has been a significant but lesser decrease in *non*-CVD deaths and in deaths from all causes (Fig. 48–5).
- Randomized clinical trials find a direct effect of CHD risk factor lowering on subsequent disease rates. Preventive trials also establish that levels of risk factors, and their associated health behaviors, can be significantly and safely modified.

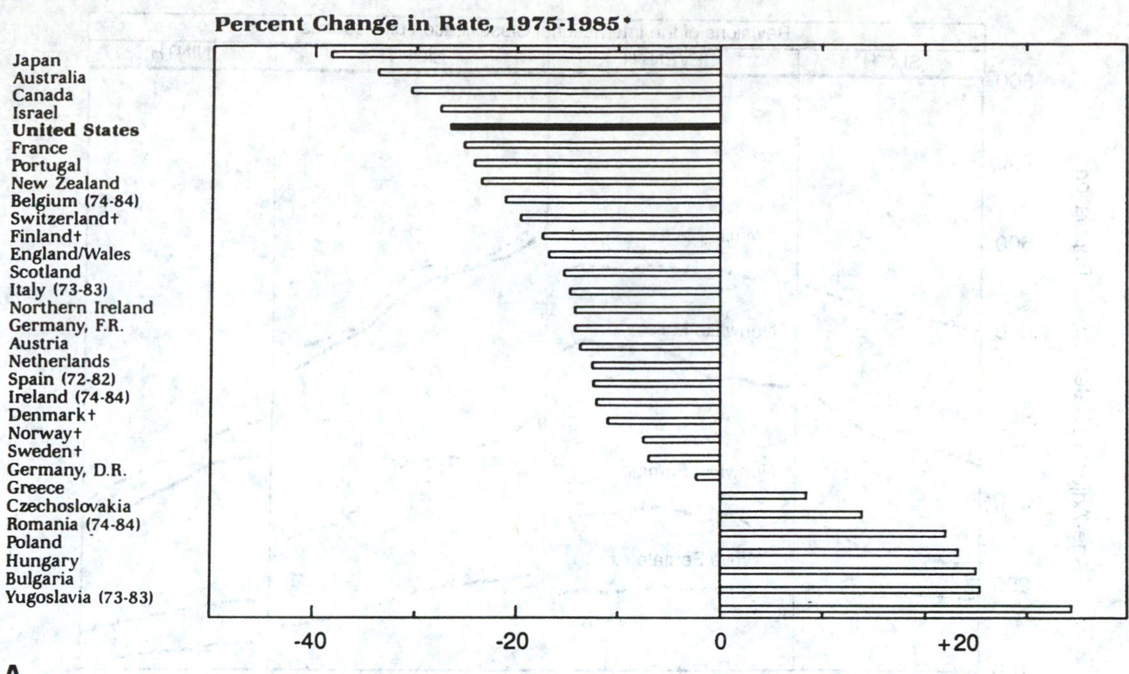

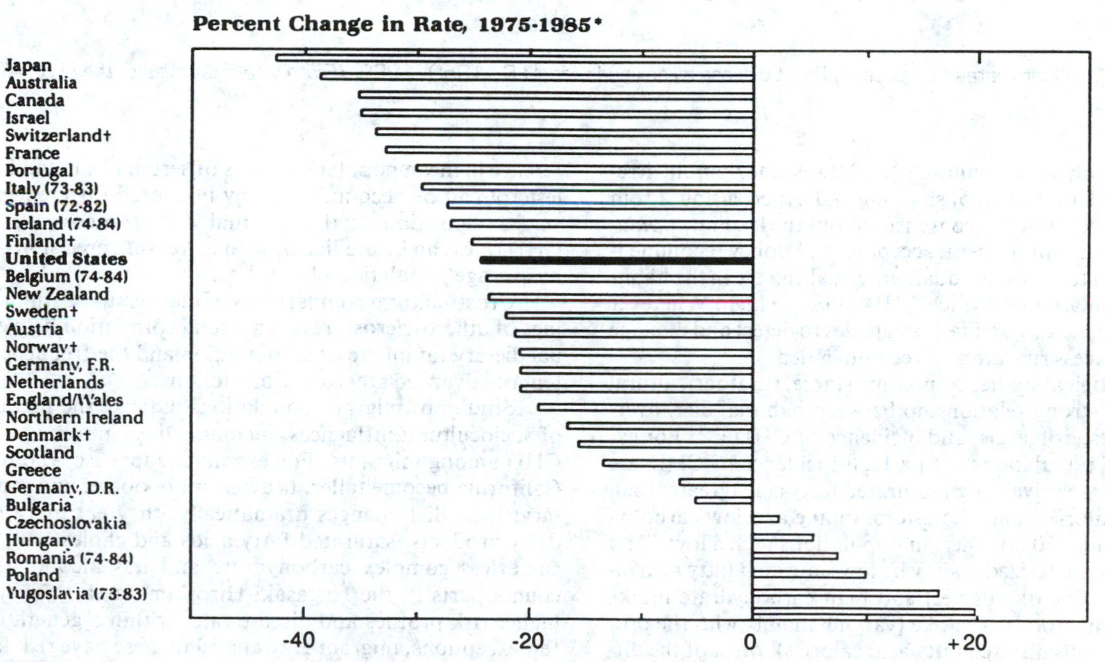

Figure 48–2. Percent change in the death rate for cardiovascular disease in men [**A**] and women [**B**] 35 to 74 years of age in selected countries, 1975–1985. Based on rates age-adjusted to the European standard population. Year range may vary as indicated. Eighth Revision of ICD for both years. *[From World Health Organization.]*

- The epidemiological evidence is generally congruent with clinical and laboratory findings about the causes and mechanisms of atherosclerosis, the process that underlies the clinical manifestations of CHD.

Diet

Diet-Disease Relationships Among Populations. There is much evidence that habitual diet in populations, a culturally determined characteristic, has an important influence on the mean levels and distribution of blood lipoproteins and, therefore, on the *population* risk and potential for prevention of CHD. Several dietary factors influence individual and population levels of low-density lipoproteins (LDL) in the blood, a leading pathogenetic factor in atherosclerosis. These include particular fatty acids and dietary cholesterol, the complex carbohydrates of starches, vegetables, fruits and their fibers, alcohol, and caloric excess. Many investigators consider that the cholesterol-raising properties of some habitual diets are essential to the development of mass atherosclerosis, leading in turn to high rates of CHD. Where average total blood cholesterol level in a population is

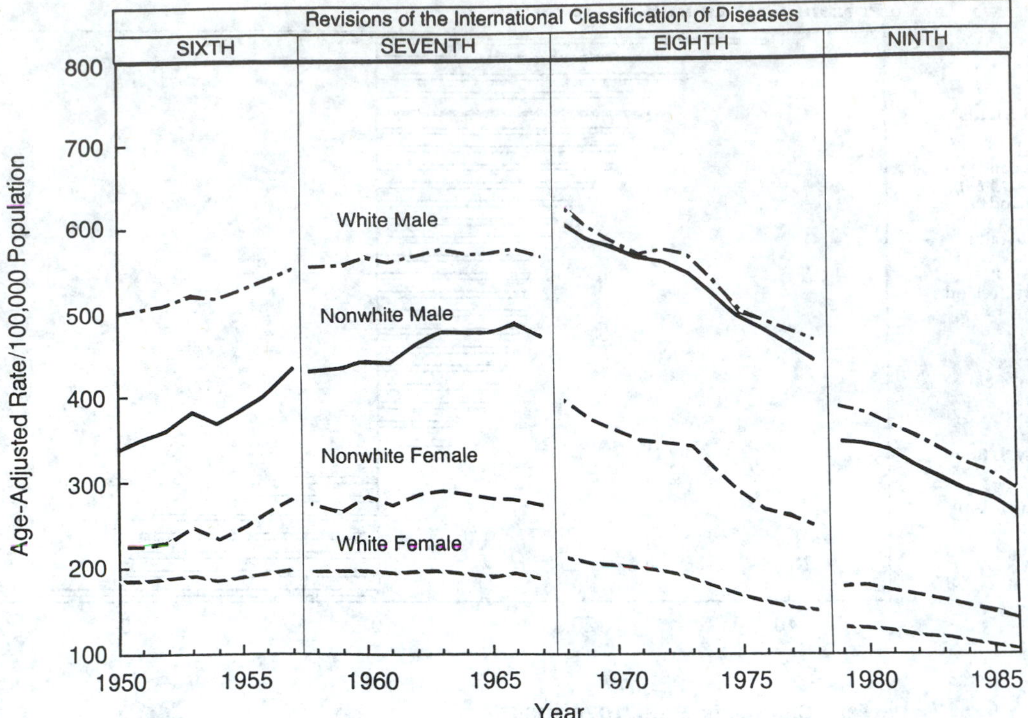

Figure 48–3. Death rates for coronary heart disease by sex and race, U.S., 1950–1986. *[From Vital Statistics of the U.S., NCHS.]*

low (<200 mg/dl, or 5.2 mmol/L), CHD is uncommon, irrespective of population levels of smoking and hypertension. From this evidence, there is now a consensus about the leading *population* causes of CHD and general acceptance of policy recommendations that lead toward a gradual, universal change in the habitual diets of populations in which CHD rates are high. Wherever economically feasible, systematic strategies to detect and manage individuals at excess risk are also recommended.

Epidemiological studies comparing stable, rural agricultural societies find a strong relationship between habitual diet, average blood cholesterol levels, and incidence of CHD.[10-12] For example, diets of populations with a high incidence of CHD are characterized by relatively high saturated fatty acid (greater than 15% of daily calories) and cholesterol intake and low carbohydrate intake (under 50%). Diets in populations with a low CHD incidence are characterized mainly by low saturated fatty acid intake (less than 10% of calories) and high carbohydrate intake but widely varying total fat intake (varying mainly with the proportion of monounsaturated fatty acid calories). Most of the difference in mean population levels of serum total (and LDL) cholesterol can be accounted for by measured differences in fatty acid composition of the habitual diet. Moreover, *population* CHD rates can be predicted, with increasing precision over time, by average population blood cholesterol levels.[13]

Cross-cultural comparisons of diet versus postmortem findings of atherosclerosis reveal a strong correlation between habitual dietary fat intake of a population and the frequency and extent of advanced atherosclerotic lesions.[14]

Studies of migrant populations indicate the predominance of sociocultural influences, including diet, in trends of risk and CHD among migrants. For example, Japanese who migrate to California become taller, heavier, more obese, and more sedentary; their diet changes dramatically; they eat more meat and dairy products, saturated fatty acids and cholesterol, and consume less complex carbohydrate and less alcohol than their counterparts in the Nagasaki-Hiroshima area.[15] They develop higher risk profiles and disease rates within a generation. With few exceptions, migrant Hawaiian Japanese have risk factor val-

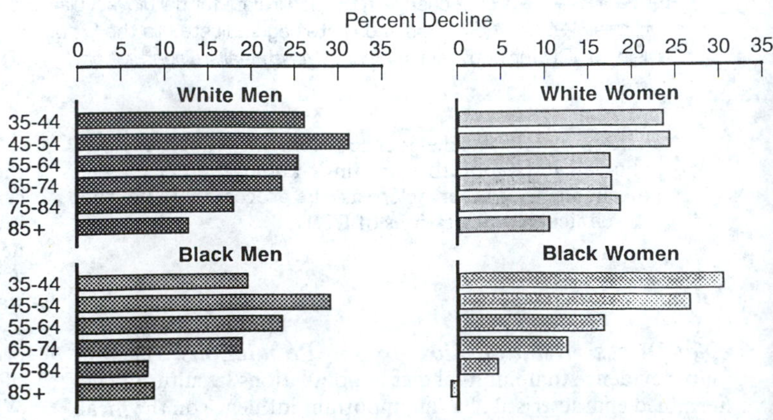

Figure 48–4. Percent decline in CHD death rates by age, race, and sex, U.S., 1979–1986. *[From Vital Statistics of the U.S., NCHS.]*

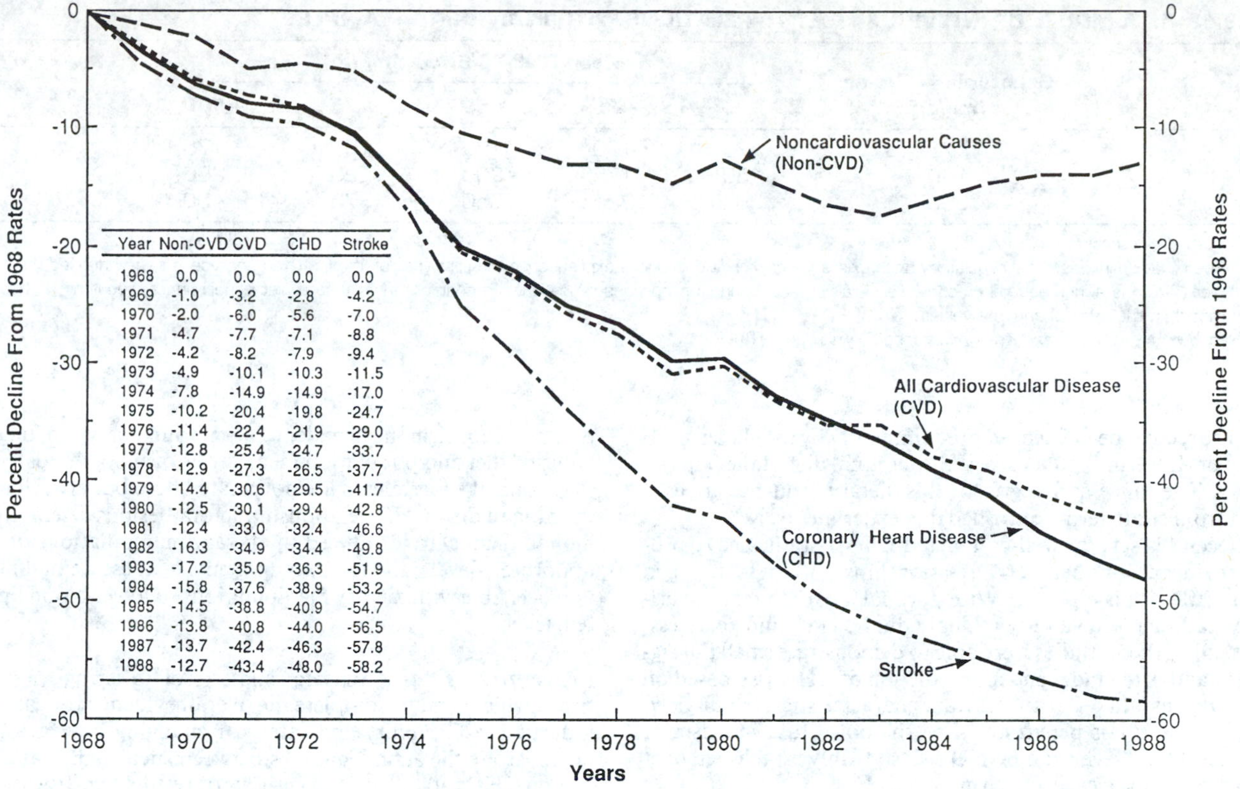

Year	Non-CVD	CVD	CHD	Stroke
1968	0.0	0.0	0.0	0.0
1969	-1.0	-3.2	-2.8	-4.2
1970	-2.0	-6.0	-5.6	-7.0
1971	-4.7	-7.7	-7.1	-8.8
1972	-4.2	-8.2	-7.9	-9.4
1973	-4.9	-10.1	-10.3	-11.5
1974	-7.8	-14.9	-14.9	-17.0
1975	-10.2	-20.4	-19.8	-24.7
1976	-11.4	-22.4	-21.9	-29.0
1977	-12.8	-25.4	-24.7	-33.7
1978	-12.9	-27.3	-26.5	-37.7
1979	-14.4	-30.6	-29.5	-41.7
1980	-12.5	-30.1	-29.4	-42.8
1981	-12.4	-33.0	-32.4	-46.6
1982	-16.3	-34.9	-34.4	-49.8
1983	-17.2	-35.0	-36.3	-51.9
1984	-15.8	-37.6	-38.9	-53.2
1985	-14.5	-38.8	-40.9	-54.7
1986	-13.8	-40.8	-44.0	-56.5
1987	-13.7	-42.4	-46.3	-57.8
1988	-12.7	-43.4	-48.0	-58.2

Figure 48–5. Percent decline in CVD and non-CVD mortality U.S., 1968–1988.

ues intermediate between mainland and California Japanese, and the CHD rate in migrants generally parallels their mean values for risk factor levels.

The rapid national trends in CHD deaths are another indication of the predominance of culture in the population causes and prevention of CHD. Nevertheless, systematic explanatory studies of trends in CHD mortality are very recent, and current attempts to estimate the relative contribution of cultural versus medical care contributions are quite tentative.[1-3,16,17] In a number of countries on an upward slope of CHD mortality, smoking and calorie and fat consumption are increasing and physical activity is decreasing, while cardiological practice is probably becoming less effective. In many other industrial countries, including the United States, decreasing CHD mortality rates parallel improved cardiac care and significant reductions in average risk characteristics.[1,2,16,18,19] Standardized measurements of risk and disease trends are not generally available for comparisons among countries, but the public health implications of these simultaneous trends in behaviors, risk, disease rates, and medical care appear to be immense.

Another feature of diet, the relative excess of calorie intake over expenditure, influences health through the metabolic maladaptations of hyperlipidemia, hyperinsulinism, and hypertension. This caloric imbalance occurs in sedentary cultures and results in mass obesity. With or without mass obesity, however, high salt intake and low potassium intake in populations appear to encourage the wide exhibition of hypertensive phenotypes. Other cations (e.g., magnesium, calcium) may also be significant dietary influences on population levels of blood pressure, while alcohol intake is clearly involved (see below).

Anthropological Aspects of Diet. Anthropology and paleontology provide insights into the probable effects of rapid cultural change, including modern diets, from the life-style to which humans adapted during earlier periods of evolution. Until 500 or so generations ago, all humans were hunters-gatherers. The habitual eating pattern very likely involved alternating scarce and abundant calories and a great variety of foods. It surely included lean wild game and usually a predominance of plant over animal calories, a relatively low sodium and high potassium intake, and of course there was universal breast feeding of infants. Observations of the eating patterns among extant hunter-gatherer tribes confirm the varied nature and the adequacy (or near adequacy) of such an eating pattern for growth and development, as well as for the potential of longevity and the absence of mass phenomena such as atherosclerosis and hypertension.[20-23] Although modern humans can scarcely return to such subsistence economies, the anthropological observations suggest that current metabolic maladaptations derived from affluent eating and exercise patterns imposed rapidly on a very different evolutionary legacy, result in the mass precursors of cardiovascular diseases found in modern society.[22]

Diet-Disease Relationships Within Populations. Despite the generally strong population (ecological) correlations between diet, blood lipid levels, and CHD rates, these correlations are often absent for individuals within high-risk industrial societies.[24] This apparent paradox does not negate the causal importance of diet in mass hypercholesterolemia and atherosclerosis. Consider, for example, the simple additive model of Table 48–1, which suggests the powerful influence, in the individual, of inherent lipid regulation. Different individual lipoprotein genotypes may develop widely different adult risk phenotypes and different serum cholesterol levels, while consuming the same U.S. type diet. Other individuals may have similar blood cholesterol levels while subsisting on very different diets. In contrast, the population model of Table 48–2 makes the assumption that the multiple genes that influence lipid metabolism are randomly and similarly distributed throughout large heterogeneous populations. Under this condition, population means and distributions of blood

TABLE 48-1. A MODEL OF INDIVIDUAL DIET-TC RELATIONS WITH INDIVIDUAL EXAMPLES

Genotypic TC Value (mg/dl)	Mean Diet-TC Effect (mg/dl)				
	0	+25	+50	+75	+100
75	75	100	125	150	175
150	150	175	200	225	250
300	300	325	350	375	400

TC = serum cholesterol.
It is assumed that an intrinsic lipid regulatory base exists for each individual and is expressed in the first year of life. On this genotype is superimposed the effect of habitual diet, which is either neutral or cholesterol-raising according to properties determined in controlled Minnesota diet experiments, resulting, in this simple additive model, in the adult phenotype values.
From Blackburn H, 1979,[25] and Keys A, Grande F, Anderson JT, 1974.[27]

lipids are seen to be influenced predominantly by the cholesterol-raising or -lowering properties of the habitual diet of the population.[25,26] The range and degree of this dietary influence are estimated from short-term controlled diet experiments.[27-29]

Recently, several well-conducted cohort studies have provided evidence of diet-CHD relationships within societies in which CHD risk is high.[30-33] With particular care to reduce variability and increase validity of individual dietary intake assessments, all of these studies were able to demonstrate small but significant and often independent prediction of CHD risk based on entry nutrient intake or other dietary characteristics. In our view, this evidence is less persuasive than the powerful synergism of diet, blood lipid levels, and CHD risk so firmly established over 30 years, but it is clearly confirmatory.[34]

With this logic, habitual diet has come to be considered the *necessary* factor in mass hypercholesterolemia and, thus, in the mass atherosclerosis that leads to high rates of CHD. The population data are, however, equally compatible with another idea, that *all three* of the major risk factors (i.e., elevated population averages of blood cholesterol, blood pressure, *and* smoking) are essential for a high population burden of CHD.

Congruence of Evidence about Diet. The relationship of habitual diet to population levels of blood lipids and blood pressure, and to CHD and CVD rates, is largely congruent with clinical and experimental observations. First, experimental modification of diet has a predictable effect on group blood lipid levels. When calories and weight are held constant in controlled diet experiments and diet composition is varied, the largest dietary contributions to serum total and LDL cholesterol level are (1) the proportion of calories consumed as saturated fatty acids, (2) dietary cholesterol, both of which raise cholesterol levels, and (3) polyunsaturated fatty acids, which have a cholesterol-lowering effect. Monounsaturates are probably neutral in that they appear to have no *specific* cholesterol-lowering effect when carbohydrate intake is used as the reference level.[27-29,34] These clinical experiments confirm the broader relation found between long-term habitual diet and population mean levels of blood lipids.[10,11]

Animal experiments are not treated here but are relevant to the human diet–CHD relationship in that lesions resembling the human plaque are produced by dietary manipulations of blood lipoprotein levels; the fatty components of these animal plaques are reversible with dietary manipulations to lower blood lipoprotein levels.

Preventive Trials. Plasma cholesterol–lowering preventive trials, which tend to complete the overall evidence for causation, indicate the feasibility and safety of changing risk factors and demonstrate the actual lagtimes between such change and its effect on CHD rates.[34,35] The synthesis of results of *all* these trials[34] and their implications for the public health are central because carrying out the "definitive diet-heart trial" is not considered feasible. Therefore, experimental "proof" of the role of diet in the primary prevention of CHD is not likely to be established.

Lipid-lowering trials demonstrate that substantial lowering of blood lipid levels is feasible, that the progress of arterial lesions is arrested, and that CHD morbidity and mortality are reduced, all in proportion to the cholesterol lowering achieved and its duration. These trials, carried out mainly in middle-aged men with moderately elevated blood lipids, have usually involved cholesterol-lowering medication *plus* diet. However, because they specifically tested the cholesterol-lowering hypothesis and because their effects are congruent with the observational evidence cited here in support of that hypothesis, these experimental findings have been extrapolated by many authorities to the potential for prevention in the broader population, including women, younger age groups, and those with lower lipid and risk levels.[34] Many consider, also, that the results of randomized clinical trials, because of their congruence with the other evidence, may be extrapolated to the larger public health, including the potential for CHD prevention by long-term change in eating patterns of the population as a whole, and, finally, to the prevention

TABLE 48-2. A MODEL OF POPULATION DIET-TC RELATIONSHIPS WITH POPULATION EXAMPLES

	Mean Diet-TC Effect (mg/dl)				
	Japan 0	Greece +25	Italy +50	U.S. +75	Finland +100
Population mean TC	150	175	200	225	250
Lower limit (2.5%)	75	100	125	150	175
Upper limit (97.5%)	225	250	275	300	325

In this oversimplified model, it is assumed that uncommon single gene effects and widespread polygenic determinants of blood cholesterol levels are randomly and usually distributed among large heterogeneous populations, such that a mean population TC value of 150 mg/dl would prevail (SD ± 37.5 mg/dl) in the presence of an habitual average diet having neutral properties in respect to cholesterol. On this mean and population distribution of intrinsic responsiveness is superposed the average habitual diet effect for a population, which is either neutral or cholesterol-raising according to the country's measured diet composition and properties, determined in controlled Minnesota diet experiments, resulting in these population means.
From Keys A, Grande F, Anderson JT, 1974,[27] and Keys, 1970[10]

of elevated risk in the first place. Because the intervention trials have concentrated on one or two risk factors only, in a disease that has multiple causal influences, because they have been carried out in middle-aged subjects with respect to a disease that develops over decades, and because they have been performed only in the fraction of the adult population at highest risk, we estimate that cholesterol lowering across the *entire* population will have a greater influence than that found in clinical trials, where it nevertheless appears relatively safe and effective within a very few years.[34,35]

Dietary Protein. International vital statistics on deaths correlated with national food-consumption data indicate that, as with fat consumption, strong ecologic correlations exist between animal protein intake and death rates from CHD, but there is little evidence that this association is causal.[34] Anitschkow[36] found originally that it was dietary lipid rather than protein that resulted in hyperlipidemia and atherosclerosis in his experimental rabbits. Controlled metabolic ward studies in men under isocaloric conditions, with fat intake held constant while protein intake was varied between 5% and 20% of daily calories, found no change in blood cholesterol level (unpublished data, Laboratory of Physiological Hygiene, University of Minnesota).

Renewed interest in protein effects has developed, however, from reports that substitution of soybean for animal protein in the diets of hypercholesterolemic persons enhances the cholesterol-lowering effect of a low-fat diet.[34] Repetition of these experiments is needed, with careful control of other nutrients and of body weight.

In our view, neither clinical, experimental, nor epidemiological evidence is now sufficient to attribute a *specific* effect of dietary protein on either blood lipid levels or CHD risk. The overall importance of the consumption of meats from domesticated animals and of fatty milk products is therefore thought to rest mainly in their saturated fatty acid content rather than their protein content, at least with respect to CHD risk.

Dietary Carbohydrate. There is generally a positive ecologic association between population intake of refined sugars and CHD mortality and a negative relationship between complex carbohydrates and CHD mortality.[34] Although these diet components are seriously confounded with other dietary factors that are strongly associated with carbohydrate intake, the effect of certain fibers, including the pectins in fruit, bran fiber, and the guar gum of numerous vegetables and legumes, on blood sugar and on blood lipid regulation has recently attracted greater interest. This is particularly so now that the fatty acid effects are well delineated; yet they fail to explain all of the observed population differences in blood lipid or all the lipid changes seen during experiments involving different nutrient composition.

More important, however, is the fact that plausible mechanisms of atherogenesis are not established for sugars. The broader issue of plant foods (fruits, vegetables, pulses, legumes, and seeds), their complex carbohydrates, protein, other nutrients, and fibers, is nevertheless of great public health interest because their consumption may affect the risk of cancers as well as of CVD.[34]

Our summary view is that the different amounts of sugars consumed in "natural diets" around the world do not account for the important differences found in population levels of blood lipids and their associated CHD risk. High carbohydrate intake is totally confounded with low fat intake (since protein intake is relatively comparable), and both are associated with low rates of CHD. More study is needed on the matter of fibers.

Alcohol. Positive correlations between alcohol consumption and blood pressure levels found for individuals in population studies appear to be dose-related and independent of body weight and smoking habits.[37,38] Evidence is also consistent with respect to the positive relationship of alcohol consumption to blood high-density lipoprotein (HDL) cholesterol level and of change in alcohol consumption to change in HDL cholesterol level. Substitution of alcohol for carbohydrates in a mixed U.S. diet results in a rise in HDL, mainly the HDL_3 subfraction, one that may not be strongly related to CHD risk.[34,39]

Experimentally, myocardial metabolism and ventricular function are affected by relatively small doses of alcohol. In addition, neurohormonal links are established between alcohol-stimulated catecholamine excretion and myocardial oxygen requirements. These effects could act as contributory factors to the clinical manifestations of ischemia.

The epidemiological evidence from longitudinal studies about the relation of alcohol to CHD risk is, however, conflicting.[40–42] Inverse relationships of alcohol intake and CHD are found in some studies, whereas a U-shaped, linear, or no relationship is found in others. Positive relationships, when found, are usually independent of tobacco, obesity, and blood pressure levels.[42]

Reasons for these inconsistent findings in the alcohol-coronary disease relationship may involve the poor (self-report) measurement for alcohol intake as well as misclassification of the cause of death among heavy drinkers who are known to die of sudden, unexplained causes. Moreover, there are many possible confounding factors, including blood pressure levels, cigarette smoking, and diet.

Preventive practice with respect to alcohol is, therefore, based on its social and public health consequences rather than on any possible direct effect, favorable or otherwise, on cardiovascular disease risk. A major concern about regular alcohol use is, however, its enhancement of overeating, underactivity, and smoking, along with its intrinsic caloric density. Given these several relationships, public health recommendations for alcohol are not indicated, in our view, in *any* quantity, as a "protective measure" for heart diseases.

Salt Intake. Salting of food, primarily for preservation, began with civilization and trade. Now salting is based mainly on acquired taste and is likely a "new" phenomenon in an evolutionary sense. Moreover, the mammalian kidney probably evolved in salt-poor regions where the predominantly plant and wild game diet was likely very low in sodium and rich in potassium. Thus survival of humans and other mammals in salt-poor environments may have rested on an evolutionarily acquired and exquisite sodium-retaining mechanism of the kidney. The physiological need for salt under ordinary circumstances is on the order of only 1 to 2 g of sodium chloride per day. It is hypothesized that this mechanism is now overwhelmed by the concentrated salt presented to modern humans in preserved meats and pickled foods, in many processed foods, and in the strong culturally acquired taste for salt.[22,43]

Clinical, experimental, and epidemiological links between salt intake and hypertension are increasingly well forged[34,43,44] (Chapter 49). Marked sodium depletion dramatically reduces blood pressure in persons with severe hypertension. Sodium restriction enables high blood pressure to be controlled with lower doses of antihypertensive drugs. In many patients, salt restriction may result in adequate control of mild to moderate hypertension without drugs. Weight reduction and salt restriction appear to be independently important in lowering high blood pressure. In summary, a culture with high salt consumption appears to encourage maximal exhibition of an inherent human susceptibility to hypertension. Because potassium tends to reduce the blood pressure–raising effects of sodium, the sodium-potassium ratio of habitual diets also may be important in the public health.[45]

Surveys consistently find strong relationships between average population blood pressure and salt intake.[44,46,47] High blood pressure is usually prevalent in high-salting cultures, irrespective of the prevalence of obesity. In contrast, hypertension is usually absent in low-salting cultures, despite frequent obesity. Moreover, rapid acculturation to greater salt intake among South Pacific islanders who migrate to industrialized countries is associated with an increased frequency of hypertension and elevated mean blood pressure.[34] Even within high-salting cultures, when special efforts are made to reduce the measurement error for blood pressure and to characterize individual sodium intake with maximum precision, significant individual salt–blood pressure correlations are usually found.[34,48,49]

Despite all this evidence, neither preventive practice nor public health policy on reduction of salting is well advanced. This may be due in part to professional skepticism, based perhaps on the relatively weak *individual* correlations of salt intake and blood pressure. Admittedly, modification of salt intake by traditional dietary counseling has not been very successful. However, when interventions are attempted in a supportive and systematic way, change in salting behavior is readily achievable.[50] In the United States, wider education has significantly and widely influenced food processing and marketing of products with lower salt content, and a great deal of voluntary public health action has been taken by food companies.

Current U.S. national dietary goals recommend no more than 4.5 to 6.0 g of salt daily.[34] For individuals, this is achievable by not salting foods at the table, by adding no salt in cooking, and by avoidance of salt-rich foods, particularly canned, processed, and pickled foods. Despite the absence of a strong policy, preventive practice and public health approaches to reduced salt consumption are increasing. Significant public health effects of such population changes might be expected in high-salting societies, in light of recent trends in blood pressure and stroke observed in Japanese populations.[51]

Soft Water and Minerals. The effects of other minerals, cations, and trace elements on cardiovascular function and disease are the subject of active research because of their important role in many basic metabolic reactions, because of the need to define their daily requirements for good nutrition, and because of the wide variation of their concentration in foods and water sources. Significant associations are found between water softness and rates of hypertension and CHD mortality. Plausible mechanisms are not established, however, and the epidemiological associations are inconsistent and confounded.[52] Leaching of minerals from the soil, composition of water supplies, and the tissue effects of minerals and trace elements are all areas of current research. Interest is centered on the intake of calcium, magnesium, manganese, lead, cadmium, the zinc-copper ratio, and selenium.

Blood Lipoproteins. Clinical, experimental, and epidemiological evidence of the relationship between certain blood lipoproteins, atherosclerosis, and incidence of CHD is strong, consistent, and congruent. Because much knowledge is available, we present here only a summary of what we regard as the salient facts in this relationship, along with a few key references. The subject was recently reviewed in detail.[53]

- Mean levels and distributions of total serum cholesterol and other blood lipids vary widely between populations.[10,11,53]
- Associations are consistently strong between mean population levels of total serum cholesterol and measured CHD incidence.[10,11]
- Associations are generally weak between mean population levels of serum triglycerides and coronary disease rates.[53–55]
- In the few instances in which it is measured, the relationship is weak between CHD incidence and mean population levels of HDL or VLDL but strong between LDL and total cholesterol levels.[53–55]
- Total serum cholesterol levels at birth have similar means and ranges in many cultures.[56]
- Average levels and distributions of total serum cholesterol differ widely for populations of school-age children.[56] They tend to parallel the differences found in adult population distributions of blood lipid levels; that is, means and distributions are found to be elevated in youth when they are elevated in adult populations.[55]
- Means and distributions of total serum cholesterol of migrants rapidly approach those of the adopted country, whether higher or lower than the country of origin.[15]
- Blood lipids measured in cohorts of healthy adults followed over time show consistently positive relationships, usually with a continuously rising individual risk of CHD according to the entry levels of total serum cholesterol (and LDL), at least until late middle age.[7,53,57,58]
- Computation of the population risk attributable to blood cholesterol levels indicates that the majority of excess CHD cases occurs in the central segment of the population distribution (generally regarded as "normal" by clinical laboratory standards), that is, 220 to 310 mg/dl, whereas only 10% derive from values above 310.[25,59]
- In healthy cohorts, a strong inverse relationship between individual HDL cholesterol level and its ratio to total cholesterol is found with subsequent CHD risk. It is relatively stronger at older ages and within populations that have a relatively high CHD risk overall.[34,60]
- Large-scale experiments indicate the feasibility and apparent safety of blood cholesterol lowering from moderate changes made in dietary composition, with and without weight loss.[9,34,61]
- A synthesis of clinical trials of lipid lowering alone in middle-aged, high-risk populations indicates a reduction of CHD risk according to the degree and duration of exposure to the lowered cholesterol level.[34]
- There has probably been a significant drop, on the order of 10% to 15%, in the U.S. mean total serum cholesterol level in the last 20 years, which is partly explained by changes in composition of the habitual diet during this period.[34]
- The downward trends observed in CHD mortality in the United States cannot be attributed directly to the lowered population levels of risk factors. The findings are compatible with causation, however, because the decline in out-of-hospital CHD mortality, a crude reflection of incidence, is proportionately greater than the decline in the number of in-hospital deaths.

The effect of improved coronary care on CHD mortality trends is documented by the decrease in hospital case-fatality from myocardial infarction and by improved long-term survival.[1,2,62,63]

Consensus from these facts has resulted in a vigorous population strategy of reduction in blood lipid level in the United States. Major recommendations are now in place for a change in eating pattern among North Americans.[34,64] Moreover, the U.S. National Cholesterol Education Program has apparently increased both public and professional awareness and has improved the medical practice of lowering blood cholesterol.[65]

Overweight and Obesity

Whatever the physiological or cosmetic disadvantages of obesity and overweight, their relationship to CVD risk and mortality remains interesting, difficult to dissect, and basically unsettled. From a clinical perspective, extreme obesity is associated with manifest physical limitations and a propensity for many disabilities and illnesses. Beyond this, however, associations with cardiovascular diseases are not consistent throughout most of the distribution of relative weight or skin fold measurements.[66]

Overweight and weight gain tend to raise risk factor levels, and correction of the many metabolic disorders that accompany obesity is prompt and substantial when weight loss is achieved, with or without an increase in physical activity. When weight loss is carried out primarily through increased physical activity, appetite is generally "self-regulated" and body fat is lost, lean body mass is better maintained, insulin activity is lowered, glucose tolerance is improved, LDL and VLDL lipoprotein levels are lowered, HDL level is raised, and cardiovascular efficiency is enhanced. As we shall review here, however, the status of obesity and weight gain and loss as risk factors for CVD is complex and uncertain.

Obesity is arbitrarily considered to be present when the fat content of the body is greater than 25% of body mass in men and 30% in women. Overweight is equally arbitrarily chosen as greater than 130 percent relative weight, according to life insurance build and mortality tables, or on a body mass index (wt/ht^2) greater than 26. "Ideal weight" criteria are often based on standards associated with the lowest mortality risk in life insurance experience. The prevalence of overweight (and obesity) in U.S. adults is variously estimated at from 20% to 50% depending on the measurement used and the definition chosen, as well as by age, sex and race classification.

A most salient fact about overweight in the United States is that average weight and relative body weight are increasing, according to national health surveys. Mean weight in men (18 to 74 years of age) has risen from 75.3 kg in 1960 to 1962 to 78.0 kg in 1976 to 1980. In women, similar changes have occurred, with mean weight in 1960 to 1962 being 63.5 kg, rising to 65.3 kg in the later survey, with no proportionate change in stature. The prevalence of extreme overweight is increasing at a greater rate than is average weight.[34] Finally, relative obesity increases with age, even in a setting of stable body weight, because, as people grow older, muscle is replaced with fat.

The causes of *mass* obesity in populations are only partly understood. Widespread abundance, availability, and low cost of foods, along with many environmental cues to appetite, encourage overeating in relation to physiologic need. These environmental "facilitators" act on an apparently widespread genetic susceptibility to obesity. This, in turn, may be an evolutionary legacy from hunter-gatherer life-styles. Moreover, there are other factors that enhance excess calorie intake relative to need. For example, dietary fat is more efficiently stored as adipose tissue than is carbohydrate under conditions of excess calorie intake.[34] Refined sugars have less satiety value than the complex carbohydrates of fruits and vegetables. And alcohol is cheap and available in many societies.

Nevertheless, a major "cause" of mass obesity in Western populations appears to be the increase of relative sedentariness. Americans are, on average, heavier now than they were earlier in this century when, in fact, they consumed significantly more calories per day.[34] The stable, rural, laboring populations that consume (and expend) more energy are, in turn, the leaner populations.[10] Unfortunately, however, sedentariness in populations is largely confounded with calorie density and other differences in eating patterns.

CHD and Obesity Among Populations. Comparisons among and within populations in the Seven Countries Study illustrate the complexity of the relationship of overweight and obesity to CHD and to death from all causes.[10,11] Among populations, CHD incidence is not correlated with any measure of obesity or overweight. The population distributions of skinfold obesity are, however, strikingly different. They almost fail to overlap, for example, between the highest skinfold values found among Serbian farmers and the lowest values among sedentary U.S. rail clerks.[10] Obesity is, therefore, a mass phenomenon and is apparently strongly determined by (a) the average energy expenditure of the population and (b) the composition (caloric density) of the diet.

CHD and Obesity Within Populations. Within populations the picture is highly variable. In East Finns, with high CHD rates, incident CHD cases are evenly distributed across the entry distribution of skin fold fatness and overweight. In another population with a high CHD incidence—U.S. railroad workers—the relationship between skin fold obesity and CHD death is weakly positive, in contrast to an insignificant and opposite relationship for relative body weight. In another population with a high CHD incidence, consisting of rural Dutch men, there is a strongly positive linear relationship between CHD incidence and overweight and obesity throughout the wide range of values found there. Among men from the southern Mediterranean regions of Italy, Greece, and Yugoslavia, there is a U-shaped relationship between overweight or obesity and CHD risk, as well as with deaths from all causes. There the thinnest individuals as well as the heaviest and fattest have the higher disease rates; lowest disease risk is found for those with intermediate weight values.[10,11]

Multivariate analysis in the Seven Countries Study, used to adjust for the many confounding variables related alike to body mass and to CHD, shows no consistent relationship of 10-year CHD incidence with either relative weight or fatness.[11] In most of these populations there is a tendency for CHD incidence to be slightly higher in the upper than in the lower half of the fatness distributions, but this tendency disappears when other variables are simultaneously considered. Similarly, except for men at the extremes of the distribution, within generally high-incidence and overweight U.S. populations, there is little relationship between obesity or overweight and risk of CHD or death in men.

Within populations, several other longitudinal studies, including the Framingham Heart Study,[67] the Evans County Study,[68] and the Manitoba Study,[69] suggest that an independent contribution of relative weight to risk in a society with high CHD incidence may be reflected only in very long-term CHD risk. In Framingham, in addition, weight gain since youth is a risk predictor for CHD.[67] Finally, in the Evans County Study, initial overweight and weight gain over time are also strongly related to the 7-year incidence of new hypertension.[68]

The ability to distinguish CVD risk according to the body distribution of obesity, usually measured as the ratio of waist to hip circumference (WHR), is relatively new.[70] WHR is positively related to risk of CHD, premature death, non-insulin-dependent diabetes mellitus, and cancers in women, as well as to established CVD risk factor levels. The finding that several diseases correlate better with fat distribution than with general measures of overweight or obesity has raised major new hypotheses about possible separate metabolic entities and about the pathogenesis, risk, and treatment of obesity.[71,72]

Results of autopsy studies are inconclusive. The International Atherosclerosis Project concluded that the degree and severity of atherosclerosis were not consistently associated with overweight and obesity.[73]

Finally, a major gap exists in our knowledge of the effect of weight reduction on disease risk in a relatively overweight society at high risk from combined CHD risk factors. This hugely confounded question, as well as the effects of weight cycling, remains to be clarified.[74]

In summary, obesity and overweight are centrally involved with the many metabolic maladaptations related to diabetes mellitus, hypertension, blood lipids, and probably atherogenesis. These maladaptations are particularly amenable to correction by weight loss, with or without increased physical activity. The epidemiological evidence indicates, however, that relative body weight and obesity have a different disease-related significance in different populations and cultures. This may be due in part to different composition of the diets by which individuals and populations become obese, as well as to coexisting elevated distributions of other CVD risk characteristics. In most societies with high CHD incidence in which the issue has been systematically studied, the relationship between overweight, obesity, and CHD risk is seen mainly at the extremes of relative weight and over the longer term. Inconsistent disease associations and the obvious and dramatic declines in CVD deaths in the United States over the last 20 years, despite the clearly increased average U.S. body mass, indicate the primary importance for population CVD risk of factors other than overweight and obesity. Less clear, but similarly downward, trends of mortality from cancers other than those of the lung, suggest the same conclusion in regard to overweight and cancer risk.[1,34]

Physical Inactivity

Two primal human activities are the obtaining and consuming of food. Only since the advent of agriculture, and more recently of urbanization and industrialization, has the sustained subsistence activity of humans changed dramatically. In affluent industrial societies with automated occupations, motorized transport, and sedentary leisure, reduced energy expenditure is one of the more profound changes in human behavior. Aside from its likely importance as a fundamental departure from evolutionary adaptations and its apparently determining effect on mass obesity, the evidence specifically linking physical activity to chronic and CVD disease risk is difficult to obtain and interpret. It defies effective analysis because, in Western society, there are simply no "unselected" active and inactive groups to compare. Moreover, a definitive, long-term controlled experiment on habitual activity with respect to CVD risk is not considered feasible.[75] We attempt here a brief synthesis of the evidence relating habitual activity to CHD risk.

The caliber of the coronary arteries at autopsy is larger in very active people, but limitations of design, method, feasibility, and cost have prevented a satisfactory study of the effect of exercise training on changes in coronary angiograms or functional measures of ischemia.

Experimental studies of the progression and regression of atherosclerosis in animal models have also revealed little evidence of a protective effect of physical activity.

In clinical trials of cardiac rehabilitation after myocardial infarction, including the effects of exercise training, samples have been too small to allow definite conclusions to be drawn. Nevertheless, Oldridge and colleagues[76] carried out a meta-analysis on the "better-designed" studies, noting first that many of the trials demonstrated an effect of exercise on levels of risk factors and exercise tolerance. They used rigorous criteria for inclusion of 10 trials in their statistical summary, which estimated a 24% reduction in deaths from all causes in patients undergoing cardiac rehabilitation and a 25% reduction in CVD mortality. Both estimates were statistically significant and clinically important. The incidence of nonfatal myocardial infarction, however, was 15% higher (not statistically significant) in all the treatment groups combined and 32% higher ($P = .058$) in the groups in which cardiac rehabilitation was begun early (i.e., within 8 weeks after infarction). Thus, cardiac rehabilitation with exercise apparently had no overall effect on risk of nonfatal infarction and, when initiated early, may even have increased the incidence of nonfatal infarction. A prudent approach, therefore, would be to avoid the premature institution (within 8 weeks) of vigorous exercise as a component of rehabilitation.[77]

The major source of information about the primary prevention of CHD is indirect, from observational studies. These usually involve attempts to identify the confounding effects of lifestyle characteristics *other* than physical activity.[77] A recent synthesis by Powell and colleagues[78] concluded that the majority of observational studies meeting their criteria found a significant and graded relationship between physical inactivity and the risk of first CHD event and that studies with a stronger design were more likely to show an effect. These authors calculated a median risk ratio of 1.9, that is, a 90% excess risk of CHD among physically inactive persons.

We analyzed the subset of 16 studies from the review of Powell et al. that measured individual levels of physical activity, and we added recent studies from the Multiple Risk Factor Intervention Trial (MRFIT) and U.S. railroad workers.[77,79,80] All 18 studies showed that habitual physical activity was inversely related to death from CHD or death from all causes. The more recent studies adjusted for confounding risks and this adjustment usually diminished, but did not abolish, the risk associated with physical inactivity. Several studies found that the relation was largely "explained" by the level of physical fitness, in that the gradient of risk with the level of physical activity largely disappeared when measures of fitness were controlled. In a cohort study, fitness measured by a maximal exercise treadmill test predicted all-cause mortality for men and women, independently of other risk characteristics.[81]

The duration, frequency, and intensity of physical activity that may be "protective" against CHD remain, nevertheless, at issue. Recent studies suggest that an energy expenditure of 150 to 300 kcal daily, in activity of moderate intensity such as walking and working around the house, is associated with lower risk, as is a moderate amount of vigorous physical activity.[79,80,82] Anthropologic observations suggest that healthy farmers and herdsmen the world over rarely work at a pace that leads to shortness of breath or exhaustion. Systematic observations in the Seven Countries Study indicate that even a substantial amount of regular, vigorous physical activity does not necessarily protect an individual or a population from CVD risk, particularly if mass hypercholesterolemia is prevalent. In that study, farmers and loggers in eastern Finland were found to be the more physically active of men, and yet they had the highest rates of CHD; there was little less risk among the more physically active within that population.[10,11]

Our interpretation of all these observations is that habitual, current physical activity very likely protects against coronary death, at least in middle-aged men. A basic uncertainty that remains is whether the apparent benefit is due to physical activity itself or to constitution (genes). People tend to exercise if they are able to and if they feel good when they exercise. Fitness, a component strongly determined by constitution, may be a major contributor to an apparently protective effect of physical activity. It is possible that fitness determines both who will be active and who will be protected from CHD.

At least two other pieces of evidence suggest that constitution is *not* the major operant. Any protective effect of having once been a college athlete, and thus presumably constitutionally superior, disappears with time after graduation, whereas current physical activity is associated with lower risk.[83] Moreover, it seems to us that constitutional factors are likely to be less important to participation in moderate exercise than to participation in vigorous exercise, but both carry a lower risk of CHD.

Finally, safety should be the foremost consideration both in prescribing exercise for individuals and in making recommendations for the public health. Siscovick et al.[84] found an excess risk of primary cardiac arrest during and shortly after strenuous exercise in all subjects, regardless of their level of habitual physical inactivity, despite a much lower overall risk of sudden coronary death in habitually active subjects. They concluded that the reduced risk of sudden death due to regular physical activity was greater than the excess risk of sudden death during vigorous activity. This view, important for the public health, would be small comfort, however, to the families of those stricken while running. The evidence suggests to us that brisk walking is the more reasonable exercise prescription, at least for sedentary and middle-aged people who have not maintained their fitness from youth.

Diabetes, Hyperglycemia, Hyperinsulinism

Since the insulin era began, enabling persons with diabetes to survive, a strong clinical impression has arisen that diabetes enhances atherosclerosis and CVD risk. In addition, there are important mechanistic interrelations between insulin-glucose regulation, lipoprotein and uric acid metabolism, obesity and hypertension, on the one hand, and atherosclerosis on the other.

The association of clinical diabetes mellitus with CHD and atherosclerotic manifestations is documented clinically, pathologically, and epidemiologically.[85,86] It is thought that hyperinsulinemia, hypoglycemic episodes, or both in treated diabetics, coupled (formerly) with the common prescription of a high-fat, low-carbohydrate, low-fiber diet, increases vascular complications. Cross-cultural comparisons suggest that the risk of atherosclerosis and CVD in diabetic patients is indeed related to factors other than the glucose-insulin disorder itself. For example, apparently low rates of atherosclerosis exist in diabetic eastern Jews, Chinese, and Southwest American Indians.[85,86] The Pima Indians of Arizona are thought to be an example of the theoretical "thrifty genotype," that is, a population only recently (in evolutionary terms) exposed to calorie abundance, that frequently (±50% of adults) develops an obese, diabetic phenotype but nevertheless manifests little CVD.[87]

In longitudinal studies among cohorts, clinical diabetes mellitus is associated with excess CHD risk and severity of CHD, and many studies confirm the excess of fatal myocardial infarction in women with diabetes.[88] The excess risk among diabetics is not always differentiated by the degree of hyperglycemia or the degree of control. Moreover, the confounding effects of insulin therapy, other drug therapy, or combined risk characteristics have not been effectively dissected. Much of the excess CHD risk in diabetics is, in fact, accounted for by associated risk variables.[85,86] More severe atherosclerosis, diabetic cardiomyopathy, and a hypercoagulable state are also thought to contribute to the excess risk of diabetes.[86]

Finally, in most autopsy studies, coronary artery disease and the frequency and severity of myocardial infarction are greater in diabetics than in controls.[85,86]

In healthy persons glucose intolerance alone is weakly and inconsistently associated with CVD risk.[86,89] However, high insulin activity was found to be a significant independent predictor of coronary events in cohorts studied in Australia, France, and Finland,[86] and it has also been proposed as a cause of excess atherosclerosis in Asian migrants.[90]

In summary, the relationship between diabetes, atherosclerosis, and coronary disease is well established among persons with clinical diabetes living under the conditions of affluent Western culture. Data from other cultures suggest, however, that other factors, such as physical activity, body weight, blood pressure, blood lipid levels, dietary composition, and smoking habits, greatly affect the risk of CHD among diabetics. This, plus evidence that the metabolic disorders of middle-aged persons with diabetes can be significantly improved through exercise and modified by diet and weight loss, provide a sound rationale for preventive practice. More study of these complex issues is needed to develop an effective preventive approach to non-insulin-dependent diabetes mellitus itself.

Elevated Blood Pressure: Hypertension

The epidemiology, control, and prevention of hypertension and its complications are discussed in detail in Chapter 49 and therefore are only summarized here.

It is estimated that hypertension contributes to more than one half of adult deaths in the United States. It is a strong and independent risk factor for CHD and stroke, and there are plausible mechanisms for its effects on atherosclerosis and vascular disease. Patients with CHD have higher average blood pressure than control subjects. Experimental atherosclerosis induced in animals is directly related to pressure levels within the arterial system. In cohort studies, elevated blood pressure is positively, continuously, and independently related to CHD risk, according to increasing level of systolic or diastolic blood pressure.[57] The relationship of elevated blood pressure to risk of cerebrovascular hemorrhage and congestive heart failure is even stronger than the relationship to risk of CHD and thrombotic stroke.

Population comparisons suggest, however, that hypertension accounts for relatively little of the great variation in CHD incidence found *among* populations, despite the fact that it is significantly related to individual CHD risk *within* populations. For example, there is a remarkable difference in CHD rates between Mediterranean populations and northern Europeans, in which average blood pressures are little different.[10,11]

The preventive potential for hypertension control is illustrated by drug trials that have demonstrated a significant decrease in rate of stroke and heart failure. Results of other trials suggest that CHD risk is lowered by control of hypertension, but most have had insufficient power to study this question.[91]

Blood pressure control has greatly improved in the United States in the last 10 to 15 years, according to surveys showing a substantial decrease in the proportion of hypertensive persons unidentified or not under control.[34,92] These trends have occurred in parallel with downward trends for both CHD and stroke mortality, although a direct relationship cannot be established. In fact, the mortality rate from stroke was diminishing long before safe and effective antihypertensive therapy was widely used. Moreover, stroke death rates in the United States fell during the 1950s and 1960s, when CHD death rates were rising sharply.[1]

Estimated changes in death rates for CHD and stroke, based on models of hypertension control, suggest a large potential for the prevention of CVD. Primary prevention of hypertension would likely have even more impressive effects on the public health.

Present challenges to preventive practice lie mainly in more effective control of elevated blood pressure in the elderly and in finding the ideal combination of drug and hygienic management for correction of mild or borderline levels of high blood pressure. The larger public health challenge lies in improvement of population-wide correlates of hypertension, such as physical inactivity, overweight, and high salt and alcohol intake. Such primary preventive and public health approaches promise to minimize the exhibition of high blood pressure, since human populations are apparently widely susceptible.

Tobacco Smoking

The broader relationship of tobacco to disease and health is detailed in Chapter 42. Much of the clinical evidence of a direct relationship between cigarette smoking and coronary disease was, until recently, anecdotal. Experimentally, ischemic pain, angiographic coronary spasm, and electrocardiographic findings are now demonstrated during smoking in patients with compromised coronary circulation.[93]

For individuals living within societies with a high CHD incidence, smoking is consistently found to be a strong and independent risk factor for myocardial infarction and sudden death, although apparently not for angina pectoris.[93-95] The risk is continuous from persons who have never smoked, to ex-smokers, to those who smoke even in small amounts and is also related to duration of the habit.[94,95] Interactions with other risk factors are also important, as indicated by the weak association of smoking with CHD risk in low-risk societies.[10,11] For example, the observed incidence of CHD in populations that do not have a base of relative mass hypercholesterolemia is much lower than the risk predicted with multiple regression equations derived from U.S. or northern European data.[94] The Japanese, for example, with a heavy prevalence of smoking and substantial amounts of hypertension, but without hypercholesterolemia, show much less coronary heart disease than would be predicted.[10,11]

As is the case with serum cholesterol level, most of the CHD cases attributable to smoking derive from the central part of the distribution, that is, light and moderate smokers; the prevalence of heavy smokers is low. A 17% population-attributable risk fraction for smoking and CHD deaths in the United States was estimated (conservatively) in the Carter Report.[96] Smoking is particularly significant in CHD risk among women.[97]

Smoking cessation is associated with lower CHD rates according to years of cessation.[98] While those who have never smoked have the best disease experience, long-term quitters approximate their rates, and even temporary quitters have a better risk experience than persistent smokers.[99] Improvement in the prognosis of survivors of myocardial infarction who quit smoking also tends to confirm the harmful cardiovascular effects of cigarettes and supports the potential for CHD prevention by reduction of tobacco use.[93,95,100]

Synthesis of this evidence, therefore, suggests that cigarette smoking is neither a primary nor a necessary factor in determining *population* rates of CHD. It is, rather, a strong and independent risk factor for CHD and vascular disease among individuals living in high-incidence populations where there is a significant background of coronary and peripheral atherosclerosis.

Mechanisms presumed to be important in CHD include the physicochemical effects of tobacco, that is, increased heart rate and myocardial contractility and greater myocardial oxygen demand due to raised catecholamine levels, decreased oxygen-carrying capacity of the blood, elevated fibrinogen levels, and platelet-aggregating effects. Other possible mechanisms include elevated fasting blood glucose levels and white blood cell counts and lower HDL levels, all found among smokers.[93,101]

A public health policy to foster so-called "safer cigarettes," at least with respect to lowering CVD risk, is not supported by the evidence of persistent high exposure to gas-phase toxins in "low-yield" cigarette users.[93] Moreover, the promotion and adoption of Western-type cigarettes and smoking patterns in developing countries augurs ill for their future CVD risk. In contrast, smoking prevalence has decreased substantially in the United States, where large numbers of educated adults in particular have stopped smoking. This is attributed to increased community awareness of the health need to stop smoking, to social pressure and legislation for "clean air" and "smoke-free" environments, and to a greater access to the support and skills needed for quitting. The downward U.S. trend in smoking is not as steep, however, among lower socioeconomic groups, and heavy smokers.[93]

Under "ideal" supportive circumstances, such as that given high-risk participants in the MRFIT, smoking cessation success rates approximate 40% in the first year, with maintenance of this rate for up to 4 years among volunteer participants. Thus a long-standing medical pessimism about helping patients stop smoking might be replaced by optimism for cessation programs that are systematically applied. Moreover, community-wide educational and legislative efforts are increasingly effective.[102,103] The results of all these efforts, and the population trends downward in smoking frequency, provide a rational basis for more public programs and for a more focused national policy to reduce cigarette smoking and tobacco production. It is equally possible that the currently declining rate of cigarette smoking will level off, unless educational programs and wider social support for nonsmoking behavior reach the lower socioeconomic classes, heavy smokers, women, and youth.

Hemostatic Factors

For decades, arguments have existed about the relative predominance of the role of blood lipids versus thrombosis in the pathogenesis of atherosclerosis and CHD. A more unified theory now joins the effects of diet and blood lipids, physical activity and smoking, and diabetes and insulin levels to atherosclerosis and to thrombosis. The interaction between chronic arterial wall disease and the blood properties leading to coagulation continues to be a major subject for research. The components of the coagulation system found so far to be of major interest are fibrin, which forms when cell walls are damaged and which contributes to fibrin platelet masses, and platelet aggregation.[104-107]

Of the several hemostatic variables measured with respect to subsequent CHD risk, fibrinogen has received the most attention. Several investigators conclude that an elevated fibrinogen level is likely to be causally associated with CHD but that its elevation overall may be due primarily to smoking.[104]

Anticoagulant trials appear to reduce short-term mortality in the hospital phase of acute myocardial infarction,[107] but long-term results are inconclusive. The reduction of reinfarction appears to be more likely than the reduction in deaths.

As for primary prevention of CHD events with low-level anticoagulation, such as with small doses of aspirin, this appears now to be established for nonfatal myocardial infarction.[108]

White Blood Cell Count

Total white blood cell count was strongly and significantly related to CHD risk, independently of smoking status, in the Multiple Risk Factor Intervention Trial.[109] A synthesis of these and other findings suggests that neutrophils are associated with CHD through their adhesive and rheological properties and through the damaging effect on endothelium of their toxic oxygen compounds.[110]

Hyperuricemia

A weak but consistent association between hyperuricemia, obesity, hypertension, hyperlipidemia, and coronary disease has been noted in clinical and epidemiological studies. Most evidence suggests that there is no significant independent association of serum uric acid level with coronary events after adequately accounting for confounding variables. A public health issue has emerged, however, in the combined effects on serum uric acid, glucose levels, and blood lipids of thiazide diuretics used widely in the control of hypertension. These drugs consistently elevate LDL and HDL levels as well as uric acid and glucose levels.[111] Preventive practice among people with hypertension now requires, therefore, careful tailoring of antihypertensive therapy with drugs *other than* thiazides or use of the lowest possible dose of diuretics, when hyperuricemia, hyperlipidemia, or glucose intolerance accompany hypertension.

Physical Environment

The weather, particularly the influx of cold fronts and rapid falls in barometric pressure, has been correlated with new hospital admissions for coronary events. Reasonable preventive practice includes advice to avoid exposure, in particular the combination of isometric work and cold, and to use light face masks to maintain a favorable personal air temperature and humidity.

Similarly, atmospheric inversions and air pollution are related to hospitalization and death rates from pulmonary and cardiovascular diseases, particularly in the elderly. Because most circumstances of the physical environment are so confounded by other risks in atherosclerosis, useful studies and preventive strategies are difficult to devise.

Behavior Pattern, Personality, and Stress

Emotional states of anger and aggression, fear and anxiety, and hyperactivity and depression are associated with overt metabolic and physiological reactions, symptoms, and signs. Pervasive popular and professional impressions are that they influence the major diseases of modern life. Causal connections between stress and behavior and coronary events and sudden death remain, however, unestablished. Laboratory study is limited by poor definition and measurement of "stress" and the components of stress reactions. Personality type, habitual behavior, and reactions to external stress have not been tied together effectively into a theoretical model susceptible of testing or amenable to preventive practice. Nevertheless, major psychosocial issues are being investigated actively, including type A behavior, hostility, and social support. Because of a long and considerable controversy in this area, and because of a wealth of new information about it, we consider these relationships here in some detail.

Type A Behavior. Type A behavior was accepted by many to be a strong psychosocial risk factor for CHD until the early 1980s. The major studies first establishing the relationship were the Western Collaborative Group Study and the Framingham Study.[112,113]

The Western Collaborative Group Study was a prospective study of more than 3000 men in whom the type A behavior pattern was assessed by its originators, using their structured interview method. The relative risk of CHD (both fatal and nonfatal incident events) among type A men was about 2.[112] The Framingham Study used a paper-and-pencil instrument to assess type A behavior in men and women, again with both fatal and nonfatal events as endpoints. The relative risk of CHD among type A persons was greater than 2 for incident events in both sexes.[113]

The relationship between type A behavior and CHD was also examined in many coronary angiographic studies in which behavior pattern was assessed before angiography. A summary of 14 such studies found about an equal balance of positive and absent associations.[114]

Several studies in the early 1980s failed to demonstrate the expected relationship to CHD.[115-118] These differed from the earlier, population-based studies on several counts: They used high-risk subgroups; for the most part, they used the Jenkins Activity Survey, another paper-and-pencil instrument; and they generally examined "harder" endpoints (CHD death or definite myocardial infarction). The MRFIT study, however, used the structured interview in a subset of participants and also found no significant relationship to risk. The Honolulu Heart Study used the Jenkins Activity Survey and found no relationship between type A behavior and incidence of disease but did find a relationship to prevalence of angina pectoris.[119]

At least one study among high-risk populations found a positive relationship between behavior pattern and CHD; the Recurrent Coronary Prevention Project reported that intervention in the behavior pattern reduced the risk of recurrent CHD.[120] These results have not been replicated.

Two recent publications based on follow-up of the original Western Collaborative Group data have also raised questions as to whether type A behavior is, in fact, a risk factor for CHD.[121,122] At present, we consider that clear evidence for a type A/B relationship to CHD risk is not established.

Hostility. Several studies have broken down type A behavior into components and attempted to examine their relationships to CHD. Both Matthews et al.[123] and Hecker et al.[124] identified hostility as a "coronary-prone" component within the Western Collaborative Group population. "Hostility" was assessed by independent raters evaluating audiotapes of baseline structured interviews.

Another approach uses the "Cook-Medley" hostility subscore of the Minnesota Multiphasic Personality Index (MMPI), a well-constructed and standardized instrument that is part of the MMPI, with data available on many populations. Six prospective studies using the Cook-Medley instrument have now been published; three have found associations of hostility with CHD and three have not.[125-130] On the other hand, hostility has been found related to CHD in several coronary angiographic studies.[131-133]

In summary, there is evidence relating hostility to CHD in men; little investigation has been carried out in women. The reasons are unclear for the discrepant results among the six methodologically similar prospective studies. Thus further investigations of hostility and CVD risk appear warranted.

Social Support

Several prospective population-based studies have established social support or "social connectedness" as a factor associated with *reduced* risk of death. Two large recent studies—one from Finland[134] and one from Sweden[135]—examined CVD disease risk. The pattern of results suggests a relationship between social support and mortality, at least in men. Whether this is a causal relationship or is attributable to a confounding variable such as baseline health or to personality characteristics such as hostility is unclear, and this line of investigation might well be continued.

Attempts have been made to change psychosocial characteristics experimentally and to measure CHD risk factors and disease changes. In our view, however, the problems of measurement, the relative absence of plausible linking mechanisms, and the limited techniques for modifying behavioral characteristics are all at a stage where a public health strategy is not feasible. Nevertheless, attempts at modifying individual behavior in preventive practice appear to be appropriate and safe.

Gender and Estrogens

The excess risk of CHD and atherosclerosis in white men is documented throughout affluent Western society. The sex differential is much less prominent, however, in nonwhite populations and in areas where the overall incidence is relatively low.[136] The particular susceptibility of men is only partly explained by their higher risk factor configurations between the ages of 25 and 60. On the other hand, the relative protection from CHD among premenopausal women is assumed to be related to hormones, although the effect of early oophorectomy, menopause, or estrogen replacement therapy on known risk factor distributions in women inadequately supports this explanation. In countries with a high incidence of CHD, where there is relative mass hyperlipidemia, much more of the plasma cholesterol is carried in the HDL fraction in women. Recent experimental evidence concerning mechanisms of LDL and HDL function, related to cell receptors and lipid transport in and out of the arterial wall, confirm this particular biological difference as a likely cause for some of the sex difference in CHD risk.

In contrast, women have a proportionately greater risk of angina pectoris than of myocardial infarction or sudden death. While they have less severe atherosclerosis in the coronary arteries, the sex difference is not as apparent in cerebral, aortic, and peripheral vessels. The male/female ratio of coronary disease prevalence and incidence is almost absent among persons with clinical diabetes.[88] Survival of women is uniformly poorer after myocardial infarction, and this, too, is largely unexplained.

Finally, trends in CHD deaths in the United States indicate that the age-specific decline in mortality is proportionately greater in women than in men.[1] Similarly, the rise in CHD death rates among women in eastern Europe, where CVD deaths overall are increasing rapidly, is proportionately greater in women and in young women.[137]

The excess risk of thromboembolism, stroke, and myocardial infarction in women taking oral contraceptives (OCs), and the interaction of OCs with age and smoking, are well established. The picture is not yet clear, however, for the effects of estrogen replacement therapy after menopause.[138] Estrogen replacement in postmenopausal women apparently raises HDL and lowers LDL cholesterol. However, young women taking OCs have systematically higher serum lipid levels, higher blood pressure, and impaired glucose tolerance compared to controls.[139]

In summary, the sex differential for atherosclerosis and cardiovascular disease events and their time trends is not adequately explained on the basis of any known effects of hormones on the level of risk factors, but it may be related in part to women's greater HDL cholesterol blood fraction. More study is needed. The widespread therapeutic use of hormones may turn out to have profound public health importance, but the issue is clear now only for the remarkable excess risk among older women smokers who are taking oral contraceptives.

Hereditary Factors

Much current work is opening up the understanding of host-environment relationships. The relative contribution of genes to disease risk of populations can be exaggerated, however, by studies of gene effects when limited to homogeneous, high-risk cultures where exposure is great and universal. Most of the lack of understanding, and much of the difficulty in identification of susceptible persons, lies in the unavailability of specific genetic markers for CVD and the incapacity of family studies to discriminate intrinsic components without such markers. Recent findings of the gene loci for apolipoprotein regulation hold great promise of an improved understanding of individual differences in blood lipoproteins and their response to diet. There is, for example, evidence of the genetic inheritance of LDL subclasses, HDL, apo B, and apo E.[140] A substantial proportion of the variation in apo B levels (43%) may be explained by a major locus.[141] A major gene controlling LDL subclasses may account for much of the familial aggregation of blood lipids and CHD risk.[142]

Most intrinsic blood lipoprotein regulation, however, is clearly polygenic and strongly interactive with the environment, especially with composition of the habitual diet. Controlled experiments in metabolically normal people suggest that there is a normal distribution of individual blood lipid responses to a known dietary change.[143]

The rare major gene effects that cause extreme manifestations of the hyperlipidemias are well characterized, but they account for only a small fraction of the mass phenomenon of hypercholesterolemia found in affluent cultures. Thus most atherosclerotic complications and most of the excess CHD events in the general population cannot be attributed to major gene effects. Nevertheless, gene-culture interactions remain important to preventive practice for better detection and individualized therapy of patients who have elevated blood lipid values. However, the majority of the excess CHD cases in the United States comes from the central part of the distribution of blood cholesterol (LDL), necessitating a population strategy of prevention.[144]

A potentially important aspect of genetically determined diet responses now under investigation is the response of individual lipoprotein fractions to specific dietary factors, mainly fatty acids and cholesterol. A wider issue, however, is the relative magnitude of the contribution of intrinsic regulation to the large population differences found for average blood lipid values and their distributions. For the time being, this contribution remains speculative.

Genetic control of CVD risk factors *other* than blood lipids is even less well known.[145] For example, not yet identified are genetic traits that might affect individual sensitivity to salt intake, to the atherogenic effect of cigarette smoking, or to the regulation of blood insulin and glucose levels, arterial wall enzymes, or personality type.

The public health view that a favorable environment assures minimal expression of phenotypic risk provides the rationale for a population approach to prevention. This rationale has not been effectively challenged, but neither has it been universally accepted.

Combined Risk Factors

Clinical, laboratory, and epidemiological studies of CVD risk factors have been oriented mainly toward determining specific causal roles for each factor. Cardiovascular diseases are clearly related, however, in both individuals and communities, to *multiple* factors operating together over time. Multiple-factor risk is firmly established and actually is quantified for both CHD and stroke. Based mainly on Framingham and Pooling Project analysis, a consistent, independent, and at least additive contribution is found for each of the major risk factors: cigarette smoking, arterial blood pressure, and total serum cholesterol level.[57] The risk ratio between highest and lowest categories for *combined* risk within populations is on the order of eight-to tenfold, in contrast to the risk ratio for single risk factors, which is on the order of two-to fourfold.

Prediction regressions derived from follow-up experience in European men, with the use of four major risk factors at baseline, when applied to men in the United States, show the multiple-risk concept to be "universal." That is, the regressions define a continuum of CHD risk among individual U.S. men in a society that has quite different CHD rates overall.[146] The slope of the relationship (regression) between the combined risk factors and disease, however, is much steeper in the United States than in the European population. At any given level of multiple risk, U.S. rates are twice those in Europe. This cultural difference in the "force" of risk factors indicates that a sizable influence on population differences in CHD risk remains unknown. Nevertheless, since these few risk factors operate universally and explain a substantial part of individual and population risk differences, public health action on that part of the difference now explained is both promising and indicated.

Still another interpretation of the evidence of combined risk of CHD is that the synergism between risk characteristics leads to a major potential for preventive effects in the population by achieving relatively small shifts in the means and distributions of the multiple risk factors. This does not exclude the possibility of a population threshold for risk factors, below which population risk is remote. That is indicated by the relative scarcity of mass atherosclerosis and CHD in societies in which average serum total cholesterol levels are less than 200 mg/dl. Nor does it exclude the concept of *necessary* versus *contributory* causes. In the absence of the presumed *necessary* factor (i.e., mass hypercholesterolemia), population risk is negligible. It may be that the departures from perfect prediction, found with the use of multiple regressions, are due in part to their failure to include the duration of exposure to, or the directionality of, a particular risk level.

ACUTE RHEUMATIC FEVER AND RHEUMATIC HEART DISEASE

Rheumatic fever and rheumatic heart disease are public health problems in parts of the world where poverty, overcrowding, malnutrition, and inadequate medical care are commonplace.[147,148] Even in industrialized societies, a relatively high prevalence of rheumatic fever persists in pockets of poverty, and outbreaks have been reported recently in affluent areas.[149] Despite the fact that rheumatic fever is demonstrably preventable and that rheumatic heart disease has declined dramatically in most industrialized nations, these conditions remain a major public health problem internationally.

For more than 40 years it has been known that β-hemolytic streptococcus infection is the cause of initial and recurrent attacks of rheumatic fever (see Chapter 7). The immunologic mechanisms and circumstances by which infection with this organism produces rheumatic fever and rheumatic heart disease and acute and chronic glomerulonephritis have been extensively investigated.[150] In as many as 3% of patients rheumatic fever develops after known streptococcal infections in epidemic circumstances.[151] This suggests that host factors significantly determine susceptibility. Age is also an obvious factor, in that infants do not have rheumatic fever even though they are susceptible to streptococcal infection and glomerulonephritis. In contrast, as many as 50% of those who have once had rheumatic fever will, if untreated, experience attacks after a subsequent streptococcal infection. Such differences in susceptibility are clearly developmental, such as the variation with age, but others may have a genetic basis. The tendency of rheumatic fever to cluster in families, however, may be explained by shared environment as well as genes.

Diagnosis

The diagnosis of acute rheumatic fever is made principally from clinical findings with the revised Jones criteria (see Chapter 7).[152] These may be insufficiently sensitive, however, to detect mild cases, particularly in Western countries where clinical patterns have changed so that arthritis is often the only presenting manifestation; chorea, subcutaneous nodules, and erythema marginatum are now rarely seen. Diagnosis may be complicated by the lack of a preceding sore throat or an apparent infection.[153]

Rapid antigen tests for the "diagnosis" of group A streptococcal throat infections are highly specific but less sensitive. A positive test indicates the need for treatment, but a negative test indicates the need for a throat culture.[154] Antibody tests can confirm a recent group A streptococcal infection (e.g., antistreptolysin O).

Epidemiology

During the 1960s, the incidence of acute rheumatic fever per 100,000 urban children 2 to 14 years of age in the United States ranged from 23 to 28 for whites and 27 to 55 for blacks. The incidence was still higher in Puerto Ricans. In Oklahoma and Connecticut the incidence was 10 to 15 per 100,000 children. Currently there are probably 5000 to 8000 first cases of acute rheumatic fever annually in the United States, most of them among the underprivileged.

In other parts of the world, lowest rates of rheumatic fever have been observed in Scandinavia, with 1.3 cases per 100,000. In underdeveloped nations, the rates are much higher. Prevalence among school-age children in South America ranges from 1% to 10%.[155]

Data on the prevalence of rheumatic heart disease in the United States are based on surveys of schoolchildren prior to 1970, with rates of from 0.5 to 5.3 per 1000. The prevalence in some socioeconomically depressed populations in the United States approaches the high rates observed in other areas of the world. Thus in Denver, Colorado, the prevalence in children 5 to 18 years of age is 1.4 per 1000 in whites and 3.4 per 1000 in blacks. In Soweto, South Africa, the prevalence in black schoolchildren 11 to 14 years of age is 10 per 1000. During the period from 1963 to 1970 the Health Examination Survey of the National Center for Health Statistics examined about 14,000 youths 6 to 19 years of age nationwide. The overall prevalence of acquired valvular heart disease in children was 7 per 1000. In youths aged 12 to 19, rheumatic heart disease was present in 11 per 1000. Although these rates appear unusually high and must be viewed with caution, it is of interest that the prevalence was higher in blacks in the southern areas of the United States, in rural areas, and in children of low-income families.

Mortality from rheumatic fever and rheumatic heart disease has fallen significantly in the United States in this century. It was 14.8 per 100,000 in 1950, 7.3 in 1970, and 2.7 in 1986, a decline of 82%.

Primary Prevention

Current recommendations for the primary prevention of acute rheumatic fever and rheumatic heart disease are as follows: Throat cultures should be made for all patients with tonsillopharyngitis, and those with a positive culture for group A streptococci should be treated when the diagnosis is made. Treatment effectively prevents rheumatic fever, even when started several days after the onset of the acute illness. The recommended treatment schedule of the American Heart Association is seen in Table 48-3. In the United States, mass throat cultures in schools have been advocated because many children with streptococcal infections have no symptoms or seek no care when symptoms are present. Such programs may be of particular value in economically depressed areas, where inaccessibility of medical care and lack of health awareness in the population are barriers to the detection and treatment of streptococcal infections.

Efficacy and Feasibility of Prevention. It has long been known that initial attacks of rheumatic fever can be prevented by adequately treating the preceding streptococcal infection. More recently, a study of the incidence of hospitalized cases of rheumatic fever among black children in Baltimore indicates that incidence decreased 60% in areas with comprehensive care clinics but remained unchanged in other areas.[151] The decline was limited to cases of rheumatic fever that followed symptomatic pharyngitis.

A program of mass throat cultures of children in the schools of Wyoming resulted in a decrease in positive culture rates for β-streptococci, from 10% positive at the beginning of each school year to below 5% at the end of the year, along with an apparent decrease in incidence of acute rheumatic fever.[156] The cost was about $1 per pupil per year.

TABLE 48-3. PRIMARY PREVENTION OF RHEUMATIC FEVER (TREATMENT OF STREPTOCOCCAL TONSILLOPHARYNGITIS)

Agent	Dose	Mode	Duration
Benzathine penicillin G	600,000 units for patients <60 lb 1,200,000 units for patients >60 lb	Intramuscular	Once
	or		
Penicillin V (phenoxymethyl penicillin)	250 mg 3 times daily	Oral	10 days
▪ For Individuals Allergic to Penicillin			
Erythromycin estolate	20–40 mg/kg per day 2–4 times daily (maximum 1 g per day)	Oral	10 days
	or		
Erythromycin ethylsuccinate	40 mg/kg per day 2–4 times daily (maximum 1 g per day)	Oral	10 days

The following agents are acceptable but are usually not recommended: amoxicillin, dicloxacillin, oral cephalosporins, and clindamycin.
The following are not acceptable: sulfonamides, trimethoprim, tetracyclines, and chloramphenicol.

Secondary Prevention

All acute streptococcal infections should be treated. Recurrent rheumatic fever can usually be prevented, and progressive valvular damage avoided, by the eradication of streptococcal infection. For long-term chemoprophylaxis, sulfadiazine given orally in a dose 1000 mg daily (500 mg for small children) has proved effective, as has oral penicillin V, 250 mg twice daily, or benzathine penicillin, 1.2 million units intramuscularly every 4 weeks. Erythromycin given orally 250 mg twice a day may be used in penicillin-sensitive individuals. The major problem with long-term chemoprophylaxis is noncompliance. Prophylaxis for patients who have had rheumatic carditis should be lifelong. In patients with a history of rheumatic fever without rheumatic carditis, prophylaxis should continue until the patient is in the early 20s and for at least 5 years after the last attack.[154]

CONGENITAL HEART DISEASE

Malformations of the cardiovascular system are among the more frequently occurring congenital defects. They result from developmental errors caused by inherent defects in the genetic material of the embryo, environmental factors, or both.[157–162]

Genetic Factors

Family studies suggest that the offspring of parents with congenital heart disease have malformation rates ranging from 1.4% to 16.1%.[163] Identical twins are both affected 25% to 30% of the time. While these and other findings of familial aggregation suggest polygenic factors, common environment may also play a role.[162] Single-gene disorders account for less than 1% of all congenital cardiovascular anomalies, and these include such defects as muscular subaortic stenosis, supravalvular aortic stenosis, endocardial fibroelastosis, and idiopathic familial myocardiopathy. In addition, there are other single-gene, noncardiac disorders that produce cardiovascular defects; these include Marfan's syndrome, Friedreich's ataxia, glycogen-storage disease, and Down's and Turner's syndromes.

Environmental Factors

Maternal viral infections during pregnancy are estimated to cause up to 10% of all congenital cardiac malformations. Rubella in the first 2 months of pregnancy is associated with congenital malformations in about 80% of live births and is thought to account for 2% to 4% of all congenital heart disease. Patent ductus arteriosus and pulmonic stenosis are the most common defects. Subclinical coxsackievirus infections may be related to congenital heart disease. Acute hypoxia, residence at high altitudes, high carboxyhemoglobin levels, and uterine vascular changes from cigarette smoking are other potential causes.[161] Maternal x-ray exposure results in an increased incidence of Down's syndrome and possibly other congenital defects.[160] Maternal metabolic defects, such as diabetes mellitus and phenylketonuria, are associated with increased incidence of congenital heart defects.

Animal investigations, which have not been substantiated in humans, indicate that dietary deficiencies in the mother may result in congenital malformations. Obstetric problems are associated with congenital heart disease, including association of advanced maternal age with Down's syndrome and a history of vaginal bleeding (threatened abortion) during the first 11 weeks of gestation with prematurity. The teratogenic potential of drugs, such as thalidomide and folic acid antagonists, is well documented. In addition, dextroamphetamines, anticonvulsants, lithium chloride, alcohol, and progesterone/estrogen are highly suspected teratogens acting in the first trimester of pregnancy, as are certain pesticides and herbicides (see Chapter 24).[164]

Epidemiology

Data on the true incidence of congenital heart disease are limited. The chief sources of information are birth certificate and hospital birth data.[158,159] Birth certificate data usually underestimate the true rate.

A U.S. multicenter collaborative study in 1970 yielded the following incidence rates for congenital heart disease: 8.1 per 1000 total births, 7.6 per 1000 live births, and 16.5 per 1000 twin births.[165] Most are correctable by modern medical and surgical methods, including cardiac transplantation; it is estimated that only one person per 1000 cannot be helped by such approaches.[166]

Although the overall incidence of congenital heart disease has apparently remained stable, the distribution of types of defects may be shifting. This includes unexplained increases in ventricular septal defects and patent ductus arteriosus. A decline in the number of infants born with rubella-caused defects may be explained by vaccination programs.[165]

Primary Prevention

Primary prevention of congenital heart disease includes the following established measures[158]:

1. Genetic counseling of potential parents and families with congenital heart disease
2. Rubella immunization programs
   a. Identification of susceptible women of child-bearing age by serologic examination
   b. Immunization of susceptible women
   c. Avoidance of pregnancy for 2 months after rubella vaccination
3. Avoidance of exposure to viral diseases during pregnancy
4. Administration of all usual vaccines to all children to eliminate reservoirs of infection
5. Avoidance of radiation during pregnancy
6. Avoidance of exposure during the first trimester of pregnancy to gas fumes, air pollution, cigarettes, alcohol, pesticides, herbicides, and high altitude
7. Avoidance of drugs of any kind during the first trimester of pregnancy, especially drugs of known or suspected teratogenic potential.

CARDIOMYOPATHIES AND MYOCARDITIS

Cardiomyopathies are a broad group of cardiac diseases that involve the heart muscle. Although less common in industrialized nations, they account for 30% or more of heart disease deaths in some countries.[167] They are of diverse etiology and are usually classified by the functional results of their effects on the myocardium: dilated or congestive, hypertrophic and restrictive. Recent recommendations suggest that the term *cardiomyopathy* be reserved for disease of unknown origin involving heart muscle.[167] However, the common use of the term still associates it with specific causal syndromes when these are known.

Some cardiomyopathies are diagnosed in their acute phase, when inflammation of the myocardium is common (myocarditis). While myocarditis is particularly difficult to categorize, diagnosis has been facilitated by the widespread use of endomyocardial biopsy.[168] These techniques have suggested that an inflammatory reaction is more common than was previously suspected. Identified causes include infectious, metabolic, toxic, allergic, and genetic factors.[169] Myocarditis and cardiomyopathy may be mild and undetected but also can be rapidly fatal through progressive heart failure.

In industrialized nations, cardiomyopathies appear to be increasing in prevalence. It is unclear whether there is an actual increase in cases or an increase in professional awareness and improved diagnostic techniques.[170] The latter include use of the echocardiogram, Doppler flow studies, and catheter-based endomyocardial biopsy. A study of death certificates in the United States in 1982 found 10,345 deaths assigned to cardiomyopathy.[170] The majority of these (87%) were coded to "other primary cardiomyopathy," with cause unspecified. Surveillance of Olmsted County, Minnesota, found an incidence of idiopathic dilated cardiomyopathy of 6 per 100,000 person years. Overall prevalence was 35.3 per 100,000 population.[171] In these and other studies, cases of cardiomyopathy are distributed evenly across ages and sexes.[172]

Alcohol abuse is an important cause of cardiomyopathy, accounting for approximately 8% of all cases in the United States.[170,173] Alcohol causes myocardial damage by several mechanisms[174,175]:

1. A direct toxic effect.
2. Effects of thiamine deficiencies.
3. Effects of additives such as cobalt in alcoholic beverages.

Abstinence from alcohol may halt or reverse the cardiomyopathy.[176]

Another major cause of cardiomyopathy in industrialized countries is viral infection, particularly coxsackie B virus, echovirus, influenza, and polio,[177] often beginning as a viral myocarditis. Subclinical viral disease is thought to be more common than was previously suspected, with many patients recovering without sequelae. More severe forms, however, result in dilated cardiomyopathy and death due to congestive heart failure or arrhythmias. Recent research has suggested an autoimmune component and indicated that immunosuppressive therapy may be helpful in modifying the disease.[178] However, early clinical trials have shown little beneficial effect for corticosteroids.[179]

Hypertrophic cardiomyopathy is less common as a cause of death.[180] Largely undiscovered until the advent of echocardiographic techniques, it is becoming increasingly clear that this condition rarely causes difficulty for patients and is usually well managed with pharmacologic therapy.[180]

In South and Central America, trypanosomiasis (Chagas' disease) is endemic; an estimated 10 million people are afflicted.[181] Extensive chronic myocarditis with heart failure may be observed years after the initial infection with the trypanosome. An acute infectious phase, characterized by fulminant and fatal myocarditis, occurs mainly in children. In most cases, however, an average of 20 years passes before Chagas' cardiomyopathy becomes clinically apparent. An autoimmune process may play some role in the disease.[182] Diagnosis is made by means of serologic study or a xenodiagnostic test. Although antiparasitic agents, such as nitroimidazole derivatives, can alter the acute infestation, there is little evidence that they are effective for the cardiomyopathy.[167]

Schistosomiasis is a major public health problem in the Nile and Yangtze basins where the parasitic infection is endemic, involving 85% of the population in certain areas. Chronic pulmonary embolization leads to pulmonary hypertension and right heart failure, but direct involvement of the myocardium is rare. New antiparasitic agents can limit the infection, but the main preventive strategy is a public health approach to control the vectors.

SYPHILITIC HEART DISEASE

Although the prevalence and patterns of syphilis worldwide have been altered significantly in the antibiotic era, it remains an important public health problem in many nations. Recent reports indicate a rise in reported cases of primary and secondary syphilis in the United States, and surveys in developing nations indicate continued high incidence and prevalence rates.[183] An increase in reported cases and a general decline in medical alertness to this condition encourage a continuing reservoir for late complications. Life-threatening tertiary syphilis is found in approximately 25% to 30% of untreated cases.[184] Approximately 10% of those are cardiovascular syphilis, manifest predominantly as uncomplicated syphilitic aortitis, aortic aneurysm, aortic valvulitis with regurgitation, and coronary ostial stenosis.[185] Although a course of antibiotic therapy is indicated when cardiovascular syphilis is diagnosed, there is little evidence that it alters the course of the cardiovascular disease.

Because syphilis remains preventable, detectable, and treatable in the early stages, continued public health approaches should lead to eradication of the late effects of syphilis, including those in the cardiovascular system.[186]

PREVENTIVE STRATEGIES

A population approach to CVD prevention has been formally outlined by the World Health Organization.[59] It embraces both the systematic practice of screening and education for high risk, where national priorities can afford such practices, and broad public health policy and programs in health promotion.

Strategies for preventive practice are now widely available. Community-based strategies, programs, and materials are becoming available. National programs are under way in blood pressure control, diet and blood lipids, and smoking. Finally, health-promotion resource centers are now established for training in the design and dissemination of preventive programs. The student and the health worker are referred to these sources: Division of Nutrition, Chronic Disease Prevention and Health Promotion at the Centers for Disease Control, Atlanta, Ga., and the Henry J. Kaiser Family Foundation, Menlo Park, Calif.

REFERENCES

1. Report of a conference on trends and determinants of coronary heart disease mortality: International comparisons. Int J Epidemiol 18(suppl 1), 1989
2. Burke GL, Sprafka JM, Folsom AR, Luepker RV, Norsted SW, Blackburn H: Trends in CHD mortality, morbidity and risk factor levels from 1960 to 1986: The Minnesota Heart Survey. Int J Epidemiol 18(suppl 1):S73–S81, 1989
3. World Health Organization MONICA Project Principal Investigators: The WHO MONICA Project: a major international collaboration. J Clin Epidemiol 41:105–114, 1988
4. World Health Organization MONICA Project. Int J Epidemiol 18(suppl 1):S29–S55, 1989
5. WHO: World Health Statistics Annual. Geneva: World Health Organization, 1986, 1987, 1988
6. Inter-Society Commission for Heart Disease Resources: Primary prevention of the atherosclerotic diseases. Circulation 42:39, 1970

7. Inter-Society Commission for Heart Disease Resources: Optimal resources for primary prevention of atherosclerotic diseases. Circulation 70:153A–205A, 1984
8. The Lipid Research Clinic Program: The lipid research clinic's coronary primary prevention trial results. II. The relationship of reduction in incidence of coronary heart disease to cholesterol lowering. JAMA 251(3):365–374, 1984
9. Multiple Risk Factor Intervention Trial Research Group: Multiple risk factor intervention trial: risk factor changes and mortality results. JAMA 248:1465–1477, 1982
10. Keys A (ed): Coronary heart disease in seven countries. Circulation 41(suppl 1):211, 1970
11. Keys A: Seven Countries: Death and Coronary Heart Disease in Ten Years. Cambridge: Harvard University Press, 1979
12. Gordon T, Garcia-Palmieri MR, Kagan A, Kannel WB, Schiffman J: Differences in coronary heart disease mortality in Framingham, Honolulu and Puerto Rico. J Chron Dis 27:329–344, 1974
13. Rose G: Incubation period of coronary heart disease. Br Med J 284:1600–1601, 1982
14. McGill HC Jr (ed): Geographic Pathology of Atherosclerosis. Baltimore: Williams & Wilkins, 1968
15. Marmot MG, Syme SL, Kagan A, et al: Epidemiologic studies of coronary heart disease and stroke in Japanese men living in Japan, Hawaii and California: prevalence of coronary and hypertensive heart disease and associated risk factors. Am J Epidemiol 102:514–525, 1975
16. Blackburn H: Trends and determinants of CHD mortality: changes in risk factors and their effects. Int J Epidemiol 18(suppl 1):S210–S215, 1989
17. Goldman L, Cook F: Decline in ischemic heart disease mortality rates. Ann Intern Med 101:825–836, 1984
18. Beaglehole R, LaRose JC, Heiss GE, et al: Serum cholesterol, diet and the decline in coronary heart disease. Prev Med 8:538–547, 1979
19. Stamler J: Life-styles, major risk factors, proof and public policy. Circulation 58:3–19, 1978
20. Lee RB, DeVore I (eds): Hunter-Gatherers: Studies of the Kung San and Their Neighbors. Cambridge, Mass: Harvard University Press, 1976
21. Truswell AS: Diet and nutrition of hunter-gatherers. In Elliott K, Whelan J (eds): Health and Disease in Tribal Societies. Ciba Foundation Symposium 49, New York: Elsevier, 1977, pp 213–22
22. Blackburn H, Prineas RJ: Diet and hypertension: anthropology, epidemiology, and public health implications. Prog Biochem Pharmacol 19:31–79, 1983
23. Eaton SB, Konner M: Paleolithic nutrition: a consideration of its nature and current implications. N Engl J Med 312:283–289, 1985
24. Jacobs DR, Anderson J, Blackburn H: Diet and serum cholesterol: do zero correlations negate the relationships? Am J Epidemiol 10:77–88, 1979
25. Blackburn H: Diet and mass hyperlipidemia: a public health view. In Levy R, Rifkind B, Dennis B, Ernest N (eds): Nutrition, Lipids, and Coronary Heart Disease. New York: Raven Press, 1979, pp 309–347
26. Blackburn H, Jacobs DR: Sources of the diet-heart controversy: confusion over population versus individual correlations. Circulation 70:775–780, 1984
27. Keys A, Grande F, Anderson JT: Bias and misrepresentation revisited—"perspective" on saturated fat. Am J Clin Nutr 27:188–212, 1974
28. Hegsted DM, McGandy RB, Myers ML, Stare FJ: Quantitative effects of dietary fat on serum cholesterol in man. Am J Clin Nutr 17:281–295, 1965
29. Connor WE, Stone DB, Hodges RE: The interrelated effects of dietary cholesterol and fat upon human serum lipid levels. J Clin Invest 43:1691–1696, 1964
30. Shekelle RB, Shryock AM, Paul O, Lepper M, Stamler J, Liu S, Raynor WJ Jr: Diet, serum cholesterol, and death from coronary heart disease: the Western Electric Study. N Engl J Med 304:65–70, 1981
31. Kromhout D, de Lezenne Coulander C: Diet, prevalence and 10-year mortality from coronary heart disease in 871 middle-aged men: the Zutphen Study. Am J Epidemiol 119:733–741, 1984
32. McGee DL, Reed DM, Yano K, Kagan A, Tillotson J: Ten-year incidence of coronary heart disease in the Honolulu Heart Program. Relationship to nutrient intake. Am J Epidemiol 119:667–676, 1984
33. Kushi LH, Lew RA, Stare FJ, Ellison CR, el Lozy M, Bourke G, Daly L, Graham I, et al: Diet and 20-year mortality from coronary heart disease: The Ireland-Boston Diet-Heart Study. N Engl J Med 312:811–818, 1985
34. National Research Council: Diet and Health: Implications for Reducing Chronic Disease Risk. Report of the Committee on Diet and Health, Food and Nutrition Board. Washington, DC: National Academy Press, 1989
35. The Lipid Research Clinic Program: The lipid research clinic's coronary primary prevention trial results. I. Reduction in incidence of coronary heart disease. JAMA 251:351–364, 1984
36. Anitschkow N: Experimental atherosclerosis in animals. In Cowdry EV (ed): Arteriosclerosis. New York: 1983, Macmillan, p 271
37. Wallace RB, Lynch CF, Pomrehn PR, Criqui MH, Heiss, G: Alcohol and hypertension: epidemiologic and experimental considerations. Circulation 64(suppl 3):41–47, 1981
38. Dyer AR, Stamler J, Paul O, et al: Alcohol, cardiovascular risk factors and mortality: the Chicago experience. Circulation 64(suppl 3):20–27, 1981
39. Haskell WL, Comargo C, Williams PT, et al: The effect of cessation and resumption of moderate alcohol intake on serum high-density lipoprotein subfractions. N Engl J Med 310:805–810, 1984
40. Kagan A, Yano K, Rhoads G, McGee D: Alcohol and cardiovascular disease: the Hawaiian experience. Circulation 64(suppl 3):27, 1981
41. Klatsky AL, Friedman GD, Siegelaub AB: Alcohol use and cardiovascular disease: the Kaiser-Permanente experience. Circulation 64:32, 1981
42. Kaelber CT, Barboriak J (eds): Symposium on alcohol and cardiovascular diseases. Circulation 64(suppl 3), 1981
43. Kare MR, Fregly MJ, Bernard RA (eds): Biological and Behavioral Aspects of Salt Intake. New York: Academic Press, 1980
44. Freis ED: Salt, volume and the prevention of hypertension. Circulation 53:589–595, 1976
45. Meneely GR, Battarbee HD: High sodium-low potassium environment and hypertension. Am J Cardiol 38:768–785, 1976
46. Gleibermann L: Blood pressure and dietary salt in human populations. Ecol Food Nutr 2:143–156, 1973
47. INTERSALT Cooperative Research Group: INTERSALT: An international study of electrolyte excretion and blood pressure: results for 24 hour urinary sodium and potassium excretion. Br Med J 297:319–328, 1988
48. Liu K, Cooper R, McKeever J, et al: Assessment of the association between habitual salt intake and high blood pressure. Am J Epidemiol 110:219–226, 1979
49. Kesteloot H, Vuylsteks M, Costenoble A: Relationship between blood pressure and sodium and potassium intake in a Belgian male population group. In Kesteloot K, Joossens J (eds): Epidemiology of Arterial Blood Pressure. The Hague: Nijhoff, 1980, pp 345–351
50. Grimm RH Jr, Kofron PM, Neaton JD, Svendsen KH, Elmer PJ, Holland L, Witte L, Clearman D, Prineas RJ: Effect of potassium supplementation combined with dietary sodium reduction on blood pressure in men taking antihypertensive medication. J Hypertens 6(suppl 4):S591–S593, 1988
51. Shimamoto T, Komachi Y, Inada H, Doi M, Iso H, Sata S, Kitamura A, et al: Trends for coronary heart disease and stroke and their risk factors in Japan. Circulation 79:503–515, 1989
52. Sharrett AR, Feinleib M: Water constituents and trace elements in relation to cardiovascular diseases. Prev Med 4:20–36, 1975
53. Wallace RB, Anderson RA. Blood lipids, lipid-related measures, and the risk of atherosclerotic cardiovascular disease. Epidemiol Rev 9:95–119, 1987

54. Hulley SB, Rosenman RH, Banol RD, Brand RJ: Epidemiology as a guide to clinical decisions: the associations between triglycerides and coronary heart disease. N Engl J Med 302:1383–1389, 1980
55. Report of a Conference on the Health Effects of Blood Lipoproteins: Optimal blood lipid levels for populations. Prev Med 8:609–759, 1979
56. Report of a Conference on Blood Lipids in Children: Optimal levels for early prevention of coronary artery disease. Prev Med 12(6):725–905, 1983
57. The Pooling Project Research Group: Relationship of blood pressure, serum cholesterol, smoking habits, relative weight and ECG abnormalities to incidence of major coronary events: final report of the Pooling Project. J Chron Dis 31:201–306, 1978
58. Stamler J, Wentworth D, Neaton JD: Is the relationship between serum cholesterol and risk of premature death from coronary heart disease continuous and graded? Findings in 356,222 primary screenees of the Multiple Risk Factor Intervention Trial (MRFIT). JAMA 256:2823–2828, 1986
59. Report of the WHO Expert Committee on Prevention of Coronary Heart Disease. Geneva: World Health Organization, Tech Ser 678, 1982
60. Gordon T, Castelli W, Hjortland MC, Kannel WB, Dawber TR: High density lipoprotein as a protective factor against coronary heart disease. Am J Med 62:707–714, 1977
61. National Diet-Heart Study Research Group: The National Diet-Heart Study: final report. Circulation 3(suppl 1):428, 1968
62. Gillum RF, Folsom AR, Blackburn H: Decline in coronary heart disease mortality. Am J Med 76:1055–1065, 1984
63. Gomez-Marin O, Folsom AR, Kottke TE, Wu SH, Jacobs DR Jr, Gillum RF, Edlvaitch SA, Blackburn H: Improved long-term survival of patients hospitalized with acute myocardial infarction, 1970–1980: the Minnesota Heart Survey. N Engl J Med 316:1353–59, 1987
64. The Surgeon General's Report on Nutrition and Health. U.S. Department of Health and Human Services, Public Health Service, DHHS (PHS) Publication No. 88-50210, 1988
65. The Expert Panel: Report of the National Cholesterol Education Program Expert Panel on detection, evaluation, and treatment of high blood cholesterol in adults. Arch Intern Med 148:36–69, 1988
66. Barrett-Connor EL: Obesity, atherosclerosis and coronary heart disease. Ann Intern Med 103:1010–1019, 1985
67. Hubert HB, Feinlieb M, McNamara PM, Castelli WP: Obesity as an independent risk factor for cardiovascular disease: a 26 year follow-up of participants in the Framingham Heart Study. Circulation 67:968–977, 1983
68. Tyroler HA, Heyden S, Hames CG: Weight and hypertension: Evans County studies of blacks and whites. In Paul O (ed): Epidemiology and Control of Hypertension. New York: Grune & Stratton, 1975
69. Rabkin SW, Mathewson FAC, Hsu PH: Relation of body weight to the development of ischemic heart disease in a cohort of young North American men after a 26-year observation period: the Manitoba study. Am J Cardiol 39:452–458, 1977
70. Larsson B, Svardsudd K, Welin L, Wilhelmsen L, Bjorntorp P, Tibblin G: Abdominal adipose tissue distribution, obesity, and risk of cardiovascular disease and death: 13 year follow-up of participants in the study of men born in 1913. Br Med J 288:1401–1404, 1984
71. Donahue RP, Abbott RD, Bloom E, Reed DM, Yano K: Central obesity and coronary heart disease in men. Lancet 1:821–824, 1987
72. Bjorntorp P: The associations between obesity, adipose tissue distribution and disease. Acta Med Scand 723(suppl):121–134, 1988
73. Montenegro MR, Solberg LA: Obesity, body weight, body length, and atherosclerosis. Lab Invest 18:594–603, 1968
74. Lissner L, Bengtsson C, Lapidus L, Larsson B, Bengtsson B, Brownell K: Body weight variability and mortality in the Goteborg prospective studies of men and women. In Bjorntorp P, Rossner S (eds): Proceedings of the European Congress of Obesity, June 1987, pp 55–60, 1989
75. Taylor HL, Buskirk ER, Remington RD: Exercise in controlled trials of the prevention of coronary heart disease. Fed Proc 32:1623–1627, 1973
76. Oldridge NB, Guyatt GH, Fischer ME, Rimm AA: Cardiac rehabilitation after myocardial infarction: combined experience of randomized clinical trials. JAMA 260:945–950, 1988
77. Blackburn H, Jacobs DR: Physical activity and the risk of coronary heart disease (editorial). N Engl J Med 319(18):1217–1219, 1988
78. Powell KE, Thompson PD, Caspersen CJ, Kendrick JS: Physical activity and the incidence of coronary heart disease. Ann Rev Public Health 8:253–287, 1987
79. Leon AS, Connett J, Jacobs DR Jr, Rauramaa R: Leisure-time physical activity levels and risk of coronary heart disease and death: the Multiple Risk Factor Intervention Trial. JAMA 258:2388–2395, 1987
80. Slattery ML, Jacobs DR Jr, Nichaman MZ: Leisure time physical activity and coronary heart disease death: the U.S. Railroad Study. Circulation 79:304–311, 1989
81. Blair SN, Kohl HW, Paffenbarger RS Jr, Clark DG, Cooper KH, Gibbons LW: Physical fitness and all-cause mortality: a prospective study of healthy men and women. JAMA 262(17)2395–2401, 1989
82. Paffenbarger RS Jr, Wing AL, Hyde RT: Physical activity as an index of heart attack risk in college alumni. Am J Epidemiol 108:161–175, 1978
83. Paffenbarger RS Jr, Hyde RT, Wing AL, Steinmetz CH: A natural history of athleticism and cardiovascular health. JAMA 252:491–495, 1984
84. Siscovick DS, Weiss NS, Fletcher RH, Lasky T: The incidence of primary cardiac arrest during vigorous exercise. N Engl J Med 311:874–877, 1984
85. West KM: Epidemiology of Diabetes and Its Vascular Lesions. New York: Elsevier, 1978, pp 375–402
86. Pyorala K, Laakso M, Uusitupa M: Diabetes and atherosclerosis: an epidemiologic view. Diabetes Metab Rev 3:463–524, 1987
87. Knowler WC, Bennett PH, Hammon RF, Miller M: Diabetes incidence and prevalence in Pima Indians: a 19-fold greater incidence than in Rochester, MN. Am J Epidemiol 108:497–505, 1978
88. Barrett-Connor E, Wingard DL: Sex differential in ischemic heart disease mortality in diabetics: a prospective population-based study. Am J Epidemiol 118:489–496, 1983
89. Stamler R, Stamler J, Lindberg HA, et al: Asymptomatic hyperglycemia and coronary heart disease in middle-aged men in two employed populations in Chicago. J Chron Dis 32:805–815, 1979
90. Hughes LO: Insulin, Indian origin and ischemic heart disease (editorial). Int J Cardiol 26:1–4, 1990
91. Hypertension Detection and Follow-Up Group: The effect of treatment on mortality in "mild" hypertension. N Engl J Med 307:976–980, 1982
92. Folsom AR, Luepker RV, Gillum RF, et al: Improvement in hypertension detection and control: the Minnesota Heart Survey experience. JAMA 250:916–921, 1983
93. Report of the Surgeon General: The Health Consequences of Smoking: Cardiovascular Disease. Rockville, Md: U.S. Department of Health and Human Services, Public Health Service, Office on Smoking and Health, 1983
94. Kannel WB, McGee DL, Castelli WP: Latest perspectives on cigarette smoking and cardiovascular disease: the Framingham Study. J Cardiovasc Rehab 4:267–277, 1984
95. Wilhelmsen L: Coronary heart disease: epidemiology of smoking and intervention studies of smoking. Am Heart J 115:242–249, 1988
96. Amler RW, Dull HB (eds): Closing the Gap: the Burden of Unnecessary Illness. New York: Oxford University Press, 1987
97. Willett WC, Green A, Stampfer MJ, et al: Relative and absolute excess risks of coronary heart disease among women who smoke cigarettes. N Engl J Med 317(21):1303–1309, 1987
98. Doll R, Hill AB: Mortality in relation to smoking: ten years' observations of British doctors. Br Med J 1(5395):1399–1410, 1964

99. Freidman GD, Petitti DB, Bawol RD, Siegelaub AB: Mortality in cigarette smokers and quitters: effect of base-line differences. N Engl J Med 304(23):1407–1410, 1981
100. Aberg A, Bergstrand J, Johansson S, et al: Cessation of smoking after myocardial infarction: effects on mortality after ten years. Br Heart J 49:416–422, 1983
101. McGill HC Jr: Potential mechanisms for the augmentation of atherosclerosis and atherosclerotic disease by cigarette smoking. Prev Med 8:390–403, 1979
102. Luepker RV, Johnson CA, Murray DM, Pechacek TF: Prevention of cigarette smoking: three year follow-up of an educational program for youth. J Behav Med 6:53–62, 1983
103. Report of the Surgeon General: Reducing the Health Consequences of Smoking: Twenty-five Years of Progress. Rockville, Md: U.S. Department of Health and Human Services, Public Health Service, Office on Smoking and Health, 1989
104. Meade TW: Clotting factors and ischemic heart disease. In Meade TW (ed): The Epidemiological Evidence From Anti-coagulants in Myocardial Infarction: A Reappraisal. New York: John Wiley & Sons, 1984
105. Wilhelmsen L, Svardsudd K, Korsan-Bengtsen K, Larsson B, Welin L, Tibblin G: Fibrinogen as a risk factor for stroke and myocardial infarction. N Engl J Med 311:501–505, 1984
106. Meade TW, Brozovich M, Chakrabarti RR, Hanes AP, Imeson JD, Mellows S, Miller JG, North RS, Sterling Y, Thompson SG: Hemostatic function and ischemic heart disease: principal results of the Northwick Park Heart Study. Lancet 2:533–537, 1986
107. Chalmers TC, Matta RJ, Smith H, Kunzler AM: Evidence favoring the use of anti-coagulants in the hospital phase of acute myocardial infarction. N Engl J Med 297:1091–1096, 1977
108. Steering Committee of the Physicians' Health Study Research Group HMS: Preliminary report: findings from the aspirin component of the ongoing Physicians' Health Study. N Engl J Med 318:262–264, 1988
109. Grimm RH Jr, Neaton JD, Ludwig W, for the MRFIT Research Group: Prognostic importance of the white blood cell count for coronary, cancer and all-cause mortality. JAMA 265:1932–1937, 1985
110. Ernst E, Hammerschmidt DE, Baagge U, Matrai A, Dormandy JA: Leukocytes and the risk of ischemic diseases. JAMA 257:2318–2324, 1987
111. Grimm RH Jr, Leon AS, Hunninghake DB, et al: Effects of thiazide diuretics on plasma lipids and lipoproteins in mildly hypertensive patients. Ann Intern Med 94:7–11, 1981
112. Rosenman RH, Brand RJ, Jenkins CD, et al: Coronary heart disease in the Western Collaborative Group Study: final follow-up experience of 8 1/2 years. JAMA 233:872–877, 1975
113. Haynes SG, Feinleib M, Kannel WB: The relationship of psychosocial factors to coronary heart disease in the Framingham Study. III. Eight-year incidence of coronary heart disease. Am J Epidemiol 111:37–58, 1980
114. Matthews KA, Haynes SG: Type A behavior pattern and coronary disease risk. Am J Epidemiol 123:923–960, 1986
115. Dimsdale JE, Gilbert J, Hutter AM, et al: Predicting cardiac morbidity based on risk factors and coronary angiographic findings. Am J Cardiol 47:73–76, 1981
116. Case RB, Heller SS, Case NB, et al: Type A behavior and survival after acute myocardial infarction. N Engl J Med 312:737–741, 1985
117. Shekelle RB, Gale M, Norusis M: Type A score (Jenkins Activity Survey) and risk of recurrent coronary heart disease in the Aspirin Myocardial Infarction Study. Am J Cardiol 56:221–225, 1985
118. Shekelle RB, Hulley SB, Neaton JD, et al: The MRFIT behavior pattern study. II. Type A behavior and incidence of coronary heart disease. Am J Epidemiol 122:559–570, 1985
119. Cohen JB, Reed D: Type A behavior and coronary heart disease among Japanese men in Hawaii. J Behav Med 8:343–352, 1985
120. Friedmann M, Thorensen CE, Gill JJ, et al: Alteration of type A behavior and reduction in cardiac recurrences in post-myocardial infarction patients. Am Heart J 108:237–248, 1984
121. Ragland DR, Brand RJ: Type A behavior and mortality from coronary heart disease. N Engl J Med 318(2):65–69, 1988
122. Ragland DR, Brand RJ: Coronary heart disease mortality in the Western Collaborative Group Study: follow-up experience of 22 years. Am J Epidemiol 127:462–475, 1988
123. Matthews KA, Glass DC, Rosenman RH, et al: Competitive drive, pattern A, and coronary heart disease: a further analysis of some data from the Western Collaborative Group Study. J Chron Dis 30:489–498, 1977
124. Hecker MHL, Chesney MA, Black GW, Frautsch N: Coronary-prone behaviors in the Western Collaborative Group Study. Psychosom Med 50:153–164, 1988
125. Barefoot JC, Dahlstrom WG, Williams RB: Hostility, CHD incidence, and total mortality: a 25-year follow-up study of 255 physicians. Psychosom Med 45:59–63, 1983
126. Shekelle RB, Gale M, Ostfeld AM, Paul O: Hostility, risk of coronary heart disease, and mortality. Psychosom Med 45:109–114, 1983
127. Barefoot JC, Williams RB, Dahlstrom WG, Dodge KA: Predicting mortality from scores on the Cook-Medley Scale: a follow-up study of 118 lawyers. Psychosom Med 49:210, 1987
128. McCranie EW, Watkins LO, Brandsma JM, Sisson BD: Hostility, coronary heart disease (CHD) incidence, and total mortality: lack of an association in a 25-year follow-up study of 478 physicians. J Behav Med 9:119–125, 1986
129. Leon GR, Finn SE, Murray D, Bailey JM: Inability to predict cardiovascular disease from hostility scores of MMPI items related to type A behavior. J Consult Clin Psychol 56:597–600, 1988
130. Hearn MD, Murray DM, Luepker RV: Hostility, coronary heart disease, and total mortality: a 33-year follow-up study of university students. J Behav Med 12(2):105–121, 1988
131. Dembroski TM, MacDougall JM, Williams RB, Haney TL, Blumenthal JA: Components of type A, hostility, and anger-in: relationship to angiographic findings. Psychosom Med 47:219–233, 1985
132. MacDougall JM, Dembroski TM, Dimsdale JE, Hackett TP: Components of type A, hostility, and anger-in: further relationship to angiographic findings. Health Psychol 4:137–152, 1985
133. Williams RB, Haney TL, Lee KL, Kong Y, Blumenthal JA, Whalen RE: Type A behavior, hostility, and coronary atherosclerosis. Psychosom Med 42:539–549, 1980
134. Kaplan GA, Salonen JT, Cohen RD, Brand RJ, Syme SL, Puska P: Social connections and mortality from all causes and from cardiovascular disease: prospective evidence from Eastern Finland. Am J Epidemiol 128:370–380, 1988
135. Orth-Gomer K, Johnson JV: Social network interaction and mortality: a six year follow-up study of a random sample of the Swedish population. J Chron Dis 40(10):949–957, 1987
136. McGill HC Jr, Stern MP: Sex and atherosclerosis. In Paoletti R, Gotto AM Jr (eds): Atherosclerosis Reviews. New York: Raven Press, 1979, vol 4, pp 157–242
137. Demirovic J: Recent trends in coronary heart disease mortality among women in Yugoslavia. CVD Epidemiol Newsletter 44:96–97, 1988
138. Bain C, Willet W, Hennekens CW, et al: Use of post-menopausal hormones and risk of myocardial infarction. Circulation 64:42–46, 1981
139. Wahl P, Walden C, Knopp R, et al: Effect of estrogen/progestin potency on lipid/lipoprotein metabolism. N Engl J Med 308:862–867, 1983
140. Austin MA, et al: Risk factors for coronary heart disease in adult female twins: genetic heritability and shared environmental influences. Am J Epidemiol 125:308–318, 1987
141. Hasstedt SJ, Wu L, Williams RR: Major locus inheritance of apolipoprotein B in Utah pedigrees. Genet Epidemiol 4:67–76, 1987
142. Austin MA, King MC, Vranizan KM, Newman B, Krauss RM: Inheritance of low-density lipoprotein subclass patterns: results of complex segregation analysis. Am J Hum Genet 43:838–846, 1988

143. Jacobs DR, Anderson JT, Hannan P, Keys A, Blackburn H: Variability in individual serum cholesterol response to change in diet. Arterosclerosis 3(4):349–356, 1983
144. Report of the WHO Expert Committee on Prevention of Coronary Heart Disease: Geneva: World Health Organization, Tech Ser 678, 1982
145. Hunt SC, Hasstedt SJ, Kuida H, Stults BM, Hopkins PN, Williams RR: Genetic heritability and common environmental components of resting and stressed blood pressures, lipids, and body mass index in Utah pedigrees and twins. Am J Epidemiol 129:625–638, 1989
146. Keys A, Aravanis C, Blackburn H, van Buchem FSP, Buzina R, Djordjevic BS, Fidanza F, Karvonen MJ, Menotti A, Puddu V, Taylor HL: Probability of middle-aged men developing coronary heart disease in five years. Circulation 45:815–828, 1972
147. Strasser T: Rheumatic fever and rheumatic heart disease in the 1970s. Public Health Rev 5:207–234, 1976
148. World Health Organization Report: Intensified program: action to prevent rheumatic fever/rheumatic heart disease. WHO Document, WHO/CVD/84.3, Geneva: World Health Organization, 1984
149. Veasy LG, Wiedmeier SE, Orsmond GS, et al: Resurgence of acute rheumatic fever in the intermountain area of the United States. N Engl J Med 316(8):421–427, 1987
150. Wannamaker LW, Matsen JM (eds): Streptococci and Streptococcal Diseases: Recognition, Understanding, and Management. New York: Academic Press, 1972
151. Gordis L, Lilienfeld A, Rodriguez R: Studies in the epidemiology and preventability of rheumatic fever: socioeconomic factors. J Chron Dis 21:655, 1969
152. American Heart Association Booklet: Jones Criteria (revised) for Guidance in the Diagnosis of Rheumatic Fever. Dallas: The Association, 1982
153. Wannamaker LW: The chain that links the heart to the throat. Circulation 48:9–18, 1973
154. Dajani AS, Bisno AL, Chung KJ, et al: Prevention of rheumatic fever: a statement for health professionals by the Committee on Rheumatic Fever, Endocarditis, and Kawasaki Disease of the Council on Cardiovascular Disease in the Young, the American Heart Association. Circulation (Special Report) 78(4):1082–1086, 1988
155. Pan American Health Organization: Fourth meeting of the Working Group on Prevention of Rheumatic Fever. Quito, Ecuador, 1970
156. Phibbs B, Taylor J, Zimmerman RA: A community-wide streptococcal control project: the Natrona County primary prevention program. JAMA 214:2018–2024, 1970
157. Elliot RS, Edwards JE: Pathology of congenital heart disease. In Hurst JW (ed): The Heart. New York: McGraw-Hill, 1978
158. Congenital Heart Disease Study Group: Primary prevention of congenital heart disease. In Wright IS, Fredrickson DT (eds): Cardiovascular Diseases, Guidelines for Prevention and Care. Reports of the Inter-Society Commission for Heart Disease Resources. Washington, DC: Government Printing Office, 1972, p 116
159. Higgins ITT: The epidemiology of congenital heart disease. J Chron Dis 18:699, 1965
160. Nora JJ: Etiologic factors in congenital heart diseases. Pediatr Clin North Am 18:1059–1074, 1971
161. Fredrich J, Alberman ED, Goldsteen H: Possible teratogenic effect of cigarette smoking. Nature (London) 231:529, 1971
162. Rose V, Gold RJM, Lindsay G, et al: A possible increase in the incidence of congenital heart defects among the offspring of affected parents. J Am Coll Cardiol 6:376–382, 1985
163. Ferencz C: Offspring of fathers with cardiovascular malformations. Am Heart J 111(6):1212–1213, 1986
164. Zierler S: Maternal drugs and congenital heart disease. Obstet Gynecol 65(2):155–165, 1985
165. NHLBI Working Group on Heart Disease Epidemiology: NIH Report 79-1667, Washington, DC: Government Printing Office, 1979
166. Bailey NA, Lay P: New horizons: infant cardiac transplantation. Heart Lung 18:172–178, 1989
167. WHO Expert Committee: Cardiomyopathies. Geneva: World Health Organization, WHO Technical Report Series 697, 1984
168. Fowles RE: Progress of research in cardiomyopathy and myocarditis in the USA. International Symposium on Cardiomyopathy and Myocarditis. Heart and Vessels (suppl. 1). Heidelberg and New York: Springer, 1985, pp 5–7
169. Olsen EGJ: What is myocarditis? International Symposium on Cardiomyopathy and Myocarditis. Heart and Vessels (suppl. 1) Heidelberg and New York: Springer, 1985, pp 1–3
170. Shabeter R: Cardiomyopathy: how far have we come in 25 years? How far yet to go? J Am Coll Cardiol 1:252–263, 1983
171. Gillum RF: Idiopathic cardiomyopathy in the United States, 1970–1982. Am Heart J 111(4):752–755, 1986
172. Codd MB, Sugrue DD, Gersh BJ, et al: Epidemiology of idiopathic dilated and hypertrophic cardiomyopathy: a population-based study in Olmsted County, MN, 1975–1984. Copyright 1988 Mayo Foundation
173. Okada R, Wakafuji S: Myocarditis in autopsy. International Symposium on Cardiomyopathy and Myocarditis. Heart and Vessels (suppl. 1), Heidelberg and New York: Springer, 1985, pp 23–29
174. Rubin E: Alcoholic myopathy in heart and skeletal muscle. N Engl J Med 301:28, 1979
175. Alexander CS: Cobalt-beer cardiomyopathy: a clinical and pathological study of twenty-eight cases. Am J Med 53:195, 1972
176. Regan TJ, Haider B, Ahmed SS, et al: Whisky and the heart. Cardiovasc Med 2:165, 1977
177. Levine HD: Virus myocarditis: a critique of the literature from clinical, electrocardiographic and pathologic standpoints. Am J Med Sci 277:132, 1979
178. McAllister HA Jr: Myocarditis: some current perspectives and future directions. Texas Heart Inst J 14(4):331–334, 1987
179. Parrillo JE, Cunnion RE, Epstein SE, et al: A prospective, randomized, controlled trial of prednisone for dilated cardiomyopathy. N Engl J Med 321(16):1061–1068, 1989
180. Wigle ED: Hypertrophic cardiomyopathy 1988. AHA-Mod Concepts Cardiovasc Dis 57(1):1–6, 1988
181. Acquatella H, Schiller NB, Puigbo JJ, et al: M-mode and two-dimensional echocardiography in chronic Chagas' heart disease: a clinical and pathologic study. Circulation 62:787, 1980
182. World Health Organization: Report of the WHO consultation on cardiomyopathies: Approaches to prevention and early detection. WHO Document, WHO/CVD/85.6, Geneva: World Health Organization, 1985
183. Centers for Disease Control: Summary of notifiable diseases—United States. MMWR 36:54–58, 1988
184. Clark EG, Danbolt N: The Oslo study of the natural course of untreated syphilis: an epidemiologic investigation based on a re-study of the Boeck-Bruusgaard material. Med Clin North Am 48:613, 1964
185. Musher DM: Syphilis. Infect Dis Clin North Am 1(1):83–95, 1987
186. Jackman JD Jr, Radolf JD: Cardiovascular syphilis. Am J Med 87:425–433, 1989

49

Hypertension

Darwin R. Labarthe

Hypertension, or high blood pressure, is a chronic condition of concern in much of the world. This concern is due to its role in the causation of coronary heart disease, stroke, and other vascular complications with a combined mortality that in some countries exceeds 50% of the total deaths. The added morbidity and the personal and societal burdens of treatment contribute further to an immense cost in compromised duration and quality of human life, as well as economic cost. Treatment is effective, however, and the detection and long-term management of those at risk pose substantial challenges.

For these reasons, hypertension and its prevention constitute important issues in public health and preventive medicine. In recent years the World Health Organization has convened expert committees whose reports provide a broad perspective on the prevention of hypertension[1] and in particular on the importance of both research and preventive programs concerning blood pressure in childhood and youth[2,3].

DEFINITION

Definitions of hypertension have varied as concepts of both its natural history and the accepted indications for its treatment have changed. Because risks of morbidity and mortality are graded continuously in relation to blood pressure levels, any demarcation to classify individuals along the continuum as "normal" or "hypertensive" is arbitrary, and persons with hypertension should no longer be viewed as a discrete subgroup.

In a committee report from the U.S. National High Blood Pressure Education Program, which appeared in 1985,[4] it was proposed that both risk and evidence of treatment response should be incorporated in a definition most appropriate for community diagnosis and for decision making about intervention; that the lowest risk in the population, rather than the average risk, should be taken as the reference or target value; and that multistage screening, which is a practical requirement for case identification before treatment, should be taken into account (see discussion of screening, below). Both systolic and diastolic pressure must be included because, although they are highly correlated, each contributes to risk. Table 49–1 reflects the resulting recommendation.

Within the United States, and perhaps elsewhere, the recommendations of the Joint National Committee on Detection, Evaluation, and Treatment of High Blood Pressure (also of the High Blood Pressure Education Program) are widely recognized. They take the same direction as that illustrated in Table 49–1 but remain closer to the more traditional (but still arbitrary) view that diastolic blood pressures below 90 mm Hg are "normal" (Table 49–2).[5]

MEASUREMENT

Definitions in terms of blood pressure values are strictly meaningful only when the measurement of blood pressure is reliable. The importance of this fact increases as refinement of the objectives of screening requires increasing stratification of populations or patients into multiple discrete classes. Accuracy of classification of the individual on any single occasion of blood pressure measurement depends on control of the potential influences of the circumstances, the equipment and procedures used, and characteristics of the observer. For many years, recommended procedures for blood pressure measurement have been published by the American Heart Association.[6] Training materials for standardization of observers in community blood pressure control programs and for multicenter research programs have also been developed[7]. It is hoped that conformity with such recommendations will eventually become the standard of clinical and public health practice.

A contemporary view of hypertension includes not only the upper extreme of the population distribution of blood pressure, where treatment has been shown effective in reducing risks, but the distribution as a whole as it varies among populations and by age and other attributes within a population. Of concern is not only the period of adulthood, where established hypertension is common, but also the period of childhood and youth, with lower absolute values but in many populations an expected progression to higher values with increasing age. Accordingly, the topics addressed here are, broadly, the natural history and effects of intervention on blood pressure, first in adulthood and then in childhood and youth.

NATURAL HISTORY IN ADULTS

Prevalence. The prevalence of hypertension in populations is assessed by cross-sectional surveys, with typical results as depicted in Figure 49–1.[8] The frequency distribution of diastolic

TABLE 49-1. DEFINITIONS OF BLOOD PRESSURE CLASSES

▪ **On the First Occasion of Measurement**	**DBP (mm Hg)**
Minimal-risk blood pressure	<80
Intermediate-risk blood pressure	80–89
Higher-risk blood pressure (to be rescreened)	≥90
▪ **On the Second Occasion of Measurement**	**DBP (mm Hg)**
Intermediate-risk blood pressure	<90
Confirmed high blood pressure	≥90
NOTE: If on the first occasion DBP is <90 but SBP is ≥160, rescreen	
▪ **Then, on the Second Occasion**	**SBP (mm Hg)**
Intermediate-risk blood pressure	<160
Confirmed high blood pressure	≥160

From Working Group on Risk and High Blood Pressure. Hypertension 7:641–651, 1985.[4]

TABLE 49-2. DEFINITIONS OF BLOOD PRESSURE CLASSES[a]

BP Range (mm Hg)	Category[b]
DBP	
<85	Normal BP
85–89	High-normal BP
90–104	Mild hypertension
105–114	Moderate hypertension
≥115	Severe hypertension
SBP, when DBP <90 mm Hg	
<140	Normal BP
140–159	Borderline isolated systolic hypertension
≥160	Isolated systolic hypertension

[a] Classification based on the average of two or more readings on two or more occasions. *BP* indicates blood pressure; *DBP*, diastolic blood pressure; and *SBP*, systolic blood pressure.

[b] A classification of borderline isolated systolic hypertension (SBP, 140 to 159 mm Hg) or isolated systolic hypertension (SBP, ≥160 mm Hg) takes precedence over high-normal BP (DBP, 85 to 89 mm Hg) when both occur in the same person. High-normal BP (DBP, 85 to 89 mm Hg) takes precedence over a classification of normal BP (SBP, <140 mm Hg) when both occur in the same person.

From 1988 Joint National Committee. Arch Intern Med 148:1023–1038, 1988.[5]

blood pressure among adults at the first stage of screening for a very large population-based trial (the Hypertension Detection and Followup Program, or HDFP) demonstrates a modal value at 80 to 84 mm Hg, and the typical skewing toward the higher values. The prevalence of "hypertension," hypothetically based on this single occasion and for diastolic pressure only, would be estimated as shown, depending on the blood pressure criterion selected. From the highest values down to 90 mm Hg, the prevalence roughly doubles for each reduction of 5 mm Hg in the criterion value. Obviously, estimates of prevalence depend on the definition used. However defined, prevalence varies among groups by age, sex, and ethnicity. For example, for blacks in the United States, prevalence of hypertension by any of these criteria is substantially greater than for the population as a whole, typically by a factor of about 2.

Screening. When surveys are conducted for the purpose of identifying candidates for possible intervention, as in the example above from the HDFP, measurement on more than one occasion is required. A scheme recommended for this screening process, according to the Working Group previously cited,[4] is illustrated on p 851.

How many persons in the United States have hypertension? On the basis of only one screening, the population would be distributed in one of the classifications shown in Table 49-3, in which the U.S. civilian, noninstitutionalized population 25 to 74 years of age based on blood pressure data for the period 1971-75, serves for illustration.

The conventional definitions of borderline and definite hypertension would include all persons with diastolic pressure of 90 mm Hg or greater or systolic pressure of 140 mm Hg or greater on a single occasion of measurement—for men and women together, a total of 37.5 million persons. The proposed definitions would identify 25.1 million persons, provisionally, as at higher risk; then, at the second stage of screening as described, approximately one third of those rescreened would not be confirmed because of the wide intraindividual variability of blood pressure readings, and the estimate would fall to between 15 and 20 million, with elevated systolic readings included (as in the scheme shown above). There are thus large differences in estimates, depending on the approach to screening and the criteria for classification. The addition of other population groups (institutionalized, military, and those beyond the 25- to 74-year age range)

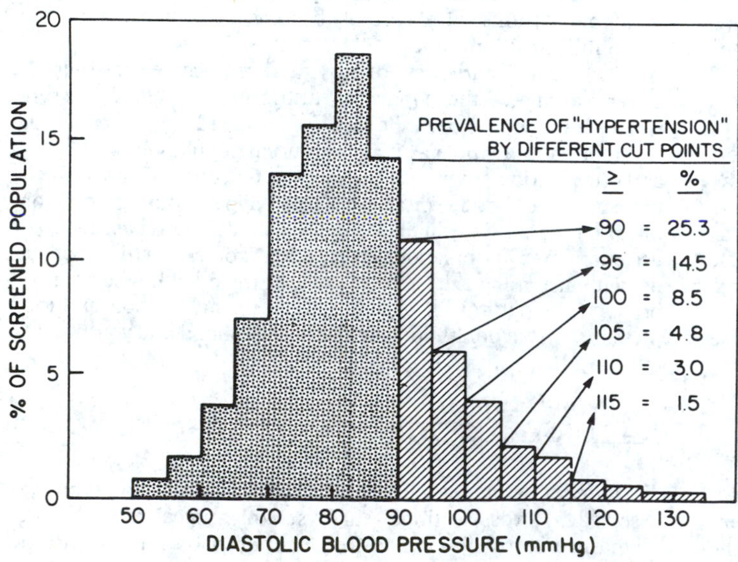

Figure 49-1. Distribution of diastolic blood pressure on single-occasion screening. *(From HDFP, 1977.[8])*

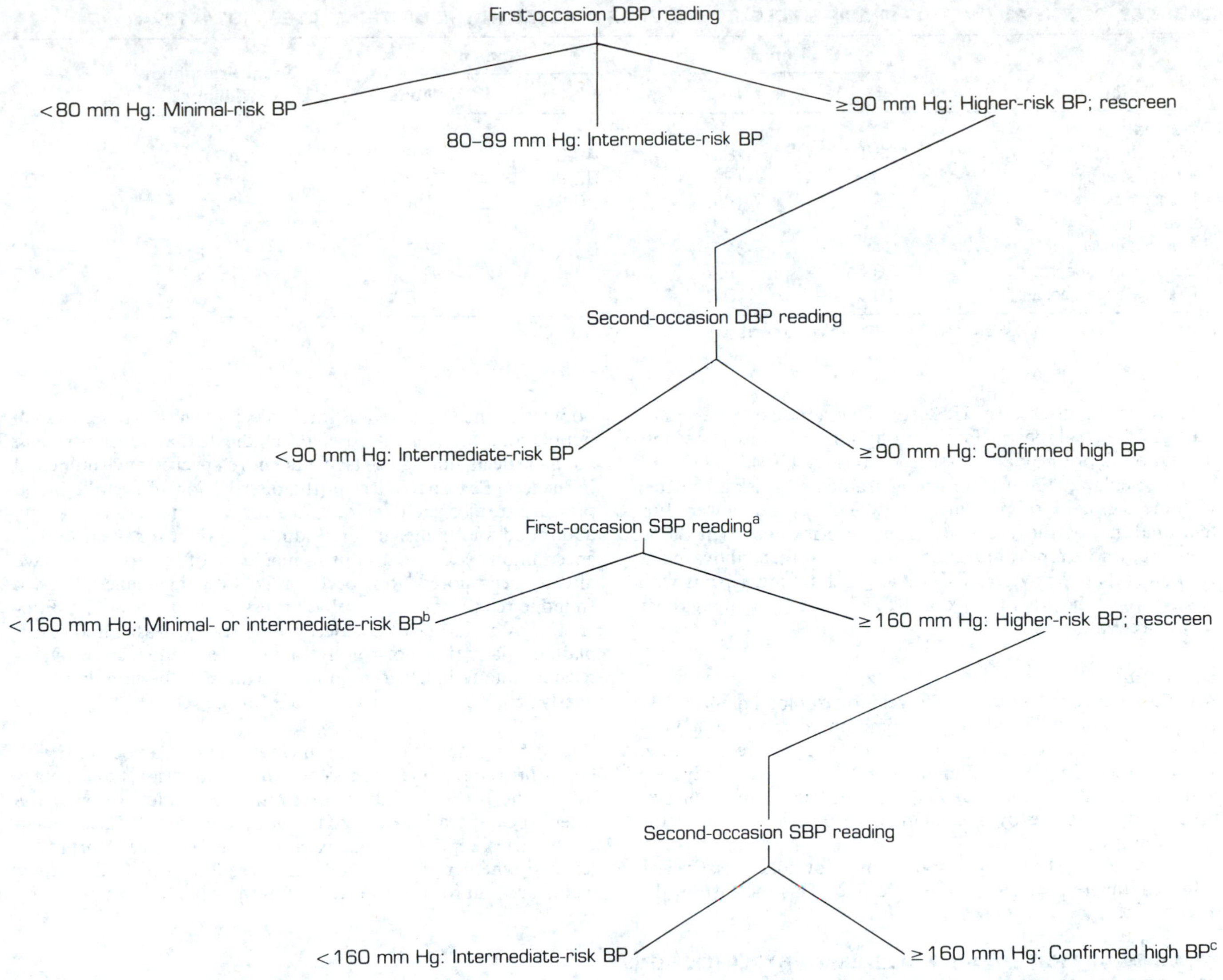

[a]Applies only to persons with DBP below 90 mm Hg.
[b]Classification with SBP below 160 is on basis of a DBP less than 80 or 80 to 89 mm Hg.
[c]Evidence currently available is insufficient to consider this risk reducible by known intervention; studies on this matter are in progress.

would, of course, increase the total number still further. The figure of 58 million given in the 1988 report by the Joint National Committee clearly reflects single-occasion screening. While it enumerates the persons with increased risk as reflected in a single casual blood pressure reading, it does not identify the subgroup of persons who would be considered eligible for treatment.[5]

Incidence. Incidence of hypertension is more difficult to estimate than prevalence. This is because changes in blood pressure levels over time must be determined in a fixed cohort, taking both inaccuracy of measurement and intraindividual variability into account. The possibility that treatment may be initiated by those who have been found hypertensive between study examinations must also be addressed. Such an investigation has been reported from the HDFP, cited above, in which persons who were not definitely hypertensive at initial screening were classified as to the presence or absence of diastolic pressures of 95 mm Hg or greater after two-stage rescreening 3 years later (Table 49–4).[9]

The overall incidence rate of 3% per year included rates of about 2% per year for white men and women and rates more than twice as great for blacks, especially black men. The incidence rates were closely related to initial blood pressure values, as would be expected, and for those with values from 80 to 94 mm Hg at initial screening the incidence was 5% per year. This result emphasizes the potential importance, for prevention of hypertension, of the early recognition of those at intermediate risk.

Incidence of hypertension was previously investigated among whites and blacks in Evans County, Georgia, and was found to relate strongly to both overweight at the time of the baseline examination and to weight gain of 10 pounds or more in the 7-year interval of analysis.[10] The greater incidence in blacks than in whites, in each class of baseline weight and weight gain, predicted the results observed in the HDFP.

Risks. The importance of high blood pressure as a public health problem results from its contribution to the risks of morbidity and mortality. Early recognition of this fact stimulated research by the Society of Actuaries, beginning early in this century, on the relation of blood pressure to mortality among life insurance policyholders. Such studies have demonstrated independent contributions to risk for both systolic and diastolic pressure (Fig. 49–2).[11]

In addition, data from several long-term cohort studies of

TABLE 49-3. PREVALENCE OF SPECIFIED BLOOD PRESSURE CLASSES IN THE UNITED STATES, 1971–1974

Definitions	Men		Women		Total Frequency (Millions)	
	%	Millions	%	Millions		
Proposed						
Minimal risk	35.6	18.0	49.3	27.6	45.6	106
Intermediate risk	36.8	18.6	30.9	17.3	35.9	
Higher risk	27.6	14.0	19.8	11.1	25.1	
Conventional						
Normotensive	61.7	31.2	67.7	37.9	69.1	106
Borderline hypertensive	18.6	9.4	15.8	8.9	18.3	
Definite hypertensive	19.7	10.0	16.5	9.2	19.2	

From Working Group on Risk and High Blood Pressure. Hypertension 7:641–651, 1985.[4]

cardiovascular diseases in U.S. adults were pooled to estimate the risk of several specific fatal or nonfatal cardiovascular events in relation to prior blood pressure levels (Fig. 49-3).[12]

These data demonstrate strong gradients of risk associated with increasing blood pressure values. The same data were further analyzed by the Working Group on Risk and High Blood Pressure, whose report indicated risks for several cardiovascular endpoints that were 1.5 to 2 times as great among persons with baseline diastolic pressures from 80 to 89 mm Hg as among those with lower values.[4]

Determinants

Age, Race, Sex, and Education. The relation of blood pressure levels to age, alluded to above, is common to most adult populations for which cross-sectional survey data are available. These observations were summarized 25 years ago by Epstein and Eckoff, who schematically represented patterns of mean systolic blood pressure by age in many populations around the world (Fig. 49-4).

Commonly, the upward slope of mean systolic pressure was a few millimeters of mercury per decade. This increase in the population mean by age was rarely absent. The existence of such populations has been interpreted to indicate that hypertension in adults reflects not aging itself but more specific environmental influences. Sex differences in the distribution of systolic blood pressure are also age-related; values for women are lower in early adulthood and higher in later adulthood than for men. Differences among sex-race groups in incidence of hypertension have already been noted.[9] Socioeconomic status has generally been found to relate inversely to blood pressure values in adults. Education, as a marker of socioeconomic status, was found to explain partially (but not wholly) the greater frequency of hypertension among blacks than among whites in the population of nearly 160,000 U.S. adults screened for the HDFP.[14]

Salt. Among specific environmental factors associated with blood pressure, none has received more attention than dietary salt in the form of sodium or sodium chloride. Recently the Intersalt Cooperative Research Group, representing 52 centers in 29 countries, reported on an extensive collaborative effort to determine whether urinary sodium excretion and other factors would account for the expected differences in blood pressure lev-

TABLE 49-4. THREE-YEAR INCIDENCE OF HYPERTENSION

	A Incidence	B % of A of Rx	C Incidence of Treated Case (A × B)	D Remaining Cases (A − C)	E Confirmation Rate (Table 4)	F Percent New Confirmed Cases (D × E)	G Two-stage Incidence of Hypertension (C + F)
Race and sex							
Black men	28.6	39.6	11.3	17.3	53.4	9.2	20.5 6.8/yr
Black women	23.3	49.5	11.5	11.8	41.8	4.9	16.4 5.5/yr
White men	8.2	53.0	4.4	3.8	47.6	1.8	6.2 2.1/yr
White women	9.6	73.1	7.0	2.6	29.8	0.8	7.8 2.6/yr
Baseline DBP (mm Hg)							
<80	5.0	65.1	3.3	1.7	29.7	0.5	3.8 1.3/yr
80–94	16.8	78.8	13.2	3.6	46.3	1.7	14.9 5.0/yr
Labiles	41.8	51.2	21.4	20.4	46.2	9.4	30.8 10.3/yr
Total	11.8	57.4	6.8	5.0	43.6	2.2	9.0 3.0/yr

From Apostolides AY et al. Prev Med 11:487–499, 1982.[9]

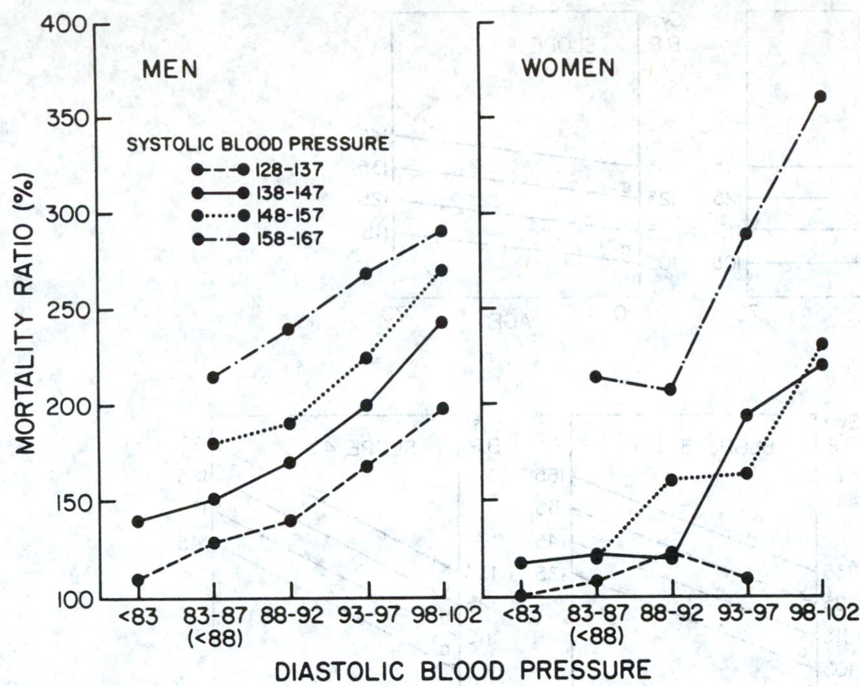

Figure 49-2. Mortality risks related to systolic and diastolic blood pressure. *[Adapted from Labarthe DR, 1977.[11]]*

els and age-related slopes within and among these populations.[15] Within populations, the urinary sodium excretion was positively correlated with systolic pressure more often than with diastolic pressure, although in some populations negative correlations were significant. In analyses between populations, the results confirmed the absence of significant blood pressure increases with age in the populations with the lowest sodium excretion. In the remaining populations, sodium excretion was related not to the median blood pressure or prevalence of hypertension but to the slope of blood pressure with age. The results may indicate a favorable influence of low salt intake on the progressive increase of blood pressure with age. The urinary sodium/potassium ratio was similarly related to the blood pressure indices in these populations.

Other Dietary Factors. Detailed and extensively documented reviews of dietary factors in relation to health have been presented recently in the United States by both the National Research Council and the Surgeon General.[16,17] In relation to blood pressure, in addition to sodium and potassium, attention is given to calcium, chloride, lead, magnesium, trace elements, carbohydrates, fiber, fat (especially polyunsaturates and the ratio of polyunsaturated to saturated fats), protein, caffeine, and overall caloric balance. Recommendations in the Surgeon General's report include improvements in food labeling, food services, food processing by manufacturers, and advice to populations at special risk of hypertension.[17] Both reports address research priorities, as many questions remain concerning the role of these specific aspects of diet and their possible implications for tailoring of dietary recommendations to the actual food sources available to particular populations.

Weight, Weight Gain, and Obesity. The relation of weight and weight gain to incidence of hypertension was discussed above

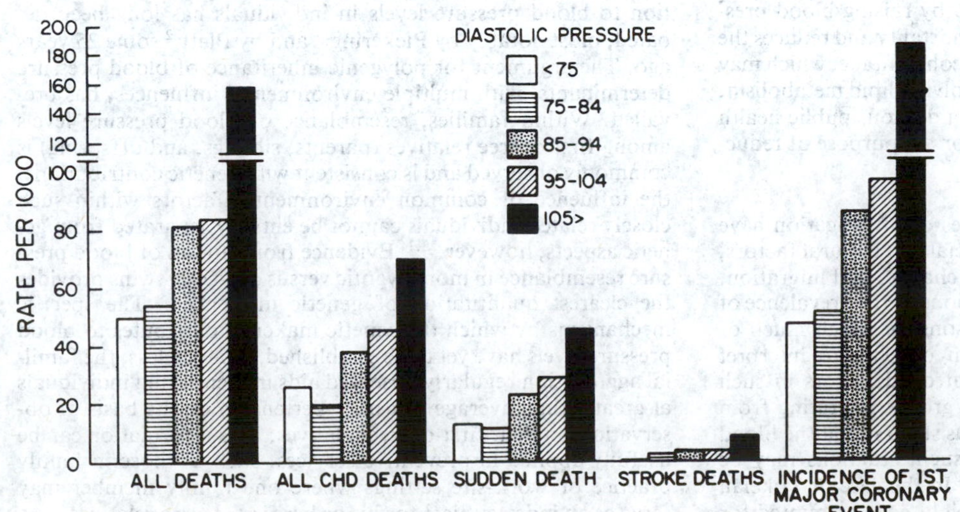

Figure 49-3. Cardiovascular risks related to diastolic blood pressure *[From the Pooling Project Research Group, 1978.[12]]*

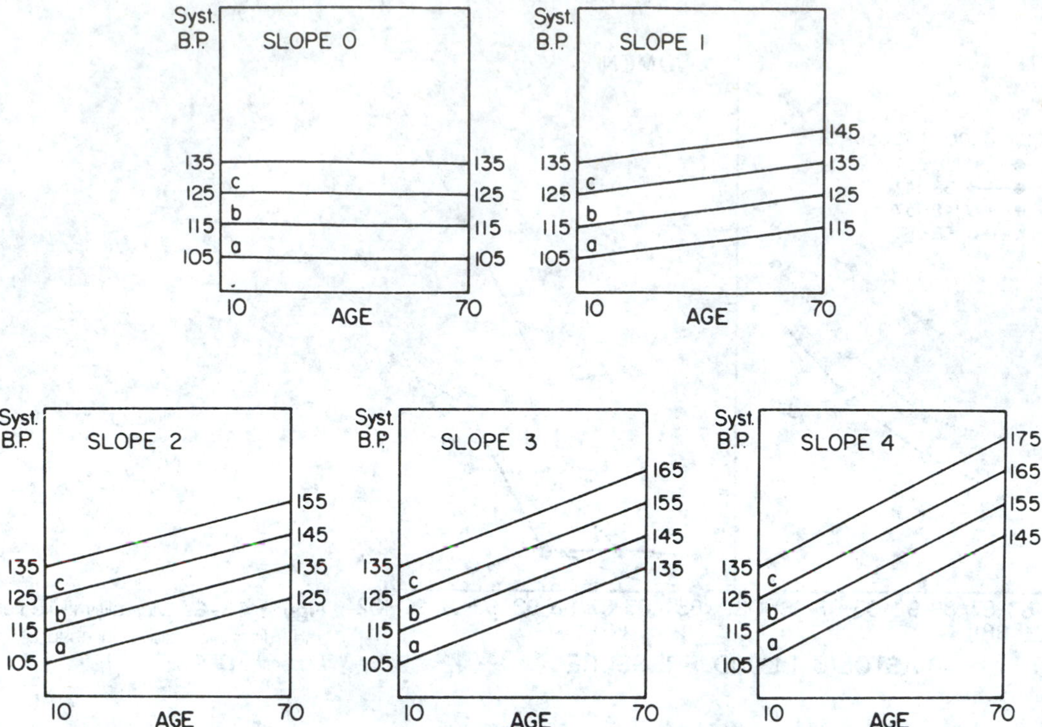

Figure 49–4. Patterns of blood pressure by age in adults. *(From Epstein FH, Eckoff RD, 1967.[13])*

and is consistent with other observations in both cross-sectional and longitudinal studies.[10] In the Intersalt Cooperative Research Group study just described, body mass index (weight in kilograms per square of height in meters) was strongly correlated with blood pressure within and across populations.[15]

Alcohol. Alcohol intake has also been found to be strongly related to blood pressure levels and is addressed in the reports cited above.[15–17] The nature of the relation between alcohol and blood pressure has been examined carefully by Criqui.[18] He demonstrates both a pressor or blood pressure–raising effect of alcohol consumption (possibly due to the alcohol-withdrawal state at the time of measurement rather than a direct effect) and the widely recognized observation that cardiovascular mortality is least not for nondrinkers but for those who report consuming about two drinks per day. It appears that alcohol, by raising blood pressure, does contribute to cardiovascular mortality and reduces the possible beneficial action of moderate alcohol intake, which may operate through a different pathway involving lipid metabolism. For this and other reasons, it would be a dubious public health policy to encourage the use of alcohol for the purpose of reducing cardiovascular disease risk.

Psychosocial and Cultural Factors. Decades of investigation have contributed abundant data on psychosocial and cultural factors, including such factors as stress, culture change, and migration, as influences on blood pressure distributions or the prevalence of hypertension. The population comparisons on which much of this evidence is based have often been difficult to interpret clearly because of the numerous uncontrolled factors in such comparisons. Two long-term studies of groups migrating from remote rural environments to urban areas suggest that the blood pressure changes previously found in such situations may be strongly determined by changes in diet. In the case of Tokelau Islanders migrating to New Zealand, weight gain accounted for most of the observed excess increase in blood pressure with age in migrating versus nonmigrating men, although for women different patterns were observed.[19] In Luo tribesmen in Kenya, migration to Nairobi was accompanied by an abrupt increase in systolic and (more gradually) in diastolic pressure, and the differences between migrating and nonmigrating men and women from their baseline values were explained largely by weight gain. This appeared to result from fluid retention caused by an increased ratio of sodium to potassium in the urine and, by inference, in the diet. In addition, however, an increase in heart rate possibly reflecting psychological factors was also observed on the first postmigration examination after only about 1 month in Nairobi.[20]

Genetics and Family History. The nature of the genetic contribution to blood pressure levels in individuals has long been debated, most notably by Pickering[21] and by Platt[22] some 25 years ago. The argument for polygenic inheritance of blood pressure determinants, with multiple environmental influences, has prevailed. Within families, resemblance of blood pressure levels among first-degree relatives (parents, siblings, and offspring) is commonly observed and is consistent with genetic contributions; the influence of common environmental factors within such closely related individuals cannot be entirely separated from genetic aspects, however.[23,24] Evidence from studies of blood pressure resemblance in monozygotic versus dizygotic twins provides the clearest quantitation of genetic influence.[25] The specific mechanisms by which the genetic makeup contributes to blood pressure levels have yet to be established. Nonetheless, the familial aggregation regularly observed aids in identifying individuals at greater than average risk of hypertension on the basis of observations in their first-degree relatives. This information can be usefully applied in preventive services, such as those in family practice or work-site settings where one family member may serve as an index subject for his or her first-degree relatives.

INTERVENTION IN ADULTS

Treatment of Established Hypertension. Evidence of the reducibility of risks of morbidity and mortality through treatment of high blood pressure has advanced greatly in the past decade. Since the late 1960s there has been little question of the importance of treatment for those with sustained diastolic blood pressures of 100 to 105 mm Hg or greater. Debate has centered on the range of diastolic pressures between 90 and 100 or 104 mm Hg, or so-called "mild hypertension," and on "isolated systolic hypertension," which refers to diastolic pressures below 90 mm Hg and systolic pressures of 160 mm Hg or greater (especially common among the elderly, see below).

The HDFP, cited above, demonstrated a significantly lower (26%) all-cause mortality in those with mild hypertension who were treated systematically (the Stepped Care Program) than in those referred to the existing sources of care in their respective communities ("referred care"), even though many of the latter also were treated.[26,27] The results of this and the other trials have been reviewed recently in relation to the policy[28] and in formal meta-analyses (e.g., Cutler et al.[29]). These results are also reflected in the current recommendations of the Joint National Committee on Detection, Evaluation, and Treatment of High Blood Pressure, which address in detail treatment through both nonpharmacologic and pharmacologic approaches for the population at large and for certain groups of special concern.[5]

Several questions continue to be investigated and will doubtless influence the further development of treatment policy. These include the long-term efficacy of nonpharmacologic therapy, either in place of or as an adjunct to drug treatment; the long-term safety of many of the newer antihypertensive drugs; the effect of blood pressure reduction specifically on risk of coronary heart disease; and the costs of blood pressure control, including programmatic alternatives in criteria for treatment eligibility, the extent of diagnostic evaluation, and the choice among available drug regimens when drug therapy is required. Such issues are addressed in the report of a recent National Heart, Lung, and Blood Institute Workshop on Antihypertensive Drug Treatment: The Benefits, Costs, and Choices.[30]

The series of Joint National Committee reports, of which the most recent appeared in 1988, together with the other public and professional educational activities of the National High Blood Pressure Education Program, are to be credited for having a major impact on the risks associated with hypertension in the United States. Community surveys before 1970 commonly showed that only a small minority of those with hypertension were detected, under treatment, and controlled, and a major public health strategy of the 1970s and 1980s was the conduct of community screening programs for case detection and for monitoring of progress in blood pressure control. The Joint National Committee now deemphasizes programs for case detection and suggests instead community services to assure follow-up of the cases already known and currently being detected so as to maintain their long-term medical management.[5]

The particular problem of blacks in the United States, and of course other population groups in many other settings, may still require special detection efforts, however, and local programs should be designed with such considerations in view. Evidence from the HDFP, based on sampling of whole communities to estimate the impact of blood pressure control, and from the North Karelia Project in East Finland demonstrates that integrated efforts to reduce the population risks attributable to hypertension can be highly effective.[26,27,31]

Primary Prevention of High Blood Pressure. Despite the importance of treatment of persons with established hypertension, the number of such persons in the United States alone reaches many millions, and the costs of care, the burden on those under treatment, and the incomplete reversal of excess risks, even with effective reduction of blood pressure, all constitute limitations of the foregoing approaches as an ultimate solution to the problem of high blood pressure in this and many other countries. The possibility of preventing the development of high blood pressure itself (the "primary prevention of hypertension") has therefore been a subject of growing interest, as reflected in an expert committee report from the World Health Organization.[1] The Joint National Committee report of 1988 notes that research in this area is in progress and that definitive recommendations cannot yet be made. The report suggests, on the basis of limited but encouraging evidence, that such nonpharmacologic measures as low sodium intake, weight reduction, and moderation of alcohol intake may be effective.[5] This direction of future policy is anticipated by the Working Group report cited above, in which the stratum of the population at "intermediate risk" is defined.[4] It is especially from this range of the blood pressure distribution that the incidence of hypertension requiring treatment occurs, as shown above. Therefore, this group is an important target for further research on the primary prevention of hypertension.

Potential Impact of Treatment and Prevention

Trends in Treatment and Drug Sales. The extent of treatment of hypertension in the United States in recent years can be estimated, albeit with wide margins of error, from surveys of use of ambulatory care and from the frequency of prescriptions for antihypertensive medications (after adjustment for the use of some of these for other conditions). Accordingly, the National Ambulatory Care Survey by the National Center for Health Statistics indicates variation from 408 to 441 visits per year per 1000 persons 45 to 64 years of age for survey periods from 1975–6 to 1985; this is more than twice the number of visits for either ischemic heart disease or diabetes—both of which, however, may also include hypertension.[32] No clear trend occurred in the frequency of visits per year over this period. Drug-use data suggest an increase in the number of prescriptions for antihypertensive medications, from approximately 128 million in 1973 to 209 million in 1985.[33] Even with allowance for population increase in this age group, greater intensity of medication is suggested by these data; this reinforces the impression that the problem of blood pressure control is one of major policy concern.

Mortality Trends in the United States. The decline in mortality from cardiovascular diseases and stroke in the United States over recent decades has been attributed in part to the improved rates of detection and control of hypertension. The change in mortality for cerebrovascular disease from 1950 to 1985 suggests a steeper downward slope from the early 1970s, when drug therapy for hypertension became increasingly common (Fig. 49–5).[34] However, stroke mortality has declined in the United States since early in the twentieth century, so that factors other than treatment of hypertension are important. Data from observational studies and from clinical and community trials all predict a beneficial impact of blood pressure reduction on these trends, but quantitation of its specific contribution to mortality trends remains uncertain.

Older Persons. The special problem of hypertension in older persons has been noted above. As characterized by the Joint National Committee report, a large proportion of persons over the age of 65 in the United States have both systolic and diastolic blood pressure elevations that warrant treatment. Available evidence suggests that older persons are likely to benefit from treatment for elevated diastolic pressure, but smaller doses of antihypertensive medications should be used initially because of possibly greater sensitivity to these agents among the elderly.[5] Early results of a successful pilot study have led to full imple-

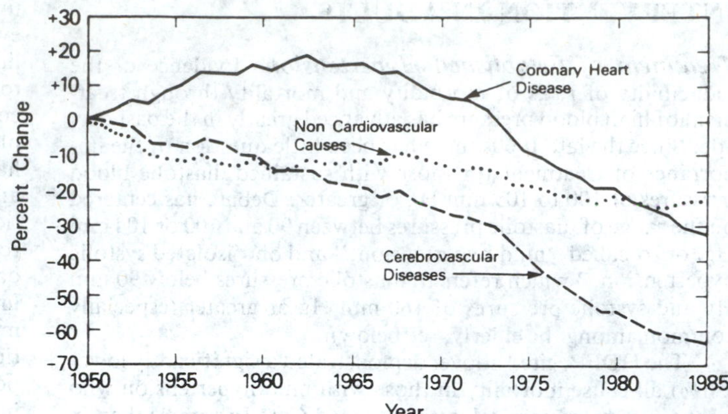

Figure 49-5. Mortality trends in the U.S. *[From Higgins MH, Luepker RV: Preface. In Higgins MH, Luepker RV (eds): Trends in Coronary Heart Disease Mortality: The Influence of Medical Care. New York, Oxford University Press, 1988.]*

mentation of a study of isolated systolic hypertension, the Systolic Hypertension in the Elderly Program (SHEP), the results of which are expected in 1991.[35] Because the elderly constitute a large and expanding segment of the Unites States population, the recommendations emerging from this and related studies will potentially have a great impact on the extent of treatment for hypertension in this country.[36]

Blacks. For blacks in the United States, as addressed earlier, the incidence and prevalence of hypertension are greater than for whites, and morbidity and mortality are correspondingly high. Although the importance of the problem of hypertension is proportionately even greater for blacks than for whites, rates of detection and effective treatment are lower, especially for black men. Similar response to treatment can be expected in blacks, although some classes of drugs are said to be less effective in blacks than in whites. The need for improved public health programs to reach this target population is evident. Whether other racial and ethnic groups similarly require special consideration in the design of programs has not been established.[5]

NATURAL HISTORY IN CHILDREN

Concepts of hypertension and of blood pressure distributions have different meanings in childhood or, more broadly, the period from birth through adolescence, from those that apply in adulthood. Although there are sometimes observed absolute levels of blood pressure that reflect true hypertension, usually due to a demonstrable pathologic condition, the primary focus of public health attention is the relative level of blood pressure and the question of its implications for the risk of essential hypertension in adulthood. The potential for early influences to determine the later development of blood pressure levels is the reason for growing interest in blood pressure in youth from the perspective of preventive medicine and public health.[1-3]

Prevalence. The distribution of blood pressure in childhood has been studied extensively. The published reports on children from around the world have been reviewed to permit comparison of the situations of childhood and adulthood in their patterns of blood pressure levels by age.[37] The results indicated that in nearly all populations the age-specific mean systolic blood pressure values by sex were within 5% of the pooled values shown in Figure 49-6. Values for boys and for girls were the same until ages corresponding to the onset of puberty, after which those for boys were consistently higher; by the late teen years the values for boys showed no further increase, while those for girls actually decreased. Similar patterns were observed for fourth-phase diastolic pressure, but much less increase by age was found for fifth-phase values, and no decrease in the later teen years was found for girls. Unlike the situation in adulthood, then, childhood populations were quite similar in their overall patterns of blood pressure increase by age, at least within the school-age period.

On the basis of such survey results, it is possible to construct curves of selected percentile values of systolic and diastolic pressure for use as reference values in assessment of individual children in screening or practice settings. For this purpose, a Task Force on Blood Pressure in Children has, for the United States,

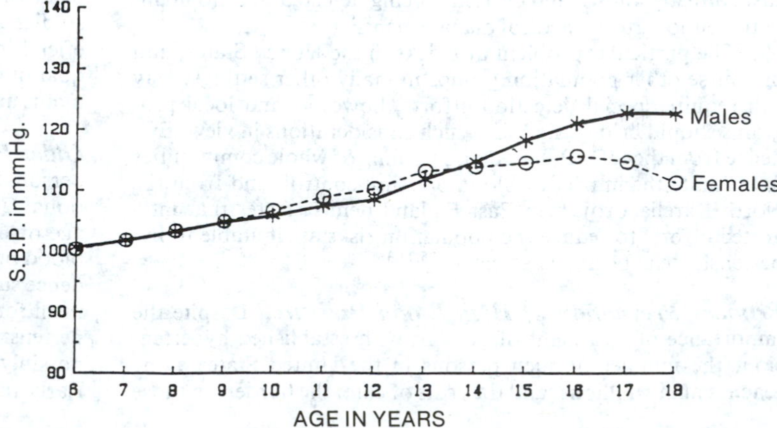

Figure 49-6. Patterns of blood pressure by age in children. *[From Brotons C, Singh P, Nishio T, Labarthe DR: Blood pressure by age in childhood and adolescence: A review of 129 studies worldwide. Int J Epidemiol 18:824-829, 1989.]*

presented reference values and detailed recommendations for detection and management of relatively high blood pressure values in children.[38] In principle, those children whose values are above the 90th or 95th percentile on repeated occasions of measurement are considered to have "hypertension" and to require special long-term management. Those in the range from the 90th to the 95th percentile who also are above the 90th percentile for height are considered to have normal blood pressure. This qualification is based on the strong relation of blood pressure to measures of growth and maturation during this period of life; hence more mature children exhibit higher levels of blood pressure.

Incidence. Just as the concept of prevalence is replaced in childhood by that of percentile rank, the concept of incidence is replaced by that of "tracking," often defined as persistence in relative blood pressure rank with increasing age. While for some purposes tracking is of interest throughout the blood pressure distribution, special attention is given to the persistence of relatively high blood pressure values, which may be predictive of hypertension in adulthood or may require intervention at current ages. A number of studies of tracking and an example of the longitudinal development of blood pressure in several successive cohorts of children are given by Szklo[39] and by Hofman,[40] respectively.

Determinants. As noted above, prominent determinants of blood pressure levels in childhood include influences of growth and maturation. One may speculate that the close resemblance of the patterns of blood pressure with age in diverse populations of children reflects predominance of these largely intrinsic influences, which are universally common to childhood and adolescence. Other factors, such as genetic differences, energy balance, and specific dietary components, are also found to contribute as in adulthood. Very early effects of diet and of general health conditions have been demonstrated or suggested by recent studies.[41,42] Further research on the natural history of blood pressure development in the perinatal period and infancy, as well as in later childhood and adolescence, is greatly needed.

INTERVENTION IN CHILDREN

Approaches to intervention in blood pressure in childhood are outlined in detail in the report of the Task Force on Blood Pressure in Children.[38] It is a generally held view that pharmacologic therapy should be used rarely in this age group. Suggested interventions are primarily related to energy balance—toward weight reduction or control of weight gain and reduction in sodium intake.

The concept that even the early development of the major risk factors for cardiovascular diseases, including blood pressure, could be averted was expressed by Strasser[43] with the term *primordial prevention*. The target of primordial prevention includes the conditions that foster development of the risk factors, such as energy imbalance leading to excess weight gain, attributable to eating and activity patterns that may accompany economic and social development. One implication of this view is that interventions may be useful for whole populations in modifying these conditions and thereby slowing, arresting, or reversing the expected undesirable shift in distributions of the risk factors.

Several studies of such interventions to modify blood pressure and other risk factors in children have been reported, most recently the Know Your Body Program of the American Health Foundation.[44] The results to date have offered some encouragement but are inconsistent and of modest degree. It may well be that longer-term evaluation, earlier and more intensive intervention, or a combination of these may be necessary to observe the expected benefits.

Potential Impact of Prevention and Treatment. It is clear from a discussion of the problem of blood pressure in adults in such places as the United States that the impact of effective prevention and, if necessary, early treatment on adult morbidity, mortality, and health care needs could be great. The United States and many other countries have experienced epidemics of cardiovascular disease related to atherosclerosis and hypertension in the twentieth century; elsewhere in the world, especially in developing countries, the complications of atherosclerosis are now expected to appear, and hypertension has already become a serious problem in some of them.[45] The concept that improved living conditions—through better-controlled development, with attendant optimization of habits related to health—could allow many populations to avert this epidemic of cardiovascular diseases poses an international public health challenge of large proportions. It remains to be seen whether current and emerging knowledge of natural history and approaches to intervention, both in adults and in children, can be joined with the necessary social and political forces to realize this goal.

REFERENCES

1. WHO Technical Report Series, No. 686: Primary prevention of essential hypertension. Geneva: World Health Organization, 1983
2. WHO Technical Report Series, No. 715: Blood pressure studies in children. Geneva: World Health Organization, 1985
3. WHO Technical Report Series, No. 792: Prevention in childhood and youth of adult cardiovascular diseases. Geneva: World Health Organization, 1990
4. Working Group on Risk and High Blood Pressure: An epidemiological approach to describing risk associated with blood pressure levels. Hypertension 7:641–651, 1985
5. 1988 Joint National Committee: The 1988 report of the Joint National Committee on Detection, Evaluation, and Treatment of High Blood Pressure. Arch Intern Med 148:1023–1038, 1988
6. Frohlich ED, Grim C, Labarthe DR, et al: Report of a special task force appointed by the Steering Committee, American Heart Association: Recommendations for human blood pressure determinations by sphygmomanometers. Hypertension 11:209A–222A, 1988
7. Curb JD, Labarthe DR, Cooper SP, et al: Training and certification of blood pressure observers. Hypertension 5:610–614, 1983.
8. Hypertension Detection and Follow-Up Program Cooperative Group: The hypertension detection and follow-up program: a progress report. Circ Res 40 (Suppl 1):106–109, 1977
9. Apostolides AY, Cutter G, Daugherty SA, et al: Three-year incidence of hypertension in 13 U.S. communities. Prev Med 11:487–499, 1982
10. Tyroler H, Heyden S, Hames C: Weight and hypertension: Evans County studies of blacks and whites. In Paul O (ed): Epidemiology and Control of Hypertension. New York: Stratton Intercontinental Medical Book Association, 1975
11. Labarthe DR: The cardiovascular complications of hypertension: natural history. In Onesti G, Klimt C (eds): Hypertension—Determinants, Complications, and Intervention. New York: Grune & Stratton, 1977
12. The Pooling Project Research Group: Relationship of blood pressure, serum cholesterol, smoking habit, relative weight and ECG abnormalities to incidence of major coronary events: final report of the Pooling Project. J Chron Dis 31:201–306, 1978
13. Epstein FH, Eckoff RD: The epidemiology of high blood pressure—geographic distributions and etiologic factors. In Stamler J, Stamler R, Pullman T (eds): The Epidemiology of Hypertension. New York: Grune & Stratton, 1967
14. Hypertension Detection and Follow-Up Program Cooperative

Group: Race, education and prevalence of hypertension. Am J Epidemiol 106:351–361, 1977

15. Intersalt Cooperative Research Group: Intersalt: an international study of electrolyte excretion and blood pressure: Results for 24 hour urinary sodium and potassium excretion. Br Med J 297:319–328, 1988
16. Committee on Diet and Health, Food and Nutrition Board, Commission on Life Sciences, National Research Council: Diet and Health: Implications for Reducing Chronic Disease. Washington, DC: National Academy Press, 1989
17. U.S. Department of Health and Human Services, Public Health Service: The Surgeon General's Report on Nutrition and Health, 1988. DHHS (PHS) Publication No. 88-50210. Washington, DC: Superintendent of Documents, U.S. Government Printing Office, 1988
18. Criqui MH: Alcohol and hypertension: new insights from population studies. Eur Heart J. 8(Suppl B):19–26, 1987
19. Salmond CE, Prior IAM, Wessen AF: Blood pressure patterns and migration: a 14-year cohort study of adult Tokelauans. Am J Epidemiol 130:37–52, 1989
20. Poulter N, Khaw KT, Mugambi M, et al: Longitudinal study of migrants from a "low blood pressure population." Abstract presented at the Second International Conference on Preventive Cardiology, Washington, D.C., June 22, 1989
21. Pickering G: The inheritance of arterial pressure. In Stamler J, Stamler R, Pullman T (eds): The Epidemiology of Hypertension. New York: Grune & Stratton, 1967
22. Platt R: The influence of heredity. In Stamler J, Stamler R, Pullman T (eds): The Epidemiology of Hypertension. New York: Grune & Stratton, 1967
23. Tyroler HA: The Detroit Project studies of blood pressure: a prologue and review of related studies and epidemiologic issues. J Chron Dis 30:659–670, 1977
24. Schull WJ, Harburg E, Schork MA, et al: Heredity, stress and blood pressure, a family set method. III. Family aggregation of hypertension. J Chron Dis 30:659–670, 1977
25. Biron P, Mongeau JG, Bertrand D: Familial aggregation of blood pressure in 558 adopted children. Can Med Assoc J 115:773–774, 1976
26. Hypertension Detection and Follow-Up Program Cooperative Group: Five year findings of the Hypertension Detection and Follow-up Program. I. Reduction in mortality of persons with high blood pressure including mild hypertension. JAMA 242:2562–2571, 1979
27. Hypertension Detection and Follow-Up Program Cooperative Group: Five year findings of the Hypertension Detection and Follow-up Program. II. Mortality by race-sex and age. JAMA 242:2572–2577, 1979
28. Labarthe, DR: Mild hypertension: the question of treatment. Ann Rev Public Health 7:193–215, 1986
29. Cutler JA, MacMahon SW, Furberg CD: Controlled clinical trials of drug treatment for hypertension: a review. Hypertension 13(suppl 1):I-36–I-44, 1989
30. Cutler JA, Horan MJ, Roccella EJ, Zusman RM (eds): The National Heart, Lung, and Blood Institute Workshop of Antihypertensive Drug Treatment: the benefits, costs, and choices. Hypertension 13(suppl 1), 1989
31. Nissinen A, Tuomilehto J, Korhonen HJ, et al: Ten-year results of hypertension care in the community: follow-up of the North Karelia Hypertension Control Program. Am J Epidemiol 127:488–499, 1988
32. Kovar MG, Collins JG, Delozier J, et al: Trends in the availability and use of medical care for coronary heart disease and related diseases. In Higgins MH, Luepker RV (eds): Trends in Coronary Heart Disease Mortality: The Influence of Medical Care. New York: Oxford University Press, 1988
33. Gross TP, Wise RP, Knapp DE: Antihypertensive drug use: trends in the United States from 1973 to 1985. Hypertension 13(Suppl I): I-113–I-118, 1989
34. Higgins MH, Luepker RV: Preface. In Higgins MH, Luepker RV (eds): Trends in Coronary Heart Disease Mortality: The Influence of Medical Care. New York: Oxford University Press, 1988
35. Hulley SB, Furberg CD, Gurland B, et al: Systolic Hypertension in the Elderly Program (SHEP): antihypertensive efficacy of chlorthanlidone. Am J Cardiol 56:913–920, 1985
36. Smith WMcF: Epidemiology of hypertension in older patients. Am J Med 85(Suppl 3B):2–6, 1988
37. Brotons C, Singh P, Nishio T, Labarthe DR: Blood pressure by age in childhood and adolescence: a review of 129 studies worldwide. Int J Epidemiol 18:824–829, 1989
38. Task Force on Blood Pressure Control in Children: Report of the Second Task Force on Blood Pressure Control in Children—1987. Pediatrics 79:1–25, 1987
39. Szklo M: Epidemiologic patterns of blood pressure in children. Epidemiol Rev 1:143–169, 1979
40. Hofman A, Valkenburg HA, Maas J, Groustra FN: The natural history of blood pressure in childhood. Int J Epidemiol 14:91–96, 1985
41. Hofman A, Hazebroek A, Valkenburg A: A randomized trial of sodium intake and blood pressure in newborn infants. JAMA 250:370–373, 1983
42. Barker DJP, Osmond C, Golding J, et al: Growth in utero, blood pressure in childhood and adult life, and mortality from cardiovascular disease. Br Med J 298:564–567, 1989
43. Strasser T: Reflections on cardiovascular diseases. Interdisc Sci Rev 3:225–230, 1978
44. Walter HJ, Hofman A, Vaughan RD, Wynder EL: Modification of risk factors for coronary heart disease: five-year results of a school-based intervention trial. N Eng J Med 318:1093–1100, 1988
45. Dodu SRA: Emergence of cardiovascular diseases in developing countries. Cardiology 75:56–64, 1988

50

Renal and Urinary Tract Diseases

Wendy E. Hoy
Stacey C. FitzSimmons

RATES AND PATTERNS

Rates and patterns of renal and urinary tract diseases differ among populations and are constantly changing. With development and industrialization, diseases related to infections, crowding, and poor nutrition recede, and those associated with affluence, aging, "overnutrition," medical interventions, drugs, addictions, and other exposures become prominent. Complex relationships between many renal and urinary tract diseases and socioeconomic, racial, cultural, and behavioral factors are becoming more apparent. The diseases of westernized societies are the main focus of this chapter, although tropical nephrology is discussed. Challah and Wing[1] provide a more comprehensive international perspective. It is not possible to cover all renal and urinary tract diseases of public health interest, and several omissions will be evident.

Rates of most renal diseases and of end-stage renal disease (ESRD) in westernized societies rise with age, and increased longevity enhances the expression of both. More males than females are affected by many renal diseases, and more males enter ESRD treatment programs. Some groups recently absorbed into westernized societies, such as U.S. blacks, North American Indians, Hispanics and Mexican Americans, urban South African blacks, Australian aborigines, Pacific Islanders, and New Zealand Maoris, have especially high rates of renal disease, in part from conditions such as hypertension and diabetes that were rare in their forebears. ESRD treatment programs themselves have produced a whole new set of clinical, economic, and sociological perspectives and concerns.

The current challenge in westernized societies, many of which have made a large commitment to life support for subjects with irreversible renal failure, is to better understand the factors that cause it. The public health perspectives of many of these diseases have been poorly defined; the distributions and natural histories of many remain obscure; specific prevention and treatment strategies have been developed for only a few; and projections of future ESRD burdens are still based on speculation.[2,3] These deficits are being repaired, however, with more population-based studies of renal diseases, more controlled intervention trials, and analyses of the efficacy and costs of screening programs, diagnostic techniques, and therapies.

Subclinical renal and urinary tract diseases may have no evidence short of biopsy or may have urinary or biochemical abnormalities that have escaped detection. Clinical renal disease may be manifested by blood, protein, or white blood cells in the urine, sometimes with hypertension. Heavy protein excretion, decreased levels of serum albumin, hyperlipidemia, and edema characterize the "nephrotic syndrome." Excretory renal function can be normal or impaired and can remain stable or progress to renal failure. Renal impairment generates, and is exacerbated by, hypertension. ESRD defines a situation of chronic irreversible renal failure in which prolonged survival is not possible without dialysis or renal transplantation.

Specific diseases are diagnosed by history and clinical findings, biochemical, serological, imaging, and urodynamic studies, and sometimes by biopsy of the kidneys, bladder, or prostate. Kidney biopsy specimens are examined by light, immunofluorescent, and electron microscopy. The serum creatinine level provides an approximate measure of renal insufficiency, although it varies with muscle mass and diet, underestimates renal insufficiency in the elderly, is relatively insensitive to loss of the first 50% of renal function, and is less sensitive to progressive loss of function in severe renal failure. Glomerular filtration rate, precisely measured by iothalamate and inulin clearances, can be estimated from the reciprocal of the serum creatinine, or by creatinine clearance. In some persons, changes in these parameters or in the logarithm of the serum creatinine follow a fairly consistent course, so that rates of renal functional deterioration can be expressed quantitatively.[4]

Although specific interventions for many diseases are not yet available, progressive renal damage might be modulated by a few standard maneuvers, thereby avoiding or postponing the development of ESRD. Control of coexisting or secondary hypertension, moderate dietary protein restriction, and in diabetics, strict control of blood glucose levels are of proven value. Other proposed mediators of progressive renal damage in a wide variety of renal diseases are hyperperfusion of surviving nephrons, high levels of blood lipids, and coagulation in glomerular capillaries; therapeutic roles have therefore been proposed for lipid-lowering agents, antiplatelet agents and nonsteroidal anti-inflammatory drugs, and for drugs that alter glomerular hemodynamics.[5–8]

Screening to define the *distribution* of selected renal and urinary tract diseases might have merit. Screening with intent to *treat* is justified in the public health setting only when the natural history of a disease is known, sensitive and specific screening tools are available, interventions are of proven benefit, and the cost/benefit ratio is favorable[9]: conditions applicable to few of these diseases at present. However, the potential to modulate

TABLE 50-1. LEADING KIDNEY AND UROLOGIC DISEASES REQUIRING VISITS TO PHYSICIANS, IN RANK ORDER AND RATE PER 100,000 PERSONS: UNITED STATES, 1985

Cause	Number	Cost in Millions
1. Urinary tract infection, including pyelonephritis and cystitis	7,991,301	$4,433
2. Other genitourinary tract infections	6,873,711	$ 454
3. Prostatitis	1,850,593	$ 293
4. Benign prostatic hyperplasia	1,790,053	$1,823
5. Urinary stone disease	944,624	$1,359
6. Obstructive uropathy	898,540	$ 766
7. Prostate cancer	887,341	$ 976
8. Hematuria	806,491	$ 444
9. Disorders of the bladder	753,229	$1,077
10. Incontinence	564,843	$ 437

From Division of Health Care Statistics, the National Center for Health Statistics, and the National Ambulatory Medical Care Survey, 1985.

progressive renal damage might justify screening for mild renal insufficiency in selected populations.

Economic Impact in United States. It is estimated that approximately 13 million people in the United States have kidney or urological disease and that most Americans will have one or more urinary tract disorders sometime during their lives. For many the affliction will be minor, self-limited, or treatable; for others it will generate significant morbidity and great cost.

Physician Visits. In 1985 there were 27 million visits to physicians for urinary tract disorders (4.9% of all visits). Table 50-1 shows the 10 leading causes.

Hospitalization Rates. In 1985, kidney and urological diseases accounted for hospitalization of more than 6 million people, 6% of hospital discharges, and 2,473,000 procedures and treatments (6.7% of the U.S. total). The 10 leading causes are shown in Table 50-2.

Mortality. In 1985, kidney and urological diseases were listed as a primary or contributing cause in 263,400 deaths, or 12.6% of all U.S. deaths. Table 50-3 shows the 10 leading causes of death and their population-adjusted rates.

Costs. In 1985 the direct and estimated indirect costs of kidney and urinary tract diseases totalled $40.3 billion. Costs were expected to exceed $50 billion by 1990. Some conditions are costly relative to their frequency; acute and chronic renal failure rank twelfth and fifth in hospitalization rates, but they rank first and second, respectively, in the average cost of each hospitalization occasioned by renal and urinary tract diseases.

SPECIFIC RENAL DISEASES

Diabetic Renal Disease

Diabetic nephropathy, a leading cause of kidney failure in the Western world, can complicate both type 1 and type 2 diabetes. It is characterized by albuminuria, hypertension, and progressive renal insufficiency. It indicates widespread diabetic vascular disease, with retinopathy the simplest marker, and is a powerful risk factor for premature death.[10,11]

In some countries maintenance therapy for diabetics with ESRD is limited by resources, but diabetics constitute the largest category of patients entering the open-access ESRD treatment program in the United States (30% in 1987)[12] and the ESRD programs in northern Europe.[13] Type 1 disease accounts for nearly all treated diabetic ESRD in the Nordic countries and more than half in the European Dialysis and Transplantation Association (EDTA) Registry.[14] In contrast, type 2 diabetes now accounts for the majority of diabetic ESRD in the United States (or 57% in 1988), and rates are rising rapidly. Because of their comorbidities, the survival rate of diabetic patients on dialysis is less than half that of most other patients with ESRD.[12]

TABLE 50-2. TEN LEADING DISCHARGE DIAGNOSES FOR HOSPITALIZATIONS FOR KIDNEY AND UROLOGIC DISEASE BY SEX: UNITED STATES, 1985.

	Number	Rate per 100,000[a]
▪ **Men**		
1. Benign prostatic hyperplasia	482,348	415
2. Urinary tract infections[b]	457,309	394
3. Urinary stone disease	295,018	254
4. Obstructive uropathy	281,074	242
5. Prostate cancer	246,201	212
6. Disorders of bladder[c]	230,211	198
7. Chronic renal failure	205,066	177
8. Essential hematuria[d]	115,495	99
9. Prostatitis	108,024	93
10. Bladder/other urinary cancer	89,108	77
▪ **Women**		
1. Urinary tract infections[b]	1,146,000	935
2. Chronic renal failure	189,000	154
3. Urinary stone disease	158,000	129
4. Incontinence	139,000	113
5. Toxemia of pregnancy	139,000	113
6. Obstructive uropathy	115,000	94
7. Disorders of bladder[c]	109,000	89
8. Hypertensive renal failure	97,000	79
9. Essential hematuria[d]	58,000	47
10. Other genitourinary tract infections	50,000	41

[a] Not age adjusted.
[b] Includes urosepsis, pyelonephritis, and cystitis.
[c] Includes neurogenic bladder and bladder hemorrhage.
[d] Probably includes undiagnosed cases of glomerulonephritis.

From Division of Health Care Statistics, National Center for Health Statistics, the National Hospital Discharge Survey, 1985, and the Veterans Administration, men only, for year ending September 30, 1986.

TABLE 50-3. LEADING CAUSES OF DEATH FROM KIDNEY AND URINARY TRACT DISEASES, IN RANK ORDER AND RATE PER 100,000 PERSONS: UNITED STATES, 1985

Cause	Number	Rate
1. Chronic renal failure	86,260	36
2. Prostate cancer[a]	36,204	31
3. Urinary tract infection, including pyelonephritis and cystitis	32,504	14
4. Acute renal failure	26,922	11
5. Hypertensive renal disease	16,135	7
6. Bladder cancer	14,636	6
7. Kidney cancer	10,709	4
8. Diabetic nephropathy	5,098	2
9. Other intrinsic/systemic[b] renal disease	4,882	2
10. Glomerulonephritis	4,529	2

[a] Rates apply only to men.
[b] Includes systemic lupus erythematosus, polyarteritis, and Wegener's glanulomatosis.

From National Center for Health Statistics: Vital Statistics of the United States, 1985, Vol II, Mortality: Part A, DHHS Publication No. 88-1102.

Glomerular filtration rate increases early in type 1 diabetes, and after 5 or more years of diabetes some subjects begin to excrete small amounts of albumin in the urine, detected only by special techniques ("microalbuminuria"). Persistent albumin excretion of >20 μg/min predicts development of overt albuminuria (>200 μg/min) several years later in 80% or more of such subjects. The cumulative risk for overt proteinuria increases rapidly 5 to 15 years after diagnosis of diabetes and then levels off, with apparent exhaustion of risk after 35 years. Renal insufficiency always follows overt proteinuria, at a mean interval of 7 to 10 years. In past studies it has afflicted 30% to 50% of all type 1 diabetics,[10,11,15] but this proportion has been falling gradually since the 1930s, a trend attributed to better patient management.[16,17]

Coexisting and superimposed hypertension and even high normal blood pressures are powerful risk factors for nephropathy in type 1 diabetes.[18-20] Other risk factors include nephropathy in diabetic siblings, male sex, poor glycemic control, and possibly cigarette smoking, diet, and physical inactivity.[21-23]

Annual screening of type 1 diabetics for "microalbuminuria" is recommended with the hope that intensified management might alter the progression of early nephropathy. Treatment includes rigorous blood pressure control and management of glycemia and body weight. The effects of meticulous control of blood glucose levels, moderate restriction of dietary protein, and inhibition of angiotensin-converting enzyme are being studied in large trials.

Nephropathy in type 2 diabetes probably develops in a similar manner, but the natural history is less well defined. Changes in renal function due to aging, hypertension, and atherosclerosis in this traditionally older group confound the discriminative and predictive value of albuminuria, and risks and attributable deaths are underestimated because of competing causes of mortality. Rates vary widely among different populations, probably because of different rates of type 2 diabetes and different renal susceptibilities.[10,12,24-31]

Rates of microalbuminuria and overt albuminuria in cross-sectional studies of type 2 diabetics equal or exceed those in type 1 diabetics.[27,28,32,33] The cumulative rate of overt proteinuria after 20 years of diabetes in one Minnesota study was 24.6%, and in the Pima Indians the rate was 50%, comparable to rates in type 1 diabetics.[26,28] Type 2 diabetes is the cause of most diabetic ESRD in some dialysis units in the United States.[24,34] Population-based rates of this form of ESRD in Mexican Americans, U.S. blacks, and American Indians are 6.1, 4, and 7 times those of non-Hispanic whites, with the differentials more marked in older subjects[12,29]; it is the leading cause of treated ESRD in Hispanics, American Indians, and Maoris, and the second leading cause in U.S. blacks and Australian aborigines.[12,24,25,35]

Hypertension is very common in type 2 diabetes and compounds the renal damage in direct relation to the height of systolic pressure.[28,30,36,37] Nephropathy risk has also been correlated with extent of glycemia, older age at onset of diabetes, duration of diabetes, insulin treatment, male gender, nephropathy in other diabetic family members, microvascular disease, and diabetic retinopathy.[38,39] Other determinants are not well defined.

Rising rates of type 2 diabetes in some populations, lower age at onset, and improved survival promise an awesome future burden of morbidity and ESRD. Over the short term, interventions similar to those in type 1 diabetes need evaluation. For the long term, the development of culturally relevant strategies to prevent type 2 diabetes and ameliorate its nephropathy are urgently needed.

Hypertensive Renal Disease

Hypertension can both produce and complicate renal disease, and its contribution to renal insufficiency is probably underestimated. Hypertensive renal disease was the most common diagnosis for blacks beginning ESRD treatment in the United States in 1987 and the second leading diagnosis for whites, constituting 36.9% and 22.7% of new ESRD cases, respectively.[12]

Primary hypertensive renal disease can be of two kinds.[40] The more common, sometimes called "nephrosclerosis," is a form of chronic renal insufficiency associated with long-standing blood pressure elevation. The second, a form of accelerated renal failure associated with malignant hypertension, is now rare where treatment of hypertension is widespread.

Race and ethnic group are powerful risk factors for hypertensive nephropathy, through mechanisms that are not yet clear. Rates of treated hypertensive ESRD in U.S. blacks are more than seven times those of whites (higher in some regional studies), although essential hypertension is only about twice as common,[12,29,41-44] and hypertensive ESRD in Texas Mexican Americans is 2.6 times more frequent than in non-Hispanic whites, although their rates of hypertension are not higher.[29] ESRD attributed to hypertension is rare in Native American groups studied to date, but blood pressure elevations in the last few decades might contribute to their high rates of renal failure from type 2 diabetes and glomerulonephritis.[45-47] Additional risk factors for nephropathy in hypertensive persons include the height of the systolic and diastolic blood pressures, the presence of diabetes, male sex, increasing age, and high normal serum creatinine levels.[42,43,48]

Although widespread treatment of hypertension has reduced other hypertensive morbidities, its effects on hypertensive renal disease are not yet clear. Two regional studies in the United States show that renal damage can progress in some treated hypertensive persons despite "adequate" blood pressure control,[43,49] and the community-based Hypertension Detection and Followup Program (HDFP) confirms this phenomenon.[48] However, most seasoned practitioners feel that blood pressure control is mitigating much hypertensive renal disease, and the HDFP suggests the superiority of aggressive control over a more relaxed treatment approach. A fall in the incidence of treated hypertensive ESRD is not yet apparent from nationwide U.S. data, but data from Jefferson County, Alabama, show that the age at onset of hypertensive ESRD in blacks has been delayed by nearly a decade over the last 15 years and that older females rather than younger males now dominate the hypertensive ESRD treatment group.[50]

The definition of "adequate" blood pressure control in this context might be critical; "safe" blood pressure limits for populations at high risk of renal disease and for those with already established renal impairment might be lower than the accepted "normal" range for the Caucasian population. Retrospective and prospective analyses of large cohorts of hypertensive subjects and comparisons of therapeutic regimens will help clarify some of these issues.

Glomerulonephritis

Glomerulonephritis (GN) encompasses several syndromes with a variety of pathological changes in the renal glomerulus. They are manifest by hematuria or proteinuria, or both, sometimes with hypertension or the nephrotic syndrome. They are variously categorized by morphological or clinical features, precipitating events, or associated conditions. Susceptibility is enhanced by infections, malnutrition, and poor living conditions, and rates fall as these conditions improve.[1] Most forms of GN are probably immunologically mediated, and genetic predispositions to some are suggested by family clusters and by associations with certain HLA types. Associations with specific infections are well established, especially in the developing world, but few precursors or etiologic factors are recognized in the common forms of GN that persist in westernized countries.

GN is the most common cause of renal failure and renal death in the developing world. It is the leading cause of treated ESRD in western Europe and Australia/New Zealand and has only recently fallen to third place in the United States, as diabetic and hypertensive nephropathies have increased.[12,13,35] Rates of ESRD and death from GN are higher in U.S. blacks, Mexican Americans, and U.S. and Canadian Indians than in their white counterparts.[12,29,41,46,51,52]

Pathological diagnosis relies on renal biopsy, which is hazardous and expensive. Little is known about the distribution or natural history of mild GN or the extent to which subclinical GN might be eroding renal function in the broader community.[53] Some European centers have estimated population-based rates of clinically recognized GN,[53–56] and a few registries for afflicted subjects have been established.[57,58]

This discussion addresses the major histological categories of idiopathic GN, idiopathic IgA nephropathy, and poststreptococcal GN (PSGN).

Chronic Idiopathic GN. The major morphological categories of idiopathic GN are minimal change disease (MCD), focal segmental glomerular sclerosis (FSGS), mesangial proliferative GN, membranous GN (MGN), and membranoproliferative GN (MPGN).[53,59,60] There are probably interfaces among these categories. Each can afflict subjects of all ages, but the distributions are dependent on age. MCD is the most common lesion in children, whereas adults have a broader distribution of all these forms of GN. MCD has the best prognosis, with remission usual before adulthood; MGN often remits but leads to renal failure after 10 to 15 years in perhaps 50% of subjects, whereas FSGS and MPGN have fewer remissions and a more relentless course. A reduction in proteinuria usually occurs with corticosteroid treatment of MCD, but response to steroids and cytotoxic drugs is less predictable in other disease.[61]

Prognostic indicators include the histological appearance of the lesion and the persistence of heavy proteinuria. Progression is rare if protein excretion remains mild or falls toward normal, whether spontaneously or with treatment. With progressive proteinuria, loss of renal function is usually detectable within 3 years.[53]

IgA Nephropathy. IgA nephropathy is one of the most common forms of GN worldwide.[62] It is probably a group of syndromes, with the common characteristic of IgA deposition in the glomerular mesangium, although a pathogenic role for IgA has not been proven. This condition constitutes 9.5% of forms of GN identified by biopsy in the United States, up to 35% in Spain, France, and Italy, high percentages in Japan, China, and Singapore, and 67% and 93% from Navajo and Zuni Indians from the southwestern United States.[46,62] Annual incidence in some European populations is estimated at 20 to 30 per million, and prevalence in one French study was 28 per 100,000.[54,62] Some cases are associated with systemic illness or liver disease, but in most cases the cause is unknown. In most series males predominate. Subjects of all ages, including children, can be affected, but most are young adults at the time of diagnosis. Family clustering is sporadic in some groups and marked in others.[46,63] Renal survival in some European groups with IgA nephropathy has been estimated at 75% at 15 years after diagnosis but is only 50% 5 years after biopsy in Navajo Indians.[46] This is the single most common GN biopsy diagnosis of Australians and American Indians with treated ESRD.[35,46]

Poststreptococcal Glomerulonephritis. The epidemiology and pathogenesis of PSGN are well defined.[64] It is characterized by the onset of hematuria, proteinuria, hypertension, and sometimes oliguria and renal insufficiency 7 to 15 days after a streptococcal upper respiratory infection and 21 to 40 days after a streptococcal skin infection. Most common in children, it can occur at all ages. Epidemic disease occurs in crowded and unhygienic living conditions and is common in tropical countries and Third World populations, especially in association with anemia, malnutrition, and intestinal parasites. It may occur in seasonal patterns and sometimes in cycles separated by several years. Epidemic disease is now uncommon in most westernized countries, although sporadic cases continue.[53] Asymptomatic disease is more common than clinical disease in most studies. Males predominate among patients with clinical but not subclinical disease. Only certain strains of streptococci have nephritogenic potential: nontypeable group A streptococci may also have that potential. It has been estimated that an average of 15% of infections with nephritogenic strains result in PSGN, with fully 90% of cases being subclinical, but the proportion varies with site of infection, the epidemic (if any), and the strain. Recurrence is uncommon.

PSGN is due to glomerular immune complex deposition, although the constituent streptococcal antigens are still being identified. A genetic predisposition is evidenced by attack rates in siblings of index cases of up to 37.8% after throat infections and 4.5% after skin infections. A streptococcal origin of acute GN is suggested if cultures or antigen tests have been positive for streptococci, or serum levels of antistreptolysin O (ASO) antibodies are elevated after throat infections (60% to 80% of cases), or if antihyaluronidase and antideoxyribonuclease antibodies are elevated after skin infections. A transient depression of serum complement helps differentiate PSGN from some other forms of GN. Renal biopsy is rarely indicated.

Prevention of PSGN involves improved nutrition, hygiene, and living conditions. Antibiotic treatment of streptococcal infections does not prevent PSGN, although it can confound the diagnosis by reducing ASO antibody production. Treatment does, however, reduce spread of streptococci to contacts and lessen their risk of getting PSGN. Prophylactic treatment for subjects at risk is recommended during epidemics and for siblings or families of patients with PSGN.

Urine abnormalities may persist for months after the acute attack. However, with follow-up limited to 10 to 15 years, studies of broad populations rather than of subjects initially hospitalized show complete recovery for most children, with rapidly progressive acute disease in less than 0.1% and chronic renal failure in less than 1%. Adults have about twice the rate of long-term urine abnormalities as children, and chronic renal failure is more common, although still exceptional. Superimposed hypertension, renal changes with aging, and the hyperperfusion phenomenon might contribute to such a course.

Autosomal Dominant Polycystic Kidney Disease

Autosomal dominant polycystic kidney disease (ADPKD)[65,66] is characterized by fluid-filled cysts in the kidney, which can compress surrounding tissue and cause renal insufficiency. It is probably part of a generalized disorder of extracellular matrix, which often includes liver and pancreatic cysts, diverticuli in the gut, berry aneurysms in the cerebral circulation, and mitral valve prolapse. Its major morbidities are renal failure and rupture of cerebral aneurysms. It probably carries an increased risk of renal cancer, sometimes bilateral.

ADPKD affects 1 of 400 to 1000 Americans, and perhaps 5 million people worldwide. It is more frequent in U.S. whites than blacks and is uncommon in American Indians studied so far.[12,45] The abnormal gene in 90% of afflicted families has been located on the short arm of chromosome 16. A 90% penetrance by the age of 90 has been estimated. The onset of clinically apparent disease is variable, with 16% diagnosed by the age of 35 and 70% by the age of 55, but it has also been diagnosed in infants and in extreme old age. The course is also quite variable: renal impairment increases most rapidly after age 40, and 50% of subjects have ESRD by age 70. ADPKD caused 3.7% of the treated incident ESRD in the United States in 1987, or 4.9 cases per million[12]; in the EDTA Registry in 1984, it caused 7.9% of incident ESRD cases under 65 years of age and 4.7% of those of 65 years or older.[14]

Imaging procedures, especially contrast-enhanced computerized tomography, can often make this diagnosis in many subjects before symptoms appear.[67] Tests for the abnormal gene through linkage markers, although complex, have recently been developed, and the gene might soon be isolated and cloned.[68] Gene typing could then be applied to genetic counseling, prenatal testing, and evaluation of potential kidney donors. Identification of the abnormal gene, however, does not predict clinical course.

Analgesic Nephropathy

Analgesic nephropathy (AN)[69-72] is a slowly progressive interstitial renal disease caused by long-term ingestion of analgesics. It mainly afflicts middle-aged women. Mechanisms are oxidant injury to the renal medulla and papillae and reduced medullary blood flow due to inhibition of prostaglandin synthesis. Phenacetin and analgesic mixtures pose the greatest risks of AN, and a synergistic effect of agents in mixtures has been proposed. A necessary minimal cumulative ingestion of at least 3 to 5 kg of these agents has been suggested. Aspirin and acetaminophen as single agents have generally been considered safe, at least until recently. Symptoms are few until preterminally, although urinary tract infections are more common. Analgesic abuse is also associated with increased rates of urothelial tumors.

The prevalence and the natural history of AN are poorly defined. Mild renal impairment due to analgesic abuse is more common than ESRD and more difficult to diagnose. Diagnosis is often circumstantial and related to the degree of suspicion. Biopsy of the renal cortex may be nonspecific, and only a portion of the cases have radiographic evidence of papillary necrosis: thus many cases might be labeled chronic renal disease of uncertain origin.

The association between analgesic abuse and nephropathy was best demonstrated in a longitudinal study of Swiss female factory workers: 5- and 10-year rates of azotemia in heavy users of analgesic agents were 5% and 6.7%, compared with rates of 0.55% and 0.9% in light users or nonusers.[73] However, several other studies have failed to demonstrate the association.[74] In the past, reported rates of suspected AN in ESRD populations have varied from 30% in Queensland, Australia, 18% in Belgium, 16.8% in West Germany, 10% in North Carolina, to only 1.7% in Philadelphia. In a 1976 poll of 30 large U.S. centers, 20% of the cases of interstitial nephritis were attributed to analgesic abuse, with a high in the southeast of 38%.[72]

Patterns of analgesic consumption, as well as differences in diagnosis and reporting, probably contribute to such variations. Rates of analgesic use are high in South African and Australian women, for example, low in some areas of the United States and very low in Welsh housewives. Low urine volume, dehydration, caffeine intake, and certain trace elements in water might facilitate renal injury.

Recent reports suggest that acetaminophen alone and modest as well as large doses of analgesics may be nephrotoxic and in a broader sense than heretofore described. A retrospective study in North Carolina described an increased risk of nephrosclerosis, diabetic nephropathy, glomerulonephritis, other forms of nephritis, and (undefined) renal insufficiency, as well as ESRD, with daily long-term use of acetaminophen alone.[75] In addition a West German study purportedly demonstrated a dose-dependent risk of ESRD from a variety of causes with cumulative use of more than 1 kg of phenacetin or acetaminophen-aspirin combinations, especially those containing caffeine.[76]

The current U.S. cost of treating subjects with AN-ESRD, estimated at 2% of the ESRD load, is $60 million per year.[69] This figure would be much higher if analgesic use indeed exacerbates other renal diseases. Additional costs are incurred in evaluating and treating hypertension, urinary tract infections, preterminal renal disease, and extrarenal manifestations of analgesic abuse.[72]

Treatment of established AN includes cessation of drug, avoidance of dehydration, management of hypertension and urinary infections, and surveillance for urothelial tumors. The extent to which the disease can be arrested is uncertain.

Analgesic nephropathy is preventable. Renal disease and ESRD due to analgesic abuse decreased dramatically in Canada, Scandinavia, and Scotland with elimination of phenacetin and with decreased availability of analgesic mixtures. Rates of AN-ESRD in Australia were not altered after 5 years of a ban on phenacetin but have fallen in the 40- to 49-year age group since mixtures of aspirin, salicylamide, and acetaminophen were restricted to prescription only.[35] The need for regulation of analgesics in the United States is still being argued.

Nephrotoxicity of nonsteroidal anti-inflammatory agents (NSAIDs) is a more recently recognized phenomenon of major concern.[69,71,76-78] It is now the most common reason for renal consultation in many centers. Fluid retention, electrolyte abnormalities, prerenal azotemia, acute renal failure, interstitial nephritis, nephrotic syndrome with minimal-change disease, and papillary necrosis have all been associated with NSAID use. These effects are recognized most frequently in elderly subjects and in those with renal compromise or hemodynamic stress, and they can occur with short-term administration of drugs in therapeutic doses. Most syndromes are reversible with cessation of the drug, but irreversible chronic renal failure, with underlying interstitial fibrosis, has been reported in several subjects taking prescribed doses.[79] The long-term toxicity of chronic NSAID use has not been defined, and some regard nonprescription access with trepidation.

Acute Renal Failure

Acute renal failure (ARF) is characterized by a sudden decline in renal function. Definitions vary (the increment in serum creatinine, the presence of oliguria, the need for dialysis, etc), which impairs comparisons of rates and outcomes. Major mechanisms are renal hypoperfusion, toxic insults, allergic reactions, and obstruction to urine flow. Recovery of renal function is usual if the patient can be supported through the acute phase.

ARF, caused by blood loss and crush injuries is common during war and natural disasters.[1,80] "Medical" and obstetric conditions make up a large proportion of ARF in tropical countries, as described later. In developed countries "surgical" ARF is more common, because of increasing numbers of complex surgical procedures on older subjects and high rates of major traumatic and industrial accidents. "Medical" causes of community-acquired ARF are not insignificant, however: they accounted for 1% of hospital admissions in one study, with 69% due to volume depletion, 12% to infections and drug toxicity, and 16% to obstruction, mostly from prostatic hypertrophy.[81]

Much ARF in the United States occurs in subjects who are already hospitalized for another reason. In one prospective study of more than 2000 hospitalized patients, ARF was documented in 4.9%.[82] Predisposing factors include renal disease or insufficiency, hypertension, and perhaps increasing age. Precipitating insults, many of them iatrogenic, include volume perturbations, heart failure and arrhythmias, surgical procedures, sepsis, nephrotoxic antibiotics and chemotherapeutic agents, radiographic contrast agents, and nonsteroidal anti-inflammatory agents. In one study, most subjects with hospital-acquired ARF had clearly identified predisposing factors, and most had more than one precipitating insult, which were additive for ARF risk and oliguria; a single insult was likely to produce ARF only in subjects with preexisting renal disease.[83]

ARF results in prolonged hospitalization, frequent tests, intensive care, sometimes dialysis, and often death. The mortality rate has classically been high (between 40% and 70%),[84] but as milder forms of ARF are recognized, survival improves, as a newer U.S. hospital-based ARF study with a mortality rate of

24.8% demonstrates.[82] Risk factors for death with ARF are pulmonary and cardiovascular complications, deep coma, severe renal injury (oliguria, anuria), jaundice, and hypercatabolism, and, in some studies, increasing age.[82,85] Accurate projections of mortality in subjects with ARF have been made by using the first four criteria.[86] Appropriately applied, such projections could minimize the great costs and suffering incurred by futile treatment.

Many nosocomial episodes of ARF can be prevented by awareness of high-risk subjects, attention to volume and hemodynamic status, judicious choice of drugs and drug combinations, and dose adjustment for renal insufficiency or advanced age. For contrast procedures, especially in diabetics with renal insufficiency, careful choice of agents and doses, avoidance of dehydration, and consideration of alternate imaging techniques are important.

Renal Disease and Illicit Drugs

Renal disease related to drug abuse[87] was described only recently, but already has great social and economic impact; in a survey reported in 1983 more than 10% of ESRD dialysis populations between 18 and 45 years in some large U.S. metropolitan areas had this diagnosis.[88] Several syndromes are recognized.

Focal segmental glomerulosclerosis (FSGS) occurs in intravenous heroin addicts, with heavy proteinuria and progression to renal failure in a few months to years.[89] There is no effective treatment. An immunologic mechanism is postulated, mediated through a response to heroin itself, to adulterants, or to infectious agents. FSGS associated with drug abuse occurs in all ethnic groups, but rates are especially high in young black males, leading to the hypothesis that parental drug abuse unmasks a genetic predisposition to FSGS in blacks. In a study from Buffalo, New York, rates of FSGS were 29 times higher in black addicts than in other blacks, and ESRD rates were 18 times higher.[88,89]

Renal deposition of amyloid, associated with chronic inflammation and infection, occurs in skin poppers.[90] Proteinuria and sometimes renal failure are diagnosed at an average age of 41 years, 10 years older than FSGS patients. In a New York City autopsy series, 5% of addicts and 26% of addicts with suppurative skin infections had unsuspected renal amyloidosis.[91]

Other renal diseases related to drug abuse include immune-complex GN associated with infectious endocarditis or hepatitis B antigenemia, necrotizing vasculitis related most strongly to amphetamine abuse, tubular dysfunction and occasionally acute renal failure in solvent sniffers, acute renal failure due to muscle breakdown, and the renal syndromes of human immunodeficiency virus infection.

Treatment of addicts with ESRD is often complicated by noncompliance, communicable diseases like hepatitis B and AIDS, and, with continued drug abuse, infection and clotting of vascular access and recurrence of disease in kidney transplants. Because of the interfaces of drug addiction with crime, some of these subjects are incarcerated. Such problems accentuate dilemmas about responsibility for personal health and allocation of limited resources.

Renal Disease and the Human Immunodeficiency Virus

Renal disease associated with infection with the human immunodeficiency virus (HIV) is also a new phenomenon.[92-94] Subjects with clinical AIDS are at risk for all the renal insults associated with critical illness, such as sepsis, volume depletion, hypotension, shock, and nephrotoxicity from therapeutic drugs. In addition, a group of syndromes appear to be distinctive for HIV infection and can occur at any time during its course. Such syndromes include mild proteinuria, the nephrotic syndrome, and heavy proteinuria with rapid progression to renal failure. Pathological findings can include severe tubulointerstitial inflammation, calcification and fibrosis, various glomerular proliferative changes, collapse of the glomerular tuft, and FSGS. Electron microscopy sometimes shows mesangial electron-dense deposits, implying immune complex deposition, cytomegalovirus and herpes simplex-like particles, and other viruslike particles.

Rates of these syndromes vary. They are lower in HIV-positive white homosexual subjects without drug abuse and more common in heterogeneous HIV-infected populations. In studies from New York and Miami, 32.4% and 43% of adult AIDS patients and 29% to 58% of HIV-positive children had significant proteinuria.[93,94] In Miami HIV infection is now the most common cause of the nephrotic syndrome in men 20 to 50 years of age. FSGS with heavy proteinuria and a relentless course is particularly common in young, black, heterosexual, HIV-positive intravenous drug abusers, and a genetic susceptibility and coinfection with other retroviruses, including HTLV-1, might influence its pathogenesis.[92]

There is no effective treatment of HIV nephropathy. Temporary dialysis is an option during episodes of ARF. Symptom-free HIV-positive subjects with chronic renal failure can do quite well on dialysis, but chronic dialysis of subjects with clinical AIDS is complicated by concomitant illness, cachexia, infectious hazards, and prolonged hospitalizations, and survival is usually short.

HIV infection in ESRD patients who are already undergoing maintenance dialysis is a somewhat different issue. Infection is usually related to drug abuse or to previous transfusions. Its prevalence is determined by patient mix and, in a limited and nonrepresentative survey of U.S. dialysis units several years ago, was estimated at somewhat more than 1%. However, some inner city dialysis populations have much higher rates: screening in the late 1980s showed a 12% prevalence at a dialysis center in Brooklyn, New York (65% of the IV drug abuse subjects undergoing dialysis), and a prevalence of 20.2% in two Miami dialysis centers[95,96]! Infected subjects without symptoms often do well, but subjects die quickly when clinical AIDS develops. Home dialysis and chronic ambulatory peritoneal dialysis are often preferred treatments to reduce in-center infectious risks. HIV screening of all ESRD patients beginning treatment is prudent and is mandatory for all potential transplant donors.

Tropical Nephrology

Patterns of renal and urinary disease in tropical countries[1,97] differ from those of westernized countries. Many diseases are associated with infections and infestations and are potentially preventable. Most countries cannot support treatment of a large number of ESRD subjects, and limited resources are better directed at prevention.

Acute renal failure is common. "Medical" conditions cause a large proportion: fluid and electrolyte depletion, infections such as schistosomiasis, malaria, leptospirosis, and typhoid fever, chemical toxins and venoms, and hemolysis from toxins or glucose-6-phosphate-dehydrogenase deficiency in the face of oxidative stresses. Obstetric ARF associated with difficult deliveries, infections, and abortions is also common.

Glomerulonephritis is very common. It is estimated that 1 of every 10,000 young adults in tropical regions gets ESRD each year as a result of GN, about 2.5 times the rate in Western countries, and in endemic malaria areas admission rates for patients with the nephrotic syndrome are 100 times those in Western countries. Rates of PSGN are high in many areas, especially in children. Etiologic factors in many other cases of GN are obscure.

GN with nephrotic syndrome is very common in subjects with quartan malaria. It is more frequent among malnourished people. It is not reversed by antimalarial or prednisone treatment but is prevented by eradication of malaria. A mild GN occurs in

20% to 50% of cases of falciparum malaria, and acute renal failure and pigmenturia (blackwater fever) can occur with heavy parasitemia, sometimes exacerbated by hemolysis due to antimalarial drugs.

Schistosomiasis causes major genitourinary morbidity, especially in Egypt and some other parts of Africa and Brazil.[1,97,98] *Schistosoma haematobium* causes fibrosis and scarring of the ureter and bladder, with obstruction, vesicoureteric reflux, urinary tract infections and squamous cell bladder cancer. In parts of Nigeria 3% of the infected population are affected, and in parts of Egypt 50% are. In addition, an immune complex GN with nephrotic syndrome occurs in the hepatosplenic form of schistosomiasis, usually in young men, many of whom have a severe course that is unaltered by treatment of the infestation. Renal amyloidosis occurs in African children with schistosomiasis but not in Egyptian and Brazilian children.

Leptospirosis causes ARF in certain tropical regions, but recovery is usual. Typhoid fever is usually accompanied by a mild temporary immune-complex GN, but severe GN or acute renal failure occur occasionally. A mild GN afflicts up to 50% of subjects with leishmaniasis, especially children and young adults, and renal function and morphology return to normal with treatment. An association between hepatitis B (HBV) and membranous GN is well recognized, especially in children, in areas with high HBV carrier rates, such as the Far East, Japan, Taiwan, sub-Saharan Africa, and some central European countries.[99] Prognosis is generally good, with high remission rates without intervention, even if HBV antigenemia persists. Membranoproliferative GN, with a more severe course, has also been reported in both adults and children with chronic HBV infection. These HBV nephropathies probably result from deposition of immune complexes containing HBV antigens in the glomerular capillary wall; membranoproliferative GN might result from direct viral infection of mesangial cells. HIV nephropathy is undoubtedly increasing in some African countries but pales in significance along side more critical issues of AIDS morbidity and control.

URINARY TRACT DISEASES

Urinary Tract Infections

Urinary tract infections (UTIs)[100-103] account for approximately 8 million physician visits and 1.6 million hospitalizations per year in the United States, at a cost of nearly $4433 million, and are the third leading cause of death due to renal and urologic diseases.[104-106] They are most frequent in young, sexually active women, and it is estimated that one in five women will have a UTI in her lifetime. UTIs are also common in preschool girls, in postmenopausal women, and in elderly men and women, especially those who are institutionalized and those with indwelling urinary catheters. UTIs in older men are often associated with urinary retention, urethral strictures, calculi, and debilitating illness. Boys and men with normal urinary tracts are not often affected, but men can acquire bacterial UTIs through heterosexual or homosexual intercourse, and recurrent UTI is the hallmark of chronic prostatitis.

Most infections are localized to the bladder and urethra, but some involve the kidneys and renal pelves (pyelonephritis), or the prostate. UTIs rarely lead to renal damage or failure unless they are associated with diabetes, pregnancy, reflux, obstruction, or neurogenic bladder. Diabetic persons with UTIs risk papillary necrosis and sepsis; abortion and other complications can result from UTIs in pregnancy; and morbidity and mortality of UTIs increase greatly in the elderly and in those with complicating conditions, such as spinal cord injury.

Most UTIs in young women are new events, are uncomplicated, and are caused by *E. coli* and other bowel organisms that enter the bladder through the short female urethra. Subjects with recurrent UTIs have increased density of bacterial receptors on epithelial cell surfaces in the vagina and bladder. Women with blood groups A and AB who are nonsecretors of blood group substance are at greater risk. Intercourse, diaphragm use, and failure to void after intercourse all increase risk. Women who have closely spaced recurrent infections with the same organisms or who have pyelonephritis should be evaluated for urinary tract abnormality, as should men with persistent infection.

In the presence of symptoms, white cells and bacteria in a clean-void midstream specimen of urine usually indicate a UTI. The usual bacterial count considered diagnostic on urine culture is >100,000/ml, but many patients have lower counts, including half of those with cystitis and most patients with urethritis syndromes. Enterobacteriaceae colony counts as low as 100/ml have a sensitivity and a specificity for UTI of 94% and 85%. An easy and relatively inexpensive dip slide urine culture technique can be performed by subjects with recurrent UTIs, and self-treatment under medical guidance can be initiated. Many uncomplicated UTIs are treated on the basis of symptoms and pyuria alone.

Screening for bacteriuria in symptom-free persons is not cost-effective and may lead to inappropriate treatment, drug reactions, and selection of resistant organisms. Treatment of asymptomatic bacteriuria is not generally recommended, except in pregnant women, diabetics, and children with vesicoureteric reflux. Symptomatic infections are treated by antimicrobials, and infections associated with sexual intercourse can usually be prevented by single-dose prophylactic therapy. Repeated or prolonged antibiotic treatment can select antibiotic-resistant organisms. Some broad-spectrum antimicrobial agents may not pose this threat and are sometimes used for prophylaxis in subjects with chronic infections.

UTIs are the leading form of nosocomial infection and are especially common in nursing homes.[103] Spread can be reduced by separation of catheterized patients from others who are debilitated or catheterized, and by washing the hands after patient contact. For subjects who require temporary catheterization, risks of infection can be reduced by aseptic insertion, curtailed duration of catheterization, and meticulous care of the patient and the drainage system. However, infection remains very common in persons with chronic indwelling catheters. The bacterial flora in the urine of catheterized subjects is in flux, colonization is often asymptomatic, and repeated courses of treatment are not advised.

Urinary Stone Disease

Urinary stone disease[1,107-115] has been recognized since antiquity. Bladder stones are common in many underdeveloped countries, especially in children, and are often related to poor nutrition. They have virtually disappeared in developed countries, while upper tract stones in adults have increased greatly. Both bladder and upper tract stones are particularly common in India, Pakistan, the British Isles, Scandinavia, the Mediterranean, Central Europe, portions of the Malay Peninsula, and in China. Rates are low in Central and South America, in Australian aborigines, Native Americans, African Bantu, North American blacks, and native-born Israelis. Stone formation is increased in mountainous and tropical areas and in dry climates.

Most stones in westernized countries are "idiopathic" and are composed of calcium oxalate, either pure (72.5%) or containing small amounts of uric acid (4% to 8%) or hydroxyapatite. A small proportion are due to such disorders as primary hyperparathyroidism, renal tubular acidosis, sarcoidosis, cystinuria, and urinary tract infection or obstruction. Idiopathic upper tract stones are more common in males, the affluent, and those with sedentary and professional occupations.

Stones occasioned nearly a million visits to physicians in the

United States in 1985.[104] Hospitalization rates for stones vary from 70 to 210 cases per 100,000 population, with a nationwide total of more than 453,000 in 1985.[105,106,112] Rates are highest in the Southeast and show seasonal variation.[108] The true and much larger frequency of stones in the United States is unknown, however, because asymptomatic stones are not recorded, some subjects do not seek medical attention with stone passage, and fewer than half of those who do are hospitalized.[108,109] It has been estimated that between 5.1% and 12% of the U.S. male population will have stones at some time in their lives. The lifetime prevalence in blacks is one half to one third that of whites, and in Orientals it is perhaps one half.[107,111]

Symptoms from stones are uncommon before the age of 15, peak at 20 to 30 years, and cause hospitalizations most often in the 45- to 64-year age group. They include pain as the stones move down the urinary tract and sometimes urinary infection and bleeding. Spontaneous passage eventually occurs in 67% to 78% of subjects, but many undergo diagnostic and urologic procedures. Intervention for impacted stones commonly includes shock-wave dissolution (lithotripsy), followed by spontaneous passage or percutaneous or ureteroscopic removal of the fragments.[115] Kidney damage occurs only occasionally, as a result of infection or obstruction, and renal failure and death are rare. Recurrence over the long term is usual, at least in older longitudinal studies; thus the tendency for idiopathic stone formation is lifelong.

Formation of idiopathic stones probably involves interaction between susceptibility and environment. Concordance for stone formation is marked among blood relatives and between spouses. Trace elements, humidity, and exposure to sunlight might all play a role. High intakes of calcium, animal protein, refined carbohydrate, salt, and oxalate, and lack of dietary fiber have been incriminated, but evidence is largely circumstantial, and dietary differences between stone formers and others are small. Precipitation of oxalate, calcium, or uric acid in the urine has been attributed to excess excretion, low urine volumes, low urine pH, or deficiencies in crystallization inhibitors, such as urinary citrate and acid mucopolysaccharide. Calcium salt deposition around a nidus of precipitated uric acid has been postulated in calcium stone formers who have high uric acid excretion. However, many studies have detected no differences in urinary composition between groups of stone formers and controls.

Regardless of the underlying predisposition, the most important modulator of stone occurrence and recurrence is urine volume. In a controlled study of new settlers in a desert environment in Israel, a high fluid intake had a strong protective effect against stone formation.[113] Increased fluid intake probably mediates the "stone clinic" effect, that is, fewer recurrences in subjects who come to clinical attention, regardless of the other components of the treatment regimen.

Management includes evaluation for risk factors and prevention of further stone formation. Increased water intake is the cornerstone of all regimens. Other interventions might include restriction of dietary calcium, oxalate and purines, increase in dietary fiber, and administration of thiazides, allopurinol, thiosulfate or pyridoxine, and supplements of inorganic phosphate or magnesium supplements. Administration of potassium citrate looks promising at the moment.[114] In evaluation of treatment efficacy, the incidence of new stones, whether passed or not, stone passage rate, and growth of existing stones should all be considered, and results should be controlled for the "stone clinic" effect.

For patients who require acute intervention, lithotripsy and percutaneous stone removal have greatly reduced costs, morbidity, and hospital stay, with savings in the United States estimated at $2,000 per case or $160 million.[108,115] Even so, direct costs for hospitalized subjects were estimated at $825 million in 1984 and more than $1 billion in 1987, and the cost of lost productivity in these subjects in 1984 was estimated at $73 million.[108] There are no cost data for the majority of patients who are treated at home. Costs will increase as the population ages and as industrialization continues. Prevention of stone recurrence is the major issue of cost containment.

Prostate Cancer

Prostate cancer is a disease of aging men,[1,116–120] with rising rates for every decade of age after 50 years. Its rates increase with urbanization and affluence. Its causes are not known.

Crude and age-adjusted rates vary greatly among countries and ethnic groups. A decade ago age-standardized incidence rates ranged from 100.2 per 100,000 black men in Alameda County, California, to 0.8 in Shanghai, China. Rates are highest in U.S. blacks, high in northern Europe and in U.S. whites, intermediate in Latin America and southern Europe, and low in eastern Europe and the Far East. Age-adjusted death rates from prostatic cancer per 100,000 men, for 1982 and 1983, ranged from 52.1 in Martinique, 32 in Sweden, 23.1 in the U.S. aggregate, to 3.3 in El Salvador.[121]

Prostate cancer is now the most common malignant disease in U.S. males and the second most common cause of male cancer deaths. There were an estimated 103,000 newly diagnosed cases in 1989, or about 75 per 100,000 men, and they accounted for 21% of all new cancers in males. There were 28,500 attributable deaths.[121] Lifetime risks for white and black males are estimated at 8.7% and 9.4%, respectively, and attributable death rates at 2.6% and 4.3%.[122] Recent relative survival rates at 5 years for U.S. whites and blacks with prostate cancer were 73% and 60%. Excess mortality continues after 5, 10, and 15 years.[122] With progressive aging of the population, a 90% increase in the number of cases and a 37% increase in attributable deaths are projected for the United States by the year 2000.[120]

There are latent and active forms of the disease. The latent form (stage A1), of generally unrecognized small and localized cancer foci, is very common in middle-aged and elderly men in almost all ethnic groups.[118] The majority never become active, rates of clinical cancer are determined by the proportion that do, and determinants of that metamorphosis are not known. In westernized societies it is estimated that about 8% of subjects with latent tumors develop distant metastases, but tumors with aggressive potential cannot be recognized, so that selective treatment of subjects with a poor prognosis is precluded. Prostate tumors of grades A2 to D are characterized by larger size, local extension, variable lymph node involvement and distant metastases, and progressively worse survival rates.

Active prostate tumors are androgen dependent, although no high-risk hormonal profiles have been identified. Expression of the *ras* p21 oncogene has been associated with the tumor and its virulence.[123] Benign prostatic hypertrophy is probably not a precursor. Some patients have a family history of prostatic cancer, but no HLA associations have been defined. Migrants from low- to high-incidence areas acquire local rates within one generation. Associations with higher socioeconomic status and level of education have been reported in Finland but not in Alameda County, California.[124,125] Associations with sexual activity, venereal disease, and prior tonsillectomy have been proposed. Correlations with consumption of animal products, animal fats, carotene, vitamin C, perhaps zinc, and with obesity or with increased lean body mass have been suggested. A 10-year prospective U.S. study associated prostate cancer risk inversely with blood levels of vitamin A. Cadmium intake, acrylonitrile exposure, and other chemicals and pollutants have been incriminated. Differences in prostate cancer death rates have been reported with different religious affiliations, and survival with prostate cancer is better in nonsmokers and in professional men.[116–119,124–130]

A tendency to treat all diagnosed cases obscures the natural history of these tumors and impedes evaluation of interventions. Treatment considerations[131] should include age and comorbidities, likelihood of death from unrelated causes, the uncertainty of the natural history of A1 tumors, and side effects and costs. Current treatment of apparently localized tumors with hope of cure involves radiation therapy and radical prostatectomy. Respective risks are radiation morbidity and impotence or urinary incontinence or both, and 10-year survivals are comparable. For disease with spread, orchiectomy or estrogens sometimes relieve symptoms but have not convincingly prolonged survival.

Screening for unsuspected disease detects more tumors, but the benefits of treating localized tumors or latent disease are not defined. By one estimate, routine digital examination of the prostate (which detects palpable tumor nodules) yields a maximum average increase in life expectancy of only 45 days per patient, at considerable expense.[132] In the U.S. multicenter National Cancer Detection Project, digital examination, transrectal ultrasound (said to be twice as sensitive as digital examination), and serum prostate-specific antigen will be evaluated as screening tools in a 5-year prospective study of 5000 men 55 to 70 years of age.[133]

Prostatic Hyperplasia

Benign prostatic hypertrophy (BPH)[134] is extremely common in older men. Clinical symptoms result from variable compression of the bladder outlet, with difficulties in urinating, and the potential for infection, complete obstruction, and bleeding. It has been estimated that by the age of 60, about 70% of men have BPH, that 85% to 95% of these have some symptoms, and that 10% to 20% undergo surgery. These are the most commonly performed surgical procedures in males in the United States (an estimated 435,000 in 1985, with annual costs exceeding $1 billion dollars).[105,120,134]

The cause of BPH is not known. Necessary conditions are the presence of androgens and aging. It is rarely identified before the age of 40, but histological examination reveals its presence in most men over 50: in 50% of those 60 years of age and 85% of those 85 years of age. No associations with sociocultural factors, sexual behavior, use of tobacco or alcohol, or other diseases have been consistently demonstrated, and there is no firm evidence that BPH is a precursor of prostate cancer.

In BPH subjects, a period of rapid prostate enlargement occurs, usually after the age of 50, followed by stabilization. The determinants of clinical symptoms are poorly understood, but they might correlate better with horizontal cross-sectional features of the prostate around the bladder neck and urethra than with total prostate weight.[135] The natural history of symptoms can vary greatly. Many subjects have mild symptoms for years, with no change, and many do not require surgical intervention.

Evaluation consists of rectal examination, blood chemistry studies, urinalysis and culture, measurement of residual urine volume after voiding, cystourethroscopy, urodynamic evaluation, and imaging or contrast studies of the kidneys and ureters. Management choices for most subjects with symptoms are prostatectomy and observation.[136,137] Indications for surgery vary, need better definition, and should be weighed against the comorbidities, complications, outcomes, and costs. Firm indications are acute urinary retention, hydronephrosis, recurrent urinary infections, severe hematuria, severe outflow obstruction, and urgency incontinence. Persistence of symptoms and impotence can result from surgery in a significant minority of subjects. Hormonal and other neuropharmacological manipulations to shorten the prostatic growth phase or to improve bladder emptying and balloon dilatation of the prostatic urethra are under evaluation as alternate forms of therapy.[136]

Interstitial Cystitis

Interstitial cystitis[138-140] is a syndrome of unknown etiology and pathogenesis, lacking uniform diagnostic criteria. It is characterized by nocturia, urgency, and suprapubic pressure and pain with bladder filling. Postulated etiologic factors have included slow virus infections, lack of protective bladder mucin, irritative substances in the urine, and allergy. Urinalysis is usually unremarkable, and cultures are usually sterile. The bladder mucosa can appear normal in early disease, show petechial hemorrhages with bladder distention in established disease, and show mucosal ulcerations in advanced disease.

This disease is 6 to 11 times more common in women than in men, but it has also been reported in children and the elderly. Its frequency and geographic and racial distributions have not been ascertained. Estimates of 20,000 to 90,000 diagnosed cases and four to five times as many undiagnosed cases were recently made in the United States, and a prevalence of 18.1 and an annual incidence of 1.2 cases per 100,000 women were estimated in Helsinki, Finland. The median age at onset of symptoms in one U.S. study was 40 to 50 years, and the duration was 7 to 10 years. Increasing proportions of young women with symptoms but with no bladder fibrosis might reflect earlier diagnosis or an increasing incidence of this disease.

Diagnosis in nonulcerative disease is often delayed, by some estimates from 30 months to 7 years, and involves many physician visits, referrals, procedures, and treatment trials. Distress from diagnostic uncertainty and intractable pain is often compounded by inferences that symptoms have a psychological basis. A recent U.S. survey revealed that 40% of patients were unable to work, 58% were unable to have intercourse, many had disrupted personal and family lives, and 55% had considered and 12% had attempted suicide. Depression and abuse of tranquillizers, analgesics, and opiates were common. Overall quality of life was well below that of white women with end-stage renal disease.[139,140]

Symptoms increase rapidly after onset but then tend to stabilize, so that most subjects can live with, although impaired by, their disease. Various topical and systemic therapies have been reported to give some relief. Desperation measures include operations to alter bladder capacity, or urinary diversion.

Costs of this condition are obscure, but the minimal cost benefit of cure based on 44,000 cases in the United States has been estimated at $428 million per year.[139]

END-STAGE RENAL DISEASE

ESRD can be caused by many renal diseases and by some urinary tract diseases when they are complicated by chronic obstruction or infection. Most descriptions are derived from subjects in ESRD treatment programs, but the full scope of ESRD is much broader. Subjects who die of untreated ESRD are probably older, sicker, and the causes of their renal failure are more poorly differentiated and multifactorial.

Rates of ESRD increase with aging and are higher in males than in females. Rates of ESRD and renal deaths are higher in some transitional populations, such as U.S. blacks, Hispanics, or Mexican Americans, North American Indians, Australian aborigines, and New Zealand Maoris than in westernized whites, and the average age at onset of ESRD is often lower.[12,35,45,46,52]

Maintenance treatment of subjects with ESRD is expensive and complex, and access is determined less by patient need than by national wealth and health policy. Registries of ESRD subjects in treatment programs are maintained in the United States, in Europe by the European Dialysis and Transplant Association (EDTA), in Japan, Canada, and Australia/New Zealand. Acceptance rates of new subjects into these programs in 1988 ranged from 46 per million (pm) population in Australia to 164 pm in the United States, and the number of patients receiving treatment at the end of that year (point prevalence) ranged from 327 pm in Australia to 726 pm in Japan (with a rate of 598 pm in the United States).[141,142] The average age of new enrollees in these programs was very similar, from 54 to 56.8 years.

Glomerulonephritis is the single most common cause of

ESRD in subjects accepted into treatment programs in Europe, Australia, and New Zealand, and the third most common in the United States. Diabetes is the leading cause in the United States and Northern Europe, and although hypertension takes second place in the United States, it is not a leading cause in Australia and Europe.[12,13,35]

Preferred treatment modes vary. Annual rates of renal transplantation range from less than 2 subjects pm in Japan to 37 pm in the United States, and subjects with functioning transplants constitute from 3.8% of the ESRD population in Japan to 57.6% in Sweden.[12,141,142] It was recently estimated that of all ESRD subjects receiving therapy worldwide, 70% were on hemodialysis, 9% on peritoneal dialysis, and 21% had functioning kidney transplants.[13,143] Transplantation is limited by national and local policies and physician and patient preferences and by the availability of donor organs. A variable proportion of grafts are donated from living donors, usually relatives. Quality of life and productivity are not fully restored by ESRD treatment, but successful transplantation of eligible subjects yields the best rehabilitation.

Recent rapid advances in this field include the wide application of high flux and bicarbonate hemodialysis, improving tolerance and efficiency of treatments, and the use of vitamin D derivatives and genetically engineered erythropoietin to combat the bone disease and the anemia of chronic renal failure. The use of cyclosporine and monoclonal antibodies against the lymphocyte mediators of rejection have improved 1-year cadaveric transplant survival to ≥80% in most centers.

Stabilizing numbers of patients in the ESRD treatment programs of some northern European countries suggest that needs have been almost met. In several western European countries, in Australia, and in the United States, accommodation of most "standard risk" subjects is approaching, and the largest annual increases are in numbers of older and "high-risk" subjects. Unmet needs of standard-risk subjects still exist in southern Europe.[12,35,142,144]

The Medicare-supported ESRD treatment program in the United States, which includes an estimated 93% of all treated ESRD patients, grew at an average annual rate of 9.8% from 1983 to 1988.[12] The number of young dialysis patients is leveling off, but increases continue in the number of older subjects, high-risk patients, and diabetics.[12,144] Blacks and males continue to be represented in relative excess. In 1988, 36,160 patients, characterized in Tables 50–4 and 50–5, started ESRD treatment in this program, and a total of 172,506 subjects received ESRD treatment at some time that year. In 1988, 8932 transplants were performed, and 36,967 patients had functioning transplants. The elderly, blacks, and females are underrepresented among transplant recipients, and graft survival is worse in blacks.[12] Successful transplantation is tending to stratify the U.S. ESRD population into potential transplant recipients less than 55 years old and older subjects likely to stay on chronic dialysis,[144] a trend mirrored elsewhere.[35,143] Current 5-year survival ranges from 67.4% for dialysis patients less than 35 years old at the start of treatment to 15.8% for those 65 and older.[12] Gross mortality rates of dialysis patients in the United States are the highest in any surveyed country and are still rising. Primary diagnosis, comorbidities, age, failure of patients to comply with scheduled treatments (also highest in the United States), and transplant rates and patterns might contribute to this phenomenon. However, widespread inadequacy of dialysis has also been incriminated, and the formal quantitation of each individual patient's dialysis needs and its rigorous prescription are strongly advocated.[145]

Direct medical payments for ESRD treatment exceeded $5.4 billion in 1988 in the United States. The estimated cost for a full year of treatment was $35,600 per patient. Of these costs, 67% to 80% were paid by the federal government. The rest was paid by other sources, including private insurance and patients and their families, who usually incurred considerable hardship. Other costs, such as those of outpatient drugs, travel for treatment, and lost productivity, are unquantitated. Average costs per patient might be stabilizing because of capitated reimbursement, technical efficiencies, marketplace competition, changes in medical practice, and increasing numbers of successful transplants. Transplantation is the most cost-effective therapy for ESRD, in spite of initially high costs and the costs of failed grafts, largely because maintenance costs of persons with functioning transplants are one third those of dialysis patients.[144]

TABLE 50-4. SUMMARY OF U.S. ESRD INCIDENT CASES IN 1988

Total	Count	Incidence per Million
	36,160	147
▪ **Age (y)**		
0–19	833	11
20–44	8,090	84
45–64	13,371	302
65–74	8,805	533
75 plus	5,061	436
▪ **Race**		
White	24,357	109
Black	10,045	404
Asian/Pacific Islander	633	121
Native American	440	415
Other	586	—
Unknown	99	—
▪ **Sex**		
Male	19,663	166
Female	16,497	116

From U.S. Renal Data System, USRDS, 1990 Annual Data Report, NIH, NIDDK.

THE FUTURE

Epidemiological and health services research in renal and urinary tract diseases is expanding rapidly. In the United States the National Institutes of Diabetes, Digestive and Kidney Diseases have collated existing data on rates, morbidities, mortalities, resource utilization, and costs. They are supporting studies on diabetic renal disease, hypertension, progressive glomerular sclerosis, progression of renal failure, urinary tract obstruction, prostatic hyperplasia, prostatic cancer screening, and urinary incontinence. They have also established research initiatives in interstitial cysti-

TABLE 50-5. U.S. ESRD INCIDENT CASES FOR 1988 ACCORDING TO PRIMARY DISEASE

Primary Disease	Count	Incidence per Million
Diabetes	11,034	43
Hypertension	9,647	37
Glomerulonephritis	5,003	19
Cystic kidney disease	1,197	5
Other urologic disease	1,995	8
Other known cause	2,048	8
Unknown cause	2,394	9
Missing data	2,843	9

From U.S. Renal Data System, USRDS, 1990 Annual Data Report, NIH, NIDDK.

tis, HIV-associated renal disease, the genetic basis of polycystic kidney disease, and renal disease and hypertension in minorities. The National Health and Nutrition Examination Survey—1988 to 1994 will yield estimates of rates of kidney stones, UTIs, interstitial cystitis, prostate disease, bladder dysfunction, microalbuminuria, and elevated serum creatinine levels. The newly established United States Renal Data System[12] promises valuable longitudinal data.

The base for such research should be expanded beyond the traditional bastions of federal agencies and academic centers to include collaborative ventures with biotechnology and pharmaceutical companies and to exploit the wealth of information and talent in clinical practice. In addition, we should move beyond the statistician-scientist-physician investigator model and establish multidisciplinary research teams to better define the social, economic, ethnic, and life-style determinants of renal and urinary tract diseases and to design realistic, cost-effective, and culturally relevant intervention strategies.

The results of these initiatives should invigorate the practice of nephrology, guide judicious apportionment of limited resources, support formulation of rational health policy, and pose a real challenge to renal and urinary tract diseases in the twenty-first century.

REFERENCES

1. Challah S, Wing AJ: The epidemiology of genitourinary disease. In Holland WW, Detels R, Knox G (eds): The Oxford Textbook of Public Health. Oxford, England: Oxford University Press, 1985, chap. 11, vol. 4
2. Plough AL: Borrowed Time—Artificial Organs and the Politics of Extending Lives. Philadelphia: Temple University Press, 1986, pp 27–35
3. Hoy WE, Watkins MA: Renal disease epidemiology: an underdeveloped discipline. Am J Kidney Dis 12:454–457, 1988
4. Levey AS, Perrone RD, Madias NE: Serum creatinine and renal function. Ann Rev Med 39:465–490, 1988
5. Hostetter TH: The hyperfiltering glomerulus. Med Clin North Am 2:387–396, 1984
6. Ihle BU, Becker GJ, Whitworth JA, et al: The effect of protein restriction on the progression of renal insufficiency. N Engl J Med 321:1773–1777, 1989
7. Avram MM: Cholesterol and lipids in renal disease. Am J Med 87:5 IN-5-2N, 1989
8. Feig PU, Rutan GH: Angiotensin converting enzyme inhibitors: the end of end stage renal disease? Ann Intern Med 111:451–453, 1989
9. Bennett PH: Microalbuminuria and diabetes, a critique: assessment of urinary albumin excretion and its role in screening for diabetic nephropathy. Am J Kidney Dis 13:29–34, 1989
10. Hawthorne VM, Herman WH: Preventing the kidney disease of diabetes mellitus: public health perspectives. Am J Kidney Dis 13:1–48, 1989
11. Kussman MJ, Goldstein HH, Gleason RE: The clinical course of diabetic nephropathy. JAMA 236:1861–1863, 1976
12. U.S. Renal Data System: USRDS 1990 Annual Data Report. Bethesda, Md: The National Institutes of Health, National Institute of Diabetes and Digestive and Kidney Diseases, August 1990
13. Brunner FP, Brynger H, Challah S, et al: Renal replacement therapy in patients with diabetic nephropathy. Nephrol Dial Transplant 3:585–594, 1988
14. Demography of dialysis and transplantation in Europe, 1984: report from the European Dialysis and Transplant Association Registry. Nephrol Dial Transplant 1:1–8, 1986
15. Anderson AR, Christiansen JS, Anderson JK, et al: Diabetic nephropathy in type 1 (insulin dependent) diabetes: an epidemiological study. Diabetologia 25:496–501, 1983
16. Kofoed-Enevoldsen A, Borch-Johnsen K, Kreiner S, et al: Declining incidence of persistent proteinuria in type 1 (insulin dependent) diabetic patients in Denmark. Diabetes 36:205–209, 1987
17. Krolewski AS, Warram JH, Christlieb AR, et al: The changing natural history of nephropathy in type 1 diabetes. Am J Med 78:785–794, 1985
18. Christlieb AR, Warram JH, Krowleski AS: Hypertension: the major risk factor in juvenile onset insulin dependent diabetics. Diabetes 30(suppl 2):90–96, 1981
19. Krolewski AS, Canessa M, Warram JH, et al: Predisposition to hypertension and susceptibility to renal disease in insulin-dependent diabetes mellitus. N Engl J Med 318:140–145, 1988
20. Chase HP, Garg SK, Harris S, et al: High normal blood pressure and early diabetic nephropathy. Arch Intern Med 150:639–641, 1990
21. Seaquist ER, Goetz FC, Rich S, et al: Familial clustering of diabetic kidney disease. N Engl J Med 320:1161–1165, 1989
22. Stegmayr B, Lithner F: Tobacco and end stage diabetic nephropathy. Br Med J 295:581–582, 1987
23. Telmer S, Sandahl Christiansen JS, Anderson AR, et al: Smoking habits and prevalence of clinical diabetic microangiopathy in insulin-dependent diabetics. Acta Med Scand 215:63–68, 1984
24. Pugh JA: The kidney disease of diabetes mellitus: end stage renal disease in Mexican Americans. Presented at the Second International Symposium on Renal Disease and Transplantation in Blacks, sponsored by Howard University and the NIDDK, Washington, DC, March 1989
25. Narva AS: End stage renal disease. IHS Primary Care Provider 10:82–85, 1985
26. Ballard DJ, Humphrey LL, Melton J, et al: Epidemiology of persistent proteinuria in type 2 diabetes mellitus: a population-based study in Rochester, Minnesota. Diabetes 37:405–412, 1988
27. Haffner SM, Mitchell BD, Pugh JA, et al: Proteinuria in Mexican Americans and nonHispanic whites with NIDDM. Diabetes Care 12:530–536, 1989
28. Kunzelman CL, Knowler WC, Pettitt DJ, et al: Incidence of proteinuria in type 2 diabetes mellitus in the Pima Indians. Kidney Int 35:681–687, 1989
29. Pugh JA, Stern MP, Haffner SM, et al: Excess incidence of treatment of end-stage renal disease in Mexican Americans. Am J Epidemiol 27:135–144, 1988
30. Nelson RG, Newman JM, Knowler WC, et al: Incidence of end-stage renal disease in type 2 (non-insulin-dependent) diabetes mellitus in Pima Indians. Diabetologia 31:730–736, 1988
31. Nelson RG, Kunzelman CL, Pettit DJ, et al: Albuminuria in type 2 (non-insulin-dependent) diabetes mellitus and impaired glucose tolerance in Pima indians. Diabetologia 32:870–876, 1989
32. Garancini P, Gallus G, Calori G, et al: Microalbuminuria and its associated risk factors in a representative sample of Italian type 2 diabetics. J Diabetic Complications 2:12–15, 1988
33. Marshall SM, Alberti KGMM: Comparison of the prevalence and associated features of abnormal albumin excretion in insulin-dependent and non-insulin-dependent diabetes. Q J Med 261:61–71, 1989
34. Gimenez L, Briefel G, Zachary J, et al: Relative contribution of type 1 and type 2 diabetics to the chronic dialysis population. Kidney Int 35:226, 1989
35. Twelfth Report of the Australia and New Zealand Combined Dialysis and Transplant Registry (ANZDATA), Woodville, South Australia, Queen Elizabeth Hospital, June 1989
36. Miller JM, Miller JM: Diabetes mellitus and hypertension in black and white populations. South Med J 79:1229, 1986
37. Tierney WM, McDonald CJ, Luft FC: Renal disease in hypertensive adults: effect of race and type 2 diabetes mellitus. Am J Kidney Dis 13:485–493, 1989
38. West KM, Erdreich LJ, Stober JA: A detailed study of risk factors for retinopathy and nephropathy in diabetes. Diabetes 29:501–508, 1980
39. Knowler WC, Bennett PH, Nelson RG. Prediabetic blood pressure predicts albuminuria after development of NIDDM. Diabetes (abstract) 37(suppl):120, 1988

40. Luke RG. Nephrosclerosis. In Schrier RW, Gottschalk CW (eds): Diseases of the Kidney, 4 edt. Boston: Little, Brown & Co, 1986, chap 54
41. Rostand SG, Kirk KA, Rutsky EA, et al: Racial differences in the incidence of treatment for end stage renal disease. N Engl J Med 306:1276–1279, 1982
42. McClellan W, Tuttle E, Issa A: Racial differences in the incidence of hypertensive end stage renal disease (ESRD) are not entirely explained by differences in the prevalence of hypertension. Am J Kidney Dis 12:285–290, 1988
43. Tierney WM, McDonald CJ, Luft FC: Renal disease in hypertensive adults: effect of race and type 2 diabetes mellitus. Am J Kidney Dis 13:485–493, 1989
44. Luft FC, Fineberg NS, Miller JZ, et al: The effects of age, race, and heredity on glomerular filtration rate following volume expansion and contraction in normal man. Am J Med Sci 279:15–24, 1980
45. Megill DM, Hoy WE, Woodruff SD: Rates and causes of end stage renal disease in Navajo Indians, 1971–1985. West J Med 149:178–182, 1988
46. Hoy WE, Megill DM: Mesangialproliferative glomerulonephritis in Southwestern Native Americans. Transplant Proc 21:3909–3912, 1989
47. Sievers ML: Historical overview of hypertension among American Indians and Alaskan Natives. Ariz Med 43:607–610, 1977
48. Schulman NB, Ford CE, Hall WD, et al: Prognostic value of serum creatinine and effect of treatment of hypertension on renal function: results from the Hypertension Detection and Follow-up Program. Hypertension 13(suppl):180–193, 1989
49. Rostand SG, Brown G, Kirk KA, et al: Renal insufficiency in treated essential hypertension. N Engl J Med 320:684–688, 1989
50. Qualheim RE, Rostand SG, Kirk KA, et al: Changing patterns of end-stage renal disease due to hypertension. Kidney Int 37:244, 1990
51. Young TK, Kaufert JM, McKenzie JK, et al: Excessive burden of end-stage renal disease among Canadian Indians: a national survey. Am J Public Health 79:756–758, 1989
52. General Mortality Statistics, Indian Health Service Chart Series Book, April 1987, pp 42–43
53. Cameron JS: The long term outcome of glomerular diseases. In Schrier RW, Gottschalk CW (eds): Diseases of the Kidney, 4 edt. Boston: Little, Brown & Co, 1986, chap 69
54. Simon P, Ramee MP, Ang KS, et al: Evolution de l'incidence annuelle des glomerulonephrites primitives dans une populations de 400,000 habitants au cours d'une periods de 10 ans (1976–1985). Nephrologie 5:185–189, 1986
55. Tiebosch ATMG, Wolters J, Frederick PFM, et al: Epidemiology of idiopathic glomerular disease: a prospective study. Kidney Int 32:112–116, 1987
56. Gonzalo A, Matesanz R, Teruel JL, et al: Incidence of membranoproliferative glomerulonephritis in a Spanish population. Clin Nephrol 26:161, 1986
57. The New Zealand Glomerulonephritis Study: Introductory report of the New Zealand Glomerulonephritis Study Group. Clin Nephrol 31:239–246, 1989
58. Central Committee of the Toronto Glomerulonephritis Registry: Regional program for the study of glomerulonephritis. Can Med Assoc J 124:158–161, 1981
59. Coggins CH: Membranous nephropathy. In Schrier RW, Gottschalk CW (eds): Diseases of the Kidney, 4 edt. Boston: Little, Brown & Co, 1986, chap 65
60. Donadio JV: Membranoproliferative Glomerulonephritis. In Schrier RW, Gottschalk CW (eds): Diseases of the Kidney, 4 edt. Boston: Little, Brown & Co, 1986, chap 66
61. Schena FP, Cameron JS: Treatment of proteinuric idiopathic glomerulonephritis in adults: a retrospective survey. Am J Med 85: 315–326, 1988
62. Levy M, Berger J: Worldwide perspectives in IgA nephropathy. Am J Kidney Dis 12:340–347, 1988
63. Julian BA, Quiggins PA, Thompson JS, et al: Familial IgA nephropathy in a Kentucky kindred: evidence of an inherited mechanism of disease. N Engl J Med 312:202–208, 1985
64. Rodriguez-Iturbe B: Acute poststreptococcal glomerulonephritis. In Schrier RW, Gottschalk CW (eds): Diseases of the Kidney, 4 edt. Boston: Little, Brown & Co, 1986, chap 63
65. Grantham JJ, Gabow PA: Polycystic kidney disease. In Schrier RW, Gottschalk CW (eds): Diseases of the Kidney, 4 edt. Boston: Little, Brown & Co, 1986, chap 18
66. Grantham JJ: Polycystic kidney disease—an old problem in a new context. N Engl J Med 19:944–946, 1988
67. Sedman A, Bell P, Manco-Johnson MM, et al: Autosomal dominant polycystic disease in childhood: a longitudinal study. Kidney Int 31:1000–1005, 1987
68. Gene testing in autosomal dominant polycystic kidney disease: results of the National Kidney Foundation Workshop. Am J Kidney Dis 13:85–87, 1989
69. Analgesic-associated kidney disease. Consensus Conference, Office of Medical Applications of Research, National Institutes of Health. JAMA 251:3123–3125, 1984
70. Goldberg M: Analgesic-associated nephropathy: an important cause of chronic renal failure in the United States? Am J Kidney Dis 7:162–163, 1986
71. Maher JF: Renal failure in America is infrequently due to analgesic abuse. Am J Kidney Dis 7:169–173, 1986
72. Buckalew VM, Schey HM: Analgesic nephropathy: a significant cause of morbidity in the United States. Am J Kidney Dis 7:164–168, 1986
73. Dubach UC, Rosner B, Pfister E: Epidemiologic study of abuse of analgesics containing phenacitin. N Engl J Med 308:357–362, 1983
74. Murray TG, Stolley PD, Anthony C, et al: Epidemiologic study of regular analgesic use and end stage renal disease. Arch Intern Med 143:1687–1693, 1983
75. Sandler DP, Smith JC, Weinberg CR, et al: Analgesic use and chronic renal disease. N Engl J Med 320:1238–1243, 1989
76. Bennett WM, DeBroe ME: Analgesic nephropathy: a preventable renal disease. N Engl J Med 320:1269–1271, 1989
77. Cooper K, Bennett WM: Nephrotoxicity of common drugs used in clinical practice. Arch Intern Med 147:1213–1217, 1987
78. Corwin HL, Bonventre JV: Renal insufficiency associated with nonsteroidal anti-inflammatory drugs. Am J Kidney Dis 4:147–152, 1984
79. Adams DH, Michael J, Bacon PA, et al: Nonsteroidal anti-inflammatory drugs and renal failure. Lancet, January 11, 1986, pp 57–60
80. Collins AJ: Kidney dialysis treatment for victims of the Armenian earthquake. N Engl J Med 320:1291–1292, 1989
81. Dhalal M, Patel B, Kaufman J: Community acquired acute renal failure. Kidney Int 37:273, 1990
82. Hou SH, Bushinsky DA, Wish JB, et al: Hospital-acquired renal insufficiency: a prospective study. Am J Med 74:243–248, 1983
83. Rasmussen HH, Ibels LS: Acute renal failure: multivariate analysis of causes and risk factors. Am J Med 73:211–218, 1982
84. Buktus DE: Persistent high mortality in acute renal failure: are we asking the right questions? Arch Intern Med 143:209–212, 1983
85. Bullock ML, Umen AJ, Finkelstein M, et al: The assessment of risk factors in 462 patients with acute renal failure. Am J Kidney Dis 5:97–103, 1985
86. Liano F, Garcia Martin F, Gallego A, et al: Easy and early prognosis in acute tubular necrosis: a forward analysis of 228 cases. Nephron 51:307–313, 1989
87. Baldwin DS, Gallo GR, Neugarten J: Drug abuse with narcotics, amphetamines and other agents. In Schrier RW, Gottschalk CW (eds): Diseases of the Kidney, 4 edt. Boston: Little, Brown & Co, 1986, chap 45
88. Cunningham EE, Zielezny MA, Venuto RC: Heroin associated nephropathy, a nationwide problem. JAMA 250:2935–2936, 1983
89. Cunningham EE, Brentjens JR, Zielezny MA, et al: Heroin nephropathy; a clinical and epidemiologic study. Am J Med 68:47–53, 1980

90. Dubrow A, Mittman N, Ghali V, et al: The changing spectrum of heroin-associated nephropathy. Am J Kidney Dis 5:36–41, 1985
91. Menchel S, Cohen D, Gross E, et al: AA protein-related renal amyloidosis in drug addicts. Am J Pathol 112:195–199, 1983
92. Schoenfeld P, Feduska NJ: Acquired immunodeficiency syndrome and renal disease: report of the National Kidney Foundation–National Institutes of Health Task Force on AIDS and Kidney Disease. Am J Kidney Dis 16:14–25, 1990
93. Pardo V, Meneses R, Jaffe DJ, et al: AIDS-related glomerulopathy: occurrence in specific risk groups. Kidney Int 31:1167–1173, 1987
94. Chander P, Sagel I, Weiss R, et al: Renal disease in human immunodeficiency virus (HIV) infected children. Kidney Int 35:368, 1989
95. Perez G, Ortiz-Interian C, Lee H, et al: Human immunodeficiency virus and human T-cell leukemia virus Type 1 in patients undergoing maintenance hemodialysis in Miami. Am J Kidney Dis 14:39–43, 1989
96. Reiser IW, Shapiro WB, Porush JG: The incidence and epidemiology of human immunodeficiency virus infection in 320 patients treated in an inner-city hemodialysis center. Am J Kidney Dis 16:26–31, 1990
97. Rastegar A, Sitprija, Rocha H: Tropical nephrology. In Schrier RW, Gottschalk CW (eds): Diseases of the Kidney. 4 edt. Boston: Little, Brown & Co, 1986, chap 85
98. Barsoum RS: Schistosomal glomerulopathy: selection factors. Nephrol Dial Transplant 2:488–497, 1987
99. Johnson RJ, Couser WG: Hepatitis B infection and renal disease: clinical, immunopathogenic and therapeutic considerations. Kidney Int 37:663–676, 1990
100. Roberts JA: Urinary tract infections. Am J Kidney Dis 4:103–117, 1984
101. Brettman LR: Pathogenesis of urinary tract infections: host susceptibility and bacterial virulence factors. Urology 32(suppl):9–11, September 1988
102. Fihn SD: Behavioral aspects of urinary tract infection. Urology 32(suppl):16–18, 1988
103. Brettman LR: Nosocomial infection is associated with short term and long term inpatient care. Urology 32(suppl):21–23, 1988
104. Division of Health Care Statistics, National Center for Health Statistics: National Ambulatory Medical Care Survey, 1985 (unpublished data).
105. National Center for Health Statistics: Detailed diagnoses and procedures for patients discharged from short stay hospitals, United States, 1985. Series B, No. 90, DHHS publication No. 87–1751, April 1987
106. Department of Veterans' Affairs, year ending Sept. 30, 1986 (unpublished data).
107. Drach GW: Urinary Lithiasis. In Walsh PC, Gittes RF, Perlmutter AD, Stamey TA (eds): Campbell's Urology. 5 edt. Philadelphia: WB Saunders Co, 1986, chap 25
108. Frangos DN, Rous SN: Incidence and economic factors in urolithiasis. In Rous SN (ed): Stone Disease: Diagnosis and Management. New York: Grune & Stratten Inc., 1987, chap 1
109. Smith LH: The medical aspects of urolithiasis: an overview. J Urol [part 2] 141:707–710, 1989
110. Rose GA: Current trends in urolithiasis research. In Rous SN (ed): Stone Disease: Diagnosis and Management. New York: Grune & Stratten Inc, 1987, chap 28
111. Office of Medical Applications of Research, National Institutes of Health: Prevention and treatment of kidney stones. JAMA 260:978–981, 1988
112. FitzSimmons SC: Self reported kidney stone disease among black and white adults: prevalence and correlates in NHANES 11(1976–1980). Presented at the 116th annual meeting of the American Public Health Association, November 1988
113. Frank M, DeVries A: Prevention of urolithiasis. Arch Environ Health 13:625–630, 1966
114. Pak CYC: Role of medical prevention. J Urol [part 2] 141:798–801, 1989
115. Segura JW: Surgical management of urinary calculi. Semin Nephrol 10:52–63, 1990
116. Catalona WJ, Scott WW: Carcinoma of the prostate. In Walsh PC, Gittes RF, Perlmutter AD, Stamey TA (eds): Campbell's Urology. 5 edt. Philadelphia: WB Saunders Co, 1986, chap 32
117. Zaridze DG, Boyle P: Cancer of the prostate: epidemiology and etiology. Br J Urol 59:493–501, 1987
118. Dohm G: Epidemiologic aspects of latent and clinically manifest carcinoma of the prostate. J Cancer Res Clin Oncol 106:210–218, 1983
119. Debre B, Geraud M, Flam T, et al: Epidemiology of prostatic cancer. J Int Med Res 18(suppl 1):3–7, 1990
120. Carter HB, Coffey DS: The prostate: an increasing medical problem. Prostate 16:39–48, 1990
121. Silverberg E, Lubera J: Cancer statistics, 1989. CA 39:1–32, 1989
122. Seidman H, Mushinski MH, Gelb SK, et al: Probabilities of eventually developing or dying of cancer—United States, 1985. CA 35:36–56, 1985
123. Viola MV, Fromowitz F, Ovarez S, et al: Expression of ras p21 oncogene in prostate cancer. N Engl J Med 314:133, 1986
124. Rimpela AH, Pukkala EI: Cancers of affluence: positive social class gradient and rising incidence trend in some cancer forms. Soc Sci Med 24:601–606, 1987
125. Ernster VL, Winkelstein W, Selvin S, et al: Race, socioeconomic status, and prostatic cancer. Cancer Treat Rep 61:187–191, 1977
126. Whittemore AS, Paffenbarger RS, Anderson K, et al: Early precursors of site-specific cancers in college men and women. J Natl Cancer Inst 74:43–51, 1985
127. Kolonel LN, Yoshizawa CN, Hankin JH: Diet and prostatic cancer: a case control study in Hawaii. Am J Epidemiol 127:999–1011, 1988
128. Severson RK, Grove JS, Nomura AMY, et al: Body mass and prostatic cancer: a prospective study. Br Med J 297:713–715, 1988
129. Chen JL, Walrath J, O'Berg MT, et al: Cancer incidence and mortality among workers exposed to acrylonitrile. Am J Ind Med 11:157–163, 1987
130. Reichman ME, Hayes RB, Ziegler RG, et al: Serum vitamin A and subsequent development of prostate cancer in the first National Health and Nutrition Examination Survey Epidemiologic Follow-up Study. Cancer Res 50:2311–2315, 1990
131. Consensus Statement: The management of clinically localized prostate cancer. NCI Monogr 7:3–6, 1988
132. Love RR, Fryback DG: A cost effectiveness analysis of screening for carcinoma of the prostate by digital examination. Med Decis Making 5:263–278, 1985
133. Lee F, Torp-Pederson ST, Littrup PJ, et al: Is ultrasound of the prostate indicated for screening purposes? J Fam Pract 27:521–524, 1988
134. Walsh PC: Benign prostatic hyperplasia. In Walsh PC, Gittes RF, Perlmutter AD, Stamey TA (eds): Campbell's Urology. 5 edt. Philadelphia: WB Saunders Co, 1986, chap 27
135. Watanabe H: Natural history of benign prostatic hypertrophy. Ultrasound Med Biol 12:567–571, 1986
136. Lepor H: Introduction: Pharmacologic Intervention in Benign Prostatic Hypertrophy. Urology 32(suppl): 3–4, 1988
137. Mebust WK: Surgical management of benign prostatic obstruction. Urology 32(suppl): 12–15, 1988
138. Messing EM: Interstitial cystitis and related syndromes. In Walsh PC, Gittes RF, Perlmutter AD, Stamey TA (eds): Campbell's Urology, 5 edt. Philadelphia: WB Saunders Co, 1986, chap 24
139. Gillenwater JY, Wein AJ: Summary of the National Institutes of Arthritis, Diabetes, Digestive and Kidney Diseases Workshop on Interstitial Cystitis, Bethesda, Maryland, August 28–29, 1987. J Urol 140:203–206, 1988
140. Ratner V: Rediscovering a "rare" disease: a patient's perspective on interstitial cystitis. Urology 29(suppl):44–45, 1987
141. Odaka M: Mortality in chronic dialysis in Japan. Am J Kidney Dis 15:410–413, 1990
142. Thirteenth Report of the Australia and New Zealand Dialysis and

Transplant Registry (ANZDATA). The Queen Elizabeth Hospital, Woodville, South Australia, June 1990

143. Demography of dialysis and transplantation in Europe in 1985 and 1986: trends over the previous decade. Nephrol Dial Transplant 3:714–727, 1988

144. Eggers PW: Effect of transplantation on the Medicare end-stage renal disease program. N Engl J Med 318:223–229, 1988

145. Hull AR, Parker TF: Introduction and summary: proceedings from the Morbidity, Mortality and Prescription of Dialysis Symposium. Am J Kidney Dis 15:375–383, 1990

51

Diabetes

Trevor J. Orchard
Ronald E. LaPorte
Janice S. Dorman

Diabetes is an important chronic disease both in terms of the number of persons affected and the considerable associated morbidity and early mortality. In this review we will focus on the epidemiology and public health implications of diabetes.

Diabetes is a chronic disease in which there is a deficiency in the action of the hormone insulin. This may result from a quantitative deficiency of insulin, an abnormal insulin, resistance to its action, or a combination of deficits. Two major forms of the disease are recognized: insulin-dependent diabetes mellitus (IDDM), which comprises about 10% of all cases, and non-insulin-dependent diabetes mellitus (NIDDM), which accounts for about 90% of the cases. The criteria for the definition of diabetes are shown in Table 51–1 and are those of the National Diabetes Data Group (NDDG).[1] Diabetes may occasionally occur as a result of other diseases: Endocrine diseases such as acromegaly and Cushing's syndrome or metabolic disorders such as hemochromatosis can cause the disease. Diabetes can also be drug induced, for example, by steroids and possibly by the thiazide diuretics and oral contraceptives. Finally, diabetes may occur secondary to disease processes directly affecting the pancreas, such as cancer or chronic pancreatitis, which destroy the insulin-producing beta cells in the pancreatic islets (of Langerhans). However, these are relatively rare causes of diabetes.

In addition to these primary and secondary types of diabetes, two further classifications of abnormalities of glucose tolerance are of note, namely, gestational diabetes and impaired glucose tolerance (IGT). Gestational diabetes occurs during pregnancy but typically remits shortly after delivery. IGT is a condition with high blood sugars after glucose challenge that are not elevated enough to be classified as diabetic but nonetheless may carry some increased risk of large vessel (e.g., coronary heart) disease.[1,2] Both gestational diabetes[3] and IGT[4] carry an increased risk for the subsequent development of NIDDM.

DIAGNOSIS

The diagnosis of IDDM, also known as type I diabetes or juvenile onset diabetes, is fairly straightforward. IDDM often, though by no means always, has its onset in childhood. Classically the child will have symptoms of excessive thirst (polydipsia), excessive urination (polyuria), and weight loss. In a child with a high blood sugar these symptoms almost invariably point to IDDM. This type of diabetes is called insulin dependent because patients lose virtually all capacity to produce insulin. Without treatment they develop severe metabolic disturbances, including ketoacidosis and dehydration, which can lead to death. As death from ketoacidosis is largely preventable, the continuing though small number of deaths from this cause represents a challenge to our preventive health services.[5,6] In a recent international study, wide variations in mortality from acute diabetes complications were noted, with high rates in Japan and low rates in Finland. This variation was thought to reflect disease incidence (low in Japan and high in Finland) and resulting availability of skilled health care.[7]

NIDDM, also known as type II, usually presents in adulthood. In the past the terms *maturity-onset* and *mild diabetes* have been used. These terms are somewhat misleading, since NIDDM may present in youth, albeit rarely, and the complications may be far from mild. Patients with NIDDM, however, produce some insulin, although its secretion is often delayed, and there is usually some resistance to its action in the peripheral tissues. This resistance is often associated with elevated concentrations of insulin, particularly in newly recognized cases. However, concentrations are now recognized to be low in many NIDDM subjects, especially after accounting for obesity and using more specific assays.[8] It is estimated that almost as many cases of NIDDM are undiagnosed as are clinically recognized. This is made clear by data from the National Health and Examination Surveys, where the overall prevalence of diabetes in the adult U.S. population (20 to 74 years old) is estimated to be about 6.7% (Table 51–2). This includes a small proportion (0.23%) who have IDDM,[9] 3.2% who are recognized to have NIDDM, and a further 3.2% of the population with undiagnosed type II diabetes. A further 4.6% of the population probably suffer from impaired glucose tolerance, whereas the remaining 0.1% of the population with diabetes have gestational diabetes. A marked increase in prevalence occurs with age such that 18% of people aged 65 to 74 years have diabetes.

In NIDDM, often the diagnosis is not made on the basis of classic diabetic symptoms but rather on the presentation of one of the complications of diabetes. Such complications can be macrovascular (accelerated atherosclerosis with coronary artery, peripheral vascular, or cerebrovascular manifestations), microvascular (with disease of the small vessels in the kidneys or the eyes), or neuropathic (which may take the form of a variety of neurological syndromes). In addition, the disease may also be

TABLE 51–1. CRITERIA FOR THE CLASSIFICATION OF DIABETES

Classification	Adults	Children
Diabetes[a]	A. Symptoms with unequivocal hyperglycemia *or* B.[b] Fasting glucose ≥ 140 mg/dl (venous plasma) or ≥ 120 mg/dl (venous or capillary whole blood) *or* C.[b] *Fasting glucose* < B, but at *2 h plus an intervening value,*[d] glucose ≥ 200 mg/dl (venous plasma or capillary whole blood) *or* ≥ 180 mg/dl (venous whole blood)	A. Symptoms with random plasma glucose ≥ 200 mg/dl *or* B.[b] Fasting glucose ≥ 140 mg/dl (venous plasma) *or* ≥ 120 mg/dl (venous/capillary whole blood) *and* *2 h plus an intervening value*[e] ≥ 200 mg/dl (venous plasma/capillary whole blood) *or* ≥ 180 mg/dl (venous whole blood)
Impaired glucose tolerance[c]	1. *Fasting glucose* < 140 mg/dl (venous plasma) *or* < 120 mg/dl (venous capillary whole blood) *and* 2. *1/2 h, 1 h, or 1 1/2 h glucose* [d] ≥ 200 mg/dl (venous plasma or capillary whole blood) *or* ≥ 180 mg/dl (venous whole blood) *and* 3. *2 h glucose*[d] between 140 and 200 mg/dl (venous plasma or capillary whole blood) *or* between 120 and 180 mg/dl (venous whole blood)	1. *Fasting glucose* < 140 mg/dl (venous plasma) *or* < 120 mg/dl (venous or capillary whole blood) *and* 2. *2 h glucose*[e] > 140 mg/dl (venous plasma) *or* > 120 mg/dl (venous or capillary whole blood)
	Two or more of the following values after a 100 g oral glucose load:	
Gestational diabetes	Fasting ≥ 105 mg/dl (venous plasma) 1 h ≥ 190 mg/dl (venous plasma) 2 h ≥ 165 mg/dl (venous plasma) 3 h ≥ 145 mg/dl (venous plasma)	90 mg/dl (venous or capillary whole blood) 170 mg/dl (venous or capillary whole blood) 145 mg/dl (venous or capillary whole blood) 125 mg/dl (venous or capillary whole blood)
Normal glucose values (nonpregnant individuals)	*Fasting* < 115 mg/dl (venous plasma) < 110 mg/dl (venous or capillary whole blood) *1/2 h,*[d] *1h,*[d] *1 1/2 h*[d] < 200 mg/dl (venous plasma/capillary whole blood) < 180 mg/dl (venous whole blood) *2 h*[d] < 140 mg/dl (venous plasma/capillary whole blood) < 120 mg/dl (venous whole blood)	*Fasting* < 130 mg/dl (venous plasma) *or* < 115 mg/dl (venous or capillary whole blood) *2 h*[e] < 140 mg/dl (venous plasma/capillary whole blood) *or* < 120 mg/dl (venous whole blood)

[a] Diabetes is subclassified as—
IDDM (type I): Insulin is needed to preserve life.
NIDDM (type II): further classed as (1) nonobese NIDDM and (2) obese NIDDM.
Gestational: diabetes or impaired glucose tolerance is first recognized during pregnancy. Usually remits postpartum.
Other: Diabetes which develops secondary to or in association with other conditions, e.g., pancreatic disease, hormonal, drug, or chemical induced, insulin receptor abnormalities, and genetic syndromes.
[b] Criteria need to be present on at least two occasions.
[c] For epidemiological purposes, an adult may be assigned to this classification if criteria 1 and 3 are met and other blood samples are not available.
[d] Following 75 g of oral glucose.
[e] Following glucose 1.5 g/kg body weight; maximum 75 g.
From National Diabetes Data Group: Criteria for the classification of diabetes. Diabetes 28:1039–1054, 1979.

recognized as a result of routine screening for elevated blood sugar or by the presence of sugar in the urine. Some cases, however, may be diagnosed because of classic diabetic symptoms.

Over the years both the diagnostic criteria and dose of glucose in the oral glucose tolerance test (OGTT) have varied. The effect of these different criteria on the prevalence of diabetes has been studied by many investigators.[10] Compared to many earlier criteria, the recent NDDG criteria (Table 51–1) represent a relatively strict set of limits requiring a higher degree of hyperglycemia before a diagnosis of diabetes is made.[11]

The reasons for choosing the current criteria are twofold. First, studies in several high-risk populations, especially among the Pima Indians,[12] have shown that the distribution of blood sugars in these populations may be bimodal rather than the unimodal pattern found in a typical U.S. white population and that the second upper distribution is characterized by plasma glucose concentrations approximately equal to the NDDG suggested limits. Second, the specific complications of diabetes, for example, retinopathy, also appeared to occur primarily among individuals who had blood sugars that exceeded these limits.

Thus in reviewing studies done in previous years, it is important to remember that the criteria of diabetes were often less stringent and that the relationship between diabetes and subsequent risk of disease may have been quite different from that based on the current definitions. Also, because of these changes in the criteria for the diagnosis of NIDDM, estimates of the prevalence and temporal trends of NIDDM are difficult if not impossible to evaluate. Furthermore, the different criteria for NIDDM

TABLE 51–2. PERCENT OF POPULATION (STANDARD ERROR) OF PREVIOUSLY DIAGNOSED AND OF UNDIAGNOSED DIABETES IN THE U.S. POPULATION AGED 20–74 YEARS (NHANES II) FROM 1976 TO 1980

	Age				
	20–74	20–44	45–54	55–64	65–74
▪ Medical History of Diabetes[a]					
All races					
Both sexes	3.4 (.14)	1.1 (.11)	4.3 (.53)	6.6 (.66)	9.3 (.45)
Male	2.9 (.25)	.6 (.12)	4.3 (.82)	5.6 (.64)	9.7 (.71)
Female	3.8 (.24)	1.5 (.22)	4.3 (.67)	7.4 (1.10)	8.9 (.56)
White					
Both sexes	3.2 (.16)	1.0 (.12)	4.2 (.55)	6.0 (.58)	8.9 (.49)
Male	2.8 (.27)	.5 (.15)	4.5 (.92)	5.3 (.66)	9.1 (.78)
Female	3.6 (.23)	1.4 (.22)	3.9 (.60)	6.6 (.91)	8.8 (.64)
Black					
Both sexes	5.2 (.49)	2.2 (.58)	5.7 (1.46)	13.1 (2.65)	13.6 (1.35)
Male	4.5 (.60)	1.8 (.63)	3.6 (1.48)	9.2 (2.55)	17.2 (2.87)
Female	5.9 (.99)	2.6 (1.00)	7.5 (2.33)	16.3 (4.03)	10.8 (1.51)
▪ Undiagnosed Diabetes (NDDG Criteria)[b]					
All races					
Both sexes	3.2 (.35)	0.9 (.31)	4.2 (.81)	6.2 (1.03)	8.4 (.85)
Male	2.8 (.41)	0.8 (.39)	3.6 (1.28)	4.0 (1.03)	9.5 (1.42)
Female	3.6 (.42)	1.0 (.38)	4.7 (1.14)	8.1 (1.68)	7.6 (.89)
White					
Both sexes	3.0 (.38)	0.7 (.31)	4.0 (.90)	5.9 (1.24)	8.0 (.85)
Male	2.5 (.36)	0.5 (.27)	3.2 (1.25)	3.8 (1.00)	9.0 (1.38)
Female	3.4 (.52)	0.8 (.40)	4.6 (1.25)	7.9 (2.08)	7.3 (.95)
Black					
Both sexes	4.4 (.91)	0.9 (.68)	7.2 (3.05)	7.7 (3.75)	12.3 (3.94)
Male	4.0 (1.72)	1.0 (.98)	7.5 (6.40)	5.2 (3.94)	12.2 (7.23)
Female	4.6 (1.35)	0.9 (.91)	7.0 (3.70)	9.1 (5.92)	12.3 (4.50)

[a] Based on a self-report that the persons had been told by a doctor that they had diabetes, plus current or past use of diabetic therapy.

[b] Based on the results of a 75 g oral glucose tolerance test conducted in the morning after an overnight 10- to 16-hour fast in persons with no medical history of diabetes.

From Harris MI, Hadden WC, Knowler WC, Bennett PH: Prevalence of diabetes and impaired glucose tolerance and plasma glucose levels in the U.S. population aged 20–74 yr. Diabetes 36(4):523–534, 1987.

used by different research groups and countries make geographical comparisons difficult. As major efforts are made to identify the specific genetic abnormalities in diabetes and to define the disease on the basis of genotypic rather than phenotypic expression, such as hyperglycemia and insulin levels, there may soon be yet another way of classifying diabetes. Furthermore the development of glycosylated hemoglobin (GHB),[13] which provides an integrated measure of hyperglycemia over the prior 2 to 3 months, represents another dimension that may add to the ability to define diabetes. For example, some patients may show a "diabetic" response to an oral glucose challenge but experience little hyperglycemia in their normal life, where such glucose loads are rare. Such patients may therefore have "diabetes" but may have normal GHB and conceivably a lower risk of complication. These developments hold great promise for the improved diagnosis, prevention, and treatment of the disease.

Heterogeneity in Primary Diabetes

Although two different primary types of diabetes have been described, the classification of diabetes into these two groups is not simple. For example, there may be varying types of insulin-dependent diabetes according to the human leukocyte antigen (HLA) types with which they are associated, particularly HLA-DR3 and HLA-DR4,[14] which are common in IDDM.[15,16] It is also possible that some cases of childhood diabetes are in fact better classified as being "maturity-onset diabetes of youth," or "Mason" type diabetes. named after the family in England first described with this variety.[17] This type of diabetes is characterized by a familial abnormality of glucose tolerance inherited in an autosomal dominant pattern, a low frequency of complications, and nondevelopment of ketoacidosis. Children in such families, however, are often treated with insulin, although they are not strictly insulin dependent. Thus there are probably further subcategories beyond the insulin- and non-insulin-dependent types, which themselves may not be totally distinct entities. For example, data from Pittsburgh[18] and from the Joslin Clinic[19] show an increased risk for the development of IDDM in families where a relative has NIDDM, suggesting that these two types of diabetes may not be totally independent of each other. Although some of this increased risk may be explained by ascertainment bias,[18] this does not seem to be the entire explanation. The possibility of an "incomplete" IDDM process of autoimmune cell destruction, which may give rise to a clinically intermediary type of diabetes, therefore exists.[20]

IDDM

One of the most important observations related to insulin-dependent diabetes is the marked geographic variability of the disease. Figure 51–1 presents the incidence of IDDM for the various registries around the world. The annual risk for developing IDDM varies from over 30/100,000 in Finland to 0.6 to 0.7/100,000 in Korea and China. Overall there is approximately a fiftyfold difference between countries for developing IDDM (Fig. 51–1).[21,22]

In the United States the risk for developing IDDM is about

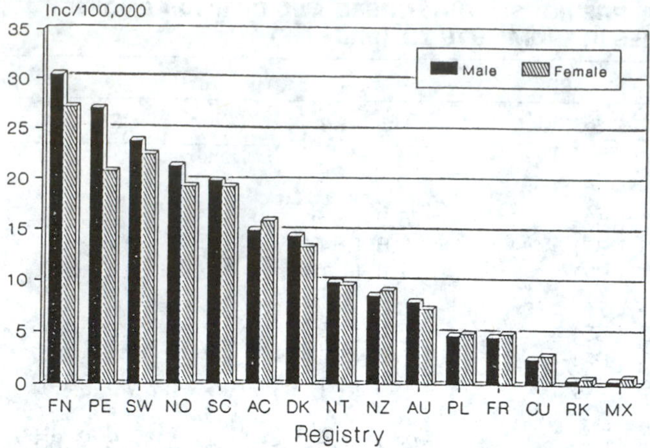

Figure 51-1. Age-standardised incidence rates of IDDM under age 15 years (per 100,000). FN, Finland; PE, Prince Edward Island, Canada; SW, Sweden; NO, Norway; SC, Scotland; AC, Allegheny County, Pennsylvania, USA; DK, Denmark; NT, The Netherlands; NZ, New Zealand; AU, Austria; PL, Poland; FR, France; CU, Cuba; RK, Republic of Korea; MX, Mexico. *(From Reivers M, LaPorte RE, King HOM, Tuomilehto J: Trends in the prevalence and incidence of diabetes: Insulin-dependent diabetes mellitus in childhood. World Health Stat Q 41:179–190, 1988.)*

15/100,000/y[23] during childhood. About 12,000 children per year develop IDDM in the United States. The estimated prevalence of IDDM is about 1.6/1000 school-age children.[24]

In addition to the marked geographic differences in incidence, IDDM has a distinctive demographic pattern. There is little difference in the overall incidence rates for males and females.[23] Whites have about 1.5 times the incidence rate of blacks. The incidence increases with age, peaking at adolescence, followed by a marked decline. This adolescent peak is likely to be related to puberty or to a growth spurt–associated phenomenon, since in females this peak occurs earlier than in males in a way similar to the onset of puberty. Although there appears to be little secular change in the incidence of IDDM in children in the United States,[25] several European countries have suggested an increase.[26] There is also a seasonal pattern of the onset of IDDM, with a consistent decline in the number of cases presenting during the summer months.[23] The pattern of seasonality has been identified in essentially all registry studies and is similar in high-risk as well as in low-risk countries.[25] The seasonality pattern has primarily been attributed to a viral cause of the disease or to an acute stress precipitating the clinical disease.[27] Recently it has been argued that the geographic patterns, seasonality, changes of incidence over time, and the migrant studies all strongly imply major environmental determinants of the disease.[28] It has been estimated that at least 70% and perhaps up to 95% of IDDM can be attributed to an environmental cause.

One of the most intriguing aspects of IDDM is the strong associations with the HLA region of chromosome 6. During the past 10 years most studies evaluating serological HLA markers have confirmed that IDDM susceptibility is highly related to specific alleles at the HLA-DR locus. Approximately 95% of all IDDM patients are HLA-DR3, HLA-DR4, or both.[15]

Children with these antigens, particularly the DR3-DR4 heterozygotes, have a greater risk of developing IDDM than individuals without the high-risk alleles have.[15,16] With the current advances in molecular biology the associations between IDDM and the HLA-D region are now being studied at the DNA level. Early restriction fragment length polymorphisms (RFLP) studies show a strong association between some HLA-DQ beta fragment patterns and IDDM.[29] The molecular HLA studies have begun to focus on the DQ locus, in search of possible "diabetogenic" genes. Recently it has been demonstrated that an amino acid other than aspartate in position 57 of the HLA-DQ beta chain (non-Asp-57) is highly associated with IDDM susceptibility, whereas an aspartic acid in this position (Asp-57) appears to protect against the development of the disease.[30,31] In a study of white probands identified from the IDDM registries in Allegheny County, Pa., 96% were homozygous for non-Asp-57, 4% were heterozygous, and none were homozygous for Asp-57. The corresponding proportions among healthy, unrelated nondiabetic controls were 19.5%, 46.3%, and 34%, respectively. Non-Asp-57 homozygosity was significantly associated with the development of IDDM, with an estimated relative risk of 107.[31]

The presence of non-Asp-57 appears to be a stronger determinant of IDDM susceptibility than DR3 or DR4.[31,32] Among diabetic non-DR3, non-DR4 haplotypes, the prevalence of non-Asp-57 was 87.5% compared to only 32.2% ($P = .001$) among nondiabetic haplotypes without DR3 or DR4.

The risk within families also appears to be associated with the presence of non-Asp-57. The differential risk of developing IDDM for the sibling of a proband depends on the number of HLA haplotypes the individual shares.[32] In normal populations, siblings have a 25% likelihood of sharing both haplotypes, a 50% likelihood of sharing only one, and a 25% probability of not sharing any haplotypes. Evaluation of DQ allele sharing in multiple-case families has revealed that 87.5% of affected sibling pairs shared both DQ alleles with the proband, 4.2% shared one, and 8.3% shared zero.[31] Among the nonaffected siblings in these families, the distribution was 27.3%, 45.4%, and 27.3%, respectively, for sharing two, one, and zero alleles with the proband. The strong associations between IDDM and the HLA-DQ beta chain genes, as well as the increase in risk for siblings who are HLA-identical with the index case, suggest that typing all siblings of an IDDM patient for the non-Asp-57 allele could provide useful information about risks among the siblings. High-risk children could then be monitored for early signs of glucose intolerance and autoimmunity.[33] However, recent studies have suggested that islet-cell antibodies may be a marker of pancreatic damage that may lead to subsequent diabetes among affected twins.[34] Sometimes these antibodies disappear without the development of IDDM.[35]

Screening the general population to identify genetically at-risk individuals is not advised. The frequency of diabetes is low even among those who are genetically susceptible. In Allegheny County, for example, the overall annual incidence of IDDM among whites is approximately 15.8/100,000.[36] However, in the general population those who are non-Asp-57 homozygous have an annual risk of 47.6/100,000/y, whereas those with at least two Asp-57 alleles have an annual risk of only 0.45/100,000/y, which approximates the incidence in Japan. Thus the risk of developing IDDM, even in those who are genetically susceptible, is only approximately 1/1000, and it would seem unlikely that a screening program, especially since there is no preventive approach, would be advantageous.

The treatment of new cases of IDDM with immunosuppressive agents such as cyclosporin is being evaluated to try to arrest the development of disease. This approach, however, is strictly experimental at present.[37]

NIDDM

NIDDM is difficult to define. The rates among and within countries vary dramatically, partially depending on the specific classification criteria used for NIDDM.

Estimates of the prevalence of NIDDM between populations vary from a low of less than 2/10,000 to a high of 4000/10,000 in the Pima Indians.[38] NIDDM occurs in all races, but the prevalence tends to be high among American Indians, Micronesians, Polynesians, U.S. black women, and Mexican

Americans.[39] The prevalence of diabetes (known and unknown) in the United States is intermediary, about 6% for whites and about 10% for blacks (Table 51–2).[40]

Certain key factors that account for these marked geographic and ethnic differences in diabetes have been suggested. One of the critical risk factors appears to be change in socioeconomic status.[39] In communities where there has been rapid economic development, such as in Korea[41] and among the Pima Indians,[38] there appears to be a marked and rapid increase in the incidence and prevalence of NIDDM.[38,39,41] Two factors have been suggested to account for this rapid rise in NIDDM. When the food sources in a population become more plentiful, a rapid rise in body weights of individuals may occur, with a corresponding increase in the rates of NIDDM. A pattern of increasing mean weight of the population and increasing prevalence of NIDDM has been noted.[42] Similarly within a population there is a strong correlation between degree of obesity and risk of NIDDM.[38,43,44] Interestingly, within a country such as the United States, one generally finds an inverse relationship between obesity and socioeconomic class,[45] as well as higher rates of NIDDM in lower socioeconomic groups.[46] Many studies have determined that obesity is independently associated with the risk of NIDDM. Approximately 80% of non-insulin-dependent diabetics are obese. Controversy is related to the specific type of calories, since there is relatively little evidence that increased sugar, per se, in the diet is a risk factor for diabetes. There are also questions about the effects of high fiber and its role in the diet and the risk of developing diabetes. Recent studies suggest there is relatively little difference in the blood sugar response to simple sugar as compared to starch among both normal individuals and those with diabetes.[47] The hypothesis that a high-fiber diet protects against diabetes remains unsubstantiated.[48] Although the value of increasing fiber in the diet to reduce the blood glucose response to food among diabetics is now fairly well established,[49] its role in preventing the development of diabetes is less clear. At present only low caloric intake and weight reduction are suggested for prevention of NIDDM.

A number of recent studies have clearly demonstrated that the distribution of body fat, independent of obesity, is a further predictor of subsequent diabetes. An increased central deposition of fat (i.e., "android" as opposed to "gynoid"), often measured as an increased waist/hip girth ratio, appears to predict not only diabetes but also cardiovascular disease (see below). Central adiposity may be associated with a different body fat composition and metabolism.[50,51]

The second primary risk factor for NIDDM associated with the increase in socioeconomic status is physical activity. As socioeconomic status increases, the overall level of physical activity generally declines, especially that related to work. Thus, at the same time that caloric intake is increasing, physical activity is decreasing, and there is an increased prevalence of obesity within the population. Recent data from the South Pacific suggest that physical activity itself may be an independent risk factor for NIDDM, separate from obesity.[52] The recognition of other risk factors is important since not all obese individuals develop NIDDM. In some populations there is little increase in the prevalence of diabetes despite a substantial increase in the degree of obesity.[39]

Genetic factors play an extremely important role in the development of NIDDM. Among a large study of twins Pyke found that the concordance rates for NIDDM among monozygotic twins was over 90% compared to 50% for IDDM.[53] Twin studies, however, do not provide the complete story. Over the past 10 years there have been numerous studies of the relationship of genetic markers to the development of NIDDM as well as of IDDM. It is now clear that the HLA system is related only to the risk of developing IDDM and not NIDDM. Several recent reports have attempted to evaluate the relationships between NIDDM and candidate genes, including the insulin gene,[54] the insulin receptor gene,[55] and the glucose transporter gene.[56] These genes, located on chromosomes 11, 19, and 1, respectively, have been cloned and are thought likely to contribute to the pathogenesis of the disease. However, population studies have been conflicting for each of these candidate genes, with some showing positive associations between particular RFLP patterns and NIDDM, and others indicating that the markers are unrelated to the development of the disease. It has been suggested that more than one gene may be necessary to determine susceptibility to NIDDM or that perhaps there is genetic heterogeneity within NIDDM. Thus family and pedigree studies are needed to determine the contribution of these genetic markers to the development of NIDDM.

The prevention of NIDDM may be possible in the future. Further analyses of the insulin gene structure and its relationship to both insulin secretion and insulin structure may provide a technique for identifying high risk individuals, at least within specific families. A consensus is growing that development of NIDDM is a two-stage process, with the first stage being resistance to insulin's action (probably exacerbated by obesity) and the second stage being failure of the pancreas to increase insulin secretion enough to compensate. This theory received support from a recent report on the Pima Indians, which showed differing predictive values of fasting and postchallenge insulin values for developing NIDDM consistent with a hyperinsulinemic phase followed by eventual insulinopenia.[57]

Weight loss is strongly recommended to improve glucose tolerance among NIDDM patients[58] and will substantially improve glucose tolerance among nondiabetic individuals.[59] As obesity is a major risk factor for NIDDM, weight loss should logically be a major goal of a prevention program. However, a study to determine the efficacy of such a program to prevent diabetes has not been completed. Similarly, there is lack of trial evidence that treating asymptomatic diabetes discovered through screening procedures improves prognosis. Thus the screening of a population either by fasting blood sugar or by the response to a glucose challenge is problematic. Furthermore, a fasting glucose has a low sensitivity for "unknown diabetes," while a postchallenge glucose is cumbersome in a screening setting.

One potential benefit of screening may be the identification of persons with impaired glucose tolerance. These individuals have an increased risk of subsequent diabetes and appear to be at increased risk for cardiovascular disease compared to individuals with normal glucose tolerance, according to the large Whitehall[2] and Paris[60] studies. However, despite an increasing body of evidence linking this subgroup with hyperinsulinemia, another CVD risk factor (see below), there is no evidence to date that intervention to correct impaired glucose tolerance is beneficial. Therefore, a major need in preventive medicine is to evaluate various preventive strategies such as weight loss in individuals at high risk for, or in the early stages of, diabetes.

MORBIDITY AND COMPLICATIONS OF DIABETES

Prior to the introduction of insulin in 1922 by Banting and Best, life expectancy of patients with IDDM was but 1 to 2 years. After the development and widespread use of insulin, there was a dramatic increase in life expectancy for patients with IDDM. Suddenly insulin-dependent diabetics could lead relatively normal lives. However, 20 to 30 years later the long-term sequelae of IDDM began to become evident.

Both IDDM and NIDDM patients are at risk for these long-term complications. These come mainly from disorders of the circulation, either macrovascular, including accelerated atherosclerosis resulting in stroke, heart disease, and peripheral vascular disease, or microvascular disorders of the kidney and retina, as well as neuropathy. The complications appear to be similar for both IDDM and NIDDM, although the prevalence may be somewhat higher in IDDM, especially of renal disease. The relationships with age and duration also vary between the two types of diabetes, partly because of the younger age of onset of IDDM (which leads to complications at a younger age) and the difficulty of determining the onset of NIDDM (which means complications are often present at the onset of known disease). The following discussion will mainly focus on IDDM, since these data are more complete.

Recently a long-term follow-up of over 2000 insulin-dependent diabetics was completed in Pittsburgh (Fig. 51-2).[5] Males with IDDM have about a fivefold greater than normal mortality risk, whereas females have about an elevenfold greater risk. In the first 10 years the primary cause of death is related to the acute complications of diabetes such as ketoacidosis. During the second decade of diabetes, renal disease becomes a major cause of death. After 20 years of diabetes the primary causes of death include both renal and cardiovascular diseases (CVDs). The mortality rate is still extraordinarily high compared to that of the general population. After 20 years of diabetes there is a twentyfold greater risk of death compared to that of the general population, with 2% of diabetic individuals dying per year.[5]

In an international study, Diabetes Epidemiology Research International (DERI), mortality in young cohorts of IDDM cases from four different countries (the United States, Israel, Japan, and Finland) is being investigated. The study shows tremendous variation in diabetes-related mortality. In addition to the high mortality from acute complications, the Japanese cohort also has a high mortality from renal disease (276/100,000/y) compared to Finland (16/100,000/y) ($P < .05$).[61] The importance of renal disease is highlighted by this recent data from the Steno Memorial Hospital in Copenhagen, which suggests that renal disease (as identified by proteinuria) is the chief risk factor for coronary disease in IDDM. Indeed, patients without proteinuria appeared to have little excess CVD risk.[62]

Mortality rates in diabetes, especially IDDM, appear to be falling.[5,62] Data from Pittsburgh suggest that cohorts who were diagnosed in the 1960s have a longer life expectancy than those diagnosed in the 1950s. Much of the decline in mortality has been the result of a reduction in deaths at onset, but there also has been an improvement in long-term life expectancy among insulin-dependent diabetics.[5,62]

Diabetic Retinopathy

After 20 years of IDDM, approximately 80% to 90% of patients show some evidence of damage to the retina called background retinopathy. Similar prevalence rates are seen in NIDDM for patients treated with insulin, although rates are lower (around 55%) for those not on insulin.[63] In addition, as many as 70% of IDDM and 30% of NIDDM on insulin may develop proliferative changes in the eyes that may lead to blindness.[63]

Diabetes is the leading cause of blindness in the 20 to 74 age group in the United States. Each year approximately 6000 diabetics become legally blind (corrected visual acuity less than 20/200 in the better eye). The prevalence of blindness due to diabetes is estimated at 40,000 individuals. Diabetes is associated with a sixfold greater risk of blindness compared to the general population.[64]

The Diabetic Retinopathy Study has demonstrated that individuals with severe diabetic retinopathy can be treated successfully and their vision preserved with laser photocoagulation therapy.[65] Currently underway is a further clinical trial related to eye disease, the Early Treatment of Diabetic Retinopathy Study (ETDRS), which is examining whether early treatment of diabetic retinopathy by photocoagulation with or without aspirin is effective in preserving vision.

As diabetic retinopathy can be detected before it threatens vision, blindness due to diabetic retinopathy can be prevented in many cases. It is thus important that patients and physicians be educated about the need for frequent eye examinations and that adequate clinical treatment for diabetic retinopathy be available in the community.

Diabetic Renal Disease

Diabetic renal disease is a major cause of morbidity and mortality among diabetics.[61,62,64,66,67] Diabetes is currently the leading cause of treatment for end stage renal disease,[64] accounting for 25% of the 4000 new end stage renal disease patients each year. About 8000 such diabetic patients are currently receiving treatment. Diabetes increases the risk of renal failure seventeen to

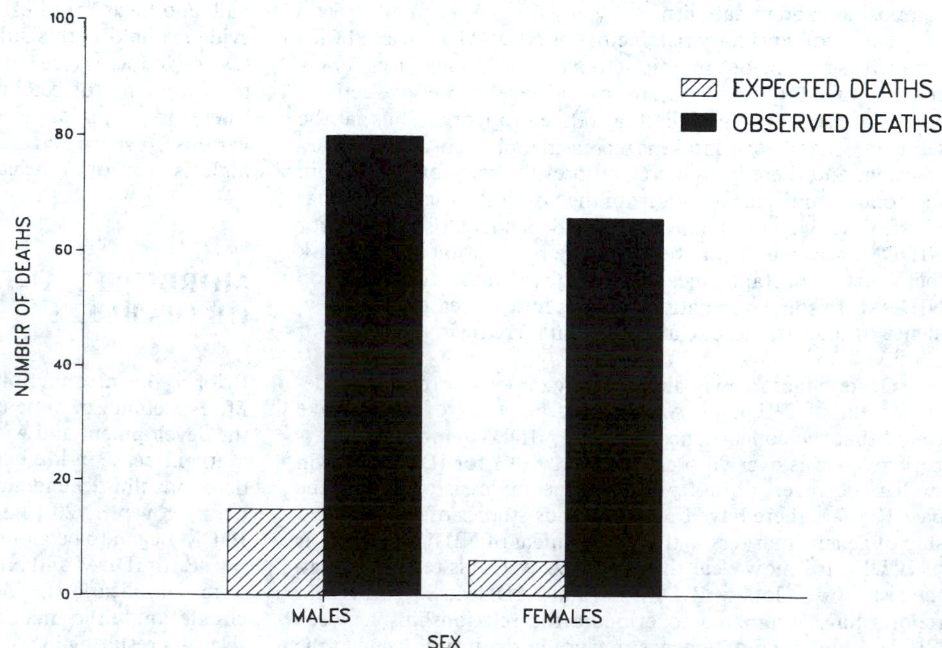

Figure 51-2. Mortality among IDDM patients compared with the U.S. population.

twenty-fold. Around 40% of patients with IDDM[62,67] eventually develop significant clinical proteinuria and renal disease.

Prevalence rates are somewhat lower in NIDDM overall, partly because the later age of onset means many patients may have died from heart disease before there has been sufficient duration to develop renal disease. The relative risk of mortality from renal disease for diabetics compared to the general population is highest for those in the 15- to 44-year age group, consistent with a higher prevalence and severity in IDDM.[66] Despite recent advances in the diagnosis and treatment of renal failure among diabetics, the problem has not been resolved. The presence of microalbuminuria (urinary albumin excretion above 30 mg/24 hours or an albumin excretion rate of 20 to 200 μg/min) appears to predict the subsequent development of diabetic nephropathy and end stage renal failure.[68] Hypertension, which may be primary or secondary to the renal disease, also accelerates the development of renal failure. Several recent reports, largely based on IDDM patients, have suggested that drug treatment of hypertension (or even mildly elevated blood pressure) or protein restriction, as well as intensified glucose control, may reduce albumin excretion in the early stages.[68] However, as the long-term value of these interventions has not been well established, screening for microalbuminuria is not, as yet, widely practiced in the United States. Thus, it is hoped that the devastating effects of diabetic renal disease may be partially preventable in the future. Meanwhile, renal transplantation and dialysis remain important needs for the diabetic community.

Neuropathy

Another major complication of diabetes is neuropathy. Clinically significant neurological disability usually does not occur until at least 5 years after the diagnosis of diabetes. The major consequences of diabetic neuropathy are pain, weakness, and loss of sensation. Parallel disorders of the autonomic nervous system may lead to problems of sexual function and urinary and gastrointestinal abnormalities. Research has focused on the metabolic causes of the nerve damage and the specific biochemical lesions that lead to neurological changes.[69] One recent epidemiological study has demonstrated both a high prevalence of distal symmetrical neuropathy in IDDM, 70% after 30 years, and a strong relationship with cardiovascular risk factors, for example, hypertension, lipid disturbances, and cigarette smoking.[70] A major problem in diabetic neuropathy is how to measure it. Multiple techniques are currently advocated.[71,72]

It has long been recognized that strict control of blood sugar may improve neural function, for example, peripheral nerve conduction.[73] The above findings concerning blood pressure and lipids suggest that studies to evaluate the benefits of controlling these factors may also be worthwhile. Another area that has been investigated recently is the role of a new group of drugs called aldose reductase inhibitors. Although the results have been variable,[74,75] most trials to date have involved late-stage neuropathy. A greater benefit might be seen if these metabolically active drugs were used earlier.

Macrovascular Disease and Atherosclerosis

Atherosclerosis, a multifactorial process, is still not clearly understood. Many of the putative risk factors, or elements in the process, are altered to varying degrees in the diverse manifestations of glucose intolerance discussed earlier. The most convincing epidemiological evidence for increased cardiovascular disease in diabetes comes from large-scale prospective studies, many of which were primarily designed to study cardiovascular disease in the general population. The reader is referred to a recent review for details.[76] Briefly, studies like Framingham[77] have demonstrated that the diabetic individual (uniquely defined in Framingham as "glucose intolerant") has a greatly enhanced risk[78,79] and that cardiovascular disease is the leading cause of death in diabetics. Diabetics have a greater than normal risk for all manifestations of atherosclerosis, including coronary, cerebrovascular, and peripheral vascular disease.[77] The latter is so common in diabetes that half of all lower extremity amputations in the United States occur in persons with diabetes.[9] In the general population women have a lower risk of coronary heart disease (CHD) than men, but this advantage is lost in women with diabetes, who have rates approaching those of men.[76,78,80] However, recently analyzed data from a mortality follow-up of individuals from a nationwide study[81] suggests that males with diabetes do have a greater risk of death from CVD than female diabetics have, although this finding is based on a reported history of diabetes that may be biased.[82] The survival of diabetic patients, especially women, after a cardiac event also appears to be less than that of the general population.[76,83]

Although when it occurs, atherosclerosis is often more extensive in diabetics[84,85] than in nondiabetics, not all studies are in agreement.[76,86] Divergent opinions also are apparent in terms of the role of blood sugar in the nondiabetic range. Some studies have shown the group with "impaired glucose tolerance" (IGT) to have a greater than normal risk of CVD.[2,60] Other studies have failed to show a relationship between blood glucose levels in the nondiabetic range and CVD.[87] Of further interest is that the IGT stage is often characterized by hyperinsulinemia and insulin resistance. In the Paris study, in multivariate analyses, insulin concentration rather than diabetic IGT status was the stronger predictor of CHD.[88] A further factor linked with hyperinsulinemia is central adiposity, which was discussed earlier as a risk factor for the development of diabetes.[50,51] Central adiposity is also a risk factor for CVD independent of obesity,[89] a finding most clearly shown in women. Consequently a male type of fat deposition (especially in women) may be associated with hyperinsulinemia[90] and thus may provide a marker for a metabolic derangement predisposing to both diabetes and CVD generally and the relatively poorer cardiovascular prognosis in diabetic women.

Unlike the diabetes complications, duration of diabetes is not strongly related to CVD in NIDDM in most studies,[79,91,92] although in Pima Indians and in IDDM a relationship with duration is seen.[93] This lack of a duration effect has led to the suggestion that diabetes per se is not a risk factor for heart disease but rather that a deranged metabolic state, which predisposes to heart disease, also leads to diabetes in some cases.[94] This hypothesis, proposed by Jarrett, is also consistent with the findings of disturbed lipoprotein concentrations in offspring of NIDDM patients with mild glucose intolerance[95] and the predictive power of CVD risk factors, notably lipoproteins, for the development of diabetes.[96] Whether insulin resistance might explain this joint predisposition to diabetes and CVD remains controversial.[97,98]

As lipoproteins are altered in diabetes, it is tempting to hypothesize that these changes account for the increased CVD risk seen in diabetes. Many studies[77,78,80] have shown that serum cholesterol levels relate to CVD risk in diabetics in a way similar to that seen in the general population. However, total and LDL-cholesterol levels are not greatly elevated in many diabetics, so the role of cholesterol in explaining the *increased* risk in diabetes is limited. Recent data from the Multiple Risk Factor Intervention Study (MRFIT), which screened over 360,000 men for CVD risk factors and subsequently followed them for mortality, suggests diabetic men had rates three times higher than nondiabetics all along the cholesterol curve.[99] The MRFIT data is exclusively NIDDM. In IDDM, as indicated earlier, it appears that the major determinant of CVD risk is proteinuria,[62] which is itself associated with lipid disturbances even in the earlier microalbuminuria stage.[100]

If cholesterol concentration has a limited role to play, other lipid measures may be of greater importance to diabetes. Two recent reports suggest that triglyceride level is an independent risk factor for CVD in diabetes.[93,101] Furthermore, alterations in

HDL concentration and lipoprotein composition occur in diabetes, which may further increase cardiovascular risk.[102] Insulin itself, beyond its effect on the lipids, can have direct effects on the arterial wall that promote atherogenicity.[103-105] Hyperinsulinemia has also been related to blood pressure elevation.[106-109] The importance of insulin is also shown by its demonstration as an independent risk factor for CVD in three prospective studies of men in the general population.[110-112]

Many studies have demonstrated altered platelet behavior in diabetes.[113] Finally, as both fibrinogen and blood pressure are increased in renal disease in diabetes,[114] these factors may provide yet another mechanism for the enhanced CVD risk in this subgroup of diabetics.[100] Thus it is abundantly clear that the diabetic has severe handicaps to face in terms of cardiovascular risk above and beyond the lipoprotein disturbances.

Diabetes and Pregnancy

Although the data concerning the prevalence of diabetic pregnancy are limited, it has been estimated that 10,000 babies are born each year to women with overt diabetes.[115] Another 90,000 babies are born to women who develop gestational diabetes, a disorder discussed earlier.[116] The sequelae of diabetes mellitus in the pregnant woman include both increased maternal and fetal morbidity and fetal wastage.[117] However, there has been substantial improvement in the treatment of the pregnant diabetic patient, with maternal morbidity and perinatal survival approaching normal. Nevertheless, an excess of birth defects still exists. Studies have generally shown that the rate of major malformations is three times higher in the diabetic compared to the nondiabetic, and fatal malformations are six times more common.[118] In the Collaborative Perinatal Project (CPP), 18% of the infants of white diabetic mothers had major malformations compared with 8% of the infants of white nondiabetics.[118] The major malformations most commonly associated with diabetes usually occur around 7 to 8 weeks of gestation.[119]

Currently the major question is whether improved metabolic control of diabetes, especially early control, will reduce or prevent the development of congenital malformations in the fetus. It is important to recognize that these malformations occur so early in fetal development that most of the women will not have sought obstetrical care at the time of highest risk.[119] Thus, if the current studies demonstrate that good metabolic control reduces the frequency of malformations (circumstantial evidence suggests this may be true[120,121]), it will be necessary to develop preventive programs that identify the IDDM women prior to pregnancy and ensure metabolic control early in the pregnancy.

In recent years the relationship between metabolic control during pregnancy and adverse pregnancy outcome has become even more muddled. Data from Cincinnati indicate that women who subsequently go on to have malformed infants have higher HbA_{1c} levels during the first trimester than do those who do not subsequently have malformed infants.[120] In contrast, the recently published data from the Diabetes and Early Pregnancy Study[121,122] reveal no increased risk for spontaneous abortion among women who have IDDM compared to nondiabetic women.[121] Women who have diabetes are at markedly increased risk for severe malformations.[122] However, there is no evidence that glycemic control early in the pregnancy is related to the increased incidence of malformations. Thus the contribution of metabolic control early in pregnancy to the incidence of severe malformations is still unclear.

Patients with gestational diabetes who enter pregnancy without clinically detectable vascular disease and who acquire no new complications during pregnancy, such as pyelonephritis and pregnancy-induced hypertension, achieve pregnancy outcomes no different from those of the nondiabetic patient.[118]

GLYCEMIC CONTROL AND PREVENTION OF COMPLICATIONS

One of the major controversies in diabetes is the role of glycemic control in determining the development of complications. This controversy has gone on for many years and remains unresolved, partly because of the inability in the past to satisfactorily measure and achieve good glycemic control.

Previous clinical trials comparing insulin and oral hypoglycemic agents to placebo among NIDDM patients in the University Group Diabetes Program (UGDP) did not demonstrate that either therapy was beneficial in reducing the morbidity and mortality from cardiovascular complications compared to placebo.[123,124] The degree of control of the blood sugar was modest at best, and the study cannot be considered a true test of the rigorous control of blood sugar among NIDDM patients. Other approaches to the prevention of macrovascular complications, such as modification of lipid and blood pressure profiles, may be more fruitful. Such trials are badly needed, for nearly all large trials have systematically excluded persons with diabetes.

The situation with regard to IDDM is more equivocal. Many diabetologists now believe that rigorous control of blood sugar and other metabolic abnormalities will reduce the risk of major microvascular, and perhaps macrovascular, complications of diabetes. New methods to deliver insulin by continuous infusion insulin pumps, improved home monitoring of blood glucose levels, and the use of glycosylated hemoglobin as a measurement of long-term hyperglycemia have substantially improved the potential to maintain tight control of blood sugar levels without serious side effects. Although reports suggest that rigorous control may reduce the early basement membrane changes seen in diabetics,[125] reports from the multicenter Kroc Collaborative Study Group[126] and Steno Group[127] show tight control of blood sugar with continuous infusion insulin does not slow the progression of retinopathy over the short term and may even accelerate it, although somewhat more encouraging results were obtained after longer follow-up.[128,129]

The Diabetes Control and Complications Trial (DCCT) is a long-term clinical trial to determine the relationship between strict glycemic control and the clinical course of microvascular complications such as diabetic retinopathy in IDDM.[130] It is hoped that this trial, which will not be completed before 1993, will provide a final answer to this important issue.

REFERENCES

1. National Diabetes Data Group: Classification and diagnosis of diabetes mellitus and other categories of glucose intolerance. Diabetes 28:57, 1979
2. Fuller JH, Shipley MJ, Rose G, Jarrett RJ, Keen H: Coronary heart disease risk and impaired glucose tolerance: the Whitehall Study. Lancet 1373–1376, 1980
3. O'Sullivan JO: Quarter century study of glucose intolerance: incidence of diabetes mellitus by USPHS, NIH and WHO criteria. In Eschevege E (ed): Advances in Diabetes Epidemiology. Amsterdam: Elsevier Biomedical Press B.O. (Inserm Symposium No. 22), 1982, pp 123–131
4. Jarrett RJ, Keen H, McCartney P: Worsening of diabetes with impaired glucose tolerance: ten-year experience in the Bedford and Whitehall Studies. In Eschevege E (ed): Advances in Diabetes Epidemiology. Amsterdam: Elsevier Biomedical Press B.O. (Inserm Symposium No. 22), 1982, pp 95–102
5. Dorman JS, LaPorte RE, Kuller LH, et al: The Pittsburgh insulin-dependent diabetes mellitus (IDDM) morbidity and mortality study: mortality results. Diabetes 33:271–276, 1984
6. Holman RC, Herron CA, Sinnock P: Epidemiologic characteristics

of mortality from disease with acidosis or coma, United States, 1970–1978. Am J Public Health 73:1169–1173, 1983

7. Diabetes Epidemiology Research International Mortality Study Group: Major cross-country differences in risk of dieing for people with IDDM. Diabetes Care 14:49–54, 1991
8. Temple RC, Carrington CA, Luzio SD, et al: Insulin deficiency in non-insulin-dependent diabetes. Lancet 1:293–295, 1989
9. Harris MI: The public health impact of diabetes. In Eschevege E (ed): Advances in Diabetes Epidemiology. Amsterdam: Elsevier Biomedical Press B.O. (Inserm Symposium No. 22), 1982, pp 17–20
10. Sasaki A: Assessment of the new criteria for diabetes mellitus according to 10-year relative survival rates: Center for Adult Diseases, Osaka, Japan. Diabetologia 20:195–198, 1981
11. Ito C, Mito K, Hara H: Review of criteria for diagnosis of diabetes mellitus based on results of follow-up study. Diabetes 32:343–351, 1983
12. Pettitt DJ, Knowler WC, Lisse JR, Bennett PH: Development of retinopathy and proteinuria in relation to plasma-glucose concentrations in Pima Indians. Lancet 1050–1052, 1980
13. Duncan BB, Heiss G: Nonenzymatic glycosylation of proteins—a new tool for assessment of cumulative hyperglycemia in epidemiologic studies, past and future. Am J Epidemiol 120:169–189, 1984
14. Rotter JI, Rimoin DL: The genetics of the glucose intolerance disorders. Am J Med 70:116–126, 1981
15. Bertrams J, Baur M: Insulin-dependent diabetes mellitus in: "Histocompatibility Testing 1984." Heidelberg: Springer-Verlag, 1984, p 348
16. Sverjgaard A, Platz P, Ryder L: HLA and disease-1982: a survey. Immunol Rev 70:193, 1983
17. Tattersall R, Pyke D, Nerup J: Genetic patterns in diabetes mellitus. Hum Pathol 11:273–283, 1980
18. Wagener D, Kuller L, Orchard T, et al: Pittsburgh Diabetes Mellitus Study. II. Secondary attack rates in families with insulin-dependent diabetes mellitus. Am J Epidemiol 5:868–878, 1982
19. Gottlieb MS: Diabetes in offspring and siblings of juvenile and maturity onset-type diabetics. J Chron Dis 33:331–339, 1979
20. Editorial: Insulin-dependent? Lancet 2:809–810, 1985
21. Diabetes Epidemiology Research International Group: Geographic patterns of childhood insulin-dependent diabetes mellitus. Diabetes 37:1113–1119, 1988
22. Rewers M, LaPorte RE, King HOM, Tuomilehto J: Trends in the prevalence and incidence of diabetes: insulin-dependent diabetes mellitus in childhood. World Health Stat 41:179–190, 1988
23. LaPorte RE, Cruickshanks KJ: Incidence and risk factors for insulin-dependent diabetes. In National Diabetes Data Group: Diabetes in America, Data Compiled 1984. Washington, D.C.: United States Department of Health and Human Services 1985: III-1-12 (NIH Publication No. 85-1468)
24. LaPorte RE, Tajima N: Prevalence of insulin-dependent diabetes. In National Diabetes Data Group: Diabetes in America, Data Compiled 1984. Washington, D.C.: United States Department of Health and Human Services 1985:V-1-8 (NIH Publication No. 85-1468)
25. Tajima N, LaPorte RE, Hibi I, Kitagawa T, Fujita H, Drash AL: A comparison of the epidemiology of youth onset insulin-dependent diabetes mellitus between Japan and the United States (Allegheny County, Pennsylvania). Diabetes Care 8(suppl 1):17–23, 1985
26. Diabetes Epidemiology Research International (DERI) Group: Secular trends in incidence of childhood insulin-dependent diabetes mellitus (IDDM) in ten countries. Diabetes 39:858–864, 1990
27. Fishbein HA, LaPorte RE, Orchard TJ, Drash AL, Kuller LH, Rabin B, Wagner DK: The Pittsburgh Insulin-Dependent Diabetes Mellitus Registry: seasonal incidence. Diabetologia 23:83–85, 1982
28. Diabetes Epidemiology Research International: Preventing insulin-dependent mellitus: the environmental challenge. Br Med J 295:479–481, 1987
29. Schreuder G, Tilanus M, Bontrop R, Bruining J, Giphart M, Van Rood J, DeVries R: HLA-DQ polymorphism associated with resistance to type I diabetes detected with monoclonal antibodies, isoelectric point differences, and restriction fragment length polymorphism. J Exp Med 164:938, 1986
30. Todd JA, Bell JI, McDevitt HO: HLA-DQ-beta gene contributes to susceptibility and resistance to insulin-dependent diabetes mellitus. Nature 329:559, 1987
31. Morel PA, Dorman JS, Todd JA, McDevitt HO, Trucco M: Aspartic acid at position 57 of the HLA-DQ-beta chain protects against type I diabetes: a family study. Proc Natl Acad Sci USA, 85:1–6, 1988
32. Cavender DE, Wagener DK, Rabin BS, et al: The Pittsburgh Insulin-Dependent Diabetes Mellitus (IDDM) Study: HLA antigens and haplotypes as risk factors for the development of IDDM in IDDM patients and their siblings. J Chron Dis 37:555–568, 1984
33. Trucco G, Fritsch R, Giorda R, Trucco M: Rapid detection of IDDM susceptibility using HLA-DQ beta alleles as markers. Diabetes 38:1617–1622, 1989
34. Srikanta S, Ganda OP, Eisenbarth GS, et al: Islet cell antibodies and beta-cell function in monozygotic triplets and twins initially discordant for type I diabetes mellitus. N Engl J Med 308(6):322–325, 1983
35. Spencer KM, Town A, Dean BM, Lister J, Bottazzo GF: Fluctuating islet-cell autoimmunity in unaffected relatives of patients with insulin-dependent diabetes. Lancet 1:764–766, 1984
36. Dorman JS, LaPorte RE, Stone RA, Trucco M: Worldwide differences in the incidence of type I diabetes are associated with amino acid variation at position 57 of the HLA DQ beta chain. Proc Natl Acad Sci 87:7370–7374, 1990
37. Lipton RB, LaPorte RE, Becker DJ, Dorman JS, Orchard TJ, Atchison J, Drash AL: Cyclosporine therapy for the prevention and cure of insulin-dependent diabetes: an epidemiologic perspective of benefits and risks. Diabetes Care 13(7):776–784, 1990
38. Bennett PH, Rushforth NB, Miller M, et al: Epidemiologic studies in diabetes in Pima Indians. Recent Prog Horm Res 32:333–376, 1976
39. Zimmet P: Epidemiology of diabetes and its macrovascular manifestations in Pacific populations: the medical effects of social progress. Diabetes Care 2:85–90, 1979
40. Harris MI, Hadden WC, Knowler WC, Bennett PH: Prevalence of diabetes and impaired glucose tolerance and plasma glucose levels in the U.S. population aged 20–74 yr. Diabetes 36:523–534, 1987
41. Min HK, Yoo HJ, Lee HK, Kim EJ: Changing patterns of the prevalence of diabetes mellitus in Korea. In Minuira A, Baba S, Goyo Y, Kobberling J (eds): Clinico-genetic Genesis of Diabetes Mellitus. Amsterdam: Excerpta Medica, 1982
42. Medalie JH: Risk factors other than hyperglycemia in diabetic macrovascular disease. Diabetes Care 2:77–84, 1979
43. Van Itallie TB: Obesity: adverse effects on health and longevity. Am J Clin Nutr 32:2723–2733, 1979
44. Keen H: The incomplete story of obesity and diabetes. In Howard A (ed): Recent Advances in Obesity Research: 1. Proceedings of the 1st International Congress on Obesity. London: Newman Publishing, 1975
45. Rimm IJ, Rimm AA: Association between socioeconomic status and obesity in 59,556 women. Prev Med 3:543–572, 1974
46. U.S. Department of Health, Education and Welfare: Diabetes Data: Compiled 1977. Washington, D.C.: DHEW Publication No. (NI 78-1468), 1978
47. Slama G, Haardt MJ, Jean-Joseph P, Costagliola D, et al: Sucrose taken during mixed meal has no additional hyperglycemic action over isocaloric amounts of starch in well-controlled diabetics. Lancet 2:122–124, 1984
48. Trowell HC: Diabetes mellitus and dietary fiber of starchy foods. Am J Clin Nutr 31:S53–57, 1978
49. American Diabetes Association: Nutritional recommendations and principles for individuals with diabetes mellitus: 1986. Diabetes Care 10:126–132, 1987
50. Ohlson LO, Larsson B, Svardsudd K, et al: The influence of body fat distribution on the incidence of diabetes mellitus: 13.5 years of

follow-up of the participants in the study of men born in 1913. Diabetes 34:1055–1058, 1985

51. Haffner SM, Stern MP, Hazuda HP, et al: Role of obesity and fat distribution in non-insulin-dependent diabetes mellitus in Mexican Americans and non-Hispanic whites. Diabetes Care 9:153–161, 1986
52. Taylor RJ, Bennett PH, LeGonidec G, et al: The prevalence of diabetes mellitus in a traditional-living Polynesian population: the Wallis Island Survey. Diabetes Care 6:334–340, 1983
53. Barnett AH, Eff C, Leslie RDG, Pyke DA: Diabetes in identical twins: a study of 200 pairs. Diabetologia 20:87–93, 1981
54. Bell GI, Karem JH, Rutter WJ: Polymorphic c DNA region adjacent to the 5′ end of the human insulin gene. Proc Natl Acad Sci 78:5759–5763, 1981
55. Elisin SC, Corsetti L, Ullrich A, Permutt MA: Multiple restriction fragment length polymorphisms at the insulin receptor locus: a highly informative marker for linkage analysis. Proc Natl Acad Sci 83:5223–5227, 1986
56. Li SR, Baroni MG, Gelbaum RS, Stock J, Galton DJ: Association of genetic variant of the glucose transporter with non-insulin-dependent diabetes mellitus. Lancet 2:368–370, 1988
57. Saad MF, Knowler WC, Pettitt DJ, Nelson RG, Mott DM: The natural history of impaired glucose tolerance in the Pima Indians. N Engl J Med 319:1500–1506, 1988
58. American Diabetes Association: The physician's guide to type II diabetes (NIDDM). New York: KPR International Media Corp., 1984.
59. Olefsky J, Reaven GM, Farquhar JW: Effects of weight reduction on obesity: studies of lipid and carbohydrate metabolism in normal and hyperlipoproteinemic subjects. J Clin Invest 53:64–76, 1974
60. Eschwege E, Ducimetiere P, Papoz L, Claude JR, Richard JL: Blood glucose and coronary heart disease. Lancet 2:472–473, 1980
61. DERI Study Group: Cause specific mortality in IDDM: a preliminary report from the Diabetes Epidemiology Research International (DERI) Study (abstr). Diabetes 38(suppl 2):145A, 1989
62. Borch-Johnsen K, Kreiner S: Proteinuria: value as predictor of cardiovascular mortality in insulin dependent diabetes mellitus. Br Med J 294:1651–1654, 1987
63. Klein R, Davis MD, Moss SE, Klein BEK, DeMets DL: The Wisconsin Epidemiologic Study of Diabetic Retinopathy: a comparison of retinopathy in younger and older onset diabetic persons. In Vranic M, Hollenberg CH, Steiner G (eds): Comparisons of type I and type II diabetes. Adv Med Biol 189:321–335, 1985
64. National Diabetes Advisory Board: Progress and promise in diabetes research. Report of the Second National Diabetes Research Conference, September 25–28, 1983. Washington, D.C.: U.S. Department of Health and Human Services, NIH Publication No. 5:84–661, March, 1984
65. Diabetic Retinopathy Study Group: Photocoagulation treatment of proliferative diabetic retinopathy. Clinical Application of Diabetic Retinopathy Study (DRS) Findings, DRS Report No. 8. Ophthalmology 88:583, 1981
66. Geiss LS, Herman WH, Teutsch SM: Diabetes and renal mortality in the United States. Am J Public Health 75(11):1325–1327, 1985
67. Knowles HC: Magnitude of the renal failure problem in diabetic patients. Kidney Int 6:52–57, 1974
68. Viberti G: Etiology and prognostic significance of albuminuria in diabetes. Diabetes Care 11:840–845, 1988
69. Winegrad AI, Morrison AD, Greene DA: Late complication of diabetes. In DeGrott LJ, Cahill GF, Martini L (eds): Endocrinology. Vol. 2. New York: Grune & Stratton, 1979
70. Maser RE, Steenkiste AE, Dorman JS, et al: The epidemiologic correlates of diabetic neuropathy: a report from the Pittsburgh Epidemiology of Diabetes Complications Study. Diabetes 38(11): 1456–1461, 1989
71. American Diabetes Association, American Academy of Neurology: Report and recommendations of the San Antonio conference on diabetic neuropathy. Diabetes Care 11:592–597, 1988
72. Maser RE, Nielsen VK, Bass EB, Manjoo Q, Dorman JS, Kelsey SF, Becker DJ, Orchard TJ: Measuring diabetic neuropathy: assessment and comparison of clinical examination and quantitative sensory testing. Diabetes Care 12:270–275, 1989
73. Ward JD, Fisher DJ, Barnes CG, Jessop JD: Improvement in nerve conduction following treatment of newly diagnosed diabetics. Lancet 1:428, 1971
74. Young RJ, Ewing DJ, Clarke BF: A controlled trial of Sorbinil, an aldose reductase inhibitor, in chronic painful diabetic neuropathy. Diabetes 32:938, 1983
75. The Sorbinil Neuropathy Study Group: Clinical response to Sorbinil treatment in diabetic neuropathy. Diabetes 38(suppl 2): 14A, 1989
76. Barrett-Conner E, Orchard TJ: Diabetes and heart disease. In Diabetes in America. Diabetes data compiled 1984: National Diabetes Data Group NIH Publication No. 85–1468, 1985
77. Kannel WB, McGee DL: Diabetes and glucose tolerance as risk factors for cardiovascular disease: The Framingham Study. Diabetes Care 2:120–126, 1979
78. Barrett-Conner E, Wingard DL: Sex differential in ischemic heart disease mortality in diabetics: a prospective population-based study. Am J Epidemiol 118:489–496, 1983
79. Panzram G: Mortality and survival in type 2 (non-insulin-dependent) diabetes mellitus. Diabetologia 30:123–131, 1987
80. Jarrett RJ, McCartney P, Keen H: The Bedford Survey: ten year mortality rates in newly diagnosed diabetics, borderline diabetics and normoglycaemic controls and risk indices for coronary heart disease in borderline diabetics. Diabetologia 22:79–84, 1982
81. Kleinman JC, Donahue RP, Harris MI, et al: Mortality among diabetics in a national sample. Am J Epidemiol 128:389–401, 1988
82. West KM: Epidemiology of diabetes in its vascular lesions. New York: Elsevier, 1978, pp 231–248
83. Abbott RD, Donahue RP, Kannel WB, et al: The impact of diabetes on survival following myocardial infarction in men vs women: The Framingham Study. JAMA 260:3456–3460, 1988
84. Waller BF, Palumbo PJ, Lie JT, et al: The heart in diabetes mellitus as viewed from a morphologic perspective. In Scott C (ed): Clinical Cardiology and Diabetes. Mount Kisco, NY: Futura Publishing Company, Inc., 1981, pp 83–125
85. Dortimer AC, Shenoy PN, Shiroff RA, et al: Diffuse coronary artery disease in diabetic patients. Circulation 57:133–336, 1978
86. Waller BF, Palumbo PJ, Lie JT, et al: Status of the coronary arteries at necropsy in diabetes mellitus with onset after age 30 years: analysis of 229 diabetic patients with and without clinical evidence of coronary heart disease and comparison to 183 control subjects. Am J Med 69:498–506, 1980
87. The International Collaborative Group: Joint discussion. J Chron Dis 32:827–829, 1979
88. Eschwege E, Richard JL, Thibult N, et al: Coronary heart disease mortality in relation with diabetes, blood glucose and plasma insulin levels: the Paris Prospective Study, ten years later. Horm Metab Res Suppl 15:41–46, 1985
89. Lapidus L, Bengtsson C, Larsson B, et al: Distribution of adipose tissue and risk of cardiovascular disease and death: a 12 year follow-up of participants in the population study of women in Gothenburg, Sweden. Br Med J 289:1257–1261, 1984
90. Peiris AN, Mueller RA, Struve MF, et al: Splanchnic insulin metabolism in obesity: influence of body fat distribution. J Clin Invest 78:1648–1658, 1986
91. Knuiman MW, Welborn TA, McCann VJ, et al: Prevalence of diabetic complications in relation to risk factors. Diabetes 35:1332–1339, 1986
92. Jarrett RJ, Shipley MJ: Type 2 (non-insulin-dependent) diabetes mellitus and cardiovascular disease - putative association via common antecedents; further evidence from the Whitehall Study. Diabetologia 31:737–740, 1988
93. Janka HU: Five-year incidence of major macrovascular complications in diabetes mellitus. Horm Metab Res Suppl 15:15–19, 1984
94. Jarrett R: Type II (non-insulin dependent) diabetes mellitus and

coronary heart disease—chicken, egg, or neither? Diabetologia 26:99–102, 1984

95. Ganda OP, Soeldner JS, Gleason RE: Alterations in plasma lipids in the presence of mild glucose intolerance in the offspring of two type II diabetic parents. Diabetes Care 8:254–260, 1985
96. Wilson PWF, Anderson KM, Kannell WB: Epidemiology of diabetes mellitus in the elderly: The Framingham Study. Am J Med 80(suppl 5A):3–9, 1986
97. Jarrett RJ: Is insulin atherogenic? Diabetologia 31:71–75, 1988
98. Orchard TJ: Is insulin atherogenic? Diabetologia 31:404–405, 1988
99. Stamler J: Epidemiology of diabetes with respect to cardiovascular diseases. Presented at Second World Conference on Diabetes Research, Monaco, March 1988
100. Jensen T, Borch-Johnsen K, Kofoed-Enevoldsen A, et al: Coronary heart disease in young type 1 (insulin-dependent) diabetic patients with and without diabetic nephropathy: incidence and risk factors. Diabetologia 30:144–148, 1987
101. West KM, Ahuja MMS, Bennett PH, et al: The role of circulating glucose and triglyceride concentrations and their interactions with other "risk factors" as determinants of arterial disease in nine diabetic population samples from the WHO Multinational Study. Diabetes Care 6:361–369, 1983
102. Howard BV: Lipoprotein metabolism in diabetes mellitus. J Lipid Res 28:613–628, 1987
103. Stout RW, Bierman EL, Ross R: Effect of insulin on the proliferation of cultured primate arterial smooth muscle cells. Circ Res 36:319–327, 1975
104. Stout RW: The effect of insulin and glucose on sterol synthesis in cultured rat arterial smooth muscle cells. Atherosclerosis 27:271–278, 1977
105. Porta M, La Selva M, Molinatti P, et al: Endothelial cell function in diabetic microangiopathy. Diabetologia 30:601–609, 1987
106. Christlieb AR, Krolewski AS, Warran JH, et al: Insulin and diastolic hypertension. Circulation 70(Suppl 2):61, 1984
107. Donahue RP, Orchard TJ, Becker DJ, et al: Sex differences in the coronary heart disease risk profile: a possible role for insulin: the Beaver County Study. Am J Epidemiol 125:650–657, 1987
108. Ferrannini E, Buzzigoli G, Bonadonna R, et al: Insulin resistance in essential hypertension. N Engl J Med 317:350–357, 1987
109. Modan M, Halkin H, Almog S, et al: Hyperinsulinemia: a link between hypertension, obesity and glucose intolerance. J Clin Invest 75:809–817, 1985
110. Ducimetiere P, Eschwege E, Papoz JL, et al: Relationship of plasma insulin levels to the incidence of myocardial infarction and coronary heart disease mortality in a middle-aged population. Diabetologia 19:205–210, 1980
111. Pyorala K: Relationship of glucose tolerance and plasma insulin in the incidence of coronary heart disease: results from two population studies in Finland. Diabetes Care 2:131–141, 1979
112. Welborn TA, Wearne K: Coronary heart disease incidence and cardiovascular mortality in Busselton with reference to glucose and insulin concentrations. Diabetes Care 2:154–160, 1979
113. Colwell JA, Winocour PD, Halushka PV: Do platelets have anything to do with diabetic microvascular disease? Diabetes 32(Suppl 2):14–19, 1983
114. Jensen T, Stender S, Deckert T: Abnormalities in plasma concentrations of lipoproteins and fibrinogen in type 1 (insulin-dependent) diabetic patients with increased urinary albumin excretion. Diabetologia 31:142–145, 1988
115. North AF, Mazumdar S, Logiullo VM: Birth weight, gestational age and perinatal deaths in 5,471 infants of diabetic mothers. J Pediatr 90:444–447, 1977
116. Freinkel N: Gestational diabetes 1979: philosophical and practical aspects of a major public health problem. Diabetes Care 3:399–401, 1980
117. Wheeler FC, Gollmar CW, Deeb LC: Diabetes and pregnancy in South Carolina: prevalence, perinatal mortality and neonatal morbidity in 1978. Diabetes Care 5:561–565, 1982
118. Chung LS, Myrianthopoulos NC: Factors affecting risk of congenital malformations. II. Effect of maternal diabetes. Birth Defects 11:10, 1975
119. Mills JL, Baker L, Goldman AS: Malformations in infants of diabetic mothers occur before the gestational week. Diabetes 28:292–293, 1979
120. Miodovnik M, Mimouni F, St. John Dignan P, Berk MA, Ballard JL, Siddiqi TA, Khoury J, Tsang RC: Major malformations in infants of IDDM women: vasculopathy and early first-trimester poor glycemic control. Diabetes Care 11:713–718, 1988
121. Mills JL, Simpson JL, Driscoll SG, Jovanovic-Peterson L, Van Allen M: Incidence of spontaneous abortion among normal women and insulin-dependent diabetic women whose pregnancies were identified within 21 days of conception. N Engl J Med 319:1617–1623, 1988
122. Mills JL, Knopp RH, Simpson JL, Jovanovic-Peterson L, Metzger BE, Holmes LB: Lack of relation of increased malformation rates in infants of diabetic mothers to glycemic control during organogenesis. N Engl J Med 318:671–676, 1988
123. A study of the effects of hypoglycemic agents on vascular complications in patients with adult-onset diabetes. II. Mortality results, University Group Diabetes Program. Diabetes 19:785–830, 1970
124. Effects of hypoglycemic agents on vascular complications in patients with adult-onset diabetes. IV. A preliminary report on phenformin results, University Group Diabetes Program. JAMA 217:777–784, 1971
125. Raskin P, Pietri AO, Unger R, Shannon WA: The effect of diabetic control in the width of skeletal-muscle capillary basement membrane in patients with type I diabetes mellitus. N Engl J Med 309:1546–1550, 1983
126. Kroc Collaborative Study Group: Near normal glycemic control does not slow progression of mild diabetic retinopathy (abstr). Diabetes 32:1–10A, 1983
127. Steno study group: Effect of six months of strict metabolic control of eye and kidney function in insulin-dependent diabetics with background retinopathy. Lancet 1:121–124, 1982
128. Lauritzen T, Frost-Larsen K, Larsen HW, et al: Effect of one year of near-normal blood glucose levels in retinopathy in insulin-dependent diabetics. Lancet 1:200–204, 1983
129. Lauritzen T, Frost-Larsen K, Larsen HW, et al: The Steno Study Group: Two-year experience with continuous subcutaneous insulin infusion in relation to retinopathy and neuropathy. Diabetes 34(Suppl 3):74–79, 1985
130. DCCT Research Group: The Diabetes Control and Complications Trial (DCCT): design and methodologic considerations for the feasibility phase. Diabetes 35:530–545, 1986

52

Respiratory Disease Prevention

David B. Coultas
Jonathan M. Samet

Diseases of the respiratory system are an important public health problem in all countries. The respiratory system, which includes the lungs and the upper airway that joins the trachea to the larynx, is exposed to a wide range of potentially injurious agents (Table 52–1). On average, an adult inhales about 5 L of air per minute; with exercise, the amount may increase twentyfold or more. With a daily inhalation of between 10,000 and 20,000 L of air, agents present even in low concentrations may be biologically significant. The respiratory system is equipped with a remarkably effective system of defense mechanisms against inhaled particles and gases. Disease may result, however, if an acute exposure overwhelms the defenses (e.g., toxic gas inhalation), if an agent is particularly toxic even at low concentrations (e.g., toluene diisocyanate), if exposure is sustained (e.g., cigarette smoking), or if the exposed person is particularly susceptible (e.g., asthmatics).

In the United States in 1986, more than 170,000 deaths were due to nonmalignant respiratory diseases (Table 52–2). Chronic obstructive pulmonary disease (COPD) and related conditions were the fifth leading cause of death, pneumonia and influenza the sixth. Chronic respiratory conditions, largely asthma and COPD, affect a significant proportion of the population, even at younger ages. Respiratory tract infections continue to cause substantial morbidity and mortality. For example, in the United States, an estimated 80.1 acute respiratory tract conditions were experienced per 100 persons,[1] and acute respiratory tract infections and influenza directly caused 69,812 deaths in 1986.[1] Worldwide, 4 to 6 million children are estimated to die annually of acute respiratory infections.[2] Environmental and occupational respiratory exposures also cause an enormous burden of potentially preventable disease. In the United States, for example, 390,000 total deaths were attributed to cigarette smoking in 1985.[3] In many countries, environmental and occupational agents that cause disease have become subject to regulation to ensure that workplaces are healthful and that neither outdoor nor indoor air causes adverse effects. Such regulations are not in place throughout the world, however, and where they do exist, enforcement and compliance are variable.

INTERNATIONAL DISTRIBUTIONS

The occurrence of respiratory system diseases varies widely around the world (Table 52–3).[4] Among children under 5 years of age, between 25% and 30% of all deaths per year, or about 4 million deaths, are due to acute respiratory tract infections; 90% of these deaths are among children from developing countries.[5] The markedly higher childhood mortality from acute respiratory tract infections in the developing countries as compared with developed countries probably reflects poorer nutrition and immunization practices and more frequent low birth weight, crowding, and indoor and outdoor air pollution.[6]

Chronic diseases of the respiratory system and respiratory tract cancer are major causes of morbidity and mortality among adults. On average, the proportion of deaths due to bronchitis, emphysema, and asthma is about 40% worldwide, but this figure varies widely, from about 7% in Thailand to 60% in Australia.[7] Internationally, the frequencies of respiratory tract cancer and of nonmalignant chronic diseases of the respiratory system can be directly related to the prevalence of cigarette smoking.[8]

PEDIATRIC RESPIRATORY DISEASES

Hyaline Membrane Disease

Hyaline membrane disease, or respiratory distress syndrome (RDS) in the newborn, results from surfactant deficiency associated with lung immaturity.[9] Because of surfactant deficiency the lung does not effectively exchange oxygen and carbon dioxide after birth and positive pressure ventilation is frequently required to maintain life. Bronchopulmonary dysplasia, characterized by persistent pulmonary dysfunction and oxygen dependence beyond the age of 1 month, occurs as a frequent sequela of RDS.[10]

It is estimated that there are 35,000 cases of RDS annually in the United States.[10] Between 1968 and 1978, RDS was the leading cause of death in the first 28 days of life, accounting for 20% of all neonatal deaths.[11] Of infants who survive RDS, estimates of the proportion in whom bronchopulmonary dysplasia develops vary from 10% to 45%.[10,12]

Several risk factors have been established for RDS, including prematurity, male sex, cesarean section, and perinatal asphyxia.[13] The incidence of RDS is inversely related to gestational age and birth weight, both measures of fetal prematurity.[9] Overall, RDS develops in 14% of newborns who weigh less than 2500 g[9] and in 29% of those who weigh 750 to 1750 g.[12]

Prevention of premature birth represents the most effective method for reducing the morbidity and mortality associated with

TABLE 52-1. MECHANISMS OF LUNG INJURY AND EXAMPLES OF INJURIOUS AGENTS AND ASSOCIATED DISEASES

Mechanism of Injury	Example	
	Agent	***Disease***
Infection	Respiratory syncytial virus	Bronchiolitis
	Streptococcus pneumonia	Pneumonia
Carcinogenesis	Cigarette smoke	Lung cancer
	Asbestos	Mesothelioma
Immunologic	Thermophilic actinomycetes	Hypersensitivity pneumonitis
Inflammation	Cigarette smoke	COPD
	Oxides of nitrogen	Silo-filler's lung
Fibrogenesis	Asbestos	Asbestosis
	Coal dust	Coal workers' pneumoconiosis
Other	Plicatic acid	Western red cedar workers' asthma
	Cotton dust	Byssinosis

RDS.[13] However, because prematurity is frequently a result of poor socioeconomic conditions, and therefore not directly amenable to medical intervention, prematurity and RDS will remain public health problems until underlying causes can be remedied.

Prenatal identification of fetuses at high risk for RDS can be accomplished by analysis of amniotic fluid phospholipids.[9] As the fetus matures, amniotic fluid lecithin concentration increases while sphingomyelin concentration remains constant. Ratios of lecithin to sphingomyelin of 2:1 or greater are associated with low risk for RDS. The "shake test" offers a rapid and inexpensive screening method for determining fetal maturity.[9]

Medical intervention may provide partial solutions for the prevention of RDS and its complications. The methods that offer the greatest promise are corticosteroids[14,15] and surfactant therapy.[12,16] The administration of corticosteroids to the mother has been shown to decrease the frequency of RDS, primarily in female neonates.[14] After the development of RDS, corticosteroids can shorten the duration of mechanical ventilation and the need for supplemental oxygen.[15] A single dose of surfactant administered immediately after birth decreases the severity of RDS in the first 24 hours, but the effects are not sustained.[16] Similarly, a single dose of surfactant administered after the development of RDS decreases the severity of the RDS for 72 hours but does not decrease mortality.[12]

TABLE 52-2. NUMBER OF DEATHS FROM RESPIRATORY DISEASES IN THE UNITED STATES IN 1986

Disease (ICD-9)[a]	Number
▪ **Diseases of Newborns**	
Respiratory distress syndrome (769)	3,408
Other respiratory conditions of newborns (770)	3,665
▪ **Nonmalignant Respiratory Diseases**	
Pneumonia and influenza (480–487)	69,812
Chronic bronchitis (491)	3,123
Emphysema (492)	14,471
Asthma (493)	3,955
Chronic airways obstruction, NEC (496)	53,513
Pneumoconioses and other lung diseases due to external agents (500–508)	8,153
Interstitial lung disease (515–516)	5,080
Pulmonary embolism (415.1)	10,516
Total disease of respiratory system (460–519)	170,938
▪ **Malignant Respiratory Diseases**	
Larynx (161)	3,611
Trachea, bronchus, lung (162)	125,522

[a] International Classification of Diseases, 9th revision.
From NCHS 1988.[1]

Cystic Fibrosis

In the United States, cystic fibrosis is the most common lethal genetic disease in whites, occurring in about 1 in 2000 live births.[17] Cystic fibrosis is transmitted as an autosomal recessive trait. The frequency of gene carriers varies widely among racial groups, with about 5% of whites and only about 2% of American blacks being carriers.

The genetic defect results in the production of an abnormally thick mucus because of the inability of epithelial cells to secrete chloride ions and, therefore, water into the mucus.[18] This defect affects the lungs, intestines, and exocrine glands and may result in diverse clinical manifestations, but patients invariably develop chronic obstructive pulmonary disease from repeated infections that destroy lung tissue. Pulmonary involvement has been reported in 94% to 100% of all patients with cystic fibrosis[19,20] and accounts for the majority of hospital admissions and nearly all of the deaths.[20]

The prognosis for patients with cystic fibrosis has improved over the last 40 years.[21,22] At two cystic fibrosis centers, one in Boston and one in Toronto, the median survival times through 1981 were 21 and 30 years, respectively. The improving prognosis of cystic fibrosis probably reflects the beneficial effects of early recognition, nutritional support, and antibiotic therapy. Because of the need for multidisciplinary management in cystic fibrosis, treatment centers have been established, although their efficacy remains controversial.[23]

Because cystic fibrosis is a fatal genetic disease, prenatal diagnosis with early termination of affected pregnancies offers the only current method for control.[24] Two techniques are available for prenatal screening, including measurement of microvillar enzymes in amniotic fluid during the second trimester and examination of DNA markers from amniotic cells or chorionic villus samples in the first or second trimester.[25] The DNA techniques are considered the method of choice because of their high accuracy.[25] However, prenatal diagnosis by DNA analysis can be offered only to the pregnant woman who has previously had a child with cystic fibrosis.[23] Since most children with the disease are born into families without a history of cystic fibrosis, current prenatal screening methods will have little impact on the incidence of the disease.[23] The recent identification of the genetic abnormality underlying the majority of cases of cystic fibrosis will undoubtedly lead to new approaches for screening.[26–28]

Effective methods of early diagnosis in newborn children may also prevent morbidity and improve survival. The identifi-

TABLE 52-3. MORTALITY RATES (PER 100,000) IN SELECTED COUNTRIES FOR VARIOUS RESPIRATORY DISEASES AGE-STANDARDIZED TO WORLD POPULATIONS

		Malignant Neoplasms of Trachea, Bronchus, and Lung (162)[a]	Diseases of the Respiratory System (460–466, 470–478, 480–519)[a]	Chronic and Unspecified Bronchitis, Emphysema, and Asthma (490–493)[a]
African Region				
Mauritius[b]	Total	10.2	90.1	39.9
	Male	17.8	116.4	55.2
	Female	4.0	68.1	29.2
Americas Region				
Guatemala[c]	Total	1.5	164.4	10.0
	Male	0.9	177.8	11.3
	Female	2.0	152.1	9.0
United States[c]	Total	36.3	37.2	5.5
	Male	56.9	54.1	7.9
	Female	20.4	26.0	3.9
European Region				
Portugal[b]	Total	13.0	40.7	11.0
	Male	24.3	58.8	16.8
	Female	4.1	27.9	7.1
England and Wales[d]	Total	38.6	56.7	15.2
	Male	64.9	83.5	25.5
	Female	19.3	41.0	9.1
Eastern Mediterranean				
Kuwait[b]	Total	14.4	40.9	7.4
	Male	20.6	45.3	9.9
	Female	7.2	37.3	4.7
Western Pacific				
Australia[d]	Total	27.8	39.8	11.0
	Male	48.0	62.0	16.4
	Female	11.5	25.5	7.5
Japan[d]	Total	16.1	38.1	7.3
	Male	27.6	56.6	11.5
	Female	7.7	26.0	4.5
Singapore[b]	Total	34.0	107.5	9.2
	Male	49.9	157.4	11.9
	Female	19.7	75.1	7.4

[a] International Classification of Diseases, 9th revision.
[b] Age-standardized to 1986 world population.
[c] Age-standardized to 1984 world population.
[d] Age-standardized to 1985 world population.
From WHO World Health Statistics Annual, 1987.[4]

cation of cases by screening of blood samples from neonates for serum trypsinogen levels may lessen morbidity in the first 2 years of life.[29] However, these methods are still being developed, and the benefits are debatable.[24,30] In a series of 622 Australian patients with cystic fibrosis, infants in whom the disorder was diagnosed before the age of 6 months had less rapid progression of lung disease, but survival was not improved when compared with those whose symptoms were diagnosed after the neonatal period.[30] The sweat chloride test is the gold standard for diagnosis of cystic fibrosis,[17] but this test is not suited for mass screening.

As noted previously, the improving survival among persons with cystic fibrosis has been attributed to better medical care. However, the relative contributions of the various components of care to the improvement cannot be readily established. The details of management of cystic fibrosis are beyond the scope of this review and have been discussed extensively elsewhere.[17,31] Two options for management that offer promise include prophylactic antibiotics[32] and corticosteroid therapy.[33] However, widespread use of these treatments should await results of larger controlled investigations currently under way. The identification of a gene for cystic fibrosis may also lead to new therapeutic approaches.

Respiratory Tract Infection

In the twentieth century, respiratory tract infections are the main cause of morbidity and mortality among children living in developing countries and, although a much less frequent cause of death, the predominant source of morbidity among children living in developed countries. Respiratory viruses are responsible for most childhood respiratory tract infections, although bacteria, *Mycoplasma,* and *Chlamydia* cause some infections at particular ages. Respiratory tract infections in childhood may plausibly have long-term sequelae, including loss of lung function after severe episodes of lower respiratory tract infection, the development of asthma, the development of bronchiectasis, and an increased risk of developing COPD in adulthood.[34]

In developed countries the predominant clinical syndromes associated with childhood respiratory tract infection include colds (infections of the upper respiratory tract), epiglottitis (infection of the epiglottis), croup or laryngeotracheobronchitis (infection of the larynx and large airways), bronchiolitis (infection of the small airways), and pneumonia (infection of the lung tissues). Rhinoviruses are most closely associated with colds, parainfluenza viruses with croup, respiratory syncytial virus with bronchiolitis, and various viruses, including respiratory syncytial virus and the parainfluenza viruses, with pneumonia.[35,36] Bacteria cause epiglottitis. Epiglottitis, croup, bronchiolitis, and pneumonia may be severe and cause death through respiratory failure. In less developed countries, measles and whooping cough may be important causes of severe respiratory tract infection.[37]

Childhood respiratory tract infections are extremely common. Surveillance data for general population samples in the United States show that children experience about six respiratory illnesses during the first year of life; by the teenage years children still have about two or three respiratory illnesses annually.[38] Mortality from childhood respiratory tract infections is low in the United States and other more developed countries, about 0.1 death annually per 1000 children from birth through the age of 5 years.[2] However, mortality rates for this same age group are more than 100 times greater in some developing countries.

Many risk factors for respiratory tract infection have been identified. In developing countries, overcrowded dwellings, poor nutrition, low birth weight, and possibly intense smoke pollution underlie the high rates.[6] Studies in developed countries have shown that males have higher rates of infection, as do younger siblings of school-age children who introduce infections into households. Children from homes of lower socioeconomic status also tend to have more respiratory infections.[36] Maternal cigarette smoking has also been causally linked to increased occurrence of respiratory tract infections during the first years of life.[39] Attendance at day care centers also increases the occurrence of respiratory tract infections among preschool children.[40,41] Some studies indicate that breast-feeding decreases risk and that use of a gas-fueled stove increases risk, but the evidence of these associations is conflicting.[42,43]

Present understanding of risk factors of respiratory tract infection in childhood indicates several approaches for primary prevention. In developing countries, improved living conditions, better nutrition, and reduction of smoke pollution indoors should reduce the burden of morbidity and mortality associated with respiratory tract infections. In developed countries, mothers should be encouraged to stop smoking or to avoid smoking in the presence of their children. We lack approaches for controlling the emerging problem of excess respiratory tract infections associated with day care. Vaccines are now available for *Haemophilus influenzae,* the bacteria that causes epiglottitis. However, effective vaccines have not yet been developed for the common respiratory viruses.

Asthma

Numerous investigations of the occurrence of asthma in children have been conducted worldwide.[44] In the United States, data from nationwide samples and survey populations indicate that asthma is a common disease in children, with an overall prevalence of about 5% (Table 52-4).[45-48] Data from Tucson, Ariz.,[46] show a sharp decline in the incidence of asthma from early childhood to adolescence (Fig. 52-1). Worldwide, data from cross-sectional surveys indicate a wide range for the prevalence of childhood asthma.[44,49] Gregg[49] summarized the findings of surveys of children and adolescents and noted that the prevalence varied from near 0 to 75%. Methodological differences among the surveys may partially explain this range, but variation in the distributions of risk factors may also be important. Prevalence estimates from developed countries are similar to those listed in Table 52-4 for the United States.[49] Generally, asthma is less common in developing countries.[44]

The natural history of childhood asthma has been described in longitudinal studies of asthmatic children; most of the studies have been conducted retrospectively in developed countries on patients from office practices or hospital clinics.[50-54] Only two longitudinal studies of children from general population samples have been carried out.[55,56] These studies have shown that between 30% and 70% of asthmatic children become symptom-free or show improvement by adolescence or early adulthood.

Many endogenous and exogenous risk factors have been identified for asthma (Table 52-5). Studies of familial aggregation of asthma[57,58] and twins[59] show a strong familial influence on the prevalence of asthma, but these studies do not separate genetic from common environmental effects. Descriptive studies of childhood asthma have consistently shown an increased prev-

TABLE 52-4. PREVALENCE OF CHILDHOOD ASTHMA IN SELECTED STUDIES IN THE UNITED STATES

Location and Date	Criterion		Findings: Males (%)	Findings: Females (%)
Tecumseh, Mich. 1962–1965[45]	Asthma or wheezing with appropriate characteristics at examination or during the last year	0–4 y	4.6	2.7
		5–9 y	5.3	3.0
		10–15 y	6.0	3.7
Tucson, Ariz. 1972–1973[46]	Report of active asthma, diagnosed by a physician	0–4 y	1.5	2.0
		5–9 y	7.3	9.5
		10–14 y	8.9	8.1
		15–19 y	8.9	6.8
			Both Sexes: Cumulative (%)	**Both Sexes: Active (%)**
National sample, 1976–1980[47]	Report of physician diagnosis of asthma	6 mo–2 y	4.0	2.3
		3–5 y	6.5	3.9
		6–11 y	7.6	3.9
		12–17 y	6.6	3.2
			Males (%)	**Females (%)**
Western Pennsylvania 1979[48]	Report of ever receiving a physician diagnosis	5–9 y	4.6	2.4
		10–14 y	4.4	2.9

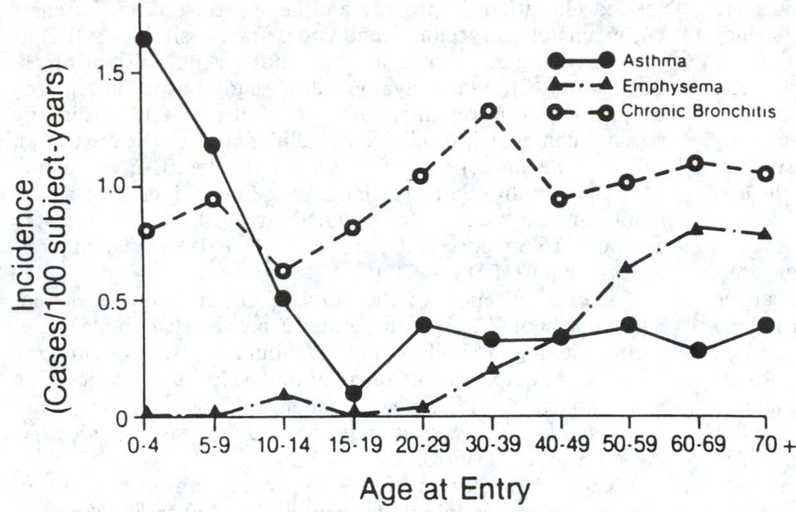

Figure 52–1. Incidence of asthma, emphysema, and chronic bronchitis according to age at entry. *(From Dodge R, Cline MG, Burrows B: Comparisons of asthma, emphysema, and chronic bronchitis diagnoses in a general population sample. Am Rev Respir Dis 133:981–986, 1986.[75])*

alence in males,[55,60] which may be explained by differences in airway geometry.[61] Atopy, defined by positive skin tests to common aeroallergens, predicts increased risk of asthma if present in the parents or child.[62] More severe episodes of lower respiratory tract infection are associated with subsequent asthma and increased airway reactivity.[63] Ambient air pollution may exacerbate asthma,[64] but it has not been established as a risk factor for childhood asthma. Similarly, environmental tobacco smoke has been shown to exacerbate asthma,[65] but its role in development of asthma is uncertain.[39]

Although risk factors for childhood asthma have been identified, preventive strategies have been directed primarily at pharmacological and other interventions to lessen morbidity. The use of bronchodilators, corticosteroids, and disodium cromoglycate greatly reduces morbidity from asthma. Speight et al.[66] found that school absenteeism, an important measure of morbidity,[67] fell tenfold after effective treatment among 31 asthmatic children who had been having more than 12 attacks per year.

Many nonpharmacological interventions have been examined, including environmental control, prevention of sensitization in infancy and childhood, immunizations, allergen immunotherapy, physical training, chest physiotherapy, and education.[68] Educational programs have been developed recently to improve self-management skills among asthmatic children.[69,70] Although children's knowledge of asthma improves with these programs, their effectiveness may be limited to children with severe asthma.[69] In the United States, a national strategy for asthma education is being developed to prevent morbidity and mortality from asthma.[71]

Death from childhood asthma, although infrequent, is well documented and potentially preventable. Childhood mortality rates from asthma vary from country to country and by age, sex, and race in the United States. Evans et al.[65] summarized U.S. vital statistics data from 1968 to 1982; age-specific mortality for children 14 years of age and younger ranged from 0.1 to 0.7 per 100,000. In 1982 rates were higher in males and in blacks.

Findings from retrospective studies suggest that clinical severity of asthma predicts risk of death.[72,73] Factors that are suspected to affect mortality include failure on the part of patients and physicians to recognize severity, behavioral patterns, underuse of corticosteroids, overuse and overdependence on nebulizers, and additive toxicity from combined use of theophylline and beta agonists.[72–74] For individual children, however, the predictive value of these factors is limited.

TABLE 52–5. RISK FACTORS FOR CHILDHOOD ASTHMA

Familial and genetic factors
Male gender
Atopy
Environmental factors
Respiratory tract infection
Ambient air pollution
Environmental tobacco smoke
Bronchial hyperreactivity

ADULT RESPIRATORY TRACT DISEASES

Asthma

Worldwide, the occurrence of asthma is lower in adults than in children.[44] Incidence is highest in children less than 5 years of age, declines during adolescence, increases slightly into early adulthood, and then remains constant (Fig. 52–1).[75] In a population-based sample of U.S. residents,[76] including 14,404 adults 25 to 74 years of age, the overall prevalence of active asthma was estimated at 2.6%. The cumulative incidence of new-onset asthma was 2.1/1000/y. In contrast to children, among adults female gender was associated with a 40% increase in incidence. However, the higher incidence in women may partly be explained by physician bias in labeling obstructive lung disease in women as asthma rather than COPD.[75]

Overall strategies for asthma management and prevention in adults differ little from those in children and incorporate pharmacological and other interventions. For adults, occupational asthma is of special concern, with more than 200 causative agents identified.[77] Early recognition of the relationship between an occupational exposure and asthma is important, since prompt removal from exposure correlates best with full resolution of asthma.[78]

Chronic Obstructive Pulmonary Disease (COPD)

COPD is a clinically applied term for persistent and generally symptomatic obstruction to airflow within the lungs. The lungs of most persons with COPD display a mixture of emphysema, enlargement and destruction of the air spaces, and inflammation and narrowing of the smaller airways, although in some persons emphysema or airway abnormalities may predominate.[79] Emphysema reduces the driving pressure for airflow, and the airway abnormalities increase the resistance to airflow.

A small number of cases of COPD, distinguished by severe emphysema, occur in smokers and nonsmokers with deficiency of alpha$_1$-antitrypsin, a substance that defends against injury by proteolytic enzymes.[79] However, most cases result from cigarette smoking[79]; occupational agents can also contribute to the development of COPD.[80] Other risk factors for COPD, including childhood respiratory tract infection[34] and hyperresponsiveness of the airways of the lung,[81] have been postulated, but the evidence is inconclusive at present.

The natural history of COPD generally follows a slow but progressive course that offers a lengthy time window for intervention. The results of epidemiological studies suggest that the development of clinically evident COPD results from sustained loss of ventilatory function beyond that expected from aging alone (Fig. 52-2).[79] The rate of decline in smokers tends to increase with the amount smoked, and former smokers generally revert to the rate of loss seen in nonsmokers. Only a minority of smokers have COPD, however. Other than alpha$_1$-antitrypsin deficiency, factors that determine susceptibility have not been identified.[79]

Clinicians make the diagnosis of COPD in patients with sufficient chronic airflow obstruction to result in shortness of breath and limitation of exercise capacity. In epidemiological studies, COPD is considered to be present if lung function tests demonstrate a specified degree of impairment or if a physician's diagnosis is reported. Although prevalence can be readily assessed with the use of these criteria, incidence cannot be described over short periods because of the slow evolution of impairment in persons developing COPD.

Epidemiological data from throughout the world show that COPD is common among adults.[79,82] For its prevalence in the United States, see Table 52-6. The prevalence is greater among men than among women and increases with the extent of smoking.

Mortality rates for COPD, although subject to well-described limitations,[84] provide another measure of occurrence. Unfortunately, procedures and codes for classifying COPD as the underlying cause of death have not been consistent across this century. Consequently, mortality trends must be interpreted cautiously. Moreover, attribution of a death to COPD ordinarily requires contact with a clinician and diagnosis of the disease. In spite of the limitations of death certificates in investigating COPD, mortality data for the United States document a dramatic increase in deaths from COPD. In 1950, 3157 deaths were attributed to categories related to COPD; by 1986 the number of deaths from COPD was 71,102.

The 1984 Report of the Surgeon General concluded that 80% to 90% of COPD in the United States is attributable to cigarette smoking.[79] Similarly high attributable risks for smoking would be anticipated for other more developed countries. The epidemiological evidence has not identified factors placing individual smokers at risk that might be used as a basis for identifying "susceptible" smokers.

The slow evolution of COPD provides an opportunity to identify and to target for intervention the smokers in whom the disease is developing. With sustained smoking, lung function in smokers, declining at a more rapid rate (Fig. 52-2), tends to drop below normal levels. Lung function testing of chronic smokers can identify individuals whose function has dropped below the range of normal values but not yet reached the degree of impairment associated with frank COPD.[85] These at-risk persons could then be targeted for intervention. The Lung Health Study, a large clinical trial incorporating these concepts, is now in progress in the United States.[86]

Adult Respiratory Distress Syndrome (ARDS)

The clinical syndrome of ARDS was originally described in the late 1960s; it represents a diffuse response of the lung to a wide variety of causative factors, including sepsis, trauma, aspiration

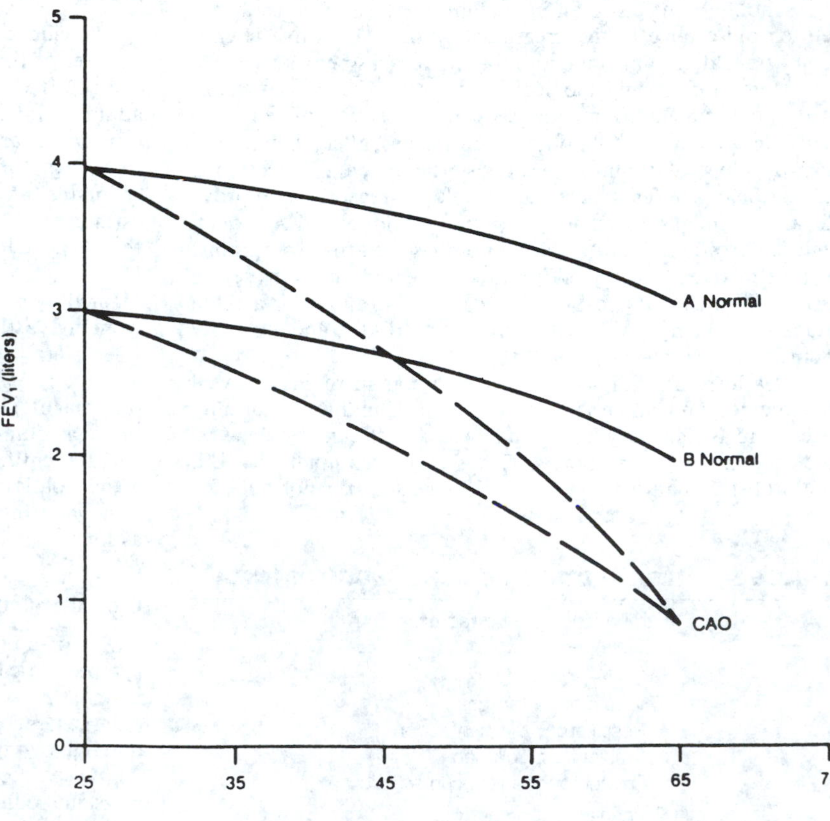

Figure 52-2. Decline of FEV$_1$ at normal rate [*solid line*] and at an accelerated rate [*dashed line*]. Note: *A*, Person who has attained a "normal" maximal FEV$_1$ during lung growth and development; *B*, person whose maximal FEV$_1$ has been reduced by childhood respiratory infection. [*From U.S. DHHS 1984.*[79]]

TABLE 52-6. PREVALENCE OF COPD IN SELECTED POPULATIONS

Population	Year of Study	Index	Prevalence (per 100)	
			Men Over 44 Years	
Tucson, Ariz.	1972–1973	Report of physician confirmed illness	Chronic bronchitis	10.2
			Emphysema	13.3
			Women Over 44 Years	
			Chronic bronchitis	9.0
			Emphysema	4.3
East Boston, Mass.	1973–1974	FEV_1 <65% of predicted	Men	5.6
			Women	3.4
Six U.S. cities	1974–1977	$FEV_1/FVC \leq 60[\%]$	Men	5.0
			Women	1.9
			Non-Hispanic Whites	
Albuquerque, N.M.	1978–1979	Physician diagnosis of current chronic bronchitis or emphysema	Men	3.6
			Women	3.4
			Hispanic Whites	
			Men	0.8
			Women	1.8
Busselton, Australia	Not given	FEV_1/FVC <70% and consistent history	Men	13.5
			Women	3.9
Tian-jin, China	Not given	Not given	Men	11.7

Adapted from Table 4 in U.S. DHHS, 1984,[79] and from Table 2 in Woolcock and Bjartveit, 1989.[83]

and other inhalational injuries, pancreatitis, multiple transfusions, and drug abuse.[87] The clinical picture comprises pulmonary edema that does not have a cardiac basis and respiratory failure. Mortality is high; about 50% of patients do not survive, but survivors tend to recover to a normal level of lung function. Little information on incidence and mortality is available. The ninth revision of the International Classification of Diseases includes a code (518.5) for "pulmonary insufficiency following trauma and surgery" including ARDS. However, this code would not capture all cases of ARDS. Approximately 150,000 cases have been estimated to occur annually in the United States.[88]

Adult respiratory distress syndrome occurs as a consequence of severe lung injury by diverse and distinct agents and often represents the most proximal cause of death. Preventive strategies must be directed toward the causative factors (e.g., motor vehicle accidents and drug abuse).

Pulmonary Thromboembolism

Each year in the United States more than 600,000 persons suffer from pulmonary thromboembolism, and about 200,000 deaths are estimated to result from pulmonary thromboembolism.[89] Despite the frequency of the problem, it is often undiagnosed[89] and, if untreated, has a mortality rate of about 30%.[89] A high index of suspicion is necessary for making the diagnosis of pulmonary thromboembolism.

Identification of risk factors for pulmonary thromboembolism (Table 52–7)[90] is the key for making a correct diagnosis.[89] In the Framingham Heart Study,[91] increased relative weight in women was the only significant predictor of major pulmonary embolism at autopsy. Among patients with angiographically confirmed thromboembolism,[92] conditions associated with pulmonary thromboembolism are common (Table 52–7). However, nearly half of the patients may have no apparent risk factors.

Because of the high frequency of pulmonary thromboembolism and the difficulties of diagnosis, prevention has been a major area of investigation. Numerous methods have been assessed for preventing venous thromboembolism in hospital patients.[93] Most information has come from surgical patients, for whom administration of subcutaneous heparin has proved efficacious.[94] Although little information is available on the use of subcutaneous heparin in nonsurgical patients, there is evidence of efficacy in patients with other medical conditions,[95] including respiratory failure, acute myocardial infarction, and acute paraplegia, quadriplegia, and stroke. Other methods that may be useful for the prevention of venous thromboembolism include intermittent pneumatic compression and aspirin.

Interstitial Lung Diseases

The interstitial lung diseases are a heterogeneous group of disorders comprising more than 130 entities that damage the pulmonary interstitium (Table 52–8).[96] About 35% of the cases are caused by identifiable factors, including occupational exposures, drugs, poisons, radiation, or infections; the remaining 65% have no known cause but have defined clinical and pathologic characteristics.[96]

In the United States, interstitial lung diseases are commonly

TABLE 52-7. RISK FACTORS FOR VENOUS THROMBOEMBOLISM

History of venous thromboembolism	Pregnancy or puerperium
Heart disease	Exogenous estrogens
Congestive heart disease	Immobility
Atrial arrhythmias	Advancing age
Mural thrombosis	
Malignant disease	
Trauma	
Major surgery	
Pelvic and lower extremity injury	

Adapted from Coon, 1984.[90]

TABLE 52-8. INTERSTITIAL LUNG DISEASES

▪ Known Causes	▪ Unknown Causes
Inorganic dusts	Idiopathic pulmonary fibrosis
Organic dusts	Collagen-vascular disorders
Gases, fumes, vapors, aerosols	Sarcoidosis
Drugs	Histiocytosis X
Poisons	Goodpasture's syndrome
Radiation	Idiopathic pulmonary hemosiderosis
Infectious agents	Wegener's granulomatosis
Chronic pulmonary edema	Vasculitides
Chronic uremia	Inherited disorders
	Lymphocytic infiltrative disorders
	Others

Adapted from Crystal et al., 1981.[96]

encountered by pulmonary physicians.[97] A 1972 Respiratory Diseases Task Force report from the National Institutes of Health[98] estimated that interstitial lung diseases accounted for about 15% of a pulmonary physician's practice. A 1980 Task Force report[99] used the Hospital Record Study, which projected the numbers of hospital admissions nationwide for 1977, and estimated that, among the respiratory diseases, interstitial lung diseases ranked second to airway obstruction as a cause of hospitalization. Although these estimates suggest that interstitial lung diseases are common, scant epidemiologic data are available.

Both endogenous and environmental factors have been proposed as determinants of interstitial lung diseases. With regard to endogenous factors, inherited interstitial lung disease,[100-102] association with human lymphocyte antigen (HLA) types,[100] and airway and lung dimensions[103] suggest that genetic factors may influence the development of some interstitial lung diseases because of altered lung clearance, lung defenses, or lung immunoregulation.

Inhalation of environmental agents and exposure to drugs account for most interstitial lung diseases of known cause, but little data are available on determinants of individual risk for disease or on the role of environmental agents in "idiopathic" interstitial lung diseases. Exposure to environmental agents may also alter risk of development of interstitial lung diseases of known or unknown cause; cigarette smoking decreases the risk of hypersensitivity pneumonitis[104,105] and increases the risk of histiocytosis X.[106] Infectious agents, viruses,[107,108] and *Mycoplasma*[109] have been implicated as causes of pulmonary fibrosis, indistinguishable from idiopathic pulmonary fibrosis, but the importance of these agents as causes of interstitial lung disease in the general population is not known.

Because of the limited epidemiologic data on risk factors for interstitial lung diseases, little specific information can be offered for prevention. For the large proportion of interstitial lung diseases of unknown cause, additional information on risk factors is needed to develop prevention strategies.

Sleep Apnea

The sleep apnea syndrome is characterized by excessive daytime sleepiness, snoring, and many episodes of cessation of breathing during sleep. In the majority of cases, the syndrome results from recurrent collapse of the pharynx with blockage of the passage of air.[110] Because of recurrent apneas, significant lack of oxygen may develop and cause fragmented sleep and secondary complications. The syndrome may result in excess mortality.[111,112]

There is limited information on the occurrence of sleep apnea syndrome in the general population. In a population-based sample of Hispanics, the prevalence of sleep apnea was 2.3% and 1.1% for males and females, respectively.[113] Among working men, Lavie[114] estimated a 1% prevalence of sleep apnea.

Little data are available on the prevention of morbidity and mortality from the sleep apnea syndrome, and the long-term benefits of treatment remain to be established.[115] Because obesity is often associated with the syndrome, weight reduction is frequently recommended but offers limited improvement unless body weight is substantially reduced.[110] Other nonsurgical (e.g., oxygen) or surgical (e.g., tracheostomy) treatments are available.[110]

CONCLUSIONS

Respiratory diseases are common causes of morbidity and mortality worldwide, and many of these diseases can be prevented. Because the occurrence of the various respiratory diseases may vary widely in different geographic locations, epidemiologic data are important for development of prevention strategies. Of particular public health concern is tobacco smoking, a major cause of avoidable respiratory disease from the prenatal period through adulthood.

REFERENCES

1. National Center for Health Statistics: Vital statistics of the United States, 1986. Volume II. Mortality, Part A. DHHS Publication No. (PHS) 88-1122. Washington, D.C.: U.S. Government Printing Office, 1988
2. Smith KR: Biofuels, Air Pollution, and Health: A Global Review. New York: Plenum Press, 1987
3. U.S. Department of Health and Human Services: Reducing the health consequences of smoking: 25 years of progress. Report of the Surgeon General. DHHS Publication No. CDC 89-8411. Rockville, Md.: Office on Smoking and Health, 1989
4. World Health Organization: World Health Statistics Annual 1987. Geneva: WHO, 1987
5. Leowski J: Mortality from acute respiratory infections in children under 5 years of age: global estimates. World Health Stat Q 39:138–144, 1986
6. Pandey MR, Boleij JSM, Smith KR, Wafula EM: Indoor air pollution in developing countries and acute respiratory infection in children. Lancet 25:427–429, February 1989
7. Bouvier MH, Guidevaux M: Mortality from disorders of the respiratory system throughout the world between 1950 and 1972. World Health Stat Q 32:174–197, 1979
8. Stanley K, Stjernsward J: Lung cancer—a worldwide health problem. Chest 96S:1S–5S, 1989
9. Farrell PM, Avery ME: Hyaline membrane disease. Am Rev Respir Dis 111:657–688, 1975
10. Bancalari E, Gerhardt T: The newborn. I. Bronchopulmonary dysplasia. Pediatr Clin North Am 33:1–23, 1986
11. Perelman RH, Farrell PM: Analysis of causes of neonatal death in the United States with specific emphasis on fatal hyaline membrane disease. Pediatrics 70:570–575, 1982
12. Horbar JD, Soll RF, Sutherland JM, et al: A multicenter randomized, placebo-controlled trial of surfactant therapy for respiratory distress syndrome. N Engl J Med 320:595–565, 1989
13. Stahlman MT: Medical complications in premature infants. Is treatment enough? (Editorial). N Engl J Med 320:1551–1553, 1989
14. Collaborative Group on Antenatal Steroid Therapy: Effect of ante-

natal dexamethasone administration on the prevention of respiratory distress syndrome. Am J Obstet Gynecol 141:276–285, 1981
15. Cummings JJ, D'Eugenio DB, Gross SJ: A controlled trial of dexamethasone in preterm infants at high risk for bronchopulmonary dysplasia. N Engl J Med 320:1505–1510, 1989
16. Kendig JW, Notter RH, Cox C, et al: Surfactant replacement therapy at birth: final analysis of a clinical trial and comparisons with similar trials. Pediatrics 82:756–762, 1988
17. Davis PB, di Sant' Agnese PA: Diagnosis and treatment of cystic fibrosis: an update. Chest 85:802–809, 1984
18. Levitan IB: The basic defect in cystic fibrosis. Science 244:1423, 1989
19. Huang NN, Schidlow DV, Szatrowski TH, Palmer J, Laraya-Causay LR, Yeung W, Hardy K, Quitell L, Fiel S: Clinical features, survival rate, and prognostic factors in young adults with cystic fibrosis. Am J Med 82:871–879, 1987
20. Penketh ARL, Wise A, Mearns MB, Hodson ME, Batten JC: Cystic fibrosis in adolescents and adults. Thorax 45:526–632, 1987
21. Warwick WJ, Pogue RE, Gerber HU, Nesbitt CJ: Survival patterns in cystic fibrosis. J Chron Dis 28:609–622, 1975
22. Corey M, McLaughlin FJ, Williams M, Levison H: A comparison of survival, growth, and pulmonary function in patients with cystic fibrosis in Boston and Toronto. J Clin Epidemiol 41:583–591, 1988
23. Geddes DM: Cystic fibrosis: future trends in care (editorial). Thorax 43:869–871, 1988
24. Dodge JA: Screening for disease: implications of the new genetics for screening for cystic fibrosis. Lancet 672–674, September 17, 1988
25. Brock DJH: Prenatal diagnosis of cystic fibrosis: Annotations. Arch Dis Child 63:701–704, 1988
26. Rommens JM, Iannuzzi MC, Kerem B, Drumm ML, Melmer G, et al: Identification of the cystic fibrosis gene: chromosome walking and jumping. Science 245:1059–1065, 1989
27. Riordan JR, Rommens JM, Kerem B, Alon N, Rozmahel R, et al: Identification of the cystic fibrosis gene: cloning and characterization of complementary DNA. Science 245:1066–1073, 1989
28. Kerem B, Rommens JM, Buchanan JA, Markiewicz D, Cox TK, et al: Identification of the cystic fibrosis gene: genetic analysis. Science 245:1073–1080, 1989
29. Bowling F, Cleghorn G, Chester A, Curran J, Griffin B, Prado J, Francis P, Shepherd R: Neonatal screening for cystic fibrosis. Arch Dis Child 63:196–198, 1988
30. Hudson I, Phelan PD: Are sex, age at diagnosis, or mode of presentation prognostic factors for cystic fibrosis? Pediatr Pulmonol 3:288–297, 1987
31. Murphy S: Cystic fibrosis in adults: diagnosis and management. Clin Chest Med 8:695–710, 1987
32. Szaff M, Høiby N, Flensborg EW: Frequent antibiotic therapy improves survival of cystic fibrosis patients with chronic *Pseudomonas aeruginosa* infection. Acta Paediatr Scand 72:651–657, 1983
33. Auerbach HS, Kirkpatrick JA, Williams M, Colten HR: Alternate-day prednisone reduces morbidity and improves pulmonary function in cystic fibrosis. Lancet, 686–688, September 28, 1985
34. Samet JM, Tager IB, Speizer FE: The relationship between respiratory illness in childhood and chronic air-flow obstruction in adulthood. Am Rev Respir Dis 127:508–523, 1983
35. Wright AL, Taussig LM, Ray CG, Harrison HR, Holberg CJ, Group Health Medical Associates: The Tucson Children's Respiratory Study. II. Lower respiratory tract illness in the first year of life. Am J Epidemiol 129:1232–1246, 1989
36. Glezen WP, Denny FW: Epidemiology of acute lower respiratory disease in children. N Engl J Med 288:498–505, 1973
37. Chretien J, Holland W, Macklem P, Murray J, Woolcock A: Acute respiratory infections in children: a global public-health problem. N Engl J Med 310:982–984, 1984
38. Monto AS, Ullman BM: Acute respiratory illness in an American community: the Tecumseh Study. JAMA 227:164–169, 1974
39. United States Department of Health and Human Services: The health consequences of involuntary smoking: report of the Surgeon General. DHHS Publication No. (CDC) 87-8398. Rockville, Md.: Office on Smoking and Health, 1986
40. Fleming DW, Cochi SL, Hightower AW, Broome CV: Childhood upper respiratory tract infections: to what degree is incidence affected by day-care attendance? Pediatrics 79:55–60, 1987
41. Anderson LJ, Parker RA, Strikas RA, Farrar JA, Gangarosa EG, Keyserling HL, Sikes RK: Day-care center attendance and hospitalization for lower respiratory tract illness. Pediatrics 82:300–308, 1988
42. Bauchner H, Leventhal JM, Shapiro ED: Studies of breast feeding and infections: how good is the evidence? JAMA 256:887–892, 1986
43. Samet JM, Marbury MC, Spengler JD: Health effects and sources of indoor air pollution. Part I. Am Rev Respir Dis 136:1486–1508, 1987
44. Cookson JB: Prevalence rates of asthma in developing countries and their comparison with those in Europe and North America. Chest 91S:97S–103S, 1987
45. Broder I, Higgins MW, Mathews KP, Keller JB: Epidemiology of asthma and allergic rhinitis in a total community, Tecumseh, Michigan. III. Second survey of the community. J Allergy Clin Immunol 53:127–138, 1974
46. Dodge RR, Burrows B: The prevalence and incidence of asthma and asthma-like symptoms in a general population sample. Am Rev Respir Dis 122:567–575, 1980
47. Evans R, Mullally D, Wilson R, Gergen P, Rosenberg H, Grauman J, Edmonds F, Feinlab M: Present evidence on mortality and morbidity of asthma. Transcript of proceedings, NIH International Workshop on Etiology of Asthma, June 25–27, Bethesda, Md., 1985
48. Schenker MB, Samet JM, Speizer FE: Risk factors for childhood respiratory disease: the effect of host factors and home environmental exposures. Am Rev Respir Dis 128:1038–1043, 1983
49. Gregg I: Epidemiological aspects. In Clark TJH, Godfrey S (eds): Asthma. London: Chapman and Hall, 1983, p 242
50. Rackemann FM, Edwards MC: Asthma in children: a follow-up study of 688 patients after an interval of twenty years. N Engl J Med 246:815–823, 1952
51. Dees SC: Development and course of asthma in children. Am J Dis Child 93:228–233, 1957
52. Ogilvie AG: Asthma: a study in prognosis of 1,000 patients. Thorax 17:183–189, 1962
53. Buffum WP, Settipane GA: Prognosis of asthma in childhood. Am J Dis Child 112:214–217, 1966
54. Blair H: Natural history of childhood asthma: 20-year follow-up. Arch Dis Child 52:613–619, 1977
55. Schachter EN, Doyle CA, Beck GJ: A prospective study of asthma in a rural community. Chest 85:623–630, 1984
56. McNicol KN, Williams HB: Spectrum of asthma in children. I. Clinical and physiological components. Br Med J 4:7–11, 1973
57. Lebowitz MD, Barbee R, Burrows B: Family concordance of IgE, atopy, and disease. J Allergy Clin Immunol 73:259–264, 1984
58. Sibbald B, Horn MEC, Gregg I: A family study of the genetic basis of asthma and wheezy bronchitis. Arch Dis Child 55:54–57, 1980
59. Hopp RJ, Bewtra AK, Watt GD, Nair NM, Townley RG: Genetic analysis of allergic disease in twins. J Allergy Clin Immunol 73:265–270, 1984
60. Horwood LJ, Fergusson DM, Shannon FT: Social and familial factors in the development of early childhood asthma. Pediatrics 75:859–868, 1985
61. Taussig LM: Maximal expiratory flows at functional residual capacity: a test of lung function for young children. 116:1031–1038, 1977
62. Weiss ST, Tager IB, Munoz A, Speizer FE: The relationship of respiratory infections in early childhood to the occurrence of increased levels of bronchial responsiveness and atopy. Am Rev Respir Dis 131:573–578, 1985
63. McConnochie KM, Roghmann KJ: Bronchiolitis as a possible cause of wheezing in childhood: new evidence. Pediatrics 74:1–10, 1984

64. American Thoracic Society: Health Effects of Air Pollution. New York: American Lung Association, 1978
65. Evans D, Levison MJ, Feldman CH, Clark NM, Wasilewski Y, Levin B, Mellins RB: The impact of passive smoking on emergency room visits of urban children with asthma. Am Rev Respir Dis 135:567–572, 1987
66. Speight ANP, Lee DA, Hey N: Underdiagnosis and undertreatment of asthma in childhood. Br Med J 286:1253–1256, 1983
67. Parcel GS, Gilman SC, Nader PR, Bunce H: A comparison of absentee rates of elementary school children with asthma and nonasthmatic school mates. Pediatrics 64:878–881, 1979
68. Meltzer EO, Orgel HA, Welch MJ, Kemp JP: Nonpharmacologic approaches to the management of asthma. In Tinkelman DG, Falliers CJ, Naspitz CK (eds): Childhood Asthma, Pathophysiology and Treatment. New York: Marcel Dekker, Inc., 1987
69. Howland J, Bauchner H, Adair R: The impact of pediatric asthma education on morbidity: assessing the evidence. Chest 94:964–969, 1988
70. Clark NM: Asthma self-management education: research and implications for clinical practice. Chest 95:1110–1113, 1989
71. Parker SR, Mellins RB, Sogn DD: Asthma education: a national strategy. Am Rev Respir Dis 140:848–853, 1989
72. Carswell F: Thirty deaths from asthma. Arch Dis Child 60:25–28, 1985
73. Strunk RC, Mrazek DA, Wolfson Fuhrmann GS, La Brecque JF: Physiologic and psychological characteristics associated with deaths due to asthma in childhood: a case-controlled study. JAMA 254:1193–1198, 1985
74. Wilson JD, Sutherland DC, Thomas AC: Has the change to beta-agonists combined with oral theophylline increased cases of fatal asthma? Lancet 1:1235–1237, 1981
75. Dodge R, Cline MG, Burrows B: Comparisons of asthma, emphysema, and chronic bronchitis diagnoses in a general population sample. Am Rev Respir Dis 133:981–986, 1986
76. McWhorter WP, Polis MA, Kaslow RA: Occurrence, predictors, and consequences of adult asthma in NHANESI and follow-up survey. Am Rev Respir Dis 139:721–724, 1989
77. Chan-Yeung M, Lam S: Occupational asthma. Am Rev Respir Dis 133:686–703, 1986
78. Chan-Yeung M: Evaluation of impairment/disability in patients with occupational asthma. Am Rev Respir Dis 135:950–951, 1987
79. United States Department of Health and Human Service: The health consequences of smoking. Chronic obstructive lung disease. Report of the Surgeon General. DHHS Publication No. (PHS) 84-50205. Rockville, Md.: Office on Smoking and Health, 1984
80. Becklake MR: Occupational pollution. Chest 96:372S–378S, 1989
81. O'Connor GT, Sparrow D, Weiss ST: The role of allergy and nonspecific airway hyperresponsiveness in the pathogenesis of chronic obstructive pulmonary disease. Am Rev Respir Dis 140:225–252, 1989
82. Murray JF: Introduction to supplementary volume on reports and recommendations of the conference on chronic airways disease held in Dubrovnik, Yugoslavia, in October 1988. Chest 96S:301S, 1989
83. Woolcock AJ, Bjartveit K: Epidemiology of chronic airways disease. Chest 96S:302S–306S, 1989
84. Feinleib M, Rosenberg HM, Collins JG, Delozier JE, Pokras R, Chevarley FM: Trends in COPD morbidity and mortality in the United States. Am Rev Respir Dis 140S:S9–S18, 1989
85. Fletcher C, Peto R: The natural history of chronic airflow obstruction. Br Med J 1645–1648, June 15, 1977
86. Anthonisen NR: Lung health study. Am Rev Respir Dis 140:871–872, 1989
87. Petty TL: Adult respiratory distress syndrome: definition and historical perspective. Clin Chest Med 3:3–7, 1982
88. Murray J, Staff of Division of Lung Diseases, National Heart, Lung and Blood Institute: Mechanisms of acute respiratory failure. Am Rev Respir Dis 115:1071–1078, 1977
89. Dalen JE, Paraskos JA, Ockene IS, Alpert JS, Hirsh J: Venous thromboembolism: scope of the problem. Chest 89:370S–373S, 1986
90. Coon WW: Venous thromboembolism: prevalence, risk factors, and prevention. Clin Chest Med 5:391–401, 1984
91. Goldhaber SZ, Savage DD, Garrison RJ, Castelli WP, Kannel WB, McNamara PM, Gherardi G, Feinleib M: Risk factors for pulmonary embolism: The Framingham Study. Am J Med 74:1023–1028, 1983
92. Bell WR, Simon TL, DeMets DL: The clinical features of submassive and massive pulmonary emboli. Am J Med 62:355–360, 1977
93. Hull RD, Raskob GE, Hirsh J: Prophylaxis of venous thromboembolism. Chest 89S:374S–383S, 1986
94. Collins R, Scrimgeour A, Jusuf S, Peto R: Reduction in fatal pulmonary embolism and venous thrombosis by perioperative administration of subcutaneous heparin; Overview of results of randomized trials in general, orthopedic, and urologic surgery. N Engl J Med 318:1162–1173, 1988
95. Hyers TM, Hull RD, Weg JG: Antithrombotic therapy for venous thromboembolic disease. Chest 89:26S–35S, 1986
96. Crystal RG, Gadek JE, Ferrans VJ, Fulmer JD, Line BR, Hunninghake GW: Interstitial lung disease: current concepts of pathogenesis, staging and therapy. Am J Med 70:542–68, 1981
97. National Institute of Health, Division of Lung Diseases, National Heart, Lung, and Blood Institute: Report of Task Force on Epidemiology of Respiratory Diseases. DHHS Publication No. (NIH) 81-2019. Washington, DC: US Government Printing Office, 1980
98. National Institute of Health, Respiratory Diseases Task Force: Report of problems, research, approaches and needs. Oct 1972. DHEW Publication No. (NIH) 76-432
99. United States Department of Health and Human Services: Tenth report of the director, National Heart, Lung and Blood Institute. Vol. 3. Lung Diseases, 1980. DHHS Publication No. (NIH) 84-2358
100. Rosenberg DM: Inherited forms of interstitial lung disease. Clin Chest Med 3:635–641, 1982
101. Bitterman PB, Rennard SI, Keogh BA, Wewers MD, Adelberg S, Crystal RG: Familial idiopathic pulmonary fibrosis: evidence of lung inflammation in unaffected family members. N Engl J Med 314:1343–1348, 1986
102. Musk AW, Zilko PJ, Manners P, Kay PH, Kamboh MI: Genetic studies in familial fibrosing alveolitis: possible linkage with immunoglobulin allotypes. Chest 89:206–210, 1986
103. Becklake MR, Toyota B, Stewart M, Hanson R, Hanley J: Lung structure as a risk factor in adverse pulmonary responses to asbestos exposure: a case-referent study in Quebec chrysotile miners and millers. Am Rev Respir Dis 128:385–388, 1983
104. Morgan DC, Smyth JT, Lister RW, Pethybridge RJ, Gilson JC, Callahan P, Thomas GO: Chest symptoms in farming communities with special reference to farmers' lung. Br J Ind Med 32:228–234, 1975
105. Boyd G, Madkour M, Middleton S, Lynch P: Effect of smoking on circulating antibody levels to avian protein in pigeon breeder's disease. Thorax 32:651, 1977
106. Hance A, Basset F, Soler P, Chollet-Martin S, Danel C, Valeyre D, Battesti JP, Chretien J, Georges R: The role of cigarette smoking in the pathogenesis of pulmonary histiocytosis X. Am Rev Respir Dis 131:A369, 1985
107. Pinsker KL, Schneyer B, Becker N, Kamholz SL: Usual interstitial pneumonia following Texas A2 influenza infection. Chest 80:123–126, 1981
108. Schooley RT, Carey RW, Miller G, Hende W, Eastman R, Mark EJ, Kenyon K, Wheeler EO: Chronic Epstein-Barr virus infection associated with fever and interstitial pneumonitis: clinical and serologic features and response to antiviral chemotherapy. Ann Intern Med 104:636–643, 1986
109. Tablau OC, Milagros PR: Chronic interstitial pulmonary fibrosis following *Mycoplasma pneumoniae* pneumonia. Am J Med 79:268–270, 1985
110. Kales A, Vela-Bueno A, Kales JD: Sleep disorders: sleep apnea and narcolepsy. Ann Intern Med 106:434–443, 1987

111. He J, Kryger MH, Zorick FJ, Conway W, Roth T: Mortality and apnea index in obstructive sleep apnea: experience in 385 male patients. Chest 94:9–14, 1988
112. Partinen M, Jamieson A, Guilleminault C: Long-term outcome for obstructive sleep apnea syndrome patients: Mortality. Chest 94:1200–1204, 1988
113. Schmidt-Nowara WW, Wiggins C, Skipper CE, Samet JM: Prevalence of sleep apnea in a population-based sample of Hispanic American adults. Am Rev Respir Dis 139:A112, 1989
114. Lavie P: Incidence of sleep apnea in a presumably healthy working population: a significant relationship with excessive daytime sleepiness. Sleep 6:312–318, 1983
115. Gonzales-Rothi RJ, Block AJ: Mortality and sleep apnea: the trouble with looking backward (editorial). Chest 94:678–679, 1988

53

Gastrointestinal Tract Disorders

Frank C. Garland
Cedric F. Garland
Edward D. Gorham

This chapter discusses recent advances in the epidemiology and prevention of four diseases of the gastrointestinal tract: duodenal ulcer, gastric ulcer, ulcerative colitis, and Crohn's disease.

There have been major changes in the epidemiology of ulcers in recent years, with a persistent decrease in hospitalization and death rates, and possibly in incidence rates. The decrease was more pronounced in men, and this has therefore resulted in a steep drop in the male to female ratio of incidence and mortality. Epidemiological studies have identified a number of important controllable risk factors such as smoking and exposure to nonsteroidal inflammatory drugs. These studies offer great promise for prevention of ulcers. More speculative associations have emerged as well, including the possibility that deficient endogenous production of various metabolites of arachidonic acid may be a precursor of ulcers, particularly in the stomach.

Chronic disorders of the lower gastrointestinal system were at one time dominated by ulcerative colitis, but the pattern has changed since the 1940s, with an increasing incidence of Crohn's disease. Part of this increase may represent better recognition of Crohn's disease, but most of the increase seems to be real. The rise in incidence rates of Crohn's disease contrasts with rates of ulcerative colitis, which recently has exhibited more stable rates (except in some population groups and regions). Certain peculiarities in incidence rates have emerged, including an apparent spike in 1973 in the incidence of ulcerative colitis in nonwhite women but not in men.

The most prominent feature of recent research is the finding in almost all studies of an inverse association between cigarette smoking and incidence of ulcerative colitis. Although smoking is not suggested as a preventive intervention (the benefit would be easily overwhelmed by increased risk of heart disease and cancer), this association opens up the possibility of better understanding the pathophysiology of ulcerative colitis. Oddly, this effect is not present for Crohn's disease; some studies discussed here have shown that smoking is associated with increased incidence of Crohn's disease.

Perhaps the most revealing paradox in the recent epidemiology of diseases of the digestive system is that factors which are positively associated with risk of peptic ulcers, especially in the stomach (such as cigarette smoking and use of aspirin and aspirin-like agents), are inversely associated with risk of ulcerative colitis.

Smoking inhibits synthesis of certain arachidonic acid metabolites such as leukotriene B_4 and prostaglandin E_2. Recent results suggest that these or other arachidonate metabolites might play a role in both peptic ulcers and ulcerative colitis in opposite directions. Some arachidonate metabolites might help to reduce the risk of gastric (and possibly duodenal) ulcers, but the same or different metabolites could adversely influence the risk of ulcerative colitis. Because synthesis of these compounds is influenced by exogenous factors such as smoking, these findings may be of possible interest in devising strategies for prevention.

GASTRIC AND DUODENAL ULCER

The traditional concepts of the epidemiology of gastric and duodenal ulcer are changing. In 1965, hospitalizations in the United States for duodenal ulcer in men were 3.4 times as frequent as for gastric ulcer; by 1981 hospitalizations for duodenal ulcer had dropped to less than those for gastric ulcer.[1,2] Gastric and duodenal ulcers are now as common in women as in men, for the most part because of the large decrease in rates in men. The male preponderance of mortality from gastric and duodenal ulcers has nearly vanished.

The possible underlying role of prostaglandins has emerged as a promising direction for epidemiological and clinical investigations.[3-7] The mechanism of action for such established risk factors as smoking and aspirin use may be related to the inhibitory effects they exert on synthesis of prostaglandins. The question of an infectious cause has been raised with the observation of the increased frequency of *Campylobacter pylori,* also known as *Helicobacter pylori,* infection in gastric and duodenal ulcers.[8-17]

Consumption of linoleic acid, once rare in the Western diet but now common because of increased consumption of polyunsaturates, has been offered as a possible explanation for the decline in rates of gastric and duodenal ulcers.[18] The role of stress is still elusive. Recent work suggests that stress in ulcer patients may not be a simple function of the burden of lifetime stressful events, but rather a unique reaction to these events that may increase risk in some individuals.[19,20]

A peptic ulcer (duodenal or gastric) is a hole in the mucosa of the digestive tract that extends through the muscularis mucosae into the submucosa and often into the muscularis propria.[21] Gastric and duodenal ulcers have a pathological factor in common: an imbalance between secretion of acid and pepsin by the stomach and the resistance of the duodenal or gastric mucosa. Factors that affect either of these, or both, may lead to ulcer. The differing epidemiology of gastric and duodenal ulcer has made the distinction between the diseases important in studying etiology and considering prospects for prevention and treatment. Diverse environmental and genetic factors contribute to the incidence of the two diseases, but only a few of these factors have been identified epidemiologically.

Trends

During the period 1950 to 1980, age-adjusted mortality rates for gastric and duodenal ulcers decreased dramatically for men and slightly for women in the United States (Fig. 53–1).[1] A large proportion of the decline in men appears to be real, but some of the decline has been attributed to changes in coding of death certificates.[5] After 1960, gastric and duodenal ulcer more often were recorded on death certificates as contributing, rather than underlying, causes of death, as they had been in the 1950s.

The reality of the decline in ulcer disease in the United States is supported by reports from Great Britain that also show a decline in mortality from ulcers over the period 1958 to 1977, with an overall decrease of about 30% for duodenal ulcer and about 34% for gastric ulcer.[23]

Sex Ratios

The notable male preponderance of gastric and duodenal ulcers has decreased over the last 30 years, with a decline in mortality rates for duodenal ulcer from 5.4 in 1950 to 2.3 in 1980 and a decline in mortality rates for gastric ulcer from 4.0 in 1950 to 1.8 in 1980 (Fig. 53–1).[1] Using data provided by the National Center for Health Statistics, Kurata and associates[1] showed that the male to female ratio for ulcer disease declined from 2.8 in 1958 to 1.0 in 1981 (Fig. 53–2).

Rates for hospitalization for duodenal ulcer dropped for both men and women, converging to drop the male to female ratio for hospitalizations from 2.2 in 1965 to 1.8 in 1981 (Fig. 53–3). Hospitalizations for gastric ulcer decreased slightly for men and increased slightly for women. The male to female ratio for gastric ulcer decreased from 1.5 in 1965 to 1.1 in 1981. However, Kurata and associates[2] observed an increase during this time period in two diagnoses closely related to gastric ulcer, gastritis and duodenitis, suggesting that changes over time in diag-

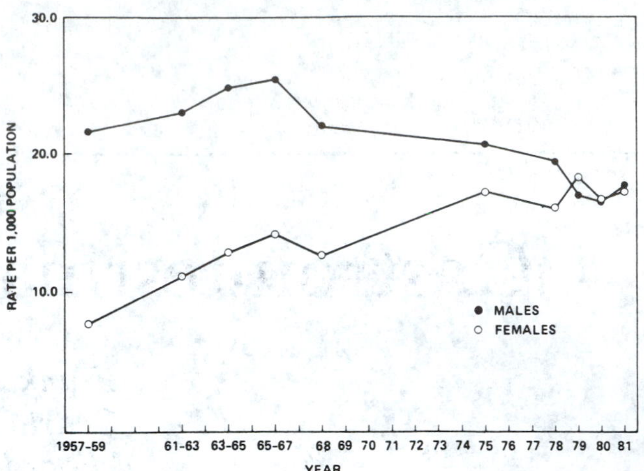

Figure 53–2. One-year period prevalence of ulcer disease in the United States, based on unpublished data from the National Health Interview Survey, National Center for Health Statistics. Prevalence was defined as condition reported as having been present during the year of the interview.[1]

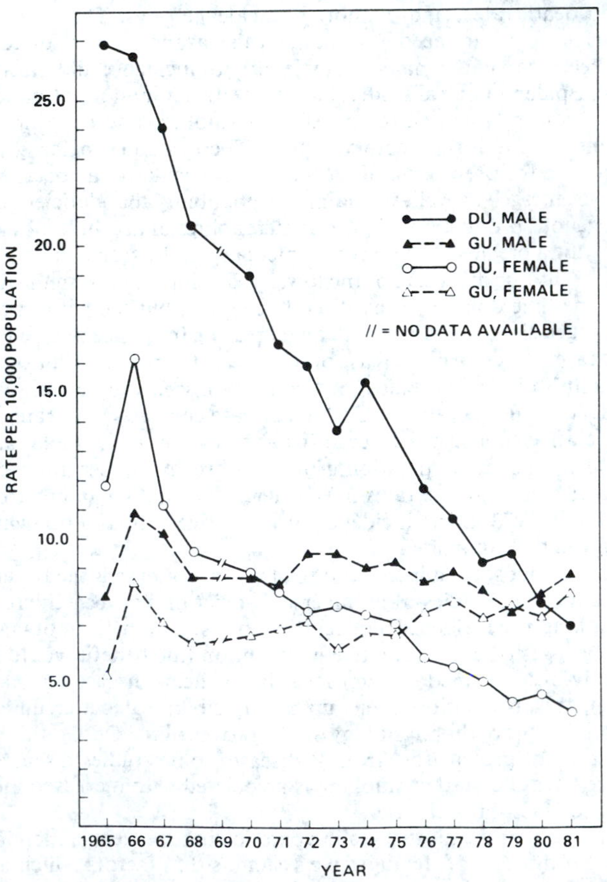

Figure 53–3. Age-adjusted hospitalization rates for gastric and duodenal ulcer as first listed diagnosis, by sex. Rates were calculated using unpublished data provided by the National Hospital Discharge Survey, National Center for Health Statistics.[1]

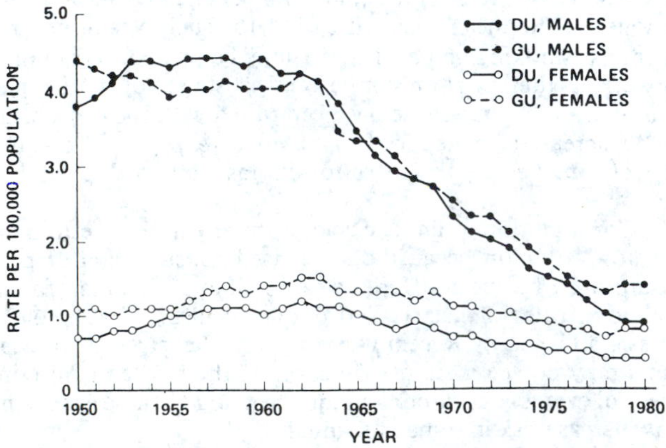

Figure 53–1. Age-adjusted mortality rates of gastric and duodenal ulcer by sex. Data for 1980 are unpublished, from the National Vital Registration System, National Center for Health Statistics.[1]

nostic methods could account for some of the changes in hospitalization rates for duodenal and gastric ulcer.

It has been postulated that the increase of ulcer disease in women may be related to increasing occupational stresses faced by women entering high-stress jobs.[1] However, this does not seem likely because the increasing prevalence in women is primarily in women 65 years old and older, an age group retired from most occupations. The increase in smoking over the past 30 years by women, on the other hand, may be an important factor.[22]

Observations of the decreasing sex ratio and a general decline in hospitalization for ulcer disease also have been made in England and Wales[23] and in West Germany.[24] Hospitalization rates for duodenal ulcer have declined for uncomplicated and hemorrhage-associated forms of the disease. However, the decline in hospitalization for uncomplicated duodenal ulcer was the most dramatic, indicating that either changes in diagnosis occurred to a greater extent in the less severe form of illness or that there was a reduced rate of hospitalization for less severe disease, perhaps because of outpatient or self-treatment.[2] The rate of patients who had perforation did not change markedly from 1970 to 1978.

Hospitalization rates for gastric ulcer over the same period showed no decline overall, nor within categories of severity of disease.[2] These findings suggest that recent changes in diagnosis or treatment have not been a major factor affecting hospitalization for gastric ulcer.

The introduction of cimetidine, a powerful H_2-receptor antagonist marketed in 1977, may have contributed to declining hospitalizations[25,26] and surgery[27-31] for duodenal ulcer. Several double-blind clinical trials in the United States and Great Britain have confirmed the effectiveness of H_2-antagonists in healing of duodenal ulcers in patients with proven ulcer crater.[32-45] The role of H_2-antagonists in gastric ulcer healing is less conclusive.[35,39]

Self-treatment with proprietary antacids also may have played some role in declining rates of hospitalization. Antacids are effective for relief of the symptoms of reflux esophagitis,[40] and very large and frequent doses of antacids also are effective in healing duodenal ulcers associated with hyperacidity.[41,42]

The combination of improved treatment, self-treatment, and the associated decline in definitive diagnostic procedures in uncomplicated cases responding to treatment may have contributed to the marked decline in rates of hospitalization and surgery for duodenal ulcer.

Population-based studies of incidence rates of peptic ulcer are less affected by changes in treatment and diagnosis. Results of these studies are inconsistent, however, and do not resolve whether there has been a decrease in the true incidence of duodenal ulcer, or whether there has been reduced severity, reduced diagnosis, or reduced need for hospitalization.

Risk Factors

Accepted risk factors for peptic ulcer include cigarette smoking, aspirin use, and family history of ulcers. Less conclusive associations have been reported for alcohol and coffee consumption, other dietary factors, infection with *Campylobacter pylori,* prostaglandin disorders, and occupational and emotional stress. The effects of these risk factors by ulcer type are summarized in Table 53–1.

Cigarette Smoking. The mortality rate for peptic ulcer is approximately twice as great among smokers as among nonsmokers, despite the presence of competing risks due to other health effects of smoking.[43-47] Several hospital- and population-based studies indicate that ulcers are also about twice as prevalent among smokers as among nonsmokers.[46-49] a dose-response relationship between peptic ulcers and cigarette exposure, as measured by number of cigarettes smoked, duration of smoking, and inhalation habits, has been established.[50] nicotine and tar levels seem less important predictors of peptic ulcer than the number of cigarettes smoked.[51]

TABLE 53–1. SUMMARY OF RISK FACTORS FOR DUODENAL AND GASTRIC ULCER

	Ulcer Type	
Risk Factor	***Duodenal***	***Gastric***
Cigarette smoking	Increases risk (RR* = 2)[50]; dose response; increases recurrence (RR = 3)[54]; retards healing.[48]	Increases risk (RR = 2)[50]; dose response; increases recurrence (RR = 3); retards healing.
Aspirin use	No established association[66].	Increased risk (RR = 2.0–6.5)
Other nonsteroidal antiinflammatory drugs	Increases risk (RR = 2 to 6) in elderly.[74-76]	Increases risk (RR = 2 to 6), especially in elderly.[50,74-76]
Camplylobacter pylori infection	Cross-sectional association not fully established, RR undetermined.[101-103]	Cross-sectional association established, but RR undetermined.[101-103]
Prostaglandin deficiency, especially prostaglandin E	No epidemiologic studies reported. Case reports and laboratory evidence suggestive of adverse effect of deficiency.[7,118,119]	No epidemiological studies reported. Case reports and laboratory evidence highly suggestive of adverse effect of deficiency.[7,118,119]
Familial aggregation	Increased risk (RR = 3).[122,130]	Increased risk (RR = 3).[122,130]
Alcohol use	No established independent association[48,50] but established association with gastritis and gastric erosion.[81]	No established independent association.[48,50]
Coffee	Equivocal.[48,50,80]	Equivocal.[48,50,80]
Diet	No established association.[81]	No established association.[81]
Emotional stress	No independent association has yet been established.[89]	No independent association has yet been established.[89]
Occupation	Reports of slight excess of peptic ulcer among foremen and executives,[93] air traffic controllers,[90,91] and shift workers.[98]	Reports of slight excess of peptic ulcer among foremen and executives,[93] air traffic controllers,[90,91] and shift workers.[98]

*RR = relative risk.

Several studies demonstrated slower healing of duodenal and gastric ulcer and greater recurrence of ulcers in smokers.[52-54] The effects of treatment with cimetidine and antacids also were diminished in smokers.[43,50,55-57] Gastric acid output is increased by smoking and is dose related,[58-60] and pancreatic bicarbonate output is reduced.[61]

Cigarette exposure also contributes to gastric ulcer by diminishing perfusion of the gastric mucosa.[60,62,63] Pyloric sphincter tone is reduced in smokers, which may cause reflux of bile acids into the stomach.[64]

Nonsteroidal Anti-inflammatory Drugs

Aspirin. Convincing epidemiological associations have been observed for aspirin use and the development of gastric, but not duodenal, ulcer.[48,65-68]

For example, Levy[66] reported a morbidity ratio of 3.4 for gastric ulcer in heavy aspirin users (four or more days a week for the preceding 12 weeks) as compared with control subjects. No association with duodenal ulcer was found. Aspirin damages the gastric mucosa, as shown endoscopically,[67,69,70] even after administration of as little as 600 mg acetylsalicylic acid (two tablets).[67] An endoscopic study of patients with rheumatic disease and no history of peptic ulcer who had been taking aspirin (2.6 g/d) for at least 3 months revealed a very high prevalence of gastric damage.[71]

Other Nonsteroidal Anti-inflammatory Drugs. Other nonsteroidal anti-inflammatory drugs have been implicated in increasing risk for gastric ulcer.[72-75] These drugs, which are prescribed primarily for the treatment of arthritis, include indomethacin and acetaminophen.

In a large case-control study in England, Somerville and associates[74] reported that nonaspirin, nonsteroidal anti-inflammatory drugs were taken more than twice as often by patients with bleeding ulcers as by population controls (estimated relative risk 2.7) or by hospital controls (estimated relative risk 3.8). The effect was present for both gastric and duodenal ulcer and in both men and women. Concurrent aspirin use, smoking, and socioeconomic status did not explain the association.

It had been thought that adrenocorticosteroid therapy also increased the risk of ulcer, bleeding, and perforation.[76] However, in a major review, Conn and Blitzer[77] grouped the findings of 42 controlled studies of 5331 patients involved in investigations of steroids or adrenocorticosteroid therapy and could find no statistically significant associations overall.

Coffee. Conclusive epidemiological evidence does not support the role of coffee in the etiology of peptic ulcer,[48] although physiological studies show that both regular and decaffeinated coffee stimulate excessive gastric acid secretion, increase esophageal reflux,[78] and exacerbate gastrointestinal symptoms (i.e., dyspepsia). Many early epidemiological studies implicating coffee consumption suffered from poor case definition or failure to control for cigarette smoking, which is strongly associated with coffee consumption.[79] A follow-up of Harvard graduates[80] found that habitual coffee consumption in college was the best predictor of peptic ulcer in later life. Information on recent changes in smoking and lifestyle was not available, however. A study of current coffee consumption among 36,656 persons in a large health maintenance organization found no relationship between coffee (or alcohol) use and history of peptic ulcer.[50]

Alcohol. Alcohol ingestion in moderate amounts does not appear to increase peptic ulcer incidence, healing time, or recurrence.[48,50,80] Patients with alcoholic cirrhosis of the liver have an excess risk of peptic ulcer, however.[57] The association between alcohol abuse and gastritis also illustrates the detrimental effect of chronic alcohol exposure on the gastric mucosa.

Physiological studies indicate that concentrated ethanol lowers mucosal resistance to gastric acid, but moderate alcohol intake suppresses gastric acid production.[81] There is no epidemiological rationale for prohibiting moderate alcohol consumption in patients with peptic ulcer.[48,81,82]

Diet and Eating Habits. Although there is no evidence suggesting that a bland diet decreases ulcer incidence, prevents recurrences, or promotes healing,[48] amelioration of symptoms in ulcer patients on a bland diet has been widely recognized.[83,84] A cohort study of Harvard alumni showed that milk consumption in college was inversely related to development of peptic ulcer in later life.[80] Current milk-drinking habits were not examined. Although heavy intake of milk increases gastric acid output 2 to 3 hours after ingestion because of acid rebound,[85] milk drinking has a soothing effect on the gastric mucosa, with relief of symptoms.[83] Because the immediate effects may be more than compensated for by acid rebound,[85] ingestion of milk is not recommended as treatment for peptic ulcer.

Surveys in India, Bangladesh, and South Africa describe elevated incidence of duodenal ulcer in areas with a high starch diet of rice[86] or yams,[87] while regions of low incidence correspond to areas producing wheat or corn. An ecological study in Israel reported a significant inverse association between dietary vitamin A and mortality from peptic ulcer.[88]

Stress and Occupation. It has not been established that psychological factors are causally related to duodenal or gastric ulcer, despite wide belief that they are important.[89] Problems with the study of psychological factors as the cause of ulcer include definition of the theoretical model, definition and measurement of psychological stress, differences in responses of individuals to "stressful" situations, and problems of blinding in experimental design.[89]

One approach to studying the role of stress in the development of ulcer has been to study occupations considered to be stressful. Air traffic controllers have been shown to have moderately elevated rates of peptic ulcer.[90,91] Foremen and executives have a higher frequency of ulcer than expected, possibly related to the role conflicts of middle management.[92,93] These studies were not controlled for cigarette smoking, which is significantly associated with self-reported subjective occupational stress indicators.[94,95] There are marked individual differences in the tendency to increase or decrease cigarette smoking in response to varying levels of stress.[94]

Adami and associates[96] in a case-control study of 132 patients with prepyloric and duodenal ulcers and 132 population controls could find no relationship between ulcers and factors such as personal worries, psychologically demanding job, or other psychiatric or somatic morbidity. Several factors associated with lower socioeconomic status such as low income, low standard of living, and low educational level attained were significantly more common in the patients than in the control subjects, as was smoking.

Sonnenberg and Haas[97] reported that manual labor as compared with sedentary labor carried a 1.6 times greater risk for gastric ulcer ($P < .001$) and a 2 times greater risk ($P < .001$) for duodenal ulcer in a survey of 73,615 German employees receiving occupational health-related medical check ups. Unfortunately, this finding was not adjusted for cigarette smoking or educational levels.

Shift workers in a large study (11,657 subjects) in Japan have been shown by Segawa and associates[98] to be at increased risk for both gastric and duodenal ulcer. For 2269 shift workers the prevalence of gastric ulcer was 2.4/100 (vs 1.4 for daytime workers), and for duodenal ulcer the prevalence was 1.4/100 (vs 0.7 for daytime workers). Segawa and associates postulated that sleep disturbances in shift workers increased ulcer risk. There was no adjustment for cigarette smoking or educational level.

It has been suggested that urbanization is an important factor in the cause of ulcer.[99] Segal and associates[100] studied the effects of urbanization in a controlled study of 100 patients with duodenal ulcer who moved from small towns in South Africa to Soweto and found no clear role for urbanization.

Feldman and associates[20] reported that peptic ulcer was not associated with the number of life events occurring in the previous year. Cross-sectionally, ulcer patients had more negative personality traits such as depression and anxiety and a diminished coping ability. Walker and associates[19] developed a theoretical model linking psychosocial and behavioral risk factors in a multifactorial concept of the cause of ulcer. They suggested that "stress in ulcer patients is not so much a function of their life events as the unique way that they react to these events."[19]

Campylobacter pylori (Helicobacter pylori). Since 1983, when Marshall and Warren[8] first reported *Campylobacter pylori* in gastric aspirates of 58 of 100 patients with gastritis, there has been a renewed interest in the possibility of an infectious etiology for ulcer.[9-14] *C. pylori,* which is also known as *Helicobacter pylori,* is a ubiquitous organism that can be found in normal gastric mucosa.[13] It is sensitive to gastric acidity and lives in mucus and between the mucous layer and the gastric mucosal surface in an area of nearly neutral pH.[15]

To date, epidemiological studies of the association of *C. pylori* and ulcer have been cross-sectional. For example, Nedenskov-Sorensen and associates,[12] in a study of 54 patients referred for upper gastrointestinal endoscopy who had antral biopsies, reported isolation of *C. pylori* significantly more frequently in patients with chronic active gastritis (21 of 25 patients) than in persons with normal mucosa (2 of 20 patients). Only 1 of 10 patients with duodenitis had *C. pylori* isolated. Generally, other investigators have documented an association of *C. pylori* with gastritis,[16,17] but the organism has been more difficult to find in duodenal tissue.[17] Yardley and Paull[14] have reviewed the work of nine investigative teams around the world and conclude that there is without exception a high degree of correlation between *C. pylori* and the presence of gastritis. However, these reviewers found the association with peptic ulcers much less clear.

Prostaglandins. Recent studies suggest that prostaglandins may play an important role in ulcers. Some risk factors for ulcer disease may be mediated by prostaglandins, and dietary changes affecting prostaglandin status may explain some of the decline in incidence and mortality rates.

Of the seven naturally occurring human prostaglandins, it is mainly the E-type (PGE) that exerts effects which inhibit ulcer development or promote its healing.[3,4] E-series prostaglandins, especially PGE_2, exert an antisecretory effect on parietal cells, inhibit gastric acid secretion,[104,105] stimulate bicarbonate production,[4] and possibly increase resistance of the gastroduodenal mucosa.[106,107] It has been hypothesized that both gastric and duodenal ulcer could be prostaglandin-deficiency diseases.[108] Synthetic forms of the hormone can reduce gastric acidity and may become useful in treating gastric[6] or duodenal[109] ulcer.

Interestingly, prostaglandins may have some relationship to established risk factors for ulcers, such as cigarette smoking and aspirin use. Cigarette smoking decreases the concentration of prostaglandins in the lumen of the stomach.[110] Prostaglandins also have been shown to protect the gastric mucosa of rats challenged with ethanol,[111-113] and chronic ethanol feeding of rats reduces tissue levels of PGE in the stomach.[114] The ability of aspirin and other necrotizing agents to induce gastric lesions in rats also was inhibited by prostaglandin administration.[115,116] Effects on prostaglandins may be an underlying mechanism through which cigarette smoking and use of aspirin increase risk of ulcer. Unfortunately, no large population-based surveys of prostaglandin status and ulcer incidence have been reported.

Clinical trials of orally administered synthetic prostaglandins have shown that these compounds can increase the healing rates of both gastric and duodenal ulcers.[6,109,117] Hollander and Tarnawski[18] have pointed out that the recent decline in ulcer disease has corresponded with an increase in linoleic acid consumption (Fig. 53-4), which is a consequence of increased use of vegetable oils. Vegetable oils are extremely rich in linoleic acid, a precursor of prostaglandins.

Genetics

Familial aggregation of peptic ulcer has been demonstrated repeatedly,[120-123] and associations with genetic markers such as blood group and secretory status are well established.[124,125] A simple mendelian inheritance pattern does not exist for all ulcer disease, however. Polygenic inheritance has been proposed,[126] but the hypothesis of genetic heterogeneity seems to better fit the observed inheritance patterns. The genetic heterogeneity hypothesis implies that peptic ulcer results from a group of distinct diseases with different etiologies and pathological mechanisms, each having both genetic and environmental components.[127-129] This concept does not preclude polygenic inheritance as one of a number of inheritance patterns.[130]

The first evidence from familial aggregation studies indicating that peptic ulcer is a group of disorders was described by Doll and Kellock in 1951.[120] They showed that first-degree relatives of patients with gastric ulcer have a threefold excess risk for gastric ulcer but no increased risk for duodenal ulcer. Similarly, first-degree relatives of patients with duodenal ulcer had a threefold excess risk for duodenal, but not gastric, ulcer. These disease-spe-

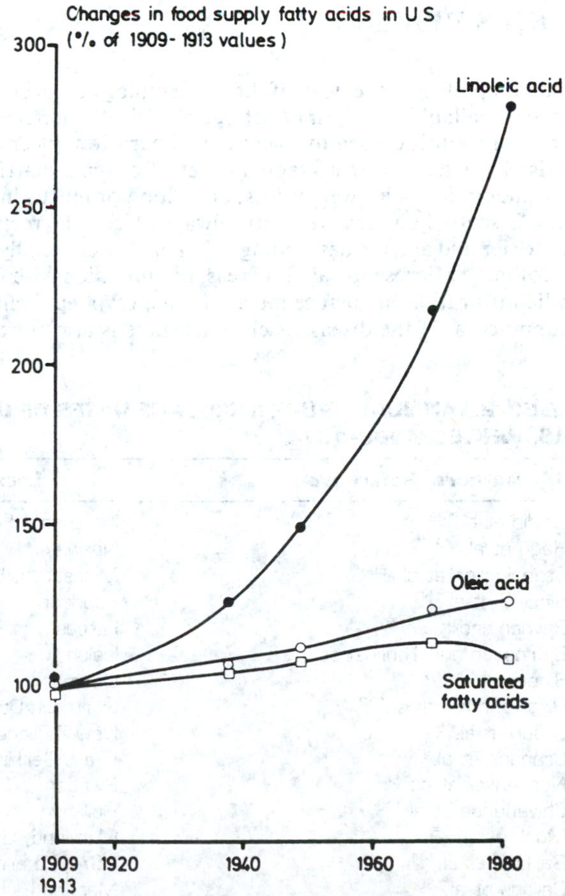

Figure 53-4. Changes in the dietary availability of linoleic and oleic acids and saturated fatty acids, United States, 1909–1980. Data are expressed as percent change from the 1909–1913 figures, which are taken as 100%.[18]

cific inheritance patterns suggest that different genetic traits influence the occurrence of the two diseases.

Further evidence for a genetic basis of familial aggregation comes from twin studies. The concordance for ulcer among monozygotic twin pairs is greater than for dizygotic twins.[131] Overall, genetic studies suggest that peptic ulcers are a number of different diseases that differ in pathogenesis and that confer differing susceptibility among individuals to environmental factors.[132,133]

Summary

Gastric and duodenal ulcers share some common pathological features; however, differing time trends in incidence, risk factors, inheritance patterns, pathogenesis, and treatment have established that duodenal and gastric ulcer are separate entities.

The dramatic decline in duodenal and gastric ulcer in the United States and elsewhere is largely unexplained. The identification of a pathogen associated with gastritis and possibly with gastric and duodenal ulcer opens up new possibilities for prevention and treatment.

The importance of reducing smoking in the prevention of ulcer cannot be overstated. All anti-inflammatory drugs currently in popular use must be prescribed with the realization that they have at least the same potential as aspirin for increasing the risk of peptic ulcers.

ULCERATIVE COLITIS AND CROHN'S DISEASE

Recent, comprehensive reviews of the epidemiology of ulcerative colitis are available.[134-140] First distinguished in the nineteenth century from colitis caused by bacteria and parasites, ulcerative colitis is characterized by a gradual onset of chronic diarrhea, colicky abdominal pain, weight loss, and blood or mucus in the stool.[134] Essentially ulcerative colitis always affects the rectum, often the sigmoid and the descending colon, and occasionally the entire colon.[134] Microscopically, there is inflammation with neutrophilic infiltration of surface mucosal cells, crypt epithelium, and submucosa. If the disease is chronic, there is also fibrosis. Detailed diagnostic guidelines have been published.[141,142] Because ulcerative colitis is an uncommon disease, most of the results described here were based on small numbers of cases. The differences reported should be considered as indicative of general trends or patterns, rather than as findings that have reached a particular criterion of statistical significance because most have not. Also, unless otherwise specified, all incidence rates are crude rates.

Ulcerative colitis is a disease of public health importance because it strikes early in life in otherwise healthy people,[141] it is difficult to treat successfully,[143,144] with a cumulative 20-year operation rate of 26%,[145] and it is a major predisposing factor to cancer of the colon.[146,147]

Incidence

The highest reported annual incidence rate of ulcerative colitis was in the North Tees district in England, 15.1 per 100,000 population (1971–1977).[148] Elsewhere, incidence rates were highest in Norway,[149] Scotland,[150] England,[151] Wales,[152] Holland,[153] Sweden,[154] Iceland,[155] the Faroes,[156] New Zealand,[157] Canada,[158] and the northern United States.[159] Intermediate rates were found in the mid-to southern United States[141,160] and in Israel.[161,162] Low rates were found in Mediterranean countries such as Italy[163] and Greece[164]; rates were also low in South Africa (in whites, colored, and blacks)[165] and in Kuwait.[166] Japan had the lowest reported incidence rate, 0.5/100,000 population,[167] despite a national research program dedicated to the ascertainment of cases of inflammatory bowel disease. The highest incidence rate, in England, was 32 times the rate in Japan.

With two notable exceptions, the incidence of ulcerative colitis appears to vary directly with latitude. The highest reported rates generally occur in areas distant from the equator (Table 53-2). The exceptions are Japan, as noted previously, which is between 31° and 45° N and has the lowest known incidence rate, and Israel, which is at 32° N, and has rates similar to those in West Germany (51° N) and New Zealand (41° S). Summary tables of incidence rates also appear in the reviews by Calkins and Mendeloff[134] and Mayberry.[135]

The geographic distribution of ulcerative colitis is highly similar to that of colorectal cancer[168]; both diseases vary directly with latitude, and both are uncommon in Japan.[167]

The apparent latitude gradient in incidence of ulcerative co-

TABLE 53-2. ANNUAL CRUDE INCIDENCE RATES OF ULCERATIVE COLITIS PER 100,000 POPULATION, SELECTED AREAS, WHITES, 1960–1974*

Authors, Reference	Location	Period	Incidence Rate
Devlin et al.[148]	Northeast England	1971–77	15.1
Haug et al.[149]	Norway	1984–85	14.8
Stonnington et al.[159]	Minnesota, USA	1960–79	13.6
Sinclair et al.[150]	Scotland	1967–76	11.3
Berner and Kiær[156]	Faroes	1983	10.7
Bjϕrnsson and Thorgeirsson[155]	Iceland	1980	7.4
Binder et al.[187]	Denmark	1962–78	7.3
Hiatt and Kaufman[172]	Northern California, USA	1971–82	5.5
Eason et al.[157]	New Zealand [whites]	1969–78	5.4
Brandes et al.[270]	West Germany	1962–75	5.1
Nordenvall et al.[154]	Sweden	1975–79	4.3
Shivananda et al.[173]	Holland	1979–83	3.6
Monk et al.[175]	Maryland, USA	1960–63	3.5
Garland et al.[141]	USA [15 areas]	1973	3.5
Calkins et al.[160]	Maryland, USA	1977–79	2.4
LaFranchi et al.[163]	Italy	1972–73	1.9
Al-Nakib et al.[166]	Kuwait	1984	1.4
Utsunomiya et al.[174]	Japan	1974	0.5

*Further detail on incidence in Jewish populations is provided in Table 53-3.

litis has not always been evident. For example, early reports of incidence of ulcerative colitis in Oxford, England, published in 1965, indicated an annual incidence rate of 6.5/100,000 population,[169] while the incidence rate reported in Norway in 1964 was only 2.0/100,000 population.[170] It appears that the rates in high-latitude countries such as Norway have climbed steeply since the 1960s.[171] The rise is especially evident in western Norway; northeastern Scotland, including the Orkney and Shetland Islands[150]; and in the Faroes, where the incidence rate rose from 2.1/100,000 population in 1964–1968 to 12.8 in 1979–1983 ($P < .01$).[156]

Incidence Rates in Jews. Incidence rates in the Jewish population show a wide range of variation (Table 53-3). In London in 1950, Paulley[178] first reported that the rate of ulcerative colitis in Jews was twice that of non-Jews. Acheson[179] later reported that four times more Jews than would be expected from the general population were discharged with a diagnosis of ulcerative colitis (and Crohn's disease) from Veterans Administration hospitals.[179] In Baltimore the incidence rate observed in the Jewish population was the highest ever reported in people of Jewish ancestry[175] and was about four times the incidence in the non-Jewish population.[180] The low rates in Israel are consistent with the latitude effect generally present for ulcerative colitis, but the high rates in Cape Town[165] are not consistent with the latitude pattern.

Trends in Incidence Rates. International secular trends in incidence of ulcerative colitis have been reviewed in detail.[160] The only longitudinal incidence data from the early half of the twentieth century are from Rochester, Minnesota,[181] where the age-adjusted incidence rate for ulcerative colitis doubled between 1935 and 1964, and from Czechoslovakia, where occurrence of ulcerative colitis also appears to have increased from 1935 to 1963.[182]

The principal recent data on trends in incidence rates of ulcerative colitis in the United States are from the Baltimore, Maryland, Standard Metropolitan Statistical Area (SMSA).[160] Annual age-adjusted incidence rates of ulcerative colitis in whites, estimated from first hospitalizations, were stable at 5.0/100,000 population in 1960–1963 and 5.1/100,000 population in 1973 but dropped to 2.3/100,000 population by 1977–1979.[160] The incidence rates in all three periods were obtained using the same diagnostic criteria and research protocols, and the medical records were reviewed by the same gastroenterologist. A review of cases from earlier periods showed that the decline in incidence rates was not due to the classification of a higher proportion of chronic colitis cases as Crohn's colitis during 1977–1979. It is possible that some of the apparent decline could have been due to increased management of mild but definite cases outside hospitals, but there are no data available to support this possibility. Trends were similar in men and women.

Age-adjusted annual incidence rates in nonwhite men in Baltimore dropped from 1.0/100,000 population in 1960–1963 to 0.7 in 1973 and then rose slightly to 1.3 in 1977–1979. The incidence rate in nonwhite women rose from 1.7 in 1960–1963 to 4.1 in 1973, then dropped slightly to 2.9 in 1977–1979.

TABLE 53-3. ANNUAL CRUDE INCIDENCE RATES OF ULCERATIVE COLITIS PER 100,000 JEWISH POPULATION, SELECTED AREAS, 1961–1984.

Wright et al.[165]	Cape Town, South Africa	1980–84	17.0
Monk et al.[175]	Maryland, USA	1960–63	13.0
Jacobsohn et al.[176]	Jerusalem, Israel	1973–80	6.3
Odes et al.[161]	Beer Sheva, Israel	1980–84	5.8
Gilat T et al.[177]	Tel-Aviv, Israel	1961–70	3.7

Only limited data on incidence rates are available elsewhere. Hiatt and Kaufman[172] reported stable first hospitalization rates for ulcerative colitis (and Crohn's disease) in a large northern California group practice during the period 1971–1982.

In Oxford, England there was a report that hospitalizations for ulcerative colitis per 100,000 population increased 72% between January 1974 and December 1983.[183] A report from a Japanese teaching hospital stated that rates remained stable at their characteristically low levels between 1954 and 1974.[184]

Migrant studies. The incidence of ulcerative colitis, like that of colon cancer, appears to be influenced by migration. For example, the incidence of ulcerative colitis was twice as high in Jews who migrated to Israel from Europe and the United States as in Jews born in Israel; the difference was most pronounced from ages 15 through 29 years, when the incidence rate in migrant Jews was three times that of resident Jews.[162] The high incidence of ulcerative colitis at these ages accounts for most of the difference between natives of Israel and those who migrated there. The vanishing difference between incidence rates of the two populations at older ages parallels the time-dependent reduction in estimated relative risk of colon cancer in new yorkers who migrated to Florida.[185] Studies performed to date cannot rule out the possibility that the observed differences might be due, at least in part, to genetic differences. A recent study of ancestry of Jews in the United States revealed that those of central European ancestry were more likely to develop ulcerative colitis (and Crohn's disease) than those of Russian or Polish ancestry.[186] However, genetic factors would not explain the similar incidence rates at older ages in migrants to Israel and natives.

RISK FACTORS

Age. Incidence of ulcerative colitis generally peaks at ages 25 through 35 years and again at ages 70 and older. Most studies of ulcerative colitis have reported bimodal age incidence,[141,148,160,161,175,187] although some studies have reported a unimodal pattern.[169,188,189]

In some areas and periods, such as early reports from Denmark[190] and more recent reports from the Faroes,[156] there appears to be a bimodal pattern in women but a unimodal pattern in men, although small sample sizes preclude a definite assessment of the data from the Faroes. Later reports from Denmark observed a bimodal pattern in both sexes.[187]

The most prominent bimodal pattern of incidence has been reported from the United States, with incidence peaks at approximately ages 25 and 75 years in men, and at 35 years and again in later life in women (Fig. 53-5).[141] By contrast, rates of first hospital admissions for ulcerative colitis per 10,000 members of a group health plan during 1971–1982 increased steadily with age in men, peaking at ages 75 and older, with the possibility of a minor early age peak at age 35 years in women and other peaks at ages 55 and 75 and older (Fig. 53-6).[171]

The most recent U.S. study, by Calkins et al.,[160] reported prominent peaks at about age 25 and 65 years in men and 35 and 70 years and above in women. A similar bimodal age distribution has been observed in multiple sclerosis.[191]

Seasonality. Self-reported relapses of ulcerative colitis have a distinct seasonality, with the greatest occurrence in fall and winter (Fig. 53-7).[192] However, admissions to emergency rooms for ulcerative colitis in Oxford, England, showed no indication of seasonality.[183]

Trauma. A case of ulcerative colitis has been described in a water skier who fell from his skis at nearly 70 km/h, wearing a

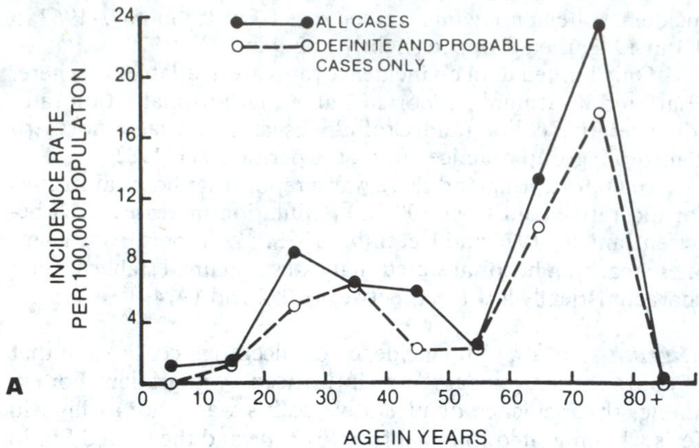

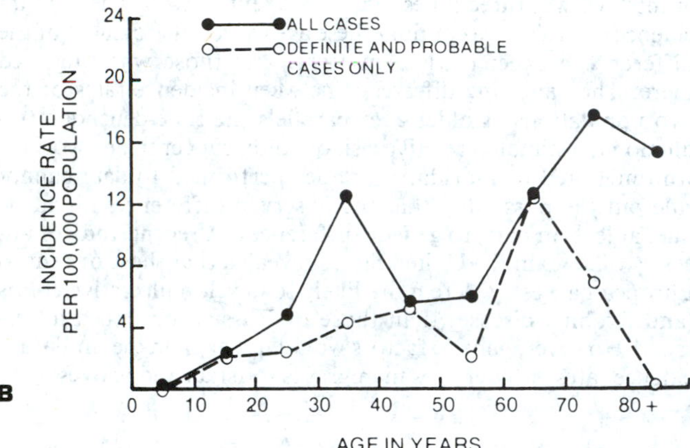

Figure 53-5. Annual age-specific incidence rates of ulcerative colitis per 100,000 population, 15 areas of the United States, 1973. **A.** White males. **B.** White females.[141]

thin bathing suit.[193] The individual was a 20-year-old man in good health, who initially reported a strong pain and surge of water into the rectum moments after taking the spill.[193] Generally, however, reports of any association between trauma and ulcerative colitis are extremely rare.

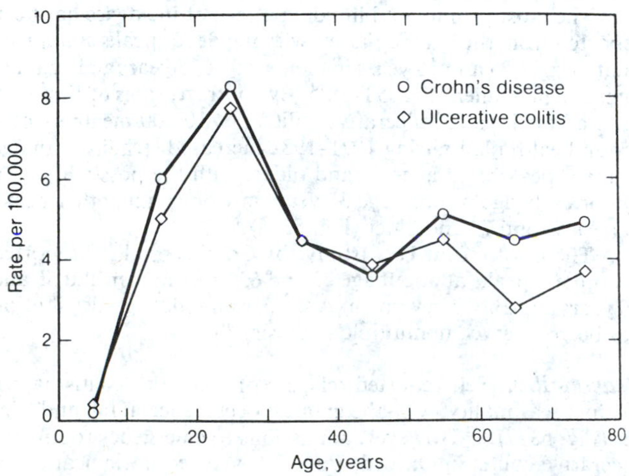

Figure 53-6. Age-specific rates of first hospitalization in the Northern California Kaiser-Permanente Medical Care Program, based on 868 cases, 1971–1982.[171]

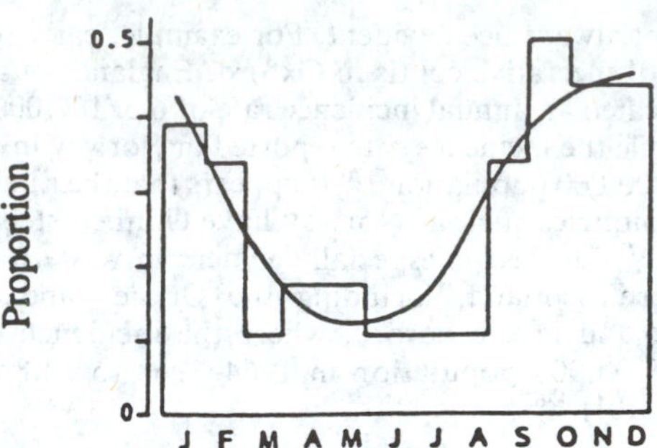

Figure 53-7. Proportion of ulcerative colitis patients in London self-reporting each month as a period when their disease was worse.[192]

Smoking. Since Heatley et al.[194] and Harries et al.[195] noticed that there were few patients with ulcerative colitis who were current smokers of cigarettes, a number of case-control studies have verified these observations.[196–214] The inverse association is strong. One study reported an odds ratio of 0.16 (95% confidence interval, 0.09 to 0.29) for current smokers at time of diagnosis compared with those who never smoked.[209] An analysis of 12 case-control studies reported a Mantel-Haenszel odds ratio of 0.25 ($P < .01$) in current smokers compared with nonsmokers.[213] The effect was also strong for smoking at the time of first diagnosis, with an odds ratio of 3.5 for nonsmokers compared to ever-smokers (95% confidence interval, 1.5 to 8.0).

In several studies it was noted that former smokers were at higher risk for ulcerative colitis than those who had never smoked or those who smoked currently.[202,207,208] One major study, based on patients in a large group practice, reported an odds ratio of 2.0 (95% confidence interval, 1.1 to 3.7) for former smokers compared with those who never smoked.[212] Another case-control study, from Italy, reported a multivariate-adjusted odds ratio of 2.7 (95% confidence interval, 1.5 to 4.9) for former smokers compared with nonsmokers.[208] A meta-analysis of 12 case-control studies reported a Mantel-Haenszel odds ratio of 1.33 for former smokers compared with those who never smoked ($P < .01$).[213] However, some studies showed former smokers to be at similar or only slightly higher risk than those who never smoked. Other studies showed associations that were not statistically significant.[209,210]

The association between not smoking and ulcerative colitis is strong and highly reproducible, suggesting that there is an agent in tobacco smoke that reduces the incidence and severity of ulcerative colitis. The agent has not yet been identified. However, advising smoking in an effort to prevent or treat ulcerative colitis would be unwise, because the incidence of lung cancer and heart disease would be increased by such a maneuver. No clinical trials of nicotinic acid or niacinamide for ulcerative colitis appear to have been reported in the literature.

A negative association also has been reported between smoking and colorectal cancer in several studies, including the Framingham, Massachusetts, heart study[215] and a 19-year prospective study of men in Chicago.[216] The results in the Chicago study did not achieve statistical significance, however.

Studies showing an inverse association between smoking and ulcerative colitis are interesting from a pathophysiological perspective. Nicotine is metabolized to its first metabolite, cotinine, through a pathway that requires arachidonic acid.[217] Arachidonic acid is a precursor of leukotriene B_4, which is elevated in the neutrophils of patients with ulcerative colitis and Crohn's disease[218] and in rectal dialysate of patients with ulcerative colitis but not colitis due to *Clostridium difficile* or Crohn's disease (except in cases of the latter with rectal ulcers).[219] Leukotriene B_4 is the major inflammatory metabolite of arachidonic acid 5-lipooxygenation, and it is the most important chemotactic agent for neutrophils in ulcerative colitis.[220,221] Leukotriene B_4 may contribute to the perpetuation of the inflammation and tissue destruction of ulcerative colitis.[222] The chemotactic response of neutrophils in inflammatory bowel disease in vitro is blocked by antisera to leukotriene B_4.[221]

It has been observed that 5-lipooxygenation is the main route of metabolism of arachidonic acid in polymorphonuclear leukocytes.[223] Arachidonic acid also is metabolized by a cyclooxygenase pathway to PGE_2 and other eicosanoids that promote inflammation in the intestine.[222] Release of PGE_2 also is associated with increased intestinal transport of electrolytes,[222] which, if protracted at abnormally enhanced levels, may be a precursor of colonic malignancy.[224] However, because indomethacin inhibits the cyclooxygenase pathway only,[225] leaving the synthesis of leukotriene B_4 intact, its inability to mitigate ulcerative colitis[226] suggests that it is the lipooxygenase pathway and not the cyclooxygenase pathway that is dominant in maintaining the inflammation associated with ulcerative colitis. Interestingly, a marked decline in synthesis of leukotriene B_4 has been reported following treatment of ulcerative colitis patients with prednisolone.[222] Two important agents in treatment of inflammatory bowel disease, sulfasalazine and 5-amino-salicylic acid, inhibit synthesis of the colonic 5-lipooxygenase product leukotriene B_4 and cyclooxygenase products such as prostaglandin E_2, respectively.[226]

Person-to-Person Transmission. Presently there is no evidence of person-to-person horizontal or vertical transmission of ulcerative colitis. Although there are rare reports of spouse pairs concordant for the disease,[227] no such pairs have been reported from large population-based studies of inflammatory bowel disease, which have included thousands of married couples.[141,171] The occurrence of ulcerative colitis (or Crohn's disease) in spouses of patients appears to be no more common than would be expected on the basis of chance.[228,229] Mother-child case pairs are no more common than other pairs of equal consanguinity,[230] suggesting that vertical transmission is uncommon or nonexistent.

There is no evidence of time or space clustering of either ulcerative colitis or Crohn's disease,[231,232] although a lymphocytotoxic antibody was reported to occur at higher levels in household contacts of patients than in relatives of equal consanguinity living outside the household.[233] There is no known relationship between any particular species of *Mycobacterium* and ulcerative colitis.[234] Attempts to culture acid-fast bacteria from tissues recovered the organisms from 9 of 19 (47%) patients with ulcerative colitis and from 18 of 27 (67%) control subjects who were free of inflammatory bowel disease. A major international case-control study of ulcerative colitis and Crohn's disease in patients who had onset of the disease before age 20 years showed that there had been no increased contact with animals or with other persons who had ulcerative colitis or other diseases. In addition, no correlation was shown with birth order, number of siblings, or a history of having been breast-fed.[235]

Genetic Factors. Genetic factors in ulcerative colitis have been reviewed previously.[134,229,230] From a genetic viewpoint, ulcerative colitis and Crohn's disease sometimes behave as a single disease.[230] The incidence of ulcerative colitis or Crohn's disease in close family members of patients (parents, siblings, or children) with inflammatory bowel disease has been reported as two to three times the expected rate. This estimate may be high, however, because some studies have accepted unvalidated reports of inflammatory bowel disease in relatives.[231] Incidence of inflammatory bowel disease appears to decrease with decreasing consanguinity to the patient.[229] Sixteen identical twin pairs in which at least one twin had ulcerative colitis were identified among 25,000 same-sex pairs in the Swedish twin registry, based on a central national diagnosis registry. Only one of the twins was concordant for the disease.[236] Twenty pairs of same-sex fraternal twins in which at least one twin had ulcerative colitis were identified, but there were no pairs in which both twins had the disease. Discordance between twins was not accounted for by differences in smoking habits.

Despite the tendency for inflammatory bowel disease to occur in families, 60% to 90% of patients have no first-degree relative with the disease,[237] and pedigree studies have failed to detect any known mendelian pattern.[230] Rapid variations in incidence of ulcerative colitis[135,149,160] suggest that although it is likely that a genetic predisposition to the disease exists, environmental factors must largely control incidence.

Religion. Although original reports suggested only a mild elevation in risk in the Jewish population,[238] a study of veterans[239] and a large-scale, population-based study reported relative risks of 3 to 4 times for ulcerative colitis in Jews compared to non-Jews.[240] A similar excess of ulcerative colitis prevalence is present in Mormons in the United Kingdom, compared to non-Mormons in the United Kingdom.[241] The excess incidence in Jews was present for both ulcerative colitis and Crohn's disease,[175] while the excess prevalence rate in Mormons was greater for ulcerative colitis (estimated Mormon/non-Mormon prevalence ratio = 4.9, $P < .0001$) than for Crohn's disease (estimated Mormon/non-Mormon prevalence ratio = 1.8, not significant).[241] This suggests that the predisposition in Jews might be due to an environmental or dietary practice or to a genetic factor more common in Jews and common to ulcerative colitis and Crohn's disease. For example, ulcerative colitis was more common among Jews of Occidental rather than Oriental birth, who differed in genetic background, diet, and latitude of origin.[242] Conversely, the incidence in Mormons may be more closely associated with rules prohibiting smoking or with dietary practices. In Utah only 10% of Mormon men and 5% of Mormon women smoked, compared with 35% and 38%, respectively, in non-Mormons in Utah.[243]

Mormon religious doctrine[244] recommends a diet including fresh fruits and vegetables and prohibits alcohol, coffee, and tea. Moderation in intake of meat is recommended. Although not all Mormons are faithful to the recommendations, it is of interest that despite their high risk of ulcerative colitis, members of the religion are apparently at low risk for appendicitis, with only 3% of British Mormons reporting having had an appendectomy,[241] compared with 12% of the non-Mormon population during roughly the same period.[245] Mormons in Utah have been reported to have a 37% lower incidence rate of colon cancer than the U.S. incidence rate.[246] Despite the lower prevalence rate of smoking in Mormons, the prevalence of Crohn's disease was slightly but nonsignificantly increased.[241]

Psychological Factors. The influence of psychological factors on ulcerative colitis has been reviewed.[140] Case-control studies have reported no correlation between the number of stressful life events and incidence of the disease, either in children[235] or in adults.[247] Although an early report[248] suggested the existence of an obsessive-compulsive, dependent personality type with restricted interpersonal relationships, more recent studies have reported no personality traits that reliably differentiate people who get ulcerative colitis from the unaffected population or from individuals with Crohn's disease.[140]

Oral Contraceptives. The incidence of ulcerative colitis appears to be about twice as high in users of oral contraceptives as in control subjects, but the small number of cases in reported series[207,249,250] and lack of statistical significance prevents a definite conclusion. Cases of ulcerative colitis or a syndrome that closely mimics it have been reported to improve on discontinuation of oral contraceptives.[251-253]

Environmental Factors. Populations with low incidence rates of ulcerative colitis generally have low incidence rates of colon and breast cancer. These include the populations of Japan,[167] China,[254] Greece,[164] black South Africans,[255] and New Zealand Maoris.[189] This suggests the possibility that environmental factors, including diet, may be important in ulcerative colitis. Although ulcerative colitis is rare in black South Africans, it is more common in black women in Baltimore than in white women.[160] However, black South Africans are of considerably different geographic origin than most American blacks, and genetic differences in susceptibility cannot be ruled out. On the other hand, the 3.5-fold increase in age-adjusted incidence of ulcerative colitis in black women in Baltimore between 1963 and 1973, if real, suggests an environmental factor introduced to black women but not to black men after 1963. Ulcerative colitis was rare in people of Asian ancestry in a prepaid medical group in northern California, suggesting the possibility of a genetic contribution to the low incidence in Asian countries.[171]

Diet. Dietary studies of ulcerative colitis and Crohn's disease have been reviewed.[256] Either a life-style factor more common in people of Jewish ancestry or a genetic predisposition is apparently associated with high incidence of ulcerative colitis, but specific dietary factors have not been identified,[240] and most dietary studies have been negative.[134] There is little evidence to date that dietary deficiency of insoluble fiber is a factor in ulcerative colitis, however, or in Crohn's disease. The people of Japan, who consume polished rice in preference to that containing bran, consume little insoluble fiber yet have the lowest known incidence rate of ulcerative colitis.[167] The hospitalization rate for ulcerative colitis in a teaching hospital in Japan remained stable at extremely low levels during 1954 to 1974, suggesting that the partial Westernization of the Japanese diet has not increased the incidence of the disease.[184] Intake of saturated fat also may not explain the geographic pattern, since New Zealand Maoris, in whom ulcerative colitis is rare,[189] appear to consume a large proportion of calories as saturated fat.[257] Intake of coffee is unrelated to risk of ulcerative colitis.[258] In people who have never smoked, decreased risk of ulcerative colitis has been reported in association with increased intake of alcohol.[258]

Cancer Risk

It has been known since 1925 that ulcerative colitis increases the risk of colorectal cancer.[259] The association has been reviewed recently in extensive detail,[146,260] and reports of incidence rates from a number of recent series are available.[261,262] A large private practice in the United States reported an incidence rate of colorectal cancer in ulcerative colitis of 7% at 26 years of age and 11% at 32 years after onset.[147]

Patients with extensive disease or with longer than a 10-year duration were at highest risk for colorectal cancer.[146] These results suggest that patients with ulcerative colitis should have colonoscopy every 1 or 2 years, with biopsies every 10 cm, including samples from normal-appearing mucosa. Although colonoscopic surveillance is recommended for patients with ulcerative colitis, colectomy may become necessary if malignancy or multifocal or persistent high-grade dysplasia is detected.[146]

Prevention

There is no known way to prevent ulcerative colitis. Attentive medical care can relieve many symptoms, minimize complications, and allow detection of colorectal cancer while it is still localized.[146] Avoidance of oral contraceptives might reduce the incidence of ulcerative colitis or of a syndrome that may mimic it. Future studies should consider whether restriction of intake of dietary arachidonic acid and its precursors such as linoleic acid, which occurs primarily in vegetable oils, might reduce incidence rates. Alternatively, increased dietary intake of nutrients that inhibit synthesis of prostaglandins may be of preventive value. These include eicosapentaenoic and docosahexaneoic fatty acids, which are present in some fatty marine fish.

CROHN'S DISEASE

Incidence rates of Crohn's disease recently have been reviewed recently.[134,135] The highest incidence rates of Crohn's disease are in the United States (Table 53-4). The rate in Spokane, Washington, is 35 times the rate in Japan, which has the lowest known incidence rate of Crohn's disease, as it does of ulcerative colitis.

Trends in incidence rates of Crohn's disease have been reviewed in detail previously, and a clear rise in incidence is evident in most studies.[134] Notably, the age-adjusted incidence rate increased 200% in Olmsted County, Minnesota, between 1945 and 1975.[269]

Incidence in Baltimore, Maryland, of Crohn's disease in white males rose from 2.6/100,000 population in 1960–1963 to 3.9 in 1973 but then declined slightly to 3.4 in 1977–1979; in white females, incidence rose from 1.3/100,000 population in 1960–1963 to 3.6 in 1973, remaining at approximately that level in 1977–1979.[160]

Crohn's disease, like ulcerative colitis, has a bimodal age distribution in most series.[134,141] Despite a persistent search for contributing factors, no risk factors other than family history,[230] a positive association with smoking,[201] and Jewish religion[179] have been identified. There is a possible adverse effect of oral contraceptives.[249]

TABLE 53-4. ANNUAL CRUDE INCIDENCE RATES OF CROHN'S DISEASE PER 100,000 POPULATION, SELECTED AREAS, WHITES (UNLESS OTHERWISE NOTED)

Authors, Reference	Location	Period	Incidence Rate
Nunes and Ahlquist[263]	USA (Washington State)	1981	8.8
Lee and Costello[264]	England (Blackpool)	1968–80	6.6
Garland et al.[141]	USA (15 areas)	1973	4.5
Dirks et al.[265]	West Germany	1980–84	4.1
Gollop et al.[266]	USA (Minnesota)	1943–82	4.0
Calkins et al.[160]	USA (Baltimore, white)	1977–79	3.5
Calkins et al.[160]	USA (Baltimore, nonwhite)	1977–79	2.7
Berner and Kiær[156]	Faroes	1964–83	1.9
Krawiec et al.[267]	Israel (Beer Sheva)	1976–80	1.8
Kimura et al.[268]	Japan	1980–81	0.25

Prevention

There is no known means of prevention of Crohn's disease, except possibly for avoidance of cigarette smoking and use of oral contraceptives. Future studies should consider whether limiting dietary intake of arachidonic acid or its precursors such as linoleic acid, which is found primarily in certain commercial vegetable (seed) oils, may have preventive value. As with ulcerative colitis, studies are needed to discover whether increased dietary intake of long-chain fatty acids, which inhibit synthesis of leukotrienes and prostanoids, may be of preventive value.

REFERENCES

1. Kurata JH, Haile BM, Elashoff JD: Sex differences in peptic ulcer disease. Gastroenterology 88:96–100, 1985
2. Kurata JH, Elashoff JD, Haile BM, Honda GD: A reappraisal of time trends in ulcer disease: Factors related to changes in ulcer hospitalization and mortality rates. Am J Public Health 73:1066–1072, 1983
3. Wilson ED: Prostaglandins in peptic ulcer disease. Postgrad Med 81:309–316, 1987
4. Aly A: Prostaglandins in the clinical treatment of gastroduodenal mucosal lesions: A review. Scand J Gastroenterol (suppl) 137:43–49, 1987
5. Fiske SC: Peptic ulcer disease, cytoprotection, and prostaglandins. Arch Intern Med 148:2112–2113, 1988
6. Rachmilewitz D: Efficacy of prostanoids in the treatment of gastric ulcer. Clin Invest Med 10:238–242, 1987
7. Hinsdale JG, Engel JJ, Wilson DE: Prostaglandin E in peptic ulcer disease. Prostaglandins 6:495, 1974
8. Marshall BJ, Warren JR: Unidentified curved bacilli in the stomach of patients with gastritis and peptic ulceration. Lancet 1:1311–1314, 1984
9. Hornick RB: Peptic ulcer disease: A bacterial infection? N Engl J Med 316:1599–1160, 1987
10. Marshall BJ: The *Campylobacter pylori* story. Scand J Gastroenterol (suppl 146)23:58–66, 1988
11. Graham DY: *Campylobacter pylori* and peptic ulcer disease. Gastroenterology 96:615–625, 1989
12. Nedenskov-Sorensen P, Björneklett A, Fausa O, Bukholm G, Aase S, Jantzen E: *Campylobacter pylori* infection and its relation to chronic gastritis. Scand J Gastroenterol 23:867–874, 1988
13. Tytgat GNJ, Rauws EAJ, de Koster E: *Campylobacter pylori:* Diagnosis and treatment. J Clin Gastroenterol 11(suppl 1):S49–S53, 1989
14. Yardley JH, Paull G: *Campylobacter pylori:* A newly recognized infectious agent in the gastrointestinal tract. Am J Surg Pathol 12(suppl 1):89–99, 1988
15. Blaser MJ: Gastric campylobacter-like organisms, gastritis, and peptic ulcer disease. Gastroenterology 93:371–383, 1987
16. Slomiany BL, Bilski J, Sarosiek J, et al: *Campylobacter pyloridis* degrades mucin and undermines gastric mucosal integrity. Biochem Biophys Res Commun 144:307–314, 1987
17. Goodwin CS, Armstrong JA, Marshall BJ: *Campylobacter pyloridis,* gastritis, and peptic ulceration. J Clin Pathol 39:353–365, 1986
18. Hollander D, Tarnawski A: Dietary essential fatty acids and the decline in peptic ulcer disease—a hypothesis. Gut 27:239–242, 1986
19. Walker P, Luther J, Samloff MI, Feldman M: Life events and stress and psychosocial factors in men with peptic ulcer disease. II. Relationships with serum pepsinogen concentrations and behavioral risk factors. Gastroenterology 94:323–330, 1988
20. Feldman M, Walker P, Green JL, Weingarden K: Life events stress and psychosocial factors in men with peptic ulcer disease: A multidimensional case-control study. Gastroenterology 91:1370–1379, 1986
21. Grossman MI: Peptic ulcer: Definition and epidemiology. In Rotter JI, Samloff IM, Rimoin DL (eds): The genetics and heterogeneity of common gastrointestinal disorders. New York: Academic Press, 1980, pp. 21–29.
22. Harrison AR, Elashoff JD, Grossman MI: Peptic ulcer disease. In Smoking and health: A report by the Surgeon General. Washington, DC.: U.S. Government Printing Office, DHEW Publication Number (PHS) 79-50066, 1979
23. Coggon D, Lambert P, Langman MJS: Twenty years of hospital admissions for peptic ulcer in England and Wales. Lancet 1:1302, 1984
24. Sonnenberg A, Fritsch A: Changing mortality of peptic ulcer disease in Germany. Gastroenterology 84:1553–1557, 1983
25. Spiro HM: H_2-blockers: How safe, how effective? J Clin Gastroenterol 5(suppl 1):143–147, 1983
26. O'Connor PC, Griffiths K, Shanks RG: Trends in peptic ulcer related diseases from 1972 to 1980: Hospital activity analysis data and general practice cimetidine prescribing levels. Eur J Clin Pharmacol 24:435–440, 1983
27. Wyllie JH, Clark CG, Alexander-Williams J, et al: Effect of cimetidine on surgery for duodenal ulcer. Lancet 2:1307–1308, 1981
28. Fineberg HV, Pearlman L: Surgical treatment of peptic ulcer in the United States. Lancet 1:1305, 1981
29. Bardhan KD, Saul DM, Edwards JL, et al: Comparison of two doses of cimetidine and placebo in the treatment of duodenal ulcer: A multicenter trial. Gut 20:68–74, 1979
30. Binder JH, Cocco A, Crossley RJ, et al: Cimetidine in the treatment of duodenal ulcer. A multicenter double blind study. Gastroenterology 74:380–388, 1978
31. Grossman MI, Kurata JH, Rotter JI, et al: Peptic ulcer: New therapies, new diseases. Ann Intern Med 95:609–627, 1981
32. Blackwood WS, Maudgal DP, Pickard RG, et al: Cimetidine in duodenal ulcer. Lancet 2:174–176, 1976
33. Gray GR, Smith IS, McKenzie I, et al: Oral cimetidine in severe duodenal ulceration. Lancet 1:4–7, 1977
34. Collen JM, Hanan MR, Maher JA, et al: Cimetidine vs. placebo in duodenal ulcer therapy. Six week controlled double-blind investigation without any antacid therapy. Dig Dis Sci 25:744–748, 1980
35. Ciclitira PJ, Machell RJ, Fathing MJ, et al: Double-blind controlled trial of cimetidine in the healing of gastric ulcer. Gut 20:730–739, 1977
36. Hetzel DJ, Hansky J, Shearman DJC, et al: Cimetidine treatment of duodenal ulceration. Gastroenterology 74:389–392, 1978
37. Schade RR, Donaldson RM Jr: How physicians use cimetidine. A survey of hospitalized patients and published cases. N Engl J Med 304:1281–1284, 1981
38. Cocco AE, Cocco DV: A survey of cimetidine prescribing. N Engl J Med 304:1281, 1981
39. Kauffman GL Jr: Drug therapy for peptic ulcer: Drugs that act on the gastric mucosa. J Clin Gastroenterol 3(suppl 2):95–101, 1981
40. Morris T, Thodes J: Progress report. Antacids and peptic ulcer—A reappraisal. Gut 20:538–545, 1979
41. Peterson WL, et al: Healing of duodenal ulcer with an antacid regimen. N Engl J Med 297:341–345, 1977
42. Ippoliti AF, Sturdevant RL, Isenberg JI, et al: Cimetidine versus intensive antacid therapy for duodenal ulcer. A multicenter trial. Gastroenterology 74:393–395, 1978
43. McCarthy DM: Smoking and ulcers—time to quit. N Engl J Med 311:726–727, 1984
44. Hammond EG: Smoking in relation to death rates of 1 million men and women. Monogr Natl Cancer Inst 13:127, 1966
45. Piper DW: The treatment of chronic peptic ulcer. Front Gastrointest Res 6:109, 1980
46. Harrison AR, Elashoff JD, Grossman MI: Peptic ulcer disease. In Smoking and Health: A report by the Surgeon General. Washington, D.C.: U.S. Government Printing Office, DHEW Publication Number (PHS) 79-50066, 1979
47. Stemmermann GN, Marcus EB, Buist AS, MacLean CJ: Relative

impact of smoking and reduced pulmonary function on peptic ulcer risk. Gastroenterology 96:1419–1424, 1989

48. Isenberg JI: Peptic ulcer: Epidemiology, nutritional aspects, drugs, smoking, alcohol, and diet. J Fam Pract 18:141–151, 1984
49. Elashoff JD, Grossman MI: Trends in hospital admissions and death rates for peptic ulcer in the United States from 1970–78. Gastroenterology 78:280–285, 1980
50. Friedman GS, Siegelaub AB, Seltzer CC: Cigarettes, alcohol, coffee, and peptic ulcer. N Engl J Med 290:469, 1974
51. Petitti DB, Friedman GD, Kahn W: Peptic ulcer disease and the tar and nicotine yield of currently smoked cigarettes. J Chron Dis 35:503–507, 1982
52. Ippoliti A, Elashoff J, Valenzuela J: Recurrent ulcer after successful treatment with cimetidine or antacid. Gastroenterology 85:875–880, 1983
53. Sonnenberg A, Muller-Lissner S, Vogel E, et al: Predictors of duodenal ulcer healing and relapse. Gastroenterology 81:1061–1067, 1981
54. Sontag S, Graham DY, Belsito A, et al: Cimetidine, cigarette smoking, and recurrence of duodenal ulcer. N Engl J Med 311:689–693, 1984
55. Korman MG, Shaw G, Hansky J, et al: Influence of smoking on healing rate of duodenal ulcer in response to cimetidine or high-dose antacid. Gastroenterology 239:39–42, 1981
56. Hasan M, Sircus W: The factors determining success or failure of cimetidine treatment of peptic ulcer. J Clin Gastroenterol 3:225–229, 1981
57. Boyd EJS, Wilson JA, Wormsley KG: Smoking impairs therapeutic gastric inhibition. Lancet 1:95–97, 1983
58. Murthy SNS, Dinoso UP, Clearfield HR, et al: Simultaneous measurement of basal pancreatic gastric acid secretion, plasma gastrin and secretin during smoking. Gastroenterology 73:758–761, 1977
59. Navis BH, Marks IN, Bank S, Sloan AW: The relation between gastric acid secretion and body habitus, blood groups, smoking, and the subsequent development of dyspepsia and duodenal ulcer. Gut 14:107–112, 1973
60. Sonnenberg A, Husmer N: Effect of nicotine on gastric musosal blood flow and acid secretion. Gut 23:532–535, 1982
61. Kikendall JW, Evaul J, Johnson LF: Effect of cigarette smoking on gastrointestinal physiology and non-neoplastic digestive disease. J Clin Gastroenterol 6:65–78, 1984
62. Hoon JR: Intragastric photographic observation of the effects of smoking on gastric mucosa. Gastrointest Endosc 15:172–174, 1969
63. Naitove A, Constantian MB, Arkins T: Gastric hemodynamic effects of smoking and nicotine. Gastroenterology 58:1058, 1970
64. Valenzuela JE, Defilippi C, Csendes A: Manometric studies on the human pyloric sphincter. Effect of cigarette smoking metoclopramide and atropine. Gastroenterology 70:481–483, 1976
65. Turnberg LA, Rees WD: Aspirin, ulcer and intestinal bleeding: What do the data show? Gastroenterology 83:726–727, 1982
66. Levy M: Aspirin use in patients with major upper gastrointestinal bleeding and peptic-ulcer disease. N Engl J Med 290:1158–1162, 1981
67. Ivey KJ: Drugs, gastritis, and peptic ulcer. J Clin Gastroenterol 3(suppl 2):29–34, 1981
68. Piper WP, Nasiry J, McIntosh, Shy CM, Pierce J, Byth K: Smoking, alcohol, analgesics, and chronic duodenal ulcer. Scand J Gastroenterol 19:1015–1021, 1984
69. Lanza FL, Royer GL, Nelson RS: Endoscopic evaluation of the effects of aspirin, buffered aspirin, and enteric-coated aspirin on gastric and duodenal mucosa. N Engl J Med 303:136–137, 1980
70. Douthwaite HA, Lintott GAM: Gastroscopic observation of the effect of aspirin and certain other substances on the stomach. Lancet 2:1222–1225, 1938
71. Silvoso GR, Ivey KS, Butt JH: Incidence of gastric lesions in patients with rheumatic disease on chronic aspirin therapy. Ann Intern Med 91:517–520, 1979
72. McIntosh JH, Fung CS, Berry G, Piper DW: Smoking, nonsteroidal anti-inflammatory drugs, and acetaminophen in gastric ulcer. Am J Epidemiol 128:761–770, 1988
73. Soll AH, Kurata J, McGuigan JE: Ulcers, nonsteroidal anti-inflammatory drugs, and related matters. Gastroenterology 96:561–568, 1989
74. Somerville K, Faulkner G, Langman MJS: Non-steroidal anti-inflammatory drugs and bleeding peptic ulcer. Lancet 1:462–464, 1986
75. Taylor RT, Huskinson EC, Whitehouse GH, et al: Gastric ulceration occurring during indomethacin therapy. Br Med J 4:734–737, 1968
76. Meltzer LE, Bockmann AA, Kanenson W, et al: The incidence of peptic ulcer among patients on long term prednisone therapy. Gastroenterology 35:351–356, 1958
77. Conn HO, Blitzer BL: Nonassociation of adrenocorticosteroid therapy and peptic ulcer. N Engl J Med 294:473–479, 1976
78. Cohen S, Booth GH: Gastric acid secretion and lower esophageal-sphincter pressure in response to coffee and caffeine. N Engl J Med 293:897, 1975
79. Kurata JH, Elashoff JD, Grossman MI: Inadequacy of the literature on the relationship between drugs, ulcers, and gastrointestinal bleeding. Gastroenterology 82:373–382, 1982
80. Paffenbarger RS, Wing AL, Hyde RT: Chronic disease in former college students. XIII. Early precursors of peptic ulcer. Am J Epidemiol 100:307–315, 1974
81. Sleisenger MD, Fordtran JS: Gastrointestinal disease; pathophysiology, diagnosis, treatment, 3 edt. Philadelphia: W.B. Saunders, 1983, p 655
82. Cooke AR: Ethanol and gastric function. Gastroenterology 62:501, 1972
83. Spiro HM: Is milk all that bad for the ulcer patient? J Clin Gastroenterol 3:219, 1981
84. Welsh J: Diet therapy and peptic ulcer disease. Gastroenterology 72:740, 1977
85. Ippoliti AF, Maxwell V, Isenberg JI: The effect of various forms of milk on gastric acid secretion in patients with duodenal ulcer and normal subjects. Ann Intern Med 84:286, 1976
86. Tovey FI: Progress report: Peptic ulcer in India and Bangladesh. Gut 20:329–347, 1979
87. Tovey FI, Tunstall M: Progress report: Duodenal ulcer in black populations in Africa south of the Sahara. Gut 16:564–576, 1975
88. Palgi A: Association between dietary changes and mortality: Israel 1949 to 1977: A trend-free regression model. Am J Clin Nutr 34:1569–1583, 1981
89. Sturdevant RAL: Epidemiology of peptic ulcer: Report of a conference. Am J Epidemiol 104:9–14, 1976
90. Cobb S, Rose RM: Hypertension, peptic ulcer and diabetes in air traffic controllers. JAMA 224:489–492, 1973
91. Grayson RR: Peptic ulcer in air traffic controllers. IMJ 142:111–152, 1972
92. Doll R, Jones FA, Bukarch MM: Occupational factors in the etiology of gastric and duodenal ulcers. Medical Research Council Special Report Series No. 76, 1951
93. Dunn JP, Cobb S: Frequency of peptic ulcer among executives, craftsmen, and foremen. J Occup Med 4:343–348, 1962
94. Conway TL, Ward HW, Vickers RR, Rahe RH: Occupational stress and variation in cigarette, coffee, and alcohol consumption. J Health Soc Behav 22:155–165, 1981
95. Cummings S: Stress, cigarettes, and ulcers. Gastroenterology 85:1232, 1983
96. Adami HO, Bergstrom R, Nyren O, et al: Is duodenal ulcer really a psychosomatic disease? Scand J Gastroenterol 22:889–896, 1987
97. Sonnenberg A, Haas J: Joint effects of occupation and nationality on the prevalence of peptic ulcer in German workers. Br J Ind Med 43:490–493, 1986
98. Segawa K, Nakazawa S, Tsukamoto Y, et al: Peptic ulcer is prevalent among shift workers. Dig Dis Sci 32:449–453, 1987
99. Susser M, Stein Z: Civilization and peptic ulcer. Lancet 1:115–118, 1962

100. Segal I, Unterhalter B, Rosenbush H: Further observations on social factors associated with duodenal ulcer in Soweto. Soc Sci Med 23:417–422, 1986
101. Marshall BJ, Armstrong JA, Mc Gechie DB, Glancy RJ: Attempt to fulfill Koch's postulates for pyloric *Campylobacter*. Med J Aust 142:436–439, 1985
102. Blaser MJ, Brown WR: Campylobacters and gastroduodenal inflammation. Adv Intern Med 34:21–42, 1989
103. Graham DY and Michaletz PA: Should I search for *Campylobacter pylori* in my patients? Much ado about not much? Gastroenterology 83:481–483, 1982
104. Robert A, Nezamis JE, Phillips JP: Inhibition of gastric secretion by prostaglandins. Dig Dis Sci 12:1073–1076, 1967
105. Karim SM, Carter DC, Bhana D, et al: Effect of orally administered prostaglandin E_2 and its 15-methyl analogues on gastric secretion. Br Med J 1:143–146, 1973
106. Chaudhury TK, Jacobson ED: Prostaglandin cytoprotection of gastric mucosa. Gastroenterology 74:58–63, 1978
107. Tarnawski A, Brzozowski T, Sarfeh IJ, et al: Prostaglandin protection of human isolated gastric glands against indomethacin and ethanol injury: Evidence for direct cellular action of prostaglandin. J Clin Invest 81:1081–1089, 1988
108. Dajani EZ: Is peptic ulcer a prostaglandin deficiency disease? Hum Pathol 17:106–107, 1986
109. Lam SK: Prostaglandins for duodenal ulcer. Clin Invest Med 10:232–237, 1987
110. Tanizawa H, Iwanaga T, Tai HH: Increase in thromboxane B_2 and decrease in prostaglandin E_2 and 6-keto-prostaglandin F_1 alpha release into rat bronchoalveolar fluid as a consequence of cigarette smoking. Prostaglandins Leukot Med 28:195–201, 1987
111. Boughton-Smith NK, Whittle BJ: Inhibition by 16,16-dimethyl PGE_2 of ethanol-induced gastric mucosal damage and leukotriene B_4 and C_4 formation. Prostaglandins 35:945–957, 1988
112. Malandrino S, Bestetti A, Fumagalli G, Borsa M, Vigano T, Tonon G: Role of endogenous prostaglandins in protection of rat gastric mucosa by tripotassium dicitrate bismuthate. Scand J Gastroenterol 22:943–948, 1987
113. Muto N, Yamamoto M, Tani S: Alteration in gastric mucosal acid protease activity induced by necrotizing agents and prevention by prostaglandin E_2. J Pharmacobiodyn 10:128–134, 1987
114. Bode C, Ito T, Rollenhagen A, Bode JC: Effect of acute and chronic alcohol feeding on prostaglandin E_2 biosynthesis in rat stomach. Dig Dis Sci 33:814–818, 1988
115. Katz LB, Genna T, Fuller BL, Tolman EL, Shriver DA: Altered susceptibility of arthritic rats to the gastric lesion-inducing effects of aspirin or ethanol and the antilesion effect of rioprostil. Agents Actions 22:134–143, 1987
116. Konturek SJ, Brzozowski T, Drozdowicz D, Beck G: Role of leukotrienes in acute gastric lesions induced by ethanol, taurocholate, aspirin, platelet-activating factor and stress in rats. Dig Dis Sci 33:806–813, 1988
117. Lauritsen K, Havelund T, Laursen LS, Bytzer P, Kjaergaard J, Rask-Madsen J: Enprostil and ranitidine in prevention of duodenal ulcer relapse: One year double blind comparative trial. Br Med J Clin Res 294:9332–9334, 1987
118. Sharon P, Cohen F, Zifroni A, et al: Prostanoid synthesis by cultured gastric and duodenal mucosa: Possible role in the pathogenesis of duodenal ulcer. Scand J Gastroenterol 18:1045–1049, 1983
119. Wright JP, Young GO, Klaff LJ, et al: Gastric mucosal prostaglandin E levels in patients with gastric ulcer disease and carcinoma. Gastroenterology 82:263–267, 1982
120. Doll R, Kellock TD: The separate inheritance of gastric and duodenal ulcers. Ann Eugen 16:231, 1951
121. Rotter JI, Rubin R, Meyer JH, et al: Rapid gastric emptying—An inherited pathophysiologic defect in duodenal ulcer? Gastroenterology 76:1229, 1979
122. Rotter JI, Jones JQ, Samloff IM, et al: Duodenal-ulcer disease associated with elevated serum pepsinogen I. An inherited autosomal dominant disorder. N Engl J Med 300:63–66, 1979
123. Taylor IL, Calan J, Rotter JI, et al: Family studies of hyperpepsinogenomic I duodenal ulcer. Ann Intern Med 95:421–425, 1981
124. Ellis A, Woodrow JC: HLA and duodenal ulcer. Gut 20:760, 1979
125. Rotter JI, Rimoin DL, Gursky JM, et al: HLA-B5 associated with duodenal ulcer. Gastroenterology 73:438, 1977
126. Rotter JI: The genetics of peptic ulcer: More than one gene, more than one disease. Prog Med Genet 4:1–58, 1980
127. Lam SK, Isenberg JI, Grossman MI, et al: Gastrin secretion is abnormally sensitive to exogenous gastrin released after peptone test meals in duodenal ulcer patients. J Clin Invest 65:555, 1980
128. Samloff IM, Liebman WM, Panitch NM: Serum group I pepsinogens by radioimmunoassay in control subjects and patients with peptic ulcer. Gastroenterology 69:83–90, 1975
129. Isenberg JI, Grossman MI, Maxwell V, Walsh JH: Increased sensitivity to stimulation of acid secretion by pentagastrin in duodenal ulcer. J Clin Invest 55:330, 1975
130. Rotter JI: Genetic aspects of ulcer disease. Compr Ther 7:16–25, 1981
131. Almy TP, Mendeloff AI, Rice D: Prevalence and significance of digestive diseases. Gastroenterology 68:1351–1371, 1975
132. Rotter JI, Rimoin DL: Peptic ulcer disease—a heterogenous group of disorders? Gastroenterology 73:604, 1977
133. Rotter JI: The genetics of gastritis and peptic ulcer. J Clin Gastroenterol 3(suppl 2):35–43, 1981
134. Calkins B, Mendeloff AI: Epidemiology of inflammatory bowel disease. Epidemiol Rev 8:60–91, 1986
135. Mayberry JF: Recent epidemiology of ulcerative colitis and Crohn's disease. Int J Colorectal Dis 4:59–66, 1989
136. Binder V: Epidemiology, course and socio-economic influence of inflammatory bowel disease. Schweiz Med Wochenschr 118:738–742, 1988
137. Sonnenberg A: Geographic variation in the incidence of and mortality from inflammatory bowel disease. Dis Colon Rectum 29:854–861, 1986
138. Mendeloff AI, Calkins B, Lilienfeld AM, Garland CF, Monk M: Inflammatory bowel disease in Baltimore, 1960–79: Hospital incidence rates, bimodality, and smoking factors. Front Gastrointest Res 11:88–93, 1986
139. Hellers G: Ulcerative colitis: Epidemiology. In Jewell DP, Gibson PR (eds): Top Gastroenterol 12:129–139, 1985
140. Zuckerman MJ, Briones DF: Inflammatory bowel disease: Overview and psychosomatics. Tex Med 85:32–36, 1989
141. Garland C, Lilienfeld AM, Mendeloff AI, Markowitz JA, Terrell KB, Garland FC: Incidence rates of ulcerative colitis and Crohn's disease in fifteen areas of the United States. Gastroenterology 81:1115–1124, 1981
142. Myren J, Bouchier AD, Watkinson G, et al: The Organization Mondiale de Gastroenterologie (OMGE) multinational inflammatory bowel disease survey 1976–1982. Scand J Gastroenterol 19(suppl 95):1–27, 1984
143. Kraft SC: Modern clinical aspects of inflammatory bowel disease. Radiol Clin North Am 25:213–220, 1987
144. Brostrom O: Ulcerative colitis in Stockholm County—a study of epidemiology, prognosis, mortality, and cancer risk with social reference to a surveillance program. Acta Chir Scand (suppl 534), 1986
145. Rötegard J, Åhsgren L, Janunger K-G: Ulcerative colitis: Mortality and surgery in an unselected population. Acta Chir Scand 154:216–220, 1988
146. Isbell G, Levin B: Ulcerative colitis and colon cancer. Gastroenterol Clin North Am 17:773–791, 1988
147. Katzka I, Brody RS, Morris E, et al: Assessment of colorectal cancer risk in patients with ulcerative colitis: Experience from a private practice. Gastroenterology 85:22–25, 1983
148. Devlin HB, Datta D, Dellipiani AW: The incidence and prevalence of inflammatory bowel disease in North Tees Health District. World J Surg 4:183–193, 1980
149. Haug K, Schrumpf E, Barstad S, Fluge G, Halvorsen JF, and the

Study Group of Inflammatory Bowel Disease in Western Norway: Epidemiology of ulcerative colitis in Western Norway. Scand J Gastroenterol 23:517–522, 1988

150. Sinclair TS, Brunt PW, Mowat NA: Nonspecific proctocolitis in Northeastern Scotland: A community study. Gastroenterology 85:1–11, 1983
151. Jones HW, Grogons J, Hoare AM: An audit of ulcerative colitis in a district general hospital (High Wycombe, England). Gut 26:A1123, 1985
152. Morris T, Rhodes J: Incidence of ulcerative colitis in the Cardiff (Wales) region, 1968–1977. Gut 26:846–848, 1977
153. Shivananda S, Hordjik ML, Pena AS, Mayberry JF: Inflammatory bowel disease: One condition or two? Digestion 38:187–192, 1987
154. Nordenvall B, Brostrom O, Berglund M, et al: Incidence of ulcerative colitis in Stockholm county, 1955–1979. Scand J Gastroenterol 20:783–790, 1985
155. Bjørnsson S, Thorgeirsson T: Colitis ulcerosa i Island (Iceland): Epidemiologisk undersokning 1950–1979. Nord Med 98:298–301, 1983
156. Berner J, Kiaer T: Ulcerative colitis and Crohn's disease on the Faroe islands 1964–83: A retrospective epidemiological survey. Scand J Gastroenterol 21:188–192, 1986
157. Eason RJ, Lee SP, Tasman-Jones C: Inflammatory bowel disease in Auckland, New Zealand. Aust NZ J Med 12:125–131, 1982
158. Pinchbeck BR, Kirdeikis J, Thompson ABR: Inflammatory bowel disease in Northern Alberta: An epidemiologic study. J Clin Gastroenterol 10:505–515, 1988
159. Stonnington CM, Phillips SF, Melton LJ, Zinsmeister AR: Chronic ulcerative colitis: Incidence and prevalence in a community (Rochester MN). Gut 28:402–409, 1987
160. Calkins BM, Lilienfeld AM, Garland CF, Mendeloff AI: Trends in incidence rates of ulcerative colitis and Crohn's disease. Dig Dis Sci 29:913–920, 1984
161. Odes HS, Fraser D, Krawiec J: Ulcerative colitis in the Jewish population of Southern Israel 1961–1985: Epidemiological and clinical study. Gut 28:1630–1636, 1987
162. Odes HS, Fraser D, Krawiec J: Incidence of idiopathic ulcerative colitis in Jewish population subgroups in the Beer Sheva region of Israel. Am J Gastroenterol 82:854–858, 1987
163. LaFranchi GA, Michelini A, Brignola C, Campieri M, Cortini C, Marzio L: Uno studio epidemiologico sulle malatie inflammatorie intestinale nella provincia di Bologna. G Clin Med 57:235–245, 1976
164. Emmanoulidis A, Manousos ON, Papadimitriou C, Triantafyllidis J: Ulcerative colitis in Greece: Course and prognostic factors. Digestion 39:181–186, 1988
165. Wright JP, Froggatt J, O'Keefe EA, et al: The epidemiology of inflammatory bowel disease in Cape Town 1980–1984. S Afr Med J 70:10–15, 1986
166. Al-Nakib B, Radhakrishnan S, Jacob GS, Al-Liddawi H, Al-Ruwaih A: Inflammatory bowel disease in Kuwait. Am J Gastroenterol 79:191–194, 1984
167. Higashi A, Watanabe Y, Ozasa K, Hayashi K, Aoike A, Kawai K: Prevalence and mortality of ulcerative colitis and Crohn's disease in Japan. Gastroenterol Jpn 23:521–526, 1988
168. Garland CF, Garland FC: Do sunlight and vitamin D reduce the risk of colon cancer. Int J Epidemiol 9:227–231, 1980
169. Evans JG, Acheson ED: An epidemiologic study of ulcerative colitis and regional enteritis in the Oxford area. Gut 6:311–324, 1965
170. Gjone E, Myren J: Colitis ulcerosa in Norge. Nord Med 71:143–145, 1964
171. Myren J, Gjone E, Hertzberg JN, et al: Epidemiology of ulcerative colitis and regional enterocolitis (Crohn's disease) in Norway. Scand J Gastroenterol 6:511–514, 1971
172. Hiatt RA, Kaufman L: Epidemiology of inflammatory bowel disease in a defined northern California population. West J Med 149:541–546, 1988
173. Shivananda S, Pena AS, Mayberry JF, et al: Epidemiology of proctocolitis in the Region of Leiden, the Netherlands: A population study from 1979 to 1983. Scand J Gastroenterol 22:993–1002, 1987
174. Utsunomiya T, et al: Incidence and prevalence of idiopathic proctocolitis in Japan. Dig Dis Sci (suppl 221):874, 1986
175. Monk M, Mendeloff AI, Siegel CI, et al: An epidemiological study of ulcerative colitis and regional enteritis among adults in Baltimore. I. Hospital incidence and prevalence. Gastroenterology 53:198–210, 1967
176. Jacobsohn WZ, Levine Y: Incidence and prevalence of ulcerative colitis in the Jewish population of Jerusalem. Isr J Med Sci 22:559–563, 1986
177. Gilat T, Ribak J, Benaroya Y, et al: Ulcerative colitis in the Jewish population of Tel Aviv-Yafo. I. Epidemiology. Gastroenterology 66:335–342, 1974
178. Paulley JW: Ulcerative colitis: A study of 173 cases. Gastroenterology 16:566, 1950
179. Acheson ED: The distribution of ulcerative colitis and regional enteritis in United States veterans with particular reference to the Jewish religion. Gut 1:91–93, 1960
180. Mendeloff AI, Monk M, Siegel CI, Lilienfeld AM: Some epidemiological features of ulcerative colitis and regional enteritis. Gastroenterology 51:748–752, 1966
181. Sedlack RE, Nobrega FR, Kurland LT, et al: Inflammatory colon disease in Rochester, Minnesota, 1935–1964. Gastroenterology 62:935–941, 1972
182. Nedbal J, Maratka Z: Ulcerative proctocolitis in Czechoslovakia. Am J Proctol 19:106–114, 1968
183. Don BAC, Goldacre MJ: Absence of seasonality in emergency room admissions for inflammatory bowel disease. Lancet 2:1156–1157, 1984
184. Ishikawa M, Watanabe H, Yamagishi G, et al: Crohn's disease, non-specific ulcers of the small intestine, and idiopathic procto-colitis in a Japanese university hospital from 1954 to 1974. Tohoku J Exp Med 118:97–109, 1976
185. Ziegler R, et al: Epidemiologic patterns of colorectal cancer. In DeVita VT, Hellman S, Rosenberg SA (eds): Important advances in oncology. New York: Lippincott Medical, 1986, pp 209–232
186. Roth MP, Petersen GM, McElree C, et al: Geographic origins of Jewish patients with inflammatory bowel disease. Gastroenterology 97:900–904, 1989
187. Binder V, Both H, Hansen PK, et al: Incidence and prevalence of ulcerative colitis and Crohn's disease in the county of Copenhagen, 1962–1978. Gastroenterology 83:563–568, 1982
188. Myren I, Gjone E, Hertzberg JN, et al: Epidemiology of ulcerative colitis and regional enteritis (Crohn's disease) in Norway. Scand J Gastroenterol 6:511–514, 1971
189. Wigley RD, MacLaurin BP: A study of ulcerative colitis in New Zealand showing a low incidence in Maoris. Br Med J 3:228–231, 1962
190. Bonnevie O, Riis R, Anthonisen P: An epidemiological study of ulcerative colitis in Copenhagen county. Scand J Gastroenterol 3:432–438, 1968
191. Fischman HR: Multiple sclerosis: A new perspective on epidemiological patterns. Neurology 32:864–870, 1982
192. Myszor M, Calam J: Seasonality of ulcerative colitis (Letter). Lancet 2:522–523, 1984
193. Bundgaard A, Jarnum S: Water ski spill and ulcerative colitis (Letter). Lancet 2:1157, 1984
194. Heatley RV, Thomas P, Prokipchuk EJ, Gauldie J, Sieniewicz DJ, Bienstock J: Pulmonary function abnormalities in patients with inflammatory bowel disease. Q J Med 203:241–250, 1982
195. Harries AD, Baird A, Rhodes J: Non-smoking: A feature of ulcerative colitis. Br Med J 284:706, 1982
196. Bures J, Fixa B, Komarkova O, Fingerland A: Cigarette smoking and ulcerative colitis. (Letter). Br Med J 285:440, 1982
197. Gyde SN, Prior P, Taylor K, Allan RN: Cigarette smoking, blood pressure, and ulcerative colitis. Gut 24:A998, 1983
198. Penny WJ, Penny E, Mayberry JF, Rhodes J: Mormons, smoking, and ulcerative colitis. Lancet 2:1315, 1983
199. Jick H, Walker AM: Cigarette smoking and ulcerative colitis. N Engl J Med 308:261–263, 1983

200. Logan R, Edmond M, Langman MJS: Is non-smoking associated with ulcerative colitis? Gut 24:A499, 1983
201. Calkins B, Lilienfeld A, Mendeloff A, Garland C: Smoking factors in ulcerative colitis and Crohn's disease (Letter). Am J Epidemiol 120:498, 1984
202. Logan RFA, Edmond M, Somerville KW, Langman MJS: Smoking and ulcerative colitis. Br Med J 288:751–753, 1984
203. Holdstock G, Savage D, Harman M, Wright R: Should patients with inflammatory bowel disease smoke? Br Med J 288:362, 1984
204. Thornton JR, Emmett PM, Heaton KW: Smoking, sugar, and inflammatory bowel disease. Br Med J 290:1786–1787, 1985
205. Tobin MV, Logan RFA, Langman MJS, McConnell RB, Gilmore IT: Smoking and inflammatory bowel disease (Abstract). Gut 26:A1155, 1985
206. Stermer E, Levy M, Heinrich I, Barkan N: Smoking, sugar, and inflammatory bowel disease (Letter). Br Med J 291:487, 1985
207. Vessey M, Jewell D, Smith A, Yeates D, McPherson K: Chronic inflammatory bowel disease, cigarette smoking, and use of oral contraceptives: Findings of a large cohort study of women of childbearing age. Br Med J 292:1101–1103, 1986
208. Franceschi S, Panza E, La Vecchia C, Parazzini F, DeCarli A, Porro GB: Nonspecific inflammatory bowel disease and smoking. Am J Epidemiol 125:445–452, 1987
209. Tobin MV, Logan RFA, Langman MJS, McConnell RB, Gilmore IT: Cigarette smoking and inflammatory bowel disease. Gastroenterology 93:316–321, 1987
210. Benoni C, Nilsson Å: Smoking habits in patients with inflammatory bowel disease. Scand J Gastroenterol 22:1130–1136, 1987
211. Motley RJ, Rhodes J, Ford GA, et al: Time relationships between cessation of smoking and onset of ulcerative colitis. Digestion 37:125–127, 1987
212. Boyko EJ, Koepsell TD, Perera DR, Inui TS: Risk of ulcerative colitis among former and current cigarette smokers. New Engl J Med 316:707–710, 1987
213. Cope GF, Heatley RV, Kelleher J, Lee PN: Cigarette smoking and inflammatory bowel disease: A review. Human Toxicol 6:189–193, 1987
214. Lindberg E, Tysk C, Andersson K, Janerot G: Smoking and inflammatory bowel disease: A case-control study. Gut 29:352–357, 1988
215. Williams RR, Sorlie PD, Feinleib M, McNamara P, Kannel WB, Dawber TR: Cancer incidence by levels of cholesterol. JAMA 245:247–252, 1981
216. Garland CF, Shekelle RB, Barrett-Connor E, Criqui MH, Rossof AH, Paul O: Dietary vitamin D and calcium and risk of colorectal cancer: A 19-year prospective study in men. Lancet 1:307–309, 1985
217. Mattamal MB, Lakshmi VM, Zenser TV, Davis BB: Lung prostaglandin H synthase and mixed-function-oxidase metabolism of nicotine. J Pharmacol Exp Ther 242:827–832, 1987
218. Nielsen OH, Ahnfelt-Ronne I, Elmgreen J: Abnormal metabolism of arachidonic acid in chronic inflammatory bowel disease: Enhanced release of leukotriene B_4 from activated neutrophils. Gut 28:181–185, 1987
219. Lauritsen K, Laursen LS, Bukhave K, et al: In vivo profiles of eicosanoids in ulcerative colitis, Crohn's colitis, and *Clostridium difficile* colitis. Gastroenterology 95:11–17, 1988
220. Goetzl EJ, Payan DG, Goldman DW: Immunopathogenic roles of leukotrienes in human diseases. J Clin Immunol 4:79–84, 1984
221. Lobos EA, Sharon P, Stenson WF: Chemotactic activity in inflammatory bowel disease: Role of leukotriene B_4. Dig Dis Sci 32:1380–1388, 1987
222. Ligumsky M, Rachmilewitz D: The role of eicosanoids in inflammatory bowel disease. In Hillier K: Eicosanoids and the gastrointestinal tract. Boston: MTP Press, 1989, pp 1–12
223. Borgeat P, Samuelsson B: Metabolism of arachidonic acid in polymorphonuclear leukocytes. J Biol Chem 254:7865–7869, 1979
224. Davies RJ, Mier L, Pempinello C, Asbun H, Funhouser W: The electrical and sodium transport characteristics of sutured premalignant mouse colon. J Surg Res 47:49–54, 1989
225. Boughton-Smith NK, Whittle BJR: Laboratory methods for studying the role of eicosanoids in inflammatory bowel disease. In Hillier K: Eicosanoids and the gastrointestinal tract. Boston: MTP Press, 1989, pp 12–17
226. Peskar DM, Dreyling KW, May B, Schaarschmidt K, Goebell H: Possible modes of action of 5-aminosalicylic acid. Dig Dis Sci 32(suppl 12):51S–56S, 1987
227. Craxi A, Olive L, Distefano G: Ulcerative colitis in a married couple. Ital J Gastroenterol 11:184–186, 1979
228. Rhodes JM, Marshall T, Hamer JD, et al: Crohn's disease in two married couples. Gut 26:1086–1087, 1985
229. Farmer RG, Michever WM, Mortimer EA: Studies of family history among patients with inflammatory bowel disease. Clin Gastroenterol 9:271–278, 1980
230. McConnell RB: Inflammatory bowel disease: Newer views of genetic influences. In Berk JE (ed): Developments in digestive diseases, Vol. 3. Philadelphia: Lea and Febiger, 1980, pp 129–137
231. Miller DS, Keighley A, Smith PG, et al: Crohn's disease in Nottingham: A search for time and space clustering. Gut 16:454–457, 1975
232. Miller DS, Keighley A, Smith PG, et al: A case-control method for seeking evidence of contagion in Crohn's disease. Gastroenterology 71:385–387, 1976
233. Krosmeyer SJ, Williams RC, Wilson ID, et al: Lymphocytotoxic antibody in inflammatory bowel disease. N Engl J Med 293:1117–1120, 1975
234. Graham DY, Markesich DC, Yoshimura HH: Mycobacteria and inflammatory bowel disease. Gastroenterology 92:436–442, 1987
235. Gilat T, Hacohen D, Lilos P, Langman MJS: Childhood factors in ulcerative colitis and Crohn's disease: An international cooperative study. Scand J Gastroenterol 22:1009–1024, 1987
236. Tysk C, Lindberg E, Jarnerot G, Floderus-Myrhed B: Ulcerative colitis and Crohn's disease in an unselected population of monozygotic and dizygotic twins: A study of heritability and the influence of smoking. Gut 29:990–996, 1988
237. Singer HC, Anderson JGO, Fischer H, et al: Familial aspects of inflammatory bowel disease. Gastroenterology 61:423–430, 1971
238. Weiner HA, Lewis CM: Some notes on the epidemiology of nonspecific ulcerative colitis: An apparent increase in incidence in Jews. Am J Dig Dis 5:406–418, 1960
239. Acheson ED, Nefzger MD: Ulcerative colitis in the United States army in 1944: Epidemiology: Comparisons between patients and controls. Gastroenterology 44:7–19, 1963
240. Garland C: Ulcerative colitis and Crohn's disease. In Motulsky A (ed): Genetic diseases in Ashkenazi Jews. New York: Raven Press, 1979, pp 401–411
241. Penny WJ, Penny E, Mayberry JF, Rhodes J: Prevalence of inflammatory bowel disease amongst Mormons in Britain and Ireland. Soc Sci Med 21:287–290, 1985
242. Birnbaum D, Groen JJ, Kallner G: Ulcerative colitis among the ethnic groups in Israel. Arch Intern Med 105:843–848, 1960
243. West DW, Lyon JL, Gardner JW: Cancer risk factors: An analysis of Utah Mormons and non-Mormons. J Natl Cancer Inst 65:1083–1095, 1980
244. Doctrine and covenants. Salt Lake City: Church of Jesus Christ of Latter Day Saints, 1957, Sections 49 and 89.
245. Ashley DB: Observations on the epidemiology of appendicitis. Gut 8:533–538, 1967
246. Lyon JL, Sorenson AW: Colon cancer in a low-risk population. Am J Clin Nutr 31:S227–S230, 1978
247. Helzer JE, Stillings WA, Chammas S, et al: A controlled study of the association between ulcerative colitis and psychiatric diagnoses. Dig Dis Sci 27:513–518, 1982
248. Engel GL: Biologic and psychologic features of the ulcerative colitis patient. Gastroenterology 40:312–322, 1961
249. Calkins BM, Mendeloff AI, Garland C: Inflammatory bowel disease in oral contraceptive users (Letter). Gastroenterology 91:523–524, 1986
250. Logan RFA, Kay CR, Scott L: The pill, smoking, and inflammatory bowel disease—Results from the Royal College of General

Practitioners (RCGP) oral contraception study. Gut 27:A1276, 1986

251. Bernardino ME, Lawson TL: Discrete colonic ulcers associated with oral contraceptives. Dig Dis Sci 21:503–506, 1976
252. Bonfils S, Hervior P, Girodet J, et al: Acute spontaneously recovering ulcerative colitis (ARUC). Am J Dig Dis 22:429–436, 1977
253. Favier D: Colite erosif chez des malades prenant des contraceptifs oraux. Nouv Presse Med 6:2074, 1977
254. Qiao LH: Clinical analysis on 1363 patients with nonspecific ulcerative colitis in China. Chin J Mod Med 7:308–311, 1987
255. Segal I, Tim LO, Hamilton DG, et al: The rarity of ulcerative colitis in South African blacks. Am J Gastroenterol 74:332–336, 1980
256. Persson PG, Ahlbom A, Hellers G: Crohn's disease and ulcerative colitis: A review of dietary studies with emphasis on methodological aspects. Scand J Gastroenterol 22:385–389, 1987
257. Garland C: Unpublished information. 1989
258. Boyko EJ, Perera DR, Koepsell TD, et al: Coffee and alcohol use and the risk of ulcerative colitis. Am J Gastroenterol 84:530–534, 1989
259. Crohn BB, Rosenberg H: The sigmoidoscopic appearance of chronic ulcerative colitis. Am J Med Sci 170:220, 1925
260. Albert MB, Nochomovitz LE: Dysplasia and cancer surveillance in inflammatory bowel disease. Gastroenterol Clin North Am 18:83–97, 1989
261. Jones HW, Grogono J, Hoare AM: Surveillance in ulcerative colitis: Burdens and benefits. Gut 29:325–331, 1988
262. Rutegård JN, Åhsgren LR, Janunger KG: Ulcerative colitis: Colorectal cancer risk in an unselected population. Ann Surg 721–724, 1988
263. Nunes GC, Ahlquist RE: Increasing incidence of Crohn's disease. Am J Surg 145:578–581, 1983
264. Lee FI, Costello FT: Crohn's disease in Blackpool—incidence and prevalence, 1968–80. Gut 26:274–278, 1985
265. Dirks E, Forster S, Goebell H: Incidence and prevalence of chronic inflammatory bowel disease in a prospective study from an industrial area in West Germany. Dig Dis Sci 31(suppl 83):323, 1986
266. Gollop JH, Phillips SF, Melton CJ, et al: Epidemiologic aspects of Crohn's disease: A population-based study in Olmsted County, Minnesota, 1943–1982. Gut 29:49–56, 1988
267. Krawiec J, Odes HS, Lasry Y, et al: Aspects of the epidemiology of Crohn's disease in the Jewish population in Beer Sheva, Israel. Isr J Med Sci 20:16–21, 1984
268. Kimura A, Sasagawa T: Incidence of Crohn's disease in Japan. In Shiratori T, Nakano H (eds): Japan Medical Research Foundation Publication 22: Inflammatory bowel disease. Tokyo: University of Tokyo Press, 1984, pp 191–200
269. Sedlack RE, Whisnant J, Elveback LR, et al: Incidence of Crohn's disease in Olmsted County, Minnesota, 1945–1975. Am J Epidemiol 112:759–763, 1980
270. Brandes JW, Lorenz-Meyer H: Epidemiologische Aspekte zur Enterocolitis regionalis Crohn und Colitis ulcerosa in Marburg Lohn (FRG) Zwischen 1962 und 1975. Z Gastroenterol 21:69–78, 1983

54
Musculoskeletal Disorders

Jennifer L. Kelsey
Marc C. Hochberg

Musculoskeletal disorders are common, affect all age groups, and are associated with a great deal of disability, impairment, and handicap. About 12 million people in the United States had their activity limited by musculoskeletal disorders in 1984, a figure greater than for any other disease category (Fig. 54–1).[1] Musculoskeletal impairments affect about 10% of the population, with the spine most commonly involved, followed by the lower extremity or hip and the upper extremity or shoulder (Table 54–1). Each year about 9% of the population in the United States experience an acute condition of the musculoskeletal system, including fractures, dislocations, sprains, and strains severe enough that medical care is sought or activity is restricted. The estimated total economic cost to the United States of musculoskeletal conditions was over $65 billion in 1984, second only to diseases of the circulatory system.[1] Indirect costs from lost earnings and services represent a particularly high proportion of this cost, since many people are affected during their most productive years.

DISORDERS PRIMARILY OF ADULTS

Low Back and Neck Pain

From 60% to 80% of the population experience low back pain at some time during their lives.[2] Most episodes of low back pain are not seriously incapacitating. Among people seeking care from family physicians for low back pain, almost 50% improve in a week, and close to 90% are better within a month, regardless of treatment.[3] The small proportion of cases that become chronic account for a high proportion of the cost; one study found that 25% of the cases accounted for 90% of the costs.[4]

In most instances the specific lesion responsible for low back pain is not known, and it is likely that the different conditions comprising the category "low back pain" (e.g., sprains and strains, disc herniations, spondylosis and spondylolisthesis, facet abnormalities) have in part different etiologies. However, until these specific conditions are identified and differentiated in epidemiological investigations, the category "low back pain" as a whole must generally be considered.

Low back pain is more common in people who do heavy manual work than in those whose work is sedentary. Jobs that involve heavy lifting (e.g., of objects weighing 25 pounds or more) are associated with an increase in risk for back pain, but there is little evidence of increased risk in most people when objects lighter than this are lifted. Factors that appear to further increase the risk for both herniated disc and low back pain include frequent lifting of heavy objects while bending and twisting the body, holding heavy objects away from the body while lifting, and failing to bend the knees while lifting.[5,6] Several studies have found an association between cigarette smoking and low back pain and between smoking and herniated disc, probably because of the pressure exerted by frequent coughing or the decreased diffusion of nutrients into the intervertebral disc, both of which are associated with smoking. Prolonged sitting in one position is also thought to increase the risk. Finally, motor vehicle driving and exposure to other forms of whole body vibration are detrimental to the spine.[7,8] Some evidence suggests that tallness is a risk factor for low back pain, that heavy body weight has little or no effect, and that a narrow spinal canal increases the risk, at least for lumbar disc herniation.[9] Although psychological factors are generally believed to play a role in the etiology of back pain, there is little firm evidence to support or refute this belief. However, one recent cohort study[9] did find a twofold increase in risk of subsequent disc herniation among people experiencing psychologically stressful symptoms.

The percentage of the population having neck pain has been found to be 40% to 80%, which is somewhat lower than those having low back pain. However, the number of neck pain cases appears to be increasing. This increase is thought to be attributable to the lower percentage of the work force participating in heavy manual work and the greater number of people sitting for long periods in front of video display terminals. Neck pain is also related to a variety of different lesions. Little is known of risk factors. Prolonged exposure to awkward postures appears to be associated with mild neck pain, and some evidence indicates that heavy lifting, cigarette smoking, frequent aquatic diving from a board, motor vehicle driving, and exposure to other sources of whole body vibration increase the risk for prolapsed cervical intervertebral disc.[10]

One important approach to the prevention of low back pain is modification of factors in the work place.[4] First, there can be careful selection of workers for jobs involving heavy manual work. Although low back x-ray and medical examinations have not proved useful as routine screening tests for worker selection, evidence suggests that selection on the basis of strength testing for specific jobs can reduce the likelihood of back injury. Training workers to bend the knees while lifting does not seem to have

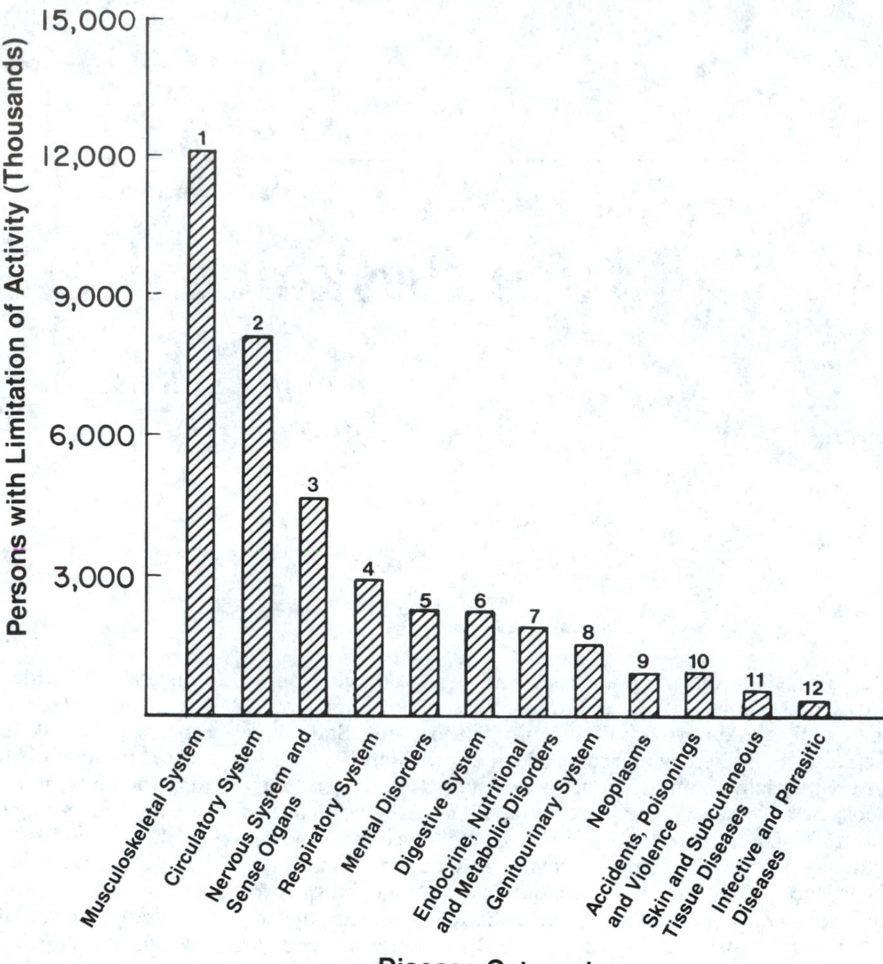

Figure 54–1. Estimated number of persons in the United States in 1984 with limitation of activity attributable to specific disease categories. *[From Holbrook TL et al, 1985, with permission.[1]]*

reduced the number of back injuries, partly because of poor compliance. Other lifting methods that workers may find more acceptable are keeping objects close to the body and lifting slowly, smoothly, and without twisting. Redesigning jobs to minimize bending and twisting motions and to reduce the amount of weight lifted can decrease the number of back injuries and also may allow an injured worker to return to work sooner.

Other methods of primary prevention are improved physical fitness, cessation of smoking, moving around from time to time in situations requiring prolonged exposure to one position, vibration dampening, and use of motor vehicles with good seat positioning and lumbar support.

As mentioned above, much back pain resolves without any specific therapy. Predictors of disability from low back pain include long duration of the pain, a history of past disability, low educational level, psychosocial factors, heavy physical demands on the job, dissatisfaction with the job, whether insurance payments are being received, and whether a lawyer has been retained.[7,11] Because surgical treatment is often unsatisfactory, conservative approaches such as physical therapy and back schools frequently are used for tertiary prevention. The primary aims of back schools are to decrease pain and illness behavior while increasing function through self-involvement and self-reliance.[12,13] Although schools have different emphases, most (1) teach patients enough about spinal mechanics so that they can use their backs effectively and avoid pain and damage, (2) try to effect attitude changes through psychological approaches, and (3) offer exercise and physical fitness programs. There have been no definitive evaluations of the efficacy of back schools, but available evidence suggests that they are effective for patients with back pain of recent onset but not for those whose pain is chronic.[14] Also important in tertiary prevention for many people is a prompt return to work, most commonly after a 2-week period of rest.[15] On first returning to work after having had an episode of low back pain, the worker should avoid lifting heavy objects, bending, twisting, sitting in a low chair, and remaining in the same position for long periods of time. Individuals should also be advised to stand close to their work and use a lumbar support and armrests while sitting.

TABLE 54–1. PREVALENCE OF MUSCULOSKELETAL IMPAIRMENTS IN THE UNITED STATES IN 1977

Type of Impairment	Estimated No. of Affected Individuals	% of Population
All musculoskeletal impairments	20,225,000	9.2
Back or spine	9,365,000	4.3
Lower extremity or hip	7,147,000	3.3
Upper extremity or shoulder	2,500,000	1.1
Other or multiple	1,213,000	0.5

Modified from Holbrook TL, et al. 1985.[1]

Osteoporosis

The reduction of bone mass in osteoporosis causes the bones to be susceptible to fracture. Fractures of the hip, vertebrae, and distal radius are particularly common. Although osteoporosis may occur secondarily to such conditions as hormonal defects, connective tissue disorders, or certain drug therapies, most cases are idiopathic.

Among adults bone loss tends to occur with age in both men and women and in blacks and whites, but the most rapid decrease occurs in white women in the years following menopause. It has been estimated that a white woman of age 50 has a 15% chance of fracturing a hip and also a forearm during the remainder of her lifetime.[16]

The relatively rapid rate of bone loss in middle-aged and older women has been related to a decrease in estrogen production. Women who have had an oophorectomy have earlier loss of bone mass than other women. Figure 54–2 shows that estrogen-replacement therapy protects against bone loss for as long as it is being administered, but loss of bone mass continues when estrogen use ceases.[17] Replacement estrogen also protects against osteoporotic fractures.[18] Thin women are at higher risk than obese women, partly because of their lower estrogen production and the lower concentration of circulating estrogens. Endogenous estrogen concentrations around the time of menopause are negatively correlated with rate of bone loss.[19] In developed countries, high parity has been associated with increased bone mass and decreased risk of fracture, possibly because of increased calcium absorption during pregnancy.[20]

Some studies have shown an association between low levels of dietary calcium and osteoporosis, with evidence suggesting that the amount of dietary calcium during childhood and the teen years is especially important. Calcium supplementation in the adult years appears to afford some protection against loss of cortical bone.[21] Adequate vitamin D intake also may be protective, but available data are contradictory. It is known that prolonged immobilization may result in osteoporosis, while the effect of moderate physical activity among healthy adults is uncertain. Again, adequate physical exercise during childhood and adolescence may be critical. Cigarette smoking probably increases the risk through a lowering of estrogen levels.[18] Heavy alcohol consumption also may increase the risk for osteoporosis and related fractures.[20,22] Use of thiazide diuretics is associated with increased bone mass and decreased risk of hip fracture.[23] Daughters of women with osteoporosis tend to have lower bone mass than other women of their age.[24]

Primary prevention includes measures that will promote adequate bone mass at an early age, such as a diet adequate in calcium, sufficient physical activity, and not smoking. Once the osteoporotic process has begun, administration of estrogens (with or without progestin) will limit further loss of bone mass, but its other benefits and risks also need to be considered. Although the effect of supplemental calcium is not nearly as strong as that of estrogen, it is believed to have no long-term detrimental effects among persons with no specific contraindications (e.g., kidney stones). Moderate physical activity, such as brisk walking, is often recommended for older people to reduce bone loss, but there is little firm evidence to support this recommendation.

In recent years there has been an increased emphasis on screening women in the perimenopausal and immediate postmenopausal period by single photon absorptiometry of the radius and, in some locales, by dual photon absorptiometry of the spine and hip; however, the value of such screening is questionable.[25,26] First, although screening of the radius by single photon absorptiometry takes only 10 minutes, it provides little information about bone density in the spine and hip. In fact, it has been reported that there is little correlation between radial bone mass and subsequent hip fracture incidence once age is taken into account.[27] Dual photon absorptiometry of the spine and hip takes about 50 minutes and is expensive. Other issues of concern are the lack of precision of single and dual photon absorptiometry, the need for serial measurements over time to estimate a woman's rate of bone loss, the uncertainty of the value of these measurements in predicting future fractures, the relatively high cost, and the problem that the advice given to women about methods of preventing further bone mass loss probably would be the same irrespective of the bone densitometry results. The development of dual energy radiography for faster and more precise measurement of bone mass may make screening more practical,[28] but to date these scanners are available in only a few specialized centers.

Reducing the likelihood of falls among those with osteoporosis may be an important way to prevent hip fracture. Possible preventive measures include balance and gait training, muscle-strengthening exercises, correction of visual and hearing problems, avoidance of long-acting sedative or centrally acting medications, and home safety improvements.[29]

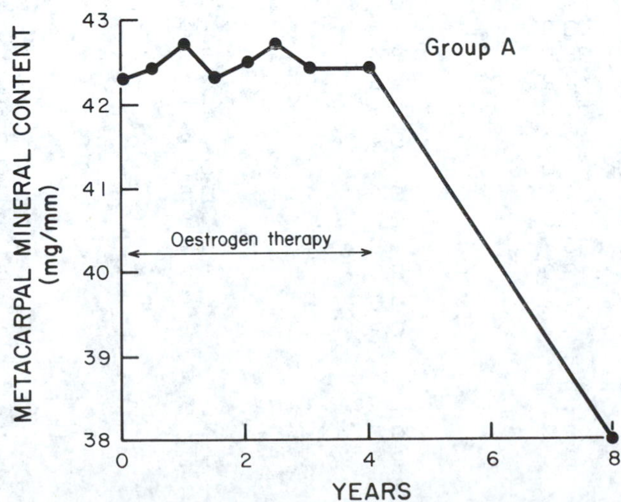

Figure 54–2. Effects of estrogen on bone mineral content of metacarpal and of withdrawal of estrogen after 4 years of active treatment. *[From Lindsay R et el, 1978, with permission.[17]]*

Arthritis

Osteoarthritis. Osteoarthritis, also known as degenerative joint disease, is characterized by degeneration of articular cartilage with proliferation and remodeling of subchondral bone. The usual clinical manifestations include pain and stiffness, accompanied by loss of function.[30] The diagnosis of osteoarthritis in most population surveys has been made using radiographic criteria as defined in the *Atlas of Standard Radiographs of Arthritis.*[31] These criteria are based on typical radiographic changes, including osteophytes, bony spurs, joint space narrowing, subchondral cysts, and bony remodeling. Recently, a new scale has been developed for grading osteoarthritis of the hands; this scale has been tested for reliability and validity in a sample of participants in the Baltimore Longitudinal Study on Aging.[32,33]

Osteoarthritis may be classified as either primary/idiopathic or secondary.[34] Subsets of the idiopathic condition include localized involvement of single joint groups as well as the syndrome of generalized osteoarthritis. Classification criteria have been developed for osteoarthritis of the knee[34] and hand[35] and are in the process of development for the hip.[36] Generalized osteoarthritis is characterized by involvement of three or more joint groups and typically affects perimenopausal and postmenopausal women.[37] Secondary osteoarthritis develops after the occurrence of an identifiable traumatic, congenital, developmental, or systemic disorder that has previously involved the joints.[38]

Approximately 30% of adults between the ages of 18 to 79 years have radiographic evidence of some degree of osteoarthritis in their hands (Table 54-2); 24% of the affected cases are classified as moderate or severe (grade III or IV).[39,40] Approximately 3.8% of adults aged 25 to 74 have osteoarthritis of the knee, and 1.3% of adult males have osteoarthritis of the hip.[39,41] Many people with radiographic evidence of osteoarthritis have no symptoms or disability. For example, in the First National Health and Nutrition Examination Survey (NHANES-1), only about half of the people with severe osteoarthritis of the hip or knee reported significant pain on most days for at least 1 month.[41] Studies in persons with osteoarthritis of the knee have identified the following factors as predictive of knee pain: severity of radiographic changes, presence of morning stiffness, crepitus on passive range of motion, and a feeling of low spirits.[42]

In general, prevalence rates of osteoarthritis and the proportion of cases that are moderate or severe increase with age.[39-41,43,44] Age-specific prevalence rates are higher in males below the age of 45 and in females above the age of 55. The pattern of joint involvement also differs between the sexes; females have a greater number of joints involved[44] and more frequent reports of morning stiffness, joint swelling, and nocturnal pain.[45] The more common occurrence of Heberden's nodes in women is believed to be related to a single autosomal gene that is dominant in females and recessive in males.[46] Recent studies using techniques of recombinant DNA analysis have demonstrated linkage of a polymorphism of the type II collagen gene (Co12A1) with generalized osteoarthritis in two families.[47] No striking racial, ethnic, regional or urban-rural differences in disease prevalence have been noted in the United States. Asian peoples, including Indians and Hong Kong Chinese, have been reported to have a lower prevalence of osteoarthritis of the hip than whites[48]; differences in life-style in addition to other ethnic and racial differences must be considered when evaluating such comparisons.

Several studies have suggested that repetitive joint trauma associated with occupational activity may predispose to osteoarthritis.[49] For instance, there are high prevalence rates of the disorder in the elbows and knees of miners,[50] in the fingers of cotton pickers,[51] and in the fingers, elbows, and knees of dock workers.[52] Anderson and Felson[53] identified significant associations of the knee-bending demands of the primary occupation with osteoarthritis of the knee in both men and women and the strength demands with osteoarthritis of the knee in men only. Davis and colleagues[54] showed that a history of unilateral knee

TABLE 54-2. PERCENT PREVALENCE PER 100 OF RADIOLOGIC CHANGES INDICATIVE OF OSTEOARTHRITIS IN HANDS, FEET, KNEES, AND HIPS, BY AGE AND SEX

Part of Body	Ages (y)	Mild, Moderate, and Severe			Moderate and Severe		
		Males	*Females*	*Total*	*Males*	*Females*	*Total*
Hands[a]	18–79	29.4	30.4	29.9	5.3	9.9	7.1
	25–74	32.0	33.0	32.5	5.4	0.2	7.9
	18–24	2.8	0.4	1.6	—	—	—
	25–34	4.8	2.1	3.4	0.1	—	—
	35–44	17.5	11.3	14.3	0.6	1.1	0.9
	45–54	39.0	34.0	36.4	1.8	5.5	3.7
	55–64	56.6	68.8	63.0	12.6	21.5	17.3
	65–74	71.0	77.1	74.5	22.4	37.0	30.7
	75–79	78.7	88.4	84.5	33.2	51.0	43.9
Feet[a]	18–79	19.8	21.3	20.6	1.5	2.9	2.2
	25–74	21.1	23.2	22.2	1.6	3.0	2.3
	18–24	4.5	1.2	2.8	—	—	—
	25–34	9.7	4.4	7.0	—	—	—
	35–44	17.3	11.2	14.1	0.4	0.4	0.4
	45–54	22.8	25.0	23.9	1.5	1.9	1.7
	55–64	29.0	44.1	36.9	3.4	6.9	5.2
	65–74	40.3	47.1	44.2	5.8	9.1	7.7
	75–79	48.6	53.1	51.3	4.8	14.6	10.7
Knees[b]	25–74	2.6	4.9	3.8	0.5	1.3	0.9
	25–34	—	0.1	0.0	—	0.0	0.0
	35–44	1.7	1.5	1.6	0.1	0.5	0.3
	45–54	2.3	3.6	3.0	0.2	0.5	0.4
	55–64	4.1	7.3	5.7	1.0	0.9	0.9
	65–74	8.3	18.0	13.8	2.0	6.6	4.6
Hips[b]	25–74	1.3	—	—	0.5	—	—
	25–34	0.4	—	—	0.2	—	—
	35–44	0.1	—	—	—	—	—
	45–54	0.7	—	—	0.1	—	—
	50–54	—	0.8	—	—	0.1	—
	55–64	2.6	2.8	2.7	0.7	1.6	1.2
	65–74	4.6	2.7	3.5	2.3	1.2	1.7
	55–74	3.5	2.8	3.1	1.4	1.4	1.4

[a] Data from the National Health Examination Survey, 1960–1962.

[b] Data from the National Health and Nutrition Examination Survey, 1971–1975.

From Lawrence RC, Hochberg MC, Kelsey JL, et al: Estimates of the prevalence of selected arthritic and musculoskeletal diseases in the United States. J Rheumatol 16:427–441, 1989, with permission.

injury was strongly associated with ipsilateral but not contralateral osteoarthritis of the knee in both sexes. However, vocational physical activity, including running, does not appear to be associated with osteoarthritis of the knees in the absence of knee injury.[55,56]

Obesity is another factor that has long been associated with osteoarthritis of the knee.[53,57–59] The association with weight has now been confirmed in data from the prospective Framingham Osteoarthritis Study,[60] in which weight at first examination was a significant predictor of osteoarthritis of the knee at examination 18 in both sexes.

Osteoarthritis of the knee is associated with excess mortality and decreased survival in persons aged 55 and older.[42] The likely explanations for this observation include the association of obesity with both osteoarthritis and mortality and possibly with adverse effects of treatment with nonsteroidal anti-inflammatory drugs (NSAIDs). One study noted excess proportionate mortality from gastrointestinal diseases in subjects with osteoarthritis,[61] while another demonstrated an increased incidence of gastroduodenal ulcers in subjects with osteoarthritis and knee pain.[42] Finally, osteoarthritis of the knee, especially with concomitant pain, is predictive of increased risk of long-term disability characterized by activity and mobility limitation.[42]

Rheumatoid Arthritis. Rheumatoid arthritis is a chronic inflammatory joint disease characterized by proliferative synovitis that results in destruction of articular cartilage and bony erosion; this gives rise to typical articular deformities.[62] The usual clinical symptoms included stiffness, pain and swelling of multiple joints, most commonly the small joints of the hands and wrists. The arthritis usually develops over time in an additive and symmetric fashion. The etiology of rheumatoid arthritis is unknown; the pathophysiology is based on a host's genetically controlled cellular and humoral immune response to a nonself antigen.[63]

Prevalence surveys of rheumatoid arthritis have relied primarily on two sets of criteria for case definition: the 1958 American Rheumatism Association (ARA) criteria[64] and the New York criteria.[65] With the 1958 ARA criteria, cases are divided into probable, definite, and classical rheumatoid arthritis. Two independent studies have noted that the majority of persons classified as having probable rheumatoid arthritis in population surveys do not have clinical rheumatoid arthritis but rather have other arthritides, most often generalized osteoarthritis.[66,67] Therefore, the following discussion will emphasize the data on definite rheumatoid arthritis, as defined by 1958 ARA criteria, with the term "definite" including classical rheumatoid arthritis as well. It should be noted that the 1958 ARA criteria have been replaced by the 1987 revised criteria (Table 54–3); the major differences are (1) the deletion of the categories of possible and probable rheumatoid arthritis, (2) the combination of definite and classical rheumatoid arthritis into a single category, and (3) the deletion of the list of exclusion diagnosis.[68] The 1987 revised criteria were just as sensitive and more specific than the 1958 criteria when tested on the study patients and controls.

Based on the U.S. Health Examination Survey of 1960 through 1962, the prevalence of definite rheumatoid arthritis is almost 1% among persons aged 18 years and older (Table 54–4).[69] A similar prevalence estimate of 0.8% was found from physical examinations done by physicians in NHANES-1 conducted from 1971 through 1975.[70]

Incidence rates of rheumatoid arthritis in the United States have been estimated over the 25-year interval from 1950 through 1974 from the Rochester Epidemiology Program Project.[71] The average annual incidence rates for persons aged 15 and older were 40, 83, and 67 per 100,000 per year for males, females, and both sexes combined, respectively. Declining incidence rates among females, but not males, were noted between the periods 1960 through 1964 and 1970 through 1974[71]; this finding was consistent with a protective effect of oral contraceptives first reported by the Royal College of General Practitioners Oral Contraceptive Study.[72] Recent analyses of data from the Second and Third National Studies of Morbidity Statistics in General Practice confirm the declining incidence of rheumatoid arthritis in females alone between 1970 and 1972 and 1980 through 1981 in the United Kingdom.[73] This analysis also found increases in prevalence rates in both sexes during the 10-year interval, most likely because of improved survival among diagnosed cases.

TABLE 54–3. THE 1987 AMERICAN RHEUMATISM ASSOCIATION REVISED CRITERIA FOR THE CLASSIFICATION OF RHEUMATOID ARTHRITIS[a]

Item	Definition
1	Morning stiffness, lasting at least 1 hour
2	Arthritis involving at least three joint groups simultaneously
3	Arthritis involving at least one area in the hands or wrists
4	Simultaneous involvement of the same joint area on both sides of the body
5	Presence of subcutaneous nodules
6	Presence of serum rheumatoid factor
7	Presence of typical radiographic features [juxta-articular osteopenia and/or erosions] on hand and wrist films

[a] Positive classification requires at least four of the seven criteria.

Modified from Arnett FC, Edworthy SM, Bloch DA, et al: 1988.[68]

In general, both prevalence and incidence rates of rheumatoid arthritis increase with age in both sexes, at least through age 65. In addition, both prevalence and incidence rates are between two and three times greater in females than in males. No striking differences in morbidity rates have been noted between American blacks and whites. However, several native American Indian tribes have particularly high prevalence rates of rheumatoid arthritis; these include the Yakima of central Washington State[74] and the Mille-Lac Band of Chippewa in Minnesota.[75] Orientals, including Japanese and Chinese, appear to have lower prevalence rates than whites.[76,77] Reasons for these differences are unknown, but they may be related to both genetic and environmental factors.

Genetic factors have an important role in the predisposition to rheumatoid arthritis. The disease exhibits familial aggregation and a higher concordance rate in monozygotic than in dizygotic twins.[78] In addition, the susceptibility to rheumatoid arthritis appears to be inherited as an autosomal dominant trait in multicase families.[79] Studies have demonstrated a strong association between the class II major histocompatibility antigen HLA-DR4 and rheumatoid arthritis; in whites, the relative risk for this association exceeds 4.0.[80,81] This association crosses ethnic and racial

TABLE 54–4. PERCENT PREVALENCE OF DEFINITE RHEUMATOID ARTHRITIS IN THE UNITED STATES: U.S. HEALTH EXAMINATION SURVEY [1960–1962]

Age (y)	Males	Females
18–24	—	—
25–34	—	—
35–44	—	0.9
45–54	0.2	1.1
55–64	1.9	2.9
≥65	1.8	4.9
Total	0.7	1.6

From National Center for Health Statistics, 1966.[69]

bounds, with just a few exceptions including the Yakima Indians of Washington State, Asian Indians, Greeks, and Israeli Jews. In whites who lack HLA-DR4 and in these other ethnic and racial groups, there is an association between rheumatoid arthritis and HLA-DR1. Recent work has identified a shared common epitope in the third hypervariable region of both DR1 and DR4[82]; this shared epitope may be involved in interactions between the antigen(s) that causes rheumatoid arthritis and other immunocompetent cells, especially T lymphocytes.

The role of infectious agents as etiological factors in rheumatoid arthritis is also under active investigation. The leading candidate at present is the Epstein-Barr virus[83]; however, it has not yet been convincingly identified as an etiologic agent, and further studies are needed. Other infectious agents, including parvovirus, are also under investigation.[84]

Finally, over the past decade, considerable attention has been directed toward the relationship of oral contraceptive use and rheumatoid arthritis, and the possible mechanism of hormonal modulation of the immune response.[85] In a meta-analysis of 11 published analytical epidemiological studies, Spector and Hochberg[86] confirmed a protective effect of oral contraceptive use on the development of rheumatoid arthritis, with a pooled relative risk of 0.70. These authors concluded, however, that it was more likely that oral contraceptives, and possibly non-contraceptive hormone replacement therapy, modified the course of rheumatoid arthritis by preventing the progression of mild to severe disease, rather than preventing the development of disease itself.

Rheumatoid arthritis is associated with excess mortality and decreased survival; the standardized mortality ratio approximates 170, and there is reduced relative survival compared to age- and sex-matched general population controls.[87,88] Causes of death that are more frequent in rheumatoid arthritis patients include respiratory and infectious diseases, gastrointestinal disorders, and complications of rheumatoid arthritis. Although the proportionate mortality from neoplastic diseases is reduced in rheumatoid arthritis, the actual incidence and mortality from non-Hodgkins lymphoma is increased compared to the general population.[89,90] It is likely that some of the excess mortality may be related to complications of therapy for the disease. Low socioeconomic status, as measured by formal educational level, is associated with increased mortality and excess disability.[91]

Gout. Gout is a metabolic disease characterized by recurrent attacks of acute arthritis, an increase in serum uric acid concentration, and deposition of sodium urate monohydrate crystals in and around joints of the extremities.[92] Because gout is relatively easy to diagnose, most reports of prevalence are based on self-reported physician diagnosis during a specified time interval. However, concern about the validity of such data have been raised,[39] and it has been suggested that classification criteria, as proposed by the American Rheumatism Association,[93] be used for case validation.

The most recent estimates of prevalence of gout are based on responses to the question "Have you had gout within the last year?" in the 1986 U.S. Health Interview Survey.[94] The prevalence rates were 13.5 per 1000 for males and 6.4 per 1000 for females. Prevalence rates increased sharply with age for both sexes and were greater in blacks than whites above age 45 (Table 54–5). Based on comparably collected data from the 1969 Health Interview Survey, the prevalence rate of gout has increased three-to-four-fold in both sexes over a 17-year period.[39] The reasons for the increase in gout prevalence include (1) a temporal increase in mean serum uric acid levels among males,[95,96] (2) increased use of drugs known to produce secondary hyperuricemia, especially diuretics in females, and (3) increased survival of persons with gout. Also, part of the apparent increase may be artifactual and attributable to incorrect diagnosis of individuals with joint pain and hyperuricemia who do not actually have gout. The most recent estimates of the annual incidence of gout in adults from the Framingham study were 3.2 per 1000 for white men and 0.5 per 1000 for white women[97]; no incidence data are available for blacks.

TABLE 54–5. PREVALENCE PER 1000 OF SELF-REPORTED GOUT IN THE UNITED STATES BY AGE, SEX, AND RACE: U.S. NATIONAL HEALTH INTERVIEW SURVEY, 1986

	Age (y)		
	18–44	***45–64***	***≥65***
Sex			
Males	2.4	34.4	51.6
Females	0.7	14.5	19.5
Race			
Whites	1.7	22.6	30.5
Blacks	1.2	38.3	49.2

From National Center for Health Statistics, 1987.[94]

A strong correlation exists between the level of serum uric acid and both the prevalence and incidence of gout[98,99] (Table 54–6). Serum uric acid levels are normally distributed with some skewing toward higher values; in the Tecumseh, Michigan, study, mean values for males were 5.1 mg/dl and for females were 4 mg/dl.[100] Male values rise during adolescence and then remain fairly constant during adult life, while values in females rise only slightly during adolescence and again after menopause to approach the levels found in males (Fig. 54–3). A serum uric acid level of 7 mg/dl or above indicates super saturation and defines physiological hyperuricemia.[92] The Maori of New Zealand, other Polynesians in the Cook Islands and on Samoa, and Filipinos have mean serum uric acid levels in excess of 6 mg/dl.[101] These high levels may in part be explained by increased socioeconomic status accompanying urbanization, alcohol intake, and a diet relatively high in protein.[102,103] Racial differences in the prevalence of gout tend to mirror those noted for hyperuricemia.

In addition to hyperuricemia and gender, several other risk factors have been identified for the development of gout. These include hypertension,[97,99,104] obesity as measured by body mass index,[97,99,104] hypercholesterolemia,[97,99] alcohol consumption[97] (especially "moonshine" whiskey[104]), renal disease,[104] occupational and environmental lead exposure,[104] and a positive family history of gout.[98]

Numerous family studies suggest a multifactorial inheritance, and it is likely that environmental factors contribute significantly to the familial aggregation.

Ankylosing Spondylitis. Ankylosing spondylitis is a form of arthritis that primarily affects the axial skeleton, producing

TABLE 54–6. INCIDENCE OF GOUT PER 1000 PERSON-YEARS BY SERUM URIC ACID LEVEL: VETERANS ADMINISTRATION NORMATIVE AGING STUDY, BOSTON

Initial Serum Uric Acid Level (mg/dl)	No. of Cases	Incidence
≤6.0	10	0.5
6.0–6.9	13	0.9
7.0–7.9	21	4.1
8.0–8.9	14	8.4
9.0–9.9	18	43.2
≥10.0	8	70.2

Modified from Campion EW, Glynn RJ, DeLabry LO: 1987.[99]

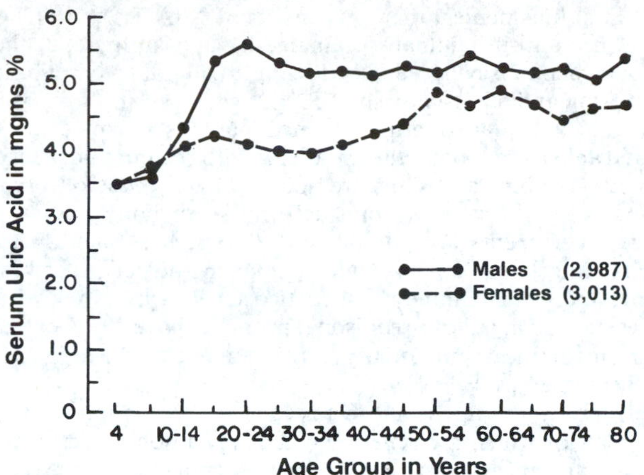

Figure 54-3. Sex-age specific mean serum uric acid in Techumseh from 1959 to 1960. *(From Mikkelsen WM et al, 1965, with permission.[100])*

symptoms of low back pain and stiffness. As the disease progresses, fusion of the sacroiliac joints and vertebrae may occur, with straightening of the lumbar spine, increased thoracic kyphosis, and decreased spinal mobility.[105] Extraspinal arthritis occurs in almost one half of patients, and involvement of the eyes, heart, lungs, and nervous system may also occur.

Three sets of diagnostic criteria have been developed for use in population surveys.[106-108] All are heavily weighted toward the radiographic diagnosis of sacroiliitis. Since radiographic sacroiliitis may exist without thoracolumbar pain, symptoms are required for diagnosis of definite ankylosing spondylitis; persons without symptoms should be designated as having asymptomatic radiographic sacroiliitis rather than probable ankylosing spondylitis.

Estimates of the prevalence of ankylosing spondylitis among white populations are quite variable (Table 54-7). These variations are attributable, at least in part, to differences in survey methods, criteria employed, and case definition. However, known marked geographic and ethnic differences in the prevalence of ankylosing spondylitis do exist.[107] Prevalence is exceedingly low among African blacks and Orientals, including Chinese and Japanese, while approaching 60 per 1000 in males among several Native American Indian tribes. These ethnic and racial differences in prevalence of ankylosing spondylitis are highly correlated with a similar variation in the phenotypic frequency of the class I histocompatibility antigen HLA-B27.[109]

For whites the age-adjusted average annual incidence rate for the period 1935 through 1973 in Rochester, Minnesota, was 11.0 per 100,000 in males and 4.0 per 100,000 in females, with the peak incidence occurring in the 25- to 35-year age group.[100] The estimated prevalence was 2 per 1000 in males and 0.7 per 1000 in females, with maximal prevalence occurring in the 55- to 64-year age group.[110] Adequate data on incidence and prevalence are not available for American blacks. The male-to-female ratio is about 4 to 1. Since the male-to-female ratio of radiographic sacroiliitis approaches unity above age 45,[111] males may have a tendency toward more frequent and more severe axial skeletal disease.[112] Alternatively, systematic underestimation of ankylosing spondylitis in females may occur because of an avoidance of pelvic radiographs in females of childbearing age and a lower index of suspicion because of the accepted male predominance.

Familial aggregation has been well documented.[113] The discovery of the association of HLA-B27 with ankylosing spondylitis was a major advance in the understanding of the genetic predisposition.[114,115] Among whites, the frequency of HLA-B27 approaches 90% in patients with ankylosing spondylitis compared to about 8% in normal controls. The association is present in all populations studied.

The evidence for a direct role of HLA-B27 in the pathogenesis of ankylosing spondylitis is summarized in Table 54-8.[116] However, since the concordance for ankylosing spondylitis in monozygotic twins is only slightly greater than 50%, and less than 20% of B27-positive individuals develop sacroiliitis, it appears that HLA-B27 is not sufficient for the development of ankylosing spondylitis. Several lines of evidence suggest that environmental triggers are important in this disease. Infectious agents, especially *Klebsiella* species colonizing the gastrointesti-

TABLE 54-7. PREVALENCE PER 1000 OF ANKYLOSING SPONDYLITIS BY RACIAL-ETHNIC GROUP

Group/Country	Prevalence (Per 1000)
Whites	
England	0.5
Norway	0.5
Netherlands	0.8
England	2.0
Hungary	2.3
Unites States	1.3
Iran	0.7
North American Indians[a]	
Haida	60.0
Bella Bella	63.0
Bella Coola	27.0
Pima	54.0
Pima	60.0
Blackfoot	6.5
Chippewa	93.0[b]
African blacks	
South Africa	0.7
West Africa	0.0
Orientals	
Japan	0.1

[a] Males only.
[b] Sacroiliitis and ankylosing spondylitis combined.
From Hochberg MC, 1984, with permission.[109]

TABLE 54-8. HLA-B27 IS CAUSALLY ASSOCIATED WITH ANKYLOSING SPONDYLITIS (AS): SUPPORTING DATA

1. AS is a disease of antiquity.
2. The frequency of HLA-B27 and the prevalence of AS parallel each other across ethnic groups.
3. The association of HLA-B27 and AS has been confirmed in all ethnic and racial populations studied.
4. HLA-B27-positive patients have a younger mean age at onset and are more likely to have acute anterior uveitis and aortic regurgitation than HLA-B27-negative patients.
5. Familial occurrence is rare in families of HLA-B27-negative patients in the absence of psoriasis or inflammatory bowel disease in relatives.
6. HLA-B27-negative patients are often B7-CREG (B7,Bw42)-positive.
7. There are no associations of AS with HLA-A, HLA-C, or HLA-D locus antigens except as explained by linkage disequilibrium (HLA-A2, HLA-Cw1, HLA-Cw2).
8. HLA-B27 has been shown to have immunologic cross-reactivity with *Klebsiella* antigens.
9. HLA-B27 has been shown to have a 6-amino-acid sequence homology with the *Klebsiella* pneumoniae nitrogenase enzyme.

Modified from Hochberg MC: 1989.[105]

nal tract, are the postulated triggers receiving the most attention at present. Increased fecal carriage of *Klebsiella* in stool cultures of patients with active ankylosing spondylitis[117] and elevated serum levels of IgA antibodies against *Klebsiella pneumoniae* have been noted.[118] In addition, immunologic cross-reactivity between certain *Klebsiella* species and HLA-B27 has been identified.[119] More recently, Schwimmbeck and colleagues[120] identified a 6-amino acid sequence homology between the *Klebsiella pneumoniae* nitrogenase enzyme and the hypervariable region of HLA-B27.[120] These observations, indirectly supported by the apparent efficacy of the antimicrobial agent sulfasalazine in the treatment of ankylosing spondylitis[121] suggest the potential use of a vaccine in B27-positive individuals.

The course of ankylosing spondylitis is characterized by exacerbations and remissions, but the overall prognosis is quite good. Most patients are able to continue work with only minimal-to-moderate disability from their disease.[122] Survivorship of community-derived cases appears to be comparable to that of the overall population.[110] Cases seen in academic referral centers appeared to have decreased long-term survival,[123,124] but this likely reflects patterns of referral or selection bias.

Prevention of Arthritic Disorders

Primary Prevention. Primary prevention requires knowledge of etiologic factors that may be the object of preventive efforts. Such knowledge is not yet available for most of the the arthritic disorders. Although groups predisposed to rheumatoid arthritis and ankylosing spondylitis may be identified through immunogenetic studies, the triggering mechanisms for these disorders are as yet unknown. Two of the arthritic disorders, osteoarthritis and gout, may be prevented to some extent.

OSTEOARTHRITIS. Although the etiology of idiopathic (primary) osteoarthritis is not known, several potentially modifiable risk factors have been identified, including obesity and repetitive joint usage and trauma. Weight loss, reduction of the number of injuries, and reduction of exposure to repetitive mechanical stress on the joints in the work place would probably be beneficial. Concerning secondary osteoarthritis, several potentially treatable diseases have been recognized as producing this condition: congenital dislocation of the hip, slipped epiphysis, and various other developmental and acquired bone and joint disorders. Early treatment of these disorders may prevent the development of or at least limit the extent of secondary osteoarthritis; however, specific studies evaluating this are not available.

GOUT. Hyperuricemia is a known necessary risk factor for the development of gout and can be readily identified in normal persons through the use of automated multichannel analysis of serum specimens. The decision as to when to treat persons with asymptomatic hyperuricemia is controversial. Liang and Fries[125] cite several practical points that militate against routine treatment, including poor compliance, high costs, and adverse drug reactions. Furthermore, these authors state that acute gouty attacks can be easily, inexpensively, and effectively treated with short courses of NSAIDs. Thus, prevention of gout in persons with asymptomatic hyperuricemia should be based on modifications in life style, such as weight reduction, control of hypertension (without the use of diuretics) and hyperlipidemia, and moderation or elimination of alcoholic intake. In addition, because of the known association of occupational lead exposure with gout, prevention efforts should also be directed at the workplace, with reduction in exposure in high-risk professions, such as painting, plumbing, shipbuilding, and steel working.

Secondary Prevention. Screening tests for the arthropathies are not available at present. Thus, secondary prevention strategies are primarily aimed at controlling the early symptoms of pain and stiffness with medical therapy. Methods of treating the arthritic disorders discussed earlier (except gout) share certain common modalities and will be described briefly; readers are referred to medical textbooks for more detailed information.[126,127]

First-line medical therapy consists of NSAIDs.[128,129] These drugs are anti-inflammatory, analgesic, and antipyretic; their mode of action is believed to be largely attributable to inhibition of prostaglandin biosynthesis. NSAIDs will be the only drugs required for adequate treatment in most patients with osteoarthritis and ankylosing spondylitis. Patients with rheumatoid arthritis whose symptoms and signs are not adequately controlled with NSAIDs or who develop joint deformities or bony erosion require other agents in addition to NSAIDs,[130,131] such as gold (oral or injectable), hydroxychloroquine, methotrexate, azathioprine, and penicillamine. Oral corticosteroids, usually given in doses of < 10 mg/d of prednisone, probably have a role in management of the rheumatoid arthritis patient as an adjunct to remittive therapy.[132]

Physical therapy is another secondary prevention strategy, the goals of which are relief of pain, prevention of deformity, and maintenance of function. Modalities employed by the therapist include rest, splinting, heat and cold, and instruction in an exercise program, including energy-conservation and joint-protection techniques and range of motion and muscle-strengthening exercises.[133] In addition, patient education and psychosocial support mechanisms are important. The physical therapy program needs to be individualized for specific diseases and for individual patients with each disorder.

Medical treatment of gout is at the stage where recurrent attacks of arthritis may be prevented through long-term use of colchicine and through reversal of hyperuricemia with agents that either increase uric acid excretion or inhibit its production.[134] In addition, the prevention strategies for gout should be used in conjunction with treatment of associated conditions such as hypertension and hyperlipidemia.

Foot Disorders in Older Adults

About three fourths of fully active older adults complain of painful feet.[135-137] Among institutionalized adults, foot problems are one fifth as common, indicating an important etiological role for stress on the feet from ordinary physical activity. Over half of noninstitutionalized older adults have corns and calluses, one fourth have bunions, one third have painful toenails, and one fourth have cold feet, often as a result of circulatory disorders. A variety of static and functional deformities of the feet, such as hallux valgus, digiti flexus, and trophic changes, are related to degenerative disease; their prevalence rates increase with age. Foot strain from walking and standing is also common. The majority of painful conditions of the foot seen by orthopedists originate in soft tissues such as muscles, ligaments, tendons, nerves, and blood vessels. Articular and skeletal disorders of the feet may result from congenital abnormalities, infections, neoplasms, or trauma,[138] as well as from osteoarthritis, rheumatoid arthritis, and, less commonly, gout.

Prevention at all levels includes wearing proper shoes, wearing socks or stockings, bathing the feet frequently, avoidance of obesity, protection against infection and trauma to the feet, and proper care of toenails.[136,139] Once foot problems occur, soft, well-padded shoes should be worn to relieve pressure in sore areas. Pads, moleskin, lamb's wool, and hammer-toe pads applied to localized areas of soreness may be helpful. In most instances, these simple methods can reduce much of the discomfort associated with foot problems.[136] In some cases, rest, application of heat and cold, specific exercises, and use of special corrective shoes may be needed.[138] Almost half of the people with foot disorders are not receiving care for the problem.[137]

Paraplegia and Quadriplegia

The most common cause of paraplegia and quadriplegia in Western countries is vertebral fractures and dislocation from trauma. Complete transection of the spinal cord results in paralysis of all muscles supplied by motor neurons below the level of the lesion and in the loss of skin sensation in all areas supplied by sensory neurons below the lesion. Because neurons in the central nervous system do not regenerate, both motor and sensory paralysis is permanent.

The effect on the patient, family, and friends is immediate and enormous. Most affected individuals were previously independent and must learn to cope with partial or complete paralysis, loss of sensation in major parts of the body, and loss of voluntary control over body functions, frequently including bowel and bladder dysfunction and loss of sexual function. The patient's work, marriage, family, and social relationships are likely to be substantially altered.[140]

In the United States about 238,000 people have traumatic spinal cord injuries, with 11,000 new cases occurring each year.[141] Spinal cord injuries occur most frequently in persons ages 15 to 20 years and are more common in males than in females and in blacks than in whites.[142] Motor vehicle accidents, especially those involving motorcycles, are by far the leading cause of these injuries. Other major causes are falls from heights, acts of violence (gunshot wounds and stabbings), and sports and recreational activities such as diving in shallow water, injuries sustained during gymnastics, and hard contact sports.[142] Nontraumatic causes include infections, vascular diseases, congenital abnormalities, tumors, intervertebral disc lesions, and neuromuscular diseases such as cerebral palsy and multiple sclerosis.[143]

The most important primary prevention measures are those that reduce the likelihood of motor vehicle accidents and lessen the risk of injury if accidents do occur. These include not driving after drinking alcoholic beverages, reduced speed limits, use of seat belts and headrests, and wearing of helmets by motorcyclists. Safety measures in occupational and recreational settings are also important. For instance, in high school and collegiate football, rules banning "spearing" or initial contact with the top of the helmet when making a tackle have markedly reduced the frequency of permanent cervical quadriplegia resulting from participation in that sport. Changes in playing techniques and equipment might reduce the frequency of such injuries in other sports as well.[144]

The number of survivors with paraplegia and quadriplegia has greatly increased because of medical and surgical advances. Since most of those injured are in their late teens and early adult years, enormous costs and very long-term severe disability ensue. In addition to psychological problems, the greatest difficulties are in self-care, locomotion, obtaining employment, and medical complications. The main object of tertiary prevention is to return the affected person to maximum physical and social functioning. Both physical and psychological adjustments are needed. Accordingly, in addition to specialists in orthopedic and neurological surgery, other specialists that should be involved in therapy of these patients include occupational and physical therapists, psychiatrists, orthotics specialists, urologists, and vocational counselors. Long leg braces, crutches, and gait training may help highly motivated paraplegics with low-level lesions return to walking and may even enable them to become self-supporting. Because many paraplegics drive cars, wheelchair accessibility of public buildings is becoming increasingly important.[145] Sexual counseling also may be helpful for many.

DISORDERS PRIMARILY OF CHILDREN

Scoliosis

Scoliosis, or abnormal lateral curvature of the spine associated with rotation of the vertebrae, is the most common cause of spinal deformity in North American children.[146] Of the various forms of scoliosis, the most common and serious is adolescent idiopathic scoliosis. About 2% to 3% of children develop curves of 10 degrees or more before growth ceases, and about 2 to 3 per 1000 children develop curves of 30 degrees or more.[147,148] Persons left with significant curvature frequently develop spinal osteoarthritis in adulthood; lung and heart complications may occur. Also, further curve progression sometimes takes place in adults.

Scoliosis is most frequently diagnosed around the ages of 11 to 14 years in girls and around 14 to 16 years in boys. The ratio of female to male cases seen at surgery is as high as 5 to 1, but mild curves of less than 15 degrees are found with almost equal frequency in both sexes. Although surgical series have indicated that scoliotic curves are most common at the thoracic level, screening programs identifying children who do not necessarily seek medical care have found that the peak frequency is at the thoracolumbar level.[149]

The risk for scoliosis in first-degree relatives of cases is about three to four times higher than in other children.[150] Little is known of other risk factors for development of the disease. Some evidence suggests that children who are skeletally more mature at the onset but not at the end of puberty are most likely to be affected, and that individuals with scoliosis tend to be taller and leaner than others of their age at the beginning but not at the end of adolescence.[151] Impaired visual and vestibular functioning, asymmetric muscle activity, unequal leg length, high concentrations of calcium in paraspinal muscles, and collagen disorders may be etiologically involved, but evidence is not conclusive.[152] Children with scoliosis appear to have mothers of older age than do other children of the same age.[150]

Some risk factors for progression of existing curves have been identified: double curves as opposed to single curves, thoracic curves as opposed to curves at lower levels, curves of greater magnitude, the female sex, absence of a sacral tilt, limb-length inequality, early chronological age, and skeletal immaturity.[153,154]

Because so little is known of the etiology of adolescent idiopathic scoliosis, primary prevention is not feasible. However, detection of early diseases by screening is being undertaken in many places; it is assumed that with early detection, affected children can be treated by conservative means and thereby avoid surgery. The traditional screening test for scoliosis has been the forward-bend test. In this test, the child's back is examined while he or she bends forward from the waist. The rotation that accompanies the lateral curvature in scoliosis results in posterior prominence of the ribs on the concave side of the curvature, so that a "rib hump" is often apparent on forward bending. In a more recently developed screening method, Moiré topography, a photograph of the back is used to measure the degree of topographic asymmetry. The forward-bend test has good specificity but fairly low sensitivity. Moiré topography has >95% sensitivity, but it picks up many minor curves.[155] The inclinometer (scoliometer), which measures trunk asymmetry as an indicator of trunk rotation, has been reported to have high sensitivity and fairly good specificity, but it has not been used much. Most school screening programs use the forward-bend test.

In the United States, school screening programs are identifying large numbers of children with possible spinal curvatures. Positive screening tests are followed up with x-ray examination for more definitive diagnosis. Curves of over 5 degrees are monitored by further x-ray examination every few months. Should a curve progress to 20 to 25 degrees, treatment is generally indicated to prevent further progression and may consist of exercises, braces, external or internal muscle stimulators, or, in severe cases, surgery.

Many questions have arisen about the desirability of widespread screening for scoliosis.[156] First, it is uncertain that school screening programs have brought about a reduction in the prevalence of severe deformities and thereby the number of operations needed. In particular, the efficacy of conservative treatment in preventing progression is uncertain. Also, many children screened as positive are not subsequently seen for definitive diagnosis. On the other hand, many false positives occur, resulting in referral of far too many children for x-ray examination. Many children incur a great deal of medical expense and anxiety and are exposed to x-rays that otherwise would have been unnecessary. In addition, not enough is known about factors that predict which curves will progress. The optimal ages for screening and whether males should be screened at all have not been determined. Criteria for referral for diagnosis and treatment should be reconsidered, and better training and evaluation of the nurses who do the screening may be needed.[148,156]

Slipped Capital Femoral Epiphysis

Slipped epiphysis of the head of the femur, in which epiphysis of the head of the femur is displaced backward and downward off the diaphysis, is primarily a disease of adolescents. It is closely related to the adolescent growth spurt and does not occur once the epiphysis is fused to the shaft of the femur. In the northeastern United States about 1 in 800 males and 1 in 2000 females will be diagnosed as having a slipped epiphysis before they reach 25 years of age.[157]

The median age at diagnosis is 13 years for males and 11 years for females, the earlier age in females corresponding to their earlier onset of puberty. Males are affected more frequently; however, the magnitude of the excess varies from one geographical area to another and appears to have decreased over time. Blacks are affected more frequently than whites. In many localities, symptoms begin more frequently in spring and summer than in fall and winter.[158,159]

A large proportion of children with slipped epiphysis are markedly overweight; about half are at or above the 95th percentile for their age (Fig. 54-4).[160] Children with slipped epiphysis tend to have undergone slower-than-average skeletal maturation and to be tall for their age at the time of diagnosis.[161] At maturity, however, their heights are almost normal for their chronological age.[159] Familial aggregation of cases has been reported,[162] but it is not clear whether this aggregation is primarily attributable to inherited characteristics or to common environmental factors.

Many of these risk factors are related either to a weakening of the epiphyseal plate, such as occurs during periods of rapid growth, or to increased shearing stress on the plate. Animal experiments indicate that a deficit of sex hormones relative to growth hormone brings about the widening of the epiphyseal plate and a reduction in the shearing force necessary to displace the epiphysis.[163] Estrogens protect against slipped epiphysis whereas androgens are protective only in large doses after prolonged exposure. Children with the unusual combination of being overweight and undergoing slow skeletal maturation would appear to be at high risk, and these children should be carefully watched for slipped epiphysis.

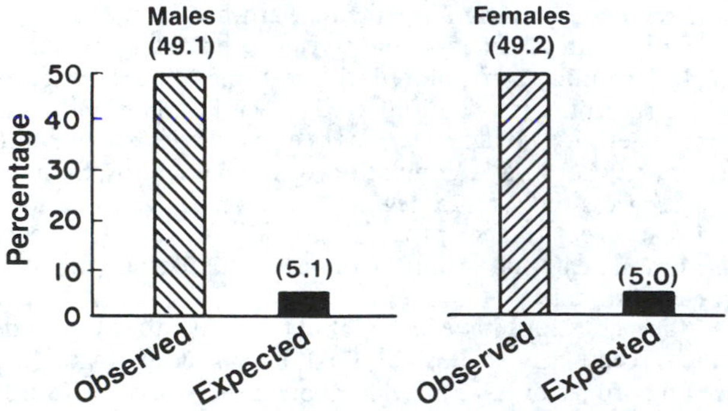

Figure 54-4. Percentage of children with slipped epiphysis with weights at or above the 95th percentile for their age. *[From Kelsey JL, Acheson RM, Keggi KJ, 1972, with permission.[160]]*

The only known means of primary prevention is prevention of obesity in adolescents. No screening tests for slipped epiphysis exist, but the diagnosis should be suspected in adolescents who have a limp and hip or knee discomfort, especially if there is restriction of internal rotation of the hip. X-ray examination should be performed immediately to confirm the diagnosis. Also, the contralateral hip of children with slipped epiphysis on one side should be carefully monitored. Slight degrees of slippage that are treated early by hip pinning have a favorable prognosis, whereas cases diagnosed late and that involve severe displacement generally are associated with early onset of osteoarthritis of the hip and permanent disability despite treatment.

Juvenile Chronic Arthritis

Juvenile chronic arthritis encompasses several distinct subsets: (1) Still's disease, which is a systemic form often complicated by rash and fever; (2) polyarthritis, seropositive for rheumatoid factor, or "true" adult rheumatoid arthritis, beginning in childhood; (3) polyarthritis, seronegative for rheumatoid factor; (4) oligoarthritis in females, usually associated with chronic iritis; and (5) oligoarthritis in males, usually associated with acute iritis, HLA-B27, and frequently developing into juvenile ankylosing spondylitis.[164] The diagnostic criteria used in population studies in the United States are those proposed by the American Rheumatism Association for juvenile rheumatoid arthritis.[165,166]

In Rochester, Minnesota,[167] prevalence of juvenile arthritis, as of January 1, 1980, was 2.0 per 1000 for females and 0.3 per 1000 for males. It should be noted that these prevalence rates include children with a previous diagnosis of juvenile arthritis but whose disease was currently inactive or in remission. The authors noted that prevalence rates for active juvenile arthritis would be substantially lower, probably 50% of that noted above. In an urban black population the prevalence as of December 31, 1980, was estimated as 0.26 per 1000 based on four subjects who are alive and under observation and fulfilled the American Rheumatism Association criteria.[168] Studies performed in Finland[169] and England[170] have reported prevalence estimates of comparable magnitude: 0.40 and 0.65 per 1000, respectively.

The average annual incidence rate of juvenile arthritis has been estimated to vary from 2.2 to 9.2 per 100,000 per year in children younger than age 17.[168,169,171,172] A recent Finnish study identified 27 incident cases in the Helsinki area over a 1-year period corresponding to an incidence rate of 18.2 per 100,000.[173] Age at onset and gender have been related to different clinical subsets of juvenile arthritis.

Genetic studies in juvenile arthritis have been reviewed.[174] The heterogeneity of juvenile arthritis is reinforced by the familial aggregations of sacroiliitis and ankylosing spondylitis in relatives of probands with sacroiliitis and of erosive arthritis in relatives of probands with seropositive polyarthritis.[175] High concordance rates of juvenile arthritis among monozygotic as compared to dizygotic twin pairs also support a role for genetic predisposition.[175] Several class I and II HLA associations, including HLA-B27, Bw35, DR5, DR8, and DPw2, have been reported with different clinical subsets of juvenile chronic arthritis.[174]

Regarding a possible infectious etiology, it has been recognized that many patients diagnosed with oligoarticular juvenile arthritis represent cases of Lyme disease.[176] Indeed, it is now accepted medical practice to obtain serologic studies for Lyme antibodies in all children presenting with features of juvenile arthritis. In children without evidence of Lyme disease the role of viral infection, particularly rubella, in the etiology of juvenile arthritis remains an area of speculation.

No methods of primary prevention are known. Aspirin and other NSAIDs approved for use in children by the Food and Drug Administration are used in treatment. Aspirin should be avoided when patients have an intercurrent viral syndrome or influenza infection because of the rare possibility of Reye's syndrome. Patients who fail to respond to these agents are treated with the same "second-line" agents as are adults with rheumatoid arthritis. Rehabilitation of patients with juvenile chronic arthritis follows the same principles and guidelines noted previously in the discussion of adult arthritic disorders. Unique features of the rehabilitation of children include educational and psychosocial development as well as the dynamic interaction in the home environment.[177] A high level of collaboration needs to be maintained between the parents, school, and rheumatology team.

Fractures

Each year almost 1 in 20 to 25 children fracture or dislocate a bone in some part of the body.[178,179] Sites fractured with high frequency in children relative to other age groups include the lower forearm, clavicle, tibia, fibula, and elbow (including supracondylar fractures and fractures of the capitulum of the humerus). A fall on an outstretched hand is a frequent cause of fractures of the clavicle, radius, ulna, and supracondylar region of the humerus; blows to the forearm frequently cause fractures of the radius and ulna; falls on the elbow may result in fractures of the capitulum of the humerus; and angulating or rotational forces are the main cause of fractures of the tibia and fibula. Motorcycle accidents, sports injuries, and accidents related to bicycles also are frequent causes of fractures of the tibia and fibula. In general, primary prevention of fractures in children depends on reducing the number of automobile and bicycle accidents, falls, child-battering injuries, sports injuries, and other childhood traumas.[180–182]

Fractures usually heal rapidly in children; the younger the age, the more rapid the healing. However, if the growth plate is involved in the fracture, growth in that bone may be adversely affected, particularly if a crushing injury has occurred. Other complications are rare but may include infection, delayed union, nonunion, avascular necrosis, and malunion. Prevention of these complications involves thorough cleansing and removal of all dead and contaminated tissue from an open (compound) fracture and competent initial treatment of the fracture.[183]

Congenital Dislocation of the Hip

In congenital dislocation of the hip the head of the femur is displaced completely or partially out of the acetabulum. Partial displacement is sometimes referred to as congenital subluxation of the hip. In about 80% of cases the diagnosis is made shortly after birth, and in the remaining cases the diagnosis is made later, especially when the child starts to walk. Although it is possible that some of these late-diagnosed cases may represent dislocations that were missed around the time of birth, there is good evidence that some dislocations actually do develop after birth.[184]

The prevalence of congenital dislocation of the hip varies considerably from one geographic area to another. Rates ranging from 1 per 1000 to 10 per 1000 births have been reported in most North American and Western European populations and in Israel, Australia, and New Zealand. Higher rates of from 10 per 1000 to 100 per 1000 have been observed in the Navajo, Apache, and Cree-Ojibwa Indians of North America, in the Lapps, and in the populations of Hungary, northern Italy, Brittany, and the Faroe Islands. Congenital dislocation of the hip is rare among blacks in South Africa, the West Indies, and Uganda, as well as among Chinese living in Hong Kong.[185] Although the frequency of congenital dislocation of the hip has been reported to be rising in recent years in certain areas, much of the apparent rise may be attributable to more extensive screening after birth and to increased awareness by physicians.[186]

In North America, girls are affected more frequently than boys in the ratio of about 6 to 1. Rates are also higher in whites than in blacks. In most areas, a greater than expected number of cases is encountered in children born in late fall and winter than in summer.[187]

Familial aggregation of cases occurs; both hereditary and environmental factors contribute to the familial excess.[188] Maternal relatives of cases have a higher risk than paternal relatives.[189] On the average, infants with congenital dislocation of the hip have had longer gestation periods than other infants and are considerably more likely to have been born by breech delivery than other infants.[187,190]

The reasons for these epidemiological characteristics are not known with certainty. Position in utero may be involved, since breech position in utero elongates the ligament of the hip joint capsule by persistent upward pressure of the greater trochanter.[191] Ligamentous and capsular laxity are probably predisposing factors also.[192] No feasible methods of primary prevention are known.

In regard to secondary prevention, examination of newborn infants for congenital dislocation of the hip is now accepted as a routine procedure. Without prompt treatment the affected leg may be shorter, the child may limp, surgery may be required, and osteoarthritis of the hip is likely to occur in young adulthood. Two screening tests are generally used: the Ortolani and the Barlow. The Ortolani test involves placing the hip in flexion and gently adducting and then abducting the hip. The test is considered positive if a palpable jerk and audible clunk are heard as the head of the femur returns to the acetabulum. Some practitioners also consider an audible click to constitute a positive test. In the Barlow test, gentle downward pressure is exerted over the lesser trochanter with the hip in flexion and adduction; the unstable hip shifts from the acetabulum, and a sensation similar to the Ortolani sign is produced. When the leg is allowed to abduct, the hip is reduced.

About half of the hips noted to be unstable at birth become stable spontaneously within 3 weeks[193]; thus, these tests are often repeated at that time. Infants showing positive results on these tests are treated with braces, splints, or harnesses for 2 to 4 months. X-ray examination of the hip is of limited value in the newborn, but is an important diagnostic tool in children past the age of 3 months. Routine checks on hips of these infants should be done until they are walking well. If the disease is diagnosed after the neonatal period, surgery is generally required, and the prognosis is poorer.[194]

Despite the routine use in many locales of screening tests for congenital dislocation of the hip, many questions have arisen in recent years regarding the effectiveness of the screening.[195,196] First, it appears that incidence rates of congenital dislocation of the hip requiring prolonged treatment are no lower now than they were before screening became widespread. Both the sensitivity and specificity of the screening tests are poor. In one recent study[195] only one third of genuine cases were detected, and the ratio of false positives to true positives was 10 to 1. Thus, for every one infant who benefits from splinting as a result of a positive test, 10 infants undergo unnecessary splinting. Furthermore, there is no consensus on indications for treatment, the timing of treatment, and the type of splint to be used. The question has arisen as to whether the screening procedures may themselves induce hip dislocation. Although these screening tests require experienced examiners for proper performance and interpretation, inexperienced examiners often are used, thus increasing both false-positive and false-negative rates. Better knowledge of which hips will spontaneously stabilize would allow better decisions about the cases that should receive immediate treatment. Disagreement exists about the significance of a soft audible or palpable click without evidence of abnormal movement between the femoral head and acetabulum.[197] Some physicians feel that such infants should be followed closely and given x-ray examination, while others feel that the likelihood of these infants actually developing congenital dislocation of the hip is too low to warrant the expense, exposure to x-rays, and anxiety. More data are needed to resolve these issues. Further use of ultrasound, which provides a defined image of the bony and cartilaginous neonatal hip for initial screening or for secondary screening in those already identified as being at high risk may alleviate some of these problems.[198,199]

CONCLUSION

The extent to which musculoskeletal disorders may be prevented varies considerably from one disorder to another. Some methods of primary prevention are available for back disorders, osteoporosis, osteoarthritis, gout, foot disorders, paraplegia and quadriplegia, slipped epiphysis, and fractures. However, these preventive measures frequently involve changes in individual behavior that are difficult to achieve. Screening tests for early detection of scoliosis, congenital dislocation of the hip, and osteoporosis are available. Although the tests for scoliosis and congenital dislocation of the hip are being widely used at present, many questions regarding their efficacy remain unresolved.

Secondary and tertiary prevention are the levels more frequently used for the major musculoskeletal disorders of adults. However, with the exception of reconstructive joint surgery, secondary and tertiary prevention for such common problems as back pain and the arthritic disorders often has met with only limited success. Because of the chronicity of most of the common musculoskeletal conditions and the frequent reliance on only partially successful secondary and tertiary prevention measures, it is not surprising that musculoskeletal disorders have such a major effect on the quality of life and are associated with such high individual and societal costs. Improving the quality of life of affected individuals and further development and evaluation of screening tests will remain important in the management of musculoskeletal disorders, but it is also hoped that more emphasis will be placed on identification of feasible ways of preventing these disorders from occurring in the first place. Since the elderly are most frequently affected by musculoskeletal disorders and since the numbers of elderly will be increasing greatly over the next several decades, development of better methods of prevention at all levels is an urgent public health concern.

REFERENCES

1. Holbrook TL, Grazier K, Kelsey JL, Stauffer RN: The Frequency of Occurrence, Impact, and Cost of Musculoskeletal Conditions in the United States. Chicago: American Academy of Orthopaedic Surgeons, 1985
2. Kelsey JL, White AA III: Epidemiology and impact of low-back pain. Spine 5:133–142, 1980
3. Dixon A St J: Progress and problems in back pain research. Rheumatol Rehabil 12:165–174, 1973
4. Snook SH: Low back pain in industry. In White AA III, Gordon SL (eds): Symposium on Idiopathic Low Back Pain. St Louis: CV Mosby, 1982
5. Andersson GB: Epidemiologic aspects of low-back pain in industry. Spine 6:53–60, 1981
6. Kelsey JL, Githens PB, White AA III, et al: An epidemiologic study of lifting and twisting on the job and risk for acute prolapsed lumbar intervertebral disc. J Orthop Res 2:61–66, 1984
7. Frymoyer JW: Back pain and sciatica. N Engl J Med 318:291–300, 1986
8. Kelsey JL, Githens PB, O'Connor T, et al: Acute prolapsed lumbar intervertebral disc: An epidemiologic study with special reference to driving automobiles and cigarette smoking. Spine 9:608–613, 1984
9. Heliovaara M: Epidemiology of sciatica and herniated lumbar intervertebral disc. Helsinki: Publications of the Social Insurance Institution, Finland, ML:76, 1988
10. Kelsey JL, Githens PB, Walter SD, et al: An epidemiologic study of acute prolapsed cervical intervertebral disc. J Bone Joint Surg 66A:907–914, 1984
11. Deyo RA, Diehl AK: Psychosocial predictors of disability in patients with low back pain. J Rheumatol 15:1557–1564, 1988
12. Fish JR, DiMonte P, Courington SM: Back schools: past, present, and future. Clin Orthop 179:18–23, 1983
13. Hall H, Iceton JA: Back school: An overview with specific reference to the Canadian back education units. Clin Orthop 179:10–17, 1983
14. Lankhurst GJ, Van de Stadt RJ, Vogelaar TW, Van de Korst JK, Prevo AJH: The effect of the Swedish back school on chronic idiopathic low back pain. Scand J Rehabil Med 15:141–145, 1983
15. Nachemson A: Work for all: Those with back pain as well. Clin Orthop 179:77–85, 1983
16. Cummings SR, Kelsey JL, Nevitt MC, O'Dowd KJ: Epidemiology of osteoporosis and osteoporotic fractures. Epidemiol Rev 7:178–208, 1985
17. Lindsay R, Hart DM, MacLean A, et al: Bone response to termination of estrogen treatment. Lancet 1:1325–1327, 1978
18. Paganini-Hill A, Ross RK, Gerkins VR, et al: Menopausal estrogen therapy and hip fractures. Ann Intern Med 95:28–31, 1981
19. Slemenda C, Hui SL, Longscope C, Johnston CC: Sex steroids and bone mass. A study of changes about the time of menopause. J Clin Invest 80:1261–1269, 1987
20. Kelsey JL: Epidemiology of osteoporosis and associated fractures. Bone Mineral Research 5:409–444, 1987
21. Riis B, Thomsen K, Christiansen C: Does calcium supplementation prevent postmenopausal bone loss? N Engl J Med 316:173–177, 1987
22. Stevenson JC, Lees B, Davenport M, Cust MP, Ganger KF: Determinants of bone density in normal women: Risk factors for future osteoporosis. Br Med J 298:924–928, 1989
23. Ray WA, Griffin MR, Downey W, Melton LJ: Long term use of thiazide diuretics and risk of hip fracture. Lancet 1:687–690, 1989
24. Seeman E, Hopper JL, Bach LA, et al: Reduced bone mass in daughters of women with osteoporosis. N Engl J Med 320:554–558, 1989
25. Cummings SR, Black D: Should perimenopausal women be screened for osteoporosis? Ann Intern Med 104:817–823, 1986
26. Health and Public Policy Committee. American College of Physicians: Bone mineral density. Ann Intern Med 107:932–936, 1987
27. Hui SL, Slemenda CW, Johnston CC Jr: Age and bone mass as predictors of fracture in a prospective study. J Clin Invest 81:1804–1809, 1988
28. Riggs BL, Wahner HW: Bone densitometry and clinical decision-making in osteoporosis (editorial). Ann Intern Med 108:293–295, 1988
29. Tinetti ME, Speechley M: Prevention of falls among the elderly. N Engl J Med 320:1055–1059, 1989
30. Hochberg MC: Osteoarthritis. Postgrad Adv Rheumatol 3:1–12, 1988
31. Council for International Organizations of Medical Sciences: The Epidemiology of Chronic Rheumatism, Vol. 20 Atlas of Standard Radiographs of Arthritis. Oxford: Blackwell, 1963
32. Kallman DA, Wigley FM, Scott WW Jr, Hochberg MC, Tobin JD: New grading scales for radiographic hand osteoarthritis: Reliability for determining prevalence and progression. Arthritis Rheum 32:1584–1591, 1989
33. Kallman DA, Wigley FM, Scott WW Jr, Hochberg MC, Tobin JD: The longitudinal course of hand osteoarthritis in a male population. Arthritis Rheum 33:1323–1332, 1990
34. Altman RD, Asch E, Bloch DA, et al: Development of criteria for the classification and reporting of osteoarthritis: Classification of osteoarthritis of the knee. Arthritis Rheum 29:1039–1049, 1986
35. Altman D, Alarcon G, Appelrouth D, et al: Development of cri-

teria for the classification and reporting of osteoarthritis of the hand. Arthritis Rheum 33:1601–1610, 1990
36. Altman RD, Bloch DA, Bole GG Jr, et al: Development of clinical criteria for osteoarthritis. J Rheumatol 14(suppl 14):3–6, 1987
37. Kellgren JH, Moore R: Generalized osteoarthritis and Heberden's nodes. Br Med J 1:181–187, 1952
38. Schumacher HR: Secondary osteoarthritis. In Moskowitz RW, Howell DS, Goldberg WM, Mankin HJ (eds): Osteoarthritis: Diagnosis and Management. Philadelphia: W.B. Saunders, 1984
39. Lawrence RC, Hochberg MC, Kelsey JL, et al: Estimates of the prevalence of selected arthritic and musculoskeletal diseases in the United States. J Rheumatol 16:427–441, 1989
40. National Center for Health Statistics: Osteoarthrosis in Adults by Selected Demographic Characteristics: United States, 1960–1962. Vital and Health Statistics, Series 2, No. 20, 1966
41. National Center for Health Statistics: Basic Data on Arthritis: Knee, Hip and Sacroiliac Joints in Adults Aged 25–74 Years: United States, 1971–1975. Vital and Health Statistics, Series 11, No. 213, 1979
42. Hochberg MC, Lawrence RC, Everett DF, Cornoni-Huntley J: Epidemiologic associations of pain in osteoarthritis of the knee. Semin Arthritis Rheum 18(suppl 2):4–9, 1989
43. Butler WJ, Hawthorne VM, Mikkelsen WM, et al: Prevalence of radiographically defined osteoarthritis in the finger and wrist joints of adult residents of Tecumseh, Michigan, 1962–65. J Clin Epidemiol 41:467–473, 1988
44. Lawrence JS, Bremner JM, Bier F: Osteoarthrosis: Prevalence in the population and relationship between symptoms and x-ray changes. Ann Rheum Dis 25:1–24, 1966
45. Acheson RM, Chan Y-K, Clemett AR: New Haven Survey of Joint Diseases. XII. Distribution and symptoms of osteoarthrosis in the hands with reference to handedness. Ann Rheum Dis 29:275–286, 1970
46. Stecher RM: Heberden's nodes: A clinical description of osteoarthritis of the finger joints. Ann Rheum Dis 14:1–10, 1955
47. Palotie A, Ott J, Elima K, et al: Predisposition to familial osteoarthrosis linked to Type II collagen gene. Lancet 1:924–927, 1989
48. Scott JC, Hochberg MC: Epidemiologic insights into the pathogenesis of hip osteoarthritis. In Hadler NM (ed): Clinical Concepts in Regional Musculoskeletal Illness. Orlando, Florida: Grune & Stratton, 1987
49. Felson DT: Epidemiology of hip and knee osteoarthritis. Epidemiol Rev 10:1–28, 1988
50. Lawrence JS: Rheumatism in coalminers. Part 3. Occupational factors. Br J Ind Med 12:249–261, 1955
51. Lawrence JS: Rheumatism in cotton operatives. Br J Ind Med 18:270–276, 1961
52. Partridge REH, Duthie JJR: Rheumatism in dockers and civil servants: A comparison of heavy manual and sedentary workers. Ann Rheum Dis 27:559–568, 1968
53. Anderson JJ, Felson DT: Factors associated with osteoarthritis of the knee in the First National Health and Nutrition Examination Survey (HANES I). Am J Epidemiol 128:179–189, 1988
54. Davis MA, Ettinger WH, Neuhaus JM, Cho SA, Hauch WW: The association of knee injury and obesity with unilateral and bilaterial osteoarthritis of the knee. Am J Epidemiol 130:278–288, 1989
55. Lane NE, Bloch DA, Jones HH, et al: Long-distance running, bone density, and osteoarthritis. JAMA 255:1147–1151, 1986
56. Panush RS, Schmidt C, Caldwell JR, et al: Is running associated with degenerative joint disease? JAMA 255:1152–1155, 1986
57. Hartz AJ, Fischer ME, Bril G, et al: The association of obesity with joint pain and osteoarthritis in the HANES data. J Chronic Dis 39:311–319, 1986
58. Davis MA, Ettinger WH, Neuhaus JM, Hauck WW: Sex differences in osteoarthritis of the knee: The role of obesity. Am J Epidemiol 127:1029–1030, 1988
59. Davis MA, Ettinger WH, Neuhaus JM: The role of metabolic factors and blood pressure in the association of obesity with osteoarthritis of the knee. J Rheumatol 15:1827–1832, 1988
60. Felson DT, Anderson JJ, Naimark A, Walker AM, Meenan RF: Obesity and knee osteoarthritis: The Framingham Study. Ann Intern Med 109:18–24, 1988
61. Monson RR, Hall AP: Mortality among arthritics. J Chron Dis 28:459–467, 1976
62. Harris ED Jr: Rheumatoid arthritis. In Kelley WN, Harris ED Jr, Ruddy S, Sledge CB (eds): Textbook of Rheumatology. Philadelphia: W.B. Saunders, 1986
63. Bennett JC: The etiology of rheumatoid arthritis. In Kelley WN, Harris ED Jr, Ruddy S, Sledge CB (eds): Textbook of Rheumatology. Philadelphia: W.B. Saunders, 1986
64. Ropes MW, Bennett GA, Cobb S, Jacox R, Jessar RA: Revision of diagnostic criteria for rheumatoid arthritis. Bull Rheum Dis 9:175–176, 1958
65. Bennett PH, Burch TA: New York symposium on population studies in the rheumatic disease: New diagnostic criteria. Bull Rheum Dis 17:453–458, 1967
66. Lawrence JS: Rheumatism in Populations. London: Heinemann Medical Books, 1977
67. O'Sullivan JB, Cathcart ES: The prevalence of rheumatoid arthritis: Follow-up examination of the effect of criteria on rates in Sudbury, Massachusetts. Ann Intern Med 76:572–577, 1972
68. Arnett FC, Edworthy SM, Bloch DA, et al: The American Rheumatism Association Revised Criteria for the Classification of Rheumatoid Arthritis, 1988
69. National Center for Health Statistics: Rheumatoid Arthritis in Adults, 1960–1962. Vital and Health Statistics, Series 11, No. 17, 1966
70. Cunningham LS, Kelsey JL: Epidemiology of musculoskeletal impairments and associated disability. Am J Public Health 74:574–579, 1984
71. Linos A, Worthington JW, O'Fallon WM, Kurland LT: The epidemiology of rheumatoid arthritis in Rochester, Minnesota: A study of incidence, prevalence and mortality. Am J Epidemiol 111:87–98, 1980
72. Wingrave S, Kay CR: Reduction in incidence of rheumatoid arthritis associated with oral contraceptives. Lancet 1:569–571, 1978
73. Hochberg MC: Contrasting trends in the incidence and prevalence of rheumatoid arthritis in England and Wales, 1970–1982. Semin Arthritis Rheum 19:294–302, 1990
74. Beasley RP, Wilkens RF, Bennett PH: High prevalence of rheumatoid arthritis in Yakima Indians. Arthritis Rheum 16:743–747, 1973
75. Harvey J, Lotze M, Arnett FC, et al: RA in a Chippewa Band: II. Field study with clinical, serologic and HLA-D correlations. J Rheumatol 10:28–32, 1983
76. Kato H, Duff IF, Russell WJ, et al: Rheumatoid arthritis and gout in Hiroshima and Nagasaki, Japan: A prevalence and incidence study. J Chronic Dis 23:659–679, 1971
77. Beasley RP, Bennett PH, Lin CC: Low prevalence of rheumatoid arthritis in Chinese: Prevalence survey in a rural community. J Rheumatol 10(suppl 10):11–15, 1983
78. del Junco DJ, Luthra HS, Annegers JF, Worthington JW, Kurland LT: The familial aggregation of rheumatoid arthritis and its relationship to the HLA-DR4 association. Am J Epidemiol 119:813–829, 1984
79. Khan MA, Kushner I, Weitkamp LR: Genetics of HLA associated diseases: rheumatoid arthritis. Tissue Antigens 22:182–185, 1983
80. Goldstein R, Arnett FC: The genetics of rheumatic disease in man. Rheum Dis Clin North Am 13:487–510, 1987
81. Grennan DM, Sanders PA: Rheumatoid arthritis. Bailliere's Clin Rheumatol 2:585–601, 1988
82. Gregersen PK, Silver J, Winchester RJ: The shared epitope hypothesis: An approach to understanding the molecular genetics of the susceptibility to rheumatoid arthritis. Arthritis Rheum 30:1205–1213, 1987
83. Vaughan JH, Carson DA, Fox RI: The Epstein-Barr virus and rheumatoid arthritis. Clin Exp Rheumatol 1:265–272, 1983
84. White DG, Woolf AD, Mortimer PP, et al: Human parvovirus arthropathy. Lancet 1:419–421, 1985

85. Silman AJ, Vandenbroucke J (eds): Female sex hormones and rheumatoid arthritis. Br J Rheumatol 28(suppl):1–73, 1989
86. Spector TD, Hochberg MC: The protective effect of oral contraceptives on the development of rheumatoid arthritis: An overview of analytic epidemiologic studies with a meta-analysis. J Clin Epidemiol 43:1221–1230, 1990
87. Kelsey JL, Hochberg MC: Epidemiology of chronic musculoskeletal disorders. Ann Rev Public Health 9:379–401, 1988
88. Kirwan JR, Silman AJ: Epidemiologic, sociological, and environmental aspects of rheumatoid arthritis and osteoarthritis. Bailliere's Clin Rheumatol 1:467–489, 1987
89. Prior P, Symmons DPM, Hawkins CF, Scott DL, Brown R: Cancer morbidity in rheumatoid arthritis. Ann Rheum Dis 43:128–131, 1984
90. Prior P, Symmons DPM, Scott DL, Brown R, Hawkins CF: Cause of death in rheumatoid arthritis. Br J Rheumatol 23:92–99, 1984
91. Pincus T, Callahan LF: Formal education as a marker for increased mortality and morbidity in rheumatoid arthritis. J Chronic Dis 38:973–984, 1985
92. Holmes EW: Clinical gout and the pathogenesis of hyperuricemia. In McCarthy DJ (ed): Arthritis and Allied Conditions. Philadelphia: Lea & Febiger, 1985
93. Wallace SL, Robinson H, Masi AT, et al: Preliminary criteria for the classification of the acute arthritis of primary gout. Arthritis Rheum 20:895–900, 1977
94. National Center for Health Statistics: Current Estimates from the National Health Interview Study, United States, 1986. Vital and Health Statistics, Series 10, No. 164, 1987
95. Glynn RJ, Campion EW, Silbert JE: Trends in serum uric acid levels, 1961–1980. Arthritis Rheum 26:87–93, 1983
96. Brand FN, McGee DL, Kannel WB, Stokes J III, Castelli WP: Hyperuricemia as a risk factor of coronary heart disease: The Framingham Study. Am J Epidemiol 121:11–18, 1985
97. Abbott RD, Brand FN, Kannel WB, Castelli WP: Gout and coronary heart disease: The Framingham Study. J Clin Epidemiol 41:237–242, 1988
98. Hall AP, Barry PE, Dawber TR, McNamara PM: Epidemiology of gout and hyperuricemia: A long-term population study. Am J Med 42:27–37, 1967
99. Campion EW, Glynn RJ, DeLabry LO: Asymptomatic hyperuricemia: Risks and consequences in the normative aging study. Am J Med 82:421–426, 1987
100. Mikkelsen WM, Dodge HJ, Valkenburg H: The distribution of serum uric acid values in a population unselected as to gout and hyperuricemia, Tecumseh, Michigan, 1959–1960. Am J Med 39:242–251, 1965
101. Prior IAM: Epidemiology of rheumatic disorders in the South Pacific with emphasis on hyperuricemia and gout. Semin Arthritis Rheum 11:213–229, 1981
102. Zimmett PZ, Whitehouse S, Jackson L, Thana K: High prevalence of hyperuricemia and gout in an urbanised Micronesian population. Br Med J 1:1237–1239, 1978
103. Prior IAM, Welby TJ, Ostbye T, Salmond CE, Stokes YM: Migration and gout: The Tokelau Island migrant study. Br Med J 295:457–459, 1987
104. Richter BS, Hochberg MC: Lead exposure and other risk factors for gout: A case-control study (abstract). Arthritis Rheum 31(suppl 4):S22, 1988
105. Hochberg MC: Ankylosing spondylitis. Semin Spine Surg 2:86–94, 1990
106. Kellgren JH, Jeffrey MR, Ball J: The Epidemiology of Chronic Rheumatism. Oxford: Blackwell Scientific, 1963
107. Bennett PH, Wood PHN: Population Studies of the Rheumatic Diseases. New York: Excerpta Medica Foundation, 1968
108. The HSG, Steven MM, van der Linden SM, Cats A: Evaluation of diagnostic criteria for ankylosing spondylitis: A comparison of the Rome, New York, and modified New York criteria in patients with a positive clinical history screening test for ankylosing spondylitis. Br J Rheumatol 24:242–249, 1985
109. Hochberg MC: Epidemiology. In Calin A (ed): Spondylarthropathies. Orlando, Florida: Grune & Stratton, 1984
110. Carter ET, McKenna CH, Brian DD, Kurland LT: Epidemiology of ankylosing spondylitis in Rochester, Minnesota: 1935–1974. Arthritis Rheum 22:365–370, 1979
111. Lawrence JS: Rheumatism in Populations. London: Heinemann Medical Books, 1977, pp 282–324
112. Resnick D, Dwosh IL, Goergen TG, et al: Clinical and radiographic abnormalities in ankylosing spondylitis: A comparison of men and women. Radiology 119:293–297, 1976
113. Hochberg MC, Bias WB, Arnett FC: Family studies in HLA-B27-associated arthritis. Medicine 57:463–475, 1978
114. Brewerton DA, Hart FD, Nicholls A, et al: Ankylosing spondylitis and HLA 27. Lancet 1:904–907, 1973
115. Schlosstein L, Terasaki PI, Bluestone R, Pearson CM: High association of an HLA antigen, W27, with ankylosing spondylitis. N Engl J Med 288:704–706, 1973
116. Ahearn JM, Hochberg MC: Epidemiology and genetics of ankylosing spondylitis. J Rheumatol 15(suppl 16):22–28, 1988
117. Ebringer R, Cooke D, Cawdell DR, Cowing P, Ebringer A: Ankylosing spondylitis: Klebsiella and HLA-B27. Rheumatol Rehabil 16:190–196, 1977
118. Trul AK, Ebringer R, Panayi GS, et al: IgA antibodies to Klebsiella pneumoniae in ankylosing spondylitis. Scand J Rheumatol 12:249–253, 1983
119. Geczy AF, Prendergast JK, Sullivan JS, et al: HLA-B27, molecular mimicry, and ankylosing spondylitis: Popular misconceptions. Ann Rheum Dis 46:171–172, 1987
120. Schwimmbeck PL, Yu DT, Oldstone MB: Autoantibodies to HLA-B27 in the sera of HLA-B27 patients with ankylosing spondylitis and Reiter's syndrome: Molecular mimicry with Klebsiella pneumoniae as a potential mechanism of autoimmune disease. J Exp Med 166:173–181, 1987
121. Nissila M, Lehtinen K, Leirisalo-Repo H, et al: Sulfasalazine in the treatment of ankylosing spondylitis: A twenty-six-week, placebo-controlled clinical trial. Arthritis Rheum 31:1111–1116, 1988
122. Carette S, Graham DC, Little HA, Rosen P: The natural disease course of ankylosing spondylitis. Arthritis Rheum 26:186–190, 1983
123. Radford EP, Doll R, Smith PG: Mortality among patients with ankylosing spondylitis not given x-ray therapy. N Engl J Med 297:572–576, 1977
124. Khan MA, Khan MK, Kushner I: Survival among patients with ankylosing spondylitis: A life table analysis. J Rheumatol 8:86–90, 1981
125. Liang MH, Fries JF: Asymptomatic hyperuricemia: The case for conservative management. Ann Intern Med 88:666–670, 1978
126. Hart FD: Drug Treatment of the Rheumatic Diseases. New York: ADIS Press, 1979
127. Trentham DEF (ed): New Directions in Antirheumatic Therapy. Rheum Dis Clin North Am 15:407–626, 1989
128. Hochberg MC: NSAIDs: Mechanisms and pathways of action. Hosp Prac 24(3):185–198, 1989
129. Hochberg MC: NSAIDs: Patterns of usage and side effects. Hosp Prac 24(5):167–174, 1989
130. Hardin JG Jr: Rheumatoid arthritis therapy: The slow-acting agents. Hosp Prac 24(6):163–178, 1989
131. Kremer JM: Methotrexate therapy in the treatment of rheumatoid arthritis. Rheum Dis Clin North Am 15:533–555, 1989
132. Weiss MM: Corticosteroids in rheumatoid arthritis. Semin Arthritis Rheum 19:9–21, 1989
133. Navarro AH: The role of the physical therapist. In Riggs GK, Gall EP (eds): Rheumatic Diseases: Rehabilitation and Management. Boston: Butterworth Publishers, 1984
134. Wallace SL, Singer JZ: Therapy in gout. Rheum Dis Clin North Am 14:441–457, 1988
135. Evanski PM: The geriatric foot. In Jahss MH (ed): Disorders of the Foot. Philadelphia: W.B. Saunders, 1982
136. Caillet R: Foot and Ankle Pain. Philadelphia: F.A. Davis, 1983

137. Elton PJ, Sanderson SP: A chiropodial survey of elderly persons over 65 years in the community. Public Health 100:219–222, 1986
138. Helfand AE: At the foot of South Mountain. A 5-year longitudinal study of foot problems and screening in an elderly population. J Am Podiatr Assoc 63:512–521, 1973
139. Edelstein JE: Foot care for the aging. Physical Ther 68:1882–1886, 1988
140. Smart CN, Sanders CR: The Costs of Motor Vehicle Related Spinal Cord Injuries. Washington, D.C.: Insurance Institute for Highway Safety, 1976
141. Ergas Z: Spinal cord injury in the United States: A statistical update. Cent Nerv Syst Trauma 2:19–32, 1985
142. Stover SL, Fine PR: The epidemiology and economics of spinal cord injury. Paraplegia 25:225–228, 1987
143. Brashear MR Jr, Raney RB Sr: Shand's Handbook of Orthopaedic Surgery. St. Louis: C.V. Mosby, 1978
144. Torg JS, Vesgo JJ, Sennett B, Das M: The National Football Head and Neck Injury Registry: 14-year report on cervical quadriplegia, 1971 through 1984. JAMA 254:3439–3443, 1985
145. Sutton RA, Bentley M, Castree B, et al: Review of the social situation of paraplegic and tetraplegic patients rehabilitated in the Hexham Regional Spinal Injury Unit in the north of England over the past four years. Paraplegia 20:71–79, 1982
146. Winter RB: Spinal problems on pediatric orthopaedics. In Lovell WW, Winters RB (eds): Pediatric Orthopaedics, Vol. 2. Philadelphia: Lippincott, 1986
147. Shands AR, Eisberg HB: The incidence of scoliosis in the state of Delaware. J Bone Joint Surg 37A:1243–1249, 1955
148. Morais T, Bernier M, Turcotte F: Age- and sex-specific prevalence of scoliosis and the value of school screening programs. Am J Public Health 75:1377–1380, 1985
149. Brooks HL, Azen SD, Gerberg E, Brooks R, Chan L: Scoliosis: A prospective epidemiological study. J Bone Joint Surg 57A:968–972, 1975
150. Wynne-Davies R: Familial (idiopathic) scoliosis. A family survey. J Bone Joint Surg 50B:24–30, 1968
151. Willner S: A Study of height, weight, and menarche in girls with idiopathic structural scoliosis. Acta Orthop Scand 46:71–83, 1975
152. Kelsey JL: Epidemiology of Musculoskeletal Disorders. New York: Oxford University Press, 1982
153. Dickson RA, Stamper P, Sharp A-M, Harker P: School screening for scoliosis: Cohort study of clinical course. Br Med J 2:265–267, 1980
154. Lonstein JR: Natural history and school screening for scoliosis. Orthop Clin North Am 19:227–237, 1988
155. Laulund T, Sojbjerg JO, Horlyck E: Moiré topography in school screening for structural scoliosis. Acta Orthop Scand 53:765–768, 1982
156. Williams JI: Criteria for screening: Are the effects predictable? Spine 13:1178–1186, 1988
157. Kelsey JL: Incidence and distribution of slipped capital femoral epiphysis in Connecticut. J Chronic Dis 23:567–587, 1971
158. Kelsey JL: Epidemiology of slipped capital femoral epiphysis: A review of the literature. Pediatrics 51:1042–1050, 1973
159. Hansson LI, Hagglund G, Ordeberg G: Slipped capital femoral epiphysis in southern Sweden, 1910–1982. Acta Orthop Scand 226:1–67, 1987
160. Kelsey JL, Acheson RM, Keggi KJ: The body builds of patients with slipped capital femoral epiphysis. Am J Dis Child 124:276–281, 1972
161. Sorenson KH: Slipped upper femoral epiphysis. Acta Orthop Scand 39:499–517, 1968
162. Rennie AM: Familial slipped upper femoral epiphysis. J Bone Joint Surg 49B:535–539, 1967
163. Morscher E: Strength and morphology of growth cartilage under hormonal influence of puberty. Reconstr Surg Traumatol 10:3–104, 1968
164. Calabro JJ: Juvenile rheumatoid arthritis. In McCarty DJ (ed): Textbook of Rheumatology. Philadelphia: Lea & Febiger, 1985
165. Cassidy JT, Levinson JE, Bass JC, et al: A study of classification criteria for a diagnosis of juvenile rheumatoid arthritis. Arthritis Rheum 29:274–281, 1986
166. Cassidy JT, Levinson JE, Brewer EJ Jr: The development of classification criteria for children with juvenile rheumatoid arthritis. Bull Rheum Dis 38(6):1–7, 1989
167. Towner SR, Michet CJ, O'Fallon WM, Nelson AM: The epidemiology of juvenile arthritis in Rochester, Minnesota, 1960–1979. Arthritis Rheum 26:1208–1213, 1983
168. Hochberg MC, Linet MS, Sills ED: The prevalence and incidence of juvenile rheumatoid arthritis in an urban black population. Am J Public Health 73:1202–1203, 1983
169. Laaksonen AL: A prognostic study of juvenile rheumatoid arthritis: Analysis of 544 cases. Acta Pediatr Scand 166:S1–S163, 1966
170. Bywaters EGL: Diagnostic criteria for Still's disease (juvenile RA). In Bennett PH, Wood PHN (eds): Population Studies of The Rheumatic Diseases. Amsterdam: Excerpta Medica Foundation, 1968, pp 235–240
171. Hill R: Juvenile arthritis in various racial groups in British Columbia. Arthritis Rheum 20:162, 1977
172. Sullivan DB, Cassidy JT, Petty RE: Pathogenic implications of age of onset in juvenile rheumatoid arthritis. Arthritis Rheum 18:251–255, 1975
173. Kunnamo I, Kallio P, Pelknonen P: Incidence of arthritis in urban Finnish children: A prospective study. Arthritis Rheum 29:1232–1238, 1988
174. Maksymowych WP, Glass DN: Population genetics and molecular biology of the childhood chronic arthropathies. Bailliere's Clin Rheumatol 2:649–671, 1988
175. Ansell BM, Bywaters EGL, Lawrence JS: Family studies in Still's disease (juvenile RA). In Bennett PH, Wood PHN (eds): Population Studies of the Rheumatic Diseases. Amsterdam: Excerpta Medica Foundation, 1968
176. Steere AC, Malawista SE: Lyme disease. In McCarty DJ (ed): Textbook of Rheumatology, 10 edt. Philadelphia: Lea & Febiger, 1985
177. Alepa FB: Juvenile rheumatoid arthritis. In Riggs GK, Gall ED (eds): Rheumatic Diseases: Rehabilitation and Management. Boston: Butterworth, 1984
178. National Center for Health Statistics. Current Estimates from the National Health Interview Survey, United States, 1987. Vital and Health Statistics, Series 10, No. 166, 1988
179. Rivara FD, Calonge N, Thompson RS: Population-based study of unintentional injury incidence and impact during childhood. Am J Public Health 79:990–994, 1989
180. Buhr AJ, Cooke AM: Fracture patterns. Lancet 1:531–536, 1959
181. Garraway WM, Stauffer RN, Kurland LT, O'Fallon WM: Limb fractures in a defined population: Frequency and distribution. Mayo Clin Proc 54:701–707, 1979
182. Rockwood CA Jr, Wilkins KE, King RE: Fractures in Children. Philadelphia: Lippincott, 1984
183. Adams JC: Outline of Fractures. Edinburgh: Churchill-Livingstone, 1978
184. Bjerkedal T: Congenital dislocation of the hip in Norway: A clinical-epidemiological study. J Oslo City Hosp 26:79–90, 1976
185. Kelsey JL: Epidemiology of Musculoskeletal Disorders. New York: Oxford University Press, 1982
186. Leck I: Rising rates of congenital dislocation of the hip. Lancet 1:372, 1976
187. Robinson GW: Birth characteristics of children with congenital dislocation of the hip. Am J Epidemiol 87:275–284, 1968
188. Record RC, Edwards JH: Environmental influences related to the aetiology of congenital dislocation of the hip. Br J Prev Soc Med 12:8–22, 1958
189. Kramer AA, Berg K, Nance WE: Familial aggregation of congenital dislocation of the hip in a Norwegian population. J Clin Epidemiol 41:91–96, 1988
190. Cyvin KB: Congenital dislocation of the hip joint. Acta Paediatr Scand 263:1–67, 1977

191. Jones DH: The early diagnosis of congenital dislocation of the hip joint. Br J Clin Pract 19:443–449, 1965
192. Carter CO, Wilkinson J: Persistent joint laxity and congenital dislocation of the hip. J Bone Joint Surg 46B:40–45, 1964
193. Katz JF, Challenor YB: Childhood orthopedic syndromes. In Downey JA, Low NL (eds): The Child with Disabling Illness. Philadelphia: W.B. Saunders, 1974
194. Cunningham KT, Beningfield SA, Moulton A, Maddock CR: A clicking hip in a newborn baby should never be ignored. Lancet 1:668–670, 1984
195. Knox EG, Armstrong EH, Lancashire RJ: Effectiveness of screening for congenital dislocation of the hip. J Epidemiol Community Health 41:283–289, 1987
196. Leck I: An epidemiological assessment of neonatal screening for dislocation of the hip. J R Coll Physicians Lond 20:56–62, 1986
197. Fulton MJ, Barer ML: Screening for congenital dislocation of the hip: An economic appraisal. Can Med Assoc J 130:1149–1156, 1984
198. MacFarlane A: Screening for congenital dislocation of the hip. Br Med J 294:1047, 1987
199. Berman L, Klenerman L: Ultrasound screening for hip abnormalities: Preliminary findings in 1001 neonates. Br Med J 293:719–722, 1986

55
Neurological Disorders

Linda D. Cowan
Alan Leviton
Karin B. Nelson

The manifestations of neurological dysfunction are multiple and diverse. This chapter considers selected chronic disorders of the central nervous system (CNS) that result in significant morbidity and disability at different ages. Included are conditions of particular importance either in pediatric populations or in adults, especially the elderly.

With the exception of cerebrovascular disease, most neurological disorders are not major causes of death. However, they do account for significant morbidity and disability. On the basis of overall estimates of the prevalence of neurological disorders,[1] and excluding headache other than migraine, approximately 12% of the U.S. population have one of the chronic neurological disorders covered in this chapter. Of the 12 chronic conditions identified from the 1983–85 National Health Interview Survey[2] as causing the highest percentage of limitation of activity, six were neurological conditions, including mental retardation, epilepsy, and multiple sclerosis.

The neurological disorders considered here have a number of common features. Diagnosis tends to be difficult for several reasons. In the absence of definitive diagnostic tests, reliance must frequently be placed on reports of subjective symptoms (e.g., headache, complex partial seizures), and for many conditions there may be no agreed-upon, uniform criteria for diagnosis. In addition, early stages of some disorders are characterized by a variable presentation (e.g., multiple sclerosis, Parkinson's disease, dementias) or by subtle signs and symptoms that are difficult to detect or that go unreported. The diagnosis of some problems in children (e.g., learning disabilities, cerebral palsy) may be delayed until the children reach the age at which deficits could reasonably be detected.

Once nervous tissue is destroyed, it cannot be replaced, and permanent deficits occur. Thus primary prevention rather than treatment is the goal. Unfortunately, the causes of most of the neurological disorders discussed in this chapter are unknown, and thus the opportunities for prevention are limited. There are also no interventions that result in cure, and available treatments have met with varying degrees of success in improving functional status or in ameliorating symptoms.

CEREBRAL PALSY

Cerebral palsy (CP) is a group of disorders in which the common denominator is abnormal control of movement or posture that begins early in life and is not the result of recognized progressive disease. The forms of CP differ according to the parts of the body affected, the specific nature of the motor difficulties of which spasticity is the most common, and the presence of other neurological disabilities, such as mental retardation, seizure disorders, and sensory problems, all of which are more common in persons with CP than in the general population.

Cerebral palsy is thought to be present in approximately 2.5 of every 1000 live births, although it is not identified with confidence until the affected child is several years old. Prevalence differs by age group, since relatively mild deficits tend to resolve spontaneously in the early years, whereas 10% to 15% of CP is acquired after the neonatal period through neurologic injury, most often infectious or traumatic. CP has been identified by early school age in 1.2 to 2.3 of every 1000 children. There is a slight excess of males among affected persons, but there are no consistent ethnic differences.

Low birth weight and immaturity at birth are among the most consistent risk factors for CP. Intrauterine infection and congenital malformations, which are independent risk factors for CP, tend to concentrate among infants of low birth weight. Not all factors that contribute to low birth weight are associated with increased risk of CP. For example, maternal cigarette smoking is a substantial risk factor for low birth weight (<2500 g), including very low birth weight (<1500 g), and yet smoking is not a risk factor for CP. Intracranial hemorrhage in premature infants and, more strikingly, necrosis of the white matter of the brain in premature infants as ascertained during the neonatal period are risk factors.

The improved survival of infants with very low birth weight who are at increased risk of CP, has been associated with an increase in CP in some population studies.[3] There has been some suggestion of a decrease in CP in large babies, but this has not been statistically significant in individual series.

Intrapartum and postnatal physical injury are potential causes of CP, as is intrauterine exposure to heavy metals, such as mercury. Marked neonatal hyperbilirubinemia, often related to Rh isoimmunization, is associated with increased risk of athetoid CP with sensorineural hearing loss and paresis of upward gaze. Recent studies have indicated a possible role of exposure to benzyl alcohol, a preservative used in solutions to flush intravascular catheters in neonatal intensive care units, in hyperbilirubinemia, intraventricular hemorrhage, and later motor and developmental disability.[4]

Severe asphyxia at birth is a risk factor for CP and may account for about 10% of all CP,[5,6] especially for the subtype spastic quadriparesis with athetosis. In clinical studies, asphyxia is measured only indirectly and by heterogeneous indicators. By all indications, however, it must be lengthy and severe to be associated with increased risk of CP. Difficult birth is associated with increased risk of CP only among children who have neurological symptoms in the neonatal period.

Population studies have identified a higher rate of cerebral and somatic malformations (both major and minor) in children with CP than in unaffected children. Noting the limited relationship of CP with obstetric factors, a recent review of the epidemiological evidence suggests: "Cerebral palsy . . . may be more akin to the congenital malformations."[7]

Some previously unreported risk factors for CP have emerged from one large correlative study[8]; among these are maternal mental retardation, seizure disorders or hyperthyroidism, and administration of certain hormonal agents during pregnancy.

Decreased incidence of isoimmunization for Rh factors has been followed by a reduction in the rate of athetoid CP. Avoidance of injury (traumatic or asphyxial) during delivery is obviously desirable, but improvements in obstetric and neonatal care and an increasing frequency of obstetric interventions have not been associated with a decrease in incidence of CP.[9,10] The paucity of information about causal factors for the majority of CP that is not attributable to birth events limits severely the development of strategies for prevention.

MENTAL RETARDATION

The prevalence rate of severe mental retardation (usually defined as an IQ below 50) is consistently found to range between 3 and 5 per 1000. On the other hand, the prevalence of mild mental retardation (diagnosed if the IQ is between 50 and 70) varies considerably, among both times and places. Indeed, the increasing prevalence of mild mental retardation during the early school years and the unchanging prevalence of severe mental retardation have led to the hypothesis that mild mental retardation is dependent in part on postnatal factors, while severe mental retardation is very much dependent on prenatal factors.

Cerebral palsy and seizures occur much more commonly in children with severe mental retardation than in children with mild mental retardation, who in turn have a higher prevalence than is found in children with IQs above 70. These findings are compatible with diffuse and severe brain damage in children with severe mental retardation and with the hypothesis that a proportion of children with milder mental retardation may also have disturbed brain structure and function. The concept that a proportion of mild mental retardation represents the consequences of social deprivation has received support from studies that show the advantages of stimulating day-care and compensatory education programs (e.g., Headstart).

More than one third of severe mental retardation has been attributed to chromosome abnormalities. With the widespread use of amniocentesis of women over 35 years of age, the occurrence of trisomy 21 has decreased prominently in recent years.[11] Improved techniques of chromosome analysis have resulted in the identification of deletions and translocations that were not diagnosable just a few years ago. The prevalence of severe mental retardation tends to be higher among males, presumably because of sex-linked chromosomal disorders such as fragile X.

Single gene disorders, such as phenylketonuria, prenatal infection (e.g., rubella, toxoplasmosis, cytomegalovirus), endocrine disorders (hypothyroidism), and toxins (e.g., alcohol, maternal phenylketonuria) are all implicated in the etiology of mild and severe mental retardation.

Severe mental retardation was diagnosed in 0.5% of the white sample and 0.7% of the black sample enrolled in the Collaborative Perinatal Project (CPP). On the other hand, mild retardation was identified in 1% of whites and 5% of blacks. Blacks may be at increased risk because of a greater frequency of adverse environmental exposures and a reduced opportunity to compensate for these adversities among the economically disadvantaged.

In the CPP the risk profile for severe retardation differed considerably from the risk profile for mild retardation.[12] Risk factors for mild retardation included socioeconomic variables, mother's nonverbal intelligence score, maternal short stature, and maternal late age at menarche. Both retardation groups included within their risk profiles the pregnancy complications of urinary tract infection, anemia, and toxemia. Infants with mild mental retardation were more likely than those with severe retardation to have low birth weight, respiratory difficulty, and low Apgar scores during the first minutes of life.

LEARNING DISABILITIES

No single definition of learning disabilities or handicaps is widely accepted. In part this reflects the heterogeneity of learning handicaps, and in part it reflects the needs of differing constituencies (government officials, teachers, investigators). The heterogeneity of what has been grouped together as learning disabilities concerns not only the multiplicity of grossly different handicaps (e.g., attention, reading, language) but also the multiplicity of disturbances that result in each of these handicaps.[13,14] Many definitions are characterized by a discrepancy between expectation and performance.

One government report classified 4% of schoolchildren as having learning handicaps (cited in reference 15). On the other hand, a Census Bureau study estimated that 9% of the adults in the United States whose native language is English are illiterate.[16] Given the problems of defining and measuring handicap, the validity of these estimates is questionable.

Boys are more likely than girls to be identified by their schools as reading disabled. By research criteria, however, the sex differential is much less obvious.

Learning handicaps do show familial clustering.[17] The finding that adoptees are overrepresented among children with learning handicaps[18] provides additional support for the influence of genetic factors in the occurrence of learning handicaps, especially those accompanied by impulsivity. The promise of chromosome and gene localization has yet to be fulfilled. Linguistic development has been related to socioeconomic status, which may account for some of the apparent familial clustering.

Although the literature dealing with birth weight as an antecedent of learning handicaps is conflicting at best,[19] treating birth weight as a continuum may miss the apparent hazards faced by low-birth-weight infants who require neonatal intensive care. Prenatal exposures to drugs, other than barbiturates, have shown little association with learning disabilities. Maternal alcohol and cigarette consumption have not been adequately evaluated. Although fetal exposure to cocaine has not yet been shown to be a risk factor for learning disabilities, an association between maternal cocaine consumption and low newborn head circumference[20] raises the possibility that children exposed in utero to cocaine and other narcotics may be at increased risk of cognitive and perceptual deficits.

Prenatal lead exposure increases the risk of early delays in perceptual motor function, but otherwise advantaged children no longer show such deficits by the age of 5 years. Postnatal lead exposure, on the other hand, is more clearly linked to persisting problems, which may interfere with a number of school-related activities, especially reading.[21]

Otitis media, which may be accompanied or followed by a fluctuating hearing loss, has been implicated as an antecedent of some language and reading handicaps, as have hearing impairments in general.

Children with inborn errors of metabolism (e.g., phenylketonuria), even when treated early and vigorously, appear to be at increased risk of language disorders. Children who were fed a chloride-deficient baby formula appear to be at increased risk of language handicap.[22]

Language delay may be the only manifestation of prenatal rubella infection. Other prenatal infections capable of damaging the brain have not been linked to isolated learning handicaps.[23]

SEIZURE DISORDERS

Epilepsy is usually defined as more than one afebrile seizure not associated with an acute CNS process.[24] There are no definitive tests that establish the diagnosis of epilepsy. Normal electroencephalographic (EEG) patterns do not exclude the diagnosis, and EEG abnormalities are observed in persons who have never had or may never have a seizure. Persons are usually diagnosed as having had a seizure solely on the basis of a description of the event provided by an observer, and, even with the best descriptions, the diagnosis may be difficult.

Prevalence rates of epilepsy in children (defined as persons less than 20 years of age) tend to be between 4 and 5 per 1000.[25] In adults, prevalence rates range from approximately 3.4 to 4.6 per 1000 before age 60 to about 1.1 to 2.7 per 1000 for those 60 years of age and older.[26] According to most estimates, the incidence of epilepsy among persons of all ages is between 30 and 55 per 100,000.[27] In children, incidence rates are approximately 70 to 80 per 100,000,[25] with highest rates in the first year of life (~1.2 to 1.4 per 1000).[24] The cumulative or lifetime incidence of epilepsy is estimated to be between 2.0% and 4.3%,[28] making epilepsy a relatively common condition, especially in infants and children.

Different types of epilepsy predominate at different ages, and some types of seizure disorder occur only in children. Specific epileptic syndromes, such as infantile spasms and Lennox-Gastaut syndrome, and certain types of seizure, such as neonatal seizures and absence (petit mal) epilepsy, occur exclusively or predominantly in children. Among children, the most prevalent types of epilepsy are tonic-clonic (grand mal), simple partial (focal motor), partial seizures secondarily generalized, complex partial (temporal lobe), and absence seizures.[29] In adults, partial seizures tend to predominate.[24,27]

Febrile seizures are unique to the pediatric age group and are the most common seizure disorder, occurring in from 2.3% to 4.6% of children. Among children with febrile seizures, factors associated with an increased risk of subsequent epilepsy are a family history of epilepsy, neurological or developmental abnormality before the onset of febrile seizures, and febrile seizures with complex features, that is, (1) focal (localized) onset, (2) lasting longer than 15 minutes, or (3) more than one seizure occurring within 24 hours.[30] Subsequent epilepsy is estimated to occur in from 11% to 17% of children with one or more of these risk factors, and in 1% to 2.5% of those without these risk factors. The decision to use anticonvulsant prophylaxis in a child who has experienced a febrile seizure should be based at least in part on the risk factor profile of the child, since there is currently no evidence that prophylaxis reduces the risk of subsequent afebrile seizures.[31]

In children, epilepsy has been attributed to perinatal insults (usually undefined), CNS infections, congenital abnormalities (e.g., cerebral palsy, microcephaly), and genetic factors. Cerebrovascular disease accounts for a small percentage of epilepsy in adults, while moderate and severe head trauma and CNS neoplasms are associated with an increased frequency of epilepsy in both children and adults. However, these known or suspected "causes" of epilepsy account for only a small fraction of all cases. From 70% to 80% of cases are considered to be idiopathic.

Remission of seizures can be achieved in the majority of persons with epilepsy. Population-based data from Rochester, Minn.,[32] showed that, over all, the net probability of remission at 10 years after diagnosis was 61% and that at 20 years after diagnosis it was 70%. The prognosis was best for persons who had generalized seizures with onset before the age of 10 years. Prognosis was less optimistic for persons with congenital neurological abnormalities and for those with complex partial seizures and adult-onset epilepsy.

HEADACHE

Headache and its accompaniments probably pose more of a burden on society than any other group of neurological disorders.[33,34] From 65% to 71% of women and from 48% to 50% of men report at least one headache per month.[35,36] In addition, headache is one of the most common symptoms prompting people to seek medical care.[33] An estimated 5.5 million days of activity restriction attributed to headache are experienced each year by adults in the United States.[37]

The incidence of migraine has been estimated mainly from prevalence studies.[34] Between age 5 and puberty the incidence probably approximates 1% per year. The incidence increases in females with the onset of menses. After about age 15 the incidence then returns to the male level and continues at about 1% until somewhere between the ages of 30 and 40 years, when the rate decreases. The greater prevalence of migraine in women persists throughout life after puberty. In both women and men, prevalence appears to decrease, beginning in the early 40s.

Although familial clustering of migraine has been reported repeatedly, the strongest evidence of a genetic contribution comes from the higher concordance in monozygotic than in dizygotic twins. If genetic factors contribute to a person's propensity to migraine, then other factors, usually exogenous, are likely to play an important role in determining the occurrence of each headache. Although some people have headaches that exhibit a predictive periodicity, for many people headache recurrence appears to be precipitated by events in their lives. For example, in women, events related to menstrual flow or the use of oral contraceptives are linked to a flare-up of their headaches. In others, ingestion of some foods (especially those containing tyramine, including chocolate and aged cheeses) or alcoholic beverages (red wines, particularly) increases the likelihood of headache in the next few hours. Apparently more common is the phenomenon of an increased headache propensity after the skipping of a meal.

Psychosocial characteristics appear to be associated with

headache (especially migraine) burden. These include perfectionism, inflexibility, and hypochondriasis, as well as propensity to anxiety and depression. "Environmental stress" and psychosocial events can also be important for some people. Excitement, even of a pleasant sort, has been linked to headache occurrence, as have "letdown" phenomena (e.g., the relaxation that follows a series of emotionally intense days) and fatigue.

Behavioral psychologists believe that an assessment searching for the antecedents and reinforcers of headache recurrence can help identify those events that, if reduced or eliminated, will help decrease headache recurrence. Relaxation training also appears to be helpful.

Although migraine is generally not viewed as a fatal disorder, people with migraine appear to be at increased risk of hypertension and atherosclerotic heart disease.[38] Very few people with migraine have what might be called seizures, but those with headaches are more likely than are people without headaches to have seizurelike phenomena (e.g., transient hemiparesis and confusional states). Linet and Stewart,[34] however, conclude that "most rigorous studies do not appear to support strongly the historically held association of epilepsy and migraine."

MULTIPLE SCLEROSIS

Multiple sclerosis is the most common of the demyelinating diseases[1] and is usually diagnosed in young to middle-aged adults. Multiple lesions in the CNS, separated by both location and time of occurrence, result in a clinical presentation that is highly variable and includes sensory, visual, and motor dysfunction. In most affected persons the disease is characterized by clinical remissions and exacerbations, although acute, progressive, and benign courses have been described.[39]

Multiple sclerosis is rarely diagnosed before the age of 15 or after the age of 60 years. The median ages at onset for cases identified in Rochester, Minn., were 34 years and 32 years for men and women, respectively.[40] Women are affected 1.5 to 2 times more frequently than men. Incidence rates are low, ranging from approximately 1 per 100,000 in low-risk areas to 3 per 100,000 in high-risk areas.[41] The median survival is estimated as 35 years, and one half of the survivors are still ambulatory 20 years after diagnosis.[41]

The most striking epidemiological feature of multiple sclerosis is the geographical distribution of prevalence rates. In the northern hemisphere, relatively distinct zones of risk have been identified, with prevalence increasing as latitude increases. High-risk areas have prevalence rates of multiple sclerosis of 30 per 100,000 or higher, while the prevalence rate in low-risk areas is less than 5 per 100,000.[42]

The causes of multiple sclerosis are unknown, although there is a general consensus that environmental factors are of primary importance in its etiology. Epidemics of multiple sclerosis are reported to have occurred in the Faroe Islands[42] and in Iceland.[42] Studies among migrants suggest that persons who move from an area of high prevalence to one of low prevalence take on the risk level of their new environment. Age at migration appears to be important, however, in that persons who move after childhood or early adolescence retain the risk level of their birthplace.[27]

The possibility that multiple sclerosis is caused by an infectious agent has been studied extensively, but no single agent has yet been identified. Measles virus and canine distemper virus have received the most attention in recent years. Infection may also serve to trigger defects in the immune response, especially in cell-mediated immunity.[39] It is unclear, however, whether the abnormalities in immunologic parameters reported in patients with multiple sclerosis have etiological significance or are a result of the disease process.[41] Other environmental risk factors that have been investigated with conflicting results include trauma, dietary fat, and exposure to trace elements and heavy metals, such as zinc and lead.[40]

A possible role for genetic factors in the etiology of multiple sclerosis has also been investigated. Blacks and Asians living in high-risk areas have lower prevalence and mortality rates than whites.[41] Familial aggregation of multiple sclerosis has been reported in numerous studies, with a six- to eightfold increased risk in siblings of affected persons.[41] Familial aggregation may reflect the influence of either a shared environment or an inherited susceptibility. Twin studies have generally found a greater concordance for multiple sclerosis among monozygotic twins than among dizygotic twins. However, concordance rates in monozygotic twins are relatively low,[39] and many of the twin studies may have been subject to selection biases.[41] Investigations of the distribution of HLA antigen phenotypes in persons with multiple sclerosis have produced contradictory results,[41] although there is some suggestion of an association with antigens of the DRw region.[39]

There is currently no definitive therapy for multiple sclerosis that affects the ultimate course of the disease. Administration of ACTH has been shown to reduce the duration of acute attacks but does not appear to influence the long-term outcome.[39]

DEMENTIAS

Dementia is a syndrome characterized by a decline in memory and other cognitive functions as compared with the person's previous level of functioning,[43,44] the decline being severe enough to compromise activities of daily living and social functioning.[45] Decrements in intellectual skills, such as judgment, comprehension, abstraction, language, and calculation, are also usually present. The diagnosis of dementia requires that cognitive changes occur in the absence of delirium or other conditions that may impair consciousness.[44] There are no uniformly accepted criteria for the diagnosis of dementia, and a number of definitions of the dementia syndrome have been proposed. The advantages and limitations of these definitions have been reviewed recently.[43]

Dementia is caused by a myriad of conditions, although most cases (52% to 72%) involve Alzheimer's disease.[45] Multi-infarct dementia accounts for 5% to 12% of the cases, followed by alcohol-related dementia (2% to 8%) and other progressive neurological disorders, such as Parkinson's disease and Huntington's disease (3% to 4%). Dementia due to metabolic factors, such as thyroid disease or intracranial lesions, is relatively rare, and the use of exhaustive diagnostic testing of all persons with signs or symptoms of dementia in an effort to find these rare causes has been questioned.

In the mid-1980s, it was recognized that acquired immunodeficiency syndrome (AIDS) can be complicated by dementia and that the neurological symptoms exhibited by some patients were related at least in part to the direct neurotoxicity of the human immunodeficiency virus (HIV).[46] "Neurologic disease" was included in the Centers for Disease Control classification of HIV infection only as recently as 1987. The symptoms of the AIDS dementia complex are highly variable and include forgetfulness, loss of concentration, inability to work and carry out complex tasks, and personality changes. The precise mechanisms of neurotoxicity, frequency of the AIDS dementia complex, clinical course, and methods of early detection are currently unknown.

The incidence and prevalence rates of dementias are highly dependent on age. Population-based incidence studies report rates of dementia of approximately 0.6% in 70- to 79-year-olds and nearly 2% in persons 80 years of age and older. In a recent meta-analysis of studies of the prevalence of dementia, Jorm et al.[47] found that overall rates of severe dementia ranged from 2% to 7.8% of persons 65 years of age and older. In all the studies they reviewed, prevalence tended to double with each 5.1-year increase in age, and no important secular trends in the prevalence of dementia were observed. The ratio of multi-infarct dementia to Alzheimer's disease varied among the populations studied, with the highest ratios being found in Japan and the Soviet Union.

At present there are few approaches available for the prevention and control of the majority of cases of dementia. A relatively small proportion of cases (approximately 5% to 10%) have potentially "reversible" causes, such as thyroid disease and normal-pressure hydrocephalus. Persons with multi-infarct dementia are more likely to have histories of hypertension and stroke than are those with other types of dementia.[45] Thus, this type of dementia should be preventable, at least in part, through interventions designed to reduce hypertension. The most consistently identified risk factors for Alzheimer's disease include a family history of dementia or Down's syndrome and severe head trauma. Only the latter factor is potentially modifiable. Numerous studies have investigated as risk factors a history of specific viral infections, immune dysfunction, occupational and environmental exposures, and CNS infection, but none of these factors has been consistently associated with risk of Alzheimer's disease. Attempts to identify a genetic marker for Alzheimer's disease are currently underway.

CEREBROVASCULAR DISEASE

Cerebrovascular disease, otherwise referred to as stroke, is primarily a condition of older persons. After the age of 50, incidence rates of first stroke double with each successive decade of age and are in the range of 10 to 20 per 1000 after the age of 75 years.[48] Stroke is the third leading cause of death in the United States, and an important cause of disability, ranking eleventh among conditions with the highest percentage of limitation in activity.[2] Strokes do occur in infants, but the risk factors and pathogenesis are considerably different from those in adults.

The major types of stroke are cerebral thrombosis, cerebral embolism, intracerebral hemorrhage and subarachnoid hemorrhage. Distinguishing among subtypes is sometimes difficult in the living patient, but improvements in accuracy of diagnosis have accompanied the development and widespread use of neuroimaging techniques. Discrimination among the types of stroke is important, since they differ with respect to risk factors,[49] treatment,[50] and prognosis.[51]

Mortality from stroke varies by country, with the highest rates reported for Japan and the lowest rates for Switzerland and Canada.[48] There are also marked differences in stroke mortality between whites and blacks in the United States. Overall death rates are approximately twice as high in blacks as in whites. The ratio of death rates in blacks compared to whites decreases with advancing age, but does not approach 1.0 until after about the age of 75 years. The difference is most marked in 35- to 44-year-old men, among whom the death rate is nearly five times higher in blacks than in whites.

As has been observed for diseases of the heart, there has been a striking decline in mortality rates for stroke in the past several decades. Reductions in mortality rates have been observed for both sexes and all race groups. The decline has been attributed primarily to a decreasing incidence of stroke due to efforts to control hypertension and, to a lesser extent, to a reduction in case fatality.

The majority of strokes can be averted through control of hypertension. Hypertension is the major risk factor for stroke and is the only factor consistently found to be related to all types of stroke.[49] Treatment of high blood pressure may be most efficacious in the primary prevention of stroke and less effective in preventing recurrent stroke.[51] In addition to hypertension, other risk factors for ischemic stroke include diabetes mellitus, transient ischemic attacks, and cardiac disease.[49] Cigarette smoking has been associated in some studies with risk of both ischemic and hemorrhagic stroke.[49] The role of alcohol consumption in increasing risk of stroke is less certain and may vary by type of stroke. One study in women found that moderate consumption of alcohol was associated with a lower risk of ischemic strokes but with an increased risk of subarachnoid hemorrhage.[52]

PARKINSON'S DISEASE

Parkinson's disease is a progressive disorder of movement that affects the elderly. The onset is insidious, progression tends to be gradual, and the course of the disease is usually prolonged. Cognitive function is generally preserved, although dementia is reported to occur in 10% to 25% of cases.

"Secondary" parkinsonism may result from exposure to toxins (e.g., carbon monoxide or manganese), drugs (e.g., phenothiazides), traumatic or vascular lesions of the brain, or tumors.[27] Arteriosclerosis, when present, is most likely a concurrent disease rather than a subtype of parkinsonism.[27,53] Postencephalitic parkinsonism is well recognized but accounts for a relatively small and decreasing proportion of all prevalent cases. The majority of cases are of unknown cause, and the term *Parkinson's disease* is frequently reserved for these idiopathic cases.

In the United States the age-adjusted death rate from Parkinson's disease is approximately 1.2 per 100,000.[54] The disease causes few deaths before the age of 45 years, but rates increase progressively after about age 50, and peak mortality rates are observed in 75- to 84-year-olds. Mortality rates are slightly higher in men than in women and three to four times higher in whites than in blacks. Kurtzke and Goldberg[54] recently reported that in the United States there is a north:south gradient in death rates from Parkinson's disease (with higher rates in the northern states) similar to that observed for multiple sclerosis. This gradient in mortality rates was seen in both whites and nonwhites and for all ages combined as well as for those 65 years of age and older.

Incidence rates for Parkinson's disease are reported to range from 6 to 19 per 100,000,[53] with the highest rates (approximately 120/100,000) in 70- to 79-year-olds.[27] Prevalence rates are low before the age of 50 years, while 1% of those over the age of 60 years and more than 2% in the oldest age groups may be affected.[27]

The cause of most cases of Parkinson's disease remains obscure. The relative importance of genetic factors is uncertain and controversial. Most studies of familial aggregation report a family history of Parkinson's disease in from 16% to 41% of idiopathic cases.[53] However, data from twin studies and from investigations of the frequency of selected histocompatibility antigens argue against genetic factors playing a major etiological role in this disease.

The importance of environmental exposures is suggested both by differences in the geographic distribution of the disease and by observations from etiological studies. Numerous studies have reported a lower risk of Parkinson's disease among cigarette smokers. Various explanations for this observation have been proposed, but whether the inverse association between cigarette smoking and risk of Parkinson's disease has biological significance or is merely an epiphenomenon remains controversial.[55]

Other potential risk factors, including exposure to toxins in well water, industrial or agricultural pollutants, head trauma, and stress, require further investigation.[55] Investigations of the effects of viruses, such as influenza, measles, and herpes simplex viruses, have not consistently demonstrated an association between past exposure and risk of Parkinson's disease. The recent observation that drug abusers exposed to the meperidine derivative MPTP sometimes have a syndrome clinically indistinguishable from advanced Parkinson's disease,[56] as well as subsequent studies using animal models of MPTP toxicity, supports the hypothesis that environmental exposures may be important in causing Parkinson's disease.

REFERENCES

1. Kurtzke JF: The current neurologic burden of illness and injury in the United States. Neurology 32:1207–1214, 1982
2. Collins JG: Prevalence of selected chronic conditions, United States, 1983–85. Advance data from vital and health statistics, No. 155. DHHS Publication No. (PHS) 88-1250. Hyattsville, Md.: Public Health Service, 1988
3. Pharoah POD, Cooke T, Rosenblood I, Cooke RWI: Trends in the birth prevalence of cerebral palsy. Arch Dis Child 62:379–389, 1987
4. Benda GI, Hiller JL, Reynolds JW: Benzyl alcohol toxicity: impact on neurologic handicaps among surviving very low birth weight infants. Pediatrics 77:507–512, 1986
5. Nelson KB, Ellenberg JH: Antecedents of cerebral palsy: multivariate analysis of risk. N Engl J Med 315:81–86, 1986
6. Blair E, Stanley FJ: Intrapartum asphyxia: a rare cause of cerebral palsy. J Pediatr 122:575–579, 1988
7. Cumming RG, Leeder SR: The changing face of neurological disease 1946–1987: an epidemiological perspective. Aust N Z J Med 18:881–889, 1988
8. Nelson KB, Ellenberg JH: Antecedents of cerebral palsy: univariate analysis of risks. Am J Dis Child 139:1031–1038, 1985
9. Stanley JK, Watson L: The cerebral palsies in Western Australia: trends, 1968 to 1981. Am J Obstet Gynecol 158:89–93, 1988
10. Emond A, Golding J, Peckham C: Cerebral palsy in two national cohort studies. Arch Dis Child 64:848–852, 1989
11. Luthy DA, Emanuel I, Hoehn H, et al: Prenatal genetic diagnosis and elective abortion in women over 35: utilization and relevant impact on the birth prevalence of Down syndrome in Washington State. Am J Med Genet 7:375–381, 1980
12. Broman S, Nichols PL, Shaughnessy P, Kennedy W: Retardation in Young Children: A Developmental Study of Cognitive Deficit. Hillsdale, N.J.: Lawrence Erlbaum Associates, 1987
13. Tallal P: Neuropsychological foundations of specific developmental disorders (language, reading, articulation). In Tallal P: Psychiatry. Philadelphia: JB Lippincott, 1985, vol 3, pp 1–15
14. Prior M, Sanson A: Attention deficit disorder with hyperactivity: a critique. J Child Psychol Psychiat 27:307–319, 1986
15. Johnson DJ: Review of research on specific reading, writing and mathematics disorders. In Kavanagh JF, Truss TJ Jr (eds): Learning Disabilities: Proceedings of the National Conference. Parkton, Md: York Press, 1988, pp 79–163
16. Werner LM: 13% of U.S. adults are illiterate in English, a federal study finds. New York Times, April 21, 1986
17. Ludlow CL, Cooper JA: Genetic aspects of speech and language disorders: current status and future directions. In Ludlow CL, Cooper JA (eds): Genetic Aspects of Speech and Language Disorders. New York: Academic Press, 1983, pp 1–18
18. Silver LB: Frequency of adoption of children and adolescents with learning disabilities. J Learn Disabil 22:325–327, 1989
19. Cohen S: Low birthweight. In Brown CC (ed): Childhood Learning Disabilities and Prenatal Risk: An Interdisciplinary Data Review for Health Care Professionals and Parents. Skillman, NJ: Johnson & Johnson, 1983, pp 70–78
20. Zuckerman B, Frank DA, Hingson R, et al: Effects of maternal marijuana and cocaine use on fetal growth. N Engl J Med 320:762–768, 1989
21. Needleman HL, Schell A, Leviton A, Allred EN, Bellinger D: Long term effects of childhood exposure to lead at low dose: an eleven-year follow-up report. N Engl J Med 322(2):83–88, 1990
22. Kaleita TA, Menkes JH, Kingbourne M: Neurologic behavioral syndrome associated with infantile dietary chloride deficiency. Clin Res 35:226a, 1987
23. Sever JL: Perinatal infections and damage to the central nervous system. In Lewis M (ed): Learning Disabilities and Prenatal Risk. Urbana: University of Illinois Press, 1986, pp 194–209
24. Hauser WA, Kurland LT: The epidemiology of epilepsy in Rochester, Minnesota, 1935 through 1967. Epilepsia 16:1–66, 1975
25. Leviton A, Cowan LD: Epidemiology of seizure disorders in children. Neuroepidemiology 1:40–83, 1982
26. Kurtzke JF: Some epidemiologic and clinical features of adult seizure disorders. J Chron Dis 21:143–156, 1968
27. Kurtzke JF, Kurland LT: The epidemiology of neurologic disease. In Baker AB, Baker LH (eds): Clinical Neurology. Philadelphia: Harper & Row, 1984, pp 1–143
28. Hauser WA: Epidemiology of epilepsy. Adv Neurol 19:313–338, 1978
29. Cowan LD, Bodensteiner JB, Leviton A, Doherty L: Prevalence of the epilepsies in children and adolescents. Epilepsia 30:94–106, 1989
30. Nelson KB, Ellenberg JH: Predictors of epilepsy in children who have experienced febrile seizures. N Engl J Med 295:1029–1033, 1976
31. National Institutes of Health Consensus Development Conference Summary: Consensus statement on febrile seizures. In Nelson KB, Ellenberg JH (eds): Febrile Seizures. New York: Raven Press, 1981, pp 301–306
32. Annegers JF, Hauser WA, Elveback LR: Remission of seizures and relapse in patients with epilepsy. Epilepsia 20:729–737, 1979
33. Leviton A: Epidemiology of headache. Adv Neurol 19:341–353, 1978
34. Linet MS, Stewart WF: Migraine headache: epidemiologic perspectives. Epidemiol Rev 6:107–139, 1984
35. Waters WE: The Pontypridd headache survey. Headache 14:81–90, 1974
36. Linet MS, Stewart WF, Celentano DD, Zieglar D, Sprecher M: An epidemiologic study of headache among adolescents and young adults. JAMA 26:2211–2216, 1989
37. National Center for Health Statistics: Acute conditions: incidence and associated disability, United States (Vital and health statistics, National Health Survey Series 10, No. 77) (DHEW publication no. (HSM)73-1503). Rockville, Md.: National Center for Health Statistics, 1972
38. Couch JR, Hassanein RS: Headache as a risk factor in atherosclerosis-related diseases. Headache 29:49–54, 1989
39. McFarlin DE, McFarland HF: Multiple sclerosis. Parts 1 and 2. N Engl J Med 307:1183–1188, 1246–1251, 1982
40. Wynn DR, Rodriguez M, O'Fallon WM, Kurland LT: Update on the epidemiology of multiple sclerosis. Mayo Clin Proc 64:808–817, 1989
41. Kurtzke JF: Neurological system. In Holland WW, Detels R, Knox G (eds): Oxford Textbook of Public Health. vol 4. Specific Applications. Oxford: Oxford University Press, 1985, pp 203–249
42. Kurtzke JF: Epidemiologic contributions to multiple sclerosis: an overview. Neurology 30:61–79, 1980
43. McLean S: Assessing dementia. Part I. Difficulties, definitions and differential diagnosis. Aust N Z J Psychiatry 21:142–174, 1987
44. McKhann G, Drachman D, Folstein M, Katzman R, Price D, Stadlan EM: Clinical diagnosis of Alzheimer's disease: report of the NINCDS-ADRDA Work Group under the auspices of Department of Health and Human Services Task Force on Alzheimer's disease. Neurology 34:939–944, 1984
45. Katzman R: Alzheimer's disease. N Engl J Med 314:964–973, 1986
46. Perry S, Marcotta RF: AIDS dementia: a review of the literature. Alzheimer Dis Assoc Disord 1:221–235, 1987
47. Jorm AF, Korten AE, Henderson AS: The prevalence of dementia: a quantitative integration of the literature. Acta Psychiatr Scand 76:465–479, 1987

48. Malmgren R, Warlow C, Bamford J, Sandercock P: Geographical and secular trends in stroke incidence. Lancet 1:1196–1200, 1987
49. Sharkness CM, Price TR, Sherwin R: Risk factors for stroke subtypes. Md Med J 37:373–377, 1988
50. Grotta JC: Current medical and surgical therapy for cerebrovascular disease. N Engl J Med 317:1505–1516, 1987
51. Meissner I, Whisnant JP, Garraway WM: Hypertension management and stroke recurrence in a community (Rochester, Minnesota, 1950–79). Stroke 19:459–463, 1988
52. Stampfer MJ, Colditz GA, Willett WC, Speizer FE, Hennekens CH: A prospective study of moderate alcohol consumption and the risk of coronary disease and stroke in women. N Engl J Med 319:267–273, 1988
53. Kessler II: Parkinson's disease in epidemiologic perspective. Adv Neurol 19:355–384, 1978
54. Kurtzke JF, Goldberg ID: Parkinsonism death rates by race, sex, and geography. Neurology 38:1558–1561, 1988
55. Tanner CM, Chen B, Wang WZ, Peng ML, Liu ZL, Liang XL, Kao LC, Gilley DW, Schoenberg BS: Environmental factors in the etiology of Parkinson's disease. Can J Neurol Sci 14:419–423, 1987
56. Kopin IJ, Markey SP: MPTP toxicity: implications for research in Parkinson's disease. Ann Rev Neurosci 11:81–96, 1988

56
Disabling Visual Disorders

Alfred Sommer

The importance of ocular disease is immediately apparent. Americans fear blindness more than any other affliction except cancer (and now AIDS), and cataract extraction is the most common major surgical procedure in the United States, with more than 1 million operations performed in 1989.[1] While the population rate may be plateauing or even in decline, cataract surgery accounts for 2 billion Medicare dollars annually.

Precise estimates of the nature and magnitude of ocular disease, disability, or even blindness were unavailable until recently. The best population-based prevalence data were limited to single diseases in isolated locales[2] or to highly selected populations.[3] A tally revealed 67 different definitions of blindness,[4] which prompted the World Health Organization to recommend a uniform classification of visual impairment (Table 56–1).[5] A recent population-based study in East Baltimore revealed that blacks are twice as likely to be blind as whites, and that rates rise rapidly in older age, reaching 12% to 14% of noninstitutionalized subjects 85 years of age and older.[6,7]

Despite the paucity of reliable data, the rate and pattern of blindness in the United States and other industrialized societies are clearly different from those of developing countries (Table 56–2).[8] There are an estimated 900,000 blind* and 3 million visually impaired individuals in the United States.[6]

WHO estimates global blindness at 20 to 40 million, the vast majority in Third World countries where prevalence rates commonly exceed 1% to 2%.[5,8-11] The high prevalence rates of blindness in developing countries can be ascribed to the presence or persistence of diseases uncommon in industrialized societies and to limited access to eye care. Trachoma, a communicable disease of impoverished populations living in dry, unsanitary environments, is thought to be responsible for blindness in 6 million people. Onchocerciasis, a parasitic disease transmitted by the bite of black flies, is responsible for 1 million blind inhabitants of Africa and a much smaller number in Latin America. Each year xerophthalmia (vitamin A deficiency) blinds 250,000 to 500,000 Asian and African children, most of whom die.[12] More than 300,000 lepers may be blind as a result of their ocular complications.[13] Cataract, a condition common to all populations, probably occurs more frequently in the "cataract belt" of Asia and is responsible for one third to one half of all blindness.

In addition to a larger number and higher incidence of blinding disorders, developing countries have more limited health care resources. The United States has 1 ophthalmic surgeon for every 20,000 people; many African and Asian countries have fewer than 1 per 1 million. The organization of health care services is almost as important as the number of ophthalmologists. India and England have roughly the same ratio of ophthalmic surgeons to population (1 per 100,000), but in India these surgeons are concentrated in the largest cities, where they are inaccessible to the predominantly impoverished rural population. In the United Kingdom greater use is made of optometric services for routine spectacle correction and case finding, and the ophthalmologists are more accessible to the population. In Peru only licensed ophthalmologists (physicians), the vast majority of whom live in the capital, can legally prescribe glasses.

Chronic degenerative conditions account for a larger proportion of blindness in developed countries because of a lower incidence of nutritional and infectious forms of blindness and because persons with chronic, potentially blinding diseases (particularly diabetes) are more likely to survive. Despite these relative differences, diseases that are important causes of blindness in the United States and other industrialized societies are also prevalent in the Third World.

REFRACTIVE ERROR

The most common chronic ocular problem is refractive error: myopia (nearsightedness), hyperopia (farsightedness), and presbyopia. While not major causes of blindness per se and correctable with appropriate spectacles or contact lenses, these conditions represent a high proportion of eye health cost. Spectacles alone are a multibillion dollar industry.

In the normal or emmetropic state, the length of the eye and the refracting power of the cornea and lens are in balance. As a result, distant objects (6 m away) are sharply focused on the retina when accommodation is relaxed. In *myopia* distant objects are focused anterior to the retina, because the eye is too long for its refracting power. Myopic persons do not see distant objects clearly, but as an object approaches the eye it is focused more posteriorly (closer to the retina) and the image improves.

**Legal definition of blindness in the United States is a visual acuity of 20/200 or less with correcting lens or a visual field of 20 degrees or less in the better eye; however, persons with "best corrected vision" of 20/50 or worse have difficulty reading regular newsprint without special aids and have difficulty obtaining an unrestricted driver's license in many states.*

TABLE 56-1. CATEGORIES OF VISUAL IMPAIRMENT

	Visual Acuity With Best Possible Correction	
	Maximum (<)	*Minimum (≥)*
▪ **Low Vision**		
1	6/18 20/70 3/10 (0.3)	6/60 20/200 1.10 (0.1)
2	6/60 20/200 1/10 (0.1)	3/60 (finger counting at 1 m) 20/400 1.20 (0.05)
▪ **Blindness**		
3	3/60 (finger counting at 3 m) 20/400 1/20 (0.05)	1/60 (finger counting at 1 m) 5/300 (20/1200) 1/50 (0.02)
4	1/60 (finger counting at 1 m) 5/300 (20/1200)	Light perception
5	No light perception	
	Undetermined or unspecified	

From World Health Organization, 1980.[5]

In literate societies the prevalence and severity of myopia increase during the first 20 to 30 years of life, eventually affecting one fifth or more of the population.[14,15] Clinicians have long suspected that environmental factors, particularly concentrated close work, contribute to its development.[16] This remains unproven.

While the vast majority of myopes are merely inconvenienced by their need for glasses, there is a direct correlation between the severity of myopia and the risk of retinal detachment. A small proportion of myopes have severe elongation of the eye and are at high risk of retinal thinning, degeneration, and detachment leading to permanent visual impairment and sometimes blindness.[17] Myopia, especially severe pathological myopia, is often associated with other congenital and developmental anomalies.

In *hyperopia* the eye is too short for its resting refractive power. Focus falls posterior to the retina. Except in rare cases of high hyperopia, the normal lenses of children and young adults can compensate by increasing accommodation (refracting power) and so achieve sharp focus. Hyperopia often goes unrecognized until middle-age, when accommodative reserves decline and lead to symptoms of brow ache, "fatigue" (asthenopia), or both. This probably accounts for many instances of "eye strain" associated with prolonged use of video display devices. Hyperopia is associated with angle-closure glaucoma and, in some young children, accommodative esotropia (crossed eyes).

Presbyopia is almost universal by the sixth decade and merely reflects an age-related reduction in accommodative function, resulting in an inability to bring near objects into sharp focus.

In the Health and Nutrition Examination Survey (HANES), the prevalence of pathological conditions causing visual impairment of 20/50 or worse in one or both eyes of persons 1 to 74 years of age was 2.8%. However, 5.9%, an excess of 3.1% (53% of the total) of the eyes were visually impaired, presumably for lack of proper spectacle correction. In the Baltimore Eye Survey[6] (BES) the presenting vision of 50% of the subjects could be improved with a new pair of spectacles; in 8% it could be improved by at least three lines.

TABLE 56-2. A COMPARISON OF CAUSES OF BLINDNESS IN THE UNITED KINGDOM AND TANZANIA

	% Blindness		Estimated Rate per 100,000	
Cause	**U.K.**	**Tanzania**	**U.K.**	**Tanzania**
Corneal opacity[a]	2	21	4	315
Cataract	23	57	41	855
Glaucoma	12	14	22	210
Retinal disorder	48	4	86	60
Other	15	4	27	60
Total	100	100	180	1500

[a] Due to blinding infections e.g., trachoma), malnutrition, measles-associated, trauma, and degenerative and dystrophic disorders.
From Foster A, 1984.[8]

BLINDING DISORDERS

Unlike mortality, "blindness" registration is largely voluntary and unregulated. Beginning in 1961, several states in the United States agreed to maintain a common registration system. Although limited to persons blind in both eyes who chose to register, data from the participating states indicate that blindness in the United States increases with age, most notably in the oldest decades, and is more common in blacks than in whites.[18] The recent BES confirmed these trends (Fig. 56-1).[6]

In the United States, Credé prophylaxis (i.e., application of silver nitrate into the eyes at birth to prevent gonococcal neonatal ophthalmia) and improved socioeconomic status have virtually eliminated infections as a major cause of blindness; increased access to surgical services has reduced the burden of cataract blindness; and recognition of the dangers of high oxygen tension among premature infants interrupted the postwar epidemic of retinopathy of prematurity (ROP). Even so, cataract is still a major cause of blindness, particularly among blacks, and with the increased survival of ever younger, more premature, and often desperately ill infants, ROP is still with us. Model reporting area (MRA) data suggest that 3% of all blindness is due to injury or poisoning and another 16% to prenatal influ-

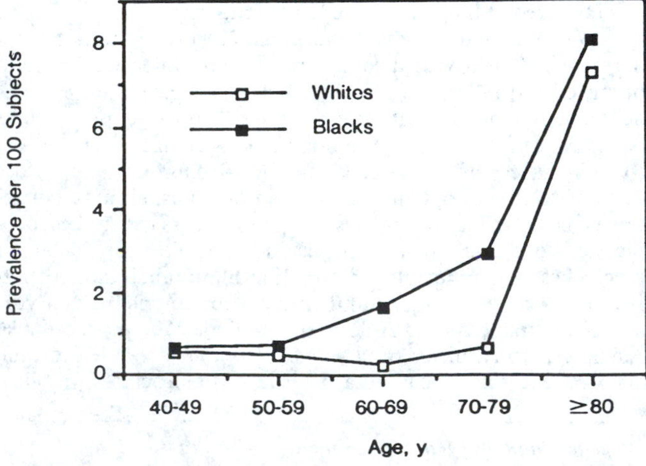

Figure 56-1. Age-specific rate of blind persons, Baltimore Eye Survey. *(From Tielsch JM, Sommer A, Witt K, et al: Blindness and visual impairment in an American urban population: The Baltimore Eye Survey. Arch Ophthalmol 108:286–290, 1990.[6])*

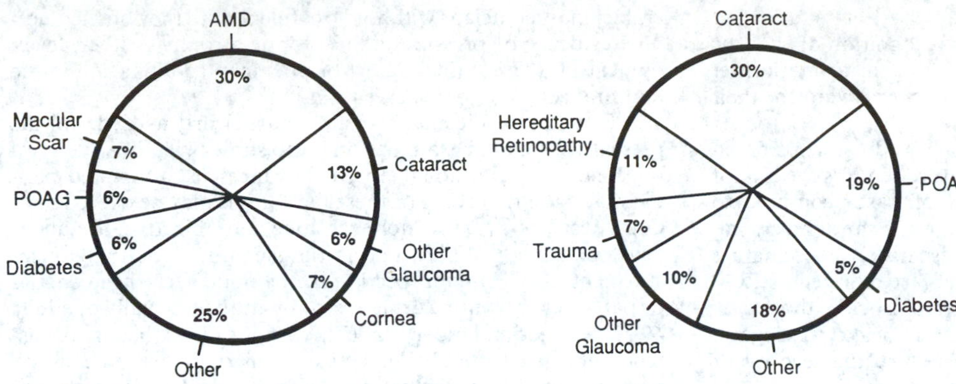

Figure 56-2. Distribution of cases of blindness, adults aged 40 and older, East Baltimore. Left figure is for whites; right figure for blacks. *[From Sommer A et al, 1990.[7]]*

ence.[18] The remainder is by and large degenerative. The major causes of blindness in the BES were untreated cataract, primary open-angle glaucoma, and age-related macular degeneration (uniquely limited to whites). Their relative importance was largely dependent on race (Fig. 56-2 and Table 56-3).[7]

Analysis of the types and causes of blindness among persons first added to the MRA rolls during 1969 and 1970 (the last years of its existence) suggest that full exploitation of existing technology would reduce the incidence of blindness by one third (Table 56-4).

PRIMARY PREVENTION

The two ocular diseases most susceptible to primary prevention are amblyopia and ROP.

Amblyopia

Most commonly both eyes are structurally normal. However, because they differ in refractive error or muscle balance during the formative stage of visual development (generally the first 6 years of life), the brain relies on one eye and fails to learn to recognize fine details with the other. Data suggest that there is hypoplasia of the lateral geniculate body subserving the amblyopic eye.[19] Because amblyopia is often mild and generally affects one eye, it rarely appears in blindness statistics. Nonetheless, as many as 1% to 4% of the population are amblyopic.[20] If detected sufficiently early, most cases can be prevented or reversed by a variety of techniques that either neutralize the disparity between the two eyes (e.g., by providing corrective spectacles) or force the person to use both eyes equally (usually by alternately "patching" one eye and then the other) until past the visually plastic stage. The critical problem is early detection; the later the diagnosis, the more difficult and less successful the therapy. This is the raison d'être for most preschool and school vision-screening programs and continues to be a major priority of the National Society to Prevent Blindness. Among older children (generally 3 to 5 years of age and up) screening depends on identifying reduced acuity in one or both eyes; among younger children, however, one must rely more heavily on tests of eye movement or fixation. Recent unpublished data from the National Society to Prevent Blindness suggest appalling sensitivity and specificity of screening tests as carried out by lay testers on preschool children and very low coverage rates.[21] Clearly, better tests, especially for preliterate young children, and more vigorous screening would have a marked impact on this eminently preventable form of visual impairment.

Retinopathy of Prematurity

Though no longer one of the major causes of blindness, ROP is particularly important because of the iatrogenic epidemic that followed World War II. The combination of new incubator design and philosophy toward oxygen use resulted in attainment of high oxygen concentrations in the immaturely vascularized infant retina, leading to vascular constriction, secondary hypoxia, and the growth of new and aberrant vessels. With time these often distorted or detached the retina. Approximately 7000 children in the United States alone were blinded by ROP between

TABLE 56-3. RATE OF ANNUAL ADDITIONS TO BLINDNESS REGISTERS BY CAUSE AND BY RACE

	Rates per 100,000		
	Nonwhite	White	Total
Retinal disease	4.4	4.2	4.2
Cataract	3.4	1.8	2.1
Glaucoma	5.1	0.8	1.5
Multiple affections	2.1	1.2	1.3
Unknown	2.5	1.6	1.8
Other	6.5	2.7	3.3

From Kahn HA, Moorhead HB, 1973.[18]

TABLE 56-4. POTENTIALLY AVOIDABLE BLINDNESS

Cause of Blindness	% of Total Blindness[a]	Proportion Potentially Avoidable[b]	% Total Blindness Avoidable
Retinal degeneration	22	0.16	3.5
Other retinal	18	0.47	8.4
Multiple affections	14	0.10	1.4
Cataract	14	0.75	10.5
Glaucoma not congenital	13	0.50	7.5
Optic nerve atrophy	8	0.18	1.4
Uveitis	4		
Myopia	3		
Other corneal/scleral	2	0.18	2.0
Retinopathy of prematurity	1		
Keratitis	1		
Total	100		34.7

[a] Excludes "unknown" and "other," 4.8% and 9.4%, respectively, of total in original tables.
[b] Based on the author's appraisal of maximal, feasible impact of new technology and research findings since 1970.
From Kahn HA, Moorhead HB, 1973, Tables 11 to 20.[18]

1943 and 1953.[22] Epidemiological insights by Patz et al,[23] and Campbell[24] were largely responsible for recognition of the true nature of the disease, which was confirmed in a multicenter trial.[25] Patz and Kinsey shared the 1956 Lasker Award for their work.

Careful monitoring of PO_2 with further adjustments based on the appearance of the retinal vasculature reduces the risk of disease. Unfortunately, large numbers of cases continue to occur. Our capacity for primary prevention is thwarted by improved survival of ever younger, more desperately ill premature infants, in whom either high oxygen levels are required or ROP develops despite oxygen tensions that remain below those previously thought to be critical.[26,27] Recent clinical trials suggest that administration of vitamin E may reduce the severity of ROP, though not necessarily its occurrence.[28]

SECONDARY PREVENTION

More than any other condition, glaucoma illustrates the interest, confusion, and frustration surrounding secondary prevention of chronic blinding disorders.[29]

Glaucoma

Glaucoma is one of the major causes of blindness in the United States,[7] particularly among blacks (Fig. 56–2, Table 56–3). In the BES, blacks 40 years of age and older were four times more likely to blinded by glaucoma than were whites,[7] confirming the higher rate of black glaucoma blindness originally suggested by the potentially biased MRA.[30]

It is generally agreed that in glaucoma, excessive intraocular pressure (IOP) leads to progressive atrophy of the optic nerve. In its most common form, chronic simple glaucoma (CSG), this occurs in the absence of any obvious structural explanation for the elevated IOP; pressures are rarely very high; and optic atrophy progresses slowly over 10 to 20 years, causing characteristic alterations in the visual field that spare central vision until the last. Patients are therefore rarely aware of the condition until most of the nerve fibers have already been lost.[31,32]

The prevalence of ocular hypertension, glaucomatous field loss, and related blindness increases with age.[7,18] To many professionals, the condition seemed (and to some still seems) ideally suited to secondary prevention: identify persons with elevated intraocular pressure, reduce their pressure by medical or surgical means, and thus prevent or retard destruction of their optic nerve.[33]

Unfortunately, there is a major problem. Although longitudinal data support the clinical impression that the risk of developing field defects characteristic of glaucomatous optic atrophy is directly related to the height of the intraocular pressure, the distribution of pressures in the general population does not provide a ready or efficient mechanism for distinguishing between those with and those without field loss.[34]

For example, the screening criterion commonly employed, 21 mm Hg, merely represents a level 2 standard deviations (SD) above the mean IOP in the population at large.[35] From the few studies that permit estimation of sensitivity, one third or more of the cases of glaucomatous field loss have a screening pressure below 21 mm Hg.[2,34,36] Specificity is generally high, on the order of 90%. With the low prevalence (0.5% to 1.5%) and poor sensitivity, however, only 1 of every 15 to 30 positive screenees will actually have established field loss.[29,30,37] Some persons with false-positive sensitivity findings will prove to have persistently elevated intraocular pressure, and some of these will ultimately experience visual field loss. As the risk of field loss in confirmed ocular hypertension is low, averaging 5 to 10 per 1000 per year, and the cost and inconvenience of long-term therapy are considerable, most clinicians withhold treatment until they observe definite evidence of pressure-induced optic atrophy—either development of a visual field defect or documented alteration in the appearance of the optic nerve head.[38,39]

Better mass screening techniques are clearly needed. For the present, visual field examination is too subjective, time-consuming, and costly, although recent advances in automated perimetry suggest that some of these limitations may be overcome.[40] Other tests, potentially more sensitive and objective, are under development.[41,42] What to do in the meantime? Certainly measurement of IOP and inspection of the optic nerve head should be part of every routine general examination, especially of adults 40 years of age and older. Patients with pressures that are persistently above 21 mm Hg, with suspicious optic nerve heads, or with a strong family history of glaucoma should be referred for definitive ophthalmological evaluation and potentially long-term follow-up.

In view of the limitations of tonometric (IOP) screening, mass screening of the general adult population may be appropriate only if local interest and resources permit. If they do not, consideration may be given to targeting screening to blacks, in whom the risk of glaucomatous blindness is clearly excessive. A full comprehensive eye examination at intervals appropriate for age, race, and other risk factors may be the most appropriate "screening test," as it is definitive and may uncover other significant disease.[29,43]

The reason blacks are at increased risk of glaucomatous blindness is uncertain. Ocular hypertension may be more prevalent in blacks. The disease has an earlier onset,[44] and blacks appear to be more refractory to standard therapeutic maneuvers.[45] Patterns of health care use and compliance may also play a role.

It is widely accepted that reduction in IOP will retard or prevent optic nerve atrophy.[34,45] While there is ample evidence that this is likely, some patients with CSG fare poorly, even when their IOP is reduced and maintained at "normal" levels.[45–47] Given the slow progression of CSG and the accepted efficacy of current therapeutic approaches, the true value of treatment will be ethically difficult to quantify.

Retinal Vascular Disease

As longevity, especially of diabetics, has increased abnormalities of the retinal blood vessels have become a leading cause of visual impairment. Abnormalities generally include loss of normal integrity of the vascular tree, ischemia, and growth of new, aberrant vessels on the surface of the retina and into the vitreous. Vision is impaired by leakage of fluid into the macula from incompetent vessels and, most severely, by complications of neovascularization (vitreous hemorrhage and retinal distortion and detachment).

The major cause of blinding retinovascular disorders is diabetes. The risk of neovascularization is greatest among type I (juvenile-onset) diabetics and increases with the duration of the diabetes (Fig. 56–3).[48,49] Because of the greater number of type II (adult-onset) diabetics, they still constitute a significant proportion of all cases blinded by diabetes, even though their risk of severe retinovascular disease is lower.

Until such time as diabetes or its effect on vascular beds can be prevented, control resides in interfering with the natural history of diabetic retinopathy, especially neovascularization. Only during the past 15 to 20 years has this become feasible.

Diabetic retinopathy is divided into three stages of increasing severity and variable duration: mild background retinopathy, which causes little if any visual impairment; more severe, preproliferative retinopathy, in which vision may be impaired, primarily from macular edema; and proliferative (neovascular) retinopathy. A multicenter controlled clinical trial of eyes with proliferative retinopathy demonstrated that panretinal photocoagulation reduced the rate of visual deterioration (Table 56–5),[50,51]

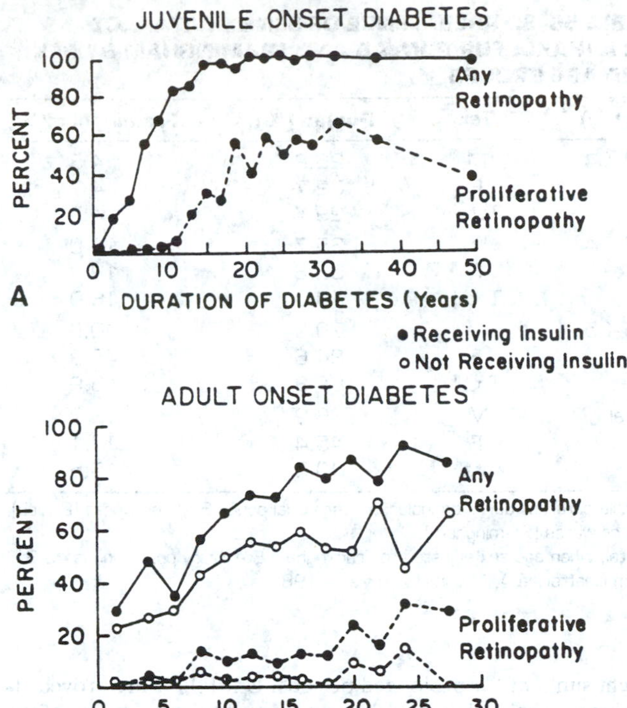

Figure 56-3. A. Frequency of retinopathy or proliferative retinopathy by duration of diabetes among individuals in whom diabetes was first diagnosed below 30 years of age. **B.** Frequency of retinopathy or proliferative retinopathy by duration for persons who were first diagnosed as having diabetes at 30 years of age or older *(From Klein R, Klein BEK, Moss SE, et al: The Wisconsin epidemiologic study of diabetic retinopathy, II and III. Arch Ophthalmol 102:520–532, 1984.[48,49])*

largely by inducing regression of established neovascular membranes and retarding the growth of new ones. The level of benefit varies with the state of the retinal vasculature (and its related risk of visually catastrophic consequences). It is assumed, but unproven, that photic destruction of ischemic retina reduces the drive (perhaps elaboration of a vasoproliferative substance) responsible for neovascularization.

A more recent collaborative trial demonstrated the value of focal photocoagulation of leaking vessels for the treatment of cystoid edema, even before it becomes symptomatic.[52]

Clearly, diabetics need regular, periodic retinal examinations to determine when and if they might benefit from photocoagulation. A recent study demonstrated that ophthalmologists were twice as likely to detect documented retinopathy as were internists,[53] suggesting that referral to and regular follow-up by an ophthalmologist is advisable. In a recent study of known diabetics in southern Wisconsin, 26% of those with younger-onset and 36% of those with older-onset diabetes had never had an ophthalmological examination.[54]

Recent modeling of the costs and benefits of careful management of diabetes indicates a substantial saving, in disability payments alone, over the costs of providing ideal ophthalmic care for all insulin-dependent diabetics.[55]

As a preventive measure, panretinal photocoagulation is less than ideal. A large amount of still-viable retina is destroyed, resulting in impaired scotopic (night) vision and a reduction in the visual fields. It is therefore not to be undertaken lightly.

Retinal Degeneration

A wide variety of conditions, far too numerous to review, result in degenerative changes in the retina, particularly the macular area. For the vast majority, the etiology is unknown. One of the most common, so-called age-related macular degeneration (AMD), is to some degree familial and increases with age, particularly after the sixth decade.[56,57]

Visual impairment in AMD arises from two different mechanisms: a dry or atrophic degeneration of retinal structures and a far more devastating vascular form in which abnormal blood vessels arising from the choroid invade the subretinal space, where they leak fluid, lipid, or blood, leading to disorganization and scarring of the overlying retina. Clinical trials demonstrate that laser obliteration of new vessels still outside the central foveal area has a beneficial effect on visual outcome (Fig. 56-4).[58,59] As dramatic and exciting as these therapeutic results are, their potential public health impact remains unclear. It will depend on the proportion of all AMD blindness that proves to be secondary to the vascular form of disease and on the proportion of individuals with the vascular form who make their way to a retinal specialist before significant damage has already occurred, with a subretinal membrane located in an area where it can still be safely treated. Only 1 of every 20 patients with AMD referred to one of the controlled trials satisfied the entry criteria[59]; 10% or fewer patients with subretinal neovascularization may be seen early enough for treatment.[60]

Ophthalmologists now warn patients with early, background changes (''drusen'') that they are at increased risk of disease and advise them to check each eye daily for reduced acuity or visual distortion and to return immediately if they detect any abnormalities.[61] Limited studies suggest that the risk of severe complications and visual impairment among persons with background drusen is roughly 2% to 15% per year, with the higher rates in patients with visual loss from AMD in the other eye.[56,62] If these risks are confirmed in large population-based studies, the role of screening will have to be seriously addressed.

TABLE 56-5. CUMULATIVE RATES OF FALL IN VISION TO LESS THAN 5/200 AMONG PATIENTS WITH DIABETIC RETINOPATHY

	Therapeutic Regimen			
	Photocoagulation		Control	
Duration of Follow-up (mo)	*No. of Eyes Followed*	*Rate of Visual Loss (per 100)*	No. of Eyes Followed	Rate of Visual Loss (per 100)
12	1588	2.5	1582	3.8
20	1200	5.3	1166	11.4
28	707	7.4	651	19.6
36	232	10.5	204	26.5

From Sommer A, 1980.[51]

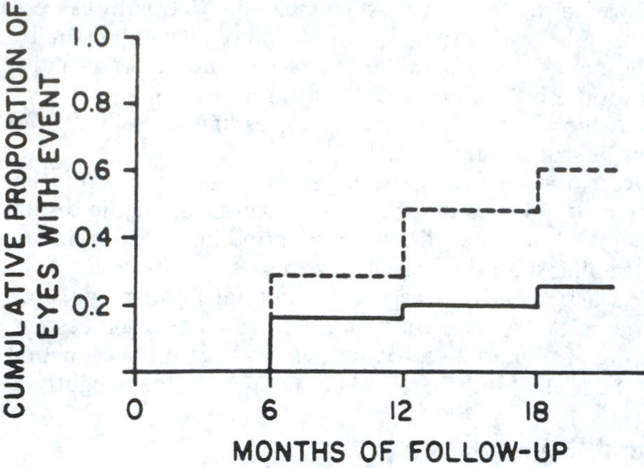

Figure 56-4. Cumulative proportion of eyes with subretinal neovascularization from macular degeneration experiencing a decrease in visual acuity of six or more lines from baseline. Solid line represents treatment group; dashed line represents control group. *(From Moorfields Macular Study Group, 1982.[58,59])*

TABLE 56-6. PREVALENCE OF SENILE CATARACT OR APHAKIA FOR PUNJAB AND FRAMINGHAM BY SEX AND AGE GROUPS[a]

Age (y)	Sex	Punjab (%)	Framingham(%)
52–64	M	26.2	4.3
	F	32.7	4.7
	Total	29.4	4.5
65–74	M	35.7	16.0
	F	52.6	19.3
	Total	43.3	18.0
75–85	M	79.3	40.9
	F	84.6	48.9
	Total	81.8	45.9
Total	M	36.2	13.2
	F	45.4	17.1
	Total	40.5[b]	15.5

[a] Senile cataract definition includes best visual acuity 6/18 or worse (Punjab), 6/9 or worse (Framingham).
[b] Total, when age-sex adjusted to Framingham Eye Study population is 43.3.
From Chatterjee A, Milton RC, Thyle S, 1982.[70]

Presumed ocular histoplasmosis syndrome (POHS) has a similar pathogenesis, though clearly a different cause. Patients with POHS are younger than those with AMD and have distinctive small chorioretinal scars in the periphery and about the disc.[63,64] The prevalence of histoplasmin skin sensitivity in this group is extremely high.[63,65] Coupled with the geographic distribution of POHS and seemingly associated risk factors,[66] it appears likely that subretinal neovascularization in these patients is related to an earlier episode of active systemic histoplasmosis. A controlled clinical trial suggests that these, too, are amenable, at least in part, to laser therapy.[67] If, in fact, the disease is related to a previous exposure to *Histoplasma capsulatum,* reducing such exposures would provide primary prevention against the disease.

Cataract

A cataract is an opacification of the lens. There are many known causes of cataract: hyperparathyroidism, juvenile-onset diabetes, galactosemia, myotonic dystrophy, prolonged use of topical steroids, exposure to high levels of ionizing radiation, and the like. These known causes and associations, however, account for only a tiny proportion of all vision-impairing cataracts. The majority go by the unenlightening term *senile.*

Senile cataracts are, in all likelihood, multifactorial in origin. They are particularly prevalent in certain geographical areas, such as the "cataract belt" cutting across India.[68,69] Although prevalence surveys using the same standardized observers in areas of presumably varied risk have not been undertaken, an attempt was made to assess a population in the Punjab with the same criteria and definitions employed in a survey in the United States (Table 56-6).[70] Results suggest a 10-year disparity between the two groups. The prevalence rate among 75- to 84-year-old inhabitants of Framingham was similar to that of 65- to 74-year-old inhabitants of the Punjab. Studies in Australia,[71] Nepal,[72] the United States,[73] and elsewhere suggest that exposure to sunlight, and in particular ultraviolet-B,[73] may play an important role (Fig. 56-5). Other studies suggest diet,[70] impaired carbohydrate metabolism,[74,75] dehydrating diarrhea,[76] and other factors (e.g., infrared radiation in "glass blowers' cataract") may be contributory.[77]

To date, none of these hypotheses or associations has been rigorously tested by an intervention trial, although some investigators have advocated ultraviolet-absorbing spectacles or shading (e.g., by wide-brimmed hats) for populations exposed to bright sunlight for prolonged periods. Until these are proved effective or until additional insights are obtained, there is little scope for the *prevention* of cataracts.

It is paradoxical that cataracts should be a major cause of blindness in the United States. Presumably, cataract blindness relates to use of health services. Surveys in developing countries repeatedly reveal that untreated cataract is the single major cause of blindness, often responsible for one half or more of all cases despite the presence of trachoma, xerophthalmia, and the like.[8,78] With the largest per capita ophthalmic force in the world, government and private health insurance, and an operation that has an extraordinary success rate, it is unclear why so many people in the United States should be blind from cataract. No doubt part of the answer is that many of the elderly (especially those living in nursing homes) fear surgery, do not realize that the costs are covered under Medical Assistance for the Elderly, and do not appreciate any need for better vision. Even if this reluctance were overcome, however, the sheer volume of cataract surgery now being performed for ever-subtler impairment of vision may contain within itself the seeds of iatrogenic "cataract" blindness of significant dimensions.[68]

In the past patients preferred distortion-free 20/60 or 20/80

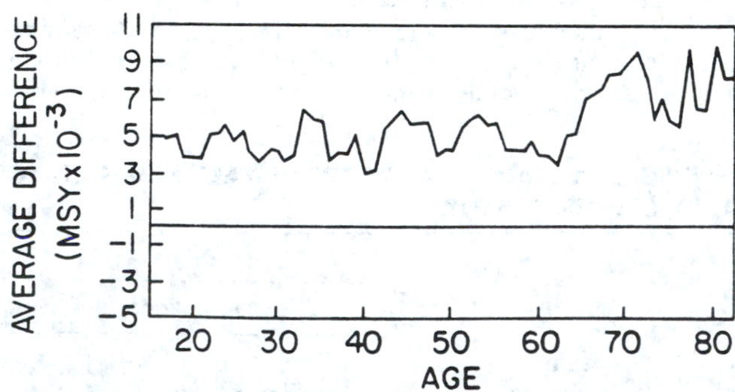

Figure 56-5. Average dose difference at each year of life between annual ultraviolet exposure among 34 watermen with cortical opacities (grade 2 or worse in the more severely affected eye) and 213 age-matched controls without this degree of cortical opacity. MSY = Maryland Sun Year. *(From Taylor HR, West SK, Rosenthal FS, et al: Effect of ultraviolet radiation on cataract formation. N Engl J Med 319:1429–1433, 1988.[73])*

cataracts to 20/20 spectacle-corrected aphakic vision. With the advent of intraocular lenses, the postcataract patient can expect distortion-free correction of the aphakic state and is now prepared to have a 20/40 or 20/60 cataract removed.[79] Even with the extraordinary success of cataract surgery, only 85% to 90% of patients achieve a corrected vision of 20/40 or better. Some of the shortfall is secondary to unrelated retinal and other problems, but a substantial proportion is directly related to the cataract surgery itself. If even 1% of the more than 1 million cataract operations performed every year (and the number is rapidly growing) ended in significant visual impairment, at least 10,000 additional eyes would become or remain impaired each year, or 100,000 eyes in 10 years, a substantial number.[68] Even with the cause of the problem apparent, we are without an obvious solution. The potential benefits of surgery are simply too great for most patients to be deterred by the low individual risk of complications.

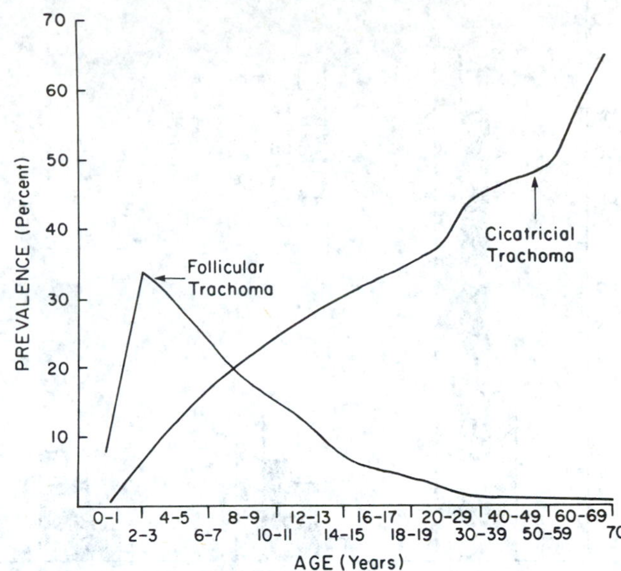

Figure 56-6. Prevalence of follicular and cicatricial trachoma by age in 61,700 Australian Aborigines. *[From Royal Australian College of Ophthalmologists, 1980.[80]]*

PREVENTION OF BLINDNESS IN DEVELOPING COUNTRIES

As already discussed, blindness is 5 to 20 times more prevalent in developing countries. Almost all of this excess blindness can be traced to rural poverty and is therefore potentially avoidable.

Untreated cataract invariably accounts for one third to one half of all blindness.[8,10,78] The problem can be attacked only by extending inexpensive surgical services to the rural population. How best to accomplish this depends upon cultural attitudes, population density, and available expertise. In Taxilla, Pakistan, and Sitapur, India, blind people will walk tens and even hundreds of miles to a hospital that provides inexpensive, high-volume cataract surgery (100 to 300 cases per day). In other areas of the Indian subcontinent, blind people will not venture outside their own village; surgery must be brought to them in the form of mobile eye camps or teams servicing satellite hospitals, which obviously makes less efficient use of the surgeon's time. Even here the ''compliant'' cases have been treated; most cataract blind are less convinced of the benefits of aphakia and increasingly demand intraocular lenses or require special inducements to encourage them to make use of newly accessible surgical services. In Africa, where the population is often widely dispersed in small, traditionally conservative communities, efficiency of volume is even harder to achieve. On cataract ''safaris,'' sometimes by light plane, commonly only two or three procedures are performed at each site.

In a very few areas, particularly in Africa, the paucity of ophthalmologists has encouraged training of general practitioners or even high school graduates to perform cataract surgery. A great deal more will have to be done along these lines if any significant impact is to be made on the backlog of existing cases. Identification and control of environmental influences, such as ultraviolet exposure and poor diet, would have an even greater impact. Estimates suggest that delaying the formation of cataracts by 10 years would halve the need for surgery.[79]

The remaining causes of excess blindness are more focally distributed. Trachoma, discussed in Chapter 7, is a chronic inflammatory disease of the tarsal conjunctiva that leads to scarring and distortion of the lids, exposure and trauma to the cornea, and ultimately corneal opacification and blindness. The prevalence and severity of inflammation is usually greatest in childhood (Fig. 56-6)[80] and is related to the frequency of reinfection by chlamydia. The poorer the hygiene, the greater the transmission of organisms, the more frequent the reinfection, and the more severe the inflammation and resultant scarring.[81] The fact that blinding trachoma (as opposed to mild inflammation leading to minimal, if any, scarring) has spontaneously disappeared from a number of areas after modest improvements in socioeconomic status (e.g., Indonesia) and the identification of specific hygiene factors (e.g., face washing) closely associated with the presence and absence of disease suggest that environmental manipulation and health education may have a more lasting impact.[82,83]

Xerophthalmia (discussed in Chapter 61), results from inadequate consumption of vitamin A, exacerbated by protein-energy malnutrition (PEM), diarrhea, respiratory disease, and especially measles.[84] Recent data suggest measles blindness, often considered the most important cause of pediatric blindness in Africa, may represent acute decompensation of xerophthalmia,[84] although immune suppression with secondary herpes infection[85] and other pathogenetic mechanisms seem to play a role.[86]

Mild vitamin A deficiency leads to night blindness and conjunctival xerosis (Bitot's spots),[87] increases susceptibility to diarrheal and respiratory disease,[88] and is associated with excess mortality on the order of 4 to 12 times background rates (Fig. 56-7).[89] Vitamin A supplementation can reduce overall childhood morbidity by 35% to 70%[90] and measles mortality by 50%.[91,92] Severe deficiency leads to corneal ulceration and necrosis (keratomalacia) with loss of the eye. The mortality rate in severely affected children is extremely high (50% to 85%).[86]

Control measures aim to increase vitamin A intake, through periodic distribution of massive dose capsules, vitamin A fortification of common dietary items, and increased consumption of natural sources of provitamin A β-carotenes (principally dark green leafy vegetables). Controlling diarrhea, PEM, and especially measles would have a significant impact not only on measles blindness in Africa but on classic keratomalacia in Asia.

Onchocerciasis is caused by the parasite *Onchocerca volvulus*. Adult worms form nodules, principally in the subcutaneous tissues, where each mature female releases 1 million or more microfilaria a year. Some of these microfilaria penetrate the eye, where they induce an inflammatory reaction that leads to optic atrophy, chorioretinal scarring, uveitis with secondary glaucoma and cataract, and corneal opacification. The risk of blindness is related to the chronicity of infection and the size of the parasitic load.[93]

As the parasite is spread by bites of black flies (*Simulium*)

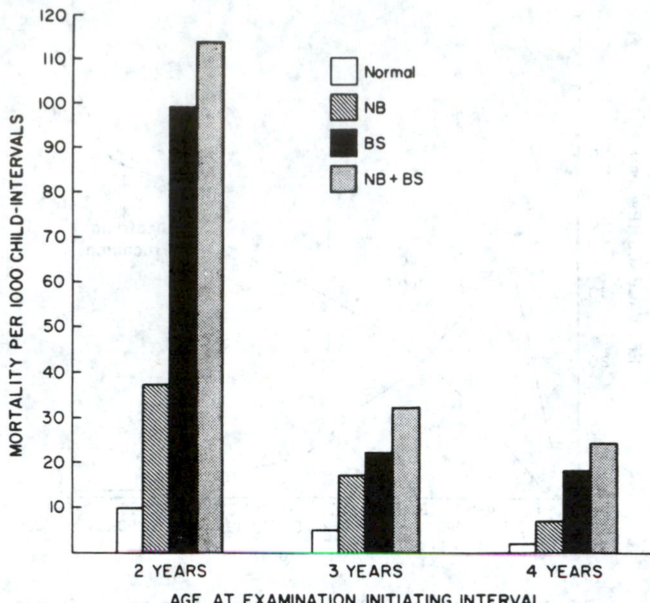

Figure 56-7. Mortality among children free of respiratory disease at the examination preceding each of the six 3-month follow-up intervals, by ocular status at the same interval-initiating examinations. NB = nightblindness; BS = Bitot's spots. *(From Sommer A et al, 1983.[89])*

which breed in fast-moving streams and rivers, the disease is classically found in fertile river valleys (principally in Africa, but also in pockets in Central and South America) and is most severe in men who work in the fields. In some intensely infected African communities, one half or more of all middle-aged men are blind from onchocerciasis.

Treatment with diethylcarbamazine or Suramin is fraught with dangers. The new "wonder drug" ivermectin (Mectizan), given annually, controls microfilarial levels and prevents ocular damage.[94] Reducing transmission through eradication or reduction of the vector, as in the ambitious vector-control program in the Volta River basin, appears to have interrupted transmission over a wide geographical area.[95] The use of ivermectin and vector control should prove a formidable combination against this recently unmanageable, devastating disease.

REFERENCES

1. Stark WJ, Sommer A, Smith RE: Changing trends in intraocular lens implantation. Arch Ophthalmol 107:1441–1444, 1989
2. Hollows FC, Graham PA: Intraocular pressure, glaucoma, and glaucoma suspects in a defined population. Br J Ophthalmol 50:570–586, 1966
3. Liebowitz HM, Krueger DE, Maunder LR, et al: The Framingham Eye Study monograph. Surv Ophthalmol 24(suppl):335–610, 1980
4. Goldman H: The Demography of Blindness Throughout the World. New York: American Foundation for the Blind, 1980
5. World Health Organization: Guidelines for Programmes for the Prevention of Blindness. Geneva: WHO, 1979, p 16
6. Tielsch JM, Sommer A, Witt K, Katz J, Royall RM: Blindness and visual impairment in an American urban population: the Baltimore Eye Survey. Arch Ophthalmol 108:286–290, 1990
7. Sommer A, Tielsch JM, Katz J, Quigley HA, Martone JF, Gottsch JD, Javitt JC, Royall RM, Witt KA, Ezrine S: The nature and causes of blindness in East Baltimore: a population-based survey. (In press.)
8. Foster A: Patterns of blindness. In Duane TD (ed): Clinical Ophthalmology, Vol 5. Philadelphia: Harper & Row, 1984, pp 1–7
9. Brilliant GE (ed): The Epidemiology of Blindness in Nepal: Report of the 1981 Nepal Blindness Survey. Chelsea, Mich: The Seva Foundation, 1988
10. Faal H, Minassian D, Sowa S, Foster A: National survey of blindness and low vision in the Gambia: results. Br J Ophthalmol 102:1766–1771, 1989
11. Malawi Ministry of Health: Blindness and Ocular Morbidity in the Lower Shire Valley, Malawi: Preliminary Report. Lilongwe, Malawi: Ministry of Health, 1984
12. Sommer A, Tarwotjo I, Hussaini G, et al: Incidence, prevalence and scale of blinding malnutrition. Lancet 1:1407–1408, 1981
13. Helen Keller International: Research Priorities for the Prevention of Blindness in Developing Countries. New York: Helen Keller International, 1983
14. Roberts J, Rowland M: Refraction status and motility defects of persons 4–74 years, U.S., 1971–1972. Vital Health Statistics Series 11, HEW Publication No. (PHS)78-1651, 1978.
15. Sperduto RD, Siegal D, Roberts J, Rowland M: Prevalence of myopia in the United States. Arch Ophthalmol 101:405–407, 1983
16. Angle J, Wissmann DA: The epidemiology of myopia. Am J Epidemiol 11:220–228, 1980
17. Curtin B, Karlin D: Axial length measurements and fundus changes in the myopic eye. Am J Ophthalmol 71:42–53, 1971
18. Kahn HA, Moorhead HB: Statistics on blindness in the model reporting area, 1969–1970. DHEW Pub. No. (NIH) 73-427. Washington, D.C., U.S. Government Printing Office, 1973
19. von Noorden GK, Middleditch PR: Histology of the monkey lateral geniculate nucleus after unilateral lid closure and experimental strabismus: further observations. Invest Ophthalmol Vis Sci 14:674–683, 1975
20. Hillis A, Flynn JT, Hawkins BS: The evolving concept of amblyopia: a challenge to epidemiologists. Am J Epidemiol 118:192–205, 1983
21. Ehrlich MI, Reinecke RD, Simons K: Preschool vision screening for amblyopia and strabismus: programs, methods, guidelines, 1983. Surv Ophthalmol 28:145–163, 1983
22. Silverman WA: Retrolental Fibroplasia: A Modern Parable. New York: Grune & Stratton, 1980, p 37
23. Patz A, Hoech LE, DelaCruz E: Studies on the effect of high oxygen administration in retrolental fibroplasia, I. Nursery observations. Am J Ophthalmol 35:1248–1253, 1952
24. Campbell K: Intensive oxygen therapy as a possible cause of retrolental fibroplasia: a clinical approach. Med J Aust 2:48–50, 1951
25. Kinsey VE: Retrolental fibroplasia: cooperative study of retrolental fibroplasia and the use of oxygen. Arch Ophthalmol 56:481–543, 1956
26. Cross KW: Cost of preventing retrolental fibroplasia? Lancet 2:954–956, 1973
27. Editorial: Retrolental fibroplasia (RLF) unrelated to oxygen therapy. Br J Ophthalmol 58:487–489, 1974
28. Hittner HM, Godio LB, Rudolph AJ, et al: Retrolental fibroplasia: efficacy of vitamin E in a double-blind clinical study of pre-term infants. N Engl J Med 305:1365–1371, 1981
29. Sommer A: Glaucoma screening: too little, too late? Frontiers in disease prevention. J Gen Intern Med 5(suppl):533–537, 1990
30. Hiller R, Kahn AH: Blindness from glaucoma. Am J Ophthalmol 80:62–69, 1975
31. Sommer A, Mill NR, Pollack I, et al: The nerve fiber layer in the diagnosis of glaucoma. Arch Ophthalmol 95:2149–2156, 1977
32. Quigley HA, Addicks EM, Green WR: Optic nerve damage in human glaucoma. III. Quantitative correlation of nerve fiber loss and visual field defect in glaucoma, ischemic neuropathy, papilledema and toxic neuropathy. Arch Ophthalmol 100:135–146, 1982
33. National Society for the Prevention of Blindness: Glaucoma Alert Program: A Guide for Community Control of Glaucoma. New York: National Society for the Prevention of Blindness, 1978

34. Sommer A: Intraocular pressure and glaucoma. Am J Ophthalmol 107:186–188, 1989
35. Leydhecker W: Zur verbreitung des glaucoma simplex in der scheinbar gesunden, augenärztlich nicht behandelten bevolkerung. Doc Ophthalmol 13:359–380, 1959
36. Kahn HA, Milton RC: Alternative definitions of open angle glaucoma: effect on prevalence and associations in the Framingham Eye Study. Arch Ophthalmol 98:2172–2177, 1980
37. Sommer A, Pollack I, Maumenee AE: Optic disc parameters and onset of glaucomatous field loss. II. Static screening criteria. Arch Ophthalmol 97:1449–1454, 1979
38. Sommer A, Pollack I, Maumenee AE: Optic disc parameters and onset of glaucomatous field loss. I. Methods and progressive changes in disc morphology. Arch Ophthalmol 97:1444–1448, 1979
39. Pederson JE, Anderson DR: The mode of progressive disc cupping in ocular hypertension and glaucoma. Arch Ophthalmol 98:490–495, 1980
40. Johnson CA, Keltner JL: Incidence of visual field loss in 20,000 eyes and its relationship to driving performance. Arch Ophthalmol 101:371–375, 1983
41. Somer A, Quigley HA, Robin AL, Miller NR, Katz J, Arkell S: Evaluation of nerve fiber layer assessment. Arch Ophthalmol 102:1766–1771, 1984
42. Caprioli J, Miller JM: Nerve fiber layer surface height in glaucoma. Ophthalmology 96:633–641, 1989
43. Quality of Care Committee: Preferred Practice Pattern: The Comprehensive Eye Evaluation. San Francisco: American Academy of Ophthalmology, 1989
44. Tielsch JM, Sommer A, Katz J, Royall RM, Quigley HA, Gotsch JD, Singh D, Javitt J, Baltimore Eye Survey Research Group: Racial variations in the prevalence of primary open angle glaucoma: the Baltimore Eye Survey (In press)
45. Grant WM, Burke JF Jr: Why do some people go blind from glaucoma? Ophthalmology 89:991–998, 1982
46. Kolker AE: Visual prognosis in advanced glaucoma: a comparison of medical and surgical therapy for retention of vision in 101 eyes with advanced glaucoma. Trans Am Ophthalmol Soc 75:539–555, 1977
47. Hart WM Jr, Becker B: The onset and evolution of glaucomatous visual field defects. Ophthalmology 89:268–279, 1982
48. Klein R, Klein BEK, Moss SE, Davis MD, DeMets DL: The Wisconsin epidemiologic study of diabetic retinopathy. II. Prevalence and risk of diabetic retinopathy when age at diagnosis is less than 30 years. Arch Ophthalmol 102:520–526, 1984
49. Klein R, Klein BEK, Moss SE, Davis MD, DeMets DL: The Wisconsin epidemiologic study of diabetic retinopathy. III. Prevalence and risk of diabetic retinopathy when age at diagnosis is 30 or more years. Arch Ophthalmol 102:527–532, 1984
50. Diabetic Retinopathy Study Research Group: Photocoagulation treatment of proliferative diabetic retinopathy, clinical application of diabetic retinopathy study findings. Ophthalmology 88:583–600, 1981
51. Sommer A: Epidemiology and Statistics for the Ophthalmologist. New York: Oxford University Press, 1980, pp 8, 13–14, 19
52. Early Treatment Diabetic Retinopathy Study Research Group: Photocoagulation for diabetic macular edema: Early Treatment Diabetic Retinopathy Study report No. 1. Arch Ophthalmol 103:1796–1806, 1985
53. Sussman EJ, Tsiaras WG, Soper KA: Diagnosis of diabetic eye disease. JAMA 247:3231–3234, 1982
54. Witkin SR, Klein R: Ophthalmologic care for people with diabetes. JAMA 251:2534–2537, 1984
55. Javitt J, Canner J, Sommer A: Cost effectiveness of current approaches to the control of retinopathy in type I diabetes. Ophthalmology 96:255–264, 1989
56. Gass JDM: Drusen and disciform macular detachment and degeneration. Arch Ophthalmol 90:206–217, 1973
57. Ferris FL III: Senile macular degeneration: a review of epidemiologic features. Am J Epidemiol 118:132–151, 1983
58. Moorfields Macular Study Group: Retinal pigment epithelial detachment in the elderly: a controlled trial of argon laser photocoagulation. Br J Ophthalmol 66:1–16, 1982
59. The Macular Photocoagulation Study Group: Argon laser photocoagulation for senile macular degeneration: results of a randomized clinical trial. Arch Ophthalmol 100:912–918, 1982
60. Berkow JW: Subretinal neovascularization in senile macular degeneration. Am J Ophthalmol 97:143–147, 1984
61. Fine SL: Further thoughts on the diagnosis and treatment of patients with macular degeneration. Arch Ophthalmol 101:1189–1190, 1983
62. Strahlman ER, Fine SL, Hillis A: The second eye of patients with senile macular degeneration. Arch Ophthalmol 101:1191–1193, 1983
63. Van Metre TE, Maumenee AE: Specific ocular uveal lesions in patients with evidence of histoplasmosis. Arch Ophthalmol 71:314–324, 1964
64. Smith RE, Ganley JP, Knox DL: Presumed ocular histoplasmosis. II. Patterns of peripheral and peripapillary scarring in persons with nonmacular disease. Arch Ophthalmol 87:251–257, 1972
65. Smith RE, Ganley JP: Presumed ocular histoplasmosis. I. Histoplasmin skin test sensitivity in cases identified during a community survey. Arch Ophthalmol 87:245–250, 1972
66. Ganley JP: Epidemiologic characteristics of presumed ocular histoplasmosis. Acta Ophthalmol 119(suppl):1–63, 1973
67. Macular Photocoagulation Study Group: Argon laser photocoagulation for ocular histoplasmosis: Results of a randomized clinical trial. Arch Ophthalmol 101:1347–1357, 1983
68. Sommer A: Cataracts as an epidemiologic problem. Am J Ophthalmol 83:334–339, 1977
69. Schwab L, Taylor HR: Cataract and delivery of surgical services in developing nations. In Duane TD (ed): Clinical Ophthalmology. Vol 5. Philadelphia: Harper & Row, 1984, Chap 53, pp 1–9
70. Chatterjee A, Milton RC, Thyle S: Cataract prevalence and etiology in the Punjab. Br J Ophthalmol 66:35–42, 1982
71. Taylor HR: The environment and the lens. Br J Ophthalmol 64:303–310, 1980
72. Brilliant LB, Grasset NC, Pokhrel RB, et al: Associations among cataract prevalence, sunlight hours, and altitude in the Himalayas. Am J Epidemiol 118:250–264, 1983
73. Taylor HR, West SK, Rosenthal FS, Munoz B, Newland HS, Abbey H, Emmett EA: Effect of ultraviolet radiation on cataract formation. N Engl J Med 319:1429–1433, 1988
74. Hiller R, Kahn HA: Senile cataract extraction and diabetes. Br J Ophthalmol 60:283–286, 1976
75. Ederer F, Hiller R, Taylor H: Senile lens changes and diabetes in two population studies. Am J Ophthalmol 91:381–395, 1981
76. Minassian DC, Mehra V, Jones BR: Dehydrational crises from severe diarrhea or heatstroke and risk of cataract. Lancet 1:751–753, 1984
77. Leske C, Sperduta RD: The epidemiology of senile cataracts: a review. Am J Epidemiol 118:152–165, 1983
78. Dawson CR, Schwab IR: Epidemiology of cataract—a major cause of preventable blindness. Bull WHO 59:493–501, 1981
79. Cairns L, Sommer A: Changing indications for cataract surgery. Trans Am Ophthalmol Soc 82:166–175, 1984
80. Royal Australian College of Ophthalmologists: The National Trachoma and Eye Health Program. Sydney, Australian College of Ophthalmologists, 1980
81. Dawson CR, Jones BR, Tarizzo ML: Guide to Trachoma Control. Geneva: WHO, 1982
82. Taylor HR, West SK, Mmbaga BBO, Katala SJ, Turner V, Lynch M, Munoz B, Rapoza PA: Hygiene factors and increased risk of trachoma in Central Tanzania. Arch Ophthalmol 107:1821–1825, 1989
83. Taylor HR, Velasco FM, Sommer A: The ecology of trachoma: an epidemiologic study of trachoma in southern Mexico. Bull WHO 63:559–567, 1985
84. Sommer A. Nutritional Blindness: Xerophthalmia and Keratomalacia. New York: Oxford University Press, 1982
85. Sandford-Smith JH, Whittle HC: Corneal ulceration following measles in Nigerian children. Br J Ophthalmol 63:720–724, 1979

86. Foster A, Sommer A: Corneal ulceration, measles and childhood blindness in Tanzania. Br J Ophthalmol 71:331–343, 1987
87. Sommer A: Field Guide to the Detection and Control of Xerophthalmia, 2 edt. Geneva: WHO, 1982
88. Sommer A, Katz J, Tarwotjo I: Increased risk of respiratory disease and diarrhea in children with pre-existing mild vitamin A deficiency. Am J Clin Nutr 40:1090–1095, 1984
89. Sommer A, Tarwotjo I, Hussaini G, Susanto D: Increased mortality in children with mild vitamin A deficiency. Lancet 2:585–588, 1983
90. Sommer A, Tarwotjo I, Djunaedi E, West KP, Loedin AA, Tilden R, Mele L: Impact of vitamin A supplementation on childhood mortality: a randomized controlled community trial. Lancet 1:1169–1173, 1986
91. Barclay AJG, Foster A, Sommer A: Vitamin A supplements and mortality related to measles: a randomized controlled community trial. Br Med J 294:294–296, 1987
92. Hussey GD, Klein M: A randomized, controlled trial of vitamin A in children with severe measles. N Engl J Med 323:160–164, 1990
93. Taylor HR: Onchocerciasis. In Duane TD (ed): Clinical Ophthalmology. Vol 5. Philadelphia: Harper & Row, 1984, Chap 62, pp 1–12
94. Taylor HR, Greene BM: The status of ivermectin in the treatment of human onchocerciasis. Am J Trop Med Hyg 41:460–466, 1989
95. Evaluation of the onchocerciasis control programme. Bull WHO 60:185–188, 1982

ADDITIONAL READING

1. Helen Keller International: Research Priorities for the Prevention of Blindness in Developing Countries. New York: Helen Keller International, 1983
2. Mburu FM, Steinkuller PG (eds): Ocular needs in Africa. Soc Sci Med 17:1683–1830, 1983
3. National Advisory Eye Council: Vision Research: A National Plan 1983–1987. HHS/NIH Publication No. 83-2469. Washington, D.C.: U.S. Public Health Service, 1983.
4. Sommer A (ed): Geographic and preventive ophthalmology section. In Duane TD (ed): Clinical Ophthalmology. Vol 5. Philadelphia: Harper & Row, 1990
5. Sommer A (guest ed): The National Eye Institute Symposium on the Epidemiology of Eye Disease and Visual Disorders. Am J Epidemiol 118:129–300, 1983
6. Sommer A (guest ed): Special Issue on Tropical Ophthalmology. Int Ophthalmol. 14(3), May 1990

57

Psychiatric Disorders

Evelyn J. Bromet
David K. Parkinson

Psychiatric disorders occur in every socioeconomic, racial, and cultural group in the world. In the United States an estimated 12% of children[1,2] and 15% of adults[3] suffer from one or more mental disorders. In the last 50 years a great deal has been learned about the distribution of psychiatric disorders in the population, factors associated with their occurrence, their prognoses, and effective treatments. For the preponderance of mental disorders, however, the specific causes are unknown and are believed to be multifactorial.

Psychiatric disorders account for a large proportion of all chronic health problems. Moreover, an individual's mental state greatly influences general health status and ability to access needed health care services. Four issues underscore the importance of mental health issues for public health: (1) quality of life is largely determined by a person's mental state; (2) a large proportion of people who need medical care have psychiatric or brain disorders; (3) many physical disorders have an important mental component; and (4) as the risk of premature death recedes, the risk of chronic impairment rises. In fact, the increase in chronic illness and disability is contributing to a crisis in public health work.[4] Given the significance of mental health problems, the search for causes is urgent. If environmental factors play a large role, prevention can be a potent force.

The methods used for psychiatric public health work are fundamentally no different from public health methods used for other disorders.[4] However, some specific features distinguish mental health from other aspects of public health. Mental disorders are not usually listed as a direct cause of death on death certificates and are not often detectable on autopsy. Thus, mortality statistics shed little light on the burden of mental disorder in the population. On the other hand, two features of mental disorders make morbidity data more accessible for statistical summaries of community diagnosis than is so for other nonfatal conditions.

First, the care of the seriously mentally ill has long been a government responsibility. Except for tuberculosis and acute communicable diseases, no other branch of medicine has such a long history of official state responsibility. Consequently, substantial data have been accumulated on the hospitalization of mentally disordered individuals. Kramer[5] developed a national system for consistent recording of hospitalization rates for mental illness and analyzed the national statistics for mental illness in the United States. These hospitalization rates are one measure of the statistics of public mental health.

A second unique feature of psychiatric epidemiology is that personal interviews can be used to obtain direct access to mental life. Questions about such experiences as depression, headaches, phobias, and hallucinations are best directed at the subjects of a population survey (although interview data can be compromised if the question has not been understood or if the respondent's memory or accuracy is flawed).

The classification of mental disorders has a long history. Current concepts are rooted in the diagnostic characterizations of Kraepelin and Bleuler.[6] The current state of classification is recorded in the American Psychiatric Association's *Diagnostic and Statistical Manual of Mental Disorders,* now in its third revised version (DSM-III-R).[7] This document reflects the "official" consensus of the types of mental disorders present throughout the life cycle and the constellation of features encompassed in each type. In making a diagnosis, a clinician depends mainly on the results of a comprehensive mental examination, which focuses on the patient's (1) intellectual ability; (2) current state of consciousness, confusion, or contact; (3) mood or affect; (4) lack of connectedness of thought patterns, hallucinations, delusions, or distortion of thoughts and ideas; (5) personality, (e.g., passivity, aggression, helplessness, rebelliousness); (6) behavior patterns; and (7) the complaint bringing the patient into treatment.

Epidemiological research aimed at establishing the incidence and prevalence of mental disorders in the United States has evolved during the twentieth century.[8] Three generations have been identified: (1) the period before World War II, during which the median prevalence rate of all mental disorders, based on information from key informants and agency records, was 3.6%; (2) World War II to the 1970s, during which the median rate was 20%, based on direct interviews with representative samples using psychological and psychosomatic symptom inventories to determine degree of "impairment"; and (3) 1970s to the present, in which lifetime rates of close to 30%[9] have been reported, based on structured diagnostic interviews and current diagnostic criteria. The latter studies, like family studies, also are important for validating clinically derived diagnostic categories in psychiatry.

This chapter focuses on findings from the recent diagnostic studies, although important earlier results and classic studies are discussed. For a more detailed historical account of the epidemiology of mental disorders, see recent reviews.[8,10,11]

It is important to review briefly the key developments in psychiatry that led to current techniques for ascertaining cases of mental disorder. First, Kramer's observation that admission rates for schizophrenia and depression differed in the United States and England[12] foreshadowed the first international study of diagnosis, demonstrating that the application of systematic interviewing techniques and comparable diagnostic criteria resulted in similar diagnostic distributions.[13] Second, systematic research on schizophrenia by the World Health Organization (WHO) supported the usefulness and importance of structured assessment of patients within[14] and outside the formal treatment network.[15] In the United States, the need to define homogeneous patient populations for clinical drug trials and multicenter collaborative research set the stage for the first systematically operationalized diagnostic method,[16] which was followed 6 years later by the Research Diagnostic Criteria[17] (RDC) and its accompanying semistructured interview schedule, the Schedule for Affective Disorders and Schizophrenia (SADS), designed for experienced clinicians.[18] The Structured Clinical Interview for Diagnosis (SCID) subsequently was created for clinically experienced raters to match DSM-III-R criteria.[19]

In the late 1970s the National Institute of Mental Health (NIMH) developed the Diagnostic Interview Schedule (DIS), a fully structured DSM-III-based schedule for lay interviewers.[20] The DIS has been administered in several community surveys, including the Epidemiologic Catchment Area (ECA) study of nearly 20,000 individuals from catchment areas in New Haven, St. Louis, Baltimore, Los Angeles, and Piedmont, North Carolina.[21] A similarly devised instrument was developed for children aged 6 to 18 years (DISC)[22] Like any tool that relies solely on respondents' memories and understanding of the questions being posed, the DIS and DISC are far from being perfectly valid diagnostic techniques.[23] On the other hand, we now have useful data on the prevalence of psychiatric disorders in the community as well as in general medical settings.

This chapter provides an overview of public health psychiatry by summarizing information on the epidemiology, treatment, and prevention of mental disorders within Morris' framework of the "uses" of epidemiology.[24]

COMMUNITY DIAGNOSIS

The prevalence and incidence rates of specific psychiatric disorders have been estimated from national probability samples and from community studies. National studies provide information on overall rates and demographic and geographic correlates. Planning mental health services for communities requires studies in more defined geographic areas.

Many prevalence studies of psychiatric disorders have been conducted (Table 57-1). Milder forms of disorder occur more frequently than more severe forms.

In the United States the first national morbidity study was conducted in the 1950s by the University of Michigan.[25] Approximately 20% of the 2460 interview subjects responded affirmatively when asked: "Have you ever felt that you were going to have a nervous breakdown?" Twenty-five percent needed psychological help at some time in their lives. National studies of drinking patterns and alcohol-related problems between 1964 and 1984 showed that 12% of the population were "heavy drinkers," defined as drinking nearly every day, with five or more drinks at a sitting at least once in a while.[26] The University of Michigan currently is undertaking the first national probability sample study of the distribution of DSM-III-R disorders.[27] Patterns of comorbidity are a major focus.

Most American morbidity research has focused on rates of disorder in specific communities, which do not necessarily reflect national rates. The first prevalence study of mental illness (insanity as it was then called) was conducted in Massachusetts in 1854 by Edward Jarvis,[28] who undertook a census of the "insane" by gathering information from general practitioners, other key informants such as clergymen, and records of mental hospitals and other official agencies. He identified 2632 "lunatics" and 1087 "idiots" needing "the care and protection of their friends or of the public for their support, restoration or custody."

The most comprehensive study using modern assessment techniques has been the ECA study of specific catchment areas in five U.S. communities. Face-to-face structured diagnostic interviews using the DIS took place at baseline and at 1-year follow-up; at the 6-month point, telephone information was obtained on interim patterns of medical and psychiatric service use.[29,30]

The 1-year incidence rates[31] and 1-month,[3] 6-month,[32] and lifetime[33] prevalence rates for selected disorders assessed in the ECA are reported in Table 57-2. Table 57-3 provides a summary of the DSM-III criteria for each disorder. The most prevalent DIS/DSM-III disorders across the five sites were substance abuse, phobias, and major depression. The least common disorders were schizophrenia, mania, and somatization. Note that the specific rates of mental disorder reported in morbidity studies depend on the diagnostic criteria used to define a "case" and on the initial and follow-up response rates.

Prevalence rates are useful when planning mental health services, and incidence data are more germane for testing etiological hypotheses. Determining incidence rates requires reliable and valid assessment procedures. For illnesses like diabetes, laboratory results are available to substantiate initial clinical findings. Psychiatric surveys depend on respondents' descriptions and, for past disorders, their memories. The difficulties with this method were illustrated in a study of reports by women of lifetime depression. The study found that over an 18-month period, women often failed to recall previous lifetime episodes that were described at the first interview, or they provided new information about lifetime episodes that had not been mentioned originally.[34] In the ECA the attempt to establish 1-year incidence rates, which requires that the population at risk be free of the disorder at the start of the period, has this inherent measurement problem. Thus, Eaton and colleagues[35] identified possible sources of measurement error and generated incidence rates for four of the ECA sites.[31] The highest incidence rates were for phobias, alcohol abuse or dependence, and major depression (Table 57-2).

The incidence rate for schizophrenia merits separate comment. Although included in Table 57-2, the reliability of the diagnosis of schizophrenia in the ECA was particularly poor. The Diagnostic Interview Schedule identified only 20% of the individuals confirmed as schizophrenic by an independent psychiatric assessment.[36] If, as Link and Dohrenwend have suggested,[37] most schizophrenic patients use formal psychiatric services, treatment data may be a more useful source of information for determining incidence. The best source of treatment data is a case registry, and several such registries exist throughout the world. Crude annual incidence rates from registries range from 0.11/1000 population in Salford, United Kingdom, to 0.70/1000 population in Maryland.[36] Similar incidence rates were found in the WHO Determinants of Outcome study of first-contact psychotic patients.[15] Based on the Present State Examination, a structured instrument developed in England, the rates per 1000 population aged 15 to 54 years range from 0.16 in Honolulu, Hawaii, to 0.42 in Chandigarh, India.

Comparative Studies. Research comparing rates of mental illness across specific areas of communities dates back to the pioneering work of Faris and Dunham,[38] which showed that hospitalization rates for schizophrenia decreased progressively with distance away from the city center. Forty-six percent of the cases were from the inner city area, compared with 13% from the outermost districts. Faris and Dunham hypothesized that the inner-city environment created the high rates of mental illness, rejecting the alternative explanation that social selection or drift had spuriously created these higher rates (see below). Since then, sev-

TABLE 57-1. MENTAL DISORDER PREVALENCE RATES PER 1000: SELECTED EARLY STUDIES

Author	Site and Date	Total Mental Disorders	Psychoses	Schizophrenia	Affective Psychoses	Neuroses	Personality Disorders	Mental Retardation	Impaired	Comments
▪ Treated Cases Plus Those Identified Through Nonmedical Records or Key Informants										
Cohen, Fairbank	Eastern Health District, 1933	44.5	8.18 [age over 15]			2.0				After Plunkett and Gordon table.
Lemkau et al.	Eastern Health District, 1936	60.5	6.6			3.10	4.61[a]			Age-adjusted rates. Population age over 10.
▪ Same Plus Intensive Survey of Subsample Population										
Rosanoff	Nassau County, 1916	13.74	2.39[a] [functional]					5.46		Intensively surveyed area's total mental disorder rate: 36.4
Roth Luton	Tennessee, 1938	69.4	6.32[a]	1.73[a]	1.65[a]	4.0[a]	37.8[a]	8.20[a]		Intensively surveyed area's total mental disorder rate: 123.7.
Lin	Formosa, 1946–48	10.8	3.8	2.1	0.7	1.2	0.5	3.4		Persons with more than one symptom pattern were counted for each, and diagnoses specific rates exceed total rate.
Leighton	Bristol, 1952	690	10			570	290	110	420	
▪ Surveys of Total Populations										
Bremer	Norway fishing village, 1939–1944	232.4	35.9			58.0	93.5	55.6	193.6 [chronic]	
Essen-Möller	Lundby, Sweden, 1947	Evident and probable, 179.0 Conceivably ill, 180	19.5[a]	7	10.2[a]	58.8[a]	Major, 64[a] Minor, 210[a]	9.8		Lifetime prevalence rates calculated on total population.
Hagnell	Lundby, Sweden, 1957		17			131		12		Lifetime prevalence rates.
Eaton, Weil	Hutterites, 1950	46.5[a]	12.4[a]	2.1	9.3	16[a]		12[a]		Base population 15 and over. Lifetime prevalence.
▪ Surveys of Probability Sample Populations										
Leighton	Stirling County, 1948–50	570							240	Population over 18.
Rennie, Srole	Midtown Manhattan, 1953–54	815							234	Interviewed population's age: 20–59.

[a] Author's calculation.

From Freedman AM, Kaplan HI, Sadock B [eds.]: Comprehensive Textbook of Psychiatry. Vol II, 2 edt. Baltimore: Williams & Wilkins, 1975.

eral studies have been conducted in other urban areas, showing the same pattern. (For a recent review, see Giggs.[39])

Urban-rural differences in rates of treated mental illness also have been studied extensively. Dohrenwend and Dohrenwend's review[40] of research before 1974 concluded that neuroses and personality disorder were more prevalent in urban areas, schizophrenia rates were similar, and other psychoses were relatively more frequent in rural areas. The pattern for schizophrenia has not been reported consistently. For example, Eaton[41] found that the hospital admission rate for schizophrenia was three times

TABLE 57-2. AVERAGE RATES OF PSYCHIATRIC DISORDER IN THE EPIDEMIOLOGICAL CATCHMENT AREA STUDY (N = 18,571), CONDUCTED IN SELECTED CATCHMENT AREAS OF NEW HAVEN, CT; DURHAM, NC; ST. LOUIS, MO; BALTIMORE MD; AND LOS ANGELES, CA

Disorder	Lifetime Prevalence	6-mo. Prevalence	1-mo. Prevalence	1-yr. Incidence
Alcohol Abuse/ Dependence	13.3	4.7	2.8	1.8
Phobia	12.5	7.7	6.2	4.0
Drug Abuse/ Dependence	5.9	2.0	1.3	1.1
Major Depressive Episode	5.8	3.0	2.2	1.6
Obsessive-compulsive	2.5	1.5	1.3	0.7
Antisocial Personality	2.5	0.8	0.5	—
Panic	1.6	0.8	0.5	0.6
Cognitive Impairment	1.3	1.3	1.3	1.2
Schizophrenia	1.3	0.8	0.6	—
Mania	0.8	0.5	0.4	—
Somatization	0.1	0.1	0.1	—

Prevalence rates adapted from Regier et al.[3] and incidence rates from Eaton et al.[31] Incidence rates do not include data from the New Haven site. Rates of cognitive impairment reflect current impairment at the time of interview only. Clinical data are based on the Diagnostic Interview Schedule and DSM III. Rates are expressed as percentages.

higher in an urban area than in a nearby rural area of Maryland. On the other hand, recent findings for neurotic disorders such as depression confirm the pattern noted above, even in untreated populations.[42–45] Two major studies have also shown that children living in urban areas have a higher risk for developing psychiatric problems than children living in rural areas.[46,47] Finally, three Scandinavian studies reported significantly lower rates of dementia in rural areas compared with urban areas.[48]

INDIVIDUAL RISKS AND CHANCES

Several nonmodifiable individual risk factors are associated with the occurrence of many psychiatric disorders; namely, gender, age, a positive family history, and for schizophrenia, season of birth.

Gender. Gender differences in rates of substance abuse, anxiety disorders, and depression have been confirmed in general population studies, in primary medical care settings, and in studies of patients with psychiatric and substance abuse. The male:female ratios are approximately 6:1 for alcoholism, 1:2 for depression, and 1:2 to 1:3 for phobias. Social and biological factors probably contribute to these differences. Gender differences in drinking habits, expressing emotional problems, social roles, and role performance, as well as professional biases in diagnosis may largely account for the differences.[49]

Among prepubertal children, psychopathology is twice as common in boys as in girls. This 2:1 sex ratio reverses itself during adolescence. A new field of developmental psychiatric epidemiology has emerged, and research is being designed to help explain why the sex ratio changes with puberty.[50]

Although there does not appear to be an overall gender difference in the prevalence of schizophrenia, the risk period occurs at an earlier age in males than in females. Men tend to be seen for treatment in their late teens and early 20s, whereas women are more likely to have their first treatment contact when they are in their late 20s or early 30s.[36]

Age. Age also has been associated with the occurrence of psychiatric disorders. For depression and anxiety disorders diag-

TABLE 57-3. A SYNOPSIS OF DSM-III CRITERIA

Disorder		Criteria
Alcohol or drug abuse	A.	Pattern of pathological use (e.g., unable to cut down; binges; blackouts; use despite serious physical disorder)
	B.	Impairment in social or occupational functioning due to alcohol or drug use
	C.	Duration at least 1 month
Alcohol or drug dependence	A.	Pattern of pathological use or impairment of social or occupational functioning
	B.	Tolerance or withdrawal
Phobia	A.	Persistent irrational fear causing avoidance of certain situations
	B.	Significant distress; recognition that fear is irrational
Major depression	A.	Depressed mood, vegetative symptoms, fatigue, impaired concentration, or suicidal ideation
	B.	Duration at least 2 weeks
Obsessive-compulsive disorder	A.	Persistent ideas, images, or impulses invade consciousness, or stereotyped behaviors are repeated compulsively
	B.	Obsessions or compulsions cause distress or interfere with functioning
Antisocial personality	A.	Childhood history of delinquency, school or family problems, or illegal behavior
	B.	Adult inability to function responsibly or within the law
Panic disorder	A.	3+ discrete periods within a 3-week period of fear, accompanied by palpitations, dizziness, faintness, and the like
Cognitive impairment	A.	Severe impairment in cognitive abilities such as orientation, attention, recall and language
Schizophrenia	A.	Delusions, hallucinations, or thought disorder accompanied by deterioration in functioning
	B.	Duration at least 6 months
Mania	A.	Elevated, expansive mood characterized by restlessness, thought racing, grandiosity, reduced need for sleep and involvement in reckless activities
	B.	Duration at least 1 week
Somatization	A.	History of complaints of multiple physical symptoms not explainable by a physician
	B.	Onset before age 30

Adapted from American Psychiatric Association: Diagnostic and Statistical Manual of Mental Disorders, Third edition, 1980.

nosed according to DSM-III criteria, the ECA found that rates were higher in those 18 to 35 years of age and lower in older populations.[33] The rate of alcoholism peaks in the early 40s. However, findings from national surveys of drinking patterns suggest that the peak period for heavy drinking, which can be associated with serious problems such as driving or fighting while intoxicated, is in the early 20s.[51] The manifestations of schizophrenia also appear to vary with age, particularly manifestations of late-onset schizophrenia-like disorder, which occurs after age 50.

Familial Aggregation of Disorder. Considerable research on familial aggregation of psychopathology is being conducted. In schizophrenia, monozygotic twins have a concordance rate for schizophrenia between 33% and 78% compared with 8% to 28% for dizygotic twins. The risk for developing schizophrenia, given the presence of an affected first-degree relative, is approximately 10% (compared with an overall prevalence of less than 1%).[52] Weissman[53] reviewed findings from family studies of depression and reported a twofold to threefold increase in major depression in first-degree adult relatives of patients with depression. Weissman's study of the offspring of depressed parents also found a threefold increase in risk for psychiatric disorder (24% with any DSM-III-R disorder compared with 8% among control subjects).[54] The preponderance of evidence regarding alcoholism deriving from family, twin, and adoption studies also points to a genetic vulnerability for developing this disease.[55] Current research is attempting to apply molecular genetics techniques in linkage studies of these disorders and in studies of bipolar disorder (manic depression)[56] and Alzheimer's disease.[57] Although promising early results on manic-depressive psychosis and schizophrenia were not confirmed in subsequent replications, the next two decades are expected to yield important advances in this area.

Season of Birth. Seasonal variation has been a well-documented phenomenon in stillbirths, neonatal deaths, and congenital rubella, although the extent of this seasonal variation has diminished over time.[58] In England, Scandinavia, and the United States, patients with schizophrenia are disproportionately likely to have been born during the winter or spring months. Possible explanations for this phenomenon include nutritional factors during pregnancy, environmental factors such as lead exposure, genetic factors, and exposure to infectious or viral agents.[59]

CAUSES

New understanding of the origins and course of mental disorder may emerge when clinical research, laboratory studies, sociological inquiries, and epidemiology interact. A dramatic illustration occurred early in the 20th century, when pellagra psychosis accounted for almost 10% of the admissions to mental hospitals. In South Carolina during the early 1920s Goldberger et al.[60] and others showed that pellagra was associated with a nutritional deficiency, although they could not identify the specific items missing from the diet. As a result of changing dietary regimens, pellagra psychosis became rare in the United States, although it remains endemic in parts of Africa and India.

Known modifiable risk factors for mental disorders fall into four groups: demographic factors, physical health, social environment factors, and agents in the physical environment. Although technically a risk factor must be presumed to exist before the onset of a disorder—that is, its presence increases the risk for developing a disorder—the insidious onset of many psychiatric disorders often makes it difficult to separate risks from consequences. Thus we have been better at detecting associations between risk factors and disorders than at demonstrating cause and effect relationships.

Demographic Factors

Age and gender are associated with the occurrence of several mental disorders. Although not modifiable, age and gender patterns have important implications for the design of preventive intervention programs. Other demographic variables associated with an increased probability of psychiatric disorders include social class (education, income, occupational attainment), ethnicity, and marital status.

Social Class. Identifying and understanding the relationship between social class and mental illness has been at the heart of the development of knowledge about the epidemiology of mental disorders. The ecological studies, starting with that of Faris and Dunham described earlier, were the first to emphasize the importance of social class. However, because such data are ecological (or aggregated), inferences about the nature and direction of the relationships could not be drawn.[61–63] That is, the alternative explanation, that vulnerable people drift into these areas and are then overrepresented in the treatment system, can be neither confirmed nor refuted with aggregated data.

The strongest support for an environmental explanation was *Social Class and Mental Illness*.[64] Among psychiatric patients, higher rates of schizophrenia occurred in the lower social classes. Most of these patients had lived in poor areas of the city all of their lives. Moreover, 90% of their families of origin were in the same social class, suggesting that downward social mobility could not explain the findings. More recent studies of individuals' social class backgrounds, however, have indicated that social selection may be the more plausible explanation. For example, in one study, the occupational attainment of schizophrenic patients was lower than that of their fathers and lower than that predicted from their school careers.[65] Currently in schizophrenia research, the preponderance of evidence indicates that social selection rather than the social or physical environment is the major contributor.

Lower social class status also is associated with increased rates of depressive symptoms, alcohol abuse or dependence, drug abuse or dependence, and antisocial personality disorder.[66] Lower social class status is a risk factor for many psychiatric disorders of both childhood[1] and old age.[67]

Ethnicity. Ethnicity can be conceptualized as an immutable individual risk factor. However, with some exceptions, its association with mental disorders is undoubtedly indirect, reflecting an array of social and physical environmental differences between the groups being compared. The exceptions to this are findings regarding higher than expected rates of schizophrenia and related psychoses in Croatia[68–70] and western Ireland,[71] which cannot be explained by differential emigration or unusual environmental circumstances.

Early prevalence studies of psychiatric patients in the United States suggested that compared with whites, blacks were disproportionately diagnosed with schizophrenia and were hospitalized at a younger age and for longer periods of time. However, the ECA data found that the lifetime prevalence rates for most of the 15 psychiatric disorders assessed were similar among black and nonblack respondents.[33] For major depression, one of the most prevalent disorders, white men tended to have higher prevalence rates than black men, but black women had higher prevalence rates than white women.[72] Comparisons of Mexican-Americans and non-Hispanic whites in the Los Angeles ECA also revealed relatively similar rates for most disorders.[73,74]

Whites of all ages have higher rates of suicide than blacks. However, age-adjusted suicide rates for Native American Indians and Chinese-Americans are higher than those for whites, whereas rates for Japanese-Americans are lower.[75] The rate among Native American Indian youths is 2.3 times that for the remainder of the U.S. population of the same age.[76]

Marital Status. Being single is associated with several psychiatric disorders, although whether it is a cause or a consequence is unknown. In schizophrenia, being single at the time of first hospital admission is associated with a poorer prognosis. However, it is usually male patients who are likely to be unmarried because, as noted earlier, males tend to be hospitalized in their late teens and early 20s, before most individuals get married.

The association between marital status and depression is more complex. The highest rates of depression occur among those recently separated and divorced,[77] suggesting that depression may be a reaction to major interpersonal stress. However, cross-sectional studies of depressive symptoms have found that married women are more symptomatic than unmarried women, whereas married men are less depressed than unmarried men.[78] Thus, being married may be a protective factor for men but not for women. The relationship between marital status and depression may also be inverse; as is true for alcoholics, depressed individuals may create conflict in the marriage and thus have higher rates of divorce.

Physical Health Status

Several sources of evidence point to a link between physical and mental health. There is a higher than expected mortality rate among psychiatrically ill individuals. In one study the adjusted death rate for psychiatric patients was two to three times higher than that for the rest of the population.[79] Another study reported that 6% of patients reporting to a psychiatric emergency service died within 2 years of the visit; the expected rate was 1.6%.[80] In a community sample aged 55 and older the odds of dying over a 15-month period was four times higher for people with affective disorder than for persons who did not have affective disorder.[81]

Hospitalized patients have high rates of psychiatric disorders. Infectious diseases may produce serious mental disorders (Table 57-4). With respect to chronic conditions, studies of patients with multiple sclerosis, cancer, diabetes mellitus, cardiovascular disease, thyroid disease, and chronic pain have reported high rates of major depression.[82] One study reported that 61% of severely ill hospital patients were depressed compared with 21% of less ill patients.[83] Whether depression is a consequence of disease or of its concomitant disability is difficult to determine. Regardless, depression is predictive of a shortened life expectancy.[81,84]

High rates of psychiatric symptoms also have been found in outpatient primary medical care populations.[82] In the ECA, 22% of respondents who had recently used a medical care facility met criteria for a DSM-III disorder compared with 17% of nonusers.[85] Affective disorders were the most common diagnoses in women, and alcohol abuse or dependence was the most common diagnosis in men. A review of British studies of psychiatric morbidity in general practice patients concluded that 20% to 25% of patients suffered from a psychiatric disturbance primarily affective in nature.[86] Despite the high prevalence of depression, patients with this disorder often are undiagnosed or are misdiagnosed, in part because both physicians and patients focus on somatic symptoms and possible physical diagnosis.[82] (For further reading, also see reference 87.)

Social Environment

One aspect of the social environment that has been linked to a variety of mental disorders is stress, defined here as a set of disruptive environmental presses or stimuli. The conceptual model most often used to explain the effects of stress on mental health is the vulnerability model, which posits that individuals who possess inadequate psychosocial resources such as poor social support are particularly likely to demonstrate adverse mental health consequences when faced with threats or significant stresses in the environment.

Three types of studies have demonstrated that higher levels of stress are associated with increased rates of psychiatric disorder and subclinical psychiatric symptoms: comparisons of geographic areas with high and low levels of stress, studies of single traumatic events such as loss of a loved one and unemployment, and research on multiple acute life events or chronic strains.

Geographic Comparisons of Environmental Stress. Community-wide stressors can expose large numbers of people to uncontrollable events and provide an opportunity to analyze both short-term and long-term psychological sequelae. Such a situation arose following the Three Mile Island (TMI) nuclear plant accident of March 1979. Like many disasters, TMI was not an acute, time-limited event but entailed a sequence of interrelated stressful occurrences that unfolded over a long period of time, including the initial crisis, intermittent radiation leaks, and difficulties surrounding the clean-up operations. It differed from other disasters, however, in that no lives were lost nor any property damaged. In a longitudinal study of mothers of preschool children living within 10 miles of the plant, the rate of major depression and generalized anxiety was double that of an unexposed comparison group during the year after the accident.[88-90] However, 2 to 3 years later the comparison site underwent widespread unemployment, and the mental health impact turned out to be remarkably similar.[90]

The psychiatric sequelae of many natural disasters such as floods, tornadoes, and earthquakes have been investigated. Recent reviews of these studies have emphasized that the only consistent psychiatric risk factor is greater involvement in terms of loss of life or property.[91,92]

Single Traumatic Events. Single traumatic events can engender short-term and long-term adverse mental health consequences, even in healthy individuals. One of the first such observations occurred during the two world wars, when soldiers prescreened for mental health often suffered from combat stress reaction when faced with extreme combat stress or deprivation. Since the Vietnam war, there has been considerable interest in establishing the prevalence of Post-Traumatic Stress Disorder among combat veterans. This disorder is defined as a response to an unusual stressor in which an individual reexperiences the traumatic event through recurrent thoughts or dreams, experiences psychic numbing, and has symptoms such as sleep disturbance, survivor guilt, difficulty concentrating, hyperalertness, avoidance of activities associated with the event, and an intensification of symptoms if reexposed to a similar event. A national study of Vietnam veterans conducted in the late 1980s reported a point prevalence rate of 15.2% and a lifetime rate of 31%.[93] These high rates have led the Veterans Administration to increase both research and treatment programs for this vulnerable group.

Other well-studied events shown to produce short-term deleterious effects in more than 50% of individuals include unemployment[90,94] and bereavement.[95] Several factors have been evaluated as potential buffers, including social support, good physical health, and preexisting financial security.

Life Events and Chronic Strains. The most extensive body of literature on environmental stress focuses on life events and chronic strains. In the general population, life events appear to play a minor and transient role in eliciting psychiatric symptoms, whereas in psychiatric patients, these events may be more important. In schizophrenia, life events may even trigger psychotic episodes, particularly in patients with inadequate social network support.[96] Adverse life events may play a causal role in the occurrence of some forms of depression.[97] Women may be particu-

TABLE 57-4. INFECTIONS PRODUCING MENTAL DISORDERS

	Agent	Reservoir	Vector	Personal Contact	Effective Immunization Active/ Passive	Effective Treatment to Prevent Brain Damage	Occurrence	Acute Symptoms	Permanent Brain Damage			Notes
									Fetal	*Childhood*	*Adult*	
Aseptic meningitis Group B Coxsackie	V	Man		PC	No	No	Common	Ac				
Chicken pox	V	Man		PC	No	No	Universal	Ac		Ch		
Smallpox	V	Man		PC	Yes		Not in United States	Ac				
Encephalitides	V	Birds?	Mosquitoes		No							
				No	See Text	No		Ac		Ch	Ad	
Eastern encephalitis	V	Wild birds	Mosquitoes	No	No	No	Sporadic or epidemic	Ac		Ch		
Western encephalitis	V	Wild birds	Mosquitoes	No	No	No	Sporadic or epidemic	Ac		Ch		
St Louis encephalitis	V	Wild birds	Mosquitoes	No	No	No	Sporadic or epidemic	Ac		Ch	Ad	
Pertussis	B	Man		PC	Active		Common	Ac		Ch		
Encephalitis lethargica					No	No	Epidemic	Ac		Ch	Ad	Apparently has disappeared from the world.
Influenza	V	Man		PC	Active	No	Epidemic	Ac	No	Ch	Ad	
Measles	V	Man		PC	Passive–gamma globulin	No	Universal	Ac		Ch	0.02%	
Meningococcus meningitis	B	Man		PC	None	Sulfas and antibiotics	Sporadic and epidemic	Ac		Ch	Ad	Especially dangerous in infants. Mental deficiency.
Mononucleosis	Unknown	Man?		PC?	None	None	Common	1% children		Ch		
Mumps	V	Man		PC	Active, lasts 2 years	None	Universal	Ac	?	Ch?	?	
Pneumococcal pneumonia	B	Man		PC	None	Sulfas and antibiotics	Common	Ac				
Rheumatic fever	?	Man		PC	None		Frequent	Ac	?	Ch?	?	Is a complication of streptococcal disease
Rubella	V	Man		PC	Passive–gamma globulin	None	Universal		F			About 10% of fetal infections in first trimester result in anomalies
Syphilis	Sp	Man		PC	None	Penicillin	Frequent		F	Ch	Ad	
Toxoplasmosis	Prot.	Many mammals		Congenital	None	Sulfonamides?	Scattered		F?			
Tuberculosis	B	Man		PC	Active	Isoniazid	Scattered			Ch	Ad	

V, virus; B, Bacterium or Bacillus; Sp, Spirochete; Prot, Protozoan; ?, Suspected; Blanks, Not known; F, fetal.

From American Public Health Association, Program Area Committee on Mental Health: Mental Disorders: A Guide to Control Methods. New York: The Association, 1962.

larly vulnerable if they lack a confiding relationship with their husbands, are not employed outside the home, have 3 or more children under the age of 6 years, and endured the loss of their own parents in childhood.[98]

Adverse effects of chronic strain at work and at home have been well studied. With regard to the work environment, employees in jobs characterized by high levels of demand, little autonomy over decision making, conflicting requirements, and ambiguity have been found to experience higher levels of psychological symptoms and alcohol abuse than employees experiencing less occupational stress.[99] The combination of high demands and low decision latitude is particularly stressful.[100,101]

Clinicians have long been aware of the links between depression and marital conflict. Empirical evidence from research on depressed patients[102] and on general populations have confirmed this association, although the causal direction is difficult to disentangle.[98,101] A stressful family environment is also a well-documented risk factor for behavioral problems in children. Children reared in families with high levels of conflict, abuse, or neglect are at high risk for a range of health problems, including depression, sleep disorders, developmental delay, generalized anxiety, school behavior problems, phobias, and antisocial behavior.[103]

Physical Environment

Four aspects of the physical environment have been studied in relation to mental health: chemical exposures in the work environment, lead exposure among children, housing characteristics, and homelessness.

Occupational Exposures. Intense exposure to lead, mercury, carbon monoxide, carbon disulfide, and the like may cause serious central nervous system (CNS) disturbances.[104] In *Alice in Wonderland,* Lewis Carroll immortalized the well-known hallucinations, delusions, and mania produced by high-level mercury exposure in the character the Mad Hatter. Since the nineteenth century, dramatic case reports have described cognitive and neurasthenic symptoms and even suicide in workers exposed to a variety of solvents. As late as the 1940s a significantly elevated suicide rate was reported in workers exposed to carbon disulfide.[105]

The issue of current public health concern is potential health effects of low-level exposure. Two neurotoxic exposures that have been investigated extensively are inorganic lead and solvents. Early studies of low-level lead exposure that often reported cognitive and psychological sequelae were based on volunteer samples, poorly matched controls, and nonblind raters, but in recent epidemiological research no significant effects on neuropsychological or psychiatric impairment were reported.[106] The findings for low-level solvent exposure are more complex. Several Scandinavian studies of male workers chronically exposed at threshold or subthreshold levels have reported significantly more CNS symptoms (headaches, fatigue, depression dizziness, memory disturbances), nonspecific somatic complaints (nausea, abdominal pain, skin problems, and aches and pains), or impaired performance on cognitive tasks compared with unexposed controls.[107-110] On the other hand, these studies have been criticized for containing serious methodological flaws.[111] The effects of low-level solvent exposure need further confirmation, particularly in women, who have been studied only rarely. Two recent studies of female workers found that low-level solvent exposure was significantly associated with increased depressive symptomatology, CNS disturbance, and an array of nonspecific somatic complaints, but more research is needed.[112,113]

The combination of low-level exposure and high occupational stress also might be especially deleterious,[114] although empirical data from male workers have not yet provided support for this compelling idea.[115,116] On the other hand, mass psychogenic illness has been described in several female work forces in which both high stress and low-level solvent exposures were present.[117]

Lead Exposure in Children. Environmental exposure to lead has been shown to have deleterious effects on children. A study using tooth samples from elementary school children showed that greater exposure was significantly related to lower intelligence test scores after controlling for 39 factors, including social class and parental IQ.[118] In an 11-year follow-up study of these children, higher dentin lead levels continued to be predictive of both school performance and whether the child dropped out of school.[119]

Housing Characteristics. After World War II, several studies examined whether specific characteristics of housing were associated with increased rates of psychiatric disturbance. Studies of effects of high-rise housing showed an association between living on higher floor levels and heightened psychological strain.[120] Apartment dwellers also have been shown to be more depressed and lonely than demographically similar residents living in single-family houses.[121]

Homelessness. The converse issue, lack of housing, has contributed in large part to the rising epidemic of homelessness. Rates of mental illness among homeless adults and children are alarmingly high. In one study, more than one quarter of homeless individuals were found to have a major chronic mental illness such as schizophrenia or substance abuse.[122] Compared with socioeconomically matched control subjects, homeless children have more overt health problems and more psychiatric risk factors such as abuse, neglect, and elevated blood lead levels.[123] In some cities, deinstitutionalization of the mentally ill from state institutions has contributed significantly to the problem of homelessness. The risk of homelessness among discharged state hospital patients was as high as 28% in a New York setting.[124] (For a detailed review of research on homelessness and mental illness, see reference 125.)

HISTORICAL TRENDS

Historical trends have been difficult to study because of temporal changes in diagnostic fashions and service provision. However, temporal changes in rates of psychosis, depression, and adolescent suicide have received considerable attention.

Psychosis

A major debate centers on whether schizophrenia has increased as a function of industrialization. A pioneering analysis by Goldhamer and Marshall[126] focused on mental hospital admission rates for psychosis from 1840 to 1940. They concluded that, although a progressive increase in hospital admissions occurred among the elderly, the rates of psychosis (primarily schizophrenia) among young and middle-aged groups changed very little. However, after extending the time period to 1970, Eaton concluded that the prevalence of psychosis had increased.[127] To date, the debate is unresolved and is perhaps unresolvable. Two pieces of recent evidence support the original conclusion of no change. First, a compelling examination of Australian mental hospital admission rates over a 130-year period concluded that admission rates were relatively stable once historical changes in diagnostic categories were taken into account.[128] Second, the WHO program of research has found similar rates of psychosis in industrialized and nonindustrialized countries.[15]

It may be impossible to settle the argument definitively. However, if rates are shown to change as a function of industrialization, research is needed to specify explanatory factors such as possible physical agents in the environment, decreased infant mortality, lifestyle changes associated with industrialization, or artifactual agents such as inclusion of milder cases into or changing availability of treatment.[129]

Depression

Evidence regarding an increase in depression since World War II is more direct. In Lundby, Sweden, a longitudinal study of a single population was initiated in 1947.[130] Direct interviews by psychiatrists, information from key informants, and medical records were all used to determine psychiatric diagnoses for the entire population. Follow-up interviews by psychiatrists were conducted in 1957 and 1972, with more than 97% success, and a significant increase in the incidence of nonpsychotic depression was found. Consistent with this important finding, an increase in hospital admission rates for affective disorder has been noted since World War II, and lower rates of lifetime depression were reported by older compared with younger community respondents in epidemiological surveys such as the ECA.[131] As with psychosis, firm conclusions about changes in depression are still difficult to draw because of artifacts like differential mortality, changes in diagnostic criteria, reporting biases, and changing attitudes about depression in society. Nevertheless, the National Institute of Mental Health became so concerned about the prevalence of depression that they instituted the Depression/Awareness, Recognition, and Treatment Program. Aimed at mental health professionals, general medical practitioners, and the general population, its ultimate aim is to reduce the level of morbidity associated with depression and to attempt to prevent its occurrence through early detection.[132]

Suicide in Adolescents and Young Adults

Between 1955 and 1980 the rate of suicide tripled in people 15 to 24 years of age, increasing from 2.6/100,000 population to 8.5/100,000 population, making suicide the second leading cause of death in this age group.[133] This increase has been seen on both national and local levels. The group at highest risk is white males. Other risk factors are prior suicide attempts, substance abuse, mental illness, and familial depression.[134–137] One study found that adolescent suicide victims with detectable blood alcohol concentrations were more likely to use firearms, a method likely to result in a completed suicide.[135] Thus it appears likely that the rising rate of substance abuse in young people is contributing to the observed increase in completed suicides.

COMPLETING THE CLINICAL PICTURE

Since most individuals with psychiatric disorders are untreated, community studies may markedly alter our understanding of the clinical signs and prognosis of some disorders. For other conditions that typically come to clinical attention, representative samples of first-episode patients may be studied longitudinally to learn more about the natural course of their condition. In fact, such follow-up studies have provided more optimistic predictions about the long-term prognosis for many disorders[138] and, conversely, also have informed us of the high medical morbidity and death rates associated with severe psychiatric illness.

The most striking contribution of epidemiology to completing the clinical picture occurred during World War II, when a large number of recruits failed to pass the Neuropsychiatric Screening Adjunct administered to enlistees. This finding emphasized just how small the tip of the iceberg was and stimulated a series of community studies on the extent of psychiatric impairment in the general population. In the late 1940s and the 1950s, diagnostic categories were regarded as unreliable, and all psychiatric disorders were believed to fall along a continuum of impairment. Using this clinical framework, community studies were carried out in New York City,[78] in Canada,[139] and with a national probability sample of the United States.[25] More than 20% of the population experienced significant symptoms and were classified as "impaired."

Recent studies applying clinical diagnostic criteria to untreated populations have helped complete the clinical picture by pointing out that the syndromes of depression and alcoholism, for example, may be different in treated and untreated groups. For example, a study of white collar employees found that 25% met DSM-III-R criteria for depression, and 10% met criteria for alcoholism.[140] Nevertheless, these individuals continued to function on their jobs, albeit with some difficulty in concentration and with occasional missed deadlines. Most of the alcohol episodes occurred long ago, and the vast majority of these people became normal drinkers with no serious legal, social, occupational, or clinical consequences. These findings suggest that community respondents meeting diagnostic criteria for depression and alcoholism may not have the significant social and occupational impairment usually noted in clinical samples, despite experiencing the same intensity of symptoms experienced by patient populations during their episodes.

Epidemiologically designed longitudinal studies of psychiatric patients provide an unbiased view of prognosis. The poor prognosis noted for conditions such as alcoholism and schizophrenia is in part because of the "clinician's illusion," which is based on treating chronic cases who stay in the service system.[138] When longitudinal studies focus on representative cohorts of first-episode cases (first-treatment contact is often the most parsimonious definition), the prognosis may be more optimistic. For example, several studies of first-episode schizophrenic patients have found that one quarter have no further signs of illness.

Another important finding is the high rate of comorbidity among individuals with psychiatric disorder. Psychiatric patients in treatment often meet criteria for more than one psychiatric disorder, sometimes labeled primary and secondary disorders. For example, patients with primary alcoholism often develop secondary depression during the course of the alcoholism. Schizophrenic patients discharged after their first lifetime admission often develop depression during the subsequent year. Patients with major depression often suffer from an accompanying anxiety disorder such as phobia or panic disorder. However, people who enter treatment often do so because they have more than one disorder (Berkson's fallacy). Recent epidemiological findings, however, have confirmed the relatively common co-occurrence of multiple psychiatric disorders in the general population. Examples of these are alcoholism with drug abuse, alcoholism with antisocial personality, obsessive-compulsive personality with panic disorder, and depression with somatization.[141]

In children, comorbidity is the rule rather than the exception. In depressed youth, anxiety disorders, conduct disorders, and drug or alcohol abuse are frequently found.[1,103] As noted earlier, adolescent suicide victims have a high prevalence of substance abuse.

IDENTIFYING NEW SYNDROMES

By systematizing clinical observations, epidemiologists can potentially identify new syndromes. Until recently, depression was viewed as an adult disorder that rarely occurred during childhood. Several factors converged to stimulate the need to define depressive disorders of childhood as a separate entity: the increasing rate of adolescent suicide and suicide attempts, the increased frequency with which childhood depressions were being noted in pediatric and psychiatric settings,[131] and the high rates of depression reported in studies of the offspring of clinically depressed parents.[54] Recent findings suggest that the rate of depression using DSM-III-R criteria is approximately 2% in prepubescent children and 5% to 10% in adolescents.[142]

Epidemiological studies of occupational exposures also have identified syndromes associated with specific toxic chemicals such as lead, cyanide, carbon monoxide, carbon disulfide, and mercury.[143] For example, the constellation of symptoms resulting from carbon monoxide (an exposure occurring in blast furnace workers, fire fighters, fork-lift truck operators, and others) includes cognitive disturbances in concentration and memory, impulsivity, and lack of insight into one's behavior. As noted, the phrase "mad as a hatter" stemmed from observations of specific types of tremors among workers in the hatting industry who were exposed to high levels of mercuric nitrate in Europe during the nineteenth century.

Although the prevalence rates are not yet known, it is now recognized that a unique type of dementia may develop in conjunction with human immunodeficiency virus (HIV) infection, and a depressive syndrome may occur in patients with Lyme disease. In one study of patients with Lyme disease the average depression symptom score was in the clinically significant range.[144] It has been estimated that in the United States in 1991, 30% of adults and 60% of children with acquired immunodeficiency syndrome (AIDS) will become demented. According to King,[145] "Although a wide variety of neuropathological findings have been reported at post-mortem in patients with HIV infection or AIDS, an encephalitis characterized by multinucleate giant cells, macrophages, microglial cells, and lymphocytes appears to be specific to HIV disease" (p.153).

MENTAL HEALTH SERVICES

Studies of the provision of mental health services help to explain why some patients are in the visible (treated) tip of the iceberg, while many others remain below the surface, undiagnosed, untreated, and unknown to treatment agencies. Evaluation of mental health services involves assessing not only ongoing treatment efforts but also preventive interventions aimed at reducing levels of morbidity in high-risk populations. This section considers three issues: a brief historical overview of American psychiatric service delivery, a discussion of factors associated with entry into treatment, and efforts to prevent mental disorders.

Historical Overview of American Psychiatric Care

In 1841, when Dorothea Lynde Dix began her crusade on behalf of the mentally ill, there were only 18 hospitals in the United States devoted exclusively to the care of the mentally ill. The vast majority of psychiatrically ill individuals were in jails and poorhouses, kept at home, boarded out, or auctioned off to the highest bidder.[146] Echoing Horace Mann's 1828 plea that the mentally ill be declared "wards of the state," Dix convinced the Massachusetts legislature that local communities had shown themselves incapable of caring for the mentally ill. Like other reformers, she did not hesitate to reinforce her arguments with the economic lure that decent treatment in state hospitals—small and geographically isolated from the stresses of daily life—would cure psychiatrically disturbed individuals quickly, making them productive members of society instead of drains on the public purse. In 1843, the legislators voted to make all of the indigent mentally ill wards of the Commonwealth of Massachusetts and to enlarge Worcester State Hospital, a mental hospital established as a result of Horace Mann's efforts a decade before.

The Dix-Mann doctrine that the mentally ill should be wards of the state reached its most explicit expression with the passage of the New York State Care Act of 1890. This legislation provided for removal of all the mentally ill from local poorhouses and jails to state hospitals, where they were to be supported and treated at state expense. The law further required each state hospital to admit all cases of mental illness in its district, regardless of prognosis. Following its inauguration in New York, other states adopted the Dix-Mann principle of complete state care for the seriously mentally ill.[147] A major consequence of this action was the isolation of mental patients and of psychiatry from the mainstream of medicine.

Although some state hospitals in the United States were established explicitly as custodial institutions, most attempted to apply moral treatment, and some closely approached that ideal (as Charles Dickens noted in 1842). Even the best-managed hospitals, however, did not long continue to function as the small, rural, therapeutic retreats that Dix and Mann had envisioned. New asylums were built as older ones overflowed, and the demand for accommodation always seemed to exceed capacity. As chronic cases accumulated and new admissions rose, overcrowding led to deterioration in the standards of care. At the turn of the century, the "cult of curability" yielded to the notion, "once insane, always insane"; moral treatment precepts were forgotten, and patients' behavior was controlled with physical restraints and seclusion.

The National Association for Mental Hygiene was founded in 1909, with the aim of improving the care and treatment of patients in mental hospitals. After World War I, the mental hygiene movement turned its attention to prevention by early detection and treatment of mental disorders, a strategy exemplified by its active support for the development of child guidance clinics and parental education.[148] The rapid growth of child guidance clinics and other outpatient psychiatric services marked the beginning of organized community-based psychiatry in the United States, which had begun in the late nineteenth century in Europe. By the mid-1930s, nearly all state mental hospitals had at least one outpatient clinic.[149]

In 1946, Congress passed the National Mental Health Act (Public Law 79-487), thereby creating the National Institute of Mental Health. For the first time, the federal government took responsibility for research, training of personnel, and assisting the states in prevention, diagnosis, and treatment of serious psychiatric disorders.

The resident patient population, having grown at a steady rate for over a century, reached an all-time high of 560,000 in 1955. The slow decline of resident mental patients that began in 1956 has been credited to three factors: the introduction of neuroleptic drugs, which accelerated management and sometimes even recovery and enabled some patients to be treated at home; the introduction of the therapeutic community, or community-oriented treatment within the hospital, which reduced the demoralization of custodial care; and the geographic decentralization of large state mental hospitals, which led to closer relationships between state hospitals and local communities.[150] Around 1960, a systematic policy of releasing patients was initiated, based on successful reforms in England, where a reduction of the patient census had preceded the use of neuroleptic drugs.[51] Criteria for both admission and release were liberalized. That is, less severe symptoms were needed for admission, and more symptoms were allowed at the time of release. Length of stay was shortened for acute admissions, and the resident patient census dropped. However, the actual number of admissions increased, in part transforming the custodial hospitals into short-term intensive therapy centers. The introduction of this "revolving door" policy highlighted the need for expanded community treatment, preferably by the hospital-based unified clinical teams' taking responsibility for inpatient and outpatient care. Mental hospital censuses decreased from 560,000 in 1955 to 150,000 in 1980.

In 1955, Congress enacted the Mental Health Study Act (Public Law 84-182) to evaluate the "human and economic problems of mental illness." This act led to the establishment of the Joint Commission on Mental Illness and Health. The Commission's final report, *Action for Mental Health,* recommended funding basic and applied research, training, and expanded services to the mentally ill. The Commission recommended establishing (a) outpatient mental health facilities in communities to provide immediate care for acutely disturbed patients, (b) one clinic per 50,000 population, (c) inpatient psychiatric units in every general hospital with 100 or more beds, (d) maximum occupancy in state mental hospitals of 1000 beds, and (e) expanded mental health education to reduce the stigma associated with mental illness. In 1963, President Kennedy delivered a message to Congress on mental illness and mental retardation in which he proposed a national federally funded program for setting up comprehensive community mental health centers and for improving care in state hospitals. This set the stage for the passage of the Community Mental Health Centers Act of October 1963. The newly mandated community mental health centers had to provide five essential services: inpatient care, outpatient care, emergency services, partial hospitalization, and consultation and education. Over time, five additional services were to be added: diagnostic services, rehabilitation services, precare and aftercare services, training, and research and evaluation. The centers were to serve geographically defined catchment areas of 75,000 to 200,000 people. By 1980, 717 community mental health centers had been funded across the country (2000 had been envisaged), with the federal government investing more than 1.5 billion dollars.

In 1977, President Carter signed an executive order establishing The President's Commission on Mental Health to review and make new recommendations on the mental health needs of the nation. Among its 100 recommendations were the following: improving linkages between community support networks and mental health facilities; expanding services to children, minorities, the elderly, and the chronically mentally ill; the continued phasing down of large state mental hospitals; and the development of a case management system by the states. In 1980, President Carter signed the resulting Mental Health Systems Act (Public Law 96-398) into law. However, the subsequent Omnibus Budget and Reconciliation Act of 1981 (Public Law 97-35) rescinded continued federal management and turned responsibility for provision of community mental health services to the states through the block grant. At present, in New York and other states, treatment of the chronically mentally ill, both young and old, is the primary focus of community mental health centers. (For a detailed discussion of the history of American psychiatric care, see references 150 and 152.)

Factors Associated With Admission

In addition to the effects of formal admission policies, distance of residence from an institution has a major impact on service utilization. In fact, this association was first described by Jarvis in the nineteenth century.[8] Even with modern transportation, Jarvis's "law of distance" still influences utilization rates, not only of psychiatric facilities, but of general hospitals and private practices as well.

When distance is controlled, rural areas tend to send fewer people to mental hospitals than do urban areas, and small cities in general have lower admission rates than do large cities.[40] Admissions within a city, as noted above, vary according to the type and conditions of the census area.

Personal characteristics of patients also affect utilization rates. In general, blacks, the poor, and the unmarried are hospitalized more frequently and remain hospitalized for longer periods. Private hospitals treat more patients from the upper socioeconomic status (SES) categories. Outpatient clinics deal with a younger and higher SES population than state hospitals. Last but not least, the nature of the psychiatric disorder for which a person is treated determines the kind of facility to which the person goes. As a rule, severely mentally ill persons without medical insurance go to public hospitals, while those who are less impaired or who have insurance go to private or general hospital inpatient psychiatric units.

Veroff and colleagues[153] conducted a national study of patterns of outpatient help seeking in the general population. They found the following characteristics to be associated with seeking professional help: being female, being younger, living in urban areas, being Jewish, having more education, attending church frequently, being divorced, residing in the Pacific states, experiencing parental divorce, and having a father who was a professional. In all, 26% of the sample reported that they sought professional help in 1976, compared with 14% in 1957. The primary sources used were clergy, physicians (other than psychiatrists), psychiatrists or psychologists, marriage counselors, mental health agencies, social service agencies, and lawyers.

Preventive Interventions

Preventive medicine divides prevention activities into primary, secondary, and tertiary categories. These divisions also are useful in identifying psychiatric problems that can be prevented totally (and thus eliminated) from those for which early detection and treatment may avert or minimize the progression of the disease. The priority assigned to each type of prevention will change as our knowledge of etiology becomes more certain.

Primary prevention can be carried out when the etiology of the disease is understood and the environmental cause is eliminated. Thus, two disorders have essentially been eradicated through primary prevention efforts: pellagra psychoses and brain damage from measles and rubella.

In the workplace, as noted earlier, high-level exposure to heavy metals such as lead and mercury resulted in psychiatric disorders. Standards such as the U.S. Occupational Safety and Health Administration's Lead Standard have reduced exposure to levels at which neuropathy or encephalopathy rarely occur. Similarly, concerns regarding childhood lead poisoning resulted in the passage of laws to reduce lead in paints, a primary source of exposure. It is important to point out, however, that in many countries in South America, Africa, Asia, and Eastern Europe, environmental exposure is poorly regulated. High levels of contaminants produce exposures comparable to those described in 19th century Europe and the United States.

In addition to environmental factors, other primary prevention efforts have focused on asymptomatic individuals in high-risk groups. For example, as a consequence of the recent increase in suicide rates in adolescents and young adults, there has been a growth in school-based programs aimed at preventing teenage suicide. Shaffer and colleagues[154] noted that in 1986, more than 100 school-based programs reaching approximately 180,000 teenagers were in operation. The goals of these programs were to heighten awareness of the problem as a primary preventive tool, to promote finding students who were at risk (a secondary prevention effort), and to provide information about mental health resources. Shaffer et al. conducted the only systematic evaluation of a school-based program, studying 1000 students 13 to 18 years old from six high schools who were exposed to one of three programs. At baseline, the teenagers were remarkably knowledgeable about the seriousness of suicidal threats and how they should be managed. Although the three programs used significantly different techniques, the authors felt that they were not differentially effective, concluding that the true value of the programs was their screening function, in which 3% of the students reported that they were suicidal and in need of professional help.

Early detection is the cornerstone of secondary prevention. The most famous example in psychiatry has been the elimination of general paresis (syphilitic psychoses) through antibiotic therapy. Secondary prevention programs have been implemented in the early phases of a variety of high-risk situations. These programs have been aimed at reducing psychological difficulties in recently separated couples; substance abuse and delinquency in young adolescents with a history of poor academic performance and disruptive behaviors; and depression in Mexican-American women, in low-income mothers, and in adults undergoing major life changes.[155]

Screening programs should be designed in accordance with sound epidemiological principles. A recent report by the U.S. Preventive Services Task Force identified several psychiatric disorders in which screening for early detection has been considered, namely, dementia, depression, suicidal intent, abnormal bereavement, and alcohol and drug abuse.[156] On the other hand, the Task Force did not recommend screening for these conditions in asymptomatic populations because of the uncertain sensitivity and specificity of available screening tools.

The workplace also has become the focal point for secondary intervention programs. Many companies have established Employee Assistance Programs to assist troubled employees. To date, there have been no systematic evaluations of their effectiveness relative to other types of interventions. However, the goal is to detect mental health problems at an early stage and offer an intervention that might avert a full-blown psychiatric episode. Similarly, health programs aimed at reducing physical symptoms (e.g., smoking, obesity, high blood pressure) also are proliferating in occupational settings, although cost-benefit analyses of their efficacy also have not been conducted.[157] In light of the significant relationship between physical and mental health, it has been suggested that these programs also will have an indirect impact on the psychological well-being of employees.

Clinical trials focused on psychotherapeutic medications or other forms of therapy are examples of tertiary prevention efforts focused on minimizing disability and handicap in patients with a history of mental illness. For example, the NIMH Depression/Awareness, Recognition and Treatment Program (a mixed secondary and tertiary prevention effort) is based on the premise that depressive disorders are treatable in 80% to 90% of cases.[132] The program is aimed at educating psychiatrists, general practitioners, and the lay public about the symptoms and treatments for affective disorders. A review of the vast psychiatric treatment literature is beyond the scope of this chapter; however, clinical drug trials currently are being conducted for an array of medications presumed to alleviate symptoms associated with schizophrenia, depression, obsessive-compulsive disorder, panic disorder, and other mental illnesses.

Two noteworthy issues have been of particular concern to public health professionals: the widespread prescribing of benzodiazepines and other tranquilizers in the general adult population and the prescribing of multiple drugs to elderly patients. Williams and his colleagues[158] have emphasized the iatrogenic effects of long-term benzodiazepine use. As a result of widespread recognition of the adverse psychiatric consequences of these practices, states such as New York have developed review procedures for targeted drugs such as benzodiazepines and narcotics.

CONCLUSION

The theme of *Mental Health Considerations in Public Health*[159] was the need to integrate mental and physical health: "Today and tomorrow community programs should encompass the mental, physical, social, and environmental aspects of health." We have yet to realize this goal. However, considerable knowledge has accumulated indicating the need for public health programs to prevent or reduce the impact of many psychiatric problems. Although the greatest progress clearly has occurred at the level of descriptive epidemiology, analytic studies currently underway and in the planning stages will be important for advancing the preventive aspects of public health psychiatry.

REFERENCES

1. Institute of Medicine: Research on Children and Adolescents with Mental, Behavioral, and Developmental Disorders: Mobilizing a National Initiative. Washington, D.C.: National Academy Press, 1989
2. Gould MS, Wunsch-Hitzig R, Dohrenwend BP: Formulation of hypotheses about the prevalence, treatment and prognostic significance of psychiatric disorders in children in the United States. In Dohrenwend BP, Dohrenwend BS, Gould MS, Link B, Neugebauer R, Wunsch-Hitzig R: Mental Illness in the United States: Epidemiological Estimates of the Scope of the Problems. New York: Praeger, 1980
3. Regier DA, Boyd JH, Burke JD, Rae DS, Myers JK, Kramer M, Robins LN, George LK, Karno M, Locke BZ: One-month prevalence of mental disorders in the United States based on five epidemiologic catchment area sites. Arch Gen Psychiatry 45:977–986, 1988
4. Gruenberg E: Mental disorders. In Last J (ed): Maxcy-Rosenau Public Health and Preventive Medicine, 11 edt. New York: Appleton-Century-Crofts, 1980.
5. Department of HHS, National Institute of Mental Health, Division of Biometry and Applied Sciences: Mental Health Statistical Notes. Washington, D.C.: GPO, various years
6. Kendall RE: The Role of Diagnosis in Psychiatry. Oxford: Blackwell Scientific Publications, 1975
7. American Psychiatric Association: Diagnostic and Statistical Manual of Mental Disorders, Third Edition, Revised. Washington D.C.: American Psychiatric Association, 1987
8. Dohrenwend BP, Dohrenwend BS: Perspectives on the past and future of psychiatric epidemiology: The 1981 Rema Lapouse Lecture. Am J Public Health 72(11):1271–1279, 1982
9. Regier D, Burke J: Psychiatric disorders in the community: The Epidemiologic Catchment Area study. In Hales R, Frances A (eds): American Psychiatric Association Annual Review, Vol 6. Washington D.C.: American Psychiatric Press, Inc., 1987, ch 27
10. Bland RC: Psychiatric epidemiology. Can J Psychiatry 33:618–625, 1988
11. Grob GN: The origins of American psychiatric epidemiology. Am J Public Health 75(3):229–236, 1985
12. Kramer M: Some problems for international research suggested by observations on differences in first admission rates to the mental hospitals of England and Wales and of the United States. In Proceedings of the Third World Congress of Psychiatry, Vol 3, Montreal, pp 153–160, 1961
13. Cooper JE, Kendell RE, Gurland BJ, Sharpe L, Copeland JRM: Psychiatric Diagnosis in New York and London: A Comparative Study of Mental Hospital Admissions. London: Oxford University Press, Institute of Psychiatry, Maudsley Monographs, No. 20, 1972
14. World Health Organization: Schizophrenia: A Multinational Study. Geneva: World Health Organization, 1975
15. Sartorius N, Jablensky A, Korten A, Ernberg G, Anker M, Cooper JE, Day R: Early manifestations and first-contact incidence of schizophrenia in different cultures: A preliminary report on the initial evaluation phase of the WHO Collaborative Study on Determinants of Outcome of Severe Mental Disorders. Psychol Med 16:909–928, 1986
16. Feighner JP, Robins E, Guze SB, et al: Diagnostic criteria for use in diagnostic research. Arch Gen Psychiatry 26:57–63, 1972
17. Spitzer R, Endicott J, Robins E: Research diagnostic criteria: Rationale and reliability. Arch Gen Psychiatry 35:773–782, 1978
18. Endicott J, Spitzer R: A diagnostic interview: The Schedule for Affective Disorders and Schizophrenia. Arch Gen Psychiatry 35:837–844, 1978
19. Spitzer R, Williams B, Gibbon M, First M: Structured Clinical Interview for DSM-III-R. New York: Biometrics Research Department, New York State Psychiatric Institute, 1987
20. Robins LN, Helzer JE, Croughan J, Ratcliff KS: National Institute of Mental Health Diagnostic Interview Schedule. Arch Gen Psychiatry 34:129–133, 1977
21. Eaton WW Jr, Kessler LG, (eds): Epidemiologic Field Methods in Psychiatry: The NIMH Epidemiologic Catchment Area Program. Orlando, Florida: Academic Press, Inc., 1985
22. Costello E, Costello A, Edelbrock C, Burns B, Dulcan M, Brent B: Psychiatric disorders in pediatric primary care. Arch Gen Psychiatry 45:1107–1116, 1988
23. Parker G: Are the lifetime prevalence estimates in the ECA Study accurate? Psychol Med 17:275–282, 1987

24. Morris JN: Uses of Epidemiology, 2 edt. London: Livingstone, 1964
25. Gurin G, Veroff J, Feld J: Americans View Their Mental Health. New York: Basic Books, 1960
26. Cahalan D: Understanding America's Drinking Problem: How to Combat the Hazards of Alcohol. San Francisco: Jossey-Bass Publishers, 1987
27. Kessler R: Epidemiological studies of persons with mental disorders that co-occur with alcoholic and drug abuse disorders. Unpublished grant proposal, 1989
28. Jarvis E: Insanity and Idiocy in Massachusetts: Report of the Commission on Lunacy, 1855. Cambridge, Mass.: Harvard University Press, 1971
29. Eaton WW Jr, Regier DA, Locke BZ, Taube CA: The Epidemiologic Catchment Area Program of the National Institute of Mental Health. Public Health 96(4):319–325, 1981
30. Regier DA, Myers JK, Kramer M, Robins LN, Blazer DG, Hough RL, Eaton WW, Locke BZ: The NIMH Epidemiologic Catchment Area Program. Arch Gen Psychiatry 41(10):934–941, 1984
31. Eaton WW Jr, Kramer M, Anthony JC, Dryman A, Shapiro S, Locke BZ: The incidence of specific DIS/DSM-III mental disorders: Data from the NIMH Epidemiologic Catchment Area Program. Acta Psychiatr Scand 79:163–178, 1989
32. Myers JK, Weissman MM, Tischler GL, Holzer CE III, Leaf PJ, Orvaschel H, Anthony JC, Boyd JH, Burke JD, Kramer M, Stoltzman R: Six-month prevalence of psychiatric disorders in three communities. Arch Gen Psychiatry 41(10):959–967, 1984
33. Robins LN, Helzer JE, Weissman MM, Orvaschel H, Gruenberg E, Burke JD Jr, Regier DA: Lifetime prevalence of specific psychiatric disorders in three sites. Arch Gen Psychiatry 41(10):949–958, 1984
34. Bromet EJ, Dunn L, Connell M, Dew MA, Schulberg HC: Long-term reliability of lifetime major depression in a community sample. Arch Gen Psychiatry 43:435–440, 1986
35. Eaton W, Kramer M, Anthony J, Chee E, Shapiro S: Conceptual and methodological problems in estimation of the incidence of mental disorders from field survey data. In Cooper B, Helgason T: Epidemiology and the Prevention of Mental Disorders. London: Routledge, 1989, ch. 7
36. Eaton WW Jr, Day R, Kramer M: The use of epidemiology for risk factor research in schizophrenia: An overview and methodologic critique. In Tsuang MT, Simpson JC (eds): Nosology, Epidemiology and Genetics of Schizophrenia. New York: Elsevier, 1988, ch. 9
37. Link B, Dohrenwend BP: Formulation of hypotheses about the ratio of untreated to treated cases in the true prevalence studies of functional psychiatric disorders in adults in the United States. In Dohrenwend BP, Dohrenwend BS, Gould MS, et al. (eds): Mental Illness in the United States: Epidemiological Estimates. New York: Praeger, 1980
38. Faris R, Dunham H: Mental Disorders in Urban Areas: An Ecological Study of Schizophrenia and Other Psychoses. New York: Hafner Publishing Co., 1939
39. Giggs JA: Mental disorders and ecological structure in Nottingham. Soc Sci Med 23(10):945–961, 1986
40. Dohrenwend BP, Dohrenwend BS: Psychiatric disorders in urban settings. In Arieti S (ed): American Handbook of Psychiatry, Volume 2: Child and Adolescent Psychiatry, Sociocultural and Community Psychiatry. New York: Basic Books, 1974
41. Eaton WW Jr: Residence, social class and schizophrenia. J Health Soc Behav 15:289–299, 1974
42. Mueller DP: The current status of urban-rural differences in psychiatric disorder: An emerging trend for depression. J Nerv Ment Dis 169(1):18–27, 1981
43. Brown GW, Davidson S, Harris T, Maclean U, Pollock S, Prudo R: Psychiatric disorder in London and North Uist. Soc Sci Med 11:367–377, 1977
44. Blazer DG, George LK, Landerman R, Pennybacker M, Melville ML, Woodbury M, Manton KG, Jordan D, Locke BZ: Psychiatric disorders: A rural/urban comparison. Arch Gen Psychiatry 42:651–656, 1985
45. Blazer DG, Crowell BA, George LK, Landerman R: Urban-rural differences in depressive disorders: Does age make a difference? In Barrett J, Rose RM (eds): Mental Disorders in the Community: Progress and Challenge. New York: The Guilford Press, 1986, ch. 3
46. Rutter M, Yule B, Quinton D, Rowlands O, Yule W, Berger M: Attainment and adjustment in two geographical areas: III. Some factors accounting for area differences. Br J Psychiatry 125:520–533, 1974
47. Offord D, Boyle M, Szatmari P, et al: Six-month prevalence of disorder and rates of service utilization. Arch Gen Psychiatry 44:832–836, 1987
48. Jorm AF, Korten A, Henderson AS: The prevalence of dementia: A quantitative integration of the literature. Acta Psychiatr Scand 76:465–479, 1987
49. Briscoe M: Sex differences in psychological well-being. Psychological Medicine Monograph Supplement 1. Cambridge, Mass: Cambridge University Press, 1982
50. Rutter M: Epidemiological approaches to developmental psychopathology. Arch Gen Psychiatry 45:486–495, 1988
51. Cahalan D, Cisin IH: American drinking practices: Summary of findings from a national probability sample. I. Extent of drinking by population subgroups. In Ward DA (ed): Alcoholism, Introduction to Theory and Treatment. Dubuque, Iowa: Kendall Hunt Publishing Co., 1980, ch. 8
52. Kendler KS: The genetics of schizophrenia: An overview. In Tsuang MT, Simpson JC (eds): Nosology, Epidemiology and Genetics of Schizophrenia. New York: Elsevier, 1988, ch. 18
53. Weissman MM: Advances in psychiatric epidemiology: Rates and risks for major depression. Am J Public Health 77(4):445–451, 1987
54. Weissman MM, Prusoff BA, Gammon GD, Merikangas KR, Leckman JF, Kidd KK: Psychopathology in the children (ages 6–18) of depressed and normal parents. J Am Acad Child Psychiatry 23(1):78–84, 1984
55. Merikangas, KR: The genetic epidemiology of alcoholism. Psychol Med 20:11–22, 1990
56. McGuffin P, Katz R: The genetics of depression and manic-depressive disorder. Br J Psychiatry 155:294–304, 1989
57. Harrison P, Pearson R: Gene expression and mental disease. Psychol Med 19:813–819, 1989
58. Hare E: Aspects of the epidemiology of schizophrenia. Br J Psychiatry 149:554–561, 1986
59. Torrey EF: Epidemiology. In Bellak L (ed): Disorders of the Schizophrenic Syndrome. New York: Basic Books, 1979, ch. 1
60. Goldberger J, Waring CH, Tanner WF: Pellagra prevention by diet in institution inmates. Public Health Rep 38:2361–2368, 1925
61. Hammond JL: Two sources of error in ecological correlations. Am Soc Rev 38:764–777, 1973
62. Morgenstern H: Uses of ecologic analysis in epidemiologic research. Am J Public Health 72(12):1336–1344, 1982
63. Robinson WS: Ecological correlations and the behavior of individuals. Am Soc Rev 15:351–357, 1950
64. Hollingshead AB, Redlich FC: Social Class and Mental Illness: A Community Study. New York: John Wiley & Sons, 1958
65. Goldberg E, Morrison S: Schizophrenia and social class. Br J Psychiatry 109:785–802, 1963
66. Schwab JJ, Schwab ME: Sociocultural Roots of Mental Illness: An Epidemiologic Survey. New York: Plenum, 1978
67. Berkman LF, Berkman CS, Kasl S, Freeman DH, Leo L, Ostfeld AM, Cornoni-Huntley J, Brody JA: Depressive symptoms in relation to physical health and functioning in the elderly. Am J Epidemiol 124:372–387, 1986
68. Lemkau PV, Kulcar Z, Crocetti GM, Kesic B: Selected aspects of the epidemiology of psychoses in Croatia, Yugoslavia: I. Background and use of psychiatric hospital statistics. Am J Epidemiology 94:112–117, 1971
69. Kulcar Z, Crocetti GM, Lemkau PV, Kesic B: Selected aspects of

the epidemiology of psychoses in Croatia, Yugoslavia: II. Pilot studies of communities. Am J Epidemiol 94:118–125, 1971

70. Crocetti GM, Lemkau PV, Kulcar Z: Selected aspects of the epidemiology of psychoses in Croatia, Yugoslavia: III. The cluster sample and the results of the pilot survey. Am J Epidemiol 94(2):126–134, 1971
71. Walsh D, O'Hare A, Blake B, Holpenny J, O'Brien P: The treated prevalence of mental illness in the Republic of Ireland—The three county case register study. Psychol Med 10:465–470, 1980
72. Somervell PD, Leaf PJ, Weissman MM, Blazer DG, Bruce ML: The prevalence of major depression in black and white adults in five United States communities. Am J Epidemiol 130(4):725–735, 1989
73. Burnam MA, Hough RL, Escobar JI, Karno M, Timbers DM, Telles CA, Locke BZ: Six-month prevalence of specific psychiatric disorders among Mexican Americans and non-Hispanic whites in Los Angeles. Arch Gen Psychiatry 44:687–694, 1987
74. Karno M, Hough RL, Burnam MA, Escobar JI, Timbers DM, Santana F, Boyd JH: Lifetime prevalence of specific psychiatric disorders among Mexican Americans and non-Hispanic whites in Los Angeles. Arch Gen Psychiatry 44:695–701, 1987
75. Kramer M, Pollack E, Redick R, Locke B: Mental Disorders/Suicide. Cambridge, Mass.: Harvard University Press, 1972
76. May P: Suicide and self-destruction among American Indian youths. American Indian and Alaska Native Mental Health Research 1:52–69, 1987
77. Leaf PJ, Weissman MM, Myers JK, Holzer CE III, Tischler GL: Psychosocial risks and correlates of major depression in one United States urban community. In Barrett J, Rose RM (eds): Mental Disorders in the Community: Findings from Psychiatric Epidemiology. New York: The Guilford Press, 1986, ch. 4
78. Srole L, Langner TS, Michael ST, Kirkpatrick P, Opler MK, Rennie TAC: Mental Health in the Metropolis: The Midtown Manhattan Study. New York: Harper & Row, 1962
79. Babigian HM, Odoroff CL: The mortality experience of a population with psychiatric illness. Am J Psychiatry 126:470–480, 1969
80. Munoz RA, Marten S, Gentry KA, et al: Mortality following a psychiatric emergency room visit: An 18-month follow-up study. Am J Psychiatry 128(2):220–224, 1971
81. Bruce ML, Leaf PJ: Psychiatric disorders and 15-month mortality in a community sample of older adults. Am J Public Health 79(6): 727–730, 1989
82. Katon W: The epidemiology of depression in medical care. Int J Psychiatry Med 17(1):93–112, 1987
83. Moffic H, Paykel E: Depression in medical inpatients. Br J Psychiatry 126:346–353, 1975
84. Wai L, Burton H, Richmond J, et al: Influence of psychosocial factors on survival of home-dialysis patients. Lancet ii: 1155–1156, 1981
85. Kessler LG, Burns BJ, Shapiro S, Tischler GL, George LK, Hough RL, Bodison D, Miller RH: Psychiatric diagnoses of medical service users: Evidence from the Epidemiologic Catchment Area Program. Am J Public Health 77(1):18–24, 1987
86. Blacker CVR, Clare AW: Depressive disorder in primary care. Br J Psychiatry 150:737–751, 1987
87. Jenkins R, Smeeton N, Shepherd M: Classification of mental disorder in primary care. Psychol Med Monogr Suppl 12, 1988
88. Bromet EJ, Parkinson D, Schulberg HC, Dunn L, Gondek PC: Mental health of residents near the TMI reactor: A comparative study of selected groups. J Prevent Psychiatry 1:225–275, 1982
89. Bromet EJ, Schulberg HC: The Three Mile Island disaster: A search for high risk groups. In Shore JH (ed): Disaster Stress Studies: New Methods and Findings. Washington, D.C.: American Psychiatric Press, 1986, ch. 1
90. Dew MA, Bromet EJ, Schulberg HC: A comparative analysis of two community stressors' long-term mental health effects. Am J Community Psychol 15:167–184, 1987
91. Bromet EJ, Schulberg HC: Epidemiologic findings from disaster research. In Hales RE, Francis AJ (eds): American Psychiatric Association Annual Review, Vol. 6. Washington, D.C.: American Psychiatric Press, 1987
92. Solomon S: Research issues in assessing disaster's effects. In Gist R, Lubin B: Psychosocial Aspects of Disaster. New York: John Wiley & Sons, 1989, ch. 12
93. Kulka RA, Schlenger WE, Fairbank JA, Hough RL, Jordan BK, Marmar CR, Weiss DS: Contractual Report of Findings from the National Vietnam Veterans Readjustment Study. Vol. I: Executive Summary, Description of Findings, and Technical Appendices. Research Triangle Park, North Carolina: Research Triangle Institute, National Vietnam Veterans Readjustment Study, 1988
94. Kates N, Greiff BS, Hagen DQ: The Psychosocial Impact of Job Loss. Washington, D.C.: American Psychiatric Press, 1990
95. Jacobs S, Hansen F, Berkman L, et al: Depressions of bereavement. Compr Psychiatry 30:218–224, 1989
96. Zubin J, Steinhauer R, Day R, van Kammen D: Schizophrenia at the crossroads: A blueprint for the 80s. Compr Psychiatry 26:217–240, 1985
97. Paykel E: Contribution of life events to causation of psychiatric illness. Psychol Med 8:245–253, 1978
98. Brown G, Harris T: Social Origins of Depression: A Study of Psychiatric Disorder in Women. New York: The Free Press, 1978
99. Kasl S: Epidemiological contributions to the study of work stress. In Cooper C, Payne R (eds): Stress at Work. New York: John Wiley & Sons, 1978, ch. 1
100. Karasek R: Job demands, job decision latitude, and mental strain: Implications for job redesign. Administrative Science Quarterly 24:285–306, 1979
101. Bromet EJ, Dew MA, Parkinson DK, Schulberg HC: Predictive effects of occupational and marital stress on the mental health of a male workforce. J Organizational Behav 9:1–13, 1988
102. Weissman MM, Paykel ES: The Depressed Woman: A Study of Social Relationships. Chicago: University of Chicago Press, 1974.
103. Garfinkel B, Carlson G, Weller E (eds): Psychiatric Disorders in Children and Adolescents. Philadelphia: W.B. Saunders Co., 1990
104. Feldman R, Ricks N, Baker E: Neuropsychological effects of industrial toxins: A review. Am J Ind Med 1:211–227, 1980
105. Mancuso T, Locke B: Carbon disulphide as a cause of suicide: Epidemiological study of viscose rayon workers. Journal Occup Med 14:595–606, 1972
106. Parkinson D, Ryan C, Bromet EJ, Connell M: A psychiatric epidemiologic study of occupational lead exposure. Am J Epidemiol 123:261–269, 1986
107. Elofsson S, Gamberale F, Hindmarsh T, et al: Exposure to organic solvents. Scand J Work Environ Health 6:239–273, 1980
108. Husman K: Symptoms of car painters with long-term exposure to a mixture of organic solvents. Scand J Work Environ Health 6:19–32, 1980
109. Larsen F, Leira H: Organic brain syndrome and long-term exposure to toluene: A clinical, psychiatric study of vocationally active printing workers. J Occup Med 30:875–878, 1988
110. Orbaek P, Risberg J, Rosen I, et al: Effects of long-term exposure to solvents in the paint industry. Scand J Work Environ Health 11(suppl 2):1–28, 1985
111. Errebo-Knudsen E, Olsen F: Organic solvents and presenile dementia (the painter's syndrome): A critical review of the Danish literature. The Sci Total Environ 48:45–67, 1986
112. Dew MA, Bromet EJ, Parkinson D, et al: Effects of solvent exposure and occupational stress on the health of blue collar women. In Ratcliffe K (ed): Women, Health and Technology. Ann Arbor, Michigan: University of Michigan Press, 1989
113. Parkinson D, Bromet EJ, Cohen S, Dunn L, Dew MA, Ryan C, Schwartz JE: Health effects of long-term solvent exposure in blue collar women. Am J Industrial Med, (In press.)
114. Ashford N: Crisis in the Workplace: Occupational Disease and Injury. Cambridge, Mass.: MIT Press, 1976
115. House J, McMichael A, Wells J, et al: Occupational stress and health among factory workers. J Health Soc Behav 20:139–160, 1979

116. Bromet EJ, Ryan CM, Parkinson DK: Psychosocial correlates of occupational lead exposure. In Lebovits AH, Baum A, Singer JE (eds): Advances in Environmental Psychology, Volume 6: Exposure to Hazardous Substances: Psychological Parameters. Hillsdale, New Jersey: Lawrence Erlbaum Associates, 1986, ch. 2
117. Colligan M, Murphy L: Mass psychogenic illness in organizations: An overview. J Occup Psychol 52:77–90, 1979
118. Needleman HL, Gunnoe C, Leviton A, Reed R, Peresie H, Maher C, Barrett P: Deficits in psychologic and classroom performance of children with elevated dentine lead levels. N Engl J Med 300(13):689–695, 1979
119. Needleman HL, Schell A, Bellinger D, Leviton A, Allred EN: The long-term effects of exposure to low doses of lead in childhood: An 11-year follow-up report. N Engl J Med 322(2):83–88, 1990
120. Gillis AR: High-rise housing and psychological strain. J Health Soc Behav 18:418–431, 1977
121. Richman N: The effects of housing on pre-school children and their mothers. Dev Med Child Neurol 16:53–58, 1974
122. Koegel P, Burnam A, Farr RK: The prevalence of specific psychiatric disorders among homeless individuals in the inner city of Los Angeles. Arch Gen Psychiatry 45:1085–1092, 1988
123. Alperstein G, Rappaport C, Flanigan JM: Health problems of homeless children in New York City. Am J Public Health 78:1232–1233, 1988
124. Susser E, Lin S, Conover S, Struening E: Homelessness in mental patients: Lifetime prevalence and childhood antecedents. Unpublished manuscript, 1990
125. Bassuk EL (ed): The Mental Health Needs of Homeless Persons. San Francisco: Jossey-Bass Publishers, 1986
126. Goldhamer H, Marshall A: Psychosis and Civilization. Glencoe, Illinois: Free Press, 1955
127. Eaton WW Jr: The Sociology of Mental Disorders. New York: Praeger, 1980
128. Krupinski J, Alexander L: Patterns of psychiatric morbidity in Victoria, Australia in relation to changes in diagnostic criteria 1848–1978. Soc Psychiatry 18:61–67, 1983
129. Hafner H: Are mental disorders increasing over time? Psychopathology 18:66–81, 1985
130. Hagnell O, Lanke J, Rorsman B, Ojesjo L: Are we entering an age of melancholy? Depressive illnesses in a prospective epidemiological study over 25 years: the Lundby Study, Sweden. Psychol Med 12:279–289, 1982
131. Klerman GL, Weissman MM: Increasing rates of depression. JAMA 261(15):2229–2235, 1989
132. Regier D, Hirschfeld R, Goodwin F, Burke J, Lazar J, Judd L: The NIMH Depression Awareness, Recognition, and Treatment Program: Structure, aims, and scientific basis. Am J Psychiatry 145:1351–1357, 1988
133. Rosenberg ML, Smith JC, Davidson LE, Conn JM: The emergence of youth suicide: An epidemiologic analysis and public health perspective. Am Rev Public Health 8:417–440, 1987
134. Brent D, Kupfer D, Bromet E, Dew MA: The assessment and treatment of patients at risk for suicide. In Frances A, Hales R: American Psychiatric Press Review of Psychiatry: Vol. 7. Washington D.C.: American Psychiatric Press, 1987
135. Brent DA, Perper JA, Allman CJ: Alcohol, firearms, and suicide among youth: Temporal trends in Allegheny County, Pennsylvania, 1960 to 1983. JAMA 257:3369–3372, 1987
136. Rich CL, Fowler RC, Young D: Substance abuse and suicide: The San Diego Study. Ann Clin Psychiatry 1:79–85, 1989
137. Rich CL, Young D, Fowler RC: San Diego Suicide Study: I. Young vs old subjects. Arch Gen Psychiatry 43:577–582, 1986
138. Cohen P, Cohen J: The clinician's illusion. Arch Gen Psychiatry 41:1178–1182, 1984
139. Leighton DC, Harding JS, Macklin D, Macmillan AM, Leighton AH: The Character of Danger. Vol. III. The Sterling County Study of Psychiatric Disorder and Socio-cultural Environment. New York: Basic Books, 1963
140. Bromet EJ, Parkinson D, Curtis EC, Schulberg H, Blane H, Dunn L, Phelan J, Dew MA, Schwartz JE: Epidemiology of depression and alcohol abuse/dependence in a managerial and professional workforce. J Occup Med 32:989–995, 1990
141. Boyd JH, Burke JD Jr, Gruenberg E, Holzer CE III, Rae DS, George LK, Karno M, Stoltzman R, McEvoy L, Nestadt G: Exclusion criteria of DSM-III. Arch Gen Psychiatry 41(10):983–989, 1984
142. Weller E, Weller R: Depressive disorders in children and adolescents. In Garfinkel B, Carlson G, Weller E (eds): Psychiatric Disorders in Children and Adolescents. Philadelphia: W.B. Saunders, 1990, ch. 1
143. Collier HE: The mental manifestations of some industrial illnesses. Occup Psychol 13:89–97, 1939
144. Krupp LB, Friedberg F, Fernquist S, Dermit S, Friedman R: Depressive symptoms in patients with chronic fatigue syndrome, Lyme disease, multiple sclerosis, lupus and controls. Presented at the 1990 meeting of the Society of Behavioral Medicine.
145. King MB: Psychological aspects of HIV infection and AIDS: What have we learned? Br J Psychiatry 156:151–156, 1990
146. Hamilton SW: The history of American mental hospitals. In Hall JK: American Psychiatric Association: One Hundred Years of American Psychiatry. New York: Columbia University Press, 1944, pp 73–166
147. Deutsch A: The Mentally Ill in America. New York: Doubleday, Doran, 1937
148. Woodward LE: The mental hygiene movement: More recent developments. In Beers C: A Mind That Found Itself (Suppl). New York: Doubleday, 1948
149. Caton CLM: Management of Chronic Schizophrenia. New York: Oxford University Press, 1984
150. Rochefort DA (ed): Handbook on Mental Health Policy in the United States. New York: Greenwood Press, 1989
151. Gruenberg EM: Mission to Britain. Int J Mental Health 11(4):24–47, 1983
152. Bloom BL: Changing Patterns of Psychiatric Care. New York: Human Sciences Press, 1975
153. Veroff J, Kulka RA, Douvan E: Mental Health in America: Patterns of Help-seeking from 1957 to 1976. New York: Basic Books, 1981
154. Shaffer D, Garland A, Gould M, Fisher P, Trautman P: Preventing teenage suicide: A critical review. Am Acad Child Adolesc Psychiatry 27(6):675–687, 1988
155. Price RH, Smith SS: A Guide to Evaluating Prevention Programs in Mental Health. Washington, D.C.: U.S. Government Printing Office, 1984
156. U.S. Preventive Services Task Force: Guide to Clinical Preventive Services: An Assessment of the Effectiveness of 169 Interventions. Baltimore: Williams & Wilkins, 1989
157. Fielding J: Effectiveness of employee health improvement programs. J Occup Med 11:907–916, 1982
158. Williams P, King M, Rodrigo E: Prevention of long-term tranquillizer use. In Cooper B, Helgason T: Epidemiology and the Prevention of Mental Disorders. London: Routledge, 1989, ch. 20
159. Goldston SE (ed): Mental Health Considerations in Public Health: A Guide for Training and Practice. Chevy Chase, Maryland: Public Health Service Pub. 1898, 1969

58

Mental Retardation

Zena A. Stein
Mervyn W. Susser

The relationship between prevention and care is nowhere more explicit than in the field of mental retardation. Scientific advances have profoundly modified both prevention and medical care, but in different directions. Prevention is expanding and offers the prospect of eliminating a number of specific disorders altogether in future generations. Medical care is increasingly effective because of these scientific advances, but it prolongs the lives of mentally retarded persons. Thus prevention reduces the *incidence* of mental retardation, and medical care, being more effective than it was, increases *prevalence*.

Another paradoxical side effect of the scientific era is the addition of new causes of mental retardation. While scientific and technological advances protect the young from physical deprivation and numerous infections, byproducts of the same technology add new hazards to the environments to which infants and children are exposed. Thus the prevention of mental retardation, the provision of medical care, and new potential causes are variously influenced by the economy and by modern technology.

DEFINITION

Mental retardation (also called mental deficiency or mental subnormality) implies an intellectual deficit that causes incompetence in the performance of social roles. The deficit is recognized in the performance of social roles and in the performance of age-appropriate tasks. The infant and the preschool child may fail to achieve developmental milestones (sitting, responding to familiar faces, walking, talking, sphincter control) at the expected ages. The schoolchild falls short of social expectations for classroom behavior and for reading, writing, and arithmetic. The adult proves incompetent in the performance of work roles within or outside the home, in communication skills, or in the understanding of money, transport, and locality.

With more severe grades of mental retardation, diagnosis can be made in the early months and years of life. Severe mental retardation is recognized by developmental delay; diagnosis depends hardly at all on cognitive performance. With mild mental retardation, on the other hand, the diagnosis leans heavily on school performance and results of intelligence tests.

Mental retardation can be described in terms of three components: *impairment* refers to an underlying biological disorder; *disability* refers to a deficit in function, usually consequent on impairment but also influenced by psychological and social factors; *handicap* refers to social role and status, the kind of social activities as well as the position in society to which a person, once defined as impaired and disabled, is assigned. Disability—the deficit in cognitive function—and handicap are common to all forms of mental retardation and can be described and measured in the same terms. Impairment, however, is heterogenous and is caused by a great variety of disorders; in mild, socially induced forms of mental retardation, it may not be detectable or, indeed, may be absent.[1]

GRADE

The severity or grade of mental defect describes the level of disability. Grade cannot be predicted accurately from knowledge of the cause; persons affected by the same disease differ considerably in grade. The performance of a child must be assessed independently of the pathological classification, and this assessment should be in terms of both intellectual function (judged by intelligence tests) and performance of social roles (usually judged informally but in some countries by a formal scale of so-called adaptive behavior). The assessment must usually be tentative in the early years. In the widely used classification drawn up by the American Association for Mental Deficiency (AAMD), four levels of mental deficiency—mild, moderate, severe, and profound—are defined. The ninth revision of the *International Classification of Diseases* (ICD-9) uses the same terminology. As shown in Table 58–1, minor differences occur among the classifications in the range of intelligence quotient (IQ) that define the grades, even when the same test is used. The use of IQ scores for assigning grade is intended to serve as a guide, not as an indicator of exact cutoff points.

The current classifications are agreed in eliminating the previously used category "borderline mental retardation." People scoring below one or another threshold but above 70 are no longer described as mentally retarded. In each classification, adaptive behavior as well as intelligence test score is taken into consideration in assessing the grade of defect.

PATHOLOGICAL CLASSIFICATION

The many causes of mental retardation belong to every category: inherited, acquired prenatally or postnatally, toxic, infective, traumatic, metabolic. The classification set out below is adapted from the AAMD[2]:

TABLE 58-1. GRADE OF MENTAL RETARDATION (SELECTED CLASSIFICATIONS)

		Stanford-Binet Cattell IQ Tests	Wechsler IQ Test	
Grade	**ICD Code**	**AAMD**	**AAMD**	**ICD**
Mild	317	52–58	55–69	50–70
Moderate	318.0	36–51	40–54	35–49
Severe	318.1	20–35	25–39	20–34
Profound	318.2	<20	<25	<20
Unspecified	319			

- *Infections and intoxications,* e.g., congenital rubella, bacterial meningitis, viral encephalitis, toxoplasmosis, congenital syphilis, cytomegalovirus
- *Trauma, physical or chemical agent,* e.g., lead, mercury, irradiation, fetal alcohol syndrome
- *Disorders of metabolism, nutrition, or both,* e.g., Hurler's, Hunter's, and Tay-Sachs diseases, phenylketonuria, iodine-deficiency diseases
- *Gross brain disease* (postnatal), e.g., subacute panencephalitis
- *Unknown prenatal influence,* e.g., hydrocephalus, microcephaly
- *Chromosomal abnormality,* e.g., Down's syndrome, fragile X syndrome
- *Gestational disorders,* e.g., premature birth, fetal growth retardation
- *Following psychiatric disorder,* e.g., infantile autism
- *Environmental influences,* e.g., cultural-familial mental retardation
- *Other*

The ICD-9 proceeds differently. Where there is an associated or underlying impairment, this condition is coded as the primary diagnosis; the mental retardation by grade is coded as the secondary diagnosis. If there is no known cause, only the grade of the mental retardation is coded. For instance, Down's syndrome is coded 758.0; in addition, the grade is coded as, say, 318.0 (moderate grade). Microcephaly is coded 742.1 and also, according to the appropriate grade of severity, under 318. As the two systems (AAMD and ICD) may coexist for some years, the differences should be kept in mind.

Although there is no one-to-one relationship between the impairment or pathological entity and the grade of disability, in general the majority of more severe grades of defect (profound, severe, moderate) are associated with organic and metabolic conditions and the majority of the mild grade are associated with sociocultural conditions. For epidemiological purposes, it is important to distinguish the mild from the more severe forms. In the rest of this chapter, "severe" will refer to a grouping of moderate, severe, and profound grades taken together.

INCIDENCE AND PREVALENCE[3-23]

Severe Mental Retardation

Incidence. Severe forms of mental retardation, usually recognized at birth or in infancy, are usually attributable to genetic or prenatal conditions. Some conditions (for instance, most cases of microcephaly or hydrocephaly) arise from no known cause, some from well-recognized mendelian or polygenic forms of inheritance that are not suspected until the first child is born, and some from trauma or from infections in prenatal, perinatal, or early postnatal life or at a later stage from encephalitis or trauma.

Strictly, one cannot speak simply of the incidence of mental retardation. Clarity is needed about what units are being counted, whether impairments, disabilities, or handicaps. Clarity is also needed about the definition of indices of frequency. Most of the impairments that underlie mental retardation arise at some point before birth, and an unknown proportion survive to be recognized. At birth and at other specified ages in the life course, one observes *point prevalence* in the survivors. The numerator of such a prevalence rate comprises cases extant at the age of observation, and the denominator comprises the surviving population at that age. One can also speak of *cumulative incidence* in a birth cohort at such specified ages: all cases recognized up to the observation point are counted in, whether or not they survived to that point, and the denominator is the birth cohort. We shall speak loosely of "incidence at birth" in this sense.

For many disorders, incidence at birth seems not to have changed much in the past half-century. For others, the incidence has declined quite sharply over this century in industrialized countries but less so in developing countries. These disorders include prolonged unassisted labor, congenital syphilis, and measles encephalitis early in childhood. Metabolic disorders of genetic origin, especially phenylketonuria, have also declined in manifest frequency in countries that have instituted newborn-screening programs and appropriate early treatment of the discovered cases. A growing number of disorders that can be detected prenatally (e.g., Down's syndrome, spina bifida, Tay-Sachs disease) can be expected to decline in frequency in the near future as screening in the prenatal period is introduced on a large scale. There is hope that prevention of neural tube defects will be achieved by a combination of specific nutrients given before conception combined with monitoring for α-fetaprotein levels during pregnancy. Iodine-deficiency diseases may be prevented entirely by the use of iodized salt, provided only that the immense problems of distribution to remote areas in the Third World are overcome. Fetal alcohol syndrome should be preventable with appropriate health education of those who are vulnerable. Data on trends of incidence, however, are sparse. In Table 58-2, clinical forms of mental retardation are categorized according to estimated potential for changes in frequency. Clearly, estimates will change as more disorders become susceptible to prevention and treatment and as techniques of prenatal diagnosis extend their range and improve in accuracy.

Additions to the list of recognized causes may follow clinical, epidemiologic, and genetic discoveries. Prader-Willi syndrome in 1956, fragile X syndrome in the late 1960s, Rett's syndrome in 1966, and inapparent perinatal cytomegalovirus infection in the 1970s are examples. These and others cannot yet be weighed quantitatively with precision. The difficulty resides partly in marked variation and partly in measurement. Neural tube defect varies with ethnicity, race, and locale; iodine deficiency disorder varies with soil and geography. Fragile X syndrome occurs twice as often in males (perhaps in 1 per 1000) as in females. Rett's syndrome occurs solely in females (1 in 25,000 in Switzerland, 1 in 15,000 in Scotland). For certain conditions measurement of frequency has proved difficult and uncertain. Thus incidence estimates are notably unstable for cytomegalovirus syndrome because of imprecise indicators of active exposure and for fetal alcohol syndromes because of weak measures, both of exposure to alcohol and of outcome in terms of definitive diagnosis.

Prevalence. Prevalence is a function of incidence and duration. In severe mental retardation, length of survival substitutes for duration. Prevalence rates at different times and places and for different age groups are shown in Table 58-3. A few of these are cohort point prevalence rates in closed populations.[6,14-16,18] Most are cross-sectional prevalence rates, which measure the fre-

TABLE 58-2. ESTIMATED CURRENT DISTRIBUTION OF SELECTED CAUSES OF SEVERE MENTAL RETARDATION IN DEVELOPED COUNTRIES AND POTENTIAL FOR CHANGES IN FREQUENCY OF CAUSES

Cause	Distribution (%) Reported	Inferred[a]	Potential for Change
Chromosomal anomaly	36	36	Reduction of births to older women; amniocentesis for older women, reduction of Down's syndrome to 1.1%; for all women, virtual elimination of Down's syndrome and perhaps fragile X syndrome
Congenital malformation syndromes with recurrence risks	20	27	Prenatal screening or prepregnancy dietary supplementation with nutrients for neural tube defects; genetic counseling; reducing consanguinity; three-fourths are unlikely to be prevented
Genetic metabolic errors	7	8	Neonatal screening and treatment eliminates PKU; carrier detection and amniocentesis could eliminate Tay-Sachs' disease; genetic counseling; research is extending possibilities for prevention
Prenatal	8	8	Most affected also have cerebral palsy; neonatal care is reducing risk in premature infants, but since more premature infants survive, prevalence of morbidity in children has not declined; the cause of growth retardation is seldom known, so the prospects for change are unpredictable; prevention of fetal alcohol syndrome will reduce frequency
Perinatal causes: birth trauma, hypoxia, hyperoxia, hyperbilirubinemia, hypoglycemia, Rh incompatibility	8	9	Improved obstetrical and neonatal care should reduce this group of causes, as it has already reduced perinatal losses
Infections: Prenatal	2	4	Treatment of syphilis and rubella immunization effective; other causes (CMV, toxoplasmosis, HIV) less well understood
Perinatal	2	5	Treatment still uncertain
Postnatal	2	3	Measles immunization eliminates measles encephalitis; immunization for pyogenic meningitides (*Streptococcus*, *Pneumococcus*) being developed; BCG reduces incidence of tuberculous meningitis; treatment of meningitides reduces sequelae

[a] Unknown causes (15%) redistributed by inference or speculation.

quency of the condition in an open population at a given point in calendar time. It is reasonable to expect a prevalence in the school-age population of 3.5 to 4.0 per 1000. There appears to have been little change in the rates over time, at least in the affluent societies of Western Europe. This seeming stability suggests that the contribution of increased survival to the prevalence rate has outweighed any reduction due to a decline in incidence. As we shall discuss, the relationship between incidence, survival, and prevalence is best illustrated by Down's syndrome, which is numerically the largest single diagnostic component of severe retardation.

TABLE 58-3. SELECTED ESTIMATES OF THE PREVALENCE OF SEVERE MENTAL RETARDATION

Location	Age Group (y)	Rate per 1000	Year of Publication
England[10]	10–14	4.35	1929
Onandaga, New York[11]	5–7	3.6	1955
Middlesex, England[12]	10–14	3.6	1962
Oregon[13]	12–14	3.3	1962
Aberdeen, Scotland[14]	8–10	3.7	1970
Quebec, Canada[5]	10	3.8	1973
Netherlands[15]	19	3.7	1976
Uppsala County, Sweden[7,8]	11–16	2.8	1977
Gothenburg, Sweden[19]	8–12	2.98	1981
Kurume City, Japan[23]	7–12	4.90	1984

Mild Mental Retardation

Mild mental retardation is often recognized on the basis of poor school performance. It follows that, in the absence of compulsory and accessible education for all children, estimates of incidence and prevalence are confounded by lack of schooling. The verbal and numerical performance on which detection rests is specific to the social role of the schoolchild in technological societies. This performance may influence out-of-school roles hardly at all. Conversely, the demands of social roles in nontechnological cultures do not stimulate these performances. These circumstances preclude valid estimates from most of the developing world and limit firm inferences about secular changes in developed countries. Evidence from Europe, however, read with all due caution, suggests that the frequency of mild mental retardation has declined with the rise in living standards since World War II.[1,19,20]

With mild mental retardation, diagnosis tends to be made first in the classroom rather than at home. Social class has a powerful effect on school performance. Frequency varies so much with social class that rates for one time or one place cannot reasonably be compared with others unless social class differences between the populations are taken into account.

The term *frequency* is used deliberately, because of the difficulty of measuring incidence in mild mental retardation. In contrast with severe mental retardation, not only is the point of onset of impairment and disability difficult to determine, but the retardation may not persist throughout life. Many persons categorized in childhood or adolescence as mildly retarded gradually become indistinguishable from the general population. Society does not universally require of adults the cognitive skills it requires of schoolchildren; at the same time, as persons with socially induced retardation mature, they develop the social and mental abilities that permit them to perform normal social roles. Thus prevalence peaks in the school years and begins to decline in young adulthood.

The validity of the criteria for the diagnosis of mild mental retardation can be questioned. IQ tests are constructed to produce a mean score of 100 and a standard deviation of 15 among the population at large. If we rely solely on the score of under 70 on such a test, then we must expect that about 2.5% of the population on whom the test has been standardized will score under 70. The first three surveys shown in Table 58–4 bear out that prediction.

On the other hand, diagnosis often rests on poor school performance followed by an ascertainment process to determine whether special schooling is appropriate. Frequency will then be much influenced by local factors, including cultural expectations of school performance, opinions about the advantages of special schooling, and availability of places. The fourth and fifth surveys in Table 58–4 exemplify variations in rates based on different modes of ascertainment.

The fourth survey in Table 58–4 covers all age groups under 50 years. The frequency of mild retardation (15 per 1000 when the diagnosis is based solely on an IQ of 50 to 69) is more than three times higher than the frequency based on two criteria taken together, namely IQ of 50 to 69 plus a low "adaptive behavior" score. The problem of diagnostic validity is further illustrated by the three frequencies given for the same total population of 400,000 19-year-old men in the Netherlands, each based on a single but different criterion.

Questions can also be raised about the usefulness of the diagnosis of mild mental retardation. To "label" a child as mentally retarded is to stigmatize and thus handicap that child in many social situations. On the other hand, it can be argued that assignment to special educational experiences may advance the verbal and numerical skills and leave the child better equipped. These are complex issues, troubling to educators and all others concerned.

TABLE 58–4. SELECTED ESTIMATES OF THE PREVALENCE OF MILD MENTAL RETARDATION

Location	Age Group (y)	Rate per 1000	Year of Publication
Oregon[13]	12–14	30.3	1962
Isles of Wight, England[16]	9–14	25.3	1970
Aberdeen, Scotland[14]	8–10	23.7	1970
Riverside, Calif.[17]	<50	15.29 (IQ 50–69) 3.86 (IQ 50–69 + Low adaptive behavior score)	1973
Netherlands[18]	19	31 (IQ <70) 55 ("clinical" diagnosis) 58 (attended special school)	1976
Gothenberg, Sweden[19,20]	8–12	3.7	1981

If one uses special school membership as the criterion, in modern cities like London, New York, or Warsaw, the rate of mild retardation in a school population is usually five to ten times that of the more severe forms. The proportion of mildly retarded is greater where the proportion of children of the poorest classes is greater (and this holds true whatever the criterion). In present-day Sweden, the prevalence of mild mental retardation differs little from that of severe mental retardation. A similar balance probably holds also among the better-off classes, for example, in Great Britain, the Netherlands, and the United States.

In fact, the most common form of mild retardation, which is unaccompanied by anatomical or physiological dysfunction, is virtually confined to families of laborers or of those in similar low-paid occupations. The intelligence of all in the sibship tends to be in the lowest range of normal, and several members besides the index case may fall into the mild retardation category. By contrast, with severe forms of mental retardation, siblings are most often of normal intelligence. If other siblings are affected, they usually have the same condition as the index case, distinctly different from unaffected siblings. There tends to be a marked preponderance of males among the mildly retarded and only a slight preponderance of males among the severely retarded. Differences in prevalence have been reported, between urban and rural areas, with higher rates of both severe and mild forms in rural areas, but these differences are not always found.

SELECTED CAUSES

Genetic Factors and Recurrence Risks

Three forms of mental retardation—phenylketonuria, Down's syndrome, and spina bifida—illustrate genetic factors and the risks of recurrence within families, which may or may not be genetic in origin. The type and degree of familial transmission are different for each condition, and so are the public health issues. The three conditions together comprise about one third of cases of severe mental retardation.

Phenylketonuria and Hyperphenylalaninemia. Phenylketonuria (PKU), first described by Folling,[24] is a rare defect of amino acid metabolism. The frequency is about 1 per 15,000 in an average white population, somewhat more common among those of Celtic origin and less so among Africans. In hyperphenylalaninemia (HPA) one or another of the enzymes involved in the breakdown of phenylalanine is deficient. Phenylalanine (or a closely related product) accumulates in the brain of the infant. No accumulation takes place in the prenatal period; the missing enzyme seems to be essential only in postnatal life, when the infants themselves must break down the protein in their diet. At later ages, in schoolchildren and adults, intellectual function seems to be less affected by high levels of circulating phenylalanine. The reason for this tolerance is not clear, but it may be related to the changing needs of the brain subsequent to its period of maximum growth.

Preventive strategies take advantage of this as yet undamaged state of the newborn child. If for the first few years of life the child can be protected from HPA by a special dietary regimen, mental retardation can be prevented. The results are satisfying and, although not perfect, PKU-preventive programs provide an outstanding model of secondary prevention.

PKU is inherited as an autosomal recessive gene, which means in practice that both parents are unaffected carriers. The probabilities are that one in four of their children will be unaffected and not carriers; half of the children, like the parents, will be unaffected carriers; one in four will inherit a gene for the defect from each parent and will show the disease.

Since an early start with the phenylalanine-free diet is needed to achieve the maximum preventive effect, the objective must be to identify every affected newborn infant as soon as possible. Delay of even a few months may lead to permanent damage. One way is to identify a family at risk after a first affected child has been discovered and then to examine carefully all subsequent children at birth, a procedure followed for several rare disorders. This method is less than ideal, since at best one child must suffer the effects of the disease. A second way is to identify parent carriers, but tests for carriers of PKU are not yet reliable. A third way is to screen all newborn infants for the sake of the rare one who can profit from the regimen. Fortunately, this is possible in countries where most births are supervised by health personnel and where testing is available, and in countries that have effective screening programs the fully developed condition is rarely seen.

The clinical syndrome of PKU is classically described (e.g., by Jervis[25]) as including severe or profound mental retardation, a tendency to seizures, light coloration of hair and skin, and a slightness of body build. Some persons with PKU have milder forms of mental retardation and, rarely, normal IQs. Since all are now treated, there is some room for doubt about the exact risk of severe retardation in untreated infants.

One new public health problem is the condition known as maternal HPA, which occurs in some women in whom PKU was successfully treated in their infancy. In maturity, they may be normal intellectually and bear children as readily as other women. Since these adult women still lack the appropriate enzyme, they have high levels of phenylalanine in the blood. These levels endanger the intrauterine growth of their offspring and increase the risk of intrauterine death and also of mental retardation in survivors. Ordinarily the children will not inherit the enzyme defect, which would interfere with their postnatal development. The problem is a far smaller one than that of PKU. The women at risk are known, and their physicians should be aware of the risks. Voluntary sterilization has been suggested by some as a remedy. Dietary restrictions before and during pregnancy have been attempted, in the hope of modifying the outcome, but the results are still unsatisfactory. From the perspective of public health, the implications are more theoretical than practical, in that they illustrate an undesirable but uncommon side effect of a preventive program.

The prevention of mental retardation associated with PKU by newborn screening has now been accepted as good public health practice in many countries, but not yet in all. It is practicable only where most births are assisted by health personnel, or where infants are examined shortly after birth; where an automated screening test system is feasible; where suspects can be followed; and where in established cases long-lasting cooperation can be sustained among parent, child, and physician. In less developed countries, such facilities are not available, and even the diet may not be regarded as affordable.

Down's Syndrome. Down's syndrome (mongolism) occurs when there is an excess of chromosomal material relating to chromosome 21. In the most common form, known as trisomy 21 or standard trisomy 21, there are three chromosomes 21 instead of the usual two; the extra chromosome is acquired because of a failure in pairing of a chromosome of one of the parental germ cells (perhaps because of nondisjunction or precocious disjunction). In rarer forms, the long arm of chromosome 21 becomes attached to another chromosome (usually 13 or 18 or another 21). Here the extra chromosome is acquired by translocation from its regular position. The rarest form is trisomy mosaic 21, in which only some of the cells are trisomic while others are normal (see Chapter 60).

The risk of bearing a child with standard trisomy 21 rises sharply with advancing maternal age, especially after the age of 35 years. Since standard trisomy 21 is by far the most common type of chromosomal rearrangement in Down's syndrome, the age pattern of childbearing in the population influences both the overall rate of Down's syndrome and the proportion of affected offspring that have one or another type of rearrangement. Thus, in the United States, a decline in incidence at birth has followed the substantial decline in childbearing among women in their 40s over the past two decades. Even with younger mothers, however, about 80% of infants with Down's syndrome will have standard trisomy, about 15% will have the translocation form, and 5% will have the mosaic form. In about one third of the translocation cases, there may be an inherited translocation detectable in one parent or the other.

As with PKU, epidemiological observations provide a strategy for prevention. This strategy is less satisfactory than that for PKU for at least three reasons. First, the method depends on amniocentesis or chorionic villus biopsy, which requires surgical skill, is not free of hazard, and is costly, and on the karyotyping of fetal cells so obtained, which with amniocentesis may not be completed by the twentieth week or later. Chorionic villus biopsy, however, can be carried out by the tenth week of gestation (compared with the fourteenth week for amniocentesis). Prenatal screening is done mostly for high-risk women as defined by maternal age or by the history of a prior Down's syndrome birth. Among women under 35 years of age, this still leaves an incidence of at least 1 case of Down's syndrome in every 850 births. Third, diagnosis of Down's syndrome at amniocentesis is preventive only if positive cases are terminated by means of induced abortion, a procedure that is not acceptable to all.

These irresolvable conflicts between prevention and care do not end with amniocentesis. In the postnatal years, survival depends heavily on advanced medical skills. Thus since World War II there has been a dramatic change in survival for persons with this condition, beginning notably with the use of antibiotics. At birth, the infant with Down's syndrome is occasionally handicapped by duodenal atresia or other forms of congenital blocking of the gastrointestinal tract, for which surgery is lifesaving. Other affected infants have congenital cardiac defects that are responsive to medical and surgical care. Recurrent infections, previously fatal, respond to antibiotics. Even the childhood leukemia that sometimes occurs with Down's syndrome can be treated. As a result, life expectancy at birth for children with Down's syndrome has been markedly influenced by scientific advances. Once the preschool period has been attained, people with Down's syndrome on average now live to the age of 40 years as often as their nonafflicted contemporaries, although they may not live as long after that age.

Although children with Down's syndrome enjoy better health than in the past, they remain mentally retarded. The majority are moderately or severely retarded, some profoundly retarded, and rarely are they only mildly retarded. Children who live with their families usually attain higher intellectual levels than children reared in institutions. Although it is possible that the selective retention of brighter children at home accounts for this superiority, such selection for placement is less likely among children placed away from home at birth, who are at the same disadvantage as those placed later. Children with Down's syndrome are like other children, therefore, in that they respond more favorably to the family environment than to that of institutions. The advantage of the family environment probably resides in the concentrated and continuous care, attention, and affection given by a few intimate adults. Children with Down's syndrome, like other children, thrive on a range of experiences and stimuli introduced at an early age.

In summary, the incidence of Down's syndrome among the

liveborn can be reduced, but the methods are costly and they create ethical problems. Meanwhile, among those born with Down's syndrome, the prognosis for a physically healthy survival grows steadily better. Given family care, community support from a early age, and a range of facilities for training and care, the prospect of a semisheltered adult life in the community, including limited occupational roles, is not unrealistic for the majority. In the absence of community facilities, increased life expectancy may lead to overcrowded residential institutions and unacceptable living standards.

Spina Bifida With or Without Hydrocephalus. In spina bifida, one among several conditions collectively termed neural tube defects, there is leakage of the cerebrospinal fluid (CSF), sometimes accompanied by herniation of meninges and cord. The defect results from incomplete closure of the embryonic neuropore, an event that usually takes place by the fourth week after conception. An affected child may have normal or low-normal intelligence but more often is mildly or moderately mentally retarded. There may be loss of function in the lower limbs as well as loss of sensation and incontinence.

Incidence varies widely among different population groups.[26] Rates are high among the Irish and probably also among Egyptians; they are lower among Africans. To the extent that inheritance occurs, its mechanism is little understood. Some consider the data compatible with polygenic transmission, others with environmental or familial factors. If either a parent or a child in a family has the condition, there is 1 chance in 20 that a subsequent child will be affected. There has been a substantial decline in the frequency of the condition in the northeastern United States over the past three decades. Time trends suggest that the rates earlier in the century were low and that they reached an epidemic peak in the period of the Great Depression in the 1930s. The risk of recurrence in sibships also declined. Thus the interaction of genetic and environmental factors appears to determine incidence.

Surgical covering of the defect is usually but not always possible, and in many cases permanent leaking of CSF persists. It is difficult, even with careful nursing, to avoid infection. Whether to operate at birth is a controversial issue. Children who had surgery had an improved life expectancy, and there was a resulting increase in prevalence. At follow-up, however, much residual disablement as well as mental retardation was found, and excessively heavy nursing chores devolved on the families of affected children. The surgeon is often unable to predict the outcome in a particular case. Fewer infants are now referred for surgery, and life expectancy is undisturbed by active intervention. In Great Britain, since the general policy of nonintervention was established, the age at death of children with neural tube defects has declined.

New tests make it possible to predict with increasing accuracy the presence of a fetus with a neural tube defect in the prenatal period. The tests depend partly on recognition of abnormalities by ultrasonography and partly on the quantitative measurement of alpha-feto protein (AFP) in amniotic fluid at about the sixteenth week of pregnancy. Several difficulties persist with the procedure, apart from those associated with amniocentesis. Even in the most experienced laboratories, the test is not entirely specific: other conditions raise AFP levels, and sometimes even with very high levels the fetus is apparently normal. The test is also not entirely sensitive; affected infants, especially those with neural tube defects that do not involve leakage but occasionally with other types too, may not be detected. Again, when a positive diagnosis is made, prevention involves induced abortion. This course may be less acceptable than with Down's syndrome, because the risk of a false-positive result (and the consequent abortion of a normal fetus) is so much higher.

Another difficulty has been that the risks of bearing affected offspring are far less well defined than for Down's syndrome (except for the few couples who have already had an affected infant). The test can be routinely performed on older women who undergo amniocentesis for Down's syndrome, but this is a hit-or-miss approach in terms of a preventive program for neural tube defects (maternal age does not predict neural tube defects). Estimation of maternal serum levels of AFP contributes to the better definition of high risk as shown by trials in which maternal sera were routinely tested when pregnancy reached 12 to 16 weeks gestation. In women judged to be at high risk on the basis of serum AFP level, amniotic fluid is obtained by amniocentesis at 16 weeks. These two tests, carried out in sequence and supplemented by ultrasonography, enhance the predictive value of AFP levels and may make possible a considerable reduction in the incidence of spina bifida. In an effective program the first test on maternal serum will have to be carried out on all women, but this is no more arduous than blood grouping and the Wassermann test. For those found to be at high risk in two tests in sequence, there is the opportunity to terminate the pregnancy.

A more satisfying target is primary prevention, and there may be a real chance of achieving this objective. For a mother who has borne an affected child supplementing the diet with multiple vitamin tablets *before conception* has seemed to reduce the incidence of the defect in subsequent births.[27–31] Several controlled trials are in progress to evaluate this strategy.

Prenatal and Perinatal Factors

Fetal Alcohol Syndrome. Adverse effects on the embryo and fetus as a result of maternal exposures to environmental factors have been documented for mercurials (Minamata disease) and possibly for lead. Heavy alcohol abuse during pregnancy has been associated with fetal alcohol syndrome (FAS), which includes mental retardation as well as low birth weight, stunting, microcephaly, flattened nasolabial facies, and narrow palpebral tissues. This form of mental retardation has not been described in detail and is likely to be mild to moderate in grade. It is not yet possible to give a useful estimate of the incidence rate of this condition. Frequency must vary with the frequency of alcohol abuse in pregnant women and perhaps with individual susceptibility. The full-blown syndrome is certainly rare, which may account for the fact that it has remained unrecognized for so long. A minimum rate of 1 in 6000 births was determined retrospectively among a consecutive series of 55,000 U.S. maternity cases in which a history of alcohol intake was not specifically sought.

Prevention is easy to prescribe but hard to execute. In view of the growing evidence that maternal drinking during pregnancy may affect the fetus adversely in a number of different ways other than mental retardation, abstinence or at least a reduction in drinking during pregnancy has become a worthwhile public health objective.

Infectious Agents. Syphilis, the first infective agent known to cause congenital defect, is now a rare cause of mental retardation. Prenatal infection with rubella virus, cytomegalovirus, and toxoplasmosis also cause grave disorders, including mental retardation, although postnatal infections with these organisms cause only minor illnesses.

Rubella was the first of these to be described. Its epidemiology is most clearly understood, and preventive measures have been used. Rubella affects the fetus only if the pregnant woman contracts the disease between the eighth and thirteenth weeks of pregnancy. Mental retardation sometimes occurs but is seldom the sole manifestation. Autism has also been reported. The attributable population risk of mental retardation from congenital rubella syndrome has varied with the timing and the extent of epidemics. Up to 1% of institutionalized cases have been attributed to this cause.

A vaccine against rubella has been effective where its use was widespread. Vaccination is not trouble free, and some vaccines can have unpleasant side effects, notably arthritis. Further, to achieve effective "herd immunity," many young people who may never undergo pregnancy must submit to vaccination even when, as in Great Britain, adolescent girls are the target. When younger children are the target, as in the United States, boys as well as girls must be vaccinated. The question has been raised whether it is appropriate that these children should be protected against a disease that is harmless to them in order to reduce the risk for a subsequent generation.

The epidemiology of some of the other infectious agents that have been connected to mental retardation, such as cytomegalovirus, is still poorly understood. Thus vaccination has been suggested as a means of protection but has not been acted upon. The problem of prenatal and perinatal infection may not yet be ripe for public health intervention on a large scale. On the other hand, in individual cases antibiotics have been promising. HIV infection in developed countries is transmitted to about one third of the offspring of infected mothers. Such children are at risk of brain syndromes, but the frequency with which they manifest mental retardation is still to be established.

Fetal Nutrients and Fetal Growth

Cretinism. Sporadic cretinism as a result of congenital hypothyroidism occurs at a rate of 1 in 78,000 births. Newborn-screening programs permit early detection and treatment of this condition. Early treatment of the infant averts the mental retardation. A well-recognized cause of endemic cretinism is severe iodine deficiency in mothers before conception and probably in early pregnancy. Endemic "nervous" cretinism, first described in India, results from a form of maternal iodine deficiency that leads to central nervous system dysfunction, which ranges from delay in motor development to cerebral palsy and mental retardation. The injection of iodized oil *before* conception provides effective prophylaxis.

Iodine deficiency has been found or suspected in many places. In the mountainous areas of Africa, Asia, and Central and South America at least 400 million people are believed to be at risk. Thus cretinism and its variants are widespread and preventable causes of mental retardation.[32–33]

Very Low Birth Weight. The incidence of mental retardation among babies of low birth weight (<2500 g) has probably been declining over the past three decades. Frequency is high in the poorer social classes. Yet the causes of many cases of low birth weight are unknown and cannot be prevented. Maternal smoking, drinking, and narcotic use affect birth weight adversely. In the developed world, maternal diet has no demonstrated effects on mental retardation. Thus low birth weight caused by prenatal undernutrition in previously well-nourished women does not lead to adult cognitive impairment.[34] In the less developed world, although severe maternal nutritional deficiencies are rife, maternal infections such as malaria are probably more important factors. Malnutrition in early childhood, in interaction with lack of social stimulation, is associated with subsequent cognitive impairment.[35] The most marked effects of malnutrition on cognition, however, are current and are observed in malnourished children before rehabilitation.

Infants born prematurely and of very low birth weight (<1500 g) have high mortality rates in the perinatal period. Survivors carry a high risk of cerebral palsy (especially spastic diplegia) and mental retardation. Mortality rates have been sharply reduced since the 1970s, but it is probable that the incidence of cerebral palsy and mental retardation in survivors has not decreased sufficiently to balance an increased prevalence of these conditions because of the survival of many more infants at high risk.

A close examination of the connections between prematurity, low birth weight, or intrauterine growth retardation on the one hand and their concomitants, such as cerebral palsy, mental retardation, and epilepsy on the other, indicates that the particular risk from these perinatal factors arises when frank neurological damage supervenes. Thus, premature delivery, intrauterine growth retardation to some degree, and perinatal hypoxia carry a high risk of cerebral palsy, mental retardation, and epilepsy in the presence of central nervous system damage. In the absence of central nervous system damage, these prenatal conditions carry a low risk, if any, of mental retardation and epilepsy. Whether low birth weight follows on premature delivery or intrauterine growth retardation or both, its causes are generally obscure. A deficient nutrient supply to the fetus is often invoked; this is a pathogenic mechanism still to be clarified.

The contribution of these perinatal factors to the prevalence of mental retardation will depend largely on the frequency of frank neurological damage. In a consecutive series of 122 retarded children (IQ <50) born in west Sweden from 1959 through 1970, mental retardation was attributed to perinatal causes (asphyxia, cerebral hemorrhage) in 7%. Some of these might have been preventable. Another 7% was attributed to intrauterine growth retardation. Among the 14% attributed to prenatal and perinatal causes, 10 of the 12 children had neurological impairment.

From such data, it seems that the greater proportion of very low birth weight infants now surviving is not likely, in the absence of manifest neurological damage, to make a large contribution to the total population of mental retardation. The situation is likely to be different where services are deficient, a contrast that points to obstetrical and neonatal care as a practical means of prevention. Where services are deficient, however, low birth weight survivors are fewer. Thus, while the risks of brain damage among these very small infants are high, not many survive to exhibit the consequences.

Postnatal Factors

Lead Absorption. Ingestion of lead by a young child leads to a severe encephalopathy, which is quite often fatal in the absence of treatment and is a cause of mental retardation in survivors. In industrial societies, lead poisoning has accounted for about 1 in 500 cases in institutions for the retarded. The most common source is lead paint on toys or cots or peeling paint from poorly maintained old housing. There is no excuse for the persistence of such cases. Exposure to lead pollution of the air has not been shown to have gross effects on mental function, although minor neurological damage cannot be excluded.

It has proved more difficult to assess the contribution to mental retardation of lesser exposures to lead. Raised blood levels have been noted in children with mild mental retardation for which no cause could be established. The levels in those children at younger ages, when the retardation was presumably induced, was not known, however. With mild and moderate retardation, it is particularly important to isolate possible sociocultural associations from those assumed to be related to lead, and few studies have been able to do this.

Nonetheless, the absorption of lead by preschool children is undoubted evidence of a health hazard. As noted, high levels cause lead encephalopathy, as well as genitourinary, gastrointestinal, behavioral, and other disturbances. These would seem sufficient reasons for outlawing exposure, without reference to the uncertain question of the effect of lower levels on mental retardation.[36]

Infections: Meningitis and Encephalitis. Turberculous meningitis, before the introduction of streptomycin, was uniformly fatal. For a few years thereafter it was a cause of mental retardation in the developed countries; a child's life could be saved, but brain damage and retardation were among the likely sequelae. Later, when isoniazid was introduced, these sequelae were seldom seen. In less developed countries, they are seen occasionally, because treatment is started late and probably because resistance is lowered by malnutrition. Pyogenic meningitides are also not uncommon causes of mental retardation in survivors in less developed countries.

Encephalitis in early childhood can cause mental retardation. For many viral forms, treatment has not proved effective. Reye's syndrome has been associated with influenza, and the treatment of fever with aspirin sharply raises the risk of occurrence. Measles encephalitis, when it complicates an episode in a very young child, leaves retardation in a proportion of survivors.

Immunization. Measles encephalitis and whooping cough encephalitis are undoubtedly causes of mental retardation. From estimates based only on notified cases of measles encephalitis, one could anticipate that one half of all survivors who were affected before the age of 2 years would be left with mental retardation. The proportion of severe cases of mental retardation attributable to measles encephalitis in the United States before widespread immunization was perhaps 1%. Immunization can prevent measles and its complications and has virtually eliminated this hazard. It has been argued that immunization against whooping cough (pertussis) causes more cases of encephalitis and residual mental retardation than the fatalities from the whooping cough it prevents. One must take note of the possibility of an adverse balance of risks, although from the evidence so far available, this is highly unlikely.[37-39]

Social Causes

Mild Mental Retardation. In young children, mild mental retardation is not easily recognized or diagnosed with certainty. We have noted that estimates of frequency depend largely on the identification of children who do not acquire skills in reading, writing, and arithmetic at the expected time,[18-40] that after leaving school the lack of scholarly skills is less evident, and that as young adults, mildly retarded persons who have the cultural-familial syndrome tend to make gains in both social adaptation and IQ. Thus for a substantial proportion the diagnosis is no longer appropriate in adulthood.

Hence age-specific incidence is low in the preschool years, rises sharply in the years after school entry, and declines in early adult life. There is a marked peak in prevalence rates based on school-age groups. The methods and standards used by different education authorities to identify mild mental retardation vary and are ruled as often by the facilities available for backward pupils as by diagnostic rationale. This is one reason for the great variability in rates between different prevalence studies. Another reason is the marked social class gradient in mild mental retardation, a gradient that is less evident with severe mental retardation. There is a concentration of cases among families at the lowest end of the scale. Thus prevalence varies according to the representation of the different social classes in the community surveyed.

Explanations for the social class gradient range from those that stress the cultural differences between classes (large families, absent fathers, immigrant status including problems of a second language, educational opportunity or values incongruent with the educational system, feelings of unworthiness) through those that stress material differences (housing, vulnerability to infections, medical care, diet) to those that stress genetic differences (separate marriage isolates).

The single cause that will explain everything is illusory. Poverty is a disadvantage to learning, and each of its undesirable components interacts with many others. This is best illustrated by the effects of malnutrition on the cognitive performance of children in the less developed world. The most careful studies find relatively small or no independent effects of early malnutrition on subsequent performance,[41] but they do show definite impairment from the interaction of poor social conditions with malnutrition.[35]

Whatever the cause of cognitive impairment, it has been shown convincingly that continuous and profound modification of the learning environment of children can markedly improve their cognitive abilities. The data come from studies of adopted children on the one hand[42] and from experimental interventions on the other.[43-45]

The Carolina Abecedarian Project[45] demonstrated a positive impact of its educational day-care program in enhancing the intellectual ability of high-risk children. The program began with the identification of pregnant women whose unborn children were at high risk of intellectual impairment. These children were randomly assigned to either the experimental day-care program or the control group. The experimental group entered the day-care program at between 6 and 12 weeks of age, for 5 days a week, 50 weeks a year. The focus of the day-care program was to promote social and cognitive growth in a structured, friendly environment. The IQ scores of the children in the experimental program, at 6 through 54 months of age, ranged from 7.9 to 20.1 points higher than those of the children in the control group when the effects of maternal retardation and home environments were controlled. At every age, a greater proportion of the children in the experimental program had normal-range IQs. Thirteen children were born to mentally retarded mothers: none of the six in the experimental program and six of the seven in the control group had IQ scores below normal.

Other studies point in the same direction and suggest that if appropriate intervention could begin early enough, continue long enough, and be executed intensively enough, the incidence of mild mental retardation without detectable handicap to learning could be radically reduced. It is not clear whether the necessary conditions will be met on a mass scale in our society. Even in the rebuilt city of Warsaw a generation after World War II, the demonstrable equality of schooling, housing, and medical care had not eliminated the social gradient in cognition among children from families of disparate education and occupation.[46] Standard educational approaches would seem to be insufficient. Perhaps workable preventive programs would have to include the parents as agents of change.[47] The demonstration that marked improvement in cognition can be produced should nevertheless be important in shaping policies and programs.

PREVENTION OF MENTAL RETARDATION

Clearly mental retardation has many causes, and preventive strategies must focus on each in turn. Sometimes, as with PKU, there are exemplary preventive programs, which can be applied wherever the administrative and economic structure can support them. Programs involving amniocentesis call for a high level of organization; for some communities, they will also involve a conflict of values. Programs that require intensification of the educational input for many children over a prolonged period call for a major allocation of funds and human resources.

Twelve recommendations for prevention were recently compiled by the Joint Commission of the International Association for the Scientific Study of Mental Deficiency and the International League of Parents of Retarded Children and accepted by the World Health Organization:

1. Genetic counseling, prenatal diagnosis, early identification, and proper treatment are important in preventing mental retardation of genetic origin.
2. Prevention of infections and parasitic diseases contributes significantly to prevention of mental retardation.
3. Monitoring the environment to protect against pollu-

tants and other chemical and physical hazards is an important part of preventive programs.

4. Safe environments for young children and the prompt treatment of injuries should reduce accidental causes of mental retardation.
5. The nutrition of mothers and children is of importance, especially in developing countries.
6. Good obstetrics and good care of the newborn reduce the incidence of mental and physical handicap. Good care includes adequate treatment of maternal illnesses, such as diabetes or toxemia; prompt recognition of obstetrical abnormalities; adequate monitoring of the fetus; immediate resuscitation of the infant; prediction, prevention, and treatment of biochemical disorders, such as respiratory distress syndrome, hypoglycemia, anoxia, and all causes of cerebral damage.
7. Social and educational stimulation is essential for proper mental growth and development. It is an important element in prevention of mental retardation, especially mild mental retardation. Suitable interventions are needed for children whose families do not provide this stimulation.
8. In more severely retarded persons, proper stimulation, modern principles of rehabilitation, and good remedial service can also reduce disability and prevent the development of secondary handicaps.
9. Improvement of living standards and the general health of the population constitutes an important element of nonspecific prevention of mental retardation. Preventive programs for mental retardation should form an integral part of all general health planning and programs.
10. The patterns of preventive programs and the speed with which they are implemented will vary according to resources, but high priority should be given to the problem in all countries.
11. International cooperation on many levels is necessary to speed up the development of effective preventive measures.
12. Research into the causes of mental retardation should be encouraged and facilitated. The effectiveness of preventive measures should be tested and monitored continuously. Special attention should be given to evaluative research in the biomedical and psychosocial spheres.

CARE: COMMUNITY SERVICES FOR MENTAL RETARDATION

Severe mental retardation shows itself in the first years of life, and the intellectual deficit is lifelong. In spite of this, many mentally retarded people achieve considerable self-reliance with maturity and training, so that the deficit is best seen as relative rather than absolute. The early years are those for which the family usually provides basic care and support, while for the later years the community does this increasingly. This distinction is preferably one of emphasis only. Interdigitation of family with community care over the life span can greatly ease the family burden and improve the outlook for mentally retarded children and adults.

A family with a mentally retarded child suffers serious effects in addition to the strain of providing for prolonged dependence. There is shock and pain when the diagnosis is imparted, and a time of emotional turbulence and readjustment to a new kind of parental role often follows. The turbulence is often compounded by concern about effects on other family members, especially siblings, painful embarrassment before friends, neighbors, and strangers, and economic strain. The strain is not limited to the early years. A mentally retarded person remains emotionally and physically dependent on parents long after the departure of other children. Dependence may continue into a phase when parents lack the physical, psychological, and economic resources to provide adequate care.

For some families, residential placement of the child at an early age is the most suitable arrangement. For many others, depending on traditions, personalities, and social circumstances, the family home is preferable. Whichever course is followed, cooperative arrangements between a family and appropriate community services work best. Types of services needed depend on the age of the child. Helpful to the family of a young child are baby-sitting, educational, and training material for use in the home and counseling or group sessions for parents and other children.

These needs for services are gradually replaced by provisions outside the home, day care, special schooling, vocational training centers, recreational centers, weekend camps, vocational facilities. In adulthood, there is a need for facilities for sheltered living that offer a range of options, depending on individual assets and limitations as well as on appropriate and congenial occupations and recreation. Families may wish to help plan these transitions, recognizing that the rights of retarded people, who cannot argue their own case, need extra protection. Increasingly, retarded adults themselves are being consulted.

SPECIAL CONCERNS OF LESS DEVELOPED COUNTRIES

Mild mental retardation tends to be invisible and ignored in societies in which universal education is not a reality.[48] In less developed countries, children who persistently fail in school tend to drop out in the primary grades. They share the handicap of a lack of academic skills with many others of their age group to whom schooling is inaccessible. Some countries have instituted remedial classes and special education in an attempt to meet at least some of their needs. Adult education may also prove beneficial.

With regard to severe mental retardation, children in these countries are affected by nearly all the same causes as children elsewhere and by other causes as well. The proportion of cases due to these additional causes (e.g., birth trauma, specific nutritional deficiencies, and infections) is not known, but while their incidence may be high their contribution to prevalence may not be great. The same circumstances that favor the operation of additional causes are also likely to shorten the lives of those affected. Little is known of the ways in which families in the poorest classes and in the rural areas of less developed countries provide for their retarded members. Among the well-off social classes, the prevalence of severe retardation and the distribution of clinical conditions seem similar to those in developed countries.

CONCLUSION

Today, the field of mental retardation involves public health in some of the most critical issues facing society. The selected issues touched on here are intended to serve as an introduction to the potential role of public health. Societal forces will shape future public health views and actions, as they have in the past. Scientific and technologic advances bring new opportunities for prevention and change the balance between incidence and prevalence. Demographic change alters population distributions, and the significance of each child in the family is enhanced as family size shrinks. In these changing circumstances, the choices societies make among the forms of prevention and care can have profound effects.

REFERENCES

1. Stein ZA, Susser MW: Changes over time in the incidence and prevalence of mental retardation. In Hellmuth J (ed): Exceptional Infant. Vol 2. Studies in Abnormalities. New York: Brunner Mazel, 1972, pp 305–340
2. Grossman HJ (ed): Classification in Mental Retardation. Washington, D.C.: American Association on Mental Deficiency, 1983
3. Drillien CM: Studies in mental handicap. II. Some obstetric factors of possible aetiological significance. Arch Dis Child 43:283, 1968
4. Kushlick A, Bunden R: The epidemiology of mental subnormality. In Clarke AM, Clarke ABD (eds): Mental Deficiency. New York: Free Press, 1974, pp 31–81
5. McDonald AD: Severely retarded children in Quebec: prevalence, cause and care. Am J Ment Defic 78:205, 1973
6. Turner G: An aetiological study of 1000 patients with an IQ assessment below 51. Med J Aust 2:927–931, 1975
7. Gustavson KH, Hagberg B, Hagberg C, Sars K: Severe mental retardation in a Swedish county. I. Epidemiology, gestational age, birth weight and associated CNS handicap in children born 1959–1970. Acta Paediatr Scan 66:373–379, 1977a
8. Gustavson KH, Hagberg B, Hagberg C, Sars K: Severe mental retardation in a Swedish county. II. Etiologic and pathologic aspects of children born 1959–1970. Neuropediatrics 8:293–304, 1977
9. Moser H, Wolf P: The nosology of mental retardation: Including the report of a survey of 1378 mentally retarded individuals at the Walter E. Fernald State School. Birth Defects 7(1), 1971
10. Lewis EO: Report of Mental Deficiency Committee. Part IV. London: Her Majesty's Stationery Office, 1929.
11. Onondaga County Survey: A Special Census of Suspected Referred Mental Retardation. Community Mental Health Research: New York State Department of Mental Hygiene Report, 1955
12. Goodman N, Tizard J: Prevalence of imbecility and idiocy among children. Br Med J 1:216–219, 1962
13. Taylor JL: Mental Retardation, Prevalence in Oregon. Oregon State Board of Health, 1962
14. Birch H, Richardson SA, Baird D, et al: Mental Subnormality in the Community. Baltimore: Williams & Wilkins, 1970
15. Stein Z, Susser M, Saenger G: Mental retardation in a national population of young men in Netherlands. I. Prevalence of severe mental retardation. Am J Epidemiol 103:477–485, 1976
16. Rutter M, Graham P, Yule W: A Neuropsychiatric Study in Childhood. Philadelphia: JB Lippincott Co., 1970
17. Mercer J: Sociobehavioral studies in mental retardation. In Eyman RK, Meyers CE, Tarjan G (eds): Sociobehavioral Studies in Mental Retardation. Monogr Am Assoc Ment Defic 1:1–18, 1973
18. Stein Z, Susser M, Saenger G: Mental retardation in a national population of young men in Netherlands. II. Prevalence of mild mental retardation. Am J Epidemiol 104:159–169, 1976
19. Hagberg B, Hagberg C, Lewerth A, Lindberg U: Mild mental retardation in Swedish school children. I. Prevalence. Acta Paediatr Scand 70:441–444, 1981
20. Hagberg B, Hagberg C, Lewerth A, Lindberg U: Mild mental retardation in Swedish schoolchildren. II. Etiologic and pathogenetic aspects. Acta Paediatr Scan 70:445–452, 1981
21. Kiely M: The prevalence of mental retardation. Epidemiol Rev 9:194–218, 1987
22. McLaren J, Bryson SE: Review of recent epidemiological studies of mental retardation: prevalence, associated disorders, and etiology. Am J Ment Retard 92:243–254, 1987
23. Shiotsuki Y, Matsuishi T, Yoshimura K, et al: The prevalence of mental retardation in Kurume City. Brain Dev 6:487–490, 1984
24. Folling A: Uber Ausscheidung von Phenylbrenztraubensaure in den Harn als Stoffwechselanomalie in Verbindung mit Imbezillitat. Hoppe Seylers Z Physiol Chem 227:169, 1934
25. Jervis GA: Phenylpyruvic oligopherenia: deficiency of phenylalanine oxidizing system. Proc Soc Exp Biol Med 82:514, 1953
26. Elwood JM, Elwood JH: Epidemiology of Anencephaly and Spina Bifida. New York: Oxford University Press, 1980
27. Smithells RW, Sheppard S, Schorah CJ, et al: Possible prevention of neural tube defects by periconceptional vitamin supplementation. Lancet 339–340, 1980
28. Mulinare J, Cordero JF, Erickson JD, Berry RJ: Periconceptional use of multivitamins and the occurrence of neural tube defects. JAMA 260:3141–3145, 1988
29. Bower C, Stanley FJ: Dietary folate as a risk factor for neural-tube defects: evidence from a case-control study in Western Australia. Med J Aust 150:613–619, 1989
30. Mills JL, Rhoads GG, Simpson JL, et al: The absence of a relationship between the periconceptional use of vitamins and neural-tube defects. N Engl J Med 321:430–435, 1989
31. Milunsky A, Jick H, Jick SS, et al: Multivitamin/folic acid supplementation in early pregnancy reduces the prevalence of neural-tube defects. JAMA 262:2847–2852, 1989
32. Hetzel BS, Pharoah POD: Endemic Cretinism. Papua, New Guinea: Institute of Human Biology, 1971
33. Hetzel BS: Iodine deficiency disorders (IDD) and their eradication. Lancet 1126–1129, 1983
34. Stein Z, Susser M, Saenger G, Marolla F: Famine and Human Development: The Dutch Hunger Winter of 1944/45. New York: Oxford University Press, 1975
35. Susser M: The challenge of causality: human nutrition, brain development and mental performance. Bull NY Acad Med 65:1032–1049, 1989
36. Lee WR, Moore MR: Low level exposure to lead. Br Med J 301:504–505, 1990
37. Hinman AR, Koplan JP: Pertussis and pertussis vaccine: reanalysis of benefits, risks and costs. JAMA 251:3109–3113, 1984
38. Hinman AR: The pertussis vaccine controversy. Public Health Rep 99 (3):255–259, 1984
39. Cody CL, Baraff LJ, Cherry JD, et al: Nature and rates of adverse reactions associated with DTP and DT immunizations in infants and children. Pediatrics 68(5):650–660, 1981
40. Tarjan G: The next decade: Expectations from the biological sciences. In Mental Retardation: A Handbook for the Primary Physician. American Medical Association on Mental Retardation. Chicago: The Association, 1964, pp 123–133
41. Lloyd-Still JD (ed): Malnutrition and Intellectual Development. England: MTP Press, 1976
42. Skodak M, Skeels HM: A final follow-up of one hundred adoptive children. J Genet Psychol 126:85–125, 1975
43. Garber HL: Intervention in infancy: a developmental approach. In Begab M, Richardson SA (eds). The Mentally Retarded and Society. Baltimore: University Park Press, 1975
44. McKay H, Sinisterra L, McKay A, Gomez H, Lloreda P: Improving cognitive ability in chronically deprived children. Science 200:270–278, 1978
45. Martin SL, Ramey CT, Ramey S: The prevention of intellectual impairment in children of impoverished families: findings of a randomized trial of educational day care. Am J Public Health 80:844–847, 1990
46. Firkowska A, Ostrowska A, Sokolowska M, et al: Cognitive development and social policy. Science 202:1357–1362, 1978
47. Brofenbrenner U: Is early intervention effective? In Guttentag M, Struening EL (eds): Handbook of Evaluation. Vol 2. Beverly Hills: Sage, 1975, pp 519–603
48. WHO, SEARO: Intercountry Workshop on Mental Retardation. New Delhi, September 1978

59

Prevention of Disability in Older Persons

William H. Barker

Increased risk of disease, disability, and death are well-known accompaniments of old age. Although disease incidence and death are the conventional indexes of a society's health status and targets of health care interventions, functional disability is perhaps the most significant index in addressing health in old age. This chapter defines the character and magnitude of disability in old age, reviews preventive and restorative approaches to specific and general causes of disability among the elderly, and examines the role of health care organizations in facilitating the delivery of such services.

DIMENSIONS OF THE PROBLEM

Concept and Measurement of Disability. Disability has been classified by the World Health Organization (WHO) as part of a continuum of measures of disease impact that include[1]:

- Impairment: the loss or abnormality of psychological, physiological, or anatomical integrity at the level of specific organ systems.
- Disability: the inability to perform an activity within the range considered normal for a human being; hence a functional limitation.
- Handicap: a disadvantage resulting from an impairment or disability that, if not addressed, limits an individual's ability to fulfill certain desired social roles.

Collectively this continuum of stages of dysfunction has been referred to as the "disablement model." Figure 59–1 depicts the conditions that characterize dysfunction at each of the three stages of the model and the types of functional assessment and medical, restorative, and social intervention appropriate to maintaining and improving function and limiting disability at each stage.

Numerous systems have been developed to measure functional ability and disability.[2] The best-known are the Activities of Daily Living (ADL) and the Instrumental Activities of Daily Living (IADL) indexes. The ADL index, first introduced by Katz and colleagues, classifies limitations in six fundamental sociobiological functions of daily living: bathing, dressing, toileting, transferring from bed or chair, continence, and feeding.[3] Lawton and others broadened the scope with the IADL concept, which incorporates measures of more complex adaptive or self-maintaining functions such as housekeeping, money management, and grocery shopping.[4] In addition to screening and care planning for individual patients, these measurement systems have been useful for describing the disability status of the elderly population, estimating community and institutional service needs, and evaluating outcomes of interventions designed to limit disability.

Magnitude of Aging and Disability. The aging or "graying" of populations is occurring in all parts of the world, most profoundly in developed areas, as illustrated in estimates compiled by the United Nations (Fig. 59–2). Furthermore, in the United States and other countries, the greatest proportionate growth is occurring among those over age 80.

The magnitude and distribution of disabled elderly Americans living both in the community and in nursing homes in the 1980s has been estimated from a variety of statistical sources, as shown in Tables 59–1 to 59–3. Some 6.3 million or 22% of older persons were disabled, 1.3 million of whom were residents of nursing homes, while more than three times as many (4.9 million) lived in the community (Table 59–1). Major disability with dependency in three or more ADLs was reported for 2.6 million older persons. Prevalence of reported disability among the elderly rises steeply with age, from about 14% among those 65 to 74 years old to 58% among those 85 and over. A higher proportion of the disabled elderly in all age groups live in the community rather than in nursing homes.

Among community-dwelling disabled elderly, the most common ADL dependencies include bathing and transferring, with dependence on assistance with eating least common. Shopping and meal preparation are the most common IADL dependencies. All domains of ADL and IADL limitation increase dramatically with age (from "young old" [65 to 74] to "old old" [85+]) and are generally more prevalent in women than men (Table 59–2).

There is a strong association between ADL limitation and the presence of chronic medical conditions, both of which increase dramatically with age in men and women.[5] With few exceptions such as stroke and hip fracture, it has been difficult to establish direct cause-and-effect relationships between specific morbidities (diseases) or combinations of morbidities and the associated disability. Nonetheless, it is reasonable to presume that a substantial amount of disability is attributable to physical and physiologic impairments caused by specific chronic diseases. In

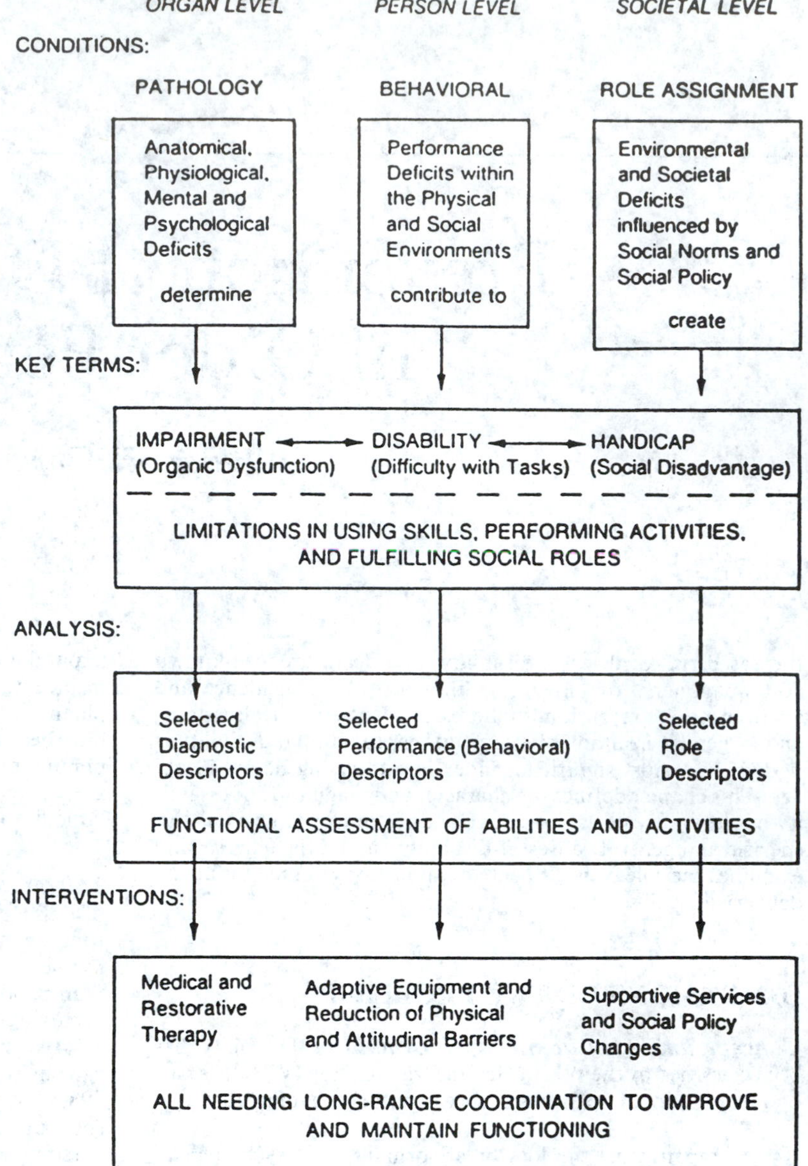

Figure 59-1. The functional approach to medical care and the disablement model. *[From Granger CV, Gresham GE: Functional Assessment in Rehabilitation Medicine. Baltimore: Williams & Wilkins, 1984, p 20.]*

turn, preventing such impairment and consequent disability would largely depend on preventing or controlling major chronic diseases using various primary and secondary preventive interventions. Disability in old age may also be explained and possibly prevented by attention to changes in physical, psychological, and social support factors related to older persons' functional integrity. Comprehensive strategies of health promotion, multidisciplinary assessment and rehabilitation, and environmental adaptation constitute the armamentarium of preventive approaches to such factors.

A further dimension of the social burden of disability in old age is the strong relationship between functional impairment and use of acute and subacute health services and long-term care. Based on the 1984 U.S. Household Health Interview Survey, dividing respondents over age 65 into those with severe impairment (major limitation in two or more ADLs), moderate impairment (some difficulty performing one or more ADLs), and no significant impairment, the average physician contacts per year were 9.9, 7.7, and 4.2, respectively, and annual hospital admission rates were 90.2, 54.6, and 22.9 per 100, respectively.[6]

Future Trends. Of great interest and consequence to the future provision of health and social services is the increased life expectancy seen in many industrialized societies in the final quarter of the twentieth century.[7] This phenomenon, along with a general decline in birth rates throughout the century, will result in an ever-increasing proportion of persons over age 65, with the largest proportionate increases involving those over age 80 (among whom functional disability is most prevalent).

These demographic developments have given rise to a number of forecasts concerning an anticipated burden of disability. At one extreme is the "compression of morbidity" thesis generated by Fries,[8] which argues that chronic disease and disability among the elderly are being postponed or prevented because of various risk-reducing and health-promoting measures. Under these circumstances, future prevalence rates of disability and chronic care needs would be expected to diminish relative to current rates. At the other extreme is the "failure of success" thesis promulgated by Gruenberg[9] and others, which argues that prolongation of life expectancy among the elderly is largely the result of advances in medical technology that prolong the average duration of certain chronic disabling conditions. This phenomenon would result in increased need for chronic care services. Others have suggested that the increased life expectancy reflects a combination of these phenomena, resulting in delayed age of onset of chronic disease and disability but not substantially reducing the overall health service burden.[10]

Although little empirical evidence exists to substantiate

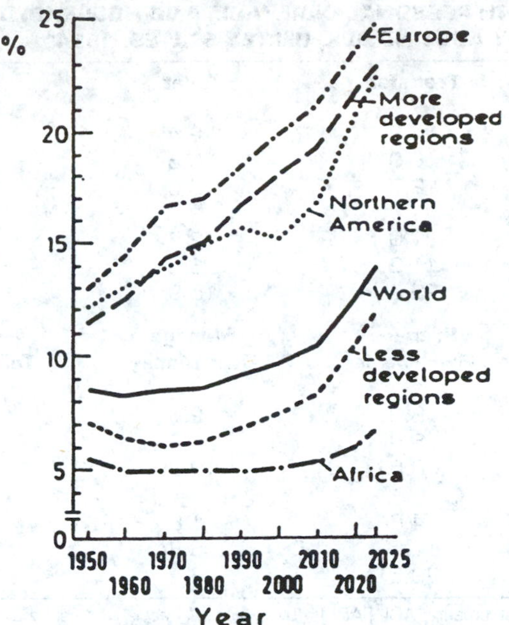

Figure 59-2. Percentage of population 60 years and over in different regions of the world. UN data and predictions 1950 to 2025. *(From Davies AM: Epidemiology and the Challenge of Aging. In Brody JA, Maddox GL (eds): Epidemiology and Aging. Copyright 1988 Springer Publishing Company, Inc., New York 10012.*

these models for forecasting future trends in disability, various longitudinal population studies are in progress in the United States,[11] Sweden,[12] and elsewhere. Common to such studies is a quest to identify and quantify determinants of disability-free aging, variably referred to as "successful aging"[13] or "active life expectancy." An example of the latter, measured in terms of remaining years of independence in activities of daily living, has been derived from data collected on a community-dwelling population of older persons in Massachusetts (see Table 59-3).

PREVENTION AND HEALTH PROMOTION

In considering approaches to preventing disability in the aging population, and indeed in the aging individual, it is important to consider several phenomena. These include, on the one hand, the biological changes of aging, pathological disease processes, and disuse or deconditioning that all contribute to disability and, on the other hand, health promotion and therapeutic, rehabilitative, and environmental intervention to prevent or reverse disability.

Impairments and Losses. Old age is associated with increased occurrence of a wide array of physiological, physical, mental, and social impairments or losses that may contribute independently or collectively to disabilities. These include elevated blood pressure; decreased immune system response; reduced visual, auditory, and olfactory acuity; loss of muscle and bone mass; fragility of the skin, slowing of mental response; decreased cognitive ability; loss of spouse and companions; reduced income; and loss of social roles and of autonomy.

Some of these changes and their consequences are intrinsic to the biology of aging. Examples include age-related decline in the individual's maximum oxygen consumption ($\dot{V}O_2max$), a fundamental index of capacity for physical activity; modifications of lens protein leading to cataract formation and loss of vision; decrease in bone density with resultant osteoporosis and heightened risk of fracture; and stiffening of arterial walls causing increased systolic blood pressure and risk of disabling cerebrovascular accident.

A growing body of evidence indicates that many physiological, physical, and mental changes, as well as virtually all social changes associated with old age, are not necessarily intrinsic to the aging process but are in part due to extrinsic or self-induced factors. The corollary is that much can be gained by identifying modifiable factors that contribute to disability and dependence and in turn developing approaches to forestalling or reversing these.

Disuse and Deconditioning. The first level of modifiable contributing factors is the discontinuation of usual activity, re-

TABLE 59-1. NUMBER AND DISTRIBUTION OF DISABLED ELDERLY, BY PLACE OF RESIDENCE, 1985

Category	Total Number of Elderly (millions)	Nursing Home		Community		Total Number (millions)	%	Disabled Elderly as a Percentage of Number of Elderly in Each Category		
		Number (millions)	%	*Number (millions)*	%			*Nursing Home*	*Community*	*All Disabled*
Age (y)										
65–74	16.9	0.2	15.4	2.1	41.9	2.3	36.5	1.3	12.3	13.6
75–84	9.1	0.5	38.5	2.0	40.9	2.5	40.0	5.6	22.1	27.7
85 and over	2.7	0.6	46.2	1.0	19.7	1.6	25.0	22.1	36.1	58.2
Sex										
Male	11.4	0.3	23.1	1.7	35.3	2.1	33.2	2.9	15.2	18.2
Female	17.2	1.0	76.9	3.3	66.2	4.3	68.0	5.7	19.1	24.8
Race										
White	25.9	1.2	92.3	4.2	84.0	5.4	85.9	4.7	16.1	20.8
Black	2.3	0.1	7.7	0.6	13.0	0.7	11.6	3.5	27.6	31.2
Number of ADL dependencies										
Fewer than three	—	0.4	28.5	3.3	67.0	3.7	58.9	1.3	11.6	12.9
Three or more	—	0.9	71.5	1.6	33.2	2.6	41.3	3.3	5.7	9.0
Total	28.6	1.3	100.0	4.9	100.0	6.3	100.0	4.6	17.3	21.9

From Rivlin AM, Wiener JM: Caring for the Disabled Elderly. Who Will Pay? Washington, D.C.: The Brookings Institution, 1988, p 6.

TABLE 59-2. PERCENTAGE OF PERSONS WHO HAVE DIFFICULTY WITH PERSONAL CARE (ADL) AND HOUSEHOLD MANAGEMENT (IADL) TASKS BECAUSE OF CHRONIC CONDITIONS, BY AGE AND SEX, UNITED STATES, 1984[a]

▪ Personal Care (ADL)	Bathe	Dress	Transfer	Toilet	Eat
Men					
65–74	5.7	4.4	4.8	2.4	1.5
75–84	9.2	7.3	6.0	3.6	2.5
85+	23.1	14.1	12.7	10.0	4.3
Women					
65–74	6.9	4.2	7.0	2.7	0.9
75–84	14.2	7.7	11.2	6.5	2.4
85+	30.1	17.7	22.2	15.9	4.4
▪ Household Management (IADL)	**Shop**	**Light Housework**	**Prepare Own Meals**	**Manage Own Money**	**Use Telephone**
Men					
65–74	4.6	3.5	3.0	2.8	3.5
75–84	9.6	6.2	6.0	5.4	7.9
85+	26.8	15.2	18.5	19.0	18.4
Women					
65–74	7.8	5.0	4.8	1.8	2.0
75–84	18.4	10.5	10.5	6.8	4.8
85+	41.6	27.4	29.5	26.2	17.1

[a] For activities of daily living (ADL), "by yourself and without using special equipment." For instrumental ADL (IADL), "by yourself." People who said they don't do an activity are in the denominator but not the numerator and are thus effectively considered nondisabled in these rates.

Data from Supplement on Aging, National Health Interview Survey, 1984. From Verbrugge LM: The iceberg of disability. In Stahl SM (ed): The Legacy of Longevity. Newbury Park, Calif.: Sage Publishing Co., 1990.

ferred to as "disuse" or "deconditioning."[14] This may occur insidiously as older persons withdraw from usual activities either voluntarily in response to a sense of "growing old" or involuntarily as a consequence of intercurrent acute illness, forced retirement from work, etc.

The best-studied model of global disuse and deconditioning, and one to which older persons are particularly prone on their own volition or their physician's or family's bidding, is extended bed rest. Going to bed for a prolonged period may lead to a litany of physiological adaptations and potentially disabling consequences (Table 59-4). Of particular concern, because they may contribute to limited mobility and lead to falls and fractures, are physiological and structural changes in muscles, bones, and joints. Rate of decrease in muscle strength may be as high as 5% per day in the bedridden individual, with leg muscles tending to lose strength faster than arm muscles. Disuse osteoporosis results from both cessation of bone synthesis and increased resorption and predominantly affects weight-bearing bones. Immobility and loss of weight-bearing forces on joints contribute to changes in both periarticular and articular tissue structure, possibly leading to joint contractures.[15]

Other possible effects of excessive bed rest are atelectasis and other pulmonary changes that predispose to pneumonia, slowing of peristalsis with resulting constipation, bladder-emptying difficulties leading to urinary incontinence, sustained pressure on fragile skin predisposing to pressure sores, and sensory deprivation leading to an array of negative affective and cognitive effects.

Clearly an essential principle is to avoid taking to bed in old age, except as necessitated by medical problems, and even then bed rest should be minimized, with emphasis on progressive mobilization of bed-bound patients, first from bed to chair, then to ambulation with or without assistance. This should include purposeful activity such as walking to the toilet or to meals and dressing in normal clothing and footwear as opposed to institutional bed clothing. These principles, well known to progressive geriatric medicine services (see below), will prevent or reverse much of the potentially disabling deconditioning associated with prolonged bed rest.

Exercise. Regular physical exercise is perhaps the most important single health promotional activity for preventing many of the dysfunctional consequences of aging. Numerous studies have demonstrated that older persons, like their younger counterparts, can significantly increase physical fitness, as reflected in $\dot{V}O_2max$, by engaging in regular aerobic exercise. Furthermore, clear experimental evidence involving older subjects shows that exercise can both retard and reverse losses of muscle mass and strength as well as bone density. Along with resultant increases in body strength and mobility, exercise has positive effects on psychological parameters, including mood and self-confidence.[16]

TABLE 59-3. LIFE EXPECTANCY IN YEARS, ACTIVE LIFE EXPECTANCY IN YEARS, AND DEPENDENT LIFE EXPECTANCY IN YEARS, MASSACHUSETTS, 1974, BY AGE

Age Group (%)	Life Expectancy	Active Life Expectancy	Dependent Life Expectancy	Age Dependency Begins	Age Dependency Ends
65–69	16.5	10.0	6.5	75.0	81.5
70–74	14.1	8.1	6.0	78.1	84.1
75–79	11.6	6.8	4.8	81.8	86.6
80–84	8.9	4.7	4.2	84.7	88.9
85+	7.3	2.9	4.4	87.9	92.3

From Katz S, Branch LG, Branson MH, et al: Active life expectancy. N Engl J Med 309:1218–1224, 1983.

TABLE 59-4. COMPLICATIONS OF BEDREST

Cardiovascular	Decreased cardiac output, contributing to decreased aerobic capacity
	Orthostatic intolerance
	Venous thrombophlebitis
Respiratory	Atelectasis
	Relative hypoxemia
	Pneumonia
Musculoskeletal	Muscle atrophy and loss of strength
	Decreased muscle oxidative capacity, contributing to decreased aerobic capacity
	Bone loss (osteoporosis)
Gastrointestinal	Constipation
Genitourinary	Incontinence
	Renal calculi
Skin	Pressure sores
Functional	Impaired ambulation
Psychological	Sensory deprivation

From Harper CM, Lyles YM: Physiology and complications of bed rest. J Am Geriatrics Soc 36:1047–1054, 1988.

The application of such experimental observations to preventing disability is captured in the concept of "threshold levels" as follows:

> Strength, aerobic power and other indices of physical ability change on continuous scales whereas functional and quality of life changes are quantal. Thus a very small strength gain may be accompanied by a considerable functional improvement if it takes the patient from being just unable to transfer independently to being just able to do so. This also applies in reverse: A gradual loss of strength may not be apparent until the patient is suddenly unable to perform a crucial function.[17]

In addition, longitudinal observations of community-dwelling elderly persons show a clear association between lack of regular exercising and subsequent decline in ability to perform certain simple physical tasks.[18]

The implication is that, barring medical contraindications, functional well-being in old age may be sustained or improved by persons engaging in regular aerobic exercise. This may consist of swimming, jogging, cycling, or walking and must be sustained for benefits to accrue.

EARLY INTERVENTION AND REHABILITATION

Despite the best efforts of primary and secondary prevention and health promotion, the majority of older persons will develop one or more potentially disabling medical conditions. Under these circumstances the goals of health care, where possible, should be early intervention, rehabilitation, or supportive care to limit disability and provide for the highest level of independence of individuals and their caregivers. Components of such tertiary prevention include both specific interventions for individual disabling conditions and comprehensive geriatric medicine services.

SELECTED DISABLING CONDITIONS

Falls and Fractures. Falls occur among some 20% to 30% of community-dwelling elderly persons per year and an even greater percentage of nursing home residents, with attendant risks of fracture, soft tissue injury, and psychological compromise to independence. Risk of falling increases with the number and type of chronic disabling conditions present. Visual and proprioceptive abnormalities, musculoskeletal and neurological diseases, depression and dementia, and hypotension-inducing conditions (biological and iatrogenic) are particularly important. A "fall risk index" comprising an inventory of chronic conditions, a performance-oriented assessment of gait and balance, and an assessment of environmental hazards can be used to identify persons predisposed to falling and to guide preventive interventions.[19]

To avoid certain secondary consequences of falls such as hypothermia from prolonged immobility, recurrent fallers should be provided with portable alarm systems as well as instructions for effectively maneuvering to right themselves following a fall.

More than a million fractures occur in older persons in the United States each year. The three most common sites are spine, hip, and distal forearm (Colles' fracture). The principal contributing factor is osteoporosis or loss of bone mass, a progressive natural process that begins in the fourth or fifth decade of life and renders aging individuals increasingly susceptible to fracture associated with relatively minor trauma. Osteoporosis is accentuated in women following menopause, and age-specific rates of osteoporotic fractures are markedly higher among older women versus men (Fig. 59-3). Osteoporosis is significantly retarded by postmenopausal estrogen replacement therapy and probably by regular exercise and supplemental calcium intake throughout adulthood.[20]

Hip fractures are associated with more deaths, disability, and medical costs than all other osteoporotic fractures combined. Over 200,000 occur annually in the United States, and the age-specific incidence of hip fracture is increasing in industrialized societies. Between 10% and 20% of patients who have fractured their hips die, and a substantial percentage of survivors are destined for long-term nursing home placement. There is, however, considerable potential for restoring mobility, if patients receive timely surgical, medical, and particularly rehabilitative care. (See below under "Geriatric Strategies.")

Incontinence. Urinary incontinence is defined as "the involuntary loss of urine so severe as to have social or hygienic consequences." A symptom with multiple causes, rather than a discrete disease process, incontinence affects 15% to 30% of community-dwelling elderly and at least half of all nursing home residents. In addition to its immense psychosocial burden on afflicted individuals and their caretakers, the costs of managing urinary incontinence in the United States are estimated at over $10 billion dollars annually. This disabling condition of old age

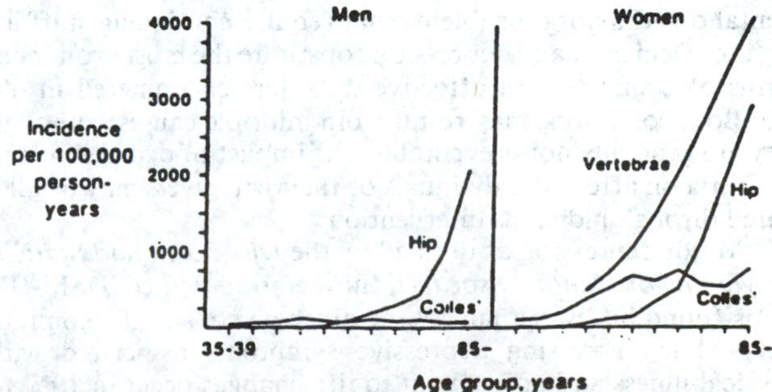

Figure 59-3. Incidence rates for the three common osteoporotic fractures (Colles', hip, and vertebral) in men and women, plotted as a function of age at the time of the fracture. *(From Riggs BL, Melton LJ: Involutional osteoporosis. N Engl J Med 314:1676–1686, 1985.)*

can in many instances be cured or effectively controlled through appropriate medical and nursing assessment and intervention.[21]

There are several subtypes of incontinence, each representing a distinctive pathophysiological mechanism. *Stress incontinence,* a particularly common form in women, occurs because dysfunction at the bladder outlet allows urine to leak whenever intra-abdominal pressure is increased (e.g., during coughing or sneezing). Pelvic muscle exercises can often help control this condition. In *urge incontinence* urine is lost because of uninhibited bladder muscle contractions, usually resulting from a neurological condition such as stroke or local bladder irritation. If treatment of a local cause, such as urinary tract infection, does not stop the incontinence, anticholinergic agents or other drugs that inhibit bladder contraction may be used. *Overflow incontinence* occurs when the bladder does not empty normally and becomes over distended because of a neurological impairment or local obstruction. Surgery (e.g., prostatectomy) may be indicated, or a program of intermittent catheter drainage instituted. *Functional incontinence* occurs when the lower urinary tract is functionally intact but impaired mobility or cognition prevents the individual from getting to toilet facilities. This variant is controllable if the person is given regular assisted access to toilet facilities.

Sensory Impairment: Hearing and Vision. The 1984 U.S. National Health Survey established prevalence rates of hearing impairment ranging from 30% to 60% among community-dwelling men over age 65 and 18% to 45% among older women. Prevalence of significantly impaired vision, including blindness, among men and women ranged from 10% at 64 to 74 years of age to 27% over age 85; 95% of the elderly population reported using glasses, most of which were prescribed.[22] In addition to potentially profound limitations in an individual's ability to communicate with others, impairments in both these sensory systems are associated with significant limitations in performing traditional ADL and IADL functions as well as with depression and cognitive difficulty.

Early detection and therapeutic intervention may reverse or delay sensory impairments attributable to certain specific degenerative disease processes, such as visual loss due to diabetic retinopathy or glaucoma. However, in large measure the task of preventing disability due to sensory loss in old age focuses on restoring the lost sense, as in surgical treatment of senile cataract or prosthetic treatment of presbycusis. Cataract surgery with lens implantation has been shown to improve physical function as well as vision.[23] Hearing aids, voice-amplifying devices, and lip reading represent the mainstays of hearing rehabilitation, which, if used effectively, can reverse physical and particularly psychosocial disability associated with hearing loss.

Depression and Dementia. Mental and psychological disability among the elderly are major societal concerns, particularly in long-term care institutions, where the majority of residents have mental or behavioral problems that require continuing staff attention. Dementia and depression constitute the most prominent forms of cognitive and affective disorders encountered in old age. Both conditions may result from multiple causes; although they are generally not preventable, the impact of depression and dementia on affected individuals or their caregivers may be alleviated through judicious intervention.

Major depression as defined by the *Diagnostic and Statistical Manual of Mental Disorders,* third edition revised (DSM-III-R), is found in fewer than 5% of older persons in the community, while distressing depressive symptoms associated with physical illness and adjustment to life changes occur in 10% to 20%.[24] A variety of antidepressant drugs as well as electroconvulsive therapy are effective in treating depression of old age, although these may cause serious side effects.[25]

Broadly defined by the DSM-III-R as "a loss of intellectual abilities sufficient to interfere with social or occupational functioning," dementia is a disabling mental condition well known to aging societies that increases dramatically in prevalence from 2% to 3% at age 65 to 30% or above at age 85 (Fig. 59-4). The most common pathological subtypes of dementia are Alzheimer's disease and multiinfarct dementia. A small percentage of cases of potentially reversible dementia occur secondary to treatable causes such as hypothyroidism, subdural hematoma, drug toxicity, and others.

A variety of intervention strategies have been developed with the twin goals of maintaining independence and dignity for dementia patients and providing social and psychological support for their caregivers. These invariably involve a multidisciplinary approach. Patient care includes continuing attention to basic medical and nursing needs, with particular emphasis on adequate nutrition, assistance with toileting and grooming, and prevention or early treatment of minor infections and skin breakdown. Regularly scheduled occupational and recreational therapy help to maintain patient morale. Support for caregivers in the community includes counseling and education about the natural course and management of dementia, particularly the highly stressful memory loss and aberrant behavior; assistance with obtaining legal, financial, and safety advice; and provision of temporary relief through day care or short-term residential respite care. For patients with advanced disease, often accompanied by wandering and verbally or physically abusive behavior, special dementia units in nursing homes are increasingly being developed.[26]

In addition to the burden suffered directly by patients and their caregivers, Alzheimer's and related disorders pose an immense monetary cost, estimated in the mid-1980s at some $30 billion annually in the United States. The largest portion of this

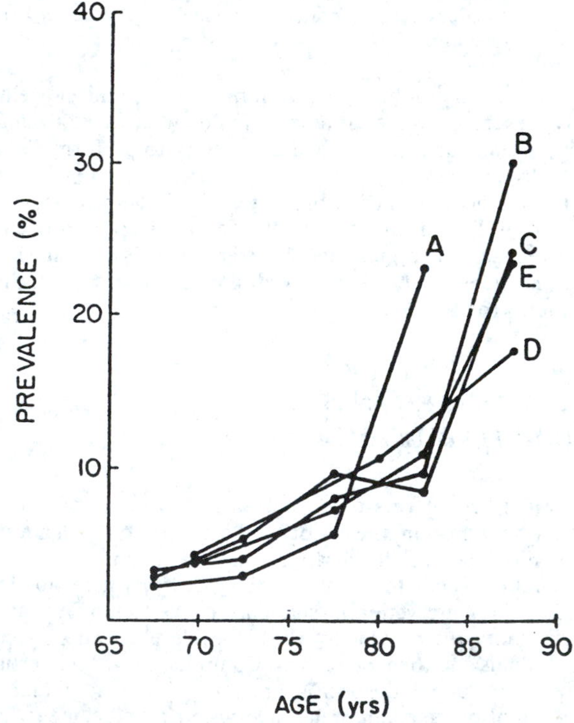

Figure 59-4. Age-specific prevalence rates for moderate or severe dementia in five studies: England [1970], United States [1978], Denmark [1963], Finland [1985], and New Zealand [1983]. *[From Mortimer JA, Hutton JT: Epidemiology and etiology of Alzheimer's disease. In Hutton JT, Kenny AD [eds]: Senile Dementia of the Alzheimer Type. New York: Alan R. Liss, 1985.]*

goes to long-term care, a component of health services not currently covered by Medicare, the universal health insurance program for elderly Americans.

Stroke and Parkinson's Disease. Stroke and Parkinson's disease are two of the most serious and common disabling neurological conditions of old age, and afflicted individuals are candidates for preventive or rehabilitative intervention.

Stroke or cerebrovascular disease comprises a heterogeneous group of pathological entities, all of which carry a high risk of residual disability. Although age-specific stroke incidence and mortality rates have declined dramatically in the past two decades, due in large part to improved control of hypertension, stroke remains the third leading cause of death and a common disabling condition of old age, with a prevalence of some 500 to 600 per 100,000 in the United States. Among the 70% to 80% of persons who survive acute strokes, up to a third require some assistance in self-care, over half experience significant depression and social isolation, and 20% to 30% are institutionalized for continuing care.[27] Multidisciplinary stroke rehabilitation programs, although not found to affect the natural recovery of motor and sensory impairment, have been shown to improve patient and family capacity to cope with residual disability and avoid institutional placement.[28]

Parkinson's disease is a degenerative condition resulting largely from deficiency of the neurotransmitter substance dopamine in the midbrain and causing generalized movement and postural abnormalities. Disabling manifestations include shuffling gait, tremulous hands, and tendency to fall, plus some cognitive decline. Increasingly common with aging, the prevalence is estimated at 500 to 1000 per 100,000 over age 60, with more than half of afflicted individuals being over 70 years of age. It is generally a disease of unknown etiology, but some parkinsonism among older persons is drug induced by neuroleptic agents and may resolve when the offending drug is discontinued. Conventional treatment to ameliorate manifest disability in Parkinson's disease consists of one of a variety of dopamine replacement regimens plus physical therapy.[29] Recent studies have demonstrated highly significant delay of progression of early disability by the antioxidative agent deprenyl, which protects against primary degeneration of the midbrain's dopamine-producing neurons.[30] Implants of fetal adrenal gland tissue may someday provide an approach to reversing the pathophysiological effects of Parkinson's disease.

Transitions: Retirement, Bereavement, and Relocation. Certain discrete transitions in social status place older persons at increased risk of onset or worsening of disabling physical and mental health problems. Most prominent among these transitions are retirement, loss of spouse, and residential relocation. These events are commonly associated with loss of autonomy and control over one's life as well as loss of the social and psychological support that contribute to one's physical and mental well-being.

Retirement may mean a reduced income and an attendant increase in various mental health problems. Loss of spouse and the accompanying experience of loneliness and bereavement are associated with the increased likelihood of nonspecific mental and physical symptoms as well as excess mortality. The excess mortality is more common in men than women and peaks during the first 6 months of bereavement. Residential relocation, particularly placement in a nursing home, represents an unusually stressful event, depriving the old person of a familiar social and physical environment as well as much of a sense of autonomy. The nursing home experience is commonly aggravated further by the excessive use of physical and chemical (psychotropic drugs) restraints that diminish or distort mental performance and increase the risk of iatrogenic illness or injury. Such untoward effects, as well as increased risk of death, tend to be concentrated in the early months following residential relocation.[13]

Reduction in the risks of ill health and increased mortality associated with social transitions may be achieved through various supportive and autonomy-enhancing interventions. Providing material assistance, medical attention as needed, and companionship are fundamental supportive approaches. Teaching, encouraging, and enabling are important autonomy-enhancing approaches, in contrast to excessive cautioning and "doing for," which may induce a sense of helplessness. A number of observations in nursing homes have demonstrated improvement in mental health and other health status indexes among residents maintained free of unnecessary restraints and encouraged to exercise initiative and choice in pursuit of daily activities.[13]

At the level of primary prevention directed to social transitions of aging, a society's or community's existing policies and practices may be altered with respect to both retirement and nursing home placement.[31] Normative, if not legally mandated, retirement age can be and has been increased in some settings. Rehabilitative and community-based services can be and have been successfully implemented as alternatives to custodial placement in nursing homes. Such continuing care alternatives have been most fully developed in societies with comprehensive health care systems.[32]

HEALTH CARE DELIVERY

The Geriatric Medicine Movement. The breadth of threats to independent functioning in old age and the potentials for preventive interventions, as reviewed above, constitute a major challenge to develop prevention-oriented health care delivery systems. In recognition of this challenge, WHO convened an expert panel in 1974 on "Planning and Organization of Geriatric Services." This body recommended that countries develop integrated health services for older persons, including "elements of medical and social prevention, multidisciplinary assessment, home and institutional curative treatment, rehabilitation, long-term care and supportive social welfare."[33] This spectrum of services, with dedicated professionals and resources, constitutes the essence of the modern geriatric medicine movement, which was pioneered in Great Britain and has now developed in many other parts of the world.[34] The principal focus of this field of medicine, captured in the motto "adding life to years," is the provision of timely interventions to treat and prevent unnecessary disease, disability, and dependency at all stages. Translating this concept into practical terms, comprehensive health services for older persons should include an array of community, hospital, and institutional continuing care elements such as found in Great Britain and summarized in Table 59–5.

Geriatric Strategies. Multidisciplinary assessment represents the core clinical activity of geriatric medicine. Practiced in inpatient and outpatient settings by geriatricians, nurses, social workers, rehabilitation therapists, and others working in collaboration, geriatric assessment identifies the vulnerable elderly patient's medical, psychosocial, and functional problems and leads to appropriate preventive, curative, rehabilitative, and long-term care.[35] In a review of 32 studies of geriatric assessment programs reported from a number of different settings, all but two programs showed significant improvement in one or more measures of patient outcome, including diagnostic and therapeutic accuracy, physical function, mental function, survival, length of hospital stay, and likelihood of nursing home placement.[36]

The need for such progressive geriatric care in the United States is particularly evident in the acute hospital sector, where older patients not only constitute the largest constituency of ad-

TABLE 59-5. SOME SPECIFIC ELEMENTS OF COMPREHENSIVE HEALTH SERVICES FOR THE ELDERLY IN GREAT BRITAIN

- **COMMUNITY**
  - **Enrollment in primary care practice**
    - General practitioner
    - Attached community nurses
    - Home visiting by general practitioners
  - **Social service liaisons**
    - Home help
    - Meals on wheels
    - Domiciliary occupational therapy
- **GENERAL HOSPITAL**
  - **Acute geriatric services**
    - Defined catchment population
    - Geriatric medicine specialists, house officers
    - Multidisciplinary teams
    - Rehabilitation emphasis
    - Home visiting
    - Day hospital
    - Respite admissions
  - **Liaison consultation with other hospital services**
    - Medicine
    - Orthopaedics
    - Psychiatry
- **INSTITUTIONAL CONTINUING CARE**
  - Medical surveillance, avoid frequent transfer to hospital
  - Multidisciplinary rehabilitation, maintenance of function
  - Social and recreational activities
- **EDUCATION**
  - Academic departments of geriatric medicine
  - Required curriculum in medical schools
  - Formal postgraduate specialty training

Barker WH: Adding Life to Years: Organized Geriatrics Services in Great Britain and Implications for the United States. Baltimore: Johns Hopkins University Press, 1987, p 170.

missions but, with increasing frequency, are inappropriately served and end up being classified as "alternate care" or "bed-blockers" awaiting nursing home placement. Emulating experience in hospital-based geriatric units in Great Britain, some general U.S. hospitals have introduced geriatric evaluation and rehabilitation programs to address this situation. Targeted to those patients most likely to benefit from geriatric assessment, such programs have been incorporated into hospitals in three ways (Fig. 59-5). The simplest approach (Fig. 59-5C) involves consultation by a multidisciplinary team, preferably early in the hospital stay, to assess the patient's potential for rehabilitation, advise on management of certain medical and medically related problems, and assist with planning for posthospital placement. Another modality (Fig. 59-5T) consists of a special hospital-based or affiliated unit to which patients are transferred for geriatric rehabilitation following acute care on a medical or surgical service. Such units have been established in a variety of hospital settings, including Veterans Administration hospitals, academic medical centers, and rehabilitation hospitals. A third modality (Fig. 59-5A) involves designating part of an inpatient medical service as an acute geriatric admitting unit.[32]

Among the documented successes of hospital-based geriatric programs, when compared with care of frail older patients by traditional medical and surgical services, two experiences are particularly illustrative.

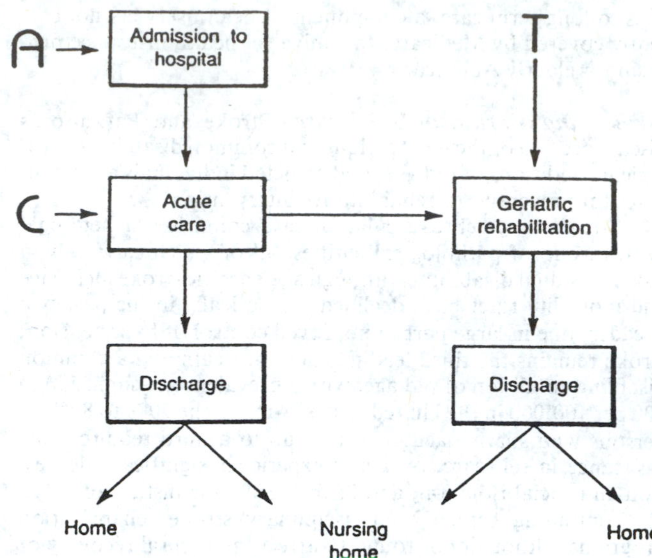

Figure 59-5. Potential intervention by special geriatrics services in the course of acute hospital admission in the United States. *A*, Admit to acute geriatrics service. *C*, Geriatric consultation on acute medical and surgical services. *T*, Postacute transfer to special geriatric rehabilitation unit. *[From Barker WH: Adding Life to Years: Organized Geriatrics Services in Great Britain and Implications for the United States. Baltimore: Johns Hopkins University Press, 1987, p 131.]*

The first of these was based at the Sepulveda Veterans Administration Medical Center in Los Angeles, a 15-bed geriatric unit operated by a full-time medical, nursing, and social work team, with part-time participation by rehabilitation therapists and other staff. The unit provides geriatric assessment to those elderly hospitalized patients who on screening are considered at high risk of deteriorating and in need of geriatric rehabilitation. In a randomized clinical trial, patients admitted to the geriatric unit, when compared with controls managed on a general medical unit, were found to experience significantly lower mortality (24% versus 49%), a reduced likelihood of nursing home admission (27% versus 47%), fewer overall acute hospital and nursing home days over a 1-year follow-up period, significantly greater improvement in functional status and morale, and lower average cost of care.[37]

The other experience involved a collaborative geriatric orthopedic rehabilitation program in Sterling, Scotland, designed to care for elderly patients with acute hip fracture during the postoperative and convalescent stage of this condition. The program involved transfer of patients postoperatively to a multidisciplinary service headed by a geriatrician. In a randomized trial comparing patients managed by the combined orthopedic-geriatrics program with those managed primarily by the orthopedic service, median length of hospital stay was shorter (24 versus 41 days), fewer patients were discharged to long-term institutional care (10% versus 32%), and more patients attained high levels of independence in activities of daily living by discharge (76% versus 46%).[38]

Comprehensive Health Services. Successful provision of geriatric assessment, rehabilitation, and continuing care with a preventive orientation is most likely to occur in a comprehensive health care program in which the various elements listed in Table 59-5 are linked together under one system of financing. Such systems are found in Great Britain, the Scandanavian countries, and a number of other societies with national health programs.[6]

In the United States, fragmentation among health care providers and payers and an excessive focus on costly institutional services (acute hospitals and nursing homes) has left many gaps in the provision of services that could prevent or alleviate disability and dependency in old age. This problem has been recognized and addressed in a number of national health policy proposals developed by health care professionals, citizens' groups, and government policymakers during the 1980s. During this same period a number of special projects as well as existing health delivery systems, including the On Lok program, the Social Health Maintenance Organization (SHMO) demonstration, and Veterans Administration health services, have developed model comprehensive programs for older persons in the United States.[32] If and when a national health program is enacted in the United States, policymakers will be well provided with these model experiences as well as those from other countries to draw on in ensuring progressive comprehensive services for society's oldest and most vulnerable members.

REFERENCES

1. World Health Organization: International Classification of Impairments, Disabilities and Handicaps (ICIDH). Geneva: World Health Organization, 1980
2. Kane RA, Kane RL: Assessing the Elderly. A Practical Guide to Measurement. Lexington, Massachusetts: Lexington, 1981
3. Katz S, Ford AB, Moskowitz RW, et al: Studies of illness in the aged. The index of ADL. JAMA 185:914–919, 1963
4. Lawton MP, Brody EM: Assessment of older people: self-maintaining and instrumental activities of daily living. The Gerontologist 9:179–186, 1969
5. Guralnik JM, LaCroix AZ, Everett DF, et al: Aging in the eighties: The prevalence of comorbidity and its association with disability. Adv Data 170:1–8, 1989
6. Rowland D, Lyons B: Disability and disease: Medical care use by the impaired elderly. The Gerontologist 29:237A, 1989
7. Heikkinen E: Health implications of population aging in Europe. World Health Statist Q 40:22–40, 1987
8. Fries JF: Aging, natural death, and the compression of morbidity. N Engl J Med 303:130–135, 1980
9. Gruenberg EM: The failures of success. Milbank Mem Fund Q 55:3–24, 1977
10. Manton KG: Changing concepts of morbidity and mortality in the elderly population. Milbank Mem Fund Q 60:183–244, 1982
11. Manton KG: A longitudinal study of functional change and mortality in the United States. J Gerontol 43:153–161, 1988
12. Svanborg A: Cohort differences in the Gothenborg studies of Swedish 70-year-olds. In Brody JA, Maddox GL (eds): Epidemiology and Aging, New York: Springer, 1988
13. Rowe JW, Kahn RL: Human aging: Usual and successful. Science 237:143–149, 1987
14. Bortz WM: Disuse and aging. JAMA 248:1203–1208, 1982
15. Harper CM, Lyles YM: Physiology and complications of bed rest. J Am Geriatrics Soc 36:1047–1054, 1988
16. Thomas GS, Rutledge JH: Fitness and exercise for elderly. In Dychtwald K (ed): Wellness and Health Promotion for the Elderly, Rockville, Maryland: Aspen, 1986
17. Young A: Exercise and physiology in geriatric practice. Acta Med Scand Suppl 711:227–232, 1986
18. Mor V, Murphy J, Masterson-Allen S, et al: Risk of functional decline among well elderly. J Clin Epidemiol 42:895–904, 1989
19. Tinetti ME, Speechley M: Prevention of falls among the elderly. N Engl J Med 320:1055–1059, 1989
20. Riggs BL, Melton LJ: Involutional osteoporosis. N Engl J Med 314:1676–1686, 1985
21. Resnick NM, Ouslander JG: Urinary incontinence: Where do we stand and where do we go from here? J Am Geriatrics Soc 38:263–264, 1990.
22. Havlik RJ: Ageing in the eighties, impaired senses for sound and light in persons age 65 years and over. Advancedata from Vital and Health Statistics, National Center for Health Statistics, 125:1–8, 1986
23. Applegate WB, Miller ST, Elam JT, et al: Impact of cataract surgery with lens implantation on vision and physical function in elderly patients. JAMA 257:1064–1066, 1987
24. Blazer D: Depression in the elderly. N Engl J Med 320:164–166, 1989
25. Gerson SC, Plotkin DA, Jarvik LF: Antidepressant drug studies, 1964 to 1986: Empirical evidence for aging patients. J Clin Psychopharmacol 8:311–322, 1988
26. Volicer L, Fibiszewski KJ, Rheaume YL, et al: Clinical Management of Alzheimer's Disease. Rockville, Md., Aspen, 1988.
27. Gresham GE, Fitzpatrick TE, Wolf PA, et al: Residual disability in survivors of stroke—the Framingham study. N Engl J Med 293:954–956, 1975.
28. Reding MJ, McDowell FH: Focused stroke rehabilitation programs improve outcome. Arch Neurol 46:700–701, 1989
29. Hildick-Smith M: Parkinson's disease. In Pathy MSJ (ed): Principles and Practice of Geriatric Medicine, Chichester, England: John Wiley & Sons, 1985
30. Parkinson Study Group: Effect of deprenyl on the progression of disability in early Parkinson's disease. N Engl J Med 321:1364–1371, 1989
31. Townsend P: The structured dependency of the elderly: A creation of social policy in the twentieth century. Ageing and Society 1:5–28, 1981
32. Barker WH: Adding Life to Years: Organized Geriatrics Services in Great Britain and Implications for the United States. Baltimore: Johns Hopkins University Press, 1987, chapters 9–11
33. World Health Organization: Planning and Organization of Geriatric Services. World Health Organizational Technical Report Series No. 548. Geneva: World Health Organization, 1974
34. Barker WH: Geriatrics internationally. In Fox R, Horan M, Puxity J (eds): Medicine in the Elderly: A Problem Solving Approach. London: Edward Arnold, 1990
35. NIA Conference on Assessment. J Geriatrics Soc 31:636–765, 1983
36. Rubenstein LZ: Geriatric assessment: An overview of its impact. Clin Geriatric Med 3:1–15, 1987
37. Rubenstein LZ, Josephson KR, Wieland GD, et al. Effectiveness of a geriatric evaluation unit: A randomized clinical trial. N Engl J Med 311:1664–1670, 1984
38. Kennie DC, Reid J, Richardson IR, Kiamari AA, Kelt C: Effectiveness of geriatric rehabilitative care after fracture of the proximal femur in elderly women: A randomized clinical trial. Br Med J 297:1083–1086, 1988

60

Genetics and the Public Health

Patricia A. Baird
Charles R. Scriver

Social policies, public health, and medicine, in that general descending order of importance, improved human well-being and longevity in the twentieth century, yet disease continues, in the form of sick populations and sick individuals,[1] and unhealthy longevity is a macroeconomic problem.[2] Naturally, there has been a response—one composed of social policies, public health, and medicine. In Canada, a major milestone in this response was the government document *A Perspective on the Health of Canadians,*[3] which outlined The Health Field Concept. Reasonable, thoughtful, and provocative, this document espoused a four-pronged attack on disease, and it welded ideas on life style, environment, health care organization, and human biology into an approach to address disease more effectively. Considerable attention has been paid to the first three but rather less has been heard about the fourth component, namely, the biological basis of disease. This chapter addresses that particular theme. Our topic is genetic determinants of disease. We believe them to be important because they explain both incidence and causes; they also explain some examples of clustering of disease in geographic regions.

Health is a state of homeostasis, and it is maintained in the face of a changing and shifting environment. The central tendencies of metrical traits (mean values) are the quantitative measures of homeostasis (e.g., level of blood glucose, cholesterol, phosphorus, osmolarity, blood pressure, and so on).[4] The polypeptide mediators of homeostasis (enzymes, transporters, channels, receptors, etc.) that are essential to this process of homeostasis are encoded by genes, descended to homo sapiens through the evolutionary process. Individuals retain health if experience does not overwhelm homeostasis or mutation does not undermine it.

In the conventional medical model, disease manifestations (symptoms and signs) are the product of a process (pathogenesis) that has an origin (cause). The manifestations of disease dominate the practice of medicine. Consideration of cause, incidence, and distribution of cases constitutes the public health focus. In medicine the emphasis is on the case; in public health it is on the population. But when adverse infectious and nutritional experiences (the major agents of genetic selection in human evolution) are well controlled, the causes of persistent disease may be of that form that undermines homeostasis rather than of the type that overwhelms it; that is, they may be intrinsic, or genetic, causes. If so the "heritability" of disease in the population has increased; further, it implies that the biological basis of disease is important and that the health care system must accommodate genetic causes of disease.

Rather than thinking of the determinants of disease as outside ourselves, our genetic individuality should be seen as a potential ingredient in the origin of health. Because each individual has a different risk for disease, progress will be optimized if this fact is recognized, taken into account, and applied. Socioeconomic and environmental factors are important determinants of health, but, given a particular environmental factor, *who* gets sick may be determined by genotype. If environmental causes of disease are examined without taking genetic predisposition into account, we not only are getting an incomplete picture but also may be missing the chance to identify, and target with preventive programs, the most "vulnerable" groups.

In this chapter we start with the premise that genetic causes of disease have implications for public health because they either explain cases or identify persons predisposed to disease under disadvantageous circumstances. Since most diseases have two histories, one biological and the other cultural, it is likely that genes have entered different populations because of those populations' different histories. This means that in some populations the genes may have reached such a frequency that they may now exhibit "clustering" of related disease. When diseases have significant genetic determinants, there is an opportunity for prevention through counseling. To explain cases and thus understand why a particular person has a particular genetic disease at a certain time, we summarize the rules of inheritance. If diseases associated with inheritance of biological determinants reach particular high frequencies in a population, it is through one or several historical mechanisms: genetic drift (founder effect), selective advantage, high mutation rate, reproductive compensation, or several genes associated with a common, shared phenotype. These mechanisms are examined in this chapter because they are relevant to public health. They are helpful in our understanding of the impact and relevance of particular population screening programs to current and future disease incidence.

A completed human gene map (both genetic and physical) is an important resource in medicine and for public health; we therefore describe its relevance. Finally, medical screening is a conventional activity in public health; genetic screening is a new form of it. The rationales, principles, and practices of genetic screening are therefore examined as well. Because innovations on the horizon (e.g., DNA tests) will change the way health care professionals view sick individuals and sick populations, we discuss the implications for public health and for society in general of the new genetic technology.

GENES IN POPULATIONS

Inheritance and Distribution

Since the beginning of Western medicine it has been recognized that physical traits and some diseases are inherited. A conceptual basis for the mechanism of inheritance was provided by Mendel,[5] and this concept of a unit of inheritance—the gene—has been richly borne out by a great deal of animal and plant experimental data as well as by empirical human data. The advent of recombinant DNA approaches has borne out the use of this concept even further.

As a species we have a long evolutionary history, and natural selection has ensured that most genes we possess are useful and advantageous. However, deleterious genes certainly exist and cause major problems for their possessors. What determines the frequency of such genes? Will modern medical care for people with deleterious genes (relaxed selection) mean that as a species we will accumulate an increasing genetic load of such mutant genes? The question of what determines the frequency of mutant genes is therefore an important one.

It has been estimated[6,7] that a human being has approximately 100,000 structural genes. In general, except for those on the sex chromosomes in males, humans have two copies of every gene, and therefore each specific function in an individual is usually coded for by two genes—one from the mother, one from the father. If both copies in a gene pair code for fully functional gene products, the individual will have normal function. If both copies code for defective products that normally are essential for life, the individual will have a lethal disease. If one member of the pair is normal and the other defective, the person's fate will depend on whether the normal gene has sufficient product to allow healthy function. Alternative forms of a given gene are called *alleles* of that gene. An individual who has identical alleles in a gene pair is said to be homozygous. If the alleles in a pair are different—that is, they code for different (although similar in structure) products—that individual is said to be heterozygous.

In thinking about the frequency of genes in a population, that population can be considered as a pool of genes, a pool from which any individual draws two alleles for each gene pair. Consider a population with random mating where a given gene may exist in the form of allele A or of allele a. The chance that a person will draw any one of three possible combinations (AA, Aa, aa) depends on the frequency of A compared with a in the gene pool.

If p is the frequency of A and q is the frequency of a, then

$$p + q = 1$$

and

$$p = 1 - q$$

and the relative proportion of the three possible combinations will be

$$p^2(AA) + 2pq\,(Aa) + q^2\,(aa)$$

This formula for the distribution of genes in a population[8,9] is known as the Hardy-Weinberg equilibrium, since this relationship only holds as long as there is no mitigating influence (e.g., AAs have twice the number of children). In the absence of any factor disturbing the equilibrium, the proportions of the genotypes will remain the same from generation to generation. Thus, if one knows how often a disease due to two defective alleles (a recessive disorder) occurs, it is possible to calculate the frequency of heterozygotes (or carriers) in the population. For example, if a given recessive disorder (aa) appears in 1 in 10,000 liveborn individuals, the frequency of carriers (Aa) in that population will be approximately 1 in 50.

It is clear from this illustration that there are far more copies of the gene in carriers than occur in affected individuals. There is a shortcut in the calculation for diseases of this kind, which have a low frequency, where P is very close to 1: the carrier frequency will be twice the square root of the disease frequency. For example, in cystic fibrosis, which occurs about 1 in 2000 births in white populations, approximately 1 in 22 individuals will carry the gene.

Changing Gene Frequencies

What may disrupt this equilibrium and change the frequency of genotypes (and resulting phenotypes) in a population? A rise in the frequency of a particular phenotype (due to changing gene frequencies) may be caused by one or more of the following five factors, which disturb the Hardy-Weinberg equilibrium.

1. Nonrandom Mating. If mating is random, the only thing determining the probability of a genotype's occurring is the relative frequency of the genes in the population pool. This condition may not be met if there is preferential mating due to traits wholly or partly genetically determined. Assortative mating (like with like) exists for several human traits.

2. Selection. A mutant allele that is harmful to the individual will be less likely to be passed on to the next generation, since its possessor is less likely to have children. In other words, it will be selected against and become less frequent. If the allele is *dominant* (i.e., just one copy of it is harmful), selection may be quite rapid, particularly if it means that all individuals with the gene are unable to reproduce; then no copies will be passed on to the next generation. In this situation, if the disorder occurs in the next generation it does so by new mutation. Thus the proportion of cases of a dominant genetic disorder that are inherited depends on the effects of the gene on the likelihood of reproduction by its possessor. Selection against *recessive* alleles is much less effective, since most copies of the gene exist in carriers who are normal and quite able to pass the mutant gene on. Even if selection is complete against reproduction in the homozygote, it would take 10 generations (about 300 years) to reduce a gene frequency of 0.10 to 0.05. The less frequent the allele, the slower the decline in frequency. From a health policy point of view, it is important to note that going in the opposite direction—that is, removing selection—acts just as slowly. Successful therapy for phenylketonuria, for example, would take many generations to raise the frequency of the gene to any appreciable extent.

If an X-linked allele affects the male so that he does not reproduce, only the genes in female carriers are passed on to the next generation. Females carry about two thirds of all such mutations. About one third of all cases of a disease are due to new mutation, with two thirds inherited. If affected males are able to have children, then a greater proportion of cases in the next generation are inherited. Treatment of males with hemophilia, for example, would be expected to cause some increase in the frequency of this condition in the absence of any other measure (such as prenatal diagnosis).

3. Mutation. A mutation is a change in the genetic material (DNA). The term can be used in a broad sense to encompass any change, including chromosomal deletions or rearrangements. However, it is usually used to mean a change in the DNA sequence of a gene so that the gene product is different (a point mutation), and that is how it is used here.

Mutations are the raw material of evolution and, in a changing environment, give a species the ability to adapt. However, most mutations cannot be expected to be beneficial, since they occur in an exquisitely coordinated system of genetic information that has taken eons to develop. A random change is not likely to be helpful. Many new dominant mutations are lethal either in utero or very early in life, so that the cases actually observed in human populations only represent a proportion of those that occur.

It is difficult to estimate with any accuracy[10] the current mutation rate in humans. It is probably quite different for different gene loci. An "average" spontaneous mutation rate in humans would be about 1 in 100,000 per locus per gamete per generation. Since mutation is usually a stochastic event, the longer the time elapsed, the greater the likelihood that a mutation will have occurred. Thus it could be predicted that parents who are older at conception would have an increased risk for a child with a dominant mutation, and this in fact is borne out by data. There is increased paternal age in fathers of children with dominant disorders (e.g., achondroplasia) that have never before occurred in the family.[11,12]

4. Heterozygote Advantage. It is possible that a gene that is harmful in the homozygous state may be advantageous in the carrier. This is the case with the genes for thalassemia and sickle-cell anemia, which in carriers may protect against malaria.[13] The gene for Tay-Sachs disease is frequent in Ashkenazi Jews, and it has been suggested that under ghetto conditions[14] it confers an advantage in the carrier. The occurrence of such genes in populations has importance in terms of health planning and in evaluating whether screening programs are appropriate for particular groups within the larger population.

5. Genetic Drift and Founder Effect. When people migrate to new regions, they may develop "new" diseases or express "old" disease at higher frequencies. This phenomenon reflects either new experiences or "old" genes expressed at altered frequencies in the settlers.[15] How many susceptible persons there are in the newly resident population after migration of the "founder" depends on the number of incoming mutant genes borne by the founders and on factors that favor their spread through the population (rates of natural increase, degree of consanguinity, and mode of inheritance). Accordingly, demographic history and structure of genetic variation may explain clustering of cases.

Methods of Measuring Mutation Rates

In theory, simply counting all individuals in a population of births who have a disease known to be due to a dominant gene, at the same time by family history evaluating how many are not inherited, should give the mutation rate for that locus. In practice, even with excellent population-based disease registries, this is extremely difficult to carry out in a large population. In addition to the logistical difficulties of collecting complete information on a large number of individuals, it is complicated by such factors as nonpaternity, mild cases that are missed, patients who die before ascertainment, and similar conditions that may be wrongly categorized. Indirect approaches to estimating the mutation rate for recessive disorders use the fact that the frequency of the recessive disease can be counted and that the reproductive "fitness" (the proportion of mutant to normal alleles passed on) can be measured in affected individuals. These are related as follows:

$$\text{Mutation rate} = (1 - \text{Fitness}) \times \text{Disease frequency}$$

These methods have yielded a range of estimates and may differ according to gene locus and sex.[16] In any case, determining frequencies in humans is difficult.[17]

INCIDENCE AND PREVALENCE OF GENETIC DISEASE

Measuring the frequency of genetically determined diseases in a population is also difficult. Onset may occur at any time in the life cycle, and there is a gradation from diseases due to genes that do not permit normal function in any environment to those in which genetic predisposition is only expressed in certain environments. Statistics are usually only available on a population for aspects such as mortality by categories of cause or hospital admissions for diseases coded to the International Classification of Disease (ICD). This classification does not allow the frequency of genetic disease to be estimated because it is not a classification by etiology. For these reasons, at present it is not possible to quantify accurately the contribution of genetic disease to death and sickness.

However, population-based registries offer a mechanism for counting the occurrence of various disorders that may be exploited to answer this question. Registries provide the basic information on disease incidence and prevalence necessary for planning health and other special programs and facilities such as health professional and other personnel needs. If a registry receives information from multiple sources over individuals' lifetime (especially if this can be linked into sibship and family groupings), some classification of disease in a population by etiology is possible. Additional coding for classification of cases by etiology is needed. With this approach it is possible to get some estimate of the relative importance of genetics to health.[18,19] Some estimates on the role of genes at different stages of life are provided:

Conception to Birth. Between 50% and 70%[20] of pregnancies in healthy women fail to produce liveborn babies. Genetic causes are a major factor in failed pregnancies, especially those during the first trimester. Chromosomal abnormalities are found in half of early spontaneous abortions.[21]

From Infancy to Young Adulthood. At least 5.3% of liveborn individuals in a large population of over a million consecutive births were found to have diseases with an important genetic component before age 25 years.[18] If congenital anomalies (some of which have a genetic cause) are also included, then 7.9% of the population has been identified by age 25 as having a genetic disorder. A sampling of over 12,000 admissions to a pediatric hospital found that 11.1% were "genetic"; 18.5% were for congenital malformations, and 2% were "probably" genetic.[22] These findings have been confirmed in other studies.[23,24]

The relative contribution of genetic disorders to all causes of disease in our population has likely increased markedly in this century for many conditions. As environmental causes of death and disease have declined, such as for infant mortality,[25] genetic causes assume more prominence. As the nutritional causes of rickets have declined, the proportion due to genetic defects in vitamin D metabolism have increased[26] and the heritability of the conditions has increased. This is but one example of several thousand different genetic diseases,[27] many of which are likely to have also increased in heritability as the environment has changed.

From Middle to Late Adulthood. We have very limited knowledge about the effects of genetic factors on the overall health of people after 25 years of age. The incidence of multifactorial disorders of late onset may be up to 60% if such conditions as diabetes, hypertension, myocardial infarction, ulcers, and thyrotoxicosis are included.[28] Including certain cancers makes this figure even higher.

If age-specific mortality rates are examined, a characteristic "U-shaped" mortality curve is obtained, with rates highest at each end of the age spectrum. The causes of death composing the two arms of the curve are not the same.[29] Those in early life are characterized by abnormal development and difficulty in adaption to life after birth. Mendelian disorders are characteristically diseases of prereproductive life,[30] with over 90% being apparent by the end of puberty. They reduce the life span and usually cause psychosocial handicaps. Those in the other "limb" of the curve are mainly diseases associated with specific environments, patterns of living, particular occupations, and advancing senescence.

The genetic variability of a cohort decreases as it moves through the life span and selection operates. The most disadaptive genes are the first to be deleted. After puberty the remaining genes contributing to disease are likely to be disadaptive only in certain environmental circumstances. In contrast, the variability of experience with environmental sources of disease determinants must increase throughout life. These reciprocal trends may be reflected in a diminution of heritability of the diseases that affect the cohort as it ages. Aging is associated with a decline in homeostatic competence of the various organ systems. This may set the stage for genes that previously had been harmless to become disadaptive. Genes are expressed differentially in ontogeny, and so new phenotypes will be revealed to selection as different stages of life are entered. This means diseases may have their own separate timetable for onset, and it will not be a general uniform decline in heritability for all diseases throughout life.

Several predictions follow from the assumption that heritability of disease declines with increasing age[29]:

1. Persons with early onset are more likely to have severe disease and to have affected first-degree relatives.
2. Age-specific age at onset should reach a peak and decline, since by some age most of those with the relevant genes will already have the disease.
3. There should be multigenic diseases that do not require a specific environment.
4. Migration, socioeconomic status, and other environmental change may change age of onset and the likelihood of the disease's clustering in families.
5. If one sex is less often affected, early onset, severity, and increased incidence in affected relatives should characterize it.
6. Concordance in monozygotic twins should be greatest when disease onset is early.
7. Patients with late-onset have milder disease that is more responsive to prevention and treatment.

For disease categories with a wide range of age of onset, monogenic forms are more likely to be found among the early-onset cases, multifactorial subtypes should characterize adult and middle age, and in the very old the disease should likely be due to environmental determinants. Single-gene disorders of early onset carry heavier burdens than those of later life and are relatively resistant to treatment.[31] There may be an irreducible minimum of genetic contribution to disease and death that feasible environmental manipulation cannot prevent, and the genetic variation in the population may determine the limits to what can be achieved by any environmental measures. However, with the advent of a greater understanding of genetic pathophysiology, it may become possible to tailor "microenvironments" to fit particular genotypes.

Determining the role of genetics in disease will require better methods of classifying disease and processing health data. Computerized record linkage will be increasingly important, not only to build longitudinal health histories on individuals but to link these into sibships and family groupings. Administrative and other health data sets that already exist can be combined to evaluate if familial clustering occurs. If familial clustering is found, then various methodologies may be used to untangle whether this is due to genetic or shared environmental factors or, more likely, an interaction between the two.

CATEGORIES OF GENETIC DISEASE

Given that genetic disease has a substantial impact on health, it is of interest to examine the various categories of genetic disease that occur in humans, their frequencies, and the strategies currently available to deal with them. Several categories may be used when thinking about genetic disease, although at some level these are artifactual and imposed to organize the reality, which is a continuum.

Chromosomal Disorders

One in 200 liveborn infants has a chromosomal error, making this a common category of disorder. All are potentially detectable by prenatal diagnosis, but since only those subgroups of women identified as being at higher risk (because of age or family history) are screened prenatally, there is only the opportunity to avoid a proportion of such conditions at present. Errors may occur in the number of chromosomes (too many or too few) or in their structure (deletions or duplications of parts of chromosomes). Two recent texts cover this topic in depth.[32,33] Many of these errors are incompatible with survival to term; for example, almost half of all recognized spontaneous abortions in the first trimester have chromosomal abnormalities.[34] The proportion of stillborn infants with chromosomal errors is about 6%.[35,36]

Autosomal Chromosome Disorders. If an extra chromosome occurs for a given pair, this is called trisomy. Trisomy has not been observed in living infants for most chromosomes, although it is compatible with life for the sex chromosomes and chromosomes 13, 15, and 21. The latter, Down's syndrome, is the most frequent trisomy in liveborn humans. It occurs approximately once in 1000 births, the exact frequency depending on the age composition of reproducing women in the population and whether prenatal diagnostic programs for its detection are in place. It is the most common recognizable cause for mental retardation in Western populations and is thus of relevance to public health and planning. Its occurrence is very strongly related to maternal age[37]; prenatal diagnostic programs are usually offered to detect chromosomal abnormalities in pregnant women over 35 years of age. Even though these programs are shown to be cost effective in terms of health resources, they can only reduce the birth incidence of Down's syndrome to a limited degree.[38] This is because even though young women have a much lower risk individually, they contribute a far greater number of births than women over 35, so that most Down's syndrome infants are born to young women. It is important that couples with an increased recurrence risk are made aware of the option of prenatal diagnosis in future pregnancies. It used to be thought that survival to adulthood in Down's syndrome was very poor, but recent data[39,40] show that over 70% of afflicted individuals survive to their thirties and about half to their late fifties. This obviously has implications for programs planning to integrate affected individuals into community, educational, vocational, and residential settings.

The other autosomal trisomies (15 and 18) are less frequent (1 in 5000 to 7000 and 1 in 8000 live births, respectively) and result in infants with multiple congenital anomalies who often fail to thrive and die relatively young. It is important to make the diagnosis so that the parents may be counselled regarding the etiology, prognosis, and recurrence risk. Deletions (or duplications) may occur in any chromosome and occur anywhere along the chromosome. The size will vary among patients and give rise to a whole array of abnormal conditions. Some correlations of particular chromosomal abnormalities with particular clinical pictures have been made, for instance, deletion of part of the short arm of chromosome 5 with the "cri du chat" syndrome. Such chromosomal abnormalities explain many infants and children who are retarded, fail to thrive, and have birth defects.

Sex Chromosome Disorders. Recognition of sex chromosome disorders is important so that there is opportunity for avoidance of abnormal offspring and so that the affected individual can receive proper management to avoid known complications. Turner's syndrome was described in 1938[41] in girls who were short and sexually immature. It was later[42] discovered that this clinical picture was found in girls missing the second X chromosome in at least some of their cells. This condition occurs once in 5000 live births and does not occur more frequently in the offspring of older mothers; the recurrence risk is negligible. Klinefelter's syndrome occurs in newborn surveys in about 1 in 500 males. This term is used to refer to males who have at least one extra X in at least some of their cells. The classic case has an XXY constitution, but there are other variants. The more Xs present, the more likely are mental retardation and additional physical stigmata. If Klinefelter's syndrome is not detected during childhood, afflicted males may learn they have the syndrome when they attend an infertility clinic as an adult.

The XYY syndrome probably occurs about 1 in 500 males. This condition was sensationalized in the lay press for a time because of a theory that the extra Y made these males taller, aggressive, and antisocial. A study in the Danish population of army inductees[43] with this condition showed that crimes of violence against another person were not higher, although the total rate of criminal convictions was greater. The intelligence and educational level of XYY individuals was lower than controls, and it is possible that they may not commit crimes more often but get caught more often. The Triple X female has been given the misnomer "superfemale" by some; however, retardation and infertility are increased in these women, although most are probably never diagnosed. If the diagnosis is made, prenatal diagnosis should be offered, since they are at increased risk for bearing XXY and XXX offspring.

Autosomal Dominant Disorders

This is the first of four categories that fall into the "single gene" disorder group. It is important to understand the mechanism of their transmission, so that opportunities for prevention can be incorporated into planning and the differing impact of preventive programs on the future frequency of these disorders be understood. About 1500 autosomal dominantly inherited conditions have been documented; another 1100 conditions are suspected to be in this category. Although individually each is uncommon, there are so many that they have *in toto* a substantial impact on the health care system.

If an allele is always expressed, whether that person is homozygous or heterozygous at that locus, it is said to be dominantly inherited. If a gene is expressed in the phenotype only when it is homozygous, that trait is said to be recessively inherited. This distinction between dominant and recessive inheritance is an operational one for convenience in many ways. As better techniques are found, more recessive genes in the heterozygote can be detected. Thus, the line between dominance and recessivity is an artificial, albeit useful, concept in practice.

What sorts of disease are inherited in an autosomal dominant fashion? Included in this category are such entities as Huntington's chorea, neurofibromatosis, achondroplasia, tuberous sclerosis, and Marfan syndrome. If the affected person reproduces, the abnormal gene will be passed on average to half his or her children, who will also be affected. If a person does not receive the gene, then that branch of the family is "in the clear" from then on. Dominant disorders can change frequency rapidly in the population with intervention, making genetic diagnosis and counseling crucial.

Several factors make counseling families for dominant disorders very difficult at a practical level, despite the seemingly simple mechanism of transmission—"like tossing a coin." Although many dominantly inherited disorders follow the pattern described, where males and females are equally likely to be affected and to pass it on, and where on average half the offspring are affected, there are also many where additional aspects must be taken into account *before* one can give accurate and informed advice. First, some dominantly inherited disorders are due to new mutations. It is important to establish if a given case is familial or due to a new mutation, since once it has occurred, it will breed true and have a 50% chance of being passed on to a child. The important practical consequence is that siblings and other relatives will not be at increased risk.

Variable expressivity must also be considered before counseling is given. Each dominantly inherited disorder has a recognized profile; one disorder may have a very narrow range clinically with little variation in expression, whereas another may typically differ between persons even within a family. If an individual has the gene for a disorder where variable expressivity is not a feature, it is safe to reassure the apparently normal sibling that his or her children will not be at increased risk. However, for dominant disorders where there is great variation in severity, such as osteogenesis imperfecta, this reassurance must be tempered with caution. If a couple asks advice about risk for children when this disorder is segregating in their family, a detailed and sophisticated examination is indicated.

Another recently identified factor is "imprinting," which is imposed on the genetic information during gametogenesis.[44,45] This imprinting persists in a stable fashion throughout DNA replication and cell division in an individual, to be erased in the germ line and then be differentially established once more in the sperm (or egg) genomes of that individual. It has the consequence that expression of a given disease gene can depend on whether it is inherited from the mother or the father. Other factors to consider are reduced penetrance (where some individuals with the gene will show no clinical effect) and variation in age of onset. All genetic disease is not congenital. Many genetic disorders do not become clinically evident until adulthood or midlife. Genetic heterogeneity is a common phenomenon that must be taken into account, not just for dominant disorders but for all categories of genetic disease. A genetic disorder that appears to be the same in different families may in fact be due to different lesions in the same gene or to a different mutation at another locus that affects the same pathway and therefore leads to a similar clinical endpoint. When a case is sporadic and no other individual in the family is affected, the clinical endpoint observed may have been reached by other means than a single gene mechanism, such as an environmental insult in development.

Autosomal Recessive Disorders

Most recessive disorders are individually rare, each with a birth prevalence of 1 in 15,000 to 100,000. However, since there are so many, they have a considerable impact, with 1 in 500 liveborn individuals being identified as having one of these disorders before age 25 years. They often have their onset in early life, and there are population screening programs at birth for several of them, based on biochemical testing. Rapid advances in DNA technology will make it possible to offer population screening programs in a public health context for some of these disorders. There are over 600 known recessive disorders in humans and another 800 conditions suspected to be due to this mechanism. Examples include phenylketonuria (which results in retardation and seizures but can be treated by diet), adenosine deaminase deficiency (which results in severe immune deficiency and early death), and cystic fibrosis, which is one of the commonest recessive disorders in white populations (approximately 1 in 22 people carry this gene).

Since genes segregate in families, the rarer the particular recessive allele for a disorder, the more likely that consanguinity is observed in the parents of an affected child case or that the individual will be born into a religious or geographical isolate. An allele for a particular recessive disorder may be so common in some subgroups that an appreciably increased risk of affected offspring occurs. It is therefore desirable to offer carrier or prenatal testing to these groups (e.g., Tay-Sach's disease in Ashkenazi Jews; thalassemia testing for populations of Mediterranean or Asian descent). For disorders with a very high carrier rate in the population (such as hemochromatosis, which has a carrier rate of about 1 in 10 people),[46] cases may appear in succeeding generations, a feature not usually observed for recessive disorders.

Just as with dominant disorders, genetic heterogeneity may occur. For example, a couple, both deaf because of being homozygous for a recessive gene that causes hearing loss, may have normal children if the genetic lesion in one parent is not allelic to that in the other. There is also variability seen in recessive disorders, just as in dominantly inherited disorders. This may be because of molecular heterogeneity—that is, the lesion in the gene is different on the two chromosomes—or because the recessive genes act on different backgrounds of other genes.

In an increasing number of recessive disorders (over 100), prenatal detection is now possible. Unfortunately, a particular couple usually does not realize the need for prenatal detection until they have had one affected child; however, they may wish to have the opportunity to avoid having another affected child. In some disorders that cause severe shortness of stature or particular morphological abnormalities, x-ray or ultrasound studies may be diagnostic. In others with a known biochemical defect, enzyme activity or other metabolites can be measured either directly in the amniotic fluid or in cultured fetal cells. In yet others, DNA diagnosis is possible. An enzyme deficiency has already been demonstrated in about a third of the known recessive disorders in humans.[27] Two alternatives that should be mentioned to couples who do not wish to take the 1 in 4 risk of an affected child and for whom prenatal diagnosis is not possible are adoption and gamete donation.

X-linked Recessive Disorders

There are more than 100 X-linked recessive disorders, and more are suspected. Some examples of X-linked single-gene disorders are hemophilia and Duchenne's muscular dystrophy. In X-linked recessive disorders, the problem gene is located on the X chromosome. Since females have two Xs, if one is normal, that female will be healthy. Since males only have one X, if this has the X-linked disease gene, the male will be affected. In these families, therefore, females may be healthy, unaffected carriers of the gene, but half of their sons will have the disease. Carrier detection tests for the female relatives of male patients are very important in giving them the option to avoid having affected sons, and prenatal diagnosis is becoming available for an increasing number.

X-linked Dominant Disorders

There are very few disorders in this category (well under 100), some examples being familial (XL) hypophosphatemia with rickets, and Alport's syndrome (hereditary nephropathy and deafness). X-linked dominant disorders occur in females as well as males, and an affected female transmits the gene to half her daughters and half her sons, whereas an affected male transmits it only to his daughters, all of whom will have the gene. There is no male-to-male transmission.

Mitochondrial Disorders

The mitochondria in human cells have circular chromosomes that contain genes that code for proteins involved in oxidative phosphorylation, providing the cell with energy. Since the mitochondria are cytoplasmic organelles, these are always inherited from the mother. A characteristic of cytoplasmic inheritance is that segregation ratios characteristic of mendelian disorders are not observed, but many offspring in the maternal line are affected. Several clinical entities have been identified with mitochondrial mutations, namely, Leber's optic atrophy, infantile bilateral striatal neurosis, and Kearns-Sayre syndrome. The situation is complex in that a wide range of abnormality is possible, depending on the numbers of abnormal mitochondria included in the egg and the differential multiplication of these organelles in different tissues.[47] They may explain some errors of development and congenital malformations.

Multifactorial Disorders

In this group, interactions between environmental factors and the genes of an individual cause disease in ways only partly understood. Some examples are common congenital malformations such as neural tube defects (spina bifida and anencephaly), congenital dislocated hips, and some adult-onset disorders such as atherosclerosis, hypertension, schizophrenia, and some cancers. It is likely that most chronic diseases of adult onset with a major impact on health care and social systems fall into this group. This is by far the largest category of genetic disease; it appears that even by age 25 at least 1 in 20 individuals in the population is affected by multifactorial disorders; over a lifetime probably a much greater number are affected.[18] The situation is not simple, and at the population level a given disease category is likely to consist of individuals who have reached that endpoint by a variety of genetic "routes," some interacting with environmental factors.

It is likely that many individuals with a common disease like Alzheimer's disease, atherosclerosis, manic depression, or diabetes have a gene that determines whether external influences will result in illness. In the future, the use of linked DNA markers will give the opportunity to prevent expression of the disease. For example, 1% to 2% of the population has a single gene type of hyperlipidemia. These individuals constitute over a quarter of individuals with heart attack at less than 60 years.[36] Such individuals may avoid this by early detection, followed by diet and medication. Since genes underlying predisposition to these "multifactorial" conditions cluster in families, there is an opportunity to identify and pull out of the larger group subsets of individuals (and members of their families) who are identifiable as being at increased risk.

Noninherited "Genetic" Disorders

Individuals who are normal at birth may acquire diseases in which clear genetic abnormalities arise in a particular type of cell. Genes may be damaged or the genome in some cells altered by environmental agents such as radiation, chemicals, or viruses. Examples of such diseases are cancer and acquired immunodeficiency syndrome (AIDS). In the future, it is also possible that many of the changes associated with aging may be found to be acquired genetic changes at the somatic cell level.

THE HUMAN GENE MAP AND GENE SEQUENCING

A detailed knowledge of the structures of genes would open the door to diagnosis and treatment of human genetic disease. A collaborative project to obtain such knowledge for all human genes, by determining the sequence of the DNA in all 23 different human chromosomes, has recently been undertaken by human and molecular geneticists worldwide.

Two remarkable technological developments have made it possible to determine the human sequence and to "map" the location of any gene. The first is "molecular cloning," the insertion of a stretch of DNA of interest from one source into another DNA molecule that can reproduce itself independently in special strains of laboratory bacteria. This allows the collection of purified DNA molecules in very large amounts that could not be obtained from their original sources. The second is "DNA sequencing," the ability to determine the order of the bases for any stretch of DNA that has been cloned. these techniques have improved to the point where one researcher could each year clone and determine the sequence of up to 20,000 bases.

Several complementary and useful approaches to developing the human gene map include somatic cell hybridization, in situ hybridization, cell sorting, deletion and duplication mapping, and linkage. These methods are even more powerful and informative when used in a complementary way.

METHODS USED IN EVALUATING THE ROLE OF GENETICS IN DISEASE

Several levels of questions can be asked about whether genetic determinants contribute to occurrence of a particular disease category or endpoint. Historically, perhaps the first question that has been asked is, "Does a given disease cluster in families?"

Various methods for assessing this question are discussed below. Given that a disease *is* found to show familial clustering, the consequent logical question to ask is whether this is caused by a common environmental exposure or a biologically inherited determinant. The second section will outline several methods that have been used in genetics to elucidate the answer to this. If in fact the disorder is found to be inherited, the next step is to clarify the particular mechanism of inheritance. Several approaches that are used in genetics to evaluate this will be discussed in the third and final section. We have taken an approach similar to that in the very useful detailed review of this topic by M.C. King et al.[48]

Evidence for Clustering in Familes

Obviously, if a disease is common, it may occur in more than one member of a family simply by chance. Several features, if present, provide evidence that the familial clustering is nonrandom:

1. Healthy individuals who have a family history of the disorder when followed over time develop that condition more often than other comparable individuals without any family history.
2. The relatives of afflicted individuals have a greater frequency of the disorder than comparable controls.
3. The relatives of afflicted individuals have a greater frequency of the disorder than is found in the general population.
4. If the trait can be quantitatively measured (e.g., blood pressure), there is a positive correlation between pairs of related individuals.

It is essential that the endpoint or disease being evaluated for familial clustering is as homogeneous as possible. If the disease being evaluated is actually a clinical picture that can be reached in several different ways (some with a genetic determinant, others where an environmental factor is the main determinant), then a very confused picture may result, with some studies finding familial clustering and others not.

There are many common diseases in adults that by the foregoing criteria have been shown to aggregate in families. For example, coronary heart disease shows familial clustering even after all known risk factors have been adjusted for (e.g., smoking, weight, serum lipids, blood pressure, diabetes, behavior pattern). There is also evidence for familial clustering of each of these risk factors.[49] Several birth defects, neurological and behavioral disorders, and cancers also cluster in families by the usual criteria. Identification of this clustering is the first step in untangling the complex web to elucidate the genetic components that determine a disease. Clustering in families may be due not to sharing of genes but to sharing of a common environment or to cultural transmission of disease determinants. Even showing that correlation in the disease frequency is greater the closer the genetic relationship is not sufficient, since shared environmental and cultural factors may also increase as the relationship gets closer.

Methods to Elucidate Cause of Familial Clustering

Usually several methods are used because they are complementary.

Twin Studies. Monozygotic (MZ) twins are genetically identical; they result from the splitting of one fertilized ovum. Dizygotic (DZ) twins are only as genetically alike as any two siblings. This allows comparison of genetically identical and genetically different individuals who are usually raised in a similar environment. It therefore makes possible an estimation of the degree of genetic influence on the disease. It is also possible to look at identical twins reared apart and together to help estimate the effect of environmental factors.

If a disease were completely determined by gene(s), then the concordance rate in MZ twins should be 100% and the concordance in DZ twins should be the same as in the other siblings of a proband. Studies in MZ and DZ twins for many common adult disorders show much higher concordance in MZ than DZ pairs. This is true for schizophrenia, multiple sclerosis, alcoholism, affective disorders, epilepsy, the neuroses, non-insulin-dependent diabetes mellitus, and allergies, clearly demonstrating a genetic contribution. However, the concordance rate in these studies in MZ twins is less than 100%, demonstrating that an environmental component is also present. Interestingly, the concordance rate for DZ twins in these studies is often greater than that shown between twin probands and their other siblings, which could reflect a greater similarity in environment of DZ twins compared with other siblings or could reflect some selection bias.

Heritability Studies. Heritability (h^2) in the narrow sense is defined as the contribution of additive genes to the phenotype of interest. It will be the proportion of variance in a population for the trait contributed by additive genes (V_A) compared with the total population variance for the phenotype (V_p).

$$h^2 - \frac{V_A}{V_p}$$

In genetic aspects of human disease this definition of heritability is usually broadened to

$$h^2 - \frac{VG}{Vp}$$

where VG refers to the total genotypic variance including nonadditive interactions, such as dominance or epistasis, between genes. (Epistasis is the synergistic effect of genes at different loci.) Estimates of heritability of a trait relate to the particular conditions under which it is measured. For example, if the environment changes, it is no longer valid. Estimates of heritability have been made for many quantitative human traits. They should be interpreted only as indicators of whether the role of genes is relatively large or small in the population and of the circumstances in which the condition is measured.[50]

Adoption Studies. If individuals are raised by adopting parents, it gives the opportunity to examine given traits or disorders in adopted individuals for resemblance to the biological and the rearing families and thus address the "nature-nurture" issues. This approach has been followed for a number of traits such as blood pressure and for disorders such as schizophrenia[51] and alcoholism.[52]

Path Analysis. Individuals give little information about causal hypotheses but analysis of pairs of relatives are much more informative (e.g., father-son pairs, brother-sister pairs). Path analysis was created by Sewall Wright as an aid in analysis of causation. It is a way of deriving consequences of linear causal assumptions and then testing these assumptions on correlation structures such as pairs of relatives.[53]

Analysis of Familial Common Environmental Exposures. Familial clustering may be due to clustering of culturally transmitted behaviors or family practices that result in particular exposures (e.g., dietary or smoking habits).[54] Kuru, for example, was a disease thought to be genetic but in reality is due to an infection perpetuated by ritual cannibalism. It is likely that diseases such as lung cancer or alcoholism involve cultural inheritance of exposure behavior as well as genetically inherited determinants.

Associations between Genotype and Susceptibility. Humans differ in an identifiable way in their HLA (human leukocyte antigen) system and their ABO blood group systems, thus allowing evaluation of existing genotypes in these systems. Different genotypes within these systems are associated with the occurrence of any one of a variety of diseases. Increasingly, recombinant DNA polymorphisms will be evaluated and correlated with a variety of disease outcomes in the same way. There are now a number of well-documented examples where having a particular identifiable genotype is associated with disease susceptibility (or resistance).

Methods for Determining Mode of Inheritance

Most common diseases that cluster in families do not show simple mendelian inheritance, since they result from an interaction of both genes and environmental factors. A number of methods elucidate the mode of inheritance of the genetic susceptibility.

Multifactorial Model Analysis. The genetic component to determination of a disease with a multifactorial etiology could be equal additive effects of many genes or a few or one gene of large effect. Either model explains why individuals could be put over a threshold in the continuum of liability and thus show disease.

The introduction of methods to detect single genes (HLA typing, DNA polymorphisms, sophisticated statistical pedigree analysis) has in recent years shown that it is likely that one or a very few genes of major effect are involved in the multifactorial pathway.[55] This finding is relevant to diabetes mellitus, rheumatoid arthritis, and some hyperlipidemias. Increasingly there will be opportunities to identify predisposed individuals, and the study of families (particularly those of early onset cases) may give the opportunity to target to clusters of higher-risk individuals. The model where many genes of small effect are relevant (polygenic) may apply to pyloric stenosis.

Segregation Analysis. If a single gene has a major effect on disease susceptibility, it is essential to clarify how it is inherited—autosomal dominant, autosomal recessive, or X-linked. These alternative modes of inheritance give different disease risks for different classes of relatives (e.g., 50% of children are affected if dominant, compared with a low risk for the children of an individual with a recessive disorder). By comparing the observed disease incidence in each class with that expected based on alternative genetic models, it is possible to see how well these agree.

Analysis of Maternal Effects. As discussed previously, the DNA of the mitochondria is inherited only from the mother. This means that diseases that appear to affect both males and females but are only transmitted by the mother are candidates for this mechanism of inheritance,[47] and data may be analyzed with this hypothesis in mind.

Linkage Analysis. If segregation analysis shows that inheritance of a single gene may be responsible for disease susceptibility, it is possible to look at whether a wide variety of genetic markers (including DNA polymorphisms) segregate along with the disease susceptibility. Already this approach has indicated that a dominant susceptibility allele may exist in linkage to particular DNA markers in certain families for Alzheimer's disease,[56] manic depression,[57,58] and breast cancer.[59]

Sibling Pair Methods. These are particularly relevant where data on genetic haplotype (usually for the HLA region) is available in siblings. On the hypothesis that there is a disease susceptibility gene close (linked) to the HLA region, this gene should usually be inherited along with a particular haplotype. Thus, siblings who share this HLA haplotype are more likely to have also both inherited the susceptibility allele. This method evaluates coinheritance of HLA haplotype and disease. Siblings who are both affected with the disease would be expected to share the same haplotype more often. With sufficient data on affected sibling pairs, it is possible to evaluate the mode of inheritance of the disease-predisposing allele.[60]

• • •

The goal of epidemiology is to understand how diseases are distributed in the population. Most common diseases today are likely due to interaction between the genotype and environmental factors, so that progress will be made by studies that control for one class of these influences while investigating the other.

Genetic methods are increasingly allowing us to identify genetically susceptible individuals. Tools from classic epidemiology can then be profitably used to compare environmental factors in affected and unaffected genetically susceptible individuals. Conversely, the other approach to disentangling the interaction is first to identify those individuals who have the environmental factor present and then compare the unaffected and affected in that group, looking for particular genetic subgroups. The new molecular genetic techniques now allow particular DNA sequences to be evaluated in patients and in controls and hold out the hope of more fruitful progress.

SCREENING

Genetic screening may serve several objectives. A program may exist to identify individuals with a particular genotype so they may receive an intervention or treatment. Newborn screening programs are of this category. A program may exist to identify individuals who are at risk of having children affected by a genetic disease. Examples of such programs are Tay-Sachs screening in Ashkenazi Jews and amniocentesis for prenatal karyotyping in women over 35 years of age. A screening program may also exist to gather needed epidemiological information. A useful review of this topic is contained in a report of a Workshop on Population Screening.[61]

Newborn Screening Programs. Screening for phenylketonuria, congenital hypothyroidism, and other inborn errors such as galactosemia is widely practiced in the Western world using a small blood spot obtained by heel stick at a few days of age. Many of these programs are mandated by law, and appropriate resources must be provided to ensure that follow-up study and counseling are available as necessary and also to ensure laboratory quality and accuracy.[62] An abnormal screening test is not diagnostic but is the signal for rapid and appropriate medical and biochemical evaluation as well as parental counseling.

Urine samples taken in the first month of life on filter paper are also used in some screening programs. The compliance rate is high, but the cost effectiveness has been questioned.[63] There is the possibility of adding neuroblastoma testing, which may make it more effective.[64] With the advent of recombinant DNA approaches a variety of additional screening tests have been suggested, including those for Duchenne's muscular dystrophy, hyperlipidemias, and cystic fibrosis. Some of the ethical and social issues raised by screening programs are discussed later.

Screening in Special Groups. Screening targeted groups is the public health response to the phenomenon of clustering that has a genetic explanation. Testing close relatives of individuals with autosomal recessive disorders may be helpful if such carrier tests are available and accurate. This is especially true for those disorders where the carrier frequency in the population is high. For example, the normal sibling of a patient in the United States with sickle-cell anemia has a two-thirds chance of being a carrier. If two married individuals are found to be carriers of the same recessive gene (e.g., by having an affected child), then they should receive counseling.

Particular genes occur in higher frequency in a number of subgroups. One such gene is that for Tay-Sachs disease in Ashkenazi Jews. Between 1970 and 1980, over 300,000 Jewish adults were voluntarily screened.[65] Screening for carrier detection for cystic fibrosis, now that the gene has been located,[66] is likely to develop rapidly. This disorder is common (1 in 2000–2500 births) in individuals of northern European extraction. Thalassemia screening is offered to people from southeast Asia and China, since the frequency of this gene is similar to that of the cystic fibrosis gene in northern Europeans. Populations of Mediterranean origin may be screened for β-thalassemia.

PRENATAL DIAGNOSIS

Prenatal diagnostic techniques are used to diagnose genetic disorders and birth defects that result in marked disability or death early in life. Although usually the option that it permits is termination of the affected fetus, in a few disorders diagnosis permits therapy *in utero* or special management during pregnancy and delivery to minimize further damage to a vulnerable infant. For example, for a fetus with methylmalonic acidemia, the mother will be given vitamin B_{12}; for a galactosemic infant, the mother may receive a low-galactose diet.

There are a number of indications for prenatal diagnosis, and the test that is done prenatally is targeted specifically to the indication for prenatal testing. For example, a mother with a previous child with Tay-Sachs disease will have hexosaminidase A measured in the amniotic fluid sample, whereas a woman who is at risk because of increased age will have chromosome analysis of the fetal cells obtained at sampling. Because some disorders are common and inexpensive to test for once a sample is obtained, they are done on any pregnant woman who is already being subject to sampling. For example, alpha-fetoprotein in the amniotic fluid sample is usually measured regardless of the indication. Several indications for prenatal screening are discussed below.

Increased Maternal Age. As maternal age increases, so does the risk of Down syndrome,[67] and this is also true for the other trisomies. For this reason many jurisdictions offer prenatal diagnosis to pregnant women 35 years and over. Such testing can decrease the birth incidence of Down syndrome by approximately 25% in most North American populations.[68]

Neural Tube Defects. These birth defects, anencephaly and spina bifida, are relatively common, occurring in approximately 1 in 700 births in many North American populations.[69] Once a couple has had an affected child, the recurrence risk in subsequent pregnancies is about 2%.[70] Other close relatives may be at increased risk.[71]

Family History of Specific Disorders. A previous child may have had a mendelian disorder, chromosome anomaly, or birth defect. Also, the family history may indicate that the woman may be a carrier for an X-linked disorder. If a test is available (biochemical, cytogenetic, or DNA) or it is possible to evaluate for abnormal morphological findings (e.g., short limbs, then this testing is offered. For example, maternal exposure to a known teratogen (e.g., valproic acid) or a maternal disorder (diabetes mellitus) may justify offering prenatal diagnosis in some cases.

GENETIC SERVICES

Genetic services, both diagnosis and counseling, are only offered to those who have been identified as in need, by their physicians or by themselves. There are two main avenues for service receipt: by having had an individual in the family with a genetic disorder or being identified as "at risk" by a population screening program.

Genetic service programs usually have arisen in association with a university or teaching hospital, fostering a research-service interaction. All province and states have at least one center, often many. However, the availability and expertise differs from one region to another. There is a useful directory of such programs published by the March of Dimes Birth Defects Foundation.[72] Many university centers also have associated training programs.[73]

The process of genetic consultation and counseling is complex and time-consuming and has not yet been well integrated into the clinical practice of medicine. Funding mechanisms for provision of this service are not satisfactory in many jurisdictions and differ from place to place, having grown in an "ad hoc" fashion. If the rapidly escalating new insights into human diseases being made in genetics are to be brought to practical use, we will need a cadre of trained individuals to deliver these services in the coming decades. Already it is not possible to offer on a population level many beneficial genetic programs (e.g., DNA diagnosis for a variety of mendelian disorders).[12]

An important principle in genetic medicine is the need for diagnostic accuracy and precision. Genetic heterogeneity is a complicating issue in many disorders. Accuracy of diagnosis may be especially difficult to achieve in the sporadic case, when the possibilities of new dominant mutations or phenocopies exist. Paternity is an issue that must be borne in mind, since in a significant proportion of cases (which will differ with the particular population) the husband cannot be assumed to be the father. This needs sensitive and empathetic handling. If the genetic mechanism leading to the particular condition diagnosed is known, it is possible to quantitate risk precisely for different relatives. If the genetic mechanism is not clear, as is the case for many "multifactorial" conditions (e.g., congenital malformations, mental retardation, schizophrenia), then if a thorough evaluation of the family history, pregnancy history, medical history, and physical findings reveals no specific etiology, empirical risk figures can be given regarding recurrence risk. These should be employed with caution, and communication of their meaning and limitations is not a simple process.

OPPORTUNITY AND DANGER: SOME SOCIAL AND ETHICAL IMPLICATIONS

We have known for a long time that many common diseases are familial, but the genetic aspects have been ill-defined. It is clear that most common diseases are genetically heterogeneous, but susceptibility is due to major genes in many cases. Genotypes relatively unusual in the population may come to make up a large proportion of those with common diseases. Individuals at risk may soon be identified by DNA testing for intervention, and there may be ample time to intervene. For example, the immunological process in diabetes can precede onset of symptoms by many years; carcinogenesis also takes many years. The phenotype of disease, what we observe clinically, is somewhat removed from the primary action of the particular gene. This means that there may be considerable modulation possible. Rather than ignore the internal genetic component of disease causation, we should evaluate the genetic input and then attempt to tailor preventive or therapeutic programs to take it into account. If the new molecular genetic capability is incorporated into health care planning, it could allow public health to enter a new era of prevention. Through this new technology, rather than exposing the whole population to the same preventive medical programs, they could be directed to those individuals at risk, with relevant health messages focussed to particular individuals.

The path to planning how the new capabilities in genetic risk identification might best be used in prevention and treatment is not simple. Although it has the potential to better the human condition, it is essential that enthusiasm for this approach be tempered with the realization that it is possible to cause great harm because we have not carefully weighed the pitfalls, ramifications, and dangers of this approach. Well-designed research projects should be undertaken before there is any implementation at the population level.[74] These should address aspects such as psychological and family impact, confidentiality, long-term outcome, compliance, safety, cost benefits, and appropriate laboratory quality control procedures. It is also important that genetic risk identification not be offered before the personnel and facilities to provide appropriate counseling and follow-up study are identified and funded.

The new capabilities raise many questions that will require scrutiny, relating, for example, to ownership of the information on genetic makeup. With regard to confidentiality, policies and procedures must be put in place on who should have access to genetic test results so that the values of personal privacy and autonomy are respected. There may be potential situations where the public good may override the value of personal confidentiality, but these must be thoroughly considered before inclusion in policy.

As we become able to identify individuals in whom the disease outcome is less clear because of unpredictable gene-environment interactions, we may need guidelines to evaluate whether such programs should be offered. We might cause harm by identifying individuals as having a genetic vulnerability. Much of illness is perception and attitude, and it is important to avoid harm by causing identified individuals to view themselves as ill. In addition to stringent guidelines regarding data confidentiality, policies to avoid possible discrimination against identified individuals are also needed.

All of us are genetically unique, and all of us have weaknesses and strengths. This realization has the potential to break down the current generally held perception of the distinction between the majority "normal" population and the small minority with "genetic diseases." A better perception—that everyone is vulnerable in his or her own way—would weaken or remove any basis for stigmatization of those with "genetic diseases." However, genetic identification could also be negative if it created a population each of whose members was aware of and continuously concerned about a particular genetic predisposition and the likelihood of becoming ill.

Some specific issues of legal and social consequence raised by DNA testing are discussed below. DNA testing can identify each individual (except for identical twins) uniquely. It can also be used to identify genetic relationships with unprecedented accuracy. These new abilities raise issues in several areas.

Paternity. The paternity tests that were previously available could disprove paternity when a child had a genetic factor that wasn't present either in the mother or in the putative father. It could not usually prove that a particular man was the father. The new DNA testing can achieve levels of probability that establish beyond any reasonable doubt (1 in 100 million) the real father, if the tests are of high quality. This has been accepted as evidence in a number of courts. At the same time it means that quality control of laboratory tests and procedures to safeguard against human error, such as mislabelled samples, are also necessary.

Immigration. In Great Britain, as in some other countries, resident immigrants can ask for resident status for certain relatives. DNA fingerprinting has been used to test if a claimed relationship is true.

Forensic Identification. DNA fingerprinting may be used to identify with great certainty whether a tissue sample found at the scene of a crime belongs to a particular suspect. DNA fingerprinting seems to provide evidence that is acceptable to British courts of law. In the United States, by mid-1989, DNA data have been considered[75] as evidence in more than 80 criminal, rape, and murder trials in 27 states. DNA testing for forensic purposes will probably increase markedly over the next decade.

Workplace Testing. DNA testing can also be used to identify persons at risk in situations where costs may be incurred, for example, by an employer or an insurance carrier. DNA testing could show predisposition to cancer, emphysema, hemolysis, ischemic artery disease, hypertension, and so on with implications for both the employer's cost and the insurance carrier's profits. For many U.S. companies, offering health benefits adds substantially to the costs of production, and this added cost is becoming important in an increasingly competitive global market. Employers may therefore wish to screen potential employees so that their medical and life insurance plan costs will be lower. Appropriate safeguards against discrimination and misuse must be put in place.

Individuals differ in the metabolic machinery they have inherited for dealing with chemicals in the home and work environments. Some individuals have genes that make them less able to handle particular pollutants, so that they are more likely to develop lung disease or other problems after exposure. This could mean that those individuals genetically vulnerable to particular exposures may be refused employment. Another danger is that a strategy of employing only "resistant" individuals may allow industries to relax expensive environmental controls.

Insurance. Laws may be needed to address how the new genetic knowledge should be limited in its application by the insurance industry as well as by employers. Guidelines or legislation may be required for medical and life insurance companies concerning genetic testing before coverage. It is possible that insurance companies could require testing before coverage and then charge higher premiums or refuse coverage to those at higher risk because of their genotype. Because the principle of insurance is to spread risk over many individuals, it seems unjust to disadvantage individuals who through no fault of their own are likely to become ill. This is not as dramatic a problem in Canada, which has a universal health care system, but it could be a very important problem in the United States. If the U.S. insurance industry is not regulated in this regard in some way, it may be necessary for government to set aside funding for health care of such noninsurable individuals.

SUMMARY AND CONCLUSIONS

It is evident that the new DNA technology will affect many areas of our society and will pose often difficult choices. It presents an opportunity and a useful tool if it is used wisely and humanely, but it is also a danger if the implications for social justice of its use are not thought through. Screening programs, in particular, if applied prematurely may cause harm and waste resources. However, if done well and with fully informed communication, they could decrease disease and better the human condition. The new DNA technology opens up questions that have wide-ranging social, ethical, and legal ramifications. Our new abilities with the technology often highlight the difficulty of balancing the individual's and the group's rights. These issues require ongoing discussion by scientists, public health practitioners, lawyers, politicians, and the public.

REFERENCES

1. Rose G: Sick individuals and sick populations. *Int J Epidemiol* 14:32–35, 1985
2. Gori GB, Richter BJ: Macroeconomics of disease. Prevention in the United States. *Science* 200:1124–1130, 1978
3. Canada Department of National Health and Welfare: A new perspective on the health of Canadians: A working document. Ottawa: Canada Department of National Health and Welfare, 1974
4. Murphy EA, Pyeritz RE: Homeostasis VII. A conspectus. *Am J Med Genet* 24:745–751, 1986
5. Mendel G: Experiments in plant hybridization. In Peters JA (ed): *Classic Papers in Genetics.* New York: Prentice-Hall, 1959
6. O'Brien SJ: On estimating functional gene number in eukaryotes. *Nature* 242:52–54, 1973
7. Bishop JO: The gene numbers game. *Cell* 2:81–85, 1974
8. Hardy GH: Mendelian proportions in a mixed population. *Science* 28:49–50, 1908
9. Weinberg W: Uber den Nachweis der Venerbungbeim Menschen jahreshefte des Vereins fur Vaterlandische. *Naturkunde in Wurttenberg* 64:368–382, 1908
10. Neel JV, Satoh C, Goriki K, Asakawa J, Fujita M, Takahashi N, Kageska T, Hazama R: Search for mutations altering protein charge and/or function in children of atomic bomb survivors: Final report. *Am J Hum Genet* 42:663–676, 1988
11. Stoll C, Roth MP, Bigel P: A reexamination of parental age effect on the occurrence of new mutations dysplasias. In Papadatos CJ, Bartsocas CS (eds): *Skeletal Dysplasias.* New York: Alan R. Liss, 1982, pp 419–426
12. Riccardi VH, Dobson CE II, Chakraborty R, Bontke C: The pathophysiology of neurofibromatosis. IX. Paternal age as a factor in the origin of new mutations. *Am J Med Genet* 18:169–176, 1984
13. Alison AC: Notes on sickle-cell polymorphism. *Ann Hum Genet* 19:39, 1954
14. Petersen GM, Rotter JI, Cantor RM, Field LL, Greenwald S, Lim JST, Roy C, Schoenfeld V, Lowden JA, Kaback MM: The Tay-Sachs disease gene in North American Jewish populations: Geographic variations and origin. *Am J Hum Genet* 35:1258–1269, 1983
15. Scriver CR: New experiences: Old genes—lessons from the Mennonites (Editorial). *Clin Invest Med* 12:142–143, 1989
16. Francke U, Felsenstein J, Gartler SM, Migeon BR, Dancis J, Seegmiller JE, Bakay F, Nyhan WL: The occurrence of new mutants in the X-linked recessive Lesch-Nyhan disease. *Am J Hum Genet* 28:123–137, 1976
17. Neel JV: Should editorials be peer-reviewed? *Am J Hum Genet* 43:981–982, 1988
18. Baird PA, Anderson TW, Newcombe HB, Lowry RB: Genetic disorders in children and young adults. *Am J Hum Genet* 42:677–693, 1988
19. Baird PA: Measuring birth defects and handicapping disorders in the population: The British Columbia Health Surveillance Registry. Can Med Assoc J 136:109–111, 1987
20. Opitz JM: *Study of the malformed fetus and infant. Pediatr Rev* 3:57–64, 1981
21. Carr DH: Detection and evaluation of pregnancy wastage. In Wilson JG, Fraser FC (eds): *Handbook of Teratology,* Vol. 3. New York: Plenum Press, 1977, pp 189–213
22. Neal JL, Saginur R, Clow A, Scriver CR: The frequency of genetic disease and congenital malformations among patients in a pediatric hospital. Can Med Assoc J 108:1111–1115, 1973
23. Day N, Holmes LB: The incidence of genetic disease in a university hospital population. *Am J Hum Genet* 25:237–246, 1973
24. Hall JE, Powers EK, McIlvaine RT, Ean VH: The frequency of familial burden of genetic disease in a pediatric hospital. *Am J Med Genet* 1:417–436, 1978
25. Kaback MM: Medial genetics. An overview. *Pediatr Clin North Am* 25:395–409, 1978
26. Scriver CR, Tenenhouse HJ: On the heritability of rickets, a common disease. (Mendel, mammals and phosphate). *Johns Hopkins Med J* 149:179–187, 1981
27. McKusick VA: Mendelian Inheritance in Man. *Catalogues of Autosomal Dominant, Autosomal Recessive, and X-Linked Phenotypes,* 8 edt. Baltimore: Johns Hopkins University Press, 1988
28. UNSCEAR Report: Genetic and somatic effects of ionizing radiation. New York: United Nations, 1986
29. Childs B, Scriver CR: Age at onset and causes of disease. *Perspect Biol Med* 29(3):437–460, 1986
30. Costa T, Scriver CR, Childs B: The effect of mendelian disease on human health: A measurement. *Am J Med Genet* 21:231–242, 1985
31. Hayes A, Costa T, Scriver CR, Childs B: The impact of mendelian disease in man. Effect of treatment: A measurement. *Am J Med Genet* 21:243–255, 1985
32. Schinzel A: *Catalogue of Unbalanced Chromosome Aberrations in Man.* Berlin: Walter de Gruyter, 1984
33. DeGrouchy J, Turleau C: *Clinical Atlas of Human Chromosomes,* 2 edt. New York: John Wiley & Sons, 1984
34. Clendenin TM, Benirschke K: Chromosome studies on spontaneous abortions. *Lab Invest* 12:1281–1291, 1963
35. Hook E: Human teratogenic and mutagenic markers in monitoring about point sources of pollution. *Environ Res* 25:178–203, 1981
36. Vogel F, Motulsky A: *Human Genetics: Problems and Approaches,* 2 edt. Berlin: Springer-Verlag, 1986
37. Trimble BK, Baird PA: Maternal age and Down syndrome. Age-specific incidence rates by single year intervals. *Am J Med Genet* 2:1–5, 1978
38. Baird PA, Sadovnick AD: Maternal age-specific rates for Down syndrome: Changes over time. *Am J Med Genet* 29:917–927, 1988
39. Baird PA, Sadovnick AD: Life expectancy in Down syndrome. *J Pediatr* 110:849–854, 1987
40. Baird PA, Sadovnick AD: Life expectancy in Down syndrome adults. *Lancet* 2:1354–1356, 1988
41. Turner HH: A syndrome of infantilism, congenital webbed neck and arbitus valgus. *Endocrinology* 25:566, 1938
42. Ford CE, Miller OJ, Polari PE, Almeida JC, de Briggs JH: A sex chromosome anomaly in a case of gonadal dysgenesis (Turner's syndrome). *Lancet* 1:886, 1959
43. Witkin HA, Sarnoff AM, Schulsinger F, Bakkestrom E, Christiansen KO, Goodenough DR, Hirschhorn K, Lundsteen C, Owen DR, Pilip J, Rubin DB, Stocking M: Criminality in XYY and XXY men. *Science* 193:547–555, 1976

44. Monk M: Genomic imprinting: Memories of mother and father. *Nature* 328:203–204, 1987
45. Reik W: Genomic imprinting and genetic disorders in man. *Trends Genet* 3:331–336, 1989
46. Bothwell TH, Charlton RW, Motulsky AG: Idiopathic hemochromatosis. In Stanbury JB, Wyngoarden JB, Fredrickson DS, Goldstein JL, Brown MS (eds): *The Metabolic Cases of Inherited Disease,* 5 edt. New York: McGraw-Hill, 1983, pp 1269–1298
47. Wallace DC: Mitochondrial DNA mutations and neuromuscular disease. *Trends Genet* 5:9–13, 1989
48. King MC, Lee GM, Spinner NB, Thomson G, Wrensch MR: Genetic epidemiology. *Ann Rev Pub Health* 5:1–52, 1984
49. Neufeld HN, Goldbourt U: Coronary heart disease: Genetic aspects. *Circulation* 67:643–654, 1983
50. Cavalli-Sforza LL, Bodmer WF: *The Genetics of Human Populations.* San Francisco: WH Freeman, 1971
51. Kety SS, Rosenthal D, Wedner PH, Schulsinger F: Studies based on a total sample of adopted individuals and their relatives: Why they were necessary, what they demonstrated and failed to demonstrate. *Schizophr Bull* 2:413–428, 1976
52. Goodwin DW: Genetic component of alcoholism. *Annu Rev Med* 32:93–99, 1981
53. Rao DC, Morton NE, Gottesman II, Lew R: Path analysis of qualitative data on pairs of relatives. Application to schizophrenia. *Hum Hered* 31:325–333, 1981
54. Cavalli-Sforza LL, Feldman MW, Chen KH, Dornbusch SM: Theory and observation in cultural transmission. *Science* 218:19–27, 1982
55. Motulsky AG: Approaches to the genetics of common disease. In Rotter JI, Samloff IM, Rimoin DL (eds): *The Genetics and Heterogeneity of Common Gastrointestinal Disorders.* New York: Academic Press, 1980, pp 3–10
56. St. George-Hyslop PH, Tanzi RE, Polinsky RJ, Haines JL, Nee L, Watkins PC, Myers CH, Feldman RB et al: The genetic defect causing familial Alzheimer's disease maps on chromosome 21. *Science* 235:885-890, 1987
57. Egeland JA, Gerhard DS, Pauls DL, Sussex JN, Kidd KK, Allen CR, Hustetter AM, Housman DE: Bipolar affective disorders linked to DNA markers on chromosome 11. *Nature* 325:783–787, 1987
58. Hodgkinson S, Sherrington R, Gurling H, Marchbanks R, Reeders S, Mallet J, McInnis M, Petursson H, Brynjolfsson J: Molecular genetic evidence for heterogeneity in manic depression. *Nature* 325:805–806, 1987
59. King MC, Go RC, Lynch HT, Elston RC, Terasaki PI, Petrakis NL, Rodgers GC, Lattanzio D, Baily-Wilson J: Genetic epidemiology of breast cancer and associated cancers in high-risk families. II Linkage analysis. *J Ant Cancer Inst* 71:463–467, 1983
60. Thomson G: A review of theoretical aspects of HLA and disease associations. *Theor Pop Biol* 20:168–201, 1981
61. Scriver CR: Population screening: Report of a workshop. *Progr Clin Biol Res* 163B:89–152, 1985
62. Scriver CR, Holtzman NA, Howell RR, Mamunes P, Nadler HL: Committee on Genetics: New issues in newborn screening for phenylketonuria and congenital hypothyroidism. *Pediatrics* 69:104–106, 1982
63. Wilcken B, Smith A, Brown DA: Urine screening for aminocidopathies: Is it beneficial? *J Pediatr* 97:492–497, 1980
64. Lemieux B, Avray-Blais C, Giguere R, Shapcott D, Scriver CR: Newborn urine screening experience with over one million infants in Quebec Network of Genetic Medicine. *J Inher Metab Dis* 2:45–55, 1988
65. Kaback MM: Heterozygote screening. In Emery AH, Remoin DL (eds): *Principles and Practice of Medical Genetics,* Vol. 2, New York: Churchill Livingstone, 1983, pp 1451–1457
66. Kerem B, Rommens JM, Buchanan JA, Markiewicz D, Cox TA, Chakravarti A, Buchwald M, Tsui LC: Identification of the cystic fibrosis gene: Genetic analysis. *Science* 245:1073–1080, 1989
67. Trimble BK, Baird PA: Maternal age and Down syndrome. Age-specific rates by single year intervals. *Am J Med Genet* 2:1-5, 1978
68. Sadovnick AD, Baird PA: The impact of prenatal chromosomal diagnosis offered to older gravidas in the population incidence of severe mental retardation. *Am J Obstet Gynecol* 143:486–487, 1982
69. Trimble BK, Baird PA: Congenital anomalies of the central nervous system. Incidence in British Columbia, 1952–72. *Teratology* 17:43–49, 1978
70. McBride M: Sib risks of anencephaly and spina bifida in British Columbia. *Am J Med Genet* 3:377–387, 1979
71. Sadovnick AD, Baird PA: A cost-benefit analysis of prenatal diagnosis for neural tube defects selectively offered to relatives of index cases. *Am J Med Genet* 12:63–73, 1982
72. Paul NW (ed): *International Directory of Genetic Services,* 8 edt. New York: March of Dimes Birth Defects Foundation, 1986
73. American Society of Human Genetics: *Guide to Human Genetics Training Programs in North America.* Bethesda, Md.: The Society, 1986
74. Baird PA: Opportunity and danger: Medical, ethical and social implications of early DNA screening for identification of genetic risk of common adult onset disorders. In Knoppers BM, Laberge CM (eds): *Genetic Screening: From Newborns to DNA Typing.* New York: Elsevier Science Publishers B.V. (Biomedical Division), 1990, pp 279–288
75. Barinaga M: Pitfalls come to light. *Science* 339:89, 1989

61

Nutrition in Public Health and Preventive Medicine

Marion Nestle

The importance of nutrition to public health and preventive medicine is self-evident: people must eat to live. Both inadequate and excessive food intake lead to adverse health consequences and contribute to the principal causes of morbidity and mortality throughout developing and industrialized nations. Because all individuals consume food, personal interest in diet makes nutrition an unusually accessible entry point into health education and service delivery systems. Because food intake is determined not only by individual choice but also by cultural norms, socioeconomic variables, and agricultural policies, public health approaches to dietary intervention should be the methods of choice.

This chapter discusses diet and nutrition within a broad public health context. It describes the health impact of dietary intake both below and above recommended levels of energy and essential nutrients. It reviews current guidelines for patterns of food intake that best meet nutritional requirements, improve nutritional status, and, therefore, promote health in the population. Finally, it suggests public health strategies to address behavioral and environmental barriers to implementation of current dietary guidelines.

DIETARY REQUIREMENTS AND ALLOWANCES

Humans require a continuous supply of external food sources of energy and essential nutrients to maintain life, to grow, and to reproduce.[1,2] By definition, essential nutrients are those that cannot be synthesized in adequate amounts by the body; their dietary or metabolically-induced deficiency causes recognizable symptoms that disappear when the nutrients are replaced. The list of nutrients essential or otherwise useful to human physiology is long, complex, and probably incomplete. It includes the more than 40 distinct substances listed in Table 61–1: sources of energy, amino acids, fatty acids, vitamins, minerals and trace elements, fiber, and water. As indicated in the table, other nutrients also may be required under certain conditions.

Malnutrition refers to excessive and unbalanced—as well as deficient—intake of essential nutrients. Fat-soluble vitamins and virtually all of the mineral elements cause disease symptoms when consumed or absorbed in excess. The adverse effects of overconsumption of energy, fat, cholesterol, sodium, sugar, and alcohol are major public health concerns. For each essential nutrient, a certain range of intake levels meets physiologic requirements but does not induce harmful symptoms.[3]

To date, however, optimal levels of intake can only be estimated. Individuals vary in nutrient requirements, and research on human nutritional requirements is incomplete. In the United States, estimates of levels of nutrient intake "adequate to meet the known nutritional needs of practically all healthy persons" are published at approximately 5-year intervals by the National Research Council as *Recommended Dietary Allowances* (RDAs).[4] The 1989 edition recommends intake levels for protein, 11 vitamins, and seven minerals according to age, body size, gender, and developmental stage. The report also presents estimates of "safe and adequate" intake ranges for seven additional nutrients for which research is too limited to define as RDA. Allowances for energy, however, reflect average needs of individuals of varying heights and weights, ages, and activity levels. The RDA levels are similar to dietary standards for other industrialized countries but typically exceed those for populations of less-developing nations.[5]

Because RDAs are used in the United States to assess dietary adequacy, interpret food consumption records, establish levels of food assistance, evaluate the nutritional status of individuals and populations, label food products, and develop nutrition education and dietary counseling guidelines,[6] their limitations require careful attention. RDAs are established at levels that exceed the requirements of 97% of the population; most individuals can meet nutrient requirements at lower levels of intake. Because they are designed to prevent deficiencies, they do not address issues of overconsumption. This omission has led to difficulties in translating RDA standards into universally applicable diet plans[7] and was the basis of the controversy responsible for a 4-year delay in publication of the most recent edition.[8]

NUTRITIONAL DEFICIENCIES: CAUSES AND CONSEQUENCES

Inadequate dietary intake is only one cause of nutrient deficiency. Symptoms also result from conditions that interfere with appetite, impair nutrient digestion, absorption, or metabolism, or substantially increase nutrient requirements or losses. Deficiencies may be manifested clinically as starvation, various forms of

TABLE 61-1. DIETARY COMPONENTS GENERALLY CONSIDERED TO BE ESSENTIAL OR BENEFICIAL FOR HUMAN HEALTH

Category	Specific Examples
Energy Sources	Carbohydrate, Fat, Protein, Alcohol[a]
Essential Amino Acids	Isoleucine, leucine, lysine, methionine, phenylalanine, threonine, tryptophan, valine, histidine[b]
Essential Fatty Acids	Linoleic acid, linolenic acid[c]
Vitamins	
Water-soluble	Ascorbic acid, biotin,[d] cobalamin, folacin, niacin, pantothenic acid, pyridoxine, riboflavin, thiamin
Fat-soluble	Vitamin A,[e] vitamin D,[f] vitamin E, and vitamine K[d]
Minerals	Calcium, chloride, magnesium, phosphate, potassium, sodium
Trace elements	Chromium, cobalt,[g] copper, fluoride, iodine, iron, manganese, molybdenum, selenium, zinc[h]
Fiber[i]	
Water	

NOTE: See references 1 and 2.
[a]Carbohydrates (starches and sugars), proteins, fat, and alcohol contribute about 4, 4, 9, and 7 kcal/g, respectively.
[b]Essential for infants; adult requirement uncertain; arginine, taurine, ornithine, and carnitine may also be required under certain circumstances.
[c]Other fatty acids in the omega-3 series may have essential functions.
[d]Synthesized by intestinal microorganisms; dietary requirement uncertain.
[e]Includes beta-carotene.
[f]Mainly synthesized from the action of sunlight on precursors of the vitamin in skin.
[g]Incorporated as part of cobalamin.
[h]Arsenic, boron, nickel, silicon, tin, and vanadium are required by certain animal species, but human requirements are uncertain.
[i]Evidence supports health benefits but no specific requirement has been determined.

protein-energy malnutrition, syndromes of deficiency of single nutrients (e.g., pellagra, scurvy, iron-deficiency anemia), or a wide range of less specific symptoms.[1,2]

The number of people throughout the world who suffer from nutritional deficiencies can only be estimated. One recent source suggests a range of 340 to 730 million (depending on the magnitude of the energy deficit used as a criterion), but this range does not include estimates from China or from any industrialized nations and is now several years out of date.[9] Most nutritional deficiencies are observed in developing countries where income, education, and housing are inadequate[10] and where water supplies are contaminated with infectious organisms that induce diarrheal diseases.[11] These problems are consequences of poverty. Except in the very poorest countries, food production is sufficient to meet the energy requirements of the population,[12] but foods cannot be obtained or used properly by those most in need.[10]

In industrialized countries, dietary deficiencies are less prevalent. Hunger, as defined by inadequate access to food assistance, has been reported to affect 20 million children and adults in the United States,[13] and surveys have identified nutrient intakes below RDA levels among poverty groups.[14] These findings are accompanied only rarely by clinical signs of nutrient deficiencies.[15] When clinical signs do occur, they are usually associated with the additional nutritional requirements of pregnancy, infancy, and early childhood[16]; illness, injury, or hospitalization[17]; aging[18]; or the toxic effects of alcohol or drug abuse.[19]

Regardless of cause, inadequate dietary intake profoundly affects human function. It induces rapid and severe losses of body weight and electrolytes, decreases blood pressure and metabolic rate, and causes electrocardiogram abnormalities, losses in muscle strength and stamina, and gastrointestinal and behavioral changes.[20] The result is a generalized lack of vigor, alertness, and vitality that reduces productivity and impairs the ability of people to escape the consequences of poverty.[9] Of special concern is the loss of immune function that accompanies starvation. Malnourished individuals lose cellular immune competence and demonstrate poor resistance to infectious disease. Infections, in turn, increase nutrient losses and requirements, and, in the absence of adequate nutrient intake, induce further malnutrition. This cycle is the principal cause of death among young children in developing countries and is an important cause of morbidity in malnourished adults.[21]

Protein-energy malnutrition is the collective term for the clinical effects of this cycle on young children. Survivors display typical effects of starvation: depression, apathy, irritability, and growth retardation.[1] Protein-energy malnutrition usually is classified into two entities—kwashiorkor and marasmus—on the basis of clinical signs and on the relative intake of protein to energy. Kwashiorkor is characterized by edema and fatty infiltration of the liver and is associated with a relative deficit of protein to energy. Marasmus is manifested as generalized wasting due to overall nutritional deprivation. In practice, these distinctions blur. Undernourished children exhibit symptoms that fall between the two extremes and similar diets contribute to either form.[22]

Numerous methods to prevent poverty-associated starvation in adults and children have been demonstrated to be effective in developing countries. Among them are programs that redistribute income, subsidize food prices, promote agricultural production, provide food supplements, and educate.[9,10,23] Improvements in sanitation and in primary health care are also essential components of programs to reduce nutritional deficiencies.[24]

DIET AND CHRONIC DISEASE

As nutritional deficiencies decline in prevalence in industrialized as well as developing countries, they are replaced rapidly by chronic conditions of dietary excess and imbalance. Two recent reports, *The Surgeon General's Report on Nutrition and Health*[25] and the National Research Council's *Diet and Health*,[26] review the entire spectrum of evidence that links diet to chronic diseases and estimate the incidence and prevalence, cost to society, and overall public health impact of these conditions in the United States. *Healthy Nutrition*, from the World Health Organization's European Regional Office, provides data on rising rates of chronic diseases in the most rapidly developing countries in this region.[27] In today's rapidly changing sociopolitical environment, populations throughout the world exhibit rising rates of chronic diseases superimposed on classic patterns of malnutrition.

In the United States, 5 of the 10 leading causes of death—coronary heart disease, cancer, stroke, diabetes, and atherosclerosis—are chronic diseases related in part to diets containing excessive energy, fat, cholesterol, or salt. Chronic liver disease and cirrhosis are associated with excessive intake of alcohol. These conditions account for nearly two thirds of the more than 2 million annual deaths.[28] When data from 32 European countries are considered together, more than half the annual deaths are due to cardiovascular and cerebrovascular diseases, cancers, and digestive diseases related in part to diet.[27] Table 61-2 lists dietary factors associated with the principal chronic diseases. These factors also are associated with hypertension, obesity, dental diseases, osteoporosis, and renal disease.

The proportion of the burden of illness attributable to diet,

TABLE 61-2. DIETARY FACTORS ASSOCIATED DIRECTLY OR INDIRECTLY WITH INCREASED CHRONIC DISEASE RISK

	Dietary Factor				
Leading Cause of Death	Excess Energy (kcal)	Excess Fat	Inadequate Fiber	Excess Sodium	Excess Alcohol
Coronary heart disease	X	X	X	X	X
Cancer	X	X	X	X	X
Stroke	X	X		X	X
Diabetes	X	X	X		
Atherosclerosis	X	X	X	X	X
Liver cirrhosis					X
Digestive diseases	X	X	X		X

Adapted from McGinnis and Nestle, 1989.[48] The evidence that supports these associations is reviewed in detail in references 25 and 26.

however, is uncertain. One estimate suggests that 30% of cancer incidence (range: 10% to 70%) is due to dietary factors and another 3% to alcohol.[29] An estimate of similar magnitude has been made for coronary heart disease.[30] Uncertainties in such estimates are due to difficulties in the design, conduct, and evaluation of research on diet and disease. Nutrition research is complicated by individual variations in dietary requirements, limitations in the ability to obtain accurate information about the dietary intake of individuals[31] or populations,[14] and by other methodologic issues reviewed in the recent reports. Proof of dietary causality is difficult to demonstrate for diseases affected by so many other genetic, environmental, and behavioral factors.

Instead, associations between diet and disease are obtained from studies of laboratory animals and from biochemical, epidemiologic, and clinical investigations in humans. Because each type of study has limitations, diet-disease associations are usually inferred from the totality of available evidence and are considered most compelling when data from all sources are consistent, strongly correlated, highly specific, dose-related, and biologically plausible.[32] Despite this difficulty, experts conclude that the preponderance of evidence supports the associations listed in Table 61-2. They consider most compelling the evidence for fat (especially saturated fat) and coronary heart disease; the evidence for the other associations, if not totally convincing, is strongly suggestive.[25,26,27]

DIETARY RECOMMENDATIONS

The ideal diet should provide energy and essential nutrients within optimal ranges from foods that are available, affordable, and palatable. Until the mid 1970s, governmental and health agencies in the United States advised the public to select diets from specific groups of foods (e.g., dairy, meat, fruits and vegetables, grains) in order to ensure adequate intake of nutrients most likely to be consumed at below-standard levels.[33] Recognition of the role of diet in chronic diseases has shifted the focus of recommendations to prevention of these highly prevalent conditions.

Dietary Goals and Guidelines. The first U.S. report to reflect this new focus established numerical targets for dietary changes to reduce chronic disease risks. Its dietary goals called for reduced intake of fat (to 30% or less of total energy), saturated fat (10%), sugar (10%), cholesterol (300 mg/d or less), and salt (5 g/d); increased intake of foods containing starch, fiber, and naturally occurring sugars (48%); moderation in alcohol intake; and balanced energy intake and expenditure to maintain appropriate body weight. To achieve these targets, the report advised the public to consume more fruits, vegetables, and grains, and to select meat and dairy foods low in fat.[34]

These recommendations incurred prolonged opposition from the food industry and certain scientific and medical groups who argued that such advice was economically unwise, unjustified by the evidence, and inappropriate for the general public.[35] Subsequently, federal dietary guidance policy omitted numerical targets when recommending dietary changes for disease prevention[36] and for development of national health objectives.[37,38] Current policy is expressed in the proposed *Dietary Guidelines for Americans:* eat a variety of foods; maintain healthy weight; choose a diet low in fat, saturated fat, and cholesterol; choose a diet with plenty of vegetables, fruits, and grain products; use sugars in moderation; use salt and sodium only in moderation; if you drink alcoholic beverages, do so in moderation.[39]

Nevertheless, more specific, numerical targets have since been recommended by agencies concerned with prevention or treatment of coronary heart disease,[40-42] cancer,[43-45] diabetes,[46] and hypertension.[47] Similar guidelines also have been issued by agencies in Canada, Australia, New Zealand, Japan,[26] and several countries in Europe.[27]

The Current Consensus. Table 61-3 summarizes the recommendations of the recent comprehensive reports. The *Surgeon General's Report* reviews research linking specific dietary factors to a wide range of chronic diseases, identifies reduction of fat intake as the primary priority for dietary change, emphasizes the consistency of the changes needed for prevention of multiple chronic diseases, and recommends far-reaching food and nutrition policies to implement these changes.[25] *Diet and Health* reaches virtually identical conclusions but extends them to include numerical targets for dietary change and recommendations for 11 daily servings of fruits, vegetables, and grains but for limitations on protein (and therefore on meat) intake.[26] The European report establishes intermediate and ultimate goals for intake of nutrients and identifies goals for individuals at risk for cardiovascular disease.[27]

These landmark reports reflect an international consensus on the scientific basis of diet-disease relationships and on the dietary changes most appropriate for chronic disease prevention. They firmly establish the need for public policies that promote implementation of current dietary recommendations.[48]

BARRIERS TO IMPLEMENTATION

Although the ultimate decisions targeted by these reports are personal food choices, individuals make such choices within the context of the social, economic, and cultural environment in which they live.[49] Adults prefer foods that taste, look, and smell

TABLE 61-3. SELECTED DIETARY RECOMMENDATIONS FOR CHRONIC DISEASE PREVENTION FROM THREE RECENT REPORTS

	Surgeon General's Report, 1988[25]	Diet and Health, 1989[26]	Healthy Nutrition, 1988[27]		
			Intermediate Goals		
			General Public	High CVD Risk	Ultimate Goals
Energy and weight control	Balance	Balance	BMI 20–25[a]	BMI 20–25	BMI 20–25
Fat, % energy	Reduce	30	35	30	20–30
Saturated fat, % energy	Reduce	10	10	10	10
Cholesterol	Reduce	300 mg/d	No rec.	300[b]	300[b]
Complex carbohydrates, Fiber, % energy	Increase	55 (11 servings per day)	40	45	45–55
Sugars, % energy	Limit (children)	No increase	10	10	10
Protein	No recommendation	Moderate	12–13	12–13	12–13
Alcohol, drinks per day	2	2	Limit	Limit	Limit
Salt, g/d	Reduce	6 (4.5 ideal)	7–8	5	5

[a] BMI = body mass index, weight in kilograms per height in meters squared; these values may not be appropriate for the developing world where the average BMI may be 18.
[b] Expressed as 100 mg/4.18 MJ or 1000 kcal.

good,[50] that are familiar,[51] and that provide variety,[52] but these preferences are influenced strongly by family and ethnic background, levels of education and income, age, and gender.[14] Food availability, advertising, and the demand for convenience are key aspects of the current culture of food choices that can create barriers to dietary change.

Food Availability. Food production, distribution, and marketing in the United States have undergone significant changes that affect food availability and, therefore, consumption patterns. Since the mid 1930s, the number of farms has declined by half, but their average size has nearly tripled. This trend has been accompanied by an increase in the proportion of foods for home use purchased in supermarkets from 6 to 67%.[53] With increased dependence on supermarkets has come an increase in the number of foods supermarkets stock. From 1978 to 1986, for example, the average number of items in a supermarket rose from under 12,000 to over 20,000.[54] In 1987, manufacturers introduced more than 10,000 new food products, among them 150 ice cream novelties and more than 1,000 candies, chewing gums, and snacks.[55]

Food Advertising. Advertising enhances the sales of such products to adults and influences the eating habits of children.[56] It promotes consumption of entire categories of foods and stimulates their production, processing, and marketing.[57] In 1987 the leading advertisers of food, candy, soft drinks, fast foods, and beer, wine, and liquor spent a total of nearly $11 billion to promote their products on the national level. McDonald's alone spent nearly $650 million on advertising that year, nearly all of it for television commercials.[58]

Demand for Convenience. From 1975 to 1988, the proportion of married women with children under 6 years of age who worked outside the home increased from 37% to 57%. In 1988, 52% of all mothers—and 72% of black mothers—of infants age 1 year or under were in the labor force.[59] This trend explains in part why convenience is so prominent a motive for food selection.[60] From 1962 to 1987, for example, the share of the U.S. food budget spent on food prepared outside the home rose from 28[61] to 46%[62]; one third of this proportion was spent on take-out meals.[63] Sales of dry-packaged dinner items increased by 19% between 1982 and 1987[64] and many of the new product introductions were foods designed to cook quickly in microwave ovens.[60] Meals consumed outside the home accounted for nearly 33% of energy and nutrient intake in adult women and 20% in their children in 1985.[65]

These trends account at least in part for observations that overall patterns of food consumption in the United States are responding slowly, if at all, to dietary recommendations.[61] Health messages to consume more fruits, vegetables, and grains must counteract these powerful societal barriers.

CONTRADICTIONS BETWEEN KNOWLEDGE OF NUTRITION AND BEHAVIOR

The U.S. public is increasingly well informed about the relationship between diet and health. In 1986, more than 90% of respondents to a telephone survey believed that reducing blood pressure, blood cholesterol levels, body weight, and intake of high-fat foods and salt might help prevent heart disease, and more than 60% believed that they could control high blood cholesterol by reducing intake of cholesterol, fat, luncheon meats, and eggs, by replacing meat with poultry and fish, and by substituting low-fat for whole milk.[66]

Despite this remarkable degree of knowledge, most consumers do not follow dietary recommendations, perhaps because alterations in dietary preferences may require deviations from accepted patterns of food intake and may be perceived as demanding increased skills, costs, or efforts in preparation.[67] In one study, only one fifth of the subjects chose diets for reasons of health; this group tended to be older, better educated, and of higher income.[68] National data on food availability and dietary intake support these results. For example, the major sources of saturated fat in the U.S. diet are meat (which contributes 35% of total saturated fat), dairy foods (20%), and fats and oils (34%).[69] Advice to consume no more than 10% of total energy as saturated fat requires consumers to eat less red meat, to select low-fat dairy foods, and to replace energy contributed by fats and oils with that from fruits, vegetables, and grains.

Food availability data (an indirect measure of dietary intake) do show increases in use of fruits and vegetables and they reveal significant replacement of whole with skim milk and butter with margarine. The level of availability of saturated fat in the U.S. food supply, however, has remained relatively constant, largely because of increased use of meat mixtures, cheese, and frozen desserts. The availability of total fat in the U.S. food supply has risen steadily throughout this century; virtually all of this increase can be accounted for by greater use of vegetable fats in salad dressings and table spreads.[69]

Trends in actual dietary intake are more difficult to evaluate due to methodologic differences among the various surveys. To the extent that determination is possible, levels of intake of total and saturated fat did not change significantly between the early 1970s and 1985.[65,70,71] One analysis has demonstrated that on a given day of dietary evaluation, more than 40% of respondents ate red meat or luncheon meats, but more than 40% ate no fruit, 15% to 25% ate no vegetables, and only 16% ate a high-fiber bread or cereal.[72]

Such observations reflect the environment of food intake in the United States. Consumers are increasingly well-informed about nutrition and health, and they will, on occasion, choose diets based on this information. On a daily basis, however, convenience in eating takes precedence over nutritional quality; meals are increasingly consumed from restaurant, fast food, and take-out establishments; and the food industry actively produces, markets, and advertises alcohol and foods high in calories, fat, cholesterol, sugar, and salt. This type of environment calls for public health approaches to needs assessment and planning and implementation of nutrition programs.

TABLE 61-4. EXAMPLES OF POPULATION SURVEY ELEMENTS FOR NUTRITIONAL STATUS EVALUATION

Nutritional History	Medical History and Physical
▪ **Dietary Intake**	▪ **Signs of Undernutrition**
Food record	Low weight-for-height
24-hour recall	Recent weight loss
Food frequency	Clinical signs of malnutrition
Diet history	Chronic or acute conditions that increase nutrient requirements or needs
Use of supplements	Medication use
Eating habits	Substance abuse
▪ **Related Social Factors**	▪ **Chronic Disease Risk**
Income	Elevated blood glucose
Educational level	High blood pressure
Ethnicity	High blood cholesterol
Use of food assistance	Overweight
Medications	
Activity levels	
Anthropometric Measurements	**Laboratory Tests**
Height	Hemoglobin, hematocrit
Weight	Iron and iron-binding
Skinfolds	Serum vitamin and mineral levels
Head circumference	Serum albumin
Elbow breadth	Blood glucose
Waist circumference	Blood cholesterol
Bioelectrical impedence	Lipoproteins

NOTE: See references 1, 76, 81, 83.

ASSESSMENT OF NUTRITIONAL STATUS

As in any other public health campaign, the first step in development of a dietary intervention is to identify the nutritional problems and therefore the needs of the population at risk. As noted earlier, malnutrition includes not only deficiency conditions resulting from chronic or specific inadequacies in food or nutrient intake but also conditions of excessive or unbalanced food or nutrient intake.[73] Evaluation of either form of malnutrition is complicated by the many genetic, medical, behavioral, and environmental factors that influence development of diet-related conditions, by the multiplicity of signs and symptoms of malnutrition, by the lack of suitable biochemical or clinical markers for many of these signs and symptoms,[1,2] and by lack of precision in available assessment methods.[74,75] Assessment is also complicated by the variety of personal, cultural, socioeconomic, health, and environmental factors that influence food intake.[14]

Assessment Methods: Individuals and Populations. At the present time, no single, independent measurement of dietary, biochemical, or clinical status has been found sufficient to indicate the nutritional status of individuals or populations. Instead, nutritional risk is defined by a combination of methods: nutritional history, medical history and physical examination, anthropometric measurements, and laboratory tests.[76] Table 61–4 lists examples of components of these methods used in population surveys. In practice, surveys rarely use the full range of nutritional assessment methods; many of them are too imprecise, inconvenient, or expensive for frequent use. Most assessments are based on clinical or professional judgment of the severity of selected nutritional risk factors.

Short of duplicate meal analysis, no ideal method exists to determine the usual dietary intake of individuals. Standard techniques produce approximations that cannot be interpreted too literally; they include a record of foods consumed during a specified time period (Food Record), retrospective recall of foods consumed within a recent time period (24-Hour Recall, or longer), and measures of the frequency of consumption of specific index foods (Food Frequencies). The nutrient content of diets described by these methods is obtained from tables of food composition and compared to standards of nutrient intake such as the RDAs[4] or to patterns of food consumption described by dietary goals[34] and guidelines.[39]

Each of these methods, used singly or in combination, has strengths and weaknesses. All yield useful, if imprecise, information.[74] Demographic and socioeconomic data are especially useful as indirect indicators of nutritional risk in community surveys where detailed diet histories, physical examinations, and laboratory tests would be impractical.

The simplest and most useful indication of undernutrition in individuals or populations is low weight for height. Other clinical signs listed in Table 61–4 are useful for assessment of the nutritional status of hospital patients.[17] Evaluation of chronic disease risk is accomplished through measurements of blood glucose, blood pressure, blood cholesterol, and body weight. The high prevalence of these risk factors is the basis of large-scale campaigns to reduce them.[47,77] The fact that no simple screen is as yet available for evaluation of diet-related cancer risk is one reason for promotion of healthier diets as a prevention strategy.[43–45]

National Nutrition Monitoring System. In the United States the prevalence of conditions of malnutrition and of dietary and other risk factors for these conditions is determined through a series of national surveys known collectively as the National Nutrition Monitoring System. This system presently includes about 40 separate surveys that measure health and nutritional status, food and nutrient consumption, food composition, dietary knowledge and attitudes, foods available for purchase, and sociodemographic and economic indicators related to dietary intake.[78] Nevertheless, the system is incomplete and fails to provide adequate data on trends in dietary intake patterns, hunger prevalence, and dietary patterns of minority groups.[79] It also has been criticized for delays in coordinating data collection and in reporting results.[80]

The most comprehensive of these surveys is the National Health and Nutrition Examination Survey (NHANES) which collects data from dietary interviews, physical examinations, and biochemical and hematological tests conducted on a large probability sample of the U.S. population. NHANES surveys were conducted in 1971 to 1974 (NHANES I) and 1976 to 1980 (NHANES II). NHANES III, which eventually will interview 40,000 persons over the age of 2 months, and examine 30,000 of them, began in 1988. When completed, it will provide data on even more data elements than those listed in Table 61–4.[81]

Community Nutrition Assessment. Methods for assessment of the nutritional needs of communities vary only slightly from conventional means of community health assessment. Table 61–5 lists the principal data elements used to evaluate the level of nutritional risk in communities. These elements include geographical, demographic, socioeconomic, and health descriptors. They also include descriptors of food and nutrition resources in the community, utilization rates for such resources, and indicators of food availability, intake, and nutritional status as obtained from nutrition monitoring surveys.

In developing countries with high rates of clinically-apparent conditions of undernutrition, investigators have selected elements from this list to develop rapid, convenient, and relatively inexpensive screening instruments to evaluate nutritional risk under field conditions.[82] These methods, which range from a graded series of bracelets to measure arm circumference to comprehensive surveys, have been used successfully to identify children at high nutritional risk who can be targeted for intervention.[83]

Since the early 1980s, more than 200 communities in the United States have correlated data on poverty levels, nonparticipation of eligible persons in food assistance programs, and the rapid expansion of private-sector soup kitchens and food pantries to document the need for expansion of federal food assistance programs.[84] Also in the United States, encouragement of local screening campaigns for high blood cholesterol is a key implementation strategy of the National Cholesterol Education Program.[77]

POLICY RECOMMENDATIONS AND IMPLEMENTATION STRATEGIES

The quantity, strength, and consistency of evidence that relates dietary factors to chronic diseases, and the substantial impact of these conditions on health, are reasons enough to promote policies to improve the availability of healthy diets. As outlined in the *Surgeon General's Report,* new policies are needed to address environmental as well as behavioral barriers to dietary change. These policies need to be directed not only to the general public and to individuals at risk of chronic disease but also to health professionals, health care service providers, the foodservice industry, food manufacturers, the government, and research investigators.[25,48]

The General Public. Education of individuals has been demonstrated to improve nutrition knowledge, attitude, and behavior[85] and to help reduce chronic disease risk factors.[67] The most effective counseling involves subjects in the design, conduct, and evaluation of their own dietary plans, employs multiple educational strategies, and uses a team approach.[86] In the United States, broad public health campaigns such as the National High Blood Pressure Education Program have proven effective[47,87]; the National Cholesterol Education Program[77] and the Kaiser Family Foundation's Project LEAN[88] also have the potential to reduce dietary risks among large segments of the population. These separate drives to reduce distinct chronic disease risk factors could well be joined into a single, universal campaign that encourages the public to follow overall dietary recommendations and to increase daily levels of physical activity.

High-Risk Groups. Pregnant women, infants, young children, and the elderly are most vulnerable to nutritional deficiencies, especially when they are poor. Members of racial and ethnic minority groups bear a disproportionate burden not only of undernutrition but also of chronic disease—largely as a consequence of poverty, inadequate access to health care, and educational disadvantage.[89] The contribution of diet to chronic disease risk in these groups is difficult to evaluate. Available data do not permit identification of consistent associations between dietary

TABLE 61–5. DATA ELEMENTS FOR COMMUNITY NUTRITION ASSESSMENT

▪ COMMUNITY DESCRIPTORS	**▪ NUTRITIONAL STATUS INDICATORS**
Geographical boundaries, area	See Table 61–4
Population within boundaries, density	
Community agencies and services	**▪ FOOD AND NUTRITION RESOURCES**
Community health care programs and services	Federal food assistance programs
Hospitals and clinics	Utilization rates
Educational institutions	Non-participation rates for eligible persons
	Community food assistance programs
▪ POPULATION DESCRIPTORS	Soup kitchens
Age, gender, racial, and ethnic distribution	Food pantries
Income level	Food banks
Educational level	Food markets
Employment level	Supermarkets
Length of time in location	Grocery stores
Primary language	Farmers' markets
Health status indicators	Food service institutions
Infant mortality	Nutrition education and training programs
Low infant birthweight	Food and nutrition advocacy groups
Life expectancy	Food assistance outreach programs
Leading causes of death	Weight control programs
Chronic disease rates	Worksite wellness programs

Adapted from Simko, Cowell, Gilbride, 1984, p 49.[76]

patterns and disease risk in minority populations; they also find few consistent differences in dietary intake patterns between minority and majority populations.[90]

Community-based, media-oriented public education ("social marketing") campaigns[91] that transmit culturally-sensitive messages[92] designed to address the needs and attitudes of specific target groups have been applied successfully to promote breast-feeding and other dietary improvements in developing countries.[93] In the United States, these techniques have been used to improve the nutritional status of low-income homemakers,[94] to increase the prevalence of breast-feeding,[95] and to improve health and function in the elderly.[96] Preliminary results of dietary intervention studies that apply these techniques to chronic disease prevention among high-risk minority groups also show promise.[97,98] In the long term, education methods that empower community members to determine their own dietary needs and interventions have been demonstrated to be most likely to prove effective.[99]

Health Professionals. Despite prolonged public, professional, and governmental demands for expanded and improved nutrition training of physicians and other health professionals, progress has been slow.[100] The necessary curriculum is well established: basic principles of nutrition, the role of diet in disease prevention, methods for assessment of nutritional status, therapeutic diets, behavioral aspects of dietary counseling, and the role of nutritionists in health care.[25] The increasing focus on disease prevention as a cost containment strategy may stimulate more rapid progress in this area.[101]

Health Care Providers. Nutrition services should be integrated into health care delivery programs as routine components of patient care. Services should include dietary counseling and prescription, referral to community nutrition and food assistance programs, and monitoring of patient progress. Programs also should address barriers that prevent access to such services[102] and that reduce the effectiveness of organization and delivery of nutritional care.[103]

The Food Service Industry. The trend toward eating meals away from home illustrates the need to shift the targets of dietary recommendations from homemakers to food providers—restaurants, schools, worksites, hospitals, nursing homes, child care centers, and other institutions. With this shift, the nutritional quality of institutional food service takes on increasing importance. Industry experts state that meals served in restaurants increasingly reflect health concerns, and they believe that this trend is likely to continue.[104] In food service institutions less driven by such market considerations, implementation of dietary recommendations may well require federal intervention or other incentives, especially since improvements are likely to require substantial education and training of kitchen personnel.

Food Manufacturers. The interest of consumers in health is one factor that motivates development of new food products,[60] but the food industry needs to be encouraged to take greater responsibility for increasing the production and marketability of foods that contribute to healthy diets. Mandatory food labeling, public education campaigns, and similar incentives ought to accelerate industry acceptance of such responsibility.

The Government

Food Labels. Because consumers rely on food labels to decide which dietary factors to choose or to avoid, mandatory nutrition labeling should encourage food manufacturers to improve their products. Labeling policies that require information about key nutrients in chronic disease prevention—energy, fat, saturated fat, cholesterol, salt, and others—are under consideration in the United States and elsewhere.[105,106] Health claims on labels have been shown to promote sales,[107] but such claims have been opposed by nutrition professionals concerned about possibilities for misleading the public.[108]

Food Assistance Programs. All individuals should have access to a sufficient and appropriate diet, and many developing countries support policies and programs that improve the availability of food to their populations.[9,10,23] In the United States, despite federal expenditures of more than $21 billion annually for USDA programs alone,[109] the demand for food assistance has increased greatly within the last decade.[110] Participation in several federal food assistance programs has been shown to result in significant health benefits.[111,112] Methods to fund expansion of these programs and to improve their accessibility and availability have been described and promoted by advocacy groups.[113]

Nutrition Monitoring. National health surveillance systems should collect more systematic data on food availability, dietary intake, and the nutritional status of the general population and of targeted high-risk groups[114] in order to establish a rational foundation for development of public policies in education, services, and research. In the United States, legislation to require coordination of the major dietary intake surveys and to focus responsibility for them, under consideration since 1984, was adopted in 1990.[79,115]

Research Investigators. The recent comprehensive reviews of research on diet and chronic disease highlight many areas in need of further investigation. Of particular public health relevance are determination of the childhood dietary pattern that best prevents chronic disease later in life, elucidation of effective methods to delay the development of chronic diseases in older adults, and identification of the most effective educational methods to help the public translate dietary messages into appropriate food choices.[25,26]

REFERENCES

1. Shils ME, Young VR (eds): Modern Nutrition in Health and Disease, 7edt. Philadelphia: Lea & Febiger, 1988
2. Passmore R, Eastwood MA: Davidson and Passmore Human Nutrition and Dietetics, 8edt. Edinburgh: Churchill-Livingstone, 1986
3. Mertz W: The essential trace elements. Science 213:1332–1338, 1981
4. National Research Council, Food and Nutrition Board: Recommended Dietary Allowances, 10edt. Washington, DC: National Academy of Sciences, 1989
5. Committee 1-5 of the International Union of Nutritional Sciences: Recommended dietary intakes around the world. Nutr Abstracts Rev 53:939–1015, 1075–1119, 1983
6. Gussow JD, Thomas PR: The Nutrition Debate: Sorting Out Some Answers. Palo Alto, Calif: Bull, 1986
7. Rosenberg IH (ed): Minisymposium: Behind and beyond the Recommended Dietary Allowances. Am J Clin Nutr 41:139–170, 1985
8. Marshall E: The Academy kills a nutrition report. Science 230:420–421, 1985
9. The World Bank: Poverty and Hunger: Issues and Options for Food Security in Developing Countries. Washington, DC: The World Bank, 1986
10. Austin JE: Nutrition Programs in the Third World: Cases and Readings. Cambridge, Mass: Oelgeschlager, Gunn & Hain, 1981
11. Chen LC: Interactions of diarrhea and malnutrition: mechanisms and interventions. In Chen LC, Scrimshaw NS (eds): Diarrhea and Malnutrition: Interactions, Mechanisms, and Interventions. New York: Plenum, 1983, pp 3–22
12. Grant JP: The State of the World's Children. New York: Oxford University Press (UNICEF), 1989
13. Brown JL: Hunger in the U.S. Sci Am 256(2):37–41, 1987

14. U.S. Department of Health and Human Services and U.S. Department of Agriculture: Nutrition Monitoring in the United States—An Update Report on Nutrition Monitoring. Washington, DC: U.S. Government Printing Office DHHS Publication No. (PHS) 89-1255, 1989
15. Petersen KE, Chen LC: Defining undernutrition for public health purposes in the United States. J Nutr 120:933–942, 1990
16. Insititute of Medicine, Committee to Study the Prevention of Low Birthweight: Preventing Low Birthweight. Washington, DC: National Academy Press, 1985
17. Roubenoff R, Roubenoff RA, Preto J, Balke CW: Malnutrition among hospitalized patients: a problem of physician awareness. Arch Intern Med 147:1462–1465, 1987
18. Letsou AP, Price LS: Health, aging, and nutrition: an overview. Clin Geriatr Med 3:253–260, 1987
19. Roe DA, Moragne L: Roles of nutrition educators in substance abuse prevention and rehabilitation programs. J Nutr Educ 19:186–189, 1987
20. Kerndt PR, Naughton JL, Driscoll CE, et al: Fasting: the history, pathophysiology, and complications. West J Med 137:379–399, 1982
21. Beisel WT: Nutrition, infection, specific immune responses, and nonspecific host defenses: a complex interaction. In Watson RR (ed): Nutrition, Disease Resistance, and Immune Function. New York: Dekker, 1984, pp 3–34
22. Coward WA, Lunn PG: The biochemistry and physiology of kwashiorkor and marasmus. Brit Med Bull 37(1):19–24, 1981
23. Scrimshaw NS, Wallerstein MB (eds): Nutrition Policy Implementation: Issues and Experience. New York: Plenum, 1982
24. Bell DE, Reich MR (eds): Health, Nutrition, and Economic Crises: Approaches to Policy in the Third World. Dover, Mass: Auburn House, 1988
25. Department of Health and Human Services, Public Health Service. The Surgeon General's Report on Nutrition and Health. Washington, DC: U.S. Government Printing Office DHHS (PHS) Publication No. 88-50210, 1988
26. National Research Council: Diet and Health: Implications for Reducing Chronic Disease Risk. Washington, DC: National Academy Press, 1989
27. James WPT: Healthy Nutrition: Preventing Nutrition-Related Diseases in Europe. WHO Regional Publications, European Series, No 24. Copenhagen: World Health Organization, 1988
28. National Center for Health Statistics: Advance report of final mortality statistics, 1988. Monthly Vital Stat Rep 37:1–10, 1988
29. Doll R, Peto R: The causes of cancer: quantitative estimates of avoidable risks of cancer in the United States today. JNCI 66:1191–1308, 1981
30. Goldman L, Cook EF: The decline in ischemic heart disease mortality rates: an analysis of the comparative effects of medical interventions and changes in life-style. Ann Intern Med 101:825–836, 1984
31. Block G: A review of validations of dietary assessment methods. Am J Epidemiol 115:492–505, 1982
32. Lilienfeld AM, Lilienfeld DE: Foundations of Epidemiology, 2edt. New York: Oxford Press, 1980
33. Houghton B, Gussow JD, Dodds JM: A historical study of the underlying assumptions for United States food guides from 1917 through the basic four food group guide. J Nutr Educ 19:169–176, 1987
34. Select Committee on Nutrition and Human Needs, United States Senate: Dietary Goals for the United States, 2edt. Washington, DC: U.S. Government Printing Office, 1977
35. Select Committee on Nutrition and Human Needs, United States Senate: Dietary Goals for the United States—Supplemental Views. Washington, DC: U.S. Government Printing Office, 1977
36. U.S. Department of Health, Education, and Welfare. Healthy People: The Surgeon General's Report on Disease Prevention and Health Promotion. Washington, DC: U.S. Government Printing Office DHEW (PHS) 79-55071, 1979
37. U.S. Department of Health and Human Services: Promoting Health/Prevention Disease: Objectives for the Nation. Washington, DC: U.S. Government Printing Office, 1980
38. Nestle M: Promoting health and preventing disease: national objectives for 1990 and 2000. Food Technol 42:103–106, 1988
39. U.S. Department of Agriculture, U.S. Department of Health and Human Services: Nutrition and Your Health: Dietary Guidelines for Americans. Washington, DC: U.S. Government Printing Office, 1990
40. American Medical Association Council on Scientific Affairs: Dietary and pharmacologic therapy for the lipid risk factors. JAMA 250:1873–1879, 1983
41. NIH Consensus Conference: Lowering blood cholesterol to prevent heart disease. JAMA 253:2080–2086, 1985
42. American Heart Association: Dietary guidelines for healthy American adults: a statement for physicians and health professionals by the Nutrition Committee, American Heart Association. Circulation. 77:721A–724A, 1988
43. National Research Council, Food and Nutrition Board: Diet, Nutrition, and Cancer. Washington, DC: National Academy Press, 1983
44. American Cancer Society: Special report: nutrition and cancer: cause and prevention. CA-Cancer J Clinicians 34 (2):121–126, 1984
45. Butrum R, Clifford CK, Lanza E: NCI dietary guidelines: rationale. Am J Clin Nutr 48:888–895, 1988
46. American Diabetes Association: Nutritional recommendations and principles for individuals with diabetes mellitus: 1986. Diabetes Care 10:126–132, 1987
47. Joint National Committee on Detection, Evaluation, and Treatment of High Blood Pressure. The 1988 report. Arch Intern Med 148:1023–1038, 1988
48. McGinnis JM, Nestle M: The Surgeon General's report on nutrition and health: policy implications and implementation strategies. Am J Clin Nutr 49:23–28, 1989
49. Axelson ML: The impact of culture on food-related behavior. Annu Rev Nutr 6:345–363, 1986
50. Rozin P, Vollmecke TA: Food likes and dislikes. Annu Rev Nutr 4:433–456, 1986
51. Pliner P: Family resemblance in food preference. J Nutr Educ 15:137–140, 1983
52. Rolls BJ: Sensory-specific satiety. Nutr Rev 44:93–101, 1986
53. Manchester A, Lipton KL: The food system: a century of transition. Natl Food Rev 28:1–6, 1985
54. Food Marketing Institute: Historical data. Washington, DC: The Institute 1987, p 207
55. Record new product intros in 1987. Food Inst Rep Jan 16:3, 1988
56. Clancy KL, Helitzer DL: Food advertising. In Weininger J, Briggs GM (eds): Nutr Update 1:357–379, 1983
57. Gallo AE, Connor JM: How advertising affects U.S. food consumption. CNI Weekly Rep 12 (42):4–5, 1982
58. Top 100 advertisers by primary business. Advertising Age; Sept 28:152, 1988
59. U.S. Department of Commerce, Bureau of Census: Statistical Abstracts of the United States, 109 edt. Washington, DC: U.S. Government Printing Office, 1989 p 386
60. Przybyla AE: Driving forces behind 1986 new food introductions. Food Engineering Apr:61–80, 1987
61. Bunch KL: Food away from home and the quality of the diet. Natl Food Rev 25:14–16, 1984
62. U.S. food marketing sales rise 4 percent. Natl Food Rev 11 (4):45, 1988
63. Price C: Take-out food in convenience stores. Natl Food Rev 11 (4):14–17, 1988
64. Best D: Shelf-stable dinner helpers. Prepared Foods Oct:152–156, 1987
65. U.S. Department of Agriculture. Nationwide Food Consumption Survey, Continuing Survey of Food Intakes by Individuals: Women 19–50 Years and Their Children 1–5 Years, 1 Day. Report 85-1. Hyattsville, Md: USDA, 1985

66. Schucker B, Bailey K, Heimbach JT et al: Change in public perspective on cholesterol and heart disease: results from two national surveys. JAMA 258:3527–3531, 1987
67. Glanz K: Nutrition education for risk factor reduction and patient education: a review. Prev Med 14:721–752, 1985
68. "What's cookin.' " Eating behavior trends revealed in Pillsbury study. Quirk's Marketing Res Rev June/July:14–44, 1988
69. U.S. Department of Agriculture: Nutrient content of the U.S. food supply. Tables of nutrients and foods provided by the U.S. food supply. Hyattsville, Md: USDA HNIS Adm Rep 299–21, 1988
70. Abraham S, Carroll MD: Fats, cholesterol, and sodium intake in the diet of persons 1–74 years: United States. NCHS Advance Data 54 (Feb 27):1–11, 1981
71. Block G, Rosenberger W, Patterson BH: Calories, fat and cholesterol: intake patterns in the U.S. population by race, sex and age. AJPH 78:1150–1155, 1988
72. Patterson BH, Block G: Food choices and the cancer guidelines. AJPH 78:282–286, 1988
73. Jelliffe DB: The Assessment of the Nutritional Status of the Community. Geneva: World Health Organization, 1966
74. Pao EM, Cypel YS: Estimation of dietary intake. In Brown ML (ed): Present Knowledge in Nutrition, 6edt. Washington, DC: International Life Sciences Institute Nutrition Foundation, 1990, pp 399–406
75. Garry PJ, Koehler KM: Problems in Interpretation of Dietary and Biochemical Data from Population Studies. In Brown ML (ed): Present Knowledge in Nutrition, 6edt. Washington, DC: International Life Sciences Institute Nutrition Foundation, 1990, pp 407–414
76. Simko MD, Cowell C, Gilbride JA: Nutrition Assessment: A Comprehensive Guide for Planning Intervention. Rockville, Md: Aspen Publishers, Inc., 1984
77. National Cholesterol Education Program: Report of the National Cholesterol Education Program expert panel on detection, evaluation, and treatment of high blood cholesterol in adults. Arch Intern Med 148:36–68, 1988
78. U.S. Department of Health and Human Services and U.S. Department of Agriculture: Nutrition Monitoring in the United States: The Directory of Federal Nutrition Monitoring Activities. Hyattsville, Md: National Center for Health Statistics DHHS Publication No. (PHS) 89–1255–1, Sept 1989
79. Nestle M: National nutrition monitoring policy: the continuing need for legislative intervention. J Nutr Educ 22:141–144, 1990
80. Woteki CE, Fanelli-Kuczmarski MT: National Nutrition Monitoring System. In Brown ML (ed): Present Knowledge in Nutrition, 6edt. Washington, DC: International Life Sciences Institute Nutrition Foundation, 1990, pp 415–429
81. Woteki CE, Briefel RR, Kuczmarski R: Contributions of the National Center for Health Statistics. Am J Clin Nutr 47:320–328, 1988
82. Rapid nutrition evaluation in drought-affected regions of Somalia—1987. JAMA 259:1928–1929, 1988
83. Beghin I, Cap M, Dujardin B: Health and Community: A Guide to Nutritional Assessment. Geneva: World Health Organization, 1988
84. Cohen BE, Burt MR: Eliminating Hunger: Food Security Policy for the 1990s. Washington, DC: The Urban Institute, 1989
85. Johnson DW, Johnson RT: Nutrition education: a model for effectiveness, a synthesis of research. J Nutr Educ 17 (2 suppl):S1–S44, 1985
86. U.S. Preventive Services Task Force: Guide to Clinical Preventive Services. Baltimore, Md: The Williams and Wilkins Company, 1989
87. Roccella EJ, Bowler AE, Ames MV, Horan MG: Hypertension knowledge, attitudes, and behavior: 1985 NHIS findings. Pub Health Rep 101:599–606, 1986
88. ProjectLEAN: The LEAN Letter. Menlo Park, Calif: Kaiser Family Foundation, Apr 1989
89. Heckler M: Report of the Secretary's Task Force on Black and Minority Health. Washington, DC: U.S. Department of Health and Human Services, 1985
90. Kumanyika S: Diet and chronic disease issues for minority populations. J Nutr Educ 22:89–96, 1990
91. Israel RC: Operational Guidelines for Social Marketing Projects in Public Health and Nutrition. Paris: UNESCO, 1987
92. U.S. Department of Agriculture and U.S. Department of Health and Human Services: Cross-cultural Counseling: A Guide for Nutrition and Health Counselors. Alexandria, Va: USDA FNS–250, 1986
93. Manoff RK: Social Marketing: New Imperative for Public Health. New York: Praeger, 1985
94. Amstutz MK, Dixon DL: Dietary changes resulting from the Expanded Food and Nutrition Education Program. J Nutr Educ 18:55–60, 1986
95. Cadwallader AA, Olson CM: Use of a breast-feeding intervention by nutrition paraprofessionals. J Nutr Educ 18:117–122, 1986
96. Maloney S: Setting the pace in geriatric health promotion. In Abdellah FG, Moore SR (eds): Surgeon General's Workshop on Health Promotion and Aging, Proceedings. Washington, DC: Office of the Surgeon General, 1988
97. Pasick RJ: Health Promotion for Minorities in California: A Report to the East Bay Area Health Education Center. Berkeley, Calif: Western Consortium for Public Health, 1987
98. Glanz K, Lewis FM, Rimer BK (eds): Health Behavior and Health Education: Theory, Research, and Practice. San Francisco: Jossey-Bass, 1990, pp 161–186, 288–313
99. Kent G: Nutrition education as an instrument of empowerment. J Nutr Educ 20:193–195, 1988
100. National Research Council: Nutrition Education in U.S. Medical Schools. Washington, DC: National Academy Press, 1985
101. Nestle M: Nutrition in medical education: new policies needed for the 1990s. J Nutr Educ 20 (1 suppl):S1–S6, 1988
102. Egan MC: Public health nutrition services: issues today and tomorrow. J Am Dietet Assoc 77:423–427, 1980
103. Vermersch J (ed): Nutrition services in state and local public health agencies. Pub Health Rep 98:7–20, 1983
104. 1990 National Restaurant Association Forecast. Washington, DC: National Restaurant Association, 1990
105. Crane NT, Behlen PM, Yetley EA, Vanderveen JE: Nutrition labeling of foods: A global perspective. Nutr Today, Jul-Aug 1990, pp 28–35
106. Nutritional labelling of foods: A rational approach to banding. Lancet 2:469, 1986
107. Levy AS, Stokes RC: Effects of a health promotion advertising campaign on sales of ready-to-eat cereals. Pub Health Rep 102:398–403, 1987
108. American Dietetic Association: Health claims on food labels. J Am Diet Assoc 86:527–528, 1988
109. Matsumoto M: Recent trends in domestic food programs. Natl Food Rev 14(1):31–32, 1991
110. House Select Committee on Hunger: Food security in the United States: the Measurement of Hunger. Washington, DC: U.S. House of Representatives, March 1989
111. Zee P, DeLeon M, Roberson P, Chen C-H: Nutritional improvement of poor urban preschool children: a 1983–1977 comparison. JAMA 253:3269–3272, 1985
112. Rush D, et al: The National WIC evaluation: evaluation of the Special Supplemental Food Program for Women, Infants, and Children. Am J Clin Nutr 48:389–519, 1988
113. Food Research and Action Center and National Anti-Hunger Coalition: Hunger in the Eighties: A Primer. Washington, DC: The Coalition, 1984
114. Anderson SA (ed): Core indicators of nutritional state for difficult-to-sample populations. J Nutr 120(11S):1555–1600
115. Shipley-Moses E, Dodds JM: Nutrition surveillance and monitoring. J Nutr Educ 19:125–127, 1987

62

Dental Public Health

R. Gary Rozier

The mouth contains a number of different tissues, some of which are found throughout the body. As a result of infection, trauma, degeneration, or neoplastic changes, these tissues can be affected by up to 265 categories of diseases or conditions.[1] Of greatest importance to oral health are two specialized tissues: the teeth and their supporting (periodontal) structures. The majority of oral health services are directed toward the prevention and control of diseases and conditions affecting these two tissues.

Oral diseases are important considerations in public health and preventive dentistry for several reasons. First, they are of almost universal prevalence. Rarely if ever does anyone go unaffected by at least one of these diseases, and most people are affected by several during their lifetimes. Second, most oral diseases do not undergo remission or termination if left untreated, as do many diseases, but accumulate a backlog of unmet needs that can ultimately end in loss of teeth. Third, these diseases usually require technically demanding, expensive, and time-consuming professional treatment. Finally, oral diseases are important for consideration in public health because they are in large measure preventable. Through a rich tradition of research and development, dentistry has at its disposal a large and sound science base for use in the prevention and control of most oral conditions, particularly dental caries and periodontal diseases. Available community and individual strategies, if fully implemented and maintained, could reduce dental caries and periodontal diseases to insignificant levels in society.

Evidence available since the mid 1970s clearly indicates that oral health promotion and disease prevention services implemented in industrialized countries beginning in the 1940s have had a dramatic effect on disease levels, particularly in children. Yet similar information suggests that further improvements in oral disease prevention are necessary to eliminate the continuing effects of disease on an excessive number of individuals.[2] These diseases have significant economic, social and health consequences. Expenditures for dental care in the United States totaled more than $29.4 billion in 1988.[3] In a given year, dental-related illnesses can account for 6.4 million days of bed disability, 14.3 million days of restricted activity, and 20.9 million lost work days.[4]

The purpose of this chapter is to review the magnitude of oral diseases and the strategies available for their prevention and control. The focus will be on dental caries, periodontal diseases and oral cancers: dental caries and periodontal diseases because of their widespread nature and the effectiveness of available prevention strategies, and oral cancers because of their devastating effects. Other oral health problems such as occlusion or problems resulting from trauma to the mouth or face are not considered in this chapter but are nevertheless important considerations in any comprehensive public health program.

DENTAL CARIES

Pathogenesis. Dental caries is generally defined as a localized destruction of teeth. The destruction of enamel, which is 95% inorganic material hydroxyapatite, is caused mainly by organic acids produced by microorganisms on the tooth surface that ferment carbohydrates, particularly sugars. In the dentin, which contains about 20% collagenlike organic material, the demineralization is accompanied by a digestion of the organic structure. These microorganisms are organized into plaque, a soft, sticky film that coats the teeth. Some microorganisms are more important than others in the pathogenesis of dental caries, supporting a specific plaque hypothesis.[5] *Streptococcus mutans* is generally associated with the initial development of coronal caries, lactobacilli with the further development of the lesion, and *Actinomyces* with root surface caries.

The interrelationships of the multiple factors involved in the etiology of dental caries are depicted in Figure 62–1.[6,7] Only when all of these three factors, a susceptible surface, caries-specific bacteria, and a substrate or diet, are present and interacting for a sufficient length of time does dental caries develop. This model should be kept firmly in mind in the prevention and control of dental caries, since prevention strategies must be directed toward one or more of these factors.

The different surfaces of the teeth are at different risks for caries attack. The occlusal, or biting surfaces of the crowns of teeth, are at high risk and are usually affected first, because microorganisms become entrapped in the pits and fissures soon after the teeth erupt into the mouth, and the microorganisms cannot be removed with oral hygiene methods. Smooth crown surfaces are affected soon thereafter and are particularly protected by fluorides. Root surface caries is generally confined to exposed root surfaces and therefore occurs later in life. The occurrence of root surface caries is dependent on previous periodontal disease causing a loss of periodontal structures and exposure of tooth cementum.

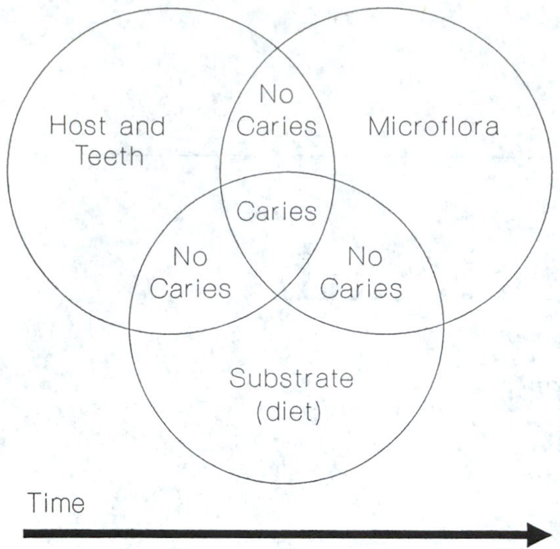

Figure 62-1. Etiologic model for dental caries. *[Adapted from Keyes, 1962,[6] and Newbrun, 1989.[7]]*

Nursing caries is a specific form of rampant decay affecting the primary teeth in preschool children.[8] Its clinical appearance is unique because the maxillary incisors show the greatest carious destruction while the mandibular incisors show the least. This pattern of decay is due in part to the protection that the tongue affords the mandibular incisors during infant sucking. Nursing caries is further characterized by very rapid development and the involvement of many primary teeth. The process results from the use of cariogenic solutions such as milk sweetened with sugar, sugared water, fruit juices, and carbonated or noncarbonated beverages in the nursing bottle or from the use of a pacifier sweetened with a substance such as honey. Nursing is usually for prolonged periods of time, particularly at night, resulting in an unremitting cariogenic attack caused by the constant supply of fermentable carbohydrates.

Epidemiology. Several exciting developments in the epidemiology of dental caries have occurred since the mid 1970s. First, and perhaps most significant, has been a decline in the prevalence of dental caries, affecting large numbers of children and young adults from around the world. The second is the increased study of various types of dental caries other than coronal caries, such as nursing caries and root surface caries. Third, with the study of the decline of coronal caries, the distribution of caries within population groups has come under closer scrutiny, resulting in the knowledge that most incidences of the disease are concentrated in a small percentage of children. With this finding has come increased attention to the study of risk indicators, beginning confirmation of some of these indicators as risk factors through longitudinal epidemiological studies, and consideration of the use of targeting for the delivery of oral health services.

Measurement of Dental Caries for Epidemiological Studies. Dental epidemiologists have developed reliable and valid clinical measures for coronal caries in the primary and permanent dentitions.[9] Dental caries is universally measured by the DMF Tooth (T) or Surface (S) Index.[10] Each of the 32 permanent tooth spaces is scored as to whether it is normal or has been diseased. If ever diseased, the tooth must exhibit one of three conditions: (1) it may be untreated (decayed); (2) show evidence of surgical treatment (missing); (3) show evidence of restorative treatment (filled). The DMF index for an individual is the sum of either teeth or surfaces having these three conditions. The index is appealing because it is nonreversible and determines someone's lifetime experience with caries. The index does become less valid in adults because teeth may be missing for reasons other than dental caries, primarily periodontal diseases and the extraction of remaining sound teeth for placement of dentures. For the primary teeth, the index is modified to include only decayed (d) and filled (f) teeth. The df tooth or surface index does not include missing teeth because of the difficulty in distinguishing primary teeth lost as a result of caries from those lost by natural exfoliation.

Compared to coronal caries, there is less consensus on diagnostic criteria and reporting for root caries.[11,12] Nevertheless, indices are available and consensus is beginning to emerge as measurement issues are debated and investigators gain more field experience in their use.[13] Reporting of the condition is generally based on the number of exposed root surfaces decayed or filled, with some consideration of the number of surfaces present in the mouth and at risk to caries.

Trends. The World Health Organization Global Oral Health Data Bank, initiated in 1969, has identified three different worldwide trends in dental caries.[14-18] The first clear trend affecting large numbers of countries was identified in 1974 and signalled an increase in caries prevalence in developing countries, particularly in urban centers. Increases were noted in countries such as American Samoa, Ethiopia, Jordan, Nigeria, Thailand, Uganda, and Zambia. For the first time ever, children in developing countries, where 80% of the world's children live, were found to have a higher prevalence of dental caries than those in industrialized countries.[19] In most Third World populations, dental caries can now be considered an ubiquitous disease.[20]

The second clear trend emerged from the WHO Data Bank in 1978 and was confirmed by other sources of data at approximately the same time. Industrialized countries, known to have high rates of dental caries, were found to be experiencing a decline. This second group of countries has received a considerable amount of study during the 1980s. At the First International Conference on the Declining Prevalence of Dental Caries, reports from nine countries (Denmark, England, Ireland, Netherlands, New Zealand, Norway, Scotland, Sweden, United States) were presented.[21] Based on this conference, our knowledge of these trends has been summarized as follows: 1) the number of decayed and missing permanent teeth has declined dramatically, while the number of filled teeth has increased moderately; 2) caries prevalence in primary teeth has also declined; 3) the percentage of caries-free children has increased; 4) the percentage reductions in decay have been as much as two to threefold greater in anterior and premolar teeth than in molars; 5) the percentage reductions in proximal and in buccal and lingual surfaces have been much greater than in occlusal surfaces; 6) caries declines have occurred in fluoride-deficient as well as fluoridated areas; and 7) significant declines have occurred in time periods as short as 3 to 5 years.[22] Additional evidence available during the 1980s provides no indication that this downward trend in caries has subsided. Since the First International Conference, further caries declines in countries represented in those proceedings as well as in other countries have occurred.[23]

In the United States, the decline in dental caries in schoolchildren, first observed nationwide in 1970–80 and estimated at 32% during the 1970s, was confirmed further by a second national epidemiological survey completed in 1987.[24] Mean DMFS scores in persons aged 5 to 17 years decreased about 36% during the interval and were evident in all ages and in all geographic regions of the country. In the 13-year period between the first national survey (National Center for Health Statistics) of 1971–74 and the 1987 survey, a 57% reduction in caries experience had occurred (Fig. 62–2).

With respect to adults, there is limited current information on caries experience. However, available data provide relatively consistent findings, suggesting that at least young adults are also

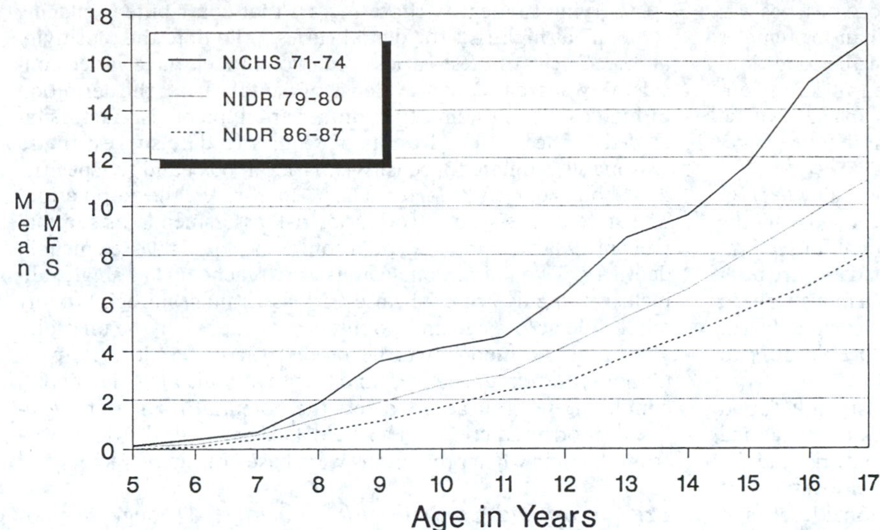

Figure 62-2. Mean DMFS scores for U.S. children aged 5–17 years, 1971–1987. *[From Brunelle JA, Carlos JP: Recent trends in dental caries in U.S. children and the effect of water fluoridation. J Dent Res 69:723–727, 1990.]*

experiencing a decline in caries prevalence. Older adults, because of high past disease experiences, have not yet attained appreciable reductions in caries. The restorative needs of older adults will continue to command considerable attention for years to come.[25]

The third worldwide trend in dental caries that has emerged, but less well documented than the other two, is that in some countries, most notably France and Japan, the prevalence of dental caries has remained unchanged.

Prevalence of Coronal Caries and Associated Factors. In 1987, 50% of U.S. children 5 to 17 years of age had never had a cavity in their permanent teeth, an increase of 4 million caries-free children since 1980, when the comparable estimate was 37%. The percent of children caries free varies inversely with age, however. By 17 years, 84% had experienced disease. Overall, the average child had 3.07 DMF surfaces, and 82% of this disease was treated with restorations; 5 to 9-year-olds had an average of 3.91 df surfaces in their primary teeth.[24] The annual increment of coronal caries in U.S. children appears to be about 1.2 DMF surfaces in fluoride-deficient communities and 0.8 DMF surfaces in fluoridated communities.[26]

With the downward trend in industrialized countries, some factors associated with dental caries appear to have changed as well, most notably socioeconomic status (SES) and race. Historically, the relationship between SES and DMF has been positive. More recent studies have reported a reversal in this relationship, and it is now generally acknowledged that caries rates are higher among children as well as young and middle-aged adults of lower social class.[27] Caries prevalence and treatment have also been strongly associated with race. For example, U.S. blacks have traditionally had a lower prevalence but more untreated disease than whites. With the overall changes in caries prevalence, this relationship, similar to SES, has reversed and blacks now have more disease than whites.[22] The net effect of trends in dental caries according to SES and race, which are most likely related, has been a shift in the burden of disease from those most able to get treatment to those least able to do so.

Traditional gender and geographic differences in caries prevalence persist. Caries prevalence is higher in males than in females in the primary dentition because of both earlier eruption and longer retention of these teeth in males. DMFS scores are higher in females than in males in the permanent dentition, most likely due to earlier eruption.[22]

To date, epidemiologists have not been able to establish a clear or consistent relationship between oral hygiene levels and dental caries prevalence.[27] Although it may be possible for an individual to prevent caries with meticulous oral hygiene, there is little epidemiological evidence that good oral hygiene actually reduces caries rates. The use of fluoride-containing dentifrices and their positive effects on dental caries makes oral hygiene easily justified, as does its effect on gingival health and personal appearance.

The consumption of sugars is probably the most important factor in the etiology of dental caries.[28] National data in the United States have indicated that the frequency of soft drinks and other sugar products between meals are related to increased caries risk, even when controlling for age, race, income, and education.[29] The correlations between dietary habits and caries increments are quickly becoming less clear, however, because of the low prevalence of caries and the relatively small differences in dietary patterns in children.[30]

In a review of physical and environmental factors associated with dental caries, Graves found that some factors, particularly past caries experience in primary and permanent teeth, have relatively strong associations with caries increments.[31] More limited data also show an association between molar occlusal morphology and caries risk—the deeper the pits and fissures, the greater the risk. Weak associations with caries appear to exist for malocclusion, nutritional levels, and genetic differences. Undoubtedly, the most important environmental factor associated with caries is past and present exposure to fluoride—systemic, topical or both—which has consistently shown an inverse relationship to caries prevalence or increment.

There is no question that caries is an infectious and transmissible disease.[32] A considerable body of data has shown a direct correlation between caries prevalence or increment and *Lactobacillus* or mutans-group streptococcal counts. In addition, some data have shown an indirect relationship between age of infection and caries risk—the younger the child at time of infection, the greater the risk. No single salivary component, such as flow rate, sugar clearance, buffering capacity, or enzyme activity has been related to caries, with the exception of extreme reduced salivary flow, consistently related to high caries risk.

Root Caries. A wide variation in root surface caries has been reported among different populations, possibly because of differences in the diagnostic methods as well as to inherent differences in the condition prevalence. When study design differences are accounted for, prevalence rates indicate that a large proportion of the adult population is affected. Recent national surveys of adult dental health have been conducted in the United States, the United Kingdom, and Ireland.[33] The percentage of U.S. working adults with at least one carious or filled root surface ranged from 7% at age 18 to 19 to 54% at age 60 and over (Fig.

62–3). The mean number of decayed and filled root surfaces was slightly higher for males (0.93 DF per person) than for females (0.55). Females had received more treatment for the condition, with about 60% of the root surface lesions being filled, in contrast to 39% in males. In seniors, 63% of males and 53% of females had at least one root surface lesion, with about 61% restored in females and 53% in males.[34]

Root caries increments appear to be low, probably averaging about one DF surface every 4 years.[35-39] Although low, the problem is much more substantial when the number of teeth at risk is taken into account. When coronal and root caries are both considered, the total caries increment for adults in industrialized countries may now be greater than coronal caries in children. Further, similar to coronal caries, a minority of people (30% to 40%) have most of the root caries.

Beyond age, there are very few variables consistently found to be related to the prevalence of root caries. Beck has suggested that those factors with the greatest potential of being risk indicators and ultimately determined to be risk factors are number of teeth, coronal caries, fluoridated water, educational level, and loss of gingival attachments.[12]

Nursing Caries. Ripa reviewed the prevalence of nursing caries from available studies in England, the United States, South Africa, Canada, Australia, and Indonesia.[8] He concluded that the prevalence of nursing caries in the United States and other Western countries is 5% or less. He also observed that some subgroups of the population, such as Native Americans, have an extremely high prevalence, as high as 67%.

Special Populations. Even with the decline in dental caries, the prevalence remains high in special subgroups of the population.[2] Included among those who need special attention through organized community and individual services are the poor, minorities, the disabled, and the institutionalized. Further, while dental caries has declined overall, some communities have very high caries rates. For example, in one statewide survey representative of all schoolchildren 5 to 17 years of age, the prevalence of dental caries varied by as much as 500% from one community to another.[40]

Caries Risk Assessment. Results of a large-scale demonstration program in the United States between 1977 and 1982 designed to evaluate a number of school-based preventive techniques emphasized the skewed distribution of dental caries among children.[41] About 20% of children were found to have 60% of the disease. These findings resulted in considerable interest in trying to identify those factors that contribute to placing someone at high risk for dental caries.[42] To date the sensitivity and specificity of these caries prediction models have varied considerably based on the prevalence of dental caries, the definition of high caries rates, and the number and type of risk factors included in the models. Results of studies to date suggest that a reasonable estimate for sensitivity is about 60% and for specificity, about 80% to 85% for a 25% high-risk child population. The state-of-the-science for caries risk assessment was summarized in 1989 at an international conference on risk assessment in dentistry. Two major conclusions were reached: (1) a single, all-inclusive, highly accurate caries risk assessment model, broadly applicable across age and population groups, may be unattainable; multiple models will be needed for different ages, populations, and circumstances; and (2) use of multifactorial models combining several factors offers the potential for making relatively good predictions. The field has progressed a long way from the time when predictions were based on single factors.[43]

Prevention and Control with Fluorides. Through years of research, systemic and topical fluorides have been proven to be effective in the prevention of dental caries. The U.S. Preventive Services Task Force, charged with reviewing methods for preventing the more common oral diseases and with making recommendations for interventions to be used by physicians, nurses, and other clinicians, judged that all major methods for providing fluorides, both systemic and topical, are well supported by scientific evidence.[44]

Mechanisms of Action. Fluoride's anticaries properties have been attributed to several characteristics. When available systemically during the years of tooth development, fluoride is incorporated into developing enamel and makes its crystalline structure less soluble during acid attack. The other mechanisms result from its topical effect. Fluoride has the ability to inhibit demineralization of the enamel and to enhance remineralization, that is, enhance repair by its presence in saliva and plaque.[45] Further, fluoride has several antibacterial properties.[46] Its concentration in plaque is sufficiently high to disrupt bacterial enzyme systems, thus resulting in less acid production and possible prevention of bacterial adhesion to the enamel surface. Most likely, fluoride works by a combination of these effects.

Fluoridation of Drinking Water. Fluoridation is the process of adding a carefully measured amount of a fluoride compound to community drinking water at a level which is optimum for the prevention of dental caries. In the United States and other tem-

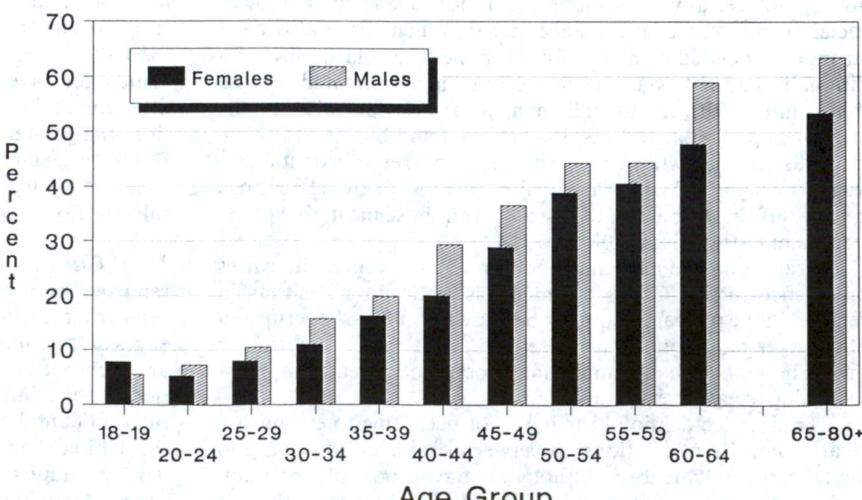

Figure 62–3. Percent of adults with at least one decayed or filled root surface by age group and gender, United States, 1985. *[From National Institute of Dental Research, 1987.[34]]*

TABLE 62-1. POPULATION SERVED BY FLUORIDE-ADJUSTED AND NATURALLY FLUORIDATED WATER, UNITED STATES, 1988

Type of Fluoridation	Population	Systems	Communities
Adjusted	124,153,775	8,874	7,867
Natural	8,812,234	3,389	1,847
Both	132,966,009	12,263	9,714

From Fluoridation Census, 1988, Table II.[49]

perate climates, the optimal fluoride levels have been determined to be between 0.7 and 1.2 parts per million, depending on a community's annual mean maximum daily air temperature.

The fluoride story represents one of the true successes in public health. The story in the United States began in 1901 when Dr. Frederick McKay arrived in Colorado Springs, Colorado, to establish his private dental practice. He immediately noticed that many of his patients, particularly those who had lived in the area all their lives, had a permanent stain on their teeth which he called mottled enamel. A desire to find the cause so that his patients could be helped led to almost 3 decades of work in which McKay developed two very important hypotheses: that the source of the etiologic agent was most likely the water supply and that those with mottling also appeared to have no increased susceptibility to dental caries, even though the enamel was defective. McKay was joined in his work in 1931 when H. Trendley Dean, a U.S. Public Health Service dentist, was assigned to full-time research on mottled enamel. By 1938, Dean and McKay had documented the prevalence of mottled enamel, which they renamed fluorosis, and provided direct evidence that fluoride in the domestic water was the primary cause.[47] Dean now set about to explore the relationship between fluoride in drinking water and dental caries. His efforts culminated in publication of the famous "21-cities study" which showed clearly the relationships between increasing fluoride concentrations and both decreasing dental caries prevalence and increasing fluorosis.[48]

The latest national data on community water fluoridation for the United States reflect the status of fluoridation as of 1988 (Table 62-1).[49] About 133 million people, or 61% of the population on public water supplies, consume water with optimal fluoride levels. Of that total, roughly 124 million people were on public water systems that were adjusting the fluoride content to optimum levels, while approximately 9 million people consumed water from community systems with adequate natural fluoride levels. To these totals can be added those special populations served by fluoridated systems, including schoolchildren benefiting through fluoridated school water supplies, American Indian and Alaska Natives on reservations with fluoridated water systems, and residents of American military bases with fluoridated systems. Of the 50 largest cities in the United States, 42 are currently fluoridated.

There has been a steady increase in the total U.S. population served by fluoridation over the first 40 years of implementation. While many states and large cities were quick to implement fluoridation programs in the 1950s and 1960s, the trend thereafter began to level off. Congress deferred fluoridation decisions to the states, which in turn largely left the responsibility to enact such measures to local governments and city councils. The net effect has been a decline in the real growth rate as compared to the earlier experience.

International statistics on community water fluoridation are difficult to obtain. According to the Federation Dentaire Internationale, 39 countries practice controlled water fluoridation. In some of these countries, such as Australia, Brazil, Canada, Czechoslovakia, Ireland, the Soviet Union, and New Zealand,[50] large segments of the population are participating.

Benefits of Water Fluoridation. The first city in the world to adjust the fluoride in its water supply to optimal levels was Grand Rapids, Michigan, USA, in 1945.[51] Grand Rapids was quickly followed by other U.S. cities: Newburgh, New York, in the same year and by Evanston, Indiana, and in Canada by Brantford, Ontario, in 1946. These four cities became part of a pioneering effort to evaluate the benefits of fluoridation. Dental caries rates in these cities were compared to matched control cities, Muskegon, Kingston, Oak Park, and Sarnia, respectively. Results at the end of the study period are presented in Table 62-2.[52]

In an extensive review of the results of 95 studies conducted between 1945 and 1978, Murray and Rugg-Gunn reported the modal percentage caries reduction following controlled water fluoridation to be 40% to 50% for primary teeth and 50% to 60% for permanent teeth.[53] Newbrun reviewed studies conducted during the 1980s, limiting his review to those with concurrent control groups because of the decline in dental caries.[54] Over 60 comparisons for fluoride-deficient and fluoridated communities, including studies in the United States, Australia, Britain, Canada, Ireland, and New Zealand, as well as several age groups, consistently demonstrated the present-day effectiveness of water fluoridation. The range of caries reductions for children and adolescents in fluoridated as compared with fluoride-deficient communities is now about 20% to 40%. Fluoridation benefits are also evident in studies of middle-aged adults and seniors, ranging from 20% to 30% and 17% to 35%, respectively. Benefits to adults and seniors include reductions in the prevalence of both coronal and root caries.

Costs and Cost-Effectiveness of Fluoridation. The smaller differences now being found in the prevalence of dental caries between those living in fluoridated compared to fluoride-deficient com-

TABLE 62-2. DMF TEETH AND MISSING TEETH PER CHILD FIRST FOUR COMMUNITY FLUORIDATION TRIALS

City	Year	DMFT	Difference (%)	MT	Difference (%)
Grand Rapids	1944	9.58		0.84	
Ages 12–14	1959	4.26	−55.5	0.29	−65.5
Evanston	1946	9.03		0.19	
Ages 12–14	1959	4.66	−48.4	0.06	−68.4
Sarnia	1959	7.46		0.75	
Brantford	1959	3.23	−56.7	0.22	−70.7
Ages 12–14					
Kingston	1960	12.46		0.92	
Newburgh	1960	3.73	−70.1	0.10	−89.1
Ages 13–14					

From Ast and Fitzgerald, 1962.[52]

munities have raised questions about the possible reduced cost-effectiveness of water fluoridation. The increase in environmental fluorides since water fluoridation was first introduced in 1945, particularly from fluoride-containing toothpastes, mouthrinses, foods and drinks, and professional sources, generally provide the basis for this issue, along with the evidence of declining caries. Water fluoridation continues to be a cost-effective strategy for caries prevention, even in those areas where the overall caries level has declined and where the cost of implementing water fluoridation has increased.[55-57]

The annual cost of fluoridation per person is estimated to be from 12 to 21 cents in large communities (>200,000), 18 to 75 cents for medium-sized communities (10,000 to 200,000), and 60 cents to $5.41 from small communities (<10,000). The larger variability in small communities is due to the high degree of sensitivity to changes in capital investment, labor, number of injection points, and type of fluoride material used. A national average cost of $3.35 per surface saved by water fluoridation has been estimated.[56]

Lessons learned from ceasing fluoridation have been painful. Studies in the United States and in Scotland have shown that when fluoridation is withdrawn, caries rates increase. In Wick, Scotland, which started water fluoridation in 1969 but stopped it in 1979, the caries prevalence in 5 to 6-year-olds increased by 27% between 1979 and 1984, despite a national decline in caries and increased availability of fluoride-containing dentifrices.[58]

Safety of Fluoridation. Over the years, fluoridation has been attacked as being part of a variety of conspiracies and the cause of numerous diseases. The most persistent question raised about the safety of fluoridation is its role in various types of cancers. Extensive reviews, expert commissions, and numerous studies have failed to find a link between fluoride and cancer.[59,60] An animal study directed by the U.S. National Toxicology Program (NTP), a unit of the National Institute of Environmental Health Sciences and charged with developing and evaluating scientific information about potentially toxic and hazardous chemicals, revived the controversy over fluoride's cancer-causing potential in 1990.[61] The results of this 2-year study were evaluated extensively by an expert panel of external reviewers and by the interested community. The panel of reviewers agreed with the final conclusion of the NTP that there was no evidence or that the evidence was too weak, depending on the gender or species of rat, to attribute any detrimental health effects to fluoride administration. The U.S. Public Health Service, along with virtually every other national organization in the United States involved with health issues, continues to support fluorides for the prevention of dental caries.[62]

Public Policy and Fluoridation. The legality of fluoridation in the United States has been thoroughly tested in our court system, and no court of last resort has ever rendered an opinion against fluoridation. The highest courts of more than a dozen states have confirmed the constitutionality of fluoridation. The U.S. Supreme Court has denied review of fluoridation on every occasion—more than 12 times—citing that no substantial federal or constitutional questions were involved.[63]

States vary considerably in their constitutional provisions on how fluoridation laws are enacted. Eight states currently mandate community water fluoridation (Connecticut, Georgia, Illinois, Michigan, Minnesota, Nebraska, Ohio, and South Dakota).[64] Five states (Delaware, Maine, Nevada, New Hampshire, and Utah) require a public vote before fluoridation can be instituted. In the remaining states, authorization to fluoridate a public water supply can be established by administrative decision, by governing body legislation, or by voter initiative. The most effective means to implementing fluoridation at the community level, in the absence of a state mandate, is to pursue promotion with the local legislative body rather than through a referendum. Of those community fluoridation decisions made during 1980–89, 78% were successful when only a governing body was involved in the decision-making, while only 37% were successful when subjected to voter referenda.[65]

School Water Fluoridation. In rural areas without a central community water supply, fluoridation of a school's drinking water is an alternative to community water fluoridation. Since children spend only 5 to 7 hours a day in school, the optimal concentration of fluoride for the school water supply is 4.5 times the optimal level recommended for community water fluoridation for that locale. Children in grades 1 to 12 attending a fluoridated school continuously from 8 years of age or younger will have approximately 40% fewer DMF surfaces.[66] As with community fluoridation, benefits from school fluoridation may now be less in the presence of already reduced levels of dental caries.

School fluoridation has been used almost exclusively in the United States. The number of fluoridated schools is currently 360,[49] down from about 500 schools involving slightly more than 200,000 children at its height.[67] These programs have many of the benefits of community fluoridation programs, yet have not been utilized extensively, primarily because of the need for personnel with water engineering skills to install and maintain equipment and the need for trained school personnel to monitor the system on a daily basis.

Conclusions. Today, community fluoridation is viewed as the single most effective public health measure available to prevent dental caries. Four and a half decades of research have proven fluoridation to be an ideal public health measure. Its characteristics can be summarized as follows: it is the least expensive and most effective way to reduce dental caries; it is eminently safe; it benefits adults as well as children; it provides benefits that last a lifetime when consumption of the water continues; it reduces the cost of children's dental treatment; it is the fairest way for everyone in a community to benefit, regardless of income, education, or the financial ability to seek dental care services; and it requires no individual effort or direct action by those who will benefit.[51] Yet, considerable work remains to be done in extending the benefits of fluoridation to all communities.

Dietary Fluoride Supplements. Dietary fluoride supplements in the form of fluoride-containing vitamins, drops, or tablets are an alternative way to provide systemic fluoride benefits to those children not benefiting from community or school water fluoridation. Fluoride supplements are taken by individuals or administered to groups of children in community programs. While there are a number of public programs that administer supplement programs, the majority of supplements are prescribed by physicians or dentists in the private-practice setting.

Over 50 reports on the effectiveness of fluoride tablets or drops have appeared in the literature indicating that their use is effective in preventing dental caries in both the primary and permanent dentitions.[68,69] Effectiveness appears to range from 40% to 80% if supplementation begins before 2 years of age. For school-based programs, effectiveness appears to be lower and more variable, with an average of approximately 30%. The costs of school programs range from U.S. 81 cents to $5.40 per child per year including material, supervisory personnel, travel, and administration.[56]

Prescribing of fluoride tablets or drops, often in association with vitamins, is widespread. Brunelle and Carlos reported that in 1986–87, 54.2% of U.S. children aged 5 to 17 years living in communities without fluoridation reported use of supplemental fluorides.[24] State and national surveys indicate that 32% to 86% of physicians and 21% to 93% of dentists prescribe supplements.[70,71] These studies also showed that some practitioners are unaware of the proper dosage guidelines for supplementation, the contraindications for their use, and the actual fluoride concentrations in water supplies where they practice. Of note was the finding that 14.8% of U.S. children 5 to 17 years of age drinking fluoridated community water also reported use of fluoride supplements.[24] Also of concern are the results of a study by Levy in which compliance by health care providers with the recommended fluoride supplement protocol was determined in patients for whom water fluoride analyses were performed prior to prescription of fluoride tablets or drops.[71] Even in patients with assay results available to the prescribing provider, one third of child patients and one half of their siblings did not receive the correct supplement dosage based on age and fluoride content of their drinking water.

Supplement Protocol. With the increased availability of fluorides from sources such as the diet, toothpaste, and the dilution of concentrated or powered baby formulas with fluoridated water, adherence to the appropriate protocol in fluoride supplementation is critical in order to provide maximum protection without risks of fluorosis. Before a fluoride supplement is prescribed, it is essential that adequate fluoride histories be taken. If the fluoride content of the patient's home or school water supply is unknown, for example, the patient drinks water from a private well or it cannot be determined if the patient is on a public water system, major sources of the patient's drinking water must be obtained and assayed for fluoride content. Natural fluorides occur in many geographic areas, and within any one area its concentration in water can be highly variable. Many state health departments and dental schools provide assay services at a nominal fee. Services are also available from commercial laboratories. Once the fluoride levels in drinking water are determined and a prescription written, the patient must be monitored to encourage compliance and to make adjustments in the dosage should the patient's fluoride exposure change.

Dosage Schedule. Dietary fluoride supplements are indicated in areas where waterborne fluoride levels are 0.7 ppm or less. Current dosage guidelines for prescribing systemic fluoride supplements recommended by the American Dental Association, the American Academy of Pediatric Dentistry, and the American Academy of Pediatrics are shown in Table 62-3. The schedules recommended by these three associations have been essentially identical since 1979 when the American Academy of Pediatrics reduced the dosage for children under 2 years of age from 0.5 mg F to the current level of 0.25 mg F.[72] This schedule has also been adopted in many other countries.[73]

Other Sources of Therapeutic Fluorides. A number of fluoride-containing gels, aqueous solutions, pastes, varnishes, and rinses are available for topical application. These fluorides fall into two categories: those applied by professionals and those that are self-applied at home or in other settings such as elementary schools, generally as part of public health programs.

TABLE 62-3. DIETARY FLUORIDE SUPPLEMENT DOSAGE SCHEDULE

Age of Child	Fluoride in Water (ppm)		
	<0.3	0.3–0.7	0.7
	Fluoride Dosage (mg/d)		
Birth to 2 y[a]	0.25	0.00	0
2 to 3 y	0.50	0.25	0
3 to 13 y	1.00	0.50	0

[a]The American Academy of Pediatrics recommends providing supplementation from 2 weeks of age through 16 years of age.

From American Dental Association: Accepted Dental Therapeutics, 40th edt. Chicago: American Dental Association, 1984.

Professionally-Applied Topical Fluorides. Pioneering efforts testing the effectiveness of solutions containing sodium fluoride, stannous fluoride, and acidulated phosphate fluoride in preventing dental caries were conducted by Bibby, Muhler, and Brudevold, respectively, beginning with Bibby's work in 1943.[74–76] Several excellent reviews of the effectiveness of these three compounds have been published.[77–80] In general, there are no clear data supporting the superiority of one of these fluoride compounds over another.

The initial use of these fluoride compounds in aqueous solutions has given way since the 1960s to gels, an aqueous solution with an added organic compound to provide increased stickiness and viscosity. Their popularity is based upon their handling characteristics, which make them easy to use in a mouth-tray or in brush-on techniques, and upon patient acceptance. There are currently two types of topical fluoride gel products available for professional use in the United States: APF and NaF compounds with 12,300 and 9,040 ppm F, respectively.[80]

The APF technique has proven to reduce dental caries in children by about 26% in fluoridated and in fluoride-deficient communities even though the absolute reduction in dental caries is less in fluoridated communities. The NaF gel has not been tested in clinical trials and has yet to be accepted by the American Dental Association. There are no completed studies testing the effects of professional applications of topical gels on dental caries in adults. Interim results of one such study have reported an indication of less root decay in an adult APF gel treatment group compared to a placebo group. The application of fluoride gels should not be performed routinely on children residing in fluoridated communities or who have had maximum exposure to fluoride supplements, but should be based on characteristics of the individual child. Children who are caries active should receive topicals, regardless of their exposure to systemic fluorides.[80] They are not currently recommended for use in school programs in countries with low caries levels.[80]

Fluoride varnishes, first introduced in 1968, are used extensively in Europe. Since varnishes adhere to the enamel surface for prolonged periods (up to 12 hours or more) there is increased contact time between the fluoride and enamel resulting in greater fluoride uptake and retention than with solutions or gels. Reviews suggest that the two available products, Duraphat and Fluor Protector, can be considered caries inhibitory, yet a firm recommendation on their use has not evolved due to design flaws in clinical trials and lack of evidence that their effectiveness compares favorably to other topicals.[80,81] Current evidence does not support the use of fluoride varnishes in school-based programs.[80]

A recent office-based fluoride topical procedure involving sequential rinses with 0.31% APF solution followed by a 0.4% SnF_2 solution has been marketed, but there is no supporting clinical data on its caries-inhibition potential, and it cannot be recommended.[80] Fluoride prophylaxis pastes, although widely used in clinical settings, have not been adequately tested in clinical trials to support their efficacy.

Self-Applied Topical Fluorides. A number of fluoride gels and rinses are likewise available for use by individuals for self-application, along with fluoride-containing dentifrices.

Fluoride rinses were developed during the 1960s as a public health measure to be used primarily in school settings. They were a direct result of the high expense associated with professional applications in school settings and the poor patient acceptance of brush-on fluoride pastes. As a result of extensive study, the three fluoride rinse systems, 0.2% sodium fluoride used once per week, 0.05% sodium fluoride used daily, and 0.2% fluoride (as acidulated phosphate fluoride) used daily, were approved by the U.S. Food and Drug Administration[82] and accepted by the American Dental Association.[83] With favorable results derived from a 17-community national demonstration project funded by the National Institute of Dental Research, as many as 12 million U.S. schoolchildren were participating in supervised weekly fluoride mouthrinse programs at their height.[84] These school-based rinse programs are popular, inexpensive, and require little time—5 to 10 minutes once every week. With the declining prevalence of dental caries becoming more pronounced in the 1980s, the cost-effectiveness of these programs is reduced. It is estimated that the annual reduction resulting from the use of fluoride rinses is no more than 0.4 DMF surfaces per child and probably half that in fluoridated communities and in other low-caries children.[85]

Fluoride-containing dentifrices are clearly an important component of efforts to prevent and control dental caries. The decline in dental caries has been attributed in part to their widespread use.[86] First marketed in the United States in 1955, they gained approval from the Council of Dental Therapeutics of the American Dental Association in 1964. The different brands containing fluoride now represent about 95% of sales in countries where dentifrices are sold. The clinical efficacy of the fluoride agents used in most dentifrices (SnF_2, Na_2PO_3F, NaF, amine F) is undisputed, and a review of clinical studies shows them to be at least similar in effectiveness. Use of these dentifrices in a fluoride-deficient community can result in reductions in dental caries of from 15% to 40%. Benefits can also be expected from their use in fluoridated communities.[87]

Of concern from a public health standpoint is the possibility of fluoride ingestion by young children when using fluoride-containing dentifrices. Since the fluoride concentration in dentifrices is approximately 1000 ppm, it is possible for a child to consume 1 mg or more of fluoride per day from inadvertent ingestion. Children who have a habit of ingesting their dentifrice and who also reside in an optimally fluoridated community or are receiving dietary fluoride supplements can have a total fluoride consumption capable of producing fluorosis. Parents should be careful to place a small amount of toothpaste on the child's brush and to supervise very small children.

Prevention and Control with Dental Sealants. Fluoride is most effective in preventing dental caries on smooth tooth surfaces and least effective on those surfaces with pits and fissures. These numerous pits and fissures, primarily on biting surfaces of the teeth, are at high risk for dental caries because they retain food debris and microorganisms and are hard to clean. Dental sealants, first introduced in the late 1960s and given full acceptance by the ADA in 1976,[88] are plastic materials that are applied as a thin coating over the pits and fissures of the teeth. They contain no therapeutic agent but provide a physical barrier, preventing microorganisms and food particles from depositing within the pits and fissures and initiating the acid conditions necessary for caries to begin.[89] To be most effective, their placement is required soon after teeth erupt, the period of time that these surfaces are most susceptible to decay. Dental sealants require no removal of tooth structure. Presently, biting surfaces represent 57% of surfaces affected with dental caries, providing a firm epidemiologic rationale for their use.[24]

In a recent review limited to those studies using newer sealant materials known to be more effective than earlier materials, median percent effectiveness in caries reductions for first molars—those teeth most susceptible to caries in children—was 83% after 1 year, declining somewhat to 66% after 7 years.[90] A single study of 10 years in duration reported a 68% reduction in caries in first molars. This review suggested an overall trend toward a more favorable long-term sealant effectiveness for fluoridated communities compared to fluoride-deficient communities. Since sealants provide only a physical barrier rather than a therapeutic effect, their effectiveness is a function of the degree to which they adhere to the tooth surface. Sealants are virtually 100% effective if fully retained on the pits and fissures. Median retention rates for first molars after one application range from 92% after 1 year to 57% after 10 years. Used in combination with fluorides, dental sealants provide optimal protection against dental caries.

Despite their proven efficacy and safety, dentists have been slow to adopt sealants for use in practice. Reasons given by dentists for not using them include a preference for amalgam restorations, concerns about retention and sealing in caries, and patients' difficulties in understanding their value; these have generally been shown to be unfounded.[91] Surveys indicated that less than 10% of U.S schoolchildren have received one or more sealants.

The use of sealants is increasing in public programs as the epidemiologic rationale for their use becomes more clear. Administrators of nine programs, primarily school-based, have reported on their experiences.[92-102] Regardless of the delivery site and personnel used for sealant application, service-oriented programs achieved retention rates similar to those reported in clinical trials. Guidelines are available providing recommendations for sealant use in both clinical practice and in public health programs.[103] These recommendations provide guidance in selecting communities, individuals, teeth, and surfaces, which help ensure cost-effectiveness of sealant programs.

Dietary Control. The public is generally aware of the potential for frequent consumption of refined carbohydrates to result in a pattern of caries typical of children and adults. There appears to be less awareness about nursing caries in toddlers. In a survey of expectant parents attending prenatal classes in the Boston area, 54% thought that a bottle of milk at other than regular feeding times would not harm the teeth of the infant, and 84% had never heard of nursing caries.[104] The main strategy for preventing nursing caries is to alert prospective parents and new parents about the condition and its causes. High-risk groups should be targeted for intervention. Education programs which can be used in these efforts have been described.[105]

PERIODONTAL DISEASES

Pathogenesis. The term *periodontal disease* is used to refer to a collection of diseases of the hard and soft tissues surrounding the teeth. The majority of adults show some signs and symptoms, ranging from swollen gums that bleed under gentle pressure to deep, bacteria-infested pockets that compromise the attachment of the teeth, or residual signs of past infection. Plaque-associated gingivitis is the most common of the periodontal diseases. It is an inflammation of the gingiva (gum tissue) and is characterized clinically by redness, gingival bleeding, edema or enlargement, and gingival sensitivity and tenderness. Periodontitis is an inflammation of the supporting tissues of the teeth, usually a progressively destructive change leading to loss of bone and periodontal ligament. Destructive periodontal diseases may be thought of as a series of infections that affect single or multiple periodontal sites within the oral cavity. Left untreated, they can result in formation of periodontal "pockets," a deepening of the space between the tooth and gums, called the gingival crevice, loosening of teeth, and ultimate loss.

The World Workshop in Clinical Periodontics identified five types of destructive periodontal diseases: adult periodontitis, early-onset periodontitis, periodontitis associated with systemic disease, necrotizing ulcerative periodontitis, and refractory periodontitis.[106] Adult periodontitis is by far the most common of these and is the one dealt with in this chapter. In their early stages, these diseases generally go unnoticed by the public because they are painless and do not interfere with function.

Etiology. Bacteria organized into plaque, the soft, sticky film that coats the tooth surface within hours of brushing, is the primary cause of gingivitis and the various forms of periodontitis.

Classic studies by Loe and his colleagues in the early 1960s demonstrated the cause-and-effect relationship between plaque and gingivitis.[107] Until the early 1960s, the amount of dental plaque rather than its composition was considered to be the most important etiologic factor in disease. Based on knowledge at the time, etiologic models of periodontal disease emphasized an overgrowth of plaque. More recently, studies suggest that the amount of plaque is less important than the specific pathogens or groups of pathogens in the plaque. Of over 300 species of microorganisms that comprise the oral microbiota, about 30 are suspected to be pathogenic of destructive disease. Difficulties in studying the microbiology of periodontal diseases have slowed progress in determining specific periodontal pathogens, but two species, *Actinobacillus actinomycetemcomitans* and *Bacteroides gingivalis,* are among those considered the most likely pathogens.[108] If left undisturbed, bacterial plaque will mineralize into hard deposits known as calculus (tartar) which can contribute to further colonization of bacteria. The body's natural defense against the effects of these bacteria can be mediated by a number of host factors (Fig. 62–4).

Progression. Gingivitis and periodontitis are two separate but related diseases. Gingivitis does not always progress to periodontitis but periodontitis has not yet been reported without a preceding gingivitis. Once periodontitis is initiated, gingivitis is not necessary for the destruction of deeper periodontal structures to continue. Data exist to support three patterns for the natural history of periodontal destruction.[106] The first, the continuous paradigm, implies slow, constant, and progressive destruction. This theory was developed primarily from cross-sectional epidemiologic studies conducted during the 1950s and 1960s. Cross-sectional data can give an impression that destruction is continuous and slowly progressive due to pooling data from groups, individuals, and sites.[109] The second pattern, the random burst theory, proposes short periods of destruction followed by periods of no destruction, occurring randomly with respect to time and sites within an individual. The final pattern, the asynchronous multiple burst theory, proposes a pattern in which destruction occurs during a defined period of life, and the disease then goes into remission. The major amount of destruction occurs over a period of a few years. The second and third theories developed out of careful longitudinal monitoring of patients.[110]

Epidemiology. The epidemiology of periodontal diseases is characterized by three eras.[111] The first era, lasting until about 1950, was distinguished by treatment of periodontitis (pyorrhea) with large numbers of tooth extractions. The prevailing thought was that the teeth with periodontitis formed a focus of infection in the body which should be dealt with through removal of the source of infection, the teeth. High rates of edentulousness were thus found during this era. The second era began with the development of the Periodontal Index in 1956 and lasted about 2 decades.[112] With this epidemiological tool in hand, the prevalence of periodontal diseases and associated sociodemographic and behavioral factors were determined worldwide. The third era began when more precise measurements of disease, many of which had been used in the clinical practice of periodontics, were adopted for use in epidemiological field studies. A renewed interest in the epidemiology of the periodontal diseases has come with this third era and is partially a result of the decline in dental caries, the retention of more teeth and the aging of the population in industrialized countries (both of which should result in more periodontal disease), and the changes in the traditional concepts of the natural history of periodontal diseases referred to before.

Measurement for Epidemiological Studies. Early indices for periodontal diseases were based on the concept that it was a single disease, with gingivitis and periodontitis representing different stages in its progression.[112,113] Indices were calculated as composite scores, usually as weighted averages of scores given to each of several signs of periodontal disease. The most common clinical signs included in these early efforts were visual signs of gingival inflammation, pocket formation, and tooth mobility as an indication of severe pocket formation. The most widely used of these indices was Russell's PI index. In response to current theories of pathogenesis of periodontal diseases, epidemiologists have taken a disaggregated approach to recording signs of disease rather than a composite one. Clinical signs, usually gingival bleeding, loss of supporting structure as a measure of past disease (recession or loss of attachment), pocket formation, and sometimes calculus as a contributing risk factor, are scored separately and presented as such. The Community Periodontal Index of Treatment Needs (CPITN) developed by the World Health Organization provides an indication of the presence of bleeding, calculus, shallow and deep pockets, as well as treatment needed for the observed conditions.[114] This index has been adopted around the world for use in hundreds of surveys in the relatively short period of time since its development. The other most common method for measuring periodontal conditions is the Extent and Severity Index (ESI) developed by the U.S. National Institute of Dental Research.[115] Combined with other companion measures of gingivitis and calculus, this index provides a comprehensive measure of information similar to that collected in clinical practice.

Prevalence and Trends. Trends in the prevalence of periodontal diseases are less clear than those occurring for dental caries and are more difficult to determine because of the different methods used in their measurement. Three U.S. national data sets, the National Center for Health Statistics (NCHS) examination surveys conducted in 1960–62 and in 1971–74, and the National Institute of Dental Research (NIDR) 1985–86 Survey of Employed and Senior Adults have been used to examine trends in periodontal diseases.[116]

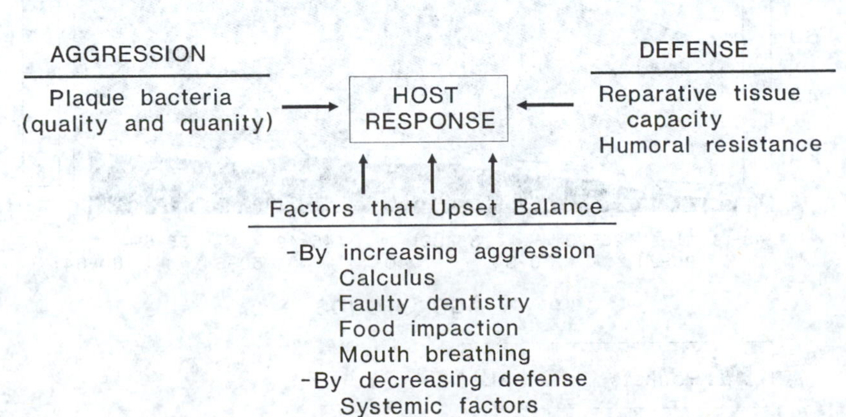

Figure 62–4. Etiologic model for periodontal diseases. *[From Bahn AN: Microbial potential in the etiology of periodontal disease. J Peridontol 41:603–610, 1970.]*

TABLE 62-4. PERCENT DISTRIBUTION OF ADULTS BY PERIODONTAL DISEASE STATUS, GENDER, AND AGE, UNITED STATES, 1960–1962 and 1971–74

Sex and Age (Years)	No Disease		Disease without Pockets		Disease with Pockets	
	1960–1962	*1971–1974*	*1960–1962*	*1971–1974*	*1960–1962*	*1971–1974*
▪ **Both Sexes**						
Total (18–79)	26.1	51.4	48.5	25.2	25.4	23.4
▪ **Males**						
Total (18–79)	20.9	51.4	49.0	28.1	30.1	26.6
18–24	29.0	45.3	60.6	42.0	10.3	7.1
25–34	26.3	50.9	51.7	30.8	22.0	15.7
35–44	22.1	53.5	48.1	25.7	29.7	30.5
45–54	15.0	39.6	48.1	22.7	36.9	37.7
55–64	15.3	37.8	39.1	15.3	45.6	46.9
65–74	5.6	27.9	36.0	13.1	58.4	58.9
75–79	6.2		33.7		60.0	
▪ **Females**						
Total (18–79)	31.0	57.1	47.9	22.5	21.0	20.4
18–24	36.8	68.6	53.6	25.6	9.6	5.8
25–34	37.6	62.0	50.2	25.9	12.3	12.1
35–44	33.3	56.4	46.2	21.4	20.5	22.2
45–54	26.6	49.0	43.7	21.3	29.6	29.7
55–64	20.8	46.1	43.6	18.1	35.5	35.8
65–74	15.2	43.3	52.0	13.8	32.8	42.9
75–79	11.0		35.3		53.8	

From Capilouto ML, Douglass CW: Trends in the prevalence and severity of periodontal diseases in the US: A public health problem? J Public Health Dent 48:245–251, 1988.

Between 1960–62 and 1971–74 there was an increase in the proportions of U.S. adults with no disease in both sexes and all ages due primarily to less gingivitis (disease without pockets). Overall there was little change in pockets but a slight trend toward a decrease in the proportions with the more severe disease (Table 62-4).

In 1985, the prevalence of gingivitis (using bleeding as the measure) was relatively high. The survey found 43.5% of the employed sample and 46.8% of seniors had gingival bleeding. This same survey indicated that the prevalence of loss of attachment was very high, with 76.6% of employed and 95.1% of seniors having attachment loss of 2 mm or greater at one or more sites (Fig. 62-5). However, the overall severity of attachment loss, expressed as the average amount of attachment loss per person for all sites examined, was relatively low for persons younger than 65 years of age: 1.93 mm per person. On the other hand, the mean attachment loss for persons older than 65 years of age, 3.13 mm, was relatively high. Approximately 15.9% of employed and 26.2% of seniors had pockets of greater than 3 mm, considered to be disease in this survey (Fig. 62-5). When using either loss of attachment or pockets as indicators of periodontal disease, the proportion of subjects with severe levels of disease was small.

In interpreting these 20 years of data, Capilouto and Douglass concluded that it was difficult to document any changes occurring in the prevalence of gingivitis; however, given the available evidence, the prevalence and severity of gingivitis has probably declined. They further concluded that periodontitis continues to affect approximately the same proportions of the overall U.S. adult population as in the past, but for those af-

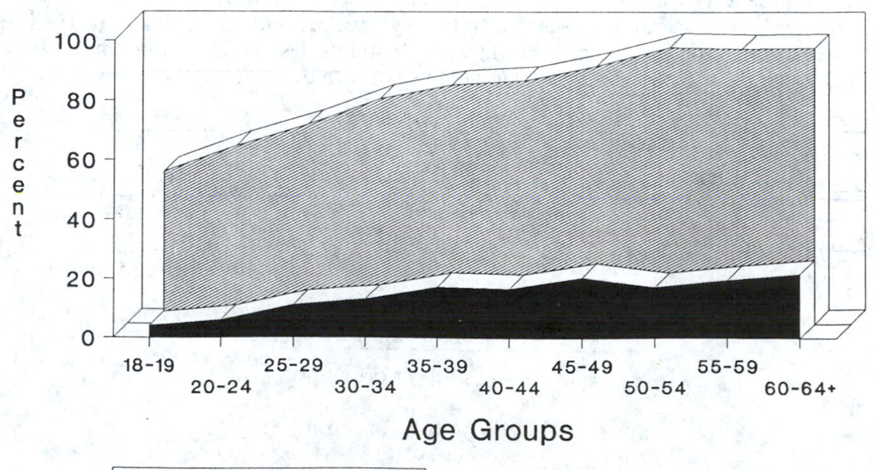

Figure 62-5. Prevalence of periodontal pockets and attachment loss, United States, 1985–1986. *(From National Institute of Dental Research, 1987.[34])*

fected, the extent and severity of the disease have declined. Finally, they concluded that older adults continue to exhibit more disease and greater levels of disease than the younger age groups. The improvements in periodontal disease levels are consistent with national trends of improved oral hygiene, improved income and education levels, increased dental care utilization, cessation of smoking habits, increased exposure to fluoride, and increased general use of systemic antibiotics.[117]

Data on the prevalence of periodontal conditions based on the CPITN and from the WHO Global Oral Health Data Bank for 35- to 44-year-olds have been presented for 34 countries.[118] Subjects with completely healthy periodontal tissues were virtually nonexistent. Calculus and shallow pocketing, periodontal conditions which require self-care combined with professional oral hygiene instruction and cleaning of teeth, were of notable magnitude in adult populations around the world. Nevertheless, with a few exceptions the percentages of persons with severe disease (deep pockets) were less than 20% (Fig. 62-6). Tooth loss because of periodontal diseases did not seem to be a frequently encountered phenomenon. Previously assumed differences between industrialized and developing countries with regard to the prevalence of severe periodontal diseases were not reflected in these survey data. For the majority of populations studied, the progress of periodontal diseases seems to have been slowed. Like dental caries, there are population groups with high levels of severe periodontal disease.

Factors Associated with Prevalence. Numerous descriptive epidemiological studies have identified factors associated with the variation of periodontal diseases. To summarize the sociodemographic characteristics, the prevalence of periodontal diseases tends to increase with age, is higher in males than in females, is higher in low socioeconomic groups compared to other groups, and is affected by race. A recent study of an elderly population found striking differences between white and black elderly, confirming similar findings in state and national surveys.[119] Multivariate analyses which controlled for socioeconomic status, education level, and last visit to the dentist explained only a small portion of the black-white differences in periodontal status. In a review of probable and potential risk factors, a large number of factors were identified as possibly related to periodontal diseases.[120] Rarely have multivariate analyses been used in analyzing epidemiologic data, and still fewer longitudinal studies have been done to confirm putative risk factors. There is accumulating evidence that smoking may be a risk factor for periodontal diseases and that it retards healing after treatment.[121]

Conclusions. The more precise measurement of periodontal diseases in the 1980s and an increase in the number of population-based surveys provide useful information in defining the epidemiology of periodontal diseases. Although periodontal diseases are still considered widespread, these new measurement techniques have allowed a clearer distinction between the prevalence of disease and its severity. While periodontal disease is very prevalent, the severity is less than once thought. Further, the disease is not as generalized within the mouth as previous measurement methods indicated. Fewer sites are affected and the estimated amount and type of treatment needed requires fewer resources based on these findings. Nevertheless, millions of individuals are affected and efforts need to be directed toward prevention and control of the disease. In the U.S. alone, a large proportion of adult Americans have experienced periodontal diseases; nearly half have gingivitis, and millions have periodontal pockets that may need treatment.[122] As with dental caries, the current epidemiology of the periodontal diseases suggests that identification of risk factors should be pursued.

Prevention. Prevention of periodontal diseases requires the control of their etiologic agent, plaque, which must be thoroughly removed on a regular basis. Plaque removal can be accomplished by physical or chemical means. Physical methods primarily include toothbrushing and flossing. Chemical methods have included antibiotics, antimicrobial agents, and enzymes, but are presently limited primarily to antimicrobial agents. Unfortunately, there are no public health interventions for the prevention and control of periodontal diseases similar to fluorides for dental caries. There have been no comprehensive community trials directed toward the prevention and control of periodontal diseases as there have been for cardiovascular diseases. As an alternative, some efforts have been directed toward dental practitioners to ensure their attention to the periodontal tissues. These efforts have met with some success, but they reach only that segment of the population who are already users of dental services.[123,124]

Physical Methods for Plaque Control. Self-care is essential for maintenance of periodontal health. A successful preventive regimen requires the thorough removal of plaque every 24 to 48

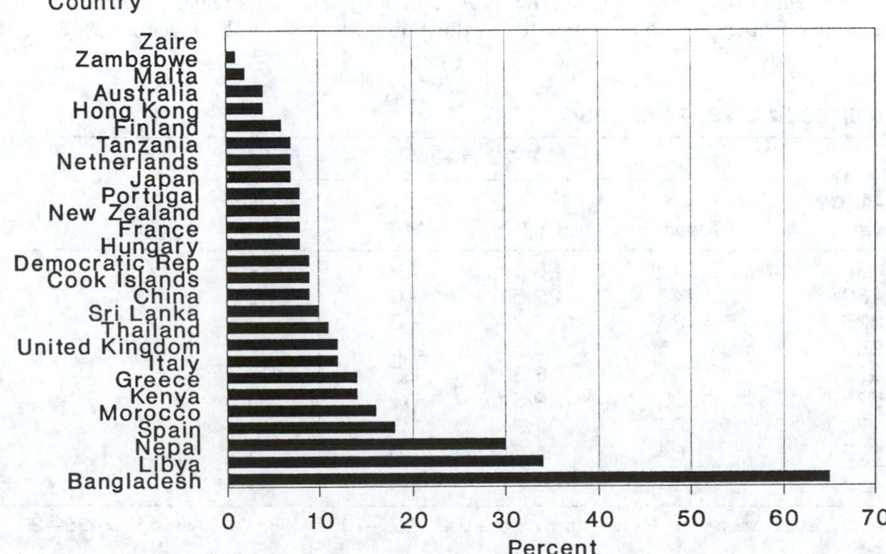

Figure 62-6. Percent with deep periodontal pockets, 35 to 44 year olds, WHO Data Bank, 1987. *(From Pilot T, Barmes DE: An update on periodontal conditions in adults, measured by CPITN. Int Dent J 37:169–172, 1987.)*

hours. The toothbrush alone cannot successfully clean all surfaces of a tooth, particularly between the teeth, and its use must be supplemented with dental floss, interproximal brush or wood point.[125]

With the confirmation of plaque as the primary etiologic agent in gingivitis, through well-designed clinical trials, efforts were made in public programs to extend plaque control to a number of groups, particularly public schoolchildren. Results of these efforts, based on supervised group brushing combined with some degree of education, proved to be equivocal.[126] While improvements in knowledge, attitudes, and behavior were achieved in these demonstration programs and clinical trials, any improvements in plaque levels and gingivitis were usually short-lived. These self-care, group plaque control strategies cannot be recommended for public health settings in the absence of more comprehensive oral or general health education programs.

Chemical Methods for Plaque Control. For more than 25 years, dental researchers have sought chemical means to control plaque: enzymes to loosen and dissolve the plaque mass so that it can be washed away, topical antibiotic rinses to eliminate certain bacteria in a narrowly focused attack, and antiseptics that work against a broad spectrum of bacteria. Unfortunately, these are of limited use in the prevention of periodontal diseases. The effectiveness of two agents for reduction of plaque and gingivitis are accepted by the Council on Dental Therapeutics of the American Dental Association: Listerine, a mixture of essential oils, and Peridex, containing 0.12% chlorhexidine gluconate as its active ingredient. In addition to being accepted by the ADA, Peridex is approved by the U.S. Food and Drug Administration. Since mouthrinses do not appreciably penetrate into the gingival crevice, their value appears to be limited to the management of plaque above the gingiva and thus to the prevention and control of gingivitis. Peridex, which has been used in Scandinavia and other European countries for 20 years, appears to be the most effective agent available for reduction of both plaque and gingivitis with short-term reductions averaging 60%. Three long-term studies have shown reductions in plaque averaging 55% and reductions in gingivitis averaging 45%. Peridex is available by prescription only, is not recommended for long-term use, and should be used only under the careful supervision of a dentist. While a number of other chemicals have been tested, results of studies with these products have been contradictory.[127] In any event, these chemical agents should be viewed as supplements to routine brushing and flossing.

Combined Personal and Professional Care. While maintenance of periodontal health depends on daily self-care, professional care is also essential, particularly when disease has caused a deepening of the periodontal crevice. Early pocket formation of 2 to 4 mm requires the removal of bacteria from the gingival crevice through professional intervention. This condition is usually responsive to scaling (removal of calculus), root planing (smoothing the root to help prevent recolonization of bacteria), and effective plaque control. As pockets deepen, scaling and root planing as well as plaque control become less effective, but still valuable for reducing inflammation and bacteria and increasing the tissue's prognosis for repair and reattachment. Clinical trials have demonstrated that regular professional tooth cleaning with individual oral hygiene can have a significant preventive effect.[128,129]

ORAL CANCERS

Epidemiology

Incidence and Mortality. In the United States, cancers of the lips, tongue, floor of the mouth, palate, gingiva, buccal mucosa, and oropharynx will account for about 31,000 new cases of cancer in 1990 and about 8400 deaths. These oral cancers are 3% of all cancers in the United States. Squamous cell carcinoma is the most common type of oral cancer, representing about 90% of those cancers that occur. About 85% of all oral cancers diagnosed between 1973 and 1984 occurred at four sites: the tongue, oropharynx, lips, and floor of the mouth (Table 62-5).[130]

Survival. Most oral cancers, exclusive of those occurring on the lip, are advanced lesions when diagnosed. According to the American Cancer Society, oral cancers in 1989 had the fifth lowest survival rate of thirteen selected sites.[130] About half of all patients with oral cancer die of their disease within 5 years. This figure would be even higher if lip cancers, 87% of which are localized when discovered, were excluded. These survival rates did not improve between 1973 and 1984, despite advances in radiation therapy, surgical management, and chemotherapy. Silverman and Gorsky underscored the importance of early diagnosis.[131] More than 79% of the oropharyngeal lesions showed regional lymph node metastases at the time of diagnosis. For cancers of the tongue, 73% were already advanced.

Risk Factors. Age is directly associated with the risk of oral cancer. The average age at diagnosis is between 60 and 65 years. As the population in industrialized countries ages, the magnitude of the problem is likely to increase. Although the overall incidence and mortality rates for oral cavity and pharyngeal cancers are decreasing, the total number of cases is increasing as are rates in some segments of the population.[131] Oral cancer is more fre-

TABLE 62-5. ORAL CANCER, SEER DATA, UNITED STATES, 1973–1984

Site	All Cases 1973–1984 Total	1979–1984 Cases	(%)	M:F	Median Age
Tongue	5,037	2,840	26.1	1.9	63
Oropharynx	4,450	2,442	22.5	2.0	62
Lip	4,395	2,138	19.7	9.0	62
Floor mouth	3,288	1,795	16.5	2.2	61
Gingiva	1,676	961	8.8	1.5	67
Buccal	577	300	2.8	1.1	70
Hard palate	376	204	1.9	1.5	66
Other mouth	316	184	1.7	2.0	66
Total	20,115	10,864	100.0	2.3	63

From Silverman S, Gorsky M: Epidemiologic and demographic update in oral cancer: California and national data 1973–1985. J Am Dent Assoc 120:495–499, 1990.

quent in males, but the male-female ratio, which was about 6:1 in 1950, is now about 2:1. The most likely explanation for this change in gender ratios is the increase in the use of tobacco among women. Differences in incidence, survival, and mortality exist according to race, with blacks having higher rates of incidence and mortality and lower rates of survival than whites. Although the incidence rate among blacks is about 30% higher than for whites, the mortality rate is twice that of whites. Race differences exist for 5-year survival as well. While 47% of whites with these cancers die within 5 years of diagnosis, 69% of blacks die within 5 years. Mortality rates for blacks have been increasing over the last 15 years.

Oral cancer is more common among persons who either smoke or use smokeless tobacco, and especially among those who are also heavy drinkers of alcohol.[132] There has been growing concern over the increased use of smokeless tobacco among American youth. User rates as high as 30 to 40% have been reported among boys in some junior and senior high schools.[133] The health effects of smokeless tobacco have been examined in a report by the U.S. Surgeon General, which concluded that far from being a safe substitute for smoking cigarettes, smokeless tobacco can cause cancer and a number of noncancerous oral conditions such as gingivitis, periodontitis, and gingival recession and can lead to nicotine addiction and dependence.[134] The excess risk of cancer of the cheek and gum may reach nearly fiftyfold among long-term users.[135]

One of the characteristic epidemiological features of oral cancer is the wide disparity in rates in different parts of the world. The disease is very common in parts of Central and Southeast Asia, where it constitutes a large percentage of all diagnosed malignancies. The geographical variation in rates reflects local conditions and habits, which influence the degree of exposure to known etiologic factors.

Prevention and Control. Programs that lead to a reduction in the use of tobacco products are important in the prevention and control of oral cancers. The role that tobacco use plays in oral cancers, as well as other cancers, should be emphasized in education programs for the public. Early detection through careful and periodic examinations is also important, and these education programs need to emphasize the importance of early detection for oral cancer. For those patients who use tobacco, at least annual visits to a dentist for early detection of premalignant or malignant lesions is recommended.[136]

Health professionals can be effective smoking cessation counselors, play an important role in oral cancer prevention, and potentially affect the smoking status of millions of patients. Dentists and dental hygienists are in a particularly unique and favorable position to modify the smoking behavior of their patients.[137] Each year more than half of the population visits a dental office, and a substantial proportion of these patients will make a series of such visits, often as a part of an ongoing relationship of several years' standing. Further, many of these patients will be adolescents, a population group under-represented in physicians' offices and the age group in which smoking usually begins. For young people some detrimental aesthetic consequences of smoking, discolored teeth and restorations, bad breath, and hairy tongue, can possibly provide more powerful motivation to stop than the fear of remote health consequences such as heart disease or cancer. The dental profession has a historically strong preventive orientation, which increases the potential for adoption of smoking cessation interventions by providers. Dental hygienists devote almost all of their treatment time to preventive procedures, of which a large portion consists of patient education. Dental providers generally have positive attitudes toward providing smoking cessation counseling in their practices, and a clinical trial has shown them to be effective counselors.[138]

CONCLUSIONS

Efforts by the public, health professionals, and researchers have all contributed to improving trends in oral health, most notably, for dental caries in children. Other conditions have improved only slightly, while some serious conditions, such as oral cancer and periodontal diseases may even be increasing in some segments of society.

Community and individual methods for the primary prevention of dental caries, periodontal diseases, oral cancer, and other conditions are available. These methods, among others, include a wide array of systemic and topical fluorides, dental sealants, regular professional care, plaque control, and avoidance of tobacco and alcohol. The scientific evidence supporting these interventions as safe and effective is in large measure overwhelming. The cost-effectiveness of some of these methods, such as community water fluoridation, are among the highest of any preventive strategies available to the public health practitioner.

Yet, much remains to be done in extending the benefits of these preventive services to larger segments of society. *Healthy People 2000: National Health Promotion and Disease Prevention Objectives* provides realistic oral health benchmarks for the end of the century.[139] This effort is complemented by *Healthy Communities 2000: Model Standards, which provides a guidebook to help communities translate Healthy People 2000* national objectives into state and local action.[140] The U.S. Preventive Services Task Force likewise provides guidance for primary care physicians, dentists, dental hygienists, nurses, and other clinicians who have numerous opportunities to prevent oral diseases.[44,136] With coordinated efforts between the public and private sectors and the translation of proven preventive technologies into practice, the public can achieve acceptable levels of oral health.

REFERENCES

1. World Health Organization: Application of the International Classification of Diseases to Dentistry and Stomatology. Geneva: World Health Organization, 1978
2. Fritz ME, Rundle DG: Dental disease. In Amler RW, Dull HB: (eds) Closing the Gap: The Burden of Unnecessary Illness. New York: Oxford University Press, 1987
3. Levit KR, Freeland MS, Waldo DR: National health care spending trends. Health Affairs 9:171–184, 1990
4. Resine S, Miller J: A longitudinal study of work loss related to dental diseases. Social Science and Medicine 21:1309–1314, 1985
5. Emilson CG, Krasse B: Support for and implications of a specific plaque hypothesis. Scand J Dent Res 93:96–104, 1985
6. Keyes PH: Recent advances in dental caries research. Bacteriology. Bacteriological findings and biological implications. Int Dent J 12:443–464, 1962
7. Newbrun E: Cariology, 3 edt. Chicago: Quintessence Publishing Co, 1989.
8. Ripa LW: Nursing caries: a comprehensive review. Pediatr Dent 10:268–282, 1988
9. World Health Organization: Oral Health Surveys: Basic Methods, 3 edt. Geneva: World Health Organization, 1987
10. Klein H, Palmer CE, Knutson JW: Studies on dental caries: I. Dental status and dental needs of elementary school children. Public Health Rep 53:751–765, 1938
11. DePaola PF, Soparkar PM, Kent RL Jr: Methodological issues relative to the quantification of root surface caries. Gerodontol 8:3–8, 1989
12. Beck J: The epidemiology of root surface caries. J Dent Res 69:1216–1221, 1990

13. Katz RV: Clinical signs of root caries: measurement issues from an epidemiologic perspective. J Dent Res 69:1211–1215, 1990
14. Barmes DE, Infirri JS: WHO activities in oral epidemiology. Community Dent Oral Epidemiol 5:22–29, 1977
15. Barmes DE: Epidemiology of dental disease. J Clin Periodontol 4:80–93, 1979
16. Infirri JS, Barmes DE: Epidemiology of oral diseases—differences in national problems. Int Dent J 29:183–190, 1979
17. Heloe LA, Haugejorden O: "The rise and fall" of dental caries: some global aspects of dental caries epidemiology. Community Dent Oral Epidemiol 9:296–299, 1981
18. Barmes DE: Indicators for oral health and their implications for developing countries. Int Dent J 33:60–66, 1982
19. Sheiham A: Changing trends in dental caries. Int J Epidemiol 13:142–147, 1984
20. Manji F, Fejerskov O: Dental caries in developing countries in relation to the appropriate use of fluoride. J Dent Res 69:733–741, 1990
21. Glass RL (ed): The first international conference on the declining prevalence of dental caries. J Dent Res 61(sp Iss):1304–1383, 1982
22. Graves RC, Bohannan HM, Disney JA, Stamm JW, Bader JD, Abernathy JR: Recent dental caries and treatment patterns in U.S. children. J Public Health Dent 46:23–29, 1986
23. Kalsbeek H, Verrips GHW: Dental caries prevalence and the use of fluorides in different European countries. J Dent Res 69:728–732, 1990
24. Brunelle JA, Carlos JP: Recent trends in dental caries in U.S. children and the effect of water fluoridation. J Dent Res 69:723–727, 1990
25. Graves RC, Stamm JW: Oral health status in the United States: prevalence of dental caries. J Dent Educ 49:341–351, 1985
26. Garcia AI: Caries incidence and costs of prevention programs. J Public Health Dent 49:259–271, 1989
27. Hunt RJ: Behavioral and sociodemographic risk factors for caries. In Bader JD (ed): Risk Assessment in Dentistry. Chapel Hill: University of North Carolina Dental Ecology, 1990, pp 29–34
28. Newbrun E: Sugar and dental caries: a review of human studies. Science 217:418–423, 1982
29. Ismail AI: Food cariogenicity in Americans aged 9 to 29 years assessed in a national cross-sectional survey, 1971–74. J Dent Res 65:1435–1440, 1986
30. Burt BA, Eklund SA, Morgan KJ, et al: The effects of sugars intake and frequency of ingestion on dental caries increment in a three-year longitudinal study. J Dent Res 67:1422–1429, 1988
31. Graves RG, Disney JA, Stamm JW, Abernathy JR, Bohannan HM: Physical and environmental risk factors in dental caries. In Bader JD (ed): Risk Assessment in Dentistry. Chapel Hill: University of North Carolina Dental Ecology, 1990, pp 37–47.
32. Krasse B: Microbiological and salivary risk factors. In Bader JD (ed): Risk Assessment in Dentistry. Chapel Hill: University of North Carolina Dental Ecology, 1990, pp 51–61
33. Aherne CA, O'Mullane D, Barrett BE: Indices of root surface caries. J Dent Res 69:1222–1226, 1990
34. Oral Health of United States Adults, The National Survey of Oral Health in U.S. Employed Adults and Seniors: 1985–86. Bethesda, Md: National Institute of Dental Research Publication No. (NIH) 87–2868, 1987
35. Banting DW, Ellen RP, Fillery ED: Longitudinal study of root caries: baseline and incidence data. J Dent Res 64:1141–1144, 1985
36. Nyvad B, Fejerskov O: Active root surface caries converted into inactive caries as a response to oral hygiene. Scand J Dent Res 94:281–284, 1986
37. Ripa LW, Leske GS, Forte F, Varma A: Effect of a 0.05% neutral NaF mouthrinse on coronal and root caries of adults. Gerodontol 6:131–136, 1987
38. Jensen ME, Kohout F: The effect of a fluoridated dentifrice on root and coronal caries in an older adult population. J Am Dent Assoc 117:829–832, 1988
39. Hand JS, Hunt RJ, Beck JD: Incidence of coronal and root caries in an older adult population. J Public Health Dent 48:14–19, 1988
40. Rozier R, Bowling M, Dudney G: Twenty-five year trends in dental caries prevalence in NC. J Dent Res 67:171, 1988
41. Bell RM, Klein SP, Bohannan HM, Graves RC, Disney JA: National Preventive Dentistry Demonstration Program: Baseline Report. R-2862-RWJ, Santa Monica, Calif: The Rand Corporation, 1982
42. Bader JD (ed): Risk Assessment in Dentistry. Chapel Hill: University of North Carolina Dental Ecology, 1990
43. Newbrun E, Leverett D: Risk assessment dental caries working group summary statement. In Bader JD (ed): Risk Assessment in Dentistry. Chapel Hill: University of North Carolina Dental Ecology, 1990, pp 304–305
44. Greene JC, Louie R, Wycoff SJ: Preventive dentistry, I: dental caries. JAMA 262:3459–3463, 1989
45. Silverstone LM: Remineralization and enamel caries: new concepts. Dental Update. 261–273, 1983
46. Eisenberg AD, Bender GR, Marquis RE: Reduction in the aciduric properties of the oral bacterium *Streptococcus mutans* GS-5 by fluoride. Arch Oral Biol 25:133–135, 1980
47. Dean HT, McKay FS: Production of mottled enamel halted by a change in common water supply. Am J Public Health 29:567–575, 1939
48. Dean HT, Arnold FA Jr, Elvove E: Domestic water and dental caries, V. Additional studies of the relation of fluoride domestic waters to dental caries experience in 4425 white children aged 12–14 years, of 13 cities in 4 states. Public Health Rep 57:1155–1179, 1942
49. Fluoridation Census, 1988: Atlanta: Centers for Disease Control, Dental Disease Prevention Activity, 1990
50. Federation Dentaire Internationale: Basic Fact Sheets. London: FDI, 1984
51. Horowitz HS: Grand Rapids: the public health story. J Public Health Dent 49:62–63, 1989
52. Ast DB, Fitzgerald B: Effectiveness of water fluoridation. J Am Dent Assoc 65:581–587, 1962
53. Murray JJ, Rugg-Gunn AJ: Fluorides and Dental Caries, 2edt. Bristol, UK: Wright, 1982
54. Newbrun E: Effectiveness of water fluoridation. J Public Health Dent 49:279–289, 1989
55. Jackson D: Has the decline of dental caries in English children made water fluoridation both unnecessary and uneconomic? Br Dent J 162:170–173, 1987
56. Burt BA (ed): Proceedings for the workshop: cost effectiveness of caries prevention in dental public health. J Public Health Dent 49:251–344, 1989
57. O'Mullane DM: The future of water fluoridation. J Dent Res 69:756–759, 1990
58. Stephen KW, McCall DR, Tallis JI: Caries prevalence in northern Scotland before, and 5 years after, water defluoridation. Br Dent J 163:324–326, 1987
59. Hoover RN, McKay FW, Fraumeni JF Jr: Fluoridated drinking water and the occurrence of cancer. J Nat Cancer Inst 57:757–768, 1976
60. Knox EG (Chairman): Fluoridation of Water and Cancer: A Review of the Epidemiological Evidence. Report of the working party. London: Her Majesty's Stationary Office, 1985
61. Marshall E: The fluoride debate: one more time. Science 247:276–277, 1990
62. Statement by James O. Mason, MD, Assistant Secretary for Health. April 26, 1990
63. Block LE: Antifluoridationists persist: the constitutional basis for fluoridation. J Public Health Dent 46:188–198, 1986
64. Easley MW, Wulf CA, Brayton KJ, Striffler DF (eds): Fluoridation: Litigation and Changing Public Policy. Proceedings of a workshop at the University of Michigan School of Public Health, Ann Arbor, 1984
65. Easley MW: The status of community water fluoridation in the United States. Public Health Rep 105:348–353, 1990

66. Horowitz HS, Heifetz SB, Law FE: Effect of school water fluoridation on dental caries: final results in Elk Lake, Pa, after 12 years. J Am Dent Assoc 84:832–838, 1972
67. Horowitz HS: The future of water fluoridation and other systemic fluorides. J Dent Res 69:760–764, 1990
68. Driscoll WS: The use of fluoride tablets for the prevention of dental caries. In Forrester DJ, Schulz EM (eds): International Workshop of Fluorides and Dental Caries Prevention. Baltimore: University of Baltimore, 1978:25–111
69. Binder K, Driscoll WS, Schutzmannsky G: Caries-preventive fluoride tablet programs. Caries Res 12 (suppl 1):22–30, 1978
70. Levy SM: Expansion of the proper use of systemic fluoride supplements. J Am Dent Assoc 112:30–34, 1986
71. Levy SM, Carrell AF: Compliance by health care providers with recommended systemic fluoride supplementation protocol. Clin Prev Dent 9:19–22, 1987
72. American Academy of Pediatrics, Committee on Nutrition: Fluoride Supplementation: Revised Dosage Schedule. Pediatrics 63:150–152, 1979
73. Dowell TB, Joyston-Bechal S: Fluoride supplements—age related dosages. Br Dent J 150:273–275, 1981
74. Bibby BG: A consideration of the effectiveness of various fluoride mixtures. J Am Dent Assoc 34:26, 1947
75. Muhler JC, Radike AW, Nebergall WH, Day HG: A comparison between the anticariogenic effect of dentifrices containing stannous fluoride and sodium fluoride. J Am Dent Assoc 51:556–559,1955
76. Brudevold F, Chilton NW: Comparative study of a fluoride dentifrice containing soluble phosphate and a calcium-free abrasive. Second year report. J Am Dent Assoc 72:889–894, 1966
77. Brudevold T, Naujoks R: Caries-preventive fluoride treatment of the individual: progress in caries prevention. Caries Res 12 (suppl 1):52–64, 1978
78. Wei SHY (ed): Clinical Uses of Fluorides. A State of the Art Conference on the Uses of Fluorides in Clinical Dentistry. Philadelphia: Lea & Febiger, 1985
79. American Dental Association: A guide to the use of fluorides for the prevention of dental caries. J Am Dent Assoc 113:506–565, 1986
80. Ripa LW: An evaluation of the use of professional (operator-applied) topical fluorides. J Dent Res 69:786–796, 1990
81. DeBruyn H, Arends J: Fluoride varnishes—a review. J Biol Buccale 15:71–82, 1987
82. Fine SD: Topical fluoride preparations for reducing incidence of dental caries. Notice of status. Fed Register 39:17245
83. Council on Dental Therapeutics: Council classifies fluoride mouthrinses. J Am Dent Assoc 91:1250–1252, 1975
84. Miller AJ, Brunelle JA: A summary of the NIDR community caries prevention demonstration program. J Am Dent Assoc 107:265–269, 1983
85. Leverett DH: Effectiveness of mouthrinsing with fluoride solutions in preventing coronal and root caries. J Public Health Dent 49:310–316, 1989
86. Renson CE, Crielaers PJA, Ibikunle SAJ, Pinto VG, Ross CB, Infirri JS, Takazoe I, Tala H: Changing patterns of oral health and implications for health manpower: part I. Int Dent J 35:235–251, 1985
87. Melberg JR, Ripa LW: Fluoride in Preventive Dentistry. Chicago: Quintessence, 1983:223–232
88. Council on Dental Materials and Devices: pit and fissure sealants. J Am Dent Assoc 93:134, 1976
89. Swift EJ: The effect of sealants on dental caries: a review. J Am Dent Assoc 116:700–704, 1988
90. Weintraub JA: The effectiveness of pit and fissure sealants. J Public Health Dent 49:317–330, 1989
91. Cohen L, Labelle A, Romberg E: The use of pit and fissure sealants in private practice: a national survey. J Public Health Dent 48:26–35, 1988
92. Whyte RJ, Leake JL, Hawkey TP: Two-year follow-up of 11,000 dental sealants in first permanent molars in the Saskatchewan Health Dental Plan. J Public Health Dent 47:177–181, 1987
93. Ismail AI, King W, Clark DC: An evaluation of the Saskatchewan pit and fissure sealant program: a longitudinal follow-up. J Public Health Dent 49:206–211, 1989
94. Calderone JJ, Mueller LA: The cost of sealant application in a state dental disease prevention program. J Public Health Dent 43:249–254, 1983
95. Hardison JR: The use of pit and fissure sealants in community public health programs in Tennessee. J Public Health Dent 43:233–239, 1983
96. Sterritt GR, Frew RA: Evaluation of a clinic-based sealant program. J Public Health Dent 48:220–224, 1988
97. Callanen VA, Weintraub JA, French DP, Connoll GN: Developing a sealant program: the Massachusetts approach. J Public Health Dent 46:141–146, 1986
98. Calderone JJ, Davis JM: The New Mexico sealant program: a progress report. J Public Health Dent 47:145–149, 1987
99. Lewis MH: Sealants for community programs. J Can Dent Assoc 51:841–846, 1985
100. Nickerson A: Sealants in a school-based preventive program: a six-month evaluation. Quintessence Int 19:565–569, 1988
101. Jones RB: The effects for recall patients of a comprehensive sealant program in a clinical dental public health setting. J Public Health Dent 46:152–155, 1986
102. Collins WJN, McCall DR, Strang R, et al: Experience with a mobile fissure sealing unit in the greater Glasgow area: results after three years. Community Dent Health 2:195–202, 1985
103. Massachusetts Department of Public Health and Massachusetts Health Research Institute, Inc: Preventing Pit and Fissure Caries: A Guide to Sealant Use. Boston, 1986
104. Tsamtsouris A, White GE: Nursing caries. J Pedod 1:198–207, 1977
105. Shelton PG, Berkowitz RJ, Forrester DJ: Nursing bottle caries. Pediatr 59:777–778, 1977
106. American Academy of Periodontology: Proceedings of the World Workshop in Clinical Periodontics. Chicago: 1989
107. Loe H, Theliade E, Jensen SB: Experimental gingivitis in man. J Periodontal 36:177–187, 1965
108. Socransky SS, Haffajee AD: Microbiological risk factors for destructive periodontal diseases. In Bader JD (ed): Risk Assessment in Dentistry. Chapel Hill: University of North Carolina Dental Ecology 1990:79–90
109. Loe H, Anerud A, Boysen H, Morrison JE: Natural history of periodontal disease in man. The rate of periodontal destruction before 40 years of age. J Periodontol 49:607–620, 1978
110. Socransky SS, Haffajee AD, Goodson JM, Lindhe J: New concepts of destructive periodontal disease. J Clin Periodontol 11:21–32, 1984
111. Burt BA: The status of epidemiological data on periodontal diseases. In Guggenheim B (ed): Periodontology Today. Basel: Karger, 1988, pp 68–76
112. Russell AL: A system of classification and scoring for prevalence surveys of periodontal disease. J Dent Res 35:350–359, 1956
113. Ramfjord SP: The periodontal disease index. J Periodontol 38 (suppl):30–38, 1967
114. Cutress TW, Ainamo J, Sardo, Infirri J: The Community Periodontal Index of Treatment Needs (CPITN) procedure for population groups and individuals. Int Dent J 37:222–233, 1987
115. Carlos JP, Wolfe MD, Kingman A: The extent and severity index: a simple method for use in epidemiological studies of periodontal disease. J Clin Periodontol 13:500–505, 1986
116. Capilouto ML, Douglass CW: Trends in the prevalence and severity of periodontal diseases in the US: a public health problem? J Public Health Dent 48:245–251, 1988
117. Douglass CW, Gillings D, Sollecito W, Gammon M: National trends in the prevalence and severity of the periodontal diseases. J Am Dent Assoc 107:403–412, 1983
118. Pilot T, Barmes DE: An update on periodontal conditions in adults, measured by CPITN. Int Dent J 37:169–172, 1987
119. Beck JD, Koch GG, Rozier RG, Tudor GE: Prevalence and risk

indicators for periodontal attachment loss in a population of older community-dwelling blacks and whites. J Periodontol 61:521–528, 1990
120. Haffajee AD, Oliver RC: Periodontal diseases working group summary and recommendations. In Bader JD (ed): Risk Assessment in Dentistry. Chapel Hill: University of North Carolina Dental Ecology, 1990, pp 306–308
121. Rivera-Hidalgo F: Smoking and periodontal health: a review of the literature. J Periodontol 57:617–624, 1986
122. Brown LJ, Oliver RC, Loe H: Evaluating periodontal status of U.S. employed adults. J Am Dent Assoc 121:226–232, 1990
123. Brown LF, Spencer AJ: Special report—continuing education in periodontology-the Adelaide study. Periodonto 10:12–13, 1989
124. Bader JD, McFall WT Jr, Rozier RG, Sams DH, Ramsey DL: Short-term change in dental providers' diagnostic data recording behavior following an educational intervention. J Cont Educat Health Professions 9:267–276, 1989
125. Federation Dentaire Internationale: The prevention of dental caries and periodontal disease. Int Dent J 34:141–158, 1984
126. Frazier JP: A new look at dental health education in community programs. Dent Hygiene 52:176–186, 1978
127. Ciancio SG: Non-surgical periodontal treatment. In Nevins M, Becker W, Kornmank (eds): Proceeding on the World Workshop in Clinical Periodontics. Chicago: American Academy of Periodontology, 1980 pp II-1–II-20
128. Knowles JW, Burgett FG, Nissle RR, et al: Results of periodontal treatment related to pocket depth and attachment level: eight years. J Periodontol 50:225–233, 1979
129. Axelsson P, Lindhe J: Effect of controlled oral hygiene procedures on caries and periodontal disease in adults: results after 6 years. J Clin Periodontol 8:239–248, 1981
130. Silverman S Jr: Oral Cancer, 3 edt. American Cancer Society, 1989
131. Silverman S, Gorsky M: Epidemiologic and demographic update in oral cancer: California and national data—1973–1985. J Am Dent Assoc 120:495–499, 1990
132. Blot WJ, McLaughlin JK, et al: Smoking and drinking in relation to oral and pharyngeal cancer. Cancer Res 48:3282–3287, 1988
133. Office of the Inspector General, Office of Analysis and Inspections: Youth Use of Smokeless Tobacco: More than a Pinch of Trouble. Dallas: Department of Health and Human Services, 1986
134. The Health Consequences of Using Smokeless Tobacco: A Report of the Advisory Committee to the Surgeon General. Bethesda, Md: Department of Health and Human Services Publication NO. (NIH) 86–2874, 1986
135. Winn DM, Blot WJ, Shy CM, Pickle LW, Toledo A, Fraumeni JR Jr: Snuff dipping and oral cancer among women in the Southern United States. N Engl J Med 304:745–749, 1981
136. Green JC, Louie R, Wycoff SJ: Preventive dentistry, II. Periodontal diseases, malocclusion, trauma, and oral cancer. JAMA 263:421–425, 1990
137. Christen AG: The dentist's role in helping patients stop smoking. J Am Dent Assoc 81:1146–1152, 1970
138. Cohn SJ, Stookey GK, Katz BP, Drook CA, Christen AG: Helping smokers quit: a randomized controlled trial with private practice dentists. J Am Dent Assoc 118:41–45, 1989
139. Healthy People 2000: National Health Promotion and Disease Prevention Objectives. Conference Edition, U.S. Department of Health and Human Services, 1990
140. Healthy Communities 2000: Model Standards Guidelines for Community Attainment of Year 2000 National Health Objectives, 3 rd edt. American Public Health Association, 1991

63

Injuries and the Public Health

Jess F. Kraus
Leon S. Robertson

This chapter is concerned with injuries that are considered unintentional. The first part of the chapter conceptualizes the causes of injuries in a public health context and presents information on the magnitude and scope of the injury problem. The second part examines countermeasure development and evaluation focusing on the variety of available strategies to reduce incidence or severity. Although space limits the breadth of the material that can be presented, the selection of illustrative topics generally corresponds with the magnitude and scope of the more common injuries.

Injuries kill and maim people, often destroy families, devastate communities, and do irreparable harm to society. Tragedies that result in great and instantaneous loss of life elicit widespread public reaction and sorrow (such as the earthquake in California during the 1989 World Series). Most people fail, however, to recognize that there is an hourly, daily, and weekly toll in death and injury, but because of the low frequency of large-loss events, the problem often is not publicized and hence is overlooked. For example, in the United States, more than 400 people die and thousands are hospitalized for treatment in an average *day* because of acute traumatic injury. Many of the injured survivors suffer lifelong disabilities, physical disfigurement, and financial ruin. One tragedy of injuries in our society is that much of the severity can be prevented with existing technology. But society, through its policy- or decision-makers, has chosen not to give the attention and resources to the problem necessary for research to determine the exposures involved or to develop (or maintain) countermeasures to reduce or eliminate injuries when the exposures are well recognized.

In addition to elected officials and policymakers, some public health professionals have not recognized that injuries represent a greater direct threat to the public's well-being than does AIDS or cancer. This lack of concern probably reflects the failure to appreciate the means available to reduce injury, plus the widely held view that injuries stem from personal behavior or irresponsible acts. It is ironic that this same view has not been openly expressed for the AIDS epidemic of the last 10 years, which, in fact, is connected directly to personal behaviors.

The traditional public health approach in disease control is to measure the occurrence of the affliction, identify the characteristics of the high-risk populations, determine the natural history and the agent of the disease, and then embark on an organized program for control. Many of the fatal infectious diseases of past centuries were greatly reduced or eliminated by focusing preventive action on the most feasible or vulnerable aspects in the chain of occurrence. This public health model has been applied to many infectious and chronic diseases, including those related to environmental exposures in the workplace, in the air we breathe, and in the food we consume. The classic model used successfully for common diseases parallels a similarly effective model to understand the ''natural history'' of injuries.

BENCHMARK CONTRIBUTIONS

Space does not permit a complete review of our evolutionary understanding of injury phenomena. However, there have been several benchmark contributions in our understanding of the nature of injuries and concepts for their control, a few of which will be cited here.

In 1971, Hugh DeHaven[1,2] survived a crash of his trainer aircraft and noted that the injuries he sustained were related to the interior design of the aircraft cabin. He surmised that the lacerations of his abdominal organs appeared to have been caused by the restraint (safety) belts, particularly the shape of the buckle where the belts attached. This observation led to broader questions of how injuries occur when humans come into contact with their physical surroundings during blunt impacts, such as car crashes and falls. Important in DeHaven's observations on falls was specifying why some people survived falls from seemingly fatal heights and others did not. The factors contributing to crash deaths or survival prompted DeHaven to explore (through the Cornell University Crash Research Project) ways in which vehicle engineering could reduce the severity of injuries during crashes. DeHaven's work prompted others to study human tolerance to energy forces during impacts of all kinds and to apply design changes that take human dynamics during car crashes into consideration.

DeHaven's efforts influenced others to explore the reasons for and the ways to control injuries during motor-vehicle crashes. For example, John Stapp[3] showed that survival without significant injury was possible in 35 to 45 *g* test-sled decelerations. These deceleration rates are similar to the ones that occur in sudden-impact motor-vehicle crashes. Stapp's sled tests illustrated the importance of the design of passenger restraints, which ultimately led to their use in automobiles.

Apparently the earliest reference to epidemiology in injury

research was in a 1949 paper by *John Gordon.*[4] Although he wrote of "accidents" and misidentified the agents, he noted that injuries were patterned by age, gender, and other demographic factors, as well as by time and place and that they were amenable to study and potential prevention, much like diseases are.

James Gibson,[5] in a 1961 paper, specified dimensions and definitions of the agent of injury—energy in its forms. His work (and that of William Haddon, Jr.[6,7]) set the foundation for the development of a conceptual formulation of injuries, their mechanism of occurrence, and strategies for control. His view that energy was the necessary and specific agent of all injuries and existed in several forms was the first of several novel illustrations of the parallel mechanism of causation between disease and injury agents.

At about the same time, *William Haddon, Jr.* recognized energy as the agent of injuries and expanded this idea to include vehicles and vectors of energy transmission and the notion of human resistance (or susceptibility) to these energy forces.[6,7] He noted two broad classes of energy-host interactions. The first was energy delivered in excess of body thresholds, such as mechanical energy in motor-vehicle crashes, and the second was insufficient energy due to metabolic interference, such as occurs in drowning or carbon monoxide poisoning.[6] His cohort and case-control studies of injuries with colleagues in the 1960s[8-10] helped establish the appropriateness and value of epidemiological approaches in injury research. He partitioned the time sequence of injuries into the preevent, event, and postevent combined with host, vehicle, and environmental factors, now called the Haddon Matrix.[10,11]

EPIDEMIOLOGICAL MODEL

Reservoirs, agents, mechanisms of transfer of the agent, and host response to the agent are traditional elements in the epidemiological analysis of almost all public health problems. This model has relevance and application to injuries as well.

The following schematic shows the elements and the manner of interchange between a susceptible host and exposure to the agent of injury via the mechanism of energy transfer.

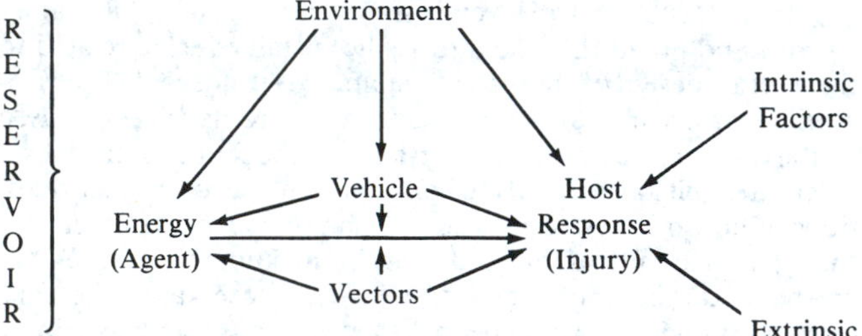

The Reservoir. In epidemiology the reservoir is that place where the agent is usually found in the environment. The concept of a "reservoir" has utility in visualizing the scheme of an energy source and the ways it is transferred. For example, generators are the reservoirs of concentrations of human-made electricity, which in turn is transmitted via electrical wires that can come into contact with the host; gasoline is a reservoir of energy converted by vehicles into kinetic energy.

The Agent. The agent is energy. Concepts of necessary and sufficient causes have some utility here, realizing that injuries are seen in a variety of different physical (clinical) ways. Energy can be delivered in such a way as to cause blunt trauma to tissues and organs, or it can be delivered in the form of projectiles, which produce penetrating wounds to those same organs. Some forms of energy damage more at the cellular or tissue level; others, at the organ or systems level. Nonetheless, without energy beyond human tolerances, there would be no trauma. The forms of energy are mechanical, electrical, chemical, radiation, and thermal forces. Understanding how energy is transmitted to the body and how it behaves at the cellular, tissue, or organ level aids in the development of preventive and treatment approaches.

Vehicles and Vectors. Vehicles are inanimate objects (motor vehicles, bullets, cigarettes, flammable fabrics) that serve to convey energy from its reservoir to potential or actual exposure of a host. An exposure may or may not result in injury, depending on whether the amount of contact between a susceptible host and the energy involved is outside the band of tissue tolerance. In day-to-day life we come into contact with small energy sources when we step into sunshine, when we bump against inanimate objects, or when we fall, as in a trip on the pavement.

The issue of threshold or tolerance level of injury is important in understanding injuries from exposure to energy.[12] A human being also can exert mechanical energy, hence becoming an animate object or a vector of energy. The kick of a horse, bite of a dog, or sting of a bee also are ways in which either mechanical or chemical energy is conveyed by vectors.

Host Response. Humans have some potential to increase their resistance to energy forces: muscle and bone strengthening among athletes and tanning for increased resistance to the sun are examples of this potential, although the risk of skin cancer is increased by the latter. Yet, there are limits beyond which energy delivered to the host cannot be absorbed or tolerated. Whether the damage is reversible and tissue integrity is restored is problematic; it depends on a number of factors, some of which are intrinsic to the host, such as changes in tissue associated with age or medical conditions. Factors extrinsic to the human are those taken in by the host that greatly influence the human's response to energy. Fatigue, alcohol, and drugs can reduce the host's ability to respond to energy forces. Likewise, proper diet and physical conditioning can improve a human's response to energy delivered in excess of whole-body threshold.

The Haddon Matrix. A refinement of the conceptual model in injury causation was advanced by Haddon over 20 years ago.[13] This model perceives injury in a time continuum; that is, factors related to exposure (preevent), to energy contact (event), and host response to the damage (postevent). It integrates the classic public health approach with the sequential steps in injury causation. Although the Haddon Matrix (Table 63-1) was initially applied to motor-vehicle crashes and countermeasures for highway safety, its use for other hazardous exposures has been established.

The first dimension of this matrix, which Haddon called phases, recognizes that damaging interactions of host and energy occurs in steps, sometimes separated only by fractions of a sec-

TABLE 63-1. THE HADDON MATRIX WITH ILLUSTRATIONS

	Factors		
Phases	***Human***	***Vehicle***	***Environment***
Preinjury	Alcohol intoxication	Instability in utility vehicles	Visibility of hazards
Injury	Resistance to energy insults	Sharp or pointed edges and surfaces	Flammable building materials
Postinjury	Hemorrhage	Rapidity of energy reduction	Emergency medical response

ond. The second dimension of the matrix is divided into human, vehicle or equipment, and environmental components. These elements or factors reflect Haddon's public health training and are comparable to the elements of the classic public health epidemiological model described earlier. In Haddon's view the matrix provided a means for identifying all hazardous interactions, resources to be allocated, and countermeasures that could be considered.[14]

INJURY OCCURRENCE

This section presents the magnitude and scope of the injury problem in the United States and is restricted largely to U.S. data. Although an exhaustive review of the magnitude of the injury problem is not possible here, we highlight some of the major problem areas and refer the reader to other resources for more in-depth treatment of the topic.

Data Sources. Gable[15] assembled information on a number of data sources on national estimates of injury occurrence. Injury counts and descriptions are found in a number of documents published routinely by the National Center for Health Statistics (NCHS). Computer data tapes are available through NCHS for additional analyses.

The most complete data base on motor-vehicle-related crash deaths is found in the Fatal Accident Reporting System (FARS) data base. Standardized crash reports from all state and local police agencies in the United States are the source of the data maintained and analyzed by the National Highway Traffic Safety Administration, which also makes data tapes available for investigator analysis.

Work-related fatal injuries, as identified through the National Traumatic Occupational Fatality Data Base in the National Institute for Occupational Safety and Health, are based on a single factor reported on the standard U.S. death certificate, namely, whether the fatal injury occurred while the person was at work. The information available on the deaths represents variables from death certificates; however, the validity of the datum to identify work-related deaths is not established.

There are a few sources of injury morbidity data available to the public health researcher. Technically, the most accurate in case identification is the hospital-discharge information from the NCHS or local hospitals. Some information is available for inpatients discharged with injury-related diagnoses, but data on circumstances is required in only a few states. The Bureau of Labor Statistics, in cooperation with the Occupational Safety and Health Administration, surveys approximately 280,000 employers each year to obtain estimates of the number and rates of occupational fatalities and injuries. The Work-Injury Annual Survey, however, has been criticized for a number of technical and administrative reasons.[16] The Bureau of Labor Statistics is moving to correct many of the difficulties, and this data source may become a more accurate and technically valuable summary of work-related fatal and nonfatal injuries. In addition, the Bureau of Labor Statistics, through state workers' compensation information, publishes reports on occupational injuries and illnesses. The workers' compensation data base extends to only 30 states in the United States and does not include populations not covered under state workers' compensation laws, such as self-employed or domestic workers.

The Consumer Product Safety Commission collects data from a national sample of U.S. hospital emergency rooms in the National Electronic Injury Surveillance System (NEISS). Unfortunately, there are fewer than 70 hospitals in the sample, and questions of representativeness and completeness of reporting based on a small sample size is of concern.

Finally, the National Highway Traffic Safety Administration collects data on nonfatal motor vehicle injuries in the National Accident Sampling System (NASS). The latter is based on an area probability sample of U.S. police-reported crashes. Gable [15] provides information on how the various data bases can be obtained.

Restriction of Data Sources. The counts of fatal injuries in the United States are virtually complete, although delayed deaths related to infection or other complications are not included in some systems. Data are substantially incomplete for those injuries not resulting in death. Since we have no nationwide surveillance system that includes circumstances and severities, it is difficult to judge their true scope, nature, and outcomes. The majority and best understood are severe injuries caused mostly by mechanical energy; however, some mortality estimates are available for poisonings, electrocutions, drownings, and injuries from other mechanisms.

Some data limitations should be noted. One concern is that most fatal-injury-counting practices are only in force for the first 30 days following an injury. With existing nosologies, a death 6 months after acute traumatic injury could be coded as a noninjury death, depending on the institution, agency, or state involved. Therefore, so-called late deaths from injury may or may not be included in statewide or national tabulations. This problem is most evident in considering late deaths in the elderly following hip fracture, where a long delay from the time of the fall to death might result in a misclassification.

Worldwide data on injury occurrences is nonexistent, although counts of fatal injuries are fairly well documented in economically developed countries. The number of worldwide hospitalized injuries and those requiring clinical or health-care-provider treatment followed by release to home or environment are also unknown. In societies where there is no system of collection of national health care data, there is little hope of valid counts of the number of persons injured, the descriptions of those injuries, and their external causes. But with today's greater emphasis on injury surveillance, by the end of this century there should be a much better appreciation of the total impact of injuries in many countries. Before long we should be able to determine, with reasonable accuracy, the number of cases each year and who is at highest risk.

INJURY FREQUENCY: DEATHS AND MORBIDITY

In 1988 there were about 150,000 men, women, and children killed from injury-related causes in the United States.[17] In 1987 more than 2.78 million people were hospitalized for treatment of injuries,[18] and the number of nonfatally injured who required some form of medical treatment during 1987 is estimated at almost 60 million individuals, or about one in every four persons in the United States.[19] There are few diseases, afflictions, or health conditions of humans that affect approximately one fourth of the population each year. Yet, the resources given to the problem are minuscule compared to their cost and societal impact.[10]

Mortality Data. Figure 63–1 shows average annual age-specific unintentional injury death rates for males and females for the United States from 1980 to 1986. Rates peak at ages 15 through 25 and in the oldest years for males and females, and males have higher death rates than females at all ages. The contribution of deaths in male teenagers and young adults (mostly from motor-vehicle crashes) and older adults (mostly from falls) accounts for a disproportionate share of the fatal injuries.

Figure 63–2 shows race-specific death rates per 100,000

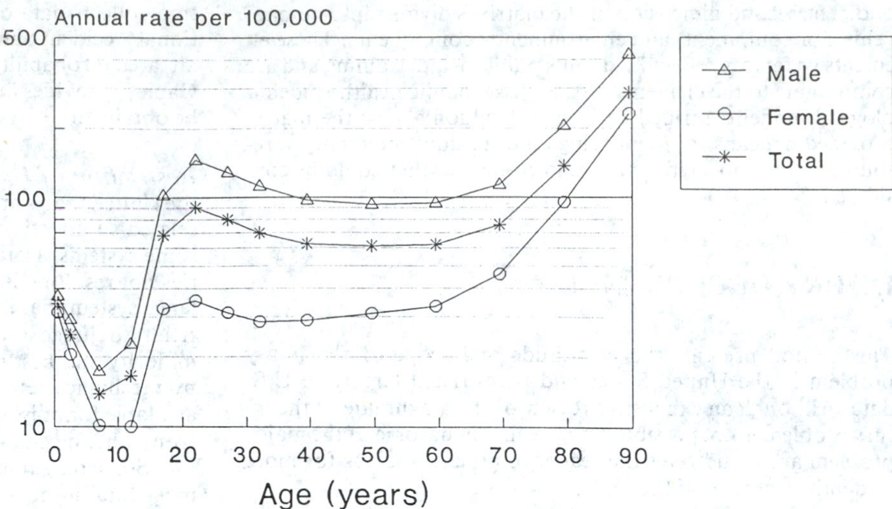

Figure 63-1. Death rate for injuries by age and sex. *[Data from Baker SP, O'Neill B, Ginsberg M: The Injury Fact Book, 2 edt. New York: Oxford University Press, 1991.]*

population by major groups of external causes, excluding intentional injuries. There are differences in death rates across the four race groups, with blacks and Native Americans having higher rates than whites and Asians in all the major categories except falls. The excessive rates for minority populations is thought to be related mainly to income and living conditions. Many of the differences in rates may be explained on the basis of exposure; for example, poor, untrained, and undereducated individuals may qualify only for the most hazardous jobs, live in the poorest housing, and drive the oldest and poorest-maintained vehicles, particularly in rural areas that have the most hazardous roads.

Deaths and Death Rates by General Circumstances. Figure 63–3 indicates types of circumstances of fatal injuries by age. Motor vehicles account for more than half of unintentional injury deaths in the United States, either as vehicle crashes or collisions of vehicles with bicyclists and pedestrians. The disparity in age-specific risks has prompted many of the countermeasures that are discussed later in this chapter. Figure 63–4 provides data proportionately for males and females. Exposure differences by gender for the age groups may account for some, but not all, of the differences in mortality patterns observed.

Figure 63–5 shows the distribution of fatal motor-vehicle-related injuries by major subgroups and age. Proportionate display is somewhat misleading because it assumes that all persons are exposed equally to all forms of exposure. The dramatic increase in death rates for adolescents reflects increases in exposure as young people become drivers of and passengers in motor vehicles. The excess includes motor-vehicle and pedestrian deaths in children, motorcycle-crash deaths in young people, and motor-vehicle–occupant deaths (beginning in the teenage years) from car or truck crashes.

Regardless of how the information on injuries is counted or displayed, injuries are the single largest cause of death in the younger segments of the U.S. population. The death rates from injuries, compared to the three leading causes of death in the United States (heart disease, cancer, and stroke), are illustrated in Figure 63–6. Throughout life, death rates vary by age, but injuries are the most obvious threat to life in the younger, most productive ages of the life cycle.

Person-Years of Life Lost. Whether measured by numbers of deaths, death rates, or as a rank of cause of death, injuries account for a tremendous toll in human life lost. Another way of describing loss is years of potential life lost, which gives age of death more substantial meaning. It has been calculated that about 5 million life years are lost each year due to injuries, and the total of life years lost for the age group 25 to 44 represents 39% of all life years lost to injury. Life years lost per death for injuries, cancer, and cardiovascular disease are illustrated in Figure 63–7.

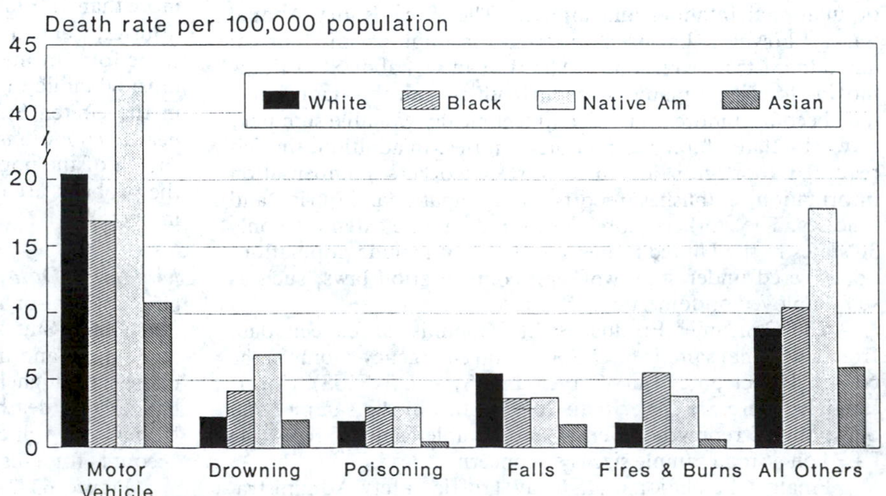

Figure 63-2. Unintentional injury death rate by external cause and race, United States, 1980–1986. *[Data from Baker SP, O'Neill B, Ginsberg M: The Injury Fact Book, 2 edt. New York: Oxford University Press, 1991.]*

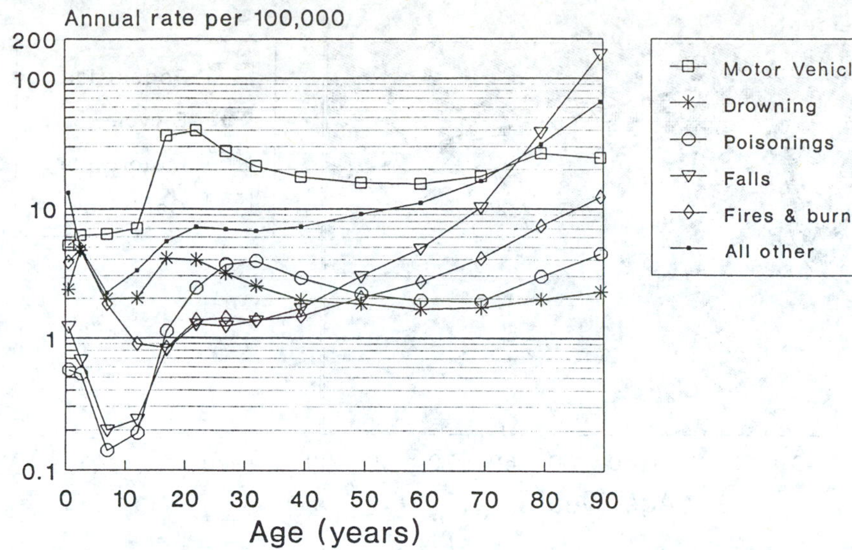

Figure 63-3. Death rate for unintentional injuries by age and external cause. *[Data from Baker SP, O'Neill B, Ginsberg M: The Injury Fact Book, 2 edt. New York: Oxford University Press, 1991.]*

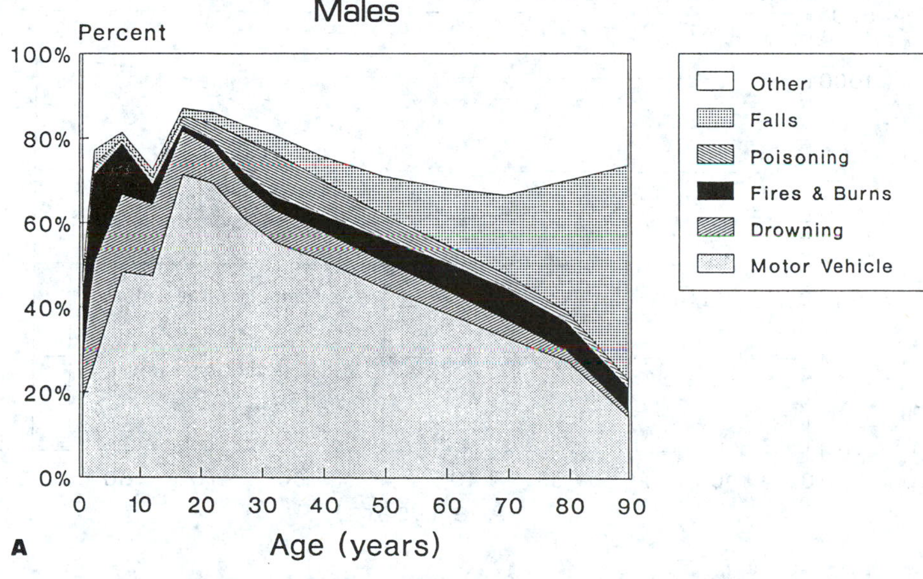

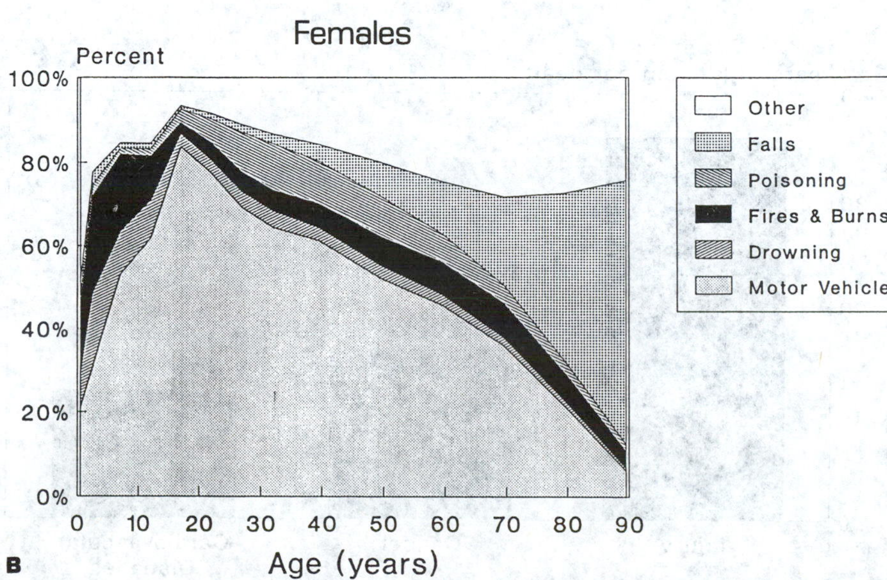

Figure 63-4. Death rate for unintentional injuries by external cause among males **[A]** and females **[B]**. *[Data from Baker SP, O'Neill B, Ginsberg M: The Injury Fact Book, 2 edt. New York: Oxford University Press, 1991.]*

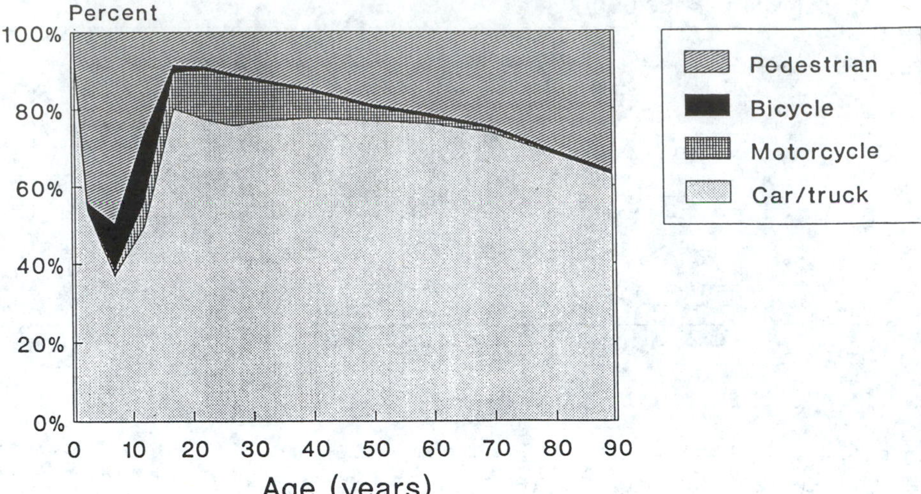

Figure 63-5. Percentage distribution of motor vehicle deaths by age and method of transport. *[Data from Baker SP, O'Neill B, Ginsberg M: The Injury Fact Book, 2 edt. New York: Oxford University Press, 1991.]*

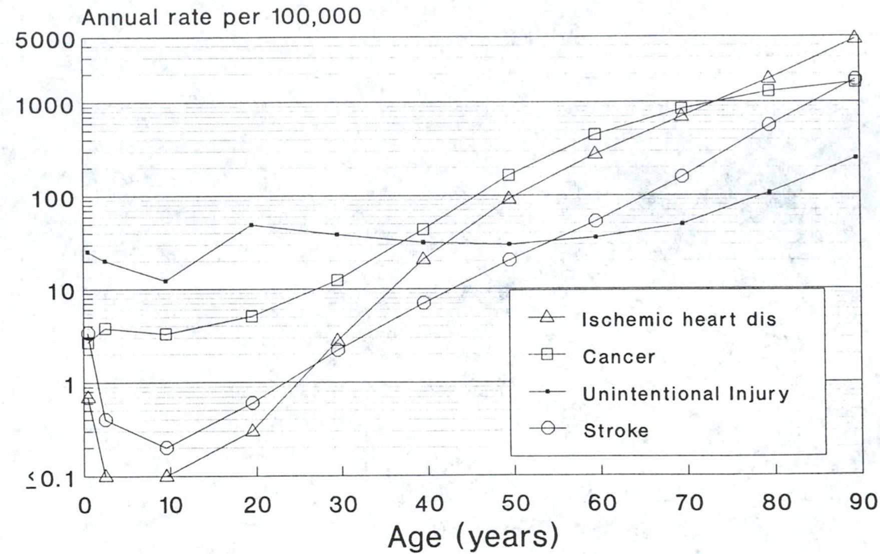

Figure 63-6. Death rate for four leading causes of death by age. *[Data from National Center for Health Statistics: Advance Report of Final Mortality Statistics, 1987. Monthly Vital Statistics Report 38[5][suppl], 1989.]*

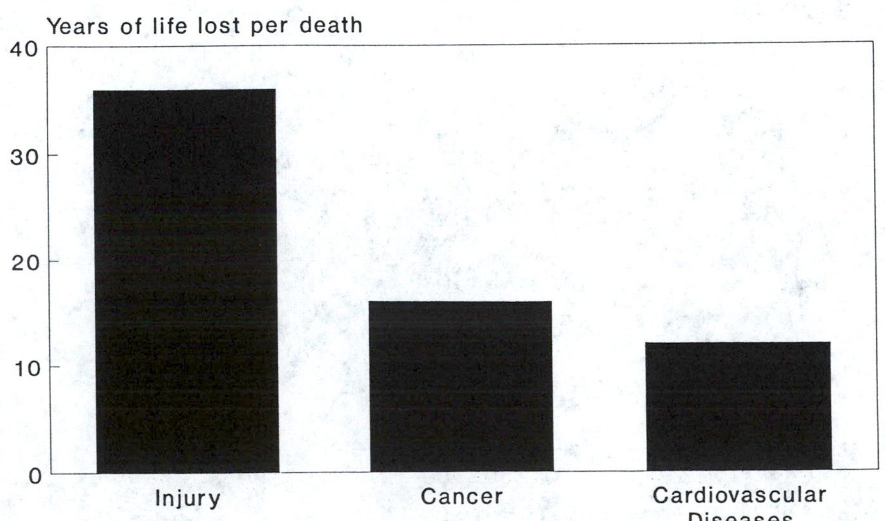

Figure 63-7. Life years lost from injury compared to other health problems. *[Data from Rice DP, MacKenzie EJ, et al: Cost of Injury in the United States. University of California and Johns Hopkins University, 1989.]*

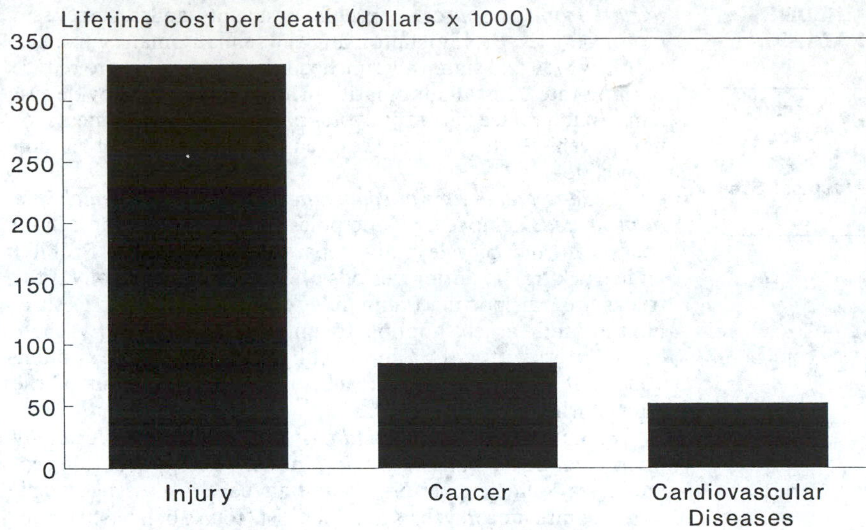

Figure 63-8. Cost of injury compared to other health problems. *[Data from Rice DP, MacKenzie EJ, et al: Cost of Injury in the United States. University of California and Johns Hopkins University, 1989.]*

Economic Costs. Direct costs are the actual expenditures related to the injury per se; they include expenses for professional medical care, institutional services, medications, and rehabilitation. Total direct costs amounted to almost $45 billion for those injured in 1985. Another way to assess costs of injuries is to compare lifetime cost per death for injuries with other causes of death, such as cancer and cardiovascular disease (Fig. 63-8). The higher lifetime costs for injuries reflect the earlier average age of onset and the longer period of time for treatment, particularly for those with severe spinal cord and brain injury.

Lifetime costs of injuries by circumstances (Fig. 63-9) show that motor-vehicle crashes account for about one third of all lifetime injury costs in the United States, while injuries from falls and firearms account for another third. Targeted and effective countermeasures on these three external causes could result in the greatest reduction in costs.

Morbidity. Although morbidity data are limited, the National Hospital Discharge Survey gives an estimate of severe injury in the U.S. population. Table 63-2 shows an annual estimate of persons hospitalized for injuries, the rates per 100,000 population, the average annual hospital days for the injuries, and the average annual length of stay per injury. Over 2.8 million people were hospitalized for an injury each year from 1983 to 1987 (about 1 per 100 population per year). This number represents more than 18 million hospital days, with an average of 6.6 days of hospital stay per person hospitalized. The table shows that spinal-cord injury, brain injury with skull fracture, and burns, while numbering 108,000 (3.8%) of the 2.8 million injuries, accounted for the highest average hospital days and the longest lengths of hospital stay. What is notable in the data is what is missing: there is little information currently available on specific types of injury associated with specific external causes.

INJURY CONTROL STRATEGIES

The conceptualization of injuries in epidemiological terms was accompanied by a rethinking of approaches to prevention. Given what we know about the contribution of kinetic energy to injury, human limitations in perception of motion, reaction time, attention spans, and addictions to alcohol and other substances makes "accident prevention" by changing human behavior far too narrow a view of the options available.[20]

Although we now often refer to "injury prevention," that too has unrealistic and unnecessary implications. Many of the most effective strategies do not prevent injuries, but they do have a major effect on severity by the control of energy or its carriers. For example, seat belts in motor vehicles seldom prevent all injuries. Cuts, contusions, and fractures, particularly to hands, arms, legs, and feet, are common among belted vehicle occupants in crashes because belts do not restrain limbs that flail around from the forces in a crash. Belts and many other approaches reduce severity—the proportion of cases in which death and disability occur. For these reasons it is more appropriate to refer to "injury control" when addressing ameliorative approaches.

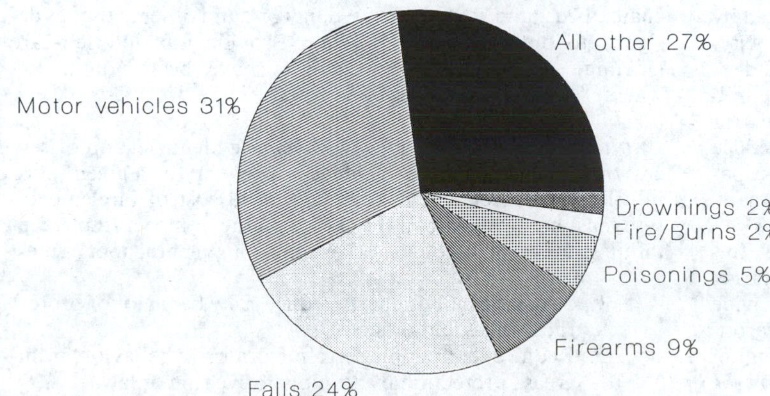

Figure 63-9. Total lifetime cost of injury by external cause, 1985. *[Data from Rice DP, MacKenzie EJ, et al: Cost of Injury in the United States. University of California and Johns Hopkins University, 1989.]*

TABLE 63-2. FIRST-LISTED DIAGNOSES OF PERSONS HOSPITALIZED FOR INJURIES IN THE UNITED STATES, 1983–1987

Condition	Average Annual Discharges (No.)	Rate/10^5	Average Annual Length of Hospital Stay (d)
Brain injury with skull fracture	19,000	8.0	11.8
Fractured skull or face without brain injury	108,000	45.4	4.5
Brain injury, no fractured skull	264,000	111.2	5.4
Spinal cord injury	16,000	6.9	23.2
Other nerve injury	9,000	3.9	3.4
Trunk fracture	166,000	70.3	9.6
Other fracture or dislocation	930,000	392.6	8.6
Internal or blood vessel injuries or open wound	377,000	159	5.1
Superficial strains or sprains	505,000	213.3	5.0
Crushing injury	10,000	4.4	5.6
Burn	73,000	30.9	10.4
Poisoning	228,000	96.2	3.7
Other	132,000	55.6	4.2
TOTAL	2,873,000	1000	6.6

From the National Center for Health Statistics, Centers for Disease Control: Data computed by the Division of Epidemiology and Health Promotion from data collected by the Division of Health Care Statistics and the U.S. Bureau of Census.

William Haddon, Jr.,[21] organized technical strategies for injury control into 10 logically distinct categories. The following is a list of the strategies, with examples relevant to some of the more commonly severe injuries:

1. *Prevent the creation of the hazard in the first place.* Do not allow the manufacture of particularly hazardous vehicles, such as motorcycles, minibikes, and "all terrain" vehicles. These vehicles are used mainly for recreation, for which there are numerous alternative and less hazardous activities.

2. *Reduce the amount of the hazard brought into being.* Require that passenger vehicles, particularly utility vehicles, have lower centers of gravity or wider track width such that track width divided by twice the height of center of gravity (T/2H) is not less than 1.2. (Vehicles with lower T/2H have 3 to 20 times as many fatal rollover crashes as those with values of 1.2 or greater, and the relative risk is strongly correlated to T/2H).[22] Require that all motor vehicles operated on a level surface be incapable of speeds greater than 65 miles per hour. (The energy generated by a vehicle in motion is an exponential function of its velocity. Limitations on maximum speed would also conserve fuel and reduce emissions). Restrict the sale of handguns to police and military units. Reduce the number of pills in a drug prescription to a number that would not kill or disable if taken all at once. Reduce flammability of clothing. Reduce maximum temperature capability of hot water heaters, which is the source of heat for many scald burns.

3. *Prevent the release of the hazard that already exists.* Improve braking capability of heavy trucks. Keep guns for target shooting at the shooting range rather than in homes. Provide canes and walkers to the elderly and handrails in their environments. Make matches and lighters less easy for children to ignite.

4. *Modify the rate or spatial distribution of release of the hazard from its source.* Use child restraints and seat belts in motor vehicles. Prohibit automatic and semiautomatic guns. Use lightly woven and smoothly finished fabrics in clothing to reduce burning rates. Install automatic sprinkler systems. Provide systems that replace air rapidly in passenger compartments of motor vehicles to prevent elevated concentrations of carbon monoxide.

5. *Separate, in time or space, the hazard and that which is to be protected.* Remove trees and poles from near roadsides. Build pedestrian and bicycle paths separated from roads. Prohibit large truck traffic during periods of congestion, especially if the trucks are transporting flammables or toxic chemicals. Restrict hunting and target shooting to unpopulated areas. Evacuate coastal areas at times of approaching hurricanes. Use cooking units that children cannot reach or keep children out of the kitchen while cooking.

6. *Separate the hazard and that which is to be protected by interposition of a material barrier.* Increase energy absorbing capability of vehicle exteriors. Install air bags in passenger vehicles. Require motorcyclists and bicyclists to use helmets. Use energy absorbing barriers on the fronts and rears of large trucks that are compatible with car bumper heights. Place energy absorbing barriers between roads and bridge abutments or other necessary rigid structures near roads. Place fences with gates that children cannot open around swimming pools and other bodies of water that are accessible to children. Install guards on boat propellers, industrial machines, and the like where moving parts can injure persons who are nearby. Use insulated firewalls in vehicles and buildings. Invent an additive to alcoholic beverages and other commonly ingested drugs that reduces absorption through the wall of the digestive track into the bloodstream as increasing amounts are ingested.

7. *Modify basic relevant qualities of the hazard.* Eliminate sharp points and edges on vehicle exteriors. Eliminate protruding knobs and "karate chop" dashboards in vehicle interiors. Use breakaway designs for utility poles and light poles along roadsides. Prohibit more than one trailer on tractor-trailer rigs. Reduce muzzle velocity of guns. Use trigger locks on guns. Apply to ammunition sold to the public the Geneva Convention regulation that prohibits flattening and fragmenting of bullets used in war. Use energy-absorbing materials of adequate depth on playground surfaces.

8. *Make what is to be protected more resistant to damage from the hazard.* Develop treatment of persons with hemophilia and osteoporosis to increase resistance to mechanical energy exchanges. Require physical conditioning before participation in sports that produce condition-related injuries.

9. *Begin to counter the damage already done by the environmental hazard.* Increase the availability of roadside emergency telephones. Place emergency response teams near areas that have relatively high injury rates. Increase the use of smoke and carbon monoxide detectors.

10. *Stabilize, repair, and rehabilitate the object of the damage.* Provide prosthetic devices for amputees, along with wheelchairs, beds, and equipment used in work and other activities designed to optimize normal living. Provide job and self-care training. Numerous other examples have been noted elsewhere.[20,21,22,24]

Implementation Strategies. Given the identification of several options to reduce the incidence or severity of a given set of injuries, the effectiveness, feasibility, and cost of implementation must be considered in the choice of one or more. Implementation strategies can be categorized into four general approaches:

1. Persuade individuals to reduce risky behavior or protect themselves and others.
2. Require that people refrain from risky behaviors or increase protection by administrative rule or law.

3. Change vehicles or environments to increase automatic protection (that is, the individual at immediate risk does not have to be changed to be protected).
4. Improve postinjury emergency and rehabilitative treatment services.

Our discussion will focus on the first three options. Usually, automatic protection is the most successful and persuasion the least successful, particularly if the persons at risk must take very frequent action for protection (e.g., use of child restraints and seat belts in cars).[25]

Persuasion. Behavior change can have negative as well as positive effects and should be subjected to the same evaluation criteria as other approaches. One of the most costly attempts to alter behavior is driver education in the public schools. According to the latest survey, 1982–83, there were 998,363 students enrolled in driver education programs. Costs per pupil among the states varied widely, but the median was $163, for a total cost to taxpayers (or parents where fees were charged) of approximately $162.7 million in that year,[26] not counting time diverted from academic subjects.

Scientific evaluation of driver education in the public schools finds that expenditure to be unjustified. Carefully controlled experiments show that driver education has little or no effect on individual risk in the aggregate.[27,28] Furthermore, it results in a large increase in licensure in an age group that has a very high crash rate.[27,29] When driver education was eliminated from the public schools in nine Connecticut school districts, there was a net 75% decline in licensure among those who would have been licensed after high school driver education compared to districts similar in population that retained the course. A parallel reduction in crashes was found in the communities that dropped the course.[30]

Involvement of several community organizations in relatively intense campaigns directed at one specific behavior has proved effective in a few instances where studied. A campaign urging use of bicycle helmets by children included distribution of coupons for a discount on helmet purchases, school and community group promotional efforts, and prizes for children wearing helmets at bicycling events. Bicycle helmet use increased from 6% to 16% among observed child bicyclists.[31]

On the basis of research regarding child "dart-out" behavior resulting in pedestrian injuries, a campaign using an animated character, "Willy Whistle," in schools and on television was studied in three cities. The researchers estimated a 20% reduction in dart-out injuries to pedestrians younger than 15 years of age and a 12% reduction in all child-pedestrian injuries.[32] The success of the campaign is dependent on use in school classrooms and on television. The television time (e.g., 380 showings in Los Angeles valued at $150,000) was contributed by local stations as a public service. Despite the effectiveness of the campaign, apparently only Miami, Florida, has used the program consistently, according to officials of the National Highway Traffic Safety Administration. While the harmful high school driver education course was retained in numerous school districts, the "Willy Whistle" videotapes and teaching materials remained on the shelves or were discarded by numerous television stations and schools to which they were sent.

Television advertisements urging belt use, even when directed at specific audiences and shown during popular programs appealing to those audiences but in the absence of other community efforts, have not been found effective when studied in controlled experiments.[33] Most such campaigns have not been subjected to outcome research. Smoke detector use increased dramatically in the 1980s, at least partly due to advertising. Numerous hospitals, foundations, institutes, safety councils, and health departments have produced and used brochures, films, and curricula aimed at changing injury-related behavior, but most have done so without careful research on the effects of the efforts.[34]

Adequately researched effects of attempts at behavior change has been mixed. The acts of simply handing out brochures or counseling by health educators has often been ineffective when it is aimed at behavior that requires frequent action (such as child-restraint use)[35] or that involves inconvenience (such as storing household articles hazardous to children).[36] The involvement of physicians in more intense counseling has been found to significantly increase child-restraint use.[37,38] Medically treated fall injuries to infants were reduced by information on falls displayed above examining tables and by physician counseling.[39]

Seat belt use has been increased by incentives in the form of lotteries[40,41] and by use of a sticker stating "seat belt use required in this car" displayed on the dash in front of passengers.[42]

In sum, certain behavior-change approaches can be demonstrated as effective scientifically, but harmful effects cannot be ruled out without good controlled research. Persons who are using or are contemplating such an approach would be well advised to test the effects in a controlled experiment before beginning widespread use. The application of this approach in a systematic, sustained way may also be problematical, even when known to be effective. The expectation that thousands of television stations, schools, communities, or physicians will adopt a given approach and use it appropriately, once the effectiveness is demonstrated, is often not realized.

Law and Individual Behavior. The effect of laws on risk reduction depends on the amount of risk associated with the targeted behavior, enforcement, and several nonlegal factors. An important nonlegal factor is augmentation of the enforcement of the law by people in the community other than police.

The legal minimum driving age is mainly enforced by parents who are unlikely to allow unlicensed drivers to use the family car. Researchers have compared fatal crash involvement of 16-year-old drivers in New Jersey where there is a 17-year-old licensing age (except for an agricultural license at age 16) with Connecticut where the licensing age is 16. A 65% to 85% reduction in fatalities where 16-year-old drivers were involved was associated with a 17-year-old minimum licensing age.[43] The study found that the fatal crash rates of drivers aged 17 to 29 years were comparable between the states, indicating no evidence that the reduction among 16-year-old drivers was offset by increased driving by 17- to 29-year-olds who were called on to transport the 16-year-old nondrivers. Also, there were no offsetting rates of 16-year-olds killed as pedestrians or bicyclists.

In 1985, 2014 people in the United States were killed in crashes where a driver was 16 years old. Since the fatality rate per mile driven of persons in the age range of the parents of 16-year-olds is 91% lower than that of their children, parent substitution for the 16-year-old driver would have prevented about 1375 deaths ($2014 \times 0.91 \times 0.75$) in 1985, if the 75% reduction in New Jersey can be generalized to other states. This is a minimal estimate because it is unlikely that every trip of a 16-year-old driver would be substituted by a parent or other adult. A survey of teenagers in Michigan, New Jersey, and New York, each state having different rates of licensure, found little effect of licensure on life-style. The increase in percentage of teenagers with jobs, comparing employment at age 15 and 16, was highest in New Jersey where licensure at 16 was prohibited except in agriculture.[44]

Similarly, laws that impose curfews on teenage driving reduce the numbers of their crashes,[45] not because police officers can identify the age of drivers at night but because the law gives parents a criterion on which to set the time of return of the teenager with the family car. The minimum legal drinking age reduces alcohol-related crashes of drivers younger than the prescribed age, primarily due to enforcement by proprietors of businesses selling alcohol.[46]

Health problems related to alcohol, including motor vehicle fatalities, are lower where alcohol taxes are higher.[47] However, alcohol taxes have not been raised to keep pace with inflation. Restoring the 1950 taxes on alcohol, adjusted for inflation, would increase the generated revenues by $20 billion per year.[48]

Observability of behavior is also an important factor in the effect of law on individual behavior. Drivers who are intoxicated can often drive well enough to avoid notice by police, who must have probable cause to obtain a breath or blood sample. The arrest rate is very low, between 1 in 200 and 1 in 2000. Laws such as administrative license suspension for driving while intoxicated (DWI) and mandatory jail sentences for DWI have been found to have small effects on fatal crashes of motor vehicles, 5% and 2%, respectively.[49]

Laws directed to more easily observable behaviors are far more successful. In association with the enactment of child-restraint use laws, infant deaths to car occupants per population in that age group declined 37% from 1980 to 1984. The reduction for children 1 to 4 years of age in 1980 to 1984 was 25% and for 5 to 9 years of age was 11%.[50] In one emergency room, head injuries to children younger than 4 years of age declined 26% from before to after the child-restraint-use law in California, while changes in less severe injuries were statistically insignificant.[51] The reductions were found despite numerous exemptions in the laws among states. About 39% of the children 0 to 5 years of age who were killed in the year preceding the law were not covered by the law because of age or other exemptions.[52]

Laws requiring motorcyclists to use easily observable helmets reduce motorcyclists' deaths about 24% to 30%.[53-55] Data on nonfatal head injuries are sparse, but one study indicates that the increase in such injuries from before to after repeal of a helmet law paralleled the increase in deaths. The nonfatal head-injury to death ratio was 3:1.[56] The number of motorcyclists' fatalities in states without helmet laws in 1985 was 2714. Therefore, based on a minimum estimate of 24% reduction from the law, it is estimated that there would have been 651 fewer deaths and 1953 fewer head injuries if these states had had helmet use laws. Such a reduction is particularly significant because it would disproportionately reduce public expenditures. A detailed analysis of the cost of treatment and rehabilitative care of motorcyclists in a major trauma center found that 63% of the costs were borne by the taxpayers, mainly through Medicaid.[57] This is in contrast to all motor vehicle injuries, for which about 19% of treatment and rehabilitative costs are paid by Medicare and Medicaid.[58]

Although seat belt use is observable, mandatory belt use laws have been less effective—about a 7% fatality reduction on average. This is at least partly because most states do not provide for a fine for nonuse per se; an individual must commit some other violation to also be cited for nonuse of belts.[59] Laws directed at individual behavior are less often used in the case of unintentional injuries unrelated to motor vehicles, and only a few have been studied. Comparison of a county with a law requiring smoke detectors in homes to a county without that requirement suggests a 25% reduction in deaths from housefires associated with the requirement.[60] In New York City, fatal falls of children crawling out windows of multistoried buildings were reduced from about 50 per year in the 1960s to about 4 per year in the 1980s in association with programs promoting use of window barriers and regulation requiring such barriers.[61,62]

Automatic Vehicle and Environmental Approaches. The success of automatic approaches to manage energy requires consideration of the options available, technical competence in design, and quality control in implementation. Also, when manufacturers resist change or continue to introduce unnecessarily hazardous products, skill in dealing with political, social, and economic issues is often required for implementation. The discussion here is confined to some approaches that have been evaluated as effective but that have not been fully implemented.

Twenty years of off-and-on regulation and a Supreme Court decision were required to implement a federal standard that specifies limits for forces on the head, chest, and legs in frontal crashes of automobiles traveling at 30 miles per hour into a barrier. To comply with the standard, some vehicles have driver-side air bags and seat belts in the right-front seat, while others have the automatic seat belts in driver and right-front passenger positions. Automatic seat belts vary in effectiveness depending on their designs and on whether they are easy to detach. In a survey of 169 new car showrooms in 1989, less than 30% of so-called automatic belts were attached in the vehicles for sale.[63] Shoulder belts mounted in the door may be less effective, allowing partial ejection of the upper torso if the door opens in a crash. The standards do not apply to trucks, utility vehicles, and vans, but rule making to do so has begun.

Estimates of the effects of various forms of compliance with an automatic restraint standard have been argued for two decades. The official regulatory analysis indicates fatality reductions of 40% to 50% for fully used lap-shoulder belts, 35% to 50% for fully used automatic belts, and 45% to 55% for air bags with full lap-shoulder belt use.[64] Because full belt use will not be accomplished even with belt use laws and automatic belts, the actual effectiveness depends on projections of belt use generally and use among people at higher risk particularly. The effect on fatalities of increased belt use as the result of use laws is not nearly as high as is predicted by the estimated effectiveness of belts.[59]

Air bag usage will probably increase as the relative effectiveness of the various technologies in actual use becomes known. The use of full front-seat air bags in cars, assuming no belt use, is estimated to reduce deaths by about 6190 (range 3780 to 8630). This would be substantially greater if vans, utility vehicles, and pickup trucks were included. Increased belt use would reduce this estimate to the extent that there is overlap in the injuries reduced by air bags and those reduced by belts. At least half of the reduction associated with belt use is in side crashes and ejections that would not overlap with the effect of air bags.

The National Highway Traffic Safety Administration (NHTSA) has proposed a rule to increase protection to occupants of passenger cars hit from the side, which accounted for 32% of car occupant fatalities in 1985.[65] The NHTSA analysis presents the effects of various degrees of protection. At the highest level of proposed protection, the estimated fatality reduction would be approximately 1200 over the life of a given model year of cars.

The federal standard for head restraints can be met by adjustable restraints or by high seat backs that reduce neck injury in rear-end crashes automatically. Despite the fact that high seat backs are probably less expensive and certainly more effective in reducing neck injuries, about 70% of new cars are equipped with adjustable restraints. High seat backs were found to reduce injuries by 17% compared to 10% for adjustable restraints and were said to cost $28 less per car.[66] Under pressure from the auto industry, NHTSA revised its cost estimate, indicating little difference in costs of the two types of restraints on average, but the costs vary depending on materials used, from $20 to $40 for adjustable restraints and from $20 to $37 for high seat backs.[67] A reduction of about 64,000 neck injuries in rear-end collisions occurred annually with a mix of 70% adjustable restraints and 30% high seat backs. If there were 100% high seat backs, the reduction would be about 85,000, a difference of 21,000.[66]

Other factors that contribute to the severity of pedestrian injuries are the points, edges, and bumper heights on motor vehicles. Analysis of vehicles in England suggested that a 30% reduction in pedestrian fatalities could be achieved if all vehicles were designed to reduce energy exchanges.[78] Because some of these changes would result in the use of less materials through the elimination of sharp points on the front corners of several large American cars, production costs of at least some vehicles would be reduced, as would injury costs. A comparison of U.S. vehicles with sharp front corners and relatively smooth front corners found a 26% higher death rate to pedestrians struck on the front corners of the sharp-cornered cars but no difference in death rates to pedestrians struck at other points on the vehicles.[69]

Increased conspicuity of motor vehicles has been found to be an important factor in multiple-vehicle crash rates. It has been estimated that the daytime use of headlamps, parking lamps, or redesigned systems would reduce daytime, multiple-vehicle crashes by 7% to 38%.[70] In Sweden there was an 11% to 13% reduction in such crashes when daytime headlamp use was required by law, despite the fact that 50% of drivers were using headlamps in daytime before the law was enacted.[71]

While crash reductions can be largely accomplished by legally requiring that drivers turn vehicle lights on, there is substantial potential for adverse reaction from people whose batteries die when they forget to turn the lights off at the end of a trip. This problem could be alleviated by an automatic relay, available in some new cars, that turns the lights and the ignition off at the same time.

Although the current use of headlamps in daylight in the United States is unknown, it probably does not exceed 5%. Therefore, even considering the differences in year-round weather and hours of daylight between Sweden and the United States, the 11% to 13% reduction in crashes in Sweden (given a 50% prelaw headlamp use) seems a minimum to expect from automatic use if such a policy were adopted in the United States. A 12% reduction in daytime multiple-vehicle collisions in 1985 would have reduced deaths by approximately 372 and prevented more than 40,000 injuries, not to mention property damage.

Comparison of large trucks with and without reflective tape defining the outline of the truck indicates a 15% reduction of car-into-truck crashes associated with reflectorization.[71] The extent of use of this approach is unknown, but trucks with striping are rarely seen on the roads. Other factors that have significant effects are changes in the road environment.

A longer yellow light phase of traffic control lights at signalized intersections is associated with a substantially lower crash rate, the degree depending on the time length of the lights.[72] An all-red interval after a green in either direction at intersections also has been associated with reduced crash rates,[73] as has the use of flashing lights at approaches to stop signs at rural intersections. One study found a 51% reduction in injuries and an 80% reduction in deaths at installation sites.[73]

Fatal crashes that occur when vehicles cross over into the paths of oncoming vehicles are reduced 85% to 90% by concrete barriers that are flared at the bottom to guide an errant vehicle back into its lane.[73] Widening of bridges is associated with an average 50% reduction in fatal crashes related to bridge width, and modifications of the road approach have also reduced bridge crashes substantially.[74] Better delineation of curves (such as edge and center stripes, and roadside and center reflectors) is associated with a 16% reduction in fatal crashes on modified roads.[73]

Curved road sections with low or absent cross slopes are particularly hazardous when wet. Congressional staff visiting one such notorious site on the Washington, D.C., beltway observed cars spinning and some that spun off the road, going over embankments or striking bridge abutments.[75] One study found an average 25% higher crash frequency per mile between sites that had no cross slope and a cross slope of 0.025 ft/ft in an area with high average rainfall.[76] Pavement grooving was also effective in reducing crashes on wet roads, but the estimates vary widely among studies: 27% reduction in Louisiana; 69% in California; and 62% in Baltimore.[77]

At intersections, lanes that channel left-turning vehicles out of the path of through traffic are associated with a 42% reduction in fatal crashes compared to intersections without this feature.[73] About 50% fewer fatal crashes occur on lighted sections of urban freeways compared to unlighted sections.[78] Studies of sight distance at intersections indicated substantial reduction of crash rates where sight distance was unimpaired, compared to areas impaired by hedges, fences, and the like.[73] Intersection crash rates at night are 25% to 86% less at lighted compared to nonlighted intersections, depending on type of intersection, type of crash, and number of lanes.[73]

The effectiveness of flashing lights and gates in preventing severe and fatal injuries in car-train crashes has been estimated at 64% to 80%.[79] Separation of motor vehicle and rail traffic by overpasses is even more effective. The numbers of deaths at railroad crossings was cut in half from 1973 through 1984 by rail-crossing modifications, while exposures increased 4%.[80]

On rural highways, crashes per mile are strongly correlated to business accesses per mile. The data suggest that an average 33% reduction of fatalities could be achieved on roads without access control if they were changed to partial access control.[81] In urban areas, changing from two-way traffic flow to one-way flow frequently results in reduced crashes and pedestrian injuries, although there is a wide variation: 10% to 50%.[82]

In 1985, almost 12,000 motor-vehicle fatalities occurred in collisions with fixed objects near roadsides: trees or shrubbery (2967); utility poles or signs (2221); guardrails (1129); and other objects (5477). Research indicates that 50% to 75% of these fatalities could be prevented by removal of trees from roadsides, the application of impact attenuators, breakaway poles and signs, or improved guardrails.[73]

The cost of applying many environmental interventions depends on the extent to which they are targeted at the higher-risk populations or sites. For example, research comparing sites of fatal crashes into fixed objects with sites 1 mile in the direction from which the vehicles traveled, indicates that the high-risk sites can be substantially identified by road characteristics. Twenty-five percent of the crash sites were within 500 feet of curves greater than 6 degrees and downhill grades greater than 2%; only 8% of the comparison sites had such characteristics. There was no difference in number of objects along the road at the fatal and comparison sites.[83] Use of such epidemiological studies to set priorities would decrease the cost of many interventions relative to the cost of the relevant injuries.

Approaches that do not require action by those to be protected have been less often studied for injuries in settings other than on the road. The following includes a few examples. The most frequent cause of house fires is a cigarette dropped on bedding or upholstered furniture, where it smolders and later produces a killing smoke or fire, often after household occupants are asleep. In response to The Cigarette Safety Act of 1984, a Technical Study Group on Cigarette and Little Cigar Safety produced a report on the feasibility and costs of modifying cigarettes to reduce the likelihood of ignition by dropped cigarettes.[84]

Experimental cigarettes manufactured on equipment currently used by the industry were tested on fabric that was standardized as to padding and geometry. The numbers of ignitions in 20 tests varied from 0 to 20 among cigarettes with 41 combinations of tobacco type, tobacco density, paper porosity, citrate added, circumference, and second paper wrapping. Lower ignitions were associated with low tobacco density, lower circumference, lower paper porosity, and no citrate added.

Subsequent tests on commercially available furniture with fabric and substrate similar to the standardized mockup produced an exceptionally strong correlation ($r = 0.86$) to results with the mockup. Although the Technical Study Group cautiously called for more work to establish performance criteria, the results of these studies indicate that reliable tests of cigarettes for potential ignition are feasible and standards for cigarette manufacture could be based on performance in such tests. Application of all the possible modifications identified would achieve up to 75% reduction in cigarette-related fire injuries.[85]

Drownings associated with children wandering into unsupervised swimming pools occurred 65% less frequently in Honolulu, where pool fencing is required, compared to Brisbane, Australia, which had no such requirement. The cities have similar weather and pool-to-household ratios.[86]

Some industries take injuries into account in adopting technology, but formal analysis of effects seldom is reported publicly. For example, in oil drilling, pipes are connected and disconnected by large tongs that work similarly to wrenches. Workers who handle the tongs experience a variety of injuries. Worker proximity to the mechanical energy in such operations can be altered by the use of "power makeup equipment." Comparison of sites with such equipment to those without, both before and after the installation of the equipment, indicated a reduction of 42% in related worker injuries per hours worked. The reduced cost of the injuries would pay for the equipment in 6 years.[87]

Such seemingly mundane injuries as fractures and other injuries caused by sliding into bases while playing softball are not without significant costs. A recent study estimated a cost of $1223 per sliding injury, whereas use of breakaway bases reduced such injuries by 95% at a cost of $48 per base.[88]

CONCLUSIONS

Data on injuries have improved as research support by governmental and private sources has increased. Much work remains to be done to provide data for more efficient targeting of countermeasures to more severe injuries and to identify newly emerging hazards before they become epidemics. Better evidence on the effectiveness and costs of injury control programs is also needed, but the lack of implementation of many injury prevention strategies is clearly not for want of evidence of effectiveness. Failure in implementation is often due to ideological factors and concentrated interests that result in opposition to certain interventions.

Although product manufacturers often claim that their opposition to safety standards is due to increased costs, the evidence suggests more complex motivation. Changes to motor vehicles, such as smooth front ends and interiors and high seat backs, would cost no more than current designs, and in many cases would cost less. Developers of a research safety vehicle that included full front-seat air bags, radar-controlled brakes, and increased exterior and interior energy absorption, have said that, in production of one million or more cars, the cost would be no more than that of compact cars.[89] In 1976 the Secretary of Transportation found that manufacturers had engaged in deceptive accounting of air bag costs in representations to the government.[90] On the basis of interviews with senior corporate executives regarding regulation generally, mostly on issues other than safety, one analyst concluded that the major factor in resistance to regulation was the executives' resentment to any limitation on their power to make decisions rather than to costs.[91]

If product manufacturers were more interested in the health of their customers than in their own power, they would welcome regulation. By applying the same standards to all like products, regulations reduce or eliminate the price advantage to a manufacturer that would otherwise seek a price advantage by making a less safe product. There appears to be little recognition of this principle in the virtually solid wall of opposition to safety regulation among firms doing business in the United States.

In the 1960s and 1970s, many legislators understood the importance of this principle and voted for the creation of regulatory agencies, such as the National Highway Traffic Safety Administration, the Consumer Product Safety Commission, and the Occupational Safety and Health Administration. However, in the 1980s the effectiveness of these agencies was eliminated or retarded by the political war on regulation. Under orders to rescind certain regulations (such as the automatic restraint standard) or to issue no new ones, and as a result of both real and inflationary budget cuts, the regulatory agencies ceased aggressive activity. While a few legislators attempted to push the agencies through the oversight process (with an occasional response such as action on certain "all-terrain" vehicles), most law-makers timidly waited for a political environment more conducive to social responsibility.

Seemingly overwhelming ideological opposition or lobbying power is not always as solid as it seems, however. Although the majority of motorcyclists were in favor of helmet use laws, a vocal minority were successful in gaining repeal in many states during the late 1970s.[92] Recently the California legislature enacted a helmet use law only to have it vetoed by an arch conservative governor. No one familiar with Tennessee politics would have expected that state to be the first to enact a child-restraint use law, but it did,[93] and other states followed. Armed with data and the commitment to reduce injuries, public health professionals have played a crucial role in these efforts.

REFERENCES

1. Baker S: Injury science comes of age. JAMA 262:2284–2285, 1989
2. DeHaven H: Beginnings of crash injury research. In Brinkhaus K (ed): Accident Pathology. Washington, D.C.: Department of Transportation Publication. FH 11-6595, 1968
3. Stapp J: Effects of mechanical force on living tissue: I. Abrupt deceleration and windblast. J Aviat Med 26:268–288, 1955
4. Gordon J: The epidemiology of accidents. Am J Public Health 39:504–515, 1949
5. Gibson J: The contribution of experimental psychology to the formulation of the problem of safety: A brief for basic science. In Behavioral Approaches to Accident Research. New York: Association for the Aid of Crippled Children, 1961
6. Haddon W Jr: A note concerning accident theory and research with special reference to motor-vehicle accidents. Ann N Y Acad Sci 107:635–646, 1963
7. Haddon W Jr, Schuman E, Klein D: Accident Research: Methods and Approaches. New York: Harper & Row, 1964
8. Haddon W Jr, Valien P, McCarrol J, Umberger C: A controlled investigation of the characteristics of adult pedestrians fatally injured by motor vehicles in Manhattan. J Chronic Dis 14:655–678, 1961
9. Haddon W Jr, Ellison E, Carroll E: Skiing injuries. Public Health Rep 77:975–985, 1962
10. Haddon W Jr: The changing approach to the epidemiology, prevention, and amelioration of trauma: The transition to approaches etiologically rather than descriptively based. Am J Public Health 58:1431–1438, 1968
11. Haddon W Jr: Options for prevention of motor-vehicle injury. Isr J Med Sci 16:45–65, 1980
12. Viano D, King A, Melvin J, Weber K: Injury biomechanics research: An essential element in the prevention of trauma. J Biomech 22:403–417, 1989
13. Haddon W Jr: A logical framework for categorizing highway safety phenomena and activity. J Trauma 12:193–207, 1972
14. Haddon W Jr: Advances in the epidemiology of injuries as a basis for public policy. Public Health Rep 95:411–421, 1980
15. Gable C: A compendium of public health data sources. Am J Epidemiol 131:381–394, 1990
16. Pollack E, Keimig D (eds): Counting Injuries and Illnesses in the Workplace: Proposals for a Better System. Washington, D.C.: National Academy Press, 1987
17. National Center for Health Statistics: Annual Summary of Births, Marriages, Divorces, and Deaths: United States, 1989
18. Graves EJ: Detailed Diagnosis and Procedures National Hospital Discharge Survey 1987. Vital Health Statistics (13), 1989
19. Adams P, Hardy A: Current Estimates from the National Health

Interview Survey: United States, 1988. Hyattsville, Md.: National Center for Health Statistics.

20. Robertson, LS: Injuries: Causes, Control Strategies, and Public Policy. Lexington: DC Heath, 1983
21. Haddon W Jr: On the escape of tigers: An ecologic note. Tech Rev 72:44, 1970
22. Robertson LS: Risk of fatal rollovers in utility vehicles relative to static stability. Am J Public Health 79:300, 1989
23. Baker SP, O'Neill B, Karpf RS: The Injury Fact Book. Lexington, Mass.: DC Heath, 1984
24. Waller JA: Injury Control: A Guide to the Causes and Prevention of Trauma. Lexington, Mass.: DC Heath, 1985
25. Robertson LS: Behavioral research and strategies in public health: A demur. Soc Sci Med 9:165, 1975
26. National Safety Council: 1982–83 Driver Education Status Report. Chicago: National Safety Council, 1985
27. Shaoul J: The Use of Accidents and Traffic Offenses as Criteria for Evaluating Courses in Driver Education. Salford, England: University of Salford, 1975
28. Lund AK, Williams AF, Zador PF: High school driver education: Further analysis of the DeKalb County study. Accid Anal Prev 18:349, 1986
29. Robertson LS, Zador PF: Driver education and fatal crash involvement of teenaged drivers. Am J Public Health 68:959, 1978
30. Robertson LS: Crash involvement of teenaged drivers when driver education is eliminated from high school. Am J Public Health 70:599, 1980
31. DiGuiseppi CG, Rivara FP, Koepsell TD, Polissar L: Bicycle helmet use by children: Evaluation of a community-wide campaign. JAMA 262:2256–2261, 1989
32. Blomberg RD, Preusser DF, Hale A, Leaf WA: Experimental Field Test of Proposed Pedestrian Safety Messages, Vol. 2. Child Messages. Washington, D.C.: U.S. Department of Transportation, 1983
33. Robertson LS, Kelley AB, O'Neill B, Wixom CW, Eiswirth RS, Haddon W Jr: A controlled study of the effect of television messages on safety belt use. Am J Public Health 64:1071–1080, 1974
34. Richards JS: Resources: A National Directory of Spinal Cord Injury Prevention Programs. Birmingham: University of Alabama, Birmingham, 1990
35. Reisinger KS, Williams AF: Evaluation of programs designed to increase protection of infants in cars. Pediatrics 62:280–287, 1978
36. Dershewitz RA, Williamson JW: Prevention of childhood household injuries: A controlled clinical trial. Am J Public Health 67:1148, 1977
37. Reisinger KS, Williams AF, Wells JAK, John CE, Roberts TR, Podgainy HJ: The effect of pediatricians' counseling on infant restraint use. Pediatrics 67:201–206, 1981
38. Berger LR, Saunders S, Armitage K, Schauer L: Promoting the use of car safety devices for infants: An intensive health education approach. Pediatrics 74:16–19, 1984
39. Kravitz H: Prevention of falls in infancy by counseling mothers. Illinois Med J 144:570–573, 1973
40. Elman D, Killebrew TJ: Incentives and seat belts: Changing a resistant behavior through extrinsic motivation. J Appl Psysiol 8:72–83, 1978
41. Geller ES: Rewarding safety belt usage at an industrial setting: Tests of treatment generality and response maintenance. J Appl Behav Anal 16:43–56, 1983
42. Geller ES: A behavioral science approach to transportation safety. Bull N Y Acad Med 64:632–661, 1988
43. Williams AF, Karpf RS, Zador PL: Variations in minimum licensing age and fatal motor vehicle crashes. Am J Public Health 73:1401–1403, 1983
44. Preusser DF, Williams AF, Lund AK: Driver licensing age and lifestyles of 16-year-olds. Am J Public Health 75:358, 1985
45. Preusser DF, Williams AF, Zador PL, Blomberg RD: The effects of curfew laws on motor vehicle crashes. Law Policy 6:115, 1984
46. Robertson LS: Blood alcohol in fatally injured drivers and the minimum legal drinking age. J Health Polit Policy Law 14:817, 1989
47. Cook PJ: The effects of liquor taxes on drinking, cirrhosis and auto accidents. In Moore MH, Gerstein DR (eds): Alcohol and Public Policy: Beyond the Shadow of Prohibition. Washington, D.C.: National Academy Press, 1981
48. Hacker G: Taxing booze for health and wealth. J Pol Anal Man 6:701, 1987
49. Zador PL, Lund AK, Fields M, Weinberg K: Fatal crash involvement and laws against alcohol-impaired driving. J Public Health Policy 10:467, 1989
50. Robertson LS: Childhood injury prevention: Some lessons learned. In Haller JA (ed): Emergency Medical Services for Children. Columbus, Ohio: Ross Laboratories, 1989
51. Agran PF, Dunkle DE, Winn DG: Effects of legislation on motor vehicle injuries to children. Am J Dis Child 141:959, 1987
52. Teret S, Jones AS, Williams AF, Wells JAK: Child restraint laws: An analysis of gaps in coverage. Am J Public Health 76:31, 1986
53. Robertson LS: An instance of effective legal regulation: Motorcyclist helmet and daytime headlamp laws. Law Soc Rev 10:456, 1976
54. Watson GF, Zador PL, Wilks A: The repeal of helmet use laws and increased motorcyclist mortality in the United States, 1975–1978. Am J Public Health 70:579, 1980
55. Hartunian NS, Smart CN, Willeman TR, Zador PL: The economics of safety deregulation: Lives and dollars lost due to repeal of motorcycle helmet laws. J Health Polit Policy Law 8:76, 1983
56. McSwain NE, Lummis M: Impact of repeal of motorcycle helmet law. Surg Gynecol Obstet 151:215, 1980
57. Rivara FP, Dicker BG, Bergman AB: The public cost of motorcycle trauma. JAMA 260:223, 1988
58. National Highway Traffic Safety Administration: The Economic Cost to Society of Motor Vehicle Accidents. Washington: D.C.: U.S. Department of Transportation, 1983
59. Williams AF, Lund AK: Mandatory seat belt use laws and occupant crash protection in the United States: Present status and future prospects. In Graham JD (ed): Preventing Automobile Injury: New Findings from Evaluation Research. Dover, Del.: Auburn House, 1988
60. McLoughlin E, Marchone M, Hanger SL, German PS, Baker SP: Smoke detector legislation: Its effect on owner-occupied homes. Am J Public Health 75:858, 1985
61. Bergner L, Mayer S, Harris D: Falls from heights: A childhood epidemic in an urban area. Am J Public Health 61:90, 1971
62. Bergner L: Environmental factors in injury control: Preventing falls from heights. In Bergman AB (ed): Preventing Childhood Injuries. Columbus, Ohio: Ross Laboratories, 1982
63. Insurance Institute for Highway Safety: Automatic belts still not attached in many showrooms. Status Report 24:1, September 23, 1989
64. National Highway Traffic Safety Administration: Final Regulatory Impact Analysis: Amendment to Federal Motor Safety Standard 208, Passenger Car Front Seat Occupant Protection. Washington, D.C.: U.S. Department of Transportation, 1984
65. National Highway Traffic Safety Administration: Preliminary Regulatory Impact Analysis: New Requirements for Passenger Cars to Meet a Dynamic Side Impact Test FMVSS 214. Washington, D.C.: U.S. Department of Transportation, 1988
66. Kahane CJ: An Evaluation of Head Restraints: Federal Motor Vehicle Safety Standard 202. Washington, D.C.: National Highway Traffic Safety Administration, 1982
67. National Highway Traffic Safety Administration: Preliminary Regulatory Evaluation: Proposed Extension of Head Restraint Requirements to Light Trucks, Buses, and Multipurpose Passenger Vehicles With Gross Vehicle Weight Rating of 10,000 Pounds or Less—FMVSS 202. Washington, D.C.: U.S. Department of Transportation, 1988
68. Ashton SJ: Vehicle design and pedestrian injuries. In Chapman AJ, Wade FM, Foot HC (eds): Pedestrian Accidents. London: John Wiley & Sons, 1982
69. Robertson LS: Car design and risk of pedestrian deaths. Am J Public Health 80:609, 1990
70. Transport Canada: Analysis of a Proposed Regulation Requiring

Daytime Running Lights for Motor Vehicles. Ottawa; Transport Canada, 1986

71. Burger WJ, Mulholland MU, Smith RL: Improved Commercial Vehicle Conspicuity and Signaling Systems - Task III. Field Test Evaluation of Vehicle Reflectorization Effectiveness. Washington, D.C.: U.S. Department of Transportation Report HS 806 923, 1986
72. Zador PL, Stein H, Shapiro S, Tarnoff P: The effect of signal timing on traffic flow and crashes at signalized intersections. Washington, D.C.: Insurance Institute for Highway Safety, 1984
73. McFarland WF, Griffin LI, Rollins JB, Stockton WR, Philips DT, Dudek CL: Assessment of Techniques for Cost-Effectiveness of Highway Accident Countermeasures. Washington, D.C.: Federal Highway Administration, 1979
74. Bissell HH, Pilkington GB, Mason JM, Woods DL: Roadway cross section and alignment. In Federal Highway Administration: Synthesis of Safety Research Related to Traffic Control and Roadway Elements, Vol. 1. Washington, D.C.: Federal Highway Administration, 1982
75. Kelley AB: Boobytrap (film). Washington, D.C.: Insurance Institute for Highway Safety, 1972
76. Dart OK Jr, Mann L Jr: Relationship of rural highway geometry to accident rates in Louisiana. Highway Research Record No. 312. Washington, D.C.: Highway Research Board, 1970
77. Reviewed in Galloway BM, Benson FC, Mounce JM, Bissell HH, Rosenbaum MJ: Pavement surface. In Federal Highway Administration: Synthesis of Safety Research Related to Traffic Control and Roadway Elements, Vol. 1. Washington, D.C.: Federal Highway Administration, 1982
78. Schwab RN, Walton NB, Mounce JM, Rosenbaum MJ: Roadway lighting. In Federal Highway Administration: Synthesis of Safety Research Related to Traffic Control and Roadway Elements. Washington, D.C.: Federal Highway Administration, 1982
79. Pinnell C, Mason JM, Berg WD, Coleman JA, Rosenbaum MJ: Railroad-highway grade crossings. In Federal Highway Administration: Synthesis of Safety Research Related to Traffic Control and Roadway Elements, Vol. 2. Washington, D.C.: Federal Highway Administration, 1982
80. Dempsey WH: Testimony. Extension of the Nation's Highway, Highway Safety, and Public Transit Programs: Hearings before the Subcommittee on Surface Transportation of the Committee on Public Works and Transportation. Washington, D.C.: U.S. House of Representatives, 1985
81. Stover VG, Tignor SC, Rosenbaum MJ: Access control and driveways. In Federal Highway Administration: Synthesis of Safety Research Related to Traffic Control and Roadway Elements. Washington, D.C.: Federal Highway Administration, 1982
82. Parsonson PS, Nehmad IR, Rosenbaum MJ: One-way streets and reversible lanes. In Federal Highway Administration: Synthesis of Safety Research Related to Traffic Control and Roadway Elements, Vol. 1. Washington, D.C.: Federal Highway Administration, 1982
83. Wright PH, Robertson LS: Priorities for roadside hazard modification: A study of 300 fatal roadside object crashes. Traf Eng 46:24, 1976
84. Technical Study Group: Toward a Less Fire-Prone Cigarette. Washington, D.C.: U.S. Consumer Product Safety Commission, 1987
85. Rueg RT, Weber SF, Lippiatt BC, Fuller SK: Improving the Fire Safety of Cigarettes: An Economic Impact Analysis. Washington, D.C.: Consumer Product Safety Commission, 1987
86. Pearn JH, Wong RYK, Brown J, Ching Y, Bart R, Hammar S: Drowning and near-drowning involving children: A five-year total population study from the city and county of Honolulu. Am J Public Health 69:450, 1979
87. Mohr DL, Clemmer DI: Evaluation of an occupational injury intervention in the petroleum drilling industry. Accid Anal Prev 21:263–271, 1989
88. Janda DH, Wojtys EM, Hankin FM, Benedict MG: Softball sliding injuries: A prospective study comparing standard and modified bases. JAMA 259:1848, 1988
89. DiNapoli N, Fitzpatrick M, Strother C, Struble D, Tanner R: Research Safety Vehicle Phase II: Comprehensive Technical Results. Springfield, Va.: National Technical Information Service, 1977
90. The Secretary's Decision Concerning Motor Vehicle Occupant Restraints. Washington, D.C.: U.S. Department of Transportation, 1976
91. Lane R: The Regulation of Businessmen. New Haven, Conn.: Yale University Press, 1954
92. Baker SP: On lobbies, liberty, and the public good. Am J Public Health 70:573, 1980
93. Sanders RS: Legislative approach to auto safety: The Tennessee experience. In Bergman AB (ed): Preventing Childhood Injuries. Columbus, Ohio: Ross Laboratories, 1982

64

Violence

Assaultive Violence

Mark L. Rosenberg
James A. Mercy

Definition of the Problem. Each year more than 20,000 people in the United States die from homicide, making this type of assaultive violence the twelfth leading cause of death and the fourth leading cause of premature mortality.[1] In 1986, homicide ranked as the third leading cause of death among persons 15 to 24 years of age and was the leading cause of death for black males 15 to 34 years of age. The lifetime risk of death from homicide is 1 in 28 for black males compared with 1 in 164 for white males.[2,3] And while homicide is the fatal outcome of assaultive behaviors, the ratio of nonfatal assaults to homicide is probably far greater than 100:1.[4]

Assaultive violence includes both nonfatal and fatal interpersonal violence where physical force by one person is used with the intent of causing harm, injury, or death to another. Homicide is death caused by injuries inflicted by one person with intent to injure or kill another by any means. Homicide can be classified as criminal or noncriminal; noncriminal homicide includes deaths caused by negligence and those committed in self-defense.

Four legal categories used to designate types of nonfatal assaultive violence are aggravated assault, simple assault, rape, and robbery. Aggravated assault is (1) an attack with a weapon, whether or not there is an injury; (2) an attack without a weapon resulting in serious injury (e.g., broken bones, loss of teeth, internal injuries, or loss of consciousness) or in undetermined injury requiring 2 or more days of hospitalization; or (3) an attempted assault with a weapon.[4] Simple assault is an attack or attempted attack without a weapon resulting either in minor injury (e.g., bruises, black eyes, cuts, scratches, or swelling) or in undetermined injury requiring less than 2 days of hospitalization.[4] Research literature generally presents assault and homicide as similar categories of behavior and considers homicide "completed" assault. Rape is carnal knowledge through the use of force or the threat of force, including attempts.[4] Robbery is a completed or attempted theft directly from a person of property or cash by force or threat of force, with or without a weapon.[4]

Assaultive violence can be categorized by different types of victim-offender relationship, setting, and circumstances. Categorizing by the nature of victim-offender relationship is helpful because both the etiology and prevention strategies vary by this relationship. Three general categories that are particularly useful are family, acquaintance, and stranger.

Assaultive violence has only recently been recognized as an important public health problem. During the past 30 years, assaultive violence was considered to be the domain of the criminal justice system alone, and control strategies focused primarily on deterrence through punishment and imprisonment. However, there have been dramatic increases in homicide rates in the United States over this same 30-year period. The public health approach suggests that homicide and other types of assault are concerns to be addressed and remedied, not as inalterable facts of life. As with other public health problems, a public health approach to the problem of assaultive violence is to establish a framework for developing relevant information through epidemiology and then to transfer that information into effective action. This approach has four steps: surveillance to collect, analyze, interpret, and disseminate relevant data; identification of risk groups and the places, times, and other circumstances associated with increased risk; identification of risk factors; and program development, implementation, and evaluation.

National Data Sources

Federal Bureau of Investigation (FBI) Uniform Crime Reports (UCR). This program receives monthly information from more than 16,000 city, county, and state law enforcement agencies. During 1986, the agencies active in the UCR program held jurisdiction over 96% of the U.S. population.[5] These law enforcement agencies report the number of actual offenses known for murder and nonnegligent manslaughter, justifiable homicide, negligent manslaughter, forcible rape, robbery, aggravated assault, burglary, larceny-theft, motor-vehicle theft, and arson. This program also uses the Supplementary Homicide Report (SHR) to collect information on the age, race, and sex of the victim and the offender; the relationship of the offender to the victim; and the crime circumstances. For cases that are "unsolved" at the time of reporting, the relationship of victim to offender is listed as "unknown." Unless specifically amended in a later report, the "relationship unknown" is counted in the final statistics for the year. Each year, data are incomplete for approximately 5% to 10% of the total number of murder and nonnegligent manslaughter cases.

A principal limitation of FBI-UCR data on aggravated assault, robbery, and rape is that these data represent only the violent offenses known to the police; however, the majority of nonfatal violent offenses do not come to the attention of law enforcement agencies.[6] In addition, the FBI-UCR program does not collect information on victim and offender characteristics or relationships for aggravated assaults, robberies, or rapes. Finally, these data are categorized by a crime hierarchy, so that if an incident occurs that includes several different types of assault, the system counts only the most serious act, with homicide ranked as the most serious, followed by rape, robbery, aggravated assault, burglary, larceny, and motor vehicle theft.

National Crime Survey (NCS). The NCS was developed by the Bureau of Justice Statistics of the U.S. Department of Justice to acquire detailed information about victims and consequences of crime, to estimate numbers and types of crimes not reported to police, and to establish uniform measures for selected types of crimes in order to permit reliable comparisons over time and between areas.[7] Focusing on rape, robbery, assault, burglary, larceny, and motor vehicle theft, these surveys collect information on physical injury, medical treatment, property loss, characteristics of the victim, relationship of the victim to the offender, and whether the police were notified.

Because it is based on interviews with victims and not on official law enforcement records, the NCS is an excellent source of information on victimization and its consequences. However, the accuracy of information on injuries and victimization caused by spouse, child, and elder abuse is questionable because interviews with household members are not conducted privately and subjects may be reluctant to speak openly in the presence of the person who victimized them. In addition, the survey asks about criminal assaults, and subjects may not perceive assaults by family members as "criminal." Groups at highest risk for serious injury from assault may be difficult to reach using the sampling and interviewing techniques of this survey. Finally, the survey uses the same crime hierarchy used in the FBI-UCR; therefore, serious crimes are more accurately estimated than crimes lower in the hierarchy.

National Center for Health Statistics (NCHS) Mortality Data. The Vital Statistics Program has compiled data from records of all death certificates filed in state vital statistics offices since 1933. The system provides annual data on homicide for the nation and each state, counties, and other local areas and monthly provisional data for the nation and each state. Rates, numbers, gender, and geographic detail for all deaths are published monthly,[8] but there is considerable delay in the publication of detailed reports on specific causes of death. Data are collected based on the *International Classification of Diseases,* 9th Revision, *Clinical Modification* (ICD-9-CM)[9] with the Supplementary External Cause (E) code for homicide. Limitations of these data include the lack of information on the victim-offender relationship and the lack of distinction between criminal homicides and homicide committed in self-defense.

Other Sources. Other national data sources could prove useful in surveillance and research on assaultive violence if modifications are made in the types of information collected. Currently the *National Health Interview Survey* (*NHIS*) staff interview persons in about 42,000 households sampled to be representative of the civilian, noninstitutionalized population each year. The survey collects data on a number of health issues including injury, but some of the information on injuries cannot be broken down by cause of injury (e.g., assaultive violence, suicidal behavior, unintentional injury) because of the small number of injuries in the sample. In addition, the considerable ambiguity in the way the questions are asked precludes detailed analysis.

The *National Hospital Discharge Survey* (*NHDS*) collects information on discharge diagnosis and type of surgical procedure performed from approximately 200,000 records each year. These records represent a sample of about 400 short-stay, nonfederal hospitals. Information is available on traumatic injury, but is of limited value because data on the cause of injury are not completely reported and vary greatly by the type of injury. Also, the sample of hospitals is based only on those that agree to cooperate with the survey.

The *National Electronic Injury Surveillance System* (*NEISS*) collects data on all injuries seen in the emergency rooms of 66 hospitals throughout the United States. These hospitals represent a stratified probability sample of all hospitals in the United States and its territories. The system collects information on all injuries seen at the emergency room that are "product related," but certain products such as automobiles and firearms are not included.

State and Local Data Sources. Thirty-nine state criminal justice agencies have mandatory reporting requirements; data from these agencies are forwarded to the FBI-UCR program. The agencies in the other 11 states report voluntarily to the UCR program. The bases for the state- and national-level UCR data are detailed reports on crime from county and city law enforcement agencies, which are a potentially rich source of information on assaultive violence.

Coroners' and medical examiners' records are also potential sources of data, and the Centers for Disease Control is assessing the feasibility of developing suicide and homicide surveillance systems based on these data. At present, these data are useful for state and local studies, but few coroners' or medical examiners' offices collect standardized information on homicide, and data from these offices are not collected or analyzed nationally. The quality of information varies considerably since few states have medical examiners in each county and records are often completed by persons acting as coroners. Data from these offices may be particularly useful for examining the relationship between alcohol and drug use and homicide victimization.

Data from medical and social service agencies such as hospitals, battered women's shelters, mental health clinics, and substance abuse treatment facilities may contain a tremendous amount of useful information concerning the circumstances and histories of persons who have been victims or perpetrators of assaultive violence. However, definitions and records have not been standardized, nor has there been any attempt to collect and analyze these data nationally.

At both the national and local levels, there is an urgent need for information on injuries resulting from nonfatal assaults and for systems that collect accurate information on the magnitude and nature of nonfatal assaultive violence between persons known to one another (e.g., family members, intimates, friends, and acquaintances). Present sources of such information have only limited use for epidemiological research and surveillance, but their utility will increase significantly when hospital discharge data routinely include information on external cause of injury (E-coding).

Causes and Risk Factors. There are many types of assaultive violence, and for each type the causes are complex and diverse. It is helpful to examine various disciplinary approaches to aspects of the problem because each contributes valuable perspectives. However, these separate approaches can obscure the complex interaction of different types of factors that contribute to assaultive violence. Ultimately, what is needed are "causal" explanations that combine biological, psychological, and sociological factors in ways that explain the occurrence of assaultive violence involving different perpetrators, victims, and circumstances.

Biological explanations of assaultive violence have examined sex, age, and certain psychiatric illnesses as important risk factors for homicide victimization and perpetration.[10] For example, greater numbers of males among perpetrators and victims may reflect the influence of male sex hormones on aggressive behavior, and the decreasing numbers of victims and perpetrators with increasing age may be a result of biological transformations associated with aging.[11]

Psychological approaches to violence include two major

theories: social learning, which posits that behavior is learned through imitation of role models and reinforced by rewards and punishments,[12] and developmental theory, which focuses on deterrents to violence through early parent-child ties of love; childhood experiences relatively free of punitive discipline or abuse; and experiences that reinforce the child's attachments, minimize frustrations, and encourage flexible inner control.[13]

Four major sociological approaches to understanding are cultural, structural, interactionist, and economic. The cultural approach views violent behavior as the result of learned and shared values and behavior specific to a given group that are applied in recognizable situations and transmitted across generations. Certain subgroups exhibit higher rates of assaultive violence because they are in a subculture that has violence as a norm. However, critics point to the frequency of violence in groups where violence is clearly not a norm (e.g., the middle class) and to the fact that this theory tends to "blame the victim."

The structural approach holds that rates of assaultive violence are largely influenced by broad-scale social forces, such as poverty or lack of opportunity. In one widely known formulation, violence and other "illegitimate" behaviors arise when persons are deprived of "legitimate" means and resources to realize culturally valued goals. This theory does not adequately explain, however, why conflicts arising from structural deprivation lead to violence in one situation and to other behaviors, passivity for instance, in other situations.[14]

The interactionist approach focuses on the nature of the interaction sequence as it escalates into violent behavior. For example, one investigator describes it as a series of offender and victim "moves" as they relate to each other and to the reaction of the audience. From this, he derived a set of time-ordered stages that most of the transactions followed.[15] Other research has shown that violence grows out of a series of provocative arguments that escalate to murder. The arguments often are threats to identity (especially sexual identity) and self-esteem.

The economic approach is the basis for many current policies aimed at reducing homicide and assault. This theory posits that decisions to engage in criminal behavior are based on a person's perception of what outcome appears more valuable.[16] Thus, some people commit assaults not because their motivation differs from that of other people but because their perceived benefits and costs differ. In order for the desired choices to be made, people must be aware of the benefits and costs of the alternatives available to them. This assumes that people have equal capability of making rational decisions under all conditions and circumstances, but the ability to make a rational judgment may be impaired, for example, if the person is under the influence of alcohol or drugs.

Specific structural factors that relate to homicide include poverty (associated with murders of friends and acquaintances, children, and spouses, and with robbery-associated murders of strangers)[17]; belief in male dominance (spouse abuse); and racial discrimination (linked with killings of strangers and friends or acquaintances).[18,19]

An interactionist factor, consumption of alcohol and drugs, has been associated with all types of homicide except child homicide. Many studies have shown that about half of all victims and perpetrators of homicides had consumed alcohol. However, without control or comparison populations, these studies have not been able to demonstrate a causal role for alcohol.[20] The same situation applies to the association between alcohol use and family violence. Some researchers suggest that the disinhibiting effect of alcohol may be more psychological than physiological and that alcohol may serve as an excuse for behavior already decided on.[21]

It may be that alcohol and drug use contributes to homicide by influencing the risk of both victimization and perpetration, for example, if it has a physiological effect on the brain that reduces inhibitions against aggressive behavior.[20] Alternatively, alcohol and drug use may be associated with homicide because their use is associated with specific situations, environments, or activities that place individuals at high risk of victimization. Moreover, individuals who take illicit drugs, distribute them, or do both may have higher risks for homicide victimization because of the high profits, criminal behaviors, and instability associated with drug dealing.[22]

Outcomes

Mortality. In 1986, homicides in the United States accounted for the loss of at least 21,731 lives based on NCHS mortality data, of which 269 (1.2%) were perpetrated by law enforcement officials in the line of duty. The United States has one of the highest homicide rates among countries of the world reporting homicide statistics to the World Health Organization.[23] Reporting methods of individual countries may differ and domestic and international wars may affect homicide rates in some areas.

Homicide is far more prevalent among minorities, males, and the young. While homicide was the twelfth leading cause of death for Americans, homicide was *the* leading cause of death for young people (15 to 34 years of age) who are black. Although the homicide rates for black males are much higher than those for all other races, it is difficult to determine the precise contribution of race to these high rates. Several studies suggest that socioeconomic status is a more important determinant than race.[24,25]

Ethnicity also appears to be an important determinant of homicide rates. For the period 1976 to 1980 in five southwestern states where more than 60% of all Hispanics in the United States reside, the overall homicide rate for Hispanics (20.5 per 100,000) was more than two and one-half times the Anglo or non-Hispanic white rate (7.9 per 100,000). This difference was most striking in the young male age groups in which the Hispanic homicide rate was almost five times that for Anglos.[26]

Of the homicides committed in the United States in 1986 and reported to the FBI, 40% involved friends and acquaintances; 15.1% were within families; and 12.5% were between strangers.[27] The percentage of homicides with an unknown relationship was 32.4%. However, data suggest that these "unknown relationship" homicides are most likely to be murders of strangers because murders between intimates are more likely to be cleared (i.e., an arrest is made) and appropriately classified.

Most family homicides involve spouses and occur in the home, frequently after many assaultive incidents.[15,21] The median age of victims is 33 years and of offenders, 32. In 38.4% of the cases, a handgun is used, followed by other guns (19.5%), knives (17.0%), and other means (25.1%).[28]

Victims of acquaintance homicide are typically younger than the victims of family homicide and are much more likely to be male and black. In 1986, 43.4% of the victims were black, and 37.3%, white. Offenders (median age, 23 years) are usually younger than their victims. Handguns were used in 44.7% of the cases; knives in 19.5%. Acquaintance homicides are most likely to occur within a private residence, although one third occur on the street, and a higher percentage occurs in bars than is true for other types of killings.[19]

In homicides among strangers, the victims and offenders are predominantly male and the median age of the victim (31 years) is higher than that of the offender (25 years). Most such killings are with firearms (49.1% with handguns, 12.2% with another type of gun). Nationally, 46.9% of killings of strangers are associated with another crime, often robbery, although the chance of being killed in a robbery remains relatively small.

In 1986, 59.1% of homicides were committed with firearms, with almost three quarters (74.1%) of these victims being killed with handguns. After firearms, cutting and piercing instruments were the next most frequently used weapon (20.3%), followed by bodily force (6.7%), and blunt objects (5.6%). Other or undetermined weapons accounted for 8.3% of homicides in 1986.

A relatively small proportion of homicides (19.4% in 1986) are committed during the perpetration of another felony or crime, such as robbery or narcotics offenses. Verbal arguments are the most frequently occurring circumstance associated with homicide (37.5% in 1986), while other nonfelony circumstances including brawls due to the influence of alcohol or narcotics, juvenile gang killings, and institutional killings accounted for 18.6% of the circumstances associated with homicide. In 22.5% of the cases, the circumstances leading to the killing were unknown.

Morbidity. For Americans over the age of 12 years, 5.5 million incidents of violent crime (i.e., excluding homicide, but including simple and aggravated assault, robbery, and rape) occurred in 1986 (2810 violent crimes per 100,000 people).[8] Simple and aggravated assaults accounted for 79.3% of these incidents; attempted and completed robbery, 18.3%; attempted and completed rape, 2.4%. Males were 1.7 times more likely to be victims than females, with men aged 16 to 19 years being at greatest risk (8120 per 100,000).[8] Blacks were at 1.2 times greater risk of being a victim of a violent crime than whites, while Hispanics were about equally likely as non-Hispanics to have been a victim.[8]

Almost one third of victims (32.2%) of robbery and assault sustained a physical injury. Given the severe emotional trauma associated with rape, all victims are considered to have been injured regardless of whether or not a physical injury was reported. Of all victims of violent crime, 7.8% received hospital care. Hospital costs (for those who survived assaults plus those who eventually died as a result of aggravated assault) totaled approximately $606 million. The cost of physician visits raised that cost to $638 million. No data are available for the costs of emergency room treatment, pharmaceuticals, extended care after initial hospitalization, or the treatment of offenders who were injured in aggravated assaults.

Aggravated assaults accounted for more than 8 million days lost from activities such as paid work (at least 4,718,200 days), school, or child rearing. The costs of disabilities, primarily psychological, sensory, and musculoskeletal, resulting from assaults cannot even be estimated.

Projections based on the National Crime Survey indicate that from 1982 to 1984 there were approximately 1.5 million incidents of assaultive violence (rape, robbery, aggravated assault, simple assault) among family members (213.8 per 100,000 U.S. population).[29] Other estimates of the number of women beaten each year range from 1.8 million[30] to 3 to 4 million.[31] Assaults within families represent at least 21,000 hospitalizations, 99,800 hospital days, 28,700 emergency room visits, and 39,900 physician visits. Health care costs incurred for domestic assaults totaled at least $44,393,700.

Assaults within families accounted for at least 175,500 days lost from paid work in 1980. Medical resources are used by abused women to a greater extent than other groups. Battered women frequently use medical services instead of other refuge; of all the emergency room visits made by women seeking treatment for injury, 19% involve battering. Primary care sites such as maternity clinics or ambulatory care services are frequent sites of visits precipitated by battering.

Assaultive violence can seriously affect the quality of life of victims, their families, and society as a whole, causing fear, anxiety, and subsequent restrictions in activities and movements. Homicide, in particular, can have a crippling effect on surviving family members that affects several generations.

Research indicates that children who are victims of violence suffer delays in physical, social, and emotional development. Many who witness violence suffer from posttraumatic stress disorders, particularly if they must participate in the court process.[32] Battered women are at risk of alcoholism, drug abuse, attempted suicide, fear of child abuse, rape, and mental health problems, including severe depression and even psychosis.[31] Family violence is often cited as a reason for divorce, which can result in economic hardship for women and children even though it may solve the immediate problem. However, being divorced or single does not necessarily protect women from subsequent battering. At one large metropolitan hospital, 72% of the women who had battering injuries were single, separated, or divorced.[31]

Society as a whole also pays for violence through expenditures for police and criminal justice intervention, social service intervention, emergency room and trauma center services, and educational services in school systems that must cope with children with academic and social problems as a result of maltreatment at home.

Interventions to Prevent Assaultive Violence. Strategies to reduce or prevent the incidence of assaultive violence must involve both broad social changes in our overall approach to violence and specific interventions aimed at cases of potential or actual violence, assault, or abuse. These specific interventions may try to reach individuals before a pattern of victimization or interpersonal violence is established, or they may attempt to minimize the consequences and costs of interpersonal violence. The recommendations discussed here are grouped for consideration as changes in general public policy, in the health and social services, in the criminal justice system, and in the environment.

Social and Cultural Changes

1. Decrease the cultural acceptance of violence particularly among and against certain groups (blacks, teenagers, women, children) and promote the notion that violent individuals are responsible for their own behavior. Of special interest in this area is the portrayal of violence in children's television programming and the role of corporal punishment at schools and in homes.
2. Reduce racial discrimination and the effects of racism associated with the low self-esteem and low valuation of human life that have been linked with violence.
3. Reduce gender inequality and support male role models that emphasize flexibility, shared decision-making, and nonviolent means of self-development and expression.
4. Reduce the consumption of alcohol and other drugs through interventions directed towards adolescents and young adults, emphasizing the benefits of dependence-free development as well as the effects of harmful substances on self-control. Prevention can also focus on environmental changes such as raising the minimum drinking age, passing stricter laws against selling alcohol to individuals already intoxicated, limiting the hours and places where alcohol can be served, and regulating alcohol advertising.

Health and Related Social Services

1. Develop educational programs to teach conflict-resolution skills. Special programs in schools, churches, and health care and other community organizations could focus on (1) the magnitude of the threat that homicide and assault pose to lives and health, (2) how to recognize volatile situations before they escalate, and (3) how to diffuse or walk away from potentially homicidal fights.[33,34]
2. Increase education for family life, family planning, and child rearing to reduce family stress and violence.[35] Information and services that reduce the incidence of unwanted or unexpected children, that identify families at risk, and provide preventive education as well as education about reporting physical and sexual abuse could reduce violence in the home, thus reducing the amount of violence learned there and later perpetrated against acquaintances and strangers. Family education about developmental difficulties might help parents identify and

seek appropriate treatments for children with aggressive and antisocial behaviors and children whose learning disabilities make it harder to learn appropriate social skills.
3. Support families with community-based support services that help to integrate individuals into the community because research indicates that individuals and families embedded in kin and community groups are less likely to be abusive than individuals who are socially or physically isolated.[21,30,36] Tax, welfare, and business policies that promote isolation and divide families should also be reexamined.
4. Address problems in the recognition of cases of violence by the medical care system by making risk profiles and a history of victimization or perpetration of violence a part of every physical examination.
5. Decrease disincentives for medical personnel to become involved by addressing the legal entanglements that surround cases of child and woman abuse and by addressing the threats of violence and inhibitions that keep health care personnel from even questioning their patients about the cause of their injuries.
6. Improve the management and treatment of victims of violence, particularly for high-risk groups, such as infants or adolescents, who may be in danger of repeated attacks or homicide.
7. Improve the ability of the health care system to recognize and treat consequences of violence other than injuries, including alcoholism, drug dependency, and psychiatric trauma. Intervention programs for children who are victims of violence as well as those who witness violence are urgently needed.[32] Witnesses of violence also need help dealing with the criminal justice system since their experience as witnesses may traumatize them further.
8. Ensure that victims can receive medical care without being dependent on a spouse for adequate medical insurance.
9. Improve the identification and treatment of perpetrators of violence by the health care system; since perpetrators are often injured, they frequently require health services.
10. Improve record-keeping and reporting for victims of interpersonal violence by health care institutions and personnel.
11. Improve communication and cooperation among health care providers, police departments, social service organizations, and schools to improve identification of individuals at risk and documentation for victims who later may decide to prosecute.
12. Develop programs to train high-risk adolescents and to make jobs available for them in order to provide clear, positive roles for adolescents in our culture.
13. Emphasize prevention in the treatment of illness related to consumption of alcohol and other drugs. Health care personnel usually concentrate on immediate problems, like bruises, overdoses, and detoxification, and fail to address prevention issues.
14. Develop health education curricula that address issues of self-directed and interpersonal violence.

Criminal Justice Changes. Changes in the criminal justice system focus on more active citizen interaction with the police and on changes that involve the courts and lawmakers, prosecutors, and prisons. Attempts to deal with homicide in this sector have usually taken two forms: *deterrence* (discouraging others by imposing sanctions) and *incapacitation* (preventing offenders from committing other crimes by physically restraining them). Despite many studies on deterrence and incapacitation, the effect of different sanctions on various crime types is mostly unknown.[37]

1. Police should treat physical assaults among family members, intimates, and acquaintances as criminal behavior.
2. Train police and citizen intervention teams to mediate disputes and refer troubled people to other social service agencies. These teams need to be very sensitive to the concerns of women and minorities if they are going to reduce rather than potentially increase violence. Crisis intervention units that are not staffed by police may be even more effective. These units may be those located within the police complex although administered by civilian personnel; located within City Hall and working in close conjunction with the police and other emergency services; or may be community-based with direct access to police and other emergency services. These groups can prevent situations from erupting into violence by providing backup to the police or support to victims.
3. Improve linkages between police and social services in response to violence.[28]
4. Initiate informal citizen surveillance and silent-witness programs.
5. Facilitate access of victims to legal services through protective orders, temporary restraining orders, and peace bonds to keep violent offenders from attacking partners or children.
6. Initiate victim- and witness-assistance programs that eliminate long waiting periods between the initial arrest and final disposition.

Environmental and Other Changes

1. Develop strategies to reduce injuries associated with firearms. Despite the magnitude and costs of injuries and mortality attributed to firearms, the role of firearms in producing injury and crime is an extremely contentious political and social issue in our society. However, if effective strategies are to be devised for preventing firearm injuries, a scientific perspective must be adopted towards this issue. Common approaches to the prevention of firearm injuries include (1) strict licensing; (2) prohibitions against buying, selling, or possessing guns; (3) prohibitions against carrying (but not owning) guns; and (4) mandatory penalties for the use of a gun in a felony and for carrying unlicensed firearms. In addition, firearms should be modified to prevent the possibility of discharge by young children. Finally, there is a tremendous need for research in the area of firearm injury to determine the magnitude, characteristics, and costs of nonfatal firearm injuries; to estimate the risks of owning or carrying a firearm; and to evaluate the effectiveness of laws, regulations, and other strategies designed to prevent firearm injuries.
2. Create safe environments through architectural and social-planning principles.
3. Define high-risk settings and occupations and determine interventions specific for them, such as bulletproof vests for police and barriers for taxicabs.

Spouse Abuse

Evan Stark
Anne H. Flitcraft

Each year in the United States, 3 to 4 million women are assaulted in their homes by their husbands, former husbands, boyfriends, or lovers. Another 3 to 4 million have been beaten in the past and remain in abusive relationships.[38,39]

Consider the health implications of these statistics. A Harris poll of Kentucky housewives reported that 17% of those who had been battered used emergency medical services.[40] This represents almost 1 million women per year nationwide. A more recent random survey estimates that in Texas alone, 358,595 women have required medical treatment at some point in their lives because of abuse.[41] Stark and colleagues[38,39] reviewed the medical records of 3676 women presenting with physical injuries at a major metropolitan hospital and determined that fully 19% were abused; these findings have been replicated elsewhere. Abuse may be the single most common source of serious injury to women, accounting for almost three times as many visits for health care as motor vehicle crashes. In Britain and Scotland, where medical care is more readily available than in the United States, as many as 80% of abused women have brought their injuries to medical attention, and 40% have done so on at least five occasions.

Even these statistics understate the problem because battering prompts a range of medical and psychosocial problems in addition to injury that also require health and social services. Although it is rarely identified as such, battering is a significant factor in rape, miscarriages and abortion, attempted suicide, alcohol and drug abuse, psychiatric disease, and child abuse.

The health professional is often the first person outside the battered woman's family that she turns to, if only because her problems require medical attention. This fact and the statistics on utilization mean that the medical system is perhaps *the* crucial point in the initial identification, treatment, and prevention of abuse.

Despite the importance of battering, Stark and associates[38] found that health care personnel accurately identified one abusive episode in 25 and failed to identify any of the psychosocial sequelae of abuse as dimensions of battering. Instead, perhaps because battering often expresses itself in multiple complaints and problems with no clear organic basis, battered women are often dismissed as "hysterics" or "crocks." Other punitive interventions include inappropriate sedation, institutionalization, and the removal of children to foster care.

Definition of the Problem. Spouse abuse involves a deliberate physical assault on an adult by another adult intimate, typically a spouse, lover, or dating partner. How severe an assault must be to constitute "abuse" and which patterns of relationship constitute "spousal" arrangements are subjects of controversy. However, regardless of these differences, in clinical settings the most effective operational definition of spouse abuse must rely on an inclusive notion of violence or control, regardless of the severity of injury inflicted or whether the presentation involves injury or psychosocial problems. Because the clinician's central concern is with future health risks, the important differentiation is between an anonymous assault, where further assault by the criminal is unlikely, and assault by any social partner regardless of gender, age, or marital status and whether or not they are present or past cohabitants. Although women are injured by abuse approximately 13 times as frequently as men, the term "spouse" is retained to indicate concern for men who also are assaulted in intimate relations.

The battering syndrome refers to the combination of medical and psychosocial problems that may follow spouse abuse and that are evoked when the victim of abuse is dominated by the assailant, a process referred to as "entrapment." Although either men or women may assault a spouse, the syndrome associated with battering has been identified only among women. Battering is a chronic problem with a low spontaneous cure rate: in the vast majority of cases where a woman has *ever* presented with an abusive injury, she appears to be still at risk.[42] The inadequacy of current protections against violence, the survivor's fear of being killed, the fear that children will be scapegoats, the lack of economic opportunity, the inappropriate and punitive responses of helping institutions, and the total control many batterers exercise over the lives of their victims all contribute to the entrapment of abused women in battering relationships. In light of these constraints, it is remarkable that as many as 65% of women eventually escape from abusive relationships.

Researchers have distinguished injuries resulting from battering not by their severity but by the accompanying history of repeated injury and visits to seek help as well as by their predictive value for subsequent assaults. In addition to a history of adult trauma and unsuccessful help-seeking, battering may present through nonspecific complaints of pain, injury during pregnancy, fear or anxiety associated with family conflict, and multiple psychosocial problems, including alcoholism, drug abuse, rape, child abuse, attempted suicide, homelessness, and mental illness. Since the increased risk of these problems among battered women appears only after a pattern of abusive injury is established, these problems appear to be the result rather than the cause of battering for these women. The problems associated with battering develop through stages brought on by increasing danger, fear, isolation, and entrapment. Assessment on these parameters can be a more important index of the emergent nature of the problem than the severity of the injury.

Data Sources. There are no periodic standardized databases from which to reliably estimate the prevalence of spouse abuse. Estimates of prevalence are based on a representative national survey and follow-up and on surveys of state and local populations.[40,41,43–48] No widely recognized procedures have been adopted to identify abuse or battering, and reporting is sporadic, even in states where it is mandated.

Gathering spouse-abuse data in health care settings for case identification is important both clinically and epidemiologically. This process begins with the patient encounter but may extend to a complete review of the patient's medical records to determine the history and extent of abuse and to document the patient's previous attempts to find aid. No attempts have yet been made to use medical records to identify interspousal violence or husband abuse.

Since physicians rarely record abuse or list it as a diagnosis in medical records, incidence data based on physician reporting seriously and consistently underestimate the magnitude of the problem. Through a critical review of the medical records, however, the trained researcher can identify both abused women and women whose medical histories suggest domestic violence. Where there is access to a consolidated medical records system, potential battered women may be identified by retrospective review of the full medical records of adult women. Women should be defined at risk if their history contains at least one episode attributed to an assault by a male intimate (positives); an assaultive episode not attributed to street crime (probables); or where the recorded alleged etiology is inconsistent with the injury presentation (suggestives). Early claims that abused women delay or fail to report injuries have not been sustained. Indeed, abusive injury is reported promptly.[39]

Frank but sensitive probing and eliciting a history of deliberate assault are the most important steps to identify abused women. The routine use of a trauma history avoids the problem of identifying abuse only after the extent and nature of injuries make the diagnosis tragically obvious.

Battering should be part of the differential diagnosis of every encounter with an injured client. Specific complaints should heighten the clinician's suspicion. These include multiple injuries, central injuries, rape, and medically insignificant trauma or injury during pregnancy. Other complaints that may be indicators of battering are headache or nonspecific pain, sleep disorders, anxiety, dysphagia, hyperventilation, or other signs of living in a stressful environment. In obstetrical and gynecological clinics a history that should prompt the clinician's suspicion of abuse includes self-induced or attempted abortions, multiple therapeutic abortions, miscarriages, and divorce or separation during pregnancy. Persistent gynecological complaints, particularly abdominal pain and dyspareunia in the context of normal physical examinations, are frequently overlooked manifestations of domestic violence. The strongest clues of abuse are the clustering and repetition of presentations and complaints rather than isolated events.

Causes and Risk Factors. The literature on domestic violence is characterized by a wealth of descriptive material and a dearth of systematic theorizing. Three explanatory models emerge from attempts to summarize this vast body of material.

According to the *interpersonal violence model,* violence arises among adults who lack the skills to cope appropriately and nonviolently with stress or conflict. Underlying behavioral or psychological causes are the focus of identification and intervention, rather than violence per se. The methods that work from this approach include individual, couples, or family systems therapy; cognitive-behavioral work with batterers or alcoholics, and programs designed to teach mothers of abused children how to parent more effectively. Three related propositions follow from this theory: that victims and assailants suffer disproportionately from psychological and behavioral problems; that these problems lead to abuse; and that batterers and their victims have a distinctive personality profile, family history, or pattern of relating that predisposes them to violence.

The disproportionate rates of various problems suffered by battered women are well documented.[38,43,49,50] However, to establish a major causal role for pathology, the numbers of victims affected by these problems must be determined as well as whether these problems precede abuse. Among battered women, disproportionate rates of problems such as attempted suicide or substance abuse typically have their onset only after a history of violence and frustrated help-seeking is established.[51] This fact highlights safety for victims and early interventions to prevent violence as steps to reduce female alcoholism, child abuse, and other problems linked to woman battering. Furthermore, most persons involved in spouse abuse are indistinguishable psychologically from "normal" populations, and researchers have failed to identify a specific personality profile that makes people "violence prone." Despite this, in combination with vigorous law enforcement and shelter for women, cognitive-behavioral therapy and court-mandated "re-education" programs are effective with many batterers.

The *family violence model,* on the other hand, emphasizes the normative support our society gives to violence as a means of resolving conflict, the special intensity of family relations as a source of such conflict, and the fact that family members who have experienced or witnessed violence in childhood or are suffering the stresses of poverty or unemployment are at particular risk.[43] By documenting the frequency of various forms of conflict in families (from spanking and sibling fights to domestic homicide), researchers hope to emphasize how, regardless of who initiates violence, all family members become enmeshed in violent patterns. While some forms of violence may receive publicity (such as child abuse or woman battering), unrecognized forms of conflict or violence (such as spanking or husband battering) are no less important for public policy. Interventions based on this model target the family unit as the client and highlight broad initiatives to challenge cultural supports for violence, particularly in the media, and to reduce violence by attacking poverty.

Survey data implicate women as well as men in assaultive behavior and homicide, lending support to the family violence approach. In addition, as the model predicts, disproportionate numbers of both batterers and their victims are abused as children, violence is linked to such indicators of stress as low income and minority status, and child abuse commonly accompanies woman battering, suggesting a "family" problem.

The major claims of this model find only weak support, however. The very different meaning, consequence, and history of violence where men are the perpetrators suggests that family treatment models should be used only after violence has ceased and the victims are safe. Most child abuse is committed by men (often the same men who are abusing the mothers),[52] and they should be held accountable, not the women. Moreover, although violence in the family of origin increases a man's propensity to abuse his wife and child, most abused children become nonviolent adults, and the vast majority of violent adults neither were abused as children nor witnessed abuse.[52] Finally, although money is a common source of conflict in violent homes, social class and racial differences in violence are relatively small.

The *gender-politics model* contends that violence in the family is merely a special instance of a pattern of male control that extends from dating relationships through parenting and marriage to economic life. Violence is one option when men feel their privileged access to scarce resources like money or sex threatened by female independence or by the personal failure of women to fulfill presumed domestic responsibilities. Women stay in abusive relationships because fear, lack of support, victim-blaming interventions, and the absence of resources combine to make mere survival more practical than escape. The gender-politics model suggests that an end to battering must begin with political choices: punishment of male violence, funding for the community-based shelter movement, and support for women's personal and economic independence.

Compelling evidence supports the argument that battering arises primarily from patterns of dominance based on gender. For instance, woman abuse is many times more common than other forms of "family violence" and is typically accompanied by forms of economic, sexual, and social control that reflect male prerogatives; women who are single, divorced, separated, or merely dating are at equal or even greater risk of abuse than married women; issues involving women's traditional responsibilities in the home are the most common source of fights in which abuse occurs; and the couples at highest risk for abuse are those in which the woman's status is higher than her partner's.

Vulnerability Factors. Battering follows no clear demographic pattern. Population surveys suggest that battering is two to three times more common among blacks than whites; however, among groups with similar income, blacks are less likely than whites to experience spousal violence.[40,43,53] Surveys report higher rates of abuse among poor, unemployed, or working-class groups. However, the difference between low-income and middle-income women may be small,[40] and extensive abuse has been identified in relatively affluent communities.

Research on domestic violence fails to establish the clear temporal sequence needed to show that personality characteristics are risk factors rather than outcomes of spouse abuse. Therefore it is best to view personality, demographic, and social factors as vulnerability factors for spouse abuse.[54] These factors may interact with the situational dynamics in domestic conflict to increase the likelihood that violence will result. Studies report few if any significant personality differences between battered and nonbattered women, and no personality profile has been identified that makes certain women "violence prone." Although some evidence suggests that battered women have low self-esteem, they generally neither blame themselves for violence nor exhibit a helplessness syndrome.[39,55–58]

Age is inversely related to domestic violence, yet teens and the elderly represent high-risk populations whose battering is often misidentified. The battering of elderly women should be clearly differentiated from the abuse of the frail elderly by a caretaker. Pregnancy is a high-risk period among abused women; between 20% and 25% of obstetrical patients are abused women,[38] an even higher percentage than in the emergency service.

Although the reported violence rates among men who use alcohol are 2 to 15 times higher than rates among abstainers, a causal role for alcohol cannot be supported. Among women, alcohol is typically the consequence rather than the cause of victimization. Although drinking is associated with higher rates of wife abuse, alcohol is not typically an immediate antecedent, nor does cessation of alcohol use appear to affect abusive behavior.[59–63]

An indicator of spouse abuse may be a profile of violent couples based on a combination of low-income, minority status, unemployment, status inconsistency, alcoholism, and an inheritance of violence. However, the lack of specificity prevents such a profile from aiding identification, particularly in medical, police, mental health, or other multiproblem caseloads. A history of victimization and of frustrating helping encounters are the best predictors of woman abuse.

Medical Response. Neglect, denial, isolation, mistreatment, and punitive interventions and referrals characterize the ongoing care of women who present with abusive injury, responses that increase a woman's risk and reinforce denial, minimization, abuse, and victim-blaming by the batterer. A failure to identify battered women in health and mental health settings has been documented from medical records. In addition, records reviews, patient interviews, and direct observations reveal that health providers are more likely to refer battered than nonbattered women to psychiatry, to apply traditional female labels or denigrating stigmata, to prescribe tranquilizers and other pain medications, and to institutionalize them in state hospitals.[38] Battered women who attempt suicide are more likely to be sent home with no follow-up than nonbattered women.[39] Battered mothers of abused children are more likely than nonbattered mothers to have the children placed in foster care. At advanced stages of battering, clinicians interpret the sequelae of abuse as its cause and may intervene to manage these secondary problems like alcoholism in ways that actually aggravate a victim's predicament.

Outcomes. Battering may be the single most common cause of injury for which women seek medical attention. Battered women are 13 times more likely than nonbattered women to be injured in the breast, chest, and abdomen, and three times as likely to be injured while pregnant.[38] Still, abusive injuries are no more likely to result in hospitalization than nonabusive injuries, suggesting that severity in itself is not a good indicator of abuse.

The greatest proportion of medical visits by battered women do not involve trauma but general medical, behavioral, and psychiatric presentations. Nontrauma medicine provides most of their care. Clearly, spouse abuse protocols should not be limited to emergency or trauma settings.

The rate of alcoholism and drug abuse among battered women is significantly greater than among nonbattered women. Therefore, battering appears to be an important risk factor for female alcoholism, possibly occurring in 50% of cases.[64] After the onset of abuse, alcoholism is 16 times as common among battered women. It is so common that abused women who develop alcohol problems have a higher rate of emergency medical utilization than any other population.[38] Unfortunately, "AOB" (alcohol on breath) is a frequent reason clinicians give for dismissing a woman's abuse. In addition, once a battered woman develops an alcohol or drug problem, the violence is seen as the consequence of the substance abuse, and interventions neglect her physical safety.

Attempted suicide, particularly multiple attempts, is a significant sequela of abuse among women, affecting 1 abused woman in 10.[38,39] Conversely, abuse may be the single most important precipitant for female suicide. As many as 50% of black women who attempt suicide have been abused. Of the battered women who attempt suicide, 85% have been seen in the hospital for at least one abusive injury prior to their first suicide attempt. This highlights the importance of abuse as a precipitating factor as well as the importance of early identification of abuse in suicide prevention.

Abuse may be the single most important precipitant of rape as well as of child abuse. Stark and Flitcraft[50,51] reported that of mothers of children suspected of being physically abused or neglected, 45% are battered women, the highest percentage of battered women identified in any client population. Although child abuse programs almost exclusively target mothers, men are three times as likely to be the abusing parents.

Severe mental health problems and disproportionate use of emergency psychiatric services are significant sequelae of abuse. The prevalence of woman abuse among mental health clients is even greater than among medical patients, approaching half of all female inpatients.[49,65] Compared to nonbattered mental health patients, battered women are less likely to manifest psychotic illness but are more likely to carry a diagnosis of situational or personality disorder and to exhibit impaired self-esteem. The most common diagnosis of abuse victims is depression (37%), but 1 abused woman in 10 suffers a psychotic break.[39] Battered women are also far more likely than others to be given a pseudopsychiatric label such as "hysteric," "hypochondriac," and "crock."

Battering has a cumulative cost and impact on health services far greater than the impact of abuse-related injury alone, often involving dozens, sometimes hundreds of medical and mental health visits. Recent evidence suggests that battering is a major cause of homelessness among women and children.[66] The combination of assault and institutional victimization constitutes the dual trauma of battering, extends male control over women's lives, and leads to an increasing sense of isolation, fear, entrapment, self-destructive behavior, and even homicidal rage among abused women. Although each of the problems associated with abuse may appear to have an independent etiology and although the multi-problem profile may seem intractable, the emergence of these problems only after a history of abuse and frustrated help-seeking is well established. This underscores the importance of early intervention at primary care sites and at each of the secondary treatment sites where the psychosocial consequences of living in a violent relationship are managed.

Interventions. Preventing spouse abuse requires protecting victims; stopping violence; expanding the resources available to victims and assailants; and early identification, referral, and public education. Thus far, emphasis has been placed on shelter, police and legal action, and legislation.

The traditional medical model provides an adequate framework for a health care response to spouse abuse for the following reasons:

- It greatly undervalues the psychological and social costs of abuse.
- It underplays the complex social origins of spouse abuse.
- It is based on outdated notions of prevention. Interventions must instead target social behaviors; health providers must form working alliances with community-based services and with disciplines outside health; and emphasis should be placed on nonmedical policies and interventions that can reduce violence and improve health. We term this *complex social prevention*.

Although the costs and benefits of these interactions have not yet been rigorously evaluated, we believe that the following nonmedical policies and practices may have the greatest bearing on health:

1. Increase our knowledge of the causes of spouse abuse and of which interventions most effectively prevent it.
2. Give national recognition to the criminal nature of spouse abuse with particular emphasis on its health consequences for women.
3. Decrease the cultural acceptance of violence against vulnerable groups.
4. Support the empowerment of women by expanding their social and economic options.
5. Make spouse abuse a top priority for all human resource and public health funding.
6. Support more flexible role models for women and men, that is, educate women and men about the destructiveness of prejudice and beliefs that certain roles, actions, modes of expression, or work are only for men or only for women.

Primary Prevention. These interventions are designed to prevent battering by enabling health institutions to respond more effectively to interpersonal conflict before it escalates:

1. Establish and implement model protocols for the early identification and referral of abuse victims in health settings.
2. Introduce model curricula on spouse abuse and gender bias into the professional education, training and continuing education of health and social service providers, school counselors, and criminal justice groups.
3. Develop and distribute public information on spouse abuse and available services for the media.

Secondary Prevention

1. Support the development of spouse abuse protocols in secondary treatment sites dealing with rape, alcohol and drug abuse, suicide prevention, emergency psychiatric problems, child abuse, and the homeless.
2. Extend the range of options available to battered women.
3. Expand the counseling, treatment, and life-style options available to violent men.

Rape and Sexual Assault

Judith M. Conn
Dean G. Kilpatrick
Ann W. Burgess
Carol R. Hartman

Definition of the Problem. Contrary to popular belief, rape is not a rare event but rather affects the lives of thousands of people each year. It has been estimated[67] that the population of the United States contains more rape victims (3,750,000) than combat veterans (2,480,544),[68] yet in our society, compared to veterans, rape victims are relatively silent and invisible. Since 1977 the rate of forcible rape has increased by 21%, the largest increase among all major crimes. Although all types of crime have harmful effects, rape has been shown to have a particularly damaging effect on its victims. Rape victims experience long-term problems in the areas of psychological functioning (fear, anxiety, depression), impaired social adjustment, and sexual dysfunction. Further, being a rape victim is associated with an increased risk of suicide.[69] In addition, the recovery rate from rape appears to be slower and may be less complete than researchers once thought.[70] Sexual assault claims many indirect victims as well. Often marriages dissolve, or victims are forced to leave their jobs or relocate to prevent retaliation after they have pressed criminal charges. Even women who have never been raped or abused restrict their daily mobility because of the fear of rape.

The human suffering contained in these facts indicates that rape is a problem of major public health importance. It is currently the most underreported violent crime, in part because of the treatment victims receive from the criminal justice system.[71] Yet without victim cooperation the criminal justice system cannot function effectively, which leaves criminals free to reoffend. If the treatment of rape victims is improved, more victims may seek help and report these crimes to authorities, thus improving the ability of the criminal justice system to prosecute offenders and ultimately prevent subsequent rapes.

Compared to other types of serious crime, rape has a number of unique characteristics. First, it is particularly difficult to know how frequently rape occurs because of the low reporting rate. Second, in contrast to other crimes, there is a subjective element in the determination of whether the sexual act occurred against the victim's will. If the victim is of unquestioned chastity and if considerable force is employed by the assailant, then the act is considered to be "real" rape. However, if a woman is forced to have sex with a man she has dated and originally met in a bar, many individuals may not construe the act as rape. Third, rape is the only serious crime in which victims are sometimes held responsible for their own assaults. Many individuals believe that women like to be overpowered sexually and say "no" when they mean "yes." Rules of evidence accepted in the courtroom have been stringent; for example, signs of resistance are required as proof of nonconsent.[72]

Part of the problem inherent in understanding rape and sexual assault is derived from its equivocal definition. From a legal perspective, rape is a criminal act. Whereas old laws viewed rape as an act of illicit sex, more recent legislation defines rape as a type of assault. As defined by the Federal Bureau of Investigation (FBI) Uniform Crime Report (UCR), forcible rape "is the carnal knowledge of a female forcibly and against her will."[73(p 13)] Although some variations between states exist, rape as legally defined generally refers to forced sexual penetration of a victim by an offender who is not the victim's spouse. Some state laws patterned after the FBI's definition limit the term "rape" to incidents in which the victim is female and in which only vaginal penetration has occurred. Many statutes have a marital exclusion rule that states that criminal sexual conduct cannot legally occur if the offender and victim are married. This rule stems from the historical legal theory that a wife is the property of her husband.[74]

Because the legal definition of forcible rape is so restrictive, the term "sexual assault" has been used to cover a wider range of sexual crimes, including any manual, genital, or oral contact with the victim's genitalia without consent and obtained by force, threat, or fraud. Most states define as illegal any type of sexual behavior with a child. Statutory rape may also be charged in cases where the victim cannot give consent because of mental deficiency, psychosis, or altered consciousness induced by sleep, drugs, illness, or intoxication. As public attention is directed toward this area of definition, there is concurrent pressure for legal reform. Reformed legislation with its increased emphasis on force, threat of force, and coercion comes closer to capturing the psychological essence of rape.

The manner in which rape is defined will have a profound impact on incidence and prevalence rates. That is, the number of sexual assaults and rape incidents both detected and reported depends on the victim's and the authority's (e.g., police, researcher) perception of what occurred. The process involved in getting a rape reported can be seen in the following elaboration.[75] First, for a rape to be reported, victims must perceive that a rape has occurred. Second, they must classify the event as an illegal activity. Third, they must decide whether to disclose it. The fourth step in this process is a redefinition on the part of the police officer (or researcher) who decides whether the disclosed event meets the definition of the illegal activity. Only if his or her classification agrees with that of the victim does the incident become recorded. The process of definition, then, is important both at the victim's or respondent's level and secondly at the inquirer's level. If there is substantial disagreement, considerable underrepresentation in victimization surveys will result. This is particularly true for those women who have been defined as "unacknowledged" victims[76]: women whose experiences meet the legal definition of rape (i.e., forced sexual penetration obtained without consent) but who do not view their experiences as criminal and do not report them as such. Often the unacknowledged victim has been assaulted by someone known to her. The public perception that rape involves a brutal attack by a stranger in a remote setting is so firmly entrenched in our society that many individuals, including the victims themselves, do not apply the label "rape" to an assault that deviates from the commonly accepted stereotype. This highlights the importance of asking about sexual assault using behavioral descriptions, thereby avoiding the subjective bias introduced by using the word "rape."

Present statistics suggest that rape comprises 7% of violent crime volume and 1% of the Crime Index total, with an estimated 87,340 assaults reported annually.[73] Geographically the highest rates of rape currently occur in the Western states, followed by the South, then the Midwest and the Northeast. The largest number of forcible rapes tend to occur in the summer; the lowest total was reported for the month of February. Most rapes involve a lone victim and a lone perpetrator and take place at night.

Data Sources. Data on rape and sexual assault are available at the national level from both the FBI UCR and the National Crime Survey (NCS). A major limitation of both of these data sets is the degree of underreporting. The UCR provides statistics on the number of forcible rapes reported annually to the police. Yet it is well known that only a small percentage of rapes are ever reported, and of those reported rapes, some proportion are deemed "unfounded" by the police and hence never become part of the UCR statistics. In addition, the UCR uses a restricted definition of rape ("carnal knowledge of a female forcibly and against her will"), thereby excluding cases involving oral or anal penetration, male victims, or wives assaulted by their husbands. Furthermore, the FBI employs a crime hierarchy in which events are classified according to the most serious crime; for instance, a case in which a victim is both raped and killed is recorded as a homicide.

The NCS reports annual victimization data based on a continuing survey of a nationally representative sample of households.[77] This data set is also limited by underreporting. It has been noted that the NCS inquires about rape in a way that decreases the likelihood that accurate information will be obtained.[78] For example, a "screen" question requires the respondent to infer that rape is being asked about. Further, questions regarding rape are embedded in a context of other violent crimes. Respondents who have been victimized by family members or other known assailants often do not know these experiences are criminal. The actual incidence for rape has been estimated to be 10 to 15 times higher than NCS estimates.[78]

In general, victimization surveys provide the most accurate statistics on both the incidence and prevalence rates of crime, although numerous methodological variables influence the reliability and validity of these data. Four major errors may occur in the retrospective measurement of victimization: ignorance of events, forgetting or not telling, inaccuracy or incomplete recall, and differential interview productivity.[79(p 11)] Ignorance of events was primarily a problem of earlier surveys when only one respondent per household was questioned about events that occurred to all household members. Recent surveys ask respondents only about crimes that have happened to them personally. Forgetting or not telling has a major impact on all victimization studies. Reverse-record-check studies prove that not all incidents reported to police are subsequently remembered and disclosed, particularly as time elapses and if the assailant is known by the victim. The third error, inaccuracy or incomplete recall, occurs when respondents provide inaccurate information about details of the incident. This may involve temporal telescoping, or placing an event at the wrong point in time. Use of short reference periods and bounded interviews produces more accurate estimates. The fourth error, differential productivity, refers to the tendency for more highly educated respondents to disclose more victimization experiences to interviewers. Since most experts believe that people with lower educational and socioeconomic status experience the bulk of criminal victimization, these findings are counterintuitive. Possible explanations include the tendency for better educated people to have greater recall and to feel more comfortable in interview situations.

Causes and Risk Factors. Two major theoretical models have been proposed to account for the commission of rape. The first centers on the psychopathology of the offender; the second views social factors as causative. The first model resulted in numerous studies in which rapists were compared with nonrapists on various psychological tests. Support for this model has been lacking, as rapists generally do not differ on these tests from prisoners who have committed nonsexual violent crimes. Further, as the percentage of rapists reported and convicted is extremely small, these studies have been criticized because of the nonrepresentativeness of the sample employed and the consequent lack of generalizability.

In contrast, the social control–social conflict model maintains that sexual aggression against females results not from diagnosable, individual pathology, but rather from the acceptance of societal attitudes that foster male dominance and dehumanize women. Numerous studies have supported this model by showing a relationship between certain attitudes (e.g., acceptance of rape myths, sex role stereotyping) and various measures of aggression.[80,81] While early research treated the two models as mutually exclusive, recent work suggests that incorporating variables from both models may be requisite.[82] Stimulated by Finkelhor's[83] work on child abuse, some authors[84] have posited a synergistic process involving variables such as internal motivation, deviant sexual arousal, and reduction of inhibition of aggression that may apply to both acquaintance rape and stranger assault.[85]

Early attempts to explain the occurrence of rape focused on identifying characteristics within the victim that would render her susceptible to assault. Three models have been proposed to explain how women become rape victims: victim precipitation, social control, and situational blame. It should be noted that all these models are, to varying degrees, ideologically related to a victim-blame perspective and have been criticized because of the lack of attention paid to offender behavior.[86] Empirical support for the victim precipitation model, which posits that specific behaviors or personality characteristics heighten susceptibility to rape,[87] has been noticeably lacking. The social control model, which also has found little empirical support, posits that victims adhere to a rape-supportive belief system that increases their vulnerability to assault. The only study to date that has directly examined victim adherence to such a belief system found no support for this hypothesis.[76] The situational blame model maintains that rape is more likely to occur in particular environmental contexts and subsequent to particular victim and perpetrator behaviors. Support for this model has generally come from studies of rape avoidance that compared the resistance strategies employed by women who avoided rape and those who failed to avoid it. The evidence to date suggests that differences in the ability to avoid rape are the result of strategies used, as opposed to demographic or background variables. To summarize, there are no reliable findings to date that distinguish rape victims from women who have not been victimized.

Outcomes. Rape victims experience significant long-term problems in the areas of psychological functioning, social adjustment, and impaired sexual functioning. Fear, anxiety, and depression are the most frequently identified psychological sequelae of rape.[88]

As the literature on crime victims has expanded, attention has shifted from simply describing symptoms to assessing symptom constellations consistent with major psychiatric diagnoses. Posttraumatic stress disorder (PTSD) has frequently been identified among victims of sexual assault.[67,88] Briefly stated, PTSD represents a characteristic set of symptoms that results from exposure to a psychologically traumatic event. The hallmark symptoms of PTSD (all of which have been documented in victims of rape)[89,90] include reexperiencing the event through persistent, intrusive, and distressing recollections; mood disturbance, including diminished responsiveness, loss of interest, and feelings of estrangement; and increased arousal (e.g., exaggerated startle response, hypervigilance) and behavioral avoidance of stimuli resembling the traumatic event.[91]

Recent evidence suggests that a history of criminal victimization is associated with an increased likelihood of several mental health disorders, including social phobia, sexual dysfunction, major depression, and obsessive-compulsive disorder.[69] Available evidence also suggests that a history of sexual assault is associated with an increased risk of suicide.[69,70,92]

Interventions. Victims of rape and sexual assault require access to a comprehensive system of resources, including emergency clinical services and counseling. These important resources should include a 24-hour rape hotline staffed by trained personnel and available trained staff to accompany victims to the hospital following an assault. Accompaniment to the hospital can also serve the much needed function of ensuring that rape victims are adequately informed regarding hospital procedures (including procedures for the collection of evidence). Because many initial police interviews are conducted at the hospital, accompaniment provides trained advocates to help victims make informed choices regarding prosecution.

Crisis counseling by mental health workers should be available after the emergency services have been completed. This type of crisis intervention focuses on the assault and its aftermath and emphasizes assisting the victim to achieve mastery over anxiety, identifying a supportive social network, and seeking self-enhancing ways of solving problems related to the rape and possible court proceedings to follow. For some victims, specialized long-term therapy is necessary. A number of effective treatment procedures have been developed to target specific rape-induced symptomatology.[93–95] With some victims, intervention with the family is helpful as well.[96,97]

Victims involved with the criminal justice system need to be oriented to courtroom procedure and kept informed about their cases. These services can be provided by the victim-witness staff of the prosecutor's office. After trial, many states allow the victim to be involved in the sentencing process by providing a victim-input statement. Other services provided by the state include victim compensation programs, which vary extensively from state to state.

Rape prevention remains the primary area for further research. Although services to rape victims have improved qualitatively and quantitatively during the last decade, no breakthrough has occurred in the prevention of sexual assault. Strategies to prevent rape vary along two dimensions: whether the strategy aims at the victim or the perpetrator and whether it aims at the individual or the societal level.

Research on victims and victimizers should take place within continued investigation of the social context that gives rise to violence and sex crimes, including violent media portrayals and pornography. Attention must also be given to the prevention of sexual aggression among acquaintances. At present, the majority of intervention programs focus on stranger rape, but given the incidence rates, this effort should be redirected. Prevention programs should target those at risk for perpetrating and suffering acquaintance rape before they begin dating. Achieving the goal of eliminating rape from society will require nothing less than radical changes in society's structure and its acceptance of stereotypical notions of the roles, duties, and needs of men and women.

Child Abuse

Eli H. Newberger

Definition of the Problem. Definitions of child abuse have broadened significantly in the last two decades. The commonsense meaning of the term "child abuse" is a situation where a caregiver, generally a parent, sets out in a systematic way to harm a defenseless child. In 1962, Professor C. Henry Kempe and his associates published an article in the *Journal of the American Medical Association* entitled "The Battered Child Syndrome"[98] that drew great attention in the professional and lay media. One of the outcomes of increased public awareness was the drafting of a model child abuse reporting statute by the Children's Bureau, the lead federal agency for children. Child abuse came to be defined in the state reporting laws as injuries inflicted by caregivers, and many believed that it could be diagnosed by physicians and medical institutions. However, Kempe's perpetrator-victim model of etiology and the notion of a syndrome of physical examination findings in the child and psychopathology in the caregiver led to several problematical consequences.

Physicians are likely to confuse the task of diagnosis with investigation (to find out who did what to whom and how). Perceptions persist that all adults who harm children in their care are mentally ill and agencies that receive the reports maintain a conflicted sense of responsibility. The perpetrator-victim model substantially inhibits the range of diagnostic and therapeutic possibilities in these agencies.

In the 1970s, laws concerning child abuse reporting were revised. Parents of abused children were seen as people who could be helped, and child abuse was perceived as related to other family disturbances with implications for the health and welfare of children. The government's role was to provide timely help to troubled families. The National Center on Child Abuse and Neglect was created in 1973. At the same time, the definition of child abuse was broadened to include child neglect, emotional injury, parental deprivation of medical care, and factors injurious to a child's moral development. The draft statute proposing this new definition also lengthened the list of professionals required by law to report child abuse to include virtually anyone responsible for the care of children. However, the draft legislation included nothing about budgeting for services. Although a dramatic increase in reports was foreseen, the people drafting the legislation assumed that state legislators would contend with the cost implications.[99] Furthermore, unless states' statutes conformed to the new model reporting statute, they would not be eligible for their share of federal monies that were stipulated to go for improving state services.

One unforeseen consequence of that effort was a changing sense of government's responsibility for children and families in trouble. With new reporting legislation and media attention came a deluge of reports of child abuse. Child welfare agencies are now overburdened in every state.

In 1985, in the reauthorization of the National Center on Child Abuse and Neglect, child abuse was conceived still more broadly to include situations where handicapped infants may be denied medical care necessary to insure their survival. Highly publicized cases of child sexual abuse in day-care centers has led to yet another initiative to expand the concept of child abuse and the role of child protection agencies.

Physicians are trained not to make judgments about the people they treat. If they are obliged to make known abuse or risks of abuse, conforming to the ethical doctrines under which physicians practice will be difficult.

Practitioners oriented to the perpetrator-victim model may restrict their field of vision to major findings, such as fractures, bruises to portions of the body that would not ordinarily occur in play, scalds, collections of blood around, above, or beneath the dense lining of the brain, poisonings, lacerations, and contusions to internal organs. These injuries evoke greater concern when children are younger or when different forms of trauma occur simultaneously or over time.[100]

A medical concept of child abuse that goes beyond the perpetrator-victim model focuses on relationships among the "pediatric social illness" (i.e., maltreatment), unintentional injuries, poisonings, and failure to thrive.[101] The child's physical symptoms are placed in an ecological framework that includes many interacting elements: developmental qualities and risk, parents' adaptations to their children's needs, psychological attributes of the family, realities and exigencies of the nurturing environment, and the favorable and unfavorable qualities of professional personnel, service programs, and institutions with which they have contact. Physicians should focus on family strengths and on prevention of abuse rather than on pathologies to be treated.

Recent attention has also been focused on two other concerns to physicians and other medical workers: the "Munchausen syndrome by proxy" and the problem of sexual victimization of children by professionals, including physicians.[102,103] The Munchausen syndrome has been used to describe the adult patient who falsifies medical history and examination findings. In its application to child abuse, the syndrome relates to the parent who endeavors to make the child ill in order to draw attention to the parent's own problems. Physicians often perceive the children's mothers as ideal, concerned parents and prefer to perform diagnostic studies rather than question the validity of the proffered history.

Data Sources. There are few data sources on child abuse that permit inferences to be drawn on prevalence, incidence, risk factors, outcomes, and the effectiveness of interventions. This is a consequence of the selective nature of case ascertainment for clinical research, limitations of study design in nearly every clinical study, and of a reluctance in the formation of national policy on child abuse to make use of standard methods of measurement and program evaluation.

The major data sets on child abuse give some useful estimates of reported prevalence, and four studies demonstrate the utility of methodologies that do not rely on case reports. The first, established by David Gil,[104] is a systematic treatment of child abuse case reports to agencies mandated by the initial wave of reporting statutes in the early and mid-1960s. From respondents in a national probability sample an incidence estimate of between 2 1/2 million cases per year was made. The study's conclusion that poverty is the principal determinant of abuse has been criticized on the grounds that demographic attributes of the reported cases reflect the class and other biases of the reporting process.

The American Humane Association (AHA) compiles official reports of child abuse and neglect[105]; however, the lack of standardized definitions, dependence on individual states' data aggregation methods, and inability to gauge the meaning of the case reports in reference to any sampling methodology hinders the usefulness of these data. As with data in the previous study, AHA describes children who get into the child protection system identified as abused or neglected. Most of these children come from indigent families, reflecting in part the bias of ascertainment that causes poor children to be reported to agencies of the state.

However, the AHA data do document how the problem of child abuse has grown. The Gil study in 1967 and 1968 documented only 6000 to 7000 cases a year; in 1986 the AHA survey yielded an estimated prevalence of 1,928,000 abused children. AHA data also document an increasing number of reported cases of child sexual victimization, perhaps prompted by media attention and increased public and professional awareness.

The first national survey of family violence by Murray Straus and his associates[106] used a scale to measure the techniques family members used to resolve conflicts among themselves. In turn, this scale provided the entry point for a series of questions about violent practices. On the basis of a national sample of families with two adults and at least one child between the ages of 3 and 17, the researchers produced the first systematic and reliable projections of the frequency of particular incidents of violence, including the use or threat to use a knife or gun in resolving conflict. There were several limitations to this survey: the sample was not representative of American families with children; infants were not represented because the investigators were interested in violence between adults and among children and adults; and neither neglect nor sexual abuse was explored.

However, the study yielded a prevalence estimate suggesting that in 1975 there were 1.4 million children aged 3 to 17 years who had been abused. Gelles and Straus[107] recently reported the findings of a second national family violence survey that yielded a much lower prevalence estimate, perhaps because their 1985 interviews were collected over the phone, thus excluding families without phones, a group more likely to experience social isolation and economic adversity. Respondents in 1985 also may have been more reluctant to report family violence than in 1975. However, the authors of the study believe that there has been a true decline in the rates of violence against children.

A national incidence study of child abuse and neglect was conducted through funding by the Children's Bureau to delineate the dimensions of the "iceberg" of child abuse, the tip of which was seen in child abuse case reports. Data were gathered from child protective agencies and other sources such as hospitals, police departments, and mental health agencies.[108] Systematic definitions were declared and a weighting system devised to generalize to the national experience. For the 26-county sample, 17,645 cases of child abuse came to attention between May 1, 1979, and April 30, 1980. It was projected that nationwide 1,151,600 cases were suspected by professionals. Of these, 562,000 were considered likely to meet the study's criteria and, therefore, to be true cases of child abuse and neglect.

This study methodology has been criticized because child sexual abuse was rarely reported at the time of the incidence study.[109] Other studies suggest a far greater frequency than the case reporting compilations would suggest. The first national incidence study data are available now and are useful for studies of agency practice.

A second national incidence study used similar methodology.[110] The data for 1986 are presented in the recently published report, along with perceived changes since the earlier study. The estimated 1986 national incidence of abuse and neglect was 1,584,700. There was a 74% increase in the incidence of abuse (to 657,000 cases), within which there was an increase of 58% for child physical abuse (to 358,300 cases) and over 300% for child sexual abuse (to 155,900 cases). No changes were noted in the incidence of emotional abuse or neglect. Physical abuse was the most frequent type of abuse identified in the study, followed by emotional abuse and by sexual abuse, with respective incidence rate estimates of 5.7, 3.4, and 2.5 cases per thousand children. With regard to the size of the child abuse "iceberg," the proportion of cases that were reported to state child protection agencies did not change, but more stringent screening standards by these agencies indicate "that some of the children who would, in the past, have had their cases substantiated (and possibly received services as a result) are now excluded as unfounded."[110(p xxv)]

Causes and Risk Factors. Early efforts to understand child abuse centered on psychological problems of the parents of the victims, focusing on distorted expectations of their children, frustrated dependency needs, personal isolation, and histories of having themselves been abused as children.[111] But many other social and cultural factors have been proposed as contributing to the causes of child abuse in addition to individual deviant behavior. The psychoanalytical approach posits that unconscious parental drives and conflicts determine abusive behavior.[112] Social learning theory suggests that abusers learn the behavior as abused children themselves. Environmental stress theory suggests that overwhelmingly stressful factors, such as poverty, unemployment, social isolation, and inadequate housing, help cause the violence or interfere with the parent's ability to care for the child. Cognitive-developmental theory suggests that immature parental understanding of the child and of the parental role are associated with abuse. By presuming social inequality, labeling theory suggests that the interests of dominant power groups are served by defining as deviant a class of socially marginal individuals (child abusers) whose problems are the concerns of helping professionals.[113]

All these theories individually explain some part of the problem, but all have clear limitations. Professionals and researchers have begun to integrate parts of these theories into interactive, multicausal theories that investigate how aspects of an individual's personality or environment interact with his or her particular experience.

Some researchers have attempted to integrate causal factors for child abuse from multiple levels: individual, family, and society.[114-117] At the individual level, one consistent finding has been the prevalence of acute or chronic illness in the abused children.[118] However, a number of long-held "causes" of child abuse are now viewed with skepticism; these include low birthweight of the infant, young maternal age, and inadequate mother-infant bond formation.[119-120]

Behavioral and social science research have not generally produced results that are applicable in clinical settings, mostly because the predominant research approach attempts to explain child abuse statistically factor by factor, thus ignoring the complexity of individual cases. Those studies that have considered the complexity of family interactions have focused on the formation of universal rules that govern behavior, while the clinician is concerned with treatment appropriate to individual cases. Interaction among clinicians and researchers is needed to develop a body of knowledge concerning etiology, therapeutic interventions, and effective intervention programs.

Outcomes. Documented medical consequences of child abuse include injuries of every organ system, which can frequently cause chronic impairment.[121] Another outcome of child abuse is homicide, which is one of the five leading causes of death for children between the ages of 1 and 18 years.[122] Sexual abuse of children resulted in venereal disease in 13% of the 409 children in one study.[123]

Because of varying definitions of abuse and problems with differing methodologies and outcome criteria, studies of long-term psychological effects of child abuse have mixed descriptions of outcome, but most agree there are profound and serious effects, including a propensity to aggression in adolescence, language disorders, and lower performance on standardized tests of intelligence. However, a sampling bias that favors selection of children from impoverished families makes it impossible to separate developmental attrition associated with low socioeconomic status from the presumed effects of abuse.[124]

Although there has been no systematic study of the immediate and long-term effects of child sexual victimization, changes that have been described from clinical case studies include hypervigilance, phobias, nightmares, feelings of guilt and shame, and changes in sleeping and eating patterns.[125-127] Psychosomatic disorders include abdominal pain, headaches, and loss of appetite. When force has been used in sexual acts, the subsequent symptoms appear to be more severe. These behavioral outcomes may reflect several variables and their interactions, such as the presence of antecedent behavioral problems, the family's support after disclosure, how much the child is blamed or stigmatized, and the nature and quality of interventions used to help the child.

Sexual abuse of boys may be associated with a propensity toward violence towards others—perhaps allowing the victim the feeling of no longer being vulnerable. Sexual abuse during childhood is a frequent finding in studies of pedophiles, rapists, and murderers.[128] Women who have been sexually abused as children appear to have an unusual frequency of depression and self-destructive behavior, as well as disturbances in adult sexual functioning and in protecting themselves from other victimizing relationships.[129-130]

Interventions. There is much disagreement about the most effective intervention for preventing child abuse. Although many consider child abuse a crime and there is a strong impulse toward retribution of abusers, most social policy in the United States has inclined toward a human service model for victims. Compounding the problem are judicial systems that may further abuse a child in the process of prosecuting an abuser and child protective services that are seriously overburdened and underfunded. Decisions to remove children from their homes are often made by personnel responsible for protecting children in haste and without sufficient attention to the strengths of families that could be maintained by providing homemakers, child care, parent aides, self-help groups, or specialized medical or psychiatric services.

Interventions must provide protection but should also develop support for the family. One study[131] of a child abuse program suggests that interdisciplinary review of individual cases with a systematic program to follow up cases with agencies designated to provide services to children and families is associated with a shorter duration of hospitalization, a lower dollar cost of treatment, and a reduction in the reinjury rate. Another study shows that lay interventional agents may be as effective as child welfare professionals.[132]

The National Clinical Evaluation Study[133] found that cost-effective treatment in child sexual abuse cases included a combination of family and group counseling for the victim, the victim's siblings, the perpetrator, and the perpetrator's spouse. In cases of child neglect, the most efficient interventions combine family counseling with parent education and basic care services such as babysitting, medical care, clothing, and housing assistance. The author of this study, noting the paucity of resources available for victims and the families of victims, also points out that treatment efforts are at best successful with only half of the clients. Given the risks of reinjury and the consequences of child abuse, the high cost of treatment services, the lack of funds, and the limited promise for remediating the consequences of maltreatment, prevention efforts may be the most efficient alternative.

Primary and secondary preventive initiatives may be organized in relation to the following theories of etiology:

Psychoanalytical Theory

- Our concept of health must include emotional as well as biological health. Physicians and others should be trained to recognize and tend to emotional issues, and third party payers should support services that support mental health.

Learning Theory

- Parents should have access to information about child development and about nonviolent methods of socializing their children.

Attachment Theory

- Elevate the parent-child relationship to an appropriate position of respect and importance by preventing prematurity through prenatal care, bringing fathers into the delivery room, emphasizing the father's supportive role, and encouraging paternity as well as maternity leaves from work.[134]

Stress Theory

- Provide hotlines for parents at times of distress.
- Make mental health services available to all children.
- Make emergency homemaker and other child care services available to families in crisis.
- Reduce social isolation by ensuring access to telephones and public transportation to facilitate social interactions.
- Support existing community organizations that offer support, a sense of community, and feelings of self-worth for their members.
- Empower women and acknowledge the extent to which male-dominated professions hold more power than professions composed mainly of women.

Labeling Theory

- Remove stigma associated with getting help by detaching protective services from public welfare systems.
- Expand public awareness of the prevalence of child abuse and domestic violence and emphasize that the potential for violence is in all of us, rather than attributing the problem to deviant and minority individuals.

Child Sexual Abuse

David Finkelhor

Definition of the Problem. Child sexual abuse is sexual contact with a child that occurs as a result of force or in a relationship where it is exploitative because of an age difference or caretaking responsibility. There is almost universal agreement that sexual contact between a child and the child's father, stepfather, mother, stepmother, another older relative, teacher, or baby-sitter constitutes sexual abuse, as does sexual contact by any adult or older person, whether known or unknown. Also included are rape and forced sexual contact at the hands of anyone, even a peer. However, not everyone uses this definition, nor is there universal agreement about the exact boundaries of various terms.

The National Center on Child Abuse and Neglect (NCCAN) and related child welfare agencies within individual states tend to restrict their definition to activity at the hands of caretakers,[135] which separates child welfare functions from criminal justice functions. Other researchers limit child sexual abuse to contacts with adults, excluding forced sex at the hands of other children.[136]

Other specific definitional disagreements include the age

range of what constitutes childhood (persons up to age 18 or 16?),[137] what is an exploitative age difference,[137] and what sexual activities are included. Most definitions of child sexual abuse include the use of children in prostitution and pornography.

State statutes vary widely in defining sexual abuse, involving a mixture of offenses including rape, statutory rape, sodomy, indecent liberties, and incest with terminology like "carnal knowledge" and "lewd and lascivious acts." All states but one include sexual abuse in their laws requiring the reporting of child abuse and neglect, but sexual abuse is rarely defined here either.

This variation in reported rates of child sexual abuse reflects a variety of factors, including the use of different definitions of sexual abuse, differences in the extent of victimization in different geographic areas and population subgroups, and the way in which investigators select subjects and ask questions about an extremely sensitive subject. The best sense of the scope of child sexual abuse comes from community surveys of adults.[138-144] Researchers have found that at least 5% of adults report sexual abuse in their childhood, but the variation among the studies is great, with the reported incidence ranging from 6% to 62% for women and from 3% to 31% for men.[145] There were an estimated 155,900 cases of child sexual abuse identified by professionals in 1986, a 221% increase over 1980. However, research on this subject is difficult, scarce, and extremely variable in quality.

Data Sources. Police, protective services, and medical facilities are the main agencies that document reports of child sexual abuse. Numerous studies have been done on samples from all these sources.[146-150] The American Association for the Protection of Children (formerly, the American Humane Association) collated state reports of child abuse and neglect including sexual abuse.[151] In addition, the NCCAN conducted two national incidence studies from counties selected to represent the country.[135,152] Another data source is mental health facilities where victims seek treatment.[153] Data on abusers come from studies mostly in prison settings,[154] and studies of adults in the "normal" population have identified individuals with histories of sexual abuse.[145]

All data sources on child abuse have serious limitations. Fear of prosecution and the shame and embarrassment associated with abuse make it difficult to obtain valid and reliable data. The national data collected by the American Association for the Protection of Children used uniform definitions and protocols, but there are relatively few variables relating to each case and the reported cases represent a fraction of all occurrences of child sexual abuse.[151] The two national incidence studies conducted by NCCAN have many of the same problems.

Data from the criminal justice system are limited by the variability of laws that define sexual abuse in the states, which make it difficult to compare data across or even within states. The FBI Uniform Crime Reports have not included the age of the victim, making it impossible to distinguish child sexual abuse from other sexual assaults. Also, cases that come to the attention of the system constitute a small percentage of actual cases.

Although studies of offenders have suggested hypotheses about the motivations for sexual abuse, many of these studies are limited by the inclusion of only incarcerated offenders, which is a small and unrepresentative fraction of offenders.[154]

Community surveys are the most representative data collection efforts because they gather information on cases never reported to an agency. However, these surveys are very expensive to conduct; there are questions concerning reliability and validity of the data gathered; there may be distortion or withholding of information because of memory loss or embarrassment; and the data may not be generalized to the current generation of children because rates and circumstances of victimization may be very different.

Developing Better Data Sources. There is a need in this field for ongoing national data collection with uniform standards and mandated participation. In addition, other data sources that should be considered are large community surveys of young adults and older adolescents who are old enough to be free from possible retaliation from their abusers but close enough to the experience to give accurate information; surveys of young dependent children (which must be combined with extremely sensitive efforts to screen for and intervene in cases of ongoing abuse discovered in the study); longitudinal studies of cohorts of children to determine which ones become victims and how this affects their development; and case-control studies of offenders and nonoffenders to discover risk sources for abusive behavior among representative samples of incarcerated and nonincarcerated abusers.

Causes and Risk Factors. Community studies are the best sources of information about the characteristics of different types of sexual abuse.[138-144] These studies suggest that abuse by fathers and stepfathers, even though it dominates reports from the child welfare system, actually constitutes no more than 7% to 8% of all abuse cases. Abuse by other family members (most frequently uncles and older brothers) make up an additional 16% to 42%. Other nonrelatives known to the child make up 32% to 60% of offenders. Abuse by strangers is substantially less common than abuse by family members or persons known to the child.

The largest category of abuse in most studies involves groping or fondling of children's bodies on top of or underneath the clothing. Only 16% to 29% of the abuse involves intercourse or attempted intercourse. Another 3% to 11% of the activities involve attempted or completed oral or anal intercourse, and 13% to 33%, manual touching of the genitals.

Community studies show that the frequency of child sexual abuse seems to peak when victims are between ages 9 and 12 and then declines somewhat during later adolescent years. Most studies show that a quarter of the incidents occur before the child is 8 years of age, and some clinicians insist that this percentage would be even greater if it were not for the occlusion of memories from these early years. Approximately 42% to 75% of experiences reported in the surveys are single events, which do not reoccur. Repeated abusive experiences occur at older ages and are associated with abuse within the family.

In addition to community surveys, compilations of "officially reported" cases have been used to generate incidence estimates and describe other characteristics of child sexual abuse. For example, the National Incidence Study II[152] projected that 155,900 new cases of sexual abuse became known to professionals in the United States in 1986. Incidence estimates based on reported cases such as these appear to overrepresent (1) abuse involving fathers and stepfathers, (2) abuse involving intercourse and other more intrusive acts, and (3) abuse perpetrated over an extended period. The ages of the victimized children also tend to be higher, since these reported cases record the age at the time of the disclosure rather than the age at onset. Compared to the community studies, there also seems to be an underreporting of the sexual abuse of boys.[140]

Community surveys have also provided information on the sociodemographic distribution of sexual abuse.[155] These studies consistently fail to find differences in rates among different social classes or races. However, other factors have been associated with risk of abuse: (1) living without one of the biological parents, (2) unavailability of the mother because of outside employment or disability or illness, (3) reports from the child stating that the parents' marriage is unhappy or full of conflict, (4) reports from the child of a poor relationship with the parents or of extremely punitive discipline or child abuse, and (5) report by the child of having a stepfather. Although few studies have examined why these factors increase risk, poor supervision, emotional turmoil, neglect, and rejection may make the child vulnerable to child molesters. With little help or support from parents, children may also find it hard to stop the abuse once it begins.

Research on Offenders. Offenders are predominantly males, which clearly distinguishes sexual abuse from other forms of child abuse and neglect. Studies of incarcerated offenders[139] have suggested a wide variety of theories that account for behavior of abusers: (1) they get powerful, developmentally induced emotional gratification from the acts; (2) they have deviant physiological sexual arousal patterns; (3) they are blocked in their capacity to meet their sexual needs in more conventional ways; and (4) they have problems in their capacity for behavioral inhibition.

Empirical support for these theories includes studies that show unusual levels of deviant sexual arousal to children among offenders,[156,157] histories of offenders who have been victims of sexual abuse (25% to 33%),[158] history of conflict over heterosexual relationships or disruption of normal adult heterosexual partnerships among offenders,[159] and use of alcohol related to the act in 19% to 70% of the offenses.

A review of studies of incestuous fathers[160] shows evidence that such men have difficulties in empathy, nurturing, and caretaking and are socially isolated and lacking in social skills. They frequently have histories of physical abuse, have poor relationships with their fathers, and are weakly identified with masculine roles. One study of incestuous fathers[161] found that these fathers had participated less actively in early care of their victim children than had a comparison group of normal fathers.

Another study found a much greater extent and variety of deviant sexual acts among child molesters and found that these histories of deviance and deviant fantasies go back to adolescence.[162]

Outcomes. Clinicians have noted many symptoms in children who have been sexually abused. These include fear, compulsivity, hyperactivity, phobias, withdrawal, guilt, depression, mood swings, suicidal ideation, fatigue, loss of appetite, somatic complaints, changes in sleeping and eating patterns, hostility, mistrust, sexual acting out, dissociative disorders, compulsive masturbation, and school problems.[163,164] However, there have been only a few systematic evaluations of large samples of sexually abused children to assess the prevalence and seriousness of these various symptoms.

In contrast to these initial effects, the long-term impact of sexual abuse has been the subject of more sophisticated studies. Various surveys of sexually abused women in the general population have all found significant, identifiable mental health impairment in victims compared to non-victims in the same samples.[163] One of the best was a survey of 344 women in Calgary using such epidemiological measures as the Middlesex Hospital Health survey and the CES-D depression scale.[138] This study found that sexually abused women, when compared to women without histories of abuse, have about twice the risk for depression, psychoneurosis, somatic anxiety, psychiatric hospitalization, and suicidal gestures. Moreover, sexual abuse was demonstrated to be a major risk for such outcomes even when controlling for other negative developmental and family background factors. However, severe levels of psychopathology were apparent in less than 25% of the sexual abuse victims. Another epidemiological survey[165] found two to three times the rate of morbidity for DSM-III-R category diagnoses among adults molested as children, men as well as women. Two other outcomes uncovered by studies in the general population are sexual problems—including frigidity, vaginismus, flashbacks, and other emotional problems related to sex—and a much higher risk of subsequent sexual victimization.[142,166]

Studies that have compared sexual abuse victims to other help-seekers in various clinical populations have also found sexual abuse victims to be more impaired on a number of dimensions[152]: victims experienced more isolation, lower self-esteem, fear of men, anxiety attacks, sleeping difficulties, nightmares, alcohol and drug abuse, and were more prone to suicide and self-mutilation. Additional research suggests connections between sexual abuse and prostitution,[167] multiple personality disorder, and eating disorders.[168] In short, these studies contribute to very rapidly mounting evidence of negative mental health outcomes for victims of child sexual abuse. None of the studies by themselves are definitive on this point, but the weight of the growing number of studies is impressive.

Given such evidence of serious effects on some individuals, researchers have now begun to look at whether certain aspects of the experience or the context of the experience may explain the degree of trauma. However, this research is still very tentative.[163] The weight of current evidence is that victims show more long-term symptoms when the abuse involves fathers and step-fathers, sexual intercourse, and force. On the other hand, studies have not been able to demonstrate consistently that abuse at any particular age is more traumatic. One study of initial effects in children[169] shows that the factors predictive of greater disturbance are (1) violence and physical injury in the abusive episode, (2) a mother's hostile attitude toward the child upon revelation of the abuse, and (3) removal of the child from his or her home subsequent to the abuse. Unfortunately, research to date does not yet provide a clear basis for designating those types of abuse that should receive priority for professional attention.

Interventions. Professional efforts to respond to the problem of sexual abuse can be grouped into five categories:

1. Public awareness: Broad campaigns to increase public and professional awareness have caused a rapid growth in the number of cases reported to authorities. This, in turn, has raised many questions about policy. No criteria exist for how to prioritize reported cases for investigation, and the cases are very difficult to confirm. There also have not been any studies assessing the reliability of various means of substantiating reports. There is considerable controversy surrounding children's credibility, and although most information regarding sexual abuse urges disclosure, it is also true that disclosure is extremely stressful on victims and families. Studies are badly needed for better understanding of effects of disclosure and for minimizing these effects.
2. Preventive education: A variety of programs are aimed at making children better able to protect themselves, to explain what sexual abuse is, to inform children that they have the right and an obligation to refuse such activity, and to encourage them to tell someone about it. Research indicates that children do learn the concepts and report incidents, but it is not known if such programs reduce the amount of victimization.
3. Treatment programs for victims and their families: Specialized programs have been established to help victims and families deal with disclosure and reduce the potential for long-term trauma. However, very little research has been done to assess the effectiveness of specific types of interventions.
4. Treatment programs for offenders: Some specialized experimental child molester treatment programs exist around the country. These use a diversity of techniques such as individual and group psychotherapy, behavior modification, social skills training, and some drug treatment.[170] Although the programs exist both within and outside the criminal justice system, it has been generally found that the threat or reality of criminal sanctions must be used to ensure participation. There are many reports of successful treatment of child molest-

ers,[171] but skepticism is still warranted because of the lack of long-term follow-up. Moreover, there are no techniques for identifying offenders who are not amenable to treatment.

5. Reforms of the criminal justice system: Changes that have been suggested include the use of videotaped testimony by children, victim advocates to assist victims and their families during the court process, diversion programs to encourage guilty pleas by offenders, restraining orders to remove offenders from the household to avoid removal of the child, expediting prosecution in sexual abuse cases, and redrafting of criminal statutes and their associated penalties. Research is needed on how these criminal justice reforms actually affect the conviction, sentencing, and recidivism of offenders, and on how often children are traumatized by the criminal justice process and which aspects of the process create trauma.

Elder Abuse

Karl Pillemer
Susan Frankel

Definition of the Problem. In the mid-1980s, the U.S. Administration on Aging funded a study in which information on reports of elder mistreatment was gathered from all 50 states. Researchers used this data to estimate the national incidence of reports of elder abuse.[172] Since state statutes vary considerably among the states, attempts to make national estimates are limited. However, given these limitations, the researchers concluded that nationally between 51,000 and 186,000 elderly persons were reported to authorities as victims of some form of elder mistreatment in 1985.

There has been wide variation in the way researchers have defined the term "elder abuse." The confusion surrounding what exactly constitutes elder abuse has made it difficult to interpret the results of studies on the subject. Some researchers have included some or all of the following dimensions in describing abusive and nonabusive relationships with the elderly: physical abuse, physical neglect, emotional abuse, emotional neglect, emotional deprivation, sexual exploitation and assault, verbal assault, medical neglect, material abuse, neglect of the elder's environment, violation of rights, and financial exploitation. Other studies have focused only on major forms of abuse such as physical abuse, psychological abuse, and neglect.

The development of better definitions of maltreatment of the elderly has become a high priority for researchers. An important aspect of the problem is the differentiation of various types of maltreatment.

Although at present it is impossible to resolve the definitional issue, there are some commonalities. All discussions of elder abuse include physical violence. There seems to be consensus among researchers that physical assault against an elder constitutes abusive behavior. Most of the research literature includes a category of psychological or emotional abuse. Material abuse, or the misuse or theft of an elder's property or financial resources, is usually included. Finally, it appears that the intentional failure of a clearly designated caregiver to meet the needs of an elder (neglect) is a form of maltreatment.

This section will focus on *violence* against the elderly (persons aged 65 and older) in domestic settings.

Data Sources. Research on the extent of elder abuse has been inconsistent because of the limited sources of data on the problem. However, there are three sources of existing data that represent different approaches to the study of elder abuse: surveys, case-control studies, and secondary sources of data.

Surveys. Surveys include random sample surveys and surveys of clinical professionals who have contact with elder abuse cases. One random sample survey of the Washington, D.C., area[173] of community agencies, elderly persons in the community, and health and human services personnel indicated that the extent of elder abuse was 4%; however, the response rate in this survey was low and the data sample was small (N = 73). Researchers estimated from a New Jersey survey that 1% of the state's elderly would report having been victimized.[174] Of 324 persons surveyed, only five reported any form of abuse, and of these five, only one reported physical maltreatment; all others reported financial exploitation. A study[175] in the Boston metropolitan area found 63 elderly persons who had been maltreated out of a stratified random sample of 2020 community-dwelling elderly persons aged 65 or older. This survey inquired about personal experiences of three types of maltreatment: physical violence, chronic verbal aggression, and neglect by family members and persons close to them. The findings of this survey translate into a rate of 32 maltreated elderly persons per 1000 or between 8647 and 13,487 abused and neglected elderly in the Boston area. A nationwide survey of the prevalence and circumstances of elder abuse in Canada[176] based on the instruments and methodology used in the Boston study found very similar rates of elder abuse.

The most common type of study is a survey of professionals who work with the elderly, which in essence shows the extent to which service professionals are familiar with elder abuse and neglect. Some surveys of professionals cited in the literature include a mail survey of 1044 professionals and paraprofessionals in Massachusetts[177] in which 55% of those surveyed (35% response rate) reported contact with a case of elder abuse. A mail survey of 302 agencies in the Detroit area[178] found a total of 77 case reports of elder mistreatment. Other researchers[179] found in interviews with 228 professionals that virtually all were familiar with domestic maltreatment of elders, while another mail survey[180] of 90 practitioners in social, medical, homemaker, and legal services found that 29 of the 30 professionals who responded indicated that they had dealt with cases of elder abuse.

A recent mail survey in two midwestern communities of police officers and social service providers[181] found that, of the police officers reporting, 33% had encountered abuse or neglect and, of the social service personnel reporting, 69% had encountered cases of elder abuse, sexual abuse, or neglect. However, this study was designed more for exploring attitudes and practices than for assessing prevalence.

Two other studies[182,183] gathered information on elder abuse from agency case records. The first study[182] found that of 404 elderly clients served in a 12-month period, nearly 10% were identified as victims of maltreatment. The second study[183] examined 39 cases of physical, psychological, or mental abuse by caseworkers at three model projects on elder abuse and then used the data to develop a characterization of the victim and perpetrator of elder abuse. Both these studies used data from professional accounts rather than from interviews with the victims themselves.

Case-Control Studies. Several recent studies go beyond previous efforts by interviewing the victims themselves and by including a control group of nonabused elderly. In one study at Wayne State University,[184] researchers tried to identify factors that placed the elderly at risk of abuse. Service providers selected abused victims and a nonabused control for each case. Researchers identified several risk factors that accurately (94%) classified cases as abused or nonabused. Interviewers in another study,[185] where cases and controls were identified by public health nurses in social service agencies, assessed the presence or absence of neglect. Flaws in the approaches used in these studies made the results questionable, however. Both studies failed to differentiate among types of maltreatment, and it is not clear what criteria were used for matching the cases and controls.

Other studies conducted in New England evaluated risk factors for elder abuse. One study focused only on physical abuse,[186] which was verified by use of the Conflict Tactics Scale developed by Straus.[187] A second study[175] compared elder abuse victims identified in a random sample survey of residents of the greater Boston area with a group of elderly control cases randomly selected from nonabused survey respondents. This study focused on three categories of maltreatment: physical abuse, neglect, and chronic verbal aggression. The findings from these studies showed that abuser characteristics are more powerful indicators of elder mistreatment than victim characteristics.

Other Sources. Several secondary sources of data that may provide important information about domestic violence against the elderly include information from law enforcement agencies, health providers, and state agencies. The FBI UCR record the relationship between the assailant and victim in cases of homicide, which would allow investigation of cases in which parents and grandparents are murdered. Other sources of criminal behavior against the elderly are the police, the courts, and the prisons. All these sources are subject to underreporting, the extent of which is unknown.

Emergency room personnel and other health care providers have been sources of data on child and wife abuse and could provide information on elder abuse as well. It is only recently that efforts have been made to collect data on elder mistreatment from health providers. As with crime statistics, such reports are valuable but subject to bias: only those cases in which abuse has resulted in serious injury are likely to be recorded.

By 1987, all states had established systems to respond to reports of elder abuse and neglect, with 43 states having legislated mandatory reporting laws. Most states also exhibited special protective service agencies to intervene in elder abuse cases. In all states, records are maintained on persons who are reported, which comprises a valuable source of data on abuse victims.

Causes and Risk Factors

Characteristics of Abuse Victims. Despite their methodological limitations, studies suggest fairly consistent findings regarding the abused elderly. Most of the studies have found that the abused individuals tend to be female (some found equal numbers of men and women,[175] usually aged 75 and older). Many found victims who were vulnerable because of illness or impairment, and abused elders tend to live with the perpetrator of abuse. These, however, are the only findings that emerge reliably from the studies. Results relating to the frequency with which abuse occurs and the types of abuse most often found are virtually impossible to compare because of the widely varying definitions employed. Also, few studies provide reliable evidence of the causes of elder abuse.

Causal Factors. Extensive research literature in the area of child and spouse abuse and on the relations between spouses and between the elderly and adult children can provide important insights into elder abuse, particularly in concert with the literature on domestic violence. Five areas have emerged from the review of the literature in these areas: intraindividual dynamics (psychopathology of the abuser), intergenerational transmission of violent behavior, dependency and exchange relations between abuser and abused, external stress, and social isolation.

Intraindividual dynamics emphasizes pathological characteristics of the abuser as the primary cause of maltreatment. The characteristics identified have included the general quality of family relationships, the presence of psychological disease, flaws in the socialization process, and alcohol and drug abuse. Critics of investigations in these areas have stressed that investigations lacked rigorous research methodologies and have failed to account for structural factors such as socioeconomic status, economic stress, and unemployment.

It should also be noted that the dynamics of elder abuse may differ from other forms of family violence. Abusers of the elderly may be more likely to suffer from well-defined psychological problems than child or wife abusers. Some research has indicated that abusers of the elderly are more likely to be developmentally disabled, mentally ill, or alcoholic.[179,182,188–190]

A number of studies concerning *intergenerational transmission of violent behavior*[191,192] have indicated that people learn to be violent in the family setting. Research evidence shows that witnessing parental violence during childhood is a strong risk factor for wife abuse as an adult, and the amount of physical punishment experienced as a child was positively associated with the rate of abusive violence to one's own children. While it is reasonable to postulate that abusers of the elderly will also be more likely to have been raised in violent homes, at present there is no evidence to support this theory. Also, the ''cycle of violence'' experienced in spouse and child abuse may take an alternative form in elderly abuse in that the formerly abused child retaliates and strikes out against the abuser.

Two competing theories relate *dependency* to elder abuse. One emphasizes the role of ''caregiver stress'' as a risk factor for maltreatment, while the second suggests that increased dependency of the abuser on his or her victim leads to maltreatment. Literature on family relations supports the notion that dependency of an old person leads to poor quality relationships with relatives. A likely reason for this is the effect of declining parental health on the prior flow of support between the generations. A number of studies[193–195] have supported this theory. Families experience ''situational inversion'' when the elderly person becomes dependent on the children for financial, physical, or emotional support,[196] and this leads to severe stress on the caregiver. As costs grow for the caregiver and rewards diminish, the exchange is perceived as unfair. If the caregivers do not have the ability to escape or improve the situation, they may become abusive. Although this theory seems plausible, there are few firm research findings to support it.

Conversely, a number of other studies[184,189,190,197,198] have found that abusers were likely to be dependent on their victims financially and in a variety of other ways. The finding that continued dependence of an adult child or spouse on an elderly victim may be related to physical violence may be explained by the social exchange theory and the concept of power.[199] It may be that the feeling of powerlessness of an adult child still dependent on a parent is particularly acute because it violates society's expectations for normal adult behavior.

The role of dependency deserves serious attention. Perhaps a better way to conceptualize the issue is to view a serious imbalance of dependency in either direction, parent or adult child, as a potential risk factor.

External stress caused by social-structural, macrolevel variables such as unemployment and economic conditions may play an important role in elder abuse, but the model alone does not explain why some families respond to stress with abuse and others do not. This appears to be an important area for future investigation.

Social isolation also has been found to be characteristic of families in which other forms of domestic violence occur.[200-203] Because behaviors considered to be illegitimate tend to be hidden, the presence of an active social network may be a particularly strong deterrent to elder abuse.

Outcomes. The concern about long-term consequences of maltreatment has important policy implications because abused victims may use health care services and depend on support services more than the nonabused elderly do. Although little is known about the consequences of elder abuse, some data do exist on the physical manifestations of abuse, such as bruises and sprains, abrasions, bone fractures, burns, and wounds.[173,177,178,183] Anecdotal evidence suggests that victimization produces negative psychological outcomes, although sound empirical findings are scarce. The literature on child abuse and wife abuse indicates negative psychological consequences that include lowered self-esteem, confusion and a sense of powerlessness and helplessness, increased dependency on others, depression, disturbed eating and sleeping patterns, and a sense of isolation.[204] The only investigator to have examined this issue in a case-control study found victims of elder abuse and neglect to be significantly more likely to be depressed.[185]

It is equally difficult to achieve documentation of the physical consequences of maltreatment because these effects may be confounded with normal physical changes that accompany aging and various physical ailments. It would also be difficult to determine which physical indicator is an antecedent or a consequence of maltreatment.

Interventions. Although over 10 years have passed since the problem of elder abuse and neglect first came to the public's attention, our ability to design prevention and intervention strategies and programs is still greatly handicapped by lack of knowledge regarding the extent, nature, and dynamics of elder abuse. In the absence of a comprehensive national policy, states and communities have designed their own programs ranging from elder protective services to family counseling and legal intervention. The different strategies adopted can be placed into three basic categories: mandatory reporting laws, protective services, and direct services. Mandatory reporting and protective services have become the favored response, but both are highly controversial. At present, one of the greatest gaps in information is the lack of evaluation data regarding various types of interventions. Evaluation of interventions is in turn dependent on knowing the incidence of a problem with and without the intervention, and such incidence data are also frequently lacking.

Mandatory Reporting Laws. All 50 states have mandatory reporting laws covering the elderly that have the goal of identifying abused people so that the state can intervene in their situations. However, there is tremendous variation from state to state. Definitions vary as to who should be classified as abused. Agencies that are designated to receive reports usually have the responsibility for investigation. Proponents of mandatory reporting argue that these laws are the best method for bringing cases to light. In contrast, opponents argue that there is no evidence that mandatory reporting is effective.[205-207] Some claim that an increased number of reports results from publicity and that penalties for not reporting are rarely enforced. Some critics note that states have failed to provide sufficient funds for services to victims and abusers, and small staffs must attempt to handle a large number of referrals in response to the law.[205] Others claim that reporting interferes with the relationship and confidentiality between professionals and clients. This presents professionals with a dilemma: either to violate the law or break trust with a client and possibly jeopardize a therapeutic relationship. Finally, other critics believe that using the child abuse model, proponents adopt a set of assumptions not applicable to older people; that is, they infantalize the elder's position in society, foster negative stereotypes of the aged, and limit the older persons' ability to control their own lives.[208(p 731)]

Thus, major controversy exists over mandatory reporting, and statutes must be carefully evaluated to determine their effectiveness. At a minimum, mandatory reporting must be accompanied by a substantial commitment of resources to the designated reporting agency.

Protective Services. Protective services are equally controversial. Most public protective services involve the use of legal surrogate options, such as guardianship or conservatorship, when the elderly person is judged to be incompetent.[209(p 3)] Critics, including members of the legal community, see such programs as an intrusion on the civil liberties of the elderly and as a way of infantalizing them. They also argue that states define abuse too broadly and allow an intrusion into families with merely the normal range of human problems.[210]

To be effective, protective service programs need to reduce tension within the legal community and reduce the ambiguity and multiplicity of tasks performed by protective service agencies. One researcher has suggested a systematic combination of specific crisis intervention and protective services strategies,[211] while another has called for the integration of the adult protective services system with human service providers.[212]

Service Options. Service options in communities tend to be based on one of two assumptions: that dependency of the victim causes maltreatment or that a relatively independent elder is abused by a dependent relative.

Based on the assumption that dependency of the victim causes maltreatment, communities have emphasized health and service needs of the elderly that are not specific to abuse. In many cases, services to relieve the burden of caregiving, such as housekeeping and meal preparation, are provided. However, research indicates that this pattern of elderly abuse occurs in only a minority of cases.

Interventions based on the assumption that the elder is abused by a dependent relative may benefit from interventions that have been effective with victims of wife abuse. Options for the elderly that relate to the wife abuse model are social support for the elderly, employing the use of self-help groups that contribute to consciousness-raising; "safe houses" or emergency shelters for elderly victims; and legal action. Research in the area of spouse abuse suggests that police intervention may reduce further episodes of wife abuse and that police can link victims with effective community services.[213] Police departments are just one type of community agency that is becoming concerned with the problem of elder abuse and neglect. Many communities have created task forces of service providers and other interested individuals who attempt to raise the consciousness of professionals and lay people regarding the needs of abused and neglected elders.

Recommendations. Given the lack of firm research, it is perhaps more appropriate to make proposals for future research than for practice and policy. The most critical need at present is information about the incidence and causes of elder abuse.

1. Investigators should design studies based on direct interviews with abused elders. While assessment data compiled by competent professionals may accurately describe certain aspects of the case, understanding the family dynamics that produced maltreatment ultimately relies on direct interviews of the parties involved.

2. Future studies must move away from agency samples toward general population surveys. A national incidence survey is needed to learn the magnitude of the problem and to describe the relationship of conflict and violence. As the initial step in developing a national surveillance system for elder abuse, a national voluntary reporting system with standards accepted by all states could provide a national profile of reported cases.
3. Control-group studies must be designed to identify the characteristics of victims.
4. Researchers should study not only the abused but the abusers.
5. Research should begin to focus to a greater degree on the consequences of abuse.
6. Investigators need to pay attention to the content of abusive acts and the specifics regarding the circumstances in which domestic violence against the elderly occurs.
7. Existing intervention programs should be systematically evaluated. A high priority must be the use of sophisticated evaluation research techniques to determine the impact of treatment programs. Without such careful consideration, funds may be wasted on inappropriate services that fail to help, or may even harm, elder abuse victims and their families.

Suicide

Patrick W. O'Carroll

Definition of the Problem. In 1987 there were 30,796 deaths from suicide in the United States, making suicide the eighth leading cause of death in this country.[214] Unlike the rates for many diseases, suicide rates are substantial among both young and old people. As a result, suicide is the fifth leading cause of premature death, as defined by years of potential life lost before age 65.[215] In past decades the rate of suicide was relatively low among adolescents and young adults but increased steadily with increasing age. However, suicide rates among younger age groups have increased dramatically in the last 3 to 4 decades.[216] In particular, the suicide rate among persons 15 to 24 years of age has almost tripled: in 1950 the suicide rate for this age group was 4.5 per 100,000; in 1988, this rate was 12.8.[217,218] Suicide has been the second or third leading cause of death among persons 15 to 24 years of age in recent years. Although most suicides occur among persons younger than 40 years of age, the highest rates occur among the elderly.[216]

In general, males are three to five times more likely to commit suicide than females. Furthermore, males are at higher risk than females across all age and race groups. White males are at the highest risk of suicide, followed by males of races other than white, white females, and females of races other than white. White males have also experienced the greatest increase in suicide rates among persons 15 to 24 years of age. In 1987 the rate of suicide in this race-sex-age group was almost twice the overall national suicide rate.[219]

For both males and females, firearms are the most frequently used method of suicide; overall, approximately 60% of all suicides are committed with firearms. Among males, hanging is the second most common method of suicide, followed by poisoning by gases (chiefly carbon monoxide). Among females, ingestion of an overdose of drugs is the second most common method. The predominance of firearms as a method of suicide is increasing among males, while it is new for females. In 1970, for example, more females committed suicide by drug ingestion than by firearms. In recent years, firearm suicides have accounted for an increasingly large proportion of all suicides among persons 15 to 24 years of age. From 1970 to 1984 the proportion of suicides committed with firearms increased 17% and 59% for males and females, respectively.[220]

Reliable information regarding morbidity from attempted (as opposed to completed) suicide is sparse. In one large, multisite survey of adults in the United States, approximately three of every 1000 reported having attempted suicide at some point during the preceding year.[221] This estimate, which is in line with previous smaller surveys, suggests that approximately 750,000 adults attempt suicide each year in the United States and that there are approximately 25 suicide attempts for each completed suicide.

Data Sources. Suicide mortality data ultimately derive from death certificate data. The determination of suicide as a cause of death, however, is not necessarily a straightforward process. Suicide has been defined fairly succinctly as death from intentionally self-inflicted injury,[222] but it can be difficult to apply this definition. In particular, determining whether a decedent intended to commit suicide necessarily involves retrospective collection of data regarding the decedent's state of mind prior to the death. The amount and quality of such information varies greatly from case to case. Moreover, until recently there were no published guidelines explicitly describing what type of data ought to be collected in a death investigation in order to make an informed determination of manner of death.[222] The great variability across the United States in the qualifications of the coroner or official responsible for medicolegal certification presents additional questions about the validity and reliability of death certificate information.[223]

Against the backdrop of these structural problems in suicide certification, there is also the social stigma associated with suicide. For religious, financial, and even political reasons, coroners and medical examiners may sometimes be reluctant to certify suicide as a cause of death. Given these limitations in the way suicide is determined as a cause of death, it is not surprising that many investigators believe official suicide statistics substantially underestimate the true suicide rate. Estimates of the true suicide rate range from a low of 1.01 to 1.8 times the official rate, but it is likely that the true rate of suicide is no more than 1.25 times the official rate.[224]

There is essentially no information at the national level concerning the magnitude of the physical and mental health consequences of attempted suicide. Indeed, the incidence estimates from surveys of adults cited above are quite limited in what they tell us about attempted suicide. For example, because attempted suicide was self-defined in these surveys, it is unclear what proportion of these "suicide attempts" resulted in injury, in a visit to an emergency health facility, or in subsequent attempted or completed suicide. There also are no national estimates of the incidence of attempted suicide among persons younger than 18 years of age, although there are indications that the attempted suicide rate in this group may be even higher than in the adult population. Without such information on a national, longitudinal basis, it is difficult to accurately estimate suicide attempt morbidity and trends or to assess the efficacy of suicide prevention programs.

Causes and Risk Factors. Even though it is common to hear people say that a person committed suicide because he was mentally ill or because he could not cope with stressful events in his life, in reality there are many factors that contribute to the causal mechanism of suicide. Certain psychiatric illnesses are, of course, both extremely important and well-recognized as risk factors. In particular, affective disorders have been clearly shown, in both retrospective case-control studies and prospective cohort studies, to increase markedly the risk of suicide.[225] For example, in a population-based cohort study of 3563 males in Sweden who were observed for 15 to 25 years, the suicide rate among men with an initial diagnosis of any mental illness was almost 39 times higher than the rate for men with no mental disorder. Men with an initial diagnosis of a depressive disorder had a suicide rate 80 times higher than men with no mental disorder.[226]

After clinical depression, alcoholism is the most commonly reported mental illness associated with suicide.[227-230] In many studies, however, no control group was used in assessing the contribution of alcohol use to suicide risk.[231-233] In addition, the independent effect of alcoholism on the suicide rate is rarely estimated; rather, the diagnosis of alcoholism among the case series is often reported along with the prevalence of affective illness, social isolation, and other factors that might themselves account for any observed increase in the risk of suicide. Most of the studies have been done using special populations, such as psychiatric inpatients[234-236] or hospitalized alcoholics,[237-239] and the findings of these studies are not necessarily applicable to alcoholics in general. Finally, little work has been done separately to assess the effects of acute exposure to alcohol (i.e., alcohol intoxication) and alcohol abuse on the risk of suicide. More research is needed to elucidate the mechanism(s) underlying the observed association between alcoholism and suicide.

Certain personality disorders (in particular, borderline and antisocial personality disorders) have also been shown to be correlated with suicidal behavior.[240] The interpretation of this correlation is problematic, however, since suicidal behavior is inherently part of the definition of certain of these disorders, such as borderline personality disorder. The strength and the predictive value of personality disorders as risk factors for suicide, as well as the mechanisms explaining the observed association between certain of these disorders and suicide, must be determined in future research.

There is an increasing body of literature addressing putative genetic and biological risk factors for suicide. Suicide has long been observed to "run in families," but such a phenomenon might either be caused by common exposure among family members to environmental-sociocultural risk factors for suicide, or by genetic factors shared by family members. Meta-analysis of twin studies, however, strongly suggests a genetically based risk for mental illness and suicide. Moreover, several Danish-American adoption studies suggest that this genetic risk may be inherited independently of major psychiatric illness, perhaps as an inability to control impulsive behavior.[241]

Certain neurotransmitter metabolites have been convincingly associated with an increased risk of suicide.[242] In particular, a clear relationship has been demonstrated between low concentrations of the serotonin metabolite 5-hydroxyindoleacetic acid (5-HIAA) in cerebrospinal fluid and an increased incidence of attempted and completed suicide in psychiatric patients. Most of the evidence for this relationship is based on studies of patients with major affective illness (particularly unipolar depression), but there is some evidence this relationship may hold for other diagnostic categories as well, particularly for personality disorders[243] and possibly for schizophrenia.[244] The mechanism that accounts for the relationship between a disturbed or inadequate serotonin system and suicidal behavior is not clear.

Recent suicide clusters among teenagers and young adults have suggested that suicides may sometimes be caused by "contagion," that is, by exposure to the suicide or suicidal behavior of others.[245,246] There is ample anecdotal evidence to suggest that, in any given suicide cluster, suicides occurring later in the cluster often appear to have been influenced by suicides occurring earlier in the cluster.[247,248] This contagion hypothesis has never been formally tested at the individual level, and the strength and public health importance of contagion as a risk factor for suicide remains to be determined. In general, contagion in the context of suicide clusters has been conceptualized as being mediated through an amalgam of imitation, identification, grief, and the highly charged emotional atmosphere common in many communities that have experienced suicide clusters. Despite uncertainty about contagion as a risk factor for suicide, many believe it is prudent to recognize the possibility of a contagious effect of suicide and to institute measures to minimize potential contagion in the context of an apparent suicide cluster.[249]

Suicide contagion may not be limited to geographically localized clusters of suicides. A number of ecological studies have been done to assess whether the incidence of suicide in the general population is increased by exposure to television news stories and movies about suicide. Some investigators have reported an increase in suicide following such exposure,[250,251] but this finding has not been seen in all studies[252,253] and has been challenged in others.[254,255] Both the nature of the exposure to suicide and the hypothesized induction period from exposure to outcome in these studies are quite different than is hypothesized for geographically localized suicide clusters. In the former the exposure is to stories, fictional or otherwise, of suicides by persons unknown to the study subjects; the induction period implied in the study designs is 1 to 2 weeks. In the case of geographically localized suicide clusters, however, the suicides to which victims of the suicide cluster were exposed were frequently those of close or intimate friends; reported suicide clusters have typically occurred over the course of 1 to 4 months[256] but have ranged from several weeks to over 1 year.[257]

There is a variety of situational risk factors for suicide. Stressful life events, such as the death of a loved one or recent loss of employment, often appear to be clear precipitants of suicide.[258] In general, stressful life events may elevate the background risk of suicide by a factor of 5 to 10, although the duration of time after exposure to these stressful events during which suicide risk remains elevated has not been well characterized.[259] A loss or disruption of normal social support mechanisms also increases the risk of suicide. Divorce, unemployment, and migration from one community to another are but three examples of factors that may lead to some disruption of social support networks; all three have been shown to be related to increased suicide rates.[225,260] Absent or inadequate social support networks presumably increase the risk of suicide through interaction with other suicide risk factors, such as clinical depression and recent stressful life events.

Another situational risk factor of potentially great importance is the ready accessibility of firearms. Unlike drug ingestions, carbon monoxide poisoning, and many other suicide methods, a suicide attempt with a firearm is often immediately lethal, leaving little or no opportunity for postattempt rescue. Moreover, if a firearm is readily accessible, little planning and time are required between the moment a person decides to commit suicide and the execution of the attempt. The accessibility of a firearm may both limit the preattempt opportunity for intervention by others and facilitate impulsive suicidal acts.[261,262] Theoretically, at least some proportion of impulsive decisions to commit suicide might never be acted on if substantial efforts were necessary to arrange for a suicide method. However, the factors that determine choice of suicide method are complex, and careful research is needed to determine whether accessibility to firearms increases the risk of suicide.

Finally, several risk factors for suicide are useful for delineating high-risk groups, although these factors do not appear to be "causal" in the traditional sense. For example, being male or elderly identifies one as belonging to a high-risk group, and having a past history of attempted suicide has also been clearly shown to increase the risk of future completed suicide.[225] These markers for increased suicide risk presumably correlate with other, causal risk factors for suicide. A past history of attempted suicide, for example, may correlate with impulsivity or with a vulnerability to affective illness.

Outcomes. In human and economic terms, the cost of suicide in the United States is enormous. In 1984 alone, suicide among persons younger than 65 years of age resulted in the loss of over 645,000 years of potential life.[263] Weinstein and Saturno[264] estimate that in 1980, suicide among persons 15 to 24 years of age alone resulted in the loss of 276,000 years of potential life and economic costs of $2.26 billion. Adding in attempted suicide among persons in this age group brought the estimated economic costs to $3.19 billion.

The emotional trauma experienced by the "survivors" of suicide—family members and friends of the victims—is enormous.[265] The process of grief and bereavement over the death of a loved one is always painful and difficult, but when the decedent has committed suicide, this process is even more difficult and traumatic. Death from suicide is usually sudden and unexpected. In addition, suicide may engender feelings of guilt or rejection in the survivors. Because of the social stigma associated with suicide, traditional mourning rituals may be avoided, and the usual social supports for the decedent's family and friends may be withdrawn or attenuated. All of these factors increase the risk of disturbed or unresolved grief reactions among the survivors.[266]

Interventions. Although a wide variety of suicide prevention programs have been devised, the strategies underlying these programs may be considered under five broad conceptual categories. The first such strategy is to improve the identification, referral, and treatment of persons at high risk of suicide by various caretakers and "gatekeepers" in the community. Increased training of primary care physicians in the recognition and treatment or referral of patients with clinical depression is one example of this approach; school-based screening programs designed to identify suicidal youth in the context of an evolving suicide cluster is another. A second suicide prevention strategy focuses on the treatment of underlying risk factors for suicide. Clinical depression, for example, is addressed through psychotherapeutic and pharmacological treatment of patients with this illness. Although alcohol rehabilitation programs are not traditionally thought of in terms of suicide prevention, they may nevertheless contribute to the prevention of suicide by addressing one of the most important risk factors—alcoholism.

A third general suicide prevention strategy is to decrease individual vulnerability to suicide through education of the general population. Affective education programs, for example, seek to help individuals understand and cope with the type of problems that can lead to suicide.[267] Other programs are designed to increase public awareness of helping resources in the community to facilitate help-seeking behavior by suicidal persons. A fourth, related suicide prevention strategy is to provide or expand the accessibility of self-referral resources for suicidal persons. Hot lines and walk-in crisis centers are the best known examples of this strategy.

A final strategy for suicide prevention seeks to limit access to lethal means of suicide, such as high places, prescription drugs, or firearms.[268] This strategy derives from the hypothesis that if substantial efforts are required by an individual to arrange for a lethal suicide method or if a less lethal method is substituted in its stead, the likelihood of a completed suicide will be diminished.

The above strategies have differing strengths and weaknesses, and each may be important in the prevention of suicide. Unfortunately, the effectiveness of many of these strategies has yet to be established. Eddy and colleagues[267] surveyed 15 suicide experts as to their judgments of the effectiveness of a variety of existing and proposed youth suicide prevention strategies. On the average these experts estimated that approximately 10% of potential youth suicides were being averted by existing prevention programs and that each of the proposed strategies to improve prevention might reduce the incidence of youth suicide by 6% to 16%, depending on the strategy. Even if all of the proposed strategies were simultaneously implemented, the expected reduction in youth suicide was estimated to range from 15% to no more than 50%. The uncertainty regarding program effectiveness and the relatively modest nature of the reduction in mortality that may be expected from our present array of interventions are not limited to youth suicide prevention programs but extend to suicide prevention in general. There is clearly an urgent need to develop a better empirical base of information regarding the effectiveness of various prevention strategies so that policy makers can make the best use of limited suicide prevention resources.

REFERENCES

1. Centers for Disease Control: Homicide surveillance: High-risk racial and ethnic groups—Blacks and Hispanics, 1970 to 1983. Atlanta: Centers for Disease Control, 1986
2. O'Carroll PW, Mercy JA: Patterns and recent trends in black homicide. In Hawkins DF (ed): Homicide Among Black Americans. Lanham, Md: University Press of America, 1986, pp 29–42
3. U.S. Department of Justice: Crime in the United States, 1981. Washington, D.C.: The Department, 1982
4. U.S. Department of Justice, Bureau of Justice Statistics: Criminal Victimization in the United States, 1986: A National Crime Survey Report. Washington, D.C.: The Department Report NCJ-111456, 1988
5. U.S. Department of Justice: Crime in the United States, 1986. Washington, D.C.: The Department, 1987
6. Barancik JI, Chatterjee BF, Greene YZ, Mekenzie EM, Fife B: Northeastern Ohio Trauma Study: I. Magnitude of the problem. Am J Public Health 73:746–751, 1983
7. U.S. Department of Justice, Bureau of Justice Statistics: National Crime Surveys: National Sample, 1973–1979. Ann Arbor, Mich: Inter-University Consortium Political and Social Research, 1981
8. Technical Notes: Hyattsville, Md: National Center for Health Statistics, 1989, (Monthly Vital Statistics Reports, appears in all issues).
9. U.S. Department of Health and Human Services. International Classification of Diseases, 9th Revision, Clinical Modification. Washington, D.C.: The Department, 1980
10. Mednick SA, Pollock V, Volavka J, Gabrielli J: Biology and violence. In Wolfgang ME, Weiner NA (eds): Criminal Violence. Beverly Hills, Calif: Sage Publications, 1982, pp 21–80
11. Wolfgang ME: Patterns in Criminal Homicide. New York: John Wiley & Sons, 1958
12. Megargee EI: Psychosocial determinants and correlates of criminal violence. In Weiner Ma (ed): Criminal Violence. Beverly Hills, Calif: Sage Publications, 1982, pp 81–170
13. Mulvihill DJ, Tunin MM (eds): Crimes of violence: A staff report

submitted to the National Commission on the Causes and Prevention of Violence. Washington, D.C.: U.S. Government Printing Office, 1969
14. Wolfgang ME, Zahn MA: Criminal homicide. In Kadish SH (ed): Encyclopedia of Crime and Justice. New York: The Free Press, 1983
15. Luckenbill DF: Criminal homicide as a situated transaction. Soc Problems 25:176–186, 1977
16. Rubin PH: The economics of crime. Atlanta Economic Review, July/August, 28(4):38–43, 1978
17. Smith MD, Parker RN: Type of homicide and variation in regional rates. Soc Forces 136–147, 1980
18. Curtis LA: Violence, Race and Culture. Lexington, Mass: D.C. Heath, 1975
19. Riedel M, Zahn MA: The Nature and Patterns of American Homicide: An Annotated Bibliography. Washington, D.C.: National Institute of Justice, 1982
20. Goodman RA, Mercy JA, Loya F, Rosenberg ML, Smith JC, Allen NH, Vargas L, Kolts R: Alcohol use and interpersonal violence: Alcohol detected in homicide victims. Am J Public Health 76:144–149, 1986
21. Gelles RJ: The Violent Home: A Study of Physical Aggression Between Husbands and Wives. Beverly Hills, Calif: Sage Publications, 1974
22. Goldstein PJ: The drugs violence nexus: A tripartite conceptual framework. Drug Issues 15:493–506, 1985
23. World Health Organization: World Health Stat Annuals. Geneva: Worth Health Organization, 1986, 1987, 1988
24. Williams KR: Economic sources of homicide: Reestimating the effects of poverty and unequality. Am Soc Rev, April 49:283–289, 1984
25. Centerwall BS: Race, socioeconomic status and domestic homicide, Atlanta, 1971–72. Am J Public Health 74:813–815, 1984
26. Smith J, Mercy J, Rosenberg M: Comparison of homicides among Anglos and Hispanics in five southwestern states. Presented at U.S.-Mexico Border Health Association Meeting, Hermosillo, Mexico, April 10, 1984
27. U.S. Department of Justice: Crime in the United States, 1986. Washington, D.C.: The Department, 1987
28. Saltzman LE, Mercy JA, Rosenberg ML, et al: Magnitude and patterns of family and intimate assault in Atlanta, Georgia, 1984. Violence and Victims 5(1):3–17, 1990
29. U.S. Department of Justice, Bureau of Justice Statistics: Violent Crime by Strangers and Nonstrangers: Bureau of Justice Statistics Special Report. Washington, D.C.: Bureau of Justice Statistics, U.S. Department of Justice Report NCJ–103702, 1987
30. Straus MA, Gelles JR, Steinmetz SK: Behind Closed Doors: Violence in the American Family. Garden City, N.Y.: Anchor Press/Doubleday, 1980
31. Stark E, Flitcraft A, Zuckerman D, et al: Wife Abuse in the Medical Settings: An Introduction for Health Personnel. Washington, D.C.: Office of Domestic Violence Monograph No. 7, 1981
32. Eth S, Pynoos RS: Bearing witness: A model of research and intervention. Presented at the American Psychiatric Association, Anaheim, California, May 10, 1984
33. Prothrow-Stith D: Primary prevention of homicide: Preliminary report of a demonstration project investigating the value of health education in the high school on anger and violence. Presented at the NASW-NIMH workshop on prevention of black homicide, Washington, D.C., June 1984
34. Prothrow-Stith D: Violence Prevention Curriculum for Adolescents. Newton, Mass: Education Development Center, 1987
35. Ross CH, Zigler E: An agenda for action. In Gerbna G, Ross CJ, Zigler E (eds): Child Abuse: An Agenda for Action. New York: Oxford University Press, 1980, pp 293–304
36. Garbarino J: The human ecology of child maltreatment. J Marriage and Family 39:412–427, 1977
37. Blumstein A, Cohen J, Nagen D (eds): Deterrence and Incapacitation: Estimating the Effects of Criminal Sanctions on Crime Rates. Washington, D.C.: National Academy of Sciences, 1978
38. Stark E, Flitcraft A, Zuckerman D, et al: Wife Abuse in the Medical Setting: An Introduction for Health Personnel. Washington, D.C.: Office of Domestic Violence Monograph No. 7, 1981
39. Stark E: The Battering Syndrome: Social Knowledge, Social Therapy and the Abuse of Women. State University of New York at Binghamton, 1984. Thesis
40. Schulman MA: Survey of spousal violence against women in Kentucky. Harris Study No. 792701, 1979
41. Teske RHC, Parker ML: Spouse Abuse in Texas: A Study of Women's Attitudes and Experiences. Huntsville, Tex: Criminal Justice Center, Sam Houston State University, 1983
42. Stark E, Flitcraft A, Frazier W: Medicine and patriarchal violence: The social construction of a "private" event. Int J Health Serv 9:461–493, 1979
43. Straus M, Gelles R, Steinmetz SK: Behind Closed Doors: A Survey of Family Violence in America. New York: Doubleday and Company, 1980
44. Hornung CA, McCullough BC, Sugimoto T: Status relationships in marriage: Risk factors in spouse abuse. J Marriage and Family 43:675–692, 1981
45. Szinovacz ME: Using couple data as a methodological tool: The case of marital violence. J Marriage and Family 45:633–644, 1983
46. Meredith WH, Abbott DA, Adams SL: Family violence: Its relation to marital and parental satisfaction and family strengths. J Family Violence 1:299–305, 1986
47. Straus MA, Gelles RJ: Violence in American families. In Chilman CC, Cox F, Nunnaly E (eds): Families in Trouble. Beverly Hills, Calif: Sage Publications, 1987
48. Genteman KM: Attitudes of North Carolina women toward the acceptance and causes of wife beating. Presented at the meeting of the Southeastern Women's Studies Association, Nashville, Tennessee, 1980
49. Carmen (Hilberman) E, Rieker P, Mills T: Victims of violence and psychiatric illness. Am J Psychiatry 141:378–383, 1984
50. Stark E, Flitcraft A: Woman-battering, child abuse and social heredity: What is the relationship? In Johnson N (ed): Marital Violence. Sociological Review Monograph No. 31. London: Routledge & Kegan Paul, 1985
51. Stark E, Flitcraft A: Violence Among Intimates: An Epidemiological Review. In Hasselt VN, et al (eds): Handbook of Family Violence. New York: Plenum Press, 1988, pp 293–318
52. Stark E, Flitcraft A: Women and children at risk: A feminist perspective on child abuse. Int J Health Serv 18:97–118, 1988
53. Casanave NA, Straus MA: Race, class, network embeddedness and family violence: A search for potent support systems. J Comparative Family Studies 10:281–299, 1979
54. Brown GW, Harris T: Social Origins of Depression—A Study of Psychiatric Disorder in Women. London: Tavistock, 1978
55. Cambell JC: A test of two explanatory models of women's response to battering. Nursing Res 38:18–24, 1989
56. Frieze IH: Causal attributions as mediators of battered women's response to battering. Washington, D.C.: National Institute of Mental Health Grant No. 1 R01 MH30193, 1980
57. Giles-Simms J: Wife-battering: A Systems Theory Approach. New York: Guilford Press, 1983
58. Walker L: The battered woman syndrome study. In Finkelhor D, et al (eds): The Dark Side of Families. Beverly Hills, Calif: Sage Publications, 1983
59. Dobash RE, Dobash R: Violence Against Wives. New York: The Free Press, 1979
60. Okun L: Woman Abuse: Facts Replacing Myths. Albany, N.Y.: State University of New York Press, 1986
61. Byles JA: Violence, alcohol problems and other problems in disintegrating families. J Stud Alcohol 39, 1979
62. Orne TC, Rimmer J: Alcoholism and child abuse: A review. J Stud Alcohol 42, 1980

63. Richardson DC, Cambell JL: Alcohol and wife abuse: The effect of alcohol on attributions of blame for wife abuse. Personality Social Psychol Bull 6:51–56, 1980
64. Hilberman E, Munson K: Sixty battered women. Victimology: An International Journal 2:460–470, 1977–78
65. Post RD, Willett AB, Franks RD, et al: A preliminary report on the prevalence of domestic violence among psychiatric inpatients. Am J Psychiatry 137:974–975, 1980
66. Bassuck EL, Rosenberg L: Why does family homelessness occur? A case-control study. J Public Health 28:783–788, 1988
67. Kilpatrick DG, Veronen LJ, Best CL: Factors predicting psychological distress among rape victims. In Figley CR (ed): Trauma and Its Wake. New York: Brunner/Mazel, 1985, pp 113–141
68. Veterans Administration. Myths and Realities: A Study of Attitudes Toward Vietnam Era Veterans. Washington, D.C.: Harris and Associates, 1980
69. Kilpatrick DG, Veronen LJ, Saunders BE, Best CL, Amick-McMullan A, Paduhovich J: The Psychological Impact of Crime: A Study of Randomly Surveyed Crime Victims. National Institute of Justice Grant No. 84-IJ-CX-0039, Final report, 1987
70. Resick PA: Psychological effects of victimization: Implications for the criminal justice system. Crime and Delinquency 33:468–478, 1987
71. Kidd RF, Chayet EF: Why victims fail to report? The psychology of criminal victimization. J Social Issues 40:34–50, 1984
72. Schwendinger JR, Schwendinger H: Rape and Inequality. Beverly Hills, Calif.: Sage Publications, 1983
73. Federal Bureau of Investigation. Crime in the United States: Uniform Crime Reports. Washington, D.C.: U.S. Department of Justice, 1986
74. Brownmiller S: Against Our Will: Men, Women and Rape. New York: Simon & Schuster, 1975
75. Sparks RF, Glenn HG, Dodd DJ: Surveying Victims. New York: John Wiley, 1977
76. Koss MP: The hidden rape victim: Personality, attitudinal and situational characteristics. Psych Women Quarterly 9:193–212, 1985
77. Bureau of Justice Statistics. Criminal Victimization in the United States, 1982. Washington, D.C.: Department of Justice Publication No. NCJ-92820, 1984
78. Koss MP, Gidycz CA, Wisniewski N: The scope of rape: Incidence and prevalence of sexual aggression and victimization in a national sample of higher education students. J Consult Clin Psychol 55:162–170, 1987
79. Skogan WG: Issues in the Measurement of Victimization. Washington, D.C.: Department of Justice, Bureau of Statistics Publication No. NCJ-74682, 1981
80. Malamuth NM, Donnerstein E (eds): Pornography and Sexual Aggression. Orlando, Fla: Academic Press, 1984
81. Koss MP, Leonard KE, Beezley DA, Oros CJ: Nonstranger sexual aggression: A discriminant analysis of the psychological characteristics of undetected offenders. Sex Roles 12:981–992, 1985
82. Rapaport K, Burkhart BR: Personality and attitudinal characteristics of sexually coercive college males. J Abnorm Psychol 93:216–221, 1984
83. Finkelhor D: Child Sexual Abuse: New Theory and Research. New York: The Free Press, 1985
84. Koss MP, Dinero TE: Predictors of sexual aggression among a national sample of male college students. Presented at the New York Academy of Sciences Conference, Human Sexual Aggression: Current Perspectives, New York City, 1987
85. Malamuth NM: Predictors of naturalistic sexual aggression. J Pers Soc Psychol 50:953–962, 1986
86. Koss MP, Harvey M: The Rape Victim: Clinical and Community Approaches to Treatment. New York: Stephen Greene Press, 1987
87. Amir M: Patterns in Forcible Rape. Chicago: University of Chicago Press, 1971
88. Steketee G, Foa EB: Rape-victims: Post-traumatic stress responses and their treatment: A review of the literature. J Anxiety Disorders 1:69–86, 1987
89. Kilpatrick DG, Veronen LJ: Assessing victims of rape: Methodological issues. Rockville, Md: National Institute for Mental Health, Grant No. 1 R01 MH38052, Final report, 1984
90. Ellis EM, Atkeson BM, Calhoun KS: An assessment of long-term reaction to rape. J Abnorm Psychol 90:263–266, 1981
91. American Psychiatric Association: Diagnostic and Statistical Manual of Mental Disorders, 3rd edt, rev. Washington, D.C.: The Association, 1987
92. Kilpatrick DG, Best CL, Veronen LJ, Amick AE, Villeponteaux LA, Ruff GA: Mental health correlates of criminal victimization: A random community survey. J Consult Clin Psychol 53:866–873, 1985
93. Veronen LJ, Kilpatrick DG: Stress management for rape victims. In Meichenbaum D, Jaremko ME (eds): Stress Reduction and Prevention. New York: Plenum Press, 1983, pp 341–373
94. Frank E, Stewart BD: Treating depression in victims of rape. Clinical Psychologist 36:95–98, 1983
95. Becker JV, Skinner LJ: Assessment and treatment of rape-related sexual dysfunctions. Clinical Psychologist 36:102–105, 1983
96. Burgess AW, Holmstrom LL: Rape: Crisis and Recovery. West Newton, Mass: Awab, 1986
97. Foley T: Family response to rape and sexual assault. In Burgess AW (ed): Rape and Sexual Assault. New York: Garland, 1985
98. Kempe CH, Silverman FN, Steele BF, et al: The battered child syndrome. JAMA 181:17–24, 1962
99. Cohen S, Sussman R: Reporting Child Abuse. Cambridge, Mass: Ballinger, 1977
100. Bittner S, Newberger EH: Pediatric understanding of child abuse and neglect. Pediatrics 2:197–207, 1981
101. Newberger EH, Hampton RL, Marx TJ, White KN: Child abuse and pediatric social illness: An epidemiological analysis and ecological reformulation. Am J Orthopsychiatry 56:589–601, 1986
102. Meadow R: Munchausen syndrome by proxy: The hinterland of child abuse. Lancet 2:343–344, 1977
103. Newberger CM, Newberger EH: When the pediatrician is a pedophile. In Burgess AW, Hartman CR (eds): Sexual Exploitation of Patients by Health Professionals. New York: Praeger, 1986, pp 99–106
104. Gil DG: Violence Against Children: Physical Child Abuse in the United States. Cambridge, Mass: Harvard University Press, 1970
105. American Humane Association. Annual Report of Official Child Abuse and Neglect Reporting. Denver: The Association, 1986
106. Straus M, Gelles RJ, Steinmetz SK: Behind Closed Doors: Violence in the American Family. New York: Doubleday, 1980
107. Gelles RJ, Straus MA: Intimate Violence. New York: Simon & Schuster, 1988
108. U.S. Department of Health and Human Services. Study Methodology: National Study of the Incidence and Severity of Child Abuse and Neglect. Washington, D.C.: DHHS Publication No. (OHDS) 81-30326, 1981
109. Finklehor D, Hotaling GT: Sexual abuse in the national incidence study of child abuse and neglect: An appraisal. Child Abuse and Neglect 8:23–27, 1984
110. U.S. Department of Health and Human Services. Study Findings: Study of National Incidence and Prevalence of Child Abuse and Neglect. Washington, D.C.: DHHS Report of Contract 105-85-1702, 1988
111. Steele BF, Pollock C: A psychiatric study of parents who abuse infants and small children. In Helfer RE, Kempe CH (eds): The Battered Child. Chicago: University of Chicago Press, 1974, pp 80–133
112. Galdston R: Violence begins at home. Am J Child Psychiatry 10:336–350, 1971
113. O'Toole R, Turbett, Nalepka C: Theories, professional knowledge, and diagnosis of child abuse. In Finkelhor D, Gelles R, Hotaling GT, Straus MA (eds): The Dark Side of Families: Current Family Violence Research. Beverly Hills, Calif: Sage Publications, 1983, pp 349–362
114. Starr RH: Controlled study of the ecology of child abuse and drug abuse. Child Abuse and Neglect 2:19–28, 1978
115. Burgess RL, Draper P: The explanation of family violence: The

role of biological, behavioral, and cultural selection. In Ohlin L, Tonry M (eds): Family Violence: Chicago: University of Chicago Press, 1989, pp 59–116
116. Garbarino J, Gilliam G: Understanding Abusive Families. Lexington, Mass: Lexington Books, 1980
117. Zuravin S: Fertility patterns: Their relationship to child physical abuse and child neglect. J Marriage and Family 50:93–99, 1988
118. Sherrod KB, O'Connor S, Vietze PM, et al: Child health and maltreatment. Child Dev 55:1174–1183, 1984
119. Leventhal JM: Risk factors for child abuse: Methodologic standards in case-control studies. Pediatrics 63:684–690, 1981
120. Egeland B, Vaughn B: Failure of "bond formation" as a cause of abuse, neglect, and maltreatment. Am J Orthopsychiatry 51:78–84, 1981
121. Ellerstein NS: Child Abuse: A Medical Reference. New York: John Wiley, 1981
122. Jason J, Gilliand JC, Tyler CW: Homicide as a cause of pediatric mortality in the United States. Pediatrics 72:191–193, 1983
123. White ST, Loda FA, Ingram DL, et al: Sexually transmitted diseases in sexually abused children. Pediatrics 72:16–21, 1983
124. Elmer E: A follow-up study of traumatized children. Pediatrics 59:273, 1977
125. Wyatt GE, Powell GJ: Lasting Effects of Child Sexual Abuse. Newbury Park, Calif: Sage Publications, 1988
126. Sedney M, Brooks B: Factors associated with a history of childhood sexual experience in a nonclinical population. J Am Acad Child Psychiatry 23:215, 1984
127. Summit R, Kryso J: Sexual abuse of children: A clinical spectrum. Am J Orthopsychiatry 48:237–251, 1978
128. Groth A, Birnbaum J: Men Who Rape: A Psychology of the Offender. New York: Plenum Press, 1979
129. Meiselman K: Incest: A Psychological Study of the Causes and Effects with Treatment Recommendations. San Francisco: Jossey-Bass, 1978
130. Newberger CM, DeVos E: Abuse and victimization: A life-span developmental perspective. Am J Orthopsychiatry 58:505–511, 1988
131. Newberger EH, Hagenbuch JJ, Ebeling NB, et al: Reducing the literal and human cost of child abuse: Impact of a new hospital management system. Pediatrics 51:840–848, 1973
132. Cohn AH: Evaluation of Child Abuse and Neglect Demonstration Projects (2 vol). Washington, D.C.: (DHHS) National Center for Health Services Research, 1978
133. Daro D: Confronting Child Abuse: Research for Effective Program Design. New York: The Free Press, 1988
134. Garbarino J: Changing hospital childbirth practices: A developmental perspective on prevention of child maltreatment. Am J Orthopsychiatry 49:588–597, 1979
135. National Center on Child Abuse and Neglect: National Study of Incidence and Severity of Child Abuse and Neglect. Washington, D.C.: The Center, 1981
136. MacFarlane K, Jones B, Jenstrom L: Sexual Abuse of Children: Selected Readings. Washington, D.C.: U.S. Department of Health and Human Services Publication No. 78-30161, 1980
137. Kocen L, Bulkley J: Analysis of criminal child sex offense statutes. In Bulkley J (ed): Child Sexual Abuse and the Law. Washington, D.C.: American Bar Association, 1981, pp 1–51
138. Bagley C, Ramsay R: Disrupted childhood and vulnerability to sexual assault: Long-term sequels with implications for consulting. Soc Work Hum Sexuality 4:33–48, 1985
139. Committee on Sexual Offenses Against Children and Youth. Sexual Offenses Against Children, Vol. 1. Ottawa: Canadian Government Publishing Centre, 1984
140. Finkelhor D: Child Sexual Abuse: New Theory and Research. New York: The Free Press, 1984
141. Kercher G, McShane M: The prevalence of child sexual abuse victimization in an adult sample of Texas residents. Child Abuse Neglect 8:495–502, 1984
142. Russell DEH: The Secret Trauma: Incest in the Lives of Girls and Women. New York: Basic Books, 1986
143. Wyatt G: The sexual abuse of Afro-American and white American women in childhood. Child Abuse Neglect 9:507–519, 1985
144. Finkelhor D, Hotaling G, Lewis I, Smith C: Sexual abuse in a national survey of adult men and women: Prevalence, characteristics and risk factors. Child Abuse Neglect 14:19–28, 1990
145. Peters S, Wyatt G, Finkelhor D: The prevalence of child sexual abuse. In Finkelhor D, et al (eds): A Sourcebook on Child Sexual Abuse. Beverly Hills, Calif: Sage Publications, 1986, pp 15–59
146. Burgess AW, Groth AN, Holstrom LL, Sgroi SM: Sexual Assault of Children and Adolescents. Lexington, MA: Lexington Books, 1978
147. DeFrancis V: Protecting the child victim of sex crimes committed by adults. Denver: American Humane Association, 1969
148. Griffith S, Anderson S, Bach C, Paperny D: Intrafamily sexual abuse of male children: An underreported problem. Presented at the Third International Congress of Child Abuse and Neglect, Amsterdam, 1981
149. Jaffe AC, Dynneson L, Ten Bensel R: Sexual abuse: An epidemiological study. Am J Dis Child 129:689–692, 1975
150. Queen's Bench Foundation. Sexual Abuse of Children. San Francisco: The Foundation, 1976
151. American Association for Protecting Children, Inc: National Study on Child Neglect and Abuse Reporting. Denver: American Humane Association, 1984
152. National Center on Child Abuse and Neglect: Study Findings: Study of the National Incidence and Prevalence of Child Abuse and Neglect. Washington, D.C.: U.S. Department of Health and Human Services, 1988
153. Briere J: The effect of childhood sexual abuse on later psychological functioning: Defining a "post-sexual-abuse syndrome." Presented at the Third National Conference on Sexual Victimization of Children, Washington, D.C., April 1984
154. Araji S, Finkelhor D: Explanations of pedophilia: Review of empirical evidence. Bull Am Acad Psychiatry Law 13:17–38, 1985
155. Finkelhor D, Baron L: High risk children. In Finkelhor D, et al. (eds). A Sourcebook on Child Sexual Abuse. Beverly Hills, Calif: Sage Publications, 1986, pp 60–88
156. Abel GG, Becker JV, Murphy WD, Falanagan B: Identifying dangerous child molesters. In Stuart RB (ed): Violent Behavior. New York: Brunner/Mazel, 1981, pp 116–137
157. Freund K: Erotic preference in pedophilia. Behav Res Ther 5:209–228, 1967
158. Hanson R, Slater S: Sexual victimization in the history of sexual abusers: A review. Ann Sex Res 1:485–499, 1988
159. Langevin R: Sexual Strands: Understanding and Treating Sexual Anomalies in Men. Hillsdale, N.J.: Erlbaum Associates, 1983
160. Williams LM, Finkelhor D: The characteristics of incestuous fathers: A review of recent studies. In Marshall W, Laws R, Barbaree H (eds): The Handbook of Sexual Assault: Issues, Theories and Treatment of the Offender. New York: Plenum Press, 1990
161. Parker H, Parker S: Father-daughter sexual abuse: An emerging perspective. Am J Orthopsychiatry 56:531–549, 1986
162. Abel GG, Cummingham-Rathner J, Becker JB, McHugh J: Motivating sex offenders for treatment with feedback of their psychophysiologic assessment. Presented at the World Congress of Behavior Therapy, Washington, D.C., December 1983
163. Browne A, Finkelhor D: The impact of child sexual abuse: Review of the research. Psych Bull 99(1):66–77, 1986
164. Gelinas DJ: The persisting negative effects of incest. Psychiatry 46:312–332, 1983
165. Stein J, et al: Long-term psychological sequelae of child sexual abuse: The Los Angeles Epidemiologic Catchment Area Study. In Wyatt G, Powell G (eds): Lasting Effects of Child Sexual Abuse. Newbury Park, Calif: Sage Publications, 1988
166. Herman JL: Father-Daughter Incest. Cambridge, Mass: Harvard University Press, 1981
167. Silbert MN, Pines AM: Sexual child abuse as an antecedent to prostitution. Child Abuse Neglect 5:407–411, 1981
168. Oppenheimer R, Palmer RL, Braden S: A clinical evaluation of

early sexually abusive experience in adult anorexic and bulimic females: Implications for preventative work in childhood. Presented at the Fifth International Conference on Child Abuse and Neglect, Montreal, 1984
169. Tufts New England Medical Center, Division of Child Psychiatry: Sexually Exploited Children: Service and Research Project. Final report for the Office of Juvenile Justice and Delinquency Prevention. Boston: U.S. Department of Justice, 1984
170. MacFarlane K, Bulkley J: Treating child sexual abuse: An overview of current program models. In Conte J, Shore D (eds). Social Work and Child Sexual Abuse. New York: Haworth, 1982, pp 69–81
171. Kelley RJ: Behavioral re-orientation of pedophiliacs: Can it be done? Clin Psychology Rev 2:387–408, 1982
172. Tatara T: Toward the development of estimates of national incidence of reports of elder abuse based on currently available state data: An exploratory study. In Filinson R, Ingman S (eds): Elder Abuse: Practice and Policy. New York: Human Services Press, 1989, pp 153–165
173. Block MR, Sinnott JD: Battered Elder Syndrome: An Exploratory Study. College Park, Md: University of Maryland, Center on Aging, 1979
174. Gioglio RG, Blakemore P: Elder Abuse in New Jersey: The Knowledge and Experience of Abuse Among Older New Jerseyans. Trenton, N.J.: N.J. Department of Human Services, 1983
175. Pillemer K, Finkelhor D: Prevalence of elder abuse: A random sample survey. Gerontologist 28:51–57, 1988
176. Podnieks E, Pillemer K: Final Report on Survey of Elder Abuse in Canada. Ottawa: Health and Welfare, Canada, 1989
177. O'Malley T, O'Malley HC, Perez R, Mitchell V, Knuepfel GM: Elder Abuse in Massachusetts: A Survey of Professionals and Paraprofessionals. Boston: Legal Research and Services for the Elderly, 1979
178. Sengstock MD, Laing J: Identifying and Characterizing Elder Abuse. Detroit: Wayne State Institute of Gerontology, 1982
179. Douglas RL, Hickey T, Noel C: A Study of Maltreatment of the Elderly and Other Vulnerable Adults. Ann Arbor, Mich: University of Michigan, Institute of Gerontology, 1980
180. Chen PN, Bell SL, Dolinsky DL, Doyle J, Dunn M: Elder abuse in domestic settings: A pilot study. J Gerontological Social Work 4:3–17, 1981
181. Dolan R, Hendricks J: An exploratory study comparing attitudes and practices of police officers and social service providers in elder abuse and neglect cases. J Elder Abuse Neglect 1:75–90, 1989
182. Lau E, Kosberg J: Abuse of the elderly by informal care providers. Aging Sept/Oct:10–15, 1979
183. Wolf R, Godkin MA, Pillemer K: Elder Abuse and Neglect: Report from Three Model Projects. Worcester, Mass: University of Massachusetts Medical Center, 1984
184. Hwalek M, Sengstock M, Lawrence R: Assessing the probability of abuse of the elderly. Presented at the Annual Meeting of the Gerontological Society of America, San Francisco, Calif: November 1984
185. Phillips LR: Abuse and neglect of the frail elderly at home: An exploration of theoretical relationships. J Advanced Nursing 8:379–392, 1983
186. Pillemer K: Risk factors in elder abuse: Results from a case-control study. In Pillemer K, Wolf RS (eds): Elder Abuse: Conflict in the Family. Dover, Mass: Auburn House, 1986, pp 239–263
187. Straus MA: Family patterns and child abuse in a nationally representative American sample. Child Abuse Neglect 3:213–225, 1979
188. Bristowe E, Collins JB: Family mediated abuse of noninstitutionalized frail elderly men and women living in British Columbia. J Elder Abuse Neglect 1:45–64, 1989
189. Pillemer K, Finkelhor D: Causes of elder abuse: Caregiver stress versus problem relatives. Am J Orthopsychiatry 59:179–187, 1989
190. Anetzberger GJ: Etiology of Elder Abuse by Adult Offspring. Springfield, Illinois: Charles C. Thomas, 1987
191. Hotaling G, Sugarman D: An analysis of risk markers in husband to wife violence: The current state of knowledge. Violence and Victims 1:101–124, 1986
192. Straus M, Gelles RJ, Steinmetz S: Behind Closed Doors: Violence in the American Family. New York: Doubleday, 1980
193. Cicirelli VG: Adult children and their parents. In Brubaker TH (ed): Family Relations in Later Life. Beverly Hills, Calif: Sage Publications, 1983
194. Cicirelli VG: Adult children's attachment and helping behavior to elderly parents: A path model. J Marriage and Family 45:815–825, 1983
195. Adams BN: Kinship in an Urban Setting. Chicago: Markham, 1968
196. Steinmetz SK, Amsden DJ: Dependency, family stress, and abuse. In Brubaker TH (ed): Family Relationships in Later Life. Beverly Hills, Calif: Sage Publications, 1983, pp 173–192
197. Wolf R, Strugnell C, Godkin M: Preliminary Findings from the Three Model Projects on Elder Abuse. Worcester, Mass: University of Massachusetts Medical Center, 1982
198. Pillemer K: The dangers of dependency: New findings on domestic violence against the elderly. Social Problems 33:146–158, 1985
199. Finkelhor D: Common features of family abuse. In Finkelhor D, Gelles RJ, Hotaling G, Straus M (eds). Dark Side of Families: Current Family Violence Research. Beverly Hills, Calif: Sage Publications, 1983, pp 17–26
200. Gil DG: Violence Against Children: Physical Abuse in the United States. Cambridge, Mass: Harvard University Press, 1971
201. Justice B, Justice R: The Abusing Family. New York: Human Services Press, 1976
202. Gelles RJ: The Violent Home. Beverly Hills, Calif: Sage Publications, 1972
203. Stark E, Flitcraft A, Zuckerman D, Gray A, Robinson J, Frazier W: Wife Abuse in the Medical Setting: An Introduction to Health Personnel. Washington, D.C.: National Clearinghouse on Domestic Violence, 1981
204. Browne A: When Battered Women Kill. New York: The Free Press, 1986
205. Crystal S: Social policy and elder abuse. In Pillemer KA, Wolf RS (eds). Elder Abuse: Conflict in the Family. Dover, Mass: Auburn House, 1986, pp 331–339
206. Faulkner LR: Mandating the reporting of suspected cases of elder abuse: An inappropriate, ineffective and ageist response to the abuse of older adults. Family Law Quarterly 16:69–91, 1982
207. Callahan JJ: Elder abuse programming: Will it help the elderly? Urban and Social Change Review 15:15–19, 1982
208. Lee D: Mandatory reporting of elder abuse: A cheap but ineffective solution to the problem. Fordham Urban Law J 14:131–139, 1986
209. Callendar W: Improving protective services for older Americans: A national guide series. Portland, Me: Center for Research and Advanced Study, University of Southern Maine, 1982
210. Callahan JJ: Elder abuse programming: Will it help the elderly? Presented at the National Conference on the Abuse of Older Persons, Boston, Mass, 1981
211. Bergman JA: Responding to abuse and neglect cases: Protective services versus crisis intervention. In Filinson R, Ingman S (eds): Elder Abuse: Practice and Policy. New York: Human Services Press, 1989, pp 94–103
212. Bergeron LR: Elder abuse prevention: A holistic approach. In Filinson R, Ingman S (eds): Elder Abuse: Practice and Policy. New York: Human Services Press, 1989, pp 218–228
213. Sherman LW, Berk RA: Minneapolis domestic violence experiment. Police Foundation Reports, Vol. 1, April 1984
214. National Center for Health Statistics: Advance Report of Final Mortality Statistics, 1987. Hyattsville, Md: National Center for Health Statistics, DHHS Publication No. (PHS)89-1120 [Monthly Vital Statistics Report 38 (5 supp)], 1989
215. Centers for Disease Control: Premature mortality due to suicide and homicide—United States, 1983. MMWR 35:357–365, 1986
216. Rosenberg ML, Smith JC, Davidson LE, Conn JM: The emergence of youth suicide: An epidemiologic analysis and public health perspective. Ann Rev Public Health 8:417–440, 1987
217. Centers for Disease Control: Youth suicide in the United States, 1970–1980. Atlanta: The Centers, 1986

218. National Center for Health Statistics: Annual Summary of Births, Marriages, Divorces, and Deaths: United States, 1988. Monthly Vital Statistics Report 37(13):21, 1989
219. National Center for Health Statistics: Unpublished final data. Table 290: Death rates for 72 selected causes, by 10-year age groups, color, and sex: United States, 1979–87:486,488
220. Saltzman LE, Levenson A, Smith JA: Suicide among persons 15–24 years of age, 1970–1984. In Centers for Disease Control: CDC Surveillance Summaries, February 1988. MMWR 37(No. SS-1):61–68, 1988
221. Moscicki EK, O'Carroll PW, Rae DS, Roy AG, Locke BZ, Regier DA: Suicidal ideation and attempts: The Epidemiologic Catchment Area study. In Alcohol, Drug Abuse and Mental Health Administration: Report of the Secretary's Task Force on Youth Suicide, Vol. 4. Strategies for the Prevention of Youth Suicide. Washington, D.C.: DHHS Publication No. (ADM)89–1624, 1989, pp 115–128
222. Rosenberg ML, Davidson LE, Smith JC, et al: Operational criteria for the determination of suicide. J Forensic Sciences 33:1445–1456, 1988
223. Nelson FL, Farberow NL, MacKinnon DR: The certification of suicide in eleven Western states: An inquiry into the validity of reported suicide rates. Suicide and Life-Threatening Behavior 8:75–88, 1978
224. O'Carroll PW: A consideration of the validity and reliability of suicide mortality data. Suicide and Life-Threatening Behavior 19:1–16, 1989
225. Monk M: Epidemiology of suicide. Epidemiologic Reviews 9:51–69, 1987
226. Hagnell O, Lanke J, Rorsman B: Suicide rates in the Lundby study: Mental illness as a risk factor for suicide. Neuropsychobiology 7:248–253, 1981
227. Murphy GE: Problems in studying suicide. Psychiatric Dev 1(4):339–350, 1983
228. Miles CP: Conditions predisposing to suicide: A review. J Nerv Ment Dis 164(4):231–246, 1977
229. Roy A, Linnoila M: Alcoholism and suicide. Suicide and Life-Threatening Behavior 16(2):244–273, 1986
230. Kendall RE: Alcohol and suicide. Substance Alcohol Actions Misuse 4(2–3):121–127, 1983
231. Fernandez-Pol B: Characteristics of 77 Puerto Ricans who attempted suicide. Am J Psychiatry 143:1460–1463, 1986
232. Kost-Grant BL: Self-inflicted gunshot wounds among Alaska Natives. Public Health Rep 98(1):72–78, 1983
233. Chynoweth R, Tonge JI, Armstrong J: Suicide in Brisbane—A retrospective psychosocial study. Aus N Z J Psychiatry 14(1):37–45, 1980
234. Morrison JR: Suicide in a psychiatric practice population. J Clin Psychiatry 43(9):348–352, 1982
235. Robbins DR, Alessi NE: Depressive symptoms and suicidal behavior in adolescents. Am J Psychiatry 142:588–592, 1985
236. Black DW, Warrack G, Winokur G: The Iowa record-linkage study: I. Suicides and accidental deaths among psychiatric patients. Arch Gen Psychiatry 42(1):71–75, 1985
237. Shuckitt MA: Primary men alcoholics with histories of suicide attempts. J Stud Alcohol 47(1):78–81, 1986
238. Bacue LO, Epstein L: Suicide attitudes and experiences of hospitalized alcoholics. Psychol Rep 47:1233–1234, 1980
239. Berglund M: Suicide in alcoholism: A prospective study of 88 suicides: I. The multidimensional diagnosis at first admission. Arch Gen Psychiatry 41(9):888–891, 1984
240. Frances A, Blumenthal S: Personality as a predictor of youthful suicide. In Alcohol, Drug Abuse and Mental Health Administration: Report of the Secretary's Task Force on Youth Suicide, Vol. 2. Risk Factors for Youth Suicide. Washington, D.C.: DHHS Publication No. (ADM)89–1624, 1989, pp 160–171
241. Roy A: Genetics and suicidal behavior. In Alcohol, Drug Abuse and Mental Health Administration: Report of the Secretary's Task Force on Youth Suicide, Vol. 2. Risk Factors for Youth Suicide. Washington, D.C.: DHHS Publication No. (ADM)89–1624, 1989, pp 247–262
242. Asberg M: Neurotransmitter monoamine metabolites in the cerebrospinal fluid as risk factors for suicidal behavior. In Alcohol, Drug Abuse and Mental Health Administration: Report of the Secretary's Task Force on Youth Suicide, Vol. 2. Risk Factors for Youth Suicide. Washington, D.C.: DHHS Publication No. (ADM)89–1624, 1989, pp 193–212
243. Traskman L, Asberg M, Bertillson L, Sjostrand L: Monoamine metabolites in CSF and suicidal behavior. Arch Gen Psychiatry 38:631–636, 1981
244. van Praag HM: CSF 5-HIAA and suicide in non-depressed schizophrenics. Lancet 2:977–978, 1983
245. Robbins D, Conroy C: A cluster of adolescent suicide attempts: Is suicide contagious? J Adolesc Health Care 3:253–255, 1983
246. Davidson L, Gould MS: Contagion as a risk factor for youth suicide. In Alcohol, Drug Abuse and Mental Health Administration: Report of the Secretary's Task Force on Youth Suicide, Vol. 2. Risk Factors for Youth Suicide. Washington, D.C.: DHHS Publication No. (ADM)89–1624, 1989, pp 88–109
247. Centers for Disease Control: Cluster of suicides and suicide attempts—New Jersey. MMWR 37:213–216, 1988
248. O'Carroll PW: An investigation of a cluster of suicide attempts. In Yufit RI (ed): Combined Proceedings of the Twentieth Annual Meeting of the American Association of Suicidology and the Nineteenth Annual Congress of the International Association of Suicide Prevention. San Francisco: American Association of Suicidology, 1987, pp 262–264
249. O'Carroll PW, Mercy JA, Steward JA: CDC recommendations for a community plan for the prevention and containment of suicide clusters. MMWR 37(suppl S6):1–12, 1988
250. Phillips DP, Carstensen LL: Clustering of teenage suicides after television news stories about suicide. N Engl J Med 315:685–689, 1986
251. Gould MS, Shaffer D: The impact of suicide in television movies: Evidence of imitation. N Engl J Med 315:690–694, 1986
252. Phillips DP, Paight DJ: The impact of televised movies about suicide: A replicative study. N Engl J Med 317:809–811, 1987
253. Berman AL: Fictional depiction of suicide in television films and imitation effects. Am J Psychiatry 145:982–986, 1988
254. Kessler RC, Stipp H: The impact of fictional television suicide stories on U.S. fatalities: A replication. Am J Sociology 90:151–167, 1984
255. Baron JN, Reiss PC: Same time, next year: Aggregate analyses of the mass media and violent behavior. Am Sociological Review 50:347–363, 1985
256. Gould MS: A study of time-space clustering: Phase I Report. Atlanta: Centers for Disease Control Contract No. RFP 200–85–0834, 1985
257. Davidson LE, Rosenberg ML, Mercy JA, et al: An epidemiologic study of risk factors in two teenage suicide clusters. JAMA 262:2687–2692, 1989
258. See, for example, Paykel ES, Prusoff BA, Myers JK: Suicide attempts and recent life events: A controlled comparison. Arch Gen Psychiatry 32:327–337, 1975
259. Paykel ES: Stress and life events. In Alcohol, Drug Abuse and Mental Health Administration: Report of the Secretary's Task Force on Youth Suicide, Vol. 2. Risk Factors for Youth Suicide. Washington, D.C.: DHHS Publication No. (ADM)89–1624, 1989, pp 110–130
260. Platt S: Unemployment and suicidal behavior: A review of the literature. Soc Sci Med 19:93–115, 1984
261. Boyd JH: The increasing rate of suicide by firearms. N Engl J Med 308:872–874, 1983
262. Sloan JH, Rivara FP, Reay DT, Ferris JAJ, Kellerman AL: Firearm regulations and community suicide rates: A comparison of two metropolitan areas. N Engl J Med 322:369–373, 1990

263. Centers for Disease Control. Premature mortality due to suicide and homicide—United States, 1984. MMWR 36:531–534, 1987
264. Weinstein MC, Saturno PJ: Economic impact of youth suicides and suicide attempts. In Alcohol, Drug Abuse and Mental Health Administration: Report of the Secretary's Task Force on Youth Suicide, Vol. 4. Strategies for the Prevention of Youth Suicide. Washington, D.C.: DHHS Publication No. (ADM)89-1624, 1989, pp 82–93
265. Dunne EJ, Dunne-Maxim K: Suicide and Its Aftermath: Understanding and Counseling the Survivors. New York: Norton, 1987
266. Hauser MJ: Special aspects of grief after a suicide. In Dunne EJ, Dunne-Maxim K: Suicide and Its Aftermath: Understanding and Counseling the Survivors. New York: Norton, 1987, pp 57–70
267. Eddy DM, Wolpert RL, Rosenberg ML: Estimating the effectiveness of interventions to prevent youth suicides. In Alcohol, Drug Abuse and Mental Health Administration: Report of the Secretary's Task Force on Youth Suicide, Vol. 4. Strategies for the Prevention of Youth Suicide. Washington, D.C.: DHHS Publication No. (ADM)89-1624, 1989, pp 37–81
268. National Committee for Injury Prevention and Control: Injury Prevention: Meeting the Challenge. New York: Oxford University Press, 1989, pp 252–260

SECTION SIX

Health Care Planning, Organization, and Evaluation

Edited by F. Douglas Scutchfield and John M. Last

65

The American Health Care System: Structure and Function

F. Douglas Scutchfield
Stephen J. Williams

This chapter reviews the organization and operation of the nation's health care system. A systems approach to health care is used to emphasize the interdependencies among the parts of the system and between the system's "hard assets" and the organizational and financial arrangements that allow the system to function. A solid understanding of the system is essential for all participants: provider, consumer, payer, and policy-maker.

SYSTEMS APPROACH

A systems approach to health care analysis creates a topology to guide the review of the components of the system and places each element in context. The system uses resources such as facilities, (e.g., hospitals), personnel, (e.g., physicians), and technology. These resources must be processed through transforming variables such as financing mechanisms and organizations to produce services to consumers.

The system is dynamic and cybernetic. There are feedback loops among the components. This allows for change in the system. The system is interdependent. Modification of one element will impact other elements. It is impossible to change one part of the system without causing modifications in other elements.

The dynamic and interactive nature of the system frequently is forgotten in policy making. Efforts to improve service to consumers often are based on modifying a single element within the system without recognizing the impact of that modification on other components. Thus each element and the system as a whole must be examined and understood.

The system does not operate in isolation from the environment within which it functions. The external environment dramatically influences the function of the health care system. For example, the changing demographic composition of the United States, with an aging population and a growing proportion of minorities, influences the location and types of services that need to be provided.

The changing nature of disease also provides a dramatic illustration of interaction with the external environment. In the early 1900s the leading causes of death were infectious diseases with acute, frequently self-limited courses (Table 65–1). In 1985, by contrast, major causes of death were the chronic diseases of an aging population. Also prevalent are diseases closely linked to life-style rather than to fundamental environmental concerns, such as water quality and sewage disposal, as in the early 1900s. Health care system managers and policy-makers must continually survey the external environment and adjust the system accordingly.

Even since 1950 dramatic changes have occurred in the patterns of disease and illness to which the system must respond. Death rates from cardiovascular and cerebrovascular disease have declined while those from certain malignant neoplasms have increased (Table 65–2). Overall, reductions in death rates have resulted in greater longevity, which in itself has placed financial and political stress on other aspects of our society, including the Social Security system, Medicare, housing, and education.

The changing nature of the external environment, patterns of illness, and of the system's necessary responses has been outlined by Torrens (Table 65–3).[1] The problems addressed by the health care system and the nature of the system's changes over the years have been dramatic. There is little doubt that the future will hold even more dramatic and rapid change.

Within the larger overall system are a multitude of subsystems. Many of these subsystems are informal, put together by the consumer or provider, and some are more formal, put together by insurers and governments. Existing subsystems range from community preventive services to personal care for illness and injury, to mental illness care, to care for aging or debilitated patients. These subsystems vary for each individual. There may be little coordination between providers of each service, and subsystems may be affected by the patient's ability to pay.

Purpose of Health Care. The universal goal of the health care system is to assure adequate access to quality care at a reasonable price. The components of this goal include access, quality, and price. Again, each of these factors cannot be dealt with in isolation. Increasing access may have a negative impact on quality and costs. Decreasing costs often have an adverse impact on access or quality.

In the best of all worlds, each component would be maximized with the goal of improving health. Our nation has a tendency to focus on each component serially while the pendulum

Portions of this chapter are adapted from Williams SJ, Torrens PR (eds): Introduction to Health Services, 3 edt. Albany, N.Y.: Delmar Publishing Co., 1988.

TABLE 65-1. DEATH RATES FOR LEADING CAUSES OF DEATH, 1900 AND 1985, UNITED STATES

Causes of Death	Crude Death Rate*
▪ 1900	
All causes	1719.0
Pneumonia, influenza	202.2
Tuberculosis	194.4
Diarrhea, enteritis and ulceration of intestine	142.7
Diseases of heart	137.4
Senility, ill defined or unknown	117.5
Intracranial lesions of vascular origin	106.9
Nephritis	88.6
All accidents	72.3
Cancer and other malignant tumors	64.0
Diphteria	40.3
▪ 1985	
All causes	874.8
Diseases of heart	325.0
Malignant neoplasms	191.7
Cerebrovascular accidents	64.0
Accidents	38.6
Chronic obstructive pulmonary diseases	31.2
Pneumonia, influenza	27.9
Diabetes mellitus	16.2
Suicide	12.0
Chronic liver disease and cirrhosis	11.2
Atherosclerosis	9.9

*Crude death rates calculated per 100,000 population per year.
From Vital Statistics of the United States. Washington, DC.: U.S. National Center for Health Statistics, August 1972; National Center for Health Statistics, Monthly Vital Statistics Report, vol. 34, September 10, 1986.

swings from one side to the other. A major concern in the 1960s was assuring access to care; the major concern in the 1980s was containing the cost of that care. We have not been successful in achieving our health care goals and at the same time adequately addressing the issues of access, quality, and cost. That is the challenge we face in the 1990s.

Against this backdrop of general considerations the system is examined. Keep in mind that each part of the system cannot be dealt with in isolation.

COMPONENTS OF THE SYSTEM

The parts of the system are discussed in the next few sections. They are both described and analyzed in their relation to the entire system. The final parts of this chapter address the integration and control of the subsystems, such as manipulation of the flow of dollars spent on care through various insurance programs, that put the pieces together into a "system."

Although not every component of the system is addressed in detail, the major parts are covered.

Institutional Care: The Hospital

The hospital is the predominant institutional health care provider. The hospital consumes the largest share of health care resources and in some respects is the most visible and central organization in modern health care.

The hospital has not always been held in high esteem. The hospital had its origins in the religious orders of medieval times who would provide care for the sick poor. In the United States the earliest hospitals were the almshouses and pesthouses, a legacy of the British tradition. They were dark, smelly facilities, unappealing and to be avoided whenever possible. Only people without homes and families were housed in them; anyone of means was cared for in their home by family.

The first modern hospital was the Pennsylvania Hospital, founded in Philadelphia in 1751. Slowly throughout the 1800s, other large facilities were built, such as the Massachusetts General Hospital. It was not until the middle 1900s, however, that the modern hospital became a common and central component of the system. The rise of the contemporary hospital resulted from changes in the way medicine was practiced.

The Changing Hospital Environment. The first influence on the growth of the modern hospital was the ability to perform surgical procedures successfully. This was the result of two important scientific advances. The first was the discovery, in the 1850s, of anesthesia. Before anesthesia, the very best surgeon was the speediest one; complicated procedures could not be performed because of the pain associated with them. The advent of anesthesia ushered in the golden age of surgery in the late 1800s.

The second major advance was the discovery of sepsis. Patients undergoing surgery frequently developed postoperative infections. With the advent of sepsis the danger of postoperative infection was reduced substantially.

TABLE 65-2. AGE-ADJUSTED DEATH RATES FOR SELECTED CAUSES OF DEATH PER 100,000 RESIDENT POPULATION, UNITED STATES, 1950, 1970, AND 1988

Cause of Death	1950	1970	1988
All causes	841.5	714.3	535.5
Diseases of heart	307.6	253.6	166.3
Malignant neoplasms	125.4	129.4	132.7
Respiratory system	12.8	28.4	39.9
Colorectal	19.0	16.8	13.9
Prostate [male]	13.4	13.3	15.2
Breast [female	22.2	23.1	23.1
Chronic obstructive pulmonary diseases	4.4	13.2	19.4
Pneumonia and influenza	26.2	22.1	14.2
Chronic liver disease and cirrhosis	8.5	14.7	9.0
Diabetes mellitus	14.3	14.1	10.1
Accidents and adverse effects	57.5	53.7	35.0
Motor vehicle accidents	23.3	27.4	19.7
Suicide	11.0	11.8	11.4
Homicide and legal intervention	5.4	9.1	9.0
Human Immunodeficiency virus infection	—	—	6.6

From National Center for Health Statistics. Health, United States, 1990. Hyattsville, Md.: U.S. Public Health Service, 1991.

TABLE 65-3. MAJOR TRENDS IN THE DEVELOPMENT OF HEALTH CARE IN THE UNITED STATES, 1850 TO PRESENT

Trends	1850–1900	1900 to World War II	World War II to Present	Future
Predominant health problems of the American people	Epidemics of acute infections	Acute events, trauma or infections affecting individuals, not groups	Chronic diseases such as heart disease, cancer, stroke	Chronic ill-health, particularly emotional and behaviorally related conditions
Technology available to handle predominant health problems	Virtually none	Beginning and rapid growth of basic medical sciences and technology	Explosive growth of medical science; technology captures the health care system	Continued growth and expansion of technology with attempts to repersonalize technology
Social organization for the use of technology	None; individuals left to their own resources or to charity	Beginning societal, governmental efforts to care for those who could not care for themselves	Health care as a right; governmental responsibility to organize and monitor health care for everyone	Greater centralization of responsibility and control in federal government; greater use of organized systems of health insurance and financing to shape, control developments within the health care system

From Torrens PR: Historical evolution and overview of health services in the United States. In Williams SJ, Torrens, PR (eds): Introduction to Health Services, 3 edt. Albany, NY: Delmar Publishing Co., 1988, chap 1.

These advances allowed surgery to become a major force in the care of patients. One need only consider that over 40% of total hospital beds are surgical beds to understand the impact of these discoveries. The more recent advances in outpatient surgical procedures probably represent another turning point in the influence of surgery on the system.

The late 1800s saw the emergence of the biological revolution. The discovery of the new sciences of microbiology ushered in a new understanding of disease. The notion of the etiologic agent as the cause of disease required fundamental rethinking of diagnosis and treatment. New technology to assist in the diagnosis and treatment of patients developed rapidly during that period. The discovery of the electrocardiograph and the x-ray illustrate the expanding role of technology.

The early laboratories and machines of this technological revolution were primitive by today's standards and were physically very large. It made sense to provide a central place, the hospital, where all physicians could have access to this new technology. To this day, the hospital continues to serve a major role as the repository of technology for the community, although presently much is being done to move this technology into noninstitutional locations.

A third major development occurred in the nursing profession. Inmates provided what nursing care was available in the early almshouses. In the mid-1800s, during the Crimean War, Florence Nightingale demonstrated the advantages of professional nursing services on mortality. She later developed nurse training programs in Britain, and hospitals in the United States followed suit. The availability of well-trained nursing personnel made hospitals much safer and more pleasant places.

The training of physicians also has changed dramatically, and this has been an important factor in the development of hospitals. Before 1900, medical education in the United States was seriously deficient. Most physicians were trained in proprietary apprenticeships, with many lectures and little exposure to patients.

The development of professional licensure was important in the reformation of American medical education. Licensing was based on an examination and graduation from an approved school. A second contributing factor was the Flexner Report. The Carnegie Foundation, at the urging of the American Medical Association, hired a nonphysician educator, Abraham Flexner, to visit the nation's medical schools and to provide recommendations for their reform. Flexner reported that the existing medical schools were grossly inadequate.

One school, however, stood out. This school, Johns Hopkins University, served as an example for the others. The positive features of this school were: (1) students were required to have a college degree before they were admitted; (2) the medical curriculum was 4 years in duration, with 2 years dedicated to basic sciences and 2 years to work with full-time clinical instructors; (3) the medical school was an integral part of a comprehensive university; and (4) faculty of the school were actively engaged in medical research. Hospitals increasingly became the training site for both medical students and residents training for a medical or surgical specialty.

Another development that was critical to the modern hospital was the increasing health insurance coverage held by the population. Health insurance was relatively unknown until the 1930s. During the 1940s, there was a rapid increase in the proportion of people who were covered.

Types of Hospitals. Hospitals can be classified by length of stay. There are short- and long-term hospitals; the dividing point is an average length of stay of 30 days. Hospitals also are characterized by type of service, the most common being the general hospital. There are also children's, eye, and other specialized hospitals. A third classification for hospitals is by ownership: governmental, not-for-profit, proprietary (also known as for-profit), or investor-owned (Table 65-4). Hospital usage trends are presented in Table 65-5.

Governmental hospitals are classified as federal, state, and local. Federal hospitals serve groups eligible as the result of some type of entitlement. Indian Health Service hospitals, for example, meet treaty obligations, and Veterans Administration hospitals serve certain eligible veterans.

State facilities generally are either mental or tuberculosis hospitals. The states share responsibility with local government as a provider of last resort for patients without resources.

Local governmental hospitals include city or county hospitals that provide care to those without the resources to pay. They are usually under local political government supervision. They are often large and overburdened, have decaying physical plants, and usually are affiliated with a medical school that provides medical staff.

Local government hospitals have gone through troubled

TABLE 65-4. SHORT-STAY HOSPITALS, BEDS, AND OCCUPANCY RATES ACCORDING TO TYPE OF OWNERSHIP: UNITED STATES

Type of Ownership	1988
▪ **Hospitals**	
All ownerships	5,892
Federal	313
Nonfederal	5,579
Nonprofit	3,256
Proprietary	790
State-local government	1,533
▪ **Beds**	
All ownerships	1,033,881
Federal	84,419
Nonfederal	949,462
Nonprofit	668,101
Proprietary	103,623
State-local government	177,738
▪ **Occupancy Rate (percent)**	
All ownerships	65.9%
Federal	71.2%
Nonfederal	65.5%
Nonprofit	68.2%
Proprietary	50.9%
State-local government	63.8%

From National Center for Health Statistics, United States, 1990. Hyattsville, Md.: U.S. Public Health Service, 1991.

times. With the advent of Medicaid it was thought that these hospitals would be abandoned by the urban poor who could then buy care elsewhere. But this did not happen, and the growth in the uninsured population has put severe stresses on these hospitals in an era of declining support.

Another type of local hospital, popular in the western United States, is the public authority hospital, which is financed in part by a hospital assessment district similar to a water or fire district. These hospitals receive tax money and are controlled by an elected board. Many of these facilities, however, serve relatively affluent suburbs.

Not-for-profit hospitals are public corporations exempt from taxation. Any excess revenue over expenses is retained to expand services. Many not-for-profit hospitals are affiliated with religious orders.

Proprietary hospitals have been around for many years. Early in the century prominent physicians would build a hospital for their own use. Although these declined in number over the years, the 1960s saw the early development of large "chains" of investor-owned facilities. These hospitals are owned by stockholders, who receive a return on their equity as in other publicly held companies. These entities saw rapid growth as the chains built, bought, or developed management contracts with an increasing number of hospitals.

There is considerable controversy regarding the relative efficiency and quality of care of not-for-profit versus for-profit hospitals.[2] Any definitive resolution of this controversy must await more research.[3,4] In general, both types of hospital ownership seem to serve the consumer adequately.

In response to the growth of these corporations and the need to have access to capital and to achieve economies of scale, other multihospital systems have developed. Some are small, some focus on rural hospitals, and many are composed of not-for-profit hospitals. As occupancy rates have fallen, hospitals have had to become more competitive. They also have diversified, adding new programs and services. Hospitals have developed market niches through specialized programs and have established joint ventures with each other and with physicians to attract dollars, physicians, and patients.

Structure of the Hospital. There are three competing sources of authority in the hospital: the governing board, the administration, and the medical staff. The governing board has the ultimate responsibility for the hospital. They set policy, hire and fire the administrator, and appoint members of the medical staff. They also have ultimate responsibility for the quality of care; many hospitals have added members of the medical staff to the board, and most have increased quality assurance activities.

In the United States there usually is not a direct financial relationship between hospitals and physicians, although physicians need a hospital to practice in and hospitals need physicians to admit patients. The mutual dependence is represented by the governing bylaws of the medical staff, which define the rules and regulations governing physician interaction with the hospital. Election and duties of the officers and committees and processes for awarding and maintaining privileges are defined.

The growth in the size and complexity of the hospital mandates a well-educated administrator who can provide leadership and professional management. The administrator now is often termed the president or chief executive officer to reflect a corporate orientation.

Challenges Facing the Hospital. The hospital faces many complex problems; these problems are especially severe for small and rural hospitals.[5,6] The rising cost of hospital care, consuming 42% of the health-care dollar, has prompted programs to control the use of hospital beds. Some of these mechanisms, such as diagnosis-related groups (DRG), have substantial impact on hospital decision-making. Employers and insurers negotiate with hospitals for discounted rates for their employees or subscribers. The federally mandated Profession Review Organizations (PRO) review care provided to recipients of Medicare benefits for appropriateness of use.

Another issue is overbedding. After World War II the Health Facilities and Planning Act (Hill-Burton) was passed. Although successful, this program and subsequent hospital construction has resulted in excess capacity. In addition, out-of-hospital care and quicker recovery of patients have shortened hospital stays. Excess capacity contributes to higher costs as the fixed costs of operating an empty bed is borne by the consumer in the filled beds.

A third, and related, issue is the changing nature of hospital use. Patients who previously would have been hospitalized now are being treated on an outpatient basis; those remaining in the hospital are sicker and require more technology and care. These increases in intensity also contribute to nursing stresses and shortages.

Ambulatory Care

Ambulatory care includes a wide range of practitioners, settings, and services for the "walking" or noninstitutionalized patient. Ambulatory care services play a central role as the initial and continuing point of contact with the system for most people. Ambulatory services provide intake for patients, serve as the point of contact for follow-up and ongoing care, and serve a broker function as the center of the referral network for specialized hospital and physician services, an especially visible role in managed-care programs.

Types of Care Provided. Primary prevention includes services designed to avoid the occurrence of disease in populations. Although these services do not involve the direct provision of health care, they are critical to the improvement of health; they include protection of the work place through accident avoidance

TABLE 65-5. DISCHARGES AND DAYS OF CARE PER 1,000 POPULATION AND AVERAGE LENGTH OF STAY IN SHORT-STAY HOSPITALS: UNITED STATES, 1964 AND 1989

Characteristics	Discharges		Days of Care		Average Length of Stay (days)	
	1964	1989	1964	1989	1964	1989
▪ Total[a,b]	109.1	92.6	970.9	646.6	8.9	7.0
▪ Age (y)						
Under 15	67.6	44.1	405.7	256.4	6.0	5.8
Under 5	94.3	76.6	731.1	506.2	7.8	6.6
5–14	53.1	26.7	229.1	122.8	4.3	4.6
15–44	100.6	67.0	760.7	371.8	7.6	5.5
45–64	146.2	130.5	1,559.3	937.5	10.7	7.2
65 and over	190.0	265.6	2,292.7	2,360.8	12.1	8.9
65–74	181.2	236.7	2,150.4	2,004.3	11.9	8.5
75 and over	206.7	311.0	2,560.4	2,918.6	12.4	9.4
▪ Sex[a]						
Male	103.8	95.0	1,010.2	690.0	9.7	7.3
Female	113.7	91.2	933.4	615.7	8.2	6.8
▪ Race[a]						
White	112.4	92.0	961.4	635.9	8.6	6.9
Black[c]	84.0	105.2	1,062.9	798.9	12.7	7.6
▪ Family Income[a,d]						
Less than $14,000	102.4	131.3	1,051.2	1,013.0	10.3	7.7
$14,000–$24,999	116.4	91.2	1,213.9	600.5	10.4	6.6
$25,000–$34,999	110.7	93.0	939.8	630.5	8.5	6.8
$35,000–$49,999	109.2	75.0	882.6	476.9	8.1	6.4
$50,000 or more	110.7	72.1	918.9	497.4	8.3	6.9
▪ Geographic Region[a]						
Northeast	98.5	80.2	993.8	589.5	10.1	7.4
Midwest	109.2	98.4	944.9	690.2	8.7	7.0
South	117.8	106.5	968.0	721.6	8.2	6.8
West	110.5	75.7	985.9	528.8	8.9	7.0

[a] Age adjusted.
[b] Includes all other races not shown separately and unknown family income.
[c] 1964 data include all other races.
[d] Family income categories for 1987.

and safety efforts and protection of the food and water supplies. Preventive health services include the direct provision of care to avoid disease. These services include smoking alleviation classes, disease screening, and immunizations and vaccinations.

Primary care includes the daily routine care that individuals receive from the health care system for diagnosis, counseling, follow-up, and therapy. More complex care is termed secondary care. Considerable secondary care is provided on an ambulatory basis. Tertiary care includes the most highly complex services, such as open-heart surgery, and is provided in sophisticated medical centers.

Historical Perspective. Historically, most medical care has been provided on an ambulatory care basis. Ambulatory care services traditionally have been provided by individual medical practitioners providing care in their offices and in patients' homes, and by public clinics operating primarily for poor and medically indigent patients. The general practitioner who made house calls and offered what treatment was available was "typical" of the primary care provider before World War II.

Since World War II, fewer physicians have been able to spend the time required traveling to the patient's home, and many can no longer carry with them the specialized resources available in the office. The growth of technology and specialization has led to the rapid expansion of newer settings for providing care, such as group practices and hospital clinics. For the poor, care often has been limited to public or philanthropic clinics or dispensaries. These public care providers eventually evolved into public hospitals and governmentally sponsored clinics.

Use of Ambulatory Care Services. Quantitative information on the use of ambulatory care resources consists mostly of data on physician use. These data reflect greater use of hospital outpatient departments by blacks than by whites, and by lower income than by higher income people (Table 65–6). This would suggest that office-based care may be less accessible to the poor and to minorities than to the nonpoor and to whites.

Most of the ambulatory care that people receive is provided in office-based practice settings, as reflected in Table 65–6. Although a significant amount of care is provided in hospital settings, the predominant source of care is the physician's office, including solo, group, and noninstitutional clinic practices.

The two predominant private settings or forms of practice are solo and group practice. Solo practice comprises a single private practitioner. Group practice is the combination of three or more practitioners in a medical or other office-based practice.

Most ambulatory care services traditionally have been provided by physicians in solo office-based practice. From the provider's perspective, solo practice offers an opportunity to

TABLE 65-6. PHYSICIAN CONTACTS: UNITED STATES, 1989

Characteristics	Number Physician Contacts per Person	Percent Distribution				
		Doctor's Office	*Hospital Outpatient Department*[a]	*Telephone*	*Home*	*Other*[b]
▪ **Total**[c,d]	5.3	59.6	13.2	12.3	1.4	13.4
▪ **Age**						
Under 15 years	4.6	62.2	11.8	14.5	*0.5	11.1
Under 5 years	6.7	61.4	9.8	15.5	*0.5	12.8
5–14 years	3.5	63.0	13.8	13.4	*0.4	9.4
15–44 years	4.6	58.1	13.5	11.4	0.6	16.3
45–64 years	6.1	59.0	14.4	12.5	1.6	12.5
65 years and over	8.9	59.6	13.3	9.4	7.5	10.3
65–74 years	8.2	58.4	15.5	10.0	4.0	12.1
75 years and over	9.9	61.1	10.4	8.7	12.0	7.9
▪ **Sex**[c]						
Male	4.8	58.1	15.0	11.2	1.2	14.5
Female	5.9	60.5	12.1	12.9	1.6	12.9
▪ **Race**[c]						
White	5.5	60.9	12.2	12.9	1.4	12.7
Black	4.9	50.6	20.4	9.3	2.0	17.8
▪ **Family Income**[c]						
Less than $14,000	6.3	48.5	18.0	10.8	2.4	20.3
$14,000–$24,999	5.2	58.9	14.3	12.9	1.4	12.5
$25,000–$34,999	5.5	61.0	12.1	12.4	0.8	13.7
$35,000–$49,999	5.2	63.1	12.1	12.9	0.6	11.4
$50,000 or more	6.0	63.4	10.7	13.6	1.7	10.7
▪ **Geographic Region**[c]						
Northeast	5.3	59.8	16.0	12.8	1.4	10.0
Midwest	5.4	57.6	13.3	12.9	1.7	14.5
South	5.3	62.5	11.1	12.3	1.6	12.5
West	5.5	57.4	13.8	11.3	0.9	16.5

[a] Includes hospital outpatient clinic, emergency room, and other hospital contacts.
[b] Includes clinics or other places outside a hospital.
[c] Age adjusted.
[d] Includes all other races not shown separately and unknown family income.

avoid organizational dependence and to be self-employed. Philosophically, solo practice is most closely aligned with the traditional economic orientations that have characterized medicine. Although solo practice still accounts for more ambulatory services than any other setting, group practice and hospital-based services are expanding dramatically. Changing lifestyles, the cost of establishing a practice, external pressures on practitioners, and governmental programs also have adversely affected the traditional dominance of solo practice.

National Ambulatory Care Survey. An ongoing national study of all private office-based physicians, the National Ambulatory Medical Care Survey (NAMCS), has been conducted by the federal government.[7] The NAMCS involves a random sample of the nation's office-based nonfederal physicians who are asked to complete a data collection form for each patient treated during a brief time period. The most common care provided is routine care, follow-up or ongoing care, and the prominence of relatively simple primary care problems is striking.

Limited examinations, laboratory tests, and blood pressure checks were the most common diagnostic services provided, whereas counseling was the most common therapeutic service provided, exclusive of drugs.

Group Practice. Group practice is an affiliation of providers, usually physicians, who share income, expenses, facilities, equipment, medical records, and support personnel in the provision of services through a formal, legally constituted organization. Some of the earliest group practices in the United States were started by industries that needed to provide care to employees in rural sites where medical care was unavailable.

The Mayo Clinic in Rochester, Minnesota, was the first successful nonindustrial group practice. The Mayo Clinic, originally organized as a single specialty group practice in 1887 and later broadened into a multispecialty group, represented a reputable model for group practice. In 1931 the Committee on the Costs of Medical Care issued a report suggesting a major role for group practice, especially those associated with hospitals, in providing comprehensive care.

Developments in medical practice, especially increasing specialization and expansion of technology, also spurred the group practice movement. More complex and expensive facilities, equipment, and personnel were needed, and group practice provided a structure for sharing costs. Multispecialty groups could provide patients with more of their health care under one roof and thus reduce problems of physical access to care. Group practice was seen by many as facilitating referral arrangements and shared after-hours coverage, providing more flexible working hours, and requiring less financial risk for the physician, while also benefiting the patient.

The American Medical Association has conducted surveys of physician-oriented medical group practices in the United

States on a periodic basis since 1965, and most recently in 1984.[8] The number of group practices nearly doubled during the 10-year period from 1974 to 1984. There are now over 15,000 group practices in the United States, two thirds of which are single-specialty groups.

Approximately 140,000 physicians in the United States are now working in group practices, which represents a marked increase from 67,000 in 1975 and 88,000 in 1980. A higher percentage of all physicians in group practice work in multispecialty groups, largely because the average multispecialty group is substantially larger (26.6 physicians on average) than the average single-specialty (5.8 physicians on average) group. The average size of all group practices in the United States in 1984 was 9.1 physicians, an increase from 7.9 physicians in 1975 and 8.2 physicians in 1980.

The geographic distribution of group practice in the United States is dominated by seven states, which account for 40% of all groups. These states are California, Pennsylvania, New York, Texas, Illinois, Florida, and Ohio.

The increasing integration of the health care system raises interesting questions regarding the affiliations of group practices with other organizations. Approximately half of all groups, and more than half of all group-practice physicians, are directly affiliated with a hospital.

From a community perspective, groups may reduce the geographic dispersion of providers and thus increase difficulties of physical access to care. In addition groups may reduce competition in the health care marketplace by consolidating what would otherwise be competing providers.

Hospital-based Ambulatory Care. An increasing number of people have sought primary care from hospitals, sometimes as a result of lack of access to other care, taxing the ability of many facilities to respond. The result has been overcrowded facilities; the wrong mix of services, equipment, and personnel to respond to patient needs; and extremely dissatisfied consumers and providers. Most hospitals have now successfully expanded outpatient services and hired full-time providers to staff redesigned hospital ambulatory facilities.

A hospital-sponsored or hospital-based group practice can provide comprehensive and accessible care and remove primary care patients from emergency rooms. These groups also increase the use of the hospital inpatient and ancillary services. Hospitals with ambulatory care resources can negotiate contracts for providing a wide range of both inpatient and outpatient services. They are also better able to control the use of services and costs.

Increasing competition is forcing many hospitals to enter this business.[9] Hospitals are becoming involved with the construction of medical office buildings and with new businesses such as joint ventures, development of health plans, and purchases of medical practices.[10] The success or failure of these ventures will not be measurable for some time, but they place the hospital at greater financial risk as hospitals become more dependent on their successful administrative and financial incorporation into other ventures.

Ambulatory Surgery Centers. A further innovation in hospital-based care has been the development of ambulatory surgery centers that provide 1-day surgical care. In the early 1970s, free-standing ambulatory surgery centers were opened independent of hospitals. Many physicians perform surgery in their offices as well; specialties such as oral surgery, plastic surgery, and ophthalmology use office-based facilities extensively.

Free-standing emergency centers also have opened in many cities. These emergency centers sometimes provide a wide range of primary care in addition to responding to urgent problems. The future of specialized ambulatory centers, in both hospitals and as free-standing facilities, will include further expansion into other areas of health care, ranging from sports medicine to women's health care. The commercial success of these organizations, however, is certainly not assured, especially as the health care marketplace becomes more competitive.

Governmental and Noninstitutional Programs. Governmental programs have been designed to increase the availability of health care resources. Neighborhood Health Centers, first funded in 1965, are free-standing group practices that predominantly serve the medically indigent in urban areas. The combination of former "free" clinics, neighborhood health centers, public agency clinics, and some hospital clinics and groups now form an informal "safety net" of providers for individuals who lack private insurance or access to other sources of care, or who simply need care. Some of these providers contract to provide care under local governmental entitlement programs.

The federal government also operates health care facilities. The Veterans Administration includes the largest health services system under a unified management structure in the United States. The military services provides health care to millions of people in the armed forces. The Indian Health Service is charged with ensuring access to medical care on Indian reservations and in other locations.

Many other services help to meet the needs of a community. The list is nearly endless. Home health services are provided by visiting nurse associations, proprietary companies, some hospitals, public health departments, and other agencies. Rural health care has required unique and innovative solutions in many communities, especially in the absence of adequate supplies of physicians and facilities, and remains a challenging test of the ingenuity and resourcefulness of the health services system. Other community health services include school health services; prison health services; vision care; dental care provided by solo, group, and institutionally based practitioners; foot care from podiatrists; and drug-dispensing from pharmacists.

Long-Term Care

Long-term care represents, along with mental health services, perhaps our greatest challenge for the future in health care. Although other countries have successfully implemented long-term care innovations, the United States has been slow to innovate and to address the underlying problems of those people in need of long-term care.

Long-term care encompasses a wide spectrum of services, termed the continuum of care. Long-term care includes skilled nursing, intermediate, and respite care; certain acute care services such as rehabilitation; ambulatory care, including both traditional services and more targeted care such as adult day care and substance abuse programs; home health care; outreach, health promotion, and recreational and housing services.[11] Among the problems our nation faces in the area of long-term care are coordination of each component of the continuum and assuring access to those services that meet the specific needs of each patient. Financing for most components of the system is inadequate at present.[12]

The nursing home is the most costly component of the continuum of care and the one that attracts the most visibility. There are nearly 1.5 million residents of the nation's more than 23,000 nursing homes (Table 65-7).[13] Most residents are over age 75, are female, have multiple health problems, and have severe mobility and independence difficulties. Although many nursing homes are small, there is an increasing trend toward larger homes and toward ownership by multihome, not-for-profit and for-profit entities.

Because Medicare generally does not cover care in nursing homes, patients must rely on their own financial resources until these are depleted and then must rely on Medicaid. Financial support for nursing home care generally is inadequate to provide the level of services, activities, physical environment, and staff

TABLE 65-7. NURSING HOME AND PERSONAL CARE HOME RESIDENTS UNITED STATES, 1963 AND 1985

	No. of Residents		Residents per 1,000 U.S. Population	
	1963	**1985**	**1963**	**1985**
▪ **Age**				
▪ **All Ages**	445,600	1,318,300	25.4	46.2
65–74 y	89,600	212,100	7.9	12.5
75–84 y	207,200	509,000	36.9	57.7
85 and over	148,700	597,300	148.4	220.3
▪ **Sex**				
Male	141,000	334,400	18.1	29.0
Female	304,500	983,900	31.1	57.9
▪ **Race**				
White	431,700	1,227,400	26.6	47.7
Black	13,800	82,000	10.3	35.0

From National Center for Health Statistics. Health, United States, 1990. Hyattsville, Md.: U.S. Public Health Services, 1991.

known to be of maximum benefit to residents from both somatic and psychosocial perspectives.

Other progress is being made in the continuum of long-term care. The hospice provides services to the terminally ill in a caring and medically supportive environment. Home health services have expanded rapidly over the past few years. Various types of retirement and "life care" communities are being developed, although some earlier attempts were not financially successful. The financing, administrative, and coordinating requirements to adequately address these long-term care needs remains far too limited.[14] The availability of increased financial support would likely lead to great success in meeting the needs of the long-term care patient.

Mental Health Services

Mental health care shares some similar characteristics with long-term care, but it also has some unique considerations. Financing is inadequate in this arena as well, and many insurers and governmental programs provide only limited reimbursement for these services. Unfortunately the trend is probably toward even further restrictions, with the possible exception of substance abuse programs.

Mental health services also lack political clout. Definitions of illness in this area often are vague and therapies are far from definitive in most cases. The extent of unmet demand for mental health care is unknown, creating great uncertainties for planning services, and the potential for use of these services is likely to be extensive.

The existing need for services is met by two systems of care. One, consisting of public hospitals and clinics, tends to the needs of the poor and underinsured. The other, primarily encompassing private practice psychiatrists, other practitioners, and private mental hospitals, cares for patients who have the ability to pay.

Nearly 2 million inpatient and close to 3 million outpatient episodes of mental health care occur annually. The deinstitutionalization of patients from state and local government mental hospitals that occurred over the past 25 years has led to a revolving door syndrome, where many people experience frequent readmissions and discharges over their lifetime. Thus although lengths of stay have been reduced dramatically, it has been at the cost of readmissions, increases in the number of homeless, and other social problems.

Mental health services present a number of other interesting features. A variety of types of practitioners, including physicians, psychologists, social workers, and nurses vie for patient care responsibility, especially in ambulatory care. Financing of services remains oriented toward short-term interventions, especially in insurance plans; government, especially at the local level, remains the provider of last resort. Complex legal and social issues related to patient rights, to the obligations of providers, and to the role of society are constantly evolving; many issues have not been adequately addressed.

As with long-term care, our society has yet to accept responsibility for solving the problems involving the mental health of our nation's citizens. Although the technology for clinical intervention is in a relatively young but hopeful stage of development, with considerable long-term progress likely, the financial, political, and administrative challenges continue to beg for attention.

HEALTH CARE PERSONNEL

The health care system is a major employer. There are numerous professions that are involved in health services. Physicians are the most powerful of these professionals, and they have the most important role in making decisions about the use of resources in the system.

The Physician. In the mid-1960s there was a perception that a shortage of physicians existed. National policy resulted in the growth of medical school classes and the building of new medical schools. Foreign medical school graduates also were viewed as a source of physicians for the United States.

In 1963 the Health Profession Educational Assistance Act was passed to provide funds to medical schools based on enrollments and for grants and loans for the construction of new medical education facilities. This legislation marked the first instance of direct federal involvement in medical education. Previous attempts by the federal government had been opposed by both organized medicine and the medical schools themselves, based on concern that government would regulate medical education.

The incentives contained in the Health Professions Assistance Act were effective in increasing the number of medical school graduates. From 1965 to 1980 the number of medical schools and graduates approximately doubled.

Immigration policy preferentially allowed foreign medical school graduates to enter the country. An influx of physicians from many foreign countries, especially from the Asian subcontinent, resulted. Many hospitals used these physicians to fill resi-

TABLE 65-8. ACTIVE PHYSICIANS: UNITED STATES AND OUTLYING U.S. AREAS, SELECTED YEARS

Year	All Active Physicians	Doctors of Medicine	Doctors of Osteopathy	Active Physicians per 10,000 Population
1950	219,900	209,000	10,900	14.1
1960	259,400	247,300	12,200	14.0
1970	326,500	314,200	12,300	15.6
1980	457,500	440,400	17,100	19.7
1990	601,100	573,300	27,800	24.0
▪ **PROJECTIONS**				
2000	721,600	682,100	39,500	26.9

From National Center for Health Statistics. Health, United States, 1990. Hyattsville, Md.: U.S. Public Health Service, 1991.

dency training programs and to staff the hospital. At its peak, foreign medical graduates received nearly half of the annual new licenses issued.

By the mid-1970s these policies may have overcorrected physician supply, and a surplus may now exist. It is projected that there will be more than 700,000 active physicians by the year 2000 (Table 65-8). In 1980 the Graduate Medical Education Advisory Committee (GMEAC) suggested that by 1990 there would be an excess of 70,000 physicians.[15] With the pendulum now swinging the other way, medical school class sizes have declined, and immigration laws no longer allow preferential treatment for foreign medical graduates.

In 1988 the Council on Graduate Medical Education (COGME) concluded that the nation had more physicians than it needed. However, there remains some controversy regarding the current balance between supply and demand (Table 65-9).

Medicine also may be declining in popularity as a professional career. There has been a significant decrease in the number of applicants to medical school over the past few years, with a corresponding increase in the acceptance ratio. The number of women choosing careers in medicine has increased. The proportion of women entering medical school has increased from 5% to 25% from the 1960s to the 1980s. Much less success has been achieved with minority enrollments.

There is also concern about specialty distribution. There is a perception of a shortage of primary care physicians. Efforts to correct specialty imbalances have included federal training grants for residency training in primary care specialties. The Council on Graduate Medical Education identified the shortage of primary care and preventive medicine specialists as a national problem. Physician reimbursement policy may be partially to blame for this maldistribution. Primary care physicians have lower incomes than physicians in procedure-oriented specialties. New approaches to provide reimbursement based on the resources required to care for patients are being developed to address this disparity.

Another issue has been physician geographic distribution. Rural and inner city areas have had difficulty attracting physicians because of income differentials, ambience, peer interaction, and other factors. The physician is a well-educated professional who wants the amenities of education, cultural opportunities, and an appealing environment for his or her family. There has been speculation that the increase in the number of physicians would result in physicians locating in shortage areas, and to some extent this has begun to occur, although deficiencies still exist.

Some states have loan programs for students who agree to practice in medically underserved areas. The Federal National Health Service Corps also was developed to support medical students who agreed to practice in shortage areas. Other programs exposed medical students and residents to rural and urban underserved areas. The Area Health Education Center program provides experiences in underserved areas. Most of these programs have had only limited success.

Nursing. The nursing profession is in transition. The development of the professional nurse contributed to the rise of the modern hospital. Florence Nightingale validated the tremendous impact of good nursing on mortality. Dorthea Dix had a similar impact on the nursing profession in the U.S. Civil War. The first nursing training programs associated with hospitals were 3 years

TABLE 65-9. PHYSICIANS, ACCORDING TO ACTIVITY AND PLACE OF MEDICAL EDUCATION: UNITED STATES AND OUTLYING U.S. AREAS

Activity and Place of Medical Education	1986
Doctors of medicine	569,160
Professionally active	505,750
Places of medical education	
U.S. medical graduates	398,314
Foreign medical graduates[a]	107,436
Activity	
Nonfederal	483,812
Patient care	436,877
Office-based practice	325,757
General and family practice	53,622
Internal medicine	52,287
Pediatrics	22,530
General surgery	23,542
Obstetrics and gynecology	23,580
Other specialty	150,196
Hospital-based practice	111,120
Residents and interns	77,618
Full-time hospital staff	33,502
Other professional activity[b]	46,935
Federal	21,938
Patient care	16,985
Office-based practice	1,221
Hospital-based practice	15,764
Residents and interns	2,858
Full-time hospital staff	12,906
Other professional activity[b]	4,953
Inactive	46,835
Not classified[c]	13,661
Unknown address	2,914

[a] Foreign medical graduates who received their medical education in schools outside the United States and Canada.
[b] Includes medical teaching, administration, research, clinical fellows, and other.
[c] Not classified established in 1970; however, complete data not available until 1972.

in length, and graduates, who received a diploma, were eligible to take state registered nurse (RN) examinations. To assist the registered nurse, another auxiliary, the licensed practical nurse, was created. The licensed practical nurse trains for about 1 year in a vocational program.

Hospital-trained diploma nurses registered by the state as RNs and 1 year licensed practical or vocational nurses were predominant until the 1950s. During the 1950s and 1960s the nursing profession sought a more professional role. The nursing profession promoted university-educated nurses who received baccalaureate degrees and could assume overall patient care responsibility. A second group were nurses trained in a 2-year technical program. Both the "professional" nurse and the "technical" nurse were eligible for the registration examination. Diploma and 1-year licensed practical nurse (LPN) programs were to be phased out.

Recently the nursing profession has suggested that only the baccalaureate nurse should be eligible for the RN examination. The number of diploma graduates has decreased, and the number of baccalaureate and associate degree nurses has increased, although these changes have not been without controversy.

Although there are more nurses than any other health professional group, many nurses have left the field because of salary and work condition constraints and other more attractive opportunities. In addition the rise in activity of hospital care has increased the demand for nursing personnel. The result has been a shortage of nurses available for patient care. Until such difficult issues as erratic hours, low pay, lack of esteem, and burnout associated with caring for ill patients are addressed adequately, nursing personnel are likely to be in short supply. Furthermore, careers previously not readily available to women, such as medicine and law, are now opening.

Dental Personnel. There are approximately 50,000 dentists licensed to practice in the United States. Dentistry has achieved great success in prevention, but also has become a troubled profession. Dentistry is largely a discretionary service and in times of economic stagnation people have a tendency to postpone using dental services. Dentistry frequently is not fully covered by insurance, increasing its price sensitivity. Advances in dentistry such as fluoridation of the public water supply and better oral hygiene have decreased the incidence of tooth decay and other oral health problems.

Dentists have changed the way they practice by using auxiliary personnel more effectively to increase the volume of services they provide. The use of four-handed dentistry also has improved productivity. Like medicine, dentistry benefited from the Health Professions Education Assistance Act, which increased the number of schools and class sizes. However, the current surplus supply of dentists has led to the closure of some schools and a downturn in the number of applicants to dental schools.

Auxiliary Personnel. During the 1960s and 1970s, in response to a perceived shortage of physicians, especially in primary care, and geographic maldistribution of physicians, various nonphysician professionals were promoted, including nurse practitioners and physician assistants. Nurse practitioners are registered nurses who receive 1 or 2 years of additional specialized clinical training leading to a certificate and sometimes a master's degree.

These programs provide the skills to do histories and physical examinations, to follow protocols for diagnosing common illnesses, and to provide limited clinical care, including prescribing certain medications. Increased access to care was intended to result from the decision of these professionals to practice in areas where a physician was unavailable or where a practice could efficiently use such practitioners.

The use of nurse practitioners and physician assistants has been limited by clinical and political struggles over where and under what conditions they can practice. State practice statutes and insurance billing procedures also have hindered their role. Finally, the increasing supply of physicians is leading to turf battles and a decreased role for some of these personnel, except in some prepaid settings and in physician practices where they can clearly increase the incomes and productivity of the physicians. Finally, the quality of care provided and patient satisfaction appear to be quite good when supervision is adequate.

FINANCING AND THE COST OF MEDICAL CARE

The United States spends over 11% of its gross national product on health care, or over 600 billion dollars per year (Table 65–10). Table 65–11 illustrates where these funds are spent. The hospital is the largest user of health care dollars. Although physicians account for under 20% of expenditures, they control many other resources. The United States spends a greater percentage of its gross national product on health care than any other nation, although the international differences have not always been so great (Table 65–12).

Questions have been raised as to whether longevity and morbidity differences between nations justify the great differences in national resources allocated to health care. The rapid escalation of health care costs and the increasing percentage of national productive resources required for health care has been a continuing serious concern throughout the twentieth century.

The largest payer of medical care expenses is government (about 40%), with private health insurance close behind (about 33%). Among governments, the federal government through the Medicare program has borne the greatest burden, although state and local resources have been stressed severely by health care costs.

A number of factors have contributed to the tremendous increase in the costs of medical care. Medical care is as sensitive as other goods and services to general inflationary pressures. The aging of the population, with elderly people using more health services, has increased costs. The growth in health insurance also has created increased use of the system because people with health insurance are more likely to use services (moral hazard in insurance terminology). Major technological innovations are now available to the consumer, such as growth in the number of intensive care beds and imaging techniques.

Reimbursement to Professionals. Physicians can be reimbursed through three mechanisms: fee-for-service, capitation, and salary. The predominant mode of reimbursement in this country is fee-for-service, where a physician renders care and the

TABLE 65-10. GROSS NATIONAL PRODUCT AND NATIONAL HEALTH EXPENDITURES: UNITED STATES

	National Health Expenditures	
Year	*Amount in Billions*	*Percent of Gross National Product*
1929	$ 3.6	3.5
1940	4.0	4.0
1950	12.7	4.4
1960	26.9	5.2
1970	75.0	7.4
1980	248.1	9.1
1988	539.9	11.1
1990 (est.)	615.0	12.1

From National Center for Health Statistics. Health, United States, 1990. Hyattsville, Md.: U.S. Public Health Service, 1991.

TABLE 65-11. NATIONAL HEALTH EXPENDITURES AND PERCENT DISTRIBUTION ACCORDING TO TYPE OF EXPENDITURE: UNITED STATES, SELECTED YEARS 1970 AND 1988

Type of Expenditure	1970	1988
Total (in billions)	$74.4	$539.9
All expenditures (percent)	100	100
Health services and supplies	93	96
Personal health care	87	89
Hospital care	38	39
Physician services	18	19
Dentist services	6	5
Nursing home care	7	8
Other professional services	2	4
Home health care	—	1
Drugs and other medical nondurables	12	8
Vision products and other medical durables	3	2
Other personal health care	2	2
Program administration net cost of health insurance	4	5
Government public health activities	2	3
Research and construction	7	4
Noncommercial research	3	2
Construction	5	2

From National Center for Health Statistics. Health, United States, 1990. Hyattsville, Md.: U.S. Public Health Service, 1991.

patient or third party (insurance company) reimburses the physician on a per service basis. This reimbursement frequently is computed based on usual, customary, and reasonable, or prevailing, fees. The physician receives a fee based on the physician's own fee history and on what other physicians in the community usually charge for the same service.

Capitation is more common in other countries.[16] In the United Kingdom the family physician receives a per capita payment based on the number of patients in their "panel." In exchange for this prospective payment the physician is obligated to provide all benefits mandated by the government. The capitation fee usually covers only primary care, with referral to hospital-based consultants for specialized and hospital care.

TABLE 65-12. TOTAL HEALTH EXPENDITURES AS A PERCENTAGE OF GROSS DOMESTIC PRODUCT: SELECTED COUNTRIES, SELECTED YEARS 1960 AND 1986

Country	1960	1986
Australia	4.6	6.8
Austria	4.6	8.0
Belgium	3.4	7.1
Canada	5.5	8.5
Denmark	3.6	6.1
Finland	4.2	7.5
France	4.2	8.5
Germany	4.7	8.1
Greece	2.9	3.9
Iceland	5.9	7.5
Ireland	4.0	7.9
Italy	3.3	6.7
Japan	3.0	6.7
Netherlands	3.9	8.3
New Zealand	4.4	6.9
Norway	3.3	6.8
Portugal	—	5.6
Spain	2.3	6.0
Sweden	4.7	9.1
Switzerland	3.3	8.0
United Kingdom	3.9	6.2
United States	5.2	11.1

A variant of capitation is used in some managed care systems in the United States under which the primary care physician receives a capitated fee to cover all of the services that an enrolled patient receives. This mechanism tends to decrease use of services by the physician, and it provides a powerful incentive to decrease the use of unnecessary or marginal services. It also may lower quality of care if physicians under use services that might otherwise be in the patients's best interest.

Salary usually is combined with some form of incentive reimbursement tied to productivity. Salary is more common outside the United States. In England the consulting physician, the hospital-based specialist, is paid on a salary. In this country many staff model Health Maintenance Organizations (HMOs) pay their physicians on a salaried basis.

Recently, physician reimbursement has received careful scrutiny.[17] The usual, customary, and reasonable fees paid by insurance carriers are based on physicians historical charge data and may over-value procedural as compared with cognitive services. In addition, some procedures that formerly were complex have become less so, but fees have not been reduced to reflect this change. Fee schedules based on the resources required to provide a specific service now have been developed. These fees consider the time and effort required, complexity of services, and any associated administrative costs. These resources-based relative value scales (RBRVS) will charge physician reimbursement by the federal government under Medicare and will likely be used by other payers as well.

Payment for preventive services such as counseling, screening procedures, and immunization frequently are not reimbursed. For example, Medicare will only reimburse the physician for pneumonia vaccination and hepatitis B vaccine in high-risk groups. It has only recently begun to reimburse for screening mammograms or pap smears, and it does not reimburse for influenza immunization, despite the demonstrated efficacy of that preventive service.

Institutional Reimbursement. Hospitals may be reimbursed based on charges. Patients (or less often insurers) receive an itemized bill representing all services obtained. Note that charges differ from costs. Hospitals cross-subsidize some services. For example, nursing care generally does not pay its way, and pharmacy, laboratory, and radiology often are "profit" generating. Patients are not charged the true costs of "hotel services," but they pay more for ancillary services to subsidize nursing. Costs reflect the institution's true cost of providing each service; charges reflect a somewhat arbitrary price assigned to service.

Under prospective payment, a facility receives a negotiated payment that is determined before services are rendered. A form of this type of payment is the reimbursement under Medicare Part A, DRGs.[18,19]

Until recently, retrospective cost reimbursement was common. Hospitals would determine their costs for providing care and would then bill insurance carriers and Medicare that proportion of total costs that carrier's subscribers incurred. This method has been criticized because it provides no incentives to contain costs.

Conversely, prospective reimbursement schemes have been praised for the incentives they provide to contain costs. The quality of care, especially as pertains to access restrictions, under utilization, and early discharge, has been inadequately addressed, however.[20]

Health Insurance. Most individuals have some health insurance. Health insurance does not easily fit the classical insurance model, which is oriented to infrequent, undesirable events. Insurance companies developed health care policies primarily so that they could offer a full line of products to customers.

The providers of health services themselves initiated the health insurance industry. The depression of the 1930s profoundly affected the hospital industry, as patients were unable to pay their bills. In response a Texas hospital developed a health insurance plan for school teachers, the forerunner of Blue Cross. This concept was adopted by other hospital associations who developed Blue Cross plans in their own states.

Medical societies adopted these hospital industry concepts to develop insurance to provide reimbursement to physicians. Blue Shield was thus developed. Blue Cross and Blue Shield, developed by the hospitals and physicians, were termed provider-sponsored plans. Although originally controlled by the providers, most provider-sponsored plans now have boards that are representative of the subscribers, with a minority representation of providers.

During World War II, prices and wages were frozen. Unions negotiated for fringe benefits rather than for wage increases. The commercial insurance companies entered the health care field marketing to companies.

Use of a plan is termed the experience of the group. Experience such as 280 bed days of hospital care per enrollee is used to compute the premium. Adverse selection occurs when a plan attracts enrollees who are unusually high users.

Premium rating based on a community experience is termed community rating. Premiums based on the experience of a specific group in the community is termed experience rating.

Financial arrangements between the enrollee, insurer, and providers vary as well. In indemnity plans, consumers (or employers) pay the premium to the plan. Providers bill the consumer who then submits a claim to the plan; there is no relationship between the plan and the provider. The provider may bill the consumer more or less than the plan will pay. The contractual relationships are between the plan and the consumer, and the consumer and the provider.

The exception is when the provider accepts assignment under which the consumer assigns the right to the claim to the provider. Under assignment, the plan pays the provider directly. The provider may agree to accept the assignment as payment in full for the service. In some instances, the providers may bill the patient for the difference between the charge and what the plan pays (balance billing).

A service plan involves a more complex contractual arrangement. The consumer (or employer) pays the premium to the plan. When the consumer visits the provider, the provider bills the plan; the plan pays the provider. Generally, the provider agrees, in advance, to accept the reimbursement as payment in full for the bill, except for any required copayments.

The Uninsured and Underinsured. Although a large proportion of the population has some health insurance coverage, currently over 30 million people are without any coverage (Table 65-13). Many of these people are employed or are dependents of employed individuals, often minimum wage earners. The problems associated with assuring financial access to care for this population is a continuing national issue.[21]

A second consideration is the extent of coverage by those who have health insurance. Hospital care is covered more frequently than outpatient physician services, which is covered more frequently than pharmacy benefits. Most plans have coinsurance requirements, a fixed portion of the bill that must be paid by the patient, or deductibles, an initial payment responsibility paid by the patient before coverage begins. Some indemnity plans leave patients responsible for fees charged in excess of

TABLE 65-13. HEALTH CARE COVERAGE (PERCENT) FOR PERSONS UNDER 65 YEARS OF AGE: UNITED STATES, 1986

Characteristics	Private Insurance	Medicaid[a]	Not Covered[b]
▪ **Total[c,d]**	75.9	5.9	15.3
▪ **Age (y)**			
Under 5	68.0	12.0	17.5
5–14	73.1	9.5	15.3
15–44	75.8	4.1	17.4
45–64	82.4	3.0	10.3
▪ **Sex**			
Male	76.4	4.8	15.8
Female	75.4	6.8	14.9
▪ **Race**			
White	79.1	4.0	14.0
Black	57.0	17.4	22.6
▪ **Family Income[c,e]**			
Less than $10,000	31.3	28.4	37.0
$10,000–14,999	58.1	.8.8	31.3
$15,000–19,999	72.6	2.7	21.2
$20,000–$34,999	88.3	1.0	8.4
$35,000 or more	93.7	0.4	3.9
▪ **Geographic Region[c]**			
Northeast	81.6	5.9	10.7
Midwest	79.7	7.6	10.9
South	71.6	5.1	19.2
West	72.9	5.1	18.8

[a] Includes persons receiving Aid to Families with Dependent Children or Supplemental Security Income or those with current Medicaid cards.
[b] Includes persons not covered by private insurance, Medicaid, Medicare, or military plans.
[c] Age adjusted.
[d] Includes all other races not shown separately and unknown family income.
[e] Family income categories for 1982 and 1986.

allowable reimbursements. About one third of all medical care costs are still paid out-of-pocket by the consumer.

Managed Care. New insurance approaches to contain costs include managed care plans. A popular managed care approach has been the HMO, which is both a financing and an organizational mechanism.[22,23] In HMOs the consumer contracts with a plan and pays a prospective monthly premium. The plan, in turn, contracts with providers (primarily hospitals and physicians) to provide care for enrolled patients. The providers often are at financial risk because the income received must cover all care needed. Thus there is a tremendous incentive to use resources wisely or to "manage patients' care." These incentives also have appealed to the government, and a number of risk-sharing prepaid contracts are now used in the Medicare program.[22]

There are two types of HMOs: closed panel or staff model and the independent practice association (IPA). In the staff model HMO the plan contracts with, or directly hires, providers who care exclusively for enrollees in the plan. The enrollees must, except in emergencies, use the providers specified by the plan.

The IPA (or open model or foundation HMO) contracts with community-based providers, who are not exclusively bound to the enrollees in the plan and who care for other patients as well. These plans often provide for financial risk-sharing arrangements with providers; usually have strong peer review systems to control "unnecessary" use; and may impose barriers to free use of services, such as prehospitalization authorization or required second opinions before surgery.

HMOs have achieved some cost advantages through decreased use of inpatient hospital services. HMOs generally have increased use of ambulatory services by patients. These plans have been especially successful in the western United States and in certain parts of the Midwest.[24,25]

A more recent type of managed care system is the Preferred Provider Organization (PPO).[26,27] In a PPO, the plan negotiates with the community-based providers to obtain discounted fees. Patients must use contracted providers for maximum coverage. If an enrollee uses other providers, the plan's reimbursement is reduced substantially. In the Exclusive Provider Organization (EPO), a variation of the PPO, the enrollee has no coverage for care provided outside the contracted care.

Governmental Insurance Programs. In addition to private insurance, two major public insurance plans operate in the United States: Title 18 (Medicare) and Title 19 (Medicaid) of the Social Security Act. These programs were enacted in 1966 with the intention of providing financial access to medical care for the nation's poor and elderly. Both programs have been revised many times in response to cost containment pressures, quality and utilization concerns, and various political factors.

Medicare is a federal program with two parts: A and B. Medicare eligibility generally includes those people aged 65 years and over, the permanently and totally disabled, and people with end-stage renal disease. Part A is financed by a Medicare trust fund composed of contributions from employers and employees. Part B is financed by a monthly premium for enrollees and general federal funds. Part A was established to resemble Blue Cross, and Part B was established to resemble Blue Shield. Originally, Part A reimbursed hospitals on a service plan basis, based on retrospective costs. In 1986 the method of reimbursement was changed to prospective payment. All diagnoses and conditions were categorized based on resource requirements for the inpatient care in nearly 500 DRGs. Hospitals are paid a prospectively determined fixed dollar amount based on a patient's DRG category. If the hospital can provide the required care for less than the reimbursement, it keeps the difference. If more money is required to care for the patient, the hospital is required to provide that care with no additional reimbursement, except for certain "outliers," or special cases of justified extra care.

Part B of Medicare reimburses physicians based on a percentage of the usual, customary, and prevailing fee, like an indemnity plan. Some physicians accept assignment as payment-in-full, except for co-payments, and this is actively encouraged by Medicare. Reimbursement of physicians is undergoing change. Medicare has begun to reimburse using Resource-based Relative Value Scales (RBRUS) instead of usual and customary reimbursement. This system will increase financial rewards for primary care physicians doing cognitive work and decrease rewards for physicians who do procedures, such as surgeons.

Because of the program's benefits, deductibles, co-insurance, and premiums, Medicare only pays for approximately 50% of the total cost of medical care for the eligible population. There is minimal coverage for nursing home care, a serious concern for this population group.

Medicaid is a joint federal-state program. The states administer and jointly fund Medicaid programs and agree to provide a minimum set of services to recipients. These services include inpatient and outpatient care, physician's office care, laboratory, x-ray, family planning services, mental health benefits, and early periodic diagnostic screening and treatment services. The federal government requires that these services be provided to the categorically needy, a determination based on income levels. The proportion of the federal government's financial participation is based on a formula that considers the state's wealth and other factors.

States may expand the scope of benefits, with the federal government paying its proportion of such costs as ambulance services, durable medical equipment, and chiropractic care. The states' eligibility levels for Medicaid benefits are subject to certain federal guidelines. States may elect to cover the medically needy as well as the categorically needy. There is limited uniformity between the states in the Medicaid programs, which has led to considerable inequity across the nation.

The categorically needy are people who receive cash payments under the Supplemental Security Income (SSI-welfare payments) program. These people include those who are blind, those who are permanently and totally disabled, the aged, and those who receive aid to families with dependent children. People in these categories who are not poor are ineligible for Medicaid; people who are poor but do not fit one of the categories also are not eligible. The medically indigent can be covered at the election of the state. This category is comprised of individuals who have more income than the official poverty level and fit one of the SSI categories, but whose medical expenses put them below the official poverty level.

The range of benefits and eligibility requirements across the country is complex and confusing. Moreover, these programs are frequently so underfunded that providers receive only limited reimbursement. These concerns, and the paperwork involved in claims, is such that many providers do not participate in Medicaid programs at all. Although these programs were intended to provide a "safety net" for the poor, their success has been somewhat limited.

THE FUTURE

It is obvious that there are problems with the health care "system." Many of these problems will require action by policymakers. The pendulum swings between the competing issues of assuring access to quality care and providing such care at a reasonable cost.[29] The major concerns of this past decade have surrounded the costs of health care.

Changes in reimbursement policy have changed how providers are doing business. Hospitals have closed, multi-hospital systems have been created, joint venture by physicians and hospitals is popular, group practice has grown, and managed care has proliferated. There will continue to be new experiments in the delivery of health care, especially to further address issues of the cost of care. But serious access problems continue to exist. The aging of the population also represents a challenge that must be dealt with, especially as regards long-term care.

Government has only relatively recently been a major player in health care, but increasingly government is being asked to solve the problems of the health care system, even in the face of government's own increasingly disturbing financial problems. Government will continue to be involved in the decision making about how health is organized, delivered, and paid for. Our nation must choose wisely to assure both high quality care and access for all of our citizens.

REFERENCES

1. Torrens P: Historical evolution and overview of health services in the United States. In Williams SJ, Torrens PR (eds): Introduction to Health Services, 3 edt. Albany, N.Y.: Delmar Publishing Co, 1988, chap 1
2. Nutter D: Access to care and the evolution of corporate for-profit medicine. N Engl J Med 311:919, 1984
3. Watt JA, Derzon RA, Renn SC, et al: The comparative economic performance of investor-owned chain and not-for-profit hospitals. N Engl J Med 314:89, 1986
4. Gray BH, McNerney WJ: For-profit enterprise in health care: The Institute of Medicine Study. N Engl J Med 314:1523–1528, 1986
5. Mullner RM, McNeil D: Rural and urban hospital closures. Health Aff 5:131–140, 1986
6. Rosenblatt R, Moscovice I: Rural Health Care. New York: Wiley, 1982
7. National Center for Health Statistics. National Ambulatory Medical Care Survey: Background and Methodology. Washington, D.C.: U.S. Department of Health, Education, and Welfare Publication No. (HRA) 76-1335, 1976
8. Hwulic PL: Medical Groups in the U.S., 1984. Chicago: American Medical Association, 1985
9. Williams SJ: Ambulatory care: Can hospitals compete? Hospital and Health Services Administration 28(5):22–34, 1983
10. Ermann D, Gabel J: The changing face of American health care: Multihospital systems, emergency centers, and surgery centers. Med Care 23:401–420, 1985
11. Evashwick C, Weiss L: Managing the Continuum of Care: A Practical Guide to Organization and Operations. Rockville, Md.: Aspen Publishers, 1987
12. Doty P, Liu K, Wiener J: An overview of long-term care. Health Care Financing Rev 6(3):69–78, 1985
13. National Center for Health Statistics: An overview of the 1982 National Master Facility Inventory Survey of nursing and related care homes. Advanced Data from Vital and Health Statistics, No. 111. DHHS Publication No. (PHS) 85-1250. Hyattsville, Md.: Public Health Service, 1985
14. Harrington C, Newcomer R, Estes C: Long-Term Care of the Elderly: Public Policy Issues. Beverly Hills, Calif.: Sage Publications, 1985
15. Report of the Graduate Medical Education Advisory Committee to the Secretary, DHHS, Vol 1: GMENAC Summary Report. Washington, D.C.: U.S. Department of Health and Human Services Publication No. (HRA) 81-653, 1980
16. Reinhardt UE: The compensation of physicians: Approaches used in foreign countries. QRB 11:366–377, 1985
17. Hadley J: How should Medicare pay physicians? Milbank Mem Fund Q 62:279–299, 1984
18. Mitchell JB: Physician DRGs. N Engl J Med 313:670–675, 1985
19. Wennberg JE, McPherson K, Caper P, et al: Will payment based on diagnosis-related groups control hospital costs? N Engl J Med 311:295–300, 1984
20. Iglehart JK: Early experience with prospective payment of hospitals. N Engl J Med 23:401–420, 1985
21. Blendon RJ, Aiken LH, Freeman HE, et al: Uncompensated care by hospitals or public insurance for the poor. N Engl J Med 314:1160–1163, 1986
22. Iglehart JK: Medicare turns to HMOs. N Engl J Med 312:132–136, 1985
23. Adamache KW, Rossiter LJ: The entry of HMOs into the Medicare market: Implications for TEFRA's mandate. Inquiry 23:349–364, 1986
24. Cromley EK, Shannon GW: The establishment of Health Maintenance Organizations: A geographical analysis. Am J Public Health 73:184–187, 1983
25. Anderson OW, Herold T, Butler R, et al: HMO Development: Patterns and Prospects. A Comparative Analysis of HMOs. Chicago: University of Chicago, Center for Health Administration Studies, 1985
26. Gabel J, Ermann D, Rice T, et al: The emergence and future of PPOs. J Health Polit Policy Law 11:305–322, 1986
27. De Lissovoy G, Rice T, Ermann D, et al: Preferred provider organizations: Today's models and tomorrow's prospects. Inquiry 23:7–15, 1986
28. Glandon GL, Morrisey MA: Redefining the hospital-physician relationship under prospective payment. Inquiry 23:166–175, 1986
29. Luft HS: Competition and regulation. Med Care 23:383–400, 1985

66

Health Planning and Evaluation

Thomas G. Rundall

Planning for health involves three types of activities: assessment of the current status, identification of the desired state in the future, and specification of interventions and other activities that will effect the necessary changes to achieve the new desired state. Planning may focus on achieving changes in the characteristics of individuals (such as knowledge, attitudes, health risk behaviors, and health status), in the characteristics of organizations (such as cost, availability, and quality of services), or in the physical, economic, legal, and social characteristics of the environments in which people work and live. In the most comprehensive of planning efforts, the focus may be broad and include all of the structures and processes described above.

These activities are central to the mission of public health. Affirmation of the importance of planning to an effective public health system is provided by the recent Institute of Medicine report *The Future of Public Health.*[1] The Committee for the Study of Public Health found that "the core functions of public health agencies at all levels of government are assessment, policy development, and assurance." To assess public health needs, the Committee recommends that every public health agency regularly and systematically collect, assemble, analyze, and make available information on the health of the community, including statistics on health status, community health needs, and epidemiological and other studies of health problems. With regard to policy development, the Committee recommends that every public health agency exercise its responsibility to serve the public interest in the development of comprehensive public policies by promoting the use of the scientific knowledge base in decision-making about public health and by leading in developing public health policy. Agencies are encouraged to take a strategic approach, developed on the basis of a positive appreciation for the democratic political process. The Institute of Medicine Committee further recommends that public health agencies assure their constituents that services necessary to achieve agreed upon goals are provided, either by encouraging actions by other entities (private or public sector), by requiring such action through regulation, or by providing services directly.

Planning for change requires a wide range of skills and insights. Assessing the status quo typically entails the use of data collection and analysis skills. Identifying the desired future state is largely a matter of values, and determining what should be done to effect the desired changes is a complicated process that requires expert knowledge of theories of social and behavioral change, technical knowledge of how organizations and health care systems operate, and in-depth understanding of a community's values, beliefs, politics, and patterns of interaction. Thus the process of health planning requires many different skills. As Shonick[2] has written:

> Many in the planning field work almost exclusively in one of these aspects. Others are involved with the entire process. For those working primarily at determining the status quo, the task mainly requires information acquisition skills, analysis technique, and availability of data. For those concerned mainly with the final outcome, value systems and views of ethics influence choices. Desired ends are usually determined mainly by the power relations within and among the groups that commission the planning, such as legislative bodies and corporate boards of all sorts. These are often affected, however, by analysis of value systems that uncover hidden implications of pursuing different goals and objectives . . . Determining approaches for achieving the desired outcomes, once these are agreed upon, often calls for considerable technical skill in areas like decision theory to help in choosing alternative ways to achieve the desired outcomes. If the planners also have responsibilities for facilitating the implementation of the adopted plan, then skills in achieving consensus are also frequently needed. . . .

It should be clear from the above discussion that the role of planning in directing and attaining social change of a specific and desired nature place it in distinct opposition to laissez faire market principles that make up the dominant political and economic value system in the United States. Although some have argued that planning is actually a preferred instrument of social change,[3] others have argued that planning inevitably distorts desirable market forces that efficiently allocate resources and should, at best, be restricted to planning how to use private interests and free markets for public purposes.[4] The middle ground on this issue is to invoke formal planning as a means to correct gross distortions in the supply or allocation of goods and services that are created when the markets for those goods and services are themselves flawed (e.g., not satisfying the requirements of a "free market").[5]

These different views of planning, often deeply embedded in political ideologies and value systems, have surrounded health planning efforts in the United States with a climate of tension, mistrust, and at times open hostility. This is not surprising, because the planning process explicitly exposes the implicit planning that often has benefited powerful professions and institutions. Hence the acceptance of broad health planning efforts by these interests and by the populations served by the health system has waxed and waned with the popularity of government intervention in social problems generally, and more specifically, with the public's concern over inequities in health and access to health services.[2]

THREE TYPES OF PLANNING

The type of planning that is done depends on who the client agency is and on what the focus of concern is. The three most common clients are official health agencies charged with representing the interests of an entire population in a specified region, specific health service institutions, and specific health programs. The planning done for these clients is designated as population-based planning, institution-based planning, and program planning, respectively.

Population-based Planning. Population-based planning attempts to study the entire population of a designated region to specify the changes in existing resources needed to meet the health service requirements of that population. This type of planning for the organization and delivery of health services began in the United States in the 1930s as voluntary efforts by hospital associations, medical societies, and other groups. The focus of these early planning efforts was the coordination of services provided by municipal public health and welfare departments and hospitals, primarily for the purpose of increasing access to health services for indigent people. Without regulatory or other enforcement powers, reform of the structure of the health care system was beyond the reach of these early planning organizations. The first organized attempt at planning for the coordination of services was initiated in the 1930s in New York City with the founding of the Hospital Council of Greater New York. During the ensuing decade a number of cities, including Rochester, New York, and Detroit, followed New York's example. These efforts were supported in large measure by philanthropies that wanted to ensure that the investments they were making in the medical care system were being put to wise use.[6]

Spurred on by the recommendations of the prestigious Committee on the Costs of Medical Care, which was formed in 1927 to study the organization, financing, and use of the U.S. health care system, health planning became more firmly established in the 1940s under the auspices of federal and state governments. The Committee specifically recommended the establishment of state and local agencies for the purposes of conducting research and developing plans for coordinating health services. It further recommended that health planning efforts adopt the concept of regionalization of health services as detailed in the Dawson Report issued 12 years earlier in the United Kingdom.[6]

Three principles emerged from this era that dominated health planning efforts through the 1970s. First is the notion that planning ought to be a participatory process that occurs within voluntary organizations. Second is that an important goal of health planning is the creation of a regionalized health system, that is, a division of functions among hospitals, clinics, and medical personnel based on vertically integrated levels of specialization. Third is that health planning should be minimally disruptive to established patterns of medical practice, a principle that was often in conflict with principle 2 but that was politically necessary to maintain the support of established medical institutions for health planning.

After World War II, concerns over the health status of the population, the maldistribution of hospitals, and the poor condition of most hospitals prompted the federal government to establish the nation's first major health services planning and construction subsidy program, The Hill-Burton Program (The Hospital Survey and Construction Act of 1946). Since the initiation of the federal government's involvement with the Hill-Burton Program, the objectives, scope, and organization of planning were largely determined by federal policy as expressed in a continuing stream of legislation, including the Regional Medical Programs; the Heart Disease, Cancer and Stroke Act of 1965 (P.L. 89–239); the Comprehensive Health Planning Program; the Partnership for Health Act of 1967 (P.L. 90–174); the Experimental Health Services Delivery Program; and the National Health Planning and Resources Development Act of 1974 (p. 329).[6]

Although each of these measures required planning efforts on the part of communities and states as a condition of receiving federal funds, planning efforts throughout the 1950s and 1960s were structurally, fiscally, and politically unable to bring about the kinds of changes that were necessary to significantly affect the cost, quality, and accessibility of health services. In the 1970s, as the primary concern of government shifted from increasing access to health services to control of health sector costs, the federal government attempted to correct the deficiencies in the health planning system, particularly the principle of noninterference with existing patterns of practice, with the passage of the National Health Planning and Resources Development Act of 1974 and subsequent amendments to this legislation.

The basic framework for planning defined by this legislation consisted of a two-tiered state and regional structure. At the regional level, health systems agencies (HSAs) were established as nonprofit corporations or government agencies with boards comprised of representatives of the general public, health care providers, third-party payers, and politicians (maintaining the principle of participatory planning). The HSA's principal mission was to develop plans for its health services area and to communicate these plans to the State Health Planning and Development Agency (SHPDA) and to the State Health Coordinating Committee (SHCC), an advisory body of the SHPDA.[6]

The National Health Planning and Resources Development Act of 1974 explicitly defined the products that each of these organizations was expected to produce. These included long-range comprehensive plans (e.g., state health facilities plans) and shorter range plans for implementing the longer range plans (e.g., annual implementation plans). All plans were supposed to be based on current quantitative information about populations' health service needs and about the cost, quality, and availability of health services.

Population-based planning as implemented as part of these local and state plans involved what Shonick[2] describes as

> estimating existing health service utilization compared with appropriate health service utilization, determining the consequent deficit or surplus in utilization, and outlining a strategy for transition from existing to appropriate levels of utilization, which may also involve a transition from existing to appropriate levels of resources.

The plans prepared by the HSAs were typically for 5-year terms with 1-year short-term plans that were revised each subsequent year based on the prior year's experience.[7]

The power to enforce health plans was largely embodied in provisions of the statute that required states to enact a certificate-of-need law and to establish within its SHPDA means for determining which proposals for new or expanded facilities conformed with needs documented in the state's health plans. The intent was for the SHPDA to deny requests for new or expanded facilities that were not needed.

Unfortunately, even this strengthened planning system was unable to achieve the long sought after twin goals of increased access to care and control of health care costs. Political opposition to the certificate-of-need facility approval process came from, among others, hospitals and other providers who wished to expand individual facilities or develop new facilities, from communities that wanted facilities that the local and state planning processes had determined were unnecessary, and from politicians who objected to having politically sensitive decisions such as governmental support for local hospital development located outside their sphere of influence. As a result the health planning system became a battleground for competing financial and political interests, resulting in numerous overrides of certificate-of-need refusals and many time-consuming and costly legal challenges. In the end the nation's confidence in the ability of the planning system to achieve its objectives, particularly the control of health care costs, eroded. With the resurgence of conservative political ideology in the 1980s and the broad movement to replace regulation in all sorts of industries with market forces as the means of making resource allocation decisions and controlling inflation, political support for health planning withered. In 1986 the U.S. Congress rejected efforts to renew the centerpiece health planning legislation, and since then the national network of planning agencies has been dismantled.

Although federal support for regional and state planning agencies was phased out during the 1980s, a few HSAs have remained active with state and local support. In addition, many state and local health departments have continued population-based planning, particularly for traditional public health services such as childhood immunizations and public health nursing. As the cost of health care continues to grow into the 1990s, population-based planning, linked to a more effective system of cost control, may once again be proposed as a means to channel development of new health services to areas in greatest need.

Institution-based Planning. Institution-based planning involves determining what types and levels of service the institution (such as a hospital, health maintenance organization, or neighborhood health center) needs to accomplish its defined mission, and then proceeding to market services to the required clientele. The major difference between population-based and institution-based planning is that the latter attempts to define only a subset of the regional population as its "market," and the institutional plan may well call for serving clients from outside the regional area.

The institutional planning tasks begin with defining the present market for the services the institution provides and estimating the future demand required to meet the service objectives adopted by the institution. The resources required to meet this projected demand are then estimated, and a work plan for transforming the existing institutional utilization level and resources to the called-for utilization and resources is the end product of the planning process.

Program Planning. Program planning incorporates aspects of both of the other types of planning. It resembles population-based planning because for each type of program service (AIDS prevention education, for example) the planning process identifies target populations, attempts to determine their needs, estimates the services required to meet those needs, and proposes an allocation of resources for providing those services. In developing the details of the plan, the methods of population-based planning often are used because the primary aim of most categorical health programs is to achieve desired changes in the health status of a population. Program planning does, however, share some characteristics with institution-based planning. The request for a program plan is almost always initiated by an institution, and it is typically the case that some changes in the services provided or in the ways in which services are provided are an integral part of a program plan designed to improve the health of a target population.

Program planning is probably the most common type of planning currently being done in the United States, and since program planning incorporates many of the features of population-based and institution-based planning, the remainder of this chapter will focus on health program planning. In the following sections the numerous steps required in the development of a program plan and in the evaluation of a health program are presented in detail.

DEVELOPING A PROGRAM PLAN

Planning activities are crucial to the success of any intervention designed to improve the health of the public. Whether the intervention focuses on health education, environmental protection, health services delivery, or any other aspect of public health and preventive medicine, a plan is critical because it provides a guide for the development of the intervention, specifying what is considered the status quo, the goals for the intervention program, and how those goals will be achieved.

The Program Planning Process. Plans for health programs include many components that are interconnected, and the process by which plans are developed, implemented, evaluated, and revised is a complicated one. Figure 66–1, adapted from Dignan and Carr,[8] depicts the program planning framework typically used in health education and health promotion programs. An extensive process of analyzing a community's health problems, prioritizing health concerns, identifying practical pathways to change, and identifying the appropriate level, or units, at which the intervention will be targeted should precede the development of the program plan. Once these important and often difficult steps are taken, the essential components of a program plan, as defined in Table 66–1, may be prepared.

The first component of a program plan is a statement of goals. More specific statements of measurable objectives, meth-

TABLE 66–1. COMPONENTS OF HEALTH PROGRAM PLANS

Program Plan Components	Definition
Statements of goals	Broad statements that define what the health program is expected to accomplish.
Objectives	Specific statements of activities and outcomes needed to reach a goal, including a time frame, a strong verb, a single purpose, and a single result or end-product.
Methods and activities	The means through which the changes will be made. Methods identify the vehicle for change, such as mass media or regulatory legislation. Activities describe the specific things that will be done to implement the change methodology.
Resources and constraints	Specific resources in the target community that may be used for the program to bring about change. Constraints are forces that are expected to work against the program.
Evaluation plan	Procedures for the collection and analysis of information to determine program performance.
Implementation plan	Procedures for introducing the program to the target group.

From Dignan MB, Carr PA: Program Planning for Health Education and Health Promotion. Philadelphia: Lea & Febiger, 1987

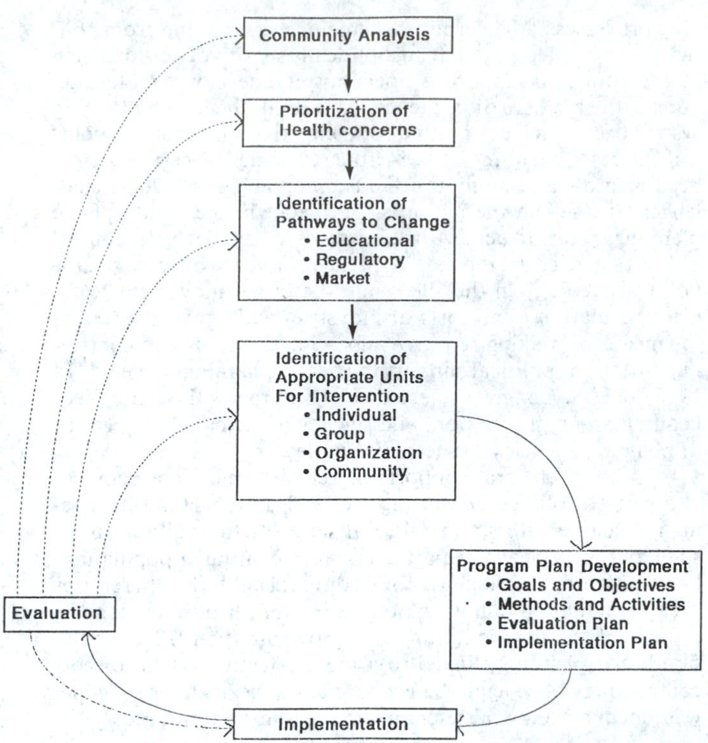

Figure 66-1. The program planning framework. *[Adapted from Dignan MB, Carr PA: Program Planning for Health Education and Health Promotion. Philadelphia: Lea & Febiger, 1987.]*

ods, activities, resources, and constraints also should be included in the plan. The evaluation of the program should be considered carefully at the outset of the planning process, and an evaluation plan should be included in the overall planning document. Finally, an implementation plan, the procedures that will be followed to introduce the program to the target group, also should be included.

Developing a health program plan obviously is a complicated task, one requiring the input of numerous individuals who have various technical skills and perspectives. It is especially important during the planning process to include the views of those who will be affected by the program. Hence, the first step in the planning process is to organize a working planning group.

Organizing a Working Planning Group. The development of a program plan is a complex and time consuming task. To make the effort manageable and to assure input into the plan from differing points of view, planning usually is done by a group rather than by a single individual.

Planning Group Membership. Planning groups may be created in any number of ways. A key member of the group, such as the project director, may appoint the other members. The make-up of the group also may be dictated by a funding source. Groups that are likely to receive the programs' services may select representatives to participate in program planning. Important prerequisites for membership on a planning group are interest in improving the health of the target population, willingness to work with other group members, good communication skills, and dependability. One very important additional consideration in creating a planning group is the inclusion of representatives from the target group. There are several advantages to including target group representatives in a planning group. These representatives provide the planning group with the viewpoint of those who will be most directly affected by the program. They bring to the planning discussions an understanding of the problems experienced by the target group, the values and belief systems that importantly affect behavior, and a sense of the limits of acceptable intervention program activities and policies. Moreover, when members of the target group participate actively in the planning process, there is a feeling of ownership of the program being planned, which facilitates implementation of the program and encourages participation.

Community Participation. As indicated above, community participation in the planning process is essential to the development of successful program plans. Occasionally, entire target groups participate in program planning. In these instances the target populations are relatively small, and virtually all members must be motivated to solve the problem under consideration. More often, individuals volunteer to serve as members of the planning group. Although this means of gaining community participation assures that planning group members will be motivated, volunteers may not always represent the view of the majority in a target population. When individuals have hidden agendas or unspoken goals, the planning process or the program itself may be misdirected. Identifying and resolving hidden agendas of planning group members is an important step in developing a successful program plan. Hidden agendas may be identified through individual sessions with planning group members, key informants, or through group process exercises with the entire planning group. Although this is a difficult process to go through, once any existing hidden agendas are resolved, the group can more readily agree on common goals for the program and the procedures to be used to develop the program plan.

Organizers of program planning groups should be wary of selecting those persons from a target group that may be most friendly or visible. It is essential to recruit persons who can communicate the felt needs of the target group to other members of the planning group. Community representatives must be familiar with the lifestyle and beliefs related to the health practices of the target group, and they must be able to provide insight into the probable reactions of the target population to the intervention program. By assuring such community participation in the program planning process, the program activities designed to improve health will be appropriate for the target group and, most importantly, will be accepted by them.

Orientation to the Task of Planning. The first step in activating the planning group is to orient the group to the process of planning a health program. Because planning groups may have members with widely varying experiences with the program planning process, it is important to familiarize all planning group members with the nature of health promotion or disease prevention programs and with the process to be followed in developing the specific program plan under consideration. Planning group members should understand that the health program is designed to meet identified needs of the target group, and that the plan must take into account the health-related practices, customs, and beliefs of the target group as well as the norms, laws, and economic conditions that prevail in the community and may affect the program. When each member understands the nature of the planning task, the roles to be played by various group members should be identified.

Role Negotiation. An important outcome of the orientation process is for each group member to understand how the planning task ahead relates to his or her own area of expertise. Each person should be asked to identify the skills and knowledge they bring to the planning process and to suggest how they may best contribute to the planning tasks. After the group has identified the activities and skills required to complete the planning process, the roles for the group members may be negotiated. Roles that frequently are found within planning groups include chairperson, recorder, treasurer, writer or editor, facilitator, meeting coordinator, data analyst, and target group representative or agency representative. Role negotiation may be an uncomfortable experience for some members of the planning group, especially for target group members who may feel that they do not bring specialized skills to the task. The importance of their contribution must be recognized formally, however, and all members of the planning group must come to feel that they have a role that is valued by the entire group.

Delegation of Responsibility. Up to the time when roles are negotiated, one or two individuals may have carried the responsibility for establishing the planning group and coordinating the program planning process. With the clarification and negotiation of roles, however, the responsibilities of the original group organizers may be delegated to others. Each member of the planning group should be encouraged to assume some specific responsibilities for the program. It is important that the bulk of responsibility not be delegated to one person, since this will only serve to overwhelm one unfortunate group member and to dilute the sense of ownership of the process among the other members.

Once role negotiation is completed and specific responsibilities have been delegated to group members, the group is ready to plan a program.

Formulating Program Goals. Goal statements typically represent the first concrete step in the process of planning programs for specific community health problems. Goals are broad statements that indicate what programs are intended to accomplish. Goals are important because they provide a vision of how the targeted community and health problem should be changed as a result of the intervention program. Planning group members must reach a consensus on a programs' goals; therefore these statements tend to be somewhat global, lacking specific details over which group members might easily disagree. Examples of goal statements for health programs include:

1. Residents of Monterey County will have a reduced prevalence of uncontrolled hypertension.
2. Cigarette smoking among students at Alexander High School will be reduced substantially.
3. Knowledge about the risk factors for infection with human immunodeficiency virus will be increased among the residents of Oak Creek City.

Goal statements need to be verified by the target population and the program sponsors. Because goals provide the framework for the rest of the program and, in particular, drive the specification of program objectives, the goals must reflect a realistic solution to the problems of the target population in terms of change that is both desirable and feasible. Acceptance of program goals by the program sponsors also is important because, ultimately, they will be asked to provide support for the program. Gaining the program sponsor's agreement on goal statements provides assurance of support before the difficult process of formulating objectives begins.

Specifying Program Objectives. Program objectives are precise statements that identify the tasks necessary to achieve the program's goal. The notion is that a number of specific objectives could be stated that describe what program activities must take place; what changes in the characteristics, organizations, and communities must occur as a result of these activities; and what specific outcomes must be observed for the goal to be achieved.

Numerous frameworks for specifying objectives have been proposed. One common approach to formulating objectives, particularly in the field of education, is to state behavioral objectives. Every behavioral objective includes a statement of a test stimulus and its intended reaction, namely, the correct response by someone who has the desired skill, knowledge, or attitude.

The form of a behavioral objective is that, given a specified stimulus, there will be a specified response. Examples of behavioral objectives in the health field include the following:

- Given a list of menu items, the dietician will identify the number of calories contained in each item.
- Given a list of modes of transmission of infectious diseases, the student will correctly identify the ways in which HIV is transmitted.
- Given six advertisements for cigarette smoking, the trained observer will identify correctly the psychological principles at work.

There are two major problems with this type of behavioral objective:

1. Behavioral objectives tend to be used only for describing ends intended by the program (outcome objectives), not means (what some have called program operation and bridging objectives).
2. Behavioral objectives tend to focus on the individual learner as that which is being evaluated rather than on the program.

These problems often are compounded when behavioral objectives are made relative: when the level of response that is considered to be satisfactory varies for each individual depending on the starting point. This often is referred to as goal attainment scaling (GAS). An example of a behavioral objective stated in the GAS Framework is

> Given a list of menu items, the dietician will correctly identify the number of calories contained in 20 items more than before the program.

The problems with GAS are

1. It is time consuming and expensive for large scale studies involving many targets.
2. It runs counter to the intervention approaches of the many programs that are concerned with consistent outcome results for the target population.
3. GAS may result in lower program effects by equating "success" with the minimal impacts achievable with each program participant.

For these reasons, behavioral objectives and GAS should be used with caution in program evaluation. Finally, it is important to note that many contemporary health promotion or disease prevention programs focus on changing characteristics of environments such as changing environmental regulations, economic incentives, and norms pertaining to risk behaviors, none of which lend themselves well to goal attainment scaling of behavioral objectives.

An alternative strategy for writing objectives, which builds on some initial suggestions by Shortell and Richardson,[9] is presented:

> Definition: A well-stated objective is a clear statement: (1) using strong verbs, (2) stating only one purpose or aim, (3) specifying a single end-product or result, and (4) specifying the expected time frame for achievement.

A strong verb is an action-oriented verb that describes an observable or measurable behavior, attitude, knowledge, or physical status that will occur; examples are "write," "increase," "identify," "start," "attend." Examples of weaker, nonspecific verbs are "promote," "enhance," "encourage," and "understand."

An objective should state only a single purpose. Two or more purposes will require different implementation and assessment strategies, making achievement of an objective difficult to determine. An example of such a dual-purpose objective is

> To begin three prenatal classes for pregnant women and provide outreach transportation services to accommodate 25 women per class.

If one purpose is accomplished but not the other, to what extent has the objective been met? It is better to break up multiple-purpose objectives into single-purpose ones.

An objective should specify a single end product or result. Sometimes an aim or purpose is stated, but there is no indication of what end product or result will serve as evidence that the aim or purpose has been achieved. Consider the following objective:

> To establish communication with the health systems agency.

Is the intended end result one phone call? Two phone calls? One phone call and one interdepartmental meeting? Also, statements such as the following specify an end product but no aim or purpose:

> To provide all monthly discharge abstracts to the Commission on Professional and Hospital Activities.

Surely this can be achieved without being sure what purpose is intended. Such activities come close to being rituals and are not the sort that one wants to devote much evaluation to. The purpose or aim describes what will be accomplished; the end product or result describes evidence that will exist when it has been done. Finally, an objective should state the time of expected achievement by specifying a target date or period.

An example of a well-stated objective for a school-based antismoking program might be

> To reduce the prevalence of serious smoking (ten or more cigarettes a month) among participants in a peer counseling program as indicated by a 50% reduction in self-reported serious smoking within 6 months.

Identification of Intervention Methods. Once the program goals and objectives have been identified, the planning group must determine how the objectives will be achieved. In some cases, the objectives explicitly state the intended method or activity to be used to produce change. In other cases the objectives may be met in any of several different ways, and the planning group must decide which method will be implemented.

Intervention methods describe how change is to be achieved in the target group. For example, smoking behavior could be affected by a number of different intervention methods including behavior modification, mass media, peer counseling, and tobacco tax reform. The choice of which method to use depends on the acceptability of the method within the target population, the literacy of the target population, convenience of use, feasibility, anticipated effectiveness, and cost. Most importantly, program planners should be able to provide a plausible rationale for their expectation that the use of a given method will result in the desired change in the target population. This rationale should be grounded in one or more theories of social or behavioral change, preferably building on the experience of prior programs that targeted similar health issues. Many intervention methods are used in health programs. Dignan and Carr[8] and Green et al.[10] provide useful summaries of commonly used health program intervention methods.

Estimating Resources and Constraints. The planning group must identify specific resources that exist within the target group and from other sources that can be used to implement the health program. Needed resources usually include money, facilities, supplies, volunteer workers, and political support. Although the program sponsor may provide most of the resources needed to implement the program, identifying other sources of support provides the potential for enriching the program's services and broadens the base of support for the program.

The program plan also should anticipate potential barriers to program success. These would include shortages of any of the resources identified above, legal and ethical limitations on program activities, organized opposition from vested interest groups, difficulty in reaching the target population, and bureaucratic red tape in acquiring the cooperation of large complex organizations.

Once resources and constraints have been identified, some revision of the program plan may be required. Goal statements, objectives, and intervention methods may have to be adjusted in light of a realistic appraisal of the resources available and the number and types of constraints the project will face.

Implementation of Program Activities. An essential step in health program planning is the development of a plan for program implementation. This plan specifies the necessary sequence of events that is required to put the program into action. Implementation plans typically cover five aspects of program implementation.

1. Personnel hiring, orientation, and training.
2. Specification of schedules and routine tasks.
3. Establishment of management systems.
4. Gaining acceptance of the program from the target group.
5. Marketing the program.

As the implementation plan is carried out, all assumptions about the availability of resources, cooperation with other agencies, accessibility of the target population, and other aspects of the program plan are tested. Some, perhaps many, of these assumptions will prove incorrect. Indeed, virtually all programs go through a period of change as program staff learn about the program's real environment and adapt their activities to the opportunities, resources, and constraints actually present.

Assessing the Effect of the Program. It is always best to consider program evaluation in detail during the planning process, when there is still time to weigh alternative evaluation strategies that may be appropriate for the program and to plan for the timely collection of data needed to assess program performance. Indeed, an evaluation plan may be a required component of the overall program plan. Increasingly, federal, state, and other agencies are requiring that evaluation be an integral component of the planning and provision of health services.[11] It is now widely accepted that before the expenditure of significant resources, the administrators of health programs should establish systems to determine the extent to which their efforts have produced desirable changes in those served by the program.[10-13] Such demands for evaluation often provoke feelings of anger or nervousness on the part of program staff, many of whom may feel threatened by the evaluation. These negative feelings can often be overcome by structuring the evaluation in such a way that it is truly helpful to the program staff. A good evaluation not only will provide the means to demonstrate the extent to which a program has achieved its goals but also will provide information to program staff on how to improve program performance as the program develops, thereby increasing the likelihood that program goals will be met.

As evaluation methodologies have developed, a number of differing schools of thought have emerged. House identifies eight different major approaches to evaluation, ranging from qualitative case studies to quantitative systems analysis (Table 66-2).[14]

One author identifies more than 50 approaches to evaluation.[15] A similar lack of consensus may be noted in descriptions of what constitutes the essential core of evaluation research. Fairweather[16] has argued that although surveys, correlational studies, and quasi-experiments have a place, "finally, for an accurate evaluation. . . . it is *absolutely essential* that an experiment be carried out with random assignment of participants." Parlette and Hamilton,[17] however, propose a radically different view of evaluation: "the researcher . . . makes no attempt to manipulate, control, or eliminate situational variables, but takes as given the complex scene he encounters. His chief task is to unravel it." Such disagreement has led to confusion over what is the "correct" approach to health program evaluation. The position taken here is that there is no one best way to evaluate health programs. The selection of a given strategy must depend on the purposes of the evaluation and the methodological opportunities available within the program setting.

EVALUATION OF HEALTH PROGRAMS

What Is Program Evaluation? Evaluation is defined here as the collection and analysis of information to determine program

TABLE 66-2. A TAXONOMY OF MAJOR EVALUATION APPROACHES

Model	Major Audiences or Reference Groups	Consensus Assumed	Methodology	Outcome	Typical Questions
Systems analysis	Economists, managers	Goals, known cause and effect, quantified variables	PPBS, linear programming, planned variation, cost-benefit analysis	Efficiency	Are the expected effects achieved? Can the effects be achieved more economically? What are the most efficient programs?
Behavioral objectives	Managers, psychologists	Prespecified objectives, quantified outcome variables	Behavioral objectives, achievement tests	Productivity, accountability	Is the program achieving the objectives? Is the program producing?
Decision-making	Decision-makers, especially administrators	General goals, criteria	Surveys, questionnaires, interviews, natural variation	Effectiveness, quality control	Is the program effective? What parts are effective?
Goal-free	Consumers	Consequences, criteria	Bias control, logical analysis, modus operandi	Consumer choice, social utility	What are all the effects?
Art criticism	Connoisseurs, consumers	Critics, standards	Critical review	Improved standards, heightened awareness	Would a critic approve this program? Is the audience's appreciation increased?
Professional review	Professionals, public	Criteria, panel, procedures	Review by panel, self-study	Professional acceptance	How would professionals rate this program?
Quasi-legal	Jury	Procedures and judges	Quasi-legal procedures	Resolution	What are the arguments for and against the program?
Case study	Client, practitioners	Negotiations, activities	Case studies, interviews, observations	Understanding diversity	What does the program look like to different people?

From House ER: Evaluating with Validity, p 23. Copyright © 1980 by Sage Publications, Inc. Reprinted by permission of Sage Publications, Inc.

performance. A program is defined here as "an organized response to eliminate or reduce one or more problems where the response includes one or more objectives, performance of one or more activities, and the expenditure of resources."[18]

Some activities are not likely to benefit from systematic evaluation because they are not programs to begin with. An example of a nonprogram is the commonly used tactic of moral persuasion. In 1981 President Reagan suggested that it would be patriotic for every business in the United States to hire one new worker. Although here a specific problem was being addressed—the alarmingly high rate of unemployment—since virtually no resources were being spent and no decision regarding the allocation of resources hinged on an assessment of the success of the President's plea, an evaluation would have been of little consequence.

Some health-related services such as a community's water supply and sewage disposal systems and institutions such as hospitals technically fall within our definition of a program, but to make the evaluation problem manageable, large systems often are broken down into their component parts for evaluation.

Suchman[19] identified the cyclical nature of health program planning and administration. Figure 66-2 presents Suchman's diagram describing the typical sequence of activities occurring through the life of a program. Five types of evaluation have been added to the diagram. Together they comprise a set of information collection and analysis tasks that help program staff make decisions regarding the program's activities. Indeed, within every successful program manager resides an inquisitive evaluation researcher.

Veney and Kaluzny,[13] following the lead of the World Health Organization (WHO), have suggested the five dimensions of program performance shown in Figure 66-2: relevance, progress, effectiveness, impact, and efficiency. These dimensions of performance also define the various purposes of evaluation information.

Dimensions of Program Performance

Relevance Evaluation. Relevance evaluation refers to activities designed to determine whether the program is needed or whether the program is targeting its efforts at the individuals in need. Other terms used to describe this type of evaluation include "formative evaluation" and "needs assessment." Historically, health services have been considered worthwhile because by their very nature they seemed beneficial. As Suchman[19] notes, "So great was the faith in service techniques that public agency and community workers usually begrudged any diversion of effort or funds away from them." But in recent years, as the cost of programs has increased, the need for and underlying rationale of health programs have become important evaluation issues.

The following are seven key questions around which relevance evaluations may be organized.

1. What problem does the program address?
2. How adequate is the definition of the problem?
3. What is the level of need for services associated with the problem?
4. How accurate is the information about the problem?
5. How adequate is the definition of the program?
6. Is the program appropriate to the defined problem?
7. Are those identified to be in need of services receiving the program?

As these questions suggest, it is typically assumed by health services evaluators that programs are most efficient and effective when the targets reached are restricted to units (often, but not

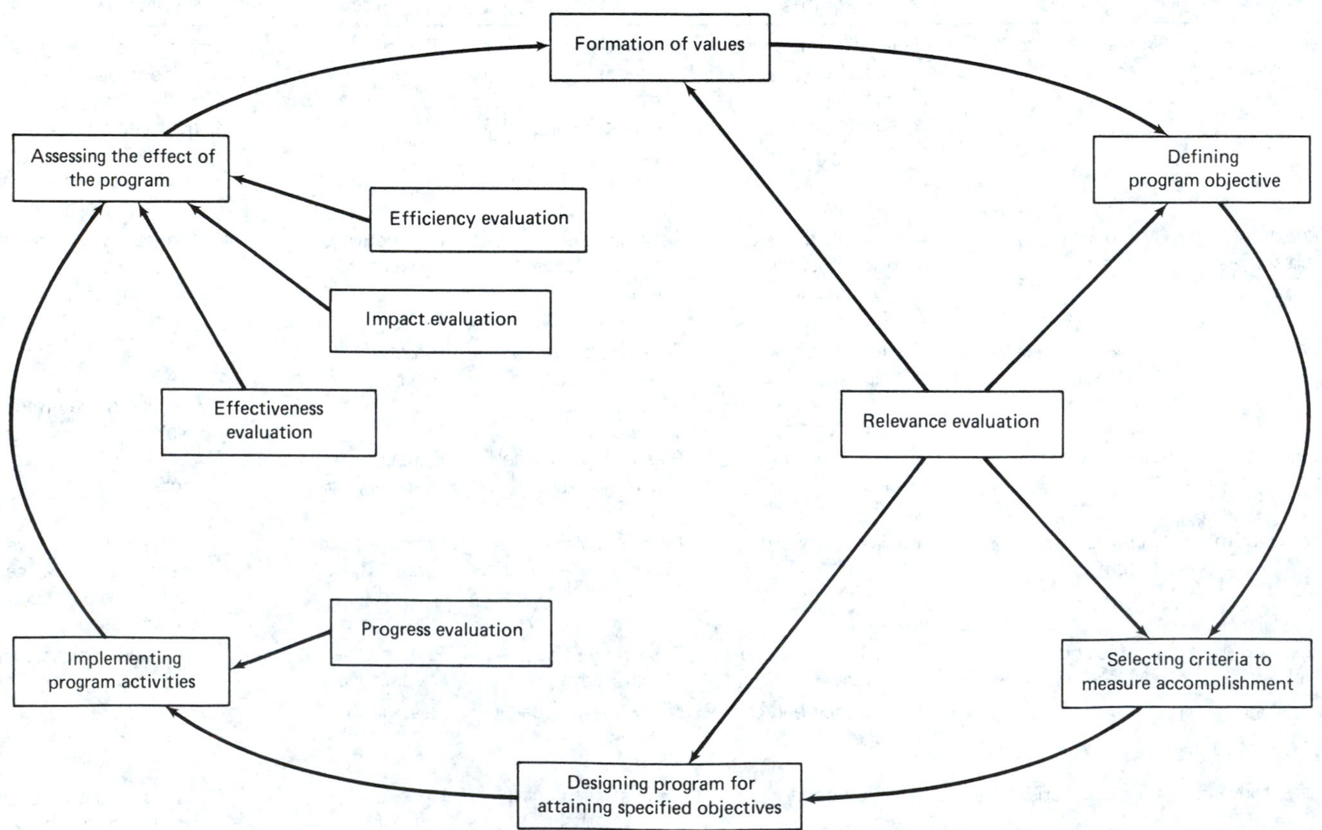

Figure 66-2. Interdependence of program planning, management, and evaluation. *[Reprinted from Edward Suchman, Evaluative Research, © 1968 Russell Sage Foundation. Used with permission of the Russell Sage Foundation.]*

always, individuals) that need the intervention; that is, when there is neither over-inclusion nor exclusion.

Progress Evaluation. Program evaluation refers to efforts made to assess how well program implementation complies with the program plan. This also is referred to as "process evaluation" and "implementation evaluation." The assessment of whether a program is being provided in a fashion consistent with planner's original intentions should be helpful to program managers in making early adjustments of the program and in making decisions concerning program continuation and expansion. This type of evaluation has always been considered a part of the management process. As many program managers have sadly discovered, a large proportion of programs that fail to show desired effects have really failed to deliver the interventions in the ways specified. There are three general forms of such failures:

- No treatment or not enough treatment is provided.
- The wrong treatment is provided.
- The treatment is provided unsystematically or varies substantially across program targets.

A progress evaluation may be organized around the following questions:

- Are the required personnel, equipment, and financial resources in place at the times and locations necessary to meet program needs?
- Do program activities clearly conform to the original plan?
- Are there any unanticipated factors influencing program implementation?
- Are the various activities or components of the program being provided to all program targets with uniform quality and quantity?

A progress evaluation is most useful early in the implementation of a health program, because that is when a reasonable chance exists for progress data to affect managerial decisions. Four types of recommendations might follow logically from a progress evaluation: terminate the project, reorganize the project, "fine tune" the project, or proceed with the project as it has been implemented.

Effectiveness Evaluation. Effectiveness evaluation refers to whether program results meet predetermined objectives. Here the emphasis is on immediate outcomes of program activities and whether these outcomes meet the objectives specified by the program planners.

- Did the program meet its stated objectives?
- Were program providers satisfied with the effects of program activities?
- Were program beneficiaries satisfied with effects of program activities?
- Is the problem reduced or eliminated as a result of the program?

Determining whether a program has met its prespecified objectives is a considerably more difficult task than might be imagined at first glance. The problem of determining the effectiveness of a program is identical to the problem of establishing that the program is the cause of some specified effect. Determining program effects essentially amounts to establishing causality; that is, demonstrating the validity of the assertion:

$$X \xrightarrow{\text{causes}} Y$$

X	Y
Participation in a health program	Change in some outcome variable

There is general agreement that five criteria must be satisfied to establish a causal relationship.

The first criterion is that an association between X and Y must exist. For a cause-effect relationship to exist, a change in one variable must be accompanied by or associated with a change in another variable. Several statistical procedures, all related basically to correlation, can be used to establish the existence of an association between two variables. If no such relationship can be found using these techniques, no cause-effect relationship can be assumed to exist; however, correlation is not enough to demonstrate causality.

An analysis of the possible relationships that may actually produce a correlation between two variables may help to make the point.

Let us assume we have a correlation where $r > 0$ is observed. There are four possible relationships that would be consistent with these data:

1. $X \rightarrow Y$. (X causes Y.)
2. $Y \rightarrow X$. (Y causes X.)
3. $Z \rightarrow X$ and Y. (Some third variable, Z, is causing both X and Y.)
4. Chance.

Demonstrating that the true causal structure reflected by $r > 0$ is $X \rightarrow Y$ requires meeting several other criteria that, in effect, rule out these other possibilities. The task of the investigator or program evaluator in testing causal relationships is to design the project so that the other criteria for claiming causal relationships are systematically met.

The second criterion is that there is proper time ordering among causes and effects. Causes must precede effects. If the effect occurred before the assumed "cause," that cause automatically would be ruled out as the real cause.

The third criterion is the elimination of alternative competing causal explanations. All other variables must be ruled out as possible causes of the association found between the two variables.

Two additional criteria often are assumed implicitly but should be made explicit. The fourth criterion is that the finding must be replicable to eliminate the possibility that an association between two variables appeared once by chance.

Finally, there must be a plausible explanation for the causal relationship that is compatible with the available data.

Campbell and Stanley[20] have helped generations of evaluators to grapple with the issue of causality with their work on specifying the various threats to internal validity (did the program cause the outcome?) and external validity (how generalizable are the results of this program demonstration?). The more prominent threats to internal and external validity in health program evaluation research are identified below.

Threats to Internal Validity

1. *History:* Extraneous events occurring during the period in which the program is implemented may affect the outcome measures.
2. *Maturation:* Physical or psychological processes associated with growing older may affect program outcomes, especially with long-term programs.
3. *Testing (reactive effects of pretest):* For some types of tests, individuals may do better on a second test; hence, posttest results may be different from pretest results.
4. *Instrumentation (different instruments/observers):* Changes in the calibration of a measurement instrument (e.g., thermometer) or changes in the observers who collect the data may themselves produce changes in the obtained measurements.
5. *Statistical regression:* A group of individuals selected

for program participation on the basis of their extreme scores on some variable (e.g., blood pressure) will have posttest scores that have regressed toward the population mean.

6. *Selection bias:* Differential selection of subjects into treatment and control groups possibly will produce differences in group pretest and posttest scores.
7. *Mortality (attrition):* Differential loss of participants from treatment or control groups also may produce differential outcome scores.

Threats to External Validity

1. *Interaction of treatment with pretesting:* Pretesting might sensitize participants to the treatment, making the participants unrepresentative of the nonpretested population.
2. *Reactive effects of testing:* Individuals who know they are being tested, observed, or otherwise assessed may react to such situations differently than the nontested population.

One of the tasks before the evaluator is to design a plan that dictates *when* and *from whom* measurements will be gathered and that minimizes the threats to internal or external validity as appropriate for the program in question. More will be said on evaluation design later.

Impact Evaluation. Impact evaluation refers to the long-term outcomes of the program. While the evaluation of effectiveness focuses on immediate program outcomes, impact evaluation considers whether the programmed intervention had any long-lasting effects on the ultimate problems that the program was intended to remedy. It is, of course, quite possible that a program may prove effective in producing short-term outcomes and yet have minimal long-term effects. For instance, increasing adolescents' knowledge of the harmful effects of smoking through an education program is no guarantee that the knowledge will be retained over months and years, nor is it a sure indication that the program participants will refrain from smoking cigarettes. Such issues are of the type principally addressed in impact evaluations. All concerns raised by effectiveness evaluations with regard to establishing causality and specifying objectives also must be considered when doing impact assessments.

Efficiency Evaluations. Efficiency evaluations attempt to relate the results obtained from a specific program to the resources expended to maintain the program. Efficiency evaluations are receiving increasingly greater attention as programs must compete for limited resources. The types of questions central to efficiency evaluation include:

- Do program benefits exceed the costs incurred?
- Are program benefits more or less costly per unit of outcome when compared with other programs designed to achieve the same objectives?

Such questions typically are addressed through cost-benefit or cost-effectiveness analyses.

STRATEGIES FOR EVALUATIVE ANALYSIS

This section describes methods and their relative strengths, limitations, and appropriateness for the five different types of evaluation—relevance, progress, effectiveness, impact, and efficiency.

Monitoring

Monitoring is the process by which information about program events or activities is recorded over time. It tells the administrator how well program tasks are being implemented. As Selby[15] has noted, monitoring involves the routine collection of data to allow an appraisal of the extent to which: (1) the designated target population is being served; (2) the quantity and quality of staff performance are satisfactory and consistent with program goals; and (3) policies comply with predesignated standards, laws, and regulations imposed on the agency by external funding sources, regulatory agencies, professional bodies, and so forth.

Monitoring takes place after the initial planning function has been completed. Once goals have been identified, target populations specified, technologies selected, and staff recruited and trained, the monitoring of program operations begins.

The data typically collected for monitoring include the following:

- *Input Data:* For example, financial/budgetary reports, personnel available and vacancies existing, transportation records, equipment and supplies purchased.
- *Process Data:* For example, specific activities carried out in completing the program, the sequence in which they are carried out, and their timing.
- *Output Data:* For example, services or goods provided (such as the number of immunizations or proportion of target population served).

Although monitoring may be accomplished without the use of any formal reporting system, for health programs of any significant complexity, it is best to adopt one. Numerous formal strategies have been proposed, including input/effort analysis, management by objectives (MBO), Gantt charts, program evaluation and review techniques (PERT), and the critical path method (CPM) of analysis.

Input/effort analysis involves monitoring the performance of program staff by calculating the percentages of time spent on various program activities. In this way the amount of time (or money, when time is capitalized into dollar amounts) budgeted for identifiable program activities may be compared with the amount of time expended by program staff to perform those activities.

MBO is a technique for managing program work that requires specific measurable objectives to be set for each member of the program staff. The work group leader and members share equally in developing the individual and work group objectives to be met over a specific time period. This approach clarifies the goals of the program at the outset and links these goals to the work performance objectives for each staff member. Work performance over the given time period is then compared with each individual's specified objectives, and feedback is provided to staff.

A Gantt chart provides a means of visually indicating the sequence of events or activities that make up the project as it proceeds through time. Typically the left vertical axis of a Gantt chart lists the major tasks to be performed by project staff over the lifetime of the project. Tasks to be completed early in the project's timetable are usually ordered at the top. The horizontal axis is marked off in time periods, and time lines are drawn in for each task to indicate how long it will take to finish and its expected date for completion. The Gantt chart provides a clear representation of the project's sequence of events and their projected timelines against which it reflects a realistic flow of program tasks and realistic estimates of the work and time to be allocated to each task.

PERT and CPM are quite similar in application. Both techniques (as with the construction of the Gantt chart) break a project down into a series of relatively self-contained activities. These activities are then arranged in a precedence table; those activities that must precede other activities are listed in order in the table. Once the precedence table is established, a PERT diagram may be produced that links discrete events such as completion of hiring of staff, initiating delivery of services, or completion of an evaluation report (often represented as circles in the diagram) with the activities required for the events to occur (represented as arrows in the diagram).

The major value of a PERT network is its ability to determine a critical path representing the sequence of activities and events that defines the longest time from the start of the project to its conclusion. There are two advantages to knowing the critical path. First, with this information it is possible to recognize the critical path activities that must be completed on time if the project is to be completed within the allowed time period. Second, given knowledge of the critical path, the project coordinator may recognize activities not on the critical path that provide a certain amount of slack to the project in terms of time and other resources.

Although the formal strategies for health program monitoring differ in how program data are arrayed and used to monitor activities, a few principles are common to virtually all programs:

1. The program is broken down into a series of relatively self-contained activities or outputs.
2. A precedence table (sometimes called a timetable or flowchart) is established for these activities and outputs. This consists of an estimate of the necessary ordering of the various activities and tasks and of their completion dates.
3. Cost estimates for each activity or output are established.
4. A data-collection system is implemented that periodically generates data on program status with regard to activities, outputs completed, and costs.

The data-collection system may range from site visit reports to detailed financial statements. An essential consideration is that the information collected must be acceptable to the user of the information. It also is essential to determine whether collecting the data is feasible and within reasonable limits of workload and cost. Figure 66–3 shows the general process of monitoring types of evaluations.

In many health programs a relatively simple "quarterly report" monitoring system meets these requirements. Figure 66–4 presents one of the key monitoring documents used by the Health Education–Risk Reduction Division of the State of California Department of Health Services, a statistical summary sheet showing the current level of performance of various risk-reduction programs. Other more detailed forms are used for monitoring timeline assessments, budgets, personnel, and unscheduled events.

Despite the importance of monitoring as an evaluation strategy, its application to health services programs is subject to several limitations. First, physicians and other health professionals sometimes object to being monitored. The practice of medical care is permeated by the notion that professionals are responsible people and that monitoring is an unnecessary interference. The more extreme proponents of this view argue that monitoring uses time and resources that should be devoted to "practice." Second, complex programs are very difficult to monitor, and there is a tendency in such situations to give only limited attention to monitoring. Third, when monitoring is considered important, there is a tendency to gather too much information in too much detail.

When properly restricted to those aspects of the program relevant to decision making, monitoring is an excellent strategy for doing a progress evaluation. Monitoring provides systematic information about whether a program is going according to plan, is on schedule, and whether activities are being carried out when and where they should be.

Monitoring also may provide important information for effectiveness and efficiency evaluations. Data on program output and costs typically are collected by monitoring and are necessary to these types of evaluations.

Monitoring is of little help, however, in relevance or impact evaluations. In the former case, monitoring is unlikely to provide much information on need, the significance of a problem, or the quality of the data being collected. In the latter case, most programs are underway for a long period of time before any assessment of impact can be made.

STEPS	ACTIONS
1. Data analyzed and conclusions made on status of project	Standardized forms are used by agency staffs to collect information on a project's activities and outputs; planned activities and outputs are compared with those reported to be actually occurring in order to identify problems warranting action
↓	↓
2. Monitoring system user makes decisions based on monitoring information	Appropriate management personnel are informed when activities specified and considered essential to project success either are not occurring as planned or are not producing the expected immediate output. Management is then responsible for deciding whether action is warranted
↓	↓
3. Management action taken in response to monitoring information	Agency assigns staff to act as trouble shooters to resolve problems identified through the monitoring system that are expected to impede achievement of project objectives and goals
↓	↓
4. Agency objectives are achieved	Monitoring system produces a final report by each project documenting activities, events, schedules, etc., to accompany project evaluation

Figure 66–3. General process of monitoring evaluations. *[Adapted from Selby, 1978.[15]]*

Agency Name ____________________
Contract Number ____________________

Quarter: 1 2 3 4

QUARTERLY STATISTICAL SUMMARY

A. UNITS OF SERVICE

1. Number of persons assessed ____________________. Cumulative total ____________________.
2. Number of persons receiving counseling regarding assessment ____________________.
3. Number of client referrals made to non-HE-RR contract health-related organizations ____________________.
4. Number of referred clients who enroll in risk reduction program (OPTIONAL) ____________________.
5. Number of persons attending non-intervention or informational presentations/seminars ____________________.
   Cumulative total ____________________.
6. Staff-organized programmatic interventions (Repeat "A–G" for each intervention):

QUARTERLY TOTALS	SMOKING	CUM. TOTAL	EXERCISE	CUM. TOTAL	WEIGHT CONTROL	CUM. TOTAL	STRESS	CUM. TOTAL	OTHER (SPECIFY)	CUM. TOTAL
A. No. of sessions/ classes offered										
B. No. who signed-up enrolled										
C. No. who drop out (2 sessions or less)										
D. No. who complete the intervention										
E. Average attendance for sessions/classes										
F. Persons receiving individual counseling										
G. No. of individual counseling sessions held										

7. Self-help interventions: (non-class) (Repeat for each intervention)
   Number of persons receiving self-help process materials or kits ____________________.

INTERVENTIONS	SMOKING	EXERCISE	WEIGHT CONTROL	STRESS	OTHER (SPECIFY)
Number of persons receiving self-help materials.					

8. List the number and kind of informational or media products developed by the program:

Figure 66-4. Quarterly statistical summary.

Case Studies

The case study is a useful means for acquiring a great deal of information about a single program. The program may be the subject of study because it is thought to be typical or because it is itself sufficiently interesting to justify an in-depth, detailed analysis.

Depth and detail of information are the hallmarks of case study analysis. Wilson[21] has suggested that descriptive case study evaluations provide a special kind of information: "They provide a sufficiently comprehensive amount of outcome and how-to information that someone interested in undertaking a similar project can make the decision wisely and even get specific help in how to go about it."

Four characteristics of a case study distinguish it from other approaches[15]:

1. *Case studies are particularistic.* They attempt to portray events as they occur in one particular situation (e.g., a specific program implemented at a specific time and place).
2. *Case studies are holistic.* They try to be comprehensive in the variables studied and often include descriptions of history and context. They also attempt to describe the interplay of different forces as they affect the issue of interest.
3. *Case studies are qualitative.* Usually they provide documentation of events, quotes, behaviors, etc. They typically use prose and literary technique to describe and analyze situations rather than summarizing quantitative data. The data often found in case studies consist of:
   - Detailed descriptions of situations, events, people, interactions, and observed behaviors
   - Direct quotations from people about their experiences, attitudes, beliefs, and thoughts
   - Excerpts from documents, correspondence, records, etc.
4. *Case studies are often* exploratory in nature. In situations where very little is known about a particular program, a case study may be the best strategy to obtain initial information. Decision-making about the program may rely on this information, or the case study may provide the basic data to help design a monitoring system or a more rigorous evaluation design.

Case studies have significant limitations. Two of the most important weaknesses are the inherent difficulties of collecting and analyzing qualitative data and the lack of a comparison between situations within which a program does or does not exist. Hence, strong statements about the causal effect of a given program are difficult to make when the evaluation relies solely on the case study technique.

Given these limitations, a case study potentially can be useful to each type of evaluation discussed in this chapter. Case studies could provide detailed analyses of the health problems in a community and of the extent to which a program is designed to meet those problems (relevance). A case study approach could provide information on the progress in a health services program and on the effectiveness, impact, and efficiency of programs. Qualitative data may be acquired using the case study approach. Typical case studies do not, however, include examinations of comparison groups or alternative treatments. It is impossible to tell whether or not the major results observed with a case study method would have prevailed without the program.

Basic Survey Designs

Survey research, as an approach to understanding social phenomena, uses data collected through questionnaires or interviews directed to a sample of persons drawn from some population of interest. To distinguish better among alternative designs it is helpful to first discuss general concepts of design.

A design is a plan that dictates when and from whom measurements will be gathered during the course of an evaluation. It is useful because

- It organizes the evaluation study: all the right people will take part in the evaluation at the right times.
- It makes explicit how comparative information will be gathered so that results from the program being evaluated can be placed within a context for judgment of their size and worth and of the extent to which it may be argued that the program actually caused those results.

The Elements of Design: Groups, Treatments, Measurements

Groups. In evaluation design the term *group* is reserved for a collection of people (or other units) defined by the treatment or program received.

The *treatment group* receives the program or treatment that is to be evaluated. The *control group* is an identified group consisting of individuals who are as similar as possible to those in the treatment group and who are measured at the same times as the treatment groups, but who do not get the treatment program. In many studies a control group may not receive any program. In other cases the control group may receive an alternative program.

As with case studies, in evaluations using a survey design where only the treatment group is measured, interpretation of the results often is difficult and unconvincing. Without any control or comparison group, it is difficult to know how good the results are, whether the results would have been as good with some other program, and whether the program had any effect on the results at all. It is therefore strongly recommended that evaluations of health programs use a comparison or control group.

The *equivalent or "true" control group* is one formed by random assignment. The evaluation designs that are strongest in internal validity are those that include true control groups. This is so because, in general, results that are apparent in the treatment group but not in the control groups are not likely to have been caused by anything other than the difference in treatment given the two groups.

For example, suppose that an evaluation has shown that program subjects (the treatment group) on average had higher posttest scores on some survey of knowledge about cigarette-related disease than subjects from the control group. The results might be attacked as unconvincing by such comments as:

- The subjects in the program were smarter.
- The parents of subjects in the program reinforce the program content to a greater extent than the parents of the control subjects.
- The control group started out lower than the treatment group.

Each of these arguments asserts a selection bias of some type. Random assignment of subjects to treatment and control groups is the most effective way of eliminating such explanations. Randomization makes it likely that factors that influence outcomes—smartness, parental background, or pretest level of achievement, for instance—will be distributed evenly between groups from the beginning.

Some people object to randomization in situations where individuals may be deprived of benefits on the basis of chance. There are some strategies for overcoming this common objection and achieving *true control groups.* One may be described as the two-new-programs strategy; program planners design two interventions and assign subjects randomly to each intervention group. A second technique is the delayed-program strategy: after the intervention group has completed the program, it is made available to the control group.

At times when random assignment of individuals to groups is impossible, a *nonequivalent control group* must be used. This is a group selected because it is similar to the treatment group. Sometimes a nonequivalent control group is called a "comparison" group.

If the treatment is selected by a particular procedure (e.g., a blood pressure test), then the comparison group should be selected by a procedure that is as nearly the same as possible. Evaluators should be prepared to document similarities and differences between the comparison and treatment groups. The credibility of one's findings will depend on one's ability to demonstrate that the treatment and comparison groups have been as alike as possible except for the difference in the programs they received.

Measurement Times. There are two major types of tests or observations to be made: pretests, given before a program or experiment starts and posttests, given at the conclusion of a program.

Experimental Designs. The classic approach in evaluation research is the experimental design. This is the standard against which other design alternatives are compared to assess their capacity to estimate the changes caused by the program. Even though true experiments seldom are conducted in health program evaluation, evaluators should be familiar with experimental designs.

Features Required of Experimental Designs

1. Random assignment of individuals (or some other unit of analysis) to experimental and control conditions
2. Systematic manipulation of the experimental group
3. Control over other important factors affecting experimental and control groups
4. Measurement of some outcome variable (after the manipulation) with which to compare the two groups

Quasi-experimental Designs. Under ideal conditions the following three designs include all features of experimental designs; that is, they all satisfy the criteria for classification as true experiments. In the real world of health programs, it usually is impossible to satisfy criterion number 3, control over other factors. Given that individuals are not confined to careful, controlled environments, it is virtually impossible to claim control over extraneous factors that might alter the outcome variables. Hence, these designs are called quasi-experimental.

The Pretest-Posttest Control Group Design

$$\begin{array}{cccc} R & O_1 & X & O_2 \\ R & O_3 & & O_4 \end{array}$$

Where R indicates random assignment to groups, X indicates exposure to the health program of interest, and O indicates data collected on outcome variables of interest. This design controls very well for most threats to internal validity, including history, maturation, testing, instrumentation, regression to the mean, selection bias, and experimental mortality (differential attrition). This design does not control for some factors affecting external validity; for example, the effects of X observed may be specific to groups "warmed up" by a pretest.

The Solomon Four-Group Design. One might want to try a design controlling for the interaction of testing and the intervention but at the same time wish to be careful not to lose internal validity. The Solomon four-group design builds in these characteristics:

$$\begin{array}{llll} R & O_1 & X & O_2 \\ R & O_3 & & O_4 \\ R & & X & O_5 \\ R & & & O_6 \end{array}$$

This design has the additional strengths (over the pretest-posttest control group design) of allowing one to determine the effects of testing and the interaction of testing and X on the generalizability of the results. In addition, the effect of the program X may be examined in four different ways:

$$O_2 \overset{?}{>} O_1 \;;\; O_2 \overset{?}{>} O_4 \;;\; O_5 \overset{?}{>} O_4 \;;\; O_5 \overset{?}{>} O_6$$

The major drawback of the Solomon four-group design is its cost. Two additional groups, one that receives the program and one that does not, and two more data-collection efforts are required.

The Posttest-Only Control Group Design. This design is strong on both internal and external validity but is surprisingly inexpensive compared with the Solomon four-group design:

$$\begin{array}{lll} R & X & O_1 \\ R & & O_2 \end{array}$$

The most adequate all-purpose assurance of lack of initial biases between groups is randomization. When reasonably large numbers of study participants may be randomly assigned to treatment and control groups, there is no need to pretest to ensure that groups are equivalent. Hence, the posttest-only control group design controls for testing as a threat to internal validity and controls for the interaction of testing and X as a threat to external validity. But, unlike the Solomon four-group design, this design does not measure these factors. Thus, the Solomon four-group design is superior to the posttest-only control group design, but the extra gains may not be worth the extra effort and cost.

Nonexperimental Designs. Many survey research designs used to establish program effects share some but not all of the characteristics of true or even quasi-experiments. Four groups of these nonexperimental designs will be introduced here: cross-sectional, trend, cohort, and panel survey studies.

Cross-Sectional Studies. A common cross-sectional research design used in health services evaluation is the *after-only design.* In this design, data are collected after the intervention at one point in time from a sample selected to represent the larger population.

$$X \quad O$$

Although there are many threats to the internal and external validity of this design (e.g., history, maturation, instrumentation, mortality, and reactive effect of the experimental situation), the fundamental problem is that there is no comparison group or even a pretest that would allow the treatment group to be compared with itself at two different time periods. Hence, although frequently used, this design is of little value when attempting to determine the causal impact of a program on some outcome variable.

An alternative cross-sectional survey design in evaluation research that avoids most of the problems of the after-only design is the *separate sample pretest–posttest design.* In this design two equivalent samples (cross sections of the population of interest) are studied. One sample is measured before experiencing a program, and the other sample is surveyed after exposure to the program.

$$\begin{array}{llll} R & O_1 & (X) & \\ R & & X & O_2 \end{array}$$

The conventional notation introduced above has been used where R indicates that each group is a random sample of the population, O_1 and O_2 indicate the administration of a survey instrument to each sample, and X indicates exposure to a program. (X) indicates that exposure to the program of the "control" group is not essential to the evaluation analysis. In terms of making causal statements regarding the program's effect, use of such a cross-sectional survey design is much superior to a case study. This is so because of the opportunity to observe situations with and without the program, because random selection of those to be studied assures that they are representative of the population (assuming the sample size is large), and because the data collection in the two groups is equivalent.

Trend Studies. These designs study changes within some general population over time. Data are collected on different samples of a general population at different points in time, before and after completion of a program targeted to the general population. Following are trend study designs:

$$(R_1g)O_1 \quad X \quad (R_2g)O_2$$
$$(R_1g)O_1 \quad (R_2g)O_2 \quad (R_3g)O_3 \quad X \quad (R_4g)O_4 \quad (R_5g)O_5 \quad (R_6g)O_6$$

The designs indicate two alternative trend study designs where (R_1g) indicates a random sample from the general population from which the first set of observations is taken. The design with multiple waves of data collection is stronger with regard to internal validity but is also more costly.

Cohort Studies. Cohort studies examine specific subpopulations as they change over time. Typically a cohort is an age group, but a cohort also can be based on some other time grouping, such as of those who got married in 1980 or women who are in their first trimester of pregnancy. The cohort design focuses on the same specific population (the group identified by the temporally related characteristic they share), although the actual samples of individuals may differ each time that the data are collected. Cohort studies may look similar to trend studies, but the samples drawn (in our case, random samples) in cohort studies are not from a general population but from a specific one (R 1s) (e.g., all women residing in San Francisco County who are in their first trimester of pregnancy). Following are cohort study designs:

$$(R_1s)O_1 \quad X \quad (R_2s)O_2$$
$$(R_1s)O_1 \quad (R_2s)O_2 \quad (R_3s)O_3 \quad X \quad (R_4s)O_4 \quad (R_5s)O_5 \quad (R_6s)O_6$$

The difference between trend and cohort designs is important because the cohort design, being restricted to a specific group, allows the evaluator to build in comparison samples taken from other presumably equivalent groupings who have not received the program in question. For example, the seventh- and eighth-grade students who are the targets of antismoking programming in one school (a) may be compared with seventh- and eighth-grade students from another school (b) in a similar social and economic environment. Such an equivalent cohort design would look as follows:

$$(R1a)O_1 \quad X \quad (R2a)O_2$$
$$(R1b)O_3 \qquad (R2b)O_4$$

Panel Studies. Panel studies are similar to trend and cohort studies except that the same set of people is studied each time. One example would be a hypertension-reduction program in which a specific group is selected for treatment and is followed over time. Following is the panel study design:

$$(P)O_1 \quad X \quad (P)O_2$$

where (P) indicates that each individual has been selected into the panel based on a sampling procedure or some criteria of interest. Of course, this design also could be expanded by adding multiple waves of observation and adding a comparison panel.

Survey research techniques are limited by the fact that interviews and questionnaires can be used to collect data on only some aspects of reality. The experience, training, and foresight of the evaluator will greatly determine the range and quality of the data. Appropriately addressing the threats to internal and external validity by carefully following planned research designs can be bothersome and expensive. As the use of survey research techniques becomes commonplace, people are becoming more wary of responding to surveys, necessitating special efforts to get reliable and valid survey data from a large population of the target sample.

Despite these limitations, survey techniques are used extensively in health services evaluation. This is in part because survey data can be useful to all types of evaluations presented here. With regard to relevance evaluation, for example, survey research may provide information on the state of the social environment or the perceived nature of the problem that a program is intended to solve. Survey research, perhaps in conjunction with a monitoring strategy, also can provide information on the state of program operations, thus fulfilling a progress evaluation function. Perceptions of efficiency also could be addressed by a survey; although subjective, such assessments are important in understanding the program.

When properly designed and executed, the survey approach is the most powerful evaluation technique available for assessing the effectiveness or impact of a given program. Its great strength is that it can determine, with reasonable certainty, whether a program has produced more in terms of a desired outcome than would have occurred in the absence of the program or with an alternative program.

SUMMARY

There is no one best way to evaluate a program. Depending on the purposes of evaluation information and the opportunities and constraints present in a given situation, various types of evaluation may be performed using one or more strategies. Clearly, some strategies are better suited to some types of evaluations than are other strategies, though all are potentially useful for more than one type of evaluation. Table 66–3 presents a summary of the major contributions of each strategy.

Relevance evaluations are best performed with case study and survey research data. The richness of data obtained with surveys and the flexibility of these two strategies make them well-suited to assessments of relevance. While progress evaluations also could be done with case study and survey techniques, monitoring is the most frequently used strategy for determining the progress of a program. For effectiveness and efficiency evaluation, any strategy could be useful. Because monitoring takes place only during the lifetime of a given program, however, it usually is not very useful for impact evaluations (except to the extent that monitoring information can help account for why long-term program effects were not observed).

Other issues related to public health program evaluation deserve further comment. Who should do program evaluations? Of course, all managers do evaluation as part of their managerial function. Managers who are intimately familiar with the program content, program staff, and the health problems being addressed by the program are a unique resource in evaluation; in fact, most relevance and progress evaluations must be done by program managers because of their detailed knowledge. However, efficiency, effectiveness, and impact evaluation often require the specialized knowledge, skills, and experience of a formally trained evaluator. An evaluation, in reality, almost always reflects a balance of inputs from the manager and an evaluator. The possibility that evaluations conducted by program staff persons may be biased is an important concern in evaluation research. Where the pressure for a given evaluation to reflect favorably on a program is so great that an unbiased evaluation by a program manager or staff evaluator will be difficult to achieve, an external evaluation consultant should be hired to conduct the evaluation.

Evaluators often are criticized for failing to provide information that is useful to program decision-makers. Two problems often found with program evaluations that justify this criticism are the length of time required to complete an evaluation and the failure of the evaluation to address questions important to program administrators as they go through the decision-making process required to direct the program. For evaluation to be useful to program decision makers, it must provide the information they view as important and must provide it when they need it. This does not mean that evaluators should ignore the formal, scientific canons of evaluation research in the name of expediency. It does mean that the evaluator must recognize the administrators' need for information that they can use as the program develops.

Evaluation research is, in the end, research. The logic of inquiry, standards for rejecting assumptions about the state of the world, and data requirements for using the vast array of qualitative and quantitative data analytic techniques are the same as those found in so-called pure or basic research enterprises. What is unique about evaluation research is that it typically takes place in an environment that we cannot control and can only dimly understand. The challenge for the evaluation researcher is to deal with the opportunities and constraints associated with a given program and to tailor an evaluation in such a way that a defensible assessment of program performance is produced.

TABLE 66–3. EVALUATION STRATEGIES AND THEIR RELATIVE STRONG POINTS

Strategies	Relevance	Progress	Effectiveness	Impact	Efficiency
Monitoring	X	X	X		X
Case study	X	X	X	X	X
Survey research	X	X	X	X	X
Cost-benefit			X	X	X
Cost-effectiveness			X	X	X

REFERENCES

1. Institute of Medicine (U.S.) Committee for the Study of the Future of Public Health: The Future of Public Health. Washington, D.C.: National Academy Press, 1988
2. Shonick W: Health planning. In Last J (ed): Maxy-Rosenau Public Health and Preventive Medicine, 12 edt. Norwalk, Conn.: Appleton-Century-Crofts, 1986
3. Blum H: Planning for Health. New York: Human Sciences Press, 1981
4. Schultz CL: The Public Use of Private Interest. Washington, D.C.: The Brookings Institution, 1977
5. Feldstein PJ: Health Care Economics. New York: John Wiley & Sons, 1979
6. Bice TW: Health services planning and regulation. In Williams SJ, Torrens PR (eds): Introduction to Health Services. New York: John Wiley & Sons, 1980
7. Shonick W: Elements of Planning for Areawide Personal Health Services. St. Louis: C.V. Mosby, 1976
8. Dignan MB, Carr PA: Program Planning for Health Education and Health Promotion. Philadelphia: Lea & Febiger, 1987
9. Shortell SM, Richardson WC: Health Program Evaluation. St. Louis: C.V. Mosby Company, 1978
10. Green LW, Kreuter MW, Deeds SG, Partridge KB: Health Education Planning: A Diagnostic Approach. Palo Alto, Calif.: Mayfield, 1980
11. Wye CG, Hatry HP (eds): Timely, Low-Cost Evaluation to the Public Sector. San Francisco: Jossey-Bass, Inc., 1988
12. Weiss CH: Evaluation Research: Methods for Assessing Program Effectiveness. Englewood Cliffs, N.J.: Prentice-Hall, 1972
13. Veney JE, Kaluzny AD: Evaluation and Decision Making for Health Services Programs. Englewood Cliffs, N.J.: Prentice-Hall, 1984
14. House ER: Evaluating With Validity. Beverly Hills, Calif.: Sage, 1980
15. Selby JM: Program Management: Evaluation and Project Monitoring. Boise, Idaho: Health Policy Analysis and Accountability Network, 1978
16. Fairweather GW: Community psychology for the 1980s and beyond. Evaluation Program Planning 3:245–250, 1980
17. Parlette M, Hamilton D: Evaluation and illumination: A new approach to the study of innovatory programs. In Hamilton D, et al (eds): Beyond the Numbers Game. Berkeley, Calif.: McCutchan, 1978
18. Kane RL, Hanson R, Deniston OL: Program evaluation: Is it worth it? In Kane RL (ed): The Challenges of Community Medicine. New York: Springer, 1974
19. Suchman EA: Evaluative Research. New York: Russell Sage Foundation, 1967
20. Campbell DT, Stanley JC: Experimental and Quasi-Experimental Designs for Research. Chicago: Rand McNally, 1963
21. Wilson S: Explorations of the usefulness of case study evaluations. Evaluation Q 3:446–459, 1979

67

Maternal and Child Health

Alan W. Cross

This chapter provides an overview of maternal and child health, highlighting the basic principles that make the health of women and children different from that of other segments of the population. Most of the details of specific aspects of maternal and child health are covered in other chapters.

HISTORY

Health services for women and children began to receive separate attention early in this century. This was in recognition of their greater vulnerability, particularly to socioeconomic and environmental forces, and the interdependence of the child's health and that of the mother. In 1909 the first White House Conference on Child Health recommended the formation of the Children's Bureau, which proceeded to investigate the causes of infant mortality (then more than 100 per 1000 live births). The first direct support of health services for mothers and children came with the Shepard-Towner Act of 1921, which resulted in complete birth registration and the establishment of maternal and child health divisions in state and local health departments.[1] Title V of the Social Security Act of 1935 extended services to crippled children and further established the principle of public responsibility for the health of mothers and children.

In the 1960s and early 1970s a host of additional programs were initiated by Congress. These included Medicaid, Early Periodic Screening, Diagnosis and Treatment (EPSDT), Neighborhood Health Centers, Maternity and Infant Care, Family Planning, Children and Youth Projects, Head Start, Title I educational assistance, the Right to Education of the Handicapped (PL 94–142), and nutrition programs (WIC and School Lunch). While these laws expanded services at the state and local levels, the resultant programs were administered by a variety of different branches of government, diffusing responsibility and often leading to poor coordination and the undermining of MCH divisions.

Maternal and Child Health (MCH) services were seriously weakened by the budget cuts of the Reagan years. Rather than cutting specific services, the programs were lumped into block grants that gave state governments greater freedom to apportion the reduced funds as they saw fit. This has begun the trend of providing greater local autonomy in the establishment and administration of health programs for women and children. This trend may hold promise for the creation of innovative programs that more precisely address the community's needs, making greater use of local resources.

Progress in MCH has been driven by the dual forces of research and advocacy. Multidisciplinary studies over the last 20 years have shed important light on the health problems of women and children and provided numerous examples of effective means to ameliorate those problems.[2] Articulate and committed individuals and organizations have played a critical role in fostering public commitment to improve the lives of mothers and children. However, that support has been significantly reduced through the 1980s. As our knowledge of what to do has continued to grow, the political will to use that knowledge has shrunk.

HEALTH INDICATORS

Various health indicators are used to assess the status of MCH. The continuous monitoring of these indicators is an essential part of evaluating our progress in improving the health status of women and children.

Maternal mortality rates, historically used as the main indicator of maternal health, have reached such a low level in the United States that they are less valuable now. Maternal health is reflected in fertility rates and birth rates as well as in pregnancy-related mortality and morbidity rates. Pregnancy outcomes have become a more important measure of maternal health and quality of maternity services provided. Miscarriage, therapeutic abortion, stillbirth, and especially low birth weight versus term birth rates can be used to assess the success of the pregnancy. Prenatal care, place of delivery, attendant at delivery, type of delivery, complications, length of stay, and cost all measure the availability and quality of maternal health services.

The infant mortality rate remains an important though crude measure of MCH. Linking infant birth and death records has provided a far more precise way of assessing factors associated with pregnancy outcome, particularly when the causes of death are grouped by pregnancy-related conditions, such as prematurity, rather than by the organ system taxonomy of the ICD-9 codes.[3] The new birth certificate form that was adopted in 1989 includes a wider array of information on both the mother and the child, offering opportunities for future exploration of the relationships between more extensive sociodemographic and medical information and various pregnancy outcomes. Childhood morbidity is less easily measured. Birth defects registries, neonatal intensive care use, discharge diagnoses, and national health surveys provide some estimates of morbidity. Immunization rates, school-based health data, and the data from such programs as EPSDT and Crippled Children are also helpful indicators of child health.

Larger social and demographic changes are also important indicators of the status of mothers and children. Over the last 20 years there have been dramatic increases in the percentage of mothers in the work force, the percentage of marriages that end in divorce, the numbers of homeless mothers and children, and the percentage of children living in poverty. These social problems contribute directly or indirectly to most of the health problems of women and children.

SERVICE DELIVERY

The goals of MCH services are (1) to encourage desired pregnancy, achieving the best possible outcome for the baby and the mother; (2) to promote healthy relationships within the family to nurture the growing child; (3) to optimize the normal developmental processes to allow the child to achieve his or her fullest potential; (4) to prevent child health problems and reduce the risks of adult health problems; and (5) to provide early intervention in the health problems of women and children so as to minimize morbidity and mortality in a cost-effective manner. To achieve these goals, attention must be paid to several basic principles of maternal and child health. These principles are a product of the nature of women and children and the problems from which they suffer and therefore are a bit different from the general principles that underlie all health service delivery.

Two Clients. Maternal services are unique in that they simultaneously provide care for two equally important clients, the mother and the fetus. Balancing the needs of both to achieve the best possible outcome requires a thorough understanding of the complex interdependence of the maternal/fetal unit and the implications of events and treatments for both mother and baby.

Family-centered Services. Because of the extreme importance of the family in the nurturing of the pregnant woman and the young child, it is essential that MCH services be delivered with attention to the family circumstances of the clients. The family influences growth, development, health-related behaviors, and life-style habits. Family resources influence the use and availability of health services and the ability to provide the care needed, particularly in chronic disease. The child is not merely the passive recipient of the influences of the family but, rather, plays an increasingly interactive role in the family, shaping in part the environment in which he or she lives.

Developmental Perspective. The fetus and the child are being continuously shaped by the normal developmental processes that result in a reasonably predictable series of changes from conception through adolescence. Progress over this course is a sensitive measure of both health and disease. These developmental forces can be potent allies in the management of chronic health problems. However, continued disruption of normal development can have a progressively magnifying effect on the fetus or child. Because of the importance of development, the dimension of time and the continuity of care over time become critical elements in the provision of MCH services. Prompt identification of problems and early intervention, therefore, hold the greatest promise for achieving the best outcome.

Health Promotion and Disease Prevention. Childhood is both a means to adulthood and an end in itself. There is great potential, therefore, for health promotion and disease prevention to benefit both the current child and the future adult. However, careful attention must be paid to the immediate implications of interventions that are aimed at preventing problems in the distant future, making sure that the desired long-term benefits are not counterbalanced by short-term hazards.

Timely, Cost-effective Treatment. The early identification and proper treatment of common health problems is a critical dimension of reducing morbidity and mortality in women and children. Simple early treatments can often prevent the development of expensive and serious problems, such as adolescent pregnancy, a premature birth, or a handicapping condition.

Integration of Principles. Perhaps the greatest challenge to delivery of MCH service is trying to integrate all the principles articulated above into the care of each client. It is difficult for the provider to simultaneously attend to the treatment and prevention needs while considering the family and development issues in the care of both the mother and the child. However, the greatest success is achieved when all these concepts are addressed together.[4]

TRENDS AND INNOVATIONS IN SERVICES

The United States lags far behind all other developed countries in the provision of most services to mothers and children. Western Europe and Japan offer extensive maternity benefits, prenatal care, day care, and well-child care to all women and children.[5] In infant mortality rates the United States ranks twentieth in the world, a fact that many attribute at least in part to the inadequate provision of maternal and infant services. The last decade has seen little progress in this arena, but some interesting innovations in the delivery of MCH services have recently emerged and warrant brief description. Many of these have not yet come into general practice but hold promise for the future, once they have been more carefully evaluated. Social trends of the last decade have also had an effect on MCH services and must be considered in the process of recommending improvements for the future.

Family Planning and Abortion. Optimum health for both mother and child has long been known to be related to maternal age, spacing of children, and the balance between family resources and family size. The ready availability of birth control and the option for abortion have provided means of achieving family planning. The recent rise in opposition to birth control, particularly for teenagers, and the moral indignation against abortion have made these services far less available to those whose health might be most benefitted by them.

Malpractice Crisis. The malpractice crisis has created a defensive, adversarial atmosphere in the practice of medicine, particularly in obstetrics. Efforts to reduce the uncertainties of practice and avoid mistakes have resulted in the establishment of a new standard of care that is more expensive and not necessarily in the best interest of the mother, the fetus, or the health care provider. Since this new standard serves as the basis for judging malpractice we have entered an escalating vicious cycle of trying to eliminate all the inherent imperfections in the practice of medicine. Pressures on state legislatures to enact tort reforms have not yet had much effect.

Preconceptional Health Promotion. Many of the critical phases of fetal development have already occurred before a woman is even aware that she is pregnant. Optimum fetal health, therefore, requires attention to maternal health and health-related behaviors even before conception. Efforts to counsel women before conception to avoid alcohol, drugs, tobacco, and other fetal hazards are being tested to determine the impact on pregnancy outcome.[6] Likewise, the efficacy of periconceptional vitamin use in preventing neural tube defects is being assessed.[7,8]

Prenatal Care. The timing of prenatal visits and the services provided were devised to detect and treat the problems that arise toward the end of pregnancy and complicate a normal delivery. It is now apparent that prematurity is a serious problem that needs to be prevented with efforts that must begin very early in gestation.[9] Several programs have tested the benefits of identifying women at risk of a preterm delivery and instituting preventive interventions. The results to date are mixed, with some showing dramatic reductions in preterm births and others showing no benefit at all.[10,11] The U.S. Public Health Service has recently released revised recommendations for prenatal care, incorporating some of the concepts and practices that have been promoted in the prematurity-prevention programs.[12] For low-income mothers it has been calculated that every dollar spent on prenatal care saves $3.38 in later costs for the medical care of preventable problems.[13]

Improving access to and quality of prenatal services continues to be a challenge with no obvious solution. Recent expansion of Medicaid to include women up to 185% of the federal poverty level in comprehensive services should make a dent in this problem. Some states have developed innovative programs to improve quality and access for the poor, and many local community-based projects have also been created with these goals in mind.

Human Immunodeficiency Virus. The accelerating spread of HIV infection through intravenous drug use and heterosexual contact has increased the numbers of infected women. Approximately one third of the babies born to such women also acquire the virus. In the large cities this has created a crisis in both maternal and infant mortality as well as in foster care.

Delivery Services. Economic pressures have continued to shorten the average length of hospital stay for an uncomplicated delivery to the point where discharge on the second day is the rule now and not the exception. This requires closer follow-up to detect problems that might occur in both the mother and the baby in the first week after delivery. When discharge occurs before the baby is 24 hours old, the results of PKU screening may not be accurate.

Home-style and at-home deliveries continue to be popular with a small segment of society. High rates of cesarean section continue to generate controversy without a clear resolution in sight.

Circumcision. For more than a decade the health benefits of circumcision have been considered to be insignificant and therefore not a reasonable justification for the procedure. Recent studies, however, have suggested that uncircumcised males are many times more likely to have urinary tract infections and that the morbidity from this relatively rare problem is sufficient to justify circumcision, as it outweighs the small risks of the surgery.[14]

Immunization. Further development of the acellular pertussis vaccine offers hope that some of the complications of the currently used vaccine might be avoided.[15] The new conjugated vaccine against *Hemophilus influenzae* has recently been approved for use in infants as young as 2 months of age. Once this vaccine is in wide use, it should significantly reduce the incidence of meningitis in infants. The high-dose Edmonston-Zagreb measles vaccine has been shown to be 98% effective in infants as young as 6 months, and there is evidence of somewhat less effectiveness in 4-month-olds.[16] This vaccine will be particularly valuable in developing countries, where measles remains a major child killer. As the hepatitis B vaccine becomes affordable, it will come into wide use in the prevention of both hepatitis and the consequent hepatic cancer—both major problems, particularly in developing countries.

Day Care. As maternal employment continues to rise, we are falling farther behind in providing adequate, affordable day care for young children. Most states provide little regulation of day-care facilities, particularly home-based centers with few children. This aggravates concerns about spread of infection, injury, and child abuse in day-care facilities.

Injury Prevention. Recognition that injuries account for more deaths after the first birthday than all other causes combined has finally drawn attention to injury prevention. The American Academy of Pediatrics has launched a major campaign against injuries, and the federal government has funded several injury-prevention research centers. Most states now have mandatory child safety restraint laws, which have clearly been shown to reduce automotive deaths. The organized effort that led to these laws is a good example of well-planned and coordinated advocacy for children.

Sexual Abuse. Over the last decade we have been forced to recognize that child sexual abuse occurs far more frequently than we would like to believe. As this problem has come out of the closet, innovative programs have been developed to teach children how to avoid sexual exploitation and to identify and treat more effectively those who are victims. Many school systems have adopted curricula in prevention of sex abuse for children as young as those in kindergarten, and the open discussion of this problem has made it easier to inquire about such incidents as a part of routine health care. Many states are also experimenting with creative ways of humanely dealing with the child witness in court without unduly infringing on the constitutional rights of the accused. However, we are probably still studying only the tip of this iceberg as we begin to explore the consequences of the more subtle forms of abuse and try to gain a better understanding of the abusers and the factors that lead to abuse in some families.

New Drugs of Abuse. The "crack" epidemic has created a crisis in the inner city. Children and teenagers are deeply involved as addicts and pushers, reaping large sums of money and suffering from the massive violence that surrounds the cocaine trade. The rewards lure children from school or legitimate employment, and addiction snuffs out future potential in these youth. Cocaine also has significant effects on the fetus; it is a major cause of low birth weight and the need for neonatal intensive care in many large cities. Efforts to stem this tide have so far had little effect.

The abuse of anabolic steroids appears to be common among teenagers, even those who are not athletes.[17] The true extent of this problem has not yet been well defined; nor have the consequences of such abuse been measured.

Community-based Social Support. Pregnant women and young children thrive best when they are surrounded by friends and relatives who provide companionship and assistance. As unwed motherhood becomes more common and the extended family further disintegrates, more young families face isolation and inadequate social supports. To remedy this, several programs have used home visitors to befriend and work closely with pregnant women and young families, offering the assistance and social support that are so often inadequate. Some of these programs have been able to demonstrate benefits in health and well-being associated with participation in the program.[18,19]

FUTURE DIRECTIONS

The 1960s and 1970s produced a number of centrally funded programs to help mothers and children. Through the 1980s the support for these programs eroded, and control over spending priorities for the diminished funding was shifted to the state capitols through block grants. Over the same period new initiatives for the elderly received increasing support. Despite renewed outcries about the plight of America's children, there seems to be little public support for pouring new money into the current MCH programs. Competition for scarce resources is not likely to succeed until a new approach can be found that assures the public that the resources are neither being abused nor inadvertently perpetuating the problems that they are designed to solve.

Shifting even more control for human service programs to the community may provide the improvements needed to garner greater support. The current system of impersonal bureaucracies overseeing categorical programs with complex rules and eligibility requirements may be too cumbersome to offer the young family opportunities to achieve greater competence and self-sufficiency. Community-controlled programs have the potential of reducing duplication, filling gaps, and engendering cooperation across agencies to make the services run more efficiently and effectively and to allow a more personalized array of assistance for those in need. Funding from state and federal taxes would still allow resource redistribution to ensure services in poorer communities. Such a trend would also return to the community the sense of responsibility that each citizen has some obligation to ensure that all the citizens have a reasonable standard of living and access to the common resources of their community.

REFERENCES

1. Schmidt WM: The development of health services for mothers and children in the United States. Am J Public Health 63:419–437, 1973
2. Schorr LB, Schorr D: Within Our Reach: Breaking the Cycle of Disadvantage. New York: Anchor Press/Doubleday, 1988
3. Dollfus C, Patetta M, Siegel E, Cross AW: Infant mortality: A practical approach to the analysis of the leading causes of death and risk factors. Pediatrics 86:176–183, 1990
4. Health Services Integration: Lessons for the 1980's. Report of a Study by the Institute of Medicine, Washington, DC: National Academy Press, 1982
5. Miller CA: Maternal Health and Infant Survival. Washington DC: National Center for Clinical Infant Programs, 1987
6. Cefalo RC, Moos M-K: Preconceptional Health Promotion: A Practical Guide. Rockville, Md: Aspen Publishers, 1988
7. Mulinare J, Cordero JF, Erickson JD, Berry RJ: Periconceptional use of multivitamins and the occurrence of neural tube defects. JAMA 260:3141–5, 1988
8. Mills JL, Rhoads GG, Simpson JL, et al: The absence of a relation between the periconceptional use of vitamins and neural tube defects. N Engl J Med 321:430–435, 1989
9. Preventing Low Birthweight. Report of the Institute of Medicine Committee to Study the Prevention of Low Birthweight. Washington, DC: National Academy Press, 1985
10. McCormick MC: The contribution of low birthweight to infant mortality and childhood morbidity. N Engl J Med 312(2):82–90, 1985
11. Buescher PA, Meis PJ, Ernest JM, Moore ML, Michielutte R, Sharp P: A comparison of women in and out of a prematurity prevention project in a North Carolina perinatal care region. Am J Public Health 78:264–267, 1988
12. Caring For Our Future: The Content of Prenatal Care. Report of the Public Health Service Expert Panel on the Content of Prenatal Care. Washington, DC: Public Health Service, Department of Health and Human Services, 1989
13. Preventing Low Birthweight. Report of the Institute of Medicine Committee to Study the Prevention of Low Birthweight. Washington, DC: National Academy Press, 1985, chap 10
14. American Academy of Pediatrics: Report of the Task Force on Circumcision. Pediatrics 84:388–391, 1989
15. Blennow M, Granstrom M, Jaatmaa E, et al: Primary immunization of infants with an acellular pertussis vaccine in a double blind randomized clinical trial. Pediatrics 82:293–299, 1988
16. Markowitz LE, Sepulveda J, Diaz-Ortega JL, et al: Immunization of six-month-old infants with different doses of Edmunston-Zagreb and Schwarz measles vaccines. N Engl J Med 322:580–587, 1990
17. Terney R, McLain LG: The use of anabolic steroids in high school students. Am J Dis Child 144:99–103, 1990
18. Chapman J, Siegel E, Cross A: Home visitors and child health: Analysis of selected programs. Pediatrics 85:1059–1068, 1990
19. Olds DL, Kitzman H: Can home visitation improve the health of women and children at environmental risk? Pediatrics 86:108–116, 1990

68

Family Planning Programs and Practices: An Epidemiological Viewpoint

Carl W. Tyler, Jr.
Herbert B. Peterson

FAMILY PLANNING PROBLEM IN PUBLIC HEALTH

Even though an estimated 94% of the world's population lives in countries with policies that favor family planning, five out of every six couples of reproductive age do not use adequate measures of fertility regulation according to the World Health Organization (WHO). Nonetheless, important advances have been made in family planning over the past 3 decades. As recently as the end of the 1960s, only four major countries in Africa and two in Latin America had official family planning policies. By the beginning of the 1980s, more than 80% of Africa's people and more than 90% of those in Latin America lived in countries that supported family planning programs.[1] Even though family planning and the control of human fertility influence health and the quality of human life throughout the world as they never have before, the benefits from family planning services have yet to be fully realized. Some areas of family planning, birth prevention, and their effects on public health remain under careful scrutiny.

The rapid changes in family planning policies have led to similar changes in health programs and have presented health professionals with areas of responsibility with which many are not yet entirely comfortable. The first area involves human values. Another focuses on the need for scientific knowledge on personal fertility control. Although the elimination of disease and disability is accepted almost universally as the goal of health programs, the limitation of fertility is not accepted in the same way. We can agree that diseases such as smallpox, measles, and polio can and should be eliminated, but we clearly do not want to reduce fertility to zero. But what level is desirable or acceptable? What means should individuals and national policy makers be permitted to use to achieve this level? Although most societies limit fertility by some means, only recently has scientific information been acquired on the determinants of fertility and on the effectiveness and safety of methods for limiting fertility. These issues have become even more difficult to address in the presence of the global epidemic of AIDS (acquired immunodeficiency syndrome), the development of RU 486, an effective antiprogestational agent, and concern about side effects of widely used contraceptives, for example, oral contraception and its possible relationship to breast cancer.

In this chapter we identify some of the important issues related to family planning, health, and human values. After identifying the relevant basic values, discussing the practice of epidemiology in relationship to family planning, and reviewing the goals, policies, and laws related to family planning programs, we describe the effectiveness and safety of current methods of fertility control. Next, we focus on specific issues of special importance to family planning, namely, teenage pregnancy, breast cancer, oral contraception, and AIDS. In closing we consider the factors that might influence personal decisions about family planning.

FAMILY PLANNING AND HUMAN VALUES

We define family planning to be the voluntary use of methods and procedures intended to affect the number and timing of pregnancies. This definition includes all the proximate determinants of fertility, including age of a person at first sexual intercourse or marriage, postpartum lactation for spacing purposes, contraception, and sterilization. Induced abortion, although not a method of family planning by this definition, is widely used to influence the timing and number of births. This method will also be addressed in this chapter. Communities (as well as states and nations) may select strategies that modify one or all of these determinants to achieve their family planning goals.

Most human value systems respect life, place a high value on the family, are pronatalist, and have strong taboos and values related to sexuality and reproduction. Nonetheless, most of them have little ethical tradition directly related to family planning and fertility control.

There are four major ethical justifications for making family planning a part of public policy and programs. Each is relevant to both community and individual decision making, and none is based on any one system of values, religion, or philosophy. These four values, which are mentioned in the preamble to the Constitution of the United States, are freedom, justice, general welfare, and security or survival.[2] The most acceptable policies might reflect all four. Controversy and debate surround family planning because of different opinions on the relative merits of these values and because some policies emphasize one value at the expense of another.

Freedom is identified in the U.S. Declaration of Independence as one of the "inalienable rights" of "life, liberty, and the pursuit of happiness." This goal provides one criterion for evaluating any public policies including those dealing with family planning information and services. International documents establish a consensus that a right to family planning exists. In 1966 the United Nations General Assembly resolved that "the size of the family should be the free choice of each individual."[3] In 1974 a consensus of 136 countries meeting in Bucharest stated in the *World Population Plan of Action* that "all couples and individuals have the basic right . . . to decide freely and responsibly the number and spacing of their children" and went on to assert that these couples should exercise their rights in a way that takes account of the future needs of children and communities.[4] A decade later, in 1984, the United Nations International Conference on Population in Mexico City reaffirmed the Bucharest plan of action but placed greater emphasis on child survival and primary health care.[5] Since the conference in Mexico City, new emphasis has been placed on the study of the relation between birth intervals and child health by both funding organizations and researchers.

Justice means equality in law. Social justice requires mutual respect among members of society and nondiscrimination in relation to human life and worth. Distributive justice means reducing the differences in health and other social problems among people of different income levels, places of residence, and ethnic and cultural backgrounds. Distributive justice is the major rationale for public health programs in the United States. The objective of these programs is to reduce health problems among those lacking resources, skills, or motivation to use private health care services for preventing or resolving health problems.

General welfare involves two precepts related to family planning. The first is that regulating fertility is as important as controlling mortality and morbidity and is an essential component of personal, social, and economic development. General welfare also includes the health rationale for family planning, which can be described in several ways. The average potential number of live births per women in most societies is approximately 15.[6] A policy of limiting fertility to replacement levels or fewer benefits society by permitting existing resources to be distributed more equitably. If each couple had two children, 13 births would be prevented, as would 86% of the maternal and infant deaths that would occur at maximum fertility levels. Preventing these births would also permit a greater allocation of health resources per person and should, therefore, lead to further improvements in the quality of services provided to those children who are born. The specific methods for limiting fertility also influence the health rationale for adopting family planning.

Postponing heterosexual activities for 5 to 10 years after reaching the age of potential childbearing, breast feeding for a lengthy interval, and using birth control services provided by health professionals can also improve health for women in their childbearing years and for their offspring.

The final rationale for family planning is security or survival. This issue relates to the survival of individuals, families, and communities and to the definition of the onset of life. The former includes concerns regarding maternal and infant welfare. The latter concerns the morality at the individual level of induced abortion and morality at the community level of having large families. The onset of human life has been variously defined as conception, quickening, birth, or viability. The definition one chooses affects one's perception of the morality of induced abortion.

EPIDEMIOLOGY

Even though family planning became part of everyday life around the world in a very short time, epidemiologists have made important and timely contributions to scientific knowledge regarding the effectiveness, safety, and acceptability of family planning programs and birth prevention technology. Studies of oral contraception,[7] intrauterine devices,[8] abortion,[9] and sterilization[10] all show how the fundamental concepts of epidemiology and its practice can be applied as effectively in fertility and family planning methods and services as they can in other health problems and programs.

Definition of Epidemiology Applied to Family Planning. The definition of epidemiology has two fundamental elements: it is "the study of the distribution and determinants of health related states and events in populations and the application of this study to the control of health problems."[11] Epidemiology is, therefore, essential to the scientific basis and the practice of public health and preventive medicine. As such, it can be applied to family planning and to family planning programs. Like all other fields of public health, the results of epidemiological studies in family planning must meet the criteria of direct, or causal, association, and those associations must not be the result of chance, bias, or confounding.

Epidemiology as a Basis for Action. The basic tasks of epidemiological practice are (1) public health surveillance, (2) investigation, (3) analysis, and (4) evaluation. Each of these tasks can be applied to the problems of family planning. Surveillance, for instance, has documented changes in the practice of induced abortion in the United States.[12] Epidemiological investigations have shown that use of intrauterine contraception devices may be related to clusters of septic spontaneous abortion[13] and that oral contraceptive use protects against ovarian cancer.[14] Epidemiological analysis showed that there was a causal association between oral contraceptive use and benign liver tumors.[15] Epidemiological evaluation demonstrated the relative benefits and hazards of different kinds of intrauterine contraceptive devices[16] and evaluated the effects of community programs on fertility change.[17]

FAMILY PLANNING PROGRAMS

Goals. The goals of national family planning programs reflect a country's aspirations. In some cases these aspirations are conceived in terms of a national need for improved economic development, improved general welfare, or enhanced rights for individuals. Beginning in the early 1960s, several Asian nations sought to improve their economic development.[18] Programs in Latin America, on the other hand, sought to improve the health of mothers and children. In Chile, for example, epidemiological studies of abortion emphasized the burden that this illegal practice placed, not only on the health of women, but also on the nationalized health and hospital service system.[19] A contraceptive service program, therefore, became acceptable because it was viewed as a campaign against abortion. The few programs based on national policies in Africa sought to improve the health of mothers and children by improved child spacing.[20] The national family planning program in the United States seeks primarily to prevent unintended pregnancies.[21,22] By 1980, national goals to reduce population growth and to improve the health of women and children, or both, were recognized as crucial in nearly every country worldwide. Moreover, most nations agreed that couples and individuals had the right to control their own fertility.[22]

The United States set specific national health objectives to be achieved by 1990 and developed new objectives for the year 2000. The national objective that addresses family planning has specific components related to prevention of teenage pregnancies and reduced sexual activity and increased use of effective contraceptives among young and unmarried individuals.[21,23]

Policy and Law. How are these goals carried out with regard to national policies and laws? Both social customs and family planning practices can influence fertility. Recognizing the importance of reducing the years during which an individual is at risk of pregnancy, many Asian countries have passed laws prohibiting child marriage and establishing a minimum age of wedlock (ranging from 12 to 25 years).[24] Paradoxically, most nations have overlooked how breast feeding improves infant nutrition and curbs fertility. They do not, therefore, have laws or policies that promote breast feeding.

Historically, many countries, including the United States, have had laws that restrict the use of most approaches to fertility control, that is, contraception, abortion, and sterilization. These restrictions on fertility control exist because of the complex deliberations inherent in the legislative processes required to make laws that serve society's current needs and values and the difficulty legislators have in developing laws at a pace that matches advances in technology.

The rapid global increase in the use of surgical sterilization has led to the enactment of legislation influencing its availability. Although some countries specifically permit voluntary surgical sterilization, this form of fertility control is legal in most countries simply because there is no law that prohibits it. Nonetheless, even where voluntary surgical sterilization is permitted, some legal constraints still exist, among which are a minimum age, specific medical indications, authorization by a spouse, or a minimum number of living children.

The legal status of voluntary induced abortion has changed substantially during the past 30 years and is likely to be further modified in the near future. In 1959 the American Law Institute proposed a model penal code that justified abortion on the following grounds: (1) a pregnancy that places at risk the life or the physical or mental health of the women, (2) a pregnancy likely to produce a child with a serious physical or mental impairment, (3) a pregnancy resulting from incest, (4) a pregnancy resulting from rape.[25] Subsequently, as states in the United States and other countries enacted laws that permitted abortion, they followed the guidance of the American Law Institute and added additional legal grounds for the voluntary interruption of pregnancy. These grounds include the effects of childbirth not only on the health and welfare of the woman but also on her existing children and the rest of the family; jeopardy to the social position of the woman or her family; failure of routinely used contraception; and at the request (usually during the first trimester of pregnancy) of the pregnant woman. Some legislative changes included special constraints such as a minimum age, a minimum period of residence in the area of jurisdiction, or a maximum duration of pregnancy.[26]

Except in China, recent laws permitting abortions require that physicians carry out the procedure. Most legislation requires that the procedure be performed in medically approved facilities such as hospitals or clinics. Moreover, these institutions may have additional requirements, such as a concurring opinion from a second physician or a committee decision and consent requirements or clauses that concern individuals who work in health facilities and that address the voluntary nature of the procedure.

In the United States, judicial action has led to important changes. In 1973 the cases of *Doe vs. Bolton* and *Roe vs. Wade* led to nationwide changes in the performance of legal abortion.[27] In 1988 the United States Supreme Court decision in *Webster vs. Reproductive Health* limited this practice. Further decisions are expected to continue this general trend, although some cases have been settled by the disputants before reaching the United States Supreme Court, and advocates of the right to choose abortion may seek legislated rather than judicial action in support of their position.[28]

Four fundamental legal principles can be used in evaluating abortion laws and their related human values. The first is the right to privacy. Decisions related to fertility regulation are generally accepted to be private matters not subject to the control of other individuals. This right of privacy conflicts with the countervailing argument that the fetus has its own right to exist. The second principle is necessity; that is, individuals who perform abortions to preserve the life or health of others should not have to fear criminal liability. Third, laws should be applied equally. If only wealthy women can evade the limitations on the practice of abortion, then laws should be changed to permit poor women access to the same service. Fourth, the physician must act on the basis of health considerations of patients for whose care he or she is responsible. The WHO defines health as a state of complete physical, mental, and social well-being, not merely the absence of disease or infirmity. The 1973 decisions made by the United States Supreme Court in *Roe vs. Wade* and *Doe vs. Bolton* relied on this WHO definition of health.[27]

Education on reproductive health and family planning, both formal and informal, is an essential component of any program for preventing unintended pregnancies. A WHO meeting on this subject declared that appropriate education on reproductive health for the general public has the highest priority because of its importance in prevention and its potential influence on the largest number of people possible.[29] This concept received reinforcement in the recommendations that resulted from the International Conference on Population held in Mexico City in 1984.

Preventing pregnancy among teenagers is a high priority in many countries throughout the world, including the United States. If sexually active adolescents are to prevent pregnancies, then access to safe, effective fertility control must be permitted. In some countries, however, contraceptives may be distributed legally only to married persons.[24] In the United States, notifying parents when adolescents plan to use contraceptive services is a topic of public debate. At present, adolescents face serious problems in acquiring the information and skills needed to defer parenting.

Services and Methods. Family planning services may be provided through hospitals, clinics, individual health professionals, or commercial facilities such as drug stores. The services may include temporary contraception or permanent surgical sterilization. In considering services and methods of fertility control, both service providers and individuals needing service are influenced by certain key facts: the characteristics of the service provider (e.g., the gender of the examining physician), facilities (e.g., hospitals, public clinics, or private physician's offices), effectiveness, prevalence, popularity, perceived risk, and scientific evidence for the safe use of each approach to limiting fertility.

CONTRACEPTION

Widespread public service programs that enable individuals and couples to limit childbearing are a recent phenomenon. In the mid-1930s, several states began to provide limited contraceptive counseling and services for poor women. In July 1969, President Nixon proposed creating a federal program to help poor women have the same access to effective contraceptive methods as the affluent. The legislation supporting that proposal, Title X of the Public Health Service Act, was passed in 1970. By 1983, nearly 5 million women were receiving family planning services in organized family planning clinics; this represents a fourfold increase since 1969.[30]

Overall, where do women obtain family planning services? The answer depends heavily on income. Of women with family incomes 1.5 times the established level of poverty who make a family planning visit, 77% are likely to see a private physician, compared with 53% of lower income women. Teenagers are less likely to visit a private physician (48%) for family planning. By contrast, family planning clinic patients are largely poor; 83% have incomes below the established level of poverty. Of family planning clinic patients, 26% are black and 11% are Hispanic.[31]

In the United States, family planning services are provided primarily by physicians, nurse family planning practitioners, and pharmacists. In other countries, successful programs have marketed contraception through the commercial sector with appropriate advertising and have distributed contraceptives through community-based family planning programs. Research shows that in at least one region, the United States–Mexico border region, most Mexican Americans and Anglos would accept family planning services from medically trained persons who are not physicians and that roughly half would accept them from trained nonmedical persons.[32]

Oral Contraception

Use. Oral contraception, "the Pill," is a popular, highly effective, and for most women a safe method of contraception. An estimated 10.7 million U.S. women were using the Pill in 1988, compared with 8.4 million in 1982.[33] Pills are the most popular method of birth control for never-married women and for all women less than 25 years old.

Effectiveness. The Pill is a highly effective method of temporary contraception; currently available preparations containing both estrogen and progestin have an efficacy approaching 100%. Because they must be used consistently and correctly, however, the actual failure rate for combined (estrogen-progestin) pills is about 3% (Fig. 68-1).[34]

Progestin-only or so-called mini-pills may be somewhat less effective than pills that combine both progestin and estrogen because ovulation is not prevented as often. Studies on the efficacy of the mini-pill are less complete than those on combined pills, and reliable estimates of efficacy are therefore lacking. Nevertheless, mini-pills are considered highly effective.[34]

Complications. The short- and long-term health effects of oral contraceptives have been studied more thoroughly than those of any other drug currently prescribed. On balance, most such studies indicate that the Pill is safe for most women. In fact, studies attempting to identify potentially harmful effects of oral contraceptives have documented important noncontraceptive health benefits. Oral contraceptive users are less likely to be hospitalized for pelvic inflammatory disease (PID), ectopic pregnancy, benign breast disease, and functional ovarian cysts. They are also less likely to have iron deficiency anemia, and they may be less likely to have uterine fibroids.[35] Finally, oral contraceptives have been shown to protect against both endometrial and ovarian cancer.[14,36] (Concerns about a potentially positive relationship between Pill use and breast cancer are sufficiently controversial that this topic will be discussed in a separate section later in this chapter.)

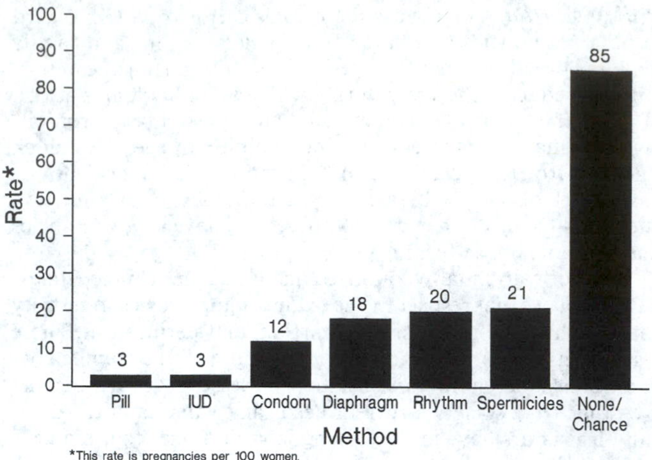

Figure 68-1. Typical accidental pregnancy rate during the first year of use by contraceptive method used in the United States. Rate is pregnancies per 100 women.

Nonetheless, the Pill is not without risk. Oral contraceptive use has been clearly associated with an increased risk of myocardial infarction, venous thrombosis, and stroke.[35] The increased risk is largely, but not exclusively, found among older women who smoke (Table 68-1).[37] Most studies report that past users have no increased risk; the increased risk appears attributable to current oral contraceptive use. Furthermore, the reported risk for cardiovascular diseases associated with oral contraceptive use may be overestimated because most reports include estimates based, in part, on use of oral contraceptive formulations no longer available. In 1988 the marketing of preparations containing $>50\ \mu g$ of estrogens was phased out after the U.S. Food and Drug Administration's Fertility and Maternal Health Drugs Advisory Committee concluded that such preparations did not have sufficient clinical advantage to warrant continued distribution. Only limited data are available to determine the risks associated with the oral contraceptives currently used. Data on whether pills containing $<50\ \mu g$ carry a reduced risk of venous thromboembolism are contradictory. Recent reports from the Group Health Cooperative of Puget Sound[38] and the Oxford Family Planning Association[39] suggest that oral contraceptives now in

TABLE 68-1. CURRENT USE OF ORAL CONTRACEPTIVES (OCs), CIGARETTE SMOKING, AND RISK OF MYOCARDIAL INFARCTION (MI)

		MIs per 100,000 Women per Year		MIs per 100,000 Current OC Users per Year	
Age (y)	**Cigarettes per Day**	***OC Users***	***Nonusers***	***Relative Risk****	***Attributable Risk***
30–39	All women	11	4	3	7
	0–14	6	2	3	4
	>15	30	11	3	19
40–44	All women	89	22	4	67
	0–14	47	12	4	35
	>15	246	61	4	185

*Relative risk of MI for OC users compared with nonusers.

From Lee N, Peterson HB, Chu SY: The health effects of contraception. In Parnell A (ed): Contraceptive Use and Controlled Fertility: Health Issues for Women and Children—Background Papers. Washington D.C.: National Academy Press, 1989.

use pose a lower risk of myocardial infarction than did those previously studied. In the former report, no deaths from cardiovascular disease were identified in the period 1977 to 1981 after approximately 55,000 woman-years of oral contraceptive use. In the latter report, no cases of myocardial infarction and only one case of angina were reported among women using oral contraceptives containing $< 50\ \mu g$ of estrogen.

Gallbladder disease and rare benign liver tumors are also occasionally associated with taking the Pill. There is controversy regarding the relationship between Pill use and development of malignant melanoma[40] and liver cancer (hepatocellular carcinoma).[41,42] Both tumors are rare in the United States, but any relationship between oral contraceptive use and malignant liver tumors could be important in developing countries where liver malignancies are more common.

The relationship between Pill use and cervical cancer continues to be controversial, in part because bias related to sexual behavior complicates the study of this association. One recent report from a study in Costa Rica[43] has also highlighted the importance of detection bias in the study of this relationship. In this report from Costa Rica, when the effects of sexual activity were adjusted for statistical control, oral contraceptive users had no greater risk of cervical cancer. Although there was an increased risk of cervical carcinoma in situ, the risk was limited to those women in whom oral contraceptive use was strongly linked to Pap smear screening, thereby suggesting bias due to the way in which information was obtained on subjects with cancer in situ.

The United States Food and Drug Administration considers the following conditions as absolute contraindications to oral contraceptive use: (1) thrombophlebitis or thromboembolic disorders, (2) a past history of deep vein thrombophlebitis or thromboembolic disorders, (3) cerebrovascular or coronary artery disease, (4) known or suspected carcinoma of the breast, (5) known or suspected estrogen-dependent neoplasia, (6) undiagnosed, abnormal genital bleeding, (7) pregnancy, (8) benign or malignant liver tumors that developed during the use of oral contraceptives or other estrogen preparations. Oral contraceptives are not usually prescribed for women who have not established a regular menstrual pattern, and estrogen-containing pills are not prescribed for women during the first 6 weeks that they are breast-feeding an infant.[44] Although no absolute upper age restriction for use has been determined, women over the age of 40 have generally been discouraged from using oral contraceptives. Recently this age limit has been questioned. The American College of Obstetricians and Gynecologists now recommends that healthy, nonsmoking women 35 to 44 years of age may continue using oral contraceptives if they do not wish to or are unable to use another reversible contraceptive method or undergo surgical sterilization.[45]

Intrauterine Devices

Use. Intrauterine contraceptive devices (IUDs) are an effective, safe method of birth control for most women. In 1982 an estimated 2.2 million women were wearing IUDs in the United States, but by 1988 only 0.7 million women were using them.[33] In other countries such as China the IUD is the most popular form of contraception.[37] In the late 1980s, manufacturers voluntarily stopped the sale of most IUDs in the United States. Sales were discontinued for marketing reasons largely attributable to the cost of litigating numerous lawsuits brought against manufacturers. Most such lawsuits alleged that IUD use resulted in pelvic infection or infertility.[46] In 1989 a new copper IUD, the Copper T 380A, was introduced to U.S. markets.

Effectiveness. The IUD is highly effective, with method failure rates of about 3% per year (Fig. 68–1). The user-effectiveness rates, which include the risk of undetected IUD expulsion, is somewhat higher, at about 6% per year.

Complications. Unlike oral contraceptives, IUDs have no documented noncontraceptive health benefits. Although pregnancy rates are low for IUD users, women who do become pregnant have a greater risk of ectopic pregnancy and of spontaneous septic abortion of an intrauterine pregnancy.[47] If the IUD is removed as soon as the pregnancy is diagnosed, most cases of septic abortion can be prevented.

In particular, IUDs have been associated with an increased risk of pelvic inflammatory disease (PID). The Dalkon Shield IUD, which is no longer available, has been associated with a high risk of PID.[48] Women using other types of IUD have been found to have risks about 1.5 to 2.0 times greater than those for women who use no contraception.[48] One recent report indicates that IUD users in mutually monogamous sexual relationships may have little increased risk of PID associated with IUD use, suggesting that much of the increased risk of PID among IUD users is confined to women at increased risk for sexually transmitted diseases.[48] Results of studies on IUD-associated infertility are difficult to interpret. Any increased risk is presumably related to an increased risk of PID. One study found that women who reported having only one sexual partner had no increased risk of tubal infertility associated with IUD use.[37]

Wearing an IUD is absolutely contraindicated for women with active pelvic infection including known or suspected gonorrheal infection or for those with uterine or cervical malignancy. Women with abnormal uterine bleeding, dysmenorrhea, distortions or congenital malformations of the uterine cavity, or impaired resistance to infection should not use IUDs. Uterine perforation is more likely to occur when an IUD is inserted into the uterus of a lactating woman.[44]

Traditional Methods

The condom, vaginal diaphragm, and spermicidal creams, foams, jellies, and suppositories are the traditional contraceptive methods in the United States. Newer related methods include the spermicide-impregnated contraceptive sponge and the cervical cap. All these methods require substantial user motivation and are likely influenced by user experience and skill at use.

Use. Traditional contraceptive methods are used by millions of American couples, despite the widespread prevalence of the Pill and IUD. Condoms were used by approximately 3.6 million United States couples in 1982; this number increased to 5.1 million (a 41% increase) in 1988.[33] The role of condoms for prevention of human immunodeficiency virus and other sexually transmitted diseases has likely led to this increased prevalence of use. In the United States during 1982, diaphragms were used by 1.9 million and spermicides by 1.5 million women; there were slight decreases in use in 1988.[33] Newly developed methods similar to the traditional methods include contraceptive sponges and cervical caps. These approaches to fertility control are used less frequently at present than are the more established traditional methods.

Effectiveness. Failure rates will be largely influenced by user determinants. Of the traditional methods, the condom is the most effective when used consistently and correctly. The estimated user-failure rate for condoms in the first year is 12% (Fig. 68–1). The diaphragm (used with spermicides) and vaginal spermicides (alone) have a 1.5 to 2.0 times greater risk of unintended pregnancy relative to the condom.

Clinical data suggest that overall, contraceptive sponges are less effective than the diaphragm. Although the failure rates for nulliparous sponge users are similar to those for diaphragm users, rates among parous women are appreciably higher. The cervical cap is estimated to be as effective as the diaphragm, although few published data are available.[49]

Complications. The risks associated with use of traditional contraceptives include the risk of unintended pregnancy and the usually minor and specific complaints associated with the method. These complaints include vaginal irritation by spermicidal jelly, discomfort from a poorly positioned diaphragm, or local response to condom lubricant. In addition, diaphragm users have a twofold to threefold greater risk of urinary tract infections compared to women who do not use contraceptives.[37] Although one report raised concern about a possible positive relationship between spermicides and the risk of congenital defects, several larger and better designed studies failed to confirm any association.[37] Contraceptive sponge users may be at increased risk for vaginal candidiasis,[50] and both sponge and diaphragm users have a relatively increased risk of toxic shock syndrome.[51] Because toxic shock syndrome is rare, however, the absolute risk associated with sponge or diaphragm use is small. Women immediately postpartum and women who have had toxic shock syndrome should not use either the sponge or diaphragm, and neither the sponge nor diaphragm should be left in the vagina for more than 30 hours.[52]

Rhythm and Fertility Awareness

Use. Rhythm and fertility awareness, or natural family planning methods, are not widely used in the United States, although their use is prevalent in some other countries. Fewer than 1 million couples used these methods in the United States in 1988.[33]

Effectiveness. The reported method failure rates for periodic abstinence is 2%, but the user failure rate is 18%; the method failure rate for withdrawal is 10%, and the user failure rates is 20%. Clearly, methods of natural family planning depend largely on user determinants, such as motivation and skill.

Complications. Other than unintended pregnancy, which occurs more frequently than with most other methods mentioned thus far, no adverse health effects are associated with these methods.

Other Approaches

Two additional methods, postcoital contraception and injectable hormones, deserve discussion even though they are infrequently used in the United States and are not fully sanctioned. One frequently recommended drug for postcoital contraception is the combination pill containing ethinylestradiol 50 μg and *dl*-norgestrel 0.5 mg (marketed in the United States as Ovral). When used for postcoital contraception, two of these tablets are taken within 3 days of unprotected intercourse (preferably within 12 to 24 hours) followed by two additional tablets taken 12 hours later. Clinical studies indicate that this regimen is highly effective.[53] Regular use of postcoital contraception is not recommended.

The injectable hormone depo-medroxyprogesterone acetate has been used extensively around the world, but it is not approved for use in the United States. The scientific basis for its lack of approval was its carcinogenic effect in experimental animals. Epidemiological studies have produced conflicting, but mostly negative, findings regarding cancer in humans.[37] The drug appears similar in efficacy to oral contraceptives. Clinical trials of other injectable progestins are currently underway.

A final method, Norplant, is a subdermal implant system of six silastic rods impregnated with a progestin (levonorgestrel), which is continuously and slowly released. Norplant has undergone extensive clinical testing and is highly effective for 5 years, after which it should be removed and replaced if desired. The most common side effect is irregular menstrual bleeding. Abnormal bleeding decreases with use but is the most frequent reason for discontinuing use of the method. Epidemiological studies of the long-term health effects of Norplant have not been conducted. Laboratory studies have generally identified no important changes in metabolic measurements, but studies of lipid metabolism have been somewhat conflicting.[54] The United States Food and Drug Administration has recently approved Norplant for use as a contraceptive in the United States.

Breast Feeding

Breast feeding is described as ''nature's contraceptive,'' and it is asserted that on a worldwide scale, more births are prevented by breast feeding than by any other method of contraception. One relatively isolated society that has no other practices that limit fertility, such as delaying the age of marriage or having a taboo against intercourse during lactation, has breast feeding as one of its most important means of limiting fertility. These people have an average completed family size of 4.7 children and an average birth interval of 4.1 years. Their use of breast feeding differs, however, from practices in the Western world in that the mother and infant are together throughout the day and night. The infant suckles frequently (on average four times per hour) for brief intervals when being carried about by the mother during the day and while the mother is sleeping at night.[55] Because breast feeding in the United States is a relatively infrequent practice, controlling fertility while lactating becomes a problem of choosing the right contraceptive during the time that a mother is breast feeding her infant. Since oral contraceptives with estrogens suppress lactation, their use should either be deferred until lactation is well established (usually until the infant is 6 weeks old and gaining weight), or some other method should be chosen. Traditional contraceptives, progestational agents, intrauterine devices, and surgical sterilization do not inhibit lactation.

Sterilization

Surgical sterilization is estimated to be the most prevalent form of contraception in the world today. Globally more than 100 million couples are using this form of birth control; an estimated 95 million women have undergone tubal sterilization—making it the most widely used contraceptive method in the world.[56] China, India, and the United States have the highest estimated numbers of sterilized couples. In 1988 an estimated 47% of United States women 35 to 44 years of age were relying on surgical sterilization (including vasectomy) of the spouse for fertility control.[33]

Female Sterilization

Use. The prevalence of tubal sterilization in the United States increased dramatically during the 1970s. The number of tubal sterilizations performed in hospitals increased from approximately 200,000 in 1970 to approximately 702,000 in 1977. Thereafter the number of procedures performed in hospitals began to decline.[57,58] This decline was at least in part attributable to an increased performance of tubal sterilization in out-of-hospital facilities. Because systematic national surveillance of outpatient tubal sterilization has not been conducted, we cannot accurately assess trends in outpatient tubal sterilization over time. A recent report, however, estimates that in 1987, 640,000 tubal sterilizations were performed in the United States, and an estimated 33% of these were performed out-of-hospital.[59] The large number of tubal sterilizations continuing to be performed in the United States is particularly remarkable given that the number of reproductive-age women who can bear children (and thus are candidates for tubal sterilization) is reduced by hysterectomy as well as by tubal sterilization. About one of every three women in the

United States will undergo a hysterectomy by the time she is 60 years old.[60] The prevalence rate for tubal sterilization in 1978 was adjusted for cumulative prevalences of hysterectomy and tubal sterilization among women of reproductive age in the United States. The corrected sterilization rates were appreciably higher than the uncorrected rates, particularly among older women.[61]

Effectiveness. Published estimates of the efficacy of tubal sterilization techniques are limited by methodological problems, including a lack of large numbers of sterilized women with long-term follow-up. Most of the methodological limitations would tend to underestimate the number of sterilization failures, and, thus, most published estimates, including the estimate of 4 per 1000 procedures, are likely underestimates. The likelihood of sterilization failure will almost certainly depend on certain physician and patient characteristics, as well as method of tubal occlusion. A more accurate picture of the relationship between these factors and sterilization failure must await further study as women are followed up over sufficient time. Data are currently available, however, to indicate that the likelihood of ectopic pregnancy when sterilization failure does occur is influenced by method of tubal occlusion: electrocoagulation failures are more likely to result in ectopic gestations than methods of mechanical occlusion are. This is a relative increase, however, because the absolute increased risk of ectopic pregnancy depends on the overall efficacy of each method of tubal occlusion, which is incompletely characterized.[62]

Complications. The short-term safety of tubal sterilization, which has been extensively studied, shows that the risk of dying from tubal sterilization in the United States is estimated to be one to two deaths per 100,000 procedures.[63] Complications from general anesthesia cause most deaths attributable to sterilization. Hemorrhage, usually associated with abdominal penetration for laparoscopy, and infection, particularly associated with thermal bowel injury following unipolar electrocoagulation, are other important causes.[64] Although case-fatality rates in developing countries have been reported to be higher than those in the United States, the major causes of death are similar. For example, in Bangladesh a case-fatality rate of 19/100,000 tubal sterilizations was identified in 1982, and complications of anesthesia were also the leading cause of death; however, in this instance, oversedation with narcotic analgesics during local anesthesia was the problem.[65] A follow-up study revealed that the case-fatality rate dropped dramatically after recommendations for lower doses of analgesics and larger doses of local anesthetics.[66]

Major morbidity from tubal sterilization is also uncommon. In the World Health Organization's Multinational Study, approximately 1600 women were randomly assigned to be sterilized by either minilaparotomy (i.e., abdominal entry via a 2 to 5 cm incision) or laparoscopy (i.e., insertion of a surgical endoscope through a 1 cm subumbilical incision). Major complications occurred in 1.5% of approximately 800 women who underwent minilaparotomy and in 0.9% of approximately 800 women who underwent laparoscopy using electrocoagulation.[67] A multicenter follow-up study of laparoscopic tubal sterilization in the United States revealed that 1.7% of women had at least one of six intraoperative or postoperative complications.[68] The most frequent (1.1%) was unintended major surgery, which sometimes occurred because of incidental pathology identified during laparoscopy or because of technical limitations of laparoscopy, not because of procedural complications per se. In that study the risk of complications was increased at least twofold by the following factors: obesity, pulmonary disease, diabetes mellitus, previous abdominal or pelvic surgery, or a history of pelvic inflammatory disease.

Although major complication rates are generally reported as being less than 2%, these rates, nevertheless, indicate that sterilization-attributable complications can and do result in serious injury. The likelihood of serious injury apparently varies by surgical approach and method of tubal occlusion. Most minilaparotomy complications are not serious; minor bleeding, minor wound infections, and uterine perforations are those most frequently reported.[56]

By contrast, complications of laparoscopy are more likely to be life threatening. Although rare, thermal bowel injuries may result from tubal occlusion by electrocoagulation, and major vessel injury or viscus perforation may result from abdominal penetration prior to insertion of the laparoscope.[68] When such complications occur, early diagnosis and intervention can be critical for a patient's survival.

The long-term safety and acceptability of tubal sterilization are less completely studied, but recently published reports are mostly reassuring, although a longer period of follow-up will be needed. The existence of a so-called postubal syndrome has been debated since the early 1950s. The debate began when menstrual disturbances were reported at varying intervals after sterilization. Most recent data suggest that such changes are not likely attributable to sterilization per se but rather to other factors, for example, cessation of oral contraceptive use. Although studies that provide the most reassurance are based on only 1 to 2 years of poststerilization follow-up, two studies[69,70] with longer follow-up were less encouraging. Thus an answer to the question of whether a "postubal syndrome" exists must await further studies with long-term follow-up.

Tubal sterilization and hysterectomy are common surgical procedures. Tubal sterilization could potentially increase the risk of subsequent hysterectomy by at least three possible mechanisms: (1) the posttubal syndrome, if real, may result in menstrual disturbances that are managed by hysterectomy; (2) the perception that the postubal syndrome exists may encourage the use of hysterectomy for managing poststerilization menstrual disturbances even if they are not attributable to sterilization per se; (3) once a woman is sterilized, she or her physician may more quickly resort to surgical management of a gynecologic problem. A cohort study in the United Kingdom, however, identified no increase among sterilized women in hospital referrals for hysterectomy at 3 and 6 years after tubal sterilization compared with wives of men who had vasectomies.[69] By contrast, a population-based study in Canada found an increased likelihood of subsequent hysterectomy that was limited to women undergoing tubal sterilization at ages 25 to 29 years.[71] Beginning with a 2-year follow-up and increasing for up to 9 years, that group had a 60% statistically significant increased risk of subsequent hysterectomy.

Most data suggest that women are satisfied with their decisions to undergo tubal sterilizations; the range of estimated dissatisfaction across studies varies widely, however, from 2% to 13%.[56] This range likely reflects, to some extent, variations of definitions of regret used for study. For example, a survey of women in the United States found that 26% responded affirmatively when asked, "If it were possible for you to have another baby, would you, yourself, like to have one?"[72] Regardless of how a study defines younger women, being young at the time of sterilization appears to be a key determinant of later regret. Most women who express regret attempt to have their sterilization reversed by surgical reanastomosis. In a U.S. follow-up study, approximately 2/1000 sterilized women had undergone tubal reanastomosis by the fifth year of poststerilization follow-up.[73] Reversal surgery is expensive, requires laparotomy, and is not always available. In general, a reported 50% to 70% of women who undergo reversal surgery achieve intrauterine pregnancy, but many factors, including method of tubal occlusion used for sterilization, influence this rate of intrauterine pregnancy.[56] Most published reports are likely overestimates, for they usually represent the selected series of highly skilled surgeons using sophisticated techniques.

Male Sterilization

Use. More than 40 million men are currently using vasectomy for contraception worldwide; most of these men live in the United States, United Kingdom, China, and India.[74] Because vasectomy is rarely performed in a hospital, the number of men who undergo this procedure each year in the United States can only be approximated. In 1987 an estimated 336,000 men in the United States underwent vasectomy.[75]

Effectiveness. Most studies of the effectiveness of vasectomy are case series done by individual physicians or institutions; they do not allow for a comparison of the methods of vas occlusion. Such studies report failure rates less than 1% with a range from 0 to 2%.[76] Those failures typically result either from unprotected coitus shortly after vasectomy or from spontaneous reanastomosis of the vas. To avoid pregnancy from unprotected coitus, clearance of sperm from the reproductive tract should be documented before intercourse is resumed. Without such documentation, additional contraception should be used for the first 15 ejaculations, or for 6 weeks, after vasectomy.[77] Most true vasectomy failures result from spontaneous reanastomosis of the vas via fistulous tracks within sperm granulomas.[76] The likelihood of spontaneous reanastomosis may vary by vasectomy technique, and coagulation occlusion is theoretically less likely than ligation to result in sperm granuloma and fistula formation at the vas occlusion site.[78] Coagulation occlusion may, however, result in a greater likelihood of epididymal sperm granuloma formation; this may impair any subsequent attempt at reversing a vasectomy.

Complications. Vasectomy is a minor surgical procedure that usually takes 5 to 20 minutes to perform. Local anesthesia without premedication is used for most vasectomies. During the procedure the vas deferens is isolated and then occluded, using either ligation, coagulation, or clip application. Ligation is the most widely used approach.

The risk of death attributable to vasectomy is quite low. The Association For Voluntary Surgical Contraception has identified only two vasectomy-attributable deaths associated with more than 160,000 procedures performed in the international programs it has supported.[77] Major morbidity is also uncommon. Although as many as 50% of men may experience minor complications, such as swelling of the scrotal tissue, bruising, and pain, these generally subside without treatment within 1 to 2 weeks after vasectomy.[76] Hematoma formation and infection occur much less frequently and generally are not serious. A 1983 survey of U.S. physicians reported a hematoma rate of 2%.[79] Infection after vasectomy is generally reported in fewer than 2% of men. Epididymitis, which is manifested by swelling and tenderness of the epididymis, is usually reported in fewer than 1% of men undergoing vasectomy.[76] "Epididymitis" may be a misnomer because bacterial infection as a cause is unusual, and much of the aching associated with epididymitis is likely to result from epididymal congestion caused by back pressure rather than from infection or inflammation. Formation of sperm granulomas at the surgical site or in the epididymis is another complication of vasectomy. Most sperm granulomas are, however, small and asymptomatic. Nonetheless, their presence may complicate any future attempt at reversing sterilization.[76]

The long-term health effects of vasectomy are now well characterized. Reports of an increased risk of atherosclerosis among cynomolgus monkeys after vasectomy caused great concern regarding the risk of atherosclerosis among men after vasectomy. This concern led to numerous epidemiological investigations in men and further laboratory studies in monkeys. All strongly suggest that vasectomy does not increase the risk of myocardial infarction or coronary heart disease in men after vasectomy.[80]

The same reports that addressed the possibility of cardiovascular disease remote from vasectomy also studied the relationship between vasectomy and a variety of other diseases. Although vasectomy was associated with an increased risk of several genitourinary tract diseases, including certain cancers, these associations were reported as isolated findings in a minority of studies and are inconsistent between studies.[80] Most studies have found no link between vasectomy and genitourinary tract disorders and no association between vasectomy and other disease outcomes. The breadth and depth of the investigations and the general lack of positive findings are broadly reassuring and suggest that little concern regarding the long-term health effects of vasectomy is warranted.[80] In sum, numerous investigations strongly support the contention that vasectomy is safe both in the short- and in the long-term.

PROGRAM EFFECTS

Family planning services and programs can have profound effects on fertility, health, and society.

Fertility Change. Family planning influences the fertility of countries and communities, as well as individuals. Taiwan was one of the first countries to undertake a nationwide family planning program, and one of the first to document a reduction in fertility. In this island nation the crude birth rate declined 48% from 37.7/1000 population in 1961 to 19.6/1000 population in 1984. The general fertility rate (live births per 1000 women aged 15 to 44) and the total fertility, both of which allow for the age structure of the women in a population, decreased even more (58% and 63%).[81] Moreover, the use of effective fertility control measures increased strikingly as fertility declined. In 1965, 41% of women aged 35 to 39 years had used contraception at some time; by 1980, 92% of the women in this age group stated that they had used some form of contraception. The number of individuals who had undergone abortion, sterilization, or both also increased. Finally, responses to questions about the preferred number of children per family reflected a decline during these years.[82]

Similar effects have been found in other nations. South Korea, Singapore, China, and Chile are countries where IUD use has played an important role. In others, such as Brazil,[83] Colombia,[84] and Puerto Rico,[85] contraceptive sterilization has played a prominent role. The effect of induced abortion on fertility change is best documented in eastern Europe.[86] The influence of organized family planning programs is presumed to be of particular importance in Costa Rico, Panama, and Mauritius.

A worldwide assessment of family planning programs in developing countries has shown that where programs make a strong effort, a decline in fertility often follows. In regions where developing countries predominate, south and east Asia include nations that make the greatest effort, whereas sub-Saharan African countries as a group make the least.[87] Nonetheless, even in countries with high fertility rates and national programs considered to be rather ineffective, areas can be found where contraceptive prevalence is comparatively higher and fertility is substantially lower than in the rest of the nation.[88]

Health Change. Family planning programs may influence health in at least four ways:

1. By permitting a woman to bear children at an age when the risk of health problems to her and her offspring is lowest.
2. By permitting a couple to choose the number of children they wish to have.
3. By permitting a couple to determine the spacing of their children.

4. By providing safe and effective measures of fertility control that are part of a service program that includes information, education, and comprehensive preventive health services.

The risk of health problems during pregnancy increases with age and with the number of pregnancies. A report from the United Kingdom states that toxemia of pregnancy is an important cause of maternal mortality for young women (less than 20 years of age) having their first child.[89] Thus the use of family planning enhances maternal health by permitting women to delay the birth of their first child and to avoid childbearing in their later reproductive years by using surgical sterilization, if so desired.[90]

Infant health will also be improved if women postpone the birth of their first child until they are at least 20 and avoid childbearing after they reach age 35. Recent data from the United States using linked birth and infant death records show high infant mortality for young mothers (age 10 to 14) and for women in their later reproductive years (age 35 or older). In addition, the risk of infant death is lowest for infants of second and third live birth order and highest for infants of birth order five and greater.[91] Birth defects, such as Down syndrome and heart malformations—most likely to affect infants of mothers who are in their mid and late 30s or older—are specific causes of death that cause particular concern. The incidence of Down syndrome in the United States has declined by 50% in the past several decades. At least half of this decline has been attributed to the use of effective family planning by women in the later years of reproductive life.[92]

Family size also influences the health of children. Not only infant death rates but also fetal death rates increase as the birth order of the pregnancy increases.[93,94] In addition, family size influences nutritional status; as the number of children per family increases, the per capita protein consumption declines, and the proportion of children who are malnourished increases.[95,96]

Birth spacing influences survival during the neonatal and postneonatal periods and throughout the years before the fifth birthday.[97] For births that occur less than 2 years apart, the risk of mortality may increase by more than 50%. Because breast feeding is an important determinant of the birth interval and because hormonal contraception may suppress lactation, the use of fertility control agents that may limit breast feeding need careful consideration. It may be desirable to postpone the use of methods such as the Pill, to use an effective, but nonhormonal method, or to consider voluntary postpartum sterilization to establish lactation and optimize family health.

Social Change. Family planning programs and services in some countries have social change as a goal. In the United States, for example, "family planning is based on the voluntary decisions and the actions of individuals. Its purpose is to enable individuals to make their own decisions regarding reproduction and to implement their decisions. Family planning includes measures, both to prevent unintended fertility and to overcome unintended infertility."[21]

Can family planning programs and services actually attain such goals? Survey research permits the analysis of fertility to separate births into specific categories: mistimed, unwanted, and planned. A mistimed birth is one that did not exceed the total number a woman wanted but that occurred at a time in the life cycle when it was not desired (e.g., before marriage). An unwanted birth is one that occurred after the last wanted birth. The sum of the mistimed and unwanted births may be termed unintended or unplanned.

In the United States, mistimed births increased between 1979–1982 and 1984–1988 for all ages except 30 to 34. Overall, the percent of mistimed births increased from 27% to 28%, and the percent for mothers whose age was from 15 through 19 years was 54% during the years 1979–1982 and 57% during 1984–1988. The percent unintended for 15- to 19-year-old mothers increased from 67% in 1979–1982 to 73% in 1984–1988.[98]

The status of unwanted fertility has been analyzed for several countries. In the United States, where family planning efforts have focused on reducing unwanted childbearing, the results of national surveys show that unwanted births declined in all race and marital status groups since 1968,[99] but the 1988 National Survey of Family Growth (NSFG) showed an increase in unwanted births since the 1982 NSFG from 10% to 12% for mothers of all ages and from 14% to 16% for those younger than 20 years of age.[98] Analysis of these trends shows that if unwanted fertility were prevented, the population increase in this country would be at replacement, assuming no changes in determinants other than fertility, that is, mortality or migration.[100]

In an analysis of the demographic and health surveys done in a selected group of developing countries, the importance of increasing the prevalence of contraceptive use in reducing unwanted fertility was emphasized if unwanted births were to be prevented.[100]

As profound as these changes are in the United States, they may fall short of the goal, as stated in the national health objectives. Persistent differences in the proportion of unwanted and mistimed pregnancies between different racial groups for women of every marital status are associated with differences in contraceptive use, including the use of surgical sterilization. A comparison of unplanned fertility and family planning services in the United States with those in other developed countries indicates that family planning services in the United States are less likely to promote the use of highly effective contraception. This approach to health promotion may help to explain the shortfall in meeting the nation's goal.

Women with a wanted pregnancy may be more likely to seek earlier prenatal care than are those with an unwanted pregnancy.[101] In addition, evidence suggests that those married women with an unwanted pregnancy are less likely to stop smoking than are those whose pregnancy is wanted.[102]

Abortion

Use and Changes in Practice. The number of legal abortions reported by official channels to the Centers for Disease Control (CDC) increased each year from 1969 through 1982, declined slightly the following year, and has remained in the range of 1.3 million each year since. Preliminary data indicate that 1.354 million abortions were performed in 1987. Most of the women undergoing legal, voluntary termination of pregnancy were younger than age 25, white, unmarried, had no previous live births, and underwent the procedure in their state of residence. Almost all the procedures were suction curettage and were done in the first 12 weeks of pregnancy.[103]

Reports from The Alan Guttmacher Institute (AGI) consistently cite numbers of abortions greater than those from the CDC. AGI states that the number of abortions performed legally is between 1.4 and 1.5 million each year since early in this decade. The AGI reports come from sources that include other than official agencies; data from the CDC probably give conservative estimates of the total number of legal abortions done in the United States each year.

Current trends in the medical practice of abortion in the United States continue to favor improved health for pregnant women. Since 1983 intrauterine saline instillation has been used for fewer than 2% of all abortions for which the procedure is known and reached its lowest level (1.3%) in 1987, the most recent year reported. Major surgical procedures, that is, hysterotomy or hysterectomy, were used for fewer than 0.05% of all procedures (fewer than 200 each year) beginning in 1984. In the late 1970s, two trends that continued into the 1980s started:

abortions were performed in the state where the woman lives and within the first 12 weeks of pregnancy.[103]

Complications. Legal abortion continues to be a safe surgical procedure for pregnant women. The CDC reports that the death-to-case rate was less than 1/100,000 procedures for every year in the 1980s and was less than 0.5 in 1985.[104] Beginning with the eighth menstrual week of gestation, the longer the pregnancy, the more likely a pregnant woman is to experience morbidity or mortality.

The risk of nonfatal complications from abortion, like the risk of mortality, increases with the length of pregnancy. In 1980 there were an estimated 4530 hospitalizations because of the complications of legal abortions. This is estimated to be half the number related to the use of oral contraceptives and IUDs.[105] Only six women died from these complications in 1985.[106]

Concern about abortion and continued differences in viewpoints on abortion in the United States have focused attention on the mental health, educational, and behavioral aspects of this approach. A review of available studies by the surgeon general of the Public Health Service led Dr. C. Everett Koop to report that the evidence regarding adverse mental health effects was insufficient and of such poor quality as to provide no information.[107] Moreover, a study of black teenage women beginning at the time they sought pregnancy testing and lasting for 2 years of follow-up found higher rates of timely high school graduation, improved economic status, and no greater anxiety, stress, or psychological problems for those who underwent abortion compared with those who carried their pregnancy to term or those who had negative pregnancy tests.[108]

KEY ISSUES

Teenage Fertility. Teenage pregnancy is an important issue to public health for at least three reasons: (1) pregnancies in very young women of reproductive age are often not intended; (2) teenage pregnancies may be at high risk of preventable health problems for both infant and mother; and (3) children born to young women may lead to unanticipated momentum in population growth by increasing total family size over a lifetime and by shortening the time between generations of future children.

The United States Department of Health and Human Services goals for 1990 and for 2000 highlight the problem of childbearing among teenagers.[21] Specifically, the 1990 national health objectives stated that (1) there should be almost no unintended births to girls 14 years of age and under; (2) the fertility rate for girls 15 years of age should be reduced to 10/1000; (3) the fertility rate for girls 16 years of age should be reduced to 25/1000; (4) the fertility rate for girls 17 years of age should be reduced to 45/1000.

Survey data showed that in 1973, nearly 60% of births to women younger than age 20 were unplanned (i.e., unwanted or mistimed); more recent data showed that in 1982, that proportion had reached nearly 80%. The number of teenage births increased nearly 8% from an estimated 361,000 in 1973 to 389,000, yet the total number of births to women in this age group declined nearly 20%. Because the national birth rates for this age group did not decline substantially between 1982 and 1988 and because the percentage of unintended births increased between the 1982 NSFG and the 1988 NSFG, there is no reason to believe this trend has changed in recent years.

This estimate deals only with live births and does not include the legal abortions (232,000 in 1973 and 418,000 in 1982) that women in this age group underwent or the births and abortions to those younger than age 15, which accounted for more than 24,000 pregnancies in 1973 and in 1982.[33] Pregnancy rates for teenagers who are of a race other than white are double the rates for those who are white, even though the proportion of unplanned pregnancies is not appreciably different for these two groups of young women.[109]

Compared with other nations for which data are available on teenage pregnancy, the United States has a rate (95/1000 women aged 15 to 19) that is among the highest.[110] The pregnancy rate for Canada (46/1000 women aged 15 to 19) is less than half that for the United States. The Netherlands has a teenage pregnancy rate of 15, the lowest reported.

The Pill and Breast Cancer. Because breast cancer is a hormonally related malignancy, we should question whether using the Pill may be related to the risk of breast cancer. Because breast cancer is both common and serious and oral contraceptive use is so widespread, any relationship would be of great importance.

Numerous epidemiological studies are now being conducted to evaluate the impact of pill use on breast cancer risk. Most studies to date suggest that overall, a woman's risk of breast cancer is not influenced by having ever used oral contraceptives. For example, a meta-analysis by Prentice and Thomas of 16 studies published through 1986 found that women who used oral contraceptives and women who did not had exactly the same risk for breast cancer (relative risk = 1.0). The authors noted, however that many of these studies were conducted in the 1970s, at a time when the long-term effects of oral contraceptive use were difficult to assess, because only 10 to 15 years had elapsed since the introduction of oral contraceptives.[111] Even studies conducted in the 1980s are constrained by having the mid-50s as an upper age limit for study participants because women older than that did not have oral contraceptives available to them during the reproductive years. No published reports have studied the risk of developing breast cancer at ages during which most women have breast cancer diagnosed, that is, in their 60s and 70s.

The Cancer and Steroid Hormone Study[112] is the largest study to date of the risk of breast cancer associated with oral contraceptive use. This study was a population-based, case-control study that was conducted from 1980 to 1982 in eight geographic regions of the United States and included study participants who were 20 to 54 years of age. It gathered detailed clinical and demographic information from 4711 women who had newly diagnosed breast cancer and 4676 women who were controls. The overall risk of breast cancer for women who had ever used oral contraceptives was no different from that for women who had never used them (relative risk = 1.0). Even women who had used them for 15 or more years had no increased risk of breast cancer. No increased risks were identified for any of the 12 most commonly used oral contraceptives in the United States, and no increased risks were identified among women considered as potentially high risk, including those with a family history of breast cancer, women with a personal history of benign breast disease, women who were never pregnant during the study period, and women who were relatively older at first term pregnancy.

Although most data suggest that the overall risk of breast cancer is not increased by oral contraceptive use, data are conflicting regarding the risk of oral contraceptive use by certain specific groups of women, including those who used the oral contraceptives for a long time, began to use them at an early age, or used them before their first term pregnancy,[113] even though the Cancer and Steroid Hormone Study found no increased risk among any of these subgroups. Even though the data are not conclusive, they suggest that the relationship of oral contraceptive use and breast cancer risk may vary by age at breast cancer diagnosis. Researchers have observed such variation for several known breast cancer risk factors such as parity. Parous women are more likely to have breast cancer diagnosed before age 35 but less likely than nulliparous women to have breast cancer diagnosed after age 35. Most studies of oral contraceptive use restricted to women with a diagnosis of breast cancer before age 45 identify slightly increased risks for women who use oral contraception relative to those who do not. By contrast, several studies have identified slightly reduced risk for breast cancer diagnosis at older ages (up to the mid-50s) for women who use oral contraception.

Whether Pill use mimics pregnancy and has a different effect on the risk of breast cancer at different ages is unclear. The public health implications of any such effects are evident, however. Because breast cancer diagnosis before age 45 is relatively uncommon, any increased risk associated with Pill use would affect a relatively small number of women; conversely, any real and persistent protective effect would influence the health of large numbers of women and would potentially lead to a decreased lifetime risk of developing breast cancer. Although further studies regarding breast cancer risk are urgently needed, the available data are broadly reassuring regarding the relationship between Pill use and lifetime breast cancer risk.

AIDS and Family Planning. Acquired immunodeficiency syndrome (AIDS), first described in 1981, is now a worldwide epidemic. Since AIDS was first identified, more than 100,000 people in the United States have contracted this disease. An estimated 1 to 1.5 million people in the United States and an estimated 5 to 10 million people worldwide are currently infected with human immunodeficiency virus (HIV).

AIDS is caused by the HIV, which was first described in 1984. There are only three routes of HIV transmission: (1) sexual, by exposure to an infected person's genital secretions, (2) exposure to infected blood or blood products, and (3) mother-to-infant (vertical or perinatal) transmission before, during, or shortly after birth. Although treatment under development promises to improve the length and quality of life for many persons with AIDS, no cure is on the horizon, and therefore prevention of AIDS remains paramount.

Family planning plays a key role in preventing AIDS because of its relation to both heterosexual and mother-to-infant transmission of HIV. Condom use—which has been considered by family planners primarily to be a method of family planning and by sexually transmitted disease (STD) personnel primarily as a method for prevention of STD—serves both important functions within the family planning–AIDS relationship.

Although the most effective strategies for preventing heterosexual transmission of HIV are abstinence or having sex with an uninfected partner in a mutually monogamous relationship, condom use continues to play an important role in preventing heterosexual transmission. Laboratory data indicate that an intact latex condom prevents HIV transmission.[114,115] Because natural membrane condoms are not manufactured, pore sizes may vary, and presumably, some may be large enough to allow passage of HIV. Because the natural membrane condoms are thus of uncertain efficacy, latex condoms should be preferentially recommended for HIV prevention.

The effectiveness of condoms in the laboratory may not necessarily reflect their effectiveness during actual use. By analogy, condom use prevents passage of sperm in the laboratory because sperm, like HIV, are too large to pass through the microscopic pores of a condom. Yet, condoms have not been considered a highly effective method of family planning.

Possible explanations for the observed discrepancy between effectiveness in the laboratory and effectiveness with actual condom use include these:

1. Breakage of the condom: Although data are limited, this event is estimated to occur in 0.7% to 0.5% of condoms used.[116,117] The age of the condom and condom storage conditions almost certainly influence breakage. Condoms should be stored in a cool, dry place. Condoms in damaged packages or those with obvious signs of age should not be used.
2. Failure to consistently and correctly use condoms: Failure to use condoms properly with each act of intercourse, failure to put the condom on before genital contact occurs, and failure to completely unroll the condom during application are more important determinants of condom efficacy than breakage. Leakage from the condom after ejaculation is likely preventable with proper use. Only water-based lubricants should be used for condoms because petroleum- or oil-based products can damage latex.[118]
3. Spermicides may not inactivate HIV: Although spermicides inactivate HIV in the laboratory,[115] the effectiveness of spermicides for preventing HIV transmission in humans has not been well studied. To be effective, spermicides would have to be dispersed adequately in sufficient concentration to destroy HIV over all exposed portions of the cervix and vagina. Spermicides cannot be considered an appropriate alternative to condom use for preventing HIV infection. Spermicides may, however, provide additional protection against HIV transmission in the event of condom breakage. In theory, if a condom broke, using intravaginal spermicides plus condoms would be more effective than using only condoms lubricated with spermicides because the intravaginal spermicides can be present in higher concentrations.

Oral contraceptives are highly effective for preventing pregnancy and thus are an important strategy for prevention of mother-to-infant transmission of HIV. The steroid hormones in oral contraceptives could theoretically increase or decrease the risk of HIV transmission; further, those hormones could potentially alter the clinical course of HIV infection favorably or unfavorably. Insufficient data exist to address those considerations, and consequently, there is no reason to change prescribing practices or use of oral contraceptives based on HIV transmission. At the same time, however, no evidence suggests that oral contraceptives protect against HIV transmission, so oral contraceptive users at risk for HIV infection must also use condoms consistently and correctly.

The relationship between other methods of family planning and HIV transmission also remains unclear. No data regarding the relationship between use of intrauterine devices, barrier methods (such as vaginal diaphragms), injectable and implantable steroid hormones, and risk of HIV transmission have been published; therefore, any such considerations are only theoretical. The relationship between male and female sterilization and HIV transmission is also unclear.

HIV infection among women of reproductive age represents a compound tragedy because of the potential for transmission of infection from infected mother to infant. The percentage of AIDS cases among women in the United States is increasing. In 1989, most of the approximately 10% of reported AIDS cases among women occurred in those of reproductive age. Most pediatric AIDS cases result from mother-to-infant transmission. Therefore, preventing AIDS in children will largely depend on the prevention of HIV infection among women of reproductive age and unintended pregnancy among women already infected. An estimated 25% to 40% of infants born to infected mothers will become HIV-infected themselves.[119]

HIV-infected women who choose not to become pregnant because of this risk of transmission or for any other reason should have highly effective birth prevention methods available. In the United States, most HIV-infected women are members of minority groups and at substantial socioeconomic disadvantage. Often, such women have reduced access to family planning services. Even when such services are available, many women who are likely to be HIV-infected fail to use them. Thus, innovative outreach programs may be needed to assure that HIV-infected women who choose not to become pregnant have the resources to support that decision.

FACTORS INFLUENCING PERSONAL CHOICE

The prediction that there will be no fundamentally new approaches to fertility control before the next century[120] seems likely to be accurate. Thus, for the foreseeable future, individuals will have to make choices about fertility control from among existing options.[105] How does one make these choices, particularly in view of the need to balance personal health needs and values, on the one hand, with the health needs and values of the community, society, and future generations on the other? Given an individual's own sense of social responsibility, the prevalent diversity of career aspirations and plans for childbearing and family life-styles, decisions about reproduction are more complicated than ever. Despite this complexity, there are three general rules that apply almost universally:

1. Almost any method of fertility control is safer and more effective than no method when pregnancy is not wanted.
2. Consistent, careful use of contraception will both increase pregnancy prevention and limit adverse side effects.
3. The better informed a person is about human reproduction and its control, the more likely the person is to make satisfactory decisions about the important issues related to fertility and his or her family.

In reflecting on personal values and responsibility to society and in going beyond these general rules, there is a series of important personal questions one might ask;

1. How do I feel about being sexually active outside of marriage?
2. Do I want children?
3. How do I feel about the importance of avoiding an unintended pregnancy?
4. Am I afraid to use birth control?
5. How do I feel about abortion?
6. How old do I want to be when I start my family?
7. Where do I want to be in terms of my career when I start my family?
8. If I have more than one child, how old do I want each one to be when the next one is born?
9. How many children are enough for me and my family?
10. Do my partner and I agree on the answers to the key questions about fertility control?
11. After I have all the children I want, how do I feel about sterilization as a permanent method of fertility control, or would I rather continue using a method of contraception that is not permanent?
12. How does my partner feel about being sterilized or about using temporary contraception?

From now into the foreseeable future, choices and recommendations regarding methods of fertility control should include the need for protection against sexually transmitted diseases, including AIDS. For individuals who are at risk because of having sexual intercourse with partners who may be infected, consistent and correct use of condoms is the only approach that can be recommended, other than abstinence. Therefore, individuals at risk of infection who choose to use methods other than condoms to prevent pregnancy will need to use condoms, in addition, to avoid the transmission of infection.

One key factor that influences choice is an individual's own intentions. Women who wish to avoid any more pregnancies are consistently more effective users of the birth control method they choose, no matter what that method may be, than are those who are only trying to delay their next conception.

REFERENCES

1. Nortman DL: Population and Family Planning Programs: A Compendium of Data Through 1981, 11 edt. New York: Population Council, 1982
2. Callahan D: Ethics and population limitation. Science 174:487–494, 1972
3. United Nations Fund for Population Activities: The United Nations and population: major resolutions and instruments. Resolution 2211 (xxi). New York: Oceana Publications, 1974, pp 81–82
4. United Nations: Report of the United Nations World Population Conference, Bucharest August 19–30, 1974. New York: Oceana Publications, 1975
5. United Nations: Report of the International Conference on Population, Mexico City, August 6–14, 1984. New York: United Nations Publication, 1984
6. Freedman R, Whelpton PK, Campbell AA: Sterility and fecundity of American families. Family Planning, Sterility, and Population Growth. New York: McGraw-Hill, 1959, pp 17–56
7. Ory HW, Cole PT, MacMahon B, Hoover R: Oral contraceptives and reduced risk of benign breast tumors. N Engl J Med 294:419–422, 1976
8. Cates W Jr, Ory HW, Rochat RW, Tyler CW Jr: The intrauterine device and deaths from spontaneous abortion. N Engl J Med 295:1155–1159, 1976
9. Centers for Disease Control. Abortion Surveillance, 1977. Public Health Service, DHHS. Atlanta, Ga. 1979
10. Peterson HB, DeStefano F, Greenspan JR. Mortality risk associated with tubal sterilization in United States hospitals. Am J Obstet Gynecol 143:125–129, 1982
11. Last JM: A Dictionary of Epidemiology, 2 edt. Oxford, England: Oxford University Press, 1988
12. Centers for Disease Control: Abortion surveillance, United States, 1982–1983. In CDC Surveillance Summaries, February 1987. MMWR 36(1ss):11ss–42ss, 1987
13. Kafrissen ME, Grimes DA, Hogue CJR, Sacks JJ: Cluster of abortion deaths at a single facility. Obstet Gynecol 68:387–389, 1986
14. Lee NC, et al: The reduction in risk of ovarian cancer associated with oral-contraceptive use. N Engl J Med 316:650–655, 1987
15. Rooks JB, Ory HW, Ishak KG, et al: Epidemiology of hepatocellular adenoma: the role of oral contraceptive use. JAMA 242:644–648, 1979
16. Tietze C, Lewit S: Evaluation of intrauterine devices: Ninth progress report of the cooperative statistical program. Stud Fam Plann 5:1–40, 1970
17. Warren, CW: Fertility determinants in Puerto Rico. Stud Fam Plann 18:42–48, 1987
18. Berelson B, Freedman R: A study in fertility control. Sci Am pp 29–44, May 1964
19. Requena M: Chilean program of abortion control and fertility planning: Present situation and forecast for the next decade. In Behrman SJ, Corsa L, Freedman R (eds): Fertility and Family Planning: A World View. Ann Arbor: University of Michigan Press, 1969, pp 478–489
20. Omran AR, Standley CC (eds): Family Formation Patterns and Health: An International Collaborative Study in India, Iran, Lebanon, Philippines, and Turkey. Geneva: World Health Organization, 1976
21. Department of Health and Human Services, Public Health Service: Family Planning. In Promoting Health/Preventing Disease: Objectives for the Nation. Washington, D.C.: Government Printing Office, 1980
22. Nortman DL, Fisher J: Government positions on population growth

and family planning in less-developed countries, 1982 (map). In Population and Family Planning Programs: A Compendium of Data Through 1981, 11 edt. New York: Population Council, 1982
23. Department of Health and Human Services, Public Health Service: The 1990 Health Objectives for the Nation: A Midcourse Review. Washington, D.C.: Government Printing Office, 1990
24. Paxman JM: Reproductive health, youth, and the law. WHO Chronicle 38:199–207, 1984
25. The American Law Institute: Model Penal Code: Proposed Official Draft: Section 230.3:189–192, Philadelphia, May 4, 1962
26. Tietze C: Induced Abortion, a World Review, 1983, 5 edt. New York: The Population Council, 1983
27. Supreme Court of the United States: The abortion experience: Psychological and medical impact. Supreme Court of the United States. Syllabus number 70–18(Roe, et al v Wade: appeal from the United States District Court for the Northern District of Texas. Decided January 22, 1973) and number 70–40 (Doe et al v Bolton: appeal from the United States District Court for the Northern District of Georgia. Decided January 22, 1973)
28. Supreme Court of the United States syllabus. Number 88-605(Webster, et al v Reproductive Health Services: appeal from the United States Court of Appeals for the Eighth Circuit. Decided July 3, 1989)
29. Magarick RH, Burkman RT (eds): Reproductive Health Education and Technology: Issues and Future Directions. Geneva: World Health Organization, 1988
30. Dryfoos JG: Family planning clinics—a study of growth and conflict. Fam Plann Perspect 20:282–287, 1988
31. Forrest JD: The delivery of family planning services in the United States. Fam Plann Perspect 20:88–98, 1988
32. Smith JC, Warren CW, Nunez JG: Attitudes toward family planning services. In the U.S. Mexico Border Survey: Contraceptive Use and Maternal Health Care in Perspective. Atlanta: United States–Mexico Border Health Association, 1983, p 21
33. Mosher WD, Pratt WF: Contraceptive use in The United States, 1973–88. Advancedata from Vital and Health Statistics of the National Center for Health Statistics. March 20, 1990
34. Trussell J, Hatcher RA, Cates W, Stewart FH, Kost K: Contraceptive failure in the United States: An update. Stud Fam Plann 21:51–54, 1990
35. Peterson HB, Lee NC: The health effects of oral contraceptives, misperceptions, controversies, and continuing good news. Clin Obstet Gynecol, 32:339–355, 1988
36. Kendrick JS, Lee NC, Wingo PA, Rubin GL: Oral contraceptive use and the risk of endometrial cancer. JAMA 257:796–800, 1987
37. Lee NC, Peterson HB, Chu SY: The health effects of contraception. In Parnell A (ed): Contraceptive Use and Controlled Fertility: Health Issues for Women and Children—Background Papers. Washington, D.C.: National Academy Press, 1989
38. Porter JB, Jick H, Walker AM: Mortality among oral contraceptive users. Obstet Gynecol 70:29–32, 1987
39. Mant D, Villard-Mackintosh L, Vessey MP, et al: Myocardial infarction and angina pectoris in young women. J Epidemiol Community Health 41:215–219, 1987
40. Stadel B: Oral contraceptives and the occurrence of disease. In Gregoire AT, Blye RG (eds): Contraceptive steroids—pharmacology and safety. New York: Plenum Press, 1986, p 3
41. Neuberger J, Forman D, Doll R, et al: Oral contraceptives and hepatocellular carcinoma. Br Med J 292:1355–1357, 1986
42. World Health Organization: Collaborative study of neoplasia and steroid contraceptives: Combined oral contraceptives and liver cancer. Int J Cancer 43:254–259, 1989
43. Irwin KL, Rosero-Bixby L, Oberle MW, et al: Oral contraceptives and cervical cancer risk in Costa Rica: Detection bias or causal association? JAMA 259:59–64, 1988
44. Physicians Desk Reference. 44th edt. Oradell, N.J.: Medical Economics Co., 1990
45. American College of Obstetricians and Gynecologists Committee on Gynecologic Practice: Contraception for women in their later reproductive years. ACOG Committee Opinion. Washington, D.C.: The College, No. 41, 1985
46. Forrest JD: The end of IUD marketing in the United States: What does it mean for American women? Fam Plann Perspect 14:52–55, 1986
47. Ory HW: The Women's Health Study: ectopic pregnancy and intrauterine contraceptive devices: New perspectives. Obstet Gynecol 57:137–141, 1981
48. Lee NC, Rubin GL, Borucki R: The intrauterine device and pelvic inflammatory disease revisited: New results from the Women's Health Study. Obstet Gynecol 712:1–6, 1988
49. Richwald GA, Greenland S, Gerber MA, et al: Effectiveness of the cavity-rim cervical cap: Results of a large clinical study. Obstet Gynecol 74:143–148, 1989
50. Rosenberg MJ, Rojanapithayakorn W, Feldblum PJ, Higgins JE: Effect of the contraceptive sponge on chlamydial infection, gonorrhea, and candidiasis. JAMA 257:2308–2312, 1987
51. Schwartz B, Gaventa S, Broome CV, et al: Nonmenstrual toxic shock syndrome associated with barrier contraceptives: Report of a case-control study. Rev Infect Dis (suppl. 1):S43–S49, 1989
52. Reingold AL: Toxic shock syndrome and the contraceptive sponge. JAMA 255:242–243, 1986
53. Yuzpe AA, Smith P, Rademaker A: A multicenter clinical investigation employing ethinyl estradiol combined with *dl*-norgestrel as a postcoital contraceptive agent. Fertil Steril 37:508–513, 1982
54. Liskin L, Blackburn R, Ghani R: Hormonal contraception: New long-acting methods. Popul Reports [K], no. 3, 1987
55. Short RV: Breast feeding. Sci Am 250:35–41, 1984
56. Liskin L, Rinehart W, Blackburn R, et al: Minilaparotomy and laparoscopy: Safe, effective, and widely used. Popul Reports [C], no. 9, 1985
57. DeStefano F, Greenspan JR, Ory HW, et al: Demographic trends in tubal sterilization: United States, 1970–1978. Am J Public Health 72:480–484, 1982
58. Centers for Disease Control: Tubal sterilization among women of reproductive age, United States, update for 1979–1980. In CDC Surveillance Summaries, MMWR 32(3ss):9–14ss, 1983
59. Schwartz D, Wingo PA, Antarsh L, Smith JC: Female sterilizations in the United States, 1987. Fam Plann Perspect 21:209–212, 1989
60. Pokras R: Hysterectomy: Past, present and future. Stat Bull Metrop Insur Co, pp 12–21, Oct–Dec, 1989
61. Nolan TF, Ory HW, Layde PM, Hughes JM, Greenspan JR: Cumulative prevalence rates and corrected incidence rates of surgical sterilization among women in the United States, 1971–1978. Am J Epidemiol 116:776–781, 1982
62. DeStefano F, Peterson HB, Layde, et al: Risk of ectopic pregnancy following tubal sterilization. Obstet Gynecol 60:326–330, 1982
63. Escobedo LG, Peterson HB, Grubb GS, Franks AL: Case-fatality rates for tubal sterilization in U.S. hospitals, 1979 to 1980. Am J Obstet Gynecol 160:147–150, 1989
64. Peterson HB, DeStefano F, Rubin GL, et al: Deaths attributable to tubal sterilization in the United States, 1977 to 1981. Am J Obstet Gynecol 146:131–136, 1983
65. Grimes DA, Peterson HB, Rosenberg MJ, et al: Sterilization-attributable deaths in Bangladesh. Int J Gynaecol Obstet 20:149–154, 1982
66. Grimes DA, Satterthwaite AP, Rochat RW, et al: Deaths from contraceptive sterilization in Bangladesh: Rates, causes, and prevention. Obstet Gynecol 60:635–640, 1982
67. World Health Organization Task Force on Female Sterilization: Minilaparotomy or laparoscopy for sterilization: A multicenter, multinational, randomized study. Am J Obstet Gynecol 143:645–652, 1982
68. DeStefano F, Greenspan JR, Dicker RC, et al: Complications of interval laparoscopic tubal sterilization. Obstet Gynecol 61:153–158, 1983
69. Vessey M, Huggins G, Lawless M, et al: Tubal sterilization: Findings in a large prospective study. Br J Obstet Gynecol 90:203–209, 1983

70. DeStefano F, Perlman JA, Peterson HB, et al: Long-term risk of menstrual disturbances after tubal sterilization. Am J Obstet Gynecol 152:835–841, 1985
71. Cohen MM: Long-term risk of hysterectomy after tubal sterilization. Am J Epidemiol 125:410–419, 1987
72. Henshaw SK, Singh S: Sterilization regret among U.S. couples. Fam Plann Perspect 18:238–240, 1986
73. Wilcox LS, Chu SY, Peterson HB: Characteristics of women who considered or obtained tubal reanastomosis: Results from a prospective study of tubal sterilization. Obstet Gynecol 75:661–665, 1990
74. Gallen ME, Liskin L, Kak N: Men—new focus for family planning programs. Popul Reports [J], no.33, 1986
75. Association for Voluntary Surgical Contraception: The 1987 estimate of U.S. sterilizations: Trend to outpatient services continues. AVSC News 27(2):1–4, 1989
76. Liskin L, Pile JM, Quillin WF: Vasectomy—safe and simple. Popul Reports [D], no.4, 1983
77. Ross JA, Hong S, Huber DH: Voluntary sterilization—an international fact book. New York: Association for Voluntary Sterilization, 1985
78. Schmidt SS: Vasectomy. JAMA 259:3176, 1988
79. Kendrick JS, Gonzales B, Huber DH, et al: Complications of vasectomies in the United States. J Fam Pract 3:245–248, 1987
80. Peterson HB, Huber DH, Belker AM: Vasectomy: An appraisal for the obstetrician-gynecologist. Obstet Gynecol 76:568–572, 1990
81. Chang C, Freedman R, Sun T: Trends in fertility, family size preferences, and family planning practice: Taiwan, 1961–85. Stud Fam Plann 18:320–337, 1987
82. Chang C, Freedman R, Sun T: Trends in fertility, family size preferences, and family planning practice: Taiwan, 1961–80. Stud Fam Plann 12:211–218, 1981
83. Rutenberg N, Ferraz EA: Measuring unmet need, female sterilization and its demographic impact in Brazil. Int Fam Plann Perspect 14:61–67, 1988
84. Prada E, Ojeda G: Fertility and contraception in Colombia: Selected findings from the demographic and health survey in Colombia, 1986. Int Fam Plann Perspect 13:116–120, 1987
85. Warren CW, Westoff CF, Herold JM, Rochat RW, Smith JC: Contraceptive sterilization in Puerto Rico. Demography 23:351–365, 1986
86. David HP: Eastern Europe: Pronatalist policies and private behavior. Popul Bull 36(6), 1982
87. Lapham RJ, Maudlin WP: Family planning program effort and birthrate decline in developing countries. Int Fam Plan Perspect 10:109–118, 1984
88. Goldberg HI, McNeil M, Spitz A; Contraceptive use and fertility decline in Chogoria, Kenya. Stud Fam Plann 20:17–25, 1989
89. Tomkinson J, Turnbull A, Robson G, et al: Report on confidential enquiries into maternal deaths in England and Wales, 1973–1975. Department of Health and Social Security, Report on Social Subjects 14. London: Her Majesty's Stationary Office, 1979
90. Fortney JA: The importance of family planning in reducing maternal mortality. Stud Fam Planning 18:109–114, 1987
91. Centers for Disease Control: National Infant Mortality Weekly Report. In CDC Surveillance Summaries. MMWR 38(3ss); Dec. 1989
92. Smith RG, Gardner RW, Steinhoff P, Chung CS, Palmore JA: The effect of induced abortion on the incidence of Down's syndrome in Hawaii. Fam Plann Persp 12:201–205, 1980
93. Lyle KC, Segal SJ, Chang C, Ch'ien L: Perinatal study in Tientsin: 1978. Int J Gynaecol Obstet 18:280–289, 1980
94. Puffer RR, Serrano CV: Birthweight, maternal age, and birth order: Three important determinants in infant mortality. Washington, D.C.: Pan American Health Organization, Scientific Publication no. 294, 1975
95. Rao KV, Gopalan C: Nutrition and family size. J Nutr Diet 6:258–266, 1969
96. Study Committee of the Office of the Foreign Secretary, National Academy of Sciences: Rapid Population Growth: Consequences and Policy Implications. Baltimore: Johns Hopkins Press, 1971
97. Pebley AR, Millman S. Birthspacing and child survival. Int Fam Plann Perspect 12:71–79, 1986
98. Forrest JD, Singh S: The sexual and reproductive behavior of American women. Fam Plann Perspect 22:206–214, 1990
99. Weller RH, Heuser RL: Wanted and unwanted childbearing in the United States. Vital Health Stat [21], no. 32, 1978
100. Westoff CF et al: The demographic impact of changes in contraceptive practice. Popul Devel Rev 15:91–106, 1989
101. Joyce TJ, Grossman M: Pregnancy wantedness and the early initiation of prenatal care. Demography 27:1–17, 1990
102. Weller RH, Eberstein IW, Bailey M: Pregnancy wantedness and maternal behavior during pregnancy. Demography 24:407–412, 1987
103. Centers for Disease Control: Abortion surveillance, United States, 1982–1983. In CDC Surveillance Summaries, February 1987. MMWR 36(1ss):11ss–42ss, 1987
104. Centers for Disease Control: Abortion surveillance, United States, 1984–1985. In CDC Surveillance Summaries, September 1989. MMWR 38(ss2):11–45, 1989
105. Ory HW, Forrest JD, Lincoln R: Making choices: Evaluating the health risks and benefits of birth control methods. Washington, D.C.: The Alan Guttmacher Institute, 1983
106. CDC Abortion Surveillance special tabulations, provided by Hani Atrash, M.D., 1990
107. Koop CE: The United States surgeon general on the health effects of abortion. Popul Devel Rev 15:172–175, 1989
108. Zabin LS, Hirsch MB, Emerson MR: When urban adolescents choose abortion: Effects on education, psychological status and subsequent pregnancy. Fam Plann Perspect 21:248–255, 1989
109. Henshaw SK, Kenney AM, Somberg D, Wan Vort J: Teenage pregnancy in the U.S.: The scope of the problem and state responses. The Alan Guttmacher Institute. New York: 1989
110. Hatcher RA et al: Contraceptive Technology, int edt. Births to teenagers and age at first marriage: The 10 most populous nations in the world plus the United Kingdom, Egypt, Turkey, and Mexico, table 4.2. Atlanta: Printed Matter, Inc. 1989, p 37
111. Prentice RL, Thomas DB: On the epidemiology of oral contraceptives and disease. Adv Cancer Res 49:285–401, 1987
112. The Cancer and Steroid Hormone Study of the Centers for Disease Control and the National Institute of Child Health and Human Development: Oral contraceptive use and the risk of breast cancer. N Engl J Med 315:405–411, 1986
113. Skegg DC: Potential for bias in case-control studies of oral contraceptives and breast cancer. Am J Epidemiol 127:205–212, 1988
114. Van de Perre P, Jacobs D, Sprecher B, Goldberger S: The latex condom, an efficient barrier against transmission of AIDS-related viruses. AIDS 1:49–52, 1987
115. Reitmeijer CAM, Krebs JW, Feorino PM, Judson F: Condoms as physical and chemical barriers against human immunodeficiency virus. JAMA 259:1851–1853, 1988
116. Consumers Union: Consumer Reports, 1989, pp 135–141
117. Richters J, Donovan B, Georgi J, Watson L: Low condom breakage rate in commercial sex. Lancet 2:1489, 1988
118. Centers for Disease Control: Condoms for prevention of sexually transmitted diseases. MMWR 37:133–137, March 11, 1988
119. Peterson HB, Rogers MF: Perinatal Transmission. In De Vita VT, Hellman S, Rosenberg SA (eds): AIDS: Etiology, Diagnosis, Treatment, and Prevention, 3d edt. Philadelphia: JB Lippincott (in press)
120. Djerassi C: The bitter pill. Science 245:356–361, 1989

69

Provision of Public Health Services

C. M. G. Buttery

Public health services are those services provided to population groups to prevent disease and to maintain health. Medical care services are covered in Chapter 65.

Public health services have long been a part of history. The Pharaohs and the ancient Hebrews were concerned about food and procreation. The ancient Greeks regarded good health as an ideal. Indeed, all societies and civilizations have practiced some sort of public health measures, however inadequate.[1]

Public health services are an important segment of the health care systems in all countries. In some countries all health services are provided to the public, without charge, by employees of the state. In others the pattern is a mixture of public and private services. In the United States, as in many other developed countries, the services are such a mixture. Medical care is provided by private practitioners, hospitals, and nursing homes except for special services to indigenous populations, such as the American Indians and Eskimos. Most of the traditional public health services are provided to prevent illness or for early identification of infectious diseases that have a significant public health consequence if care is not provided. Most public health services are delivered at the community level and are required by laws passed under the police powers of the state or nation. The basic programs, present in many communities since the early 1900s, are vital statistics, control of communicable disease, environmental sanitation, maternal and child health, health education, and public health laboratory support.

HISTORY IN THE UNITED STATES

Public health services started early in the United States. One of the public health laws enacted by the first Congress was to provide care for sailors and to prevent importation of such diseases as cholera, smallpox, and yellow fever. This was provided by the forerunner of the U.S. Public Health Service (USPHS), the Marine Hospital Services. A Commissioned Corps was instituted in 1889 and the name was changed to the USPHS in 1912.

Initially, other than the program for sailors, most public health activities were local, community based, and developed for environmental purposes. A milestone in development of community public health services was reached with the publication of the Shattuck report in 1850 by the Massachusetts Sanitary Commission.[1] The Shattuck report was the first significant public health plan to improve health. It focused on environmental services to remove and dispose of sewage and provide potable drinking water.

In New York concern about abuse of children as laborers in the clothing industry and the need to care for pregnant women led to the first of many White House Conferences on Child Health in 1909. At this time infant death rates were 10% of live births. After several years of discussion, the first clinical public health service supported by the federal government was enacted by the 1921 Sheppard-Towner Act[1] to provide maternal and child health services. It focused on poor women and their children. This act lapsed after 8 years but was revived in 1935 with the introduction of the Social Security Act. This act reinstated children's programs and added a "crippled children's" program as well as funds for demonstration programs.

In the period between the two World Wars control of tuberculosis became a public health clinical focus with development of sanatoriums to provide quarantine and care for people with pulmonary tuberculosis.

After World War II, the use of penicillin and sulfonamides was expected to revolutionize control of communicable diseases of concern to the public health services. Emphasis was placed on control and eradication of gonorrhea and syphilis. However, despite penicillin and newer antibiotics, these diseases were not eradicated and their control still requires concentrated case finding followed by contact tracing. Control of these diseases remains a major challenge.

The value of preventing infectious diseases during the war stimulated protection from common childhood infectious diseases through immunization, starting in the 1950s. In the late 1950s, after the poliomyelitis epidemic of the early 1950s, poliomyelitis vaccines were developed. Then new vaccines for measles, rubella, and mumps were introduced in the mid 1960s. The use of these vaccines, along with use of sulfonamides, penicillin, and a number of first-generation broad-spectrum antibiotics, was accompanied by a major reduction in infant deaths and morbidity. Within 15 years from the end of World War II improvement in feeding of children, improvement in provision of safe drinking water, widespread use of vaccines for childhood infections, and use of penicillin for treating streptococcal infections resulted in dramatic improvements in child health. Hospitals for the treatment of children's infectious diseases were converted to other uses.

While childhood infections were controlled with vaccines,

new antibiotics were used by public health departments to make dramatic changes in the treatment of tuberculosis, with reduction of new infections by the use of chemical prophylaxis. Hospitals previously used for tuberculosis patients were turned over to other agencies by the mid 1980s.

Maternal and child health continued to be an important concern for national and state public health agencies. Most of the incentives for improvement came in the form of grants from the federal government to the states. The grants were passed on to interested local communities to assist in direct prevention of infant deaths and reduction of infant and childhood morbidity. Most of these grants were restricted to major cities. It was only in the mid 1980s that separate states in the United States started to take the need for prenatal care and for health care of infants seriously and to extend programs to improve maternal and infant care across states into rural areas. This is in contrast to the efforts of most other countries, particularly the poorer countries, that placed emphasis on care of women and children at the forefront of their public health efforts. This same emphasis has been promoted by the World Health Organization (WHO), which also promotes primary care services as a public health measure—another contrast to the United States, where the emphasis is on tertiary care.

Since the mid 1970s national public health attention has also been focused on chemical pollution of the environment, whereas previously the concern had been on potable water and sewage disposal.

FEDERAL PROGRAMS

Public health services in the United States have developed into three fairly well-separated levels—national, state, and local.

National programs were developed by the federal government to promote specific policies, such as the care of pregnant women and children, the control of infectious diseases, and the protection of the environment. These programs aim to achieve equity among the states. Because many governmental policies are restricted to the states by the U.S. Constitution, the federal government can only offer incentives such as grants-in-aid or make policy statements. It cannot force states to carry out activities unless the U.S. Congress specifically provides resources in a way that does not violate the separation of federal and state rights.

The federal government has a particular interest in dealing with problems that cross state boundaries, such as pollution of the air, water, and ground. It also has a particular interest in protecting the rights of all citizens to equal treatment under law by ensuring certain basic levels of support. It performs functions that protect the health of all citizens who may be placed in danger from interstate commerce. An example of this is the work of the Food and Drug Administration, which has the responsibility to set standards for drugs, cosmetics, and food that are sold across state boundaries.

The federal authority passes from the President through a group of cabinet officers (ministers) selected by the President and approved by the Senate. A cabinet secretary for the Department of Health and Human (social) Services (DHHS) has the responsibility for overseeing the majority of the federal health programs through a deputy secretary for health. Health services are provided by two major branches of the DHHS. One function of the DHHS is to provide funds for clinical services for the poor, the aged, and the totally disabled through the *Health Care Financing Administration (HCFA)*.

The other major functional branch for health services is the *Public Health Service (PHS)*. The PHS carries out its public health functions, similar to those of other countries, through a group of technically oriented branches. It is responsible for evaluation of safe food and drugs through the Food and Drug Administration (FDA), the science of preventive medicine through basic and applied research (including vital data collection) in the Centers for Disease Control (CDC), research into treatment of major categories of diseases through the National Institutes of Health (NIH), for maternal and child health (MCH) services through the Health Resources & Services Administration (HRSA), for mental health and behavioral intervention through the Alcohol, Drug Abuse and Mental Health Agency (ADAMHA), for services to indigenous populations (native Indians and Eskimos) through the Indian Health Services, and registration of hazardous chemicals through the Agency for Toxic Substances and Disease Registry. Other than providing funds to states and localities, the branches of the PHS carry out technical research and develop regulations for control of health-related activities by aggregating groups of highly technical specialists into national resources that could not be funded or attracted at the state level.

The Centers for Disease Control. After World War II the USPHS developed a Communicable Disease Center (CDC) for research into control of communicable diseases. This has grown into the Centers for Disease Control, a major national and international asset to prevent and treat diseases and, more recently, to foster epidemiologic and health education techniques to control chronic diseases by primary prevention. These centers, all branches of the CDC within the PHS, have special importance for the day-to-day activity of local health departments and public health in general. Although there are counterparts in many countries and some larger states, few have the scope in breadth and depth of expertise that has developed at the CDC over the last 45 years. Many on the staff of the CDC are loaned to state and local health departments and foreign governments to provide consultation in development and administration of public health programs. These consultants are found in every field of public health. Many programs of the World Health Organization in Geneva have core staffs assigned from the CDC.

In all countries the basis of public health is good data. *The National Center for Health Statistics (NCHS)* gathers population-based public health data. It has developed a series of continuing population- and institution-based surveys to provide data on the health status of the population, as well as the volume and types of health services delivered (see Chapter 2). Because each series of surveys is distinguished by the color of its covers, this is often known as the "rainbow series" of surveys. While all are important for development of national health policy, those that are most helpful for state and community policy development are the health interview, health examination, health and nutrition, and ambulatory medical care surveys. The health interview surveys are repeated cross-sectional surveys of a representative sample of the national population, which describe health status as reported by the individual. The health examination surveys represent a similar cross section but include physical, physiological, and biochemical measurements. The health and nutrition surveys measure growth, development, and intake of food and selected nutrients. The ambulatory medical care surveys measure the numbers of visits by diagnosis, medications, and treatments prescribed by physicians. No single state or community can afford to develop surveys of similar depth, breadth, detail, and credibility. The NCHS has consulted with other countries and the WHO to standardize data-collection instruments and allow comparability of data with other countries.

The National Institute for Occupational Safety and Health (NIOSH) is one of the newer centers for preventive medicine and public health. National interest in occupational medicine started before 1950 and accelerated with recognition of "black lung disease" as a compensable work-related disease. In the 1960s concern developed for other chronic diseases that were not initially seen as work related. The first emphasis was on asbestosis and lung cancer in shipyard workers, who during the war had worked in confined spaces installing asbestos-insulated pipes in warships. Their exposure became a major cause of death and disability 20 to 30 years later (see Chapter 17). The large numbers of people affected by asbestos increased interest in "work-associated" disease and led to enactment of an Occupational Health and Safety Act. This encouraged the Department of Labor, assisted by NIOSH, to focus epidemiological techniques on the work site. An important function of NIOSH is to provide advice on human effects and hazards in the workplace by use of epidemiologic techniques.

The Center for Infectious Diseases influences immunization policy and conducts research on infections of national and worldwide importance. Development of new vaccines against childhood infections spurred an increased emphasis on prevention, linking the USPHS more closely to the states through the CDC. Federal funding allows the states to develop programs to immunize all children against several common childhood diseases. One problem with immunizations in the United States is their price. The United States requires that all children be immunized (e.g., against measles). The cost of basic vaccines in the United States is higher than in other countries because of the cost of litigation and of protection against litigation. The extent of litigation is unique to the United States.

The Center for Environmental Health and Injury Control was developed in response to the problems of contamination of the environment by chemicals, such as occurred at Love Canal in New York and at Triani in Alabama. The staff of this center is concerned with developing a science base for assessing the potentially harmful effects of chemical compounds on people, as opposed to flora and fauna. The work of the center will help to determine the true public health risks of environmental contamination, rather than the theoretical risks extrapolated from animal and cell studies, usually performed for purposes other than assessment of human population risk. This center is also responsible for epidemiological evaluation of non-work-related injuries, such as vehicular accidents and homicide.

The Center for Chronic Disease Prevention and Prevention Services was developed in response to the federal long-range plans to promote a healthy population by deterring disease resulting from personal behaviors. This center funds a series of behavioral risk-factor surveys of the population currently used by 25 of the 50 states. The surveys are used to measure the effectiveness of the health education strategies adopted by the various states.

Other branches of the PHS cover program areas that are the responsibility of similar agencies in many other countries and act as a base for similar programs at the state level.

The *Food and Drug Administration* helps set standards for food service inspections in restaurants and evaluates the quality of drugs produced for public consumption.

The *Agency for Toxic Substances and Disease Registry* keeps a registry of toxic substances with data to establish an epidemiological link between chemicals and diseases.

The *Alcohol, Drug Abuse and Mental Health Administration (ADAMHA)* is responsible for planning for delivery of mental health, mental retardation, and substance abuse services, which in most states have been placed in agencies outside the state public health agency. During the second half of the twentieth century, as more knowledge and ways to control diseases affecting behavior came under control by medical interventions, national programs for mental health and alcohol, tobacco, and other forms of drug abuse were combined into the *Alcohol, Drug Abuse and Mental Health Administration.* Because of the associated problems of mental retardation and developmental disabilities, cooperative links have developed between ADAMHA and the various national maternal and child health programs.

The *National Institutes of Health* is the research arm of the DHHS. As epidemiology became applied to solving noninfectious disease problems, some of the centers of the NIH have become more focused on prevention. The NIH-funded programs for research into heart disease and stroke now center on nutrition, exercise, and behavior to prevent disease, moving personal clinical services into the realm of public prevention of communicable disease. In the late 1950s prospective epidemiological studies such as the Framingham Heart Disease Study were started.[2,3]

The Health Resources and Services Administration (HRSA) is linked to the public health system through its *Bureau of Maternal and Child Health and Resources Development Programs.* Maternal and child health (MCH) programs are at the core of clinical care provided through state and local departments of public health. For many years the focus of these agencies has been on health maintenance of mothers and children. This focus continues today. Over the last 20 years there has been increasing interest in reduction of infant mortality and funding of prenatal and child health care. The focus became clearer in the late 1980s and is accentuated because of invidious comparisons of infant death rates in the United States with those of other developed countries.[4] Despite the United States' world leadership in medical technology, little concern had been shown for cheaper, simpler, less glamorous interventions to ensure good health and outcome for poor women and children. To quote a 1988 Institute of Medicine report entitled *Prenatal Care—Reaching Mothers, Reaching Infants,*[5] "The maternity system—as part of the health care system in the U.S.—is fundamentally flawed, fragmented, and overly complex. Unlike many European nations, the United States has no direct, straightforward system for easy access to maternity services. Although well-insured, affluent women can be reasonably certain of receiving appropriate health care during pregnancy and childbirth, many women cannot share this experience." The problems of high-quality MCH programs have been a basic public health service in almost every other country in the world than the USA, despite the poverty of many of these countries.

Recent federal laws are starting to help the United States catch up with other countries. Because states failed to accept their responsibility, the federal government mandated that state and local public school systems must provide special educational and health services for all children 2 or more years of age. The federal government expects all states to plan services for this age group. Typical of the U.S. "high tech" approach to solving problems, Congress mandated expensive care of affected children but put no effort into *preventing* the occurrence of developmental disability by providing quality prenatal care initially. In fact, by 1990, only one or two states had developed comprehensive plans to prevent neonatal disability.

Although many other countries provide nutritional programs for their children as part of their social support systems, the public health effort is fragmented in the United States. In the United States these programs are provided at the federal level by the Department of Agriculture (DA), primarily for the benefit of the farming industry. The DA does this through several different uncoordinated programs. A special program for women and children at nutritional risk provides screening of pregnant women, infants, and children for entry into the Women, Infant and Children's nutritional program (WIC). In most states and localities this program is carried out by the local public health departments. Additional nutritional programs for children include the National School Lunch and Breakfast Programs delegated to local schools

Data from the NCHS, as well as from state health departments, have shown that the differences in infant mortality between communities are related to socioeconomic factors. The difference in infant mortality between white and black women is 100%. Infant mortality rates (IMRs) for white women are 8 to 10 per 1000 live births (LBs); those for black women are 18 to 20 per 1000 LBs. In neighborhoods containing the highest-income, best-educated families, the IMRs may be as low as 3 to 4 per 1000

LBs, while in the neighborhoods with the lowest-income, most poorly educated families the IMRs are often 20 to 25 per 1000 LBs, almost a 1000% difference. These differences have been well publicized since 1980. There has been momentum and an increasing willingness in Congress, but not in the states, to fund maternal and child health care. This is done by a combination of grants from the PHS and by reimbursement for MCH services through the Medicaid program. Medicaid is a federally supervised program that provides payment for medical services provided to poor people (see Chapter 65). In 1989 Congress allowed the states to pay for care of pregnant women and their children below 6 years of age if their income is no more than 180% of the federal poverty level. It mandated that they pay for care of women, and children up to 1 year of age, living in households with an income at or below 100% of the poverty level. In addition to these medical services, the Medicaid program also pays for prevention services for children up to 18 years of age through an Early Periodic Screening Diagnosis and Treatment program (EPSDT). Although Congress has enacted this program, because it requires matching funds from state governments, few states have enacted the total approved program. Part of the reason is that the federal government, in its concern for children and families, enacted a large number of mandated services and required the states to pay for them.

Funds for prenatal, infant, and child health care come from a combination of federal health, social service, education, and agricultural agencies. Each agency has different eligibility and accounting standards, which makes delivery of services unnecessarily complicated and duplicative and reduces funds available to provide service. In most countries a single agency is responsible for services to children. This problem is further complicated by the different state and local agencies, each required to coordinate a spectrum of services from different state agencies. These programs provided $534 million to the states in 1988. The method of providing these funds to the states, and their accountability, keeps changing. For example, after the election of President Reagan various funds were pulled together in one block for MCH services. This included funds that were previously categorical line item funds for handicapped children, basic MCH grants, the supplemental security programs, genetic disease, hemophilia, and adolescent pregnancy programs. This block method of providing funds should allow more flexible delivery at the state and local levels. Proponents of various advocacy groups were concerned that this reduced the visibility of their special interests and would be detrimental to continuation of services. Over the last few years, with concerns about lack of prenatal and early childhood care, there has been a swing back to a categorical approach. However, the categories are still fairly general and now require a complete range of primary care services for children, within the limits of funds available.

Studies of the cost benefits of the prenatal portions of the MCH program alone have shown that each $1 spent on prenatal care saves at least $3 in medical care in neonatal intensive care units. If the analysis were carried through the lifetime of the child born after good prenatal care, the costs saved by avoiding a need for special educational and mental health support programs would be much higher, in the range of thousands of dollars saved after birth and during the ensuing lifetime for each dollar spent on prenatal care.

A program complementary to the MCH programs is the family planning program. Family planning programs are intended to ensure that all children born are both wanted and cared for. Women need to know about their own reproductive processes and to decide when to become pregnant, rather than having unplanned, undesired pregnancies. Just as the MCH programs are cost effective so are family planning programs which have also been shown to save the public at least $3 for each $1 invested.[6] If lifetime analyses, rather than analyses through just 18 years of age, were performed the cost benefits would be even more striking.

Issues of policy development for MCH programs at the national level continue to focus on leadership and assessment of problems, as well as on needs and resources, on the basis of effective planning. Leaders in the field are concerned with development of national minimal standards of care, quality assurance, public education, and development of useful data systems that can relate funding to improved prenatal and perinatal outcome. Research is necessary to develop better evaluation techniques, reduce barriers between agencies, and encourage coordination in development of objectives and delivery of services. More will be said about this in the discussion of state and local responsibilities.

The HCFA has grown increasingly important to the function of state and local departments of public health because of funds available for clinical services from Medicaid and Medicare. It has also raised the visibility of state health departments that have been given the responsibility to administer state Medicaid programs. A few states have given this responsibility to their social service agencies, whereas others have created a separate state agency. Many health departments that provide both general and categorical clinical services (such as the MCH programs) obtain revenue from Medicaid. Health departments that operate home health services obtain funds from both Medicaid and Medicare. The multiple funding sources needed to develop public health services in the United States require a large bureaucracy compared with other countries whose socialized health care systems provide this care through a single agency and a single program.

The Year 2000 Goals. The 1990 goals, the National Health Objectives,[7,8] defined a set of national priorities for public health.[9-11] These are grouped into three major foci: prevention, protection, and promotion. Each of these is subdivided into five goals (Table 69-1). The 1990 goals themselves arose from an earlier study, *Healthy People—The Surgeon General's Report on Health Promotion and Disease Prevention,*[11] published in 1979. These goals and their enabling objectives are in the process of redefinition for a set of "Year 2000 Goals," which were published in 1991 to guide us throughout the present decade.[12]

TABLE 69-1. HEALTH STRATEGY TARGETS

- **HEALTH PROMOTION FOR POPULATION GROUPS**

Smoking cessation
Alcohol and drug abuse reduction
Improved nutrition
Exercise and fitness
Stress control

- **HEALTH PROTECTION FOR POPULATION GROUPS**

Toxic agent control
Occupational health and safety
Accidental injury control
Community water supply fluoridation
Infectious agent control

- **PREVENTIVE HEALTH SERVICES FOR INDIVIDUALS**

Family planning
Pregnancy and infant care
Immunizations
Sexually transmissible diseases services
High blood pressure control

STATE HEALTH DEPARTMENTS

State public health policy is made by the state legislature, which enacts laws and appropriates funds. The legislature gets its advice from a secretary, if the state has a cabinet form of government, as well as from local health department employees, the state board of health, district advisory boards, and the state public health director. The state health department should develop its budget, manpower, and capital resources needs on the basis of a long-range plan covering 5 to 6 years, with the plan starting in each health district. The district budgets are consolidated into a single statewide budget by the state health department's budget and planning directors. This approach encourages each district to work as part of a team to convince local elected officials of the benefits to be gained from supporting the local health department's budget.

Activities carried out by state health departments are a subset of those carried out by the federal government. They combine in one agency the programs found in the CDC and the HRSA at the federal level. Few states have technical resources similar to those of the federal government. Figure 69–1 shows an organizational chart locating the major programs found in a typical state health department. In many states, because of concern for the governor's span of control, a secretarial cabinet has been developed to provide operational control of the multitude of state agencies. Cabinet members are called "secretaries," as are their counterparts in the federal government. In many state cabinets a single secretary has responsibility for a myriad of health and social services agencies.

In a typical state (Fig. 69–2) 16 agencies report to a secretary for health and human resources. Six are most important: public health, mental health, rehabilitation, health professional licensing, medical assistance services (Medicaid), and social services. There is a host of small specialized agencies with a few employees (usually fewer than 20), such as a department for volunteerism, a department for children, a department for aging, a department for the blind, and a department for the hard of hearing. Many of these small agencies tie into healthrelated programs and provide a special visibility and accountability not otherwise available.

In some states all health programs report to the governor through a commissioner or secretary for health, while the social service agencies report through a separate channel. Mental health services have been separated from "health" services in most states because they are seen more as social (counseling) and housing programs than as disease-oriented, curative, or prevention services.

The state health agency has a primary responsibility to plan for health services. It should plan delivery of a complete range of health services to all citizens, even though the delivery of the service may be carried out by the private sector. The range of services should include both public and private services, whether institutionally based or not.

Organizationally, state health services are usually separated into divisions based on technical functions. Both state and local health departments manage the traditional health programs of environmental health, vital data, communicable disease, maternal and child health, and health education. Laboratories exist at both the state and local health department levels, depending on the complexity and frequency of tests performed. In some states, in an effort to improve effectiveness and efficiency, a central laboratory consolidates services to all state agencies (not just health agencies) at a single facility.

State health departments, in addition to routine administrative functions of personnel, fiscal, supply, and data management, are funded by the PHS to be the state facility licensor and guarantor of quality care in hospitals and nursing homes. They may also license and set standards for individuals involved in emergency medical services and manage health-related grants provided by the federal government.

The Medicaid program may be part of either the state health department or the social service department, or it may be a separate agency, depending on whether the emphasis is on eligibility, medical services, or financial accountability. Medicaid budgets have become so big that they dwarf state health department budgets and compete for funds needed to improve basic public health services. In most states the Medicaid budget is second only to highway and education budgets, and will soon be second to none. This detracts from the public health approach, which combines primary care and prevention services targeted toward the poor. Without an increase in preventive services, such as the MCH programs, associated social support, educational, and mental health services have to increase far faster than necessary. When lawmakers look at Medicaid budgets, if these budgets are part of the state health department's budget, all other state public health programs may lose money to pay for the rapidly increasing cost of Medicaid.

Where it is separate, the Medicaid agency frequently works closely with the state health department. The Medicaid program has the task of managing financial resources to deliver health care to poor citizens. The health department has the responsibility to monitor the quality of care and, through its planning function, ensure appropriate distribution of resources.

The health care services (HCS) management area is responsible for managing federal categorical funds for maternal and child health services, handicapped child services, genetic services, developmental disability services, family planning, dental health, health education, and public relations. In addition to these health delivery components, the manager overseeing family health services is also responsible for health education, communicable disease, epidemiology, and toxicology programs.

The HCS manager is responsible for passing the federal MCH, handicapped child, and WIC funds to the local health departments. These funds, their proper allocation, and standards of performance and organization are an important link between national and state policies and actual delivery of services to people. States have an interest in good MCH programs. State leaders have begun to see the correlation between lack of pre-, peri-, and postnatal services and increased expenditures in social, mental, and educational support services. Much of this awareness has come about as states have tried to control problems of family abuse, alcoholism, teenage pregnancy, illegitimacy, poor school performance, care of children with developmental disabilities and the increasing cost of medical services, which have resulted in dramatic cases of indigent pregnant women being refused care at their local community hospitals.

MCH policies at the state level, although similar to those at the national level, are usually more sharply focused. They are concerned with high infant death rates and childhood morbidity. Because of the U.S. social structure and funding focused on income MCH programs focus on disparity among the minority populations as well as problems of increased incidence of families headed by single females. They are concerned about the effects of substance abuse, particularly use of intravenous drugs, and the associated problems of hepatitis B and human immunodeficiency virus infections. Learning disabilities, suicide, and homicide are an increasing problem. There is concern about lack of proper hygiene in day-care centers, which leads to transmission of communicable diseases, including vaccine-preventable diseases.

The MCH programs focus on preconception, antepartum, intrapartum, and postpartum services to ensure an appropriate range of services to pregnant women.

In the preconceptual phase the focus is on education, genetic screening, contraception and other family planning ser-

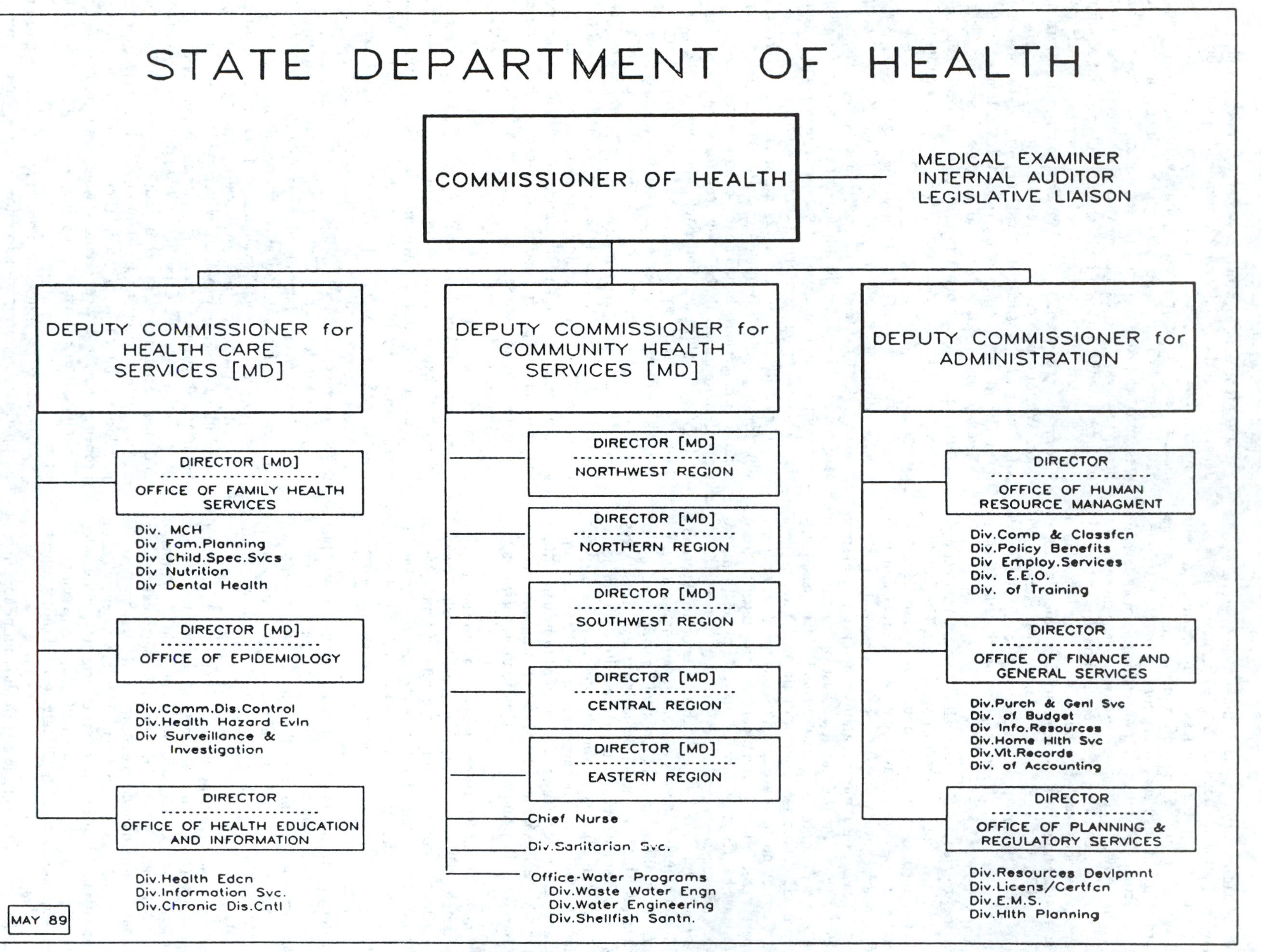

STATE DEPARTMENT OF HEALTH
COMMISSIONER OF HEALTH
MEDICAL EXAMINER
INTERNAL AUDITOR
LEGISLATIVE LIAISON
DEPUTY COMMISSIONER for HEALTH CARE SERVICES [MD]
DIRECTOR [MD]
OFFICE OF FAMILY HEALTH SERVICES
Div. MCH
Div Fam.Planning
Div Child.Spec.Svcs
Div Nutrition
Div Dental Health
DIRECTOR [MD]
OFFICE OF EPIDEMIOLOGY
Div.Comm.Dis.Control
Div.Health Hazard Evln
Div Surveillance & Investigation
DIRECTOR
OFFICE OF HEALTH EDUCATION AND INFORMATION
Div.Health Edcn
Div.Information Svc.
Div.Chronic Dis.Cntl
MAY 89
DEPUTY COMMISSIONER for COMMUNITY HEALTH SERVICES [MD]
DIRECTOR [MD]
NORTHWEST REGION
DIRECTOR [MD]
NORTHERN REGION
DIRECTOR [MD]
SOUTHWEST REGION
DIRECTOR [MD]
CENTRAL REGION
DIRECTOR [MD]
EASTERN REGION
Chief Nurse
Div.Sanitarian Svc.
Office-Water Programs
Div.Waste Water Engn
Div.Water Engineering
Div.Shellfish Santn.
DEPUTY COMMISSIONER for ADMINISTRATION
DIRECTOR
OFFICE OF HUMAN RESOURCE MANAGMENT
Div.Comp & Classfcn
Div.Policy Benefits
Div Employ.Services
Div. E.E.O.
Div. of Training
DIRECTOR
OFFICE OF FINANCE AND GENERAL SERVICES
Div.Purch & Genl Svc
Div. of Budget
Div Info.Resources
Div.Home Hlth Svc
Div.Vlt.Records
Div. of Accounting
DIRECTOR
OFFICE OF PLANNING & REGULATORY SERVICES
Div.Resources Devlpmnt
Div.Licens/Certfcn
Div.E.M.S.
Div.Hlth Planning

Figure 69-1. Organization Chart, Model State Health Department.

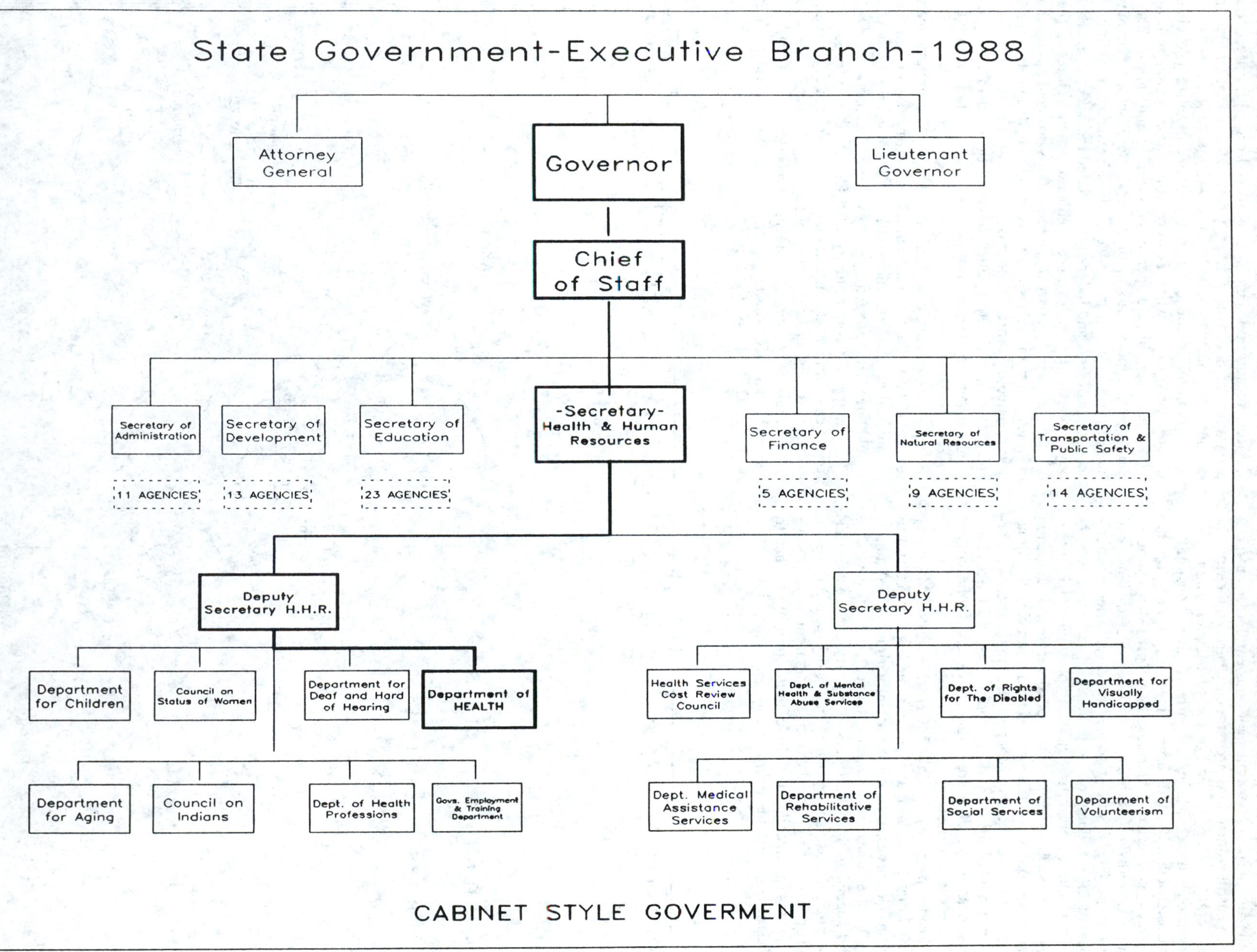

Figure 69-2. Cabinet form of State Government.

vices, nutrition, prevention of sexually transmissible diseases (STDs), and prevention of rape and violence in the home.

In the antepartum phase the programs emphasize outreach services to enroll women into prenatal care early in their pregnancy (preferably before the end of the first trimester) and risk assessment to ensure that high-risk patients have a consultation with an obstetrician. They determine levels of care appropriate to the patient's level of maternal risk as provided by nurse practitioners, midwives, family physicians, obstetricians, and perinatologists. They ensure good medical care, review the quality of local nutrition education programs, and assist in determining family psychosocial status. They are coordinated with other state agencies, such as Medicaid, social service, and mental health agencies to develop case management and care coordination with home visiting, provision of homemaker services, arranging for transportation, and development of substance abuse strategies, whether for abuse of legal drugs such as tobacco and alcohol or of illegal drugs.

In the intrapartum period the MCH staff ensures continuity of care and develops regional plans and methods of referral to provide services necessary for the patient with identified maternal risk. This includes evaluation of the neonatal intensive care units and special perinatal services in tertiary care centers. Finally, during the postpartum period they work with families to promote breast-feeding, home visiting, and parental education.

Programs for all children include finding appropriate health care, access to affordable primary and acute care, immunization, screening for conditions consistent with a child's age, dental care, developmental screening, school health, and nutrition services. In addition, emphasis is placed on injury-prevention programs from birth, with provision of car seats when the mother goes home from the hospital with her new baby.

A continuing concern is maintenance of current levels of service. Many of these programs rely on primary care physicians to provide the clinical supervision and personal care, either in local health departments or on referral. Because of a combination of low payments from Medicaid, increased medical liability costs, fear of suit, and federally mandated record keeping, these physicians are refusing to see Medicaid patients either in their offices or at health department clinics. This problem has reached crisis level in many states where women living distant from tertiary care medical centers cannot obtain prenatal care, even if they are Medicaid recipients. They have to turn up in emergency rooms when they are ready to deliver, having had no prenatal care.

Most states have a separate division for community health services (CHS), like that in the model department which consists of 36 health districts, each with a minimum population of 100,000 people, managed by five regional directors (Fig. 69-3). The manager for community health services is also responsible for the environmental consultants and a consultant representing the field nursing services, the chief nurse.

Because of concern by the fishery services in some states, as well as concerns for wetlands, marine, stream and lake ecology,

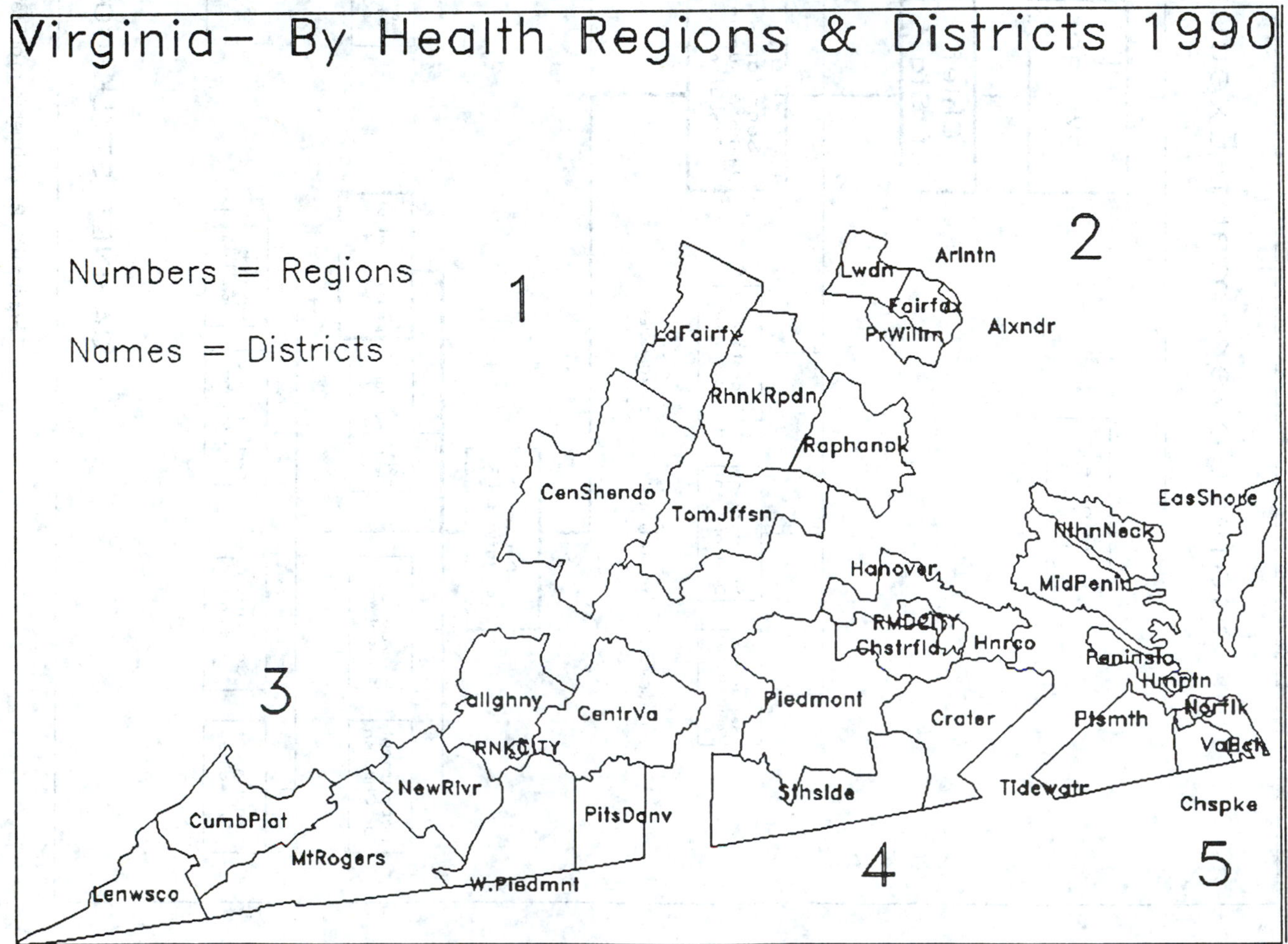

Figure 69-3. State divided by regions and districts.

environmental programs (except those that need medical supervision or that relate to the environment of the individual homeowner) have been pulled together under a secretary for the environment. Air and water pollution problems are managed by engineers and ecologists in the environmental secretariat, as are solid waste problems. Permitting of individual homesite sewage disposal and well systems frequently remains a responsibility of the state and local health departments. The health department is usually responsible for shellfish evaluation and engineering services for construction of drinking water and sewage disposal systems. The inflow and output are usually controlled by a state water control board.

When agencies cooperate, such division of responsibility works well. The department of health provides consultation from its epidemiology and toxicology staff to help the air, water, and solid waste programs determine the potential for human harm. These other agencies perform the actual licensing, development, and monitoring.

In some states, all local health departments are part of a state system that is supervised and run by state employees. This results in statewide standards that can be enforced equitably across the state, bearing in mind the vagaries of individuals. Funding of local health departments differs. For some states there is a mix of state and local funding. The locality's share is determined by a formula that takes into account tax capability and net worth of the community, as well as current efforts and use of resources. In other states the state health department may provide a series of grants and contracts, with performance standards to enhance funds provided by local government. Elsewhere the state is basically a regulatory and data-collection agency, and all the service and funds are local.

LOCAL HEALTH DEPARTMENT

The local health department is the action arm of the national and state public health agencies. The staff of the local health department carries out the day-to-day provision of clinical care, environmental review, and staff support to ensure that the agency meets its goals. The staff usually includes nurses, sanitarians, office support staff, laboratory technicians, health educators, dentists, animal control officers, engineers, administrators, nutritionists, and others who, under the direction of the local health director, plan, budget for, and ensure the department's success.

At the national level the CDC, the American Public Health Association (APHA), the U.S. Conference of Local Health Officials, and the National Association of County Officials are completing a third version of *Model Standards, A Guide for Community Preventive Services.*[13] This document provides a framework for examining the goals and objectives of both local and state health departments and contains model goals and objectives, rather than standards. It also suggests data sources to use for measuring the outcome of the various goals and objectives. In addition to the *Model Standards* the same group has been working on a self-evaluation tool for local health departments, known as APEX/PH,[14] which has recently become available for use by state and local health departments.

In many respects, just as the state health department is a smaller version of the federal public health services, the local health department is a limited and smaller version of the state system. In most states, facility licensure is operated out of the state office. In a few of the largest cities this function may be delegated to a local health department. Just as certain programs are operated by the federal government because of a need for a few very well-trained staff that cannot reasonably be replicated in each state, the state similarly performs certain functions centrally. Facility licensure requires special competencies that cannot be replicated in each community or region.

The three major administrative groups seen at the state level are usually different at the local level (compare Figs. 69-1 and 69-4). States tend to group their activities and span of control by three functional areas: local health department support, federal and special programs, and administration (including fiscal, planning, and licensure). The local health department is more likely to group its functions by clinical, environmental, and support services.

Clinical Services. Clinical services encompass most program areas found in the state agency. The main difference in the local department is that a specific individual may work in several program areas. These services prevent disease, promote health, and in some departments provide treatment for categorical diseases, such as tuberculosis and STDs, and also provide primary medical care for the community's medically indigent in urban areas.

Programs provided for many years include maternal and child health, immunization and sexually transmitted disease services. Within the last 10 to 15 years many departments have extended their clinical services to include family planning, chronic disease screening, and the WIC nutrition program.

The risk of high blood levels of lead and mental retardation in young children is particularly high in inner city areas. As a result, many city health departments now perform lead screening. They refer homes of children with positive tests to their environmental health sections. Larger cities also provide specialty clinics, usually in cooperation with state agencies, for developmental disabilities and genetic screening for enzyme defects and sickle cell disease. They also conduct clinics to evaluate handicapped children who need surgery or prostheses or those with chronic diseases, such as cystic fibrosis.

Communicable Disease Prevention. Communicable disease programs focus on vaccine-preventable diseases, sexually transmissible diseases, and monitoring for vector-borne diseases such as encephalitis. Tuberculosis, which had been under reasonable control for several years, has increased in incidence and prevalence since immigration from southeast Asia has increased and as a result of the increase in AIDs. Local health department staffs, often supplemented by CDC investigators, are also responsible for investigation and follow-up of reported waterborne diseases such as hepatitis A; foodborne outbreaks of shigellosis, hepatitis A, or streptococcal food poisoning, as well as rarer epidemics among newborn infants in hospital nurseries and evaluation of zoonotic diseases such as plague, Lyme disease, and rabies.

School entry immunization levels are surveyed regularly to determine coverage against diphtheria, tetanus, whooping cough, poliomyelitis, rubella, measles, and mumps. *Haemophilus influenzae* B immunizations are now recommended for children beginning at age 2 months. In the last few years health departments have had to cope with measles outbreaks in college populations, where immunization levels have been low or where primary immunization may have been improperly timed for maximum effect.[15]

Chronic Disease Programs. Research has demonstrated the value of screening, detection, and early intervention and treatment for such chronic diseases as hypertension, atherosclerotic heart disease, diabetes, and emphysema. Many local health departments have hired health educators and developed health education programs for entire communities. In addition to education, they are involved in screening, and referral to community physicians, of persons with asymptomatic hypertension, smokers with early hypertension, obese persons with non-insulin-dependent diabetes, and those with high serum cholesterol levels.

Many health departments developed home health service

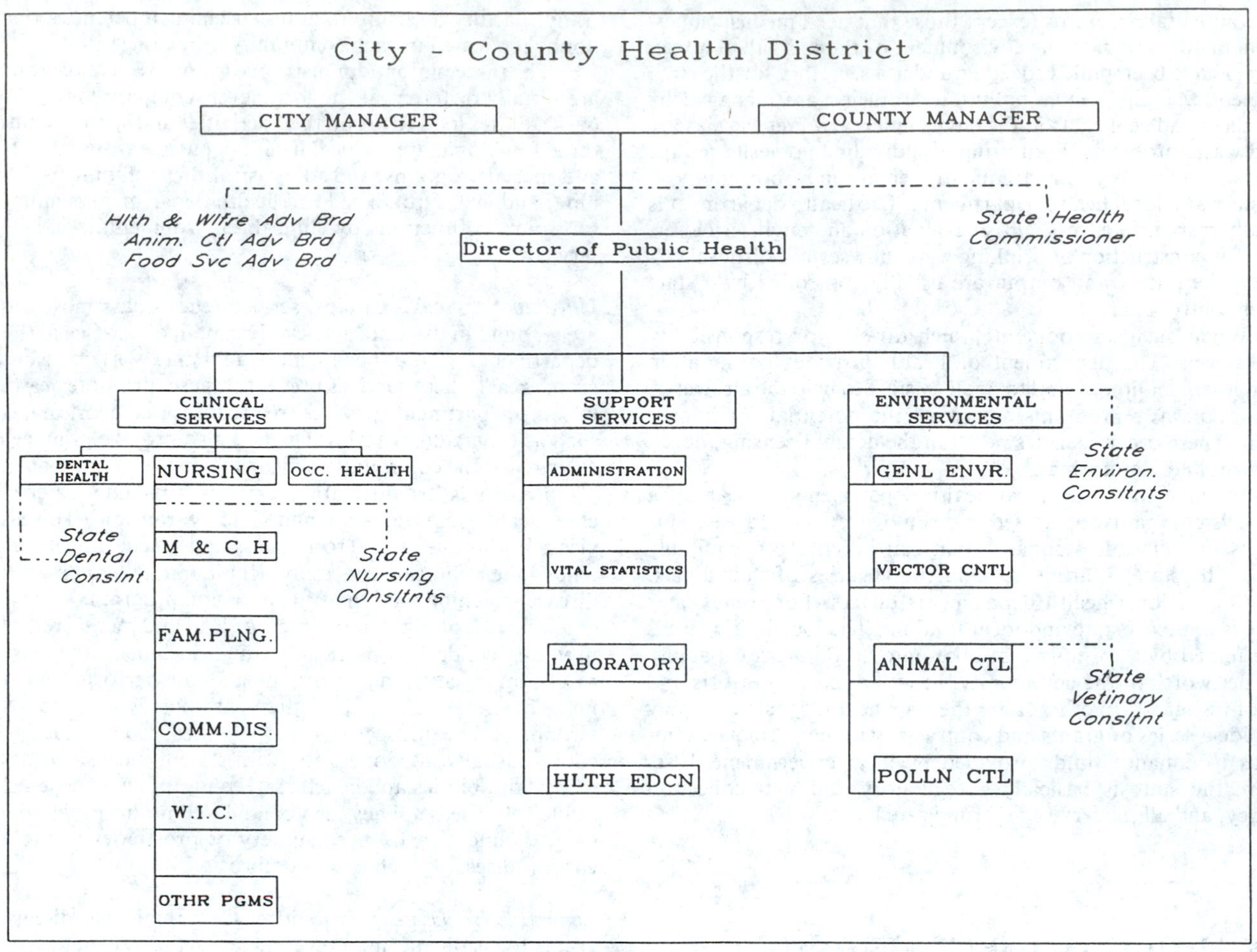

Figure 69–4. Organization chart—model local health department.

agencies in the late 1960s and early 1970s, after Medicare was enacted to pay for care of older persons in their own homes. The gap in services to the elderly who are unable to carry out activities of daily living because of chronic diseases was filled by local public health departments. This program has been taken over by private providers in some communities. The case management approach of public health nurses, however, has been preferred by many private practitioners, who still refer their patients to local health department home health services rather than to private profit-making groups.

A New Role in Primary Care. As the result of medical care cost-containment programs aimed at hospitals, patients are being discharged earlier and sicker. They need more community support systems, including home health services and primary care. This earlier discharge has placed increasing pressures on local communities to care for these patients, who are often elderly and often poor, particularly those returning home to rural and inner city communities.

An increasing number of local health departments, because of the dwindling supply of rural and inner city primary care physicians, find their governing bodies asking them to take on the responsibility for delivering primary care for at least the indigent citizens.

In countries other than the United States, primary care and public health services may be provided in physician's offices. Only the United States among developed countries has failed to provide financial access to primary care for all its citizens.

Emergency Medical Services. Areas with few primary physicians are also the ones where emergency medical services may be distant. Serious accidents require highly technical stabilization and transportation skills. Rural areas may not have a large enough tax base to match federal funds to buy and stock an emergency vehicle or have enough people willing to acquire and maintain skills beyond the emergency medical technician level to staff emergency service programs. In a number of state legislatures there is a move to reduce requirements for demonstration of competency. This is being done because people will not join the rescue squads. In larger cities either the local or the state health departments frequently regulate and inspect emergency squads to ensure minimum performance levels. In other countries emergency services are part of the health system, and their availability is built into regional health service funds.

Occupational Health. An increasing number of local health departments are developing expertise in occupational health. This is particularly true where the local health director is a physician. As OSHA and EPA increasingly enforce minimal work standards and place increasing emphasis on national environmental standards, local government looks to the local health director for guidance on health hazard assessment and toxicological analysis. Local government often finds that application of occupational medicine and epidemiology quickly provides benefits by ensuring a fitter work force, a reduction in injuries, and faster return to work when people are injured, thus increasing efficiency and effectiveness of the labor force. This is another compelling reason for local health departments to consider an increased role in primary care delivery.

Environmental Services. Environmental services were formerly focused on preventing the spread of enteric diseases, but now they are increasingly used to prevent exposure to toxic chemicals and particles in the air and water, as well as to improve the quality of housing.

Traditional environmental services ensure proper disposal and treatment of human waste and provision of potable water. Only a few years ago disposal of human waste took place in pit privies, through septic tank and drain field systems (individual sewage-disposal systems), and through public sewage-disposal systems. Research provided standards for installation based on the percolation rate and number of bedrooms. As land has become scarcer, as septic systems have failed in increasing numbers, as concern for pollution of rivers and shellfish beds has increased, and as wells and aquifers have become polluted, the standards for installation of private waste-disposal systems have changed. Now the presence of neighbors, the percolation rate, the likelihood of surface discharge of effluent, the level of water in the soil, and the ability of the soil to absorb and treat waste found in the bottom of septic tanks are all taken into account. In addition to advice from sanitarians and local health departments, realtors now employ engineers and soil scientists and are likely to appeal denials of septic tank installation. Some communities want to tighten up septic tank regulations, not as public health policy but to deter future growth.

Today's sanitarian, or environmental specialist, has to know not only about septic tanks but all about soil profiles and consistency, the names and meanings of various types of soil, and soil's ability to treat waste found in the bottom of septic tanks but also about the use of sand filters, low-pressure, soil-injection systems, spray irrigation, various types of packaged waste-disposal systems, and how to apply for national pollutant discharge elimination system permits if other than a standard septic tank and drain field is being used.

In addition to waste discharge the sanitarian has to know the standards needed to install wells to obtain groundwater and be able to explain to homeowners the need for casing and grouting a well. The sanitarian also has to know how to place the well so that it is separated from the waste discharge system and will not contaminate the aquifer from which it draws water.

Food service control has become increasingly important. Improper storage, handling, preparation, holding, and serving of food can contribute to the development and spread of foodborne diseases. The sanitarian needs to be able to inspect, explain, and teach about food handling to managers, operators, and staffs of food service facilities. This often requires an understanding of different cultural practices and of how to prevent ingrained cultural behavior from causing food poisoning.

The environmentalists may also be responsible not just for evaluation of building codes for rented or reoccupied housing but also for inspections of day-care premises, group homes, summer camps, and recreational facilities to make sure their food service, drinking water, and waste-disposal facilities meet minimum standards.

Animal control is a responsibility of many local health departments. In urban centers animal control is also seen as necessary to prevent spread of disease from dog and cat feces. Animal control requires knowledge about animal behavior and the ability to instruct the public in safe keeping, rearing, and public contact of their pets. The majority of animal bites come from dogs, although more cats are rabid. Pets have the ability to pass a number of vectorborne diseases. It is also necessary to limit contact between pets, raccoons, and skunks to prevent the spread of rabies.

Support Services. The central services that support the field staff include laboratory, vital data, and administrative services. Laboratory services at the local level depend on the programs supported. The federal Clinical Laboratory Improvement Act requires evidence of quality control in laboratories. For certain procedures where immediate results are not necessary, many states have developed centralized services. Typical examples are unusual services, such as evaluation of animal tissues for presence of rabies, complex analyses that require careful monitoring, or testing where clinical cases are few and procedures are time consuming. In major metropolitan areas the local health department often has a laboratory for clinical testing, including serologic studies, gonorrhea cultures, blood sugar testing, urinalyses, and simple hematology analyses. Some may even perform their own milk and water testing or serve as regional branches of a central state laboratory.

Different states and localities handle vital data collection differently. Vital data on births and deaths, with additional data itemizing complications and preexisting or contributing conditions, are essential for public health analysis of community health status. Many health departments also collect vital data related to marriage and divorce.

Administrative services provide support for hiring, payroll, leave administration, standard procurement policies, fiscal planning and analysis, and budgetary guidance to all other staffs of the health department.

Staffing. A clear understanding of the role and responsibilities of the local health director is essential to the understanding of leadership necessary for planning, programming, budgeting, and communication with other local, state, and federal agencies and local elected officials.

The local health director, in those states and communities in which this is a full-time position, is usually a physician. In other communities the director is often a nonphysician with administrative and management skills. In states with an integrated personnel system the staff comprises state employees supervised from the state health commissioner's office. In other states the health director and staff will be local government employees supervised by a nonphysician, often a deputy or assistant city manager. In either case, there may be a conflict of interest that the director has to live with. The director will often be the only physician in local government; if there are others, they will report to the director. The physician who is a local employee usually serves as a delegated enforcer of state health policy by agreement with the state health commissioner and usually holds a warrant for enforcement of state regulations, even when those regulations may compete with the desire of local government. When the local director is a direct employee of the state, he or she would be wise to act as though an employee of local government. The director should attend all of the department head meetings of local government and not place too much emphasis on the special skills of a physician but provide counseling to the city/county executive, whether appointed or elected, and act as a staff specialist. This balance, which is difficult and often treacherous for new appointees, can most easily be developed where there is close supervision of new health directors by a veteran who is used to the pull, tug, and sensitivities of local politics. The new director has to be specially sensitive to the respect many of the community will have for the health department staff, who may have worked in the community for years. The new director, before rushing out to bring the community up to the best standards, should spend the first year developing credibility and making changes only where his or her expertise can be demonstrated.

One way for the health director to develop credibility in the medical community, if a physician, is to join the local medical society and the local hospital staff(s), attend staff meetings, professional meetings, and take the opportunity to participate in debate. It is advisable to start in areas of competence, such as immunization, infectious disease epidemiology, environmental hazard analysis, or interpretation of state and federal policy.

The outstanding health department and its leaders show certain common traits. They have both long- and short-range plans. They are good fiscal managers with budgets that relate to plans. Staff members provide the community with environmental assessments based on "state-of-the-art" knowledge of biology, chemistry, physics, geology, and hydrology as a minimum. The staff should communicate well with the public. Their services, goals, and accomplishments are known to the community. They have contacts throughout the governmental agencies as well as with the for-profit and not-for-profit voluntary health agencies in the community. The first place these communities look for expertise as it relates to people's health is the health department, which is known for giving accurate, clear, reliable advice in an easily understood format. The written and electronic media will look to the department to interpret national and state health trends. The local staff will be consulted by the local physicians, hospitals, and health-related organizations before they look outside the community to state or national resources. Probably most important, everyone in the community, from the highest elected person to those whose home is the street or low-income housing, sees the health department and its staff as advocates of good health and health services.

To function effectively, the health director must be a delegator whose interest is service above self. Except for major policy decisions, such as whether the department will deliver primary care services or provide services to intravenous drug addicts, the director should let field and program supervisors make day-to-day decisions for the department. They are closer to the action and usually know the public and its feeling better. The director should ensure spans of control of less than eight per supervisor at all levels and should lead by example and by the appropriate use of public health skills of epidemiology, biostatistics, toxicology, pharmacology, physiology, biology, radiation physics, general medicine, cultural anthropology, and systems analysis. The director and staff must form an integrated team that melds together the total skills of the organization to respond to the local elected officials, county/city executives, local boards of health (never be without one), United Way agencies, welfare groups and their representatives, and the various health activists.

If the staff consists of more than 25 persons, an administrator trained in either business or public administration, should be obtained. When the staff approaches 100 in size, the administrator and administrative staff will need special skills in budgeting, fiscal management, systems development, computer applications, and program evaluation. The chief administrator should have at least a master's degree in business or public administration, health care, or hospital administration. The administrator will need the assistance of accountants, personnel managers, supply clerks, statisticians, and computer technicians.

Clinical divisions of many larger local health departments are headed by nurses with masters' or doctoral degrees in nursing administration. In the smaller departments the clinical division is headed by a nurse with a baccalaureate or master's degree. Staffing depends not only on total population but on the number of fertile females, the poverty level, the geographic distribution of the population, population density in different areas, travel time, public transportation, and the range of programs provided. Because of the high cost of physicians and the lack of primary care physicians, a number of departments are successfully using nurse practitioners who have specialized in family planning, obstetrics, and primary care.

Those health departments that provide dental care employ dentists, dental hygienists, and dental assistants. The dentists and the dental hygienists teach in the school, screen to determine need for dental care, and provide therapeutic services in the office. The dentist performs the more difficult procedures, while the hygienist concentrates on application of fluoride and sealants to prevent cavity formation and ensure development of cavity-free permanent teeth.

Where there is an occupational health program either a full-time or consultant occupational health physician with training in health hazard evaluation and special knowledge about teratogenesis, oncogenesis, cytogenesis, and mutagenesis is needed. This physician will need consultant backup from environmental hygienists and toxicologists.

Except in the smallest departments, the environmental division should be managed by an environmentalist with a master's degree in environmental sciences or civil engineering and additional training in environmental biology and chemistry. If the major programs deal with individual homesites and food service, more emphasis should be placed on an environmental science background. If there are many industries, rivers, or waterfront areas, the need is for someone from an engineering background who can provide policy analysis for potential air and water pollution and be familiar with development and planning of waste-disposal systems from the community and industrial standpoints. In either case the environmental manager will need the backup of sanitarians trained in soil sciences and food management. The environmental group should be proactive in development of community environmental policy and not wait for the general public to raise issues. They have a responsibility to educate the elected officials, other county/city agency heads, and the public.

The support staff should include the laboratory director and laboratory technicians trained in either biology or chemistry, depending on the range of programs found in the department. Smaller departments may only need one or two technicians to test for common STDs, evaluate milk and water composition, and perform a few clinical services. The vital statisticians can be trained on site. In the larger department it helps if one or two staff members have been trained in nosology in a hospital records department, because the work they do in classifying births and deaths is crucial to community analysis.

All the staff members discussed have to be welded into a well-functioning team by the health director and senior managers. This takes time and effort. It does not happen by itself. Development of such a team takes planning and thought. It takes a combination of incentives and sometimes a few disciplinary actions. Members of the health care team should have cross-training so they can recognize when to call in members from other programs. Just as a nurse should be able to call a sanitarian on observation of unsafe wiring, lack of food-storage facilities, and lack of heat in the winter, a sanitarian who observes apparent disease or disability going untreated should be able to call on the nurses. Team building starts at the top. The leadership of the health director is important in setting a pattern for the rest of the staff. The health director needs to be a role model for leadership as well as a role model for health. The staff members need to develop formal and informal ties to the other health care providers in the community to develop teams with them. Remember that one will never have all the resources needed and must learn to make maximum use of the resources already in the community.

Development of Policy. Local health directors are responsible for educating city/county executives and elected officials about important health policies. Resources for health and medical care services must compete with those for education, transportation, housing, food, clothing, and capital investment to produce new jobs. Demographic variables affect these changes and their impact in the future. The community needs to understand the effect of changes in diet, exercise, and smoking that lead to increased longevity and less disability. It needs to understand the impact of changes in incidence and prevalence of chronic disease, the increase in the population over 65 years of age, changes in development of new and expensive medical technology, the problem of excess fertility, lack of prenatal services and their effects on the cost of health care in the next 10 years.

Planning activities and resulting policy must consider the needs of people, industry, and the environment as separate, interactive, concurrent developing systems.

It is necessary to sell public health programs to the community. A family planning program may be funded by the state, the federal government, Planned Parenthood, or a combination of all three. It may be provided by the health department, hospital clinics, private physicians, or Planned Parenthood, or a mixture of all of these. Its effectiveness is measured by fertility rates, age at first pregnancy, numbers of grand multiparity, the marital status of the user, and evidence of unplanned births. Each program will draw detractors. Combinations of programs, if properly presented to the community, will have wide endorsement. Linking family planning programs to prenatal care, and reduced infant mortality helps sell programs that might otherwise be controversial.

Provision of primary health care is a problem if the department diverts funds that would have been used to prevent disease rather than finding additional funds. A policy for providing primary health care is important in the United States and will become increasingly so in the future, particularly as it supports programs to reduce chronic disease.

Policy options frequently focus on whether to fund programs through the public or private sector. First, it is necessary to determine whether there are data to show effectiveness. If a program is not effective, there is no point worrying about efficiency. With good planning, clear options, careful data analysis, and involvement of all sectors of the community, good policies can be developed and will have lasting effect.

Collecting Data for Planning, Evaluating, and Budgeting. Epidemiology is a core skill of public health planning and evaluation, supported by skills in biostatistics. Depending on the size of the department, and program involvement, you may gather data by hand or have it collected by computer. Ideally, no single piece of data should be collected more than once. Computers can link different data systems together to minimize repetitious collection of data.

Timely, valid, accurate, easily accessible data are essential to the development of good health policy. Good data, presented clearly, promote development of rational health policy and reasonable choices when resources are short. Health education based on local data is usually more effective than that based on national trends. Citizens find data about their community more compelling than data about what is happening in the world or nation. Data on categorical diseases are essential to winning the help of the cancer, diabetes, and heart associations. It is easier to obtain coordinated approaches from the different groups with good data. Such data allow comparison of local, state, and national health outcomes and show how good outcomes improve everyone's health.

Examples of the kinds of data that are useful in program planning and analysis are census data gathered either in the decennial census or by an interval census made by various local, state, and national agencies. Information about geographic or spatial epidemiology describing the numbers, composition, location, race, age, and economic levels of households throughout the community is particularly helpful. Such data provide the denominator to develop disease, disability, and death rates. There is a host of data in the community and in your own files that, once accessed, is invaluable for planning, evaluating success, and analyzing future programs and policies. Compare rates in your community with state data from the NCHS data series. Make synthetic estimates of expected occurrences of disease and deaths in your community to compare to data from the NCHS surveys.

Geographic epidemiology is particularly useful. With current software, it is easy to turn data collected by census tracts into maps. Comparison of different events allows one to select areas in the community for concentrated effort. Deaths, for instance, can be mapped by census tract; births by age of mother and date of first prenatal visit. Particularly interesting work was done to identify the potential for lead poisoning in children by mapping the plumes of effluent from a lead smelter in El Paso.[16]

Program Analysis and Budget Preparation. Program data must be analyzed to develop the budget as a statement of program priorities (goals and objectives). The budget describes the resources needed to meet a department's short-term objectives, the next fiscal year. A single-year budget serves as the first year of a locality's long range (5- to 6-year) plans.

Information required to set objectives consists of specific outcome and process data elements. Outcome tells us what happened. Process tells us what we had to do to make it happen. Process data may be a nursing visit, an immunization, restaurant inspection, or yards of ditches sprayed for mosquito larvae.

Objectives are specific measurable endpoints you expect to reach in a defined time. *Goals* are midterm (commonly 5-year) statements of desires stated in general terms.

An example of a health department goal is a general statement such as "maintenance of present efforts to improve health status." It is a goal rather than an objective, because it cannot be measured in a specific time by specific measurements. A goal is usually a policy statement based on your community charter. Your department will have subsets of its overall goal for each of three major avenues of service: clinical, environmental, and support services.

An example of a clinical objective follows. Many additional examples can be found in the "model standards" document described earlier.

Examples. Changes in childhood vaccine-preventable diseases could have a number of objectives, such as the following:

1. "No more than one case of rubella or rubeola in the next 12 months."
2. "Immunization of 100% of children prior to school entry."
3. "Immunization of children to be 100% by 2 years of age."

For the first objective, the *outcome* is the number of cases of disease, while the *process* is the number of immunizations given. For the second, the *outcome* is the proportion of children fully immunized, while the *process* data include the number of immunizations given, the number of clinics held, and the number of doses spoiled. The third objective, however, illustrates problems of measurement as well as enforcement, a common occurrence in public health. It is impossible to enforce immunization of all children by the time they reach the age of 2 years, let alone measure the results. It is possible to enforce immunization on school entry because a certificate of vaccination can be required as one criterion for school entry. There are legal remedies if parents fail to enroll and ensure attendance of their children. There is no satisfactory tool or surrogate to measure immunization levels at 2 years of age. An *outcome that cannot be measured should not be used.* It reduces credibility, one of your most important assets. The ability of a local health department to set realistic measurable outcome contrasts with social programs whose measurable outcomes (e.g., reduced substance abuse rates or recidivism rates) may have other causes than program intervention and may be uncontrollable by the agency. This is a problem for many social goals, which are not nearly as clear cut as most health-related goals. The public health goals that are most difficult to set and measure with clear objectives are behaviorally related health education goals that look for changes in smoking, eating, and exercising habits and can be influenced over time by many causes other than health department intervention.

Environmental health objectives were used by one local health department to improve its food sanitation program. It used process measures such as number of persons tested for communicable disease, number of food handlers' cards issued, restaurants inspected, and permits issued. The *outcome data* included incidence of tuberculosis and syphilis and inspection report scores that averaged in the low 70s. The program was not effective, let alone cost-effective or efficient.

The staff changed both the processes and the outcome. The *new outcomes* became "90% of restaurants to have scores greater than 85 percent, less than 5 percent to score below 70 percent." *Process measures* included food managers trained, food handlers educated, and numbers of inspections per restaurant per year.

During the next 2 years, more than 16,000 food handlers and more than 3000 food managers were trained in a community of approximately 270,000 persons, augmented significantly in the summer months by vacationers. Average inspection scores rose to 85%; in fact, 80% of the restaurants scored more than 90 out of a possible 100 points. Only 12 of the 970 restaurants scored less than 75 points.

The sums of individual program objectives add up to accomplishment of program goals. If you provide the public (legislators, council persons, boards of supervisors) with program objectives as well as goals, they can choose between programs to support reduced infant deaths, prevention of teenage pregnancies, prevention of childhood lead poisoning, or prevention of disabilities from infectious diseases such as measles, rather than choosing between a sanitarian and a nurse. This approach shifts the focus from line items to outcomes. An objective to "hire one more nurse" is less defensible than—and will not have the impact of—an objective to "reduce infant deaths and disabilities." The latter objective should have more impact than "resurfacing 2 miles of road."

One community's approach to analyzing infant mortality and planning changes is shown as another example of public health program evaluation.

Data for several preceding years was mapped to provide a clear visual pattern for both the department and the public. It included city population by census tract and socioeconomic level, infant deaths and death rates totaled for 5-year periods by census tracts, births by number and rate, fertility rates, and maternity clinic attendance by clinic site and census tract of patients in relation to clinic site, as well as immunizations given by clinic site and staff/client ratios for the preceding 15 years.

The infant death rate for the preceding 5 years was 50% higher than for the state or the nation. Over the preceding 6 years total births increased from 5300 to 6000, with teenage births representing 20% of the total. The total population had increased by 40,000 since the previous national census. Attendance at prenatal clinics had increased from 980 to 2300. Waiting time for first visits to the maternity clinic had increased to 8 weeks. MCH staff available to give care had dropped from 31 to 29 over the past 10 years, despite addition of many new activities to the maternal health program.

The data were presented to the city council, county commissioners, minority groups, state legislators, and the media. The progress and distribution of resources over the past 15 years were reviewed. Major changes in health status were discussed; these included the significant drop in immunization-preventable communicable diseases, improved immunization levels on entry to school, reduced attendance at storefront immunization clinics, introduction of the WIC program, and changes in clinic attendance by location of clinics.

The city council and county supervisors were given several options:

1. Maintain all status quo (do nothing).
2. Close all neighborhood storefront clinics and redistribute nursing staff to maternity clinics.
3. Fund a staff increase to match patient/staff ratios present 10 years ago.

The city council and the county commissioners endorsed a goal "to ensure referral of maternity patients to the appropriate level of care and fund sufficient staff so that clients would not have a waiting period of longer than 2 weeks to enter maternity clinics." They also agreed to:

1. Close six of the nine neighborhood immunization clinics immediately.
2. Evaluate two of the other three for 6 months and close them if attendance did not improve.
3. Keep the remaining clinic open because of its remote location but to reduce the time it is open to 1 hour a month.
4. Ask the state health department MCH program for funds to hire three public health nurses and two clerks.
5. Refer all high-risk patients (based on a clinical protocol) to the hospital district obstetric clinic funded by the county.

In addition, it was agreed that:

6. The county commissioners would fund a new nurse-midwife position for the health department.
7. The hospital district obstetric clinic would refer normal pregnancies to the health department.
8. The community pediatric hospital would continue developing neonatal intensive care programs.

Results of these actions included a 100% increase in patient contact hours, reduction of waiting time to enter the prenatal clinics to 10 days, and decline in infant death rate from 14 deaths to 7.8 per 1000 live births.

Many programs are funded only when process data (number of patients visits, number of shots) as well as outcome data (fertility rate, number of infant deaths) can be related to money provided by funding agencies. Budget requests backed up by good data, rather than philosophy, are far more likely to get funded.

Modern managers expect budgets to be based on resources needed to attain realistic, measurable, achievable objectives during the upcoming budget period. This is usually 1 year at the local level, 2 years at the state level, and 5 years at the federal level.

Good program objectives approved by a policy-making board of health can attract media coverage and help policy makers choose between 20 additional infant deaths, 100 more children born with developmental disabilities, 50 more cases of hepatitis B, 200 more illegitimate births to teenagers, or reduction of home health services to elderly adults, forcing them out of their own homes and into nursing homes. Mayors, city councils, chairmen, and county boards of supervisors in local communities have to balance outcomes against the needs for additional sewers, paving of roads, housing for the indigent, and additional schoolteachers. Clear objectives help a community to define its values. This feedback allows you to clarify your need to change priorities or to provide additional information to help the community change its values.

When money is short, elected officials may require across-the-board reductions of 20% from each line of your budget. They are more likely to support you if given the chance to choose from outcome measures, such as reducing infant deaths or developmental disabilities, than among different staffing levels. You cannot cut 10% of a doctor or nurse practitioner. With a line item cut you may be forced to cut a whole program rather than to readjust priorities between programs.

Budget Preparation. In the United States many local departments serve multiple jurisdictions, such as cities and counties. They often have to agree to perform minimal levels of service to obtain financial support from the state health agency. In some states a joint contract outlining expected services is signed annually by local and state agencies. An agency with multiple funding is typical of many local health agencies but few other local governmental agencies in the U.S. Even in states where the local departments are branches of the state agency, and part of their personnel system, the local health departments usually have additional funds for local programs provided by the local jurisdictions, which they administer separately.

In some local departments staffs in nursing, environmental health, and support services are found on the payrolls and personnel systems of each of the partners to the annual agreement. In such instances the staff in each program, whatever the paycheck/personnel system origin, performs similar duties for different salaries and different fringe benefits. Funding may be further complicated by grants from the federal government or from private foundations. Each funding agent may, and usually does, have different fiscal years and accounting procedures. The department's total budget package has to be presented as a single unit to each partner at different times of the year, usually in different formats. Development of a budget in which all the programs are integrated under a single set of goals and objectives helps each funding agency see how it contributes to the community as a whole.

This "performance budget" allows the department to be held accountable to the community as a whole, identifies the expected benefits, and allows each partner to work with the others for the good of the whole.

The constraints of multiple funding and accountability make budget analysis, projection, and preparation a continual time-consuming task for the local health department. The use of computerized spreadsheets can cut budget-preparation time by 90% by reducing the retyping and the repeated iterations needed in such preparation. A budget that used to take 3 to 4 weeks of typing and retyping now takes no more than 3 to 4 hours.

Budget planning starts by evaluating the current goals and objectives and their associated costs. This is used as a base to plan increases or reductions for the coming year. Successful programs may reduce health hazards to the point where the program is no longer needed. It should never be assumed automatically that all programs should be continued at the same or increased levels, or even funded from the same source.

A number of communities require that each program within a budget be evaluated from scratch each year, with restatement of the objectives, analysis of expected outcomes, projection of costs to reach the objectives, and then statement of priorities among the programs. By setting outcome objectives, such as "inspecting all food service places quarterly and re-inspecting all places with a score below 75 weekly until attaining that score," the agency can determine the staffing needed.

A local base staffing standard has to be used because there are no current national standards. The closest definition to a local health department standard is the *Model Standards,* which, as noted previously, provides a description of goals and objectives that should be found in state and local health departments, not of legally accountable standards. Most local officials expect part of budget preparation to involve evaluation of performance against measurable standards. Some agencies evaluate their outcome only in term of process data (number of patients seen), rather than outcome (number of infant deaths prevented).

Many state and local health departments are modifying goals, objectives, and fiscal management systems to provide better evaluation. Some state agencies are making plans to develop written contracts that state outcomes desired from local health departments on the basis of resources provided. Unfortunately, the *Model Standards* provides no guides to staffing or financing of the objectives described. The Assessment Protocol for Excellence in Public Health has already been described. It was developed because of this need to measure local department performance. It is a voluntary self-assessment protocol for determining local health department strengths and weaknesses in areas of community assessment, public health skills, and management capacity. It puts its major emphasis on peer review by a similar-sized agency from a similar community. As local health departments take part in the APEX/PH system, it should stimulate improved management, use and distribution of public health resources, and improvement in health outcomes across the nation, as well as better budgeting. This should lead after a number of assessments to definition of staffing options for various public health programs.[14]

Although a department often has several funding sources, one is usually primary. It is simplest to use the fiscal year of the major partner for your annual budget and to fit everyone else in. Start planning your budget at least 6 months before you have to submit it. Base your budget on the preceding 18 months' expenditures. Then plan 18 months into the future, thus covering the preceding 18 months plus the 6 months left in the current fiscal year plus the full 12 months of the fiscal year you are planning. A budget evaluation thus covers at least 36 months.

When developing your budget be careful to examine how changes in one program affect other programs. Changes in a maternity program can result in women being referred to the WIC program earlier in their pregnancy. Earlier detection of prenatal problems can result in earlier referral to a high-risk OB clinic. As more women come into the prenatal program, you may need to add a pediatric nurse practitioner to your infant and child health programs, at additional cost. Every time you make changes in one program, you should examine the entire system to look for potential linkage to other programs, as well as potential costs, savings, or both.

In times of declining resources it is even more important to get the maximum use out of each dollar. Plan the cash flow of your budget so you can use your money when it has the most useful effect. A piece of equipment bought early in the year provides more benefit than one bought in the last quarter. Budgeted funds do not have to be spent equally in each month or quarter. Your expenditure plan is just as important as developing the budget. If you have mosquito programs, most of your funds may be spent in the spring and fall, when rains are heaviest. If you have a light rain in the fall, you may want to use oil and insecticide funds for another environmental program, such as picking up stray animals. If the rains are heavier the next year, you will already have made inroads into the unowned pet populations and can reduce activity in that program, then shift money and buy additional oil. This planning for periodic spurts and declines in spending is vital to good money management.

Budget Presentation and Program Evaluation. When you have collected your data, set priorities, and developed a budget, you still have to get the elected officials to accept your recommendations. This is just as true at the national and state levels as at the local level. However, if you cannot sell a budget at the local level you are unlikely to sell the same budget at the state or national level, where the players are far more sophisticated. Consider the political, technical, organizational, and financial environment in which your health department exists. Identify all the players, particularly those who are technically knowledgeable, such as the medical society, hospitals, schools of health science, and categorical health agencies, such as the heart and cancer societies. Also consider social agencies, such as departments of social services, mental health, voluntary health agencies, rural and central city agencies, poverty agencies such as the community action agencies, minority group representatives, and the special purpose activist groups who may want to endorse special objectives within your overall program. Together they represent a formidable support group.

Do not hurt your funding chances by torpedoing programs of special interest to your elected officials: though they do not make good public health sense, they may make good political sense. Determine how to use support of services of interest to these officials in return for your high-priority programs. County commissioners in some areas have little visibility except when they serve on mosquito commissions and obtain these services for their districts. It may be effective to disperse a fine invisible mist of insecticide. Adding a little diesel oil may not reduce the effectiveness, but the resulting visible emission may make your local commissioner look as though he or she is doing something special. You can often have your cake and eat it with a little give, take, and innovation.

Look for support from umbrella agencies, such as Councils of Governments (COGs), that believe they should be arbiters of what is important. These groups are frequently required to endorse local proposals that are applications for state or federal funds. Involve and educate these agencies early in the process so that they become supporters rather than critics.

Computer systems[17-20] are becoming essential to efficient and effective use of resources as well as development of budgets and data bases to evaluate effectiveness. Computers can tell the story of the health department in pictures (graphics) without employing artists.

The changes in ease of use and availability of a multitude of excellent software have improved the ability of local health departments to adapt their use to data collection and improved evaluation. This is the result of better operating systems, the part of the system that makes the hardware work and transfers data between the floppy or hard disks, the monitor, and the printers as well as performing the computations.

It is difficult for a community that spent $10 million 5 years ago on a mainframe that has still not been paid off to accept the same work being done on a $15,000 personal computer. Local and state governments are just starting to catch up with private industry in development of data systems. Because health departments have joined the computer milieu late, they are well placed to use cheaper and better computers.

Some local governments provide every sanitarian with a portable computer to make restaurant inspections, print reports for the food services manager, and dump the reports into a PC back at the department when the day is over. In other departments the environmentalist can evaluate a homesite with a topographic contour-based plot on a screen before going out to the site. After returning to the office, the same sanitarian can draw the sewage system and well location onto the screen with a light pen. The data are then transferred to the planning department's data base and can be called up as necessary.

In summary, the local department is a small version of the state health department, which itself is a condensed version of the federal agencies. Public health agencies focus on programs that prevent disease and maintain the quality of life. At each higher level agencies perform more tasks of a limited and specialized nature, using more highly trained personnel. The national programs tend to focus on issues that transcend state boundary lines and plan programs to equalize different capabilities to provide public services between the states.

REFERENCES

1. Rosen G: A History of Public Health. New York: MD Publications, 1958
2. Kannell WB, Wolf PA, Verter J: Manifestations of coronary disease predisposing to stroke. JAMA 250:2942–2946, 1983
3. Anderson KM, Castelli WP, Levy D: Cholesterol and mortality—30 years of follow-up from the Framingham study. JAMA 252:2176–2180, 1987
4. Nabrit SM (ed): Infant Death: An Analysis by Maternal Risk and Health Care. Contrasts in Health Status. Panel on Health Services Research, Institute of Medicine, National Academy of Sciences, 1973
5. Brown SS (ed): Prenatal Care: Reaching Mothers, Reaching Infants. Committee to Study Outreach for Prenatal Care, Institute of Medicine, National Academy of Sciences, 1988
6. Chamie M, Henshaw SR: The costs and benefits of governmental expenditures for family planning programs. Fam Plann Perspect 13(9), 1981
7. Prospects for a Healthier America: Achieving the Nation's Health Promotion Objectives. Washington, D.C.: US Department of HHS, PHS, November 1984
8. The 1990 Health Objectives for The Nation: A Midcourse Review. Washington, D.C.: US Department of HHS, PHS, November 1986
9. Forward Plan for Health, FY 1978–82. Washington, D.C.: US Department of HEW, PHS, August 1976
10. Promoting Health, Preventing Disease—Objectives for the Nation. Washington, D.C.: US Department of HEW, August 1979
11. Healthy People. The Surgeon General's Report on Health Promotion and Disease Prevention. Washington, D.C.: US Department of HEW, PHS, 1979
12. Healthy People 2000. National Health Promotion and Disease Prevention Objectives. DHHS Pub. No. (PHS) 91-50212, 1991
13. Model Standards, A Guide for Community Preventive Services, 2 edt. Atlanta: Centers for Disease Control, 1985
14. Wasserman MP: APEX/PH: Self-Assessment for local health departments. Public Health Macroview 2(3), 1989
15. Gustavson TL, Lievans AW, Buttery CM, et al: Measles outbreak in a fully immunized secondary-school population. N Engl J Med 316:771–774, 1987
16. Landrigan PA, et al: Epidemic lead absorption near an ore smelter. N Engl J Med 292(3):123–129, 1975
17. Peterson HH: Developing Computer Solutions for Your Personal Business Problems. Englewood Cliffs, NJ: Prentice Hall, 1982
18. Curry JW: How to Find and Buy Good Software. Englewood Cliffs, NJ: Prentice Hall, 1983
19. Orthnor FO, Blum BI (eds): Implementing Health Care Information Systems. New York: Springer Verlag, 1989
20. McDonough FA (ed): Managing Microcomputers in Large Organizations. Commission on Engineering and Technical Systems, National Research Council, National Academy of Sciences

70

International Health

John M. Last

When we use the term *international health,* we recognise that health problems have no national boundaries. An outbreak of influenza A or paralytic poliomyelitis in Bangladesh concerns people who live in Belgium or the Bronx; a toxic spill into the Mississippi River can affect people who eat fish caught off the coast of Africa; cocaine from Colombia kills American teenagers; tobacco from the United States kills people in all the countries to which it is exported; acid emissions from factory chimneys in England kill forests in Scandinavia, and this ultimately harms human health; drought and the depletion of trees in Africa not only threaten human health locally but also are changing the climate and could disrupt global ecology. Dangers to health anywhere on earth are dangers to health everywhere.

It has long been realized that epidemic infectious disease is not stopped by national frontiers. International conferences aimed at standardizing quarantine regulations and procedures have been held at intervals since 1851, and such conferences led to the establishment of the Office International d'Hygiěne Publique (OIHP) in 1907, which was the precursor of the Health Office of the League of Nations. In 1948 the functions of the Health Office were assumed by the World Health Organization (WHO), which soon became the most important international health agency.

A CLASSIFICATION OF NATIONS

Terms such as *developing* and *developed country* are loosely used. The World Bank[1] divides developing countries into those with a gross national product (GNP) in 1987 of $480 U.S. or less per person, and a second category of middle income countries with GNPs of more than $480 U.S. per person but less than $6000 U.S.; these are further subdivided into a lower group (below $1940 U.S.) and an upper group. High income countries are all those with per capita incomes of $6000 or more. The distinction formerly made between Eastern European nonmarket economy nations and Western European market nations, Japan, the United States and Canada, and Australia and New Zealand has been dropped, along with categorizing into oil-importing and oil-exporting nations. About 2.7 billion people—over half the world's population—live in countries in the poorest group, which includes China and India. A further 1.4 billion live in the ''lower middle'' income nations of the developing world. About 750 million people live in the affluent industrial nations, which are affluent at least in part because they extract resources such as oil, minerals, and food from the poorer nations. To put it another way, 75% of the world's people live in developing nations, which collectively have about 20% of the world's wealth and productive capacity. Moreover, the gap between rich and poor nations is getting wider.

Another term sometimes used to describe the developing nations is the *third world;* this originated in French (*tiers monde*) and evokes memories of the era just after the end of World War II when our planet became divided along ideological grounds into the so-called ''free world,'' the communist and socialist nations that were politically aligned with the Soviet Union, and the rest, the ''third world,'' also known as nonaligned nations. The Brandt Commission[2] gave us another concept, a division of the world into the ''North,'' the industrially developed nations, nearly all in the northern hemisphere, and the ''South,'' comprising almost all of Africa, Latin America, and the south, southeast, and southwest parts of Asia, all of which are industrially and economically less developed or undeveloped. All descriptive terms for the nations of the world clearly have limitations.

Economic and social development and health improvement is taking place to varying degrees among the developing nations. In the early 1990s, some nations, notably those in Africa south of the Sahara, are deteriorating; some are suffering because of inadequate natural resources that have to be shared among too many people, some because of poor planning and use of available resources, and some because of political or military turmoil. The prospects for short-term improvement are not bright for the worst-off nations.

WHY BE CONCERNED ABOUT INTERNATIONAL HEALTH?

There are several reasons why we should be concerned about international health. The most obvious is self-interest. The world is afflicted with problems that endanger us all. Those of us who live in the affluent industrial nations can easily become complacent or indifferent to the poverty, the malnutrition and starvation, the widespread disease, and the premature death of children and of women in the reproductive years that occur in many developing countries. Of course similar problems exist in parts of some rich nations. These deplorable conditions influence the health and well-being of us all, wherever we may live. These conditions are at the roots of much of the tension that constantly threatens the world with new outbreaks of hostilities, and they extend breeding grounds of disease that can be exported to other nations, as well as of disease that threatens people from rich and favored nations when they travel to or work in the developing world. Political unrest and warfare in parts of the third world disrupt routine preventive measures and so add to the risk that dangerous communicable diseases will occur and spread. Other reasons for international health programs include the scientific challenge of unsolved health problems and the altruistic impulse that leads some people to devote their lives to improving the lot of those less fortunate than themselves. This has been a motive for medical missionaries, and even when religious conversion is not a priority, hospitals and clinics run by missionaries sometimes provide the only health care available in some communities in developing countries.

Ideas that advance the human condition move in all directions among the nations of the world. Vaccines and nutritional supplements from the North enhance the lives of infants and mothers in the South; efficacious traditional remedies and herbal medications from many developing countries have been adopted with benefit in Europe and North America; urban automobile exhaust pollution is being tackled in Nigeria and Mexico by limiting circulation of cars on certain days, a way to control traffic congestion that could usefully be adopted in many affluent industrial cities. Methods of disease surveillance that originated in the Eastern European bloc could be used to advantage in the west.

AGENCIES INVOLVED IN INTERNATIONAL HEALTH

International and national agencies under the control of governments, nongovernmental organizations (NGOs), and private voluntary organizations are all active in international health. The government-sponsored international agencies include several United Nations (UN) organizations, the best known of which is WHO. Other UN agencies with important health-related roles are the United Nations Children's Fund (UNICEF), the United Nations Development Programme (UNDP), the Food and Agriculture Organization (FAO), the United Nations Fund for Population Activities (UNFPA), the Office of the UN High Commissioner for Refugees (UNHCR), the UN Fund for Drug Abuse Control (UNFDAC), and the International Bank for Reconstruction and Development, better known as the World Bank. The most important international nongovernmental organization is probably the International Commission of the Red Cross/Red Crescent (ICRC).

Most affluent industrial nations support bilateral or multilateral agencies by providing financial and logistic support for health-related activities. Included in this category are the U.S. Agency for International Development (USAID) and similar agencies of the Swedish, British, Canadian, German, and other Western European governments, and those of newly rich nations such as Japan and the Arab oil states, especially Saudi Arabia. Many governmental agencies and NGOs have affiliations with WHO; examples include the Centers for Disease Control, the Public Health Laboratory Service in Britain, the Addiction Research Foundation in Canada, and many national and international professional associations in the health field.

The NGOs and private voluntary organizations raise funds for international health work of many kinds, mainly by voluntary subscriptions and donations. Many churches and missionary groups also play a prominent role; their activities include general and specific programs, such as hospital and community-based therapeutic and preventive services, aid for persons with specific diseases such as leprosy, trachoma, cataract, and aid for destitute children. Several philanthropic foundations, for example, the Rockefeller Foundation and the Ford Foundation, have made important contributions to the advance of medical research and education in developing countries.

THE WORK OF WHO

WHO is supported by all nations and is concerned with all aspects of human health. Its achievements since 1948 have been impressive. WHO has been responsible for at least one contribution of lasting historical importance, the eradication of smallpox; this was accomplished in 1979 after an international collaborative effort that was coordinated and directed by WHO.[3] If WHO had done nothing else, the eradication of this disease, one of the great scourges of humanity since prehistoric times, would have justified its existence. Given enough money, material and manpower, WHO could similarly eradicate other diseases, as well as improve the human condition in many other ways.

Communicable disease control is much emphasized among the activities of WHO[4]; there are programs aimed at controlling all the principal communicable diseases of developing and tropical countries—malaria, schistosomiasis, onchocerciasis, leishmaniasis, trypanosomiasis, leprosy, yaws, tuberculosis, yellow fever, parasitic diseases, sexually transmitted diseases, viral hemorrhagic fevers, zoonoses. Since the mid-1980s, the Global Programme on AIDS (GPA) has become one of the most prominent activities of WHO. WHO programs focus on maternal and child health, nutritional deficiency diseases, occupational and environmental health problems, mental disorders, etc. Other programs deal with education and training of health workers, information and technology transfer, and quality control of biological products and pharmaceutical preparations. A section is concerned with epidemiologic surveillance, health status and health trend assessment and world health statistics, disease classification systems, etc. An activity that is often done in collaboration with organizations such as ICRC and UNHCR is emergency and disaster relief, when natural or manmade disasters displace large numbers of people, rendering them homeless and depriving them of means to subsist and survive. In the late 1980s an estimated 15 million people lived in refugee communities in various parts of the world.[5] Another 50 million have been displaced by natural disasters such as drought or by political or military action, without being technically classified as refugees. It is difficult to find any aspect of health affairs that is not dealt with somewhere within the scope of work of WHO.

The work of WHO is conducted at the headquarters in Geneva, in the six regional offices,[6] at country offices, and in the field. All regional offices have specialized permanent staff, reinforced by temporary advisers, short-term consultants, technical experts, etc. The six regions are defined by geographic and political criteria, and within each there is considerable economic and cultural diversity; this may both help and hinder the collaborative efforts of countries within a region. The rich nations can help the poor, but cultural and ideological differences sometimes impede understanding and cooperation.

The early postwar activities of WHO were dominated by programs to control specific diseases such as malaria, smallpox, and yellow fever. World health strategies took a new direction after a resolution approved by the World Health Assembly in 1977 and an international conference in Alma-Ata, USSR, in 1978.[7] At this conference it was agreed that a realistic target to aim for would be the provision of primary health care for all the world's people by the year 2000. This inspired the slogan "Health for all by the year 2000"—a slogan, not a goal—and the slogan in turn has inspired much effort and thought about ways to achieve better health for people everywhere who now face many impediments to good health. At a series of working conferences, experts on every aspect of health and disease have considered how to achieve the goals of "health for all." Many strategies and tactics have been formulated at national, regional, and international levels, and action has begun on many of them. Within the regions of WHO, specific objectives have been set, relating to the existing health problems and health resources. The targets of the European region,[8] for instance, give precedence to health promotion initiatives, in which respect they differ from those of the United States,[9] where the emphasis is more on disease prevention, and those of Southeast Asia, where the emphasis remains on control of communicable diseases.

THE STATE OF THE WORLD IN THE 1990s

Much of the improvement in health since the beginning of the twentieth century is attributable to advances of medical science and the application of public health measures such as sanitation and clean water. Some formidable obstacles to health and well-being, however, still exist. Wars and political instability are at the heart of some of the most intractable problems. Others in the industrially developed, affluent nations are due to uncontrolled excesses in exploiting the environment, destroying what was naturally present, and poisoning vegetation, wildlife, and even human communities.[10] It is important to bear these problems in mind while we consider the health problems of the developing world, which are the main concern of this chapter. We cannot separate the developed from the developing world, and consider their problems in isolation from each other.

Population Growth. As we entered the 1990s the world's population passed 5.2 billion; by the beginning of the twenty-first century, it will have passed 6 billion; the latest billion will be added in just 12 years.

Throughout history and as far as we can determine, since long before recorded history began, the growth rate of human numbers was linear, save for occasional disruptions such as the epidemics of plague in the fourteenth century, which killed about a third of the population of Europe and large numbers in Asia. But at varying times from the late eighteenth century onward, the rate of growth became exponential. This exponential growth has occurred all over the world, beginning in the late eighteenth century in Western Europe, the early nineteenth century in Eastern Europe, and the early twentieth century in Africa, in south and Southeast Asia, and Latin America.[11] In North America the pattern is distorted by migrations, discussed below; birth rates began to greatly exceed death rates, however, early in the nineteenth century in the United States.

The causes of this surge in human numbers have been much debated.[12] Some demographers believe that improved nutrition, related to changes in climatic conditions and the opening up to agriculture of vast areas in the Americas and Australasia, was the principal determinant. Others believe the reasons are more complex, including reduced risks of infant death from infections due to ecological changes, and subtle changes in attitudes towards family size that influenced traditional methods used to limit the numbers of offspring (see Chapter 3). Since the change to an exponential growth rate preceded most of the modern advances of medical science, it is not due to control of infectious disease by antibiotics and immunization programs, although these did play a part in accelerating the trend in some countries.

This exponential increase in the numbers of humanity cannot continue indefinitely. Other living creatures fluctuate in numbers according to the supply of needed nutriment and pressure from predators. Humans are subject to the same biological laws, and like bacterial colonies, flour beetles, field mice, shoals of herring, and roving herds of caribou, we must strike a balance between reproductive rates and the supply of food and other essentials. The difference between humans and the other life forms whose reproductive performance has been studied is that humans have greater capacity to adapt to a wide range of environmental conditions. This has made it possible for humans to settle all over the planet on a scale unmatched by any other species; but it has also meant that almost no part of the earth's surface has remained untouched (and unspoilt) by human occupation. Humans have transformed the planetary ecology as a result. The ultimate consequences of this cannot be determined or predicted, but there is a growing consensus that there will be serious adverse effects on the global environment, probably soon. We might pay a heavy price for our reproductive success (see Chapter 39).

Other Population Problems—Migrations and Rural-Urban Shifts. Several times in human history there have been massive movements of large numbers of people about the earth, great redistributions, probably related to imbalance between numbers and the supply of needed resources of food, fuel, raw materials, or valued commodities. There is evidence from archeological digs and folklore of much movement between Asia and southeastern Europe about 2000 B.C.; there was another mass movement about the time of the fall of the Roman Empire (c. A.D. 200–600) when tribes of people from Asiatic Russia invaded Europe. Another movement began with the earliest European colonization of the Americas, gathered momentum towards the end of the nineteenth century with large-scale migration from Europe to the Americas and Australasia, and continues until the present, interrupted only by the two world wars.[13] This movement includes not only massive flow of people from many European nations to other parts of the world, but also at least as much movement, perhaps more, between Asian nations, from Asia to Europe and the Americas, and within Africa. Much of the migration is not documented in detail, though the approximate numbers and their origins and destinations are known. This migration is a poorly understood feature of modern times that has had and continues to have profound effects on the well-being and the health of huge numbers of people in many countries. Population pressure and acute shortages of land, food, water, and natural resources are obliging huge numbers of people to move in the late twentieth century, but many have nowhere to go. This imbalance could have explosive consequences.

Within many developing nations (and also within the industrially developed nations) there has been considerable redistribution from rural to urban areas. In the late 1970s, it was estimated by the UN Statistical Office that by the year 2000 the proportion of people living in urban areas would exceed the proportion in rural areas. By the early 1980s, about 40% of the world population already was urbanized.[14] Some of this rural-urban movement has been due to drought or other natural disasters that have led people to flee from the land in search of work in cities. On the Indian subcontinent, in Southeast Asia (especially in Indochina), and in several Latin American and African countries, rural-urban movement has been due at least in part to economic and political disturbances often aggravated by warfare or rural banditry. Dispossessed subsistence farmers and displaced or unwanted rural agricultural laborers have moved in huge numbers to squalid shantytowns on the outskirts of cities, swelling the urban populations and overloading already inadequate water supply and sanitary services. Whenever they can, people living

TABLE 70-1. URBAN AGGLOMERATIONS WITH MORE THAN 10 MILLION INHABITANTS: 1950, 1975, AND 2000

▪ 1950	Millions		Millions
New York, northeastern New Jersey	12.2	London	10.4
▪ 1975			
New York, northeastern New Jersey	19.8	Tokyo, Yokohama	17.7
Mexico City	11.9	Shanghai	11.6
Los Angeles, Long Beach	10.8	São Paulo	10.7
		London	10.4
▪ 2000			
Mexico City	31.0	São Paulo	25.8
Tokyo, Yokohama	24.2	New York, northeastern New Jersey	22.8
Shanghai	22.7	Rio de Janeiro	19.0
Beijing	19.9	Calcutta	16.7
Greater Bombay	17.1	Seoul	14.2
Jakarta	16.6	Cairo, Giza, Imbaba	13.1
Los Angeles, Long Beach	14.2	Manila	12.3
Madras	12.9	Bangkok, Thonburi	11.9
Greater Buenos Aires	12.1	Delhi	11.7
Karachi	11.8	Paris	11.3
Bogotá	11.7	Istanbul	11.2
Tehran	11.3	Osaka, Kobe	11.2
Baghdad	11.1		

From World Bank World Development Report, 1984, and U.N. Statistical Reports.

under such conditions as these seek to escape by migrating—legally or illegally—to industrially developed nations.

The growth of cities, especially in the developing nations, is an awe-inspiring problem. The population expected to be living in cities of 11 million or more by the year 2000 is shown in Table 70–1; even cities in affluent industrial nations are unlikely to function well or to be pleasant places in which to live when they reach such numbers as these. In most developing nations, food supplies, sanitary services, fuel, and shelter will almost certainly be inadequate to cope with the projected numbers. Moreover, the rural areas of many of the nations in which these cities are located will be experiencing equal or greater rates of population growth, and they will not have much if any spare to contribute to the food supply.

HEALTH PROBLEMS OF DEVELOPING NATIONS

A useful way to arrange and classify the nations of the world, suggested by UNICEF Director General James Grant, is according to their prevailing infant mortality rates.[15] Infant mortality rates correlate closely with levels of economic development, literacy, housing conditions, access to pure water supplies, and several other variables dependent upon economic development; the availability of health care is not directly related to infant mortality rates, although it is often related to the level of economic development.

Table 70–2, which arranges selected nations in order of under-age-5 mortality, also shows the nations' infant mortality rates, total population, annual growth rates, per capita GNP, literacy levels, and life expectancy. But the table does not offer any potential solution to problems of underdevelopment. The World Bank's recognition of the relationship between economic development and health is an important contribution to the solution. Many developing nations are caught in a vicious circle of unrelieved poverty that causes or contributes to much of the ill-health, which in turn aggravates the poverty. Development assistance that relieves the poverty may be the first step towards improvement of health. The low status of women, leading to female illiteracy and thus to poor understanding of ways to protect their infants' health, must also be dealt with.

Interaction of Infection, Malnutrition and Population Growth. The traditional health problems of the developing world arise from the interaction of three forces: infectious diseases (especially affecting infants and young children), malnutrition, and uncontrolled population growth.

Infectious diseases take a terrible toll. There are about a billion cases each year of some of the common infectious diseases—diarrhea, respiratory infections, malaria, schistosomiasis, tuberculosis, intestinal parasites. In Africa about a million deaths occur each year from malaria alone. About 4 million children die each year from diarrhea, 2 to 3 million die from respiratory infections, and another 4 million die from a combination of malnutrition and vaccine-preventable diseases, especially measles. About another million deaths are due to neonatal tetanus. There are also about half a million maternal deaths each year in the developing world, and many of these, leaving infants motherless, are followed by the death of these infants.[16]

Malnutrition is almost universal in some of the poorest nations, notably those affected by the widespread droughts and famine in Africa. All forms of malnutrition occur—marasmus, protein-calorie shortage, vitamin deficiency diseases. Malnutrition increases susceptibility to infection, and infection enhances metabolic demand for protein and calorie intake, so there is a vicious circle in the infection/malnutrition complex that causes so many premature deaths in the poorer developing countries.

Children continue to die of measles and diarrhea, despite the fact that there are inexpensive ways to prevent and treat these diseases. As part of the "Health for All" strategy, the Expanded Programme on Immunization has set targets to be achieved by the year 2000 in immunization coverage of infants and children against important communicable diseases. Considerable progress has been made in some regions and countries, but this must be a continuing effort, for new generations of susceptible infants

TABLE 70-2. BASIC INDICATORS OF NATIONAL HEALTH

	Under 5 Mortality Rate		Infant Mortality Rate (under 1)		Total Population (millions)	Percentage Increase of Population per annum	GNP per Capita (US $)	Life Expectancy at Birth (years)	Total Adult Literacy Rate
	1960	**1988**	**1960**	**1988**	**1988**		**1987**	**1988**	**1985**
▪ **Very High U5MR Countries (over 170)**									
Median	**314**	**203**	**190**	**127**	**489T**	**. .**	**275**	**48**	**33**
1 Afghanistan	380	300	215	171	15.1	n.a.	. .	42	24
2 Mozambique	330	298	190	172	14.8	n.a.	170	47	39
3 Mali	370	292	210	168	8.8	. .	210	44	17
4 Angola	346	292	208	172	9.5	2.7	470	45	41
5 Sierra Leone	386	266	219	153	3.9	. .	300	41	30
6 Malawi	364	262	206	149	7.9	. .	160	47	42
7 Ethiopia	294	259	175	153	44.7	3.9	130	41	66
8 Guinea	346	248	208	146	6.5	. .	. .	42	29
9 Burkina Faso	362	233	205	137	8.5	. .	190	47	14
10 Niger	320	228	191	134	6.7	. .	260	45	14
11 Chad	326	223	195	131	5.4	. .	150	46	26
12 Central African Rep.	308	223	183	131	2.8	. .	330	46	41
13 Somalia	294	221	175	131	7.1	. .	290	45	12
14 Mauritania	320	220	191	126	1.9	. .	440	46	17
15 Rwanda	248	206	146	121	6.8	. .	300	49	47
16 Kampuchea	218	199	146	127	7.9	. .	. .	49	75
17 Yemen Dem.	378	197	214	118	2.3	. .	420	51	42
18 Nepal	297	197	186	127	18.2	2.4	160	51	26
19 Bhutan	297	197	186	127	1.5	. .	150	48	. .
20 Yemen	378	190	214	115	7.5	. .	590	51	25
21 Burundi	258	188	152	111	5.1	. .	250	49	34
22 Bangladesh	262	188	156	118	109.6	2.6	160	51	33
23 Benin	310	185	185	109	4.4	. .	310	47	27
24 Madagascar	364	184	219	119	11.2	. .	210	54	68
25 Sudan	293	181	170	107	23.8	3.0	330	50	24
26 Tanzania	248	176	146	105	25.4	3.2	180	53	91
27 Namibia	262	176	155	105	1.8	. .	. .	56	. .
28 Nigeria	318	174	190	104	105.5	3.3	370	51	43
29 Bolivia	282	172	167	109	6.9	. .	580	53	75
30 Haiti	294	171	197	116	6.3	. .	360	55	38
▪ **High U5MR Countries (95–170)**									
Median	**241**	**125**	**153**	**83**	**1486T**	**. .**	**580**	**57**	**59**
31 Uganda	224	169	133	102	17.2	3.3	260	51	58
32 Gabon	288	169	171	102	1.1	. .	2700	52	62
33 Pakistan	277	166	163	108	114.9	2.5	350	57	30
34 Laos	232	159	155	109	3.8	. .	170	49	84
35 Togo	305	153	182	93	3.2	. .	290	53	41
36 Cameroon	275	153	163	93	10.7	. .	970	51	56
37 India	282	149	165	98	818.8	1.5	300	58	43
38 Liberia	258	147	153	86	2.4	. .	450	55	35
39 Ghana	224	146	132	89	14.1	. .	390	54	54
40 Côte d'Ivoire	264	142	165	95	11.6	. .	740	53	42
41 Zaire	251	138	148	83	33.8	3.1	150	53	62
42 Senegal	313	136	180	80	7.0	. .	520	46	28
43 Lesotho	208	136	149	99	1.7	. .	370	56	73
44 Zambia	228	127	135	79	7.9	. .	250	54	76
45 Egypt	300	125	179	83	51.5	1.7	680	61	45
46 Peru	233	123	142	87	21.3	1.9	1470	62	85
47 Morocco	265	119	163	80	23.9	. .	610	61	34
48 Libyan Arab Jamahiriya	268	119	160	80	4.2	. .	5460	61	66
49 Indonesia	235	119	139	84	175.0	1.5	450	56	74
50 Congo	241	114	143	72	1.9	. .	870	49	63
51 Zimbabwe	182	113	110	71	9.1	. .	580	59	74
52 Kenya	208	113	124	71	23.1	4.1	330	59	60
53 Honduras	232	107	144	68	4.8	. .	810	64	59

(continued)

TABLE 70-2. BASIC INDICATORS OF NATIONAL HEALTH (Continued)

	Under 5 Mortality Rate		Infant Mortality Rate (under 1)		Total Population (millions)	Percentage Increase of Population per annum	GNP per Capita (US $)	Life Expectancy at Birth (years)	Total Adult Literacy Rate
	1960	1988	1960	1988	1988		1987	1988	1985
▪ **High U5MR Countries (95–170) Median**	**241**	**125**	**153**	**83**	**1486T**	**. .**	**580**	**57**	**59**
54 Algeria	270	107	168	73	23.8	. .	2680	63	50
55 Guatemala	230	99	125	58	8.7	. .	950	62	55
56 Saudi Arabia	292	98	170	70	13.1	. .	6200	64	51
57 South Africa	192	95	135	71	33.7	. .	1890	61	. .
58 Nicaragua	210	95	140	61	3.6	. .	830	64	88
59 Myanmar	229	95	153	69	40.0	. .	200	60	84
▪ **Middle U5MR Countries (31–94) Median**	**155**	**63**	**111**	**44**	**2170T**	**. .**	**1400**	**66**	**84**
60 Iraq	222	94	139	68	17.7	2.9	3020	64	89
61 Turkey	258	93	190	74	53.5	1.6	1210	64	74
62 Botswana	174	92	119	66	1.2	2.5	1050	59	71
63 Iran, Islamic Rep. of	254	90	169	61	53.1	2.0	. .	66	51
64 Viet Nam	233	88	156	63	64.2	. .	. .	62	84
65 Ecuador	183	87	124	62	10.2	. .	1040	66	83
66 Brazil	160	85	116	62	144.4	1.5	2020	65	78
67 El Salvador	206	84	142	58	5.0	. .	860	63	72
68 Tunisia	255	83	159	58	7.8	. .	1180	66	55
69 Papua New Guinea	247	81	165	57	3.8	. .	700	54	45
70 Dominican Rep.	200	81	125	64	6.9	. .	730	66	78
71 Philippines	135	73	80	44	59.5	1.7	590	64	86
72 Guyana	94	71	69	56	1.0	. .	390	70	96
73 Mexico	140	68	92	46	84.9	1.9	1830	69	90
74 Colombia	148	68	93	46	30.6	1.6	1240	65	82
75 Syria	218	64	135	47	11.6	. .	1640	65	60
76 Oman	378	64	214	40	1.4	. .	5810	56	30
77 Paraguay	134	62	86	42	4.0	. .	990	67	88
78 Mongolia	158	59	109	44	2.1	. .	. .	64	93
79 Jordan	218	57	135	43	3.9	. .	1560	66	75
80 Lebanon	92	51	68	39	2.8	. .	. .	67	78
81 Thailand	149	49	103	38	54.1	1.5	850	65	91
82 Venezuela	114	44	81	36	18.8	. .	3230	70	87
83 Sri Lanka	113	43	70	32	16.8	1.4	400	70	87
84 China	202	43	150	31	1104.0	1.0	290	70	69
85 Argentina	75	37	61	32	31.5	1.0	2390	71	95
86 Panama	105	34	69	23	2.3	. .	2240	72	89
87 Albania	151	34	112	28	3.1	. .	. .	72	. .
88 Korea Dem.	120	33	85	24	21.9	. .	. .	69	. .
89 Korea Rep.	120	33	85	24	42.6	1.1	2690	69	92
90 United Arab Emirates	239	32	145	25	1.5	. .	15830	71	. .
91 Malaysia	106	32	73	24	16.6	. .	1810	70	74
92 USSR	53	32	38	25	283.7	0.7	4550	70	. .
93 Uruguay	56	31	50	27	3.1	. .	2190	71	95
▪ **Low U5MR Countries (30 and under) Median**	**44**	**12**	**37**	**10**	**950T**	**. .**	**7940**	**75**	**93**
94 Mauritus	104	29	70	22	1.1	. .	1490	69	83
95 Yugoslavia	113	28	92	25	23.6	0.9	2480	72	91
96 Romania	82	28	69	22	23.0	1.8	2560	70	. .
97 Chile	142	26	114	19	12.7	1.1	1310	72	97
98 Trinidad and Tobago	67	23	54	20	1.2	. .	4210	70	96
99 Kuwait	128	22	89	19	1.9	. .	14610	73	70
100 Jamaica	88	22	62	18	2.4	. .	940	74	. .
101 Costa Rica	121	22	84	18	2.9	. .	1610	75	93
102 Bulgaria	69	20	49	15	9.0	. .	4150	72	. .
103 Hungary	57	19	51	17	10.6	0.7	2240	70	. .

(continued)

TABLE 70-2. BASIC INDICATORS OF NATIONAL HEALTH (Continued)

	Under 5 Mortality Rate		Infant Mortality Rate (under 1)		Total Population (millions)	Percentage Increase of Population per annum	GNP per Capita (US $)	Life Expectancy at Birth (years)	Total Adult Literacy Rate
	1960	1988	1960	1988	1988		1987	1988	1985
▪ **Low U5MR Countries (30 and under) Median**	**44**	**12**	**37**	**10**	**950T**	**. .**	**7940**	**75**	**93**
104 Poland	70	18	62	16	38.0	0.9	2070	71	. .
105 Cuba	87	18	62	15	10.2	. .	. .	74	96
106 Greece	84	18	53	13	10.0	. .	4020	76	92
107 Portugal	112	17	81	14	10.2	. .	2830	73	84
108 Czechoslovakia	32	15	26	12	15.6	0.6	5820	71	. .
109 Israel	40	14	33	11	4.4	. .	6800	75	95
110 USA	30	13	26	10	245.4	0.7	18530	75	. .
111 Belgium	35	13	31	10	9.9	. .	11480	75	. .
112 Germany Dem.	44	12	37	8	16.6	. .	7180	73	. .
113 Singapore	50	12	36	9	2.6	. .	7940	73	86
114 New Zealand	27	12	23	10	3.3	. .	7750	75	. .
115 Spain	56	12	46	9	39.1	0.7	6010	77	94
116 Denmark	25	11	22	8	5.1	0.1	14930	75	. .
117 United Kingdom	27	11	23	9	56.8	0.1	10420	75	. .
118 Italy	50	11	44	10	57.3	0.1	10350	76	97
119 Australia	25	10	21	9	16.4	1.0	11100	76	. .
120 Germany Fed.	40	10	33	8	60.7	−0.1	14400	75	. .
121 Hong Kong	65	10	44	8	5.7	. .	8070	76	88
122 Austria	43	10	37	8	7.5	. .	11980	74	. .
123 Norway	23	10	19	8	4.2	. .	17190	77	. .
124 France	34	10	29	8	55.8	0.4	12790	76	. .
125 Ireland	36	9	31	7	3.7	. .	6120	74	. .
126 Netherlands	22	8	18	8	14.6	. .	11860	77	. .
127 Canada	33	8	28	7	26.1	1.0	15160	77	. .
128 Japan	40	8	31	5	122.4	0.6	15760	78	. .
129 Switzerland	27	8	22	7	6.5	0.1	21330	77	. .
130 Sweden	20	7	16	6	8.3	0.1	15550	77	. .
131 Finland	28	7	22	6	5.0	0.1	14470	75	. .

Data from UNICEF and World Bank reports, recent years.

are added each year.[17] Some countries lag far behind in immunization coverage, while in others impressive progress is being made.

Oral rehydration therapy—a simple and inexpensive supplement that replaces fluid and electrolytes lost during bouts of diarrhea—has saved many lives; this technique is easily taught even to illiterate village women. International health agencies have justifiably invested much effort in teaching about oral rehydration therapy, and the benefits are apparent in many rural communities in the third world. The program has the virtue of being easily applied by minimally trained health workers.

The fact that so many children now live who previously would have died helps to convince parents that fewer children have to be conceived to provide the workforce needed to maintain farms or paddy fields. Protecting and preserving the lives of infants and children is the first step towards dealing with the most urgent and frightening problem of all, the problem of uncontrolled human reproduction. Much effort is necessary, however, to educate parents and thus accelerate the transition from high to reduced birth rates; without this effort, the consequence is greatly increased population pressure on land that is already overcrowded.

The rate of population growth is influenced by complex cultural factors, religious beliefs, levels of education and literacy, especially literacy of women, which depends upon the status of women in society. Once they are able to read, women are better able to understand the basic principles of contraception; they are also better able to understand that disease and premature death are not inevitable facts of life.[18] The education that is needed to change traditional values is another urgent priority. Perhaps television can play its most valuable role in human affairs by contributing to the education and value changes needed to improve the status of women. This situation, however, is changing in regions such as much of sub-Saharan Africa where HIV infection is highly prevalent among young adults and their offspring.

Special efforts are needed in some developing nations to improve the status of women. In many rural agrarian societies, women's lives are determined for them by the elders of the family or tribe; most are destined to spend their lives in a combination of childbearing and heavy manual labor, working crops, carrying fuel or water long distances, and crouching over smoky cooking fires inhaling toxic fumes.[19] They may be denied access to modern education, so they have no way to learn how much they are missing by reading about the better situation of women and their families in other lands.

High density of population contributes to the spread of communicable diseases, so population pressure not only drains food resources and leads to widespread malnutrition, but also sets the stage for epidemics. These three problems, population pressure, malnutrition, and infection, thus constantly reinforce one another. Economic development may best help to break these vicious circles by concentrating on the control of infections, but in turn the control of infections cannot achieve much without opportunities for employment of the increasing numbers of survivors—which requires improved education and higher levels of literacy. Clearly the solution is as complex as the problem.

New Problems. The combination of population pressure, malnutrition, and infection has sapped the vitality of the developing nations for generations. Now new problems are being added. Industrial development, often without the restraining laws and regulations of the affluent industrial nations, is causing serious environmental damage and occupational diseases. And some of the worst dangers to health of the industrial nations, notably cigarette smoking and traffic injury, are increasingly common.

Industrial development is needed in the third world, but unfortunately many multinational corporations are attracted to the idea of setting up petrochemical plants, textile mills, and factories, not by the desire to assist these nations towards economic development, but by the supply of cheap labor and the desire to avoid laws and regulations that have been enacted in the industrially developed nations to protect the health of workers and to preserve environmental quality. Factories in the developing nations frequently employ children and women for low wages, have no workers' compensation, and few if any industrial safety standards. Workers who are injured on the job can be dismissed without compensation and their places filled by others from the virtually unlimited available pool of unemployed workers among the rural and new urban poor. Environmental quality is often damaged by unrestrained discharge of toxic waste products into the air and water.

In some regions of the developing world the ecosystems are being gravely jeopardized by a combination of population pressure on former wilderness areas and of unsound agricultural practices, such as the slash-and-burn approach that is endangering much of the Amazon rain forest to create pasture for cattle that will ultimately be slaughtered for meat—an ecologically unsound means of providing protein foods. Hydroelectric development programs that flood wide areas of tropical rain forest make this situation even more serious (See chapter 39).

The habits and customs we increasingly recognise as harmful to health are eagerly embraced by people in third world nations, who often perceive them as outward signs of their own emergence into better times. Women are persuaded that artificial formula is more desirable than breast-feeding; for some years the multinational infant formula manufacturers engaged in a persuasive advertising campaign to promote infant formulas, even though it was well known that mothers in rural villages lacked the means to purchase, sterilize, or store formula under safe and hygienic conditions. Despite pressure from UNICEF and other representatives of the international community, persuasion to use infant formula rather than breast milk continues in some third world nations.[20]

The adoption of cigarette smoking is probably the worst of the unhealthy practices of industrially developed nations. The tobacco companies are able to promote their deadly product without restraint in most developing nations; advertising often is directed specifically at children. The use of cigarettes is equated with social and economic success, with the result that in some developing nations about half the child population of both sexes is already addicted to cigarettes.[21] Just as bad, tobacco has become firmly established as a lucrative cash crop, displacing badly needed subsistence agriculture; moreover, trees are being depleted to provide fuel for flue-curing tobacco to make into cigarettes.

Another problem that reflects low standards of ethical and moral conduct by some multinational corporations is the export to developing countries of pharmaceutical preparations that have been denied a license in the country where they were originally developed, usually because of doubts about their safety or efficacy or both.[22] In some developing countries, for example, in Latin America and Southeast Asia, these drugs are sold in open stalls in marketplaces. Apart from the harm they may do, some of these drugs are broad-spectrum antibiotic combinations that help to produce resistant strains of pathogenic microorganisms.

There has always been a heavy toll of accidental death and injury in developing countries from such causes as burns and scalds that commonly occur when cooking is done over open fires. With the influx of automobiles, often on roads never built to carry them and with drivers who have never been properly taught to drive, the toll of traffic injury and premature death is also rising. The density of traffic is already high in the cities in many developing countries and will undoubtedly continue to rise, but it is unlikely that adequate roads will be constructed for many years and still less likely that cars will be separated from pedestrians, cyclists, and carts drawn by animals. Industrial accidents also occur with increasing frequency because untrained workers and unsafe machinery are a dangerous combination. For all these reasons, the burden of accidental death and injury is rapidly increasing.

Failures of Planning and Organization. The solution of many of the health problems in developing nations is elusive at least in part because of poor planning, inadequate organization, and faulty values. These human factors cause or contribute to several problems, of which the following are the most obvious, although this is not an all-inclusive list.

Unequal Access to Health Care. The poor, especially the rural poor, often have difficulty gaining access to any form of health care except perhaps traditional village healers. Health care services of all kinds tend to be concentrated in the cities, and frequently those who use them are required to pay a fee. While the small numbers of well-to-do people in the cities may have abundant health care of good quality, the rest of the population may lack even the most elementary health services.

Treatment Gets Higher Priority Than Prevention. Of course this problem is not unique to developing countries. In developing countries, however, expensively equipped modern hospitals to treat complex and difficult medical and surgical cases can actually do harm because they attract not only an unfair share of the small budget available for health services but also a disproportionate share of skilled and well-trained health care workers. Moreover, they often contribute to the "brain drain": in order to acquire the necessary skills to work in specialized health care settings it is necessary for bright young graduates to get their training abroad—and many never return to their homeland.[23] Meanwhile training for primary care and public health workers may be underfunded or nonexistent.

Unsuitable Distribution Among the Health Professions. In many countries there is a serious maldistribution among the branches of health care practice. There may be a surplus of physicians and a shortage of nurses, as well as greater numbers of specialists than generalized physicians. This problem is particularly acute in nations where the low status of women leads to high female illiteracy rates, low rates of recruitment into the nursing profession, and thus to a situation in which there may be several practicing doctors to each nurse, rather than the other way around. Another factor is that nursing is viewed as a low-status occupation, akin to domestic service; midwifery, on the other hand, may have high status, even when practiced by traditional village midwives who lack proper professional training. There may also be serious shortages of certain classes of technicians, for example, medical laboratory assistants.

Inappropriate Investment in High Technology. Political decisions may lead to investment in expensive technical devices such as electron microscopes and diagnostic imaging equipment that not only is expensive in itself and requires expensively trained technical staff to work it but also is even more expensive to maintain; but there may be no funds for maintenance of equipment or persons qualified to do repairs.

Inappropriate Training Programs. Although many international planning groups sponsored by WHO and other agencies have recommended emphasis on training primary health care workers, national pride, tradition, and reluctance to change established educational systems may lead to continuation of training programs in a pattern set along the lines of the United States or Western Europe. The graduates of such training programs are attracted towards nations where they can practice the kind of medicine or nursing that they have been taught, and they are reluctant to work in the rural areas of their own countries where there is great need for their services. This can be a particularly difficult problem for health planners and policy makers, for there is an understandable reluctance to train indigenous health workers to supposedly lower standards than those prevailing in the rich nations. What is needed here is a change in values, an acceptance of the fact that training programs for primary health care workers are not of a lower but of a different standard.

Lack of Health Information. Sometimes the numbers of the people are not accurately known, let alone their diseases and causes of death. One of the highest priorities—recognized in the strategies for the "Health for All" programs—is to establish and maintain comprehensive health information systems, or if this is not possible, at the very least to set up registration areas in which the numbers of persons and health-related states and events can be accurately and continuously ascertained. Only when this is done can health planners argue persuasively for an adequate allocation from the national budget that will enable them to begin dealing with the prevailing health problems.

Administrative Deficiencies. Frequently there is no trained cadre of administrators. Some former colonies of European nations were left with no civil service at all when the colonists departed; many of these nations have been plagued by political and military unrest, and their health services, as well as all other essential services, are led by untrained office staff or members of the armed forces, among whom a common view is that "anyone can be an administrator." In some countries the administration is corrupt, further aggravating the situation.

Breakdown of Communication. All forms of communication may be faulty—transportation services from the center to the periphery, the postal and telephone services, even contact between professionals in different sections of the service. Thus it can happen that someone who encounters a problem is unaware that another professional elsewhere in the same country, even the same city or the same building, possesses the solution (or it may be in the library, to which access may be restricted).

Wrong Priorities. National budgets are meager at best, but often the funds are misallocated. There is an obscene imbalance between expenditures on social and health services and on military weapons in many developing countries, indeed in the world as a whole.[24] Since the 1960s, the scale of expenditure on armed services, and imports of sophisticated armaments from the industrial nations to the developing nations, has sharply increased. The wars in various parts of the world are all in developing countries, and often are surrogate conflicts in which the geopolitical designs of the great powers are worked out with the lives and over the land of people in some of the poorest and most backward nations on earth.

Getting Priorities Right. The independent Commission on Health Research for Development, comprising some 20 distinguished health scientists and politicians from developed and developing nations, issued a report and recommendations in 1990[25] calling for expanded research in developing countries on several well-defined priority problems as a new initiative aimed at enhancing the capacity of developing countries to solve their most pressing health problems. This Commission pointed out that the goal of Health for All is slipping out of our reach as the developing nations are beset by a daunting combination of problems, the double burden of old and new diseases, insufficient human and institutional capabilities to deal with these problems, the crippling burden of debt, and the near impossibility of developing cost-effective health services. In addition to the debt crisis, the problems include population growth (aggravated by the sluggish effort of developed nations to help establish effective family planning programs), pervasive poverty, displacement of rural subsistence populations by warfare, agrarian developments—a combination of difficulties that seem insurmountable.

HEALTH PROBLEMS OF INDUSTRIAL NATIONS

The preceding account could be misleading unless balanced by a brief summary of problems afflicting the industrial nations that, like those already described, are mainly manmade.[26] Industrial societies show signs of processes resembling the sequence that Durkheim called *anomie.* People do not know or care about neighbors, even blood relations, who sometimes are abandoned when they most need help. Young people numb their minds with addictive drugs, alcohol, and other substances. Children are reared increasingly often in homes with but a single parent. Life in the high-rise tenements of densely packed city slums offers the pablum of television but no constructive suggestions about ways to improve the human situation. Health and social problems sometimes are attributed vaguely to dissatisfaction with modern urban living; we seek solutions to substance abuse, vandalism, and mindless violence, but these are probably symptoms of deeper underlying social pathology.

We are looting the earth's nonrenewable resources without thought for generations that will come after us and leaving a trail of poisoned regions in our wake. These world health problems are as challenging and as difficult to deal with as the health problems of the third world. It is an indictment of our way of life when we do nothing about these health problems.

PROBLEM SOLVING IN THE DEVELOPING WORLD

Probably because the problems are tangible rather than a reflection of social values, progress towards solutions is sometimes faster and more convincing in developing nations than in industrial nations. There is much to inspire confidence and hope.

The Alma-Ata conference gave a focus to what had previously been somewhat aimless efforts. The Expanded Programme on Immunization and the oral rehydration program have achieved measurable results; the tropical disease research program, chasing seemingly will-o'-the-wisp goals such as vaccines against malaria and schistosomiasis, has achieved more than optimists could have hoped for a few years ago. Less glamorous but just as important, the underpinning of primary care services and health information systems in developing countries is beginning to work. Instrumental in this is the collaboration among WHO, other official agencies, and NGOs, which have responded to the challenge of meeting specific goals with finite deadlines.

Perhaps the most significant achievement has been the way the international agencies have shifted the emphasis of leadership to local communities, giving control over their own health affairs back to the people who will directly benefit, in contrast to preserving the traditional approach in which expatriate advisers, with varying degrees of paternalism, made all the decisions and implemented all the plans. A central feature of this reorientation of aims and methods has been the development of primary health care—a direct and explicit reaction to the "Health for All" initiatives. A few years ago, many developing countries had virtually no primary health care workers other than traditional healers; now increasingly there are battalions of rural health workers. Trained for a few months in first aid, health education, and elementary principles of personal preventive medicine, these health workers are concerned mainly with promoting better health and only secondarily with treatment of incidental illnesses and injuries that afflict the people in the villages where they work. Part of this approach is to upgrade the skills of traditional healers. A valuable form of development assistance that industrial nations can offer to the third world is to help with these training programs for primary health care workers.

Other priorities include promoting the concept of global interdependence, the recognition that actions of groups, communities, and nations in one part of the world affect those who live at a distance and ultimately react on all of us wherever we may live.

Another priority is to focus our attention on a few major problems, rather than attempting to deal superficially with a great many at once, including some of little consequence.[27] Programs that protect the lives of infants and children are the highest priorities.

CAREERS IN INTERNATIONAL HEALTH

The above discussion should convey an idea of what it takes to be an effective international health worker. The knowledge, skills, and attitudes that make a competent public health worker are all needed: knowledge and skills in infectious disease control, nutrition, population dynamics, environmental health, behavioral sciences, including an understanding of anthropology, and perhaps most important, methods of surveillance epidemiology. Some special surveillance methods include the ability to identify the situations where important diseases can flourish, for example, the existence of anopheline breeding sites. The ability to examine thick blood films for malaria parasites is also required. Other kinds of surveillance have been added, for example, the use of a simple tape measure to record upper arm circumference in growth monitoring programs as a clue to nutritional status. This is a skill that can easily be taught to village health workers so that enthusiastic assistants at the periphery reinforce the thin ranks of experts.

Managerial skills are equally important: without good organization, the service cannot be efficient. The international health worker's training must include attention to management and administration; evaluation is an integral part of this. It is useless to have plans unless there is provision for a method by which their success can be objectively evaluated.

International health attracts a special kind of health worker with unusual commitment and dedication to endure hard work, uncomfortable, even dangerous working conditions, and uncertain long-term career prospects. Health workers from industrially developed nations may be able to work for an international agency such as WHO or UNICEF, or through the aid programs sponsored by their own national government, or through a nongovernmental organization, missionary society, etc.

Although international health work may not include active clinical involvement, the health professional who undertakes work in a developing country without possessing good clinical skills is at hazard. It is essential to be able to demonstrate the qualities that accompany good clinical skills, high among which is a capacity for making swift—and correct—decisions. Emergencies may require wide-ranging ability, and it is likely that there will be occasions calling for the use of dental forceps, a spatula to remove foreign bodies from the eye, and the ability to recognize exanthemata and the peculiar odor of diphtheria. Outbreaks of disease must be recognised early and controlled effectively. The health worker who cannot cope with these everyday situations has little credibility when attempting to promote health and prevent disease.

REFERENCES

1. World Bank: World Development Report. New York: Oxford University Press, 1989
2. Brandt Commission: Reports, e.g. Common Crisis; North-South Cooperation for World Recovery. London: Pan Books, 1983
3. Fenner F, Henderson DA, Arita I, Jezek Z, Ladnyi ID: Smallpox and its Eradication. Geneva: WHO, 1988
4. The Work of WHO 1988–89: Biennial Report of the Director General. Geneva: WHO, 1990
5. World Health Organization: Global Estimates for Health Situation Assessment and Projections, 1990. Geneva: WHO/HST/90.2
6. World Health Organization: Evaluation of the strategy for health for all by the year 2000; Seventh Report of the world health situation (six volumes). Geneva: WHO, 1986
7. Primary Health Care. Geneva, New York: WHO and UNICEF, 1978
8. Targets for Health for All. Copenhagen: World Health Organization Regional Office for Europe, 1985
9. Healthy People; the Surgeon General's Report on health promotion and disease prevention. Washington, DC: USDHHS, 1979
10. United Nations: Our Common Future; the Report of the World Commission on Environment and Development (The Bruntland Report). Oxford, New York: Oxford University Press, 1988
11. McEvedy C, Jones R: Atlas of world population history. London: Allen Lane, Penguin Books, 1977
12. McKeown T, Record RG: Reasons for the decline in mortality in England and Wales during the nineteenth century. Population Studies 1962, 16:94–122, and subsequent exchanges
13. Taylor G: Environment, race and migration. Toronto: University of Toronto Press, 1949
14. UN Statistical Office: Population Estimates, 1988. New York: United Nations
15. The State of the World's Children. New York: Oxford University Press (annual reports of UNICEF)
16. UNICEF: State of the World's Children, 1990. New York: Oxford University Press, 1990
17. World Health Organization: Expanded Programme on Immunization. Status Report, 1990. Geneva: WHO, 1990
18. Women, health and development; a report by the Director General. WHO Offset Publication No. 90. Geneva: World Health Organization, 1985
19. de Koning H, Smith KR, Last JM: Biomass fuel combustion and health. Bull WHO 63:1:11–26, 1985
20. WHO/UNICEF Meeting on Infant and Young Child Feeding. WHO Chronicle 33:435–443, 1979
21. World Health Organization: Tobacco Alert. Geneva: WHO, 1990
22. Silverman M, Lee PR, Lydecker M: Prescriptions for death; the

drugging of the third world. Berkeley: University of California Press, 1982
23. Mejia A, Pizvrki H, Royston E: Physician and nurse migration; analysis and policy implications. Geneva: WHO, 1979
24. Sivard RL: World Military and Social Expenditures. Washington: World Priorities Inc., 1990
25. Commission on Health Research for Development: Report. New York: Oxford University Press, 1990
26. O'Neill PD: Health Crisis 2000. Copenhagen: WHO Regional Office for Europe, 1982
27. Walsh JA: Establishing health priorities in the developing world. New York: UNDP, 1988

71 Military Medicine

Llewellyn J. Legters
Craig H. Llewellyn

"Military medicine" is not a well-defined specialty and lacks a certifying board examination; however, armed forces physicians generally recognize that there is a body of knowledge peculiar to the medical problems and needs of military units and that this knowledge base is different from that required in ordinary medical practice. The latter, as accomplished in military settings, does not differ in any significant aspect from clinic or hospital practice in civilian communities, whereas military medicine deals with risk ("threat") assessment, prevention, and medical evacuation and clinical management of diseases and injuries resulting from military occupational exposures.

This is not to suggest that the environmental hazards to which military members may be exposed are completely unfamiliar in civilian occupations; rather, it is the manner and degree of the military occupational exposures that are unique. Thus, while civilian workers certainly may be at risk of hearing loss from exposure to noise, few are at risk of exposure to the high blast overpressures generated by artillery pieces and other explosive weapons.[1] Armored vehicle crewmen operating in the confined, sometimes poorly-ventilated spaces of their vehicles, may receive short, intermittent, high-level exposures to a variety of toxic gases, including carbon monoxide, from weapons firing and engine exhaust[2]—conditions of exposure seldom duplicated in any civilian occupation. Forces deployed in tropical third world countries may be exposed in nature to a variety of infectious diseases capable of producing catastrophic morbidity, such as malaria,[3] diarrhea,[4] hepatitis,[5] and leptospirosis,[6] to mention a few—diseases that only rarely produce morbidity in civilian work forces on a scale comparable to that frequently seen in military operations. To these examples, one may add exposures to very high altitudes, either in aircraft or mountainous terrain, various undersea environments, and extreme conditions of cold and heat. Finally, the injuries inflicted by modern conventional weapons, not to mention those capable of being produced by chemical, biological, and nuclear weapons, represent the hazards one usually thinks of as being associated with military service.

The military medicine specialist, then, besides having technical competence in general medicine, must have additional skills and knowledge in the specialty areas of preventive medicine, trauma management, behavioral sciences, environmental medicine, and tropical infectious diseases. Besides being able to move comfortably between fixed and field medical facilities and to provide quality medical care in both,[7] in combat units, the military physician sometimes must serve as staff "surgeon," providing medical recommendations to the military unit commander on matters concerning the health of the command.

At least three other categories of basic knowledge under the rubric Military Leadership and Management are essential to successful performance in this latter capacity, namely, knowledge of operational environments, military operations, and military organizational structure. A similar knowledge base is required in civilian occupational medicine practice, albeit one peculiar to the industry being served. On several counts, then, one might argue that military medicine is a unique brand of occupational medicine, one that deals with the prevention and treatment of diseases and injuries resulting from work in military occupations and military operational environments.

MISSION OF SERVICE MEDICAL DEPARTMENTS

The military medical system has two major missions within the Department of Defense (DoD): (1) maintenance of medical readiness and (2) provision of health care to eligible beneficiaries. The medical readiness mission includes delivery of preventive and curative services to active duty military populations and maintenance of the capability to provide medical support of U.S. forces during contingency deployments and combat operations anywhere in the world. The delivery of health care to other eligible beneficiaries besides active duty personnel, that is, dependents of active duty personnel and military retirees and their dependents, is accomplished in military medical facilities, as space, medical staff, and time permit, or is purchased from civilian sources through the Civilian Health and Medical Program of the Uniformed Services (CHAMPUS), which is a reimbursement program similar to civilian health insurance.

The readiness mission has two principal objectives: (1) in peacetime to maintain military forces "fit to fight" and (2) in combat to "conserve the fighting strength," through countermeasures directed at the prevention of disease and injury and through treatment at the lowest possible echelon of care, with a view toward rapid return to duty of sick or injured individuals. Attainment of these objectives requires special medical organizations able to accompany and support military units as they carry out their missions and special military and medical training for medical personnel.

The second mission, the provision of health care to eligible beneficiaries, was mandated in the Congressional Health Benefit Act of 1966.[8] Beneficiary care has represented the major demand on the military health care system since World War II. At present, the care provided to eligible beneficiaries other than active duty personnel comprises approximately 70% of the daily military medical system workload.[9] The medical practice involved in carrying out this latter mission is virtually indistinguishable from general civilian outpatient and inpatient medicine.

Paradoxically, the workloads engendered by the medical readiness mission and the active duty medical care requirement (30% of the daily workload) are the primary criteria used by the DoD and Congress to determine size and composition of the Medical Corps, medical facilities, and training programs. This paradox is complicated by rapid shifts in policy, which may from time to time direct that more Medical Corps personnel be deployed to support operational forces, while simultaneously directing that more eligible beneficiaries be treated in military medical facilities. Analysts have observed that except for World War II, the military medical system has never had resources adequate to successfully accomplish both missions. This produces programmatic competition and enormously complicates the resource allocation task of system managers.

SCOPE OF MEDICAL SERVICES AND ACTIVITIES

The U.S. military medical system is one of the largest in the world, with a $10 billion a year budget, providing health care to more than 10 million eligible beneficiaries (21% of whom are active duty military personnel) in 168 hospitals and 936 clinics and dispensaries around the world. The system employs more than 170,000 doctors, dentists, nurses, and support personnel, who manage nearly 1 million inpatient admissions and nearly 50 million outpatient visits per year. Table 71-1 shows the medical workload by category of beneficiary. The entire spectrum of care, from routine outpatient services to highly sophisticated subspecialty tertiary care, is available within a global system, which is linked by a medical evacuation system.[10]

TABLE 71-1. DOD MEDICAL WORKLOAD, FY 1985[9,10]

	Outpatient Visits	Beds Occupied (Daily Average)	Admissions Worldwide
Active duty	18,460,524 (37.9%)	21,516 (36.7%)	283,976 (29.5%)
Retired	4,596,094 (9.4%)	9,765 (16.7%)	114,945 (11.9%)
Active duty dependent	16,580,578 (34%)	16,810 (28.7%)	412,312 (42.8%)
Retired dependent	5,876,412 (12.1%)	8,263 (14.1%)	118,390 (12.3%)
Other*	3,169,445 (6.5%)	2,153 (3.7%)	32,727 (3.4%)
Total	48,703,053	58,507	962,350

*Includes Public Health Service, Coast Guard, and National Oceanic and Atmospheric Administration.

The focus of the peacetime military medical system is the military communities in the United States and abroad, which are the support bases for various military units. These bases provide dependent housing, schools, stores, and recreational resources very similar to those found in civilian communities, along with a similar mixture of medical, dental, preventive medicine, and public health services. Within the military units at these bases, one finds the so-called "organic" medical elements belonging to the units, which provide primary care and preventive medicine support to unit personnel. These elements of the field medical system are organizationally separate from the community-based military health care system but in practice frequently provide personnel augmentation to the military community hospitals.

When military units deploy from their bases for exercises or war, the organic medical elements accompany them and are augmented by additional field medical units: medical companies and battalions, preventive medicine detachments, field laboratories, and a mixture of field hospitals such as mobile surgical hospitals, evacuation hospitals, and combat support hospitals. All of these are mobile, enabling them to accompany the units they support in deployments around the globe. Since most of these units are far below required personnel strength before deployment, they are brought up to strength by personnel taken from the fixed facility, community-based hospital system. The community-based hospital system must continue to carry on its normal function, while also preparing to accept casualties from the deployed units and to support recently mobilized Reserve and National Guard units assigned to the base. Active duty military medical forces are insufficient to meet both the base and field medical support requirements. Reserve medical forces are expected to provide 60% to 70% of military medical personnel required in wartime[11]; however, activation of Reserve forces would require a Presidential Order.

Dental Activities

Dental care is provided to active duty personnel through a system of military community-based dental activities and field dental units that parallels the medical care system. The full spectrum of services, including preventive dentistry and dental specialty care, is available to active duty personnel. Dental fitness of military personnel has a high priority in maintaining a force "fit to fight." Field dental units and detachments are separate from this system and must also be prepared to accompany deployed troops.

Preventive Medicine

> A corps of Medical Officers was not established solely for the purpose of attending the wounded and sick; the proper treatment of these sufferers is certainly a matter of very great importance, and is an imperative duty, but the labors of Medical Officers cover a more extended field. The *leading idea,* which should be constantly kept in view, is to strengthen the hands of the Commanding General by keeping his army in the most vigorous health, thus rendering it, in the highest degree, efficient for enduring fatigue and privation and for fighting. (Dr. Jonathan Letterman, Surgeon, Army of the Potomac, 1862–1864.)[12]

Preventive medicine programs for military units and personnel are designed to preserve and promote health and to prevent physical and mental diseases and disabilities. Knowledge of the environment in which these programs are to be applied is essential in order to recognize situations that require modifications to civilian preventive medicine practice or that represent unique hazards. Most importantly, military preventive medicine officers must serve as advisors to military commanders, upon whom rests final responsibility for the health of their commands. Through the performance of its advisory, inspectorial, and regulatory duties, military preventive medicine is concerned with the administration of the whole force. In military units the scope of preventive medicine responsibility and authority exceeds that of all other medical specialties.

Military preventive medicine incorporates all the subspecialty areas of preventive medicine and public health: general preventive medicine, aviation medicine, undersea medicine, occupational medicine, community health nursing, sanitary engineering, environmental science, entomology, parasitology, and veterinary medicine. Preventive medicine activities are found in all military units and communities. Regulations require each company-size Army unit (150 to 200 men) engaged in field operations to have a field sanitation team. From this "grass roots" level through higher command echelons, preventive medicine personnel are assigned as staff advisors to commanders on matters relating to the health and welfare of their personnel. Also available to assist commanders are special resources, such as epidemiology and environmental sanitation detachments and teams, and regional resources, such as area laboratories (e.g., the Navy environmental and preventive medicine units), and highly sophisticated, centrally directed technical assistance organizations (e.g., the Army epidemiologic consultation service of Walter Reed Army Institute of Research and the U.S. Army Environmental Hygiene Agency at Edgewood Arsenal, Maryland). Because of the extraordinary variety of industrial operations found in military units and support activities, occupational medicine and industrial hygiene represent major areas of military preventive medicine activity.

Health Promotion

The impetus for development of health promotion programs in the U.S. armed forces, as in the civilian sector, derives from the recognition that health risks are not entirely work related and that failure to take measures directed at risk reduction outside the work environment represents poor stewardship of the organization's training investment. In civilian industry the determination of whether an illness or injury is work related depends on whether the exposure or the accident occurred at work. In contrast, in the U.S. military, servicemen are considered to be on duty 24 hours a day; the only question that must be addressed in determining if an illness or injury is service connected is whether it resulted from the individual's misconduct. Philosophically then, even though the services obviously do not exercise 24-hour control over their members, tacitly they do assume 24-hour responsibility for a member's welfare. Moreover, as noted elsewhere in this chapter, the services maintain complete "company towns" around the world, in which the military provides virtually total support. Such communities, isolated and self-sufficient as they are in many cases, offer excellent opportunities to establish effective programs of health education and health promotion.

This is not to say that the U.S. armed services have pioneered in this area, because in fact the emphasis on health promotion is relatively recent. Contrast, for example, policies that endorsed the inclusion of cigarettes in combat rations until well after the Korean War with those that now forbid smoking at all in Army basic combat training.

The Army Health Promotion Program, called Fit To Win, involves a wide range of activities aimed at "enhancing the quality of life of soldiers, Army civilians, family members and retirees; and encouraging lifestyles to improve and protect physical, emotional, and spiritual health."[13] Components include an antitobacco program, physical conditioning, weight control, nutrition, stress management, alcohol and drug abuse prevention and control, early identification of hypertension, suicide prevention, spiritual fitness, and oral health. The overall program goal is to maximize readiness, combat efficiency, and work performance. The program is command directed, meaning that it is not exclusively a medical program; at the installation level the installation commander himself chairs a health promotion council. The installation "surgeon" is a principal advisor to the commander on health promotion matters, but program implementation involves the coordinated efforts of a large number of nonmedical staff. The linkage being made in the Army program between health promotion and the capacity of individual soldiers to accomplish the readiness mission (Fit To Fight), over time, should result in institutionalization of wellness behaviors as the cultural norm.

Veterinary Activities

The veterinary medical services focus on food inspection services, handling and storage of food and rations, veterinary care of government-owned animals, and the prevention of endemic zoonotic diseases. By interactions with logistics, engineer, transportation, and quartermaster officers, veterinarians play a pivotal role in protecting military personnel from diseases transmitted through food.

Medical Staff Advice to Line Commanders

By congressional statute the military commander is responsible for the health of his command. A command surgeon serves as his medical staff advisor. The military physician, in the role as staff surgeon, is responsible for participating in the development of all command plans and policies, advising the commander on relevant medical issues, and working with other staff officers to insure medical support of both garrison and field operations.

This essential relationship between the commander and the command surgeon has been recognized since the American Revolution. As Dr. Benjamin Rush wrote in 1798 to the physician general of the United States:

> I admit with General Washington in a letter to President Adams that the physician general of an army should be one of the limbs of a commander in chief. He should reside in his family. No order for marching, encamping, eating, drinking or even fighting (as far as it relates to the time of a battle) should be issued without his knowledge and concurrence.[14]

Thus, as a unit surgeon, the military physician must understand military operations, military staff planning and administrative processes, the enormously varied military work environments, and the natural and manmade hazards that military personnel may encounter. The military physician must be proficient in medical planning and the employment of the various elements of the field medical system. As the medical advisor to a base or camp commander, the military physician must be able to oversee the medical activities required to support the military community, such as schools, recreational facilities, eating establishments, crisis action, and immunization programs. Interaction is required with the post engineer, safety officer, quartermaster, provost marshall, quartermaster and commissary activities, DoD school principals, and neighboring civilian community medical and public health authorities.

Medical Education and Training

Schools of military medicine were established in Russia and Prussia during the eighteenth century and in England after the

Crimean War in 1860. In 1893 the U.S. Army Medical School, the first school of preventive medicine in the United States, was established in Washington, D.C., by the surgeon general, George Miller Sternberg, who was an internationally known microbiologist. At present more than 70 countries have schools of military medicine.

Medical education and training programs in the United States armed forces include entry level training of corpsmen and technicians and extend across the spectrum of undergraduate medical education (through the Health Professions Scholarship Program and the Uniformed Services University of the Health Sciences [USUHS] School of Medicine) and graduate medical education, including residency and fellowship training in most specialties and subspecialties.

The U.S. military establishment operates the largest training system for medical support personnel in the United States. Courses cover the complete array of paraprofessional medical fields (laboratory, x-ray, operating room, preventive medicine) and military-unique areas, such as combat medical technician, navy independent duty corpsman, and aviation medical technician. As noted, the needs of both the community-based medical system and the field medical system, in many cases, must be met by the same personnel, who will transfer from one system to the other in times of deployment or hostilities. Attainment of these different training objectives and the maintenance of proficiency in both spheres of activity is a daunting task.

Medical Research and Development

Military medical research is conducted in both the community-based and field medical care systems. Clinical research programs are conducted in military community hospitals and the tertiary care medical centers and generally focus on the same issues as clinical research programs in civilian institutions. These programs are centrally supervised, reviewed, and funded.

Field and operational medical problems are addressed by the medical research and development establishments of each of the military services and generally target issues specific to the particular service. These mission-oriented research programs are organized in four general research areas: (1) infectious and tropical diseases, (2) combat casualty care, (3) health hazards of military systems and operations, and (4) medical defense against nuclear, biological, and chemical weapons.

Military medical research traditionally has focused on the prevention and control of epidemic and endemic diseases in troops. Throughout military history, these problems have been the greatest cause of military noneffectiveness and medical workload. From the work of Walter Reed on typhoid fever and yellow fever, through more recent programs directed at development of malaria chemoprophylactic drugs and vaccines, HIV infection and AIDS (for example), military medical research has made significant contributions to the understanding and control of a wide range of infectious diseases.

As new weapons systems have begun to exceed the boundaries of human tolerance and performance, and as new materials have been introduced that present unknown toxic risks, the study of health hazards posed by the equipment and materials that troops use has become increasingly important. New weapons and their effects require studies on prevention and treatment of resulting injuries. Equally important is the need to adapt emerging diagnostic and therapeutic technology to combat casualty care under austere battlefield conditions. The nuclear, biological, and chemical weapons threat must be understood in order to provide for prophylaxis, diagnosis, and treatment. Effective medical protection against chemical agents would greatly reduce their potential for use during hostilities and assist in forcing treaty agreements for their reduction or elimination.

MILITARY MEDICAL SYSTEM ORGANIZATION AND MANAGEMENT

The DoD and the component military services (Army, Navy, and Air Force) each have civilian political appointees as service secretaries and a military staff that is subordinate to them. The military medical system likewise follows this model.

The assistant secretary of defense for health affairs (ASD [HA]) is the highest level of medical systems management within the DoD. The ASD(HA), a civilian political appointee, is supported by a staff of military personnel from each of the three military services and career civil servants. He has advisory, planning, and supervisory responsibilities for the medical readiness and health care missions carried out by the three military service medical departments.[15] In addition, the ASD(HA) chairs the Defense Health Council, composed of the surgeons general of the Army, Navy, Air Force, and Public Health Service; the medical director of the Veterans Administration; the president of the Uniformed Services University of the Health Sciences; the assistant secretaries for personnel of the Army, Navy, and Air Force; and a representative from the Office of the Joint Chiefs of Staff. This forum provides the highest level of medical policy and program development, review, and coordination among the separate military services, the Department of Defense, the Department of Health and Human Services, and the Veterans Administration.

The Office of the Joint Chiefs of Staff also has triservice medical representation in the logistics (J-4) section. This group provides medical advice to the Joint Chiefs in its function of policy development for mobilization and strategic planning support.

The Army, Navy, and Air Force medical departments are organized in consonance with the component services they support. Each military service is under the control of a civilian secretary. The senior military officer in each service (chief of staff, Army; chief of naval operations; chief of staff, Air Force) has a surgeon general on his staff. The surgeons general have authorities and responsibilities defined by congressional statute to provide medical support within their respective services. Under their supervision, medical command structures, organized regionally, geographically, or by major command, operate the fixed facility, community-based medical care system in the continental United States. Figure 71-1 depicts these relationships.

Triservice coordination for mutual support in the provision of medical care is accomplished regionally in order to maximize access to medical care for all personnel regardless of their service. Thus, patients from each military service may receive medical care in the regional medical centers and the military community hospitals. In some areas, regional medical centers are jointly staffed and operated. Beneficiary care is often provided through civilian contract outpatient clinics or by contract physicians working in military medical facilities. A recent initiative, the CHAMPUS (Civilian Health and Medical Program Uniformed Services) Reform Program, involves contracting with civilian for-profit medical organizations to provide medical care for eligible beneficiaries along the lines of the Health Maintenance Organization (HMO) model in an attempt to reduce costs and improve access to care.

As noted above, the field medical system is separate from the fixed facility, community-based system and is generally only partially staffed. When deployed for operations, field medical units must be substantially augmented with officers and enlisted personnel drawn from the community-based system, impacting negatively on the latter's capability to provide care. In addition, since these "filler" personnel have full-time clinical jobs, it is extremely difficult to free them for the recurrent training required to develop and maintain proficiency in the field medical system.

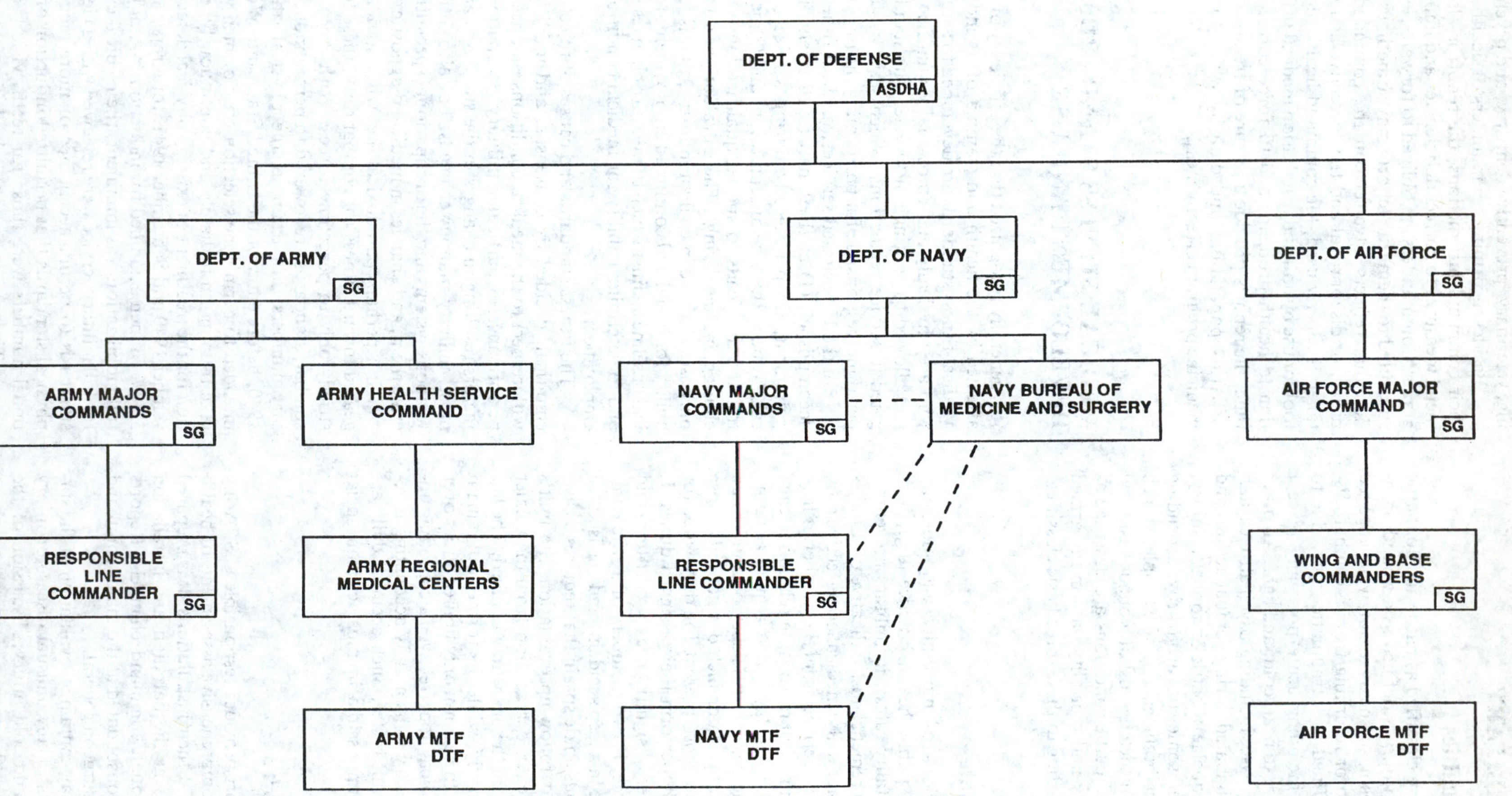

Figure 71–1. Peacetime Organization of Military Health Care System in the United States. ASD(HA), assistant secretary of defense for health affairs. SG, surgeon general, staff medical advisor. MTF, medical treatment facility: hospital, dispensary, clinic. DTF, dental treatment facility. – –, technical support responsibility. ——, command responsibility.

HEALTH STATUS MEASURES UNIQUE TO THE MILITARY

Classes of Military Casualties

Casualties in military units are classified as battle and nonbattle injuries, and disease. Battle injury is defined as a wound or injury incurred as the direct result of enemy action while engaged in combat, or while going to or returning from a combat mission; nonbattle injury is defined as a traumatic injury due to causes other than combat, including acute poisoning (except food poisoning), and exposure to heat, cold, and light. All other casualties are classified as disease, including psychiatric casualties (even if the condition originated during combat action) and patients readmitted for the sequelae of battle or nonbattle injury. Some conditions are classified somewhat arbitrarily, depending on the circumstances of their occurrence. For example, trench foot and accidental and self-inflicted gunshot wounds sustained either in combat or under nonbattle conditions are classified as nonbattle injuries. Morbidity and mortality data in the armed services are maintained according to these three basic classifications.[16]

Medical Noneffective Rate

In addition to the expressions of morbidity and mortality customarily used in civilian public health practice (e.g., incidence, prevalence, and mortality rates), in military preventive medicine practice, the measurement most indicative of a unit's true health status is the (average daily) medical noneffective rate. This is a point prevalence ratio derived from the number of men not present for *full* duty for medical reasons, in relation to each 1000 men assigned to the unit per day.[16] It is a more accurate measure of disability and the combat efficiency of a unit than any other rate, because the numerator includes not only those admitted to hospital but also those present for duty who, for medical reasons, cannot fully perform their assigned duties. It attaches an appropriate degree of significance to short-term and partial disability. For example, if two members of a rifle company on the Korean DMZ are in a jeep accident, and one is killed and the other sustains a serious ankle sprain that requires a cast, crutches, physiotherapy, and follow-up evaluation, the unit's combat efficiency suffers greater degradation from the soldier with the ankle injury than from the one who was killed. The latter will be replaced fairly quickly, while the former will remain with the unit but may be able to perform only limited duties over an extended period. The medical noneffective rate also has unusual precision, since in military units a daily accounting is required of each man on the unit roster. Such accurate daily accounting is impractical or impossible in most civilian social organizations.

Command Health Report[17]

The Command Health Report provides responsible U.S. Army commanders with periodic comprehensive assessments of health conditions in their units and at their installations. It is prepared monthly by medical officers at the battalion and installation level and is transmitted through command channels. Reports from subordinate units are consolidated at the major command level for transmission to the surgeon general.

Any particular report may contain an evaluation of the status of troop hygiene; reports of any unusual disease or injury occurrence, including heat and cold injury; discussion of the installation's occupational health program; information about environmental sanitation problems, including any that involve the water supply, liquid and solid waste disposal, insect and rodent control, housing, and food service; observations on troop nutritional status; and information about the community nursing, veterinary, preventive dentistry, and psychiatry programs.

Besides informing commanders of health conditions within their command jurisdictions, the report is also used to recommend measures to correct deficiencies and improve existing programs. Commanders are obliged to forward reports as originally submitted to them (the reports may sometimes contain information that reflects adversely on the command), indicating approval or disapproval and the corrective actions that are being taken. Properly used, the command health report is a powerful tool for use by unit and installation medical officers to call attention to health problems and to force corrective actions. Over time, the reports provide a picture of trends in the health status of Army populations and data by which to assess preventive medicine program effectiveness.

MEDICAL FITNESS STANDARDS: DEVELOPMENT AND USE

It is generally recognized that the efficiency of an armed force is affected by the health and stamina of its individual members. Medical fitness standards are developed to assure that only those who are physically and emotionally qualified are accepted for and allowed to continue in service. The standards are promulgated in service regulations, which serve as guides for medical personnel responsible for performing the physical evaluations.

In the U.S. armed services, medical fitness evaluations are accomplished (1) at the time of enlistment, induction, or appointment, (2) periodically during service ("retention physicals") and at the time of separation, and (3) before admission to training that leads to special qualifications (e.g., flying, parachuting, marine diving). These evaluations serve much the same purposes as those in civilian industry, that is, to determine suitability for initial and continued employment, to establish a medical baseline against which to measure changes in physical status, and to determine liability for medical conditions resulting from employment.

The fitness standards and causes of rejection for service are empirical, decided by consensus, and modified by experience with respect to the medical conditions that preclude satisfactory performance in particular military occupations. The principal factors resulting in changes in the standards are, first and foremost, military manpower needs, but also introduction of new weapons systems and the occupational specialties required to operate them, and changes in medical diagnostic technology.

It is perhaps paradoxical that while standards generally are geared toward fitness for combat duty, these tend to be applied strictly only to peacetime forces. With the outbreak of actual combat, standards are lowered to permit induction of the necessary numbers. For example, the physical standards in use in 1940, before entry of the United States into World War II, were intended to permit the selection only of men who could undertake training immediately and continuously, without interruption for the treatment of existing physical defects.[18] Between November 1940 and September 1941, total rejections ran as high as 52.8% of men examined for induction.[19] As it became clear that full mobilization was imminent, the medical causes of rejection for full military service were reviewed with a view to lowering the standards to permit acceptance of more men. The changes in physical standards that permitted induction of the largest additional numbers were those for teeth, vision, and venereal diseases.[20] The present Army standards[21] are not markedly different from those in use at the end of World War II. These apparently have adequately served the needs of the armed services in the procurement of required numbers of physically qualified men and women since World War II, during periods of both universal conscription and voluntary service.

SPECIAL DISEASE PROBLEMS IN RECRUIT CAMPS

The high incidence of respiratory-borne diseases among recruits in military training camps has been widely reported. This phenomenon is the result of person-to-person spread of a number of viral and bacterial agents among susceptibles assembled under barracks living conditions that permit frequent close contact. Historically, the respiratory-borne diseases of primary importance in military recruit camps have included acute respiratory diseases due to adenoviruses types 4 and 7,[22] meningococcal disease,[23,24] and streptococcal disease.[16] The advent and use in recent years of specific vaccines effective against the predominant adenovirus types and meningococcal serogroups, and of specific antibiotic prophylaxis in circumstances of high streptococcal disease incidence have yielded remarkable reductions in medical noneffectiveness from these causes.

Acute Respiratory Disease (ARD)

During the years of World War II, 1942–1945, the so-called "common respiratory diseases" and influenza accounted for over 4 million admissions to hospital and quarters in the U.S. Army alone, which represented 22% of admissions for all causes.[16,22] Epidemics of ARD occurred during the winter months in recruits but not in "seasoned" troops, and disease appeared to confer immunity.[25,26] In the early 1950s, viruses originally recovered from human adenoidal tissues by Rowe et al.[27] were subsequently isolated from the throat washings of patients with ARD during a 1953 epidemic of acute respiratory disease among recruits at Fort Leonard Wood, Missouri.[28,29] These viruses were etiologically related to those causing ARD among recruits at Fort Bragg in the 1940s.[30] In many subsequent studies it has been amply demonstrated that adenovirus types 4 and 7 are the principal causes of ARD among U.S. military recruits, although types 3 and 21 have been implicated very occasionally.[22,31,32]

Before effective vaccines became available, the impact of ARD on recruits and the basic training program was considerable. Table 71-2 shows the incidence of ARD in one carefully studied platoon of recruits at Fort Dix, New Jersey, in the winter of 1965, which was a typical incidence pattern at northern training posts in the winter. Nineteen of the 24 severe cases and 7 of 13 mild febrile cases were due to type 4 adenovirus; 24 (50%) of the 48 soldiers in the platoon were incapacitated and required hospitalization. Most of the illnesses and admissions occurred during the first 3 weeks of training. The loss of 50% of the men necessitated establishment of an additional training program by the cadre, and in some cases, the "recycling" of hospitalized trainees to make up for lost training time.[33]

Adenovirus type 4 and 7 vaccines both are currently administered to Army, Navy, and Marine recruits as soon as possible after arrival at basic training posts.[34] No other adenoviruses appear to have emerged to replace adenoviruses 4 and 7 as major causes of ARD in immunized recruits.

Meningococcal Disease

Outbreaks of meningococcal disease have invariably accompanied periods of mobilization. World War II was associated with a severe outbreak of meningococcal disease in both U.S. civilian and military populations. From July 1941 to June 1943, of over 5000 cases recorded, 67% occurred among recruits who had been in the service for 3 months or less.[16]

World War II ushered in the use of sulfadiazine as prophylaxis to control dissemination of meningococci under conditions of troop crowding and during outbreaks,[35,36] and sulfadiazine prophylaxis continued to be used successfully to abort meningococcal disease outbreaks among recruits until early 1963. At that time the drug failed to control outbreaks at both San Diego Naval Training Center[37] and Fort Ord, California.[23] (Table 71-3).

Since the 1960s, localized outbreaks in recruit camps have been due predominantly to serogroups B,[23] C,[24] and Y,[38] though in World War II, 91% of isolates from military cases were Group A.[39] The emergence of sulfadiazine-resistant meningococci led to the successful development, at Walter Reed Army Institute of Research, of polysaccharide vaccines effective against various meningococcal serogroups, first, group C, and subsequently, groups A, Y, and W-135. The polyvalent vaccine containing antigens from these four serogroups is administered to U.S. recruits in all the services within the first 3 days of arrival at the training centers.[34]

Other environmental and administrative measures that have been more or less continuously employed at training camps to control ARD as well as meningococcal disease include a "liberal admissions policy" for recruits, permitting the early diagnosis and treatment of cases of meningococcal disease,[24] and the reduction of crowding and the provision of adequate ventilation of living and sleeping quarters.[40]

Hemolytic Streptococcal Infections

Before World War II, disease caused by the hemolytic streptococci was not recognized as an important military problem. During World War II, from 1942 to 1945, 29,512 cases of scarlet fever and 18,339 cases of rheumatic fever were reported in the U.S. Army.[16] During the same period, 59,448 cases of scarlet fever and 21,209 cases of rheumatic fever, plus 14,150 cases of

TABLE 71-2. INCIDENCE OF ACUTE RESPIRATORY DISEASE CLASSIFIED AS TO CLINICAL SEVERITY IN A PLATOON OF RECRUITS AT FORT DIX, N.J., BY WEEK OF BASIC TRAINING[33]

	Week of Basic Training									
Illness	**0**	**1**	**2**	**3**	**4**	**5**	**6**	**7**	**8**	**Total**
Total strength	48	48	48	48	46	41	40	39	39	
Afebrile URI[a]	10	16	13	11	1	0	0	0	0	51
Mild febrile	0	6	3	3	2	0	0	1	1	17
Severe febrile	1	1	17	13	0	0	0	0	0	24
Total	11	23	23	27	3	3	0	1	1	92
Admitted to hospital	0	3	7	11	0	2	0	1	0	24

[a] Upper respiratory infection

TABLE 71-3. INCIDENCE OF MENINGOCOCCAL DISEASE AT FORT ORD, CALIF., 1962–1963, BY WEEK OF TRAINING[23]

Week	Cases: Number	Cases: Percent
▪ **Basic Training**		
0	0	
1	5	5.4
2	12	12.9
3	20	21.5
4	10	10.8
5	11	11.8
6	11	11.8
7	11	11.8
8	9	9.7
▪ **Advanced Training**		
9	0	
10	0	
11	1	1.1
12	1	1.1
13	0	
14	1	1.1
15	0	
16	0	
Cadre	1	1.1
Total	93	100.0

acute arthritis which may have been acute rheumatic fever, were reported in the U.S. Navy.[41]

As with ARD and meningococcal disease, the highest rates of streptococcal disease were recorded in recruit camps in the northern United States.[16] High streptococcal disease rates were also recorded among "seasoned" troops when such personnel were brought together in geographic regions of high incidence[42]; even so, the limited data available suggest that under similar conditions of exposure, new recruits were far more susceptible to infection than seasoned troops.[16]

Since approximately 1959, benzathine penicillin G (BPG), usually administered in a single dose at the beginning of recruit training, has been the primary method used to control streptococcal pharyngitis outbreaks in Navy and Marine training centers. In 1979, prompted by a marked decline in the incidence of acute rheumatic fever among recruits, year-round BPG prophylaxis was discontinued. However, the recent resurgence of streptococcal disease at some Navy and Marine recruit centers has resulted in reinstitution of either year-round or seasonal BPG prophylaxis, depending on the experience at each installation.[43] Recent outbreaks (1988) of streptococcal disease followed by cases of acute rheumatic fever at the Navy Training Center, San Diego, and the Army basic training center at Fort Leonard Wood, Missouri, demonstrate that streptococcal disease remains a significant military medicine problem and underscore the need for surveillance programs that will rapidly detect increases in streptococcal disease incidence at installations where BPG prophylaxis is not routinely used.[44]

IMMUNIZATION PROGRAMS

Immunizations represent a direct and specific approach to disease prevention and control in the armed services. In military settings, effective vaccines are among the most efficient means of disease prevention, because in contrast to environmental controls and other individual preventive measures (e.g., antimalarial drugs and the application of insect repellants to prevent malaria), their use requires no conscious effort by the individuals in whom protection is sought.

General Policies and Practices[34]

Immunization policies and guidelines are established for the respective services by the surgeons general of the Army, Navy (for the Navy and Marine Corps), and Air Force and the chief, Coast Guard Office of Health Services. With some exceptions, vaccine schedules and dosages for armed services personnel follow the recommendations of the Advisory Committee on Immunization Practices (ACIP) of the U.S. Public Health Service; however, the surgeons general have authority to mandate administration of additional unlicensed vaccines to armed services personnel in national emergencies and under special operational conditions (see below). Vaccines administered under such circumstances must be approved by the appropriate armed services Investigational Drug Review Board.

Immunizations prescribed by the surgeons general are mandatory for armed services personnel; exceptions are granted only for documented allergies to specific vaccines and for religious objections. Exceptions granted for religious reasons may be revoked if the disease risk posed by failure to immunize is judged to threaten military mission accomplishment. If necessary, immunizations can be forcibly administered. These policies ensure high rates of compliance with immunization requirements, and they have been especially effective in preventing significant outbreaks of the various vaccine-preventable respiratory-borne diseases commonly experienced in recruit camps before specific vaccines became available (see Special Disease Problems in Recruit Camps above).

Immunizations recommended by the ACIP are also provided by the medical services of the armed forces to dependents of military personnel, including immunizations required for overseas travel and attendance at school and day-care centers. Federal civilian employees are offered free services for immunizations required for overseas travel and to prevent diseases to which they may be occupationally exposed (e.g., hepatitis B among health care workers). Such services include annual administration of the influenza vaccine.

History of Armed Services Immunization Program

The routine use of smallpox vaccine among American military personnel antedates the use of any other and is said to have begun during the Revolutionary War.[45] This was followed by typhoid-paratyphoid vaccine in 1911 and tetanus toxoid in 1941. During World War II these three vaccines became known for administrative purposes as the "routine immunizations."[46]

In January 1941, yellow fever vaccine was made mandatory for military personnel stationed in the tropical regions of the western hemisphere. An epidemic of over 50,000 cases of jaundice resulted from administration of certain vaccine lots[46,47] and is now known to have been due to hepatitis B virus contaminating the human serum used to stabilize the vaccine.

Additional vaccines developed or placed in limited use during World War II included cholera, plague, typhus, influenza, and Japanese (B) encephalitis.[46] The current armed forces immunization program has been built on this World War II foundation.

Current Immunization Requirements[34]

Table 71-4 shows present mandatory immunizations for military personnel by service and the circumstances of their required ad-

TABLE 71-4. IMMUNIZATION REQUIREMENTS FOR MILITARY PERSONNEL[40]

Immunizing Agent	Army	Navy	Air Force	Marine Corps	Coast Guard
Adenovirus types 4 and 7	B	B	B	B	H
Cholera	F	F	F	F	F
Hepatitis B	E,G,H	E,G,H	E,G,H	E,G,H	G,H
Influenza	A,B,X	A,B,R	A,B,R	A,B,R	B,C,H
Measles	B,G	B,G	B,G	B,G	B,G
Meningococcal (A,C,Y,W135)	B,H	B,H	B,H	B,H	B,H
Mumps	G,H	G,H	G,H	G,H	G
Plague	C,D,E,G	D,G	E	A,G	E
Polio	A,R	A,R	A,R	A,R	A
Rabies	D,G,H	D,G,H	D,G,H	D,G,H	H
Rubella	B,G	B,G	B,G	B,G	B
Smallpox	B,H	B,H	B,H	B,H	B,H
Tetanus-diphtheria	A,B,R	A,B,R	A,B,R	A,B,R	A,B
Typhoid	C,E,H	H	C,E,H	H	E
Yellow fever	C,D,E	A,R	C,E	A,R	B,E

A, all active duty personnel. B, recruits. C, alert forces. D, special operating forces components. E, when deploying or traveling to high risk areas. F, only when required by host country for entry. G, high risk occupational groups. H, as directed by the applicable surgeon general; Commander, NAVMEDCOM; or Chief, Coast Guard Office of Health Services. R, reserve components. X, reserve component personnel on active duty for 30 days or more during the influenza season.

ministration. For practical purposes, vaccine dosages are as recommended by the ACIP and contained in the USPHS publication *Health Information for International Travel.*[48]

Vaccines are administered to recruits for three main purposes:

1. To prevent epidemics of respiratory-borne diseases during recruit training (adenovirus, influenza, measles,* meningococcal disease, and rubella*)
2. To boost antibody titers against disease agents for which recruits may have been fully or partially immunized earlier (measles,* polio, rubella,* tetanus-diphtheria)
3. To initiate a primary vaccine series in recruits who lack a reliable history of previous immunizations (tetanus-diphtheria)

Smallpox vaccine is also administered to new inductees, but to avoid the risk of vaccine in unimmunized contacts, it is given only in situations where contact with unvaccinated individuals can be avoided for at least 2 weeks after vaccination. The requirement for smallpox vaccination is based on the presumption that smallpox virus represents a potential, highly effective biological warfare agent and that the best insurance against its use by an opposing force is "herd" immunity in one's own.

The various immunizations remaining after initial induction and training are administered primarily to prevent specific diseases in military units and personnel deployed or travelling in overseas areas and in individuals at high risk of occupational exposure. Forces with the potential for rapid commitment anywhere in the world (Army Alert Forces and Marines) and units with predesignated missions in geographic areas where there is a known high risk of exposure to specific diseases, such as plague, typhoid, and yellow fever, are required to maintain high levels of immunity against these diseases continuously among assigned personnel. In addition, several special vaccines still in an investigational new drug status are available and could be authorized for use by the surgeons general in deployments to geographic areas where surveillance indicates a high risk of transmission. Such vaccines include Rift Valley fever, Q fever, Venezuelan equine encephalitis, and Japanese encephalitis.

**Female personnel are tested for pregnancy and rubella antibody, and measles antibody if a CDC-approved test is used; nonpregnant susceptible females are immunized selectively based on test results.*

FIELD AND COMBAT OPERATIONS

Mission

The mission of the armed forces is to carry out national policy by maintaining the ability to use or, on direction, by using the force of arms. In this context the mission of the medical elements supporting the combat forces is fourfold:

1. To prepare for deployments through the conduct of individual and unit training programs
2. To provide primary medical care, resuscitation, initial surgery, and evacuation
3. To maintain disease and injury surveillance
4. To carry out programs directed at primary and secondary disease and injury prevention in supported units

Organization

The field medical units are organized to support the tactical military forces in the theater of operations. The echelons of medical support, that is, in the battalion, division, and corps support areas, and the communications zone (COMMZ), extend rearward from the forward edge of the battle area, through the COMMZ, in an integrated and continuous system to the zone of interior (ZI) in the United States. Figure 71-2 depicts these levels of health service support for U.S. Army forces and the connecting evacuation systems. The health service support functions provided by the field medical system include environmental health and preventive medicine; collection of the sick and wounded; treatment; evacuation; medical logistics and maintenance; dental, veterinary, and laboratory services; medical information and intelligence; medical administration; command and control; and reinforcement of lower echelons of the field medical system.

These echelons of medical care are also known as the The-

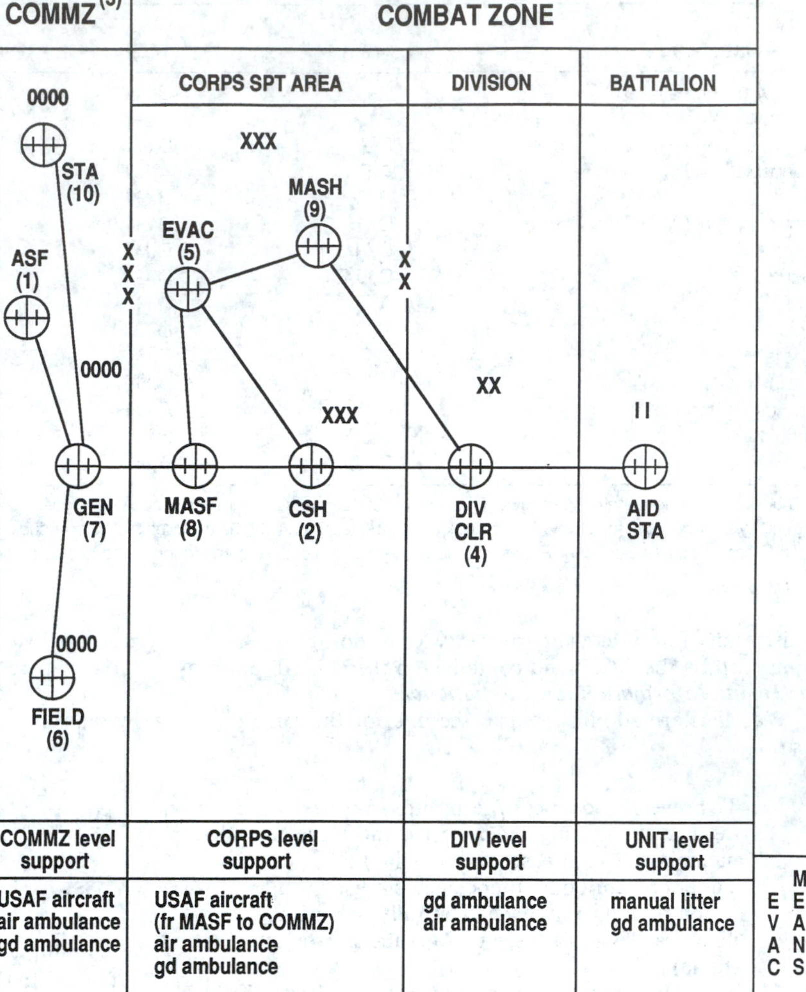

Figure 71-2. Theater of operations medical system. (1) ASF, aeromedical staging facility (USAF). (2) CSH, combat support hospital. (3) COMMZ, communications zone. (4) DIV CLR, division clearing station. (5) EVAC, evacuation hospital. (6) FIELD, field hospital. (7) GEN, general hospital. (8) MASF, mobile aeromedical staging facility (USAF). (9) MASH, mobile army surgical hospital. (10) STA, station hospital. USAF aircraft is the preferred mode of evacuation from corps support area and COMMZ. NOTE: Critically injured or ill patients requiring life- or limb-saving treatment or surgical procedures may be evacuated by air from point of injury or illness to the nearest facility that can best satisfy their needs.

ater Medical System, the organization of which is shown for the separate services in Figure 71-3. The various functions performed at each echelon are as follows:

Echelon 1. Environmental health and preventive medicine activities; collection of the sick and wounded; first aid; emergency medical treatment; routine outpatient care; and evacuation from the point of injury or illness to the unit aid station. (The Air Force has no medical personnel at echelon 1; treatment functions are limited to self-aid and buddy care at this echelon.)

Echelon 2. Environmental health and preventive medicine activities; evacuation of patients from forward unit level aid stations; emergency and resuscitative care in a clearing station staffed by physicians; and evaluation for return to duty, admission (1 to 2 days) at the aid station or clearing company, or onward evacuation for hospitalization at higher echelons.

Echelon 3. Treatment in a mobile medical facility staffed and equipped to provide resuscitation, initial wound surgery, postoperative treatment, and preparation for further evacuation for definitive care, rehabilitation or convalescence, and return to duty.

Echelon 4. Treatment in a general hospital located in the COMMZ, which is the support area for the combat zone, staffed and equipped to provide definitive care. Casualties are rehabilitated for return to duty or onward evacuation to the United States.

In addition, echelons 3 and 4 contain units that provide laboratory, dental, preventive medicine, blood, optometry, veterinary, and medical logistics support.

The echelonment of medical care was first employed by Jonathan Letterman during the Civil War to provide the highest level of field medical support possible, as close to the combat action as possible.[12] Each medical echelon is designed to function within the operational environment characteristic of the tactical echelon. Each higher level contains the same treatment capabilities as those levels forward of it, plus still more sophisticated treatment capabilities.

Medical Threats

The nature and magnitude of the medical threats faced by a deploying military force depend primarily on the geographic area of deployment, the mission and composition of the force, and the level (intensity) of the conflict. The major disease and injury problems among U.S. forces in past wars have resulted from naturally occurring infectious diseases, from environmental hazards, including extremes of heat, cold, and altitude, and hazards from machines, especially motor vehicles, and from weapons.

The factors that influence the number and types of casual-

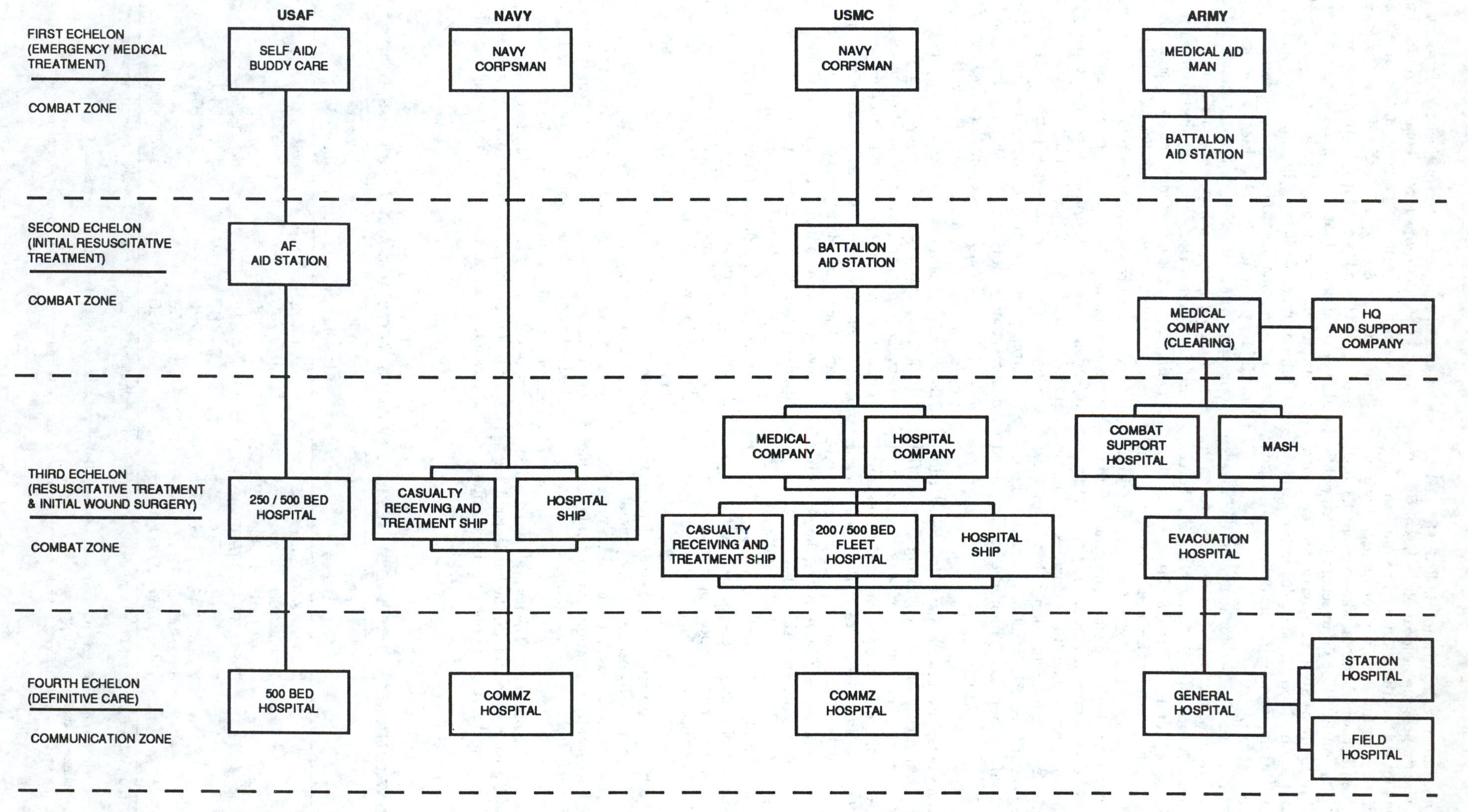

Figure 71–3. Echelonment of health services support in a theater of operations.

ties in any particular conflict are inextricably linked. The medical threats associated with the geographic location of the conflict are determined by climate and weather, altitude, terrain, endemic diseases, and distance from logistical support bases. However, the intensity of the conflict, whether total war waged on a global scale or "low intensity conflict" fought to secure limited political objectives, will certainly be affected by geographic factors. And the mission and composition of the deployed force will be decided based both on estimates of enemy capabilities in the area of operations and on geography.

The U.S. armed intervention in Grenada in 1983 will serve to illustrate the effect of these factors on the medical threat and their interrelationships. A force of U.S. Army, Navy, Air Force, and Marines conducted a "no-notice" raid and rescue operation in Grenada against light opposition. Eighteen U.S. servicemen were killed and 116 wounded in action. However, the rapid tempo of the operation, the high ambient temperature and humidity, and the very heavy combat loads carried produced large numbers of heat and physical exhaustion casualties during the first 48 hours. Because of the brief duration of hostilities, most disease problems (primarily enteric infections, including hookworm) emerged only after troops had left Grenada and returned to their home bases.[49]

Weapons Effects. Weapons effects have increased enormously during the twentieth century, even ignoring the potential effects of nuclear weapons. Automatic, high-velocity personal weapons have increased the amount of tissue damage sustained from a hit and at the same time have increased the probability of multiple hits per casualty. Improved conventional artillery munitions possess greatly increased explosive power and produce larger numbers of fragments per explosion, also increasing the probability of multiple hits. Fuel-air explosives kill and wound over a large area through blast effects alone. So-called "smart weapons" increase the probability of target hits. Lasers used as aiming devices and antipersonnel weapons pose a new array of battlefield hazards. As armies increasingly ride to battle in armored vehicles, the protection afforded from small-caliber bullets and fragments is being offset by munitions that pierce armor and may wound an entire crew by producing fragmentation inside the vehicle and secondary fires. All such weapons effects must be considered in casualty estimation and medical planning for treatment and evacuation.

Natural Battlefield Environment. The natural battlefield environment may pose greater hazards than the battle itself. High temperatures and inadequate water supplies will incapacitate or vastly reduce the combat effectiveness of troops. Historically, cold and wet conditions have frequently routed unprepared armies. Moreover, armies operating in the same locations under similar conditions may have vastly different experiences depending on the availability of proper clothing and on the effectiveness of issued equipment and command-directed prevention programs. For example, during the Italian Campaign of World War II in the winter of 1943–44, British troops had one cold injury per 45 battle casualties, while U.S. troops suffered a ratio of one cold injury per four battle casualties.[50,51] Again, in northern Europe in the winter of 1944–45, the British had 206 cases of nonfreezing cold injury, while the Americans experienced 71,000 during the same period.[50,51] Recognition of the threat, planning, training, and discipline enforced by command would have greatly reduced American casualties from this cause.

While the proportion of hospital admissions due to disease, nonbattle injury, and battle injury has varied from war to war, *infectious diseases* have invariably produced higher admission rates and, until World War II, higher mortality rates than either nonbattle or battle injuries (see Table 71-5).[16,52,53] The tactical and strategic importance of disease in military forces has been documented by many authors, such as Prinzing in *Epidemics Resulting from Wars,*[54] Zinsser in *Rats, Lice and History,*[55] and Gordon in *Preventive Medicine in World War II* (volume IV).[16] Historically, respiratory diseases have accounted for the largest numbers of hospital admissions in virtually all military forces, especially during periods of mobilization and especially in recruit populations (see *Special Disease Problems in Recruit Camps,* above). Diarrheal diseases and dysentery frequently become important disease problems among invading forces immediately following their introduction, when insufficient attention is paid to environmental sanitation.[4] Arthropodborne diseases, especially malaria and a wide range of arthropodborne viruses, such as sandfly fever and dengue, have invariably represented major disease hazards during combat operations in tropical and semitropical areas.[3,56] Common skin infections, including the various dermatophytoses, have often become major causes of attrition in combat units, most recently during U.S. operations in Vietnam.[57]

Venereal diseases represent a special infectious disease problem that has plagued armies everywhere throughout recorded history.[58] In the U.S. Army in World War I the "venereal diseases" (gonorrhea, syphilis, chancroid, lymphogranuloma venereum, and granuloma inguinale) were second only to influenza as causes of disability and time lost from duty.[59] In World War II, incidence rates varied considerably between the United States and overseas areas and among the various overseas the-

TABLE 71-5. DEATHS FROM DISEASE AND BATTLE INJURY IN U.S. WARS, U.S. ARMY,[a] 1846–1975[15,68,69]

War	Dates	Disease (D)	Battle Injury (BI)[b]	D:BI[c]
Mexican War	25 Apr 1846–5 Jul 1848	11,155	1,721	6.48:1
Civil War (North)	15 Apr 1861–1 Aug 1865	199,720	138,154	1.45:1
Spanish-American War	1 May 1898–31 Aug 1898	1,939	369	5:25:1
Philippine Insurrection	Feb 1899–Dec 1902	4,356	1,061	4.11:1
World War I	1 Apr 1917–31 Dec 1918	51,447	50,510	1.02:1
World War II	7 Dec 1941–31 Dec 1945	15,779	234,874	0.07:1
Korean War	Jul 1950–Jul 1953	509	27,704	0.02:1
Vietnam War	1 Jan 1961–30 Apr 1975	1,433	30,900	0.05:1[d]

[a] Before World War I, the U.S. Army sustained the vast majority of deaths from battle injury; for consistency of comparisons between wars, only U.S. Army data are used throughout.

[b] Includes individuals declared dead from missing in action and those who died of nonbattle causes while captured or missing.

[c] Ratio of deaths from disease to deaths from battle injury.

[d] As of 30 April 1985; personnel are still dying of wounds incurred during the war and bodies are still being recovered and identified.

aters; however, from January 1942 to June 1945 the overall incidence rate from all venereal diseases was 37.0 per thousand per year.[60] In the Korean War, from 1951 to 1955, the comparable rate was 184.0 per thousand per year,[61] and in Vietnam, from 1963 to June 1972, 312.1 per thousand per year.[56] While incidence rates generally have increased during periods of conflict since World War II, time lost from duty as a result of these conditions has decreased because of the advent of effective treatments. During World War II the policy of punishment by loss of pay or by having to make up for "bad time" for acquiring a venereal disease was repealed. Sexually transmitted disease control programs in the armed forces now feature the measures of education, prophylaxis, early detection and treatment, and suppression of prostitution.

Nonbattle Injuries. Nonbattle injuries, mostly due to vehicle accidents and accidental explosions and fires, have often nearly equalled battle casualties. As military forces have become increasingly mechanized and equipment operation and maintenance more complex, the risk of nonbattle injury has assumed greater importance.

Psychological Stress. Finally, combat and even the threat of combat can produce temporarily incapacitating psychological stress, a condition recognized in armies since antiquity. Known as "nostalgia" in the American Civil War, "shell shock" in World War I, "combat exhaustion" in World War II, and currently called "battle fatigue" or "combat stress," this exaggeration of the normal response to frightening experiences is associated with all combat environments. The incidence of the condition is directly proportional to the intensity of combat as measured by the rate of wounded in action.[62,63] In recent wars the Israeli Defense Forces experienced rates of stress casualties to wounded of 30:100, and in some units, the ratio was as high as 86:100.[64] Good leadership, high unit cohesion, and realistic training strongly influence prevention and recovery. Appropriate early medical intervention at echelon 2 in a nonpatient status consists of rest, warm food and drink, professional support and reassurance to bolster individual defenses, and creation of the expectation that the situation is temporary. Experience has shown that this approach results in the return to duty of 80% to 85% of such casualties within 3 days and that only 7% have a recurrence. Of those admitted to hospital for treatment, less than 25% will fully recover.[65]

Casualty Management and Evacuation

The "conservation of fighting strength" is the primary goal of the field medical system in combat. This is accomplished by maintaining health and preventing attrition due to disease and injury. Equally important is the provision of a system for the timely collection, treatment, and evacuation of casualties from the battlefield, which is a significant contributor to high morale and willingness to fight.

The organization of the field medical system depends on the intensity of the conflict, the qualitative and quantitative aspects of the casualty load, and the available medical personnel and logistical capabilities. Care must be brought to the casualty or the casualty moved to care. The battlefield system is inevitably a compromise between what is best for the casualty and what is logistically supportable. Sophisticated hospitals are bulky, immobile, and create a large logistical burden; therefore they are inappropriate for the combat zone. More austere and mobile units are required in forward areas, linked by evacuation means from the front to facilities in the rear.

Ground evacuation by litter carry, armored tracked ambulance, or other available ground transport is the rule forward of the first hospital. Helicopter evacuation is unlikely to be employed at this echelon because of the ground-to-air missile threat. From the forward hospitals (echelon 3), both fixed and rotary-wing evacuation are employed to the maximum possible extent, and trains, buses, and river barges may also be used. Evacuation is never a substitute for treatment. Provision must be made for stabilization and care enroute. The whole must be an integrated system under central regulation to achieve good results.

An essential element of this system is the practice of triage, or sorting, which is based on the principal of accomplishing the greatest good for the greatest number under the circumstances. Decisions are based on the need for resuscitation and emergency surgery and the futility of surgery for individuals with intrinsically lethal wounds. Triage, therefore, establishes the priorities for treatment and evacuation. Only through the use of triage can mass casualty situations, which otherwise would overwhelm available medical resources, be managed. *Triage categories* are as follows:

1. *Urgent:* Injuries requiring urgent intervention, possibly including airway establishment, chest tubes, hemorrhage control, intravenous volume replacement, and emergency surgery to prevent death. The hopelessly wounded should not be included.
2. *Immediate:* Life-threatening wounds requiring procedures of short duration with a high probability of survival. These casualties are temporarily stable but would become unstable if surgery were delayed.
3. *Delayed:* Injuries that will tolerate delay prior to operative intervention without significant compromise of a successful outcome; casualties may be held 8 to 10 hours until the urgent and immediate cases have been treated.
4. *Minimal:* Superficial wounds requiring minor surgery or casting, or observation for evolution of radiation sickness.
5. *Expectant:* Mortal wounds, so severe that even if all medical resources were applied, survival would be unlikely.

Triage is a highly dynamic process and must be repeated at each echelon of care subsequent to initial treatment. Treatment is focused first on saving life and secondly on preserving limbs and function.

A second major consideration in the operation of the field medical system is the *evacuation policy,* which establishes the maximum period, in days, that casualties are permitted to be held within the Theater of Operations before being returned to duty. A patient who is not expected to return to duty within this specified period is evacuated to the United States or some other safe area outside the theater. The evacuation policy is a tool that permits medical planners to structure the field medical system for a particular operation, to calculate the number of hospital beds, medical units, supplies and equipment required, and to estimate aeromedical evacuation requirements. A short evacuation policy requires fewer beds and medical units in the theater but increases the requirement for aeromedical evacuation, hospital beds in the United States, and personnel replacements. A long evacuation policy, on the other hand, increases the requirement for beds, medical units, and medical logistics in the theater but decreases the requirements for aeromedical evacuation, beds outside the theater, and replacements. The evacuation policy is established by the secretary of defense on the recommendation of the theater commander and his senior medical advisor, with advice from the Joint Chiefs of Staff. It results from an analysis of the nature of the combat operations, the estimated number and types of casualties, the evacuation means, the availability of replacements, and the availability of resources in the theater of operations. No matter what the evacuation policy, the selection of patients for evacuation is based on physicians' assessments of a patient's ability to tolerate movement to the next echelon of care.

Additional principles that guide medical planners in decisions about the organization of the field medical system are (1) that casualties are evacuated no further to the rear than their clinical condition and the tactical situation warrant; (2) in forward hospitals, that only surgery be done that is necessary to render the casualty transportable to rear area hospitals for reparative surgery; (3) that casualties be returned to duty from the lowest possible echelon of care; and (4) that medical evacuation is an integral element of medical care, not a logistics function, and must be under medical regulation and control.

Disease and Injury Prevention

There are four key components of the strategy for disease and injury prevention in field and combat operations:

1. Determining the nature and magnitude of the disease and injury threats in the planned area of operations before force deployment
2. Identifying the principal countermeasures that must be emphasized to reduce the threats to some acceptable level
3. Training individuals in the use of these countermeasures
4. Rigorous command enforcement of these countermeasures in the operational area

While initial threat evaluations and countermeasures may become modified by later experience, a large part of the preventive medicine effort is expended before any actual deployment. To a large extent the health of the force, indeed, the success of the operation, may depend on the skill and thoroughness with which this work is accomplished.

Medical Threat Assessments. The purpose of medical threat assessments is to help decide on the specific preventive measures that must be planned for use by the force. Medical threat assessments are derived using information from a variety of sources, such as statistical reports of national and international health agencies, publications in the open medical literature, medical historical data from previous operations, and the unpublished observations of health care personnel and epidemiologists working or visiting in the geographical areas of interest. In addition, the DoD maintains medical research facilities in a number of widely dispersed geographic areas dedicated to the study of the epidemiology and prevention of regional medical problems of potential military importance. The collection and evaluation of medical information from these various sources and the preparation of reports on the medical threats for particular regions are accomplished for the DoD by the Armed Forces Medical Intelligence Center. The Armed Forces Pest Management Board* also maintains a worldwide data base on the arthropod vectors of infectious diseases of military importance.

Generally, medical threat assessments are qualitative because the data are seldom available to predict with accuracy specific disease and injury rates for anticipated deployments. Gross estimates of admission rates for specific diseases and injuries based on historical data and expert opinion were recently developed at the U.S. Army Academy of Health Sciences, for the purpose of estimating medical resource requirements for various combat scenarios.* In addition, there are ongoing efforts directed at development of quantitative malaria incidence models for forces deployed in various countries,† but these have never been verified under conditions of actual deployment.

Forest Glen Section, Walter Reed Army Medical Center, Washington, D.C.

At a minimum, medical threat assessments should address the following general categories of information:

1. Incidence and prevalence of infectious diseases among indigenous populations that have the potential to produce significant morbidity and mortality in the force
2. Arthropod vectors and animal reservoirs of major endemic diseases, and other insects, animals, and plants of medical importance
3. Topography and climate
4. Social and economic determinants of disease
5. Conditions of environmental sanitation
6. Estimates of the potential effectiveness of available countermeasures against the important endemic diseases

Identifying the Principal Countermeasures. In military operations there are two general approaches to disease and injury control: individual prophylactic methods and environmental controls. Individual prophylactic methods are those that alter the individual in some way to increase refractoriness to the risk, such as immunizations, chemoprophylaxis, insect repellants, protective clothing, and safety equipment. Environmental controls are those directed at removal or attenuation of environmental risk factors, such as engineering design of machines and equipment, chlorination of unit water supplies, and application of insecticides for disease vector control.

The efficiency of individual prophylactic methods, as a rule, is inversely proportional to the effort demanded of the individual. In the case of immunizations the individual's participation is passive. Chemoprophylaxis by daily or weekly dosage requires minimal individual effort, while the use of insect repellants and protective clothing and equipment requires more conscious effort on the part of the individual, usually with less consistently reliable results. If an individual prophylactic method involves making significant changes in routine behavior, a great deal of training time will be required, and even then, continuous reinforcement by unit leaders may be necessary for such methods to work effectively. Nevertheless, in the highly mobile tactical operations characteristic of modern warfare it is frequently necessary to place virtually total reliance for disease and injury prevention on the use of individual prophylactic methods applied under the supervision of leaders of small tactical units.

In more stable tactical situations it is possible to place heavier reliance on environmental controls accomplished by the units themselves or by combat service support units on an area basis. The reduction of environmental risks through the efforts of a few specialized personnel has the advantage of saving the training time that would be required if individuals had to cope on their own. In field situations, environmental controls are directed mainly at the provision of potable water and sanitary food supplies, the sanitary disposal of wastes, and the control of vectors and animal reservoirs of disease. Besides the function of disease vector control, which is accomplished by specialized preventive medicine units, environmental controls are the responsibility

Combat Developments Branch, U.S. Army Academy of Health Sciences, Fort Sam Houston, Tex.

†*Insects Affecting Man and Animals Research Laboratory, P.O. Box 14565, Gainesville, Fla.*

of nonmedical personnel and units (engineers and quartermaster). Medical personnel retain responsibility for technical inspections to ensure compliance with prescribed standards.

Malaria is perhaps the best example of a highly significant military disease problem that would receive the careful attention of preventive medicine planners during preparations for deployment to an endemic area. Decisions about the countermeasures to be used against malaria by the force would be written into the medical annexes to operations orders, which have the authority of command directives. These decisions would also represent the basis for procurement of medical supply items, such as drugs for the prophylaxis and treatment of malaria, and insecticides and insecticide dispersal equipment for mosquito control.

The primary consideration would be the malaria chemoprophylactic regimen used by the force, the determination of which would depend on information about malaria prevalence in the region, the predominant infecting species, and the prevalence of drug-resistant *Plasmodium falciparum.* Other individual prophylactic methods that would be addressed include use of the standard-issue insect repellant (DEET), used in conjunction with the permethrin-impregnated battle dress uniform (BDU), the proper wearing of the uniform ("shirts on, collars buttoned, sleeves rolled down, from dusk to dawn"), and the use of bed nets. Determinations of specific insecticide products and stockage levels to accompany the force would depend on the revelations of the medical threat assessment; however, mosquito control programs in the operational area, including insecticide dispersal methods, would be devised based upon on-site professional entomological surveys conducted to elicit the principal malaria vector species, their breeding sites, and adult biting and resting habits. Additional environmental controls that might be addressed in command directives include policies regarding campsite selection in relation to native villages, whose inhabitants might represent a reservoir of malaria infection, the use of indigenes as a labor force, and medical civic action programs directed at reduction of the size of the reservoir through identification and treatment of infected individuals.

Training Personnel to Use Countermeasures. As noted, it is frequently necessary to rely almost totally on individual prophylactic methods for disease and injury prevention, especially in the early phases of a deployment. During this period the combat service support units responsible for environmental controls may not have arrived in the area, as the combat elements invariably will have been given priority for movement. The medical personnel that are present will be those assigned to the combat elements, and of necessity, they may be more preoccupied with combat casualty care than with the institution of environmental controls. Moreover, it is during this period, in the disorganization of battle and before the construction of any permanent facilities, that troops are most vulnerable to arthropodborne infections, such as malaria, dengue, and sandfly fever, that have the potential to produce catastrophic outbreaks. While the onset of epidemic disease will not be immediate, should it coincide with the inevitable counterattack by opposing forces, the success of the operation could be seriously jeopardized. Under such circumstances, faithful universal application of available individual prophylactic methods can be seen to be crucial.

The individual prophylactic methods determined to be necessary for use by the force must be integrated into predeployment training programs. Through repetition and constant reinforcement by the noncommissioned officers (NCOs) at squad and platoon level, it is to be expected that the use of prescribed methods will become second nature among the troops, as much as any other required soldierly skill. The organizational mechanism for instilling this kind of "military discipline" is well-developed in the U.S. armed services. The principal prerequisite to the successful incorporation of the desired behaviors into the troops' repertoire is to convince the NCO leaders of small tactical units that the measures are important to the success of the mission.

Rigorous Command Enforcement of Countermeasures. Enforcement of the use of countermeasures is a command function. The appearance in a unit of cases of a specific disease that is preventable by the countermeasures in force (e.g., cases of vivax or chloroquine-sensitive falciparum malaria when weekly chloroquine is the prescribed regimen) should result in an epidemiological investigation to determine if the outbreak is the result of a breakdown in unit "malaria discipline" or unexpected failure of the measure to prevent cases. If the investigation shows that it is due to the latter, better methods must be identified and put in place quickly. If due to the former, command-directed disciplinary action may be warranted. In this connection, Field Marshall Sir William Slim, commander of the British Army in Burma in World War II, in his personal history of the period, stated:

> Good doctors are no use without discipline. More than half the battle against disease is fought, not by doctors, but by the regimental officers. . . . When mepacrine was first introduced . . . often the little tablet was not swallowed. An individual medical test in almost all cases will show whether it has been taken or not. . . . I, therefore, had surprise checks of whole units, every man being examined. If the overall result was less than ninety-five per cent positive I sacked the commanding officer. I only had to sack three; by then the rest had got my meaning.[66]

REFERENCES

1. Gaydos JC: A historical view of occupational health for the soldier. Medical Bulletin of the U.S. Army Medical Department PB 8-88-2:4–10, 1988
2. Dalton BA: Carbon monoxide in U.S. Army tactical vehicles. Ibid, 2:11–13, 1988
3. Nowosiwsky T: The epidemic curve of *Plasmodium falciparum* in a nonimmune population. American troops in Vietnam, 1965 and 1966. Am J Epidemiol 86:461–467, 1967
4. Hurewitz S: Military medical problems of the Lebanon crisis. Military Med 125:26–35, 1960
5. Gauld RL: Epidemiological field studies of infectious hepatitis in the Mediterranean theatre of operations. II. A. Epidemic patterns; B. Outbreaks with distinctive features. Am J Hygiene 43:255, 1946
6. U.S. Army Medical Research Unit, Institute for Medical Research: Annual Progress Report, 1 July 1961–30 June 1962. Kuala Lumpur, Malaysia, 1962
7. Baker TS, Cowan ML, Llewellyn CH: USUHS: Military medical education. U.S. Navy Medicine 77:7–11, March-April 1986
8. U.S. Congress, House: Dept of Defense Appropriation Bill 1985, Report of Committee on Appropriations, p. 67, September 26, 1984
9. Washington Headquarters Services Directorate for Information, Operations and Reports: Department of Defense. Selected Medical Care Statistics for the Quarter Ending March 31, 1989. Washington, DC: Superintendent of Documents, U.S. Government Printing Office
10. Cooper CD: Military Medicine—A new perspective. The Retired Officer 21:24–28, 1986
11. U.S. Army Medicine. Army Magazine 36:41–43, 1986
12. Letterman J: Medical Recollections of the Army of the Potomac. New York: D. Appleton and Co., 1866
13. Headquarters, Department of the Army: Army Regulation 600–63, Personnel—General, Army Health Promotion. Washington, DC, 17 November 1987
14. Bayne-Jones S: The Evolution of Preventive Medicine in the United

States Army, 1607–1939. Washington, DC: Office of the Surgeon General, Department of the Army, 1968

15. Ginn RVN: Organization of the military health care system. Military Med 151:299–305, 1986
16. Coates JB Jr, Hoff EC, Hoff PM (eds): Preventive Medicine in World War II. Volume IV. Communicable Diseases Transmitted Chiefly Through Respiratory and Alimentary Tracts. Washington, DC: Medical Department, United States Army, 1958
17. Headquarters, Department of the Army: Army Regulation 40-5, Medical Services, Preventive Medicine. Washington, DC, 1 June 1985
18. War Department: Mobilization Regulations1-9. Standards of Physical Examination During Mobilization. Washington, DC, August 31, 1940
19. National Headquarters, Selective Service System: Medical Statistics Bulletin No. 2. Washington, DC, 1 August 1943
20. Anderson RS, Wiltsie CM (eds): Physical Standards in World War II. Medical Department, United States Army, Washington, DC, 1967
21. Headquarters, Department of the Army: Army Regulation 40-501, Medical Services, Standards of Medical Fitness. Washington, DC, 1 July 1987
22. Hilleman MR: Epidemiology of adenovirus respiratory infections in military recruit populations. Ann NY Acad Sci 67:262–272, 1957
23. Gauld JR, Nitz RE, Hunter DH, Rust JH, Gauld RL: Epidemiology of meningococcal meningitis at Fort Ord. Am J Epidemiol 82:56–72, 1965
24. Bartley JD: Natural history of meningococcal disease in basic training at Fort Dix, NJ. Military Med 137:373–380, 1972
25. Commission on Acute Respiratory Diseases: Clinical patterns of undifferentiated and other acute respiratory diseases in Army recruits. Medicine 26:441–464, 1947
26. Sartwell PE: Common respiratory disease in recruits. Am J Hyg 53:224–235, 1951
27. Rowe WP, Huebner RJ, Gilmore LK, Parrott RH, Ward TG: Isolation of a cytopathogenic agent from human adenoids undergoing spontaneous degeneration in tissue culture. Proc Soc Exp Biol Med 84:570–573, 1953
28. Hilleman MR, Werner JH: Recovery of new agent from patients with acute respiratory illness. Proc Soc Exp Biol Med 85:183–188, 1954
29. Hilleman MR, Werner JH, Stewart MT: Grouping and occurrence of RI (prototype RI-67) viruses. Proc Soc Exp Biol Med 90:555–562, 1955
30. Dingle JH, Ginsberg HS, Badger GF, Jordan WS, Katz S: Evidence for the specific etiology of acute respiratory disease (ARD). Trans Assoc Am Physicians 67:149–154, 1954
31. Van der Veen J, Oei KG, Abarbanel MFW: Patterns of infections with adenovirus types 4, 7 and 21 in military recruits during a 9-year survey. J Hyg (Camb) 67:255–267, 1969
32. Kurian PV, Roshan L, Pandit V: Adenovirus infections in Indian Army personnel. Ind J Med Res 54:812–818, 1966
33. Top FH Jr: Control of adenovirus acute respiratory disease in U.S. Army trainees. Yale J Biol Med 48:185–195, 1975
34. Headquarters, Departments of the Army, the Navy, the Air Force and Transportation: Army Regulation 40-562, NAVMEDCOMINST 6230.3, AFR 161–13, CG COMDINST M6230.4D. Washington DC, 7 October 1988
35. Fairbrother RW: Cerebrospinal meningitis. .. use of sulfonamide derivatives in prophylaxis. Brit Med J 2:859–862, 1940
36. Kuhns DM, Nelson CT, Feldman HA, Kuhn LR: The prophylactic value of sulfadiazine in the control of meningococci meningitis. JAMA 123:335–339, 1943
37. Millar JW, Siess EC, Feldman HA, Silverman C, Frank P: *In vivo* and *in vitro* resistance to sulfadiazine in strains of *Neisseria meningitidis*. JAMA 186:139–141, 1963
38. Koppes GM, Ellenbogen C, Gebhart RJ: Group Y meningococcal disease in United States Air Force recruits. Am J Med 62:661–666, 1977
39. Phair JJ, Schoenbach EB: The dynamics of meningococcal infections and the effect of chemotherapy. Am J Hyg 40:318–344, 1944
40. Brodkey C, Gaydos JC: United States Army guidelines for troop living space: A historical review. Military Med 145:418–421, 1980
41. Coburn AF, Young DC: The Epidemiology of Hemolytic Streptococcus During World War II in the United States Navy. Baltimore: Williams and Wilkins, 1949
42. Rantz LA, Rantz HH, Boisvert PJ, Spink WW: Streptococcic and nonstreptococcic disease of the respiratory tract; epidemiologic observations. Arch Intern Med 77:121–131, 1946
43. Thomas RJ, Conwill DE, Morton DE, Brooks TJ, Holmes CK, Mahaffey WB: Penicillin prophylaxis for streptococcal infections in United States Navy and Marine Corps recruit camps, 1951–1985. Rev Infect Dis 10:125–130, 1988
44. Sampson GL, Williams RG, House MD, Wetzel NE, Brundage JF, NcNeil JG, Magruder CD, Gray GC: Acute rheumatic fever among Army trainees - Fort Leonard Wood, Missouri, 1987–1988. MMWR 37(34):519–522, 1988
45. Hume EE: Victories of Army Medicine. Philadelphia: JP Lippincott, 1943
46. Coates JB Jr, Hoff EC (eds): Preventive Medicine in World War II. Volume III. Personal Health Measures and Immunizations. Washington, DC: Office of the Surgeon General, Department of the Army, 1955
47. Walker DW: Some epidemiological aspects of infectious hepatitis in the U.S. Army. Am J Trop Med Hyg 25:75–82, 1945
48. United States Department of Health and Human Services, Public Health Service, Centers for Disease Control: Health Information for International Travel. Washington, DC: Superintendent of Documents, U.S. Government Printing Office, 1989
49. Fry MT, Kayler RS: Health Service Support in Joint Operation. Operation Urgent Fury. Executive Research Project 525, Industrial College of the Armed Forces, Ft McNair, Washington, DC, 1988
50. Francis TJR: Non-freezing cold injury: A historical review. J R Navy Med Serv 70:139–143, 1984
51. Whayne TF, DeBakey ME: Cold Injury: General Type. Washington, DC: Office of the Surgeon General, U.S. Army, 1958
52. Reister FA: Battle Casualties and Medical Statistics. U.S. Army Experience in the Korean War. Washington, DC: The Surgeon General, Department of the Army
53. Washington Headquarters Services Directorate for Information, Operations and Reports: Department of Defense. U.S. Casualties in Southeast Asia. Statistics as of April 30, 1985. Washington, DC: Superintendent of Documents, U.S. Government Printing Office
54. Prinzing F: Epidemics Resulting from Wars. London: Carnegie Endowment for International Peace, Oxford Clarendon Press, 1916
55. Zinsser H: Rats, Lice and History. Boston: Little Brown & Co., 1935
56. Ognibene AJ, Barrett O'N Jr (eds): Internal Medicine in Vietnam. II. General Medicine and Infectious Diseases. Washington, DC: Office of the Surgeon General and Center of Military History, United States Army, 1982
57. Allen AM: Internal Medicine in Vietnam. I. Skin Diseases in Vietnam, 1965–72. Washington, DC: Office of the Surgeon General and Center of Military History, United States Army, 1977
58. Garrison FH: Notes on the History of Military Medicine. New York: G. Olms Verlag, 1970
59. Dunham GC: Venereal diseases in the American Army. Army Med Bull 6:152–92, 1923
60. Coates JB Jr, Hoff EB, Hoff PM (eds): Preventive Medicine in World War II. Volume V. Communicable Diseases Transmitted by Contact or by Unknown Means. Medical Department, United States Army, Washington, DC, 1960
61. Greenberg JH: Venereal disease in the armed forces. Med Clin North Am 56:1087–1100, Sept 1972
62. Glass AJ: Observations Upon the Epidemiology of Mental Illness in Troops During Warfare. Symposium on Preventive and Social Psychiatry. Washington, DC: Walter Reed Army Institute of Research, 1957
63. Glass AJ (ed): Neuropsychiatry in World War II. Volume I. Zone of

the Interior. Washington, DC: Office of the Surgeon General, U.S. Army, 1957
64. Levin S: Models for Prediction of Neuropsychiatric Casualties in High Intensity Combat. Contract Regrant BLI-CR-556. Aberdeen Proving Ground, Maryland: U.S. Army Ballistic Research Laboratory, 1986
65. Bilenkey GL, Tyner FC, Soditz FJ: Israeli Battle Shock Casualties: 1973 and 1982. Report WRAIR NP-83-5. Washington, DC: Walter Reed Army Institute of Research, 1983
66. Slim, Field-Marshall Sir W: Defeat Into Victory. London: Cassell and Company, Ltd., 1956

72
Prison Health

Jonathan B. Weisbuch

The population confined behind bars in the United States in 1988 was in excess of 750,000.[1] More than 8 million Americans are processed through the correctional system, city and county jails, houses of correction, state prisons, juvenile facilities, and federal penitentiaries, in any one year.[2] In most systems, new inmates receive a summary health examination; those who remain a week or more behind bars, receive a more complete physical examination from a physician, nurse practitioner, or physician's assistant. On any day of the week 75,000 to 80,000 visits to sick call are evaluated by prison health care personnel. The total annual cost of providing health care to prisoners is estimated to be $1 to $1.5 billion.

The prison health care system is big—big medicine, big business, and often a big problem for correctional officials whose primary responsibility is security and not the provision of health care. Prisoners carry a much greater burden of illness than other members of society; they harbor diseases that are determined both by the environment out of which they come and by the prison in which they live. The unusual nature of prison medicine and its attendant pathology stimulated Tauxe and Patterson[3] to recommend the use of the term *desmoteric medicine* (from the Greek word *desmoterion,* "prison") to describe conditions related to this branch of medicine. The term is an appropriate addition to the medical lexicon; more than 1000 physicians and 2500 to 3000 other health professionals spend all or part of their working day serving a unique population with unusual health problems in a distinct setting removed from the mainstream of medical care.

The problems faced by the prison practitioner are legion. Desmotologists must be familiar with the latest medical information on many diseases that are infrequently seen in community practice: problems of severe substance abuse, tuberculosis, trauma and violence, unusual neuropsychiatric diseases, epilepsy, the manifestations of stress, and of course AIDS and HIV infection. They must consider that patients may use the medical encounter for secondary gain unrelated to signs or symptoms. They realize that medical recommendations have an impact on the health and security of others both within the system and outside it, and they know that litigation is not the only outcome to fear if patients are dissatisfied with their care: riots have been provoked by poor medical care.

Prison medicine often involves a balancing act between the conflicting priorities that are inherent to a prison environment: security, social rehabilitation, and medical service (Fig. 72–1). The shaded regions, where priorities overlap, create dilemmas for the prison physician, described by Thornburn[4] as a frustrating conflict between service to the system and service to the patient. If serving the needs of the patient is to remain the first priority, the practitioner must acquire skills not generally taught in medical school or residency.

Desmotologists must be skilled in medical administration and interpersonal diplomacy and must understand well the varied and complex social systems that exist within prisons. Prison clinicians must also practice prevention and health promotion. They must apply epidemiology to determine patterns of prison illness, they must be able to recognize and reduce environmental health hazards, they must be willing to struggle with suicide and mental illness, substance abuse, violence, stress, and other dysfunctional behaviors that are inevitably manifested by patients within the prison context. When appointed as medical director of a prison health system, the physician must add management, budgeting, planning, personnel organization, and leadership to his or her clinical skills. Prison physicians must provide clinical care, prevention, occupational medicine, and medical management. They are specialists in clinical preventive medicine in the broadest definition of that term.

EXPANSION AND IMPROVEMENT

Before the late 1960s, neither public health nor organized medicine was much concerned with the medical services provided in American prisons and jails. The deplorable state of American prison health care before 1970 has been well documented by the litigation of that period,[5-8] and by the report of the American Medical Association on the status of health care in prisons and jails.[9] As a result of the judicial decrees and the efforts of organized medicine,[10] health care in most American prisons has improved. Prisoners now receive medical examinations on admittance and have reasonable access to health services while incarcerated.

In 1977, as this revolution began, Weisbuch[11] urged public health professionals to participate in the development and improvement of prison health care. In some jurisdictions, state and local health departments have worked with the prisons to assure quality of care for prisoners,[12,13] but most of the 3000 state and local health agencies still remain aloof from the prison population. Prison health care managers have had to work on their own to define standards and develop methods to assure quality.

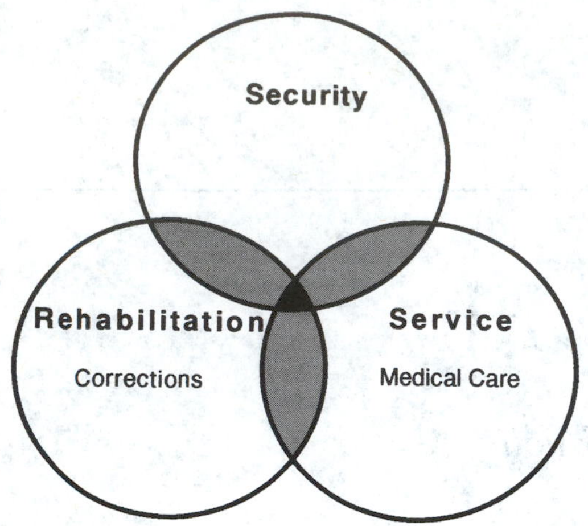

Figure 72-1 Overlapping priorities in corrections.

The process has been successful. Prison health care is improving. Wardens no longer hire a part-time physician and a nurse or two to provide, reluctantly, the medical care demanded by prisoners. During the 1980s, state correctional systems organized health services under medical supervision. Some programs employed physicians as medical directors to supervise prison medical care. Others contracted with private corporations to provide health services to the prison population.[14] The recognition by states and large cities and counties of the need for medical direction has increased the number of skilled health care providers in prisons. Assurance of quality is not universal, however; few systems monitor quality routinely.

Assessment standards do exist, nevertheless. In 1977 the American Public Health Association published the first set of standards for prison and jail health care.[15] These were updated in 1983. The APHA standards provide guidelines for building a system of services that include prevention, primary and secondary care, special care for women and other minority groups, dental care, environmental health, pharmacy, and the organization of the medical record system. Legal issues and the determination of quality are also included in the standards. A prison health care system designed to the standards of the APHA should provide an optimal level of care for inmates.

A less comprehensive approach to prison health care standards was published in 1978 by the American Medical Association.[16] These guidelines were organized to provide a framework for prison health service accreditation, similar to the methods of the Joint Commission on Hospital Accreditation of that time. As an accreditation tool, the AMA standards were used successfully to accredit more than 250 jail health systems in the early 1980s. Revised in January 1987, and published under the independent authority of the Board of the National Commission on Correctional Health Care (NCCHC), the AMA standards were improved and expanded.[17] Nearly 350 jails and prison systems are now accredited under NCCHC jail and prison standards.

The publication of standards, the judicial mandate for better prison health care, the provision of contract services, and the accreditation of prison health systems have reduced public health's direct responsibility for providing quality medical care in prisons. These developments, however, do not exempt public health professionals from their mission to assure a healthy environment for all citizens. Infectious diseases cross prison walls. The prevention and management of trauma and violence must have a broad focus, which includes the prison. The enforcement of environmental health regulations requires public health professionals. The promotion of health, the reduction of drug and alcohol abuse, the control of sexually transmitted diseases, early prenatal care, and the assurance of quality health care are all public health imperatives. They are not tasks for jailors. Public health responsibilities do not stop when people are jailed, any more than they do when children attend school or workers enter a factory.

THE PRISON ENVIRONMENT AND THE PUBLIC'S HEALTH

Prisons and jails are conduits through which the pathology of our society is funneled. Significant public health problems (e.g., substance abuse, AIDS, hepatitis, trauma, violence, tuberculosis, suicide, mental illness, and venereal disease, to mention only a few) are concentrated in American correctional facilities. Whether measured by the frequency of positive responses on an intake medical questionnaire[18] or by the frequency of complaints at sick call,[19,20] the prevalence of these and many other illnesses among prisoners is excessive. The surfeit of prisoner health problems increases the demand for medical care, the need for specialty referral services, and the cost of prison health care above that which might be expected from another population consisting primarily of young males. A few examples of health problems found most frequently among prisoners are discussed below.

Substance Abuse, Alcohol, and Drugs

Substance abuse—with its public and private medical, social, legal, and criminal ramifications—may be the most significant sociomedical problem facing the United States. In the general population of young adults in 1986, alcohol was used with regularity by 30% to 42%, cocaine at least once a year by 13% to 21%, and heroin by fewer than 0.2%.[21] While comparable statistics are not available for the entire prison and jail population, a 1979 nationwide survey of substance abuse among state prisoners, reported by Miller,[22] emphasized that 33% of males and 29% of females were drunk when they committed the offense for which they were currently imprisoned and that 8.5% of males and 13.7% of females admitted to daily intravenous heroin use at the time of incarceration.

In most parts of the nation, repeat convictions for driving under the influence of alcohol (DWI) are punishable with incarceration; many alcoholics await trial or have been sentenced for this offense.

Substance abusers bring into the prisons and jails all the infirmities associated with their addictions: AIDS, hepatitis B, withdrawal syndromes, emotional illness, suicidal behavior, traumatic injuries, and the manifestations of violence. All must be managed by prison clinicians. After acute treatment and even a minimal amount of counseling, these patients will return to the community and their addictive life-style. The carousel goes around and around; its outcome is human suffering, disease, and death, much of which must be handled by providers of prison health care.

A 1988 report by the AMA's Board of Trustees[23] emphasizes that substance abusers in the United States will not be reduced in number through the interdiction of supply and enforcement of tougher laws. Only through the expansion of treatment programs and the education of users and potential users will addiction decline. These are public health functions. Within the prison system, addicts are easily recognized. These inmates can be enrolled immediately in substance abuse programs if the programs have been instituted.

Well-managed programs within the prisons and jails decrease prison drug abuse and increase the chance that inmates, when discharged, will enter community treatment programs and remain drug free. Unpublished data from the states of New Jersey, Delaware, and New York also show a decrease in prison recidivism of drug abusers who have participated in a well-run prison treatment program. Treatment programs within the prison environment, managed, directed, and financed by the public health system, should reduce program costs and improve quality. Any degree of success in reducing addictive behavior will increase the chance that the inmate will remain drug free on discharge or parole and will ultimately lower the probability of his or her returning to the prison system.

AIDS

The national AIDs epidemic has created an additional crisis for an overburdened American correctional system. In state and federal prisons in 1988 the incidence of AIDS, 75 per 100,000 prisoners,[24] was more than five times the national rate of 13.7 per 100,000. Prison incidence varies by region, however; in 1988 it was zero in Iowa and Nebraska and 536 per 100,000 in New York.

Risk factors among inmates are changing also. In 1984 and 1985 homosexuality was the predominant risk factor; by 1988, in New York City more than half of new AIDs cases were associated with intravenous (IV) drug abuse. At the Rikers Island jail in New York City, approximately half of the 150,000 prisoners admitted in 1988 were drug users; 35% to 40% of these were HIV-positive.[24] In Baltimore, where similar trends have been identified, the HIV prevalence among new admissions was 7% in 1988.[25]

This high seroprevalence on intake does not, however, appear to result in a high rate of seroconversion among inmates whose ELISA/Western Blot tests were negative when they were admitted to the system. In a study of Baltimore inmates, 4.1 conversions to HIV-positive status were detected for every 1000 inmate-years of exposure.[25] Whether this conversion rate was a function of high-risk inmate behavior or a delay in conversion of individuals who had already been infected with HIV at the time of admission cannot be determined because viral cultures of inmates' blood were not performed. The work of Imagawa and his coworkers in Los Angeles[26] has shown that up to 23% of drug abusers and homosexuals who are seronegative for HIV by standard tests may still harbor a silent infection with the virus, which may not be manifest in a positive ELISA/Western Blot examination for years.

Grave problems confront the desmotologist responsible for the management of HIV infection in the prison system. Should new inmates be tested for HIV?[27,28] Should only those who are homosexual or IV drug users be tested? Should those at high risk who are found to be HIV-negative by the standard ELISA/Western Blot process be further evaluated for silent viral infection by lymphocyte culture? What housing arrangements are appropriate for HIV-positive inmates? Who should be informed of the prisoner's HIV status? Should contact tracing both inside the prison and in the outside community be initiated? By whom? Can confidentiality be maintained in the prison setting? What are the implications for individuals' health when their HIV status is known? Should patients with clinical AIDS be discharged from the jail or prison? Should zidovudine treatment be given? Who should pay for it? Who should be responsible for providing counseling to the patients? Who shall attempt to allay fear of the disease among inmates and correctional staff? Should drug abusers, regardless of their HIV status, be enrolled in prison treatment programs? The list goes on ad infinitum.

These questions have ramifications well beyond the prison walls. The public health implications deserve input from those public health experts who manage the AIDS problem in the community. Decisions concerning the prison population at risk of HIV infection should not be made in a vacuum.

Most prison systems do have a written AIDS policy to answer some or all of these questions. Occasionally state or local health departments were consulted in the development of the policy. Implementation of these policies remains a problem, however. Medical resources are limited. Prison bed space for isolation is nonexistent in most systems. Confidentiality is impossible. Fear of AIDS places inmates who carry the virus at risk of injury and even death. Public health professionals have a clear role in this situation.

Decisions concerning HIV testing must involve the health department. Pretest and posttest counseling requires trained professionals. The education of inmates and correctional staff deserves more than the distribution of informational pamphlets. Contact tracing, maintenance of confidentiality,[29] the support of family and friends, treatment in the terminal phase of the illness, and the referral of HIV-positive prisoners to appropriate community resources on release from prison are all health department functions that demand coordination and cooperation between health and corrections authorities.

Hepatitis

Hepatitis B, another disease in which high prevalence among prisoners is related to IV drug use, poses a health threat both while the patient is in prison and when he or she is returned to the community. Prevalence studies of new inmates indicate that 20% to 50% were exposed to the hepatitis B virus before incarceration[30,31]; HBV (hepatitis B surface antigen [HBsAg]) carrier rates of between 0.4% and 4.1% are reported.[32,33] Tucker et al.,[34] studying all new admissions to the Virginia prison system, identified 1.3% who carried the delta agent and 33% who had been exposed to HBsAg. Virtually all of these prisoners were IV drug abusers.

Even though exposure to HBsAg is common among inmates, correctional systems have shown less concern for the illness than they have for AIDS. The incidence of hepatitis B in prisons is low.[35] Viral transmission among prisoners is 8 to 14 cases per 1000 inmate-years of exposure.[35,36] Treatment is inexpensive, moreover, and mortality is not perceived as a problem. From the perspective of the prison, vaccination of inmates with expensive vaccine appears not to be worth the marginal benefit.

From a public health perspective, however, recognizing that most prisoners will return to their communities, Anda and his coworkers[31] suggest that all drug users who have not been exposed to HBsAg be started on a vaccination program while in prison. The current episode of imprisonment may be the only chance society has to protect these persons before they become infected, break down with disease, or infect others. In Anda's Wisconsin study population, fewer than 20% of prisoners admitted were both IV drug abusers and uninfected with HBV. Therefore the cost of vaccination would be less than $25 per prison admission. Whether these costs would reduce the treatment cost of the 300,000 cases of hepatitis B in the nonprison community can be evaluated only when transmission rates outside prisons are known.

Tuberculosis

Tuberculosis (TB) is another public health problem that might be eliminated if public health and prison health authorities would work together. The incidence of TB among prisoners has long been recognized as a significant problem.[37] In 1985 the incidence of tuberculosis in 29 state correctional systems was three times higher than for nonincarcerated adults 15 to 64 years of age.[38] Since 1985 the problem of active TB has been exacerbated by the increasing prevalence of HIV.[39–41] In 1987 TB rates among prison inmates were 80.3 per 100,000 in California, 105.5 per 100,000 in New York, and 109.9 per 100,000 in New Jersey.[41] The national rate in that year, according to the Centers for Disease Control statistics, was 9.4 per 100,000.[42]

Most prisons have policies for testing all new inmates for TB, and for treating those who are found to be PPD-positive. These programs suffer, however, from lack of input, inadequate communication, and poor coordination with the public health community. Surveillance, containment, and assessment are sophisticated tasks that require experts in TB control, who are generally found in city, county, and state health departments but not among prison health providers.

The appropriate treatment of a Mantoux-positive prisoner depends on HIV status.[43] When returned to the community, the patient must be followed by public health workers to assure the continuation of therapy. Close associates should be tested and treated in order to close the ring.

Collaboration between corrections and health personnel improves the chance that new cases are registered, that contacts are identified and tested, and that appropriate prophylaxis and treatment are initiated and maintained.

The resurgence of tuberculosis in the United States will not be stopped in the prisons by prison health officials; it will be arrested by trained public health professionals in the community carrying out appropriate testing and treatment. To find new cases, however, public health professionals must work closely with their colleagues in prison health.

Suicide

Suicide in prisons and jails constitutes a major problem, which accounts for the largest number of years of life lost of any medical problem in most jurisdictions. Estimates vary, but a nationwide survey[44] of the problem indicates that suicide rates in jails are as high as 100 per 100,000 inmates, which is five times the rate for nonprisoners.[45,46] As many as 1% of all inmates admitted to British jails attempt self-destruction.[47]

Jail suicides differ in a number of significant ways from those that occur in long-term penitentiaries. Suicides in jails or city lockups usually occur within 24 hours of incarceration.[48] They are usually not associated with the alleged crime but are related to the stress of acute incarceration and often to alcohol intoxication.[49] Suicides in prisons after sentencing often occur after months of confinement and are associated with long sentences and serious crimes.[50]

A problem of this magnitude is a public health concern. To prevent this human loss, corrections, mental health, and public health professionals must work together. The jail authorities must provide a suicide-prevention area and train their officers in suicide prevention.[51] Departments of mental health should participate in training the correctional staff, reviewing the protocols, and providing the psychiatric backup for inmates with profound emotional problems. Public health professionals can create the reporting system and integrate substance-abuse programs into the prevention process.

Other Public Health Problems Associated With Prisons and Jails

The items noted above constitute only the tip of the prison health iceberg. Public health responsibility in the prison extends to dental problems, the prevention and treatment of traumatic injury, the array of health problems faced by women prisoners, and concern for the management of mental health problems other than suicide that confront prison authorities on a daily basis.

Public health, under its licensure authority, assures that quality medical care is provided in institutions that serve the public. Prisons serve the public. The standard of medical care provided to prisoners must be acceptable. Therefore, licensure of health services provided in jails and prisons should be a public health responsibility. Accreditation by national agencies such as the National Commission for Correctional Health Care (NCCHC), or the Joint Commission for the Accreditation of Health Care Organizations (JCAHCO), may be allowed as a substitute for the assessment of facilities by local public inspectors. However, the public health agency should require a regular review process to assure that prison health services meet minimal standards. The unregulated system now in effect should be terminated.

Education, research, epidemiology of prison health problems, and the monitoring of environmental health in correctional facilities are also duties that public health departments should perform for the prison system. The list can be lengthened, as can the tale of problems. Prison medicine needs public health guidance to assure that its future is focused on preventing illness as well as providing first-rate care.

The mission of public health is to assure society that the conditions in which people live and work are healthful.[52] Neglecting the health of the 8 million citizens who pass through prisons annually and the well-being of those in close contact with them before, during, and after incarceration is perilous to society. The prison population is a vector for disease. When public health resources are brought to bear on it, the community will be served and diseases that burden American society will be controlled, if not eliminated.

REFERENCES

1. United States Justice Department: Statistics on Criminal Justice, 1989
2. Bureau of Justice Statistics on Jail Inmates, 1986. Doc. No. NCJ-107123. Washington, D.C.: US Department of Justice, October 1987
3. Tauxe RV, Patterson CB: A word about prisons: "desmoteric." N Engl J Med 317:1669–1670, 1988
4. Thornburn KM: Croaker's dilemma: should prison physicians serve prisons or prisoners? West J Med 134:457–461, 1981
5. Estelle v Gamble, 97 S. Ct. 285, 429 US 97
6. Newman v Alabama, 349F. Supp 278,503 F.2d 1320, 5th Cir. (1974). cert. denied 421 US 948 (1975)
7. Todaro v Ward. 565 F.2d 48, 52 (2 Cir. 1977)
8. *Charles Street Jail, Inmates of Suffolk County Jail v Eisenstadt,* 360 F Supp 676 (D. Mass. 1973)
9. Medical Care in US Jails—A 1972 Survey. Chicago: American Medical Association, 1973
10. Anno BJ: The role of organized medicine in correctional health care. JAMA 247:2923–2925, 1982
11. Weisbuch JB: Public health professionals and prison health care needs. Am J Public Health 67(8):720–722, 1977
12. Granthan EV, Sandler ES, Block MJ: Treatment of correctional center inmates at a public health department: a cooperative venture. J Public Health Dent 42:251–255, 1982
13. Rice D: Judicial involvement in Colorado prison health care reform. J Health Polit Policy Law 6:315–320, 1981
14. Prout C, Ross RN: Care and Punishment. Pittsburgh: University of Pittsburgh Press, 1988, pp 117–126
15. Standards for Health Care in Correction Institutions, Jails and Prisons, 1983, American Public Health Association
16. Standards for Health Services in Jails, Prisons, and Juvenile Homes. Chicago: National Commission on Correctional Health Care, 1987
17. Standards for Health Services in Jails (81 pp) and Standards for Health Services in Prisons (83 pp) Chicago: National Commission on Correctional Health Care, 1986
18. Shapiro S, Shapiro MF: Identification of health care problems in a county jail. J Community Health 12:23–30, 1987
19. Shep SB, Schechter MT, Prefontain RG: Prison health services: a utilization study. J Community Health 12:4–21, 1987
20. Freeman RW, Gollub RE, Wolski M, Gschwend JA, Al-Ibrahim MS, Hawthorn PR, Golden AS, Kamka G, Kelly GB: Planning

health services for a city jail: impact of contractual services on men's sick call. Med Care 19:410–418, 1981
21. O'Malley PM, Bachman JG, Johnston LD: Period, age, and cohort effects on substance use among young Americans: a decade of change. 1976–86. Am J Public Health 78:1315–1321, 1988
22. Miller RE: Nationwide profile of female inmate substance involvement. J Psychoactive Drugs 16:319–326, 1984
23. American Medical Association: Proceedings of the House of Delegates, 137th annual meeting, June 26–30, 1988, Board of Trustees Report NNN, "Drug Abuse in the United States: A Policy Report," pp 236–250
24. Hammett TM: 1988 Update: AIDS in Correctional Facilities, Doc No. NCJ-115522. Washington, DC: U.S. Department of Justice, National Institute of Justice, 1989
25. Brewer TF, Taylor E, Munoz A: Transmission of human immunodeficiency virus type 1 (HIV-1) within a statewide prison system. AIDS 2:263–368, 1988
26. Imagawa DT, Lee MH, Wolinsky SM, Sano K, Morales F, Kwok S, Sninsky JJ, Nishanian PG, Giorgi J, Bahey HL, Dudley J, Visschere BR, Detels R: Human immunodeficiency virus type 1 infection in homosexual men who remain seronegative for prolonged periods. N Engl J Med 320:1458–1462, 1989
27. Policy statement on Intake Testing for HIV in Prisons and Jails. National Commission on Correctional Health Care, April 1988
28. American Medical Association: Proceedings of the House of Delegates, Board of Trustees Report UU, Chicago, June 1987
29. Vernon T: Partner Notification. JAMA 260:3274, 1988
30. Bader TF: Hepatitis in prisons. Biomed Pharmacother 40:248–251, 1986
31. Anda RF, Perlman SB, D'Alessio DJ, Davis JP, Dodson VN: Hepatitis B in Wisconsin male prisoners: considerations for serologic screening and vaccination. Am J Public Health 75:1182–1185, 1985
32. Brewer, F: J Prison Jail Health 5:102–107, 1985
33. Kibby T, Devine J, Love C: Prevalence of hepatitis B among men admitted to a federal prison. N Engl J Med 306:175, 1982
34. Tucker RM, Geffey MJ, Fisch MJ, Kaiser DL. Guerranct RL, Normansell DE: Seroepidemiology of hepatitis D (delta agent) and hepatitis B among Virginia state prisoner. Clin Ther 9:622–628, 1987
35. Decker MD, Vaughn WK, Brodie JS, et al: Incidence of hepatitis B in Tennessee prisoners. J Infect Dis 152:214–217, 1985
36. Hull HF, Lyons LF, Mann JM, Hadler SC, et al: Incidence of hepatitis B in the penitentiary of New Mexico. Am J Public Health 75:1213–1214, 1985
37. Stead WW: Undetected tuberculosis in prison (source of infection for the community at large). JAMA 240:2544–2547, 1978
38. Centers for Disease Control: Prevention and control of tuberculosis in correctional institutions: recommendations of the Advisory Committee for the Elimination of Tuberculosis. MMWR 38:313–325, 1989
39. Selwyn PA, Hartel D, Lewis VA, Schoenbaum EE, Vermund SH, Klein RS, Walker AT, Friedland GH: A prospective study of the risk of tuberculosis among intravenous drug users with human immunodeficiency virus infection. N Engl J Med 320:545–550, 1989
40. Salive M, Brewer TF: Tuberculosis and human immunodeficiency virus infection: an emerging problem in inmates. J Prison Jail Health, 1988
41. Braun MM, Truman BI, Maguire B, DiFerninando GT Jr, Wormser G, Broaddus R, Morse DL: Increasing incidence of tuberculosis in a prison inmate population: associated with HIV infection. JAMA 261:393–397, 1989
42. Reider HL, Cauthen GM, Kelly GD, Bloch AB, Snider DE: JAMA 262:385–389, 1989
43. Centers for Disese Control: MMWR 38:313–325, 1989
44. National Study of Jail Suicides: Seven Years Later. Alexandria, Va: The National Center on Institutions and Alternatives, 1988
45. Tuskan JJ, Thase ME: Suicides in jails and prisons. J Psychosoc Nurs Ment Health Serv 21:29–33, 1983
46. Burtch BE: Prisoner suicides reconsidered. Int J Law Psychiatry 2:407–413, 1979
47. Wool RJ, Dooley E: A study of attempted suicides in prisons. Med Sci Law 27:297–300, 1987
48. Brackett SA: Suicide in Scottish prisons. Br J Psychiatry 151:218–221, 1987
49. Jordan FB, Schmeckpeper K, Strope M: Jail suicides by hanging: an epidemiological review and recommendations for prevention. Am J Forensic Med Psych 8:27–31, 1987
50. Salive ME, Smith GS, Brewer TF: Suicide mortality in the Maryland state prison system, 1979–87. JAMA 262:365–369, 1989
51. Rowan JR, Hayes LM: Training curriculum on suicide detection and prevention in jails and lockups. The Jail Suicide Prevention Information Task Force, National Center on Institutions and Alternatives, in cooperation with Juvenile and Criminal Justice International, Inc. and the National Sheriffs' Association.
52. The Institute of Medicine: The Future of Public Health. Washington DC: National Academy Press, p 223, 1988.

73

Health Policy and the Politics of Health

Philip R. Lee
George A. Silver
A. E. Benjamin

Health policy and the politics of health deal with the way a society makes decisions about the health of its people and the services they receive. The term *policy* derives from the conceptualization by Lasswell and Kaplan[1] of policy as consensus, that is, a "projected program of goal values and practices." They saw the policy process as the "formulation, promulgation, and application of identifications, demands and expectations."[1]

Public policy is a reflection, however dim, of a society's values or ideals. Values or ideals (e.g., access to good health care, a sound education, responsible government) determine, in part, what we want and how we act. They influence social choices and actions.

Policies, plans, and programs are strategies to achieve goals. Policies are usually stated in terms of goals, guiding principles, or a course of action to be followed by government, as in party platforms, budget statements, reports of commissions, and decisions by international assemblies. Plans and programs define more specifically how the goals will be achieved in terms of direct actions and operating rules. These strategies—including health policy—are normally developed through political processes. Policies may be made by the legislative, executive, or judicial branches of the federal, state, or local governments to implement or interpret laws enacted by the legislative branches.

The policy-making process moves through at least three stages:

1. Agenda setting: the process by which issues come to public attention and are placed on the agenda for government action.
2. Policy adoption: the legislative process through which elected officials decide the broad outlines of policy.
3. Policy implementation: the process by which administrators develop policy by addressing the numerous issues not addressed by legislation.[2,3]

The importance of agenda setting has been described by political reporter Hedrick Smith[4] in *The Power Game: How Washington Works:*

> In the grand scheme of American government, the paramount task and power of the president is to articulate the national purpose: to fix the nation's agenda. Of all the big games at the summit of American politics, the agenda game must be won first.

As one moves from agenda setting and policy adoption to implementation, the roles of elected officials become more remote and that of administrators more important. The roles of administrators are particularly important when legislators are not specific in defining policies. The term *intentional ambiguity* has been used to denote legislative and administrative mandates that are deliberately vague and nonspecific. Intentional ambiguity is also often the aim of those who draft federal legislation. Since the law will have to be applied in 53 different jurisdictions, legislators intend that each jurisdiction should be in a position to apply the law with its own legislative and judicial structure in mind. By being broad or very general, policies provide wide latitude for program administrators in determining program goals and in developing specific strategies for achieving the goals. Estes[2] notes:

> Intentional ambiguity is likely to characterize legislation or program implementation when (1) there is little apparent national consensus on the nature of the problem to be addressed, the goals to be achieved, or the methods used in implementing policy; (2) suggested alternative policies are thought to be politically controversial, make it risky to establish an unambiguous policy choice; or (3) a measure passed by one political party is then implemented during the administration of another party with differing policies and priorities.

There are various examples of legislative ambiguity. The problems associated with the Older Americans Act have been described in detail by Estes.[2]

A central theme of Lowi's "interest group liberalism" is the growing role of administrators in politics.[3] As federal programs expanded dramatically in the 1960s, administrative agencies assumed a larger role. Often the agencies were dominated by major organized interests. Interest groups dominate the policy process, Lowi argues, not only through their influence on the legislative process (policy adoption) but also through their influence on the administration of programs (policy implementation). Recently, Smith[4] has described the role and the power of special interests in influencing federal policy decisions.

Health policy may mean defining the social objective itself, ordering priorities, or selecting the process for its implementation. Health policy is what society intends to do about all the circumstances that lead to or detract from health, that foster or prevent disease. In effect, health policy is the sum of legislative and budgeting actions that express the social will and intent to promote, maintain, or restore health and provide care for the sick and disabled.

Health policy also encompasses the measures that government adopts to achieve a variety of public health goals—in health promotion and disease prevention, in care and treatment, or in rehabilitation of the sick and disabled. To achieve these goals, government may want to influence the availability of resources through support of research, education and training of health care personnel, or the supply of health care facilities (e.g., hospitals) and equipment. The support of these activities is usually through a subsidy strategy, such as the support of biomedical research by the National Institutes of Health.[5]

However, in the light of what is customarily referred to as "health," policy goals have to do largely with obtaining preventive or curative services from the medical care establishment. For all practical purposes, health policy in this country usually means medical care policy. Other aspects of social policy are partitioned off into wage and employment policies, child care policies, educational policies, nutritional policies, environmental policies, and so on.

In addition to determination of the objective as policy, there is also selection of the route as policy. All parties and interest groups may agree on a policy objective—better access to medical care services, for example—but action may be blocked by disagreement on the way in which this should be accomplished. Policy implementation may also be characterized by bureaucratic policymaking, in that the intent of the Congress may be deflected or frustrated in the regulations adopted by the officials charged with implementation. This practice was refined by the Nixon and Reagan administrations when the Democrats dominated congressional law-making.

Brown[5] has observed that the chronological sequence of policy development in the United States in recent years has been subsidy (1945-), financing (1965-), reorganization (1970-), and regulation (1972-). Today, Brown[5] notes, "federal health policy is the sum of these four strategies of intervention, each constituting a distinct political and policy 'arena'; policy options are mainly variations on those established strategic and programmatic themes." The subsidy period began with the federal-state program of hospital planning and construction after World War II (the Hill-Burton program). Later, the support of biomedical research in universities and teaching hospitals and the development of regional medical programs in the 1960s fostered creation of tertiary care hospitals and, to a limited extent, regionalization of care. Additional efforts have included federal support for community (neighborhood) health centers, community mental health centers, and, more recently, health maintenance organizations. The big change in the federal and state roles in health care financing followed the enactment of the Medicare and Medicaid programs in 1965.

Health planning, regulation, and financial incentives have been used to affect both the supply of resources (e.g., hospital beds) and the behavior of providers (e.g., hospitals, physicians). A variety of regulatory mechanisms have been used in the past 15 years, including comprehensive health-planning agencies, professional standards review organizations, and prospective payment of hospitals by Medicare. In the early 1970s, President Nixon froze wages and prices in the health sector in order to curb inflation in health care. From 1984 through 1986, physician payments in the Medicare program were frozen by Congress to slow the growth of health expenditures.

Finally, since the goal of social-health policy is not merely to replace individual solutions with bureaucratic solutions but also to adjust social action (e.g., public programs, governmental legislation) to changing conceptions of the social role, there arises the question of where the initiative for policy begins. What triggers examination of, and decisions on, policies? It ends, obviously, with legislative action or lack of it. One can assume a "top down" pattern of the formulation of health policy, in which the initiative is taken by the Congress, or a "bottom up" pattern, in which local grievances are transformed into local mandates for action, becoming national policies over time.

CHARACTERISTICS OF THE POLICY PROCESS

To understand health policy and the politics of health in the United States, it is important to appreciate the social, political, cultural, and economic factors that shape health policy.

In the United States, more than in any other western industrialized democracy, the role of government has been to support and subsidize the private sector. The primary economic justification for government intervention has been to remedy market failure. In spite of the enormous changes in the United States in the past 200 years, that basic justification remains. Certainly, there is ample evidence of market failure in public health and medical care.

Government policies and programs at the federal, state, and local levels play a major role in the planning, development, financing, organization, and regulation of health care. Public programs account for an increasing share of the nation's personal health care expenditures. Most physicians and health care workers have been trained at public expense, most nonprofit community and university hospitals have been built or modernized with government subsidies, and the bulk of all health research and development funds are provided by the government.[6] Government supports the functioning of the private sector more often than it serves as a provider of care, although that does occur when the market fails, as in the care of the poor.

There are aspects of the American scene—history, traditions, popular attitudes, and socioeconomic patterns—that make unique contributions to the development of public policy, factors that distinguish the American policy possibilities from those of other nations. The special factors that shape public policy in the United States include (1) the American character, (2) federalism, (3) pluralism, and (4) incrementalism.

The American Character. "National character" is not an inherited quality. Climate, geography, cultural and traditional approaches to education, and upbringing foster similarities in response and social behavior among the majority of a country's citizens. The American character embodies a distrust of government, an independent nature, and an entrepreneurial focus, along with an emphasis on the primacy of the private sector, even in public policy. The American character also combines idealism with practical realism, compassion with hardheadedness when it comes to solving problems. "Americans are proud and loud, daring and caring. They extol individuality but always pitch in when it comes to helping others . . . they are industrious, hospitable, brash, confident, outspoken and resourceful" (de Tocqueville).[7] Typical American traits described by various authors are paradoxical: Americans are both entrepreneurial and cooperative, competitive and collaborative, individualistic and communal, loners and teamworkers, selfish and altruistic. Americans have a social conscience, believing in equality and social justice, in community action. But, at the same time, Americans are "me-first individualists" who relish competition, value hard work, and jealously guard their own property.[8]

There is a marked difference in the way Americans react to social demand. American responses are different from European responses in general, even as the European countries differ from one another. Lynn Payer[9] describes the differences in approach to diagnosis and treatment of disease in various countries. The

United States, she writes, "shows a . . . frontier mentality and orientation toward aggressive action linked to the aggressiveness and impatience of American physicians and their radical orientation to the use of many surgical interventions." The use of medical services also varies from country to country, reflecting differing views about the role of medical care. The average number of physician visits per patient in different countries varies widely—an average of 12 to 15 visits a year per person in Israel, 10 to 12 visits in Germany, 4 to 5 visits in the United States and England, and 2 to 3 visits in Scandinavia."[9]

Today's Americans, separated by hundreds of years from the forces that have molded their attitudes and values, continue to exhibit contradictory social attitudes. Public opinion polls are so paradoxical as to call forth a diagnosis of "schizophrenia." Despite a commitment to help one another, to use the great powers of the American nation to promote quality, Americans "continue to oppose the use of government to achieve necessary social objectives."[10] This opposition to collective action by government has deep roots in the origins of the republic.[11]

In essence, American attitudes toward government make a difference in how Americans go about making public policy. There is in this the ambivalence Americans feel about government involvement in personal matters. This is coupled with the scorn Americans usually express about the ineptitude of government actions and the sluggish or inappropriate response to public-social needs. European countries tend to assign social welfare policies (including health) to the governmental sector. The United States has always been reluctant to begin with governmental action and has tended to pick and choose among social responsibilities before responding with a public program. Individual, family, or private charitable resources are considered to be the appropriate response mechanisms in the first instance. Government is the succor of last resort.

This duality of the American character is what accounts for the cyclical shifts in election returns and public policies. The rhetoric of political leadership determines which aspects of the divided self will be called forth for public expression. Since each person manages to contain within himself or herself these contradictory characteristics, the leadership that strongly supports social action calls forth that part of the character; support of inaction may be equally evoked. Leadership determines the response.

Federalism. Federalism is another powerful determinant of health policy, largely overlooked in consideration of policy formulation. "Federalism represents a form of governance that differs both from a unitary state, where regional and local authority derive legally from the central government, and from a confederation, in which the national government has limited authority and does not reach individual citizens directly."[12]

The concept of federalism remains a point of political and constitutional controversy and debate, as it has over much of the nation's 200-year history.[13] Federalism was originally a legal concept that defined the division of authority between the federal government and the states. The concept stressed the independence of each level of government from the other and incorporated the idea that some functions (e.g., foreign policy, defense) were the exclusive province of the central government, while other functions (e.g., education, police protection) were the responsibility of state and local government.[14] Both public health and medical care were long thought to be primarily the responsibility of state and local government and the private sector, including the individual who must pay out of pocket.

Formally, national legislation (the effect of policymaking) is a result of the interaction of the national government and the participant governing bodies in the states and localities. Dominance and division of responsibility among governmental levels in the public sector represent the federalist influence. At different times in American history different elements have dominated the policy process, and the division of responsibility has rarely, if ever, been equal.

From its inception, the eighteenth century independence movement was sharply divided between those who sought autonomy for the individual states (states' rights advocates) and proponents of central authority. The budding American republic required the united confidence of these opposing factions. The Constitution indulged in an ambiguity of phrasing, language intended to satisfy both sides and thus prevent early dissolution of the union. While much of the conflict was discreetly compromised away in the Constitution, the opposing views continued—and still continue—to trouble the political process. In Article 6 of the Constitution (the "supremacy clause") the central authority is proclaimed to enunciate "the supreme law of the land." The Tenth Amendment (adopted 4 years later as part of the Bill of Rights) states, however, that "the powers not delegated to the United States by the Constitution, nor prohibited by it to the states, are reserved to the states respectively, or to the people." In this way, neither states nor central authority could claim absolute authority. The compromise meant that American federalism would eternally guarantee friction and competition between the protagonists of state sovereignty against those of federal dominance. Bitter rivalries persisted—and continue to this day—among politicians of both persuasions.

In addition to the ambiguity generated at the structural level by this uncertainly defined concept of federalism, there is a similar ambiguity at the functional level. If federalism allots to the states those powers not specifically assigned to the federal government in the Constitution, is it not also appropriate to assume that all matters relating to welfare will originate and be implemented and supervised at the state level? On the other hand, if we are all equally citizens of the United States, is it not the responsibility of the central government to protect us in these matters as well as against a foreign foe? Elazar[15] considered this dual federalism—"two separate federal and state streams flowing in distinct but closely parallel channels"—to be the earliest dominant mode and a true reflection of postcolonial sentiments. Within this framework, the federal government and the states operate more or less in parallel, neither yielding to nor imposing on the other.

Although the concept of separation of functions within the federal system continues today, there is a complex web of relationships among federal, state, and local governments and the private sector with respect to domestic social programs. The relationships are further complicated because federal fiscal, monetary, defense, and foreign policies have a profound effect on state and local governments and their capacity to meet social needs.[16] What seems to matter most in the structure of relationships within federalism is not so much the distribution of activities among levels of governments but the relationships among them.[17]

The differing views about the concept of federalism are clearly illustrated in the contrasting policies of Roosevelt's New Deal and Reagan's New Federalism. The Great Depression inaugurated a sharp change in attitudes about the role of the federal government. President Franklin D. Roosevelt spelled it out in his first inaugural address: "The emergency was national because of the 'interdependence of the various elements in, and parts of, the United States.' The mode of action must be national."[18] Once the New Deal had demonstrated the necessity for federal action in meeting national social emergencies (as well as staving off economic collapse), a period of federal dominance and control over the states was initiated. "Federalism" came to mean the way the states reacted to federal initiatives. The New Deal "revolution" overlooked, or downgraded, the useful aspects of the states' strengths. In particular, the danger of losing the states' innovative contribution was overlooked.

After 50 years of a type of federalism in which the federal government called the tune to which the states danced, a variety of social, economic, and military forces combined to change popular attitudes about this condition. Ronald Reagan was elected President with an apparent mandate to end the overwhelming dominance of the national political establishment. The backbone of the Reagan New Federalism effort to divest the federal government of its responsibilities was based on one traditional interpretation of the federalism thesis—that the states are constitutionally responsible for providing health and welfare policies and programs. The Reagan administration's vision of federalism emphasized the devolution of responsibilities to governments that are closer to the people.

Reagan's New Federalism had as its "ultimate goal . . . to sort out functional responsibilities between the federal and state governments and to turn back appropriate revenue sources and decision-making authority to the states."[19]

If, however, the role of federalism includes the need for states to initiate policy, neither those who support the Reagan doctrine nor those who attack the principle, are dealing with the crucial defect of the New Federalism. It has come to mean the sloughing off of federal responsibility. While states initiate policy and test social programs, the federal government should be supplementing and complementing the state effort.

Brizius,[20] reviewing the influence of federalism in achieving a national purpose, contrasts the trend toward centralization with the important factors that counsel decentralization. While equity and efficiency, for example, might urge centralized efforts, these are not necessarily the sole product of centralization, and the need for diversity, accountability, and competition might well outweigh other considerations.

The argument about centralization and decentralization has not been settled, despite vigorous debate in recent years. No agreement has been reached on the vital question of the distribution of authority and responsibility among various levels of government. While the federal government finances or regulates certain health activities (e.g., hospital and medical services for the elderly through Medicare, biomedical research, the entry of new drugs into the market, and environmental/occupational health measures), both state and local governments are mandated by higher levels of government—either by regulation or by court order—to provide services or implement various environmental health or occupational health and safety regulations.

States spend a large portion of their general fund budgets on health care for the poor (Medicaid), on mental health services, on the support of a range of public health programs, and on the education and training of health professionals. However, state governments often depend on local governments (counties, cities, special districts) to deliver the necessary health services (e.g., hospital, outpatient, and emergency care for the poor, mental health and substance abuse services, and a variety of public health services). To further complicate the problem of intergovernmental responsibility and authority, local governments may deal directly with the federal government in connection with grant-in-aid programs. Local governments, particularly in recent years, have often been ahead of the federal government and state governments in responding to local needs. Local health agencies also differ in their relationships with the private sector.

The Advisory Committee on Intergovernmental Relations has three proposals for reforming federalism:

1. Decongestion or a better assignment and reordering of government functions, urging a centralization of fiscal and administrative responsibilities for a "cluster of national responsibilities, chiefly welfare programs and income and employment security."
2. Full devolution of a range of other program responsibilities in which the federal government role is fiscally modest or in which the federal aid outlay is small.
3. Consolidation into block grants those remaining categorical grants that operate in program areas that are of an intergovernmental nature.[21]

Although the choices may seem clear, the effects of the choices on health policies are not so clear. It also is not at all certain how the attempts by the Reagan administration to alter the federal role in domestic health programs will fare in the long run. Nor is it clear what the alternatives proposed by the Advisory Committee on Intergovernmental Relations would do in terms of equity, effectiveness of program implementation, and costs.

Pluralism. The ideology of pluralism has greatly influenced the shape, scope, and effectiveness of health policies in the United States. It allows for simultaneous reliance on public and private sector initiatives and permits acquiescence to market forces and competition along with governmental involvement in the same field. For instance, legislative action depends on consensus among ethnic, religious, political, and social groups, and majority policy decisions may mean acknowledging demands of all participants in the consensus. The result may be the creation of plural programs—duplicative, competitive, and presumably complementary, though not necessarily cooperative.[22] For example, the neighborhood health centers, created by the Office of Economic Opportunity in the 1960s and 1970s, were supported with federal funds and paid in part by Medicaid. At the same time, Medicaid was paying private practitioners and hospital clinics for services to the same clientele. All were presumably reaching out to the same pool of clients, but there was no attempt to organize or rationalize service commitments.

The concept of pluralism posits that a variety of actors have a place at the policy table. The result has been the extraordinary influence exerted by special interests on health policy in the United States. Ginzberg[23] identified four power centers in the health care field that influence the nature of health care and the role of government: (1) physicians, (2) large insurance organizations, (3) hospitals, and (4) a highly diversified group of participants in profit-making activities within the health care arena. These interest groups, with governmental executives and congressional committees, are major actors in what Cater[24] described as a "new form of federalism." He noted,

> In the politics of modern America, a new form of federalism has emerged, more relevant to the distribution of power than the old. The old federalism which ordered power according to geographic hegemonies—national, state, and local—no longer adequately describes the governing arrangement. New subgovernmental arrangements have grown up, by which much of the pressing domestic business is ordered.

Health has become one of the largest and most powerful subgovernments, with growing influence by provider interests. Although the broad goals of federal and state health policies have been fairly clear, the proliferation of categorical programs has tended to respond to the needs of particular interests rather than contribute to the broader public interest.

Pluralism is a prime characteristic of the American health care system and the process by which domestic social policy decisions are made. As Lewis[25] noted, "Pluralism has come to mean a system of government where everybody is in charge, and nobody is in charge." In this pluralistic system of interest group influence, government has become only another actor at the bargaining table.

Incrementalism. The best descriptions of the policy process are in Lindblom's concepts of "muddling through" and "incrementalism." Lindblom[26] writes of the American scene: "Policymaking is a process of successive approximation of some desired objectives in which what is desired itself continues to change under reconsideration.'' He calls this process the ''science of muddling through.''

A closely allied concept, unique in American policymaking, is one he calls incrementalism, ''a method of social action that takes existing reality as one alternative and compares the probable gains and losses of closely related alternatives by making relatively small adjustments in existing reality, or making larger adjustments about whose consequences approximately as much is known as about the consequences of existing reality, or both.'' This politically effective process offers excellent scope for compromise, because both parties recognize its impermanence. ''Policy is not made once and for all. It is made and remade endlessly.''[26]

The incremental model posits that policy is made in small steps (increments) and that policy is rarely modified in dramatic ways. Prior policy becomes the basis for most subsequent policy decisions. Since major policy decisions often have unintended consequences, policymakers usually opt for gradual modifications to avoid the risks of major change.

An example of incremental change was the gradual evolution of the National Institutes of Health from a small federal laboratory conducting biomedical research in the 1930s to a multibillion dollar research enterprise. The addition of new institutes took place over a 50-year period. Budgets also grew gradually, beginning after World War II. Even when major health policy initiatives such as Medicare and Medicaid were adopted, the change was in the source of funds to pay for medical care for the elderly and the poor, not in the organization or provision of medical care.

European countries that practice a parliamentary rather than representative democracy can effect larger changes more swiftly. In the parliamentary form of government, party policies are implemented speedily because the winning party practices bloc voting. Delay occurs only when there is inability to achieve power. In representative governments, the parties cannot manage the discipline necessary to enforce party loyalty to programs or policies because elected representatives owe more (or at least as much) to their personal appeal than to party designation.

THE EVOLUTION OF HEALTH POLICY IN THE UNITED STATES

The Bases for Federal, State, and Local Involvement in Health Policy. The basis for federal involvement in health policy rests on the interpretation of the commerce clause and the welfare clause of the Constitution by the U.S. Congress, the Executive Branch, and, ultimately, the U.S. Supreme Court. While the Constitution granted primary responsibility for the health of the public to the states, four developments have significantly expanded the federal role. First, the Supreme Court decision in 1813 established the doctrine of implied powers, which expanded the powers beyond those specifically delegated in the Constitution to those reasonably implied by the delegated powers.[27] Second, the passage in 1913 of the Sixteenth Amendment authorizing a national income tax significantly expanded the revenue-raising capacity of the federal government, permitting it to deal with domestic social needs. Third, in 1937 the Supreme Court upheld the constitutionality of the Social Security Act on the basis of the general welfare clause of the Constitution, interpreting it broadly enough to permit a wide range of federal interventions previously deemed the domain of the states. Finally, the Civil Rights Act of 1964 provided the means to assure equal treatment of all citizens.

The role of state governments in health policy is based on federal and state legislation, state constitutions, and rulings by federal and state courts. In 1824 the U.S. Supreme Court ruled that ''inspection laws, quarantine laws, health laws of every description'' were the responsibility of states because they were not specifically assigned to the federal government by the Constitution.[28] And local governments draw their authority from the states.

States as Sources of Authority and Innovation. The evolution of policymaking in the United States has been profoundly influenced by the ''doctrine that the states are the source of authority from which all other governments are derived.''[29] During the evolution of social policy building, the states met their own social needs.

American politicians and foreign observers in the nineteenth century agreed that the key to effective social action was state action. Lord Bryce[30] observed that initiating action at the state level allows ''people to try experiments in legislation and administration which could not safely be tried in a large centralized country. A comparatively small commonwealth like an American state easily makes and unmakes its laws; mistakes are not serious, for they are soon corrected; other states profit by the experience of a law or a method which has worked well or ill in the state that has tried it.''

Justice Brandeis,[31] in a famous dissent, made an even more cogent statement in that connection, suggesting that state initiatives might actually be requirements for eventual national action. ''It is one of the happy incidents of the federal system that a single courageous state may, if its citizens so choose, serve as a laboratory and try novel social and economic experiments without risk to the rest of the country.'' It can be argued that, without previous state models, federal legislation may be inexpertly drawn, so as to require reexamination and revision soon after passage and frequently thereafter—as in the case of Medicare—because the inherent errors of legislating de novo need constant correction. If the principle goes through the molding process of trials in one or more states, the eventual national legislation might be more prudently drawn and more likely to stand up to the exigencies of implementation.

The Committee for the Study of the Future of Public Health/Institute of Medicine[27] identified two key ingredients in the state role in public health:

- Statewide assessment, policy development, and assurance that the functions and services necessary to meet the needs throughout the state are in place. The functions may be carried out through local government, the private sector, or the state government.
- Designation of a lead agency for public health in the state to assure that the functions of assessment, policy development, and assurance are properly carried out.

States first exercised their public health authority through special committees or commissions to control communicable diseases. Louisiana established the first state department of health in 1855. Massachusetts followed in 1869. By 1915 public health agencies had been established in every state. Today there are state health agencies in every state, the District of Columbia, and the six U.S. territories. In addition, there are more than 3000 local health departments within the United States. The authority of the local agencies to protect the public health derives from the authority that resides in the state constitution. Over the years many federal policies (e.g., child health, old age assistance) had their origins in state policy.

A half dozen states—including New York, Maryland, Connecticut, and Massachusetts—were the first to initiate health care regulation, using their constitutional powers to establish vigorous certificate-of-need and hospital rate-setting programs independent of federal mandates. National health-planning legislation and a variety of cost-control measures, including review of professional activities, followed state models.[19]

After the Civil War, state control began to slip and social welfare began to be recognized as something of a federal responsibility as well as a state one.[32] Growing affluence, along with increased population growth and migration, made it difficult for the states to operate completely on their own. The period of cooperative federalism began.[15] Initially, however, the federal government played only a limited role in public health.

Expansion of the Federal Role. In the early years of the republic, the federal government played a limited role in health policy, which was left largely to the jurisdiction of the states and the private sector. Private charity shouldered the responsibility for the care of the poor, including the medical care that was provided. Although the federal government did provide for care of sick and disabled seamen as early as 1798 and imposed a quarantine on ships entering U.S. ports, it did not play a significant role in public health until the twentieth century.

When the national government did enter into legislation of social measures, it first undertook to give national exposure to what had been state pioneering efforts. The Social Security Act embodied pieces of previously enacted state legislation.[33] The Act established the principle of federal aid to the states for public health, maternal and child health, and welfare assistance. It also provided the structure for old age insurance, unemployment insurance, and disability insurance. It was to be the basis, 30 years later, for Medicare and Medicaid.

The involvement of the national government in health services—largely financial initiatives toward structural reform—was a New Deal development. The needs were great, the capabilities of the states clearly inadequate, and national action was obviously the only solution. The Great Depression changed people's attitudes toward government, toward social policy, and toward themselves.

In the 1930s and 1940s there was a gradual expansion of the federal role, particularly in support of biomedical research, in hospital planning and construction, and in the provision of hospital care for veterans. However, when the emergency generated by the Great Depression abated and the incredible level of unemployment declined, many of the old attitudes toward governmental intervention returned. Incrementalism was the order of the day.

The 1960s brought a period of renewed faith in the federal government. The Kerr-Mills Act of 1960 was a major watershed; for the first time, the federal government authorized grants-in-aid to the states for medical services for a class of citizens with no federal connections whatever—the aged. The election of President Johnson in 1964 saw a rapid expansion of the federal role. During the Johnson presidency the traditional federal-state relationship was expanded to include direct federal support for local government, as well as for a wide range of nonprofit and proprietary institutions enlisted to carry out health policy, education, employment and training, housing and community development, and other federal objectives. There was the Civil Rights Act in 1964; federal aid to the schools, which provided for added support for health services for schoolchildren; the Economic Opportunity Act, which introduced far-reaching federal intervention into personal health matters as federal concerns; and the Health Professions Education Assistance Act of 1963, which brought the federal government into medical education. More than 200 categorical grant-in-aid programs were enacted during the Johnson presidency.[6] This was a period of growing concern about inequities in access to health care and growing acceptance of a larger role of the public sector in health care. Subsidies to expand resources were provided and new financing mechanisms (Medicare, Medicaid) were introduced to assure the elderly and the poor access to health care. Brown[5] stated it succinctly: "Equity was at the heart of the period's public philosophy."

With the rapid growth of categorical grants-in-aid during the 1960s, there was growing concern on the part of state and local government officials about excessive federal direction and control. This concern resulted in two separate approaches—block grants and revenue sharing in the 1970s. Block grants were given for broader purposes than categorical grants-in-aid but were limited to a particular area, such as mental health, child health, or public health. Revenue sharing, in contrast, simply turned over to state and local governments federal revenues that could be used for broad purposes at the discretion of the state and local governments. Revenue sharing disappeared in the 1980s because of the rapid increase in the federal deficit.

In the 1970s more health legislation came into being, aimed at improving the organization of the medical care system and regulating medical practice. At about this time, both the Congress and the Executive Branch began to worry about unplanned growth and associated uncontrollable costs, duplication, and waste. Planning was seen as necessary to control costs. The Hospital Survey and Construction Act (1946) and the Regional Medical Programs and the Comprehensive Health Planning Act (1965) had been only cautious intrusions into planning. The National Health Planning and Resources Act (1974) proved to be equally toothless. Inflation continued.

Between 1963 and 1983, more than 50 federally sponsored and supported programs involving medical care services came into being. In that interval, the federal contribution to the overall payments for medical care rose from 12% to 40% and the total expenditures for medical care rose from $3 billion to almost $500 billion, a rate of increase far in excess of the rate of increase in the gross national product.

Unwilling to enact a comprehensive national medical care program, yet beset by simultaneous demands for additional services and mounting and uncontrollable inflation of costs (and associated tax-funding requirements), legislators seized on bits and pieces of legislative action in desperate efforts to expand services and at the same time control costs.

There followed a period of growing conviction in the marketplace about the role of the private sector in dealing with the pressing public health and medical care issues of the day. The priorities shifted from equity and access to cost containment and efficiency. Both Presidents Nixon and Reagan advocated New Federalism with decentralization of authority and responsibility from the federal government to state and local governments and to the private sector.

The experience of almost 50 years of a national hegemony in the financing and control of public services so dominated our lives that we think of that national role as "traditional." The concept of federalism as a philosophy of shared powers, of cooperative efforts by the state and the federal governments, and the loss of either partner as a fatal blow to the national purpose was almost erased.

Need for a New Partnership. The federal establishment is too cumbersome to allow for detailed operative supervision. A multiplicity of projects in the same general area may be funded by many different agencies, and even departments, with no overall control of the interaction or complementarity of the projects. A congressional committee reported that, in addition to 11 different health programs, there were 12 income-maintenance programs, 9 nutrition programs, 19 social service programs, 12 education and training programs, 4 housing programs, and 4 tax programs specifically addressing children's issues. These were lodged in 13 independent offices and cabinet departments, each of which is represented by several agencies.[34] It has been noted by Berkelhamer, Noyes, and Chen[35]: "Within the vast federal bureaucracy there is no single voice focussing on the long-term needs of the maternal and child population in any kind of comprehensive framework. There are more than a hundred voices scattered through six Cabinet departments, each of which competes for its own priorities with its own justifications.''[35] In the area of aging, there are more than 80 federal programs.[2] Congressional oversight is, of course, situated in a correspondingly diverse number of committees of the House and Senate, not to mention administration and oversight in the associated state and local bureaus, offices, and legislative committees. This has led to a patchwork of programs and fragmentation, which results in a multiplication of administrative costs and responsibility and even failure of the overall effort to meet the desired goals.

It appears that the pendulum is swinging back to state initiatives. In fact, the actions of the Reagan and Bush administrations have forced the states to invent and make do to meet their responsibilities as help from the federal government has dwindled. To an extent, this ''growth through struggle'' has succeeded in stimulating the states to understake their traditional tasks. In some states, the legislatures and governors have risen to the occasion and either found funds to maintain the defunded federal programs or even found ways of starting additional ones.[36]

The Brandeis thesis that innovation should be encouraged inasmuch as the states are ''laboratories of democracy'' is central to the argument for devolution: democratic values embrace pluralism and popular sovereignty. In addition, there are checks and balances in such a sharing, so that ''hasty, ill-considered and possibly unconstitutional actions by one level of government can be challenged by other levels.''[20]

The federal government needs to use its capabilities and authority to stimulate the states, using grants and other federal support, to seek new and imaginative answers to pressing national social and health problems. The policies that emerge from one or more state models can serve as templates for national solutions. Schultze[37] urges ''market analogues''—public funding of competing public programs, so as to allow selection of the most efficient, economical, and satisfactory one—which such encouragement of multiple state experimentation would permit.[37]

The failure of the United States to legislate a broad-based national health program derives, at least in part, from a failure to recognize traditional American practice in health policy formulation. The lack of state models in advance of national action and attempts to initiate action at the federal level have obstructed national policy development. In effect, the failure to follow the pattern of employing state initiatives on which to base federal action has not only delayed the inauguration of a national health policy, it has so complicated the issue that wholly new approaches may be required.

Of course, the transformation in medical care objectives and professional attitudes was not solely the result of the federalization of policymaking that began in the 1930s. A great deal has been learned about the capability and effectiveness of a dynamic federal role. There have been necessary and desirable accomplishments as a result of federal intervention and command. A new approach will have to partake of both past and present concepts of federalism, giving states back their proper role of initiation but supplying a federal role parallel to and supportive of state initiative.

The 1990s have dawned on a continuing cost crisis in health care, with a growing number of uninsured persons (now approximately 31 million), a rising number of persons with AIDS who require costly and often intensive levels of care, and an epidemic of drug abuse, particularly involving cocaine, that is sweeping the urban areas of the country with a devastating effect on pregnant women and their infants. Incremental change and pluralistic solutions may not suffice in the face of these growing challenges. Already state developments in Medicaid reform, programs for the uninsured and underinsured, global budgeting for hospitals, and rudimentary comprehensive and compulsory health insurance programs suggest that the traditional American approach to national health and welfare programming—state initiatives—is gathering strength. Incremental change has been too slow, and as dissatisfaction and frustration mount, different state approaches may make it possible for a national program to rise out of the lessons learned from the mistakes and successes of these state efforts.

REFERENCES

1. Lasswell HD, Kaplan A: Power and Society. New Haven: Yale University Press, 1950, p 71
2. Estes CL: The Aging Enterprise. San Francisco: Jossey-Bass Publishers, 1980, pp 61–74
3. Lowi TJ: The End of Liberalism: The Second Republic of the United States. New York: WW Norton, 1979
4. Smith H: The Power Game: How Washington Works. New York: Random House, 1988
5. Brown LD: Health Policy in the United States: Issues and Options. (Occasional Paper #4, Ford Foundation Project on Social Welfare and the American Future). New York: Ford Foundation, 1988, pp 3–8, 49–56
6. Lee PR, Benjamin AE: Health policy and the politics of health care. In Williams SJ, Torrens PR (eds): Introduction of Health Services, 3 edt. New York: John Wiley, 1988, p 459
7. Atlantic Monthly, May 1986, p 33
8. Hummel RP, Isaak RA: The Real American Politics. Englewood Cliffs, NJ: Prentice-Hall, 1986, p 26
9. Payer L: Medicine and Culture: Varieties of Treatment in the United States, England, West Germany and France. New York: Henry Holt, 1988
10. Free LA, Cantril H: The Political Beliefs of Americans. New Brunswick, NJ: Rutgers University Press, 1967, pp 178–180
11. Chisman FP, Pifer A: Government for the People—The Federal Social Role: What It Is, What It Should Be. New York: WW Norton, 1987, pp 47–58
12. Vladeck BC: The design of failure: health policy and the structure of federalism. J Health Polit Policy Law 4:522–535, 1979
13. Walker D: Toward a Functioning Federalism. Cambridge, Mass: Winthrop Publishers Inc., 1981
14. Reagan M, Sanzone JG: The New Federalism, 2 edt. New York: Oxford University Press, 1981, p 7
15. Elazar DJ: The American Partnership. Chicago: University of Chicago Press, 1962
16. Reagan MD: The New Federalism. New York: Oxford University Press, 1972
17. Clarke GJ: The role of the states in the delivery of health services. Am J Public Health 71(suppl):59–69, 1981
18. Advisory Committee on Intergovernmental Relations: Breakdown of constitutional restraints: Interpretive variations from the first constitutional revolution to the ''fourth.'' In The Condition of Contemporary Federalism (Report #A-78). Washington, DC: The Committee, August 1981, chap. 2
19. Greenberg G, Feldman P: New federalism and state support of technology assessment. In Institute of Medicine, Assessing Medical Technologies. Appendix B. Washington DC: National Academy of Science Press, 1986, pp 542–553
20. Brizius JA: Federalism and National Purpose (Working Paper #2). Washington DC: Project on the Federal Social Role, July 26, 1984, pp 72–98
21. Advisory Committee on Intergovernmental Relations: The Transformation in American Politics: Implications for Federalism (Report #A-106). Washington DC: The Committee, August 1986
22. Bankowski Z, Bryant J: Health Policy, Ethics and Human Values. Geneva: CIOMS, 1985, p 22
23. Ginzberg E (ed): Regionalization and Health Policy. Washington DC: U.S. Government Printing Office, 1977

24. Cater D: An overview. In Cater D, Lee PR (eds): Politics of Health. New York: Medcom Press, 1972, p 4
25. Lewis IJ: Evolution of federal policy on access to health care, 1965–80. Presentation to New York Academy of Medicine, 1982
26. Lindblom CE: The science of "muddling through." Public Adm Rev 10:79–88, 1959
27. Institute of Medicine, Committee for the Study of the Future of Public Health: The Future of Public Health. Washington DC: National Academy Press, 1988, pp 35–55
28. Lashof J, Lepper M: Federal-state-local partnership in health. In Health in America, 1776–1976. DHEW Publication No. (HRA) 76-616. Washington DC: U.S. Government Printing Office, 1976, p 123
29. Kaufman H: Politics and Policies in State and Local Governments. Englewood Cliffs, NJ: Prentice-Hall, 1963, p 30
30. Bryce J: The American Commonwealth. New York: Putnam, 1959, pp 81–88
31. Brandeis LD: New State Ice Company v Liebman (285 U.S. 262), 1932
32. Grob GN: Mental Illness and American Society, 1875–1940. Princeton, NJ: Princeton University Press, 1983, p 106
33. Jacob H, Vines KN: Politics in the American States. Boston: Little Brown, 1971, p 389
34. U.S. Congress, Select Committee on Children, Youth, and Families: Federal Programs Affecting Children. Washington DC: U.S. Government Printing Office, 1984
35. Berkehamer JE, Noyes EJ, Chen RT: Child health policy—an overview of federal involvement. In Year Book of Pediatrics, Chicago: Yearbook Medical Publishers, 1982, p 211
36. Palmer JL, Sawhill IV (eds): The Reagan Experiment. Washington DC: Urban Institute Press, 1982
37. Schultze CL: The public use of private interest. Harper's, May 1977, pp 43–62

74

Public Health Responses to Natural and Human-made Disasters

Victor W. Sidel
Erol Onel
H. Jack Geiger
Jennifer Leaning
William H. Foege

Disasters are a major cause of premature death, impaired health status, and diminished quality of life. Indeed, the direct effect on humans, on the environment, or on physical structures important to humans usually defines whether a phenomenon will be viewed as a "disaster"[1,2] (Table 74–1). The importance of disasters has been recognized by the designation of the 1990s as the "International Decade for Natural Disaster Reduction" by the United Nations.[3]

In approximate order of the importance of their effects on humans, the most destructive natural disasters are climatological (e.g., floods, storms) rather than geological (e.g., earthquakes, volcanic eruptions, and tsunami) (Table 74–2). Climatological disasters are more frequent than geological disasters. Whether measured by economic loss or by deaths and injuries, Asia is most prone to natural disasters; Latin America and Africa are intermediate; and North America, Europe, and Australia are least prone. For each major natural disaster in Europe and Australia, there are 10 in Latin America and Africa and 15 in Asia.[1]

There are many types of disaster beyond those usually considered "natural." While the consequences of geological and climatological disasters are often exacerbated by preceding human activities, with the exception of certain forms of flood and drought, they are unlikely to be caused by humans. In contrast, many other disasters have large elements of human causation, either accidental or intended. We can classify them into three types: (1) sudden disasters, (2) insidious disasters, and (3) war and civil conflict (Table 74–2).

Examples of sudden disaster in which human factors rather than natural factors bear the major responsibility include the release of methyl isocyanate at a pesticide plant in Bhopal, India,[4,5] in 1984 and of radioactive substances following an explosion at the Chernobyl nuclear power reactor in the Soviet Union in 1986.[6] Even sudden disasters that are considered natural are often caused by preceding human activities. For example, disastrous flooding may be the result of deforestation or of construction of dams.[7]

Examples of insidious and continuing disasters include the leakage of toxic chemicals from a dump site at Love Canal in Buffalo, N.Y.,[8,9] the tainting of the soil in Times Beach, Mo., with dioxin in oils sprayed on the roads,[10] and the leakage of radioactive materials from nuclear weapons production facilities.[11] Some natural phenomena, such as prolonged drought, may be considered continuing disasters. Other forms of long-term and continuing human-made disasters include global warming (the "greenhouse effect") caused by heat-trapping gases in the atmosphere released by burning of fossil fuels, depletion of the ozone layer due to the use of aerosolized chlorofluorohydrocarbons, and acid precipitation (see Chapter 39).

In many ways the most pernicious human-made disasters are wars and civil conflicts. In 1981 the World Health Assembly[12] stated that "The role of physicians and other health workers in the prevention of war and promotion of peace is the most significant factor for the attainment of health for all."

PUBLIC HEALTH CONSEQUENCES OF DISASTERS

Disasters can cause short-term morbidity, mortality, and damage to quality of life as well as long-term environmental changes that will increase morbidity, premature death, and diminished quality of life in the future. The causes of short-term morbidity and mortality can be classified into four types: injuries, emotional stress, epidemics, and increase in indigenous diseases. Injuries usually exceed deaths in storms, explosions, fires, famines, and epidemics, and deaths frequently exceed injuries in earthquakes, landslides, avalanches, volcanic eruptions, tidal waves, and floods.

Serious epidemics might be classified as disasters, but they may also be the result of disasters. Epidemic or enhanced endemic diseases that may follow a disaster include food-and waterborne illnesses (e.g., typhoid and cholera), vectorborne illnesses (e.g., plague and malaria), and diseases spread by person-to-person contact (e.g., hepatitis A and shigellosis) or by the respiratory route (e.g., measles and influenza).[13]

Improvements in environmental sanitation, immunization, disease surveillance, and other aspects of public health and preventive medicine have led to a significant reduction in the threat

TABLE 74–1. SHORT-TERM HEALTH EFFECTS OF NATURAL DISASTERS

	Earthquakes	Hurricanes High Winds	Volcanic Eruptions	Floods	Tidal Wave Flash Flood
Deaths	Many	Few	Varies	Few	Many
Severe injuries requiring intensive medical care	Overwhelming	Moderate	Varies	Few	Few
Increased risk of infectious disease	Potential problem in all major disasters (probability rises with overcrowding and deteriorating sanitation)				
Food scarcity	Rare (may occur because of factors other than food shortages)	Rare	Common	Common	Common
Major population movements	Rare (may occur in heavily damaged urban areas)	Rare	Common	Common	Common

From Pan American Health Organization. International Health Relief Assistance: *A Guide for Effective Aid.* Washington, D.C.: The Organization, 1990, p 12.

of disease after disasters. People in Europe and North America are usually at risk of relatively few diseases that might follow disasters, such as food poisoning, sewage poisoning, nonspecific diarrhea, hepatitis A, shigellosis, and influenza. The low risk of other diseases is due to their disappearance from the population (e.g., smallpox, plague), high immunity levels produced by vaccines (e.g., measles, whooping cough, tetanus), availability of antimicrobial agents (e.g., streptococcal disease, tuberculosis), and a significant reduction in the prevalence of the illnesses (e.g., typhoid fever).[13] Disasters are often followed by increases in the prevalence of diseases indigenous to the area because of the disruption of health facilities and programs.

Disaster survivors often exhibit emotional stress, the "disaster shock" syndrome: successive stages of shock, suggestibility, euphoria, and frustration. These stages may vary in extent and duration.[13] A wide range of psychological reactions to disaster, many requiring assistance, have been reported (Table 74–3).

Public health measures can prevent much of the death, injury, and economic disruption due to disasters. *Primary prevention* represents efforts to prevent the occurrence of the disaster, and *secondary prevention* covers efforts to mitigate disaster consequences by preparing for them in advance by early recognition of the disaster and countermeasures to reduce the consequences after the disaster has occurred.

Sudden Disasters

Climatological Disasters. Flash floods and more predictable coastal and river floods destroy water purification and sewage-disposal systems, cause overflow of toxic waste sites, enhance vector-breeding conditions, and rupture underground pipelines and storage tanks. Long-term effects reported to be associated with floods include increased infectious diseases and toxic effects and increases in hypertensive disease, leukemia, lymphoma, and psychological disorders.[14]

The most frequent cause of death in water-based storms is drowning. Winds can also cause trauma and death. Human shelter is particularly vulnerable in poor countries. Sewage systems and water supplies may be disrupted, and serious psychological trauma can occur.[15] In land-based storms injuries and deaths are largely due to physical trauma rather than to drowning, but the long-term effects may be similar to those of water-based storms.[16]

Geological Disasters. Physical injuries associated with earthquakes are usually caused by collapsing structures. Damage usually includes disruption of sewage systems and water supplies, as well as damage to such structures as bridges and highways that contribute to human well-being and to the economy. Social consequences include homelessness and loss of employment.[17]

Volcanic eruptions may constitute both an immediate public health hazard and a long-term environmental hazard. The principal long-term dangers include ash and larger fragments (occasionally contaminated with fibrogenic crystalline silica, as in the 1980 Mount Saint Helens eruption) raining from an explosion cloud, as well as mudflows, lava flows, and the concentration of volcanic gases in topographic depressions.[18]

Psychosocial stress is an important component of the consequences of geological disasters. After earthquakes devastated Thessaloniki, Greece, in 1978, the relative risk of atherosclerotic heart disease increased three fold, leading to an increase in stress-related cardiac deaths.[19] Serious psychological and psychosomatic disorders were noted after a 1987 avalanche in Armero, California, and after the Mount Saint Helens disaster in Washington.[20]

Catastrophic Events. Catastrophic events include fires, explosions, crashes, and spills, with or without the release of toxic materials. Burning of large populated communities rarely occurs in industrialized countries, but it remains a threat in poor countries. Fires in hospitals, institutions, or large office or residential structures may occur anywhere. Fires and explosions may injure hundreds, even thousands, of people and yet—unless a toxic substance is released—may have few public health consequences beyond the immediate casualties.[21]

Massive oil spills, with major ecological effects, have little public health impact other than economic and undetermined other long-term effects. Human health may be adversely affected after oil spills by the release of volatile hydrocarbons, such as benzene.

Sudden Chemical Exposures. Industrial disasters are an important source of sudden chemical exposure.[22,23] In Seveso, Italy, in 1976 an explosion in a chemical plant released 2,3,7,8-TCDD (dioxin) into the air. Almost 5000 acres of land were contaminated and 100,000 animals were killed; some 760 people were evacuated.[23] In Bhopal, India, in 1984 an explosion in a pesticide plant storage tank released tons of methyl isocyanate into the air. Wind conditions and an atmospheric inversion, along with delayed warnings and a population that had not been taught the nature of the risks and the appropriate response, increased the impact. Among the 200,000 people exposed to methyl isocyanate, nearly 3000 had died by 1988, and an additional 1700 were expected to die by 1995 as a result of the release.[4,5] In Basel, Switzerland, in 1985, 33 tons of pesticides were released into the Rhine River from a chemical warehouse.[24] The public health consequences of such releases range from the immediate and long-term toxic effects at Sevesco and Bhopal to the largely unknown long-term effects.

TABLE 74-2. "NATURAL" AND "HUMAN-CAUSED" DISASTERS

Type	Recent Examples
▪ **"Natural" Disasters**	
Climatological	
Floods	Shandong, China [1969]
	Northern Italy [1985]
	Bolivia and Colombia [1986]
	Bangladesh [1991]
Storms	
Water-based	Caribbean [hurricanes]
	Indian Ocean [cyclones]
	Pacific [typhoons]
	Philippines
Land-based	Midwestern United States [tornadoes]
Geological	
Earthquakes	Tangshan, China [1976]
	Mexico City [1985]
	Chile [1987]
	Philippines [1987]
	Ecuador [1988]
	Armenia [1988]
	San Francisco [1989]
Volcanic eruptions	Mount Saint Helens, Washington, [1980]
	Colombia [1983]
	Mount Pinatubo, Phillipines, [1991]
	Mount Unzen, Japan, [1991]
Tsunami [seismic sea waves]	Honshu, Japan [1983]
▪ **"Human-Caused" Disasters**[a]	
Sudden	
Explosions	Mexico City [butane storage facility] [1984]
	Pasadena, Texas [petrochemical plant] [1989]
Fires	Las Vegas, Nevada [hotel] [1980]
	São Paulo, Brazil [shanty town] [1984]
	Torrance, California [oil refinery] [1989]
Crashes	Mt. Ogura, Japan [airliner] [1985]
	Lockerbie, Scotland [airliner] [1989]
Spills	Prince William Sound, Alaska [oil] [1989]
	Gulf of Mexico, Texas [oil] [1990]
Chemical exposures	Seveso, Italy [dioxin] [1976]
	Bhopal, India [methyl isocyanate] [1984]
	Basel, Switzerland [pesticides] [1987]
Radiation exposures	Three Mile Island, Pennsylvania [1979]
	Chernobyl, Soviet Union [1986]
▪ **Insidious and Continuing**	
Drought and famine	The Sahel, Africa [1968–73]
Chemical exposures	Love Canal, Buffalo, New York [toxic chemicals]
	Times Beach, Missouri [dioxin]
Radiation exposures	Rocky Flats, Colorado
	Hanford, Washington
▪ **War and Civil Conflict**	During 1987, 27 wars causing 2,500,000 deaths

[a] Data from Hoffman MS [ed]: The World Almanac and Book of Facts 1989. New York: Pharos Books, 1989, pp 523–529.

Sudden Radiation Exposures. The principal peacetime source of risk of sudden and dangerous radiation exposure to large populations is the global network of nuclear power reactors.[25] A partial meltdown of the reactor core at Three Mile Island, near Harrisburg, Pa., in 1979—an event that nuclear engineers had repeatedly described as virtually impossible—released about 13 curies of radioactive material. It posed only small health risks[26] but revealed the inadequacy of emergency evacuation planning, the risk of human error involving complex technologies, and the problem of effective and credible communication to populations at risk.[27-30] Many of the same problems are evident in other dangerous U.S. reactor accidents that were not disclosed to the public at the time.

The disaster potential of large nuclear reactors was more fully realized by the accident at reactor 4 of the Chernobyl nuclear power station in the Soviet Union on April 26, 1986, which resulted in the largest reported accidental release of radioactive material in the history of nuclear power. It deposited more than 7 million curies of iodine 131, cesium 134 and 137, strontium 90, and other isotopes throughout the northern hemisphere, exposing almost 3 billion people to excess radiation.[6]

TABLE 74-3. PSYCHOLOGICAL REACTIONS TO A DISASTER

People of different age groups tend to react to a disaster in different ways, although appetite and sleep disturbances are common at all ages. Other common reactions in each group include:

Preschool (1 to 5 years old)
- Fearfulness
- Night terrors
- Clinging to parents

Early Childhood (5 to 11 years old)
- Night terrors, nightmares, fear of the dark
- Aggressive behavior at home or at school
- Stomachaches, headaches
- Clinging or whining
- Poor concentration in school

Preadolescence (11 to 14 years old)
- Rebellion in the home, such as refusal to do chores
- Stomachaches or headaches
- Loss of interest in friends
- School problems, such as loss of interest or attention-seeking behavior

Adolescence (14 to 18 years old)
- Loss of interest in dating
- Irresponsible and/or delinquent behavior
- Poor concentration
- Hypochondria

Adulthood
- Distressing, intrusive memories of the disaster; flashbacks of upsetting feelings: intense distress at reminders
- Irritability
- Being easily startled
- Blunting of feelings
- Lack of interest in pleasures
- Estrangement from people
- Troubling dreams
- Insomnia
- Poor concentration

From Fisher LM: The California quake: Children live with fear. In *New York Times*, Oct. 24, 1989, p. B12. Based on material from the Center for the Study of Psychological Trauma and the American Psychiatric Association: *Diagnostic and Statistical Manual of Mental Disorders, third edition, revised.* 1987.

This disaster caused 237 cases of acute radiation sickness, including 31 deaths, mostly among plant workers.[31] The long-term risks—leukemia, cancer, genetic defects, and mental retardation—are concentrated among the 115,000 most heavily exposed people who were evacuated from the 30 km zone around Chernobyl but may also affect other areas of the Ukraine and Byelorussia. The evacuated population can expect a doubling of the risk of leukemia (with a 150% increased risk for the 4000 persons whose average dose was 2 Gy [200 rads]).[32]

The radioactive plume reached Scandinavia, the United Kingdom, eastern Europe, and southern Europe within a few days. Estimates of the long-term effects remain a matter of scientific disagreement, ranging from a low of 17,000 additional fatal cancers in Europe to a high of more than 100,000 over many decades (an increment of 0.02% to 1.0% over the 123 million normally expected). Current estimates conservatively predict small increments of genetic disorders and severe mental retardation (1500 and 500 additional cases, respectively) for all of Europe and the Soviet Union. The estimated financial cost of this single accident is $14 billion[6]; less quantifiable are the psychological stresses and social costs of fear and population relocation, environmental and food survellance, decontamination, and medical care.

Insidious and Continuing Disasters

Drought and Famine. Many scientific definitions of "drought" depend on measuring quantities of rainfall, which leads to classification of drought as a climatological disaster. The causes of drought are so manifold and the needs for water so varied that the Niger Ministry of Agriculture now uses another definition: "Not as much water as the people need." Another definition has been developed for Tanzania: A "major" drought is one that diminishes crop yields by as much as 30%; a "severe" drought reduces crop and animal production by about 8%.[1]

Drought can have a relatively sudden onset, usually as a result of lack of seasonable rainfall, or it can have an insidious onset because of long-term change in rainfall or because rainfall is ineffective when water runs off too rapidly and does not benefit crops and pastures. The latter condition can be produced by slash-and-burn agriculture or deforestation; the lack of vegetation and the eventual lack of topsoil prevent the land from retaining water.[1]

In the 1968-1973 Sahel drought, which most directly affected Chad, Mali, Mauritania, Niger, Senegal, and Burkina-Faso, between 50,000 and 150,000 people died. By 1974 some 200,000 people in Niger (5% of the population) were completely dependent on food distribution; 250,000 people in Mauritania (20%) were completely destitute; and in Mali another 250,000 people (5%) were totally dependent on aid. In 1984 more than 150 million people in 24 western, eastern, and southern African nations were "on the brink of starvation" because of drought.[33] In 1990 the threat of severe drought and famine returned to some of these regions.

Insidious Chemical Exposure. Times Beach, Mo., was a summer resort about 20 miles southwest of St. Louis. Its soil was contaminated in the late 1960s and early 1970s by oil tainted with dioxin that was sprayed on the unpaved streets to keep down dust. Dioxin is suspected of causing disorders of the nervous system, liver, kidneys, and bladder and has been linked to cancer in laboratory animals. The dioxin in the soil was discovered in 1972; the U.S. government responded by purchasing all of the town's 801 homes and businesses and moving all the residents out.[10]

Insidious Radiation Exposure. Recent investigations have defined a new source of radiation exposure to large civilian populations: the nuclear weapons production factories, research laboratories, and underground testing facilities of the nuclear powers. Releases of radioactive substances (uranium, plutonium, tritium, and others, many with long half-lives) into air, soil, and groundwater near these facilities have been documented in the United States, the United Kingdom, and the Soviet Union. Because these releases have been poorly documented, occurred over several decades, and sometimes resulted from unanticipated events, such as fires or explosions, they are often poorly quantified and characterized, making accurate dose-reconstruction efforts difficult or impossible. Long latency periods for cancer effects (other than for the leukemias), the mobility of populations, and the relative absence of morbidity (as opposed to mortality) studies will complicate epidemiological follow-up investigations.[32]

War and Civil Conflict

"Conventional" War. Since 1700 there have been 471 "wars" (defined as conflicts with deaths of 1000 or more per year), resulting in more than 100 million fatalities. More than 90% of the war deaths of these 3 centuries have occurred in the twentieth century.[34] Since World War II there have been 127 wars and 21.8 million war-related deaths (Table 74-4).[35]

TABLE 74-4. WARS AND WAR-RELATED DEATHS, 1945–1989

	Number of Deaths		
	Civilian[a]	*Military*[a]	Total
Latin America	448,000	211,000	668,000
Europe	—	11,000	176,000
Middle East	474,000	1,038,000	1,813,000
South Asia	2,510,000	593,000	3,103,000
Far East	5,974,000	3,448,000	10,645,000
Sub-Saharan Africa	3,818,000	1,490,000	5,490,000
Other Africa	95,000	19,000	114,000
Total	13,319,000	6,810,000	21,809,000

[a] Incomplete because breakdown on civilian and military deaths not available in all cases.

Data from Sivard RL: World Military and Social Expenditures 1989. Washington, D.C.: World Priorities, 1989, p. 22.

In the eighteenth, nineteenth, and most of the twentieth century, civilians represented about 50% of war-related deaths. Recently the proportion of civilians among the dead has been increasing. Of the more than 20 million citizens of the Soviet Union killed during World War II, two thirds were civilians. In the 1950s and 1960s civilians accounted for approximately 50% of war deaths; in the 1970s and in the 1980s, more than 75%.[36] A high percentage of those dying in recent wars were children. Air power and the wide-ranging nature of modern war put entire populations at risk, disrupting food production and supply routes, imperiling fragile ecosystems, and forcing refugees by the hundreds of thousands to flee the fighting. More than half the civilian deaths in current hostilities resulted from war-related famine.

The geography of warfare has also changed radically. Europe was the principal site of wars and war deaths over the 3-century span, but since World War II only one war (in Hungary) has taken place in Europe. All other wars have been fought in developing countries. They have not, however, been without the involvement of the major powers; through most of the 1980s this involvement, often indirect and covert, appears to have increased.[35]

In 1987, 27 wars were under way, the highest number since 1700. The death toll up to 1987 in these wars was 2,477,000. Civilians accounted for approximately 85% of the recorded deaths.[36] It is possible that 1987 represented a peak in the number of wars and that the dramatic reduction in tension between the superpower blocs at the end of the 1980s will lead to a diminution in the number and extent of wars.[36]

As for "causes" of wars, the most frequent objectives were territory and independence. However, civil wars, representing power conflicts within nations, have increased sharply in the twentieth century, and are now by far the major form of warfare. Many of these are classified as "civil conflicts" or "civil disturbances," but powerful weaponry may be used, and the casualties and public health risks may be high.[37] In some of these conflicts, large amounts of tear gas have been used, with resulting casualties.[38] In others, the civil conflict has led to the cessation of public health programs, such as immunization, further endangering the population, especially infants and children.

Nuclear Weapons

Consequences of Production and Testing. The *production* of nuclear weapons, conducted for more than 40 years in the name of national security, has created massive environmental contamination by radioactive and toxic wastes that pose serious risks to the health of large populations. In the United States a study of the Department of Energy's 17 nuclear weapons production, research, and testing facilities[39] found that groundwater beneath the Hanford Reservation in the state of Washington, the Savannah River plant in South Carolina, the Rocky Flats plant near Denver, the Feed Materials Production Center near Cincinnati, and the Lawrence Livermore Laboratory near San Francisco is contaminated with radioactive substances at levels hundreds and in some instances thousands of times above drinking water standards. At the Hanford facility, more than 200 billion gallons of radioactive and chemical wastes—enough to cover Manhattan to a depth of 40 feet—have been dumped into unlined pits and trenches, the tanks filled with highly radioactive liquid wastes have leaked enough plutonium into the ground to build 50 Nagasaki-sized bombs.[34] The Department of Energy[40] identified and ranked 121 contaminated sites requiring cleanup (more properly called "risk containment," in view of the centuries-long half-lives of many of the radioactive contaminants) at an estimated total cost of $130 billion, or $2.1 million for every nuclear weapon the United States has produced. The health effects may not be known precisely for years, if ever; tedious and difficult dose-reconstruction efforts are just beginning. Radioactive iodine released at Hanford exposed nearly 14,000 persons to an organ-specific dose of 33 rads to the thyroid, and a small number of infants and children to a thyroid dose of 2900 rads—the equivalent of 100 diagnostic thyroid nuclear scans for each.

The health risks are greatest and best understood for the workers at these facilities, a population of nearly 600,000 persons who have been employed by the Department of Energy and its predecessor agencies since the 1940s. Recent epidemiological studies of these workers have noted apparent excesses of brain cancers, leukemias, multiple myeloma, and other radiogenic tumors,[41,42] but free scientific inquiry has been blocked by governmental insistence on the secrecy of the workforce's radiation-exposure records and morbidity and mortality data.[43]

These problems afflict all the nuclear weapons-producing nations, not just the United States. Accidents and fires at the Sellafield facility in the United Kingdom have been widely reported, and a recent case study found an association between the incidence of childhood leukemia and the preconception external radiation dose received by fathers who worked at the plant.[44]

Consequences of Use. A massive and unprecedented change in the potential consequences of war began with the development of nuclear weapons. In the years since their use on Hiroshima and Nagasaki in 1945 the number of nuclear weapons in the world's arsenals has grown to more than 50,000. Public health and other scientists have estimated the direct effects of a large-scale nuclear exchange; the totals of the profoundly injured and the dead would exceed 2.25 billion, almost half the world's population.[45] The survivors would experience longer, slower but massive population damage and deterioration because of epidemic disease, starvation, radiation-induced cancer and genetic defects, infant mortality, and reproductive impairment on a scale sufficient to threaten demographic stability, even in populations far removed from the initial destruction.[46–49]

Nuclear war would irreparably rupture the social fabric on which human life depends, rendering it inadequate to support the most basic human activities—finding food, water, and shelter, or maintaining family units.

The scope and magnitude of nuclear warfare are presented by consideration of a nationwide attack. One such attack, envisioned by U.S. civil defense planners and totaling 6559 megatons, would kill 86 million people in the first few hours. In the ensuing months, fatalities would rise to 133 million, and of 93 million survivors, some 32 million would have been injured.[50] Approximately 80% of U.S. medical resources—hospital beds and personnel, blood, drugs and medical supplies—would be destroyed. There would be only one hospital bed available for every 64 trauma and burn victims requiring hospitalization, only one surviving physician for every 633 injured patients, only

14,000 available units of blood when 64 million units would be needed.[51]

During the postattack period, tens of thousands of people would be packed together in radiation shelters that would usually lack adequate water and food supplies and systems for heating, cooling, ventilation, or waste disposal. Since full-time shelter occupancy would be necessary in many areas for 5 to 30 days and part-time occupancy or as long as 9 months, the risks of dehydration, malnutrition, and epidemic viral and bacterial disease would be extreme. In the postshelter survival period the epidemic potential would continue, made more intense by malnutrition and lack of protection against infectious diseases. Communicable disease death rates as high as 25% have been predicted.[51]

To these consequences must be added the effects of a potential "nuclear winter," a precipitous drop in surface temperatures on a hemispheric or global scale as a result of millions of metric tons of soot injected by mass fires into the upper atmosphere, blocking sunlight and absorbing heat.[52–55]

Chemical Weapons. The Hague Declaration of 1899 outlawed use of "poison gases" in war; yet chlorine, phosgene, mustard gas, and "tear gas" were used extensively in World War I, accounting for more than 1 million casualties. In Geneva in 1925 a "Protocol For the Prohibition of the Use in War of Asphyxiating, Poisonous or Other Gases and of All Analagous Liquids, Materials or Devices and of Bacteriological Methods of Warfare"—the Geneva Protocol—was concluded. Some nations that signed the protocol reserve the right to respond in kind after attack with chemical weapons, so the Geneva Protocol is a "no first use" treaty and does nothing to hinder research, development, production, or storage of such weapons or their use to retaliate in kind.

Despite the Protocol, Italy used mustard gas in its invasion of Abyssinia (Ethiopia) in 1936 and Japan used mustard and tear gas in China, starting in 1937. Germany, with its excellent dye industry and facilities for pesticide production, developed the cholinesterase inhibitors known as the "nerve gases" during World War II and used them in its extermination camps but not in open warfare.

The United States used tear gases and herbicides in the war in Indochina,[56] and there are detailed reports of the use by Korea and Israel of tear gases in large quantities in civil disturbances.[38] These countries argued that their use of these weapons was not prohibited by the Geneva Protocol. Mustard gas and possibly other chemical weapons were used in the 1980s in the Iran-Iraq War and by Iraq against its own Kurdish people.[57]

The types of chemical weapons are shown in Table 74–5.[58–60] Since it is virtually impossible to protect civilian populations adequately against chemical weapons, they are viewed by many as specifically anticivilian weapons. The United States and other countries are doing extensive work on the development and production of chemical weapons, at the same time they are initiating the destruction of outdated weapons.[61]

Since some poor nations consider chemical weapons (and, in some cases, biological weapons) to be the "poor nations' nuclear weapons," they may object to arms-control measures that do not also include controls on nuclear weapons. These weapons (and biological weapons) can also potentially be used by terrorists.

Biological Weapons. When the Geneva Protocol was negotiated in 1925, prohibition of "bacteriological methods" of warfare was added to what had originally been envisaged as a chemical weapons treaty. Nonetheless, these weapons were allegedly used in the 1930s and 1940s. It is alleged that when Japan attacked China in the 1930s, rice and wheat grain were mixed with fleas carrying plague, resulting in plague in areas of China that had not had plague before. According to testimony at the Nuremberg trials, prisoners at German concentration camps were infected in tests of biological weapons. The British released anthrax spores on Gruinard Island off the coast of Scotland; it remained uninhabitable for many years. Churchill is said to have considered attacking German livestock with anthrax, but this was never carried out. In the United States, work on anthrax and brucellosis as weapons was performed. There have also been reports of Soviet research on biological weapons during World War II.[62]

In the 1950s and 1960s the University of Utah, under contract, conducted secret experiments at the U.S. Army Dugway Proving Ground involving large-scale field testing of some of the most infectious and toxic biological warfare agents, including tularemia, Rocky Mountain spotted fever, plague, and Q fever. In September 1950, U.S. Navy mine sweepers released aerosolized *Serratia marsescens* in sufficient quantities to contaminate 117 square miles of the San Francisco area. This presumably harmless species is believed by some analysts to have been a cause of infections and deaths and to be a particular threat to immunologically compromised persons. During the 1950s and 1960s the United States conducted 239 top-secret open-air disseminations involving such areas as the subways of New York City and Washington National Airport.[63]

In 1969 the Nixon administration announced that the United States would unilaterally dismantle its biological weapons program, and in 1972 the Convention on the Prohibition of the Development, Prevention and Stockpiling of Bacteriological (Biological) and Toxin Weapons and on Their Destruction was concluded. This "Biological Weapons Convention" was ratified by the U.S. Senate in 1975 (the same year it belatedly ratified the Geneva Protocol of 1925), and more than 100 nations are party to it. The convention prohibits (except for "prophylactic, protective, and other peaceful purposes") the development, or acquisition of biological agents or toxins, as well as weapons and means of production, stockpiling, transfer, and delivery. Examples of potential weapons are given in Table 74–5.

TABLE 74–5. CHEMICAL AND POTENTIAL BIOLOGICAL[a] WEAPONS

▪ CHEMICAL WEAPONS	▪ POTENTIAL BIOLOGICAL WEAPONS
Incapacitating Agents	**Bacteria**
CN (tear gas)	Anthrax
CS (tear gas)	Dysentery
BZ (psychoactive)	Meningitis
Blister Agents	Plague
Sulfur mustard	Tularemia
Nitrogen mustard	Typhoid fever
Lewisite	**Viruses**
Choking Agents	Dengue fever
Phosgene	Encephalitis
Chlorine	Influenza
Chloropicrin	Smallpox
Blood Agents	Yellow fever
Hydrogen cyanide	**Sources of Toxins**
Cyanogen chloride	Cobras
Nerve Agents	Rattlesnakes
Tabun GA	Scorpions
Sarin GB	Shellfish
VX	
Toxin Agents	
Botulin X, A	
Saxitoxin TZ	
Enterotoxin B	

[a] Data from Thatcher G: Poison On the Wind: The New Threat of Chemical and Biological Weapons. Boston: Christian Science Monitor Publishing Society, 1988, pp. 11, 32.
Based on U.S. Department of Defense materials.

Funding for the U.S. Army Biological Defense Research Program (BDRP) quadrupled from 1981 to 1988. Much of this research is medical, including the development of immunizations or treatment against organisms that might be used as weapons. Hazardous infectious organisms, aerosols, and genetic engineering techniques are used.[64]

Concerns have been raised about this research, which many view as ambiguous and provocative, for two reasons: (1) risk of release of virulent organisms into the environment with the danger of infection of people or animals and (2) escalating development, production, and stockpiling of biological weapons with the danger of use of these weapons in war or terrorism or of their accidental dissemination.

Concern has been expressed about the militarization of genetic engineering and of biology in general, much as physics and chemistry were militarized during World War II. Biological weapons have been characterized as "public health in reverse."[65]

Public Health Costs of Preparation for War. Since World War II an estimated $16 trillion has been spent on the world's military forces; military expenditures have climbed to more than $900 billion each year, an amount in constant dollars about 2.5 times the level of 1960. The rate of increase in world military expenditures has far exceeded the increase in GNP per capita since 1960. Since 1945 some $4 trillion has been spent on nuclear weapons alone.[66]

Several of the world's industrialized nations, the United States and the Soviet Union in particular, spend large amounts of their resources on arms. The expenditures lead to economic problems that affect health and human services as well as specific diminution of governmental funding for services to promote health and human welfare.

Along with the diversion of revenue to military research, arms spending diverts scientists from working to improve health and the quality of life to supporting military functions. World expenditures on weapons research exceed the combined spending on development of new energy technologies, improvement of human health, increased agriculture productivity, and control of pollutants.

The developed countries spend about 20 times as much on military programs as on foreign economic aid. Compounding this tragedy, even small conversions of the funds being spent on arms into spending on health could produce enormous benefits:

- The cost of 1 hour's world spending on arms is equivalent to the entire cost of the successful 20-year effort to eradicate smallpox from the earth.
- The cost of 2 hours of the arms race would pay for the World Health Organization's entire annual budget.
- The cost of ½ day of world arms spending could pay for the full immunization of all the children in the world against the common infectious diseases.
- The cost of 4 days of world military spending would pay for a 5-year program to control malaria.
- The cost of 3 weeks of world arms spending would pay for primary health care for every child in the poor countries of the world, including safe water supplies and full immunizations.
- The cost of 6 months of world arms spending would pay for a 10-year program providing health and food needs in developing countries.

Overall, the military outlay of developing nations is as large as all their public investment in the education and health care of their 3 billion people.

This use of resources—financial and scientific and technical—for military purposes clearly causes mortality, morbidity, and destruction of the quality of life even if the weapons are never used. It has been termed "destruction before detonation."[67]

PUBLIC HEALTH RESPONSES TO DISASTERS

Primary Prevention (Prevention of the Occurrence of the Disaster)

Sudden Disasters. We do not know how to prevent climatological and geological disasters, although methods for mitigating their consequence are known but generally underused. On the other hand, much can be done to prevent flood and drought. Much can also be done to prevent not only the consequences but also the occurrence of fires, explosions, crashes, spills, and sudden chemical and radiation exposures.

Most of these opportunities for the primary prevention of sudden disasters (as well as for the primary prevention of insidious disasters) lie in the political realm. These include active support of legislation for tighter regulation of chemical plants and other hazardous facilities and insistence that new nuclear power reactors or chemical plants cannot be built near dense population areas or geologic fault lines. Controversial regulations demanding personnel testing in companies that transport chemicals, nuclear waste, oil, and other potentially dangerous substances must be examined from the view of protection of public health.

Insidious and Continuing Disasters. Insidious disasters should be primarily prevented or at least detected and reversed at the earliest possible time. This requires strong regulation and surveillance by public health authorities.

In the cases of nuclear power plants, nuclear weapons production facilities, and the management of nuclear wastes from these and other sources, the necessary public health mechanisms already exist in the form of careful elaborated state and federal environmental standards and regulations. What is needed is a clear, independent, and exclusive mandate—especially in the case of nuclear weapons plants, which until recently have been exempt from such outside regulation—for public health and environmental authorities, rather than those who produce and transport the wastes, to apply these standards.

However, these standards provide only relatively short-term protection. No satisfactory method of treatment or storage of radionuclides with half-lives of hundreds to thousands of years has been demonstrated; yet they continue to be produced.

War and Civil Conflict. Although the sequelae of war—famine, malnutrition, exposure, epidemic disease, and environmental contamination—are classic concerns of public health, war itself has rarely been addressed as a public health problem. War has been seen, instead, as a "social," "political," or "military" problem, beyond the expertise of physicians and other public health practitioners.

Others, however, point to the long "political" involvement of physicians in efforts to reduce childhood poisonings, control the lead content of gasoline, legislate the use of automobile seat belts, and lobby for gun control and insist that prevention of war is an extention—albeit awesomely magnified—of the dictum that, for health workers, health outcome must be the primary concern of all policy decisions.

The role of health professionals in the prevention of nuclear war has been a subject of legitimate and ongoing debate. Many health professionals have insisted that nuclear weapons and nuclear war are a health issue as well as a political issue and that their expertise is relevant to both aspects of the problem. Much credit may be claimed by the decades-long campaign by physicians for the lessening of tensions and the prevention of nuclear war—efforts that were recognized by the awarding of the Nobel Prize for Peace to the International Physicians for the Prevention of Nuclear War in 1985.

Secondary Prevention (Mitigation of Disaster Consequences)

Sudden Disasters

Land Use and Building Codes. Stringent building codes and land-use management problems in the United States and other industrialized countries have led to decreased morbidity and mortality after hurricanes, earthquakes, and fires. However, many older structures and communities remain vulnerable. In countries without stringent codes, structures and people remain at high risk.

Public Education. Education of the public is important in preventing disasters, both before the disaster occurs and as it is happening. Before the event, people must know how to prepare for a disaster (e.g., store food reserves, obtain an emergency radio) and must have information more specific to their situation (e.g., standing in a doorway when an earthquake occurs). Evacuation alternatives for hurricanes and tornadoes should be discussed in the media well in advance of the event, including the alternatives under certain circumstances of not leaving current shelter.

One disaster provides an example of the application of this procedure. On April 10, 1979, a series of tornadoes occurred in Wichita Falls, Tex., resulting in 44 dead, 1871 injured, 6000 families left homeless, and more than $300 million in damages.[68] Of the 25 persons whose deaths were associated with passenger vehicles, 16 had gotten into their cars specifically to avoid the tornado; the homes of 11 of these persons escaped major damage.

An analysis of the relative risk of various protective measures revealed that those who sought shelter indoors were at little risk of fatal injuries, even when their homes were hit by a tornado. In contrast, persons in the open or in vehicles were at a higher risk.[68] Some deaths associated with tornadoes may be prevented by ensuring that people know to stay in their homes or other structures, even if the structure is in the path of the tornado. In the less developed world, unfortunately, public education on disasters is even less common than in industrialized countries.

Preparation of Relief Plan. The Pan American Health Organization has developed a series of guides for surveillance, health management, environmental health management, and vector control after natural disasters.[69] The United Nations High Commissioner for Refugees has developed a *Handbook for Emergencies,*[70] and the National Governors Association has provided a manual for emergency management.[71] Disaster managers now have thoughtful and helpful aids to help avoid repeating past mistakes.

A relief plan might include some or all of the following activities:

1. Rescue of victims
2. Provision of emergency medical care
3. Elimination of physical dangers (e.g., fires and gas leaks)
4. Evacuation of the population (chemical and nuclear emergencies)
5. Provision of preventive and routine medical care
6. Provision of water
7. Provision of food
8. Provision of clothing
9. Provision of shelter
10. Disposal of human waste
11. Control of vectorborne disease
12. Disposal of human bodies
13. Disposal of solid waste

To ensure that the above activities could be carried out, a relief plan would also need to address the following support activities:

1. Coordination of volunteer assistance
2. Management of facilities
3. Storage and distribution of material
4. Management of communication systems
5. Management of transportation
6. Management of public information and rumor-control services
7. Management of registration inquiry services
8. Traffic and crowd control

Early Warning. During the disaster an early warning system may be helpful in notifying residents of what to do. For specific types of climatological disasters, for example, early warning may prevent significant morbidity and mortality. In the United States the National Weather Service and its National Severe Storms Forecast Center are responsible for warning of land-based storms such as tornadoes. A thunderstorm or tornado *watch* is an alert that conditions exist for its formation; a *warning* indicates that the storm is already occurring. One of the problems with such a warning system is that predicting the formation of tornadoes is an inexact science. Reliance on the system can lead both to expensive and perhaps hazardous responses to false alarms and to potentially costly and dangerous absence of advance warning of an actual storm. Doppler radar systems can improve the accuracy of the prediction, but such systems are expensive and their installation in the United States has been slow.

In the United States the National Hurricane Center of the National Oceanic and Atmospheric Administration is responsible for tracking water-based storms such as hurricanes. Identifying and tracking hurricanes with the use of satellites, radar, and aircraft is more sophisticated than predicting tornadoes, and the accuracy of predicting the landfall and severity of hurricanes in the United States has been excellent. Most coastal areas at high-risk of hurricanes in the United States have emergency contingency plans for orderly evacuation and adequate shelter capacity for evacuees, but road conditions may make rapid evacuation difficult, and it is often impossible to secure complete compliance with evacuation orders. In the less developed countries early warning systems and provisions for emergency shelter are far less likely to be available.

War and Civil Conflict

Civil Defense. During the first half of the twentieth century, two world wars and many regional conflicts provided the incentive and the experience for governments to develop civil defense programs.

The introduction of nuclear weapons reshaped civil defense programs. Governments have defined the principal threat as a massive air attack, occurring with little warning, and the explosion of nuclear weapons.

Among nations assumed to be targets of nuclear weapons, the effects against which civil defense must protect have been considered to be blast, fire, and radioactive fallout. Among non-targeted nations, protection only against radioactive fallout has been assumed to be necessary.

The aims of civil defense programs in this context of the threat of nuclear war have been to create the perception that the country is prepared to defend itself against attack and to contribute as much as possible to making that perception a reality.

The public health implications of civil defense plans for nuclear war have been described from two perspectives: (1) the extent to which these plans support the health of the public after nuclear war and (2) the extent to which these plans distract attention and divert resources from efforts that might have greater positive impact on the public health. Short-term survival would constitute a minimum end point by which to assess the efficacy of civil defense plans. Integration of issues such as the numbers of people surviving over time and their overall quality of life would constitute more robust and realistic assessments.

The debate over civil defense has persisted for more than 40 years. As the weapons have increased in ferocity and their effects have become more widely understood, advocates of civil defense have found it increasingly difficult to claim that any population-based option could forestall the deaths of millions of people or massive destruction of the environment.[72]

This evolution in the civil defense discussion has paralleled an easing in superpower tensions, which in turn has rendered less relevant the strategic and psychological justifications for civil defense.

As a consequence of these changes in public knowledge and world politics, by the end of the 1980s in the United States there was general acknowledgment that civil defense had little role in protecting or ensuring the public health in the event of nuclear war.

Preparation for War. In the latter half of the twentieth century some of the most difficult ethical dilemmas for physicians have arisen not with regard to conduct during war but with conduct in preparation for war. The development of weapons of mass destruction and the links between this development and the civilian scientific and medical communities have contributed to this state of affairs.

Weapons of mass destruction are indiscriminate, killing and injuring civilians as well as military personnel and destroying and contaminating ecosystems over wide areas. Medical response after the use of such weapons in war could not restore life to the millions who would be killed, salvage life for the millions who would be injured, or recreate the biological and physical environment. Confronting the consequences of such a war, many physicians around the world have turned toward efforts to stop the arms race and prevent nuclear war. Such efforts against what appears to be the ultimate threat to public health have frequently put physicians in conflict with government policies endorsing the development, production, and deployment of increasing numbers of these weapons.

Assessment and Surveillance

Measurement Criteria. Investigation and analyses of past disasters have led to the use of numerous objective measurement criteria. These tools can be employed to ascertain how a current disaster compares with others in the past and how the disaster and its effects are changing over time.[73,74]

Physical measurements, such as the height of a river above flood stage, the level of pollutants in the air, the amount of toxic material in food or water, or the levels of radiation in areas surrounding the site of a nuclear accident, can be used to assess the magnitude of a disaster. The Richter scale is used to specify the intensity of earthquakes. Other items measure the biological effects of a disaster. Age-specific case and death rates over time are standard measures. Laboratory typing of organisms, biochemical testing of affected individuals, and environmental tests may all be necessary. The extent and intensity of a famine can be determined by calculating height/weight ratios for children in the affected areas. These tools and others permit objective assessment of the effects of a disaster and the meaningful communication and comparison of those effects.

An effective plan for public health and other personnel during a disaster situation would outline activities designed to minimize the effects. These efforts can be summarized as situation analysis and response; the two types of activity are closely interrelated. Although many relief workers may be needed to obtain surveillance information, analyze the data, provide relief services, evaluate results, and provide information to the public, it is essential that a single person with managerial experience be placed in absolute charge of the entire disaster relief operation.[75]

After a disaster the desire to provide immediate relief may lead to hasty decisions that are not based on the actual needs of the affected population. To determine the actual needs of the population and make responsible relief decisions, disaster relief managers must have reliable information on problems occurring in the disaster-stricken area, relief resources available, and relief activities already in progress. Thus, surveillance systems must be set up immediately.

The object of surveillance in a disaster situation is to obtain information required for making decisions. The specific information required will vary from disaster to disaster, but a basic three-step process includes (1) collection of data, (2) analysis of data, and (3) response to data.[76]

The collection of data involves obtaining denominator as well as numerator data (e.g., the number of people at risk of injury as well as the number of people injured). Without denominator data, one cannot realistically determine the magnitude of a problem. One hundred deaths in a city of 1 million would be interpreted quite differently from 100 deaths in a small town.

The analysis involves collating and interpreting the data, and can include asking such questions as the following:

- What problems are occurring? Why are they occurring?
- Where are problems occurring?
- Who is affected?
- What problems are causing the greatest morbidity and mortality?
- What problems are increasing or decreasing?
- What problems will subside on their own? When?
- What problems will increase if unattended?
- What relief resources are available?
- How can relief resources be used most efficiently?
- What relief activities are in progress?
- Are relief activities meeting relief needs?
- What additional information is needed for decision making?[75]

After answering such questions, one can proceed with the third step in the process: planning an appropriate response to the situation described in the surveillance data. In developing this plan, one will decide what types of relief response are appropriate and what the relative priorities are among the relief activities.

Analysis consists of measuring the results of various relief activities and determining how these relief responses should be updated to better address the changing disaster situation. The analysis also includes identifying information to be collected in order to evaluate the modified responses. This three-step process of data collection, analysis, and response can be described as a closed feedback system involving reevaluation of relief needs and their effects. Surveillance after a disaster evolves in phases: (1) immediate assessment ("quick and dirty"), (2) short-term assessment, and (3) ongoing surveillance. The surveillance cycle applies to each of these phases; however, the information obtained in each phase differs in reliability and level of detail, largely because of the speed with which the initial assessments must be conducted. Each phase builds upon the previous one. The information obtained in the immediate phase is analyzed to determine the forms of relief needed immediately and the information required as part of the short-term assessment. The information collected during the short-term assessment is used not only to make relief decisions but also to determine further surveillance needs. The later surveillance indicates with more precision how relief activities should be maintained or changed.

Immediate Assessment ("Quick and Dirty"). The object of this phase of surveillance is to obtain as quickly as possible as much general information as possible. The most basic information needed is the following: (1) the geographic extent of the disaster-stricken area, (2) the major problems occurring in the area, and (3) the number of people affected. This information can be obtained by whatever means seems most efficient. Asking questions and listening carefully to the replies is often the best way to begin.

An aerial survey may be useful in defining the geographic extent of the disaster-stricken area and in observing major damage and destruction. Census data can be examined to determine how many people previously lived in the disaster-stricken area and thus were at risk. Hospitals, clinics, and morgues that are in operation may be able to obtain numbers of known deaths and injuries. It is useful to determine the most frequent causes of death and types of injury in order to predict whether demands for medical care will be increasing or decreasing.

Some problems likely to occur after a disaster can be predicted by past experience. For example, disruption of water supplies has often been a problem after earthquakes. New types of disaster, such as chemical emergencies and nuclear accidents, still present many unknowns. As more disaster research is done, disaster relief managers will become better equipped to predict the types of problem likely to result from different kinds of disaster.

When a general picture of the disaster situation has been obtained, a rapid analysis should be made. There are two major questions to be answered: (1) Is the information already obtained sufficient to determine immediate relief needs? (2) What additional information is needed for further decision making?

The initial assessment may not have yielded enough information to warrant an immediate decision as to what relief resources must be ordered or what relief activities must take place. If fires are raging and threatening to spread, the fires must be extinguished. But if one knows only that crops have been destroyed, one would collect more information before deciding whether to provide food relief. Whatever relief decisions are made at this point, further decisions must also be made to determine what additional information is needed. At this point or sooner, it will be important to respond to inquiries from the press.[77]

Short-term Assessment. The short-term assessment involves more systematic methods of collecting data than the "quick-and-dirty" approach and is likely to result in more detailed, reliable information on problems, relief resources, and relief activities in progress. One way to organize data collection during this phase of assessment is to divide the disaster-stricken area into smaller areas ("blocks") to be surveyed simultaneously by different workers. Simple reporting forms can be developed and workers can be sent out to survey the different areas and report at a specified time.

Following is a list of the kinds of information that may be needed before relief decisions can be made. Only items that are truly needed should be requested from the data gatherers.

1. The geographic extent of the affected area as defined by streets or other clear boundaries.
2. The number of persons known to be dead, possibly according to age group and sex.
3. The estimated number of persons who are severely injured and require medical care, possibly according to age group, sex, and type of injury or medical problem.
4. Estimated numbers of homes destroyed, homes uninhabitable, and homes that are still habitable.
5. Location and condition of schools, churches, public buildings, etc.
6. Condition and extent of water supply.
7. Condition and extent of food supply.
8. Condition of roads, bridges, communication facilities, and public utilities.
9. Location and condition of health facilities.
10. Estimates of medical personnel, equipment, and supplies.
11. Descriptions of relief activities already in progress (e.g., search and rescue, first aid, food relief).

To simplify and speed up the data collection and analysis, the information requested during this phase should be as brief and as specific as possible. Every item on every reporting form should have a purpose. For example, the purpose of determining the condition of schools and churches is to ascertain what facilities in the area could be used as shelters.

The types of information needed and the simplicity of reporting forms are only two factors that influence the amount of time that must be allowed for short-term assessment. Other factors are as follows:

- The size and terrain of the disaster-stricken area and the distances between areas to be surveyed.
- The types and numbers of personnel available to obtain and analyze the needed information.
- The methods of communication and transportation available and usable in the area.

Depending on such factors as the above, short-term assessment may take as little as 4 to 5 hours or as much as 2 to 3 days. A reasonable reporting time should be estimated and set so that data will be returned and analyzed as quickly as possible.

As early as possible, relief priorities should be determined, resources ordered, and full-scale relief activities initiated. All channels of public information should be used to disseminate the information obtained and explain the relief actions to be taken. The information to be obtained during the next phase of surveillance depends largely on the nature and extent of problems caused by the disaster, as well as the relief decisions made at this point. For example, if it was decided to provide hot meals at churches in three of the affected areas, one would need to set up a system of monitoring the food relief provided and determining the effects of a relief action.

Ongoing Surveillance. Once the short-term assessment is complete and appropriate relief is in progress, surveillance becomes an ongoing program. Efforts at this time are directed at monitoring disaster-associated problems, determining the effects of relief activities on those problems, and deciding how the overall program of relief should be altered to correspond to the current situation.

During this phase of surveillance, several methods of data collection can be used. Monitoring of relief facilities and activities has already been mentioned. In addition, a system of rumor control may be set up, house-to-house or random surveys may be conducted as needed, and data on the predisaster situation may be examined more thoroughly than was previously possible.

When relief facilities such as clinics, hospitals, or food distribution centers are being monitored, it may be best to assign someone already working at the facility to report regularly. An inspector can be sent from time to time to double-check the reports or to investigate problems that are reported. For example, if a shelter reported a case of measles, an investigation and possibly immunizations would be required. Investigation should also take place if no reports are received from a facility. A rumor-control system involves the screening of rumors reported by the public or by officials and the investigation of those that seem most prevalent or serious.

When information obtained by ongoing surveillance is analyzed, new problems may become apparent and require investigation. The cycle of data collection, analysis, and response continues. One response that becomes very important is the distribution of a regular surveillance report. Through these reports the data collectors can be provided with the feedback they need to continue reporting carefully and regularly. Surveillance reports should be sent to the data collectors and also to the decision makers involved in the different relief activities. The surveillance report is one way of coordinating different agencies and preventing duplication of relief efforts. As part of the ongoing phase of the surveillance cycle, the relief efforts in progress would be evaluated and perhaps modified.

Implementation of Disaster Relief

Sudden Disasters. All of the relevant elements of the relief plan discussed earlier should be implemented as rapidly as possible. The quick-and-dirty assessment of a disaster situation must simultaneously see the beginnings of disaster relief. Priority must be placed on the treatment of trauma cases. Medical teams must be able to improvise their handling of different disasters, and the use of radiology has proved instrumental in identification of the victims. Treatment may need to be provided in impromptu settings (e.g., schools that have large enough auditoriums that they can serve as hospital areas); thus surveying of the area for these facilities is also necessary. The importation of needed medical supplies and personnel must be accomplished quickly, because within 48 hours most trauma victims will have either stabilized or died. Responses may include provision of shelter (both short-term and long-term rebuilding) and ensuring adequate nutrition. Repairs in sewage systems or the building of temporary substitutes may be necessary. In industrialized countries immunization programs are rarely needed as a specific postdisaster measure, but they may be required in developing countries.

Treatment of the survivors must include attending to their mental injuries as well as their physical ones. Accordingly, personnel brought into treat the victims must be alert to the psychosocial stresses. In sum, the effective management of people—both the victims and the relief personnel—must be high on the list of skills needed to cope with a sudden disaster.

Finally, the disaster itself must be confronted. If fires are raging or an oil slick is expanding, it is important to contain the hazard. Care must be taken that this containment does not, in and of itself, cause additional harm to the area (e.g., the long-term effects of natural deforestation).

The nuclear accidents in Chernobyl and at Three Mile Island have shown the necessity for well-organized, efficient health care delivery. The Soviets used three levels of care—rescue and first aid at the emergency site, emergency treatment at regional hospitals, and definitive evaluation and treatment in Moscow—all the while focusing on diagnosis, triage, patient disposition, attendant exposure, and preventive actions.

Insidious and Continuing Disasters. Secondary prevention of insidious disasters lies in early detection and in prompt amelioration of the threat to public health. Usually these disasters are unrecognized until their health consequences or extraordinary or serendipitous surveillance causes them to be recognized. The event that precipitates recognition may be the crossing of a "toxic threshold" for chemicals or radiation released. Once the newly labeled disaster is brought to the public eye, public health professionals and disaster relief personnel must be quickly involved. At this point the insidious disaster may be handled like a sudden disaster, with quick-and-dirty and long-term assessments carried out under the supervision of a trained disaster relief manager who has a well-thought-out disaster relief plan. Education of the population on the potential risks, including those involved in the use of water and food, is of prime importance. Provision for moving the population to housing away from the source of risk was important in the initial response to the Love Canal disaster. Finally, compensation for those affected may be appropriate. Most important, public health officials must find ways to work cooperatively with citizens groups concerned about the impact of and the response to the disaster.

War and Civil Conflict. Secondary prevention in times of conflict can cause ethical dilemmas for health workers. Military medical personnel carry out triage and care for the sick and injured in such a manner as to maintain maximum fighting efficiency; this may lead to different decisions from those that would be made if the primary goal were to minimize suffering and disability. The military medical goals might simply make war more bearable and prevention of war more difficult.[78]

Some health workers specifically eschew military service and aim to bring relief from outside the sphere of battle. Red Cross, Red Crescent, conscientious objectors, and pacifist organizations such as the American Friends Service Committee provide essential drugs, medical supplies, and food supplies to sustain the victims of war, military and civilian alike. Sometimes it has been possible for such groups to arrange a truce (e.g., in the "low-intensity" war in El Salvador when hostilities were suspended for a time so that children could be immunized).

Evaluation of Public Health Response. Evaluation of any endeavor should consist of comparing what actually happened with what was intended and should be an integral part of the entire relief operation. In the case of disaster management, the evaluator would be looking at the "actual" versus the "desired" on two levels—the overall outcome of disaster management efforts and the impact of each discrete category of relief efforts (e.g., provision of food and shelter, management of communications).

A critical step in the management of any disaster relief effort is the setting of objectives that specify the intended outcome of the relief. The general objectives for disaster management (i.e., the elimination of unnecessary morbidity, mortality, and economic loss directly attributable to mismanagement of disaster relief efforts) could be made more specific for a particular disaster situation by estimating the levels of morbidity, mortality, and economic loss that would be consistent with appropriate management of disaster relief and the current levels of scientific, technical, and operational knowledge.

Specific and measurable objectives can be established for each of the operational categories of disaster relief. For example, those responsible for providing food in a particular disaster might specify an objective of providing a specific number of people with a specified minimum amount of food in a specified amount of time. Once these objectives have been stated, evaluation requires the gathering of the information necessary to assess whether they were met. This information is obtained as part of surveillance.

The comparison of actual with desired is the first critical step of evaluation. If the objectives were not met, it is desirable for those conducting the evaluation to continue with the evaluative process, identify the reason for the discrepancy, and suggest corrective action. Only in this way can such deviations from the intended effects be prevented in the future. In many cases, simulated disaster operations should be undertaken to test the various components before actual needs arise.

The elimination of morbidity, mortality, and economic loss resulting from mismanagement of relief is of primary public health concern since the consequences of mismanagement are totally amenable to prevention. Public health authorities also need to prevent losses directly attributable to disasters.

Existing knowledge that might reduce the undesirable effects of disasters is often not applied. Hurricane and tornado warning systems, legislation to prevent building in floodplains and to require mobile home tiedowns or tornado cellars in mobile home parks, aseismic housing codes for earthquake-prone areas, and other similar procedures are frequently underused.

The difficulties of implementing these procedures (e.g., cost, lack of legislation) are readily apparent. The benefits, however, remain largely unknown because of insufficient studies of past disasters to identify and quantify avoidable situations that have led to injury, illness, death, and economic loss.

A surveillance procedure has been suggested for managing disaster relief. This same basic procedure can be applied to increase the probability that the preventable effects of disaster do not occur. Data on the problem can be gathered, analyzed, and interpreted, and actions in response to the situation described can be developed and implemented.

Individuals and organizations in public health can contribute by collecting data on morbidity, mortality, and economic loss, as well as the causes of those adverse consequences, after each disaster. By analyzing these data, investigators can determine the degree to which such adverse consequences could have been prevented. They can also identify geographic areas (e.g., fault areas, floodplains, coastal areas) and populations (e.g., the aged, individuals living alone, mobile home dwellers, those dependent on life-support systems) at greatest risk of losses from disasters. Specific interventions (e.g., aseismic housing codes, early warning, preparation, and evacuation procedures) can then be suggested to mitigate the negative consequences of disasters for these high-risk populations and areas.

Once these specific activities have been identified, public health professionals can assist other governmental authorities in implementing the recommendations. Subsequent assessment of the impact of these interventions can lead to actions that are even more effective in preventing morbidity, mortality, and economic loss directly attributable to disasters.

Refugees. Large-scale disasters disrupt housing and often force people to move away from their previous place of shelter. At any given time, there are an estimated 15 to 18 million refugees in the world. Another 40 to 50 million who are not technically classified as refugees have been forced to move by natural or human-made disasters, commonly military or political turmoil. Most people in both categories present a combination of problems that stretch conventional public health services to the limit and are best dealt with by specialized refugee community health services.[79] The problems that have to be dealt with include provision of emergency shelter, clothing and food, social services aimed at reuniting scattered family members, tracing missing family members, and usually organizing medical and public health services for large refugee populations that often settle in semipermanent communities, as on the border of Thailand and Kampuchea, in Eritrea and the Sudan, Gaza and the West Bank of the River Jordan, parts of Lebanon, Mozambique, and Angola, and in several parts of the Indian subcontinent. In Central America and parts of South America, refugees from political and military turbulence and rural banditry have often tended to head north toward the United States, where many have settled as legal or illegal immigrants and have been absorbed, more or less, into American society and social and health care systems. Elsewhere in the world, special services have almost always been required to meet the needs of refugee communities.

These needs include the provision of basic public health services as well as care for emergency and routine medical and surgical conditions, pregnancy and childbirth, etc. Refugee communities tend to be established in inhospitable environments and often also remain under threat of political repression, military action, or both. Under these trying conditions, it is difficult but essential to establish and maintain basic sanitary services, to provide immunization programs, growth monitoring, health education, nutrition supplements, and communicable disease control programs, and to make long-term plans for resettlement and restoration of some hope for better conditions for many people whose lives have been shattered.

Epidemiological assessment is an essential step in long-term planning for refugee health care. It provides baseline data on existing emergency needs and subsequently is the basis for program evaluation. Long-term planning is needed because experience has repeatedly demonstrated that "temporary" refugee communities often become permanent settlements. For this reason, plans should include provision for education of children so that they, at least, might have some hope of escape to a better life.

PUBLIC HEALTH CONSEQUENCES OF MISMANAGEMENT OF DISASTER RELIEF

Ideally, attempts to mitigate the results of a disaster would not add to the negative consequences. In many instances, however, inappropriate or incomplete management actions taken after a disaster have contributed to unnecessary morbidity, mortality, and resource wastage. According to the United Nations Economic and Social Council, many of the casualties and much of the destruction occurring in a natural disaster are due to ignorance and neglect on the part of individuals and public authorities.

Many publications describe the inappropriate actions taken to manage past disasters. The same mismanagement problems tend to recur. Physicians and nurses have been sent into disaster areas in numbers far exceeding actual need.[80,81] Medical and paramedical personnel have often been hampered by the lack of specific supplies they need to apply their skills. In some cases available supplies have not been inventoried until well after the disaster; this has resulted in the importation of material that was neither used nor needed.[81]

The Peruvian earthquake of 1970[80] and the Nicaraguan earthquake of 1972[81] provide two examples of inappropriate actions taken in managing disaster relief operations. After both earthquakes, disaster relief hospitals (portable, prefabricated facilities) were provided, although they were not needed. Relief goods were sent to the countries, but no provisions were made to transport them to the specific areas where they were needed.[82] It is likely that this failure to transport relief supplies to needy areas resulted in unnecessary morbidity and mortality.

Many volunteers who went to Peru after the 1970 earthquake neither spoke Spanish nor had any disaster relief experience. They added to, rather than reduced, the problems of the Peruvian authorities.[80] Personnel from more than 70 volunteer and official agencies went to Managua after the Nicaraguan earthquake of 1972, but there was no coordination and little cooperation among these groups.

Inappropriate timing of the response to a disaster was evident after the hurricanes in British Honduras, Yucatan, and Tampico in 1955. Supplies with which to treat casualties were brought into the disaster area 48 hours after the disaster. By that time, victims with traumatic injuries had either already been cared for or had already died.[82]

In a study of past disaster mismanagement problems and their causes,[83,84] the following problems were categorized:

1. Inadequate appraisal of damages
2. Inadequate problem ranking
3. Inadequate identification of resources
4. Inadequate location of resources
5. Inadequate transportation of resources
6. Inadequate utilization of resources.

Among 22 U.S. disasters in this study, 93 instances of inappropriate management activities were identified. Some individual disasters were accompanied by more than 20 such instances.

Most disaster mismanagement problems occurred because relief managers did not know what all of the relief activities were or how they should be accomplished. Although extensive information is available on the various components of disaster relief and a variety of disaster relief plans exist, only in recent years have the good regional and global guidelines described in the previous sections been available.

REFERENCES

1. Wijkman A, Timberlake L: Natural Disasters: Acts of God or Acts of Man? Washington, DC: The International Institute for Environment and Development (Earthscan Paperback), 1984
2. Gregg MB (ed): The Public Health Consequences of Disaster 1989. Atlanta: Centers for Disease Control, 1989
3. United Nations General Assembly: Resolution 44/236, 1989
4. Weir D: The Bhopal Syndrome. San Francisco: Sierra Club Books, 1987
5. Bhopal Working Group: APHA technical report. The public health implications of the Bhopal disaster; report to the Program Development Board, American Public Health Association. Am Public Health 77:230–236, 1987
6. Anspaugh LR, Catlin RJ, Goldman M: The global impact of the Chernobyl reactor accident. Science 242:1513–1519, 1988
7. Adams P, Solomon L: In the Name of Progress: The Underside of Foreign Aid. Toronto: Energy Probe Research Foundation, 1985
8. Stone RA, Levine AG: Reactions to collective stress: correlates of active citizen participation at Love Canal. Special Issue: Beyond the individual: Environmental approaches and prevention. Prevention Human Services 4(1-2): 153–177, Fall-Winter 1985-86
9. Freudenberg N: Not In Our Backyards! Community Action for Health and the Environment. New York: Monthly Review Press, 1984, pp 42–59
10. Stehr-Green PA, Andrews JS Jr, Hoffman RE, Schram WF: An overview of the Missouri dioxin studies. Arch Environ Health 43(2): 174–177, 1988
11. Deadly Defense: Military Radioactive Landfills, New York: Radioactive Waste Campaign, 1988
12. World Health Assembly: Resolution 34.28, 1981
13. Western K: The Epidemiology of Natural and Manmade Disasters: The Present State of the Art. Dissertation, London School of Hygiene and Tropical Medicine. University of London, 1972
14. French JG, Holt KW: Floods. In Gregg,[2] pp 69–78
15. French JG: Hurricanes. In Gregg,[2] pp 33–37
16. Sanderson LM: Tornadoes. In Gregg,[2] pp 39–49
17. Stratton JW: Earthquakes. In Gregg,[2] pp 13–24
18. Baxter PJ: Volcanoes. In Gregg,[2] pp 25–32
19. Katsouyanni K, Kogevinas M, Trichopoulos D: Earthquake-related stress and cardiac mortality. Int J Epidemiol 15(3):326–330, 1986
20. Shore JH, Tatum EL, Vollmer W: Evolution of mental effects of disaster, Mount St. Helens eruption. Am J Public Health 76(3 suppl):76–83, 1986
21. Sanderson LM: Fires. In Gregg,[2] pp 103–115
22. Melius J, Binder S: Industrial disasters. In Gregg,[2] pp 97–102
23. Withers J: Major Industrial Hazards: Their Appraisal and Control. New York: Halsted Press, 1988
24. Eheman CR: Nuclear reactor incidents. In Gregg,[2] pp 117–127
25. Hatch MC, Byea J, Nieves JW, Susser M: Cancer near the Three Mile Island nuclear plant: radiation emissions. Am J Epidemiol 132(3):397–412, 1990
26. Upton AC: Health Impact of the Three Mile Island Accident. In Moss TH, Sills DL (eds): The Three Mile Island Nuclear Accident: Lessons and Implications. New York: New York Academy of Sciences, 1981, pp 63–75
27. Mileti DS, Hartsough D, Madson P, Hufnagel R: The Three Mile Island incident: a study of behavioral indicators of human stress. Int Mass Emerg Disast 2:89–114, 1984
28. Wolf CP: The accident at Three Mile Island: social science perspectives. Soc Sci Res Council Items 33(3/4):56–61, 1979
29. Beyea J: Emergency planning for reactor accidents. Bull Atomic Sci 36(10):40–45, 1980
30. Geiger HJ: The accident at Chernobyl and the medical response. JAMA 256:609–612, 1986
31. Illyin LA: Ecological features and biomedical consequences of the accident at Chernobyl. J Radiol Protect 10(13), 1990
32. Subcommittee on Oversight and Investigations of the Committee on Energy and Commerce, U.S. House of Representatives: Health and Safety at the Department of Energy's Nuclear Weapons Facilities. Committee Print 101-H. Washington, DC: U.S. Government Printing Office, 1989
33. Toole MJ, Foster S: Famines. In Gregg,[2] pp 79–89
34. Sivard RL: World Military and Social Expenditures 1987-88. Washington, DC: World Priorities, 1987, pp 28–31
35. Sivard RL: World Military and Social Expenditures 1989. Washington, DC: World Priorities, 1989, p 23
36. Stockholm International Peace Research Institute: Yearbook 1989. Uppsala: Uppsala University, 1989
37. Leaning J, Barron RA, Rumack BH: Bloody Sunday: "Trauma in Tbilisi." Report of a Medical Mission to Soviet Georgia. Boston: Physicians for Human Rights, 1990
38. Hu H, Fine J, Epstein P, Kelsey K, Reynolds P, Walker B: Tear gas harassing agent or toxic chemical weapons? JAMA 262:660–663, 1989
39. General Accounting Office: Environmental Issues at DOE's Nuclear Facilities, GAO/RCED-86-192. Washington, DC: U.S. Government Printing Office, September 1986
40. US Department of Energy: Environmental Survey: Preliminary Summary Report of the Defense Production Facilities. Washington, DC: U.S. Government Printing Office, 1988
41. Wilkinson GS, Tietjen GL, Wiggs LD, et al: Mortality among plutonium and other radiation workers at a plutonium weapons facility. Am J Epidemiol 125:231–250, 1987
42. Cragle DL, McLain RW, et al: Mortality among workers at a nuclear fuels production facility. Am J Ind Med 14 (4):379–401, 1988
43. Geiger HJ: Testimony Before the Committee on Energy and Natural Resources, U.S. Senate, November 17, 1989. Washington DC: Physicians for Social Responsibility, 1989
44. Gardner MW, Snee MP, Hall AJ: Results of case-control study of leukemia and lymphoma among young people near Sellafeld nuclear plant. Br Med J 300:423–429, 1990
45. Nathan DC, Geiger JH, Sidel VW, Lown B: The medical consequences of thermonuclear war. N Engl J Med 266:1126–1155, 1962
46. Leaf A: New perspectives on the medical consequences of nuclear war. N Engl J Med 315:905–912, 1986
47. Leaning J: Civil defense in the nuclear age: What purpose does it serve and what survival does it promise? In Cassel C, McCally M, Abraham H (eds): Nuclear Weapons and Nuclear War: A Source Book for Health Professionals. New York: Prager, 1984, pp 406–437
48. World Health Organization: Effects of Nuclear War on Health and Health Services. Report of the WHO Management Group on Follow-up of Resolution WHA36.28: The Role of Physicians and Other Health Workers in the Preservation and Promotion of Peace. Geneva: World Health Organizations, 1987
49. Geiger HJ: The medical effects of a nuclear attack. In Dennis J (ed): Nuclear Almanac: Confronting the Atom in War and Peace. Reading, Mass: Addison-Wesley, 1984, p 112
50. Abrams HL: Medical resources after nuclear war. JAMA 252:653–658, 1984
51. Abrams HL, Von Kaenel WE: Medical problems of survivors of nuclear war: infection and spread of communicable disease. N Engl J Med 305:1226–1232, 1981
52. Turco RP, et al: Nuclear winter: global consequences of multiple nuclear explosions. Science 222:1283–1292, 1983
53. Geiger JH, Leaning J: Nuclear winter with long-term consequences of nuclear war. Prev Med 16:309–318, 1987

54. Ehrlich PR, et al: Long-term biological consequences of nuclear war. Science 222:1293–1300, 1983
55. Turco RP, Toon OB, Ackerman TP, Pollack JB, Sagan C: Climate and smoke: an appraisal of nuclear winter. Science 247:166–176, 1990
56. Sidel VW, Goldwyn R: Chemical and biological weapons—a primer. N Eng J Med 274:21–27, 1966
57. Hu H, Cook-Deegan R, Shukri A: The use of chemical weapons: conducting an investigation using survey epidemiology. JAMA 262:640–643, 1989
58. Sidel VW: Weapons of mass destruction: the greatest threat to public health. JAMA 262:680–682, 1989
59. Thatcher G: Poison on the Wind: The New Threat of Chemical and Biological Weapons. Boston: Christian Science Monitor Publishing Society, 1988
60. World Health Organization: Health Aspects of Chemical and Biological Weapons. Geneva: World Health Organizations, 1970
61. Carnes SA, Watson AP: Disposing of the US chemicals weapons stockpile: an approaching reality. JAMA 262:653–659, 1989
62. Wright S (ed): Preventing a Biological Arms Race. Cambridge, Mass: MIT Press, 1990
63. Cole LA: Clouds of Secrecy: The Army's Germ Warfare Tests Over Populated Areas. Totawa, NJ: Rowman & Littlefield, 1988
64. Jacobson JA, Rosenberg BH: Biological defense research: charting a safer course. JAMA 262:675–676, 1989
65. Sidel VW: Proliferation of biological weapons. Public Health Comments 3(11):4–6, 1989
66. Mitcham C, Siekevitz P (eds): Ethical issues associated with scientific and technological research for the military. Ann N Y Acad Sci vol 577, Dec 29, 1989
67. Sidel VW: Destruction before detonation: the health and social costs of the arms race. Health Med 1(4):6–15, 1983
68. U.S. Department of Health, Education, and Welfare, Public Health Service, Centers for Disease Control: MMWR, May 4, 1979
69. Pan American Health Organization: Emergency Preparedness and Disaster Relief Coordination Program Scientific Publications: Emergency Health Management After Natural Disaster (No. 407, 1981); Emergency Vector Control After Natural Disaster (No. 419, 1982); Epidemiologic Surveillance After Natural Disaster (No. 420, 1982); Environmental Health Management After Natural Disasters (No. 430, 1982); Medical Supply Management After Natural Disaster (No. 438, 1983); Health Services Organization in the Event of Disaster (No. 443, 1983). Washington, DC: World Health Organization
70. United Nations High Commissioner for Refugees: Handbook for Emergencies. Part One: Field Operations. Geneva: United Nations, 1982
71. Whittaker H (ed): 1978 Emergency Preparedness Project, National Governors' Association. Final Report (No. 008-040-00080-0). Washington, DC: U.S. Government Printing Office, 1979
72. Leaning J, Keyes L (eds): The Counterfeit Ark: Crisis Relocation for Nuclear War. Cambridge, Mass: Ballinger Publishing Co, 1984
73. Gregg MB: Surveillance and Epidemiology. In Gregg,[2] pp 3–4
74. Gunn SWA: Multilingual Dictionary of Disaster Medicine and International Relief. Dordrecht, The Netherlands: Kluwer Academic Publishers, 1989
75. Walsh MC: Disasters: Current Planning and Recent Experience. London: Edward Arnold, 1989
76. Foege WH: Epidemiologic surveillance of protein calories malnutrition and of specific deficiencies. Paper presented at Prince Leopold Institute of Tropical Medicine, Antwerp, Belgium, Dec. 6, 1975
77. Gregg MB: Working with the news media. In Gregg,[2] pp 5–6
78. Sidel VW: Quid est amor patriae? PSR Q vol 2, June 1991 (Physicians for Social Responsibility, publisher)
79. Simmonds S, Vaughn P, Gunn SW (eds): Refugee Community Care. Oxford, England: Oxford Medical Publications, 1983
80. Rennie D: After the earthquake. Lancet 2:704–707, 1970
81. Faich GA: Earthquake Disaster Assessment, Managua, Nicaragua; Memorandum. Atlanta: Centers for Disease Control, Jan. 8, 1973
82. Kroger E: International assistance in natural disasters: experiences and proposals (dissertation). London, London School of Hygiene and Tropical Medicine, University of London, 1971
83. Sweeney EC: Medical department participation in disaster relief. Med Tech Bull 7:93–102
84. U.S. Department of Health Education and Welfare, Public Health Service, Centers for Disease Control: Disaster Management: A Study of the Problem and Its Causes. July 9, 1974

75

Ethics and Public Health Policy

John M. Last

Ethics is a set of philosophical beliefs and practices concerned with the distinction between right and wrong, with moral values, and with rights, duties, and obligations. All societies distinguish between acceptable and unacceptable conduct. There is a high degree of consistency among human communities regarding some aspects of conduct, illustrated by the almost universal taboo against incest. In other respects, such as infanticide, abortion, capital punishment, slavery, and child labor, values, behavior, and policies have differed widely over time and among civilized societies. In western industrial nations, many aspects of acceptable conduct derive ultimately from ancient roots such as the Ten Commandments, whence evolved laws that have been codified to protect society from harm due to violations.

ETHICS, MORALITY, VALUES, AND LAW

There is close concordance between ethics and morality. The distinction is based mainly on the intellectual and emotional level at which we accept or reject standards of conduct; we may be upset by a person's conduct if it offends our moral values, but if that conduct can be explained, it may be seen to conform to ethical standards. An undercover policeman gathering evidence against a criminal might behave in a way that would outrage law-abiding citizens unaware of reasons for this behavior, but the same people might approve if they knew the reasons. The moral values of society are the basis for many of our laws, whether these laws are enacted by a legislative body or based on judgments rendered in a court of law.

Community standards are also influenced by social values, which fluctuate more than moral values do. For example, changing American attitudes toward alcohol led to the constitutional amendment on prohibition and then to its repeal. Health-related social values have changed remarkably in the past 100 years. Epidemiological evidence that has become part of general knowledge and popular culture has influenced social values, thereby leading to many important changes in public health policy and law. Examples include improved standards of personal hygiene and public food handling, safer working conditions and labor laws, altered dietary and exercise habits, and transformation of attitudes and behavior about tobacco smoking. Many communities have restricted smoking in public places, such as cinemas and restaurants, often with backing of laws or regulations.

In general, laws uphold the values of society. Some actions may be legal but unethical. A man who holds an elected office in government may legally advise his wife about investments on the basis of privileged information that he possesses, unless this is proscribed by rules relating to conflict of interest; but although it may be legal for him to offer such advise, it is unethical. On the other hand, it is illegal to assist a suicidal act, but it is ethical for a physician to act in such a way as to avoid needlessly prolonging the distress sometimes associated with the process of dying. (This dilemma has been the subject of much legal and ethical debate.)

PRINCIPLES OF BIOMEDICAL ETHICS

In western industrial nations, many principles of ethics have descended to us from Aristotle,[1] whose *Ethics* (fourth century BC) discussed many actions aimed at achieving some good or desirable end. Aristotle's concepts of ethics resemble in some ways the biblical precepts of the Old Testament and the teachings of Jesus of Nazareth. Aristotle's philosophy and the Judeo-Christian beliefs were modified by John Stuart Mill and Immanuel Kant, whose names are associated, respectively, with theories of ethics called utilitarian (''greatest good for the greatest number'') and deontological (recognizing rights and duties to behave in certain ways, generally because they conform to religious beliefs or other widely held moral values).

Much of medical ethics is founded on four basic principles: respect for autonomy, nonmaleficence, beneficence, and justice.

Respect for autonomy means concern about human dignity and freedom, the fundamental rights of the individual.

Nonmaleficence is the principle of not harming, derived from the ancient medical maxim, *primum non nocere* (first do no harm); this may have had greater force in former times when medical care was often hazardous, but it remains relevant today.

Beneficence is the principle of doing good, which members of the professions related to public health practice often believe to be the main function of health care.

Justice in the ethical sense means natural justice, distributive justice—fairness, equity, and impartiality.

These four principles are upheld as far as possible in all aspects of health care, but they are sometimes in conflict. For example, we must sometimes restrict individual freedom (autonomy) in the interest of justice. In decisions about resource allocation, expensive high-technology care of individual patients is often regarded by clinicians as the highest priority, whereas public health specialists seek a larger share of health budgets for health promotion and disease prevention. Entirely new situations have arisen in modern medical practice. Some are a consequence of advancing medical science (e.g., the problems presented by organ and tissue transplants, intensive care life support systems, genetic engineering, and new reproductive technologies). Others are a result of changing social values. An example of changing social values with important implications for medical ethics relates to female reproductive behavior and health. Should women have imposed on them the view that it is sinful to interfere with natural reproductive processes, whether to reduce the risk of pregnancy or to terminate an unwanted pregnancy? There is great variation in the extent to which individuals and groups in society regard interference with pregnancy as tolerable, sinful, or criminal; the variation is related to conflict between a moral value ("right to life") and a social value ("freedom of choice").

In the discussion that follows, applying the principles of biomedical ethics can help us reach "correct" decisions when we are faced with dilemmas or ambiguous situations in public health practice and research. Some of the ambiguities are as difficult to resolve as the ethical dilemmas of clinical practice. There is not always a "right" answer, so it is preferable to apply logically the principles of biomedical ethics rather than to rely on ex cathedra statements of "expert" opinion. However eminent the experts may be, ex cathedra statements are often flawed.

RIGHTS AND NEEDS: COMMUNICABLE DISEASE CONTROL

The concept of contagion has been recognized for centuries. Many communities have reacted by identifying persons with "contagious" diseases and sometimes by segregating or isolating them. These customs date back to the leper's bell and the lazaretto. Since the fourteenth century the practice of quarantine has arisen; this led to development of procedures aimed at restricting freedom of movement of apparently healthy people in contact with persons thought to be suffering from certain infectious diseases. These procedures were codified by Johann Peter Frank[2] and subsequently reinforced by laws and regulations in organized societies all over the world.

Identifying persons with communicable diseases means that they are labeled, and in practice this has sometimes stigmatized them. Isolation and quarantine, of course, restrict freedom. Individuals, families, even entire communities may be identified and stigmatized, isolated, or quarantined. These practices are widely accepted features of communicable disease control and are often held to be necessary to benefit society as a whole.

Until recently there has been little objection to these measures aimed at control of communicable diseases. The need of society for protection has been considered paramount over the rights of the individual case or contact. When smallpox, cholera, poliomyelitis, and diphtheria were prevalent, few people questioned the actions of public health authorities who notified and isolated cases, quarantined contacts, and sometimes severely infringed the freedom and dignity of entire families. Some diseases (e.g., tuberculosis, syphilis) carried considerable social stigma.

Reactions to essentially the same phenomena when they arise in relation to cases of AIDS and HIV infection have been rather different. The first wave of the AIDS epidemic in the United States hit hardest at an already stigmatized group, male homosexuals, who had only recently been able to break free from age-old prejudices. The hostile reaction toward persons with AIDS among many members of "respectable" society was aggravated by homophobia and by exaggerated fears about the mode of transmission of AIDS. Combined with the rising demand for equity and justice in dealing with minority groups in society, it heightened awareness of the need to provide health care services with justice and equity for all. Widely publicized instances of victimization of AIDS patients—homosexual men hounded out of their jobs, hemophiliac children rejected by schools and even communities—have aroused public opinion on the side of compassionate and humane management of these patients. A second wave of the epidemic affected intravenous drug abusers who shared needles. This group has not attracted the sympathy of many people, but their infants who are infected with HIV have generally been recognized as innocent victims. Even if somebody gets AIDS or HIV infection as a consequence of behavior that some members of the health professions might regard with disgust, we all have an obligation to apply our professional skills helpfully, impartially, and nonjudgmentally.

The social reactions to AIDS and HIV infection have led to much discussion about the ethics of management and control. The diagnosis of HIV infection is widely regarded as a virtual death sentence and an irrevocable edict against promiscuous sexual behavior. The diagnosis must not be lightly made; nor should the test for HIV antibody be lightly undertaken. Both voluntary testing and communication of the results of a positive test must be accompanied by careful counseling of all persons concerned and of their sexual partners.[3] Health workers have an obligation not to discriminate against persons who are HIV antibody positive or who suffer from AIDS. The obligation of physicians and nurses to care for patients with HIV infection is no less than the obligation to care for patients with any other communicable disease. Moreover, HIV infection is considerably less contagious than conditions such as tuberculosis or streptococcal infection, from which in former times many physicians and nurses died after being infected by patients.

For epidemiological surveillance, public health authorities need data on the prevalence of HIV infection. The World Health Organization and many national authorities agree that unlinked anonymous HIV testing is the best way to generate prevalence data.[4] Aliquots of blood taken for other purposes are tested for HIV antibody after all personal identifiers have been removed. Suitable populations for surveillance include pregnant women and newborn infants. Until recently in the United Kingdom and The Netherlands, it has been held that anonymous unlinked testing is unethical, because identifying and counseling infected persons and their sexual partners was regarded as a higher moral responsibility than determining community-wide prevalence trends. In some African nations where prevalence of HIV infection is high, public health authorities believe that the need for prevalence data is urgent enough to justify compulsory testing. However, as neither treatment nor counseling is feasible, results of the tests are sometimes withheld even from persons found to be HIV antibody positive.

The rules that have evolved for testing and reporting of AIDS and HIV infection are a variant of rules and procedures for identifying, notifying, and initiating control measures for other sexually transmitted diseases or, indeed, for many other forms of communicable disease. These rules are not draconian. With the exception of Cuba, where HIV antibody–positive persons are subject to enforced quarantine, there have been no serious intrusions on personal liberty. There are, however, other severe sanctions, notably restrictions on medical and life insurance, employment, freedom to move from one nation to another. For example, although it makes no epidemiological sense and violates human rights, most HIV-positive persons are denied entry visas to many countries, including the United States[5]. There have been many discussions and publications on AIDS and HIV-antibody testing.[6]

INDIVIDUAL RIGHTS AND COMMUNITY NEEDS: ENVIRONMENTAL HEALTH

The rights of individuals have to be balanced against the needs of communities in other respects besides control of communicable diseases. Most orderly societies have laws or regulations aimed at protecting people from tainted foodstuffs, unsafe working conditions, and unsatisfactory housing, although the strength of such laws and regulations is variable and enforcement is often lax. It may be necessary for aggrieved parties to resort to litigation before an issue can be resolved. Community values and standards have lately shifted toward greater control over environmental hazards to health, reflecting growing concern about our deteriorating environment. In Canada the Law Reform Commission proposed laws to protect the public from the consequences of "crimes against the environment,"[7] but adherence to environmental ethics would be a better solution. Those who pollute the environment harm themselves as well as others; it is in everybody's interest to uphold standards such as those proposed in the European Charter on Environment and Health.[8]

Sometimes health is adversely affected by environmental conditions, but correcting these conditions may have unpleasant economic repercussions, such as massive unemployment, and may be opposed by the people whose health is threatened. Public health specialists then are in the situation portrayed by Dr. Stockmann in Ibsen's play *An Enemy of the People*—reviled for actions aimed at protecting health. It can be difficult to decide the best course of action in such situations, but a useful guideline is to consider the ethical principles of beneficent truth telling, distributive justice, and nonmaleficence: what is the truth about the situation and which of the competing priorities will harm the fewest people over the longest period?

RISKS AND BENEFITS

Faced with an outbreak of smallpox in 1947, the public health authorities of the city of New York vaccinated about 5 million people in a brief period of 6 weeks or so. The human costs of this were 45 known cases of postvaccinal encephalitis and four deaths[9]—an acceptable risk in view of the enormous benefit, the safety of a city of 8 million among whom thousands would have died had the epidemic struck, but a heavy price for the victims of vaccination accidents and their next of kin.

Similar risk-to-benefit ratios have to be calculated for every immunizing agent, indeed for all forms of health care. Consider measles; there may be a risk somewhere between 1 in 1 million and 1 in 5 million of subacute sclerosing panencephalitis (SSPE) as an adverse effect of measles vaccination.[10] Measles is close to elimination from North America (despite recent flare-ups). If we continue to immunize infants against measles after the disease is eliminated, there will be occasional unpleasant adverse consequences, perhaps an occurrence of many cases of septicemia from a contaminated batch of vaccine. This fact and the cost of measles vaccination in the face of competing claims for other uses of the same funds will be incentives to stop using measles vaccine. However, stopping the immunizations will entail the risk that epidemic measles may return at some later date, perhaps not until there is a large population of unvaccinated susceptible persons. History could repeat itself: mortality rates up to 40% occurred when measles was introduced into the Americas by European colonists. High death rates would be unlikely in the era of antibiotics, but the morbidity and complication rates would be troublesome in an unimmunized population.

The risks of adverse reactions to other immunizing agents are all greater than the risks of reactions to measles vaccine, but the risks of not immunizing are almost always greater[11] (Table 75-1).

One duty of all who conduct immunization campaigns is to ensure that everybody is aware of the risks as well as the benefits; in short, informed consent is an indispensable prerequisite. This becomes especially important when children are not admitted to school until their parents or guardians can show evidence of immunization (i.e., when immunization is mandatory rather than voluntary).

In the United States and some other countries the threat of litigation in the event of vaccination mishaps is a deterrent to immunization procedures, even a threat to the manufacturers of vaccines. However, health care providers can be sued for negligence if they fail to immunize vulnerable persons or groups, as well as for damages if there are adverse reactions—a Hobson's choice. In Great Britain, France, Switzerland, New Zealand, and some other countries the threat of litigation has been removed by legislation providing for a standard scale of compensation for accidents and mishaps associated with use of immunizing agents. A bill with similar provisions was enacted by the United States Congress in 1986 and began to be implemented in 1990.

Acceptable Risks. In many other situations we trade risks against benefits. The use of diagnostic x-rays is an example. The epidemiological evidence demonstrates that a single diagnostic dose of x-ray can harm the developing human fetus,[12] but there are medical conditions in which this small and distant future risk is acceptable because the alternative is a larger and more immediate risk, such as serious complications of untreated renal disease. Diagnostic imaging techniques, such as ultrasound, have removed what was previously a difficult clinical decision when x-rays were the only resort of the obstetrician who suspected fetal malposition or disproportion, but x-rays remain the best diagnostic tool for some conditions.

Health administrations and hospital staff members also ac-

TABLE 75-1. ESTIMATED RATES OF ADVERSE REACTIONS TO IMMUNIZATIONS

Vaccine	Reaction	Rate per 100,000
BCG	Disseminated infection	<0.1
	Osteomyelitis	<0.1–30
	Suppurative adenitis	100–4,000
DPT	Convulsions	0.3–90
	Encephalitis	0.1–3
	Brain damage	0.2–0.6
	Death	0.2
Measles	Convulsions	30
	Encephalitis	0.0–0.03

▪ ADVERSE OUTCOMES OF PERTUSSIS AND IMMUNIZATION

	Cases per million	
	With Immunization	**Without**
Effect (Birth–6 months)		
Hospitalization	1,060	11,098
Death	12.5	130.6
Encephalitis	2.4	25.5
Residual defect	0.8	8.5
(6 months–5 years)		
Cases of pertussis	34,048	356,566
Hospitalizations	6,529	38,787
Deaths	44	457
Encephalitis	162	87
Residual defects	54	29

From USDHHS Task Force, 1986.[11]

cept the small risk of malignant disease among radiographers and other health workers who are occupationally exposed to x-rays and the risk of fetal loss among operating room staff exposed to waste anesthetic gases. However, not all the occupationally exposed individuals are informed of this admittedly small risk.

Mass Medication. Risk-benefit calculations are required for all forms of mass medication, not only for immunizations. The possibility of adverse effects or idiosyncratic reaction always exists. Opposition to fluoridation of drinking water is based in part on the unfounded fear that fluoride can cause cancer or some other terrible disease. Epidemiological analysis shows no association between fluoridation and cancer,[13] although the occurrence of osteosarcoma among rats exposed to fluoride salts[14] has reopened debate. Opposition to fluoridation of drinking water is really more a political than a public health issue, in which the catchphrase of the antifluoridation movement—"keep the water pure"—is difficult to rebut. Other political arguments rest on the claim that fluoridation is a paternalist measure, inflicted on the population whether they like it or not. The antipaternalist argument is that individuals in a free society should be able to choose for themselves whether they want to drink fluoridated water. Responsible adults can choose, but for infants and small children, fluoridated drinking water makes all the difference between healthy and carious teeth. Using the ethical principle of beneficence, public health authorities argue that infants and small children should receive fluoride in sufficient quantity to ensure that their dental enamel can resist cariogenic bacteria.

Some people have a genuine conscientious objection to mass medication such as fluoridation of drinking water or immunization of their children against communicable diseases. Opting out can be difficult. Opting out of fluoridation means the trouble and expense of using special supplies of bottled water. Opting out of immunization can mean exclusion of one's children from schools that make entry conditional on a certificate testifying to successful immunization against measles, poliomyelitis, etc. The argument in favor of immunization is strengthened by reports of epidemics of paralytic poliomyelitis among children of members of religious sects that oppose immunization.[15] Children, it can be argued, should not be exposed to risks because of their parents' beliefs. In many jurisdictions, courts have intervened to save lives of infants and children requiring blood transfusions that their parents object to for religious reasons. The circumstances are different when immunizations are offered to healthy children with the aim of protecting them against diseases that are rare anyway. This is a difficult dilemma when the immunizing agent has adverse effects. The principles of beneficence and nonmaleficence appear to cancel each other out. There remains another argument based on the principle of distributive justice: all infants deserve the protection of vaccines, even though a few may be harmed by untoward consequences.

PRIVACY AND HEALTH STATISTICS

Many people are troubled by the thought that intimate information about them is stored in computers, accessible in theory to anyone who can operate the keyboard. Of course the same information has long existed in narrative form in medical charts where it was as easily accessible to unauthorized readers as it now allegedly is to unauthorized computer operators. As many as 100 people are authorized to make entries in the hospital chart of the average patient in an acute short-stay general hospital bed, and all must read the chart if their entries are to make sense in context. In this respect, the confidentiality of the doctor-patient relationship, the cornerstone of the argument for privacy, is a myth.[16]

Computer storage and retrieval of health-related information greatly enhance the power of analysis to reveal significant associations between exposures and outcomes. Much of our recently acquired knowledge about many causal relationships has come from routine analyses of health statistics and from epidemiological studies that have made use of existing medical records. Examples include the association between rubella and birth defects, cigarette smoking and cancer, exposure to ionizing radiation and cancer, adverse drug reactions such as the thromboembolic effects of the oral contraceptive pill, and excess deaths due to use of certain antiasthmatic drugs (see Chapter 2). Community benefit outweighs any harm attributable to invasion of privacy, especially as that harm is theoretical; confidentiality and personal integrity, if not autonomy, remain intact. In some nations (e.g. Sweden, Australia) government-appointed guardians of privacy oversee the uses of medical and other records when these are requested for research purposes.

Resistance to use of routinely collected medical records for epidemiological analysis has come not only from guardians of privacy but also from special interest groups who would prefer that inconvenient facts not be disclosed. Industrial corporations sometimes have tried to prevent disclosure of the adverse effects of occupational or environmental exposures, which it has not been in their financial interest to have widely known. Even governments that ought to have the public interest as their first priority have been known to suppress information derived from analyses of health statistics when it is politically inconvenient for such information to be publicized. Public health workers and epidemiologists must be alert to the risk of these forms of "censorship" and must be prepared to defend access to sources of health-related information.

Applying the principle of beneficence, it is desirable not only to maintain data files of health-related information but to expand them; available ideas as well as available information should be used for the common good. Statistical analysis of health-related information has been so convincingly demonstrated to be in the public interest that there is no rational argument against continuing on our present course and expanding further the scope of these activities. This argument applies with particular force to the use of linked medical records, potentially the most powerful method of studying diseases that are rare or have very long incubation times.

Health workers have a moral obligation to respect the confidentiality of the records that they use. Irresponsible disclosure of confidential details that can harm individuals is not only unethical but can arouse public opinion against collection and use of such material. Properly used, health statistics and the records from which they are derived do not invade individual privacy. Indeed, as Black[17] has pointed out, the argument that individual rights are infringed in the interest of the community is an example of a "false antithesis"—the rights of the individual are congruent with, not in conflict with, the needs of the community because, as a member of the community, every individual benefits from the analyses that are based on individual health records.

Generally the law reinforces this ethical position while upholding autonomy by safeguarding privacy. For example, a U.S. Court of Appeals ruled in favor of preserving the confidentiality of medical records used by the Centers for Disease Control in an epidemiological study of toxic shock syndrome attributed to the use of certain varieties of vaginal tampon. Lawyers for the manufacturer of these tampons had tried to subpoena the records so that they could call the women as witnesses and presumably challenge their testimony. The court ruled that it would not be in the public interest to establish a precedent in which records of epidemiological importance could be used in this sort of adversarial situation, because this would be a deterrent both to those aspiring to conduct future epidemiological studies and to participants in such studies.[18] However, in 1989 a U.S. Circuit Court granted a tobacco company access to clinical records (albeit stripped of personal identifiers) that had been the basis of another epidemiological study.[19] The issue of confidentiality of medical records, and their subsequent use for epidemiological analysis, remains open; the potential threat that courts may allow access by hostile interest groups could become a deterrent to future aspiring epidemiologists unless this matter can be clarified. In 1990 the Society for Epidemiologic Research agreed, after much debate, that research data should be shared with outside parties who might wish to reanalyze raw data.[20] Reasons for reanalysis should not influence the right of access.

ETHICAL GUIDELINES FOR EPIDEMIOLOGISTS

The preceding discussions have alluded to several problems that have preoccupied many epidemiologists who have been defining ethical issues and formulating appropriate responses. Groups that have developed guidelines on ethics include the Society for Epidemiologic Research, the Industrial Epidemiology Forum,[21] the Swedish Society of Public Health Research Workers, and the International Epidemiological Association.[22] The Council for International Organizations of the Medical Sciences (CIOMS), which had already developed *Guidelines for Ethical Review of Research Involving Human Subjects,*[23] has drafted similar guidelines for ethical review of epidemiological practice and research.[24] National research-funding agencies also have been concerned about these issues, and several (e.g., the National Health and Medical Research Council in Australia,[25] the Canadian Medical Research Council,[26] and the European Medical Research Councils) have prepared position papers. The National Institutes of Health discussed a checklist of ethical questions for epidemiological research in the early 1970s.[27]

All epidemiological studies, whether for public health surveillance or for research, involve human subjects and must therefore abide by the Helsinki Declaration[28] and its revisions, respecting human dignity. Research and surveillance must not harm people,[29] and informed consent is usually a sine qua non.

Informed Consent. Informed consent to all medical interventions is both a legal requirement and an ethical imperative. The process and procedures for obtaining informed consent[30] should be clearly understood by all health workers. The process consists of transfer of information and understanding of its significance to all subjects of medical interventions, followed by explicit consent of the subjects (or responsible proxies) to the intervention. The task of informing is important; it should be conducted by someone senior and responsible and not delegated to a junior nurse or a medical student. Consent is usually active (i.e., agreement to take part); sometimes it is passive (i.e., people are regarded as taking part unless they explicitly refuse). Consent need not be written; the act of offering an arm and a vein for withdrawal of a sample of blood implies consent; the essential feature is understanding the purpose for which the blood is taken. Concepts of autonomy vary. In some cultures patients regard their personal physicians as responsible for decisions about participation; in other cultures a village headman, a tribal elder, or a religious leader is considered to have responsibility for the group, in which individuals may not all perceive themselves as autonomous. Nevertheless, each individual in such a group should be asked to give consent to whatever procedure is being performed as part of a public health intervention or epidemiological research project.

Obligations of Epidemiologists. The obligation of epidemiologists to respect the Helsinki Declaration is inviolable. However, sometimes epidemiologists study large populations and it is not feasible to obtain the informed consent of every individual whose records contribute to the statistical analysis.[31] Sometimes the records are those of deceased persons. Epidemiologists are then expected to abide by a code of conduct such as that formulated by the International Statistical Institute for official statisticians.[32] This is made formal in many nations by requiring those who work with official records to take an oath of secrecy. In some countries (e.g., Sweden, France, Germany) there have been public and political concerns about access to and use of official statistics, such as death certificate and hospital discharge data. There have even been proposals to respect the privacy of the dead by withholding from death certificates the cause of death when this cause carries a stigma, such as AIDS.

Although respect for privacy is a paramount concern of epidemiologists in surveillance and research, sometimes privacy must be invaded (e.g., when sexual partners must be traced as part of control measures for sexually transmitted diseases). Individual integrity, if not autonomy, is respected by obtaining informed consent whenever possible to these invasions of privacy.

Impartiality and Advocacy. Epidemiology, like all science, is objective, so it ought to be impartial. Quite often, however, epidemiological findings reveal dangers to health that require activist campaigns aimed at changing the status quo, sometimes in direct opposition to established custom and social, economic, commercial, industrial, and political interests and institutions. The discovery that smoking causes lung cancer is a good example; some of the epidemiologists who identified this massive public health problem became advocates for better health and opponents of the tobacco industry and of the many institutions of society that encouraged the use of tobacco. Advocacy and scientific objectivity are uneasy bedfellows, and epidemiology is not "value-neutral." In many situations since the early days of the controversy about smoking and lung cancer (long ago resolved, no longer a controversy) public health workers in general and epidemiologists in particular have had to wrestle with the problem of reconciling impartiality with advocacy of measures to enhance health.

Research Ethics. Consider the data shown in Table 75-2. Such distributions could come from a case-control study or a randomized controlled trial. The distributions in Table 75-2B just reach a level of statistical significance at the 5% level; the distributions in Table 75-2A do not. A public health (or any other) scientist eager to achieve a "significant" result might yield to the temptation to find reasons for excluding one of the observations, perhaps on the grounds that it is an outlier, or reasons for moving an observation from one cell to another in the table.

TABLE 75-2. HOW TO ACHIEVE "STATISTICAL SIGNIFICANCE"

	A. "Not Significant" Differences		B. "Significant" Differences	
	+	–	+	–
+	20	30	20	31
–	30	20	30	19
Total	50	50	50	50
	$P > .05$ [= 0.072]		$P < .05$ [= 0.045]	
	+	–	+	–
+	6	14	5	14
–	44	36	45	36
Total	50	50	50	50
	$P > .05$ [= 0.080]		$P < .05$ [= 0.041]	

NOTE: In each of the distributions, moving one observation achieves a level of "statistical significance" at the 5% level.

This may seem to be almost a venial sin; it is to be hoped that it is an uncommon one. It becomes more serious when data are altered after the fact or when some observations in a series are discarded. Even more serious violations of research ethics are coming to light increasingly often. These range from sloppy research design to gross varieties of scientific fraud and misrepresentation. There has been enough concern about serious violations to prompt the Institute of Medicine of the National Academy of Science[33] to issue guidelines that include a mandatory requirement for rigorously observing protocols, maintaining and preserving research logbooks, and other measures aimed at reducing such unethical conduct to a minimum.

Conflicts of Interest. Conflicts of interest have worried several professional associations, especially in the United States. Concern has arisen because of several episodes. For example, research that had been completed and submitted for publication has been "leaked" to an industrial corporation or pharmaceutical company, which has then hired its own scientists and paid a fee to encourage criticism aimed at discrediting the work even before it is published. In at least two recent instances pressure was applied with the aim of preventing publication of results that might have proved to be damaging to commercial interests. It is not known how often original research has been "censored" (i.e., withheld from publication) because of intimidation, bribery, or more subtle pressure. This and related problems have preoccupied biomedical science editors at recent conferences.[34] The problems may be more widespread and more serious than the high-profile crimes of scientific fraud and plagiarism.

POPULATION SCREENING

Screening is the application of diagnostic tests or procedures to apparently healthy people with the aim of sorting them into those who may have a condition that would benefit from early intervention and those who do not. An ideal screening test would sort people into two groups—those who definitely have and those who definitely do not have the condition. In our imperfect world, screening tests sometimes yield false-positive or false-negative results. A false-positive test exposes individuals to the anxiety, costs, and risks of further investigation and perhaps unnecessary treatment and imposes economic burdens on the health care system that would better be avoided. A false-negative screening test result could have disastrous consequences if, for example, persons suffering from early cancer are incorrectly reassured that there is nothing wrong with them. An important use for epidemiology is the calculation of false-positive and false-negative rates and the predictive power of screening tests; these calculations must be borne in mind when one is deciding whether it is ethical to apply a particular test as a population-screening procedure. For example, if a condition has a prevalence of less than 1 in 1000, the test costs $3 per person, and the predictive power of a positive test is less than 80%, we could question whether the use of resources for the screening test is ethically as well as economically acceptable. The cost of confirmatory tests as well as the feasibility of treatment must be taken into account. For example, interviews can be used to screen populations for evidence of Alzheimer's disease, but the confirmatory tests (diagnostic imaging, etc.) are expensive, so it is important to determine ahead of time who will pay for these.

Screening for evidence of inapparent disease implies and can lead to interventions that will change the lives of people who previously thought themselves to be well. Such persons may react in several ways to the knowledge that they have a disease or a condition that requires treatment; they may assume a sick role—develop symptoms, lose time from work, and become unduly worried about themselves.[35] Some people who previously considered themselves to be healthy may perceive as gratuitous or paternalist the intervention of the well-meaning specialist who found something wrong, especially if the intervention makes them feel worse, as treatment for hypertension may. Questions of medical etiquette as well as ethics can arise. Screening programs are often conducted by staff members in public health rather than personal health care services. It is essential for public health workers to communicate results to personal physicians responsible for the care of individuals with positive tests. At the very least, a positive test result can arouse anxiety (though it can also allay anxiety); it often leads to inconvenience, expense, sometimes to discomfort, and distress. A false-positive test result can lead to needless anxiety and expense. Counseling must be carefully planned and built into screening programs to minimize anxiety. This is an ethical imperative.

More complex questions and moral ambiguities arise in genetic screening and counseling. It is now feasible to screen for Huntington's disease, Tay-Sachs disease, and Duchenne muscular dystrophy among other conditions. In Huntington's disease, a positive screening test result has appalling implications for the person concerned, although early experience with volunteers from high-risk families has suggested that some, at least, prefer to know than not to know their status.[36] If Tay-Sachs disease or Duchenne muscular dystrophy are detected by screening early in pregnancy, termination of the pregnancy is regarded by many authorities as the most humane action (see Chapter 60).

HEALTH EDUCATION

Public health workers regard health education with enthusiasm. What could be more beneficent than providing information about risks to health and actions that can be taken to reduce these risks? Such actions encourage all to take greater responsibility for their own health. Often laws or regulations act synergistically with such forms of health education as advice about immunizations and admonitions against tobacco addiction. But other issues arise when health educators, with or without the help of laws or regulations, seek to control addiction to tobacco or alcohol use. Some civil libertarians hold that everyone has a right to use alcohol or tobacco. This may be true, so long as their use does not harm others, such as children of smoking parents or road users who may be killed or maimed by impaired drivers—which, unhappily, is all too often the case. At the other extreme are those who would prohibit alcohol use altogether and would indict smoking parents or pregnant women for child abuse. Economic interests and well-being of communities dependent on the alcohol and tobacco industries, it is argued, also have to be taken into account in deciding how to deal with the public health problems associated with tobacco and alcohol use. These are complex economic and political and ethical questions. No cash crop is as lucrative as tobacco, and in many parts of the developing world as well as in the United States, tobacco has replaced food crops; in Africa, trees are being destroyed to provide fuel for flue-cured tobacco, contributing to the advance of deserts.[37] These facts, and the annual worldwide toll of tobacco-related premature deaths, provide strong support for the argument that the economic well-being of tobacco-producing communities is best safeguarded by converting to food crops as rapidly as possible. The ethical principles here are beneficence and justice.

POPULATION POLICIES AND FAMILY PLANNING PROGRAMS

All nations have population policies, sometimes explicit but more often implicit. These policies range from encouragement of couples to have or refrain from having children, commonly with related laws or regulations on access to and use of contraceptives, to vaguely visualized policies implied by the appearance in newspapers and women's magazines of articles on birth control that contain statements about the efficacy of contraceptive methods. Most western nations provide funds from taxation or other revenue for support of family planning clinics that are accessible without charge to low-income women, although not always to sexually active unmarried teenage girls.

There are numerous international variations in the constraints on access to such clinics by girls around the age of puberty who are, or may soon become, sexually active. There are also great variations in the nature and extent of sex education, especially education about contraception, and in access to effective contraceptive methods. Predictably, these variations are associated with corresponding international variations in pregnancy rates (Figure 75-1).[38]

Some nations, notably the two most populous (India and China) and one of the most crowded (Singapore), have provided strong economic incentives or even introduced coercive measures, such as enforced sterilization or abortion, aimed at restricting the perceived alarming rate of population growth. Other nations have adopted pronatalist policies (e.g., because of a perceived threat of being overwhelmed by extraneous population groups).

In all nations that have government-supported family planning programs, public health workers are responsible for management and have the task of implementing government policies. Even if these policies are implicit rather than explicit, their general direction is usually clear. In a free society, public health workers have a moral obligation to consider each patient or client as an individual with his or her own unique life situation, problems, and requests and not just a "case" to which the official policies necessarily apply. The aspirations of women and couples to have or refrain from having children are powerful and very personal. Staff members of family planning clinics have an obligation to offer advice and treatment and an equally important obligation not to enforce their own or official views on individual clients.

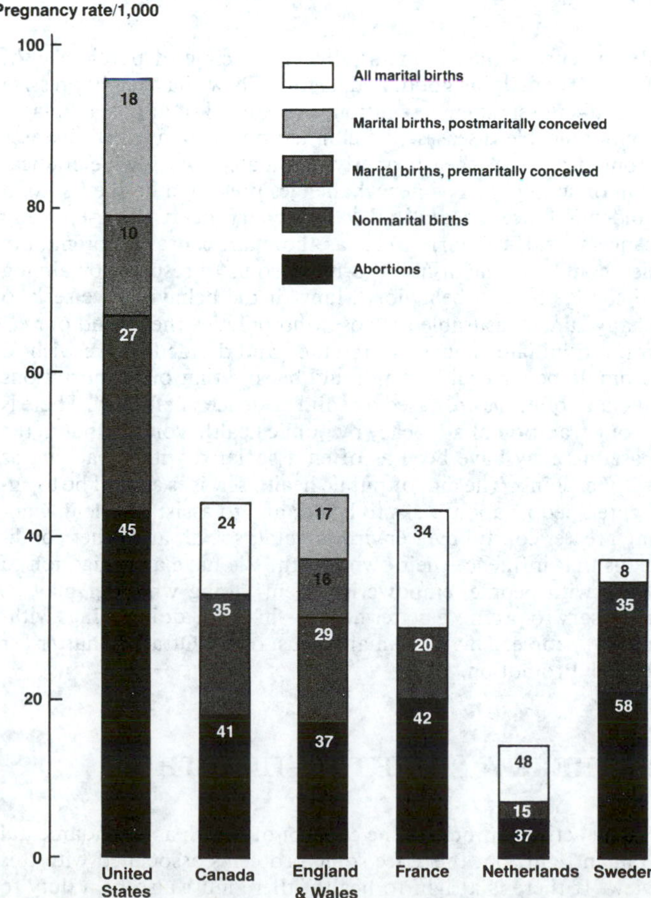

Figure 75-1. Pregnancy rates at ages 15 to 19 in selected countries. Rates are lowest in countries with effective educational programs in human sexuality for schoolchildren and easy access to contraceptives. *[From Jones EF et al: Teenage Pregnancy in Industrialized Countries. New Haven, Conn.: Yale University Press, 1986.]*

EQUITY AND JUSTICE IN RESOURCE ALLOCATION

Public health is inherently concerned with social justice, with fair and equitable distribution of scarce resources to protect, preserve, and restore health. Public health workers therefore frequently become advocates for health care systems that provide access to needed services without economic or other barriers. Historically, public health workers have often provided the impetus to establish a social security system with unimpeded access to health care for all members of society, regardless of income, with access based only on need. In almost every nation that has social security, public health workers are prominent among the organizers and administrators. Moreover, if health services are offered to population groups that do not attract fee-for-service practice, these are often run by staff members from public health services. When analysis of health statistics reveals regions or districts and population groups that have unmet needs, public health workers often take the initiative to meet these needs.

The principles of equity and justice go further. The allocation of funds for health care is often based on political or emotional grounds and on the ability of eloquent and aggressive spokesmen for glamorous high-technology diagnostic and therapeutic services to promote these interests. Funds sometimes are allocated for expensive equipment and devices, perhaps on dubious grounds, while much-needed public health services, such as water-purification plants in need of renovation or logistic support for immunization programs, go without funds. It is an ethical imperative for public health workers to be as aggressive as circumstances require in obtaining an equitable share of resources and funds for public health services.

OCCUPATIONAL HEALTH

The specialist in occupational health or industrial medicine is responsible for safeguarding the health or workers, is often employed by management, answerable also to government regulatory agencies, and subjected to pressure from labor unions and public interest groups. Preserving impartiality among such potentially and often actually adversarial groups can be very difficult. Cognizant of this, in 1976 the American Occupational Medical Association adopted a *Code of Conduct*[39] (Table 75-3); in 1990 the International Commission on Occupational Health circulated a similar draft code of ethics. The latter is intended for all occupational health workers, not just physicians. Neither code explicitly recognizes the needs of such vulnerable groups as pregnant women and underage workers, which may be a problem especially in developing countries.

INTERNATIONAL HEALTH

International health is concerned with the interlocking and interdependent relationships among all people and nations on earth (see Chapter 70). For many years the rich nations have provided

TABLE 75-3. CODE OF ETHICAL CONDUCT FOR PHYSICIANS PROVIDING OCCUPATIONAL MEDICAL SERVICES (ADOPTED BY THE BOARD OF DIRECTORS OF THE AMERICAN OCCUPATIONAL MEDICAL ASSOCIATION, JULY 23, 1976)

These principles are intended to aid physicians in maintaining ethical conduct in providing occupational medical service. They are standards to guide physicians in their relationships with the individuals they serve, with employers and workers' representatives, with colleagues in the health professions, and with the public.

Physicians should:

1. accord highest priority to the health and safety of the individual in the workplace
2. practice on a scientific basis with objectivity and integrity
3. make or endorse only statements which reflect their observations or honest opinion
4. actively oppose and strive to correct unethical conduct in relation to occupational health service
5. avoid allowing their medical judgment to be influenced by any conflict of interest
6. strive conscientiously to become familiar with the medical fitness requirements, the environment and the hazards of the work done by those they serve, and with the health and safety aspects of the products and operations involved
7. treat as confidential whatever is learned about individuals served, releasing information only when required by law or by over-riding public health considerations, or to other physicians at the request of the individual according to traditional medical ethical practice; and should recognize that employers are entitled to counsel about the medical fitness of individuals in relation to work, but are not entitled to diagnoses or details of a specific nature
8. strive continually to improve medical knowledge, and should communicate information about health hazards in timely and effective fashion to individuals or groups potentially affected, and make appropriate reports to the scientific community
9. communicate understandably to those they serve any significant observations about their health, recommending further study, counsel, or treatment when indicated
10. seek consultation concerning the individual or the workplace whenever indicated
11. cooperate with governmental health personnel and agencies, and foster and maintain sound ethical relationships with other members of the health professions
12. avoid solicitation of the use of their services by making claims, offering testimonials, or implying results which may not be achieved, but they may appropriately advise colleagues and others of services available

support for health care, public health, and medical research in the poorer nations. Until recently few questioned the rightness of this; it was regarded as mutually beneficial. There has been concern about the "brain drain"—the hemorrhage of talent from poorer nations that send their best and brightest young people abroad for advanced training and lose them permanently to the rich nations. This has been regarded as a necessary price to pay for assistance in development. Now other difficulties are perceived. Questions have been raised about the appropriateness of technology transfer from rich to poor countries, about the use by research workers from rich countries of the large populations and of the challenging unsolved health problems, with the aim of addressing priorities as perceived in rich countries but without regard for perceived problems and priorities in the poorer nations. This has been described as "ethical imperialism."[40]

Other problems are associated with the disparity between rich and poor nations. These include the export from rich nations to poor nations of problems that are attributable to affluence and industrial development—tobacco addiction, traffic injuries, exploitation of workers (often women and children who work for starvation wages), and environmental pollution.

Other problems arise from differing values and behaviors that prevail in some developing nations. The status of women may be quite different from that in western industrial nations, and such customs as female circumcision, child marriage, and infanticide may be found. Sometimes developing nations are ruled by a repressive military dictatorship without regard for equity in health care. International health workers who encounter such phenomena are in a difficult situation. Speaking out against customs that they deplore or against the actions of repressive rulers is unlikely to help the people of the country and may expose the health workers to the risk of being deported or, worse, arrested, tortured, or imprisoned. Yet it is morally repugnant to remain silent.

International health workers should be able to speak out more forcefully against health-harming exported practices of the industrial nations, such as promotion of infant formula in societies that lack facilities to sterilize infant feeds, dumping of drugs that have not been approved for use in industrial nations, and advertising of tobacco.

PATERNALISM AND PUBLIC HEALTH

Beneficence is the dominant ethical principle of public health. We believe in doing good, and historically we have an impressive record—the sanitary revolution, the control of almost all major communicable diseases, the elimination of many such diseases from large areas they formerly dominated, worldwide eradication of smallpox. The new challenges presented by the "second epidemiological revolution"[41]—coronary heart disease, many cancers, traffic injuries, etc. as the main causes of premature death and chronic disability—have led us to respond by aiming to change human behavior. Many of the behaviors we seek to change are pleasurable to those who practice them, and our efforts to initiate change are resented and derided. If we wish to promote better health, we should be sure that our exhortations and admonitions are based on solid evidence of efficacy. There is a long tradition of advocacy by public health workers, but in the past this may have been as often associated with preaching as with teaching. The aim of public health services should be to enlighten people about risks to health and to assist people in gaining greater control over environmental, social, and other conditions that influence their own health. We have an obligation to work with people, empowering them, doing whatever may be necessary to promote better health—in short, doing things with, not to, people. This is the main thrust of the Ottawa Charter for Health Promotion.[42]

IS THERE A "RIGHT TO HEALTH"?

Social activists proclaim the concept of health as a fundamental human right, but there are some problems associated with this view. If there is a right to health, there must also be a duty to provide this right. Whose duty is it? The answer may be that it is the duty of the individual whose health is the "right" in question, but this leads to the idea of blaming the victim when health is impaired. A further difficulty arises when we try to define what is meant by *health*. There is often confusion between health and quality of life. Nobody would describe the theoretical physicist Stephen Hawking as healthy; he has been slowly dying of amyotrophic lateral sclerosis for many years, but they have been immensely productive years and, judging from his own testimony,[43] they have been happy years. There are many other examples of severely disabled people whose lives have been happy and productive—just as there are examples of "healthy" people who lead miserable lives. Probably it is wise for public health workers to avoid getting drawn into discussions of the supposed right to health. Even so, there is clear justification on grounds of beneficence for public health workers to strive for economic, environmental, social, and political conditions that will maximize the prospects for good health. This is clearly stated in the Ottawa Charter for Health Promotion, in the "Targets" document of the European Region of WHO,[44] and in many similar manifestos.

METHODS IN ETHICS

How should we deal with the moral dilemmas and ethical ambiguities that arise in public health practice and research? The answer is essentially the same in public health as in clinical practice. Several monographs provide some guidance.[45] Enough has been said to make clear the fact that often there is no easy answer. Sometimes we must choose with the certain knowledge that not all parties will be satisfied with the decision. Decisions can be extremely difficult. An orderly, systematic approach is helpful.

First, we should clearly identify the problem(s). We should identify the available options and decide whose problem(s) we are dealing with—particular persons, communities, health care workers, organizations, institutions, etc. We must gather all the available information and evaluate it carefully, trying as far as possible to set priorities among the options that have to be considered. We must also consider the consequences of the decisions that have to be taken, relating these to prevailing values, beliefs, community standards, etc. Having done all this, we must choose among the options and act. Finally, we must evaluate or review the consequences, often on an ongoing basis, remembering that often there is no "right answer" but a series of alternatives that are in some way both satisfactory and unsatisfactory. One of the most difficult aspects of biomedical ethics is that the more securely we may think we can grasp the philosophical principles, the harder it may become to arrive at a satisfactory answer to the problem. Indeed, there may not be an answer.

THE PHILOSOPHICAL BASIS FOR PUBLIC HEALTH

All public health workers should ask themselves: "Why am I doing this?" The aims of public health are to promote and preserve good health, to restore health, and to relieve suffering and distress. We often judge our success by reduction of infant mortality rates and increases in life expectancy but seldom try to measure, record, and analyze data on relief of distress (e.g., associated with chronic unemployment or homelessness). Clinicians responsible for intensive care services and for care of the elderly have been obliged to consider the question of quality of life now that life-prolonging measures are so widely used. There is growing concern about the quality of death as well as the quality of life.[46] In public health practice, we require a similar reorienting of focus to consider some less tangible measures of outcome than infant mortality rates and life expectancy. Included in this is the need to consider the impact of "improved" human reproductive performance on other living creatures with which we share planet earth.[47] Human reproductive success is endangering planetary ecology and therefore our own survival as a species; health must be a sustainable state for all, not merely for selected humans.[48]

This is especially necessary in developing nations, where spectacular reductions in infant mortality have been achieved from the expanded program on immunization, oral rehydration therapy, growth monitoring, etc. Innumerable infants and small children who would have died just a few years ago are being kept alive. What will become of them? Will they starve now, because there are so many more mouths to feed? Will they get an education? Will they have a lifetime of meaningful work? Will they die eventually, rich in years and experience, surrounded by a loving family? The answers to these difficult questions will depend on our response to challenges more subtle than reduction of infant and child mortality rates. The goals of the programs that are part of the strategy of *Targets for Health for All by the Year 2000* refer in places to the quality of life, but the supporting documents do not say how to sustain or enhance the quality of life. The search for ways to accomplish this has high priority among the aims of public health in the 1990s and beyond the year 2000.

Ethics and morality are based on the most fundamental values of our culture, derived from many centuries of tradition. We can trace beliefs that have descended from biblical lore and from the ancient Greek philosophers, reinforced by ideas from the great monotheistic religions, Judaism, Christianity, and Islam. We can trace the influence of rapidly advancing knowledge and changing values in our time. Some of our beliefs are enshrined in codes of conduct, others are poorly defined but firmly held and vary in relation to customs and traditions handed on from one generation to the next.

This review gives some idea of the range and complexity of the ethical issues that arise in public health practice and research. It does not address the nature of the relationship between person-oriented and population-oriented ethics. These are intermingled in a complex pattern and often reflect dissonance in our value system. We spare no effort or expense in striving to prolong lives of infants with incurable liver disease by finding donors for liver transplants; we maintain indefinitely on life-support systems some patients who are in a persistent vegetative state from which they cannot recover.[49] Yet we do little to prevent many diseases that commonly take the lives of or destroy the joy of life for much larger numbers of people, such as infants who are the victims of fetal alcohol syndrome and young adults whose brains are permanently damaged by serious injuries in traffic crashes. We spend large amounts and invest much effort in heroic interventions for advanced coronary heart disease but spend relatively little intellectual effort or money on measures that might reduce the magnitude of this public health problem.

This raises philosophical questions about the meaning of our culture, questions similar in nature to those raised by thoughtful critics of the arms race who wonder whether our huge investments in weapons to preserve our freedom are enslaving us in fear and paranoia and critics of our environmental development policies that rely on exploitation rather than on learning to live an interdependent existence with all the other living creatures on our planet.

REFERENCES

1. Aristotle: Ethics (translated by Thomson JAK, translation revised by Tredennick H). New York: Viking Penguin, 1976
2. Frank JP: A System of Complete Medical Police (translated by Lesky E). Baltimore: Johns Hopkins, 1976
3. WHO AIDS Series, No. 8: Guidelines for counselling about HIV infection and disease. Geneva: World Health Organization, 1990

4. Global programme on AIDS: Guidelines for Monitoring HIV Infection in Populations. Geneva: World Health Organization, 1989
5. Duckett M, Orkin AJ: AIDS-related migration and travel policies and restrictions; a global survey. AIDS 3 (Suppl): S231–S252, 1989
6. Kaslow RA, Francis DP (eds): The Epidemiology of AIDS. New York: Oxford University Press, 1989
7. Law Reform Commission of Canada: Crimes against the environment. Working Paper No. 44. Ottawa, 1985
8. European Charter on Environment and Health. Copenhagen: World Health Organization, Regional Office for Europe, 1989
9. Greenberg M, Appelbaum E: Postvaccinian encephalitis; a report of 45 cases in New York City. Am J Med Sci 216:565–570, 1948
10. WHO Weekly Epidemiological Record 3:13–15, 1984
11. USDHHS Task Force: Pertussis: CPS, a case study. In Determining Risks to Health—Federal Policy and Practice. Dover, Mass: Auburn, 1986
12. Meyer MB, Tonascia J: Long-term effects of prenatal x-ray of human females. Am J Epidemiol 114:304–336, 1981
13. Kinlen L: Cancer incidence in relation to fluoride level in water supplies. Br Dent J 138:221–224, 1975
14. Marshall E: The fluoride debate; one more time. Science 247:276–277, 1990
15. White FMM, Lacey BA, Constance PDA: An outbreak of poliomyelitis infection in Alberta, 1978. Can J Public Health, 72:239–244, 1981
16. Siegler M: Confidentiality in medicine; a decrepit concept. N Engl J Med 307:1518–1521, 1982
17. Black D: An Anthology of False Antitheses. London: Nuffield Provincial Hospitals Trust, 1984
18. Curran WJ: Protecting confidentiality in epidemiologic investigations by the Centers for Disease Control. N Engl J Med 314:1027–1028, 1986
19. U.S. Court of Appeals, Second Circuit 89-7317: American Tobacco Company, RJ Reynolds Tobacco Company, and Philip Morris Inc. versus Mount Sinai School of Medicine and the American Cancer Society.
20. Epidemiology Monitor 11(5):1–2, 1990 (See also Marshall E: A clash over standards for scientific records. Science 247:544–545, 1990
21. Cook R, Beauchamp T, Fayerweather W: A code of ethics for epidemiologists. J Clin Epidemiol 44(suppl 5):151S–169S, 1991
22. Last JM: Guidelines on ethics for epidemiologists. Int J Epidemiol 19:226–229, 1990
23. Proposed International Guidelines for Biomedical Research Involving Human Subjects. Geneva: Council for International Organizations of the Medical Services, 1982
24. Proposed International Guidelines for Ethical Review of Epidemiological Studies. Geneva: Council for International Organizations of the Medical Sciences, 1990 (Fifth Draft, July 1991)
25. Commonwealth of Australia, National Health and Medical Research Council, Medical Research Ethics Committee: Report on ethics in epidemiological research. Canberra, 1985
26. Medical Research Council of Canada: Guidelines on research involving human subjects. Ottawa, 1987
27. Last JM: Epidemiology; questions of science, ethics, morality and law. Am J Epidemiol 130:1073, 1989
28. World Medical Association: Declaration of Helsinki, adopted by the 18th World Medical Assembly, Helsinki, Finland, June 1964, amended by the 29th World Medical Assembly, Tokyo, Japan, October 1975, the 35th World Medical Assembly, Venice, Italy, October 1983, and the 41st World Medical Assembly, Hong Kong, September 1989.
29. Last JM: Obligations of epidemiologists to research subjects. J Clin Epidemiol 44(suppl 5):95S–101S, 1991
30. Faden RR, Beauchamp TL: A history and theory of informed consent. New York: Oxford University Press, 1986
31. Last JM: Epidemiology and ethics. Background paper for the CIOMS Guidelines on Ethics for Epidemiologists. Geneva: Council for International Organizations of the Medical Sciences, 1990
32. International Statistical Institute: Declaration on professional ethics. Int Stat Rev 54:227–242, 1986
33. Institute of Medicine, National Academy of Sciences: Report of a Study on the Responsible Conduct of Research in the Health Sciences (Chairman: A.H. Rubenstein). Washington DC: National Academy 1989; reprinted in part in Clin Res 37(2):179–191, 1989
34. First International Congress on Peer Review in Biomedical Publication. Published as "Guarding the Guardians" in JAMA 263:1317–1441, 1990 (entire issue)
35. Haynes RB, Sackett DL, Taylor DW, et al: Increased absenteeism from work after detection and labeling of hypertensive patients. N Engl J Med 299:741–747, 1978
36. Turner DR, Willoughby JO: Ethical issues in Huntington disease presymptomatic testing. Aust N Z J Med 20:545–547, 1990
37. McNamara RS: The challenges for Sub-Saharan Africa. Washington DC: Consultative Group on International Agricultural Research, 1985
38. Jones EF, et al: Teenage Pregnancy in Industrialized Countries. New Haven: Yale University Press, 1986
39. Code of ethical conduct for physicians providing occupational medical services. Washington DC: American Occupational Medical Association, 1976
40. Angell M: Ethical imperialism? ethics in international collaborative research. N Engl J Med 319:1081–1083, 1988
41. Terris M: The changing relationship of epidemiology and society. J Public Health Pol 6:15–36, 1985
42. World Health Organization: A charter for health promotion (The Ottawa Charter). Can J Public Health 77:425–430, 1986
43. Hawking S: A brief history of time. New York: Bantam, 1988
44. Targets for Health for All 2000. Copenhagen: World Health Organization Regional Office for Europe, 1985
45. Gillon R: Philosophical medical ethics. London: Wiley, 1985
46. Feinstein AR: The state of the art. JAMA 255:1488, 1986
47. Last JM, et al: Homo sapiens—a suicidal species? World Health Forum 12(2), 1991
48. King M: Health is a sustainable state. Lancet 336:664–667, 1990
49. Annas GJ, et al: Bioethicists' Statement on the U.S. Supreme Court's Cruzan Decision. N Engl J Med 323:686–687, 1990

INDEX